# How to use this book

This book provides information about prescription and over-the-counter medicines. It is written in everyday language, making it a valuable reference guide for consumers.

On this page, you'll find general information about how to use this book. An illustration showing how the listings are organized appears on the back of this page

## About the monographs

The drug entries are arranged alphabetically like an encyclopedia. *If you already know what entry the drug belongs to,* you can turn directly to it.

*If you know only the drug's generic or brand name,* the best way to find your information is to use the index at the front of this book. It will tell you what entry includes that drug and the page number on which the entry starts.

## For more information

For general guidelines about medicines, see *To the Reader* (page v), which also discusses this book's content and USP in depth. In addition to the entries, this book has a glossary plus a four-color medicine chart and the following supplemental appendixes:

▶ *Appendix 1* General Information About Use of Medicines

▶ *Appendix 2* USP People

▶ *Appendix 3* Additional Products and Uses

▶ *Appendix 4* Athletes Precautions

*See illustration on the back of this page.*

# Sample entry

**Title section:** lists the drug's commonly used brand names in both the United States and Canada.

**Proper use of this medicine:** tells how to store and use the drug, including usual doses and information such as what to do if you miss a dose.

**Precautions:** tells you what to avoid or be careful of when using the drug, and when medical supervision is required.

**Additional Information:** when necessary, gives details about other uses that are not shown in the product labeling.

---

## PYRAZINAMIDE   Systemic

Some commonly used brand names in Canada are pms-Pyrazinamide and Tebrazid.
Available in the U.S. as generic name product.

### Description

Pyrazinamide (peer-a-ZIN-a-mide) belongs to the family of medicines called anti-infectives. It is used, along with other medicines, to treat tuberculosis (TB).

*To help clear up your tuberculosis (TB) completely, you must keep taking this medicine for the full time of treatment, even if you begin to feel better. This is very important. It is also important that you do not miss any doses.*

Pyrazinamide is available only with your doctor's prescription, in the following dosage form:

*Oral*
- Tablets (U.S. and Canada)

### Before Using This Medicine

In deciding to use a medicine, the risks of taking the medicine must be weighed against the good it will do. This is a decision you and your doctor will make. For pyrazinamide, the following should be considered:

**Allergies**—Tell your doctor if you have ever had any unusual or allergic reaction to pyrazinamide or to ethionamide (e.g., Trecator-SC), isoniazid (e.g., INH, Nydrazid), or niacin (e.g., Nicobid, nicotinic acid). Also tell your health care professional if you are allergic to any other substances, such as foods, preservatives, or dyes.

**Pregnancy**—Studies on effects in pregnancy have not been done in either humans or animals.

**Breast-feeding**—Pyrazinamide passes into the breast milk in small amounts.

**Children**—Pyrazinamide has been used in children and, in effective doses, has not been reported to cause different side effects or problems in children than it does in adults.

**Older adults**—Many medicines have not been studied specifically in older people. Therefore, it may not be known whether they work exactly the same way they do in younger adults. Although there is no specific information comparing pyrazinamide in the elderly with use in other age groups, this medicine is not expected to cause different side effects or problems in older people than it does in younger adults.

**Other medicines**—Although certain medicines should not be used together at all, in other cases two different medicines may be used together even if an interaction might occur. In these cases, your doctor may want to change the dose, or other precautions may be necessary. Tell your health care professional if you are taking any other prescription or nonprescription (over-the-counter [OTC]) medicine.

**Other medical problems**—The presence of other medical problems may affect the use of pyrazinamide. Make sure you tell your doctor if you have any other medical problems, especially:
- Gout (history of)—Pyrazinamide may worsen or cause a gout attack in patients with a history of gout
- Liver disease (severe)—Patients with severe liver disease who take pyrazinamide may have an increase in side effects

### Proper Use of This Medicine

To help clear up your TB completely, *it is important that you keep taking this medicine for the full time of treatment*, even if you begin to feel better after a few weeks. *It is important that you do not miss any doses.*

**Dosing**—The dose of pyrazinamide will be different for different patients. *Follow your doctor's orders or the directions on the label.* The following information includes only the average doses of pyrazinamide. *If your dose is different, do not change it unless your doctor tells you to do so.*

- For *oral* dosage form (tablets):
  —For tuberculosis (TB):
  - Adults and children—Dose is based on body weight. The usual dose is 15 to 30 milligrams (mg) of pyrazinamide per kilogram (kg) (6.8 to 13.6 mg per pound) of body weight once a day; or 50 to 70 mg per kg (22.7 to 31.8 mg per pound) two times a week or three times a week, depending on the schedule your doctor chooses for you. This medicine must be taken along with other medicines used to treat TB.

**Missed dose**—If you do miss a dose of this medicine, take it as soon as possible. However, if it is almost time for your next dose, skip the missed dose and go back to your regular dosing schedule. Do not double doses.

**Storage**—To store this medicine:
- Keep out of the reach of children.
- Store away from heat and direct light.
- Do not store in the bathroom, near the kitchen sink, or in other damp places. Heat or moisture may cause the medicine to break down.
- Do not keep outdated medicine or medicine no longer needed. Be sure that any discarded medicine is out of the reach of children.

### Precautions While Using This Medicine

It is very important that your doctor check your progress at regular visits.

If your symptoms do not improve within 2 to 3 weeks, or if they become worse, check with your doctor.

For diabetic patients:
- *This medicine may cause false test results with urine ketone tests.* Check with your doctor before changing your diet or the dosage of your diabetes medicine.

### Side Effects of This Medicine

Along with its needed effects, a medicine may cause some unwanted effects. Although not all of these side effects may occur, if they do occur they may need medical attention.

*Check with your doctor immediately* if any of the following side effects occur:
*More common*
  Pain in large and small joints

*Rare*
  Loss of appetite; pain and swelling of joints, especially big toe, ankle, and knee; tense, hot skin over affected joints; unusual tiredness or weakness; yellow eyes or skin

Other side effects may occur that usually do not need medical attention. These side effects may go away during treatment as your body adjusts to the medicine. However, check with your doctor if any of the following side effects continue or are bothersome:
*Rare*
  Itching; skin rash

Other side effects not listed above may also occur in some patients. If you notice any other effects, check with your doctor.

Revised: 05/02/94

---

**Before using this medicine:** explains what you and your health care professional should consider in advance, such as allergies and special diet restrictions.

**Description:** tells how to pronounce the drug's name, what the drug is used for, what dosage forms are available, and if a doctor must prescribe the drug.

**Side effects:** lists both common and rare side effects of the drug and whether they require medical attention.

# COMPLETE DRUG REFERENCE

## 1995 Edition

United States Pharmacopeia

Consumer Reports Books
A Division of Consumers Union

Yonkers, New York

Published simultaneously by USPC, Inc., under the title *USP DI, Volume II (Advice for the Patient)*, Fifteenth Edition, 1995. Previous editions of this book appeared under the title *United States Pharmacopeia Drug Information for the Consumer*.

*Complete Drug Reference*, 1995 Edition, is a Consumer Reports Book published by Consumers Union, the nonprofit organization that publishes *Consumer Reports*, the monthly magazine of test reports, product Ratings, and buying guidance. Established in 1936, Consumers Union is chartered under the Not-For-Profit Corporation Law of the State of New York.

The purposes of Consumers Union, as stated in its charter, are to provide consumers with information and counsel on consumer goods and services, to give information on all matters relating to the expenditure of the family income, and to initiate and to cooperate with individual and group efforts seeking to create and maintain decent living standards.

Consumers Union derives its income solely from the sale of *Consumer Reports* and other publications. In addition, expenses of occasional public service efforts may be met, in part, by nonrestrictive, noncommercial contributions, grants, and fees. Consumers Union accepts no advertising or product samples and is not beholden in any way to any commercial interest. Its Ratings and reports are solely for the use of the readers of its publications. Neither the Ratings nor the reports nor any Consumers Union publications, including this book, may be used in advertising or for any commercial purpose. Consumers Union will take all steps open to it to prevent such uses of its material, its name, or the name of *Consumer Reports*.

Check
the INDEX first.
It's on page 1.

# Contents

# Complete Drug Reference

# Foreword to the
# Consumer Reports Books Edition

For 175 years, the United States Pharmacopeia has set official standards of strength, quality, purity, packaging, and labeling for medical products in the United States. And for 59 years Consumers Union, through its magazine *Consumer Reports,* has served as this country's foremost source for authoritative, reliable, and unbiased product testing and buying guidance. It thus seems only natural that these two organizations, both dedicated to the consumer's well-being, should join forces to publish a layman's guide to prescription and over-the-counter drugs.

At one time or another, most of us find it necessary to use some type of medical drug. In fact, many people feel that medical treatment is only effective when it includes drug therapy. It's not surprising, then, that in 1994 it is estimated that Americans will spend $49.2 billion on prescription drugs, and another $28 billion on nonprescription drugs. Moreover, studies show that up to 50 percent of all prescriptions are taken incorrectly, and as many as 70 percent of all patients receive little or no counseling about drug usage, including, interactions with food or other drugs, and possible side effects. It is apparent that there is a grave need for a straightforward, objective guide to drugs that cautions and informs the consumer about the role of prescription drugs as a routine part of medical care.

*Complete Drug Reference* lists almost every medicine, prescription and nonprescription, available in the United States and Canada. It provides consumers with up-to-date information about drug usage and potential side effects. Organized alphabetically by generic or family name, each entry includes different dosage forms and common brand names—over 9,000 different brand and generic entries in all. It is well indexed according to both generic and brand names, making it easy to look up any medication. Most important, unlike other drug information books available to the consumer, notably the *Physicians' Desk Reference,* the information presented in this guide is not controlled by drug manufacturers or anyone connected with the drug industry. Rather, *Complete Drug Reference* is a consensus book put together by many experts—physicians, pharmacists, pharmacologists, dentists, nurses, chemists, microbiologists, and other individuals particularly qualified to judge drugs—and is supported by 33 advisory panels representing differing medical specialties, health professionals, and consumers. The guide is reviewed by so many experts that it is constantly in revision, with the result that it may contain the latest precautions and side effects of a particular drug before the information is readily available elsewhere.

We believe that the therapeutic use of drugs deserves much closer scrutiny by physicians, pharmacists, and patients than is usually the case. Even the exacting approval process undertaken by the Food and Drug Administration (FDA) cannot possibly guarantee that all drugs on the market are totally safe and effective. Post-marketing surveillance by physicians and patients should therefore be an integral part of drug usage. It is also important that patients report the side effects of drugs to their physicians and that the physicians relay that information to the FDA, if only so that future editions of *Complete Drug Reference* may reflect that new knowledge and experience.

The material contained in this book is presented in a direct, factual manner with a refreshing absence of editorial opinion or biased discussions about the relative merits of one drug over another. Each profile of a specific drug lists indications, proper usage, precautions, and side effects. The language is easily understood and targeted specifically to the patient. *Complete Drug Reference* is the most comprehensive drug information book available to the public, and we are proud to present it to our readers.

# To The Reader

When purchasing a medicine, whether over-the-counter (nonprescription) or with a doctor's prescription, you may have questions about its usefulness to you, the best way to take it, possible side effects, and precautions to take to avoid complications. For instance, some medicines should be taken with meals, others between meals. Some may make you drowsy while others may tend to keep you awake. Alcoholic or other beverages, other medicines, certain foods, or smoking may affect the way your medicine works. As for side effects, some are merely bothersome and may go away while others may require medical attention.

*Complete Drug Reference* contains information which may provide general answers to some of your questions as well as suggestions for the correct use of your medicine. *It is important to remember, however, that the human body is very complex and medicines may act differently on different people—and even in the same person at different times. If you want additional information about your medicine or its possible side effects, ask your doctor, nurse, or pharmacist. They are there to help you.*

## How to Use This Book

*Complete Drug Reference* contains a section of general information about the correct use of any medicine, as well as individual discussions of a wide variety of commonly and not so commonly used medicines. *You should read both the general information and the information specific to the medicine you are taking.* See Appendix I for this general information.

Each medicine has a generic name that all manufacturers who make that medicine must use. Some manufacturers also create a brand name to put on the label and to use in advertising. *Look in the index* for the generic name or the brand name of the medicine about which you have questions. We have put the generic names and common brand names in the same index, so you do not have to know whether the name you have is a generic name or a brand name. However, it is a good idea for you to learn both the generic and the brand names of the medicines you are using and to write them down and keep them for future use.

Although the informational monographs generally appear in alphabetical order by generic name, there are numerous occasions when closely related medicines are grouped under a family name. Therefore, the surest way to quickly find the page number of the information about each medicine is to *look in the index first.*

The information for each medicine is presented according to the area of the body which is affected. As a general rule, information for one type of use will not be the same as for other types of use. For example, if you take tetracycline capsules by mouth for their systemic effect in treating an infection, the information will not be the same as for tetracycline ointment, which is applied directly to the skin for its topical effects. And both of these will be different from the information for tetracyclines used in the eye. The common divisions used in this publication are:

- *BUCCAL*—For general effects throughout the body when a medicine is placed in the cheek pocket and slowly absorbed.
- *DENTAL*—For local effects when applied to the teeth or gums.
- *INHALATION*—For local, and in some cases systemic, effects when inhaled into the lungs.
- *INTRA-AMNIOTIC*—For local effects when a medicine is injected into the sac that contains the fetus and amniotic fluid.
- *INTRACAVERNOSAL*—For local effects in the penis when a medicine is given by injection.
- *LINGUAL*—For general effects throughout the body when a medicine is absorbed through the lining of the mouth.
- *MUCOSAL*—For local effects when applied directly to mucous membranes (for example, the inside of the mouth).
- *NASAL*—For local effects when used in the nose.
- *OPHTHALMIC*—For local effects when applied directly to the eyes.

- *ORAL-LOCAL*—For local effects in the gastrointestinal tract when taken by mouth (i.e., not absorbed into the body).
- *OTIC*—For local effects when used in the ear.
- *PARENTERAL-LOCAL*—For local effects in a specific area of the body when given by injection.
- *RECTAL*—For local, and in some cases systemic, effects when used in the rectum.
- *SUBLINGUAL*—For general effects throughout the body when a medicine is placed under the tongue and slowly absorbed.
- *SYSTEMIC*—For general effects throughout the body; applies to most medicines when taken by mouth or given by injection.
- *TOPICAL*—For local effects when applied directly to the skin.
- *VAGINAL*—For local, and in some cases systemic, effects when used in the vagina.

---

## Notice

The information about the drugs contained herein is general in nature and is intended to be used in consultation with your health care providers. It is not intended to replace specific instructions or directions or warnings given to you by your physician or other prescriber or accompanying a particular product. The information is selective and it is not claimed that it includes all known precautions, contraindications, effects, or interactions possibly related to the use of a drug. The information may differ from that contained in the product labeling which is required by law. The information is not sufficient to make an evaluation as to the risks and benefits of taking a particular drug in a particular case and is not medical advice for individual problems and should not alone be relied upon for these purposes. Since the inclusion or exclusion of particular information about a drug is judgmental in nature and since opinion as to drug usage may differ, you may wish to consult additional sources. Should you desire additional information or if you have any questions as to how this information may relate to you in particular, ask your doctor, nurse, pharmacist, or other health care provider.

Since new drugs are constantly being marketed and since previously unreported side effects, newly recognized precautions, or other new information for any given drug may come to light at any time, continuously updated drug information sources should be consulted as necessary.

There are many brands of drugs on the market. The listing of selected brand names is intended only for ease of reference. The inclusion of a brand name does not mean the USP or Consumers Union has any particular knowledge that the brand listed has properties different from other brands of the same drug, nor should it be interpreted as an endorsement by the USPC or Consumers Union. Similarly, the fact that a brand name has not been included does not indicate that that particular brand has been judged to be unsatisfactory or unacceptable.

*If any of the information in this book causes you special concern, do not decide against taking any medicine prescribed for you without first checking with your doctor.*

## About USP

The information in this volume is prepared by the United States Pharmacopeia (USP), the organization that sets the official standards of strength, quality, purity, packaging, and labeling for medical products used in the United States.

The United States Pharmacopeia is an independent, not-for-profit corporation composed of delegates from the accredited colleges of medicine and pharmacy in the U.S.; state medical and pharmaceutical associations; many national associations concerned with medicines, such as the American Medical Association, the American Nurses Association, the American Dental Association, the National Association of Retail Druggists, and the American Pharmaceutical Association; and various departments of the federal government, including the Food and Drug Administration. In addition, four members have been appointed by the Board of Trustees specifically to represent the public. USP was established 175 years ago, and is the only national body that represents the professions of both pharmacy and medicine.

The first convention came into being on January 1, 1820, and within the year published the first national drug formulary of the United States. The *U.S. Pharmacopeia* of 1820 contained 217 drug names, divided into two groups according to the level of general acceptance and usage.

When Congress passed the first major drug safety law in 1906, the standards recognized by that statute were those set forth in the *United States Pharmacopeia* and in the *National Formulary*. Today, the *USP* and *NF* continue to be the official U.S. compendia for standards for drugs and for the inactive ingredients in drug dosage forms. The *United States Pharmacopeia* is the world's oldest regularly revised national pharmacopeia and is generally accepted as being the most influential.

The work of the USP is carried out by the Committee of Revision. This committee of experts is elected by the members and currently consists of 114 outstanding physicians, pharmacists, dentists, nurses, chemists, microbiologists, and other individuals particularly qualified to judge the merits of drugs and the standards and information that should apply to them. Committee members serve without pay and are assisted by numerous advisory panels, other outside reviewers, and USP staff.

# Index

Brand names are in *italics*. There are many brands and different manufacturers of drugs and the listing of selected American and Canadian brand names and manufacturers is intended only for ease of reference. There are additional brands and manufacturers that have not been included. The inclusion of a brand name does not mean the USPC has any particular knowledge that the brand listed has properties different from other brands of the same drug, nor should it be interpreted as an endorsement by the USP. Similarly, the fact that a particular brand has not been included does not indicate that the product has been judged to be unsatisfactory or unacceptable. The page numbers MC-1 to MC-24 refer to the product identification photographs in The Medicine Chart.

## A

*Abbokinase*—Urokinase—*See* Thrombolytic Agents (Systemic), 1604

*Abbokinase Open-Cath*—Urokinase—*See* Thrombolytic Agents (Systemic), 1604

*Abenol*—Acetaminophen (Systemic), 161

*Abitrate*—Clofibrate (Systemic), 572

*A/B Otic*—Antipyrine and Benzocaine (Otic), 334

*A.C.&C.*—Aspirin, Codeine, and Caffeine—*See* Narcotic Analgesics and Aspirin (Systemic), 1185

*Accupep HPF*—Enteral Nutrition Formula, Monomeric (Elemental)—*See* Enteral Nutrition Formulas (Systemic), 769

*Accupril*—Quinapril—*See* Angiotensin-converting Enzyme (ACE) Inhibitors (Systemic), 245, MC-20

*Accutane*—Isotretinoin (Systemic), 997, MC-12

*Accutane Roche*—Isotretinoin (Systemic), 997

Acebutolol—*See* Beta-adrenergic Blocking Agents (Systemic), 404

ACE Inhibitors—*See* Angiotensin-converting Enzyme (ACE) Inhibitors (Systemic), 245

ACE Inhibitors and Hydrochlorothiazide—*See* Angiotensin-converting Enzyme (ACE) Inhibitors and Hydrochlorothiazide (Systemic), 249

*Acel-Imune*—Diphtheria and Tetanus Toxoids and Pertussis Vaccine Adsorbed (Systemic), 728

Acellular DTP—*See* Diphtheria and Tetanus Toxoids and Pertussis Vaccine Adsorbed (Systemic), 728

Acenocoumarol (Systemic), 1745

*Acetaco*—Acetaminophen and Codeine—*See* Narcotic Analgesics and Acetaminophen (Systemic), 1181

*Aceta with Codeine*—Acetaminophen and Codeine—*See* Narcotic Analgesics and Acetaminophen (Systemic), 1181

*Aceta Elixir*—Acetaminophen (Systemic), 161

Acetaminophen (Systemic), 161

Acetaminophen and Aspirin—*See* Acetaminophen and Salicylates (Systemic), 164

Acetaminophen, Aspirin, and Caffeine—*See* Acetaminophen and Salicylates (Systemic), 164

Acetaminophen, Aspirin, and Caffeine, Buffered—*See* Acetaminophen and Salicylates (Systemic), 164

Acetaminophen, Aspirin, and Salicylamide, Buffered—*See* Acetaminophen and Salicylates (Systemic), 164

Acetaminophen, Aspirin, Salicylamide, and Caffeine—*See* Acetaminophen and Salicylates (Systemic), 164

Acetaminophen and Caffeine—*See* Acetaminophen (Systemic), 161

Acetaminophen and Codeine—*See* Narcotic Analgesics and Acetaminophen (Systemic), 1181, MC-1

Acetaminophen, Codeine, and Caffeine—*See* Narcotic Analgesics and Acetaminophen (Systemic), 1181

Acetaminophen and Salicylamide—*See* Acetaminophen and Salicylates (Systemic), 164

Acetaminophen, Salicylamide, and Caffeine—*See* Acetaminophen and Salicylates (Systemic), 164

Acetaminophen and Salicylates (Systemic), 164

Acetaminophen, Sodium Bicarbonate, and Citric Acid (Systemic), 169

*Acetaminophen Uniserts*—Acetaminophen (Systemic), 161

*Aceta Tablets*—Acetaminophen (Systemic), 161

*Acetazolam*—Acetazolamide—*See* Carbonic Anhydrase Inhibitors (Systemic), 488

Acetazolamide—*See* Carbonic Anhydrase Inhibitors (Systemic), 488

Acetazolamide (Systemic), 1745

*Acetest*—Nitroprusside Urine Ketone Test—*See* Urine Glucose and Ketone Test Kits for Home Use, 1644

Acetohexamide—*See* Antidiabetics, Oral (Systemic), 283

Acetohydroxamic Acid (Systemic), 172

Acetophenazine—*See* Phenothiazines (Systemic), 1330

*Acetoxyl 2.5 Gel*—Benzoyl Peroxide (Topical), 397

*Acetoxyl 5 Gel*—Benzoyl Peroxide (Topical), 397

*Acetoxyl 10 Gel*—Benzoyl Peroxide (Topical), 397

*Acetoxyl 20 Gel*—Benzoyl Peroxide (Topical), 397

Acetylcysteine (Inhalation), 174

Acetylsalicylic acid—Aspirin—*See* Salicylates (Systemic), 1473

*Achromycin*—Tetracycline—*See* Tetracyclines (Ophthalmic), 1568; Tetracyclines (Systemic), 1570; Tetracyclines (Topical), 1574

*Achromycin V*—Tetracycline—*See* Tetracyclines (Systemic), 1570, MC-22

Aciclovir—*See* Acyclovir (Systemic), 175; Acyclovir (Topical), 178

Acitretin (Systemic), 1745

*Aclophen*—Chlorpheniramine, Phenylephrine, and Acetaminophen—*See* Antihistamines, Decongestants, and Analgesics (Systemic), 316

*Aclovate*—Alclometasone—*See* Corticosteroids—Low Potency (Topical), 624

*Acne Aid 10 Cream*—Benzoyl Peroxide (Topical), 397

*Allergy Cold*—Triprolidine and Pseudoephedrine—*See* Antihistamines and Decongestants (Systemic), 311

*Allergy Drops*—Naphazoline (Ophthalmic), 1174

*Allergy Formula Sinutab*—Dexbrompheniramine and Pseudoephedrine—*See* Antihistamines and Decongestants (Systemic), 311

*Allergy Relief Medicine*—Chlorpheniramine and Phenylpropanolamine—*See* Antihistamines and Decongestants (Systemic), 311

*AllerMax Caplets*—Diphenhydramine—*See* Antihistamines (Systemic), 304

*Aller-med*—Diphenhydramine—*See* Antihistamines (Systemic), 304

*Allerphed*—Triprolidine and Pseudoephedrine—*See* Antihistamines and Decongestants (Systemic), 311

*All-Nite Cold Formula*—Doxylamine, Pseudoephedrine, Dextromethorphan, and Acetaminophen—*See* Cough/Cold Combinations (Systemic), 637

Allopurinol (Systemic), 187, MC-1

*Almacone*—Alumina, Magnesia, and Simethicone—*See* Antacids (Oral), 253

*Almacone II*—Alumina, Magnesia, and Simethicone—*See* Antacids (Oral), 253

*Alma-Mag Improved*—Alumina, Magnesia, and Simethicone—*See* Antacids (Oral), 253

*Almay Anti-itch Lotion*—Pramoxine and Menthol—*See* Anesthetics (Topical), 240

*Alomide*—Lodoxamide (Ophthalmic), 1047

*Alophen*—Phenolphthalein—*See* Laxatives (Oral), 1017

Alpha$_1$-antitrypsin—*See* Alpha$_1$-proteinase Inhibitor, Human (Systemic), 190

*Alphacaine*—Lidocaine—*See* Anesthetics (Topical), 240

*Alphaderm*—Hydrocortisone—*See* Corticosteroids—Low Potency (Topical), 624

*Alphamine*—Hydroxocobalamin—*See* Vitamin B$_{12}$ (Systemic), 1667

*Alphamul*—Castor Oil—*See* Laxatives (Oral), 1017

*AlphaNine*—Factor IX (Systemic), 823

*AlphaNine SD*—Factor IX (Systemic), 823

Alpha$_1$-proteinase Inhibitor, Human (Systemic), 190

*Alpha-Tamoxifen*—Tamoxifen (Systemic), 1559

Alpha tocopherol—*See* Vitamin E (Systemic), 1674

*Alphatrex*—Betamethasone—*See* Corticosteroids—Medium to Very High Potency (Topical), 626

*Alphosyl*—Coal Tar (Topical), 589

Alprazolam—*See* Benzodiazepines (Systemic), 389, MC-1

*Alprazolam Intensol*—Alprazolam—*See* Benzodiazepines (Systemic), 389

Alprostadil (Intracavernosal), 191

*Altace*—Ramipril—*See* Angiotensin-converting Enzyme (ACE) Inhibitors (Systemic), 245, MC-21

Alteplase, Recombinant—*See* Thrombolytic Agents (Systemic), 1604

*AlternaGEL*—Aluminum Hydroxide—*See* Antacids (Oral), 253

Altretamine (Systemic), 192

*Alu-Cap*—Aluminum Hydroxide—*See* Antacids (Oral), 253

*Aludrox*—Alumina, Magnesia, and Simethicone—*See* Antacids (Oral), 253

*Alumadrine*—Chlorpheniramine, Phenylpropanolamine, and Acetaminophen—*See* Antihistamines, Decongestants, and Analgesics (Systemic), 316

Alumina and Magnesia—*See* Antacids (Oral), 253

Alumina, Magnesia, and Calcium Carbonate—*See* Antacids (Oral), 253

Alumina, Magnesia, Calcium Carbonate, and Simethicone—*See* Antacids (Oral), 253

Alumina, Magnesia, and Simethicone—*See* Antacids (Oral), 253

Alumina and Magnesium Carbonate—*See* Antacids (Oral), 253

Alumina and Magnesium Trisilicate—*See* Antacids (Oral), 253

Alumina, Magnesium Trisilicate, and Sodium Bicarbonate—*See* Antacids (Oral), 253

Aluminum Carbonate, Basic—*See* Antacids (Oral), 253

Aluminum Hydroxide—*See* Antacids (Oral), 253

*Alupent*—Metaproterenol—*See* Bronchodilators, Adrenergic (Inhalation), 430; Bronchodilators, Adrenergic (Oral/Injection), 436

*Alurate*—Aprobarbital—*See* Barbiturates (Systemic), 370

*Alu-Tab*—Aluminum Hydroxide—*See* Antacids (Oral), 253

*Amacodone*—Hydrocodone and Acetaminophen—*See* Narcotic Analgesics and Acetaminophen (Systemic), 1181

Amantadine (Systemic), 194, MC-1

*Amaphen*—Butalbital, Acetaminophen, and Caffeine—*See* Butalbital and Acetaminophen (Systemic), 453

*Amaril D*—Chlorpheniramine, Phenyltoloxamine, Phenylephrine, and Phenylpropanolamine—*See* Antihistamines and Decongestants (Systemic), 311

*Amaril D Spantab*—Chlorpheniramine, Phenyltoloxamine, Phenylephrine, and Phenylpropanolamine—*See* Antihistamines and Decongestants (Systemic), 311

*Ambay Cough*—Bromodiphenhydramine and Codeine—*See* Cough/Cold Combinations (Systemic), 637

Ambenonium—*See* Antimyasthenics (Systemic), 332

*Ambenyl Cough*—Bromodiphenhydramine and Codeine—*See* Cough/Cold Combinations (Systemic), 637

*Ambenyl-D Decongestant Cough Formula*—Pseudoephedrine, Dextromethorphan, and Guaifenesin—*See* Cough/Cold Combinations (Systemic), 637

*Ambien*—Zolpidem (Systemic), 1694, MC-24

*Ambophen Expectorant*—Bromodiphenhydramine, Diphenhydramine, Codeine, Ammonium Chloride, and Potassium Guaiacolsulfonate—*See* Cough/Cold Combinations (Systemic), 637

Amcinonide—*See* Corticosteroids—Medium to Very High Potency (Topical), 626

*Amcort*—Triamcinolone—*See* Corticosteroids/Corticotropin—Glucocorticoid Effects (Systemic), 630

*Amen*—Medroxyprogesterone—*See* Progestins (Systemic), 1402

*Americaine Hemorrhoidal*—Benzocaine—*See* Anesthetics (Rectal), 237

*Americaine Topical Anesthetic First Aid Ointment*—Benzocaine—*See* Anesthetics (Topical), 240

*Americaine Topical Anesthetic Spray*—Benzocaine—*See* Anesthetics (Topical), 240

*A-methaPred*—Methylprednisolone—*See* Corticosteroids/Corticotropin—Glucocorticoid Effects (Systemic), 630

Amethocaine—Tetracaine—*See* Anesthetics (Dental), 229; Anesthetics (Ophthalmic), 234; Anesthetics (Rectal), 237; Anesthetics (Topical), 240

Amethopterin—*See* Methotrexate—For Cancer (Systemic), 1102; Methotrexate—For Noncancerous Conditions (Systemic), 1105

Amfebutamone—*See* Bupropion (Systemic), 446

Amfepramone—Diethylpropion—*See* Appetite Suppressants (Systemic), 339

Amfetamine—Amphetamine—*See* Amphetamines (Systemic), 209

*Amgenal Cough*—Bromodiphenhydramine and Codeine—*See* Cough/Cold Combinations (Systemic), 637

*Amicar*—Aminocaproic Acid—*See* Antifibrinolytic Agents (Systemic), 290

*Amidate*—Etomidate—*See* Anesthetics, General (Systemic), 243

*Amidrine*—Isometheptene, Dichloralphenazone, and Acetaminophen (Systemic), 990

*Ami-Drix*—Dexbrompheniramine and Pseudoephedrine—*See* Antihistamines and Decongestants (Systemic), 311

*Amigesic*—Salsalate—*See* Salicylates (Systemic), 1473

Amikacin—*See* Aminoglycosides (Systemic), 201

*Amikin*—Amikacin—*See* Aminoglycosides (Systemic), 201

Amiloride—*See* Diuretics, Potassium-sparing (Systemic), 742

Amiloride and Hydrochlorothiazide—*See* Diuretics, Potassium-sparing and Hydrochlorothiazide (Systemic), 745, MC-1

*Amin-aid*—Enteral Nutrition Formula, Disease-specific—*See* Enteral Nutrition Formulas (Systemic), 769

Aminobenzoate Potassium (Systemic), 197

Aminocaproic Acid—*See* Antifibrinolytic Agents (Systemic), 290

*Aminofen*—Acetaminophen (Systemic), 161

*Aminofen Max*—Acetaminophen (Systemic), 161

Aminoglutethimide (Systemic), 199

Aminoglycosides (Systemic), 201

*Amino-Opti-E*—Vitamin E (Systemic), 1674

Aminophylline—*See* Bronchodilators, Xanthine-derivative (Systemic), 442

Aminosalicylate Sodium (Systemic), 204

5-aminosalicylic acid—*See* Mesalamine (Rectal), 1097

Amiodarone (Systemic), 206, MC-1

*Ami Rax*—Theophylline, Ephedrine, and Hydroxyzine (Systemic), 1580

*Ami-Tex LA*—Phenylpropanolamine and Guaifenesin—*See* Cough/Cold Combinations (Systemic), 637

*Amitone*—Calcium Carbonate—*See* Antacids (Oral), 253

Amitriptyline—*See* Antidepressants, Tricyclic (Systemic), 277, MC-1

Amlodipine (Systemic), 207, MC-1

Ammonia N 13—*See* Radiopharmaceuticals (Diagnostic), 1439

Ammonium Molybdate—*See* Molybdenum Supplements (Systemic), 1153

Amobarbital—*See* Barbiturates (Systemic), 370

*Amogel PG*—Kaolin, Pectin, Belladonna Alkaloids, and Opium (Systemic), 1005

*Amonidrin*—Guaifenesin (Systemic), 892

Amoxapine—*See* Antidepressants, Tricyclic (Systemic), 277

Amoxicillin—*See* Penicillins (Systemic), 1299, MC-1, MC-2

Amoxicillin and Clavulanate—*See* Penicillins and Beta-lactamase Inhibitors (Systemic), 1306, MC-2

*Amoxil*—Amoxicillin—*See* Penicillins (Systemic), 1299, MC-1

Amphetamine—*See* Amphetamines (Systemic), 209

Amphetamines (Systemic), 209

*Amphojel*—Aluminum Hydroxide—*See* Antacids (Oral), 253

*Amphojel 500*—Alumina and Magnesia—*See* Antacids (Oral), 253

*Amphojel Plus*—Alumina, Magnesia, and Simethicone—*See* Antacids (Oral), 253; Simethicone, Alumina, Magnesium Carbonate, and Magnesia—*See* Antacids (Oral), 253

Amphotericin B (Systemic), 213

Amphotericin B (Topical), 214

Ampicillin—*See* Penicillins (Systemic), 1299, MC-2

Ampicillin and Sulbactam—*See* Penicillins and Beta-lactamase Inhibitors (Systemic), 1306

*Ampicin*—Ampicillin—*See* Penicillins (Systemic), 1299

Amsacrine (Systemic), 1745

*Amsa P-D*—Amsacrine (Systemic), 1745

Amyl Nitrite (Systemic), 216

*Amytal*—Amobarbital—*See* Barbiturates (Systemic), 370

Anabolic Steroids (Systemic), 218

*Anacin*—Aspirin and Caffeine—*See* Salicylates (Systemic), 1473

*Anacin-3*—Acetaminophen (Systemic), 161

*Anacin with Codeine*—Aspirin, Codeine, and Caffeine—*See* Narcotic Analgesics and Aspirin (Systemic), 1185

*Anacin-3 Extra Strength*—Acetaminophen (Systemic), 161

*Anacobin*—Cyanocobalamin—*See* Vitamin $B_{12}$ (Systemic), 1667

*Anadrol-50*—Oxymetholone—*See* Anabolic Steroids (Systemic), 218

*Anafranil*—Clomipramine—*See* Antidepressants, Tricyclic (Systemic), 277, MC-5

*Ana-Guard*—Epinephrine—*See* Bronchodilators, Adrenergic (Oral/Injection), 436

*Analgesic Ear Drops*—Antipyrine and Benzocaine (Otic), 334

*Anamine*—Chlorpheniramine and Pseudoephedrine—*See* Antihistamines and Decongestants (Systemic), 311

*Anamine HD*—Chlorpheniramine, Phenylephrine, and Hydrocodone—*See* Cough/Cold Combinations (Systemic), 637

*Anamine T.D.*—Chlorpheniramine and Pseudoephedrine—*See* Antihistamines and Decongestants (Systemic), 311

*Anandron*—Nilutamide (Systemic), 1751

*Anaplex*—Chlorpheniramine and Pseudoephedrine—*See* Antihistamines and Decongestants (Systemic), 311

*Anaplex HD*—Chlorpheniramine, Phenylephrine, and Hydrocodone—*See* Cough/Cold Combinations (Systemic), 637

*Anaplex S.R.*—Chlorpheniramine and Pseudoephedrine—*See* Antihistamines and Decongestants (Systemic), 311

*Anapolon 50*—Oxymetholone—*See* Anabolic Steroids (Systemic), 218

*Anaprox*—Naproxen—*See* Nonsteroidal Anti-inflammatory Drugs (Systemic), 1229, MC-16

*Anaprox DS*—Naproxen—*See* Nonsteroidal Anti-inflammatory Drugs (Systemic), 1229

*Anaspaz*—Hyoscyamine—*See* Anticholinergics/Antispasmodics (Systemic), 258

*Anatuss*—Chlorpheniramine, Phenylephrine, Phenylpropanolamine, Dextromethorphan, Guaifenesin, and Acetaminophen—*See* Cough/Cold Combinations (Systemic), 637

*Anatuss with Codeine*—Chlorpheniramine, Phenylpropanolamine, Codeine, Guaifenesin, and Acetaminophen—*See* Cough/Cold Combinations (Systemic), 637

*Anatuss DM*—Pseudoephedrine, Dextromethorphan, and Guaifenesin—*See* Cough/Cold Combinations (Systemic), 637

*Anatuss LA*—Pseudoephedrine and Guaifenesin—*See* Cough/Cold Combinations (Systemic), 637

*Anbesol, Baby*—Benzocaine—*See* Anesthetics (Dental), 229

*Anbesol Baby Jel*—Benzocaine—*See* Anesthetics (Dental), 229

*Anbesol Gel*—Benzocaine and Phenol—*See* Anesthetics (Dental), 229

*Anbesol Liquid*—Benzocaine and Phenol—*See* Anesthetics (Dental), 229

*Anbesol Maximum Strength Gel*—Benzocaine—*See* Anesthetics (Dental), 229

*Anbesol Maximum Strength Liquid*—Benzocaine—*See* Anesthetics (Dental), 229; Benzocaine and Phenol—*See* Anesthetics (Dental), 229

*Anbesol Regular Strength Gel*—Benzocaine and Phenol—*See* Anesthetics (Dental), 229

*Anbesol Regular Strength Liquid*—Benzocaine and Phenol—*See* Anesthetics (Dental), 229

*Ancalixir*—Phenobarbital—*See* Barbiturates (Systemic), 370

*Ancasal 8*—Aspirin, Codeine, and Caffeine—*See* Narcotic Analgesics and Aspirin (Systemic), 1185

*Ancasal 15*—Aspirin, Codeine, and Caffeine—*See* Narcotic Analgesics and Aspirin (Systemic), 1185

*Ancasal 30*—Aspirin, Codeine, and Caffeine—*See* Narcotic Analgesics and Aspirin (Systemic), 1185

*Ancef*—Cefazolin—*See* Cephalosporins (Systemic), 498

*Ancobon*—Flucytosine (Systemic), 842

*Ancotil*—Flucytosine (Systemic), 842

*Andrest 90-4*—Testosterone and Estradiol—*See* Androgens and Estrogens (Systemic), 225

*Andro 100*—Testosterone—*See* Androgens (Systemic), 221

*Androcur*—Cyproterone (Systemic), 1747

*Andro-Cyp 100*—Testosterone—*See* Androgens (Systemic), 221

*Andro-Cyp 200*—Testosterone—*See* Androgens (Systemic), 221

*Andro-Estro 90-4*—Testosterone and Estradiol—*See* Androgens and Estrogens (Systemic), 225

Androgens (Systemic), 221

Androgens and Estrogens (Systemic), 225

*Androgyn L.A.*—Testosterone and Estradiol—*See* Androgens and Estrogens (Systemic), 225

*Android-10*—Methyltestosterone—*See* Androgens (Systemic), 221

*Android-25*—Methyltestosterone—*See* Androgens (Systemic), 221

*Android-F*—Fluoxymesterone—*See* Androgens (Systemic), 221

*Andro L.A. 200*—Testosterone—*See* Androgens (Systemic), 221

*Andronate 100*—Testosterone—*See* Androgens (Systemic), 221

*Andronate 200*—Testosterone—*See* Androgens (Systemic), 221

*Andropository 100*—Testosterone—*See* Androgens (Systemic), 221

*Andryl 200*—Testosterone—*See* Androgens (Systemic), 221

*Anergan 25*—Promethazine—*See* Antihistamines, Phenothiazine-derivative (Systemic), 325

*Anergan 50*—Promethazine—*See* Antihistamines, Phenothiazine-derivative (Systemic), 325

Anesthetics (Dental), 229

Anesthetics (Ophthalmic), 234

Anesthetics (Parenteral-Local), 235

Anesthetics (Rectal), 237

Anesthetics (Topical), 240

Anesthetics, General (Systemic), 243

*Anexate*—Flumazenil (Systemic), 1748

*Anexsia*—Hydrocodone and Acetaminophen—*See* Narcotic Analgesics and Acetaminophen (Systemic), 1181

*Anexsia 7.5*—Hydrocodone and Acetaminophen—*See* Narcotic Analgesics and Acetaminophen (Systemic), 1181

Angiotensin-converting Enzyme (ACE) Inhibitors (Systemic), 245

*Anhydron*—Cyclothiazide—*See* Diuretics, Thiazide (Systemic), 749

Anileridine (Systemic), 1745

Aniline violet—*See* Methylene Blue (Systemic), 1117

Anisindione—*See* Anticoagulants (Systemic), 262

Anisotropine—*See* Anticholinergics/Antispasmodics (Systemic), 258

Anisoylated plasminogen-streptokinase activator complex—Anistrelplase—*See* Thrombolytic Agents (Systemic), 1604

Anistreplase—*See* Thrombolytic Agents (Systemic), 1604

*Anodynos DHC*—Hydrocodone and Acetaminophen—*See* Narcotic Analgesics and Acetaminophen (Systemic), 1181

*Anolor-300*—Butalbital, Acetaminophen, and Caffeine—*See* Butalbital and Acetaminophen (Systemic), 453

*Anolor DH 5*—Hydrocodone and Acetaminophen—*See* Narcotic Analgesics and Acetaminophen (Systemic), 1181

*Anoquan*—Butalbital, Acetaminophen, and Caffeine—*See* Butalbital and Acetaminophen (Systemic), 453

*Anorex SR*—Phendimetrazine—*See* Appetite Suppressants (Systemic), 339

*Ansaid*—Flurbiprofen—*See* Nonsteroidal Anti-inflammatory Drugs (Systemic), 1229, MC-10

*Answer*—Pregnancy Test Kits for Home Use, 1385

*Answer Ovulation*—Ovulation Prediction Test Kits for Home Use, 1265

*Answer Plus*—Pregnancy Test Kits for Home Use, 1385

*Answer Plus II*—Pregnancy Test Kits for Home Use, 1385

*Answer Quick & Simple*—Pregnancy Test Kits for Home Use, 1385

*Antabuse*—Disulfiram (Systemic), 736

Antacids (Oral), 253

*AntaGel*—Alumina, Magnesia, and Simethicone—*See* Antacids (Oral), 253

*AntaGel-II*—Alumina, Magnesia, and Simethicone—*See* Antacids (Oral), 253

*Anthra-Derm*—Anthralin (Topical), 256

*Anthraforte 1*—Anthralin (Topical), 256

*Anthraforte 2*—Anthralin (Topical), 256

*Anthraforte 3*—Anthralin (Topical), 256

*Apo-Diclo*—Diclofenac—*See* Nonsteroidal Anti-inflammatory Drugs (Systemic), 1229

*Apo-Diflunisal*—Diflunisal—*See* Nonsteroidal Anti-inflammatory Drugs (Systemic), 1229

*Apo-Diltiaz*—Diltiazem—*See* Calcium Channel Blocking Agents (Systemic), 467

*Apo-Dimenhydrinate*—Dimenhydrinate—*See* Antihistamines (Systemic), 304

*Apo-Dipyridamole*—Dipyridamole (Diagnostic), 731; Dipyridamole (Therapeutic), 732

*Apo-Doxy*—Doxycycline—*See* Tetracyclines (Systemic), 1570

*Apo-Erythro*—Erythromycin Base—*See* Erythromycins (Systemic), 786

*Apo-Erythro E-C*—Erythromycin Base—*See* Erythromycins (Systemic), 786

*Apo-Erythro-ES*—Erythromycin Ethylsuccinate—*See* Erythromycins (Systemic), 786

*Apo-Erythro-S*—Erythromycin Stearate—*See* Erythromycins (Systemic), 786

*Apo-Ferrous Gluconate*—Ferrous Gluconate—*See* Iron Supplements (Systemic), 986

*Apo-Ferrous Sulfate*—Ferrous Sulfate—*See* Iron Supplements (Systemic), 986

*Apo-Fluphenazine*—Fluphenazine—*See* Phenothiazines (Systemic), 1330

*Apo-Flurazepam*—Flurazepam—*See* Benzodiazepines (Systemic), 389

*Apo-Flurbiprofen*—Flurbiprofen—*See* Nonsteroidal Anti-inflammatory Drugs (Systemic), 1229

*Apo-Folic*—Folic Acid (Vitamin B$_9$) (Systemic), 857

*Apo-Furosemide*—Furosemide—*See* Diuretics, Loop (Systemic), 738

*Apo-Glyburide*—Glyburide—*See* Antidiabetics, Oral (Systemic), 283

*Apo-Guanethidine*—Guanethidine (Systemic), 898

*Apo-Haloperidol*—Haloperidol (Systemic), 910

*Apo-Hydro*—Hydrochlorothiazide—*See* Diuretics, Thiazide (Systemic), 749

*Apo-Hydroxyzine*—Hydroxyzine—*See* Antihistamines (Systemic), 304

*Apo-Ibuprofen*—Ibuprofen—*See* Nonsteroidal Anti-inflammatory Drugs (Systemic), 1229

*Apo-Imipramine*—Imipramine—*See* Antidepressants, Tricyclic (Systemic), 277

*Apo-Indomethacin*—Indomethacin—*See* Nonsteroidal Anti-inflammatory Drugs (Systemic), 1229

*Apo-ISDN*—Isosorbide Dinitrate—*See* Nitrates—Oral (Systemic), 1218; Nitrates—Sublingual, Chewable, or Buccal (Systemic), 1221

*Apo-K*—Potassium Chloride—*See* Potassium Supplements (Systemic), 1373

*Apo-Keto*—Ketoprofen—*See* Nonsteroidal Anti-inflammatory Drugs (Systemic), 1229

*Apo-Keto-E*—Ketoprofen—*See* Nonsteroidal Anti-inflammatory Drugs (Systemic), 1229

*Apo-Lorazepam*—Lorazepam—*See* Benzodiazepines (Systemic), 389

*Apo-Meprobamate*—Meprobamate (Systemic), 1089

*Apo-Methyldopa*—Methyldopa (Systemic), 1111

*Apo-Metoclop*—Metoclopramide (Systemic), 1123

*Apo-Metoprolol*—Metoprolol—*See* Beta-adrenergic Blocking Agents (Systemic), 404

*Apo-Metoprolol (Type L)*—Metoprolol—*See* Beta-adrenergic Blocking Agents (Systemic), 404

*Apo-Metronidazole*—Metronidazole (Systemic), 1125

*Apo-Napro-Na*—Naproxen—*See* Nonsteroidal Anti-inflammatory Drugs (Systemic), 1229

*Apo-Napro-Na DS*—Naproxen—*See* Nonsteroidal Anti-inflammatory Drugs (Systemic), 1229

*Apo-Naproxen*—Naproxen—*See* Nonsteroidal Anti-inflammatory Drugs (Systemic), 1229

*Apo-Nifed*—Nifedipine—*See* Calcium Channel Blocking Agents (Systemic), 467

*Apo-Nitrofurantoin*—Nitrofurantoin (Systemic), 1227

*Apo-Oxazepam*—Oxazepam—*See* Benzodiazepines (Systemic), 389

*Apo-Oxtriphylline*—Oxtriphylline—*See* Bronchodilators, Xanthine-derivative (Systemic), 442

*Apo-Pen-VK*—Penicillin V—*See* Penicillins (Systemic), 1299

*Apo-Perphenazine*—Perphenazine—*See* Phenothiazines (Systemic), 1330

*Apo-Phenylbutazone*—Phenylbutazone—*See* Nonsteroidal Anti-inflammatory Drugs (Systemic), 1229

*Apo-Piroxicam*—Piroxicam—*See* Nonsteroidal Anti-inflammatory Drugs (Systemic), 1229

*Apo-Prednisone*—Prednisone—*See* Corticosteroids/Corticotropin—Glucocorticoid Effects (Systemic), 630

*Apo-Primidone*—Primidone (Systemic), 1388

*Apo-Propranolol*—Propranolol—*See* Beta-adrenergic Blocking Agents (Systemic), 404

*Apo-Quinidine*—Quinidine (Systemic), 1428

*Apo-Ranitidine*—Ranitidine—*See* Histamine H$_2$-receptor Antagonists (Systemic), 925

*Apo-Sulfamethoxazole*—Sulfamethoxazole—*See* Sulfonamides (Systemic), 1542

*Apo-Sulfatrim*—Sulfamethoxazole and Trimethoprim (Systemic), 1529

*Apo-Sulfatrim DS*—Sulfamethoxazole and Trimethoprim (Systemic), 1529

*Apo-Sulfinpyrazone*—Sulfinpyrazone (Systemic), 1538

*Apo-Sulin*—Sulindac—*See* Nonsteroidal Anti-inflammatory Drugs (Systemic), 1229

*Apo-Tetra*—Tetracycline—*See* Tetracyclines (Systemic), 1570

*Apo-Thioridazine*—Thioridazine—*See* Phenothiazines (Systemic), 1330

*Apo-Timol*—Timolol—*See* Beta-adrenergic Blocking Agents (Systemic), 404

*Apo-Timop*—Timolol—*See* Beta-adrenergic Blocking Agents (Ophthalmic), 402

*Apo-Tolbutamide*—Tolbutamide—*See* Antidiabetics, Oral (Systemic), 283

*Apo-Triazide*—Triamterene and Hydrochlorothiazide—*See* Diuretics, Potassium-sparing and Hydrochlorothiazide (Systemic), 745

*Apo-Triazo*—Triazolam—*See* Benzodiazepines (Systemic), 389

*Apo-Trifluoperazine*—Trifluoperazine—*See* Phenothiazines (Systemic), 1330

*Apo-Trihex*—Trihexyphenidyl—*See* Antidyskinetics (Systemic), 287

*Apo-Trimip*—Trimipramine—*See* Antidepressants, Tricyclic (Systemic), 277

*Apo-Verap*—Verapamil—*See* Calcium Channel Blocking Agents (Systemic), 467

*Apo-Zidovudine*—Zidovudine (Systemic), 1689

*Appecon*—Phendimetrazine—*See* Appetite Suppressants (Systemic), 339

Appetite Suppressants (Systemic), 339

Apraclonidine (Ophthalmic), 342

*Apresazide*—Hydralazine and Hydrochlorothiazide (Systemic), 933, MC-11

*Apresoline*—Hydralazine (Systemic), 931, MC-11

*Apresoline-Esidrix*—Hydralazine and Hydrochlorothiazide (Systemic), 933

Aprobarbital—*See* Barbiturates (Systemic), 370

*Aprodine with Codeine*—Triprolidine, Pseudoephedrine, and Codeine—*See* Cough/Cold Combinations (Systemic), 637

*Aprodrine*—Triprolidine and Pseudoephedrine—*See* Antihistamines and Decongestants (Systemic), 311

*Aprozide*—Hydralazine and Hydrochlorothiazide (Systemic), 933

APSAC—Anistreplase—*See* Thrombolytic Agents (Systemic), 1604

*Aquachloral Supprettes*—Chloral Hydrate (Systemic), 509

*AquaMEPHYTON*—Phytonadione—*See* Vitamin K (Systemic), 1676

*Aquaphyllin*—Theophylline—*See* Bronchodilators, Xanthine-derivative (Systemic), 442

*Aquasol A*—Vitamin A (Systemic), 1664

*Aquasol E*—Vitamin E (Systemic), 1674

*Aquatar*—Coal Tar (Topical), 589

*Aquatensen*—Methyclothiazide—*See* Diuretics, Thiazide (Systemic), 749

*Aqueous Charcodote*—Charcoal, Activated (Oral), 504

*Aquest*—Estrone—*See* Estrogens (Systemic), 795

Ara-A—*See* Vidarabine (Ophthalmic), 1658

Arabinoside—*See* Vidarabine (Ophthalmic), 1658

Ara-C—*See* Cytarabine (Systemic), 673

*Aralen*—Chloroquine (Systemic), 529

*Aralen HCl*—Chloroquine (Systemic), 529

*Arcet*—Butalbital, Acetaminophen, and Caffeine—*See* Butalbital and Acetaminophen (Systemic), 453

*Aredia*—Pamidronate (Systemic), 1281

*Aristocort*—Triamcinolone—*See* Corticosteroids/Corticotropin—Glucocorticoid Effects (Systemic), 630; Corticosteroids—Medium to Very High Potency (Topical), 626

*Aristocort A*—Triamcinolone—*See* Corticosteroids—Medium to Very High Potency (Topical), 626

*Aristocort C*—Triamcinolone—*See* Corticosteroids—Medium to Very High Potency (Topical), 626

*Aristocort D*—Triamcinolone—*See* Corticosteroids—Medium to Very High Potency (Topical), 626

*Aristocort Forte*—Triamcinolone—*See* Corticosteroids/Corticotropin—Glucocorticoid Effects (Systemic), 630

*Aristocort Intralesional*—Triamcinolone—*See* Corticosteroids/Corticotropin—Glucocorticoid Effects (Systemic), 630

*Aristocort R*—Triamcinolone—*See* Corticosteroids—Medium to Very High Potency (Topical), 626

*Aristospan Intra-articular*—Triamcinolone—*See* Corticosteroids/Corticotropin—Glucocorticoid Effects (Systemic), 630

*Aristospan Intralesional*—Triamcinolone—*See* Corticosteroids/Corticotropin—Glucocorticoid Effects (Systemic), 630

*Arlidin*—Nylidrin (Systemic), 1242

*Arlidin Forte*—Nylidrin (Systemic), 1242

*Arm-a-Med Isoetharine*—Isoetharine—*See* Bronchodilators, Adrenergic (Inhalation), 430

*Arm-a-Med Metaproterenol*—Metaproterenol—*See* Bronchodilators, Adrenergic (Inhalation), 430

*Arm and Hammer Pure Baking Soda*—Sodium Bicarbonate (Systemic), 1499

*A.R.M. Maximum Strength Caplets*—Chlorpheniramine and Phenylpropanolamine—*See* Antihistamines and Decongestants (Systemic), 311

*Armour Thyroid*—Thyroid—*See* Thyroid Hormones (Systemic), 1606

*Arrestin*—Trimethobenzamide (Systemic), 1626

*Artane*—Trihexyphenidyl—*See* Antidyskinetics (Systemic), 287

*Artane Sequels*—Trihexyphenidyl—*See* Antidyskinetics (Systemic), 287

*Arthrinol*—Aspirin—*See* Salicylates (Systemic), 1473

*Arthrisin*—Aspirin—*See* Salicylates (Systemic), 1473

*Arthritis Pain Formula*—Aspirin, Alumina, and Magnesia—*See* Salicylates (Systemic), 1473

*Arthropan*—Choline Salicylate—*See* Salicylates (Systemic), 1473

*Articulose-50*—Prednisolone—*See* Corticosteroids/Corticotropin—Glucocorticoid Effects (Systemic), 630

*Articulose-L.A.*—Triamcinolone—*See* Corticosteroids/Corticotropin—Glucocorticoid Effects (Systemic), 630

*Artria S.R.*—Aspirin—*See* Salicylates (Systemic), 1473

ASA—Aspirin—*See* Salicylates (Systemic), 1473

5-ASA—*See* Mesalamine (Rectal), 1097

*Asacol*—Mesalamine (Rectal), 1751, MC-14

*Asasantine*—Dipyridamole and Aspirin (Systemic), 1748

*Asbron G*—Theophylline and Guaifenesin (Systemic), 1586

*Asbron G Inlay-Tabs*—Theophylline and Guaifenesin (Systemic), 1586

*Ascabiol*—Benzyl Benzoate (Topical), 400

*Ascomp with Codeine No.3*—Butalbital, Aspirin, Caffeine, and Codeine—*See* Barbiturates, Aspirin, and Codeine (Systemic), 376

Ascorbic Acid (Vitamin C) (Systemic), 344

*Ascorbicap*—Ascorbic Acid (Vitamin C) (Systemic), 344

*Ascriptin*—Aspirin, Buffered—*See* Salicylates (Systemic), 1473

*Ascriptin A/D*—Aspirin, Buffered—*See* Salicylates (Systemic), 1473

*Asendin*—Amoxapine—*See* Antidepressants, Tricyclic (Systemic), 277

*A-200 Shampoo Concentrate*—Pyrethrins and Piperonyl Butoxide (Topical), 1417

*Asmalix*—Theophylline—*See* Bronchodilators, Xanthine-derivative (Systemic), 442

Asparaginase (Systemic), 347

*A-Spas*—Dicyclomine—*See* Anticholinergics/Antispasmodics (Systemic), 258

*Aspergum*—Aspirin—*See* Salicylates (Systemic), 1473
*Aspirin*—Aspirin—*See* Salicylates (Systemic), 1473
Aspirin—*See* Salicylates (Systemic), 1473
Aspirin, Alumina, and Magnesia—Aspirin, Buffered—*See* Salicylates (Systemic), 1473
Aspirin and Caffeine—*See* Salicylates (Systemic), 1473
Aspirin, Caffeine, and Dihydrocodeine—*See* Narcotic Analgesics and Aspirin (Systemic), 1185, MC-2
Aspirin and Codeine—*See* Narcotic Analgesics and Aspirin (Systemic), 1185, MC-2
Aspirin, Codeine, and Caffeine—*See* Narcotic Analgesics and Aspirin (Systemic), 1185
Aspirin, Codeine, and Caffeine, Buffered—*See* Narcotic Analgesics and Aspirin (Systemic), 1185
*Aspirin Free Anacin Maximum Strength Caplets*—Acetaminophen (Systemic), 161
*Aspirin Free Anacin Maximum Strength Gel Caplets*—Acetaminophen (Systemic), 161
*Aspirin Free Anacin Maximum Strength Tablets*—Acetaminophen (Systemic), 161
*Aspirin-Free Excedrin Caplets*—Acetaminophen and Caffeine—*See* Acetaminophen (Systemic), 161
Aspirin, Sodium Bicarbonate, and Citric Acid (Systemic), 349
Astemizole—*See* Antihistamines (Systemic), 304, MC-2
*AsthmaHaler Mist*—Epinephrine—*See* Bronchodilators, Adrenergic (Inhalation), 430
*AsthmaNefrin*—Racepinephrine—*See* Bronchodilators, Adrenergic (Inhalation), 430
*Astramorph*—Morphine—*See* Narcotic Analgesics—For Pain Relief (Systemic), 1176; Narcotic Analgesics—For Surgery and Obstetrics (Systemic), 1179
*Astramorph PF*—Morphine—*See* Narcotic Analgesics—For Pain Relief (Systemic), 1176; Narcotic Analgesics—For Surgery and Obstetrics (Systemic), 1179
*Astrin*—Aspirin—*See* Salicylates (Systemic), 1473
*Atabrine*—Quinacrine (Systemic), 1427
*Atarax*—Hydroxyzine—*See* Antihistamines (Systemic), 304, MC-11
*Atasol-8*—Acetaminophen, Codeine, and Caffeine—*See* Narcotic Analgesics and Acetaminophen (Systemic), 1181
*Atasol-15*—Acetaminophen, Codeine, and Caffeine—*See* Narcotic Analgesics and Acetaminophen (Systemic), 1181
*Atasol-30*—Acetaminophen, Codeine, and Caffeine—*See* Narcotic Analgesics and Acetaminophen (Systemic), 1181
*Atasol Caplets*—Acetaminophen (Systemic), 161
*Atasol Drops*—Acetaminophen (Systemic), 161
*Atasol Forte Caplets*—Acetaminophen (Systemic), 161
*Atasol Forte Tablets*—Acetaminophen (Systemic), 161
*Atasol Oral Solution*—Acetaminophen (Systemic), 161
*Atasol Tablets*—Acetaminophen (Systemic), 161
Atenolol—*See* Beta-adrenergic Blocking Agents (Systemic), 404, MC-2
Atenolol and Chlorthalidone—*See* Beta-adrenergic Blocking Agents and Thiazide Diuretics (Systemic), 410, MC-2
*Ativan*—Lorazepam—*See* Benzodiazepines (Systemic), 389, MC-14
Atovaquone (Systemic), 353, MC-2
*Atrofed*—Triprolidine and Pseudoephedrine (Systemic), 1754

*Atrohist Pediatric*—Chlorpheniramine, Pyrilamine, and Phenylephrine—*See* Antihistamines and Decongestants (Systemic), 311
*Atrohist Plus*—Chlorpheniramine, Phenylephrine, Phenylpropanolamine, Atropine, Hyoscyamine, and Scopolamine—*See* Antihistamines, Decongestants, and Anticholinergics (Systemic), 322
*Atrohist Sprinkle*—Brompheniramine, Phenyltoloxamine, and Phenylephrine—*See* Antihistamines and Decongestants (Systemic), 311
*Atromid-S*—Clofibrate (Systemic), 572
*Atropair*—Atropine—*See* Atropine/Homatropine/Scopolamine (Ophthalmic), 354
Atropine—*See* Anticholinergics/Antispasmodics (Systemic), 258; Atropine/Homatropine/Scopolamine (Ophthalmic), 354
*Atropine Care*—Atropine—*See* Atropine/Homatropine/Scopolamine (Ophthalmic), 354
Atropine/Homatropine/Scopolamine (Ophthalmic), 354
Atropine, Hyoscyamine, Methenamine, Methylene Blue, Phenyl Salicylate, and Benzoic Acid (Systemic), 357
Atropine, Hyoscyamine, Scopolamine, and Phenobarbital—*See* Belladonna Alkaloids and Barbiturates (Systemic), 382, MC-2
Atropine and Phenobarbital—*See* Belladonna Alkaloids and Barbiturates (Systemic), 382
*Atropine Sulfate S.O.P.*—Atropine—*See* Atropine/Homatropine/Scopolamine (Ophthalmic), 354
*Atropisol*—Atropine—*See* Atropine/Homatropine/Scopolamine (Ophthalmic), 354
*Atrosept*—Atropine, Hyoscyamine, Methenamine, Methylene Blue, Phenyl Salicylate, and Benzoic Acid (Systemic), 357
*Atrovent*—Ipratropium (Inhalation), 980; Ipratropium (Nasal), 984
*A/T/S*—Erythromycin (Topical), 782
*Attain*—Enteral Nutrition Formula, Polymeric—*See* Enteral Nutrition Formulas (Systemic), 769
Attapulgite (Oral), 359
*Attenuvax*—Measles Virus Vaccine Live (Systemic), 1069
*Augmentin*—Amoxicillin and Clavulanate—*See* Penicillins and Beta-lactamase Inhibitors (Systemic), 1306, MC-2
*Aurafair*—Antipyrine and Benzocaine (Otic), 334
*Auralgan*—Antipyrine and Benzocaine (Otic), 334
Auranofin—*See* Gold Compounds (Systemic), 884, MC-2
*Aureomycin*—Chlortetracycline—*See* Tetracyclines (Ophthalmic), 1568; Tetracyclines (Topical), 1574
*Aurodex*—Antipyrine and Benzocaine (Otic), 334
Aurothioglucose—*See* Gold Compounds (Systemic), 884
*Aut*—Pyrantel (Oral), 1414
*AVC*—Sulfanilamide—*See* Sulfonamides (Vaginal), 1545; Sulfanilamide, Aminacrine, and Allantoin—*See* Sulfonamides (Vaginal), 1545
*Aveeno Acne Bar*—Salicylic Acid and Sulfur (Topical), 1481
*Aveeno Cleansing Bar*—Salicylic Acid and Sulfur (Topical), 1481
*Aventyl*—Nortriptyline—*See* Antidepressants, Tricyclic (Systemic), 277
*Avirax*—Acyclovir (Systemic), 175
*Avlosulfon*—Dapsone (Systemic), 687
*Axid*—Nizatidine—*See* Histamine H$_2$-receptor Antagonists (Systemic), 925, MC-16

# B

*Bayer Select Flu Relief Caplets*—Chlorpheniramine, Pseudoephedrine, Dextromethorphan, and Acetaminophen—*See* Cough/Cold Combinations (Systemic), 637

*Bayer Select Head and Chest Cold Caplets*—Pseudoephedrine, Dextromethorphan, Guaifenesin, and Acetaminophen—*See* Cough/Cold Combinations (Systemic), 637

*Bayer Select Head Cold Caplets*—Pseudoephedrine and Acetaminophen—*See* Decongestants and Analgesics (Systemic), 691

*Bayer Select Ibuprofen Caplets*—Ibuprofen—*See* Nonsteroidal Anti-inflammatory Drugs (Systemic), 1229

*Bayer Select Maximum Strength Headache Pain Relief Formula*—Acetaminophen and Caffeine—*See* Acetaminophen (Systemic), 161

*Bayer Select Maximum Strength Sinus Pain Relief Caplets*—Pseudoephedrine and Acetaminophen—*See* Decongestants and Analgesics (Systemic), 691, 1753

*Bayer Select Night Time Cold Caplets*—Triprolidine, Pseudoephedrine, Dextromethorphan, and Acetaminophen—*See* Cough/Cold Combinations (Systemic), 637

*Bayer Timed-Release Arthritic Pain Formula*—Aspirin—*See* Salicylates (Systemic), 1473

*Bayhistine DH*—Chlorpheniramine, Pseudoephedrine, and Codeine—*See* Cough/Cold Combinations (Systemic), 637

*Bayhistine Expectorant*—Pseudoephedrine, Codeine, and Guaifenesin—*See* Cough/Cold Combinations (Systemic), 637

*Baytussin AC*—Codeine and Guaifenesin—*See* Cough/Cold Combinations (Systemic), 637

*Baytussin DM*—Dextromethorphan and Guaifenesin—*See* Cough/Cold Combinations (Systemic), 637

*BC Cold Powder*—Chlorpheniramine, Phenylpropanolamine, and Aspirin (Systemic), 1746

*BC Cold Powder Non-Drowsy Formula*—Phenylpropanolamine and Aspirin—*See* Decongestants and Analgesics (Systemic), 691

*BC Multi Symptom Cold Powder*—Chlorpheniramine, Phenylpropanolamine, and Aspirin—*See* Antihistamines, Decongestants, and Analgesics (Systemic), 316

BCNU—*See* Carmustine (Systemic), 494

*Beben*—Betamethasone—*See* Corticosteroids—Medium to Very High Potency (Topical), 626

*Bebulin VH*—Factor IX (Systemic), 823

*Because*—Nonoxynol 9—*See* Spermicides (Vaginal), 1512

*Beclodisk*—Beclomethasone—*See* Corticosteroids (Inhalation), 611

*Becloforte*—Beclomethasone—*See* Corticosteroids (Inhalation), 611

Beclometasone—Beclomethasone—*See* Corticosteroids (Inhalation), 611; Corticosteroids (Nasal), 617; Corticosteroids—Medium to Very High Potency (Topical), 626

Beclometasone dipropionate—Beclomethasone—*See* Corticosteroids (Inhalation), 611

Beclomethasone—*See* Corticosteroids (Inhalation), 611; Corticosteroids (Nasal), 617; Corticosteroids—Medium to Very High Potency (Topical), 626

Beclomethasone dipropionate—Beclomethasone—*See* Corticosteroids (Inhalation), 611

*Beclovent*—Beclomethasone—*See* Corticosteroids (Inhalation), 611

*Beclovent Rotacaps*—Beclomethasone—*See* Corticosteroids (Inhalation), 611

*Beconase*—Beclomethasone—*See* Corticosteroids (Nasal), 617

*Beconase AQ*—Beclomethasone—*See* Corticosteroids (Nasal), 617

*Bedoz*—Cyanocobalamin—*See* Vitamin $B_{12}$ (Systemic), 1667

*Beepen-VK*—Penicillin V—*See* Penicillins (Systemic), 1299

*Beesix*—Pyridoxine (Vitamin $B_6$) (Systemic), 1419

*Beldin*—Diphenhydramine—*See* Antihistamines (Systemic), 304

*Belix*—Diphenhydramine—*See* Antihistamines (Systemic), 304

Belladonna—*See* Anticholinergics/Antispasmodics (Systemic), 258

Belladonna Alkaloids and Barbiturates (Systemic), 382

Belladonna and Butabarbital—*See* Belladonna Alkaloids and Barbiturates (Systemic), 382

Belladonna and Phenobarbital—*See* Belladonna Alkaloids and Barbiturates (Systemic), 382

*Bellalphen*—Atropine, Hyoscyamine, Scopolamine, and Phenobarbital—*See* Belladonna Alkaloids and Barbiturates (Systemic), 382

*Bell/ans*—Sodium Bicarbonate (Systemic), 1499

*Bellergal*—Ergotamine, Belladonna Alkaloids, and Phenobarbital (Systemic), 778

*Bellergal-S*—Ergotamine, Belladonna Alkaloids, and Phenobarbital (Systemic), 778

*Bellergal Spacetabs*—Ergotamine, Belladonna Alkaloids, and Phenobarbital (Systemic), 778

*Bena-D 10*—Diphenhydramine—*See* Antihistamines (Systemic), 304

*Bena-D 50*—Diphenhydramine—*See* Antihistamines (Systemic), 304

*Benadryl*—Diphenhydramine—*See* Antihistamines (Systemic), 304, MC-7

*Benadryl 25*—Diphenhydramine—*See* Antihistamines (Systemic), 304

*Benadryl Allergy/Sinus Headache Caplets*—Diphenhydramine, Pseudoephedrine, and Acetaminophen (Systemic), 1748

*Benadryl Cold*—Diphenhydramine, Pseudoephedrine, and Acetaminophen—*See* Antihistamines, Decongestants, and Analgesics (Systemic), 316

*Benadryl Cold Nighttime Liquid*—Diphenhydramine, Pseudoephedrine, and Acetaminophen—*See* Antihistamines, Decongestants, and Analgesics (Systemic), 316

*Benadryl Decongestant*—Diphenhydramine and Pseudoephedrine—*See* Antihistamines and Decongestants (Systemic), 311

*Benadryl Kapseals*—Diphenhydramine—*See* Antihistamines (Systemic), 304

*Benahist 10*—Diphenhydramine—*See* Antihistamines (Systemic), 304

*Benahist 50*—Diphenhydramine—*See* Antihistamines (Systemic), 304

*Ben-Allergin-50*—Diphenhydramine—*See* Antihistamines (Systemic), 304

*Ben-Aqua-2½ Gel*—Benzoyl Peroxide (Topical), 397

*Ben-Aqua-5 Gel*—Benzoyl Peroxide (Topical), 397

*Ben-Aqua-10 Gel*—Benzoyl Peroxide (Topical), 397

*Betapen-VK*—Penicillin V—*See* Penicillins (Systemic), 1299

*Betaseron*—Interferon Beta-1b (Systemic), 1750

*Betatrex*—Betamethasone—*See* Corticosteroids—Medium to Very High Potency (Topical), 626

*Beta-Val*—Betamethasone—*See* Corticosteroids—Medium to Very High Potency (Topical), 626

*Betaxin*—Thiamine (Vitamin B₁) (Systemic), 1591

Betaxolol—*See* Beta-adrenergic Blocking Agents (Ophthalmic), 402, 1745; Beta-adrenergic Blocking Agents (Systemic), 404, MC-3

Bethanechol (Systemic), 418

*Betnelan*—Betamethasone—*See* Corticosteroids/Corticotropin—Glucocorticoid Effects (Systemic), 630

*Betnesol*—Betamethasone—*See* Corticosteroids (Ophthalmic), 620; Corticosteroids (Otic), 622; Corticosteroids/Corticotropin—Glucocorticoid Effects (Systemic), 630; Betamethasone (Dental), 1745

*Betnovate*—Betamethasone—*See* Corticosteroids—Medium to Very High Potency (Topical), 626

*Betnovate-½*—Betamethasone—*See* Corticosteroids—Medium to Very High Potency (Topical), 626

*Betoptic*—Betaxolol—*See* Beta-adrenergic Blocking Agents (Ophthalmic), 402, 1745

*Betoptic S*—Betaxolol—*See* Beta-adrenergic Blocking Agents (Ophthalmic), 402

*Bewon*—Thiamine (Vitamin B₁) (Systemic), 1591

*Bexophene*—Propoxyphene, Aspirin, and Caffeine—*See* Narcotic Analgesics and Aspirin (Systemic), 1185

*Biamine*—Thiamine (Vitamin B₁) (Systemic), 1591

*Biaxin*—Clarithromycin (Systemic), 559, MC-5

*Bicillin L-A*—Penicillin G—*See* Penicillins (Systemic), 1299

*Bicitra*—Sodium Citrate and Citric Acid—*See* Citrates (Systemic), 554

*BiCNU*—Carmustine (Systemic), 494

*Bifenabid*—Probucol (Systemic), 1395

*Bilagog*—Magnesium Sulfate—*See* Laxatives (Oral), 1017

*Bilax*—Dehydrocholic Acid and Docusate—*See* Laxatives (Oral), 1017

*Bilivist*—Ipodate—*See* Cholecystographic Agents, Oral (Diagnostic), 536

*Bilopaque*—Tyropanoate—*See* Cholecystographic Agents, Oral (Diagnostic), 536

*Biloptin*—Ipodate—*See* Cholecystographic Agents, Oral (Diagnostic), 536

*Biltricide*—Praziquantel (Systemic), 1378

*BioCal*—Calcium Carbonate—*See* Calcium Supplements (Systemic), 472

*Bio-Gan*—Trimethobenzamide (Systemic), 1626

*Bio-Syn*—Fluocinolone—*See* Corticosteroids—Medium to Very High Potency (Topical), 626

*Biotel/diabetes*—Glucose Oxidase Urine Glucose Test—*See* Urine Glucose and Ketone Test Kits for Home Use, 1644

Biotin (Systemic), 420

*Biotirmone*—Dextrothyroxine (Systemic), 702

*Bio-Tn*—Biotin (Systemic), 420

*Bio-Well*—Lindane (Topical), 1042

Biperiden—*See* Antidyskinetics (Systemic), 287

*Biphetane DC Cough*—Brompheniramine, Phenylpropanolamine, and Codeine—*See* Cough/Cold Combinations (Systemic), 637

*Bisac-Evac*—Bisacodyl—*See* Laxatives (Oral), 1017

Bisacodyl—*See* Laxatives (Oral), 1017; Laxatives (Rectal), 1023

Bisacodyl and Docusate—*See* Laxatives (Oral), 1017

*Bisacolax*—Bisacodyl—*See* Laxatives (Oral), 1017; Laxatives (Rectal), 1023

*Bisco-Lax*—Bisacodyl—*See* Laxatives (Rectal), 1023

*Bismatrol*—Bismuth Subsalicylate (Oral), 421

*Bismatrol Extra Strength*—Bismuth Subsalicylate (Oral), 421

*Bismed*—Bismuth Subsalicylate (Oral), 421

Bismuth Subsalicylate (Oral), 421

*Bisodol*—Calcium Carbonate and Magnesia—*See* Antacids (Oral), 253; Magnesium Carbonate and Sodium Bicarbonate—*See* Antacids (Oral), 253

Bisoprolol—*See* Beta-adrenergic Blocking Agents (Systemic), 404, MC-3

Bisprolol and Hydrochlorothiazide—*See* Beta-adrenergic Blocking Agents and Thiazide Diuretics (Systemic), 410, MC-3

Bitolterol—*See* Bronchodilators, Adrenergic (Inhalation), 430

*Black-Draught*—Casanthranol—*See* Laxatives (Oral), 1017

*Black-Draught Lax-Senna*—Senna—*See* Laxatives (Oral), 1017

*Blanex*—Orphenadrine (Systemic), 1260

*Blenoxane*—Bleomycin (Systemic), 424

Bleomycin (Systemic), 424

*Bleph-10*—Sulfacetamide—*See* Sulfonamides (Ophthalmic), 1540

*Blocadren*—Timolol—*See* Beta-adrenergic Blocking Agents (Systemic), 404, MC-23

*Blue*—Pyrethrins and Piperonyl Butoxide (Topical), 1417

*Bonamine*—Meclizine—*See* Meclizine/Buclizine/Cyclizine (Systemic), 1079

*Bonine*—Meclizine—*See* Meclizine/Buclizine/Cyclizine (Systemic), 1079

*Bontril PDM*—Phendimetrazine—*See* Appetite Suppressants (Systemic), 339

*Bontril Slow-Release*—Phendimetrazine—*See* Appetite Suppressants (Systemic), 339

*Botox*—Botulinum Toxin Type A (Parenteral-Local), 426

Botulinum Toxin Type A (Parenteral-Local), 426

*BQ Cold*—Chlorpheniramine, Phenylpropanolamine, and Acetaminophen—*See* Antihistamines, Decongestants, and Analgesics (Systemic), 316

*Breonesin*—Guaifenesin (Systemic), 892

*Brethaire*—Terbutaline—*See* Bronchodilators, Adrenergic (Inhalation), 430

*Brethine*—Terbutaline—*See* Bronchodilators, Adrenergic (Oral/Injection), 436, MC-22

*Brevicon*—Norethindrone and Ethinyl Estradiol—*See* Estrogens and Progestins (Oral Contraceptives) (Systemic), 804

*Brevicon 0.5/35*—Norethindrone and Ethinyl Estradiol—*See* Estrogens and Progestins (Oral Contraceptives) (Systemic), 804

*Brevicon 1/35*—Norethindrone and Ethinyl Estradiol—*See* Estrogens and Progestins (Oral Contraceptives) (Systemic), 804

*Brevital*—Methohexital—*See* Anesthetics, General (Systemic), 243

*Brevoxyl 4 Gel*—Benzoyl Peroxide (Topical), 397

*Broncholate*—Ephedrine and Guaifenesin—*See* Cough/Cold Combinations (Systemic), 637

*Broncomar-GG*—Theophylline and Guaifenesin (Systemic), 1586

*Brondelate*—Oxtriphylline and Guaifenesin (Systemic), 1270

*Bronitin Mist*—Epinephrine—*See* Bronchodilators, Adrenergic (Inhalation), 430

*Bronkaid Mist*—Epinephrine—*See* Bronchodilators, Adrenergic (Inhalation), 430

*Bronkaid Mistometer*—Epinephrine—*See* Bronchodilators, Adrenergic (Inhalation), 430

*Bronkephrine*—Ethylnorepinephrine—*See* Bronchodilators, Adrenergic (Oral/Injection), 436

*Bronkodyl*—Theophylline—*See* Bronchodilators, Xanthine-derivative (Systemic), 442

*Bronkolixir*—Theophylline, Ephedrine, Guaifenesin, and Phenobarbital (Systemic), 1577

*Bronkometer*—Isoetharine—*See* Bronchodilators, Adrenergic (Inhalation), 430

*Bronkosol*—Isoetharine—*See* Bronchodilators, Adrenergic (Inhalation), 430

*Bronkotabs*—Theophylline, Ephedrine, Guaifenesin, and Phenobarbital (System), 1577

*Bronkotuss Expectorant*—Chlorpheniramine, Ephedrine, and Guaifenesin—*See* Cough/Cold Combinations (Systemic), 637

*Brotane DX Cough*—Brompheniramine, Pseudoephedrine, and Dextromethorphan—*See* Cough/Cold Combinations (Systemic), 637

*Bucet*—Butalbital and Acetaminophen (Systemic), 453

*Bucladin-S Softabs*—Buclizine—*See* Meclizine/Buclizine/Cyclizine (Systemic), 1079

*Buclizine*—*See* Meclizine/Buclizine/Cyclizine (Systemic), 1079

Budesonide—*See* Corticosteroids (Inhalation), 611; Corticosteroids (Nasal), 617

Budesonide (Rectal-Local), 1745

Bufexamac (Topical), 1745

*Buffaprin*—Aspirin, Buffered—*See* Salicylates (Systemic), 1473

Buffered Aspirin—*See* Salicylates (Systemic), 1473

*Bufferin*—Aspirin, Buffered—*See* Salicylates (Systemic), 1473

*Buffets II*—Acetaminophen, Aspirin, and Caffeine, Buffered—*See* Acetaminophen and Salicylates (Systemic), 164

*Buffinol*—Aspirin, Buffered—*See* Salicylates (Systemic), 1473

*Buf-Puf Acne Cleansing Bar with Vitamin E*—Salicylic Acid (Topical), 1478

Bumetanide—*See* Diuretics, Loop (Systemic), 738, MC-3

*Bumex*—Bumetanide—*See* Diuretics, Loop (Systemic), 738, MC-3

Bupivacaine—*See* Anesthetics (Parenteral-Local), 235

*Buprenex*—Buprenorphine—*See* Narcotic Analgesics—For Pain Relief (Systemic), 1176; Narcotic Analgesics—For Surgery and Obstetrics (Systemic), 1179

Buprenorphine—*See* Narcotic Analgesics—For Pain Relief (Systemic), 1176; Narcotic Analgesics—For Surgery and Obstetrics (Systemic), 1179

Bupropion (Systemic), 446, MC-3

*Buscopan*—Scopolamine—*See* Anticholinergics/Antispasmodics (Systemic), 258

Buserelin (Systemic), 447

*Busodium*—Butabarbital—*See* Barbiturates (Systemic), 370

*BuSpar*—Buspirone (Systemic), 449, MC-3

Buspirone (Systemic), 449, MC-3

Busulfan (Systemic), 450

Butabarbital—*See* Barbiturates (Systemic), 370

*Butace*—Butalbital, Acetaminophen, and Caffeine—*See* Butalbital and Acetaminophen (Systemic), 453

*Butalan*—Butabarbital—*See* Barbiturates (Systemic), 370

Butalbital-AC—Butalbital, Aspirin, and Caffeine—*See* Butalbital and Aspirin (Systemic), 456

Butalbital and Acetaminophen (Systemic), 453

Butalbital, Acetaminophen, and Caffeine—*See* Butalbital and Acetaminophen (Systemic), 453, MC-3

Butalbital and Aspirin (Systemic), 456

Butalbital, Aspirin, and Caffeine—*See* Butalbital and Aspirin (Systemic), 456, MC-3

Butalbital, Aspirin, Caffeine, and Codeine—*See* Barbiturates, Aspirin, and Codeine (Systemic), 376, MC-3

Butalbital compound—Butalbital, Aspirin, and Caffeine—*See* Butalbital and Aspirin (Systemic), 456

*Butalbital Compound with Codeine*—Butalbital, Aspirin, Caffeine, and Codeine—*See* Barbiturates, Aspirin, and Codeine (Systemic), 376

*Butalgen*—Butalbital, Aspirin, and Caffeine—*See* Butalbital and Aspirin (Systemic), 456

Butamben—*See* Anesthetics (Topical), 240

*Butazolidin*—Phenylbutazone—*See* Nonsteroidal Anti-inflammatory Drugs (Systemic), 1229

*Butesin Picrate*—Butamben—*See* Anesthetics (Topical), 240

*Butibel*—Belladonna and Butabarbital—*See* Belladonna Alkaloids and Barbiturates (Systemic), 382

*Butinal with Codeine No.3*—Butalbital, Aspirin, Caffeine, and Codeine—*See* Barbiturates, Aspirin, and Codeine (Systemic), 376

*Butisol*—Butabarbital—*See* Barbiturates (Systemic), 370

Butoconazole—*See* Antifungals, Azole (Vaginal), 296

Butorphanol—*See* Narcotic Analgesics—For Pain Relief (Systemic), 1176, 1745; Narcotic Analgesics—For Surgery and Obstetrics (Systemic), 1179, 1745

Butyl aminobenzoate—Butamben—*See* Anesthetics (Topical), 240

*Bydramine Cough*—Diphenhydramine—*See* Antihistamines (Systemic), 304

# C

*C2*—Aspirin and Caffeine—*See* Salicylates (Systemic), 1473

566C80—*See* Atovaquone (Systemic), 353

*Cafergot*—Ergotamine and Caffeine—*See* Headache Medicines, Ergot Derivative-containing (Systemic), 914, MC-9

*Cafergot-PB*—Ergotamine, Caffeine, Belladonna Alkaloids, and Pentobarbital—*See* Headache Medicines, Ergot Derivative-containing (Systemic), 914

*Cafertine*—Ergotamine and Caffeine—*See* Headache Medicines, Ergot Derivative-containing (Systemic), 914

*Calmylin Expectorant*—Guaifenesin (Systemic), 1749

*Calmylin Pediatric*—Pseudoephedrine and Dextromethorphan (Systemic), 1753

*Calphosan*—Calcium Glycerophosphate and Calcium Lactate—*See* Calcium Supplements (Systemic), 472

*Calsan*—Calcium Carbonate—*See* Calcium Supplements (Systemic), 472

*Caltrate 300*—Calcium Carbonate—*See* Calcium Supplements (Systemic), 472

*Caltrate 600*—Calcium Carbonate—*See* Calcium Supplements (Systemic), 472

*Caltrate Chewable*—Calcium Carbonate—*See* Calcium Supplements (Systemic), 472

*Cama Arthritis Pain Reliever*—Aspirin, Alumina, and Magnesium Oxide—*See* Salicylates (Systemic), 1473

*Camalox*—Alumina, Magnesia, and Calcium Carbonate—*See* Antacids (Oral), 253

*Cam-Ap-Es*—Reserpine, Hydralazine, and Hydrochlorothiazide (Systemic), 1449

Camphorated Opium Tincture—Paregoric—*See* Opium Preparations (Systemic), 1258

*Canesten*—Clotrimazole—*See* Antifungals, Azole (Vaginal), 296

*Canesten 1*—Clotrimazole—*See* Antifungals, Azole (Vaginal), 296

*Canesten 3*—Clotrimazole—*See* Antifungals, Azole (Vaginal), 296

*Canesten Cream*—Clotrimazole (Topical), 583

*Canesten Solution*—Clotrimazole (Topical), 583

*Canesten Solution with Atomizer*—Clotrimazole (Topical), 583

*Cantil*—Mepenzolate—*See* Anticholinergics/Antispasmodics (Systemic), 258

*Capastat*—Capreomycin (Systemic), 476

*Capen*—Tiopronin (Systemic), 1612

*Capital with Codeine*—Acetaminophen and Codeine—*See* Narcotic Analgesics and Acetaminophen (Systemic), 1181

*Capitrol*—Chloroxine (Topical), 532

*Capoten*—Captopril—*See* Angiotensin-converting Enzyme (ACE) Inhibitors (Systemic), 245, MC-3

*Capozide*—Captopril and Hydrochlorothiazide—*See* Angiotensin-converting Enzyme (ACE) Inhibitors and Hydrochlorothiazide (Systemic), 249, MC-3

Capreomycin (Systemic), 476

Capsaicin (Topical), 477

*Captimer*—Tiopronin (Systemic), 1612

Captopril—*See* Angiotensin-converting Enzyme (ACE) Inhibitors (Systemic), 245, MC-3

Captopril and Hydrochlorothiazide—*See* Angiotensin-converting Enzyme (ACE) Inhibitors and Hydrochlorothiazide (Systemic), 249, MC-3

*Carafate*—Sucralfate (Oral), 1522, MC-21

Carbachol (Ophthalmic), 479

*Carbacot*—Methocarbamol—*See* Skeletal Muscle Relaxants (Systemic), 1495

Carbamazepine (Systemic), 481, MC-3, MC-4

Carbamide—*See* Urea (Intra-amniotic), 1643

Carbamylcholine—*See* Carbachol (Ophthalmic), 479

Carbenicillin—*See* Penicillins (Systemic), 1299, MC-4

Carbidopa and Levodopa—*See* Levodopa (Systemic), 1033, MC-4

Carbinoxamine—*See* Antihistamines (Systemic), 304

*Carbinoxamine Compound*—Carbinoxamine, Pseudoephedrine, and Dextromethorphan—*See* Cough/Cold Combinations (Systemic), 637

*Carbinoxamine Compound-Drops*—Carbinoxamine, Pseudoephedrine, and Dextromethorphan—*See* Cough/Cold Combinations (Systemic), 637

Carbinoxamine and Pseudoephedrine—*See* Antihistamines and Decongestants (Systemic), 311

Carbinoxamine, Pseudoephedrine, and Dextromethorphan—*See* Cough/Cold Combinations (Systemic), 637

Carbinoxamine, Pseudoephedrine, and Guaifenesin—*See* Cough/Cold Combinations (Systemic), 637

*Carbiset*—Carbinoxamine and Pseudoephedrine—*See* Antihistamines and Decongestants (Systemic), 311

*Carbiset-TR*—Carbinoxamine and Pseudoephedrine—*See* Antihistamines and Decongestants (Systemic), 311

*Carbocaine*—Mepivacaine—*See* Anesthetics (Parenteral-Local), 235

*Carbocaine with Neo-Cobefrin*—Mepivacaine—*See* Anesthetics (Parenteral-Local), 235

*Carbodec*—Carbinoxamine and Pseudoephedrine—*See* Antihistamines and Decongestants (Systemic), 311

*Carbodec DM Drops*—Carbinoxamine, Pseudoephedrine, and Dextromethorphan—*See* Cough/Cold Combinations (Systemic), 637

*Carbodec TR*—Carbinoxamine and Pseudoephedrine—*See* Antihistamines and Decongestants (Systemic), 311

Carbohydrates and Electrolytes (Systemic), 484

Carbol-Fuchsin (Topical), 487

*Carbolith*—Lithium (Systemic), 1044

Carbonic Anhydrase Inhibitors (Systemic), 488

Carboplatin (Systemic), 491

Carboprost (Systemic), 493

Carboxymethylcellulose (Ophthalmic), 1746

Carboxymethylcellulose, Casanthranol, and Docusate—*See* Laxatives (Oral), 1017

Carboxymethylcellulose and Docusate—*See* Laxatives (Oral), 1017

*Cardec DM*—Carbinoxamine, Pseudoephedrine, and Dextromethorphan—*See* Cough/Cold Combinations (Systemic), 637

*Cardec DM Drops*—Carbinoxamine, Pseudoephedrine, and Dextromethorphan—*See* Cough/Cold Combinations (Systemic), 637

*Cardec DM Pediatric*—Carbinoxamine, Pseudoephedrine, and Dextromethorphan—*See* Cough/Cold Combinations (Systemic), 637

*Cardec-S*—Carbinoxamine and Pseudoephedrine—*See* Antihistamines and Decongestants (Systemic), 311

*Cardene SR*—Nicardipine—*See* Calcium Channel Blocking Agents (Systemic), 467, MC-16

*Cardilate*—Erythrityl Tetranitrate—*See* Nitrates—Oral (Systemic), 1218; Nitrates—Sublingual, Chewable, or Buccal (Systemic), 1221

*Cardioquin*—Quinidine (Systemic), 1428

*Cardizem*—Diltiazem—*See* Calcium Channel Blocking Agents (Systemic), 467, MC-7

*Cardizem CD*—Diltiazem—*See* Calcium Channel Blocking Agents (Systemic), 467, MC-7

*Cardizem SR*—Diltiazem—*See* Calcium Channel Blocking Agents (Systemic), 467, MC-7

*Cardura*—Doxazosin (Systemic), 756, MC-8

Carisoprodol—*See* Skeletal Muscle Relaxants (Systemic), 1495, MC-4

Carisoprodol and Aspirin (Systemic), MC-4

Carisoprodol, Aspirin, and Codeine (Systemic), MC-4

*Cari-Tab*—Vitamins A, D, and C and Fluoride—*See* Vitamins and Fluoride (Systemic), 1678

*Carmol-HC*—Hydrocortisone Acetate—*See* Corticosteroids—Low Potency (Topical), 624

Carmustine (Systemic), 494

*Carnation Follow-Up Formula*—Infant Formulas, Milk-based—*See* Infant Formulas (Systemic), 958

*Carnation Good Start*—Infant Formulas, Milk-based—*See* Infant Formulas (Systemic), 958

*Carnation Instant Breakfast*—Enteral Nutrition Formula, Milk-based—*See* Enteral Nutrition Formulas (Systemic), 769

*Carnation Instant Breakfast No Sugar Added*—Enteral Nutrition Formula, Milk-based—*See* Enteral Nutrition Formulas (Systemic), 769

*Carnitor*—Levocarnitine (Systemic), 1032

*Caroid Laxative*—Cascara Sagrada and Phenolphthalein—*See* Laxatives (Oral), 1017

Carteolol—*See* Beta-adrenergic Blocking Agents (Ophthalmic), 402; Beta-adrenergic Blocking Agents (Systemic), 404, MC-4

*Carter's Little Pills*—Bisacodyl—*See* Laxatives (Oral), 1017

*Cartrol*—Carteolol—*See* Beta-adrenergic Blocking Agents (Systemic), 404, MC-4

Casanthranol—*See* Laxatives (Oral), 1017

Casanthranol and Docusate—*See* Laxatives (Oral), 1017

Cascara Sagrada—*See* Laxatives (Oral), 1017

Cascara Sagrada and Aloe—*See* Laxatives (Oral), 1017

Cascara Sagrada and Phenolphthalein—*See* Laxatives (Oral), 1017

*Casec*—Enteral Nutrition Formula, Modular—*See* Enteral Nutrition Formulas (Systemic), 769

*Castellani Paint*—*See* Carbol-Fuchsin (Topical), 487

*Castel Plus*—Carbol-Fuchsin (Topical), 487

Castor Oil—*See* Laxatives (Oral), 1017

*Cataflam*—Diclofenac—*See* Nonsteroidal Anti-inflammatory Drugs (Systemic), 1229

*Catapres*—Clonidine (Systemic), 576, MC-5

*Catapres-TTS*—Clonidine (Systemic), 576

*C2 Buffered*—Aspirin, Buffered, and Caffeine—*See* Salicylates (Systemic), 1473

*C2 Buffered with Codeine*—Aspirin, Codeine, and Caffeine, Buffered—*See* Narcotic Analgesics and Aspirin (Systemic), 1185

CCNU—*See* Lomustine (Systemic), 1048

*C2 with Codeine*—Aspirin, Codeine, and Caffeine—*See* Narcotic Analgesics and Aspirin (Systemic), 1185

2-CdA—*See* Cladribine (Systemic), 557

*Cebid Timecelles*—Ascorbic Acid (Vitamin C) (Systemic), 344

*Ceclor*—Cefaclor—*See* Cephalosporins (Systemic), 498, MC-4

*Cecon*—Ascorbic Acid (Vitamin C) (Systemic), 344

*Cedocard-SR*—Isosorbide Dinitrate—*See* Nitrates—Oral (Systemic), 1218

*Cee-500*—Ascorbic Acid (Vitamin C) (Systemic), 344

*CeeNU*—Lomustine (Systemic), 1048

Cefaclor—*See* Cephalosporins (Systemic), 498, MC-4

Cefadroxil—*See* Cephalosporins (Systemic), 498, MC-4

*Cefadyl*—Cephapirin—*See* Cephalosporins (Systemic), 498

Cefamandole—*See* Cephalosporins (Systemic), 498

*Cefanex*—Cephalexin—*See* Cephalosporins (Systemic), 498

Cefazolin—*See* Cephalosporins (Systemic), 498

Cefixime—*See* Cephalosporins (Systemic), 498, MC-4

*Cefizox*—Ceftizoxime—*See* Cephalosporins (Systemic), 498

Cefmetazole—*See* Cephalosporins (Systemic), 498

*Cefobid*—Cefoperazone—*See* Cephalosporins (Systemic), 498

Cefonicid—*See* Cephalosporins (Systemic), 498

Cefoperazone—*See* Cephalosporins (Systemic), 498

*Cefotan*—Cefotetan—*See* Cephalosporins (Systemic), 498

Cefotaxime—*See* Cephalosporins (Systemic), 498

Cefotetan—*See* Cephalosporins (Systemic), 498

Cefoxitin—*See* Cephalosporins (Systemic), 498

Cefpodoxime—*See* Cephalosporins (Systemic), 498

Cefprozil—*See* Cephalosporins (Systemic), 498, MC-4

Ceftazidime—*See* Cephalosporins (Systemic), 498

*Ceftin*—Cefuroxime—*See* Cephalosporins (Systemic), 498, MC-4

Ceftizoxime—*See* Cephalosporins (Systemic), 498

Ceftriaxone—*See* Cephalosporins (Systemic), 498

Cefuroxime—*See* Cephalosporins (Systemic), 498, MC-4

*Cefzil*—Cefprozil—*See* Cephalosporins (Systemic), 498, MC-4

*Celestoderm-V*—Betamethasone—*See* Corticosteroids—Medium to Very High Potency (Topical), 626

*Celestoderm-V/2*—Betamethasone—*See* Corticosteroids—Medium to Very High Potency (Topical), 626

*Celestone*—Betamethasone—*See* Corticosteroids/Corticotropin—Glucocorticoid Effects (Systemic), 630

*Celestone Phosphate*—Betamethasone—*See* Corticosteroids/Corticotropin—Glucocorticoid Effects (Systemic), 630

*Celestone Soluspan*—Betamethasone—*See* Corticosteroids/Corticotropin—Glucocorticoid Effects (Systemic), 630

*Cellufresh*—Carboxymethylcellulose (Ophthalmic), 1746

Cellulose Sodium Phosphate (Systemic), 496

*Celluvisc*—Carboxymethylcellulose (Ophthalmic), 1746

*Celontin*—Methsuximide—*See* Anticonvulsants, Succinimide (Systemic), 271

*Cemill*—Ascorbic Acid (Vitamin C) (Systemic), 344

*Cenafed*—Pseudoephedrine (Systemic), 1412

*Cenafed Plus*—Triprolidine and Pseudoephedrine—*See* Antihistamines and Decongestants (Systemic), 311

*Cena-K*—Potassium Chloride—*See* Potassium Supplements (Systemic), 1373

*Cenocort A-40*—Triamcinolone—*See* Corticosteroids/Corticotropin—Glucocorticoid Effects (Systemic), 630

*Cenocort Forte*—Triamcinolone—*See* Corticosteroids/Corticotropin—Glucocorticoid Effects (Systemic), 630

*Cenolate*—Sodium Ascorbate—*See* Ascorbic Acid (Vitamin C) (Systemic), 344

*Centrax*—Prazepam—*See* Benzodiazepines (Systemic), 389

*Ceo-Two*—Potassium Bitartrate and Sodium Bicarbonate—*See* Laxatives (Rectal), 1023

Cephalexin—*See* Cephalosporins (Systemic), 498, MC-4

Cephalosporins (Systemic), 498

Cephalothin—*See* Cephalosporins (Systemic), 498

Cephapirin—*See* Cephalosporins (Systemic), 498

Cephradine—*See* Cephalosporins (Systemic), 498, MC-4

*Ceptaz*—Ceftazidime—*See* Cephalosporins (Systemic), 498

*Ceredase*—Alglucerase (Systemic), 186

*Cerespan*—Papaverine (Systemic), 1289

*Cerose-DM*—Chlorpheniramine, Phenylephrine, and Dextromethorphan—*See* Cough/Cold Combinations (Systemic), 637

*Cerubidine*—Daunorubicin (Systemic), 689

Cervical Cap, Cavity-rim, 1746

*C.E.S.*—Conjugated Estrogens—*See* Estrogens (Systemic), 795

*Cesamet*—Nabilone (Systemic), 1165

*Cetacort*—Hydrocortisone—*See* Corticosteroids—Low Potency (Topical), 624

*Cetamide*—Sulfacetamide—*See* Sulfonamides (Ophthalmic), 1540

*Cetane*—Ascorbic Acid (Vitamin C) (Systemic), 344

*Cetane 500*—Ascorbic Acid (Vitamin C) (Systemic), 344

Cetirizine—*See* Antihistamines (Systemic), 304

*Cevalin*—Ascorbic Acid (Vitamin C) (Systemic), 344

*Cevi-Bid*—Ascorbic Acid (Vitamin C) (Systemic), 344

*Ce-Vi-Sol*—Ascorbic Acid (Vitamin C) (Systemic), 344

*Charac-50*—Charcoal, Activated (Oral), 504

*Charac-tol 50*—Charcoal, Activated, and Sorbitol—*See* Charcoal, Activated (Oral), 504

*Charcoaid*—Charcoal, Activated, and Sorbitol—*See* Charcoal, Activated (Oral), 504

Charcoal, Activated (Oral), 504

Charcoal, Activated, and Sorbitol—*See* Charcoal, Activated (Oral), 504

*Charcocaps*—Charcoal, Activated (Oral), 504

*Charcodote*—Charcoal, Activated, and Sorbitol—*See* Charcoal, Activated (Oral), 504

*Charcodote TFS*—Charcoal, Activated, and Sorbitol—*See* Charcoal, Activated (Oral), 504

*Chardonna-2*—Belladonna and Phenobarbital—*See* Belladonna Alkaloids and Barbiturates (Systemic), 382

*Chemet*—Succimer (Systemic), 1520

*Chemstrip K*—Nitroprusside Urine Ketone Test—*See* Urine Glucose and Ketone Test Kits for Home Use, 1644

*Chemstrip uG*—Glucose Oxidase Urine Glucose Test—*See* Urine Glucose and Ketone Test Kits for Home Use, 1644

*Chemstrip uGK*—Urine Glucose and Ketone (Combined) Test—*See* Urine Glucose and Ketone Test Kits for Home Use, 1644

Chenodeoxycholic acid—*See* Chenodiol (Systemic), 506

Chenodiol (Systemic), 506

*Cheracol*—Codeine and Guaifenesin—*See* Cough/Cold Combinations (Systemic), 637

*Cheracol D Cough*—Dextromethorphan and Guaifenesin—*See* Cough/Cold Combinations (Systemic), 637

*Cheracol Nasal Spray*—Oxymetazoline (Nasal), 1274

*Cheracol Nasal Spray Pump Cherry Scented*—Oxymetazoline (Nasal), 1274

*Cheracol Plus*—Chlorpheniramine, Phenylpropanolamine, and Dextromethorphan—*See* Cough/Cold Combinations (Systemic), 637

*Cheracol Sinus*—Dexbrompheniramine and Pseudoephedrine—*See* Antihistamines and Decongestants (Systemic), 311

*Cherapas*—Reserpine, Hydralazine, and Hydrochlorothiazide (Systemic), 1449

*Chibroxin*—Norfloxacin (Ophthalmic), 1241

*Children's Benylin DM-D*—Pseudoephedrine and Dextromethorphan (Systemic), 1753

*Children's Dramamine*—Dimenhydrinate—*See* Antihistamines (Systemic), 304

*Children's Formula Cough*—Dextromethorphan and Guaifenesin—*See* Cough/Cold Combinations (Systemic), 637

*Children's Hold*—Dextromethorphan (Systemic), 701

*Children's NyQuil*—Chlorpheniramine and Pseudoephedrine (Systemic), 1747

*Children's Tylenol Cold*—Chlorpheniramine, Pseudoephedrine, and Acetaminophen—*See* Antihistamines, Decongestants, and Analgesics (Systemic), 316

*Children's Tylenol Cold Multi Symptom Plus Cough*—Chlorpheniramine, Pseudoephedrine, Dextromethorphan, and Acetaminophen—*See* Cough/Cold Combinations (Systemic), 637

*Children's Vicks NyQuil Cold/Cough Relief*—Chlorpheniramine, Pseudoephedrine, and Dextromethorphan—*See* Cough/Cold Combinations (Systemic), 637

*Chlo-Amine*—Chlorpheniramine—*See* Antihistamines (Systemic), 304

Chlophedianol (Systemic), 507

*Chlor-100*—Chlorpheniramine—*See* Antihistamines (Systemic), 304

*Chloracol Ophthalmic Solution*—Chloramphenicol (Ophthalmic), 514

*Chlorafed*—Chlorpheniramine and Pseudoephedrine—*See* Antihistamines and Decongestants (Systemic), 311

*Chlorafed H.S. Timecelles*—Chlorpheniramine and Pseudoephedrine—*See* Antihistamines and Decongestants (Systemic), 311

*Chlorafed Timecelles*—Chlorpheniramine and Pseudoephedrine—*See* Antihistamines and Decongestants (Systemic), 311

Chloral Hydrate (Systemic), 509

Chlorambucil (Systemic), 511

Chloramphenicol (Ophthalmic), 514

Chloramphenicol (Otic), 516

Chloramphenicol (Systemic), 517

Chloramphenicol (Topical), 519

*Chloraseptic Lozenges*—Benzocaine and Menthol—*See* Anesthetics (Dental), 229

*Chloraseptic Lozenges Cherry Flavor*—Benzocaine and Menthol—*See* Anesthetics (Dental), 229

*Chloraseptic Lozenges, Children's*—Benzocaine—*See* Anesthetics (Dental), 229

*Chlorate*—Chlorpheniramine—*See* Antihistamines (Systemic), 304

Chlordiazepoxide—*See* Benzodiazepines (Systemic), 389, MC-4

Chlordiazepoxide and Amitriptyline (Systemic), 520, MC-4

Chlordiazepoxide and Clidinium (Systemic), 523, MC-4

*Chlordrine S.R.*—Chlorpheniramine and Pseudoephedrine—*See* Antihistamines and Decongestants (Systemic), 311

*Clysodrast*—Bisacodyl—*See* Laxatives (Rectal), 1023

*CoActifed*—Triprolidine, Pseudoephedrine, and Codeine—*See* Cough/Cold Combinations (Systemic), 637

*CoActifed Expectorant*—Triprolidine, Pseudoephedrine, Codeine, and Guaifenesin—*See* Cough/Cold Combinations (Systemic), 637

*CoAdvil Caplets*—Pseudoephedrine and Ibuprofen—*See* Decongestants and Analgesics (Systemic), 691

Coal Tar (Topical), 589

*Co-Apap*—Chlorpheniramine, Pseudoephedrine, Dextromethorphan, and Acetaminophen—*See* Cough/Cold Combinations (Systemic), 637

*Cobantril*—Pyrantel (Oral), 1414

*Cobex*—Cyanocobalamin—*See* Vitamin B$_{12}$ (Systemic), 1667

*Cobiron*—Neomycin, Polymyxin B, and Hydrocortisone (Ophthalmic), 1203

Cocaine (Mucosal-Local), 591

*Codalan No.1*—Acetaminophen, Codeine, and Caffeine—*See* Narcotic Analgesics and Acetaminophen (Systemic), 1181

*Codalan No.2*—Acetaminophen, Codeine, and Caffeine—*See* Narcotic Analgesics and Acetaminophen (Systemic), 1181

*Codalan No.3*—Acetaminophen, Codeine, and Caffeine—*See* Narcotic Analgesics and Acetaminophen (Systemic), 1181

*Codamin #2*—Acetaminophen, Codeine, and Caffeine—*See* Narcotic Analgesics and Acetaminophen (Systemic), 1181

*Codamin #3*—Acetaminophen, Codeine, and Caffeine—*See* Narcotic Analgesics and Acetaminophen (Systemic), 1181

*Codamine*—Phenylpropanolamine and Hydrocodone—*See* Cough/Cold Combinations (Systemic), 637

*Codamine Pediatric*—Phenylpropanolamine and Hydrocodone—*See* Cough/Cold Combinations (Systemic), 637

*Codaminophen*—Acetaminophen, Codeine, and Caffeine—*See* Narcotic Analgesics and Acetaminophen (Systemic), 1181

*Codan*—Hydrocodone and Homatropine—*See* Cough/Cold Combinations (Systemic), 637

*Codegest Expectorant*—Phenylpropanolamine, Codeine, and Guaifenesin—*See* Cough/Cold Combinations (Systemic), 637

*Codehist DH*—Chlorpheniramine, Pseudoephedrine, and Codeine—*See* Cough/Cold Combinations (Systemic), 637

Codeine—*See* Narcotic Analgesics—For Pain Relief (Systemic), 1176

Codeine and Calcium Iodide—*See* Cough/Cold Combinations (Systemic), 637

Codeine and Guaifenesin—*See* Cough/Cold Combinations (Systemic), 637

Codeine and Iodinated Glycerol—*See* Cough/Cold Combinations (Systemic), 637

*Codiclear DH*—Hydrocodone and Guaifenesin—*See* Cough/Cold Combinations (Systemic), 637

*Codimal*—Chlorpheniramine, Pseudoephedrine, and Acetaminophen—*See* Antihistamines, Decongestants, and Analgesics (Systemic), 316

*Codimal-A*—Brompheniramine—*See* Antihistamines (Systemic), 304

*Codimal DH*—Pyrilamine, Phenylephrine, and Hydrocodone—*See* Cough/Cold Combinations (Systemic), 637

*Codimal DM*—Pyrilamine, Phenylephrine, and Dextromethorphan—*See* Cough/Cold Combinations (Systemic), 637

*Codimal Expectorant*—Phenylpropanolamine and Guaifenesin—*See* Cough/Cold Combinations (Systemic), 637

*Codimal-L.A.*—Chlorpheniramine and Pseudoephedrine—*See* Antihistamines and Decongestants (Systemic), 311

*Codimal PH*—Pyrilamine, Phenylephrine, and Codeine—*See* Cough/Cold Combinations (Systemic), 637

*Codistan No. 1*—Dextromethorphan and Guaifenesin—*See* Cough/Cold Combinations (Systemic), 637

Coenzyme R—*See* Biotin (Systemic), 420

*Cogentin*—Benztropine—*See* Antidyskinetics (Systemic), 287, MC-3

*Co-Gesic*—Hydrocodone and Acetaminophen—*See* Narcotic Analgesics and Acetaminophen (Systemic), 1181

*Cognex*—Tacrine (Systemic), 1557, MC-21

*Colace*—Docusate—*See* Laxatives (Oral), 1017

*Colaspase*—*See* Asparaginase (Systemic), 347

*Colax*—Docusate and Phenolphthalein—*See* Laxatives (Oral), 1017

*ColBenemid*—Probenecid and Colchicine (Systemic), 1392

Colchicine (Systemic), 593

*Coldrine*—Pseudoephedrine and Acetaminophen—*See* Decongestants and Analgesics (Systemic), 691

*Colebrin*—Iocetamic Acid—*See* Cholecystographic Agents, Oral (Diagnostic), 536

*Colebrina*—Iocetamic Acid—*See* Cholecystographic Agents, Oral (Diagnostic), 536

*Colegraf*—Iopanoic Acid—*See* Cholecystographic Agents, Oral (Diagnostic), 536

*Colestid*—Colestipol (Oral), 597

Colestipol (Oral), 597

*Colfed-A*—Chlorpheniramine and Pseudoephedrine—*See* Antihistamines and Decongestants (Systemic), 311

Colistin, Neomycin, and Hydrocortisone (Otic), 599

*ColoCare*—Fecal Occult Blood Test Kits—*See* Fecal Occult Blood Test Kits, 826

*Cologel*—Methylcellulose—*See* Laxatives (Oral), 1017

Colony Stimulating Factors (Systemic), 600

*Colo-Rectal Test*—Fecal Occult Blood Test Kits—*See* Fecal Occult Blood Test Kits, 826

*Color Ovulation Test*—Ovulation Prediction Test Kits for Home Use, 1265

*ColoScreen*—Fecal Occult Blood Test Kits—*See* Fecal Occult Blood Test Kits, 826

*ColoScreen III*—Fecal Occult Blood Test Kits—*See* Fecal Occult Blood Test Kits, 826

*ColoScreen Self-Test*—Fecal Occult Blood Test Kits—*See* Fecal Occult Blood Test Kits, 826

*Colovage*—Polyethylene Glycol and Electrolytes (Local), 1369

*Col-Probenecid*—Probenecid and Colchicine (Systemic), 1392

*Coltab Children's*—Chlorpheniramine and Phenylephrine—*See* Antihistamines and Decongestants (Systemic), 311

*Coly-Mycin Otic*—Colistin, Neomycin, and Hydrocortisone (Otic), 599

*Coly-Mycin S Otic*—Colistin, Neomycin, and Hydrocortisone (Otic), 599

*Colyte*—Polyethylene Glycol and Electrolytes (Local), 1369

*Colyte-flavored*—Polyethylene Glycol and Electrolytes (Local), 1369

*Combantrin*—Pyrantel (Oral), 1414

*Combipres*—Clonidine and Chlorthalidone (Systemic), 579, MC-6

*Comfort Eye Drops*—Naphazoline (Ophthalmic), 1174

*Comhist*—Chlorpheniramine, Phenyltoloxamine, and Phenylephrine—*See* Antihistamines and Decongestants (Systemic), 311

*Comhist LA*—Chlorpheniramine, Phenyltoloxamine, and Phenylephrine—*See* Antihistamines and Decongestants (Systemic), 311

*Compal*—Dihydrocodeine, Acetaminophen, and Caffeine—*See* Narcotic Analgesics and Acetaminophen (Systemic), 1181

*Compa-Z*—Prochlorperazine—*See* Phenothiazines (Systemic), 1330

*Compazine*—Prochlorperazine—*See* Phenothiazines (Systemic), 1330, MC-20

*Compazine Spansule*—Prochlorperazine—*See* Phenothiazines (Systemic), 1330, MC-20

*Compleat Modified*—Enteral Nutrition Formula, Blenderized—*See* Enteral Nutrition Formulas (Systemic), 769

*Compleat Regular*—Enteral Nutrition Formula, Blenderized—*See* Enteral Nutrition Formulas (Systemic), 769

*Comply*—Enteral Nutrition Formula, Polymeric—*See* Enteral Nutrition Formulas (Systemic), 769

*Compound W Gel*—Salicylic Acid (Topical), 1478

*Compound W Liquid*—Salicylic Acid (Topical), 1478

*Compoz*—Diphenhydramine—*See* Antihistamines (Systemic), 304

*Comtrex A/S*—Chlorpheniramine, Pseudoephedrine, and Acetaminophen—*See* Antihistamines, Decongestants, and Analgesics (Systemic), 316

*Comtrex A/S Caplets*—Chlorpheniramine, Pseudoephedrine, and Acetaminophen—*See* Antihistamines, Decongestants, and Analgesics (Systemic), 316

*Comtrex Cough Formula*—Pseudoephedrine, Dextromethorphan, Guaifenesin, and Acetaminophen—*See* Cough/Cold Combinations (Systemic), 637

*Comtrex Daytime Caplets*—Pseudoephedrine, Dextromethorphan, and Acetaminophen—*See* Cough/Cold Combinations (Systemic), 637

*Comtrex Daytime Maximum Strength Cold, Cough, and Flu Relief*—Pseudoephedrine, Dextromethorphan, and Acetaminophen—*See* Cough/Cold Combinations (Systemic), 637

*Comtrex Daytime Maximum Strength Cold and Flu Relief*—Pseudoephedrine, Dextromethorphan, and Acetaminophen—*See* Cough/Cold Combinations (Systemic), 637

*Comtrex Hot Flu Relief*—Chlorpheniramine, Pseudoephedrine, Dextromethorphan, and Acetaminophen—*See* Cough/Cold Combinations (Systemic), 637

*Comtrex Maximum Strength LiquiGels*—Chlorpheniramine, Phenylpropanolamine, Dextromethorphan, and Acetaminophen—*See* Cough/Cold Combinations (Systemic), 637

*Comtrex Multi-Symptom Cold Reliever*—Chlorpheniramine, Phenylpropanolamine, Dextromethorphan, and Acetaminophen—*See* Cough/Cold Combinations (Systemic), 637

*Comtrex Multi-Symptom Hot Flu Relief*—Chlorpheniramine, Pseudoephedrine, Dextromethorphan, and Acetaminophen (Systemic), 1747

*Comtrex Multi-Symptom Non-Drowsy Caplets*—Pseudoephedrine, Dextromethorphan, and Acetaminophen—*See* Cough/Cold Combinations (Systemic), 637

*Comtrex Nighttime*—Chlorpheniramine, Pseudoephedrine, Dextromethorphan, and Acetaminophen—*See* Cough/Cold Combinations (Systemic), 637

*Comtrex Nighttime Maximum Strength Cold, Cough, and Flu Relief*—Chlorpheniramine, Pseudoephedrine, Dextromethorphan, and Acetaminophen—*See* Cough/Cold Combinations (Systemic), 637

*Comtrex Nighttime Maximum Strength Cold and Flu Relief*—Chlorpheniramine, Pseudoephedrine, Dextromethorphan, and Acetaminophen—*See* Cough/Cold Combinations (Systemic), 637

*Conceive Ovulation Predictor*—Ovulation Prediction Test Kits for Home Use, 1265

*Concentrated Phillips' Milk of Magnesia*—Magnesium Hydroxide—*See* Magnesium Supplements (Systemic), 1060

*Concentrin*—Pseudoephedrine, Dextromethorphan, and Guaifenesin—*See* Cough/Cold Combinations (Systemic), 637

*Conceptrol Contraceptive Inserts*—Nonoxynol 9—*See* Spermicides (Vaginal), 1512

*Conceptrol Gel*—Nonoxynol 9—*See* Spermicides (Vaginal), 1512

*Conceptrol Shields*—Latex Condoms—*See* Condoms, 602

*Conceptrol Supreme*—Latex Condoms—*See* Condoms, 602

Condoms, 602

*Condrin-LA*—Chlorpheniramine and Phenylpropanolamine—*See* Antihistamines and Decongestants (Systemic), 311

*Condylox*—Podofilox (Topical), 1752

*Conex*—Phenylpropanolamine and Guaifenesin—*See* Cough/Cold Combinations (Systemic), 637

*Conex with Codeine Liquid*—Phenylpropanolamine, Codeine, and Guaifenesin—*See* Cough/Cold Combinations (Systemic), 637

*Conex D.A.*—Chlorpheniramine and Phenylpropanolamine—*See* Antihistamines and Decongestants (Systemic), 311

*Congespirin for Children Cold Tablets*—Phenylephrine and Acetaminophen—*See* Decongestants and Analgesics (Systemic), 691

*Congespirin for Children Liquid Cold Medicine*—Phenylpropanolamine and Acetaminophen—*See* Decongestants and Analgesics (Systemic), 691

*Congess JR*—Pseudoephedrine and Guaifenesin—*See* Cough/Cold Combinations (Systemic), 637

*Congess SR*—Pseudoephedrine and Guaifenesin—*See* Cough/Cold Combinations (Systemic), 637

*Congest*—Conjugated Estrogens—*See* Estrogens (Systemic), 795

*Congestac Caplets*—Pseudoephedrine and Guaifenesin—*See* Cough/Cold Combinations (Systemic), 637

*Congestant D*—Chlorpheniramine, Phenylpropanolamine, and Acetaminophen—*See* Antihistamines, Decongestants, and Analgesics (Systemic), 316

*Conjec-B*—Brompheniramine—*See* Antihistamines (Systemic), 304

Conjugated estrogens—Estrogens, Conjugated—*See* Estrogens (Systemic), 795

Conjugated estrogens and methyltestosterone—Estrogens, Conjugated, and Methyltestosterone—*See* Androgens and Estrogens (Systemic), 225

*Cruex Antifungal Cream*—Undecylenic Acid, Compound (Topical), 1639

*Cruex Antifungal Powder*—Undecylenic Acid, Compound (Topical), 1639

*Cruex Antifungal Spray Powder*—Undecylenic Acid, Compound (Topical), 1639

*Cruex Cream*—Undecylenic Acid, Compound (Topical), 1639

*Cruex Powder*—Undecylenic Acid, Compound (Topical), 1639

*Crystamine*—Cyanocobalamin—*See* Vitamin $B_{12}$ (Systemic), 1667

*Crysti-12*—Cyanocobalamin—*See* Vitamin $B_{12}$ (Systemic), 1667

*Crysticillin 300 A.S.*—Penicillin G—*See* Penicillins (Systemic), 1299

*Crystodigin*—Digitoxin—*See* Digitalis Medicines (Systemic), 716

*C-Tussin Expectorant*—Pseudoephedrine, Codeine, and Guaifenesin—*See* Cough/Cold Combinations (Systemic), 637

*Cuplex Gel*—Salicylic Acid (Topical), 1478

Cupric sulfate—Copper Sulfate—*See* Copper Supplements (Systemic), 608

*Cuprimine*—Penicillamine (Systemic), 1297

*Curretab*—Medroxyprogesterone—*See* Progestins (Systemic), 1402

*Cutar Water Dispersible Emollient Tar*—Coal Tar (Topical), 589

*Cuticura Acne 5 Cream*—Benzoyl Peroxide (Topical), 397

*Cuticura Ointment*—Sulfur (Topical), 1550

*Cutivate*—Fluticasone—*See* Corticosteroids—Medium to Very High Potency (Topical), 626

*Cyanide Antidote Package*—Sodium Thiosulfate (Systemic), 1509

Cyanocobalamin—*See* Vitamin $B_{12}$ (Systemic), 1667

Cyanocobalamin Co 57—*See* Radiopharmaceuticals (Diagnostic), 1439

*Cyanoject*—Cyanocobalamin—*See* Vitamin $B_{12}$ (Systemic), 1667

Cyclandelate (Systemic), 661

*Cyclen*—Norgestimate and Ethinyl Estradiol—*See* Estrogens and Progestins (Oral Contraceptives) (Systemic), 804

Cyclizine—*See* Meclizine/Buclizine/Cyclizine (Systemic), 1079

Cyclobenzaprine (Systemic), 662, MC-6

*Cyclocort*—Amcinonide—*See* Corticosteroids—Medium to Very High Potency (Topical), 626

*Cyclogyl*—Cyclopentolate (Ophthalmic), 664

*Cyclomen*—Danazol (Systemic), 681

Cyclopentolate (Ophthalmic), 664

Cyclophosphamide (Systemic), 666

Cycloserine (Systemic), 669

*Cyclospasmol*—Cyclandelate (Systemic), 661

Cyclosporin A—*See* Cyclosporine (Systemic), 671

Cyclosporine (Systemic), 671, MC-6

Cyclothiazide—*See* Diuretics, Thiazide (Systemic), 749

*Cycoflex*—Cyclobenzaprine (Systemic), 662

*Cycrin*—Medroxyprogesterone—*See* Progestins (Systemic), 1402

*Cyklokapron*—Tranexamic Acid—*See* Antifibrinolytic Agents (Systemic), 290

*Cylert*—Pemoline (Systemic), 1295

*Cylert Chewable*—Pemoline (Systemic), 1295

*Cyomin*—Cyanocobalamin—*See* Vitamin $B_{12}$ (Systemic), 1667

Cyproheptadine—*See* Antihistamines (Systemic), 304

Cyproterone (Systemic), 1747

*Cysticide*—Praziquantel (Systemic), 1378

*Cystospaz*—Hyoscyamine—*See* Anticholinergics/Antispasmodics (Systemic), 258

*Cystospaz-M*—Hyoscyamine—*See* Anticholinergics/Antispasmodics (Systemic), 258

*Cytadren*—Aminoglutethimide (Systemic), 199

Cytarabine (Systemic), 673

*Cytomel*—Liothyronine—*See* Thyroid Hormones (Systemic), 1606

*Cytosar*—Cytarabine (Systemic), 673

*Cytosar-U*—Cytarabine (Systemic), 673

Cytosine arabinoside—*See* Cytarabine (Systemic), 673

*Cytotec*—Misoprostol (Systemic), 1144, MC-15

*Cytovene*—Ganciclovir (Systemic), 868

*Cytoxan*—Cyclophosphamide (Systemic), 666

# D

Dacarbazine (Systemic), 677

*D.A. Chewable*—Chlorpheniramine, Phenylephrine, and Methscopolamine—*See* Antihistamines, Decongestants, and Anticholinergics (Systemic), 322

*Dacodyl*—Bisacodyl—*See* Laxatives (Oral), 1017; Laxatives (Rectal), 1023

Dactinomycin (Systemic), 679

*Dagenan*—Sulfapyridine (Systemic), 1532

*Daisy 2*—Pregnancy Test Kits for Home Use, 1385

*Dalacin C*—Clindamycin (Systemic), 561

*Dalacin C Palmitate*—Clindamycin (Systemic), 561

*Dalacin C Phosphate*—Clindamycin (Systemic), 561

*Dalacin T Topical Solution*—Clindamycin (Topical), 563

*Dalalone*—Dexamethasone—*See* Corticosteroids/Corticotropin—Glucocorticoid Effects (Systemic), 630

*Dalalone D.P.*—Dexamethasone—*See* Corticosteroids/Corticotropin—Glucocorticoid Effects (Systemic), 630

*Dalalone L.A.*—Dexamethasone—*See* Corticosteroids/Corticotropin—Glucocorticoid Effects (Systemic), 630

*Dalcaine*—Lidocaine—*See* Anesthetics (Parenteral-Local), 235

*Dalgan*—Dezocine (Systemic), 704

*Dallergy*—Chlorpheniramine, Phenylephrine, and Methscopolamine—*See* Antihistamines, Decongestants, and Anticholinergics (Systemic), 322

*Dallergy Caplets*—Chlorpheniramine, Phenylephrine, and Methscopolamine—*See* Antihistamines, Decongestants, and Anticholinergics (Systemic), 322

*Dallergy-D*—Chlorpheniramine and Phenylephrine—*See* Antihistamines and Decongestants (Systemic), 311; Chlorpheniramine and Pseudoephedrine—*See* Antihistamines and Decongestants (Systemic), 311

*Dallergy Jr.*—Brompheniramine and Pseudoephedrine—*See* Antihistamines and Decongestants (Systemic), 311

*Dalmane*—Flurazepam—*See* Benzodiazepines (Systemic), 389, MC-10

*Damason-P*—Hydrocodone, Aspirin, and Caffeine—*See* Narcotic Analgesics and Aspirin (Systemic), 1185

Danazol (Systemic), 681, MC-6

*Danex*—Pyrithione (Topical), 1424

*Dan-Gard*—Pyrithione (Topical), 1424

*Danocrine*—Danazol (Systemic), 681, MC-6

Danthron and Docusate—*See* Laxatives (Oral), 1017

*Dantrium*—Dantrolene (Systemic), 683, MC-6

*Dantrium Intravenous*—Dantrolene (Systemic), 683

Dantrolene (Systemic), 683, MC-6

*Dapa*—Acetaminophen (Systemic), 161

*Dapacin Cold*—Chlorpheniramine, Phenylpropanolamine, and Acetaminophen—*See* Antihistamines, Decongestants, and Analgesics (Systemic), 316

*Dapa X-S*—Acetaminophen (Systemic), 161

Dapiprazole (Ophthalmic), 686

Dapsone (Systemic), 687

*Daranide*—Dichlorphenamide—*See* Carbonic Anhydrase Inhibitors (Systemic), 488

*Daraprim*—Pyrimethamine (Systemic), 1421

*Darbid*—Isopropamide—*See* Anticholinergics/Antispasmodics (Systemic), 258

*Daricon*—Oxyphencyclimine—*See* Anticholinergics/Antispasmodics (Systemic), 258

*Dartal*—Thiopropazate—*See* Phenothiazines (Systemic), 1330

*Darvocet-N 50*—Propoxyphene and Acetaminophen—*See* Narcotic Analgesics and Acetaminophen (Systemic), 1181, MC-20

*Darvocet-N 100*—Propoxyphene and Acetaminophen—*See* Narcotic Analgesics and Acetaminophen (Systemic), 1181, MC-20

*Darvon*—Propoxyphene—*See* Narcotic Analgesics—For Pain Relief (Systemic), 1176

*Darvon with A.S.A.*—Propoxyphene and Aspirin—*See* Narcotic Analgesics and Aspirin (Systemic), 1185

*Darvon Compound*—Propoxyphene, Aspirin, and Caffeine—*See* Narcotic Analgesics and Aspirin (Systemic), 1185

*Darvon Compound-65*—Propoxyphene, Aspirin, and Caffeine—*See* Narcotic Analgesics and Aspirin (Systemic), 1185

*Darvon-N*—Propoxyphene—*See* Narcotic Analgesics—For Pain Relief (Systemic), 1176

*Darvon-N with A.S.A.*—Propoxyphene and Aspirin—*See* Narcotic Analgesics and Aspirin (Systemic), 1185

*Darvon-N Compound*—Propoxyphene, Aspirin, and Caffeine—*See* Narcotic Analgesics and Aspirin (Systemic), 1185

*Datril Extra-Strength*—Acetaminophen (Systemic), 161

Daunorubicin (Systemic), 689

*Daypro*—Oxaprozin (Systemic)—*See* Nonsteroidal Anti-inflammatory Drugs (Systemic), 1229, MC-17

*DayQuil Multi-Sympton Cold/Flu LiquiCaps*—Pseudoephedrine, Dextromethorphan, Guaifenesin, and Acetaminophen—*See* Cough/Cold Combinations (Systemic), 637

*DayQuil Non-Drowsy Cold/Flu*—Pseudoephedrine, Dextromethorphan, Guaifenesin, and Acetaminophen—*See* Cough/Cold Combinations (Systemic), 637, 1753

*DayQuil Non-Drowsy Sinus Pressure and Pain Relief Caplets*—Pseudoephedrine and Acetaminophen—*See* Decongestants and Analgesics (Systemic), 691

*DayQuil Sinus Pressure and Congestion Relief Caplets*—Phenylpropanolamine and Guaifenesin—*See* Cough/Cold Combinations (Systemic), 637

*Dayto Himbin*—Yohimbine (Systemic), 1684

*Dazamide*—Acetazolamide—*See* Carbonic Anhydrase Inhibitors (Systemic), 488

2'DCF—*See* Pentostatin (Systemic), 1314

*DDAVP*—Desmopressin (Systemic), 699

*DDAVP Nasal Spray*—Desmopressin (Systemic), 699

*DDAVP Rhinal Tube*—Desmopressin (Systemic), 699

*DDAVP Rhinyle Drops*—Desmopressin (Systemic), 699

ddC—*See* Zalcitabine (Systemic), 1687

ddI—*See* Didanosine (Systemic), 709

DDS—*See* Dapsone (Systemic), 687

*Debetrol*—Dextrothyroxine (Systemic), 702

Debrisoquine (Systemic), 1747

*Decaderm*—Dexamethasone—*See* Corticosteroids—Low Potency (Topical), 624

*Decadrol*—Dexamethasone—*See* Corticosteroids/Corticotropin—Glucocorticoid Effects (Systemic), 630

*Decadron*—Dexamethasone—*See* Corticosteroids (Ophthalmic), 620; Corticosteroids (Otic), 622; Corticosteroids/Corticotropin—Glucocorticoid Effects (Systemic), 630, MC-6; Corticosteroids—Low Potency (Topical), 624

*Decadron-LA*—Dexamethasone—*See* Corticosteroids/Corticotropin—Glucocorticoid Effects (Systemic), 630

*Decadron Phosphate*—Dexamethasone—*See* Corticosteroids/Corticotropin—Glucocorticoid Effects (Systemic), 630

*Decadron Respihaler*—Dexamethasone—*See* Corticosteroids (Inhalation), 611

*Decadron Turbinaire*—Dexamethasone—*See* Corticosteroids (Nasal), 617

*Deca-Durabolin*—Nandrolone—*See* Anabolic Steroids (Systemic), 218

*Decaject*—Dexamethasone—*See* Corticosteroids/Corticotropin—Glucocorticoid Effects (Systemic), 630

*Decaject-L.A.*—Dexamethasone—*See* Corticosteroids/Corticotropin—Glucocorticoid Effects (Systemic), 630

*Decaspray*—Dexamethasone—*See* Corticosteroids—Low Potency (Topical), 624

*Decholin*—Dehydrocholic Acid—*See* Laxatives (Oral), 1017

*Declinax*—Debrisoquine (Systemic), 1747

*Declomycin*—Demeclocycline—*See* Tetracyclines (Systemic), 1570

*Decofed*—Pseudoephedrine (Systemic), 1412

*Decohistine DH*—Chlorpheniramine, Pseudoephedrine, and Codeine—*See* Cough/Cold Combinations (Systemic), 637

*De-Comberol*—Testosterone and Estradiol—*See* Androgens and Estrogens (Systemic), 225

*Deconamine*—Chlorpheniramine and Pseudoephedrine—*See* Antihistamines and Decongestants (Systemic), 311

*Deconamine SR*—Chlorpheniramine and Pseudoephedrine—*See* Antihistamines and Decongestants (Systemic), 311

*Decongestabs*—Chlorpheniramine, Phenyltoloxamine, Phenylephrine, and Phenylpropanolamine—*See* Antihistamines and Decongestants (Systemic), 311

Decongestants and Analgesics (Systemic), 691

*Deconsal II*—Pseudoephedrine and Guaifenesin—*See* Cough/Cold Combinations (Systemic), 637

*Deconsal Pediatric*—Pseudoephedrine, Codeine, and Guaifenesin—*See* Cough/Cold Combinations (Systemic), 637

*Deconsal Sprinkle*—Phenylephrine and Guaifenesin—*See* Cough/Cold Combinations (Systemic), 637

*Decylenes Powder*—Undecylenic Acid, Compound (Topical), 1639

Deferoxamine (Systemic), 696

*Deficol*—Bisacodyl—*See* Laxatives (Oral), 1017; Laxatives (Rectal), 1023

*Degest 2*—Naphazoline (Ophthalmic), 1174

*Dehist*—Brompheniramine—*See* Antihistamines (Systemic), 304; Chlorpheniramine and Phenylpropanolamine—*See* Antihistamines and Decongestants (Systemic), 311

Dehydrocholic Acid—*See* Laxatives (Oral), 1017

Dehydrocholic Acid and Docusate—*See* Laxatives (Oral), 1017

Dehydrocholic Acid, Docusate, and Phenolphthalein—*See* Laxatives (Oral), 1017

*Delacort*—Hydrocortisone—*See* Corticosteroids—Low Potency (Topical), 624

*Deladiol-40*—Estradiol—*See* Estrogens (Systemic), 795

*Deladumone*—Testosterone and Estradiol—*See* Androgens and Estrogens (Systemic), 225

*Del-Aqua-5 Gel*—Benzoyl Peroxide (Topical), 397

*Del-Aqua-10 Gel*—Benzoyl Peroxide (Topical), 397

*Delatest*—Testosterone—*See* Androgens (Systemic), 221

*Delatestadiol*—Testosterone and Estradiol—*See* Androgens and Estrogens (Systemic), 225

*Delatestryl*—Testosterone—*See* Androgens (Systemic), 221

*Delaxin*—Methocarbamol—*See* Skeletal Muscle Relaxants (Systemic), 1495

*Delestrogen*—Estradiol—*See* Estrogens (Systemic), 795

*Delfen*—Nonoxynol 9—*See* Spermicides (Vaginal), 1512

*Delsym*—Dextromethorphan (Systemic), 701

*Delta-Cortef*—Prednisolone—*See* Corticosteroids/Corticotropin—Glucocorticoid Effects (Systemic), 630

*Deltalin*—Ergocalciferol—*See* Vitamin D and Related Compounds (Systemic), 1669

*Deltasone*—Prednisone—*See* Corticosteroids/Corticotropin—Glucocorticoid Effects (Systemic), 630, MC-19

Delta-9-tetrahydrocannabinol (THC)—*See* Dronabinol (Systemic), 760

*Delta-Tritex*—Triamcinolone—*See* Corticosteroids—Medium to Very High Potency (Topical), 626

*Demadex*—Torsemide (Systemic), 1754

*Demazin*—Chlorpheniramine and Phenylpropanolamine—*See* Antihistamines and Decongestants (Systemic), 311

*Demazin Repetabs*—Chlorpheniramine and Phenylpropanolamine—*See* Antihistamines and Decongestants (Systemic), 311

Demecarium—*See* Antiglaucoma Agents, Cholinergic, Long-acting (Ophthalmic), 299

Demeclocycline—*See* Tetracyclines (Systemic), 1570

*Demerol*—Meperidine—*See* Narcotic Analgesics—For Pain Relief (Systemic), 1176, MC-14; Meperidine—for Surgery and Obstetrics—*See* Narcotic Analgesics—For Surgery and Obstetrics (Systemic), 1179

*Demerol-APAP*—Meperidine and Acetaminophen—*See* Narcotic Analgesics and Acetaminophen (Systemic), 1181

*Demi-Regroton*—Reserpine and Chlorthalidone—*See* Rauwolfia Alkaloids and Thiazide Diuretics (Systemic), 1445, MC-21

*Demser*—Metyrosine (Systemic), 1134

*Demulen 1/35*—Ethynodiol Diacetate and Ethinyl Estradiol—*See* Estrogens and Progestins (Oral Contraceptives) (Systemic), 804, MC-9

*Demulen 1/50*—Ethynodiol Diacetate and Ethinyl Estradiol—*See* Estrogens and Progestins (Oral Contraceptives) (Systemic), 804, MC-9

*Demulen 30*—Ethynodiol Diacetate and Ethinyl Estradiol—*See* Estrogens and Progestins (Oral Contraceptives) (Systemic), 804

*Demulen 50*—Ethynodiol Diacetate and Ethinyl Estradiol—*See* Estrogens and Progestins (Oral Contraceptives) (Systemic), 804

*Denorex*—Coal Tar (Topical), 589

*Denorex Extra Strength Medicated Shampoo*—Coal Tar (Topical), 589

*Denorex Extra Strength Medicated Shampoo with Conditioners*—Coal Tar (Topical), 589

*Denorex Medicated Shampoo*—Coal Tar (Topical), 589

*Denorex Medicated Shampoo and Conditioner*—Coal Tar (Topical), 589

*Denorex Mountain Fresh Herbal Scent Medicated Shampoo*—Coal Tar (Topical), 589

*Dentapaine*—Benzocaine—*See* Anesthetics (Dental), 229

*Dentocaine*—Benzocaine—*See* Anesthetics (Dental), 229

*Dent-Zel-Ite*—Benzocaine—*See* Anesthetics (Dental), 229

2'-deoxycoformycin—*See* Pentostatin (Systemic), 1314

*Depakene*—Valproic Acid (Systemic), 1651, MC-24

*Depakote*—Divalproex—*See* Valproic Acid (Systemic), 1651, MC-8

*Depakote Sprinkle*—Divalproex—*See* Valproic Acid (Systemic), 1651, MC-8

*depAndro 100*—Testosterone—*See* Androgens (Systemic), 221

*depAndro 200*—Testosterone—*See* Androgens (Systemic), 221

*depAndrogyn*—Testosterone and Estradiol—*See* Androgens and Estrogens (Systemic), 225

*Depen*—Penicillamine (Systemic), 1297

*depGynogen*—Estradiol—*See* Estrogens (Systemic), 795

*depMedalone 40*—Methylprednisolone—*See* Corticosteroids/Corticotropin—Glucocorticoid Effects (Systemic), 630

*depMedalone 80*—Methylprednisolone—*See* Corticosteroids/Corticotropin—Glucocorticoid Effects (Systemic), 630

*Depo-Estradiol*—Estradiol—*See* Estrogens (Systemic), 795

*Depogen*—Estradiol—*See* Estrogens (Systemic), 795

*Depoject-40*—Methylprednisolone—*See* Corticosteroids/Corticotropin—Glucocorticoid Effects (Systemic), 630

*Depoject-80*—Methylprednisolone—*See* Corticosteroids/Corticotropin—Glucocorticoid Effects (Systemic), 630

*Depo-Medrol*—Methylprednisolone—*See* Corticosteroids/Corticotropin—Glucocorticoid Effects (Systemic), 630

*Deponit*—Nitroglycerin—*See* Nitrates—Topical (Systemic), 1224

*Depopred-40*—Methylprednisolone—*See* Corticosteroids/Corticotropin—Glucocorticoid Effects (Systemic), 630

*Depopred-80*—Methylprednisolone—*See* Corticosteroids/Corticotropin—Glucocorticoid Effects (Systemic), 630

Diatrizoates—*See* Radiopaque Agents (Diagnostic), 1436; Radiopaque Agents (Diagnostic, Mucosal), 1438

*Diazemuls*—Diazepam—*See* Benzodiazepines (Systemic), 389

Diazepam—*See* Benzodiazepines (Systemic), 389, MC-6

*Diazepam Intensol*—Diazepam—*See* Benzodiazepines (Systemic), 389

Diazoxide (Oral), 706

*Dibenzyline*—Phenoxybenzamine (Systemic), 1340

Dibucaine—*See* Anesthetics (Rectal), 237; Anesthetics (Topical), 240

*Dicarbosil*—Calcium Carbonate—*See* Antacids (Oral), 253; Calcium Supplements (Systemic), 472

Dichlorphenamide—*See* Carbonic Anhydrase Inhibitors (Systemic), 488

Diclofenac—*See* Anti-inflammatory Agents, Nonsteroidal (Ophthalmic), 330; Nonsteroidal Anti-inflammatory Drugs (Systemic), 1229, MC-7

Diclofenamide—Dichlorphenamide—*See* Carbonic Anhydrase Inhibitors (Systemic), 488

Dicloxacillin—*See* Penicillins (Systemic), 1299, MC-7

Dicoumarol—Dicumarol—*See* Anticoagulants (Systemic), 262

Dicumarol—*See* Anticoagulants (Systemic), 262

Dicyclomine—*See* Anticholinergics/Antispasmodics (Systemic), 258, MC-7

Dicycloverine—Dicyclomine—*See* Anticholinergics/Antispasmodics (Systemic), 258

Didanosine (Systemic), 709, MC-7

*Didrex*—Benzphetamine—*See* Appetite Suppressants (Systemic), 339, MC-3

*Didronel*—Etidronate (Systemic), 814

Dienestrol—*See* Estrogens (Vaginal), 801

*Diet-Aid Maximum Strength*—Phenylpropanolamine (Systemic), 1347

Diethylamine Salicylate (Topical), 1748

Diethylcarbamazine (Systemic), 712

Diethylpropion—*See* Appetite Suppressants (Systemic), 339, MC-7

Diethylstilbestrol—*See* Estrogens (Systemic), 795

Diethylstilbestrol and Methyltestosterone—*See* Androgens and Estrogens (Systemic), 225

Difenidol—*See* Diphenidol (Systemic), 723

Difenoxin and Atropine (Systemic), 713

Diflorasone—*See* Corticosteroids—Medium to Very High Potency (Topical), 626

*Diflucan*—Fluconazole—*See* Antifungals, Azole (Systemic), 292, MC-10

Diflucortolone—*See* Corticosteroids—Medium to Very High Potency (Topical), 626

Diflunisal—*See* Nonsteroidal Anti-inflammatory Drugs (Systemic), 1229, MC-7

Difluorophate—Isoflurophate—*See* Antiglaucoma Agents, Cholinergic, Long-acting (Ophthalmic), 299

*Di-Gel*—Alumina, Magnesia, and Simethicone—*See* Antacids (Oral), 253

*Digitaline*—Digitoxin—*See* Digitalis Medicines (Systemic), 716

Digitalis Medicines (Systemic), 716

Digitoxin—*See* Digitalis Medicines (Systemic), 716

*DigiWipe*—Fecal Occult Blood Test Kits—*See* Fecal Occult Blood Test Kits, 826

Digoxin—*See* Digitalis Medicines (Systemic), 716, MC-7

*Dihistine*—Chlorpheniramine and Phenylephrine—*See* Antihistamines and Decongestants (Systemic), 311

*Dihistine DH*—Chlorpheniramine, Pseudoephedrine, and Codeine—*See* Cough/Cold Combinations (Systemic), 637

*Dihistine Expectorant*—Pseudoephedrine, Codeine, and Guaifenesin—*See* Cough/Cold Combinations (Systemic), 637

Dihydrocodeine, Acetaminophen, and Caffeine—*See* Narcotic Analgesics and Acetaminophen (Systemic), 1181

Dihydrocodeine compound—Aspirin, Caffeine, and Dihydrocodeine—*See* Narcotic Analgesics and Aspirin (Systemic), 1185

Dihydroergotamine—*See* Headache Medicines, Ergot Derivative–containing (Systemic), 914

*Dihydroergotamine-Sandoz*—Dihydroergotamine—*See* Headache Medicines, Ergot Derivative–containing (Systemic), 914

Dihydromorphinone—Hydromorphone—*See* Narcotic Analgesics—For Pain Relief (Systemic), 1176

Dihydrotachysterol—*See* Vitamin D and Related Compounds (Systemic), 1669

Dihydroxyaluminum Aminoacetate—*See* Antacids (Oral), 253

Dihydroxyaluminum Sodium Carbonate—*See* Antacids (Oral), 253

Diiodohydroxyquin—*See* Iodoquinol (Oral), 977

*Dilacor-XR*—Diltiazem—*See* Calcium Channel Blocking Agents (Systemic), 467

*Dilacor XR*—Diltiazem (Systemic), MC-7

*Dilantin*—Phenytoin—*See* Anticonvulsants, Hydantoin (Systemic), 267

*Dilantin-30*—Phenytoin—*See* Anticonvulsants, Hydantoin (Systemic), 267

*Dilantin-125*—Phenytoin—*See* Anticonvulsants, Hydantoin (Systemic), 267

*Dilantin Infatabs*—Phenytoin—*See* Anticonvulsants, Hydantoin (Systemic), 267, MC-18

*Dilantin Kapseals*—Phenytoin—*See* Anticonvulsants, Hydantoin (Systemic), 267, MC-18

*Dilatair*—Phenylephrine (Ophthalmic), 1345

*Dilatrate-SR*—Isosorbide Dinitrate—*See* Nitrates—Oral (Systemic), 1218, MC-12

*Dilaudid*—Hydromorphone—*See* Narcotic Analgesics—For Pain Relief (Systemic), 1176, MC-11

*Dilaudid Cough*—Hydromorphone and Guaifenesin—*See* Cough/Cold Combinations (Systemic), 637

*Dilaudid-HP*—Hydromorphone—*See* Narcotic Analgesics—For Pain Relief (Systemic), 1176

*Dilocaine*—Lidocaine—*See* Anesthetics (Parenteral-Local), 235

*Dilor*—Dyphylline—*See* Bronchodilators, Xanthine-derivative (Systemic), 442

*Dilor-400*—Dyphylline—*See* Bronchodilators, Xanthine-derivative (Systemic), 442

Diloxanide (Systemic), 718

Diltiazem—*See* Calcium Channel Blocking Agents (Systemic), 467, MC-7

Diphenhydramine—*See* Antihistamines (Systemic), 304, MC-7

Diphenhydramine, Codeine, and Ammonium Chloride—*See* Cough/Cold Combinations (Systemic), 637

Diphenhydramine, Dextromethorphan, and Ammonium Chloride (Systemic), 1748

Diphenhydramine, Phenylpropanolamine, and Aspirin—*See* Antihistamines, Decongestants, and Analgesics (Systemic), 316

Diphenhydramine and Pseudoephedrine—*See* Antihistamines and Decongestants (Systemic), 311

Diphenhydramine, Pseudoephedrine, and Acetaminophen—*See* Antihistamines, Decongestants, and Analgesics (Systemic), 316, 1748

Diphenhydramine, Pseudoephedrine, Dextromethorphan, and Acetaminophen—*See* Cough/Cold Combinations (Systemic), 637

Diphenidol (Systemic), 723

Diphenoxylate and Atropine (Systemic), 725, MC-7

*Diphenylan*—Phenytoin—*See* Anticonvulsants, Hydantoin (Systemic), 267

*Diphenylhydantoin*—Phenytoin—*See* Anticonvulsants, Hydantoin (Systemic), 267

Diphenylpyraline—*See* Antihistamines (Systemic), 304

Diphenylpyraline, Phenylephrine, and Dextromethorphan—*See* Cough/Cold Combinations (Systemic), 637

Diphenylpyraline, Phenylephrine, and Hydrocodone—*See* Cough/Cold Combinations (Systemic), 637

Diphenylpyraline, Phenylephrine, Hydrocodone, and Guaifenesin—*See* Cough/Cold Combinations (Systemic), 637

Diphtheria and Tetanus Toxoids and Pertussis Vaccine Adsorbed (Systemic), 728

Dipivefrin (Ophthalmic), 729

*Dipivefrine*—*See* Dipivefrin (Ophthalmic), 729

*Dipridacot*—Dipyridamole (Diagnostic), 731; Dipyridamole (Therapeutic), 732

*Diprivan*—Propofol—*See* Anesthetics, General (Systemic), 243

*Diprolene*—Betamethasone—*See* Corticosteroids—Medium to Very High Potency (Topical), 626

*Diprolene AF*—Betamethasone—*See* Corticosteroids—Medium to Very High Potency (Topical), 626

*Diprosone*—Betamethasone—*See* Corticosteroids—Medium to Very High Potency (Topical), 626

Dipyridamole (Diagnostic), 731

Dipyridamole (Therapeutic), 732, MC-7, MC-8

Dipyridamole and Aspirin (Systemic), 1748

*Diquinol*—Iodoquinol (Oral), 977

*Disalcid*—Salsalate—*See* Salicylates (Systemic), 1473

*Disanthrol*—Casanthranol and Docusate—*See* Laxatives (Oral), 1017

*Disipal*—Orphenadrine (Systemic), 1260

*Disobrom*—Dexbrompheniramine and Pseudoephedrine—*See* Antihistamines and Decongestants (Systemic), 311

*Disolan*—Docusate and Phenolphthalein—*See* Laxatives (Oral), 1017

*Disolan Forte*—Carboxymethylcellulose, Casanthranol, and Docusate—*See* Laxatives (Oral), 1017

*Disonate*—Docusate—*See* Laxatives (Oral), 1017

*Disophrol*—Dexbrompheniramine and Pseudoephedrine—*See* Antihistamines and Decongestants (Systemic), 311

*Disophrol Chronotabs*—Dexbrompheniramine and Pseudoephedrine—*See* Antihistamines and Decongestants (Systemic), 311

*Disoplex*—Carboxymethylcellulose and Docusate—*See* Laxatives (Oral), 1017

Disopyramide (Systemic), 734, MC-8

*Di-Sosul*—Docusate—*See* Laxatives (Oral), 1017

*Di-Sosul Forte*—Casanthranol and Docusate—*See* Laxatives (Oral), 1017

*Di-Spaz*—Dicyclomine—*See* Anticholinergics/Antispasmodics (Systemic), 258

Disulfiram (Systemic), 736

*Dithranol*—*See* Anthralin (Topical), 256

*Ditropan*—Oxybutynin (Systemic), 1272, MC-17

*Diucardin*—Hydroflumethiazide—*See* Diuretics, Thiazide (Systemic), 749

*Diuchlor H*—Hydrochlorothiazide—*See* Diuretics, Thiazide (Systemic), 749

*Diulo*—Metolazone—*See* Diuretics, Thiazide (Systemic), 749

*Diupres*—Reserpine and Chlorothiazide—*See* Rauwolfia Alkaloids and Thiazide Diuretics (Systemic), 1445

*Diurese-R*—Reserpine and Trichlormethiazide—*See* Rauwolfia Alkaloids and Thiazide Diuretics (Systemic), 1445

Diuretics, Loop (Systemic), 738

Diuretics, Potassium-sparing (Systemic), 742

Diuretics, Potassium-sparing, and Hydrochlorothiazide (Systemic), 745

Diuretics, Thiazide (Systemic), 749

*Diurigen with Reserpine*—Reserpine and Chlorothiazide—*See* Rauwolfia Alkaloids and Thiazide Diuretics (Systemic), 1445

*Diuril*—Chlorothiazide—*See* Diuretics, Thiazide (Systemic), 749

*Diutensen-R*—Reserpine and Methyclothiazide—*See* Rauwolfia Alkaloids and Thiazide Diuretics (Systemic), 1445

*Divalproex*—*See* Valproic Acid (Systemic), 1651, MC-8

*Dixarit*—Clonidine (Systemic), 576

DMSA—*See* Succimer (Systemic), 1520

DMSO—*See* Dimethyl Sulfoxide (Mucosal), 720

*DM Syrup*—Dextromethorphan (Systemic), 701

DNase I—*See* Dornase Alfa (Inhalation), 754

*Doak Oil*—Coal Tar (Topical), 589

*Doak Oil Forte*—Coal Tar (Topical), 589

*Doak Oil Forte Therapeutic Bath Treatment*—Coal Tar (Topical), 589

*Doak Oil Therapeutic Bath Treatment For All-Over Body Care*—Coal Tar (Topical), 589

*Doak Tar Lotion*—Coal Tar (Topical), 589

*Doak Tar Shampoo*—Coal Tar (Topical), 589

*Doan's*—Magnesium Salicylate—*See* Salicylates (Systemic), 1473

*Doctar Hair & Scalp Shampoo and Conditioner*—Coal Tar (Topical), 589

*Doctar Shampoo*—Coal Tar (Topical), 589

*Docucal-P*—Docusate and Phenolphthalein—*See* Laxatives (Oral), 1017

*Docu-K Plus*—Casanthranol and Docusate—*See* Laxatives (Oral), 1017

Docusate—*See* Laxatives (Oral), 1017; Laxatives (Rectal), 1023

Docusate and Phenolphthalein—*See* Laxatives (Oral), 1017

---

*Dramocen*—Dimenhydrinate—*See* Antihistamines (Systemic), 304

*Dramoject*—Dimenhydrinate—*See* Antihistamines (Systemic), 304

*Drenison*—Flurandrenolide—*See* Corticosteroids—Medium to Very High Potency (Topical), 626

*Drenison-¼*—Flurandrenolide—*See* Corticosteroids—Low Potency (Topical), 624

*D-Rex 65*—Propoxyphene and Acetaminophen—*See* Narcotic Analgesics and Acetaminophen (Systemic), 1181

D(Rh$_0$) immune globulin—*See* RH$_0$(D) Immune Globulin (Systemic), 1456

*Drisdol*—Ergocalciferol—*See* Vitamin D and Related Compounds (Systemic), 1669

*Dristan*—Chlorpheniramine, Phenylpropanolamine, Aspirin, and Caffeine—*See* Antihistamines, Decongestants, and Analgesics (Systemic), 316

*Dristan Allergy Caplets*—Brompheniramine and Pseudoephedrine—*See* Antihistamines and Decongestants (Systemic), 311

*Dristan Cold*—Chlorpheniramine, Phenylephrine, and Acetaminophen (Systemic), 1746

*Dristan Cold Caplets*—Pseudoephedrine and Acetaminophen—*See* Decongestants and Analgesics (Systemic), 691

*Dristan Cold and Flu*—Chlorpheniramine, Pseudoephedrine, Dextromethorphan, and Acetaminophen—*See* Cough/Cold Combinations (Systemic), 637, 1747

*Dristan Cold Maximum Strength Caplets*—Brompheniramine, Pseudoephedrine, and Acetaminophen—*See* Antihistamines, Decongestants, and Analgesics (Systemic), 316

*Dristan Cold Multi-Symptom Formula*—Chlorpheniramine, Phenylephrine, and Acetaminophen—*See* Antihistamines, Decongestants, and Analgesics (Systemic), 316

*Dristan Formula P*—Pyrilamine, Phenylephrine, Aspirin, and Caffeine—*See* Antihistamines, Decongestants, and Analgesics (Systemic), 316

*Dristan 12-Hr Nasal Spray*—Oxymetazoline (Nasal), 1274

*Dristan Juice Mix-in Cold, Flu, and Cough*—Pseudoephedrine, Dextromethorphan, and Acetaminophen—*See* Cough/Cold Combinations (Systemic), 637, 1753

*Dristan Sinus Caplets*—Pseudoephedrine and Ibuprofen—*See* Decongestants and Analgesics (Systemic), 691

*Drithocreme*—Anthralin (Topical), 256

*Drithocreme HP*—Anthralin (Topical), 256

*Dritho-Scalp*—Anthralin (Topical), 256

*Drixoral*—Brompheniramine and Pseudoephedrine—*See* Antihistamines and Decongestants (Systemic), 311; Dexbrompheniramine and Pseudoephedrine—*See* Antihistamines and Decongestants (Systemic), 311

*Drixoral Cold and Allergy*—Dexbrompheniramine and Pseudoephedrine—*See* Antihistamines and Decongestants (Systemic), 311

*Drixoral Cold and Flu*—Dexbrompheniramine, Pseudoephedrine, and Acetaminophen—*See* Antihistamines, Decongestants, and Analgesics (Systemic), 316

*Drixoral Cough Liquid Caps*—Dextromethorphan (Systemic), 701

*Drixoral Non-Drowsy Formula*—Pseudoephedrine (Systemic), 1412

*Drixoral Sinus*—Dexbrompheniramine, Pseudoephedrine, and Acetaminophen—*See* Antihistamines, Decongestants, and Analgesics (Systemic), 316

*Drixtab*—Dexbrompheniramine and Pseudoephedrine—*See* Antihistamines and Decongestants (Systemic), 311

*Drize*—Chlorpheniramine and Phenylpropanolamine—*See* Antihistamines and Decongestants (Systemic), 311

Drocode, acetaminophen, and caffeine—Dihydrocodeine, Acetaminophen, and Caffeine—*See* Narcotic Analgesics and Acetaminophen (Systemic), 1181

Drocode and aspirin—Aspirin, Caffeine, and Dihydrocodeine—*See* Narcotic Analgesics and Aspirin (Systemic), 1185

Dronabinol (Systemic), 760

*Dry and Clear Double Strength 10 Cream*—Benzoyl Peroxide (Topical), 397

*Dry and Clear 5 Lotion*—Benzoyl Peroxide (Topical), 397

*Dryox 5 Gel*—Benzoyl Peroxide (Topical), 397

*Dryox 10 Gel*—Benzoyl Peroxide (Topical), 397

*Dryox 20 Gel*—Benzoyl Peroxide (Topical), 397

*Dryox Wash 5*—Benzoyl Peroxide (Topical), 397

*Dryox Wash 10*—Benzoyl Peroxide (Topical), 397

*DSMC Plus*—Casanthranol and Docusate—*See* Laxatives (Oral), 1017

*D-S-S*—Docusate—*See* Laxatives (Oral), 1017

*D-S-S plus*—Casanthranol and Docusate—*See* Laxatives (Oral), 1017

*DTaP*—*See* Diphtheria and Tetanus Toxoids and Pertussis Vaccine Adsorbed (Systemic), 728

*DTIC*—Dacarbazine (Systemic), 677

*DTIC-Dome*—Dacarbazine (Systemic), 677

*DTP*—*See* Diphtheria and Tetanus Toxoids and Pertussis Vaccine Adsorbed (Systemic), 728

*DTwP*—*See* Diphtheria and Tetanus Toxoids and Pertussis Vaccine Adsorbed (Systemic), 728

*Duadacin*—Chlorpheniramine, Phenylpropanolamine, and Acetaminophen—*See* Antihistamines, Decongestants, and Analgesics (Systemic), 316

*Dulcodos*—Bisacodyl and Docusate—*See* Laxatives (Oral), 1017

*Dulcolax*—Bisacodyl—*See* Laxatives (Oral), 1017; Laxatives (Rectal), 1023

*Duocet*—Hydrocodone and Acetaminophen—*See* Narcotic Analgesics and Acetaminophen (Systemic), 1181

*Duo-Cyp*—Testosterone and Estradiol—*See* Androgens and Estrogens (Systemic), 225

*Duofilm*—Salicylic Acid (Topical), 1478

*Duo-Gen L.A.*—Testosterone and Estradiol—*See* Androgens and Estrogens (Systemic), 225

*Duogex L.A.*—Testosterone and Estradiol—*See* Androgens and Estrogens (Systemic), 225

*Duo-Medihaler*—Isoproterenol and Phenylephrine (Systemic), 995

*Duoplant Topical Solution*—Salicylic Acid (Topical), 1478

*Duoprin*—Acetaminophen and Salicylamide—*See* Acetaminophen and Salicylates (Systemic), 164

*Duosol*—Docusate—*See* Laxatives (Oral), 1017

*Duotrate*—Pentaerythritol Tetranitrate—*See* Nitrates—Oral (Systemic), 1218

*Duphalac*—Lactulose—*See* Laxatives (Oral), 1017

# E

Ecothiopate—Echothiopate—*See* Antiglaucoma Agents, Cholinergic, Long-acting (Ophthalmic), 299

*Ecotrin*—Aspirin—*See* Salicylates (Systemic), 1473

*Ectosone Mild*—Betamethasone—*See* Corticosteroids—Medium to Very High Potency (Topical), 626

*Ectosone Regular*—Betamethasone—*See* Corticosteroids—Medium to Very High Potency (Topical), 626

*Ectosone Scalp Lotion*—Betamethasone—*See* Corticosteroids—Medium to Very High Potency (Topical), 626

*E-Cypionate*—Estradiol—*See* Estrogens (Systemic), 795

*Ed A-Hist*—Chlorpheniramine and Phenylephrine—*See* Antihistamines and Decongestants (Systemic), 311

*Ed-Bron G*—Theophylline and Guaifenesin (Systemic), 1586

*Edecrin*—Ethacrynic Acid—*See* Diuretics, Loop (Systemic), 738

*ED-TLC*—Chlorpheniramine, Phenylephrine, and Hydrocodone—*See* Cough/Cold Combinations (Systemic), 637

*ED Tuss HC*—Chlorpheniramine, Phenylephrine, and Hydrocodone—*See* Cough/Cold Combinations (Systemic), 637

*E.E.S.*—Erythromycin Ethylsuccinate—*See* Erythromycins (Systemic), 786, MC-9

*Efed II Yellow*—Phenylpropanolamine (Systemic), 1347

*Effective Strength Cough Formula*—Chlorpheniramine and Dextromethorphan—*See* Cough/Cold Combinations (Systemic), 637

*Effective Strength Cough Formula with Decongestant*—Pseudoephedrine and Dextromethorphan—*See* Cough/Cold Combinations (Systemic), 637

*Effer-K*—Potassium Bicarbonate and Potassium Citrate—*See* Potassium Supplements (Systemic), 1373

*Effer-syllium*—Psyllium Hydrophilic Mucilloid—*See* Laxatives (Oral), 1017

*Effexor*—Venlafaxine (Systemic), MC-24

*Efficol Cough Whip (Cough Suppressant/Decongestant)*—Phenylpropanolamine and Dextromethorphan—*See* Cough/Cold Combinations (Systemic), 637

*Efficol Cough Whip (Cough Suppressant/Decongestant/Antihistamine)*—Chlorpheniramine, Phenylpropanolamine, and Dextromethorphan—*See* Cough/Cold Combinations (Systemic), 637

*Efficol Cough Whip (Cough Suppressant/Expectorant)*—Dextromethorphan and Guaifenesin—*See* Cough/Cold Combinations (Systemic), 637

*Efidac/24*—Pseudoephedrine (Systemic), 1412

Eflornithine (Systemic), 764

*Efudex*—Fluorouracil (Topical), 852

*E/Gel*—Erythromycin (Topical), 1748

*EHDP*—*See* Etidronate (Systemic), 814

*E-200 I.U. Softgels*—Vitamin E (Systemic), 1674

*E-1000 I.U. Softgels*—Vitamin E (Systemic), 1674

*E-400 I.U. in a Water Soluble Base*—Vitamin E (Systemic), 1674

*Elavil*—Amitriptyline—*See* Antidepressants, Tricyclic (Systemic), 277, MC-1

*Elavil Plus*—Perphenazine and Amitriptyline (Systemic), 1322

*Eldepryl*—Selegiline (Systemic), 1485, MC-21

*Eldisine*—Vindesine (Systemic), 1755

*Elementra*—Enteral Nutrition Formula, Modular—*See* Enteral Nutrition Formulas (Systemic), 769

*Elimite*—Permethrin (Topical), 1752

*Elixomin*—Theophylline—*See* Bronchodilators, Xanthine-derivative (Systemic), 442

*Elixophyllin*—Theophylline—*See* Bronchodilators, Xanthine-derivative (Systemic), 442

*Elixophyllin-GG*—Theophylline and Guaifenesin (Systemic), 1586

*Elixophyllin SR*—Theophylline—*See* Bronchodilators, Xanthine-derivative (Systemic), 442

*Elocom*—Mometasone—*See* Corticosteroids—Medium to Very High Potency (Topical), 626

*E-Lor*—Propoxyphene and Acetaminophen—*See* Narcotic Analgesics and Acetaminophen (Systemic), 1181

*Elspar*—Asparaginase (Systemic), 347

*Eltor 120*—Pseudoephedrine (Systemic), 1412

*Eltroxin*—Levothyroxine—*See* Thyroid Hormones (Systemic), 1606

*Embrace*—Latex Condoms—*See* Condoms, 602

*Emcodeine No.2*—Aspirin and Codeine—*See* Narcotic Analgesics and Aspirin (Systemic), 1185

*Emcodeine No.3*—Aspirin and Codeine—*See* Narcotic Analgesics and Aspirin (Systemic), 1185

*Emcodeine No.4*—Aspirin and Codeine—*See* Narcotic Analgesics and Aspirin (Systemic), 1185

*Emcyt*—Estramustine (Systemic), 793

*Emetrol*—Fructose, Dextrose, and Phosphoric Acid (Oral), 861

*Emex*—Metoclopramide (Systemic), 1123

*Emgel*—Erythromycin (Topical), 1748

*Eminase*—Anistreplase—*See* Thrombolytic Agents (Systemic), 1604

*Emko*—Nonoxynol 9—*See* Spermicides (Vaginal), 1512

*EMLA*—Lidocaine and Prilocaine (Topical), 1038

*Emo-Cort*—Hydrocortisone—*See* Corticosteroids—Low Potency (Topical), 624

*Emo-Cort Scalp Solution*—Hydrocortisone—*See* Corticosteroids—Low Potency (Topical), 624

*Empirin*—Aspirin—*See* Salicylates (Systemic), 1473

*Empirin with Codeine No.2*—Aspirin and Codeine—*See* Narcotic Analgesics and Aspirin (Systemic), 1185, MC-2

*Empirin with Codeine No.3*—Aspirin and Codeine—*See* Narcotic Analgesics and Aspirin (Systemic), 1185, MC-2

*Empirin with Codeine No.4*—Aspirin and Codeine—*See* Narcotic Analgesics and Aspirin (Systemic), 1185, MC-2

*Empracet-30*—Acetaminophen and Codeine—*See* Narcotic Analgesics and Acetaminophen (Systemic), 1181

*Empracet-60*—Acetaminophen and Codeine—*See* Narcotic Analgesics and Acetaminophen (Systemic), 1181

*Emtec-30*—Acetaminophen and Codeine—*See* Narcotic Analgesics and Acetaminophen (Systemic), 1181

*Emulsoil*—Castor Oil—*See* Laxatives (Oral), 1017

*E-Mycin*—Erythromycin Base—*See* Erythromycins (Systemic), 786, MC-9

Enalapril—*See* Angiotensin-converting Enzyme (ACE) Inhibitors (Systemic), 245, MC-8

Enalaprilat—*See* Angiotensin-converting Enzyme (ACE) Inhibitors (Systemic), 245

Enalapril and Hydrochlorothiazide—*See* Angiotensin-converting Enzyme (ACE) Inhibitors and Hydrochlorothiazide (Systemic), 249, 1748, MC-8

Encainide (Systemic), 766

*Encare*—Nonoxynol 9—*See* Spermicides (Vaginal), 1512

Ephedrine and Guaifenesin—*See* Cough/Cold Combinations (Systemic), 637

Ephedrine and Potassium Iodide—*See* Cough/Cold Combinations (Systemic), 637

*Epiclase*—Phenacemide (Systemic), 1325

*Epifoam*—Hydrocortisone Acetate—*See* Corticosteroids—Low Potency (Topical), 624

*Epifrin*—Epinephrine (Ophthalmic), 771

*Epimorph*—Morphine—*See* Narcotic Analgesics—For Pain Relief (Systemic), 1176; Narcotic Analgesics—For Surgery and Obstetrics (Systemic), 1179

*Epinal*—Epinephryl Borate—*See* Epinephrine (Ophthalmic), 771

Epinephrine—*See* Bronchodilators, Adrenergic (Inhalation), 430; Bronchodilators, Adrenergic (Oral/Injection), 436

Epinephrine (Ophthalmic), 771

Epinephryl Borate—*See* Epinephrine (Ophthalmic), 771

*EpiPen Auto-Injector*—Epinephrine—*See* Bronchodilators, Adrenergic (Oral/Injection), 436

*EpiPen Jr. Auto-Injector*—Epinephrine—*See* Bronchodilators, Adrenergic (Oral/Injection), 436

Epirubicin (Systemic), 1748

*Epistatin*—Simvastatin—*See* HMG-CoA Reductase Inhibitors (Systemic), 929

*Epitol*—Carbamazepine (Systemic), 481

*Epival*—Divalproex—*See* Valproic Acid (Systemic), 1651

EPO—*See* Epoetin (Systemic), 773

Epoetin (Systemic), 773

*Epogen*—Epoetin (Systemic), 773

*Eppy/N*—Epinephryl Borate—*See* Epinephrine (Ophthalmic), 771

*Eprex*—Epoetin (Systemic), 773

*Epromate-M*—Meprobamate and Aspirin (Systemic), 1091

Epsom salts—Magnesium Sulfate—*See* Laxatives (Oral), 1017

Eptastatin—Pravastatin—*See* HMG-CoA Reductase Inhibitors (Systemic), 929

*e.p.t. Quick Stick*—Pregnancy Test Kits for Home Use, 1385

*Equagesic*—Meprobamate and Aspirin (Systemic), 1091

*Equalactin*—Polycarbophil—*See* Laxatives (Oral), 1017

*Equanil*—Meprobamate (Systemic), 1089

*Equibron G*—Theophylline and Guaifenesin (Systemic), 1586

*Equilet*—Calcium Carbonate—*See* Antacids (Oral), 253

*Ercaf*—Ergotamine and Caffeine—*See* Headache Medicines, Ergot Derivative–containing (Systemic), 914

*Ergamisol*—Levamisole (Systemic), 1029

*Ergo-Caff*—Ergotamine and Caffeine—*See* Headache Medicines, Ergot Derivative–containing (Systemic), 914

Ergocalciferol—*See* Vitamin D and Related Compounds (Systemic), 1669

*Ergodryl*—Ergotamine, Caffeine, and Diphenhydramine—*See* Headache Medicines, Ergot Derivative–containing (Systemic), 914

Ergoloid Mesylates (Systemic), 775, MC-9

*Ergomar*—Ergotamine—*See* Headache Medicines, Ergot Derivative–containing (Systemic), 914

Ergometrine—Ergonovine—*See* Ergonovine/Methylergonovine (Systemic), 776

Ergonovine—*See* Ergonovine/Methylergonovine (Systemic), 776

Ergonovine/Methylergonovine (Systemic), 776

*Ergostat*—Ergotamine—*See* Headache Medicines, Ergot Derivative–containing (Systemic), 914

Ergot alkaloids, dihydrogenated—*See* Ergoloid Mesylates (Systemic), 775

Ergotamine—*See* Headache Medicines, Ergot Derivative–containing (Systemic), 914

Ergotamine, Belladonna Alkaloids, and Phenobarbital (Systemic), 778

Ergotamine and Caffeine—*See* Headache Medicines, Ergot Derivative–containing (Systemic), 914, MC-9

Ergotamine, Caffeine, and Belladonna Alkaloids—*See* Headache Medicines, Ergot Derivative–containing (Systemic), 914

Ergotamine, Caffeine, Belladonna Alkaloids, and Pentobarbital—*See* Headache Medicines, Ergot Derivative–containing (Systemic), 914

Ergotamine, Caffeine, and Cyclizine—*See* Headache Medicines, Ergot Derivative–containing (Systemic), 914

Ergotamine, Caffeine, and Dimenhydrinate—*See* Headache Medicines, Ergot Derivative–containing (Systemic), 914

Ergotamine, Caffeine, and Diphenhydramine—*See* Headache Medicines, Ergot Derivative–containing (Systemic), 914

*Ergotrate*—Ergonovine—*See* Ergonovine/Methylergonovine (Systemic), 776

*Ergotrate Maleate*—Ergonovine—*See* Ergonovine/Methylergonovine (Systemic), 776

*Eridium*—Phenazopyridine (Systemic), 1327

Eritrityl tetranitrate—Erythrityl Tetranitrate—*See* Nitrates—Oral (Systemic), 1218; Nitrates—Sublingual, Chewable, or Buccal (Systemic), 1221

*Erybid*—Erythromycin Base—*See* Erythromycins (Systemic), 786

*ERYC*—Erythromycin Base—*See* Erythromycins (Systemic), 786, MC-9

*ERYC-250*—Erythromycin Base—*See* Erythromycins (Systemic), 786

*ERYC-333*—Erythromycin Base—*See* Erythromycins (Systemic), 786

*Erycette*—Erythromycin (Topical), 782

*EryDerm*—Erythromycin (Topical), 782

*Erygel*—Erythromycin (Topical), 782

*Erymax*—Erythromycin (Topical), 782

*EryPed*—Erythromycin Ethylsuccinate—*See* Erythromycins (Systemic), 786, MC-9

*Ery-Sol*—Erythromycin (Topical), 782

*Ery-Tab*—Erythromycin Base—*See* Erythromycins (Systemic), 786, MC-9

Erythritol tetranitrate—Erythrityl Tetranitrate—*See* Nitrates—Oral (Systemic), 1218; Nitrates—Sublingual, Chewable, or Buccal (Systemic), 1221

Erythrityl Tetranitrate—*See* Nitrates—Oral (Systemic), 1218; Nitrates—Sublingual, Chewable, or Buccal (Systemic), 1221

*Erythro*—Erythromycin Ethylsuccinate—*See* Erythromycins (Systemic), 786

*Erythrocin*—Erythromycin Lactobionate—*See* Erythromycins (Systemic), 786; Erythromycin Stearate—*See* Erythromycins (Systemic), 786, MC-9

*Erythrocot*—Erythromycin Stearate—*See* Erythromycins (Systemic), 786

*Eudal-SR*—Pseudoephedrine and Guaifenesin—*See* Cough/Cold Combinations (Systemic), 637

*Euflex*—Flutamide (Systemic), 856

*Euglucon*—Glyburide—*See* Antidiabetics, Oral (Systemic), 283

*Eulexin*—Flutamide (Systemic), 856

*Eulipos*—Dextrothyroxine (Systemic), 702

*Eumovate*—Clobetasone—*See* Corticosteroids—Medium to Very High Potency (Topical), 626

*Eurax Cream*—Crotamiton (Topical), 659

*Eurax Lotion*—Crotamiton (Topical), 659

*Evac-U-Gen*—Phenolphthalein—*See* Laxatives (Oral), 1017

*Evac-U-Lax*—Phenolphthalein—*See* Laxatives (Oral), 1017

*Everone*—Testosterone—*See* Androgens (Systemic), 221

*E-Vista*—Hydroxyzine—*See* Antihistamines (Systemic), 304

*E-Vitamin Succinate*—Vitamin E (Systemic), 1674

*Excedrin Caplets*—Acetaminophen and Caffeine—*See* Acetaminophen (Systemic), 161

*Excedrin Extra-Strength Caplets*—Acetaminophen, Aspirin, and Caffeine—*See* Acetaminophen and Salicylates (Systemic), 164

*Excedrin Extra Strength Caplets*—Acetaminophen and Caffeine—*See* Acetaminophen (Systemic), 161

*Excedrin Extra-Strength Tablets*—Acetaminophen, Aspirin, and Caffeine—*See* Acetaminophen and Salicylates (Systemic), 164

*Excedrin IB*—Ibuprofen—*See* Nonsteroidal Anti-inflammatory Drugs (Systemic), 1229

*Excedrin IB Caplets*—Ibuprofen—*See* Nonsteroidal Anti-inflammatory Drugs (Systemic), 1229

*Excita Extra*—Latex Condoms and Nonoxynol 9—*See* Condoms, 602

*Excita Fiesta*—Latex Condoms—*See* Condoms, 602

*Exdol*—Acetaminophen (Systemic), 161

*Exdol-8*—Acetaminophen, Codeine, and Caffeine—*See* Narcotic Analgesics and Acetaminophen (Systemic), 1181

*Exdol-15*—Acetaminophen, Codeine, and Caffeine—*See* Narcotic Analgesics and Acetaminophen (Systemic), 1181

*Exdol-30*—Acetaminophen, Codeine, and Caffeine—*See* Narcotic Analgesics and Acetaminophen (Systemic), 1181

*Exdol Strong*—Acetaminophen (Systemic), 161

*Exelderm*—Sulconazole (Topical), 1523

*Exgest LA*—Phenylpropanolamine and Guaifenesin—*See* Cough/Cold Combinations (Systemic), 637

*Ex-Lax*—Phenolphthalein—*See* Laxatives (Oral), 1017

*Ex-Lax Maximum Relief Formula*—Phenolphthalein—*See* Laxatives (Oral), 1017

*Ex-Lax Pills*—Phenolphthalein—*See* Laxatives (Oral), 1017

*Exna*—Benzthiazide—*See* Diuretics, Thiazide (Systemic), 749

*Exsel Lotion Shampoo*—Selenium Sulfide (Topical), 1487

*Extendryl*—Chlorpheniramine, Phenylephrine, and Methscopolamine—*See* Antihistamines, Decongestants, and Anticholinergics (Systemic), 322

*Extendryl JR*—Chlorpheniramine, Phenylephrine, and Methscopolamine—*See* Antihistamines, Decongestants, and Anticholinergics (Systemic), 322

*Extendryl SR*—Chlorpheniramine, Phenylephrine, and Methscopolamine—*See* Antihistamines, Decongestants, and Anticholinergics (Systemic), 322

*Extra Action Cough*—Dextromethorphan and Guaifenesin—*See* Cough/Cold Combinations (Systemic), 637

*Extra Gentle Ex-Lax*—Docusate and Phenolphthalein—*See* Laxatives (Oral), 1017

*Extra Strength Gas-X*—Simethicone (Oral), 1494

*EZ Detect*—Fecal Occult Blood Test Kits—*See* Fecal Occult Blood Test Kits, 826

*Ezol*—Butalbital, Acetaminophen, and Caffeine—*See* Butalbital and Acetaminophen (Systemic), 453

# F

*4-Way Cold*—Chlorpheniramine, Phenylpropanolamine, and Acetaminophen—*See* Antihistamines, Decongestants, and Analgesics (Systemic), 316

*4-Way Long Acting Nasal Spray*—Oxymetazoline (Nasal), 1274

5-aminosalicylic acid—*See* Mesalamine (Rectal), 1097

5-ASA—*See* Mesalamine (Rectal), 1097

5-FC—*See* Flucytosine (Systemic), 842

5-Fluorocytosine—*See* Flucytosine (Systemic), 842

5-FU—*See* Fluorouracil (Systemic), 850; Fluorouracil (Topical), 852

566C80—*See* Atovaquone (Systemic), 353

Factor IX (Systemic), 823

Factor VIII—*See* Antihemophilic Factor (Systemic), 302

*Fact Plus*—Pregnancy Test Kits for Home Use, 1385

*Factrel*—Gonadorelin (Systemic), 887

Famotidine—*See* Histamine $H_2$-receptor Antagonists (Systemic), 925, MC-9

*Fansidar*—Sulfadoxine and Pyrimethamine (Systemic), 1525

*Fastin*—Phentermine—*See* Appetite Suppressants (Systemic), 339

Fat Emulsions (Systemic), 825

*Father John's Medicine Plus*—Chlorpheniramine, Phenylephrine, Dextromethorphan, Guaifenesin, and Ammonium Chloride—*See* Cough/Cold Combinations (Systemic), 637

FBM—*See* Felbamate (Systemic), 828

5-FC—*See* Flucytosine (Systemic), 842

Fecal Occult Blood Test Kits, 826

*Fedahist*—Chlorpheniramine and Pseudoephedrine—*See* Antihistamines and Decongestants (Systemic), 311

*Fedahist Decongestant*—Chlorpheniramine and Pseudoephedrine—*See* Antihistamines and Decongestants (Systemic), 311

*Fedahist Gyrocaps*—Chlorpheniramine and Pseudoephedrine—*See* Antihistamines and Decongestants (Systemic), 311

*Fedahist Timecaps*—Chlorpheniramine and Pseudoephedrine—*See* Antihistamines and Decongestants (Systemic), 311

*Feen-a-Mint*—Docusate and Phenolphthalein—*See* Laxatives (Oral), 1017

*Feen-a-Mint Gum*—Phenolphthalein—*See* Laxatives (Oral), 1017

*Feen-a-Mint Pills*—Docusate and Phenolphthalein—*See* Laxatives (Oral), 1017

Felbamate (Systemic), 828, MC-9

*Felbatol*—Felbamate (Systemic), 828, MC-9

*Flavored Alka-Seltzer Effervescent Pain Reliever and Antacid*—Aspirin, Sodium Bicarbonate, and Citric Acid (Systemic), 349
Flavoxate (Systemic), 837
Flecainide (Systemic), 838
*Fleet Babylax*—Glycerin—*See* Laxatives (Rectal), 1023
*Fleet Bisacodyl*—Bisacodyl—*See* Laxatives (Rectal), 1023
*Fleet Bisacodyl Prep*—Bisacodyl—*See* Laxatives (Rectal), 1023
*Fleet Enema*—Sodium Phosphates—*See* Laxatives (Rectal), 1023
*Fleet Enema Mineral Oil*—Mineral Oil—*See* Laxatives (Rectal), 1023
*Fleet Flavored Castor Oil*—Castor Oil—*See* Laxatives (Oral), 1017
*Fleet Laxative*—Bisacodyl—*See* Laxatives (Oral), 1017; Laxatives (Rectal), 1023
*Fleet Phospho-Soda*—Sodium Phosphate—*See* Laxatives (Oral), 1017
*Fleet Relief*—Pramoxine—*See* Anesthetics (Rectal), 237
*Fletcher's Castoria*—Senna—*See* Laxatives (Oral), 1017
*Flexagin*—Orphenadrine (Systemic), 1260
*Flexain*—Orphenadrine (Systemic), 1260
*Flexeril*—Cyclobenzaprine (Systemic), 662, MC-6
*Flexoject*—Orphenadrine (Systemic), 1260
*Flexon*—Orphenadrine (Systemic), 1260
*Flint SSD*—Silver Sulfadiazine (Topical), 1492
Floctafenine—*See* Nonsteroidal Anti-inflammatory Drugs (Systemic), 1229
*Florinef*—Fludrocortisone (Systemic), 845
*Florone*—Diflorasone—*See* Corticosteroids—Medium to Very High Potency (Topical), 626
*Florone E*—Diflorasone—*See* Corticosteroids—Medium to Very High Potency (Topical), 626
*Floropryl*—Isoflurophate—*See* Antiglaucoma Agents, Cholinergic, Long-acting (Ophthalmic), 299
*Floxin*—Ofloxacin—*See* Fluoroquinolones (Systemic), 847, MC-17
*Floxin IV*—Ofloxacin—*See* Fluoroquinolones (Systemic), 847
Floxuridine (Systemic), 840
*Fluanxol*—Flupenthixol—*See* Thioxanthenes (Systemic), 1601
*Fluanxol Depot*—Flupenthixol—*See* Thioxanthenes (Systemic), 1601
*Fluclox*—Flucloxacillin—*See* Penicillins (Systemic), 1299
Flucloxacillin—*See* Penicillins (Systemic), 1299
Fluconazole—*See* Antifungals, Azole (Systemic), 292, MC-10
Flucytosine (Systemic), 842
*Fludara*—Fludarabine (Systemic), 843
Fludarabine (Systemic), 843
Fludeoxyglucose F 18—*See* Radiopharmaceuticals (Diagnostic), 1439
Fludrocortisone (Systemic), 845
Fludroxycortide—Flurandrenolide—*See* Corticosteroids—Medium to Very High Potency (Topical), 626
*Flu-Imune*—Influenza Virus Vaccine (Systemic), 959
*Flumadine*—Rimantadine (Systemic), 1467
Flumazenil (Systemic), 1748
Flumetasone—Flumethasone—*See* Corticosteroids—Low Potency (Topical), 624

Flumethasone—*See* Corticosteroids—Low Potency (Topical), 624
Flunarizine—*See* Calcium Channel Blocking Agents (Systemic), 467
Flunisolide—*See* Corticosteroids (Inhalation), 611; Corticosteroids (Nasal), 617
*Fluocet*—Fluocinolone—*See* Corticosteroids—Medium to Very High Potency (Topical), 626
*Fluocin*—Fluocinonide—*See* Corticosteroids—Medium to Very High Potency (Topical), 626
Fluocinolone—*See* Corticosteroids—Medium to Very High Potency (Topical), 626
Fluocinonide—*See* Corticosteroids—Medium to Very High Potency (Topical), 626, 1748
Fluocinonide, Procinonide, and Ciprocinonide (Topical), 1748
*Fluoderm*—Fluocinolone—*See* Corticosteroids—Medium to Very High Potency (Topical), 626
*Fluogen*—Influenza Virus Vaccine (Systemic), 959
*Fluolar*—Fluocinolone—*See* Corticosteroids—Medium to Very High Potency (Topical), 626
*Fluonid*—Fluocinolone—*See* Corticosteroids—Medium to Very High Potency (Topical), 626
*Fluonide*—Fluocinolone—*See* Corticosteroids—Medium to Very High Potency (Topical), 626
*Fluor-A-Day*—Sodium Fluoride (Systemic), 1502
*Fluoritab*—Sodium Fluoride (Systemic), 1502
5-Fluorocytosine—*See* Flucytosine (Systemic), 842
*Fluorodex*—Sodium Fluoride (Systemic), 1502
Fluorometholone—*See* Corticosteroids (Ophthalmic), 620
*Fluor-Op*—Fluorometholone—*See* Corticosteroids (Ophthalmic), 620
*Fluoroplex*—Fluorouracil (Topical), 852
Fluorouracil (Systemic), 850
Fluorouracil (Topical), 852
*Fluothane*—Halothane—*See* Anesthetics, General (Systemic), 243
*Fluotic*—Sodium Fluoride (Systemic), 1502
Fluoxetine (Systemic), 854, 1750, MC-10
Fluoxymesterone—*See* Androgens (Systemic), 221, MC-10
Fluoxymesterone and Ethinyl Estradiol—*See* Androgens and Estrogens (Systemic), 225
Flupenthixol—*See* Thioxanthenes (Systemic), 1601
Flupentixol—Flupenthixol—*See* Thioxanthenes (Systemic), 1601
Fluphenazine—*See* Phenothiazines (Systemic), 1330, MC-10
*Flura*—Sodium Fluoride (Systemic), 1502
*Flura-Drops*—Sodium Fluoride (Systemic), 1502
Flurandrenolide—*See* Corticosteroids—Low Potency (Topical), 624; Corticosteroids—Medium to Very High Potency (Topical), 626
Flurazepam—*See* Benzodiazepines (Systemic), 389, MC-10
Flurbiprofen—*See* Anti-inflammatory Agents, Nonsteroidal (Ophthalmic), 330; Nonsteroidal Anti-inflammatory Drugs (Systemic), 1229, MC-10
*Flurosyn*—Fluocinolone—*See* Corticosteroids—Medium to Very High Potency (Topical), 626
*FluShield*—Influenza Virus Vaccine (Systemic), 959
Fluspirilene (Systemic), 1749
Flutamide (Systemic), 856
*Flutex*—Triamcinolone—*See* Corticosteroids—Medium to Very High Potency (Topical), 626

Fluticasone—*See* Corticosteroids—Medium to Very High Potency (Topical), 626

Flu vaccine—*See* Influenza Virus Vaccine (Systemic), 959

Fluvastatin (Systemic), MC-10

*Fluviral*—Influenza Virus Vaccine (Systemic), 959

*Fluzone*—Influenza Virus Vaccine (Systemic), 959

*FML Forte*—Fluorometholone—*See* Corticosteroids (Ophthalmic), 620

*FML Liquifilm*—Fluorometholone—*See* Corticosteroids (Ophthalmic), 620

*FML S.O.P.*—Fluorometholone—*See* Corticosteroids (Ophthalmic), 620

*Foamicon*—Alumina and Magnesium Trisilicate—*See* Antacids (Oral), 253

*Foille*—Neomycin, Polymyxin B, and Bacitracin (Topical), 1200

*FoilleCort*—Hydrocortisone Acetate—*See* Corticosteroids—Low Potency (Topical), 624

*Foldan*—Thiabendazole (Systemic), 1588

*Folex*—Methotrexate—For Cancer (Systemic), 1102; Methotrexate—For Noncancerous Conditions (Systemic), 1105

*Folex PFS*—Methotrexate—For Cancer (Systemic), 1102; Methotrexate—For Noncancerous Conditions (Systemic), 1105

Folic Acid (Vitamin B$_9$) (Systemic), 857

Folinic acid—*See* Leucovorin (Systemic), 1025

Follicle-stimulating hormone—*See* Urofollitropin (Systemic), 1646

*Folvite*—Folic Acid (Vitamin B$_9$) (Systemic), 857

*Forane*—Isoflurane—*See* Anesthetics, General (Systemic), 243

*Formulex*—Dicyclomine—*See* Anticholinergics/Antispasmodics (Systemic), 258

*Fortabs*—Butalbital, Aspirin, and Caffeine—*See* Butalbital and Aspirin (Systemic), 456

*Fortaz*—Ceftazidime—*See* Cephalosporins (Systemic), 498

*222 Forte*—Aspirin, Codeine, and Caffeine—*See* Narcotic Analgesics and Aspirin (Systemic), 1185

*222 Forte*—Aspirin, Codeine, and Caffeine—*See* Narcotic Analgesics and Aspirin (Systemic), 1185

*Fortel*—Ovulation Prediction Test Kits for Home Use, 1265

*Fortel Midstream*—Pregnancy Test Kits for Home Use, 1385

*Fortel Plus*—Pregnancy Test Kits for Home Use, 1385

Foscarnet (Systemic), 860

*Foscavir*—Foscarnet (Systemic), 860

Fosinopril—*See* Angiotensin-converting Enzyme (ACE) Inhibitors (Systemic), 245, MC-10

*Fostex 10 Bar*—Benzoyl Peroxide (Topical), 397

*Fostex CM*—Sulfur (Topical), 1550

*Fostex 10 Cream*—Benzoyl Peroxide (Topical), 397

*Fostex 5 Gel*—Benzoyl Peroxide (Topical), 397

*Fostex 10 Gel*—Benzoyl Peroxide (Topical), 397

*Fostex Medicated Cleansing Bar*—Salicylic Acid and Sulfur (Topical), 1481

*Fostex Medicated Cleansing Cream (for face and scalp)*—Salicylic Acid and Sulfur (Topical), 1481

*Fostex Medicated Cleansing Liquid*—Salicylic Acid and Sulfur (Topical), 1481

*Fostex Regular Strength Medicated Cleansing Bar*—Salicylic Acid and Sulfur (Topical), 1481

*Fostex Regular Strength Medicated Cleansing Cream (for face and scalp)*—Salicylic Acid and Sulfur (Topical), 1481

*Fostex Regular Strength Medicated Cover-Up*—Sulfur (Topical), 1550

*Fostex 10 Wash*—Benzoyl Peroxide (Topical), 397

*Fostril Cream*—Sulfur (Topical), 1550

*Fostril Lotion*—Sulfur (Topical), 1550

*Fototar*—Coal Tar (Topical), 589

*Fourex Natural Skins*—Lamb Cecum Condoms—*See* Condoms, 602

*Fowler's Diarrhea Tablets*—Attapulgite (Oral), 359

Framycetin (Ophthalmic), 1749

Framycetin (Topical), 1749

Framycetin and Gramicidin (Topical), 1749

Framycetin, Gramicidin, and Dexamethasone (Ophthalmic), 1751

Framycetin, Gramicidin, and Dexamethasone (Otic), 1749

*Freezone*—Salicylic Acid (Topical), 1478

*Frisium*—Clobazam (Systemic), 1747

*Froben*—Flurbiprofen—*See* Nonsteroidal Anti-inflammatory Drugs (Systemic), 1229

*Froben SR*—Flurbiprofen—*See* Nonsteroidal Anti-inflammatory Drugs (Systemic), 1229

Fructose, Dextrose, and Phosphoric Acid (Oral), 861

FSH—*See* Urofollitropin (Systemic), 1646

5-FU—*See* Fluorouracil (Systemic), 850; Fluorouracil (Topical), 852

*Fucidin*—Fusidic Acid (Systemic), 1749; Fusidic Acid (Topical), 1749

*FUDR*—Floxuridine (Systemic), 840

*Fulvicin P/G*—Griseofulvin (Systemic), 889

*Fulvicin-U/F*—Griseofulvin (Systemic), 889

*Fulvicin U/F*—Griseofulvin (Systemic), 889

*Fumasorb*—Ferrous Fumarate—*See* Iron Supplements (Systemic), 986

*Fumerin*—Ferrous Fumarate—*See* Iron Supplements (Systemic), 986

*Fungizone*—Amphotericin B (Topical), 214

*Fungizone Intravenous*—Amphotericin B (Systemic), 213

*Furadantin*—Nitrofurantoin (Systemic), 1227

*Furalan*—Nitrofurantoin (Systemic), 1227

*Furamide*—Diloxanide (Systemic), 718

*Furatoin*—Nitrofurantoin (Systemic), 1227

Furazolidone (Oral), 863

Furosemide—*See* Diuretics, Loop (Systemic), 738, MC-10

*Furoside*—Furosemide—*See* Diuretics, Loop (Systemic), 738

*Furoxone*—Furazolidone (Oral), 863

*Furoxone Liquid*—Furazolidone (Oral), 863

Fusidic Acid (Systemic), 1749

Fusidic Acid (Topical), 1749

*Fynex*—Diphenhydramine—*See* Antihistamines (Systemic), 304

# G

Gabapentin (Systemic), 1749, MC-10

Gadodiamide (Diagnostic)—*See* MRI Contrast Agents (Diagnostic), 1158

Gadopentetate (Diagnostic)—*See* MRI Contrast Agents (Diagnostic), 1158

Gadoteridol (Diagnostic)—*See* MRI Contrast Agents (Diagnostic), 1158

Gallium Citrate Ga 67—*See* Radiopharmaceuticals (Diagnostic), 1439

Gallium Nitrate (Systemic), 867

*Gamimune N*—Immune Globulin Intravenous (Human) (Systemic), 954

Gamma benzene hexachloride—*See* Lindane (Topical), 1042

*Gammagard*—Immune Globulin Intravenous (Human) (Systemic), 954

*Gammar–IV*—Immune Globulin Intravenous (Human) (Systemic), 954

*Gamulin Rh*—RH$_0$(D) Immune Globulin (Systemic), 1456

Ganciclovir (Systemic), 868

*Ganite*—Gallium Nitrate (Systemic), 867

*Gantanol*—Sulfamethoxazole—*See* Sulfonamides (Systemic), 1542

*Gantrisin*—Sulfisoxazole—*See* Sulfonamides (Ophthalmic), 1540; Sulfonamides (Systemic), 1542

*Garamycin*—Gentamicin—*See* Aminoglycosides (Systemic), 201; Gentamicin (Ophthalmic), 872; Gentamicin (Topical), 874

*Garamycin Otic Solution*—Gentamicin (Otic), 873

*Gas-is-gon*—Alumina, Magnesium Trisilicate, and Sodium Bicarbonate—*See* Antacids (Oral), 253

*Gas Relief*—Simethicone (Oral), 1494

*Gastrocrom*—Cromolyn (Oral), 658, MC-6

*Gastrolyte*—Oral Rehydration Salts—*See* Carbohydrates and Electrolytes (Systemic), 484

*Gastrosed*—Hyoscyamine—*See* Anticholinergics/Antispasmodics (Systemic), 258

*Gastrozepin*—Pirenzepine—*See* Anticholinergics/Antispasmodics (Systemic), 258

*Gas-X*—Simethicone (Oral), 1494

*Gaviscon*—Alumina and Magnesium Carbonate—*See* Antacids (Oral), 253; Alumina and Magnesium Trisilicate—*See* Antacids (Oral), 253; Aluminum Hydroxide—*See* Antacids (Oral), 253

*Gaviscon-2*—Alumina and Magnesium Trisilicate—*See* Antacids (Oral), 253

*Gaviscon Extra Strength Relief Formula*—Alumina and Magnesium Carbonate—*See* Antacids (Oral), 253

*GBH*—Lindane (Topical), 1042

G-CSF—Filgrastim—*See* Colony Stimulating Factors (Systemic), 600

*2/G-DM Cough*—Dextromethorphan and Guaifenesin—*See* Cough/Cold Combinations (Systemic), 637

*Gee-Gee*—Guaifenesin (Systemic), 892

*Gelamal*—Alumina and Magnesia—*See* Antacids (Oral), 253

*Gelpirin*—Acetaminophen, Aspirin, and Caffeine, Buffered—*See* Acetaminophen and Salicylates (Systemic), 164

*Gelusil*—Alumina and Magnesia—*See* Antacids (Oral), 253; Alumina, Magnesia, and Simethicone—*See* Antacids (Oral), 253

*Gelusil Extra Strength*—Alumina and Magnesia—*See* Antacids (Oral), 253

Gemfibrozil (Systemic), 870, MC-10

*Gemnisyn*—Acetaminophen and Aspirin—*See* Acetaminophen and Salicylates (Systemic), 164

*Gemonil*—Metharbital—*See* Barbiturates (Systemic), 370

*Genabid*—Papaverine (Systemic), 1289

*Genac*—Triprolidine and Pseudoephedrine—*See* Antihistamines and Decongestants (Systemic), 311

*Genagesic*—Propoxyphene and Acetaminophen—*See* Narcotic Analgesics and Acetaminophen (Systemic), 1181

*Genahist*—Diphenhydramine—*See* Antihistamines (Systemic), 304

*Gen-Allerate*—Chlorpheniramine—*See* Antihistamines (Systemic), 304

*Genamin*—Chlorpheniramine and Phenylpropanolamine—*See* Antihistamines and Decongestants (Systemic), 311

*Genapap Children's Elixir*—Acetaminophen (Systemic), 161

*Genapap Children's Tablets*—Acetaminophen (Systemic), 161

*Genapap Extra Strength Caplets*—Acetaminophen (Systemic), 161

*Genapap Extra Strength Tablets*—Acetaminophen (Systemic), 161

*Genapap, Infants'*—Acetaminophen (Systemic), 161

*Genapap Regular Strength Tablets*—Acetaminophen (Systemic), 161

*Genapax*—Gentian Violet (Vaginal), 877

*Genaphed*—Pseudoephedrine (Systemic), 1412

*Genaspore Cream*—Tolnaftate (Topical), 1617

*Genatap*—Brompheniramine and Phenylpropanolamine—*See* Antihistamines and Decongestants (Systemic), 311

*Genaton*—Alumina and Magnesium Trisilicate—*See* Antacids (Oral), 253

*Genatuss*—Guaifenesin (Systemic), 892

*Genatuss DM*—Dextromethorphan and Guaifenesin—*See* Cough/Cold Combinations (Systemic), 637

*Gencalc*—Calcium Carbonate—*See* Calcium Supplements (Systemic), 472

*Gen-Cefazolin*—Cefazolin—*See* Cephalosporins (Systemic), 498

*GenCept 0.5/35*—Norethindrone and Ethinyl Estradiol—*See* Estrogens and Progestins (Oral Contraceptives) (Systemic), 804

*GenCept 1/35*—Norethindrone and Ethinyl Estradiol—*See* Estrogens and Progestins (Oral Contraceptives) (Systemic), 804

*GenCept 10/11*—Norethindrone and Ethinyl Estradiol—*See* Estrogens and Progestins (Oral Contraceptives) (Systemic), 804

*Gencold*—Chlorpheniramine and Phenylpropanolamine—*See* Antihistamines and Decongestants (Systemic), 311

*Gendecon*—Chlorpheniramine, Phenylephrine, and Acetaminophen—*See* Antihistamines, Decongestants, and Analgesics (Systemic), 316

*Gen-D-phen*—Diphenhydramine—*See* Antihistamines (Systemic), 304

*Genebs Extra Strength Caplets*—Acetaminophen (Systemic), 161

*Genebs Regular Strength Tablets*—Acetaminophen (Systemic), 161

*Genebs X-Tra*—Acetaminophen (Systemic), 161

*Generlac*—Lactulose—*See* Laxatives (Oral), 1017

*Genex*—Phenylpropanolamine and Acetaminophen—*See* Decongestants and Analgesics (Systemic), 691

*Gen-Glybe*—Glyburide—*See* Antidiabetics, Oral (Systemic), 283

*Genite*—Doxylamine, Pseudoephedrine, Dextromethorphan, and Acetaminophen—*See* Cough/Cold Combinations (Systemic), 637

*Gen-K*—Potassium Chloride—*See* Potassium Supplements (Systemic), 1373

*Genoptic Liquifilm*—Gentamicin (Ophthalmic), 872

*Genoptic S.O.P.*—Gentamicin (Ophthalmic), 872

*Genora 0.5/35*—Norethindrone and Ethinyl Estradiol—*See* Estrogens and Progestins (Oral Contraceptives) (Systemic), 804, MC-17

*Genora 1/35*—Norethindrone and Ethinyl Estradiol—*See* Estrogens and Progestins (Oral Contraceptives) (Systemic), 804, MC-17

*Genora 1/50*—Norethindrone and Mestranol—*See* Estrogens and Progestins (Oral Contraceptives) (Systemic), 804, MC-17

*Genpril*—Ibuprofen—*See* Nonsteroidal Anti-inflammatory Drugs (Systemic), 1229

*Genpril Caplets*—Ibuprofen—*See* Nonsteroidal Anti-inflammatory Drugs (Systemic), 1229

*Gen-Salbutamol*—Albuterol—*See* Bronchodilators, Adrenergic (Inhalation), 430

*Gentacidin*—Gentamicin (Ophthalmic), 872

*Gentafair*—Gentamicin (Ophthalmic), 872

*Gentak*—Gentamicin (Ophthalmic), 872

*Gentamar*—Gentamicin (Topical), 874

Gentamicin—*See* Aminoglycosides (Systemic), 201

Gentamicin (Ophthalmic), 872

Gentamicin (Otic), 873

Gentamicin (Topical), 874

Gentamycin—Gentamicin—*See* Aminoglycosides (Systemic), 201; Gentamicin (Ophthalmic), 872

Gentian Violet (Topical), 875

Gentian Violet (Vaginal), 877

*Gen-Timolol*—Timolol—*See* Beta-adrenergic Blocking Agents (Ophthalmic), 402

*Gentlax S*—Senna and Docusate—*See* Laxatives (Oral), 1017

*Gentle Nature*—Sennosides—*See* Laxatives (Oral), 1017

*Gentrasul*—Gentamicin (Ophthalmic), 872

*Gen-Triazolam*—Triazolam—*See* Benzodiazepines (Systemic), 389

*Gen-XENE*—Clorazepate—*See* Benzodiazepines (Systemic), 389

*Geocillin*—Carbenicillin—*See* Penicillins (Systemic), 1299, MC-4

*Geopen*—Carbenicillin—*See* Penicillins (Systemic), 1299

*Geopen Oral*—Carbenicillin—*See* Penicillins (Systemic), 1299

*Gerber Baby Formula*—Infant Formulas, Milk-based—*See* Infant Formulas (Systemic), 958

*Gerber Soy Formula*—Infant Formulas, Soy-based—*See* Infant Formulas (Systemic), 958

*Geridium*—Phenazopyridine (Systemic), 1327

*Gerimal*—Ergoloid Mesylates (Systemic), 775

*Gesterol 50*—Progesterone—*See* Progestins (Systemic), 1402

*GG-CEN*—Guaifenesin (Systemic), 892

GH—Somatrem—*See* Growth Hormone (Systemic), 891; Somatropin—*See* Growth Hormone (Systemic), 891

*Glaucon*—Epinephrine (Ophthalmic), 771

Glibenclamide—Glyburide—*See* Antidiabetics, Oral (Systemic), 283

Glipizide—*See* Antidiabetics, Oral (Systemic), 283, 1749, MC-10

*Glo-Sel*—Selenium Sulfide (Topical), 1487

Glucagon (Systemic), 878

*Glucagon Emergency Kit*—Glucagon (Systemic), 878

*Glucerna*—Enteral Nutrition Formula, Disease-specific—*See* Enteral Nutrition Formulas (Systemic), 769

*Glucophage*—Metformin (Systemic), 1751

*Glucose & Ketone Urine Test*—Urine Glucose and Ketone (Combined) Test—*See* Urine Glucose and Ketone Test Kits for Home Use, 1644

Glucose Oxidase Urine Glucose Test—*See* Urine Glucose and Ketone Test Kits for Home Use, 1644

*Glucotrol*—Glipizide—*See* Antidiabetics, Oral (Systemic), 283, 1749, MC-10

*Glucotrol XL*—Glipizide (Systemic), MC-10

Glutethimide (Systemic), 881

*Glyate*—Guaifenesin (Systemic), 892

Glyburide—*See* Antidiabetics, Oral (Systemic), 283, MC-11

*Glycate*—Calcium Carbonate—*See* Antacids (Oral), 253

Glycerin—*See* Laxatives (Rectal), 1023

Glycerin (Systemic), 882

Glyceryl guaiacolate—*See* Guaifenesin (Systemic), 892

*Glyceryl-T*—Theophylline and Guaifenesin (Systemic), 1586

Glyceryl trinitrate—Nitroglycerin—*See* Nitrates—Lingual Aerosol (Systemic), 1216; Nitrates—Oral (Systemic), 1218; Nitrates—Sublingual, Chewable, or Buccal (Systemic), 1221; Nitrates—Topical (Systemic), 1224

*Glycofed*—Pseudoephedrine and Guaifenesin—*See* Cough/Cold Combinations (Systemic), 637

Glycopyrrolate—*See* Anticholinergics/Antispasmodics (Systemic), 258

Glycopyrronium bromide—Glycopyrrolate—*See* Anticholinergics/Antispasmodics (Systemic), 258

*Gly-Cort*—Hydrocortisone—*See* Corticosteroids—Low Potency (Topical), 624

*Glycotuss*—Guaifenesin (Systemic), 892

*Glycotuss-dM*—Dextromethorphan and Guaifenesin—*See* Cough/Cold Combinations (Systemic), 637

*Glydeine Cough*—Codeine and Guaifenesin—*See* Cough/Cold Combinations (Systemic), 637

*Glynase PresTab*—Glyburide—*See* Antidiabetics, Oral (Systemic), 283

*Glyrol*—Glycerin (Systemic), 882

*Glysennid*—Sennosides—*See* Laxatives (Oral), 1017

*Glytuss*—Guaifenesin (Systemic), 892

GM-CSF—Sargramostim—*See* Colony Stimulating Factors (Systemic), 600

*G-Mycin*—Gentamicin—*See* Aminoglycosides (Systemic), 201

*G-Myticin*—Gentamicin (Topical), 874

GnRH—*See* Gonadorelin (Systemic), 887

*Gold Circle Coin*—Latex Condoms—*See* Condoms, 602

Gold Compounds (Systemic), 884

Gold Sodium Thiomalate—*See* Gold Compounds (Systemic), 884

*GoLYTELY*—Polyethylene Glycol and Electrolytes (Local), 1369

Gonadorelin (Systemic), 887, 1749

Gonadotropin-releasing hormone—*See* Gonadorelin (Systemic), 887

*Gonak*—Hydroxypropyl Methylcellulose (Ophthalmic), 941

*Goniosol*—Hydroxypropyl Methylcellulose (Ophthalmic), 941

*Goody's Extra Strength Tablets*—Acetaminophen, Aspirin, and Caffeine—*See* Acetaminophen and Salicylates (Systemic), 164

*Goody's Headache Powders*—Acetaminophen, Aspirin, and Caffeine—*See* Acetaminophen and Salicylates (Systemic), 164

*Gordochom Solution*—Undecylenic Acid, Compound (Topical), 1639

*Gordofilm*—Salicylic Acid (Topical), 1478

Goserelin (Systemic), 888, 1749

*Gotamine*—Ergotamine and Caffeine—*See* Headache Medicines, Ergot Derivative–containing (Systemic), 914

*GP-500*—Pseudoephedrine and Guaifenesin—*See* Cough/Cold Combinations (Systemic), 637

*Gramcal*—Calcium Lactate-Gluconate and Calcium Carbonate—*See* Calcium Supplements (Systemic), 472

Granisetron (Systemic), 1749

Granulocyte colony stimulating factor—Filgrastim—*See* Colony Stimulating Factors (Systemic), 600

Granulocyte-macrophage colony stimulating factor—Sargramostim—*See* Colony Stimulating Factors (Systemic), 600

*Gravergol*—Ergotamine, Caffeine, and Dimenhydrinate—*See* Headache Medicines, Ergot Derivative–containing (Systemic), 914

*Gravol*—Dimenhydrinate—*See* Antihistamines (Systemic), 304

*Gravol L/A*—Dimenhydrinate—*See* Antihistamines (Systemic), 304

*Great Shake*—Enteral Nutrition Formula, Milk-based—*See* Enteral Nutrition Formulas (Systemic), 769

*Grifulvin V*—Griseofulvin (Systemic), 889, MC-11

*Grisactin*—Griseofulvin (Systemic), 889

*Grisactin Ultra*—Griseofulvin (Systemic), 889

Griseofulvin (Systemic), 889, MC-11

*Grisovin-FP*—Griseofulvin (Systemic), 889

*Gris-PEG*—Griseofulvin (Systemic), 889

Growth Hormone (Systemic), 891

*Guaifed*—Pseudoephedrine and Guaifenesin—*See* Cough/Cold Combinations (Systemic), 637

*Guaifed-PD*—Pseudoephedrine and Guaifenesin—*See* Cough/Cold Combinations (Systemic), 637

Guaifenesin (Systemic), 892, 1749

*GuaiMAX-D*—Pseudoephedrine and Guaifenesin—*See* Cough/Cold Combinations (Systemic), 637, 1753

*Guaipax*—Phenylpropanolamine and Guaifenesin—*See* Cough/Cold Combinations (Systemic), 637

*Guaiphed*—Theophylline, Ephedrine, Guaifenesin, and Phenobarbital (Systemic), 1577

*Guaitab*—Pseudoephedrine and Guaifenesin—*See* Cough/Cold Combinations (Systemic), 637

Guanabenz (Systemic), 894, MC-11

Guanadrel (Systemic), 896

Guanethidine (Systemic), 898

Guanethidine and Hydrochlorothiazide (Systemic), 900

Guanfacine (Systemic), 903, MC-11

*GuiaCough CF*—Phenylpropanolamine, Dextromethorphan, and Guaifenesin—*See* Cough/Cold Combinations (Systemic), 637

*GuiaCough PE*—Pseudoephedrine and Guaifenesin—*See* Cough/Cold Combinations (Systemic), 637

*Guiamid D.M. Liquid*—Dextromethorphan and Guaifenesin—*See* Cough/Cold Combinations (Systemic), 637

*Guiatuss*—Guaifenesin (Systemic), 892

*Guiatuss A.C.*—Codeine and Guaifenesin—*See* Cough/Cold Combinations (Systemic), 637

*Guiatuss CF*—Phenylpropanolamine, Dextromethorphan, and Guaifenesin—*See* Cough/Cold Combinations (Systemic), 637

*Guiatuss DAC*—Pseudoephedrine, Codeine, and Guaifenesin—*See* Cough/Cold Combinations (Systemic), 637

*Guiatuss-DM*—Dextromethorphan and Guaifenesin—*See* Cough/Cold Combinations (Systemic), 637

*Guiatussin with Codeine Liquid*—Codeine and Guaifenesin—*See* Cough/Cold Combinations (Systemic), 637

*Guiatussin DAC*—Pseudoephedrine, Codeine, and Guaifenesin—*See* Cough/Cold Combinations (Systemic), 637

*Guiatussin w/Dextromethorphan*—Dextromethorphan and Guaifenesin—*See* Cough/Cold Combinations (Systemic), 637

*Guiatuss PE*—Pseudoephedrine and Guaifenesin—*See* Cough/Cold Combinations (Systemic), 637

*G-well*—Lindane (Topical), 1042

*Gynecort*—Hydrocortisone Acetate—*See* Corticosteroids—Low Potency (Topical), 624

*Gynecort 10*—Hydrocortisone Acetate—*See* Corticosteroids—Low Potency (Topical), 624, 1750

*Gyne-Lotrimin*—Clotrimazole—*See* Antifungals, Azole (Vaginal), 296

*Gynergen*—Ergotamine—*See* Headache Medicines, Ergot Derivative–containing (Systemic), 914

*Gyne-T*—Copper-T 200 IUD—*See* Copper Intrauterine Devices (IUDs), 605

*Gyne-T 380 Slimline*—Copper-T 380S IUD—*See* Copper Intrauterine Devices (IUDs), 605

*Gynogen L.A. 20*—Estradiol—*See* Estrogens (Systemic), 795

*Gynogen L.A. 40*—Estradiol—*See* Estrogens (Systemic), 795

*Gynol II Extra Strength Contraceptive Jelly*—Nonoxynol 9—*See* Spermicides (Vaginal), 1512

*Gynol II Original Formula Contraceptive Jelly*—Nonoxynol 9—*See* Spermicides (Vaginal), 1512

*Gyno-Trosyd*—Tioconazole—*See* Antifungals, Azole (Vaginal), 296

# H

*Habitrol*—Nicotine (Systemic), 1212

Haemophilus b Conjugate Vaccine (HbOC—Diphtheria $CRM_{197}$ Protein Conjugate)—*See* Haemophilus b Conjugate Vaccine (Systemic), 905

Haemophilus b Conjugate Vaccine (PRP-D—Diphtheria Toxoid Conjugate)—*See* Haemophilus b Conjugate Vaccine (Systemic), 905

*Hexadrol*—Dexamethasone—*See* Corticosteroids/Corticotropin—Glucocorticoid Effects (Systemic), 630

*Hexadrol Phosphate*—Dexamethasone—*See* Corticosteroids/Corticotropin—Glucocorticoid Effects (Systemic), 630

*Hexalen*—Altretamine (Systemic), 192

*Hexalol*—Atropine, Hyoscyamine, Methenamine, Methylene Blue, Phenyl Salicylate, and Benzoic Acid (Systemic), 357

Hexamethylmelamine—*See* Altretamine (Systemic), 192

*Hexastat*—Altretamine (Systemic), 192

*Hexit*—Lindane (Topical), 1042

Hib CPS—*See* Haemophilus b Polysaccharide Vaccine (Systemic), 907

Hib polysaccharide vaccine—*See* Haemophilus b Polysaccharide Vaccine (Systemic), 907

*Hibtiter*—Haemophilus b Conjugate Vaccine (HbOC—Diphtheria CRM$_{197}$ Protein Conjugate)—*See* Haemophilus b Conjugate Vaccine (Systemic), 905

*Hi-Cor 1.0*—Hydrocortisone—*See* Corticosteroids—Low Potency (Topical), 624

*Hi-Cor 2.5*—Hydrocortisone—*See* Corticosteroids—Low Potency (Topical), 624

*Hiprex*—Methenamine (Systemic), 1100

*Hip-Rex*—Methenamine (Systemic), 1100

*Hismanal*—Astemizole—*See* Antihistamines (Systemic), 304, MC-2

*Histafed C*—Triprolidine, Pseudoephedrine, and Codeine—*See* Cough/Cold Combinations (Systemic), 637

*Histagesic Modified*—Chlorpheniramine, Phenylephrine, and Acetaminophen—*See* Antihistamines, Decongestants, and Analgesics (Systemic), 316

*Histaject Modified*—Brompheniramine—*See* Antihistamines (Systemic), 304

*Histalet*—Chlorpheniramine and Pseudoephedrine—*See* Antihistamines and Decongestants (Systemic), 311

*Histalet Forte*—Chlorpheniramine, Pyrilamine, Phenylephrine, and Phenylpropanolamine—*See* Antihistamines and Decongestants (Systemic), 311

*Histalet X*—Pseudoephedrine and Guaifenesin—*See* Cough/Cold Combinations (Systemic), 637

*Histamic*—Chlorpheniramine, Phenyltoloxamine, Phenylephrine, and Phenylpropanolamine—*See* Antihistamines and Decongestants (Systemic), 311

Histamine (Diagnostic), 924

Histamine H$_2$-receptor Antagonists (Systemic), 925

*Histantil*—Promethazine—*See* Antihistamines, Phenothiazine-derivative (Systemic), 325

*Histatab Plus*—Chlorpheniramine and Phenylephrine—*See* Antihistamines and Decongestants (Systemic), 311

*Histatan*—Chlorpheniramine, Pyrilamine, and Phenylephrine—*See* Antihistamines and Decongestants (Systemic), 311

*Histatuss Pediatric*—Chlorpheniramine, Ephedrine, Phenylephrine, and Carbetapentane—*See* Cough/Cold Combinations (Systemic), 637

*Hista-Vadrin*—Chlorpheniramine, Phenylephrine, and Phenylpropanolamine—*See* Antihistamines and Decongestants (Systemic), 311

*Histerone-50*—Testosterone—*See* Androgens (Systemic), 221

*Histerone-100*—Testosterone—*See* Androgens (Systemic), 221

*Histine DM*—Brompheniramine, Phenylpropanolamine, and Dextromethorphan—*See* Cough/Cold Combinations (Systemic), 637

*Histor-D*—Chlorpheniramine and Phenylephrine—*See* Antihistamines and Decongestants (Systemic), 311

*Histor-D Timecelles*—Chlorpheniramine, Phenylephrine, and Methscopolamine—*See* Antihistamines, Decongestants, and Anticholinergics (Systemic), 322

*Histosal*—Pyrilamine, Phenylpropanolamine, Acetaminophen, and Caffeine—*See* Antihistamines, Decongestants, and Analgesics (Systemic), 316

Histrelin (Systemic), 1749

*Histussin HC*—Chlorpheniramine, Phenylephrine, and Hydrocodone—*See* Cough/Cold Combinations (Systemic), 637

*HIVID*—Zalcitabine (Systemic), 1687

HMG—*See* Menotropins (Systemic), 1087

HMG-CoA Reductase Inhibitors (Systemic), 929

*HMS Liquifilm*—Medrysone—*See* Corticosteroids (Ophthalmic), 620

*Hold*—Dextromethorphan (Systemic), 701

*Homapin*—Homatropine—*See* Anticholinergics/Antispasmodics (Systemic), 258

Homatropine—*See* Anticholinergics/Antispasmodics (Systemic), 258; Atropine/Homatropine/Scopolamine (Ophthalmic), 354

*Honvol*—Diethylstilbestrol—*See* Estrogens (Systemic), 795

*8-Hour Bayer Timed-Release*—Aspirin—*See* Salicylates (Systemic), 1473

*12-Hour Cold*—Chlorpheniramine and Phenylpropanolamine—*See* Antihistamines and Decongestants (Systemic), 311

*H$_2$Oxyl 2.5 Gel*—Benzoyl Peroxide (Topical), 397

*H$_2$Oxyl 5 Gel*—Benzoyl Peroxide (Topical), 397

*H$_2$Oxyl 10 Gel*—Benzoyl Peroxide (Topical), 397

*H$_2$Oxyl 20 Gel*—Benzoyl Peroxide (Topical), 397

*H.P. Acthar Gel*—Corticotropin—*See* Corticosteroids/Corticotropin—Glucocorticoid Effects (Systemic), 630

HRIG—*See* Rabies Immune Globulin (Systemic), 1433

Human chorionic gonadotropin—*See* Chorionic Gonadotropin (Systemic), 540

Human erythropoietin, recombinant—*See* Epoetin (Systemic), 773

Human growth hormone (hGH)—Somatrem—*See* Growth Hormone (Systemic), 891; Somatropin—*See* Growth Hormone (Systemic), 891

Human menopausal gonadotropins—*See* Menotropins (Systemic), 1087

*Humate-P*—Antihemophilic Factor (Systemic), 302

*Humatrope*—Somatropin—*See* Growth Hormone (Systemic), 891

*Humibid DM*—Dextromethorphan and Guaifenesin—*See* Cough/Cold Combinations (Systemic), 637

*Humibid DM Sprinkle*—Dextromethorphan and Guaifenesin—*See* Cough/Cold Combinations (Systemic), 637

*Humibid L.A.*—Guaifenesin (Systemic), 892

*Humibid Sprinkle*—Guaifenesin (Systemic), 892

*Humorsol*—Demecarium—*See* Antiglaucoma Agents, Cholinergic, Long-acting (Ophthalmic), 299

*Humulin 10/90*—Insulin, Isophane, Human, and Insulin Human—*See* Insulin (Systemic), 961

*Humulin 20/80*—Insulin, Isophane, Human, and Insulin Human—*See* Insulin (Systemic), 961

*Humulin 30/70*—Insulin, Isophane, Human, and Insulin Human—*See* Insulin (Systemic), 961

*Humulin 40/60*—Insulin, Isophane, Human, and Insulin Human—*See* Insulin (Systemic), 961

*Humulin 50/50*—Insulin, Isophane, Human, and Insulin Human—*See* Insulin (Systemic), 961

*Humulin 70/30*—Insulin, Isophane, Human, and Insulin Human—*See* Insulin (Systemic), 961

*Humulin-L*—Insulin Zinc, Human—*See* Insulin (Systemic), 961

*Humulin L*—Insulin Zinc, Human—*See* Insulin (Systemic), 961

*Humulin-N*—Insulin, Isophane, Human—*See* Insulin (Systemic), 961

*Humulin N*—Insulin, Isophane, Human—*See* Insulin (Systemic), 961

*Humulin-R*—Insulin Human—*See* Insulin (Systemic), 961

*Humulin R*—Insulin Human—*See* Insulin (Systemic), 961

*Humulin-U*—Insulin Zinc, Extended, Human—*See* Insulin (Systemic), 961

*Humulin U Ultralente*—Insulin, Zinc, Extended, Human—*See* Insulin (Systemic), 961

*Hurricaine*—Benzocaine—*See* Anesthetics (Dental), 229

*HY-5*—Hydrocodone and Acetaminophen—*See* Narcotic Analgesics and Acetaminophen (Systemic), 1181

*Hyate:C*—Antihemophilic Factor (Systemic), 302

*Hybolin Decanoate*—Nandrolone—*See* Anabolic Steroids (Systemic), 218

*Hybolin-Improved*—Nandrolone—*See* Anabolic Steroids (Systemic), 218

*Hycodan*—Hydrocodone—*See* Narcotic Analgesics—For Pain Relief (Systemic), 1176; Hydrocodone and Homatropine—*See* Cough/Cold Combinations (Systemic), 637

*Hycomed*—Hydrocodone and Acetaminophen—*See* Narcotic Analgesics and Acetaminophen (Systemic), 1181

*Hycomine*—Phenylpropanolamine and Hydrocodone—*See* Cough/Cold Combinations (Systemic), 637; Pyrilamine, Phenylephrine, Hydrocodone, and Ammonium Chloride—*See* Cough/Cold Combinations (Systemic), 637

*Hycomine Compound*—Chlorpheniramine, Phenylephrine, Hydrocodone, Acetaminophen, and Caffeine—*See* Cough/Cold Combinations (Systemic), 637

*Hycomine Pediatric*—Phenylpropanolamine and Hydrocodone—*See* Cough/Cold Combinations (Systemic), 637

*Hycomine-S Pediatric*—Pyrilamine, Phenylephrine, Hydrocodone, and Ammonium Chloride—*See* Cough/Cold Combinations (Systemic), 637

*Hycopap*—Hydrocodone and Acetaminophen—*See* Narcotic Analgesics and Acetaminophen (Systemic), 1181

*Hyco-Pap*—Hydrocodone and Acetaminophen—*See* Narcotic Analgesics and Acetaminophen (Systemic), 1181

*Hycotuss Expectorant*—Hydrocodone and Guaifenesin—*See* Cough/Cold Combinations (Systemic), 637

*Hydeltrasol*—Prednisolone—*See* Corticosteroids/Corticotropin—Glucocorticoid Effects (Systemic), 630

*Hydeltra T.B.A.*—Prednisolone—*See* Corticosteroids/Corticotropin—Glucocorticoid Effects (Systemic), 630

*Hydergine*—Ergoloid Mesylates (Systemic), 775, MC-9

*Hydergine LC*—Ergoloid Mesylates (Systemic), 775, MC-9

*Hyderm*—Hydrocortisone Acetate—*See* Corticosteroids—Low Potency (Topical), 624

Hydralazine (Systemic), 931, MC-11

Hydralazine and Hydrochlorothiazide (Systemic), 933, MC-11

*Hydramine*—Diphenhydramine—*See* Antihistamines (Systemic), 304

*Hydramine Cough*—Diphenhydramine—*See* Antihistamines (Systemic), 304

*Hydramyn*—Diphenhydramine—*See* Antihistamines (Systemic), 304

*Hydrate*—Dimenhydrinate—*See* Antihistamines (Systemic), 304

*Hydra-zide*—Hydralazine and Hydrochlorothiazide (Systemic), 933

*Hydrea*—Hydroxyurea (Systemic), 943

*Hydrex*—Benzthiazide—*See* Diuretics, Thiazide (Systemic), 749

*Hydril*—Diphenhydramine—*See* Antihistamines (Systemic), 304

*Hydrisalic*—Salicylic Acid (Topical), 1478

*Hydrobexan*—Hydroxocobalamin—*See* Vitamin $B_{12}$ (Systemic), 1667

*Hydrocet*—Hydrocodone and Acetaminophen—*See* Narcotic Analgesics and Acetaminophen (Systemic), 1181

*Hydro-chlor*—Hydrochlorothiazide—*See* Diuretics, Thiazide (Systemic), 749

Hydrochlorothiazide—*See* Diuretics, Thiazide (Systemic), 749, MC-11

*Hydrocil Instant*—Psyllium Hydrophilic Mucilloid—*See* Laxatives (Oral), 1017

*Hydro-Cobex*—Hydroxocobalamin—*See* Vitamin $B_{12}$ (Systemic), 1667

Hydrocodone—*See* Narcotic Analgesics—For Pain Relief (Systemic), 1176

Hydrocodone and Acetaminophen—*See* Narcotic Analgesics and Acetaminophen (Systemic), 1181, MC-11

Hydrocodone with APAP—Hydrocodone and Acetaminophen—*See* Narcotic Analgesics and Acetaminophen (Systemic), 1181

Hydrocodone and Aspirin—*See* Narcotic Analgesics and Aspirin (Systemic), 1185

Hydrocodone, Aspirin, and Caffeine—*See* Narcotic Analgesics and Aspirin (Systemic), 1185

Hydrocodone and Guaifenesin—*See* Cough/Cold Combinations (Systemic), 637

Hydrocodone and Homatropine—*See* Cough/Cold Combinations (Systemic), 637

Hydrocodone and Potassium Guaiacolsulfonate—*See* Cough/Cold Combinations (Systemic), 637

Hydrocortisone—*See* Corticosteroids (Dental), 610; Corticosteroids (Ophthalmic), 620; Corticosteroids (Otic), 622; Corticosteroids/Corticotropin—Glucocorticoid Effects (Systemic), 630, MC-11; Corticosteroids—Low Potency (Topical), 624, 1750

Hydrocortisone (Rectal), 936

Hydrocortisone Acetate—*See* Corticosteroids—Low Potency (Topical), 624, 1750

Hydrocortisone and Acetic Acid—*See* Corticosteroids and Acetic Acid (Otic), 629

Hydrocortisone Butyrate—*See* Corticosteroids—Medium to Very High Potency (Topical), 626

Hydrocortisone and Urea (Topical), 1750

Hydrocortisone Valerate—*See* Corticosteroids—Medium to Very High Potency (Topical), 626

*Hydrocortone*—Hydrocortisone—*See* Corticosteroids/Corticotropin—Glucocorticoid Effects (Systemic), 630

*Hydrocortone Acetate*—Hydrocortisone—*See* Corticosteroids/Corticotropin—Glucocorticoid Effects (Systemic), 630

*Hydrocortone Phosphate*—Hydrocortisone—*See* Corticosteroids/Corticotropin—Glucocorticoid Effects (Systemic), 630

*Hydro-Crysti-12*—Hydroxocobalamin—*See* Vitamin $B_{12}$ (Systemic), 1667

*Hydro-D*—Hydrochlorothiazide—*See* Diuretics, Thiazide (Systemic), 749

*HydroDIURIL*—Hydrochlorothiazide—*See* Diuretics, Thiazide (Systemic), 749, MC-11

Hydroflumethiazide—*See* Diuretics, Thiazide (Systemic), 749

*Hydrogesic*—Hydrocodone and Acetaminophen—*See* Narcotic Analgesics and Acetaminophen (Systemic), 1181

*Hydromet*—Hydrocodone and Homatropine—*See* Cough/Cold Combinations (Systemic), 637

*Hydromine*—Phenylpropanolamine and Hydrocodone—*See* Cough/Cold Combinations (Systemic), 637

*Hydromine Pediatric*—Phenylpropanolamine and Hydrocodone—*See* Cough/Cold Combinations (Systemic), 637

Hydromorphone—*See* Narcotic Analgesics—For Pain Relief (Systemic), 1176, MC-11

Hydromorphone and Guaifenesin—*See* Cough/Cold Combinations (Systemic), 637

*Hydromox*—Quinethazone—*See* Diuretics, Thiazide (Systemic), 749

*Hydromycin*—Neomycin, Polymyxin B, and Hydrocortisone (Ophthalmic), 1203

*Hydropane*—Hydrocodone and Homatropine—*See* Cough/Cold Combinations (Systemic), 637

*Hydrophed*—Theophylline, Ephedrine, and Hydroxyzine (Systemic), 1580

*Hydrophen*—Phenylpropanolamine and Hydrocodone—*See* Cough/Cold Combinations (Systemic), 637

*Hydropine*—Reserpine and Hydroflumethiazide—*See* Rauwolfia Alkaloids and Thiazide Diuretics (Systemic), 1445

*Hydropine H.P.*—Reserpine and Hydroflumethiazide—*See* Rauwolfia Alkaloids and Thiazide Diuretics (Systemic), 1445

*Hydropres*—Reserpine and Hydrochlorothiazide—*See* Rauwolfia Alkaloids and Thiazide Diuretics (Systemic), 1445

*Hydrosine*—Reserpine and Hydrochlorothiazide—*See* Rauwolfia Alkaloids and Thiazide Diuretics (Systemic), 1445

*Hydrotensin*—Reserpine and Hydrochlorothiazide—*See* Rauwolfia Alkaloids and Thiazide Diuretics (Systemic), 1445

*Hydro-Tex*—Hydrocortisone—*See* Corticosteroids—Low Potency (Topical), 624

*Hydroxacen*—Hydroxyzine—*See* Antihistamines (Systemic), 304

Hydroxocobalamin—*See* Vitamin $B_{12}$ (Systemic), 1667

Hydroxychloroquine (Systemic), 937, MC-11

Hydroxyprogesterone—*See* Progestins (Systemic), 1402

Hydroxypropyl Cellulose (Ophthalmic), 940

Hydroxypropyl Methylcellulose (Ophthalmic), 941

Hydroxyurea (Systemic), 943

Hydroxyzine—*See* Antihistamines (Systemic), 304, MC-11, MC-12

*Hy/Gestrone*—Hydroxyprogesterone—*See* Progestins (Systemic), 1402

*Hygroton*—Chlorthalidone—*See* Diuretics, Thiazide (Systemic), 749, MC-5

*Hylorel*—Guanadrel (Systemic), 896

*Hylutin*—Hydroxyprogesterone—*See* Progestins (Systemic), 1402

Hyoscine—Scopolamine—*See* Atropine/Homatropine/Scopolamine (Ophthalmic), 354

Hyoscine hydrobromide—Scopolamine—*See* Anticholinergics/Antispasmodics (Systemic), 258

Hyoscine methobromide—Methscopolamine—*See* Anticholinergics/Antispasmodics (Systemic), 258

Hyoscyamine—*See* Anticholinergics/Antispasmodics (Systemic), 258

Hyoscyamine and Phenobarbital—*See* Belladonna Alkaloids and Barbiturates (Systemic), 382

*Hyosophen*—Atropine, Hyoscyamine, Scopolamine, and Phenobarbital—*See* Belladonna Alkaloids and Barbiturates (Systemic), 382

*Hyperab*—Rabies Immune Globulin (Systemic), 1433

*HY-PHEN*—Hydrocodone and Acetaminophen—*See* Narcotic Analgesics and Acetaminophen (Systemic), 1181

*HypRho-D Full Dose*—$RH_0(D)$ Immune Globulin (Systemic), 1456

*HypRho-D Mini-Dose*—$RH_0(D)$ Immune Globulin (Systemic), 1456

Hypromellose—*See* Hydroxypropyl Methylcellulose (Ophthalmic), 941

*Hyrexin-50*—Diphenhydramine—*See* Antihistamines (Systemic), 304

*Hytakerol*—Dihydrotachysterol—*See* Vitamin D and Related Compounds (Systemic), 1669

*Hytinic*—Iron-Polysaccharide—*See* Iron Supplements (Systemic), 986

*Hytone*—Hydrocortisone—*See* Corticosteroids—Low Potency (Topical), 624

*Hytrin*—Terazosin (Systemic), 1561, MC-22

*Hytuss*—Guaifenesin (Systemic), 892

*Hytuss-2X*—Guaifenesin (Systemic), 892

*Hyzine-50*—Hydroxyzine—*See* Antihistamines (Systemic), 304

# I

*Ibifon 600 Caplets*—Ibuprofen—*See* Nonsteroidal Anti-inflammatory Drugs (Systemic), 1229

*Ibren*—Ibuprofen—*See* Nonsteroidal Anti-inflammatory Drugs (Systemic), 1229

*Ibu*—Ibuprofen—*See* Nonsteroidal Anti-inflammatory Drugs (Systemic), 1229

*Ibu-200*—Ibuprofen—*See* Nonsteroidal Anti-inflammatory Drugs (Systemic), 1229

*Isuprel Glossets*—Isoproterenol—*See* Bronchodilators, Adrenergic (Oral/Injection), 436

*Isuprel Mistometer*—Isoproterenol—*See* Bronchodilators, Adrenergic (Inhalation), 430

Itraconazole—*See* Antifungals, Azole (Systemic), 292, MC-13

*I-Tropine*—Atropine—*See* Atropine/Homatropine/Scopolamine (Ophthalmic), 354

*Iveegam*—Immune Globulin Intravenous (Human) (Systemic), 954

IVIG—*See* Immune Globulin Intravenous (Human) (Systemic), 954

*I.V. Persantine*—Dipyridamole (Diagnostic), 731


# J

Japanese Encephalitis Virus Vaccine (Systemic), 1001

*Jectofer*—Iron Sorbitol—*See* Iron Supplements (Systemic), 986

*Jenamicin*—Gentamicin—*See* Aminoglycosides (Systemic), 201

*Jenest*—Norethindrone and Ethinyl Estradiol—*See* Estrogens and Progestins (Oral Contraceptives) (Systemic), 804

*Je-Vax*—Japanese Encephalitis Virus Vaccine (Systemic), 1001

*Jevity*—Enteral Nutrition Formula, Fiber-containing—*See* Enteral Nutrition Formulas (Systemic), 769

*Jopanonsyre*—Iopanoic Acid—*See* Cholecystographic Agents, Oral (Diagnostic), 536

*Jumex*—Selegiline (Systemic), 1485

*Jumexal*—Selegiline (Systemic), 1485

*Juprenil*—Selegiline (Systemic), 1485

*Just Tears*—Hydroxypropyl Methylcellulose (Ophthalmic), 941


# K

*K-10*—Potassium Chloride—*See* Potassium Supplements (Systemic), 1373

*K+ 10*—Potassium Chloride—*See* Potassium Supplements (Systemic), 1373

*Kabikinase*—Streptokinase—*See* Thrombolytic Agents (Systemic), 1604

*Kabolin*—Nandrolone—*See* Anabolic Steroids (Systemic), 218

*Kalcinate*—Calcium Gluconate—*See* Calcium Supplements (Systemic), 472

*Kalium Durules*—Potassium Chloride—*See* Potassium Supplements (Systemic), 1373

*Kamu Jay*—Ascorbic Acid (Vitamin C) (Systemic), 344

Kanamycin—*See* Aminoglycosides (Systemic), 201

Kanamycin (Oral), 1003

*Kantrex*—Kanamycin—*See* Aminoglycosides (Systemic), 201; Kanamycin (Oral), 1003

*Kaochlor-10*—Potassium Chloride—*See* Potassium Supplements (Systemic), 1373

*Kaochlor 10%*—Potassium Chloride—*See* Potassium Supplements (Systemic), 1373

*Kaochlor-20*—Potassium Chloride—*See* Potassium Supplements (Systemic), 1373

*Kaochlor-Eff*—Potassium Chloride, Potassium Bicarbonate, and Potassium Citrate—*See* Potassium Supplements (Systemic), 1373

*Kaochlor S-F 10%*—Potassium Chloride—*See* Potassium Supplements (Systemic), 1373

Kaolin and Pectin (Oral), 1004

Kaolin, Pectin, Belladonna Alkaloids, and Opium (Systemic), 1005

Kaolin, Pectin, and Paregoric (Systemic), 1008

*Kaon*—Potassium Gluconate—*See* Potassium Supplements (Systemic), 1373

*Kaon-Cl*—Potassium Chloride—*See* Potassium Supplements (Systemic), 1373

*Kaon-Cl-10*—Potassium Chloride—*See* Potassium Supplements (Systemic), 1373

*Kaon-Cl 20% Liquid*—Potassium Chloride—*See* Potassium Supplements (Systemic), 1373

*Kaopectate*—Attapulgite (Oral), 359

*Kaopectate Advanced Formula*—Attapulgite (Oral), 359

*Kaopectate II Caplets*—Loperamide (Oral), 1750

*Kaopectate Maximum Strength*—Attapulgite (Oral), 359

*Kao-Spen*—Kaolin and Pectin (Oral), 1004

*Kapectolin*—Kaolin and Pectin (Oral), 1004

*Kapectolin with Paregoric*—Kaolin, Pectin, and Paregoric (Systemic), 1008

*Kapectolin PG*—Kaolin, Pectin, Belladonna Alkaloids, and Opium (Systemic), 1005

*Karacil*—Psyllium Hydrophilic Mucilloid—*See* Laxatives (Oral), 1017

*Karidium*—Sodium Fluoride (Systemic), 1502

*Kasof*—Docusate—*See* Laxatives (Oral), 1017

*Kato*—Potassium Chloride—*See* Potassium Supplements (Systemic), 1373

*Kay Ciel*—Potassium Chloride—*See* Potassium Supplements (Systemic), 1373

*Kaylixir*—Potassium Gluconate—*See* Potassium Supplements (Systemic), 1373

*K+ Care*—Potassium Chloride—*See* Potassium Supplements (Systemic), 1373

*K+ Care ET*—Potassium Bicarbonate—*See* Potassium Supplements (Systemic), 1373

*KCL 5%*—Potassium Chloride—*See* Potassium Supplements (Systemic), 1373

*K-Dur*—Potassium Chloride—*See* Potassium Supplements (Systemic), 1373, MC-19

*Keep Alert*—Caffeine (Systemic), 463

*Keflex*—Cephalexin—*See* Cephalosporins (Systemic), 498, MC-4

*Keflin*—Cephalothin—*See* Cephalosporins (Systemic), 498

*Keftab*—Cephalexin—*See* Cephalosporins (Systemic), 498, MC-4

*Kefurox*—Cefuroxime—*See* Cephalosporins (Systemic), 498

*Kefzol*—Cefazolin—*See* Cephalosporins (Systemic), 498

*Kellogg's Castor Oil*—Castor Oil—*See* Laxatives (Oral), 1017

*Kemadrin*—Procyclidine—*See* Antidyskinetics (Systemic), 287

*Kenac*—Triamcinolone—*See* Corticosteroids—Medium to Very High Potency (Topical), 626

*Kenacort*—Triamcinolone—*See* Corticosteroids/Corticotropin—Glucocorticoid Effects (Systemic), 630

*Kenacort Diacetate*—Triamcinolone—*See* Corticosteroids/Corticotropin—Glucocorticoid Effects (Systemic), 630

*Kenaject-40*—Triamcinolone—*See* Corticosteroids/Corticotropin—Glucocorticoid Effects (Systemic), 630

*Kenalog*—Triamcinolone—*See* Corticosteroids—Medium to Very High Potency (Topical), 626

*Kenalog-10*—Triamcinolone—*See* Corticosteroids/Corticotropin—Glucocorticoid Effects (Systemic), 630

*Kenalog-40*—Triamcinolone—*See* Corticosteroids/Corticotropin—Glucocorticoid Effects (Systemic), 630

*Kenalog-H*—Triamcinolone—*See* Corticosteroids—Medium to Very High Potency (Topical), 626

*Kenalog in Orabase*—Triamcinolone—*See* Corticosteroids (Dental), 610

*Kenonel*—Triamcinolone—*See* Corticosteroids—Medium to Very High Potency (Topical), 626

*Keralyt*—Salicylic Acid (Topical), 1478

*Keratex Gel*—Salicylic Acid (Topical), 1478

*Kerlone*—Betaxolol—*See* Beta-adrenergic Blocking Agents (Systemic), 404, MC-3

*Kestrone-5*—Estrone—*See* Estrogens (Systemic), 795

*Ketalar*—Ketamine—*See* Anesthetics, General (Systemic), 243

Ketamine—*See* Anesthetics, General (Systemic), 243

Ketazolam—*See* Benzodiazepines (Systemic), 389

Ketoconazole—*See* Antifungals, Azole (Systemic), 292, MC-13

Ketoconazole (Topical), 1010

*Keto-diastix*—Urine Glucose and Ketone (Combined) Test—*See* Urine Glucose and Ketone Test Kits for Home Use, 1644

Ketoprofen—*See* Nonsteroidal Anti-inflammatory Drugs (Systemic), 1229

Ketorolac (Ophthalmic), 1012

Ketorolac (Systemic), 1013, MC-13

*KetoStix*—Nitroprusside Urine Ketone Test—*See* Urine Glucose and Ketone Test Kits for Home Use, 1644

Ketotifen (Systemic), 1750

*Key-Pred 25*—Prednisolone—*See* Corticosteroids/Corticotropin—Glucocorticoid Effects (Systemic), 630

*Key-Pred 50*—Prednisolone—*See* Corticosteroids/Corticotropin—Glucocorticoid Effects (Systemic), 630

*Key-Pred SP*—Prednisolone—*See* Corticosteroids/Corticotropin—Glucocorticoid Effects (Systemic), 630

*K-Flex*—Orphenadrine (Systemic), 1260

*K-G Elixir*—Potassium Gluconate—*See* Potassium Supplements (Systemic), 1373

KI—*See* Potassium Iodide (Systemic), 1371

*Kiddy Koff*—Phenylpropanolamine, Dextromethorphan, and Guaifenesin—*See* Cough/Cold Combinations (Systemic), 637

*K-Ide*—Potassium Bicarbonate—*See* Potassium Supplements (Systemic), 1373; Potassium Chloride—*See* Potassium Supplements (Systemic), 1373

*Kidrolase*—Asparaginase (Systemic), 347

*KIE*—Ephedrine and Potassium Iodide—*See* Cough/Cold Combinations (Systemic), 637

*Kildane*—Lindane (Topical), 1042

*Kimono*—Latex Condoms—*See* Condoms, 602

*Kimono Plus*—Latex Condoms and Nonoxynol 9—*See* Condoms, 602

*Kinesed*—Atropine, Hyoscyamine, Scopolamine, and Phenobarbital—*See* Belladonna Alkaloids and Barbiturates (Systemic), 382

*Klavikordal*—Nitroglycerin—*See* Nitrates—Oral (Systemic), 1218

*K-Lease*—Potassium Chloride—*See* Potassium Supplements (Systemic), 1373

*Klerist-D*—Chlorpheniramine and Pseudoephedrine—*See* Antihistamines and Decongestants (Systemic), 311

*K-Long*—Potassium Chloride—*See* Potassium Supplements (Systemic), 1373

*Klonopin*—Clonazepam—*See* Benzodiazepines (Systemic), 389

*K-Lor*—Potassium Chloride—*See* Potassium Supplements (Systemic), 1373

*Klor-Con 8*—Potassium Chloride—*See* Potassium Supplements (Systemic), 1373, MC-19

*Klor-Con 10*—Potassium Chloride—*See* Potassium Supplements (Systemic), 1373, MC-19

*Klor-Con/EF*—Potassium Bicarbonate—*See* Potassium Supplements (Systemic), 1373

*Klor-Con Powder*—Potassium Chloride—*See* Potassium Supplements (Systemic), 1373

*Klor-Con/25 Powder*—Potassium Chloride—*See* Potassium Supplements (Systemic), 1373

*Klorvess*—Potassium Bicarbonate and Potassium Chloride—*See* Potassium Supplements (Systemic), 1373

*Klorvess Effervescent Granules*—Potassium Bicarbonate and Potassium Chloride—*See* Potassium Supplements (Systemic), 1373

*Klorvess 10% Liquid*—Potassium Chloride—*See* Potassium Supplements (Systemic), 1373

*Klotrix*—Potassium Chloride—*See* Potassium Supplements (Systemic), 1373, MC-19

*K-Lyte*—Potassium Bicarbonate—*See* Potassium Supplements (Systemic), 1373

*K-Lyte/Cl*—Potassium Bicarbonate and Potassium Chloride—*See* Potassium Supplements (Systemic), 1373

*K-Lyte/Cl 50*—Potassium Bicarbonate and Potassium Chloride—*See* Potassium Supplements (Systemic), 1373

*K-Lyte/Cl Powder*—Potassium Chloride—*See* Potassium Supplements (Systemic), 1373

*K-Lyte DS*—Potassium Bicarbonate and Potassium Citrate—*See* Potassium Supplements (Systemic), 1373

*K-Norm*—Potassium Chloride—*See* Potassium Supplements (Systemic), 1373

*Koate-HP*—Antihemophilic Factor (Systemic), 302

*Koffex*—Dextromethorphan (Systemic), 701

*Kogenate*—Antihemophilic Factor (Systemic), 302

*Kolephrin*—Chlorpheniramine, Phenylephrine, Acetaminophen, Salicylamide, and Caffeine—*See* Antihistamines, Decongestants, and Analgesics (Systemic), 316

*Kolephrin/DM Caplets*—Chlorpheniramine, Phenylpropanolamine, Dextromethorphan, and Aspirin—*See* Cough/Cold Combinations (Systemic), 637; Chlorpheniramine, Pseudoephedrine, Dextromethorphan, Acetaminophen, and Caffeine—*See* Cough/Cold Combinations (Systemic), 637

*Kolephrin GG/DM*—Dextromethorphan and Guaifenesin—*See* Cough/Cold Combinations (Systemic), 637

*Kolephrin NN Liquid*—Pyrilamine, Phenylpropanolamine, Dextromethorphan, and Sodium Salicylate—*See* Cough/Cold Combinations (Systemic), 637

*Kolyum*—Potassium Gluconate and Potassium Chloride—*See* Potassium Supplements (Systemic), 1373

*Konakion*—Phytonadione—*See* Vitamin K (Systemic), 1676

*Kondremul*—Mineral Oil—*See* Laxatives (Oral), 1017

*Kondremul with Cascara*—Mineral Oil and Cascara Sagrada—*See* Laxatives (Oral), 1017

*Kondremul with Phenolphthalein*—Mineral Oil and Phenolphthalein—*See* Laxatives (Oral), 1017

*Kondremul Plain*—Mineral Oil—*See* Laxatives (Oral), 1017

*Konsyl*—Psyllium—*See* Laxatives (Oral), 1017

*Konsyl-D*—Psyllium Hydrophilic Mucilloid—*See* Laxatives (Oral), 1017

*Konsyl-Orange*—Psyllium Hydrophilic Mucilloid—*See* Laxatives (Oral), 1017

*Konyne 80*—Factor IX (Systemic), 823

*Kophane*—Chlorpheniramine, Phenylpropanolamine, Dextromethorphan, and Ammonium Chloride—*See* Cough/Cold Combinations (Systemic), 637

*Kophane Cough and Cold Formula*—Chlorpheniramine, Phenylpropanolamine, and Dextromethorphan—*See* Cough/Cold Combinations (Systemic), 637

*Koromex Cream*—Octoxynol 9—*See* Spermicides (Vaginal), 1512

*Koromex Crystal Clear Gel*—Nonoxynol 9—*See* Spermicides (Vaginal), 1512

*Koromex Foam*—Nonoxynol 9—*See* Spermicides (Vaginal), 1512

*Koromex Jelly*—Nonoxynol 9—*See* Spermicides (Vaginal), 1512

*Koromex with Nonoxynol 9*—Latex Condoms and Nonoxynol 9—*See* Condoms, 602

*K-P*—Kaolin and Pectin (Oral), 1004

KPAB—*See* Aminobenzoate Potassium (Systemic), 197

*K-Pek*—Attapulgite (Oral), 359

*K-Phos M. F.*—Potassium and Sodium Phosphates—*See* Phosphates (Systemic), 1349

*K-Phos Neutral*—Potassium and Sodium Phosphates—*See* Phosphates (Systemic), 1349

*K-Phos No. 2*—Potassium and Sodium Phosphates—*See* Phosphates (Systemic), 1349

*K-Phos Original*—Potassium Phosphates—*See* Phosphates (Systemic), 1349

*Kronofed-A Jr. Kronocaps*—Chlorpheniramine and Pseudoephedrine—*See* Antihistamines and Decongestants (Systemic), 311

*Kronofed-A Kronocaps*—Chlorpheniramine and Pseudoephedrine—*See* Antihistamines and Decongestants (Systemic), 311

Krypton Kr 81m—*See* Radiopharmaceuticals (Diagnostic), 1439

*K-Tab*—Potassium Chloride—*See* Potassium Supplements (Systemic), 1373, MC-19

*Kudrox Double Strength*—Alumina, Magnesia, and Simethicone—*See* Antacids (Oral), 253

*Ku-Zyme HP*—Pancrelipase (Systemic), 1284

*Kwelcof Liquid*—Hydrocodone and Guaifenesin—*See* Cough/Cold Combinations (Systemic), 637

*Kwell*—Lindane (Topical), 1042

*Kwellada*—Lindane (Topical), 1042

*Kwildane*—Lindane (Topical), 1042

*Kytril*—Granisetron (Systemic), 1749

# L

*LA-12*—Hydroxocobalamin—*See* Vitamin $B_{12}$ (Systemic), 1667

Labetalol—*See* Beta-adrenergic Blocking Agents (Systemic), 404, MC-13

*Lacril*—Hydroxypropyl Methylcellulose (Ophthalmic), 941

*Lacrisert*—Hydroxypropyl Cellulose (Ophthalmic), 940

*LactiCare-HC*—Hydrocortisone—*See* Corticosteroids—Low Potency (Topical), 624

*Lactisol*—Salicylic Acid (Topical), 1478

*Lactofree*—Infant Formulas, Milk-based—*See* Infant Formulas (Systemic), 958

*Lactulax*—Lactulose—*See* Laxatives (Oral), 1017

Lactulose—*See* Laxatives (Oral), 1017

*Lady Protex with Spermicidal Lubricant*—Latex Condoms and Nonoxynol 9—*See* Condoms, 602

*Lady Protex Ultra-Thin*—Latex Condoms—*See* Condoms, 602

*Lagol*—Benzocaine—*See* Anesthetics (Topical), 240

*Lamisil*—Terbinafine (Topical), 1563

*Lamprene*—Clofazimine (Systemic), 570

*Lanacort*—Hydrocortisone Acetate—*See* Corticosteroids—Low Potency (Topical), 624

*Lanacort 10*—Hydrocortisone Acetate—*See* Corticosteroids—Low Potency (Topical), 624, 1750

*Lanatuss Expectorant*—Chlorpheniramine, Phenylpropanolamine, Guaifenesin, Sodium Citrate, and Citric Acid—*See* Cough/Cold Combinations (Systemic), 637

*Laniazid*—Isoniazid (Systemic), 992

*Laniroif*—Butalbital, Aspirin, and Caffeine—*See* Butalbital and Aspirin (Systemic), 456

*Lanophyllin*—Theophylline—*See* Bronchodilators, Xanthine-derivative (Systemic), 442

*Lanorinal*—Butalbital, Aspirin, and Caffeine—*See* Butalbital and Aspirin (Systemic), 456

*Lanoxicaps*—Digoxin—*See* Digitalis Medicines (Systemic), 716, MC-7

*Lanoxin*—Digoxin—*See* Digitalis Medicines (Systemic), 716, MC-7

*Lansoÿl*—Mineral Oil—*See* Laxatives (Oral), 1017

*Lanvis*—Thioguanine (Systemic), 1596

*Largactil*—Chlorpromazine—*See* Phenothiazines (Systemic), 1330

*Largactil Liquid*—Chlorpromazine—*See* Phenothiazines (Systemic), 1330

*Largactil Oral Drops*—Chlorpromazine—*See* Phenothiazines (Systemic), 1330

*Largon*—Propiomazine (Systemic), 1410

*Lariam*—Mefloquine (Systemic), 1081

*Larodopa*—Levodopa (Systemic), 1033

*Lasan*—Anthralin (Topical), 256

*Lasan 0.1*—Anthralin (Topical), 256

*Lasan 0.2*—Anthralin (Topical), 256

*Lasan 0.4*—Anthralin (Topical), 256

Lidocaine and Prilocaine (Topical), 1038

Lidocaine—For Self-Injection (Systemic), 1036

*Lidoject-1*—Lidocaine—*See* Anesthetics (Parenteral-Local), 235

*Lidoject-2*—Lidocaine—*See* Anesthetics (Parenteral-Local), 235

*LidoPen*—Lidocaine—For Self-Injection (Systemic), 1036

*Lidox*—Chlordiazepoxide and Clidinium (Systemic), 523

*Lidoxide*—Chlordiazepoxide and Clidinium (Systemic), 523

*LifeStyles Extra Strength with Spermicide*—Latex Condoms and Nonoxynol 9—*See* Condoms, 602

*LifeStyles Form Fitting*—Latex Condoms—*See* Condoms, 602

*LifeStyles Lubricated*—Latex Condoms—*See* Condoms, 602

*LifeStyles Spermicidally Lubricated*—Latex Condoms and Nonoxynol 9—*See* Condoms, 602

*LifeStyles Ultra Sensitive*—Latex Condoms—*See* Condoms, 602

*LifeStyles Vibra-Ribbed*—Latex Condoms—*See* Condoms, 602

Lignocaine—Lidocaine—*See* Anesthetics (Dental), 229; Anesthetics (Parenteral-Local), 235; Anesthetics (Topical), 240

*Limbitrol*—Chlordiazepoxide and Amitriptyline (Systemic), 520, MC-4

*Limbitrol DS*—Chlordiazepoxide and Amitriptyline (Systemic), 520, MC-4

*Lincocin*—Lincomycin (Systemic), 1040

Lincomycin (Systemic), 1040

*Lincorex*—Lincomycin (Systemic), 1040

Lindane (Topical), 1042

*Lioresal*—Baclofen (Systemic), 368, MC-2

Liothyronine—*See* Thyroid Hormones (Systemic), 1606, 1750

Liotrix—*See* Thyroid Hormones (Systemic), 1606

Lipancreatin—*See* Pancrelipase (Systemic), 1284

*Lipisorb*—Enteral Nutrition Formula, Disease-specific—*See* Enteral Nutrition Formulas (Systemic), 769

*Liposyn II*—Fat Emulsions (Systemic), 825

*Liposyn III*—Fat Emulsions (Systemic), 825

*Liquaemin*—Heparin (Systemic), 920

*Liqui-Char*—Charcoal, Activated (Oral), 504

*Liqui-Doss*—Mineral Oil—*See* Laxatives (Oral), 1017

Liquid petrolatum—Mineral Oil—*See* Laxatives (Oral), 1017

*Liquid Pred*—Prednisone—*See* Corticosteroids/Corticotropin—Glucocorticoid Effects (Systemic), 630

*Liqui-E*—Vitamin E (Systemic), 1674

*Liquimat Creamy Beige*—Alcohol and Sulfur (Topical), 183

*Liquimat Dark*—Alcohol and Sulfur (Topical), 183

*Liquimat Light*—Alcohol and Sulfur (Topical), 183

*Liquimat Medium*—Alcohol and Sulfur (Topical), 183

*Liquimat Natural Beige*—Alcohol and Sulfur (Topical), 183

*Liquiprin Children's Elixir*—Acetaminophen (Systemic), 161

*Liquiprin Infants' Drops*—Acetaminophen (Systemic), 161

*Liquor Carbonis Detergens*—Coal Tar (Topical), 589

Lisinopril—*See* Angiotensin-converting Enzyme (ACE) Inhibitors (Systemic), 245, MC-13

Lisinopril and Hydrochlorothiazide—*See* Angiotensin-converting Enzyme (ACE) Inhibitors and Hydrochlorothiazide (Systemic), 249, MC-13

*Lisolipin*—Dextrothyroxine (Systemic), 702

*Listerex Golden Scrub Lotion*—Salicylic Acid (Topical), 1478

*Listerex Herbal Scrub Lotion*—Salicylic Acid (Topical), 1478

*Lite Pred*—Prednisolone—*See* Corticosteroids (Ophthalmic), 620

*Lithane*—Lithium (Systemic), 1044

Lithium (Systemic), 1044, MC-13

*Lithizine*—Lithium (Systemic), 1044

*Lithobid*—Lithium (Systemic), 1044

*Lithonate*—Lithium (Systemic), 1044

*Lithostat*—Acetohydroxamic Acid (Systemic), 172

*Lithotabs*—Lithium (Systemic), 1044

*Livostin*—Levocabastine (Nasal), 1750; (Ophthalmic), 1030

*Locacorten*—Flumethasone—*See* Corticosteroids—Low Potency (Topical), 624

*Locacorten Vioform*—Clioquinol and Flumethasone (Otic), 1747; Clioquinol and Flumethasone (Topical), 1747

*Locoid*—Hydrocortisone Butyrate—*See* Corticosteroids—Medium to Very High Potency (Topical), 626

*Lodine*—Etodolac (Systemic)—*See* Nonsteroidal Anti-inflammatory Drugs (Systemic), 1229, MC-9

Lodoxamide (Ophthalmic), 1047

Lodoxamide trometamol—*See* Lodoxamide (Ophthalmic), 1047

*Lodrane LD*—Brompheniramine and Pseudoephedrine—*See* Antihistamines and Decongestants (Systemic), 311

*Loestrin 1/20*—Norethindrone Acetate and Ethinyl Estradiol—*See* Estrogens and Progestins (Oral Contraceptives) (Systemic), 804, MC-17

*Loestrin 1.5/30*—Norethindrone Acetate and Ethinyl Estradiol—*See* Estrogens and Progestins (Oral Contraceptives) (Systemic), 804, MC-17

*Loestrin Fe 1/20*—Norethindrone Acetate/Ethinyl Estradiol and Ferrous Fumarate (Systemic), MC-17

*Loestrin Fe 1.5/30*—Norethindrone Acetate/Ethinyl Estradiol and Ferrous Fumarate (Systemic), MC-17

*Lofene*—Diphenoxylate and Atropine (Systemic), 725

*Loftran*—Ketazolam—*See* Benzodiazepines (Systemic), 389

*Logen*—Diphenoxylate and Atropine (Systemic), 725

*Lombriareu*—Pyrantel (Oral), 1414

Lomefloxacin—*See* Fluoroquinolones (Systemic), 847, MC-13

*Lomine*—Dicyclomine—*See* Anticholinergics/Antispasmodics (Systemic), 258

*Lomocot*—Diphenoxylate and Atropine (Systemic), 725

*Lomotil*—Diphenoxylate and Atropine (Systemic), 725, MC-7

Lomustine (Systemic), 1048

*Lonalac*—Enteral Nutrition Formula, Milk-based—*See* Enteral Nutrition Formulas (Systemic), 769

*Loniten*—Minoxidil (Systemic), 1140, MC-15

*Lonox*—Diphenoxylate and Atropine (Systemic), 725

*Lo-Ovral*—Norgestrel and Ethinyl Estradiol—*See* Estrogens and Progestins (Oral Contraceptives) (Systemic), 804, MC-17

Loperamide (Oral), 1050, 1750, MC-13

*Lopid*—Gemfibrozil (Systemic), 870, MC-10

*Lopresor*—Metoprolol—*See* Beta-adrenergic Blocking Agents (Systemic), 404

*Lopresor SR*—Metoprolol—*See* Beta-adrenergic Blocking Agents (Systemic), 404

# M

*Magnaprin Arthritis Strength*—Aspirin, Alumina, and Magnesia—*See* Salicylates (Systemic), 1473

Magnesium Carbonate and Sodium Bicarbonate—*See* Antacids (Oral), 253

Magnesium Chloride—*See* Magnesium Supplements (Systemic), 1060

Magnesium Citrate—*See* Laxatives (Oral), 1017; Magnesium Supplements (Systemic), 1060

Magnesium Gluceptate—*See* Magnesium Supplements (Systemic), 1060

Magnesium glucoheptonate—Magnesium Gluceptate—*See* Magnesium Supplements (Systemic), 1060

Magnesium Gluconate—*See* Magnesium Supplements (Systemic), 1060

Magnesium Hydroxide—*See* Antacids (Oral), 253; Laxatives (Oral), 1017; Magnesium Supplements (Systemic), 1060

Magnesium Lactate—*See* Magnesium Supplements (Systemic), 1060

Magnesium Oxide—*See* Antacids (Oral), 253; Laxatives (Oral), 1017; Magnesium Supplements (Systemic), 1060

Magnesium Pidolate—*See* Magnesium Supplements (Systemic), 1060

Magnesium pyroglutamate—Magnesium Pidolate—*See* Magnesium Supplements (Systemic), 1060

*Magnesium-Rougier*—Magnesium Gluceptate—*See* Magnesium Supplements (Systemic), 1060

Magnesium Salicylate—*See* Salicylates (Systemic), 1473

Magnesium Sulfate—*See* Laxatives (Oral), 1017; Magnesium Supplements (Systemic), 1060

Magnesium Supplements (Systemic), 1060

*Magnolax*—Milk of Magnesia, Mineral Oil, and Glycerin—*See* Laxatives (Oral), 1017

*Magnum Lubricated*—Latex Condoms—*See* Condoms, 602

*Magnum with Spermicidal Lubricant*—Latex Condoms and Nonoxynol 9—*See* Condoms, 602

*Mag-Ox*—Magnesium Oxide—*See* Magnesium Supplements (Systemic), 1060

*Mag-Ox 400*—Magnesium Oxide—*See* Antacids (Oral), 253; Laxatives (Oral), 1017

*Mag-Tab SR*—Magnesium Lactate—*See* Magnesium Supplements (Systemic), 1060

*Majeptil*—Thioproperazine—*See* Phenothiazines (Systemic), 1330

*Malatal*—Atropine, Hyoscyamine, Scopolamine, and Phenobarbital—*See* Belladonna Alkaloids and Barbiturates (Systemic), 382

Malathion (Topical), 1063

*Mallamint*—Calcium Carbonate—*See* Antacids (Oral), 253; Calcium Supplements (Systemic), 472

*Mallopres*—Reserpine and Hydrochlorothiazide—*See* Rauwolfia Alkaloids and Thiazide Diuretics (Systemic), 1445

*Malogen*—Testosterone—*See* Androgens (Systemic), 221

*Malogex*—Testosterone—*See* Androgens (Systemic), 221

*Malotuss*—Guaifenesin (Systemic), 892

Malt Soup Extract—*See* Laxatives (Oral), 1017

Malt Soup Extract and Psyllium—*See* Laxatives (Oral), 1017

*Maltsupex*—Malt Soup Extract—*See* Laxatives (Oral), 1017

*Mandelamine*—Methenamine (Systemic), 1100

*Mandol*—Cefamandole—*See* Cephalosporins (Systemic), 498

Manganese Gluconate—*See* Manganese Supplements (Systemic), 1065

Manganese Sulfate—*See* Manganese Supplements (Systemic), 1065

Manganese Supplements (Systemic), 1065

*Mannest*—Estrogens, Conjugated (Systemic), 1748

*Maolate*—Chlorphenesin—*See* Skeletal Muscle Relaxants (Systemic), 1495

*Maox*—Magnesium Oxide—*See* Antacids (Oral), 253; Laxatives (Oral), 1017; Magnesium Supplements (Systemic), 1060

*Mapap Cold Formula*—Chlorpheniramine, Pseudoephedrine, Dextromethorphan, and Acetaminophen—*See* Cough/Cold Combinations (Systemic), 637

*Maprin*—Aspirin, Alumina, and Magnesia—*See* Salicylates (Systemic), 1473

*Maprin I-B*—Aspirin, Alumina, and Magnesia—*See* Salicylates (Systemic), 1473

Maprotiline (Systemic), 1066, MC-14

*Marax*—Theophylline, Ephedrine, and Hydroxyzine (Systemic), 1580

*Marax-DF*—Theophylline, Ephedrine, and Hydroxyzine (Systemic), 1580

*Marbaxin*—Methocarbamol—*See* Skeletal Muscle Relaxants (Systemic), 1495

*Marblen*—Calcium and Magnesium Carbonates—*See* Antacids (Oral), 253

*Marcaine*—Bupivacaine—*See* Anesthetics (Parenteral-Local), 235

*Marcaine Spinal*—Bupivacaine—*See* Anesthetics (Parenteral-Local), 235

*Marcof Expectorant*—Hydrocodone and Potassium Guaiacolsulfonate—*See* Cough/Cold Combinations (Systemic), 637

*Marezine*—Cyclizine—*See* Meclizine/Buclizine/Cyclizine (Systemic), 1079

*Marflex*—Orphenadrine (Systemic), 1260

*Margesic A-C*—Propoxyphene, Aspirin, and Caffeine—*See* Narcotic Analgesics and Aspirin (Systemic), 1185

*Marinol*—Dronabinol (Systemic), 760

*Marmine*—Dimenhydrinate—*See* Antihistamines (Systemic), 304

*Marnal*—Butalbital, Aspirin, and Caffeine—*See* Butalbital and Aspirin (Systemic), 456

*Marplan*—Isocarboxazid—*See* Antidepressants, Monoamine Oxidase (MAO) Inhibitor (Systemic), 274

*Marvelon*—Desogestrel and Ethinyl Estradiol—*See* Estrogens and Progestins (Oral Contraceptives) (Systemic), 804

*Marzine*—Cyclizine—*See* Meclizine/Buclizine/Cyclizine (Systemic), 1079

*Matulane*—Procarbazine (Systemic), 1399

*Maxair*—Pirbuterol—*See* Bronchodilators, Adrenergic (Inhalation), 430

*Maxaquin*—Lomefloxacin—*See* Fluoroquinolones (Systemic), 847, MC-13

*Max-Caro*—Beta-carotene—For Dietary Supplement (Vitamin) (Systemic), 415; Beta-carotene—For Photosensitivity (Systemic), 417

*Maxenal*—Pseudoephedrine (Systemic), 1412

*Maxeran*—Metoclopramide (Systemic), 1123

*Maxidex*—Dexamethasone—*See* Corticosteroids (Ophthalmic), 620

*Maxiflor*—Diflorasone—*See* Corticosteroids—Medium to Very High Potency (Topical), 626

*Maximum Strength Cortaid*—Hydrocortisone—*See* Corticosteroids—Low Potency (Topical), 624

*Maximum Strength Gas Relief*—Simethicone (Oral), 1494

*Maximum Strength Phazyme*—Simethicone (Oral), 1494

*Maximum Strength Tylenol Allergy Sinus Caplets*—Chlorpheniramine, Pseudoephedrine, and Acetaminophen—*See* Antihistamines, Decongestants, and Analgesics (Systemic), 316

*Maxivate*—Betamethasone—*See* Corticosteroids—Medium to Very High Potency (Topical), 626

*MAXX*—Latex Condoms—*See* Condoms, 602

*MAXX Plus*—Latex Condoms and Nonoxynol 9—*See* Condoms, 602

*Maxzide*—Triamterene and Hydrochlorothiazide—*See* Diuretics, Potassium-sparing and Hydrochlorothiazide (Systemic), 745, MC-24

*Mazanor*—Mazindol—*See* Appetite Suppressants (Systemic), 339

Mazindol—*See* Appetite Suppressants (Systemic), 339

*MCT Oil*—Enteral Nutrition Formula, Modular—*See* Enteral Nutrition Formulas (Systemic), 769

Measles Virus Vaccine Live (Systemic), 1069

*Measurin*—Aspirin—*See* Salicylates (Systemic), 1473

*Mebaral*—Mephobarbital—*See* Barbiturates (Systemic), 370

*Mebendacin*—Mebendazole (Systemic), 1070

Mebendazole (Systemic), 1070

*Mebutar*—Mebendazole (Systemic), 1070

Mecamylamine (Systemic), 1073

Mechlorethamine (Systemic), 1075

Mechlorethamine (Topical), 1077

*Meclan*—Meclocycline—*See* Tetracyclines (Topical), 1574

Meclizine—*See* Meclizine/Buclizine/Cyclizine (Systemic), 1079, MC-14

Meclizine/Buclizine/Cyclizine (Systemic), 1079

Meclocycline—*See* Tetracyclines (Topical), 1574

Meclofenamate—*See* Nonsteroidal Anti-inflammatory Drugs (Systemic), 1229, MC-14

Meclofenamic acid—Meclofenamate—*See* Nonsteroidal Anti-inflammatory Drugs (Systemic), 1229

*Meclomen*—Meclofenamate—*See* Nonsteroidal Anti-inflammatory Drugs (Systemic), 1229, 1753, MC-14

*Meda Syrup Forte*—Chlorpheniramine, Phenylephrine, Dextromethorphan, and Guaifenesin—*See* Cough/Cold Combinations (Systemic), 637

*Medi-Flu*—Chlorpheniramine, Pseudoephedrine, Dextromethorphan, and Acetaminophen—*See* Cough/Cold Combinations (Systemic), 637

*Medi-Flu Caplets*—Chlorpheniramine, Pseudoephedrine, Dextromethorphan, and Acetaminophen—*See* Cough/Cold Combinations (Systemic), 637

*Medigesic*—Butalbital, Acetaminophen, and Caffeine—*See* Butalbital and Acetaminophen (Systemic), 453

*Medihaler-Epi*—Epinephrine—*See* Bronchodilators, Adrenergic (Inhalation), 430

*Medihaler Ergotamine*—Ergotamine—*See* Headache Medicines, Ergot Derivative–containing (Systemic), 914

*Medihaler-Iso*—Isoproterenol—*See* Bronchodilators, Adrenergic (Inhalation), 430

*Medilax*—Phenolphthalein—*See* Laxatives (Oral), 1017

*Mediplast*—Salicylic Acid (Topical), 1478

*Medipren*—Ibuprofen—*See* Nonsteroidal Anti-inflammatory Drugs (Systemic), 1229

*Medipren Caplets*—Ibuprofen—*See* Nonsteroidal Anti-inflammatory Drugs (Systemic), 1229

*Mediquell*—Dextromethorphan (Systemic), 701

*Mediquell Decongestant Formula*—Pseudoephedrine and Dextromethorphan—*See* Cough/Cold Combinations (Systemic), 637

*Medotar*—Coal Tar (Topical), 589

*Medralone-40*—Methylprednisolone—*See* Corticosteroids/Corticotropin—Glucocorticoid Effects (Systemic), 630

*Medralone-80*—Methylprednisolone—*See* Corticosteroids/Corticotropin—Glucocorticoid Effects (Systemic), 630

*Medrol*—Methylprednisolone—*See* Corticosteroids/Corticotropin—Glucocorticoid Effects (Systemic), 630, MC-15

*Medrol Enpak*—Methylprednisolone—*See* Corticosteroids/Corticotropin—Glucocorticoid Effects (Systemic), 630, MC-15

Medroxyprogesterone—*See* Progestins (Systemic), 1402, MC-14

Medrysone—*See* Corticosteroids (Ophthalmic), 620

*Med Tamoxifen*—Tamoxifen (Systemic), 1559

Mefenamic Acid—*See* Nonsteroidal Anti-inflammatory Drugs (Systemic), 1229

Mefloquine (Systemic), 1081

*Mefoxin*—Cefoxitin—*See* Cephalosporins (Systemic), 498

*Mega-Cal*—Calcium Carbonate—*See* Calcium Supplements (Systemic), 472

*Megace*—Megestrol—*See* Progestins (Systemic), 1402

*Megace Oral Suspension*—Megestrol (Systemic), 1751

*Megacillin*—Penicillin G—*See* Penicillins (Systemic), 1299

*Megagesic*—Hydrocodone and Acetaminophen—*See* Narcotic Analgesics and Acetaminophen (Systemic), 1181

Megestrol—*See* Progestins (Systemic), 1402, 1751

*Megral*—Ergotamine, Caffeine, and Cyclizine—*See* Headache Medicines, Ergot Derivative–containing (Systemic), 914

*MelATE*—Antihemophilic Factor (Systemic), 302

*Melfiat-105 Unicelles*—Phendimetrazine—*See* Appetite Suppressants (Systemic), 339

*Mellaril*—Thioridazine—*See* Phenothiazines (Systemic), 1330, MC-23

*Mellaril Concentrate*—Thioridazine—*See* Phenothiazines (Systemic), 1330

*Mellaril-S*—Thioridazine—*See* Phenothiazines (Systemic), 1330

Melphalan (Systemic), 1083, 1751

Menadiol—*See* Vitamin K (Systemic), 1676

*Menaval-20*—Estradiol—*See* Estrogens (Systemic), 795

*Menest*—Esterified Estrogens—*See* Estrogens (Systemic), 795

*Meni-D*—Meclizine—*See* Meclizine/Buclizine/Cyclizine (Systemic), 1079

Meningococcal Polysaccharide Vaccine (Systemic), 1086

*Menoject-L.A.*—Testosterone and Estradiol—*See* Androgens and Estrogens (Systemic), 225

*Menomune*—Meningococcal Polysaccharide Vaccine (Systemic), 1086

Menotropins (Systemic), 1087

*Mentor Lubricated*—Latex Condoms—*See* Condoms, 602

*Mentor Plus Spermicidal Lubricant*—Latex Condoms and Nonoxynol 9—*See* Condoms, 602

*Menu Magic Instant Breakfast*—Enteral Nutrition Formula, Milk-based—*See* Enteral Nutrition Formulas (Systemic), 769

*Menu Magic Milk Shake*—Enteral Nutrition Formula, Milk-based—*See* Enteral Nutrition Formulas (Systemic), 769

Mepacrine—*See* Quinacrine (Systemic), 1427

Mepenzolate—*See* Anticholinergics/Antispasmodics (Systemic), 258

Meperidine—*See* Narcotic Analgesics—For Pain Relief (Systemic), 1176, MC-14; Narcotic Analgesics—For Surgery and Obstetrics (Systemic), 1179

Meperidine and Acetaminophen—*See* Narcotic Analgesics and Acetaminophen (Systemic), 1181

Mephenytoin—*See* Anticonvulsants, Hydantoin (Systemic), 267

Mephobarbital—*See* Barbiturates (Systemic), 370

*Mephyton*—Phytonadione—*See* Vitamin K (Systemic), 1676

Mepivacaine—*See* Anesthetics (Parenteral-Local), 235

Meprobamate (Systemic), 1089

Meprobamate and Aspirin (Systemic), 1091

*Meprogesic*—Meprobamate and Aspirin (Systemic), 1091

*Meprogesic Q*—Meprobamate and Aspirin (Systemic), 1091

*Meprolone*—Methylprednisolone—*See* Corticosteroids/Corticotropin—Glucocorticoid Effects (Systemic), 630

*Mepron*—Atovaquone (Systemic), 353, MC-2

*Meprospan 200*—Meprobamate (Systemic), 1089

*Meprospan-400*—Meprobamate (Systemic), 1089

*Meprospan 400*—Meprobamate (Systemic), 1089

Mepyramine—Pyrilamine—*See* Antihistamines (Systemic), 304

Mercaptopurine (Systemic), 1094

*Meritene*—Enteral Nutrition Formula, Milk-based—*See* Enteral Nutrition Formulas (Systemic), 769

*Meruvax II*—Rubella Virus Vaccine Live (Systemic), 1470

Mesalamine (Rectal), 1097, 1751, MC-14

Mesalazine—*See* Mesalamine (Rectal), 1097

*Mesantoin*—Mephenytoin—*See* Anticonvulsants, Hydantoin (Systemic), 267

Mesna (Systemic), 1098

*MESNEX*—Mesna (Systemic), 1098

Mesoridazine—*See* Phenothiazines (Systemic), 1330

*Mestinon*—Pyridostigmine—*See* Antimyasthenics (Systemic), 332

*Mestinon-SR*—Pyridostigmine—*See* Antimyasthenics (Systemic), 332

*Mestinon Timespans*—Pyridostigmine—*See* Antimyasthenics (Systemic), 332

Mesuximide—Methsuximide—*See* Anticonvulsants, Succinimide (Systemic), 271

*Metaderm Mild*—Betamethasone—*See* Corticosteroids—Medium to Very High Potency (Topical), 626

*Metaderm Regular*—Betamethasone—*See* Corticosteroids—Medium to Very High Potency (Topical), 626

*Metahydrin*—Trichlormethiazide—*See* Diuretics, Thiazide (Systemic), 749

Meta-iodobenzylguanidine—*See* Iobenguane, Radioiodinated (Therapeutic), 972

Metamfetamine—Methamphetamine—*See* Amphetamines (Systemic), 209

*Metamucil*—Psyllium Hydrophilic Mucilloid—*See* Laxatives (Oral), 1017

*Metamucil Apple Crisp Fiber Wafers*—Psyllium Hydrophilic Mucilloid—*See* Laxatives (Oral), 1017

*Metamucil Cinnamon Spice Fiber Wafers*—Psyllium Hydrophilic Mucilloid—*See* Laxatives (Oral), 1017

*Metamucil Instant Mix, Orange Flavor*—Psyllium Hydrophilic Mucilloid—*See* Laxatives (Oral), 1017

*Metamucil Orange Flavor*—Psyllium Hydrophilic Mucilloid—*See* Laxatives (Oral), 1017

*Metamucil Sugar Free*—Psyllium Hydrophilic Mucilloid—*See* Laxatives (Oral), 1017

*Metamucil Sugar-Free, Lemon-Lime Flavor*—Psyllium Hydrophilic Mucilloid—*See* Laxatives (Oral), 1017

*Metamucil Sugar-Free, Orange Flavor*—Psyllium Hydrophilic Mucilloid—*See* Laxatives (Oral), 1017

*Metamucil Sunrise Smooth, Citrus Flavor*—Psyllium Hydrophilic Mucilloid—*See* Laxatives (Oral), 1017

*Metamucil Sunrise Smooth, Orange Flavor*—Psyllium Hydrophilic Mucilloid—*See* Laxatives (Oral), 1017

*Metamucil Sunrise Smooth Sugar-Free, Citrus Flavor*—Psyllium Hydrophilic Mucilloid—*See* Laxatives (Oral), 1017

*Metamucil Sunrise Smooth Sugar-Free, Orange Flavor*—Psyllium Hydrophilic Mucilloid—*See* Laxatives (Oral), 1017

*Metamucil Sunrise Smooth Sugar-Free, Regular Flavor*—Psyllium Hydrophilic Mucilloid—*See* Laxatives (Oral), 1017

*Metandren*—Methyltestosterone—*See* Androgens (Systemic), 221

*Metaprel*—Metaproterenol—*See* Bronchodilators, Adrenergic (Inhalation), 430; Bronchodilators, Adrenergic (Oral/Injection), 436

Metaproterenol—*See* Bronchodilators, Adrenergic (Inhalation), 430; Bronchodilators, Adrenergic (Oral/Injection), 436, MC-14

*Metastron*—Strontium 89 Chloride (Therapeutic), 1519

*Metatensin*—Reserpine and Trichlormethiazide—*See* Rauwolfia Alkaloids and Thiazide Diuretics (Systemic), 1445

Metaxalone—*See* Skeletal Muscle Relaxants (Systemic), 1495

*Meted Maximum Strength Anti-Dandruff Shampoo with Conditioners*—Salicylic Acid and Sulfur (Topical), 1481

Metformin (Systemic), 1751

Methacholine (Inhalation), 1099

Methadone—*See* Narcotic Analgesics—For Pain Relief (Systemic), 1176

*Methadose*—Methadone—*See* Narcotic Analgesics—For Pain Relief (Systemic), 1176

Methamphetamine—*See* Amphetamines (Systemic), 209

Methantheline—*See* Anticholinergics/Antispasmodics (Systemic), 258

Methanthelinium—Methantheline—*See* Anticholinergics/Antispasmodics (Systemic), 258

Metharbital—*See* Barbiturates (Systemic), 370

Midazolam (Systemic), 1138

*Midchlor*—Isometheptene, Dichloralphenazone, and Acetaminophen (Systemic), 990

*Midol IB*—Ibuprofen—*See* Nonsteroidal Anti-inflammatory Drugs (Systemic), 1229

*Midrin*—Isometheptene, Dichloralphenazone, and Acetaminophen (Systemic), 990

*Migergot*—Ergotamine and Caffeine—*See* Headache Medicines, Ergot Derivative–containing (Systemic), 914

*Migquin*—Isometheptene, Dichloralphenazone, and Acetaminophen (Systemic), 990

*Migrapap*—Isometheptene, Dichloralphenazone, and Acetaminophen (Systemic), 990

*Migratine*—Isometheptene, Dichloralphenazone, and Acetaminophen (Systemic), 990

*Migrazone*—Isometheptene, Dichloralphenazone, and Acetaminophen (Systemic), 990

*Migrend*—Isometheptene, Dichloralphenazone, and Acetaminophen (Systemic), 990

*Migrex*—Isometheptene, Dichloralphenazone, and Acetaminophen (Systemic), 990

*Milkinol*—Mineral Oil—*See* Laxatives (Oral), 1017

Milk of Magnesia and Mineral Oil—*See* Laxatives (Oral), 1017

Milk of Magnesia, Mineral Oil, and Glycerin—*See* Laxatives (Oral), 1017

*Milontin*—Phensuximide—*See* Anticonvulsants, Succinimide (Systemic), 271

*Milophene*—Clomiphene (Systemic), 574

*Miltown*—Meprobamate (Systemic), 1089

*'Miltown'-200*—Meprobamate (Systemic), 1089

*'Miltown'-400*—Meprobamate (Systemic), 1089

*'Miltown'-600*—Meprobamate (Systemic), 1089

Mineral Oil—*See* Laxatives (Oral), 1017; Laxatives (Rectal), 1023

Mineral Oil and Cascara Sagrada—*See* Laxatives (Oral), 1017

Mineral Oil, Glycerin, and Phenolphthalein—*See* Laxatives (Oral), 1017

Mineral Oil and Phenolphthalein—*See* Laxatives (Oral), 1017

*Minestrin 1/20*—Norethindrone Acetate and Ethinyl Estradiol—*See* Estrogens and Progestins (Oral Contraceptives) (Systemic), 804

*Mini-Gamulin Rh*—RH₀(D) Immune Globulin (Systemic), 1456

*Minims Atropine*—Atropine—*See* Atropine/Homatropine/Scopolamine (Ophthalmic), 354

*Minims Cyclopentolate*—Cyclopentolate (Ophthalmic), 664

*Minims Homatropine*—Homatropine—*See* Atropine/Homatropine/Scopolamine (Ophthalmic), 354

*Minims Phenylephrine*—Phenylephrine (Ophthalmic), 1345

*Minims Pilocarpine*—Pilocarpine (Ophthalmic), 1355

*Minims Tetracaine*—Tetracaine—*See* Anesthetics (Ophthalmic), 234

*Minims Tropicamide*—Tropicamide (Ophthalmic), 1634

*Minipress*—Prazosin (Systemic), 1380, MC-19

*Minizide*—Prazosin and Polythiazide (Systemic), 1382, MC-19

*Minocin*—Minocycline—*See* Tetracyclines (Systemic), 1570, MC-15

Minocycline—*See* Tetracyclines (Systemic), 1570, MC-15

*Min-Ovral*—Levonorgestrel and Ethinyl Estradiol—*See* Estrogens and Progestins (Oral Contraceptives) (Systemic), 804

Minoxidil (Systemic), 1140, MC-15

Minoxidil (Topical), 1142

*Mintezol*—Thiabendazole (Systemic), 1588

*Mintox*—Alumina and Magnesia—*See* Antacids (Oral), 253

*Mintox Plus*—Alumina, Magnesia, and Simethicone—*See* Antacids (Oral), 253

*Minzolum*—Thiabendazole (Systemic), 1588

*Miocarpine*—Pilocarpine (Ophthalmic), 1355

*Miostat*—Carbachol (Ophthalmic), 479

*Miradon*—Anisindione—*See* Anticoagulants (Systemic), 262

Misoprostol (Systemic), 1144, MC-15

*Mithracin*—Plicamycin (Systemic), 1362

Mithramycin—*See* Plicamycin (Systemic), 1362

Mitomycin (Systemic), 1145

Mitotane (Systemic), 1147

Mitoxantrone (Systemic), 1149

*Mitride*—Isometheptene, Dichloralphenazone, and Acetaminophen (Systemic), 990

*Mitrolan*—Polycarbophil—*See* Laxatives (Oral), 1017

*Moban*—Molindone (Systemic), 1151

*Moban Concentrate*—Molindone (Systemic), 1151

*Mobenol*—Tolbutamide—*See* Antidiabetics, Oral (Systemic), 283

*Mobidin*—Magnesium Salicylate—*See* Salicylates (Systemic), 1473

*Mobiflex*—Tenoxicam—*See* Nonsteroidal Anti-inflammatory Drugs (Systemic), 1229

*Moctanin*—Monooctanoin (Local), 1155

*Modane*—Phenolphthalein—*See* Laxatives (Oral), 1017

*Modane Bulk*—Psyllium Hydrophilic Mucilloid—*See* Laxatives (Oral), 1017

*Modane Soft*—Docusate—*See* Laxatives (Oral), 1017

*Modecate*—Fluphenazine—*See* Phenothiazines (Systemic), 1330

*Modecate Concentrate*—Fluphenazine—*See* Phenothiazines (Systemic), 1330

*ModiCon*—Norethindrone and Ethinyl Estradiol—*See* Estrogens and Progestins (Oral Contraceptives) (Systemic), 804

Modified Shohl's solution—Sodium Citrate and Citric Acid—*See* Citrates (Systemic), 554

*Moditen Enanthate*—Fluphenazine—*See* Phenothiazines (Systemic), 1330

*Moditen HCl*—Fluphenazine—*See* Phenothiazines (Systemic), 1330

*Moditen HCl-H.P.*—Fluphenazine—*See* Phenothiazines (Systemic), 1330

*Modrastane*—Trilostane (Systemic), 1625

*Modical*—Enteral Nutrition Formula, Modular—*See* Enteral Nutrition Formulas (Systemic), 769

*Moduret*—Amiloride and Hydrochlorothiazide—*See* Diuretics, Potassium-sparing and Hydrochlorothiazide (Systemic), 745

*Moduretic*—Amiloride and Hydrochlorothiazide—*See* Diuretics, Potassium-sparing and Hydrochlorothiazide (Systemic), 745, MC-1

*Mogadon*—Nitrazepam—*See* Benzodiazepines (Systemic), 389

*Mycotussin*—Pseudoephedrine and Hydrocodone—*See* Cough/Cold Combinations (Systemic), 637
*Mydfrin*—Phenylephrine (Ophthalmic), 1345
*Mydriacyl*—Tropicamide (Ophthalmic), 1634
*Mydriafair*—Tropicamide (Ophthalmic), 1634
*My-E*—Erythromycin Stearate—*See* Erythromycins (Systemic), 786
*Myfedrine*—Pseudoephedrine (Systemic), 1412
*Mygel*—Alumina, Magnesia, and Simethicone—*See* Antacids (Oral), 253
*Mygel II*—Alumina, Magnesia, and Simethicone—*See* Antacids (Oral), 253
*Myhistine DH*—Chlorpheniramine, Pseudoephedrine, and Codeine—*See* Cough/Cold Combinations (Systemic), 637
*Myhistine Expectorant*—Pseudoephedrine, Codeine, and Guaifenesin—*See* Cough/Cold Combinations (Systemic), 637
*Myhydromine*—Phenylpropanolamine and Hydrocodone—*See* Cough/Cold Combinations (Systemic), 637
*Myhydromine Pediatric*—Phenylpropanolamine and Hydrocodone—*See* Cough/Cold Combinations (Systemic), 637
*Myidil*—Triprolidine—*See* Antihistamines (Systemic), 304
*Myidone*—Primidone (Systemic), 1388
*Mykacet*—Nystatin and Triamcinolone (Topical), 1247
*Mykacet II*—Nystatin and Triamcinolone (Topical), 1247
*Mykrox*—Metolazone—*See* Diuretics, Thiazide (Systemic), 749, MC-15
*Mylanta*—Alumina, Magnesia, and Simethicone—*See* Antacids (Oral), 253; Calcium and Magnesium Carbonates—*See* Antacids (Oral), 253
*Mylanta-II*—Alumina, Magnesia, and Simethicone—*See* Antacids (Oral), 253
*Mylanta Double Strength*—Alumina, Magnesia, and Simethicone—*See* Antacids (Oral), 253
*Mylanta Double Strength Plain*—Alumina and Magnesia—*See* Antacids (Oral), 253
*Mylanta Extra Strength*—Alumina, Magnesia, and Simethicone—*See* Antacids (Oral), 253
*Mylanta Gas*—Simethicone (Oral), 1494
*Mylanta Gas Maximum Strength*—Simethicone (Oral), 1494
*Mylanta Gas Regular Strength*—Simethicone (Oral), 1494
*Myleran*—Busulfan (Systemic), 450
*Mylicon Drops*—Simethicone (Oral), 1494
*Mymethasone*—Dexamethasone—*See* Corticosteroids/Corticotropin—Glucocorticoid Effects (Systemic), 630
*Myminic Expectorant*—Phenylpropanolamine and Guaifenesin—*See* Cough/Cold Combinations (Systemic), 637
*Myminicol*—Chlorpheniramine, Phenylpropanolamine, and Dextromethorphan—*See* Cough/Cold Combinations (Systemic), 637
*Myochrysine*—Gold Sodium Thiomalate—*See* Gold Compounds (Systemic), 884
*Myoflex*—Triethanolamine Salicylate (Topical), 1754
*Myolin*—Orphenadrine (Systemic), 1260
*Myotrol*—Orphenadrine (Systemic), 1260
*Myphetane DC Cough*—Brompheniramine, Phenylpropanolamine, and Codeine—*See* Cough/Cold Combinations (Systemic), 637
*Myphetane DX Cough*—Brompheniramine, Pseudoephedrine, and Dextromethorphan—*See* Cough/Cold Combinations (Systemic), 637

*Myphetapp*—Brompheniramine and Phenylpropanolamine—*See* Antihistamines and Decongestants (Systemic), 311
*Myproic Acid*—Valproic Acid (Systemic), 1651
*Myrosemide*—Furosemide—*See* Diuretics, Loop (Systemic), 738
*Mysoline*—Primidone (Systemic), 1388
*Mytelase Caplets*—Ambenonium—*See* Antimyasthenics (Systemic), 332
*Mytrex*—Nystatin and Triamcinolone (Topical), 1247
*Mytussin*—Guaifenesin (Systemic), 892
*Mytussin AC*—Codeine and Guaifenesin—*See* Cough/Cold Combinations (Systemic), 637
*Mytussin DAC*—Pseudoephedrine, Codeine, and Guaifenesin—*See* Cough/Cold Combinations (Systemic), 637
*Mytussin DM*—Dextromethorphan and Guaifenesin—*See* Cough/Cold Combinations (Systemic), 637

# N

*9-1-1*—Hydrocortisone Acetate—*See* Corticosteroids—Low Potency (Topical), 624
Nabilone (Systemic), 1165
Nabumetone—*See* Nonsteroidal Anti-inflammatory Drugs (Systemic), 1229, MC-15
Nadolol—*See* Beta-adrenergic Blocking Agents (Systemic), 404, MC-16
Nadolol and Bendroflumethiazide—*See* Beta-adrenergic Blocking Agents and Thiazide Diuretics (Systemic), 410, MC-16
*Nadopen-V*—Penicillin V—*See* Penicillins (Systemic), 1299
*Nadopen-V 200*—Penicillin V—*See* Penicillins (Systemic), 1299
*Nadopen-V 400*—Penicillin V—*See* Penicillins (Systemic), 1299
*Nadostine*—Nystatin (Oral), 1243; Nystatin (Topical), 1245; Nystatin (Vaginal), 1246
*Nadrothyron-D*—Dextrothyroxine (Systemic), 702
Nafarelin (Systemic), 1166, 1751
*Nafazair*—Naphazoline (Ophthalmic), 1174
*Nafcil*—Nafcillin—*See* Penicillins (Systemic), 1299
Nafcillin—*See* Penicillins (Systemic), 1299
*Nafrine Decongestant Nasal Drops*—Oxymetazoline (Nasal), 1274
*Nafrine Decongestant Nasal Spray*—Oxymetazoline (Nasal), 1274
*Nafrine Decongestant Pediatric Nasal Spray/Drops*—Oxymetazoline (Nasal), 1274
Naftifine (Topical), 1168
*Naftin*—Naftifine (Topical), 1168
Nalbuphine—*See* Narcotic Analgesics—For Pain Relief (Systemic), 1176; Narcotic Analgesics—For Surgery and Obstetrics (Systemic), 1179
*Nalcrom*—Cromolyn (Oral), 658
*Naldecon*—Chlorpheniramine, Phenyltoloxamine, Phenylephrine, and Phenylpropanolamine—*See* Antihistamines and Decongestants (Systemic), 311, MC-4
*Naldecon-CX Adult Liquid*—Phenylpropanolamine, Codeine, and Guaifenesin—*See* Cough/Cold Combinations (Systemic), 637

*Naldecon-DX Adult Liquid*—Phenylpropanolamine, Dextromethorphan, and Guaifenesin—*See* Cough/Cold Combinations (Systemic), 637

*Naldecon-DX Children's Syrup*—Phenylpropanolamine, Dextromethorphan, and Guaifenesin—*See* Cough/Cold Combinations (Systemic), 637

*Naldecon-DX Pediatric Drops*—Phenylpropanolamine, Dextromethorphan, and Guaifenesin—*See* Cough/Cold Combinations (Systemic), 637

*Naldecon-EX*—Phenylpropanolamine and Guaifenesin—*See* Cough/Cold Combinations (Systemic), 637

*Naldecon-EX Pediatric Drops*—Phenylpropanolamine and Guaifenesin—*See* Cough/Cold Combinations (Systemic), 637

*Naldecon Pediatric Drops*—Chlorpheniramine, Phenyltoloxamine, Phenylephrine, and Phenylpropanolamine—*See* Antihistamines and Decongestants (Systemic), 311

*Naldecon Pediatric Syrup*—Chlorpheniramine, Phenyltoloxamine, Phenylephrine, and Phenylpropanolamine—*See* Antihistamines and Decongestants (Systemic), 311

*Naldecon Senior DX*—Dextromethorphan and Guaifenesin—*See* Cough/Cold Combinations (Systemic), 637

*Naldecon Senior EX*—Guaifenesin (Systemic), 892

*Naldegesic*—Pseudoephedrine and Acetaminophen—*See* Decongestants and Analgesics (Systemic), 691

*Naldelate*—Chlorpheniramine, Phenyltoloxamine, Phenylephrine, and Phenylpropanolamine—*See* Antihistamines and Decongestants (Systemic), 311

*Naldelate DX Adult*—Phenylpropanolamine, Dextromethorphan, and Guaifenesin—*See* Cough/Cold Combinations (Systemic), 637

*Naldelate Pediatric Syrup*—Chlorpheniramine, Phenyltoloxamine, Phenylephrine, and Phenylpropanolamine—*See* Antihistamines and Decongestants (Systemic), 311

*Nalfon*—Fenoprofen—*See* Nonsteroidal Anti-inflammatory Drugs (Systemic), 1229, MC-10

*Nalfon 200*—Fenoprofen—*See* Nonsteroidal Anti-inflammatory Drugs (Systemic), 1229, MC-10

*Nalgest*—Chlorpheniramine, Phenyltoloxamine, Phenylephrine, and Phenylpropanolamine—*See* Antihistamines and Decongestants (Systemic), 311

*Nalgest Pediatric*—Chlorpheniramine, Phenyltoloxamine, Phenylephrine, and Phenylpropanolamine—*See* Antihistamines and Decongestants (Systemic), 311

Nalidixic Acid (Systemic), 1170, MC-16

*Nallpen*—Nafcillin—*See* Penicillins (Systemic), 1299

Naltrexone (Systemic), 1172

Nandrolone—*See* Anabolic Steroids (Systemic), 218

Naphazoline (Ophthalmic), 1174

*Naphcon*—Naphazoline (Ophthalmic), 1174

*Naphcon Forte*—Naphazoline (Ophthalmic), 1174

*Napril*—Chlorpheniramine and Pseudoephedrine—*See* Antihistamines and Decongestants (Systemic), 311

*Naprosyn*—Naproxen—*See* Nonsteroidal Anti-inflammatory Drugs (Systemic), 1229, MC-16

*Naprosyn-E*—Naproxen—*See* Nonsteroidal Anti-inflammatory Drugs (Systemic), 1229

*Naprosyn-SR*—Naproxen—*See* Nonsteroidal Anti-inflammatory Drugs (Systemic), 1229

Naproxen—*See* Nonsteroidal Anti-inflammatory Drugs (Systemic), 1229, MC-16

*Naqua*—Trichlormethiazide—*See* Diuretics, Thiazide (Systemic), 749

*Naquival*—Reserpine and Trichlormethiazide—*See* Rauwolfia Alkaloids and Thiazide Diuretics (Systemic), 1445

Narcotic Analgesics and Acetaminophen (Systemic), 1181

Narcotic Analgesics and Aspirin (Systemic), 1185

Narcotic Analgesics—For Pain Relief (Systemic), 1176

Narcotic Analgesics—For Surgery and Obstetrics (Systemic), 1179

*Nardil*—Phenelzine—*See* Antidepressants, Monoamine Oxidase (MAO) Inhibitor (Systemic), 274

*Nasacort*—Triamcinolone—*See* Corticosteroids (Nasal), 617

*Nasahist*—Chlorpheniramine, Phenylephrine, and Phenylpropanolamine—*See* Antihistamines and Decongestants (Systemic), 311

*Nasahist B*—Brompheniramine—*See* Antihistamines (Systemic), 304

*Nasalcrom*—Cromolyn (Nasal), 654

*Nasalide*—Flunisolide—*See* Corticosteroids (Nasal), 617

*Nasatab LA*—Pseudoephedrine and Guaifenesin—*See* Cough/Cold Combinations (Systemic), 637

*Natacyn*—Natamycin (Ophthalmic), 1189

Natamycin (Ophthalmic), 1189

*Natulan*—Procarbazine (Systemic), 1399

*Naturacil*—Psyllium—*See* Laxatives (Oral), 1017

*Naturalyte*—Dextrose and Electrolytes—*See* Carbohydrates and Electrolytes (Systemic), 484

*Nature's Remedy*—Cascara Sagrada and Aloe—*See* Laxatives (Oral), 1017

*Naturetin*—Bendroflumethiazide—*See* Diuretics, Thiazide (Systemic), 749, MC-3

*Nauseatol*—Dimenhydrinate—*See* Antihistamines (Systemic), 304

*Navane*—Thiothixene—*See* Thioxanthenes (Systemic), 1601, MC-23

*Naxen*—Naproxen—*See* Nonsteroidal Anti-inflammatory Drugs (Systemic), 1229

*ND Clear T.D.*—Chlorpheniramine and Pseudoephedrine—*See* Antihistamines and Decongestants (Systemic), 311

*ND-Gesic*—Chlorpheniramine, Pyrilamine, Phenylephrine, and Acetaminophen—*See* Antihistamines, Decongestants, and Analgesics (Systemic), 316

*ND-Stat Revised*—Brompheniramine—*See* Antihistamines (Systemic), 304

*Nebcin*—Tobramycin—*See* Aminoglycosides (Systemic), 201

*NebuPent*—Pentamidine (Inhalation), 1311

Nedocromil (Inhalation), 1191

*N.E.E. 1/35*—Norethindrone and Ethinyl Estradiol—*See* Estrogens and Progestins (Oral Contraceptives) (Systemic), 804

*N.E.E. 1/50*—Norethindrone and Ethinyl Estradiol—*See* Estrogens and Progestins (Oral Contraceptives) (Systemic), 804

*NegGram*—Nalidixic Acid (Systemic), 1170, MC-16

*Nelova 10/11*—Norethindrone and Ethinyl Estradiol—*See* Estrogens and Progestins (Oral Contraceptives) (Systemic), 804

*Nelova 0.5/35E*—Norethindrone and Ethinyl Estradiol—*See* Estrogens and Progestins (Oral Contraceptives) (Systemic), 804

*Nelova 1/35E*—Norethindrone and Ethinyl Estradiol—*See* Estrogens and Progestins (Oral Contraceptives) (Systemic), 804

*Nelova 1/50M*—Norethindrone and Mestranol—*See* Estrogens and Progestins (Oral Contraceptives) (Systemic), 804

*Nelulen 1/35E*—Ethynodiol Diacetate and Ethinyl Estradiol—*See* Estrogens and Progestins (Oral Contraceptives) (Systemic), 804

*Nelulen 1/50E*—Ethynodiol Diacetate and Ethinyl Estradiol—*See* Estrogens and Progestins (Oral Contraceptives) (Systemic), 804

*Nemasole*—Mebendazole (Systemic), 1070

*Nemasol Sodium*—Aminosalicylate Sodium (Systemic), 204

*Nembutal*—Pentobarbital—*See* Barbiturates (Systemic), 370

*Neo-Calglucon*—Calcium Glubionate—*See* Calcium Supplements (Systemic), 472

*Neocidin Ophthalmic Ointment*—Neomycin, Polymyxin B, and Bacitracin (Ophthalmic), 1199

*Neocidin Ophthalmic Solution*—Neomycin, Polymyxin B, and Gramicidin (Ophthalmic), 1201

*NeoCitran A*—Pheniramine and Phenylephrine—*See* Antihistamines and Decongestants (Systemic), 311

*NeoCitran Colds and Flu Calorie Reduced*—Pheniramine, Phenylephrine, and Acetaminophen—*See* Antihistamines, Decongestants, and Analgesics (Systemic), 316

*NeoCitran DM Coughs & Colds*—Pheniramine, Phenylephrine, and Dextromethorphan (Systemic), 1752

*NeoCitran Extra Strength Colds and Flu*—Pheniramine, Phenylephrine, and Acetaminophen—*See* Antihistamines, Decongestants, and Analgesics (Systemic), 316

*Neo Citran Extra Strength Sinus*—Phenylephrine and Acetaminophen—*See* Decongestants and Analgesics (Systemic), 691

*Neo-Codema*—Hydrochlorothiazide—*See* Diuretics, Thiazide (Systemic), 749

*Neocontrast*—Iopanoic Acid—*See* Cholecystographic Agents, Oral (Diagnostic), 536

*Neo-Cultol*—Mineral Oil—*See* Laxatives (Oral), 1017

*Neocyten*—Orphenadrine (Systemic), 1260

*Neo-DM*—Dextromethorphan (Systemic), 701

*Neo-Durabolic*—Nandrolone—*See* Anabolic Steroids (Systemic), 218

*Neo-Estrone*—Esterified Estrogens—*See* Estrogens (Systemic), 795

*Neo-Fer*—Ferrous Fumarate—*See* Iron Supplements (Systemic), 986

*Neo-K*—Potassium Bicarbonate and Potassium Chloride—*See* Potassium Supplements (Systemic), 1373

*Neolax*—Dehydrocholic Acid and Docusate—*See* Laxatives (Oral), 1017

*Neoloid*—Castor Oil—*See* Laxatives (Oral), 1017

*Neomycin*—*See* Aminoglycosides (Systemic), 201

Neomycin (Ophthalmic), 1193

Neomycin (Oral), 1194

Neomycin (Topical), 1196

Neomycin and Polymyxin B (Topical), 1197

Neomycin, Polymyxin B, and Bacitracin (Ophthalmic), 1199

Neomycin, Polymyxin B, and Bacitracin (Topical), 1200

Neomycin, Polymyxin B, and Gramicidin (Ophthalmic), 1201

Neomycin, Polymyxin B, and Hydrocortisone (Ophthalmic), 1203

Neomycin, Polymyxin B, and Hydrocortisone (Otic), 1204

*Neopap*—Acetaminophen (Systemic), 161

*Neo-Pause*—Testosterone and Estradiol—*See* Androgens and Estrogens (Systemic), 225

*Neoquess*—Dicyclomine—*See* Anticholinergics/Antispasmodics (Systemic), 258; Hyoscyamine—*See* Anticholinergics/Antispasmodics (Systemic), 258

*Neosar*—Cyclophosphamide (Systemic), 666

*Neosporin Cream*—Neomycin and Polymyxin B (Topical), 1197

*Neosporin Maximum Strength Ointment*—Neomycin, Polymyxin B, and Bacitracin (Topical), 1200

*Neosporin Ointment*—Neomycin, Polymyxin B, and Bacitracin (Topical), 1200

*Neosporin Ophthalmic Ointment*—Neomycin, Polymyxin B, and Bacitracin (Ophthalmic), 1199

*Neosporin Ophthalmic Solution*—Neomycin, Polymyxin B, and Gramicidin (Ophthalmic), 1201

Neostigmine—*See* Antimyasthenics (Systemic), 332

*Neo-Synephrine*—Phenylephrine (Ophthalmic), 1345

*Neo-Synephrine 12 Hour Nasal Spray*—Oxymetazoline (Nasal), 1274

*Neo-Synephrine 12 Hour Nasal Spray Pump*—Oxymetazoline (Nasal), 1274

*Neo-Synephrine II Long Acting Nasal Spray Adult Strength*—Xylometazoline (Nasal), 1681

*Neo-Synephrine II Long Acting Nose Drops Adult Strength*—Xylometazoline (Nasal), 1681

*Neo-Synephrine Nasal Drops*—Phenylephrine (Nasal), 1343

*Neo-Synephrine Nasal Jelly*—Phenylephrine (Nasal), 1343

*Neo-Synephrine Nasal Spray*—Phenylephrine (Nasal), 1343

*Neo-Synephrine Pediatric Nasal Drops*—Phenylephrine (Nasal), 1343

*Neotal*—Neomycin, Polymyxin B, and Bacitracin (Ophthalmic), 1199

*Neothylline*—Dyphylline—*See* Bronchodilators, Xanthine-derivative (Systemic), 442

*Neo-Zol Cream*—Clotrimazole (Topical), 583

*Nephro-Calci*—Calcium Carbonate—*See* Calcium Supplements (Systemic), 472

*Nephron*—Racepinephrine—*See* Bronchodilators, Adrenergic (Inhalation), 430

*Nephrox*—Aluminum Hydroxide—*See* Antacids (Oral), 253

*Nepro*—Enteral Nutrition Formula, Disease-specific—*See* Enteral Nutrition Formulas (Systemic), 769

*Neptazane*—Methazolamide—*See* Carbonic Anhydrase Inhibitors (Systemic), 488

*Nerisone*—Diflucortolone—*See* Corticosteroids—Medium to Very High Potency (Topical), 626

*Nerisone Oily*—Diflucortolone—*See* Corticosteroids—Medium to Very High Potency (Topical), 626

*Nervine*—Aspirin and Caffeine—*See* Salicylates (Systemic), 1473

*Nervine Nighttime Sleep-Aid*—Diphenhydramine—*See* Antihistamines (Systemic), 304

*Nervocaine*—Lidocaine—*See* Anesthetics (Parenteral-Local), 235

*Nesacaine*—Chloroprocaine—*See* Anesthetics (Parenteral-Local), 235

*Nesacaine-CE*—Chloroprocaine—*See* Anesthetics (Parenteral-Local), 235

*Nesacaine-MPF*—Chloroprocaine—*See* Anesthetics (Parenteral-Local), 235
Netilmicin—*See* Aminoglycosides (Systemic), 201
*Netromycin*—Netilmicin—*See* Aminoglycosides (Systemic), 201
*Neuleptil*—Pericyazine—*See* Phenothiazines (Systemic), 1330
*Neupogen*—Filgrastim—*See* Colony Stimulating Factors (Systemic), 600
*Neurontin*—Gabapentin (Systemic), 1749, MC-10
*Neutralca-S*—Alumina and Magnesia—*See* Antacids (Oral), 253
*Neutra-Phos*—Potassium and Sodium Phosphates—*See* Phosphates (Systemic), 1349
*Neutra-Phos-K*—Potassium Phosphates—*See* Phosphates (Systemic), 1349
*NeuTrexin*—Trimetrexate (Systemic), 1630
*Neutrogena Acne Mask 5*—Benzoyl Peroxide (Topical), 397
*New-Decongestant Pediatric*—Chlorpheniramine, Phenyltoloxamine, Phenylephrine, and Phenylpropanolamine—*See* Antihistamines and Decongestants (Systemic), 311
*New-Decongest Pediatric Syrup*—Chlorpheniramine, Phenyltoloxamine, Phenylephrine, and Phenylpropanolamine—*See* Antihistamines and Decongestants (Systemic), 311
*N3 Gesic*—Orphenadrine, Aspirin, and Caffeine—*See* Orphenadrine and Aspirin (Systemic), 1262
*N3 Gesic Forte*—Orphenadrine, Aspirin, and Caffeine—*See* Orphenadrine and Aspirin (Systemic), 1262
*Nia-Bid*—Niacin—For High Cholesterol (Systemic), 1206; Niacin (Vitamin B$_3$) (Systemic), 1208
*Niac*—Niacin—For High Cholesterol (Systemic), 1206; Niacin (Vitamin B$_3$) (Systemic), 1208
*Niacels*—Niacin—For High Cholesterol (Systemic), 1206; Niacin (Vitamin B$_3$) (Systemic), 1208
Niacinamide—*See* Niacin (Vitamin B$_3$) (Systemic), 1208, MC-16
Niacin—For High Cholesterol (Systemic), 1206, MC-16
Niacin (Vitamin B$_3$) (Systemic), 1208, MC-16
*Niacor*—Niacin—For High Cholesterol (Systemic), 1206; Niacin (Vitamin B$_3$) (Systemic), 1208
Nicardipine—*See* Calcium Channel Blocking Agents (Systemic), 467, MC-16
*Niclocide*—Niclosamide (Oral), 1210
Niclosamide (Oral), 1210
*Nico-400*—Niacin—For High Cholesterol (Systemic), 1206; Niacin (Vitamin B$_3$) (Systemic), 1208
*Nicobid Tempules*—Niacin—For High Cholesterol (Systemic), 1206, MC-16; Niacin (Vitamin B$_3$) (Systemic), 1208, MC-16
*Nicoderm*—Nicotine (Systemic), 1212
*Nicolar*—Niacin—For High Cholesterol (Systemic), 1206, MC-16; Niacin (Vitamin B$_3$) (Systemic), 1208, MC-16
*Nicorette*—Nicotine (Systemic), 1212, MC-16
*Nicorette DS*—Nicotine (Systemic), 1212
Nicotinamide (Topical), 1751
Nicotine (Systemic), 1212, MC-16
*Nicotinex Elixir*—Niacin—For High Cholesterol (Systemic), 1206; Niacin (Vitamin B$_3$) (Systemic), 1208
Nicotinic acid—*See* Niacin—For High Cholesterol (Systemic), 1206; Niacin (Vitamin B$_3$) (Systemic), 1208
Nicotinyl Alcohol (Systemic), 1215

*Nicotrol*—Nicotine (Systemic), 1212
*Nico-Vert*—Dimenhydrinate—*See* Antihistamines (Systemic), 304
*Nidryl*—Diphenhydramine—*See* Antihistamines (Systemic), 304
Nifedipine—*See* Calcium Channel Blocking Agents (Systemic), 467, MC-16
*Niferex*—Iron-Polysaccharide—*See* Iron Supplements (Systemic), 986
*Niferex-150*—Iron-Polysaccharide—*See* Iron Supplements (Systemic), 986
*Night Cast R*—Salicylic Acid and Sulfur (Topical), 1481
*Night Cast Regular Formula Mask-lotion*—Salicylic Acid and Sulfur (Topical), 1481
*Night Cast Special Formula Mask-lotion*—Resorcinol and Sulfur (Topical), 1454
*Night-Time Effervescent Cold*—Diphenhydramine, Phenylpropanolamine, and Aspirin—*See* Antihistamines, Decongestants, and Analgesics (Systemic), 316
*Nilstat*—Nystatin (Oral), 1243; Nystatin (Topical), 1245; Nystatin (Vaginal), 1246
Nilutamide (Systemic), 1751
Nimodipine—*See* Calcium Channel Blocking Agents (Systemic), 467, MC-16
*Nimotop*—Nimodipine—*See* Calcium Channel Blocking Agents (Systemic), 467, MC-16
*Niong*—Nitroglycerin—*See* Nitrates—Oral (Systemic), 1218
*Nipent*—Pentostatin (Systemic), 1314
N-IPV—Poliovirus Vaccine Inactivated Enhanced Potency—*See* Poliovirus Vaccine (Systemic), 1367
*Nisaval*—Pyrilamine—*See* Antihistamines (Systemic), 304
Nitrates—Lingual Aerosol (Systemic), 1216
Nitrates—Oral (Systemic), 1218
Nitrates—Sublingual, Chewable, or Buccal (Systemic), 1221
Nitrates—Topical (Systemic), 1224
Nitrazepam—*See* Benzodiazepines (Systemic), 389
*Nitro-Bid*—Nitroglycerin—*See* Nitrates—Topical (Systemic), 1224
*Nitrocap*—Nitroglycerin—*See* Nitrates—Oral (Systemic), 1218
*Nitrocap T.D.*—Nitroglycerin—*See* Nitrates—Oral (Systemic), 1218
*Nitrodisc*—Nitroglycerin—*See* Nitrates—Topical (Systemic), 1224
*Nitro-Dur*—Nitroglycerin—*See* Nitrates—Topical (Systemic), 1224
*Nitro-Dur II*—Nitroglycerin—*See* Nitrates—Topical (Systemic), 1224
*Nitrofuracot*—Nitrofurantoin (Systemic), 1227
Nitrofurantoin (Systemic), 1227, 1751, MC-16
*Nitrogard*—Nitroglycerin—*See* Nitrates—Sublingual, Chewable, or Buccal (Systemic), 1221
*Nitrogard SR*—Nitroglycerin—*See* Nitrates—Sublingual, Chewable, or Buccal (Systemic), 1221
Nitrogen mustard—*See* Mechlorethamine (Systemic), 1075; Mechlorethamine (Topical), 1077
Nitroglycerin—*See* Nitrates—Lingual Aerosol (Systemic), 1216; Nitrates—Oral (Systemic), 1218, MC-16; Nitrates—Sublingual, Chewable, or Buccal (Systemic), 1221, MC-16; Nitrates—Topical (Systemic), 1224

*Nitroglyn*—Nitroglycerin—*See* Nitrates—Oral (Systemic), 1218

*Nitrol*—Nitroglycerin—*See* Nitrates—Topical (Systemic), 1224

*Nitrolin*—Nitroglycerin—*See* Nitrates—Oral (Systemic), 1218

*Nitrolingual*—Nitroglycerin—*See* Nitrates—Lingual Aerosol (Systemic), 1216

*Nitronet*—Nitroglycerin—*See* Nitrates—Oral (Systemic), 1218

*Nitrong*—Nitroglycerin—*See* Nitrates—Oral (Systemic), 1218; Nitrates—Topical (Systemic), 1224

*Nitrong SR*—Nitroglycerin—*See* Nitrates—Oral (Systemic), 1218

Nitroprusside Urine Ketone Test—*See* Urine Glucose and Ketone Test Kits for Home Use, 1644

*Nitrospan*—Nitroglycerin—*See* Nitrates—Oral (Systemic), 1218

*Nitrostat*—Nitroglycerin—*See* Nitrates—Sublingual, Chewable, or Buccal (Systemic), 1221, MC-16; Nitrates—Topical (Systemic), 1224

Nitrous Oxide—*See* Anesthetics, General (Systemic), 243

*Nix Cream Rinse*—Permethrin (Topical), 1320, 1752

*Nix Dermal Cream*—Permethrin (Topical), 1752

Nizatidine—*See* Histamine $H_2$-receptor Antagonists (Systemic), 925, MC-16

*Nizoral*—Ketoconazole—*See* Antifungals, Azole (Systemic), 292, MC-13

*Nizoral Cream*—Ketoconazole (Topical), 1010

*Nizoral Shampoo*—Ketoconazole (Topical), 1010

*NoDoz*—Caffeine (Systemic), 463

*NoDoz Maximum Strength Caplets*—Caffeine (Systemic), 463

*Nolahist*—Phenindamine—*See* Antihistamines (Systemic), 304

*Nolamine*—Chlorpheniramine, Phenindamine, and Phenylpropanolamine—*See* Antihistamines and Decongestants (Systemic), 311

*Nolex LA*—Phenylpropanolamine and Guaifenesin—*See* Cough/Cold Combinations (Systemic), 637

*Nolvadex*—Tamoxifen (Systemic), 1559, MC-21

*Nolvadex-D*—Tamoxifen (Systemic), 1559

Nonoxinol 9—Nonoxynol 9—*See* Spermicides (Vaginal), 1512

Nonoxynol 9—*See* Spermicides (Vaginal), 1512

Nonsteroidal Anti-inflammatory Drugs (Systemic), 1229

*Noradex*—Orphenadrine (Systemic), 1260

*Noradryl*—Diphenhydramine—*See* Antihistamines (Systemic), 304

*Noralac*—Calcium and Magnesium Carbonates—*See* Antacids (Oral), 253

*Noraminic*—Chlorpheniramine and Phenylpropanolamine—*See* Antihistamines and Decongestants (Systemic), 311

*Noratuss II Liquid*—Pseudoephedrine, Dextromethorphan, and Guaifenesin—*See* Cough/Cold Combinations (Systemic), 637

*Norcet*—Hydrocodone and Acetaminophen—*See* Narcotic Analgesics and Acetaminophen (Systemic), 1181

*Norcet 7.5*—Hydrocodone and Acetaminophen—*See* Narcotic Analgesics and Acetaminophen (Systemic), 1181

*Nordette*—Levonorgestrel and Ethinyl Estradiol—*See* Estrogens and Progestins (Oral Contraceptives) (Systemic), 804, MC-13

*Nordryl*—Diphenhydramine—*See* Antihistamines (Systemic), 304

*Nordryl Cough*—Diphenhydramine—*See* Antihistamines (Systemic), 304

*Norel Plus*—Chlorpheniramine, Phenyltoloxamine, Phenylpropanolamine, and Acetaminophen—*See* Antihistamines, Decongestants, and Analgesics (Systemic), 316

Norethindrone—*See* Progestins (Systemic), 1402

Norethindrone Acetate and Ethinyl Estradiol—*See* Estrogens and Progestins (Oral Contraceptives) (Systemic), 804, MC-17

Norethindrone Acetate/Ethinyl Estradiol and Ferrous Fumarate (Systemic), MC-17

Norethindrone and Ethinyl Estradiol—*See* Estrogens and Progestins (Oral Contraceptives) (Systemic), 804, MC-16, MC-17

Norethindrone and Mestranol—*See* Estrogens and Progestins (Oral Contraceptives) (Systemic), 804, MC-17

*Norethin 1/35E*—Norethindrone and Ethinyl Estradiol—*See* Estrogens and Progestins (Oral Contraceptives) (Systemic), 804

*Norethin 1/50M*—Norethindrone and Mestranol—*See* Estrogens and Progestins (Oral Contraceptives) (Systemic), 804

Norethisterone—Norethindrone—*See* Progestins (Systemic), 1402

*Norfemac*—Bufexamac (Topical), 1745

*Norflex*—Orphenadrine (Systemic), 1260

Norfloxacin—*See* Fluoroquinolones (Systemic), 847, MC-17

Norfloxacin (Ophthalmic), 1241

*Norfranil*—Imipramine—*See* Antidepressants, Tricyclic (Systemic), 277

*Norgesic*—Orphenadrine, Aspirin, and Caffeine—*See* Orphenadrine and Aspirin (Systemic), 1262

*Norgesic Forte*—Orphenadrine, Aspirin, and Caffeine—*See* Orphenadrine and Aspirin (Systemic), 1262

Norgestimate and Ethinyl Estradiol—*See* Estrogens and Progestins (Oral Contraceptives) (Systemic), 804

Norgestrel—*See* Progestins (Systemic), 1402

Norgestrel and Ethinyl Estradiol—*See* Estrogens and Progestins (Oral Contraceptives) (Systemic), 804, MC-17

*Norinyl 1/50*—Norethindrone and Mestranol—*See* Estrogens and Progestins (Oral Contraceptives) (Systemic), 804

*Norinyl 1+35*—Norethindrone and Ethinyl Estradiol—*See* Estrogens and Progestins (Oral Contraceptives) (Systemic), 804

*Norinyl 1+50*—Norethindrone and Mestranol—*See* Estrogens and Progestins (Oral Contraceptives) (Systemic), 804

*Norlutate*—Norethindrone—*See* Progestins (Systemic), 1402

*Norlutin*—Norethindrone—*See* Progestins (Systemic), 1402

*Normatane*—Brompheniramine, Phenylephrine, and Phenylpropanolamine—*See* Antihistamines and Decongestants (Systemic), 311

*Normatane DC*—Brompheniramine, Phenylpropanolamine, and Codeine—*See* Cough/Cold Combinations (Systemic), 637

*Normodyne*—Labetalol—*See* Beta-adrenergic Blocking Agents (Systemic), 404, MC-13

*Noroxin*—Norfloxacin—*See* Fluoroquinolones (Systemic), 847, MC-17; Norfloxacin (Ophthalmic), 1241

*Norpace*—Disopyramide (Systemic), 734, MC-8

*Norpace CR*—Disopyramide (Systemic), 734, MC-8

*Norpanth*—Propantheline—*See* Anticholinergics/Antispasmodics (Systemic), 258

*Norphadrine*—Orphenadrine, Aspirin, and Caffeine—*See* Orphenadrine and Aspirin (Systemic), 1262

*Norphadrine Forte*—Orphenadrine, Aspirin, and Caffeine—*See* Orphenadrine and Aspirin (Systemic), 1262

*Norpramin*—Desipramine—*See* Antidepressants, Tricyclic (Systemic), 277, MC-6

*Nor-Pred T.B.A.*—Prednisolone—*See* Corticosteroids/Corticotropin—Glucocorticoid Effects (Systemic), 630

*Nor-QD*—Norethindrone—*See* Progestins (Systemic), 1402

Nortriptyline—*See* Antidepressants, Tricyclic (Systemic), 277, MC-17

*Nortussin*—Guaifenesin (Systemic), 892

*Nortussin with Codeine*—Codeine and Guaifenesin—*See* Cough/Cold Combinations (Systemic), 637

*Norvasc*—Amlodipine (Systemic), 207, MC-1

*Norwich Aspirin*—Aspirin—*See* Salicylates (Systemic), 1473

*Norwood Sunburn Spray*—Lidocaine—*See* Anesthetics (Topical), 240

*Norzine*—Thiethylperazine (Systemic), 1594

*Nostrilla Long-Acting Nasal Decongestant*—Oxymetazoline (Nasal), 1274

*Nostril Spray Pump*—Phenylephrine (Nasal), 1343

*Nostril Spray Pump Mild*—Phenylephrine (Nasal), 1343

*Novafed*—Pseudoephedrine (Systemic), 1412

*Novafed A*—Chlorpheniramine and Pseudoephedrine—*See* Antihistamines and Decongestants (Systemic), 311

*Novagest Expectorant w/Codeine*—Pseudoephedrine, Codeine, and Guaifenesin—*See* Cough/Cold Combinations (Systemic), 637

*Novahistex*—Chlorpheniramine and Pseudoephedrine—*See* Antihistamines and Decongestants (Systemic), 311

*Novahistex C*—Phenylephrine and Codeine—*See* Cough/Cold Combinations (Systemic), 637

*Novahistex DH*—Phenylephrine and Hydrocodone—*See* Cough/Cold Combinations (Systemic), 637

*Novahistex DH Expectorant*—Diphenylpyraline, Phenylephrine, Hydrocodone, and Guaifenesin—*See* Cough/Cold Combinations (Systemic), 637

*Novahistex DM*—Diphenylpyraline, Phenylephrine, and Dextromethorphan—*See* Cough/Cold Combinations (Systemic), 637

*Novahistine*—Chlorpheniramine and Phenylephrine—*See* Antihistamines and Decongestants (Systemic), 311

*Novahistine DH*—Diphenylpyraline, Phenylephrine, and Hydrocodone—*See* Cough/Cold Combinations (Systemic), 637

*Novahistine DH Expectorant*—Diphenylpyraline, Phenylephrine, Hydrocodone, and Guaifenesin—*See* Cough/Cold Combinations (Systemic), 637

*Novahistine DH Liquid*—Chlorpheniramine, Pseudoephedrine, and Codeine—*See* Cough/Cold Combinations (Systemic), 637

*Novahistine DMX Liquid*—Pseudoephedrine, Dextromethorphan, and Guaifenesin—*See* Cough/Cold Combinations (Systemic), 637

*Novahistine Expectorant*—Pseudoephedrine, Codeine, and Guaifenesin—*See* Cough/Cold Combinations (Systemic), 637

*Novamoxin*—Amoxicillin—*See* Penicillins (Systemic), 1299

*Novantrone*—Mitoxantrone (Systemic), 1149

*Nova Rectal*—Pentobarbital—*See* Barbiturates (Systemic), 370

*Novasen*—Aspirin—*See* Salicylates (Systemic), 1473

*Nova-T*—Copper-T 200Ag IUD—*See* Copper Intrauterine Devices (IUDs), 605

*Novo-Alprazol*—Alprazolam—*See* Benzodiazepines (Systemic), 389

*Novo-Ampicillin*—Ampicillin—*See* Penicillins (Systemic), 1299

*Novo-Atenol*—Atenolol—*See* Beta-adrenergic Blocking Agents (Systemic), 404

*Novo-AZT*—Zidovudine (Systemic), 1689

*Novobetamet*—Betamethasone—*See* Corticosteroids—Medium to Very High Potency (Topical), 626

*Novo-Butamide*—Tolbutamide—*See* Antidiabetics, Oral (Systemic), 283

*Novocain*—Procaine—*See* Anesthetics (Parenteral-Local), 235

*Novocarbamaz*—Carbamazepine (Systemic), 481

*Novo-Chlorhydrate*—Chloral Hydrate (Systemic), 509

*Novochlorocap*—Chloramphenicol (Systemic), 517

*Novo-Chlorpromazine*—Chlorpromazine—*See* Phenothiazines (Systemic), 1330

*Novocimetine*—Cimetidine—*See* Histamine H$_2$-receptor Antagonists (Systemic), 925

*Novo-Clopate*—Clorazepate—*See* Benzodiazepines (Systemic), 389

*Novo-Cloxin*—Cloxacillin—*See* Penicillins (Systemic), 1299

*Novo-Difenac*—Diclofenac—*See* Nonsteroidal Anti-inflammatory Drugs (Systemic), 1229

*Novo-Difenac SR*—Diclofenac—*See* Nonsteroidal Anti-inflammatory Drugs (Systemic), 1229

*Novo-Diflunisal*—Diflunisal—*See* Nonsteroidal Anti-inflammatory Drugs (Systemic), 1229

*Novodigoxin*—Digoxin—*See* Digitalis Medicines (Systemic), 716

*Novo-Diltazem*—Diltiazem—*See* Calcium Channel Blocking Agents (Systemic), 467

*Novo-Dimenate*—Dimenhydrinate—*See* Antihistamines (Systemic), 304

*Novodipam*—Diazepam—*See* Benzodiazepines (Systemic), 389

*Novodipiradol*—Dipyridamole (Diagnostic), 731; Dipyridamole (Therapeutic), 732

*Novodoparil*—Methyldopa and Hydrochlorothiazide—*See* Methyldopa and Thiazide Diuretics (Systemic), 1114

*Novo-Doxepin*—Doxepin—*See* Antidepressants, Tricyclic (Systemic), 277

*Novodoxylin*—Doxycycline—*See* Tetracyclines (Systemic), 1570

*Novoferrogluc*—Ferrous Gluconate—*See* Iron Supplements (Systemic), 986

*Novoferrosulfa*—Ferrous Sulfate—*See* Iron Supplements (Systemic), 986

*Novofibrate*—Clofibrate (Systemic), 572

*Novoflupam*—Flurazepam—*See* Benzodiazepines (Systemic), 389

*Novo-Flurazine*—Trifluoperazine—*See* Phenothiazines (Systemic), 1330

*Novo-Flurprofen*—Flurbiprofen—*See* Nonsteroidal Anti-inflammatory Drugs (Systemic), 1229

*Novo-Folacid*—Folic Acid (Vitamin $B_9$) (Systemic), 857

*Novofumar*—Ferrous Fumarate—*See* Iron Supplements (Systemic), 986

*Novogesic C8*—Acetaminophen, Codeine, and Caffeine—*See* Narcotic Analgesics and Acetaminophen (Systemic), 1181

*Novogesic C15*—Acetaminophen, Codeine, and Caffeine—*See* Narcotic Analgesics and Acetaminophen (Systemic), 1181

*Novogesic C30*—Acetaminophen, Codeine, and Caffeine—*See* Narcotic Analgesics and Acetaminophen (Systemic), 1181

*Novo-Glyburide*—Glyburide—*See* Antidiabetics, Oral (Systemic), 283

*Novo-Hydrazide*—Hydrochlorothiazide—*See* Diuretics, Thiazide (Systemic), 749

*Novohydrocort*—Hydrocortisone Acetate—*See* Corticosteroids—Low Potency (Topical), 624

*Novo-Hydroxyzin*—Hydroxyzine—*See* Antihistamines (Systemic), 304

*Novo-Hylazin*—Hydralazine (Systemic), 931

*Novo-Keto-EC*—Ketoprofen—*See* Nonsteroidal Anti-inflammatory Drugs (Systemic), 1229

*Novolente-K*—Potassium Chloride—*See* Potassium Supplements (Systemic), 1373

*Novo-Lexin*—Cephalexin—*See* Cephalosporins (Systemic), 498

*Novolin 70/30*—Insulin, Isophane, Human, and Insulin Human—*See* Insulin (Systemic), 961

*Novolin ge 10/90*—Insulin, Isophane, Human, and Insulin Human—*See* Insulin (Systemic), 961

*Novolin ge 20/80*—Insulin, Isophane, Human, and Insulin Human—*See* Insulin (Systemic), 961

*Novolin ge 30/70*—Insulin, Isophane, Human, and Insulin Human—*See* Insulin (Systemic), 961

*Novolin ge 40/60*—Insulin, Isophane, Human, and Insulin Human—*See* Insulin (Systemic), 961

*Novolin ge 50/50*—Insulin, Isophane, Human, and Insulin Human—*See* Insulin (Systemic), 961

*Novolin ge Lente*—Insulin Zinc, Human—*See* Insulin (Systemic), 961

*Novolin ge NPH*—Insulin, Isophane, Human—*See* Insulin (Systemic), 961

*Novolin ge Toronto*—Insulin Human—*See* Insulin (Systemic), 961

*Novolin ge Ultralente*—Insulin Zinc, Extended, Human—*See* Insulin (Systemic), 961

*Novolin L*—Insulin Zinc, Human—*See* Insulin (Systemic), 961

*Novolin N*—Insulin, Isophane, Human—*See* Insulin (Systemic), 961

*Novolin R*—Insulin Human—*See* Insulin (Systemic), 961

*Novo-Lorazem*—Lorazepam—*See* Benzodiazepines (Systemic), 389

*Novomedopa*—Methyldopa (Systemic), 1111

*Novo-Methacin*—Indomethacin—*See* Nonsteroidal Anti-inflammatory Drugs (Systemic), 1229

*Novometoprol*—Metoprolol—*See* Beta-adrenergic Blocking Agents (Systemic), 404

*Novo-Naprox*—Naproxen—*See* Nonsteroidal Anti-inflammatory Drugs (Systemic), 1229

*Novo-Naprox Sodium*—Naproxen—*See* Nonsteroidal Anti-inflammatory Drugs (Systemic), 1229

*Novo-Naprox Sodium DS*—Naproxen—*See* Nonsteroidal Anti-inflammatory Drugs (Systemic), 1229

*Novo-Niacin*—Niacin—For High Cholesterol (Systemic), 1206; Niacin (Vitamin $B_3$) (Systemic), 1208

*Novonidazol*—Metronidazole (Systemic), 1125

*Novo-Nifedin*—Nifedipine—*See* Calcium Channel Blocking Agents (Systemic), 467

*Novopentobarb*—Pentobarbital—*See* Barbiturates (Systemic), 370

*Novo-Pen-VK*—Penicillin V—*See* Penicillins (Systemic), 1299

*Novo-Peridol*—Haloperidol (Systemic), 910

*Novo-Pheniram*—Chlorpheniramine—*See* Antihistamines (Systemic), 304

*Novo-Pindol*—Pindolol—*See* Beta-adrenergic Blocking Agents (Systemic), 404

*Novo-Pirocam*—Piroxicam—*See* Nonsteroidal Anti-inflammatory Drugs (Systemic), 1229

*Novopoxide*—Chlordiazepoxide—*See* Benzodiazepines (Systemic), 389

*Novopramine*—Imipramine—*See* Antidepressants, Tricyclic (Systemic), 277

*Novopranol*—Propranolol—*See* Beta-adrenergic Blocking Agents (Systemic), 404

*Novo-Profen*—Ibuprofen—*See* Nonsteroidal Anti-inflammatory Drugs (Systemic), 1229

*Novo-Propamide*—Chlorpropamide—*See* Antidiabetics, Oral (Systemic), 283

*Novopropoxyn*—Propoxyphene—*See* Narcotic Analgesics—For Pain Relief (Systemic), 1176

*Novopropoxyn Compound*—Propoxyphene, Aspirin, and Caffeine—*See* Narcotic Analgesics and Aspirin (Systemic), 1185

*Novopyrazone*—Sulfinpyrazone (Systemic), 1538

*Novoquinidin*—Quinidine (Systemic), 1428

*Novoquinine*—Quinine (Systemic), 1430

*Novoreserpine*—Reserpine—*See* Rauwolfia Alkaloids (Systemic), 1442

*Novo-Ridazine*—Thioridazine—*See* Phenothiazines (Systemic), 1330

*Novo-Rythro*—Erythromycin Ethylsuccinate—*See* Erythromycins (Systemic), 786

*Novo-rythro*—Erythromycin Estolate—*See* Erythromycins (Systemic), 786; Erythromycin Stearate—*See* Erythromycins (Systemic), 786

*Novo-rythro Encap*—Erythromycin Base—*See* Erythromycins (Systemic), 786

*Novo-Salmol*—Albuterol—*See* Bronchodilators, Adrenergic (Inhalation), 430; Bronchodilators, Adrenergic (Oral/Injection), 436

*Novosecobarb*—Secobarbital—*See* Barbiturates (Systemic), 370

*Novosemide*—Furosemide—*See* Diuretics, Loop (Systemic), 738

*Novosorbide*—Isosorbide Dinitrate—*See* Nitrates—Oral (Systemic), 1218

*Novosoxazole*—Sulfisoxazole—*See* Sulfonamides (Systemic), 1542

*Novospiroton*—Spironolactone—*See* Diuretics, Potassium-sparing (Systemic), 742

*Novo-Spirozine*—Spironolactone and Hydrochlorothiazide—*See* Diuretics, Potassium-sparing and Hydrochlorothiazide (Systemic), 745

*Novo-Sundac*—Sulindac—*See* Nonsteroidal Anti-inflammatory Drugs (Systemic), 1229

*Novo-Tamoxifen*—Tamoxifen (Systemic), 1559

*Novo-Terfenadine*—Terfenadine—*See* Antihistamines (Systemic), 304

*Novotetra*—Tetracycline—*See* Tetracyclines (Systemic), 1570

*Novo-Thalidone*—Chlorthalidone—*See* Diuretics, Thiazide (Systemic), 749

*Novo-Timol*—Timolol—*See* Beta-adrenergic Blocking Agents (Systemic), 404

*Novo-Tolmetin*—Tolmetin—*See* Nonsteroidal Anti-inflammatory Drugs (Systemic), 1229

*Novo-Triamzide*—Triamterene and Hydrochlorothiazide—*See* Diuretics, Potassium-sparing and Hydrochlorothiazide (Systemic), 745

*Novotrimel*—Sulfamethoxazole and Trimethoprim (Systemic), 1529

*Novotrimel DS*—Sulfamethoxazole and Trimethoprim (Systemic), 1529

*Novo-Triolam*—Triazolam—*See* Benzodiazepines (Systemic), 389

*Novotriphyl*—Oxtriphylline—*See* Bronchodilators, Xanthine-derivative (Systemic), 442

*Novo-Tripramine*—Trimipramine—*See* Antidepressants, Tricyclic (Systemic), 277

*Novotriptyn*—Amitriptyline—*See* Antidepressants, Tricyclic (Systemic), 277

*Novo-Veramil*—Verapamil—*See* Calcium Channel Blocking Agents (Systemic), 467

*Novoxapam*—Oxazepam—*See* Benzodiazepines (Systemic), 389

*Noxzema Anti-Acne Gel*—Salicylic Acid (Topical), 1478

*Noxzema Anti-Acne Pads Maximum Strength*—Salicylic Acid (Topical), 1478

*Noxzema Anti-Acne Pads Regular Strength*—Salicylic Acid (Topical), 1478

*Noxzema Clear-ups Maximum Strength 10 Lotion*—Benzoyl Peroxide (Topical), 397

*Noxzema Clear-ups On-The-Spot 10 Lotion*—Benzoyl Peroxide (Topical), 397

*Nozinan*—Methotrimeprazine—*See* Phenothiazines (Systemic), 1330

*Nozinan Liquid*—Methotrimeprazine—*See* Phenothiazines (Systemic), 1330

*Nozinan Oral Drops*—Methotrimeprazine—*See* Phenothiazines (Systemic), 1330

*NP-27 Cream*—Tolnaftate (Topical), 1617

*NPH Iletin*—Insulin, Isophane—*See* Insulin (Systemic), 961

*NPH Iletin I*—Insulin, Isophane—*See* Insulin (Systemic), 961

*NPH Iletin II*—Insulin, Isophane—*See* Insulin (Systemic), 961

*NPH Insulin*—Insulin, Isophane—*See* Insulin (Systemic), 961

NPH insulin—Insulin, Isophane—*See* Insulin (Systemic), 961

*NPH-N*—Insulin, Isophane—*See* Insulin (Systemic), 961

*NP-27 Powder*—Tolnaftate (Topical), 1617

*NP-27 Solution*—Tolnaftate (Topical), 1617

*NP-27 Spray Powder*—Tolnaftate (Topical), 1617

*NTS*—Nitroglycerin—*See* Nitrates—Topical (Systemic), 1224

*NTZ Long Acting Decongestant Nasal Spray*—Oxymetazoline (Nasal), 1274

*NTZ Long Acting Decongestant Nose Drops*—Oxymetazoline (Nasal), 1274

*Nu-Alpraz*—Alprazolam—*See* Benzodiazepines (Systemic), 389

*Nu-Amoxi*—Amoxicillin—*See* Penicillins (Systemic), 1299

*Nu-Ampi*—Ampicillin—*See* Penicillins (Systemic), 1299

*Nubain*—Nalbuphine—*See* Narcotic Analgesics—For Pain Relief (Systemic), 1176; Narcotic Analgesics—For Surgery and Obstetrics (Systemic), 1179

*Nu-Cal*—Calcium Carbonate—*See* Calcium Supplements (Systemic), 472

*Nu-Cephalex*—Cephalexin—*See* Cephalosporins (Systemic), 498

*Nu-Cloxi*—Cloxacillin—*See* Penicillins (Systemic), 1299

*Nucochem*—Pseudoephedrine and Codeine—*See* Cough/Cold Combinations (Systemic), 637

*Nucochem Expectorant*—Pseudoephedrine, Codeine, and Guaifenesin—*See* Cough/Cold Combinations (Systemic), 637

*Nucochem Pediatric Expectorant*—Pseudoephedrine, Codeine, and Guaifenesin—*See* Cough/Cold Combinations (Systemic), 637

*Nucofed*—Pseudoephedrine and Codeine—*See* Cough/Cold Combinations (Systemic), 637

*Nucofed Expectorant*—Pseudoephedrine, Codeine, and Guaifenesin—*See* Cough/Cold Combinations (Systemic), 637

*Nucofed Pediatric Expectorant*—Pseudoephedrine, Codeine, and Guaifenesin—*See* Cough/Cold Combinations (Systemic), 637

*Nu-Cotrimox*—Sulfamethoxazole and Trimethoprim (Systemic), 1529

*Nu-Cotrimox DS*—Sulfamethoxazole and Trimethoprim (Systemic), 1529

*Nucotuss Expectorant*—Pseudoephedrine, Codeine, and Guaifenesin—*See* Cough/Cold Combinations (Systemic), 637

*Nucotuss Pediatric Expectorant*—Pseudoephedrine, Codeine, and Guaifenesin—*See* Cough/Cold Combinations (Systemic), 637

*Nu-Diclo*—Diclofenac—*See* Nonsteroidal Anti-inflammatory Drugs (Systemic), 1229

*Nu-Diltiaz*—Diltiazem—*See* Calcium Channel Blocking Agents (Systemic), 467

*Nu-Flurbiprofen*—Flurbiprofen—*See* Nonsteroidal Anti-inflammatory Drugs (Systemic), 1229

*Nu-Ibuprofen*—Ibuprofen—*See* Nonsteroidal Anti-inflammatory Drugs (Systemic), 1229

*Nu-Indo*—Indomethacin—*See* Nonsteroidal Anti-inflammatory Drugs (Systemic), 1229

*Nu-Iron*—Iron-Polysaccharide—*See* Iron Supplements (Systemic), 986

*Nu-Iron 150*—Iron-Polysaccharide—*See* Iron Supplements (Systemic), 986

*Nujol*—Mineral Oil—*See* Laxatives (Oral), 1017

*Nu-Loraz*—Lorazepam—*See* Benzodiazepines (Systemic), 389

*Nulytely*—Polyethylene Glycol and Electrolytes (Local), 1369

*Nu-Medopa*—Methyldopa (Systemic), 1751

*Nu-Metop*—Metoprolol (Systemic), 1751

*Numorphan*—Oxymorphone—*See* Narcotic Analgesics—For Pain Relief (Systemic), 1176

*Numzident*—Benzocaine—*See* Anesthetics (Dental), 229

*Num-Zit Gel*—Benzocaine—*See* Anesthetics (Dental), 229

*Num-Zit Lotion*—Benzocaine—*See* Anesthetics (Dental), 229

*Nu-Naprox*—Naproxen—*See* Nonsteroidal Anti-inflammatory Drugs (Systemic), 1229

*Nu-Nifed*—Nifedipine—*See* Calcium Channel Blocking Agents (Systemic), 467

*Nu-Pen-VK*—Penicillin V—*See* Penicillins (Systemic), 1299

*Nupercainal*—Dibucaine—*See* Anesthetics (Rectal), 237

*Nupercainal Cream*—Dibucaine—*See* Anesthetics (Topical), 240

*Nupercainal Ointment*—Dibucaine—*See* Anesthetics (Topical), 240

*Nu-Pirox*—Piroxicam—*See* Nonsteroidal Anti-inflammatory Drugs (Systemic), 1229

*Nuprin*—Ibuprofen—*See* Nonsteroidal Anti-inflammatory Drugs (Systemic), 1229

*Nuprin Caplets*—Ibuprofen—*See* Nonsteroidal Anti-inflammatory Drugs (Systemic), 1229

*Nursoy*—Infant Formulas, Soy-based—*See* Infant Formulas (Systemic), 958

*Nu-Sulindac*—Sulindac—*See* Nonsteroidal Anti-inflammatory Drugs (Systemic), 1229

*Nu-Tetra*—Tetracycline—*See* Tetracyclines (Systemic), 1570

*Nutracort*—Hydrocortisone—*See* Corticosteroids—Low Potency (Topical), 624

*Nutramigen*—Infant Formulas, Hypoallergenic—*See* Infant Formulas (Systemic), 958

*Nutren 1.0*—Enteral Nutrition Formula, Polymeric—*See* Enteral Nutrition Formulas (Systemic), 769

*Nutren 1.5*—Enteral Nutrition Formula, Polymeric—*See* Enteral Nutrition Formulas (Systemic), 769

*Nutren 2.0*—Enteral Nutrition Formula, Polymeric—*See* Enteral Nutrition Formulas (Systemic), 769

*Nutren 1.0 with Fiber*—Enteral Nutrition Formula, Fiber-containing—*See* Enteral Nutrition Formulas (Systemic), 769

*Nu-Triazo*—Triazolam—*See* Benzodiazepines (Systemic), 389

*NutriHep*—Enteral Nutrition Formula, Disease-specific—*See* Enteral Nutrition Formulas (Systemic), 769

*Nutrilan*—Enteral Nutrition Formula, Polymeric—*See* Enteral Nutrition Formulas (Systemic), 769

*NutriSource*—Enteral Nutrition Formula, Fiber-containing—*See* Enteral Nutrition Formulas (Systemic), 769

*NutriSource HN*—Enteral Nutrition Formula, Fiber-containing—*See* Enteral Nutrition Formulas (Systemic), 769

*NutriVent*—Enteral Nutrition Formula, Disease-specific—*See* Enteral Nutrition Formulas (Systemic), 769

*Nu-Verap*—Verapamil—*See* Calcium Channel Blocking Agents (Systemic), 467

*Nyaderm*—Nystatin (Topical), 1245; Nystatin (Vaginal), 1246

*Nydrazid*—Isoniazid (Systemic), 992

Nylidrin (Systemic), 1242

Nystatin (Oral), 1243

Nystatin (Topical), 1245

Nystatin (Vaginal), 1246

Nystatin and Triamcinolone (Topical), 1247

*Nystex*—Nystatin (Oral), 1243; Nystatin (Topical), 1245

*Nytcold Medicine*—Doxylamine, Pseudoephedrine, Dextromethorphan, and Acetaminophen—*See* Cough/Cold Combinations (Systemic), 637

*Nytilax*—Sennosides—*See* Laxatives (Oral), 1017

*Nytime Cold Medicine Liquid*—Doxylamine, Pseudoephedrine, Dextromethorphan, and Acetaminophen—*See* Cough/Cold Combinations (Systemic), 637

*Nytol with DPH*—Diphenhydramine—*See* Antihistamines (Systemic), 304

*Nytol Maximum Strength*—Diphenhydramine—*See* Antihistamines (Systemic), 304

# O

*OB*—Testosterone and Estradiol—*See* Androgens and Estrogens (Systemic), 225

*Obalan*—Phendimetrazine—*See* Appetite Suppressants (Systemic), 339

*Obe-Nix*—Phentermine—*See* Appetite Suppressants (Systemic), 339

*Obezine*—Phendimetrazine—*See* Appetite Suppressants (Systemic), 339

*Occlucort*—Betamethasone (Topical), 1745

*Occlusal-HP Topical Solution*—Salicylic Acid (Topical), 1478

*Occlusal Topical Solution*—Salicylic Acid (Topical), 1478

*OCL*—Polyethylene Glycol and Electrolytes (Local), 1369

*Octamide*—Metoclopramide (Systemic), 1123

*Octamide PFS*—Metoclopramide (Systemic), 1123

*Octatropine*—Anisotropine—*See* Anticholinergics/Antispasmodics (Systemic), 258

*Octicair*—Neomycin, Polymyxin B, and Hydrocortisone (Otic), 1204

*Octocaine*—Lidocaine—*See* Anesthetics (Parenteral-Local), 235

*Octocaine-50*—Lidocaine—*See* Anesthetics (Parenteral-Local), 235

*Octocaine-100*—Lidocaine—*See* Anesthetics (Parenteral-Local), 235

Octoxinol—Octoxynol 9—*See* Spermicides (Vaginal), 1512

Octoxynol 9—*See* Spermicides (Vaginal), 1512

Octreotide (Systemic), 1251

*Ocu-Caine*—Proparacaine—*See* Anesthetics (Ophthalmic), 234

*Ocu-Carpine*—Pilocarpine (Ophthalmic), 1355

*Ocu-Chlor Ophthalmic Ointment*—Chloramphenicol (Ophthalmic), 514

*Ocu-Chlor Ophthalmic Solution*—Chloramphenicol (Ophthalmic), 514

*OcuClear*—Oxymetazoline (Ophthalmic), 1276

*Ocu-Dex*—Dexamethasone—*See* Corticosteroids (Ophthalmic), 620

*Ocufen*—Flurbiprofen—*See* Anti-inflammatory Agents, Nonsteroidal (Ophthalmic), 330

*Ocuflox*—Ofloxacin (Ophthalmic), 1252

*Ocugestrin*—Phenylephrine (Ophthalmic), 1345

*Ocu-Mycin*—Gentamicin (Ophthalmic), 872

*Ocu-Pentolate*—Cyclopentolate (Ophthalmic), 664

*Ocu-Phrin Sterile Eye Drops*—Phenylephrine (Ophthalmic), 1345

*Ocu-Phrin Sterile Ophthalmic Solution*—Phenylephrine (Ophthalmic), 1345

*Ocu-Pred*—Prednisolone—*See* Corticosteroids (Ophthalmic), 620

*Ocu-Pred-A*—Prednisolone—*See* Corticosteroids (Ophthalmic), 620

*Ocu-Pred Forte*—Prednisolone—*See* Corticosteroids (Ophthalmic), 620

*Ocupress*—Carteolol—*See* Beta-adrenergic Blocking Agents (Ophthalmic), 402

*Ocusert Pilo-20*—Pilocarpine (Ophthalmic), 1355

*Ocusert Pilo-40*—Pilocarpine (Ophthalmic), 1355

*Ocu-Spor-B*—Neomycin, Polymyxin B, and Bacitracin (Ophthalmic), 1199

*Ocu-Spor-G*—Neomycin, Polymyxin B, and Gramicidin (Ophthalmic), 1201

*Ocusporin*—Neomycin, Polymyxin B, and Bacitracin (Ophthalmic), 1199

*Ocu-Sul-10*—Sulfacetamide—*See* Sulfonamides (Ophthalmic), 1540

*Ocu-Sul-15*—Sulfacetamide—*See* Sulfonamides (Ophthalmic), 1540

*Ocu-Sul-30*—Sulfacetamide—*See* Sulfonamides (Ophthalmic), 1540

*Ocusulf-10*—Sulfacetamide—*See* Sulfonamides (Ophthalmic), 1540

*Ocutricin HC*—Neomycin, Polymyxin B, and Hydrocortisone (Ophthalmic), 1203

*Ocutricin Ophthalmic Ointment*—Neomycin, Polymyxin B, and Bacitracin (Ophthalmic), 1199

*Ocutricin Ophthalmic Solution*—Neomycin, Polymyxin B, and Gramicidin (Ophthalmic), 1201

*Ocu-Tropic*—Tropicamide (Ophthalmic), 1634

*Ocu-Tropine*—Atropine—*See* Atropine/Homatropine/Scopolamine (Ophthalmic), 354

*Ocu-Zoline Sterile Ophthalmic Solution*—Naphazoline (Ophthalmic), 1174

*Oestrilin*—Estrone—*See* Estrogens (Vaginal), 801

*Off-Ezy Topical Solution Corn & Callus Remover Kit*—Salicylic Acid (Topical), 1478

*Off-Ezy Topical Solution Wart Removal Kit*—Salicylic Acid (Topical), 1478

*O-Flex*—Orphenadrine (Systemic), 1260

Ofloxacin—*See* Fluoroquinolones (Systemic), 847, MC-17

Ofloxacin (Ophthalmic), 1252

*Ogen*—Estropipate—*See* Estrogens (Systemic), 795; (Vaginal), 801

*Ogen .625*—Estropipate—*See* Estrogens (Systemic), 795

*Ogen 1.25*—Estropipate—*See* Estrogens (Systemic), 795

*Ogen 2.5*—Estropipate—*See* Estrogens (Systemic), 795

*Oligo-CRM*—Haemophilus b Conjugate Vaccine (HbOC—Diphtheria CRM$_{197}$ Protein Conjugate)—*See* Haemophilus b Conjugate Vaccine (Systemic), 905

Olsalazine (Oral), 1254

Omeprazole (Systemic), 1255, MC-17

*Omnicol*—Chlorpheniramine, Phenindamine, Phenylephrine, Dextromethorphan, Acetaminophen, Salicylamide, Caffeine, and Ascorbic Acid—*See* Cough/Cold Combinations (Systemic), 637

*OMNIhist L.A.*—Chlorpheniramine, Phenylephrine, and Methscopolamine—*See* Antihistamines, Decongestants, and Anticholinergics (Systemic), 322

*Omnipen*—Ampicillin—*See* Penicillins (Systemic), 1299, MC-2

*Omnipen-N*—Ampicillin—*See* Penicillins (Systemic), 1299

*Omni-Tuss*—Chlorpheniramine, Phenyltoloxamine, Ephedrine, Codeine, and Guaiacol Carbonate—*See* Cough/Cold Combinations (Systemic), 637

*Oncaspar*—Pegaspargase (Systemic), 1751

*Oncovin*—Vincristine (Systemic), 1662

Ondansetron (Systemic), 1257, 1751, MC-17

*One-Alpha*—Alfacalcidol—*See* Vitamin D and Related Compounds (Systemic), 1669

*Ophthacet*—Sulfacetamide—*See* Sulfonamides (Ophthalmic), 1540

*Ophthaine*—Proparacaine—*See* Anesthetics (Ophthalmic), 234

*Ophthalmic*—Neomycin, Polymyxin B, and Bacitracin (Ophthalmic), 1199

*Ophthetic*—Proparacaine—*See* Anesthetics (Ophthalmic), 234

*Ophtho-Chloram Ophthalmic Solution*—Chloramphenicol (Ophthalmic), 514

*Ophthochlor Ophthalmic Solution*—Chloramphenicol (Ophthalmic), 514

*Ophtho-Dipivefrin*—Dipivefrin (Ophthalmic), 729

*Ophtho-Tate*—Prednisolone—*See* Corticosteroids (Ophthalmic), 620

Opium Injection—*See* Narcotic Analgesics—For Pain Relief (Systemic), 1176

Opium Preparations (Systemic), 1258

Opium Tincture—*See* Opium Preparations (Systemic), 1258

*Opticrom*—Cromolyn (Ophthalmic), 656

*Optimine*—Azatadine—*See* Antihistamines (Systemic), 304

*OptiPranolol*—Metipranolol—*See* Beta-adrenergic Blocking Agents (Ophthalmic), 402

*OPV*—Poliovirus Vaccine Live Oral—*See* Poliovirus Vaccine (Systemic), 1367

*Orabase, Baby*—Benzocaine—*See* Anesthetics (Dental), 229

*Orabase-B with Benzocaine*—Benzocaine—*See* Anesthetics (Dental), 229

*Orabase-HCA*—Hydrocortisone—*See* Corticosteroids (Dental), 610

---

© 1994  The United States Pharmacopeial Convention, Inc.

*Oracit*—Sodium Citrate and Citric Acid—*See* Citrates (Systemic), 554

*Oracort*—Triamcinolone—*See* Corticosteroids (Dental), 610

*Oradexon*—Dexamethasone—*See* Corticosteroids/Corticotropin—Glucocorticoid Effects (Systemic), 630

*Oragrafin Calcium*—Ipodate—*See* Cholecystographic Agents, Oral (Diagnostic), 536

*Oragrafin Sodium*—Ipodate—*See* Cholecystographic Agents, Oral (Diagnostic), 536

*Orajel, Baby*—Benzocaine—*See* Anesthetics (Dental), 229

*Orajel Extra Strength*—Benzocaine—*See* Anesthetics (Dental), 229

*Orajel Liquid*—Benzocaine—*See* Anesthetics (Dental), 229

*Orajel Maximum Strength*—Benzocaine—*See* Anesthetics (Dental), 229

*Orajel Nighttime Formula, Baby*—Benzocaine—*See* Anesthetics (Dental), 229

*Oralone*—Triamcinolone—*See* Corticosteroids (Dental), 610

Oral Rehydration Salts—*See* Carbohydrates and Electrolytes (Systemic), 484

*Oraminic II*—Brompheniramine—*See* Antihistamines (Systemic), 304

*Oraminic Spancaps*—Chlorpheniramine and Phenylpropanolamine—*See* Antihistamines and Decongestants (Systemic), 311

*Orap*—Pimozide (Systemic), 1357

*Oraphen-PD*—Acetaminophen (Systemic), 161

*Orasone 1*—Prednisone—*See* Corticosteroids/Corticotropin—Glucocorticoid Effects (Systemic), 630

*Orasone 5*—Prednisone—*See* Corticosteroids/Corticotropin—Glucocorticoid Effects (Systemic), 630

*Orasone 10*—Prednisone—*See* Corticosteroids/Corticotropin—Glucocorticoid Effects (Systemic), 630

*Orasone 20*—Prednisone—*See* Corticosteroids/Corticotropin—Glucocorticoid Effects (Systemic), 630

*Orasone 50*—Prednisone—*See* Corticosteroids/Corticotropin—Glucocorticoid Effects (Systemic), 630

*Oratect Gel*—Benzocaine—*See* Anesthetics (Dental), 229

*Orazinc*—Zinc Sulfate—*See* Zinc Supplements (Systemic), 1691

*Orbenin*—Cloxacillin—*See* Penicillins (Systemic), 1299

*Orciprenaline*—Metaproterenol—*See* Bronchodilators, Adrenergic (Inhalation), 430; Bronchodilators, Adrenergic (Oral/Injection), 436

*Ordrine AT*—Phenylpropanolamine and Caramiphen—*See* Cough/Cold Combinations (Systemic), 637

*Oretic*—Hydrochlorothiazide—*See* Diuretics, Thiazide (Systemic), 749, MC-11

*Oreticyl*—Deserpidine and Hydrochlorothiazide—*See* Rauwolfia Alkaloids and Thiazide Diuretics (Systemic), 1445

*Oreticyl Forte*—Deserpidine and Hydrochlorothiazide—*See* Rauwolfia Alkaloids and Thiazide Diuretics (Systemic), 1445

*Oreton*—Methyltestosterone—*See* Androgens (Systemic), 221

*Orflagen*—Orphenadrine (Systemic), 1260

*Orfro*—Orphenadrine (Systemic), 1260

*Orimune*—Poliovirus Vaccine Live Oral—*See* Poliovirus Vaccine (Systemic), 1367

*Orinase*—Tolbutamide—*See* Antidiabetics, Oral (Systemic), 283, MC-23

*Ormazine*—Chlorpromazine—*See* Phenothiazines (Systemic), 1330

*Ornade*—Chlorpheniramine and Phenylpropanolamine—*See* Antihistamines and Decongestants (Systemic), 311

*Ornade-A.F.*—Chlorpheniramine and Phenylpropanolamine—*See* Antihistamines and Decongestants (Systemic), 311

*Ornade-DM 10*—Chlorpheniramine, Phenylpropanolamine, and Dextromethorphan—*See* Cough/Cold Combinations (Systemic), 637

*Ornade-DM 15*—Chlorpheniramine, Phenylpropanolamine, and Dextromethorphan—*See* Cough/Cold Combinations (Systemic), 637

*Ornade-DM 30*—Chlorpheniramine, Phenylpropanolamine, and Dextromethorphan—*See* Cough/Cold Combinations (Systemic), 637

*Ornade Expectorant*—Chlorpheniramine, Phenylpropanolamine, and Guaifenesin—*See* Cough/Cold Combinations (Systemic), 637

*Ornade Spansules*—Chlorpheniramine and Phenylpropanolamine—*See* Antihistamines and Decongestants (Systemic), 311, MC-4

*Ornex•DM 15*—Dextromethorphan (Systemic), 701

*Ornex•DM 30*—Dextromethorphan (Systemic), 701

*Ornex Maximum Strength Caplets*—Pseudoephedrine and Acetaminophen—*See* Decongestants and Analgesics (Systemic), 691

*Ornex No Drowsiness Caplets*—Pseudoephedrine and Acetaminophen—*See* Decongestants and Analgesics (Systemic), 691

*Ornex Severe Cold No Drowsiness Caplets*—Pseudoephedrine, Dextromethorphan, and Acetaminophen—*See* Cough/Cold Combinations (Systemic), 637

*Ornidyl*—Eflornithine (Systemic), 764

Orphenadrine (Systemic), 1260

Orphenadrine and Aspirin (Systemic), 1262

Orphenadrine, Aspirin, and Caffeine—*See* Orphenadrine and Aspirin (Systemic), 1262

*Orphenagesic*—Orphenadrine, Aspirin, and Caffeine—*See* Orphenadrine and Aspirin (Systemic), 1262

*Orphenagesic Forte*—Orphenadrine, Aspirin, and Caffeine—*See* Orphenadrine and Aspirin (Systemic), 1262

*Orphenate*—Orphenadrine (Systemic), 1260

ORS-bicarbonate—Oral Rehydration Salts—*See* Carbohydrates and Electrolytes (Systemic), 484

ORS-citrate—Oral Rehydration Salts—*See* Carbohydrates and Electrolytes (Systemic), 484

*Ortega Otic-M*—Neomycin, Polymyxin B, and Hydrocortisone (Otic), 1204

*Ortho 0.5/35*—Norethindrone and Ethinyl Estradiol—*See* Estrogens and Progestins (Oral Contraceptives) (Systemic), 804

*Ortho 1/35*—Norethindrone and Ethinyl Estradiol—*See* Estrogens and Progestins (Oral Contraceptives) (Systemic), 804

*Ortho 7/7/7*—Norethindrone and Ethinyl Estradiol—*See* Estrogens and Progestins (Oral Contraceptives) (Systemic), 804

*Ortho 10/11*—Norethindrone and Ethinyl Estradiol—*See* Estrogens and Progestins (Oral Contraceptives) (Systemic), 804

*Oxy Clean Extra Strength Medicated Pads*—Salicylic Acid (Topical), 1478

*Oxy Clean Extra Strength Skin Cleanser Topical Solution*—Salicylic Acid (Topical), 1478

*Oxy Clean Medicated Cleanser*—Salicylic Acid (Topical), 1478

*Oxy Clean Medicated Pads Maximum Strength*—Salicylic Acid (Topical), 1478

*Oxy Clean Medicated Pads Regular Strength*—Salicylic Acid (Topical), 1478

*Oxy Clean Medicated Pads Sensitive Skin*—Salicylic Acid (Topical), 1478

*Oxy Clean Medicated Soap*—Salicylic Acid (Topical), 1478

*Oxy Clean Regular Strength Medicated Cleanser Topical Solution*—Salicylic Acid (Topical), 1478

*Oxy Clean Regular Strength Medicated Pads*—Salicylic Acid (Topical), 1478

*Oxy Clean Sensitive Skin Cleanser Topical Solution*—Salicylic Acid (Topical), 1478

*Oxy Clean Sensitive Skin Pads*—Salicylic Acid (Topical), 1478

*Oxycocet*—Oxycodone and Acetaminophen—*See* Narcotic Analgesics and Acetaminophen (Systemic), 1181

*Oxycodan*—Oxycodone and Aspirin—*See* Narcotic Analgesics and Aspirin (Systemic), 1185

Oxycodone—*See* Narcotic Analgesics—For Pain Relief (Systemic), 1176, MC-18

Oxycodone and Acetaminophen—*See* Narcotic Analgesics and Acetaminophen (Systemic), 1181, MC-18

Oxycodone with APAP—Oxycodone and Acetaminophen—*See* Narcotic Analgesics and Acetaminophen (Systemic), 1181

Oxycodone and Aspirin—*See* Narcotic Analgesics and Aspirin (Systemic), 1185, MC-18

*Oxy 10 Daily Face Wash*—Benzoyl Peroxide (Topical), 397

*Oxyderm 5 Lotion*—Benzoyl Peroxide (Topical), 397

*Oxyderm 10 Lotion*—Benzoyl Peroxide (Topical), 397

*Oxyderm 20 Lotion*—Benzoyl Peroxide (Topical), 397

Oxymetazoline (Nasal), 1274

Oxymetazoline (Ophthalmic), 1276

Oxymetholone—*See* Anabolic Steroids (Systemic), 218

Oxymorphone—*See* Narcotic Analgesics—For Pain Relief (Systemic), 1176

*Oxy Night Watch Maximum Strength Lotion*—Salicylic Acid (Topical), 1478

*Oxy Night Watch Night Time Acne Medication Extra Strength Lotion*—Salicylic Acid (Topical), 1478

*Oxy Night Watch Night Time Acne Medication Regular Strength Lotion*—Salicylic Acid (Topical), 1478

*Oxy Night Watch Sensitive Skin Lotion*—Salicylic Acid (Topical), 1478

Oxyphencyclimine—*See* Anticholinergics/Antispasmodics (Systemic), 258

*Oxy Sensitive Skin Vanishing Formula Lotion*—Salicylic Acid (Topical), 1478

Oxytetracycline—*See* Tetracyclines (Systemic), 1570

*Oxy 5 Tinted Lotion*—Benzoyl Peroxide (Topical), 397

*Oxy 10 Tinted Lotion*—Benzoyl Peroxide (Topical), 397

Oxytocin (Systemic), 1277

*Oxy 5 Vanishing Formula Lotion*—Benzoyl Peroxide (Topical), 397

*Oxy 5 Vanishing Lotion*—Benzoyl Peroxide (Topical), 397

*Oxy 10 Vanishing Lotion*—Benzoyl Peroxide (Topical), 397

*Oysco*—Calcium Carbonate—*See* Calcium Supplements (Systemic), 472

*Oysco 500 Chewable*—Calcium Carbonate—*See* Calcium Supplements (Systemic), 472

*Oyst-Cal 500*—Calcium Carbonate—*See* Calcium Supplements (Systemic), 472

*Oyst-Cal 500 Chewable*—Calcium Carbonate—*See* Calcium Supplements (Systemic), 472

*Oystercal 500*—Calcium Carbonate—*See* Calcium Supplements (Systemic), 472

# P

*Pacaps*—Butalbital, Acetaminophen, and Caffeine—*See* Butalbital and Acetaminophen (Systemic), 453

Paclitaxel (Systemic), 1279, 1751

*P-A-C Revised Formula*—Aspirin and Caffeine—*See* Salicylates (Systemic), 1473

*Palafer*—Ferrous Fumarate—*See* Iron Supplements (Systemic), 986

*Palafer Pediatric Drops*—Ferrous Fumarate—*See* Iron Supplements (Systemic), 986

*Palmiron*—Ferrous Fumarate—*See* Iron Supplements (Systemic), 986

*Paludrine*—Proguanil (Systemic), 1406

*Pamelor*—Nortriptyline—*See* Antidepressants, Tricyclic (Systemic), 277, MC-17

Pamidronate (Systemic), 1281

*Pamine*—Methscopolamine—*See* Anticholinergics/Antispasmodics (Systemic), 258

P-aminoclonidine—*See* Apraclonidine (Ophthalmic), 342

*Pamprin-IB*—Ibuprofen—*See* Nonsteroidal Anti-inflammatory Drugs (Systemic), 1229

*Panadol*—Acetaminophen (Systemic), 161

*Panadol, Children's*—Acetaminophen (Systemic), 161

*Panadol Extra Strength*—Acetaminophen (Systemic), 161

*Panadol, Infants'*—Acetaminophen (Systemic), 161

*Panadol Junior Strength Caplets*—Acetaminophen (Systemic), 161

*Panadol Maximum Strength Caplets*—Acetaminophen (Systemic), 161

*Panadol Maximum Strength Tablets*—Acetaminophen (Systemic), 161

*Pancoate*—Pancrelipase (Systemic), 1284

*Pancrease*—Pancrelipase (Systemic), 1284, MC-18

*Pancrease MT 4*—Pancrelipase (Systemic), 1284

*Pancrease MT 10*—Pancrelipase (Systemic), 1284

*Pancrease MT 16*—Pancrelipase (Systemic), 1284

Pancreatin, Pepsin, Bile Salts, Hyoscyamine, Atropine, Scopolamine, and Phenobarbital (Systemic), 1282

Pancrelipase (Systemic), 1284, MC-18

*Panectyl*—Trimeprazine—*See* Antihistamines, Phenothiazine-derivative (Systemic), 325

*Panesclerina*—Probucol (Systemic), 1395

*Panmycin*—Tetracycline—*See* Tetracyclines (Systemic), 1570, MC-22

*PanOxyl AQ 2½ Gel*—Benzoyl Peroxide (Topical), 397

*PanOxyl AQ 5 Gel*—Benzoyl Peroxide (Topical), 397
*PanOxyl AQ 10 Gel*—Benzoyl Peroxide (Topical), 397
*PanOxyl 5 Bar*—Benzoyl Peroxide (Topical), 397
*PanOxyl 10 Bar*—Benzoyl Peroxide (Topical), 397
*PanOxyl 5 Gel*—Benzoyl Peroxide (Topical), 397
*PanOxyl 10 Gel*—Benzoyl Peroxide (Topical), 397
*PanOxyl 15 Gel*—Benzoyl Peroxide (Topical), 397
*PanOxyl 20 Gel*—Benzoyl Peroxide (Topical), 397
*Panshape M*—Phentermine—*See* Appetite Suppressants (Systemic), 339
*Pantopon*—Opium—*See* Narcotic Analgesics—For Pain Relief (Systemic), 1176
Pantothenic Acid (Vitamin B₅) (Systemic), 1286
*Panwarfin*—Warfarin—*See* Anticoagulants (Systemic), 262
*Papaveretum*—Opium—*See* Narcotic Analgesics—For Pain Relief (Systemic), 1176
Papaverine (Intracavernosal), 1287
Papaverine (Systemic), 1289
*Paplex*—Salicylic Acid (Topical), 1478
*Paplex Ultra*—Salicylic Acid (Topical), 1478
*Papulex*—Nicotinamide (Topical), 1751
Paracetamol—*See* Acetaminophen (Systemic), 161
*Paradione*—Paramethadione—*See* Anticonvulsants, Dione (Systemic), 265
*Paraflex*—Chlorzoxazone—*See* Skeletal Muscle Relaxants (Systemic), 1495
*Parafon Forte*—Chlorzoxazone and Acetaminophen (Systemic), 533
*Parafon Forte DSC*—Chlorzoxazone—*See* Skeletal Muscle Relaxants (Systemic), 1495, MC-5
*ParaGard-T 380A*—Copper-T 380A IUD—*See* Copper Intrauterine Devices (IUDs), 605
*Para-Hist HD*—Chlorpheniramine, Phenylephrine, and Hydrocodone—*See* Cough/Cold Combinations (Systemic), 637
*Paral*—Paraldehyde (Systemic), 1290
Paraldehyde (Systemic), 1290
Paramethadione—*See* Anticonvulsants, Dione (Systemic), 265
*Parapectolin*—Attapulgite (Oral), 359
*Paraplatin*—Carboplatin (Systemic), 491
*Paraplatin-AQ*—Carboplatin (Systemic), 491
*Parathar*—Teriparatide (Systemic), 1564
*Par Decon*—Chlorpheniramine, Phenyltoloxamine, Phenylephrine, and Phenylpropanolamine (Systemic), 1746
*Par-Drix*—Dexbrompheniramine and Pseudoephedrine—*See* Antihistamines and Decongestants (Systemic), 311
Paregoric—*See* Opium Preparations (Systemic), 1258
*Parepectolin*—Kaolin, Pectin, and Paregoric (Systemic), 1008
*Parfenac*—Bufexamac (Topical), 1745
*Parhist SR*—Chlorpheniramine and Phenylpropanolamine—*See* Antihistamines and Decongestants (Systemic), 311
*Parlodel*—Bromocriptine (Systemic), 427, MC-3
*Parnate*—Tranylcypromine—*See* Antidepressants, Monoamine Oxidase (MAO) Inhibitor (Systemic), 274, MC-23
Paroxetine (Systemic), 1293, MC-18
*Parsidol*—Ethopropazine—*See* Antidyskinetics (Systemic), 287
*Parsitan*—Ethopropazine—*See* Antidyskinetics (Systemic), 287

*Partapp*—Brompheniramine and Phenylpropanolamine—*See* Antihistamines and Decongestants (Systemic), 311
*Partapp TD*—Brompheniramine, Phenylephrine, and Phenylpropanolamine—*See* Antihistamines and Decongestants (Systemic), 311
*Partuss LA*—Phenylpropanolamine and Guaifenesin—*See* Cough/Cold Combinations (Systemic), 637
*Parzine*—Phendimetrazine—*See* Appetite Suppressants (Systemic), 339
PAS—*See* Aminosalicylate Sodium (Systemic), 204
*Pathilon*—Tridihexethyl—*See* Anticholinergics/Antispasmodics (Systemic), 258
*Pathocil*—Dicloxacillin—*See* Penicillins (Systemic), 1299
*Pavabid*—Papaverine (Systemic), 1289
*Pavabid HP*—Papaverine (Systemic), 1289
*Pavacels*—Papaverine (Systemic), 1289
*Pavacot*—Papaverine (Systemic), 1289
*Pavagen*—Papaverine (Systemic), 1289
*Pavarine*—Papaverine (Systemic), 1289
*Pavased*—Papaverine (Systemic), 1289
*Pavatine*—Papaverine (Systemic), 1289
*Pavatym*—Papaverine (Systemic), 1289
*Paveral*—Codeine—*See* Narcotic Analgesics—For Pain Relief (Systemic), 1176
*Paverolan*—Papaverine (Systemic), 1289
*Paxil*—Paroxetine (Systemic), 1293, MC-18
*Paxipam*—Halazepam—*See* Benzodiazepines (Systemic), 389
PBZ—Tripelennamine—*See* Antihistamines (Systemic), 304
PBZ-SR—Tripelennamine—*See* Antihistamines (Systemic), 304
PCE—Erythromycin Base—*See* Erythromycins (Systemic), 786, MC-9
*PediaCare Allergy Formula*—Chlorpheniramine—*See* Antihistamines (Systemic), 304
*PediaCare Children's Cough-Cold*—Chlorpheniramine, Pseudoephedrine, and Dextromethorphan—*See* Cough/Cold Combinations (Systemic), 637
*PediaCare Cold Formula*—Chlorpheniramine and Pseudoephedrine—*See* Antihistamines and Decongestants (Systemic), 311
*PediaCare Cough-Cold*—Chlorpheniramine, Pseudoephedrine, and Dextromethorphan—*See* Cough/Cold Combinations (Systemic), 637
*PediaCare Infants' Oral Decongestant Drops*—Pseudoephedrine (Systemic), 1412
*PediaCare Night Rest Cough-Cold Liquid*—Chlorpheniramine, Pseudoephedrine, and Dextromethorphan—*See* Cough/Cold Combinations (Systemic), 637
*Pediacof Cough*—Chlorpheniramine, Phenylephrine, Codeine, and Potassium Iodide—*See* Cough/Cold Combinations (Systemic), 637
*Pediaflor*—Sodium Fluoride (Systemic), 1502
*Pedialyte*—Dextrose and Electrolytes—*See* Carbohydrates and Electrolytes (Systemic), 484
*Pediapred*—Prednisolone—*See* Corticosteroids/Corticotropin—Glucocorticoid Effects (Systemic), 630
*Pediasure*—Enteral Nutrition Formula, Polymeric—*See* Enteral Nutrition Formulas (Systemic), 769
*Pediasure with Fiber*—Enteral Nutrition Formula, Fiber-containing—*See* Enteral Nutrition Formulas (Systemic), 769

Pericyazine—*See* Phenothiazines (Systemic), 1330

*Peridex*—Chlorhexidine (Dental), 526

*Peridol*—Haloperidol (Systemic), 910

*PerioGard*—Chlorhexidine (Dental), 1745

*Peritrate*—Pentaerythritol Tetranitrate—*See* Nitrates—Oral (Systemic), 1218

*Peritrate Forte*—Pentaerythritol Tetranitrate—*See* Nitrates—Oral (Systemic), 1218

*Peritrate SA*—Pentaerythritol Tetranitrate—*See* Nitrates—Oral (Systemic), 1218

*Permapen*—Penicillin G—*See* Penicillins (Systemic), 1299

*Permax*—Pergolide (Systemic), 1319

Permethrin (Topical), 1320, 1752

*Permitil*—Fluphenazine—*See* Phenothiazines (Systemic), 1330

*Permitil Concentrate*—Fluphenazine—*See* Phenothiazines (Systemic), 1330

*Pernox Lemon Medicated Scrub Cleanser*—Salicylic Acid and Sulfur (Topical), 1481

*Pernox Lotion Lathering Abradant Scrub Cleanser*—Salicylic Acid and Sulfur (Topical), 1481

*Pernox Lotion Lathering Scrub Cleanser*—Salicylic Acid and Sulfur (Topical), 1481

*Pernox Regular Medicated Scrub Cleanser*—Salicylic Acid and Sulfur (Topical), 1481

Perphenazine—*See* Phenothiazines (Systemic), 1330

Perphenazine and Amitriptyline (Systemic), 1322, MC-18

*Persa-Gel 5*—Benzoyl Peroxide (Topical), 397

*Persa-Gel 10*—Benzoyl Peroxide (Topical), 397

*Persa-Gel W 5*—Benzoyl Peroxide (Topical), 397

*Persa-Gel W 10*—Benzoyl Peroxide (Topical), 397

*Persantine*—Dipyridamole (Diagnostic), 731; Dipyridamole (Therapeutic), 732, MC-7

*Pertofrane*—Desipramine—*See* Antidepressants, Tricyclic (Systemic), 277

*Pertussin All Night CS*—Dextromethorphan and Guaifenesin—*See* Cough/Cold Combinations (Systemic), 637

*Pertussin All Night PM*—Doxylamine, Pseudoephedrine, Dextromethorphan, and Acetaminophen—*See* Cough/Cold Combinations (Systemic), 637

*Pertussin Cough Suppressant*—Dextromethorphan (Systemic), 701

*Pertussin CS*—Dextromethorphan (Systemic), 701

*Pertussin ES*—Dextromethorphan (Systemic), 701

Pethidine—Meperidine—*See* Narcotic Analgesics—For Pain Relief (Systemic), 1176; Narcotic Analgesics—For Surgery and Obstetrics (Systemic), 1179

P.E.T.N.—Pentaerythritol Tetranitrate—*See* Nitrates—Oral (Systemic), 1218

*Petrogalar Plain*—Mineral Oil—*See* Laxatives (Oral), 1017

PFA—*See* Foscarnet (Systemic), 860

*Pfeiffer's Allergy*—Chlorpheniramine—*See* Antihistamines (Systemic), 304

*Pfizerpen*—Penicillin G—*See* Penicillins (Systemic), 1299

*Pfizerpen-AS*—Penicillin G—*See* Penicillins (Systemic), 1299

PGE$_1$—*See* Alprostadil (Intracavernosal), 191

*Phanadex*—Pyrilamine, Phenylpropanolamine, Dextromethorphan, Guaifenesin, Potassium Citrate, and Citric Acid—*See* Cough/Cold Combinations (Systemic), 637

*Phanatuss*—Dextromethorphan and Guaifenesin—*See* Cough/Cold Combinations (Systemic), 637

*Pharma-Cort*—Hydrocortisone Acetate—*See* Corticosteroids—Low Potency (Topical), 624

*Pharmagesic*—Butalbital, Acetaminophen, and Caffeine—*See* Butalbital and Acetaminophen (Systemic), 453

*Pharmatex*—Benzalkonium Chloride—*See* Spermicides (Vaginal), 1512

*Pharmorubicin PFS*—Epirubicin (Systemic), 1748

*Pharmorubicin RDF*—Epirubicin (Systemic), 1748

*Phazyme*—Simethicone (Oral), 1494

*Phazyme 55*—Simethicone (Oral), 1494

*Phazyme 95*—Simethicone (Oral), 1494

Phenacemide (Systemic), 1325

Phenacetylcarbamide—*See* Phenacemide (Systemic), 1325

*Phenahist-TR*—Chlorpheniramine, Phenylephrine, Phenylpropanolamine, Atropine, Hyoscyamine, and Scopolamine—*See* Antihistamines, Decongestants, and Anticholinergics (Systemic), 322

*Phenameth DM*—Promethazine and Dextromethorphan—*See* Cough/Cold Combinations (Systemic), 637

*Phenameth VC with Codeine*—Promethazine, Phenylephrine, and Codeine—*See* Cough/Cold Combinations (Systemic), 637

*PhenAPAP No. 2*—Phenylpropanolamine and Acetaminophen—*See* Decongestants and Analgesics (Systemic), 691

*Phenapap Sinus Headache & Congestion*—Chlorpheniramine, Pseudoephedrine, and Acetaminophen—*See* Antihistamines, Decongestants, and Analgesics (Systemic), 316

*Phenaphen Caplets*—Acetaminophen (Systemic), 161

*Phenaphen-650 with Codeine*—Acetaminophen and Codeine—*See* Narcotic Analgesics and Acetaminophen (Systemic), 1181, MC-1

*Phenaphen with Codeine No.2*—Acetaminophen and Codeine—*See* Narcotic Analgesics and Acetaminophen (Systemic), 1181, MC-1; Phenobarbital, Aspirin, and Codeine—*See* Barbiturates, Aspirin, and Codeine (Systemic), 376

*Phenaphen with Codeine No.3*—Acetaminophen and Codeine—*See* Narcotic Analgesics and Acetaminophen (Systemic), 1181, MC-1; Phenobarbital, Aspirin, and Codeine—*See* Barbiturates, Aspirin, and Codeine (Systemic), 376

*Phenaphen with Codeine No.4*—Acetaminophen and Codeine—*See* Narcotic Analgesics and Acetaminophen (Systemic), 1181, MC-1; Phenobarbital, Aspirin, and Codeine—*See* Barbiturates, Aspirin, and Codeine (Systemic), 376

*Phenate T.D.*—Chlorpheniramine, Phenylpropanolamine, and Acetaminophen—*See* Antihistamines, Decongestants, and Analgesics (Systemic), 316

*Phenazine 25*—Promethazine—*See* Antihistamines, Phenothiazine-derivative (Systemic), 325

*Phenazine 50*—Promethazine—*See* Antihistamines, Phenothiazine-derivative (Systemic), 325

*Phenazo*—Phenazopyridine (Systemic), 1327

*Phenazodine*—Phenazopyridine (Systemic), 1327

Phenazopyridine (Systemic), 1327

*Phencen-50*—Promethazine—*See* Antihistamines, Phenothiazine-derivative (Systemic), 325

*Phenchlor SHA*—Chlorpheniramine, Phenylephrine, Phenylpropanolamine, Atropine, Hyoscyamine, and Scopolamine—*See* Antihistamines, Decongestants, and Anticholinergics (Systemic), 322

*Phendiet*—Phendimetrazine—*See* Appetite Suppressants (Systemic), 339

*Phendiet-105*—Phendimetrazine—*See* Appetite Suppressants (Systemic), 339

*Phendimet*—Phendimetrazine—*See* Appetite Suppressants (Systemic), 339

Phendimetrazine—*See* Appetite Suppressants (Systemic), 339

*Phendry*—Diphenhydramine—*See* Antihistamines (Systemic), 304

*Phendry Children's Allergy Medicine*—Diphenhydramine—*See* Antihistamines (Systemic), 304

Phenelzine—*See* Antidepressants, Monoamine Oxidase (MAO) Inhibitor (Systemic), 274

*Phenergan*—Promethazine—*See* Antihistamines, Phenothiazine-derivative (Systemic), 325, MC-20

*Phenergan with Codeine*—Promethazine and Codeine—*See* Cough/Cold Combinations (Systemic), 637

*Phenergan with Dextromethorphan*—Promethazine and Dextromethorphan—*See* Cough/Cold Combinations (Systemic), 637

*Phenergan Fortis*—Promethazine—*See* Antihistamines, Phenothiazine-derivative (Systemic), 325

*Phenergan Plain*—Promethazine—*See* Antihistamines, Phenothiazine-derivative (Systemic), 325

*Phenergan VC*—Promethazine and Phenylephrine—*See* Antihistamines and Decongestants (Systemic), 311

*Phenergan VC with Codeine*—Promethazine, Phenylephrine, and Codeine—*See* Cough/Cold Combinations (Systemic), 637

*Phenerzine*—Promethazine—*See* Antihistamines, Phenothiazine-derivative (Systemic), 325

*Phenetron*—Chlorpheniramine—*See* Antihistamines (Systemic), 304

*Phenetron Lanacaps*—Chlorpheniramine—*See* Antihistamines (Systemic), 304

*Phenhist DH w/Codeine*—Chlorpheniramine, Pseudoephedrine, and Codeine—*See* Cough/Cold Combinations (Systemic), 637

*Phenhist Expectorant*—Pseudoephedrine, Codeine, and Guaifenesin—*See* Cough/Cold Combinations (Systemic), 637

Phenindamine—*See* Antihistamines (Systemic), 304

Phenindamine, Hydrocodone, and Guaifenesin—*See* Cough/Cold Combinations (Systemic), 637

Pheniramine, Codeine, and Guaifenesin—*See* Cough/Cold Combinations (Systemic), 637

Pheniramine and Phenylephrine—*See* Antihistamines and Decongestants (Systemic), 311

Pheniramine, Phenylephrine, and Acetaminophen—*See* Antihistamines, Decongestants, and Analgesics (Systemic), 316

Pheniramine, Phenylephrine, Codeine, Sodium Citrate, Sodium Salicylate, and Caffeine Citrate—*See* Cough/Cold Combinations (Systemic), 637

Pheniramine, Phenylephrine, and Dextromethorphan (Systemic), 1752

Pheniramine, Phenylephrine, Phenylpropanolamine, Hydrocodone, and Guaifenesin—*See* Cough/Cold Combinations (Systemic), 637

Pheniramine, Phenylephrine, Phenylpropanolamine, Hydrocodone, and Guaifenesin—*See* Antihistamines and Decongestants (Systemic), 311

Pheniramine, Phenylephrine, Sodium Salicylate, and Caffeine—*See* Antihistamines, Decongestants, and Analgesics (Systemic), 316

Pheniramine, Phenyltoloxamine, Pyrilamine, and Phenylpropanolamine—*See* Antihistamines and Decongestants (Systemic), 311

Pheniramine, Pyrilamine, Hydrocodone, and Potassium Citrate—*See* Cough/Cold Combinations (Systemic), 637

Pheniramine, Pyrilamine, Hydrocodone, Potassium Citrate, and Ascorbic Acid—*See* Cough/Cold Combinations (Systemic), 637

Pheniramine, Pyrilamine, Phenylephrine, Phenylpropanolamine, and Hydrocodone—*See* Cough/Cold Combinations (Systemic), 637, 1752

Pheniramine, Pyrilamine, and Phenylpropanolamine—*See* Antihistamines and Decongestants (Systemic), 311

Pheniramine, Pyrilamine, Phenylpropanolamine, and Codeine—*See* Cough/Cold Combinations (Systemic), 637

Pheniramine, Pyrilamine, Phenylpropanolamine, Codeine, Acetaminophen, and Caffeine—*See* Cough/Cold Combinations (Systemic), 637

Pheniramine, Pyrilamine, Phenylpropanolamine, and Dextromethorphan—*See* Cough/Cold Combinations (Systemic), 637

Pheniramine, Pyrilamine, Phenylpropanolamine, Dextromethorphan, and Ammonium Chloride—*See* Cough/Cold Combinations (Systemic), 637

Pheniramine, Pyrilamine, Phenylpropanolamine, Dextromethorphan, and Guaifenesin—*See* Cough/Cold Combinations (Systemic), 637

Pheniramine, Pyrilamine, Phenylpropanolamine, and Guaifenesin—*See* Cough/Cold Combinations (Systemic), 637

Pheniramine, Pyrilamine, Phenylpropanolamine, and Hydrocodone—*See* Cough/Cold Combinations (Systemic), 637

Pheniramine, Pyrilamine, Phenylpropanolamine, Hydrocodone, and Guaifenesin—*See* Cough/Cold Combinations (Systemic), 637

Phenobarbital—*See* Barbiturates (Systemic), 370, MC-18

Phenobarbital, Aspirin, and Codeine—*See* Barbiturates, Aspirin, and Codeine (Systemic), 376

*Phenoject-50*—Promethazine—*See* Antihistamines, Phenothiazine-derivative (Systemic), 325

*Phenolax*—Phenolphthalein—*See* Laxatives (Oral), 1017

Phenolphthalein—*See* Laxatives (Oral), 1017

*Phenolphthalein Petrogalar*—Mineral Oil and Phenolphthalein—*See* Laxatives (Oral), 1017

Phenol red—*See* Phenolsulfonphthalein (Diagnostic), 1328

Phenolsulfonphthalein (Diagnostic), 1328

Phenothiazines (Systemic), 1330

Phenoxybenzamine (Systemic), 1340

Phensuximide—*See* Anticonvulsants, Succinimide (Systemic), 271

*Phentercot*—Phentermine—*See* Appetite Suppressants (Systemic), 339

Phentermine—*See* Appetite Suppressants (Systemic), 339, MC-18

Phentolamine and Papaverine (Intracavernosal), 1341

*Phentride*—Phentermine—*See* Appetite Suppressants (Systemic), 339

*Phenurone*—Phenacemide (Systemic), 1325

Phenylalanine mustard—*See* Melphalan (Systemic), 1083

Phenylbutazone—*See* Nonsteroidal Anti-inflammatory Drugs (Systemic), 1229

*Phenyldrine*—Phenylpropanolamine (Systemic), 1347

Phenylephrine (Nasal), 1343

Phenylephrine (Ophthalmic), 1345

Phenylephrine and Acetaminophen—*See* Decongestants and Analgesics (Systemic), 691

Phenylephrine and Codeine—*See* Cough/Cold Combinations (Systemic), 637

Phenylephrine, Dextromethorphan, and Guaifenesin—*See* Cough/Cold Combinations (Systemic), 637

Phenylephrine and Guaifenesin—*See* Cough/Cold Combinations (Systemic), 637

Phenylephrine, Guaifenesin, Acetaminophen, Salicylamide, and Caffeine—*See* Cough/Cold Combinations (Systemic), 637

Phenylephrine and Hydrocodone—*See* Cough/Cold Combinations (Systemic), 637

Phenylephrine, Hydrocodone, and Guaifenesin—*See* Cough/Cold Combinations (Systemic), 637

Phenylephrine, Phenylpropanolamine, Carbetapentane, and Potassium Guaiacolsulfonate—*See* Cough/Cold Combinations (Systemic), 637

Phenylephrine, Phenylpropanolamine, Carbetapentane,and Potassium Guaiacolsulfonate—*See* Cough/Cold Combinations (Systemic), 637

Phenylephrine, Phenylpropanolamine, and Guaifenesin—*See* Cough/Cold Combinations (Systemic), 637, 1752, MC-18

*Phenylfenesin L.A.*—Phenylpropanolamine and Guaifenesin—*See* Cough/Cold Combinations (Systemic), 637

Phenylpropanolamine (Systemic), 1347

Phenylpropanolamine and Acetaminophen—*See* Decongestants and Analgesics (Systemic), 691

Phenylpropanolamine, Acetaminophen, and Aspirin—*See* Decongestants and Analgesics (Systemic), 691

Phenylpropanolamine, Acetaminophen, Salicylamide, and Caffeine—*See* Decongestants and Analgesics (Systemic), 691

Phenylpropanolamine and Aspirin—*See* Decongestants and Analgesics (Systemic), 691

Phenylpropanolamine and Caramiphen—*See* Cough/Cold Combinations (Systemic), 637, MC-18

Phenylpropanolamine, Codeine, and Guaifenesin—*See* Cough/Cold Combinations (Systemic), 637

Phenylpropanolamine and Dextromethorphan—*See* Cough/Cold Combinations (Systemic), 637

Phenylpropanolamine, Dextromethorphan, and Acetaminophen—*See* Cough/Cold Combinations (Systemic), 637

Phenylpropanolamine, Dextromethorphan, and Guaifenesin—*See* Cough/Cold Combinations (Systemic), 637, 1752

Phenylpropanolamine and Guaifenesin—*See* Cough/Cold Combinations (Systemic), 637, 1752, MC-18

Phenylpropanolamine and Hydrocodone—*See* Cough/Cold Combinations (Systemic), 637

Phenylpropanolamine, Hydrocodone, Guaifenesin,and Salicylamide—*See* Cough/Cold Combinations (Systemic), 637

Phenyltoloxamine and Hydrocodone—*See* Cough/Cold Combinations (Systemic), 637

Phenyltoloxamine, Phenylpropanolamine, and Acetaminophen—*See* Antihistamines, Decongestants, and Analgesics (Systemic), 316

*Phenytex*—Phenytoin—*See* Anticonvulsants, Hydantoin (Systemic), 267

Phenytoin—*See* Anticonvulsants, Hydantoin (Systemic), 267, MC-18

*Pherazine w/Codeine*—Promethazine and Codeine—*See* Cough/Cold Combinations (Systemic), 637

*Pherazine DM*—Promethazine and Dextromethorphan—*See* Cough/Cold Combinations (Systemic), 637

*Pherazine VC*—Promethazine and Phenylephrine—*See* Antihistamines and Decongestants (Systemic), 311

*Pherazine VC with Codeine*—Promethazine, Phenylephrine, and Codeine—*See* Cough/Cold Combinations (Systemic), 637

*Pheryl-E*—Vitamin E (Systemic), 1674

*Phetylureum*—Phenacemide (Systemic), 1325

*Phillips' Gelcaps*—Docusate and Phenolphthalein—*See* Laxatives (Oral), 1017

*Phillips' LaxCaps*—Docusate and Phenolphthalein—*See* Laxatives (Oral), 1017

*Phillips' Magnesia Tablets*—Magnesium Hydroxide—*See* Laxatives (Oral), 1017

*Phillips' Milk of Magnesia*—Magnesium Hydroxide—*See* Antacids (Oral), 253; Laxatives (Oral), 1017; Magnesium Supplements (Systemic), 1060

*pHisoAc BP 10 Cream*—Benzoyl Peroxide (Topical), 397

Phosphates (Systemic), 1349

*Phosphocol P 32*—Chromic Phosphate P 32 (Therapeutic), 542

*Phospholine Iodide*—Echothiophate—*See* Antiglaucoma Agents, Cholinergic, Long-acting (Ophthalmic), 299

Phosphonoformic acid—*See* Foscarnet (Systemic), 860

*Phrenilin*—Butalbital and Acetaminophen (Systemic), 453

*Phrenilin Forte*—Butalbital and Acetaminophen (Systemic), 453

*Phyllocontin*—Aminophylline—*See* Bronchodilators, Xanthine-derivative (Systemic), 442

*Phyllocontin-350*—Aminophylline—*See* Bronchodilators, Xanthine-derivative (Systemic), 442

Physostigmine (Ophthalmic), 1353

Phytomenadione—Phytonadione—*See* Vitamin K (Systemic), 1676

Phytonadione—*See* Vitamin K (Systemic), 1676

*Pilagan*—Pilocarpine (Ophthalmic), 1355

*Pilocar*—Pilocarpine (Ophthalmic), 1355

Pilocarpine (Ophthalmic), 1355

Pilocarpine (Systemic), 1752

*Pilokair*—Pilocarpine (Ophthalmic), 1355

*Pilopine HS*—Pilocarpine (Ophthalmic), 1355

*Piloptic-1*—Pilocarpine (Ophthalmic), 1355

*Piloptic-2*—Pilocarpine (Ophthalmic), 1355

*Piloptic-4*—Pilocarpine (Ophthalmic), 1355

*Pilostat*—Pilocarpine (Ophthalmic), 1355

*Pima*—Potassium Iodide (Systemic), 1371

Pimaricin—*See* Natamycin (Ophthalmic), 1189

Pimozide (Systemic), 1357

Pindolol—*See* Beta-adrenergic Blocking Agents (Systemic), 404, MC-19

Pindolol and Hydrochlorothiazide—*See* Beta-adrenergic Blocking Agents and Thiazide Diuretics (Systemic), 410

Piperacillin—*See* Penicillins (Systemic), 1299

Piperacillin and Tazobactam—*See* Penicillins and Beta-lactamase Inhibitors (Systemic), 1306

Piperazine (Systemic), 1359

Piperazine estrone sulfate—Estropipate—*See* Estrogens (Systemic), 795; Estrogens (Vaginal), 801

*Piportil L₄*—Pipotiazine—*See* Phenothiazines (Systemic), 1330

Pipotiazine—*See* Phenothiazines (Systemic), 1330

*Pipracil*—Piperacillin—*See* Penicillins (Systemic), 1299

*Pirbuterol*—*See* Bronchodilators, Adrenergic (Inhalation), 430

Pirenzepine—*See* Anticholinergics/Antispasmodics (Systemic), 258

Piroxicam—*See* Nonsteroidal Anti-inflammatory Drugs (Systemic), 1229, MC-19

*Pitocin*—Oxytocin (Systemic), 1277

*Pitressin*—Vasopressin (Systemic), 1657

*Pitrex Cream*—Tolnaftate (Topical), 1617

Pivampicillin—*See* Penicillins (Systemic), 1299

Pivmecillinam—*See* Penicillins (Systemic), 1299

Pizotyline (Systemic), 1752

*Placidyl*—Ethchlorvynol (Systemic), 810

*Plaquenil*—Hydroxychloroquine (Systemic), 937, MC-11

Plasma thromboplastin component (PTC)—*See* Factor IX (Systemic), 823

*Platinol*—Cisplatin (Systemic), 551

*Platinol-AQ*—Cisplatin (Systemic), 551

*Plegine*—Phendimetrazine—*See* Appetite Suppressants (Systemic), 339

*Plendil*—Felodipine—*See* Calcium Channel Blocking Agents (Systemic), 467, MC-10

Plicamycin (Systemic), 1362

*PMS Benztropine*—Benztropine—*See* Antidyskinetics (Systemic), 287

*PMS-Bismuth Subsalicylate*—Bismuth Subsalicylate (Oral), 421

*PMS-Chloral Hydrate*—Chloral Hydrate (Systemic), 509

*PMS Diazepam*—Diazepam—*See* Benzodiazepines (Systemic), 389

*PMS-Dimenhydrinate*—Dimenhydrinate—*See* Antihistamines (Systemic), 304

*PMS Dopazide*—Methyldopa and Hydrochlorothiazide—*See* Methyldopa and Thiazide Diuretics (Systemic), 1114

*PMS Egozinc*—Zinc Sulfate—*See* Zinc Supplements (Systemic), 1691

*PMS Ferrous Sulfate*—Ferrous Sulfate—*See* Iron Supplements (Systemic), 986

*PMS Haloperidol*—Haloperidol (Systemic), 910

*PMS Isoniazid*—Isoniazid (Systemic), 992

*PMS Levazine*—Perphenazine and Amitriptyline (Systemic), 1322

*PMS-Levothyroxine Sodium*—Levothyroxine—*See* Thyroid Hormones (Systemic), 1606

*PMS Lindane*—Lindane (Topical), 1042

*PMS-Methylphenidate*—Methylphenidate (Systemic), 1118

*PMS Nylidrin*—Nylidrin (Systemic), 1242

*PMS Nystatin*—Nystatin (Oral), 1243

*PMS-Oxtriphylline*—Oxtriphylline—*See* Bronchodilators, Xanthine-derivative (Systemic), 442

*PMS Perphenazine*—Perphenazine—*See* Phenothiazines (Systemic), 1330

*PMS Primidone*—Primidone (Systemic), 1388

*PMS Prochlorperazine*—Prochlorperazine—*See* Phenothiazines (Systemic), 1330

*PMS Procyclidine*—Procyclidine—*See* Antidyskinetics (Systemic), 287

*PMS-Progesterone*—Progesterone—*See* Progestins (Systemic), 1402

*pms Propranolol*—Propranolol—*See* Beta-adrenergic Blocking Agents (Systemic), 404

*pms-Pyrazinamide*—Pyrazinamide (Systemic), 1416

*PMS Sulfasalazine*—Sulfasalazine (Systemic), 1535

*PMS Sulfasalazine E.C.*—Sulfasalazine (Systemic), 1535

*PMS Theophylline*—Theophylline—*See* Bronchodilators, Xanthine-derivative (Systemic), 442

*PMS Thioridazine*—Thioridazine—*See* Phenothiazines (Systemic), 1330

*PMS Trifluoperazine*—Trifluoperazine—*See* Phenothiazines (Systemic), 1330

*PMS Trihexyphenidyl*—Trihexyphenidyl—*See* Antidyskinetics (Systemic), 287

*PMS-Yohimbine*—Yohimbine (Systemic), 1684

Pneumococcal Vaccine Polyvalent (Systemic), 1364

*Pneumomist*—Guaifenesin (Systemic), 892

*Pneumopent*—Pentamidine (Inhalation), 1311

*Pneumotussin HC*—Hydrocodone and Guaifenesin—*See* Cough/Cold Combinations (Systemic), 637

*Pneumovax 23*—Pneumococcal Vaccine Polyvalent (Systemic), 1364

*P.N. Ophthalmic*—Neomycin, Polymyxin B, and Gramicidin (Ophthalmic), 1201

*Pnu-Imune 23*—Pneumococcal Vaccine Polyvalent (Systemic), 1364

*Podocon-25*—Podophyllum (Topical), 1365

Podofilox (Topical), 1752

*Podofin*—Podophyllum (Topical), 1365

Podophyllum (Topical), 1365

*Poladex T.D.*—Dexchlorpheniramine—*See* Antihistamines (Systemic), 304

*Polaramine*—Dexchlorpheniramine—*See* Antihistamines (Systemic), 304

*Polaramine Expectorant*—Dexchlorpheniramine, Pseudoephedrine, and Guaifenesin—*See* Cough/Cold Combinations (Systemic), 637

*Polaramine Repetabs*—Dexchlorpheniramine—*See* Antihistamines (Systemic), 304

Poliovirus Vaccine (Systemic), 1367

Poliovirus Vaccine Inactivated—*See* Poliovirus Vaccine (Systemic), 1367

Poliovirus Vaccine Inactivated Enhanced Potency—*See* Poliovirus Vaccine (Systemic), 1367

Poliovirus Vaccine Live Oral—*See* Poliovirus Vaccine (Systemic), 1367

*Polocaine*—Mepivacaine—*See* Anesthetics (Parenteral-Local), 235

*Polocaine-MPF*—Mepivacaine—*See* Anesthetics (Parenteral-Local), 235

*Poloxalkol*—Poloxamer 188—*See* Laxatives (Oral), 1017

*Poloxamer 188*—*See* Laxatives (Oral), 1017

*Polycarbophil*—*See* Laxatives (Oral), 1017

*Polycillin*—Ampicillin—*See* Penicillins (Systemic), 1299

*Polycillin-N*—Ampicillin—*See* Penicillins (Systemic), 1299

*Polycitra-K*—Potassium Citrate and Citric Acid—*See* Citrates (Systemic), 554

*Polycitra-K Crystals*—Potassium Citrate and Citric Acid—*See* Citrates (Systemic), 554

*Polycitra-LC*—Tricitrates—*See* Citrates (Systemic), 554

*Polycitra Syrup*—Tricitrates—*See* Citrates (Systemic), 554

*Polycose*—Enteral Nutrition Formula, Modular—*See* Enteral Nutrition Formulas (Systemic), 769

Polyethylene Glycol and Electrolytes (Local), 1369

*Polygam*—Immune Globulin Intravenous (Human) (Systemic), 954

*Polygesic*—Hydrocodone and Acetaminophen—*See* Narcotic Analgesics and Acetaminophen (Systemic), 1181

*Poly-Histine-CS*—Brompheniramine, Phenylpropanolamine, and Codeine—*See* Cough/Cold Combinations (Systemic), 637

*Poly-Histine-D*—Pheniramine, Phenyltoloxamine, Pyrilamine, and Phenylpropanolamine—*See* Antihistamines and Decongestants (Systemic), 311

*Poly-Histine-DM*—Brompheniramine, Phenylpropanolamine, and Dextromethorphan—*See* Cough/Cold Combinations (Systemic), 637

*Poly-Histine-D Ped*—Pheniramine, Phenyltoloxamine, Pyrilamine, and Phenylpropanolamine—*See* Antihistamines and Decongestants (Systemic), 311

*Polymox*—Amoxicillin—*See* Penicillins (Systemic), 1299

Polymyxin B (Ophthalmic), 1753

*Polythiazide*—*See* Diuretics, Thiazide (Systemic), 749

*Poly-Vi-Flor*—Multiple Vitamins and Fluoride—*See* Vitamins and Fluoride (Systemic), 1678

*Ponderal*—Fenfluramine (Systemic), 830

*Ponderal Pacaps*—Fenfluramine (Systemic), 830

*Pondimin*—Fenfluramine (Systemic), 830

*Pondocillin*—Pivampicillin—*See* Penicillins (Systemic), 1299

*Ponstan*—Mefenamic Acid—*See* Nonsteroidal Anti-inflammatory Drugs (Systemic), 1229

*Ponstel*—Mefenamic Acid—*See* Nonsteroidal Anti-inflammatory Drugs (Systemic), 1229

*Pontocaine*—Tetracaine—*See* Anesthetics (Ophthalmic), 234; Anesthetics (Parenteral-Local), 235

*Pontocaine Cream*—Tetracaine—*See* Anesthetics (Rectal), 237; Anesthetics (Topical), 240

*Pontocaine Ointment*—Tetracaine and Menthol—*See* Anesthetics (Rectal), 237; Anesthetics (Topical), 240

*Portalac*—Lactulose—*See* Laxatives (Oral), 1017

*Postacne*—Alcohol and Sulfur (Topical), 183

*Posture*—Tribasic Calcium Phosphate—*See* Calcium Supplements (Systemic), 472

*Potaba*—Aminobenzoate Potassium (Systemic), 197

*Potaba Envules*—Aminobenzoate Potassium (Systemic), 197

*Potaba Powder*—Aminobenzoate Potassium (Systemic), 197

*Potage*—Potassium Chloride—*See* Potassium Supplements (Systemic), 1373

*Potasalan*—Potassium Chloride—*See* Potassium Supplements (Systemic), 1373

Potassium Acetate—*See* Potassium Supplements (Systemic), 1373

Potassium aminobenzoate—*See* Aminobenzoate Potassium (Systemic), 197

Potassium Bicarbonate—*See* Potassium Supplements (Systemic), 1373

Potassium Bicarbonate and Potassium Chloride—*See* Potassium Supplements (Systemic), 1373

Potassium Bicarbonate and Potassium Citrate—*See* Potassium Supplements (Systemic), 1373

Potassium Bitartrate and Sodium Bicarbonate—*See* Laxatives (Rectal), 1023

Potassium Chloride—*See* Potassium Supplements (Systemic), 1373, MC-19

Potassium Chloride, Potassium Bicarbonate, and Potassium Citrate—*See* Potassium Supplements (Systemic), 1373

Potassium Citrate—*See* Citrates (Systemic), 554

Potassium Citrate and Citric Acid—*See* Citrates (Systemic), 554

Potassium Citrate and Sodium Citrate—*See* Citrates (Systemic), 554

Potassium citrate, sodium citrate, and citric acid—Tricitrates—*See* Citrates (Systemic), 554

Potassium Gluconate—*See* Potassium Supplements (Systemic), 1373

Potassium Gluconate and Potassium Chloride—*See* Potassium Supplements (Systemic), 1373

Potassium Gluconate and Potassium Citrate—*See* Potassium Supplements (Systemic), 1373

Potassium Iodide (Systemic), 1371

Potassium para-aminobenzoate—*See* Aminobenzoate Potassium (Systemic), 197

Potassium Phosphates—*See* Phosphates (Systemic), 1349

Potassium and Sodium Phosphates—*See* Phosphates (Systemic), 1349

*Potassium-Rougier*—Potassium Gluconate—*See* Potassium Supplements (Systemic), 1373

*Potassium-Sandoz*—Potassium Bicarbonate and Potassium Chloride—*See* Potassium Supplements (Systemic), 1373

Potassium Supplements (Systemic), 1373

Potassium triplex—Trikates—*See* Potassium Supplements (Systemic), 1373

*Poxi*—Chlordiazepoxide—*See* Benzodiazepines (Systemic), 389

PPA—*See* Phenylpropanolamine (Systemic), 1347

*Pramegel*—Pramoxine and Menthol—*See* Anesthetics (Topical), 240

Pramocaine—Pramoxine—*See* Anesthetics (Rectal), 237; Anesthetics (Topical), 240

Pramoxine—*See* Anesthetics (Rectal), 237; Anesthetics (Topical), 240

Pramoxine and Menthol—*See* Anesthetics (Topical), 240

*Pravachol*—Pravastatin—*See* HMG-CoA Reductase Inhibitors (Systemic), 929, MC-19

Pravastatin—*See* HMG-CoA Reductase Inhibitors (Systemic), 929, MC-19

*Prax*—Pramoxine—*See* Anesthetics (Topical), 240

Prazepam—*See* Benzodiazepines (Systemic), 389

Praziquantel (Systemic), 1378

Prazosin (Systemic), 1380, MC-19

Prazosin and Polythiazide (Systemic), 1382, MC-19

*Pre-Attain*—Enteral Nutrition Formula, Polymeric—*See* Enteral Nutrition Formulas (Systemic), 769

*Precision HN*—Enteral Nutrition Formula, Polymeric—*See* Enteral Nutrition Formulas (Systemic), 769

*Precision Isotonic Diet*—Enteral Nutrition Formula, Polymeric—*See* Enteral Nutrition Formulas (Systemic), 769

*Precision Low Residue*—Enteral Nutrition Formula, Polymeric—*See* Enteral Nutrition Formulas (Systemic), 769

*Predair*—Prednisolone—*See* Corticosteroids (Ophthalmic), 620

*Predair A*—Prednisolone—*See* Corticosteroids (Ophthalmic), 620

*Predair Forte*—Prednisolone—*See* Corticosteroids (Ophthalmic), 620

*Predaject-50*—Prednisolone—*See* Corticosteroids/Corticotropin—Glucocorticoid Effects (Systemic), 630

*Predalone 50*—Prednisolone—*See* Corticosteroids/Corticotropin—Glucocorticoid Effects (Systemic), 630

*Predalone T.B.A.*—Prednisolone—*See* Corticosteroids/Corticotropin—Glucocorticoid Effects (Systemic), 630

*Predate 50*—Prednisolone—*See* Corticosteroids/Corticotropin—Glucocorticoid Effects (Systemic), 630

*Predate S*—Prednisolone—*See* Corticosteroids/Corticotropin—Glucocorticoid Effects (Systemic), 630

*Predate TBA*—Prednisolone—*See* Corticosteroids/Corticotropin—Glucocorticoid Effects (Systemic), 630

*Predcor-25*—Prednisolone—*See* Corticosteroids/Corticotropin—Glucocorticoid Effects (Systemic), 630

*Predcor-50*—Prednisolone—*See* Corticosteroids/Corticotropin—Glucocorticoid Effects (Systemic), 630

*Predcor-TBA*—Prednisolone—*See* Corticosteroids/Corticotropin—Glucocorticoid Effects (Systemic), 630

*Pred Forte*—Prednisolone—*See* Corticosteroids (Ophthalmic), 620

*Predicort-50*—Prednisolone—*See* Corticosteroids/Corticotropin—Glucocorticoid Effects (Systemic), 630

*Predicort-RP*—Prednisolone—*See* Corticosteroids/Corticotropin—Glucocorticoid Effects (Systemic), 630

*Pred Mild*—Prednisolone—*See* Corticosteroids (Ophthalmic), 620

*Prednicen-M*—Prednisone—*See* Corticosteroids/Corticotropin—Glucocorticoid Effects (Systemic), 630

Prednisolone—*See* Corticosteroids (Ophthalmic), 620; Corticosteroids/Corticotropin—Glucocorticoid Effects (Systemic), 630

Prednisone—*See* Corticosteroids/Corticotropin—Glucocorticoid Effects (Systemic), 630, MC-19

*Prednisone Intensol*—Prednisone—*See* Corticosteroids/Corticotropin—Glucocorticoid Effects (Systemic), 630

*Preemie SMA 20*—Infant Formulas, Milk-based—*See* Infant Formulas (Systemic), 958

*Preemie SMA 24*—Infant Formulas, Milk-based—*See* Infant Formulas (Systemic), 958

*Pre-Fil*—Nonoxynol 9—*See* Spermicides (Vaginal), 1512

*Prefrin Liquifilm*—Phenylephrine (Ophthalmic), 1345

*Pregestimil*—Infant Formulas, Hypoallergenic—*See* Infant Formulas (Systemic), 958

Pregnancy Test Kits for Home Use, 1385

*Pregnyl*—Chorionic Gonadotropin (Systemic), 540

*Prehist*—Chlorpheniramine and Phenylephrine—*See* Antihistamines and Decongestants (Systemic), 311

*Prehist D*—Chlorpheniramine, Phenylephrine, and Methscopolamine—*See* Antihistamines, Decongestants, and Anticholinergics (Systemic), 322

*Prelone*—Prednisolone—*See* Corticosteroids/Corticotropin—Glucocorticoid Effects (Systemic), 630

*Prelu-2*—Phendimetrazine—*See* Appetite Suppressants (Systemic), 339

*Premarin*—Conjugated Estrogens—*See* Estrogens (Systemic), 795, MC-9; Estrogens (Vaginal), 801

*Premarin Intravenous*—Conjugated Estrogens—*See* Estrogens (Systemic), 795

*Premarin with Methyltestosterone*—Conjugated Estrogens and Methyltestosterone—*See* Androgens and Estrogens (Systemic), 225

*Prentif*—Cervical Cap, Cavity-rim, 1746

*Prepidil*—Dinoprostone (Cervical/Vaginal), 722

*Prepulsid*—Cisapride (Systemic), 550

*Presalin*—Acetaminophen, Aspirin, and Salicylamide, Buffered—*See* Acetaminophen and Salicylates (Systemic), 164

*Pressyn*—Vasopressin (Systemic), 1657

*Prevex B*—Betamethasone—*See* Corticosteroids—Medium to Very High Potency (Topical), 626

*Prevex HC*—Hydrocortisone—*See* Corticosteroids—Low Potency (Topical), 624, 1750

Prilocaine—*See* Anesthetics (Parenteral-Local), 235

*Prilosec*—Omeprazole (Systemic), 1255, MC-17

Primaquine (Systemic), 1386

*Primatene Mist*—Epinephrine—*See* Bronchodilators, Adrenergic (Inhalation), 430

*Primatene Mist Suspension*—Epinephrine—*See* Bronchodilators, Adrenergic (Inhalation), 430

*Primatuss Cough Mixture 4*—Chlorpheniramine and Dextromethorphan—*See* Cough/Cold Combinations (Systemic), 637

*Primatuss Cough Mixture 4D*—Pseudoephedrine, Dextromethorphan, and Guaifenesin—*See* Cough/Cold Combinations (Systemic), 637

*Primaxin*—Imipenem and Cilastatin (Systemic), 953

*Primaxin IM*—Imipenem and Cilastatin (Systemic), 953

*Primaxin IV*—Imipenem and Cilastatin (Systemic), 953

*Primazine*—Promazine—*See* Phenothiazines (Systemic), 1330

Primidone (Systemic), 1388

*Principen*—Ampicillin—*See* Penicillins (Systemic), 1299, MC-2

*Prinivil*—Lisinopril—*See* Angiotensin-converting Enzyme (ACE) Inhibitors (Systemic), 245, MC-13

*Prinzide*—Lisinopril and Hydrochlorothiazide—*See* Angiotensin-converting Enzyme (ACE) Inhibitors and Hydrochlorothiazide (Systemic), 249, MC-13

*Pro-50*—Promethazine—*See* Antihistamines, Phenothiazine-derivative (Systemic), 325

*Pro-Air*—Procaterol—*See* Bronchodilators, Adrenergic (Inhalation), 430

*Probalan*—Probenecid (Systemic), 1390

*Pro-Banthine*—Propantheline—*See* Anticholinergics/Antispasmodics (Systemic), 258, MC-20

*Probate*—Meprobamate (Systemic), 1089

Proben-C—Probenecid and Colchicine (Systemic), 1392

Probenecid (Systemic), 1390

Probenecid and Colchicine (Systemic), 1392

Probucol (Systemic), 1395, MC-19

Procainamide (Systemic), 1396, MC-19

Procaine—See Anesthetics (Parenteral-Local), 235

Pro-Cal-Sof—Docusate—See Laxatives (Oral), 1017

Procan SR—Procainamide (Systemic), 1396, MC-19

Procarbazine (Systemic), 1399

Procardia—Nifedipine—See Calcium Channel Blocking Agents (Systemic), 467, MC-16

Procardia XL—Nifedipine—See Calcium Channel Blocking Agents (Systemic), 467, MC-16

Procaterol—See Bronchodilators, Adrenergic (Inhalation), 430

Prochlorperazine—See Phenothiazines (Systemic), 1330, MC-20

Procrit—Epoetin (Systemic), 773

Proctocort—Hydrocortisone (Rectal), 936

ProctoFoam/non-steroid—Pramoxine—See Anesthetics (Rectal), 237

Procyclid—Procyclidine—See Antidyskinetics (Systemic), 287

Procyclidine—See Antidyskinetics (Systemic), 287

Procythol—Selegiline (Systemic), 1485

Procytox—Cyclophosphamide (Systemic), 666

Pro-Depo—Hydroxyprogesterone—See Progestins (Systemic), 1402

Prodiem—Psyllium Hydrophilic Mucilloid and Senna—See Laxatives (Oral), 1017

Prodiem Plain—Psyllium Hydrophilic Mucilloid—See Laxatives (Oral), 1017

Prodrox—Hydroxyprogesterone—See Progestins (Systemic), 1402

Profasi—Chorionic Gonadotropin (Systemic), 540

Profasi HP—Chorionic Gonadotropin (Systemic), 540

Profenal—Suprofen—See Anti-inflammatory Agents, Nonsteroidal (Ophthalmic), 330

Profenamine—Ethopropazine—See Antidyskinetics (Systemic), 287

Profene—Propoxyphene—See Narcotic Analgesics—For Pain Relief (Systemic), 1176

Profiber—Enteral Nutrition Formula, Fiber-containing—See Enteral Nutrition Formulas (Systemic), 769

Profilate OSD—Antihemophilic Factor (Systemic), 302

Profilnine Heat-Treated—Factor IX (Systemic), 823

Progestasert—Progesterone (Intrauterine), 1753

Progesterone (Intrauterine), 1753

Progesterone—See Progestins (Systemic), 1402

Progestins (Systemic), 1402

Proglycem—Diazoxide (Oral), 706

Proguanil (Systemic), 1406

Prohibit—Haemophilus b Conjugate Vaccine (PRP-D—Diphtheria Toxoid Conjugate)—See Haemophilus b Conjugate Vaccine (Systemic), 905

Prohim—Yohimbine (Systemic), 1684

Prolamine—Phenylpropanolamine (Systemic), 1347

Prolastin—Alpha₁-proteinase Inhibitor, Human (Systemic), 190

Pro-Lax—Psyllium Hydrophilic Mucilloid—See Laxatives (Oral), 1017

Proleukin—Aldesleukin (Systemic), 184

Prolixin—Fluphenazine—See Phenothiazines (Systemic), 1330, MC-10

Prolixin Concentrate—Fluphenazine—See Phenothiazines (Systemic), 1330

Prolixin Decanoate—Fluphenazine—See Phenothiazines (Systemic), 1330

Prolixin Enanthate—Fluphenazine—See Phenothiazines (Systemic), 1330

Prolopa—Levodopa and Benserazide (Systemic), 1750

Proloprim—Trimethoprim (Systemic), 1628, MC-24

Promacot—Promethazine—See Antihistamines, Phenothiazine-derivative (Systemic), 325

Promazine—See Phenothiazines (Systemic), 1330

Pro-Med 50—Promethazine—See Antihistamines, Phenothiazine-derivative (Systemic), 325

Promet—Promethazine—See Antihistamines, Phenothiazine-derivative (Systemic), 325

Prometa—Metaproterenol—See Bronchodilators, Adrenergic (Oral/Injection), 436

Promethazine—See Antihistamines, Phenothiazine-derivative (Systemic), 325, MC-20

Promethazine and Codeine—See Cough/Cold Combinations (Systemic), 637

Promethazine and Dextromethorphan—See Cough/Cold Combinations (Systemic), 637

Promethazine DM—Promethazine and Dextromethorphan—See Cough/Cold Combinations (Systemic), 637

Promethazine and Phenylephrine—See Antihistamines and Decongestants (Systemic), 311

Promethazine, Phenylephrine, and Codeine—See Cough/Cold Combinations (Systemic), 637

Promethazine VC—Promethazine and Phenylephrine—See Antihistamines and Decongestants (Systemic), 311

Promethazine VC w/ Codeine—Promethazine, Phenylephrine, and Codeine—See Cough/Cold Combinations (Systemic), 637

Prometh w/ Dextromethorphan—Promethazine and Dextromethorphan—See Cough/Cold Combinations (Systemic), 637

Promethist w/Codeine—Promethazine, Phenylephrine, and Codeine—See Cough/Cold Combinations (Systemic), 637

Prometh VC with Codeine—Promethazine, Phenylephrine, and Codeine—See Cough/Cold Combinations (Systemic), 637

Prometh VC Plain—Promethazine and Phenylephrine—See Antihistamines and Decongestants (Systemic), 311

Promine—Procainamide (Systemic), 1396

Prominic Expectorant—Phenylpropanolamine and Guaifenesin—See Cough/Cold Combinations (Systemic), 637

Prominicol Cough—Pheniramine, Pyrilamine, Phenylpropanolamine, Dextromethorphan, and Ammonium Chloride—See Cough/Cold Combinations (Systemic), 637

Promist HD Liquid—Chlorpheniramine, Pseudoephedrine, and Hydrocodone—See Cough/Cold Combinations (Systemic), 637

ProMod—Enteral Nutrition Formula, Modular—See Enteral Nutrition Formulas (Systemic), 769

Promote—Enteral Nutrition Formula, Polymeric—See Enteral Nutrition Formulas (Systemic), 769

*Prompt*—Psyllium Hydrophilic Mucilloid and Sennosides—*See* Laxatives (Oral), 1017
*Pronestyl*—Procainamide (Systemic), 1396, MC-19
*Pronestyl-SR*—Procainamide (Systemic), 1396, MC-19
*Pronto Lice Killing Shampoo Kit*—Pyrethrins and Piperonyl Butoxide (Topical), 1417
*Propac*—Enteral Nutrition Formula, Modular—*See* Enteral Nutrition Formulas (Systemic), 769
*Propacet 100*—Propoxyphene and Acetaminophen—*See* Narcotic Analgesics and Acetaminophen (Systemic), 1181
*Propaderm*—Beclomethasone—*See* Corticosteroids—Medium to Very High Potency (Topical), 626
Propafenone (Systemic), 1408, MC-20
*Propagest*—Phenylpropanolamine (Systemic), 1347
*Propain-HC*—Hydrocodone and Acetaminophen—*See* Narcotic Analgesics and Acetaminophen (Systemic), 1181
*Propanthel*—Propantheline—*See* Anticholinergics/Antispasmodics (Systemic), 258
Propantheline—*See* Anticholinergics/Antispasmodics (Systemic), 258, MC-20
*Propa P.H. 10 Acne Cover Stick*—Benzoyl Peroxide (Topical), 397
*Propa P.H. 10 Liquid Acne Soap*—Benzoyl Peroxide (Topical), 397
*Propa pH Medicated Acne Cream Maximum Strength*—Salicylic Acid (Topical), 1478
*Propa pH Medicated Cleansing Pads Maximum Strength*—Salicylic Acid (Topical), 1478
*Propa pH Medicated Cleansing Pads Sensitive Skin*—Salicylic Acid (Topical), 1478
*Propa pH Perfectly Clear Skin Cleanser Topical Solution Normal/Combination Skin*—Salicylic Acid (Topical), 1478
*Propa pH Perfectly Clear Skin Cleanser Topical Solution Oily Skin*—Salicylic Acid (Topical), 1478
*Propa pH Perfectly Clear Skin Cleanser Topical Solution Sensitive Skin Formula*—Salicylic Acid (Topical), 1478
Proparacaine—*See* Anesthetics (Ophthalmic), 234
*Propine C Cap B.I.D.*—Dipivefrin (Ophthalmic), 729
Propiomazine (Systemic), 1410
*Proplex T*—Factor IX (Systemic), 823
Propofol—*See* Anesthetics, General (Systemic), 243
*Pro Pox*—Propoxyphene—*See* Narcotic Analgesics—For Pain Relief (Systemic), 1176
*Pro Pox with APAP*—Propoxyphene and Acetaminophen—*See* Narcotic Analgesics and Acetaminophen (Systemic), 1181
*Pro Pox Plus*—Propoxyphene, Aspirin, and Caffeine—*See* Narcotic Analgesics and Aspirin (Systemic), 1185
Propoxycaine and Procaine—*See* Anesthetics (Parenteral-Local), 235
*Propoxycon*—Propoxyphene—*See* Narcotic Analgesics—For Pain Relief (Systemic), 1176
Propoxyphene—*See* Narcotic Analgesics—For Pain Relief (Systemic), 1176
Propoxyphene and Acetaminophen—*See* Narcotic Analgesics and Acetaminophen (Systemic), 1181, MC-20
Propoxyphene with APAP—Propoxyphene and Acetaminophen—*See* Narcotic Analgesics and Acetaminophen (Systemic), 1181

Propoxyphene and Aspirin—*See* Narcotic Analgesics and Aspirin (Systemic), 1185
Propoxyphene, Aspirin, and Caffeine—*See* Narcotic Analgesics and Aspirin (Systemic), 1185
Propoxyphene hydrochloride compound—Propoxyphene, Aspirin, and Caffeine—*See* Narcotic Analgesics and Aspirin (Systemic), 1185
Propranolol—*See* Beta-adrenergic Blocking Agents (Systemic), 404, MC-20
Propranolol and Hydrochlorothiazide—*See* Beta-adrenergic Blocking Agents and Thiazide Diuretics (Systemic), 410, MC-20
*Propulsid*—Cisapride (Systemic), MC-5
Propylthiouracil—*See* Antithyroid Agents (Systemic), 336
*Propyl-Thyracil*—Propylthiouracil—*See* Antithyroid Agents (Systemic), 336
*Prorazin*—Prochlorperazine—*See* Phenothiazines (Systemic), 1330
*Prorex-25*—Promethazine—*See* Antihistamines, Phenothiazine-derivative (Systemic), 325
*Prorex-50*—Promethazine—*See* Antihistamines, Phenothiazine-derivative (Systemic), 325
*Proscar*—Finasteride (Systemic), 835, MC-10
*Prosed/DS*—Atropine, Hyoscyamine, Methenamine, Methylene Blue, Phenyl Salicylate, and Benzoic Acid (Systemic), 357
*Pro-Sobee*—Infant Formulas, Soy-based—*See* Infant Formulas (Systemic), 958
*Pro-Sof*—Docusate—*See* Laxatives (Oral), 1017
*Pro-Sof Liquid Concentrate*—Docusate—*See* Laxatives (Oral), 1017
*Pro-Sof Plus*—Casanthranol and Docusate—*See* Laxatives (Oral), 1017
*ProSom*—Estazolam—*See* Benzodiazepines (Systemic), 389, MC-9
*Pro-Span*—Hydroxyprogesterone—*See* Progestins (Systemic), 1402
Prostaglandin E₁—*See* Alprostadil (Intracavernosal), 191
*Prostaphlin*—Oxacillin—*See* Penicillins (Systemic), 1299, MC-17
*ProStep*—Nicotine (Systemic), 1212
*Prostigmin*—Neostigmine—*See* Antimyasthenics (Systemic), 332
*Prostin E₂*—Dinoprostone (Cervical/Vaginal), 722
*Prostin F₂ Alpha*—Dinoprost (Intra-amniotic), 721
*Prostin/15M*—Carboprost (Systemic), 493
*Prostin VR*—Alprostadil (Intracavernosal), 191
*Prostin VR Pediatric*—Alprostadil (Intracavernosal), 191
*Protain XL*—Enteral Nutrition Formula, Disease-specific—*See* Enteral Nutrition Formulas (Systemic), 769
*Protex Arouse*—Latex Condoms—*See* Condoms, 602
*Protex Contracept Plus with Spermicidal Lubricant*—Latex Condoms and Nonoxynol 9—*See* Condoms, 602
*Protex Secure*—Latex Condoms—*See* Condoms, 602
*Protex Touch*—Latex Condoms—*See* Condoms, 602
*Prothazine*—Promethazine—*See* Antihistamines, Phenothiazine-derivative (Systemic), 325
*Prothazine Plain*—Promethazine—*See* Antihistamines, Phenothiazine-derivative (Systemic), 325
Prothrombin complex concentrate (PCC)—*See* Factor IX (Systemic), 823

Pyrilamine, Phenylephrine, and Codeine—*See* Cough/Cold Combinations (Systemic), 637

Pyrilamine, Phenylephrine, and Dextromethorphan—*See* Cough/Cold Combinations (Systemic), 637

Pyrilamine, Phenylephrine, Dextromethorphan, and Acetaminophen—*See* Cough/Cold Combinations (Systemic), 637

Pyrilamine, Phenylephrine, and Hydrocodone—*See* Cough/Cold Combinations (Systemic), 637

Pyrilamine, Phenylephrine, Hydrocodone, and Ammonium Chloride—*See* Cough/Cold Combinations (Systemic), 637

Pyrilamine, Phenylpropanolamine, Acetaminophen, and Caffeine—*See* Antihistamines, Decongestants, and Analgesics (Systemic), 316

Pyrilamine, Phenylpropanolamine, Dextromethorphan, Guaifenesin, Potassium Citrate, and Citric Acid—*See* Cough/Cold Combinations (Systemic), 637

Pyrilamine, Phenylpropanolamine, Dextromethorphan, and Sodium Salicylate—*See* Cough/Cold Combinations (Systemic), 637

Pyrilamine, Pseudoephedrine, Dextromethorphan, and Acetaminophen (Systemic), AI-637

Pyrimethamine (Systemic), 1421

*Pyrinyl*—Pyrethrins and Piperonyl Butoxide (Topical), 1417

Pyrithione (Topical), 1424, 1754

*Pyrroxate Extra Strength*—Chlorpheniramine, Phenylpropanolamine, and Acetaminophen —*See* Antihistamines, Decongestants, and Analgesics (Systemic), 316

Pyrvinium (Oral), 1425

PZI insulin—Insulin, Protamine Zinc—*See* Insulin (Systemic), 961

# Q

*Q-test*—Ovulation Prediction Test Kits for Home Use, 1265; Pregnancy Test Kits for Home Use, 1385

*Quadra-Hist*—Chlorpheniramine, Phenyltoloxamine, Phenylephrine, and Phenylpropanolamine—*See* Antihistamines and Decongestants (Systemic), 311

*Quadra-Hist Pediatric*—Chlorpheniramine, Phenyltoloxamine, Phenylephrine, and Phenylpropanolamine—*See* Antihistamines and Decongestants (Systemic), 311

*Quarzan*—Clidinium—*See* Anticholinergics/Antispasmodics (Systemic), 258

Quazepam—*See* Benzodiazepines (Systemic), 389, MC-20

*Quelidrine Cough*—Chlorpheniramine, Ephedrine, Phenylephrine, Dextromethorphan, Ammonium Chloride, and Ipecac—*See* Cough/Cold Combinations (Systemic), 637

*Questran*—Cholestyramine (Oral), 538

*Questran Light*—Cholestyramine (Oral), 538

*Quiagel PG*—Kaolin, Pectin, Belladonna Alkaloids, and Opium (Systemic), 1005

*Quibron*—Theophylline and Guaifenesin (Systemic), 1586, MC-22

*Quibron-300*—Theophylline and Guaifenesin (Systemic), 1586

*Quibron-T Dividose*—Theophylline—*See* Bronchodilators, Xanthine-derivative (Systemic), 442, MC-22

*Quibron-T/SR*—Theophylline—*See* Bronchodilators, Xanthine-derivative (Systemic), 442

*Quibron-T/SR Dividose*—Theophylline—*See* Bronchodilators, Xanthine-derivative (Systemic), 442, MC-22

*Quick Pep*—Caffeine (Systemic), 463

*Quiess*—Hydroxyzine—*See* Antihistamines (Systemic), 304

*Quin-260*—Quinine (Systemic), 1430

Quinacrine (Systemic), 1427

*Quinaglute Dura-tabs*—Quinidine (Systemic), 1428, MC-20

*Quinalan*—Quinidine (Systemic), 1428

*Quin-amino*—Quinine (Systemic), 1430

*Quinamm*—Quinine (Systemic), 1430

Quinapril—*See* Angiotensin-converting Enzyme (ACE) Inhibitors (Systemic), 245, MC-20

*Quinate*—Quinidine (Systemic), 1428

*Quindan*—Quinine (Systemic), 1430

Quinestrol—*See* Estrogens (Systemic), 795

Quinethazone—*See* Diuretics, Thiazide (Systemic), 749

*Quinidex Extentabs*—Quinidine (Systemic), 1428, MC-20

Quinidine (Systemic), 1428, MC-20

Quinine (Systemic), 1430

*Quinora*—Quinidine (Systemic), 1428

*Quiphile*—Quinine (Systemic), 1430

*Q-vel*—Quinine (Systemic), 1430

# R

*RA*—Resorcinol (Topical), 1453

Rabies Immune Globulin (Systemic), 1433

Rabies Vaccine (Systemic), 1434

Rabies Vaccine Adsorbed—*See* Rabies Vaccine (Systemic), 1434

Rabies Vaccine, Human Diploid Cell—*See* Rabies Vaccine (Systemic), 1434

Racepinephrine—*See* Bronchodilators, Adrenergic (Inhalation), 430

*Radanil*—Benznidazole (Systemic), 387

Radioiodinated Albumin—*See* Radiopharmaceuticals (Diagnostic), 1439

Radiopaque Agents (Diagnostic), 1436

Radiopaque Agents (Diagnostic, Mucosal), 1438

Radiopharmaceuticals (Diagnostic), 1439

*Radiostol Forte*—Ergocalciferol—*See* Vitamin D and Related Compounds (Systemic), 1669

Ramipril—*See* Angiotensin-converting Enzyme (ACE) Inhibitors (Systemic), 245, MC-21

*Ramses Contraceptive Foam*—Nonoxynol 9—*See* Spermicides (Vaginal), 1512

*Ramses Contraceptive Vaginal Jelly*—Nonoxynol 9—*See* Spermicides (Vaginal), 1512

*Ramses Crystal Clear Gel*—Nonoxynol 9—*See* Spermicides (Vaginal), 1512

*Ramses Extra*—Latex Condoms and Nonoxynol 9—*See* Condoms, 602

*Ramses Extra-15*—Latex Condoms and Nonoxynol 9—*See* Condoms, 602

*Ramses Extra with Spermicidal Lubricant*—Latex Condoms and Nonoxynol 9—*See* Condoms, 602

*Ramses Non-lubricated*—Latex Condoms—*See* Condoms, 602

*Ramses Non-Lubricated Reservoir End*—Latex Condoms—*See* Condoms, 602

*Ramses NuFORM*—Latex Condoms—*See* Condoms, 602

*Ramses Ribbed*—Latex Condoms and Nonoxynol 9—*See* Condoms, 602

*Ramses Sensitol*—Latex Condoms—*See* Condoms, 602

*Ramses Sensitol Lubricated*—Latex Condoms—*See* Condoms, 602

*Ramses Ultra*—Latex Condoms—*See* Condoms, 602

*Ramses Ultra-15*—Latex Condoms and Nonoxynol 9—*See* Condoms, 602

Ranitidine—*See* Histamine $H_2$-receptor Antagonists (Systemic), 925, MC-21

*Rapolyte*—Oral Rehydration Salts—*See* Carbohydrates and Electrolytes (Systemic), 484

*Raudixin*—Rauwolfia Serpentina—*See* Rauwolfia Alkaloids (Systemic), 1442

*Rauval*—Rauwolfia Serpentina—*See* Rauwolfia Alkaloids (Systemic), 1442

*Rauverid*—Rauwolfia Serpentina—*See* Rauwolfia Alkaloids (Systemic), 1442

Rauwolfia Alkaloids (Systemic), 1442

Rauwolfia Alkaloids and Thiazide Diuretics (Systemic), 1445

Rauwolfia Serpentina—*See* Rauwolfia Alkaloids (Systemic), 1442

Rauwolfia Serpentina and Bendroflumethiazide—*See* Rauwolfia Alkaloids and Thiazide Diuretics (Systemic), 1445

*Rauzide*—Rauwolfia Serpentina and Bendroflumethiazide—*See* Rauwolfia Alkaloids and Thiazide Diuretics (Systemic), 1445

*Ravocaine and Novocain with Levophed*—Propoxycaine and Procaine—*See* Anesthetics (Parenteral-Local), 235

*Ravocaine and Novocain with Neo-Cobefrin*—Propoxycaine and Procaine—*See* Anesthetics (Parenteral-Local), 235

*R & C*—Pyrethrins and Piperonyl Butoxide (Topical), 1417

*RCF*—Infant Formulas, Soy-based—*See* Infant Formulas (Systemic), 958

*Reabilan*—Enteral Nutrition Formula, Monomeric (Elemental)—*See* Enteral Nutrition Formulas (Systemic), 769

*Reabilan HN*—Enteral Nutrition Formula, Monomeric (Elemental)—*See* Enteral Nutrition Formulas (Systemic), 769

*Reactine*—Cetirizine—*See* Antihistamines (Systemic), 304

*Reclomide*—Metoclopramide (Systemic), 1123

*Recombinate*—Antihemophilic Factor (Systemic), 302

*Recombivax HB*—Hepatitis B Vaccine Recombinant (Systemic), 922

*Recombivax HB Dialysis Formulation*—Hepatitis B Vaccine Recombinant (Systemic), 922

*Rectocort*—Hydrocortisone (Rectal), 936

*Rederm*—Hydrocortisone—*See* Corticosteroids—Low Potency (Topical), 624

*Redutemp*—Acetaminophen (Systemic), 161

*Reese's Pinworm Medicine*—Pyrantel (Oral), 1414

*Regitine*—Phentolamine—*See* Phentolamine and Papaverine (Intracavernosal), 1341

*Reglan*—Metoclopramide (Systemic), 1123, MC-15

*Regonol*—Pyridostigmine—*See* Antimyasthenics (Systemic), 332

*Regroton*—Reserpine and Chlorthalidone—*See* Rauwolfia Alkaloids and Thiazide Diuretics (Systemic), 1445, MC-21

*Regulace*—Casanthranol and Docusate—*See* Laxatives (Oral), 1017

*Regular (Concentrated) Iletin II, U-500*—Insulin—*See* Insulin (Systemic), 961

*Regular Iletin*—Insulin—*See* Insulin (Systemic), 961

*Regular Iletin I*—Insulin—*See* Insulin (Systemic), 961

*Regular Iletin II*—Insulin—*See* Insulin (Systemic), 961

*Regular Insulin*—Insulin—*See* Insulin (Systemic), 961

Regular insulin—Insulin—*See* Insulin (Systemic), 961

*Regulax SS*—Docusate—*See* Laxatives (Oral), 1017

*Regulex*—Docusate—*See* Laxatives (Oral), 1017

*Regulex-D*—Danthron and Docusate—*See* Laxatives (Oral), 1017

*Reguloid Natural*—Psyllium Hydrophilic Mucilloid—*See* Laxatives (Oral), 1017

*Reguloid Orange*—Psyllium Hydrophilic Mucilloid—*See* Laxatives (Oral), 1017

*Regutol*—Docusate—*See* Laxatives (Oral), 1017

*Rehydralyte*—Dextrose and Electrolytes—*See* Carbohydrates and Electrolytes (Systemic), 484

*Rela*—Carisoprodol—*See* Skeletal Muscle Relaxants (Systemic), 1495

*Relafen*—Nabumetone (Systemic)—*See* Nonsteroidal Anti-inflammatory Drugs (Systemic), 1229, MC-15

*Relaxadon*—Atropine, Hyoscyamine, Scopolamine, and Phenobarbital—*See* Belladonna Alkaloids and Barbiturates (Systemic), 382

*Relefact TRH*—Protirelin (Diagnostic), 1411

*Relief Eye Drops for Red Eyes*—Phenylephrine (Ophthalmic), 1345

*Remcol-C*—Chlorpheniramine, Dextromethorphan, and Acetaminophen—*See* Cough/Cold Combinations (Systemic), 637

*Remcol Cold*—Chlorpheniramine, Phenylpropanolamine, and Acetaminophen—*See* Antihistamines, Decongestants, and Analgesics (Systemic), 316

*Renedil*—Felodipine—*See* Calcium Channel Blocking Agents (Systemic), 467

*Renese*—Polythiazide—*See* Diuretics, Thiazide (Systemic), 749

*Renese-R*—Reserpine and Polythiazide—*See* Rauwolfia Alkaloids and Thiazide Diuretics (Systemic), 1445

*Renoquid*—Sulfacytine—*See* Sulfonamides (Systemic), 1542

*Rentamine Pediatric*—Chlorpheniramine, Ephedrine, Phenylephrine, and Carbetapentane—*See* Cough/Cold Combinations (Systemic), 637

*Repan*—Butalbital, Acetaminophen, and Caffeine—*See* Butalbital and Acetaminophen (Systemic), 453

*Replete*—Enteral Nutrition Formula, Polymeric—*See* Enteral Nutrition Formulas (Systemic), 769

*Replete with Fiber*—Enteral Nutrition Formula, Fiber-containing—*See* Enteral Nutrition Formulas (Systemic), 769

*Rep-Pred 40*—Methylprednisolone—*See* Corticosteroids/Corticotropin—Glucocorticoid Effects (Systemic), 630

*Rep-Pred 80*—Methylprednisolone—*See* Corticosteroids/Corticotropin—Glucocorticoid Effects (Systemic), 630

*Resaid S.R.*—Chlorpheniramine and Phenylpropanolamine—*See* Antihistamines and Decongestants (Systemic), 311

*Rescaps-D S.R.*—Phenylpropanolamine and Caramiphen—*See* Cough/Cold Combinations (Systemic), 637

*Rescon*—Chlorpheniramine and Phenylpropanolamine—*See* Antihistamines and Decongestants (Systemic), 311; Chlorpheniramine and Pseudoephedrine—*See* Antihistamines and Decongestants (Systemic), 311

*Rescon-DM*—Chlorpheniramine, Pseudoephedrine, and Dextromethorphan—*See* Cough/Cold Combinations (Systemic), 637

*Rescon-ED*—Chlorpheniramine and Pseudoephedrine—*See* Antihistamines and Decongestants (Systemic), 311

*Rescon-GG*—Phenylephrine and Guaifenesin—*See* Cough/Cold Combinations (Systemic), 637

*Rescon JR*—Chlorpheniramine and Pseudoephedrine—*See* Antihistamines and Decongestants (Systemic), 311

*Reserfia*—Reserpine—*See* Rauwolfia Alkaloids (Systemic), 1442

Reserpine—*See* Rauwolfia Alkaloids (Systemic), 1442

Reserpine and Chlorothiazide—*See* Rauwolfia Alkaloids and Thiazide Diuretics (Systemic), 1445

Reserpine and Chlorthalidone—*See* Rauwolfia Alkaloids and Thiazide Diuretics (Systemic), 1445, MC-21

Reserpine, Hydralazine, and Hydrochlorothiazide (Systemic), 1449, MC-21

Reserpine and Hydrochlorothiazide—*See* Rauwolfia Alkaloids and Thiazide Diuretics (Systemic), 1445

Reserpine and Hydroflumethiazide—*See* Rauwolfia Alkaloids and Thiazide Diuretics (Systemic), 1445

Reserpine and Methyclothiazide—*See* Rauwolfia Alkaloids and Thiazide Diuretics (Systemic), 1445

Reserpine and Polythiazide—*See* Rauwolfia Alkaloids and Thiazide Diuretics (Systemic), 1445

Reserpine and Trichlormethiazide—*See* Rauwolfia Alkaloids and Thiazide Diuretics (Systemic), 1445

*Resol*—Dextrose and Electrolytes—*See* Carbohydrates and Electrolytes (Systemic), 484

Resorcinol (Topical), 1453

Resorcinol and Sulfur (Topical), 1454

*Resource*—Enteral Nutrition Formula, Polymeric—*See* Enteral Nutrition Formulas (Systemic), 769

*Resource Plus*—Enteral Nutrition Formula, Polymeric—*See* Enteral Nutrition Formulas (Systemic), 769

*Respaire-60 SR*—Pseudoephedrine and Guaifenesin—*See* Cough/Cold Combinations (Systemic), 637

*Respaire-120 SR*—Pseudoephedrine and Guaifenesin—*See* Cough/Cold Combinations (Systemic), 637

*Respalor*—Enteral Nutrition Formula, Disease-specific (Systemic), 1748

*Respbid*—Theophylline—*See* Bronchodilators, Xanthine-derivative (Systemic), 442

*Restoril*—Temazepam—*See* Benzodiazepines (Systemic), 389, MC-22

*Resyl*—Guaifenesin (Systemic), 892

*Retin-A*—Tretinoin (Topical), 1620

*Retin-A Regimen Kit*—Tretinoin (Topical), 1620

Retinoic acid—*See* Tretinoin (Topical), 1620

Retinol—*See* Vitamin A (Systemic), 1664

*Retrovir*—Zidovudine (Systemic), 1689, MC-24

*Rev-Eyes*—Dapiprazole (Ophthalmic), 686

*Rexigen Forte*—Phendimetrazine—*See* Appetite Suppressants (Systemic), 339

*Rezamid Acne Treatment*—Resorcinol and Sulfur (Topical), 1454

*Rezamid Lotion*—Resorcinol and Sulfur (Topical), 1454

RH₀(D) Immune Globulin (Systemic), 1456

RhD immune globulin—*See* RH₀(D) Immune Globulin (Systemic), 1456

Rh₀(D) immune human globulin—*See* RH₀(D) Immune Globulin (Systemic), 1456

rhDNase—*See* Dornase Alfa (Inhalation), 754

*Rheaban*—Attapulgite (Oral), 359

*Rheumatrex*—Methotrexate—For Noncancerous Conditions (Systemic), 1105, 1751

Rh-IG—*See* RH₀(D) Immune Globulin (Systemic), 1456

Rh immune globulin—*See* RH₀(D) Immune Globulin (Systemic), 1456

*Rhinalar*—Flunisolide—*See* Corticosteroids (Nasal), 617

*Rhinall*—Phenylephrine (Nasal), 1343

*Rhinall-10 Children's Flavored Nose Drops*—Phenylephrine (Nasal), 1343

*Rhinatate*—Chlorpheniramine, Pyrilamine, and Phenylephrine—*See* Antihistamines and Decongestants (Systemic), 311

*Rhinocaps*—Phenylpropanolamine, Acetaminophen, and Aspirin—*See* Decongestants and Analgesics (Systemic), 691

*Rhinocort Aqua*—Budesonide—*See* Corticosteroids (Nasal), 617

*Rhinocort Turbuhaler*—Budesonide—*See* Corticosteroids (Nasal), 617

*Rhinogesic*—Chlorpheniramine, Phenylephrine, Acetaminophen, and Salicylamide—*See* Antihistamines, Decongestants, and Analgesics (Systemic), 316

*Rhinolar*—Chlorpheniramine, Phenylpropanolamine, and Methscopolamine—*See* Antihistamines, Decongestants, and Anticholinergics (Systemic), 322

*Rhinolar-EX*—Chlorpheniramine and Phenylpropanolamine—*See* Antihistamines and Decongestants (Systemic), 311

*Rhinolar-EX 12*—Chlorpheniramine and Phenylpropanolamine—*See* Antihistamines and Decongestants (Systemic), 311

*Rhinosyn*—Chlorpheniramine and Pseudoephedrine—*See* Antihistamines and Decongestants (Systemic), 311

*Rhinosyn-DM*—Chlorpheniramine, Pseudoephedrine, and Dextromethorphan—*See* Cough/Cold Combinations (Systemic), 637

*Rhinosyn-DMX Expectorant*—Dextromethorphan and Guaifenesin—*See* Cough/Cold Combinations (Systemic), 637

*Rhinosyn-PD*—Chlorpheniramine and Pseudoephedrine—*See* Antihistamines and Decongestants (Systemic), 311

*Rhinosyn-X*—Pseudoephedrine, Dextromethorphan, and Guaifenesin—*See* Cough/Cold Combinations (Systemic), 637

*Rhodis*—Ketoprofen—*See* Nonsteroidal Anti-inflammatory Drugs (Systemic), 1229

*Rhodis-EC*—Ketoprofen—*See* Nonsteroidal Anti-inflammatory Drugs (Systemic), 1229

*RhoGAM*—RH₀(D) Immune Globulin (Systemic), 1456

*Rhotrimine*—Trimipramine—*See* Antidepressants, Tricyclic (Systemic), 277

r-HuEPO—*See* Epoetin (Systemic), 773

*Rhulicort*—Hydrocortisone Acetate—*See* Corticosteroids—Low Potency (Topical), 624
Ribavirin (Systemic), 1457
Riboflavin (Vitamin B₂) (Systemic), 1458
Rice Syrup Solids and Electrolytes—*See* Carbohydrates and Electrolytes (Systemic), 484
*Rid*—Pyrethrins and Piperonyl Butoxide (Topical), 1417
*Rid-A-Pain*—Benzocaine—*See* Anesthetics (Dental), 229
*Rid-A-Pain Compound*—Acetaminophen, Salicylamide, and Caffeine—*See* Acetaminophen and Salicylates (Systemic), 164
*Ridaura*—Auranofin—*See* Gold Compounds (Systemic), 884, MC-2
Rifabutin (Systemic), 1460
*Rifadin*—Rifampin (Systemic), 1461
*Rifadin IV*—Rifampin (Systemic), 1461
*Rifamate*—Rifampin and Isoniazid (Systemic), 1464
*Rifampicin*—*See* Rifampin (Systemic), 1461
*Rifampicin and isoniazid*—*See* Rifampin and Isoniazid (Systemic), 1464
Rifampin (Systemic), 1461
Rifampin and Isoniazid (Systemic), 1464
*RIG*—*See* Rabies Immune Globulin (Systemic), 1433
*Rimactane*—Rifampin (Systemic), 1461
Rimantadine (Systemic), 1467
*Rimso-50*—Dimethyl Sulfoxide (Mucosal), 720
*Rinade B.I.D.*—Chlorpheniramine and Pseudoephedrine—*See* Antihistamines and Decongestants (Systemic), 311
*Riopan*—Magaldrate—*See* Antacids (Oral), 253
*Riopan Extra Strength*—Magaldrate—*See* Antacids (Oral), 253
*Riopan Plus*—Magaldrate and Simethicone—*See* Antacids (Oral), 253
*Riopan Plus 2*—Magaldrate and Simethicone—*See* Antacids (Oral), 253
*Riopan Plus Extra Strength*—Magaldrate and Simethicone—*See* Antacids (Oral), 253
*Riphen*—Aspirin—*See* Salicylates (Systemic), 1473
*Risperdal*—Risperidone (Systemic), 1754, MC-21
Risperidone (Systemic), 1754, MC-21
*Ritalin*—Methylphenidate (Systemic), 1118, MC-15
*Ritalin-SR*—Methylphenidate (Systemic), 1118, MC-15
Ritodrine (Systemic), 1468
*Rivotril*—Clonazepam—*See* Benzodiazepines (Systemic), 389
*RMS Uniserts*—Morphine—*See* Narcotic Analgesics—For Pain Relief (Systemic), 1176
*Ro7-1051*—Benznidazole (Systemic), 387
*Robafen AC Cough*—Codeine and Guaifenesin—*See* Cough/Cold Combinations (Systemic), 637
*Robafen CF*—Phenylpropanolamine, Dextromethorphan, and Guaifenesin—*See* Cough/Cold Combinations (Systemic), 637
*Robafen DAC*—Pseudoephedrine, Codeine, and Guaifenesin—*See* Cough/Cold Combinations (Systemic), 637
*Robafen DM*—Dextromethorphan and Guaifenesin—*See* Cough/Cold Combinations (Systemic), 637
*Robalate*—Dihydroxyaluminum Aminoacetate—*See* Antacids (Oral), 253
*Robamol*—Methocarbamol—*See* Skeletal Muscle Relaxants (Systemic), 1495

*Robaxin*—Methocarbamol—*See* Skeletal Muscle Relaxants (Systemic), 1495, MC-14
*Robaxisal*—Methocarbamol and Aspirin (Systemic), MC-14
*Robidex*—Dextromethorphan (Systemic), 701
*Robidone*—Hydrocodone—*See* Narcotic Analgesics—For Pain Relief (Systemic), 1176
*Robidrine*—Pseudoephedrine (Systemic), 1412
*Robigesic*—Acetaminophen (Systemic), 161
*Robinul*—Glycopyrrolate—*See* Anticholinergics/Antispasmodics (Systemic), 258
*Robinul Forte*—Glycopyrrolate—*See* Anticholinergics/Antispasmodics (Systemic), 258
*Robitet*—Tetracycline—*See* Tetracyclines (Systemic), 1570
*Robitussin*—Guaifenesin (Systemic), 892
*Robitussin A-C*—Codeine and Guaifenesin—*See* Cough/Cold Combinations (Systemic), 637; Pheniramine, Codeine, and Guaifenesin—*See* Cough/Cold Combinations (Systemic), 637
*Robitussin-CF*—Phenylpropanolamine, Dextromethorphan, and Guaifenesin—*See* Cough/Cold Combinations (Systemic), 637
*Robitussin with Codeine*—Pheniramine, Codeine, and Guaifenesin—*See* Cough/Cold Combinations (Systemic), 637
*Robitussin Cold and Cough Liqui-Gels*—Pseudoephedrine, Dextromethorphan, and Guaifenesin—*See* Cough/Cold Combinations (Systemic), 637
*Robitussin Cough Calmers*—Dextromethorphan (Systemic), 701
*Robitussin-DAC*—Pseudoephedrine, Codeine, and Guaifenesin—*See* Cough/Cold Combinations (Systemic), 637
*Robitussin-DM*—Dextromethorphan and Guaifenesin—*See* Cough/Cold Combinations (Systemic), 637
*Robitussin Maximum Strength Cough and Cold*—Pseudoephedrine and Dextromethorphan—*See* Cough/Cold Combinations (Systemic), 637, 1753
*Robitussin Maximum Strength Cough Suppressant*—Dextromethorphan (Systemic), 701
*Robitussin Night Relief*—Pyrilamine, Pseudoephedrine, Dextromethorphan, and Acetaminophen—*See* Cough/Cold Combinations (Systemic), 637
*Robitussin Night Relief Colds Formula Liquid*—Pyrilamine, Phenylephrine, Dextromethorphan, and Acetaminophen—*See* Cough/Cold Combinations (Systemic), 637
*Robitussin-PE*—Pseudoephedrine and Guaifenesin—*See* Cough/Cold Combinations (Systemic), 637
*Robitussin Pediatric*—Dextromethorphan (Systemic), 701
*Robitussin Pediatric Cough & Cold*—Pseudoephedrine and Dextromethorphan—*See* Cough/Cold Combinations (Systemic), 637
*Robitussin Severe Congestion Liqui-Gels*—Pseudoephedrine and Guaifenesin—*See* Cough/Cold Combinations (Systemic), 637
*Robomol*—Methocarbamol—*See* Skeletal Muscle Relaxants (Systemic), 1495
*Rocaltrol*—Calcitriol—*See* Vitamin D and Related Compounds (Systemic), 1669, MC-3
*Rocephin*—Ceftriaxone—*See* Cephalosporins (Systemic), 498
*Rochagan*—Benznidazole (Systemic), 387
*Rodex*—Pyridoxine (Vitamin B₆) (Systemic), 1419
*Rofact*—Rifampin (Systemic), 1461

*Roferon-A*—Interferon Alfa-2a, Recombinant—*See* Interferons, Alpha (Systemic), 968

*Rogaine*—Minoxidil (Topical), 1142

*Rogesic No.3*—Hydrocodone and Acetaminophen—*See* Narcotic Analgesics and Acetaminophen (Systemic), 1181

*Rogitine*—Phentolamine—*See* Phentolamine and Papaverine (Intracavernosal), 1341

*Rolaids*—Dihydroxyaluminum Sodium Carbonate—*See* Antacids (Oral), 253

*Rolaids Calcium Rich*—Calcium Carbonate—*See* Antacids (Oral), 253; Calcium Supplements (Systemic), 472

*Rolaids Extra Strength with Simethicone*—Calcium Carbonate and Simethicone—*See* Antacids (Oral), 253

*Rolatuss Expectorant*—Chlorpheniramine, Phenylephrine, Codeine, and Ammonium Chloride (Systemic)—*See* Cough/Cold Combinations (Systemic), 637

*Rolatuss w/Hydrocodone*—Pheniramine, Pyrilamine, Phenylephrine, Phenylpropanolamine, and Hydrocodone—*See* Cough/Cold Combinations (Systemic), 637

*Rolatuss Plain*—Chlorpheniramine and Phenylephrine—*See* Antihistamines and Decongestants (Systemic), 311

*Romazicon*—Flumazenil (Systemic), 1748

*Rondamine-DM Drops*—Carbinoxamine, Pseudoephedrine, and Dextromethorphan—*See* Cough/Cold Combinations (Systemic), 637

*Rondec*—Carbinoxamine and Pseudoephedrine—*See* Antihistamines and Decongestants (Systemic), 311

*Rondec-DM*—Carbinoxamine, Pseudoephedrine, and Dextromethorphan—*See* Cough/Cold Combinations (Systemic), 637

*Rondec-DM Drops*—Carbinoxamine, Pseudoephedrine, and Dextromethorphan—*See* Cough/Cold Combinations (Systemic), 637

*Rondec Drops*—Carbinoxamine and Pseudoephedrine—*See* Antihistamines and Decongestants (Systemic), 311

*Rondec-TR*—Carbinoxamine and Pseudoephedrine—*See* Antihistamines and Decongestants (Systemic), 311

*Roniacol*—Nicotinyl Alcohol (Systemic), 1215

*Roubac*—Sulfamethoxazole and Trimethoprim (Systemic), 1529

*Rounox*—Acetaminophen (Systemic), 161

*Rounox and Codeine 15*—Acetaminophen and Codeine—*See* Narcotic Analgesics and Acetaminophen (Systemic), 1181

*Rounox and Codeine 30*—Acetaminophen and Codeine—*See* Narcotic Analgesics and Acetaminophen (Systemic), 1181

*Rounox and Codeine 60*—Acetaminophen and Codeine—*See* Narcotic Analgesics and Acetaminophen (Systemic), 1181

*Rowasa*—Mesalamine (Rectal), 1097

*Roxanol*—Morphine—*See* Narcotic Analgesics—For Pain Relief (Systemic), 1176

*Roxanol 100*—Morphine—*See* Narcotic Analgesics—For Pain Relief (Systemic), 1176

*Roxanol SR*—Morphine—*See* Narcotic Analgesics—For Pain Relief (Systemic), 1176

*Roxicet*—Oxycodone and Acetaminophen—*See* Narcotic Analgesics and Acetaminophen (Systemic), 1181, MC-18

*Roxicet 5/500*—Oxycodone and Acetaminophen—*See* Narcotic Analgesics and Acetaminophen (Systemic), 1181

*Roxicodone*—Oxycodone—*See* Narcotic Analgesics—For Pain Relief (Systemic), 1176, MC-18

*Roxiprin*—Oxycodone and Aspirin—*See* Narcotic Analgesics and Aspirin (Systemic), 1185, MC-18

*Roychlor-10%*—Potassium Chloride—*See* Potassium Supplements (Systemic), 1373

*Royflex*—Triethanolamine Salicylate (Topical), 1754

*R-Tannamine*—Chlorpheniramine, Pyrilamine, and Phenylephrine—*See* Antihistamines and Decongestants (Systemic), 311

*R-Tannamine Pediatric*—Chlorpheniramine, Pyrilamine, and Phenylephrine—*See* Antihistamines and Decongestants (Systemic), 311

*R-Tannate*—Chlorpheniramine, Pyrilamine, and Phenylephrine—*See* Antihistamines and Decongestants (Systemic), 311

*R-Tannate Pediatric*—Chlorpheniramine, Pyrilamine, and Phenylephrine—*See* Antihistamines and Decongestants (Systemic), 311

rt-PA—Alteplase, Recombinant—*See* Thrombolytic Agents (Systemic), 1604

Rubella Virus Vaccine Live (Systemic), 1470

*Rubesol-1000*—Cyanocobalamin—*See* Vitamin B$_{12}$ (Systemic), 1667

*Rubex*—Doxorubicin (Systemic), 758

Rubidium Rb 82—*See* Radiopharmaceuticals (Diagnostic), 1439

*Rubion*—Cyanocobalamin—*See* Vitamin B$_{12}$ (Systemic), 1667

*Rubramin*—Cyanocobalamin—*See* Vitamin B$_{12}$ (Systemic), 1667

*Rubramin PC*—Cyanocobalamin—*See* Vitamin B$_{12}$ (Systemic), 1667

*Rufen*—Ibuprofen—*See* Nonsteroidal Anti-inflammatory Drugs (Systemic), 1229, MC-12

*Rulox*—Alumina and Magnesia—*See* Antacids (Oral), 253

*Rulox No. 1*—Alumina and Magnesia—*See* Antacids (Oral), 253

*Rulox No. 2*—Alumina and Magnesia—*See* Antacids (Oral), 253

*Rum-K*—Potassium Chloride—*See* Potassium Supplements (Systemic), 1373

*Ru-Tuss*—Chlorpheniramine and Phenylephrine—*See* Antihistamines and Decongestants (Systemic), 311; Chlorpheniramine, Phenylephrine, Phenylpropanolamine, Atropine, Hyoscyamine, and Scopolamine—*See* Antihistamines, Decongestants, and Anticholinergics (Systemic), 322

*Ru-Tuss II*—Chlorpheniramine and Phenylpropanolamine—*See* Antihistamines and Decongestants (Systemic), 311

*Ru-Tuss DE*—Pseudoephedrine and Guaifenesin—*See* Cough/Cold Combinations (Systemic), 637

*Ru-Tuss Expectorant*—Pseudoephedrine, Dextromethorphan, and Guaifenesin—*See* Cough/Cold Combinations (Systemic), 637

*Ru-Tuss with Hydrocodone Liquid*—Pheniramine, Pyrilamine, Phenylephrine, Phenylpropanolamine, and Hydrocodone—*See* Cough/Cold Combinations (Systemic), 637

*Ru-Vert M*—Meclizine—*See* Meclizine/Buclizine/Cyclizine (Systemic), 1079

RVA—Rabies Vaccine Adsorbed—*See* Rabies Vaccine (Systemic), 1434

*Rymed*—Phenylephrine, Phenylpropanolamine, and Guaifenesin—*See* Cough/Cold Combinations (Systemic), 637;

Pseudoephedrine and Guaifenesin—*See* Cough/Cold Combinations (Systemic), 637
*Rymed Liquid*—Pseudoephedrine and Guaifenesin—*See* Cough/Cold Combinations (Systemic), 637
*Rymed-TR Caplets*—Pseudoephedrine and Guaifenesin—*See* Cough/Cold Combinations (Systemic), 637
*Ryna*—Chlorpheniramine and Pseudoephedrine—*See* Antihistamines and Decongestants (Systemic), 311
*Ryna-C Liquid*—Chlorpheniramine, Pseudoephedrine, and Codeine—*See* Cough/Cold Combinations (Systemic), 637
*Rynacrom*—Cromolyn (Nasal), 654
*Ryna-CX Liquid*—Pseudoephedrine, Codeine, and Guaifenesin—*See* Cough/Cold Combinations (Systemic), 637
*Rynatan*—Chlorpheniramine, Pyrilamine, and Phenylephrine—*See* Antihistamines and Decongestants (Systemic), 311, MC-18
*Rynatan Pediatric*—Chlorpheniramine, Pyrilamine, and Phenylephrine—*See* Antihistamines and Decongestants (Systemic), 311
*Rynatan-S Pediatric*—Chlorpheniramine, Pyrilamine, and Phenylephrine—*See* Antihistamines and Decongestants (Systemic), 311
*Rynatuss*—Chlorpheniramine, Ephedrine, Phenylephrine, and Carbetapentane—*See* Cough/Cold Combinations (Systemic), 637
*Rynatuss Pediatric*—Chlorpheniramine, Ephedrine, Phenylephrine, and Carbetapentane—*See* Cough/Cold Combinations (Systemic), 637
*Rythmodan*—Disopyramide (Systemic), 734
*Rythmodan-LA*—Disopyramide (Systemic), 734
*Rythmol*—Propafenone (Systemic), 1408, MC-20

# S

*S-2*—Racepinephrine—*See* Bronchodilators, Adrenergic (Inhalation), 430
*6-MP*—*See* Mercaptopurine (Systemic), 1094
*642*—Propoxyphene—*See* Narcotic Analgesics—For Pain Relief (Systemic), 1176
*692*—Propoxyphene, Aspirin, and Caffeine—*See* Narcotic Analgesics and Aspirin (Systemic), 1185
Sabin vaccine—Poliovirus Vaccine Live Oral—*See* Poliovirus Vaccine (Systemic), 1367
*S-A-C*—Acetaminophen, Salicylamide, and Caffeine—*See* Acetaminophen and Salicylates (Systemic), 164
*Safe Tussin 30*—Dextromethorphan and Guaifenesin—*See* Cough/Cold Combinations (Systemic), 637
*Salac*—Salicylic Acid (Topical), 1478
*Salacid*—Salicylic Acid (Topical), 1478
*Sal-Acid Plaster*—Salicylic Acid (Topical), 1478
*Salactic Film Topical Solution*—Salicylic Acid (Topical), 1478
*Sal-Adult*—Aspirin—*See* Salicylates (Systemic), 1473
*Salagen*—Pilocarpine (Systemic), 1752
*Salazide*—Reserpine and Hydroflumethiazide—*See* Rauwolfia Alkaloids and Thiazide Diuretics (Systemic), 1445
*Salazopyrin*—Sulfasalazine (Systemic), 1535
*Salazopyrin EN-Tabs*—Sulfasalazine (Systemic), 1535
Salazosulfapyridine—*See* Sulfasalazine (Systemic), 1535

Salbutamol—Albuterol—*See* Bronchodilators, Adrenergic (Inhalation), 430; Bronchodilators, Adrenergic (Oral/Injection), 436
*Sal-Clens Plus Shampoo*—Salicylic Acid (Topical), 1478
*Sal-Clens Shampoo*—Salicylic Acid (Topical), 1478
*Salcylic Acid*—Salsalate—*See* Salicylates (Systemic), 1473
*Saleto*—Acetaminophen, Aspirin, Salicylamide, and Caffeine—*See* Acetaminophen and Salicylates (Systemic), 164
*Saleto-CF*—Phenylpropanolamine, Dextromethorphan, and Acetaminophen—*See* Cough/Cold Combinations (Systemic), 637
*Saleto D*—Phenylpropanolamine, Acetaminophen, Salicylamide, and Caffeine—*See* Decongestants and Analgesics (Systemic), 691
*Salflex*—Salsalate—*See* Salicylates (Systemic), 1473
*Salgesic*—Salsalate—*See* Salicylates (Systemic), 1473
*Sal hepatica*—Sodium Phosphate—*See* Laxatives (Oral), 1017
Salicylates (Systemic), 1473
Salicylazosulfapyridine—*See* Sulfasalazine (Systemic), 1535
Salicylic Acid (Topical), 1478
Salicylic Acid and Sulfur (Topical), 1481, 1754
Salicylic Acid, Sulfur, and Coal Tar (Topical), 1483
Salicylsalicylic acid—Salsalate—*See* Salicylates (Systemic), 1473
*Saligel*—Salicylic Acid (Topical), 1478
*Sal-Infant*—Aspirin—*See* Salicylates (Systemic), 1473
Salk vaccine—Poliovirus Vaccine Inactivated—*See* Poliovirus Vaccine (Systemic), 1367
*Salofalk*—Mesalamine (Rectal), 1097
*Salonil*—Salicylic Acid (Topical), 1478
*Salphenyl*—Chlorpheniramine, Phenylephrine, Acetaminophen, and Salicylamide—*See* Antihistamines, Decongestants, and Analgesics (Systemic), 316
*Sal-Plant Gel Topical Solution*—Salicylic Acid (Topical), 1478
Salsalate—*See* Salicylates (Systemic), 1473
*Salsitab*—Salsalate—*See* Salicylates (Systemic), 1473
*Saluron*—Hydroflumethiazide—*See* Diuretics, Thiazide (Systemic), 749
*Salutensin*—Reserpine and Hydroflumethiazide—*See* Rauwolfia Alkaloids and Thiazide Diuretics (Systemic), 1445
*Salutensin-Demi*—Reserpine and Hydroflumethiazide—*See* Rauwolfia Alkaloids and Thiazide Diuretics (Systemic), 1445
*Sandimmune*—Cyclosporine (Systemic), 671, MC-6
*Sandoglobulin*—Immune Globulin Intravenous (Human) (Systemic), 954
*Sandomigran*—Pizotyline (Systemic), 1752
*Sandomigran DS*—Pizotyline (Systemic), 1752
*Sandostatin*—Octreotide (Systemic), 1251
*Sani-Supp*—Glycerin—*See* Laxatives (Rectal), 1023
*Sanorex*—Mazindol—*See* Appetite Suppressants (Systemic), 339
*Sans-Acne*—Erythromycin (Topical), 782
*Sansert*—Methysergide (Systemic), 1121
Sargramostim—*See* Colony Stimulating Factors (Systemic), 600
*Sarisol No. 2*—Butabarbital—*See* Barbiturates (Systemic), 370

Sarna HC 1.0%—Hydrocortisone—See Corticosteroids— Low Potency (Topical), 624

S.A.S.-500—Sulfasalazine (Systemic), 1535

S.A.S. Enteric-500—Sulfasalazine (Systemic), 1535

Sastid (AL) Scrub—Salicylic Acid and Sulfur (Topical), 1481

Sastid Plain Shampoo and Acne Wash—Salicylic Acid and Sulfur (Topical), 1481

Sastid Soap—Salicylic Acid and Sulfur (Topical), 1481

Saxon Ribbed Lubricated—Latex Condoms—See Condoms, 602

Saxon Spermicidal—Latex Condoms and Nonoxynol 9—See Condoms, 602

Saxon Ultra Thin—Latex Condoms—See Condoms, 602

Saxon Wet Lubricated—Latex Condoms—See Condoms, 602

Scabene—Lindane (Topical), 1042

Scopolamine—See Anticholinergics/Antispasmodics (Systemic), 258; Atropine/Homatropine/Scopolamine (Ophthalmic), 354

Scot-tussin—Guaifenesin (Systemic), 892

Scot-Tussin DM—Chlorpheniramine and Dextromethorphan—See Cough/Cold Combinations (Systemic), 637

Scot-tussin Original 5-Action Cold Formula—Pheniramine, Phenylephrine, Sodium Salicylate, and Caffeine—See Antihistamines, Decongestants, and Analgesics (Systemic), 316

Scot-tussin Original 5-Action Cold Medicine—Pheniramine, Phenylephrine, Sodium Salicylate, and Caffeine—See Antihistamines, Decongestants, and Analgesics (Systemic), 316

SD Deprenyl—Selegiline (Systemic), 1485

Seba-Nil Liquid Cleanser—Alcohol and Acetone (Topical), 182

Sebasorb Liquid—Salicylic Acid and Sulfur (Topical), 1481

Sebex—Pyrithione (Topical), 1424; Salicylic Acid and Sulfur (Topical), 1481

Sebex-T Tar Shampoo—Salicylic Acid, Sulfur, and Coal Tar (Topical), 1483

Sebucare—Salicylic Acid (Topical), 1478

Sebulex Antiseborrheic Treatment and Conditioning Shampoo—Salicylic Acid and Sulfur (Topical), 1481

Sebulex Antiseborrheic Treatment Shampoo—Salicylic Acid and Sulfur (Topical), 1481

Sebulex Conditioning Suspension Shampoo—Salicylic Acid and Sulfur (Topical), 1481

Sebulex Cream Medicated Shampoo—Salicylic Acid and Sulfur (Topical), 1481

Sebulex Lotion Shampoo—Salicylic Acid and Sulfur (Topical), 1481

Sebulex Medicated Dandruff Shampoo with Conditioners— Salicylic Acid and Sulfur (Topical), 1481

Sebulex Medicated Shampoo—Salicylic Acid and Sulfur (Topical), 1481

Sebulex Regular Medicated Dandruff Shampoo—Salicylic Acid and Sulfur (Topical), 1481

Sebulon—Pyrithione (Topical), 1424

Sebutone—Salicylic Acid, Sulfur, and Coal Tar (Topical), 1483

Secobarbital—See Barbiturates (Systemic), 370

Secobarbital and Amobarbital—See Barbiturates (Systemic), 370

Seconal—Secobarbital—See Barbiturates (Systemic), 370

Sectral—Acebutolol—See Beta-adrenergic Blocking Agents (Systemic), 404

Sedapap—Butalbital and Acetaminophen (Systemic), 453

Sedatuss—Dextromethorphan (Systemic), 701

Seldane—Terfenadine—See Antihistamines (Systemic), 304, MC-22

Seldane Caplets—Terfenadine—See Antihistamines (Systemic), 304

Seldane-D—Terfenadine and Pseudoephedrine—See Antihistamines and Decongestants (Systemic), 311, MC-22

Selegiline (Systemic), 1485, MC-21

Selenious Acid—See Selenium Supplements (Systemic), 1489

Selenium—See Selenium Supplements (Systemic), 1489

Selenium Sulfide (Topical), 1487

Selenium Supplements (Systemic), 1489

Sele-Pak—Selenious Acid—See Selenium Supplements (Systemic), 1489

Selepen—Selenious Acid—See Selenium Supplements (Systemic), 1489

Selestoject—Betamethasone—See Corticosteroids/Corticotropin—Glucocorticoid Effects (Systemic), 630

Selexid—Pivmecillinam—See Penicillins (Systemic), 1299

Selsun—Selenium Sulfide (Topical), 1487

Selsun Blue—Selenium Sulfide (Topical), 1487

Selsun Blue Dry Formula—Selenium Sulfide (Topical), 1487

Selsun Blue Extra Conditioning Formula—Selenium Sulfide (Topical), 1487

Selsun Blue Extra Medicated Formula—Selenium Sulfide (Topical), 1487

Selsun Blue Oily Formula—Selenium Sulfide (Topical), 1487

Selsun Blue Regular Formula—Selenium Sulfide (Topical), 1487

Semicid—Nonoxynol 9—See Spermicides (Vaginal), 1512

Semilente Insulin—Insulin Zinc, Prompt—See Insulin (Systemic), 961

Semilente insulin—Insulin Zinc, Prompt—See Insulin (Systemic), 961

Semprex-D—Acrivastine and Pseudoephedrine—See Antihistamines and Decongestants (Systemic), 311, MC-1

Senefen III—Hydrocodone and Acetaminophen—See Narcotic Analgesics and Acetaminophen (Systemic), 1181

Senexon—Senna—See Laxatives (Oral), 1017

Senna—See Laxatives (Oral), 1017; Laxatives (Rectal), 1023

Senna and Docusate—See Laxatives (Oral), 1017

Sennosides—See Laxatives (Oral), 1017

Senokot—Senna—See Laxatives (Oral), 1017; Laxatives (Rectal), 1023

Senokot-S—Senna and Docusate—See Laxatives (Oral), 1017

Senolax—Senna—See Laxatives (Oral), 1017

SensoGARD Canker Sore Relief—Benzocaine—See Anesthetics (Dental), 229

Sensorcaine—Bupivacaine—See Anesthetics (Parenteral-Local), 235

Sensorcaine-MPF—Bupivacaine—See Anesthetics (Parenteral-Local), 235

Sensorcaine-MPF Spinal—Bupivacaine—See Anesthetics (Parenteral-Local), 235

*Sine-Aid Maximum Strength Gelcaps*—Pseudoephedrine and Acetaminophen—*See* Decongestants and Analgesics (Systemic), 691

*Sinemet*—Carbidopa and Levodopa—*See* Levodopa (Systemic), 1033, MC-4

*Sinemet CR*—Carbidopa and Levodopa—*See* Levodopa (Systemic), 1033

*Sine-Off Maximum Strength Allergy/Sinus Formula Caplets*—Chlorpheniramine, Pseudoephedrine, and Acetaminophen—*See* Antihistamines, Decongestants, and Analgesics (Systemic), 316

*Sine-off Maximum Strength No Drowsiness Formula Caplets*—Pseudoephedrine and Acetaminophen—*See* Decongestants and Analgesics (Systemic), 691

*Sine-Off Sinus Medicine*—Chlorpheniramine, Phenylpropanolamine, and Aspirin—*See* Antihistamines, Decongestants, and Analgesics (Systemic), 316

*Sinequan*—Doxepin—*See* Antidepressants, Tricyclic (Systemic), 277, MC-8

*Singlet*—Chlorpheniramine, Pseudoephedrine, and Acetaminophen—*See* Antihistamines, Decongestants, and Analgesics (Systemic), 316

*Sintrom*—Acenocoumarol (Systemic), 1745

*Sinucon Pediatric Drops*—Chlorpheniramine, Phenyltoloxamine, Phenylephrine, and Phenylpropanolamine—*See* Antihistamines and Decongestants (Systemic), 311

*Sinufed Timecelles*—Pseudoephedrine and Guaifenesin—*See* Cough/Cold Combinations (Systemic), 637

*Sinulin*—Chlorpheniramine, Phenylpropanolamine, and Acetaminophen—*See* Antihistamines, Decongestants, and Analgesics (Systemic), 316

*Sinumist-SR*—Guaifenesin (Systemic), 892

*Sinupan*—Phenylephrine and Guaifenesin—*See* Cough/Cold Combinations (Systemic), 637

*Sinus Excedrin Extra Strength*—Pseudoephedrine and Acetaminophen—*See* Decongestants and Analgesics (Systemic), 691

*Sinus Excedrin Extra Strength Caplets*—Pseudoephedrine and Acetaminophen—*See* Decongestants and Analgesics (Systemic), 691

*Sinus-Relief*—Pseudoephedrine and Acetaminophen—*See* Decongestants and Analgesics (Systemic), 691

*Sinutab Without Drowsiness*—Pseudoephedrine and Acetaminophen—*See* Decongestants and Analgesics (Systemic), 691

*Sinutab Without Drowsiness Extra Strength*—Pseudoephedrine and Acetaminophen—*See* Decongestants and Analgesics (Systemic), 691

*Sinutab Extra Strength*—Chlorpheniramine, Pseudoephedrine, and Acetaminophen—*See* Antihistamines, Decongestants, and Analgesics (Systemic), 316

*Sinutab II Maximum Strength*—Pseudoephedrine and Acetaminophen—*See* Decongestants and Analgesics (Systemic), 691

*Sinutab Maximum Strength Without Drowsiness*—Pseudoephedrine and Acetaminophen—*See* Decongestants and Analgesics (Systemic), 691

*Sinutab Maximum Strength Without Drowsiness Caplets*—Pseudoephedrine and Acetaminophen—*See* Decongestants and Analgesics (Systemic), 691

*Sinutab Maximum Strength Sinus Allergy*—Chlorpheniramine, Pseudoephedrine, and Acetaminophen—*See* Antihistamines, Decongestants, and Analgesics (Systemic), 316

*Sinutab Maximum Strength Sinus Allergy Caplets*—Chlorpheniramine, Pseudoephedrine, and Acetaminophen—*See* Antihistamines, Decongestants, and Analgesics (Systemic), 316

*Sinutab Regular*—Chlorpheniramine, Pseudoephedrine, and Acetaminophen—*See* Antihistamines, Decongestants, and Analgesics (Systemic), 316

*Sinutab SA*—Phenyltoloxamine, Phenylpropanolamine, and Acetaminophen—*See* Antihistamines, Decongestants, and Analgesics (Systemic), 316

*Sinutrex Extra Strength*—Chlorpheniramine, Pseudoephedrine, and Acetaminophen—*See* Antihistamines, Decongestants, and Analgesics (Systemic), 316

*SINUvent*—Phenylpropanolamine and Guaifenesin—*See* Cough/Cold Combinations (Systemic), 637

*Skelaxin*—Metaxalone—*See* Skeletal Muscle Relaxants (Systemic), 1495

Skeletal Muscle Relaxants (Systemic), 1495

*Skelex*—Methocarbamol—*See* Skeletal Muscle Relaxants (Systemic), 1495

*Sleep-Eze 3*—Diphenhydramine—*See* Antihistamines (Systemic), 304

*Slo-Bid*—Theophylline—*See* Bronchodilators, Xanthine-derivative (Systemic), 442

*Slo-bid Gyrocaps*—Theophylline—*See* Bronchodilators, Xanthine-derivative (Systemic), 442, MC-22

*Slo-Niacin*—Niacin—For High Cholesterol (Systemic), 1206, MC-16; Niacin (Vitamin $B_3$) (Systemic), 1208, MC-16

*Slo-Phyllin*—Theophylline—*See* Bronchodilators, Xanthine-derivative (Systemic), 442, MC-22

*Slo-Phyllin GG*—Theophylline and Guaifenesin (Systemic), 1586

*Slo-Phyllin Gyrocaps*—Theophylline—*See* Bronchodilators, Xanthine-derivative (Systemic), 442, MC-22

*Slow Fe*—Ferrous Sulfate—*See* Iron Supplements (Systemic), 986

*Slow-K*—Potassium Chloride—*See* Potassium Supplements (Systemic), 1373, MC-19

*Slow-Mag*—Magnesium Chloride—*See* Magnesium Supplements (Systemic), 1060

*Slow-Trasicor*—Oxprenolol—*See* Beta-adrenergic Blocking Agents (Systemic), 404

*SMA 13*—Infant Formulas, Milk-based—*See* Infant Formulas (Systemic), 958

*SMA 20*—Infant Formulas, Milk-based—*See* Infant Formulas (Systemic), 958

*SMA 24*—Infant Formulas, Milk-based—*See* Infant Formulas (Systemic), 958

*SMA 27*—Infant Formulas, Milk-based—*See* Infant Formulas (Systemic), 958

*SMA Lo-Iron 13*—Infant Formulas, Milk-based—*See* Infant Formulas (Systemic), 958

*SMA Lo-Iron 20*—Infant Formulas, Milk-based—*See* Infant Formulas (Systemic), 958

*SMA Lo-Iron 24*—Infant Formulas, Milk-based—*See* Infant Formulas (Systemic), 958

SMZ-TMP—*See* Sulfamethoxazole and Trimethoprim (Systemic), 1529

*Snaplets-D*—Chlorpheniramine and Phenylpropanolamine—*See* Antihistamines and Decongestants (Systemic), 311

*Snaplets-DM*—Phenylpropanolamine and Dextromethorphan—*See* Cough/Cold Combinations (Systemic), 637

*Snaplets-EX*—Phenylpropanolamine and Guaifenesin—*See* Cough/Cold Combinations (Systemic), 637

*Snaplets-FR*—Acetaminophen (Systemic), 161

*Snaplets-Multi*—Chlorpheniramine, Phenylpropanolamine, and Dextromethorphan—*See* Cough/Cold Combinations (Systemic), 637

*Soda Mint*—Sodium Bicarbonate (Systemic), 1499

Sodium Ascorbate—*See* Ascorbic Acid (Vitamin C) (Systemic), 344

Sodium aurothiomalate—Gold Sodium Thiomalate—*See* Gold Compounds (Systemic), 884

Sodium azodisalicylate—*See* Olsalazine (Oral), 1254

Sodium Benzoate and Sodium Phenylacetate (Systemic), 1498

Sodium Bicarbonate (Systemic), 1499

Sodium Chloride (Intra-amniotic), 1501

Sodium Chromate Cr 51—*See* Radiopharmaceuticals (Diagnostic), 1439

Sodium Citrate and Citric Acid—*See* Citrates (Systemic), 554

Sodium cromoglycate—*See* Cromolyn (Inhalation), 650; Cromolyn (Nasal), 654; Cromolyn (Ophthalmic), 656; Cromolyn (Oral), 658

Sodium Fluoride (Systemic), 1502

Sodium Iodide (Systemic), 1505

Sodium Iodide I 123—*See* Radiopharmaceuticals (Diagnostic), 1439

Sodium Iodide I 131—*See* Radiopharmaceuticals (Diagnostic), 1439

Sodium Iodide I 131 (Therapeutic), 1507

Sodium Iopodate—Ipodate—*See* Cholecystographic Agents, Oral (Diagnostic), 536

Sodium Pertechnetate Tc 99m—*See* Radiopharmaceuticals (Diagnostic), 1439

Sodium Phosphate—*See* Laxatives (Oral), 1017

Sodium Phosphate P 32 (Therapeutic), 1508

Sodium Phosphates—*See* Laxatives (Rectal), 1023; Phosphates (Systemic), 1349

Sodium Salicylate—*See* Salicylates (Systemic), 1473

*Sodium Sulamyd*—Sulfacetamide—*See* Sulfonamides (Ophthalmic), 1540

Sodium Thiosulfate (Systemic), 1509

Sodium Tyropanoate—Tyropanoate—*See* Cholecystographic Agents, Oral (Diagnostic), 536

*Sodol*—Carisoprodol—*See* Skeletal Muscle Relaxants (Systemic), 1495

*Sofarin*—Warfarin—*See* Anticoagulants (Systemic), 262

*Sofracort Eye-Ear Drops*—Framycetin, Gramicidin, and Dexamethasone (Ophthalmic), 1749; Framycetin, Gramicidin, and Dexamethasone (Otic), 1749

*Sofracort Eye-Ear Ointment*—Framycetin, Gramicidin, and Dexamethasone (Ophthalmic), 1749; Framycetin, Gramicidin, and Dexamethasone (Otic), 1749

*Soframycin*—Framycetin (Ophthalmic), 1749; Framycetin and Gramicidin (Topical), 1749

*Sofra-Tulle*—Framycetin (Topical), 1749

*Solatene*—Beta-carotene—For Dietary Supplement (Vitamin) (Systemic), 415; Beta-carotene—For Photosensitivity (Systemic), 417

*Solazine*—Trifluoperazine—*See* Phenothiazines (Systemic), 1330

*Solfoton*—Phenobarbital—*See* Barbiturates (Systemic), 370

*Solganal*—Aurothioglucose—*See* Gold Compounds (Systemic), 884

*Solium*—Chlordiazepoxide—*See* Benzodiazepines (Systemic), 389

*Solu-Cortef*—Hydrocortisone—*See* Corticosteroids/Corticotropin—Glucocorticoid Effects (Systemic), 630

*Solu-Flur*—Sodium Fluoride (Systemic), 1502

*Solu-Medrol*—Methylprednisolone—*See* Corticosteroids/Corticotropin—Glucocorticoid Effects (Systemic), 630

*Solu-Phyllin*—Theophylline—*See* Bronchodilators, Xanthine-derivative (Systemic), 442

*Solurex*—Dexamethasone—*See* Corticosteroids/Corticotropin—Glucocorticoid Effects (Systemic), 630

*Solurex-LA*—Dexamethasone—*See* Corticosteroids/Corticotropin—Glucocorticoid Effects (Systemic), 630

*Soma*—Carisoprodol—*See* Skeletal Muscle Relaxants (Systemic), 1495, MC-4

*Soma Compound*—Carisoprodol and Aspirin (Systemic), MC-4

*Soma Compound with Codeine*—Carisoprodol, Aspirin, and Codeine (Systemic), MC-4

Somatrem—*See* Growth Hormone (Systemic), 891

Somatropin—*See* Growth Hormone (Systemic), 891

*Sominex Formula 2*—Diphenhydramine—*See* Antihistamines (Systemic), 304

*Somnol*—Flurazepam—*See* Benzodiazepines (Systemic), 389

*Somnothane*—Halothane—*See* Anesthetics, General (Systemic), 243

*Somophyllin-12*—Theophylline—*See* Bronchodilators, Xanthine-derivative (Systemic), 442

*Sopamycetin*—Chloramphenicol (Otic), 516

*Sopamycetin Ophthalmic Ointment*—Chloramphenicol (Ophthalmic), 514

*Sopamycetin Ophthalmic Solution*—Chloramphenicol (Ophthalmic), 514

*Soprodol*—Carisoprodol—*See* Skeletal Muscle Relaxants (Systemic), 1495

*Sorbitrate*—Isosorbide Dinitrate—*See* Nitrates—Oral (Systemic), 1218, MC-12; Nitrates—Sublingual, Chewable, or Buccal (Systemic), 1221, MC-12

*Soriatane*—Acitretin (Systemic), 1745

*Soridol*—Carisoprodol—*See* Skeletal Muscle Relaxants (Systemic), 1495

*Sotacor*—Sotalol—*See* Beta-adrenergic Blocking Agents (Systemic), 404

Sotalol—*See* Beta-adrenergic Blocking Agents (Systemic), 404, MC-21

*Soyalac*—Infant Formulas, Soy-based—*See* Infant Formulas (Systemic), 958

*Span-FF*—Ferrous Fumarate—*See* Iron Supplements (Systemic), 986

*Sparine*—Promazine—*See* Phenothiazines (Systemic), 1330

*Spaslin*—Atropine, Hyoscyamine, Scopolamine, and Phenobarbital—*See* Belladonna Alkaloids and Barbiturates (Systemic), 382

Streptozocin (Systemic), 1517

*Stresstein*—Enteral Nutrition Formula, Disease-specific—*See* Enteral Nutrition Formulas (Systemic), 769

*Stri-Dex Dual Textured Pads Maximum Strength*—Salicylic Acid (Topical), 1478

*Stri-Dex Dual Textured Pads Regular Strength*—Salicylic Acid (Topical), 1478

*Stri-Dex Dual Textured Pads Sensitive Skin*—Salicylic Acid (Topical), 1478

*Stri-Dex Maximum Strength Pads*—Salicylic Acid (Topical), 1478

*Stri-Dex Maximum Strength Treatment 10 Cream*—Benzoyl Peroxide (Topical), 397

*Stri-Dex Regular Strength Pads*—Salicylic Acid (Topical), 1478

*Stri-Dex Super Scrub Pads*—Salicylic Acid (Topical), 1478

*217 Strong*—Aspirin and Caffeine—*See* Salicylates (Systemic), 1473

Strong iodine tincture—*See* Iodine (Topical), 974

Strontium 89 Chloride (Therapeutic), 1519

*Stulex*—Docusate—*See* Laxatives (Oral), 1017

*Sublimaze*—Fentanyl—*See* Narcotic Analgesics—For Surgery and Obstetrics (Systemic), 1179

Succimer (Systemic), 1520

Sucralfate (Oral), 1522, MC-21

*Sucrets, Children's*—Dyclonine—*See* Anesthetics (Dental), 229

*Sucrets Cough Control Formula*—Dextromethorphan (Systemic), 701

*Sucrets Maximum Strength*—Dyclonine—*See* Anesthetics (Dental), 229

*Sucrets Regular Strength*—Dyclonine—*See* Anesthetics (Dental), 229

*Sudafed*—Pseudoephedrine (Systemic), 1412

*Sudafed Cold & Cough Liquid Caps*—Pseudoephedrine, Dextromethorphan, Guaifenesin, and Acetaminophen—*See* Cough/Cold Combinations (Systemic), 637

*Sudafed Cough*—Pseudoephedrine, Dextromethorphan, and Guaifenesin—*See* Cough/Cold Combinations (Systemic), 637

*Sudafed DM*—Pseudoephedrine and Dextromethorphan—*See* Cough/Cold Combinations (Systemic), 637

*Sudafed Expectorant*—Pseudoephedrine and Guaifenesin—*See* Cough/Cold Combinations (Systemic), 637

*Sudafed 12 Hour*—Pseudoephedrine (Systemic), 1412

*Sudafed Liquid, Children's*—Pseudoephedrine (Systemic), 1412

*Sudafed Plus*—Chlorpheniramine and Pseudoephedrine—*See* Antihistamines and Decongestants (Systemic), 311

*Sudafed Severe Cold Formula Caplets*—Pseudoephedrine, Dextromethorphan, and Acetaminophen—*See* Cough/Cold Combinations (Systemic), 637

*Sudafed Sinus Maximum Strength*—Pseudoephedrine and Acetaminophen—*See* Decongestants and Analgesics (Systemic), 691

*Sudafed Sinus Maximum Strength Caplets*—Pseudoephedrine and Acetaminophen—*See* Decongestants and Analgesics (Systemic), 691

*Sufedrin*—Pseudoephedrine (Systemic), 1412

*Sufenta*—Sufentanil—*See* Narcotic Analgesics—For Surgery and Obstetrics (Systemic), 1179

Sufentanil—For Surgery and Obstetrics—*See* Narcotic Analgesics—For Surgery and Obstetrics (Systemic), 1179

*Sul-Azo*—Sulfisoxazole and Phenazopyridine—*See* Sulfonamides and Phenazopyridine (Systemic), 1547

Sulconazole (Topical), 1523

*Sulcrate*—Sucralfate (Oral), 1522

*Suleo-M*—Malathion (Topical), 1063

*Sulf-10*—Sulfacetamide—*See* Sulfonamides (Ophthalmic), 1540

Sulfacetamide—*See* Sulfonamides (Ophthalmic), 1540

Sulfacytine—*See* Sulfonamides (Systemic), 1542

Sulfadiazine—*See* Sulfonamides (Systemic), 1542

Sulfadiazine and Trimethoprim (Systemic), 1754

Sulfadoxine and Pyrimethamine (Systemic), 1525

Sulfafurazole—Sulfisoxazole—*See* Sulfonamides (Ophthalmic), 1540; Sulfonamides (Systemic), 1542

*Sulfa-Gyn*—Triple Sulfa—*See* Sulfonamides (Vaginal), 1545

*Sulfair*—Sulfacetamide—*See* Sulfonamides (Ophthalmic), 1540

*Sulfair 10*—Sulfacetamide—*See* Sulfonamides (Ophthalmic), 1540

*Sulfair 15*—Sulfacetamide—*See* Sulfonamides (Ophthalmic), 1540

*Sulfair Forte*—Sulfacetamide—*See* Sulfonamides (Ophthalmic), 1540

Sulfamethizole—*See* Sulfonamides (Systemic), 1542

*Sulfamethoprim*—Sulfamethoxazole and Trimethoprim (Systemic), 1529

*Sulfamethoprim DS*—Sulfamethoxazole and Trimethoprim (Systemic), 1529

Sulfamethoxazole—*See* Sulfonamides (Systemic), 1542

Sulfamethoxazole and Phenazopyridine—*See* Sulfonamides and Phenazopyridine (Systemic), 1547

Sulfamethoxazole and Trimethoprim (Systemic), 1529, MC-21

*Sulfamide*—Sulfacetamide—*See* Sulfonamides (Ophthalmic), 1540

*Sulfamylon*—Mafenide (Topical), 1059

Sulfanilamide—*See* Sulfonamides (Vaginal), 1545

Sulfanilamide, Aminacrine, and Allantoin—*See* Sulfonamides (Vaginal), 1545

*Sulfaprim*—Sulfamethoxazole and Trimethoprim (Systemic), 1529

*Sulfaprim DS*—Sulfamethoxazole and Trimethoprim (Systemic), 1529

Sulfapyridine (Systemic), 1532

Sulfasalazine (Systemic), 1535, MC-21

Sulfathiazole, sulfacetamide, and sulfabenzamide—Triple Sulfa—*See* Sulfonamides (Vaginal), 1545

*Sulfatrim*—Sulfamethoxazole and Trimethoprim (Systemic), 1529

*Sulfatrim DS*—Sulfamethoxazole and Trimethoprim (Systemic), 1529

*Sulfex*—Sulfacetamide—*See* Sulfonamides (Ophthalmic), 1540

*Sulfimycin*—Erythromycin and Sulfisoxazole (Systemic), 790

Sulfinpyrazone (Systemic), 1538

Sulfisoxazole—*See* Sulfonamides (Ophthalmic), 1540; Sulfonamides (Systemic), 1542

Sulfisoxazole and Phenazopyridine—*See* Sulfonamides and Phenazopyridine (Systemic), 1547

Sulfonamides (Ophthalmic), 1540

Sulfonamides (Systemic), 1542

Sulfonamides (Vaginal), 1545

Sulfonamides and Phenazopyridine (Systemic), 1547

*Sulforcin*—Resorcinol and Sulfur (Topical), 1454

*Sulfoxaprim*—Sulfamethoxazole and Trimethoprim (Systemic), 1529

*Sulfoxaprim DS*—Sulfamethoxazole and Trimethoprim (Systemic), 1529

Sulfur (Topical), 1550

Sulfurated Lime (Topical), 1552

Sulindac—*See* Nonsteroidal Anti-inflammatory Drugs (Systemic), 1229, MC-21

*Sulnac*—Triple Sulfa—*See* Sulfonamides (Vaginal), 1545

Sulphacetamide—Sulfacetamide—*See* Sulfonamides (Ophthalmic), 1540

Sulphafurazole—Sulfisoxazole—*See* Sulfonamides (Ophthalmic), 1540

*Sulpho-Lac*—Sulfur (Topical), 1550

*Sulsal Soap*—Salicylic Acid and Sulfur (Topical), 1481

*Sulten-10*—Sulfacetamide—*See* Sulfonamides (Ophthalmic), 1540

*Sultrin*—Triple Sulfa—*See* Sulfonamides (Vaginal), 1545

*Sumacal*—Enteral Nutrition Formula, Modular—*See* Enteral Nutrition Formulas (Systemic), 769

Sumatriptan (Systemic), 1554

*Sumycin*—Tetracycline—*See* Tetracyclines (Systemic), 1570, MC-22

*Sunkist*—Ascorbic Acid (Vitamin C) (Systemic), 344

*Supac*—Acetaminophen, Aspirin, and Caffeine, Buffered—*See* Acetaminophen and Salicylates (Systemic), 164

*Supasa*—Aspirin—*See* Salicylates (Systemic), 1473

*Super Calcium 1200*—Calcium Carbonate—*See* Calcium Supplements (Systemic), 472

*Superlipid*—Probucol (Systemic), 1395

*Supeudol*—Oxycodone—*See* Narcotic Analgesics—For Pain Relief (Systemic), 1176

*Suplena*—Enteral Nutrition Formula, Disease-specific—*See* Enteral Nutrition Formulas (Systemic), 769

*Suppap-120*—Acetaminophen (Systemic), 161

*Suppap-325*—Acetaminophen (Systemic), 161

*Suppap-650*—Acetaminophen (Systemic), 161

*Supprelin*—Histrelin (Systemic), 1749

*Supracaine*—Tetracaine—*See* Anesthetics (Dental), 229

*Suprane*—Desflurane (Inhalation-Systemic), 697

*Suprax*—Cefixime—*See* Cephalosporins (Systemic), 498, MC-4

*Suprefact*—Buserelin (Systemic), 447

*Supres*—Methyldopa and Chlorothiazide—*See* Methyldopa and Thiazide Diuretics (Systemic), 1114

Suprofen—*See* Anti-inflammatory Agents, Nonsteroidal (Ophthalmic), 330

*SureCell hCG-Urine Test*—Pregnancy Test Kits for Home Use, 1385

*Surfak*—Docusate—*See* Laxatives (Oral), 1017

*Surgam*—Tiaprofenic Acid—*See* Nonsteroidal Anti-inflammatory Drugs (Systemic), 1229

*Surgam SR*—Tiaprofenic Acid—*See* Nonsteroidal Anti-inflammatory Drugs (Systemic), 1229

*Surmontil*—Trimipramine—*See* Antidepressants, Tricyclic (Systemic), 277, MC-24

*Susano*—Atropine, Hyoscyamine, Scopolamine, and Phenobarbital—*See* Belladonna Alkaloids and Barbiturates (Systemic), 382

*Sus-Phrine*—Epinephrine—*See* Bronchodilators, Adrenergic (Oral/Injection), 436

*Sustacal*—Enteral Nutrition Formula, Polymeric—*See* Enteral Nutrition Formulas (Systemic), 769

*Sustacal 8.8*—Enteral Nutrition Formula, Polymeric—*See* Enteral Nutrition Formulas (Systemic), 769

*Sustacal with Fiber*—Enteral Nutrition Formula, Fiber-containing—*See* Enteral Nutrition Formulas (Systemic), 769

*Sustacal HC*—Enteral Nutrition Formula, Polymeric—*See* Enteral Nutrition Formulas (Systemic), 769

*Sustacal Plus*—Enteral Nutrition Formula, Polymeric (Systemic), 1748

*Sustagen*—Enteral Nutrition Formula, Milk-based—*See* Enteral Nutrition Formulas (Systemic), 769

*Sutilan*—Tiopronin (Systemic), 1612

*Syllact*—Psyllium—*See* Laxatives (Oral), 1017

*Syllamalt*—Malt Soup Extract and Psyllium—*See* Laxatives (Oral), 1017

*Symadine*—Amantadine (Systemic), 194

*Symmetrel*—Amantadine (Systemic), 194, MC-1

*Synacort*—Hydrocortisone—*See* Corticosteroids—Low Potency (Topical), 624

*Synalar*—Fluocinolone—*See* Corticosteroids—Medium to Very High Potency (Topical), 626

*Synalar-HP*—Fluocinolone—*See* Corticosteroids—Medium to Very High Potency (Topical), 626

*Synalgos-DC*—Aspirin, Caffeine, and Dihydrocodeine—*See* Narcotic Analgesics and Aspirin (Systemic), 1185, MC-2

*Synamol*—Fluocinolone—*See* Corticosteroids—Medium to Very High Potency (Topical), 626

*Synarel*—Nafarelin (Systemic), 1166, 1751

*Syn-Clonazepam*—Clonazepam—*See* Benzodiazepines (Systemic), 389

*Syn-Diltiazem*—Diltiazem—*See* Calcium Channel Blocking Agents (Systemic), 467

*Synemol*—Fluocinolone—*See* Corticosteroids—Medium to Very High Potency (Topical), 626

*Synflex*—Naproxen—*See* Nonsteroidal Anti-inflammatory Drugs (Systemic), 1229

*Synflex DS*—Naproxen—*See* Nonsteroidal Anti-inflammatory Drugs (Systemic), 1229

*Synkayvite*—Menadiol—*See* Vitamin K (Systemic), 1676

*Syn-Nadolol*—Nadolol—*See* Beta-adrenergic Blocking Agents (Systemic), 404

*Synophylate-GG*—Theophylline and Guaifenesin (Systemic), 1586

*Synphasic*—Norethindrone and Ethinyl Estradiol—*See* Estrogens and Progestins (Oral Contraceptives) (Systemic), 804

*Syn-Pindolol*—Pindolol—*See* Beta-adrenergic Blocking Agents (Systemic), 404

*Synthroid*—Levothyroxine—*See* Thyroid Hormones (Systemic), 1606, MC-13

*Syntocinon*—Oxytocin (Systemic), 1277

Synvinolin—Simvastatin—*See* HMG-CoA Reductase Inhibitors (Systemic), 929

*Syprine*—Trientine (Systemic), 1622

*Syracol Liquid*—Phenylpropanolamine and Dextromethorphan—*See* Cough/Cold Combinations (Systemic), 637

# T

*Test-Estro Cypionate*—Testosterone and Estradiol—*See* Androgens and Estrogens (Systemic), 225

*Testex*—Testosterone—*See* Androgens (Systemic), 221

*Testoderm*—Testosterone—*See* Androgens (Systemic), 221

*Testoject-50*—Testosterone—*See* Androgens (Systemic), 221

*Testoject-LA*—Testosterone—*See* Androgens (Systemic), 221

Testolactone (Systemic), 1565

*Testone L.A. 100*—Testosterone—*See* Androgens (Systemic), 221

*Testone L.A. 200*—Testosterone—*See* Androgens (Systemic), 221

*Testopel*—Testosterone (Systemic), 1754

Testosterone—*See* Androgens (Systemic), 221, 1754

Testosterone and Estradiol—*See* Androgens and Estrogens (Systemic), 225

*Testred*—Methyltestosterone—*See* Androgens (Systemic), 221

*Testred Cypionate 200*—Testosterone—*See* Androgens (Systemic), 221

*Testrin-P.A.*—Testosterone—*See* Androgens (Systemic), 221

Tetanus Toxoid (Systemic), 1567

Tetracaine—*See* Anesthetics (Dental), 229; Anesthetics (Ophthalmic), 234; Anesthetics (Parenteral-Local), 235; Anesthetics (Rectal), 237; Anesthetics (Topical), 240

Tetracaine and Menthol—*See* Anesthetics (Rectal), 237; Anesthetics (Topical), 240

Tetracycline—*See* Tetracyclines (Ophthalmic), 1568; Tetracyclines (Systemic), 1570, MC-22; Tetracyclines (Topical), 1574

Tetracyclines (Ophthalmic), 1568

Tetracyclines (Systemic), 1570

Tetracyclines (Topical), 1574

*Tetracyn*—Tetracycline—*See* Tetracyclines (Systemic), 1570

Tetrahydroaminoacridine—*See* Tacrine (Systemic), 1557

Tetramethylthionine chloride—*See* Methylene Blue (Systemic), 1117

*Texacort*—Hydrocortisone—*See* Corticosteroids—Low Potency (Topical), 624

*T-Gel*—Coal Tar (Topical), 589

*T/Gel Therapeutic Conditioner*—Coal Tar (Topical), 589

*T/Gel Therapeutic Shampoo*—Coal Tar (Topical), 589

*T-Gen*—Trimethobenzamide (Systemic), 1626

THA—*See* Tacrine (Systemic), 1557

*Thalitone*—Chlorthalidone—*See* Diuretics, Thiazide (Systemic), 749, MC-5

Thallous Chloride Tl 201—*See* Radiopharmaceuticals (Diagnostic), 1439

*Theo-24*—Theophylline—*See* Bronchodilators, Xanthine-derivative (Systemic), 442, MC-22

*Theo 250*—Theophylline—*See* Bronchodilators, Xanthine-derivative (Systemic), 442

*Theobid Duracaps*—Theophylline—*See* Bronchodilators, Xanthine-derivative (Systemic), 442

*Theobid Jr. Duracaps*—Theophylline—*See* Bronchodilators, Xanthine-derivative (Systemic), 442

*Theochron*—Theophylline—*See* Bronchodilators, Xanthine-derivative (Systemic), 442

*Theoclear-80*—Theophylline—*See* Bronchodilators, Xanthine-derivative (Systemic), 442

*Theoclear L.A.-130*—Theophylline—*See* Bronchodilators, Xanthine-derivative (Systemic), 442

*Theoclear L.A.-260*—Theophylline—*See* Bronchodilators, Xanthine-derivative (Systemic), 442

*Theocon*—Oxtriphylline and Guaifenesin (Systemic), 1270

*Theodrine*—Theophylline, Ephedrine, and Phenobarbital (Systemic), 1583

*Theo-Dur*—Theophylline—*See* Bronchodilators, Xanthine-derivative (Systemic), 442, MC-22

*Theofedral*—Theophylline, Ephedrine, and Phenobarbital (Systemic), 1583

*Theolair*—Theophylline—*See* Bronchodilators, Xanthine-derivative (Systemic), 442

*Theolair-SR*—Theophylline—*See* Bronchodilators, Xanthine-derivative (Systemic), 442

*Theolate*—Theophylline and Guaifenesin (Systemic), 1586

*Theomar*—Theophylline—*See* Bronchodilators, Xanthine-derivative (Systemic), 442

*Theomax DF*—Theophylline, Ephedrine, and Hydroxyzine (Systemic), 1580

*Theophedrital*—Theophylline, Ephedrine, and Phenobarbital (Systemic), 1583

Theophylline—*See* Bronchodilators, Xanthine-derivative (Systemic), 442, MC-22

Theophylline, Ephedrine, Guaifenesin, and Phenobarbital (Systemic), 1577

Theophylline, Ephedrine, and Hydroxyzine (Systemic), 1580

Theophylline, Ephedrine, and Phenobarbital (Systemic), 1583

Theophylline and glyceryl guaiacolate—*See* Theophylline and Guaifenesin (Systemic), 1586

Theophylline and Guaifenesin (Systemic), 1586, MC-22

*Theo-Sav*—Theophylline—*See* Bronchodilators, Xanthine-derivative (Systemic), 442

*Theospan-SR*—Theophylline—*See* Bronchodilators, Xanthine-derivative (Systemic), 442

*Theo-SR*—Theophylline—*See* Bronchodilators, Xanthine-derivative (Systemic), 442

*Theostat 80*—Theophylline—*See* Bronchodilators, Xanthine-derivative (Systemic), 442

*Theotal*—Theophylline, Ephedrine, and Phenobarbital (Systemic), 1583

*Theo-Time*—Theophylline—*See* Bronchodilators, Xanthine-derivative (Systemic), 442

*Theovent Long-Acting*—Theophylline—*See* Bronchodilators, Xanthine-derivative (Systemic), 442

*Theo-X*—Theophylline—*See* Bronchodilators, Xanthine-derivative (Systemic), 442

*Therac Lotion*—Salicylic Acid and Sulfur (Topical), 1481

*TheraCys*—Bacillus Calmette-Guérin (BCG) Live (Mucosal-Local), 367

*TheraFlu/Flu, Cold and Cough Medicine*—Chlorpheniramine, Pseudoephedrine, Dextromethrophan, and Acetaminophen—*See* Cough/Cold Combinations (Systemic), 637

*TheraFlu/Flu and Cold Medicine*—Chlorpheniramine, Pseudoephedrine, and Acetaminophen—*See* Antihistamines, Decongestants, and Analgesics (Systemic), 316

*TheraFlu Maximum Strength Non-Drowsy Formula Flu, Cold, and Cough Medicine*—Pseudoephedrine, Dextromethorphan, and Acetaminophen—*See* Cough/Cold Combinations (Systemic), 637

*Tisit Blue*—Pyrethrins and Piperonyl Butoxide (Topical), 1417

*Tisit Shampoo*—Pyrethrins and Piperonyl Butoxide (Topical), 1417

Tissue-type plasminogen activator (recombinant)—Alteplase, Recombinant—*See* Thrombolytic Agents (Systemic), 1604

*Titralac*—Calcium Carbonate—*See* Antacids (Oral), 253; Calcium Supplements (Systemic), 472

*Titralac Extra Strength*—Calcium Carbonate—*See* Antacids (Oral), 253

*Titralac Plus*—Calcium Carbonate and Simethicone—*See* Antacids (Oral), 253

*T-Koff*—Chlorpheniramine, Phenylephrine, Phenylpropanolamine, and Codeine—*See* Cough/Cold Combinations (Systemic), 637

Tobramycin—*See* Aminoglycosides (Systemic), 201

Tobramycin (Ophthalmic), 1613

*Tobrex*—Tobramycin (Ophthalmic), 1613

Tocainide (Systemic), 1615, MC-23

*Today*—Nonoxynol 9—*See* Spermicides (Vaginal), 1512

*Today with Spermicidal Lubricant*—Latex Condoms and Nonoxynol 9—*See* Condoms, 602

*Tofranil*—Imipramine—*See* Antidepressants, Tricyclic (Systemic), 277, MC-12

*Tofranil-PM*—Imipramine—*See* Antidepressants, Tricyclic (Systemic), 277, MC-12

*Tolamide*—Tolazamide—*See* Antidiabetics, Oral (Systemic), 283

Tolazamide—*See* Antidiabetics, Oral (Systemic), 283, MC-23

Tolbutamide—*See* Antidiabetics, Oral (Systemic), 283, MC-23

*Tolectin 200*—Tolmetin—*See* Nonsteroidal Anti-inflammatory Drugs (Systemic), 1229, MC-23

*Tolectin 400*—Tolmetin—*See* Nonsteroidal Anti-inflammatory Drugs (Systemic), 1229

*Tolectin 600*—Tolmetin—*See* Nonsteroidal Anti-inflammatory Drugs (Systemic), 1229, MC-23

*Tolectin DS*—Tolmetin—*See* Nonsteroidal Anti-inflammatory Drugs (Systemic), 1229, MC-23

*Tolerex*—Enteral Nutrition Formula, Monomeric (Elemental)—*See* Enteral Nutrition Formulas (Systemic), 769

*Tolinase*—Tolazamide—*See* Antidiabetics, Oral (Systemic), 283, MC-23

Tolmetin—*See* Nonsteroidal Anti-inflammatory Drugs (Systemic), 1229, MC-23

Tolnaftate (Topical), 1617

*Tol-Tab*—Tolbutamide—*See* Antidiabetics, Oral (Systemic), 283

*Tolu-Sed Cough*—Codeine and Guaifenesin—*See* Cough/Cold Combinations (Systemic), 637

*Tolu-Sed DM*—Dextromethorphan and Guaifenesin—*See* Cough/Cold Combinations (Systemic), 637

*Tonocard*—Tocainide (Systemic), 1615, MC-23

*Topex 5 Lotion*—Benzoyl Peroxide (Topical), 397

*Topex 10 Lotion*—Benzoyl Peroxide (Topical), 397

*Topicaine*—Benzocaine—*See* Anesthetics (Dental), 229

*Topicort*—Desoximetasone—*See* Corticosteroids—Medium to Very High Potency (Topical), 626

*Topicort LP*—Desoximetasone—*See* Corticosteroids—Medium to Very High Potency (Topical), 626

*Topicort Mild*—Desoximetasone—*See* Corticosteroids—Medium to Very High Potency (Topical), 626

*Topicycline*—Tetracycline—*See* Tetracyclines (Topical), 1574

*Topilene*—Betamethasone—*See* Corticosteroids—Medium to Very High Potency (Topical), 626

*Topisone*—Betamethasone—*See* Corticosteroids—Medium to Very High Potency (Topical), 626

*Topisporin*—Neomycin, Polymyxin B, and Bacitracin (Topical), 1200

*Toprol-XL*—Metoprolol—*See* Beta-adrenergic Blocking Agents (Systemic), 404, MC-15

*Topsyn*—Fluocinonide—*See* Corticosteroids—Medium to Very High Potency (Topical), 626

TOPV—Poliovirus Vaccine Live Oral—*See* Poliovirus Vaccine (Systemic), 1367

*Toradol*—Ketorolac (Systemic), 1013, MC-13

*Toradol*^(IM)—Ketorolac (Systemic), 1013

*Toradol*^(ORAL)—Ketorolac (Systemic), 1013

*Torecan*—Thiethylperazine (Systemic), 1594

*Tornalate*—Bitolterol—*See* Bronchodilators, Adrenergic (Inhalation), 430

Torsemide (Systemic), 1754

*Totacillin*—Ampicillin—*See* Penicillins (Systemic), 1299; Ampicillin (Systemic), MC-2

*Totacillin-N*—Ampicillin—*See* Penicillins (Systemic), 1299

*Touro A&H*—Brompheniramine and Pseudoephedrine—*See* Antihistamines and Decongestants (Systemic), 311

*Touro Ex*—Guaifenesin (Systemic), 892

*Touro LA Caplets*—Pseudoephedrine and Guaifenesin—*See* Cough/Cold Combinations (Systemic), 637

t-PA—Alteplase, Recombinant—*See* Thrombolytic Agents (Systemic), 1604

*T-Phyl*—Theophylline—*See* Bronchodilators, Xanthine-derivative (Systemic), 442

*Trac Tabs 2X*—Atropine, Hyoscyamine, Methenamine, Methylene Blue, Phenyl Salicylate, and Benzoic Acid (Systemic), 357

*Trancopal Caplets*—Chlormezanone (Systemic), 528

*Trancot*—Meprobamate (Systemic), 1089

*Trandate*—Labetalol—*See* Beta-adrenergic Blocking Agents (Systemic), 404, MC-13

Tranexamic Acid—*See* Antifibrinolytic Agents (Systemic), 290

*Transact*—Alcohol and Sulfur (Topical), 183

*Transderm-Nitro*—Nitroglycerin—*See* Nitrates—Topical (Systemic), 1224

*Transderm-Scōp*—Scopolamine—*See* Anticholinergics/Antispasmodics (Systemic), 258

*Transderm-V*—Scopolamine—*See* Anticholinergics/Antispasmodics (Systemic), 258

*Trans-Plantar*—Salicylic Acid (Topical), 1478

*Trans-Ver-Sal*—Salicylic Acid (Topical), 1478

*Tranxene*—Clorazepate—*See* Benzodiazepines (Systemic), 389

*Tranxene-SD*—Clorazepate—*See* Benzodiazepines (Systemic), 389, MC-6

*Tranxene T-Tab*—Clorazepate—*See* Benzodiazepines (Systemic), 389, MC-6

Tranylcypromine—*See* Antidepressants, Monoamine Oxidase (MAO) Inhibitor (Systemic), 274, MC-23

*Trasicor*—Oxprenolol—*See* Beta-adrenergic Blocking Agents (Systemic), 404

*TraumaCal*—Enteral Nutrition Formula, Disease-specific—*See* Enteral Nutrition Formulas (Systemic), 769

*Traum-Aid HBC*—Enteral Nutrition Formula, Disease-specific—*See* Enteral Nutrition Formulas (Systemic), 769

*Travamine*—Dimenhydrinate—*See* Antihistamines (Systemic), 304

*Travasorb Hepatic Diet*—Enteral Nutrition Formula, Disease-specific—*See* Enteral Nutrition Formulas (Systemic), 769

*Travasorb HN*—Enteral Nutrition Formula, Monomeric (Elemental)—*See* Enteral Nutrition Formulas (Systemic), 769

*Travasorb Renal Diet*—Enteral Nutrition Formula, Disease-specific—*See* Enteral Nutrition Formulas (Systemic), 769

*Travasorb STD*—Enteral Nutrition Formula, Monomeric (Elemental)—*See* Enteral Nutrition Formulas (Systemic), 769

*Traveltabs*—Dimenhydrinate—*See* Antihistamines (Systemic), 304

Trazodone (Systemic), 1618, MC-23

*Trazon*—Trazodone (Systemic), 1618

*Trecator-SC*—Ethionamide (Systemic), 812

*Trendar*—Ibuprofen—*See* Nonsteroidal Anti-inflammatory Drugs (Systemic), 1229

*Trental*—Pentoxifylline (Systemic), 1316, MC-18

Tretinoin (Topical), 1620

*Trexan*—Naltrexone (Systemic), 1172

*Triacet*—Triamcinolone—*See* Corticosteroids—Medium to Very High Potency (Topical), 626

*Triacin C Cough*—Triprolidine, Pseudoephedrine, and Codeine—*See* Cough/Cold Combinations (Systemic), 637

*Triad*—Butalbital, Acetaminophen, and Caffeine—*See* Butalbital and Acetaminophen (Systemic), 453

*Triadapin*—Doxepin—*See* Antidepressants, Tricyclic (Systemic), 277

*Triaderm*—Triamcinolone—*See* Corticosteroids—Medium to Very High Potency (Topical), 626

*Triafed*—Triprolidine and Pseudoephedrine—*See* Antihistamines and Decongestants (Systemic), 311

*Triafed w/Codeine*—Triprolidine, Pseudoephedrine, and Codeine—*See* Cough/Cold Combinations (Systemic), 637

*Trialodine*—Trazodone (Systemic), 1618

*Triam-A*—Triamcinolone—*See* Corticosteroids/Corticotropin—Glucocorticoid Effects (Systemic), 630

Triamcinolone—*See* Corticosteroids (Dental), 610; Corticosteroids (Inhalation), 611; Corticosteroids (Nasal), 617; Corticosteroids/Corticotropin—Glucocorticoid Effects (Systemic), 630; Corticosteroids—Medium to Very High Potency (Topical), 626

*Triam-Forte*—Triamcinolone—*See* Corticosteroids/Corticotropin—Glucocorticoid Effects (Systemic), 630

*Triaminic*—Chlorpheniramine and Phenylpropanolamine—*See* Antihistamines and Decongestants (Systemic), 311; Pheniramine, Pyrilamine, and Phenylpropanolamine—*See* Antihistamines and Decongestants (Systemic), 311

*Triaminic-12*—Chlorpheniramine and Phenylpropanolamine—*See* Antihistamines and Decongestants (Systemic), 311

*Triaminic Allergy*—Chlorpheniramine and Phenylpropanolamine—*See* Antihistamines and Decongestants (Systemic), 311

*Triaminic Chewables*—Chlorpheniramine and Phenylpropanolamine—*See* Antihistamines and Decongestants (Systemic), 311

*Triaminic Cold*—Chlorpheniramine and Phenylpropanolamine—*See* Antihistamines and Decongestants (Systemic), 311

*Triaminic-DM Cough Formula*—Phenylpropanolamine and Dextromethorphan—*See* Cough/Cold Combinations (Systemic), 637

*Triaminic-DM Daytime*—Phenylpropanolamine, Dextromethorphan, and Guaifenesin (Systemic), 1752

*Triaminic-DM Expectorant*—Pheniramine, Pyrilamine, Phenylpropanolamine, Dextromethorphan, and Guaifenesin—*See* Cough/Cold Combinations (Systemic), 637

*Triaminic DM Night time for Children*—Chlorpheniramine, Pseudoephedrine, and Dextromethorphan (Systemic), 1747

*Triaminic Expectorant*—Pheniramine, Pyrilamine, Phenylpropanolamine, and Guaifenesin—*See* Cough/Cold Combinations (Systemic), 637; Phenylpropanolamine and Guaifenesin—*See* Cough/Cold Combinations (Systemic), 637

*Triaminic Expectorant with Codeine*—Phenylpropanolamine, Codeine, and Guaifenesin—*See* Cough/Cold Combinations (Systemic), 637

*Triaminic Expectorant DH*—Pheniramine, Pyrilamine, Phenylpropanolamine, Hydrocodone, and Guaifenesin—*See* Cough/Cold Combinations (Systemic), 637

*Triaminicin with Codeine*—Pheniramine, Pyrilamine, Phenylpropanolamine, Codeine, Acetaminophen, and Caffeine—*See* Cough/Cold Combinations (Systemic), 637

*Triaminicin Cold, Allergy, Sinus*—Chlorpheniramine, Phenylpropanolamine, and Acetaminophen—*See* Antihistamines, Decongestants, and Analgesics (Systemic), 316

*Triaminic Nite Light*—Chlorpheniramine, Pseudoephedrine, and Dextromethorphan—*See* Cough/Cold Combinations (Systemic), 637

*Triaminicol DM*—Pheniramine, Pyrilamine, Phenylpropanolamine, and Dextromethorphan—*See* Cough/Cold Combinations (Systemic), 637

*Triaminicol Multi-Symptom Relief*—Chlorpheniramine, Phenylpropanolamine, and Dextromethorphan—*See* Cough/Cold Combinations (Systemic), 637

*Triaminicol Multi-Sympton Relief Colds with Cough*—Chlorpheniramine, Phenylpropanolamine, and Dextromethorphan—*See* Cough/Cold Combinations (Systemic), 637

*Triaminic Oral Infant Drops*—Pheniramine, Pyrilamine, and Phenylpropanolamine—*See* Antihistamines and Decongestants (Systemic), 311

*Triaminic Sore Throat Formula*—Pseudoephedrine, Dextromethorphan, and Acetaminophen—*See* Cough/Cold Combinations (Systemic), 637

*Triaminic TR*—Pheniramine, Pyrilamine, and Phenylpropanolamine—*See* Antihistamines and Decongestants (Systemic), 311

*Triamolone 40*—Triamcinolone—*See* Corticosteroids/Corticotropin—Glucocorticoid Effects (Systemic), 630

*Triamonide 40*—Triamcinolone—*See* Corticosteroids/Corticotropin—Glucocorticoid Effects (Systemic), 630

Triamterene—*See* Diuretics, Potassium-sparing (Systemic), 742

Triamterene and Hydrochlorothiazide—*See* Diuretics, Potassium-sparing and Hydrochlorothiazide (Systemic), 745, MC-23, MC-24

*Trianide Mild*—Triamcinolone—*See* Corticosteroids—Medium to Very High Potency (Topical), 626

*Trianide Regular*—Triamcinolone—*See* Corticosteroids—Medium to Very High Potency (Topical), 626

*Triaphen*—Aspirin—*See* Salicylates (Systemic), 1473

*Triaprin*—Butalbital and Acetaminophen (Systemic), 453

*Triasox*—Thiabendazole (Systemic), 1588

*Triavil*—Perphenazine and Amitriptyline (Systemic), 1322, MC-18

Triazolam—*See* Benzodiazepines (Systemic), 389, MC-24

*Triazole*—Sulfamethoxazole and Trimethoprim (Systemic), 1529

*Triazole DS*—Sulfamethoxazole and Trimethoprim (Systemic), 1529

*Triban*—Trimethobenzamide (Systemic), 1626

*Tribavirin*—*See* Ribavirin (Systemic), 1457

*Tribenzagan*—Trimethobenzamide (Systemic), 1626

*Tribiotic*—Neomycin, Polymyxin B, and Gramicidin (Ophthalmic), 1201

*Trichlorex*—Trichlormethiazide—*See* Diuretics, Thiazide (Systemic), 749

Trichlormethiazide—*See* Diuretics, Thiazide (Systemic), 749

Tricitrates—*See* Citrates (Systemic), 554

*Tricodene Cough & Cold*—Pyrilamine and Codeine—*See* Cough/Cold Combinations (Systemic), 637

*Tricodene Forte*—Chlorpheniramine, Phenylpropanolamine, and Dextromethorphan—*See* Cough/Cold Combinations (Systemic), 637

*Tricodene NN*—Chlorpheniramine, Phenylpropanolamine, and Dextromethorphan—*See* Cough/Cold Combinations (Systemic), 637

*Tricodene Pediatric*—Phenylpropanolamine and Dextromethorphan—*See* Cough/Cold Combinations (Systemic), 637

*Tricodene Sugar Free*—Chlorpheniramine and Dextromethorphan—*See* Cough/Cold Combinations (Systemic), 637

*Tricom Caplets*—Chlorpheniramine, Pseudoephedrine, and Acetaminophen—*See* Antihistamines, Decongestants, and Analgesics (Systemic), 316

*Tricosal*—Choline and Magnesium Salicylates—*See* Salicylates (Systemic), 1473

*Tri-Cyclen*—Norgestimate and Ethinyl Estradiol—*See* Estrogens and Progestins (Oral Contraceptives) (Systemic), 804

*Triderm*—Triamcinolone—*See* Corticosteroids—Medium to Very High Potency (Topical), 626

*Tridesilon*—Desonide—*See* Corticosteroids—Low Potency (Topical), 624

Tridihexethyl—*See* Anticholinergics/Antispasmodics (Systemic), 258

*Tridione*—Trimethadione—*See* Anticonvulsants, Dione (Systemic), 265

*Tridione Dulcets*—Trimethadione—*See* Anticonvulsants, Dione (Systemic), 265

*Trien*—*See* Trientine (Systemic), 1622

Trientine (Systemic), 1622

Triethanolamine Salicylate (Topical), 1754

*Trifed*—Triprolidine and Pseudoephedrine—*See* Antihistamines and Decongestants (Systemic), 311

*Trifed-C Cough*—Triprolidine, Pseudoephedrine, and Codeine—*See* Cough/Cold Combinations (Systemic), 637

Trifluoperazine—*See* Phenothiazines (Systemic), 1330, MC-24

Trifluorothymidine—*See* Trifluridine (Ophthalmic), 1623

Triflupromazine—*See* Phenothiazines (Systemic), 1330

Trifluridine (Ophthalmic), 1623

*Trihexane*—Trihexyphenidyl—*See* Antidyskinetics (Systemic), 287

*Trihexy*—Trihexyphenidyl—*See* Antidyskinetics (Systemic), 287

Trihexyphenidyl—*See* Antidyskinetics (Systemic), 287

*Tri-Hydroserpine*—Reserpine, Hydralazine, and Hydrochlorothiazide (Systemic), 1449

*Tri-Immunol*—Diphtheria and Tetanus Toxoids and Pertussis Vaccine Adsorbed (Systemic), 728

*Tri-K*—Trikates—*See* Potassium Supplements (Systemic), 1373

*Trikacide*—Metronidazole (Systemic), 1125

Trikates—*See* Potassium Supplements (Systemic), 1373

*Tri-Kort*—Triamcinolone—*See* Corticosteroids/Corticotropin—Glucocorticoid Effects (Systemic), 630

*Trilafon*—Perphenazine—*See* Phenothiazines (Systemic), 1330

*Trilafon Concentrate*—Perphenazine—*See* Phenothiazines (Systemic), 1330

*Trilax*—Dehydrocholic Acid, Docusate, and Phenolphthalein—*See* Laxatives (Oral), 1017

*Tri-Levlen*—Levonorgestrel and Ethinyl Estradiol—*See* Estrogens and Progestins (Oral Contraceptives) (Systemic), 804, MC-13

*Trilisate*—Choline and Magnesium Salicylates—*See* Salicylates (Systemic), 1473

*Trilog*—Triamcinolone—*See* Corticosteroids/Corticotropin—Glucocorticoid Effects (Systemic), 630

*Trilombrin*—Pyrantel (Oral), 1414

*Trilone*—Triamcinolone—*See* Corticosteroids/Corticotropin—Glucocorticoid Effects (Systemic), 630

Trilostane (Systemic), 1625

Trimeprazine—*See* Antihistamines, Phenothiazine-derivative (Systemic), 325

Trimethadione—*See* Anticonvulsants, Dione (Systemic), 265

Trimethobenzamide (Systemic), 1626, MC-24

Trimethoprim (Systemic), 1628, MC-24

*Trimeth-Sulfa*—Sulfamethoxazole and Trimethoprim (Systemic), 1529

Trimetrexate (Systemic), 1630

*Triminol Cough*—Chlorpheniramine, Phenylpropanolamine, and Dextromethorphan—*See* Cough/Cold Combinations (Systemic), 637

Trimipramine—*See* Antidepressants, Tricyclic (Systemic), 277, MC-24

*Trimox*—Amoxicillin—*See* Penicillins (Systemic), 1299, MC-1

*Trimpex*—Trimethoprim (Systemic), 1628

*Trinalin Repetabs*—Azatadine and Pseudoephedrine—*See* Antihistamines and Decongestants (Systemic), 311, MC-2

*Trind*—Chlorpheniramine and Phenylpropanolamine—*See* Antihistamines and Decongestants (Systemic), 311

*Tri-Nefrin Extra Strength*—Chlorpheniramine and Phenyl-propanolamine—*See* Antihistamines and Decongestants (Systemic), 311

*Trinex*—Chlorpheniramine, Pseudoephedrine, and Guaifene-sin—*See* Cough/Cold Combinations (Systemic), 637

*Tri-Norinyl*—Norethindrone and Ethinyl Estradiol—*See* Estrogens and Progestins (Oral Contraceptives) (Systemic), 804

*Triofed*—Triprolidine and Pseudoephedrine—*See* Antihistamines and Decongestants (Systemic), 311

*Tri-Ophthalmic*—Neomycin, Polymyxin B, and Gramicidin (Ophthalmic), 1201

*Triostat*—Liothyronine (Systemic), 1750

*Triotann*—Chlorpheniramine, Pyrilamine, and Phenyleph-rine—*See* Antihistamines and Decongestants (Systemic), 311

*Triotann Pediatric*—Chlorpheniramine, Pyrilamine, and Phenylephrine—*See* Antihistamines and Decongestants (Systemic), 311

Trioxsalen (Systemic), 1632

Trioxysalen—*See* Trioxsalen (Systemic), 1632

*Tri-Pain Caplets*—Acetaminophen, Aspirin, Salicylamide, and Caffeine—*See* Acetaminophen and Salicylates (Systemic), 164

*Tripalgen Cold*—Chlorpheniramine and Phenylpropanol-amine—*See* Antihistamines and Decongestants (Systemic), 311

*Tripedia*—Diphtheria and Tetanus Toxoids and Pertussis Vaccine Adsorbed (Systemic), 728

Tripelennamine—*See* Antihistamines (Systemic), 304

*Triphasil*—Levonorgestrel and Ethinyl Estradiol—*See* Estrogens and Progestins (Oral Contraceptives) (Systemic), 804, MC-13

*Tri-Phen-Chlor*—Chlorpheniramine, Phenyltoloxamine, Phenylephrine, and Phenylpropanolamine—*See* Antihistamines and Decongestants (Systemic), 311

*Tri-Phen-Chlor Pediatric*—Chlorpheniramine, Phenyltolox-amine, Phenylephrine, and Phenylpropanolamine—*See* Antihistamines and Decongestants (Systemic), 311

*Tri-Phen-Chlor T.R.*—Chlorpheniramine, Phenyltoloxamine, Phenylephrine, and Phenylpropanolamine—*See* Antihistamines and Decongestants (Systemic), 311

*Triphenyl*—Chlorpheniramine and Phenylpropanolamine—*See* Antihistamines and Decongestants (Systemic), 311

*Triphenyl Expectorant*—Phenylpropanolamine and Guaifene-sin—*See* Cough/Cold Combinations (Systemic), 637

*Triphenyl T.D.*—Pheniramine, Pyrilamine, and Phenylpropa-nolamine—*See* Antihistamines and Decongestants (Systemic), 311

*Triple-Gen*—Neomycin, Polymyxin B, and Hydrocortisone (Ophthalmic), 1203

Triple Sulfa—*See* Sulfonamides (Vaginal), 1545

*Triple X*—Pyrethrins and Piperonyl Butoxide (Topical), 1417

*Triposed*—Triprolidine and Pseudoephedrine—*See* Antihistamines and Decongestants (Systemic), 311

Triprolidine—*See* Antihistamines (Systemic), 304

Triprolidine and Pseudoephedrine—*See* Antihistamines and Decongestants (Systemic), 311, 1754

Triprolidine, Pseudoephedrine, and Acetaminophen—*See* Antihistamines, Decongestants, and Analgesics (Systemic), 316

Triprolidine, Pseudoephedrine, and Codeine—*See* Cough/Cold Combinations (Systemic), 637

Triprolidine, Pseudoephedrine, Codeine, and Guaifenesin—*See* Cough/Cold Combinations (Systemic), 637

Triprolidine, Pseudoephedrine, and Dextromethorphan—*See* Cough/Cold Combinations (Systemic), 637

Triprolidine, Pseudoephedrine, Dextromethorphan, and Acetaminophen—*See* Cough/Cold Combinations (Systemic), 637

*Triptil*—Protriptyline—*See* Antidepressants, Tricyclic (Systemic), 277

*Triptone Caplets*—Dimenhydrinate—*See* Antihistamines (Systemic), 304

*Triquilar*—Levonorgestrel and Ethinyl Estradiol—*See* Estrogens and Progestins (Oral Contraceptives) (Systemic), 804

*Trisoralen*—Trioxsalen (Systemic), 1632

*Tristatin II*—Nystatin and Triamcinolone (Topical), 1247

*Tristoject*—Triamcinolone—*See* Corticosteroids/Corticotro-pin—Glucocorticoid Effects (Systemic), 630

*Trisulfam*—Sulfamethoxazole and Trimethoprim (Systemic), 1529

*Trisyn*—Fluocinonide, Procinonide, and Ciprocinonide (Topical), 1748

*Tritann*—Chlorpheniramine, Pyrilamine, and Phenyleph-rine—*See* Antihistamines and Decongestants (Systemic), 311

*Tri-Tannate*—Chlorpheniramine, Pyrilamine, and Phenyleph-rine—*See* Antihistamines and Decongestants (Systemic), 311

*Tri-Tannate Pediatric*—Chlorpheniramine, Pyrilamine, and Phenylephrine—*See* Antihistamines and Decongestants (Systemic), 311

*Tri-Tannate Plus Pediatric*—Chlorpheniramine, Ephedrine, Phenylephrine, and Carbetapentane—*See* Cough/Cold Combinations (Systemic), 637

*Tritann Pediatric*—Chlorpheniramine, Pyrilamine, and Phenylephrine—*See* Antihistamines and Decongestants (Systemic), 311

*Tri-Vi-Flor*—Vitamins A, D, and C and Fluoride—*See* Vitamins and Fluoride (Systemic), 1678

*Trobicin*—Spectinomycin (Systemic), 1511

*Trocal*—Dextromethorphan (Systemic), 701

*Trojan-Enz*—Latex Condoms—*See* Condoms, 602

*Trojan-Enz Large Lubricated*—Latex Condoms—*See* Condoms, 602

*Trojan-Enz Large with Spermicidal Lubricant*—Latex Condoms and Nonoxynol 9—*See* Condoms, 602

*Trojan-Enz Lubricated*—Latex Condoms—*See* Condoms, 602

*Trojan-Enz with Spermicidal Lubricant*—Latex Condoms and Nonoxynol 9—*See* Condoms, 602

*Trojan Extra Strength Lubricated*—Latex Condoms—*See* Condoms, 602

*Trojan Kling-Tite Naturalamb*—Lamb Cecum Condoms—*See* Condoms, 602

*Trojan Naturalube Ribbed*—Latex Condoms—*See* Condoms, 602

*Trojan Plus*—Latex Condoms—*See* Condoms, 602

*Trojan Plus 2*—Latex Condoms and Nonoxynol 9—*See* Condoms, 602

*Trojan Ribbed*—Latex Condoms—*See* Condoms, 602

*Ty-Tab with Codeine No.3*—Acetaminophen and Codeine—*See* Narcotic Analgesics and Acetaminophen (Systemic), 1181

*Ty-Tab with Codeine No.4*—Acetaminophen and Codeine—*See* Narcotic Analgesics and Acetaminophen (Systemic), 1181

# U

*UAA*—Atropine, Hyoscyamine, Methenamine, Methylene Blue, Phenyl Salicylate, and Benzoic Acid (Systemic), 357

*Ucephan*—Sodium Benzoate and Sodium Phenylacetate (Systemic), 1498

*Ulone*—Chlophedianol (Systemic), 507

*ULR-LA*—Phenylpropanolamine and Guaifenesin—*See* Cough/Cold Combinations (Systemic), 637, 1752

*ULTRAbrom PD*—Brompheniramine and Pseudoephedrine—*See* Antihistamines and Decongestants (Systemic), 311

*Ultracal*—Enteral Nutrition Formula, Fiber-containing—*See* Enteral Nutrition Formulas (Systemic), 769

*Ultracef*—Cefadroxil—*See* Cephalosporins (Systemic), 498

*Ultragesic*—Hydrocodone and Acetaminophen—*See* Narcotic Analgesics and Acetaminophen (Systemic), 1181

*Ultralan*—Enteral Nutrition Formula, Polymeric—*See* Enteral Nutrition Formulas (Systemic), 769

*Ultralente Insulin*—Insulin Zinc, Extended—*See* Insulin (Systemic), 961

Ultralente insulin—Insulin Zinc, Extended—*See* Insulin (Systemic), 961

*Ultralente U*—Insulin Zinc, Extended—*See* Insulin (Systemic), 961

*Ultra MOP*—Methoxsalen (Systemic), 1107

*UltraMOP Lotion*—Methoxsalen (Topical), 1110

*Ultra Pep-Back*—Caffeine (Systemic), 463

*Ultra Pred*—Prednisolone—*See* Corticosteroids (Ophthalmic), 620

*Ultrase MT 12*—Pancrelipase (Systemic), 1284

*Ultrase MT 20*—Pancrelipase (Systemic), 1284

*Ultra Tears*—Hydroxypropyl Methylcellulose (Ophthalmic), 941

*Ultravate*—Halobetasol—*See* Corticosteroids—Medium to Very High Potency (Topical), 626

*Ultrazine-10*—Prochlorperazine—*See* Phenothiazines (Systemic), 1330

*Unasyn*—Ampicillin and Sulbactam—*See* Penicillins and Beta-lactamase Inhibitors (Systemic), 1306

Undecylenic Acid, Compound (Topical), 1639

*Uni-Bent Cough*—Diphenhydramine—*See* Antihistamines (Systemic), 304

*Uni-Bronchial*—Theophylline and Guaifenesin (Systemic), 1586

*Unicort*—Hydrocortisone—*See* Corticosteroids—Low Potency (Topical), 624

*Uni-Decon*—Chlorpheniramine, Phenyltoloxamine, Phenylephrine, and Phenylpropanolamine—*See* Antihistamines and Decongestants (Systemic), 311

*Uni-Lom*—Diphenoxylate and Atropine (Systemic), 725

*Unipen*—Nafcillin—*See* Penicillins (Systemic), 1299

*Uniphyl*—Theophylline—*See* Bronchodilators, Xanthine-derivative (Systemic), 442

*Unipres*—Reserpine, Hydralazine, and Hydrochlorothiazide (Systemic), 1449

*Unisom Nighttime Sleep Aid*—Doxylamine—*See* Antihistamines (Systemic), 304

*Unisom SleepGels Maximum Strength*—Diphenhydramine—*See* Antihistamines (Systemic), 304

*Uni-tussin*—Guaifenesin (Systemic), 892

*Uni-tussin DM*—Dextromethorphan and Guaifenesin—*See* Cough/Cold Combinations (Systemic), 637

*Unproco*—Dextromethorphan and Guaifenesin—*See* Cough/Cold Combinations (Systemic), 637

*Urabeth*—Bethanechol (Systemic), 418

*Uracel*—Sodium Salicylate—*See* Salicylates (Systemic), 1473

Uracil Mustard (Systemic), 1640

Urea (Intra-amniotic), 1643

*Ureaphil*—Urea (Intra-amniotic), 1643

*Urecholine*—Bethanechol (Systemic), 418

*Urex*—Methenamine (Systemic), 1100

*Uridon*—Chlorthalidone—*See* Diuretics, Thiazide (Systemic), 749

*Uridon Modified*—Atropine, Hyoscyamine, Methenamine, Methylene Blue, Phenyl Salicylate, and Benzoic Acid (Systemic), 357

*Urimed*—Atropine, Hyoscyamine, Methenamine, Methylene Blue, Phenyl Salicylate, and Benzoic Acid (Systemic), 357

*Urinary Antiseptic No. 2*—Atropine, Hyoscyamine, Methenamine, Methylene Blue, Phenyl Salicylate, and Benzoic Acid (Systemic), 357

Urine Glucose and Ketone (Combined) Test—*See* Urine Glucose and Ketone Test Kits for Home Use, 1644

Urine Glucose and Ketone Test Kits for Home Use, 1644

*Urised*—Atropine, Hyoscyamine, Methenamine, Methylene Blue, Phenyl Salicylate, and Benzoic Acid (Systemic), 357

*Uriseptic*—Atropine, Hyoscyamine, Methenamine, Methylene Blue, Phenyl Salicylate, and Benzoic Acid (Systemic), 357

*Urispas*—Flavoxate (Systemic), 837

*Uritab*—Atropine, Hyoscyamine, Methenamine, Methylene Blue, Phenyl Salicylate, and Benzoic Acid (Systemic), 357

*Uritin*—Atropine, Hyoscyamine, Methenamine, Methylene Blue, Phenyl Salicylate, and Benzoic Acid (Systemic), 357

*Uritol*—Furosemide—*See* Diuretics, Loop (Systemic), 738

*Urocit-K*—Potassium Citrate—*See* Citrates (Systemic), 554

*Urodine*—Phenazopyridine (Systemic), 1327

Urofollitropin (Systemic), 1646

*Urogesic*—Phenazopyridine (Systemic), 1327

Urokinase—*See* Thrombolytic Agents (Systemic), 1604

*Uro-KP-Neutral*—Potassium and Sodium Phosphates—*See* Phosphates (Systemic), 1349

*Urolene Blue*—Methylene Blue (Systemic), 1117

*Uro-Mag*—Magnesium Oxide—*See* Antacids (Oral), 253; Magnesium Supplements (Systemic), 1060

*Uromitexan*—Mesna (Systemic), 1098

*Uroplus DS*—Sulfamethoxazole and Trimethoprim (Systemic), 1529

*Uroplus SS*—Sulfamethoxazole and Trimethoprim (Systemic), 1529

*Uro-Ves*—Atropine, Hyoscyamine, Methenamine, Methylene Blue, Phenyl Salicylate, and Benzoic Acid (Systemic), 357

*Urozide*—Hydrochlorothiazide—*See* Diuretics, Thiazide (Systemic), 749

*Ursinus Inlay*—Pseudoephedrine and Aspirin—*See* Decongestants and Analgesics (Systemic), 691

Ursodeoxycholic acid—*See* Ursodiol (Systemic), 1647

Ursodiol (Systemic), 1647, MC-24

*Ursofalk*—Ursodiol (Systemic), 1647

*Utex-S.R.*—Phenylpropanolamine and Guaifenesin—*See* Cough/Cold Combinations (Systemic), 637

*Uticort*—Betamethasone—*See* Corticosteroids—Medium to Very High Potency (Topical), 626

# V

*Vagistat-1*—Tioconazole—*See* Antifungals, Azole (Vaginal), 296

*Vagitrol*—Sulfanilamide—*See* Sulfonamides (Vaginal), 1545

*Valergen-10*—Estradiol—*See* Estrogens (Systemic), 795

*Valergen-20*—Estradiol—*See* Estrogens (Systemic), 795

*Valergen-40*—Estradiol—*See* Estrogens (Systemic), 795

*Valertest No. 1*—Testosterone and Estradiol—*See* Androgens and Estrogens (Systemic), 225

*Valertest No. 2*—Testosterone and Estradiol—*See* Androgens and Estrogens (Systemic), 225

*Valisone*—Betamethasone—*See* Corticosteroids—Medium to Very High Potency (Topical), 626

*Valisone Reduced Strength*—Betamethasone—*See* Corticosteroids—Medium to Very High Potency (Topical), 626

*Valisone Scalp Lotion*—Betamethasone—*See* Corticosteroids—Medium to Very High Potency (Topical), 626

*Valium*—Diazepam—*See* Benzodiazepines (Systemic), 389, MC-6

*Valnac*—Betamethasone—*See* Corticosteroids—Medium to Very High Potency (Topical), 626

*Valorin*—Acetaminophen (Systemic), 161

*Valorin Extra*—Acetaminophen (Systemic), 161

*Valpin 50*—Anisotropine—*See* Anticholinergics/Antispasmodics (Systemic), 258

Valproic Acid (Systemic), 1651, MC-24

*Valrelease*—Diazepam—*See* Benzodiazepines (Systemic), 389, MC-6

*Vancenase*—Beclomethasone—*See* Corticosteroids (Nasal), 617

*Vancenase AQ*—Beclomethasone—*See* Corticosteroids (Nasal), 617

*Vanceril*—Beclomethasone—*See* Corticosteroids (Inhalation), 611

*Vancocin*—Vancomycin (Oral), 1654; Vancomycin (Systemic), 1655

*Vancoled*—Vancomycin (Systemic), 1655

Vancomycin (Oral), 1654

Vancomycin (Systemic), 1655

*Vanex Expectorant*—Pseudoephedrine, Hydrocodone, and Guaifenesin—*See* Cough/Cold Combinations (Systemic), 637

*Vanex Forte Caplets*—Chlorpheniramine, Pyrilamine, Phenylephrine, and Phenylpropanolamine—*See* Antihistamines and Decongestants (Systemic), 311

*Vanex-HD*—Chlorpheniramine, Phenylephrine, and Hydrocodone—*See* Cough/Cold Combinations (Systemic), 637

*Vanex-LA*—Phenylpropanolamine and Guaifenesin—*See* Cough/Cold Combinations (Systemic), 637

*Vanoxide 5 Lotion*—Benzoyl Peroxide (Topical), 397

*Vanquin*—Pyrvinium (Oral), 1425

*Vanquish Caplets*—Acetaminophen, Aspirin, and Caffeine, Buffered—*See* Acetaminophen and Salicylates (Systemic), 164

*Vanseb Cream Dandruff Shampoo*—Salicylic Acid and Sulfur (Topical), 1481

*Vanseb Lotion Dandruff Shampoo*—Salicylic Acid and Sulfur (Topical), 1481

*Vanseb-T*—Salicylic Acid, Sulfur, and Coal Tar (Topical), 1483

*Vansil*—Oxamniquine (Systemic), 1267

*Vantin*—Cefpodoxime—*See* Cephalosporins (Systemic), 498

*Vapocet*—Hydrocodone and Acetaminophen—*See* Narcotic Analgesics and Acetaminophen (Systemic), 1181

*Vaponefrin*—Racepinephrine—*See* Bronchodilators, Adrenergic (Inhalation), 430

*Vascor*—Bepridil—*See* Calcium Channel Blocking Agents (Systemic), 467, MC-3

*Vaseretic*—Enalapril and Hydrochlorothiazide—*See* Angiotensin-converting Enzyme (ACE) Inhibitors and Hydrochlorothiazide (Systemic), 249, 1748, MC-8

*VasoClear*—Naphazoline (Ophthalmic), 1174

*VasoClear A*—Naphazoline (Ophthalmic), 1174

*Vasocon*—Naphazoline (Ophthalmic), 1174

*Vasocon Regular*—Naphazoline (Ophthalmic), 1174

*Vasodilan*—Isoxsuprine (Systemic), 999

Vasopressin (Systemic), 1657

*Vasotec*—Enalapril—*See* Angiotensin-converting Enzyme (ACE) Inhibitors (Systemic), 245, MC-8; Enalaprilat—*See* Angiotensin-converting Enzyme (ACE) Inhibitors (Systemic), 245

*VCF*—Nonoxynol 9—*See* Spermicides (Vaginal), 1512

*V-Cillin K*—Penicillin V—*See* Penicillins (Systemic), 1299, MC-18

*V-Dec-M*—Pseudoephedrine and Guaifenesin—*See* Cough/Cold Combinations (Systemic), 637

*Veetids*—Penicillin V—*See* Penicillins (Systemic), 1299, MC-18

*Veganin*—Acetaminophen, Codeine, and Caffeine—*See* Narcotic Analgesics and Acetaminophen (Systemic), 1181

*Velban*—Vinblastine (Systemic), 1660

*Velbe*—Vinblastine (Systemic), 1660

*Velosef*—Cephradine—*See* Cephalosporins (Systemic), 498, MC-4

*Velosulin Human*—Insulin Human—*See* Insulin (Systemic), 961

*Velsar*—Vinblastine (Systemic), 1660

*Veltane*—Brompheniramine—*See* Antihistamines (Systemic), 304

*Veltap*—Brompheniramine, Phenylephrine, and Phenylpropanolamine—*See* Antihistamines and Decongestants (Systemic), 311

Venlafaxine (Systemic), MC-24

*Venoglobulin-I*—Immune Globulin Intravenous (Human) (Systemic), 954

# W

*WinGel*—Alumina and Magnesia—*See* Antacids (Oral), 253

*Winpred*—Prednisone—*See* Corticosteroids/Corticotropin—Glucocorticoid Effects (Systemic), 630

*WinRho SD*—RH$_0$(D) Immune Globulin (Systemic), 1456

*Winstrol*—Stanozolol—*See* Anabolic Steroids (Systemic), 218

*Wintrocin*—Erythromycin Stearate—*See* Erythromycins (Systemic), 786

*Wolfina*—Rauwolfia Serpentina—*See* Rauwolfia Alkaloids (Systemic), 1442

*Wycillin*—Penicillin G—*See* Penicillins (Systemic), 1299

*Wygesic*—Propoxyphene and Acetaminophen—*See* Narcotic Analgesics and Acetaminophen (Systemic), 1181

*Wymox*—Amoxicillin—*See* Penicillins (Systemic), 1299, MC-2

*Wytensin*—Guanabenz (Systemic), 894, MC-11

# X

*Xanax*—Alprazolam—*See* Benzodiazepines (Systemic), 389, MC-1

*Xanax TS*—Alprazolam—*See* Benzodiazepines (Systemic), 389

Xenon Xe 127—*See* Radiopharmaceuticals (Diagnostic), 1439

Xenon Xe 133—*See* Radiopharmaceuticals (Diagnostic), 1439

*Xerac*—Alcohol and Sulfur (Topical), 183

*Xerac BP 5 Gel*—Benzoyl Peroxide (Topical), 397

*Xerac BP 10 Gel*—Benzoyl Peroxide (Topical), 397

*X-Prep Liquid*—Senna—*See* Laxatives (Oral), 1017

*X-Seb*—Salicylic Acid (Topical), 1478

*Xylocaine*—Lidocaine—*See* Anesthetics (Dental), 229; Anesthetics (Parenteral-Local), 235; Anesthetics (Topical), 240

*Xylocaine with Glucose*—Lidocaine—*See* Anesthetics (Parenteral-Local), 235

*Xylocaine-MPF*—Lidocaine—*See* Anesthetics (Parenteral-Local), 235

*Xylocaine-MPF with Glucose*—Lidocaine—*See* Anesthetics (Parenteral-Local), 235

*Xylocaine Test Dose*—Lidocaine—*See* Anesthetics (Parenteral-Local), 235

*Xylocaine Viscous*—Lidocaine—*See* Anesthetics (Dental), 229

Xylometazoline (Nasal), 1681

# Y

Yellow Fever Vaccine (Systemic), 1683

*YF-Vax*—Yellow Fever Vaccine (Systemic), 1683

*Yocon*—Yohimbine (Systemic), 1684

*Yodoquinol*—Iodoquinol (Oral), 977

*Yodoxin*—Iodoquinol (Oral), 977

*Yohimar*—Yohimbine (Systemic), 1684

Yohimbine (Systemic), 1684

*Yohimex*—Yohimbine (Systemic), 1684

*Yoman*—Yohimbine (Systemic), 1684

*Yovital*—Yohimbine (Systemic), 1684

*Yutopar*—Ritodrine (Systemic), 1468

# Z

*Zaditen*—Ketotifen (Systemic), 1750

Zalcitabine (Systemic), 1687

*Zanosar*—Streptozocin (Systemic), 1517

*Zantac*—Ranitidine—*See* Histamine H$_2$-receptor Antagonists (Systemic), 925, MC-21

*Zantac-C*—Ranitidine—*See* Histamine H$_2$-receptor Antagonists (Systemic), 925

*Zantryl*—Phentermine—*See* Appetite Suppressants (Systemic), 339

*Zarontin*—Ethosuximide—*See* Anticonvulsants, Succinimide (Systemic), 271

*Zaroxolyn*—Metolazone—*See* Diuretics, Thiazide (Systemic), 749, MC-15

*Zeasorb-AF*—Miconazole (Topical), 1137

*Zeasorb-AF Powder*—Tolnaftate (Topical), 1617

*Zebeta*—Bisoprolol—*See* Beta-adrenergic Blocking Agents (Systemic), 404, MC-3

*Zebrax*—Chlordiazepoxide and Clidinium (Systemic), 523

*Zefazone*—Cefmetazole—*See* Cephalosporins (Systemic), 498

*Zentel*—Albendazole (Systemic), 179

*Zephrex*—Pseudoephedrine and Guaifenesin—*See* Cough/Cold Combinations (Systemic), 637

*Zephrex-LA*—Pseudoephedrine and Guaifenesin—*See* Cough/Cold Combinations (Systemic), 637

*Zeroxin-5 Gel*—Benzoyl Peroxide (Topical), 397

*Zeroxin-10 Gel*—Benzoyl Peroxide (Topical), 397

*Zestoretic*—Lisinopril and Hydrochlorothiazide—*See* Angiotensin-converting Enzyme (ACE) Inhibitors and Hydrochlorothiazide (Systemic), 249, MC-13

*Zestril*—Lisinopril—*See* Angiotensin-converting Enzyme (ACE) Inhibitors (Systemic), 245, MC-13

*Zetar Emulsion*—Coal Tar (Topical), 589

*Zetar Medicated Antiseborrheic Shampoo*—Coal Tar (Topical), 589

*Zetar Shampoo*—Coal Tar (Topical), 589

*Zetran*—Diazepam—*See* Benzodiazepines (Systemic), 389

*Ziac*—Bisoprolol and Hydrochlorothiazide—*See* Beta-adrenergic Blocking Agents and Thiazide Diuretics (Systemic), 410, MC-3

Zidovudine (Systemic), 1689, MC-24

*Zilactin-L*—Lidocaine—*See* Anesthetics (Dental), 229

*Zinacef*—Cefuroxime—*See* Cephalosporins (Systemic), 498

*Zinc-220*—Zinc Sulfate—*See* Zinc Supplements (Systemic), 1691

*Zincate*—Zinc Sulfate—*See* Zinc Supplements (Systemic), 1691

Zinc Chloride—*See* Zinc Supplements (Systemic), 1691

Zinc Gluconate—*See* Zinc Supplements (Systemic), 1691

*Zincon Dandruff Lotion Shampoo*—Pyrithione (Topical), 1424

Zinc Sulfate—*See* Zinc Supplements (Systemic), 1691

Zinc Supplements (Systemic), 1691

*Zinkaps-220*—Zinc Sulfate—*See* Zinc Supplements (Systemic), 1691

# The Medicine Chart

*The Medicine Chart* presents photographs of the most frequently prescribed medicines in the United States. In general, commonly used brand name products and a representative sampling of generic products have been included. The pictorial listing is not intended to be inclusive and does not represent all products on the market. Only selected solid oral dosage forms (capsules and tablets) have been included. The inclusion of a product does not mean the USPC has any particular knowledge that the product included has properties different from other products, nor should it be interpreted as an endorsement by USPC. Similarly, the fact that a particular product has not been included does not indicate that the product has been judged by the USPC to be unsatisfactory or unacceptable.

The drug products in *The Medicine Chart* are listed alphabetically by generic name of active ingredient(s). To quickly locate a particular medicine, check the product listing index that follows. This listing provides brand and generic names and directs the user to the appropriate page and chart location. In addition, any identifying code found on the surface of a capsule or tablet that might be useful in making a correct identification is included in the parentheses that follow the product's index entry. Please note that these codes may change as manufacturers reformulate or redesign their products. In addition, some companies may not manufacture all of their own products. In some of these cases, the imprinting on the tablet or capsule may be that of the actual manufacturer and not of the company marketing the product.

Brand names are in *italics*. An asterisk next to the generic name of the active ingredient(s) indicates that the solid oral dosage forms containing the ingredient(s) are available only from a single source with no generic equivalents currently available in the U.S. Where multiple source products are shown, it must be kept in mind that other products may also be available.

The size and color of the products shown are intended to match the actual product as closely as possible; however, there may be some differences due to variations caused by the photographic process. Also, manufacturers may occasionally change the color, imprinting, or shape of their products, and for a period of time both the "old" and the newly changed dosage form may be on the market. Such changes may not occur uniformly throughout the different dosages of the product. These types of changes will be incorporated in subsequent versions of the chart as they are brought to our attention.

---

Use of this chart is limited to serving as an initial guide in identifying drug products. The identity of a product should be verified further before any action is taken.

---

Erythromycin *(continued)*
  Abbott Tablets—
    250 mg (EB) . . . . . . . . . . . MC-9, A7
    500 mg (EA) . . . . . . . . . . . MC-9, A7
  Barr Delayed-release Capsules—
    250 mg (584) . . . . . . . . . . . MC-9, B3
  Erythromycin Estolate . . . . MC-9, B6–7
  Erythromycin Ethylsuccinate . . . MC-9, C1–3
  Barr Tablets—
    400 mg (259) . . . . . . . . . . . MC-9, C3
  Erythromycin Stearate . . . . . . . . MC-9, C4
*Esidrix* Tablets—
  25 mg (22) . . . . . . . . . . . . . . MC-11, C3
  50 mg (46) . . . . . . . . . . . . . . MC-11, C3
  100 mg (192) . . . . . . . . . . . . MC-11, C3
*Eskalith*
  Capsules—
    300 mg . . . . . . . . . . . . . . . . MC-13, D1
*Eskalith CR* Extended-release Tablets—
  450 mg (J10) . . . . . . . . MC-13, D2
Estazolam . . . . . . . . . . . . . . . . MC-9, C5
*Estrace* Tablets—
  1 mg (MJ 755) . . . . . . . . . . . MC-9, C6
  2 mg (MJ 756) . . . . . . . . . . . MC-9, C6
Estradiol . . . . . . . . . . . . . . . . . MC-9, C6
Estrogens, Conjugated . . . . . . MC-9, C7–D1
Estropipate . . . . . . . . . . . . . . MC-9, D2
*Ethmozine* Tablets—
  200 mg (200) . . . . . . . . . . . MC-15, D5
  250 mg (250) . . . . . . . . . . . MC-15, D5
  300 mg (300) . . . . . . . . . . . MC-15, D6
Ethynodiol Diacetate and Ethinyl
  Estradiol . . . . . . . . . . . . . . MC-9, D3–4
Etodolac . . . . . . . . . . . . . . . . . MC-9, D5
Famotidine . . . . . . . . . . . . . . . MC-9, D6
Felbamate . . . . . . . . . . . . . . . . MC-9, D7
*Felbatol* Tablets—
  400 mg (04 30) . . . . . . . . . . MC-9, D7
  600 mg (04 31) . . . . . . . . . . MC-9, D7
*Feldene* Capsules—
  10 mg (322) . . . . . . . . . . . . MC-19, A4
  20 mg (323) . . . . . . . . . . . . MC-19, A4
Felodipine . . . . . . . . . . . . . . . MC-10, A1
Fenoprofen . . . . . . . . . . . . . . MC-10, A2–7
  Geneva
    Capsules—
      200 mg (GG 558) . . . . . . MC-10, A4
      300 mg (GG 559) . . . . . . MC-10, A4
    Tablets—
      600 mg (GG 254) . . . . . . MC-10, A5
  Purepac Tablets—
    600 mg (317) . . . . . . . . . . MC-10, A6
  Schein/Danbury Tablets—
    600 mg (5704) . . . . . . . . . MC-10, A7
Ferrous Sulfate . . . . . . . . . . . . MC-10, B1
  Upsher-Smith Tablets—
    300 mg . . . . . . . . . . . . . . . . MC-10, B1
Finasteride . . . . . . . . . . . . . . . MC-10, B2
*Fioricet* Tablets—
  50/325/40 mg (78-84) . . . . . . MC-3, C2
*Fiorinal*
  Capsules—
    50/325/40 mg (78-103) . . . . MC-3, C4
  Tablets—
    50/325/40 mg (78-104) . . . . MC-3, C5
*Fiorinal with Codeine* Capsules—
  50/325/30/40 mg (78-107) . . . MC-3, C6
*Flagyl* Tablets—
  250 mg (1831) . . . . . . . . . . . MC-15, C5
  500 mg (500) . . . . . . . . . . . MC-15, C5
*Flexeril* Tablets—
  10 mg (MSD 931) . . . . . . . . MC-6, B6
*Floxin* Tablets—
  200 mg (200 mg) . . . . . . . . MC-17, C3
  300 mg (300 mg) . . . . . . . . MC-17, C3
  400 mg (400 mg) . . . . . . . . MC-17, C3

Fluconazole . . . . . . . . . . . . . . . MC-10, B3
Fluoxetine . . . . . . . . . . . . . . . . MC-10, B4
Fluoxymesterone . . . . . . . . . . . MC-10, B5
Fluphenazine . . . . . . . . . . . MC-10, B6–C1
  Mylan Tablets—
    1 mg (4) . . . . . . . . . . . . . . . MC-10, B7
    2.5 mg (9) . . . . . . . . . . . . . MC-10, B7
    5 mg (74) . . . . . . . . . . . . . . MC-10, C1
    10 mg (97) . . . . . . . . . . . . MC-10, C1
Flurazepam . . . . . . . . . . . . MC-10, C2–C5
  Barr Capsules—
    15 mg (377) . . . . . . . . . . . MC-10, C2
    30 mg (378) . . . . . . . . . . . MC-10, C2
  Purepac Capsules—
    15 mg (R021) . . . . . . . . . MC-10, C3
    30 mg (R022) . . . . . . . . . MC-10, C3
  Schein/Danbury Capsules—
    15 mg (DAN 5614) . . . . . . MC-10, C5
    30 mg (DAN 5615) . . . . . . MC-10, C5
Flurbiprofen . . . . . . . . . . . . . . MC-10, C6
Fluvastatin . . . . . . . . . . . . . . . MC-10, C7
Fosinopril . . . . . . . . . . . . . . . . MC-10, D1
Furosemide . . . . . . . . . . . . . MC-10, D2–4
  Barr Tablets—
    20 mg (170) . . . . . . . . . . . MC-10, D2
    40 mg (555 169) . . . . . . . MC-10, D2
    80 mg (555 196) . . . . . . . MC-10, D2
  Schein/Danbury Tablets—
    20 mg (M2) . . . . . . . . . . . MC-10, D4
    40 mg (5575) . . . . . . . . . . MC-10, D4
    80 mg (302) . . . . . . . . . . . MC-10, D4
Gabapentin . . . . . . . . . . . . . . . MC-10, D5
*Gastrocrom* Capsules—
  100 mg (101) . . . . . . . . . . . MC-6, B5
Gemfibrozil . . . . . . . . . . . . . . MC-10, D6
*Genora 0.5/35-21* Tablets—
  0.5/0.035 mg (0.5/35) . . . . . MC-17, A2
*Genora 1/35-28* Tablets—
  1/0.035 mg (1/35) . . . . . . . . MC-17, A3
  Inert . . . . . . . . . . . . . . . . . MC-17, A3
*Genora 1/50-28* Tablets—
  1/0.05 mg (1/50) . . . . . . . . MC-17, B2
  Inert . . . . . . . . . . . . . . . . . MC-17, B2
*Geocillin* Tablets—
  382 mg (143) . . . . . . . . . . . MC-4, A2
Glipizide . . . . . . . . . . . . . . . . MC-10, D7
*Glucotrol XL* Extended-release Tablets—
  5 mg (5) . . . . . . . . . . . . . . . MC-10, D7
  10 mg (10) . . . . . . . . . . . . MC-10, D7
Glyburide . . . . . . . . . . . . . . MC-11, A1–2
*Grifulvin V* Tablets—
  250 mg (211) . . . . . . . . . . . MC-11, A3
  500 mg (214) . . . . . . . . . . . MC-11, A3
Griseofulvin . . . . . . . . . . . . . . MC-11, A3
Guanabenz . . . . . . . . . . . . . . . MC-11, A4
Guanfacine . . . . . . . . . . . . . . . MC-11, A5
*Halcion* Tablets—
  0.125 mg (0.125) . . . . . . . . MC-24, A4
  0.25 mg (0.25) . . . . . . . . . . MC-24, A4
*Haldol* Tablets—
  0.5 mg (½) . . . . . . . . . . . . . MC-11, B2
  1 mg (1) . . . . . . . . . . . . . . . MC-11, B2
  2 mg (2) . . . . . . . . . . . . . . . MC-11, B2
  5 mg (5) . . . . . . . . . . . . . . . MC-11, B2
  10 mg (10) . . . . . . . . . . . . MC-11, B2
  20 mg (20) . . . . . . . . . . . . MC-11, B2
Haloperidol . . . . . . . . . . . . MC-11, A6–B4
  Barr Tablets—
    0.5 mg (477) . . . . . . . . . . MC-11, A6
    1 mg (478) . . . . . . . . . . . MC-11, A6
    2 mg (479) . . . . . . . . . . . MC-11, A6
    5 mg (480) . . . . . . . . . . . MC-11, A6
    10 mg (481) . . . . . . . . . . MC-11, A7
    20 mg (482) . . . . . . . . . . MC-11, A7

Haloperidol *(continued)*
  Geneva Tablets—
    0.5 mg (105) . . . . . . . . . . MC-11, B1
    1 mg (123) . . . . . . . . . . . MC-11, B1
    2 mg (GG 124) . . . . . . . . MC-11, B1
    5 mg (GG 125) . . . . . . . . MC-11, B1
    10 mg (GG 126) . . . . . . . MC-11, B1
    20 mg (GG 134) . . . . . . . MC-11, B1
  Mylan Tablets—
    0.5 mg (351) . . . . . . . . . . MC-11, B3
    1 mg (257) . . . . . . . . . . . MC-11, B3
    2 mg (214) . . . . . . . . . . . MC-11, B3
    5 mg (327) . . . . . . . . . . . MC-11, B3
  Purepac Tablets—
    0.5 mg (289) . . . . . . . . . . MC-11, B4
    1 mg (280) . . . . . . . . . . . MC-11, B4
    2 mg (281) . . . . . . . . . . . MC-11, B4
    5 mg (282) . . . . . . . . . . . MC-11, B4
    10 mg (286) . . . . . . . . . . MC-11, B4
    20 mg (287) . . . . . . . . . . MC-11, B4
*Halotestin* Tablets—
  2 mg (2) . . . . . . . . . . . . . . . MC-10, B5
  5 mg (5) . . . . . . . . . . . . . . . MC-10, B5
  10 mg (10) . . . . . . . . . . . . MC-10, B5
*Hismanal* Tablets—
  10 mg (Ast 10) . . . . . . . . . . MC-2, B2
*Hydergine*
  Tablets—
    1 mg . . . . . . . . . . . . . . . . MC-9, A3
  Sublingual Tablets—
    0.5 mg . . . . . . . . . . . . . . MC-9, A4
    1 mg . . . . . . . . . . . . . . . . MC-9, A4
*Hydergine LC* Capsules—
  1 mg (78-101) . . . . . . . . . . MC-9, A2
Hydralazine . . . . . . . . . . . . . MC-11, B5–6
  Lederle Tablets—
    25 mg (H11) . . . . . . . . . . MC-11, B6
    50 mg (H12) . . . . . . . . . . MC-11, B6
Hydralazine and
  Hydrochlorothiazide . . . . . . . MC-11, B7
Hydrochlorothiazide . . . . . . . MC-11, C1–5
  Barr Tablets—
    25 mg (555 19) . . . . . . . . MC-11, C2
    50 mg (555 20) . . . . . . . . MC-11, C2
    100 mg (555 192) . . . . . . . MC-11, C2
  Geneva Tablets—
    25 mg (GG 28) . . . . . . . . MC-11, C4
    50 mg (GG 27) . . . . . . . . MC-11, C4
Hydrocodone and
  Acetaminophen . . . . . . . . . MC-11, C6–D1
Hydrocortisone . . . . . . . . . . . MC-11, D2
*HydroDIURIL* Tablets—
  25 mg (MSD 42) . . . . . . . . MC-11, C5
  50 mg (MSD 105) . . . . . . . . MC-11, C5
  100 mg (MSD 410) . . . . . . . MC-11, C5
Hydromorphone . . . . . . . . . . . MC-11, C3
Hydroxychloroquine . . . . . . . . MC-11, D4
Hydroxyzine . . . . . . MC-11, D5–MC-12, A2
  Geneva Tablets—
    10 mg (37) . . . . . . . . . . . MC-11, D5
    25 mg (38) . . . . . . . . . . . MC-11, D5
    50 mg (39) . . . . . . . . . . . MC-11, D5
  Rugby Tablets—
    10 mg (3874) . . . . . . . . . MC-12, A1
    25 mg (3875) . . . . . . . . . MC-12, A1
    50 mg (3876) . . . . . . . . . MC-12, A1
  Schein/Danbury Tablets—
    10 mg (5522) . . . . . . . . . MC-12, A2
    25 mg (5523) . . . . . . . . . MC-12, A2
    50 mg (5565) . . . . . . . . . MC-12, A2
*Hygroton* Tablets—
  25 mg (22 (R)) . . . . . . . . . . MC-5, B3
  50 mg (20 (R)) . . . . . . . . . . MC-5, B3
  100 mg (21) . . . . . . . . . . . MC-5, B3

*Hytrin* Tablets—
  1 mg (DF)................ MC-22, A5
  2 mg (DH)................ MC-22, A5
  5 mg (DJ)................ MC-22, A5
  10 mg (DI)................ MC-22, A5
Ibuprofen................ MC-12, A3–B4
  Barr Tablets—
    400 mg (419)........... MC-12, A3
    600 mg (420)........... MC-12, A3
    800 mg (499)........... MC-12, A3
  Boots Laboratories Tablets—
    400 mg (IBU 400)....... MC-12, A4
    600 mg (IBU 600)....... MC-12, A4
    800 mg (IBU 800)....... MC-12, A4
  Rugby Tablets—
    400 mg (3977).......... MC-12, A6
    600 mg (3978).......... MC-12, A6
    800 mg (3979).......... MC-12, A7
  Schein/Danbury Tablets—
    200 mg (5585).......... MC-12, B1
    400 mg (5584).......... MC-12, B1
    600 mg (5586).......... MC-12, B2
    800 mg (5644).......... MC-12, B2
*Ilosone*
  Capsules—
    250 mg (H09)........... MC-9, B6
  Chewable Tablets—
    125 mg (U05)........... MC-9, B7
    250 mg (U25)........... MC-9, B7
Imipramine........... MC-12, B5–7
*Imodium* Capsules—
  2 mg.................. MC-13, D5
*Imuran* Tablets—
  50 mg (50)............. MC-2, D4
Indapamide............ MC-12, C1
*Inderal* Tablets—
  10 mg (10)............. MC-20, C3
  20 mg (20)............. MC-20, C3
  40 mg (40)............. MC-20, C3
  60 mg (60)............. MC-20, C3
  80 mg (80)............. MC-20, C3
*Inderal LA* Extended-release Capsules—
  60 mg (60)............. MC-20, C1
  80 mg (80)............. MC-20, C1
  120 mg (120)........... MC-20, C2
  160 mg (160)........... MC-20, C2
*Inderide* Tablets—
  40/25 mg (40/25)....... MC-20, D1
  80/25 mg (80/25)....... MC-20, D1
*Inderide LA* Extended-release Capsules—
  80/50 mg (80/50)....... MC-20, C6
  120/50 mg (120/50)..... MC-20, C6
  160/50 mg (160/50)..... MC-20, C7
*Indocin* Capsules—
  25 mg (MSD 25)........ MC-12, C3
  50 mg (MSD 50)........ MC-12, C3
*Indocin SR* Extended-release Capsules—
  75 mg (MSD 693)....... MC-12, C4
Indomethacin.............. MC-12, C2–4
  Geneva Capsules—
    25 mg (GG 517)....... MC-12, C2
    50 mg (GG 518)....... MC-12, C2
*Ionamin* Capsules—
  15 mg (15)............. MC-18, D2
  30 mg (30)............. MC-18, D2
*ISMO* Tablets—
  20 mg (20)............. MC-12, D6
*Isoptin* Tablets—
  40 mg (40)............. MC-24, B7
  80 mg (80)............. MC-24, B7
  120 mg (120).......... MC-24, B7
*Isoptin SR*
  Extended-release Tablets—
    120 mg (120 SR)....... MC-24, C1
    180 mg (180 MG)....... MC-24, C2
    240 mg................ MC-24, C2

*Isordil*
  Tablets—
    5 mg (4152)............ MC-12, C6
    10 mg (4153)........... MC-12, C6
    20 mg (4154)........... MC-12, C6
    30 mg (4159)........... MC-12, C6
    40 mg (4192)........... MC-12, C6
  Extended-release Tablets—
    40 mg (4125)........... MC-12, C7
  Sublingual Tablets—
    2.5 mg (25)............ MC-12, D1
    5 mg (5)............... MC-12, D1
    10 mg (10)............. MC-12, D1
Isosorbide Dinitrate....... MC-12, C5–D5
Isosorbide Mononitrate.... MC-12, D6
Isotretinoin.............. MC-12, D7
Isradipine............... MC-13, A1
Itraconazole.............. MC-13, A2
*K-Dur* Extended-release Tablets—
  750 mg (10)............ MC-19, A7
  1500 mg (20)........... MC-19, A7
*Keflex* Capsules—
  250 mg (H69)........... MC-4, C3
  500 mg (H71)........... MC-4, C3
*Keftab* Tablets—
  250 mg (250)........... MC-4, C4
  500 mg (500)........... MC-4, C4
*Kerlone* Tablets—
  10 mg (10)............. MC-3, B1
  20 mg (20)............. MC-3, B1
Ketoconazole.............. MC-13, A3
Ketorolac................. MC-13, A4
*Klor-Con* Extended-release Tablets—
  600 mg (8)............. MC-19, B3
  750 mg (10)............ MC-19, B3
*Klotrix* Extended-release Tablets—
  750 mg (MJ 10 mEq 770)... MC-19, A6
*K-Tab* Extended-release Tablets—
  750 mg................ MC-19, A5
Labetalol................ MC-13, A5–6
*Lanoxicaps* Capsules—
  0.05 mg (A2C)......... MC-7, B6
  0.1 mg (B2C).......... MC-7, B6
  0.2 mg (C2C).......... MC-7, B6
*Lanoxin* Tablets—
  0.125 mg (Y3B)......... MC-7, B7
  0.25 mg (X3A)......... MC-7, B7
  0.5 mg (T9A).......... MC-7, B7
*Lasix* Tablets—
  20 mg................. MC-10, D3
  40 mg (40)............. MC-10, D3
  80 mg (80)............. MC-10, D3
*Ledercillin VK* Tablets—
  250 mg (L 10).......... MC-18, B7
  500 mg (L 9).......... MC-18, B7
*Lescol* Capsules—
  20 mg (20)............. MC-10, C7
  40 mg (40)............. MC10, C7
*Levatol* Tablets—
  20 mg (22)............. MC-18, B4
*Levlen 21 and 28* Tablets—
  0.15/0.03 mg (21)...... MC-13, A7
  Inert (28)............. MC-13, A7
Levonorgestrel and Ethinyl
  Estradiol.............. MC-13, A7–B3
Levothyroxine............ MC-13, B4–C1
  Rugby Tablets—
    0.1 mg (3952).......... MC-13, C1
    0.15 mg (3953)......... MC-13, C1
    0.2 mg (4381).......... MC-13, C1
    0.3 mg (3958).......... MC-13, C1
*Levoxine* Tablets—
  0.025 mg (dp 25)....... MC-13, B6
  0.05 mg (dp 50)........ MC-13, B6
  0.075 mg (dp 75)....... MC-13, B6
  0.088 mg (dp 88)....... MC-13, B6
  0.1 mg (dp 100)........ MC-13, B6

*Levoxine* Tablets *(continued)*
  0.112 mg (dp 112)........ MC-13, B7
  0.125 mg (dp 125)........ MC-13, B7
  0.15 mg (dp 150)........ MC-13, B7
  0.175 mg (dp 175)....... MC-13, B7
  0.2 mg (dp 200)......... MC-13, B7
  0.3 mg (dp 300)......... MC-13, B7
*Librax* Capsules—
  5/2.5 mg............... MC-4, D5
*Libritabs* Tablets—
  5 mg (5)............... MC-4, D2
  25 mg (25)............. MC-4, D2
*Librium* Capsules—
  5 mg (5)............... MC-4, D1
  10 mg (10)............. MC-4, D1
  25 mg (25)............. MC-4, D1
*Limbitrol* Tablets—
  5/12.5 mg............. MC-4, D4
  10/25 mg............. MC-4, D4
*Lioresal* Tablets—
  10 mg (23)............. MC-2, D6
  20 mg (33)............. MC-2, D6
Lisinopril................. MC-13, C2–3
Lisinopril and
  Hydrochlorothiazide....... MC-13, C4–5
Lithium.................. MC-13, C6–D3
  Roxane
    Capsules—
      150 mg (54 213)....... MC-13, C6
      300 mg (54 463)....... MC-13, C6
      600 mg (54 702)....... MC-13, C6
    Tablets—
      300 mg (54 452)....... MC-13, C7
  Solvay Capsules—
    300 mg (0665 4160)..... MC-13, D3
*Lodine* Capsules—
  200 mg (200 mg)........... MC-9, D5
  300 mg (300 mg)........... MC-9, D5
*Loestrin 21 1/20* Tablets—
  1/0.02 mg (P-D 915).... MC-17, A4
*Loestrin 21 1.5/30* Tablets—
  1.5/0.03 mg (P-D 916).... MC-17, A5
*Loestrin Fe 1/20* Tablets—
  1/0.02 mg (P-D 915).... MC-17, A6
  75 mg (P-D 622)........ MC-17, A6
*Loestrin Fe 1.5/30* Tablets—
  1.5/0.03 mg (P-D 916)... MC-17, A7
  75 mg (P-D 622)........ MC-17, A7
Lomefloxacin.............. MC-13, D4
*Lomotil* Tablets—
  2.5/0.025 mg (61).......... MC-7, D5
*Loniten* Tablets—
  2.5 mg (U 121)......... MC-15, D3
  10 mg (10)............. MC-15, D3
*Lo-Ovral-21 and -28* Tablets—
  0.3/0.03 mg (78)....... MC-17, B4
  Inert (486)............ MC-17, B4
Loperamide................ MC-13, D5
*Lopid* Tablets—
  600 mg................ MC-10, D6
*Lopressor* Tablets—
  50 mg (51 51).......... MC-15, B6
  100 mg (71 71).......... MC-15, B6
*Lopressor HCT* Tablets—
  50/25 mg (35 35)....... MC-15, C1
  100/25 mg (53 53)...... MC-15, C1
  100/50 mg (73 73)...... MC-15, C1
*Lopurin* Tablets—
  100 mg (0051).......... MC-1, B3
  300 mg (0052).......... MC-1, B3
*Lorabid* Capsules—
  200 mg (3170).......... MC-13, D6
Loracarbef................ MC-13, D6
Loratadine................ MC-13, D7

*Neurontin* Capsules—
  100 mg (100 mg) .......... MC-10, D5
  300 mg (300 mg) .......... MC-10, D5
  400 mg (400 mg) .......... MC-10, D5
Niacin ................... MC-16, B1–4
Nicardipine ............... MC-16, B5
*Nicobid* Extended-release Capsules—
  125 mg (125 mg) ......... MC-16, B1
  250 mg (250 mg) ......... MC-16, B1
  500 mg (500) ............ MC-16, B2
*Nicolar* Tablets—
  500 mg (NE) ............. MC-16, B3
*Nicorette* Chewing Gum Tablets—
  2 mg. ................... MC-16, B6
Nicotine. ................. MC-16, B6
Nifedipine ............. MC-16, B7–C4
  Purepac Capsules—
   10 mg (R 497) ........ MC-16, C3
   20 mg (R 530) ........ MC-16, C3
  Schein Capsules—
   10 mg (10-0364). ..... MC-16, C4
   20 mg (20-0364). ..... MC-16, C4
Nimodipine ............... MC-16, C5
*Nimotop* Capsules—
  30 mg (855) ............. MC-16, C5
Nitrofurantoin. ....... MC-16, C6–D1
  Schein/Danbury Capsules—
   25 mg (25 mg DAN). ..... MC-16, D1
   50 mg (50 mg DAN). ..... MC-16, D1
   100 mg (100 mg DAN) ... MC-16, D1
Nitroglycerin. .......... MC-16, D2–3
  Geneva Extended-release Capsules—
   2.5 mg (GG 511) ....... MC-16, D2
   6.5 mg (GG 501) ....... MC-16, D2
   9 mg (GG 512) ........ MC-16, D2
*Nitrostat* Sublingual Tablets—
  0.3 mg. ................. MC-16, D3
  0.4 mg. ................. MC-16, D3
  0.6 mg. ................. MC-16, D3
Nizatidine ................ MC-16, D4
*Nizoral* Tablets—
  200 mg. ................. MC-13, A3
*Nolvadex* Tablets—
  10 mg (600) ............. MC-21, D7
*Nordette-21 and -28* Tablets—
  0.15/0.03 mg (75) ....... MC-13, B2
  Inert (486). ............. MC-13, B2
Norethindrone and Ethinyl
  Estradiol ........ MC-16, D5–A3
Norethindrone Acetate and Ethinyl
  Estradiol ......... MC-17, A4–5
Norethindrone Acetate/Ethinyl Estradiol
  and Ferrous Fumarate..... MC-17, A6–7
Norethindrone and
  Mestranol .......... MC-17, B1–2
Norfloxacin. .............. MC-17, B3
Norgestrel and Ethinyl
  Estradiol ......... MC-17, B4–5
*Normodyne* Tablets—
  100 mg (244) ........... MC-13, A6
  200 mg (752) ........... MC-13, A6
  300 mg (438) ........... MC-13, A6
*Noroxin* Tablets—
  400 mg (MSD 705). ........ MC-17, B3
*Norpace* Capsules—
  100 mg (2752) ........... MC-8, A5
  150 mg (2762) ........... MC-8, A5
*Norpace CR* Extended-release Capsules—
  100 mg (2732) ........... MC-8, A6
  150 mg (2742) ........... MC-8, A6
*Norpramin* Tablets—
  10 mg (68-7). ........... MC-6, C6
  25 mg (25) .............. MC-6, C6
  50 mg (50) .............. MC-6, C6
  75 mg (75) .............. MC-6, C7
  100 mg (100) ............ MC-6, C7
  150 mg (150) ............ MC-6, C7

Nortriptyline............. MC-17, B6–C2
  Schein/Danbury Capsules—
   10 mg (DAN 10mg) ...... MC-17, C1
   25 mg (DAN 25mg) ...... MC-17, C1
   50 mg (DAN 50mg) ...... MC-17, C2
   75 mg (DAN 75mg) ...... MC-17, C2
*Norvasc* Tablets—
  2.5 mg (2.5) ............. MC-1, D4
  5 mg (5) ................. MC-1, D4
  10 mg (10) ............... MC-1, D4
Ofloxacin. ................ MC-17, C3
Omeprazole. ............... MC-17, C4
*Omnipen* Capsules—
  250 mg (53) .............. MC-2, A6
  500 mg (309) ............. MC-2, A6
Ondansetron ............... MC-17, C5
*Oretic* Tablets—
  25 mg. .................. MC-11, C1
  50 mg. .................. MC-11, C1
*Orinase* Tablets—
  250 mg (250) ............ MC-23, C2
  500 mg (500) ............ MC-23, C2
*Ornade* Extended-release Capsules—
  75/12 mg (SKF) ........... MC-4, D6
*Ortho-Est* Tablets—
  0.625 mg (1801). .......... MC-9, D2
  1.25 mg (1800). ........... MC-9, D2
*Ortho-Novum 1/35-21 and -28* Tablets—
  1/0.035 mg (135). ........ MC-16, D7
  Inert. .................. MC-16, D7
*Ortho-Novum 1/50-21 and -28* Tablets—
  1/0.05 mg (150). .......... MC-17, B1
  Inert. ................... MC-17, B1
*Ortho-Novum 7/7/7-21 and -28* Tablets—
  0.5/0.035 mg (535). ....... MC-17, A1
  0.75/0.035 mg (75) ........ MC-17, A1
  1/0.035 mg (135). ......... MC-17, A1
  Inert. ................... MC-17, A1
*Ovcon 35-21 and -28* Tablets—
  0.4/0.035 mg (583). ...... MC-16, D5
  Inert (850). ............ MC-16, D5
*Ovcon 50-21 and -28* Tablets—
  1/0.05 mg (584). ........ MC-16, D6
  Inert (850). ............ MC-16, D6
*Ovral-21 and -28* Tablets—
  0.5/0.05 mg (56) ......... MC-17, B5
  Inert (445). ............. MC-17, B5
Oxacillin ................. MC-17, C6
Oxaprozin ................. MC-17, C7
Oxazepam .............. MC-17, D1–6
  Barr
   Capsules—
    10 mg (374) .......... MC-17, D1
    15 mg (375) .......... MC-17, D1
    30 mg (376) .......... MC-17, D1
   Tablets—
    15 mg (373) .......... MC-17, D2
  Purepac Capsules—
   10 mg (067) ........... MC-17, D3
   15 mg (069) ........... MC-17, D3
   30 mg (073) ........... MC-17, D3
  Schein/Danbury Capsules—
   10 mg (DAN 5617). ..... MC-17, D4
   15 mg (DAN 5616). ..... MC-17, D4
   30 mg (DAN 5618). ..... MC-17, D4
Oxybutynin ................ MC-17, D7
Oxycodone. ................ MC-18, A1
Oxycodone and Aceta-
  minophen. ............ MC-18, A2–4
Oxycodone and Aspirin..... MC-18, A5–7
*Pamelor* Capsules—
  10 mg (78-86). .......... MC-17, B6
  25 mg (78-87). .......... MC-17, B6
  50 mg (78-78). .......... MC-17, B7
  75 mg (78-79). .......... MC-17, B7

*Pancrease* Delayed-release Capsules—
  4/12/12*. ............... MC-18, B1
  4/20/25* (MT 4). ........ MC-18, B1
  10/30/30* (MT 10). ...... MC-18, B1
  16/48/48* (MT 16). ...... MC-18, B2
  25/75/75* (MT 25). ...... MC-18, B2
Pancrelipase .............. MC-18, B1–2
*Panmycin* Capsules—
  250 mg (250 mg). ........ MC-22, B7
*Parafon Forte DSC* Tablets—
  500 mg. ................. MC-5, B5
*Parlodel*
  Capsules—
   5 mg (78-102). ......... MC-3, B4
  Tablets—
   2.5 mg (78-17) ......... MC-3, B5
*Parnate* Tablets—
  10 mg. .................. MC-23, D1
Paroxetine ................ MC-18, B3
*Paxil* Tablets—
  20 mg (20) .............. MC-18, B3
  30 mg (30) .............. MC-18, B3
*PCE* Tablets—
  333 mg. .................. MC-9, B2
  500 mg (EK) .............. MC-9, B2
Penbutolol ................ MC-18, B4
*Penetrex* Tablets—
  200 mg (5100) ............ MC-9, A1
  400 mg (5140) ............ MC-9, A1
Penicillin V ............. MC-18, B5–C2
  Biocraft Tablets—
   250 mg Round (15) ..... MC-18, B6
   250 mg Oval (16). ..... MC-18, B6
   500 mg Round (17). .... MC-18, B6
   500 mg Oval (49). ..... MC-18, B6
Pentazocine and
  Acetaminophen. .......... MC-18, C3
Pentazocine and Naloxone .... MC-18, C4
Pentoxifylline ............ MC-18, C5
*Pen-Vee K* Tablets—
  250 mg (59) ............. MC-18, C2
  500 mg (390) ............ MC-18, C2
*Pepcid* Tablets—
  20 mg (MSD 963) .......... MC-9, D6
  40 mg (MSD 964) .......... MC-9, D6
*Percocet* Tablets—
  5/325 mg ................ MC-18, A2
*Percodan* Tablets—
  4.88/325 mg ............. MC-18, A5
*Percodan-Demi* Tablets—
  2.44/325 mg ............. MC-18, A6
Perphenazine and
  Amitriptyline ........... MC-18, C6–7
*Persantine* Tablets—
  25 mg (BI 17). ........... MC-7, D7
  50 mg (BI 18). ........... MC-7, D7
  75 mg (BI 19). ........... MC-7, D7
*Phenaphen with Codeine* Capsules—
  325/15 mg (AHR 6242). ..... MC-1, A3
  325/30 mg (AHR 6257). ..... MC-1, A3
*Phenergan* Tablets—
  12.5 mg (19). ........... MC-20, A3
  25 mg (27) .............. MC-20, A3
  50 mg (227) ............. MC-20, A3
Phenobarbital ............. MC-18, D1
  Warner Chilcott Tablets—
   15 mg (WC 699) ........ MC-18, D1
   30 mg (WC 700) ........ MC-18, D1
   60 mg (WC 607) ........ MC-18, D1
   100 mg (WC 698) ....... MC-18, D1
Phentermine ............... MC-18, D2
Phenylephrine, Chlorpheniramine, and
  Pyrilamine .............. MC-18, D3
Phenylephrine, Phenylpropanolamine, and
  Guaifenesin. ............ MC-18, D4
Phenylpropanolamine and
  Guaifenesin. ............ MC-18, D5

Phenytoin. . . . . . . . . . . . . . . . . . MC-18, D6
Phenytoin Sodium . . . . . . . . . . . MC-18, D7
Pindolol . . . . . . . . . . . . . . . . . . MC-19, A1–2
  Mutual Tablets—
    5 mg (MP 178) . . . . . . . . . MC-19, A1
    10 mg (MP 183) . . . . . . . . MC-19, A1
Piroxicam . . . . . . . . . . . . . MC-19, A3–4
  Mutual Capsules—
    10 mg (165) . . . . . . . . . . . . MC-19, A3
    20 mg (166) . . . . . . . . . . . . MC-19, A3
*Plaquenil* Tablets—
  200 mg. . . . . . . . . . . . . . . . . MC-11, D4
*Plendil* Tablets—
  5 mg (MSD 451) . . . . . . . . . . MC-10, A1
  10 mg (MSD 452) . . . . . . . . . MC-10, A1
Potassium Chloride . . . . . . . MC-19, A5–B3
*Pravachol* Tablets—
  10 mg (10) . . . . . . . . . . . . . MC-19, B4
  20 mg (20) . . . . . . . . . . . . . MC-19, B4
  40 mg (40) . . . . . . . . . . . . . MC-19, B4
Pravastatin . . . . . . . . . . . . . . MC-19, B4
Prazosin. . . . . . . . . . . . . . . . . . MC-19, A5–7
  Purepac Capsules—
    1 mg (500) . . . . . . . . . . . . MC-19, B6
    2 mg (501) . . . . . . . . . . . . MC-19, B6
    5 mg (502) . . . . . . . . . . . . MC-19, B6
  Schein/Danbury Capsules—
    1 mg (DAN 5697) . . . . . . . MC-19, B7
    2 mg (DAN 5696) . . . . . . . MC-19, B7
    5 mg (DAN 5693) . . . . . . . MC-19, B7
Prazosin and Polythiazide. . . . . MC-19, C1
Prednisone. . . . . . . . . . . . . . . . . MC-19, C2–4
  Roxane Tablets—
    1 mg (54 092). . . . . . . . . . . MC-19, C2
    2.5 mg (54 339). . . . . . . . . MC-19, C2
    5 mg (54 612). . . . . . . . . . . MC-19, C2
    10 mg (54 899). . . . . . . . . . MC-19, C2
    20 mg (54 760). . . . . . . . . . MC-19, C2
    50 mg (54 343). . . . . . . . . . MC-19, C2
  Rugby Tablets—
    5 mg. . . . . . . . . . . . . . . . MC-19, C3
    10 mg (4325) . . . . . . . . . . . MC-19, C3
    20 mg (4326) . . . . . . . . . . . MC-19, C3
    50 mg. . . . . . . . . . . . . . . MC-19, C3
*Premarin* Tablets—
  0.3 mg (0.3) . . . . . . . . . . MC-9, C7
  0.625 mg (0.625) . . . . . . . MC-9, C7
  0.9 mg (0.9) . . . . . . . . . . MC-9, C7
  1.25 mg (1.25) . . . . . . . . . MC-9, D1
  2.5 mg (2.5) . . . . . . . . . . MC-9, D1
*Prilosec* Delayed-release Capsules—
  20 mg (MSD 742) . . . . . . . . . MC-17, C4
*Principen* Capsules—
  250 mg (7992) . . . . . . . . . . . MC-2, A4
  500 mg (7993) . . . . . . . . . . . MC-2, A4
*Prinivil* Tablets—
  5 mg (MSD 19) . . . . . . . . . . MC-13, C2
  10 mg (MSD 106) . . . . . . . . . MC-13, C2
  20 mg (MSD 207) . . . . . . . . . MC-13, C2
  40 mg (MSD 237) . . . . . . . . . MC-13, C2
*Prinzide* Tablets—
  20/12.5 mg (MSD 140) . . . MC-13, C4
  20/25 mg (MSD 142) . . . . . . MC-13, C4
*Pro-Banthine* Tablets—
  7.5 mg (611) . . . . . . . . . . . MC-20, A5
  15 mg (601) . . . . . . . . . . . . MC-20, A5
Probucol . . . . . . . . . . . . . . . MC-19, C5
Procainamide . . . . . . . . . . . MC-19, C6–D7
  Geneva
    Capsules—
      250 mg (GG 551) . . . . . MC-19, C6
      375 mg (GG 552) . . . . . MC-19, C6
      500 mg (GG 553) . . . . . MC-19, C6
    Extended-release Tablets—
      250 mg (GG 472) . . . . . MC-19, C7
      500 mg (GG 473) . . . . . MC-19, C7
      750 mg (GG 474) . . . . . MC-19, C7

Procainamide *(continued)*
  Schein/Danbury
    Capsules—
      250 mg (DAN 5026). . . . MC-19, D6
      375 mg (DAN 5350). . . . MC-19, D6
      500 mg (DAN 5333). . . . MC-19, D6
    Extended-release Tablets—
      250 mg (5562) . . . . . . . MC-19, D7
      500 mg (55 63). . . . . . . MC-19, D7
      750 mg (55 64). . . . . . . MC-19, D7
*Procan SR* Extended-release Tablets—
  500 mg (P-D 204) . . . . . . . . MC-19, D1
  750 mg (P-D 205) . . . . . . . . MC-19, D2
  1 gram (P-D 207). . . . . . . . . MC-19, D2
*Procardia* Capsules—
  10 mg (260) . . . . . . . . . . . . MC-16, C1
  20 mg (261) . . . . . . . . . . . . MC-16, C1
*Procardia XL* Extended-release Tablets—
  30 mg (30) . . . . . . . . . . . . . MC-16, C2
  60 mg (60) . . . . . . . . . . . . . MC-16, C2
  90 mg (90) . . . . . . . . . . . . . MC-16, C2
Prochlorperazine. . . . . . . . . . . MC-20, A1–2
*Prolixin* Tablets—
  1 mg (PPP 863) . . . . . . . . . MC-10, B6
  2.5 mg (PPP 864) . . . . . . . . MC-10, B6
  5 mg (PPP 877) . . . . . . . . . MC-10, B6
  10 mg (PPP 956) . . . . . . . . . MC-10, B6
*Proloprim* Tablets—
  100 mg (09A) . . . . . . . . . . . MC-24, B1
  200 mg (200) . . . . . . . . . . . MC-24, B1
Promethazine . . . . . . . . . . . . MC-20, A3
*Pronestyl*
  Capsules—
    250 mg (758) . . . . . . . . . MC-19, D3
    375 mg (756) . . . . . . . . . MC-19, D3
    500 mg (757) . . . . . . . . . MC-19, D3
  Tablets—
    250 mg (431) . . . . . . . . . MC-19, D4
    375 mg (434) . . . . . . . . . MC-19, D4
    500 mg (438) . . . . . . . . . MC-19, D4
*Pronestyl-SR* Extended-release Tablets—
  500 mg (PPP 775) . . . . . . . . MC-19, D5
Propafenone . . . . . . . . . . . . . MC-20, A4
Propantheline . . . . . . . . . . . . MC-20, A5
Propoxyphene Napsylate and
  Acetaminophen. . . . . . . . MC-20, A6–B2
  Barr Tablets—
    50/325 mg (317) . . . . . . . MC-20, A6
    100/650 mg Pink
      (470) . . . . . . . . . . . . . . MC-20, A6
    100/650 mg White
      (318) . . . . . . . . . . . . . . MC-20, A6
  Mylan Tablets—
    100/650 mg Pink
      (155) . . . . . . . . . . . . . . MC-20, B1
    100/650 mg White
      (521) . . . . . . . . . . . . . . MC-20, B1
  Purepac Tablets—
    100/650 mg (085) . . . . . . MC-20, B2
Propranolol . . . . . . . . . . . . MC-20, B3–C3
  Geneva Tablets—
    10 mg (GG 71) . . . . . . . . MC-20, B3
    20 mg (GG 72) . . . . . . . . MC-20, B3
    40 mg (GG 73) . . . . . . . . MC-20, B3
    60 mg (GG 74) . . . . . . . . MC-20, B3
    80 mg (GG 75) . . . . . . . . MC-20, B3
  Lederle Tablets—
    10 mg (P 44) . . . . . . . . . MC-20, B4
    20 mg (P 45) . . . . . . . . . MC-20, B4
    40 mg (P 46) . . . . . . . . . MC-20, B4
    60 mg (P 65) . . . . . . . . . MC-20, B4
    80 mg (P 47) . . . . . . . . . MC-20, B4
  Purepac Tablets—
    10 mg (27) . . . . . . . . . . . MC-20, B5
    20 mg (29) . . . . . . . . . . . MC-20, B5
    40 mg (331) . . . . . . . . . . MC-20, B5

Propranolol
  Purepac Tablets *(continued)*
    60 mg (321) . . . . . . . . . . . MC-20, B5
    80 mg (333) . . . . . . . . . . . MC-20, B5
  Rugby Tablets—
    10 mg (4309) . . . . . . . . . . MC-20, B6
    20 mg (4313) . . . . . . . . . . MC-20, B6
    40 mg (4314) . . . . . . . . . . MC-20, B6
    60 mg (4315) . . . . . . . . . . MC-20, B6
    80 mg (4316) . . . . . . . . . . MC-20, B6
  Schein/Danbury Tablets—
    10 mg (DAN 5554) . . . . . . MC-20, B7
    20 mg (DAN 5555) . . . . . . MC-20, B7
    40 mg (DAN 5556) . . . . . . MC-20, B7
    60 mg (127) . . . . . . . . . . . MC-20, B7
    80 mg (DAN 5557) . . . . . . MC-20, B7
Propranolol and
  Hydrochlorothiazide. . . . . MC-20, C4–D1
  Purepac Tablets—
    40/25 mg (358) . . . . . . . . MC-20, C4
    80/25 mg (360) . . . . . . . . MC-20, C4
  Rugby Tablets—
    40/25 mg (4402) . . . . . . . MC-20, C5
    80/25 mg (4403) . . . . . . . MC-20, C5
*Propulsid* Tablets—
  10 mg (P10) . . . . . . . . . . . . MC-5, C4
  20 mg (P20) . . . . . . . . . . . . MC-5, C4
*Proscar* Tablets—
  5 mg (MSD 72) . . . . . . . . . . MC-10, B2
*ProSom* Tablets—
  1 mg (UC) . . . . . . . . . . . . . MC-9, C5
  2 mg (UD) . . . . . . . . . . . . . MC-9, C5
*Prostaphlin* Capsules—
  250 mg (7977) . . . . . . . . . . MC-17, C6
  500 mg (7982) . . . . . . . . . . MC-17, C6
*Proventil* Extended-release Tablets—
  4 mg (431) . . . . . . . . . . . . MC-1, B2
*Provera* Tablets—
  2.5 mg (2.5) . . . . . . . . . . . MC-14, B5
  5 mg (5) . . . . . . . . . . . . . . MC-14, B5
  10 mg (10) . . . . . . . . . . . . . MC-14, B5
*Prozac* Capsules—
  20 mg (3105) . . . . . . . . . . . MC-10, B4
Pseudoephedrine and
  Guaifenesin. . . . . . . . . . . . MC-20, D2
Quazepam . . . . . . . . . . . . . . MC-20, D3
*Quibron* Capsules—
  150/90 mg (516) . . . . . . . . . MC-22, D3
  300/180 mg (515) . . . . . . . . MC-22, D3
*Quibron-T Dividose* Tablets—
  300 mg (BL 512) . . . . . . . . . MC-22, C2
*Quibron-T/SR Dividose* Extended-release
  Tablets—
    300 mg (BL 519) . . . . . . . . MC-22, C3
*Quinaglute Dura-Tabs* Extended-release
  Tablets—
    324 mg. . . . . . . . . . . . . . MC-20, D5
Quinapril. . . . . . . . . . . . . . . . . MC-20, D4
*Quinidex* Extended-release Tablets—
  300 mg (AHR). . . . . . . . . . . MC-20, D7
Quinidine Gluconate . . . . . . . MC-20, D5–6
  Schein/Danbury Extended-release
    Tablets—
      324 mg (5538) . . . . . . . MC-20, D6
Quinidine Sulfate. . . . . . . . . . . MC-20, D7
Ramipril . . . . . . . . . . . . . . . . MC-21, A1
Ranitidine . . . . . . . . . . . . . . . MC-21, A2
*Reglan* Tablets—
  5 mg (5) . . . . . . . . . . . . . . MC-15, A7
  10 mg (AHR 10) . . . . . . . . . MC-15, A7
*Regroton* Tablets—
  0.25/50 mg (31). . . . . . . . . . MC-21, A4
*Relafen* Tablets—
  500 mg (500) . . . . . . . . . . . MC-15, D7
  750 mg (750) . . . . . . . . . . . MC-15, D7

Reserpine and
  Chlorthalidone ........... MC-21, A3–4
Reserpine, Hydralazine, and
  Hydrochlorothiazide........ MC-21, A5
*Restoril* Capsules—
  7.5 mg (7.5 mg) ............ MC-22, A4
  15 mg (78-98) .............. MC-22, A4
  30 mg (78-99)............... MC-22, A4
*Retrovir* Capsules—
  100 mg (Y9C 100)........ MC-24, D6
*Ridaura* Capsules—
  3 mg............................. MC-2, D2
*Risperdal* Tablets—
  1 mg (R1)................... MC-21, A6
  2 mg (R2)................... MC-21, A6
  3 mg (R3)................... MC-21, A6
  4 mg (R4)................... MC-21, A6
Risperidone .................. MC-21, A6
*Ritalin* Tablets—
  5 mg (7) .................... MC-15, A2
  10 mg (3) ................... MC-15, A2
  20 mg (34) ................. MC-15, A2
*Ritalin-SR* Extended-release Tablets—
  20 mg (16) ................. MC-15, A3
*Robaxin* Tablets—
  500 mg (AHR)............. MC-14, C4
  750 mg (750) .............. MC-14, C4
*Robaxisal* Tablets—
  400/325 mg (AHR)........ MC-14, C5
*Rocaltrol* Capsules—
  0.25 mcg (.25) ............. MC-3, C7
  0.5 mcg (.5) ................ MC-3, C7
*Roxicet* Tablets—
  5/325 mg (543) ............ MC-18, A4
  5/500 mg (54 730) ........ MC-18, A4
*Roxicodone* Tablets—
  5 mg (54 582) ............. MC-18, A1
*Roxiprin* Tablets—
  4.88/325 mg (54 902) ..... MC-18, A7
*Rufen* Tablets—
  400 mg (400) .............. MC-12, A5
  600 mg (6) ................. MC-12, A5
  800 mg (8) ................. MC-12, A5
*Rynatan* Tablets—
  25/8/25 mg (37-0713) ...... MC-18, D3
*Rythmol* Tablets—
  150 mg (150) ............... MC-20, A4
  300 mg (300) ............... MC-20, A4
*Sandimmune SGC* Capsules—
  25 mg (78 240).............. MC-6, C2
  100 mg (78 241) ........... MC-6, C2
*Seldane* Tablets—
  60 mg........................ MC-22, A7
*Seldane-D* Tablets—
  60/120 mg ................. MC-22, B1
Selegiline ................... MC-21, A7
*Semprex-D* Capsules—
  8/60 mg .................... MC-1, A4
*Septra* Tablets—
  400/80 mg (Y2B) .......... MC-21, C4
  800/160 mg (DS 02C) ...... MC-21, C4
*Ser-Ap-Es* Tablets—
  0.1/25/15 mg (71)......... MC-21, A5
*Serax*
  Capsules—
    10 mg (51) ............... MC-17, D5
    15 mg (6) ................ MC-17, D5
    30 mg (52) ............... MC-17, D5
  Tablets—
    15 mg (317) .............. MC-17, D6
Sertraline................... MC-21, B1
Simvastatin.................. MC-21, B2
*Sinemet* Tablets—
  10/100 mg (647) ........... MC-4, A3
  25/100 mg (650) ........... MC-4, A3
  25/250 mg (654) ........... MC-4, A3

*Sinequan* Capsules—
  10 mg (534) ................ MC-8, B5
  25 mg (535) ................ MC-8, B5
  50 mg (536) ................ MC-8, B5
  75 mg (539) ................ MC-8, B6
  100 mg (538) ............... MC-8, B6
  150 mg (537) ............... MC-8, B6
*Slo-bid* Extended-release Capsules—
  50 mg (50) ................. MC-22, C5
  75 mg (75 mg) .............. MC-22, C5
  100 mg (100 mg) ........... MC-22, C5
  125 mg (125 mg) ........... MC-22, C6
  200 mg (200 mg) ........... MC-22, C6
  300 mg (300 mg) ........... MC-22, C6
*Slo-Niacin* Extended-release Tablets—
  250 mg (250) ............... MC-16, B4
  500 mg (500) ............... MC-16, B4
  750 mg (750) ............... MC-16, B4
*Slo-Phyllin*
  Extended-release Capsules—
    60 mg (WHR 1354) ...... MC-22, C7
    125 mg (125 mg) ........ MC-22, C7
    250 mg (WHR 1356) ..... MC-22, C7
  Tablets—
    100 mg (rPr 351) ........ MC-22, D1
    200 mg (rPr 352) ........ MC-22, D1
*Slow-K* Extended-release Tablets—
  600 mg........................ MC-19, B2
*Soma* Tablets—
  350 mg (37-2001)............ MC-4, A4
*Soma Compound* Tablets—
  200/325 mg (2103) .......... MC-4, A5
*Soma Compound with Codeine* Tablets—
  200/325/16 mg (2403) ...... MC-4, A6
*Sorbitrate*
  Tablets—
    5 mg (770) ............... MC-12, D2
    10 mg (780) .............. MC-12, D2
    20 mg (820) .............. MC-12, D2
    30 mg (773) .............. MC-12, D3
    40 mg (774) .............. MC-12, D3
  Chewable Tablets—
    5 mg (810) ............... MC-12, D4
    10 mg (815) .............. MC-12, D4
  Sublingual Tablets—
    2.5 mg (853).............. MC-12, D5
    5 mg (760) ............... MC-12, D5
    10 mg (761) .............. MC-12, D5
Sotalol ..................... MC-21, B3
Spironolactone ............ MC-21, B4–6
  Geneva Tablets—
    25 mg (GG 85) .......... MC-21, B4
  Purepac Tablets—
    25 mg (388) ............. MC-21, B5
Spironolactone and
  Hydrochlorothiazide..... MC-21, B7–C2
  Geneva Tablets—
    25/25 mg (GG 95) ..... MC-21, B7
  Schein/Danbury Tablets—
    25/25 mg (5496) ....... MC-21, C1
*Sporanox* Capsules—
  100 mg (100) .............. MC-13, A2
*Stelazine* Tablets—
  2 mg (S04) ................ MC-24, A6
Sucralfate................... MC-21, C3
Sulfamethoxazole and
  Trimethoprim ............ MC-21, C4–6
  Schein/Danbury Tablets—
    400/80 mg (5546) ...... MC-21, C6
    800/160 mg (5547) ..... MC-21, C6
Sulfasalazine............. MC-21, C7–D1
Sulindac................. MC-21, D2–5
  Mutual Tablets—
    150 mg (MP 112) ........ MC-21, D3
    200 mg (MP 116) ........ MC-21, D3

Sulindac *(continued)*
  Schein/Danbury Tablets—
    150 mg (5661) .......... MC-21, D4
    200 mg (5660) .......... MC-21, D4
  Warner Chilcott Tablets—
    150 mg (WC 773) ....... MC-21, D5
    200 mg (WC 774) ....... MC-21, D5
*Sumycin*
  Capsules—
    250 mg (655) ........... MC-22, B2
    500 mg (763) ........... MC-22, B2
  Tablets—
    250 mg (663) ........... MC-22, B3
    500 mg (603) ........... MC-22, B3
*Suprax* Tablets—
  200 mg (LL 200) .......... MC-4, B4
  400 mg (400) ............. MC-4, B4
*Surmontil* Capsules—
  25 mg (4132) .............. MC-24, B2
  50 mg (4133) .............. MC-24, B2
  100 mg (4158) ............. MC-24, B2
*Symmetrel* Capsules—
  100 mg........................ MC-1, C4
*Synalgos-DC* Capsules—
  356.4/30/16 mg (4191) .... MC-2, A7
*Synthroid* Tablets—
  0.025 mg (25) ............. MC-13, B4
  0.05 mg (50) .............. MC-13, B4
  0.075 mg (75) ............. MC-13, B4
  0.1 mg (100) .............. MC-13, B4
  0.112 mg (112) ............ MC-13, B4
  0.125 mg (125) ............ MC-13, B5
  0.15 mg (150).............. MC-13, B5
  0.175 mg (175) ............ MC-13, B5
  0.2 mg (200)............... MC-13, B5
  0.3 mg (300)............... MC-13, B5
Tacrine....................... MC-21, D6
*Tagamet* Tablets—
  200 mg (200 SKF).......... MC-5, B7
  300 mg (300 SKF).......... MC-5, B7
  400 mg (400 SKF).......... MC-5, C1
  800 mg (800 SKF).......... MC-5, C1
*Talacen* Tablets—
  25/650 mg (T37).......... MC-18, C3
*Talwin-Nx* Tablets—
  50/0.5 mg (T 51).......... MC-18, C4
Tamoxifen.................... MC-21, D7
*Tavist* Tablets—
  1.34 mg (78-75) ........... MC-5, C6
  2.68 mg (78-72) ........... MC-5, C6
*Tegretol*
  Tablets—
    200 mg (27 27)............ MC-3, D5
  Chewable Tablets—
    100 mg (52) .............. MC-3, D6
Temazepam................ MC-22, A1–4
  Barr Capsules—
    15 mg (487) ............. MC-22, A1
    30 mg (488) ............. MC-22, A1
  Mylan Capsules—
    15 mg (4010) ............ MC-22, A2
    30 mg (5050) ............ MC-22, A2
  Purepac Capsules—
    15 mg (076) ............. MC-22, A3
    30 mg (077) ............. MC-22, A3
*Tenex* Tablets—
  1 mg (1) .................. MC-11, A5
  2 mg (2) .................. MC-11, A5
*Tenoretic* Tablets—
  50/25 mg (115) ............ MC-2, C4
  100/25 mg (117) ........... MC-2, C4
*Tenormin* Tablets—
  25 mg (107) ............... MC-2, C1
  50 mg (105) ............... MC-2, C1
  100 mg (101) .............. MC-2, C1

**Tenuate**
Tablets—
25 mg (25) .............. MC-7, B3
Extended-release Tablets—
75 mg (75) ............. MC-7, B4
Terazosin.................. MC-22, A5
Terbutaline ................ MC-22, A6
Terfenadine ................ MC-22, A7
Terfenadine and
Pseodoephedrine........... MC-22, B1
Tetracycline ............. MC-22, B2–C1
Purepac Capsules—
250 mg (404) .......... MC-22, B5
500 mg (406) .......... MC-22, B5
Schein Capsules—
250 mg Blue/Yellow
(H 214) ............ MC-22, B6
250 mg Orange/Yellow
(DAN 5162)........... MC-22, B6
500 mg (H 203) ......... MC-22, B6
Warner Chilcott Capsules—
250 mg (WC 407) .... MC-22, C1
500 mg (WC 697) ....... MC-22, C1
**Thalitone** Tablets—
25 mg (76) ............. MC-5, B2
**Theo-24** Extended-release Capsules—
100 mg (2832) ........ MC-22, D2
200 mg (2842) ........ MC-22, D2
300 mg (2852) ........ MC-22, D2
**Theo-Dur** Extended-release Tablets—
100 mg (100) ......... MC-22, C4
200 mg (200) ......... MC-22, C4
300 mg (300) ......... MC-22, C4
Theophylline ........... MC-22, C2–D2
Theophylline and Guaifenesin . MC-22, D3
Thioridazine ...... MC-22, D4–MC-23, A4
Barr Tablets—
10 mg (260) .......... MC-22, D4
25 mg (261) .......... MC-22, D4
50 mg (262) .......... MC-22, D4
100 mg (263) ......... MC-22, D4
150 mg (327) ......... MC-22, D5
200 mg (328) ......... MC-22, D5
Geneva Tablets—
150 mg (GG 35) ....... MC-22, D6
200 mg (GG 36) ........ MC-22, D6
Mylan Tablets—
10 mg (M 54).......... MC-22, D7
25 mg (M 58) ......... MC-22, D7
50 mg (M 59).......... MC-22, D7
100 mg (M 61).......... MC-22, D7
Schein/Danbury Tablets—
10 mg (5566) ......... MC-23, A3
25 mg (5542) ......... MC-23, A3
50 mg (5568) ......... MC-23, A3
100 mg (5569) ........ MC-23, A4
150 mg (5580) ........ MC-23, A4
200 mg (5581) ........ MC-23, A4
Thiothixene............. MC-23, A5–B1
Geneva Capsules—
1 mg (GG 589) ........ MC-23, A5
2 mg (GG 596) ........ MC-23, A5
5 mg (GG 597) ........ MC-23, A5
10 mg (GG 598) ........ MC-23, A5
Schein/Danbury Capsules—
1 mg (5593) .......... MC-23, B1
2 mg (5592) .......... MC-23, B1
5 mg (5595) .......... MC-23, B1
10 mg (5594) ......... MC-23, B1
**Thorazine**
Extended-release Capsules—
75 mg (T64) .......... MC-5, A3
Tablets—
25 mg (T74) ........... MC-5, A4
**Ticlid** Tablets—
250 mg (250) .......... MC-23, B2

Ticlopidine ............... MC-23, B2
**Tigan** Capsules—
100 mg (100) .......... MC-24, A7
250 mg (250) .......... MC-24, A7
Timolol ............... MC-23, B3–5
Mylan Tablets—
5 mg (M 55)........... MC-23, B4
10 mg (M 221).......... MC-23, B4
20 mg (715) .......... MC-23, B4
Schein/Danbury Tablets—
5 mg (5736) .......... MC-23, B5
10 mg (5737) ......... MC-23, B5
20 mg (5738) ......... MC-23, B5
Tocainide................. MC-23, B6
**Tofranil** Tablets—
10 mg (32) ............ MC-12, B7
25 mg (140) .......... MC-12, B7
50 mg (136) .......... MC-12, B7
**Tofranil-PM** Capsules—
75 mg (20) ........... MC-12, B5
100 mg (40) .......... MC-12, B5
125 mg (45) .......... MC-12, B6
150 mg (22) .......... MC-12, B6
Tolazamide .............. MC-23, B7–C1
Geneva Tablets—
100 mg (GG 270) ...... MC-23, B7
250 mg (GG 271) ...... MC-23, B7
500 mg (GG 272) ...... MC-23, B7
Tolbutamide ............ MC-23, C2
**Tolectin** Tablets—
200 mg (200) ......... MC-23, C4
600 mg (600) ......... MC-23, C4
**Tolectin DS** Capsules—
400 mg.............. MC-23, C3
**Tolinase** Tablets—
100 mg (100) ......... MC-23, C1
250 mg (250) ......... MC-23, C1
500 mg (500) ......... MC-23, C1
Tolmetin ............... MC-23, C3–7
Mutual
Capsules—
400 mg (179) ........ MC-23, C5
Tablets—
200 mg (MP 50) ...... MC-23, C6
Purepac Capsules—
400 mg (R 520) ........ MC-23, C7
**Tonocard** Tablets—
400 mg (MSD 707) ...... MC-23, B6
600 mg (MSD 709) ........ MC-23, B6
**Toprol XL** Extended-release Tablets—
50 mg (MO) ......... MC-15, B5
100 mg (MS) .......... MC-15, B5
200 mg (MY) ......... MC-15, B5
**Toradol** Tablets—
10 mg............. MC-13, A4
**Totacillin** Capsules—
250 mg (BMP 140) ....... MC-2, A5
500 mg (BMP 141) ....... MC-2, A5
**Trandate** Tablets—
100 mg (100) ......... MC-13, A5
200 mg (200) ......... MC-13, A5
300 mg (300) ......... MC-13, A5
**Tranxene SD** Tablets—
11.25 mg (TX) ........ MC-6, A6
22.5 mg (TY) ......... MC-6, A6
**Tranxene T-Tab** Tablets—
3.75 mg (TL) ......... MC-6, A7
7.5 mg (TM).......... MC-6, A7
15 mg (TN) .......... MC-6, A7
Tranylcypromine............. MC-23, D1
Trazodone ............... MC-23, D2–5
Mutual Tablets—
50 mg (MP 118) ........ MC-23, D3
100 mg (MP 114) ....... MC-23, D3
Purepac Tablets—
50 mg (439) .......... MC-23, D4
100 mg (441) .......... MC-23, D4

Trazodone *(continued)*
Schein/Danbury Tablets—
50 mg (5600) ......... MC-23, D5
100 mg (5599) .......... MC-23, D5
**Trental** Extended-release Tablets—
400 mg.................. MC-18, C5
Triamterene and Hydrochlorothiazide ......... MC-23, D6–MC-24, A3
Barr Tablets—
75/50 mg (555 444) .... MC-23, D6
Geneva Tablets—
75/50 mg (GG 172) .... MC-23, D7
Schein/Danbury Tablets—
75/50 mg
(DAN 5682) ........ MC-24, D2
**Triavil** Tablets—
2/10 mg (MSD 914)........ MC-18, C6
2/25 mg (MSD 921)........ MC-18, C6
4/10 mg (MSD 934)........ MC-18, C6
4/25 mg (MSD 946)........ MC-18, C7
4/50 mg (MSD 517)........ MC-18, C7
Triazolam ............... MC-24, A4
Trifluoperazine............. MC-24, A5–6
Geneva Tablets—
1 mg (GG 51) ........... MC-24, A5
2 mg (GG 53) .......... MC-24, A5
5 mg (GG 55)........... MC-24, A5
10 mg (GG 58) ........ MC-24, A5
*Tri-Levlen 21 and 28* Tablets—
0.05/0.03 mg (95) ....... MC-13, B1
0.075/0.04 mg (96) ...... MC-13, B1
0.125/0.03 mg (97) ...... MC-13, B1
Inert (11)................. MC-13, B1
Trimethobenzamide........... MC-24, A7
Trimethoprim ............. MC-24, B1
Trimipramine ............... MC-24, B2
**Trimox** Capsules—
250 mg (7278) ........ MC-1, D5
500 mg (7279) ........ MC-1, D5
**Trinalin** Extended-release Tablets—
1/120 mg (PAA or 703)...... MC-2, D3
*Triphasil-21 and -28* Tablets—
0.05/0.03 mg (641) ........ MC-13, B3
0.075/0.04 mg (642) ....... MC-13, B3
0.125/0.03 mg (643) ....... MC-13, B3
Inert (650)................. MC-13, B3
**Tylenol with Codeine** Tablets—
300/7.5 mg (1) .............. MC-1, A1
300/15 mg (2) ............. MC-1, A1
300/30 mg (3) ............. MC-1, A2
300/60 mg (4) ............. MC-1, A2
**Tylox** Capsules—
5/500 mg .............. MC-18, A3
Ursodiol................ MC-24, B3
**Valium** Tablets—
2 mg (2) ................. MC-6, D7
5 mg (5) ............... MC-6, D7
10 mg (10) ............. MC-6, D7
Valproic Acid............ MC-24, B4
**Valrelease** Extended-release Capsules—
15 mg (15) ............. MC-6, D6
**Vascor** Tablets—
200 mg (200) ............. MC-3, A7
300 mg (300) ............. MC-3, A7
400 mg (400) ............. MC-3, A7
**Vaseretic** Tablets—
10/25 mg (MSD 720)....... MC-8, D7
**Vasotec** Tablets—
2.5 mg (MSD 14) ....... MC-8, D6
5 mg (MSD 712).......... MC-8, D6
10 mg (MSD 713)........ MC-8, D6
20 mg (MSD 714)........ MC-8, D6
**V-Cillin K** Tablets—
125 mg (125) ......... MC-18, C1
250 mg (250) ......... MC-18, C1
500 mg (500) ......... MC-18, C1

*Veetids* Tablets—
  250 mg (684) . . . . . . . . . . . . MC-18, B5
  500 mg (648) . . . . . . . . . . . . MC-18, B5
*Velosef* Capsules—
  250 mg (113) . . . . . . . . . MC-4, C5
  500 mg (114) . . . . . . . . . MC-4, C5
Venlafaxine . . . . . . . . . . . . . MC-24, B5
*Ventolin* Tablets—
  2 mg (2) . . . . . . . . . . . MC-1, A7
  4 mg (4) . . . . . . . . . . . MC-1, A7
Verapamil . . . . . . . . . . . MC-24, B6–D1
  Barr Tablets—
    80 mg (425) . . . . . . . . . MC-24, B6
    120 mg (455) . . . . . . . . . MC-24, B6
  Geneva Tablets—
    80 mg (GG 132) . . . . . . . . MC-24, C3
    120 mg (GG 133) . . . . . . . . MC-24, C3
  Purepac Tablets—
    80 mg (473) . . . . . . . . . MC-24, C6
    120 mg (475) . . . . . . . . . MC-24, C6
  Rugby Tablets—
    80 mg (4812) . . . . . . . . . MC-24, C7
    120 mg (4932) . . . . . . . . . MC-24, C7
  Schein/Danbury Tablets—
    80 mg (5601) . . . . . . . . . MC-24, D1
    120 mg (5602) . . . . . . . . . MC-24, D1
*Verelan* Extended-release Capsules—
  120 mg (V8) . . . . . . . . . . MC-24, C4
  180 mg (V7) . . . . . . . . . . MC-24, C4
  240 mg (V9) . . . . . . . . . . MC-24, C5
*Vibramycin* Capsules—
  50 mg (094) . . . . . . . . . . MC-8, C6
  100 mg (095) . . . . . . . . . . MC-8, C6
*Vibra-Tabs* Tablets—
  100 mg (099) . . . . . . . . . . MC-8, C7
*Vicodin* Tablets—
  5/500 mg . . . . . . . . . . . MC-11, C6

*Vicodin ES* Tablets—
  7.5/750 mg . . . . . . . . . . . MC-11, C7
*Videx* Tablets—
  25 mg (25) . . . . . . . . . . . MC-7, B2
*Visken* Tablets—
  5 mg (78-111) . . . . . . . . . MC-19, A2
  10 mg (78-73) . . . . . . . . . MC-19, A2
*Vistaril* Capsules—
  25 mg (541) . . . . . . . . . . MC-11, D6
  50 mg (542) . . . . . . . . . . MC-11, D6
  100 mg (543) . . . . . . . . . . MC-11, D6
*Voltaren* Tablets—
  25 mg (25) . . . . . . . . . . . MC-7, A2
  50 mg (50) . . . . . . . . . . . MC-7, A2
  75 mg (75) . . . . . . . . . . . MC-7, A2
Warfarin Sodium . . . . . . . . . MC-24, D4–5
*Wellbutrin* Tablets—
  75 mg (75) . . . . . . . . . . . MC-3, B7
  100 mg (100) . . . . . . . . . . MC-3, B7
*Wymox* Capsules—
  250 mg (559) . . . . . . . . . . MC-2, A1
  500 mg (560) . . . . . . . . . . MC-2, A1
*Wytensin* Tablets—
  4 mg (73) . . . . . . . . . . . MC-11, A4
  8 mg (74) . . . . . . . . . . . MC-11, A4
*Xanax* Tablets—
  0.25 mg (0.25) . . . . . . . . . MC-1, C3
  0.5 mg (0.5) . . . . . . . . . . MC-1, C3
  1 mg (1.0) . . . . . . . . . . . MC-1, C3
  2 mg (2) . . . . . . . . . . . MC-1, C3
*Zantac* Tablets—
  150 mg (150) . . . . . . . . . . MC-21, A2
  300 mg (300) . . . . . . . . . . MC-21, A2
*Zaroxolyn* Tablets—
  2.5 mg (2½) . . . . . . . . . . MC-15, B4
  5 mg (5) . . . . . . . . . . . MC-15, B4
  10 mg (10) . . . . . . . . . . . MC-15, B4

*Zebeta* Tablets—
  5 mg (B 1) . . . . . . . . . . MC-3, B2
  10 mg (B 3) . . . . . . . . . . MC-3, B2
*Zestoretic* Tablets—
  20/12.5 mg (142) . . . . . . . . MC-13, C5
  20/25 mg (145) . . . . . . . . . MC-13, C5
*Zestril* Tablets—
  5 mg (130) . . . . . . . . . . MC-13, C3
  10 mg (131) . . . . . . . . . . MC-13, C3
  20 mg (132) . . . . . . . . . . MC-13, C3
  40 mg (134) . . . . . . . . . . MC-13, C3
*Ziac* Tablets—
  2.5/6.25 mg (B 12) . . . . . . . MC-3, B3
  5/6.25 mg (B 13) . . . . . . . . MC-3, B3
  10/6.25 mg (B 14) . . . . . . . MC-3, B3
Zidovudine . . . . . . . . . . . . MC-24, D6
*Zithromax* Capsules—
  250 mg (305) . . . . . . . . . . MC-2, D5
*Zocor* Tablets—
  5 mg (MSD 726) . . . . . . . . . MC-21, B2
  10 mg (MSD 735) . . . . . . . . MC-21, B2
*Zofran* Tablets—
  4 mg (4) . . . . . . . . . . . MC-17, C5
  8 mg (8) . . . . . . . . . . . MC-17, C5
*Zoloft* Tablets—
  50 mg (50 MG) . . . . . . . . . MC-21, B1
  100 mg (100 MG) . . . . . . . . MC-21, B1
Zolpidem . . . . . . . . . . . MC-24, D7
*Zovirax*
  Capsules—
    200 mg (200) . . . . . . . . . MC-1, A5
  Tablets—
    400 mg . . . . . . . . . . . MC-1, A6
    800 mg (800) . . . . . . . . . MC-1, A6
*Zyloprim* Tablets—
  100 mg (100) . . . . . . . . . . MC-1, B4
  300 mg (300) . . . . . . . . . . MC-1, B4

*In thousands of units of lipase/amylase/protease, respectively.

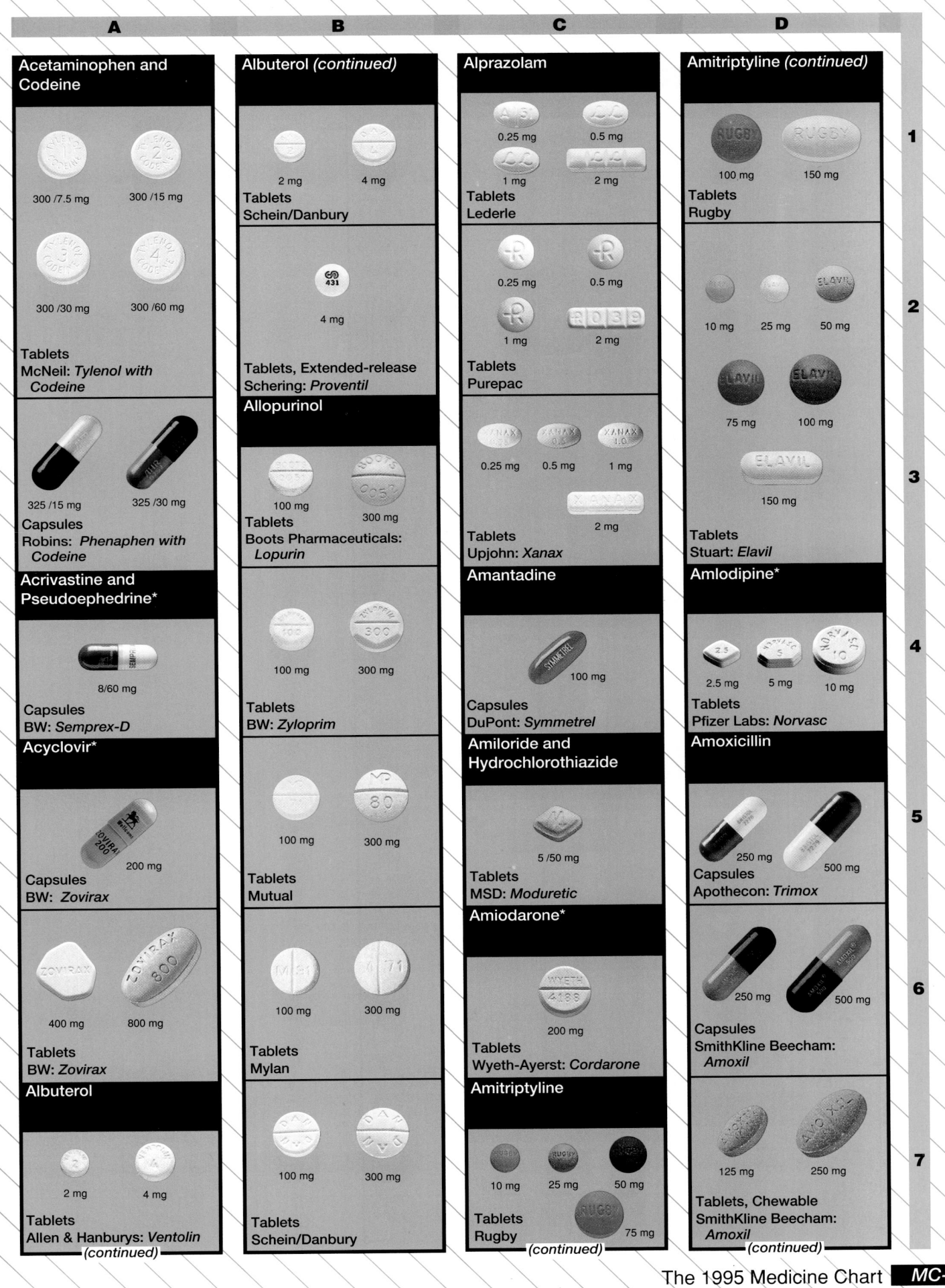

## A

**Acetaminophen and Codeine**

300 /7.5 mg  300 /15 mg
300 /30 mg  300 /60 mg

Tablets
McNeil: *Tylenol with Codeine*

325 /15 mg  325 /30 mg

Capsules
Robins: *Phenaphen with Codeine*

**Acrivastine and Pseudoephedrine***

8/60 mg

Capsules
BW: *Semprex-D*

**Acyclovir***

200 mg

Capsules
BW: *Zovirax*

400 mg  800 mg

Tablets
BW: *Zovirax*

**Albuterol**

2 mg  4 mg

Tablets
Allen & Hanburys: *Ventolin*
*(continued)*

## B

**Albuterol** *(continued)*

2 mg  4 mg

Tablets
Schein/Danbury

4 mg

Tablets, Extended-release
Schering: *Proventil*

**Allopurinol**

100 mg  300 mg

Tablets
Boots Pharmaceuticals: *Lopurin*

100 mg  300 mg

Tablets
BW: *Zyloprim*

100 mg  300 mg

Tablets
Mutual

100 mg  300 mg

Tablets
Mylan

100 mg  300 mg

Tablets
Schein/Danbury

## C

**Alprazolam**

0.25 mg  0.5 mg
1 mg  2 mg

Tablets
Lederle

0.25 mg  0.5 mg
1 mg  2 mg

Tablets
Purepac

0.25 mg  0.5 mg  1 mg

2 mg

Tablets
Upjohn: *Xanax*

**Amantadine**

100 mg

Capsules
DuPont: *Symmetrel*

**Amiloride and Hydrochlorothiazide**

5 /50 mg

Tablets
MSD: *Moduretic*

**Amiodarone***

200 mg

Tablets
Wyeth-Ayerst: *Cordarone*

**Amitriptyline**

10 mg  25 mg  50 mg
75 mg

Tablets
Rugby
*(continued)*

## D

**Amitriptyline** *(continued)*

100 mg  150 mg

Tablets
Rugby

10 mg  25 mg  50 mg
75 mg  100 mg
150 mg

Tablets
Stuart: *Elavil*

**Amlodipine***

2.5 mg  5 mg  10 mg

Tablets
Pfizer Labs: *Norvasc*

**Amoxicillin**

250 mg  500 mg

Capsules
Apothecon: *Trimox*

250 mg  500 mg

Capsules
SmithKline Beecham: *Amoxil*

125 mg  250 mg

Tablets, Chewable
SmithKline Beecham: *Amoxil*
*(continued)*

1
2
3
4
5
6
7

The 1995 Medicine Chart **MC-1**

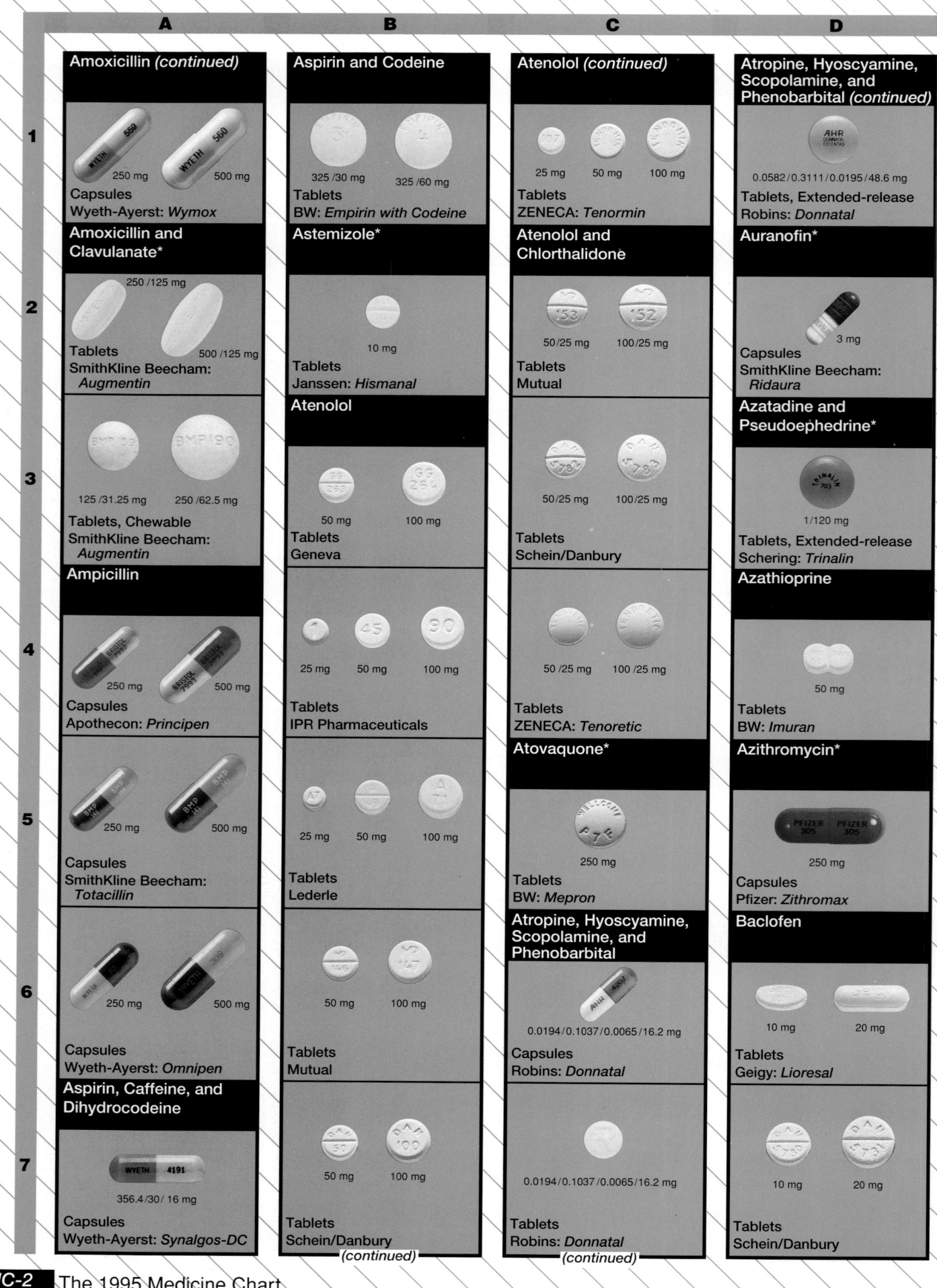

**A**

**Amoxicillin** *(continued)*

250 mg · 500 mg
Capsules
Wyeth-Ayerst: *Wymox*

**Amoxicillin and Clavulanate***

250 /125 mg
500 /125 mg
Tablets
SmithKline Beecham: *Augmentin*

125 /31.25 mg · 250 /62.5 mg
Tablets, Chewable
SmithKline Beecham: *Augmentin*

**Ampicillin**

250 mg · 500 mg
Capsules
Apothecon: *Principen*

250 mg · 500 mg
Capsules
SmithKline Beecham: *Totacillin*

250 mg · 500 mg
Capsules
Wyeth-Ayerst: *Omnipen*

**Aspirin, Caffeine, and Dihydrocodeine**

356.4 /30/ 16 mg
Capsules
Wyeth-Ayerst: *Synalgos-DC*

**B**

**Aspirin and Codeine**

325 /30 mg · 325 /60 mg
Tablets
BW: *Empirin with Codeine*

**Astemizole***

10 mg
Tablets
Janssen: *Hismanal*

**Atenolol**

50 mg · 100 mg
Tablets
Geneva

25 mg · 50 mg · 100 mg
Tablets
IPR Pharmaceuticals

25 mg · 50 mg · 100 mg
Tablets
Lederle

50 mg · 100 mg
Tablets
Mutual

50 mg · 100 mg
Tablets
Schein/Danbury
*(continued)*

**C**

**Atenolol** *(continued)*

25 mg · 50 mg · 100 mg
Tablets
ZENECA: *Tenormin*

**Atenolol and Chlorthalidone**

50 /25 mg · 100 /25 mg
Tablets
Mutual

50 /25 mg · 100 /25 mg
Tablets
Schein/Danbury

50 /25 mg · 100 /25 mg
Tablets
ZENECA: *Tenoretic*

**Atovaquone***

250 mg
Tablets
BW: *Mepron*

**Atropine, Hyoscyamine, Scopolamine, and Phenobarbital**

0.0194/0.1037/0.0065/16.2 mg
Capsules
Robins: *Donnatal*

0.0194/0.1037/0.0065/16.2 mg
Tablets
Robins: *Donnatal*
*(continued)*

**D**

**Atropine, Hyoscyamine, Scopolamine, and Phenobarbital** *(continued)*

0.0582/0.3111/0.0195/48.6 mg
Tablets, Extended-release
Robins: *Donnatal*

**Auranofin***

3 mg
Capsules
SmithKline Beecham: *Ridaura*

**Azatadine and Pseudoephedrine***

1/120 mg
Tablets, Extended-release
Schering: *Trinalin*

**Azathioprine**

50 mg
Tablets
BW: *Imuran*

**Azithromycin***

250 mg
Capsules
Pfizer: *Zithromax*

**Baclofen**

10 mg · 20 mg
Tablets
Geigy: *Lioresal*

10 mg · 20 mg
Tablets
Schein/Danbury

The 1995 Medicine Chart
© 1994 The United States Pharmacopeial Convention, Inc.

*Single source product for solid oral dosage forms in the U.S.

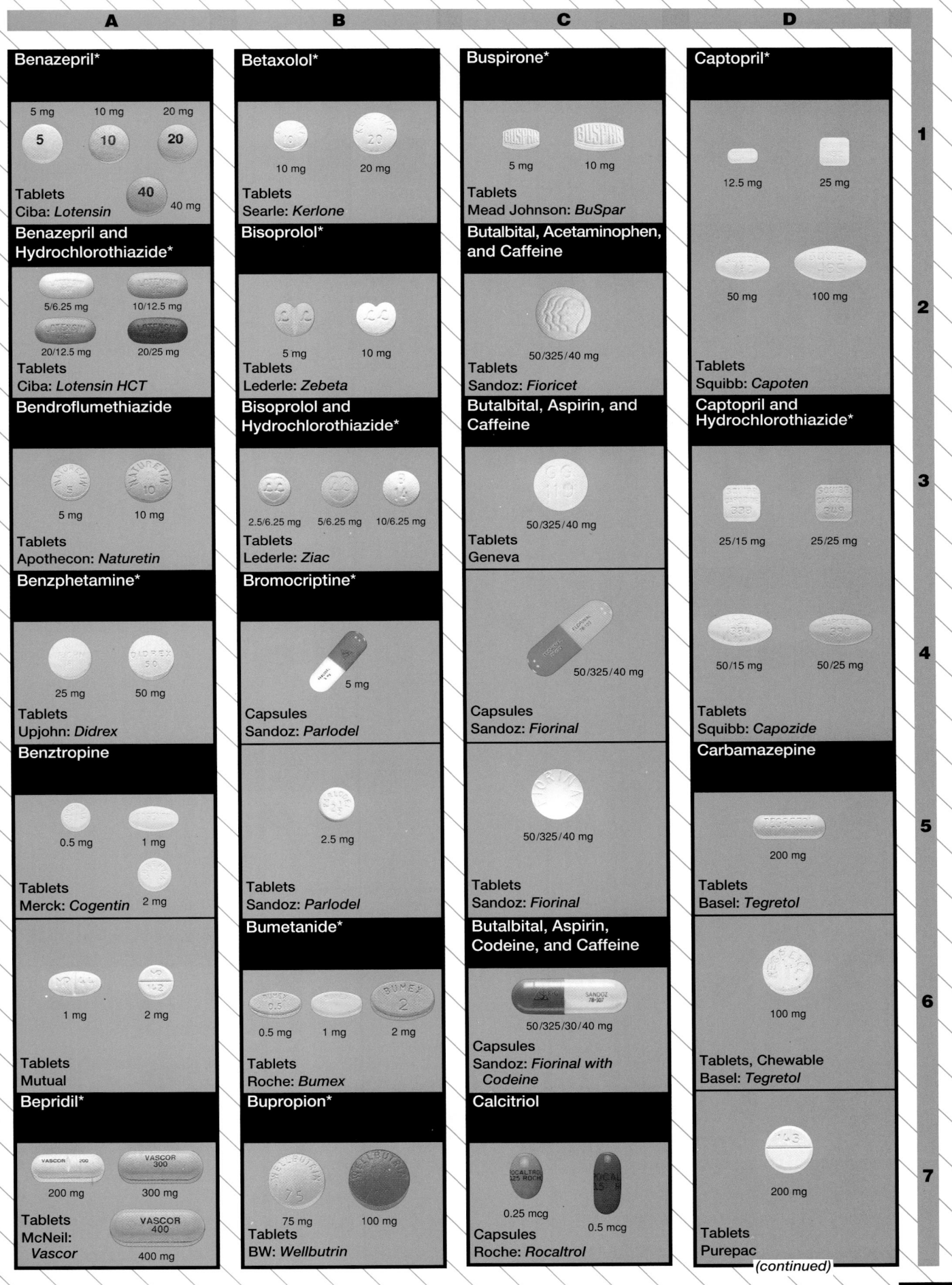

## A

**Benazepril***

5 mg  10 mg  20 mg

**5**  **10**  **20**

**40** 40 mg

Tablets
Ciba: *Lotensin*

**Benazepril and Hydrochlorothiazide***

5/6.25 mg  10/12.5 mg
20/12.5 mg  20/25 mg

Tablets
Ciba: *Lotensin HCT*

**Bendroflumethiazide**

5 mg  10 mg

Tablets
Apothecon: *Naturetin*

**Benzphetamine***

25 mg  50 mg

Tablets
Upjohn: *Didrex*

**Benztropine**

0.5 mg  1 mg
2 mg

Tablets
Merck: *Cogentin*

1 mg  2 mg

Tablets
Mutual

**Bepridil***

200 mg  300 mg
400 mg

Tablets
McNeil:
*Vascor*

## B

**Betaxolol***

10 mg  20 mg

Tablets
Searle: *Kerlone*

**Bisoprolol***

5 mg  10 mg

Tablets
Lederle: *Zebeta*

**Bisoprolol and Hydrochlorothiazide***

2.5/6.25 mg  5/6.25 mg  10/6.25 mg

Tablets
Lederle: *Ziac*

**Bromocriptine***

5 mg

Capsules
Sandoz: *Parlodel*

2.5 mg

Tablets
Sandoz: *Parlodel*

**Bumetanide***

0.5 mg  1 mg  2 mg

Tablets
Roche: *Bumex*

**Bupropion***

75 mg  100 mg

Tablets
BW: *Wellbutrin*

## C

**Buspirone***

5 mg  10 mg

Tablets
Mead Johnson: *BuSpar*

**Butalbital, Acetaminophen, and Caffeine**

50/325/40 mg

Tablets
Sandoz: *Fioricet*

**Butalbital, Aspirin, and Caffeine**

50/325/40 mg

Tablets
Geneva

50/325/40 mg

Capsules
Sandoz: *Fiorinal*

50/325/40 mg

Tablets
Sandoz: *Fiorinal*

**Butalbital, Aspirin, Codeine, and Caffeine**

50/325/30/40 mg

Capsules
Sandoz: *Fiorinal with Codeine*

**Calcitriol**

0.25 mcg  0.5 mcg

Capsules
Roche: *Rocaltrol*

## D

**Captopril***

12.5 mg  25 mg

50 mg  100 mg

Tablets
Squibb: *Capoten*

**Captopril and Hydrochlorothiazide***

25/15 mg  25/25 mg

50/15 mg  50/25 mg

Tablets
Squibb: *Capozide*

**Carbamazepine**

200 mg

Tablets
Basel: *Tegretol*

100 mg

Tablets, Chewable
Basel: *Tegretol*

200 mg

Tablets
Purepac

*(continued)*

The 1995 Medicine Chart

1  2  3  4  5  6  7

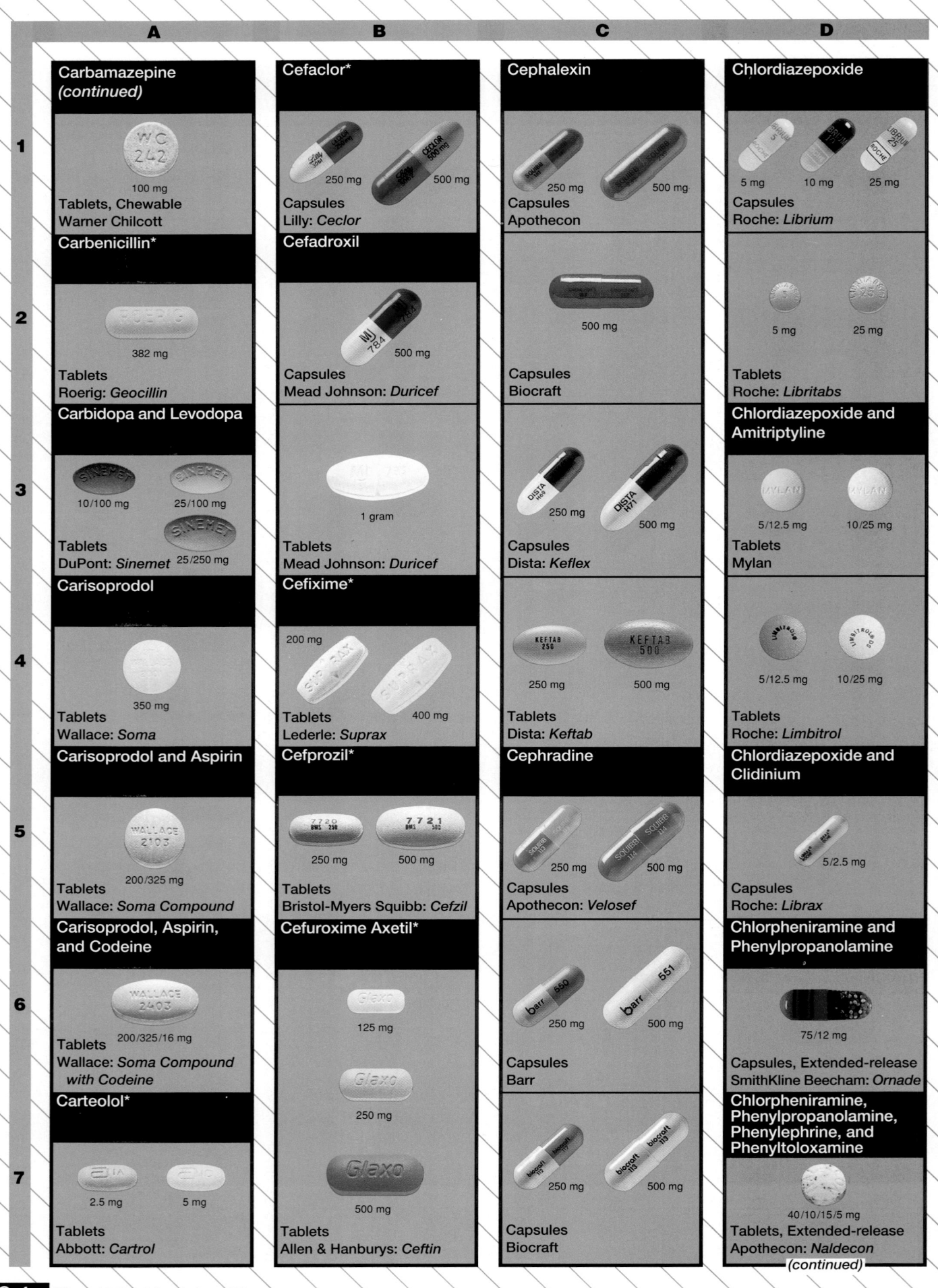

**A**

## Carbamazepine
*(continued)*

**1**
WC 242
100 mg
Tablets, Chewable
Warner Chilcott

## Carbenicillin*

**2**
ROERIG
382 mg
Tablets
Roerig: *Geocillin*

## Carbidopa and Levodopa

**3**
SINEMET 10/100 mg    SINEMET 25/100 mg
SINEMET 25/250 mg
Tablets
DuPont: *Sinemet*

## Carisoprodol

**4**
350 mg
Tablets
Wallace: *Soma*

## Carisoprodol and Aspirin

**5**
WALLACE 2103
200/325 mg
Tablets
Wallace: *Soma Compound*

## Carisoprodol, Aspirin, and Codeine

**6**
WALLACE 2403
200/325/16 mg
Tablets
Wallace: *Soma Compound with Codeine*

## Carteolol*

**7**
2.5 mg    5 mg
Tablets
Abbott: *Cartrol*

---

**B**

## Cefaclor*

**1**
250 mg    500 mg
Capsules
Lilly: *Ceclor*

## Cefadroxil

**2**
MJ 784
500 mg
Capsules
Mead Johnson: *Duricef*

**3**
MJ 787
1 gram
Tablets
Mead Johnson: *Duricef*

## Cefixime*

**4**
200 mg
SUPRAX    SUPRAX
400 mg
Tablets
Lederle: *Suprax*

## Cefprozil*

**5**
7720 BMS 250    7721 BMS 500
250 mg    500 mg
Tablets
Bristol-Myers Squibb: *Cefzil*

## Cefuroxime Axetil*

**6**
Glaxo
125 mg

Glaxo
250 mg

**7**
Glaxo
500 mg
Tablets
Allen & Hanburys: *Ceftin*

---

**C**

## Cephalexin

**1**
250 mg    500 mg
Capsules
Apothecon

**2**
500 mg
Capsules
Biocraft

**3**
DISTA H69 250 mg    DISTA H71 500 mg
Capsules
Dista: *Keflex*

**4**
KEFTAB 250    KEFTAB 500
250 mg    500 mg
Tablets
Dista: *Keftab*

## Cephradine

**5**
SQUIBB 500 113    SQUIBB 114
250 mg    500 mg
Capsules
Apothecon: *Velosef*

**6**
barr 550    barr 551
250 mg    500 mg
Capsules
Barr

**7**
biocraft 112    biocraft 113
250 mg    500 mg
Capsules
Biocraft

---

**D**

## Chlordiazepoxide

**1**
5 mg    10 mg    25 mg
Capsules
Roche: *Librium*

**2**
5 mg    25 mg
Tablets
Roche: *Libritabs*

## Chlordiazepoxide and Amitriptyline

**3**
5/12.5 mg    10/25 mg
Tablets
Mylan

**4**
5/12.5 mg    10/25 mg
Tablets
Roche: *Limbitrol*

## Chlordiazepoxide and Clidinium

**5**
5/2.5 mg
Capsules
Roche: *Librax*

## Chlorpheniramine and Phenylpropanolamine

**6**
75/12 mg
Capsules, Extended-release
SmithKline Beecham: *Ornade*

## Chlorpheniramine, Phenylpropanolamine, Phenylephrine, and Phenyltoloxamine

**7**
40/10/15/5 mg
Tablets, Extended-release
Apothecon: *Naldecon*
*(continued)*

---

The 1995 Medicine Chart
© 1994 The United States Pharmacopeial Convention, Inc.

*Single source product for solid oral dosage forms in the U.S.

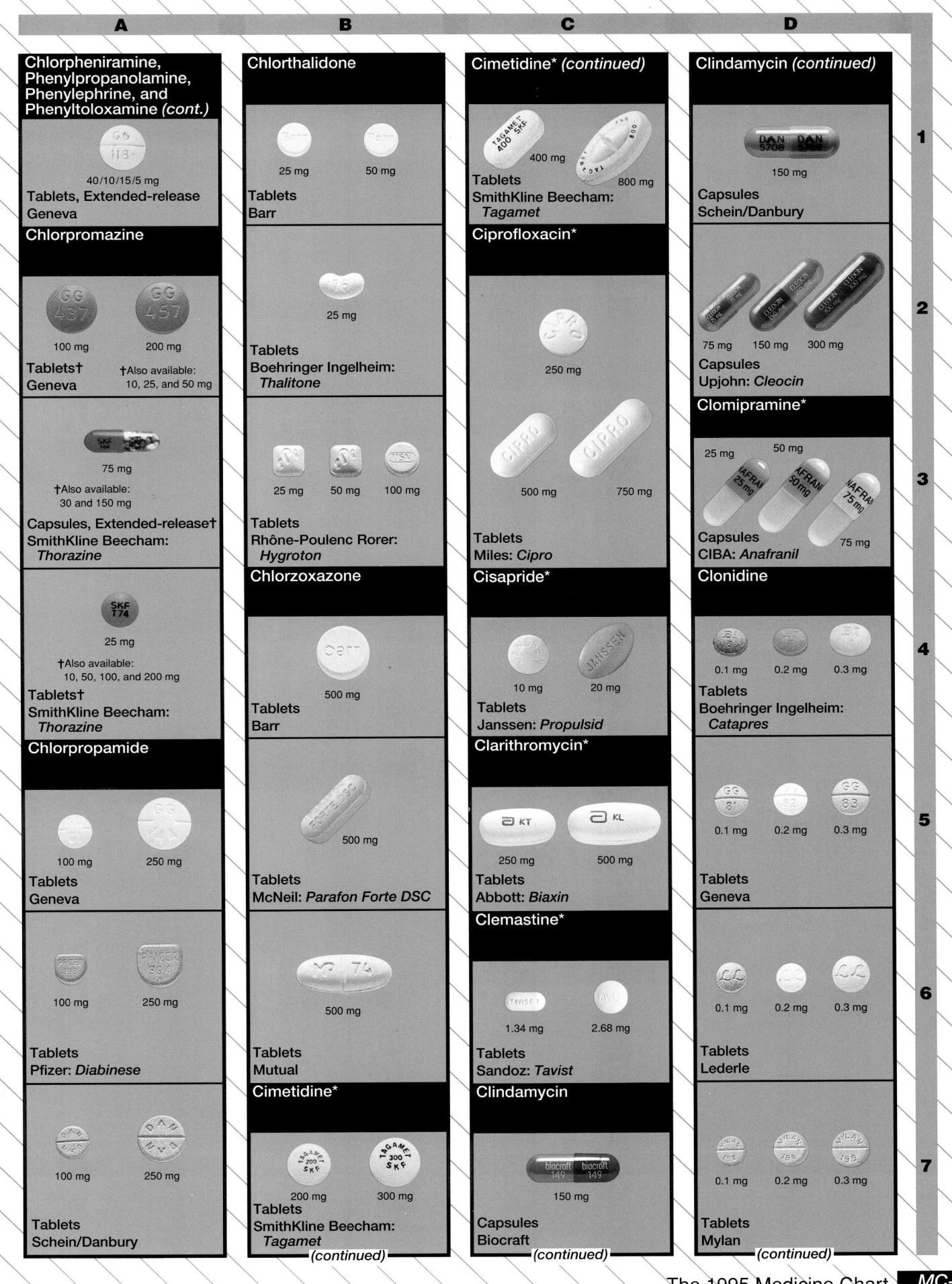

**A**

## Chlorpheniramine, Phenylpropanolamine, Phenylephrine, and Phenyltoloxamine *(cont.)*

40/10/15/5 mg
Tablets, Extended-release
Geneva

## Chlorpromazine

100 mg · 200 mg
Tablets†     †Also available:
Geneva       10, 25, and 50 mg

75 mg
†Also available:
30 and 150 mg
Capsules, Extended-release†
SmithKline Beecham:
*Thorazine*

25 mg
†Also available:
10, 50, 100, and 200 mg
Tablets†
SmithKline Beecham:
*Thorazine*

## Chlorpropamide

100 mg · 250 mg
Tablets
Geneva

100 mg · 250 mg
Tablets
Pfizer: *Diabinese*

100 mg · 250 mg
Tablets
Schein/Danbury

**B**

## Chlorthalidone

25 mg · 50 mg
Tablets
Barr

25 mg
Tablets
Boehringer Ingelheim:
*Thalitone*

25 mg · 50 mg · 100 mg
Tablets
Rhône-Poulenc Rorer:
*Hygroton*

## Chlorzoxazone

500 mg
Tablets
Barr

500 mg
Tablets
McNeil: *Parafon Forte DSC*

500 mg
Tablets
Mutual

## Cimetidine*

200 mg · 300 mg
Tablets
SmithKline Beecham:
*Tagamet*
*(continued)*

**C**

## Cimetidine* *(continued)*

400 mg · 800 mg
Tablets
SmithKline Beecham:
*Tagamet*

## Ciprofloxacin*

250 mg

500 mg · 750 mg
Tablets
Miles: *Cipro*

## Cisapride*

10 mg · 20 mg
Tablets
Janssen: *Propulsid*

## Clarithromycin*

250 mg · 500 mg
Tablets
Abbott: *Biaxin*

## Clemastine*

1.34 mg · 2.68 mg
Tablets
Sandoz: *Tavist*

## Clindamycin

150 mg
Capsules
Biocraft
*(continued)*

**D**

## Clindamycin *(continued)*

150 mg
Capsules
Schein/Danbury

75 mg · 150 mg · 300 mg
Capsules
Upjohn: *Cleocin*

## Clomipramine*

25 mg · 50 mg
75 mg
Capsules
CIBA: *Anafranil*

## Clonidine

0.1 mg · 0.2 mg · 0.3 mg
Tablets
Boehringer Ingelheim:
*Catapres*

0.1 mg · 0.2 mg · 0.3 mg
Tablets
Geneva

0.1 mg · 0.2 mg · 0.3 mg
Tablets
Lederle

0.1 mg · 0.2 mg · 0.3 mg
Tablets
Mylan
*(continued)*

1 2 3 4 5 6 7

*Single source product for solid oral dosage forms in the U.S.    © 1994 The United States Pharmacopeial Convention, Inc.

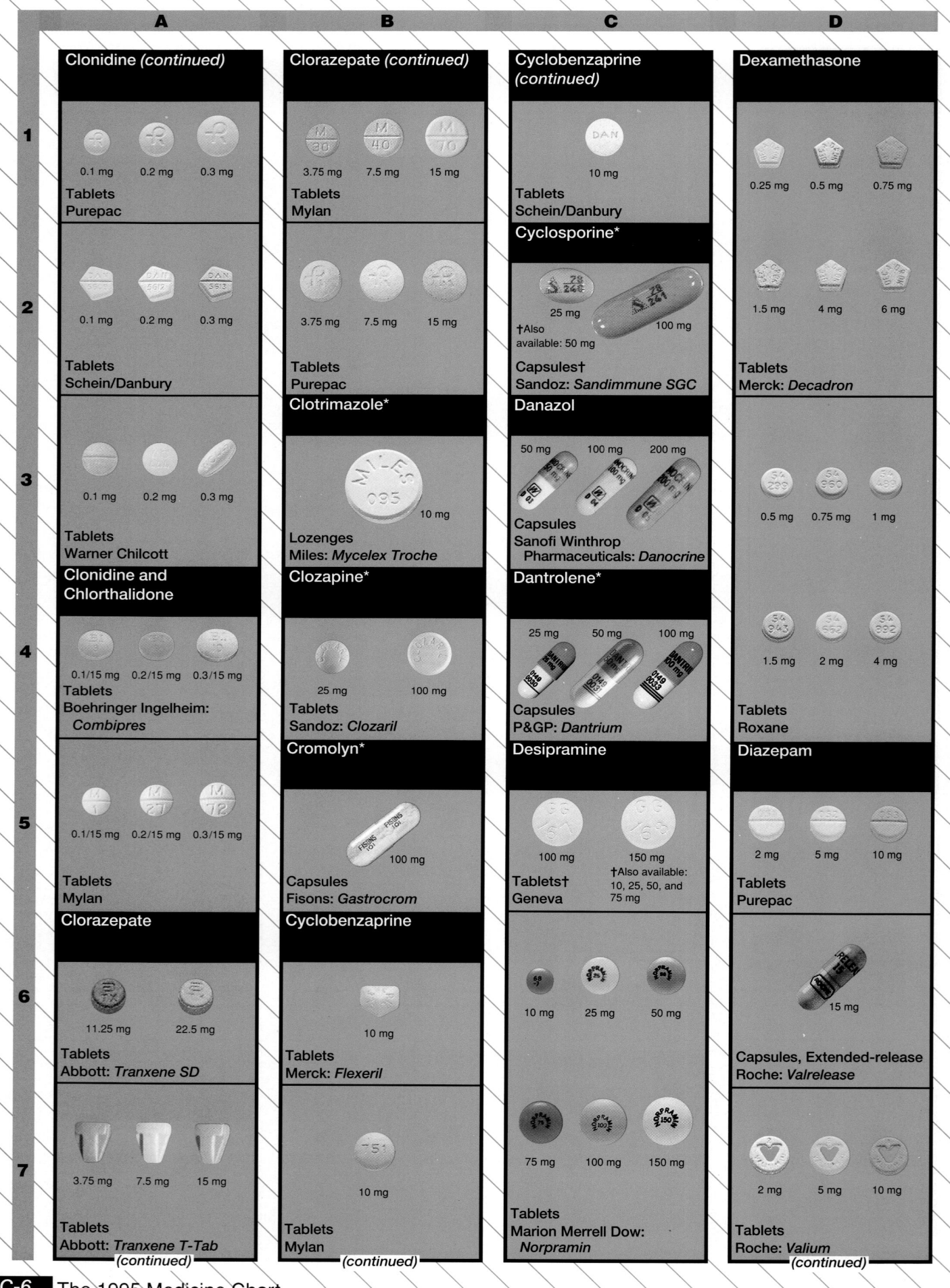

**A**

## Clonidine (continued)

**1** — 0.1 mg, 0.2 mg, 0.3 mg
Tablets
Purepac

**2** — 0.1 mg, 0.2 mg, 0.3 mg
Tablets
Schein/Danbury

**3** — 0.1 mg, 0.2 mg, 0.3 mg
Tablets
Warner Chilcott

## Clonidine and Chlorthalidone

**4** — 0.1/15 mg, 0.2/15 mg, 0.3/15 mg
Tablets
Boehringer Ingelheim: *Combipres*

**5** — 0.1/15 mg, 0.2/15 mg, 0.3/15 mg
Tablets
Mylan

## Clorazepate

**6** — 11.25 mg, 22.5 mg
Tablets
Abbott: *Tranxene SD*

**7** — 3.75 mg, 7.5 mg, 15 mg
Tablets
Abbott: *Tranxene T-Tab*
*(continued)*

**B**

## Clorazepate (continued)

**1** — 3.75 mg, 7.5 mg, 15 mg
Tablets
Mylan

**2** — 3.75 mg, 7.5 mg, 15 mg
Tablets
Purepac

## Clotrimazole*

**3** — 10 mg
Lozenges
Miles: *Mycelex Troche*

## Clozapine*

**4** — 25 mg, 100 mg
Tablets
Sandoz: *Clozaril*

## Cromolyn*

**5** — 100 mg
Capsules
Fisons: *Gastrocrom*

## Cyclobenzaprine

**6** — 10 mg
Tablets
Merck: *Flexeril*

**7** — 10 mg
Tablets
Mylan
*(continued)*

**C**

## Cyclobenzaprine (continued)

**1** — 10 mg
Tablets
Schein/Danbury

## Cyclosporine*

**2** — 25 mg, 100 mg
†Also available: 50 mg
Capsules†
Sandoz: *Sandimmune SGC*

## Danazol

**3** — 50 mg, 100 mg, 200 mg
Capsules
Sanofi Winthrop Pharmaceuticals: *Danocrine*

## Dantrolene*

**4** — 25 mg, 50 mg, 100 mg
Capsules
P&GP: *Dantrium*

## Desipramine

**5** — 100 mg, 150 mg
†Also available: 10, 25, 50, and 75 mg
Tablets†
Geneva

**6** — 10 mg, 25 mg, 50 mg

**7** — 75 mg, 100 mg, 150 mg
Tablets
Marion Merrell Dow: *Norpramin*

**D**

## Dexamethasone

**1** — 0.25 mg, 0.5 mg, 0.75 mg

**2** — 1.5 mg, 4 mg, 6 mg
Tablets
Merck: *Decadron*

**3** — 0.5 mg, 0.75 mg, 1 mg

**4** — 1.5 mg, 2 mg, 4 mg
Tablets
Roxane

## Diazepam

**5** — 2 mg, 5 mg, 10 mg
Tablets
Purepac

**6** — 15 mg
Capsules, Extended-release
Roche: *Valrelease*

**7** — 2 mg, 5 mg, 10 mg
Tablets
Roche: *Valium*
*(continued)*

The 1995 Medicine Chart
© 1994 The United States Pharmacopeial Convention, Inc.

*Single source product for solid oral dosage forms in the U.S.

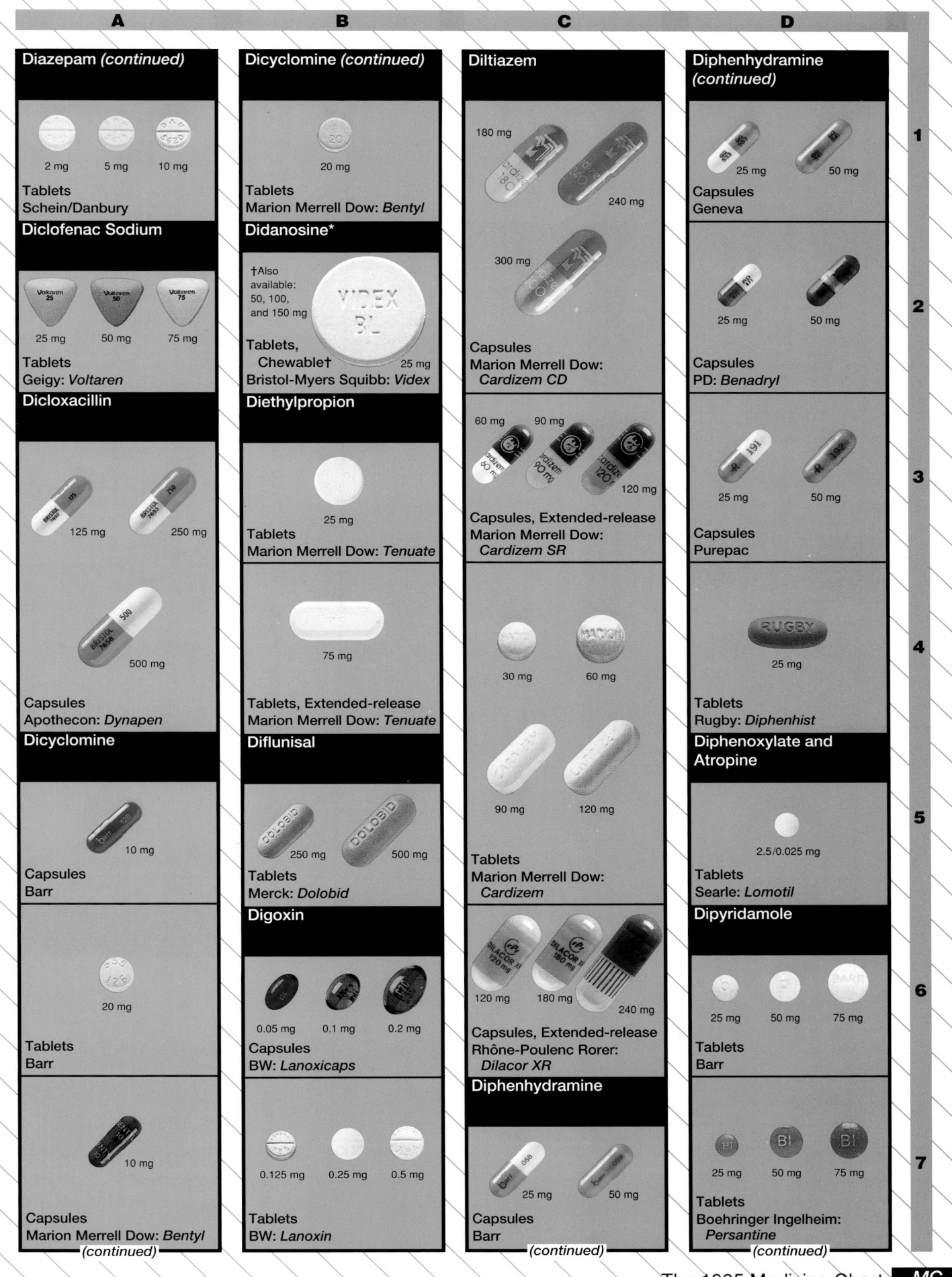

**A**

**Diazepam** *(continued)*

2 mg  5 mg  10 mg
Tablets
Schein/Danbury

**Diclofenac Sodium**

Voltaren 25  Voltaren 50  Voltaren 75
25 mg  50 mg  75 mg
Tablets
Geigy: *Voltaren*

**Dicloxacillin**

125 mg  250 mg
500 mg
Capsules
Apothecon: *Dynapen*

**Dicyclomine**

10 mg
Capsules
Barr

20 mg
Tablets
Barr

10 mg
Capsules
Marion Merrell Dow: *Bentyl*
*(continued)*

**B**

**Dicyclomine** *(continued)*

20 mg
Tablets
Marion Merrell Dow: *Bentyl*

**Didanosine***

†Also available: 50, 100, and 150 mg

VIDEX B'L

Tablets, Chewable†      25 mg
Bristol-Myers Squibb: *Videx*

**Diethylpropion**

25 mg
Tablets
Marion Merrell Dow: *Tenuate*

75 mg
Tablets, Extended-release
Marion Merrell Dow: *Tenuate*

**Diflunisal**

250 mg  500 mg
Tablets
Merck: *Dolobid*

**Digoxin**

0.05 mg  0.1 mg  0.2 mg
Capsules
BW: *Lanoxicaps*

0.125 mg  0.25 mg  0.5 mg
Tablets
BW: *Lanoxin*

**C**

**Diltiazem**

180 mg  240 mg
300 mg
Capsules
Marion Merrell Dow:
*Cardizem CD*

60 mg  90 mg  120 mg
Capsules, Extended-release
Marion Merrell Dow:
*Cardizem SR*

30 mg  60 mg
90 mg  120 mg
Tablets
Marion Merrell Dow:
*Cardizem*

120 mg  180 mg  240 mg
Capsules, Extended-release
Rhône-Poulenc Rorer:
*Dilacor XR*

**Diphenhydramine**

25 mg  50 mg
Capsules
Barr
*(continued)*

**D**

**Diphenhydramine** *(continued)*

25 mg  50 mg
Capsules
Geneva

25 mg  50 mg
Capsules
PD: *Benadryl*

25 mg  50 mg
Capsules
Purepac

RUGBY
25 mg
Tablets
Rugby: *Diphenhist*

**Diphenoxylate and Atropine**

2.5/0.025 mg
Tablets
Searle: *Lomotil*

**Dipyridamole**

25 mg  50 mg  75 mg
Tablets
Barr

25 mg  50 mg  75 mg
Tablets
Boehringer Ingelheim:
*Persantine*
*(continued)*

1  2  3  4  5  6  7

*Single source product for solid oral dosage forms in the U.S.

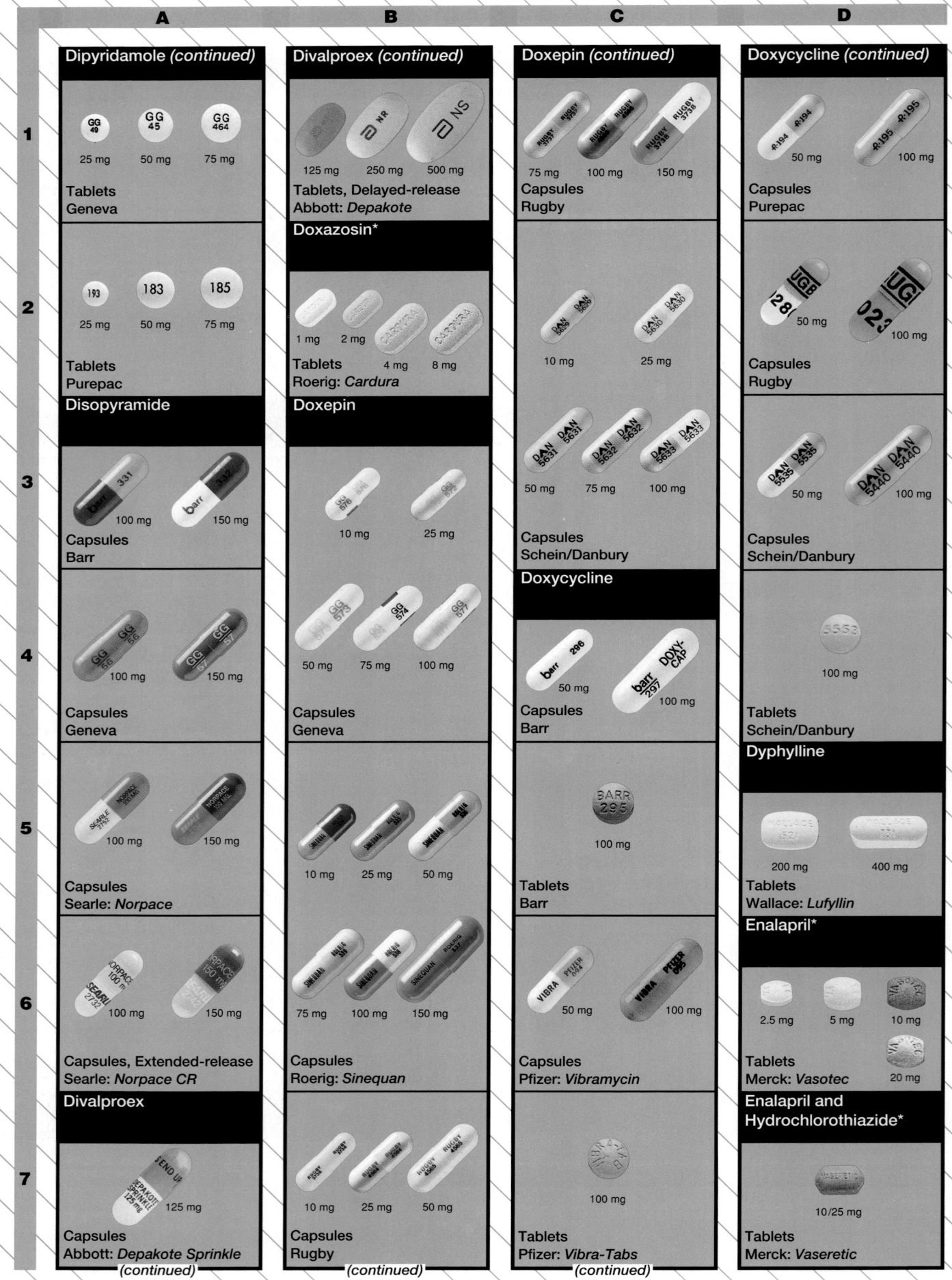

**A**

**Dipyridamole** (*continued*)

GG 49 — 25 mg
GG 45 — 50 mg
GG 464 — 75 mg

Tablets
Geneva

193 — 25 mg
183 — 50 mg
185 — 75 mg

Tablets
Purepac

**Disopyramide**

barr 331 — 100 mg
barr 332 — 150 mg

Capsules
Barr

GG 56 — 100 mg
GG 57 — 150 mg

Capsules
Geneva

NORPACE 100 mg — 100 mg
NORPACE 150 mg — 150 mg

Capsules
Searle: *Norpace*

NORPACE 100 mg — 100 mg
NORPACE 150 mg — 150 mg

Capsules, Extended-release
Searle: *Norpace CR*

**Divalproex**

DEPAKOTE SPRINKLE 125 mg — 125 mg

Capsules
Abbott: *Depakote Sprinkle*
(*continued*)

**B**

**Divalproex** (*continued*)

125 mg
NR — 250 mg
NS — 500 mg

Tablets, Delayed-release
Abbott: *Depakote*

**Doxazosin\***

1 mg
2 mg
CARDURA — 4 mg
CARDURA — 8 mg

Tablets
Roerig: *Cardura*

**Doxepin**

GG 676 — 10 mg
GG 672 — 25 mg

GG 673 — 50 mg
GG 574 — 75 mg
GG 677 — 100 mg

Capsules
Geneva

SINEQUAN — 10 mg
SINEQUAN — 25 mg
SINEQUAN — 50 mg

SINEQUAN — 75 mg
SINEQUAN — 100 mg
SINEQUAN — 150 mg

Capsules
Roerig: *Sinequan*

RUGBY — 10 mg
RUGBY — 25 mg
RUGBY 4365 — 50 mg

Capsules
Rugby
(*continued*)

**C**

**Doxepin** (*continued*)

RUGBY 3737 — 75 mg
RUGBY 3737 — 100 mg
RUGBY 3738 — 150 mg

Capsules
Rugby

DAN 5665 — 10 mg
DAN 5630 — 25 mg

DAN 5631 — 50 mg
DAN 5632 — 75 mg
DAN 5633 — 100 mg

Capsules
Schein/Danbury

**Doxycycline**

barr 296 — 50 mg
barr 297 DOXY-CAP — 100 mg

Capsules
Barr

BARR 295 — 100 mg

Tablets
Barr

VIBRA PFIZER 094 — 50 mg
VIBRA PFIZER 095 — 100 mg

Capsules
Pfizer: *Vibramycin*

VIBRA-TABS — 100 mg

Tablets
Pfizer: *Vibra-Tabs*
(*continued*)

**D**

**Doxycycline** (*continued*)

P-194 P-194 — 50 mg
P-195 P-195 — 100 mg

Capsules
Purepac

UGB 28 — 50 mg
UGB 023 — 100 mg

Capsules
Rugby

DAN 5535 — 50 mg
DAN 5440 — 100 mg

Capsules
Schein/Danbury

5553 — 100 mg

Tablets
Schein/Danbury

**Dyphylline**

WALLACE 521 — 200 mg
WALLACE 771 — 400 mg

Tablets
Wallace: *Lufyllin*

**Enalapril\***

2.5 mg
5 mg
VASOTEC — 10 mg
VASOTEC — 20 mg

Tablets
Merck: *Vasotec*

**Enalapril and Hydrochlorothiazide\***

VASERETIC — 10/25 mg

Tablets
Merck: *Vaseretic*

The 1995 Medicine Chart
© 1994 The United States Pharmacopeial Convention, Inc.

\*Single source product for solid oral dosage forms in the U.S.

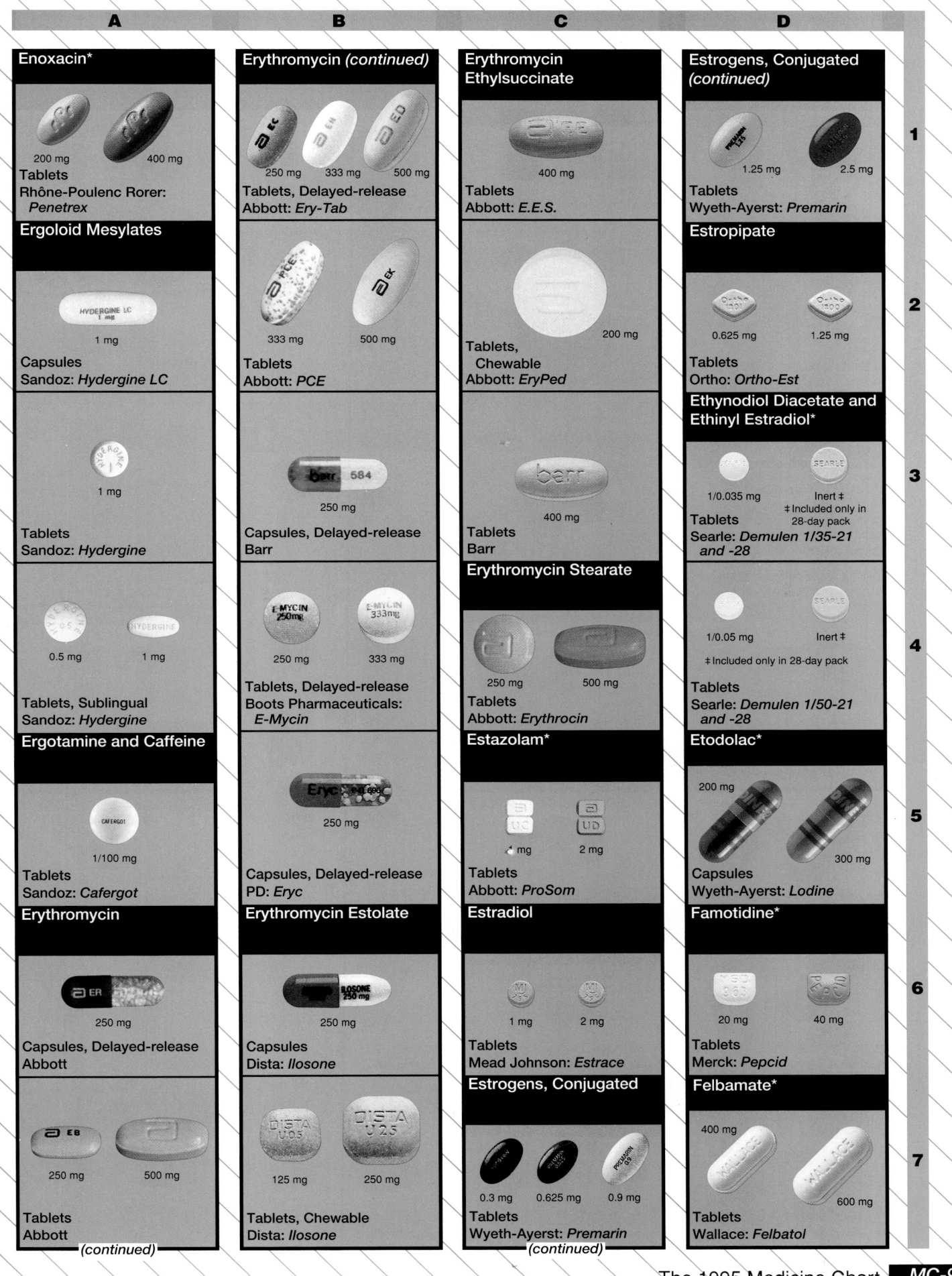

## Column A

**Enoxacin***

200 mg — 400 mg
Tablets
Rhône-Poulenc Rorer: *Penetrex*

**Ergoloid Mesylates**

1 mg
Capsules
Sandoz: *Hydergine LC*

1 mg
Tablets
Sandoz: *Hydergine*

0.5 mg — 1 mg
Tablets, Sublingual
Sandoz: *Hydergine*

**Ergotamine and Caffeine**

1/100 mg
Tablets
Sandoz: *Cafergot*

**Erythromycin**

250 mg
Capsules, Delayed-release
Abbott

250 mg — 500 mg
Tablets
Abbott
*(continued)*

## Column B

**Erythromycin** *(continued)*

250 mg — 333 mg — 500 mg
Tablets, Delayed-release
Abbott: *Ery-Tab*

333 mg — 500 mg
Tablets
Abbott: *PCE*

250 mg
Capsules, Delayed-release
Barr

250 mg — 333 mg
Tablets, Delayed-release
Boots Pharmaceuticals: *E-Mycin*

250 mg
Capsules, Delayed-release
PD: *Eryc*

**Erythromycin Estolate**

250 mg
Capsules
Dista: *Ilosone*

125 mg — 250 mg
Tablets, Chewable
Dista: *Ilosone*

## Column C

**Erythromycin Ethylsuccinate**

400 mg
Tablets
Abbott: *E.E.S.*

200 mg
Tablets, Chewable
Abbott: *EryPed*

400 mg
Tablets
Barr

**Erythromycin Stearate**

250 mg — 500 mg
Tablets
Abbott: *Erythrocin*

**Estazolam***

1 mg — 2 mg
Tablets
Abbott: *ProSom*

**Estradiol**

1 mg — 2 mg
Tablets
Mead Johnson: *Estrace*

**Estrogens, Conjugated**

0.3 mg — 0.625 mg — 0.9 mg
Tablets
Wyeth-Ayerst: *Premarin*
*(continued)*

## Column D

**Estrogens, Conjugated** *(continued)*

1.25 mg — 2.5 mg
Tablets
Wyeth-Ayerst: *Premarin*

**Estropipate**

0.625 mg — 1.25 mg
Tablets
Ortho: *Ortho-Est*

**Ethynodiol Diacetate and Ethinyl Estradiol***

1/0.035 mg — Inert ‡
‡ Included only in 28-day pack
Tablets
Searle: *Demulen 1/35-21 and -28*

1/0.05 mg — Inert ‡
‡ Included only in 28-day pack
Tablets
Searle: *Demulen 1/50-21 and -28*

**Etodolac***

200 mg — 300 mg
Capsules
Wyeth-Ayerst: *Lodine*

**Famotidine***

20 mg — 40 mg
Tablets
Merck: *Pepcid*

**Felbamate***

400 mg — 600 mg
Tablets
Wallace: *Felbatol*

The 1995 Medicine Chart    **MC-9**

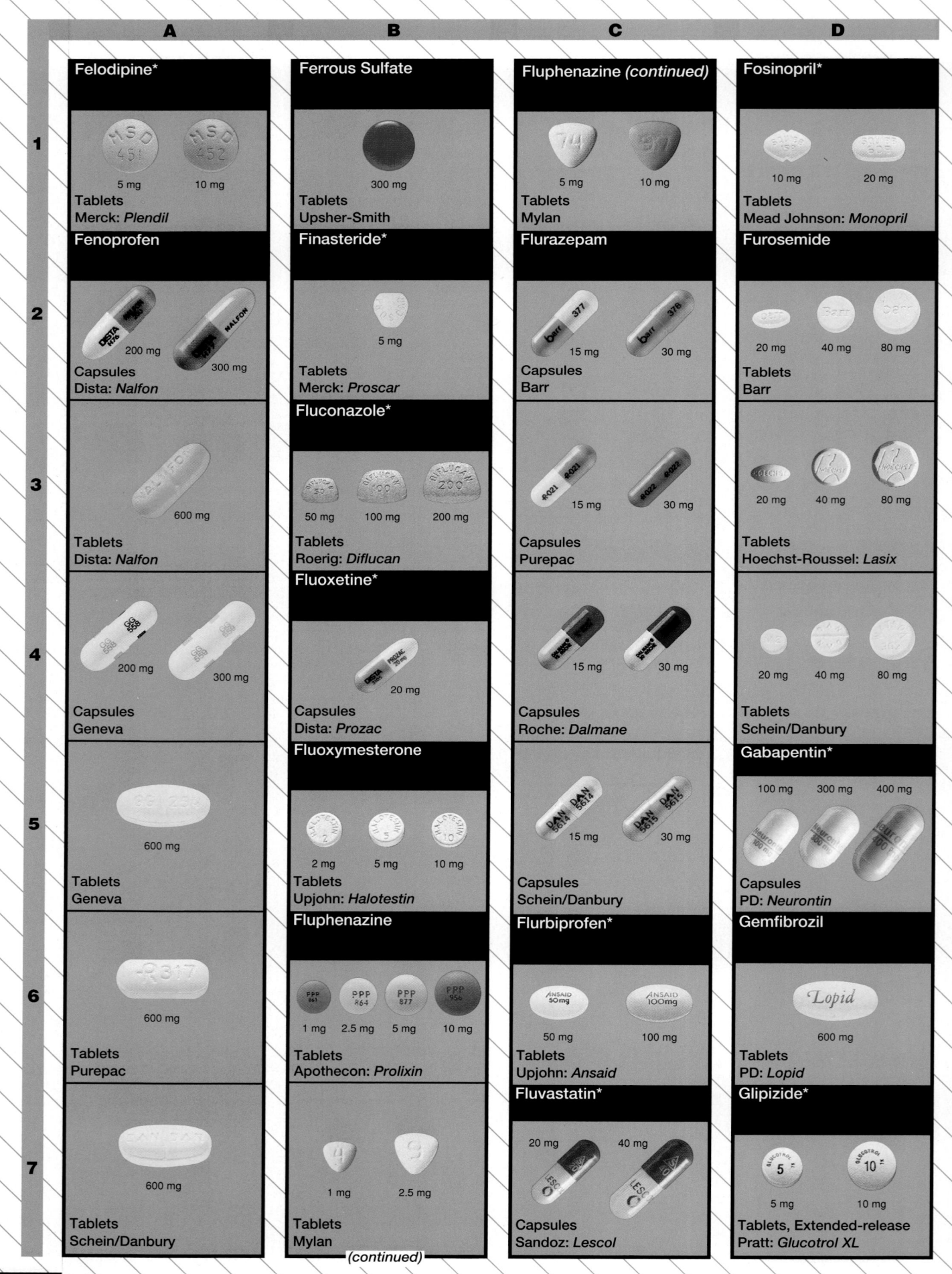

| | **A** | **B** | **C** | **D** |
|---|---|---|---|---|
| | **Felodipine*** | **Ferrous Sulfate** | **Fluphenazine** *(continued)* | **Fosinopril*** |
| **1** | 5 mg  10 mg  Tablets  Merck: *Plendil* | 300 mg  Tablets  Upsher-Smith | 5 mg  10 mg  Tablets  Mylan | 10 mg  20 mg  Tablets  Mead Johnson: *Monopril* |
| | **Fenoprofen** | **Finasteride*** | **Flurazepam** | **Furosemide** |
| **2** | 200 mg  300 mg  Capsules  Dista: *Nalfon* | 5 mg  Tablets  Merck: *Proscar* | 15 mg  30 mg  Capsules  Barr | 20 mg  40 mg  80 mg  Tablets  Barr |
| | | **Fluconazole*** | | |
| **3** | 600 mg  Tablets  Dista: *Nalfon* | 50 mg  100 mg  200 mg  Tablets  Roerig: *Diflucan* | 15 mg  30 mg  Capsules  Purepac | 20 mg  40 mg  80 mg  Tablets  Hoechst-Roussel: *Lasix* |
| | | **Fluoxetine*** | | |
| **4** | 200 mg  300 mg  Capsules  Geneva | 20 mg  Capsules  Dista: *Prozac* | 15 mg  30 mg  Capsules  Roche: *Dalmane* | 20 mg  40 mg  80 mg  Tablets  Schein/Danbury |
| | | **Fluoxymesterone** | | **Gabapentin*** |
| **5** | 600 mg  Tablets  Geneva | 2 mg  5 mg  10 mg  Tablets  Upjohn: *Halotestin* | 15 mg  30 mg  Capsules  Schein/Danbury | 100 mg  300 mg  400 mg  Capsules  PD: *Neurontin* |
| | | **Fluphenazine** | **Flurbiprofen*** | **Gemfibrozil** |
| **6** | 600 mg  Tablets  Purepac | 1 mg  2.5 mg  5 mg  10 mg  Tablets  Apothecon: *Prolixin* | 50 mg  100 mg  Tablets  Upjohn: *Ansaid* | 600 mg  Tablets  PD: *Lopid* |
| | | | **Fluvastatin*** | **Glipizide*** |
| **7** | 600 mg  Tablets  Schein/Danbury | 1 mg  2.5 mg  Tablets  Mylan | 20 mg  40 mg  Capsules  Sandoz: *Lescol* | 5 mg  10 mg  Tablets, Extended-release  Pratt: *Glucotrol XL* |

*(continued)*

The 1995 Medicine Chart

*Single source product for solid oral dosage forms in the U.S.

## A

### Glyburide

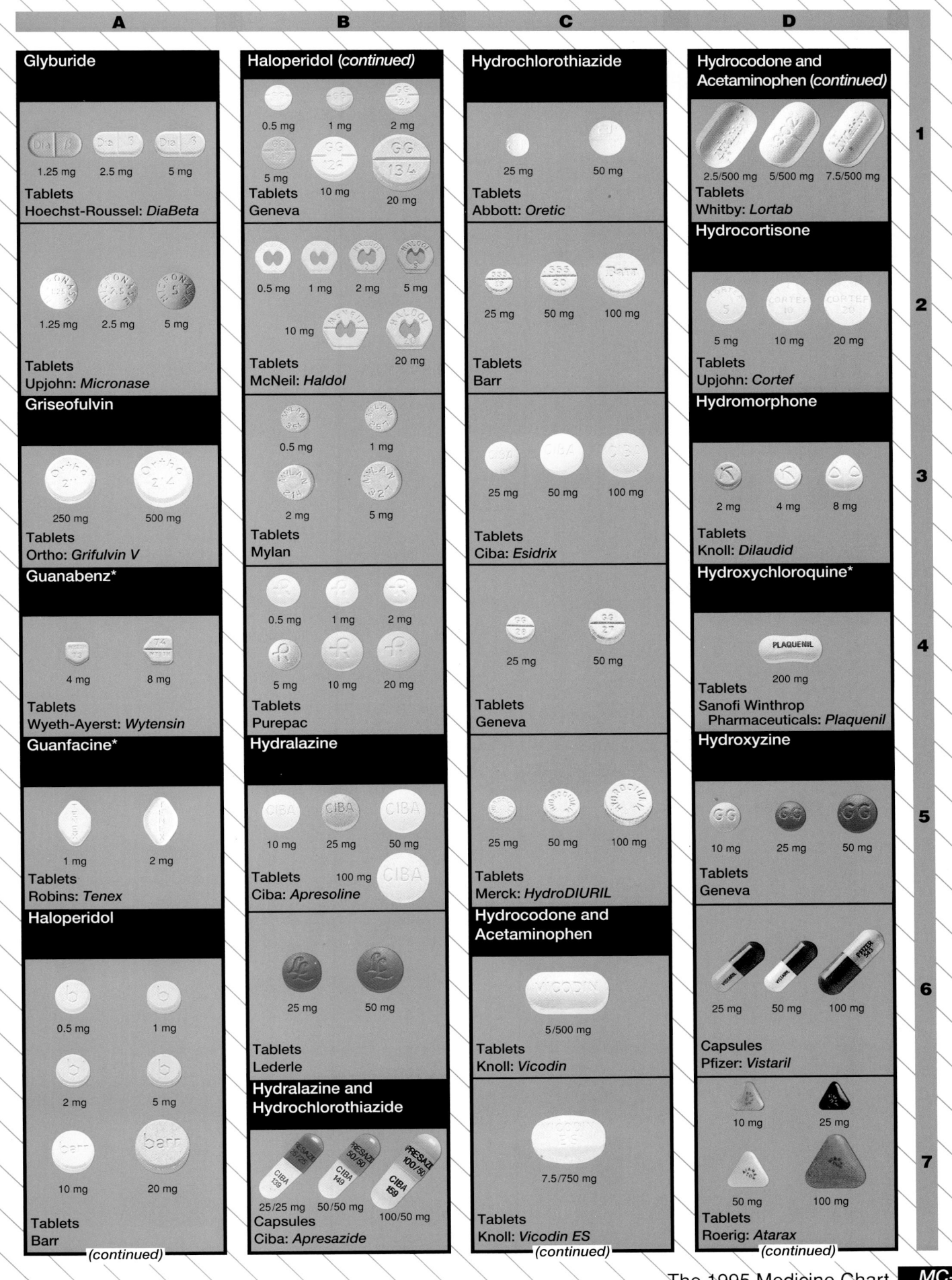

1.25 mg   2.5 mg   5 mg

Tablets
Hoechst-Roussel: *DiaBeta*

1.25 mg   2.5 mg   5 mg

Tablets
Upjohn: *Micronase*

### Griseofulvin

250 mg   500 mg

Tablets
Ortho: *Grifulvin V*

### Guanabenz*

4 mg   8 mg

Tablets
Wyeth-Ayerst: *Wytensin*

### Guanfacine*

1 mg   2 mg

Tablets
Robins: *Tenex*

### Haloperidol

0.5 mg   1 mg

2 mg   5 mg

10 mg   20 mg

Tablets
Barr

*(continued)*

## B

### Haloperidol (continued)

0.5 mg   1 mg   2 mg

5 mg   10 mg   20 mg

Tablets
Geneva

0.5 mg   1 mg   2 mg   5 mg

10 mg   20 mg

Tablets
McNeil: *Haldol*

0.5 mg   1 mg

2 mg   5 mg

Tablets
Mylan

0.5 mg   1 mg   2 mg

5 mg   10 mg   20 mg

Tablets
Purepac

### Hydralazine

10 mg   25 mg   50 mg

100 mg

Tablets
Ciba: *Apresoline*

25 mg   50 mg

Tablets
Lederle

### Hydralazine and Hydrochlorothiazide

25/25 mg   50/50 mg   100/50 mg

Capsules
Ciba: *Apresazide*

## C

### Hydrochlorothiazide

25 mg   50 mg

Tablets
Abbott: *Oretic*

25 mg   50 mg   100 mg

Tablets
Barr

25 mg   50 mg   100 mg

Tablets
Ciba: *Esidrix*

25 mg   50 mg

Tablets
Geneva

25 mg   50 mg   100 mg

Tablets
Merck: *HydroDIURIL*

### Hydrocodone and Acetaminophen

5/500 mg

Tablets
Knoll: *Vicodin*

7.5/750 mg

Tablets
Knoll: *Vicodin ES*
*(continued)*

## D

### Hydrocodone and Acetaminophen (continued)

2.5/500 mg   5/500 mg   7.5/500 mg

Tablets
Whitby: *Lortab*

### Hydrocortisone

5 mg   10 mg   20 mg

Tablets
Upjohn: *Cortef*

### Hydromorphone

2 mg   4 mg   8 mg

Tablets
Knoll: *Dilaudid*

### Hydroxychloroquine*

200 mg

Tablets
Sanofi Winthrop
Pharmaceuticals: *Plaquenil*

### Hydroxyzine

10 mg   25 mg   50 mg

Tablets
Geneva

25 mg   50 mg   100 mg

Capsules
Pfizer: *Vistaril*

10 mg   25 mg

50 mg   100 mg

Tablets
Roerig: *Atarax*
*(continued)*

The 1995 Medicine Chart   **MC-1**

| A | B | C | D |
|---|---|---|---|

## A

### Hydroxyzine (continued)

10 mg  25 mg  50 mg

**Tablets**
**Rugby**

10 mg  25 mg  50 mg

**Tablets**
**Schein/Danbury**

### Ibuprofen

400 mg  600 mg
800 mg

**Tablets**
**Barr**

IBU 400  IBU 600
400 mg  600 mg
800 mg  IBU 800

**Tablets**
**Boots**
**Laboratories**

RUFEN 6
600 mg
400 mg  RUFEN 8
800 mg

**Tablets**
**Boots Pharmaceuticals: Rufen**

RUGBY
400 mg

RUGBY
600 mg

RUGBY
800 mg

**Tablets**
**Rugby**
(continued)

## B

### Ibuprofen (continued)

DAN  DAN
200 mg  400 mg

DAN  DAN
600 mg  800 mg

**Tablets**
**Schein/Danbury**

MOTRIN 300mg  MOTRIN
300 mg  400 mg

MOTRIN 600mg  MOTRIN 800mg
600 mg  800 mg

**Tablets**
**Upjohn: Motrin**

### Imipramine

Geigy 20  Geigy 40
75 mg  100 mg

Geigy 45  Geigy 22
125 mg  150 mg

**Capsules**
**Geigy: Tofranil-PM**

GEIGY  GEIGY  GEIGY
10 mg  25 mg  50 mg

**Tablets**
**Geigy: Tofranil**

## C

### Indapamide*

R  R
1.25 mg  2.5 mg

**Tablets**
**Rhône-Poulenc Rorer: Lozol**

### Indomethacin

25 mg  50 mg

**Capsules**
**Geneva**

MSD 25 INDOCIN  MSD 50 INDOCIN
25 mg  50 mg

**Capsules**
**Merck: Indocin**

INDOCIN
75 mg

**Capsules, Extended-release**
**Merck: Indocin SR**

### Isosorbide Dinitrate

ITC 0920
40 mg

**Capsules, Extended-release**
**Reed & Carnrick:**
**Dilatrate-SR**

5 mg  10 mg  20 mg

4133  4192
30 mg  40 mg

**Tablets**
**Wyeth-Ayerst: Isordil**

40 mg

**Tablets, Extended-release**
**Wyeth-Ayerst: Isordil**
(continued)

## D

### Isosorbide Dinitrate (continued)

2.5 mg  5 mg  10 mg

**Tablets, Sublingual**
**Wyeth-Ayerst: Isordil**

S  S
5 mg  10 mg

S
20 mg

S  S
30 mg  40 mg

**Tablets**
**ZENECA: Sorbitrate**

S  S
5 mg  10 mg

**Tablets, Chewable**
**ZENECA: Sorbitrate**

2.5 mg  5 mg  10 mg

**Tablets, Sublingual**
**ZENECA: Sorbitrate**

### Isosorbide Mononitrate*

ISMO 20
20 mg

**Tablets**
**Wyeth-Ayerst: ISMO**

### Isotretinoin*

ACCUTANE 10 ROCHE  ACCUTANE 20 ROCHE  ACCUTANE 40 ROCHE
10 mg  20 mg  40 mg

**Capsules**
**Roche: Accutane**

The 1995 Medicine Chart

*Single source product for solid oral dosage forms in the U.S.

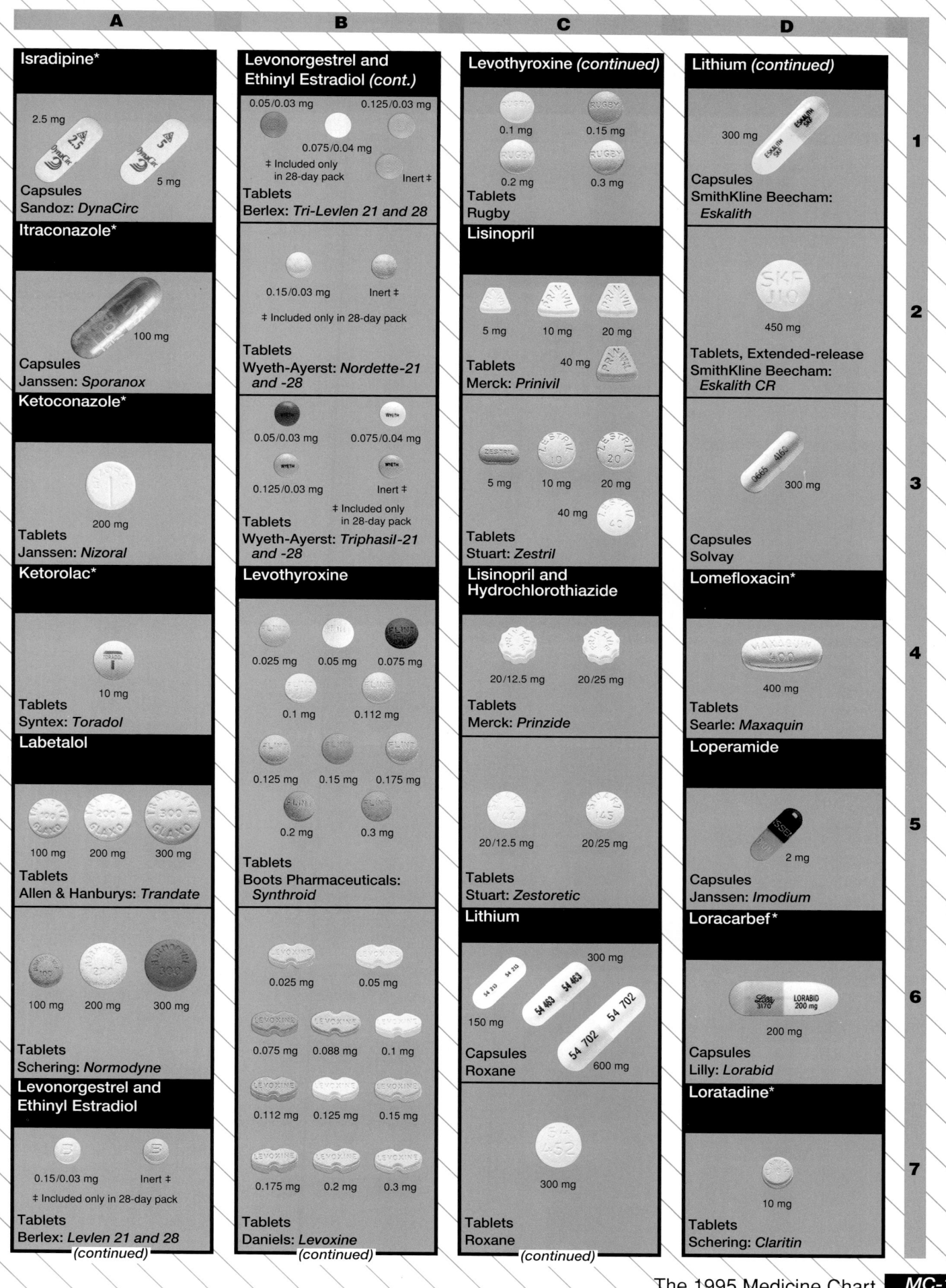

**A**

## Isradipine*

2.5 mg
5 mg

Capsules
Sandoz: *DynaCirc*

## Itraconazole*

100 mg

Capsules
Janssen: *Sporanox*

## Ketoconazole*

200 mg

Tablets
Janssen: *Nizoral*

## Ketorolac*

10 mg

Tablets
Syntex: *Toradol*

## Labetalol

100 mg    200 mg    300 mg

Tablets
Allen & Hanburys: *Trandate*

100 mg    200 mg    300 mg

Tablets
Schering: *Normodyne*

## Levonorgestrel and Ethinyl Estradiol

0.15/0.03 mg    Inert ‡

‡ Included only in 28-day pack

Tablets
Berlex: *Levlen 21 and 28*
(continued)

---

**B**

## Levonorgestrel and Ethinyl Estradiol (cont.)

0.05/0.03 mg    0.125/0.03 mg

0.075/0.04 mg

‡ Included only
in 28-day pack    Inert ‡

Tablets
Berlex: *Tri-Levlen 21 and 28*

0.15/0.03 mg    Inert ‡

‡ Included only in 28-day pack

Tablets
Wyeth-Ayerst: *Nordette-21 and -28*

0.05/0.03 mg    0.075/0.04 mg

0.125/0.03 mg    Inert ‡

‡ Included only
in 28-day pack

Tablets
Wyeth-Ayerst: *Triphasil-21 and -28*

## Levothyroxine

0.025 mg    0.05 mg    0.075 mg

0.1 mg    0.112 mg

0.125 mg    0.15 mg    0.175 mg

0.2 mg    0.3 mg

Tablets
Boots Pharmaceuticals:
*Synthroid*

0.025 mg    0.05 mg

0.075 mg    0.088 mg    0.1 mg

0.112 mg    0.125 mg    0.15 mg

0.175 mg    0.2 mg    0.3 mg

Tablets
Daniels: *Levoxine*
(continued)

---

**C**

## Levothyroxine (continued)

0.1 mg    0.15 mg

0.2 mg    0.3 mg

Tablets
Rugby

## Lisinopril

5 mg    10 mg    20 mg

40 mg

Tablets
Merck: *Prinivil*

5 mg    10 mg    20 mg

40 mg

Tablets
Stuart: *Zestril*

## Lisinopril and Hydrochlorothiazide

20/12.5 mg    20/25 mg

Tablets
Merck: *Prinzide*

20/12.5 mg    20/25 mg

Tablets
Stuart: *Zestoretic*

## Lithium

300 mg

150 mg

54 463 54 463

54 702 54 702

54 702 54 702
600 mg

Capsules
Roxane

300 mg

Tablets
Roxane
(continued)

---

**D**

## Lithium (continued)

300 mg

Capsules
SmithKline Beecham:
*Eskalith*

450 mg

Tablets, Extended-release
SmithKline Beecham:
*Eskalith CR*

300 mg

Capsules
Solvay

## Lomefloxacin*

400 mg

Tablets
Searle: *Maxaquin*

## Loperamide

2 mg

Capsules
Janssen: *Imodium*

## Loracarbef*

200 mg

Capsules
Lilly: *Lorabid*

## Loratadine*

10 mg

Tablets
Schering: *Claritin*

---

1
2
3
4
5
6
7

*Single source product for solid oral dosage forms in the U.S.

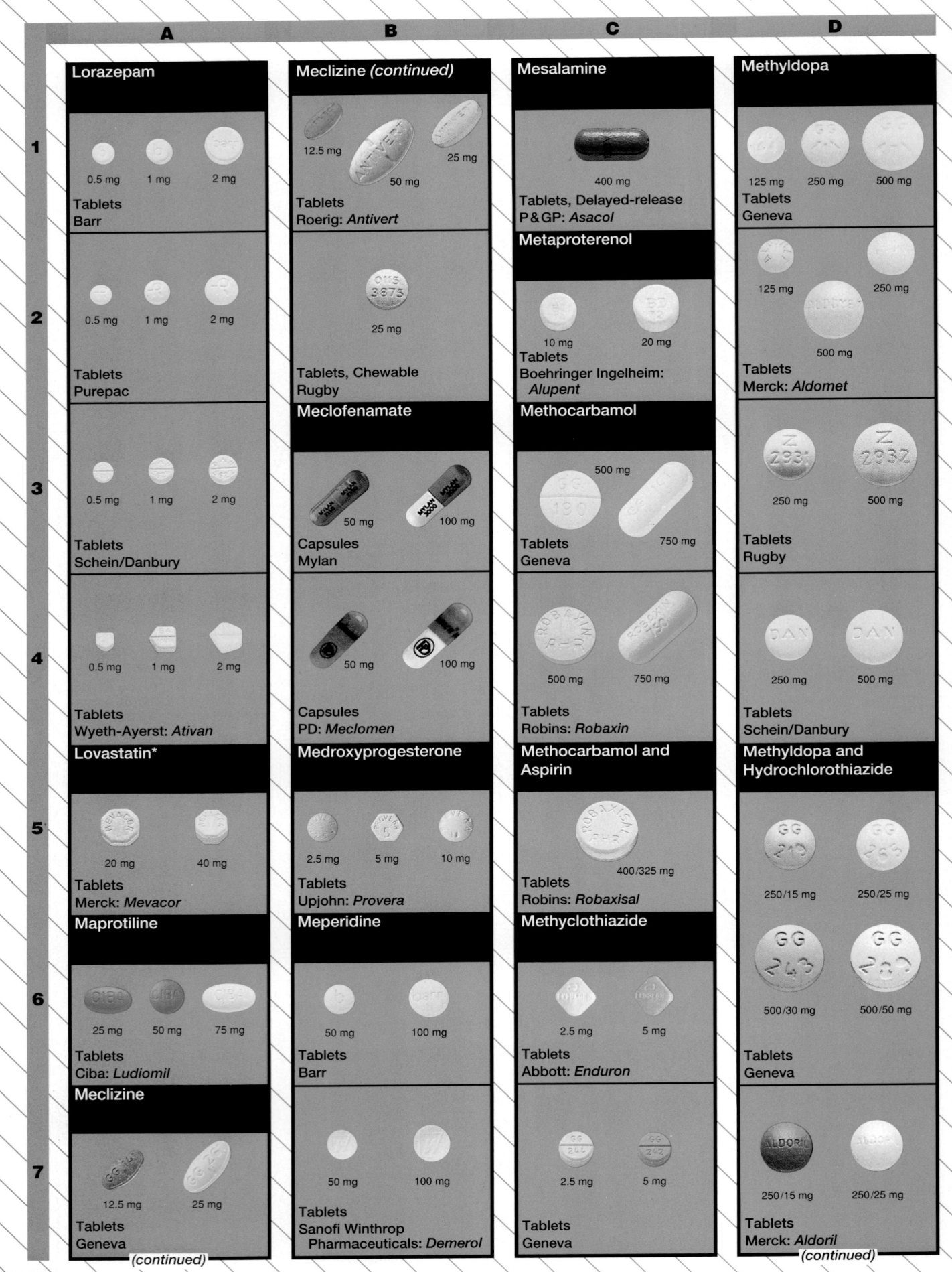

**A**

## Lorazepam

0.5 mg  1 mg  2 mg
Tablets
Barr

0.5 mg  1 mg  2 mg
Tablets
Purepac

0.5 mg  1 mg  2 mg
Tablets
Schein/Danbury

0.5 mg  1 mg  2 mg
Tablets
Wyeth-Ayerst: *Ativan*

## Lovastatin*

20 mg  40 mg
Tablets
Merck: *Mevacor*

## Maprotiline

25 mg  50 mg  75 mg
Tablets
Ciba: *Ludiomil*

## Meclizine

12.5 mg  25 mg
Tablets
Geneva
(continued)

**B**

## Meclizine (continued)

12.5 mg  50 mg  25 mg
Tablets
Roerig: *Antivert*

25 mg
Tablets, Chewable
Rugby

## Meclofenamate

50 mg  100 mg
Capsules
Mylan

50 mg  100 mg
Capsules
PD: *Meclomen*

## Medroxyprogesterone

2.5 mg  5 mg  10 mg
Tablets
Upjohn: *Provera*

## Meperidine

50 mg  100 mg
Tablets
Barr

50 mg  100 mg
Tablets
Sanofi Winthrop
 Pharmaceuticals: *Demerol*

**C**

## Mesalamine

400 mg
Tablets, Delayed-release
P&GP: *Asacol*

## Metaproterenol

10 mg  20 mg
Tablets
Boehringer Ingelheim:
 *Alupent*

## Methocarbamol

500 mg
750 mg
Tablets
Geneva

500 mg  750 mg
Tablets
Robins: *Robaxin*

## Methocarbamol and Aspirin

400/325 mg
Tablets
Robins: *Robaxisal*

## Methyclothiazide

2.5 mg  5 mg
Tablets
Abbott: *Enduron*

2.5 mg  5 mg
Tablets
Geneva

**D**

## Methyldopa

125 mg  250 mg  500 mg
Tablets
Geneva

125 mg  250 mg
500 mg
Tablets
Merck: *Aldomet*

Z 293?  Z 2932
250 mg  500 mg
Tablets
Rugby

250 mg  500 mg
Tablets
Schein/Danbury

## Methyldopa and Hydrochlorothiazide

GG 210  GG 263
250/15 mg  250/25 mg

GG 243  GG 280
500/30 mg  500/50 mg
Tablets
Geneva

250/15 mg  250/25 mg
Tablets
Merck: *Aldoril*
(continued)

The 1995 Medicine Chart
© 1994 The United States Pharmacopeial Convention, Inc.

*Single source product for solid oral dosage forms in the U.S.

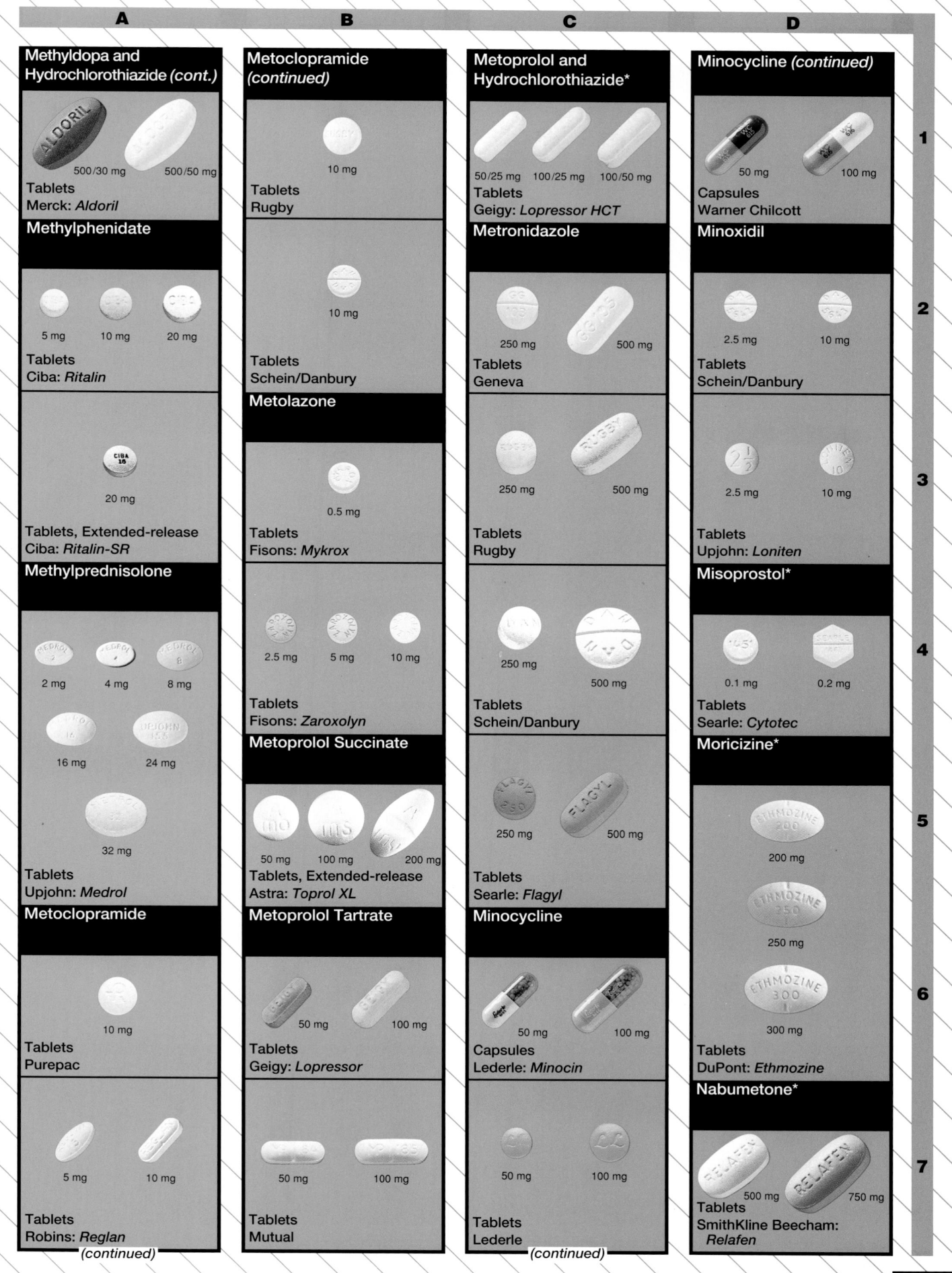

| A | B | C | D |
|---|---|---|---|

**A**

## Methyldopa and Hydrochlorothiazide *(cont.)*

500/30 mg     500/50 mg
Tablets
Merck: *Aldoril*

## Methylphenidate

5 mg    10 mg    20 mg
Tablets
Ciba: *Ritalin*

20 mg
Tablets, Extended-release
Ciba: *Ritalin-SR*

## Methylprednisolone

2 mg    4 mg    8 mg

16 mg    24 mg

32 mg
Tablets
Upjohn: *Medrol*

## Metoclopramide

10 mg
Tablets
Purepac

5 mg    10 mg
Tablets
Robins: *Reglan*
*(continued)*

**B**

## Metoclopramide *(continued)*

10 mg
Tablets
Rugby

10 mg
Tablets
Schein/Danbury

## Metolazone

0.5 mg
Tablets
Fisons: *Mykrox*

2.5 mg    5 mg    10 mg
Tablets
Fisons: *Zaroxolyn*

## Metoprolol Succinate

50 mg    100 mg    200 mg
Tablets, Extended-release
Astra: *Toprol XL*

## Metoprolol Tartrate

50 mg    100 mg
Tablets
Geigy: *Lopressor*

50 mg    100 mg
Tablets
Mutual

**C**

## Metoprolol and Hydrochlorothiazide*

50/25 mg   100/25 mg   100/50 mg
Tablets
Geigy: *Lopressor HCT*

## Metronidazole

250 mg    500 mg
Tablets
Geneva

250 mg    500 mg
Tablets
Rugby

250 mg    500 mg
Tablets
Schein/Danbury

250 mg    500 mg
Tablets
Searle: *Flagyl*

## Minocycline

50 mg    100 mg
Capsules
Lederle: *Minocin*

50 mg    100 mg
Tablets
Lederle
*(continued)*

**D**

## Minocycline *(continued)*

50 mg    100 mg
Capsules
Warner Chilcott

## Minoxidil

2.5 mg    10 mg
Tablets
Schein/Danbury

2.5 mg    10 mg
Tablets
Upjohn: *Loniten*

## Misoprostol*

0.1 mg    0.2 mg
Tablets
Searle: *Cytotec*

## Moricizine*

200 mg

250 mg

300 mg
Tablets
DuPont: *Ethmozine*

## Nabumetone*

500 mg    750 mg
Tablets
SmithKline Beecham:
*Relafen*

The 1995 Medicine Chart   **MC-15**

*Single source product for solid oral dosage forms in the U.S.

© 1994 The United States Pharmacopeial Convention, Inc.

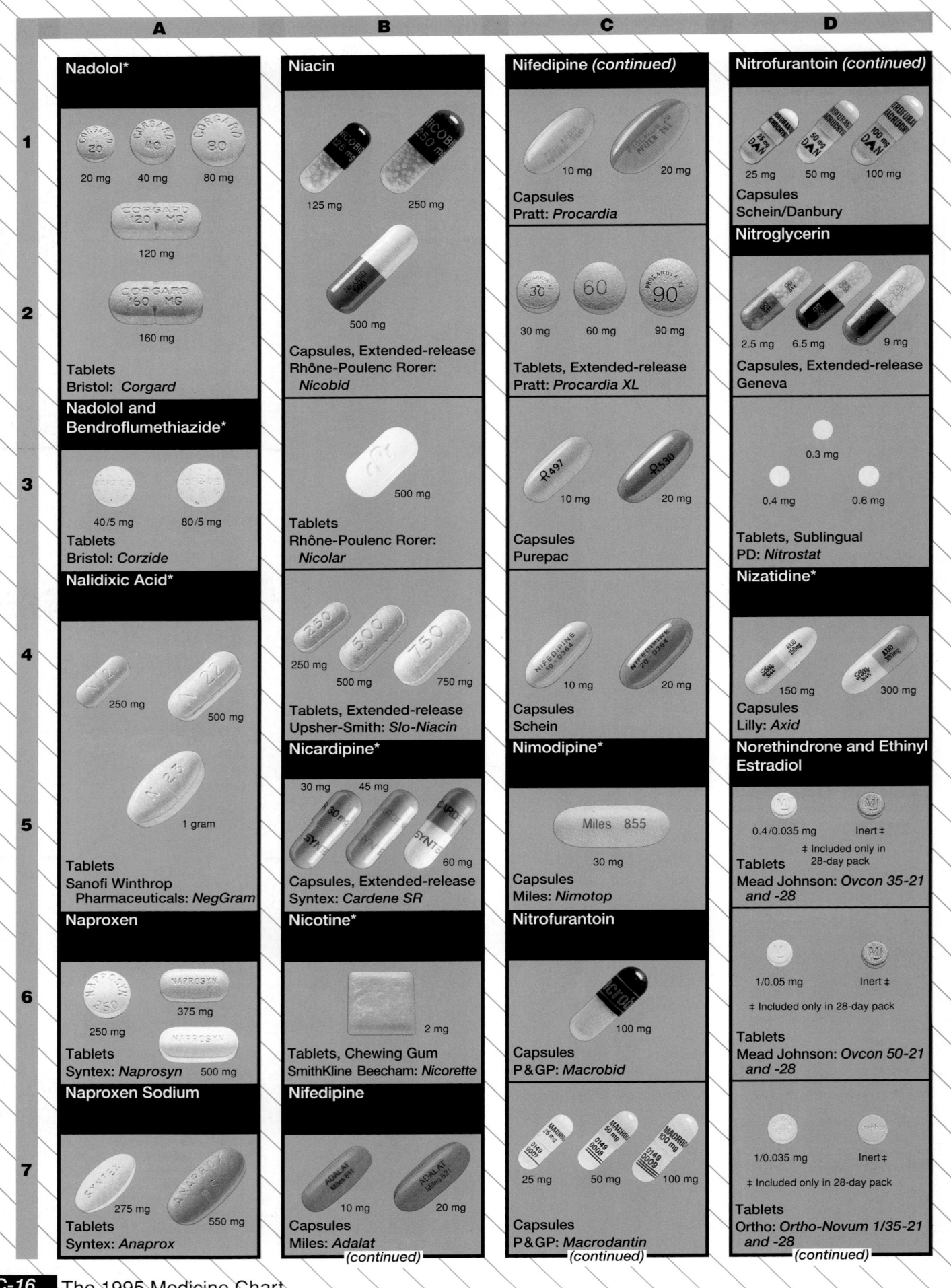

**A**

## Nadolol*

20 mg    40 mg    80 mg

120 mg

160 mg

Tablets
Bristol: *Corgard*

## Nadolol and Bendroflumethiazide*

40/5 mg     80/5 mg

Tablets
Bristol: *Corzide*

## Nalidixic Acid*

250 mg     500 mg

1 gram

Tablets
Sanofi Winthrop
   Pharmaceuticals: *NegGram*

## Naproxen

375 mg

250 mg

500 mg

Tablets
Syntex: *Naprosyn*

## Naproxen Sodium

275 mg     550 mg

Tablets
Syntex: *Anaprox*

---

**B**

## Niacin

125 mg     250 mg

500 mg

Capsules, Extended-release
Rhône-Poulenc Rorer:
   *Nicobid*

500 mg

Tablets
Rhône-Poulenc Rorer:
   *Nicolar*

250 mg    500 mg    750 mg

Tablets, Extended-release
Upsher-Smith: *Slo-Niacin*

## Nicardipine*

30 mg    45 mg

60 mg

Capsules, Extended-release
Syntex: *Cardene SR*

## Nicotine*

2 mg

Tablets, Chewing Gum
SmithKline Beecham: *Nicorette*

## Nifedipine

10 mg     20 mg

Capsules
Miles: *Adalat*
*(continued)*

---

**C**

## Nifedipine *(continued)*

10 mg     20 mg

Capsules
Pratt: *Procardia*

30 mg    60 mg    90 mg

Tablets, Extended-release
Pratt: *Procardia XL*

10 mg     20 mg

Capsules
Purepac

10 mg     20 mg

Capsules
Schein

## Nimodipine*

Miles 855

30 mg

Capsules
Miles: *Nimotop*

## Nitrofurantoin

100 mg

Capsules
P & GP: *Macrobid*

25 mg    50 mg    100 mg

Capsules
P & GP: *Macrodantin*
*(continued)*

---

**D**

## Nitrofurantoin *(continued)*

25 mg    50 mg    100 mg

Capsules
Schein/Danbury

## Nitroglycerin

2.5 mg    6.5 mg    9 mg

Capsules, Extended-release
Geneva

0.3 mg

0.4 mg     0.6 mg

Tablets, Sublingual
PD: *Nitrostat*

## Nizatidine*

150 mg     300 mg

Capsules
Lilly: *Axid*

## Norethindrone and Ethinyl Estradiol

0.4/0.035 mg     Inert ‡

‡ Included only in
   28-day pack

Tablets
Mead Johnson: *Ovcon 35-21
and -28*

1/0.05 mg     Inert ‡

‡ Included only in 28-day pack

Tablets
Mead Johnson: *Ovcon 50-21
and -28*

1/0.035 mg     Inert ‡

‡ Included only in 28-day pack

Tablets
Ortho: *Ortho-Novum 1/35-21
and -28*
*(continued)*

---

The 1995 Medicine Chart
© 1994 The United States Pharmacopeial Convention, Inc.

*Single source product for solid oral dosage forms in the U.S.

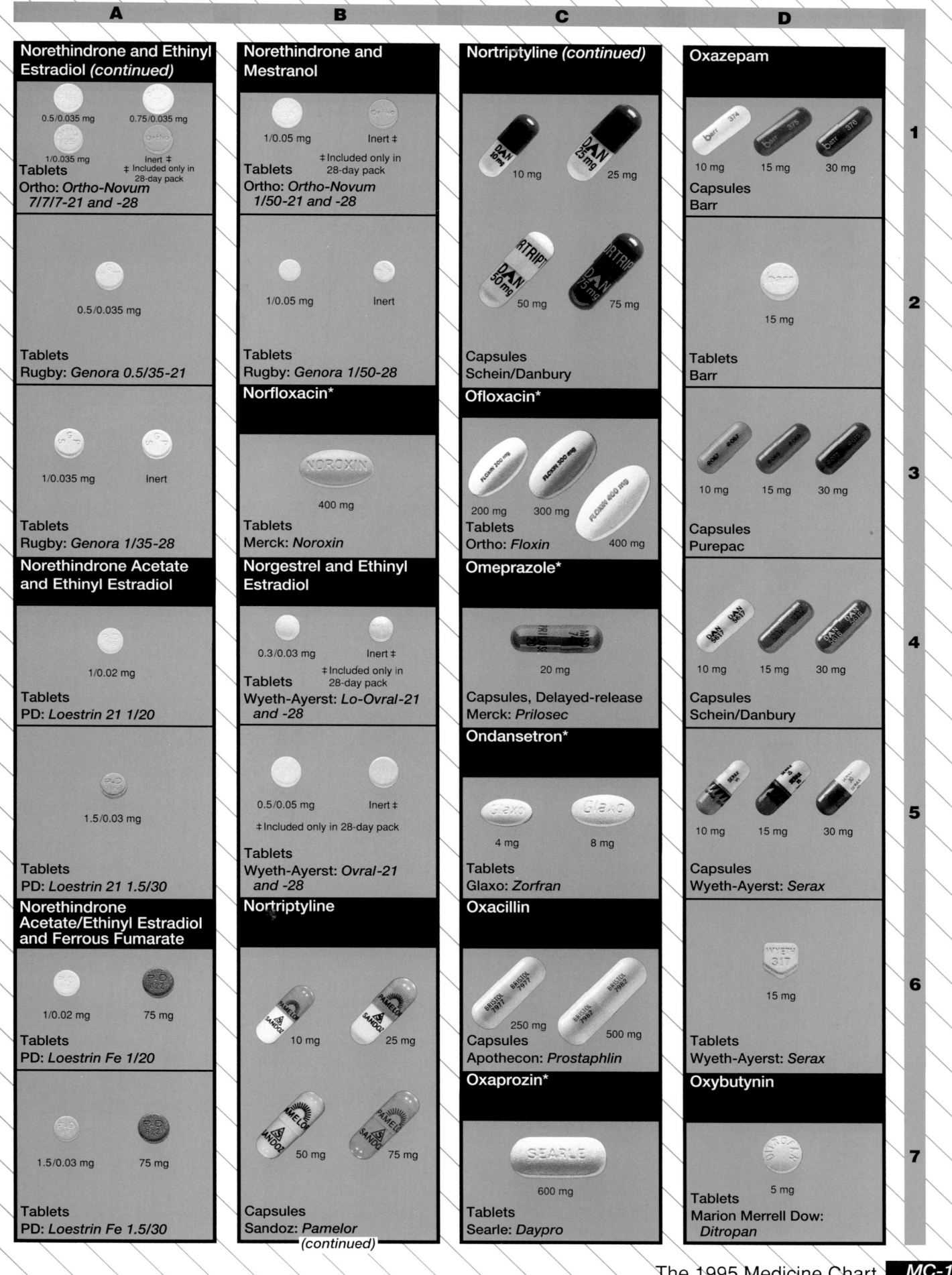

**A**

### Norethindrone and Ethinyl Estradiol *(continued)*

0.5/0.035 mg — 0.75/0.035 mg
1/0.035 mg — Inert ‡
‡ Included only in 28-day pack
**Tablets**
Ortho: *Ortho-Novum 7/7/7-21 and -28*

0.5/0.035 mg
**Tablets**
Rugby: *Genora 0.5/35-21*

1/0.035 mg — Inert
**Tablets**
Rugby: *Genora 1/35-28*

### Norethindrone Acetate and Ethinyl Estradiol

1/0.02 mg
**Tablets**
PD: *Loestrin 21 1/20*

1.5/0.03 mg
**Tablets**
PD: *Loestrin 21 1.5/30*

### Norethindrone Acetate/Ethinyl Estradiol and Ferrous Fumarate

1/0.02 mg — 75 mg
**Tablets**
PD: *Loestrin Fe 1/20*

1.5/0.03 mg — 75 mg
**Tablets**
PD: *Loestrin Fe 1.5/30*

**B**

### Norethindrone and Mestranol

1/0.05 mg — Inert ‡
‡ Included only in 28-day pack
**Tablets**
Ortho: *Ortho-Novum 1/50-21 and -28*

1/0.05 mg — Inert
**Tablets**
Rugby: *Genora 1/50-28*

### Norfloxacin*

NOROXIN
400 mg
**Tablets**
Merck: *Noroxin*

### Norgestrel and Ethinyl Estradiol

0.3/0.03 mg — Inert ‡
‡ Included only in 28-day pack
**Tablets**
Wyeth-Ayerst: *Lo-Ovral-21 and -28*

0.5/0.05 mg — Inert ‡
‡ Included only in 28-day pack
**Tablets**
Wyeth-Ayerst: *Ovral-21 and -28*

### Nortriptyline

10 mg — 25 mg
50 mg — 75 mg
**Capsules**
Sandoz: *Pamelor*
*(continued)*

**C**

### Nortriptyline *(continued)*

10 mg — 25 mg
50 mg — 75 mg
**Capsules**
Schein/Danbury

### Ofloxacin*

200 mg — 300 mg
400 mg
**Tablets**
Ortho: *Floxin*

### Omeprazole*

20 mg
**Capsules, Delayed-release**
Merck: *Prilosec*

### Ondansetron*

4 mg — 8 mg
**Tablets**
Glaxo: *Zorfran*

### Oxacillin

250 mg — 500 mg
**Capsules**
Apothecon: *Prostaphlin*

### Oxaprozin*

600 mg
**Tablets**
Searle: *Daypro*

**D**

### Oxazepam

10 mg — 15 mg — 30 mg
**Capsules**
Barr

15 mg
**Tablets**
Barr

10 mg — 15 mg — 30 mg
**Capsules**
Purepac

10 mg — 15 mg — 30 mg
**Capsules**
Schein/Danbury

10 mg — 15 mg — 30 mg
**Capsules**
Wyeth-Ayerst: *Serax*

15 mg
**Tablets**
Wyeth-Ayerst: *Serax*

### Oxybutynin

5 mg
**Tablets**
Marion Merrell Dow: *Ditropan*

**1**

**2**

**3**

**4**

**5**

**6**

**7**

The 1995 Medicine Chart **MC-17**

*Single source product for solid oral dosage forms in the U.S.

© 1994 The United States Pharmacopeial Convention, Inc.

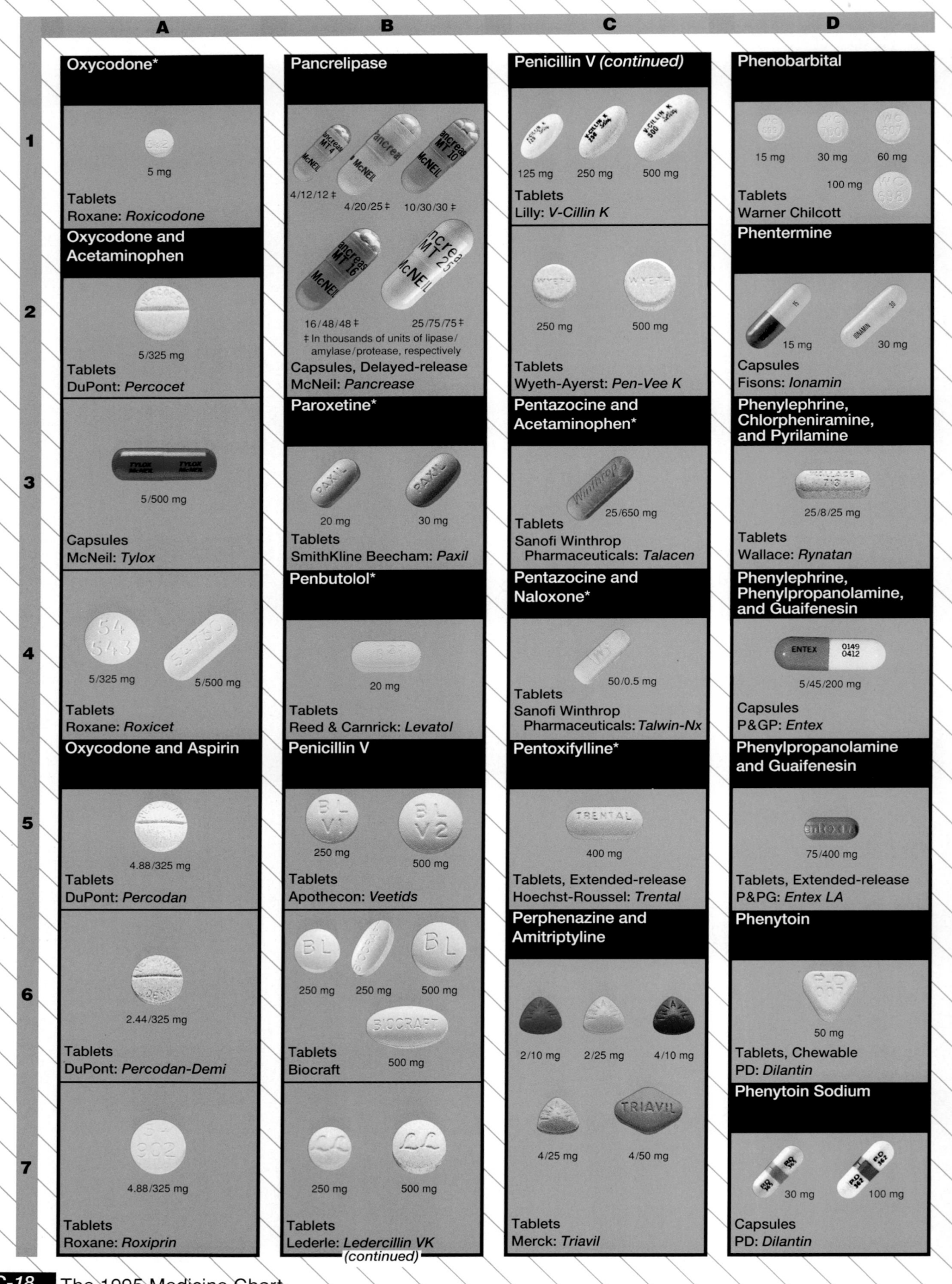

| **A** | **B** | **C** | **D** |
|---|---|---|---|

### A

**Oxycodone\***

5 mg

Tablets
Roxane: *Roxicodone*

**Oxycodone and Acetaminophen**

5/325 mg

Tablets
DuPont: *Percocet*

5/500 mg

Capsules
McNeil: *Tylox*

54 543 — 5/325 mg        5/500 mg

Tablets
Roxane: *Roxicet*

**Oxycodone and Aspirin**

4.88/325 mg

Tablets
DuPont: *Percodan*

2.44/325 mg

Tablets
DuPont: *Percodan-Demi*

4.88/325 mg

Tablets
Roxane: *Roxiprin*

### B

**Pancrelipase**

4/12/12 ‡        4/20/25 ‡        10/30/30 ‡

16/48/48 ‡        25/75/75 ‡
‡ In thousands of units of lipase/
amylase/protease, respectively

Capsules, Delayed-release
McNeil: *Pancrease*

**Paroxetine\***

20 mg        30 mg

Tablets
SmithKline Beecham: *Paxil*

**Penbutolol\***

20 mg

Tablets
Reed & Carnrick: *Levatol*

**Penicillin V**

250 mg        500 mg

Tablets
Apothecon: *Veetids*

250 mg    250 mg    500 mg

500 mg

Tablets
Biocraft

250 mg        500 mg

Tablets
Lederle: *Ledercillin VK*
(continued)

### C

**Penicillin V** *(continued)*

125 mg    250 mg    500 mg

Tablets
Lilly: *V-Cillin K*

250 mg        500 mg

Tablets
Wyeth-Ayerst: *Pen-Vee K*

**Pentazocine and Acetaminophen\***

25/650 mg

Tablets
Sanofi Winthrop
  Pharmaceuticals: *Talacen*

**Pentazocine and Naloxone\***

50/0.5 mg

Tablets
Sanofi Winthrop
  Pharmaceuticals: *Talwin-Nx*

**Pentoxifylline\***

400 mg

Tablets, Extended-release
Hoechst-Roussel: *Trental*

**Perphenazine and Amitriptyline**

2/10 mg    2/25 mg    4/10 mg

4/25 mg        4/50 mg

Tablets
Merck: *Triavil*

### D

**Phenobarbital**

15 mg    30 mg    60 mg
100 mg

Tablets
Warner Chilcott

**Phentermine**

15 mg        30 mg

Capsules
Fisons: *Ionamin*

**Phenylephrine, Chlorpheniramine, and Pyrilamine**

25/8/25 mg

Tablets
Wallace: *Rynatan*

**Phenylephrine, Phenylpropanolamine, and Guaifenesin**

5/45/200 mg

Capsules
P&GP: *Entex*

**Phenylpropanolamine and Guaifenesin**

75/400 mg

Tablets, Extended-release
P&PG: *Entex LA*

**Phenytoin**

50 mg

Tablets, Chewable
PD: *Dilantin*

**Phenytoin Sodium**

30 mg        100 mg

Capsules
PD: *Dilantin*

The 1995 Medicine Chart
© 1994 The United States Pharmacopeial Convention, Inc.                \*Single source product for solid oral dosage forms in the U.S.

**A**

## Pindolol

5 mg     10 mg

Tablets
Mutual

5 mg     10 mg

Tablets
Sandoz: *Visken*

## Piroxicam

10 mg     20 mg

Capsules
Mutual

10 mg     20 mg

Capsules
Pratt: *Feldene*

## Potassium Chloride

750 mg

Tablets, Extended-release
Abbott: *K-Tab*

750 mg

Tablets, Extended-release
Apothecon: *Klotrix*

750 mg     1500 mg

Tablets, Extended-release
Key: *K-Dur*
*(continued)*

**B**

## Potassium Chloride *(cont.)*

600 mg     750 mg

Capsules, Extended-release
Robins: *Micro-K*

Slow-K

600 mg

Tablets, Extended-release
Summit: *Slow-K*

KLOR-CON 8     KLOR-CON 10

600 mg     750 mg

Tablets, Extended-release
Upsher-Smith: *Klor-Con*

## Pravastatin

10 mg    20 mg    40 mg

Tablets
Squibb: *Pravachol*

## Prazosin

1 mg     2 mg

5 mg

Capsules
Pfizer: *Minipress*

1 mg     2 mg

5 mg

Capsules
Purepac

1 mg     2 mg

5 mg

Capsules
Schein/Danbury

**C**

## Prazosin and Polythiazide*

1/0.5 mg    2/0.5 mg

5/0.5 mg

Capsules
Pfizer: *Minizide*

## Prednisone

1 mg    2.5 mg    5 mg

10 mg    20 mg    50 mg

Tablets
Roxane

5 mg    10 mg    20 mg

50 mg

Tablets
Rugby

2.5 mg    5 mg    10 mg

20 mg     50 mg

Tablets
Upjohn: *Deltasone*

## Probucol*

250 mg     500 mg

Tablets
Marion Merrell Dow: *Lorelco*

## Procainamide

250 mg    375 mg

500 mg

Capsules
Geneva

GG 472   GG 473   750 mg

GG 474

250 mg    500 mg

Tablets, Extended-release
Geneva
*(continued)*

**D**

## Procainamide *(continued)*

500 mg

750 mg     1 gram

Tablets, Extended-release
PD: *Procan SR*

250 mg     375 mg

500 mg

Capsules
Apothecon: *Pronestyl*

250 mg    375 mg    500 mg

Tablets
Apothecon: *Pronestyl*

500 mg

Tablets, Extended-release
Apothecon: *Pronestyl-SR*

250 mg    375 mg    500 mg

Capsules
Schein/Danbury

250 mg     500 mg

750 mg

Tablets, Extended-release
Schein/Danbury

1   2   3   4   5   6   7

The 1995 Medicine Chart   **MC-19**

*Single source product for solid oral dosage forms in the U.S.    © 1994 The United States Pharmacopeial Convention, Inc.

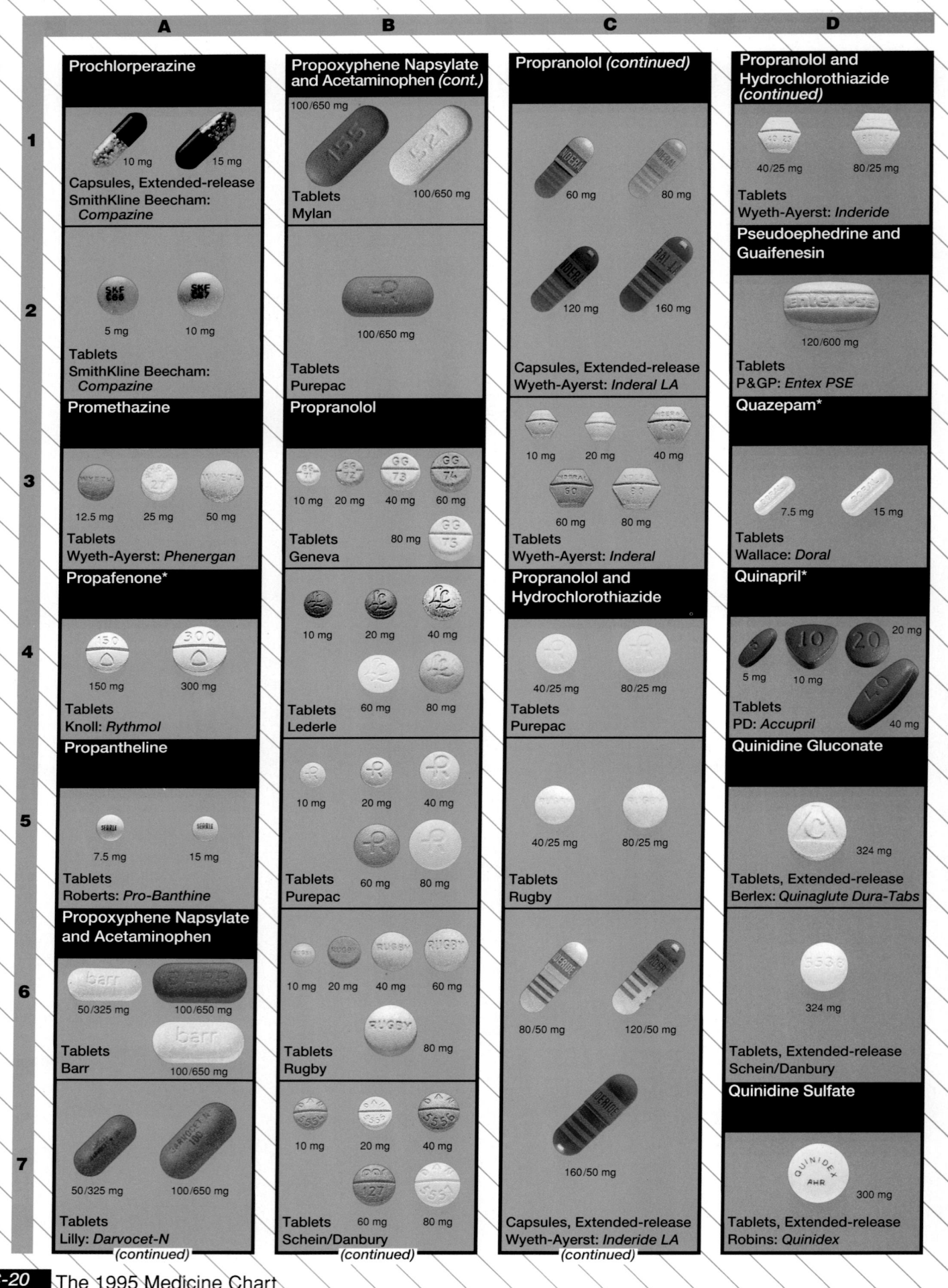

**Column A**

### Prochlorperazine

10 mg    15 mg

Capsules, Extended-release
SmithKline Beecham: *Compazine*

5 mg    10 mg

Tablets
SmithKline Beecham: *Compazine*

### Promethazine

12.5 mg    25 mg    50 mg

Tablets
Wyeth-Ayerst: *Phenergan*

### Propafenone*

150 mg    300 mg

Tablets
Knoll: *Rythmol*

### Propantheline

7.5 mg    15 mg

Tablets
Roberts: *Pro-Banthine*

### Propoxyphene Napsylate and Acetaminophen

50/325 mg    100/650 mg
100/650 mg

Tablets
Barr

50/325 mg    100/650 mg

Tablets
Lilly: *Darvocet-N*
*(continued)*

**Column B**

### Propoxyphene Napsylate and Acetaminophen *(cont.)*

100/650 mg

100/650 mg

Tablets
Mylan

100/650 mg

Tablets
Purepac

### Propranolol

10 mg   20 mg   40 mg   60 mg

80 mg

Tablets
Geneva

10 mg   20 mg   40 mg

60 mg   80 mg

Tablets
Lederle

10 mg   20 mg   40 mg

60 mg   80 mg

Tablets
Purepac

10 mg   20 mg   40 mg   60 mg

80 mg

Tablets
Rugby

10 mg   20 mg   40 mg

60 mg   80 mg

Tablets
Schein/Danbury
*(continued)*

**Column C**

### Propranolol *(continued)*

60 mg    80 mg

120 mg    160 mg

Capsules, Extended-release
Wyeth-Ayerst: *Inderal LA*

10 mg   20 mg   40 mg

60 mg   80 mg

Tablets
Wyeth-Ayerst: *Inderal*

### Propranolol and Hydrochlorothiazide

40/25 mg    80/25 mg

Tablets
Purepac

40/25 mg    80/25 mg

Tablets
Rugby

80/50 mg    120/50 mg

160/50 mg

Capsules, Extended-release
Wyeth-Ayerst: *Inderide LA*
*(continued)*

**Column D**

### Propranolol and Hydrochlorothiazide *(continued)*

40/25 mg    80/25 mg

Tablets
Wyeth-Ayerst: *Inderide*

### Pseudoephedrine and Guaifenesin

120/600 mg

Tablets
P&GP: *Entex PSE*

### Quazepam*

7.5 mg    15 mg

Tablets
Wallace: *Doral*

### Quinapril*

5 mg   10 mg   20 mg
40 mg

Tablets
PD: *Accupril*

### Quinidine Gluconate

324 mg

Tablets, Extended-release
Berlex: *Quinaglute Dura-Tabs*

324 mg

Tablets, Extended-release
Schein/Danbury

### Quinidine Sulfate

300 mg

Tablets, Extended-release
Robins: *Quinidex*

The 1995 Medicine Chart
© 1994 The United States Pharmacopeial Convention, Inc.

*Single source product for solid oral dosage forms in the U.S.

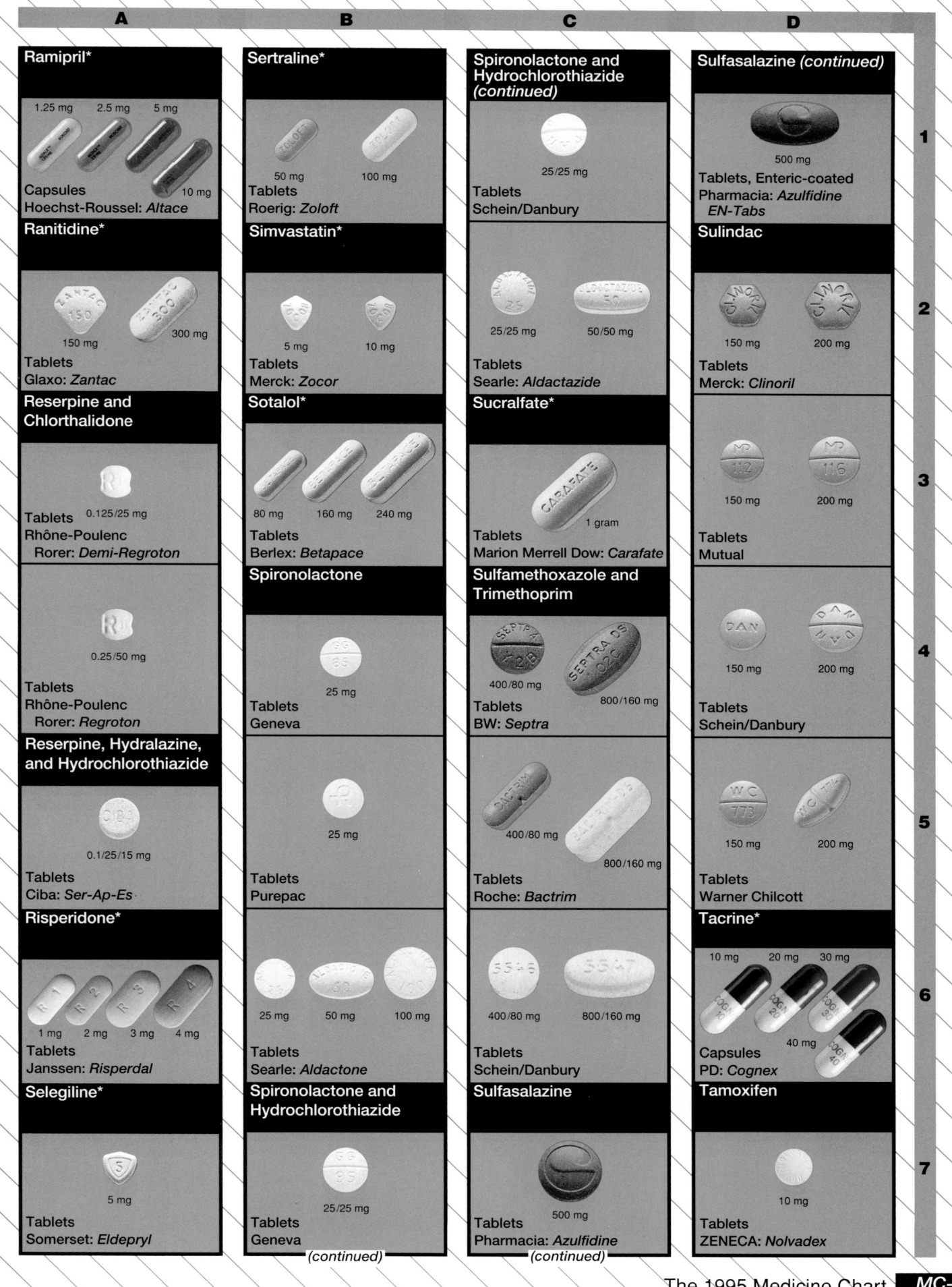

## A

**Ramipril***

1.25 mg  2.5 mg  5 mg  10 mg

Capsules
Hoechst-Roussel: *Altace*

**Ranitidine***

150 mg  300 mg

Tablets
Glaxo: *Zantac*

**Reserpine and Chlorthalidone**

0.125/25 mg

Tablets
Rhône-Poulenc Rorer: *Demi-Regroton*

0.25/50 mg

Tablets
Rhône-Poulenc Rorer: *Regroton*

**Reserpine, Hydralazine, and Hydrochlorothiazide**

0.1/25/15 mg

Tablets
Ciba: *Ser-Ap-Es*

**Risperidone***

1 mg  2 mg  3 mg  4 mg

Tablets
Janssen: *Risperdal*

**Selegiline***

5 mg

Tablets
Somerset: *Eldepryl*

## B

**Sertraline***

50 mg  100 mg

Tablets
Roerig: *Zoloft*

**Simvastatin***

5 mg  10 mg

Tablets
Merck: *Zocor*

**Sotalol***

80 mg  160 mg  240 mg

Tablets
Berlex: *Betapace*

**Spironolactone**

25 mg

Tablets
Geneva

25 mg

Tablets
Purepac

25 mg  50 mg  100 mg

Tablets
Searle: *Aldactone*

**Spironolactone and Hydrochlorothiazide**

25/25 mg

Tablets
Geneva

*(continued)*

## C

**Spironolactone and Hydrochlorothiazide** *(continued)*

25/25 mg

Tablets
Schein/Danbury

25/25 mg  50/50 mg

Tablets
Searle: *Aldactazide*

**Sucralfate***

1 gram

Tablets
Marion Merrell Dow: *Carafate*

**Sulfamethoxazole and Trimethoprim**

400/80 mg  800/160 mg

Tablets
BW: *Septra*

400/80 mg  800/160 mg

Tablets
Roche: *Bactrim*

400/80 mg  800/160 mg

Tablets
Schein/Danbury

**Sulfasalazine**

500 mg

Tablets
Pharmacia: *Azulfidine*

*(continued)*

## D

**Sulfasalazine** *(continued)*

500 mg

Tablets, Enteric-coated
Pharmacia: *Azulfidine EN-Tabs*

**Sulindac**

150 mg  200 mg

Tablets
Merck: *Clinoril*

150 mg  200 mg

Tablets
Mutual

150 mg  200 mg

Tablets
Schein/Danbury

150 mg  200 mg

Tablets
Warner Chilcott

**Tacrine***

10 mg  20 mg  30 mg  40 mg

Capsules
PD: *Cognex*

**Tamoxifen**

10 mg

Tablets
ZENECA: *Nolvadex*

1  2  3  4  5  6  7

The 1995 Medicine Chart  **MC-21**

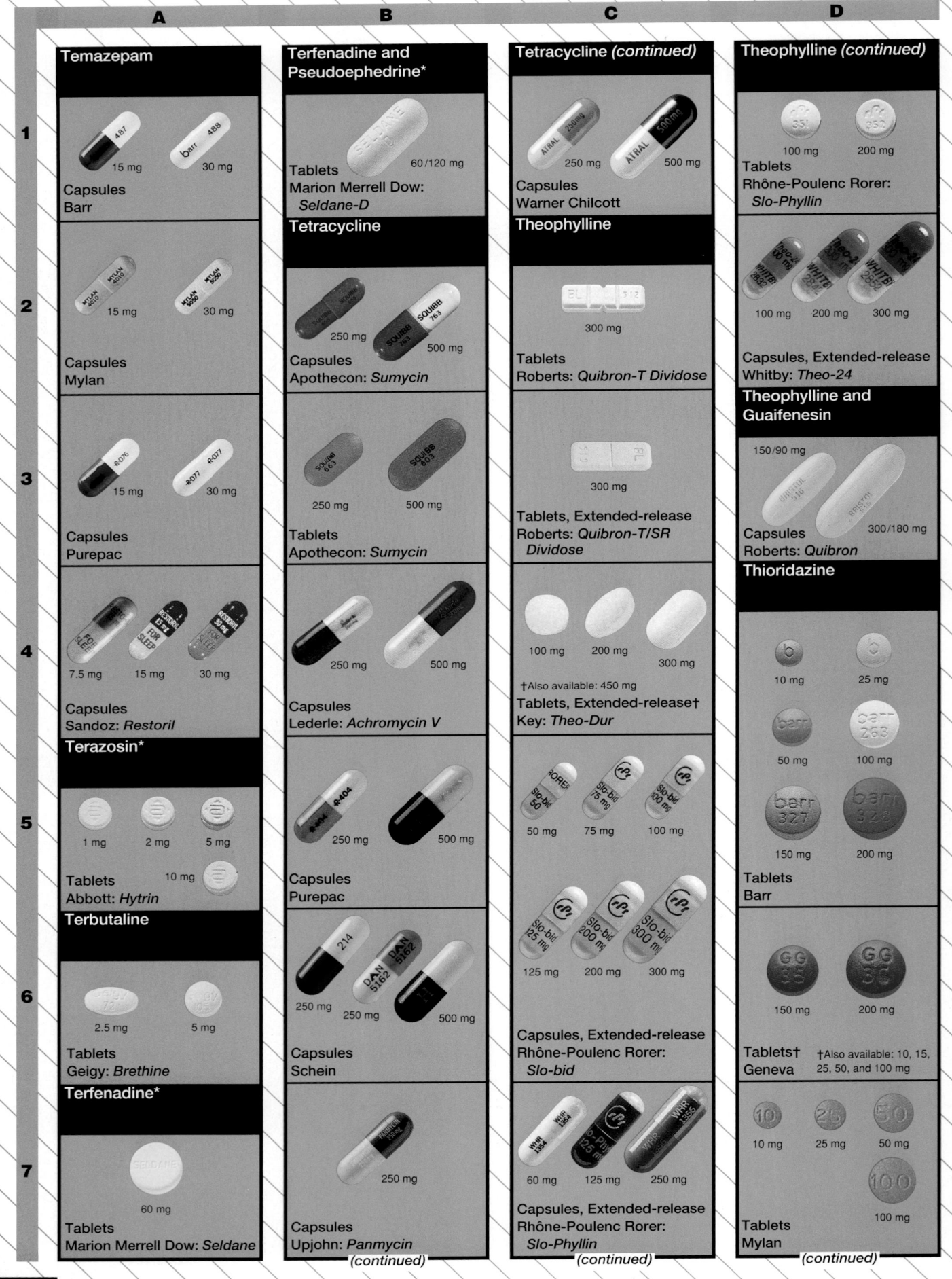

**A**

### Temazepam

15 mg    30 mg
Capsules
Barr

15 mg    30 mg
Capsules
Mylan

15 mg    30 mg
Capsules
Purepac

7.5 mg   15 mg   30 mg
Capsules
Sandoz: *Restoril*

### Terazosin*

1 mg   2 mg   5 mg
10 mg
Tablets
Abbott: *Hytrin*

### Terbutaline

2.5 mg   5 mg
Tablets
Geigy: *Brethine*

### Terfenadine*

60 mg
Tablets
Marion Merrell Dow: *Seldane*

---

**B**

### Terfenadine and Pseudoephedrine*

60 /120 mg
Tablets
Marion Merrell Dow:
*Seldane-D*

### Tetracycline

250 mg   500 mg
Capsules
Apothecon: *Sumycin*

250 mg   500 mg
Tablets
Apothecon: *Sumycin*

250 mg   500 mg
Capsules
Lederle: *Achromycin V*

250 mg   500 mg
Capsules
Purepac

250 mg   250 mg   500 mg
Capsules
Schein

250 mg
Capsules
Upjohn: *Panmycin*

*(continued)*

---

**C**

### Tetracycline *(continued)*

250 mg   500 mg
Capsules
Warner Chilcott

### Theophylline

300 mg
Tablets
Roberts: *Quibron-T Dividose*

300 mg
Tablets, Extended-release
Roberts: *Quibron-T/SR Dividose*

100 mg   200 mg   300 mg

†Also available: 450 mg
Tablets, Extended-release†
Key: *Theo-Dur*

50 mg   75 mg   100 mg
125 mg   200 mg   300 mg
Capsules, Extended-release
Rhône-Poulenc Rorer:
*Slo-bid*

60 mg   125 mg   250 mg
Capsules, Extended-release
Rhône-Poulenc Rorer:
*Slo-Phyllin*

*(continued)*

---

**D**

### Theophylline *(continued)*

100 mg   200 mg
Tablets
Rhône-Poulenc Rorer:
*Slo-Phyllin*

100 mg   200 mg   300 mg
Capsules, Extended-release
Whitby: *Theo-24*

### Theophylline and Guaifenesin

150 /90 mg
300 /180 mg
Capsules
Roberts: *Quibron*

### Thioridazine

10 mg   25 mg
50 mg   100 mg
150 mg   200 mg
Tablets
Barr

150 mg   200 mg
Tablets†   †Also available: 10, 15, 25, 50, and 100 mg
Geneva

10 mg   25 mg   50 mg
100 mg
Tablets
Mylan

*(continued)*

---

The 1995 Medicine Chart
© 1994 The United States Pharmacopeial Convention, Inc.
*Single source product for solid oral dosage forms in the U.S.

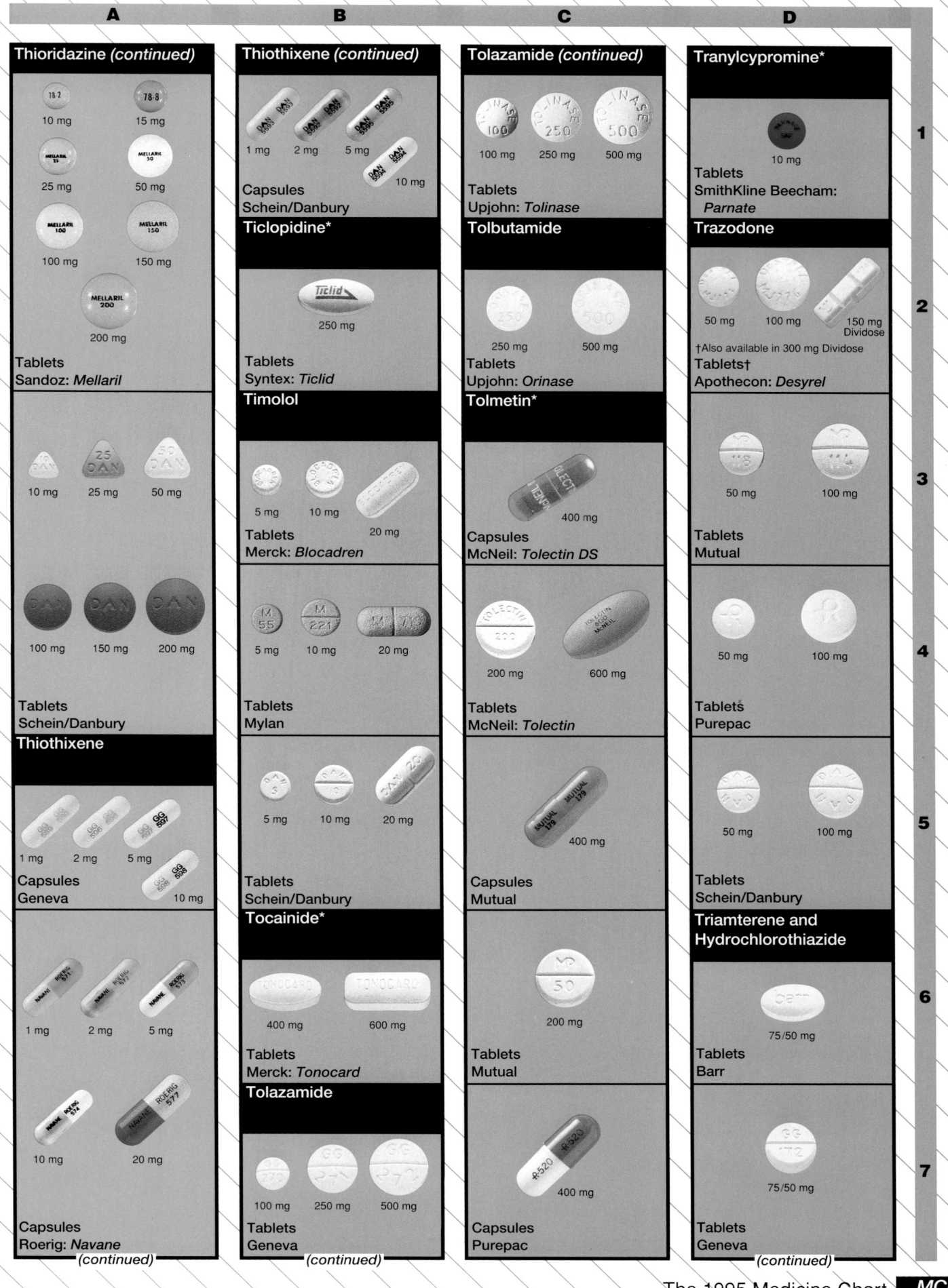

## A

### Thioridazine *(continued)*

78·2 — 10 mg
78·8 — 15 mg
MELLARIL 25 — 25 mg
MELLARIL 50 — 50 mg
MELLARIL 100 — 100 mg
MELLARIL 150 — 150 mg
MELLARIL 200 — 200 mg

Tablets
Sandoz: *Mellaril*

10 mg
25 mg
50 mg

100 mg
150 mg
200 mg

Tablets
Schein/Danbury

### Thiothixene

GG 596 — 1 mg
GG 593 — 2 mg
GG 597 — 5 mg
GG 598 — 10 mg

Capsules
Geneva

NAVANE ROERIG 571 — 1 mg
NAVANE ROERIG 572 — 2 mg
NAVANE ROERIG 573 — 5 mg
NAVANE ROERIG 574 — 10 mg
NAVANE ROERIG 577 — 20 mg

Capsules
Roerig: *Navane*
*(continued)*

## B

### Thiothixene *(continued)*

DAN 5591 — 1 mg
DAN 5592 — 2 mg
DAN 5593 — 5 mg
DAN 5594 — 10 mg

Capsules
Schein/Danbury

### Ticlopidine*

Ticlid — 250 mg

Tablets
Syntex: *Ticlid*

### Timolol

5 mg
10 mg
20 mg

Tablets
Merck: *Blocadren*

M 55 — 5 mg
M 221 — 10 mg
M — 20 mg

Tablets
Mylan

DAN 5 — 5 mg
DAN 10 — 10 mg
DAN 20 — 20 mg

Tablets
Schein/Danbury

### Tocainide*

TONOCARD — 400 mg
TONOCARD — 600 mg

Tablets
Merck: *Tonocard*

### Tolazamide

GG — 100 mg
GG 271 — 250 mg
GG 270 — 500 mg

Tablets
Geneva
*(continued)*

## C

### Tolazamide *(continued)*

TOLINASE 100 — 100 mg
TOLINASE 250 — 250 mg
TOLINASE 500 — 500 mg

Tablets
Upjohn: *Tolinase*

### Tolbutamide

250 mg
500 mg

Tablets
Upjohn: *Orinase*

### Tolmetin*

TOLECTIN DS MCNEIL — 400 mg

Capsules
McNeil: *Tolectin DS*

TOLECTIN 200 — 200 mg
TOLECTIN 600 MCNEIL — 600 mg

Tablets
McNeil: *Tolectin*

MUTUAL 179 — 400 mg

Capsules
Mutual

MP 50 — 200 mg

Tablets
Mutual

P-520 — 400 mg

Capsules
Purepac

## D

### Tranylcypromine*

SKF — 10 mg

Tablets
SmithKline Beecham:
*Parnate*

### Trazodone

50 mg
100 mg
MJ 778 — 150 mg Dividose

†Also available in 300 mg Dividose

Tablets†
Apothecon: *Desyrel*

MP 118 — 50 mg
MP — 100 mg

Tablets
Mutual

PR — 50 mg
PR — 100 mg

Tablets
Purepac

DAN — 50 mg
DAN — 100 mg

Tablets
Schein/Danbury

### Triamterene and Hydrochlorothiazide

barr — 75/50 mg

Tablets
Barr

GG 172 — 75/50 mg

Tablets
Geneva
*(continued)*

---

1
2
3
4
5
6
7

The 1995 Medicine Chart **MC-23**

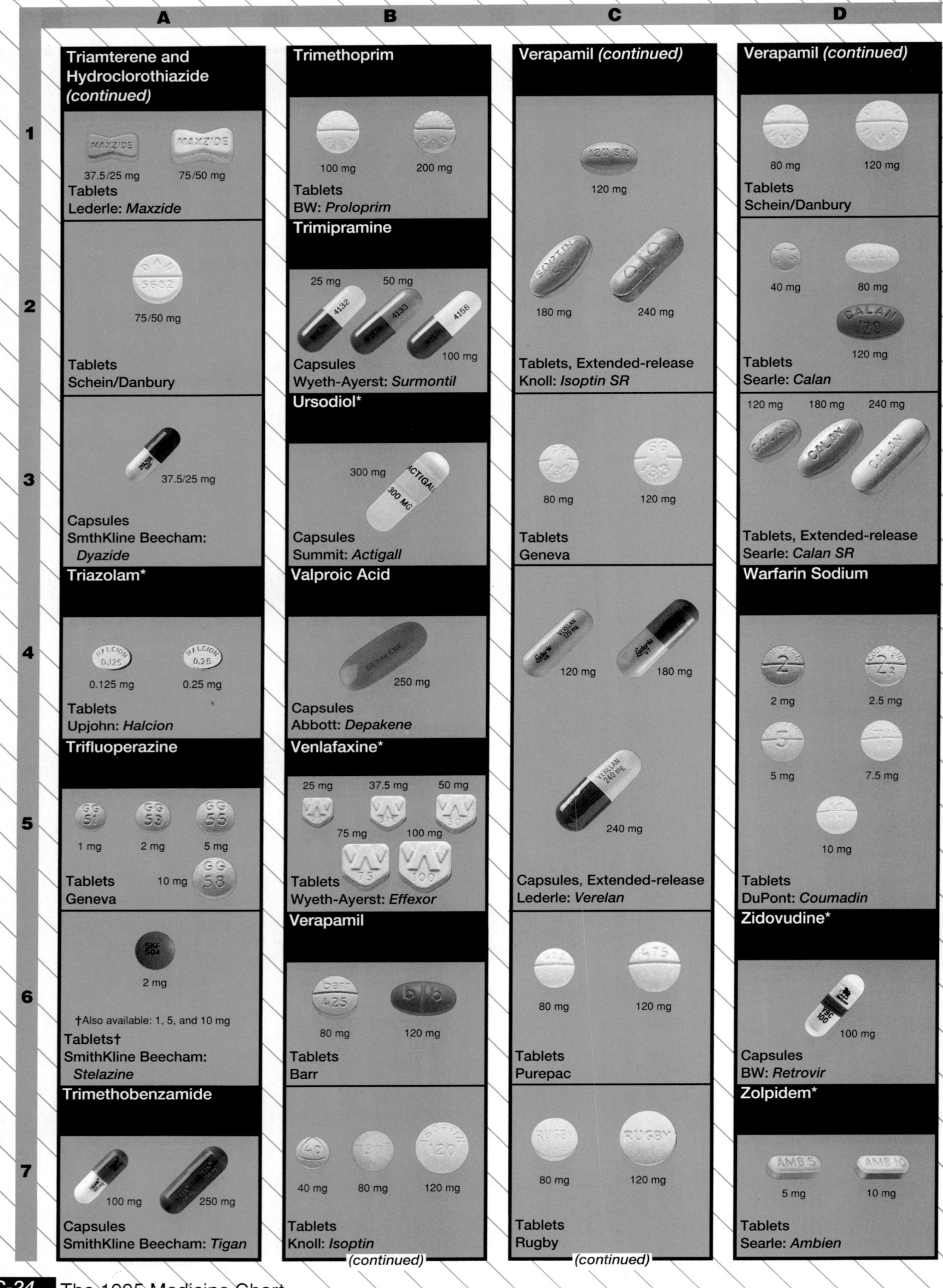

**A**

### Triamterene and Hydroclorothiazide *(continued)*

MAXZIDE 37.5/25 mg   MAXZIDE 75/50 mg
Tablets
Lederle: *Maxzide*

DAN 5582   75/50 mg
Tablets
Schein/Danbury

37.5/25 mg
Capsules
SmthKline Beecham: *Dyazide*

### Triazolam*

HALCION 0.125   0.125 mg    HALCION 0.25   0.25 mg
Tablets
Upjohn: *Halcion*

### Trifluoperazine

GG 51   1 mg    GG 53   2 mg    GG 55   5 mg    GG 56   10 mg

SKF 504   2 mg

†Also available: 1, 5, and 10 mg
Tablets†
SmithKline Beecham: *Stelazine*

### Trimethobenzamide

100 mg    250 mg
Capsules
SmithKline Beecham: *Tigan*

**B**

### Trimethoprim

100 mg    200 mg
Tablets
BW: *Proloprim*

### Trimipramine

25 mg   4132    50 mg   4133    4158   100 mg
Capsules
Wyeth-Ayerst: *Surmontil*

### Ursodiol*

300 mg   ACTIGALL 300 MG
Capsules
Summit: *Actigall*

### Valproic Acid

DEPAKENE   250 mg
Capsules
Abbott: *Depakene*

### Venlafaxine*

25 mg    37.5 mg    50 mg    75 mg    100 mg
Tablets
Wyeth-Ayerst: *Effexor*

### Verapamil

barr 425   80 mg    5|6   120 mg
Tablets
Barr

40 mg    80 mg    ISOPTIN 120   120 mg
Tablets
Knoll: *Isoptin*
*(continued)*

**C**

### Verapamil *(continued)*

120 SR   120 mg

ISOPTIN SR   180 mg    240 mg
Tablets, Extended-release
Knoll: *Isoptin SR*

GG 732   80 mg    GG 733   120 mg
Tablets
Geneva

VERELAN 120 mg   120 mg    VERELAN   180 mg    VERELAN 240 mg   240 mg
Capsules, Extended-release
Lederle: *Verelan*

474   80 mg    475   120 mg
Tablets
Purepac

RUGBY   80 mg    RUGBY   120 mg
Tablets
Rugby
*(continued)*

**D**

### Verapamil *(continued)*

80 mg    120 mg
Tablets
Schein/Danbury

40 mg    CALAN   80 mg    CALAN 120   120 mg
Tablets
Searle: *Calan*

CALAN 120 mg    CALAN 180 mg    CALAN 240 mg
Tablets, Extended-release
Searle: *Calan SR*

### Warfarin Sodium

COUMADIN 2   2 mg    COUMADIN 2 1/2   2.5 mg    5   5 mg    7 1/2   7.5 mg    10   10 mg
Tablets
DuPont: *Coumadin*

### Zidovudine*

Y9C 50C   100 mg
Capsules
BW: *Retrovir*

### Zolpidem*

AMB 5   5 mg    AMB 10   10 mg
Tablets
Searle: *Ambien*

The 1995 Medicine Chart
© 1994 The United States Pharmacopeial Convention, Inc.

*Single source product for solid oral dosage forms in the U.S.

# ACETAMINOPHEN  Systemic

Some commonly used brand names are:

**In the U.S.—**

| | |
|---|---|
| Aceta Elixir[1] | Liquiprin Children's Elixir[1] |
| Aceta Tablets[1] | Liquiprin Infants' Drops[1] |
| Acetaminophen Uniserts[1] | Neopap[1] |
| Actamin[1] | Oraphen-PD[1] |
| Actamin Extra[1] | Panadol, Children's[1] |
| Actamin Super[2] | Panadol, Infants'[1] |
| Aminofen[1] | Panadol Junior Strength |
| Aminofen Max[1] | Caplets[1] |
| Apacet Capsules[1] | Panadol Maximum Strength |
| Apacet Elixir[1] | Caplets[1] |
| Apacet Extra Strength | Panadol Maximum Strength |
| Caplets[1] | Tablets[1] |
| Apacet Extra Strength | Phenaphen Caplets[1] |
| Tablets[1] | Redutemp[1] |
| Apacet, Infants'[1] | Snaplets-FR[1] |
| Apacet Regular Strength | St. Joseph Aspirin-Free |
| Tablets[1] | Fever Reducer for |
| Aspirin Free Anacin | Children[1] |
| Maximum | Suppap-120[1] |
| Strength Caplets[1] | Suppap-325[1] |
| Aspirin Free Anacin | Suppap-650[1] |
| Maximum | Tapanol Extra Strength |
| Strength Gel Caplets[1] | Caplets[1] |
| Aspirin Free Anacin | Tapanol Extra Strength |
| Maximum | Tablets[1] |
| Strength Tablets[1] | Tempra[1] |
| Aspirin-Free Excedrin | Tempra D.S.[1] |
| Caplets[2] | Tempra, Infants'[1] |
| Banesin[1] | Tempra Syrup[1] |
| Bayer Select Maximum | Tylenol Children's Chewable |
| Strength Headache Pain | Tablets[1] |
| Relief Formula[2] | Tylenol Children's Elixir[1] |
| Dapa[1] | Tylenol Children's Suspension |
| Dapa X-S[1] | Liquid[1] |
| Datril Extra-Strength[1] | Tylenol Extra-Strength Adult |
| Feverall, Children's[1] | Liquid Pain Reliever[1] |
| Feverall, Infants'[1] | Tylenol Extra Strength |
| Feverall Junior Strength[1] | Caplets[1] |
| Feverall Sprinkle Caps, | Tylenol Extra Strength |
| Children's[1] | Gelcaps[1] |
| Feverall Sprinkle Caps | Tylenol Extra Strength |
| Junior Strength[1] | Tablets[1] |
| Genapap Children's Elixir[1] | Tylenol Infants' Drops[1] |
| Genapap Children's Tablets[1] | Tylenol Infants' Suspension |
| Genapap Extra Strength | Drops[1] |
| Caplets[1] | Tylenol Junior Strength |
| Genapap Extra Strength | Caplets[1] |
| Tablets[1] | Tylenol Junior Strength |
| Genapap, Infants'[1] | Chewable Tablets[1] |
| Genapap Regular Strength | Tylenol Regular Strength |
| Tablets[1] | Caplets[1] |
| Genebs Extra Strength | Tylenol Regular Strength |
| Caplets[1] | Tablets[1] |
| Genebs Regular Strength | Valorin[1] |
| Tablets[1] | Valorin Extra[1] |
| Genebs X-Tra[1] | |

**In Canada—**

| | |
|---|---|
| Abenol[1] | Apo-Acetaminophen[1] |
| Actimol Chewable Tablets[1] | Atasol Caplets[1] |
| Actimol Children's | Atasol Drops[1] |
| Suspension[1] | Atasol Forte Caplets[1] |
| Actimol Infants' Suspension[1] | Atasol Forte Tablets[1] |
| Actimol Junior Strength | Atasol Oral Solution[1] |
| Caplets[1] | Atasol Tablets[1] |
| Anacin-3[1] | Excedrin Caplets[2] |
| Anacin-3 Extra Strength[1] | |

Excedrin Extra Strength
   Caplets[2]
Exdol[1]
Exdol Strong[1]
Panadol[1]
Panadol Extra Strength[1]
Robigesic[1]
Rounox[1]
Tempra Caplets[1]
Tempra Chewable Tablets[1]
Tempra Drops[1]
Tempra Syrup[1]
Tylenol Caplets[1]
Tylenol Children's Chewable
   Tablets[1]
Tylenol Drops[1]
Tylenol Elixir[1]
Tylenol Gelcaps[1]
Tylenol Junior Strength
   Caplets[1]
Tylenol Tablets[1]

Other commonly used names are APAP and paracetamol.

This information applies to the following medicines:

1. Acetaminophen (a-seat-a-MIN-oh-fen)‡§
2. Acetaminophen and Caffeine (kaf-EEN)

---

‡Generic name product may also be available in the U.S.
§Generic name product may also be available in Canada.

---

## Description

Acetaminophen is used to relieve pain and reduce fever. Unlike aspirin, it does not relieve the redness, stiffness, or swelling caused by rheumatoid arthritis. However, it may relieve the pain caused by mild forms of arthritis.

This medicine is available without a prescription; however, your medical doctor or dentist may have special instructions on the proper dose of acetaminophen for your medical condition.

Acetaminophen is available in the following dosage forms:

*Oral*

Acetaminophen
- Capsules (U.S.)
- Oral granules (in packets) (U.S.)
- Oral liquid (drops) for babies (U.S. and Canada)
- Oral liquid for children (U.S. and Canada)
- Oral liquid for adults (U.S.)
- Oral powders (in capsules) (U.S.)
- Oral suspension (drops) for babies (U.S. and Canada)
- Oral suspension (liquid) for children (U.S. and Canada)
- Tablets (U.S. and Canada)
- Chewable tablets (U.S. and Canada)

Acetaminophen and Caffeine
- Tablets (U.S. and Canada)

*Rectal*

Acetaminophen
- Suppositories (U.S. and Canada)

---

## Before Using This Medicine

If you are taking this medicine without a prescription, carefully read and follow any precautions on the label. For acetaminophen, the following should be considered:

**Allergies**—Tell your doctor if you have ever had any unusual or allergic reaction to acetaminophen or aspirin. Also tell your health care professional if you are allergic to any other substances, such as foods, preservatives, or dyes.

**Pregnancy**—Although studies have not been done in pregnant women, acetaminophen has not been reported to cause birth defects or other problems.

**Breast-feeding**—Although acetaminophen passes into the breast milk in small amounts, it has not been reported to cause problems in nursing babies.

**Children**—This medicine has been tested in children and has not been shown to cause different side effects or problems than it does in adults. However, some children's products containing acetaminophen also contain aspartame, which may be dangerous if it is given to children with phenylketonuria.

**Older adults**—Acetaminophen has been tested and has not been shown to cause different side effects or problems in older people than it does in younger adults.

**Other medicines**—Although certain medicines should not be used together at all, in other cases two different medicines may be used together even if an interaction might occur. In these cases, your doctor may want to change the dose, or other precautions may be necessary. Tell your health care professional if you are taking any other prescription or nonprescription (over-the-counter [OTC]) medicine.

**Other medical problems**—The presence of other medical problems may affect the use of acetaminophen. Make sure you tell your doctor if you have any other medical problems, especially:

- Alcohol abuse or
- Kidney disease (severe) or
- Hepatitis or other liver disease—The chance of serious side effects may be increased
- Phenylketonuria—Some brands of acetaminophen contain aspartame, which can make your condition worse

## Proper Use of This Medicine

*Unless otherwise directed by your medical doctor or dentist:*

- *Do not take more of this medicine than is recommended on the package label.* If too much is taken, liver and kidney damage may occur.
- *Children up to 12 years of age should not take this medicine more than 5 times a day.*

To use *acetaminophen oral granules* (e.g., Snaplets-FR):

- Just before the medicine is to be taken, open the number of packets needed for one dose. Mix the granules inside of the packets with a small amount of soft food, such as applesauce, ice cream, or jam. Eat the acetaminophen granules along with the food.

To use *acetaminophen oral powders* (e.g., Feverall Sprinkle Caps [Children's or Junior Strength]):

- These capsules are not intended to be swallowed whole. Instead, just before the medicine is to be taken, open the number of capsules needed for one dose. Empty the powder from each capsule into 1 teaspoonful of water or other liquid. Drink the medicine along with the liquid. You may drink more liquid after taking the medicine. You may also mix the powder with a small amount of soft food, such as applesauce, ice cream, or jam. Eat the acetaminophen powder along with the food.

For patients using *acetaminophen suppositories:*

- If the suppository is too soft to insert, chill it in the refrigerator for 30 minutes or run cold water over it before removing the foil wrapper.
- To insert the suppository:

   —First remove the foil wrapper and moisten the suppository with cold water. Lie down on your side and use your finger to push the suppository well up into the rectum.

**Dosing**—The dose of acetaminophen will be different for different patients. *Follow your doctor's orders or the directions on the label.* The following information includes only the average doses of acetaminophen. *If your dose is different, do not change it* unless your doctor tells you to do so.

The number of capsules, tablets, teaspoonfuls of oral solution or suspension that you take, the amount of oral granules or powders that you take, or the number of suppositories that you use, depends on the strength of the medicine. Also, the number of doses you use each day and the time allowed between doses depend on the strength of the medicine.

- For *oral* dosage forms (capsules, granules, powders, solution, suspension, or tablets) and *rectal* dosage forms (suppositories):

   —For pain or fever:

   - Adults and teenagers—325 or 500 milligrams (mg) every three or four hours, 650 mg every four to six hours, or 1000 mg every six hours as needed. For short-term treatment (up to ten days), the total dose should not be more than 4000 mg (for example, eight 500-mg tablets) a day. For long-term treatment, the total dose should not be more than 2600 mg (for example, eight 325-mg tablets) a day.
   - Children—Acetaminophen dose is based on the child's age.

      —Infants up to 3 months of age: 40 mg every four hours as needed.

      —Infants 4 to 12 months of age: 80 mg every four hours as needed.

      —Children 1 to 2 years of age: 120 mg every four hours as needed.

      —Children 2 to 4 years of age: 160 mg every four hours as needed.

      —Children 4 to 6 years of age: 240 mg every four hours as needed.

      —Children 6 to 9 years of age: 320 mg every four hours as needed.

      —Children 9 to 11 years of age: 320 to 400 mg every four hours as needed.

      —Children 11 to 12 years of age: 320 to 480 mg every four hours as needed.

**Storage**—To store this medicine:
- Keep out of the reach of children.
- Store away from heat and direct light.
- Do not store acetaminophen tablets (including caplets and gelcaps), capsules, or granules in the bathroom, near the kitchen sink, or in other damp places. Heat or moisture may cause the medicine to break down.
- Keep the liquid and suppository forms of this medicine from freezing.
- Do not keep outdated medicine or medicine no longer needed. Be sure that any discarded medicine is out of the reach of children.

## Precautions While Using This Medicine

If you will be taking this medicine for a long time, especially in high doses (more than eight 325-mg or five 500-mg doses a day), your doctor should check your progress at regular visits.

Check with your medical doctor or dentist:
- If you are taking this medicine to relieve pain, including arthritis pain, and the pain lasts for more than 10 days for adults or 5 days for children or if the pain gets worse, new symptoms occur, or the painful area is red or swollen. These could be signs of a serious condition that needs medical or dental treatment.
- If you are taking this medicine to bring down a fever, and the fever lasts for more than 3 days or returns, the fever gets worse, new symptoms occur, or redness or swelling is present. These could be signs of a serious condition that needs treatment.
- If you are taking this medicine for a sore throat, and the sore throat is very painful, lasts for more than 2 days, or occurs together with or is followed by fever, headache, skin rash, nausea, or vomiting.

*Check the labels of all prescription and nonprescription (over-the-counter [OTC]) medicines you now take. If any contain acetaminophen, check with your health care professional.* Taking them together with this medicine may cause an overdose.

If you will be taking more than an occasional 1 or 2 doses of acetaminophen, *do not drink alcoholic beverages.* To do so may increase the chance of liver damage, especially if you drink large amounts of alcoholic beverages regularly, if you take more acetaminophen than is recommended on the package label, or if you take it regularly for a long time.

Taking certain other medicines together with acetaminophen may increase the chance of unwanted effects. The risk will depend on how much of each medicine you take every day, and on how long you take the medicines together. If your medical doctor or dentist directs you to take these medicines together on a regular basis, follow his or her directions carefully. However, *do not take any of the following medicines together with acetaminophen*

*for more than a few days, unless your doctor has directed you to do so and is following your progress:*

Aspirin or other salicylates
Diclofenac (e.g., Voltaren)
Diflunisal (e.g., Dolobid)
Etodolac (e.g., Lodine)
Fenoprofen (e.g., Nalfon)
Floctafenine (e.g., Idarac)
Flurbiprofen, oral (e.g., Ansaid)
Ibuprofen (e.g., Motrin)
Indomethacin (e.g., Indocin)
Ketoprofen (e.g., Orudis)
Ketorolac (e.g., Toradol)
Meclofenamate (e.g., Meclomen)
Mefenamic acid (e.g., Ponstel)
Nabumetone (e.g., Relafen)
Naproxen (e.g., Naprosyn)
Oxaprozin (e.g., Daypro)
Phenylbutazone (e.g., Butazolidin)
Piroxicam (e.g., Feldene)
Sulindac (e.g., Clinoril)
Tenoxicam (e.g., Mobiflex)
Tiaprofenic acid (e.g., Surgam)
Tolmetin (e.g., Tolectin)

Acetaminophen may interfere with the results of some medical tests. Before you have any medical tests, tell the person in charge if you have taken acetaminophen within the past 3 or 4 days. If possible, it is best to call the laboratory where the test will be done about 4 days ahead of time, to find out whether this medicine may be taken during the 3 or 4 days before the test.

For *diabetic patients:*
- Acetaminophen may cause false results with some blood glucose (sugar) tests. If you notice any change in your test results, or if you have any questions about this possible problem, check with your health care professional. This is especially important if your diabetes is not well-controlled.

For patients taking one of the products that contain *caffeine* in addition to acetaminophen:
- Caffeine may interfere with the results of a test that uses adenosine (e.g., Adenocard) or dipyridamole (e.g., Persantine) to help find out how well your blood is flowing through certain blood vessels. Therefore, you should not have any caffeine for 8 to 12 hours before the test.

*If you think that you or anyone else may have taken an overdose of acetaminophen, get emergency help at once, even if there are no signs of poisoning.* Signs of severe poisoning may not appear for 2 to 4 days after the overdose is taken, but treatment to prevent liver damage or death must be started as soon as possible. Treatment started more than 24 hours after the overdose is taken may not be effective.

## Side Effects of This Medicine

Along with its needed effects, a medicine may cause some unwanted effects. Although not all of these side effects may occur, if they do occur they may need medical attention.

*Check with your doctor immediately* if any of the following side effects occur:

*Rare*

   Yellow eyes or skin

*Symptoms of overdose*

   Diarrhea; increased sweating; loss of appetite; nausea or vomiting; stomach cramps or pain; swelling, pain, or tenderness in the upper abdomen or stomach area

Also, check with your doctor as soon as possible if any of the following side effects occur:

*Rare*

   Bloody or black, tarry stools; bloody or cloudy urine; fever with or without chills (not present before treatment and not caused by the condition being treated); pain in lower back and/or side (severe and/or sharp); pinpoint red spots on skin; skin rash, hives, or itching; sores, ulcers, or white spots on lips or in mouth; sore throat (not present before treatment and not caused by the condition being treated); sudden decrease in amount of urine; unusual bleeding or bruising; unusual tiredness or weakness

Other side effects not listed above may also occur in some patients. If you notice any other effects, check with your doctor.

Revised: 07/12/94

---

# ACETAMINOPHEN AND SALICYLATES   Systemic

Some commonly used brand names are:

**In the U.S.—**

| | |
|---|---|
| Buffets II[3] | Goody's Headache Powders[2] |
| Duoprin[6] | Presalin[5] |
| Duradyne[2] | Rid-A-Pain Compound[7] |
| Excedrin Extra-Strength | S-A-C[7] |
| Caplets[2] | Saleto[4] |
| Excedrin Extra-Strength | Supac[3] |
| Tablets[2] | Tri-Pain Caplets[4] |
| Gelpirin[3] | Vanquish Caplets[3] |
| Gemnisyn[1] | |
| Goody's Extra Strength | |
| Tablets[2] | |

Note: In Canada, Excedrin contains acetaminophen and caffeine, but no aspirin.

This information applies to the following medicines:

1. Acetaminophen and Aspirin (a-seat-a-MIN-oh-fen and AS-pir-in)[†]
2. Acetaminophen, Aspirin, and Caffeine (kaf-EEN)[†]
3. Acetaminophen, Aspirin, and Caffeine, Buffered[†]
4. Acetaminophen, Aspirin, Salicylamide (sal-i-SILL-a-mide), and Caffeine[†]
5. Acetaminophen, Aspirin, and Salicylamide, Buffered[†]
6. Acetaminophen and Salicylamide[†]
7. Acetaminophen, Salicylamide, and Caffeine[†]

   [†]Not commercially available in Canada.

## Description

Acetaminophen and salicylate combination medicines relieve pain and reduce fever. They may be used to relieve occasional pain caused by mild inflammation or arthritis (rheumatism). However, neither acetaminophen nor salicylamide is as effective as aspirin for treating chronic or severe pain, or other symptoms, caused by inflammation or arthritis. Some of these combination medicines do not contain any aspirin. Even those that do contain aspirin may not contain enough to be effective in treating these conditions.

A few reports have suggested that acetaminophen and salicylates used together may cause kidney damage or cancer of the kidney or urinary bladder. This may occur if large amounts of both medicines are taken together for a very long time. However, taking usual amounts of these combination medicines for a short time has not been shown to cause these unwanted effects. Also, these effects are not likely to occur with either acetaminophen or a salicylate used alone, even if large amounts have been taken for a long time. Therefore, for long-term use, it may be best to use either acetaminophen or a salicylate, but not both, unless you are under a doctor's care.

*Before giving any of these combination medicines to a child, check the package label very carefully. Some of these medicines are too strong for use in children.* If you are not certain whether a specific product can be given to a child, or if you have any questions about the amount to give, check with your health care professional.

These medicines are available without a prescription. However, your doctor may have special instructions on the proper dose of these medicines for your medical condition.

These medicines are available in the following dosage forms:

*Oral*

   Acetaminophen and Aspirin
   • Tablets (U.S.)
   Acetaminophen, Aspirin, and Caffeine
   • Oral powders (U.S.)
   • Tablets (U.S.)
   Acetaminophen, Aspirin, and Caffeine, Buffered
   • Tablets (U.S.)
   Acetaminophen, Aspirin, Salicylamide, and Caffeine
   • Tablets (U.S.)
   Acetaminophen, Aspirin, and Salicylamide, Buffered
   • Tablets (U.S.)
   Acetaminophen and Salicylamide
   • Capsules (U.S.)
   Acetaminophen, Salicylamide, and Caffeine
   • Capsules (U.S.)
   • Tablets (U.S.)

# Before Using This Medicine

If you are taking this medicine without a prescription, carefully read and follow any precautions on the label. For acetaminophen and salicylate combinations, the following should be considered:

**Allergies**—Tell your doctor if you have ever had any unusual or allergic reaction to acetaminophen, aspirin or other salicylates including methyl salicylate (oil of wintergreen), or to any of the following medicines:

Diclofenac (e.g., Voltaren)
Diflunisal (e.g., Dolobid)
Etodolac (e.g., Lodine)
Fenoprofen (e.g., Nalfon)
Floctafenine (e.g., Idarac)
Flurbiprofen, oral (e.g., Ansaid)
Ibuprofen (e.g., Motrin)
Indomethacin (e.g., Indocin)
Ketoprofen (e.g., Orudis)
Ketorolac (e.g., Toradol)
Meclofenamate (e.g., Meclomen)
Mefenamic acid (e.g., Ponstel)
Nabumetone (e.g., Relafen)
Naproxen (e.g., Naprosyn)
Oxaprozin (e.g., Daypro)
Oxyphenbutazone (e.g., Tandearil)
Phenylbutazone (e.g., Butazolidin)
Piroxicam (e.g., Feldene)
Sulindac (e.g., Clinoril)
Suprofen (e.g., Suprol)
Tenoxicam (e.g., Mobiflex)
Tiaprofenic acid (e.g., Surgam)
Tolmetin (e.g., Tolectin)
Zomepirac (e.g., Zomax)

Also tell your health care professional if you are allergic to any other substances, such as foods, preservatives, or dyes.

**Pregnancy**—

- *For Acetaminophen*: Studies on birth defects have not been done in humans. However, acetaminophen has not been reported to cause birth defects or other problems.

- *For Aspirin*: Studies in humans have not shown that aspirin causes birth defects. However, aspirin has been shown to cause birth defects in animals.

  *Do not take aspirin during the last 3 months of pregnancy unless it has been ordered by your doctor.* Some reports have suggested that too much use of aspirin late in pregnancy may cause a decrease in the newborn's weight and possible death of the fetus or newborn infant. However, the mothers in these reports had been taking much larger amounts of aspirin than are usually recommended. Studies of mothers taking aspirin in the doses that are usually recommended did not show these unwanted effects. However, there is a chance that regular use of aspirin late in pregnancy may cause unwanted effects on the heart or blood flow in the fetus or newborn infant.

  Use of aspirin during the last 2 weeks of pregnancy may cause bleeding problems in the fetus before or during delivery, or in the newborn infant. Also, too much use of aspirin during the last 3 months of pregnancy may increase the length of pregnancy, prolong labor, cause other problems during delivery, or cause severe bleeding in the mother before, during, or after delivery.

- *For Salicylamide*: Studies on birth defects have not been done in humans.

- *For Caffeine*: Studies in humans have not shown that caffeine causes birth defects. However, use of large amounts of caffeine by the mother during pregnancy may cause problems with the heart rhythm of the fetus and may affect the growth of the fetus. Studies in animals have shown that caffeine causes birth defects when given in very large doses (amounts equal to the amount of caffeine in 12 to 24 cups of coffee a day).

**Breast-feeding**—

- *For Acetaminophen and for Aspirin:* Acetaminophen and aspirin pass into the breast milk; however, they have not been reported to cause problems in nursing babies.

- *For Caffeine:* Caffeine (contained in some of these combination medicines) passes into the breast milk in small amounts. Taking caffeine in the amounts present in these medicines has not been reported to cause problems in nusing babies. However, studies have shown that babies may appear jittery and have trouble in sleeping when their mothers drink large amounts of caffeine-containing beverages. Therefore, breast-feeding mothers who use these medicines should probably limit the amount of caffeine they take in from other medicines or from beverages.

**Children**—

- *For Acetaminophen*: Acetaminophen has been tested in children and, in effective doses, has not been shown to cause different side effects or problems than it does in adults.

- *For Aspirin and for Salicylamide: Do not give a medicine containing aspirin or salicylamide to a child with symptoms of a virus infection, especially flu or chickenpox, without first discussing its use with your child's doctor.* This is very important because aspirin may cause a serious illness called Reye's syndrome in children with fever caused by a virus infection, especially flu or chickenpox. Children who do not have a virus infection may also be more sensitive to the effects of aspirin, especially if they have a fever or have lost large amounts of body fluid because of vomiting, diarrhea, or sweating. This may increase the chance of side effects during treatment.

- *For Caffeine*: There is no specific information comparing use of caffeine in children up to 12 years of age with use in other age groups. However, caffeine is not expected to cause different side effects or problems in children than it does in adults.

**Teenagers**—*Teenagers with fever or other symptoms of a virus infection, especially flu or chickenpox, should check with a doctor before taking this medicine. Aspirin* and salicylamide may cause a serious illness called Reye's syndrome in teenagers with fever caused by a virus infection, especially flu or chickenpox.

**Older adults**—Elderly people may be more likely than younger adults to develop serious kidney problems if they take large amounts of these combination medicines for a long time. Therefore, it is best that elderly people not take this medicine for more than 5 days in a row unless they are under a doctor's care.

- *For Acetaminophen*: Acetaminophen has been tested and, in effective doses, has not been shown to cause different side effects or problems in older people than it does in younger adults.
- *For Aspirin*: People 60 years of age and older are especially sensitive to the effects of aspirin. This may increase the chance of side effects during treatment.
- *For Caffeine*: Many medicines have not been studied specifically in older people. Therefore, it may not be known whether they work exactly the same way they do in younger adults or if they cause different side effects or problems in older people. There is no specific information comparing use of caffeine in the elderly with use in other age groups.

**Other medicines**—Although certain medicines should not be used together at all, in other cases two different medicines may be used together even if an interaction might occur. In these cases, your doctor may want to change the dose, or other precautions may be necessary. When you are taking an acetaminophen and salicylate combination, it is especially important that your health care professional know if you are taking any of the following:

- Anticoagulants (blood thinners) or
- Carbenicillin by injection (e.g., Geopen) or
- Cefamandole (e.g., Mandol) or
- Cefoperazone (e.g., Cefobid) or
- Cefotetan (e.g., Cefotan) or
- Dipyridamole (e.g., Persantine) or
- Divalproex (e.g., Depakote) or
- Heparin or
- Inflammation or pain medicine, except narcotics, or
- Pentoxifylline (e.g., Trental) or
- Plicamycin (e.g., Mithracin) or
- Ticarcillin (e.g., Ticar) or
- Valproic acid (e.g., Depakene)—Taking these medicines together with aspirin (present in some of these combination medicines) may increase the chance of serious bleeding
- Antidiabetics, oral (diabetes medicine you take by mouth)—Aspirin (present in some of these combination medicines) may increase the effects of the antidiabetic medicine; a change in dose may be needed if aspirin is taken regularly
- Ciprofloxacin (e.g., Cipro) or
- Enoxacin (e.g., Penetrex) or
- Itraconazole (e.g., Sporanox) or
- Ketoconazole (e.g., Nizoral) or
- Lomefloxacin (e.g., Maxaquin) or
- Norfloxacin (e.g., Noroxin) or
- Ofloxacin (e.g., Floxin) or
- Tetracyclines (medicine for infection), taken by mouth—Antacids (present in buffered forms of acetaminophen and salicylate combination medicines) can keep these other medicines from working properly if the medicines are taken too close together
- Methotrexate (e.g., Mexate)—Taking aspirin (present in some of these combination medicines) together with methotrexate may increase the chance of serious side effects
- Probenecid (e.g., Benemid)—Aspirin (present in some of these combination medicines) can keep probenecid from working properly for treating gout
- Sulfinpyrazone (e.g., Anturane)—Aspirin (present in some of these combination medicines) can keep sulfinpyrazone from working properly for treating gout; also, taking aspirin together with sulfinpyrazone may increase the chance of bleeding
- Urinary alkalizers (medicine that makes the urine less acid, such as acetazolamide [e.g., Diamox], calcium- and/or magnesium-containing antacids, dichlorphenamide [e.g., Daranide], methazolamide [e.g., Neptazane], potassium or sodium citrate and/or citric acid, sodium bicarbonate [baking soda])—These medicines may make aspirin (present in some of these combination medicines) less effective by causing it to be removed from the body more quickly

**Other medical problems**—The presence of other medical problems may affect the use of acetaminophen and salicylate combinations. Make sure you tell your doctor if you have any other medical problems, especially:

- Alcohol abuse or
- Asthma, allergies, and nasal polyps (history of) or
- Hepatitis or other liver disease or
- Kidney disease—The chance of serious side effects may be increased
- Anemia or
- Stomach ulcer or other stomach problems—Aspirin (present in some of these combination medicines) may make these conditions worse
- Gout—Aspirin (present in some of these combination medicines) can make this condition worse and can also lessen the effects of some medicines used to treat gout
- Heart disease—Caffeine (present in some of these combination medicines) can make your condition worse
- Hemophilia or other bleeding problems—Aspirin (present in some of these combination medicines) increases the chance of serious bleeding

## Proper Use of This Medicine

*Take this medicine with food or a full glass (8 ounces) of water* to lessen the chance of stomach upset.

Unless otherwise directed by your doctor:

- *Do not take more of this medicine than directed on the package label.* Taking too much acetaminophen may cause liver damage or lead to other medical problems because of an overdose. Also, taking too much aspirin can cause stomach problems or lead to other medical problems because of an overdose.
- *Children up to 12 years of age should not take this medicine more often than 5 times a day.*

*Check with your doctor before taking one of these combination medicines to treat severe or chronic inflammation or arthritis (rheumatism). These combination* medicines may not relieve the severe pain, redness, swelling, or stiffness caused by these conditions unless very large amounts are taken for a long time. *It is best not to take acetaminophen and salicylate combination medicines in large amounts for a long time* unless you are under a doctor's care.

*If a combination medicine containing aspirin has a strong vinegar-like odor, do not use it.* This odor means the medicine is breaking down. If you have any questions about this, check with your pharmacist.

**Dosing**—The dose of acetaminophen and salicylate combination medicines will be different for different patients. *Follow your doctor's orders or the directions on the label.* The following information includes only the average doses of these combination medicines. *If your dose is different, do not change it* unless your doctor tells you to do so.

The number of capsules, tablets (including caplets), or packets of oral powders that you take depends on the total amount of acetaminophen and salicylate (aspirin and/or salicylamide) in one capsule, tablet, or packet of oral powder. Also, the number of doses you take each day and the time allowed between doses depend on the strength of the medicine.

- For *oral capsule or tablet (including caplet)* dosage forms:
  —For pain, fever, or mild arthritis symptoms:
    - Adults and teenagers—The usual dose is 1 or 2 capsules or tablets every three, four, or six hours, depending on the strength of the product. Do not take any of these combination medicines for more than ten days, unless otherwise directed by your doctor.
    - Children—Use and dose must be determined by your doctor.
- For *oral powder* dosage form:
  —For pain, fever, or mild arthritis symptoms:
    - Adults and teenagers—This medicine is very strong. Each packet of powder contains 260 mg of acetaminophen and 500 mg of aspirin (a total of 760 mg of both medicines). The usual dose is one packet of powder every six hours. Do not take this medicine for more than ten days, unless otherwise directed by your doctor.
    - Children—The oral powder dosage form is too strong to use in children 12 years of age or younger.

**Storage**—To store this medicine:
- Keep out of the reach of children. Overdose of the salicylates in these combination medicines is very dangerous in young children.
- Store away from heat and direct light.
- Do not store tablets (including caplets), capsules, or powders in the bathroom, near the kitchen sink, or in other damp places. Heat or moisture may cause the medicine to break down.

- Do not keep outdated medicine or medicine no longer needed. Be sure that any discarded medicine is out of the reach of children.

---

## Precautions While Using This Medicine

If you will be taking this medicine for a long time, or in high doses, *your doctor should check your progress at regular visits.* This is especially important for elderly people, who may be more likely than younger adults to develop serious kidney problems if they take large amounts of this medicine for a long time.

Check with your doctor:
- If you are taking this medicine to relieve pain and the pain lasts for more than 10 days (5 days for children), if the pain gets worse, if new symptoms occur, or if the painful area is red or swollen. These could be signs of a serious condition that needs treatment.
- If you are taking this medicine to bring down a fever, and the fever lasts for more than 3 days or returns, if your fever gets worse, if new symptoms occur, or if redness or swelling is present. These could be signs of a serious condition that needs treatment.
- If you are taking this medicine for a sore throat, and the sore throat is very painful, lasts for more than 2 days, or occurs together with or is followed by fever, headache, skin rash, nausea, or vomiting.

Do not take any of the combination medicines containing aspirin for 5 days before any surgery, including dental surgery, unless otherwise directed by your medical doctor or dentist. Taking aspirin during this time may cause bleeding problems.

*Check the label of all over-the-counter (OTC), nonprescription, and prescription medicines you now take.* If any of them contain acetaminophen, aspirin, other salicylates such as bismuth subsalicylate (e.g., Pepto Bismol) or magnesium salicylate (e.g., Nuprin Backache Caplets), or salicylic acid (present in some shampoos and skin products), *check with your health care professional. Using any of them together with this medicine may cause an overdose.*

*If you will be taking more than an occasional 1 or 2 doses of this medicine, do not drink alcoholic beverages.* Stomach problems may be more likely to occur if you drink alcoholic beverages while you are taking aspirin. Also, liver damage may be more likely to occur if you drink large amounts of alcoholic beverages while you are taking acetaminophen.

Taking certain other medicines together with acetaminophen and salicylates may increase the chance of unwanted effects. The risk will depend on how much of each medicine you take every day, and on how long you take the medicines together. If your medical doctor or dentist directs you to take these medicines together on a regular basis, follow his or her directions carefully. However, *do not take any of the following medicines together with any of these combination medicines for more than a few days, unless your doctor has directed you to do so and is following your progress:*

Diclofenac (e.g., Voltaren)
Diflunisal (e.g., Dolobid)
Etodolac (e.g., Lodine)
Fenoprofen (e.g., Nalfon)
Floctafenine (e.g., Idarac)
Flurbiprofen, oral (e.g., Ansaid)
Ibuprofen (e.g., Motrin)
Indomethacin (e.g., Indocin)
Ketoprofen (e.g., Orudis)
Ketorolac (e.g., Toradol)
Meclofenamate (e.g., Meclomen)
Mefenamic acid (e.g., Ponstel)
Nabumetone (e.g., Relafen)
Naproxen (e.g., Naprosyn)
Oxaprozin (e.g., Daypro)
Phenylbutazone (e.g., Butazolidin)
Piroxicam (e.g., Feldene)
Sulindac (e.g., Clinoril)
Tenoxicam (e.g., Mobiflex)
Tiaprofenic acid (e.g., Surgam)
Tolmetin (e.g., Tolectin)

The antacid present in buffered forms of these combination medicines can keep other medicines from working properly. If you need to take a buffered form of this medicine, and you are also taking one of the following medicines, *be sure to take the buffered acetaminophen and salicylate combination medicine:*

- *At least 6 hours before or 2 hours after taking ciprofloxacin (e.g., Cipro) or lomefloxacin (e.g., Maxaquin).*
- *At least 8 hours before or 2 hours after taking enoxacin (e.g., Penetrex).*
- *At least 2 hours after taking itraconazole (e.g., Sporanox).*
- *At least 3 hours before or after taking ketoconazole (e.g., Nizoral).*
- *At least 2 hours before or after taking norfloxacin (e.g., Noroxin) or ofloxacin (e.g., Floxin).*
- *At least 3 or 4 hours before or after taking a tetracycline antibiotic by mouth.*
- *At least 1 or 2 hours before or after taking any other medicine by mouth.*

If you are taking a laxative containing cellulose, do not take it within 2 hours of taking this medicine. Taking the laxative and this medicine close together may make this medicine less effective by preventing the salicylate in it from being absorbed by your body.

Acetaminophen and salicylate combinations may interfere with the results of some medical tests. Before you have any medical tests, tell the person in charge if you have taken any of these combination medicines within the past 3 or 4 days. If possible, it is best to call the laboratory where the test will be done about 4 days ahead of time, to find out whether the medicine may be taken during the 3 or 4 days before the test.

For diabetic patients:

- Acetaminophen and salicylate combinations may cause false results with some blood and urine glucose (sugar) tests. If you notice any change in your test results, or if you have any questions about this possible problem, check with your health care professional. This is especially important if your diabetes is not well-controlled.

For patients taking one of the products that contain *caffeine:*

- Caffeine may interfere with the results of a test that uses adenosine (e.g., Adenocard) or dipyridamole (e.g., Persantine) to help find out how well your blood is flowing through certain blood vessels. Therefore, you should not have any caffeine for 8 to 12 hours before the test.

*If you think that you or anyone else may have taken an overdose of this medicine, get emergency help at once.* Taking an overdose of a salicylate may cause unconsciousness or death. The first symptom of an aspirin overdose may be ringing or buzzing in the ears. Other signs include convulsions (seizures), hearing loss, confusion, severe drowsiness or tiredness, severe excitement or nervousness, and unusually fast or deep breathing. Signs of severe acetaminophen overdose may not appear until 2 to 4 days after the overdose is taken, but treatment to prevent liver damage or death must be started within 24 hours or less after the overdose is taken.

---

## Side Effects of This Medicine

Along with its needed effects, a medicine may cause some unwanted effects. Although not all of these side effects may occur, if they do occur they may need medical attention.

*Check with your doctor immediately if any of the following side effects occur:*

*Less common or rare*

Difficulty in swallowing; dizziness, lightheadedness, or feeling faint (severe); flushing, redness, or other change in skin color; shortness of breath, troubled breathing, tightness in chest, or wheezing; sudden decrease in amount of urine; swelling of eyelids, face, or lips

*Signs and symptoms of overdose*

Agitation, anxiety, excitement, irritability, nervousness, or restlessness; any loss of hearing; bloody urine; confusion or delirium; convulsions (seizures); diarrhea (severe or continuing); dizziness or lightheadedness; drowsiness (severe); fast or deep breathing; fast or irregular heartbeat (for medicines containing caffeine); frequent urination (for medicines containing caffeine); hallucinations (seeing, hearing, or feeling things that are not there); headache (severe or continuing); increased sensitivity to touch or pain (for medicines containing caffeine); increased sweating; increased thirst; loss of appetite; muscle trembling or twitching (for medicines containing caffeine); nausea or vomiting (continuing, sometimes with blood); ringing or buzzing in ears (continuing); seeing flashes of "zig-zag" lights (for medicines containing caffeine);

stomach cramps or pain (severe or continuing); swelling, pain, or tenderness in the upper abdomen or stomach area; trouble in sleeping (for medicines containing caffeine); uncontrollable flapping movements of the hands, especially in elderly patients; unexplained fever; vision problems

*Signs of overdose in children*

Changes in behavior; drowsiness or tiredness (severe); fast or deep breathing

Also, check with your doctor as soon as possible if any of the following side effects occur:

*Less common or rare*

Bloody or black, tarry stools; bloody or cloudy urine; fever with or without chills (not present before treatment and not caused by the condition being treated); pain in lower back and/or side (severe and/or sharp); pinpoint red spots on skin; skin rash, hives, or itching; sores, ulcers, or white spots on lips or in mouth; sore throat (not present before treatment and not caused by the condition being treated); swelling of face, fingers, feet, or lower legs; unusual bleeding or bruising; unusual tiredness or weakness; vomiting of blood or material that looks like coffee grounds; weight gain; yellow eyes or skin

Other side effects may occur that usually do not need medical attention. These side effects may go away during treatment as your body adjusts to the medicine. However, check with your doctor if any of the following side effects continue or are bothersome:

*More common*

Heartburn or indigestion (for medicines containing aspirin); nausea, vomiting, or stomach pain (for medicines containing aspirin)

*Less common*

Drowsiness (for medicines containing salicylamide); trouble in sleeping, nervousness, or jitters (for medicines containing caffeine)

Some side effects may occur after you have stopped taking these combination medicines, especially if you have taken large amounts of them for a long time. *Check with your doctor immediately* if any of these side effects occur after you have stopped taking these medicines:

*Rare*

Bloody or cloudy urine; decreased urination; swelling of face, fingers, feet, or lower legs; weight gain

Other side effects not listed above may also occur in some patients. If you notice any other effects, check with your doctor.

Revised: 07/12/94

# ACETAMINOPHEN, SODIUM BICARBONATE, AND CITRIC ACID   Systemic†

A commonly used brand name in the U.S. is Bromo-Seltzer.

†Not commercially available in Canada.

## Description

Acetaminophen, sodium bicarbonate, and citric acid (a-seat-a-MIN-oh-fen, SOE-dee-um bi-KAR-boe-nate, and SI-trik AS-id) combination is used to relieve pain occurring together with heartburn, sour stomach, or acid indigestion. The acetaminophen in this combination medicine is the pain reliever. The sodium bicarbonate in this medicine is an antacid. It neutralizes stomach acid by combining with it to form a new substance that is not an acid.

This medicine is available without a prescription; however, your doctor may have special instructions on the proper dose for your medical condition.

Acetaminophen, sodium bicarbonate, and citric acid combination is available in the following dosage form:

*Oral*

• Effervescent granules (U.S.)

## Before Using This Medicine

If you are taking this medicine without a prescription, carefully read and follow any precautions on the label. For acetaminophen, sodium bicarbonate, and citric acid combination, the following should be considered:

**Allergies**—Tell your doctor if you have ever had any unusual or allergic reaction to acetaminophen or aspirin, or to sodium bicarbonate. Also tell your health care professional if you are allergic to any other substances, such as foods, preservatives, or dyes.

**Diet**—Make certain your health care professional knows if you are on a low-sodium, low-sugar, or any other special diet. This medicine contains a large amount of sodium (more than 750 mg for each 325 mg of acetaminophen).

**Pregnancy**—Although studies on birth defects have not been done in humans, the ingredients in this combination medicine have not been reported to cause birth defects in humans. However, you should avoid this medicine if you tend to retain (keep) body water because the sodium in it can cause the body to hold water. This can result in swelling and weight gain.

**Breast-feeding**—Acetaminophen passes into the breast milk in small amounts. However, acetaminophen, sodium bicarbonate, and citric acid have not been reported to cause problems in nursing babies.

**Children**—Acetaminophen has been tested in children and has not been shown to cause different side effects or problems than it does in adults. However, sodium bicarbonate should not be given to young children (under 6 years of age) unless ordered by their doctor. Small children with stomach problems usually cannot describe their symptoms very well. They should be checked by a doctor, because they may have a condition that needs other treatment.

**Older adults**—Acetaminophen has been tested and has not been shown to cause different side effects or problems in older people than it does in younger adults. However, the large amount of sodium in this combination medicine can be harmful to some elderly people. Therefore, it is best that older people not use this medicine for more than 5 days in a row, unless otherwise directed by their doctor.

**Other medicines**—Although certain medicines should not be used together at all, in other cases two different medicines may be used together even if an interaction might occur. In these cases, your doctor may want to change the dose, or other precautions may be necessary. When you are taking this combination medicine, it is especially important that your health care professional know if you are taking any of the following:

- Alcohol—The chance of liver damage may be increased
- Ciprofloxacin (e.g., Cipro) or
- Enoxacin (e.g., Penetrex) or
- Itraconazole (e.g., Sporanox) or
- Ketoconazole (e.g., Nizoral) or
- Lomefloxacin (e.g., Maxaquin) or
- Methenamine (e.g., Mandelamine) or
- Norfloxacin (e.g., Noroxin) or
- Ofloxacin (e.g., Floxin) or
- Tetracyclines (medicine for infection), taken by mouth— Sodium bicarbonate can keep these medicines from working properly
- Mecamylamine (e.g., Inversine)—Sodium bicarbonate can increase the risk of unwanted effects by causing mecamylamine to stay in your body longer than usual

**Other medical problems**—The presence of other medical problems may affect the use of acetaminophen, sodium bicarbonate, and citric acid combination. Make sure you tell your doctor if you have any other medical problems, especially:

- Alcohol abuse or
- Hepatitis or other liver disease—The chance of serious side effects, including liver damage, may be increased
- Appendicitis (symptoms of, such as stomach or lower abdominal pain, cramping, bloating, soreness, nausea, or vomiting)—Sodium bicarbonate can make your condition worse; also, people who may have appendicitis need medical attention and should not try to treat themselves
- Edema (swelling of face, fingers, feet, or lower legs caused by too much water in the body) or
- Heart disease or
- High blood pressure or
- Toxemia of pregnancy—The sodium in this combination medicine can make these conditions worse

- Kidney disease—The chance of serious side effects may be increased

## Proper Use of This Medicine

*Unless otherwise directed by your doctor, do not take more of this medicine than is recommended on the package label.* If too much is taken, liver damage or other serious side effects may occur.

To use this medicine:

- This medicine must be taken in the form of a liquid that is made from the effervescent granules. Do not swallow the granules themselves.
- To make the liquid, pour the amount of effervescent granules directed on the package into a glass. Then add ½ glass (4 ounces) of cool water.
- Drink all of the liquid. You may drink the liquid while it is still fizzing or after the fizzing stops.
- Add a little more water to the glass and drink that, to make sure that you get the full amount of the medicine.

**Dosing**—The dose of this combination medicine will be different for different people. *Follow your doctor's orders or the directions on the label.* The following information includes only the average doses of the acetaminophen in this combination medicine. *If your dose is different, do not change it* unless your doctor tells you to do so.

- For *oral* dosage form (effervescent granules):
    —For pain and upset stomach:
    - Adults and teenagers—325 to 650 milligrams (mg) of acetaminophen, dissolved in water, every four hours as needed. The bottle cap can be used to measure the dose. There are 325 mg of acetaminophen in three-fourths of a capful.
    - Children—Use and dose must be determined by your doctor.

**Missed dose**—If your doctor has directed you to take this medicine according to a regular schedule and you miss a dose, take it as soon as you remember. However, if it is almost time for your next dose, skip the missed dose and go back to your regular dosing schedule. Do not double doses.

**Storage**—To store this medicine:

- Keep out of the reach of children.
- Store away from heat and direct light.
- Do not store this medicine in the bathroom, near the kitchen sink, or in other damp places. Heat or moisture may cause the medicine to break down.
- Do not keep outdated medicine or medicine no longer needed. Be sure that any discarded medicine is out of the reach of children.

## Precautions While Using This Medicine

If you will be taking this medicine for a long time (more than 10 days in a row), your doctor should check your progress at regular visits.

Check with your doctor if your pain and/or upset stomach last for more than 10 days or if they get worse, if new symptoms occur, or if the painful area is red or swollen. These could be signs of a serious condition that needs medical treatment.

The sodium bicarbonate in this combination medicine can keep other medicines from working properly if the 2 medicines are taken too close together. *Always take this medicine:*

- *At least 6 hours before or 2 hours after taking ciprofloxacin (e.g., Cipro) or lomefloxacin (e.g., Maxaquin).*
- *At least 8 hours before or 2 hours after taking enoxacin (e.g., Penetrex).*
- *At least 2 hours after taking itraconazole (e.g., Sporanox).*
- *At least 3 hours before or after taking ketoconazole (e.g., Nizoral).*
- *At least 2 hours before or after taking norfloxacin (e.g., Noroxin) or ofloxacin (e.g., Floxin).*
- *At least 3 or 4 hours before or after taking a tetracycline antibiotic by mouth.*
- *At least 1 or 2 hours before or after taking any other medicine by mouth.*

*Check the labels of all nonprescription (over-the-counter [OTC]) and prescription medicines you now take. If any contain acetaminophen or sodium, check with your health care professional.* Taking them together with this medicine may cause an overdose.

Taking certain other medicines together with acetaminophen may increase the chance of unwanted effects. The risk will depend on how much of each medicine you take every day, and on how long you take the medicines together. If your medical doctor or dentist directs you to take these medicines together on a regular basis, follow his or her directions carefully. However, *do not take any of the following medicines together with acetaminophen for more than a few days, unless your doctor has directed you to do so and is following your progress:*

Aspirin or other salicylates
Diclofenac (e.g., Voltaren)
Diflunisal (e.g., Dolobid)
Etodolac (e.g., Lodine)
Fenoprofen (e.g., Nalfon)
Floctafenine (e.g., Idarac)
Flurbiprofen, oral (e.g., Ansaid)
Ibuprofen (e.g., Motrin)
Indomethacin (e.g., Indocin)
Ketoprofen (e.g., Orudis)
Ketorolac (e.g., Toradol)
Meclofenamate (e.g., Meclomen)
Mefenamic acid (e.g., Ponstel)
Nabumetone (e.g., Relafen)
Naproxen (e.g., Naprosyn)
Oxaprozin (e.g., Daypro)
Phenylbutazone (e.g., Butazolidin)
Piroxicam (e.g., Feldene)
Sulindac (e.g., Clinoril)
Tenoxicam (e.g., Mobiflex)
Tiaprofenic acid (e.g., Surgam)
Tolmetin (e.g., Tolectin)

If you will be taking more than an occasional 1 or 2 doses of this medicine:

- *Do not drink alcoholic beverages.* Drinking alcoholic beverages while you are taking acetaminophen may increase the chance of liver damage, especially if you drink large amounts of alcoholic beverages regularly, if you take more acetaminophen than is recommended on the package label, or if you take it regularly for a long time.
- *Do not also drink a lot of milk or eat a lot of milk products.* To do so may increase the chance of side effects.
- To prevent side effects caused by too much sodium in the body, you may need to limit the amount of sodium in the foods you eat. Some foods that contain large amounts of sodium are canned soup, canned vegetables, pickles, ketchup, green and ripe (black) olives, relish, frankfurters and other sausage-type meats, soy sauce, and carbonated beverages. If you have any questions about this, check with your health care professional.

Acetaminophen may interfere with the results of some medical tests. Before you have any medical tests, tell the person in charge if you have taken acetaminophen within the past 3 or 4 days. If possible, it is best to call the laboratory where the test will be done about 4 days ahead of time, to find out whether this medicine may be taken during the 3 or 4 days before the test.

For diabetic patients:

- Acetaminophen may cause false results with some blood glucose (sugar) tests. If you notice any change in your test results, or if you have any questions about this possible problem, check with your health care professional. This is especially important if your diabetes is not well-controlled.

*If you think that you or anyone else may have taken an overdose of this medicine, get emergency help at once, even if there are no signs of poisoning.* Signs of severe acetaminophen poisoning may not appear for 2 to 4 days after the overdose is taken, but treatment to prevent liver damage or death must be started as soon as possible. Treatment started more than 24 hours after the overdose is taken may not be effective.

## Side Effects of This Medicine

Along with its needed effects, a medicine may cause some unwanted effects. Although the following side effects occur very rarely when 1 or 2 doses of this combination medicine is taken occasionally, they may be more likely to occur if:

- too much medicine is taken.
- the medicine is taken several times a day.
- the medicine is taken for more than a few days in a row.

*Check with your doctor immediately* if any of the following side effects occur:

*Rare*
Yellow eyes or skin

*Symptoms of overdose*
Diarrhea; increased sweating; loss of appetite; nausea or vomiting; stomach cramps or pain; swelling, pain, or tenderness in the upper abdomen or stomach area

Also, check with your doctor as soon as possible if any of the following side effects occur:

*Less common or rare*
Bloody or black, tarry stools; bloody or cloudy urine, frequent urge to urinate, or sudden decrease in amount of urine; fever with or without chills (not present before treatment and not caused by the condition being treated); headache (continuing); increased blood pressure; mood or mental changes; muscle pain or twitching; nervousness or restlessness; pain (severe and/or sharp) in lower back and/or side; skin rash, hives, or itching; slow breathing; sores, ulcers, or white spots on lips or in mouth; sore throat (not present before treatment and not caused by the condition being treated); swelling of face, fingers, ankles, feet, or lower legs; unpleasant taste; unusual bleeding or bruising; unusual tiredness or weakness; weight gain

Other side effects may occur that usually do not need medical attention. These side effects may go away during treatment as your body adjusts to the medicine. However, check with your doctor if any of the following side effects continue or are bothersome:

*Less common*
Increased thirst

Other side effects not listed above may also occur in some patients. If you notice any other effects, check with your doctor.

Revised: 07/12/94

# ACETOHYDROXAMIC ACID   Systemic†

A commonly used brand name in the U.S. is Lithostat.

†Not commercially available in Canada.

## Description

Acetohydroxamic acid (a-SEE-toe-hye-drox-AM-ik AS-id) is used to keep kidney stones from forming and to stop the growth of existing stones. Such stone build-up is often caused by certain bacterial infections.

The bacteria produce an enzyme that makes the urine too alkaline. Under such conditions, kidney stones tend to form and, once formed, to grow in size. Acetohydroxamic acid stops the enzyme action and so reduces the chance for stones to form. This medicine is not used to dissolve existing stones and is not used in place of surgery. It is sometimes used to make antibiotics or similar medicines work better when treating kidney or urinary tract infections.

Acetohydroxamic acid is available only with your doctor's prescription, in the following dosage form:

*Oral*
• Tablets (U.S.)

## Before Using This Medicine

In deciding to use a medicine, the risks of taking the medicine must be weighed against the good it will do. This is a decision you and your doctor will make. For acetohydroxamic acid, the following should be considered:

**Allergies**—Tell your doctor if you have ever had any unusual or allergic reaction to acetohydroxamic acid. Also tell your health care professional if you are allergic to any other substances, such as foods, preservatives, or dyes.

**Pregnancy**—Acetohydroxamic acid should not be used during pregnancy since it has been shown to cause serious birth defects in animals. Effective methods of contraception (birth control) must be used during treatment with this medicine to prevent a pregnancy that could result in birth defects. Be sure you have discussed this with your doctor.

**Breast-feeding**—It is not known whether acetohydroxamic acid passes into the breast milk. Although no problems have been reported in nursing babies, its use in breast-feeding mothers is not recommended.

**Children**—Although there is no specific information comparing use of acetohydroxamic acid in children with use in other age groups, it is not expected to cause different side effects or problems in children than it does in adults.

**Older adults**—Many medicines have not been studied specifically in older people. Therefore, it may not be known whether they work exactly the same way they do in younger adults or if they cause different side effects or problems in older people. There is no specific information comparing use of acetohydroxamic acid in the elderly with use in other age groups.

**Other medicines**—Although certain medicines should not be used together at all, in many cases two different medicines may be used together even if an interaction might occur. In these cases, your doctor may want to change the dose, or other precautions may be necessary. When you are taking acetohydroxamic acid it is especially important that your health care professional know if you are taking the following:

- Iron supplements or any other medicine containing iron, taken by mouth—Use with acetohydroxamic acid may decrease effects of both medicines; iron supplements by injection may be needed

**Other medical problems**—The presence of other medical problems may affect the use of acetohydroxamic acid. Make sure you tell your doctor if you have any other medical problems, especially:

- Anemia or other blood disorders or
- Blood clots (history of) or
- Phlebitis (vein inflammation)—If you have one of these conditions, use of acetohydroxamic acid increases the risk of problems occurring
- Other kidney disorders—Higher blood levels of acetohydroxamic acid may result and a change in your dose may be needed

## Proper Use of This Medicine

*Acetohydroxamic acid works best when taken on an empty stomach.* Take the medicine 1 hour before or 2 hours after meals if possible.

*Take this medicine exactly as ordered by your doctor.* This is especially important because it is used along with antibiotics or other medicine to clear up the infection.

*Do not miss any doses.* Skipped doses may delay treatment progress and your recovery. When too many doses are missed, stone formation and growth may start again. Remember that this medicine is intended to prevent kidney stones and the surgery that is sometimes required to remove them.

**Dosing**—The dose of acetohydroxamic acid will be different for different patients. *Follow your doctor's orders or the directions on the label.* The following information includes only the average doses of acetohydroxamic acid. *If your dose is different, do not change it* unless your doctor tells you to do so.

- *To prevent kidney stones:*
  —For *oral* dosage form (tablets):
  - Adults—250 milligrams (mg) taken every six to eight hours. The dose is usually not more than 1500 mg a day.
  - Children—Dose is based on body weight and must be determined by your doctor. The dose is usually 10 mg per kilogram (kg) (4.5 mg per pound) of body weight a day.

**Missed dose**—If you miss a dose of acetohydroxamic acid, take it as soon as possible. Then go back to your regular dosing schedule. Do not double doses.

**Storage**—To store this medicine:

- Keep out of the reach of children.
- Store away from heat and direct light.
- Do not store in the bathroom, near the kitchen sink, or in other damp places. Heat or moisture may cause the medicine to break down.
- Do not keep outdated medicine or medicine no longer needed. Be sure that any discarded medicine is out of the reach of children.

## Precautions While Using This Medicine

Your doctor should check your progress at regular visits to make sure that this medicine is working properly and does not cause unwanted effects.

*Do not take any form of iron by mouth while you are taking acetohydroxamic acid.* Taking the 2 medicines together will keep both medicines from working properly.

*Do not drink alcoholic beverages while you are taking acetohydroxamic acid.* To do so may cause a rash to appear on the arms and face about 30 to 45 minutes after you drink the alcohol. Also, the skin may become flushed and feel warm and tingling. This reaction lasts about 30 minutes and can be very strong in some patients.

*If you suspect you may have become pregnant during treatment with acetohydroxamic acid, stop taking the medicine immediately and check with your doctor.*

## Side Effects of This Medicine

Along with its needed effects, a medicine may cause some unwanted effects. The following side effects may be caused by blood clots. If they occur, they need immediate medical attention. *Stop taking this medicine and get emergency help immediately* if any of the following side effects occur:

*More common*

Headache (severe or sudden); loss of coordination (sudden); pains in chest, groin, or legs (especially in calves of legs); shortness of breath (sudden); slurred speech (sudden); vision changes (sudden)

Other side effects may occur that require medical attention. Check with your doctor as soon as possible if any of the following side effects occur:

*More common*

Anxiety, confusion, or mental depression; loss of appetite; nausea or vomiting; nervousness, shakiness, or tremors; unusual tiredness or weakness

Other side effects may occur that usually do not need medical attention. These side effects may go away during treatment as your body adjusts to the medicine. However,

check with your doctor if any of the following side effects continue or are bothersome:

*More common*
    General feeling of discomfort or illness; headache (mild)
*Less common*
    Hair loss; skin rash (non-itching) on arms and face

Other side effects not listed above may also occur in some patients. If you notice any other effects, check with your doctor at once.

Revised: 12/11/92
Interim revision: 06/13/94

# ACETYLCYSTEINE   Inhalation

Some commonly used brand names are:
**In the U.S.—**
    Mucomyst                    Mucosil-10
    Mucomyst-10                 Mucosil-20
    Generic name product may also be available.
**In Canada—**
    Mucomyst

## Description

Acetylcysteine (a-se-teel-SIS-teen) belongs to the group of medicines called mucolytics (medicines that destroy or dissolve mucus). It is usually given by inhalation but may be given in other ways in a hospital.

Acetylcysteine is used to help make breathing easier in conditions such as bronchitis, emphysema, tuberculosis, and other lung diseases. It may also be used in patients with a tracheostomy. Acetylcysteine liquefies (thins) or dissolves mucus so that it may be coughed up. Sometimes the mucus may have to be removed by suction.

This medicine is available only with your doctor's prescription, in the following dosage form:

*Inhalation*
    • Solution (U.S. and Canada)

## Before Using This Medicine

In deciding to use a medicine, the risks of taking the medicine must be weighed against the good it will do. This is a decision you and your doctor will make. For acetylcysteine, the following should be considered:

**Allergies**—Tell your doctor if you have ever had any unusual or allergic reaction to acetylcysteine. Also tell your health care professional if you are allergic to any other substances, such as foods, preservatives, or dyes.

**Pregnancy**—Acetylcysteine has not been studied in pregnant women. However, acetylcysteine has not been shown to cause birth defects or other problems in animal studies when given in doses larger than the recommended human dose.

**Breast-feeding**—It is not known whether acetylcysteine passes into the breast milk. Although most medicines pass into breast milk in small amounts, many of them may be used safely while breast-feeding. Mothers who are taking

this medicine and who wish to breast-feed should discuss this with their doctor.

**Children**—Although there is no specific information comparing use of acetylcysteine in children with use in other age groups, this medicine is not expected to cause different side effects or problems in children than it does in adults.

**Older adults**—Many medicines have not been studied specifically in older people. Therefore, it may not be known whether they work exactly the same way they do in younger adults or if they cause different side effects or problems in older people. There is no specific information comparing use of acetylcysteine in the elderly with use in other age groups.

**Other medical problems**—The presence of other medical problems may affect the use of acetylcysteine. Make sure you tell your doctor if you have any other medical problems, especially:
    • Asthma or
    • Other lung disease—Acetylcysteine may make the condition worse

## Proper Use of This Medicine

*Use acetylcysteine only as directed*. Do not use more of it and do not use it more often than your doctor ordered. To do so may increase the chance of side effects.

If you are using this medicine at home, make sure you understand exactly how to use it. If you have any questions about this, check with your doctor.

After using acetylcysteine, try to cough up the loosened or thinned mucus. If this does not work, it may have to be suctioned out. This will prevent too much mucus from building up in the lungs. If you have any questions about this, check with your doctor.

**Dosing**—The dose of acetylcysteine will be different for different patients. *Follow your doctor's orders or the directions on the label.* The following information includes only the average doses of acetylcysteine. *If your dose is different, do not change it* unless your doctor tells you to do so.

The amount of solution that you use depends on the strength of the medicine and the method of inhalation used. Also, *the number of doses you use each day, the time allowed between doses, and the length of time you use the medicine depend on the medical problem for which you are using acetylcysteine.*

- For *inhalation* dosage form (solution):
    —To thin or dissolve mucus in lung diseases:
    - Adults and children—
        —3 to 5 milliliters (mL) of a 20% solution or 6 to 10 mL of a 10% solution used in a nebulizer three or four times a day. The medicine is inhaled through a face mask, mouth piece, or tracheostomy.
        —The 10 or 20% solution may be used for inhalation as a heavy mist in a tent or croupette.
        —Sometimes the 10 or 20% solution is placed directly into the trachea or through a catheter into the trachea for certain conditions.
    —For use in tests to diagnose lung problems:
    - Adults and children—1 to 2 mL of a 20% solution or 2 to 4 mL of a 10% solution used for inhalation or placed directly into the trachea for two or three times before the test.

**Missed dose**—If you miss a dose of this medicine, use it as soon as possible. Then use any remaining doses for that day at regularly spaced intervals.

**Storage**—To store this medicine:
- Keep out of the reach of children.
- Before the container is opened, store it away from heat and direct light.
- After the container is opened, store it in the refrigerator. However, keep the medicine from freezing. The opened container should be discarded after 96 hours.
- Do not keep outdated medicine or medicine no longer needed. Be sure that any discarded medicine is out of the reach of children.

## Precautions While Using This Medicine

*If your condition does not improve or if it becomes worse, check with your doctor.*

## Side Effects of This Medicine

Along with its needed effects, a medicine may cause some unwanted effects. Although not all of these side effects may occur, if they do occur they may need medical attention.

Check with your doctor as soon as possible if any of the following side effects occur:

*Less common*
    Spitting up blood; wheezing, tightness in chest, or difficulty in breathing (especially in asthma patients)

*Rare*
    Skin rash or other irritation

Other side effects may occur that usually do not need medical attention. These side effects may go away during treatment as your body adjusts to the medicine. However, check with your doctor if any of the following side effects continue or are bothersome:

*Less common*
    Clammy skin; fever; increase in amount of mucus in lungs; irritation or soreness of mouth, throat, or lungs; nausea or vomiting; runny nose

For patients using a face mask for inhalation of acetylcysteine:
- The mask may leave a stickiness on your face. This can be removed with water.

When you use acetylcysteine, you may notice that the medicine has an unpleasant odor at first. However, this smell will go away soon after you use the medicine.

Other side effects not listed above may also occur in some patients. If you notice any other effects, check with your doctor.

Revised: 08/03/93
Interim revision: 04/29/94

# ACYCLOVIR   Systemic

Some commonly used brand names are:
**In the U.S.—**
    Zovirax
**In Canada—**
    Avirax                          Zovirax
Other commonly used names are aciclovir.

## Description

Acyclovir (ay-SYE-kloe-veer) belongs to the family of medicines called antivirals, which are used to treat infections caused by viruses. Usually these medicines work for only one kind or group of virus infections.

Acyclovir is used to treat the symptoms of herpes virus infections of the genitals (sex organs), the skin, the brain, and mucous membranes (lips and mouth). Acyclovir is also used to treat chickenpox and shingles. Although acyclovir will not cure herpes, it does help relieve the pain and discomfort and helps the sores (if any) heal faster.

Acyclovir may also be used for other virus infections as determined by your doctor. However, it does not work in treating certain viruses, such as the common cold.

Acyclovir is available only with your doctor's prescription, in the following dosage forms:

*Oral*
- Capsules (U.S. and Canada)
- Oral suspension (U.S. and Canada)
- Tablets (U.S. and Canada)

*Parenteral*
- Injection (U.S. and Canada)

## Before Using This Medicine

In deciding to use a medicine, the risks of taking the medicine must be weighed against the good it will do. This is a decision you and your doctor will make. For acyclovir, the following should be considered:

**Allergies**—Tell your doctor if you have ever had any unusual or allergic reaction to acyclovir or ganciclovir. Also tell your health care professional if you are allergic to any other substances, such as foods, sulfites or other preservatives, or dyes.

**Pregnancy**—Acyclovir has been used in pregnant women and has not been reported to cause birth defects or other problems. However, studies have not been done in humans. Studies in rabbits have shown that acyclovir given by injection may keep the fetus from becoming attached to the lining of the uterus (womb). However, acyclovir has not been shown to cause birth defects or other problems in mice given many times the usual human dose, or in rats or rabbits given several times the usual human dose.

**Breast-feeding**—Acyclovir passes into the breast milk. However, it has not been reported to cause problems in nursing babies.

**Children**—A limited number of studies have been done using oral acyclovir in children, and it has not caused different effects or problems in children than it does in adults.

**Older adults**—Acyclovir has been used in the elderly and has not been shown to cause different side effects or problems in older people than it does in younger adults.

**Other medicines**—Although certain medicines should not be used together at all, in many cases two different medicines may be used together even if an interaction might occur. In these cases, changes in dose or other precautions may be necessary. If you are receiving acyclovir by injection it is especially important that your health care professional know if you are taking any of the following:
- Carmustine (e.g., BiCNU) or
- Cisplatin (e.g., Platinol) or
- Combination pain medicine containing acetaminophen and aspirin (e.g., Excedrin) or other salicylates or
- Cyclosporine (e.g., Sandimmune) or
- Deferoxamine (e.g., Desferal) (with long-term use) or
- Gold salts (medicine for arthritis) or
- Inflammation or pain medicine, except narcotics, or
- Lithium (e.g., Lithane) or
- Methotrexate (Mexate) or
- Other medicine for infection or
- Penicillamine (e.g., Cuprimine) or

- Plicamycin (e.g., Mithracin) or
- Streptozocin (e.g., Zanosar) or
- Tiopronin (Thiola)—Concurrent use of these medicines with acyclovir by injection may increase the chance for side effects, especially when kidney disease is present

**Other medical problems**—The presence of other medical problems may affect the use of acyclovir. Make sure you tell your doctor if you have any other medical problems, especially:
- Kidney disease—Kidney disease may increase blood levels of acyclovir, increasing the chance of side effects
- Nerve disease—Acyclovir by injection may increase the chance for nervous system side effects

## Proper Use of This Medicine

Patient information about the treatment of herpes is available with this medicine. Read it carefully before using this medicine.

Acyclovir is best used as soon as possible after the symptoms of herpes infection (for example, pain, burning, blisters) begin to appear.

Acyclovir capsules, tablets, and oral suspension may be taken with meals.

If you are taking acyclovir for the *treatment of chickenpox*, it is best to start taking acyclovir as soon as possible after the first sign of the chickenpox rash, usually within one day.

If you are using *acyclovir oral suspension*, use a specially marked measuring spoon or other device to measure each dose accurately. The average household teaspoon may not hold the right amount of liquid.

Acyclovir is best taken with a full glass (8 ounces) of water.

To help clear up your herpes infection, *keep taking acyclovir for the full time of treatment*, even if your symptoms begin to clear up after a few days. *Do not miss any doses.* However, *do not use this medicine more often or for a longer time than your doctor ordered.*

**Dosing**—The dose of acyclovir will be different for different patients. *Follow your doctor's orders or the directions on the label.* The following information includes only the average doses of acyclovir. Your dose may be different if you have kidney disease. *If your dose is different, do not change it* unless your doctor tells you to do so.

The number of capsules or tablets or teaspoonfuls of suspension that you take depends on the strength of the medicine. Also, *the number of doses you take each day, the time allowed between doses, and the length of time you take the medicine depend on the medical problem for which you are taking acyclovir.*
- For *oral* dosage forms (capsules, oral suspension, or tablets):
  —For treatment of herpes of the genitals or mucous membranes, or for shingles:
    - Adults and children 12 years of age and older— 200 to 800 milligrams (mg) two to five times a day for up to ten days.

- Children younger than 12 years of age—Use and dose must be determined by the doctor.
  —For treatment of chickenpox:
  - Adults and children 2 years of age and older—Dose is based on body weight. The usual dose is 20 mg per kilogram (kg) of body weight, up to 800 mg, four times a day for five days.
  - Children younger than 2 years of age—Use and dose must be determined by the doctor.
- For *injection* dosage form:
  —For treatment of herpes of the genitals or mucous membranes, or for shingles:
  - Adults and children 12 years of age and older—Dose is based on body weight. The usual dose is 5 to 10 mg of acyclovir per kg (2.3 to 4.6 mg per pound) of body weight, injected slowly into a vein over at least a one-hour period, and repeated every eight hours for five to ten days.
  - Children younger than 12 years of age—Dose is based on body weight or body size. The medicine is injected slowly into a vein over at least a one-hour period and repeated every eight hours for five to ten days.

**Missed dose**—If you do miss a dose of this medicine, take it as soon as possible. However, if it is almost time for your next dose, skip the missed dose and go back to your regular dosing schedule. Do not double doses.

**Storage**—To store this medicine:
- Keep out of the reach of children.
- Store away from heat and direct light.
- Do not store the capsule or tablet form of this medicine in the bathroom, near the kitchen sink, or in other damp places. Heat or moisture may cause the medicine to break down.
- Do not keep outdated medicine or medicine no longer needed. Be sure that any discarded medicine is out of the reach of children.

## Precautions While Using This Medicine

*Women with genital herpes may be more likely to get cancer of the cervix (entrance to the womb).* Therefore, it is very important that a Pap test be taken at least once a year to check for cancer. Cervical cancer can be cured if found and treated early.

If your symptoms do not improve within a few days, or if they become worse, check with your doctor.

The areas affected by herpes should be kept as clean and dry as possible. Also, wear loose-fitting clothing to avoid irritating the sores (blisters).

*It is important to remember that acyclovir will not keep you from spreading herpes to others.*

Herpes infection of the genitals can be caught from or spread to your partner during any sexual activity. Even though you may get herpes if your partner has no symptoms, the infection is more likely to be spread if sores are present. This is true until the sores are completely healed and the scabs have fallen off. *Therefore, it is best to avoid any sexual activity if either you or your sexual partner has any symptoms of herpes.* The use of a latex condom ("rubber") may help prevent the spread of herpes. However, spermicidal (sperm-killing) jelly or a diaphragm will probably not help.

## Side Effects of This Medicine

Along with its needed effects, a medicine may cause some unwanted effects. Although not all of these side effects may occur, if they do occur they may need medical attention.

*Check with your doctor immediately* if any of the following side effects occur:
*For acyclovir injection only*
  *More common*
    Pain, swelling, or redness at place of injection
  *Less common (more common with rapid injection)*
    Abdominal or stomach pain; decreased frequency of urination or amount of urine; increased thirst; loss of appetite; nausea or vomiting; unusual tiredness or weakness
  *Rare*
    Confusion; convulsions (seizures); hallucinations (seeing, hearing, or feeling things that are not there); trembling

Other side effects may occur that usually do not need medical attention. These side effects may go away during treatment as your body adjusts to the medicine. However, check with your doctor if any of the following side effects continue or are bothersome:
*For oral acyclovir only*
  *Less common (especially seen with long-term use or high doses)*
    Diarrhea; headache; lightheadedness; nausea or vomiting

Other side effects not listed above may also occur in some patients. If you notice any other effects, check with your doctor.

## Additional Information

Once a medicine has been approved for marketing for a certain use, experience may show that it is also useful for other medical problems. Although not specifically included in product labeling, acyclovir by injection is used in certain patients with the following medical conditions:
- Disseminated neonatal herpes simplex (widespread infection in the newborn)
- Herpes simplex (prevention of repeated infections)

Other than the above information, there is no additional information relating to proper use, precautions, or side effects for these uses.

Revised: 06/22/94

# ACYCLOVIR   Topical

A commonly used brand name in the U.S. and Canada is Zovirax. Other commonly used names are aciclovir and acycloguanosine.

## Description

Acyclovir (ay-SYE-kloe-veer) belongs to the family of medicines called antivirals. Antivirals are used to treat infections caused by viruses. Usually they work for only one kind or group of virus infections.

Topical acyclovir is used to treat the symptoms of herpes simplex virus infections of the skin, mucous membranes, and genitals (sex organs). Although topical acyclovir will not cure herpes simplex, it may help relieve the pain and discomfort and may help the sores (if any) heal faster. Topical acyclovir may also be used for other conditions as determined by your doctor.

Acyclovir is available only with your doctor's prescription, in the following dosage form:

*Topical*
- Ointment (U.S. and Canada)

## Before Using This Medicine

In deciding to use a medicine, the risks of using the medicine must be weighed against the good it will do. This is a decision you and your doctor will make. For acyclovir, the following should be considered:

**Allergies**—Tell your doctor if you have ever had any unusual or allergic reaction to acyclovir. Also tell your health care professional if you are allergic to any other substances, such as preservatives or dyes.

**Pregnancy**—Topical acyclovir has not been studied in pregnant women. However, this medication has not been shown to cause birth defects or other problems in animal studies using mice, rats, or rabbits.

**Breast-feeding**—It is not known whether topical acyclovir passes into the breast milk. However, acyclovir ointment has not been reported to cause problems in nursing babies, even though small amounts of topical acyclovir are absorbed through the mother's skin and mucous membranes.

**Children**—Although there is no specific information comparing the use of topical acyclovir in children with use in other age groups, this medicine is not expected to cause different side effects or problems in children than it does in adults.

**Older adults**—Many medicines have not been studied specifically in older people. Therefore, it may not be known whether they work exactly the same way they do in younger adults. Although there is no specific information comparing the use of topical acyclovir in the elderly with use in other age groups, this medicine is not expected to cause different side effects or problems in older people than it does in younger adults.

**Other medicines**—Although certain medicines should not be used together at all, in other cases two different medicines may be used together even if an interaction might occur. In these cases, your doctor may want to change the dose, or other precautions may be necessary. Tell your health care professional if you are using any other topical prescription or nonprescription (over-the-counter [OTC]) medicine that is to be applied to the same area of the skin.

## Proper Use of This Medicine

Acyclovir may come with patient information about herpes simplex infections. Read this information carefully. If you have any questions, check with your health care professional.

*Do not use this medicine in the eyes.*

*Acyclovir is best used as soon as possible after the symptoms of herpes infection (for example, pain, burning, or blisters) begin to appear.*

*Use a finger cot or rubber glove when applying this medicine. This will help keep you from spreading the infection to other areas of your body.* Apply enough medicine to completely cover all the sores (blisters). A 1.25-cm (approximately ½-inch) strip of ointment applied to each area of the affected skin measuring 5 × 5 cm (approximately 2 × 2 inches) is usually enough, unless otherwise directed by your doctor.

To help clear up your herpes infection, *continue using acyclovir for the full time of treatment,* even if your symptoms begin to clear up after a few days. *Do not miss any doses.* However, *do not use this medicine more often or for a longer time than your doctor ordered.*

**Dosing**—The dose of topical acyclovir will be different for different patients. *Follow your doctor's orders or the directions on the label.* The following information includes only the average dose of topical acyclovir. *If your dose is different, do not change it* unless your doctor tells you to do so.

- For *topical* dosage form (ointment):
  —For herpes simplex infection:
    - Adults and children—Apply to the affected area(s) of the skin and mucous membranes, every three hours, for a total of six times a day, for seven days.

**Missed dose**—If you miss a dose of this medicine, apply it as soon as possible. However, if it is almost time for your next dose, skip the missed dose and go back to your regular dosing schedule.

**Storage**—To store this medicine:
- Keep out of the reach of children.
- Store away from heat and direct light.
- Keep the medicine from freezing.

- Do not keep outdated medicine or medicine no longer needed. Be sure that any discarded medicine is out of the reach of children.

## Precautions While Using This Medicine

*Women with genital herpes may be more likely to get cancer of the cervix (opening to the womb). Therefore, it is very important that Pap tests be taken at least once a year to check for cancer. Cervical cancer can be cured if found and treated early.*

If your symptoms do not improve within 1 week, or if they become worse, check with your doctor.

The areas affected by herpes should be kept as clean and dry as possible. Also, wear loose-fitting clothing to avoid irritating the sores (blisters).

Herpes infection of the genitals can be caught from or spread to your partner during any sexual activity. Although you may get herpes even though your sexual partner has no symptoms, the infection is more likely to be spread if sores are present. This is true until the sores are completely healed and the scabs have fallen off. The use of a condom (prophylactic) may help prevent the spread of herpes. However, spermicidal (sperm-killing) jelly or a diaphragm will not help prevent the spread of herpes. *Therefore, it is best to avoid any sexual activity if either you or your partner has any symptoms of herpes. It is also important to remember that acyclovir will not keep you from spreading herpes to others.*

## Side Effects of This Medicine

Along with its needed effects, a medicine may cause some unwanted effects. The following side effects may go away during treatment as your body adjusts to the medicine. However, check with your doctor if any of these effects continue or are bothersome:

*More common*
  Mild pain, burning, or stinging
*Less common*
  Itching
*Rare*
  Skin rash

Other side effects not listed above may also occur in some patients. If you notice any other effects, check with your doctor.

Revised: 01/15/92
Interim revision: 05/10/94

# ALBENDAZOLE    Systemic*†

Some commonly used brand names are Eskazole and Zentel.

*Not commercially available in the U.S.
†Not commercially available in Canada.

## Description

Albendazole (al-BEN-da-zole) is used to treat worm infections. Albendazole works by keeping the worm from absorbing sugar (glucose), so that the worm loses energy and dies.

Albendazole is used to treat:
- Common roundworms (ascariasis);
- Hookworms (ancylostomiasis and necatoriasis);
- Hydatid disease (echinococcosis);
- Pinworms (enterobiasis or oxyuriasis);
- Tapeworms (taeniasis);
- Threadworms (strongyloidiasis);
- Whipworms (trichuriasis).

This medicine may also be used for other worm infections as determined by your doctor.

Albendazole is available only with your doctor's prescription, in the following dosage forms:
*Oral*
  - Oral suspension (United Kingdom)
  - Tablets (United Kingdom)

## Before Using This Medicine

In deciding to use a medicine, the risks of taking the medicine must be weighed against the good it will do. This is a decision you and your doctor will make. For albendazole, the following should be considered:

**Allergies**—Tell your doctor if you have ever had any unusual or allergic reaction to albendazole. Also tell your health care professional if you are allergic to any other substances, such as foods, preservatives, or dyes.

**Pregnancy**—Albendazole has not been studied in pregnant women. However, studies in animals have shown that albendazole can cause birth defects or other problems. Before taking this medicine, make sure your doctor knows if you are pregnant or if you may become pregnant.

Women of childbearing age (15 to 40 years) should take the medicine within 7 days of the start of their period (menstrual cycle). Birth control must be used during treatment and for one month after stopping treatment with albendazole.

**Breast-feeding**—It is not known whether albendazole passes into human breast milk. Although most medicines pass into breast milk in small amounts, many of them may be used safely while breast-feeding. Mothers who are taking this medicine and who wish to breast-feed should discuss this with their doctor.

**Children**—Although there is no specific information comparing use of albendazole in children with use in other age groups, this medicine is not expected to cause different side effects or problems in children than it does in adults.

**Older adults**—Many medicines have not been studied specifically in older people. Therefore, it may not be known whether they work exactly the same way they do in younger adults or if they cause different side effects or problems in older people. There is no specific information comparing use of albendazole in the elderly with use in other age groups.

**Other medical problems**—The presence of other medical problems may affect the use of albendazole. Make sure you tell your doctor if you have any other medical problems, especially:
- Liver disease—Patients with liver disease may have an increased chance of side effects

## Proper Use of This Medicine

No special preparations (fasting, laxatives, or enemas) are necessary before, during, or immediately after treatment with albendazole.

Albendazole is best taken with meals, especially with food containing fat, to help your body absorb the medicine better.

For patients taking the *tablet form* of albendazole:
- Tablets may be chewed, swallowed whole with a small amount of liquid, or crushed and mixed with food.

To help clear up your infection completely, *take this medicine exactly as directed by your doctor for the full time of treatment*. In some infections, a second treatment in 2 to 3 weeks with this medicine may be needed to clear up the infection completely. *Do not miss any doses.*

Pinworms may be easily passed from one person to another, especially among persons in the same household. Therefore, all household members may have to be treated at the same time to prevent their infection or reinfection.

**Dosing**—The dose of albendazole will be different for different patients. *Follow your doctor's orders or the directions on the label.* The following information includes only the average doses of albendazole. *If your dose is different, do not change it* unless your doctor tells you to do so.

The number of tablets or teaspoonfuls of suspension that you take depends on the strength of the medicine. Also, *the number of doses you take each day, the time allowed between doses, and the length of time you take the medicine depend on the medical problem for which you are taking albendazole*.
- For *oral* dosage forms (oral suspension and tablets):
  —For common roundworms, hookworms, pinworms, and whipworms:
    • Adults and children over 2 years of age—400 milligrams (mg) once a day for one day. Treatment may need to be repeated in 3 weeks.

    • Children up to 2 years of age—200 mg once a day for one day. Treatment may need to be repeated in 3 weeks.
  —For tapeworms and threadworms:
    • Adults and children over 2 years of age—400 mg once a day for three days in a row. Treatment may need to be repeated in 3 weeks.
    • Children up to 2 years of age—200 mg once a day for three days in a row. Treatment may need to be repeated in 3 weeks.
  —For hydatid disease:
    • Adults—800 mg per day for twenty-eight days. Treatment may be repeated when necessary or in 2 weeks.
    • Children up to 6 years of age—Dosage has not been established.
    • Children 6 years of age and over—Dose is based on body weight and must be determined by your doctor. However, the usual dose is 12 mg of albendazole per kilogram (5.5 milligrams per pound) of body weight per day for 28 days. Treatment may be repeated when necessary.

**Missed dose**—If you miss a dose of this medicine, take it as soon as possible. However, if it is almost time for your next dose, skip the missed dose and go back to your regular dosing schedule. Do not double doses.

**Storage**—To store this medicine:
- Keep out of the reach of children.
- Store away from heat and direct light.
- Do not store in the bathroom, near the kitchen sink, or in other damp places. Heat or moisture may cause the medicine to break down.
- Keep the suspension form of this medicine from freezing.
- Do not keep outdated medicine or medicine no longer needed. Be sure that any discarded medicine is out of the reach of children.

## Precautions While Using This Medicine

It is important that your doctor check your progress after treatment. This is to make sure that the infection is cleared up completely, and to allow your doctor to check for any unwanted effects.

If your symptoms do not improve after you have taken this medicine for the full course of treatment, or if they become worse, check with your doctor.

While you are taking albendazole, it is important that you use birth control, since this medicine can cause birth defects or other problems.

For patients taking albendazole for *hookworms:*
- In hookworm infections, anemia may occur. Therefore, your doctor may want you to take iron supplements. If so, it is important to take iron every day while you are being treated for hookworm infection. Do not miss any doses. Your doctor may also want

you to keep taking iron supplements for at least 3 to 6 months after you stop taking albendazole. If you have any questions about this, check with your doctor.

For patients taking albendazole for *hydatid disease:*
- Avoid contacts with infected dogs; animal waste should be burned or buried to prevent reinfection of dogs.

For patients taking albendazole for *pinworms:*
- In some patients, pinworms may return after treatment with albendazole. Wear pajamas and underwear to sleep, take a bath every day, and wash (not shake) all bedding and nightclothes (pajamas) after treatment to help prevent reinfection. Treatment may be repeated after 3 weeks.
- Pinworms may be easily passed from one person to another, especially among persons in the same household. Therefore, all household members may have to be treated at the same time to prevent their infection or reinfection.

For patients taking albendazole for *roundworms* and *whipworms:*
- Good health habits, such as proper disposal of waste, are required to help prevent reinfection.

For patients taking albendazole for *tapeworms*:
- Check or inspect the meat carefully.
- Cook all pork and beef thoroughly before eating. You may also freeze, or refrigerate and salt, the meat for a long period of time. All of these measures will destroy or kill the worm that may be present in the meat and will help prevent reinfection.

For patients taking albendazole for *threadworms:*
- Cook vegetables thoroughly before eating. This will destroy or kill the worm that may be present in the vegetables and will help prevent reinfection.

## Side Effects of This Medicine

Along with its needed effects, a medicine may cause some unwanted effects. Although not all of these side effects may occur, if they do occur they may need medical attention.

Check with your doctor as soon as possible if any of the following side effects occur:
*Rare*
Fever; skin rash or itching; sore throat; unusual tiredness and weakness

Other side effects may occur that usually do not need medical attention. These side effects may go away during treatment as your body adjusts to the medicine. However, check with your doctor if any of the following side effects continue or are bothersome:
*Less common*
Abdominal or stomach upset or pain; diarrhea; dizziness; headache; nausea; vomiting
*Rare*
Thinning or loss of hair

Other side effects not listed above may also occur in some patients. If you notice any other effects, check with your doctor.

## Additional Information

Once a medicine has been approved for marketing for a certain use, experience may show that it is also useful for other medical problems. Although these uses are not included in product labeling, albendazole is used in certain patients with the following infections:
- Capillariasis
- Clonorchiasis
- Giardiasis
- Neurocysticercosis
- Trichinosis
- Trichostrongyliasis

For patients taking this medicine for *giardiasis:*
- Household contacts and sexual partners of infected patients should be seen by the doctor to prevent spread of infection to others. After treatment, it is important that your doctor check to see whether or not the infection in your body has been cleared up completely.

Other than the above information, there is no additional information relating to proper use, precautions, or side effects for these uses.

Revised: 8/18/93

# ALCOHOL AND ACETONE    Topical†

Some commonly used brand names in the U.S. are Seba-Nil Liquid Cleanser, Tyrosum Liquid, and Tyrosum Packets.

†Not commercially available in Canada.

## Description

Alcohol and acetone (AL-koe-hol and A-se-tone) combination is used to clean oily or greasy skin associated with acne or other oily skin conditions.

This medicine is available without a prescription; however, your doctor may have special instructions on the proper use of this medicine for your medical condition.

Alcohol and acetone combination is available in the following dosage forms:

*Topical*
- Detergent lotion (U.S.)
- Pledgets (U.S.)

## Before Using This Medicine

If you are using this medicine without a prescription, carefully read and follow any precautions on the label. For alcohol and acetone combination, the following should be considered:

**Allergies**—Tell your doctor if you have ever had any unusual or allergic reaction to alcohol or acetone. Also tell your health care professional if you are allergic to any other substances, such as preservatives or dyes.

**Pregnancy**—Topical alcohol and acetone combination has not been shown to cause birth defects or other problems in humans.

**Breast-feeding**—Topical alcohol and acetone combination has not been reported to cause problems in nursing babies.

**Children**—This medicine should not be used on children up to 8 years of age. In older children, although there is no specific information comparing use of alcohol and acetone with use in other age groups, this medicine is not expected to cause different side effects or problems in older children than it does in adults.

**Older adults**—Many medicines have not been tested in older people. Therefore, it may not be known whether they work exactly the same way they do in younger adults. Although there is no specific information comparing use of alcohol and acetone in the elderly with use in other age groups, this medicine is not expected to cause different side effects or problems in older people than it does in younger adults.

**Other medicines**—Although certain medicines should not be used together at all, in other cases two different medicines may be used together even if an interaction might occur. In these cases, your doctor may want to change the dose, or other precautions may be necessary. Tell your health care professional if you are using any other topical prescription or nonprescription (over-the-counter [OTC]) medicine that is to be applied to the same area of the skin.

**Other medical problems**—The presence of other medical problems may affect the use of alcohol and acetone combination. Make sure you tell your doctor if you have any other medical problems, especially:

- Burns or wounds—Alcohol and acetone combination may cause severe irritation if applied to burns or wounds.

## Proper Use of This Medicine

*Keep this medicine away from the eyes, the inside of the nose, and the lips.*

This medicine is flammable. Do not use near heat, near open flame, or while smoking.

To use the *lotion form* of this medicine:

- Put a small amount of this medicine on a gauze pad or cotton ball and apply by wiping or rubbing over the face and other affected areas to remove dirt and surface oil.

To use the *pledget form* of this medicine:

- Apply by wiping or rubbing over the face and other affected areas to remove dirt and surface oil.

After applying this medicine, do not rinse the affected areas with water, since this will remove the medicine.

**Dosing**—The dose of topical alcohol and acetone combination will be different for different patients. *Follow your doctor's orders or the directions on the label.* The following information includes only the average dose of topical alcohol and acetone combination. *If your dose is different, do not change it* unless your doctor tells you to do so.

- For *topical* dosage forms (detergent lotion or pledgets):
  —For acne or oily skin:
    - Adults and children 8 years of age and older— Apply to the affected area(s) of the skin two to four times a day as needed.
    - Children up to 8 years of age—Use is not recommended.

**Missed dose**—If you are using this medicine on a regular schedule and you miss a dose, apply it as soon as possible. Then go back to your regular dosing schedule.

**Storage**—To store this medicine:
- Keep out of the reach of children.
- Store away from heat and direct light.
- Keep the lotion form of this medicine from freezing.
- Do not keep outdated medicine or medicine no longer needed. Be sure that any discarded medicine is out of the reach of children.

## Precautions While Using This Medicine

*When using alcohol and acetone combination, do not use any of the following preparations on the same affected area*, unless otherwise directed by your doctor:

    Abrasive soaps or cleaners
    Any other topical acne preparation or preparation containing a peeling agent (for example, benzoyl peroxide, resorcinol, salicylic acid, sulfur, or tretinoin [vitamin A acid])
    Cosmetics or soaps that dry the skin
    Medicated cosmetics
    Other alcohol-containing preparations
    Other topical medicine for the skin

To use any of the above preparations on the same affected area as this medicine may cause severe irritation of the skin

## Side Effects of This Medicine

Along with its needed effects, a medicine may cause some unwanted effects. Although not all of these side effects may occur, if they do occur they may need medical attention.

Check with your doctor as soon as possible if any of the following side effects occur:

    Irritation, pain, redness, or swelling of skin; skin infection

Other side effects may occur that usually do not need medical attention. These side effects may go away during treatment as your body adjusts to the medicine. However, check with your health care professional if the following side effect continues or is bothersome:

    Burning or stinging of skin

Other side effects may also occur in some patients. If you notice any other effects, check with your health care professional.

Revised: 01/15/92
Interim revision: 06/08/94

# ALCOHOL AND SULFUR    Topical

Some commonly used brand names are:

**In the U.S.—**
    Liquimat Creamy Beige    Liquimat Natural Beige
    Liquimat Dark    Transact
    Liquimat Light    Xerac
    Liquimat Medium

**In Canada—**
    Postacne

## Description

Alcohol and sulfur (AL-koe-hol and SUL-fur) combination is used in the treatment of acne and oily skin. Some of the products are tinted a flesh color and can be used as a makeup or cover-up.

This medicine is available without a doctor's prescription; however, your doctor may have special instructions on the proper use of this medicine for your medical condition.

Alcohol and sulfur combination is available in the following dosage forms:

*Topical*
- Gel (U.S.)
- Lotion (U.S. and Canada)

## Before Using This Medicine

If you are using this medicine without a prescription, carefully read and follow any precautions on the label. For alcohol and sulfur combination, the following should be considered:

**Allergies**—Tell your doctor if you have ever had any unusual or allergic reaction to alcohol or sulfur. Also tell your health care professional if you are allergic to any other substances, such as preservatives or dyes.

**Pregnancy**—Topical alcohol and sulfur combination has not been shown to cause birth defects or other problems in humans.

**Breast-feeding**—Topical alcohol and sulfur combination has not been reported to cause problems in nursing babies.

**Children**—This medicine should not be used for children up to 8 years of age. In older children, although there is no specific information comparing use of alcohol and sulfur with use in other age groups, this medicine is not expected to cause different side effects or problems than it does in adults.

**Older adults**—Many medicines have not been studied specifically in older people. Therefore, it may not be known whether they work exactly the same way they do in younger adults. Although there is no specific information comparing use of alcohol and sulfur in the elderly with use in other age groups, this medicine is not expected to cause different side effects or problems in older people than it does in younger adults.

**Other medicines**—Although certain medicines should not be used together at all, in other cases two different medicines may be used together even if an interaction might occur. In these cases, your doctor may want to change the dose, or other precautions may be necessary. Tell your health care professional if you are using any other topical prescription or nonprescription (over-the-counter [OTC]) medicine that is to be applied to the same area of the skin.

## Proper Use of This Medicine

Before using this medicine, wash or cleanse the affected areas thoroughly and gently pat dry. Then apply a small amount of this medicine to the affected areas and rub in gently.

*Keep this medicine away from the eyes, the inside of the nose, and the lips.* If you accidentally get some in your eyes, flush them thoroughly with water.

This medicine is flammable. Do not use near heat, near open flame, or while smoking.

*Use this medicine only as directed.* Do not use it more often than recommended on the label, unless otherwise directed by your doctor.

**Dosing**—The dose of alcohol and sulfur combination will be different for different patients. *Follow your doctor's orders or the directions on the label.* The following information includes only the average doses of alcohol and sulfur combination. *If your dose is different, do not change it* unless your doctor tells you to do so.

- For acne or oily skin:
  —For *gel* dosage form:
    - Adults and children 8 years of age and older—Apply to the affected area(s) of the skin one to three times a day.
    - Children up to 8 years of age—Use is not recommended.
  —For *lotion* dosage form:
    - Adults and children 8 years of age and older—Apply to the affected area(s) of the skin one or two times a day.
    - Children up to 8 years of age—Use is not recommended.

**Missed dose**—If you miss a dose of this medicine, apply it as soon as possible. Then go back to your regular dosing schedule.

**Storage**—To store this medicine:
- Keep out of the reach of children.
- Store away from heat and direct light.
- Keep the medicine from freezing.
- Do not keep outdated medicine or medicine no longer needed. Be sure that any discarded medicine is out of the reach of children.

## Precautions While Using This Medicine

*When using alcohol and sulfur combination, do not use any of the following preparations on the same affected area*, unless otherwise directed by your doctor.

Abrasive soaps or cleansers
Any other topical acne preparation or preparation containing a peeling agent (for example, benzoyl peroxide, resorcinol, salicylic acid, or tretinoin [vitamin A acid])
Cosmetics or soaps that dry the skin
Medicated cosmetics
Other alcohol-containing preparations
Other topical medicine for the skin

To use any of the above preparations on the same affected area as this medicine may cause severe irritation of the skin.

*Do not use any topical mercury-containing preparation, such as ammoniated mercury ointment, on the same affected area as this medicine.* To do so may cause a foul odor, may be irritating to the skin, and may stain the skin black. If you have any questions about this, check with your health care professional.

## Side Effects of This Medicine

Along with its needed effects, a medicine may cause some unwanted effects. Although not all of these side effects may occur, if they do occur they may need medical attention.

Check with your doctor as soon as possible if the following side effect occurs:

Skin irritation not present before use of this medicine

Other side effects may occur that usually do not need medical attention. These side effects may go away during treatment as your body adjusts to the medicine. However, check with your health care professional if any of the following side effects continue or are bothersome:

Burning or stinging of skin; dryness or peeling of skin (may occur after a few days)

Other side effects not listed above may also occur in some patients. If you notice any other effects, check with your health care professional.

Revised: 01/15/92
Interim revision: 05/18/94

# ALDESLEUKIN   Systemic†

A commonly used brand name in the U.S. is Proleukin. Other commonly used names are interleukin-2 and IL-2.

†Not commercially available in Canada.

## Description

Aldesleukin (al-des-LOO-kin) is a synthetic (man-made) version of a substance called interleukin-2. Interleukins are produced naturally by cells in the body to help white blood cells work. Aldesleukin is used to treat cancer of the kidney.

Aldesleukin causes some other very serious effects in addition to its helpful effects. Some effects can be fatal. For that reason, aldesleukin is given only in the hospital. If severe side effects occur, which is common, treatment in an intensive care unit (ICU) may be necessary. Other effects may not be serious but may cause concern. Before you begin treatment with aldesleukin, you and your doctor should talk about the good this medicine will do as well as the risks of using it.

Aldesleukin is to be administered only by or under the immediate supervision of your doctor. It is available in the following dosage form:

*Parenteral*
  • Injection (U.S.)

## Before Using This Medicine

In deciding to use a medicine, the risks of taking the medicine must be weighed against the good it will do. This is a decision you and your doctor will make. For aldesleukin, the following should be considered:

**Allergies**—Tell your doctor if you have ever had any unusual or allergic reaction to aldesleukin.

**Pregnancy**—Aldesleukin has not been studied in humans or in animals. However, because this medicine may cause serious side effects, use during pregnancy is usually not recommended.

Be sure that you have discussed this with your doctor before receiving this medicine.

**Breast-feeding**—It is not known whether aldesleukin passes into breast milk.

**Children**—There is no specific information comparing use of aldesleukin in children with use in other age groups.

**Older adults**—Many medicines have not been studied specifically in older people. Therefore, it may not be known whether they work exactly the same way they do in younger adults. There is no specific information comparing use of aldesleukin in the elderly with use in other age groups.

**Other medicines**—Although certain medicines should not be used together at all, in other cases two different medicines may be used together even if an interaction might occur. In these cases, your doctor may want to change the dose, or other precautions may be necessary. Tell your health care professional if you are taking *any* other medicine.

**Other medical problems**—The presence of other medical problems may affect the use of aldesleukin. Make sure you tell your doctor if you have any other medical problems, especially:
  • Chickenpox (including recent exposure) or
  • Herpes zoster (shingles)—Risk of severe disease affecting other parts of the body

  • Heart disease or
  • Immune system problems or
  • Liver disease or
  • Lung disease or
  • Psoriasis or
  • Underactive thyroid—May be worsened by aldesleukin
  • Infection—Aldesleukin may decrease your body's ability to fight infection
  • Kidney disease—Effects of aldesleukin may be increased because of slower removal from the body
  • Mental problems—Aldesleukin may make them worse
  • Seizures (history of)—Aldesleukin can cause seizures

## Proper Use of This Medicine

**Dosing**—The dose of aldesleukin will be different for different patients. The dose that is used may depend on a number of things, including what the medicine is being used for, the patient's weight, and whether or not other medicines are also being taken. Because this medicine can cause very serious side effects, your doctor will be watching your dose very carefully and may change it as needed. If you have any questions about the proper dose of aldesleukin, ask your doctor.

## Precautions While Using This Medicine

Aldesleukin can temporarily affect the white blood cells in your blood, increasing the chance of getting an infection. It can also lower the number of platelets, which are necessary for proper blood clotting. If this occurs, there are certain precautions you can take, especially when your blood count is low, to reduce the risk of infection or bleeding:
  • If you can, avoid people with infections. *Check with your doctor immediately* if you think you are getting an infection or if you get a fever or chills, cough or hoarseness, lower back or side pain, or painful or difficult urination.
  • *Check with your doctor immediately* if you notice any unusual bleeding or bruising; black, tarry stools; blood in urine or stools; or pinpoint red spots on your skin.
  • Be careful when using a regular toothbrush, dental floss, or toothpick. Your medical doctor, dentist, or nurse may recommend other ways to clean your teeth and gums. Check with your medical doctor before having any dental work done.
  • Do not touch your eyes or the inside of your nose unless you have just washed your hands and have not touched anything else in the meantime.
  • Be careful not to cut yourself when you are using sharp objects such as a safety razor or fingernail or toenail cutters.
  • Avoid contact sports or other situations where bruising or injury could occur.

## Side Effects of This Medicine

Along with its needed effects, a medicine may cause some unwanted effects. Some side effects will have signs or symptoms that you can see or feel. Your doctor may watch for others by doing certain tests.

*Check with your doctor or nurse immediately* if any of the following side effects occur:

*More common*
Fever or chills; shortness of breath

*Less common*
Black, tarry stools; blisters on skin; blood in urine; bloody vomit; chest pain; cough or hoarseness; lower back or side pain; painful or difficult urination; pinpoint red spots on skin; stomach pain (severe); unusual bleeding or bruising

Check with your health care professional as soon as possible if any of the following side effects occur:

*More common*
Agitation; confusion; diarrhea; dizziness; drowsiness; mental depression; nausea and vomiting; sores in mouth and on lips; tingling of hands or feet; unusual decrease in urination; unusual tiredness; weight gain of 5 to 10 pounds or more

*Less common*
Bloating and stomach pain; blurred or double vision; faintness; fast or irregular heartbeat; loss of taste; rapid breathing; redness, swelling, and soreness of tongue; trouble in speaking; yellow eyes and skin

*Rare*
Changes in menstrual periods; clumsiness; coldness; convulsions (seizures); listlessness; muscle aches; pain or redness at site of injection; sudden inability to move; swelling in the front of the neck; swelling of feet or lower legs; weakness

This medicine may also cause the following side effects that your doctor will watch for:

*More common*
Anemia; heart problems; kidney problems; liver problems; low blood pressure; low platelet counts in blood; low white blood cell counts; other blood problems; underactive thyroid

Other side effects may occur that usually do not need medical attention. These side effects may go away during treatment as your body adjusts to the medicine. Also, your health care professional may be able to tell you about ways to prevent or reduce some of these side effects. Check with your health care professional if any of the following side effects continue or are bothersome or if you have any questions about them:

*More common*
Dry skin; loss of appetite; skin rash or redness with burning or itching, followed by peeling; unusual feeling of discomfort or illness

*Less common*
Constipation; headache; joint pain; muscle pain

Other side effects not listed above may also occur in some patients. If you notice any other effects, check with your doctor.

Developed: 09/15/93
Interim revision: 08/08/94

# ALGLUCERASE   Systemic

A commonly used brand name in the U.S. and Canada is Ceredase.

## Description

Alglucerase (al-GLOO-ser-ace) is used to treat Gaucher's disease caused by the lack of a certain enzyme, glucocerebrosidase, in the body. This enzyme is necessary for your body to use fats.

Alglucerase is made from human placenta tissue that is collected after a baby is born. Before it is used, the tissue is tested for hepatitis and human immunodeficiency virus (HIV). This is similar to the testing that a blood bank does on donated blood before it is given to anyone else.

Alglucerase is available with your doctor's prescription, in the following dosage form:

*Parenteral*
• Injection (U.S. and Canada)

## Before Receiving This Medicine

In deciding to use a medicine, the risks of receiving the medicine must be weighed against the good it will do.

This is a decision you and your doctor will make. For alglucerase, the following should be considered:

**Allergies**—Tell your doctor if you have ever had any unusual or allergic reaction to alglucerase. Also tell your health care professional if you are allergic to any other substances, such as foods, preservatives, or dyes.

**Pregnancy**—Studies have not been done in either humans or animals.

**Breast-feeding**—It is not known whether alglucerase passes into human breast milk.

**Children**—This medicine has been tested in a limited number of children. In effective doses, the medicine has not been shown to cause different side effects or problems than it does in adults.

**Older adults**—Many medicines have not been studied specifically in older people. Therefore, it may not be known whether they work exactly the same way they do in younger adults or if they cause different side effects or problems in older people. There is no specific information

comparing use of alglucerase in the elderly with use in other age groups.

**Other medicines**—Although certain medicines should not be used together at all, in other cases two different medicines may be used together even if an interaction might occur. In these cases, your doctor may want to change the dose, or other precautions may be necessary. Tell your health care professional if you are taking any other prescription or nonprescription (over-the-counter [OTC]) medicines.

## Proper Use of This Medicine

This medicine will not cure Gaucher's disease but it does help control it. Therefore, you must continue to receive it if you expect to keep your condition under control. You may have to receive alglucerase for the rest of your life. If Gaucher's disease is not treated, it can cause serious blood, liver, skeletal, or spleen problems.

**Dosing**—The dose of alglucerase will be different for different patients. *Follow your doctor's orders*. The following information includes only the average doses of alglucerase.

- For Gaucher's disease:
  —For *injection* dosage form:
    - Adults and children—The dose is based on body weight. The usual dose is 60 Units per kilogram (kg) (27 Units per pound) of body weight injected into a vein over one to two hours. The dose may be repeated once every other day to once every four weeks, depending on your condition. Later your doctor may lower your dose. A dose

of 2.3 Units per kg (1 Unit per pound) three times a week may be used.

## Precautions While Receiving This Medicine

It is important that your doctor check your progress while you are receiving alglucerase to make sure that the dosage is correct for you.

## Side Effects of This Medicine

Since alglucerase is made from human tissue, it is possible that diseases caused by viruses could be passed on. Examples of such diseases are hepatitis and HIV infection. These problems have not been reported to date, however, and are unlikely since the tissue is tested before being used. If you have questions or concerns about this, check with your doctor.

Along with its needed effects, a medicine may cause some unwanted effects. The following side effects may go away during treatment as your body adjusts to the medicine. However, check with your doctor if any of these effects continue or are bothersome:

*Less common*
   Abdominal discomfort; chills; fever; nausea and vomiting; swelling at place of injection

Other side effects not listed above may also occur in some patients. If you notice any other effects, check with your doctor.

Revised: 01/18/93
Interim revision: 06/06/94

# ALLOPURINOL    Systemic

Some commonly used brand names are:
**In the U.S.—**
   Lopurin                                    Zyloprim
   Generic name product may also be available.
**In Canada—**
   Apo-Allopurinol                            Zyloprim
   Purinol

## Description

Allopurinol (al-oh-PURE-i-nole) is used to treat chronic gout (gouty arthritis). This condition is caused by too much uric acid in the blood.

This medicine works by causing less uric acid to be produced by the body. Allopurinol will not relieve a gout attack that has already started. Also, it does not cure gout, but it will help prevent gout attacks. However, it works only after you have been taking it regularly for a few months. Allopurinol will help prevent gout attacks only as long as you continue to take it.

Allopurinol is also used to prevent or treat other medical problems that may occur if too much uric acid is present in the body. These include certain kinds of kidney stones or other kidney problems.

Certain medicines or medical treatments can greatly increase the amount of uric acid in the body. This can cause gout or kidney problems in some people. Allopurinol is also used to prevent these problems.

Allopurinol is available only with your doctor's prescription in the following dosage form:
*Oral*
   - Tablets (U.S. and Canada)

## Before Using This Medicine

In deciding to use a medicine, the risks of taking the medicine must be weighed against the good it will do.

This is a decision you and your doctor will make. For allopurinol, the following should be considered:

**Allergies**—Tell your doctor if you have ever had any unusual or allergic reaction to allopurinol. Also tell your health care professional if you are allergic to any other substances, such as foods, preservatives, or dyes.

**Pregnancy**—Although studies on birth defects have not been done in pregnant women, allopurinol has not been reported to cause problems in humans. In one study in mice, large amounts of allopurinol caused birth defects and other unwanted effects. However, allopurinol did not cause birth defects or other problems in rats or rabbits given doses up to 20 times the amount usually given to humans.

**Breast-feeding**—Allopurinol passes into the breast milk. Mothers who are taking this medicine and who wish to breast-feed should discuss this with their doctor.

**Children**—This medicine has been tested in children and, in effective doses, has not been shown to cause different side effects or problems than it does in adults.

**Older adults**—Many medicines have not been studied specifically in older people. Therefore, it may not be known whether they work exactly the same way they do in younger adults or if they cause different side effects or problems in older people. There is no specific information comparing use of allopurinol in the elderly with use in other age groups.

**Other medicines**—Although certain medicines should not be used together at all, in other cases two different medicines may be used together even if an interaction might occur. In these cases, your doctor may want to change the dose, or other precautions may be necessary. When you are taking allopurinol, it is especially important that your doctor and pharmacist know if you are taking any of the following:
- Anticoagulants (blood thinners)—Allopurinol may increase the chance of bleeding; changes in the dose of the anticoagulant may be needed, depending on blood test results
- Azathioprine (e.g., Imuran) or
- Mercaptopurine (e.g., Purinethol)—Allopurinol may cause higher blood levels of azathioprine or mercaptopurine, leading to an increased chance of serious side effects

**Other medical problems**—The presence of other medical problems may affect the use of allopurinol. Make sure you tell your doctor if you have any other medical problems, especially:
- Congestive heart disease or
- Diabetes mellitus (sugar diabetes) or
- High blood pressure or
- Kidney disease—There is an increased risk of severe allergic reactions or other serious effects; a change in the dose of allopurinol may be needed

## Proper Use of This Medicine

If this medicine upsets your stomach, it may be taken after meals. If stomach upset (indigestion, nausea, vomiting, diarrhea, or stomach pain) continues, check with your doctor.

*In order for this medicine to help you, it must be taken regularly as ordered by your doctor.*

To help prevent kidney stones while taking allopurinol, adults should drink at least 10 to 12 full glasses (8 ounces each) of fluids each day unless otherwise directed by their doctor. Check with the doctor about the amount of fluids that children should drink each day while receiving this medicine. Also, your doctor may want you to take another medicine to make your urine less acid. It is important that you follow your doctor's instructions very carefully.

For patients taking allopurinol for *chronic gout:*
- After you begin to take allopurinol, gout attacks may continue to occur for a while. However, if you take this medicine regularly as directed by your doctor, the attacks will gradually become less frequent and less painful. After you have been taking allopurinol regularly for several months, the attacks may stop completely.
- Allopurinol is used to help prevent gout attacks. It will not relieve an attack that has already started. *Even if you take another medicine for gout attacks, continue to take this medicine also.*

**Dosing**—The dose of allopurinol will be different for different patients. *Follow your doctor's orders or the directions on the label.* The following information includes only the average doses of allopurinol. *If your dose is different, do not change it* unless your doctor tells you to do so.

The number of tablets that you take each day and the number of times that you take the medicine every day depend on the strength of the medicine, on the dose that you need, and on the reason you are taking allopurinol. Up to 300 milligrams (mg) of allopurinol can be taken at one time. Doses larger than 300 mg a day should be divided into smaller amounts that are taken two, three, or even four times a day.
- For the *oral* dosage form (tablets):
  —For gout:
    • Adults—At first, most people will take 100 mg a day. After about a week, your doctor will probably increase the dose gradually until the amount of uric acid in your blood has been lowered to normal levels. The total amount of allopurinol is usually not more than 800 mg a day. After the uric acid has remained at normal levels for a while, your doctor may lower your dose gradually until you are taking the smallest amount of medicine that will keep the uric acid from increasing again.
    • Children and teenagers—Use and dose must be determined by the doctor.
  —For kidney stones:
    • Adults—100 to 800 mg a day, depending on the kind of kidney stones.
    • Children and teenagers—Use and dose must be determined by the doctor.

—For preventing or treating medical problems that may occur if certain treatments increase the amount of uric acid in the blood:

- Adults—600 to 800 mg a day, starting one to three days before the treatment.
- Children—The dose depends on the child's age.
    —Children up to 6 years of age: 50 mg (one-half of a 100-mg tablet) three times a day.
    —Children 6 to 10 years of age: One 100-mg tablet three times a day or one 300-mg tablet a day.
    —Children 11 years of age and older: The dose may be the same as for adults.

**Missed dose**—If you miss a dose of this medicine, take it as soon as possible. However, if it is almost time for your next dose, skip the missed dose and go back to your regular dosing schedule. Do not double doses.

**Storage**—To store this medicine:

- Keep out of the reach of children.
- Store away from heat and direct light.
- Do not store this medicine in the bathroom, near the kitchen sink, or in other damp places. Heat or moisture may cause the medicine to break down.
- Do not keep outdated medicine or medicine no longer needed. Be sure that any discarded medicine is out of the reach of children.

## Precautions While Using This Medicine

Your doctor should check your progress at regular visits. Blood tests may be needed to make sure that this medicine is working properly and is not causing unwanted effects.

Drinking too much alcohol may increase the amount of uric acid in the blood and lessen the effects of allopurinol. Therefore, people with gout and other people with too much uric acid in the body should be careful to limit the amount of alcohol they drink.

Taking too much vitamin C may make the urine more acidic and increase the possibility of kidney stones forming while you are taking allopurinol. Therefore, check with your doctor before you take vitamin C while taking this medicine.

*Check with your doctor immediately:*

- *If you notice a skin rash, hives, or itching while you are taking allopurinol.*
- *If chills, fever, joint pain, muscle aches or pains, sore throat, or nausea or vomiting occur, especially if they occur together with or shortly after a skin rash.*

Very rarely, these effects may be the first signs of a serious reaction to the medicine.

Allopurinol may cause some people to become drowsy or less alert than they are normally. *Make sure you know how you react to this medicine before you drive, use machines, or do anything else that could be dangerous if you are not alert.*

## Side Effects of This Medicine

Along with its needed effects, a medicine may cause some unwanted effects. Although not all of these side effects may occur, if they do occur they may need medical attention.

*Stop taking this medicine and check with your doctor immediately* if any of the following side effects occur:

*More common*
   Skin rash or sores, hives, or itching

*Rare*
   Black, tarry stools; bleeding sores on lips; blood in urine or stools; chills, fever, muscle aches or pains, nausea, or vomiting—especially if occurring with or shortly after a skin rash; difficult or painful urination; pinpoint red spots on skin; redness, tenderness, burning, or peeling of skin; red and/or irritated eyes; red, thickened, or scaly skin; shortness of breath, troubled breathing, tightness in chest, or wheezing; sores, ulcers, or white spots in mouth or on lips; sore throat and fever; sudden decrease in amount of urine; swelling in upper abdominal (stomach) area; swelling of face, fingers, feet, or lower legs; swollen and/or painful glands; unusual bleeding or bruising; unusual tiredness or weakness; weight gain (rapid); yellow eyes or skin

Also, check with your doctor as soon as possible if any of the following side effects occur:

*Rare*
   Loosening of fingernails; numbness, tingling, pain, or weakness in hands or feet; pain in lower back or side; unexplained nosebleeds

Other side effects may occur that usually do not need medical attention. These side effects may go away during treatment as your body adjusts to the medicine. However, check with your doctor if any of the following side effects continue or are bothersome:

*Less common or rare*
   Diarrhea; drowsiness; headache; indigestion; nausea or vomiting occurring without a skin rash or other side effects; stomach pain occurring without other side effects; unusual hair loss

Other side effects not listed above may also occur in some patients. If you notice any other effects, check with your doctor.

Revised: 08/25/94

# ALPHA$_1$-PROTEINASE INHIBITOR, HUMAN   Systemic

A commonly used brand name in the U.S. and Canada is Prolastin. Another commonly used name is alpha$_1$-antitrypsin.

## Description

Alpha$_1$-proteinase (AL-fa wun PRO-teen-ayce) inhibitor (alpha$_1$-PI) is used to treat emphysema caused by the lack of a certain protein, alpha$_1$-antitrypsin, in the body. This medicine replaces the protein when the body does not produce enough by itself.

Alpha$_1$-PI is prepared from human blood received from many donors. Each donor's blood is tested for human immunodeficiency virus (HIV) and hepatitis B virus before it is used to prepare this medicine. Also, alpha$_1$-PI is treated with heat to further reduce the risk of transmission of virus infections. However, no procedure has been found to be totally effective in removing viruses from blood products.

There have not been any reports of hepatitis developing in any patients receiving alpha$_1$-PI. However, as a precaution, before you receive this medicine, you should be vaccinated with hepatitis B vaccine. This will help prevent infection by any hepatitis virus that may have been in the blood used to prepare alpha$_1$-PI. In some cases, there may not be enough time for the vaccine to take effect before the alpha$_1$-PI is given. Therefore, you may be given hepatitis B immune globulin at the same time that you receive the hepatitis B vaccine.

Alpha$_1$-PI is given once a week. Your doctor may want you to receive this medicine regularly for a long time. However, it is not known what the effects of this medicine are when it is used regularly to treat emphysema caused by lack of alpha$_1$-antitrypsin. Be sure you have discussed this with your doctor.

Alpha$_1$-PI is administered only by or under the immediate supervision of your doctor. It is available in the following dosage form:

*Parenteral*
- Injection (U.S. and Canada)

## Before Receiving This Medicine

In deciding to use a medicine, the risks of using the medicine must be weighed against the good it will do. This is a decision you and your doctor will make. For alpha$_1$-proteinase inhibitor, the following should be considered:

**Allergies**—Tell your doctor if you have ever had any unusual or allergic reaction to alpha$_1$-proteinase inhibitor. Also tell your health care professional if you are allergic to any other substances, such as foods, preservatives, or dyes.

**Pregnancy**—Studies on effects in pregnancy have not been done in either humans or animals.

**Breast-feeding**—It is not known whether alpha$_1$-proteinase inhibitor passes into breast milk. Although most medicines pass into breast milk in small amounts, many of them may be used safely while breast-feeding. Mothers who are taking this medicine and who wish to breast-feed should discuss this with their doctor.

**Children**—Studies on this medicine have been done only in adult patients, and there is no specific information comparing use of alpha$_1$-proteinase inhibitor in children with use in other age groups.

**Older adults**—Many medicines have not been studied specifically in older people. Therefore, it may not be known whether they work exactly the same way they do in younger adults or if they cause different side effects or problems in older people. There is no specific information comparing use of alpha$_1$-proteinase inhibitor in the elderly with use in other age groups.

**Other medicines**—Although certain medicines should not be used together at all, in other cases two different medicines may be used together even if an interaction might occur. In these cases, your doctor may want to change the dose, or other precautions may be necessary. Tell your health care professional if you are taking any other prescription or nonprescription (over-the-counter [OTC]) medicine.

## Proper Use of This Medicine

*In order for alpha$_1$-proteinase inhibitor (alpha$_1$-PI) to work properly, it is important that you receive this medicine once a week on a regular schedule.* If you have any questions about this, check with your doctor.

**Dosing**—The dose of alpha$_1$-proteinase inhibitor will be different for different patients. *Follow your doctor's orders or the directions on the label.* The following information includes only the average dose of alpha$_1$-proteinase inhibitor. *If your dose is different, do not change it unless your doctor tells you to do so.*

- For *emphysema caused by lack of the protein alpha$_1$-antitrypsin in the body:*
  —For *injection* dosage form:
    - Adults—Dose is based on body weight and must be determined by your doctor. The usual dose is 60 milligrams (mg) per kilogram (kg) (27 mg per pound) of body weight, slowly injected into a vein over a period of several minutes. This dose is given once a week.
    - Children—Use and dose must be determined by your doctor.

## Side Effects of This Medicine

Along with its needed effects, a medicine may cause some unwanted effects. The following side effects usually do not require medical attention. However, check with your doctor if any of these effects continue or are bothersome:

*Less common or rare*

Chills and fever; dizziness or lightheadedness; fever up to 102 °F (38.9 °C)

Note: Chills and fever may occur several hours after you receive this medicine but are usually mild and only temporary. Also, fever up to 102 °F (38.9 °C) may occur up to 12 hours after you receive this medicine and will disappear within about 24 hours.

Other side effects not listed above may also occur in some patients. If you notice any other effects, check with your doctor.

---

Revised: 08/09/94

---

# ALPROSTADIL   Intracavernosal

Some commonly used brand names are:

**In the U.S.—**
  Prostin VR Pediatric

**In Canada—**
  Prostin VR

Other commonly used names are PGE₁ and prostaglandin E₁.

## Description

Alprostadil (al-PROSS-ta-dil) belongs to the group of medicines called vasodilators. Vasodilators cause blood vessels to expand, thereby increasing blood flow. Alprostadil is used to produce erections in some impotent men. When alprostadil is injected into the penis (intracavernosal), it increases blood flow to the penis, which results in an erection.

Alprostadil injection should not be used as a sexual aid by men who are not impotent. If the medicine is not used properly, permanent damage to the penis and loss of the ability to have erections could result.

Alprostadil is available only with your doctor's prescription, in the following dosage form:

*Parenteral*
  • Injection (U.S. and Canada)

## Before Using This Medicine

In deciding to use a medicine, the risks of taking the medicine must be weighed against the good it will do. This is a decision you and your doctor will make. For alprostadil, the following should be considered:

**Allergies**—Tell your doctor if you have ever had any unusual or allergic reaction to alprostadil. Also tell your health care professional if you are allergic to any other substances, such as foods, preservatives, or dyes.

**Older adults**—Many medicines have not been studied specifically in older people. Therefore, it may not be known whether they work exactly the same way they do in younger adults or if they cause different side effects or problems in older people. There is no specific information comparing the use of alprostadil in the elderly with use in other age groups.

**Other medicines**—Although certain medicines should not be used together at all, in other cases two different medicines may be used together even if an interaction might occur. In these cases, your doctor may want to change the dose, or other precautions may be necessary. Tell your health care professional if you are taking any other prescription or nonprescription (over-the-counter [OTC]) medicine.

**Other medical problems**—The presence of other medical problems may affect the use of alprostadil. Make sure you tell your doctor if you have any other medical problems, especially:

  • Bleeding problems or
  • Liver disease—These conditions increase the risk of bleeding at the place of injection
  • Priapism (history of) or
  • Sickle cell disease—Patients with these conditions have an increased risk of priapism (erection lasting longer than 4 hours) while using alprostadil

## Proper Use of This Medicine

To give *alprostadil injection*:

  • Cleanse the injection site with alcohol. Using a sterile needle, *inject the medicine slowly and directly into the base of the penis as instructed by your doctor. Alprostadil should not be injected just under the skin.* The injection is usually not painful. If the injection is very painful or you notice bruising or swelling at the place of injection, that means you have been injecting the medicine under the skin. Stop, withdraw the needle, and reposition it properly before continuing with the injection.
  • After you have completed the injection, put pressure on the place of injection to prevent bruising. Then massage your penis as instructed by your doctor. This helps the medicine spread to all parts of the penis, so that the medicine will work better.

This medicine usually begins to work in about 5 to 10 minutes. You should attempt intercourse within 10 to 30 minutes after injecting the medicine.

Do not use the same injection site each time you use alprostadil. Rather, rotate injection sites with each use, to prevent skin problems.

**Dosing**—The dose of alprostadil will be different for different patients. *Follow your doctor's orders or the directions on the label.* The following information includes only the average doses of alprostadil. *If your dose is different, do not change it* unless your doctor tells you to do so.

- For *injection* dosage form:
  —For the treatment of impotence:
    - Adults—2.5 to 20 micrograms (mcg) (0.0025 to 0.02 milligrams [mg]), mixed with 0.5 to 3 milliliters (mL) 0.9% sodium chloride injection in your syringe. Inject this medicine very slowly into the area of your penis as directed by your doctor. Allow one or two minutes to completely inject the dose. Do not inject more than one dose in a day. Also, do not use this medicine more than two days in a row or more than three times a week.

**Storage**—To store this medicine:
- Keep out of the reach of children.
- Refrigerate. Keep the medicine from freezing.

## Precautions While Using This Medicine

*Use alprostadil injection exactly as directed by your doctor.* Do not use more of it and do not use it more often than ordered. If too much is used, the erection lasts too long and does not reverse when it should. This condition is called priapism, and it can be very dangerous. If the erection is not reversed, the blood supply to the penis may be cut off and permanent damage may occur.

*Contact your doctor immediately if the erection lasts for longer than 4 hours or if it becomes painful.* This may be a sign of priapism and must be treated right away to prevent permanent damage.

If you notice bleeding at the site when you inject alprostadil, put pressure on the spot until the bleeding stops. If it doesn't stop, check with your doctor.

## Side Effects of This Medicine

Along with its needed effects, a medicine may cause some unwanted effects. Although not all of these side effects may occur, if they do occur they may need medical attention.

*Check with your doctor immediately* if the following side effect occurs:

*Rare*
> Erection continuing for more than 4 hours

Other side effects may occur that usually do not need medical attention. These side effects may go away during treatment as your body adjusts to the medicine. However, check with your doctor if any of the following side effects continue or are bothersome:

*More common*
> Pain at place of injection; pain during erection (burning or aching)

*Rare*
> Bruising or bleeding at place of injection; swelling at place of injection

Other side effects not listed above may also occur in some patients. If you notice any other effects, check with your doctor.

Revised: 04/08/92
Interim revision: 06/29/94

---

# ALTRETAMINE  Systemic

Some commonly used brand names are:
**In the U.S.**
  Hexalen
**In Canada**
  Hexastat
Another commonly used name is hexamethylmelamine.

## Description

Altretamine (al-TRET-a-meen) belongs to the group of medicines called antineoplastics. It is used to treat cancer of the ovaries.

Altretamine interferes with the growth of cancer cells, which are eventually destroyed. Since the growth of normal body cells may also be affected by altretamine, other effects will also occur. Some of these may be serious and must be reported to your doctor. Other effects may not

be serious but may cause concern. Some effects may not occur for months or years after the medicine is used.

Before you begin treatment with altretamine, you and your doctor should talk about the good this medicine will do as well as the risks of using it.

Altretamine is available only with your doctor's prescription in the following dosage form:

*Oral*
- Capsules (U.S. and Canada)

## Before Using This Medicine

In deciding to use a medicine, the risks of taking the medicine must be weighed against the good it will do.

This is a decision you and your doctor will make. For altretamine, the following should be considered:

**Allergies**—Tell your doctor if you have ever had any unusual or allergic reaction to altretamine.

**Pregnancy**—There is a chance that this medicine may cause birth defects if either the male or female is taking it at the time of conception or if it is taken during pregnancy. In addition, many cancer medicines may cause sterility which could be permanent. Although sterility has not been reported with this medicine, it does occur in animals and the possibility should be kept in mind.

Be sure that you have discussed this with your doctor before taking this medicine. It is best to use some kind of birth control while you are taking altretamine. Tell your doctor right away if you think you have become pregnant while taking altretamine.

**Breast-feeding**—Because altretamine may cause serious side effects, breast-feeding is generally not recommended while you are taking it.

**Children**—There is no specific information comparing use of altretamine in children with use in other age groups.

**Older adults**—Many medicines have not been studied specifically in older people. Therefore, it may not be known whether they work exactly the same way they do in younger adults. Although there is no specific information comparing use of altretamine in the elderly with use in other age groups, this medicine is not expected to cause different side effects or problems in older people than it does in younger adults.

**Other medicines**—Although certain medicines should not be used together at all, in other cases two different medicines may be used together even if an interaction might occur. In these cases, your doctor may want to change the dose, or other precautions may be necessary. When you are taking altretamine, it is especially important that your health care professional know if you are taking any of the following:
- Amphotericin B by injection (e.g., Fungizone) or
- Antithyroid agents (medicine for overactive thyroid) or
- Azathioprine (e.g., Imuran) or
- Chloramphenicol (e.g., Chloromycetin) or
- Colchicine or
- Flucytosine (e.g., Ancobon) or
- Ganciclovir (e.g., Cytovene) or
- Interferon (e.g., Intron A, Roferon-A) or
- Plicamycin (e.g., Mithracin) or
- Zidovudine (e.g., AZT, Retrovir) or
- If you have ever been treated with radiation or cancer medicines—Altretamine may increase the effects of these medicines or radiation therapy on the blood
- Monoamine oxidase (MAO) inhibitors (furazolidone [e.g., Furoxone], isocarboxazid [e.g., Marplan], phenelzine [e.g., Nardil], procarbazine [e.g., Matulane], selegiline [e.g., Eldepryl], tranylcypromine [e.g., Parnate])—Taking altretamine while you are taking MAO inhibitors may cause a severe drop in blood pressure

**Other medical problems**—The presence of other medical problems may affect the use of altretamine. Make sure you tell your doctor if you have any other medical problems, especially:
- Chickenpox (including recent exposure) or
- Herpes zoster (shingles)—Risk of severe disease affecting other parts of the body
- Nervous system problems—May be worsened by altretamine
- Infection—Altretamine may decrease your body's ability to fight infection
- Kidney disease—Effects of altretamine may be increased because of slower removal from the body
- Liver disease—Effects may be changed because altretamine is activated and cleared from the body by the liver

## Proper Use of This Medicine

This medicine often causes nausea and vomiting. However, it is very important that you continue to receive the medicine even if you begin to feel ill. Taking this medicine after meals will lessen stomach upset. Ask your health care professional for other ways to lessen these effects.

**Dosing**—The dose of altretamine will be different for different patients. The dose that is used may depend on a number of things, including what the medicine is being used for, the patient's size, and whether or not other medicines are also being taken. *If you are taking altretamine at home, follow your doctor's orders or the directions on the label.* If you have any questions about the proper dose of altretamine, ask your doctor.

**Missed dose**—If you miss a dose of this medicine, take it as soon as possible. However, if it is almost time for your next dose, skip the missed dose and go back to your regular dosing schedule. Do not double doses.

**Storage**—To store this medicine:
- Keep out of the reach of children.
- Store away from heat and direct light.
- Do not store in the bathroom, near the kitchen sink, or in other damp places. Heat or moisture may cause the medicine to break down.
- Do not keep outdated medicine or medicine no longer needed. Be sure that any discarded medicine is out of the reach of children.

## Precautions While Using This Medicine

*It is very important that your doctor check your progress at regular visits* to make sure that this medicine is working properly and to check for unwanted effects.

While you are being treated with altretamine, and after you stop treatment with it, *do not have any immunizations (vaccinations) without your doctor's approval.* Altretamine may lower your body's resistance and there is a chance you might get the infection the immunization is meant to prevent. In addition, other persons living in your household should not take oral polio vaccine since there is a chance they could pass the polio virus on to you. Also, avoid persons who have taken oral polio vaccine. Do not get close to them and do not stay in the same room with them for very long. If you cannot take these precautions, you should consider wearing a protective face mask that covers the nose and mouth.

Altretamine can temporarily lower the number of white blood cells in your blood, increasing the chance of getting an infection. It can also lower the number of platelets, which are necessary for proper blood clotting. If this occurs, there are certain precautions you can take, especially when your blood count is low, to reduce the risk of infection or bleeding:

- If you can, avoid people with infections. *Check with your doctor immediately* if you think you are getting an infection or if you get a fever or chills, cough or hoarseness, lower back or side pain, or painful or difficult urination.
- *Check with your doctor immediately* if you notice any unusual bleeding or bruising; black, tarry stools; blood in urine or stools; or pinpoint red spots on your skin.
- Be careful when using a regular toothbrush, dental floss, or toothpick. Your medical doctor, dentist, or nurse may recommend other ways to clean your teeth and gums. Check with your medical doctor before having any dental work done.
- Do not touch your eyes or the inside of your nose unless you have just washed your hands and have not touched anything else in the meantime.
- Be careful not to cut yourself when you are using sharp objects such as a safety razor or fingernail or toenail cutters.
- Avoid contact sports or other situations where bruising or injury could occur.

## Side Effects of This Medicine

Along with its needed effects, a medicine may cause some unwanted effects. Although not all of these side effects may occur, if they do occur they may need medical attention.

Also, because of the way these medicines act on the body, there is a chance that they might cause other unwanted

effects that may not occur until months or years after the medicine is used. These delayed effects may include certain types of cancer, such as leukemia. Discuss these possible effects with your doctor.

*Check with your doctor or nurse immediately* if any of the following side effects occur:

*Less common or rare*
    Black, tarry stools; blood in urine or stools; cough or hoarseness; fever or chills; lower back or side pain; painful or difficult urination; pinpoint red spots on skin; unusual bleeding or bruising; unusual tiredness

Check with your doctor as soon as possible if any of the following side effects occur:

*More common*
    Anxiety; clumsiness; confusion; dizziness; mental depression; numbness in arms or legs; weakness

*Rare*
    Convulsions (seizures); skin rash or itching

Other side effects may occur that usually do not need medical attention. These side effects may go away during treatment as your body adjusts to the medicine. Also, your health care professional may be able to tell you about ways to prevent or reduce some of these side effects. Check with your doctor if any of the following side effects continue or are bothersome or if you have any questions about them:

*More common*
    Nausea and vomiting

*Less common*
    Diarrhea; loss of appetite; stomach cramps

Other side effects not listed above may also occur in some patients. If you notice any other effects, check with your doctor.

Revised: 07/23/92
Interim revision: 04/29/94

---

# AMANTADINE  Systemic

Some commonly used brand names are:
**In the U.S.—**
    Symadine
    Symmetrel
    Generic name product may also be available.
**In Canada—**
    Symmetrel

## Description

Amantadine (a-MAN-ta-deen) is an antiviral. It is used to prevent or treat certain influenza (flu) infections (type

A). It may be given alone or along with flu shots. Amantadine will not work for colds, other types of flu, or other virus infections.

Amantadine also is an antidyskinetic. It is used to treat Parkinson's disease, sometimes called paralysis agitans or shaking palsy. It may be given alone or with other medicines for Parkinson's disease. By improving muscle control and reducing stiffness, this medicine allows more normal movements of the body as the disease symptoms are reduced. Amantadine is also used to treat stiffness and shaking caused by certain medicines used to treat nervous, mental, and emotional conditions.

Amantadine may be used for other conditions as determined by your doctor.

Amantadine is available only with your doctor's prescription, in the following dosage forms:

*Oral*
- Capsules (U.S. and Canada)
- Syrup (U.S. and Canada)

## Before Using This Medicine

In deciding to use a medicine, the risks of taking the medicine must be weighed against the good it will do. This is a decision you and your doctor will make. For amantadine, the following should be considered:

**Allergies**—Tell your doctor if you have ever had any unusual or allergic reaction to amantadine. Also tell your health care professional if you are allergic to any other substances, such as foods, preservatives, or dyes.

**Pregnancy**—Studies have not been done in humans. However, studies in some animals have shown that amantadine is harmful to the fetus and causes birth defects.

**Breast-feeding**—Amantadine passes into breast milk. However, the effects of amantadine in newborn babies and infants are not known.

**Children**—This medicine has been tested in children over one year of age and has not been shown to cause different side effects or problems in these children than it does in adults. There is no specific information comparing the use of amantadine in children under one year of age with use in other age groups.

**Older adults**—Elderly people are especially sensitive to the effects of amantadine. Confusion, difficult urination, blurred vision, constipation, and dry mouth, nose, and throat may be especially likely to occur.

**Other medicines**—Although certain medicines should not be used together at all, in other cases two different medicines may be used together even if an interaction might occur. In these cases, your doctor may want to change the dose, or other precautions may be necessary. When you are taking amantadine, it is especially important that your health care professional know if you are taking any of the following:
- Amphetamines or
- Appetite suppressants (diet pills), except fenfluramine (e.g., Pondimin), or
- Caffeine (e.g., NoDoz) or
- Chlophedianol (e.g., Ulone) or
- Cocaine or
- Medicine for asthma or other breathing problems or
- Medicine for colds, sinus problems, or hay fever or other allergies (including nose drops or sprays) or
- Methylphenidate (e.g., Ritalin) or
- Nabilone (e.g., Cesamet) or
- Pemoline (e.g., Cylert)—The use of amantadine with these medicines may increase the chance of unwanted effects

such as nervousness, irritability, trouble in sleeping, and possibly seizures or irregular heartbeat
- Anticholinergics (medicine for abdominal or stomach spasms or cramps)—The use of amantadine with these medicines may increase the chance of unwanted effects such as blurred vision, dryness of the mouth, confusion, hallucinations, and nightmares

**Other medical problems**—The presence of other medical problems may affect the use of amantadine. Make sure you tell your doctor if you have any other medical problems, especially:
- Eczema (recurring)—Amantadine may cause or worsen eczema
- Epilepsy or other seizures (history of)—Amantadine may increase the frequency of convulsions (seizures) in patients with a seizure disorder
- Heart disease or other circulation problems or
- Swelling of feet and ankles—Amantadine may increase the chance of swelling of the feet and ankles, and may worsen heart disease or circulation problems
- Kidney disease—Amantadine is removed from the body by the kidneys; patients with kidney disease will need to receive a lower dose of amantadine
- Mental or emotional illness—Higher doses of amantadine may cause confusion, hallucinations, and nightmares

## Proper Use of This Medicine

For patients *taking amantadine to prevent or treat flu infections:*
- Talk to your doctor about the possibility of getting a flu shot if you have not had one yet.
- This medicine is *best taken before exposure, or as soon as possible after exposure,* to people who have the flu.
- To help keep yourself from getting the flu, *keep taking this medicine for the full time of treatment.* Or if you already have the flu, continue taking this medicine for the full time of treatment even if you begin to feel better after a few days. This will help to clear up your infection completely. If you stop taking this medicine too soon, your symptoms may return. This medicine should be taken for at least 2 days after all your flu symptoms have disappeared.
- This medicine works best when there is a constant amount in the blood. *To help keep the amount constant, do not miss any doses. Also, it is best to take the doses at evenly spaced times day and night.* For example, if you are to take 2 doses a day, the doses should be spaced about 12 hours apart. If this interferes with your sleep or other daily activities, or if you need help in planning the best times to take your medicine, check with your health care professional.
- If you are using the oral liquid form of amantadine, use a specially marked measuring spoon or other device to measure each dose accurately. The average household teaspoon may not hold the right amount of liquid.

For patients *taking amantadine for Parkinson's disease or movement problems* caused by certain medicines used to treat nervous, mental, and emotional conditions:

- *Take this medicine exactly as directed by your doctor.* Do not miss any doses and do not take more medicine than your doctor ordered.
- Improvement in the symptoms of Parkinson's disease usually occurs in about 2 days. However, in some patients this medicine must be taken for up to 2 weeks before full benefit is seen.

**Dosing**—The dose of amantadine will be different for different patients. *Follow your doctor's orders or the directions on the label.* The following information includes only the average doses of amantadine. Your dose may be different if you have kidney disease. *If your dose is different, do not change it* unless your doctor tells you to do so.

- The number of capsules or teaspoonfuls of suspension that you take depends on the strength of the medicine. Also, *the number of doses you take each day, the time allowed between doses, and the length of time you take the medicine depend on the medical problem for which you are taking amantadine.*
- For the *treatment or prevention of flu:*
    —Older adults: 100 milligrams once a day.
    —Adults and children 12 years of age and older: 200 milligrams once a day, or 100 milligrams two times a day.
    —Children 9 to 12 years of age: 100 milligrams two times a day.
    —Children 1 to 9 years of age: Dose is based on body weight and must be determined by the doctor.
- For the *treatment of Parkinson's disease or movement problems:*
    —Older adults: 100 milligrams once a day to start. The dose may be increased slowly over time, if needed.
    —Adults: 100 milligrams one or two times a day.
    —Children: Dose has not been determined.

**Missed dose**—If you miss a dose of this medicine, take it as soon as possible. This will help to keep a constant amount of medicine in the blood. However, if it is almost time for your next dose, skip the missed dose and go back to your regular dosing schedule. Do not double doses.

**Storage**—To store this medicine:

- Keep out of the reach of children.
- Store away from heat and direct light.
- Do not store the capsule form of this medicine in the bathroom, near the kitchen sink, or in other damp places. Heat or moisture may cause the medicine to break down.
- Keep the oral liquid form of this medicine from freezing.
- Do not keep outdated medicine or medicine no longer needed. Be sure that any discarded medicine is out of the reach of children.

## Precautions While Using This Medicine

Drinking alcoholic beverages while taking this medicine may cause increased side effects such as circulation problems, dizziness, lightheadedness, fainting, or confusion. Therefore, *do not drink alcoholic beverages while you are taking this medicine.*

This medicine may cause some people to become dizzy, confused, or lightheaded, or to have blurred vision or trouble concentrating. *Make sure you know how you react to this medicine before you drive, use machines, or do anything else that could be dangerous if you are dizzy or are not alert or able to see well.* If these reactions are especially bothersome, check with your doctor.

Getting up suddenly from a lying or sitting position may also be a problem because of the dizziness, lightheadedness, or fainting that may be caused by this medicine. Getting up slowly may help. If this problem continues or gets worse, check with your doctor.

Amantadine may cause dryness of the mouth, nose, and throat. For temporary relief of mouth dryness, use sugarless candy or gum, melt bits of ice in your mouth, or use a saliva substitute. However, if your mouth continues to feel dry for more than 2 weeks, check with your doctor or dentist. Continuing dryness of the mouth may increase the chance of dental disease, including tooth decay, gum disease, and fungus infections.

This medicine may cause purplish red, net-like, blotchy spots on the skin. This problem occurs more often in females and usually occurs on the legs and/or feet after this medicine has been taken regularly for a month or more. Although the blotchy spots may remain as long as you are taking this medicine, they usually go away gradually within 2 to 12 weeks after you stop taking the medicine. If you have any questions about this, check with your doctor.

For patients *taking amantadine to prevent or treat flu infections:*

- If your symptoms do not improve within a few days, or if they become worse, check with your doctor.

For patients *taking amantadine for Parkinson's disease or movement problems* caused by certain medicines used to treat nervous, mental, and emotional conditions:

- *Patients with Parkinson's disease must be careful not to overdo physical activities as their condition improves and body movements become easier* since injuries resulting from falls may occur. Such activities must be gradually increased to give your body time to adjust to changing balance, circulation, and coordination.
- Some patients may notice that this medicine gradually loses its effect while they are taking it regularly for a few months. If you notice this, check with your doctor. Your doctor may want to adjust the dose or stop the medicine for a while and then restart it to restore its effect.

• *Do not suddenly stop taking this medicine without first checking with your doctor* since your Parkinson's disease may get worse very quickly. Your doctor may want you to reduce your dose gradually before stopping the medicine completely.

## Side Effects of This Medicine

Along with its needed effects, a medicine may cause some unwanted effects. Although not all of these side effects may occur, if they do occur they may need medical attention.

*Check with your doctor immediately* if any of the following side effects occur:

*Less common*
> Blurred vision; confusion (especially in elderly patients); difficult urination (especially in elderly patients); fainting; hallucinations (seeing, hearing, or feeling things that are not there)

*Rare*
> Convulsions (seizures); decreased vision or any change in vision; difficulty in coordination; irritation and swelling of the eye; mental depression; skin rash; swelling of feet or lower legs; unexplained shortness of breath

Other side effects may occur that usually do not need medical attention. These side effects may go away during treatment as your body adjusts to the medicine. However, check with your doctor if any of the following side effects continue or are bothersome:

*More common*
> Difficulty concentrating; dizziness or lightheadedness; headache; irritability; loss of appetite; nausea; nervousness; purplish red, net-like, blotchy spots on skin; trouble in sleeping or nightmares

*Less common or rare*
> Constipation; dryness of the mouth, nose, and throat; vomiting

Other side effects not listed above may also occur in some patients. If you notice any other effects, check with your doctor.

## Additional Information

Once a medicine has been approved for marketing for a certain use, experience may show that it is also useful for other medical problems. Although this use is not included in product labeling, amantadine is used in certain patients with the following medical condition:

• Unusual tiredness or weakness associated with multiple sclerosis

Other than the above information, there is no additional information relating to proper use, precautions, or side effects for this use.

Revised: 02/23/93

# AMINOBENZOATE POTASSIUM   Systemic

Some commonly used brand names in the U.S. and Canada are Potaba, Potaba Envules, and Potaba Powder.

Other commonly used names are KPAB, potassium aminobenzoate, and potassium para-aminobenzoate.

## Description

Aminobenzoate potassium (a-mee-noe-BEN-zoe-ate poe-TAS-ee-um) is used to treat fibrosis, a condition in which the skin and underlying tissues tighten and become less flexible. This condition occurs in such diseases as dermatomyositis, morphea, Peyronie's disease, scleroderma, and linear scleroderma.

Aminobenzoate potassium is also used to treat a certain type of inflammation (nonsuppurative inflammation) that occurs in such diseases as dermatomyositis, pemphigus, and Peyronie's disease.

This medicine is available only with your doctor's prescription in the following dosage forms:

*Oral*
- Capsules (U.S. and Canada)
- Powder for oral solution (U.S. and Canada)
- Tablets (U.S. and Canada)

## Before Using This Medicine

In deciding to use a medicine, the risks of taking the medicine must be weighed against the good it will do. This is a decision you and your doctor will make. For aminobenzoate potassium, the following should be considered:

**Allergies**—Tell your doctor if you have ever had any unusual or allergic reaction to aminobenzoate potassium or aminobenzoic acid (PABA). Also tell your health care professional if you are allergic to any other substances, such as foods, preservatives, or dyes.

**Diet**—Make certain your health care professional knows if you are on any special diet, such as a low-sodium or low-sugar diet.

**Pregnancy**—Studies on effects in pregnancy have not been done in either humans or animals.

**Breast-feeding**—Aminobenzoate potassium has not been reported to cause problems in nursing babies.

**Children**—Although there is no specific information comparing use of aminobenzoate potassium in children with use in other age groups, this medicine is not expected to cause different side effects or problems in children than it does in adults.

**Older adults**—Elderly people may be more sensitive to certain symptoms of the low blood sugar side effect. These symptoms include confusion, difficulty in concentration, and headache. In addition, these symptoms may be harder to detect in elderly persons than in younger adults. This may increase the chance of problems during treatment with this medicine.

**Other medicines**—Although certain medicines should not be used together at all, in other cases two different medicines may be used together even if an interaction might occur. In these cases, your doctor may want to change the dose, or other precautions may be necessary. When you are taking aminobenzoate potassium, it is especially important that your health care professional know if you are taking any of the following:

- Aminosalicylates or
- Sulfonamides (sulfa medicine)—Aminobenzoate potassium may decrease the effects of these medicines

**Other medical problems**—The presence of other medical problems may affect the use of aminobenzoate potassium. Make sure you tell your doctor if you have any other medical problems, especially:

- Diabetes mellitus (sugar diabetes) or
- Hypoglycemia (low blood sugar)—The risk of the medicine causing hypoglycemia (low blood sugar) may be increased
- Kidney disease—Aminobenzoate potassium is removed from the body by the kidneys; higher blood levels of the medicine may occur if kidney disease is present, which may increase the chance of side effects

---

## Proper Use of This Medicine

Take this medicine with meals or snacks to lessen the possibility of stomach upset. If stomach upset continues, check with your doctor.

For patients taking the *capsule or tablet form* of aminobenzoate potassium:

- Take each dose with a full glass (8 ounces) of water or milk to lessen the possibility of stomach upset.
- Patients using the tablets should dissolve them in water before taking. This will help lessen the possibility of stomach upset.

For patients using the *powder form* of this medicine:

- This medicine should never be taken in its dry form. Instead, always mix it with water or citrus juice, as directed.
- To cover up the taste of aminobenzoate potassium, you may dissolve the powder in citrus drinks instead of in water. However, if you do dissolve the powder in water, drinking a citrus juice or a carbonated beverage immediately after each dose of medicine will also help cover up the taste.
- The flavor of this medicine is improved if the solution is chilled before you take it.

- For patients using the *two-gram individual packets of powder*:
  —Dissolve one packet (2 grams) of aminobenzoate potassium in a full glass (8 ounces) of water or citrus juice.
  —Stir well to dissolve the powder.
- For patients using the *bulk powder form* of this medicine:
  —Use a specially marked measuring spoon or other device to measure out the correct amount of medicine. Your health care professional can help you with this.
  —To make a 10-percent solution of this medicine:
  - Choose a container that is resistant to light, such as an amber glass container, a metal container, or a plastic container that you cannot see through. Make sure the container is large enough to measure one liter (approximately one quart).
  - Place 100 grams (approximately 3 ounces) of aminobenzoate potassium powder in the container.
  - Add enough water or citrus juice to make one liter (approximately one quart) of solution and stir well.
  - Store the solution in a container that is resistant to light, such as an amber glass container, a metal container, or a plastic container that you cannot see through.
  - Keep the solution refrigerated. Stir well before pouring each dose. Discard the unused portion after one week.

*For this medicine to be effective, it must be taken every day* as ordered by your doctor. It may take 3 or more months before you begin to see an improvement in your condition.

**Dosing**—The dose of aminobenzoate potassium will be different for different patients. *Follow your doctor's orders or the directions on the label*. The following information includes only the average dose of aminobenzoate potassium. *If your dose is different, do not change it* unless your doctor tells you to do so.

- For *oral dosage forms* (capsules, powder for oral solution, and tablets):
  —For fibrosis:
  - Adults—12 grams a day, divided into four to six doses and taken with meals or snacks.
  - Children—Dose is based on body weight and must be determined by your doctor. The usual dose is 220 milligrams (mg) per kilogram (kg) (100 mg per pound) of body weight a day. This is divided into four to six doses and taken with meals or snacks.

**Missed dose**—If you miss a dose of this medicine, take it as soon as possible. However, if it is within 2 hours of your next dose, skip the missed dose and go back to your regular dosing schedule. Do not double doses.

**Storage**—To store this medicine:

- Keep out of the reach of children.
- Store away from heat and direct light.
- Do not store the medicine in the bathroom, near the kitchen sink, or in other damp places. Heat or moisture may cause the medicine to break down.
- Store the liquid form of this medicine in the refrigerator. However, keep the medicine from freezing. Store the liquid form of this medicine in a container that is resistant to light, such as an amber glass container, a metal container, or a plastic container that you cannot see through.
- Discard the unused portion of the liquid form of this medicine after one week.
- Do not keep outdated medicine or medicine no longer needed. Be sure that any discarded medicine is out of the reach of children.

## Precautions While Using This Medicine

While you are taking this medicine, it is important that your doctor check your progress at regular visits.

*Check with your doctor right away if you cannot eat normally while taking this medicine* because of nausea, loss of appetite, or for any other reason. Taking this medicine when you have not been eating normally for several days may cause low blood sugar (hypoglycemia).

*If symptoms of low blood sugar (hypoglycemia) appear, stop taking this medicine, eat or drink something containing sugar, and check with your doctor right away.* Good sources of sugar are table sugar mixed in water, sugar cubes, orange juice, corn syrup, or honey. One popular source of sugar is a glassful of orange juice containing 2 or 3 teaspoonfuls of table sugar.

- *Tell someone ahead of time to take you to your doctor or to a hospital right away if you begin to feel that you may pass out. If you do pass out, emergency help should be gotten at once.*

- *Even if you correct the symptoms of low blood sugar by eating or drinking something with sugar, it is very important to call your doctor right away. The effects this medicine has on low blood sugar may last for a few days, and the symptoms may return often during this period of time.*

## Side Effects of This Medicine

Along with its needed effects, a medicine may cause some unwanted effects. Although not all of these side effects may occur, if they do occur they may need medical attention.

Check with your doctor as soon as possible if any of the following side effects occur:

*Less common or rare*
    Chills; fever; skin rash; sore throat
*Symptoms of low blood sugar*
    Anxiety; chills; cold sweats; confusion; cool pale skin; difficulty in concentration; drowsiness; excessive hunger; fast heartbeat; headache; nervousness; shakiness; unsteady walk; unusual tiredness or weakness

Other side effects may occur that usually do not need medical attention. These side effects may go away during treatment as your body adjusts to the medicine. However, check with your doctor if either of the following side effects continues or is bothersome:

*More common*
    Loss of appetite; nausea

Other side effects not listed above may also occur in some patients. If you notice any other effects, check with your doctor.

Revised: 07/06/94

# AMINOGLUTETHIMIDE   Systemic

A commonly used brand name in the U.S. and Canada is Cytadren.

## Description

Aminoglutethimide (a-mee-noe-gloo-TETH-i-mide) acts on a part of the body called the adrenal cortex. It affects production of steroids and also has some other effects. Aminoglutethimide is used to treat some kinds of tumors that affect the adrenal cortex. Also, it is sometimes used when the adrenal cortex is overactive without being cancerous.

In addition, aminoglutethimide is sometimes used to treat certain other conditions as determined by your doctor.

Aminoglutethimide is available only with your doctor's prescription, in the following dosage form:

*Oral*
- Tablets (U.S. and Canada)

## Before Using This Medicine

In deciding to use a medicine, the risks of taking the medicine must be weighed against the good it will do. This is a decision you and your doctor will make. For aminoglutethimide, the following should be considered:

**Allergies**—Tell your doctor if you have ever had any unusual or allergic reaction to glutethimide or aminoglutethimide. Also tell your health care professional if you are allergic to any other substances, such as foods, preservatives, or dyes.

**Pregnancy**—Aminoglutethimide has been shown to cause birth defects in humans and animals. However, this medicine may be needed in serious diseases or in other situations that threaten the mother's life. Be sure you have discussed this with your doctor before taking this medicine.

**Breast-feeding**—It is not known whether aminoglutethimide passes into breast milk. However, this medicine has not been reported to cause problems in nursing babies.

**Children**—There is no specific information comparing use of aminoglutethimide in children with use in other age groups. However, there is a chance that aminoglutethimide could cause premature growth and sexual development in males or development of male features in females.

**Older adults**—Lack of energy is more likely to occur in the elderly, who are usually more sensitive to the effects of aminoglutethimide.

**Other medicines**—Although certain medicines should not be used together at all, in other cases two different medicines may be used together even if an interaction might occur. In these cases, your doctor may want to change the dose, or other precautions may be necessary. When you are taking aminoglutethimide it is especially important that your health care professional know if you are taking any of the following:

- Dexamethasone (e.g., Decadron)—Aminoglutethimide increases the rate at which dexamethasone is removed from the body

**Other medical problems**—The presence of other medical problems may affect the use of aminoglutethimide. Make sure you tell your doctor if you have any other medical problems, especially:

- Chickenpox (including recent exposure) or
- Herpes zoster (shingles)—Risk of severe disease affecting other parts of the body
- Infection—May affect the adrenal cortex. If a steroid supplement is being used, a change in dose may be needed
- Kidney disease or
- Liver disease—Effects of aminoglutethimide may be increased because of slower removal from the body
- Underactive thyroid—Aminoglutethimide can cause underactive thyroid

## Proper Use of This Medicine

*Take this medicine only as directed by your doctor.* Do not take more or less of it, and do not take it more often than your doctor ordered.

This medicine sometimes causes nausea and vomiting. This effect usually goes away or lessens after you have taken the medicine for a while. It is very important that you continue to use this medicine even if you begin to feel ill. Ask your health care provider for ways to lessen these effects. *Do not stop taking this medicine without first checking with your doctor.*

If you vomit shortly after taking a dose of aminoglutethimide, check with your doctor. You will be told whether to take the dose again or to wait until the next scheduled dose.

**Dosing**—The dose of aminoglutethimide will be different for different patients. The dose that is used may depend on a number of things, including what the medicine is being used for, the patient's weight, and whether or not other medicines are also being taken. *If you are taking aminoglutethimide at home, follow your doctor's orders or the directions on the label.* If you have any questions about the proper dose of aminoglutethimide, ask your doctor.

**Missed dose**—If you miss a dose of this medicine and remember within 2 to 4 hours of the missed dose, take it as soon as possible. Then go back to your regular dosing schedule. However, if it is almost time for your next dose, skip the missed dose and go back to your regular dosing schedule. Do not double doses.

**Storage**—To store this medicine:

- Keep out of the reach of children.
- Store away from heat and direct light.
- Do not store in the bathroom, near the kitchen sink, or in other damp places. Heat or moisture may cause the medicine to break down.
- Do not keep outdated medicine or medicine no longer needed. Be sure that any discarded medicine is out of the reach of children.

## Precautions While Using This Medicine

*It is very important that your doctor check your progress at regular visits* to make sure that the medicine is working properly and does not cause unwanted effects.

Your doctor may want you to carry a medical identification card or wear a bracelet stating that you are taking this medicine.

Before you have any kind of surgery (including dental surgery) or emergency treatment, tell the medical doctor or dentist in charge that you are taking this medicine. Because this medicine affects the adrenal gland, extra steroids may be needed.

*Check with your doctor right away if you get an injury, infection, or illness of any kind.* This medicine may weaken your body's defenses against infection or inflammation.

This medicine may cause some people to become dizzy, drowsy, or less alert than they are normally. *Make sure you know how you react to this medicine before you drive, use machines, or do anything else that could be dangerous if you are dizzy or are not alert.*

## Side Effects of This Medicine

Along with its needed effects, a medicine may cause some unwanted effects. Some side effects will have signs or symptoms that you can see or feel. Your doctor may watch for others by doing certain tests. Some of the unwanted effects that may be caused by aminoglutethimide are listed below. Although not all of these side effects may occur, if they do occur they may need medical attention.

*Check with your doctor immediately* if any of the following side effects occur:

*Rare*

Black, tarry stools; blood in urine or stools; cough or hoarseness; fever or chills; lower back or side pain; painful or difficult urination; pinpoint red spots on skin; unusual bleeding or bruising; yellow eyes or skin

Check with your doctor as soon as possible if the following side effects occur:

*Less common*

Darkening of skin; mental depression

*Rare*

Neck tenderness or swelling

This medicine may also cause the following side effects that your doctor will watch for:

*More common*

Low red blood cell count; low white blood cell count

Other side effects may occur that usually do not need medical attention. These side effects may go away during treatment as your body adjusts to the medicine. However, check with your health care professional if any of the following side effects continue or are bothersome:

*More common*

Clumsiness; dizziness or lightheadedness (especially when getting up from a lying or sitting position); drowsiness;

lack of energy; loss of appetite; measles-like skin rash or itching on face and/or palms of hands; nausea; uncontrolled eye movements

*Less common or rare*

Deepening of voice in females; headache; increased hair growth in females; irregular menstrual periods; mental depression; muscle pain; vomiting

Other side effects not listed above may also occur in some patients. If you notice any other effects, check with your doctor.

## Additional Information

Once a medicine has been approved for marketing for a certain use, experience may show that it is also useful for other medical problems. Although these uses are not included in product labeling, aminoglutethimide is used in certain patients with the following medical conditions:

• Breast cancer
• Prostate cancer

Other than the above information, there is no additional information relating to proper use, precautions, or side effects for these uses.

Revised: 04/09/93
Interim revision: 04/29/94

# AMINOGLYCOSIDES   Systemic

Some commonly used brand names are:

**In the U.S.—**

| | |
|---|---|
| Amikin[1] | Kantrex[3] |
| Garamycin[2] | Nebcin[7] |
| G-Mycin[2] | Netromycin[5] |
| Jenamicin[2] | |

**In Canada—**

| | |
|---|---|
| Amikin[1] | Nebcin[7] |
| Cidomycin[2] | Netromycin[5] |
| Garamycin[2] | |

Note: For quick reference, the following aminoglycosides are numbered to match the corresponding brand names.
This information applies to the following medicines:

1. Amikacin (am-i-KAY-sin)‡
2. Gentamicin (jen-ta-MYE-sin)‡
3. Kanamycin (kan-a-MYE-sin)†‡
4. Neomycin (nee-oh-MYE-sin)†‡
5. Netilmicin (ne-til-MYE-sin)
6. Streptomycin (strep-toe-MYE-sin)‡§
7. Tobramycin (toe-bra-MYE-sin)‡

†Not commercially available in Canada.
‡Generic name product may also be available in the U.S.
§Generic name product may also be available in Canada.

## Description

Aminoglycosides (a-mee-noe-GLYE-koe-sides) are used to treat serious bacterial infections. They work by killing bacteria or preventing their growth.

Aminoglycosides are given by injection to treat serious bacterial infections in many different parts of the body. In addition, some aminoglycosides may be given by irrigation (applying a solution of the medicine to the skin or mucous membranes or washing out a body cavity) or by inhalation into the lungs. Streptomycin may also be given for tuberculosis (TB). These medicines may be given with 1 or more other medicines for bacterial infections, or they may be given alone. Aminoglycosides may also be used for other conditions as determined by your doctor. However, aminoglycosides will not work for colds, flu, or other virus infections.

Aminoglycosides given by injection are usually used for serious bacterial infections for which other medicines may not work. However, aminoglycosides may also cause some serious side effects, including damage to your hearing, sense of balance, and kidneys. These side effects may be more likely to occur in elderly patients and newborn infants. *You and your doctor should talk about the good these medicines may do as well as the risks of receiving them.*

Aminoglycosides are to be administered only by or under the immediate supervision of your doctor. They are available in the following dosage forms:

*Inhalation*
Amikacin
- Inhalation solution (U.S.)
Gentamicin
- Inhalation solution (U.S.)
Kanamycin
- Inhalation solution (U.S.)
Tobramycin
- Inhalation solution (U.S.)

*Irrigation*
Kanamycin
- Irrigation solution (U.S.)

*Parenteral*
Amikacin
- Injection (U.S. and Canada)
Gentamicin
- Injection (U.S. and Canada)
Kanamycin
- Injection (U.S.)
Neomycin
- Injection (U.S.)
Netilmicin
- Injection (U.S. and Canada)
Streptomycin
- Injection (U.S. and Canada)
Tobramycin
- Injection (U.S. and Canada)

## Before Receiving This Medicine

In deciding to use a medicine, the risks of taking the medicine must be weighed against the good it will do. This is a decision you and your doctor will make. For aminoglycosides, the following should be considered:

**Allergies**—Tell your doctor if you have ever had any unusual or allergic reaction to any of the aminoglycosides. Also tell your health care professional if you are allergic to any other substances, such as foods, sulfites, or other preservatives.

**Pregnancy**—Studies on most of the aminoglycosides have not been done in pregnant women. Some reports have shown that aminoglycosides, especially streptomycin and tobramycin, may cause damage to the infant's hearing, sense of balance, and kidneys if the mother was receiving the medicine during pregnancy. However, this medicine may be needed in serious diseases or other situations that threaten the mother's life. Be sure you have discussed this with your doctor.

**Breast-feeding**—Aminoglycosides pass into breast milk in small amounts. However, they are not absorbed very much when taken by mouth. To date, aminoglycosides have not been reported to cause problems in nursing babies.

**Children**—Children are especially sensitive to the effects of aminoglycosides. Damage to hearing, sense of balance, and kidneys is more likely to occur in premature infants and neonates.

**Older adults**—Elderly people are especially sensitive to the effects of aminoglycosides. Serious side effects, such as damage to hearing, sense of balance, and kidneys may occur in elderly patients.

**Other medicines**—Although certain medicines should not be used together at all, in other cases two different medicines may be used together even if an interaction might occur. In these cases, your doctor may want to change the dose, or other precautions may be necessary. When you are receiving aminoglycosides it is especially important that your health care professional knows if you are taking any of the following:

- Aminoglycosides, used on the skin or mucous membranes and by injection at the same time; or more than one aminoglycoside at a time or
- Anti-infectives by mouth or by injection (medicine for infection) or
- Capreomycin (e.g., Capastat) or
- Carmustine (e.g., BiCNU) or
- Chloroquine (e.g., Aralen) or
- Cisplatin (e.g., Platinol) or
- Combination pain medicine containing acetaminophen and aspirin (e.g., Excedrin) or other salicylates (with large amounts taken regularly) or
- Cyclosporine (e.g., Sandimmune) or
- Deferoxamine (e.g., Desferal) (with long-term use) or
- Gold salts (medicine for arthritis) or
- Hydroxychloroquine (e.g., Plaquenil) or
- Inflammation or pain medicine, except narcotics, or
- Lithium (e.g., Lithane) or
- Methotrexate (e.g., Mexate) or
- Penicillamine (e.g., Cuprimine) or
- Plicamycin (e.g., Mithracin) or
- Quinine (e.g., Quinamm) or
- Streptozocin (e.g., Zanosar) or
- Tiopronin (e.g., Thiola)—Use of any of these medicines with aminoglycosides may increase the chance of hearing, balance, or kidney side effects

**Other medical problems**—The presence of other medical problems may affect the use of the aminoglycosides. Make sure you tell your doctor if you have any other medical problems, especially:

- Kidney disease—Patients with kidney disease may have increased aminoglycoside blood levels and increased chance of side effects
- Loss of hearing and/or balance (eighth-cranial-nerve disease)—High aminoglycoside blood levels may cause hearing loss or balance disturbances
- Myasthenia gravis or
- Parkinson's disease—Aminoglycosides may cause muscular problems, resulting in further muscle weakness

## Proper Use of This Medicine

To help clear up your infection completely, *aminoglycosides must be given for the full time of treatment,* even if you begin to feel better after a few days. Also, this medicine works best when there is a certain amount in the blood or urine. To help keep the correct level, aminoglycosides must be given on a regular schedule.

**Dosing**—The dose of aminoglycosides will be different for different patients. *Follow your doctor's orders or the directions on the label.* The following information includes only the average doses of aminoglycosides. Your dose may be different if you have kidney disease. *If your dose is different, do not change it* unless your doctor tells you to do so.

The dose of most aminoglycosides is based on body weight and must be determined by your doctor. The medicine is injected into a muscle or vein. Depending on the aminoglycoside prescribed, doses are given at different times and for different lengths of time. These times are as follows:

*For amikacin*
- For *all* dosage forms:
  —Adults and children: The dose is given every eight or twelve hours for seven to ten days.
  —Newborn babies: The dose is given every twelve hours for seven to ten days.
  —Premature babies: The dose is given every eighteen to twenty-four hours for seven to ten days.

*For gentamicin*
- For *all* dosage forms:
  —Adults and children: The dose is given every eight hours for seven to ten days or more.
  —Infants: The dose is given every eight to sixteen hours for seven to ten days or more.
  —Premature and full-term newborn babies: The dose is given every twelve to twenty-four hours for seven to ten days or more.

*For kanamicin*
- For *all* dosage forms:
  —Adults and children: The dose is given every eight or twelve hours for seven to ten days.

*For netilmicin*
- For *all* dosage forms:
  —Adults and children: The dose is given every eight or twelve hours for seven to fourteen days.

*For tobramycin*
- For *all* dosage forms:
  —Adults and adolescents: The dose is given every six to eight hours for seven to ten days or more.

  —Older infants and children: The dose is given every six to sixteen hours.
  —Premature and full-term newborn babies: The dose is given every twelve to twenty-four hours.

*For streptomycin*
- For *all* dosage forms—The dose of streptomycin is often not based on body weight and the amount given depends on the disease being treated.
  —*Treatment of tuberculosis (TB):*
    - Adults and adolescents: 1 gram injected into a muscle once a day. This will be reduced to two or three times a week, if possible. This medicine must be given with other medicines for tuberculosis (TB).
    - Children: Dose is based on body weight and must be determined by your doctor. This dose is injected into a muscle once a day. This medicine must be given with other medicines for tuberculosis (TB).
  —*Treatment of bacterial infections:*
    - Adults and adolescents: 250 milligrams to 1 gram of streptomycin is injected into a muscle every six to twelve hours.
    - Children: Dose is based on body weight and must be determined by your doctor. This dose is injected into a muscle every six to twelve hours.

## Side Effects of This Medicine

Along with its needed effects, a medicine may cause some unwanted effects. Although not all of these side effects may occur, if they do occur they may need medical attention.

*Check with your health care professional immediately* if any of the following side effects occur:

*More common*
　　Any loss of hearing; clumsiness or unsteadiness; dizziness; greatly increased or decreased frequency of urination or amount of urine; increased thirst; loss of appetite; nausea or vomiting; numbness, tingling, or burning of face or mouth (streptomycin only); muscle twitching, or convulsions (seizures); ringing or buzzing or a feeling of fullness in the ears

*Less common*
　　Any loss of vision (streptomycin only); skin rash, itching, redness, or swelling

*Rare*
　　Difficulty in breathing; drowsiness; weakness

In addition, leg cramps, skin rash, fever, and convulsions (seizures) may occur when gentamicin is given by injection into the muscle or a vein, and into the spinal fluid.

For up to several weeks after you stop receiving this medicine, it may still cause some side effects that need medical attention. Check with your doctor if you notice any of the following side effects or if they get worse:

  Any loss of hearing; clumsiness or unsteadiness; dizziness; greatly increased or decreased frequency of urination or amount of urine; increased thirst; loss of appetite; nausea or vomiting; ringing or buzzing or a feeling of fullness in the ears

Other side effects not listed above may also occur in some patients. If you notice any other effects, check with your doctor.

Revised: 02/23/93

---

# AMINOSALICYLATE SODIUM    Systemic

Some commonly used brand names are:

**In the U.S.—**
  Tubasal
**In Canada—**
  Nemasol Sodium
Another commonly used name is PAS.

---

## Description

Aminosalicylate sodium (a-mee-noe-sal-I-si-late soe-dee-um) belongs to the family of medicines called anti-infectives. It is used with other medicines, to help the body overcome tuberculosis (TB). It will not work for colds, flu, or other virus infections.

*To help clear up your tuberculosis (TB) completely, you must keep taking this medicine for the full time of treatment, even if you begin to feel better. This is very important. It is also important that you do not miss any doses.*

Aminosalicylate sodium is available only with your doctor's prescription, in the following dosage form:
  *Oral*
  • Tablets (U.S. and Canada)

---

## Before Using This Medicine

In deciding to use a medicine, the risks of taking the medicine must be weighed against the good it will do. This is a decision you and your doctor will make. For aminosalicylate sodium, the following should be considered:

**Allergies**—Tell your doctor if you have ever had any unusual or allergic reaction to aminosalicylate sodium, aspirin or other salicylates, including methyl salicylate (oil of wintergreen), or to other related medicines such as sulfonamides (sulfa medicine). Also tell your health care professional if you are allergic to any other substances, such as foods, preservatives, or dyes.

**Pregnancy**—In one study where aminosalicylates were taken with other medicines for tuberculosis, there was an increase in birth defects. However, other studies have not shown aminosalicylates to cause birth defects.

**Breast-feeding**—Aminosalicylate sodium passes into the breast milk. However, this medicine has not been reported to cause problems in nursing babies.

**Children**—There is no specific information comparing use of aminosalicylate sodium in children with use in other age groups.

**Older adults**—Many medicines have not been studied specifically in older people. Therefore, it may not be known whether they work exactly the same way they do in younger adults or if they cause different side effects or problems in older people. There is no specific information comparing use of aminosalicylate sodium in the elderly with use in other age groups.

**Other medicines**—Although certain medicines should not be used together at all, in other cases two different medicines may be used together even if an interaction might occur. In these cases, your doctor may want to change the dose, or other precautions may be necessary. When you are taking aminosalicylate sodium, it is especially important that your health care professional know if you are taking any of the following:

  • Aminobenzoates (e.g., Potaba)—Use of aminosalicylate sodium with aminobenzoates may decrease the effectiveness of aminosalicylate sodium

**Other medical problems**—The presence of other medical problems may affect the use of aminosalicylate sodium. Make sure you tell your doctor if you have any other medical problems, especially:

  • Glucose-6-phosphate dehydrogenase (G6PD) deficiency—Aminosalicylate sodium may cause or worsen this blood problem
  • Heart disease or other circulation problems—The sodium in aminosalicylate sodium may cause or worsen heart or circulation problems
  • Kidney disease (severe)—Patients with kidney disease may have an increase in side effects
  • Liver disease (severe)—Patients with severe liver disease may have an increase in side effects
  • Stomach ulcer—Aminosalicylate sodium may cause stomach irritation

---

## Proper Use of This Medicine

Aminosalicylate sodium may be taken with or after meals or with an antacid if it upsets your stomach.

To help clear up your tuberculosis (TB) completely, *it is important that you keep taking this medicine for the full time of treatment* even if you begin to feel better after a few weeks. Since TB may take a long time to clear up, you may have to take the medicine every day for as long as 1 to 2 years or more. If you stop taking this medicine too soon, your symptoms may return.

This medicine works best when there is a constant amount in the blood. *To help keep the amount constant, do not miss any doses. Also, it is best to take the doses at evenly spaced times day and night.* For example, if you are to take 3 doses a day, doses should be spaced about 8 hours apart. If this interferes with your sleep or other daily activities, or if you need help in planning the best times to take your medicine, check with your health care professional.

**Dosing**—The dose of aminosalicylate sodium will be different for different patients. *Follow your doctor's orders or the directions on the label.* The following information includes only the average doses of aminosalicylate sodium. This medicine comes in tablets as aminosalicylate sodium (the salt form), but your doctor bases the dose on the amount of aminosalicylate acid (the acid form of the medicine) in the tablet. *If your dose is different, do not change it* unless your doctor tells you to do so.

- For the *tablet* dosage form:
  —For the treatment of tuberculosis:
  - Adults and children 12 years of age and older— 3.3 to 4 grams (aminosalicylate acid) every eight hours, or 5 to 6 grams (aminosalicylate acid) every twelve hours. This medicine must be taken with other medicines used to treat tuberculosis (TB).
  - Younger children—The dose is based on body weight and must be determined by the doctor. Depending on the size of the dose, the medicine may be given every six or eight hours. This medicine must be taken with other medicines used to treat tuberculosis (TB).

**Missed dose**—If you do miss a dose of this medicine, take it as soon as possible. This will help to keep a constant amount of medicine in the blood. However, if it is almost time for your next dose, skip the missed dose and go back to your regular dosing schedule. Do not double doses.

**Storage**—To store this medicine:
- Keep out of the reach of children.
- Store away from heat and direct light.
- Do not store in the bathroom, near the kitchen sink, or in other damp places. Heat or moisture may cause the medicine to break down.
- Do not keep outdated medicine or medicine no longer needed. Be sure that any discarded medicine is out of the reach of children.

## Precautions While Using This Medicine

If your symptoms do not improve within 2 to 3 weeks, or if they become worse, check with your doctor.

Do not take aminosalicylate sodium within 6 hours of taking rifampin. Taking the 2 medicines too close together may keep rifampin from working properly.

For diabetic patients:
- *This medicine may cause false test results with some urine sugar tests.* Check with your doctor before changing your diet or the dosage of your diabetes medicine.

## Side Effects of This Medicine

Along with its needed effects, a medicine may cause some unwanted effects. Although not all of these side effects may occur, if they do occur they may need medical attention.

*Check with your doctor immediately* if any of the following side effects occur:
  *More common*
    Fever; joint pains; skin rash or itching; unusual tiredness or weakness
  *Less common*
    Abdominal pain (severe); backache; headache; lower back pain; pain or burning while urinating; paleness of skin; sore throat; yellow eyes or skin

Check with your doctor as soon as possible if any of the following side effects occur:
  *Less common—with long-term, high-dose therapy*
    Changes in menstrual periods; decreased sexual ability in males; dry, puffy skin; swelling of front part of neck; weight gain (unusual)

Other side effects may occur that usually do not need medical attention. These side effects may go away during treatment as your body adjusts to the medicine. However, check with your doctor if any of the following side effects continue or are bothersome:
  *More common*
    Diarrhea; loss of appetite; nausea and vomiting; stomach pain (mild)

Other side effects not listed above may also occur in some patients. If you notice any other effects, check with your doctor.

Revised: 05/02/94

# AMIODARONE Systemic

A commonly used brand name in the U.S. and Canada is Cordarone.

## Description

Amiodarone (am-ee-OH-da-rone) belongs to the group of medicines known as antiarrhythmics. It is used to correct irregular heartbeats to a normal rhythm.

Amiodarone produces its helpful effects by slowing nerve impulses in the heart and acting directly on the heart tissues.

This medicine is available only with your doctor's prescription, in the following dosage form:

*Oral*
- Tablets (U.S. and Canada)

## Before Using This Medicine

In deciding to use a medicine, the risks of taking the medicine must be weighed against the good it will do. This is a decision you and your doctor will make. For amiodarone, the following should be considered:

**Allergies**—Tell your doctor if you have ever had any unusual or allergic reaction to amiodarone. Also tell your health care professional if you are allergic to any other substances, such as foods, preservatives, or dyes.

**Pregnancy**—Amiodarone has been shown to cause thyroid problems in babies whose mothers took amiodarone when pregnant. In addition, there is concern that amiodarone could cause slow heartbeat in the newborn. However, this medicine may be needed in serious situations that threaten the mother's life. Be sure you have discussed this with your doctor before taking this medicine.

**Breast-feeding**—Although amiodarone passes into breast milk, it has not been shown to cause problems in nursing babies. However, amiodarone has been shown to cause growth problems in rats. It may be necessary for you to stop breast-feeding during treatment. Be sure you have discussed the risks and benefits of the medicine with your doctor.

**Children**—Amiodarone can cause serious side effects in any patient. Therefore, it is especially important that you discuss with the child's doctor the good that this medicine may do as well as the risks of using it.

**Older adults**—Elderly patients may be more likely to get thyroid problems with this medicine. Also, difficulty in walking and numbness, tingling, trembling, or weakness in hands or feet are more likely to occur in the elderly.

**Other medicines**—Although certain medicines should not be used together at all, in other cases two different medicines may be used together even if an interaction might occur. In these cases, your doctor may want to change the dose, or other precautions may be necessary. When you are taking amiodarone, it is especially important that

your health care professional knows if you are taking any of the following:
- Anticoagulants (blood thinners) or
- Other heart medicine or
- Phenytoin (e.g., Dilantin)—Effects may be increased

**Other medical problems**—The presence of other medical problems may affect the use of amiodarone. Make sure you tell your doctor if you have any other medical problems, especially:
- Liver disease—Effects may be increased because of slower removal from the body
- Thyroid problems—Risk of overactive or underactive thyroid is increased

## Proper Use of This Medicine

*Take amiodarone exactly as directed by your doctor even though you may feel well.* Do not take more medicine than ordered and do not miss any doses.

**Dosing**—The dose of amiodarone will be different for different patients. *Follow your doctor's orders or the directions on the label.* The following information includes only the average doses of amiodarone. *If your dose is different, do not change it* unless your doctor tells you to do so:
- For *oral* dosage form (tablets):
  —For treatment of *ventricular arrhythmias:*
    - Adults—At first, 800 to 1600 milligrams (mg) per day taken in divided doses. Then, 600 to 800 mg per day for one month. Then, 400 mg per day.
    - Children—Dose is based on body weight and must be determined by your doctor. The dose for the first ten days is usually 10 mg per kilogram (4.55 mg per pound) of body weight per day. Then, the dose is decreased to 5 mg per kilogram (2.27 mg per pound) of body weight per day. After several weeks, the dose is then decreased to 2.5 mg per kilogram (1.14 mg per pound) of body weight per day.

**Missed dose**—If you do miss a dose of this medicine, do not take the missed dose at all and do not double the next one. Instead, go back to your regular dosing schedule. If you miss two or more doses in a row, check with your doctor.

**Storage**—To store this medicine:
- Keep out of the reach of children.
- Store away from heat and direct light.
- Do not store in the bathroom, near the kitchen sink, or in other damp places. Heat or moisture may cause the medicine to break down.
- Do not keep outdated medicine or medicine no longer needed. Be sure that any discarded medicine is out of the reach of children.

## Precautions While Using This Medicine

It is important that your doctor check your progress at regular visits to make sure the medicine is working properly. This will allow for changes to be made in the amount of medicine you are taking, if necessary.

Your doctor may want you to carry a medical identification card or bracelet stating that you are taking this medicine.

*Before having any kind of surgery (including dental surgery) or emergency treatment, tell the medical doctor or dentist in charge that you are taking this medicine.*

Amiodarone increases the sensitivity of your skin to sunlight; too much exposure could cause a serious burn. Your skin may continue to be sensitive to sunlight for several months after treatment with this medicine is stopped. A burn can occur even through window glass or thin cotton clothing. If you must go out in the sunlight, *cover your skin and wear a wide-brimmed hat. A special sun-blocking cream should also be used;* it must contain zinc or titanium oxide because other sunscreens will not work. *In case of a severe burn, check with your doctor.*

After you have taken this medicine for a long time, it may cause a blue-gray color to appear on your skin, especially in areas exposed to the sun, such as your face, neck, and arms. This color will usually fade after treatment with amiodarone has ended, although it may take several months. However, check with your doctor if this effect occurs.

## Side Effects of This Medicine

Along with its needed effects, a medicine may cause some unwanted effects. Although not all of these side effects may occur, if they do occur they may need medical attention. Also, some side effects may not appear until several weeks or months, or even years, after you start taking amiodarone.

*Check with your doctor immediately* if any of the following side effects occur:

*More common*
Cough; painful breathing; shortness of breath

Check with your doctor as soon as possible if any of the following side effects occur:

*More common*
Fever (slight); numbness or tingling in fingers or toes; sensitivity of skin to sunlight; trembling or shaking of hands; trouble in walking; unusual and uncontrolled movements of the body; weakness of arms or legs

*Less common*
Blue-gray coloring of skin on face, neck, and arms; blurred vision or blue-green halos seen around objects; coldness; dry eyes; dry, puffy skin; fast or irregular heartbeat; nervousness; pain and swelling in scrotum; sensitivity of eyes to light; sensitivity to heat; slow heartbeat; sweating; swelling of feet or lower legs; trouble in sleeping; unusual tiredness; weight gain or loss

*Rare*
Skin rash; yellow eyes or skin

Other side effects may occur that usually do not need medical attention. These side effects may go away during treatment as your body adjusts to the medicine. However, check with your doctor if any of the following side effects continue or are bothersome:

*More common*
Constipation; headache; loss of appetite; nausea and vomiting

*Less common*
Bitter or metallic taste; decreased sexual ability in males; decrease in sexual interest; dizziness; flushing of face

After you stop using this medicine, your body may need time to adjust. The length of time this takes depends on the amount of medicine you were using and how long you used it. During this period of time check with your doctor if you notice any of the following side effects:

Cough; fever (slight); painful breathing; shortness of breath

Other side effects not listed above may also occur in some patients. If you notice any other effects, check with your doctor.

Revised: 04/13/93

# AMLODIPINE    Systemic†

A commonly used brand name in the U.S. is Norvasc.

†Not commercially available in Canada.

## Description

Amlodipine (am-LOE-di-peen) is a calcium channel blocker used to treat angina (chest pain) and high blood pressure. Amlodipine affects the movement of calcium into the cells of the heart and blood vessels. As a result, amlodipine relaxes blood vessels and increases the supply of blood and oxygen to the heart while reducing its workload.

High blood pressure adds to the workload of the heart and arteries. If it continues for a long time, the heart and arteries may not function properly. This can damage the blood vessels of the brain, heart, and kidneys, resulting in a stroke, heart failure, or kidney failure. High blood pressure may also increase the risk of heart attacks. These problems may be less likely to occur if blood pressure is controlled.

This medicine is available only with your doctor's prescription, in the following dosage form:

*Oral*
- Tablets (U.S.)

## Before Using This Medicine

In deciding to use a medicine, the risks of taking the medicine must be weighed against the good it will do. This is a decision you and your doctor will make. For amlodipine, the following should be considered:

**Allergies**—Tell your doctor if you have ever had any unusual or allergic reaction to amlodipine. Also tell your health care professional if you are allergic to any other substances, such as foods, preservatives, or dyes.

**Pregnancy**—Amlodipine has not been studied in pregnant women. However, studies in animals have shown that, at very high doses, amlodipine may cause fetal death. Before taking this medicine, make sure your doctor knows if you are pregnant or if you may become pregnant.

**Breast-feeding**—It is not known whether amlodipine passes into breast milk. Although most medicines pass into breast milk in small amounts, many of them may be used safely while breast-feeding. Mothers who are taking this medicine and who wish to breast-feed should discuss this with their doctor.

**Children**—Studies on this medicine have been done only in adult patients, and there is no specific information comparing use of amlodipine in children with use in other age groups.

**Older adults**—Elderly people may be especially sensitive to the effects of amlodipine. This may increase the chance of side effects during treatment.

**Other medicines**—Although certain medicines should not be used together at all, in other cases two different medicines may be used together even if an interaction might occur. In these cases, your doctor may want to change the dose, or other precautions may be necessary. Tell your health care professional if you are using any other prescription or nonprescription (over-the-counter [OTC]) medicine.

**Other medical problems**—The presence of other medical problems may affect the use of amlodipine. Make sure you tell your doctor if you have any other medical problems, especially:
- Congestive heart failure—There is a small chance that amlodipine may make this condition worse
- Liver disease—Higher blood levels of amlodipine may result and a smaller dose may be needed
- Very low blood pressure—Amlodipine may make this condition worse

## Proper Use of This Medicine

*Take this medicine exactly as directed* even if you feel well and do not notice any chest pain. Do not take more of this medicine and do not take it more often than your doctor ordered. Do not miss any doses.

For patients taking this medicine *for high blood pressure:*
- In addition to the use of the medicine your doctor has prescribed, treatment for your high blood pressure may include weight control and care in the types of food you eat, especially foods high in sodium (salt). Your doctor will tell you which of these are most important for you. You should check with your doctor before changing your diet.
- Many patients who have high blood pressure will not notice any signs of the problem. In fact, many may feel normal. It is very important that you *take your medicine exactly as directed* and that you keep your appointments with your doctor even if you feel well.
- Remember that this medicine will not cure your high blood pressure but it does help control it. Therefore, you must continue to take it as directed if you expect to lower your blood pressure and keep it down. *You may have to take high blood pressure medicine for the rest of your life.* If high blood pressure is not treated, it can cause serious problems such as heart failure, blood vessel disease, stroke, or kidney disease.

**Dosing**—The dose of amlodipine will be different for different patients. *Follow your doctor's orders or the directions on the label.* The following information includes only the average doses of amlodipine. *If your dose is different, do not change it* unless your doctor tells you to do so.

The number of tablets that you take depends on the strength of the medicine.
- For *oral* dosage form (tablets):
  —For angina (chest pain):
  - Adults—5 to 10 milligrams (mg) once a day.
  - Children—Use must be determined by your doctor.
  —For high blood pressure:
  - Adults—2.5 to 10 mg once a day.
  - Children—Use must be determined by your doctor.

**Missed dose**—If you miss a dose of this medicine, take it as soon as possible. However, if it is almost time for your next dose, skip the missed dose and go back to your regular dosing schedule. Do not double doses.

**Storage**—To store this medicine:
- Keep out of the reach of children.
- Store away from heat and direct light.
- Do not store in the bathroom, near the kitchen sink, or in other damp places. Heat or moisture may cause the medicine to break down.
- Keep the medicine from freezing. Do not refrigerate.

- Do not keep outdated medicine or medicine no longer needed. Be sure that any discarded medicine is out of the reach of children.

## Precautions While Using This Medicine

It is important that your doctor check your progress at regular visits. This will allow your doctor to make sure the medicine is working properly and to change the dosage if needed.

If you have been using this medicine regularly for several weeks, do not suddenly stop using it. Stopping suddenly may cause your chest pain or high blood pressure to come back or get worse. Check with your doctor for the best way to reduce gradually the amount you are taking before stopping completely.

Chest pain resulting from exercise or physical exertion usually is reduced or prevented by this medicine. This may tempt you to be too active. *Make sure you discuss with your doctor a safe amount of exercise for your medical problem.*

After taking a dose of this medicine you may get a headache that lasts for a short time. This should become less noticeable after you have taken this medicine for a while. If this effect continues, or if the headaches are severe, check with your doctor.

In some patients, tenderness, swelling, or bleeding of the gums may appear soon after treatment with this medicine is started. Brushing and flossing your teeth carefully and regularly and massaging your gums may help prevent this. *See your dentist regularly* to have your teeth cleaned. Check with your medical doctor or dentist if you have any questions about how to take care of your teeth and gums, or if you notice any tenderness, swelling, or bleeding of your gums.

For patients taking this medicine *for high blood pressure:*
- *Do not take other medicines unless they have been discussed with your doctor.* This especially includes over-the-counter (nonprescription) medicines for appetite control, asthma, colds, cough, hay fever, or sinus problems, since they may tend to increase your blood pressure.

## Side Effects of This Medicine

Along with its needed effects, a medicine may cause some unwanted effects. Although not all of these side effects may occur, if they do occur they may need medical attention.

Check with your doctor as soon as possible if any of the following side effects occur:
*More common*
Swelling of ankles or feet
*Less common*
Dizziness; pounding heartbeat
*Rare*
Chest pain; dizziness or lightheadedness when getting up from a lying or sitting position; slow heartbeat

Other side effects may occur that usually do not need medical attention. These side effects may go away during treatment as your body adjusts to the medicine. However, check with your doctor if any of the following side effects continue or are bothersome:
*More common*
Flushing; headache
*Less common*
Nausea; unusual tiredness or weakness

Other side effects not listed above may also occur in some patients. If you notice any other effects, check with your doctor.

Revised: 08/12/93

---

# AMPHETAMINES  Systemic

Some commonly used brand names are:

**In the U.S.—**
Desoxyn[3]                     Dexedrine Spansule[2]
Desoxyn Gradumet[3]            DextroStat[2]
Dexedrine[2]

**In Canada—**
Dexedrine[2]
Dexedrine Spansule[2]

Note: For quick reference, the following amphetamines are numbered to match the corresponding brand names.

This information applies to the following medicines:
1. Amphetamine (am-FET-a-meen)[†‡]
2. Dextroamphetamine (dex-troe-am-FET-a-meen)[‡]
3. Methamphetamine (meth-am-FET-a-meen)[†]

[†]Not commercially available in Canada.
[‡]Generic name product may also be available in the U.S.
[§]Generic name product may also be available in Canada.

## Description

Amphetamines (am-FET-a-meens) belong to the group of medicines called central nervous system (CNS) stimulants. They are used to treat attention-deficit hyperactivity disorder (ADHD). Amphetamines increase attention and decrease restlessness in patients who are overactive, unable to concentrate for very long or are easily distracted, and have unstable emotions. These medicines are used as part of a total treatment program that also includes social, educational, and psychological treatment.

Amphetamine and dextroamphetamine are also used in the treatment of narcolepsy (uncontrollable desire for sleep or sudden attacks of deep sleep).

Amphetamines should not be used for weight loss or weight control or to combat unusual tiredness or weakness or replace rest. When used for these purposes, they may be dangerous to your health.

Amphetamines may also be used for other conditions as determined by your doctor.

These medicines are available only with a doctor's prescription. Prescriptions cannot be refilled. A new prescription must be obtained from your doctor each time you or your child needs this medicine.

Amphetamines are available in the following dosage forms:

*Oral*

Amphetamine
- Tablets (U.S.)

Dextroamphetamine
- Extended-release capsules (U.S. and Canada)
- Tablets (U.S. and Canada)

Methamphetamine
- Tablets (U.S.)
- Extended-release tablets (U.S.)

## Before Using This Medicine

In deciding to use a medicine, the risks of taking the medicine must be weighed against the good it will do. This is a decision you and your doctor will make. For amphetamines, the following should be considered:

**Allergies**—Tell your doctor if you have ever had any unusual or allergic reaction to amphetamine, dextroamphetamine, ephedrine, epinephrine, isoproterenol, metaproterenol, methamphetamine, norepinephrine, phenylephrine, phenylpropanolamine, pseudoephedrine, or terbutaline. Also tell your health care professional if you are allergic to any other substances, such as foods, preservatives, or dyes.

**Pregnancy**—Studies have not been done in humans. However, animal studies have shown that amphetamines may increase the chance of birth defects if taken during the early months of pregnancy.

In addition, overuse of amphetamines during pregnancy may increase the chances of a premature delivery and of having a baby with a low birth weight. Also, the baby may become dependent on amphetamines and experience withdrawal effects such as agitation and drowsiness.

**Breast-feeding**—Amphetamines pass into breast milk. Although this medicine has not been reported to cause problems in nursing babies, it is best not to breast-feed while you are taking an amphetamine. Be sure you have discussed this with your doctor.

**Children**—When amphetamines are used for long periods of time in children, they may cause unwanted effects on behavior and growth. Before these medicines are given to a child, you should discuss their use with your child's doctor.

**Older adults**—Many medicines have not been studied specifically in older people. Therefore, it may not be known whether they work exactly the same way they do in younger adults or if they cause different side effects or problems in older people. There is no specific information comparing use of amphetamines in the elderly with use in other age groups.

**Other medicines**—Although certain medicines should not be used together at all, in many cases 2 different medicines may be used together even if an interaction might occur. In these cases, changes in dose or other precautions may be necessary. When you are taking amphetamines, it is especially important that your health care professional know if you are taking any of the following:

- Amantadine (e.g., Symmetrel) or
- Caffeine (e.g., NoDoz) or
- Chlophedianol (e.g., Ulone) or
- Methylphenidate (e.g., Ritalin) or
- Nabilone (e.g., Cesamet) or
- Pemoline (e.g., Cylert)—Use of these medicines may increase the CNS stimulation effects of amphetamines and cause unwanted effects such as nervousness, irritability, trouble in sleeping, and possibly convulsions (seizures)
- Appetite suppressants (diet pills), except fenfluramine (e.g., Pondimin), or
- Medicine for asthma or other breathing problems or
- Medicine for colds, sinus problems, or hay fever or other allergies (including nose drops or sprays)—Use of these medicines may increase the CNS stimulation effects of amphetamines and cause unwanted effects such as nervousness, irritability, trouble in sleeping, and possibly convulsions (seizures), as well as unwanted effects on the heart and blood vessels
- Beta-adrenergic blocking agents (acebutolol [e.g., Sectral], atenolol [e.g., Tenormin], betaxolol [e.g., Kerlone], carteolol [e.g., Cartrol], labetalol [e.g., Normodyne], metoprolol [e.g., Lopressor], nadolol [e.g., Corgard], oxprenolol [e.g., Trasicor], penbutolol [e.g., Levatol], pindolol [e.g., Visken], propranolol [e.g., Inderal], sotalol [e.g., Sotacor], timolol [e.g., Blocadren]—Use of amphetamines with beta-blocking agents may increase the chance of high blood pressure and heart problems
- Cocaine—Use by persons taking amphetamines may cause a severe increase in blood pressure and other unwanted effects, including nervousness, irritability, trouble in sleeping, and possible convulsions (seizures)
- Digitalis glycosides (heart medicine)—Amphetamines may cause additive effects, resulting in irregular heartbeat
- Meperidine—Use of meperidine by persons taking amphetamines is not recommended because the chance of serious side effects (such as high fever, convulsions, and coma) may be increased
- Monoamine oxidase (MAO) inhibitors (furazolidone [e.g., Furoxone], isocarboxazid [e.g., Marplan], phenelzine [e.g., Nardil], procarbazine [e.g., Matulane], selegiline [e.g., Eldepryl], tranylcypromine [e.g., Parnate])—Taking amphetamines while you are taking or within 2 weeks of taking monoamine oxidase (MAO) inhibitors may increase the chance of serious side effects such as sudden and severe high blood pressure or fever
- Thyroid hormones—The effects of either these medicines or amphetamines may be increased; unwanted effects may occur in patients with heart or blood vessel disease
- Tricyclic antidepressants (amitriptyline [e.g., Elavil], amoxapine [e.g., Asendin], clomipramine [e.g., Anafranil], desipramine [e.g., Pertofrane], doxepin [e.g., Sinequan], imipramine [e.g., Tofranil], nortriptyline [e.g.,

Aventyl], protriptyline [e.g., Vivactil], trimipramine [e.g., Surmontil])—Although tricyclic antidepressants may be used with amphetamines to help make them work better, using the 2 medicines together may increase the chance of fast or irregular heartbeat, severe high blood pressure, or high fever

**Other medical problems**—The presence of other medical problems may affect the use of amphetamines. Make sure you tell your doctor if you have any other medical problems, especially:

- Anxiety or tension (severe) or
- Drug abuse or dependence, (history of) or
- Glaucoma or
- Heart or blood vessel disease or
- High blood pressure or
- Mental illness (severe), especially in children, or
- Overactive thyroid or
- Tourette's syndrome (history of) or other tics—Amphetamines may make the condition worse

## Proper Use of This Medicine

*Take this medicine only as directed by your doctor.* Do not take more or less of it, do not take it more often, and do not take it for a longer time than your doctor ordered. If too much is taken, it may become habit-forming (causing mental or physical dependence).

If you think this medicine is not working properly after you have taken it for several weeks, *do not increase the dose.* Instead, check with your doctor.

**For patients taking** *the short-acting form* of this medicine:

- Take the last dose for each day at least 6 hours before bedtime to help prevent trouble in sleeping.

For patients taking *the long-acting form* of this medicine:

- Take the daily dose about 10 to 14 hours before bedtime to help prevent trouble in sleeping.
- These capsules or tablets should be swallowed whole. Do not break, crush, or chew them before swallowing.

Amphetamines may be taken with or without food or on a full or empty stomach. However, if your doctor tells you to take the medicine a certain way, take it exactly as directed.

**Dosing**—The dose of amphetamines will be different for different patients. *Follow your doctor's orders or the directions on the label.* The following information includes only the average doses of amphetamines. *If your dose is different, do not change it* unless your doctor tells you to do so.

The number of capsules or tablets that you take depends on the strength of the medicine. Also, *the number of doses you take each day, the time allowed between doses, and the length of time you take the medicine depend on the medical problem for which you are taking amphetamines.*

*For amphetamine*

- For *oral* dosage form (tablets):
  —For attention-deficit hyperactivity disorder:
    - Adults—At first, 5 milligrams (mg) one to three times a day. Your doctor may increase your dose if needed.
    - Children 6 years of age and over—At first, 5 mg one or two times a day. Your doctor may increase your dose if needed.
    - Children 3 to 6 years of age—At first, 2.5 mg once a day. Your doctor may increase your dose if needed.
    - Children up to 3 years of age—Use is not recommended.
  —For narcolepsy:
    - Adults—At first, 5 mg one to three times a day. Your doctor may increase your dose if needed.
    - Children 12 years of age and over—At first, 5 mg two times a day. Your doctor may increase your dose if needed.
    - Children 6 to 12 years of age—At first, 2.5 mg two times a day. Your doctor may increase your dose if needed.
    - Children up to 6 years of age—Dose must be determined by your doctor.

*For dextroamphetamine*

- For *oral extended-release capsule* dosage form:
  —For attention-deficit hyperactivity disorder:
    - Adults—5 to 60 milligrams (mg) a day.
    - Children 6 years of age and over—At first, 5 mg one or two times a day. Your doctor may increase your dose if needed.
    - Children 3 to 6 years of age—At first, 2.5 mg a day. Your doctor may increase your dose if needed.
    - Children up to 3 years of age—Use is not recommended.
  —For narcolepsy:
    - Adults—5 to 60 mg a day.
    - Children 12 years of age and over—At first, 10 mg a day. Your doctor may increase your dose if needed.
    - Children 6 to 12 years of age—At first, 5 mg a day. Your doctor may increase your dose if needed.
    - Children 3 to 6 years of age—Dose must be determined by your doctor.
    - Children up to 3 years of age—Use is not recommended.
- For *oral tablet* dosage form:
  —For attention-deficit hyperactivity disorder:
    - Adults—5 to 60 mg a day.
    - Children 6 years of age and over—At first, 5 mg one or two times a day. Your doctor may increase your dose if needed.

- Children 3 to 5 years of age—At first, 2.5 mg a day. Your doctor may increase your dose if needed.
- Children up to 3 years of age—Use is not recommended.

—For narcolepsy:

- Adults—5 to 60 mg a day.
- Children 12 years of age and over—At first, 10 mg a day. Your doctor may increase your dose if needed.
- Children 6 to 12 years of age—At first, 5 mg a day. Your doctor may increase your dose if needed.
- Children up to 6 years of age—Dose must be determined by your doctor.

*For methamphetamine*

- For *oral tablet* dosage form:

—For attention-deficit hyperactivity disorder:

- Children 6 years of age and over—At first, 5 milligrams (mg) one or two times a day. Your doctor may increase your dose if needed.
- Children up to 6 years of age—Use is not recommended.

- For *oral extended-release tablet* dosage form:

—For attention-deficit hyperactivity disorder:

- Children 6 years of age and over—20 to 25 mg a day.
- Children up to 6 years of age—Use is not recommended.

**Missed dose**—If you miss a dose of this medicine and your dosing schedule is:

- One dose a day—Take the missed dose as soon as possible, but not later than stated above, to prevent trouble in sleeping. However, if you do not remember the missed dose until the next day, skip it and go back to your regular dosing schedule. Do not double doses.
- Two or three doses a day—If you remember within an hour or so of the missed dose, take the dose right away. However, if you do not remember until later, skip it and go back to your regular dosing schedule. Do not double doses.

**Storage**—To store this medicine:

- Keep out of the reach of children.
- Store away from heat and direct light.
- Do not store the capsule or tablet form of this medicine in the bathroom, near the kitchen sink, or in other damp places. Heat or moisture may cause the medicine to break down.
- Keep the liquid form of this medicine from freezing.
- Do not keep outdated medicine or medicine no longer needed. Be sure that any discarded medicine is out of the reach of children.

## Precautions While Using This Medicine

Your doctor should check your progress at regular visits to make sure that this medicine does not cause unwanted effects.

If you will be taking this medicine in large doses for a long time, *do not stop taking it without first checking with your doctor.* Your doctor may want you to reduce gradually the amount you are taking before stopping completely.

This medicine may cause some people to feel a false sense of well-being or to become dizzy, lightheaded, or less alert than they are normally. *Make sure you know how you react to this medicine before you drive, use machines, or do anything else that could be dangerous if you are dizzy or are not alert.*

Before you have any medical tests, tell the medical doctor in charge that you are taking this medicine. The results of the metyrapone test may be affected by this medicine.

*If you have been using this medicine for a long time and you think you may have become mentally or physically dependent on it, check with your doctor.* Some signs of dependence on amphetamines are:

- A strong desire or need to continue taking the medicine.
- A need to increase the dose to receive the effects of the medicine.
- Withdrawal effects (for example, mental depression, nausea or vomiting, stomach cramps or pain, trembling, unusual tiredness or weakness) occurring after the medicine is stopped.

## Side Effects of This Medicine

Along with its needed effects, a medicine may cause some unwanted effects. Although not all of these side effects may occur, if they do occur they may need medical attention.

Check with your doctor as soon as possible if any of the following side effects occur:

*More common*
    Irregular heartbeat
*Rare*
    Chest pain; fever, unusually high; skin rash or hives; uncontrolled movements of head, neck, arms, and legs
*With long-term use or high doses*
    Difficulty in breathing; dizziness or feeling faint; increased blood pressure; mood or mental changes; pounding heartbeat; unusual tiredness or weakness

Other side effects may occur that usually do not need medical attention. These side effects may go away during treatment as your body adjusts to the medicine. However, check with your doctor if any of the following side effects continue or are bothersome:

*More common*
   False sense of well-being; irritability; nervousness; restlessness; trouble in sleeping
Note: After these stimulant effects have worn off, drowsiness, trembling, unusual tiredness or weakness, or mental depression
   may occur.

*Less common*
   Blurred vision; changes in sexual desire or decreased sexual ability; constipation; diarrhea; dizziness or lightheadedness; dryness of mouth or unpleasant taste; fast
   or pounding heartbeat; headache; increased sweating;
   loss of appetite; nausea or vomiting; stomach cramps
   or pain; weight loss

After you stop using this medicine, your body may need
time to adjust. The length of time this takes depends on
the amount of medicine you were using and how long
you used it. During this period of time check with your
doctor if you notice any of the following side effects:

   Mental depression; nausea or vomiting; stomach cramps or
   pain; trembling; unusual tiredness or weakness

Other side effects not listed above may also occur in some
patients. If you notice any other effects check with your
doctor.

Revised: 08/18/94

# AMPHOTERICIN B    Systemic

A commonly used brand name in the U.S. and Canada is Fungizone
   Intravenous.
Generic name product may also be available in the U.S.

## Description

Amphotericin (am-foe-TER-i-sin) B is an antifungal. It
is used to help the body overcome serious fungus infections. It may also be used for other problems as determined by your doctor.

Amphotericin B is available only with your doctor's prescription. It is available in the following dosage form:

*Parenteral*
   • Injection (U.S. and Canada)

## Before Receiving This Medicine

In deciding to use a medicine, the risks of taking the
medicine must be weighed against the good it will do.
This is a decision you and your doctor will make. For
amphotericin B, the following should be considered:

**Allergies**—Tell your doctor if you have ever had any unusual or allergic reaction to amphotericin B. Also tell
your health care professional if you are allergic to any
other substances, such as foods, preservatives, or dyes.

**Pregnancy**—Amphotericin B has not been reported to
cause birth defects or other problems in humans.

**Breast-feeding**—Amphotericin B has not been reported
to cause problems in nursing babies.

**Children**—Although there is no specific information comparing use of amphotericin B in children with use in other
age groups, this medicine is not expected to cause different side effects or problems in children than it does
in adults.

**Older adults**—Many medicines have not been studied specifically in older people. Therefore, it may not be known
whether they work exactly the same way they do in

younger adults or if they cause different side effects or
problems in older people. There is no specific information
comparing use of amphotericin B in the elderly with use
in other age groups.

**Other medicines**—Although certain medicines should not
be used together at all, in other cases two different medicines may be used together even if an interaction might
occur. In these cases, your doctor may want to change
the dose, or other precautions may be necessary. When
you are taking amphotericin B, it is especially important
that your health care professional knows if you are taking
any of the following:

• Antineoplastics (cancer medicine) or
• Antithyroid agents (medicine for overactive thyroid) or
• Azathioprine (e.g., Imuran) or
• Chloramphenicol (e.g., Chloromycetin) or
• Colchicine or
• Cyclophosphamide (e.g., Cytoxan) or
• Flucytosine (e.g., Ancobon) or
• Ganciclovir (e.g., Cytovene) or
• Interferon (e.g., Intron A, Roferon-A) or
• Mercaptopurine (e.g., Purinethol) or
• Zidovudine (e.g., AZT, Retrovir) or
• X-ray treatment—Use of amphotericin B with any of these
   medicines or x-ray treatment may increase the chance of
   side effects affecting the blood
• Bumetanide (e.g., Bumex) or
• Carmustine (e.g., BiCNU) or
• Cisplatin (e.g., Platinol) or
• Combination pain medicine containing acetaminophen and
   aspirin (e.g., Excedrin) or other salicylates (with large
   amounts taken regularly) or
• Cyclosporine (e.g., Sandimmune) or
• Deferoxamine (e.g., Desferal) (with long-term use) or
• Ethacrynic acid (e.g., Edecrin) or
• Furosemide (e.g., Lasix) or
• Gold salts (medicine for arthritis) or
• Indapamide (e.g., Lozol) or
• Inflammation or pain medicine, except narcotics, or
• Lithium (e.g., Lithane) or
• Other medicine for infection or
• Plicamycin (e.g., Mithracin) or

- Streptozocin (e.g., Zanosar) or
- Tiopronin (e.g., Thiola) or
- Thiazide diuretics (water pills)—Using these medicines with amphotericin B may increase the risk of side effects affecting the kidneys
- Corticosteroids (cortisone-like medicine) or
- Corticotropin (ACTH)—Use of amphotericin B with these medicines may cause changes in the blood that may increase the chance for heart problems
- Digitalis glycosides (heart medicine)—Use of amphotericin B with digitalis medicines (such as digoxin) may cause changes in the blood that may increase the chance of heart problems
- Methotrexate (e.g., Mexate) or
- Penicillamine (e.g., Cuprimine)—Using these medicines with amphotericin B may increase the risk of side effects affecting the blood and the kidneys

**Other medical problems**—The presence of other medical problems may affect the use of amphotericin B. Make sure you tell your doctor if you have any other medical problems, especially:

- Kidney disease—Amphotericin B may cause side effects affecting the kidneys

---

## Proper Use of This Medicine

**Dosing**—The dose of amphotericin B will be different for different patients. The following information includes only the average doses of amphotericin B. Your dose may be different if you have kidney disease.

- For the *injection* dosage form:
  —Adults and children: A small test dose is usually given first to see how you react to the medicine. The dose is then slowly increased, depending on what your infection is and how well you tolerate the medicine. The dose must be determined by your doctor.

---

## Side Effects of This Medicine

Along with its needed effects, a medicine may cause some unwanted effects. Although not all of these side effects may occur, if they do occur they may need medical attention.

*Check with your health care professional immediately* if any of the following side effects occur:

*More common*
*With intravenous injection*
Fever and chills; headache; increased or decreased urination; irregular heartbeat; muscle cramps or pain; nausea; pain at the place of injection; unusual tiredness or weakness; vomiting

*Less common or rare*
*With intravenous injection*
Blurred or double vision; convulsions (seizures); numbness, tingling, pain, or weakness in hands or feet; shortness of breath, troubled breathing, wheezing, or tightness in chest; skin rash or itching; sore throat and fever; unusual bleeding or bruising

*With spinal injection*
Blurred vision or any change in vision; difficult urination; numbness, tingling, pain, or weakness

Other side effects may occur that usually do not need medical attention. These side effects may go away during treatment as your body adjusts to the medicine. However, check with your doctor if any of the following side effects continue or are bothersome:

*More common*
*With intravenous injection*
Diarrhea; headache; indigestion; loss of appetite; nausea or vomiting; stomach pain

*Less common*
*With spinal injection*
Back, leg, or neck pain; dizziness or lightheadedness; headache; nausea or vomiting

Other side effects not listed above may also occur in some patients. If you notice any other effects, check with your doctor.

---

Revised: 02/23/93

---

# AMPHOTERICIN B    Topical†

A commonly used brand name in the U.S. is Fungizone.

†Not commericialy available in Canada.

## Description

Amphotericin (am-foe-TER-i-sin) B belongs to the family of medicines called antifungals. Amphotericin B topical preparations are used to treat fungus infections.

Amphotericin B is available only with your doctor's prescription, in the following dosage forms:

*Topical*
- Cream (U.S.)
- Lotion (U.S.)
- Ointment (U.S.)

## Before Using This Medicine

In deciding to use a medicine, the risks of using the medicine must be weighed against the good it will do.

---

© 1994   The United States Pharmacopeial Convention, Inc.

This is a decision you and your doctor will make. For amphotericin B, the following should be considered:

**Allergies**—Tell your doctor if you have ever had any unusual or allergic reaction to amphotericin B. Also tell your health care professional if you are allergic to any other substances, such as preservatives or dyes.

**Pregnancy**—Amphotericin B topical preparations have not been shown to cause birth defects or other problems in humans.

**Breast-feeding**—Amphotericin B topical preparations have not been reported to cause problems in nursing babies.

**Children**—Although there is no specific information comparing use of amphotericin B topical preparations in children with use in other age groups, this medicine is not expected to cause different side effects or problems in children than it does in adults.

**Older adults**—Many medicines have not been studied specifically in older people. Therefore, it may not be known whether they work exactly the same way they do in younger adults. Although there is no specific information comparing use of topical amphotericin B preparations in the elderly with use in other age groups, these preparations are not expected to cause different side effects or problems in older people than they do in younger adults.

**Other medicines**—Although certain medicines should not be used together at all, in other cases two different medicines may be used together even if an interaction might occur. In these cases, your doctor may want to change the dose, or other precautions may be necessary. Tell your health care professional if you are using any other topical prescription or nonprescription (over-the-counter [OTC]) medicine that is to be applied to the same area of the skin.

## Proper Use of This Medicine

Apply enough amphotericin B to cover the affected areas, and rub in gently.

*Do not apply an occlusive dressing (airtight covering such as kitchen plastic wrap) over this medicine* since it may cause irritation of the skin. If you have any questions about this, check with your doctor.

To help clear up your infection completely, *it is very important that you keep using this medicine for the full time of treatment,* even if your symptoms begin to clear up after a few days. Since fungus infections may be very slow to clear up, you may have to continue using this medicine every day for several months or longer. If you stop using this medicine too soon, your symptoms may return. *Do not miss any doses.*

**Dosing**—The dose of topical amphotericin B will be different for different patients. *Follow your doctor's orders*

*or the directions on the label.* The following information includes only the average doses of topical amphotericin B. *If your dose is different, do not change it* unless your doctor tells you to do so.

- For *topical* dosage forms (cream, lotion, and ointment):
  —For fungus infections:
    • Adults and children—Apply to the affected area(s) of the skin two to four times a day.

**Missed dose**—If you miss a dose of this medicine, apply it as soon as possible. Then go back to your regular dosing schedule.

**Storage**—To store this medicine:
- Keep out of the reach of children.
- Store away from heat and direct light.
- Keep the medicine from freezing.
- Do not keep outdated medicine or medicine no longer needed. Be sure that any discarded medicine is out of the reach of children.

## Precautions While Using This Medicine

If your skin problem does not improve within 1 to 2 weeks, or if it becomes worse, check with your doctor.

When amphotericin B is rubbed into the affected skin areas, it may stain the skin slightly, especially if it is applied to areas on or around the nails. It may also stain the nails.

For patients using the *cream or lotion form* of this medicine:
- If either of these forms stain your clothing, the stain may be removed by hand-washing the clothing with soap and warm water.

For patients using the *ointment form* of this medicine:
- If this form stains your clothing, the stain may be removed with a standard cleaning fluid.

## Side Effects of This Medicine

Along with its needed effects, a medicine may cause some unwanted effects. Although not all of these side effects may occur, if they do occur they may need medical attention.

Check with your doctor as soon as possible if any of the following side effects occur:
*Less common*
   Burning, itching, redness, or other sign of irritation not present before use of this medicine
   *Rare*
   Skin rash

Other side effects may occur that usually do not need medical attention. These side effects may go away during treatment as your body adjusts to the medicine. However,

check with your doctor if the following side effect continues or is bothersome:

*Less common—for cream only*
    Dryness of skin

Other side effects not listed above may also occur in some patients. If you notice any other effects, check with your doctor.

---

Revised: 07/25/94

---

# AMYL NITRITE    Systemic

Generic name product available in the U.S. and Canada.

---

## Description

Amyl nitrite (AM-il NYE-trite) is related to the nitrate medicines and is used by inhalation to relieve the pain of angina attacks. It works by relaxing blood vessels and increasing the supply of blood and oxygen to the heart while reducing its work load.

Amyl nitrite may also be used for other conditions as determined by your doctor.

This medicine comes in a glass capsule covered by a protective cloth. The cloth covering allows you to crush the glass capsule between your fingers without cutting yourself.

On the street, this medicine and others like it are sometimes called "poppers." They have been used by some people to cause a "high" or to improve sex. Use in this way is not recommended. Amyl nitrite can cause serious harmful effects if too much is inhaled.

Amyl nitrite is available only with your doctor's prescription, in the following dosage form:

*Inhalation*
- Glass capsules (U.S. and Canada)

---

## Before Using This Medicine

In deciding to use a medicine, the risks of taking the medicine must be weighed against the good it will do. This is a decision you and your doctor will make. For amyl nitrite, the following should be considered:

**Allergies**—Tell your doctor if you have ever had any unusual or allergic reaction to amyl nitrite or nitrates. Also tell your health care professional if you are allergic to any other substances, such as foods or dyes.

**Pregnancy**—Studies on effects in pregnancy have not been done in either humans or animals. However, use of amyl nitrite is not recommended during pregnancy because it could cause serious problems in the unborn baby.

**Breast-feeding**—It is not known whether amyl nitrite passes into breast milk. However, use of amyl nitrite is not recommended during breast-feeding, because it may cause unwanted effects in nursing babies.

**Children**—Studies on this medicine have been done only in adult patients and there is no specific information comparing use of amyl nitrite in children with use in other age groups.

**Older adults**—Dizziness or lightheadedness may be more likely to occur in the elderly, who are usually more sensitive to the effects of amyl nitrite.

**Other medicines**—Although certain medicines should not be used together at all, in other cases two different medicines may be used together even if an interaction might occur. In these cases, your doctor may want to change the dose, or other precautions may be necessary. When you are taking amyl nitrite, it is especially important that your health care professional knows if you are taking any of the following:

- Amantadine (e.g., Symmetrel) or
- Antidepressants (medicine for depression) or
- Antihypertensives (high blood pressure medicine) or
- Antipsychotics (medicine for mental illness) or
- Bromocriptine (e.g., Parlodel) or
- Diuretics (water pills) or
- Levodopa (e.g., Dopar) or
- Medicine for heart disease or
- Nabilone (e.g., Cesamet)—in high doses or
- Narcotic pain medicine or
- Nimodipine (e.g., Nimotop) or
- Pentamidine (e.g., Pentam) or
- Pimozide (e.g., Orap) or
- Promethazine (e.g., Phenergan) or
- Trimeprazine (e.g., Temaril)—May increase dizziness or lightheadedness when getting up from a lying or sitting position

It is also important that your health care professional knows if you are using any of the following medicines in the eye:

- Levobunolol (e.g., Betagan) or
- Metipranolol (e.g., Optipranolol) or
- Timolol (e.g., Timoptic)—May increase dizziness or lightheadedness when getting up from a lying or sitting position

**Other medical problems**—The presence of other medical problems may affect the use of amyl nitrite. Make sure you tell your doctor if you have any other medical problems, especially:

- Anemia (severe)
- Glaucoma—Amyl nitrite may make this condition worse

- Overactive thyroid
- Recent stroke, heart attack, or head injury

## Proper Use of This Medicine

To use amyl nitrite:

- *When you begin to feel an attack of angina starting (chest pains or a tightness or squeezing in the chest), sit down. Then crush the cloth-covered glass capsule containing amyl nitrite between your finger and thumb. Pass it back and forth close to your nose and inhale the vapor several (1 to 6) times.* Since you may become dizzy, lightheaded, or faint soon after using amyl nitrite, it is best to sit or lie down rather than stand while the medicine is working. If you become dizzy or faint while sitting, take several deep breaths of air and either bend forward with your head between your knees or lie down with your feet elevated.
- Remain calm and you should feel better in a few minutes.

*Use this medicine exactly as directed by your doctor*, and do not use more than your doctor ordered. Using too much amyl nitrite may cause a dangerous overdose. If the medicine does not seem to be working as well after you have used it for a while, check with your doctor. *Do not increase the dose on your own.*

**Dosing**—*Follow your doctor's orders or the directions on the label.* The following information includes only the average doses of amyl nitrite:

- For *inhalation* dosage form:
  —Adults: 0.18 or 0.3 milliliter (1 ampul) taken by inhaling the vapor of amyl nitrite through the nose. Dose may be repeated within 1 to 5 minutes if pain is not relieved. *If you still have chest pain after a total of 2 doses in a 10-minute period, contact your doctor or have someone take you to a hospital emergency room without delay.*

**Storage**—To store this medicine:

- Keep out of the reach of children.
- Store away from heat and direct light.
- Do not store in the bathroom or in the kitchen. Heat may cause the medicine to break down.
- Do not keep outdated medicine or medicine no longer needed. Be sure that any discarded medicine is out of the reach of children.

## Precautions While Using This Medicine

*Amyl nitrite is extremely flammable.* Keep it away from heat or any open flame, especially when crushing the capsule. Amyl nitrite can catch fire very easily and cause serious burns.

*Dizziness or lightheadedness may occur*, especially when you get up from a lying or sitting position. Getting up slowly may help, but if the problem continues or gets worse, check with your doctor.

*Drinking alcohol while you are taking this medicine may make the dizziness or lightheadedness worse and may cause a serious drop in blood pressure.* Check with your doctor before drinking alcoholic beverages.

After using a dose of amyl nitrite, you may get a mild headache that lasts for a short time. This is a common side effect and is no cause for alarm. However, if this effect continues, or if the headaches are severe, check with your doctor.

## Side Effects of This Medicine

Along with its needed effects, a medicine may cause some unwanted effects. Although not all of these side effects may occur, if they do occur they may need medical attention.

Check with your doctor as soon as possible if any of the following side effects occur:

*Rare*
 Skin rash; unusual tiredness or weakness
*Signs and symptoms of overdose*
 Bluish-colored lips, fingernails, or palms of hands; dizziness (extreme) or fainting; feeling of extreme pressure in head; shortness of breath; unusual tiredness or weakness; weak and fast heartbeat

Other side effects may occur that usually do not need medical attention. These side effects may go away during treatment as your body adjusts to the medicine. However, check with your doctor if any of the following side effects continue or are bothersome:

*More common*
 Dizziness or lightheadedness, especially when getting up from a lying or sitting position; fast pulse; flushing of face and neck; headache (mild); nausea or vomiting; restlessness

Other side effects not listed above may also occur in some patients. If you notice any other effects, check with your doctor.

Revised: 04/12/93

# ANABOLIC STEROIDS   Systemic

Some commonly used brand names are:

**In the U.S.—**

| | |
|---|---|
| Anadrol-50[3] | Kabolin[1] |
| Deca-Durabolin[1] | Neo-Durabolic[1] |
| Durabolin[1] | Oxandrin[2] |
| Hybolin Decanoate[1] | Winstrol[4] |
| Hybolin-Improved[1] | |

**In Canada—**

| | |
|---|---|
| Anapolon 50[3] | Durabolin[1] |
| Deca-Durabolin[1] | |

Note: For quick reference, the following anabolic steroids are numbered to match the corresponding brand names.

This information applies to the following medicines:

1. Nandrolone (NAN-droe-lone)‡
2. Oxandrolone (ox-AN-droe-lone)†
3. Oxymetholone (ox-i-METH-oh-lone)
4. Stanozolol (stan-OH-zoe-lole)†

---

†Not commercially available in Canada.
‡Generic name product may also be available in the U.S.

---

## Description

This medicine belongs to the group of medicines known as anabolic (an-a-BOL-ik) steroids. They are related to testosterone, a male sex hormone. Anabolic steroids help to rebuild tissues that have become weak because of serious injury or illness. A diet high in proteins and calories is necessary with anabolic steroid treatment.

Anabolic steroids are used for several reasons:

- to help patients gain weight after a severe illness, injury, or continuing infection. They also are used when patients fail to gain or maintain normal weight because of unexplained medical reasons.
- to treat certain types of anemia.
- to treat certain kinds of breast cancer in some women.
- to treat hereditary angioedema, which causes swelling of the face, arms, legs, throat, windpipe, bowels, or sexual organs.

Anabolic steroids may also be used for other conditions as determined by your doctor.

Anabolic steroids are available only with your doctor's prescription, in the following dosage forms:

*Oral*

Oxandrolone
- Tablets (U.S.)

Oxymetholone
- Tablets (U.S. and Canada)

Stanozolol
- Tablets (U.S.)

*Parenteral*

Nandrolone
- Injection (U.S. and Canada)

---

## Before Using This Medicine

In deciding to use a medicine, the risks of taking the medicine must be weighed against the good it will do.

This is a decision you and your doctor will make. For anabolic steroids, the following should be considered:

**Allergies**—Tell your doctor if you have ever had any unusual or allergic reaction to anabolic steroids or androgens (male sex hormones). Also tell your health care professional if you are allergic to any other substances, such as foods, preservatives, or dyes.

**Pregnancy**—Anabolic steroids are not recommended during pregnancy. They may cause the development of male features in the female fetus and premature growth and development of male features in the male fetus. Be sure you have discussed this with your doctor.

**Breast-feeding**—It is not known whether anabolic steroids can cause problems in nursing babies. There is very little experience with their use in mothers who are breast-feeding.

**Children**—Anabolic steroids may cause children to stop growing. In addition, they may make male children develop too fast sexually and may cause male-like changes in female children.

**Older adults**—When elderly male patients are treated with anabolic steroids, they may have an increased risk of enlarged prostate or cancer of the prostate.

**Other medicines**—Although certain medicines should not be used together at all, in other cases two different medicines may be used together even if an interaction might occur. In these cases, your doctor may want to change the dose, or other precautions may be necessary. When you are taking anabolic steroids, it is especially important that your health care professional know if you are taking any of the following:

- Acetaminophen (e.g., Tylenol) (with long-term, high-dose use) or
- Amiodarone (e.g., Cordarone) or
- Androgens (male hormones) or
- Anti-infectives by mouth or by injection (medicine for infection) or
- Antithyroid agents (medicine for overactive thyroid) or
- Carbamazepine (e.g., Tegretol) or
- Carmustine (e.g., BiCNU) or
- Chloroquine (e.g., Aralen) or
- Dantrolene (e.g., Dantrium) or
- Daunorubicin (e.g., Cerubidine) or
- Disulfiram (e.g., Antabuse) or
- Divalproex (e.g., Depakote) or
- Estrogens (female hormones) or
- Etretinate (e.g., Tegison) or
- Gold salts (medicine for arthritis) or
- Hydroxychloroquine (e.g., Plaquenil) or
- Mercaptopurine (e.g., Purinethol) or
- Methotrexate (e.g., Mexate) or
- Methyldopa (e.g., Aldomet) or
- Naltrexone (e.g., Trexan) (with long-term, high-dose use) or
- Oral contraceptives (birth control pills) containing estrogen or

- Phenothiazines (acetophenazine [e.g., Tindal], chlorpromazine [e.g., Thorazine], fluphenazine [e.g., Prolixin], mesoridazine [e.g., Serentil], perphenazine [e.g., Trilafon], prochlorperazine [e.g., Compazine], promazine [e.g., Sparine], promethazine [e.g., Phenergan], thioridazine [e.g., Mellaril], trifluoperazine [e.g., Stelazine], triflupromazine [e.g., Vesprin], trimeprazine [e.g., Temaril]) or
- Phenytoin (e.g., Dilantin) or
- Plicamycin (e.g., Mithracin) or
- Valproic acid (e.g., Depakene)—Taking anabolic steroids with any of these medicines may increase the chances of liver damage. Your doctor may want you to have extra blood tests to check for this if you must take both medicines
- Anticoagulants, oral (blood thinners you take by mouth)—Anabolic steroids can increase the effect of these medicines and possibly cause excessive bleeding

**Other medical problems**—The presence of other medical problems may affect the use of anabolic steroids. Make sure you tell your doctor if you have any other medical problems, especially:

- Breast cancer (in males and some females) or
- Diabetes mellitus (sugar diabetes)—Anabolic steroids can decrease blood sugar levels
- Enlarged prostate or
- Prostate cancer—Anabolic steroids may make these conditions worse by causing more enlargement of the prostate or more growth of a tumor
- Heart or blood vessel disease—Anabolic steroids can worsen these conditions by increasing blood cholesterol levels
- Kidney disease
- Liver disease
- Too much calcium in the blood (or history of) (in females)—Anabolic steroids may worsen this condition by raising the amount of calcium in the blood even more

## Proper Use of This Medicine

*Take this medicine only as directed.* Do not take more of it and do not take it more often than your doctor ordered. To do so may increase the chance of side effects.

*In order for this medicine to work properly, it is important that you follow a diet high in proteins and calories.* If you have any questions about this, check with your health care professional.

**Dosing**—The dose of these medicines will be different for different patients. *Follow your doctor's orders or the directions on the label.* The following information includes only the average doses of these medicines. *If your dose is different, do not change it* unless your doctor tells you to do so.

The number of tablets that you take depends on the strength of the medicine. Also, *the number of doses you take each day, the time allowed between doses, and the length of time you take the medicine depend on the medical problem for which you are taking the anabolic steroid.*

*For nandrolone decanoate*
- For *injection* dosage form:
  —For treatment of certain types of anemia:
    - Women and girls 14 years of age and older—50 to 100 milligrams (mg) injected into a muscle every one to four weeks.
    - Men and boys 14 years of age and older—50 to 200 mg injected into a muscle every one to four weeks.
    Your doctor may want to continue treatment for up to twelve weeks. After a four-week rest period without receiving this medicine, your doctor may want you to repeat the cycle.
    - Children up to 2 years of age—Dose must be determined by your doctor.
    - Children 2 to 13 years of age—25 to 50 mg injected into a muscle every three to four weeks.

*For nandrolone phenpropionate*
- For *injection* dosage form:
  —For treatment of certain breast cancers in women:
    - Adults—25 to 100 milligrams (mg) injected into a muscle once a week for up to twelve weeks. After a four-week rest period without receiving this medicine, your doctor may want you to repeat the cycle.
    - Children—Dose must be determined by your doctor.

*For oxandrolone*
- For *oral* dosage form (tablets):
  —For treatment in rebuilding tissue after a serious illness or injury:
    - Adults and teenagers—2.5 milligrams (mg) two to four times a day for up to four weeks. Your doctor may increase your dose up to 20 mg a day.
    - Children—Dose is based on body weight and must be determined by your doctor. The usual dose is 0.25 mg per kilogram (kg) (0.11 mg per pound) of body weight a day.

*For oxymetholone*
- For *oral* dosage form (tablets):
  —For treatment of certain types of anemia:
    - Adults, teenagers, children, and older infants —Dose is based on body weight and must be determined by your doctor. The usual dose is 1 to 5 milligrams (mg) per kilogram (kg) (0.45 to 2.3 mg per pound) of body weight a day.
    - Premature and newborn infants—Dose is based on body weight or size and must be determined by your doctor. The usual dose is 0.175 mg per kg (0.08 mg per pound) of body weight once a day.

*For stanozolol*
- For *oral* dosage form (tablets):
  —To prevent hereditary angioedema, which causes swelling of the face, arms, legs, throat, windpipe, bowels, or sexual organs:

- Adults and teenagers—At first, 2 milligrams (mg) three times a day to 4 mg four times a day for five days. Then, your doctor may slowly lower the dose to 2 mg once a day or once every other day.

**Missed dose**—If you miss a dose of this medicine and your dosing schedule is:

- One dose a day—Take the missed dose as soon as possible. However, if you do not remember it until the next day, skip the missed dose and go back to your regular dosing schedule. Do not double doses.
- More than one dose a day—Take the missed dose as soon as possible. However, if it is almost time for your next dose, skip the missed dose and go back to your regular dosing schedule. Do not double doses.

If you have any questions about this, check with your doctor.

**Storage**—To store this medicine:

- Keep out of the reach of children.
- Store away from heat and direct light.
- Do not store the tablet form of this medicine in the bathroom, near the kitchen sink, or in other damp places. Heat or moisture may cause the medicine to break down.
- Keep the liquid form of this medicine from freezing.
- Do not keep outdated medicine or medicine no longer needed. Be sure that any discarded medicine is out of the reach of children.

## Precautions While Using This Medicine

Your doctor should check your progress at regular visits to make sure that this medicine does not cause unwanted effects.

For diabetic patients:

- This medicine may affect blood sugar levels. If you notice a change in the results of your blood or urine sugar tests or if you have any questions, check with your doctor.

## Side Effects of This Medicine

Tumors of the liver, liver cancer, or peliosis hepatis, a form of liver disease, have occurred during long-term, high-dose therapy with anabolic steroids. Although these effects are rare, they can be very serious and may cause death. Discuss these possible effects with your doctor.

Along with its needed effects, a medicine may cause some unwanted effects. Although not all of these side effects may occur, if they do occur they may need medical attention.

*Check with your doctor immediately if any of the following side effects occur:*

*For both females and males*
*Less common*
Yellow eyes or skin

*Rare (with long-term use)*
Black, tarry, or light-colored stools; dark-colored urine; purple- or red-colored spots on body or inside the mouth or nose; sore throat and/or fever; vomiting of blood

Also, check with your doctor as soon as possible if any of the following side effects occur:

*For both females and males*
*Less common*
Bone pain; nausea or vomiting; sore tongue; swelling of feet or lower legs; unusual bleeding; unusual weight gain

*Rare (with long-term use)*
Abdominal or stomach pain; feeling of discomfort (continuing); headache (continuing); hives; loss of appetite (continuing); unexplained weight loss; unpleasant breath odor (continuing)

*For females only*
*More common*
Acne or oily skin; enlarging clitoris; hoarseness or deepening of voice; irregular menstrual periods; unnatural hair growth; unusual hair loss

*Less common*
Mental depression; unusual tiredness

*For young males (boys) only*
*More common*
Acne; enlarging penis; increased frequency of erections; unnatural hair growth

*Less common*
Unexplained darkening of skin

*For sexually mature males only*
*More common*
Enlargement of breasts or breast soreness; frequent or continuing erections; frequent urge to urinate

*For elderly males only*
*Less common*
Difficult or frequent urination

Other side effects may occur that usually do not need medical attention. These side effects may go away during treatment as your body adjusts to the medicine. However, check with your doctor if any of the following side effects continue or are bothersome:

*For both females and males*
*Less common*
Chills; diarrhea; feeling of abdominal or stomach fullness; muscle cramps; trouble in sleeping; unusual decrease or increase in sexual desire

*For males only*
*More common*
Acne

*Less common*
Decreased sexual ability

Other side effects not listed above may also occur in some patients. If you notice any other effects, check with your doctor.

## Additional Information

Once a medicine has been approved for marketing for a certain use, experience may show that it is also useful for other medical problems. Although these uses are not included in product labeling, anabolic steroids may be used in certain patients with the following medical conditions:

- Certain blood clotting diseases
- Growth failure

- Turner's syndrome

Other than the above information, there is no additional information relating to proper use, precautions, or side effects for these uses.

Revised: 06/20/92
Interim revision: 06/08/94

# ANDROGENS    Systemic

Some commonly used brand names are:

**In the U.S.—**

| | |
|---|---|
| Andro 100[3] | Everone[3] |
| Andro-Cyp 100[3] | Halotestin[1] |
| Andro-Cyp 200[3] | Histerone-50[3] |
| Andro L.A. 200[3] | Histerone-100[3] |
| Andronate 100[3] | Oreton[2] |
| Andronate 200[3] | T-Cypionate[3] |
| Andropository 100[3] | Testa-C[3] |
| Andryl 200[3] | Testamone 100[3] |
| Android-10[2] | Testaqua[3] |
| Android-25[2] | Testex[3] |
| Android-F[1] | Testoderm[3] |
| Delatest[3] | Testoject-50[3] |
| Delatestryl[3] | Testoject-LA[3] |
| depAndro 100[3] | Testone L.A. 100[3] |
| depAndro 200[3] | Testone L.A. 200[3] |
| Depotest[3] | Testred[2] |
| Depo-Testosterone[3] | Testred Cypionate 200[3] |
| Duratest-100[3] | Testrin P.A.[3] |
| Duratest-200[3] | Virilon[2] |
| Durathate-200[3] | Virilon IM[3] |

**In Canada—**

| | |
|---|---|
| Delatestryl[3] | Malogen[3] |
| Depo-Testosterone Cypionate[3] | Malogex[3] |
| Halotestin[1] | Metandren[2] |

Note: For quick reference, the following androgens are numbered to match the corresponding brand names.

This information applies to the following medicines:
1. Fluoxymesterone (floo-ox-i-MES-te-rone)‡
2. Methyltestosterone (meth-ill-tess-TOSS-te-rone)‡
3. Testosterone (tess-TOSS-te-rone)‡

‡Generic name product may also be available in the U.S.

## Description

Androgens (AN-droe-jens) are male hormones. Some androgens are naturally produced in the body and are necessary for the normal sexual development of males.

Androgens are used for several reasons, such as:
- to replace the hormone when the body is unable to produce enough on its own.
- to stimulate the beginning of puberty in certain boys who are late starting puberty naturally.
- to treat certain types of breast cancer in females.

In addition, some of these medicines may be used for other conditions as determined by your doctor.

Androgens are available only with your doctor's prescription, in the following dosage forms:

*Oral*
　Fluoxymesterone
　　• Tablets (U.S. and Canada)
　Methyltestosterone
　　• Capsules (U.S.)
　　• Buccal tablets (U.S. and Canada)
　　• Oral tablets (U.S. and Canada)

*Parenteral*
　Testosterone
　　• Injection (U.S. and Canada)

*Topical*
　Testosterone
　　• Ointment
　　• Transdermal system (stick-on patch) (U.S.)

## Before Using This Medicine

In deciding to use a medicine, the risks of taking the medicine must be weighed against the good it will do. This is a decision you and your doctor will make. For androgens, the following should be considered:

**Allergies**—Tell your doctor if you have ever had any unusual or allergic reaction to androgens or anabolic steroids. Also tell your health care professional if you are allergic to any other substances, such as foods, preservatives, or dyes.

**Pregnancy**—Androgens are not recommended during pregnancy. They have been shown to cause the development of male features in female babies and premature (too early) development of male features in male babies in humans.

**Breast-feeding**—Use is not recommended in nursing mothers, since androgens may pass into the breast milk and may cause unwanted effects in the nursing baby, such as premature (too early) sexual development in males and development of male features in female babies.

**Children**—Androgens may cause children to stop growing. In addition, androgens may make male children develop too fast sexually and may cause male-like changes in female children.

**Older adults**—When elderly male patients are treated with androgens, they may have an increased risk of enlarged prostate or growth of cancer of the prostate. For this reason, a prostate examination and a blood test to check for prostate cancer is often done before androgens are prescribed for men over the age of 50 years. These examinations may be repeated during treatment.

**Other medicines**—Although certain medicines should not be used together at all, in other cases two different medicines may be used together even if an interaction might occur. In these cases, your doctor may want to change the dose, or other precautions may be necessary. When you are taking androgens, it is especially important that your health care professional know if you are taking any of the following:

- Acetaminophen (e.g., Tylenol) (with long-term, high-dose use) or
- Amiodarone (e.g., Cordarone) or
- Anabolic steroids (nandrolone [e.g., Anabolin], oxandrolone [e.g., Anavar], oxymetholone [e.g., Anadrol], stanozolol [e.g., Winstrol]) or
- Anti-infectives by mouth or by injection (medicine for infection) or
- Antithyroid agents (medicine for overactive thyroid) or
- Carbamazepine (e.g., Tegretol) or
- Carmustine (e.g., BiCNU) or
- Chloroquine (e.g., Aralen) or
- Dantrolene (e.g., Dantrium) or
- Daunorubicin (e.g., Cerubidine) or
- Disulfiram (e.g., Antabuse) or
- Divalproex (e.g., Depakote) or
- Estrogens (female hormones) or
- Etretinate (e.g., Tegison) or
- Gold salts (medicine for arthritis) or
- Hydroxychloroquine (e.g., Plaquenil) or
- Mercaptopurine (e.g., Purinethol) or
- Methotrexate (e.g., Mexate) or
- Methyldopa (e.g., Aldomet) or
- Naltrexone (e.g., Trexan) (with long-term, high-dose use) or
- Oral contraceptives (birth control pills) containing estrogen or
- Phenothiazines (acetophenazine [e.g., Tindal], chlorpromazine [e.g., Thorazine], fluphenazine [e.g., Prolixin], mesoridazine [e.g., Serentil], perphenazine [e.g., Trilafon], prochlorperazine [e.g., Compazine], promazine [e.g., Sparine], promethazine [e.g., Phenergan], thioridazine [e.g., Mellaril], trifluoperazine [e.g., Stelazine], triflupromazine [e.g., Vesprin], trimeprazine [e.g., Temaril]) or
- Phenytoin (e.g., Dilantin) or
- Plicamycin (e.g., Mithracin) or
- Valproic acid (e.g., Depakene)—All of these medicines and androgens can cause liver damage. Your doctor may want you to have extra blood tests that tell about your liver, while you are taking any of these medicines with an androgen.
- Anticoagulants (blood thinners)—Androgens can increase the effect of these medicines and possibly cause excessive bleeding

**Other medical problems**—The presence of other medical problems may affect the use of androgens. Make sure you tell your doctor if you have any other medical problems, especially:

- Breast cancer (in males) or
- Prostate cancer—Androgens can cause growth of these tumors
- Diabetes mellitus (sugar diabetes)—Androgens can increase blood sugar levels. Careful monitoring of blood glucose should be done
- Edema (swelling of face, hands, feet, or lower legs) or
- Kidney disease or
- Liver disease—These conditions can be worsened by the fluid retention (keeping too much body water) that can be caused by androgens. Also, liver disease can prevent the body from getting the medicine out of the bloodstream as fast as it normally would. This could increase the chance of side effects
- Enlarged prostate—Androgens can cause further enlargement of the prostate
- Heart or blood vessel disease—Androgens can make these conditions worse because androgens may increase blood cholesterol levels. Also, androgens can cause fluid retention (keeping too much body water), which also can worsen heart or blood vessel disease

## Proper Use of This Medicine

For patients taking *fluoxymesterone* or the *capsule or regular tablet form of methyltestosterone*:

- Take this medicine with food to lessen possible stomach upset, unless otherwise directed by your doctor.

For patients using the *buccal tablet form of methyltestosterone*:

- *This medicine should not be swallowed whole.* It is meant to be absorbed through the lining of the mouth. Place the tablet in the upper or lower pouch between your gum and the side of your cheek. Let the tablet slowly dissolve there. Do not eat, drink, chew, or smoke while the tablet is dissolving. It is important that you brush your teeth or thoroughly rinse out your mouth after the tablet has completely dissolved and you can no longer taste it. This will help prevent tooth decay and cavities from the sugar in the tablet, as well as mouth irritation or soreness.

*Take this medicine only as directed. Do not take more of it and do not take it more often than your doctor ordered.* To do so may increase the chance of side effects.

For patients using the *skin patch form of testosterone:*

- You must apply the patch to the scrotum because the medicine easily passes into your body at this area. Other areas of your skin are too thick for the medicine to work properly.
- This medicine comes with patient directions. Read them carefully before using this medicine.
- Wash and dry your hands thoroughly before and after handling.
—Before applying the patch:
  - Clean and dry your scrotum.
  - You should also dry-shave this area once a week by using a shaver only (no soap or water). To dry-shave, stretch the skin of your scrotum with your

fingers. Use short gentle strokes with no pressure on the razor to remove the hair. Do not use shaving cream or hair-removing creams (e.g., Nair).

- You may sit with your legs apart or stand while applying the patch.

—To apply the patch:

- Open the wrapper containing the patch at the point shown on the package.
- Carefully remove the patch from its protective plastic liner by peeling the patch from the liner starting at the corner.
- Warm your scrotum for a few seconds before applying the patch for best results. Stretch the skin of your scrotum gently to remove the folds by pulling the penis up and to the side. Use your first and middle fingers to stretch the skin of the scrotum. Another way is to pull your scrotum down. Use your first and middle fingers to stretch the skin of your scrotum.
- Place the shiny side of the patch onto the warm stretched skin of your scrotum.
- Press the shiny side of the patch firmly in place with the palm of your hand for about 10 seconds. Make sure there is good contact, especially around the edges. The patch should stick to your scrotum and show the natural wrinkles of your scrotum.
- Put on comfortable close-fitting briefs (underwear) immediately.
- If a patch becomes loose or falls off, you may reapply it or discard it and apply a new patch.

—To remove the skin patch:

- Gently peel the patch from the skin.
- If the wearing period is over, throw the patch away.
- You may reuse the patch after removing it for swimming, bathing, or showering. First, remove the patch and place the shiny (sticky) side up on a counter. Be sure the skin on your scrotum is dry. Then, follow the directions to reapply the patch.

**Dosing**—The dose of these medicines will be different for different patients. *Follow your doctor's orders or the directions on the label.* The following information includes only the average doses of these medicines. *If your dose is different, do not change it* unless your doctor tells you to do so.

The number of capsules, buccal tablets, or oral tablets that you take depends on the strength of the medicine. Also, *the number of doses you take each day, the time allowed between doses, and the length of time you take the medicine depend on the medical problem for which you are taking the androgen.*

*For fluoxymesterone*

- For *oral* dosage form (oral tablets):
  —For androgen hormone replacement in men:
  - Adults—5 milligrams (mg) one to four times a day.
  —For treatment of breast cancer in women:
  - Adults—20 to 50 mg a day.

—For treatment of delayed sexual development in boys:

- Children—2.5 to 10 mg a day for four to six months.

*For methyltestosterone*

- For *oral* dosage forms (capsules or oral tablets):
  —For androgen hormone replacement:
  - Adults—10 to 50 milligrams (mg) a day.
  —For treatment of breast cancer in women:
  - Adults—50 mg one to four times a day. Your doctor may decrease your dose to 50 mg two times a day after two to four weeks.
  —For treatment of delayed sexual development in boys:
  - Children—5 to 25 mg a day for four to six months.
- For *oral* dosage form (buccal tablets):
  —For androgen hormone replacement in men:
  - Adults—5 to 25 milligrams (mg) a day dissolved in the side of your cheek.
  —For treatment of breast cancer in women:
  - Adults—25 mg one to four times a day dissolved in the side of your cheek. Your doctor may decrease your dose to 25 mg two times a day after two to four weeks.
  —For treatment of delayed sexual development in boys:
  - Children—2.5 to 12.5 mg a day dissolved in the side of your cheek for up to four to six months.

*For testosterone*

- For *injection* dosage form:
  —For androgen hormone replacement in men:
  - Adults—25 to 50 milligrams (mg) injected into a muscle two or three times a week.
  —For treatment of breast cancer in women:
  - Adults—50 to 100 mg injected into a muscle three times a week.
  —For treatment of delayed sexual development in boys:
  - Children—Up to 100 mg injected into a muscle once a month for four to six months.

*For testosterone cypionate* or *testosterone enanthate*

- For *injection* dosage form:
  —For androgen hormone replacement:
  - Adults—50 to 400 milligrams (mg) injected into a muscle every two to four weeks.
  —For treatment of breast cancer in women:
  - Adults—200 to 400 mg injected into a muscle every two to four weeks.
  —For treatment of delayed sexual development in boys:
  - Children—Up to 100 mg injected into a muscle once a month for four to six months.

*For testosterone propionate*
- For *injection* dosage form:
  - —For androgen hormone replacement:
    - Adults—25 to 50 milligrams (mg) injected into a muscle two or three times a week.
  - —For treatment of breast cancer in women:
    - Adults—50 to 100 mg injected into a muscle three times a week.
  - —For treatment of delayed sexual development in boys:
    - Children—Up to 100 milligrams (mg) injected into a muscle once a month for four to six months.
- For *topical* dosage form (ointment):
  - —For treatment of skin irritation of the vulva (a part of the female genitals):
    - Adults—Apply to your vulva two times a day for six weeks or until the itching stops.
  - —For treatment of an unusually small penis in certain children:
    - Children—Apply to your penis two times day for three months.
- For *topical* dosage form (patch):
  - —For androgen hormone replacement:
    - Adults—One transdermal system (skin patch) (4 to 6 milligrams [mg]) applied to your scrotum once a day. The patch should be worn at least 22 of the 24 hours in a day.
    - Children and teenagers—Use and dose must be determined by your doctor.

**Missed dose**—If you miss a dose of this medicine and your dosing schedule is:
- One dose a day—Take, use, or apply the missed dose as soon as possible. However, if you do not remember it until the next day, skip the missed dose and go back to your regular dosing schedule. Do not double doses.
- More than one dose a day—Take or use the missed dose as soon as possible. However, if it is almost time for your next dose, skip the missed dose and go back to your regular dosing schedule. Do not double doses.

If you have any questions about this, check with your doctor.

**Storage**—To store this medicine:
- Keep out of the reach of children.
- Store away from heat and direct light.
- Do not store in the bathroom, near the kitchen sink, or in other damp places. Heat or moisture may cause the medicine to break down.
- Keep the injection form of this medicine from freezing.
- Do not keep outdated medicine or medicine no longer needed. Be sure that any discarded medicine is out of the reach of children.

## Precautions While Using This Medicine
Your doctor should check your progress at regular visits to make sure this medicine does not cause unwanted effects.

For *diabetic patients:*
- This medicine may affect blood sugar levels. If you notice a change in the results of your blood or urine sugar tests or if you have any questions, check with your doctor.

For *patients using the skin patch:*
- In some cases, this medicine can pass from you to your sexual partner. Tell your doctor if your female sex partner complains of a great increase in acne. Also, tell your doctor if her hair begins to grow in odd places like her upper lip, chest, or back.

## Side Effects of This Medicine
Discuss these possible effects with your doctor:
- Tumors of the liver, liver cancer, or peliosis hepatis (a form of liver disease), have occurred during long-term, high-dose therapy with androgens. Although these effects are rare, they can be very serious and may cause death.
- When androgens are used in women, especially in high doses, male-like changes may occur, such as hoarseness or deepening of the voice, unnatural hair growth, or unusual hair loss. Most of these changes will go away if the medicine is stopped as soon as the changes are noticed. However, some changes, such as voice changes or enlarged clitoris, may not go away.
- When androgens are used in high doses in males, they interfere with the production of sperm. This effect is usually temporary and only happens during the time you are taking the medicine. However, discuss this possible effect with your doctor if you are planning on having children.

Along with its needed effects, a medicine may cause some unwanted effects. Although not all of these side effects appear very often, when they do occur they may require medical attention.

*Check with your doctor immediately* if any of the following side effects occur:
*For both females and males*
  *Less common*
    Itching of skin; yellow eyes or skin
  *Rare (with long-term use and/or high doses)*
    Black, tarry, or light-colored stools; dark-colored urine; purple- or red-colored spots on body or inside the mouth or nose; sore throat or fever; vomiting of blood

Also, check with your doctor as soon as possible if any of the following side effects occur:
*For both females and males*
  *Less common*
    Changes in skin color; confusion; constipation; dizziness; flushing or redness of skin; headache (frequent or continuing); increased thirst; increase in urination; mental depression; nausea or vomiting; swelling of feet or lower legs; unusual bleeding; unusual tiredness; weight gain (rapid)

*Rare (with long-term use and/or high doses)*

Abdominal or stomach pain (continuing); feeling of discomfort (continuing); hives; loss of appetite (continuing); pain, tenderness, or swelling in the upper abdominal or stomach area; unpleasant breath odor (continuing)

*For females only*
*More common*

Acne or oily skin; decreased breast size; enlarged clitoris; hoarseness or deepening of voice; irregular menstrual periods; male type of baldness; unnatural and excessive hair growth

*For males only*
*More common*

Breast soreness; enlargement of breasts; frequent or continuing erections; frequent urge to urinate

*Less common*

Chills; difficult urination; pain in scrotum or groin

*For prepubertal boys only*
*Less common*

Acne; early growth of pubic hair; enlargement of penis; increased frequency of erections

Other side effects may occur that usually do not need medical attention. These side effects may go away during treatment as your body adjusts to the medicine. However, check with your doctor if any of the following side effects continue or are bothersome:

*For both females and males*
*Less common*

Acne (mild); diarrhea; increase in pubic hair growth; infection, redness, pain, or other irritation at the place of injection (for patients receiving testosterone by injection); irritation or soreness of mouth or unusual watering of mouth (for patients taking buccal tablet form of methyltestosterone); stomach pain; trouble in sleeping; unusual decrease or increase in sexual desire

*For males only*
*Less common*

Decrease in testicle size; impotence; infection, itching, redness, or other skin irritation of the scrotum

Other side effects not listed above may also occur in some patients. If you notice any other effects, check with your doctor.

## Additional Information

Once a medicine has been approved for marketing for a certain use, experience may show that it is also useful for other medical problems. Although these uses are not included in product labeling, androgens are used in certain patients with the following medical conditions:

- Anemias (some types of blood diseases)
- Delayed growth spurt
- Development of male features in transsexuals
- Microphallus (under-development of the penis)
- Lichen sclerosus (a skin problem of the vulva)

Other than the above information, there is no additional information relating to proper use, precautions, or side effects for these uses.

Revised: 08/23/94

# ANDROGENS AND ESTROGENS   Systemic

Some commonly used brand names are:

**In the U.S.—**

| | |
|---|---|
| Andrest 90-4[5] | Estratest[3] |
| Andro-Estro 90-4[5] | Estratest H.S.[3] |
| Androgyn L.A.[5] | Halodrin[4] |
| De-Comberol[5] | Menoject-L.A.[5] |
| Deladumone[5] | OB[5] |
| Delatestadiol[5] | Premarin with |
| depAndrogyn[5] | Methyltestosterone[2] |
| Depo-Testadiol[5] | Teev[5] |
| Depotestogen[5] | Tes Est Cyp[5] |
| Duo-Cyp[5] | Test-Estro Cypionate[5] |
| Duo-Gen L.A.[5] | Tylosterone[1] |
| Dura-Dumone 90/4[5] | Valertest No. 1[5] |
| Duratestin[5] | Valertest No. 2[5] |

**In Canada—**

| | |
|---|---|
| Climacteron[5] | Premarin with |
| Duogex L.A.[5] | Methyltestosterone[2] |
| Neo-Pause[5] | |

Another commonly used name for diethylstilbestrol is DES.

Note: For quick reference, the following androgens and estrogens are numbered to match the corresponding brand names.

This information applies to the following medicines:

1. Diethylstilbestrol (dye-eth-il-stil-BESS-trole) and Methyltestosterone (meth-il-tes-TOSS-ter-one)
2. Estrogens, Conjugated (ESS-troe-jenz, CON-ju-gate-ed), and Methyltestosterone
3. Estrogens, Esterified (ess-TAIR-i-fyed), and Methyltestosterone
4. Fluoxymesterone (floo-ox-e-MESS-ter-own) and Ethinyl Estradiol (ETH-in-il ess-tra-DYE-ole)
5. Testosterone (tess-TOSS-ter-own) and Estradiol‡

‡Generic name product may also be available in the U.S.

## Description

Androgens (AN-droe-jens) and estrogens (ESS-troe-jens) are hormones. Estrogens are produced by the body in greater amounts in females. They are necessary for normal sexual development of the female and for regulation of the menstrual cycle during the childbearing years. Androgens are produced by the body in greater amounts in males. However, androgens are also present in females in small amounts.

The ovaries and adrenal glands begin to produce less of these hormones after menopause. This combination product is prescribed to make up for this lower production of hormones. This may relieve signs of menopause, such as hot flashes and unusual sweating, chills, faintness, or dizziness.

Androgens and estrogens may also be used for other conditions as determined by your doctor.

There is no medical evidence to support the belief that the use of estrogens (contained in this combination medicine) will keep the patient feeling young, keep the skin soft, or delay the appearance of wrinkles. Nor has it been proven that the use of estrogens during the menopause will relieve emotional and nervous symptoms, unless these symptoms are caused by other menopausal symptoms, such as hot flashes.

*A paper called "Information for the Patient" should be given to you with your prescription. Read this carefully.* Also, before you use an androgen and estrogen product, you and your doctor should discuss the good that it will do as well as the risks of using it.

This medicine is available only with your doctor's prescription, in the following dosage forms:

*Oral*
    Diethylstilbestrol and Methyltestosterone
        • Tablets (U.S.)
    Estrogens, Conjugated, and Methyltestosterone
        • Tablets (U.S. and Canada)
    Estrogens, Esterified, and Methyltestosterone
        • Tablets (U.S.)
    Fluoxymesterone and Ethinyl Estradiol
        • Tablets (U.S.)
*Parenteral*
    Testosterone and Estradiol
        • Injection (U.S. and Canada)

---

## Before Using This Medicine

In deciding to use a medicine, the risks of taking the medicine must be weighed against the good it will do. This is a decision you and your doctor will make. For androgen and estrogen combination products, the following should be considered:

**Allergies**—Tell your doctor if you have ever had any unusual or allergic reaction to androgens, anabolic steroids, or estrogens. Also tell your health care professional if you are allergic to any other substances, such as foods, preservatives, or dyes.

**Pregnancy**—Estrogens (contained in this combination medicine) are not recommended for use during pregnancy, since some estrogens have been shown to cause serious birth defects in humans. Some daughters of women who took diethylstilbestrol (DES) during pregnancy have developed reproductive (genital) tract problems and, rarely, cancer of the vagina and/or uterine cervix when they reached childbearing age. Some sons of women who took DES during pregnancy have developed urinary-genital tract problems.

Androgens (contained in this combination medicine) should not be used during pregnancy because they may cause male-like changes in a female baby.

**Breast-feeding**—Use of this medicine is not recommended in nursing mothers. Estrogens pass into the breast milk and their possible effect on the baby is not known. It is not known if androgens pass into breast milk. However, androgens may cause unwanted effects in nursing babies such as too early sexual development in males or male-like changes in females.

**Older adults**—This medicine has been tested and has not been shown to cause different side effects or problems in older women than it does in younger females.

**Other medicines**—Although certain medicines should not be used together at all, in other cases two different medicines may be used together even if an interaction might occur. In these cases, your doctor may want to change the dose, or other precautions may be necessary. When you are taking an androgen and estrogen combination product, it is especially important that your health care professional know if you are taking any of the following:

• Acetaminophen (e.g., Tylenol) (with long-term, high-dose use) or
• Amiodarone (e.g., Cordarone) or
• Anabolic steroids (nandrolone [e.g., Anabolin], oxandrolone [e.g., Anavar], oxymetholone [e.g., Anadrol], stanozolol [e.g., Winstrol]) or
• Anti-infectives by mouth or by injection (medicine for infection) or
• Antithyroid agents (medicine for overactive thyroid) or
• Carbamazepine (e.g., Tegretol) or
• Carmustine (e.g., BiCNU) or
• Chloroquine (e.g., Aralen) or
• Dantrolene (e.g., Dantrium) or
• Daunorubicin (e.g., Cerubidine) or
• Disulfiram (e.g., Antabuse) or
• Divalproex (e.g., Depakote) or
• Etretinate (e.g., Tegison) or
• Gold salts (medicine for arthritis) or
• Hydroxychloroquine (e.g., Plaquenil) or
• Mercaptopurine (e.g., Purinethol) or
• Methotrexate (e.g., Mexate) or
• Methyldopa (e.g., Aldomet) or
• Naltrexone (e.g., Trexan) (with long-term, high-dose use) or
• Phenothiazines (acetophenazine [e.g., Tindal], chlorpromazine [e.g., Thorazine], fluphenazine [e.g., Prolixin], mesoridazine [e.g., Serentil], perphenazine [e.g., Trilafon], prochlorperazine [e.g., Compazine], promazine [e.g., Sparine], promethazine [e.g., Phenergan], thioridazine [e.g., Mellaril], trifluoperazine [e.g., Stelazine], triflupromazine [e.g., Vesprin], trimeprazine [e.g., Temaril]) or
• Phenytoin (e.g., Dilantin) or
• Plicamycin (e.g., Mithracin) or
• Valproic acid (e.g., Depakene)—Androgens, estrogens, and all of these medicines can cause liver damage. Your doctor may want you to have extra blood tests that tell about your liver, while you are taking any of these medicines with an androgen and estrogen combination product.
• Anticoagulants (blood thinners)—Androgens can cause an increased effect of blood thinners, which could lead to uncontrolled or excessive bleeding
• Cyclosporine (e.g., Sandimmune)—Estrogens can increase the chances of toxic effects to the kidney or liver from cyclosporine because estrogens can interfere with the

body's ability to get the cyclosporine out of the bloodstream as it normally would

**Other medical problems**—The presence of other medical problems may affect the use of androgen and estrogen combination products. Make sure you tell your doctor if you have any other medical problems, especially:

- Blood clots (or history of during previous estrogen therapy)—Estrogens may worsen blood clots or cause new clots to form
- Breast cancer (active or suspected)—Estrogens may cause growth of the tumor
- Changes in vaginal bleeding of unknown causes—Some irregular vaginal bleeding is a sign that the lining of the uterus is growing too much or is a sign of cancer of the uterus lining; estrogens may make these conditions worse
- Diabetes mellitus (sugar diabetes)—Androgens can decrease blood sugar levels
- Edema (swelling of feet or lower legs caused by retaining [keeping] too much body water) or
- Heart or circulation disease or
- Kidney disease or
- Liver disease—Androgens can worsen these conditions because androgens cause the body to retain extra fluid (keep too much body water). Also, heart or circulation disease can be worsened by androgens because androgens may increase blood cholesterol levels
- Endometriosis—Estrogens may worsen endometriosis by causing growth of endometriosis implants
- Fibroid tumors of the uterus—Estrogens may cause fibroid tumors to increase in size
- Gallbladder disease or gallstones (or history of)—There is no clear evidence as to whether estrogens increase the risk of gallbladder disease or gallstones
- Jaundice (or history of during pregnancy)—Estrogens use may worsen or cause jaundice in these patients
- Liver disease—Toxic drug effects may occur in patients with liver disease because the body is not able to get this medicine out of the bloodstream as it normally would
- Porphyria—Estrogens can worsen porphyria

## Proper Use of This Medicine

For patients taking any of the androgen and estrogen products by mouth:

- *Take this medicine only as directed by your doctor. Do not take more of it and do not take it for a longer time than your doctor ordered.*
- Try to take the medicine at the same time each day to reduce the possibility of side effects and to allow it to work better.
- Nausea may occur during the first few weeks after you start taking estrogens. This effect usually disappears with continued use. If the nausea is bothersome, it can usually be prevented or reduced by taking each dose with food or immediately after food.

**Dosing**—The dose of these medicines will be different for different patients. *Follow your doctor's orders or the directions on the label.* The following information includes only the average doses of these medicines. *If your dose is different, do not change it* unless your doctor tells you to do so.

The number of tablets that you take depends on the strength of the medicine. Also, *the number of doses you take each day, the time allowed between doses, and the length of time you take the medicine depend on the medical problem for which you are taking combinations of androgen and estrogen.*

*For diethylstilbestrol and methyltestosterone*

- For *oral* dosage form (tablets):
  —For treatment of certain signs of menopause, such as hot flashes and unusual sweating, chills, faintness, or dizziness:
  - Adults—0.25 milligrams (mg) of diethylstilbestrol and 5 mg of methyltestosterone once a day for twenty-one days. Stop the medicine for seven days, then repeat the twenty-one day cycle. After a while, your doctor may decrease your dose to 0.125 mg of diethylstilbestrol and 2.5 mg of methyltestosterone once a day for twenty-one days. Again, after stopping for seven days, you will then repeat the cycle.

*For conjugated estrogens and methyltestosterone*

- For *oral* dosage form (tablets):
  —For treatment of certain signs of menopause, such as hot flashes and unusual sweating, chills, faintness, or dizziness:
  - Adults—1.25 milligrams (mg) of conjugated estrogens and 10 mg of methyltestosterone once a day for twenty-one days. Stop the medicine for seven days, then repeat the twenty-one day cycle.

*For esterified estrogens and methyltestosterone*

- For *oral* dosage form (tablets):
  —For treatment of certain signs of menopause, such as hot flashes and unusual sweating, chills, faintness, or dizziness:
  - Adults—0.625 to 2.5 mg of esterified estrogens and 1.25 to 5 mg of methyltestosterone once a day for twenty-one days. Stop the medicine for seven days, then repeat the twenty-one day cycle.

*For fluoxymesterone and ethinyl estradiol*

- For *oral* dosage form (tablets):
  —For treatment of certain signs of menopause, such as hot flashes and unusual sweating, chills, faintness, or dizziness:
  - Adults—1 to 2 milligrams (mg) of fluoxymesterone and 0.02 to 0.04 mg of ethinyl estradiol two times a day for twenty-one days. Stop the medicine for seven days, then repeat the twenty-one day cycle.

*For testosterone cypionate and estradiol cypionate*

- For *injection* dosage form:
  —For treatment of certain signs of menopause, such as hot flashes and unusual sweating, chills, faintness, or dizziness:
  - Adults—50 milligrams (mg) of testosterone cypionate and 2 mg of estradiol cypionate injected into a muscle once every four weeks.

*For testosterone enanthate and estradiol valerate*

- For *injection* dosage form:
    —For treatment of certain signs of menopause, such as hot flashes and unusual sweating, chills, faintness, or dizziness:
    - Adults—90 milligrams (mg) of testosterone enanthate and 4 mg of estradiol valerate injected into a muscle once every four weeks.

*For testosterone enanthate benzilic acid hydrazone, estradiol dienanthate, and estradiol benzoate*

- For *injection* dosage form:
    —For treatment of bone loss (osteoporosis) or certain signs of menopause, such as hot flashes and unusual sweating, chills, faintness, or dizziness:
    - Adults—150 milligrams (mg) of testosterone enanthate benzilic acid hydrazone, 7.5 mg of estradiol dienanthate, and 1 mg of estradiol benzoate injected into a muscle once every four to eight weeks or less.

**Missed dose**—If you miss a dose of this medicine and your dosing schedule is:

- One dose a day—Take the missed dose as soon as possible. However, if you do not remember it until the next day, skip the missed dose and go back to your regular dosing schedule. Do not double doses.
- More than one dose a day—Take the missed dose as soon as possible. However, if it is almost time for your next dose, skip the missed dose and go back to your regular dosing schedule. Do not double doses.

If you have any questions about this, check with your doctor.

**Storage**—To store this medicine:

- Keep out of the reach of children.
- Store away from heat and direct light.
- Do not store in the bathroom medicine cabinet because the heat or moisture may cause the medicine to break down.
- Keep the injectable form of this medicine from freezing.
- Do not keep outdated medicine or medicine no longer needed. Be sure that any discarded medicine is out of the reach of children.

## Precautions While Using This Medicine

*It is very important that your doctor check your progress at regular visits to make sure this medicine does not cause unwanted effects.* These visits will usually be every 6 to 12 months, but many doctors require them more often.

It is not yet known whether the use of estrogen increases the risk of breast cancer in women. Therefore, it is very important that you regularly check your breasts for any unusual lumps or discharge. You should also have a mammogram (x-ray picture of the breasts) done if your doctor recommends it.

In some patients using estrogens, tenderness, swelling, or bleeding of the gums may occur. Brushing and flossing your teeth carefully and regularly and massaging your gums may help prevent this. See your dentist regularly to have your teeth cleaned. Check with your medical doctor or dentist if you have any questions about how to take care of your teeth and gums, or if you notice any tenderness, swelling, or bleeding of your gums.

For diabetic patients:

- This medicine may affect blood sugar levels. If you notice a change in the results of your blood or urine sugar tests or if you have any questions, check with your doctor.

*If you think that you may have become pregnant, check with your doctor immediately.* Continued use of this medicine during pregnancy may cause birth defects or future health problems in the child.

In studies with oral contraceptives (birth control pills) containing estrogens, cigarette smoking during the use of estrogens was shown to cause an increased risk of serious side effects affecting the heart or blood circulation, such as dangerous blood clots, heart attack, or stroke. The risk increased as the amount of smoking and the age of the smoker increased. Women aged 35 and over were at greatest risk when they smoked while using oral contraceptives containing estrogens. It is not known if this risk exists with the use of androgens and estrogens for symptoms of menopause. However, smoking may make estrogens less effective.

Do not give this medicine to anyone else. Your doctor has prescribed it specifically for you after studying your health record and the results of your physical examination. Androgens and estrogens may be dangerous for some people because of differences in their health and body chemistry.

## Side Effects of This Medicine

Discuss these possible effects with your doctor:

- Tumors of the liver, liver cancer, and peliosis hepatis (a form of liver disease) have occurred during long-term, high-dose therapy with androgens. Although these effects are rare, they can be very serious and may cause death.
- When androgens are used in women, especially in high doses, male-like changes may occur, such as hoarseness or deepening of the voice, unnatural hair growth, or unusual hair loss. Most of these changes will go away if the medicine is stopped as soon as the changes are noticed. However, some changes, such as voice changes, may not go away.
- The prolonged use of estrogens has been reported to increase the risk of endometrial cancer (cancer of the uterus lining) in women after menopause. The risk seems to increase as the dose and the length of use increase. When estrogens are used in low doses for less than one year, there is less risk. The risk is also reduced if a progestin (another female hormone)

is added to, or replaces part of, your estrogen dose. If the uterus has been removed by surgery (total hysterectomy), there is no risk of endometrial cancer.

• It is not yet known whether the use of estrogens increases the risk of breast cancer in women. Although some large studies show an increased risk, most studies and information gathered to date do not support this idea.

Along with its needed effects, a medicine may cause some unwanted effects. Although not all of these side effects may occur, if they do occur they may need medical attention.

*Check with your doctor immediately* if any of the following side effects occur:

*Less common*
Yellow eyes or skin

*Rare*
Uncontrolled jerky muscle movements; vomiting of blood (with long-term use or high doses)

Also, check with your doctor as soon as possible if any of the following side effects occur:

*More common*
Acne or oily skin (severe); breast pain or tenderness; changes in vaginal bleeding (spotting, breakthrough bleeding, prolonged or heavier bleeding, or complete stoppage of bleeding); enlarged clitoris; enlargement or decrease in size of breasts; hoarseness or deepening of voice; swelling of feet or lower legs; unnatural hair growth; unusual hair loss; weight gain (rapid)

*Less common or rare*
Confusion; dizziness; flushing or redness of skin; headaches (frequent or continuing); hives (especially at place of injection); shortness of breath (unexplained); skin rash, hives, or itching; unusual bleeding; unusual tiredness or drowsiness

*With long-term use or high doses*
Black, tarry, or light-colored stools; dark-colored urine; general feeling of discomfort or illness (continuing); hives (frequent or continuing); loss of appetite (continuing); lump in, or discharge from breast; nausea (severe); pain, swelling, or tenderness in stomach or upper abdomen (continuing); purple- or red-colored spots on body or inside the mouth or nose; sore throat or fever (continuing); unpleasant breath odor (continuing); vomiting (severe)

Other side effects may occur that usually do not need medical attention. These side effects may go away during treatment as your body adjusts to the medicine. However, check with your doctor if any of the following side effects continue or are bothersome:

*More common*
Bloating of abdomen or stomach; cramps of abdomen or stomach; loss of appetite (temporary); nausea (mild); stomach pain (mild); unusual increase in sexual desire; vomiting (mild)

*Less common*
Constipation; diarrhea (mild); dizziness (mild); headaches (mild); infection, redness, pain, or other irritation at place of injection; migraine headaches; problems in wearing contact lenses; trouble in sleeping

Also, many women who are taking a progestin (another type of female hormone) with this medicine will begin to have monthly vaginal bleeding again, similar to menstrual periods. This effect will continue for as long as this medicine is used. However, monthly bleeding will not occur in women who have had the uterus removed by surgery (total hysterectomy).

Other side effects not listed above may also occur in some patients. If you notice any other effects, check with your doctor.

Revised: 06/30/92
Interim revision: 06/21/94

# ANESTHETICS  Dental

Some commonly used brand names are:

**In the U.S.—**
Anbesol, Baby[1]
Anbesol Maximum Strength Gel[1]
Anbesol Maximum Strength Liquid[1]
Anbesol Regular Strength Gel[3]
Anbesol Regular Strength Liquid[3]
Benzodent[1]
Chloraseptic Lozenges[2]
Chloraseptic Lozenges, Children's[1]
Dentapaine[1]
Dent-Zel-Ite[1]
Hurricaine[1]
Numzident[1]
Num-Zit Gel[1]
Num-Zit Lotion[1]

Orabase, Baby[1]
Orabase-B with Benzocaine[1]
Orajel, Baby[1]
Orajel Maximum Strength[1]
Orajel Nighttime Formula, Baby[1]
Oratect Gel[1]
Rid-A-Pain[1]
SensoGARD Canker Sore Relief[1]
Spec-T Sore Throat Anesthetic[1]
Sucrets, Children's[4]
Sucrets Maximum Strength[4]
Sucrets Regular Strength[4]
Xylocaine[5]
Xylocaine Viscous[5]
Zilactin-L[5]

**In Canada—**
Anbesol Baby Jel[1]
Anbesol Gel[3]
Anbesol Liquid[3]
Anbesol Maximum Strength Liquid[3]
Chloraseptic Lozenges Cherry Flavor[2]
Dentocaine[1]

Orajel, Baby[1]
Orajel Extra Strength[1]
Orajel Liquid[1]
Supracaine[6]*
Topicaine[1]
Xylocaine[5]
Xylocaine Viscous[5]

Other commonly used names are:
amethocaine[6]
dyclocaine[4]
ethyl aminobenzoate[1]
lignocaine[5]

Note: For quick reference, the following anesthetics are numbered to match the corresponding brand names.

This information applies to the following medicines:
1. Benzocaine (BEN-zoe-kane)
2. Benzocaine and Menthol (MEN-thole)
3. Benzocaine and Phenol (FEE-nole)
4. Dyclonine (DYE-kloe-neen)
5. Lidocaine (LYE-doe-kane)‡
6. Tetracaine (TET-ra-kane)

*Not commercially available in the U.S.
‡Generic name product may also be available in the U.S.

# Description

Dental anesthetics (an-ess-THET-iks) are used in the mouth to relieve pain or irritation caused by many conditions. Examples include toothache, teething, and sores in or around the mouth, such as cold sores, canker sores, and fever blisters. Also, some of these medicines are used to relieve pain or irritation caused by dentures or other dental appliances, including braces. However, if you have an infection or a lot of large sores in your mouth, check with your medical doctor or dentist before using a dental anesthetic because other kinds of treatment may be needed. Also, the chance of side effects is increased.

One form of lidocaine is also used to relieve pain caused by certain throat conditions. Some forms of benzocaine, benzocaine and menthol combination, and dyclonine are also used to relieve sore throat pain.

Some of these medicines are available only with your medical doctor's or dentist's prescription. Others are available without a prescription; however, your medical doctor or dentist may have special instructions on the proper use and dose for your medical problem. Some nonprescription (over-the-counter [OTC]) aerosols, gels, liquids, or ointments that contain a local anesthetic are not meant to be used in or around the mouth. If you have any questions about which product to use, check with your pharmacist.

These medicines are available in the following dosage forms:

*Dental*

Benzocaine
• Aerosol spray (U.S.)
• Dental paste (U.S.)
• Film-forming gel (U.S.)
• Gel (U.S. and Canada)
• Lozenges (U.S.)
• Ointment (U.S. and Canada)
• Solution (liquid) (U.S. and Canada)
Benzocaine and Menthol
• Lozenges (U.S. and Canada)
Benzocaine and Phenol
• Gel (U.S. and Canada)
• Solution (liquid) (U.S. and Canada)
Dyclonine
• Lozenges (U.S.)
Lidocaine
• Aerosol spray (U.S. and Canada)
• Ointment (U.S. and Canada)
• Solution (U.S. and Canada)
• Viscous (very thick) solution (U.S. and Canada)
Tetracaine
• Aerosol spray (Canada)

# Before Using This Medicine

If you are taking this medicine without a prescription, carefully read and follow any precautions on the label. For dental anesthetics, the following should be considered:

**Allergies**—Tell your doctor if you have ever had any unusual or allergic reaction to a local anesthetic, especially one that was applied to any part of the body as a liquid, cream, ointment, or spray. Also tell your health care professional if you are allergic to any other substances, such as foods, preservatives, or dyes.

**Pregnancy**—Dental anesthetics have not been reported to cause birth defects or other problems in humans.

**Breast-feeding**—Dental anesthetics have not been reported to cause problems in nursing babies.

**Children**—Children may be especially sensitive to the effects of dental anesthetics. This may increase the chance of unwanted effects, some of which can be serious, during treatment. When using a dental anesthetic for a child, be very careful not to use more of the medicine than directed on the label, unless otherwise directed by your health care professional. Teething medicines that contain benzocaine may be used in babies 4 months of age and older. One product that contains benzocaine (Orabase-B with Benzocaine) may be used in children 6 years of age and older. Most of the other nonprescription (over-the-counter [OTC]) medicines that contain a dental anesthetic may be used in children 2 years of age and older. However, these other nonprescription products should not be used in infants or children younger than 2 years of age unless prescribed by a health care professional.

**Older adults**—Elderly people are especially sensitive to the effects of many local anesthetics. This may increase the chance of side effects during treatment, especially with lidocaine. Nonprescription (over-the-counter [OTC]) products containing local anesthetics are not likely to cause problems. However, elderly people should be especially careful not to use more medicine than directed on the package label, unless otherwise directed by a medical doctor or a dentist.

**Other medicines**—Although certain medicines should not be used together at all, in other cases two different medicines may be used together even if an interaction might occur. In these cases, your doctor may want to change the dose, or other precautions may be necessary. Before you use a dental anesthetic, check with your medical doctor, dentist, or pharmacist if you are taking any other prescription or nonprescription (over-the-counter [OTC]) medicine.

# Proper Use of This Medicine

For safe and effective use of this medicine:
• Follow your medical doctor's or dentist's instructions if this medicine was prescribed.
• Follow the manufacturer's package directions if you are treating yourself.

- *Do not use more of this medicine, do not use it more often, and do not use it for a longer time than directed.* To do so may increase the chance of absorption into the body and the risk of side effects. This is particularly important for young children and elderly patients, especially with lidocaine.
- Dental anesthetics should be used only for conditions being treated by your medical doctor or dentist or for problems listed in the package directions. *Do not use any of them for other problems without first checking with your medical doctor or dentist.* These medicines should not be used if certain kinds of infections are present.

To use *the viscous (very thick) liquid form of lidocaine* (e.g., Xylocaine Viscous):

- This medicine may cause serious side effects if too much of it is swallowed. Be certain that you understand exactly how you are to use this medicine, and whether or not you are to swallow it. Follow your medical doctor's or dentist's directions very carefully. Also, *be very careful to measure the exact amount of medicine that you are to use.* Use a special measuring spoon to measure the amount; regular household teaspoons or soup spoons that you use at the table may not measure the amount correctly. These measures are especially important when this medicine is used for young children, who are especially sensitive to its effects.
- If you are using this medicine for a problem in the mouth, you may apply it to the sore places with a cotton-tipped applicator. Or, you may swish the measured amount of medicine around in your mouth until you are certain that it has reached all of the sore places. *Do not swallow the medicine unless your medical doctor or dentist has told you to do so.*
- If you are using this medicine for a problem in the throat, gargle with the measured amount of medicine as directed by your doctor. *Do not swallow the medicine unless your doctor has told you to do so.*

To use *benzocaine film-forming gel* (e.g., Oratect Gel):

- Children may find it difficult to apply this medicine correctly. They should be helped by an adult.
- First, dry the area where the medicine is needed, using a swab included in the package.
- Apply the gel to a second swab. Then roll the swab over the dried area.
- Keep your mouth open and dry for about 30 to 60 seconds after applying the medicine. A film will form where you placed the medicine.
- Do not remove the film. It will slowly disappear and should be gone about 6 hours after the medicine was applied.

To use *other gel or liquid forms of a dental anesthetic:*

- Apply the medicine to the sore places with a clean finger, a cotton-tipped applicator, or a piece of gauze.

- When relieving pain caused by dentures or other dental appliances, *do not apply this medicine directly to the appliance, and do not place the appliance in your mouth while the medicine is there,* unless directed to do so by your dentist. Instead, apply the medicine to the sore areas in your mouth and wait until the pain is relieved. Then rinse your mouth with water before replacing the appliance.

To use *benzocaine dental paste* (e.g., Orabase-B with Benzocaine):

- Use a cotton-tipped applicator to dab small amounts of the medicine onto the sore places. Do not rub or try to spread the medicine with your finger while you are applying it, because the medicine will become crumbly and gritty.

To use *aerosol or spray forms of a dental anesthetic:*

- To help prevent unwanted effects, be very careful not to inhale (breathe in) the medicine. Also, do not spray the back of your mouth or throat with it unless your medical doctor or dentist directs you to do so.

To use *lozenge forms of benzocaine, benzocaine and menthol, or dyclonine:*

- These lozenges should be dissolved slowly in the mouth. Do not bite or chew them or swallow them whole. Before giving a lozenge to a young child, be sure that the child understands these directions and will follow them.

**Dosing**—The dose of these medicines will be different for different patients. *Follow your health care professional's orders or the directions on the label.* The following information includes only the average doses of these medicines. *If your dose is different, do not change it* unless your medical doctor or dentist tells you to do so.

*For benzocaine*

- For *dental paste* dosage form:
  —For sores in and around the mouth, sore gums, or pain caused by dental appliances:
  - Adults, teenagers, and children 6 years of age and older—Apply a small amount of the medicine to the painful areas.
  - Children up to 6 years of age—Use and dose must be determined by your health care professional.
- For *film-forming gel, liquid, and ointment* dosage forms:
  —For sores in and around the mouth, toothache, sore gums, or pain caused by dental appliances:
  - Adults, teenagers, and children 2 years of age and older—Apply a small amount of medicine to the painful areas up to four times a day.
  - Children up to 2 years of age—Use and dose must be determined by your health care professional.

- For *gel* dosage form:
  —For sores in and around the mouth, toothache, sore gums, or pain caused by dental appliances:
    • Adults, teenagers, and children 2 years of age and older—Apply a small amount of medicine to the painful areas up to four times a day.
    • Children up to 2 years of age—Use and dose must be determined by your health care professional.
  —For teething pain:
    • Infants up to 4 months of age—Use and dose must be determined by your health care professional.
    • Infants and children 4 months to 2 years of age—Apply a small amount of the 7.5% or 10% benzocaine gel to sore gums up to four times a day.
    • Children 2 years of age and older—Apply any strength of benzocaine gel to sore gums up to four times a day.
- For *lozenge* dosage form:
  —For pain in the mouth or throat:
    • Adults and teenagers—One lozenge, dissolved slowly in the mouth every two hours as needed.
    • Children up to 2 years of age—Use and dose must be determined by your health care professional.
    • Children 2 years of age and older—One children's strength (5-milligram [mg]) lozenge, dissolved slowly in the mouth every two hours as needed.
- For *aerosol spray* dosage form:
  —For pain in the mouth:
    • Adults and teenagers—One or 2 sprays, pointed at the sore places. Each spray should last about one second.
    • Children—Use and dose must be determined by your dentist.

*For benzocaine and menthol combination*
- For *lozenge* dosage form:
  —For pain in the mouth or throat:
    • Adults, teenagers, and children 2 years of age and older—One lozenge, dissolved slowly in the mouth every two hours as needed.
    • Children up to 2 years of age—Use and dose must be determined by your health care professional.

*For benzocaine and phenol combination*
- For *gel* dosage form:
  —For sores in and around the mouth, teething, toothache, sore gums, or pain caused by dental appliances:
    • Adults, teenagers, and children 2 years of age and older—Apply a small amount of medicine to the painful areas up to four times a day.

    • Children up to 2 years of age—Use and dose must be determined by your health care professional.
- For *liquid* dosage form:
  —For sores in and around the mouth, toothache, sore gums, or pain caused by dental appliances:
    • Adults, teenagers, and children 2 years of age and older—Apply a small amount of medicine to the painful areas up to four times a day.
    • Children up to 2 years of age—Use and dose must be determined by your health care professional.

*For dyclonine*
- For *lozenge* dosage form:
  —For pain in the mouth or throat:
    • Adults and teenagers—One 2-milligram (mg) or 3-mg lozenge, dissolved slowly in the mouth every two hours as needed.
    • Children up to 2 years of age—Use and dose must be determined by your health care professional.
    • Children 2 years of age and older—One children's strength (1.2-mg) lozenge, dissolved slowly in the mouth every two hours as needed.

*For lidocaine*
- For *dental liquid* dosage form (e.g., Zilactin-L):
  —For sores on the lips and around the mouth:
    • Adults and teenagers—Apply to sores every one or two hours for the first three days. Then apply as needed.
    • Children—Dose must be determined by your health care professional.
- For *dental ointment* dosage form:
  —For gum pain:
    • Adults—Apply a small amount of medicine to the sore places. Do not apply the ointment directly to dentures, braces, or other dental appliances, unless your dentist has directed you to do so.
    • Children—Use and dose must be determined by your health care professional.
- For *aerosol spray* dosage form:
  —For pain in the mouth:
    • Adults and teenagers—Two sprays, pointed at the sore places. Do not use more than twenty sprays a day.
    • Children—Use and dose must be determined by your health care professional.
- For *viscous (very thick) solution* dosage form (e.g., Xylocaine Viscous):
  —For pain in the mouth:
    • Adults and teenagers—One tablespoonful of medicine (or less), swished around in the mouth, then spit out. Or, apply a total of 1 tablespoonful (or less) to the sore places with a cotton-tipped

applicator. This medicine should not be used more often than every three hours.

- Infants and children up to 3 years of age—Apply a total of one-fourth of a teaspoonful (or less) to the sore places with a cotton-tipped applicator. This medicine should not be used more often than every three hours.
- Children 3 years of age and older—Apply a small amount of medicine to the sore places with a cotton-tipped applicator. The largest amount that can be used must be determined by your health care professional.

—For sore throat pain:

- Adults and teenagers—One tablespoonful, used as a gargle. Swallow after gargling only if directed to do so by your doctor. Otherwise, spit out the medicine after gargling with it.
- Children—Dose must be determined by your doctor.

*For tetracaine*

- For *aerosol spray* dosage form:
  —For pain in the mouth:
  - Adults and teenagers—Two sprays, pointed at the sore places.
  - Children—Dose must be determined by your health care professional.

**Missed dose**—If your health care professional has directed you to use this medicine on a regular schedule, and you miss a dose, use it as soon as possible. However, if it is almost time for your next dose, skip the missed dose and go back to your regular dosing schedule. Do not double doses.

**Storage**—To store this medicine:

- Keep out of the reach of children.
- Store away from heat and direct light.
- Do not store throat lozenge forms of benzocaine, benzocaine and menthol combination, or dyclonine in the bathroom, near the kitchen sink, or in other damp places. Heat or moisture may cause the medicine to break down.
- Keep the medicine from freezing.
- Do not puncture, break, or burn aerosol containers, even when they are empty.
- Do not keep outdated medicine or medicine no longer needed. Be sure that any discarded medicine is out of the reach of children.

## Precautions While Using This Medicine

*Check with your medical doctor:*

- If you are using this medicine for a sore throat and your sore throat is severe or lasts for more than 2 days.
- If other symptoms, such as fever, headache, skin rash, swelling, nausea, or vomiting, are also present.

You may have a condition that needs other treatment.

*Check with your health care professional:*

- If you are using this medicine for pain or sores in or around the mouth and your condition does not get better within 7 days or gets worse.
- If you notice other symptoms, such as swelling, rash, or fever.

You may have a condition that needs other treatment.

*Check with your dentist:*

- If you are using this medicine for a toothache. This medicine should not be used for a long time. It is meant to relieve toothache pain temporarily, until the problem causing the toothache can be corrected. Arrange for treatment as soon as possible.
- If you are using this medicine to relieve pain caused by new dentures or other dental appliances. An adjustment to your appliance may be needed to prevent more soreness. Also, if your dentist has ordered you to apply this medicine to the appliance before inserting it or to keep the appliance in your mouth while using the medicine, he or she will want to make sure that the medicine is not causing any unwanted effects.

False test results may occur if benzocaine, lidocaine, or tetracaine is present in your body when a certain laboratory test is done. This test uses a medicine called bentiromide (e.g., Chymex) to show how well your pancreas is working. You should not use any products containing benzocaine, lidocaine, or tetracaine for about 72 hours (3 days) before this test is done.

If you are using this medicine in the back of the mouth, or in the throat, *do not eat or drink anything for one hour after using it*. When this medicine is applied to these areas, it may interfere with swallowing and cause choking.

*Do not chew gum or food while your mouth or throat feels numb after you use this medicine.* To do so may cause an injury. You may accidentally bite your tongue or the inside of your cheeks.

## Side Effects of This Medicine

Along with its needed effects, a medicine may cause some unwanted effects. Although not all of these side effects may occur, if they do occur they may need medical attention.

*Stop using this medicine and check with your medical doctor or dentist immediately* if any of the following side effects occur:

*Less common*

Large swellings that look like hives on skin or in mouth or throat

*Signs and symptoms of too much medicine being absorbed by the body*

Blurred or double vision; confusion; convulsions (seizures); dizziness or lightheadedness; drowsiness; feeling hot, cold, or numb; headache; increased sweating; ringing or buzzing in the ears; shivering or trembling;

slow or irregular heartbeat; troubled breathing; unusual anxiety, excitement, nervousness, or restlessness; unusual paleness; unusual tiredness or weakness

Also, check with your health care professional as soon as possible if any of the following side effects occur:

*Less common*
> Burning, stinging, swelling, or tenderness not present before treatment; skin rash, redness, itching, or hives in or around the mouth

Other side effects not listed above may also occur in some patients. If you notice any other effects, check with your medical doctor or dentist.

Revised: 09/01/94

# ANESTHETICS   Ophthalmic

Some commonly used brand names are:
**In the U.S.—**
| | |
|---|---|
| Ak-Taine[1] | Ophthaine[1] |
| Ak-T-Caine[2] | Ophthetic[1] |
| Alcaine[1] | Pontocaine[2] |
| Ocu-Caine[1] | Spectro-Caine[1] |

**In Canada—**
| | |
|---|---|
| Alcaine[1] | Ophthetic[1] |
| Diocaine[1] | Pontocaine[2] |
| Minims Tetracaine[2] | |

Other commonly used names are:
Amethocaine[2]
Proxymetacaine[1]

Note: For quick reference, the following anesthetics are numbered to match the corresponding brand names.

This information applies to the following medicines:
1. Proparacaine (proe-PARE-a-kane)‡
2. Tetracaine (TET-ra-kane)‡§

‡Generic name product may also be available in the U.S.
§Generic name product may also be available in Canada.

## Description

Proparacaine and tetracaine are local anesthetics that are used in the eye to cause numbness or loss of feeling. They are used before certain procedures such as measuring of eye pressure, removing foreign objects or sutures (stitches) from the eye, and performing certain eye examinations.

These medicines are to be administered only by or under the immediate supervision of your doctor. They are available in the following dosage forms:

*Ophthalmic*
Proparacaine
• Ophthalmic solution (U.S. and Canada)
Tetracaine
• Ophthalmic ointment (U.S.)
• Ophthalmic solution (U.S. and Canada)

## Before Receiving This Medicine

In deciding to use a medicine, the risks of using the medicine must be weighed against the good it will do. This is a decision you and your doctor will make. For local anesthetics used in the eye, the following should be considered:

**Allergies**—Tell your doctor if you have ever had any unusual or allergic reaction after use of a local anesthetic in the eye. Such a reaction may include severe itching,

pain, redness, or swelling of the eye or eyelid, or severe and continuing watering of the eyes.

Also, tell your doctor if you have ever had any unusual or allergic reaction to tetracaine or other local anesthetics, such as benzocaine, butacaine, butamben, chloroprocaine, procaine, or propoxycaine, when given by injection or applied to the skin.

In addition, tell your doctor if you have ever had an allergic reaction to aminobenzoic acid (also called para-aminobenzoic acid [PABA]), or if you are allergic to any other substances, such as foods, preservatives, or dyes.

**Pregnancy**—Although studies on effects in pregnancy have not been done in either humans or animals, proparacaine and tetracaine have not been reported to cause birth defects or other problems in humans.

**Breast-feeding**—It is not known whether proparacaine or tetracaine passes into breast milk. Although most medicines pass into breast milk in small amounts, many of them may be used safely while breast-feeding. Mothers who receive this medicine and who wish to breast-feed should discuss this with their doctor.

**Children**—Although there is no specific information comparing use of ophthalmic anesthetics in children with use in other age groups, these medicines are not expected to cause different side effects or problems in children than they do in adults.

**Older adults**—Many medicines have not been studied specifically in older people. Therefore, it may not be known whether they work exactly the same way they do in younger adults. Although there is no specific information comparing use of ophthalmic anesthetics in the elderly with use in other age groups, these medicines are not expected to cause different side effects or problems in older people than they do in younger adults.

**Other medicines**—Although certain medicines should not be used together at all, in other cases two different medicines may be used together even if an interaction might occur. In these cases, your doctor may want to change the dose, or other precautions may be necessary. Before receiving a local anesthetic in the eye, tell your doctor if you are taking any other prescription or nonprescription (over-the-counter [OTC]) medicine.

**Other medical problems**—The presence of other medical problems may affect the use of local anesthetics in the eye. Make sure you tell your doctor if you have any other medical problems, especially:

- Allergies—The risk of unwanted effects may be increased

## Proper Use of This Medicine

**Dosing**—The dose of proparacaine or tetracaine will be different for different people. It will depend on the reason the anesthetic is being used. Your health care professional will apply the medicine.

*For proparacaine or tetracaine*
- For *ophthalmic drops* dosage form (eye drops):
  —For causing loss of feeling in the eye:
  - Adults and teenagers—For most procedures, one or two drops will be all that is needed. However, for some other procedures, several applications of the medicine may be needed, usually five or ten minutes apart.
  - Children—Use and dose must be determined by the doctor.

*For tetracaine*
- For *ophthalmic ointment* dosage form (eye ointment):
  —For causing loss of feeling in the eye:
  - Adults and teenagers—Your health care professional will apply a small amount of the ointment to the lower eyelid.
  - Children—Use and dose must be determined by the doctor.

## Precautions After Receiving This Medicine

After a local anesthetic is applied to the eye, *do not rub or wipe the eye until the anesthetic has worn off and feeling in the eye returns*. To do so may cause injury or damage to the eye. The effects of these medicines usually last for about 20 minutes. However, if more than one dose is applied, the effects may last longer.

If you get one of these medicines on your fingers, it may cause a rash with dryness and cracking of the skin. If you touch your eye after this medicine has been applied, wash your hands as soon as possible.

## Side Effects of This Medicine

Along with its needed effects, a medicine may cause some unwanted effects. Although not all of these side effects may occur, if they do occur they may need medical attention.

*Tell your doctor immediately* if any of the following side effects occur shortly after this medicine has been applied:
*Symptoms of too much medicine being absorbed into the body—very rare*
    Dizziness or drowsiness; increased sweating; irregular heartbeat; muscle twitching or trembling; nausea or vomiting; shortness of breath or troubled breathing; unusual excitement, nervousness, or restlessness; unusual tiredness or weakness

Other side effects may occur that usually do not need medical attention. Mild stinging or eye irritation may occur as soon as tetracaine is applied or up to several hours after proparacaine is applied. Although these side effects usually are not serious, *check with your doctor as soon as possible if any of the following side effects are severe,* because you may be having an allergic reaction to the medicine. Also, check with your doctor if any of these effects continue or are bothersome:
*Less common*
    Burning, stinging, redness, or other irritation of eye
*Rare*
    Itching, pain, redness, or swelling of the eye or eyelid; watering of eyes

Other side effects not listed above may also occur in some patients. If you notice any other effects, check with your doctor.

Revised: 08/25/94

# ANESTHETICS    Parenteral-Local

Some commonly used brand names are:
**In the U.S.—**
| | |
|---|---|
| Carbocaine[5] | Lidoject-2[4] |
| Carbocaine with Neo-Cobefrin[5] | Marcaine[1] |
| | Marcaine Spinal[1] |
| Citanest Forte[6] | Nervocaine[4] |
| Citanest Plain[6] | Nesacaine[2] |
| Dalcaine[4] | Nesacaine-MPF[2] |
| Dilocaine[4] | Novocain[7] |
| Duranest[4] | Octocaine[4] |
| Duranest-MPF[3] | Polocaine[5] |
| Isocaine[5] | Polocaine-MPF[5] |
| L-Caine[4] | Pontocaine[9] |
| Lidoject-1[4] | Ravocaine and Novocain with Levophed[8] |

| | |
|---|---|
| Ravocaine and Novocain with Neo-Cobefrin[8] | Sensorcaine-MPF Spinal[1] |
| Sensorcaine[1] | Xylocaine[4] |
| Sensorcaine-MPF[1] | Xylocaine-MPF[4] |
| | Xylocaine-MPF with Glucose[4] |
| **In Canada—** | |
| Carbocaine[5] | Octocaine-50[4] |
| Citanest Forte[6] | Octocaine-100[4] |
| Citanest Plain[6] | Polocaine[5] |
| Isocaine 2%[5] | Pontocaine[9] |
| Isocaine 3%[5] | Xylocaine[4] |
| Marcaine[1] | Xylocaine with Glucose[4] |
| Nesacaine-CE[2] | Xylocaine Test Dose[4] |
| Novocain[7] | |

Another commonly used name for lidocaine is lignocaine.

Note: For quick reference, the following anesthetics are numbered to match the corresponding brand names.

This information applies to the following medicines:

1. Bupivacaine (byoo-PIV-a-kane)‡
2. Chloroprocaine (klor-oh-PROE-kane)‡
3. Etidocaine (e-TI-doe-kane)
4. Lidocaine (LYE-doe-kane)‡§
5. Mepivacaine (me-PIV-a-kane)‡
6. Prilocaine (PRIL-oh-kane)§
7. Procaine (PROE-kane)‡
8. Propoxycaine and Procaine (proe-POX-i-kane)
9. Tetracaine (TET-ra-kane)

‡Generic name product may also be available in the U.S.
§Generic name product may also be available in Canada.

## Description

Parenteral-local anesthetics (an-ess-THET-iks) are given by injection to cause loss of feeling before and during surgery, dental procedures (including dental surgery), or labor and delivery. These medicines do not cause loss of consciousness.

These medicines are given only by or under the immediate supervision of a medical doctor or dentist, or by a specially trained nurse, in the doctor's office or in a hospital.

These medicines are available in the following dosage forms:

*Parenteral*

Bupivacaine
• Injection (U.S. and Canada)
Chloroprocaine
• Injection (U.S. and Canada)
Etidocaine
• Injection (U.S.)
Lidocaine
• Injection (U.S. and Canada)
Mepivacaine
• Injection (U.S. and Canada)
Prilocaine
• Injection (U.S. and Canada)
Procaine
• Injection (U.S. and Canada)
Propoxycaine and Procaine
• Injection (U.S.)
Tetracaine
• Injection (U.S. and Canada)

## Before Receiving This Medicine

In deciding to use a medicine, the risks of using the medicine must be weighed against the good it will do. This is a decision you and your medical doctor, dentist, or nurse will make. For local anesthetics, the following should be considered:

**Allergies**—Tell your medical doctor, dentist, or nurse if you have ever had any unusual or allergic reaction to a local anesthetic or to epinephrine (e.g., Adrenalin). Also tell your medical doctor, dentist, nurse, or pharmacist if you are allergic to any other substances, such as sulfites or other preservatives, especially aminobenzoic acid (also called para-aminobenzoic acid [PABA]).

**Pregnancy**—Local anesthetics have not been reported to cause birth defects in humans.

Use of a local anesthetic during labor and delivery may rarely cause unwanted effects. These medicines may increase the length of labor by making it more difficult for the mother to bear down (push). They may also cause unwanted effects in the fetus or newborn baby, especially if certain medical problems are present at the time of delivery. Before receiving a local anesthetic for labor and delivery, you should discuss with your doctor the good that this medicine will do as well as the risks of receiving it.

**Breast-feeding**—It is not known whether local anesthetics pass into the breast milk. However, these medicines have not been reported to cause problems in nursing babies.

**Children**—Children may be especially sensitive to the effects of parenteral-local anesthetics. This may increase the chance of side effects.

**Older adults**—Elderly people are especially sensitive to the effects of parenteral-local anesthetics. This may increase the chance of side effects.

**Other medicines**—Although certain medicines should not be used together at all, in other cases two different medicines may be used together even if an interaction might occur. In these cases, your medical doctor, dentist, or nurse may want to change the dose, or other precautions may be necessary. It is very important that you tell the person in charge if you are taking:

• Any other medicine, prescription or nonprescription (over-the-counter [OTC]), or
• "Street" drugs, such as amphetamines ("uppers"), barbiturates ("downers"), cocaine (including "crack"), marijuana, phencyclidine (PCP, "angel dust"), and heroin or other narcotics—Serious side effects may occur if anyone gives you a local anesthetic without knowing that you have taken another medicine

**Other medical problems**—The presence of other medical problems may affect the use of local anesthetics. Make sure you tell your medical doctor, dentist, or nurse if you have *any* other medical problems, especially:

• Malignant hyperthermia (very high fever, fast and irregular heartbeat, muscle spasms or tightness, and breathing problems occurring during, or soon after, use of an anesthetic) (history of, in yourself or in any close relative)—The chance of an attack of malignant hyperthermia is increased. Some anesthetics are more likely than others to cause this unwanted effect. Your medical doctor, dentist, or nurse will want to avoid using them

## Proper Use of This Medicine

**Dosing**—The dose of a local anesthetic will be different for different patients. Your health care professional will decide on the right amount for you, depending on:

• Your age;
• Your general physical condition;
• The reason the local anesthetic is being given; and

- Other medicines you are taking or will receive before or after the local anesthetic is given.

## Precautions After Receiving This Medicine

For patients going home before the numbness or loss of feeling caused by a local anesthetic wears off:

- During the time that the injected area feels numb, serious injury can occur without your knowing about it. Be especially careful to avoid injury until the anesthetic wears off or feeling returns to the area.
- If you have received a local anesthetic injection in your mouth, do not chew gum or food while your mouth feels numb. You may injure yourself by biting your tongue or the inside of your cheeks.

## Side Effects of This Medicine

Along with its needed effects, a medicine may cause some unwanted effects. Although not all of these side effects may occur, if they do occur they may need medical attention. While you are in the hospital or your medical doctor's or dentist's office, your medical doctor, dentist, or nurse will carefully follow the effects of any medicine you have received. However, some effects may not be noticed until later.

*Check with your doctor immediately* if any of the following side effects occur:
> *Less common or rare*
>> Skin rash, hives, or itching

Also, check with your dentist if you have received a local anesthetic for dental work, and the feeling of numbness or tingling in your lips and mouth does not go away within a few hours, or if you have difficulty in opening your mouth.

Other side effects not listed above may also occur in some patients. If you notice any other effects, check with your medical doctor or dentist.

Revised: 01/30/92
Interim revision: 08/14/94

# ANESTHETICS  Rectal

Some commonly used brand names are:

**In the U.S.—**
Americaine Hemorrhoidal[1]  Pontocaine Ointment[5]
Nupercainal[2]  ProctoFoam/non-steroid[3]
Fleet Relief[3]  Tronolane[3]
Pontocaine Cream[4]†  Tronothane[3]

**In Canada—**
Nupercainal[2]
Tronothane[3]

Other commonly used names are:
amethocaine[4]  ethyl aminobenzoate[1]
cinchocaine[2]  pramocaine[3]

Note: For quick reference, the following anesthetics are numbered to match the corresponding brand names.
This information applies to the following medicines:

1. Benzocaine (BEN-zoe-kane)
2. Dibucaine (DYE-byoo-kane)‡
3. Pramoxine (pra-MOX-een)
4. Tetracaine (TET-ra-kane)
5. Tetracaine and Menthol (MEN-thol)

†Not commercially available in Canada.
‡Generic name product may also be available in the U.S.

## Description

Rectal anesthetics (an-ess-THET-iks) are used to relieve the pain and itching of hemorrhoids (piles) and other problems in the rectal area. However, if you have hemorrhoids that bleed, especially after a bowel movement, check with your doctor before using this medicine. Bleeding may mean that you have a condition that needs other treatment.

These medicines are available without a prescription; however, your doctor may have special instructions on the proper use and dose for your medical problem.

These medicines are available in the following dosage forms:
> *Rectal*
>> Benzocaine
>> - Ointment (U.S.)
>> Dibucaine
>> - Ointment (U.S. and Canada)
>> Pramoxine
>> - Aerosol foam (U.S.)
>> - Cream (U.S. and Canada)
>> - Ointment (U.S.)
>> Tetracaine
>> - Cream (U.S.)
>> Tetracaine and Menthol
>> - Ointment (U.S.)

## Before Using This Medicine

If you are using this medicine without a prescription, carefully read and follow any precautions on the label. For rectal anesthetics, the following should be considered:

**Allergies**—Tell your doctor if you have ever had any unusual or allergic reaction to a local anesthetic, especially one that was applied to any part of the body as a liquid, cream, ointment, or spray. Also tell your health care professional if you are allergic to any other substances, such as foods, preservatives, or dyes.

**Pregnancy**—Rectal anesthetics have not been reported to cause birth defects or other problems in humans.

**Breast-feeding**—Rectal anesthetics have not been reported to cause problems in nursing babies.

**Children**—Children may be especially sensitive to the effects of local anesthetics. This may increase the chance of side effects during treatment.

**Older adults**—Elderly people are especially sensitive to the effects of local anesthetics. This may increase the chance of side effects during treatment.

**Other medicines**—Although certain medicines should not be used together at all, in other cases two different medicines may be used together even if an interaction might occur. In these cases, your doctor may want to change the dose, or other precautions may be necessary. Before you use a rectal anesthetic, check with your health care professional if you are taking any other prescription or nonprescription (over-the-counter [OTC]) medicine.

**Other medical problems**—The presence of other medical problems may affect the use of rectal anesthetics. Make sure you tell your doctor if you have any other medical problems, especially:

- Infection at or near place of treatment or
- Large sores, broken skin, or severe injury at or near place of treatment—The chance of unwanted effects may be increased

---

## Proper Use of This Medicine

For safe and effective use of this medicine:

- Rectal anesthetics usually come with patient directions. Read them carefully before using the medicine, even if it was prescribed by your doctor. Check with your pharmacist if you have any questions about how to use the product.
- Follow your doctor's instructions if this medicine was prescribed.
- Follow the manufacturer's package directions if you are treating yourself.
- *Do not use more of this medicine, do not use it more often, and do not use it for a longer time than directed.* To do so may increase the chance of absorption into the body and the chance of unwanted effects.

This medicine should be used only for conditions being treated by your doctor or for problems listed on the package label. *Do not use it for other problems without first checking with your doctor.* This medicine should not be used if certain kinds of infections are present.

For *applying a rectal anesthetic to the area around the rectum:*

- First, clean the area, using mild soap and water or a cleansing wipe. Rinse the area carefully and dry it gently with a soft towel or toilet paper.
- Apply a small amount of medicine to the sore area, using a piece of gauze, a tissue, or a "finger cot."

For *inserting a rectal cream or ointment inside the rectum:*

- Use only products that come packaged in pre-filled applicators or that come packaged with a special inserter called a rectal tube.
- If you are using a product that has an inserter (rectal tube) packaged separately from the tube of cream or ointment:
  —Remove the cap from the tube of cream or ointment. Attach the inserter to the top of the tube. Squeeze the tube until a little cream or ointment comes out on the inserter. Then spread the cream or ointment over the inserter.
  —Place the inserter into your rectum and squeeze the tube until a small amount of medicine comes out. Then remove the inserter from your body.
  —Remove the inserter from the tube and replace the cap. Then wash the applicator carefully.
- If you are using the product that comes in pre-filled applicators:
  —Follow the manufacturer's directions for using the applicator and inserting the medicine. Each applicator is meant to be used only once. Throw the applicator away after using it.

For *inserting the rectal aerosol foam (e.g., Proctofoam/nonsteroid) into the rectum:*

- Do not insert the container itself into your rectum. Use the applicator provided.
- To fill the container—First, shake the container hard for several seconds. Then, holding the container upright, insert it into the applicator. Press the cap of the container until the foam reaches the fill line of the applicator. Remove the applicator from the container.
- To use the medicine—Place a small amount of foam on the tip of the applicator. Insert the applicator into your rectum, then push the plunger as far as possible. Remove the applicator. Then take it apart and wash it carefully.

**Dosing**—The dose of rectal anesthetics will be different for different patients. *Follow your doctor's orders or the directions on the label.* The following information includes only the average doses of these medicines. *If your dose is different, do not change it* unless your doctor tells you to do so.

*For benzocaine*

- For pain and itching of hemorrhoids or other problems in the rectal area:
  —For *rectal ointment* dosage form:
    - Adults—Apply a small amount of ointment to the area around the rectum up to six times a day.
    - Children—Use and dose must be determined by the doctor.

*For dibucaine*

- For pain and itching of hemorrhoids or other problems in the rectal area:
  —For *rectal ointment* dosage form:
    - Adults—Insert a small amount of ointment into the rectum three or four times a day, in the morning, in the evening, and after bowel movements.

Or, apply a small amount of ointment to the area around the rectum three or four times a day.
- Children—Use and dose must be determined by the doctor.

*For pramoxine*
- For pain and itching of hemorrhoids or other problems in the rectal area:
  —For *rectal cream* dosage form:
  - Adults—Apply a small amount to the area around the rectum up to five times a day, in the morning, in the evening, and after bowel movements.
  - Children—Use and dose must be determined by the doctor.
  —For *rectal ointment* dosage form:
  - Adults—Insert a small amount of ointment into the rectum up to five times a day, in the morning, in the evening, and after bowel movements. Or, apply a small amount to the area around the rectum up to five times a day, in the morning, in the evening, and after bowel movements.
  —For the *rectal aerosol foam* dosage form:
  - Adults—Insert 1 applicatorful into the rectum two or three times a day. Or, apply a small amount to the area around the rectum two or three times a day.
  - Children—Use and dose must be determined by the doctor.

*For tetracaine and for tetracaine and menthol*
- For pain and itching of hemorrhoids or other problems in the rectal area:
  —For the *rectal cream* or *rectal ointment* dosage form:
  - Adults—Insert a small amount into the rectum up to six times a day. Or, apply a small amount to the area around the rectum up to six times a day.
  - Children—Use and dose must be determined by the doctor.

**Missed dose**—If your doctor has directed you to use this medicine on a regular schedule and you miss a dose, use it as soon as possible. However, if it is almost time for your next dose, skip the missed dose and go back to your regular dosing schedule.

**Storage**—To store this medicine:
- Keep out of the reach of children.
- Store away from heat and direct light.
- Keep the medicine from freezing.

- Do not puncture, break, or burn the pramoxine aerosol foam container, even after it is empty.
- Do not keep outdated medicine or medicine no longer needed. Be sure that any discarded medicine is out of the reach of children.

## Precautions While Using This Medicine

Check with your doctor:
- If your condition does not improve after you have been using this medicine regularly for 7 days, or if it becomes worse.
- If any bleeding from the rectum occurs.
- If you notice any rash, redness, or irritation that was not present before you started using this medicine.

False test results may occur if benzocaine or tetracaine is present in your body when a certain laboratory test is done. This test uses a medicine called bentiromide (e.g., Chymex) to show how well your pancreas is working. You should not use any products containing benzocaine or tetracaine for about 72 hours (3 days) before this test is done.

## Side Effects of This Medicine

Along with its needed effects, a medicine may cause some unwanted effects. Although not all of these side effects may occur, if they do occur they may need medical attention.

*Stop using this medicine and check with your doctor immediately* if any of the following side effects occur:
  *Signs and symptoms of too much medicine being absorbed by the body*
    Blurred or double vision; confusion; convulsions (seizures); dizziness or lightheadedness; drowsiness; feeling hot, cold, or numb; increased sweating; ringing or buzzing in ears; shivering or trembling; slow or irregular heartbeat; unusual anxiety, excitement, nervousness, or restlessness; unusual paleness

Also, check with your doctor as soon as possible if any of the following side effects occur:
  *Less common*
    Burning, stinging, swelling, or tenderness not present before treatment; skin rash, redness, itching, or hives at or near place of application

Other side effects not listed above may also occur in some patients. If you notice any other effects, check with your doctor.

Revised: 09/01/94

# ANESTHETICS   Topical

Some commonly used brand names are:

**In the U.S—**

| | |
|---|---|
| Almay Anti-itch Lotion[7] | Nupercainal Cream[4] |
| Americaine Topical Anesthetic First Aid Ointment[1] | Nupercainal Ointment[4] |
| | Pontocaine Cream[8] |
| Americaine Topical Anesthetic Spray[1] | Pontocaine Ointment[9] |
| | Pramegel[7] |
| Butesin Picrate[3] | Prax[6] |
| DermaFlex[5] | Tronothane[6] |
| Dermoplast[2] | Xylocaine[5] |
| Lagol[1] | |

**In Canada—**

| | |
|---|---|
| After Burn Double Strength Gel[5] | Endocaine[1] |
| | Norwood Sunburn Spray[5] |
| After Burn Double Strength Spray[5] | Nupercainal Ointment[4] |
| | Pramegel[7] |
| After Burn Gel[5] | Shield Burnasept Spray[1] |
| After Burn Spray[5] | Tronothane[6] |
| Alphacaine[5] | Xylocaine[5] |
| Dermoplast[2] | |

Other commonly used names are:

| | |
|---|---|
| Amethocaine[8] | Ethyl aminobenzoate[1] |
| Butyl aminobenzoate[2] | Lignocaine[5] |
| Cinchocaine[4] | Pramocaine[6] |

Note: For quick reference, the following anesthetics are numbered to match the corresponding brand names.

This information applies to the following medicines:

1. Benzocaine (BEN-zoe-kane)‡
2. Benzocaine and Menthol (MEN-thol)
3. Butamben (byoo-TAM-ben)
4. Dibucaine (DYE-byoo-kane)‡
5. Lidocaine (LYE-doe-kane)‡
6. Pramoxine (pra-MOX-een)
7. Pramoxine and Menthol
8. Tetracaine (TET-ra-kane)
9. Tetracaine and Menthol

‡Generic name product may also be available in the U.S.

# Description

This medicine belongs to a group of medicines known as topical local anesthetics (an-ess-THET-iks). Topical anesthetics are used to relieve pain and itching caused by conditions such as sunburn or other minor burns, insect bites or stings, poison ivy, poison oak, poison sumac, and minor cuts and scratches.

Topical anesthetics deaden the nerve endings in the skin. They do not cause unconsciousness as do general anesthetics used for surgery.

Most topical anesthetics are available without a prescription; however, your doctor may have special instructions on the proper use and dose for your medical problem.

These medicines are available in the following dosage forms:

*Topical*

Benzocaine
- Cream (U.S.)
- Ointment (U.S.)
- Topical aerosol (U.S.)
- Topical spray solution (Canada)

Benzocaine and Menthol
- Lotion (U.S.)
- Topical aerosol solution (U.S. and Canada)

Butamben
- Ointment (U.S.)

Dibucaine
- Cream (U.S.)
- Ointment (U.S. and Canada)

Lidocaine
- Film-forming gel (U.S.)
- Jelly (Canada)
- Ointment (U.S. and Canada)
- Topical aerosol (Canada)
- Topical spray solution (Canada)

Pramoxine
- Cream (U.S. and Canada)
- Lotion (U.S.)

Pramoxine and Menthol
- Gel (U.S. and Canada)
- Lotion (U.S.)

Tetracaine
- Cream (U.S.)

Tetracaine and Menthol
- Ointment (U.S.)

# Before Using This Medicine

If you are using this medicine without a prescription, carefully read and follow any precautions on the label. For topical anesthetics, the following should be considered:

**Allergies**—Tell your doctor if you have ever had any unusual or allergic reaction to a local anesthetic, especially when applied to the skin or other areas of the body. Also tell your health care professional if you are allergic to any other substances, such as foods, preservatives, or dyes, especially aminobenzoic acid (also called para-amino-benzoic acid [PABA]), to parabens (preservatives in many foods and medicines), or to paraphenylenediamine (a hair dye).

**Pregnancy**—Although studies on effects in pregnancy have not been done in humans, topical anesthetics have not been reported to cause problems in humans. Lidocaine has not been shown to cause birth defects or other problems in animal studies. Other topical anesthetics have not been studied in animals.

**Breast-feeding**—Topical anesthetics have not been reported to cause problems in nursing babies.

**Children**—Benzocaine may be absorbed through the skin of young children and cause unwanted effects. There is no specific information comparing use of other topical anesthetics in children with use in other age groups, but it is possible that they may also cause unwanted effects in young children. Check with your doctor before using any product that contains a topical anesthetic for a child younger than 2 years of age.

**Older adults**—Many medicines have not been studied specifically in older people. Therefore, it may not be known

whether they work exactly the same way they do in younger adults or if they cause different side effects or problems in older people. There is no specific information comparing use of topical anesthetics in the elderly with use in other age groups.

**Other medicines**—Although certain medicines should not be used together at all, in other cases two different medicines may be used together even if an interaction might occur. In these cases, your doctor may want to change the dose, or other precautions may be necessary. Tell your health care professional if you are taking any other prescription or nonprescription (over-the-counter [OTC]) medicine.

**Other medical problems**—The presence of other medical problems may affect the use of topical anesthetics. Before using a topical anesthetic, check with your health care professional if you have any other medical problems, especially:

- Infection at or near the place of application or
- Large sores, broken skin, or severe injury at the area of application—The chance of side effects may be increased

## Proper Use of This Medicine

For safe and effective use of this medicine:

- Follow your doctor's instructions if this medicine was prescribed.
- Follow the manufacturer's package directions if you are treating yourself.
- Unless otherwise directed by your doctor, *do not use this medicine on large areas, especially if the skin is broken or scraped. Also, do not use it more often than directed on the package label, or for more than a few days at a time.* To do so may increase the chance of absorption through the skin and the chance of unwanted effects. This is especially important when benzocaine is used for children younger than 2 years of age.

This medicine should be used only for problems being treated by your doctor or conditions listed in the package directions. *Check with your doctor before using it for other problems, especially if you think that an infection may be present.* This medicine should not be used to treat certain kinds of skin infections or serious problems, such as severe burns.

Read the package label very carefully to see if the product contains any alcohol. Alcohol is flammable and can catch on fire. *Do not use any product containing alcohol near a fire or open flame, or while smoking. Also, do not smoke after applying one of these products until it has completely dried.*

If you are using this medicine on your face, *be very careful not to get it in your eyes, mouth, or nose.* If you are using an aerosol or spray form of this medicine, do not spray it directly on your face. Instead, use your hand or an applicator (for example, a sterile gauze pad or a cotton swab) to apply the medicine.

For patients using *butamben:*

- Butamben may stain clothing and discolor hair. It may not be possible to remove the stains. To avoid this, do not touch your clothing or your hair while applying the medicine. Also, cover the treated area with a loose bandage after applying butamben, to protect your clothes.

To use *lidocaine film-forming gel* (e.g., DermaFlex):

- First dry the area with a clean cloth or a piece of gauze. Then apply the medicine. The medicine should dry, forming a clear film, after about 1 minute.

**Dosing**—The dose of a topical anesthetic will be different for different patients. *Follow your doctor's orders or the directions on the label.* The following information includes only the average doses of these medicines. *If your dose is different, do not change it* unless your doctor tells you to do so.

*For benzocaine and for benzocaine and menthol combination*

- For *topical* dosage forms (aerosol solution, cream, lotion, ointment, and spray solution):
  —For pain and itching caused by minor skin conditions:
    - Adults and children 2 years of age and older—Apply to the affected area three or four times a day as needed.
    - Children younger than 2 years of age—Dose must be determined by your doctor.

*For butamben*

- For *topical* dosage form (ointment):
  —For pain and itching caused by minor skin conditions:
    - Adults—Apply to the affected area three or four times a day as needed.
    - Children—Dose must be determined by your doctor.

*For dibucaine*

- For *topical cream* dosage form:
  —For pain and itching caused by minor skin conditions:
    - Adults and children 2 years of age and older—Apply to the affected area three or four times a day as needed.
    - Children up to 2 years of age—Dose must be determined by your doctor.
- For *topical ointment* dosage form:
  —For pain and itching caused by minor skin conditions:
    - Adults—Apply to the affected area three or four times a day as needed. The largest amount that may be used in a twenty-four-hour period is 30 grams, but much smaller amounts are usually enough.
    - Children 2 years of age and older—Apply to the affected area three or four times a day as

needed. Do not use more than 7.5 grams in a twenty-four-hour period.

- Children up to 2 years of age—Dose must be determined by your doctor.

*For lidocaine*

- For *topical* dosage forms (aerosol solution, film-forming gel, jelly, ointment, and spray solution):

  —For pain and itching caused by minor skin conditions:

  - Adults—Apply to the affected area three or four times a day as needed.
  - Children—Dose must be determined by your doctor.

*For pramoxine and for pramoxine and menthol combination*

- For *topical* dosage forms (cream, gel, and lotion):

  —For pain and itching caused by minor skin conditions:

  - Adults and children 2 years of age and older—Apply to the affected area three or four times a day as needed.
  - Children younger than 2 years of age—Dose must be determined by your doctor.

*For tetracaine and for tetracaine and menthol combination*

- For *topical* dosage forms (cream and ointment):

  —For pain and itching caused by minor skin conditions:

  - Adults and teenagers—Apply to the affected area three or four times a day as needed. The largest amount that may be used in a twenty-four-hour period is 30 grams (a whole tube of the medicine), but much smaller amounts are usually enough.
  - Children 2 years of age and older—Apply to the affected area three or four times a day as needed. Do not use more than 7 grams (about one-fourth of a tube of the medicine) in a twenty-four-hour period.
  - Children younger than 2 years of age—Dose must be determined by your doctor.

**Missed dose**—If your doctor has ordered you to use this medicine according to a regular schedule and you miss a dose, use it as soon as possible. However, if it is almost time for your next dose, skip the missed dose and use your next dose at the regularly scheduled time.

**Storage**—To store this medicine:

- Keep out of the reach of children.
- Store away from heat and direct light.
- Keep the medicine from freezing.

- Do not puncture, break, or burn aerosol containers, even when they are empty.
- Do not keep outdated medicine or medicine no longer needed. Be sure that any discarded medicine is out of the reach of children.

## Precautions While Using This Medicine

After applying this medicine to the skin of a child, *watch the child carefully to make sure that he or she does not get any of the medicine into his or her mouth.* Topical anesthetics can cause serious side effects, especially in children, if any of the medicine gets into the mouth or is swallowed.

*Stop using this medicine and check with your doctor:*

- *If your condition does not improve within 7 days, or if it gets worse.*
- *If the area you are treating becomes infected.*
- *If you notice a skin rash, burning, stinging, swelling, or any other sign of irritation that was not present when you began using this medicine.*
- *If you swallow any of the medicine.*

## Side Effects of This Medicine

Along with its needed effects, a medicine may cause some unwanted effects. Although not all of these side effects may occur, if they do occur they may need medical attention.

*Check with your doctor immediately* if any of the following side effects occur:

*Less common*

Large swellings that look like hives on the skin or in the mouth or throat

*Symptoms of too much medicine being absorbed by the body—very rare*

Blurred or double vision; confusion; convulsions (seizures); dizziness or lightheadedness; drowsiness; feeling hot, cold, or numb; headache; increased sweating; ringing or buzzing in the ears; shivering or trembling; slow or irregular heartbeat; troubled breathing; unusual anxiety, excitement, nervousness, or restlessness; unusual paleness; unusual tiredness or weakness

Also, check with your doctor as soon as possible if any of the following side effects occur:

Burning, stinging, or tenderness not present before treatment; skin rash, redness, itching, or hives

Other side effects not listed above may also occur in some patients. If you notice any other effects, check with your doctor.

Revised: 08/29/94

# ANESTHETICS, GENERAL  Systemic

Some commonly used brand names are:

**In the U.S.—**

| Amidate[2] | Forane[4] |
|---|---|
| Brevital[6] | Ketalar[5] |
| Diprivan[9] | Penthrane[7] |
| Ethrane[1] | Pentothal[10] |
| Fluothane[3] | |

**In Canada—**

| Brietal[6] | Forane[4] |
|---|---|
| Diprivan[9] | Ketalar[5] |
| Ethrane[1] | Pentothal[10] |
| Fluothane[3] | Somnothane[3] |

Other commonly used names are:
Methohexitone[6]
Thiopentone[10]

Note: For quick reference, the following general anesthetics are numbered to match the corresponding brand names.

This information applies to the following medicines:

1. Enflurane (EN-floo-rane)‡
2. Etomidate (e-TOM-i-date)†
3. Halothane (HA-loe-thane)‡
4. Isoflurane (eye-soe-FLURE-ane)
5. Ketamine (KEET-a-meen)
6. Methohexital (meth-oh-HEX-i-tal)
7. Methoxyflurane (meth-ox-ee-FLOO-rane)
8. Nitrous (NYE-trus) Oxide‡§
9. Propofol (PROE-po-fole)
10. Thiopental (thye-oh-PEN-tal)‡

---

†Not commercially available in Canada.
‡Generic name product may also be available in the U.S.
§Generic name product may also be available in Canada.

---

## Description

General anesthetics (an-ess-THET-iks) are normally used to produce loss of consciousness before and during surgery. However, for obstetrics (labor and delivery) or certain minor procedures, an anesthetic may be given in small amounts to relieve anxiety or pain without causing unconsciousness. Also, some of the anesthetics may be used for certain procedures in a medical doctor's or dentist's office.

Thiopental is also sometimes used to control convulsions (seizures) caused by certain medicines or seizure disorders. Thiopental may be used to reduce pressure on the brain in certain conditions. Thiopental may also be used for other conditions as determined by your doctor.

General anesthetics are usually given by inhalation or by injection into a vein. However, certain anesthetics may be given rectally to help produce sleep before surgery or certain procedures. Although most general anesthetics can be used by themselves in producing loss of consciousness, some are often used together. This allows for more effective anesthesia in certain patients.

*General anesthetics are given only by or under the immediate supervision of a medical doctor or dentist trained to use them.* If you will be receiving a general anesthetic during surgery, your doctor or anesthesiologist will give you the medicine and closely follow your progress.

General anesthetics are available in the following dosage forms:

*Inhalation*

Enflurane
 • Inhalation (U.S. and Canada)
Halothane
 • Inhalation (U.S. and Canada)
Isoflurane
 • Inhalation (U.S. and Canada)
Methoxyflurane
 • Inhalation (U.S.)
Nitrous oxide
 • Inhalation (U.S. and Canada)

*Parenteral*

Etomidate
 • Injection (U.S.)
Ketamine
 • Injection (U.S. and Canada)
Methohexital
 • Injection (U.S. and Canada)
Propofol
 • Injection (U.S. and Canada)
Thiopental
 • Injection (U.S. and Canada)

*Rectal*

Methohexital
 • Rectal solution (U.S. and Canada)
Thiopental
 • Rectal solution (U.S. and Canada)
 • Rectal suspension (U.S.)

---

## Before Receiving This Medicine

In deciding to use a medicine, the risks of taking the medicine must be weighed against the good it will do. This is a decision you and your doctor will make. For general anesthetics, the following should be considered:

**Allergies**—Tell your doctor if you have ever had any unusual or allergic reaction to barbiturates or general anesthetics. Also tell your health care professional if you are allergic to any other substances, such as foods, preservatives, or dyes.

**Pregnancy—**

• *For barbiturate anesthetics (methohexital and thiopental)*—Methohexital has not been studied in pregnant women. However, it has not been shown to cause birth defects or other problems in animal studies. Studies on effects in pregnancy with thiopental have not been done in either humans or animals. However, use of barbiturate anesthetics during pregnancy may affect the nervous system in the fetus.

• *For etomidate*—Etomidate has not been studied in pregnant women. Although studies in animals have not shown etomidate to cause birth defects, it has been shown to cause other unwanted effects in the animal fetus when given in doses usually many times the human dose.

- *For inhalation anesthetics (enflurane, halothane, isoflurane, methoxyflurane, and nitrous oxide)*— Enflurane, halothane, isoflurane, methoxyflurane, and nitrous oxide have not been studied in pregnant women. However, studies in animals have shown that inhalation anesthetics may cause birth defects or other harm to the fetus.

  When used as an anesthetic for an abortion, enflurane, halothane, or isoflurane may cause increased bleeding.

  When used in small doses to relieve pain during labor and delivery, halothane may slow delivery and increase bleeding in the mother after the baby is born. These effects do not occur with small doses of enflurane, isoflurane, or methoxyflurane. However, they may occur with large doses of these anesthetics.

- *For ketamine*—Ketamine has not been studied in pregnant women. Studies in animals have not shown that ketamine causes birth defects, but it caused damage to certain tissues when given in large amounts for a long period of time.

- *For propofol*—Propofol has not been studied in pregnant women. Although studies in animals have not shown propofol to cause birth defects, it has been shown to cause deaths in nursing mothers and their offspring when given in doses usually many times the human dose.

General anesthetics may cause unwanted effects, such as drowsiness, in the newborn baby if large amounts are given to the mother during labor and delivery.

**Breast-feeding**—Barbiturate anesthetics (methohexital and thiopental), halothane, and propofol pass into the breast milk. However, general anesthetics have not been reported to cause problems in nursing babies.

**Children**—Anesthetics given by inhalation and ketamine have been tested in children and have not been shown to cause different side effects or problems in children than they do in adults.

Although there is no specific information comparing use of barbiturate anesthetics (methohexital and thiopental), etomidate, or propofol in children with use in other age groups, these medicines are not expected to cause different side effects or problems in children than they do in adults.

**Older adults**—Elderly people are especially sensitive to the effects of the barbiturate anesthetics (methohexital and thiopental), etomidate, propofol, and anesthetics given by inhalation. This may increase the chance of side effects.

Ketamine has not been shown to cause different side effects or problems in older people than it does in younger adults.

**Other medicines**—Although certain medicines should not be used together at all, in other cases 2 different medicines may be used together even if an interaction might occur. In these cases, your doctor may want to change

the dose, or other precautions may be necessary. When you are receiving general anesthetics, it is especially important that your health care professional know if you are taking *any other medicine*, including any of the following:

- "Street" drugs, such as amphetamines ("uppers"), barbiturates ("downers"), cocaine, marijuana, phencyclidine (PCP or "angel dust"), and heroin or other narcotics— Serious, possibly fatal, side effects may occur if your medical doctor or dentist gives you an anesthetic without knowing that you have taken another medicine

**Other medical problems**—The presence of other medical problems may affect the use of general anesthetics. Make sure you tell your doctor if you have any other medical problems, especially:

- Malignant hyperthermia, during or shortly after receiving an anesthetic (history of, or family history of). Signs of malignant hyperthermia include very high fever, fast and irregular heartbeat, muscle spasms or tightness, and breathing problems—This side effect may occur again

---

## Proper Use of This Medicine

**Dosing**—The dose of a general anesthetic will be different for different patients. Your doctor will decide on the right amount for you. The dose will depend on:

- Your age;
- Your general physical condition;
- The kind of surgery or other procedure you are having; and
- Other medicines you are taking or will receive before and during surgery.

---

## Precautions After Receiving This Medicine

For patients going home within 24 hours after receiving a general anesthetic:

- General anesthetics may cause you to feel drowsy, tired, or weak for up to a few days after they have been given. They may also cause problems with coordination and your ability to think. Therefore, for at least 24 hours (or longer if necessary) after receiving a general anesthetic, *do not drive, use machines, or do anything else that could be dangerous if you are not alert.*

- Unless otherwise directed by your medical doctor or dentist, *do not drink alcoholic beverages or take other CNS depressants (medicines that slow down the nervous system, possibly causing drowsiness) for about 24 hours after you have received a general anesthetic.* To do so may add to the effects of the anesthetic. Some examples of CNS depressants are antihistamines or medicine for hay fever, other allergies, or colds; other sedatives, tranquilizers, or sleeping medicine; prescription pain medicine or narcotics; other barbiturates; medicine for seizures; and muscle relaxants.

## Side Effects of This Medicine

Along with its needed effects, a medicine may cause some unwanted effects. Although not all of these side effects may occur, if they do occur they may need medical attention. While you are receiving a general anesthetic, your doctor will closely follow its effects. However, some effects may not be noticed until later.

Check with your doctor as soon as possible if any of the following side effects occur within 2 weeks after you have received an anesthetic:

*Rare*

Abdominal or stomach pain; back or leg pain; black or bloody vomit; fever; headache (severe); increase or decrease in amount of urine; loss of appetite; nausea (severe); pale skin; unusual tiredness or weakness; weakness of wrist and fingers; weight loss (unusual); yellow eyes or skin

Other side effects may occur that usually do not need medical attention. The following side effects should go away as the effects of the anesthetic wear off. However, check with your doctor if any of the following side effects continue or are bothersome:

*More common*

Shivering or trembling

*Less common*

Blurred or double vision or other vision problems; dizziness, lightheadedness, or feeling faint; drowsiness; headache; mood or mental changes; nausea (mild) or vomiting; nightmares or unusual dreams

Other side effects not listed above may also occur in some patients. If you notice any other effects, check with your doctor.

## Additional Information

Once a medicine has been approved for marketing for a certain use, experience may show that it is also useful for other medical problems. Although these uses are not included in product labeling, thiopental is used in certain patients with the following medical conditions:

- Hypoxia, cerebral (shortage of oxygen supplied to the brain)
  or
- Ischemia, cerebral (shortage of blood supplied to the brain)

Other than the above information, there is no additional information relating to proper use, precautions, or side effects for these uses.

Revised: 08/26/94

# ANGIOTENSIN-CONVERTING ENZYME (ACE) INHIBITORS   Systemic

Some commonly used brand names are:

**In the U.S.—**

| | |
|---|---|
| Accupril[7] | Monopril[5] |
| Altace[8] | Prinivil[6] |
| Capoten[2] | Vasotec[3,4] |
| Lotensin[1] | Zestril[6] |

**In Canada—**

| | |
|---|---|
| Capoten[2] | Vasotec[3,4] |
| Prinivil[6] | Zestril[6] |

Note: For quick reference, the following angiotensin-converting enzyme (ace) inhibitors are numbered to match the corresponding brand names.

This information applies to the following medicines:

1. Benazepril (ben-AY-ze-pril)†
2. Captopril (KAP-toe-pril)
3. Enalapril (e-NAL-a-pril)
4. Enalaprilat (e-NAL-a-pril-at)
5. Fosinopril (foe-SIN-oh-pril)†
6. Lisinopril (lyse-IN-oh-pril)
7. Quinapril (KWIN-a-pril)†
8. Ramipril (ra-MI-pril)†

†Not commercially available in Canada.

## Description

ACE inhibitors belong to the class of medicines called high blood pressure medicines (antihypertensives). They are used to treat high blood pressure (hypertension).

High blood pressure adds to the work load of the heart and arteries. If it continues for a long time, the heart and arteries may not function properly. This can damage the blood vessels of the brain, heart, and kidneys, resulting in a stroke, heart failure, or kidney failure. High blood pressure may also increase the risk of heart attacks. These problems may be less likely to occur if blood pressure is controlled.

Captopril is used in some patients after a heart attack. After a heart attack, some of the heart muscle is damaged and weakened. The heart muscle may continue to weaken as time goes by. This makes it more difficult for the heart to pump blood. Captopril helps slow down the further weakening of the heart.

Captopril is also used to treat kidney problems in some diabetic patients who use insulin to control their diabetes. Over time, these kidney problems may get worse. Captopril may help slow down the further worsening of kidney problems.

In addition, some ACE inhibitors are used to treat congestive heart failure, or may be used for other conditions as determined by your doctor.

The exact way that these medicines work is not known. They block an enzyme in the body that is necessary to produce a substance that causes blood vessels to tighten. As a result, they relax blood vessels. This lowers blood pressure and increases the supply of blood and oxygen to the heart.

These medicines are available only with your doctor's prescription, in the following dosage forms:

*Oral*

Benazepril
- Tablets (U.S.)

Captopril
- Tablets (U.S. and Canada)

Enalapril
- Tablets (U.S. and Canada)

Fosinopril
- Tablets (U.S.)

Lisinopril
- Tablets (U.S. and Canada)

Quinapril
- Tablets (U.S.)

Ramipril
- Capsules (U.S.)

*Parenteral*

Enalaprilat
- Injection (U.S. and Canada)

## Before Using This Medicine

In deciding to use a medicine, the risks of taking the medicine must be weighed against the good it will do. This is a decision you and your doctor will make. For the angiotensin-converting enzyme (ACE) inhibitors, the following should be considered:

**Allergies**—Tell your doctor if you have ever had any unusual or allergic reaction to benazepril, captopril, enalapril, fosinopril, lisinopril, quinapril, or ramipril. Also tell your health care professional if you are allergic to any other substances, such as foods, preservatives, or dyes.

**Pregnancy**—Use of angiotensin-converting enzyme (ACE) inhibitors during pregnancy, especially in the second and third trimesters (after the first three months) can cause low blood pressure, severe kidney failure, too much potassium, or even death in the newborn. *Therefore, it is important that you check with your doctor immediately if you think that you may be pregnant.* Be sure that you have discussed this with your doctor before taking this medicine. In addition, if you are taking:

- *Benazepril*—Benazepril has not been shown to cause birth defects in animals when given in doses more than 3 times the highest recommended human dose.
- *Captopril*—Studies in rabbits and rats at doses up to 400 times the recommended human dose have shown that captopril causes an increase in deaths of the fetus and newborn. Also, captopril has caused deformed skulls in the offspring of rabbits given doses 2 to 70 times the recommended human dose.
- *Enalapril*—Studies in rats at doses many times the recommended human dose have shown that use of enalapril causes the fetus to be smaller than normal. Studies in rabbits have shown that enalapril causes an increase in fetal death. Enalapril has not been shown to cause birth defects in rats or rabbits.
- *Fosinopril*—Studies in rats have shown that fosinopril causes the fetus to be smaller than normal. Studies in rabbits have shown that fosinopril causes

fetal death, probably due to extremely low blood pressure. In rats, birth defects such as skeletal and facial deformities were seen. However, it is not clear that the deformities were related to fosinopril. Birth defects were not seen in rabbits.

- *Lisinopril*—Studies in mice and rats at doses many times the recommended human dose have shown that use of lisinopril causes a decrease in successful pregnancies, a decrease in the weight of infants, and an increase in infant deaths. It has also caused a decrease in successful pregnancies and abnormal bone growth in rabbits. Lisinopril has not been shown to cause birth defects in mice, rats, or rabbits.
- *Quinapril*—Studies in rats have shown that quinapril causes lower birth weights and changes in kidney structure of the fetus. However, birth defects were not seen in rabbits given quinapril.
- *Ramipril*—Studies in animals have shown that ramipril causes lower birth weights.

**Breast-feeding**—

- *Benazepril, captopril, and fosinopril*—These medicines pass into breast milk.
- *Enalapril, lisinopril, quinapril, or ramipril*—It is not known whether these medicines pass into breast milk. However, these medicines have not been reported to cause problems in nursing babies.

**Children**—Children may be especially sensitive to the blood pressure–lowering effect of ACE inhibitors. This may increase the chance of side effects or other problems during treatment. Therefore, it is especially important that you discuss with the child's doctor the good that this medicine may do as well as the risks of using it.

**Older adults**—This medicine has been tested in a limited number of patients 65 years of age or older and has not been shown to cause different side effects or problems in older people than it does in younger adults.

**Other medicines**—Although certain medicines should not be used together at all, in other cases two different medicines may be used together even if an interaction might occur. In these cases, your doctor may want to change the dose, or other precautions may be necessary. When you are taking or receiving ACE inhibitors it is especially important that your health care professional know if you are taking any of the following:

- Diuretics (water pills)—Effects on blood pressure may be increased. In addition, some diuretics make the increase in potassium in the blood caused by ACE inhibitors even greater
- Potassium-containing medicines or supplements or
- Salt substitutes or
- Low-salt milk—Use of these substances with ACE inhibitors may result in an unusually high potassium level in the blood, which can lead to heart rhythm and other problems

**Other medical problems**—The presence of other medical problems may affect the use of the ACE inhibitors. Make sure you tell your doctor if you have any other medical problems, especially:

- Diabetes mellitus (sugar diabetes)—Increased risk of potassium levels in the body becoming too high
- Heart or blood vessel disease or
- Heart attack or stroke (recent)—Lowering blood pressure may make problems resulting from these conditions worse
- Kidney disease or
- Liver disease—Effects may be increased because of slower removal of medicine from the body
- Kidney transplant—Increased risk of kidney disease caused by ACE inhibitors
- Systemic lupus erythematosus (SLE)—Increased risk of blood problems caused by ACE inhibitors
- Previous reaction to any ACE inhibitor involving hoarseness; swelling of face, mouth, hands, or feet; or sudden trouble in breathing—Reaction is more likely to occur again

## Proper Use of This Medicine

To help you remember to take your medicine, try to get into the habit of taking it at the same time each day.

For patients taking *captopril:*

- This medicine is best taken on an empty stomach 1 hour before meals, unless you are otherwise directed by your doctor.

For patients taking this medicine *for high blood pressure:*

- In addition to the use of the medicine your doctor has prescribed, treatment for your high blood pressure may include weight control and care in the types of foods you eat, especially foods high in sodium. Your doctor will tell you which of these are most important for you. You should check with your doctor before changing your diet.
- Many patients who have high blood pressure will not notice any signs of the problem. In fact, many may feel normal. It is very important that you *take your medicine exactly as directed* and that you keep your appointments with your doctor even if you feel well.
- Remember that this medicine will not cure your high blood pressure but it does help control it. Therefore, you must continue to take it as directed if you expect to lower your blood pressure and keep it down. *You may have to take high blood pressure medicine for the rest of your life.* If high blood pressure is not treated, it can cause serious problems such as heart failure, blood vessel disease, stroke, or kidney disease.

**Dosing**—The dose of the ACE inhibitor will be different for different patients. *Follow your doctor's orders or the directions on the label.* The following information includes only the average doses. *If your dose is different, do not change it* unless your doctor tells you to do so.

The number of capsules or tablets that you take depends on the strength of the medicine. Also, *the number of doses you take each day, the time allowed between doses, and the length of time you take the medicine depend on the* medical problem for which you are taking the ACE inhibitor.

*For benazepril*

- For *oral* dosage form (tablets):
  —For high blood pressure:
  - Adults—10 milligrams (mg) once a day at first. Then, your doctor may increase your dose to 20 to 40 mg a day taken as a single dose or divided into two doses.
  - Children—Use and dose must be determined by your doctor.

*For captopril*

- For *oral* dosage form (tablets):
  —For congestive heart failure:
  - Adults—12.5 to 100 mg two or three times a day.
  - Children—Dose must be determined by your doctor.
  —For high blood pressure:
  - Adults—12.5 to 25 mg two or three times a day.
  - Children—Dose must be determined by your doctor.
  —For kidney problems related to diabetes:
  - Adults—25 mg three times a day.
  —For treatment after a heart attack:
  - Adults—12.5 to 50 mg three times a day.

*For enalapril*

- For *oral* dosage form (tablets):
  —For congestive heart failure:
  - Adults—2.5 mg once a day or two times a day at first. Your doctor may increase your dose to 5 to 20 mg a day taken as a single dose or divided into two doses.
  - Children—Use and dose must be determined by your doctor.
  —For high blood pressure:
  - Adults—5 mg once a day at first. Then, your doctor may increase your dose to 10 to 40 mg a day taken as a single dose or divided into two doses.
  - Children—Use and dose must be determined by your doctor.
  —For treating weakened heart muscle:
  - Adults—2.5 mg two times a day at first. Then, your doctor may increase your dose up to 20 mg a day taken in divided doses.
- For *injection* dosage form:
  —For high blood pressure:
  - Adults—1.25 mg every six hours injected into a vein.
  - Children—Use and dose must be determined by your doctor.

*For fosinopril*
- For *oral* dosage form (tablets):
  —For high blood pressure:
    - Adults—10 to 40 mg once a day.
    - Children—Use and dose must be determined by your doctor.

*For lisinopril*
- For *oral* dosage form (tablets):
  —For congestive heart failure:
    - Adults—2.5 to 20 mg once a day.
    - Children—Use and dose must be determined by your doctor.
  —For high blood pressure:
    - Adults—10 to 40 mg once a day.
    - Children—Use and dose must be determined by your doctor.

*For quinapril*
- For *oral* dosage form (tablets):
  —For high blood pressure:
    - Adults—10 mg once a day at first. Then, your doctor may increase your dose to 20 to 80 mg a day taken as a single dose or divided into two doses.
    - Children—Use and dose must be determined by your doctor.

*For ramipril*
- For *oral* dosage form (capsules):
  —For high blood pressure:
    - Adults—2.5 mg once a day at first. Then, your doctor may increase your dose up to 20 mg a day taken as a single dose or divided into two doses.
    - Children—Use and dose must be determined by your doctor.

**Missed dose**—If you miss a dose of this medicine, take it as soon as possible. However, if it is almost time for your next dose, skip the missed dose and go back to your regular dosing schedule. Do not double doses.

**Storage**—To store this medicine:
- Keep out of the reach of children.
- Store away from heat and direct light.
- Do not store in the bathroom, near the kitchen sink, or in other damp places. Heat or moisture may cause the medicine to break down.
- Do not keep outdated medicine or medicine no longer needed. Be sure that any discarded medicine is out of the reach of children.

## Precautions While Using This Medicine

It is important that your doctor check your progress at regular visits to make sure that this medicine is working properly and to check for unwanted effects.

For patients taking this medicine *for high blood pressure:*
- *Do not take other medicines unless they have been discussed with your doctor.* This especially includes over-the-counter (nonprescription) medicines for appetite control, asthma, colds, cough, hay fever, or sinus problems, since they may tend to increase your blood pressure.

Dizziness or lightheadedness may occur after the first dose of this medicine, especially if you have been taking a diuretic (water pill). Make sure you know how you react to this medicine before you drive, use machines, or do anything else that could be dangerous if you are dizzy.

Check with your doctor right away if you become sick while taking this medicine, especially with severe or continuing nausea and vomiting or diarrhea. These conditions may cause you to lose too much water and lead to low blood pressure.

Dizziness, lightheadedness, or fainting may also occur if you exercise or if the weather is hot. Heavy sweating can cause loss of too much water and low blood pressure. Use extra care during exercise or hot weather.

*Avoid alcoholic beverages until you have discussed their use with your doctor.* Alcohol may make the low blood pressure effect worse and/or increase the possibility of dizziness or fainting.

Before having any kind of surgery (including dental surgery) or emergency treatment, tell the medical doctor or dentist in charge that you are taking this medicine.

For patients taking *captopril or fosinopril:*
- Before you have any medical tests, tell the doctor in charge that you are taking this medicine. The results of some tests may be affected by this medicine.

## Side Effects of This Medicine

Along with its needed effects, a medicine may cause some unwanted effects. Although not all of these side effects may occur, if they do occur they may need medical attention.

*Check with your doctor immediately* if any of the following side effects occur:

*Rare*
Fever and chills; hoarseness; swelling of face, mouth, hands, or feet; trouble in swallowing or breathing (sudden); stomach pain, itching of skin, or yellow eyes or skin

Check with your doctor as soon as possible if any of the following side effects occur:

*Less common*
Dizziness, lightheadedness, or fainting; skin rash, with or without itching, fever, or joint pain

*Rare*
Abdominal pain, abdominal distention, fever, nausea, or vomiting; chest pain

*Signs and symptoms of too much potassium in the body*

Confusion; irregular heartbeat; nervousness; numbness or tingling in hands, feet, or lips; shortness of breath or difficulty breathing; weakness or heaviness of legs

Other side effects may occur that usually do not need medical attention. These side effects may go away during treatment as your body adjusts to the medicine. However, check with your doctor if any of the following side effects continue or are bothersome:

*More common*

Cough (dry, continuing)

*Less common*

Diarrhea; headache; loss of taste; nausea; unusual tiredness

Other side effects not listed above may also occur in some patients. If you notice any other effects, check with your doctor.

## Additional Information

Once a medicine has been approved for marketing for a certain use, experience may show that it is also useful for other medical problems. Although these uses are not included in product labeling, ACE inhibitors are used in certain patients with the following medical conditions:

- Hypertension in scleroderma (high blood pressure in patients with hardening and thickening of the skin)
- Renal crisis in scleroderma (kidney problems in patients with hardening and thickening of the skin)

Other than the above information, there is no additional information relating to proper use, precautions, or side effects for these uses.

Revised: 07/12/92
Interim revision(s): 08/04/93; 07/12/94

# ANGIOTENSIN-CONVERTING ENZYME (ACE) INHIBITORS AND HYDROCHLOROTHIAZIDE   Systemic†

Some commonly used brand names are:

**In the U.S.—**

| Capozide[1] | Vaseretic[2] |
| Prinzide[3] | Zestoretic[3] |

Note: For quick reference, the following medicines are numbered to match the corresponding brand names.

This information applies to the following medicines:

1. Captopril (KAP-toe-pril) and Hydrochlorothiazide (hye-droe-klor-oh-THYE-a-zide)†
2. Enalapril (e-NAL-a-pril) and Hydrochlorothiazide†
3. Lisinopril (lyse-IN-oh-pril) and Hydrochlorothiazide†

†Not commercially available in Canada.

## Description

This combination belongs to the class of medicines called high blood pressure medicines (antihypertensives). It is used to treat high blood pressure (hypertension).

High blood pressure adds to the workload of the heart and arteries. If it continues for a long time, the heart and arteries may not function properly. This can damage the blood vessels of the brain, heart, and kidneys, resulting in a stroke, heart failure, or kidney failure. High blood pressure may also increase the risk of heart attacks. These problems may be less likely to occur if blood pressure is controlled.

The exact way in which captopril, enalapril, and lisinopril work is not known. They block an enzyme in the body that is necessary to produce a substance that causes blood vessels to tighten. As a result, they relax blood vessels. This lowers blood pressure and increases the supply of blood and oxygen to the heart. Hydrochlorothiazide helps reduce the amount of salt and water in the body by acting

on the kidneys to increase the flow of urine; this also helps to lower blood pressure.

This combination may also be used for other conditions as determined by your doctor.

This medicine is available only with doctor's prescription, in the following dosage forms:

*Oral*

Captopril and Hydrochlorothiazide
- Tablets (U.S.)

Enalapril and Hydrochlorothiazide
- Tablets (U.S.)

Lisinopril and Hydrochorothiazide
- Tablets (U.S.)

## Before Using This Medicine

In deciding to use a medicine, the risks of taking the medicine must be weighed against the good it will do. This is a decision you and your doctor will make. For the angiotensin-converting enzyme (ACE) inhibitors and hydrochlorothiazide, the following should be considered:

**Allergies**—Tell your doctor if you have ever had any unusual or allergic reaction to enalapril, captopril, lisinopril, sulfonamides (sulfa drugs), bumetanide, furosemide, acetazolamide, dichlorphenamide, or methazolamide or to hydrochlorothiazide or any of the other thiazide diuretics (water pills). Also tell your health care professional if you are allergic to any other substances, such as foods, sulfites or other preservatives, or dyes.

**Pregnancy**—Studies with this combination medicine have not been done in pregnant women. However, use of any of the ACE inhibitors (captopril, enalapril, lisinopril) during pregnancy, especially in the second and third trimesters (after the first three months) can cause low blood pressure, kidney failure, too much potassium, or even death in newborns. *Therefore, it is important that you check with your doctor immediately if you think that you may be pregnant.* Be sure that you have discussed this with your doctor before taking this medicine. In addition, if your medicine contains:

- *Captopril*—Studies in rabbits and rats at doses up to 400 times the recommended human dose have shown that captopril causes an increase in death of the fetus and newborn. Also, captopril has caused deformed skulls in the offspring of rabbits given doses 2 to 70 times the recommended human dose.
- *Enalapril*—Studies in rats at doses many times the recommended human dose have shown that use of enalapril causes the fetus to be smaller than normal. Studies in rabbits have shown that enalapril causes an increase in fetal death. Enalapril has not been shown to cause birth defects in rats or rabbits.
- *Lisinopril*—Studies in mice and rats at doses many times the recommended human dose have shown that use of lisinopril causes a decrease in successful pregnancies, a decrease in the weight of infants, and an increase in infant deaths. It has also caused a decrease in successful pregnancies and abnormal bone growth in rabbits. Lisinopril has not been shown to cause birth defects in mice, rats, or rabbits.
- *Hydrochlorothiazide*—Hydrochlorothiazide has not been shown to cause birth defects or other problems in animal studies. However, when hydrochlorothiazide is used during pregnancy, it may cause side effects including jaundice, blood problems, and low potassium in the newborn baby.

**Breast-feeding—**
- *Captopril*—Passes into breast milk. However, this medicine has not been reported to cause problems in nursing babies.
- *Enalapril or lisinopril*—It is not known whether enalapril or lisinopril passes into breast milk. However, these medicines have not been reported to cause problems in nursing babies.
- *Hydrochlorothiazide*—Passes into breast milk. However, this medicine has not been reported to cause problems in nursing babies.

**Children—**Children may be especially sensitive to the blood pressure–lowering effect of ACE inhibitors. This may increase the chance of side effects or other problems during treatment. Extra caution may be necessary when using hydrochlorothiazide in infants with jaundice because it can make this condition worse. Therefore, it is especially important that you discuss with the child's doctor the good that this medicine may do as well as the risks of using it.

**Older adults—**Dizziness or lightheadedness and symptoms of too much potassium loss may be more likely to

occur in the elderly, who may be more sensitive to the effects of this medicine.

**Other medicines—**Although certain medicines should not be used together at all, in other cases two different medicines may be used together even if an interaction might occur. In these cases, your doctor may want to change the dose, or other precautions may be necessary. When taking ACE inhibitors and hydrochlorothiazide it is especially important that your health care professional know if you are taking any of the following:

- Cholestyramine or
- Colestipol—Use with thiazide diuretics may prevent the diuretic from working properly; the diuretic should be taken at least 1 hour before or 4 hours after cholestyramine or colestipol
- Digitalis glycosides (heart medicine)—If potassium levels in the body are decreased, symptoms of digitalis toxicity may occur
- Diuretics (water pills)—Effects on blood pressure may be increased
- Lithium (e.g., Lithane)—Risk of lithium overdose, even at low doses, may be increased
- Potassium-containing medicines or supplements or
- Salt substitutes or
- Low-salt milk—Use of these substances with ACE inhibitors may result in an unusually high potassium level in the blood, which can lead to heart rhythm and other problems

**Other medical problems—**The presence of other medical problems may affect the use of the ACE inhibitors. Make sure you tell your doctor if you have any other medical problems, especially:

- Diabetes mellitus (sugar diabetes)—Increased risk of potassium levels in the body becoming too high
- Gout (or history of)—Hydrochlorothiazide may increase the amount of uric acid in the body, which can lead to gout
- Heart or blood vessel disease or
- Heart attack or stroke (recent)—Lowering blood pressure may make problems resulting from these conditions worse
- Kidney disease or
- Liver disease—Effects may be increased because of slower removal from the body
- Kidney transplant—Increased risk of kidney disease caused by ACE inhibitors
- Pancreatitis (inflammation of the pancreas)—Hydrochlorothiazide can make this condition worse
- Systemic lupus erythematosus (SLE) (or history of)—Hydrochlorothiazide may worsen the condition, and there is an increased risk of blood problems caused by ACE inhibitors
- Previous reaction to captopril, enalapril, or lisinopril involving hoarseness; swelling of face, mouth, hands, or feet; or sudden trouble in breathing—Reaction is more likely to occur again

## Proper Use of This Medicine

To help you remember to take your medicine, try to get into the habit of taking it at the same time each day.

For patients taking *captopril and hydrochlorothiazide:*
- This medicine is best taken on an empty stomach 1 hour before meals, unless you are otherwise directed by your doctor.

For patients taking this medicine *for high blood pressure:*
- In addition to the use of the medicine your doctor has prescribed, treatment for your high blood pressure may include weight control and care in the types of foods you eat, especially foods high in sodium. Your doctor will tell you which of these are most important for you. You should check with your doctor before changing your diet.
- Many patients who have high blood pressure will not notice any signs of the problem. In fact, many may feel normal. It is very important that you *take your medicine exactly as directed* and that you keep your appointments with your doctor even if you feel well.
- Remember that this medicine will not cure your high blood pressure but it does help control it. Therefore, you must continue to take it as directed if you expect to lower your blood pressure and keep it down. *You may have to take high blood pressure medicine for the rest of your life.* If high blood pressure is not treated, it can cause serious problems such as heart failure, blood vessel disease, stroke, or kidney disease.

This medicine may cause you to have an unusual feeling of tiredness when you begin to take it. You may also notice an increase in the amount of urine or in your frequency of urination. After you have taken the medicine for a while, these effects should lessen. In general, to keep the increase in urine from affecting your sleep:
- If you are to take a single dose a day, take it in the morning after breakfast.
- If you are to take more than one dose a day, take the last dose no later than 6 p.m., unless otherwise directed by your doctor.

However, it is best to plan your dose or doses according to a schedule that will least affect your personal activities and sleep. Ask your health care professional to help you plan the best time to take this medicine.

**Dosing**—The dose of these medicines will be different for different patients. *Follow your doctor's orders or the directions on the label.* The following information includes only the average doses of these medicines. *If your dose is different, do not change it* unless your doctor tells you to do so.

The number of tablets that you take depends on the strength of the medicine.

*For captopril and hydrochlorothiazide combination*
- For *oral* dosage form (tablets):
  —For high blood pressure:
  - Adults—1 tablet two or three times a day.
  - Children—Dose is based on body weight and must be determined by your doctor.

*For enalapril and hydrochlorothiazide combination*
- For *oral* dosage form (tablets):
  —For high blood pressure:
  - Adults—1 tablet once a day.
  - Children—Dose is based on body weight and must be determined by your doctor.

*For lisinopril and hydrochlorothiazide combination*
- For *oral* dosage form (tablets):
  —For high blood pressure:
  - Adults—1 or 2 tablets once a day.
  - Children—Dose must be determined by your doctor.

**Missed dose**—If you miss a dose of this medicine, take it as soon as possible. However, if it is almost time for your next dose, skip the missed dose and go back to your regular dosing schedule. Do not double doses.

**Storage**—To store this medicine:
- Keep out of the reach of children.
- Store away from heat and direct light.
- Do not store in the bathroom, near the kitchen sink, or in other damp places. Heat or moisture may cause the medicine to break down.
- Do not keep outdated medicine or medicine no longer needed. Be sure that any discarded medicine is out of the reach of children.

## Precautions While Using This Medicine

It is important that your doctor check your progress at regular visits to make sure that this medicine is working properly and to check for unwanted effects.

Dizziness or lightheadedness may occur, especially after the first dose of this medicine. Make sure you know how you react to the medicine before you drive, use machines, or do anything else that could be dangerous if you are dizzy.

Check with your doctor right away if you become sick while taking this medicine, especially with severe or continuing nausea and vomiting or diarrhea. These conditions may cause you to lose too much water and lead to low blood pressure.

Dizziness, lightheadedness, or fainting may also occur if you exercise or if the weather is hot. Heavy sweating can cause loss of too much water and low blood pressure. Use extra care during exercise or hot weather.

*Avoid alcoholic beverages until you have discussed their use with your doctor.* Alcohol may make the low blood pressure effect worse and/or increase the possibility of dizziness or fainting.

Before having any kind of surgery (including dental surgery) or emergency treatment, tell the medical doctor or dentist in charge that you are taking this medicine.

For patients taking *captopril and hydrochlorothiazide:*
- Before you have any medical tests, tell the doctor in charge that you are taking this medicine. The results of some tests may be affected by this medicine.

For patients taking this medicine *for high blood pressure:*
- *Do not take other medicines unless they have been discussed with your doctor.* This especially includes over-the-counter (nonprescription) medicines for appetite control, asthma, colds, cough, hay fever, or sinus problems, since they may tend to increase your blood pressure.

For *diabetic patients:*
- Hydrochlorothiazide (contained in this combination medicine) may raise blood sugar levels. While you are taking this medicine, be especially careful in testing for sugar in your urine.

Hydrochlorothiazide (contained in this combination medicine) may cause your skin to be more sensitive to sunlight than it is normally. Exposure to sunlight, even for brief periods of time, may cause a skin rash, itching, redness or other discoloration of the skin, or a severe sunburn. When you first begin taking this medicine:
- Stay out of direct sunlight, especially between the hours of 10:00 a.m. and 3:00 p.m., if possible.
- Wear protective clothing, including a hat. Also, wear sunglasses.
- Apply a sun block product that has a skin protection factor (SPF) of at least 15. Some patients may require a product with a higher SPF number, especially if they have a fair complexion. If you have any questions about this, check with your health care professional.
- Apply a sun block lipstick that has an SPF of at least 15 to protect your lips.
- Do not use a sunlamp or tanning bed or booth.

If you have a severe reaction from the sun, check with your doctor.

Before you have any medical tests, tell the doctor in charge that you are taking this medicine. The results of some tests may be affected by this medicine.

## Side Effects of This Medicine

Along with its needed effects, a medicine may cause some unwanted effects. Although not all of these side effects may occur, if they do occur they may need medical attention.

*Check with your doctor immediately* if any of the following side effects occur:

*Rare*

Fever and chills; hoarseness; swelling of face, mouth, hands, or feet; trouble in swallowing or breathing (sudden)

Check with your doctor as soon as possible if any of the following side effects occur:

*Less common*

Dizziness, lightheadedness, or fainting; skin rash, with or without itching, fever, or joint pain

*Rare*

Chest pain; joint pain; lower back or side pain; stomach pain (severe) with nausea and vomiting; unusual bleeding or bruising; yellow eyes or skin

*Signs and symptoms of too much or too little potassium in the body*

Dryness of mouth; increased thirst; irregular heartbeats; mood or mental changes; muscle cramps or pain; numbness or tingling in hands, feet, or lips; weakness or heaviness of legs; weak pulse

Other side effects may occur that usually do not need medical attention. These side effects may go away during treatment as your body adjusts to the medicine. However, check with your doctor if any of the following side effects continue or are bothersome:

*More common*

Cough (dry, continuing)

*Less common*

Diarrhea; headache; increased sensitivity of skin to sunlight (skin rash, itching, redness or other discoloration of skin or severe sunburn after exposure to sunlight); loss of appetite; loss of taste; stomach upset; unusual tiredness

Other side effects not listed above may also occur in some patients. If you notice any other effects, check with your doctor.

## Additional Information

Once a medicine has been approved for marketing for a certain use, experience may show that it is also useful for other medical problems. Although this use is not included in product labeling, ACE inhibitors and hydrochlorothiazide are used in certain patients with the following medical condition:
- Congestive heart failure

Other than the above information, there is no additional information relating to proper use, precautions, or side effects for this use.

Revised: 07/28/92
Interim revision: 06/29/94

# ANTACIDS Oral

Some commonly used brand names are:

**In the U.S.—**

| | | | |
|---|---|---|---|
| Advanced Formula Di-Gel[12] | Creamalin[1] | Maalox HRF Heartburn Relief Formula[5] | Rolaids[17] |
| Alamag[1] | Dialume[9] | Maalox Plus, Extra Strength[4] | Rolaids Calcium Rich[10] |
| Algenic Alka[5] | Dicarbosil[10] | Maalox TC[1] | Rolaids Extra Strength with Simethicone[15] |
| Algicon[5] | Di-Gel[4] | Magnagel[5] | Rulox[1] |
| Alka-Mints[10] | Equilet[10] | Mag-Ox 400[22] | Rulox No. 1[1] |
| Alkets[14] | Foamicon[6] | Mallamint[10] | Rulox No. 2[1] |
| Almacone[4] | Gas-is-gon[7] | Maox[22] | Simaal Gel[4] |
| Almacone II[4] | Gaviscon[5 6] | Marblen[13] | Simaal 2 Gel[4] |
| Alma-Mag Improved[4] | Gaviscon-2[6] | Mi-Acid[4] | Spastosed[13] |
| AlternaGEL[9] | Gaviscon Extra Strength Relief Formula[5 24] | Mintox[1] | Tempo[3] |
| Alu-Cap[9] | | Mintox Plus[4] | Titralac[10] |
| Aludrox[4] | Gelamal[1] | Mygel[4] | Titralac Extra Strength[10] |
| Alu-Tab[9] | Gelusil[4] | Mygel II[4] | Titralac Plus[15] |
| Amitone[10] | Genaton[6] | Mylanta[4 13] | Tums[10] |
| Amphojel[9] | Glycate[10] | Mylanta-II[4] | Tums E-X[10] |
| AntaGel[4] | Kudrox Double Strength[1] | Nephrox[9] | Tums Liquid Extra Strength[10] |
| AntaGel-II[4] | | Noralac[13] | Tums Liquid Extra Strength with Simethicone[15] |
| Basaljel[8] | Losotron Plus[19] | Phillips' Milk of Magnesia[21] | |
| Bisodol[11 20] | Lowsium[18] | Riopan[18] | Uro-Mag[22] |
| Calglycine[10] | Lowsium Plus[19] | Riopan Plus[19] | WinGel[1] |
| Camalox[2] | Maalox[1] | Riopan Plus 2[19] | |
| Chooz[10] | Maalox Extra Strength[1] | | |

**In Canada—**

| | | | |
|---|---|---|---|
| Algicon[5] | Diovol Ex[1] | Maalox Plus, Extra Strength[4] | Phillips' Milk of Magnesia[21] |
| Alu-Tab[9] | Diovol Plus[4 24] | Maalox TC[1] | Riopan[18] |
| Amphojel[9] | Gaviscon[6 9] | Mylanta[4] | Riopan Extra Strength[18] |
| Amphojel 500[1] | Gelusil[1] | Mylanta Double Strength[4] | Riopan Plus[19] |
| Amphojel Plus[4 24] | Gelusil Extra Strength[1] | Mylanta Extra Strength[4] | Riopan Plus Extra Strength[19] |
| Basaljel[9] | Maalox[1] | Mylanta Double Strength Plain[1] | |
| Diovol[1] | Maalox Plus[4] | Neutralca-S[1] | Robalate[16] |

Note: For quick reference the following antacids are numbered to match the corresponding brand names.

This information applies to the following medicines:

1. Alumina (a-LOO-mi-na) and Magnesia (mag-NEE-zha)
2. Alumina, Magnesia, and Calcium Carbonate (KAL-see-um KAR-boe-nate)
3. Alumina, Magnesia, Calcium Carbonate, and Simethicone (Si-METH-i-kone)†
4. Alumina, Magnesia, and Simethicone
5. Alumina and Magnesium Carbonate (mag-NEE-zhum).
6. Alumina and Magnesium Trisilicate (trye-SILL-i-kate)
7. Alumina, Magnesium Trisilicate, and Sodium Bicarbonate (SOE-dee-um bi-KAR-boe-nate)
8. Aluminum Carbonate (a-LOO-mi-num), Basic
9. Aluminum Hydroxide (hye-DROX-ide)*†
10. Calcium Carbonate*
11. Calcium Carbonate and Magnesia
12. Calcium Carbonate, Magnesia, and Simethicone
13. Calcium and Magnesium Carbonates
14. Calcium and Magnesium Carbonates and Magnesium Oxide (mag-NEE-zhum OX-ide)
15. Calcium Carbonate and Simethicone
16. Dihydroxyaluminum Aminoacetate (dye-hye-DROX-ee-a-LOO-mi-num a-mee-noe-ASS-e-tate)
17. Dihydroxyaluminum Sodium Carbonate
18. Magaldrate (MAG-al-drate)*
19. Magaldrate and Simethicone
20. Magnesium Carbonate and Sodium Bicarbonate
21. Magnesium Hydroxide*†
22. Magnesium Oxide

23. Simethicone, Alumina, Magnesium Carbonate, and Magnesia
24. Alumina, Magnesium Carbonate, and Sodium Bicarbonate

---

*Generic name product may also be available in U.S.
†Generic name product available in Canada.

---

## Description

Antacids are taken by mouth to relieve heartburn, sour stomach, or acid indigestion. They work by neutralizing excess stomach acid. Some antacid combinations also contain simethicone, which may relieve the symptoms of excess gas. Antacids alone or in combination with simethicone may also be used to treat the symptoms of stomach or duodenal ulcers.

With larger doses than those used for the antacid effect, magnesium hydroxide (magnesia) and magnesium oxide antacids produce a laxative effect. The information that follows applies only to their use as an antacid.

Some antacids, like aluminum carbonate and aluminum hydroxide, may be prescribed with a low-phosphate diet to treat hyperphosphatemia (too much phosphate in the blood). Aluminum carbonate and aluminum hydroxide may also be used with a low-phosphate diet to prevent the formation of some kinds of kidney stones. Aluminum hydroxide may also be used for other conditions as determined by your doctor.

These medicines are available without a prescription. However, your doctor may have special instructions on the proper use and dose of these medicines for your medical problem. They are available in the following dosage forms:

*Oral*

Alumina and Magnesia
- Oral suspension (U.S. and Canada)
- Tablets (Canada)
- Chewable tablets (U.S. and Canada)

Alumina, Magnesia, and Calcium Carbonate
- Oral suspension (U.S.)
- Chewable tablets (U.S.)

Alumina, Magnesia, and Simethicone
- Oral suspension (U.S. and Canada)
- Chewable tablets (U.S. and Canada)

Alumina, Magnesia, Calcium Carbonate, and Simethicone
- Chewable tablets (U.S.)

Alumina and Magnesium Carbonate
- Oral suspension (U.S. and Canada)
- Chewable tablets (U.S. and Canada)

Alumina and Magnesium Trisilicate
- Chewable tablets (U.S. and Canada)

Alumina, Magnesium Trisilicate, and Sodium Bicarbonate
- Chewable tablets (U.S.)

Aluminum Carbonate, Basic
- Capsules (U.S.)
- Gel (U.S.)
- Tablets (U.S.)

Aluminum Hydroxide
- Capsules (U.S. and Canada)
- Gel (U.S. and Canada)
- Tablets (U.S. and Canada)

Calcium Carbonate
- Chewing gum (U.S.)
- Oral suspension (U.S.)
- Tablets (U.S.)
- Chewable tablets (U.S.)

Calcium Carbonate and Magnesia
- Chewable tablets (U.S.)

Calcium Carbonate, Magnesia, and Simethicone
- Tablets (U.S.)

Calcium and Magnesium Carbonates
- Oral suspension (U.S.)
- Tablets (U.S.)
- Chewable tablets (U.S.)

Calcium and Magnesium Carbonates and Magnesium Oxide
- Tablets (U.S.)

Calcium Carbonate and Simethicone
- Oral suspension (U.S.)
- Chewable tablets (U.S.)

Dihydroxyaluminum Aminoacetate
- Tablets (Canada)

Dihydroxyaluminum Sodium Carbonate
- Chewable tablets (U.S.)

Magaldrate
- Oral suspension (U.S. and Canada)
- Tablets (U.S.)
- Chewable tablets (U.S. and Canada)

Magaldrate and Simethicone
- Oral suspension (U.S. and Canada)
- Chewable tablets (U.S. and Canada)

Magnesium Carbonate and Sodium Bicarbonate
- For oral suspension (U.S.)

Magnesium Hydroxide
- Milk of magnesia (U.S. and Canada)
- Tablets (U.S. and Canada)
- Chewable Tablets (U.S. and Canada)

Magnesium Oxide
- Capsules (U.S.)
- Tablets (U.S.)

Simethicone, Alumina, Magnesium Carbonate, and Magnesia
- Chewable tablets (U.S. and Canada)

## Before Using This Medicine

If you are taking this medicine without a prescription, carefully read and follow any precautions on the label. For antacids, the following should be considered:

**Allergies**—Tell your health care professional if you have ever had any unusual or allergic reaction to aluminum-, calcium-, magnesium-, simethicone-, or sodium bicarbonate–containing medicines. Also tell your health care professional if you are allergic to any other substances, such as foods, preservatives, or dyes.

**Diet**—Make certain your health care professional knows if you are on a low-sodium diet. Some antacids contain large amounts of sodium.

**Pregnancy**—Studies have not been done in either humans or animals. However, there have been reports of antacids causing side effects in babies whose mothers took antacids for a long time, especially in high doses during pregnancy. Also, sodium-containing medicines should be avoided if you tend to retain (keep) body water.

**Breast-feeding**—These medicines have not been reported to cause problems in nursing babies.

**Children**—Antacids should not be given to young children (under 6 years of age) unless ordered by their doctor. Since children cannot usually describe their symptoms very well, a doctor should first check the child. The child may have a condition that needs other treatment. If so, antacids will not help and may even cause unwanted effects or make the condition worse. In addition, aluminum- or magnesium-containing medicines should not be given to premature or very young children because they may cause serious side effects, especially when given to children who have kidney disease or who are dehydrated.

**Older adults**—Aluminum-containing antacids should not be used by elderly persons with bone problems or with Alzheimer's disease. The aluminum may cause their condition to get worse.

**Other medicines**—Although certain medicines should not be used together at all, in other cases two different medicines may be used together even if an interaction might occur. In these cases, your doctor may want to change the dose, or other precautions may be necessary. When you are taking antacids, it is especially important that your health care professional know if you are taking any of the following:
- Cellulose sodium phosphate (e.g., Calcibind)—Calcium-containing antacids may decrease the effects of cellulose

sodium phosphate; use with magnesium-containing antacids may prevent either medicine from working properly; antacids should not be taken within 1 hour of cellulose sodium phosphate

- Ciprofloxacin or
- Lomefloxacin or
- Norfloxacin or
- Ofloxacin—Antacids may decrease the effects of these medicines; the antacid should be taken 4 hours before or 2 hours after these medicines
- Isoniazid taken by mouth (e.g., INH)—Aluminum-containing antacids may decrease the effects of isoniazid; isoniazid should be taken at least 1 hour before or after the antacid
- Ketoconazole (e.g., Nizoral) or
- Methenamine (e.g., Mandelamine)—Antacids may decrease the effects of ketoconazole or methenamine; these medicines should be taken 3 hours before the antacid
- Mecamylamine (e.g., Inversine)—Antacids may increase the effects and possibly the side effects of mecamylamine
- Sodium polystyrene sulfonate resin (SPSR) (e.g., Kayexalate)—This medicine may decrease the effects of antacids
- Tetracyclines (medicine for infection) taken by mouth—Use with antacids may decrease the effects of both medicines; antacids should not be taken within 3 to 4 hours of tetracyclines

**Other medical problems**—The presence of other medical problems may affect the use of antacids. Make sure you tell your doctor if you have any other medical problems, especially:

- Alzheimer's disease (for aluminum-containing antacids only) or
- Appendicitis (or signs of) or
- Bone fractures or
- Colitis or
- Constipation (severe and continuing) or
- Hemorrhoids or
- Inflamed bowel or
- Intestinal blockage or
- Intestinal or rectal bleeding—Antacids may make these conditions worse
- Colostomy or
- Ileostomy—Use of antacids may cause the body to retain (keep) water and electrolytes such as sodium and/or potassium
- Diarrhea (continuing)—Aluminum-containing antacids may cause the body to lose too much phosphorus; magnesium-containing antacids may make diarrhea worse
- Edema (swelling of feet or lower legs) or
- Heart disease or
- Liver disease or
- Toxemia of pregnancy—Use of sodium-containing antacids may cause the body to retain (keep) water
- Kidney disease—Antacids may cause higher blood levels of aluminum, calcium, or magnesium, which may increase the risk of serious side effects
- Sarcoidosis—Use of calcium-containing antacids may cause kidney problems or too much calcium in the blood
- Underactive parathyroid glands—Use with calcium-containing antacids may cause too much calcium in the blood

## Proper Use of This Medicine

For patients taking the *chewable tablet form* of this medicine:

- Chew the tablets well before swallowing. This is to allow the medicine to work faster and be more effective.

For patients taking this medicine for a *stomach or duodenal ulcer:*

- Take it exactly as directed and for the full time of treatment as ordered by your doctor, to obtain maximum relief of your symptoms.
- Take it 1 and 3 hours after meals and at bedtime for best results, unless otherwise directed by your doctor.

For patients taking *aluminum carbonate* or *aluminum hydroxide* to *prevent kidney stones:*

- Drink plenty of fluids for best results, unless otherwise directed by your doctor.

For patients taking *aluminum carbonate* or *aluminum hydroxide* for *hyperphosphatemia* (too much phosphate in the blood):

- Your doctor may want you to follow a low-phosphate diet. If you have any questions about this, check with your doctor.

**Dosing**—The dose of an antacid will be different for different patients. *Follow your doctor's orders or the directions on the label.*

**Missed dose**—If your doctor has told you to take this medicine on a regular schedule and you miss a dose, take it as soon as possible. However, if it is almost time for your next dose, skip the missed dose and go back to your regular dosing schedule. Do not double doses.

**Storage**—To store this medicine:

- Keep out of the reach of children.
- Store away from heat and direct light.
- Do not store the capsule, tablet, or powder form of this medicine in the bathroom, near the kitchen sink, or in other damp places. Heat or moisture may cause the medicine to break down.
- Keep the liquid form of this medicine from freezing.
- Do not keep outdated medicine or medicine no longer needed. Be sure that any discarded medicine is out of the reach of children.

## Precautions While Using This Medicine

If this medicine has been ordered by your doctor and you will be taking it in large doses, or for a long time, your doctor should check your progress at regular visits. This is to make sure the medicine does not cause unwanted effects.

Some tests may be affected by this medicine. Tell the doctor in charge that you are taking this medicine before you have any tests to determine how much acid your stomach produces.

*Do not take this medicine:*

- *if you have any signs of appendicitis or inflamed bowel* (such as stomach or lower abdominal pain, cramping, bloating, soreness, nausea, or vomiting). Instead, check with your doctor as soon as possible.
- *within 1 to 2 hours or more of taking other medicine by mouth.* To do so may keep the other medicine from working properly.

For patients on a *sodium-restricted diet:*

- Some antacids (especially sodium bicarbonate–containing ones) contain a large amount of sodium. If you have any questions about this, check with your health care professional.

For patients taking this medicine for increased stomach acid:

- Do not take it for more than 2 weeks unless otherwise directed by your doctor. Antacids should be used only for occasional relief.
- If your stomach problem is not helped by the antacid or if it keeps coming back, check with your doctor.
- Using magnesium- or sodium bicarbonate–containing antacids too often, or in high doses, may produce a laxative effect. This happens fairly often and depends on the individual's sensitivity to the medicine.

For patients taking *aluminum-containing antacids* (including magaldrate):

- Before you have any test in which a radiopharmaceutical will be used, tell the doctor in charge that you are taking this medicine. The results of the test may be affected by aluminum-containing antacids.

For patients taking *calcium-* or *sodium bicarbonate–containing antacids:*

- *Do not take the antacid with large amounts of milk or milk products.* To do so may increase the chance of side effects.

## Side Effects of This Medicine

Along with its needed effects, a medicine may cause some unwanted effects. Although the following side effects occur very rarely when this medicine is taken as recommended, they may be more likely to occur if:

- too much medicine is taken.
- it is taken in large doses.
- it is taken for a long time.

- it is taken by patients with kidney disease.

Check with your doctor as soon as possible if any of the following side effects (which may be signs of overdose) occur:

*For aluminum-containing antacids (including magaldrate)*

Bone pain; constipation (severe and continuing); feeling of discomfort (continuing); loss of appetite (continuing); mood or mental changes; muscle weakness; swelling of wrists or ankles; weight loss (unusual)

*For calcium-containing antacids*

Constipation (severe and continuing); difficult or painful urination; frequent urge to urinate; headache (continuing); loss of appetite (continuing); mood or mental changes; muscle pain or twitching; nausea or vomiting; nervousness or restlessness; slow breathing; unpleasant taste; unusual tiredness or weakness

*For magnesium-containing antacids (including magaldrate)*

Difficult or painful urination (with magnesium trisilicate); dizziness or lightheadedness; feeling of discomfort (continuing); irregular heartbeat; loss of appetite (continuing); mood or mental changes; muscle weakness; unusual tiredness or weakness; weight loss (unusual)

*For sodium bicarbonate–containing antacids*

Frequent urge to urinate; headache (continuing); loss of appetite (continuing); mood or mental changes; muscle pain or twitching; nausea or vomiting; nervousness or restlessness; slow breathing; swelling of feet or lower legs; unpleasant taste; unusual tiredness or weakness

Other side effects may occur that usually do not need medical attention. These side effects may go away during treatment as your body adjusts to the medicine. However, check with your doctor if any of the following side effects continue or are bothersome:

*More common*

Chalky taste

*Less common*

Constipation (mild); diarrhea or laxative effect; increased thirst; speckling or whitish discoloration of stools; stomach cramps

Other side effects not listed above may also occur in some patients. If you notice any other effects, check with your doctor.

Revised: 07/15/93

# ANTHRALIN   Topical

Some commonly used brand names are:

**In the U.S.—**

| | |
|---|---|
| Anthra-Derm | Lasan 0.1 |
| Drithocreme | Lasan 0.2 |
| Drithocreme HP | Lasan 0.4 |
| Dritho-Scalp | Lasan HP-1 |
| Lasan | |

**In Canada—**

| | |
|---|---|
| Anthraforte 1 | Anthranol 0.2 |
| Anthraforte 2 | Anthranol 0.4 |
| Anthraforte 3 | Anthrascalp |
| Anthranol 0.1 | |

Another commonly used name is dithranol.

## Description

Anthralin (AN-thra-lin) is used to treat psoriasis. It may also be used to treat other skin conditions as determined by your doctor.

In the U.S., this medicine is available only with your doctor's prescription. In Canada, this medicine should be used only on the advice of your doctor.

This medicine is available in the following dosage forms:

*Topical*
- Cream (U.S. and Canada)
- Ointment (U.S. and Canada)

## Before Using This Medicine

In deciding to use a medicine, the risks of using the medicine must be weighed against the good it will do. This is a decision you and your doctor will make. For anthralin, the following should be considered:

**Allergies**—Tell your doctor if you have ever had any unusual or allergic reaction to anthralin. Also tell your health care professional if you are allergic to any other substances, such as preservatives or dyes.

**Pregnancy**—Anthralin may be absorbed through the skin. However, studies on effects in pregnancy have not been done in either humans or animals.

**Breast-feeding**—Anthralin may be absorbed through the mother's skin. It is not known whether anthralin passes into the breast milk. However, this medicine has not been reported to cause problems in nursing babies.

**Children**—Studies on this medicine have been done only in adult patients, and there is no specific information comparing use of anthralin in children with use in other age groups.

**Older adults**—Many medicines have not been studied specifically in older people. Therefore, it may not be known whether they work exactly the same way they do in younger adults or if they cause different side effects or problems in older people. There is no specific information comparing use of anthralin in the elderly with use in other age groups.

**Other medicines**—Although certain medicines should not be used together at all, in other cases two different medicines may be used together even if an interaction might occur. In these cases, your doctor may want to change the dose, or other precautions may be necessary. Tell your health care professional if you are using any other prescription or nonprescription (over-the-counter [OTC]) medicine.

**Other medical problems**—The presence of other medical problems may affect the use of anthralin. Make sure you tell your doctor if you have any other medical problems, especially:
- Skin diseases or problems (other)—Anthralin may make the condition worse

## Proper Use of This Medicine

*Keep this medicine away from the eyes and other mucous membranes, such as the mouth and the inside of the nose.*

*Do not apply this medicine to blistered, raw, or oozing areas of the skin or scalp.*

*Do not use this medicine on your face or sex organs or in the folds and creases of your skin.* If you have any questions about this, check with your doctor.

*Use this medicine only as directed.* Do not use more of it, do not use it more often, and do not use it for a longer time than your doctor ordered. To do so may increase the chance of side effects.

Anthralin may be used in different ways. In some cases, it is applied at night and allowed to remain on the affected areas overnight, then washed off the next morning or before the next application. In other cases, it may be applied and allowed to remain on the affected areas for a short period of time (usually 10 to 30 minutes), then washed off. (This is called short contact treatment.) Make sure you understand exactly how you are to use this medicine. If you have any questions about this, check with your doctor.

Anthralin may cause irritation of normal skin. If it does, petrolatum may be applied to the skin or scalp around the affected areas for protection.

Apply a thin layer of anthralin to only the affected area of the skin or scalp and rub in gently.

Immediately after applying this medicine, wash your hands to remove any medicine that may be on them.

For patients using *anthralin for short contact* (usually 10 to 30 minutes) treatment:
- After applying anthralin, allow the medicine to remain on the affected area for 10 to 30 minutes or as directed by your doctor. Then remove the medicine by bathing, if the anthralin was applied to the skin, or by shampooing, if it was applied to the scalp.

For patients using the *cream form* of anthralin for overnight treatment:
- If anthralin cream is applied to the skin, any medicine remaining on the affected areas the next morning should be removed by bathing.
- If anthralin cream is applied to the scalp, shampoo to remove the scales and any medicine remaining on the affected areas from the previous application. Dry the hair and, after parting, rub the cream into the affected areas. Check with your doctor to see when the cream should be removed.

For patients using the *ointment form* of anthralin for overnight treatment:
- If anthralin ointment is applied to the skin at night, any ointment remaining on the affected areas the next morning should be removed with warm liquid petrolatum followed by bathing.

• If anthralin ointment is applied to the scalp at night, use a shampoo the next morning to clean the scalp.

**Dosing**—The dose of anthralin will be different for different patients. *Follow your doctor's orders or the directions on the label.* The following information includes only the average doses of anthralin. *If your dose is different, do not change it* unless your doctor tells you to do so.

• For psoriasis:
—For *cream* dosage form:
• Adults—Apply to the affected area(s) of the skin once a day.
• Children—Use and dose must be determined by your doctor.
—For *ointment* dosage form:
• Adults—Apply to the affected area(s) of the skin one or two times a day.
• Children—Use and dose must be determined by your doctor.

**Missed dose**—If you miss a dose of this medicine, apply it as soon as possible. However, if it is almost time for your next dose, skip the missed dose and go back to your regular dosing schedule. Do not double doses.

**Storage**—To store this medicine:
• Keep out of the reach of children.
• Store away from heat and direct light.
• Keep the medicine from freezing.
• Do not keep outdated medicine or medicine no longer needed. Be sure that any discarded medicine is out of the reach of children.

## Precautions While Using This Medicine

*Anthralin may stain the skin, hair, fingernails, clothing, bed linens, or bathtub or shower:*
• Avoid getting the medicine on your clothing or on bed linens. Protective dressings may be used, unless you have been otherwise directed by your doctor.
• The stain on the skin or hair will wear off in several weeks after you stop using this medicine.
• To prevent staining of your hands, you may wear plastic gloves when you apply this medicine.

• If the medicine is applied to the scalp at night, check with your doctor to see if you may wear a plastic cap to prevent staining of the pillow.
• To remove any medicine on the surface of the bathtub or shower, wash it with hot water immediately after bathing or showering. Then use a household cleanser to remove any remaining deposit of the medicine on the bathtub or shower.

## Side Effects of This Medicine

Anthralin has been shown to cause tumors (some cancerous) in animals. However, there have been no reports of anthralin causing tumors in humans.

Along with its needed effects, a medicine may cause some unwanted effects. Although not all of these side effects may occur, if they do occur they may need medical attention.

Check with your doctor as soon as possible if any of the following side effects occur:
*More common*
Redness or other skin irritation not present before use of this medicine
*Rare*
Skin rash

Other side effects not listed above may also occur in some patients. If you notice any other effects, check with your doctor.

## Additional Information

Once a medicine has been approved for marketing for a certain use, experience may show that it is also useful for other medical problems. Although this use is not included in product labeling, anthralin is used in certain patients with the following medical condition:
• Alopecia areata (a certain type of baldness)

Other than the above information, there is no additional information relating to proper use, precautions, or side effects for this use.

Revised: 01/15/92
Interim revision 07/01/94

# ANTICHOLINERGICS/ANTISPASMODICS   Systemic

Some commonly used brand names are:
In the U.S.—

| | | | |
|---|---|---|---|
| Anaspaz[8] | Cystospaz-M[8] | Levsinex Timecaps[8] | Pro-Banthine[15] |
| Antispas[5] | Darbid[9] | Levsin S/L[8] | Quarzan[4] |
| A-Spas[5] | Daricon[13] | Neoquess[5,8] | Robinul[6] |
| Banthine[11] | Di-Spaz[5] | Norpanth[15] | Robinul Forte[6] |
| Bentyl[5] | Gastrosed[8] | Or-Tyl[5] | Spasmoject[5] |
| Cantil[10] | Homapin[7] | Pamine[12] | Transderm-Scōp[16] |
| Cystospaz[8] | Levsin[8] | Pathilon[17] | Valpin 50[1] |

In Canada—
Bentylol[5]                          Pro-Banthine[15]
Buscopan[16]                         Propanthel[15]
Formulex[5]                          Robinul[6]
Gastrozepin[14]                      Robinul Forte[6]
Levsin[8]                            Spasmoban[5]
Lomine[5]                            Transderm-V[16]

Other commonly used names are:
dicycloverine[5]                     hyoscine methobromide[12]
glycopyrronium bromide[6]            methanthelinium[11]
hyoscine hydrobromide[16]            octatropine[1]

Note: For quick reference, the following anticholinergics/antispasmodics are numbered to match the corresponding brand names.

This information applies to the following medicines:
1. Anisotropine (an-iss-oh-TROE-peen)†‡
2. Atropine (A-troe-peen)‡§
3. Belladonna (bell-a-DON-a)†‡
4. Clidinium (kli-DI-nee-um)†
5. Dicyclomine (dye-SYE-kloe-meen)‡
6. Glycopyrrolate (glye-koe-PYE-roe-late)‡
7. Homatropine (hoe-MA-troe-peen)†
8. Hyoscyamine (hye-oh-SYE-a-meen)
9. Isopropamide (eye-soe-PROE-pa-mide)†
10. Mepenzolate (me-PEN-zoe-late)†
11. Methantheline (meth-AN-tha-leen)†
12. Methscopolamine (meth-skoe-POL-a-meen)†
13. Oxyphencyclimine (ox-i-fen-SYE-kli-meen)†
14. Pirenzepine (peer-EN-ze-peen)*
15. Propantheline (proe-PAN-the-leen)‡
16. Scopolamine (scoe-POL-a-meen)‡
17. Tridihexethyl (trye-dye-hex-ETH-il)†

---

*Not commercially available in the U.S.
†Not commercially available in Canada.
‡Generic name product may also be available in the U.S.
§Generic name product may also be available in Canada.

---

# Description

The anticholinergics/antispasmodics are a group of medicines that include the natural belladonna alkaloids (atropine, belladonna, hyoscyamine, and scopolamine) and related products.

The anticholinergics/antispasmodics are used to relieve cramps or spasms of the stomach, intestines, and bladder. Some are used together with antacids or other medicine in the treatment of peptic ulcer. Others are used to prevent nausea, vomiting, and motion sickness.

Anticholinergics/antispasmodics are also used in certain surgical and emergency procedures. In surgery, some are given by injection before anesthesia to help relax you and to decrease secretions, such as saliva. During anesthesia and surgery, atropine, glycopyrrolate, hyoscyamine, and scopolamine are used to help keep the heartbeat normal. Atropine is also given by injection to help relax the stomach and intestines for certain types of examinations. Some anticholinergics are also used to treat poisoning caused by medicines such as neostigmine and physostigmine, certain types of mushrooms, and poisoning by "nerve" gases or organic phosphorous pesticides (for example, demeton [Systox], diazinon, malathion, parathion, and ronnel [Trolene]). Also, anticholinergics can be used for painful menstruation, runny nose, and to prevent urination during sleep.

These medicines may also be used for other conditions as determined by your doctor.

The anticholinergics/antispasmodics are available only with your doctor's prescription in the following dosage forms:

*Oral*
Anisotropine
• Tablets (U.S.)
Atropine
• Tablets (U.S.)
• Soluble tablets (U.S.)
Belladonna
• Tincture (U.S.)
Clidinium
• Capsules (U.S.)
Dicyclomine
• Capsules (U.S. and Canada)
• Syrup (U.S. and Canada)
• Tablets (U.S. and Canada)
• Extended-release Tablets (Canada)
Glycopyrrolate
• Tablets (U.S. and Canada)
Homatropine
• Tablets (U.S.)
Hyoscyamine
• Extended-release capsules (U.S.)
• Elixir (U.S.)
• Oral solution (U.S. and Canada)
• Tablets (U.S.)
Isopropamide
• Tablets (U.S.)
Mepenzolate
• Tablets (U.S.)
Methantheline
• Tablets (U.S.)
Methscopolamine
• Tablets (U.S.)
Oxyphencyclimine
• Tablets (U.S.)
Pirenzepine
• Tablets (Canada)
Propantheline
• Tablets (U.S. and Canada)
Scopolamine
• Tablets (Canada)
Tridihexethyl
• Tablets (U.S.)

*Parenteral*
Atropine
• Injection (U.S. and Canada)
Dicyclomine
• Injection (U.S. and Canada)
Glycopyrrolate
• Injection (U.S. and Canada)
Hyoscyamine
• Injection (U.S. and Canada)
Scopolamine
• Injection (U.S. and Canada)

*Rectal*
Scopolamine
• Suppositories (Canada)

*Transdermal*
Scopolamine
• Transdermal disk (U.S. and Canada)

---

## Before Using This Medicine

In deciding to use a medicine, the risks of taking the medicine must be weighed against the good it will do. This is a decision you and your doctor will make. For anticholinergics/antispasmodics the following should be considered:

**Allergies**—Tell your doctor if you have ever had any unusual or allergic reaction to any of the natural belladonna alkaloids (atropine, belladonna, hyoscyamine, and scopolamine), iodine or iodides, or any related products. Also, tell your health care professional if you are allergic to any other substances, such as foods, preservatives, or dyes.

**Pregnancy**—If you are pregnant or if you may become pregnant, make sure your doctor knows if your medicine contains any of the following:

- *Atropine*—Atropine has not been shown to cause birth defects or other problems in animals. However, when injected into humans during pregnancy, atropine has been reported to increase the heartbeat of the fetus.
- *Belladonna*—Studies on effects in pregnancy have not been done in either humans or animals.
- *Clidinium*—Clidinium has not been studied in pregnant women. However, clidinium has not been shown to cause birth defects or other problems in animal studies.
- *Dicyclomine*—Dicyclomine has been associated with a few cases of human birth defects but dicyclomine has not been confirmed as the cause.
- *Glycopyrrolate*—Glycopyrrolate has not been studied in pregnant women. However, glycopyrrolate did not cause birth defects in animal studies, but did decrease the chance of becoming pregnant and in the newborn's chance of surviving after weaning.
- *Hyoscyamine*—Studies on effects in pregnancy have not been done in either humans or animals. However, when injected into humans during pregnancy, hyoscyamine has been reported to increase the heartbeat of the fetus.
- *Isopropamide*—Studies on effects in pregnancy have not been done in either humans or animals.
- *Mepenzolate*—Mepenzolate has not been studied in pregnant women. However, studies in animals have not shown that mepenzolate causes birth defects or other problems.
- *Propantheline*—Studies on effects in pregnancy have not been done in either humans or animals.
- *Scopolamine*—Studies on effects in pregnancy have not been done in either humans or animals.

**Breast-feeding**—Although these medicines may pass into the breast milk, they have not been reported to cause problems in nursing babies. However, the flow of breast milk may be reduced in some patients. The use of dicyclomine in nursing mothers has been reported to cause breathing problems in infants.

**Children**—Unusual excitement, nervousness, restlessness, or irritability and unusual warmth, dryness, and flushing of skin are more likely to occur in children, who are usually more sensitive to the effects of anticholinergics. Also, when anticholinergics are given to children during hot weather, a rapid increase in body temperature may occur. In infants and children, especially those with spastic paralysis or brain damage, this medicine may be more likely to cause severe side effects. Shortness of breath or difficulty in breathing has occurred in children taking dicyclomine.

**Older adults**—Confusion or memory loss; constipation; difficult urination; drowsiness; dryness of mouth, nose, throat, or skin; and unusual excitement, nervousness, restlessness, or irritability may be more likely to occur in the elderly, who are usually more sensitive than younger adults to the effects of anticholinergics. Also, eye pain may occur, which may be a sign of glaucoma.

**Other medicines**—Although certain medicines should not be used together at all, in other cases two different medicines may be used together even if an interaction might occur. In these cases, your doctor may want to change the dose, or other precautions may be necessary. When you are taking anticholinergics/antispasmodics, it is especially important that your health care professional know if you are taking any of the following:

- Antacids or
- Diarrhea medicine containing kaolin or attapulgite or
- Ketoconazole (e.g., Nizoral)—Using these medicines with an anticholinergic may lessen the effects of the anticholinergic
- Central nervous system (CNS) depressants (medicines that cause drowsiness)—Taking scopolamine with CNS depressants may increase the effects of either medicine
- Other anticholinergics (medicine for abdominal or stomach spasms or cramps) or
- Tricyclic antidepressants (amitriptyline [e.g., Elavil], amoxapine [e.g., Asendin], clomipramine [e.g., Anafranil], desipramine [e.g., Pertofrane], doxepin [e.g., Sinequan], imipramine [e.g., Tofranil], nortriptyline [e.g., Aventyl], protriptyline [e.g., Vivactil], trimipramine [e.g., Surmontil])—Taking anticholinergics with tricyclic antidepressants or other anticholinergics may cause an increase in the effects of the anticholinergic
- Potassium chloride (e.g., Kay Ciel)—Using this medicine with an anticholinergic may make gastrointestinal problems caused by potassium worse

**Other medical problems**—The presence of other medical problems may affect the use of anticholinergics/antispasmodics. Make sure you tell your doctor if you have any other medical problems, especially:

- Bleeding problems (severe)—These medicines may increase heart rate, which would make bleeding problems worse
- Brain damage (in children)—May increase the CNS effects of this medicine
- Colitis (severe) or
- Dryness of mouth (severe and continuing) or
- Enlarged prostate or
- Fever or
- Glaucoma or

- Heart disease or
- Hernia (hiatal) or
- High blood pressure (hypertension) or
- Intestinal blockage or other intestinal problems or
- Lung disease (chronic) or
- Myasthenia gravis or
- Toxemia of pregnancy or
- Urinary tract blockage or difficult urination—These medicines may make these conditions worse
- Down's syndrome (mongolism)—These medicines may cause an increase in pupil dilation and heart rate
- Kidney disease or
- Liver disease—Higher blood levels may occur and cause an increase in side effects
- Overactive thyroid—These medicines may further increase heart rate
- Spastic paralysis (in children)—This condition may increase the effects of the anticholinergic

## Proper Use of This Medicine

*Take this medicine only as directed.* Do not take more of it, do not take it more often, and do not take it for a longer time than your doctor ordered. To do so may increase the chance of side effects.

**Missed dose**—If you miss a dose of this medicine, take it as soon as possible. However, if it is almost time for your next dose, skip the missed dose and go back to your regular dosing schedule. Do not double doses.

For patients *taking any of these medicines by mouth:*
- Take this medicine 30 minutes to 1 hour before meals unless otherwise directed by your doctor.

To use the *rectal suppository* form of *scopolamine:*
- If the suppository is too soft to insert, chill it in the refrigerator for 30 minutes or run cold water over it before removing the foil wrapper.
- To insert the suppository: First remove the foil wrapper and moisten the suppository with cold water. Lie down on your side and use your finger to push the suppository well up into the rectum.

To use the *transdermal disk* form of *scopolamine:*
- This medicine usually comes with patient directions. Read them carefully before using this medicine.
- Wash and dry your hands thoroughly before and after handling.
- Apply the disk to the hairless area of skin behind the ear. Do not place over any cuts or irritations.

**Storage**—To store this medicine:
- Keep out of the reach of children. Overdose is especially dangerous in young children.
- Store away from heat and direct light.
- Do not store the capsule or tablet form of this medicine in the bathroom, near the kitchen sink, or in other damp places. Heat or moisture may cause the medicine to break down.
- Keep the liquid form of this medicine tightly closed and keep it from freezing. Do not refrigerate the syrup form of this medicine.
- Do not keep outdated medicine or medicine no longer needed. Be sure that any discarded medicine is out of the reach of children.

## Precautions While Using This Medicine

*If you think you or someone else may have taken an overdose, get emergency help at once.* Taking an overdose of any of the belladonna alkaloids or taking scopolamine with alcohol or other CNS depressants may lead to unconsciousness and possibly death. Some signs of overdose are clumsiness or unsteadiness; dizziness; severe drowsiness; fever; hallucinations (seeing, hearing, or feeling things that are not there); confusion; shortness of breath or troubled breathing; slurred speech; unusual excitement, nervousness, restlessness, or irritability; fast heartbeat; and unusual warmth, dryness, and flushing of skin.

These medicines may make you sweat less, causing your body temperature to increase. *Use extra care not to become overheated during exercise or hot weather while you are taking this medicine,* since overheating may result in heat stroke. Also, hot baths or saunas may make you dizzy or faint while you are taking this medicine.

*Check with your doctor before you stop using this medicine.* Your doctor may want you to reduce gradually the amount you are using before stopping completely. Stopping this medicine may cause withdrawal side effects such as vomiting, sweating, and dizziness.

Anticholinergics may cause some people to have blurred vision. *Make sure your vision is clear before you drive or do anything else that could be dangerous if you are not able to see well.* These medicines may also cause your eyes to become more sensitive to light than they are normally. Wearing sunglasses may help lessen the discomfort from bright light.

These medicines, especially in high doses, may cause some people to become dizzy or drowsy. *Make sure you know how you react to this medicine before you drive, use machines, or do anything else that could be dangerous if you are dizzy or are not alert.*

Dizziness, lightheadedness, or fainting may occur, especially when you get up from a lying or sitting position. Getting up slowly may help lessen this problem.

These medicines may cause dryness of the mouth, nose, and throat. For temporary relief of mouth dryness, use sugarless candy or gum, melt bits of ice in your mouth, or use a saliva substitute. However, if your mouth continues to feel dry for more than 2 weeks, check with your medical doctor or dentist. Continuing dryness of the mouth may increase the chance of dental disease, including tooth decay, gum disease, and fungus infections.

For patients taking *isopropamide:*
- Make sure your doctor knows if you are planning to have any future thyroid tests. The results of the thyroid test may be affected by the iodine in this medicine.

For patients taking *scopolamine:*
* This medicine will add to the effects of alcohol and other CNS depressants (medicines that slow down the nervous system, possibly causing drowsiness). Some examples of CNS depressants are antihistamines or medicine for hay fever, other allergies, or colds; sedatives, tranquilizers, or sleeping medicine; prescription pain medicine or narcotics; barbiturates; medicine for seizures; muscle relaxants; or anesthetics, including some dental anesthetics. *Check with your doctor before taking any of the above while you are using this medicine.*

For patients *taking any of these medicines by mouth:*
* Do not take this medicine within 2 or 3 hours of taking antacids or medicine for diarrhea. Taking antacids or antidiarrhea medicines and this medicine too close together may prevent this medicine from working properly.

## Side Effects of This Medicine

Along with its needed effects, a medicine may cause some unwanted effects. Although not all of these side effects may occur, if they do occur they may need medical attention.

Check with your doctor as soon as possible if any of the following side effects occur:

*Rare*
> Confusion (especially in the elderly); dizziness, lightheadedness (continuing), or fainting; eye pain; skin rash or hives

*Symptoms of overdose*
> Blurred vision (continuing) or changes in near vision; clumsiness or unsteadiness; confusion; convulsions (seizures); difficulty in breathing, muscle weakness (severe), or tiredness (severe); dizziness; drowsiness (severe); dryness of mouth, nose, or throat (severe); fast heartbeat; fever; hallucinations (seeing, hearing, or feeling things that are not there); slurred speech; unusual excitement, nervousness, restlessness, or irritability; unusual warmth, dryness, and flushing of skin

Other side effects may occur that usually do not need medical attention. These side effects may go away during treatment as your body adjusts to the medicine. However, check with your doctor if any of the following side effects continue or are bothersome:

*More common*
> Constipation (less common with hyoscyamine); decreased sweating; dryness of mouth, nose, throat, or skin

*Less common or rare*
> Bloated feeling; blurred vision; decreased flow of breast milk; difficult urination; difficulty in swallowing; drowsiness (more common with high doses of any of these medicines and with usual doses of scopolamine when given by mouth or by injection); false sense of well-being (for scopolamine only); headache; increased sensitivity of eyes to light; lightheadedness (with injection); loss of memory; nausea or vomiting; redness or other signs of irritation at place of injection; trouble in sleeping (for scopolamine only); unusual tiredness or weakness

For patients using *scopolamine:*
* After you stop using scopolamine, your body may need time to adjust. The length of time this takes depends on the amount of scopolamine you were using and how long you used it. During this period of time check with your doctor if you notice any of the following side effects:
> Anxiety; irritability; nightmares; trouble in sleeping

For patients using the *transdermal disk* of *scopolamine:*
* While using the disk or even after removing it, your eyes may become more sensitive to light than usual. You may also notice the pupil in one eye is larger than the other. Check with your doctor if this side effect continues or is bothersome.

Other side effects not listed above may also occur in some patients. If you notice any other effects, check with your doctor.

## Additional Information

Once a medicine has been approved for marketing for a certain use, experience may show that it is also useful for other medical problems. Although these uses are not included in product labeling, anticholinergics/antispasmodics are used in certain patients with the following medical conditions:
* Diarrhea
* Excessive watering of mouth

Other than the above information, there is no additional information relating to proper use, precautions, or side effects for these uses.

Revised: 01/29/92

---

# ANTICOAGULANTS  Systemic

Some commonly used brand names are:

**In the U.S.—**
| | |
|---|---|
| Coumadin[3] | Panwarfin[3] |
| Miradon[1] | Sofarin[3] |

**In Canada—**
| | |
|---|---|
| Coumadin[3] | Warfilone[3] |

Note: For quick reference, the following anticoagulants are numbered to match the corresponding brand names.

This information applies to the following medicines:
1. Anisindione (an-iss-in-DYE-one)[†]
2. Dicumarol (dye-KOO-ma-role)[†‡]
3. Warfarin (WAR-far-in)[‡]

This information does *not* apply to heparin.

[†]Not commercially available in Canada.
[‡]Generic name product may also be available in the U.S.

# Description

Anticoagulants decrease the clotting ability of the blood and therefore help to prevent harmful clots from forming in the blood vessels. These medicines are sometimes called blood thinners, although they do not actually thin the blood. They also will not dissolve clots that already have formed, but they may prevent the clots from becoming larger and causing more serious problems. They are often used as treatment for certain blood vessel, heart, and lung conditions.

In order for an anticoagulant to help you without causing serious bleeding, it must be used properly and all of the precautions concerning its use must be followed exactly. Be sure that you have discussed the use of this medicine with your doctor. It is very important that you understand all of your doctor's orders and that you are willing and able to follow them exactly.

Anticoagulants are available only with your doctor's prescription, in the following dosage forms:

*Oral*
   Anisindione
   • Tablets (U.S.)
   Dicumarol
   • Tablets (U.S.)
   Warfarin
   • Tablets (U.S. and Canada)
*Parenteral*
   Warfarin
   • Injection (U.S.)

# Before Using This Medicine

In deciding to use a medicine, the risks of taking the medicine must be weighed against the good it will do. This is a decision you and your doctor will make. For anticoagulants, the following should be considered:

**Allergies**—Tell your doctor if you have ever had any unusual or allergic reaction to an anticoagulant. Also tell your health care professional if you are allergic to any other substances, such as foods, preservatives, or dyes.

**Pregnancy**—Anticoagulants may cause birth defects. They may also cause other problems affecting the physical or mental growth of the fetus or newborn baby. In addition, use of this medicine during the last 6 months of pregnancy may increase the chance of severe, possibly fatal, bleeding in the fetus. If taken during the last few weeks of pregnancy, anticoagulants may cause severe bleeding in both the fetus and the mother before or during delivery and in the newborn infant.

*Do not begin taking this medicine during pregnancy, and do not become pregnant while taking it,* unless you have first discussed the possible effects of this medicine with your doctor. Also, if you suspect that you may be pregnant and you are already taking an anticoagulant, check with your doctor at once. Your doctor may suggest that you take a different anticoagulant that is less likely to harm the fetus or the newborn infant during all or part of your pregnancy. Anticoagulants may also cause severe

bleeding in the mother if taken soon after the baby is born.

**Breast-feeding**—Warfarin is not likely to cause problems in nursing babies. Other anticoagulants may pass into the breast milk. A blood test can be done to see if unwanted effects are occurring in the nursing baby. If necessary, another medicine that will overcome any unwanted effects of the anticoagulant can be given to the baby.

**Children**—Very young babies may be especially sensitive to the effects of anticoagulants. This may increase the chance of bleeding during treatment.

**Older adults**—Elderly people are especially sensitive to the effects of anticoagulants. This may increase the chance of bleeding during treatment.

**Other medicines**—Although certain medicines should not be used together at all, in other cases two different medicines may be used together even if an interaction might occur. In these cases, your doctor may want to change the dose, or other precautions may be necessary. *Many different medicines can affect the way anticoagulants work in your body.* Therefore, it is very important that your health care professional knows if you are taking *any* other prescription or nonprescription (over-the-counter [OTC]) medicine, even aspirin, laxatives, vitamins, or antacids.

**Other medical problems**—The presence of other medical problems may affect the use of anticoagulants. Make sure you tell your doctor if you have *any* other medical problems, or if you are now being treated by any other medical doctor or dentist. Many medical problems and treatments will affect the way your body responds to this medicine.

Also, it is important that you tell your doctor if you have recently had any of the following conditions or medical procedures:

   • Childbirth or
   • Falls or blows to the body or head or
   • Fever lasting more than a couple of days or
   • Heavy or unusual menstrual bleeding or
   • Insertion of intrauterine device (IUD) or
   • Medical or dental surgery or
   • Severe or continuing diarrhea or
   • Spinal anesthesia or
   • X-ray (radiation) treatment—The risk of serious bleeding may be increased

# Proper Use of This Medicine

*Take this medicine only as directed by your doctor.* Do not take more or less of it, do not take it more often, and do not take it for a longer time than your doctor ordered. This is especially important for elderly patients, who are especially sensitive to the effects of anticoagulants.

*Your doctor should check your progress at regular visits.* A blood test must be taken regularly to see how fast your blood is clotting. This will help your doctor decide on the proper amount of anticoagulant you should be taking each day.

**Dosing**—The dose of these medicines will be different for different patients. *Follow your doctor's orders or the directions on the label.* The following information includes only the average doses of these medicines. *If your dose is different, do not change it* unless your doctor tells you to do so.

*For anisindione*
- For *oral* dosage form (tablets):
  —For preventing harmful blood clots:
    • Adults and teenagers—The usual dose is 25 to 250 milligrams (mg) per day.
    • Children—Dose must be determined by your doctor.

*For dicumarol*
- For *oral* dosage form (tablets):
  —For preventing harmful blood clots:
    • Adults and teenagers—The usual dose is 25 to 200 milligrams (mg) per day.
    • Children—Dose must be determined by your doctor.

*For warfarin*
- For *oral* dosage form (tablets):
  —For preventing harmful blood clots:
    • Adults and teenagers—The starting dose is usually 10 to 15 milligrams (mg) per day for two to four days. Then, your doctor may decrease the dose to 2 to 10 mg per day, depending on your condition.
    • Children—Dose must be determined by your doctor.
- For *injection* dosage form:
  —For preventing harmful blood clots:
    • Adults and teenagers—The starting dose is usually 10 to 15 mg, injected into a muscle or a vein, once a day for two to four days. Then, your doctor may decrease the dose to 2 to 10 mg per day, depending on your condition.
    • Children—Dose must be determined by your doctor.

**Missed dose**—If you miss a dose of this medicine, take it as soon as possible. Then go back to your regular dosing schedule. If you do not remember until the next day, do not take the missed dose at all and do not double the next one. *Doubling the dose may cause bleeding.* Instead, go back to your regular dosing schedule. It is recommended that you keep a record of each dose as you take it to avoid mistakes. Also, be sure to give your doctor a record of any doses you miss. If you have any questions about this, check with your doctor.

**Storage**—To store this medicine:
- Keep out of the reach of children.
- Store away from heat and direct light.
- Do not store this medicine in the bathroom, near the kitchen sink, or in other damp places. Heat or moisture may cause the medicine to break down.
- Do not keep outdated medicine or medicine no longer needed. Be sure that any discarded medicine is out of the reach of children.

## Precautions While Using This Medicine

*Tell all medical doctors, dentists, and pharmacists you go to that you are taking this medicine.*

*Check with your health care professional before you start or stop taking any other medicine.* This includes any nonprescription (over-the-counter [OTC]) medicine, even aspirin or acetaminophen. Many medicines change the way this medicine affects your body. You may not be able to take the other medicine, or the dose of your anticoagulant may need to be changed.

*It is important that you carry identification stating that you are using this medicine.* If you have any questions about what kind of identification to carry, check with your health care professional.

While you are taking this medicine, it is very important that you avoid sports and activities that may cause you to be injured. Report to your doctor any falls, blows to the body or head, or other injuries, since serious internal bleeding may occur without your knowing about it.

Be careful to avoid cutting yourself. This includes taking special care in brushing your teeth and in shaving. Use a soft toothbrush and floss gently. Also, it is best to use an electric shaver rather than a blade.

Drinking too much alcohol may change the way this anticoagulant affects your body. You should not drink regularly on a daily basis or take more than 1 or 2 drinks at any time. If you have any questions about this, check with your doctor.

The foods that you eat may also affect the way this medicine affects your body. Eat a normal, balanced diet while you are taking this medicine. Do not go on a reducing diet, make other changes in your eating habits, start taking vitamins, or begin using other nutrition supplements unless you have first checked with your health care professional. Also, check with your doctor if you are unable to eat for several days or if you have continuing stomach upset, diarrhea, or fever. These precautions are important because the effects of the anticoagulant depend on the amount of vitamin K in your body. Therefore, it is best to have the same amount of vitamin K in your body every day. Some multiple vitamins and some nutrition supplements contain vitamin K. Vitamin K is also present in meats, dairy products (such as milk, cheese, and yogurt), and green, leafy vegetables (such as broccoli, cabbage, collard greens, kale, lettuce, and spinach). It is especially important that you do not make large changes in the amounts of these foods that you eat every day while you are taking an anticoagulant.

After you stop taking this medicine, your body will need time to recover before your blood clotting ability returns to normal. Your health care professional can tell you how long this will take depending on which anticoagulant you were taking. Use the same caution during this period of time as you did while you were taking the anticoagulant.

## Side Effects of This Medicine

Along with its needed effects, a medicine may cause some unwanted effects. Although not all of these side effects may occur, if they do occur they may need medical attention.

*Check with your doctor immediately* if any of the following side effects occur:

*Less common or rare*
> Blue or purple color of toes and pain in toes; cloudy or dark urine; difficult or painful urination; sores, ulcers, or white spots in mouth or throat; sore throat and fever or chills; sudden decrease in amount of urine; swelling of face, feet, or lower legs; unusual tiredness or weakness; unusual weight gain; yellow eyes or skin

Since many things can affect the way your body reacts to this medicine, you should always watch for signs of unusual bleeding. Unusual bleeding may mean that your body is getting more medicine than it needs. *Check with your doctor immediately if any of the following signs of overdose occur:*

> Bleeding from gums when brushing teeth; unexplained bruising or purplish areas on skin; unexplained nosebleeds; unusually heavy bleeding or oozing from cuts or wounds; unusually heavy or unexpected menstrual bleeding

*Signs and symptoms of bleeding inside the body*
> Abdominal or stomach pain or swelling; back pain or backaches; blood in urine; bloody or black tarry stools; constipation; coughing up blood; dizziness; headache (severe or continuing); joint pain, stiffness, or swelling; vomiting blood or material that looks like coffee grounds

Also, check with your doctor as soon as possible if any of the following side effects occur:

*Less common or rare*
> Diarrhea (more common with dicumarol); nausea or vomiting; skin rash, hives, or itching; stomach cramps or pain

For patients taking *anisindione* (e.g., Miradon):
- Depending on your diet, this medicine may cause your urine to turn orange. Since it may be hard to tell the difference between blood in the urine and this normal color change, check with your doctor if you notice any color change in your urine.

Other side effects may occur that usually do not need medical attention. These side effects may go away during treatment as your body adjusts to the medicine. However, check with your doctor if any of the following side effects continue or are bothersome:

*More common*
> Bloated feeling or gas (with dicumarol)

*Less common*
> Blurred vision or other vision problems (with anisindione); loss of appetite; unusual hair loss

Other side effects not listed above may also occur in some patients. If you notice any other effects, check with your doctor.

Revised: June 1990
Interim revision: 07/28/94

# ANTICONVULSANTS, DIONE  Systemic†

Some commonly used brand names are:
**In the U.S.—**
Paradione[1]     Tridione Dulcets[2]
Tridione[2]

Note: For quick reference, the following dione anticonvulsants are numbered to match the corresponding brand names.
This information applies to the following medicines:
1. Paramethadione (par-a-meth-a-DYE-one)†
2. Trimethadione (trye-meth-a-DYE-one)†

†Not commercially available in Canada.

## Description

Dione anticonvulsants are used to control certain types of seizures in the treatment of epilepsy. These medicines act on the central nervous system (CNS) to reduce the number of seizures.

This medicine is available only with your doctor's prescription in the following dosage forms:
*Oral*
Paramethadione
- Capsules (U.S.)

Trimethadione
- Capsules (U.S.)
- Oral solution (U.S.)
- Tablets (U.S.)

## Before Using This Medicine

In deciding to use a medicine, the risks of taking the medicine must be weighed against the good it will do. This is a decision you and your doctor will make. For dione anticonvulsants, the following should be considered:

**Allergies**—Tell your doctor if you have ever had any unusual or allergic reaction to anticonvulsant medicines. Also tell your health care professional if you are allergic to any other substances, such as foods, preservatives, or dyes.

**Pregnancy**—There have been reports of increased birth defects when dione anticonvulsants were used during pregnancy. The use of an effective method of birth control is recommended during treatment with dione anticonvulsants. Be sure you have discussed this with your doctor before taking this medicine. Dione anticonvulsants may also cause a bleeding problem in the mother during delivery and in the newborn. Doctors can help prevent this by giving vitamin K to the mother during delivery, and to the baby immediately after birth.

**Breast-feeding**—It is not known whether this medicine passes into breast milk.

**Children**—Although there is no specific information comparing use of dione anticonvulsants in children with use in other age groups, these medicines are not expected to cause different side effects or problems in children than they do in adults.

**Older adults**—Many medicines have not been studied specifically in older people. Therefore, it may not be known whether they work exactly the same way they do in younger adults. Although there is no specific information comparing use of dione anticonvulsants in the elderly with use in other age groups, these medicines are not expected to cause different side effects or problems in older people than they do in younger adults.

**Other medicines**—Although certain medicines should not be used together at all, in other cases 2 different medicines may be used together even if an interaction might occur. In these cases, your doctor may want to change the dose, or other precautions may be necessary. When you are taking dione anticonvulsants, it is especially important that your health care professional know if you are taking any of the following:

- Central nervous system (CNS) depressants (medicine that causes drowsiness) or
- Tricyclic antidepressants (medicine for depression)—Using these medicines together may increase the CNS depressant effects

**Other medical problems**—The presence of other medical problems may affect the use of the dione anticonvulsants. Make sure you tell your doctor if you have any other medical problems, especially:

- Blood disease (severe) or
- Diseases of the eye or optic nerve or
- Kidney disease (severe) or
- Liver disease (severe)—Dione anticonvulsants may make the condition worse
- Porphyria—Trimethadione may make the condition worse

## Proper Use of This Medicine

For patients taking *paramethadione capsules:*

- Swallow the capsules whole. Do not crush, chew, or break them before swallowing.

For patients taking *trimethadione tablets:*

- The tablets may be chewed or crushed and dissolved in a small amount of water before they are swallowed.

If this medicine upsets your stomach, take it with a small amount of food or milk unless otherwise directed by your doctor.

*This medicine must be taken every day in regularly spaced doses as ordered by your doctor.*

**Dosing**—The dose of dione anticonvulsants will be different for different patients. *Follow your doctor's orders or the directions on the label.* The following information includes only the average doses of paramethadione and trimethadione. *If your dose is different, do not change it* unless your doctor tells you to do so.

*For paramethadione*

- For *oral* dosage forms (capsules):
  —Adults and adolescents: To start, 300 milligrams three or four times a day. Your doctor may increase your dose by 300 milligrams every week until seizures are controlled or side effects appear.
  —Children 6 years of age and over: 300 milligrams three times a day.
  —Children 2 to 6 years of age: 200 milligrams three times a day.
  —Children up to 2 years of age: 100 milligrams three times a day.

*For trimethadione*

- For *oral* dosage forms (capsules, solution, tablets):
  —Adults and adolescents: To start, 300 milligrams three or four times a day. Your doctor may increase your dose by 300 milligrams every week until seizures are controlled or side effects appear.
  —Children 6 years of age and over: 300 milligrams three or four times a day.
  —Children 2 to 6 years of age: 200 milligrams three times a day.
  —Children up to 2 years of age: 100 milligrams three times a day.

**Missed dose**—If you miss a dose of this medicine, take it as soon as possible. However, if it is almost time for your next dose, skip the missed dose and go back to your regular dosing schedule. If only one dose is missed, it may be taken at bedtime.

**Storage**—To store this medicine:

- Keep out of the reach of children.
- Store away from heat and direct light.
- Do not store the capsule or tablet form of this medicine in the bathroom, near the kitchen sink, or in other damp places. Heat or moisture may cause the medicine to break down.
- Keep the liquid form of this medicine from freezing.
- Do not keep outdated medicine or medicine no longer needed. Be sure that any discarded medicine is out of the reach of children.

## Precautions While Using This Medicine

*It is very important that your doctor check your progress at regular visits, especially during the first few months of treatment with this medicine.*

*If you have been taking this medicine regularly, do not stop taking it without first checking with your doctor.* Your doctor may want you to reduce gradually the amount you are taking before stopping completely. Stopping this medicine suddenly may cause seizures.

This medicine may cause your eyes to become more sensitive to bright light than they are normally, making it difficult for you to see well. Wearing sunglasses and avoiding too much exposure to bright light may help lessen the discomfort. You may also have difficulty seeing in light that changes in brightness. If you notice this effect, be especially careful when driving at night.

This medicine will add to the effects of alcohol and other CNS depressants (medicines that slow down the nervous system, possibly causing drowsiness). Some examples of CNS depressants are antihistamines or medicine for hay fever, other allergies, or colds; sedatives, tranquilizers, or sleeping medicine; prescription pain medicine or narcotics; barbiturates; medicine for seizures; muscle relaxants; or anesthetics, including some dental anesthetics. *Check with your doctor before taking any of the above while you are using this medicine.*

This medicine may cause some people to become drowsy or less alert than they are normally. *Make sure you know how you react to this medicine before you drive, use machines, or do anything else that could be dangerous if you are not alert.* After you have taken this medicine for a while, this effect may not be so bothersome.

*Before having any kind of surgery, dental treatment, or emergency treatment, tell the medical doctor or dentist in charge that you are taking this medicine.* Taking dione anticonvulsants together with medicines that are used during surgery or dental or emergency treatments may increase the CNS depressant effects.

*Be sure to tell your doctor as soon as possible if you have a sore throat, fever, or general feeling of tiredness, or if you notice any unusual bleeding or bruising,* such as reddish or purplish spots on the skin, or recurring nosebleeds or bleeding gums.

*Check with your doctor as soon as possible if you suspect you have become pregnant.*

## Side Effects of This Medicine

Along with its needed effects, a medicine may cause some unwanted effects. Although not all of these side effects may occur, if they do occur they may need medical attention.

Check with your doctor as soon as possible if any of the following side effects occur:

*More common*
> Changes in vision, such as glare or snowy image, caused by bright light, or double vision

*Rare*
> Confusion; convulsions (seizures); dark or cloudy urine; dizziness; fever; loss of appetite or weight; muscle weakness (severe), especially drooping eyelids, difficulty in chewing, swallowing, talking, or breathing, and unusual tiredness; nausea or vomiting; pain in abdomen or joints; skin rash or itching; sore throat and fever; swelling of face, hands, legs, and feet; swollen glands; unusual bleeding or bruising, such as recurring nosebleeds, bleeding gums, or vaginal bleeding, or red or purple spots on skin; unusual tiredness or weakness; yellow eyes or skin

*Symptoms of overdose*
> Clumsiness or unsteadiness; dizziness (severe); drowsiness (severe); nausea (severe)

Other side effects may occur that usually do not need medical attention. These side effects may go away during treatment as your body adjusts to the medicine. However, check with your doctor if any of the following side effects continue or are bothersome:

*More common*
> Dizziness; drowsiness; headache; increased sensitivity of eyes to light; irritability

*Less common*
> Behavior or mood changes; blood pressure changes; hair loss; hiccups; stomach pain or upset; tingling, burning, or prickly sensations; trouble in sleeping

Other side effects not listed above may also occur in some patients. If you notice any other effects, check with your doctor.

Revised: 01/29/93

# ANTICONVULSANTS, HYDANTOIN  Systemic

Some commonly used brand names are:

**In the U.S.—**

| | |
|---|---|
| Dilantin[3] | Diphenylan[3] |
| Dilantin-125[3] | Mesantoin[2] |
| Dilantin Infatabs[3] | Peganone[1] |
| Dilantin Kapseals[3] | Phenytex[3] |

**In Canada—**

| | |
|---|---|
| Dilantin[3] | Dilantin Infatabs[3] |
| Dilantin-30[3] | Mesantoin[2] |
| Dilantin-125[3] | |

Another commonly used name for phenytoin is diphenylhydantoin.

Note: For quick reference, the following hydantoin anticonvulsants are numbered to match the corresponding brand names.

This information applies to the following medicines:

1. Ethotoin (ETH-oh-toyn)†
2. Mephenytoin (me-FEN-i-toyn)
3. Phenytoin (FEN-i-toyn)‡

†Not commercially available in Canada.
‡Generic name product may also be available in the U.S.

# Description

Hydantoin anticonvulsants (hye-DAN-toyn an-tye-kon-VUL-sants) are used most often to control certain convulsions or seizures in the treatment of epilepsy. Phenytoin may also be used for other conditions as determined by your doctor.

In seizure disorders, these medicines act on the central nervous system (CNS) to reduce the number and severity of seizures. Hydantoin anticonvulsants may also produce some unwanted effects. These depend on the patient's individual condition, the amount of medicine taken, and how long it has been taken. It is important that you know what the side effects are and when to call your doctor if they occur.

Hydantoin anticonvulsants are available only with your doctor's prescription, in the following dosage forms:

*Oral*
Ethotoin
- Tablets (U.S.)
Mephenytoin
- Tablets (U.S. and Canada)
Phenytoin
- Extended capsules (U.S. and Canada)
- Prompt capsules (U.S.)
- Oral suspension (U.S. and Canada)
- Chewable tablets (U.S. and Canada)

*Parenteral*
Phenytoin
- Injection (U.S. and Canada)

# Before Using This Medicine

In deciding to use a medicine, the risks of taking the medicine must be weighed against the good it will do. This is a decision you and your doctor will make. For hydantoin anticonvulsants, the following should be considered:

**Allergies**—Tell your doctor if you have ever had any unusual or allergic reaction to any hydantoin anticonvulsant medicine. Also tell your health care professional if you are allergic to any other substance, such as foods, preservatives, or dyes.

**Pregnancy**—Although most mothers who take medicine for seizure control deliver normal babies, there have been reports of increased birth defects when these medicines were used during pregnancy. It is not definitely known if any of these medicines are the cause of such problems.

Also, pregnancy may cause a change in the way hydantoin anticonvulsants are absorbed in your body. You may have more seizures, even though you are taking your medicine regularly. Your doctor may need to increase the anticonvulsant dose during your pregnancy.

In addition, when taken during pregnancy, this medicine may cause a bleeding problem in the mother during delivery and in the newborn. This may be prevented by giving vitamin K to the mother during delivery, and to the baby immediately after birth.

**Breast-feeding**—Ethotoin and phenytoin pass into the breast milk in small amounts. It is not known whether mephenytoin passes into breast milk. Be sure you have discussed the risks and benefits of the medicine with your doctor.

**Children**—Some side effects, especially bleeding, tender, or enlarged gums and enlarged facial features, are more likely to occur in children and young adults. Also, unusual and excessive hair growth may occur, which is more noticeable in young girls. In addition, some children may not do as well in school after using high doses of this medicine for a long time.

**Older adults**—Some medicines may affect older patients differently than they do younger patients. Overdose is more likely to occur in elderly patients and in patients with liver disease.

**Other medicines**—Although certain medicines should not be used together at all, in other cases 2 different medicines may be used together even if an interaction might occur. In these cases, your doctor may want to change the dose, or other precautions may be necessary. When you are taking or receiving hydantoin anticonvulsants, it is especially important that your health care professional know if you are taking any of the following:

- Alcohol or
- Central nervous system (CNS) depressants (medicine that causes drowsiness)—Long-term use of alcohol may decrease the blood levels of hydantoin anticonvulsants, resulting in decreased effects; use of hydantoin anticonvulsants in cases where a large amount of alcohol is consumed may increase the blood levels of the hydantoin, resulting in an increased risk of side effects
- Aminophylline (e.g., Somophyllin) or
- Caffeine (e.g., NoDoz) or
- Oxtriphylline (e.g., Choledyl) or
- Theophylline (e.g., Somophyllin-T)—Hydantoin anticonvulsants may make these medicines less effective
- Amiodarone (e.g., Cordarone)—Use with phenytoin and possibly with other hydantoin anticonvulsants may increase blood levels of the hydantoin, resulting in an increase in serious side effects
- Antacids or
- Medicine containing calcium—Use of antacids or calcium supplements may decrease the absorption of phenytoin; doses of antacids and phenytoin or calcium supplements and phenytoin should be taken 2 to 3 hours apart
- Anticoagulants (blood thinners) or
- Chloramphenicol (e.g., Chloromycetin) or
- Cimetidine (e.g., Tagamet) or
- Disulfiram (e.g., Antabuse) (medicine for alcoholism) or
- Isoniazid (INH) (e.g., Nydrazid) or
- Fluconazole (e.g., Diflucan) or
- Fluoxetine (e.g., Prozac) or
- Phenylbutazone (e.g., Butazolidin) or
- Sulfonamides (sulfa drugs)—Blood levels of hydantoin anticonvulsants may be increased, increasing the risk of serious side effects; hydantoin anticonvulsants may increase the effects of the anticoagulants at first, but with continued use may decrease the effects of these medicines

- Corticosteroids (cortisone-like medicines) or
- Estrogens (female hormones) or
- Oral contraceptives (birth-control pills) containing estrogens—Hydantoin anticonvulsants may decrease the effects of these medicines; use of hydantoin anticonvulsants with oral, estrogen-containing contraceptives may result in breakthrough bleeding and contraceptive failure; the amount of estrogen in the oral contraceptive may need to be increased to stop the bleeding and decrease the risk of pregnancy
- Diazoxide (e.g., Proglycem)—Use with hydantoin anticonvulsants may decrease the effects of both medicines; therefore, these medicines should not be taken together
- Lidocaine—Risk of slow heartbeat may be increased. Other effects of lidocaine may be decreased because hydantoin anticonvulsants may cause it to be removed from the body more quickly
- Methadone (e.g., Dolophine, Methadose)—Long-term use of phenytoin may bring on withdrawal symptoms in patients being treated for drug dependence
- Phenacemide (e.g., Phenurone)—Use with hydantoin anticonvulsants may increase the risk of serious side effects
- Rifampin (e.g., Rifadin)—Use with phenytoin may decrease the effects of phenytoin; your doctor may need to adjust your dosage
- Streptozocin (e.g., Zanosar)—Phenytoin may decrease the effects of streptozocin; therefore, these medicines should not be used together
- Sucralfate (e.g., Carafate)—Use of sucralfate may decrease the absorption of hydantoin anticonvulsants
- Valproic acid (e.g., Depakene, Depakote)—Use with phenytoin, and possibly other hydantoin anticonvulsants, may increase seizure frequency and increase the risk of serious liver side effects, especially in infants

**Other medical problems**—The presence of other medical problems may affect the use of hydantoin anticonvulsants. Make sure you tell your doctor if you have any other medical problems, especially:

- Alcohol abuse—Blood levels of phenytoin may be decreased, decreasing its effects
- Blood disease—Risk of serious infections rarely may be increased by hydantoin anticonvulsants
- Diabetes mellitus (sugar diabetes) or
- Porphyria or
- Systemic lupus erythematosus—Hydantoin anticonvulsants may make the condition worse
- Fever above 101 °F for longer than 24 hours—Blood levels of hydantoin anticonvulsants may be decreased, decreasing the medicine's effects
- Heart disease—Administration of phenytoin by injection may change the rhythm of the heart
- Kidney disease or
- Liver disease—Blood levels of hydantoin anticonvulsants may be increased, leading to an increase in serious side effects
- Thyroid disease—Blood levels of thyroid hormones may be decreased

## Proper Use of This Medicine

For patients taking the *liquid form* of this medicine:
- Shake the bottle well before using.

- Use a specially marked measuring spoon, a plastic syringe, or a small measuring cup to measure each dose accurately. The average household teaspoon may not hold the right amount of liquid.

For patients taking the *chewable tablet form* of this medicine:
- Tablets may be chewed or crushed before they are swallowed, or may be swallowed whole.

For patients taking the *capsule form* of this medicine:
- Swallow the capsule whole.

If this medicine upsets your stomach, take it with food, unless otherwise directed by your doctor. The medicine should always be taken at the same time in relation to meals to make sure that it is absorbed in the same way.

To control your medical problem, *take this medicine every day* exactly as ordered by your doctor. Do not take more or less of it than your doctor ordered. To help you remember to take the medicine at the correct times, try to get into the habit of taking it at the same time each day.

**Dosing**—The dose of hydantoin anticonvulsants will be different for different patients. *Follow your doctor's orders or the directions on the label.* The following information includes only the average doses of ethotoin, mephenytoin, and phenytoin. *If your dose is different, do not change it* unless your doctor tells you to do so.

The number of capsules or tablets or teaspoonfuls of suspension that you take depends on the strength of the medicine. Also, *the number of doses you take each day, the time allowed between doses, and the length of time you take the medicine depend on the medical problem for which you are using an hydantoin anticonvulsant.*

*For ethotoin*
- For *oral* dosage form (tablets):
  —As an anticonvulsant:
    - Adults and teenagers—To start, 125 to 250 milligrams (mg) four to six times a day. Your doctor may increase your dose gradually over several days if needed. However, the dose is usually not more than 3000 mg a day.
    - Children—To start, up to 750 mg a day, based on the age and weight of the child. The doctor may increase the dose gradually if needed.

*For mephenytoin*
- For *oral* dosage form (tablets):
  —As an anticonvulsant:
    - Adults and teenagers—To start, 50 to 100 milligrams (mg) once a day. Your doctor may increase your dose by 50 to 100 mg a day at weekly intervals if needed. However, the dose is usually not more than 1200 mg a day.
    - Children—To start, 25 to 50 mg once a day. The doctor may increase the dose by 25 to 50 mg a day at weekly intervals if needed. However, the dose is usually not more than 400 mg a day.

*For phenytoin*
- For *oral* dosage forms (capsules, chewable tablets, or suspension):
  —As an anticonvulsant:
    - Adults and teenagers—To start, 100 to 125 milligrams (mg) three times a day. Your doctor may adjust your dose at intervals of seven to ten days if needed.
    - Children—Dose is based on body weight or body surface area. The usual dose is 5 mg of phenytoin per kilogram (kg) (2.3 mg per pound) of body weight to start. The doctor may adjust the dose if needed.
    - Older adults—Dose is based on body weight. The usual dose is 3 mg per kg (1.4 mg per pound) of body weight. The doctor may need to adjust the dose based on your response to the medicine.
- For *injection* dosage form:
  —As an anticonvulsant:
    - Adults and children—Dose is based on illness being treated, and body weight or body surface area of the patient. The medicine is usually injected into a vein.

**Missed dose**—*If you miss a dose of this medicine* and your dosing schedule is:
- One dose a day—Take the missed dose as soon as possible. However, if you do not remember the missed dose until the next day, skip it and go back to your regular dosing schedule. Do not double doses.
- More than one dose a day—Take the missed dose as soon as possible. However, if it is within 4 hours of your next dose, skip the missed dose and go back to your regular dosing schedule. Do not double doses.

If you miss doses for 2 or more days in a row, check with your doctor.

**Storage**—To store this medicine:
- Keep out of the reach of children.
- Store away from heat and direct light.
- Do not store in the bathroom, near the kitchen sink, or in other damp places. Heat or moisture may cause the medicine to break down.
- Keep the liquid form of this medicine from freezing. Do not refrigerate.
- Do not keep outdated medicine or medicine no longer needed. Be sure any discarded medicine is out of the reach of children.

## Precautions While Using This Medicine

*Your doctor should check your progress at regular visits,* especially during the first few months of treatment with this medicine. During this time the amount of medicine you are taking may have to be changed often to meet your individual needs.

*Do not start or stop taking any other medicine without your doctor's advice. Other medicines may affect the way this medicine works.*

This medicine will add to the effects of alcohol and other CNS depressants (medicines that slow down the nervous system, possibly causing drowsiness). Some examples of CNS depressants are antihistamines or medicine for hay fever, other allergies, or colds; sedatives, tranquilizers, or sleeping medicine; prescription pain medicine or narcotics; barbiturates; other medicine for seizures; muscle relaxants; or anesthetics, including some dental anesthetics. *Check with your doctor before taking any of the above while you are using this medicine.*

Do not take this medicine within 2 to 3 hours of taking antacids or medicine for diarrhea. Taking these medicines and hydantoin anticonvulsants too close together may make the hydantoins less effective.

Do not change brands or dosage forms of phenytoin without first checking with your doctor. Different products may not work the same way. If you refill your medicine and it looks different, check with your pharmacist.

*If you have been taking this medicine regularly for several weeks or more, do not suddenly stop taking it.* Your doctor may want you to reduce gradually the amount you are taking before stopping completely.

Your doctor may want you to carry a medical identification card or bracelet stating that you are taking this medicine.

For diabetic patients:
- This medicine may affect blood sugar levels. If you notice a change in the results of your blood or urine sugar tests or if you have any questions, check with your doctor.

Before you have any medical tests, tell the doctor in charge that you are taking this medicine. The results of some tests (including the dexamethasone, metyrapone, or Schilling tests, and certain thyroid function tests) may be affected by this medicine.

*Before having any kind of surgery, dental treatment, or emergency treatment, tell the medical doctor or dentist in charge that you are taking this medicine.* Taking hydantoin anticonvulsants together with medicines that are used during surgery or dental or emergency treatments may cause increased side effects.

This medicine may cause some people to become dizzy, lightheaded, drowsy, or less alert than they are normally. After you have taken this medicine for a while, this effect may not be so bothersome. However, *make sure you know how you react to this medicine before you drive, use machines, or do anything else that could be dangerous if you are dizzy or are not alert.*

*Oral contraceptives (birth control pills) containing estrogen may not work properly if you take them while you are taking hydantoin anticonvulsants. Unplanned pregnancies may occur. You should use a different or additional means of birth control while you are taking hydantoin anticonvulsants.* If you have any questions about this, check with your health care professional.

For patients taking *phenytoin* or *mephenytoin*:
- In some patients (usually younger patients), tenderness, swelling, or bleeding of the gums (gingival hyperplasia) may appear soon after phenytoin or mephenytoin treatment is started. To help prevent this, brush and floss your teeth carefully and regularly and massage your gums. Also, *see your dentist every 3 months to have your teeth cleaned. If you have any questions about how to take care of your teeth and gums, or if you notice any tenderness, swelling, or bleeding of your gums, check with your doctor or dentist.*

## Side Effects of This Medicine

Along with its needed effects, a medicine may cause some unwanted effects. Although not all of these side effects may occur, if they do occur they may need medical attention.

Check with your doctor as soon as possible if any of the following side effects or signs of overdose occur:

*More common*
> Bleeding, tender, or enlarged gums (rare with ethotoin); clumsiness or unsteadiness; confusion; continuous, uncontrolled back-and-forth and/or rolling eye movements—may be sign of overdose; enlarged glands in neck or underarms; fever; increase in seizures; mood or mental changes; muscle weakness or pain; skin rash or itching; slurred speech or stuttering—may be sign of overdose; sore throat; trembling—may be sign of overdose; unusual excitement, nervousness, or irritability

*Rare*
> Bone malformations; burning pain at place of injection; chest discomfort; chills and fever; dark urine; dizziness; frequent breaking of bones; headache; joint pain; learning difficulties—in children taking high doses for a long time; light gray–colored stools; loss of appetite; nausea or vomiting; pain of penis on erection; restlessness or agitation; slowed growth; stomach pain (severe); troubled or quick, shallow breathing; uncontrolled jerking or twisting movements of hands, arms, or legs; uncontrolled movements of lips, tongue, or cheeks; unusual bleeding (such as nosebleeds) or bruising; unusual tiredness or weakness; weight loss (unusual); yellow eyes or skin

*Rare (with long-term use of phenytoin)*
> Numbness, tingling, or pain in hands or feet

*Symptoms of overdose*
> Blurred or double vision; clumsiness or unsteadiness (severe); confusion (severe); dizziness or drowsiness (severe); staggering walk

Other side effects may occur that usually do not need medical attention. These side effects may go away during treatment as your body adjusts to the medicine. However, check with your doctor if any of the following side effects continue or are bothersome:

*More common*
> Constipation; dizziness (mild); drowsiness (mild)

*Less common*
> Diarrhea (with ethotoin); enlargement of jaw; muscle twitching; swelling of breasts—in males; thickening of lips; trouble in sleeping; unusual and excessive hair growth on body and face (more common with phenytoin); widening of nose tip

Other side effects not listed above may also occur in some patients. If you notice any other effects, check with your doctor.

## Additional Information

Once a medicine has been approved for marketing for a certain use, experience may show that it is also useful for other medical problems. Although these uses are not included in product labeling, phenytoin is used in certain patients with the following medical conditions:
- Cardiac arrhythmias (changes in your heart rhythm) caused by digitalis medicine
- Episodic dyscontrol (certain behavior disorders)
- Myotonia congenita or
- Myotonic muscular dystrophy or
- Neuromyotonia (certain muscle disorders)
- Paroxysmal choreoathetosis (certain movement disorders)
- Tricyclic antidepressant poisoning
- Trigeminal neuralgia (tic douloureux)

Other than the above information, there is no additional information relating to proper use, precautions, or side effects for these uses.

Revised: 03/09/93
Interim revision: 03/24/94; 04/29/94; 05/13/94

# ANTICONVULSANTS, SUCCINIMIDE   Systemic

Some commonly used brand names are:

**In the U.S.—**
Celontin[2]                        Zarontin[1]
Milontin[3]

**In Canada—**
Celontin[2]
Zarontin[1]

Note: For quick reference, the following succinimide anticonvulsants are numbered to match the corresponding brand names.

This information applies to the following medicines:
1. Ethosuximide (eth-oh-SUX-i-mide)‡
2. Methsuximide (meth-SUX-i-mide)
3. Phensuximide (fen-SUX-i-mide)†

†Not commercially available in Canada.
‡Generic name product may also be available in the U.S.

# Description

Succinimide anticonvulsants are used to control certain seizures in the treatment of epilepsy. These medicines act on the central nervous system (CNS) to reduce the number and severity of seizures.

This medicine is available only with your doctor's prescription, in the following dosage forms:

*Oral*
Ethosuximide
- Capsules (U.S. and Canada)
- Syrup (U.S. and Canada)
Methsuximide
- Capsules (U.S. and Canada)
Phensuximide
- Capsules (U.S.)

# Before Using This Medicine

In deciding to use a medicine, the risks of taking the medicine must be weighed against the good it will do. This is a decision you and your doctor will make. For succinimide anticonvulsants, the following should be considered:

**Allergies**—Tell your doctor if you have ever had any unusual or allergic reaction to anticonvulsant medicines. Also tell your health care professional if you are allergic to any other substances, such as foods, preservatives, or dyes.

**Pregnancy**—Although succinimide anticonvulsants have not been shown to cause problems in humans, there have been unproven reports of increased birth defects associated with the use of other anticonvulsant medicines.

**Breast-feeding**—Ethosuximide passes into breast milk. It is not known whether methsuximide or phensuximide passes into breast milk. However, these medicines have not been reported to cause problems in nursing babies.

**Children**—Succinimide anticonvulsants are not expected to cause different side effects or problems in children than they do in adults.

**Older adults**—Many medicines have not been studied specifically in older people. Therefore, it may not be known whether they work exactly the same way they do in younger adults. Although there is no specific information comparing use of succinimide anticonvulsants in the elderly to use in other age groups, they are not expected to cause different side effects or problems in older people than they do in younger adults.

**Other medicines**—Although certain medicines should not be used together at all, in other cases two different medicines may be used together even if an interaction might occur. In these cases, your doctor may want to change the dose, or other precautions may be necessary. When you are taking succinimide anticonvulsants, it is especially important that your health care professional know if you are taking any of the following:

- Central nervous system (CNS) depressants (medicines that cause drowsiness)—Using these medicines together may increase CNS depressant effects

- Haloperidol (e.g., Haldol)—A change in the pattern and/or the frequency of seizures may occur; the dose of either medicine may need to be changed

**Other medical problems**—The presence of other medical problems may affect the use of succinimide anticonvulsants. Make sure you tell your doctor if you have any other medical problems, especially:

- Blood disease or
- Intermittent porphyria or
- Kidney disease (severe) or
- Liver disease—Succinimide anticonvulsants may make the condition worse

# Proper Use of This Medicine

*This medicine must be taken every day in regularly spaced doses as ordered by your doctor.* Do not take more or less of it than your doctor ordered.

If this medicine upsets your stomach, take it with food or milk unless otherwise directed by your doctor.

**Dosing**—The dose of succinimide anticonvulsants will be different for different patients. *Follow your doctor's orders or the directions on the label.* The following information includes only the average doses of ethosuximide, methsuximide, and phensuximide. *If your dose is different, do not change it* unless your doctor tells you to do so.

The number of capsules or teaspoonfuls of syrup that you take depends on the strength of the medicine. Also, *the number of doses you take each day, the time allowed between doses, and the length of time you take the medicine depend on the medical problem for which you are taking a succinimide anticonvulsant.*

*For ethosuximide*
- For *oral* dosage form (capsules or syrup):
  —As an anticonvulsant:
    - Adults and children 6 years of age and over—To start, 250 milligrams (mg) twice a day. Your doctor may increase your dose gradually if needed. However, the dose is usually not more than 1500 mg a day.
    - Children up to 6 years of age—To start, 250 mg once a day. Your doctor may increase your dose gradually if needed. However, the dose is usually not more than 1000 mg a day.

*For methsuximide*
- For *oral* dosage form (capsules):
  —As an anticonvulsant:
    - Adults, teenagers, and children—To start, 300 milligrams (mg) once a day. Your doctor may increase your dose gradually if needed. However, the dose is usually not more than 1200 mg a day.

*For phensuximide*
- For *oral* dosage form (capsules):
  —As an anticonvulsant:
    - Adults, teenagers, and children—To start, 500 milligrams (mg) two or three times a day.

Your doctor may increase your dose gradually if needed. However, the dose is usually not more than 3000 mg a day.

**Missed dose**—If you miss a dose of this medicine, take it as soon as possible. However, if it is within 4 hours of your next dose, skip the missed dose and go back to your regular dosing schedule. Do not double doses.

**Storage**—To store this medicine:
- Keep out of the reach of children.
- Store away from heat and direct light.
- Do not store the capsule form of this medicine in the bathroom, near the kitchen sink, or in other damp places. Heat or moisture may cause the medicine to break down.
- Keep the liquid form of this medicine from freezing. Do not refrigerate.
- Do not keep outdated medicine or medicine that is no longer needed. Be sure any discarded medicine is out of the reach of children.

## Precautions While Using This Medicine

*Your doctor should check your progress at regular visits,* especially during the first few months of treatment with this medicine. During this time the amount of medicine you are taking may have to be changed often to meet your individual needs.

*If you have been taking a succinimide anticonvulsant regularly, do not stop taking it without first checking with your doctor.* Your doctor may want you to reduce gradually the amount you are taking before stopping completely. Stopping this medicine suddenly may cause seizures.

*Do not start or stop taking any other medicine without your doctor's advice.* Other medicines may affect the way this medicine works.

This medicine will add to the effects of alcohol and other CNS depressants (medicines that slow down the nervous system, possibly causing drowsiness). Some examples of CNS depressants are antihistamines or medicine for hay fever, other allergies, or colds; sedatives, tranquilizers, or sleeping medicine; prescription pain medicine or narcotics; barbiturates; medicine for seizures; muscle relaxants; or anesthetics, including some dental anesthetics. *Check with your doctor before taking any of the above while you are using this medicine.*

This medicine may cause some people to become drowsy or less alert than they are normally. *Make sure you know how you react to this medicine before you drive, use machines, or do anything else that could be dangerous if you are not alert.* After you have taken this medicine for a while, this effect may lessen.

*Before having any kind of surgery, dental treatment, or emergency treatment, tell the medical doctor or dentist in charge that you are taking this medicine.* Taking succinimide anticonvulsants together with medicines that are used during surgery or dental or emergency treatments may increase the CNS depressant effects.

Your doctor may want you to carry a medical identification card or bracelet stating that you are taking this medicine.

For patients taking *methsuximide*:
- Do not use capsules that are not full or in which the contents have melted, because they may not work properly.

## Side Effects of This Medicine

Along with its needed effects, a medicine may cause some unwanted effects. Although not all of these side effects may occur, if they do occur they may need medical attention.

Check with your doctor as soon as possible if any of the following side effects occur:

*More common*
  Muscle pain; skin rash and itching; swollen glands; sore throat and fever

*Less common*
  Aggressiveness; difficulty in concentration; mental depression; nightmares

*Rare*
  Chills; increased chance of certain types of seizures; mood or mental changes; nosebleeds or other unusual bleeding or bruising; shortness of breath; sores, ulcers, or white spots on lips or in mouth; unusual tiredness or weakness; wheezing, tightness in chest, or troubled breathing

*Symptoms of overdose*
  Drowsiness (severe); nausea and vomiting (severe); troubled breathing

Other side effects may occur that usually do not need medical attention. These side effects may go away during treatment as your body adjusts to the medicine. However, check with your doctor if any of the following side effects continue or are bothersome:

*More common*
  Clumsiness or unsteadiness; dizziness; drowsiness; headache; hiccups; loss of appetite; nausea or vomiting; stomach cramps

*Less common*
  Irritability

Phensuximide may cause the urine to turn pink, red, or red-brown. This is harmless and is to be expected while you are taking this medicine.

Other side effects not listed above may also occur in some patients. If you notice any other effects, check with your doctor.

Revised: 05/23/94

# ANTIDEPRESSANTS, MONOAMINE OXIDASE (MAO) INHIBITOR   Systemic

Some commonly used brand names are:

**In the U.S.—**
Marplan[1]                              Parnate[3]
Nardil[2]

**In Canada—**
Marplan[1]                              Parnate[3]
Nardil[2]

Note: For quick reference, the following antidepressants are numbered to match the corresponding brand names.

This information applies to the following medicines:
1. Isocarboxazid (eye-soe-kar-BOX-a-zid)
2. Phenelzine (FEN-el-zeen)
3. Tranylcypromine (tran-ill-SIP-roe-meen)

Note: This information does *not* apply to furazolidone, procarbazine, or selegiline.

## Description

Monoamine oxidase (MAO) inhibitors are used to relieve certain types of mental depression. They work by blocking the action of a chemical substance known as monoamine oxidase (MAO) in the nervous system.

Although these medicines are very effective for certain patients, they may also cause some unwanted reactions if not taken in the right way. It is very important to avoid certain foods, beverages, and medicines while you are being treated with an MAO inhibitor. Your health care professional will help you obtain a list to carry in your wallet or purse as a reminder of which products you should avoid.

MAO inhibitors are available only with your doctor's prescription, in the following dosage forms:

*Oral*
Isocarboxazid
  • Tablets (U.S. and Canada)
Phenelzine
  • Tablets (U.S. and Canada)
Tranylcypromine
  • Tablets (U.S. and Canada)

## Before Using This Medicine

In deciding to use a medicine, the risks of taking the medicine must be weighed against the good it will do. This is a decision you and your doctor will make. For monoamine oxidase (MAO) inhibitors, the following should be considered:

**Allergies**—Tell your doctor if you have ever had any unusual or allergic reaction to any MAO inhibitor. Also tell your health care professional if you are allergic to any other substances, such as foods, preservatives, or dyes.

**Diet**—Dangerous reactions such as sudden high blood pressure may result when MAO inhibitors are taken with certain foods or drinks. The following foods should be avoided:

  • Foods that have a high tyramine content (most common in foods that are aged or fermented to increase their flavor), such as cheeses; fava or broad bean pods; yeast or meat extracts; smoked or pickled meat, poultry, or fish; fermented sausage (bologna, pepperoni, salami, summer sausage) or other fermented meat; sauerkraut; or any overripe fruit. If a list of these foods and beverages is not given to you, ask your health care professional to provide one.
  • Alcoholic beverages or alcohol-free or reduced-alcohol beer and wine.
  • Large amounts of caffeine-containing food or beverages such as coffee, tea, cola, or chocolate.

**Pregnancy**—A limited study in pregnant women showed an increased risk of birth defects when these medicines were taken during the first 3 months of pregnancy. In animal studies, MAO inhibitors caused a slowing of growth and increased excitability in the newborn when very large doses were given to the mother during pregnancy.

**Breast-feeding**—Tranylcypromine passes into the breast milk; it is not known whether isocarboxazid or phenelzine passes into breast milk. Problems in nursing babies have not been reported.

**Children**—Studies on these medicines have been done only in adult patients, and there is no specific information comparing use of MAO inhibitors in children with use in other age groups. However, animal studies have shown that these medicines may slow growth in the young. Therefore, be sure to discuss with your doctor the use of these medicines in children.

**Older adults**—Dizziness or lightheadedness may be especially likely to occur in elderly patients, who are usually more sensitive than younger adults to these effects of MAO inhibitors.

**Other medicines**—Although certain medicines should not be used together at all, in other cases 2 different medicines may be used together even if an interaction might occur. In these cases, your doctor may want to change the dose, or other precautions may be necessary. When you are taking MAO inhibitors, it is especially important that your health care professional know if you are taking any of the following:
  • Amphetamines or
  • Antihypertensives (high blood pressure medicine) or
  • Appetite suppressants (diet pills) or
  • Cyclobenzaprine (e.g., Flexeril) or
  • Fluoxetine (e.g., Prozac) or
  • Levodopa (e.g., Dopar, Larodopa) or
  • Maprotiline (e.g., Ludiomil) or
  • Medicine for asthma or other breathing problems or
  • Medicines for colds, sinus problems, or hay fever or other allergies (including nose drops or sprays) or
  • Meperidine (e.g., Demerol) or
  • Methylphenidate (e.g., Ritalin) or
  • Monoamine oxidase (MAO) inhibitors, other, including furazolidone (e.g., Furoxone), procarbazine (e.g., Matulane), or selegiline (e.g., Eldepryl), or
  • Paroxetine (e.g., Paxil), or

- Sertraline (e.g., Zoloft), or
- Tricyclic antidepressants (amitriptyline [e.g., Elavil], amoxapine [e.g., Asendin], clomipramine [e.g., Anafranil], desipramine [e.g., Pertofrane], doxepin [e.g., Sinequan], imipramine [e.g., Tofranil], nortriptyline [e.g., Aventyl], protriptyline [e.g., Vivactil], trimipramine [e.g., Surmontil])—Using these medicines while you are taking or within 2 weeks of taking MAO inhibitors may cause serious side effects such as sudden rise in body temperature, extremely high blood pressure, severe convulsions, and death; however, sometimes certain of these medicines may be used with MAO inhibitors under close supervision by your doctor
- Antidiabetics, oral (diabetes medicine you take by mouth) or
- Insulin—MAO inhibitors may change the amount of antidiabetic medicine you need to take
- Bupropion (e.g., Wellbutrin)—Using bupropion while you are taking or within 2 weeks of taking MAO inhibitors may cause serious side effects such as seizures
- Buspirone (e.g., BuSpar)—Use with MAO inhibitors may cause high blood pressure
- Carbamazepine (e.g., Tegretol)—Use with MAO inhibitors may increase seizures
- Central nervous system (CNS) depressants (medicines that cause drowsiness)—Using these medicines with MAO inhibitors may increase the CNS and other depressant effects
- Cocaine—Cocaine use by persons taking MAO inhibitors, including furazolidone and procarbazine, may cause a severe increase in blood pressure
- Dextromethorphan—Use with MAO inhibitors may cause excitement, high blood pressure, and fever
- Trazodone or
- Tryptophan used as a food supplement or a sleep aid—Use of these medicines by persons taking MAO inhibitors, including furazolidone and procarbazine, may cause mental confusion, excitement, shivering, trouble in breathing, or fever

**Other medical problems**—The presence of other medical problems may affect the use of MAO inhibitors. Make sure you tell your doctor if you have any other medical problems, especially:

- Alcohol abuse—Drinking alcohol while you are taking an MAO inhibitor may cause serious side effects
- Angina (chest pain) or
- Headaches (severe or frequent)—These conditions may interfere with warning signs of serious side effects of MAO inhibitors
- Asthma or bronchitis—Some medicines used to treat these conditions may cause serious side effects when used while you are taking an MAO inhibitor
- Diabetes mellitus (sugar diabetes)—These medicines may change the amount of insulin or oral antidiabetic medication that you need
- Epilepsy—Seizures may occur more often
- Heart or blood vessel disease or
- Liver disease or
- Mental illness (or history of) or
- Parkinson's disease or
- Recent heart attack or stroke—MAO inhibitors may make the condition worse
- High blood pressure—Condition may be affected by these medicines

- Kidney disease—Higher blood levels of MAO inhibitors may occur, which increases the chance of side effects
- Overactive thyroid or
- Pheochromocytoma (PCC)—Serious side effects may occur

## Proper Use of This Medicine

*Sometimes this medicine must be taken for several weeks before you begin to feel better. Your doctor should check your progress at regular visits, especially during the first few months of treatment, to make sure that this medicine is working properly and to check for unwanted effects.*

*Take this medicine only as directed by your doctor.* Do not take more of it, do not take it more often, and do not take it for a longer time than your doctor ordered.

MAO inhibitors may be taken with or without food or on a full or empty stomach. However, if your doctor tells you to take the medicine a certain way, take it exactly as directed.

**Dosing**—The dose of MAO inhibitors will be different for different patients. *Follow your doctor's orders or the directions on the label.* The following information includes only the average doses of isocarboxazid, phenelzine, and tranylcypromine. *If your dose is different, do not change it* unless your doctor tells you to do so.

The number of tablets that you take depends on the strength of the medicine. Also, *the number of doses you take each day, the time allowed between doses, and the length of time you take the medicine depend on the medical problem for which you are using an MAO inhibitor.*

*For isocarboxazid*
- For *oral* dosage form (tablets):
  —For treatment of depression:
  - Adults—To start, 30 milligrams (mg) a day. Your doctor may decrease or increase your dose as needed. However, the dose is usually not more than 60 mg a day.
  - Children up to 16 years of age—Use and dose must be determined by the doctor.

*For phenelzine*
- For *oral* dosage form (tablets):
  —For treatment of depression:
  - Adults—Dose is based on your body weight. To start, the usual dose is 1 milligram (mg) per kilogram (kg) of body weight (0.45 mg per pound) a day. Your doctor may decrease or increase your dose as needed. However, the dose is usually not more than 90 mg a day.
  - Children up to 16 years of age—Use and dose must be determined by the doctor.
  - Older adults—To start, 15 mg in the morning. Your doctor may increase your dose gradually as needed. However, the dose is usually not more than 60 mg a day.

*For tranylcypromine*
- For *oral* dosage form (tablets):
  —For treatment of depression:
    - Adults—To start, 30 milligrams (mg) a day. Your doctor may increase your dose gradually as needed. However, the dose is usually not more than 60 mg a day.
    - Children up to 16 years of age—Use and dose must be determined by the doctor.
    - Older adults—To start, 2.5 to 5 mg a day. The doctor may increase your dose as needed. However, the dose is usually not more than 45 mg a day.

**Missed dose**—If you miss a dose of this medicine, take it as soon as possible. However, if it is within 2 hours of your next dose, skip the missed dose and go back to your regular dosing schedule. Do not double doses.

**Storage**—To store this medicine:
- Keep out of the reach of children.
- Store away from heat and direct light.
- Do not store in the bathroom, near the kitchen sink, or in other damp places. Heat or moisture may cause the medicine to break down.
- Do not keep outdated medicine or medicine no longer needed. Be sure that any discarded medicine is out of the reach of children.

## Precautions While Using This Medicine

When taken with certain foods, drinks, or other medicines, MAO inhibitors can cause very dangerous reactions such as sudden high blood pressure (also called hypertensive crisis). To avoid such reactions, *obey the following rules of caution:*
- Do not eat foods that have a high tyramine content (most common in foods that are aged or fermented to increase their flavor), such as cheeses; fava or broad bean pods; yeast or meat extracts; smoked or pickled meat, poultry, or fish; fermented sausage (bologna, pepperoni, salami, and summer sausage) or other fermented meat; sauerkraut; or any overripe fruit. If a list of these foods is not given to you, ask your health care professional to provide one.
- Do not drink alcoholic beverages or alcohol-free or reduced-alcohol beer and wine.
- Do not eat or drink large amounts of caffeine-containing food or beverages such as coffee, tea, cola, or chocolate.
- Do not take any other medicine unless approved or prescribed by your doctor. This especially includes nonprescription (over-the-counter [OTC]) medicine, such as that for colds (including nose drops or sprays), cough, asthma, hay fever, and appetite control; "keep awake" products; or products that make you sleepy.

This medicine will add to the effects of alcohol and other CNS depressants (medicines that slow down the nervous system, possibly causing drowsiness). Some examples of CNS depressants are antihistamines or medicine for hay fever, other allergies, or colds; sedatives, tranquilizers, or sleeping medicine; prescription pain medicine or narcotics; barbiturates; medicine for seizures; muscle relaxants; or anesthetics, including some dental anesthetics. *Check with your doctor before taking any of the above while you are using this medicine.*

*Check with your doctor or hospital emergency room immediately* if severe headache, stiff neck, chest pains, fast heartbeat, or nausea and vomiting occur while you are taking this medicine. These may be symptoms of a serious side effect that should have a doctor's attention.

*Do not stop taking this medicine without first checking with your doctor.* Your doctor may want you to reduce gradually the amount you are using before stopping completely.

*Dizziness, lightheadedness, or fainting may occur,* especially when you get up from a lying or sitting position. *Getting up slowly may help.* When you get up from lying down, sit on the edge of the bed with your feet dangling for 1 or 2 minutes. Then stand up slowly. If the problem continues or gets worse, check with your doctor.

This medicine may cause blurred vision or make some people drowsy or less alert than they are normally. *Make sure you know how you react to this medicine before you drive, use machines, or do anything else that could be dangerous if you are unable to see well or are not alert.*

*Before having any kind of surgery, dental treatment, or emergency treatment, tell the medical doctor or dentist in charge that you are using this medicine or have used it within the past 2 weeks.* Taking MAO inhibitors together with medicines that are used during surgery or dental or emergency treatments may increase the risk of serious side effects.

Your doctor may want you to carry an identification card stating that you are using this medicine.

For patients with *angina* (chest pain):
- This medicine may cause you to have an unusual feeling of good health and energy. However, *do not suddenly increase the amount of exercise you get without discussing it with your doctor.* Too much activity could bring on an attack of angina.

For *diabetic* patients:
- This medicine may affect blood sugar levels. While you are using this medicine, be especially careful in testing for sugar in your blood or urine. If you have any questions about this, check with your doctor.

*After you stop using this medicine, you must continue to obey the rules of caution for at least 2 weeks* concerning food, drink, and other medicine, since these things may continue to react with MAO inhibitors.

## Side Effects of This Medicine

Along with its needed effects, a medicine may cause some unwanted effects. Although not all of these side effects may occur, if they do occur they may need medical attention.

*Stop taking this medicine and get emergency help immediately* if any of the following side effects occur:

*Symptoms of unusually high blood pressure (hypertensive crisis)*

Chest pain (severe); enlarged pupils; fast or slow heartbeat; headache (severe); increased sensitivity of eyes to light; increased sweating (possibly with fever or cold, clammy skin); nausea and vomiting; stiff or sore neck

Check with your doctor as soon as possible if any of the following side effects occur:

*More common*

Dizziness or lightheadedness (severe), especially when getting up from a lying or sitting position

*Less common*

Diarrhea; fast or pounding heartbeat; swelling of feet or lower legs; unusual excitement or nervousness

*Rare*

Dark urine; fever; skin rash; slurred speech; sore throat; staggering walk; yellow eyes or skin

*Symptoms of overdose*

Anxiety (severe); confusion; convulsions (seizures); cool, clammy skin; dizziness (severe); drowsiness (severe); fast and irregular pulse; fever; hallucinations (seeing, hearing, or feeling things that are not there); headache (severe); high or low blood pressure; muscle stiffness; sweating; troubled breathing; trouble in sleeping (severe); unusual irritability

Other side effects may occur that usually do not need medical attention. These side effects may go away during treatment as your body adjusts to the medicine. However, check with your doctor if any of the following side effects continue or are bothersome:

*More common*

Blurred vision; decreased amount of urine; decreased sexual ability; dizziness or lightheadedness (mild), especially when getting up from a lying or sitting position; drowsiness; headache (mild); increased appetite (especially for sweets) or weight gain; increased sweating; muscle twitching during sleep; restlessness; shakiness or trembling; tiredness and weakness; trouble in sleeping

*Less common or rare*

Chills; constipation; decreased appetite; dryness of mouth

Other side effects not listed above may also occur in some patients. If you notice any other effects, check with your doctor.

## Additional Information

Once a medicine has been approved for marketing for a certain use, experience may show that it is also useful for other medical problems. Although these uses are not included in product labeling, phenelzine and tranylcypromine are used in certain patients with the following medical conditions:

- Headache
- Panic disorder

Other than the above information, there is no additional information relating to proper use, precautions, or side effects for these uses.

Revised: 05/23/94

---

# ANTIDEPRESSANTS, TRICYCLIC   Systemic

Some commonly used brand names are:

**In the U.S.—**

| | |
|---|---|
| Anafranil[3] | Pamelor[7] |
| Asendin[2] | Sinequan[5] |
| Aventyl[7] | Surmontil[9] |
| Elavil[1] | Tipramine[6] |
| Endep[1] | Tofranil[6] |
| Enovil[1] | Tofranil-PM[6] |
| Norfranil[6] | Vivactil[8] |
| Norpramin[4] | |

**In Canada—**

| | |
|---|---|
| Anafranil[3] | Novopramine[6] |
| Apo-Amitriptyline[1] | Novo-Tripramine[9] |
| Apo-Imipramine[6] | Novotriptyn[1] |
| Apo-Trimip[9] | Pertofrane[4] |
| Asendin[2] | Rhotrimine[9] |
| Aventyl[7] | Sinequan[5] |
| Elavil[1] | Surmontil[9] |
| Impril[6] | Tofranil[6] |
| Levate[1] | Triadapin[5] |
| Norpramin[4] | Triptil[8] |
| Novo-Doxepin[5] | |

Note: For quick reference, the following tricyclic antidepressants are numbered to match the corresponding brand names.

This information applies to the following medicines:

1. Amitriptyline (a-mee-TRIP-ti-leen)‡§
2. Amoxapine (a-MOX-a-peen)‡
3. Clomipramine (cloe-MIP-ra-meen)
4. Desipramine (dess-IP-ra-meen)‡§
5. Doxepin (DOX-e-pin)‡
6. Imipramine (im-IP-ra-meen)‡§
7. Nortriptyline (nor-TRIP-ti-leen)‡
8. Protriptyline (proe-TRIP-ti-leen)
9. Trimipramine (trye-MIP-ra-meen)‡

‡Generic name product may also be available in the U.S.
§Generic name product may also be available in Canada.

## Description

Tricyclic antidepressants are used to relieve mental depression.

One form of this medicine (imipramine) is also used to treat enuresis (bedwetting) in children. Another form (clomipramine) is used to treat obsessive-compulsive disorders. Tricyclic antidepressants may be used for other conditions as determined by your doctor.

These medicines are available only with your doctor's prescription, in the following dosage forms:

*Oral*

Amitriptyline
- Syrup (Canada)
- Tablets (U.S. and Canada)

Amoxapine
- Tablets (U.S. and Canada)

Clomipramine
- Capsules (U.S.)
- Tablets (Canada)

Desipramine
- Tablets (U.S. and Canada)

Doxepin
- Capsules (U.S. and Canada)
- Oral solution (U.S.)

Imipramine
- Capsules (U.S.)
- Tablets (U.S. and Canada)

Nortriptyline
- Capsules (U.S. and Canada)
- Oral solution (U.S.)

Protriptyline
- Tablets (U.S. and Canada)

Trimipramine
- Capsules (U.S. and Canada)
- Tablets (Canada)

*Parenteral*

Amitriptyline
- Injection (U.S.)

Imipramine
- Injection (U.S.)

---

## Before Using This Medicine

In deciding to use a medicine, the risks of taking the medicine must be weighed against the good it will do. This is a decision you and your doctor will make. For tricyclic antidepressants, the following should be considered:

**Allergies**—Tell your doctor if you have ever had any unusual or allergic reaction to any tricyclic antidepressant or to carbamazepine, maprotiline, or trazodone. Also tell your health care professional if you are allergic to any other substances, such as foods, preservatives, or dyes.

**Pregnancy**—Studies have not been done in pregnant women. However, there have been reports of newborns suffering from muscle spasms and heart, breathing, and urinary problems when their mothers had taken tricyclic antidepressants immediately before delivery. Also, studies in animals have shown that some tricyclic antidepressants may cause unwanted effects in the fetus.

**Breast-feeding**—Tricyclic antidepressants pass into the breast milk. Doxepin has been reported to cause drowsiness in the nursing baby.

**Children**—Children are especially sensitive to the effects of this medicine. This may increase the chance of side effects during treatment. However, side effects in children taking this medicine for bedwetting usually disappear upon continued use. The most common of these are nervousness, sleeping problems, tiredness, and mild stomach upset. If these side effects continue or are bothersome, check with your doctor.

**Older adults**—Drowsiness, dizziness, confusion, vision problems, dryness of mouth, constipation, and problems in urinating are more likely to occur in elderly patients, who are usually more sensitive than younger adults to the effects of tricyclic antidepressants.

**Other medicines**—Although certain medicines should not be used together at all, in other cases 2 different medicines may be used together even if an interaction might occur. In these cases, your doctor may want to change the dose, or other precautions may be necessary. When you are taking a tricyclic antidepressant, it is especially important that your health care professional know if you are taking any of the following:

- Amphetamines or
- Appetite suppressants (diet pills) or
- Ephedrine or
- Epinephrine (e.g., Adrenalin) or
- Isoproterenol (e.g., Isuprel) or
- Medicine for asthma or other breathing problems or
- Medicine for colds, sinus problems, or hay fever or other allergies or
- Phenylephrine (e.g., Neo-Synephrine)—Using these medicines with tricyclic antidepressants may increase the risk of serious effects on the heart
- Antipsychotics (medicine for mental illness) or
- Clonidine (e.g., Catapres)—Using these medicines with tricyclic antidepressants may increase the CNS depressant effects and increase the chance of serious side effects
- Antithyroid agents (medicine for overactive thyroid) or
- Cimetidine (e.g., Tagamet)—Using these medicines with tricyclic antidepressants may increase the chance of serious side effects
- Central nervous system (CNS) depressants (medicine that causes drowsiness)—Using these medicines with tricyclic antidepressants may increase the CNS depressant effects
- Guanadrel (e.g., Hylorel) or
- Guanethidine (e.g., Ismelin)—Tricyclic antidepressants may keep these medicines from working as well
- Methyldopa (e.g., Aldomet) or
- Metoclopramide (e.g., Reglan) or
- Metyrosine (e.g., Demser) or
- Pemoline (e.g., Cylert) or
- Pimozide (e.g., Orap) or
- Promethazine (e.g., Phenergan) or
- Rauwolfia alkaloids (alseroxylon [e.g., Rauwiloid], deserpidine [e.g., Harmonyl], rauwolfia serpentina [e.g., Raudixin], reserpine [e.g., Serpasil]) or
- Trimeprazine (e.g., Temaril)—Tricyclic antidepressants may cause certain side effects to be more severe and occur more often
- Metrizamide—The risk of seizures may be increased
- Monoamine oxidase (MAO) inhibitors (furazolidone [e.g., Furoxone], isocarboxazid [e.g., Marplan], phenelzine [e.g., Nardil], procarbazine [e.g., Matulane], selegiline [e.g., Eldepryl], tranylcypromine [e.g., Parnate])—Taking tricyclic antidepressants while you are taking or within 2 weeks of taking MAO inhibitors may cause sudden high

body temperature, extremely high blood pressure, severe convulsions, and death; however, sometimes certain of these medicines may be used together under close supervision by your doctor

**Other medical problems**—The presence of other medical problems may affect the use of tricyclic antidepressants. Make sure you tell your doctor if you have any other medical problems, especially:

- Alcohol abuse (or history of)—Drinking alcohol may cause increased CNS depressant effects
- Asthma or
- Bipolar disorder (manic-depressive illness) or
- Blood disorders or
- Convulsions (seizures) or
- Difficult urination or
- Enlarged prostate or
- Glaucoma or increased eye pressure or
- Heart disease or
- High blood pressure (hypertension) or
- Schizophrenia—Tricyclic antidepressants may make the condition worse
- Kidney disease or
- Liver disease—Higher blood levels of tricyclic antidepressants may result, increasing the chance of side effects
- Overactive thyroid or
- Stomach or intestinal problems—Tricyclic antidepressants may cause an increased chance of serious side effects

## Proper Use of This Medicine

To lessen stomach upset, take this medicine with food, even for a daily bedtime dose, unless your doctor has told you to take it on an empty stomach.

*Take this medicine only as directed by your doctor,* to benefit your condition as much as possible. Do not take more of it, do not take it more often, and do not take it for a longer time than your doctor ordered.

*Sometimes this medicine must be taken for several weeks before you begin to feel better.* Your doctor should check your progress at regular visits.

To use *doxepin oral solution:*

- This medicine is to be taken by mouth even though it comes in a dropper bottle. The amount you should take should be measured with the dropper provided with your prescription and diluted just before you take each dose. Dilute each dose with about one-half glass (4 ounces) of water, milk, citrus fruit juice, tomato juice, or prune juice. Do not mix this medicine with grape juice or carbonated beverages since these may decrease the medicine's effectiveness.
- Doxepin oral solution must be mixed immediately before you take it. Do not prepare it ahead of time.

**Dosing**—The dose of tricyclic antidepressants will be different for different patients. *Follow your doctor's orders or the directions on the label.* The following information includes only the average doses of tricyclic antidepressants. *If your dose is different, do not change it* unless your doctor tells you to do so.

The number of capsules or tablets, or the amount of solution or syrup that you take depends on the strength of the medicine. Also, *the number of doses you take each day, the time allowed between doses, and the length of time you take the medicine depend on the medical problem for which you are taking tricyclic antidepressants.*

*For amitriptyline*
- For *tablet* dosage form:
  —For depression:
    • Adults—At first, 25 milligrams (mg) two to four times a day. Your doctor may increase your dose gradually as needed. However, the dose is usually not more than 150 mg a day, unless you are in the hospital. Some hospitalized patients may need higher doses.
    • Teenagers—At first, 10 mg three times a day, and 20 mg at bedtime. Your doctor may increase your dose gradually as needed. However, the dose is usually not more than 100 mg a day.
    • Children 6 to 12 years of age—10 to 30 mg a day.
    • Children up to 6 years of age—Use and dose must be determined by your doctor.
    • Older adults— At first, 25 mg at bedtime. Your doctor may increase your dose gradually as needed. However, the dose is usually not more than 100 mg a day.
- For *syrup* dosage form:
  —For depression:
    • Adults—At first, 25 mg two to four times a day. Your doctor may increase your dose gradually as needed.
    • Teenagers—At first, 10 mg three times a day, and 20 mg at bedtime. Your doctor may increase your dose gradually as needed. However, the dose is usually not more than 100 mg a day.
    • Children 6 to 12 years of age—10 to 30 mg a day.
    • Children up to 6 years of age—Use and dose must be determined by your doctor.
    • Older adults—At first, 10 mg three times a day, and 20 mg at bedtime. Your doctor may increase your dose gradually as needed. However, the dose is usually not more than 100 mg a day.
- For *injection* dosage form:
  —For depression:
    • Adults—20 to 30 mg four times a day, injected into a muscle.
    • Children up to 12 years of age—Use and dose must be determined by your doctor.

*For amoxapine*
- For *tablet* dosage form:
  —For depression:
    • Adults—At first, 50 milligrams (mg) two to three times a day. Your doctor may increase your dose gradually as needed.

- Children up to 16 years of age—Use and dose must be determined by your doctor.
- Older adults—At first, 25 mg two to three times a day. Your doctor may increase your dose gradually as needed.

*For clomipramine*
- For *capsule or tablet* dosage forms:
  —For obsessive-compulsive disorders:
    - Adults—At first, 25 milligrams (mg) once a day. Your doctor may increase your dose gradually as needed. However, the dose is usually not more than 250 mg a day, unless you are in the hospital. Some hospitalized patients may need higher doses.
    - Teenagers and children 10 years of age and over—At first, 25 mg once a day. Your doctor may increase your dose gradually as needed. However, the dose is usually not more than 200 mg a day.
    - Children up to 10 years of age—Use and dose must be determined by your doctor.
    - Older adults—At first, 20 to 30 mg a day. Your doctor may increase your dose gradually as needed.

*For desipramine*
- For *tablet* dosage form:
  —For depression:
    - Adults—100 to 200 milligrams (mg) a day. Your doctor may increase your dose gradually as needed. However, the dose is usually not more than 300 mg a day.
    - Teenagers—25 to 50 mg a day. Your doctor may increase your dose gradually as needed. However, the dose is usually not more than 100 mg a day.
    - Children 6 to 12 years of age—10 to 30 mg a day.
    - Older adults—25 to 50 mg a day. Your doctor may increase your dose gradually as needed. However, the dose is usually not more than 150 mg a day.

*For doxepin*
- For *capsule or solution* dosage forms:
  —For depression:
    - Adults—At first, 25 milligrams (mg) three times a day. Your doctor may increase your dose gradually as needed. However, the dose is usually not more than 150 mg a day, unless you are in the hospital. Some hospitalized patients may need higher doses.
    - Children up to 12 years of age—Use and dose must be determined by your doctor.
    - Older adults—At first, 25 to 50 mg a day. Your doctor may increase your dose gradually as needed.

*For imipramine*
- For *tablet* dosage form:
  —For depression:
    - Adults—25 to 50 milligrams (mg) three to four times a day. Your doctor may increase your dose gradually as needed. However, the dose is usually not more than 200 mg a day, unless you are in the hospital. Some hospitalized patients may need higher doses.
    - Adolescents—25 to 50 mg a day. Your doctor may increase your dose gradually as needed. However, the dose is usually not more than 100 mg a day.
    - Children 6 to 12 years of age—10 to 30 mg a day.
    - Children up to 6 years of age—Use and dose must be determined by your doctor.
    - Older adults—At first, 25 mg at bedtime. Your doctor may increase your dose gradually as needed. However, the dose is usually not more than 100 mg a day.
  —For bedwetting:
    - Children—25 mg once a day, taken one hour before bedtime. Your doctor may increase the dose as needed, based on the child's age.
- For *capsule* dosage form:
  —For depression:
    - Adults—At first, 75 mg a day taken at bedtime. Your doctor may increase your dose gradually as needed. However, the dose is usually not more than 200 mg a day, unless you are in the hospital. Some hospitalized patients may need higher doses.
    - Children up to 12 years of age—Use and dose must be determined by your doctor.
- For *injection* dosage form:
  —For depression:
    - Adults—Dose must be determined by your doctor. It is injected into a muscle. The dose is usually not more than 300 mg a day.
    - Children up to 12 years of age—Use and dose must be determined by your doctor.

*For nortriptyline*
- For *capsule or solution* dosage forms:
  —For depression:
    - Adults—25 milligrams (mg) three to four times a day. Your doctor may increase your dose gradually as needed. However, the dose is usually not more than 150 mg a day.
    - Teenagers—25 to 50 mg a day. Your doctor may increase your dose gradually as needed.
    - Children 6 to 12 years of age—10 to 20 mg a day.
    - Older adults—30 to 50 mg a day. Your doctor may increase your dose gradually as needed.

*For protriptyline*
- For *tablet* dosage form:
  —For depression:
  - Adults—At first, 5 to 10 milligrams (mg) three to four times a day. Your doctor may increase your dose gradually as needed. However, the dose is usually not more than 60 mg a day.
  - Teenagers—At first, 5 mg three times a day. Your doctor may increase your dose gradually as needed.
  - Children up to 12 years of age—Use and dose must be determined by your doctor.
  - Older adults—At first, 5 mg three times a day. Your doctor may increase your dose gradually as needed.

*For trimipramine*
- For *capsule or tablet* dosage forms:
  —For depression:
  - Adults—At first, 75 milligrams (mg) a day. Your doctor may increase your dose as needed. However, the dose is usually not more than 200 mg a day, unless you are hospitalized. Some hospitalized patients may need higher doses.
  - Teenagers—At first, 50 mg a day. Your doctor may increase your dose gradually as needed. However, the dose is usually not more than 100 mg a day.
  - Children up to 12 years of age—Use and dose must be determined by your doctor.
  - Older adults—At first, 50 mg a day. Your doctor may increase your dose gradually as needed. However, the dose is usually not more than 100 mg a day.

**Missed dose**—If you miss a dose of this medicine and your dosing schedule is:
- One dose a day at bedtime—Do not take the missed dose in the morning since it may cause disturbing side effects during waking hours. Instead, check with your doctor.
- More than one dose a day—Take the missed dose as soon as possible. However, if it is almost time for your next dose, skip the missed dose, and go back to your regular dosing schedule. Do not double doses.

If you have any questions about this, check with your doctor.

**Storage**—To store this medicine:
- Keep out of the reach of children. Overdose of this medicine is very dangerous in young children.
- Store away from heat and direct light.
- Do not store the tablet or capsule form of this medicine in the bathroom, near the kitchen sink, or in other damp places. Heat or moisture may cause the medicine to break down.
- Keep the liquid form of this medicine from freezing.

- Do not keep outdated medicine or medicine no longer needed. Be sure that any discarded medicine is out of the reach of children.

## Precautions While Using This Medicine

It is very important that your doctor check your progress at regular visits to allow dosage adjustments and to help reduce side effects.

This medicine will add to the effects of alcohol and other CNS depressants (medicines that make you drowsy or less alert). Some examples of CNS depressants are antihistamines or medicine for hay fever, other allergies, or colds; sedatives, tranquilizers, or sleeping medicine; prescription pain medicine or narcotics; barbiturates; medicine for seizures; muscle relaxants; or anesthetics, including some dental anesthetics. *Check with your medical doctor or dentist before taking any of the above while you are taking this medicine.*

This medicine may cause some people to become drowsy. *If this occurs, do not drive, use machines, or do anything else that could be dangerous if you are not alert.*

*Dizziness, lightheadedness, or fainting may occur,* especially when you get up from a lying or sitting position. Getting up slowly may help. If this problem continues or gets worse, check with your doctor.

*This medicine may cause dryness of the mouth. For temporary relief, use sugarless gum or candy, melt bits of ice in your mouth, or use a saliva substitute.* However, if your mouth continues to feel dry for more than 2 weeks, check with your medical doctor or dentist. Continuing dryness of the mouth may increase the chance of dental disease, including tooth decay, gum disease, and fungus infections.

Tricyclic antidepressants may cause your skin to be more sensitive to sunlight than it is normally. Exposure to sunlight, even for brief periods of time, may cause a skin rash, itching, redness or other discoloration of the skin, or a severe sunburn. When you begin taking this medicine:
- Stay out of direct sunlight, especially between the hours of 10:00 a.m. and 3:00 p.m., if possible.
- Wear protective clothing, including a hat. Also, wear sunglasses.
- Apply a sun block product that has a skin protection factor (SPF) of at least 15. Some patients may require a product with a higher SPF number, especially if they have a fair complexion. If you have any questions about this, check with your health care professional.
- Apply a sun block lipstick that has an SPF of at least 15 to protect your lips.
- Do not use a sunlamp or tanning bed or booth.

*If you have a severe reaction from the sun, check with your doctor.*

Before you have any medical tests, tell the medical doctor in charge that you are taking this medicine. The results of the metyrapone test may be affected by this medicine.

*Before having any kind of surgery, dental treatment, or emergency treatment, tell the medical doctor or dentist in charge that you are using this medicine.* Taking tricyclic antidepressants together with medicines used during surgery or dental or emergency treatments may increase the risk of side effects.

*For diabetic patients:*
- This medicine may affect blood sugar levels. If you notice a change in the results of your blood or urine sugar tests or if you have any questions, check with your doctor.

*Do not stop taking this medicine without first checking with your doctor.* Your doctor may want you to reduce gradually the amount you are using before stopping completely. This may help prevent a possible worsening of your condition and reduce the possibility of withdrawal symptoms such as headache, nausea, and/or an overall feeling of discomfort.

*The effects of this medicine may last for 3 to 7 days after you have stopped taking it.* Therefore, all the precautions stated here must be observed during this time.

*For patients taking protriptyline:*
- If taken late in the day, protriptyline may interfere with nighttime sleep.

---

## Side Effects of This Medicine

Along with its needed effects, a medicine may cause some unwanted effects. Although not all of these side effects may occur, if they do occur they may need medical attention.

*Stop taking this medicine and get emergency help immediately* if any of the following side effects occur:
*Reported for amoxapine only—rare*
Convulsions (seizures); difficult or fast breathing; fever with increased sweating; high or low (irregular) blood pressure; loss of bladder control; muscle stiffness (severe); pale skin; unusual tiredness or weakness

Check with your doctor as soon as possible if any of the following side effects occur:
*Less common*
Blurred vision; confusion or delirium; constipation (especially in the elderly); decreased sexual ability (more common with amoxapine and clomipramine); difficulty in speaking or swallowing; eye pain; fainting; fast or irregular heartbeat (pounding, racing, skipping); hallucinations; loss of balance control; mask-like face; nervousness or restlessness; problems in urinating; shakiness or trembling; shuffling walk; slowed movements; stiffness of arms and legs
*Reported for amoxapine only (in addition to the above)—less common*
Lip smacking or puckering; puffing of cheeks; rapid or worm-like movements of tongue; uncontrolled chewing

movements; uncontrolled movements of hands, arms, or legs
*Rare*
Anxiety; breast enlargement in both males and females; hair loss; inappropriate secretion of milk—in females; increased sensitivity to sunlight; irritability; muscle twitching; red or brownish spots on skin; ringing, buzzing, or other unexplained sounds in the ears; seizures (more common with clomipramine); skin rash and itching; sore throat and fever; swelling of face and tongue; swelling of testicles (more common with amoxapine); trouble with teeth or gums (more common with clomipramine); weakness; yellow eyes or skin
*Symptoms of acute overdose*
Confusion; convulsions (seizures); disturbed concentration; drowsiness (severe); enlarged pupils; fast, slow, or irregular heartbeat; fever; hallucinations (seeing, hearing, or feeling things that are not there); restlessness and agitation; shortness of breath or troubled breathing; unusual tiredness or weakness (severe); vomiting

Other side effects may occur that usually do not need medical attention. These side effects may go away during treatment as your body adjusts to the medicine. However, check with your doctor if any of the following side effects continue or are bothersome:
*More common*
Dizziness; drowsiness; dryness of mouth; headache; increased appetite (may include craving for sweets); nausea; tiredness or weakness (mild); unpleasant taste; weight gain
*Less common*
Diarrhea; heartburn; increased sweating; trouble in sleeping (more common with protriptyline, especially when taken late in the day); vomiting

Certain side effects of this medicine may occur after you have stopped taking it. Check with your doctor if you notice any of the following effects:
Headache; irritability; nausea, vomiting, or diarrhea; restlessness; trouble in sleeping, with vivid dreams; unusual excitement
*Reported for amoxapine only (in addition to the above)*
Lip smacking or puckering; puffing of cheeks; rapid or worm-like movements of the tongue; uncontrolled chewing movements; uncontrolled movements of arms or legs

Other side effects not listed above also may occur in some patients. If you notice any other effects, check with your doctor.

---

## Additional Information

Once a medicine has been approved for marketing for a certain use, experience may show that it is also useful for other medical problems. Although these uses are not included in product labeling, tricyclic antidepressants are used in certain patients with the following medical conditions:
- Attention deficit hyperactivity disorder (hyperactivity in children) (desipramine, imipramine, and protriptyline)

- Bulimia (uncontrolled eating, followed by vomiting) (amitriptyline, clomipramine, desipramine, and imipramine)
- Cocaine withdrawal (desipramine and imipramine)
- Headache prevention (for certain types of frequent or continuing headaches) (most tricyclic antidepressants)
- Itching with hives due to cold temperature exposure (doxepin)
- Narcolepsy (extreme tendency to fall asleep suddenly) (clomipramine, desipramine, imipramine, and protriptyline)
- Neurogenic pain (a type of continuing pain) (amitriptyline, clomipramine, desipramine, doxepin, imipramine, nortriptyline, and trimipramine)

- Panic disorder (clomipramine, desipramine, doxepin, nortriptyline, and trimipramine)
- Stomach ulcer (amitriptyline, doxepin, and trimipramine)
- Urinary incontinence (imipramine)

Other than the above information, there is no additional information relating to proper use, precautions, or side effects for these uses.

Revised: 05/22/92
Interim revision(s): 06/1/92; 03/01/93; 04/29/94

# ANTIDIABETICS, ORAL  Systemic

Some commonly used brand names are:

**In the U.S.—**

| | |
|---|---|
| DiaBeta[4] | Micronase[4] |
| Diabinese[2] | Orinase[6] |
| Dymelor[1] | Tolamide[5] |
| Glucotrol[3] | Tolinase[5] |
| Glynase PresTab[4] | Tol-Tab[6] |

**In Canada—**

| | |
|---|---|
| Albert Glyburide[4] | Euglucon[4] |
| Apo-Chlorpropamide[2] | Gen-Glybe[4] |
| Apo-Glyburide[4] | Mobenol[6] |
| Apo-Tolbutamide[6] | Novo-Butamide[6] |
| DiaBeta[4] | Novo-Glyburide[4] |
| Diabinese[2] | Novo-Propamide[2] |
| Dimelor[1] | Orinase[6] |

Another commonly used name for glyburide is glibenclamide.

Note: For quick reference, the following oral antidiabetics are numbered to match the corresponding brand names.

This information applies to the following medicines:

1. Acetohexamide (a-set-oh-HEX-a-mide)‡
2. Chlorpropamide (klor-PROE-pa-mide)‡§
3. Glipizide (GLIP-i-zide)†
4. Glyburide (GLYE-byoo-ride)
5. Tolazamide (tole-AZ-a-mide)†‡
6. Tolbutamide (tole-BYOO-ta-mide)‡§

†Not commercially available in Canada.
‡Generic name product may also be available in the U.S.
§Generic name product may also be available in Canada.

## Description

Oral antidiabetics (diabetes medicine you take by mouth) may help reduce the amount of sugar in the blood by causing your pancreas gland to make more insulin. They are used to treat certain types of diabetes mellitus (sugar diabetes).

Oral antidiabetics can usually be used only by adults who develop diabetes after 30 years of age and who do not require insulin shots (or who usually do not require more than 20 Units of insulin a day) to control their condition. This type of diabetic patient is said to have non–insulin-dependent diabetes mellitus (or NIDDM), sometimes known as maturity-onset or Type II diabetes. Oral antidiabetics do not help diabetic patients who have insulin-dependent diabetes mellitus (or IDDM), sometimes known as juvenile-onset or Type I diabetes.

Chlorpropamide may also be used for other conditions as determined by your doctor.

Oral antidiabetic medicines do not help diabetic patients who are insulin-dependent (type I). However, non–insulin-dependent (type II) diabetic patients who are taking oral antidiabetics may have to temporarily switch to insulin if they:

- develop diabetic coma or ketoacidosis.
- have a severe injury or burn.
- develop a severe infection.
- are to have major surgery.
- are pregnant.

Before you begin treatment with this medicine, you and your doctor should talk about the good the medicine will do as well as the risks of using it. You should also find out about other possible ways to treat your diabetes such as by diet alone or by diet plus insulin.

Oral antidiabetics are available only with your doctor's prescription, in the following dosage forms:

*Oral*

Acetohexamide
- Tablets (U.S. and Canada)

Chlorpropamide
- Tablets (U.S. and Canada)

Glipizide
- Tablets (U.S.)

Glyburide
- Tablets (U.S. and Canada)

Tolazamide
- Tablets (U.S.)

Tolbutamide
- Tablets (U.S. and Canada)

## Before Using This Medicine

In deciding to use a medicine, the risks of taking the medicine must be weighed against the good it will do. This is a decision you and your doctor will make. For oral antidiabetic medicines, the following should be considered:

**Allergies**—Tell your doctor if you have ever had any unusual or allergic reaction to oral antidiabetic medicines, or to sulfonamide-type (sulfa) medications, including thiazide diuretics (a certain type of water pill). Also tell your health care professional if you are allergic to any other substances, such as foods, preservatives, or dyes.

**Diet**—If you have non–insulin-dependent (type II) diabetes, your doctor may try to control your condition by prescribing a personal meal plan for you before prescribing medicine. Such a diet is low in refined carbohydrates (foods such as sugar and candy used for quick energy) and fat. The daily number of calories in this meal plan should be adjusted by a dietitian to help you reach and maintain a proper body weight. Oral antidiabetics are less effective if you are greatly overweight. It may be very important for you to follow a planned weight reduction diet. In addition, meals and snacks are arranged to meet the energy needs of your body at different times of the day.

Many people with type II diabetes are able to control their diabetes by carefully following their prescribed meal and exercise plan. Oral antidiabetics are prescribed only when additional help is needed.

**Pregnancy**—Oral antidiabetics should not be used during pregnancy. Insulin may be needed to keep blood sugar levels as close to normal as possible. Poor control of blood sugar levels may cause birth defects or death of the fetus. In addition, use of oral antidiabetics during pregnancy may cause the newborn baby to have low blood sugar levels. This may last for several days following birth.

**Breast-feeding**—Chlorpropamide passes into the breast milk and its use is not recommended because it could cause low blood sugar in the baby. Although it is not known if the other oral antidiabetics pass into breast milk and these medicines have not been shown to cause problems in humans, the chance always exists.

**Children**—There is little information about the use of oral antidiabetic agents in children. Type II diabetes is unusual in this age group.

**Older adults**—The elderly may be more sensitive than younger adults to the effects of oral antidiabetics. Also, elderly patients who take chlorpropamide are more likely to retain (keep) too much body water.

**Other medicines**—Although certain medicines should not be used together at all, in other cases two different medicines may be used together even if an interaction might occur. In these cases, your doctor may want to change the dose, or other precautions may be necessary. *Do not take any other medicine, unless prescribed or approved by your doctor.* When you are taking oral antidiabetic drugs, it is especially important that your health care professional know if you are taking any of the following:

- Anticoagulants (blood thinners)—The effect of either the blood thinner or the antidiabetic medicine may be increased or decreased if the 2 medicines are used together

- Appetite control medicines or
- Asthma medicines or
- Cough or cold medicines or
- Hay fever or allergy medicines—Many medicines (including nonprescription [over-the-counter]) products can affect the control of your blood glucose (sugar)
- Aspirin or other salicylates or
- Chloramphenicol (e.g., Chloromycetin) or
- Guanethidine (e.g., Ismelin) or
- Sulfonamides (sulfa medicine)—These medicines may increase the chances of low blood sugar
- Beta-blockers (acebutolol [e.g., Sectral], atenolol [e.g., Tenormin], carteolol [e.g., Cartrol], labetalol [e.g., Normodyne], metoprolol [e.g., Lopressor], nadolol [e.g., Corgard], oxprenolol [e.g., Trasicor], penbutolol [e.g., Levatol], pindolol [e.g., Visken], propranolol [e.g., Inderal], sotalol [e.g., Sotacor], timolol [e.g., Blocadren])—Beta-blockers may increase the risk of high or low blood sugar occurring. They can also block symptoms of low blood sugar (such as fast heartbeat or high blood pressure). Because of this, a diabetic patient might not know that he or she had low blood sugar and might not immediately take the proper steps to raise the blood sugar level. Beta-blockers can also cause low blood sugar to last longer
- Monoamine oxidase (MAO) inhibitors (furazolidone [e.g., Furoxone], isocarboxazid [e.g., Marplan], pargyline [e.g., Eutonyl], phenelzine [e.g., Nardil], procarbazine [e.g., Matulane], or tranylcypromine [e.g., Parnate])—Taking oral antidiabetic medicines while you are taking (or within 2 weeks of taking) monoamine oxidase (MAO) inhibitors may increase the chances of low blood sugar occurring

**Other medical problems**—The presence of other medical problems may affect the use of the oral antidiabetic medicines. Make sure you tell your doctor if you have any other medical problems, especially:

- Heart disease—Chlorpropamide causes some patients to retain (keep) more body water than usual. Heart disease may be worsened by this extra body water
- Infection (severe)—Insulin may be needed temporarily to control diabetes in patients with severe infection because changes in blood sugar may occur rapidly and without much warning
- Kidney disease or
- Liver disease—Low blood sugar may be more likely to occur because the kidney or liver is not able to get the medicine out of the blood stream as it normally would. Also, people with kidney disease who take chlorpropamide are more likely to retain (keep) too much body water
- Thyroid disease
- Underactive adrenal glands (untreated) or
- Underactive pituitary gland (untreated)—Patients with these conditions may be more likely to develop low blood sugar (hypoglycemia) while taking oral antidiabetic medicines

## Proper Use of This Medicine

*Follow carefully your special meal plan, since this is the most important part of controlling your diabetes and is necessary if the medicine is to work properly.*

*Take your oral antidiabetic medicine only as directed by your doctor.* Do not take more or less of it than your doctor ordered, and take it at the same time each day. This will help to control your blood sugar levels.

**Dosing**—The dose of these medicines will be different for different patients. *Follow your doctor's orders or the directions on the label.* The following information includes only the average doses of these medicines. *If your dose is different, do not change it* unless your doctor tells you to do so.

The number of tablets that you take depends on the strength of the medicine. Also, *the number of doses you take each day, the time allowed between doses, and the length of time you take the medicine depend on the amount of sugar in your blood or urine.*

For *acetohexamide*
- For *oral* dosage form (tablets):
  —For treating sugar diabetes (diabetes mellitus):
  - Adults—At first, 250 milligrams (mg) once a day. Some elderly people may need a lower dose of 125 to 250 mg a day at first. Then, your doctor may change your dose at little at a time if needed. The dose is usually not more than 1.5 grams a day. If your dose is 1 gram or more, the dose is usually divided into two doses. These doses are taken before the morning and evening meals.
  - Children—The type of diabetes treated with this medicine is rare in children. However, if a child needs this medicine, the dose would have to be determined by the doctor.

For *chlorpropamide*
- For *oral* dosage form (tablets):
  —For treating sugar diabetes (diabetes mellitus):
  - Adults—At first, 250 milligrams (mg) once a day. Some elderly people may need a lower dose of 100 to 125 mg a day at first. Then, your doctor may change your dose a little at a time if needed. The dose is usually not more than 750 mg a day.
  - Children—The type of diabetes treated with this medicine is rare in children. However, if a child needs this medicine, the dose would have to be determined by the doctor.

For *glipizide*
- For *oral* dosage form (tablets):
  —For treating sugar diabetes (diabetes mellitus):
  - Adults—At first, 5 milligrams (mg) once a day. Some elderly people may need a lower dose of 2.5 mg a day at first. Then, your doctor may change your dose a little at a time if needed. The dose is usually not more than 40 mg a day. If your dose is 15 mg or more, the dose is usually divided into two doses. These doses are taken before the morning and evening meals.
  - Children—The type of diabetes treated with this medicine is rare in children. However, if a child needs this medicine, the dose would have to be determined by the doctor.

For *glyburide*
- For *oral* dosage form (tablets):
  —For treating sugar diabetes (diabetes mellitus):
  - Adults—At first, 2.5 to 5 milligrams (mg) once a day. Some elderly people may need a lower dose of 1.25 to 2.5 mg a day at first. Then, your doctor may change your dose a little at a time if needed. The dose is usually not more than 20 mg a day. If your dose is 10 mg or more, the dose is usually divided into two doses. These doses are taken before the morning and evening meals.
  - Children—The type of diabetes treated with this medicine is rare in children. However, if a child needs this medicine, the dose would have to be determined by the doctor.

For *tolazamide*
- For *oral* dosage form (tablets):
  —For treating sugar diabetes (diabetes mellitus):
  - Adults—At first, 100 to 250 milligrams (mg) once a day in the morning. Then, your doctor may change your dose a little at a time if needed. The dose is usually not more than 1 gram a day. If your dose is 500 mg or more, the dose is usually divided into two doses. These doses are taken before the morning and evening meals.
  - Children—The type of diabetes treated with this medicine is rare in children. However, if a child needs this medicine, the dose would have to be determined by the doctor.

For *tolbutamide*
- For *oral* dosage form (tablets):
  —For treating sugar diabetes (diabetes mellitus):
  - Adults—At first, 500 milligrams (mg) to 2 grams a day. Some elderly people may need lower doses to start. The dose is usually divided into two doses. These doses are taken before the morning and evening meals. Your doctor may change your dose a little at a time if needed. The dose is usually not more than 3 grams a day.
  - Children—The type of diabetes treated with this medicine is rare in children. However, if a child needs this medicine, the dose would have to be determined by the doctor.

**Missed dose**—If you miss a dose of this medicine, take it as soon as possible. However, if it is almost time for your next dose, skip the missed dose and go back to your regular dosing schedule. Do not double doses.

**Storage**—To store this medicine:
- Keep out of the reach of children.
- Store away from heat and direct light.
- Do not store in the bathroom, near the kitchen sink, or in other damp places. Heat or moisture may cause the medicine to break down.
- Do not keep outdated medicine or medicine no longer needed. Be sure that any discarded medicine is out of the reach of children.

## Precautions While Using This Medicine

Your doctor will want to check your progress at regular visits, especially during the first few weeks that you take this medicine.

Test for sugar in your blood or urine as directed by your doctor. This is important in making sure your diabetes is being controlled and provides an early warning when it is not.

*Do not take any other medicines, unless prescribed or approved by your doctor.* This especially includes non-prescription (over-the-counter [OTC]) medicines such as those for colds, cough, asthma, hay fever, or appetite control.

*Avoid drinking alcoholic beverages until you have discussed their use with your doctor.* Some patients who drink alcohol while taking this medicine may suffer stomach pain, nausea, vomiting, dizziness, pounding headache, sweating, or flushing (redness of face and skin). In addition, alcohol may produce hypoglycemia (low blood sugar).

Oral antidiabetic medicines may cause your skin to be more sensitive to sunlight than it is normally. Exposure to sunlight, even for brief periods of time, may cause a skin rash, itching, redness or other discoloration of the skin, or a severe sunburn.

When you begin taking this medicine:
• Stay out of direct sunlight, especially between the hours of 10:00 a.m. and 3:00 p.m., if possible.
• Wear protective clothing, including a hat. Also, wear sunglasses.
• Apply a sun block product that has a skin protection factor (SPF) of at least 15. Some patients may require a product with a higher SPF number, especially if they have a fair complexion. If you have any questions about this, check with your health care professional.
• Apply a sun block lipstick that has an SPF of at least 15 to protect your lips.
• Do not use a sunlamp or tanning bed or booth.

*If you have a severe reaction from the sun, check with your doctor.*

*Eat or drink something containing sugar and check with your doctor right away if mild symptoms of low blood sugar (hypoglycemia) appear.* Good sources of sugar are glucose tablets or gel or fruit juice, corn syrup, honey, non-diet soft drinks, or sugar cubes or table sugar (dissolved in water). It is a good idea also to check your blood sugar to confirm that it is low.

• *If severe symptoms such as convulsions (seizures) or unconsciousness occur, diabetics should not eat or drink anything.* There is a chance that they could choke from not swallowing correctly. Emergency medical help should be obtained immediately.

• *Symptoms of low blood sugar (hypoglycemia) are:*
Abdominal or stomach pain (mild)
Anxious feeling
Chills (continuing)
Cold sweats
Confusion
Convulsions (seizures)
Cool pale skin

Difficulty in concentration
Drowsiness
Excessive hunger
Fast heartbeat
Headache (continuing)
Nausea or vomiting (continuing)
Nervousness
Shakiness
Unconsciousness
Unsteady walk
Unusual tiredness or weakness
Vision changes

• Different people may have different symptoms of hypoglycemia. It is important that you learn your own signs of low blood sugar so that you can treat it quickly.
• *These symptoms may occur if you:*
—delay or miss a scheduled meal or snack.
—exercise much more than usual.
—cannot eat because of nausea and vomiting.
—drink a significant amount of alcohol.
• *Tell someone to take you to your doctor or to a hospital right away if the symptoms do not improve after eating or drinking a sweet food.*
• Even if you correct these symptoms by eating sugar, it is very important to call your doctor or hospital emergency service right away, since the blood sugar–lowering effects of this medicine may last for days and the symptoms may return often during this time.

Before having any kind of surgery, dental treatment, or emergency treatment, tell the medical doctor or dentist in charge that you are taking this medicine.

You should wear a medical I.D. bracelet or chain at all times. In addition, you should carry an identification card that says you have diabetes and that lists your medications.

## Side Effects of This Medicine

The use of oral antidiabetics has been reported to increase the risk of death from heart and blood vessel disease. A report based on a study by the University Group Diabetes Program (UGDP) compared the use of one of the oral medicines (tolbutamide) to the use of diet alone or diet plus insulin. Although only tolbutamide was studied, other oral antidiabetics may cause a similar effect since all these medicines are related chemically and in the way they work.

Along with their needed effects, oral antidiabetics may cause some unwanted effects. Although not all of these side effects may occur, if they do occur they may need medical attention.

Check with your doctor as soon as possible if any of the following side effects occur:
*Rare*
Chest pain; chills; coughing up blood; dark urine; fever; general feeling of illness; increased amounts of sputum (phlegm); increased sweating; itching of the skin; light-colored stools; shortness of breath; sore throat; unusual

bleeding or bruising; unusual tiredness or weakness (continuing and unexplained); yellow eyes or skin

*Symptoms of overdose (hypoglycemia)*

Abdominal or stomach pain (mild); anxious feeling; chills (continuing); cold sweats; confusion; convulsions (seizures); cool, pale skin; difficulty in concentration; drowsiness; excessive hunger; fast heartbeat; headache (continuing); nausea or vomiting (continuing); nervousness; shakiness; unconsciousness; unsteady walk; unusual tiredness or weakness; vision changes

Other side effects may occur that usually do not need medical attention. These side effects may go away during treatment as your body adjusts to the medicine. However, check with your doctor if any of the following side effects continue or are bothersome:

*More common*

Changes in taste (for tolbutamide); constipation; diarrhea; dizziness; drowsiness (mild); headache; heartburn; increased or decreased appetite; nausea; vomiting; stomach pain, fullness, or discomfort

*Less common or rare*

Hives; increased sensitivity of skin to sun; skin redness, itching, or rash

For patients taking chlorpropamide:

• Some patients who take chlorpropamide may retain (keep) more body water than usual. Check with your

doctor as soon as possible if any of the following signs occur:

Breathing difficulty; shortness of breath

Other side effects not listed above may also occur in some patients. If you notice any other effects, check with your doctor.

## Additional Information

Once a medicine has been approved for marketing for a certain use, experience may show that it is also useful for other medical problems. Although this use is not included in product labeling, chlorpropamide is used in certain patients with the following medical condition:

• Diabetes insipidus (water diabetes)

If you are taking this medicine for water diabetes, the advice listed above that relates to diet and urine testing for patients with *sugar* diabetes *does not apply to you*. However, the advice about hypoglycemia (low blood sugar) does apply to you. Call your doctor right away if you feel any of the symptoms described.

Revised: July 1990
Interim revision: 06/30/94

# ANTIDYSKINETICS Systemic

Some commonly used brand names are:

**In the U.S.—**
Akineton[2]          Kemadrin[4]
Artane[5]            Parsidol[3]
Artane Sequels[5]    Trihexane[5]
Cogentin[1]          Trihexy[5]

**In Canada—**
Akineton[2]          Kemadrin[4]
Apo-Benztropine[1]   Parsitan[3]
Apo-Trihex[5]        PMS Benztropine[1]
Artane[5]            PMS Procyclidine[4]
Artane Sequels[5]    PMS Trihexyphenidyl[5]
Cogentin[1]          Procyclid[4]

Other commonly used names are:
Benzatropine[1]          Profenamine[3]

Note: For quick reference, the following antidyskinetics are numbered to match the corresponding brand names.

This information applies to the following medicines:
1. Benztropine (BENZ-troe-peen)‡§
2. Biperiden (bye-PER-i-den)
3. Ethopropazine (eth-oh-PROE-pa-zeen)
4. Procyclidine (proe-SYE-kli-deen)
5. Trihexyphenidyl (trye-hex-ee-FEN-i-dill)‡

Note: This information does *not* apply to Amantadine, Carbidopa and Levodopa, Diphenhydramine, Haloperidol, and Levodopa.

‡Generic name product may also be available in the U.S.
§Generic name product may also be available in Canada.

## Description

Antidyskinetics are used to treat Parkinson's disease, sometimes referred to as "shaking palsy." By improving muscle control and reducing stiffness, this medicine allows more normal movements of the body as the disease symptoms are reduced. It is also used to control severe reactions to certain medicines such as reserpine (e.g., Serpasil) (medicine to control high blood pressure) or phenothiazines, chlorprothixene (e.g., Taractan), thiothixene (e.g., Navane), loxapine (e.g., Loxitane), and haloperidol (e.g., Haldol) (medicines for nervous, mental, and emotional conditions).

Antidyskinetics may also be used for other conditions as determined by your doctor.

These medicines are available only with your doctor's prescription in the following dosage forms:

*Oral*
Benztropine
• Tablets (U.S. and Canada)
Biperiden
• Tablets (U.S. and Canada)
Ethopropazine
• Tablets (U.S. and Canada)
Procyclidine
• Elixir (Canada)
• Tablets (U.S. and Canada)

Trihexyphenidyl
- Extended-release capsules (U.S. and Canada)
- Elixir (U.S. and Canada)
- Tablets (U.S. and Canada)

*Parenteral*
Benztropine
- Injection (U.S. and Canada)
Biperiden
- Injection (U.S.)

## Before Using This Medicine

In deciding to use a medicine, the risks of taking the medicine must be weighed against the good it will do. This is a decision you and your doctor will make. For antidyskinetics, the following should be considered:

**Allergies**—Tell your doctor if you have ever had any unusual or allergic reaction to antidyskinetics. Also tell your health care professional if you are allergic to any other substances, such as foods, preservatives, or dyes.

**Pregnancy**—Studies on effects in pregnancy have not been done in either humans or animals. However, antidyskinetics have not been shown to cause problems in humans.

**Breast-feeding**—It is not known if antidyskinetics pass into breast milk. Although most medicines pass into breast milk in small amounts, many of them may be used safely while breast-feeding. Mothers who are taking these medicines and who wish to breast-feed should discuss this with their doctor.

Since antidyskinetics tend to decrease the secretions of the body, it is possible that the flow of breast milk may be reduced in some patients.

**Children**—Children may be especially sensitive to the effects of antidyskinetics. This may increase the chance of side effects during treatment.

**Older adults**—Agitation, confusion, disorientation, hallucinations, memory loss, and mental changes are more likely to occur in elderly patients, who are usually more sensitive to the effects of antidyskinetics.

**Other medicines**—Although certain medicines should not be used together at all, in other cases 2 different medicines may be used together even if an interaction might occur. In these cases, your doctor may want to change the dose, or other precautions may be necessary. When you are taking an antidyskinetic, it is especially important that your health care professional know if you are taking any of the following:

- Anticholinergics (medicine for abdominal or stomach spasms or cramps) or
- Central nervous system (CNS) depressants (medicine that causes drowsiness) or
- Tricyclic antidepressants (medicine for depression)—Using these medicines together with antidyskinetics may result in additive effects, increasing the chance of unwanted effects

**Other medical problems**—The presence of other medical problems may affect the use of antidyskinetics. Make sure you tell your doctor if you have any other medical problems, especially:

- Difficult urination or
- Enlarged prostate or
- Glaucoma or
- Heart or blood vessel disease or
- High blood pressure or
- Intestinal blockage or
- Myasthenia gravis or
- Uncontrolled movements of hands, mouth, or tongue—Antidyskinetics may make the condition worse
- Kidney disease or
- Liver disease—Higher blood levels of the antidyskinetics may result, increasing the chance of side effects

## Proper Use of This Medicine

*Take this medicine only as directed by your doctor.* Do not take more of it, do not take it more often, and do not take it for a longer period of time than your doctor ordered. To do so may increase the chance of side effects.

To lessen stomach upset, take this medicine with meals or immediately after meals, unless otherwise directed by your doctor.

**Dosing**—The dose of antidyskinetics will be different for different patients. *Follow your doctor's orders or the directions on the label.* The following information includes only the average doses of benztropine, biperiden, ethopropazine, procyclidine, and trihexyphenidyl. *If your dose is different, do not change it* unless your doctor tells you to do so.

The number of capsules, tablets, or teaspoonfuls of elixir that you take depends on the strength of the medicine. Also, *the number of doses you take each day, the time allowed between doses, and the length of time you take the medicine depend on the medical problem for which you are taking antidyskinetics.*

*For benztropine*
- For *oral* dosage forms (tablets):
  —For Parkinson's disease or certain severe side effects caused by some other medicines:
    - Adults—To start, 0.5 to 4 milligrams (mg) a day, depending on your condition. Your doctor will adjust your dose as needed; however, the dose is usually not more than 6 mg a day.
    - Children—Use and dose must be determined by your doctor.
- For *injection* dosage form:
  —For Parkinson's disease or certain severe side effects caused by some other medicines:
    - Adults—1 to 4 mg a day, depending on your condition. Your doctor will adjust your dose as needed; however, the dose is usually not more than 6 mg a day.
    - Children—Use and dose must be determined by your doctor.

*For biperiden*
- For *oral* dosage forms (tablets):
  —For Parkinson's disease or certain severe side effects caused by some other medicines:
    - Adults—2 mg up to four times a day. Your doctor will adjust your dose, depending on your condition; however, the dose is usually not more than 16 mg a day.
    - Children—Use and dose must be determined by your doctor.
- For *injection* dosage form:
  —For Parkinson's disease or certain severe side effects caused by some other medicines:
    - Adults—2 mg, injected into a muscle or vein. The dose may be repeated if needed; however, the dose is usually not given more than four times a day.
    - Children—Use and dose is based on body weight and must be determined by your doctor.

*For ethopropazine*
- For *oral* dosage forms (tablets):
  —For Parkinson's disease or certain severe side effects caused by some other medicines:
    - Adults—50 mg one or two times a day. Your doctor will adjust your dose as needed; however, the dose is usually not more than 600 mg a day.
    - Children—Use and dose must be determined by your doctor.

*For procyclidine*
- For *oral* dosage forms (elixir or tablets):
  —For Parkinson's disease or certain severe side effects caused by some other medicines:
    - Adults—To start, 2.5 mg three times a day after meals. Your doctor may need to adjust your dose, depending on your condition.
    - Children—Use and dose must be determined by your doctor.

*For trihexyphenidyl*
- For *extended-release oral* dosage forms (extended-release capsules):
  —For Parkinson's disease or certain severe side effects caused by some other medicines:
    - Adults—5 mg after breakfast. Your doctor may add another 5 mg dose to be taken twelve hours later, depending on your condition.
    - Children: Use and dose must be determined by your doctor.
- For other *oral* dosage forms (elixir or tablets):
  —For Parkinson's disease or certain severe side effects caused by some other medicines:
    - Adults—To start, 1 to 2 mg a day. Your doctor may adjust your dose as needed; however, the dose is usually not more than 15 mg a day.
    - Children—Use and dose must be determined by your doctor.

**Missed dose**—If you miss a dose of this medicine, take it as soon as possible. However, if it is within 2 hours of your next dose, skip the missed dose and go back to your regular dosing schedule. Do not double doses.

**Storage**—To store this medicine:
- Keep out of the reach of children.
- Store away from heat and direct light.
- Do not store the capsule or tablet form of this medicine in the bathroom, near the kitchen sink, or in other damp places. Heat or moisture may cause the medicine to break down.
- Keep the liquid form of this medicine from freezing.
- Do not keep outdated medicine or medicine no longer needed. Be sure that any discarded medicine is out of the reach of children.

## Precautions While Using This Medicine

Your doctor should check your progress at regular visits, especially for the first few months you take this medicine. This will allow your dosage to be changed as necessary to meet your needs.

Your doctor may want you to have your eyes examined by an ophthalmologist (eye doctor) before and also sometime later during treatment.

*Do not stop taking this medicine without first checking with your doctor.* Your doctor may want you to reduce gradually the amount you are taking before stopping completely, to prevent side effects or the worsening of your condition.

This medicine will add to the effects of alcohol and other CNS depressants (medicines that slow down the nervous system, possibly causing drowsiness). Some examples of CNS depressants are antihistamines or medicine for hay fever, other allergies, or colds; sedatives, tranquilizers, or sleeping medicine; prescription pain medicine or narcotics; barbiturates; medicine for seizures; muscle relaxants; or anesthetics, including some dental anesthetics. *Check with your doctor before taking any of the above while you are using this medicine.*

Do not take this medicine within 1 hour of taking medicine for diarrhea. Taking these medicines too close together will make this medicine less effective.

If you think you or anyone else has taken an overdose of this medicine, get emergency help at once. Taking an overdose of this medicine may lead to unconsciousness. Some signs of an overdose are clumsiness or unsteadiness; seizures; severe drowsiness; severe dryness of mouth, nose and throat; fast heartbeat; hallucinations (seeing, hearing, or feeling things that are not there); mood or mental changes; shortness of breath or troubled breathing; trouble in sleeping; and unusual warmth, dryness, and flushing of skin.

This medicine may cause your eyes to become more sensitive to light than they are normally. Wearing sunglasses and avoiding too much exposure to bright light may help lessen the discomfort.

This medicine may cause some people to have blurred vision or to become drowsy, dizzy, or less alert than they are normally. *Make sure you know how you react to this medicine before you drive, use machines, or do anything else that could be dangerous if you are dizzy or are not alert or able to see well.*

Dizziness, lightheadedness, or fainting may occur, especially when you get up from lying or sitting. Getting up slowly may help. If the problem continues or gets worse, check with your doctor.

This medicine may make you sweat less, causing your body temperature to increase. *Use extra care to avoid becoming overheated during exercise or hot weather while you are taking this medicine, since overheating may result in heat stroke.* Also, hot baths or saunas may make you feel dizzy or faint while you are taking this medicine.

This medicine may cause dryness of the mouth. For temporary relief, use sugarless candy or gum, melt bits of ice in your mouth, or use a saliva substitute. However, if your mouth continues to feel dry for more than 2 weeks, check with your medical doctor or dentist. Continuing dryness of the mouth may increase the chance of dental disease, including tooth decay, gum disease, and fungus infections.

## Side Effects of This Medicine

Along with its needed effects, a medicine may cause some unwanted effects. Although not all of these side effects may occur, if they do occur they may need medical attention.

Check with your doctor as soon as possible if any of the following side effects occur:

*Rare*
    Confusion (more common in the elderly or with high doses); eye pain; skin rash

*Symptoms of overdose*
    Clumsiness or unsteadiness; drowsiness (severe); dryness of mouth, nose, or throat (severe); fast heartbeat; hallucinations (seeing, hearing, or feeling things that are

not there); mood or mental changes; seizures; shortness of breath or troubled breathing; trouble in sleeping; warmth, dryness, and flushing of skin

Other side effects may occur that usually do not need medical attention. These side effects may go away during treatment as your body adjusts to the medicine. However, check with your doctor if any of the following side effects continue or are bothersome:

*More common*
    Blurred vision; constipation; decreased sweating; difficult or painful urination (especially in older men); drowsiness; dryness of mouth, nose, or throat; increased sensitivity of eyes to light; nausea or vomiting

*Less common or rare*
    Dizziness or lightheadedness when getting up from a lying or sitting position; false sense of well-being (especially in the elderly or with high doses); headache; loss of memory (especially in the elderly); muscle cramps; nervousness; numbness or weakness in hands or feet; soreness of mouth and tongue; stomach upset or pain; unusual excitement (more common with large doses of trihexyphenidyl)

After you stop using this medicine, your body may need time to adjust. The length of time this takes depends on the amount of medicine you were using and how long you used it. During this period of time check with your doctor if you notice any of the following side effects:

    Anxiety; difficulty in speaking or swallowing; dizziness or lightheadedness when getting up from a lying or sitting position; fast heartbeat; loss of balance control; mask-like face; muscle spasms, especially of face, neck, and back; restlessness or desire to keep moving; shuffling walk; stiffness of arms or legs; trembling and shaking of hands and fingers; trouble in sleeping; twisting movements of body

Other side effects not listed above may also occur in some patients. If you notice any other effects, check with your doctor.

Revised: 05/11/93

# ANTIFIBRINOLYTIC AGENTS   Systemic

Some commonly used brand names are:
**In the U.S.—**
    Amicar[1]
    Cyklokapron[2]
**In Canada—**
    Amicar[1]
    Cyklokapron[2]
Another commonly used name for aminocaproic acid is epsilon-aminocaproic acid.
This information applies to the following medicines:
1. Aminocaproic Acid (a-mee-noe-ka-PROE-ik ASS-id)‡
2. Tranexamic Acid (tran-ex-AM-ik ASS-id)

‡Generic name product may also be available in the U.S.

## Description

Antifibrinolytic (an-tee-fye-bri-noh-LIT-ik) agents are used to treat serious bleeding, especially when the bleeding occurs after dental surgery or certain other kinds of surgery. These medicines are also sometimes given before an operation to prevent serious bleeding in patients with hemophilia or other medical problems that increase the chance of serious bleeding.

Antifibrinolytic agents may also be used for other conditions as determined by your doctor.

Antifibrinolytic agents are available only with your doctor's prescription, in the following dosage forms:

*Oral*
    Aminocaproic acid
      • Syrup (U.S. and Canada)
      • Tablets (U.S. and Canada)
    Tranexamic acid
      • Tablets (U.S. and Canada)

*Parenteral*
    Aminocaproic acid
      • Injection (U.S. and Canada)
    Tranexamic acid
      • Injection (U.S. and Canada)

## Before Using This Medicine

In deciding to use a medicine, the risks of taking the medicine must be weighed against the good it will do. This is a decision you and your doctor will make. For antifibrinolytic agents, the following should be considered:

**Allergies**—Tell your doctor if you have ever had any unusual or allergic reaction to aminocaproic acid or tranexamic acid. Also tell your health care professional if you are allergic to any other substances, such as foods, preservatives, or dyes.

**Pregnancy**—Studies on birth defects have not been done in humans. However, these medicines have been given to pregnant women without causing birth defects or other problems.

Studies on effects of aminocaproic acid in pregnancy have not been done in animals. Tranexamic acid has not been shown to cause birth defects or other problems in animal studies.

**Breast-feeding**—These medicines have not been reported to cause problems in nursing babies. However, small amounts of tranexamic acid pass into the breast milk.

**Children**—Although there is no specific information comparing use of aminocaproic acid or tranexamic acid in children with use in other age groups, these medicines are not expected to cause different side effects or problems in children than they do in adults.

**Older adults—**
• *For aminocaproic acid*: Although there is no specific information comparing use of aminocaproic acid in the elderly with use in other age groups, this medicine is not expected to cause different side effects or problems in older people than it does in younger adults.
• *For tranexamic acid*: Tranexamic acid has been tested and has not been shown to cause different side effects or problems in older people than it does in younger adults.

**Other medicines**—Although certain medicines should not be used together at all, in other cases two different medicines may be used together even if an interaction might occur. In these cases, your doctor may want to change

the dose, or other precautions may be necessary. Tell your health care professional if you are taking any other prescription or nonprescription (over-the-counter [OTC]) medicine.

**Other medical problems**—The presence of other medical problems may affect the use of antifibrinolytic agents. Make sure you tell your doctor if you have any other medical problems, especially:
• Blood clots or a history of medical problems caused by blood clots or
• Blood in the urine or
• Color vision problems or
• Heart disease or
• Kidney disease or
• Liver disease—The chance of side effects may be increased

## Proper Use of This Medicine

*Take this medicine only as directed by your doctor.* Do not take more or less of it, do not take it more often, and do not take it for a longer time than your doctor ordered. To do so may increase the chance of unwanted effects.

**Dosing**—The dose of these medicines will be different for different patients. *Follow your doctor's orders or the directions on the label.* The following information includes only the average doses of these medicines. *If your dose is different, do not change it* unless your doctor tells you to do so.

*For aminocaproic acid*
• To prevent or treat serious bleeding:
  —For *oral* dosage forms (syrup or tablets):
    • Adults—For the first hour, the dose is 5 grams. Then the dose is 1 or 1.25 grams per hour for eight hours.
    • Children—Dose is based on body weight or size and must be determined by your doctor. For the first hour, the dose is usually 100 milligrams (mg) per kilogram (kg) (45.4 mg per pound) of body weight. Then the dose is 33.3 mg per kg (15.1 mg per pound) of body weight per hour.
  —For *injection* dosage form:
    • Adults—At first, the dose is 4 to 5 grams injected into a vein, over a period of one hour. Then the dose is 1 gram per hour, injected into a vein over a period of eight hours.
    • Children—Dose is based on body weight or size and must be determined by your doctor. At first, the dose is usually 100 mg per kg (45.4 mg per pound) of body weight, injected into a vein over a period of one hour. Then the dose is 33.3 mg per kg (15.1 mg per pound) of body weight per hour, injected into a vein..

*For tranexamic acid*
• To prevent or treat serious bleeding after dental surgery:
  —For *oral* dosage form (tablets):
    • Adults and children—Dose is based on body weight and must be determined by your doctor.

The dose is usually 25 milligrams (mg) per kilogram (kg) (11.4 mg per pound) of body weight three or four times a day, beginning one day before surgery. After surgery, the dose is usually 25 mg per kg (11.4 mg per pound) of body weight three or four times a day for two to eight days.

—For *injection* dosage form:
- Adults and children—Dose is based on body weight and must be determined by your doctor. The dose is usually 10 mg per kg (4.5 mg per pound) of body weight, injected into a vein just before surgery. After surgery, the dose is usually 10 mg per kg (4.5 mg per pound) of body weight, injected into a vein three or four times a day for two to eight days.

**Missed dose—**
- *For aminocaproic acid* (e.g., Amicar): If you miss a dose, take it as soon as possible. However, if you do not remember until it is almost time for your next dose, double the next dose. Then go back to your regular dosing schedule.
- *For tranexamic acid* (e.g., Cyklokapron): If you miss a dose, take it as soon as possible. Then take any remaining doses for the day at regularly spaced times. Do not double doses. If you have any questions about this, check with your doctor.

**Storage—**To store this medicine:
- Keep out of the reach of children.
- Store away from heat and direct light.
- Do not store the tablet form of this medicine in the bathroom, near the kitchen sink, or in other damp places. Heat or moisture may cause the medicine to break down.
- Do not keep outdated medicine or medicine no longer needed. Be sure that any discarded medicine is out of the reach of children.

## Precautions While Using This Medicine

If you will be taking tranexamic acid for longer than several days, your doctor may want you to have your eyes checked regularly by an ophthalmologist (eye doctor). This will allow your doctor to check for unwanted effects that may be caused by this medicine.

## Side Effects of This Medicine

Along with its needed effects, a medicine may cause some unwanted effects. Although not all of these side effects may occur, if they do occur they may need medical attention.

The same effect that makes aminocaproic acid or tranexamic acid help prevent or stop bleeding also may cause blood clots that could be dangerous. Check with your doctor immediately if any of the following possible signs and symptoms of blood clots occur:

*Less common or rare*
Headache (severe and sudden); loss of coordination (sudden); pains in chest, groin, or legs, especially the calves; shortness of breath (sudden); slurred speech (sudden); vision changes (sudden); weakness or numbness in arm or leg

Also, check with your doctor as soon as possible if any of the following side effects occur:

*Less common or rare*
*For aminocaproic acid*
Dizziness; headache; muscle pain or weakness (severe and continuing); red or bloodshot eyes; ringing or buzzing in ears; skin rash; slow or irregular heartbeat—with the injection only; stomach cramps or pain; stuffy nose; sudden decrease in amount of urine; swelling of face, feet, or lower legs; unusual tiredness or weakness; weight gain (rapid)

*For tranexamic acid*
Blurred vision or other changes in vision; dizziness or lightheadedness; unusual tiredness or weakness

Other side effects may occur that usually do not need medical attention. These side effects may go away during treatment as your body adjusts to the medicine. However, check with your doctor if any of the following side effects continue or are bothersome:

Diarrhea; dry ejaculation; nausea or vomiting; unusual menstrual discomfort

Other side effects not listed above may also occur in some patients. If you notice any other effects, check with your doctor.

Revised: 08/15/94

---

# ANTIFUNGALS, AZOLE  Systemic

Some commonly used brand names are:

**In the U.S.—**
Diflucan[1]          Nizoral[3]
Monistat i.v.[4]     Sporanox[2]

**In Canada—**
Diflucan[1]          Sporanox[2]
Nizoral[3]

Note: For quick reference, the following antifungals are numbered to match the corresponding brand names.

This information applies to the following medicines:
1. Fluconazole (floo-KOE-na-zole)
2. Itraconazole (i-tra-KOE-na-zole)
3. Ketoconazole (kee-toe-KON-a-zole)
4. Miconazole (mi-KON-a-zole)†

†Not commercially available in Canada.

# Description

Azole antifungals are used to treat serious fungus infections that may occur in different parts of the body. These medicines may also be used for other problems as determined by your doctor.

Azole antifungals are available only with your doctor's prescription, in the following dosage forms:

*Oral*
Fluconazole
- Oral suspension (U.S.)
- Tablets (U.S. and Canada)
Itraconazole
- Capsules (U.S. and Canada)
Ketoconazole
- Oral suspension (Canada)
- Tablets (U.S. and Canada)

*Parenteral*
Fluconazole
- Injection (U.S. and Canada)
Miconazole
- Injection (U.S.)

# Before Using This Medicine

In deciding to use a medicine, the risks of taking the medicine must be weighed against the good it will do. This is a decision you and your doctor will make. For the azole antifungals, the following should be considered:

**Allergies**—Tell your doctor if you have ever had any unusual or allergic reaction to any of the azole antifungals. Also tell your health care professional if you are allergic to any other substances, such as foods, preservatives, or dyes.

**Pregnancy**—Studies have not been done in pregnant women. However, studies in some animals have shown that azole antifungals, taken in high doses, may cause harm to the mother and the fetus. They have caused birth defects in animals. Before taking these medicines, make sure your doctor knows if you are pregnant or if you may become pregnant.

**Breast-feeding**—Azole antifungals pass into breast milk. Mothers who are taking these medicines and who wish to breast-feed should discuss this with their doctors.

**Children**—A small number of children have been safely treated with azole antifungals. Be sure to discuss with your child's doctor the use of these medicines in children.

**Older adults**—Many medicines have not been studied specifically in older people. Therefore, it may not be known whether they work exactly the same way they do in younger adults or if they cause different side effects or problems in older people. There is no specific information comparing use of azole antifungals in the elderly with use in other age groups.

**Other medicines**—Although certain medicines should not be used together at all, in other cases 2 different medicines may be used together even if an interaction might occur. In these cases, your doctor may want to change

the dose, or other precautions may be necessary. When you are taking azole antifungals, it is especially important that your health care professional know if you are taking any of the following:

- Acetaminophen (e.g., Tylenol) (with long-term, high-dose use) or
- Amiodarone (e.g., Cordarone) or
- Anabolic steroids (nandrolone [e.g., Anabolin], oxandrolone [e.g., Anavar], oxymetholone [e.g., Anadrol], stanozolol [e.g., Winstrol]) or
- Androgens (male hormones) or
- Antithyroid agents (medicine for overactive thyroid) or
- Carmustine (e.g., BiCNU) or
- Chloroquine (e.g., Aralen) or
- Dantrolene (e.g., Dantrium) or
- Daunorubicin (e.g., Cerubidine) or
- Disulfiram (e.g., Antabuse) or
- Divalproex (e.g., Depakote) or
- Estrogens (female hormones) or
- Etretinate (e.g., Tegison) or
- Gold salts (medicine for arthritis) or
- Hydroxychloroquine (e.g., Plaquenil) or
- Mercaptopurine (e.g., Purinethol) or
- Methotrexate (e.g., Mexate) or
- Methyldopa (e.g., Aldomet) or
- Naltrexone (e.g., Trexan) (with long-term, high-dose use) or
- Oral contraceptives (birth control pills) containing estrogen or
- Other anti-infectives by mouth or by injection (medicine for infection) or
- Phenothiazines (acetophenazine [e.g., Tindal], chlorpromazine [e.g., Thorazine], fluphenazine [e.g., Prolixin], mesoridazine [e.g., Serentil], perphenazine [e.g., Trilafon], prochlorperazine [e.g., Compazine], promazine [e.g., Sparine], promethazine [e.g., Phenergan], thioridazine [e.g., Mellaril], trifluoperazine [e.g., Stelazine], triflupromazine [e.g., Vesprin], trimeprazine [e.g., Temaril]) or
- Plicamycin (e.g., Mithracin) or
- Valproic acid (e.g., Depakene)—Use of these medicines with azole antifungals may increase the chance of side effects affecting the liver
- Amantadine (e.g., Symmetrel) or
- Antacids or
- Anticholinergics (medicine for abdominal or stomach spasms or cramps) or
- Antidepressants (medicine for depression) or
- Antidyskinetics (medicine for Parkinson's disease or other conditions affecting control of muscles) or
- Antihistamines or
- Antipsychotics (medicine for mental illness) or
- Buclizine (e.g., Bucladin) or
- Cimetidine (e.g., Tagamet) or
- Cyclizine (e.g., Marezine) or
- Cyclobenzaprine (e.g., Flexeril) or
- Disopyramide (e.g., Norpace) or
- Famotidine (e.g., Pepcid) or
- Flavoxate (e.g., Urispas) or
- Ipratropium (e.g., Atrovent) or
- Meclizine (e.g., Antivert) or
- Methylphenidate (e.g., Ritalin) or
- Nizatidine (e.g., Axid) or
- Omeprazole (e.g., Prilosec) or
- Orphenadrine (e.g., Norflex) or
- Oxybutynin (e.g., Ditropan) or
- Procainamide (e.g., Pronestyl) or

- Promethazine (e.g., Phenergan) or
- Quinidine (e.g., Quinidex) or
- Ranitidine (e.g., Zantac) or
- Sucralfate (e.g., Carafate) or
- Trimeprazine (e.g., Temaril)—Use of these medicines may decrease the effects of itraconazole and ketoconazole; these medicines should be taken at least 2 hours after itraconazole or ketoconazole
- Antidiabetic agents, oral (chlorpropamide [e.g., Diabinese], glipizide [e.g., Glucotrol], glyburide [e.g., DiaBeta, Micronase], tolbutamide [e.g., Orinase]) or
- Cyclosporine (e.g., Sandimmune) or
- Digoxin (e.g., Lanoxin) or
- Warfarin (e.g., Coumadin)—Fluconazole may increase the effects of these medicines, which may increase the chance of side effects
- Astemizole (e.g., Hismanal) or
- Terfenadine (e.g., Seldane)—These medications should not be taken with itraconazole or ketoconazole; these azole antifungals may increase the chance of serious side effects of astemizole or terfenadine
- Carbamazepine (e.g., Tegretol) or
- Isoniazid or
- Rifampin (e.g., Rifadin)—These medicines may decrease the effects of azole antifungals
- Didanosine (e.g., ddI, Videx)—Use of didanosine with itraconazole or ketoconazole may decrease the effects of both itraconazole and ketoconazole, as well as didanosine. Itraconazole and ketoconazole should be taken at least 2 hours before or 2 hours after didanosine is given
- Phenytoin (e.g., Dilantin)—Use of phenytoin with azole antifungals may increase the effects of the azole antifungals, increase side effects of azole antifungals affecting the liver, and increase the chance of phenytoin side effects

**Other medical problems**—The presence of other medical problems may affect the use of azole antifungals. Make sure you tell your doctor if you have any other medical problems, especially:

- Achlorhydria (absence of stomach acid) or
- Hypochlorhydria (decreased amount of stomach acid)—Itraconazole and ketoconazole may not be absorbed from the stomach as well in patients who have low levels of or no stomach acid
- Alcohol abuse (or history of) or
- Liver disease—Alcohol abuse or liver disease may increase the chance of side effects caused by azole antifungals
- Kidney disease—The effects of fluconazole may be increased in patients with kidney disease

---

## Proper Use of This Medicine

Itraconazole and ketoconazole should be taken with a meal or a snack.

For patients taking the *oral liquid form of ketoconazole:*

- Use a specially marked measuring spoon or other device to measure each dose accurately. The average household teaspoon may not hold the right amount of liquid.

*If you have achlorhydria (absence of stomach acid) or hypochlorhydria (decreased amount of stomach acid), and you are taking itraconazole or ketoconazole,* your doctor may want you to take your medicine with an acidic

drink. You may dissolve your medicine in cola or seltzer water and drink the solution, or your may take your medicine with a glass of cola or seltzer water. Your doctor may suggest that you dissolve each capsule or tablet in a teaspoonful of weak hydrochloric acid solution to help you absorb the medicine better. Your health care professional can prepare the solution for you. After you dissolve the tablet in the acid solution, add this mixture to a small amount (1 or 2 teaspoonfuls) of water in a glass. Drink the mixture through a plastic or glass drinking straw. Place the straw behind your teeth, as far back in your mouth as you can. This will keep the acid from harming your teeth. Be sure to drink all the liquid to get the full dose of medicine. Next, swish around in your mouth about ½ glass of water and then swallow it. This will help wash away any acid that may remain in your mouth or on your teeth.

To help clear up your infection completely, *it is very important that you keep taking this medicine for the full time of treatment,* even if your symptoms begin to clear up or you begin to feel better after a few days. Since fungus infections may be very slow to clear up, you may have to continue taking this medicine every day for as long as 6 months to a year or more. Some fungus infections never clear up completely and require continuous treatment. If you stop taking this medicine too soon, your symptoms may return.

This medicine works best when there is a constant amount in the blood. *To help keep the amount constant, do not miss any doses. Also, it is best to take each dose at the same time every day.* If you need help in planning the best time to take your medicine, check with your health care professional.

**Dosing**—The dose of azole antifungals may be different for different patients. *Follow your doctor's orders or the directions on the label.* The following information includes only the average doses of azole antifungals. Your dose of fluconazole may be different if you have kidney disease. *If your dose is different, do not change it* unless your doctor tells you to do so.

The number of capsules, tablets, or the amount of oral suspension that you take depends on the strength of the medicine. Also, *the number of doses you take each day, the time allowed between doses, and the length of time you take the medicine depend on the medical problem for which you are taking azole antifungals.*

*For fluconazole*

- For fungus infections
  —For *oral* dosage form (oral suspension and tablets):
  - Adults and teenagers—200 to 400 milligrams (mg) on the first day, then 100 to 400 mg once a day for weeks or months, depending on the medical problem being treated.
  - Children up to 14 years of age—Dose must be determined by your doctor.

—For *injection* dosage form:
- Adults and teenagers—200 to 400 mg on the first day, then 100 to 400 mg once a day, injected into a vein, for weeks or months, depending on the medical problem being treated.
- Children up to 14 years of age—Dose must be determined by your doctor.

*For itraconazole*
- For fungus infections
  —For *oral* dosage form (capsules):
  - Adults and teenagers—200 milligrams (mg) once a day, which may be increased up to 400 mg once a day for weeks or months, depending on the medical problem being treated.
  —Children up to 16 years of age: Dose must be determined by your doctor.

*For ketoconazole*
- For fungus infections
  —For *oral* dosage form (oral suspension and tablets):
  - Adults and teenagers—200 to 400 milligrams (mg) once a day for weeks or months, depending on the medical problem being treated.
  —Children up to 2 years of age: Dose must be determined by your doctor.
  —Children over 2 years of age: 3.3 to 6.6 mg per kilogram (kg) (1.5 to 3 mg per pound) of body weight once a day for weeks or months, depending on the medical problem being treated.

*For miconazole*
- For fungus infections
  —For *injection* dosage form:
  - Adults and teenagers—200 milligrams (mg) to 1.2 gram three times a day, injected into a vein, for weeks or months, depending on the medical problem being treated.
  - Children up to 1 year of age—Dose must be determined by your doctor.
  - Children 1 year of age and over—20 to 40 mg per kilogram (kg) (9.1 to 18.2 mg per pound) of body weight per day, given in two or three doses, for weeks or months, depending on the medical problem being treated.

**Missed dose**—If you miss a dose of this medicine, take it as soon as possible. This will help to keep a constant amount of medicine in the blood. However, if it is almost time for your next dose, skip the missed dose and go back to your regular dosing schedule. Do not double doses.

**Storage**—To store this medicine:
- Keep out of the reach of children.
- Store away from heat and direct light.
- Do not store the capsule or tablet form of this medicine in the bathroom, near the kitchen sink, or in other damp places. Heat or moisture may cause the medicine to break down.
- Keep the oral liquid form of this medicine from freezing.
- Do not keep outdated medicine or medicine no longer needed. Be sure that any discarded medicine is out of the reach of children.

## Precautions While Using This Medicine

It is important that your doctor check your progress at regular visits. This will allow your doctor to check for any unwanted effects.

If your symptoms do not improve within a few weeks (or months for some infections), or if they become worse, check with your doctor.

*Itraconazole and ketoconazole should **not** be taken with astemizole (e.g., Hismanal) or terfenadine (e.g., Seldane).* Doing so may increase the risk of serious side effects affecting the heart.

Liver problems may be more likely to occur if you drink alcoholic beverages while you are taking this medicine. Alcoholic beverages may also cause stomach pain, nausea, vomiting, headache, or flushing or redness of the face. Other alcohol-containing preparations (for example, elixirs, cough syrups, tonics) may also cause problems. These problems may occur for at least a day after you stop taking ketoconazole. Therefore, *you should not drink alcoholic beverages or use alcohol-containing preparations while you are taking this medicine and for at least a day after you stop taking it.*

*If you are taking antacids, cimetidine (e.g., Tagamet), famotidine (e.g., Pepcid), nizatidine (e.g., Axid), omeprazole (e.g., Prilosec), or ranitidine (e.g., Zantac) while you are taking itraconazole or ketoconazole, take the other medicine at least 2 hours after you take itraconazole or ketoconazole.* If you take these medicines at the same time that you take itraconazole or ketoconazole, they will keep your antifungal medicine from working properly.

Ketoconazole may cause your eyes to become more sensitive to light than they are normally. Wearing sunglasses and avoiding too much exposure to bright light may help lessen the discomfort.

## Side Effects of This Medicine

Along with its needed effects, a medicine may cause some unwanted effects. Although not all of these effects may occur, if they do occur they may need medical attention.

*Check with your doctor immediately* if any of the following side effects occur:

*More common*
  Redness, swelling, or pain at the place of injection—for miconazole

*Less common*
  Fever and chills, skin rash or itching

*Rare*
  Dark or amber urine; fever and sore throat; loss of appetite; pale stools; reddening, blistering, peeling, or

loosening of skin and mucous membranes; stomach pain; unusual bleeding or bruising; unusual tiredness or weakness; yellow eyes or skin

Other side effects may occur that usually do not need medical attention. These side effects may go away during treatment as your body adjusts to the medicine. However, check with your doctor if any of the following side effects continue or are bothersome:

*Less common*

Constipation; diarrhea; dizziness; drowsiness; flushing or redness of the face or skin; headache; nausea; vomiting

*Rare—for ketoconazole*

Decreased sexual ability in males; enlargement of the breasts in males; increased sensitivity of the eyes to light; menstrual irregularities

Other side effects not listed above may also occur in some patients. If you notice any other effects, check with your doctor.

Revised: 05/20/94

# ANTIFUNGALS, AZOLE     Vaginal

Some commonly used brand names are:

**In the U.S.—**

| | |
|---|---|
| FemCare[2] | Monistat 7[4] |
| Femizole-7[2] | Mycelex-G[2] |
| Femstat[1] | Mycelex-7[2] |
| Femstat Prefill[1] | Terazol 3[5] |
| Gyne-Lotrimin[2] | Terazol 7[5] |
| Miconazole-7[4] | Vagistat-1[6] |
| Monistat 3[4] | |

**In Canada—**

| | |
|---|---|
| Canesten[2] | Monistat[4] |
| Canesten 1[2] | Monistat 3[4] |
| Canesten 3[2] | Monistat 7[4] |
| Clotrimaderm[2] | Myclo[2] |
| Ecostatin[3] | Terazol 3[5] |
| Gyno-Trosyd[6] | Terazol 7[5] |

Note: For quick reference, the following azole antifungals are numbered to match the corresponding brand names.

This information applies to the following medicines:

1. Butoconazole (byoo-toe-KOE-na-zole)†
2. Clotrimazole (kloe-TRIM-a-zole)‡
3. Econazole (e-KONE-a-zole)*
4. Miconazole (mi-KON-a-zole)‡
5. Terconazole (ter-KONE-a-zole)
6. Tioconazole (tye-oh-KONE-a-zole)

---

*Not commercially available in the U.S.
†Not commercially available in Canada.
‡Generic name product may also be available in the U.S.

---

## Description

Vaginal azoles (A-zoles) are used to treat fungus (yeast) infections of the vagina.

Most vaginal azoles are available only with your doctor's prescription, in the following dosage forms:

*Vaginal*

Butoconazole
- Cream (U.S.)

Clotrimazole
- Cream (U.S. and Canada)
- Tablets (U.S. and Canada)

Econazole
- Suppositories (Canada)

Miconazole
- Cream (U.S. and Canada)
- Suppositories (U.S. and Canada)

Terconazole
- Cream (U.S. and Canada)
- Suppositories (U.S. and Canada)

Tioconazole
- Ointment (U.S. and Canada)

## Before Using This Medicine

In deciding to use a medicine, the risks of using the medicine must be weighed against the good it will do. This is a decision you and your doctor will make. For vaginal azoles, the following should be considered:

**Allergies**—Tell your doctor if you have ever had any unusual or allergic reaction to any of the azoles. Also tell your health care professional if you are allergic to any other substances, such as foods, preservatives, or dyes.

**Pregnancy**—Studies have not been done in humans during the first trimester of pregnancy. Vaginal azoles have not been shown to cause birth defects or other problems in humans when used during the second and third trimesters.

**Breast-feeding**—It is not known whether vaginal azoles pass into the breast milk. However, these medicines have not been shown to cause problems in nursing babies.

**Children**—Studies on these medicines have been done only in adult patients, and there is no specific information comparing use of vaginal azoles in children with use in other age groups.

**Older adults**—Many medicines have not been studied specifically in older people. Therefore, it may not be known whether they work exactly the same way they do in younger adults. Although there is no specific information comparing use of vaginal azoles in the elderly with use in other age groups, they are not expected to cause different side effects or problems in older people than they do in younger adults.

**Other medicines**—Although certain medicines should not be used together at all, in other cases two different medicines may be used together even if an interaction might occur. In these cases, your doctor may want to change

the dose, or other precautions may be necessary. Tell your health care professional if you are using any other vaginal prescription or nonprescription (over-the-counter [OTC]) medicine.

## Proper Use of This Medicine

Vaginal azoles usually come with patient directions. Read them carefully before using this medicine.

Use this medicine at bedtime, unless otherwise directed by your doctor. The vaginal tampon form of miconazole should be left in the vagina overnight and removed the next morning.

This medicine is usually inserted into the vagina with an applicator. However, if you are pregnant, check with your doctor before using the applicator.

To help clear up your infection completely, *it is very important that you keep using this medicine for the full time of treatment,* even if your symptoms begin to clear up after a few days. If you stop using this medicine too soon, your symptoms may return. *Do not miss any doses.* Also, *do not stop using this medicine if your menstrual period starts during the time of treatment.*

**Dosing**—The dose of these medicines will be different for different patients. *Follow your doctor's orders or the directions on the label.* The following information includes only the average doses of these medicines. *If your dose is different, do not change it* unless your doctor tells you to do so.

*For butoconazole nitrate*
- For fungus infection:
  —For *vaginal cream* dosage form:
  - Adults and teenagers:
    —Women who are not pregnant: 100 milligrams (mg) (one applicatorful) of 2% cream inserted into the vagina at bedtime for three nights in a row.
    —Pregnant women, after the third month: 100 mg (one applicatorful) of 2% cream inserted into the vagina at bedtime for six nights in a row.
  - Children—Dose must be determined by your doctor.
  —For *vaginal suppository* dosage form:
  - Adults and teenagers:
    —Women who are not pregnant: 100 mg (one suppository) inserted into the vagina at bedtime for three nights in a row.

*For clotrimazole*
- For fungus infection:
  —For *vaginal cream* dosage form:
  - Adults and teenagers—The dose depends on the strength of the cream.
    —1% cream: 50 mg (one applicatorful) inserted into the vagina at bedtime for six to fourteen nights in a row.

—2% cream: 100 mg (one applicatorful) inserted into the vagina at bedtime for three nights in a row.
    —10% cream: 500 mg (one applicatorful) inserted into the vagina at bedtime for one night only.
  - Children—Dose must be determined by your doctor.
  —For *vaginal tablet* dosage form:
  - Adults and teenagers—The dose depends on the strength of the vaginal tablet.
    —Women who are not pregnant:
    - 100-mg tablet: Insert one tablet into the vagina at bedtime for six or seven nights in a row.
    - 200-mg tablet: Insert one tablet into the vagina at bedtime for three nights in a row.
    - 500-mg tablet: Insert one tablet into the vagina at bedtime as a single dose.
    —Pregnant women: 100 mg (one vaginal tablet) inserted into the vagina at bedtime for seven nights in a row.
  - Children—Dose must be determined by your doctor.

*For econozole nitrate*
- For fungus infection:
  —For *vaginal suppository* dosage form:
  - Adults and teenagers—150 milligrams (mg) (one vaginal suppository) inserted into the vagina at bedtime for three nights in a row.
  - Children—Dose must be determined by your doctor.

*For miconazole nitrate*
- For fungus infection:
  —For *vaginal cream* dosage form:
  - Adults and teenagers—One applicatorful inserted into the vagina at bedtime for seven or fourteen nights in a row.
  - Children—Dose must be determined by your doctor.
  —For *vaginal suppository* dosage form:
  - Adults and teenagers—The dose depends on the strength of the suppository.
    —100-mg suppository: Insert one vaginal suppository into the vagina at bedtime for seven nights in a row.
    —200-mg suppository or
    —400-mg suppository: Insert one vaginal suppository into the vagina at bedtime for three nights in a row.
  - Children—Dose must be determined by your doctor.
  —For *tampon* dosage form:
  - Adults and teenagers—100 mg (one tampon) inserted into the vagina at bedtime and then removed the next morning. This is repeated every night for five nights in a row.

• Children—Dose must be determined by your doctor.

*For terconazole*

• For fungus infection:
  —For *vaginal cream* dosage form:
    • Adults and teenagers—The dose depends on the strength of the cream.
      —0.4% cream: 20 mg (one applicatorful) inserted into the vagina at bedtime for seven nights in a row.
      —0.8% cream: 40 mg (one applicatorful) inserted into the vagina at bedtime for three nights in a row.
    • Children—Dose must be determined by your doctor.
  —For *vaginal suppository* dosage form:
    • Adults and teenagers—80 mg (one vaginal suppository) inserted into the vagina at bedtime for three nights in a row.
    • Children—Dose must be determined by your doctor.

*For tioconazole*

• For fungus infection:
  —For *vaginal ointment* dosage form:
    • Adults and teenagers—300 mg (one applicatorful) of 6.5% ointment inserted into the vagina at bedtime as a single dose.
    • Children—Dose must be determined by your doctor.
  —For *vaginal suppository* dosage form:
    • Adults and teenagers—300 mg (one vaginal suppository) inserted into the vagina at bedtime.
    • Children—Dose must be determined by your doctor.

**Missed dose**—If you miss a dose of this medicine, insert it as soon as possible. However, if it is almost time for your next dose, skip the missed dose and go back to your regular dosing schedule.

**Storage**—To store this medicine:

• Keep out of the reach of children.
• Store away from heat and direct light.
• Do not store the vaginal suppository or vaginal tablet form of this medicine in the bathroom, near the kitchen sink, or in other damp places. Heat or moisture may cause the medicine to break down.
• Keep the vaginal cream, ointment, and suppository forms of this medicine from freezing.
• Do not keep outdated medicine or medicine no longer needed. Be sure that any discarded medicine is out of the reach of children.

## Precautions While Using This Medicine

If your symptoms do not improve within a few days, or if they become worse, check with your doctor.

Vaginal medicines usually will come out of the vagina during treatment. To keep the medicine from getting on your clothing, wear a minipad or sanitary napkin. The use of nonmedicated tampons (like those used for menstrual periods) is not recommended since they may soak up the medicine.

*To help clear up your infection completely and to help make sure it does not return,* good health habits are also required.

• Wear cotton panties (or panties or pantyhose with cotton crotches) instead of synthetic (for example, nylon or rayon) panties.
• Wear only clean panties.

If you have any questions about this, check with your health care professional.

Many vaginal infections are spread by having sex. A male sexual partner may carry the fungus on or in his penis. While you are using this medicine, it may be a good idea for your partner to wear a condom during sex to avoid re-infection. Also, it may be necessary for your partner to be treated. *Do not stop using this medicine if you have sex during treatment.*

Certain brands of vaginal azoles contain oils in the cream bases the medicine is put in. Oils can weaken latex rubber condoms, diaphragms, or cervical caps. This increases the chances of a condom breaking during sexual intercourse. The rubber in cervical caps or diaphragms may break down faster and wear out sooner. Check with your health care professional to make sure the vaginal azole product you are using can be used with latex rubber birth control devices.

Some women may want to use a douche before the next dose. Some doctors will allow the use of a vinegar and water douche or other douche. However, others do not allow any douching. If you do use a douche, *do not overfill the vagina.* To do so may push the douche up into the uterus and possibly cause inflammation or infection. Also, *do not douche if you are pregnant since this may harm the fetus.* If you have any questions about this, check with your health care professional.

## Side Effects of This Medicine

Along with its needed effects, a medicine may cause some unwanted effects. Although not all of these side effects may occur, if they do occur they may need medical attention.

Check with your doctor as soon as possible if any of the following side effects occur:

*Less common*
  Vaginal burning, itching, discharge, or other irritation not present before use of this medicine

*Rare*
  Skin rash or hives

Other side effects may occur that usually do not need medical attention. These side effects may go away during treatment as your body adjusts to the medicine. However,

check with your doctor if any of the following side effects continue or are bothersome:

*Less common or rare*

Abdominal or stomach cramps or pain; burning or irritation of penis of sexual partner; headache

Other side effects not listed above may also occur in some patients. If you notice any other effects, check with your doctor.

Revised: 04/21/92
Interim revision: 07/23/92; 07/12/94

# ANTIGLAUCOMA AGENTS, CHOLINERGIC, LONG-ACTING    Ophthalmic

Some commonly used brand names are:

**In the U.S.—**
Floropryl[3]        Phospholine Iodide[2]
Humorsol[1]

**In Canada—**
Phospholine Iodide[2]

Other commonly used names are:

DFP[3]             dyflos[3]
difluorophate[3]   ecothiopate[2]

Note: For quick reference, the following medicines are numbered to match the corresponding brand names.

This information applies to the following medicines:

1. Demecarium (dem-e-KARE-ee-um)
2. Echothiophate (ek-oh-THYE-oh-fate)
3. Isoflurophate (eye-soe-FLURE-oh-fate)

## Description

Demecarium, echothiophate, and isoflurophate are used in the eye to treat certain types of glaucoma and other eye conditions, such as accommodative esotropia. They may also be used in the diagnosis of certain eye conditions, such as accommodative esotropia.

These medicines are available only with your doctor's prescription, in the following dosage forms:

*Ophthalmic*

Demecarium
• Ophthalmic solution (eye drops) (U.S.)
Echothiophate
• Ophthalmic solution (eye drops) (U.S. and Canada)
Isoflurophate
• Ophthalmic ointment (eye ointment) (U.S.)

## Before Using This Medicine

In deciding to use a medicine, the risks of taking the medicine must be weighed against the good it will do. This is a decision you and your doctor will make. For demecarium, echothiophate, or isoflurophate, the following should be considered:

**Allergies**—Tell your doctor if you have ever had any unusual or allergic reaction to demecarium, echothiophate, or isoflurophate. Also tell your health care professional if you are allergic to any other substances, such as preservatives.

**Pregnancy**—Because of the toxicity of these medicines in general, demecarium, echothiophate, and isoflurophate are not recommended during pregnancy.

**Breast-feeding**—Demecarium, echothiophate, and isoflurophate may be absorbed into the body. These medicines are not recommended during breast-feeding, because they may cause unwanted effects in nursing babies. It may be necessary for you to use another medicine or to stop breast-feeding during treatment. Be sure you have discussed the risks and benefits of the medicine with your doctor.

**Children**—Demecarium, echothiophate, or isoflurophate can cause serious side effects in any patient. When this medicine is used for a long time, eye cysts may occur. These eye cysts occur more often in children than in adults. Therefore, it is especially important that you discuss with the child's doctor the good that this medicine may do as well as the risks of using it.

**Older adults**—Many medicines have not been studied specifically in older people. Therefore, it may not be known whether they work exactly the same way they do in younger adults or if they cause different side effects or problems in older people. There is no specific information comparing use of these medicines in the elderly with use in other age groups. However, demecarium, echothiophate, or isoflurophate can cause serious side effects in any patient.

**Other medicines**—Although certain medicines should not be used together at all, in other cases two different medicines may be used together even if an interaction might occur. In these cases, your doctor may want to change the dose, or other precautions may be necessary. When you are taking demecarium, echothiophate, or isoflurophate, it is especially important that your health care professional know if you are taking any of the following:

• Amantadine (e.g., Symmetrel) or
• Anticholinergics (medicine for abdominal or stomach spasms or cramps) or
• Antidepressants (medicine for depression) or
• Antidyskinetics (medicine for Parkinson's disease or other conditions affecting control of muscles) or
• Antihistamines or
• Antimyasthenics (ambenonium [e.g., Mytelase], neostigmine [e.g., Prostigmin], pyridostigmine [e.g., Mestinon]) or
• Antipsychotics (medicine for mental illness) or
• Buclizine (e.g., Bucladin) or
• Carbamazepine (e.g., Tegretol) or
• Cyclizine (e.g., Marezine) or
• Cyclobenzaprine (e.g., Flexeril) or

- Disopyramide (e.g., Norpace) or
- Flavoxate (e.g., Urispas) or
- Ipratropium (e.g., Atrovent) or
- Meclizine (e.g., Antivert) or
- Methylphenidate (e.g., Ritalin) or
- Orphenadrine (e.g., Norflex) or
- Oxybutynin (e.g., Ditropen) or
- Procainamide (e.g., Pronestyl) or
- Promethazine (e.g., Phenergan) or
- Quinidine (e.g., Quinidex) or
- Trimeprazine (e.g., Temaril)—May increase the possibility of side effects or toxic effects; use of these medicines with demecarium, echothiophate, or isoflurophate is not recommended except under close supervision by your doctor
- Malathion (topical) (e.g., Prioderm)—May increase the possibility of side effects or toxic effects, especially if large amounts of malathion are used

**Pesticides or insecticides**—Make sure you tell your doctor if you have been exposed recently to pesticides or insecticides.

**Other medical problems**—The presence of other medical problems may affect the use of demecarium, echothiophate, or isoflurophate. Make sure you tell your doctor if you have any other medical problems, especially:

- Asthma or
- Epilepsy or
- Heart disease or
- High blood pressure or
- Myasthenia gravis or
- Overactive thyroid or
- Parkinsonism or
- Stomach ulcer or other stomach problems or
- Urinary tract blockage—If this medicine is absorbed into the body, it may make the condition worse
- Down's syndrome (mongolism)—This medicine may cause these children to become hyperactive
- Eye disease or problems (other)—May increase absorption of this medicine into the body or this medicine may make the condition worse

## Proper Use of This Medicine

To use the *ophthalmic solution (eye drops) form* of this medicine:

- First, wash your hands. Tilt the head back and, pressing your finger gently on the skin just beneath the lower eyelid, pull the lower eyelid away from the eye to make a space. Drop the medicine into this space. Let go of the eyelid and gently close the eyes. Do not blink. Keep the eyes closed and apply pressure to the inner corner of the eye with your finger for 1 or 2 minutes to allow the medicine to be absorbed by the eye.
- Remove any excess solution around the eye with a clean tissue, being careful not to touch the eye.
- Immediately after using the eye drops, wash your hands to remove any medicine that may be on them.
- To keep the medicine as germ-free as possible, do not touch the applicator tip to any surface (including the eye). Also, keep the container tightly closed.

To use the *ophthalmic ointment (eye ointment) form* of this medicine:

- First, wash your hands. Tilt the head back and, pressing your finger gently on the skin just beneath the lower eyelid, pull the lower eyelid away from the eye to make a space. Squeeze a thin strip of ointment into this space. A ½-cm (approximately ¼-inch) strip of ointment is usually enough, unless you have been told by your doctor to use a different amount. Let go of the eyelid and gently close the eyes. Keep the eyes closed for 1 to 2 minutes to allow the medicine to be absorbed by the eye.
- Immediately after using the eye ointment, wash your hands to remove any medicine that may be on them.
- Since isoflurophate loses its effectiveness when exposed to moisture, do not wash the tip of the ointment tube or allow it to touch any moist surface (including the eye).
- To keep the medicine as germ-free as possible, do not touch the applicator tip to any surface (including the eye). After using this eye ointment, wipe the tip of the ointment tube with a clean tissue and keep the tube tightly closed.
- Since an eye ointment usually causes blurred vision for a short time after you use it, ask your doctor if the dose (or one of the doses if you use more than 1 dose a day) can be used at bedtime.

*It is very important that you use this medicine only as directed.* Do not use more of it and do not use it more often than your doctor ordered. To do so may increase the chance of too much medicine being absorbed into the body and the chance of side effects.

**Dosing**—The doses of these medicines will be different for different patients. *Follow your doctor's orders or the directions on the label.* The following information includes only the average doses of these medicines. *If your dose is different, do not change it* unless your doctor tells you to do so.

*For demecarium*

- For *ophthalmic solution (eye drops)* dosage form:
  —For glaucoma:
    - Adults and older children—Use one drop in the eye one or two times a day.
    - Infants and young children—Use and dose must be determined by your doctor.
  —For treatment of accommodative esotropia:
    - Adults and older children—Use one drop in the eye once a day for two to three weeks, then one drop in the eye once every two days for three to four weeks, then use as determined by the doctor.
    - Infants and young children—Use and dose must be determined by your doctor.
  —For diagnosis of accommodative esotropia:
    - Adults and older children—Use one drop in the eye once a day for two weeks, then one drop

in the eye once every two days for two to three weeks.

- Infants and young children—Use and dose must be determined by your doctor.

*For echothiophate*

- For *ophthalmic solution (eye drops)* dosage form:
  —For glaucoma:
  - Adults and older children—Use one drop in the eye one or two times a day.
  - Infants and younger children—Use and dose must be determined by your doctor.
  —For treatment of accommodative esotropia:
  - Adults and older children—Use one drop in the eye once a day or one drop in the eye once every two days.
  - Infants and young children—Use and dose must be determined by your doctor.
  —For diagnosis of accommodative esotropia:
  - Adults and older children—Use one drop in the eye once a day at bedtime for two to three weeks.
  - Infants and young children—Use and dose must be determined by your doctor.

*For isoflurophate*

- For *ophthalmic ointment* dosage form:
  —For glaucoma:
  - Adults and older children—Use the ointment in the eyes once every three days or as often as three times a day as directed by the doctor.
  - Infants and young children—Use and dose must be determined by your doctor.
  —For treatment of accommodative esotropia:
  - Adults and older children—Use the ointment in the eyes once a day at bedtime for two weeks, then once a week or as often as once every two days as directed by the doctor.
  - Infants and young children—Use and dose must be determined by your doctor.
  —For diagnosis of accommodative esotropia:
  - Adults and older children—Use the ointment in the eyes once a day at bedtime for two weeks.
  - Infants and young children—Use and dose must be determined by your doctor.

**Missed dose**—If you miss a dose of this medicine and your dosing schedule is:

- One dose every other day—Use the missed dose as soon as possible if you remember it on the day it should be used. However, if you do not remember the missed dose until the next day, use it at that time. Then skip a day and start your dosing schedule again. Do not double doses.
- One dose a day—Use the missed dose as soon as possible. However, if you do not remember the missed dose until the next day, skip the missed dose and go back to your regular dosing schedule. Do not double doses.

- More than one dose a day—Use the missed dose as soon as possible. However, if it is almost time for your next dose, skip the missed dose and go back to your regular dosing schedule. Do not double doses.

If your dosing schedule is different from all of the above and you miss a dose of this medicine, or if you have any questions about this, check with your doctor.

**Storage**—To store this medicine:

- Keep out of the reach of children. Overdose of demecarium, echothiophate, or isoflurophate is very dangerous in young children.
- Store away from heat and direct light.
- Keep this medicine from freezing.
- Do not keep outdated medicine or medicine no longer needed. Be sure that any discarded medicine is out of the reach of children.

## Precautions While Using This Medicine

If you are using this medicine for glaucoma, your doctor should check your eye pressure at regular visits to make sure the medicine is working.

If you will be using this medicine for a long time, your doctor should examine your eyes at regular visits to make sure this medicine does not cause unwanted effects.

*Before you have any kind of surgery (including eye surgery), dental treatment, or emergency treatment,* tell the medical doctor or dentist in charge and the anesthesiologist or anesthetist (the person who puts you to sleep) that you are using this medicine or have used it within the past month.

*Avoid breathing in even small amounts of carbamate- or organophosphate-type insecticides or pesticides* (for example, carbaryl [Sevin], demeton [Systox], diazinon, malathion, parathion, ronnel [Trolene], or TEPP). They may add to the effects of this medicine. Farmers, gardeners, residents of communities undergoing insecticide or pesticide spraying or dusting, workers in plants manufacturing such products, or other persons exposed to such poisons should protect themselves by wearing a mask over the nose and mouth, changing clothes frequently, and washing hands often.

*Make sure your vision is clear before you drive, use machines, or do anything else that could be dangerous if you are not able to see well.* This is because:

- After you apply this medicine to your eyes, your pupils may become unusually small. This may cause you to see less well at night or in dim light.
- After you begin using this medicine, your vision may be blurred or there may be a change in your near or distance vision.
- The eye ointment form of this medicine usually causes blurred vision for a short time after you apply it.

## Side Effects of This Medicine

Along with its needed effects, a medicine may cause some unwanted effects. Although not all of these side effects

may occur, if they do occur they may need medical attention.

*Check with your doctor immediately* if any of the following side effects occur:

*Rare*

Veil or curtain appearing across part of vision

*Symptoms of too much medicine being absorbed into the body*

Increased sweating; loss of bladder control; muscle weakness; nausea, vomiting, diarrhea, or stomach cramps or pain; shortness of breath, tightness in chest, or wheezing; slow or irregular heartbeat; unusual tiredness or weakness; watering of mouth

Note: The most common of these symptoms, especially in children, are nausea, vomiting, diarrhea, and stomach cramps or pain. Too much medicine being absorbed is rare with the eye ointment form of this medicine.

Check with your doctor as soon as possible if any of the following side effects occur:

*Rare*

Burning, redness, stinging, or other eye irritation; eye pain

Other side effects may occur that usually do not need medical attention. These side effects may go away during treatment as your body adjusts to the medicine. However, check with your doctor if any of the following side effects continue or are bothersome:

Blurred vision or change in near or distance vision; difficulty in seeing at night or in dim light; headache or browache; twitching of eyelids; watering of eyes

Other side effects not listed above may also occur in some patients. If you notice any other effects, check with your doctor.

Revised: 06/21/94

# ANTIHEMOPHILIC FACTOR   Systemic

Some commonly used brand names are:

**In the U.S.—**

| | |
|---|---|
| Hemofil M | MelATE |
| Humate-P | Monoclate-P |
| Hyate:C | Profilate OSD |
| Koate-HP | Recombinate |
| Kogenate | |

Generic name product may also be available.

**In Canada—**
Koate-HP
Recombinate

Other commonly used names are AHF and factor VIII.

## Description

Antihemophilic (an-tee-hee-moe-FIL-ik) factor (AHF) is a protein produced naturally in the body. It helps the blood form clots to stop bleeding.

Hemophilia A, also called classical hemophilia, is a condition in which the body does not make enough AHF. If you do not have enough AHF and you become injured, your blood will not form clots as it should, and you may bleed into and damage your muscles and joints. One type of AHF is used to treat another condition called von Willebrand disease, in which there is a risk of bleeding. AHF also may be used for other conditions as determined by your doctor.

The AHF that your doctor will give you is obtained naturally from human or pig blood, or artificially by a man-made process.

AHF obtained from human blood has been treated. It is not likely to contain harmful viruses such as hepatitis B virus; non-A, non-B hepatitis; or human immunodeficiency virus (HIV), the virus that causes acquired immunodeficiency syndrome (AIDS). The man-made and pork AHF products do not contain these viruses.

AHF is available only with your doctor's prescription, in the following dosage form:

*Parenteral*
• Injection (U.S. and Canada)

## Before Using This Medicine

In deciding to use a medicine, the risks of taking the medicine must be weighed against the good it will do. This is a decision you and your doctor will make. For antihemophilic factor (AHF), the following should be considered:

**Allergies**—Tell your doctor if you have ever had any unusual or allergic reaction to AHF. Also tell your health care professional if you are allergic to any other substances, such as foods, preservatives, or dyes.

**Pregnancy**—Studies on effects in pregnancy have not been done in either humans or animals.

**Breast-feeding**—It is not known whether AHF passes into breast milk. Although most medicines pass into breast milk in small amounts, many of them may be used safely while breast-feeding. Mothers who are using this medicine and who wish to breast-feed should discuss this with their doctor.

**Children**—This medicine has been tested in children and, in effective doses, has not been shown to cause different side effects or problems than it does in adults.

**Older adults**—This medicine has been tested and has not been shown to cause different side effects or problems in older people than it does in younger adults.

**Other medicines**—Although certain medicines should not be used together at all, in other cases two different medicines may be used together even if an interaction might occur. In these cases, your doctor may want to change the dose, or other precautions may be necessary. Tell your health care professional if you are using any other prescription or nonprescription (over-the-counter [OTC]) medicine.

**Other medical problems**—The presence of other medical problems may affect the use of AHF. Make sure you tell your doctor if you have any other medical problems.

## Proper Use of This Medicine

Some medicines given by injection may sometimes be given at home to patients who do not need to be in the hospital. If you are using this medicine at home, your health care professional will teach you how to prepare and inject the medicine. You will have a chance to practice preparing and injecting it. *Be certain that you understand exactly how the medicine is to be prepared and injected.*

To prepare this medicine:
- Take the dry medicine and the liquid (diluent) out of the refrigerator or freezer and bring them to room temperature, as directed by your doctor.
- When injecting the liquid (diluent) into the dry medicine, *aim the stream of liquid (diluent) against the wall of the container of dry medicine* to prevent foaming.
- *Swirl the container gently to dissolve the medicine. Do not shake the container.*

*Use this medicine right away.* It should not be kept longer than 1 or 3 hours after it has been prepared, as directed on the package or by your doctor.

*A plastic disposable syringe and filter needle must be used with this medicine.* The medicine may stick to the inside of a glass syringe, and you may not receive a full dose.

*Do not reuse syringes and needles. Put used syringes and needles in a puncture-resistant disposable container*, or dispose of them as directed by your health care professional.

**Dosing**—The dose of antihemophilic factor (AHF) will be different for different patients. The dose you receive will be based on:
- Your body weight.
- The amount of AHF your body is able to make.
- How much, how often, and where in your body you are bleeding.
- Whether or not your body has built up a defense (antibody) against this medicine.

Your dose of this medicine may even be different at different times. It is important that you *follow your doctor's orders.*

**Missed dose**—If you miss a dose of this medicine, check with your doctor as soon as possible for instructions. If you cannot reach your doctor, use your usual dose as soon as you remember.

**Storage**—To store this medicine:
- Keep out of the reach of children.
- Some AHF products must be stored in the refrigerator and some in the freezer. However, some of them may be kept at room temperature for short periods of time. Store this medicine as directed by your doctor or by the manufacturer.
- Do not keep outdated medicine or medicine no longer needed. Be sure that any discarded medicine is out of the reach of children.

## Precautions While Using This Medicine

If you were recently diagnosed with hemophilia A, you should receive hepatitis B vaccine to reduce even further your risk of getting hepatitis B from antihemophilic factor.

*It is recommended that you carry identification stating that you have hemophilia A, and what medicine you are using.* If you have any questions about what kind of identification to carry, check with your health care professional.

After a while, your body may build up a defense (antibody) against this medicine. *Tell your doctor if this medicine seems to be less effective than usual.*

## Side Effects of This Medicine

Along with its needed effects, a medicine may cause some unwanted effects. Some side effects will have signs or symptoms that you can see or feel. Your doctor may watch for others by doing certain tests.

*Check with your doctor immediately* if any of the following side effects occur, because they may mean that you are having a serious allergic reaction to the medicine:

*Less common or rare*
  Changes in facial skin color; fast or irregular breathing; puffiness or swelling of the eyelids or around the eyes; shortness of breath, troubled breathing, tightness in chest, and/or wheezing; skin rash, hives, and/or itching

Also, check with your doctor as soon as possible if any of the following occur:

*Less common or rare*
  Chills; fever; nausea; tenderness, pain, swelling, warmth, skin discoloration, and noticeable veins over affected area; unusual bleeding or bruising; unusual tiredness or weakness

Other side effects may occur that usually do not need medical attention. These side effects may go away during

treatment as your body adjusts to the medicine. However, check with your doctor if any of the following side effects continue or are bothersome:

*Less common*

Burning, stinging, or swelling at place of injection; dizziness or lightheadedness; dry mouth or bad taste in mouth; headache; nosebleed; redness of face; vomiting

Other side effects not listed above may also occur in some patients. If you notice any other effects, check with your doctor.

Developed: 07/30/93

---

# ANTIHISTAMINES   Systemic

Some commonly used brand names are:

**In the U.S.—**

| | | | |
|---|---|---|---|
| Aller-Chlor[8] | Chlor-Trimeton Allergy[8] | Gen-Allerate[8] | Phendry[13] |
| AllerMax Caplets[13] | Chlor-Trimeton Repetabs[8] | Gen-D-phen[13] | Phendry Children's Allergy |
| Aller-med[13] | Claritin[17] | Hismanal[2] | Medicine[13] |
| Anxanil[16] | Codimal-A[5] | Histaject Modified[5] | Phenetron[8] |
| Atarax[16] | Compoz[13] | Hydramine[13] | Phenetron Lanacaps[8] |
| Banophen[13] | Conjec-B[5] | Hydramine Cough[13] | Poladex T.D.[11] |
| Banophen Caplets[13] | Contac 12 Hour Allergy[9] | Hydramyn[13] | Polaramine[11] |
| Beldin[13] | Cophene-B[5] | Hydrate[12] | Polaramine Repetabs[11] |
| Belix[13] | Dehist[5] | Hydril[13] | Quiess[16] |
| Bena-D 10[13] | Dexchlor[11] | Hydroxacen[16] | Seldane[20] |
| Bena-D 50[13] | Diamine T.D.[5] | Hyrexin-50[13] | Siladryl[13] |
| Benadryl[13] | Dimetabs[12] | Hyzine-50[16] | Silphen Cough Syrup[13] |
| Benadryl 25[13] | Dimetane[5] | Marmine[12] | Sleep-Eze 3[13] |
| Benadryl Kapseals[13] | Dimetane Extentabs[5] | Myidil[22] | Sominex Formula 2[13] |
| Benahist 10[13] | Dimetapp Allergy[5] | Nasahist B[5] | Tavist[9] |
| Benahist 50[13] | Dimetapp Allergy Liqui-Gels[5] | ND-Stat Revised[5] | Tavist-1[9] |
| Ben-Allergin-50[13] | Dinate[12] | Nervine Nighttime Sleep-Aid[13] | Tega-Vert[12] |
| Benoject-10[13] | Diphenacen-50[13] | Nico-Vert[12] | Telachlor[8] |
| Benoject-50[13] | Diphenadryl[13] | Nidryl[13] | Teldrin[8] |
| Benylin Cough[13] | Diphen Cough[13] | Nisaval[19] | Triptone Caplets[12] |
| Bromphen[5] | Diphenhist[13] | Nolahist[18] | Trymegen[8] |
| Bydramine Cough[13] | Diphenhist Captabs[13] | Noradryl[13] | Tusstat[13] |
| Calm X[12] | Dommanate[12] | Nordryl[13] | Twilite Caplets[13] |
| Children's Dramamine[12] | Dormarex 2[13] | Nordryl Cough[13] | Uni-Bent Cough[13] |
| Chlo-Amine[8] | Dormin[13] | Nytol with DPH[13] | Unisom Nighttime Sleep Aid[15] |
| Chlor-100[8] | Dramamine[12] | Nytol Maximum Strength[13] | Unisom SleepGels Maximum |
| Chlorate[8] | Dramamine Chewable[12] | Optimine[3] | Strength[13] |
| Chlor-Niramine[8] | Dramamine Liquid[12] | Oraminic II[5] | Veltane[5] |
| Chlorphed[5] | Dramanate[12] | PBZ[21] | Vertab[12] |
| Chlor-Pro[8] | Dramocen[12] | PBZ-SR[21] | Vistaject-25[16] |
| Chlor-Pro 10[8] | Dramoject[12] | PediaCare Allergy Formula[8] | Vistaject-50[16] |
| Chlorspan-12[8] | Dymenate[12] | Pelamine[21] | Vistaril[16] |
| Chlortab-4[8] | E-Vista[16] | Periactin[10] | Vistazine 50[16] |
| Chlortab-8[8] | Fynex[13] | Pfeiffer's Allergy[8] | Wehdryl-10[13] |
| Chlor-Trimeton[8] | Genahist[13] | | Wehdryl-50[13] |

**In Canada—**

| | | | |
|---|---|---|---|
| Allerdryl[13] | Dimetane Extentabs[5] | Novo-Dimenate[12] | Polaramine Repetabs[11] |
| Apo-Dimenhydrinate[12] | Dommanate[12] | Novo-Hydroxyzin[16] | Pyribenzamine[21] |
| Apo-Hydroxyzine[16] | Gravol[12] | Novo-Pheniram[8] | Reactine[7] |
| Atarax[16] | Gravol L/A[12] | Nova-Terfendadine[20] | Seldane[20] |
| Benadryl[13] | Hismanal[2] | Optimine[3] | Seldane Caplets[20] |
| Chlor-Tripolon[8] | Insomnal[13] | Periactin[10] | Tavist[9] |
| Claritin[17] | Multipax[16] | PMS-Dimenhydrinate[12] | Travamine[12] |
| Dimetane[5] | Nauseatol[12] | Polaramine[11] | Traveltabs[12] |

Note: For quick reference, the following antihistamines are numbered to match the corresponding brand names.

This information applies to the following medicines:

1. Acrivastine (AK-ri-vas-teen)
2. Astemizole (a-STEM-mi-zole)
3. Azatadine (a-ZA-ta-deen)
4. Bromodiphenhydramine (broe-moe-dye-fen-HYE-dra-meen)‡
5. Brompheniramine (brome-fen-EER-a-meen)‡
6. Carbinoxamine (kar-bi-NOX-a-meen)‡
7. Cetirizine (se-TI-ra-zeen)*
8. Chlorpheniramine (klor-fen-EER-a-meen)‡

9. Clemastine (KLEM-as-teen)‡
10. Cyproheptadine (si-proe-HEP-ta-deen)‡
11. Dexchlorpheniramine (dex-klor-fen-EER-a-meen)‡
12. Dimenhydrinate (dye-men-HYE-dri-nate)‡§
13. Diphenhydramine (dye-fen-HYE-dra-meen)‡§
14. Diphenylpyraline (dye-fen-il-PEER-a-leen)§
15. Doxylamine (dox-ILL-a-meen)†
16. Hydroxyzine (hye-DROX-i-zeen)‡§
17. Loratadine (lor-AT-a-deen)
18. Phenindamine (fen-IN-da-meen)†
19. Pyrilamine (peer-ILL-a-meen)†‡

20. Terfenadine (ter-FEN-a-deen)
21. Tripelennamine (tri-pel-ENN-a-meen)‡
22. Triprolidine (trye-PROE-li-deen)†‡

---

\*Not commercially available in the U.S.
†Not commercially available in Canada.
‡Generic name product may also be available in the U.S.
§Generic name product may also be available in Canada.

---

# Description

Antihistamines are used to relieve or prevent the symptoms of hay fever and other types of allergy. They work by preventing the effects of a substance called histamine, which is produced by the body. Histamine can cause itching, sneezing, runny nose, and watery eyes. Also, in some persons histamine can close up the bronchial tubes (air passages of the lungs) and make breathing difficult.

Some of the antihistamines are also used to prevent motion sickness, nausea, vomiting, and dizziness. In patients with Parkinson's disease, diphenhydramine may be used to decrease stiffness and tremors. Also, the syrup form of diphenhydramine is used to relieve the cough due to colds or hay fever. In addition, since antihistamines may cause drowsiness as a side effect, some of them may be used to help people go to sleep.

Hydroxyzine is used in the treatment of nervous and emotional conditions to help control anxiety. It can also be used to help control anxiety and produce sleep before surgery.

Antihistamines may also be used for other conditions as determined by your doctor.

Some antihistamine preparations are available only with your doctor's prescription. Others are available without a prescription. However, your doctor may have special instructions on the proper dose of the medicine for your medical condition.

These medicines are available in the following dosage forms:

*Oral*
Astemizole
• Oral suspension (Canada)
• Tablets (U.S. and Canada)
Azatadine
• Tablets (U.S. and Canada)
Brompheniramine
• Capsules (U.S.)
• Elixir (U.S. and Canada)
• Tablets (U.S. and Canada)
• Extended-release tablets (U.S. and Canada)
Cetirizine
• Tablets (Canada)
Chlorpheniramine
• Extended-release capsules (U.S.)
• Syrup (U.S. and Canada)
• Tablets (U.S. and Canada)
• Chewable tablets (U.S.)
• Extended-release tablets (U.S. and Canada)
Clemastine
• Syrup (U.S. and Canada)
• Tablets (U.S. and Canada)

Cyproheptadine
• Syrup (U.S. and Canada)
• Tablets (U.S. and Canada)
Dexchlorpheniramine
• Syrup (U.S. and Canada)
• Tablets (U.S. and Canada)
• Extended-release tablets (U.S. and Canada)
Dimenhydrinate
• Capsules (U.S.)
• Extended-release capsules (Canada)
• Elixir (U.S. and Canada)
• Syrup (U.S.)
• Tablets (U.S. and Canada)
• Chewable tablets (U.S.)
Diphenhydramine
• Capsules (U.S. and Canada)
• Elixir (U.S. and Canada)
• Syrup (U.S.)
• Tablets (U.S.)
Doxylamine
• Tablets (U.S.)
Hydroxyzine
• Capsules (U.S. and Canada)
• Oral suspension (U.S.)
• Syrup (U.S. and Canada)
• Tablets (U.S.)
Loratadine
• Syrup (Canada)
• Tablets (U.S. and Canada)
Phenindamine
• Tablets (U.S.)
Pyrilamine
• Tablets (U.S.)
Terfenadine
• Oral suspension (Canada)
• Tablets (U.S. and Canada)
Tripelennamine
• Elixir (U.S.)
• Tablets (U.S. and Canada)
• Extended-release tablets (U.S.)
Triprolidine
• Syrup (U.S.)

*Parenteral*
Brompheniramine
• Injection (U.S.)
Chlorpheniramine
• Injection (U.S. and Canada)
Dimenhydrinate
• Injection (U.S. and Canada)
Diphenhydramine
• Injection (U.S. and Canada)
Hydroxyzine
• Injection (U.S. and Canada)

*Rectal*
Dimenhydrinate
• Suppositories (Canada)

---

# Before Using This Medicine

In deciding to use a medicine, the risks of taking the medicine must be weighed against the good it will do. This is a decision you and your doctor will make. For antihistamines, the following should be considered:

**Allergies**—Tell your doctor if you have ever had any unusual or allergic reaction to antihistamines. Also tell your

health care professional if you are allergic to any other substances, such as foods, preservatives, or dyes.

**Diet**—Make certain your health care professional knows if you are on a low-sodium, low-sugar, or any other special diet. Most medicines contain more than their active ingredient, and many liquid medicines contain alcohol.

**Pregnancy**—Most antihistamines have not been studied in pregnant women. Although these antihistamines have not been shown to cause problems in humans, studies in animals have shown that some other antihistamines, such as meclizine (e.g., Antivert) and cyclizine (e.g., Marezine), may cause birth defects.

Also, studies in animals have shown that terfenadine, when given in doses several times the human dose, lowers the birth weight and increases the risk of death of the offspring.

Cetirizine and hydroxyzine are not recommended for use in the first months of pregnancy since they have been shown to cause birth defects in animal studies when given in doses many times higher than the usual human dose. Be sure you have discussed this with your doctor.

**Breast-feeding**—Small amounts of antihistamines pass into the breast milk. Use is not recommended since babies are more susceptible to the side effects of antihistamines, such as unusual excitement or irritability. Also, since these medicines tend to decrease the secretions of the body, it is possible that the flow of breast milk may be reduced in some patients. It is not known yet whether astemizole, cetirizine, loratadine, and terfenadine cause these same side effects.

**Children**—Serious side effects, such as convulsions (seizures), are more likely to occur in younger patients and would be of greater risk to infants than to older children or adults. In general, children are more sensitive to the effects of antihistamines. Also, nightmares or unusual excitement, nervousness, restlessness, or irritability may be more likely to occur in children.

**Older adults**—Elderly patients are usually more sensitive to the effects of antihistamines. Confusion; difficult or painful urination; dizziness; drowsiness; feeling faint; or dryness of mouth, nose, or throat may be more likely to occur in elderly patients. Also, nightmares or unusual excitement, nervousness, restlessness, or irritability may be more likely to occur in elderly patients.

**Other medicines**—Although certain medicines should not be used together at all, in other cases different medicines may be used together even if an interaction might occur. In these cases, your doctor may want to change the dose, or other precautions may be necessary. When you are taking antihistamines it is especially important that your health care professional knows if you are taking any of the following:

- Anticholinergics (medicine for abdominal or stomach spasms or cramps)—Side effects, such as dryness of mouth, of antihistamines or anticholinergics may be more likely to occur

- Azithromycin (e.g., Zithromax) or
- Clarithromycin (e.g., Biaxin) or
- Erythromycin (e.g., E-Mycin) or
- Itraconazole (e.g., Sporanox) or
- Ketoconazole (e.g., Nizoral)—Use of these medicines with astemizole and terfenadine may cause heart problems, such as an irregular heartbeat; these medicines should not be used together
- Bipridil (e.g., Vascor) or
- Disopyramide (e.g., Norpace) or
- Maprotiline (e.g., Ludiomil) or
- Phenothiazines (acetophenazine [e.g., Tindal], chlorpromazine [e.g., Thorazine], fluphenazine [e.g., Prolixin], mesoridazine [e.g., Serentil], perphenazine [e.g., Trilafon], prochlorperazine [e.g., Compazine], promazine [e.g., Sparine], promethazine [e.g., Phenergan], thioridazine [e.g. Mellaril], trifluoperazine [e.g., Stelazine], triflupromazine [e.g., Vesprin], trimeprazine [e.g., Temaril]) or
- Pimozide (e.g., Orap) or
- Procainamide (e.g., Pronestyl) or
- Quinidine (e.g., Quinaglute Dura-tabs) or
- Tricyclic antidepressants (amitriptyline [e.g., Elavil], amoxapine [e.g., Asendin], clomipramine [e.g., Anafranil], desipramine [e.g., Pertofrane], doxepin [e.g., Sinequan], imipramine [e.g., Tofranil], nortriptyline [e.g., Aventyl], protriptyline [e.g., Vivactil], trimipramine [e.g., Surmontil])—Use of these medicines with astemizole or terfenadine may increase the risk of heart rhythm problems
- Central nervous system (CNS) depressants—Effects, such as drowsiness, of CNS depressants or antihistamines may be worsened; also, taking maprotiline or tricyclic antidepressants may cause some side effects of either of these medicines, such as dryness of mouth, to become more severe
- Monoamine oxidase (MAO) inhibitors (furazolidone [e.g., Furoxone], isocarboxazid [e.g., Marplan], phenelzine [e.g., Nardil], procarbazine [e.g., Matulane], tranylcypromine [e.g., Parnate])—If you are now taking, or have taken within the past 2 weeks, any of the MAO inhibitors, the side effects of the antihistamines, such as drowsiness and dryness of mouth, may become more severe; these medicines should not be used together

**Other medical problems**—The presence of other medical problems may affect the use of antihistamines. Make sure you tell your doctor if you have any other medical problems, especially:

- Enlarged prostate or
- Urinary tract blockage or difficult urination—Antihistamines may make urinary problems worse
- Glaucoma—These medicines may cause a slight increase in inner eye pressure that may make the condition worse
- Heart rhythm problems (history of) or
- Low potassium blood levels—Use of astemizole or terfenadine can cause serious heart rhythm problems
- Liver disease—Higher blood levels of astemizole or terfenadine may result, which may increase the chance of heart problems

## Proper Use of This Medicine

*Antihistamines are used to relieve or prevent the symptoms of your medical problem. Take them only as directed. Do not take more of them and do not take them more often than recommended on the label, unless otherwise directed by your doctor. To do so may increase the chance of side effects.*

**Dosing**—The dose of an antihistamine will be different for different patients. *Follow your doctor's orders or the directions on the label.* The following information includes only the average doses of antihistamines. *If your dose is different, do not change it* unless your doctor tells you to do so.

The number of capsules or tablets or teaspoonfuls of liquid that you take or the number of suppositories you use depends on the strength of the medicine. Also, *the number of doses you take each day and the time between doses depends on whether you are taking a short-acting or long-acting form of antihistamine.*

- For use as an antihistamine:

  *For astemizole*
  - For *oral* dosage forms (tablets or liquid):
    —Adults and teenagers: 10 milligrams (mg) once a day.
    —Children younger than 6 years of age: 0.2 mg per kilogram (kg) (0.1 mg per pound) of body weight once a day.
    —Children 6 to 12 years of age: 5 mg once a day.

  *For azatadine*
  - For *oral* dosage form (tablets):
    —Adults: 1 to 2 milligrams (mg) every eight to twelve hours as needed.
    —Children younger than 12 years of age: Use and dose must be determined by your doctor.
    —Children 12 years of age and older: 0.5 mg to 1 mg two times a day as needed.

  *For brompheniramine*
  - For *regular (short-acting) oral* dosage forms (capsules, tablets, or liquid):
    —Adults and teenagers: 4 milligrams (mg) every four to six hours as needed.
    —Children 2 to 6 years of age: 1 mg every four to six hours as needed.
    —Children 6 to 12 years of age: 2 mg every four to six hours as needed.
  - For *long-acting oral* dosage form (tablets):
    —Adults: 8 milligrams (mg) every eight or twelve hours, or 12 mg every twelve hours as needed.
    —Children younger than 6 years of age: Use and dose must be determined by your doctor.
    —Children 6 years of age and older: 8 or 12 mg every twelve hours as needed.
  - For *injection* dosage form:
    —Adults and teenagers: 10 milligrams (mg) injected into a muscle, under the skin, or into a vein every eight to twelve hours.
    —Children younger than 12 years of age: 0.125 mg per kilogram (0.06 mg per pound) of body weight injected into a muscle, under the skin, or into a vein three or four times a day as needed.

  *For cetirizine*
  - For *oral* dosage form (tablets):
    —Adults: 5 to 10 milligrams (mg) once a day.
    —Children: Use and dose must be determined by your doctor.

  *For chlorpheniramine*
  - For *regular (short-acting) oral* dosage forms (tablets or liquid):
    —Adults and teenagers: 4 milligrams (mg) every four to six hours as needed.
    —Children younger than 6 years of age: Use and dose must be determined by your doctor.
    —Children 6 to 12 years of age: 2 mg three or four times a day as needed.
  - For *long-acting oral* dosage forms (capsules or tablets):
    —Adults: 8 or 12 milligrams (mg) every eight to twelve hours as needed.
    —Children younger than 12 years of age: Use and dose must be determined by your doctor.
    —Children 12 years of age and older: 8 mg every twelve hours as needed.
  - For *injection* dosage form:
    —Adults: 5 to 40 milligrams (mg) injected into a muscle, into a vein, or under the skin.
    —Children: 0.0875 mg per kilogram (0.04 mg per pound) of body weight injected under the skin every six hours as needed.

  *For clemastine*
  - For *oral* dosage forms (tablets or liquid):
    —Adults and teenagers: 1.34 milligrams (mg) two times a day or 2.68 mg one to three times a day as needed.
    —Children younger than 6 years of age: Use and dose must be determined by your doctor.
    —Children 6 to 12 years of age: 0.67 to 1.34 mg two times a day.

  *For cyproheptadine*
  - For *oral* dosage forms (tablets or liquid):
    —Adults and children 14 years of age and older: 4 milligrams (mg) every eight hours. The doctor may increase the dose if needed.
    —Children 2 to 6 years of age: 2 mg every eight to twelve hours as needed.
    —Children 6 to 14 years of age: 4 mg every eight to twelve hours as needed.

  *For dexchlorpheniramine*
  - For *regular (short-acting) oral* dosage forms (tablets or liquid):
    —Adults and teenagers: 2 milligrams (mg) every four to six hours as needed.
    —Children 2 to 5 years of age: 0.5 mg every four to six hours as needed.
    —Children 5 to 12 years of age: 1 mg every four to six hours as needed.
  - For *long-acting oral* dosage form (tablets):
    —Adults: 4 or 6 milligrams (mg) every eight to twelve hours as needed.
    —Children: Use and dose must be determined by your doctor.

*For diphenhydramine*
* For *oral* dosage forms (capsules, tablets, or liquid):
    —Adults and teenagers: 25 to 50 milligrams (mg) mg every four to six hours as needed.
    —Children younger than 6 years of age: 6.25 to 12.5 mg every four to six hours.
    —Children 6 to 12 years of age: 12.5 to 25 mg every four to six hours.
* For *injection* dosage form:
    —Adults: 10 to 50 milligrams (mg) injected into a muscle or into a vein.
    —Children: 1.25 mg per kg (0.6 mg per pound) of body weight injected into a muscle four times a day.

*For doxylamine*
* For *oral* dosage form (tablets):
    —Adults and teenagers: 12.5 to 25 milligrams (mg) every four to six hours as needed.
    —Children younger than 6 years of age: Use and dose must be determined by your doctor.
    —Children 6 to 12 years of age: 6.25 to 12.5 mg every four to six hours as needed.

*For hydroxyzine*
* For *oral* dosage forms (capsules, tablets, or liquid):
    —Adults and teenagers: 25 to 100 milligrams (mg) three or four times a day as needed.
    —Children younger than 12 years of age: 0.5 mg per kg (0.2 mg per pound) of body weight every six hours as needed.

*For loratadine*
* For *oral* dosage forms (tablets or liquid):
    —Adults and children 10 years of age and older: 10 milligrams (mg) once a day on an empty stomach.
    —Children 2 to 9 years of age: 5 mg once a day on an empty stomach.

*For phenindamine*
* For *oral* dosage form (tablets):
    —Adults and teenagers: 25 milligrams (mg) every four to six hours as needed.
    —Children younger than 6 years of age: Use and dose must be determined by your doctor.
    —Children 6 to 12 years of age: 12.5 mg every four to six hours as needed.

*For pyrilamine*
* For *oral* dosage form (tablets):
    —Adults: 25 to 50 milligrams (mg) every eight hours as needed.
    —Children 2 to 6 years of age: Use and dose must be determined by your doctor.
    —Children 6 years of age and older: 12.5 to 25 mg every eight hours as needed.

*For terfenadine*
* For *oral* dosage forms (tablets or liquid):
    —Adults and teenagers: 60 milligrams (mg) every twelve hours.
    —Children 3 to 6 years of age: 15 mg every twelve hours as needed.

    —Children 7 to 12 years of age: 30 mg every twelve hours as needed.

*For tripelennamine*
* For *regular (short-acting) oral* dosage forms (tablets or liquid):
    —Adults: 25 to 50 milligrams (mg) every four to six hours as needed.
    —Children: 1.25 mg per kilogram (kg) (0.6 mg per pound) of body weight every six hours as needed.
* For *long-acting oral* dosage form (tablets):
    —Adults: 100 milligrams (mg) every eight to twelve hours as needed.
    —Children: Use and dose must be determined by your doctor.

*For triprolidine*
* For *oral* dosage forms (liquid):
    —Adults and teenagers: 2.5 milligrams (mg) every four to six hours as needed.
    —Children 4 months to 2 years of age: 0.312 mg (1/4 teaspoonful) every six to eight hours as needed.
    —Children 2 to 4 years of age: 0.625 mg (1/2 teaspoonful) every six to eight hours as needed.
    —Children 4 to 6 years of age: 0.937 mg (3/4 teaspoonful) every six to eight hours as needed.
    —Children 6 to 12 years of age: 1.25 mg (1 teaspoonful) every six to eight hours as needed.

* For nausea, vomiting, and vertigo (only dimenhydrinate and diphenhydramine are used for vertigo):

*For dimenhydrinate*
* For *regular (short-acting) oral* dosage forms (capsules, tablets, or liquid):
    —Adults and teenagers: 50 to 100 milligrams (mg) every four hours as needed.
    —Children 2 to 6 years of age: 12.5 to 25 mg every six to eight hours as needed.
    —Children 6 to 12 years of age: 25 to 50 mg every six to eight hours as needed.
* For *long-acting oral* dosage form (capsules):
    —Adults: 1 capsule (contains 25 milligrams [mg] for immediate action and 50 mg for long action) every twelve hours.
    —Children: Use and dose must be determined by your doctor.
* For *injection* dosage form:
    —Adults: 50 milligrams (mg) injected into a muscle or into a vein every four hours as needed.
    —Children: 1.25 mg per kg (0.6 mg per pound) of body weight injected into a muscle or into a vein every six hours as needed.
* For *suppository* dosage form:
    —Adults: 50 to 100 milligrams (mg) inserted into the rectum every six to eight hours as needed.

—Children younger than 6 years of age: Use and dose must be determined by your doctor.
—Children 6 to 8 years of age: 12.5 to 25 mg inserted into the rectum every eight to twelve hours as needed.
—Children 8 to 12 years of age: 25 to 50 mg inserted into the rectum every eight to twelve hours as needed.
—Children 12 years of age and older: 50 mg inserted into the rectum every eight to twelve hours as needed.

*For diphenhydramine*
- For *oral* dosage forms (capsules, tablets, or liquid):
—Adults: 25 to 50 milligrams (mg) every four to six hours as needed.
—Children: 1 to 1.5 mg per kg (0.45 to 0.7 mg per pound) of body weight every four to six hours as needed.
- For *injection* dosage form:
—Adults: 10 milligrams (mg) injected into a muscle or into a vein. Dose may be increased to 25 to 50 mg every two to three hours.
—Children: 1 to 1.5 mg per kg (0.45 to 0.68 mg per pound) of body weight injected into a muscle every six hours.

*For hydroxyzine*
- For *oral* dosage forms (capsules, tablets, or liquid):
—Adults: 25 to 100 milligrams (mg) three or four times a day as needed.
—Children younger than 6 years of age: 12.5 mg every six hours as needed.
—Children 6 years of age and older: 12.5 to 25 mg every six hours as needed.
- For *injection* dosage form:
—Adults: 25 to 100 milligrams (mg) injected into a muscle.
—Children: 1 mg per kg (0.45 mg per pound) of body weight injected into a muscle.

- For Parkinson's disease:
*For diphenhydramine*
- For *oral* dosage forms (capsules, tablets, or liquid):
—Adults: 25 milligrams (mg) three times a day when starting treatment. Your doctor may increase the dose gradually later if needed.
- For *injection* dosage form:
—Adults: 10 to 50 milligrams (mg) injected into a muscle or into a vein.
—Children: 1.25 mg per kg (0.6 mg per pound) of body weight four times a day injected into a muscle.

- For use as a sedative (to help sleep):
*For diphenhydramine*
- For *oral* dosage forms (capsules, tablets, or liquid):
—Adults: 50 milligrams (mg) twenty to thirty minutes before bedtime if needed.

*For doxylamine*
- For *oral* dosage form (tablets):
—Adults: 25 milligrams (mg) thirty minutes before bedtime if needed.
—Children: Use and dose must be determined by your doctor.

*For hydroxyzine*
- For *oral* dosage forms (capsules, tablets, or liquid):
—Adults: 50 to 100 milligrams (mg).
—Children: 0.6 mg per kg (0.3 mg per pound) of body weight.
- For *injection* dosage form:
—Adults: 50 milligrams (mg) injected into a muscle.

- For cough:
*For diphenhydramine*
- For *oral* dosage form (liquid):
—Adults and teenagers: 25 milligrams (mg) every four to six hours.
—Children younger than 2 years of age: Use and dose must be determined by your doctor.
—Children 2 to 6 years of age: 6.25 mg (1/2 teaspoonful) every four to six hours as needed.
—Children 6 to 12 years of age: 12.5 mg (1 teaspoonful) every four to six hours as needed.

- For anxiety:
*For hydroxyzine*
- For *oral* dosage forms (capsules, tablets, or liquid):
—Adults: 50 to 100 milligrams (mg).
—Children: 0.6 mg per kilogram (0.3 mg per pound) of body weight.
- For *injection* dosage form:
—Adults: 50 to 100 milligrams (mg) injected into a muscle every four to six hours as needed.
—Children: 1 mg per kilogram (0.45 mg per pound) of body weight injected into a muscle.

**Missed dose**—If you are taking this medicine regularly and you miss a dose, take it as soon as possible. However, if it is almost time for your next dose, skip the missed dose and go back to your regular dosing schedule. Do not double doses.

For patients *taking this medicine by mouth:*
- Antihistamines can be taken with food or a glass of water or milk to lessen stomach irritation if necessary. However, food may change the amounts of astemizole and loratadine that are absorbed. For this reason, astemizole and loratadine should be taken on an empty stomach.
- If you are taking the extended-release tablet form of this medicine, swallow the tablets whole. Do not break, crush, or chew before swallowing.

For patients taking *dimenhydrinate or diphenhydramine for motion sickness:*
- Take this medicine at least 30 minutes or, even better, 1 to 2 hours before you begin to travel.

For patients using the *suppository form of this medicine:*

- To insert suppository: First remove the foil wrapper and moisten the suppository with cold water. Lie down on your side and use your finger to push the suppository well up into the rectum. If the suppository is too soft to insert, chill the suppository in the refrigerator for 30 minutes or run cold water over it before removing the foil wrapper.

For patients using the *injection form of this medicine:*

- If you will be giving yourself the injections, make sure you understand exactly how to give them. If you have any questions about this, check with your health care professional.

**Storage**—To store this medicine:

- Keep out of the reach of children, since overdose may be very dangerous in children.
- Store away from heat and direct light.
- Do not store the capsule or tablet form of this medicine in the bathroom medicine cabinet, near the kitchen sink, or in other damp places. Heat or moisture may cause the medicine to break down.
- Keep the liquid form of this medicine from freezing.
- Do not keep outdated medicine or medicine no longer needed. Be sure that any discarded medicine is out of the reach of children.

## Precautions While Using This Medicine

Before you have any skin tests for allergies, tell the doctor in charge that you are taking this medicine. The results of the test may be affected by this medicine.

When taking antihistamines on a regular basis, make sure your doctor knows if you are taking large amounts of aspirin at the same time (as for arthritis or rheumatism). Effects of too much aspirin, such as ringing in the ears, may be covered up by the antihistamine.

Antihistamines will add to the effects of alcohol and other CNS depressants (medicines that slow down the nervous system, possibly causing drowsiness). Some examples of CNS depressants are sedatives, tranquilizers, or sleeping medicine; prescription pain medicine or narcotics; barbiturates; medicine for seizures; muscle relaxants; or anesthetics, including some dental anesthetics. *Check with your doctor before taking any of the above while you are using this medicine.*

This medicine may cause some people to become drowsy or less alert than they are normally. Even if taken at bedtime, it may cause some people to feel drowsy or less alert on arising. Some antihistamines are more likely to cause drowsiness than others. Drowsiness is less likely with cetirizine, and rare with astemizole, loratadine, and terfenadine. *Make sure you know how you react to the antihistamine you are taking before you drive, use machines, or do anything else that could be dangerous if you are not alert.*

Antihistamines may cause dryness of the mouth, nose, and throat. Some antihistamines are more likely to cause

dryness of the mouth than others (astemizole, cetirizine, loratadine, and terfenadine, for example, rarely produce this effect). For temporary relief of mouth dryness, use sugarless candy or gum, melt bits of ice in your mouth, or use a saliva substitute. However, if your mouth continues to feel dry for more than 2 weeks, check with your medical doctor or dentist. Continuing dryness of the mouth may increase the chance of dental disease, including tooth decay, gum disease, and fungus infections.

For patients using *dimenhydrinate, diphenhydramine, or hydroxyzine:*

- This medicine controls nausea and vomiting. For this reason, it may cover up the signs of overdose caused by other medicines or the symptoms of appendicitis. This will make it difficult for your doctor to diagnose these conditions. Make sure your doctor knows that you are taking this medicine if you have other symptoms of appendicitis such as stomach or lower abdominal pain, cramping, or soreness. Also, if you think you may have taken an overdose of any medicine, tell your doctor that you are taking this medicine.

For patients using *diphenhydramine or doxylamine as a sleeping aid:*

- If you are already taking a sedative or tranquilizer, do not take this medicine without consulting your doctor first.

## Side Effects of This Medicine

Along with its needed effects, a medicine may cause some unwanted effects. Although not all of these side effects may occur, if they do occur they may need medical attention.

*Check with your doctor immediately* if the following side effect occurs:

> Less common or rare—with high doses of astemizole or terfenadine only
> > Fast or irregular heartbeat

Also, check with your doctor as soon as possible if any of the following side effects occur:

> *Less common or rare*
> > Sore throat and fever; unusual bleeding or bruising; unusual tiredness or weakness

> *Symptoms of overdose*
> > Clumsiness or unsteadiness; convulsions (seizures); drowsiness (severe); dryness of mouth, nose, or throat (severe); feeling faint; flushing or redness of face; hallucinations (seeing, hearing, or feeling things that are not there); shortness of breath or troubled breathing; trouble in sleeping

Other side effects may occur that usually do not need medical attention. These side effects may go away during treatment as your body adjusts to the medicine. However, check with your health care professional if any of the following side effects continue or are bothersome:

> *More common—less common with cetirizine; rare with astemizole, loratadine, and terfenadine*
> > Drowsiness; thickening of mucus

*Less common or rare*

> Blurred vision or any change in vision; confusion; difficult or painful urination; dizziness; dryness of mouth, nose, or throat; fast heartbeat; increased sensitivity of skin to sun; increased sweating; loss of appetite (increased appetite with astemizole, cetirizine, cyproheptadine, loratadine, and terfenadine); nightmares; ringing or buzzing in ears; skin rash; stomach upset or stomach pain (more common with pyrilamine and tripelennamine); unusual excitement, nervousness, restlessness, or irritability; weight gain (with astemizole and cyproheptadine only)

Other side effects not listed above may also occur in some patients. If you notice any other effects, check with your health care professional.

## Additional Information

Once a medicine has been approved for marketing for a certain use, experience may show that it is also useful for other medical problems. Although this use is not included in product labeling, astemizole, cetirizine, loratadine, and terfenadine are used in certain patients with asthma together with asthma medicines. The antihistamine is used before and during exposure to substances that cause reactions, to prevent or reduce bronchospasm (wheezing or difficulty in breathing).

Other than the above information, there is no additional information relating to proper use, precautions, or side effects for this use.

Revisd: 07/26/94

---

# ANTIHISTAMINES AND DECONGESTANTS   Systemic

Some commonly used brand names are:

**In the U.S.—**

Actagen[25]
Actifed[25]
Actifed Head Cold
   and Allergy Medicine[25]
Alamine[11]
Alersule[9]
Allent[6]
Allercon[25]
Allerest[11]
Allerest, Children's[11]
Allerest 12 Hour[11]
Allerest 12 Hour
   Caplets[11]
Allerest Maximum Strength[14]
Allerfrim[25]
Allerfrin[25]
Allergy Cold[25]
Allergy Formula Sinutab [18]
Allergy Relief Medicine[11]
Allerphed[25]
Amaril D[13]
Amaril D Spantab[13]
Ami-Drix[18]
Anamine[14]
Anamine T.D.[14]
Anaplex[14]
Anaplex S.R.[14]
Aprodrine[25]
A.R.M. Maximum
   Strength Caplets[11]
Atrohist Pediatric[15]
Atrohist Sprinkle[5]
Benadryl Decongestant[19]
Benylin Decongestant[19]
Brexin L.A.[14]
Brofed[6]
Bromaline[4]
Bromanate[4]
Bromatap[4]
Bromatapp[4]
Bromfed[6]

Bromfed-PD[6]
Bromophen T.D.[3]
Bromphen[4]
Brompheril[18]
Carbiset[7]
Carbiset-TR[7]
Carbodec[7]
Carbodec TR[7]
Cardec-S[7]
Cenafed Plus[25]
Cheracol Sinus[18]
Chlorafed[14]
Chlorafed H.S. Timecelles[14]
Chlorafed Timecelles[14]
Chlordrine S.R.[14]
Chlorphedrine SR[14]
Chlor-Rest[11]
Chlor-Trimeton 4 Hour
   Relief[14]
Chlor-Trimeton 12 Hour
   Relief[14]
Codimal-L.A.[14]
Colfed-A[14]
Coltab Children's[9]
Comhist[12]
Comhist LA[12]
Condrin-LA[11]
Conex D.A.[11]
Contac 12-Hour[11]
Contac Maximum Strength
   12-Hour Caplets[11]
Cophene No.2[14]
Co-Pyronil 2[14]
Dallergy-D[9] [14]
Dallergy Jr.[6]
Deconamine[14]
Deconamine SR[14]
Decongestabs[13]
Dehist[11]
Demazin[11]
Demazin Repetabs[11]

Dexaphen SA[18]
Dexophed[18]
Dihistine[9]
Dimaphen[4]
Dimaphen S.A.[3]
Dimetane
   Decongestant[2]
Dimetane
   Decongestant Caplets[2]
Dimetapp[4]
Dimetapp Cold
   and Allergy[4]
Dimetapp Extentabs[4]
Dimetapp 4-Hour
   Liqui-gels Maximum
   Strength[4]
Disobrom[18]
Disophrol[18]
Disophrol Chronotabs[18]
Dorcol Children's Cold
   Formula[14]
Dristan Allergy[6]
Drixoral[6] [18]
Drixoral Cold
   and Allergy[18]
Drize[11]
Duralex[14]
Dura-Tap PD[14]
Dura-Vent/A[11]
Ed A-Hist[9]
Endafed[6]
E.N.T[4]
Fedahist[14]
Fedahist
   Decongestant[14]
Fedahist Gyrocaps[14]
Fedahist Timecaps[14]
Genac[25]
Genamin[11]
Genatap[4]
Gencold[11]

Hayfebrol[14]
Histalet[14]
Histalet Forte[16]
Histamic[13]
Histatab Plus[9]
Histatan[15]
Hista-Vadrin[10]
Histor-D[9]
12-Hour Cold[11]
Isoclor[14]
Isoclor Timesules[14]
Klerist-D[14]
Kronofed-A Jr. Kronocaps[14]
Kronofed-A Kronocaps[14]
Lodrane LD[6]
Myphetapp[4]
Naldecon[13]
Naldecon Pediatric Drops[13]
Naldecon Pediatric Syrup[13]
Naldelate[13]
Naldelate Pediatric Syrup [13]
Nalgest[13]
Nalgest Pediatric[13]
Napril[14]
Nasahist[10]
ND Clear T.D.[14]
New-Decongest
   Pediatric Syrup[13]
New-Decongestant
   Pediatric[13]
Nolamine[8]
Noraminic[11]
Normatane[3]
Novafed A[14]
Novahistine[9]
Oraminic Spancaps[11]
Ornade Spansules[11]
Par-Drix[18]
Parhist SR[11]
Partapp[4]
Partapp TD[3]

PediaCare Cold Formula[14]
Phenergan VC[22]
Pherazine VC[22]
Poly-Histine-D[20]
Poly-Histine-D Ped[20]
Prehist[9]
Prometh VC Plain[22]
Promethazine VC[22]
Pseudo-Chlor[14]
Pseudo-gest Plus[14]
Quadra-Hist[13]
Quadra-Hist Pediatric[13]
Resaid S.R.[11]
Rescon[11] [14]
Rescon-ED[14]
Rescon JR[14]
Rhinatate[15]
Rhinolar-EX[11]
Rhinolar-EX 12[11]
Rhinosyn[14]
Rhinosyn-PD[14]
Rinade B.I.D.[14]

Rolatuss Plain[9]
Rondec[7]
Rondec Drops[7]
Rondec-TR[7]
R-Tannamine[15]
R-Tannamine Pediatric[15]
R-Tannate[15]
R-Tannate Pediatric[15]
Ru-Tuss[9]
Ru-Tuss II[11]
Ryna[14]
Rynatan[15]
Rynatan Pediatric[15]
Rynatan-S Pediatric[15]
Seldane-D[24]
Semprex-D[1]
Sinucon Pediatric
   Drops[13]
Snaplets-D[11]
Sudafed Plus[14]
Tamine S.R.[3]
Tanoral[15]
Tavist-D[17]

T-Dry[14]
T-Dry Junior[14]
Temazin Cold[11]
Touro A & H[6]
Triafed[25]
Triaminic-12[11]
Triaminic Allergy[11]
Triaminic Chewables[11]
Triaminic Cold[11]
Triaminic Oral
   Infant Drops[21]
Triaminic TR[21]
Trifed[25]
Trinalin Repetabs[1a]
Trind[11]
Tri-Nefrin
   Extra Strength[11]
Triofed[25]
Triotann[15]
Triotann Pediatric[15]
Tripalgen Cold[11]
Tri-Phen-Chlor[13]

Tri-Phen-Chlor Pediatric[13]
Tri-Phen-Chlor T.R.[13]
Triphenyl[11]
Triphenyl T.D.[21]
Triposed[25]
Tritann[15]
Tritann Pediatric[15]
Tri-Tannate[15]
Tri-Tannate Pediatric[15]
Tussanil Plain[9]
ULTRAbrom PD[6]
Uni-Decon[13]
Vanex Forte Caplets[16]
Veltap[3]
Vicks Children's
   NyQuil Allergy/Head
   Cold[14]
Vicks DayQuil
   4 Hour Allergy
   Relief[4]
Vicks DayQuil
   12 Hour Allergy
   Relief[4]

In Canada—

Actifed[25]
Benylin Cold[14]
Chlor-Tripolon
   Decongestant[11] [14]
Chlor-Tripolon
   Decongestant Extra
   Strength[14]

Chlor-Tripolon
   Decongestant Repetabs[14]
Claritin Extra[19a]
Corsym[11]
Dimetapp[3]
Dimetapp Extentabs[3]
Dimetapp Oral
   Infant Drops[3]

Drixoral[18]
Drixtab[18]
NeoCitran A[19b]
Novahistex[14]
Ornade[11]
Ornade-A.F.[11]

Ornade Spansules[11]
Triaminic[11] [21]
Triaminic Oral
   Infant Drops[21]
Trinalin Repetabs[1]

Note: For quick reference the following antihistamine and decongestant combinations are numbered to match the corresponding brand names.

This information applies to the following medicines:

1. Acrivastine (AK-ri-vas-teen) and Pseudoephedrine (soo-doe-e-FED-rin)
1a. Azatadine (a-ZA-ta-deen) and Pseudoephedrine
2. Brompheniramine (brome-fen-EER-a-meen) and Phenylephrine (fen-ill-EF-rin)
3. Brompheniramine, Phenylephrine, and Phenylpropanolamine (fen-ill-proe-pa-NOLE-a-meen)
4. Brompheniramine and Phenylpropanolamine
5. Brompheniramine, Phenyltoloxamine (fen-ill-toe-LOX-a-meen), and Phenylephrine
6. Brompheniramine and Pseudoephedrine
7. Carbinoxamine (kar-bi-NOX-a-meen) and Pseudoephedrine
8. Chlorpheniramine (klor-fen-EER-a-meen), Phenindamine (fen-IN-da-meen), and Phenylpropanolamine
9. Chlorpheniramine and Phenylephrine
10. Chlorpheniramine, Phenylephrine, and Phenylpropanolamine
11. Chlorpheniramine and Phenylpropanolamine
12. Chlorpheniramine, Phenyltoloxamine, and Phenylephrine
13. Chlorpheniramine, Phenyltoloxamine, Phenylephrine, and Phenylpropanolamine
14. Chlorpheniramine and Pseudoephedrine
15. Chlorpheniramine, Pyrilamine (peer-ILL-a-meen), and Phenylephrine
16. Chlorpheniramine, Pyrilamine, Phenylephrine, and Phenylpropanolamine
17. Clemastine (KLEM-as-teen) and Phenylpropanolamine
18. Dexbrompheniramine (dex-brom-fen-EER-a-meen) and Pseudoephedrine
19. Diphenhydramine (dye-fen-HYE-dra-meen) and Pseudoephedrine
19a. Loratadine (lor-AT-a-deen) and Pseudoephedrine
19b. Pheniramine (fen-EER-a-meen) and Phenylephrine
20. Pheniramine, Phenyltoloxamine, Pyrilamine, and Phenylpropanolamine
21. Pheniramine, Pyrilamine, and Phenylpropanolamine

22. Promethazine (proe-METH-a-zeen) and Phenylephrine
23. No product available
24. Terfenadine (ter-FEN-a-deen) and Pseudoephedrine
25. Triprolidine (trye-PROE-li-deen) and Pseudoephedrine

## Description

Antihistamine and decongestant combinations are used to treat the nasal congestion (stuffy nose), sneezing, and runny nose caused by colds and hay fever.

Antihistamines work by preventing the effects of a substance called histamine, which is produced by the body. Histamine can cause itching, sneezing, runny nose, and watery eyes. Antihistamines contained in these combinations are: acrivastine, azatadine, brompheniramine, carbinoxamine, chlorpheniramine, clemastine, dexbrompheniramine, diphenhydramine, loratadine, pheniramine, phenyltoloxamine, promethazine, pyrilamine, terfenadine, and triprolidine.

The decongestants, such as phenylephrine, phenylpropanolamine (also known as PPA), and pseudoephedrine, produce a narrowing of blood vessels. This leads to clearing of nasal congestion, but it may also cause an increase in blood pressure in patients who have high blood pressure.

Some of these combinations are available only with your doctor's prescription. Others are available without a prescription; however, your doctor may have special instructions on the proper dose of the medicine for your medical condition. They are available in the following dosage forms:

*Oral*

Acrivastine and Pseudoephedrine
- Capsules (U.S.)

Azatadine and Pseudoephedrine
- Extended-release tablets (U.S. and Canada)

Brompheniramine and Phenylephrine
- Elixir (U.S.)
- Tablets (U.S.)

Brompheniramine, Phenylephrine, and Phenylpropanolamine
- Elixir (U.S. and Canada)
- Oral solution (Canada)
- Tablets (Canada)
- Extended-release tablets (U.S. and Canada)

Brompheniramine and Phenylpropanolamine
- Capsules (U.S.)
- Elixir (U.S.)
- Tablets (U.S.)
- Chewable tablets (U.S.)
- Extended-release tablets (U.S.)

Brompheniramine, Phenyltoloxamine, and Phenylephrine
- Extended-release capsules (U.S.)

Brompheniramine and Pseudoephedrine
- Extended-release capsules (U.S.)
- Elixir (U.S.)
- Syrup (U.S.)
- Tablets (U.S.)

Carbinoxamine and Pseudoephedrine
- Oral solution (U.S.)
- Syrup (U.S.)
- Tablets (U.S.)
- Extended-release tablets (U.S.)

Chlorpheniramine, Phenindamine, and Phenylpropanolamine
- Extended-release tablets (U.S.)

Chlorpheniramine and Phenylephrine
- Extended-release capsules (U.S.)
- Elixir (U.S.)
- Oral solution (U.S.)
- Syrup (U.S.)
- Tablets (U.S.)
- Chewable tablets (U.S.)

Chlorpheniramine, Phenylephrine, and Phenylpropanolamine
- Extended-release capsules (U.S.)
- Tablets (U.S.)

Chlorpheniramine and Phenylpropanolamine
- Extended-release capsules (U.S. and Canada)
- Granules (U.S.)
- Oral solution (U.S. and Canada)
- Extended-release oral suspension (Canada)
- Syrup (U.S. and Canada)
- Tablets (U.S.)
- Chewable tablets (U.S.)
- Extended-release tablets (U.S.)

Chlorpheniramine, Phenyltoloxamine, and Phenylephrine
- Extended-release capsules (U.S.)
- Tablets (U.S.)

Chlorpheniramine, Phenyltoloxamine, Phenylephrine, and Phenylpropanolamine
- Extended-release capsules (U.S.)
- Oral solution (U.S.)
- Syrup (U.S.)
- Extended-release tablets (U.S.)

Chlorpheniramine and Pseudoephedrine
- Capsules (U.S. and Canada)
- Extended-release capsules (U.S. and Canada)
- Oral solution (U.S.)
- Syrup (U.S.)
- Tablets (U.S. and Canada)
- Extended-release tablets (U.S. and Canada)

Chlorpheniramine, Pyrilamine, and Phenylephrine
- Oral suspension (U.S.)
- Tablets (U.S.)
- Extended-release tablets (U.S.)

Chlorpheniramine, Pyrilamine, Phenylephrine, and Phenylpropanolamine
- Tablets (U.S.)

Clemastine and Phenylpropanolamine
- Extended-release tablets (U.S.)

Dexbrompheniramine and Pseudoephedrine
- Extended-release capsules (Canada)
- Syrup (Canada)
- Tablets (U.S.)
- Extended-release tablets (U.S. and Canada)

Diphenhydramine and Pseudoephedrine
- Capsules (U.S.)
- Oral solution (U.S.)
- Tablets (U.S.)

Loratadine and Pseudoephedrine
- Tablets (Canada)

Pheniramine and Phenylephrine
- for Oral solution (Canada)

Pheniramine, Phenyltoloxamine, Pyrilamine, and Phenylpropanolamine
- Extended-release capsules (U.S.)
- Elixir (U.S.)

Pheniramine, Pyrilamine, and Phenylpropanolamine
- Oral solution (U.S. and Canada)
- Extended-release tablets (U.S. and Canada)

Promethazine and Phenylephrine
- Syrup (U.S.)

Terfenadine and Pseudoephedrine
- Extended-release tablets (U.S.)

Triprolidine and Pseudoephedrine
- Capsules (U.S.)
- Syrup (U.S. and Canada)
- Tablets (U.S. and Canada)

## Before Using This Medicine

If you are taking this medicine without a prescription, carefully read and follow any precautions on the label. For antihistamine and decongestant combinations, the following should be considered:

**Allergies**—Tell your doctor if you have ever had any unusual or allergic reaction to antihistamines or to amphetamine, dextroamphetamine (e.g., Dexedrine), ephedrine (e.g., Ephed II), epinephrine (e.g., Adrenalin), isoproterenol (e.g., Isuprel), metaproterenol (e.g., Alupent), methamphetamine (e.g., Desoxyn), norepinephrine (e.g., Levophed), phenylephrine (e.g., Neo-Synephrine), pseudoephedrine (e.g., Sudafed), PPA (e.g., Dexatrim), or terbutaline (e.g., Brethine).

**Pregnancy**—The occasional use of antihistamine and decongestant combinations is not likely to cause problems in the fetus or in the newborn baby. However, when these medicines are used at higher doses and/or for a long time, the chance that problems might occur may increase. For the individual ingredients of these combinations, the following apply:

- *Alcohol*—Some of these combination medicines contain alcohol. Too much use of alcohol during pregnancy may cause birth defects.
- *Antihistamines*—Antihistamines have not been shown to cause problems in humans.
- *Phenylephrine*—Studies on birth defects have not been done in either humans or animals with phenylephrine.
- *Phenylpropanolamine*—Studies on birth defects have not been done in either humans or animals with phenylpropanolamine. However, it seems that women who take phenylpropanolamine in the weeks following delivery are more likely to suffer mental or mood changes.
- *Promethazine*—Phenothiazines, such as promethazine (contained in some of these combination medicines [e.g., Phenergan-D]), have been shown to cause jaundice and muscle tremors in a few newborn infants whose mothers received phenothiazines during pregnancy. Also, the newborn baby may have blood clotting problems if promethazine is taken by the mother within 2 weeks before delivery.
- *Pseudoephedrine*—Studies on birth defects with pseudoephedrine have not been done in humans. In animal studies pseudoephedrine did not cause birth defects but did cause a decrease in average weight, length, and rate of bone formation in the animal fetus when administered in high doses.

**Breast-feeding**—Small amounts of antihistamines and decongestants pass into the breast milk. Use is not recommended since the chances are greater for this medicine to cause side effects, such as unusual excitement or irritability, in the nursing baby. Also, since antihistamines tend to decrease the secretions of the body, it is possible that the flow of breast milk may be reduced in some patients. It is not known yet whether loratadine or terfenadine causes these same side effects.

**Children**—Very young children are usually more sensitive to the effects of this medicine. Increases in blood pressure, nightmares or unusual excitement, nervousness, restlessness, or irritability may be more likely to occur in children. Also, mental changes may be more likely to occur in young children taking combination medicines that contain phenylpropanolamine. *Before giving any of these combination medicines to a child, check the package label very carefully. Some of these medicines are too strong for use in children.* If you are not certain whether a specific product can be given to a child, or if you have any questions about the amount to give, check with your health care professional.

**Older adults**—Confusion, difficult and painful urination, dizziness, drowsiness, dryness of mouth, or convulsions (seizures) may be more likely to occur in the elderly, who are usually more sensitive to the effects of this medicine. Also, nightmares or unusual excitement, nervousness,

restlessness, or irritability may be more likely to occur in elderly patients.

**Other medicines**—Although certain medicines should not be used together at all, in other cases different medicines may be used together even if an interaction might occur. In these cases, your doctor may want to change the dose, or other precautions may be necessary. When you are taking antihistamines it is especially important that your health care professional know if you are taking any of the following:

- Anticholinergics (medicine for abdominal or stomach spasms or cramps)—Side effects, such as dryness of mouth, of antihistamines or anticholinergics may be more likely to occur
- Azithromycin (e.g., Zithromax) or
- Clarithromycin (e.g., Biaxin) or
- Erythromycin (e.g., E-Mycin) or
- Itraconazole (e.g., Sporanox) or
- Ketoconazole (e.g., Nizoral)—Use of these medicines with the terfenadine-containing combination may cause heart problems, such as an irregular heartbeat; these medicines should not be used together
- Central nervous system (CNS) depressants—Effects, such as drowsiness, of CNS depressants or antihistamines may be worsened
- Maprotiline (e.g., Ludiomil) or
- Tricyclic antidepressants (amitriptyline [e.g., Elavil], amoxapine [e.g., Asendin], clomipramine [e.g., Anafranil], desipramine [e.g., Pertofrane], doxepin [e.g., Sinequan], imipramine [e.g., Tofranil], nortriptyline [e.g., Aventyl], protriptyline [e.g., Vivactil], trimipramine [e.g., Surmontil])—Effects, such as drowsiness, of CNS depressants or antihistamines may be worsened; also, taking these medicines together may cause some of their side effects, such as dryness of mouth, to become more severe
- Monoamine oxidase (MAO) inhibitors (furazolidone [e.g., Furoxone], isocarboxazid [e.g., Marplan], phenelzine [e.g., Nardil], procarbazine [e.g., Matulane], selegiline [e.g., Eldepryl], tranylcypromine [e.g., Parnate])—If you are now taking, or have taken within the past 2 weeks, any of the MAO inhibitors, the side effects of the antihistamines may become more severe; these medicines should not be used together
- Rauwolfia alkaloids (alseroxylon [e.g., Rauwiloid], deserpidine [e.g., Harmonyl], rauwolfia serpentina [e.g., Raudixin], reserpine [e.g., Serpasil])—These medicines may increase or decrease the effect of the decongestant

Also, if you are taking one of the combinations containing phenylpropanolamine or pseudoephedrine and are also taking:

- Amantadine (e.g., Symmetrel) or
- Amphetamines or
- Appetite suppressants (diet pills), except fenfluramine (e.g., Pondimin) or
- Caffeine (e.g., NoDoz) or
- Chlophedianol (e.g., Ulone) or
- Medicine for asthma or other breathing problems or
- Medicine for colds, sinus problems, or hay fever or other allergies (including nose drops or sprays) or
- Methylphenidate (e.g., Ritalin) or
- Nabilone (e.g., Cesamet) or
- Pemoline (e.g., Cylert)—Using any of these medicines together with an antihistamine and decongestant combination may cause excessive stimulant side effects, such

as difficulty in sleeping, heart rate problems, nervousness, and irritability

- Beta-adrenergic blocking agents (acebutolol [e.g., Sectral], atenolol [e.g., Tenormin], betaxolol [e.g., Kerlone], bisoprolol [e.g., Zebeta], carteolol [e.g., Cartrol], labetalol [e.g., Normodyne], metoprolol [e.g., Lopressor], nadolol [e.g., Corgard], oxprenolol [e.g., Trasicor], penbutolol [e.g., Levatol], pindolol [e.g., Visken], propanolol [e.g., Inderal], sotalol [e.g., Sotacor], timolol [e.g., Blocadren])—Using any of these medicines together with an antihistamine and decongestant combination may cause high blood pressure and heart problems (e.g., unusually slow heartbeat)

**Other medical problems**—The presence of other medical problems may affect the use of antihistamine and decongestant combinations. Make sure you tell your doctor if you have any other medical problems, especially:

- Diabetes mellitus (sugar diabetes)—The decongestant in this medicine may put diabetic patients at a greater risk of having heart or blood vessel disease
- Enlarged prostate or
- Urinary tract blockage or difficult urination—Some of the effects of antihistamines may make urinary problems worse
- Glaucoma—A slight increase in inner eye pressure may occur
- Heart or blood vessel disease or
- High blood pressure—The decongestant in this medicine may cause the blood pressure to increase and may also speed up the heart rate
- Liver disease—Higher blood levels of terfenadine may result, which may increase the chance of heart problems (for terfenadine-containing combination only)
- Overactive thyroid—If the overactive thyroid has caused a fast heart rate, the decongestant in this medicine may cause the heart rate to speed up further

## Proper Use of This Medicine

*Take this medicine only as directed. Do not take more of it and do not take it more often than recommended on the label, unless otherwise directed by your doctor. To do so may increase the chance of side effects.*

If this medicine irritates your stomach, you may take it with food or a glass of water or milk, to lessen the irritation.

For patients *taking the extended-release capsule or tablet form of this medicine:*

- Swallow it whole.
- Do not crush, break, or chew before swallowing.
- If the capsule is too large to swallow, you may mix the contents of the capsule with applesauce, jelly, honey, or syrup and swallow without chewing.

**Dosing**—There is a large variety of antihistamines and decongestants combination products on the market. Some products are for use in adults only, while others may be used in children. If you have any questions about this, check with your health care professional.

The dose of antihistamines and decongestants will be different for different products. The number of capsules or tablets or teaspoonfuls of liquid or granules that you take depends on the strengths of the medicines. Also, *the number of doses you take each day and the time between doses depends on whether you are taking a short-acting or long-acting form of antihistamine and decongestant. Follow your doctor's orders if this medicine was prescribed. Or, follow the directions on the box if you are buying this medicine without a prescription.*

**Missed dose**—If you are taking this medicine regularly and you miss a dose, take it as soon as possible. However, if it is almost time for your next dose, skip the missed dose and go back to your regular dosing schedule. Do not double doses.

**Storage**—To store this medicine:

- Keep out of the reach of children.
- Store away from heat and direct light.
- Do not store in the bathroom, near the kitchen sink, or in other damp places. Heat or moisture may cause the medicine to break down.
- Keep the liquid form of this medicine from freezing.
- Do not keep outdated medicine or medicine no longer needed. Be sure that any discarded medicine is out of the reach of children.

## Precautions While Using This Medicine

Before you have any skin tests for allergies, tell the doctor in charge that you are taking this medicine. The results of the test may be affected by the antihistamine in this medicine.

When taking antihistamines (contained in this combination medicine) on a regular basis, make sure your doctor knows if you are taking large amounts of aspirin at the same time (as for arthritis or rheumatism). Effects of too much aspirin, such as ringing in the ears, may be covered up by the antihistamine.

The antihistamine in this medicine will add to the effects of alcohol and other CNS depressants (medicines that slow down the nervous system, possibly causing drowsiness). Some examples of CNS depressants are other antihistamines or medicine for hay fever, other allergies, or colds; sedatives, tranquilizers, or sleeping medicine; prescription pain medicine or narcotics; barbiturates; medicine for seizures; muscle relaxants; or anesthetics, including some dental anesthetics. *Check with your doctor before taking any of the above while you are taking this medicine.*

The antihistamine in this medicine may cause some people to become drowsy, dizzy, or less alert than they are normally. *Some antihistamines are more likely to cause drowsiness than others (loratadine and terfenadine, for example, rarely produce this effect). Make sure you know how you react before you drive, use machines, or do anything else that could be dangerous if you are dizzy or are not alert.*

The decongestant in this medicine may add to the central nervous system (CNS) stimulant and other effects of phenylpropanolamine (PPA)-containing diet aids. *Do not use medicines for diet or appetite control while taking this medicine unless you have checked with your doctor.*

The decongestant in this medicine may cause some people to be nervous or restless or to have trouble in sleeping. If you have trouble in sleeping, *take the last dose of this medicine for each day a few hours before bedtime.* If you have any questions about this, check with your doctor.

Antihistamines may cause dryness of the mouth, nose, and throat. Some antihistamines are more likely to cause dryness of the mouth than others (loratadine and terfenadine, for example, rarely produce this effect). For temporary relief, use sugarless candy or gum, melt bits of ice in your mouth, or use a saliva substitute. However, if your mouth continues to feel dry for more than 2 weeks, check with your dentist. Continuing dryness of the mouth may increase the chance of dental disease, including tooth decay, gum disease, and fungus infections.

For patients *using promethazine-containing medicine:*
- This medicine controls nausea and vomiting. For this reason, it may cover up the signs of overdose caused by other medicines or the symptoms of intestinal blockage. This will make it difficult for your doctor to diagnose these conditions. Make sure your doctor knows that you are taking this medicine if you have other symptoms such as stomach or lower abdominal pain, cramping, or soreness. Also, if you think you may have taken an overdose of any medicine, tell your doctor that you are taking this medicine.

---

### Side Effects of This Medicine

Along with its needed effects, a medicine may cause some unwanted effects. Although serious side effects occur rarely when this medicine is taken as recommended, they may be more likely to occur if:
- too much medicine is taken.
- it is taken in large doses.
- it is taken for a long period of time.

*Get emergency help immediately if any of the following symptoms of overdose occur:*

Clumsiness or unsteadiness; convulsions (seizures); drowsiness (severe); dryness of mouth, nose, or throat (severe); flushing or redness of face; hallucinations (seeing, hearing, or feeling things that are not there); headache (continuing); shortness of breath or troubled breathing; slow, fast, or irregular heartbeat; trouble in sleeping

*For promethazine only*

Muscle spasms (especially of neck and back); restlessness; shuffling walk; tic-like (jerky) movements of head and face; trembling and shaking of hands

Also, check with your doctor as soon as possible if any of the following side effects occur:

*Rare*

Mood or mental changes; sore throat and fever; tightness in chest; unusual bleeding or bruising; unusual tiredness or weakness

Other side effects may occur that usually do not need medical attention. These side effects may go away during treatment as your body adjusts to the medicine. However, check with your health care professional if any of the following side effects continue or are bothersome:

*More common—rare with loratadine- or terfenadine-containing combination*

Drowsiness; thickening of the bronchial secretions

*Less common—more common with high doses*

Blurred vision; confusion; difficult or painful urination; dizziness; dryness of mouth, nose, or throat; headache; loss of appetite; nightmares; pounding heartbeat; ringing or buzzing in ears; skin rash; stomach upset or pain (more common with pyrilamine and tripelennamine); unusual excitement, nervousness, restlessness, or irritability

Other side effects not listed above may also occur in some patients. If you notice any other effects, check with your doctor.

---

Revised: 07/19/94

---

# ANTIHISTAMINES, DECONGESTANTS, AND ANALGESICS    Systemic

Some commonly used brand names are:

**In the U.S.—**

| | |
|---|---|
| Aclophen[5] | Alumadrine[8] |
| Actifed Plus[23] | BC Multi Symptom Cold |
| Actifed Plus Caplets[23] |    Powder[10] |
| Actifed Sinus Nighttime | Benadryl Cold[18] |
|    Caplets[18] | Benadryl Cold Nighttime |
| Alka-Seltzer Plus Cold[10] |    Liquid[18] |
| Alka-Seltzer Plus | BQ Cold[8] |
|    Maximum Strength | Bromaline Plus[2] |
|    Sinus Allergy Medicine[3] | Children's Tylenol Cold[13] |
| Alka-Seltzer Plus | Chlor-Trimeton Sinus |
|    Nighttime Cold[17] |    Caplets[8] |
| Allerest Headache | Codimal[13] |
|    Strength[8] | Comtrex A/S[13] |
| Allerest Sinus Pain | Comtrex A/S Caplets[13] |
|    Formula[8] | Congestant D[8] |

| | |
|---|---|
| Contac Allergy/Sinus Night | Histagesic Modified[5] |
|    Caplets[18] | Histosal[22] |
| Coricidin Demilets[8] | Kolephrin[7] |
| Coricidin Maximum | Maximum Strength Tylenol |
|    Strength Sinus |    Allergy Sinus Caplets[13] |
|    Headache[8] | ND-Gesic[14] |
| Covangesic[15] | Night-Time Effervescent |
| Dapacin Cold[8] |    Cold[17] |
| Dimetapp Cold and Flu | Norel Plus[12] |
|    Caplets[2] | Phenapap Sinus Headache |
| Dristan Cold Maximum |    & Congestion[13] |
|    Strength Caplets[4] | Phenate T.D.[8] |
| Dristan Cold Multi Symptom | Pyrroxate Extra Strength[8] |
|    Formula[5] | Remcol Cold[8] |
| Drixoral Cold and Flu[16] | Rhinogesic[6] |
| Drixoral Sinus[16] | Salphenyl[6] |
| Duadacin[8] | |
| Gendecon[5] | |

Scot-tussin Original 5-Action
    Cold Formula[19]
Scot-tussin Original 5-Action
    Cold Medicine[19]
Simplet[13]
Sinapils[9]
Sinarest[8]
Sinarest Sinus[13]
Sine-Off Maximum Strength
    Allergy/Sinus Formula
    Caplets[13]
Sine-Off Sinus Medicine[10]
Singlet[13]
Sinulin[8]
Sinutab Extra Strength[13]

Sinutab Maximum
    Strength Sinus Allergy[13]
Sinutab Maximum Strength
    Sinus Allergy Caplets[13]
Sinutrex Extra Strength[13]
TheraFlu/Flu and Cold
    Medicine[13]
Triaminicin Cold,
    Allergy, Sinus[8]
Tricom Caplets[13]
Tylenol Allergy Sinus
    Night Time Maximum
    Strength Caplets[18]
Tylenol Cold Medication[8]
Tylenol Cold Night Time[18]
4-Way Cold[8]

**In Canada—**
Actifed A[24]
Coricidin 'D'[10]
Dimetapp-A[1]
Dimetapp-A Pediatric[1]
Dristan[11]
Dristan Formula P[22]

NeoCitran Colds and Flu
    Calorie Reduced[19]
NeoCitran Extra Strength
    Colds and Flu[19]
Sinutab Extra Strength[13]
Sinutab Regular[13]
Sinutab SA[21]

Note: For quick reference, the following antihistamine, decongestants, and analgesics are numbered to match the corresponding brand names.

This information applies to the following medicines:
1. Brompheniramine (brom-fen-EER-a-meen), Phenylephrine (fen-ill-ef-rin), Phenylpropanolamine (fen-ill-proe-pa-nole-a-meen), and Acetaminophen (a-seat-a-min-oh-fen)
2. Brompheniramine, Phenylpropanolamine, and Acetaminophen
3. Brompheniramine, Phenylpropanolamine, and Aspirin (AS-pir-in)
4. Brompheniramine, Pseudoephedrine (soo-doe-e-FED-rin), and Acetaminophen
5. Chlorpheniramine (klor-fen-EER-a-meen), Phenylephrine, and Acetaminophen†
6. Chlorpheniramine, Phenylephrine, Acetaminophen, and Salicylamide (sal-i-sill-a-mide)
7. Chlorpheniramine, Phenylephrine, Acetaminophen, Salicylamide, and Caffeine (kaf-EEN)
8. Chlorpheniramine, Phenylpropanolamine, and Acetaminophen
9. Chlorpheniramine, Phenylpropanolamine, Acetaminophen, and Caffeine
10. Chlorpheniramine, Phenylpropanolamine, and Aspirin
11. Chlorpheniramine, Phenylpropanolamine, Aspirin, and Caffeine
12. Chlorpheniramine, Phenyltoloxamine (fen-ill-tole-OX-a-meen), Phenylpropanolamine, and Acetaminophen
13. Chlorpheniramine, Pseudoephedrine, and Acetaminophen
14. Chlorpheniramine, Pyrilamine (peer-ILL-a-meen), Phenylephrine, and Acetaminophen
15. Chlorpheniramine, Pyrilamine, Phenylephrine, Phenylpropanolamine, and Acetaminophen
16. Dexbrompheniramine (dex-brome-fen-EER-a-meen), Pseudoephedrine, and Acetaminophen
17. Diphenhydramine (dye-fen-HYE-dra-meen), Phenylpropanolamine, and Aspirin
18. Diphenhydramine, Pseudoephedrine, and Acetaminophen
19. Pheniramine (fen-EER-a-meen), Phenylephrine, and Acetaminophen
20. Pheniramine, Phenylephrine, Sodium Salicylate (SOE-dee-um sa-LI-si-late), and Caffeine
21. Phenyltoloxamine, Phenylpropanolamine, and Acetaminophen
22. Pyrilamine, Phenylephrine, Aspirin, and Caffeine
23. Pyrilamine, Phenylpropanolamine, Acetaminophen, and Caffeine
24. Triprolidine (trye-PROE-li-deen), Pseudoephedrine, and Acetaminophen

*Not commercially available in the U.S.
†Not commercially available in Canada.

## Description

Antihistamine, decongestant, and analgesic combinations are taken by mouth to relieve the sneezing, runny nose, sinus and nasal congestion (stuffy nose), fever, headache, and aches and pain, of colds, influenza, and hay fever. These combinations do not contain any ingredient to relieve coughs.

Antihistamines are used to relieve or prevent the symptoms of hay fever and other types of allergy. They may also help relieve some symptoms of the common cold, such as sneezing and runny nose. They work by preventing the effects of a substance called histamine, which is produced by the body. Antihistamines contained in these combinations are: brompheniramine, chlorpheniramine, dexbrompheniramine, diphenhydramine, pheniramine, phenyltoloxamine, pyrilamine, and triprolidine.

Decongestants, such as phenylephrine, phenylpropanolamine (also known as PPA), and pseudoephedrine, produce a narrowing of blood vessels. This leads to clearing of nasal congestion, but it may also cause an increase in blood pressure in patients who have high blood pressure.

Analgesics, such as acetaminophen and salicylates (e.g., aspirin, salicylamide, sodium salicylate), are used in these combination medicines to help relieve fever, headache, aches, and pain.

Some of these medicines are available without a prescription. However, your doctor may have special instructions on the proper dose of these medicines for your medical condition. These medicines are available in the following dosage forms:

*Oral*
    Brompheniramine, Phenylephrine, Phenylpropanolamine, and Acetaminophen
    • Oral solution (Canada)
    • Tablets (Canada)
    Brompheniramine, Phenylpropanolamine, and Acetaminophen
    • Tablets (U.S.)
    Brompheniramine, Phenylpropanolamine, and Aspirin
    • Effervescent tablets (U.S.)
    Brompheniramine, Pseudoephedrine, and Acetaminophen
    • Tablets (U.S.)
    Chlorpheniramine, Phenylephrine, and Acetaminophen
    • Tablets (U.S.)
    Chlorpheniramine, Phenylephrine, Acetaminophen, and Salicylamide
    • Capsules (U.S.)
    • Tablets (U.S.)
    Chlorpheniramine, Phenylephrine, Acetaminophen, Salicylamide, and Caffeine
    • Capsules (U.S.)
    Chlorpheniramine, Phenylpropanolamine, and Acetaminophen
    • Capsules (U.S.)
    • Tablets (U.S.)
    • Chewable tablets (U.S.)
    • Effervescent tablets (U.S.)
    • Extended-release tablets (U.S.)
    Chlorpheniramine, Phenylpropanolamine, Acetaminophen, and Caffeine
    • Tablets (U.S.)
    Chlorpheniramine, Phenylpropanolamine, and Aspirin
    • For oral solution (U.S.)
    • Tablets (U.S. and Canada)

Chlorpheniramine, Phenylpropanolamine, Aspirin, and Caffeine
- Capsules (Canada)
- Tablets (Canada)

Chlorpheniramine, Phenyltoloxamine, Phenylpropanolamine, and Acetaminophen
- Capsules (U.S.)

Chlorpheniramine, Pseudoephedrine, and Acetaminophen
- Capsules (U.S. and Canada)
- For oral solution (U.S.)
- Oral solution (U.S.)
- Tablets (U.S. and Canada)
- Chewable tablets (U.S.)

Chlorpheniramine, Pyrilamine, Phenylephrine, and Acetaminophen
- Tablets (U.S.)

Chlorpheniramine, Pyrilamine, Phenylephrine, Phenylpropanolamine, and Acetaminophen
- Tablets (U.S.)

Dexbrompheniramine, Pseudoephedrine, and Acetaminophen
- Extended-release tablets (U.S.)

Diphenhydramine, Phenylpropanolamine, and Aspirin
- Tablets (U.S.)
- Effervescent tablets (U.S.)

Diphenhydramine, Pseudoephedrine, and Acetaminophen
- Oral solution (U.S.)
- Tablets (U.S.)

Pheniramine, Phenylephrine, and Acetaminophen
- For oral solution (Canada)

Pheniramine, Phenylephrine, Sodium Salicylate, and Caffeine
- Oral solution (U.S.)
- Syrup (U.S.)

Phenyltoloxamine, Phenylpropanolamine, and Acetaminophen
- Extended-release tablets (Canada)

Pyrilamine, Phenylephrine, Aspirin, and Caffeine
- Tablets (Canada)

Pyrilamine, Phenylpropanolamine, Acetaminophen, and Caffeine
- Tablets (U.S.)

Triprolidine, Pseudoephedrine, and Acetaminophen
- Tablets (U.S. and Canada)

---

## Before Using This Medicine

If you are taking this medicine without a prescription, carefully read and follow any precautions on the label. For antihistamine, decongestant, and analgesic combinations, the following should be considered:

**Allergies**—Tell your doctor if you have ever had any unusual or allergic reaction to any of the ingredients contained in this medicine. If this medicine contains *aspirin* or *another salicylate*, before taking it, check with your doctor if you have ever had any unusual or allergic reaction to any of the following medicines:

Diclofenac (e.g., Voltaren)
Diflunisal (e.g., Dolobid)
Etodolac (e.g., Lodine)
Fenoprofen (e.g., Nalfon)
Floctafenine
Flurbiprofen, by mouth (e.g., Ansaid)
Ibuprofen (e.g., Motrin)

Indomethacin (e.g., Indocin)
Ketoprofen (e.g., Orudis)
Meclofenamate (e.g., Meclomen)
Mefenamic acid (e.g., Ponstel)
Methyl salicylate (oil of wintergreen)
Nabumetone (e.g., Relafen)
Naproxen (e.g., Naprosyn)
Oxaprozin (e.g., Daypro)
Oxyphenbutazone (e.g., Tandearil)
Phenylbutazone (e.g., Butazolidin)
Piroxicam (e.g., Feldene)
Sulindac (e.g., Clinoril)
Suprofen (e.g., Suprol)
Tenoxicam (e.g., Mobiflex)
Tiaprofenic acid (e.g., Surgam)
Tolmetin (e.g., Tolectin)
Zomepirac (e.g., Zomax)

Also tell your health care professional if you are allergic to any other substances, such as foods, preservatives, or dyes.

**Pregnancy**—The occasional use of antihistamine, decongestant, and analgesic combinations is not likely to cause problems in the fetus or in the newborn baby. However, when these medicines are used at higher doses and/or for a long time, the chance that problems might occur may increase. For the individual ingredients of these combinations, the following apply:

- *Acetaminophen*—Acetaminophen has not been shown to cause birth defects or other problems in humans. However, studies on birth defects have not been done in humans.

- *Alcohol*—Some of these combination medicines contain large amounts of alcohol. Too much use of alcohol during pregnancy may cause birth defects.

- *Antihistamines*—Antihistamines have not been shown to cause problems in humans.

- *Caffeine*—Studies in humans have not shown that caffeine causes birth defects. However, studies in animals have shown that caffeine causes birth defects when given in very large doses (amounts equal to the amount of caffeine contained in 12 to 24 cups of coffee a day).

- *Phenylephrine*—Studies on birth defects have not been done in either humans or animals with phenylephrine.

- *Phenylpropanolamine*—Studies on birth defects have not been done in either humans or animals with phenylpropanolamine. However, it seems that women who take phenylpropanolamine in the weeks following delivery are more likely to suffer mental or mood changes.

- *Pseudoephedrine*—Studies on birth defects with pseudoephedrine have not been done in humans. In animal studies pseudoephedrine did not cause birth defects but did cause a decrease in average weight, length, and rate of bone formation in the animal fetus when administered in high doses.

- *Salicylates (e.g., aspirin)*—Salicylates have not been shown to cause birth defects in humans. Studies on birth defects in humans have been done with aspirin

---

but not with salicylamide. However, salicylates have been shown to cause birth defects in animals.

Regular use of salicylates late in pregnancy may cause unwanted effects on the heart or blood flow in the fetus or newborn baby. Use of salicylates during the last 2 weeks of pregnancy may cause bleeding problems in the fetus before or during delivery, or in the newborn baby. Also, too much use of salicylates during the last 3 months of pregnancy may increase the length of pregnancy, prolong labor, cause other problems during delivery, or cause severe bleeding in the mother before, during, or after delivery. *Do not take aspirin during the last 3 months of pregnancy unless it has been ordered by your doctor.*

**Breast-feeding**—If you are breast-feeding the chance that problems might occur depends on the ingredients of the combination. For the individual ingredients of these combinations, the following apply:

- *Acetaminophen*—Acetaminophen passes into the breast milk. However, it has not been shown to cause problems in nursing babies.
- *Alcohol*—Alcohol passes into the breast milk. However, the amount of alcohol in recommended doses of this medicine does not usually cause problems in nursing babies.
- *Antihistamines*—Use is not recommended since the chances are greater for this medicine to cause side effects, such as unusual excitement or irritability, in the nursing baby. Also, since antihistamines tend to decrease the secretions of the body, it is possible that the flow of breast milk may be reduced in some women.
- *Caffeine*—Small amounts of caffeine pass into the breast milk and may build up in the nursing baby. However, the amount of caffeine in recommended doses of this medicine does not usually cause problems in nursing babies.
- *Decongestants (e.g., phenylephrine, phenylpropanolamine, pseudoephedrine)*—Decongestants may pass into the breast milk and may cause unwanted effects in nursing babies of mothers taking this medicine.
- *Salicylates (e.g., aspirin, salicylamide, sodium salicylate)*—Salicylates pass into the breast milk. Although salicylates have not been reported to cause problems in nursing babies, it is possible that problems may occur if large amounts are taken regularly.

**Children**—Very young children are usually more sensitive to the effects of this medicine. Increases in blood pressure, nightmares, unusual excitement, nervousness, restlessness, or irritability may be more likely to occur in children. Also, mental changes may be more likely to occur in young children taking these combination medicines.

*Before giving any of these combination medicines to a child, check the package label very carefully. Some of these medicines are too strong for use in children.* If you are not certain whether a specific product can be given to a child, or if you have any questions about the amount to give, check with your health care professional.

*Do not give aspirin or other salicylates to a child with a fever or other symptoms of a virus infection, especially flu or chickenpox, without first discussing their use with your child's doctor.* This is very important because salicylates may cause a serious illness called Reye's syndrome in children with fever caused by a virus infection, especially flu or chickenpox. Also, children may be more sensitive to the aspirin or other salicylates contained in some of these medicines, especially if they have a fever or have lost large amounts of body fluid because of vomiting, diarrhea, or sweating.

**Teenagers**—*Do not give aspirin or other salicylates to a teenager with a fever or other symptoms of a virus infection, especially flu or chickenpox, without first discussing their use with your child's doctor.* This is very important because salicylates may cause a serious illness called Reye's syndrome in teenagers with fever caused by a virus infection, especially flu or chickenpox.

**Older adults**—The elderly are usually more sensitive to the effects of this medicine. Confusion, difficult or painful urination, dizziness, drowsiness, feeling faint, or dryness of mouth, nose, or throat may be more likely to occur in elderly patients. Also, nightmares or unusual excitement, nervousness, restlessness, or irritability may be more likely to occur in the elderly.

**Other medicines**—Although certain medicines should not be used together at all, in other cases two different medicines may be used together even if an interaction might occur. In these cases, your doctor may want to change the dose, or other precautions may be necessary. When you are taking antihistamine, decongestant, and analgesic combinations it is especially important that your health care professional know if you are taking *any* other prescription or nonprescription (over-the-counter [OTC]) medicine, for example, aspirin or other medicine for allergies. Some medicines may change the way this medicine affects your body. Also, the effect of other medicines may be increased or reduced by some of the ingredients in this medicine.

**Other medical problems**—The presence of other medical problems may affect the use of antihistamine, decongestant, and analgesic combinations. Make sure you tell your doctor if you have any other medical problems, especially:

- Alcohol abuse—Acetaminophen-containing medicines increase the chance of liver damage
- Anemia—Taking a salicylate-containing medicine may make the anemia worse
- Asthma, allergies, and nasal polyps, history of, or
- Asthma attacks—Taking a salicylate-containing medicine may cause an allergic reaction in which breathing becomes difficult; also, although antihistamines open tightened bronchial passages, other effects of the antihistamines may cause secretions to become thick so that during an asthma attack it might be difficult to cough them up

- Diabetes mellitus (sugar diabetes)—The decongestant in this medicine may put the patient with diabetes at a greater risk of having heart or blood vessel disease
- Enlarged prostate or
- Urinary tract blockage or difficult urination—Some of the effects of antihistamines may cause urinary problems to get worse
- Glaucoma—A slight increase in inner eye pressure may occur
- Gout—Aspirin- or sodium salicylate–containing medicine may make the gout worse and reduce the benefit of the medicines used for gout
- Hemophilia or other bleeding problems—Aspirin- or sodium salicylate–containing medicine increase the chance of bleeding
- Hepatitis or other liver disease—There is a greater chance of side effects because the medicine is not broken down and may build up in the body; also, if liver disease is severe there is a greater chance that aspirin-containing medicine may cause bleeding
- Heart or blood vessel disease or
- High blood pressure—The decongestant in this medicine may cause the blood pressure to increase and may also speed up the heart rate; also, caffeine-containing medicine, if taken in large amounts, may have a similar effect on the heart
- Kidney disease (severe)—The kidneys may be affected, especially if too much of this medicine is taken for a long time
- Overactive thyroid—If the overactive thyroid has caused a fast heart rate, the decongestant in this medicine may cause the heart rate to speed up further
- Stomach ulcer or other stomach problems—Salicylate-containing medicine may make the ulcer worse or cause bleeding of the stomach

## Proper Use of This Medicine

*Take this medicine only as directed.* Do not take more of it and do not take it more often than recommended on the label, unless otherwise directed by your doctor. To do so may increase the chance of side effects.

If this medicine irritates your stomach, you may take it with food or a glass of water or milk, to lessen the irritation.

For patients taking the extended-release tablet form of this medicine:

- Swallow the tablets whole.
- Do not crush, break, or chew before swallowing.

*If a combination medicine containing aspirin has a strong vinegar-like odor, do not use it.* This odor means the medicine is breaking down. If you have any questions about this, check with your pharmacist.

**Dosing**—The dose of these combination medicines will be different for different products. *Follow the the directions on the box if you are taking this medicine without a prescription. Or, follow your doctor's orders if this medicine was prescribed.* The following information includes only the average doses for these combinations.

The number of capsules or tablets or teaspoonfuls of liquid that you take depends on the strength of the medicine.

There are a large variety of antihistamine, decongestant, and analgesic combination products on the market. Some products are for use in adults only, while others may be used in children. If you have any questions about this, check with your health care professional.

For cold symptoms and sinus pain and congestion:

- For *regular (short-acting) oral* dosage forms (chewable tablets, capsules, liquid, or tablets):
  —Adults and children 12 years of age and older: Usually the dose is 1 to 2 capsules or tablets, or 1 teaspoonful of liquid, every four to six hours.
  —Children 6 to 12 years of age: Usually the dose is 1 tablet, 4 chewable tablets, or 1 to 2 teaspoonfuls of liquid every four hours.
  —Children up to 6 years of age: Use and dose must be determined by your doctor.
- For *oral* dosage forms that *must be dissolved* (effervescent tablets or powder):
  —Adults and children 12 years of age and older: Usually the dose is 2 effervescent tablets or the contents of 1 packet of powder dissolved as directed on the package.
  —Children up to 12 years of age: Use and dose must be determined by your doctor.
- For *long-acting oral* dosage form (tablets):
  —Adults and children 12 years of age and older: Usually the dose is 1 to 2 tablets every 12 hours.
  —Children up to 12 years of age: Use and dose must be determined by your doctor.

**Missed dose**—If you must take this medicine regularly and you miss a dose, take it as soon as possible. However, if it is almost time for your next dose, skip the missed dose and go back to your regular dosing schedule. Do not double doses.

**Storage**—To store this medicine:

- Keep this medicine out of the reach of children. Overdose is very dangerous in young children.
- Store away from heat and direct light.
- Do not store the capsule or tablet form of this medicine in the bathroom, near the kitchen sink, or in other damp places. Heat or moisture may cause the medicine to break down.
- Keep the liquid form of this medicine from freezing.
- Do not keep outdated medicine or medicine no longer needed. Be sure that any discarded medicine is out of the reach of children.

## Precautions While Using This Medicine

Before you have any skin tests for allergies, tell the doctor in charge that you are taking this medicine. The results of the test may be affected by the antihistamine in this medicine.

Check with your doctor if your symptoms do not improve or become worse, or if you have a high fever.

The antihistamine in this medicine will add to the effects of alcohol and other central nervous system (CNS) depressants (medicines that slow down the nervous system, possibly causing drowsiness). Some examples of CNS depressants are other antihistamines or medicine for hay fever, other allergies, or colds; sedatives, tranquilizers, or sleeping medicine; prescription pain medicine or narcotics; barbiturates; medicine for seizures; muscle relaxants; or anesthetics, including some dental anesthetics. *Check with your doctor before taking any of the above while you are taking this medicine.*

Also, stomach problems may be more likely to occur if you drink alcoholic beverages while taking a medicine that contains aspirin. In addition, drinking large amounts of alcoholic beverages while taking a medicine that contains acetaminophen may cause liver damage.

The antihistamine in this medicine may cause some people to become drowsy, dizzy, or less alert than they are normally. *Make sure you know how you react to this medicine before you drive, use machines, or do anything else that could be dangerous if you are dizzy or are not alert.*

The decongestant in this medicine may cause some people to become nervous or restless or to have trouble in sleeping. If you have trouble in sleeping, *take the last dose of this medicine for each day a few hours before bedtime.* If you have any questions about this, check with your doctor.

Also, this medicine may add to the CNS stimulant and other effects of phenylpropanolamine (PPA)-containing diet aids. *Do not use medicines for diet or appetite control while taking this medicine unless you have checked with your doctor.*

Before having any kind of surgery (including dental surgery) or emergency treatment, tell the medical doctor or dentist in charge that you are taking this medicine.

Antihistamines may cause dryness of the mouth, nose, and throat. For temporary relief of mouth dryness, use sugarless candy or gum, melt bits of ice in your mouth, or use a saliva substitute. However, if your mouth continues to feel dry for more than 2 weeks, check with your dentist. Continuing dryness of the mouth may increase the chance of dental disease, including tooth decay, gum disease, and fungus infections.

*Check the label of all over-the-counter (OTC), nonprescription, and prescription medicines you now take.* If any contain acetaminophen or aspirin or other salicylates, including diflunisal or bismuth subsalicylate (e.g., Pepto-Bismol), be especially careful. This combination medicine contains acetaminophen and/or a salicylate. Therefore, taking it while taking any other medicine that contains these drugs may lead to overdose. If you have any questions about this, check with your health care professional.

For patients taking *aspirin-containing medicine*:
- Do not take aspirin-containing medicine within 5 days before any surgery, including dental surgery, unless otherwise directed by your medical doctor or dentist. Taking aspirin during this time may cause bleeding problems.

For diabetic patients taking *salicylate-containing medicine,* false urine sugar test results may occur:
- If you take 8 or more 325-mg (5-grain) doses of aspirin every day for several days in a row.
- If you take 8 or more 325-mg (5-grain), or 4 or more 500-mg (10-grain), doses of sodium salicylate a day.

Smaller doses or occasional use usually will not affect urine sugar tests. If you have any questions about this, check with your health care professional, especially if your diabetes is not well controlled.

## Side Effects of This Medicine

Along with its needed effects, a medicine may cause some unwanted effects. Although serious side effects occur rarely when this medicine is taken as recommended, they may be more likely to occur if:
- too much medicine is taken.
- it is taken in large doses.
- it is taken for a long time.

*Get emergency help immediately if any of the following symptoms of overdose occur:*
*For all combinations*
Clumsiness or unsteadiness; convulsions (seizures); drowsiness (severe); dryness of mouth, nose, or throat (severe); fast heartbeat; flushing or redness of face; hallucinations (seeing, hearing, or feeling things that are not there); headache (continuing and/or severe); increased sweating; nausea or vomiting (severe or continuing); shortness of breath or troubled breathing; stomach cramps or pain (severe or continuing); trouble in sleeping

*For acetaminophen-containing only*
Diarrhea; loss of appetite; swelling or tenderness in the upper abdomen or stomach area
Note: Signs of severe acetaminophen overdose may not appear until 2 to 4 days after the overdose is taken, but treatment to prevent liver damage or death must be started within 24 hours or less after the overdose is taken.

*For salicylate-containing only*
Any loss of hearing; bloody urine; changes in behavior (in children); confusion; diarrhea (severe or continuing); drowsiness or tiredness (severe, especially in children); fast or deep breathing (especially in children); fever; ringing or buzzing in ears (continuing); uncontrollable flapping movements of the hands (especially in elderly patients); unusual thirst; vision problems

Also, check with your doctor as soon as possible if any of the following side effects occur:
*More common*
Nausea or vomiting; stomach pain (mild)

*Less common or rare*
Bloody or black tarry stools; changes in urine or problems with urination; skin rash, hives, or itching; sore throat and fever; swelling of face, feet, or lower legs; tightness in chest; unusual bleeding or bruising; unusual tiredness or weakness; vomiting of blood or material that looks like coffee grounds; weight gain (unusual); yellow eyes or skin

Other side effects may occur that usually do not need medical attention. These side effects may go away during treatment as your body adjusts to the medicine. However, check with your doctor if any of the following side effects continue or are bothersome:

*More common*
Drowsiness; heartburn or indigestion (for salicylate-containing medicines); thickening of mucus

*Less common—more common with high doses*
Blurred vision; confusion; difficult or painful urination; dizziness; dryness of mouth, nose, or throat; headache;

loss of appetite; nightmares; pounding heartbeat; ringing or buzzing in ears; skin rash; stomach upset or stomach pain; unusual excitement, nervousness, restlessness, or irritability

Not all of the side effects listed above have been reported for each of these medicines, but they have been reported for at least one of them. There are some similarities among these combination medicines, so many of the above side effects may occur with any of these medicines.

Other side effects not listed above may also occur in some patients. If you notice any other effects, check with your doctor.

Revised: 08/30/94

# ANTIHISTAMINES, DECONGESTANTS, AND ANTICHOLINERGICS   Systemic†

Some commonly used brand names are:

**In the U.S.—**

| | |
|---|---|
| AH-chew[1] | Histor-D Timecelles[1] |
| Atrohist Plus[2] | OMNIhist L.A.[1] |
| D.A. Chewable[1] | Phenahist-TR[2] |
| Dallergy[1] | Phenchlor SHA[2] |
| Dallergy Caplets[1] | Prehist D[1] |
| Dura-Vent/DA[1] | Rhinolar[3] |
| Extendryl[1] | Ru-Tuss[2] |
| Extendryl JR[1] | Stahist[2] |
| Extendryl SR[1] | |

Note: For quick reference the following antihistamine, decongestant, and anticholinergic combinations are numbered to match the corresponding brand names.

This information applies to the following medicines:
1. Chlorpheniramine (klor-fen-EER-a-meen), Phenylephrine (fen-ill-EF-rin), and Methscopolamine (meth-skoe-POL-a-meen)†
2. Chlorpheniramine, Phenylephrine, Phenylpropanolamine (fen-ill-proe-pa-NOLE-a-meen), Atropine (A-troe-peen)†, Hyoscyamine (hye-oh-SYE-a-meen), and Scopolamine (skoe-POL-a-meen)†
3. Chlorpheniramine, Phenylpropanolamine, and Methscopolamine†

†Not commercially available in Canada.

## Description

Antihistamine, decongestant, and anticholinergic combinations are used to treat the nasal congestion (stuffy nose) and runny nose caused by allergies.

Antihistamines work by preventing the effects of a substance called histamine, which is produced by the body. Histamine can cause itching, sneezing, runny nose, and watery eyes. The antihistamine contained in these combinations is chlorpheniramine.

The decongestants in these combinations, phenylephrine and phenylpropanolamine (also known as PPA), produce

a narrowing of blood vessels. This leads to clearing of nasal congestion, but it may also cause an increase in blood pressure in patients who have high blood pressure.

Anticholinergics, such as atropine, hyoscyamine, methscopolamine, and scopolamine may help produce a drying effect in the nose and chest.

These combinations are available only with your doctor's prescription in the following dosage forms:

*Oral*
Chlorpheniramine, Phenylephrine, and Methscopolamine
- Extended-release capsules (U.S.)
- Syrup (U.S.)
- Tablets (U.S.)
- Chewable tablets (U.S.)
- Extended-release tablets (U.S.)

Chlorpheniramine, Phenylephrine, Phenylpropanolamine, Atropine, Hyoscyamine, and Scopolamine
- Extended-release tablets (U.S.)

Chlorpheniramine, Phenylpropanolamine, and Methscopolamine
- Extended-release capsules (U.S.)

## Before Using This Medicine

In deciding to use a medicine, the risks of taking the medicine must be weighed against the good it will do. This is a decision you and your doctor will make. For antihistamine, decongestant, and anticholinergic combinations, the following should be considered:

**Allergies**—Tell your doctor if you have ever had any unusual or allergic reaction to antihistamines or anticholinergics, or to amphetamine, dextroamphetamine (e.g., Dexedrine), ephedrine (e.g., Ephed II), epinephrine (e.g.,

Adrenalin), isoproterenol (e.g., Isuprel), metaproterenol (e.g., Alupent), methamphetamine (e.g., Desoxyn), norepinephrine (e.g., Levophed), phenylephrine (e.g., Neo-Synephrine), phenylpropanolamine [PPA] (e.g., Dexatrim), pseudoephedrine (e.g., Sudafed), or terbutaline (e.g., Brethine). Also, tell your health care professional if you are allergic to any other substances, such as foods, preservatives, or dyes.

**Pregnancy**—For the individual ingredients of these combinations, the following apply:
- *Antihistamines*—Antihistamines have not been shown to cause problems in humans.
- *Atropine*—Studies on effects in pregnancy have not been done in humans. Atropine has not been shown to cause birth defects or other problems in animals.
- *Hyoscyamine*—Studies on effects in pregnancy have not been done in either humans or animals.
- *Methscopolamine*—Studies on effects in pregnancy have not been done in either humans or animals.
- *Phenylephrine*—Studies on birth defects have not been done in either humans or animals.
- *Phenylpropanolamine*—Studies on birth defects have not been done in either humans or animals. However, it seems that some women who take phenylpropanolamine in the weeks following delivery are more likely to suffer mental or mood changes.
- *Scopolamine*—Studies on effects in pregnancy have not been done in pregnant women. However, studies in animals at doses many times the human dose have shown that scopolamine causes a small increase in the number of fetal deaths.

**Breast-feeding**—Small amounts of antihistamines, decongestants, and anticholinergics may pass into the breast milk. Use is not recommended since this medicine may cause side effects, such as unusual excitement or irritability, in the nursing baby. Also, since this medicine tends to decrease the secretions of the body, it is possible that the flow of breast milk may be reduced in some women.

**Children**—Very young children are usually more sensitive than adults to the effects of this medicine. Increases in blood pressure, nightmares or unusual excitement, nervousness, restlessness, or irritability may be more likely to occur in children. Also, mental changes may be more likely to occur in young children taking combination medicines that contain phenylpropanolamine. Also, when anticholinergics are given to children during hot weather, a rapid increase in body temperature may occur, which may lead to heat stroke. In infants and children, especially those with spastic paralysis or brain damage, this medicine may be especially likely to cause severe side effects.

**Older adults**—Confusion or memory loss, difficult and painful urination, dizziness, drowsiness, dryness of mouth, or convulsions (seizures) may be more likely to occur in the elderly, who are usually more sensitive than younger adults to the effects of this medicine. Also, nightmares or unusual excitement, nervousness, restlessness, or irritability may be more likely to occur in elderly patients.

In addition, eye pain may occur, which may be a sign of glaucoma.

**Other medicines**—Although certain medicines should not be used together at all, in other cases different medicines may be used together even if an interaction might occur. In these cases, your doctor may want to change the dose, or other precautions may be necessary. When you are taking this medicine it is especially important that your health care professional know if you are taking any of the following:
- Amantadine (e.g., Symmetrel) or
- Amphetamines or
- Appetite suppressants (diet pills), except fenfluramine (e.g., Pondimin), or
- Beta-adrenergic blocking agents (acebutolol [e.g., Sectral], atenolol [e.g., Tenormin], betaxolol [e.g., Kerlone], bisoprolol [e.g., Zebeta], carteolol [e.g., Cartrol], labetalol [e.g., Normodyne], metoprolol [e.g., Lopressor], nadolol [e.g., Corgard], oxprenolol [e.g., Trasicor], penbutolol [e.g., Levatol], pindolol [e.g., Visken], propranolol [e.g., Inderal], sotalol [e.g., Sotacor], timolol [e.g., Blocadren]) or
- Caffeine (e.g., NoDoz) or
- Chlophedianol (e.g., Ulone) or
- Cocaine or
- Digitalis medicine (heart medicine) or
- Medicine for asthma or other breathing problems or
- Medicine for colds, sinus problems, or hay fever or other allergies (including nose drops or sprays) or
- Methylphenidate (e.g., Ritalin) or
- Nabilone (e.g., Cesamet) or
- Pemoline (e.g., Cylert)—Using any of these medicines together with a decongestant-containing combination may cause excessive stimulant side effects, such as difficulty in sleeping, heart rate problems, nervousness, and irritability
- Central nervous system (CNS) depressants—Using these combinations with CNS depressants may worsen the effects (e.g., drowsiness) of CNS depressants or antihistamines
- Monoamine oxidase (MAO) inhibitors (furazolidone [e.g., Furoxone], isocarboxazid [e.g., Marplan], phenelzine [e.g., Nardil], procarbazine [e.g., Matulane], selegiline [e.g., Eldepryl], tranylcypromine [e.g., Parnate])—Taking an antihistamine, decongestant, and anticholinergic combination while you are taking or within 2 weeks of taking MAO inhibitors, may make the side effects of the antihistamines, decongestants, and anticholinergics more severe; these medicines should not be used together
- Other anticholinergics (medicine for abdominal or stomach spasms or cramps)—Side effects of antihistamines or anticholinergics, such as dryness of mouth, may be more likely to occur
- Potassium chloride (e.g., Kay Ciel)—Using this medicine with an anticholinergic-containing medicine may make gastrointestinal problems caused by potassium worse
- Rauwolfia alkaloids (alseroxylon [e.g., Rauwiloid], deserpidine [e.g., Harmonyl], rauwolfia serpentina [e.g., Raudixin], reserpine [e.g., Serpasil])—These medicines may increase or decrease the effect of the decongestant in this medicine
- Tricyclic antidepressants (amitriptyline [e.g., Elavil], amoxapine [e.g., Asendin], clomipramine [e.g., Anafranil], desipramine [e.g., Pertofrane], doxepin [e.g., Sinequan], imipramine [e.g., Tofranil], nortriptyline [e.g.,

Aventyl], protriptyline [e.g., Vivactil], trimipramine [e.g., Surmontil])—Effects, such as drowsiness, may be worsened; also, taking these medicines together may make some of the anticholinergic side effects, such as dryness of mouth, more severe

**Other medical problems**—The presence of other medical problems may affect the use of antihistamine, decongestant, and anticholinergic combinations. Make sure you tell your doctor if you have any other medical problems, especially:

- Brain damage in children or
- Down's syndrome or
- Dryness of mouth (severe and continuing) or
- Enlarged prostate or
- Fever or
- Glaucoma or
- Intestinal blockage or other intestinal problems or
- Kidney disease or
- Liver disease or
- Lung disease or
- Mental or emotional problems or
- Myasthenia gravis or
- Toxemia of pregnancy or
- Urinary tract blockage or difficult urination—These medicines may make these conditions worse
- Diabetes mellitus (sugar diabetes)—The decongestant in this medicine may put diabetic patients at greater risk of having heart or blood vessel disease
- Heart or blood vessel disease or
- High blood pressure—The decongestant and anticholinergic in this medicine may cause the blood pressure to increase and may also speed up the heart rate
- Overactive thyroid—If the overactive thyroid has caused a fast heartbeat, the decongestant and anticholinergic in this medicine may cause the heart rate to speed up further

## Proper Use of This Medicine

*Take this medicine only as directed.* Do not take more of it and do not take it more often than recommended on the label, unless otherwise directed by your doctor. To do so may increase the chance of side effects.

If this medicine irritates your stomach, you may take it with food or a glass of water or milk, to lessen the irritation.

For patients *taking the extended-release capsule or extended-release tablet form of this medicine:*

- Swallow the capsule or tablet whole.
- Do not crush, break, or chew before swallowing.
- If the capsule is too large to swallow, you may mix the contents of the capsule with applesauce, jelly, honey, or syrup and swallow without chewing.

**Dosing**—The dose of these combination medicines will be different for different patients. *Follow your doctor's orders or the directions on the label.* The following information includes only the average doses for these combinations. *If your dose is different, do not change it* unless your doctor tells you to do so.

The number of capsules or tablets or teaspoonfuls of syrup that you take depends on the strength of the medicine.

Also, the number of doses you take each day and the time between doses depend on whether you are taking a short-acting or a long-acting form of this medicine.

- For *regular (short-acting)* dosage forms (syrup, tablets, or chewable tablets):
  - —For allergy and cold symptoms:
    - Adults and children 12 years of age and older— 1 or 2 tablets or chewable tables, or 1 to 2 teaspoonfuls of syrup every four to six hours.
    - Children up to 6 years of age—Use and dose must be determined by your doctor.
    - Children 6 to 12 years of age—1 chewable tablet or 1 teaspoonful of syrup every four hours.
- For *long-acting* dosage forms (extended-release capsules or tablets):
  - —For allergy and cold symptoms:
    - Adults and children 12 years of age and older— 1 capsule or tablet every twelve hours.
    - Children up to 12 years of age—Use and dose must be determined by your doctor.

**Missed dose**—If you miss a dose of this medicine, take it as soon as possible. However, if it is almost time for your next dose, skip the missed dose and go back to your regular dosing schedule. Do not double doses.

**Storage**—To store this medicine:

- Keep out of the reach of children.
- Store away from heat and direct light.
- Do not store in the bathroom, near the kitchen sink, or in other damp places. Heat or moisture may cause the medicine to break down.
- Keep the liquid form of this medicine from freezing.
- Do not keep outdated medicine or medicine no longer needed. Be sure that any discarded medicine is out of the reach of children.

## Precautions While Using This Medicine

Check with your doctor if your symptoms do not improve or become worse, or if you have a high fever.

Before you have any skin tests for allergies, tell the doctor in charge that you are taking this medicine. The results of the test may be affected by the antihistamine in this medicine.

These medicines may make you sweat less, causing your body temperature to increase. *Use extra care not to become overheated during exercise or hot weather while you are taking this medicine,* since overheating may result in heat stroke. Also hot baths or saunas may make you dizzy or faint while you are taking this medicine.

The anticholinergic contained in this medicine may cause some people to have blurred vision. *Make sure your vision is clear before you drive or do anything else that could be dangerous if you are not able to see well.* These medicines may also cause your eyes to become more sensitive to light than they are normally. Wearing sunglasses may help lessen the discomfort from bright light.

These medicines may cause some people to become dizzy or drowsy. *Make sure you know how you react to this medicine before you drive, use machines, or do anything else that could be dangerous if you are dizzy or are not alert.*

The decongestant in this medicine may cause some people to be nervous or restless or to have trouble in sleeping. If you have trouble in sleeping, *take the last dose of this medicine for each day a few hours before bedtime.* If you have any questions about this, check with your doctor.

The decongestant in this medicine may add to the central nervous system (CNS) stimulant and other effects of phenylpropanolamine (PPA)-containing diet aids. *Do not use medicines for diet or appetite control while taking this medicine unless you have checked with your doctor.*

Before having any kind of surgery (including dental surgery) or emergency treatment, tell the medical doctor or dentist in charge that you are taking this medicine.

This medicine may cause dryness of the mouth, nose, and throat. For temporary relief, use sugarless candy or gum, melt bits of ice in your mouth, or use a saliva substitute. However, if your mouth continues to feel dry for more than 2 weeks, check with your dentist. Continuing dryness of the mouth may increase the chance of dental disease, including tooth decay, gum disease, and fungus infections.

*If you think you or someone else may have taken an overdose, get emergency help at once.* Taking an overdose of this medicine or taking this medicine with alcohol or other CNS depressants may lead to unconsciousness and possibly death.

---

## Side Effects of This Medicine

Along with its needed effects, a medicine may cause some unwanted effects. Although not all of these side effects

may occur, if they do occur they may need medical attention.

*Get emergency help immediately if any of the following symptoms of overdose occur:*
> Clumsiness or unsteadiness; convulsions (seizures); drowsiness (severe); dryness of mouth, nose, or throat (severe); fast heartbeat; flushing or redness of face; hallucinations (seeing, hearing, or feeling things that are not there); headache (continuing); shortness of breath or troubled breathing; trouble in sleeping

Also, check with your doctor as soon as possible if any of the following side effects occur:
*Rare*
> Mood or mental changes; skin rash, hives, or itching; sore throat and fever; tightness in chest; unusual bleeding or bruising; unusual tiredness or weakness

Other side effects may occur that usually do not need medical attention. These side effects may go away during treatment as your body adjusts to the medicine. However, check with your health care professional if any of the following side effects continue or are bothersome:
*More common*
> Drowsiness; thickening of mucus

*Less common—more common with high doses*
> Blurred vision; confusion; difficult or painful urination; dizziness; dryness of mouth, nose, or throat; headache; loss of appetite; nightmares; pounding heartbeat; ringing or buzzing in ears; unusual excitement, nervousness, restlessness, or irritability

Other side effects not listed above may also occur in some patients. If you notice any other effects, check with your doctor.

---

Revised: 07/19/94

---

# ANTIHISTAMINES, PHENOTHIAZINE-DERIVATIVE   Systemic

Some commonly used brand names are:
**In the U.S.—**

| | |
|---|---|
| Anergan 25[2] | Promacot[2] |
| Anergan 50[2] | Pro-Med 50[2] |
| Antinaus 50[2] | Promet[2] |
| Pentazine[2] | Prorex-25[2] |
| Phenazine 25[2] | Prorex-50[2] |
| Phenazine 50[2] | Prothazine[2] |
| Phencen-50[2] | Prothazine Plain[2] |
| Phenergan[2] | Shogan[2] |
| Phenergan Fortis[2] | Tacaryl[1] |
| Phenergan Plain[2] | Temaril[3] |
| Phenerzine[2] | V-Gan-25[2] |
| Phenoject-50[2] | V-Gan-50[2] |
| Pro-50[2] | |

**In Canada—**

| | |
|---|---|
| Histantil[2] | Phenergan[2] |
| Panectyl[3] | |

Another commonly used name for trimeprazine is alimemazine.

Note: For quick reference, the following antihistamines, are numbered to match the corresponding brand names.
This information applies to the following medicines:
1. Methdilazine (meth-DILL-a-zeen)†
2. Promethazine (proe-METH-a-zeen)‡§
3. Trimeprazine (trye-MEP-ra-zeen)‡

†Not commercially available in Canada.
‡Generic name product may also be available in the U.S.
§Generic name product may also be available in Canada.

---

## Description

Phenothiazine (FEE-noe-THYE-a-zeen)-derivative antihistamines are used to relieve or prevent the symptoms of hay fever and other types of allergy. They work by preventing the effects of a substance called histamine, which is produced by the body. Histamine can cause itching, sneezing, runny nose, and watery eyes. Also, in some persons histamine can close up the bronchial tubes (air passages of the lungs) and make breathing difficult.

Some of these antihistamines are also used to prevent motion sickness, nausea, vomiting, and dizziness. In addition, some of them may be used to help people go to sleep and control their anxiety before or after surgery.

Phenothiazine-derivative antihistamines may also be used for other conditions as determined by your doctor.

In the U.S. these antihistamines are available only with your doctor's prescription. In Canada some are available without a prescription. However, your doctor may have special instructions on the proper dose of the medicine for your medical condition.

These medicines are available in the following dosage forms:

*Oral*

Methdilazine
- Syrup (U.S.)
- Tablets (U.S.)
- Chewable tablets (U.S.)

Promethazine
- Syrup (U.S. and Canada)
- Tablets (U.S. and Canada)

Trimeprazine
- Extended-release capsules (U.S.)
- Syrup (U.S. and Canada)
- Tablets (U.S. and Canada)

*Parenteral*

Promethazine
- Injection (U.S. and Canada)

*Rectal*

Promethazine
- Suppositories (U.S.)

## Before Using This Medicine

In deciding to use a medicine, the risks of taking the medicine must be weighed against the good it will do. This is a decision you and your doctor will make. For phenothiazine-derivative antihistamines, the following should be considered:

**Allergies**—Tell your doctor if you have ever had any unusual or allergic reaction to these medicines or to phenothiazines. Also tell your health care professional if you are allergic to any other substances, such as foods, preservatives, or dyes.

**Pregnancy**—Methdilazine, promethazine, and trimeprazine have not been studied in pregnant women. In animal studies, promethazine has not been shown to cause birth defects. However, other phenothiazine medicines caused jaundice and muscle tremors in a few newborn babies whose mothers received these medicines during pregnancy. Also, the newborn baby may have blood clotting problems if promethazine is taken by the mother within 2 weeks before delivery.

**Breast-feeding**—Small amounts of antihistamines pass into the breast milk. Use by nursing mothers is not recommended since babies are more sensitive to the side effects of antihistamines, such as unusual excitement or irritability. Also, with the use of phenothiazine-derivative antihistamines there is the chance that the nursing baby may be more at risk of having difficulty in breathing while sleeping or of the sudden infant death syndrome (SIDS). However, more studies are needed to confirm this.

In addition, since these medicines tend to decrease the secretions of the body, it is possible that the flow of breast milk may be reduced in some patients.

**Children**—Serious side effects, such as convulsions (seizures), are more likely to occur in younger patients and would be of greater risk to infants than to older children or adults. In general, children are more sensitive to the effects of antihistamines. Also, nightmares or unusual excitement, nervousness, restlessness, or irritability may be more likely to occur in children. *The use of phenothiazine-derivative antihistamines is not recommended in children who have a history of difficulty in breathing while sleeping, or a family history of sudden infant death syndrome (SIDS).*

Children who show signs of Reye's syndrome should not be given phenothiazine-derivative antihistamines, especially by injection. Uncontrolled movements that may occur with phenothiazine-derivative antihistamines may be mistakenly confused with symptoms of Reye's syndrome.

**Adolescents**—Adolescents who show signs of Reye's syndrome should not be given phenothiazine-derivative antihistamines, especially by injection. Uncontrolled movements that may occur with phenothiazine-derivative antihistamines may be mistakenly confused with symptoms of Reye's syndrome.

**Older adults**—Elderly patients are especially sensitive to the effects of antihistamines. Confusion; difficult or painful urination; dizziness; drowsiness; feeling faint; or dryness of the mouth, nose, or throat may be more likely to occur in elderly patients. Also, nightmares or unusual excitement, nervousness, restlessness, or irritability may be more likely to occur in elderly patients. In addition, uncontrolled movements may be more likely to occur in elderly patients taking phenothiazine-derivative antihistamines.

**Other medicines**—Although certain medicines should not be used together at all, in other cases two different medicines may be used together even if an interaction might occur. In these cases, your doctor may want to change the dose, or other precautions may be necessary. When taking phenothiazine-derivative antihistamines, it is especially important that your health care professional know if you are taking/receiving any of the following:

- Amoxapine (e.g., Asendin) or
- Antipsychotics (medicine for mental illness) or
- Methyldopa (e.g., Aldomet) or
- Metoclopramide (e.g., Reglan) or

- Metyrosine (e.g., Demser) or
- Pemoline (e.g., Cylert) or
- Pimozide (e.g., Orap) or
- Rauwolfia alkaloids (alseroxylon [e.g., Rauwiloid], deserpidine [e.g., Harmonyl], rauwolfia serpentina [e.g., Raudixin], reserpine [e.g., Serpasil])—Side effects of these medicines, such as uncontrolled body movements, may become more severe and frequent if they are used together with phenothiazine-derivative antihistamines
- Anticholinergics (medicine for abdominal or stomach spasms or cramps)—Side effects of phenothiazine-derivative antihistamines or anticholinergics, such as dryness of mouth, may be more likely to occur
- Central nervous system (CNS) depressants (medicines that cause drowsiness) or
- Maprotiline or
- Tricyclic antidepressants (medicine for depression)—Effects of CNS depressants or antihistamines, such as drowsiness, may become more severe; also, taking maprotiline or tricyclic antidepressants may cause some side effects of antihistamines, such as dryness of mouth, to become more severe
- Contrast agent, injected into spinal canal—If you are having an x-ray test of the head, spinal canal, or nervous system for which you are going to receive an injection into the spinal canal, phenothiazine-derivative antihistamines may increase the chance of seizures; stop taking any phenothiazine-derivative antihistamine 48 hours before the test and do not start taking it until 24 hours after the test
- Levodopa—When used together with phenothiazine-derivative antihistamines, the levodopa may not work as it should
- Monoamine oxidase (MAO) inhibitors (furazolidone [e.g., Furoxone], isocarboxazid [e.g., Marplan], phenelzine [e.g., Nardil], procarbazine [e.g., Matulane], selgiline [e.g., Eldepryl], tranylcypromine [e.g., Parnate])—If you are now taking or have taken within the past 2 weeks any of the MAO inhibitors, the side effects of the phenothiazine-derivative antihistamines may become more severe; these medicines should not be used together

**Other medical problems**—The presence of other medical problems may affect the use of antihistamines. Make sure you tell your doctor if you have any other medical problems, especially:

- Blood disease or
- Heart or blood vessel disease—These medicines may cause more serious conditions to develop
- Enlarged prostate or
- Urinary tract blockage or difficult urination—Phenothiazine-derivative antihistamines may cause urinary problems to become worse
- Epilepsy—Phenothiazine-derivative antihistamines, especially promethazine given by injection, may increase the chance of seizures
- Glaucoma—These medicines may cause a slight increase in inner eye pressure that may worsen the condition
- Jaundice—Phenothiazine-derivative antihistamines may make the condition worse
- Liver disease—Phenothiazine-derivative antihistamines may build up in the body, which may increase the chance of side effects such as muscle spasms

- Reye's syndrome—Phenothiazine-derivative antihistamines, especially promethazine given by injection, may increase the chance of uncontrolled movements

## Proper Use of This Medicine

*Antihistamines are used to relieve or prevent the symptoms of your medical problem. Take them only as directed.* Do not take more of them and do not take them more often than recommended on the label, unless otherwise directed by your doctor. To do so may increase the chance of side effects.

For patients *taking this medicine by mouth:*

- Antihistamines can be taken with food or a glass of water or milk to lessen stomach irritation if necessary.
- If you are taking the *extended-release capsule* form of this medicine, swallow it whole. Do not break, crush, or chew before swallowing.

For patients taking *promethazine for motion sickness:*

- Take this medicine 30 minutes to 1 hour before you begin to travel.

For patients using the *suppository form of this medicine:*

- To insert suppository: First remove the foil wrapper and moisten the suppository with cold water. Lie down on your side and use your finger to push the suppository well up into the rectum. If the suppository is too soft to insert, chill the suppository in the refrigerator for 30 minutes or run cold water over it before removing the foil wrapper.

For patients using the *injection form of this medicine:*

- If you will be giving yourself the injections, make sure you understand exactly how to give them. If you have any questions about this, check with your health care professional.

**Dosing**—The dose of an antihistamine will be different for different patients. *Follow your doctor's orders or the directions on the label.* The following information includes only the average doses of antihistamines. *If your dose is different, do not change it* unless your doctor tells you to do so.

The number of capsules or tablets or teaspoonfuls of liquid that you take depends on the strength of the medicine. Also, *the number of doses you take each day and the time between doses depends on whether you are taking a short-acting or long-acting form of antihistamine.*

*For methdilazine*

- For *regular (short-acting) oral* dosage forms (tablets or liquid):
  —For allergy symptoms:
  - Adults and teenagers—8 milligrams (mg) every six to twelve hours as needed.
  - Children younger than 3 years of age—Use and dose must be determined by your doctor.
  - Children 3 to 12 years of age—4 mg every six to twelve hours as needed.

*For promethazine*

- For *regular (short-acting) oral* dosage forms (tablets or liquid):
  - —For allergy symptoms:
    - Adults and teenagers—10 to 12.5 mg four times a day before meals and at bedtime; or 25 mg at bedtime as needed.
    - Children younger than 2 years of age—Use and dose must be determined by your doctor.
    - Children 2 years of age and older—Your doctor will determine dose based on the weight and/or size of the child. Children usually are given 5 to 12.5 mg three times a day or 25 mg at bedtime as needed.
  - —For nausea and vomiting:
    - Adults and teenagers—25 mg for the first dose, then 10 to 25 mg every four to six hours if needed.
    - Children younger than 2 years of age—Use and dose must be determined by your doctor.
    - Children 2 years of age and older—Your doctor will determine dose based on the weight and/or size of the child. Children usually are given 10 to 25 mg every four to six hours as needed.
  - —For prevention of motion sickness:
    - Adults and teenagers—25 mg taken one-half to one hour before traveling. The dose may be repeated eight to twelve hours later if needed.
    - Children younger than 2 years of age—Use and dose must be determined by your doctor.
    - Children 2 years of age and older—Your doctor will determine dose based on the weight and/or size of the child. Children usually are given 10 to 25 mg one-half to one hour before traveling. The dose may be repeated eight to twelve hours later if needed.
  - —For vertigo (dizziness):
    - Adults and teenagers—25 mg two times a day as needed.
    - Children younger than 2 years of age—Use and dose must be determined by your doctor.
    - Children 2 years of age and older—Your doctor will determine dose based on the weight and/or size of the child. Children usually are given 10 to 25 mg two times a day as needed.
  - —For use as a sedative:
    - Adults and teenagers—25 to 50 mg.
    - Children younger than 2 years of age—Use and dose must be determined by your doctor.
    - Children 2 years of age and older—Your doctor will determine dose based on the weight and/or size of the child. Children usually are given 10 to 25 mg.
- For *injection* dosage form:
  - —For allergy symptoms:
    - Adults and teenagers—25 mg injected into a muscle or into a vein.
    - Children younger than 2 years of age—Use and dose must be determined by your doctor.
    - Children 2 years of age and older—Your doctor will determine dose based on the weight and/or size of the child. Children usually are given 6.25 to 12.5 mg injected into a muscle three times a day or 25 mg at bedtime as needed.
  - —For nausea and vomiting:
    - Adults and teenagers—12.5 to 25 mg injected into a muscle or into a vein every four hours as needed.
    - Children younger than 2 years of age—Use and dose must be determined by your doctor.
    - Children 2 years of age and older—Your doctor will determine dose based on the weight and/or size of the child. Children usually are given 12.5 to 25 mg injected into a muscle every four to six hours as needed.
  - —For use as a sedative:
    - Adults and teenagers—25 to 50 mg injected into a muscle or into a vein.
    - Children younger than 2 years of age—Use and dose must be determined by your doctor.
    - Children 2 years of age and older—Your doctor will determine dose based on the weight and/or size of the child. Children usually are given 12.5 to 25 mg injected into a muscle.
- For *suppository* dosage form:
  - —For allergy symptoms:
    - Adults and teenagers—25 mg inserted in rectum. Another 25-mg suppository may be inserted two hours later if needed.
    - Children younger than 2 years of age—Use and dose must be determined by your doctor.
    - Children 2 years of age and older—Your doctor will determine dose based on the weight and/or size of the child. Children usually are given 6.25 to 12.5 mg inserted into the rectum three times a day or 25 mg at bedtime as needed.
  - —For nausea and vomiting:
    - Adults and teenagers—25 mg inserted into the rectum for the first dose, then 12.5 to 25 mg every four to six hours if needed.
    - Children younger than 2 years of age—Use and dose must be determined by your doctor.
    - Children 2 years of age and older—Your doctor will determine dose based on the weight and/or size of the child. Children usually are given 12.5 to 25 mg inserted into the rectum every four to six hours as needed.
  - —For vertigo (dizziness):
    - Adults and teenagers—25 mg inserted into the rectum, two times a day as needed.
    - Children younger than 2 years of age—Use and dose must be determined by your doctor.
    - Children 2 years of age and older—Your doctor will determine dose based on the weight and/

or size of the child. Children usually are given 12.5 to 25 mg inserted into the rectum two times a day as needed.

—For use as a sedative:

• Adults and teenagers—25 to 50 mg inserted into the rectum.

• Children younger than 2 years of age—Use and dose must be determined by your doctor.

• Children 2 years of age and older—Your doctor will determine dose based on the weight and/or size of the child. Children usually are given 12.5 to 25 mg inserted into the rectum.

*For trimeprazine*

• For *regular (short-acting) oral* dosage forms (tablets or liquid):

—For allergy symptoms:

• Adults and teenagers—2.5 mg four times a day as needed.

• Children younger than 2 years of age—Use and dose must be determined by your doctor.

• Children 2 to 3 years of age—1.25 mg at bedtime or three times a day as needed.

• Children 3 to 12 years of age—2.5 mg at bedtime or three times a day as needed.

• For *long-acting oral* dosage forms (extended-release capsules):

—For allergy symptoms:

• Adults and teenagers—5 mg every twelve hours as needed.

• Children younger than 6 years of age—Use and dose must be determined by your doctor.

• Children 6 to 12 years of age—5 mg once a day as needed.

**Missed dose**—If you are taking this medicine regularly and you miss a dose, take it as soon as possible. However, if it is almost time for your next dose, skip the missed dose and go back to your regular dosing schedule. Do not double doses.

**Storage**—To store this medicine:

• Keep out of the reach of children, since overdose may be very dangerous in children.

• Store away from heat and direct light.

• Do not store the capsule or tablet form of this medicine in the bathroom medicine cabinet, near the kitchen sink, or in other damp places. Heat or moisture may cause the medicine to break down.

• Keep the liquid form of this medicine from freezing.

• Do not keep outdated medicine or medicine no longer needed. Be sure that any discarded medicine is out of the reach of children.

## Precautions While Using This Medicine

Tell the doctor in charge that you are taking this medicine before you have any skin tests for allergies. The results of the tests may be affected by this medicine.

When taking phenothiazine-derivative antihistamines on a regular basis, make sure your doctor knows if you are taking large amounts of aspirin at the same time (as for arthritis or rheumatism). Effects of too much aspirin, such as ringing in the ears, may be covered up by the antihistamine.

Phenothiazine-derivative antihistamines will add to the effects of alcohol and other CNS depressants (medicines that slow down the nervous system, possibly causing drowsiness). Some examples of CNS depressants are sedatives, tranquilizers, or sleeping medicine; prescription pain medicine or narcotics; barbiturates; medicine for seizures; muscle relaxants; or anesthetics, including some dental anesthetics. *Check with your doctor before taking any of the above while you are using this medicine.*

This medicine may cause some people to become drowsy or less alert than they are normally. Even if taken at bedtime, it may cause some people to feel drowsy or less alert on arising. *Make sure you know how you react to the phenothiazine-derivative antihistamine you are taking before you drive, use machines, or do anything else that could be dangerous if you are not alert.*

Phenothiazine-derivative antihistamines may cause dryness of the mouth, nose, and throat. For temporary relief of mouth dryness, use sugarless candy or gum, melt bits of ice in your mouth, or use a saliva substitute. However, if your mouth continues to feel dry for more than 2 weeks, check with your medical doctor or dentist. Continuing dryness of the mouth may increase the chance of dental disease, including tooth decay, gum disease, and fungus infections.

This medicine controls nausea and vomiting. For this reason, it may cover up some of the signs of overdose caused by other medicines or the symptoms of appendicitis. This will make it difficult for your doctor to diagnose these conditions. Make sure your doctor knows that you are taking this medicine if you have other symptoms of appendicitis such as stomach or lower abdominal pain, cramping, or soreness. Also, if you think you may have taken an overdose of any medicine, tell your doctor that you are taking this medicine.

## Side Effects of This Medicine

Along with its needed effects, a medicine may cause some unwanted effects. Although not all of these side effects may occur, if they do occur they may need medical attention.

Check with your doctor as soon as possible if any of the following side effects occur:

*Less common or rare*

Sore throat and fever; unusual bleeding or bruising; unusual tiredness or weakness

*Symptoms of overdose*

Clumsiness or unsteadiness; convulsions (seizures); drowsiness (severe); dryness of mouth, nose, or throat (severe); feeling faint; flushing or redness of face; hallucinations (seeing, hearing, or feeling things that are not there); muscle spasms (especially of neck and back);

restlessness; shortness of breath or troubled breathing; shuffling walk; tic-like (jerky) movements of head and face; trembling and shaking of hands; trouble in sleeping

Other side effects may occur that usually do not need medical attention. These side effects may go away during treatment as your body adjusts to the medicine. However, check with your health care professional if any of the following side effects continue or are bothersome:

*More common*
Drowsiness (less common with methdilazine); thickening of mucus

*Less common or rare*
Blurred vision or any change in vision; burning or stinging of rectum (with rectal suppository); confusion; difficult or painful urination; dizziness; dryness of mouth, nose, or throat; fast heartbeat; feeling faint; increased sensitivity of skin to sun; increased sweating; loss of appetite; nightmares; ringing or buzzing in ears; skin rash; unusual excitement, nervousness, restlessness, or irritability

Other side effects not listed above may also occur in some patients. If you notice any other effects, check with your health care professional.

Revised: 07/26/94

# ANTI-INFLAMMATORY AGENTS, NONSTEROIDAL   Ophthalmic

Some commonly used brand names are:

**In the U.S.—**
Ocufen[2]                           Voltaren Ophthalmic[1]
Profenal[4]

**In Canada—**
Indocid[3]                          Voltaren Ophtha[1]
Ocufen[2]

Another commonly used name for indomethacin is indometacin.

Note: For quick reference, the following nonsteroidal anti-inflammatory agents are numbered to match the corresponding brand names.

This information applies to the following medicines:

1. Diclofenac (dye-KLOE-fen-ak)
2. Flurbiprofen (flure-BI-proe-fen)
3. Indomethacin (in-doe-METH-a-sin)*
4. Suprofen (soo-PROE-fen)

*Not commercially available in the U.S.

## Description

Ophthalmic anti-inflammatory medicines are used in the eye to lessen problems that can occur during or after some kinds of eye surgery. Sometimes, the pupil of the eye gets smaller during an operation. This makes it more difficult for the surgeon to reach some areas of the eye. Some of these medicines are used to help prevent this. Also, some of them are used after eye surgery, to relieve effects such as inflammation or edema (too much fluid in the eye).

These medicines may also be used for other conditions, as determined by your ophthalmologist (eye doctor).

These medicines are available only with your doctor's prescription, in the following dosage forms:

*Ophthalmic*
Diclofenac
• Ophthalmic solution (U.S. and Canada)
Flurbiprofen
• Ophthalmic solution (U.S. and Canada)

Indomethacin
• Ophthalmic suspension (Canada)
Suprofen
• Ophthalmic solution (U.S.)

## Before Using This Medicine

In deciding to use a medicine, the risks of taking the medicine must be weighed against the good it will do. This is a decision you and your doctor will make. For ophthalmic anti-inflammatory medicines, the following should be considered:

**Allergies**—Tell your doctor if you have ever had any unusual or allergic reaction to one of the ophthalmic anti-inflammatory medicines or other serious reactions, especially asthma or wheezing, runny nose, or hives, to any of the following medicines:

Aspirin or other salicylates
Diclofenac (e.g., Voltaren)
Diflunisal (e.g., Dolobid)
Etodolac (e.g., Lodine)
Fenoprofen (e.g., Nalfon)
Floctafenine (e.g., Idarac)
Flurbiprofen, oral (e.g., Ansaid)
Ibuprofen (e.g., Motrin)
Indomethacin (e.g., Indocin)
Ketoprofen (e.g., Orudis)
Ketorolac (e.g., Toradol)
Meclofenamate (e.g., Meclomen)
Mefenamic acid (e.g., Ponstel)
Nabumetone (e.g., Relafen)
Naproxen (e.g., Naprosyn)
Oxyphenbutazone (e.g., Tandearil)
Phenylbutazone (e.g., Butazolidin)
Piroxicam (e.g., Feldene)
Sulindac (e.g., Clinoril)
Suprofen (e.g., Suprol)
Tenoxicam (e.g., Mobiflex)
Tiaprofenic acid (e.g., Surgam)
Tolmetin (e.g., Tolectin)
Zomepirac (e.g., Zomax)

Also tell your health care professional if you are allergic to any other substances, such as foods, preservatives, or dyes.

**Pregnancy**—Although studies on birth defects have not been done in pregnant women after use of these medicines in the eye, ophthalmic anti-inflammatory medicines have not been reported to cause birth defects or other problems. Studies have been done in animals receiving anti-inflammatory medicines by mouth in amounts that are much greater than the amounts used in the eye. These medicines did not cause birth defects in these studies. However, they decreased the weight or slowed the growth of the fetus and caused other, more serious, harmful effects on the fetus when they were given in amounts that were large enough to cause harmful effects in the mother. Also, when these medicines were given to animals late in pregnancy, they increased the length of pregnancy or prolonged labor.

**Breast-feeding**—It is not known whether any of these medicines pass into the breast milk after they are placed in the eye. Diclofenac, indomethacin, and suprofen pass into the breast milk when they are are taken by mouth. It is not known whether flurbiprofen passes into the breast milk when it is taken by mouth. However, these medicines have not been shown to cause problems in nursing babies.

**Children**—These medicines have been studied only in adults, and there is no specific information about their use in children.

**Older adults**—These medicines have been tested and have not been shown to cause different side effects or problems in older people than they do in younger adults.

**Other medical problems**—The presence of other medical problems may affect the use of these medicines. Make sure you tell your doctor if you have any other medical problems, especially:
- Hemophilia or other bleeding problems—The possibility of bleeding may be increased

## Proper Use of This Medicine

*To use:*
- First, wash your hands. Tilt the head back and with the index finger of one hand, press gently on the skin just beneath the lower eyelid and pull the lower eyelid away from the eye to make a space. Drop the medicine into this space. Let go of the eyelid and gently close the eyes. Do not blink. Keep the eyes closed and apply pressure to the inner corner of the eye with your finger for 1 or 2 minutes, to allow the medicine to be absorbed.
- Remove any excess solution around the eye with a clean tissue, being careful not to touch the eye.
- Immediately after using the eye drops, wash your hands to remove any medicine that may be on them.
- To keep the medicine as germ-free as possible, do not touch the applicator tip to any surface (including the eye). Also, always keep the container tightly closed.

*Do not use this medicine more often or for a longer time than your doctor ordered.* To do so may increase the chance of side effects.

*Do not use any leftover medicine for future eye problems without first checking with your doctor.* If certain kinds of infection are present, using this medicine may make the infection worse and possibly lead to eye damage.

**Dosing**—The dose of these medicines will be different for different patients. *Follow your doctor's orders or the directions on the label.* The following information includes only the average doses of these medicines. *If your dose is different, do not change it* unless your doctor tells you to do so.
*For diclofenac*
- Adults:
  —For use before an eye operation: Your doctor or nurse will probably give you the medicine before your operation.
  —To relieve inflammation or edema in the eye: 1 drop in the eye 3 to 5 times a day.
- Children: To be determined by the doctor.

*For flurbiprofen*
- Adults:
  —For use before an eye operation: Your health care professional will probably give you the medicine before your operation.
  —To relieve inflammation: 1 drop in the eye every 4 hours.
- Children: To be determined by the doctor.

*For indomethacin*
- Adults:
  —For use before an eye operation: Your health care professional will probably give you the medicine before your operation.
  —To relieve inflammation or edema in the eye: 1 drop in the eye 4 times a day.
- Children: To be determined by the doctor.

*For suprofen*
- Adults:
  —For use before an eye operation: Your health care professional will probably give you the medicine before your operation.
  —To relieve inflammation or edema in the eye: To be determined by the doctor.
- Children: To be determined by the doctor.

**Missed dose**—If you miss a dose of this medicine, apply it as soon as possible. But if it is almost time for your next dose, skip the missed dose and go back to your regular dosing schedule.

**Storage**—To store this medicine:
- Keep out of the reach of children.
- Store away from heat and direct light.
- Keep the medicine from freezing.

- Do not keep outdated medicine or medicine no longer needed. Be sure that any discarded medicine is out of the reach of children.

## Precautions While Using This Medicine

Wearing soft (hydrogel) contact lenses during treatment with diclofenac has caused severe irritation (redness and itching) in some people. Therefore, *do not wear soft contact lenses during the time that you are being treated with diclofenac.*

## Side Effects of This Medicine

Along with its needed effects, a medicine may cause some unwanted effects. Check with your doctor as soon as possible if any of the following side effects occur:

*Less common or rare*
   Bleeding in the eye or redness or swelling of the eye or the eyelid (not present before you started using this

medicine or becoming worse while you are using this medicine); itching or tearing

Other side effects may occur that usually do not need medical attention. The following side effects usually do not need medical attention. However, check with your doctor if they continue or are bothersome.

*More common*
   Burning or stinging after application

Other side effects not listed above may also occur in some patients. If you notice any other effects, check with your doctor.

Revised: 09/08/92
Interim revision: 08/17/93

# ANTIMYASTHENICS   Systemic

Some commonly used brand names are:
**In the U.S.—**
   Mestinon[3]                Prostigmin[2]
   Mestinon Timespans[3]      Regonol[3]
   Mytelase Caplets[1]
**In Canada—**
   Mestinon[3]                Prostigmin[2]
   Mestinon-SR[3]             Regonol[3]

Note: For quick reference, the following antimyasthenics are numbered to match the corresponding brand names.

This information applies to the following medicines:
1. Ambenonium (am-be-NOE-nee-um)†
2. Neostigmine (nee-oh-STIG-meen)‡
3. Pyridostigmine (peer-id-oh-STIG-meen)

†Not commercially available in Canada.
‡Generic name product may also be available in the U.S.

## Description

Antimyasthenics are given by mouth or by injection to treat myasthenia gravis. Neostigmine may also be given by injection as a test for myasthenia gravis. Sometimes neostigmine is given by injection to prevent or treat certain urinary tract or intestinal disorders. In addition, neostigmine or pyridostigmine may be given by injection as an antidote to certain types of muscle relaxants used in surgery.

These medicines are available only with your doctor's prescription in the following dosage forms:

*Oral*
   Ambenonium
   • Tablets (U.S.)
   Neostigmine
   • Tablets (U.S. and Canada)
   Pyridostigmine
   • Syrup (U.S.)
   • Tablets (U.S. and Canada)
   • Extended-release tablets (U.S. and Canada)

*Parenteral*
   Neostigmine
   • Injection (U.S. and Canada)
   Pyridostigmine
   • Injection (U.S. and Canada)

## Before Using This Medicine

In deciding to use a medicine, the risks of taking the medicine must be weighed against the good it will do. This is a decision you and your doctor will make. For the antimyasthenics, the following should be considered:

**Allergies**—Tell your doctor if you have ever had any unusual or allergic reaction to ambenonium, bromides, neostigmine, or pyridostigmine. Also tell your health care professional if you are allergic to any other substances, such as foods, preservatives, or dyes.

**Pregnancy**—Antimyasthenics have not been reported to cause birth defects; however, muscle weakness has occurred temporarily in some newborn babies whose mothers took antimyasthenics during pregnancy.

**Breast-feeding**—Antimyasthenics have not been reported to cause problems in nursing babies.

**Children**—Although there is no specific information comparing use of antimyasthenics in children with use in other age groups, these medicines are not expected to cause different side effects or problems in children than they do in adults.

**Older adults**—Many medicines have not been studied specifically in older people. Therefore, it may not be known whether they work exactly the same way they do in younger adults. Although there is not much information comparing use of antimyasthenics in the elderly with use in other age groups, these medicines are not expected to cause different side effects or problems in older people than they do in younger adults.

**Other medicines**—Although certain medicines should not be used together at all, in other cases 2 different medicines may be used together even if an interaction might occur. In these cases, your doctor may want to change the dose, or other precautions may be necessary. When you are taking an antimyasthenic, it is especially important that your health care professional knows if you are using any of the following:

- Demecarium (e.g., Humorsol) or
- Echothiophate (e.g., Phospholine Iodide) or
- Isoflurophate (e.g., Floropryl) or
- Malathion (e.g., Prioderm)—Using these medicines with antimyasthenics may result in serious side effects
- Guanadrel (e.g., Hylorel) or
- Guanethidine (e.g., Ismelin) or
- Mecamylamine (e.g., Inversine) or
- Procainamide (e.g., Pronestyl) or
- Trimethaphan (e.g., Arfonad)—The effects of these medicines may interfere with the actions of the antimyasthenics

**Other medical problems**—The presence of other medical problems may affect the use of the antimyasthenics. Make sure you tell your doctor if you have any other medical problems, especially:

- Intestinal blockage or
- Urinary tract blockage or
- Urinary tract infection—These medicines may make the condition worse

## Proper Use of This Medicine

Your doctor may want you to take this medicine with food or milk to help lessen the chance of side effects. If you have any questions about how you should be taking this medicine, check with your doctor.

*Take this medicine only as directed.* Do not take more of it, do not take it more often, and do not take it for a longer time than your doctor ordered. To do so may increase the chance of side effects.

If you are taking this medicine *for myasthenia gravis*:

- When you first begin taking this medicine, your doctor may want you to keep a daily record of:
  —the time you take each dose.
  —how long you feel better after taking each dose.
  —how long you feel worse.
  —any side effects that occur.

This is to help your doctor decide whether the dose of this medicine should be increased or decreased and how often the medicine should be taken in order for it to be most effective in your condition.

**Dosing**—The dose of these medicines will be different for different patients. *Follow your doctor's orders or the directions on the label.* The following information includes only the average doses of these medicines. *If your dose is different, do not change it* unless your doctor tells you to do so.

The number of tablets or teaspoonfuls of syrup that you take depends on the strength of the medicine. Also, *the number of doses you take each day, the time allowed between doses, and the length of time you take the medicine depend on the medical problem for which you are taking these medicines.*

*For ambenonium*

- For *oral* dosage form (tablets):
  —For myasthenia gravis:
    - Adults and teenagers—At first, the dose is 5 milligrams (mg) three or four times per day. Then, if needed, the dose will be adjusted by your doctor.
    - Children—The dose is based on body weight or size and must be determined by your doctor. The total daily dose is usually 300 micrograms (mcg) per kilogram (kg) (136 mcg per pound) of body weight or 10 mg per square meter of body surface area. This dose may be divided into three or four smaller doses. If needed, the total daily dose will be increased to 1.5 mg per kg (0.68 mg per pound) of body weight or 50 mg per square meter of body surface area. This dose may be divided into three or four smaller doses.

*For neostigmine*

- For *oral* dosage form (tablets):
  —For myasthenia gravis:
    - Adults and teenagers—At first, the dose is 15 milligrams (mg) every three or four hours. Then, the dose is 150 mg taken over a twenty-four-hour period.
    - Children—The dose is based on body weight or size and must be determined by your doctor. The total daily dose is usually 2 mg per kilogram (kg) (0.91 mg per pound) of body weight or 60 mg per square meter of body surface area. This dose may be divided into six to eight smaller doses.
- For *injection* dosage form:
  —For myasthenia gravis:
    - Adults and teenagers—The usual dose is 500 micrograms (mcg) injected into a muscle or under the skin.
    - Children—The dose is based on body weight and must be determined by your doctor. It is usually 10 to 40 mcg per kg (4.5 to 18.2 mcg per pound) of body weight, injected into a muscle or under the skin, every two or three hours.
  —For urinary tract or intestinal disorders:
    - Adults and teenagers—The usual dose is 250 to 500 mcg, injected into a muscle or under the skin, as needed.
    - Children—Use and dose must be determined by your doctor.

*For pyridostigmine*

- For *oral* dosage forms (syrup and tablets):
  —For myasthenia gravis:
    - Adults and teenagers—At first, the dose is 30 to 60 milligrams (mg) every three or four hours.

Then, the dose is 60 mg to 1.5 grams (usually 600 mg) per day.

- Children—The dose is based on body weight or size and must be determined by your doctor. The total daily dose is usually 7 mg per kilogram (kg) (3.2 mg per pound) of body weight or 200 mg per square meter of body surface area. This dose may be divided into five or six smaller doses.

- For *long-acting oral* dosage form (extended-release tablets):
  —For myasthenia gravis:
  - Adults and teenagers—The usual dose is 180 to 540 mg one or two times per day.
  - Children—Dose must be determined by your doctor.

- For *injection* dosage form:
  —For myasthenia gravis:
  - Adults and teenagers—The usual dose is 2 mg, injected into a muscle or vein, every two or three hours.
  - Children—The dose is based on body weight and must be determined by your doctor. It is usually 50 to 150 micrograms (mcg) per kg (22.7 to 68.1 mcg per pound) of body weight, injected into a muscle every four to six hours.

**Missed dose**—If you miss a dose of this medicine, take it as soon as you remember. However, if it is almost time for your next dose, skip the missed dose and go back to your regular dosing schedule. Do not double doses.

**Storage**—To store this medicine:
- Keep out of the reach of children.
- Store away from heat and direct light.
- Do not store the tablet form of this medicine in the bathroom, near the kitchen sink, or in other damp places. Heat or moisture may cause the medicine to break down.
- Keep the syrup form of pyridostigmine from freezing.
- Do not keep outdated medicine or medicine no longer needed. Be sure that any discarded medicine is out of the reach of children.

## Side Effects of This Medicine

Along with its needed effects, a medicine may cause some unwanted effects. Although not all of these side effects may occur, if they do occur they may need medical attention.

*Check with your doctor immediately* if any of the following side effects occur:
*Symptoms of overdose*
Blurred vision; clumsiness or unsteadiness; confusion; convulsions (seizures); diarrhea (severe); increase in bronchial secretions or watering of mouth (excessive); increasing muscle weakness (especially in the arms, neck, shoulders, and tongue); muscle cramps or twitching; nausea or vomiting (severe); shortness of breath, troubled breathing, wheezing, or tightness in chest; slow heartbeat; slurred speech; stomach cramps or pain (severe); unusual irritability, nervousness, restlessness, or fear; unusual tiredness or weakness

Also, check with your doctor as soon as possible if any of the following side effects occur:
*Rare*
Redness, swelling, or pain at place of injection (for pyridostigmine injection only); skin rash (does not apply to ambenonium)

Other side effects may occur that usually do not need medical attention. These side effects may go away during treatment as your body adjusts to the medicine. However, check with your doctor if any of the following side effects continue or are bothersome:
*More common*
Diarrhea; increased sweating; increased watering of mouth; nausea or vomiting; stomach cramps or pain
*Less common*
Frequent urge to urinate; increase in bronchial secretions; unusually small pupils; unusual watering of eyes

Other side effects not listed above may also occur in some patients. If you notice any other effects, check with your doctor.

Revised: 09/30/91
Interim revision: 07/18/94

# ANTIPYRINE AND BENZOCAINE    Otic

Some commonly used brand names are:
**In the U.S.—**

| | |
|---|---|
| A/B Otic | Dolotic |
| Allergen | Earocol |
| Antiben | Otipyrin |
| Aurafair | Oto |
| Auralgan | Otocalm |
| Aurodex | |

**In Canada—**

| | |
|---|---|
| Analgesic Ear Drops | Earache Drops |
| Auralgan | |

Another commonly used name for antipyrine is phenazone. Another commonly used name for benzocaine is ethyl aminobenzoate.

## Description

Antipyrine (an-tee-PYE-reen) and benzocaine (BEN-zoe-kane) combination is used in the ear to help relieve the pain, swelling, and congestion of some ear infections. It will not cure the infection itself. An antibiotic will be needed to treat the infection. This medicine is also used to soften earwax so that the earwax can be washed away more easily.

In the U.S., this medicine is available only with your doctor's prescription. In Canada, this medicine is available without a prescription. However, your doctor may have special instructions on the proper dose for your ear problem. This medicine is available in the following dosage form:

*Otic*
- Otic solution (U.S. and Canada)

## Before Using This Medicine

In deciding to use a medicine, the risks of using the medicine must be weighed against the good it will do. This is a decision you and your doctor will make. For antipyrine and benzocaine combination, the following should be considered:

**Allergies**—Tell your doctor if you have ever had any unusual or allergic reaction to antipyrine or benzocaine or other local anesthetics. Also tell your health care professional if you are allergic to any other substances, such as foods, preservatives, or dyes.

**Pregnancy**—Although studies on effects in pregnancy have not been done in either humans or animals, this medicine has not been reported to cause problems in humans.

**Breast-feeding**—It is not known whether this medicine passes into the breast milk. Although most medicines pass into breast milk in small amounts, many of them may be used safely while breast-feeding. Mothers who are using this medicine and who wish to breast-feed should discuss this with their doctor.

**Children**—Infants, especially if they are 3 months of age or younger, may be especially sensitive to the effects of the benzocaine in this combination medicine. This may increase the chance of side effects. However, this medicine is not expected to cause different side effects or problems in older children than it does in adults.

**Older adults**—Many medicines have not been studied specifically in older people. Therefore, it may not be known whether they work exactly the same way they do in younger adults. Although there is no specific information comparing use of antipyrine and benzocaine in the elderly with use in other age groups, this medicine is not expected to cause different side effects or problems in older people than it does in younger adults.

**Other medical problems**—The presence of other medical problems may affect the use of antipyrine and benzocaine combination. Make sure you tell your doctor if:
- Your ear is draining—The chance of unwanted effects may be increased

## Proper Use of This Medicine

You may warm the ear drops to body temperature (37 °C or 98.6 °F) by holding the bottle in your hand for a few minutes before applying the drops.

To use:
- Lie down or tilt the head so that the affected ear faces up. Gently pull the earlobe up and back for adults (down and back for children) to straighten the ear canal. Drop the medicine into the ear canal. Keep the ear facing up for about 5 minutes to allow the medicine to be absorbed. A sterile cotton plug may be moistened with a few drops of this medicine and gently inserted into the ear opening to prevent the medicine from leaking out.
- To keep the medicine as germ-free as possible, do not touch the dropper to any surface (including the ear).
- *Do not rinse the dropper after use.* Wipe the tip of the dropper with a clean tissue and keep the container tightly closed.

If you are using this medicine to help remove earwax, the ear should be flushed with warm water after you have used this medicine for 2 or 3 days. This is usually done by your doctor. If you have been directed to flush the ear out yourself, make sure that you have learned how to do it correctly. Follow the instructions carefully.

**Dosing**—The dose of this medicine will be different for different patients. *Follow your doctor's orders or the directions on the label.* The following information includes only the average amounts of this medicine. *If your dose is different, do not change it* unless your doctor tells you to do so.
- For *otic* dosage form (ear drops):
  —Adults and children:
    - For ear pain caused by an infection—Use enough medicine to fill the entire ear canal every one or two hours until the pain is relieved.
    - For softening earwax before removal—Use enough medicine to fill the entire ear canal three times a day for two or three days.

**Missed dose**—If you miss a dose of this medicine, use it as soon as you remember. However, if it is almost time for your next dose, skip the missed dose and go back to your regular dosing schedule.

**Storage**—To store this medicine:
- Keep out of the reach of children.
- Store away from heat and direct light.
- Keep the medicine from freezing.
- Do not keep outdated medicine or medicine no longer needed. Be sure that any discarded medicine is out of the reach of children.

## Side Effects of This Medicine

Along with its needed effects, a medicine may cause some unwanted effects. The following side effects may mean that you are having an allergic reaction to the medicine.

Stop using the medicine right away if any of them occur. Check with your doctor if any of the following effects continue or are bothersome:

Itching, burning, redness, or oozing sores in the ear

Other side effects not listed above may also occur in some patients. If you notice any other effects, check with your doctor.

Revised: 02/23/94
Interim revision: 06/02/94

# ANTITHYROID AGENTS   Systemic

Some commonly used brand names are:

**In the U.S.—**
Tapazole[1]

**In Canada—**
Propyl-Thyracil[2]      Tapazole[1]

Another commonly used name for methimazole is thiamazole.

Note: For quick reference, the following antithyroid agents are numbered to match the corresponding brand names.

This information applies to the following medicines:

1. Methimazole (meth-IM-a-zole)
2. Propylthiouracil (proe-pill-thye-oh-YOOR-a-sill)‡

‡Generic name product may also be available in the U.S.

## Description

Methimazole and propylthiouracil are used to treat conditions in which the thyroid gland produces too much thyroid hormone.

These medicines work by making it harder for the body to use iodine to make thyroid hormone. They do not block the effects of thyroid hormone that was made by the body before their use was begun.

Methimazole and propylthiouracil are available only with your doctor's prescription, in the following dosage forms:

*Oral*

Methimazole
• Tablets (U.S. and Canada)
Propylthiouracil
• Tablets (U.S. and Canada)

## Before Using This Medicine

In deciding to use a medicine, the risks of taking the medicine must be weighed against the good it will do. This is a decision you and your doctor will make. For antithyroid agents, the following should be considered:

**Allergies**—Tell your doctor if you have ever had any unusual or allergic reaction to methimazole or propylthiouracil. Also tell your health care professional if you are allergic to any other substances, such as foods, preservatives, or dyes.

**Pregnancy**—Use of too large a dose during pregnancy may cause problems in the fetus. However, use of the proper dose, with careful monitoring by the doctor, is not likely to cause problems.

**Breast-feeding**—These medicines pass into breast milk. (Methimazole passes into breast milk more freely and in higher amounts than propylthiouracil.) However, your doctor may allow you to continue to breast-feed, if your dose is low and the infant gets frequent check-ups. If you are taking a large dose, it may be necessary for you to stop breast-feeding during treatment.

**Children**—This medicine has been used in children and, in effective doses, has not been shown to cause different side effects or problems in children than it does in adults.

**Teenagers**—This medicine has been used in teenagers and, in effective doses, has not been shown to cause different side effects or problems in teenagers than it does in adults.

**Older adults**—Elderly people may have an increased chance of certain side effects during treatment. Your doctor may need to take special precautions while you are taking this medicine.

**Other medicines**—Although certain medicines should not be used together at all, in other cases two different medicines may be used together even if an interaction might occur. In these cases, your doctor may want to change the dose, or other precautions may be necessary. When you are taking antithyroid agents, it is especially important that your health care professional know if you are taking any of the following:

• Amiodarone or
• Iodinated glycerol or
• Potassium iodide (e.g., Pima)—The use of these medicines may change the effect of antithyroid agents
• Anticoagulants (blood thinners)—The use of antithyroid agents may affect the way anticoagulants work in your body
• Digitalis glycosides—The use of antithyroid agents may affect the amount of digitalis glycosides in the bloodstream

**Other medical problems**—The presence of other medical problems may affect the use of antithyroid agents. Make sure you tell your doctor if you have any other medical problems, especially:

• Liver disease—The body may not get this medicine out of the bloodstream at the usual rate, which may increase the chance of side effects

## Proper Use of This Medicine

*Use this medicine only as directed by your doctor.* Do not use more or less of it and do not use it more often or for a longer time than your doctor ordered. To do so may increase the chance of side effects.

This medicine works best when there is a constant amount in the blood. *To help keep the amount constant, do not miss any doses. Also, if you are taking more than one dose a day, it is best to take the doses at evenly spaced times day and night.* For example, if you are to take 3 doses a day, the doses should be spaced about 8 hours apart. If this interferes with your sleep or other daily activities, or if you need help in planning the best times to take your medicine, check with your health care professional.

Food in your stomach may change the amount of methimazole that is able to enter the bloodstream. To make sure that you always get the same effects, try to take methimazole at the same time in relation to meals every day. That is, always take it with meals or always take it on an empty stomach.

**Dosing**—The dose of these medicines will be different for different patients. *Follow your doctor's orders or the directions on the label.* The following information includes only the average doses of these medicines. *If your dose is different, do not change it* unless your doctor tells you to do so.

The number of tablets that you take or the number of suppositories that you use depends on the strength of the medicine. Also, *the number of doses you take each day, the time allowed between doses, and the length of time you take the medicine depend on the medical problem for which you are taking antithyroid agents.*

*For methimazole*

- For *oral* dosage form (tablets):
  —For treatment of hyperthyroidism (overactive thyroid):
    - Adults and teenagers—At first, 15 to 60 milligrams (mg) a day for up to six to eight weeks. Later, your doctor may want to lower your dose to 5 to 30 mg a day. This may be taken once a day or it may be divided into two doses a day.
    - Children—Dose is based on body weight and must be determined by your doctor. The usual dose is 0.4 mg per kilogram (kg) (0.18 mg per pound) of body weight a day. Later, your doctor may want to lower the dose to 0.2 mg per kg (0.09 mg per pound) of body weight a day. The dose may be taken once a day or it may be divided into two doses a day.
  —For treatment of thyrotoxicosis (a thyroid emergency):
    - Adults and teenagers—15 to 20 mg every four hours.

- For *rectal* dosage form (suppositories):
  —For treatment of thyrotoxicosis (a thyroid emergency):
    - Adults and teenagers—15 to 20 mg inserted into the rectum every four hours. Your doctor may change your dose as needed.
    - Children—The dose is based on body weight and must be determined by your doctor. The usual dose is 0.4 mg per kg (0.18 mg per pound) of body weight inserted into the rectum a day. This may be used as a single dose or or it may be divided into two doses a day.

*For propylthiouracil*

- For *oral* dosage form (tablets):
  —For treatment of hyperthyroidism (overactive thyroid):
    - Adults and teenagers—At first, 300 to 900 milligrams (mg) a day. Some people may need up to 1200 mg a day. This may be taken as a single dose or it may be divided into two to four doses in a day. Later, your doctor may lower your dose to 50 to 600 mg a day.
    - Children 6 to 10 years of age—At first, 50 to 150 mg a day. This may be taken as a single dose or it may be divided into two to four doses in a day. Later, your doctor may change your dose as needed.
    - Children 10 years of age and older—At first, 50 to 300 mg a day. This may be taken as a single dose or it may be divided into two to four doses in a day. Then, your doctor may change your dose as needed.
  —For treatment of thyrotoxicosis (a thyroid emergency):
    - Adults and teenagers—200 to 400 mg every four hours. Your doctor will lower your dose as needed.
    - Newborn infants—Dose is based on body weight and must be determined by your doctor. The usual dose is 10 mg per kilogram (kg) (4.5 mg per pound) of body weight a day. This is usually divided into more than one dose a day.

- For *rectal* dosage forms (enemas or suppositories):
  —For treatment of thyrotoxicosis (a thyroid emergency):
    - Adults and teenagers—200 to 400 mg inserted into the rectum every four hours. Your doctor may change your dose as needed.
    - Children 6 to 10 years of age—50 to 150 mg inserted into the rectum a day. This dose may be used as a single dose or it may be divided into two to four doses in a day. Your doctor may change your dose as needed.
    - Children 10 years of and older—50 to 300 mg inserted into the rectum a day. This dose may be used as a single dose or it may be divided into two to four doses in a day. Your doctor may change your dose as needed.

• Newborn infants—Dose is based on body weight and must be determined by your doctor. The usual dose is 10 mg per kg (4.5 mg per pound) of body weight inserted into the rectum. This is usually divided into more than one dose a day. Your doctor may change your dose as needed.

**Missed dose**—If you miss a dose of this medicine, take it as soon as possible. If it is almost time for your next dose, take both doses together. Then go back to your regular dosing schedule. If you miss more than one dose or if you have any questions about this, check with your doctor.

**Storage**—To store this medicine:
• Keep out of the reach of children.
• Store away from heat and direct light.
• Do not store in the bathroom, near the kitchen sink, or in other high-moisture areas. Heat or moisture may cause the medicine to break down.
• Do not keep outdated medicine or medicine no longer needed. Be sure that any discarded medicine is out of the reach of children.

## Precautions While Using This Medicine

*It is very important that your doctor check your progress at regular visits* to make sure that this medicine is working properly and to check for unwanted effects.

It may take several days or weeks for this medicine to work. However, *do not stop taking this medicine without first checking with your doctor*. Some medical problems may require several years of continuous treatment.

Before having any kind of surgery (including dental surgery) or emergency treatment, *tell the medical doctor or dentist in charge that you are taking this medicine.*

*Check with your doctor right away if you get an injury, infection, or illness of any kind.* Your doctor may want you to stop taking this medicine or change the amount you are taking.

While you are being treated with antithyroid agents, and after you stop treatment with it, *do not have any immunizations (vaccinations) without your doctor's approval.* Antithyroid agents may lower your body's resistance and there is a chance you might get the infection the immunization is meant to prevent. In addition, other persons living in your household should not take or have recently taken oral polio vaccine since there is a chance they could pass the polio virus on to you. Also, avoid other persons who have taken oral polio vaccine. Do not get close to them, and do not stay in the same room with them for very long. If you cannot take these precautions,

you should consider wearing a protective face mask that covers the nose and mouth.

Before you have any medical tests, tell the doctor in charge that you are taking this medicine. The results of some tests may be affected by this medicine.

## Side Effects of This Medicine

Along with its needed effects, a medicine may cause some unwanted effects. Although not all of these side effects may occur, if they do occur they may need medical attention.

*Check with your doctor immediately* if any of the following side effects occur:
*Less common*
Cough; fever or chills (continuing or severe); general feeling of discomfort, illness or weakness; hoarseness; mouth sores; pain, swelling, or redness in joints; throat infection
*Rare*
Yellow eyes or skin

Check with your doctor as soon as possible if any of the following side effects occur:
*More common*
Fever (mild and temporary); skin rash or itching
*Rare*
Backache; black, tarry stools; blood in urine or stools; shortness of breath; increase in bleeding or bruising; increase or decrease in urination; numbness or tingling of fingers, toes, or face; pinpoint red spots on skin; swelling of feet or lower legs; swollen lymph nodes; swollen salivary glands
*Symptoms of overdose*
Changes in menstrual periods; coldness; constipation; dry, puffy skin; headache; listlessness or sleepiness; muscle aches; swelling in the front of the neck; unusual tiredness or weakness; weight gain (unusual)

Other side effects may occur that usually do not need medical attention. These side effects may go away during treatment as your body adjusts to the medicine. However, check with your doctor if any of the following side effects continue or are bothersome:
*Less common*
Dizziness; loss of taste (for methimazole); nausea; stomach pain; vomiting

Other side effects not listed above may also occur in some patients. If you notice any other effects, check with your doctor.

Revised: 04/21/92
Interim revision: 06/03/94

# APPETITE SUPPRESSANTS   Systemic

Some commonly used brand names are:

**In the U.S.—**

| | |
|---|---|
| Adipex-P[5] | Phendiet-105[4] |
| Adipost[4] | Phendimet[4] |
| Anorex SR[4] | Phentercot[5] |
| Appecon[4] | Phentride[5] |
| Bontril PDM[4] | Plegine[4] |
| Bontril Slow-Release[4] | Prelu-2[4] |
| Didrex[1] | PT 105[4] |
| Fastin[5] | Rexigen Forte[4] |
| Ionamin[5] | Sanorex[3] |
| Mazanor[3] | T-Diet[5] |
| Melfiat-105 Unicelles[4] | Tenuate[2] |
| Obalan[4] | Tenuate Dospan[2] |
| Obe-Nix[5] | Tepanil Ten-Tab[2] |
| Obezine[4] | Teramine[5] |
| Panshape M[5] | Wehless[4] |
| Parzine[4] | Wehless-105 Timecelles[4] |
| Phendiet[4] | Zantryl[5] |

*In Canada—*

| | |
|---|---|
| Fastin[5] | Tenuate[2] |
| Ionamin[5] | Tenuate Dospan[2] |
| Sanorex[3] | |

Other commonly used brand names are:
Amfepramone[2]
Benzfetamine[1]

Note: For quick reference, the following appetite suppressants are numbered to match the corresponding brand names.

This information applies to the following medicines:
1. Benzphetamine (benz-FET-a-meen)†
2. Diethylpropion (dye-eth-il-PROE-pee-on)‡
3. Mazindol (MAY-zin-dole)
4. Phendimetrazine (fen-dye-MET-ra-zeen)†‡
5. Phentermine (FEN-ter-meen)‡

Note: This information does *not* apply to Fenfluramine or Phenylpropanolamine.

†Not commercially available in Canada.
‡Generic name product may also be available in the U.S.

## Description

Appetite suppressants are used in the short-term treatment of obesity. For a few weeks, these medicines in combination with dieting, exercise, and changes in eating habits can help obese patients lose weight. However, since their appetite-reducing effect is only temporary, they are useful only for the first few weeks of dieting until new eating habits are established.

These medicines are available only with your doctor's prescription, in the following dosage forms:

*Oral*

Benzphetamine
• Tablets (U.S.)
Diethylpropion
• Tablets (U.S. and Canada)
• Extended-release tablets (U.S. and Canada)
Mazindol
• Tablets (U.S. and Canada)
Phendimetrazine
• Capsules (U.S.)
• Extended-release capsules (U.S.)
• Tablets (U.S.)
• Extended-release tablets (U.S.)

Phentermine
• Capsules (U.S. and Canada)
• Resin capsules (U.S. and Canada)
• Tablets (U.S.)

## Before Using This Medicine

In deciding to use a medicine, the risks of taking the medicine must be weighed against the good it will do. This is a decision you and your doctor will make. For appetite suppressants, the following should be considered:

**Allergies**—Tell your doctor if you have ever had any unusual or allergic reaction to this medicine or amphetamine, dextroamphetamine, ephedrine, epinephrine, isoproterenol, metaproterenol, methamphetamine, norepinephrine, phenylephrine, phenylpropanolamine, pseudoephedrine, terbutaline, or other appetite suppressants. Also tell your health care professional if you are allergic to any other substances, such as foods, preservatives, or dyes.

**Pregnancy—**

• *Benzphetamine*—Benzphetamine must not be used during pregnancy because it may harm the fetus. Be sure you have discussed this with your doctor. If you think you may have become pregnant during treatment with benzphetamine, tell your doctor immediately.

• *Diethylpropion*—Diethylpropion has not been reported to cause birth defects or other problems in human and animal studies.

• *Mazindol*—Studies in animals have shown that mazindol increases the chance of rib malformations, and also increases the chance of death in the newborn when given in large doses.

• *Phendimetrazine* and *phentermine*—These medicines have not been shown to cause birth defects or other problems in humans.

**Breast-feeding**—Diethylpropion and benzphetamine pass into breast milk. It is not known if other appetite suppressants pass into breast milk. However, problems in nursing babies have not been reported.

**Children**—Appetite suppressants should not be used by children up to 12 years of age.

**Older adults**—Many medicines have not been studied specifically in older people. Therefore, it may not be known whether they work exactly the same way they do in younger adults or if they cause different side effects or problems in older people. There is no specific information comparing use of appetite suppressants in the elderly to use in other age groups.

**Other medicines**—Although certain medicines should not be used together at all, in other cases two different medicines may be used together even if an interaction might occur. In these cases, your doctor may want to change the dose, or other precautions may be necessary. When

you are taking appetite suppressants, it is especially important that your health care professional know if you are taking any of the following:

- Amantadine (e.g., Symmetrel) or
- Amphetamines or
- Caffeine (e.g., NoDoz) or
- Chlophedianol (e.g., Ulone) or
- Cocaine or
- Medicine for asthma or other breathing problems or
- Medicine for colds, sinus problems, or hay fever or other allergies (including nose drops or sprays) or
- Methylphenidate (e.g., Ritalin) or
- Nabilone (e.g., Cesamet) or
- Other appetite suppressants (diet pills) or
- Pemoline (e.g., Cylert)—Using these medicines with appetite suppressants may increase the CNS stimulant effects
- Monoamine oxidase (MAO) inhibitors (furazolidone [e.g., Furoxone], isocarboxazid [e.g., Marplan], phenelzine [e.g., Nardil], procarbazine [e.g., Matulane], selegiline [e.g., Eldepryl], tranylcypromine [e.g., Parnate])—Taking appetite suppressants while you are taking or within 2 weeks of taking monoamine oxidase (MAO) inhibitors may cause sudden extremely high blood pressure; at least 14 days should be allowed between stopping treatment with one medicine and starting treatment with the other

**Other medical problems**—The presence of other medical problems may affect the use of appetite suppressants. Make sure you tell your doctor if you have any other medical problems, especially:

- Alcohol abuse (or history of) or
- Drug abuse or dependence (or history of)—Dependence on appetite suppressants may develop
- Diabetes mellitus (sugar diabetes)—The amount of insulin or oral antidiabetic medicine that you need to take may change
- Epilepsy—Diethylpropion may increase the risk of seizures
- Glaucoma or
- Heart or blood vessel disease or
- High blood pressure or
- Mental illness (severe) or
- Overactive thyroid—Appetite suppressants may make the condition worse
- Kidney disease—Higher blood levels of mazindol may occur, increasing the chance of serious side effects

## Proper Use of This Medicine

For patients taking the *short-acting form* of this medicine:

- Take the last dose for each day about 4 to 6 hours before bedtime to help prevent trouble in sleeping.

For patients taking the *long-acting form* of this medicine:

- Take the daily dose about 10 to 14 hours before bedtime to help prevent trouble in sleeping.
- These capsules or tablets are to be swallowed whole. Do not break, crush, or chew before swallowing.

For patients taking *mazindol:*

- To help prevent trouble in sleeping, if you are taking this medicine in a:
  —*1-mg tablet,* take the last dose for each day about 4 to 6 hours before bedtime.
  —*2-mg tablet,* take the dose once each day about 10 to 14 hours before bedtime.

*Take this medicine only as directed by your doctor.* Do not take more of it, do not take it more often, and do not take it for a longer time than your doctor ordered. If too much is taken, it may become habit-forming.

If you think this medicine is not working properly after you have taken it for a few weeks, *do not increase the dose*. Instead, check with your doctor.

**Dosing**—The dose of appetite suppressants will be different for different patients. *Follow your doctor's orders or the directions on the label.* The following information includes only the average doses of appetite suppressants. *If your dose is different, do not change it* unless your doctor tells you to do so.

*For benzphetamine*

- For *oral* dosage form (tablets):
  —For appetite suppression:
    - Adults—At first, 25 to 50 milligrams (mg) once a day, taken at midmorning or midafternoon. Your doctor may need to adjust your dose.
    - Children up to 12 years of age—Use is not recommended.

*For diethylpropion*

- For *oral tablet* dosage form:
  —For appetite suppression:
    - Adults—25 milligrams (mg) three times a day, taken one hour before meals.
    - Children up to 12 years of age—Use is not recommended.
- For *oral extended-release tablet* dosage form:
  —For appetite suppression:
    - Adults—75 mg once a day, taken at midmorning.
    - Children up to 12 years of age—Use is not recommended.

*For mazindol*

- For *oral* dosage form (tablets):
  —For appetite suppression:
    - Adults—At first, 1 milligram (mg) once a day, taken one hour before your first meal of the day. Your doctor may need to adjust your dose.
    - Children up to 12 years of age—Use is not recommended.

*For phendimetrazine*

- For *oral capsule* dosage form:
  —For appetite suppression:
    - Adults—35 milligrams (mg) two or three times a day, taken one hour before meals.
    - Children up to 12 years of age—Use is not recommended.

- For *oral extended-release capsule or tablet* dosage forms:
  —For appetite suppression:
    - Adults—105 mg once a day, taken thirty to sixty minutes before the morning meal.
    - Children up to 12 years of age—Use is not recommended.
- For *oral tablet* dosage form:
  —For appetite suppression:
    - Adults—17.5 to 35 mg two or three times a day, taken one hour before meals.
    - Children up to 12 years of age—Use is not recommended.

*For phentermine*
- For *oral capsule* dosage form:
  —For appetite suppression:
    - Adults—15 to 37.5 milligrams (mg) once a day, taken before breakfast or one to two hours after breakfast.
    - Children up to 12 years of age—Use is not recommended.
- For *oral tablet* dosage form:
  —For appetite suppression:
    - Adults—15 to 37.5 mg once a day, taken before breakfast or one to two hours after breakfast. Instead of taking it once a day, your doctor may tell you to take a smaller dose thirty minutes before meals.
    - Children up to 12 years of age—Use is not recommended.
- For *oral resin capsule* dosage form:
  —For appetite suppression:
    - Adults—15 to 30 mg once a day, taken before breakfast.
    - Children up to 12 years of age—Use is not recommended.

**Storage**—To store this medicine:
- Keep out of the reach of children.
- Store away from heat and direct light.
- Do not store in the bathroom, near the kitchen sink, or in other damp places. Heat or moisture may cause the medicine to break down.
- Do not keep outdated medicine or medicine no longer needed. Be sure that any discarded medicine is out of the reach of children.

## Precautions While Using This Medicine

Your doctor should check your progress at regular visits to make sure that this medicine does not cause unwanted effects.

This medicine may cause some people to feel a false sense of well-being or to become dizzy, lightheaded, drowsy, or less alert than they are normally. *Make sure you know how you react to this medicine before you drive, use*

machines, or do anything else that could be dangerous if you are dizzy or are not alert.

*Before having any kind of surgery, dental treatment, or emergency treatment, tell the medical doctor or dentist in charge that you are using this medicine.* Taking appetite suppressants together with medicines that are used during surgery or dental or emergency treatments may cause serious side effects.

If you have been taking this medicine for a long time or in large doses and *you think you may have become mentally or physically dependent on it, check with your doctor.*
- Some signs of dependence on appetite suppressants are:
  —a strong desire or need to continue taking the medicine.
  —a need to increase the dose to receive the effects of the medicine.
  —withdrawal side effects (for example, mental depression, nausea or vomiting, stomach cramps or pain, trembling, unusual tiredness or weakness when you stop taking the medicine).

For *diabetic patients:*
- This medicine may affect blood sugar levels. If you notice a change in the results of your urine or blood sugar test or if you have any questions, check with your doctor.

If you have been taking this medicine in large doses for a long time, *do not stop taking it without first checking with your doctor.* Your doctor may want you to reduce gradually the amount you are taking before stopping completely.

## Side Effects of This Medicine

Along with its needed effects, a medicine may cause some unwanted effects. Although not all of these side effects may occur, if they do occur they may need medical attention.

Check with your doctor as soon as possible if any of the following side effects occur:
*More common*
  Increased blood pressure
*Less common or rare*
  Confusion or mental depression; mental illness; skin rash or hives; sore throat and fever; unusual bleeding or bruising
*Symptoms of overdose*
  Abdominal or stomach cramps; diarrhea (severe); fast breathing; fever; hallucinations (seeing, hearing or feeling things that are not there); high or low blood pressure; hostility; irregular heartbeat; nausea or vomiting (severe); panic state; restlessness; tremor

Other side effects may occur that usually do not need medical attention. These side effects may go away during treatment as your body adjusts to the medicine. However,

check with your doctor if any of the following side effects continue or are bothersome:

*More common*
False sense of well-being; irritability; nervousness or restlessness; trouble in sleeping

Note: After these stimulant effects have worn off, drowsiness, trembling, unusual tiredness or weakness, or mental depression may occur.

*Less common or rare*
Blurred vision; changes in sexual desire or decreased sexual ability; constipation; diarrhea; difficult or painful urination; dizziness or lightheadedness; drowsiness; dryness of mouth; fast or pounding heartbeat; frequent urge to urinate or increased urination; headache; increased sweating; nausea or vomiting; stomach cramps or pain; unpleasant taste

Although not all of the side effects listed above have been reported for all of these medicines, they have been reported for at least one of them. However, since all of the appetite suppressants are very similar, any of the above side effects may occur with any of these medicines.

After you stop using this medicine, your body may need time to adjust. The length of time this takes depends on the amount of medicine you were using and how long you used it. During this time check with your doctor if you notice any of the following side effects:

Mental depression; nausea or vomiting; stomach cramps or pain; trembling; unusual tiredness or weakness

Other side effects not listed above may also occur in some patients. If you notice any other effects, check with your doctor.

Revised: 08/29/94

# APRACLONIDINE   Ophthalmic

A commonly used brand name in the U.S. and Canada is Iopidine. Other commonly used names are aplonidine and p-aminoclonidine.

## Description

Apraclonidine (a-pra-KLOE-ni-deen) 0.5% is used to treat glaucoma when the medications you have been using for glaucoma do not reduce your eye pressure enough.

Apraclonidine 1% is used just before and after certain types of eye surgery (argon laser trabeculoplasty, argon laser iridotomy, and Nd:YAG laser posterior capsulotomy). The medicine is used to control or prevent a rise in pressure within the eye (ocular hypertension) that can occur after this type of surgery.

Apraclonidine 0.5% is available only with your doctor's prescription. Apraclonidine 1% is given in the hospital at the time of the surgery. This medicine is available in the following dosage form:

*Ophthalmic*
• Ophthalmic solution (eye drops) (U.S. and Canada)

## Before Receiving This Medicine

In deciding to use a medicine, the risks of using the medicine must be weighed against the good it will do. This is a decision you and your doctor will make. For apraclonidine, the following should be considered:

**Allergies**—Tell your doctor if you have ever had any unusual or allergic reaction to apraclonidine or clonidine. Also tell your health care professional if you are allergic to any other substances, such as preservatives.

**Pregnancy**—Apraclonidine has not been studied in pregnant women. However, apraclonidine has been shown to cause death of the fetus when given by mouth to pregnant rabbits in doses that are many times larger than the human dose. Before using this medicine, make sure your doctor knows if you are pregnant or if you may become pregnant.

**Breast-feeding**—It is not known whether apraclonidine passes into the breast milk. Although most medicines pass into breast milk in small amounts, many of them may be used safely while breast-feeding. Mothers who are using 0.5% apraclonidine and who wish to breast-feed should discuss this with their doctor. For mothers who are to be treated with 1% apraclonidine during eye surgery, your doctor may want you to stop breast-feeding during the day of your surgery.

**Children**—Studies on this medicine have been done only in adult patients, and there is no specific information comparing use of apraclonidine in children with use in other age groups.

**Older adults**—Many medicines have not been studied specifically in older people. Therefore, it may not be known whether they work exactly the same way they do in younger adults or if they cause different side effects or problems in older people. There is no specific information comparing use of apraclonidine in the elderly with use in other age groups.

**Other medicines**—Although certain medicines should not be used together at all, in other cases two different medicines may be used together even if an interaction might occur. In these cases, your doctor may want to change the dose, or other precautions may be necessary. Tell your health care professional if you are using any other prescription or nonprescription (over-the-counter [OTC]) medicine.

**Other medical problems**—The presence of other medical problems may affect the use of apraclonidine. Make sure you tell your doctor if you have any other medical problems, especially:

- Depression or
- Heart or blood vessel disease or
- High blood pressure—Apraclonidine may make the condition worse
- Kidney disease or
- Liver disease—Higher blood levels of apraclonidine may result, which may lead to increased side effects
- Unusual reaction to a medicine that reduces the pressure within the eye—Apraclonidine is a strong reducer of eye pressure and could also cause this reaction
- Vasovagal attack (history of)—The signs and symptoms are paleness, nausea, sweating, slow heartbeat, sudden and severe tiredness or weakness, and possibly fainting, usually brought on by emotional stress caused by fear or pain. Apraclonidine may cause this reaction to happen again

## Proper Use of This Medicine

If your doctor ordered two different eye drops to be used together, wait at least 10 minutes between the times you apply the medicines. This will help to keep the second medicine from "washing out" the first one.

To use the *eye drops:*

- First, wash your hands. Tilt the head back and, pressing your finger gently on the skin just beneath the lower eyelid, pull the lower eyelid away from the eye to make a space. Drop the medicine into this space. Let go of the eyelid and gently close the eyes. Do not blink. Keep the eyes closed and apply pressure to the inner corner of the eye with your finger for 1 or 2 minutes to allow the medicine to be absorbed by the eye.
- If you think you did not get the drop of medicine into your eye properly, use another drop.
- To keep the medicine as germ-free as possible, do not touch the applicator tip to any surface (including the eye). Also, keep the container tightly closed.

*Use this medicine only as directed.* Do not use more of it and do not use it more often than your doctor ordered. To do so may increase the chance of too much medicine being absorbed into the body and the chance of side effects.

*It is important that your doctor check your progress at regular visits.* This is to make sure the medicine is working properly.

**Dosing**—The dose of ophthalmic apraclonadine will be different for different patients. *Follow the doctor's orders or the directions on the label.* The following information includes only the average doses of ophthalmic apraclonadine. *If your dose is different, do not change it unless your doctor tells you to do so.*

- For *ophthalmic solution (eye drops)* dosage form:
  —For glaucoma (0.5% apraclonidine):
    - Adults—Use one drop in each eye three times a day.
    - Children—Use and dose must be determined by your doctor.
  —For preventing ocular hypertension before and after eye surgery (1% apraclonidine):
    - Adults—One drop is placed in the affected eye one hour before surgery, then one drop in the same eye immediately after surgery.
    - Children—Use and dose must be determined by your doctor.

**Missed dose**—If you are using this medicine regularly and you miss a dose, use it as soon as possible. However, if it is almost time for your next dose, skip the missed dose and go back to your regular dosing schedule. Do not double doses.

**Storage**—To store this medicine:

- Keep out of the reach of children.
- Store away from heat and direct light.
- The 0.5% eye drops may be stored in the refrigerator. However, keep the medicine from freezing.
- Do not keep outdated medicine or medicine no longer needed. Be sure that any discarded medicine is out of the reach of children.

## Precautions While Using This Medicine

This medicine may cause some people to become dizzy, drowsy, or less alert than they are normally. *Make sure you know how you react to this medicine before you drive, use machines, or do anything else that could be dangerous if you are not alert.*

Apraclonidine may cause your eyes to become more sensitive to light than they are normally. Wearing sunglasses and avoiding too much exposure to bright light may help lessen the discomfort.

## Side Effects of This Medicine

Along with its needed effects, a medicine may cause some unwanted effects. Although not all of these side effects may occur, if they do occur they may need medical attention.

Check with your health care professional as soon as possible if the following side effects occur:

*For 0.5% apraclonidine*
  *More common*
    Allergic reaction (redness, itching, tearing of eye)
  *Less common or rare*
    Blurred vision or change in vision; chest pain; clumsiness or unsteadiness; depression; dizziness; eye discharge, irritation, or pain; irregular heartbeat; numbness or tingling in fingers or toes; raising of upper eyelid; rash around eyes; redness of eyelid, or inner lining of eyelid; swelling of eye, eyelid, or

inner lining of eyelid; swelling of face, hands, or feet; wheezing or troubled breathing

*For 1% apraclonidine*
  *Less common or rare*
    Allergic reaction (redness of eye or inner lining of eyelid, swelling of eyelid, watering of eye); irregular heartbeat

Check with your health care professional if any of the following side effects continue or are bothersome:

*For 0.5% apraclonidine*
  *More common*
    Dryness of mouth; eye discomfort

  *Less common or rare*
    Change in taste or smell; constipation; crusting or scales on eyelid or corner of eye; discoloration of white part of eye; drowsiness or sleepiness; dry nose or eyes; general feeling of discomfort or illness; headache; increased sensitivity of eyes to light; muscle aches; nausea; nervousness; paleness of eye or inner lining of eyelid; runny nose; sore throat; tiredness or weakness; trouble in sleeping

*For 1% apraclonidine*
  *More common*
    Increase in size of pupil of eye; paleness of eye or inner lining of eyelid; raising of upper eyelid

  *Less common or rare*
    Runny nose

Other side effects not listed above may also occur in some patients. If you notice any other effects, check with your health care professional.

Revised: 06/21/94

# ASCORBIC ACID   (Vitamin C)   Systemic

Some commonly used brand names are:

**In the U.S.—**

| | |
|---|---|
| Ascorbicap | Cetane 500 |
| Cebid Timecelles | Cevalin |
| Cecon | Cevi-Bid |
| Cee-500 | Ce-Vi-Sol |
| Cemill | Flavorcee |
| Cenolate | Sunkist |
| Cetane | |

Generic name product may also be available.

**In Canada—**

| | |
|---|---|
| Apo-C | Kamu Jay |
| Ce-Vi-Sol | Sunkist |

Generic name product may also be available.

## Description

Vitamins (VYE-ta-mins) are compounds that you *must* have for growth and health. They are needed in small amounts only and are usually available in the foods that you eat. Ascorbic (a-SKOR-bik) acid, also known as vitamin C, is necessary for healthy bones and teeth as well as the general make-up of the body; it may have other effects as well.

Lack of vitamin C can lead to a condition called scurvy, which causes muscle weakness, swollen and bleeding gums, loss of teeth, and bleeding under the skin, as well as tiredness and depression. Wounds also do not heal easily. Your doctor may treat scurvy by prescribing vitamin C for you.

Patients with the following conditions may be more likely to have a deficiency of ascorbic acid:

- Alcoholism
- Burns
- Cancer
- Diarrhea (prolonged)
- Fever (prolonged)
- Infection (prolonged)
- Intestinal diseases
- Overactive thyroid (hyperthyroidism)
- Stomach ulcer
- Stress (continuing)
- Surgical removal of stomach
- Tuberculosis

Also, the following groups of people may have a deficiency of ascorbic acid:

- Infants receiving unfortified formulas
- Smokers
- Patients using an artificial kidney (on hemodialysis)
- Individuals who do heavy manual labor on a daily basis
- Patients who undergo surgery
- Individuals who are exposed to long periods of cold temperatures

If any of these conditions apply to you, you should take ascorbic acid supplements only on the advice of your doctor after need has been established.

Ascorbic acid may be used for other conditions as determined by your doctor.

Claims that vitamin C is effective for preventing senility and the common cold, and for treating asthma, some mental problems, cancer, hardening of the arteries, allergies, eye ulcers, blood clots, gum disease, and pressure sores have not been proven. Although vitamin C is being used to prevent certain types of cancer, there is not enough information to show that this is effective.

Most strengths of vitamin C are available without a prescription. However, it may be a good idea to check with your doctor before taking vitamin C on your own.

Vitamin C is available in the following dosage forms:
*Oral*
- Extended-release capsules (U.S. and Canada)
- Oral solution (U.S. and Canada)
- Syrup (U.S.)
- Tablets (U.S. and Canada)
- Chewable tablets (U.S. and Canada)
- Effervescent tablets (U.S.)
- Extended-release tablets (U.S. and Canada)

*Parenteral*
- Injection (U.S. and Canada)

## Importance of Diet

Ascorbic acid supplements should be taken only if you cannot get enough vitamins in your diet; however, some diets may not contain all of the vitamins you need. This may occur with rapid weight loss, unusual diets (such as some reducing diets in which choice of foods is limited), prolonged intravenous feeding, or malnutrition. A balanced diet should provide all the vitamins you normally need.

In order to get enough vitamins and minerals in your diet, it is important that you eat a balanced and varied diet. Follow carefully any diet program your doctor may recommend. For your specific vitamin and/or mineral needs, ask your doctor or dietitian for a list of appropriate foods.

Ascorbic acid is found in various foods, including citrus fruits (oranges, lemons, grapefruit), green vegetables (peppers, broccoli, cabbage), tomatoes, and potatoes. It is best to eat fresh fruits and vegetables whenever possible since they contain the most vitamins. Food processing may destroy some of the vitamins. For example, exposure to air, drying, salting, or cooking (especially in copper pots), mincing of fresh vegetables, or mashing potatoes may reduce the amount of ascorbic acid in foods. Freezing does not usually cause loss of vitamin C unless foods are stored for a very long time.

Vitamins alone will not take the place of a good diet and will not provide energy. Your body also needs other substances found in food such as protein, minerals, carbohydrates, and fat. Vitamins themselves often cannot work without the presence of other foods.

In some cases, it may not be possible for you to get enough food to supply you with the proper vitamins. In other cases, the amount of vitamins you need may be increased above normal. Therefore, a vitamin supplement may be needed.

Experts have developed a list of recommended dietary allowances (RDA) for most of the vitamins. The RDA are not an exact number but a general idea of how much you need. They do not cover amounts needed for problems caused by a serious lack of vitamins.

The RDA for ascorbic acid are:
Infants and children—
Birth to 6 months of age: 30 milligrams (mg) per day.
6 months to 1 year of age: 35 mg per day.
1 to 3 years of age: 40 mg per day.
4 to 10 years of age: 45 mg per day.
Adolescent and adult males—
11 to 14 years of age: 50 mg per day.
15 years of age and over: 60 mg per day.
Adolescent and adult females—
11 to 14 years of age: 50 mg per day.
15 years of age and over: 60 mg per day.
Pregnant females—70 mg per day.
Breast-feeding females—
First 6 months: 95 mg per day.
Second 6 months: 90 mg per day.
Smokers—100 mg per day.

Remember:
- The total amount of each vitamin that you get every day includes what you get from the foods that you eat *and* what you may take as a supplement.
- Your total amount should not be greater than the RDA, unless ordered by your doctor. Taking too much ascorbic acid over a period of time may cause harmful effects.

## Before Using This Dietary Supplement

In deciding to use a dietary supplement, the risks of taking the dietary supplement must be weighed against the good it will do. This is a decision you and your doctor will make. For ascorbic acid, the following should be considered:

**Allergies**—Tell your doctor if you have ever had any unusual or allergic reaction to ascorbic acid. Also, tell your health care professional if you are allergic to any other substances, such as foods, sulfites or other preservatives, or dyes.

**Pregnancy**—It is especially important that you are receiving enough vitamins when you become pregnant and that you continue to receive the right amount of vitamins throughout your pregnancy. Healthy fetal growth and development depend on a steady supply of nutrients from mother to fetus.

However, taking too much vitamin C may not be good for the fetus and may cause your baby to need more than the usual amount after birth.

**Breast-feeding**—It is especially important that you receive the right amounts of vitamins so that your baby will also get the vitamins needed to grow properly. You should also check with your doctor if you are giving your baby an unfortified formula. In that case, the baby must get the vitamins needed some other way. However, taking large amounts of a dietary supplement while breast-feeding may be harmful to the mother and/or baby and should be avoided.

**Children**—Normal daily requirements vary according to age. It is especially important that children receive enough vitamins in their diet for healthy growth and development. Although there is no specific information about the use of vitamins in children in doses higher than the normal daily requirements, it is not expected to cause different side effects or problems in children than in adults.

**Older adults**—It is important that older people continue to receive enough vitamins in their diet for good health. Although there is no specific information about the use of vitamins in older people in doses higher than the normal daily requirements, it is not expected to cause different side effects or problems in older people than in younger adults.

**Medicines or other dietary supplements**—Although certain medicines or dietary supplements should not be used together at all, in other cases they may be used together even if an interaction might occur. In these cases, your doctor may want to change the dose, or other precautions may be necessary. Tell your health care professional if you are taking any other dietary supplement or any prescription or nonprescription (over-the-counter [OTC]) medicine.

**Other medical problems**—The presence of other medical problems may affect the use of ascorbic acid. Make sure you tell your doctor if you have any other medical problems, especially:

- Diabetes mellitus (sugar diabetes)—Very high doses of ascorbic acid may interfere with tests for sugar in the urine
- Glucose-6-phosphate dehydrogenase (G6PD) deficiency—High doses of ascorbic acid may cause hemolytic anemia
- Kidney stones (history of)—High doses of ascorbic acid may increase risk of kidney stones in the urinary tract
- Sickle cell anemia or other blood problems—High doses of ascorbic acid may bring on a crisis

## Proper Use of This Dietary Supplement

Do not take more than the recommended daily amount. Vitamin C is not stored in the body. If you take more than you need, the extra will pass into your urine. There is a chance that high doses could cause stones to form in your urinary tract. Very large doses may also interfere with tests for sugar in diabetics and with tests for blood in the stool. Some people believe that taking very large doses of vitamins (called megadoses or megavitamin therapy) is useful for treating certain medical problems. Studies have not proven this. Large doses should be taken only under the direction of your doctor after need has been identified.

For patients taking the *oral liquid form* of ascorbic acid:
- This preparation is to be taken by mouth even though it comes in a dropper bottle.

- This dietary supplement may be dropped directly into the mouth or mixed with cereal, fruit juice, or other food.

**Dosing**—The dose of ascorbic acid for prevention of ascorbic acid deficiency is based on the Recommended Dietary Allowances (RDA). See the *Importance of Diet* section for the RDA for ascorbic acid.

**Missed dose**—If you miss taking a vitamin for one or more days there is no cause for concern, since it takes some time for your body to become seriously low in vitamins. However, if your doctor has recommended that you take this vitamin, try to remember to take it as directed every day.

**Storage**—To store this dietary supplement:
- Keep out of the reach of children.
- Store away from heat and direct light.
- Do not store in the bathroom, near the kitchen sink, or in other damp places. Heat or moisture may cause the dietary supplement to break down.
- Keep the oral liquid form of this dietary supplement from freezing.
- Do not keep outdated dietary supplements or those no longer needed. Be sure that any discarded dietary supplement is out of the reach of children.

## Side Effects of This Dietary Supplement

Along with its needed effects, a dietary supplement may cause some unwanted effects. Although not all of these side effects may occur, if they do occur, they may need medical attention.

Check with your doctor as soon as possible if the following side effect occurs:

*Less common or rare—with high doses*
   Side or lower back pain

Other side effects may occur that usually do not need medical attention. These side effects may go away during treatment as your body adjusts to the dietary supplement. However, check with your health care professional as soon as possible if any of the following side effects continue or are bothersome:

*Less common or rare—with high doses*
   Diarrhea; dizziness or faintness (with the injection only); flushing or redness of skin; headache; increase in urination (mild); nausea or vomiting; stomach cramps

Other side effects not listed above may also occur in some patients. If you notice any other effects, check with your health care professional.

## Additional Information

Once a medicine or dietary supplement has been approved for marketing for a certain use, experience may show that it is also useful for other medical problems. Although these uses are not included in product labeling, ascorbic acid is used in certain patients with the following medical conditions:

- Overdose of iron (to help another drug in decreasing iron levels in the body)
- Methemoglobinemia (a blood disease)

Other than the above information, there is no additional information relating to proper use, precautions, or side effects for these uses.

Revised: 04/14/92
Interim revision: 08/09/94

# ASPARAGINASE    Systemic

Some commonly used brand names are:

**In the U.S.—**
Elspar

**In Canada—**
Kidrolase

Another commonly used name is colaspase.

## Description

Asparaginase (a-SPARE-a-gin-ase) belongs to the group of medicines known as enzymes. It is used to treat some kinds of cancer.

All cells need a chemical called asparagine to stay alive. Normal cells can make this chemical for themselves, while cancer cells cannot. Asparaginase breaks down asparagine in the body. Since the cancer cells cannot make more asparagine, they die.

Before you begin treatment with asparaginase, you and your doctor should talk about the good this medicine will do as well as the risks of using it.

Asparaginase is to be administered only by or under the supervision of your doctor. It is available in the following dosage form:

*Parenteral*
- Injection (U.S. and Canada)

## Before Using This Medicine

In deciding to use a medicine, the risks of taking the medicine must be weighed against the good it will do. This is a decision you and your doctor will make. For asparaginase, the following should be considered:

**Allergies—**Tell your doctor if you have ever had any unusual or allergic reaction to asparaginase.

**Pregnancy—**Asparaginase has not been studied in pregnant women. However, studies in mice and rats have shown that asparaginase in doses 5 times the usual human dose slows the weight gain of infants and may also increase the risk of birth defects or cause a decrease in successful pregnancies. In addition, doses slightly less than the human dose have caused birth defects in rabbits.

It is best to use some kind of birth control while you are receiving asparaginase. Tell your doctor right away if you think you have become pregnant while receiving asparaginase.

**Breast-feeding—**It is not known whether asparaginase passes into breast milk. However, because asparaginase may cause serious side effects, breast-feeding is generally not recommended while you are receiving it.

**Children—**This medicine has been tested in children and has not been shown to cause different side effects or problems than it does in adults. In fact, the side effects of this medicine seem to be less severe in children than in adults.

**Older adults—**Many medicines have not been studied specifically in older people. Therefore, it may not be known whether they work exactly the same way they do in younger adults or if they cause different side effects or problems in older people. There is no specific information comparing use of asparaginase in the elderly with use in other age groups.

**Other medicines—**Although certain medicines should not be used together at all, in other cases two different medicines may be used together even if an interaction might occur. In these cases, your doctor may want to change the dose, or other precautions may be necessary. When you are receiving asparaginase it is especially important that your health care professional know if you are taking any of the following:

- Probenecid (e.g., Benemid) or
- Sulfinpyrazone (e.g., Anturane)—Asparaginase may raise the concentration of uric acid in the blood. Since these medicines are used to lower uric acid levels, they may not work as well in patients receiving asparaginase
- If you have ever been treated with radiation or cancer medicines—Asparaginase may increase the total effects of these medications and radiation therapy

**Other medical problems—**The presence of other medical problems may affect the use of asparaginase. Make sure you tell your doctor if you have any other medical problems, especially:

- Chickenpox (including recent exposure) or
- Herpes zoster (shingles)—Risk of severe disease affecting other parts of the body
- Diabetes mellitus (sugar diabetes)—Asparaginase may increase glucose (sugar) in the blood
- Gout or
- Kidney stones—Asparaginase may increase levels of uric acid in the body, which can cause gout or kidney stones
- Infection—Asparaginase can reduce your body's ability to fight infection

- Liver disease—Asparaginase may worsen the condition
- Pancreatitis (inflammation of the pancreas)—Asparaginase may cause pancreatitis

## Proper Use of This Medicine

This medicine is usually given together with certain other medicines. If you are using a combination of medicines, it is important that you receive each one at the proper time. If you are taking some of these medicines by mouth, ask your health care professional to help you plan a way to remember to take them at the right times.

While you are using this medicine, your doctor may want you to drink extra fluids so that you will pass more urine. This will help prevent kidney problems and keep your kidneys working well.

This medicine often causes nausea, vomiting, and loss of appetite. However, it is very important that you continue to receive the medicine, even if you begin to feel ill. After several doses, your stomach upset should lessen. Ask your health care professional for ways to lessen these effects.

**Dosing**—The dose of asparaginase will be different for different patients. The dose that is used may depend on a number of things, including what the medicine is being used for, the patient's weight, and whether or not other medicines are also being taken. *If you are receiving asparaginase at home, follow your doctor's orders or the directions on the label.* If you have any questions about the proper dose of asparaginase, ask your doctor.

## Precautions While Using This Medicine

*It is very important that your doctor check your progress at regular visits* to make sure that this medicine is working properly and to check for unwanted effects.

While you are being treated with asparaginase, and after you stop treatment with it, *do not have any immunizations (vaccinations) without your doctor's approval.* Asparaginase may lower your body's resistance and there is a chance you might get the infection the immunization is meant to prevent. In addition, other persons living in your household should not take oral polio vaccine since there is a chance they could pass the polio virus on to you. Also, avoid persons who have taken oral polio vaccine. Do not get close to them, and do not stay in the same room with them for very long. If you cannot take these precautions, you should consider wearing a protective face mask that covers the nose and mouth.

Before you have any medical tests, tell the medical doctor in charge that you are receiving this medicine. The results of thyroid tests may be affected by this medicine.

## Side Effects of This Medicine

Along with its needed effects, a medicine may cause some unwanted effects. Some side effects will have signs or symptoms that you can see or feel. Your doctor may watch for others by doing certain tests. Some of the unwanted effects that may be caused by asparaginase are listed below. Although not all of these effects may occur, if they do occur, they may need medical attention.

Also, because of the way these medicines act on the body, there is a chance that they might cause other unwanted effects that may not occur until months or years after the medicine is used. These delayed effects may include certain types of cancer, such as leukemia. Discuss these possible effects with your doctor.

*Check with your doctor or nurse immediately* if any of the following side effects occur:
*More common*
    Joint pain; puffy face; skin rash or itching; stomach pain (severe) with nausea and vomiting; trouble in breathing
*Rare*
    Fever or chills; headache (severe); inability to move arm or leg; unusual bleeding or bruising

Check with your health care professional as soon as possible if any of the following side effects occur:
*Less common*
    Confusion; drowsiness; frequent urination; hallucinations (seeing, hearing, or feeling things that are not there); lower back or side pain; mental depression; nervousness; sores in mouth or on lips; swelling of feet or lower legs; unusual thirst; unusual tiredness
*Rare*
    Convulsions (seizures); pain in lower legs

This medicine may also cause the following side effect that your doctor will watch for:
*More common*
    Liver problems

Other side effects may occur that usually do not need medical attention. These side effects may go away during treatment as your body adjusts to the medicine. Also, your health care professional may be able to tell you about ways to prevent or reduce some of these side effects. Check with your health care professional if any of the following side effects continue or are bothersome or if you have any questions about them:
*More common*
    Headache (mild); loss of appetite; nausea or vomiting; stomach cramps; weight loss

After you stop receiving asparaginase, it may still produce some side effects that need attention. During this period of time, *check with your doctor or nurse immediately* if any of the following side effects occur:
    Headache (severe); inability to move arm or leg; stomach pain (severe) with nausea and vomiting

Other side effects not listed above may also occur in some patients. If you notice any other effects, check with your health care professional.

Revised: 04/09/93
Interim revision: 04/29/94

# ASPIRIN, SODIUM BICARBONATE, AND CITRIC ACID   **Systemic**

Some commonly used brand names in the U.S. and Canada are Alka-Seltzer Effervescent Pain Reliever and Antacid and Flavored Alka-Seltzer Effervescent Pain Reliever and Antacid.

Other commonly used names for aspirin are acetylsalicylic acid and ASA. Because Aspirin is a brand name in Canada, ASA is the term that commonly appears on Canadian product labels.

## Description

Aspirin, sodium bicarbonate, and citric acid (AS-pir-in, SOE-dee-um bye-KAR-boe-nate, and SI-trik AS-id) combination is used to relieve pain occurring together with heartburn, sour stomach, or acid indigestion.

The aspirin in this combination is the pain reliever. Aspirin belongs to the group of medicines known as salicylates (sa-LISS-ih-lates) and to the group of medicines known as anti-inflammatory analgesics. The sodium bicarbonate in this medicine is an antacid. It neutralizes stomach acid by combining with it to form a new substance that is not an acid.

Aspirin, sodium bicarbonate, and citric acid combination may also be used to lessen the chance of heart attack, stroke, or other problems that may occur when a blood vessel is blocked by blood clots. The aspirin in this medicine helps prevent dangerous blood clots from forming. However, this effect of aspirin may increase the chance of serious bleeding in some people. Therefore, aspirin should be used for this purpose only when your doctor decides, after studying your medical condition and history, that the danger of blood clots is greater than the risk of bleeding. *Do not take aspirin to prevent blood clots or a heart attack unless it has been ordered by your doctor.*

This combination medicine is available without a prescription. However, your doctor may have special instructions on the proper dose for your medical condition.

Aspirin, sodium bicarbonate, and citric acid combination is available in the following dosage form:

*Oral*
  • Effervescent tablets (U.S. and Canada)

## Before Using This Medicine

If you are taking this medicine without a prescription, carefully read and follow any precautions on the label. For aspirin, sodium bicarbonate, and citric acid combination, the following should be considered:

**Allergies**—Tell your doctor if you have ever had any unusual or allergic reaction to aspirin or other salicylates, including methyl salicylate (oil of wintergreen), or to any of the following medicines:

  Diclofenac (e.g., Voltaren)
  Diflunisal (e.g., Dolobid)
  Etodolac (e.g., Lodine)
  Fenoprofen (e.g., Nalfon)
  Floctafenine (e.g., Idarac)
  Flurbiprofen, oral (e.g., Ansaid)

  Ibuprofen (e.g., Motrin)
  Indomethacin (e.g., Indocin)
  Ketoprofen (e.g., Orudis)
  Ketorolac (e.g., Toradol)
  Meclofenamate (e.g., Meclomen)
  Mefenamic acid (e.g., Ponstel)
  Nabumetone (e.g., Relafen)
  Naproxen (e.g., Naprosyn)
  Oxaprozin (e.g., Daypro)
  Oxyphenbutazone (e.g., Tandearil)
  Phenylbutazone (e.g., Butazolidin)
  Piroxicam (e.g., Feldene)
  Sulindac (e.g., Clinoril)
  Suprofen (e.g., Suprol)
  Tenoxicam (e.g., Mobiflex)
  Tiaprofenic acid (e.g., Surgam)
  Tolmetin (e.g., Tolectin)
  Zomepirac (e.g., Zomax)

Also tell your health care professional if you are allergic to any other substances, such as foods, preservatives, or dyes.

**Diet**—Make certain your health care professional knows if you are on any special diet, such as a low-sodium or low-sugar diet. This medicine contains a large amount of sodium (more than 500 mg in each tablet).

**Pregnancy**—Studies in humans have not shown that aspirin causes birth defects in humans. However, it has been shown to cause birth defects in animal studies.

*Do not take aspirin during the last 3 months of pregnancy unless it has been ordered by your doctor.* Some reports have suggested that too much use of aspirin late in pregnancy may cause a decrease in the newborn's weight and possible death of the fetus or newborn infant. However, the mothers in these reports had been taking much larger amounts of aspirin than are usually recommended. Studies of mothers taking aspirin in the doses that are usually recommended did not show these unwanted effects. However, there is a chance that regular use of aspirin late in pregnancy may cause unwanted effects on the heart or blood flow in the fetus or in the newborn infant.

Use of aspirin during the last 2 weeks of pregnancy may cause bleeding problems in the fetus before or during delivery or in the newborn infant. Also, too much use of aspirin during the last 3 months of pregnancy may increase the length of pregnancy, prolong labor, cause other problems during delivery, or cause severe bleeding in the mother before, during, or after delivery.

The sodium in this combination medicine can cause your body to hold water. This may result in swelling and weight gain. Therefore, you should not use this combination medicine if you tend to hold body water.

**Breast-feeding**—Aspirin passes into the breast milk. However, aspirin (in the amounts used to relieve pain or prevent blood clots), sodium bicarbonate, and citric acid have not been reported to cause problems in nursing babies.

**Children**—*Do not give any medicine containing aspirin to a child with fever or other symptoms of a virus infection, especially flu or chickenpox, without first discussing its use with your child's doctor.* This is very important because aspirin may cause a serious illness called Reye's syndrome in children with fever caused by a virus infection, especially flu or chickenpox. Children who do not have a virus infection may also be more sensitive to the effects of aspirin, especially if they have a fever or have lost large amounts of body fluid because of vomiting, diarrhea, or sweating. This may increase the chance of side effects during treatment.

**Teenagers**—*Teenagers with fever or other symptoms of a virus infection, especially flu or chickenpox, should check with a doctor before taking this medicine.* The aspirin in this combination medicine may cause a serious illness called Reye's syndrome in teenagers with fever caused by a virus infection, especially flu or chickenpox.

**Older adults**—People 60 years of age and older are especially sensitive to the effects of aspirin. This may increase the chance of side effects during treatment. Also, the sodium in this combination medicine can be harmful to some elderly people, especially if large amounts of the medicine are taken regularly. Therefore, it is best that older people not use this medicine for more than 5 days in a row, unless otherwise directed by their doctor.

**Other medicines**—Although certain medicines should not be used together at all, in other cases two different medicines may be used together even if an interaction might occur. In these cases, your doctor may want to change the dose, or other precautions may be necessary. When you are taking this combination medicine, it is especially important that your health care professional know if you are taking any of the following:

- Anticoagulants (blood thinners) or
- Carbenicillin by injection (e.g., Geopen) or
- Cefamandole (e.g., Mandol) or
- Cefoperazone (e.g., Cefobid) or
- Cefotetan (e.g., Cefotan) or
- Dipyridamole (e.g., Persantine) or
- Divalproex (e.g., Depakote) or
- Heparin or
- Pentoxifylline (e.g., Trental) or
- Plicamycin (e.g., Mithracin) or
- Ticarcillin (e.g., Ticar) or
- Valproic acid (e.g., Depakene)—Use of these medicines together with aspirin may increase the chance of bleeding
- Antidiabetics, oral (diabetes medicine you take by mouth)—Aspirin may increase the effects of these medicines; a change in dose may be needed
- Ciprofloxacin (e.g., Cipro) or
- Enoxacin (e.g., Penetrex) or
- Itraconazole (e.g., Sporanox) or
- Ketoconazole (e.g., Nizoral) or
- Lomefloxacin (e.g., Maxaquin) or
- Methenamine (e.g., Mandelamine) or
- Norfloxacin (e.g., Noroxin) or

- Ofloxacin (e.g., Floxin) or
- Tetracyclines (medicine for infection), taken by mouth—Sodium bicarbonate can keep these medicines from working properly
- Mecamylamine (e.g., Inversine)—Sodium bicarbonate may increase the chance of unwanted effects by causing mecamylamine to stay in your body longer than usual
- Medicine for pain and/or inflammation (except narcotics) or
- Methotrexate (e.g., Mexate) or
- Vancomycin (e.g., Vancocin)—The chance of serious side effects may be increased
- Probenecid (e.g., Benemid) or
- Sulfinpyrazone (e.g., Anturane)—Aspirin can keep these medicines from working properly when they are used to treat gout

**Other medical problems**—The presence of other medical problems may affect the use of this combination medicine. Make sure you tell your doctor if you have any other medical problems, especially:

- Anemia or
- Stomach ulcer or other stomach problems—Aspirin can make these conditions worse
- Appendicitis (symptoms of, such as stomach or lower abdominal pain, cramping, bloating, soreness, nausea, or vomiting)—Sodium bicarbonate can make your condition worse; also, people who may have appendicitis need medical attention and should not try to treat themselves
- Asthma, allergies, and nasal polyps (history of) or
- Kidney disease or
- Liver disease—The chance of serious side effects may be increased
- Edema (swelling of face, fingers, feet, or lower legs caused by too much water in the body) or
- Heart disease or
- High blood pressure or
- Toxemia of pregnancy—The sodium in this combination medicine can make these conditions worse
- Gout—Aspirin can make this condition worse and can also keep some medicines used to treat gout from working properly
- Hemophilia or other bleeding problems—Aspirin increases the chance of serious bleeding

## Proper Use of This Medicine

*Unless otherwise directed by your doctor, do not take more of this medicine than is recommended on the package label.* If too much is taken, serious side effects may occur.

To use this medicine:

- The tablets must be dissolved in water before taking. Do not swallow the tablets or any pieces of the tablets.
- Place the number of tablets needed for one dose (1 or 2 tablets) into a glass. Then add ½ glass (4 ounces) of cool water.
- Check to be sure that the tablets have disappeared completely. This shows that all of the medicine is in the liquid. Then drink all of the liquid. You may drink the liquid while it is still fizzing or after the fizzing stops.

- Add a little more water to the glass and drink that, to make sure that you get the full amount of the medicine.

**Dosing**—The dose of this combination medicine will be different for different people. *Follow your doctor's orders or the directions on the label.* The following information includes only the average doses of this combination medicine. *If your dose is different, do not change it* unless your doctor tells you to do so.

- For *oral* dosage forms (effervescent tablets):
  —For pain and upset stomach:
  - Adults and teenagers—One or two regular-strength (325-milligram [mg]) tablets every four to six hours as needed, one extra-strength (500-mg) tablet every four to six hours as needed, or two extra-strength (500-mg) tablets every six hours as needed, dissolved in water. Elderly people should not take more than four regular-strength or extra-strength tablets a day. Other adults and teenagers should not take more than 6 regular-strength flavored tablets, 8 regular-strength unflavored tablets, or 7 extra-strength tablets a day.
  - Children—The dose depends on the child's age.
    —Children younger than 3 years of age: Use and dose must be determined by your doctor.
    —Children 3 to 5 years of age: One-half of a regular-strength (325-mg) tablet, dissolved in water, every four to six hours as needed.
    —Children 6 to 12 years of age: One regular-strength (325-mg) tablet, dissolved in water, every four to six hours as needed.
  —For reducing the chance of heart attack, stroke, or other problems that may occur when a blood vessel is blocked by blood clots:
  - Adults—One regular-strength (325-mg) tablet a day, dissolved in water.
  - Children and teenagers—Use and dose must be determined by your doctor.

**Missed dose**—If your doctor has ordered you to take this medicine according to a regular schedule and you miss a dose, take it as soon as you remember. However, if it is almost time for your next dose, skip the missed dose and go back to your regular dosing schedule. Do not double doses.

**Storage**—To store this medicine:

- Keep out of the reach of children. Overdose is very dangerous in young children.
- Store away from heat and direct light.
- Do not store in the bathroom, near the kitchen sink, or in other damp places. Heat or moisture may cause the medicine to break down.
- Do not keep outdated medicine or medicine no longer needed. Be sure that any discarded medicine is out of the reach of children.

## Precautions While Using This Medicine

If you will be taking this medicine for a long time (more than 5 days in a row for children or 10 days in a row for adults), your doctor should check your progress at regular visits.

Check with your doctor if your pain and/or upset stomach last for more than 10 days for adults or 5 days for children or if they get worse, if new symptoms occur, or if the painful area is red or swollen. These could be signs of a serious condition that needs medical treatment.

The sodium bicarbonate in this combination medicine can keep other medicines from working properly if the 2 medicines are taken too close together. *Always take this medicine:*

- *At least 6 hours before or 2 hours after taking ciprofloxacin (e.g., Cipro) or lomefloxacin (e.g., Maxaquin).*
- *At least 8 hours before or 2 hours after taking enoxacin (e.g., Penetrex).*
- *At least 2 hours after taking itraconazole (e.g., Sporanox).*
- *At least 3 hours before or after taking ketoconazole (e.g., Nizoral).*
- *At least 2 hours before or after taking norfloxacin (e.g., Noroxin) or ofloxacin (e.g., Floxin).*
- *At least 3 or 4 hours before or after taking a tetracycline antibiotic by mouth.*
- *At least 1 or 2 hours before or after taking any other medicine by mouth.*

If you are also taking a laxative that contains cellulose, take this combination medicine at least 2 hours before or after you take the laxative. Taking the medicines too close together may lessen the effects of aspirin.

*Check the labels of all nonprescription (over-the-counter [OTC]) and prescription medicines you now take.* If any contain aspirin or other salicylates, including bismuth subsalicylate (e.g., Pepto-Bismol), magnesium salicylate (e.g., Nuprin Backache Caplets), or salsalate (e.g., Disalcid); if any contain salicylic acid (present in some shampoos or medicines for your skin); or if any contain sodium, *check with your health care professional.* Taking other salicylate-containing or other sodium-containing products together with this medicine may cause an overdose.

Do not take aspirin for 5 days before any surgery, including dental surgery, unless otherwise directed by your medical doctor or dentist. Taking aspirin during this time may cause bleeding problems.

For patients taking this medicine to lessen the chance of a heart attack, stroke, or other problems caused by blood clots:

- *Take only the amount of aspirin ordered by your doctor.* If you need a medicine to relieve pain, a fever, or arthritis, your doctor may not want you to take extra aspirin. It is a good idea to discuss this with your doctor, so that you will know ahead of time what medicine to take.

- *Do not stop taking this medicine for any reason without first checking with the doctor who directed you to take it.*

Taking certain other medicines together with a salicylate may increase the chance of unwanted effects. The risk will depend on how much of each medicine you take every day, and on how long you take the medicines together. If your doctor directs you to take these medicines together on a regular basis, follow his or her directions carefully. However, *do not take any of the following medicines together with a salicylate for more than a few days, unless your doctor has directed you to do so and is following your progress:*

Acetaminophen (e.g., Tylenol)
Diclofenac (e.g., Voltaren)
Diflunisal (e.g., Dolobid)
Etodolac (e.g., Lodine)
Fenoprofen (e.g., Nalfon)
Floctafenine (e.g., Idarac)
Flurbiprofen, oral (e.g., Ansaid)
Ibuprofen (e.g., Motrin)
Indomethacin (e.g., Indocin)
Ketoprofen (e.g., Orudis)
Ketorolac (e.g., Toradol)
Meclofenamate (e.g., Meclomen)
Mefenamic acid (e.g., Ponstel)
Nabumetone (e.g., Relafen)
Naproxen (e.g., Naprosyn)
Oxaprozin (e.g., Daypro)
Phenylbutazone (e.g., Butazolidin)
Piroxicam (e.g., Feldene)
Sulindac (e.g., Clinoril)
Tenoxicam (e.g., Mobiflex)
Tiaprofenic acid (e.g., Surgam)
Tolmetin (e.g., Tolectin)

If you will be taking more than an occasional 1 or 2 doses of this medicine:

- *Do not drink alcoholic beverages.* Drinking alcoholic beverages while you are taking aspirin, especially if you take aspirin regularly or in large amounts, may increase the chance of stomach problems.

- *Do not drink a lot of milk or eat a lot of milk products.* To do so may increase the chance of side effects.

- To prevent side effects caused by too much sodium in the body, you may need to limit the amount of sodium in the foods you eat. Some foods that contain large amounts of sodium are canned soup, canned vegetables, pickles, ketchup, green and ripe (black) olives, relish, frankfurters and other sausage-type meats, soy sauce, and carbonated beverages. If you have any questions about this, check with your health care professional.

Before you have any medical tests, tell the person in charge that you are taking this medicine. The results of some tests may be affected by the aspirin in this combination medicine.

For *diabetic patients:*

- Aspirin can cause false urine glucose (sugar) test results if you regularly take 8 or more 324-mg, or 4 or more 500-mg (extra-strength), tablets a day. Smaller amounts or occasional use of aspirin usually will not affect the test results. However, check with your health care professional if you notice any change in your urine glucose test results. This is especially important if your diabetes is not well-controlled.

*If you think that you or anyone else may have taken an overdose, get emergency help at once.* Taking an overdose of aspirin may cause unconsciousness or death, especially in young children. Signs of overdose include convulsions (seizures), hearing loss, confusion, ringing or buzzing in the ears, severe drowsiness or tiredness, severe excitement or nervousness, and fast or deep breathing.

## Side Effects of This Medicine

Along with its needed effects, a medicine may cause some unwanted effects. Although the following side effects occur very rarely when 1 or 2 doses of this combination medicine is taken occasionally, they may be more likely to occur if:

- too much medicine is taken.
- the medicine is taken several times a day.
- the medicine is taken for more than a few days in a row.

*Get emergency help immediately* if any of the following side effects occur:

Any loss of hearing; bloody urine; confusion; convulsions (seizures); diarrhea (severe or continuing); difficulty in swallowing; dizziness, lightheadedness, or feeling faint (severe); drowsiness (severe); excitement or nervousness (severe); fast or deep breathing; flushing, redness, or other change in skin color; hallucinations (seeing, hearing, or feeling things that are not there); nausea or vomiting (severe or continuing); shortness of breath, troubled breathing, tightness in chest, or wheezing; stomach pain (severe or continuing); swelling of eyelids, face, or lips; unexplained fever; uncontrollable flapping movements of the hands (especially in elderly patients); vision problems

*Signs of overdose in children*

Changes in behavior; drowsiness or tiredness (severe); fast or deep breathing

Also, check with your doctor as soon as possible if any of the following side effects occur:

*Less common or rare*

Bloody or black, tarry stools; frequent urge to urinate; headache (severe or continuing); increased blood pressure; loss of appetite (continuing); mood or mental changes; muscle pain or twitching; ringing or buzzing in ears (continuing); skin rash, hives, or itching; slow breathing; swelling of face, fingers, ankles, feet, or lower legs; unpleasant taste; unusual tiredness or weakness; vomiting of blood or material that looks like coffee grounds; weight gain (unusual)

Other side effects may occur that usually do not need medical attention. These side effects may go away during treatment as your body adjusts to the medicine. However,

check with your health care professional if any of the following side effects continue or are bothersome:

Heartburn or indigestion; increased thirst; nausea or vomiting; stomach pain (mild)

Other side effects not listed above may also occur in some patients. If you notice any other effects, check with your doctor.

Revised: 08/29/94

---

# ATOVAQUONE   Systemic

A commonly used brand name in the U.S. and Canada is Mepron. Another commonly used name is 566C80.

## Description

Atovaquone (a-TOE-va-kwone) is used to treat *Pneumocystis* (noo-moe-SISS-tis) *carinii* pneumonia (PCP), a very serious kind of pneumonia. This particular kind of pneumonia occurs commonly in patients whose immune systems are not working normally, such as cancer patients, transplant patients, and patients with acquired immune deficiency syndrome (AIDS).

This medicine is available only with your doctor's prescription, in the following dosage form:

*Oral*
  • Tablets (U.S. and Canada)

## Before Receiving This Medicine

In deciding to use a medicine, the risks of taking the medicine must be weighed against the good it will do. This is a decision you and your doctor will make. For atovaquone, the following should be considered:

**Allergies**—Tell your doctor if you have ever had any unusual or allergic reaction to atovaquone. Also tell your health care professional if you are allergic to any other substances, such as foods, preservatives, or dyes.

**Diet**—Make certain your health care professional knows if you are on any special diet, such as a low-fat diet. This medicine must be taken with high-fat foods so that it can work properly.

**Pregnancy**—Atovaquone has not been studied in pregnant women. However, studies in rabbits have shown an increase in miscarriages and other harmful effects in the mother and fetus. Before taking this medicine, make sure your doctor knows if you are pregnant or if you may become pregnant.

**Breast-feeding**—It is not known whether atovaquone passes into human breast milk. However, it was found in the milk of rats. Be sure you have discussed the risks and benefits of atovaquone with your doctor.

**Children**—Atovaquone has been tested in a limited number of children 5 months of age to 13 years old. It is not known if this medicine causes different side effects or problems in children than it does in adults.

**Older adults**—Many medicines have not been studied specifically in older people. Therefore, it may not be known whether they work exactly the same way they do in younger adults or if they cause different side effects or problems in older people. There is no specific information comparing use of atovaquone in the elderly with use in other age groups.

**Other medicines**—Although certain medicines should not be used together at all, in other cases two different medicines may be used together even if an interaction might occur. In these cases, your doctor may want to change the dose, or other precautions may be necessary. Tell your health care professional if you are taking any other prescription or nonprescription (over-the-counter [OTC]) medicine.

**Other medical problems**—The presence of other medical problems may affect the use of atovaquone. Make sure you tell your doctor if you have any other medical problems, especially:

  • Stomach or intestinal disorders—Atovaquone may not work properly in patients with some kinds of stomach or intestinal problems

## Proper Use of This Medicine

It is *important that you take atovaquone with a high-fat meal.* This is to make sure the medicine is fully absorbed into the body and will work properly.

Atovaquone tablets may be crushed if necessary to make it easier to swallow the tablets.

To help clear up your infection completely, *keep taking your medicine for the full time of treatment,* even if you begin to feel better after a few days. If you stop taking this medicine too soon, your symptoms may return.

Atovaquone works best when there is a constant amount in the blood. *To help keep the amount constant, do not miss any doses.*

**Dosing**—The dose of atovaquone may be different for different patients. *Follow your doctor's orders or the directions on the label.* The following information includes only the average doses of atovaquone. *If your dose is different, do not change it* unless your doctor tells you to do so.

- For the *oral* dosage form (capsules):
  —For treatment of *Pneumocystis carinii* pneumonia (PCP):
    - Adults and teenagers—750 milligrams (mg) taken with a high-fat meal three times a day for twenty-one days.
    - Children—Use and dose must be determined by your doctor.

**Missed dose**—If you miss a dose of this medicine, take it as soon as possible. This will help to keep a constant amount of medicine in the blood. However, if it is almost time for your next dose, skip the missed dose and go back to your regular dosing schedule. Do not double doses.

**Storage**—To store this medicine:
- Keep out of the reach of children.
- Store away from heat and direct light.
- Do not store in the bathroom, near the kitchen sink, or in other damp places. Heat or moisture may cause the medicine to break down.
- Do not keep outdated medicine or medicine no longer needed. Be sure that any discarded medicine is out of the reach of children.

## Precautions While Using This Medicine

If your symptoms do not improve within a few days, or if they become worse, check with your doctor.

## Side Effects of This Medicine

Along with its needed effects, a medicine may cause some unwanted effects. Although not all of these side effects may occur, if they do occur they may need medical attention.

*Check with your doctor immediately* if any of the following side effects occur:

*More common*
  Fever; skin rash

Other side effects may occur that usually do not need medical attention. These side effects may go away during treatment as your body adjusts to the medicine. However, check with your doctor if any of the following side effects continue or are bothersome:

*More common*
  Cough; diarrhea; headache; nausea; trouble in sleeping; vomiting

Other side effects not listed above may also occur in some patients. If you notice any other effects, check with your doctor.

Revised: 07/22/94

---

# ATROPINE/HOMATROPINE/SCOPOLAMINE    Ophthalmic

Some commonly used brand names are:

**In the U.S.—**

| | |
|---|---|
| AK-Homatropine[2] | Isopto Atropine[1] |
| Atropair[1] | Isopto Homatropine[2] |
| Atropine Care[1] | Isopto Hyoscine[3] |
| Atropine Sulfate S.O.P.[1] | I-Tropine[1] |
| Atropisol[1] | Ocu-Tropine[1] |
| I-Homatrine[2] | Spectro-Homatropine[2] |

**In Canada—**

| | |
|---|---|
| Atropisol[1] | Minims Atropine[1] |
| Isopto Atropine[1] | Minims Homatropine[2] |
| Isopto Homatropine[2] | |

Another commonly used name for scopolamine is hyoscine.

Note: For quick reference, the following medicines are numbered to match the corresponding brand names.

This information applies to the following medicines:
1. Atropine (A-troe-peen)‡§
2. Homatropine (hoe-MA-troe-peen)‡§
3. Scopolamine (skoe-POL-a-meen)†

---

†Not commercially available in Canada.
‡Generic name product may also be available in the U.S.
§Generic name product may also be available in Canada.

---

## Description

Ophthalmic atropine, homatropine, and scopolamine are used to dilate (enlarge) the pupil of the eye. They are used before eye examinations, before and after eye surgery, and to treat certain eye conditions, such as uveitis or posterior synechiae.

These medicines are available only with your doctor's prescription, in the following dosage forms:

*Ophthalmic*
  Atropine
    - Ophthalmic ointment (U.S. and Canada)
    - Ophthalmic solution (eye drops) (U.S. and Canada)
  Homatropine
    - Ophthalmic solution (eye drops) (U.S. and Canada)
  Scopolamine
    - Ophthalmic solution (eye drops) (U.S.)

---

## Before Using This Medicine

In deciding to use a medicine, the risks of using the medicine must be weighed against the good it will do. This is a decision you and your doctor will make. For ophthalmic atropine, homatropine, and scopolamine, the following should be considered:

**Allergies**—Tell your doctor if you have ever had any unusual or allergic reaction to atropine, homatropine, or scopolamine. Also tell your health care professional if you are allergic to any other substances, such as certain preservatives.

**Pregnancy**—Studies on effects in pregnancy have not been done in either humans or animals. However, these medicines may be absorbed into the body.

**Breast-feeding**—These medicines may be absorbed into the body. Atropine passes into the breast milk in very small amounts and may cause side effects, such as fast pulse, fever, or dry skin, in babies of nursing mothers using ophthalmic atropine. It is not known whether homatropine or scopolamine passes into breast milk. Although most medicines pass into breast milk in small amounts, many of them may be used safely while breast-feeding. Mothers who are using one of these medicines and who wish to breast-feed should discuss this with their doctor.

**Children**—Infants and young children and children with blond hair or blue eyes may be especially sensitive to the effects of atropine, homatropine, or scopolamine. This may increase the chance of side effects during treatment.

**Older adults**—Elderly people are especially sensitive to the effects of atropine, homatropine, or scopolamine. This may increase the chance of side effects during treatment.

**Other medicines**—Although certain medicines should not be used together at all, in other cases two different medicines may be used together even if an interaction might occur. In these cases, your doctor may want to change the dose, or other precautions may be necessary. Tell your health care professional if you are using any other prescription or nonprescription (over-the-counter [OTC]) medicine.

**Other medical problems**—The presence of other medical problems may affect the use of ophthalmic atropine, homatropine, or scopolamine. Make sure you tell your doctor if you have any other medical problems, especially:

- Brain damage (in children) or
- Down's syndrome (mongolism) (in children and adults) or
- Glaucoma or
- Other eye diseases or problems or
- Spastic paralysis (in children)—Use of ophthalmic atropine, homatropine, or scopolamine may make the condition worse

## Proper Use of This Medicine

To use the ophthalmic solution *(eye drops) form* of this medicine:

- First, wash your hands. Tilt the head back and, pressing your finger gently on the skin just beneath the lower eyelid, pull the lower eyelid away from the eye to make a space. Drop the medicine into this space. Let go of the eyelid and gently close the eyes. Do not blink. Keep the eyes closed and apply pressure to the inner corner of the eye with your finger for 2 or 3 minutes to allow the medicine to be absorbed by the eye.
- Immediately after using the eye drops, wash your hands to remove any medicine that may be on them.

If you are using the eye drops for an infant or child, be sure to wash his or her hands immediately afterwards also, and do not let any of the medicine get in his or her mouth. In addition, wipe off any medicine that may have accidentally gotten on the infant or child, including his or her face or eyelids.

- To keep the medicine as germ-free as possible, do not touch the applicator tip to any surface (including the eye). Also, keep the container tightly closed.

To use the *ointment form* of this medicine:

- First, wash your hands. Tilt the head back and, pressing your finger gently on the skin just beneath the lower eyelid, pull the lower eyelid away from the eye to make a space. Squeeze a thin strip of ointment into this space. A ⅓- to ½-cm (approximately ⅛-inch in infants and young children and ¼-inch in older children and adults) strip of ointment is usually enough, unless you have been told by your doctor to use a different amount. Let go of the eyelid and gently close the eyes. Keep the eyes closed for 1 or 2 minutes to allow the medicine to be absorbed by the eye.
- Immediately after using the eye ointment, wash your hands to remove any medicine that may be on them. If you are using the eye ointment for an infant or child, be sure to wash his or her hands immediately afterwards also, and do not let any of the medicine get in his or her mouth. In addition, wipe off any medicine that may have accidentally gotten on the infant or child, including his or her face or eyelids.
- To keep the medicine as germ-free as possible, do not touch the applicator tip to any surface (including the eye). After using the eye ointment, wipe the tip of the ointment tube with a clean tissue and keep the tube tightly closed.

*Use this medicine only as directed.* Do not use more of it and do not use it more often than your doctor ordered. To do so may increase the chance of too much medicine being absorbed into the body and the chance of side effects. *This is especially important when this medicine is used in infants and children, since overdose is very dangerous in infants and children.*

**Dosing**—The doses of these medicines will be different for different patients. *Follow your doctor's orders or the directions on the label.* The following information includes only the average doses of these medicines. *If your dose is different, do not change it* unless your doctor tells you to do so.

The number of doses you use each day, the time allowed between doses, and the length of time you use the medicine depend on the medical problem for which you are using atropine, homatropine, or scopolamine.

*For atropine*

- For *ophthalmic ointment* dosage form:
  —For uveitis:
  - Adults—Use a thin strip of the ointment in the eye one or two times a day.

- Children—Use a thin strip of the ointment in the eye one to three times a day.
  —For eye examinations:
    - Adults—Use and dose must be determined by your doctor.
    - Children—Use a thin strip of the ointment in the eye three times a day for one to three days before the examination.
- For *ophthalmic solution (eye drops)* dosage form:
  —For uveitis:
    - Adults—Use one drop in the eye one or two times a day.
    - Children—Use one drop in the eye one to three times a day.
  —For eye examinations:
    - Adults—Use and dose must be determined by your doctor.
    - Children—Use one drop in the eye two times a day for one to three days before the examination.

*For homatropine*

- For *ophthalmic solution (eye drops)* dosage form:
  —For uveitis:
    - Adults and children—Use one drop in the eye two or three times a day.
  —For eye examinations:
    - Adults—Use one drop in the eye. May be repeated every five to ten minutes for two or three doses.
    - Children—Use one drop in the eye every ten minutes for two or three doses.

*For scopolamine*

- For *ophthalmic solution (eye drops)* dosage form:
  —For uveitis:
    - Adults and children—Use one drop in the eye up to four times a day.
  —For eye examinations:
    - Adults—Use one drop in the eye one hour before the examination.
    - Children—Use one drop in the eye two times a day for two days before the examination.
  —For posterior synechiae:
    - Adults—Use one drop in the eye every ten minutes for three doses.
    - Children—Use and dose must be determined by your doctor.
  —For use before and after surgery:
    - Adults and children—Use one drop in the eye one to four times a day.

**Missed dose**—If you miss a dose of this medicine and your dosing schedule is:

- One dose a day—Apply the missed dose as soon as possible. However, if you do not remember the missed dose until the next day, skip the missed dose and go back to your regular dosing schedule. Do not double doses.
- More than one dose a day—Apply the missed dose as soon as possible. However, if it is almost time for your next dose, skip the missed dose and go back to your regular dosing schedule. Do not double doses.

**Storage**—To store this medicine:

- Keep out of the reach of children. Overdose of this medicine is very dangerous for infants and children.
- Store away from heat and direct light.
- Keep this medicine from freezing.
- Do not keep outdated medicine or medicine no longer needed. Be sure that any discarded medicine is out of the reach of children.

## Precautions While Using This Medicine

After you apply this medicine to your eyes:

- Your pupils will become unusually large and you will have blurring of vision, especially for close objects. *Make sure your vision is clear before you drive, use machines, or do anything else that could be dangerous if you are not able to see well.*
- Your eyes will become more sensitive to light than they are normally. *Wear sunglasses to protect your eyes from sunlight and other bright lights.*

These effects may continue for several days after you stop using this medicine. However, check with your doctor if they continue longer than:

- 14 days if you are using atropine.
- 3 days if you are using homatropine.
- 7 days if you are using scopolamine.

## Side Effects of This Medicine

Along with its needed effects, a medicine may cause some unwanted effects. Although not all of these side effects may occur, if they do occur they may need medical attention.

*Check with your doctor immediately* if any of the following side effects occur:

*Symptoms of too much medicine being absorbed into the body*

Clumsiness or unsteadiness; confusion or unusual behavior; dizziness; dryness of skin; fast or irregular heartbeat; fever; flushing or redness of face; hallucinations (seeing, hearing, or feeling things that are not there); skin rash; slurred speech; swollen stomach in infants; thirst or unusual dryness of mouth; unusual drowsiness, tiredness, or weakness

Other side effects may occur that usually do not need medical attention. These side effects may go away during treatment as your body adjusts to the medicine. However, check with your doctor if any of the following side effects continue or are bothersome:

> Blurred vision; eye irritation not present before use of this medicine; increased sensitivity of eyes to light; swelling of the eyelids

Other side effects not listed above may also occur in some patients. If you notice any other effects, check with your doctor.

---

Revised: 06/21/94

---

# ATROPINE, HYOSCYAMINE, METHENAMINE, METHYLENE BLUE, PHENYL SALICYLATE, AND BENZOIC ACID  Systemic†

Some commonly used brand names are:

**In the U.S.—**

| | |
|---|---|
| Atrosept | Urimed |
| Dolsed | Urinary Antiseptic No. 2 |
| Hexalol | Urised |
| Prosed/DS | Uriseptic |
| Trac Tabs 2X | Uritab |
| UAA | Uritin |
| Uridon Modified | Uro-Ves |

---

†Not commercially available in Canada.

---

## Description

Atropine (A-troe-peen), hyoscyamine (hye-oh-SYE-a-meen), methenamine (meth-EN-a-meen), methylene (METH-i-leen) blue, phenyl salicylate (FEN-ill sa-LI-si-late), and benzoic acid (ben-ZOE-ik AS-id) combination medicine is an anticholinergic, anti-infective, and analgesic. It is given by mouth to help relieve the discomfort caused by urinary tract infections; however, it will not cure the infection itself. This combination medicine may also be used for other conditions as determined by your doctor.

This medicine is available only with your doctor's prescription in the following dosage form:

*Oral*
- Tablets (U.S.)

---

## Before Using This Medicine

In deciding to use a medicine, the risks of taking the medicine must be weighed against the good it will do. This is a decision you and your doctor will make. For this combination medicine, the following should be considered:

**Allergies**—Tell your doctor if you have ever had any unusual or allergic reaction to any of the belladonna alkaloids such as atropine, hyoscyamine, and scopolamine, or to aspirin or other salicylates. Also tell your health care professional if you are allergic to any other substances, such as foods, preservatives, or dyes.

**Diet**—While you are taking this combination medicine, it is important for your urine to be acidic. To do this, your doctor may recommend that you eat more protein and such foods as cranberries (especially cranberry juice with vitamin C added), plums, or prunes. You should avoid foods that make the urine more alkaline, such as most fruits (especially citrus fruits and juices), milk, and other dairy products.

**Pregnancy**—Studies have not been done in either humans or animals.

**Breast-feeding**—Although methenamine and very small amounts of atropine and hyoscyamine (contained in this combination medicine) pass into the breast milk, this medicine has not been reported to cause problems in nursing babies.

**Children**—Unusual excitement, nervousness, restlessness or irritability, and unusual warmth, dryness, and flushing of skin are more likely to occur in children, who are usually more sensitive to the effects of atropine and hyoscyamine (contained in this combination medicine). Also, when atropine and hyoscyamine are given to children during hot weather, a rapid increase in body temperature may occur. In infants and children, especially those with spastic paralysis or brain damage, this medicine may be more likely to cause severe side effects.

**Older adults**—Confusion or memory loss, constipation, difficult urination, excitement, agitation, drowsiness, or dryness of mouth may be more likely to occur in elderly patients, who are usually more sensitive than younger adults to the effects of atropine and hyoscyamine. Also, this combination medicine may cause eye pain in patients who have untreated glaucoma.

**Other medicines**—Although certain medicines should not be used together at all, in other cases two different medicines may be used together even if an interaction might occur. In these cases, your doctor may want to change the dose, or other precautions may be necessary. When you are taking this combination medicine, it is especially important that your health care professional know if you are taking any of the following:

- Antacids or
- Diarrhea medicine containing kaolin or attapulgite or
- Thiazide diuretics (water pills) or
- Urinary alkalizers (medicine that makes the urine less acid, such as acetazolamide [e.g., Diamox], calcium- and/or magnesium-containing antacids, dichlorphenamide [e.g., Daranide], methazolamide [e.g., Neptazone], potassium

or sodium citrate and/or citric acid, sodium bicarbonate [baking soda])—Use with these medicines may decrease the effects of this combination medicine
- Ketoconazole (e.g., Nizoral)—Use with this combination medicine may reduce the effects of ketoconazole
- Other anticholinergics (medicine for abdominal or stomach spasms or cramps)—Use with these medicines may increase the effects of atropine and hyoscyamine
- Potassium chloride (e.g., Slow K or K-Dur)—May worsen or cause an increase in lesions (sores) of the stomach or intestine
- Sulfonamides (sulfa medicine)—Use with this combination medicine may increase the risk of crystals forming in the urine

**Other medical problems**—The presence of other medical problems may affect the use of this combination medicine. Make sure you tell your doctor if you have any other medical problems, especially:
- Bleeding problems (severe)—This combination medicine may increase heart rate, which would make bleeding problems worse
- Brain damage (in children)—May increase the central nervous system (CNS) effects of this combination medicine
- Colitis (severe) or
- Dryness of mouth (severe or continuing) or
- Enlarged prostate or
- Fever or
- Glaucoma or
- Heart disease or
- Hernia (hiatal) or
- High blood pressure or
- Intestinal blockage or other intestinal or stomach problems or
- Lung disease or
- Myasthenia gravis or
- Toxemia of pregnancy or
- Urinary tract blockage or difficult urination—This combination medicine may make these conditions worse
- Dehydration or
- Kidney disease or
- Liver disease—Higher levels of medicine may result and increase the risk of side effects
- Overactive thyroid—May increase the heart rate

## Proper Use of This Medicine

*Take this medicine only as directed.* Do not take more of it, do not take it more often, and do not take it for a longer time than your doctor ordered. To do so may increase the chance of side effects.

Each dose should be taken with a full glass (8 ounces) of water or other liquid (except citrus juices and milk). Drink plenty of water or other liquids every day, unless otherwise directed by your doctor. Drinking enough liquids will help your kidneys work better and lessen your discomfort.

To help clear up your infection completely, *keep taking this medicine for the full time of treatment* even if you begin to feel better after a few days. *Do not miss any doses.*

*In order for this medicine to work well, your urine must be acid (pH 5.5 or below).* To make sure that your urine is acid:
- Before you start taking this medicine, check your urine with phenaphthazine paper or another test to see if it is acid. If you have any questions about this, check with your health care professional.
- You may need to change your diet; however, check with your doctor first if you are on a special diet (for example, for diabetes). To help make your urine more acid you should avoid most fruits (especially citrus fruits and juices), milk and other dairy products, and other foods which make the urine more alkaline. Eating more protein and foods such as cranberries (especially cranberry juice with vitamin C added), plums, or prunes may also help. If your urine is still not acid enough, check with your doctor.

**Dosing**—The dose of this combination medicine will be different for different patients. *Follow your doctor's orders or the direction on the label.* The following information includes only the average doses of this combination medicine. *If your dose is different, do not change it* unless your doctor tells you to do so.
- For *oral* dosage form (tablets):
  —For relief of urinary tract symptoms:
    • Adults and children 12 years of age and older— 1 to 2 tablets four times a day.
    • Children 6 to 12 years of age—Dose must be determined by the doctor.
    • Children up to 6 years of age—Use is not recommended.

**Missed dose**—If you miss a dose of this medicine, take it as soon as possible. However, if it is almost time for your next dose, skip the missed dose and go back to your regular dosing schedule. Do not double doses.

**Storage**—To store this medicine:
- Keep out of the reach of children.
- Store away from heat and direct light.
- Do not store this medicine in the bathroom, near the kitchen sink, or in other damp places. Heat or moisture may cause the medicine to break down.
- Do not keep outdated medicine or medicine no longer needed. Be sure that any discarded medicine is out of the reach of children.

## Precautions While Using This Medicine

If your symptoms do not improve within a few days or if they become worse, check with your doctor.

These medicines may make you sweat less, causing your body temperature to increase. *Use extra care not to become overheated during exercise or hot weather while you are taking this medicine,* since overheating may result in heat stroke. Also, hot baths or saunas may make you dizzy or faint while you are taking this medicine.

This medicine may cause some people to have blurred vision. *Make sure you know how you react to this medicine before you drive, use machines, or do anything else that could be dangerous if you are not able to see well. If your vision continues to be blurred, check with your doctor.*

This medicine may cause dryness of the mouth. For temporary relief, use sugarless candy or gum, melt bits of ice in your mouth, or use a saliva substitute. However, if your mouth continues to feel dry for more than 2 weeks, check with your dentist. Continuing dryness of the mouth may increase the chance of dental disease, including tooth decay, gum disease, and fungus infections.

Do not take this medicine within 2 or 3 hours of taking antacids or medicine for diarrhea. Taking antacids or antidiarrhea medicines and this medicine too close together may prevent this medicine from working properly.

## Side Effects of This Medicine

Along with its needed effects, a medicine may cause some unwanted effects. Although not all of these side effects may occur, if they do occur they may need medical attention.

Check with your doctor as soon as possible if any of the following side effects occur:

*Less common or rare*
> Blurred vision; eye pain; skin rash or hives

*Symptoms of overdose*
> Blood in urine and/or stools; diarrhea; dizziness; drowsiness (severe); fast heartbeat; flushing or redness of face; headache (severe or continuing); lower back pain; pain or burning while urinating; ringing or buzzing in the ears; shortness of breath or troubled breathing; sweating; unusual tiredness or weakness

Other side effects may occur that usually do not need medical attention. These side effects may go away during treatment as your body adjusts to the medicine. However, check with your doctor if any of the following side effects continue or are bothersome:

*Less common*
> Difficult urination (more common with large doses taken over a prolonged period of time); dryness of mouth, nose, or throat; nausea or vomiting; stomach upset or pain (more common with large doses taken over a prolonged period of time)

This medicine may cause your urine and/or stools to turn blue or blue-green. This is to be expected while you are taking this medicine.

Other side effects not listed above may also occur in some patients. If you notice any other effects, check with your doctor.

Revised: 05/11/93

---

# ATTAPULGITE Oral

Some commonly used brand names are:

**In the U.S.—**

| | |
|---|---|
| Diar-Aid | Kaopectate Maximum |
| Diasorb | Strength |
| Donnagel | K-Pek |
| Kaopectate | Parepectolin |
| Kaopectate Advanced Formula | Rheaban |

**In Canada—**

| | |
|---|---|
| Fowler's Diarrhea Tablets | Kaopectate |

## Description

Attapulgite (at-a-PULL-gite) is taken by mouth to treat diarrhea. Attapulgite is a clay-like powder believed to work by adsorbing the bacteria or germ that may be causing the diarrhea.

This medicine is available without a prescription; however, the product's directions and warnings should be carefully followed. In addition, your doctor may have special instructions on the proper dose or use of attapulgite medicine for your medical condition.

Attapulgite is available in the following dosage forms:

*Oral*
> Attapulgite
> • Oral suspension (U.S. and Canada)
> • Tablets (U.S. and Canada)
> • Chewable tablets (U.S. and Canada)

## Before Using This Medicine

If you are taking this medicine without a prescription, carefully read and follow any precautions on the label. For attapulgite, the following should be considered:

**Pregnancy**—This medicine is not absorbed into the body and is not likely to cause problems.

**Breast-feeding**—This medicine is not absorbed into the body and is not likely to cause problems.

**Children**—The fluid loss caused by diarrhea may result in a severe condition. For this reason, antidiarrheals must not be given to young children (under 3 years of age) without first checking with their doctor. In older children with diarrhea, antidiarrheals may be used, but it is also very important that a sufficient amount of liquids be given to replace the fluid lost by the body. If you have any questions about this, check with your health care professional.

**Older adults**—The fluid loss caused by diarrhea may result in a severe condition. For this reason, elderly persons with diarrhea, in addition to using an antidiarrheal, must receive a sufficient amount of liquids to replace the fluid lost by the body. If you have any questions about this, check with your health care professional.

**Other medicines**—Although certain medicines should not be used together at all, in other cases two different medicines may be used together even if an interaction might occur. In these cases, your doctor may want to change the dose, or other precautions may be necessary. *If you are taking any other medicine, do not take it within 2 to 3 hours of attapulgite.* Taking the medicines at the same time may prevent the other medicine from being absorbed by your body. If you have any questions about this, check with your health care professional.

**Other medical problems**—The presence of other medical problems may affect the use of attapulgite. Make sure you tell your doctor if you have any other medical problems, especially:

- Dysentery—This condition may get worse; a different kind of treatment may be needed

## Proper Use of This Medicine

*Do not use attapulgite to treat your diarrhea if you have a fever or if there is blood or mucus in your stools.* Contact your doctor.

Take this medicine after each loose bowel movement following the directions in the product package, unless otherwise directed by your doctor.

*Importance of diet and fluid intake while treating diarrhea:*

- *In addition to using medicine for diarrhea, it is very important that you replace the fluid lost by the body and follow a proper diet.* For the first 24 hours you should eat gelatin and drink plenty of clear liquids, such as ginger ale, decaffeinated cola, decaffeinated tea, and broth. During the next 24 hours you may eat bland foods, such as cooked cereals, bread, crackers, and applesauce. Fruits, vegetables, fried or spicy foods, bran, candy, and caffeine and alcoholic beverages may make the condition worse.
- If too much fluid has been lost by the body due to the diarrhea a serious condition may develop. Check with your doctor as soon as possible if any of the following occurs:
  Decreased urination
  Dizziness and lightheadedness
  Dryness of mouth
  Increased thirst
  Wrinkled skin

**Dosing**—The dose of attapulgite will be different for different patients. *Follow your doctor's orders or the directions on the label.* The following information includes only the average doses of attapulgite.

The number of tablets or teaspoonfuls of suspension that you take depends on the strength of the medicine.

- For diarrhea:
  —For *oral* dosage form (suspension):
  - Adults and children 12 years of age and older—The usual dose is 1200 to 1500 milligrams (mg) taken after each loose bowel movement. No more than 9000 mg should be taken in twenty-four hours.
  - Children 6 to 12 years of age—The usual dose is 600 mg taken after each loose bowel movement. No more than 4200 mg should be taken in twenty-four hours.
  - Children 3 to 6 years of age—The usual dose is 300 mg taken after each loose bowel movement. No more than 2100 mg should be taken in twenty-four hours.
  - Children up to 3 years of age—Use and dose must be determined by your doctor.
  —For *oral* dosage form (tablets):
  - Adults and children 12 years of age and older—The usual dose is 1200 to 1500 mg taken after each loose bowel movement. No more than 9000 mg should be taken in twenty-four hours.
  - Children 6 to 12 years of age—The usual dose is 750 mg taken after each loose bowel movement. No more than 4500 mg should be taken in twenty-four hours.
  - Children 3 to 6 years of age—The oral suspension dosage form should be used in this age group.
  —For *oral* dosage form (chewable tablets):
  - Adults and children 12 years of age and older—The usual dose is 1200 mg taken after each loose bowel movement. No more than 8400 mg should be taken in twenty-four hours.
  - Children 6 to 12 years of age—The usual dose is 600 mg taken after each loose bowel movement. No more than 4200 mg should be taken in twenty-four hours.
  - Children 3 to 6 years of age—The usual dose is 300 mg taken after each loose bowel movement. No more than 2100 mg should be taken in twenty-four hours.
  - Children up to 3 years of age—Use and dose must be determined by your doctor.

**Storage**—To store this medicine:
- Keep out of the reach of children.
- Store away from heat and direct light.
- Keep the liquid form of this medicine from freezing.
- Do not keep outdated medicine or medicine no longer needed. Be sure that any discarded medicine is out of the reach of children.

## Precautions While Using This Medicine

*Check with your doctor if your diarrhea does not stop after 1 or 2 days or if you develop a fever.*

## Side Effects of This Medicine

Along with its needed effects, a medicine may cause some unwanted effects. No serious side effects have been reported for this medicine. However, constipation may occur in some patients, especially if they take a lot of it. Check with your doctor as soon as possible if constipation continues or is bothersome.

Other side effects not listed above may also occur in some patients. If you notice any other effects, check with your doctor.

Revised: 08/12/94

---

# AZATHIOPRINE  Systemic

A commonly used brand name in the U.S. and Canada is Imuran.

## Description

Azathioprine (ay-za-THYE-oh-preen) belongs to the group of medicines known as immunosuppressive agents. It is used to reduce the body's natural immunity in patients who receive organ transplants. It is also used to treat rheumatoid arthritis. Azathioprine may also be used for other conditions as determined by your doctor.

Azathioprine is a very strong medicine. You and your doctor should talk about the need for this medicine and its risks. Even though azathioprine may cause side effects that could be very serious, remember that it may be required to treat your medical problem.

Azathioprine is available only with your doctor's prescription, in the following dosage forms:

*Oral*
- Tablets (U.S. and Canada)

*Parenteral*
- Injection (U.S. and Canada)

## Before Using This Medicine

In deciding to use a medicine, the risks of taking the medicine must be weighed against the good it will do. This is a decision you and your doctor will make. For azathioprine, the following should be considered:

**Allergies**—Tell your doctor if you have ever had any unusual or allergic reaction to azathioprine. Also tell your health care professional if you are allergic to any other substances, such as foods, preservatives, or dyes.

**Pregnancy**—Use of azathioprine is not recommended during pregnancy. It may cause birth defects if either the male or the female is using it at the time of conception. The use of birth control methods is recommended. If you have any questions about this, check with your doctor.

**Breast-feeding**—Azathioprine passes into breast milk. Because this medicine may cause serious side effects, breast-feeding is generally not recommended while you are using it.

**Children**—This medicine has been tested in children and, in effective doses, has not been shown to cause different side effects or problems than it does in adults.

**Older adults**—Many medicines have not been studied specifically in older people. Therefore, it may not be known whether they work exactly the same way they do in younger adults. Although there is no specific information comparing use of azathioprine in the elderly with use in other age groups, this medicine is not expected to cause different side effects or problems in older people than it does in younger adults.

**Other medicines**—Although certain medicines should not be used together at all, in other cases two different medicines may be used together even if an interaction might occur. In these cases, your doctor may want to change the dose, or other precautions may be necessary. When you are taking or receiving azathioprine it is especially important that your health care professional know if you are taking any of the following:
- Allopurinol (e.g., Zyloprim)—May interfere with removal of azathioprine from the body; effects of azathioprine (including toxicity) may be increased
- Chlorambucil (e.g., Leukeran) or
- Corticosteroids (cortisone-like medicine) or
- Cyclophosphamide (e.g., Cytoxan) or
- Cyclosporine (e.g., Sandimmune) or
- Mercaptopurine (e.g., Purinethol) or
- Muromonab-CD3 (monoclonal antibody) (e.g., Orthoclone OKT3)—There may be an increased risk of infection and cancer because azathioprine reduces the body's ability to fight them

**Other medical problems**—The presence of other medical problems may affect the use azathioprine. Make sure you tell your doctor if you have any other medical problems, especially:
- Chickenpox (including recent exposure) or
- Herpes zoster (shingles)—Risk of severe disease affecting other parts of the body
- Gout—Allopurinol (used to treat gout) may increase wanted and unwanted effects of azathioprine
- Infection—Azathioprine decreases your body's ability to fight infection
- Kidney disease or
- Liver disease—Effects of azathioprine may be increased because of slower removal from the body

• Pancreatitis (inflammation of the pancreas)—Azathioprine can cause pancreatitis

## Proper Use of This Medicine

*Use this medicine only as directed by your doctor.* Do not use more or less of it, and do not use it more often than your doctor ordered. The exact amount of medicine you need has been carefully worked out. Taking too much may increase the chance of side effects, while taking too little may not properly treat your condition.

This medicine is sometimes given together with certain other medicines. If you are using a combination of medicines, make sure that you take each one at the proper time and do not mix them up. Ask your health care professional to help you plan a way to remember to take your medicines at the right times.

*Do not stop taking this medicine without first checking with your doctor.*

Azathioprine sometimes causes nausea or vomiting. Taking this medicine after meals or at bedtime may lessen stomach upset. Ask your health care professional for other ways to lessen these effects.

If you vomit shortly after taking a dose of azathioprine, check with your doctor. You will be told whether to take the dose again or to wait until the next scheduled dose.

**Dosing**—The dose of azathioprine will be different for different patients. Follow your doctor's orders or the directions on the label. The following information includes only the average doses of azathioprine. *If your dose is different, do not change it* unless your doctor tells you to do so.

*The number of doses you take each day, the time allowed between doses, and the length of time you take the medicine depend on the medical problem for which you are taking azathioprine.*

• For *oral* dosage form (tablets):
  —For transplant rejection:
    • Adults, teenagers, and children: Dose is based on body weight or size. The usual beginning dose is 3 to 5 milligrams (mg) per kilogram (kg) (1.5 to 2 mg per pound) of body weight a day. As time goes on, your doctor may lower your dose to 1 to 2 mg per kg (0.5 to 1 mg per pound) a day.
  —For rheumatoid arthritis:
    • Adults, teenagers, and children: Dose is based on body weight or size. The usual beginning dose is 1 mg per kg (0.5 mg per pound) of body weight a day. Your doctor will increase this dose as needed. The highest dose is usually not more than 2.5 mg per kg (1 mg per pound) a day. Your doctor may then lower your dose as needed.
• For *injection* dosage form:
  —For transplant rejection:
    • Adults, teenagers, and children: Dose is based on body weight or size. The usual beginning dose is 3 to 5 milligrams (mg) per kilogram (kg) (1.5 to 2 mg per pound) of body weight a day. As time goes on, your doctor may lower your dose to 1 to 2 mg per kg (0.5 to 1 mg per pound) a day.

**Missed dose**—If you miss a dose of this medicine and your dosing schedule is:

• One dose a day—Do not take the missed dose at all and do not double the next one. Instead, go back to your regular dosing schedule and check with your doctor.
• More than one dose a day—Take the missed dose as soon as you remember it. If it is time for your next dose, take both doses together, then go back to your regular dosing schedule. If you miss more than one dose, check with your doctor.

**Storage**—To store this medicine:
• Keep out of the reach of children.
• Store away from heat and direct light.
• Do not store in the bathroom, near the kitchen sink, or in other damp places. Heat or moisture may cause the medicine to break down.
• Do not keep outdated medicine or medicine no longer needed. Be sure that any discarded medicine is out of the reach of children.

## Precautions While Using This Medicine

*It is very important that your doctor check your progress at regular visits* to make sure that this medicine is working properly and to check for unwanted effects.

While you are being treated with azathioprine, and after you stop treatment with it, *do not have any immunizations (vaccinations) without your doctor's approval.* Azathioprine lowers your body's resistance and there is a chance you might get the infection the immunization is meant to prevent. In addition, other persons living in your household should not take oral polio vaccine since there is a chance they could pass the polio virus on to you. Also, avoid persons who have recently taken oral polio vaccine. Do not get close to them, and do not stay in the same room with them for very long. If you cannot take these precautions, you should consider wearing a protective face mask that covers the nose and mouth.

Azathioprine can temporarily lower the number of white blood cells in your blood, increasing the chance of getting an infection. It can also lower the number of platelets, which are necessary for proper blood clotting. If this occurs, there are certain precautions you can take, especially when your blood count is low, to reduce the risk of infection or bleeding:

• If you can, avoid people with infections. *Check with your doctor immediately* if you think you are getting an infection or if you get a fever or chills, cough or hoarseness, lower back or side pain, or painful or difficult urination.
• *Check with your doctor immediately* if you notice any unusual bleeding or bruising; black, tarry stools;

blood in urine or stools; or pinpoint red spots on your skin.

- Be careful when using a regular toothbrush, dental floss, or toothpick. Your medical doctor, dentist, or nurse may recommend other ways to clean your teeth and gums. Check with your health care professional before having any dental work done.
- Do not touch your eyes or the inside of your nose unless you have just washed your hands and have not touched anything else in the meantime.
- Be careful not to cut yourself when you are using sharp objects such as a safety razor or fingernail or toenail cutters.
- Avoid contact sports or other situations where bruising or injury could occur.

## Side Effects of This Medicine

Along with its needed effects, a medicine may cause some unwanted effects. Some side effects will have signs or symptoms that you can see or feel. Your doctor will watch for others by doing certain tests.

Also, because of the way these medicines act on the body, there is a chance that they might cause other unwanted effects that may not occur until months or years after the medicine is used. These delayed effects may include certain types of cancer, such as leukemia, lymphoma, or skin cancer. However, the risk of cancer seems to be lower in people taking azathioprine for arthritis. Discuss these possible effects with your doctor.

*Check with your doctor immediately* if any of the following side effects occur:

*More common*
Unusual tiredness or weakness

*Less common*
Cough or hoarseness; fever or chills; lower back or side pain; painful or difficult urination

*Rare*
Black, tarry stools; blood in urine or stools; fast heartbeat; fever (sudden); muscle or joint pain; nausea, vomiting, and diarrhea (severe); pinpoint red spots on skin; redness or blisters on skin; stomach pain (severe) with nausea and vomiting; unusual bleeding or bruising; unusual feeling of discomfort or illness (sudden)

Check with your doctor as soon as possible if any of the following side effects occur:

*Rare*
Shortness of breath; sores in mouth and on lips; stomach pain; swelling of feet or lower legs

This medicine may also cause the following side effect that your doctor will watch for:

*Less common*
Liver problems

For patients taking this medicine *for rheumatoid arthritis:*

- Signs and symptoms of blood problems (black, tarry stools; blood in urine or stools; cough or hoarseness;

fever or chills; lower back or side pain; painful or difficult urination; pinpoint red spots on skin; unusual tiredness or weakness; or unusual bleeding or bruising) are less likely to occur in patients taking azathioprine for rheumatoid arthritis than for transplant rejection. This is because lower doses are often used.

Other side effects may occur that usually do not need medical attention. These side effects may go away during treatment as your body adjusts to the medicine. However, check with your doctor if any of the following side effects continue or are bothersome:

*More common*
Loss of appetite; nausea or vomiting

*Less common*
Skin rash

After you stop using this medicine, it may still produce some side effects that need attention. During this period of time *check with your doctor immediately* if you notice any of the following:

Black, tarry stools; blood in urine; cough or hoarseness; fever or chills; lower back or side pain; painful or difficult urination; pinpoint red spots on skin; unusual bleeding or bruising

Other side effects not listed above may also occur in some patients. If you notice any other effects, check with your doctor.

## Additional Information

Once a medicine has been approved for marketing for a certain use, experience may show that it is also useful for other medical problems. Although these uses are not included in product labeling, azathioprine is used in certain patients with the following medical conditions:

- Bowel disease, inflammatory
- Hepatitis, chronic active
- Cirrhosis, biliary
- Lupus erythematosus, systemic
- Glomerulonephritis
- Nephrotic syndrome
- Myopathy, inflammatory
- Myasthenia gravis
- Dermatomyositis, systemic
- Pemphigoid
- Pemphigus

Other than the above information, there is no additional information relating to proper use, precautions, or side effects for these uses.

Revised: 05/06/93
Interim revision: 04/29/94

# AZITHROMYCIN   Systemic

A commonly used brand name in the U.S. and Canada is Zithromax.

## Description

Azithromycin (az-ith-roe-MYE-sin) is used to treat bacterial infections in many different parts of the body. It works by killing bacteria or preventing their growth. However, this medicine will not work for colds, flu, or other virus infections. Azithromycin may be used for other problems as determined by your doctor.

Azithromycin is available only with your doctor's prescription, in the following dosage form:

*Oral*
- Capsules (U.S. and Canada)

## Before Using This Medicine

In deciding to use a medicine, the risks of taking the medicine must be weighed against the good it will do. This is a decision you and your doctor will make. For azithromycin, the following should be considered:

**Allergies**—Tell your doctor if you have ever had any unusual or allergic reaction to azithromycin or to any related medicines such as erythromycin. Also tell your health care professional if you are allergic to any other substances, such as foods, preservatives, or dyes.

**Pregnancy**—Azithromycin has not been studied in pregnant women. However, azithromycin has not been shown to cause birth defects or other problems in animal studies.

**Breast-feeding**—It is not known whether azithromycin passes into breast milk. Although most medicines pass into breast milk in small amounts, many of them may be used safely while breast-feeding. Mothers who are taking this medicine and who wish to breast-feed should discuss this with their doctor.

**Children**—This medicine has been tested in a limited number of children up to the age of 16. In effective doses, the medicine has not been shown to cause different side effects or problems than it does in adults.

**Older adults**—This medicine has been tested in a limited number of elderly patients and has not been shown to cause different side effects or problems in older people than it does in younger adults.

**Other medicines**—Although certain medicines should not be used together at all, in other cases two different medicines may be used together even if an interaction might occur. In these cases, your doctor may want to change the dose, or other precautions may be necessary. When you are taking azithromycin, it is especially important that your health care professional know if you are taking any of the following:

- Antacids, aluminum- and magnesium-containing—Antacids may decrease the amount of azithromycin in the blood, which may decrease its effects. To avoid problems,

azithromycin should be taken at least 1 hour before or at least 2 hours after antacids

**Other medical problems**—The presence of other medical problems may affect the use of azithromycin. Make sure you tell your doctor if you have any other medical problems, especially:

- Liver disease—Patients with severe liver disease may have an increased chance of side effects

## Proper Use of This Medicine

Azithromycin should be taken at least one hour before or at least 2 hours after meals. Taking azithromycin with food may decrease the amount of medicine that gets into your blood and keep the medicine from working properly.

To help clear up your infection completely, *keep taking azithromycin for the full time of treatment,* even if you begin to feel better after a few days. If you stop taking this medicine too soon, your symptoms may return.

**Dosing**—The dose of azithromycin will be different for different patients. *Follow your doctor's orders or the directions on the label.* The following information includes only the average doses of azithromycin. *If your dose is different, do not change it* unless your doctor tells you to do so.

The number of capsules that you take depends on the medical problem for which you are taking azithromycin.

- For *oral* dosage form (capsules):
  —For bronchitis, strep throat, pneumonia, and skin infections:
    - Adults and children 16 years of age and older—500 milligrams (mg) on the first day, then 250 mg once a day on the second through fifth days.
    - Children up to 16 years of age—Use and dose must be determined by your doctor.
  —For chlamydia infections:
    - Adults and children 16 years of age and older—1000 mg taken once as a single dose.
    - Children up to 16 years of age—Use and dose must be determined by your doctor.

**Missed dose**—If you miss a dose of this medicine, take it as soon as possible. However, if it is almost time for your next dose, skip the missed dose and go back to your regular dosing schedule. Do not double doses.

**Storage**—To store this medicine:
- Keep out of the reach of children.
- Store away from heat and direct light.
- Do not store in the bathroom, near the kitchen sink, or in other damp places. Heat or moisture may cause the medicine to break down.
- Do not keep outdated medicine or medicine no longer needed. Be sure that any discarded medicine is out of the reach of children.

## Precautions While Using This Medicine

If your symptoms do not improve within a few days, or if they become worse, check with your doctor.

## Side Effects of This Medicine

Along with its needed effects, a medicine may cause some unwanted effects. Although not all of these side effects may occur, if they do occur they may need medical attention.

*Stop taking this medicine and get emergency help immediately if any of the following side effects occur:*

*Rare*
Difficulty in breathing; fever; joint pain; skin rash; swelling of face, mouth, neck, hands, and feet

Other side effects may occur that usually do not need medical attention. These side effects may go away during treatment as your body adjusts to the medicine. However, check with your doctor if any of the following side effects continue or are bothersome:

*Less common*
Diarrhea; nausea; stomach pain or discomfort; vomiting

*Rare*
Dizziness; headache

Other side effects not listed above may also occur in some patients. If you notice any other effects, check with your doctor.

## Additional Information

Once a medicine has been approved for marketing for a certain use, experience may show that it is also useful for other medical problems. Although this use is not included in product labeling, azithromycin is used in certain patients with the following medical condition:

* Mycoplasmal pneumonia

Other than the above information, there is no additional information relating to proper use, precautions, or side effects for this use.

Revised: 05/27/94
Interim revision: 06/28/94

---

# AZTREONAM Systemic†

A commonly used brand name in the U.S. is Azactam.

†Not commercially available in Canada.

## Description

Aztreonam (az-TREE-oh-nam) is an antibiotic that is used to treat infections caused by bacteria. It works by killing bacteria or preventing their growth.

Aztreonam is used to treat bacterial infections in many different parts of the body. It is sometimes given with other antibiotics. This medicine will not work for colds, flu, or other virus infections.

This medicine is available only with your doctor's prescription. It is available in the following dosage form:

*Parenteral*
* Injection (U.S.)

## Before Receiving This Medicine

In deciding to use a medicine, the risks of taking the medicine must be weighed against the good it will do. This is a decision you and your doctor will make. For aztreonam, the following should be considered:

**Allergies**—Tell your doctor if you have ever had any unusual or allergic reaction to aztreonam. Also tell your health care professional if you are allergic to any other substances, such as foods, preservatives, or dyes.

**Pregnancy**—Studies have not been done in humans. However, aztreonam has not been shown to cause birth defects or other problems in studies in rabbits and rats given up to 15 times the highest human daily dose.

**Breast-feeding**—Aztreonam passes into the breast milk in small amounts. However, this medicine is not absorbed when taken by mouth, and problems have not been seen in nursing babies.

**Children**—This medicine has been tested in a limited number of children up to 12 years of age and has not been shown to cause different side effects or problems in children than it does in adults.

**Older adults**—Aztreonam has been tested in a limited number of patients 65 years of age or older and has not been shown to cause different side effects or problems in older people than it does in younger adults.

**Other medicines**—Although certain medicines should not be used together at all, in other cases two different medicines may be used together even if an interaction might occur. In these cases, your doctor may want to change the dose, or other precautions may be necessary. Tell your health care professional if you are taking any other prescription or nonprescription (over-the-counter [OTC]) medicine.

**Other medical problems**—The presence of other medical problems may affect the use of aztreonam. Make sure

you tell your doctor if you have any other medical problems, especially:

- Cirrhosis (liver disease)—Patients receiving high doses of aztreonam for a long time, who also have severe liver disease, may have an increased chance of side effects
- Kidney disease—Patients with kidney disease may have an increased chance of side effects

## Proper Use of This Medicine

To help clear up your infection completely, *aztreonam must be given for the full time of treatment,* even if you begin to feel better after a few days. Also, this medicine works best when there is a constant amount in the blood or urine. To help keep the amount constant, aztreonam must be given on a regular schedule.

**Dosing**—The dose of aztreonam will be different for different patients. *Follow your doctor's orders or the directions on the label.* The following information includes only the average doses of aztreonam. Your dose may be different if you have kidney disease. *If your dose is different, do not change it* unless your doctor tells you to do so.

- For *injection* dosage form:
  —Adults and children 12 years of age and older: 1 to 2 grams injected slowly into a vein over a twenty- to sixty-minute period. This is repeated every six to twelve hours.
  —Children up to 12 years of age: Dosage is based on body weight and must be determined by your doctor.

## Side Effects of This Medicine

Along with its needed effects, a medicine may cause some unwanted effects. Although not all of these side effects may occur, if they do occur they may need medical attention.

*Check with your doctor immediately* if any of the following side effects occur:
  *Less common*
    Pain, swelling, or redness at place of injection; skin rash, redness, or itching

Other side effects may occur that usually do not need medical attention. These side effects may go away during treatment as your body adjusts to the medicine. However, check with your doctor if any of the following side effects continue or are bothersome:
  *Less common or rare*
    Abdominal or stomach cramps; nausea, vomiting, or diarrhea

Other side effects not listed above may also occur in some patients. If you notice any other effects, check with your doctor.

Revised: 02/23/93

# BACILLUS CALMETTE-GUÉRIN (BCG) LIVE    Mucosal-Local

Some commonly used brand names are:

**In the U.S.—**
TheraCys
TICE BCG

**In Canada—**
ImmuCyst

## Description

Bacillus Calmette-Guérin (BCG) is used as a solution that is run through a tube (instilled through a catheter) into the bladder to treat bladder cancer. The exact way it works against cancer is not known, but it may work by stimulating the body's immune system.

BCG is to be administered only by or under the immediate supervision of your doctor. It is available in the following dosage form:

*Mucosal-Local*
• Bladder instillation (U.S. and Canada)

## Before Receiving This Medicine

In deciding to use a medicine, the risks of taking the medicine must be weighed against the good it will do. This is a decision you and your doctor will make. For BCG, the following should be considered:

**Allergies**—Tell your doctor if you have ever had any unusual or allergic reaction to BCG.

**Pregnancy**—BCG has not been studied in pregnant women or animals. Make sure your doctor knows if you are pregnant or if you may become pregnant before receiving BCG.

**Breast-feeding**—It is not known whether BCG passes into the breast milk.

**Children**—There is no specific information comparing use of BCG for treatment of cancer in children with use in other age groups.

**Older adults**—This medicine has been tested and has not been shown to cause different side effects or problems in older people than it does in younger adults.

**Other medicines**—Although certain medicines should not be used together at all, in other cases two different medicines may be used together even if an interaction might occur. In these cases, your doctor may want to change the dose, or other precautions may be necessary. When receiving BCG it is especially important that your health care professional know if you are taking any of the following:
• Amphotericin B by injection (e.g., Fungizone) or
• Antineoplastics (cancer medicine) or
• Antithyroid agents (medicine for overactive thyroid) or
• Azathioprine (e.g., Imuran) or
• Chlorambucil (e.g., Leukeran) or
• Chloramphenicol (e.g., Chloromycetin) or
• Colchicine or
• Corticosteroids (cortisone-like medicine) or

• Cyclophosphamide (e.g., Cytoxan) or
• Cyclosporine (e.g., Sandimmune) or
• Flucytosine (e.g., Ancobon) or
• Ganciclovir (e.g., Cytovene) or
• Interferon (e.g., Intron A, Roferon-A) or
• Mercaptopurine (e.g., Purinethol) or
• Methotrexate (e.g., Mexate) or
• Muromonab-CD3 (e.g., Orthoclone OKT3) or
• Plicamycin (e.g., Mithracin) or
• Zidovudine (e.g., AZT, Retrovir)—Because these medicines reduce the body's natural immunity, they may prevent BCG from stimulating the immune system and will cause it to be less effective. In addition, the risk of infection may be increased

**Other medical problems**—The presence of other medical problems may affect the use of BCG. Make sure you tell your doctor if you have any other medical problems, especially:
• Fever—Infection may be present and could cause problems
• Immunity problems—BCG treatment is less effective and there is a risk of infection
• Urinary tract infection—Infection and irritation of the bladder may occur

## Proper Use of This Medicine

Your doctor will ask you to empty your bladder completely before the solution is instilled into it.

*Follow your doctor's instructions carefully about how long to hold the solution in your bladder:*
• The solution should be held in your bladder for 2 hours. If you think you cannot hold it, tell your health care professional.
• During the first hour, your doctor may have you lie for 15 minutes each on your stomach, back, and each side.
• When you do empty your bladder, you should be sitting down.

*It is important that you drink extra fluids for several hours after each treatment with BCG* so that you will pass more urine. Also, empty your bladder frequently. This will help prevent bladder problems.

BCG is a live product. In other words, it contains active bacteria that can cause infection. Some bacteria will be present for several hours in urine that you pass after each treatment with BCG. Any urine that you pass during the first 6 hours after each treatment should be disinfected with an equal amount (usually about 1 cup) of undiluted household bleach. After the bleach is added to the urine, it should be allowed to sit for 15 minutes before it is flushed. If you have any questions about this, check with your doctor.

**Dosing**—The dose of BCG will be different for different patients. The dose that is used may depend on a number of things. *If you are receiving BCG at home, follow your doctor's orders or the directions on the label.* If you have any questions about the proper dose of BCG, ask your doctor.

## Precautions While Using This Medicine

While you are being treated with BCG, and for 6 to 12 weeks after you stop treatment with it, avoid contact with people who have tuberculosis. If you think you have been exposed to someone with tuberculosis, tell your doctor.

While you are being treated with BCG and for a few weeks after you stop treatment with it, do not have any immunizations (vaccinations) without your doctor's approval.

## Side Effects of This Medicine

Along with its needed effects, a medicine may cause some unwanted effects. Although not all of these side effects may occur, if they do occur they may need medical attention.

Check with your doctor as soon as possible if any of the following side effects occur:

*More common*
> Blood in urine; fever and chills; frequent urge to urinate; increased frequency of urination; joint pain; nausea and vomiting; painful urination (severe or continuing)

*Rare*
> Cough; skin rash

Other side effects may occur that usually do not need medical attention. These side effects may go away during treatment as your body adjusts to the medicine. However, check with your doctor if any of the following side effects continue or are bothersome or if you have any questions about them:

*More common*
> Burning during first urination after treatment

After you stop using this medicine, your body may need time to adjust. The length of time this takes depends on the amount of medicine you were using and how long you used it. During this period of time (up to 6 months after treatment with BCG) check with your doctor if you notice any of the following side effects:

> Cough; fever

Other side effects not listed above may also occur in some patients. If you notice any other effects, check with your doctor.

Revised: 07/11/94

# BACLOFEN   Systemic

A commonly used brand name in the U.S. and Canada is Lioresal. Generic name product may also be available in the U.S.

## Description

Baclofen (BAK-loe-fen) is used to help relax certain muscles in your body. It relieves the spasms, cramping, and tightness of muscles caused by medical problems such as multiple sclerosis or certain injuries to the spine. Baclofen does not cure these problems, but it may allow other treatment, such as physical therapy, to be more helpful in improving your condition.

Baclofen acts on the central nervous system (CNS) to produce its muscle relaxant effects. Its actions on the CNS may also cause some of the medicine's side effects. Baclofen may also be used to relieve other conditions as determined by your doctor.

This medicine is available only with your doctor's prescription, in the following dosage form:
*Oral*
- Tablets (U.S. and Canada)

## Before Using This Medicine

In deciding to use a medicine, the risks of taking the medicine must be weighed against the good it will do.

This is a decision you and your doctor will make. For baclofen, the following should be considered:

**Allergies**—Tell your doctor if you have ever had any unusual or allergic reaction to baclofen. Also tell your health care professional if you are allergic to any other substances, such as foods, preservatives, or dyes.

**Pregnancy**—Studies on birth defects with baclofen have not been done in humans. However, studies in animals have shown that baclofen, when given in doses several times the human dose, increases the chance of hernias and incomplete or slow development of bones in the fetus, and of lower birth weight.

**Breast-feeding**—Baclofen passes into the breast milk. However, this medicine has not been reported to cause problems in nursing babies.

**Children**—Studies on this medicine have been done only in adult patients, and there is no specific information comparing use of baclofen in children with use in other age groups.

**Older adults**—Side effects such as hallucinations, confusion or mental depression, other mood or mental changes, and severe drowsiness may be especially likely to occur in elderly patients, who are usually more sensitive than younger adults to the effects of baclofen.

**Other medicines**—Although certain medicines should not be used together at all, in other cases two different medicines may be used together even if an interaction might occur. In these cases, your doctor may want to change the dose, or other precautions may be necessary. When you are taking baclofen, it is especially important that your health care professional know if you are taking any of the following:

- Antidepressants, tricyclic (amitriptyline [e.g., Elavil]), amoxapine [e.g., Asendin], clomipramine [e.g., Anafranil], desipramine [e.g., Pertofrane], doxepin [e.g., Sinequan], imipramine [e.g., Tofranil], nortriptyline [e.g., Aventyl], protriptyline [e.g., Vivactil], trimipramine [e.g., Surmontil]) or
- Central nervous system (CNS) depressants—The chance of side effects may be increased

**Other medical problems**—The presence of other medical problems may affect the use of baclofen. Make sure you tell your doctor if you have any other medical problems, especially:

- Diabetes mellitus (sugar diabetes)—Baclofen may raise blood sugar levels
- Epilepsy or
- Kidney disease or
- Mental or emotional problems or
- Stroke or other brain disease—The chance of side effects may be increased

## Proper Use of This Medicine

**Missed dose**—If you miss a dose of this medicine, and you remember within an hour or so of the missed dose, take it as soon as you remember. However, if you do not remember until later, skip the missed dose and go back to your regular dosing schedule. Do not double doses.

**Storage**—To store this medicine:

- Keep out of the reach of children.
- Store away from heat and direct light.
- Do not store in the bathroom, near the kitchen sink, or in other damp places. Heat or moisture may cause the medicine to break down.
- Do not keep outdated medicine or medicine no longer needed. Be sure that any discarded medicine is out of the reach of children.

## Precautions While Using This Medicine

*Do not suddenly stop taking this medicine.* Unwanted effects may occur if the medicine is stopped suddenly. Check with your doctor for the best way to reduce gradually the amount you are taking before stopping completely.

This medicine will add to the effects of alcohol and other CNS depressants (medicines that slow down the nervous system, possibly causing drowsiness). Some examples of CNS depressants are antihistamines or medicine for hay fever, other allergies, or colds; sedatives, tranquilizers, or sleeping medicine; prescription pain medicine or narcotics; barbiturates; medicine for seizures; other muscle relaxants; or anesthetics, including some dental anesthetics.

*Check with your doctor before taking any of the above while you are using baclofen.*

This medicine may cause drowsiness, dizziness, vision problems, or clumsiness or unsteadiness in some people. *Make sure you know how you react to this medicine before you drive, use machines, or do anything else that could be dangerous if you are not alert, well-coordinated, and able to see well.*

For *diabetic patients:*

- This medicine may cause your blood sugar levels to rise. If you notice a change in the results of your blood or urine sugar test or if you have any questions about this, check with your doctor.

## Side Effects of This Medicine

Along with its needed effects, a medicine may cause some unwanted effects. Although not all of these side effects may occur, if they do occur they may need medical attention.

Check with your doctor as soon as possible if any of the following side effects occur:

*Rare*
  Bloody or dark urine; chest pain; fainting; hallucinations (seeing or hearing things that are not there); mental depression or other mood changes; ringing or buzzing in the ears; skin rash or itching

*Symptoms of overdose*
  Blurred or double vision; convulsions (seizures); muscle weakness (severe); shortness of breath or unusually slow or troubled breathing; vomiting

Other side effects may occur that usually do not need medical attention. These side effects may go away during treatment as your body adjusts to the medicine. However, check with your doctor if any of the following side effects continue or are bothersome:

*More common*
  Confusion; dizziness or lightheadedness; drowsiness; nausea; unusual weakness, especially muscle weakness

*Less common or rare*
  Abdominal or stomach pain or discomfort; clumsiness, unsteadiness, trembling, or other problems with muscle control; constipation; diarrhea; difficult or painful urination or decrease in amount of urine; false sense of well-being; frequent urge to urinate or uncontrolled urination; headache; loss of appetite; low blood pressure; muscle or joint pain; numbness or tingling in hands or feet; pounding heartbeat; sexual problems in males; slurred speech or other speech problems; stuffy nose; swelling of ankles; trouble in sleeping; unexplained muscle stiffness; unusual excitement; unusual tiredness; weight gain

Some side effects may occur after you have stopped taking this medicine, especially if you stop taking it suddenly. *Check with your doctor immediately* if any of the following effects occur:

  Convulsions (seizures); hallucinations (seeing or hearing things that are not there); increase in muscle spasm, cramping, or tightness; mood or mental changes; unusual nervousness or restlessness

Other side effects not listed above may also occur in some patients. If you notice any other effects, check with your doctor.

## Additional Information

Once a medicine has been approved for marketing for a certain use, experience may show that it is also useful for other medical problems. Although this use is not included in product labeling, baclofen is used in certain patients with trigeminal neuralgia (severe burning or stabbing pain along the nerves in the face); also called "tic douloureux."

There is no additional information relating to proper use, precautions, or side effects for this use of baclofen.

Revised: 07/09/91

# BARBITURATES   Systemic

Some commonly used brand names are:

**In the U.S.—**

| | |
|---|---|
| Alurate[2] | Mebaral[4] |
| Amytal[1] | Nembutal[6] |
| Barbita[7] | Sarisol No. 2[3] |
| Busodium[3] | Seconal[8] |
| Butalan[3] | Solfoton[7] |
| Butisol[3] | Tuinal[9] |
| Luminal[7] | |

**In Canada—**

| | |
|---|---|
| Amytal[1] | Nova Rectal[6] |
| Ancalixir[7] | Novopentobarb[6] |
| Butisol[3] | Novosecobarb[8] |
| Mebaral[4] | Seconal[8] |
| Nembutal[6] | Tuinal[9] |

**In other countries—**
Gemonil[5]

Note: For quick reference, the following barbiturates are numbered to match the corresponding brand names.

This information applies to the following medicines:
1. Amobarbital (am-oh-BAR-bi-tal)‡
2. Aprobarbital (a-proe-BAR-bi-tal)†
3. Butabarbital (byoo-ta-BAR-bi-tal)‡
4. Mephobarbital (me-foe-BAR-bi-tal)
5. Metharbital (meth-AR-bi-tal)*†
6. Pentobarbital (pen-toe-BAR-bi-tal)‡
7. Phenobarbital (fee-noe-BAR-bi-tal)‡§
8. Secobarbital (see-koe-BAR-bi-tal)‡
9. Secobarbital and Amobarbital (see-koe-BAR-bi-tal and am-oh-BAR-bi-tal)

\*Not commercially available in the U.S.
†Not commercially available in Canada.
‡Generic name product may also be available in the U.S.
§Generic name product may also be available in Canada.

## Description

Barbiturates (bar-BI-tyoo-rates) belong to the group of medicines called central nervous system (CNS) depressants (medicines that cause drowsiness). They act on the brain and CNS to produce effects that may be helpful or harmful. This depends on the individual patient's condition and response and the amount of medicine taken.

Some of the barbiturates may be used before surgery to relieve anxiety or tension. In addition, some of the barbiturates are used as anticonvulsants to help control seizures in certain disorders or diseases, such as epilepsy.

Barbiturates may also be used for other conditions as determined by your doctor.

The barbiturates have been used to treat insomnia (trouble in sleeping); but if they are used regularly (for example, every day) for insomnia, they are usually not effective for longer than 2 weeks. The barbiturates have also been used to relieve nervousness or restlessness during the daytime. However, the barbiturates have generally been replaced by safer medicines for the treatment of insomnia and daytime nervousness or tension.

If too much of a barbiturate is used, it may become habit-forming.

Barbiturates should not be used for anxiety or tension caused by the stress of everyday life.

These medicines are available only with your doctor's prescription, in the following dosage forms:

*Oral*

Amobarbital
- Capsules (U.S. and Canada)
- Tablets (U.S. and Canada)

Aprobarbital
- Elixir (U.S.)

Butabarbital
- Capsules (U.S.)
- Elixir (U.S.)
- Tablets (U.S. and Canada)

Mephobarbital
- Tablets (U.S. and Canada)

Metharbital
- Tablets (Other countries)

Pentobarbital
- Capsules (U.S. and Canada)
- Elixir (U.S.)

Phenobarbital
- Capsules (U.S.)
- Elixir (U.S. and Canada)
- Tablets (U.S. and Canada)

Secobarbital
- Capsules (U.S. and Canada)

Secobarbital and Amobarbital
- Capsules (U.S. and Canada)

*Parenteral*
Amobarbital
- Injection (U.S. and Canada)

Pentobarbital
- Injection (U.S. and Canada)

Phenobarbital
- Injection (U.S. and Canada)

Secobarbital
- Injection (U.S.)

*Rectal*
Pentobarbital
- Suppositories (U.S. and Canada)

## Before Using This Medicine

In deciding to use a medicine, the risks of taking the medicine must be weighed against the good it will do. This is a decision you and your doctor will make. For barbiturates, the following should be considered:

**Allergies**—Tell your doctor if you have ever had any unusual or allergic reaction to barbiturates. Also tell your health care professional if you are allergic to any other substances, such as foods, preservatives, or dyes.

**Pregnancy**—Barbiturates have been shown to increase the chance of birth defects in humans. However, this medicine may be needed in serious diseases or other situations that threaten the mother's life. Be sure you have discussed this and the following information with your doctor:

- Taking barbiturates regularly during pregnancy may cause bleeding problems in the newborn infant. In addition, taking barbiturates regularly during the last 3 months of pregnancy may cause the baby to become dependent on the medicine. This may lead to withdrawal side effects in the baby after birth.
- One study in humans has suggested that barbiturates taken during pregnancy may increase the chance of brain tumors in the baby.
- Barbiturates taken for anesthesia during labor and delivery may reduce the force and frequency of contractions of the uterus; this may prolong labor and delay delivery.
- Use of barbiturates during labor may cause breathing problems in the newborn infant.

**Breast-feeding**—Barbiturates pass into the breast milk and may cause drowsiness, slow heartbeat, shortness of breath, or troubled breathing in babies of nursing mothers taking this medicine.

**Children**—Unusual excitement may be more likely to occur in children, who are usually more sensitive than adults to the effects of barbiturates.

**Older adults**—Confusion, mental depression, and unusual excitement may be more likely to occur in the elderly, who are usually more sensitive than younger adults to the effects of barbiturates.

**Other medicines**—Although certain medicines should not be used together at all, in other cases 2 different medicines may be used together even if an interaction might

occur. In these cases, your doctor may want to change the dose, or other precautions may be necessary. When you are taking a barbiturate, it is especially important that your health care professional know if you are taking any of the following:

- Adrenocorticoids (cortisone-like medicine) or
- Anticoagulants (blood thinners) or
- Carbamazepine or
- Corticotropin (ACTH)—Barbiturates may decrease the effects of these medicines
- Central nervous system (CNS) depressants (medicines that cause drowsiness)—Using these medicines with barbiturates may result in increased CNS depressant effects
- Divalproex sodium or
- Valproic acid—Using these medicines with barbiturates may change the amount of either medicine that you need to take
- Oral contraceptives (birth control pills) containing estrogens—Barbiturates may decrease the effectiveness of these oral contraceptives, and you may need to change to a different type of birth control

**Other medical problems**—The presence of other medical problems may affect the use of barbiturates. Make sure you tell your doctor if you have any other medical problems, especially:

- Alcohol abuse (or history of) or
- Drug abuse or dependence (or history of)—Dependence on barbiturates may develop
- Anemia (severe) or
- Asthma (history of), emphysema, or other chronic lung disease or
- Diabetes mellitus (sugar diabetes) or
- Hyperactivity (in children) or
- Mental depression or
- Overactive thyroid or
- Porphyria (or history of)—Barbiturates may make the condition worse
- Kidney disease or
- Liver disease—Higher blood levels of barbiturates may result, increasing the chance of side effects
- Pain—Barbiturates may cause unexpected excitement or mask important symptoms of more serious problems
- Underactive adrenal gland—Barbiturates may interfere with the effects of other medicines needed for this condition

## Proper Use of This Medicine

For patients taking the *extended-release capsule or tablet form* of this medicine:

- These capsules or tablets are to be swallowed whole. Do not break, crush, or chew before swallowing.

For patients using the *rectal suppository form* of this medicine:

- To insert the suppository: First remove the foil wrapper and moisten the suppository with cold water. Lie down on your side and use your finger to push the suppository well up into the rectum.
- Wash your hands with soap and water.

*Use this medicine only as directed by your doctor.* Do not use more of it, do not use it more often, and do not use it for a longer time than your doctor ordered. If too much is used, it may become habit-forming (causing mental or physical dependence).

If you think this medicine is not working properly after you have taken it for a few weeks, *do not increase the dose*. To do so may increase the chance of your becoming dependent on the medicine. Instead, check with your doctor.

*If you are taking this medicine for epilepsy, it must be taken every day in regularly spaced doses as ordered by your doctor in order for it to control your seizures.* This is necessary to keep a constant amount of medicine in the blood. To help keep the amount constant, do not miss any doses.

**Dosing**—The dose of barbiturates will be different for different patients. *Follow your doctor's orders or the directions on the label.* The following information includes only the average doses of barbiturates. *If your dose is different, do not change it* unless your doctor tells you to do so.

The number of capsules, tablets, or teaspoonfuls of elixir that you take, the number of suppositories you use, or the number of injections you receive depends on the strength of the medicine. Also, *the number of doses you take each day, the time allowed between doses, and the length of time you take the medicine depend on the medical problem for which you are taking barbiturates.*

*For amobarbital*
- For *oral* dosage form (tablets or capsules):
  —For trouble in sleeping:
    - Adults—65 to 200 milligrams (mg) at bedtime.
    - Children—Dose must be determined by your doctor.
  —For daytime sedation:
    - Adults—50 to 300 mg, taken in smaller doses during the day.
    - Children—Dose is based on body weight or size and must be determined by your doctor. The usual dose is 2 mg per kilogram (kg) (0.9 mg per pound) of body weight taken three times a day.
  —For sedation before surgery:
    - Adults—200 mg taken one to two hours before surgery.
    - Children—Dose is based on body weight and must be determined by your doctor. The usual dose is 2 to 6 mg per kg (0.9 to 2.7 mg per pound) of body weight, taken before surgery. However, the dose is usually not more than 100 mg.
  —For sedation during labor:
    - Adults—200 to 400 mg every one to three hours if needed. However, the total dose is usually not more than 1000 mg.

- For *injection* dosage form:
  —For trouble in sleeping:
    - Adults—65 to 200 mg, injected into a muscle or vein.
    - Children up to 6 years of age—Dose is based on body weight and must be determined by your doctor. The usual dose is 2 to 3 mg per kg (0.9 to 1.4 mg per pound) of body weight, injected into a muscle.
    - Children 6 years of age and over—Dose is based on body weight and must be determined by your doctor. The usual dose is 2 to 3 mg per kg (0.9 to 1.4 mg per pound) of body weight, injected into a muscle, or 65 to 500 mg injected into a vein.
  —For daytime sedation:
    - Adults—30 to 50 mg two or three times a day, injected into a muscle or vein.
  —For sedation before surgery:
    - Children—Dose is based on body weight and must be determined by your doctor. The usual dose is 3 to 5 mg per kg (1.4 to 2.3 mg per pound) of body weight or 65 to 500 mg per dose, injected into a vein.
  —For control of seizures:
    - Adults and children 6 years of age and over—65 to 500 mg per dose, injected into a vein.
    - Children up to 6 years of age—Dose is based on body weight or size and must be determined by your doctor. The usual dose is 3 to 5 mg per kg (1.4 to 2.3 mg per pound) of body weight, injected into a muscle or vein.

*For aprobarbital*
- For *oral* dosage form (elixir):
  —For trouble in sleeping:
    - Adults—40 to 160 milligrams (mg) at bedtime.
    - Children—Dose must be determined by your doctor.
  —For daytime sedation:
    - Adults—40 mg three times a day.
    - Children—Dose must be determined by your doctor.

*For butabarbital*
- For *oral* dosage form (elixir or tablets):
  —For trouble in sleeping:
    - Adults—50 to 100 milligrams (mg) at bedtime.
    - Children—Dose must be determined by your doctor.
  —For daytime sedation:
    - Adults—15 to 30 mg three or four times a day.
    - Children—Dose is based on body weight or size and must be determined by your doctor. The usual dose is 2 mg per kilogram (kg) (0.9 mg per pound) of body weight three times a day.

—For sedation before surgery:
- Adults—50 to 100 mg sixty to ninety minutes before surgery.
- Children—Dose is based on body weight and must be determined by your doctor. The usual dose is 2 to 6 mg per kg (0.9 to 2.7 mg per pound) of body weight. However, the dose is usually not more than 100 mg.

*For mephobarbital*
- For *oral* dosage form (tablets):
  —For daytime sedation:
  - Adults—32 to 100 milligrams (mg) three or four times a day.
  - Children—16 to 32 mg three or four times a day.
  —For control of seizures:
  - Adults—200 to 600 mg a day, taken in smaller doses during the day.
  - Children up to 5 years of age—16 to 32 mg three or four times a day.
  - Children 5 years of age and over—32 to 64 mg three or four times a day.

*For metharbital*
- For *oral* dosage form (tablets):
  —For control of seizures:
  - Adults—At first, 100 milligrams (mg) one to three times a day. Your doctor may increase your dose if needed. However, the dose is usually not more than 800 mg a day.
  - Children—50 mg one to three times a day.

*For pentobarbital*
- For *oral* dosage form (elixir or capsules):
  —For trouble in sleeping:
  - Adults—100 milligrams (mg) at bedtime.
  - Children—Dose must be determined by your doctor.
  —For daytime sedation:
  - Adults—20 mg three or four times a day.
  - Children—Dose is based on body weight and must be determined by your doctor. The usual dose is 2 to 6 mg per kilogram (kg) (0.9 to 2.7 mg per pound) of body weight per day.
  —For sedation before surgery:
  - Adults—100 mg before surgery.
  - Children—Dose is based on body weight and must be determined by your doctor. The usual dose is 2 to 6 mg per kilogram (0.9 to 2.7 mg per pound) of body weight, taken before surgery. However, the dose is usually not more than 100 mg.
- For *injection* dosage form:
  —For trouble in sleeping:
  - Adults—150 to 200 mg, injected into a muscle. Or, 100 mg injected into a vein, with additional small doses given if needed. However, the dose is usually not more than 500 mg.

- Children—Dose is based on body weight and must be determined by your doctor. The usual dose is 2 to 6 mg per kg (0.9 to 2.7 mg per pound) of body weight, injected into a muscle. Or, 50 mg injected into a vein, with additional small doses given if needed.
  —For sedation before surgery:
  - Adults—150 to 200 mg, injected into a muscle.
  - Children—Dose is based on body weight and must be determined by your doctor. The usual dose is 2 to 6 mg per kg (0.9 to 2.7 mg per pound) of body weight, injected into a muscle. However, the dose is usually not more than 100 mg.
  —For control of seizures:
  - Adults—At first, 100 mg injected into a vein. Additional small doses may be given if needed. However, the dose is usually not more than 500 mg.
  - Children—At first, 50 mg injected into a muscle or vein. Additional small doses may be given if needed.
- For *rectal* dosage form (suppositories):
  —For trouble in sleeping:
  - Adults—120 to 200 mg inserted into the rectum at bedtime.
  - Children up to 2 months of age—Dose must be determined by your doctor.
  - Children 2 months to 1 year of age—30 mg inserted into the rectum at bedtime.
  - Children 1 to 4 years of age—30 or 60 mg inserted into the rectum at bedtime.
  - Children 5 to 12 years of age—60 mg inserted into the rectum at bedtime.
  - Children 12 to 14 years of age—60 or 120 mg inserted into the rectum at bedtime.
  —For daytime sedation:
  - Adults—30 mg inserted into the rectum two to four times a day.
  - Children—Dose is based on body weight or size and must be determined by your doctor. The usual dose is 2 mg per kg (0.9 mg per pound) of body weight, inserted into the rectum three times a day.
  —For sedation before surgery:
  - Children up to 2 months of age—Dose must be determined by your doctor.
  - Children 2 months to 1 year of age—30 mg inserted into the rectum.
  - Children 1 to 4 years of age—30 or 60 mg inserted into the rectum.
  - Children 5 to 12 years of age—60 mg inserted into the rectum.
  - Children 12 to 14 years of age—60 or 120 mg inserted into the rectum.

*For phenobarbital*

- For *oral* dosage form (elixir, capsules, or tablets):
  - —For trouble in sleeping:
    - Adults—100 to 320 milligrams (mg) at bedtime.
    - Children—Dose must be determined by your doctor.
  - —For daytime sedation:
    - Adults—30 to 120 mg a day, taken in smaller doses two or three times during the day.
    - Children—Dose is based on body weight or size and must be determined by your doctor. The usual dose is 2 mg per kilogram (kg) (0.9 mg per pound) of body weight three times a day.
  - —For sedation before surgery:
    - Children—Dose is based on body weight and must be determined by your doctor. The usual dose is 1 to 3 mg per kg (0.45 to 1.4 mg per pound) of body weight.
  - —For control of seizures:
    - Adults—60 to 250 mg a day.
    - Children—Dose is based on body weight and must be determined by your doctor. The usual dose is 1 to 6 mg per kg (0.45 to 2.7 mg per pound) of body weight a day.
- For *injection* dosage form:
  - —For trouble in sleeping:
    - Adults—100 to 325 mg, injected into a muscle or vein, or under the skin.
    - Children—Dose must be determined by your doctor.
  - —For daytime sedation:
    - Adults—30 to 120 mg a day, injected into a muscle or a vein, or under the skin, in smaller doses two or three times during the day,
    - Children—Dose must be determined by your doctor.
  - —For sedation before surgery:
    - Adults—130 to 200 mg, injected into a muscle sixty to ninety minutes before surgery.
    - Children—Dose is based on body weight and must be determined by your doctor. The usual dose is 1 to 3 mg per kg (0.45 to 1.4 mg per pound) of body weight, injected into a muscle or vein sixty to ninety minutes before surgery.
  - —For control of seizures:
    - Adults—100 to 320 mg injected into a vein. The dose may be repeated if needed, but is usually not more than 600 mg a day. However, higher doses may be needed for certain types of continuing seizures.
    - Children—Dose is based on body weight and must be determined by your doctor. At first, the usual dose is 10 to 20 mg per kg (4.5 to 9 mg per pound) of body weight, injected into a vein. Later, 1 to 6 mg per kg (0.45 to 2.7 mg per pound)

of body weight a day, injected into a vein. Higher doses may be needed for certain types of continuing seizures.

*For secobarbital*

- For *oral* dosage form (capsules):
  - —For trouble in sleeping:
    - Adults—100 milligrams (mg) at bedtime.
    - Children—Dose must be determined by your doctor.
  - —For daytime sedation:
    - Adults—30 to 50 mg three or four times a day.
    - Children—Dose is based on body weight or size and must be determined by your doctor. The usual dose is 2 mg per kilogram (kg) (0.9 mg per pound) of body weight three times a day.
  - —For sedation before surgery:
    - Adults—200 to 300 mg one or two hours before surgery.
    - Children—Dose is based on body weight and must be determined by your doctor. The usual dose is 2 to 6 mg per kg (0.9 to 2.7 mg per pound) of body weight one or two hours before surgery. However, the dose is usually not more than 100 mg.
- For *injection* dosage form:
  - —For trouble in sleeping:
    - Adults—100 to 200 mg injected into a muscle, or 50 to 250 mg injected into a vein.
    - Children—Dose is based on body weight or size and must be determined by your doctor. The usual dose is 3 to 5 mg per kg (1.4 to 2.3 mg per pound) of body weight, injected into a muscle. However, the dose is usually not more than 100 mg.
  - —For sedation before dental procedures:
    - Adults—Dose is based on body weight and must be determined by your doctor. The usual dose is 1.1 to 2.2 mg per kg (0.5 to 1 mg per pound) of body weight, injected into a muscle ten to fifteen minutes before the procedure.
    - Children—Dose must be determined by your dentist.
  - —For sedation before a nerve block:
    - Adults—100 to 150 mg, injected into a vein.
  - —For sedation before surgery:
    - Children—Dose is based on body weight and must be determined by your doctor. The usual dose is 4 to 5 mg per kg (1.8 to 2.3 mg per pound) of body weight, injected into a muscle.
  - —For seizures from tetanus:
    - Adults—Dose is based on body weight and must be determined by your doctor. The usual dose is 5.5 mg per kg (2.5 mg per pound) of body weight, injected into a muscle or vein. Dose may be repeated every three to four hours if needed.

- Children—Dose is based on body weight and must be determined by your doctor. The usual dose is 3 to 5 mg per kg (1.4 to 2.3 mg per pound) of body weight, injected into a muscle or vein.

*For secobarbital and amobarbital combination*
- For *oral* dosage form (capsules):
  —For trouble in sleeping:
  - Adults—1 capsule at bedtime.
  - Children—Dose must be determined by your doctor.
  —For sedation before surgery:
  - Adults—1 capsule taken one hour before surgery.
  - Children—Dose must be determined by your doctor.

**Missed dose**—If you are taking this medicine regularly (for example, every day as in epilepsy) and you do miss a dose, take it as soon as possible. However, if it is almost time for your next dose, skip the missed dose and go back to your regular dosing schedule. Do not double doses.

**Storage**—To store this medicine:
- Keep out of the reach of children since overdose is especially dangerous in children.
- Store away from heat and direct light.
- Do not store the capsule or tablet form of this medicine in the bathroom, near the kitchen sink, or in other damp places. Heat or moisture may cause the medicine to break down.
- Keep the liquid form of this medicine from freezing.
- Store the suppository form of this medicine in the refrigerator.
- Do not keep outdated medicine or medicine no longer needed. Be sure that any discarded medicine is out of the reach of children.

---

## Precautions While Using This Medicine

If you will be using this medicine regularly for a long time:
- Your doctor should check your progress at regular visits.
- Do not stop using it without first checking with your doctor. Your doctor may want you to reduce gradually the amount you are using before stopping completely.

This medicine will add to the effects of alcohol and other CNS depressants (medicines that slow down the nervous system, possibly causing drowsiness). Some examples of CNS depressants are antihistamines or medicine for hay fever, other allergies, or colds; sedatives, tranquilizers, or sleeping medicine; prescription pain medicine or narcotics; medicine for seizures; muscle relaxants; or anesthetics, including some dental anesthetics. *Check with your doctor before taking any of the above while you are using this medicine.*

Before you have any medical tests, tell the medical doctor in charge that you are taking this medicine. The results of the metyrapone test may be affected by this medicine.

*If you have been using this medicine for a long time and you think that you may have become mentally or physically dependent on it, check with your doctor.* Some signs of mental or physical dependence on barbiturates are:
- a strong desire or need to continue taking the medicine.
- a need to increase the dose to receive the effects of the medicine.
- withdrawal side effects (for example, anxiety or restlessness, convulsions [seizures], feeling faint, nausea or vomiting, trembling of hands, trouble in sleeping) occurring after the medicine is stopped.

*If you think you or someone else may have taken an overdose of this medicine, get emergency help at once.* Taking an overdose of a barbiturate or taking alcohol or other CNS depressants with the barbiturate may lead to unconsciousness and possibly death. Some signs of an overdose are severe drowsiness, severe confusion, severe weakness, shortness of breath or slow or troubled breathing, slurred speech, staggering, and slow heartbeat.

This medicine may cause some people to become dizzy, lightheaded, drowsy, or less alert than they are normally. Even if taken at bedtime, it may cause some people to feel drowsy or less alert on arising. *Make sure you know how you react to this medicine before you drive, use machines, or do anything else that could be dangerous if you are dizzy or are not alert.*

*Oral contraceptives (birth control pills) containing estrogen may not work properly if you take them while you are taking barbiturates. Unplanned pregnancies may occur. You should use a different or additional means of birth control while you are taking barbiturates.* If you have any questions about this, check with your health care professional.

---

## Side Effects of This Medicine

Along with its needed effects, a medicine may cause some unwanted effects. Although not all of these side effects may occur, if they do occur they may need medical attention.

*Check with your doctor immediately* if any of the following side effects occur:
*Rare*
  Bleeding sores on lips; chest pain; fever; muscle or joint pain; red, thickened, or scaly skin; skin rash or hives; sores, ulcers, or white spots in mouth (painful); sore throat and/or fever; swelling of eyelids, face, or lips; wheezing or tightness in chest

Also, check with your doctor as soon as possible if any of the following side effects occur:
*Less common*
  Confusion; mental depression; unusual excitement

*Rare*

Hallucinations (seeing, hearing, or feeling things that are not there); unusual bleeding or bruising; unusual tiredness or weakness

*With long-term or chronic use*

Bone pain, tenderness, or aching; loss of appetite; muscle weakness; weight loss (unusual); yellow eyes or skin

*Symptoms of overdose*

Confusion (severe); decrease in or loss of reflexes; drowsiness (severe); fever; irritability (continuing); low body temperature; poor judgment; shortness of breath or slow or troubled breathing; slow heartbeat; slurred speech; staggering; trouble in sleeping; unusual movements of the eyes; weakness (severe)

Other side effects may occur that usually do not need medical attention. These side effects may go away during treatment as your body adjusts to the medicine. However, check with your doctor if any of the following side effects continue or are bothersome:

*More common*

Clumsiness or unsteadiness; dizziness or lightheadedness; drowsiness; "hangover" effect

*Less common*

Anxiety or nervousness; constipation; feeling faint; headache; irritability; nausea or vomiting; nightmares or trouble in sleeping

For very ill patients:

• Confusion, mental depression, and unusual excitement may be more likely to occur in very ill patients.

After you stop using this medicine, your body may need time to adjust. If you took this medicine in high doses or for a long time, this may take up to about 15 days. During this period of time check with your doctor if any of the following side effects occur (usually occur within 8 to 16 hours after medicine is stopped):

Anxiety or restlessness; convulsions (seizures); dizziness or lightheadedness; feeling faint; hallucinations (seeing, hearing, or feeling things that are not there); muscle twitching; nausea or vomiting; trembling of hands; trouble in sleeping, increased dreaming, or nightmares; vision problems; weakness

Other side effects not listed above may also occur in some patients. If you notice any other effects, check with your doctor.

## Additional Information

Once a medicine has been approved for marketing for a certain use, experience may show that it is also useful for other medical problems. Although this use is not included in product labeling, phenobarbital is used in certain patients with the following medical condition:

• Hyperbilirubinemia (high amount of bile pigments in the blood that may lead to jaundice)

Other than the above information, there is no additional information relating to proper use, precautions, or side effects for these uses.

Revised: 01/27/92
Interim revision: 08/29/94

# BARBITURATES, ASPIRIN, AND CODEINE    Systemic

Some commonly used brand names are:

**In the U.S.—**

| | |
|---|---|
| Ascomp with Codeine No.3[1] | Fiorinal with Codeine No.3[1] |
| Butalbital Compound with Codeine[1] | Idenal with Codeine[1] |
| | Isollyl with Codeine[1] |
| Butinal with Codeine No.3[1] | |

**In Canada—**

| | |
|---|---|
| Fiorinal-C ¼[1] | Phenaphen with Codeine No.4[2] |
| Fiorinal-C ½[1] | Tecnal-C ¼[1] |
| Phenaphen with Codeine No.2[2] | Tecnal-C ½[1] |
| Phenaphen with Codeine No.3[2] | |

Note: For quick reference, the following corticosteroids are numbered to match the corresponding brand names.

This information applies to the following medicines:

1. Butalbital (byoo-TAL-bi-tal), Aspirin (AS-pir-in), and Codeine (KOE-deen)‡
2. Phenobarbital (fee-noe-BAR-bi-tal), Aspirin, and Codeine*‡

*Not commercially available in the U.S.
‡In Canada, *Aspirin* is a brand name. Acetylsalicylic acid is the generic name in Canada. ASA, a synonym for acetylsalicylic acid, is the term that commonly appears on Canadian product labels.

## Description

Barbiturate (bar-BI-tyoo-rate), aspirin, and codeine combinations are used to relieve headaches and other kinds of pain. These combination medicines may provide better pain relief than either aspirin or codeine used alone. In some cases, relief of pain may come at lower doses of each medicine.

Codeine is a narcotic analgesic (nar-KOT-ik an-al-JEE-zik) that acts in the central nervous system (CNS) to relieve pain. Many of its side effects are also caused by actions in the CNS. Butalbital and phenobarbital belong to the group of medicines called barbiturates. Barbiturates also act in the CNS to produce their effects.

When you use a barbiturate or codeine for a long time, your body may get used to the medicine so that larger amounts are needed to produce the same effects. This is called tolerance to the medicine. Also, barbiturates and codeine may become habit-forming (causing mental or physical dependence) when they are used for a long time or in large doses. Physical dependence may lead to withdrawal symptoms when you stop taking the medicine. In patients who get headaches, the first symptom of withdrawal may be new (rebound) headaches.

The butalbital, aspirin, and codeine combination also contains caffeine (kaf-EEN). Caffeine may help to relieve headaches. However, caffeine can also cause physical dependence when it is used for a long time. This may lead to withdrawal (rebound) headaches when you stop taking it.

Aspirin is not a narcotic and does not cause physical dependence. However, it may cause other unwanted effects if too much is taken.

These combination medicines are available only with your doctor's prescription, in the following dosage forms:

*Oral*

Butalbital, Aspirin, Caffeine, and Codeine
- Capsules (U.S. and Canada)
- Tablets (U.S.)

Phenobarbital, Aspirin, and Codeine
- Capsules (Canada)

---

## Before Using This Medicine

In deciding to use a medicine, the risks of taking the medicine must be weighed against the good it will do. This is a decision you and your doctor will make. For barbiturate, aspirin, and codeine combinations, the following should be considered:

**Allergies**—Tell your doctor if you have ever had any unusual or allergic reaction to aspirin or other salicylates including methyl salicylate (oil of wintergreen); butalbital, phenobarbital, or other barbiturates; caffeine; codeine; or any of the following medicines:

Diclofenac (e.g., Voltaren)
Diflunisal (e.g., Dolobid)
Etodolac (e.g., Lodine)
Fenoprofen (e.g., Nalfon)
Floctafenine (e.g., Idarac)
Flurbiprofen, oral (e.g., Ansaid)
Ibuprofen (e.g., Motrin)
Indomethacin (e.g., Indocin)
Ketoprofen (e.g., Orudis)
Ketorolac (e.g., Toradol)
Meclofenamate (e.g., Meclomen)
Mefenamic acid (e.g., Ponstel)
Nabumetone (e.g., Relafen)
Naproxen (e.g., Naprosyn)
Oxaprozin (e.g., Daypro)
Oxyphenbutazone (e.g., Tandearil)
Phenylbutazone (e.g., Butazolidin)
Piroxicam (e.g., Feldene)
Sulindac (e.g., Clinoril)
Suprofen (e.g., Suprol)
Tenoxicam (e.g., Mobiflex)
Tiaprofenic acid (e.g., Surgam)
Tolmetin (e.g., Tolectin)
Zomepirac (e.g., Zomax)

Also tell your health care professional if you are allergic to any other substances, such as foods, preservatives, or dyes.

**Pregnancy**—

- *For butalbital or phenobarbital:* Barbiturates have been shown to increase the chance of birth defects in humans. Also, one study in humans has suggested that barbiturates taken during pregnancy may increase the chance of brain tumors in the baby. Barbiturates may cause breathing problems in the newborn baby if taken just before or during delivery.

- *For aspirin:* Although studies in humans have not shown that aspirin causes birth defects, aspirin has caused birth defects in animal studies.

  *Do not take aspirin during the last 3 months of pregnancy unless it has been ordered by your doctor.* Some reports have suggested that use of aspirin late in pregnancy may cause a decrease in the newborn's weight and possible death of the fetus or newborn baby. However, the mothers in these reports had been taking much larger amounts of aspirin than are usually recommended. Studies of mothers taking aspirin in the doses that are usually recommended did not show these unwanted effects.

  There is a chance that regular use of aspirin late in pregnancy may cause unwanted effects on the heart or blood flow in the fetus or in the newborn baby. Also, use of aspirin during the last 2 weeks of pregnancy may cause bleeding problems in the fetus before or during delivery or in the newborn baby. In addition, too much use of aspirin during the last 3 months of pregnancy may increase the length of pregnancy, prolong labor, cause other problems during delivery, or cause severe bleeding in the mother before, during, or after delivery.

- *For codeine:* Although studies on birth defects with codeine have not been done in pregnant women, it has not been reported to cause birth defects. However, it may cause breathing problems in the newborn baby if taken just before or during delivery. Codeine did not cause birth defects in animal studies, but it caused slower development of bones and other harmful effects in the fetus.

- *For caffeine:* Studies in humans have not shown that caffeine causes birth defects. However, use of large amounts of caffeine during pregnancy may cause problems with the heart rhythm and the growth of the fetus. Also, studies in animals have shown that caffeine causes birth defects when given in very large doses (amounts equal to those in 12 to 24 cups of coffee a day).

**Breast-feeding**—Although this combination medicine has not been reported to cause problems, the chance always exists, especially if the medicine is taken for a long time or in large amounts.

- *For butalbital or phenobarbital:* Barbiturates pass into the breast milk and may cause drowsiness, unusually slow heartbeat, shortness of breath, or troubled breathing in nursing babies.

- *For aspirin:* Aspirin passes into the breast milk. However, taking aspirin in the amount present in these combination medicines has not been reported to cause problems in nursing babies.

- *For codeine:* Codeine passes into the breast milk in small amounts. However, it has not been reported to cause problems in nursing babies.
- *For caffeine:* The caffeine in the butalbital, aspirin, and codeine combination medicine passes into the breast milk in small amounts. Taking caffeine in the amounts present in this combination medicine has not been reported to cause problems in nursing babies. However, studies have shown that nursing babies may appear jittery when their mothers drink large amounts of caffeine-containing beverages. Therefore, breast-feeding mothers who use caffeine-containing medicines should probably limit the amount of caffeine they take in from other medicines or from beverages.

**Children—**

- *For butalbital or phenobarbital:* Although barbiturates often cause drowsiness, some children become excited after taking them.
- *For aspirin: Do not give a medicine containing aspirin to a child with fever or other symptoms of a virus infection, especially flu or chickenpox, without first discussing its use with your child's doctor.* This is very important because aspirin may cause a serious illness called Reye's syndrome in children with fever caused by a virus infection, especially flu or chickenpox. Children who do not have a virus infection may also be more sensitive to the effects of aspirin, especially if they have a fever or have lost large amounts of body fluid because of vomiting, diarrhea, or sweating. This may increase the chance of side effects during treatment.
- *For caffeine:* There is no specific information comparing use of caffeine in children up to 12 years of age with use in other age groups. However, caffeine is not expected to cause different side effects or problems in children than it does in adults.

**Teenagers—***Teenagers with fever or other symptoms of a virus infection, especially flu or chickenpox, should check with a doctor before taking this medicine.* The aspirin in this combination medicine may cause a serious illness called Reye's syndrome in teenagers with fever caused by a virus infection, especially flu or chickenpox.

**Older adults—**

- *For butalbital or phenobarbital:* Confusion, depression, or excitement may be especially likely to occur in elderly patients, who are usually more sensitive than younger adults to the effects of barbiturates.
- *For aspirin:* Elderly patients are more sensitive than younger adults to the effects of aspirin. This may increase the chance of side effects during treatment.
- *For codeine:* Breathing problems may be especially likely to occur in elderly patients, who are usually more sensitive than younger adults to the effects of codeine.

- *For caffeine:* Many medicines have not been studied specifically in older people. Therefore, it may not be known whether they work exactly the same way they do in younger adults or if they cause different side effects or problems in older people. There is no specific information comparing use of caffeine in the elderly with use in other age groups.

**Other medicines—**Although certain medicines should not be used together at all, in other cases two different medicines may be used together even if an interaction might occur. In these cases, your doctor may want to change the dose, or other precautions may be necessary. When you are taking this combination medicine, it is especially important that your health care professional know if you are taking any of the following:

- Antacids, large amounts taken regularly, especially calcium- and/or magnesium-containing antacids or sodium bicarbonate (baking soda), or
- Urinary alkalizers (medicine that makes the urine less acid, such as acetazolamide [e.g., Diamox], dichlorphenamide [e.g., Daranide], methazolamide [e.g., Neptazane], potassium or sodium citrate and/or citric acid)—These medicines may cause aspirin to be removed from the body faster than usual, which may shorten the length of time that aspirin is effective; acetazolamide, dichlorphenamide, and methazolamide may also increase the chance of side effects when taken together with aspirin
- Anticoagulants (blood thinners) or
- Heparin—Use of these medicines together with aspirin may increase the chance of bleeding; also, barbiturates, especially phenobarbital, may decrease the effects of anticoagulants
- Antidepressants, tricyclic (amitriptyline [e.g., Elavil], amoxapine [e.g., Asendin], clomipramine [e.g., Anafranil], desipramine [e.g., Pertofrane], doxepin [e.g., Sinequan], imipramine [e.g., Tofranil], nortriptyline [e.g., Aventyl], protriptyline [e.g., Vivactil], trimipramine [e.g., Surmontil]) or
- Central nervous system (CNS) depressants (medicines that often cause drowsiness)—These medicines may add to the effects of barbiturates and codeine and increase the chance of drowsiness or other side effects
- Carbamazepine or
- Contraceptives, oral (birth control pills) containing estrogens or
- Corticosteroids (cortisone-like medicines) or
- Corticotropin (ACTH)—Barbiturates, especially phenobarbital, may make these medicines less effective
- Divalproex (e.g., Depakote) or
- Methotrexate (e.g., Mexate) or
- Valproic acid (e.g., Depakene) or
- Vancomycin (e.g., Vancocin)—The chance of serious side effects may be increased
- Naltrexone (e.g., Trexan)—Naltrexone blocks the pain-relieving effect of codeine
- Probenecid (e.g., Benemid) or
- Sulfinpyrazone (e.g., Anturane)—Aspirin can keep these medicines from working properly for treating gout

**Other medical problems—**The presence of other medical problems may affect the use of butalbital, aspirin, and codeine combination. Make sure you tell your doctor if you have any other medical problems, especially:

- Alcohol abuse (or history of) or
- Drug abuse or dependence (or history of)—Dependence on barbiturates and/or codeine may develop
- Asthma, especially if occurring together with other allergies and nasal polyps (history of), or
- Brain disease or head injury or
- Colitis or
- Convulsions (seizures) (history of) or
- Emphysema or other chronic lung disease or
- Enlarged prostate or problems with urination or
- Gallbladder disease or gallstones or
- Hyperactivity (in children) or
- Kidney disease or
- Liver disease—The chance of serious side effects may be increased
- Diabetes mellitus (sugar diabetes) or
- Mental depression or
- Overactive thyroid or
- Porphyria (or history of)—Barbiturates can make these conditions worse
- Gout—Aspirin can make this condition worse and can also lessen the effects of some medicines used to treat gout
- Heart disease (severe)—The caffeine in the butalbital, aspirin, and codeine combination can make some kinds of heart disease worse
- Hemophilia or other bleeding problems or
- Vitamin K deficiency—Aspirin increases the chance of serious bleeding
- Stomach ulcer, especially with a history of bleeding, or other stomach problems—Aspirin can make your condition worse

## Proper Use of This Medicine

*Take this medicine with food or a full glass (8 ounces) of water* to lessen stomach irritation.

*Do not take this medicine if it has a strong vinegar-like odor.* This odor means the aspirin in it is breaking down. If you have any questions about this, check with your health care professional.

*Take this medicine only as directed by your doctor.* Do not take more of it, do not take it more often, and do not take it for a longer time than your doctor ordered. If a barbiturate or codeine is taken regularly (for example, every day), it may become habit-forming (causing mental or physical dependence). Regular use of caffeine can also cause physical dependence. Dependence is especially likely to occur in people who take these medicines to relieve frequent headaches. Also, taking too much of this combination medicine may cause stomach problems or other medical problems.

This medicine will relieve a headache best if you *take it as soon as the headache begins*. If you get warning signs of a migraine, take this medicine as soon as you are sure that the migraine is coming. This may even stop the headache pain from occurring. *Lying down in a quiet, dark room for a while after taking the medicine also helps to relieve headaches.*

People who get a lot of headaches may need to take a different medicine to help prevent headaches. *It is important that you follow your doctor's directions about taking the other medicine, even if your headaches continue to occur.* Headache-preventing medicines may take several weeks to start working. Even after they do start working, your headaches may not go away completely. However, your headaches should occur less often, and they should be less severe and easier to relieve than before. This will reduce the amount of headache relievers that you need. If you do not notice any improvement after several weeks of headache-preventing treatment, check with your doctor.

**Dosing**—The dose of these medicines will be different for different patients. *Follow your doctor's orders or the directions on the label.* The following information includes only the average doses of these medicines. *If your dose is different, do not change it* unless your doctor tells you to do so.

The number of capsules or tablets that you take depends on the strength of the medicine.

*For Butalbital, Aspirin, and Codeine combination*
- For *oral* dosage forms (capsules and tablets):
  —For relieving pain:
    - Adults—One or 2 capsules or tablets every four hours as needed. You should not take more than six capsules or tablets a day.
    - Children—Dose must be determined by your doctor.

*For Phenobarbital, Aspirin, and Codeine combination*
- For *oral* dosage form (capsules):
  —For relieving pain:
    - Adults—One or 2 capsules every three or four hours as needed.
    - Children—Dose must be determined by your doctor.

**Missed dose**—If your doctor has ordered you to take this medicine according to a regular schedule and you miss a dose, take it as soon as you remember. However, if it is almost time for your next dose, skip the missed dose and go back to your regular dosing schedule. Do not double doses.

**Storage**—To store this medicine:
- Keep out of the reach of children. Overdose is especially dangerous in young children.
- Store away from heat and direct light.
- Do not store this medicine in the bathroom, near the kitchen sink, or in other damp places. Heat or moisture may cause the medicine to break down.
- Do not keep outdated medicine or medicine no longer needed. Be sure that any discarded medicine is out of the reach of children.

## Precautions While Using This Medicine

*Check with your doctor:*
- If the medicine stops working as well as it did when you first started using it. This may mean that you

are in danger of becoming dependent on the medicine. *Do not try to get better pain relief by increasing the dose.*

- *If you are having headaches more often than you did before you started using this medicine.* This is especially important if a new headache occurs within 1 day after you took your last dose of headache medicine, headaches begin to occur every day, or a headache continues for several days in a row. This may mean that you are dependent on the headache medicine. *Continuing to take this medicine will cause even more headaches later on.* Your doctor can give you advice on how to relieve the headaches.

*Check the labels of all nonprescription (over-the-counter [OTC]) and prescription medicines you now take. If any contain a narcotic, a barbiturate, aspirin, or other salicylates, including diflunisal, check with your doctor or pharmacist.* Taking them together with this medicine may cause an overdose.

The barbiturate and the codeine in this medicine will add to the effects of alcohol and other CNS depressants (medicines that slow down the nervous system, possibly causing drowsiness). Some examples of CNS depressants are antihistamines or medicine for hay fever, other allergies, or colds; sedatives, tranquilizers, or sleeping medicine; other prescription pain medicine or narcotics; other barbiturates; medicine for seizures; muscle relaxants; or anesthetics, including some dental anesthetics. Also, stomach problems may be more likely to occur if you drink alcoholic beverages while you are taking aspirin. Therefore, *do not drink alcoholic beverages, and check with your doctor before taking any of the medicines listed above, while you are using this medicine.*

This medicine may cause some people to become drowsy, dizzy, or lightheaded, or to feel a false sense of well-being. *Make sure you know how you react to this medicine before you drive, use machines, or do anything else that could be dangerous if you are dizzy or are not alert and clearheaded.*

Dizziness, lightheadedness, or fainting may occur, especially when you get up suddenly from a lying or sitting position. Getting up slowly may help lessen this problem. Lying down for a while may relieve these effects.

Nausea or vomiting may occur, especially after the first couple of doses. This effect may go away if you lie down for a while. However, if nausea or vomiting continues, check with your doctor.

Before having any kind of surgery (including dental surgery) or emergency treatment, tell the medical doctor or dentist in charge that you are taking this medicine. Serious side effects can occur if your medical doctor or dentist gives you certain medicines without knowing that you have taken a barbiturate or codeine.

Do not take this medicine for 5 days before any planned surgery, including dental surgery, unless otherwise directed by your medical doctor or dentist. Taking aspirin during this time may cause bleeding problems.

Before you have any medical tests, tell the person in charge that you are taking this medicine. The caffeine in the butalbital, aspirin, and codeine combination interferes with the results of certain tests that use dipyridamole (e.g., Persantine) to help show how well blood is flowing to your heart. Caffeine should not be taken for 8 to 12 hours before the test. The results of some other tests may also be affected by this medicine.

If you have been taking large amounts of this medicine, or if you have been taking it regularly for several weeks or more, *do not suddenly stop using it without first checking with your doctor.* Your doctor may want you to reduce gradually the amount you are taking before stopping completely, to lessen the chance of withdrawal side effects.

*If you think you or anyone else may have taken an overdose of this medicine, get emergency help at once.* Taking an overdose of this medicine or taking alcohol or CNS depressants with this medicine may lead to unconsciousness or death. Signs of overdose of this medicine include convulsions (seizures); hearing loss; confusion; ringing or buzzing in the ears; severe excitement, nervousness, or restlessness; severe dizziness; severe drowsiness; unusually slow or troubled breathing; and severe weakness.

## Side Effects of This Medicine

Along with its needed effects, a medicine may cause some unwanted effects. Although not all of these side effects may occur, if they do occur they may need medical attention.

*The following side effects may mean that a serious allergic reaction is occurring. Check with your doctor or get emergency help immediately* if they occur, especially if several of them occur at the same time.

*Less common or rare*
> Bluish discoloration or flushing or redness of skin (occurring together with other effects listed in this section); coughing, shortness of breath, troubled breathing, tightness in chest, or wheezing; difficulty in swallowing; dizziness or feeling faint (severe); hive-like swellings (large) on eyelids, face, lips, or tongue; skin rash, itching, or hives; stuffy nose (occurring together with other effects listed in this section)

*Also check with your doctor immediately* if any of the following side effects occur, especially if several of them occur together:

*Rare*
> Bleeding or crusting sores on lips; chest pain; fever with or without chills; red, thickened, or scaly skin; sores, ulcers, or white spots in mouth (painful); sore throat (unexplained); tenderness, burning, or peeling of skin

*Symptoms of overdose*
> Anxiety, confusion, excitement, irritability, nervousness, restlessness, or trouble in sleeping (severe, especially with products containing caffeine); cold, clammy skin; convulsions (seizures); diarrhea (severe or continuing); dizziness, lightheadedness, drowsiness, or weakness (severe); frequent urination (for products containing caffeine); hallucinations (seeing, hearing, or feeling

things that are not there); increased sensitivity to touch or pain (for products containing caffeine); increased thirst; low blood pressure; muscle trembling or twitching (for products containing caffeine); nausea or vomiting (severe or continuing), sometimes with blood; pinpoint pupils of eyes; ringing or buzzing in ears (continuing) or hearing loss; seeing flashes of "zigzag" lights (for products containing caffeine); slow, fast, or irregular heartbeat; slow, fast, irregular, or troubled breathing; slurred speech; staggering; stomach pain (severe); uncontrollable flapping movements of the hands (especially in elderly patients); unusual movements of the eyes; vision problems

Also, check with your doctor as soon as possible if any of the following side effects occur:

*Less common or rare*
    Bloody or black, tarry stools; bloody urine; confusion or mental depression; pinpoint red spots on skin; skin rash, hives, or itching (without other signs of an allergic reaction to aspirin listed above); sore throat and fever; stomach pain (severe); swollen or painful glands; trembling or uncontrolled muscle movements; unusual

bleeding or bruising; unusual excitement (mild); unusual tiredness or weakness (mild)

Other side effects may occur that usually do not need medical attention. These side effects may go away during treatment as your body adjusts to the medicine. However, check with your doctor if any of the following side effects continue or are bothersome:

*More common*
    Bloated or "gassy" feeling; dizziness, lightheadedness, or drowsiness (mild); heartburn or indigestion; nausea, vomiting, or stomach pain (occurring without other symptoms of overdose)

Other side effects not listed above may also occur in some patients. If you notice any other effects, check with your doctor.

Revised: 07/14/92
Interim revision: 07/19/94

# BARIUM SULFATE    Diagnostic

## Description

Barium sulfate is a radiopaque agent. Radiopaque agents are used to help diagnose certain medical problems. Since radiopaque agents are opaque to (block) x-rays, the areas of the body in which they are localized will appear white on the x-ray film. This creates the needed distinction, or contrast, between one organ and other tissues. The contrast will help the doctor see any special conditions that may exist in that organ or part of the body.

Barium sulfate is taken by mouth or given rectally by enema. If taken by mouth, it makes the esophagus, the stomach, and/or the small intestine opaque to the x-rays so that they can be "photographed." If it is given by enema, the colon and/or the small intestine can be seen and photographed by x-rays.

The dose of barium sulfate will be different for different patients and depends on the type of test. The strength of the suspension and tablet is determined by how much barium they contain. Different tests will require a different strength and amount of suspension (some may require the tablet form), depending on the age of the patient, the contrast needed, and the x-ray equipment used.

Barium sulfate is to be used only by or under the direct supervision of a doctor.

## Before Having This Test

In deciding to use a diagnostic test, any risks of the test must be weighed against the good it will do. This is a decision you and your doctor will make. Also, test results

may be affected by other things. For barium sulfate, the following should be considered:

**Allergies**—Tell your doctor if you have ever had any unusual or allergic reaction to barium sulfate. Also, tell your doctor if you are allergic to any other substances, such as foods, preservatives, or dyes.

**Pregnancy**—X-rays of the abdomen are usually not recommended during pregnancy. This is to avoid exposing the fetus to radiation. Be sure you have discussed this with your doctor.

**Breast-feeding**—Barium sulfate does not pass into the breast milk. This medicine has not been reported to cause problems in nursing babies.

**Children**—Although there is no specific information comparing use of barium sulfate in children with use in other age groups, this agent is not expected to cause different side effects or problems in children than it does in adults.

**Older adults**—This contrast agent has been used in older people and has not been shown to cause different side effects or problems in them than it does in younger adults.

**Other medical problems**—The presence of other medical problems may affect the use of barium sulfate. Make sure you tell your doctor if you have any other medical problems, especially:

• Asthma, hay fever, or other allergies (history of)—If you have a history of these conditions, the risk of having a reaction, such as an allergic reaction to the additives in the barium sulfate preparation, is greater
• Cystic fibrosis—The risk of blockage in the small bowel is greater

- Dehydration—Barium sulfate may cause severe constipation
- Intestinal blockage or perforation—Barium sulfate may make this condition worse

## Preparation For This Test

Your doctor may have special instructions for you in preparation for your test. If you have not received such instructions or if you do not understand them, check with your doctor in advance.

For some tests your doctor may tell you not to eat after 8 the evening before the test. You may be allowed to drink small amounts of clear liquids until midnight; however, check first with your doctor. For other tests you may need to eat meals free of fiber and bulk the day before the test. You may also need to use a laxative.

## Precautions After Having This Test

Make sure to drink plenty of liquids after the test. Otherwise, barium sulfate may cause severe constipation.

## Side Effects of This Medicine

Along with its needed effects, a radiopaque agent may cause some unwanted effects. Although not all of these side effects may occur, if they do occur they may need medical attention.

*Check with your doctor immediately* if any of the following side effects occur:

*Rare*
> Bloating; constipation (severe, continuing); cramping (severe); nausea or vomiting; stomach or lower abdominal pain; tightness in chest or troubled breathing; wheezing

Other side effects may occur that usually do not need medical attention. These side effects may go away as your body adjusts to this agent. However, check with your doctor if any of the following side effects continue or are bothersome:

*More common*
> Constipation or diarrhea; cramping

Other side effects not listed above may also occur in some patients. If you notice any other effects, check with your doctor.

Revised: 07/26/94

---

# BELLADONNA ALKALOIDS AND BARBITURATES   Systemic

Some commonly used brand names are:
**In the U.S.—**

| | |
|---|---|
| Antrocol[2] | Donphen[1] |
| Barbidonna[1] | Hyosophen[1] |
| Barbidonna No. 2[1] | Kinesed[1] |
| Barophen[1] | Levsin-PB[5] |
| Bellalphen[1] | Levsin with Phenobarbital[5] |
| Butibel[3] | Malatal[1] |
| Chardonna-2[4] | Relaxadon[1] |
| Donnamor[1] | Spaslin[1] |
| Donnapine[1] | Spasmolin[1] |
| Donnatal[1] | Spasmophen[1] |
| Donnatal Extentabs[1] | Spasquid[1] |
| Donnatal No. 2[1] | Susano[1] |

**In Canada—**

| | |
|---|---|
| Donnatal[1] | Donnatal Extentabs[1] |

Note: For quick reference, the following belladonna alkaloids and barbiturates are numbered to match the corresponding brand names.

This information applies to the following medicines:

1. Atropine (A-troe-peen), Hyoscyamine (hye-oh-SYE-a-meen), Scopolamine (skoe-POL-a-meen), and Phenobarbital (fee-noe-BAR-bi-tal)†
2. Atropine and Phenobarbital†
3. Belladonna and Butabarbital (byoo-ta-BAR-bi-tal)†
4. Belladonna and Phenobarbital†
5. Hyoscyamine and Phenobarbital†

---

†Not commercially available in Canada.
‡Generic name product may also be available in the U.S.
§Generic name product may also be available in Canada.

## Description

Belladonna alkaloids and barbiturates are combination medicines taken to relieve cramping and spasms of the stomach and intestines. They are used also to decrease the amount of acid formed in the stomach.

These medicines are available only with your doctor's prescription in the following dosage forms:

*Oral*
> Atropine, Hyoscyamine, Scopolamine, and Phenobarbital
> - Capsules (U.S.)
> - Elixir (U.S. and Canada)
> - Tablets (U.S. and Canada)
> - Chewable tablets (U.S.)
> - Extended-release tablets (U.S. and Canada)
>
> Atropine and Phenobarbital
> - Capsules (U.S.)
> - Elixir (U.S.)
> - Tablets (U.S.)
>
> Belladonna and Butabarbital
> - Elixir (U.S.)
> - Tablets (U.S.)
>
> Belladonna and Phenobarbital
> - Tablets (U.S.)
>
> Hyoscyamine and Phenobarbital
> - Elixir (U.S.)
> - Oral solution (U.S.)
> - Tablets (U.S.)

## Before Using This Medicine

In deciding to use a medicine, the risks of taking the medicine must be weighed against the good it will do. This is a decision you and your doctor will make. For belladona alkaloids and barbiturates, the following should be considered:

**Allergies**—Tell your doctor if you have ever had any unusual or allergic reaction to belladonna alkaloids (atropine, belladonna, hyoscyamine, and scopolamine) or to barbiturates (butabarbital, phenobarbital). Also, tell your health care professional if you are allergic to any other substances, such as foods, preservatives, or dyes.

**Pregnancy**—Belladonna alkaloids have not been shown to cause problems in humans. However, barbiturates (contained in this medicine) have been shown to increase the chance of birth defects in humans. Also, when taken during pregnancy, barbiturates may cause bleeding problems in the newborn baby. Be sure that you have discussed this with your doctor before taking this medicine.

**Breast-feeding**—Belladonna alkaloids or barbiturates have not been shown to cause problems in nursing babies. However, traces of the belladonna alkaloids and barbiturates pass into the breast milk. Also, because the belladonna alkaloids tend to decrease the secretions of the body, it is possible that the flow of breast milk may be reduced in some patients.

**Children**—Severe side effects may be more likely to occur in infants and children, especially those with spastic paralysis or brain damage. Unusual excitement, nervousness, restlessness, or irritability and unusual warmth, dryness, and flushing of skin are more likely to occur in children, who are usually more sensitive to the effects of belladonna alkaloids. Also, when belladonna alkaloids are given to children during hot weather, a rapid increase in body temperature may occur. In addition, the barbiturate in this medicine could cause some children to become hyperactive.

**Older adults**—Confusion or memory loss; constipation; difficult urination; drowsiness; dryness of mouth, nose, throat, or skin; and unusual excitement, nervousness, restlessness, or irritability may be more likely to occur in the elderly, who are usually more sensitive than younger adults to the effects of belladonna alkaloids and barbiturates. Also, eye pain may occur, which may be a sign of glaucoma.

**Other medicines**—Although certain medicines should not be used together at all, in other cases two different medicines may be used together even if an interaction might occur. In these cases, your doctor may want to change the dose, or other precautions may be necessary. When you are taking belladonna alkaloids and barbiturates, it is especially important that your health care professional know if you are taking any of the following:

- Adrenocorticoids (cortisone-like medicine) or
- Corticotropin (ACTH)—Belladonna alkaloids and barbiturates may decrease the response to these medicines

- Antacids or
- Diarrhea medicine containing kaolin or attapulgite—These medications may decrease the response to belladonna alkaloids
- Anticholinergics (medicine for abdominal or stomach spasms or cramps)—Belladonna alkaloids and barbiturates may increase the response to anticholinergics
- Anticoagulants (blood thinners)—Belladonna alkaloids and barbiturates may decrease the effect of this medicine
- Central nervous system (CNS) depressants (medicines that cause drowsiness)—The CNS effects of either medicine could be increased
- Ketoconazole (e.g., Nizoral)—Using ketoconazole with this combination medicine may lessen the effects of ketoconazole and barbiturates
- Monoamine oxidase (MAO) inhibitors (furazolidone [e.g., Furoxone], isocarboxazid [e.g., Marplan], phenelzine [e.g., Nardil], procarbazine [e.g., Matulane], selegiline [Eldepryl]; tranylcypromine [e.g., Parnate])—Taking belladonna alkaloids and barbiturates while you are taking or within 2 weeks of taking monoamine oxidase inhibitors may increase the effects of the barbiturates
- Potassium chloride (e.g., Slow K or K-Dur)—May cause an increase in lesions (sores) of the stomach or intestine

**Other medical problems**—The presence of other medical problems may affect the use of belladonna alkaloids and barbiturates. Make sure you tell your doctor if you have any other medical problems, especially:

- Asthma, emphysema, or other chronic lung disease or
- Dryness of mouth (severe and continuing) or
- Enlarged prostate or
- Glaucoma or
- Heart disease or
- Hyperactivity (in children) or
- Intestinal blockage or other intestinal problems or
- Urinary tract blockage or difficult urination—Belladonna alkaloids and barbiturates may make these conditions worse
- Brain damage (in children) or
- Spastic paralysis (in children)—These conditions may increase the effects of the medicine
- Down's syndrome (mongolism)—This condition may increase the side effects of the medicine
- Kidney disease or
- Liver disease—Higher levels of the belladonna alkaloid and barbiturate may result, possibly leading to increased side effects

## Proper Use of This Medicine

Take this medicine about ½ to 1 hour before meals, unless otherwise directed by your doctor.

*Take this medicine only as directed.* Do not take more or less of it, do not take it more often, and do not take it for a longer time than your doctor ordered. To do so may increase the chance of side effects.

**Dosing**—The dose of belladonna alkaloids and barbiturates combination will be different for different patients. *Follow your doctor's orders or the directions on the label.* The following information includes only the average doses of these combination medicines. *If your dose is different, do not change it* unless your doctor tells you to do so.

The number of capsules or tablets or the amount of solution you take depends on the strength of the medicine. Also, *the number of doses you take each day, the time allowed between doses, and the length of time you take the medicine depend on the medical problem for which you are taking these combination products.*

*For atropine, hyoscyamine, scopolamine, and phenobarbital combination*

- For stomach or intestine problems:
  —For *oral* dosage form (capsules or tablets):
    - Older adults, adults, and teenagers—1 or 2 capsules two to four times a day. Your doctor may change the dose if needed.
    - Children—Dose must be determined by your doctor.
  —For *oral* dosage form (solution):
    - Adults and teenagers—The usual dose is 1 to 2 teaspoonfuls (5 to 10 milliliters [mL]) three or four times a day. Your doctor may change the dose if needed.
    - Children—Dose is based on body weight and must be determined by your doctor. The usual dose is 0.5 to 7.5 mL every four to six hours. Your doctor may change the dose if needed.
  —For *oral* dosage form (chewable tablets):
    - Older adults, adults, and teenagers—Chew 1 or 2 tablets three or four times a day. Your doctor may change the dose if needed.
    - Children up to 2 years of age—Use is not recommended.
    - Children 2 to 12 years of age—½ to 1 tablet three or four times a day. Your doctor may change the dose if needed.
  —For *oral* dosage form (extended-release tablets):
    - Older adults, adults, and teenagers—1 tablet every eight to twelve hours. Your doctor may change the dose if needed.
    - Children—Use is not recommended.

*For atropine and phenobarbital*

- For stomach or intestine problems:
  —For *oral* dosage form (capsules or tablets):
    - Older adults, adults, and teenagers—1 or 2 capsules or tablets two to four times a day. Your doctor may change the dose if needed.
    - Children—Dose must be determined by your doctor.
  —For *oral* dosage form (solution):
    - Older adults, adults, and teenagers—1 to 2 teaspoonfuls (5 to 10 milliliters [mL]) three or four times a day. Your doctor may change the dose if needed.
    - Children—Dose is based on body weight and must be determined by your doctor. The usual dose is 0.5 to 3 mL every four to six hours. Your doctor may change the dose if needed.

*For belladonna and butabarbital*

- For stomach or intestine problems:
  —For *oral* dosage form (solution):
    - Older adults, adults and teenagers—1 to 2 teaspoonfuls (5 to 10 milliliters [mL]) three or four times a day. Your doctor may change the dose if needed.
    - Children up to 6 years of age—1.25 to 2.5 mL three or four times a day. Your doctor may change the dose if needed.
    - Children 6 to 12 years of age—2.5 to 5 mL three or four times a day. Your doctor may change the dose if needed.
  For *oral* dosage form (tablets):
    - Older adults, adults, and teenagers—1 or 2 tablets three or four times a day. Your doctor may change the dose if needed.
    - Children—Dose must be determined by your doctor.

*For belladonna and phenobarbital*

- For stomach or intestine problems:
  —For *oral* dosage form (tablets):
    - Older adults, adults, and teenagers—1 or 2 tablets two to four times a day. Your doctor may change the dose if needed.
    - Children—Dose must be determined by your doctor.

*For hyoscyamine and phenobarbital*

- For stomach or intestine problems:
  —For *oral* dosage form (elixir):
    - Older adults, adults, and children older than 10 years of age—The usual dose is 1 to 2 teaspoonfuls (5 to 10 milliliters [mL]) every four hours. Your doctor may change the dose if needed.
    - Children up to 2 years of age—1.25 to 2.5 mL every four hours. Your doctor may change the dose if needed.
    - Children 2 to 10 years of age—2.5 to 5 mL every four hours. Your doctor may change the dose if needed
  —For *oral* dosage form (solution):
    - Older adults, adults, and children over 10 years of age—1 to 2 mL every four hours. Your doctor may change the dose if needed.
    - Children up to 1 year of age—0.1 to 0.5 mL every four hours. Your doctor may change the dose if needed.
    - Children 1 to 10 years of age—0.5 to 1 mL every four hours. Your doctor may change the dose if needed.
  —For *oral* dosage form (tablets):
    - Older adults, adults, and teenagers—1 or 2 tablets three or four times a day. Your doctor may change the dose if needed.

- Children—Dose must be determined by your doctor.

**Missed dose**—If you miss a dose of this medicine, take it as soon as possible. However, if it is almost time for your next dose, skip the missed dose and go back to your regular dosing schedule. Do not double doses.

**Storage**—To store this medicine:
- Keep this medicine out of the reach of children. Overdose of belladonna alkaloids and barbiturates is especially dangerous in young children.
- Store away from heat and direct light.
- Do not store the capsule or tablet form of this medicine in the bathroom, near the kitchen sink, or in other damp places. Heat or moisture may cause the medicine to break down.
- Keep the liquid form of this medicine from freezing.
- Do not keep outdated medicine or medicine no longer needed. Be sure that any discarded medicine is out of the reach of children.

## Precautions While Using This Medicine

This medicine will add to the effects of alcohol and other CNS depressants (medicines that slow down the nervous system, possibly causing drowsiness). Some examples of CNS depressants are antihistamines or medicine for hay fever, other allergies, or colds; sedatives, tranquilizers, or sleeping medicine; prescription pain medicine or narcotics; barbiturates; medicine for seizures; muscle relaxants; or anesthetics, including some dental anesthetics. *Check with your doctor before taking any of the above while you are taking this medicine.*

Do not take this medicine within 1 hour of taking antacids or medicine for diarrhea. Taking them too close together will make the belladonna alkaloids less effective.

Belladonna alkaloids will often make you sweat less, causing your body temperature to increase. *Use extra care not to become overheated during exercise or hot weather while you are taking this medicine,* as overheating could possibly result in heat stroke. This is especially important in children taking belladonna alkaloids.

This medicine may cause your eyes to become more sensitive to light than they are normally. Wearing sunglasses and avoiding too much exposure to bright light may help lessen the discomfort.

This medicine may cause some people to have blurred vision or to become drowsy, dizzy, or less alert than they are normally. *Make sure you know how you react to this medicine before you drive, use machines, or do anything else that could be dangerous if you are not alert or able to see well.*

This medicine may cause dryness of the mouth, nose, and throat. For temporary relief of mouth dryness, use sugarless candy or gum, melt bits of ice in your mouth, or use a saliva substitute. However, if your mouth continues to feel dry for more than 2 weeks, check with your dentist. Continuing dryness of the mouth may increase the chance of dental disease, including tooth decay, gum disease, and fungus infections.

## Side Effects of This Medicine

Along with its needed effects, a medicine may cause some unwanted effects. Although not all of these side effects may occur, if they do occur they may need medical attention.

Check with your doctor as soon as possible if any of the following side effects occur:

*Rare*
> Eye pain; skin rash or hives; sore throat and fever; unusual bleeding or bruising; yellow eyes or skin

*Symptoms of overdose*
> Blurred vision (continuing) or changes in near vision; clumsiness or unsteadiness; confusion; convulsions (seizures); dizziness (continuing); drowsiness (severe); dryness of mouth, nose, or throat (severe); fast heartbeat; fever; hallucinations (seeing, hearing, or feeling things that are not there); shortness of breath or troubled breathing; slurred speech; unusual excitement, nervousness, restlessness, or irritability; unusual warmth, dryness, and flushing of skin

Other side effects may occur that usually do not need medical attention. These side effects may go away during treatment as your body adjusts to the medicine. However, check with your doctor if any of the following side effects continue or are bothersome:

*More common*
> Constipation; decreased sweating; dizziness; drowsiness; dryness of mouth, nose, throat, or skin

*Less common or rare*
> Bloated feeling; blurred vision; decreased flow of breast milk; difficult urination; difficulty in swallowing; headache; increased sensitivity of eyes to sunlight; loss of memory; nausea or vomiting; unusual tiredness or weakness

Other side effects not listed above may also occur in some patients. If you notice any other effects, check with your doctor.

Revised: 01/13/92
Interim revision(s): 08/29/94

# BENTIROMIDE   Diagnostic†

A commonly used brand name in the U.S. is Chymex.

†Not commercially available in Canada.

## Description

Bentiromide (ben-TEER-oh-mide) is used to help find out if the pancreas is working the way it should. The pancreas helps break down the bentiromide almost the same way it helps to break down food.

After bentiromide is broken down, a part of it appears in the urine. By measuring how much appears in the urine, your doctor can tell how well your pancreas is working.

How the test is done: Bentiromide is given by mouth as a single dose. After you take bentiromide, all of your urine is collected for the next six hours. The total amount is measured and a small sample is saved and examined. Your doctor may repeat the test after seven days.

Bentiromide is to be used only under the supervision of a doctor. It is available in the following dosage form:

*Oral*
• Oral solution (U.S.)

## Before Having This Test

In deciding to use a diagnostic test, any risks of the test must be weighed against the good it will do. This is a decision you and your doctor will make. Also, test results may be affected by other things. For the test using bentiromide, the following should be considered:

**Allergies**—Tell your doctor if you have ever had any unusual or allergic reaction to bentiromide. Also tell your doctor if you are allergic to any other substances, such as foods, preservatives, or dyes.

**Diet**—Eating prunes or cranberries shortly before the bentiromide test period starts will affect test results. Avoid these foods for 3 days before the test.

**Pregnancy**—Studies with bentiromide have not been done in pregnant women. However, in animal studies bentiromide has not been shown to cause birth defects or other problems.

**Breast-feeding**—It is not known whether bentiromide passes into the breast milk. However, this medicine has not been reported to cause problems in nursing babies.

**Children**—Studies on this medicine have been done only in older children and adult patients, and there is no specific information comparing use of bentiromide in children up to 6 years of age with use in other age groups.

**Older adults**—Many medicines have not been studied specifically in older people. Therefore, it may not be known whether they work exactly the same way they do in younger adults or if they cause different side effects or problems in older people. There is no specific information comparing use of bentiromide in the elderly with use in other age groups.

**Other medicines**—Although certain medicines should not be used together at all, in other cases two different medicines may be used together even if an interaction might occur. In these cases, your doctor may want to change the dose, or other precautions may be necessary. When you are taking bentiromide it is especially important that your doctor know if you are taking or using any of the following:

• Acetaminophen (e.g., Tylenol) or
• Chloramphenicol (e.g., Chloromycetin) or
• Local anesthetics (e.g., benzocaine and lidocaine) or
• Para-aminobenzoic acid (PABA)-containing preparations (e.g., sunscreens and some multivitamins) or
• Procainamide (e.g., Pronestyl) or
• Sulfonamides (sulfa medicines) or
• Thiazide diuretics (water pills)—Use of these medicines during the test period will affect the test results
• Pancreatic supplements (e.g., pancrelipase)—Use of pancreatic supplements may give false test results

**Other medical problems**—The presence of other medical problems may affect the results of the test. Make sure you tell your doctor if you have any other medical problems, especially:

• Disease of the stomach and intestines or
• Kidney disease or
• Liver disease (severe)—These medical problems may cause false test results

## Preparation For This Test

Your doctor may ask you to avoid certain medicines or foods for at least 72 hours before this test is done. *Follow your doctor's instructions carefully.* Otherwise, this test may not work and may have to be done again.

Unless otherwise directed by your doctor:

• Do not eat anything after midnight the night before the test. Some foods may affect the results of the test.
• Urinate before taking bentiromide. You should have an empty bladder when you take the test.
• After taking bentiromide, drink a large glass of water (at least 8 ounces). Drink another large glass of water in 2 hours and then 2 more glasses of water in the next 4 hours. This will help increase the amount of urine, which is needed for testing.

## Side Effects of This Medicine

Along with its needed effects, a medicine may cause some unwanted effects. Although not all of these side effects may occur, if they do occur they may need medical attention.

*Check with your health care professional immediately* if either of the following side effects occurs:
*Rare*
Shortness of breath or troubled breathing

Other side effects may occur that usually do not need medical attention. These side effects should go away as the effects of the medicine wear off. However, check with your doctor if any of the following side effects continue or are bothersome:
*More common*
Diarrhea; headache

*Less common or rare*
Gas; nausea and vomiting; weakness

Other side effects not listed above may also occur in some patients. If you notice any other effects, check with your doctor.

---

Revised: 12/02/92
Interim revision: 06/16/94

---

# BENZNIDAZOLE    Systemic*†

Some commonly used brand names in other countries are: Radanil; Rochagan; and Ro7-1051.

---

*Not commercially available in the U.S.
†Not commercially available in Canada.

---

## Description

Benznidazole (benz-NYE-da-zole) belongs to a group of medicines called antiprotozoals. It is used to treat an infection called American trypanosomiasis (Chagas disease). Benznidazole works by killing the protozoa (tiny, one-celled animals).

Benznidazole is available only with your doctor's prescription in the following dosage form:
*Oral*
• Tablets (Brazil)

## Before Using This Medicine

In deciding to use a medicine, the risks of taking the medicine must be weighed against the good it will do. This is a decision you and your doctor will make. For benznidazole, the following should be considered:

**Allergies**—Tell your doctor if you have ever had any unusual or allergic reaction to benznidazole. Also tell your health care professional if you are allergic to any other substances, such as foods, preservatives, or dyes.

**Pregnancy**—Studies have not been done in pregnant women. The World Health Organization (WHO) does not recommend the use of benznidazole during the first 3 months of pregnancy. However, this medicine has not been shown to cause birth defects or other problems in animal studies.

**Breast-feeding**—It is not known whether benznidazole passes into breast milk. Although most medicines pass into breast milk in small amounts, many of them may be used safely while breast-feeding. Mothers who are taking this medicine and who wish to breast-feed should discuss this with their doctor.

**Children**—Although there is no specific information comparing use of benznidazole in children with use in other age groups, this medicine is not expected to cause different side effects or problems in children than it does in adults.

**Older adults**—Many medicines have not been studied specifically in older people. Therefore, it may not be known whether they work exactly the same way they do in younger adults or if they cause different side effects or problems in older people. There is no specific information comparing use of benznidazole in the elderly with use in other age groups.

**Other medicines**—Although certain medicines should not be used together at all, in other cases two different medicines may be used together even if an interaction might occur. In these cases, your doctor may want to change the dose, or other precautions may be necessary. When you are taking benznidazole, it is especially important that your health care professional know if you are taking any of the following:
• Alcohol—Taking alcohol with benznidazole may cause unwanted effects such as stomach cramps, nausea, vomiting, headache, or redness of face
• Inflammation or pain medicine, except narcotics, such as aspirin, or
• Anticoagulants (blood thinners), such as warfarin (e.g., Coumadin, Panwarfarin, Warfilone)—Taking aspirin or anticoagulants with benznidazole may increase the chance of bleeding

**Other medical problems**—The presence of other medical problems may affect the use of benznidazole. Make sure you tell your doctor if you have any other medical problems, especially:
• Blood disease or
• Kidney disease or
• Liver disease—Patients with these conditions may have an increased chance of side effects

## Proper Use of This Medicine

Take this medicine with meals, preferably after breakfast and after supper, to decrease the chance of stomach upset. If you get an upset stomach (diarrhea, nausea, stomach pain, or vomiting) and it continues, check with your doctor.

To help clear up your infection, *take this medicine exactly as directed by your doctor for the full time of treatment.*

**Dosing**—The dose of benznidazole will be different for different patients. *Follow your doctor's orders or the directions on the label.* The following information includes only the average doses of benznidazole. *If your dose is different, do not change it* unless your doctor tells you to do so.

- For *oral* dosage form (tablets):
  —For Chagas disease:
    - Adults and children 12 years of age and over—Dose is based on body weight and must be determined by your doctor. The usual dose is 5 to 7 milligrams (mg) per kilogram (kg) (2.2 to 3.1 mg per pound) of body weight per day. Treatment should continue for thirty to sixty days.
    - Children up to 12 years of age—Dose is based on body weight and must be determined by your doctor. The usual dose is 10 mg per kg (4.5 mg per pound) of body weight per day. Treatment should continue for thirty to sixty days.

**Missed dose**—If you miss a dose of this medicine, take it as soon as possible. However, if it is almost time for your next dose, skip the missed dose and go back to your regular dosing schedule. Do not double doses.

**Storage**—To store this medicine:
- Keep out of the reach of children.
- Store away from heat and direct light.
- Do not store in the bathroom, near the kitchen sink, or in other damp places. Heat or moisture may cause the medicine to break down.
- Do not keep outdated medicine or medicine no longer needed. Be sure that any discarded medicine is out of the reach of children.

## Precautions While Using This Medicine

It is important that your doctor check your progress at regular visits. This is to help make sure that the infection is cleared up completely.

*If your symptoms become worse, check with your doctor.*

*Benznidazole can rarely lower the number of white blood cells in your blood, increasing your chance of getting an infection. It also can rarely lower the number of platelets, which are necessary for proper blood clotting.*

- *Check with your doctor immediately* if you think you are getting an infection or if you get a fever or chills.
- *Check with your doctor immediately* if you notice any unusual bleeding or bruising; black, tarry stools; blood in urine or stools; or pinpoint red spots on your skin.

Drinking alcoholic beverages while taking this medicine may cause stomach pain, nausea, vomiting, headache, flushing or redness of the face. Other alcohol-containing preparations (for example, elixirs, cough syrups, tonics) may also cause problems. Therefore, *do not drink alcoholic beverages or take other alcohol-containing preparations while you are taking benznidazole.*

## Side Effects of This Medicine

Along with its needed effects, a medicine may cause some unwanted effects. Although not all of these side effects may occur, if they do occur they may need medical attention.

*Check with your doctor as soon as possible if any of the following side effects occur:*

*More common*
  Convulsions (seizures); numbness, tingling pain, or weakness in hands or feet; reddish discoloration of skin

*Rare*
  Fever or chills; pinpoint red spots on skin; skin rash; sore throat; unusual bleeding or bruising

Other side effects may occur that usually do not need medical attention. These side effects may go away during treatment as your body adjusts to the medicine. However, check with your doctor if any of the following side effects continue or are bothersome:

*More common*
  Abdominal or stomach pain; diarrhea; nausea; vomiting

*Rare*
  Confusion; dizziness; headache; restlessness; temporary loss of memory; trouble in sleeping; difficulty concentrating; unusual tiredness or weakness

Other side effects not listed above may also occur in some patients. If you notice any other effects, check with your doctor.

Developed: 08/31/94

# BENZODIAZEPINES   Systemic

Some commonly used brand names are:

**In the U.S.—**

| | |
|---|---|
| Alprazolam Intensol[1] | Lorazepam Intensol[11] |
| Ativan[11] | Paxipam[9] |
| Centrax[14] | Poxi[3] |
| Dalmane[8] | ProSom[7] |
| Diazepam Intensol[6] | Restoril[16] |
| Doral[15] | Serax[13] |
| D-Val[6] | Tranxene-SD[5] |
| Gen-XENE[5] | Tranxene T-Tab[5] |
| Halcion[17] | Valium[6] |
| Klonopin[4] | Valrelease[6] |
| Libritabs[3] | Xanax[1] |
| Librium[3] | Zetran[6] |

**In Canada—**

| | |
|---|---|
| Apo-Alpraz[1] | Novoflupam[8] |
| Apo-Chlordiazepoxide[3] | Novo-Lorazem[11] |
| Apo-Clorazepate[5] | Novopoxide[3] |
| Apo-Diazepam[6] | Novo-Triolam[17] |
| Apo-Flurazepam[8] | Novoxapam[13] |
| Apo-Lorazepam[11] | Nu-Alpraz[1] |
| Apo-Oxazepam[13] | Nu-Loraz[11] |
| Apo-Triazo[17] | Nu-Triazo[17] |
| Ativan[11] | PMS-Diazepam[6] |
| Dalmane[8] | Restoril[16] |
| Diazemuls[6] | Rivotril[4] |
| Gen-Triazolam[17] | Serax[13] |
| Halcion[17] | Solium[3] |
| Lectopam[2] | Somnol[8] |
| Librium[3] | Syn-Clonazepam[4] |
| Loftran[10] | Tranxene[5] |
| Mogadon[12] | Valium[6] |
| Novo-Alprazol[1] | Vivol[6] |
| Novo-Clopate[5] | Xanax[1] |
| Novodipam[6] | Xanax TS[1] |

Note: For quick reference, the following benzodiazepines are numbered to match the corresponding brand names.

This information applies to the following medicines:

1. Alprazolam (al-PRAZ-oh-lam)‡§
2. Bromazepam (broe-MA-ze-pam)*
3. Chlordiazepoxide (klor-dye-az-e-POX-ide)‡
4. Clonazepam (kloe-NA-ze-pam)
5. Clorazepate (klor-AZ-e-pate)‡
6. Diazepam (dye-AZ-e-pam)‡
7. Estazolam (ess-TA-zoe-lam)†
8. Flurazepam (flure-AZ-e-pam)‡
9. Halazepam (hal-AZ-e-pam)†
10. Ketazolam (kee-TAY-zoe-lam)*
11. Lorazepam (lor-AZ-e-pam)‡
12. Nitrazepam (nye-TRA-ze-pam)*
13. Oxazepam (ox-AZ-e-pam)‡
14. Prazepam (PRAZ-e-pam)†‡
15. Quazepam (KWA-ze-pam)†
16. Temazepam (tem-AZ-e-pam)‡
17. Triazolam (trye-AY-zoe-lam)§

*Not commercially available in the U.S.
†Not commercially available in Canada.
‡Generic name product may also be available in the U.S.
§Generic name product may also be available in Canada.

## Description

Benzodiazepines (ben-zoe-dye-AZ-e-peens) belong to the group of medicines called central nervous system (CNS) depressants (medicines that slow down the nervous system).

Some benzodiazepines are used to relieve nervousness or tension. Others are used in the treatment of insomnia (trouble in sleeping). However, if used regularly (for example, every day) for insomnia, they are usually not effective for more than a few weeks.

One of the benzodiazepines, diazepam, is also used to help relax muscles or relieve muscle spasm. Another benzodiazepine, alprazolam, is also used in the treatment of panic disorder. Clonazepam, clorazepate, and diazepam are also used to treat certain convulsive (seizure) disorders, such as epilepsy. The benzodiazepines may also be used for other conditions as determined by your doctor.

Benzodiazepines should not be used for nervousness or tension caused by the stress of everyday life.

These medicines are available only with your doctor's prescription, in the following dosage forms:

*Oral*

Alprazolam
- Oral solution (U.S.)
- Tablets (U.S. and Canada)

Bromazepam
- Tablets (Canada)

Chlordiazepoxide
- Capsules (U.S. and Canada)
- Tablets (U.S.)

Clonazepam
- Tablets (U.S. and Canada)

Clorazepate
- Capsules (U.S. and Canada)
- Tablets (U.S.)

Diazepam
- Extended-release capsules (U.S.)
- Oral solution (U.S. and Canada)
- Tablets (U.S. and Canada)

Estazolam
- Tablets (U.S.)

Flurazepam
- Capsules (U.S. and Canada)
- Tablets (Canada)

Halazepam
- Tablets (U.S.)

Ketazolam
- Capsules (Canada)

Lorazepam
- Oral solution (U.S.)
- Tablets (U.S. and Canada)
- Sublingual tablets (Canada)

Nitrazepam
- Tablets (Canada)

Oxazepam
- Capsules (U.S.)
- Tablets (U.S. and Canada)

Prazepam
- Capsules (U.S.)
- Tablets (U.S.)

Quazepam
- Tablets (U.S.)

Temazepam
- Capsules (U.S. and Canada)
- Tablets (U.S.)

Triazolam
  • Tablets (U.S. and Canada)
*Parenteral*
Chlordiazepoxide
  • Injection (U.S. and Canada)
Diazepam
  • Injection (U.S. and Canada)
Lorazepam
  • Injection (U.S. and Canada)
*Rectal*
Diazepam
  • For rectal solution (U.S. and Canada)

## Before Using This Medicine

In deciding to use a medicine, the risks of taking the medicine must be weighed against the good it will do. This is a decision you and your doctor will make. For benzodiazepines, the following should be considered:

**Allergies**—Tell your doctor if you have ever had any unusual or allergic reaction to benzodiazepines. Also tell your health care professional if you are allergic to any other substances, such as foods, preservatives, or dyes.

**Pregnancy**—Chlordiazepoxide and diazepam have been reported to increase the chance of birth defects when used during the first 3 months of pregnancy. Although similar problems have not been reported with the other benzodiazepines, the chance always exists since all of the benzodiazepines are related.

Studies in animals have shown that clonazepam, lorazepam, and temazepam cause birth defects or other problems, including death of the animal fetus.

Too much use of benzodiazepines during pregnancy may cause the baby to become dependent on the medicine. This may lead to withdrawal side effects after birth. Also, use of benzodiazepines during pregnancy, especially during the last weeks, may cause drowsiness, slow heartbeat, shortness of breath, or troubled breathing in the newborn infant.

Benzodiazepines given just before or during labor may cause weakness in the newborn infant. When diazepam is given in high doses (especially by injection) within 15 hours before delivery, it may cause breathing problems, muscle weakness, difficulty in feeding, and body temperature problems in the newborn infant.

**Breast-feeding**—Benzodiazepines may pass into the breast milk and cause drowsiness, slow heartbeat, shortness of breath, or troubled breathing in nursing babies of mothers taking this medicine.

**Children**—Most of the side effects of these medicines are more likely to occur in children, especially the very young. These patients are usually more sensitive than adults to the effects of benzodiazepines.

When clonazepam is used for long periods of time in children, it may cause unwanted effects on physical and mental growth. These effects may not be noticed until many years later. Before this medicine is given to children for long periods of time, you should discuss its use with your child's doctor.

**Older adults**—Most of the side effects of these medicines are more likely to occur in the elderly, who are usually more sensitive to the effects of benzodiazepines.

Taking benzodiazepines for trouble in sleeping may cause more daytime drowsiness in elderly patients than in younger adults. In addition, falls and related injuries may be more likely to occur in elderly patients taking benzodiazepines.

**Other medicines**—Although certain medicines should not be used together at all, in other cases 2 different medicines may be used together even if an interaction might occur. In these cases, your doctor may want to change the dose, or other precautions may be necessary. When you are taking or receiving benzodiazepines it is especially important that your health care professional know if you are taking any of the following:

  • Central nervous system (CNS) depressants (medicine that causes drowsiness)—The CNS depressant effects of either these medicines or benzodiazepines may be increased; your doctor may want to change the dose of either or both medicines

**Other medical problems**—The presence of other medical problems may affect the use of benzodiazepines. Make sure you tell your doctor if you have any other medical problems, especially:

  • Alcohol abuse (or history of) or
  • Drug abuse or dependence (or history of)—Dependence on benzodiazepines may develop
  • Brain disease—CNS depression and other side effects of benzodiazepines may be more likely to occur
  • Difficulty in swallowing (in children) or
  • Emphysema, asthma, bronchitis, or other chronic lung disease or
  • Glaucoma or
  • Hyperactivity or
  • Mental depression or
  • Mental illness (severe) or
  • Myasthenia gravis or
  • Porphyria or
  • Sleep apnea (temporarily stopping of breathing during sleep)—Benzodiazepines may make the condition worse
  • Epilepsy or history of seizures—Although clonazepam and diazepam are used in treating epilepsy, starting or suddenly stopping treatment with these medicines may increase seizures
  • Kidney or liver disease—Higher blood levels of benzodiazepines may result, increasing the chance of side effects

## Proper Use of This Medicine

For patients taking *diazepam extended-release capsules:*
  • Swallow capsules whole.
  • Do not crush, break, or chew the capsules before swallowing.

For patients taking *lorazepam oral solution:*
  • Each dose may be diluted with water, soda or soda-like beverages, or semisolid food, such as applesauce or pudding.

For patients taking *lorazepam sublingual tablets:*
- Do not chew or swallow the tablet. This medicine is meant to be absorbed through the lining of the mouth. Place the tablet under your tongue (sublingual) and let it slowly dissolve there. Do not swallow for at least 2 minutes.

*Take this medicine only as directed by your doctor.* Do not take more of it, do not take it more often, and do not take it for a longer time than your doctor ordered. If too much is taken, it may become habit-forming (causing mental or physical dependence).

If you think this medicine is not working properly after you have taken it for a few weeks, *do not increase the dose.* Instead, check with your doctor.

For patients taking this medicine *for epilepsy or other seizure disorder:*
- *In order for this medicine to control your seizures, it must be taken every day in regularly spaced doses as ordered by your doctor.* This is necessary to keep a constant amount of the medicine in the blood. To help keep the amount constant, do not miss any doses.

For patients taking this medicine *for insomnia:*
- *Do not take this medicine when your schedule does not permit you to get a full night's sleep (7 to 8 hours).* If you must wake up before this, you may continue to feel drowsy and may experience memory problems, because the effects of the medicine have not had time to wear off.

For patients taking *flurazepam:*
- *When you begin to take this medicine, your sleeping problem will improve somewhat the first night. However, 2 or 3 nights may pass before you receive the full effects of this medicine.*

**Dosing**—The dose of benzodiazepines will be different for different patients. *Follow your doctor's orders or the directions on the label.* The following information includes only the average doses of benzodiazepines. *If your dose is different, do not change it* unless your doctor tells you to do so.

The number of capsules or tablets, or the amount of solution that you take, or the number of injections you receive, depends on the strength of the medicine. Also, *the number of doses you take each day, the time allowed between doses, and the length of time you take the medicine depend on the medical problem for which you are taking benzodiazepines.*

*For alprazolam*
- For *oral* dosage form (solution or tablets):
  —For anxiety:
    - Adults—At first, 0.25 to 0.5 milligrams (mg) three times a day. Your doctor may increase your dose if needed. However, the dose is usually not more than 4 mg a day.
    - Children up to 18 years of age—Use and dose must be determined by your doctor.

- Older adults—At first, 0.25 mg two to three times a day. Your doctor may increase your dose if needed.
  —For panic disorder:
    - Adults—At first, 0.5 mg three times a day. Your doctor may increase your dose if needed. However, the dose is usually not more than 10 mg a day.
    - Children up to 18 years of age—Use and dose must be determined by your doctor.

*For bromazepam*
- For *oral* dosage form (tablets):
  —For anxiety:
    - Adults—6 to 30 milligrams (mg) a day, taken in smaller doses during the day.
    - Children up to 18 years of age—Use and dose must be determined by your doctor.
    - Older adults—At first, up to 3 mg a day. Your doctor may change your dose if needed.

*For chlordiazepoxide*
- For *oral* dosage form (capsules or tablets):
  —For anxiety:
    - Adults—5 to 25 milligrams (mg) three or four times a day.
    - Children 6 years of age and over—5 mg two to four times a day. Your doctor may increase your dose if needed.
    - Children up to 6 years of age—Use and dose must be determined by your doctor.
    - Older adults—At first, 5 mg two to four times a day. Your doctor may increase your dose if needed.
  —For sedation during withdrawal from alcohol:
    - Adults—At first, 50 to 100 mg, repeated if needed. However, the dose is usually not more than 400 mg a day.
    - Children—Use and dose must be determined by your doctor.
- For *injection* dosage form:
  —For anxiety:
    - Adults—At first, 50 to 100 mg, injected into a muscle or vein. Then, if needed, 25 to 50 mg three or four times a day.
    - Teenagers—25 to 50 mg, injected into a muscle or vein.
    - Children up to 12 years of age—Use and dose must be determined by your doctor.
    - Older adults—25 to 50 mg, injected into a muscle or vein.
  —For sedation during withdrawal from alcohol:
    - Adults—At first, 50 to 100 mg, injected into a muscle or vein. If needed, the dose may be repeated in two to four hours.
    - Children—Use and dose must be determined by your doctor.

*For clonazepam*
- For *oral* dosage form (tablets):
  —For control of seizures:
    - Adults—At first, 0.5 milligrams (mg) three times a day. Your doctor may increase your dose if needed. However, the dose is usually not more than 20 mg a day.
    - Infants and children up to 10 years of age— Dose is based on weight and must be determined by your doctor.

*For clorazepate*
- For *oral* dosage form (capsules or tablets):
  —For anxiety:
    - Adults and teenagers—7.5 to 15 milligrams (mg) two to four times a day. Or your doctor may want you to start by taking 15 mg at bedtime.
    - Children up to 12 years of age—Use and dose must be determined by your doctor.
    - Older adults—At first, 3.75 to 15 mg a day. Your doctor may increase your dose if needed.
  —For sedation during withdrawal from alcohol:
    - Adults and teenagers—At first, 30 mg. Your doctor will set up a schedule that will gradually reduce your dose.
    - Children up to 12 years of age—Use and dose must be determined by your doctor.
  —For control of seizures:
    - Adults and teenagers—At first, up to 7.5 mg taken three times a day. Your doctor may increase your dose if needed. However, the dose is usually not more than 90 mg a day.
    - Children 9 to 12 years of age—At first, 7.5 mg two times a day. Your doctor may increase your dose if needed. However, the dose is usually not more than 60 mg a day.
    - Children up to 9 years of age—Use and dose must be determined by your doctor.

*For diazepam*
- For *oral* dosage form (extended-release capsules):
  —For anxiety:
    - Adults—15 to 30 milligrams (mg) once a day.
    - Children 6 months of age and over—15 mg once a day.
    - Children up to 6 months of age—Use is not recommended.
    - Older adults—15 mg once a day.
  —For relaxing muscles:
    - Adults—15 to 30 mg once a day.
    - Children 6 months of age and over—15 mg once a day.
    - Children up to 6 months of age—Use is not recommended.
    - Older adults—15 mg once a day.

- For *oral* dosage form (solution or tablets):
  —For anxiety:
    - Adults—2 to 10 mg two to four times a day.
    - Children 6 months of age and over—Dose is based on body weight or size and must be determined by your doctor.
    - Children up to 6 months of age—Use is not recommended.
    - Older adults—2 to 2.5 mg one or two times a day. Your doctor may increase your dose if needed.
  —For sedation during withdrawal from alcohol:
    - Adults—At first, 10 mg three or four times a day. Your doctor will set up a schedule that will gradually decrease your dose.
    - Children—Use and dose must be determined by your doctor.
  —For control of seizures:
    - Adults—2 to 10 mg taken two to four times a day.
    - Children 6 months of age and over—Dose is based on body weight or size and must be determined by your doctor.
    - Children up to 6 months of age—Use is not recommended.
    - Older adults—2 to 2.5 mg one or two times a day. Your doctor may increase your dose if needed.
  —For relaxing muscles:
    - Adults—2 to 10 mg three or four times a day.
    - Children 6 months of age and over—Dose is based on body weight or size and must be determined by your doctor.
    - Children up to 6 months of age—Use is not recommended.
    - Older adults—2 to 2.5 mg one or two times a day. Your doctor may increase your dose if needed.
- For *injection* dosage form:
  —For anxiety:
    - Adults—2 to 10 mg, injected into a muscle or vein.
    - Children—Use and dose must be determined by your doctor.
    - For older adults—2 to 5 mg, injected into a muscle or vein.
  —For sedation during withdrawal from alcohol:
    - Adults—At first, 10 mg injected into a muscle or vein. If needed, 5 to 10 mg may be given three or four hours later.
    - Children—Use and dose must be determined by your doctor.
  —For sedation before surgery or other procedures:
    - Adults—5 to 20 mg, injected into a muscle or vein.

- Children—Use and dose must be determined by your doctor.
- Older adults—2 to 5 mg, injected into a muscle or vein.
- —For control of seizures:
  - Adults—At first, 5 to 10 mg, usually injected into a vein. If needed, the dose may be repeated.
  - Children 5 years of age and older—At first, 1 mg injected into a vein every two to five minutes. The dose may need to be repeated.
  - Infants over 30 days of age and children up to 5 years of age—At first, 0.2 to 0.5 mg injected into a vein every two to five minutes. The dose may need to be repeated.
  - Newborns and infants up to 30 days of age: Use and dose must be determined by your doctor.
  - Older adults—2 to 5 mg, injected into a muscle or vein.
- —For relaxing muscle spasms:
  - Adults—At first, 5 to 10 mg injected into a muscle or vein. The dose may be repeated in three or four hours.
  - Children: Use and dose must be determined by your doctor.
  - Older adults—2 to 5 mg, injected into a muscle or vein.
- —For relaxing muscles in tetanus:
  - Adults—At first, 5 to 10 mg injected into a muscle or vein. Your doctor may increase your dose if needed.
  - Children 5 years of age and older—5 to 10 mg, injected into a muscle or vein. The dose may be repeated every three to four hours if needed.
  - Infants over 30 days of age and children up to 5 years of age—1 to 2 mg, injected into a muscle or vein. The dose may be repeated every three to four hours if needed.
  - Newborns and infants up to 30 days of age: Use and dose must be determined by your doctor.
- For *rectal* dosage form (solution):
  - —For control of seizures:
    - Adults and teenagers—Dose is based on body weight and must be determined by your doctor.
    - Children—Dose is based on body weight and must be determined by your doctor.

*For estazolam*
- For *oral* dosage form (tablets):
  - —For trouble in sleeping:
    - Adults—1 milligram (mg) at bedtime.
    - Children up to 18 years of age—Use and dose must be determined by your doctor.

*For flurazepam*
- For *oral* dosage form (capsules or tablets):
  - —For trouble in sleeping:
    - Adults—15 or 30 milligrams (mg) at bedtime.
    - Children up to 15 years of age—Use and dose must be determined by your doctor.
    - Older adults—At first, 15 mg at bedtime. Your doctor may increase your dose if needed.

*For halazepam*
- For *oral* dosage form (tablets):
  - —For anxiety:
    - Adults—20 to 40 milligrams (mg) three or four times a day.
    - Children up to 18 years of age—Use and dose must be determined by your doctor.
    - Older adults—20 mg one or two times a day.

*For ketazolam*
- For *oral* dosage form (capsules):
  - —For anxiety:
    - Adults—15 milligrams (mg) one or two times a day. Your doctor may increase your dose if needed.
    - Children up to 18 years of age—Use and dose must be determined by your doctor.
    - Infants—Use is not recommended.
    - Older adults—15 mg once a day.

*For lorazepam*
- For *oral* dosage form (solution or tablets):
  - —For anxiety:
    - Adults—1 to 3 milligrams (mg) two or three times a day.
    - Children up to 12 years of age—Use and dose must be determined by your doctor.
    - Older adults—0.5 to 2 mg a day, taken in smaller doses during the day.
  - —For trouble in sleeping:
    - Adults—2 to 4 mg taken at bedtime.
    - Children up to 12 years of age—Use and dose must be determined by your doctor.
- For *sublingual tablet* dosage form:
  - —For anxiety:
    - Adults—2 to 3 mg a day, in smaller doses placed under the tongue during the day. Your doctor may increase your dose if needed. However, the dose is usually not more than 6 mg a day.
    - Children 6 to 18 years of age—Use and dose must be determined by your doctor.
    - Children up to 6 years of age—Use is not recommended.
    - Older adults—At first, 0.5 mg a day. Your doctor may increase your dose if needed.
  - —For sedation before surgery:
    - Adults—Dose is based on body weight and is usually 0.05 mg per kilogram (0.023 mg per

pound) of body weight, placed under the tongue, one to two hours before surgery. The dose is usually not more than 4 mg.
- Children—Use and dose must be determined by your doctor.
- For *injection* dosage form:
  —For sedation before surgery or other procedures:
  - Adults—Dose is based on body weight and will be determined by your doctor. However, the dose is usually not more than 4 mg, injected into a muscle or vein.
  - Children up to 18 years of age—Use and dose must be determined by your doctor.

*For nitrazepam*
- For *oral* dosage form (tablets):
  —For trouble in sleeping:
  - Adults—5 to 10 milligrams (mg) at bedtime.
  - Children—Use and dose must be determined by your doctor.
  - Older adults—At first, 2.5 mg taken at bedtime. Your doctor may increase your dose if needed.
  —For control of seizures:
  - Children up to 30 kilograms (66 pounds) of body weight—Dose is based on body weight and is usually 0.3 to 1 mg per kilogram (0.14 to 0.45 mg per pound) of body weight per day, taken in smaller doses three times during the day. Your doctor may increase your dose if needed.

*For oxazepam*
- For *oral* dosage form (capsules or tablets):
  —For anxiety:
  - Adults—10 to 30 milligrams (mg) three or four times a day.
  - Children 6 to 12 years of age—Use and dose must be determined by your doctor.
  - Children up to 6 years of age—Use is not recommended.
  - Older adults—At first, 10 mg three times a day. Your doctor may increase your dose if needed. However, the dose is usually not more than 15 mg taken four times a day.
  —For sedation during withdrawal from alcohol:
  - Adults—15 to 30 mg three or four times a day.
  - Children—Use and dose must be determined by your doctor.

*For prazepam*
- For *oral* dosage form (capsules or tablets):
  —For anxiety:
  - Adults—10 milligrams (mg) three times a day, or 20 to 40 mg taken at bedtime.
  - Children—Use and dose must be determined by your doctor.
  - Older adults—At first, 10 to 15 mg a day, taken in smaller doses during the day. Your doctor may increase your dose if needed.

*For quazepam*
- For *oral* dosage form (tablets):
  —For trouble in sleeping:
  - Adults—7.5 to 15 milligrams (mg) taken at bedtime.
  - Children up to 18 years of age—Use and dose must be determined by your doctor.

*For temazepam*
- For *oral* dosage form (capsules or tablets):
  —For trouble in sleeping:
  - Adults—15 milligrams (mg) taken at bedtime.
  - Children up to 18 years of age—Use and dose must be determined by your doctor.
  - Older adults—At first, 7.5 mg at bedtime. Your doctor may increase your dose if needed.

*For triazolam*
- For *oral* dosage form (tablets):
  —For trouble in sleeping:
  - Adults—125 to 250 micrograms (mcg) taken at bedtime.
  - Children up to 18 years of age—Use and dose must be determined by your doctor.
  - Older adults—At first, 125 mcg at bedtime. Your doctor may increase your dose if needed.

**Missed dose**—If you are taking this medicine regularly (for example, every day as for epilepsy) and you miss a dose, take it right away if you remember within an hour or so of the missed dose. However, if you do not remember until later, skip the missed dose and go back to your regular dosing schedule. Do not double doses.

**Storage**—To store this medicine:
- Keep out of the reach of children. Overdose of benzodiazepines may be especially dangerous in children.
- Store away from heat and direct light.
- Do not store the capsule or tablet form of this medicine in the bathroom, near the kitchen sink, or in other damp places. Heat or moisture may cause the medicine to break down.
- Keep the liquid form of this medicine from freezing.
- Do not keep outdated medicine or medicine no longer needed. Be sure that any discarded medicine is out of the reach of children.

## Precautions While Using This Medicine

If you will be *taking this medicine regularly for a long time:*
- Your doctor should check your progress at regular visits to make sure that this medicine does not cause unwanted effects. If you are taking clonazepam, this is also important during the first few months of treatment.
- If you are taking this medicine for nervousness or tension or for panic disorder, check with your doctor

at least every 4 months to make sure you need to continue taking this medicine.

- If you are taking estazolam, flurazepam, quazepam, temazepam, or triazolam for insomnia (trouble in sleeping), and you think you need this medicine for more than 7 to 10 days, be sure to discuss it with your doctor. Insomnia that lasts longer than this may be a sign of another medical problem.

If you will be taking this medicine in large doses or for a long time, do not stop taking it without first checking with your doctor. Your doctor may want you to reduce gradually the amount you are taking before stopping completely. Stopping this medicine suddenly may cause withdrawal side effects. Also, if you are taking this medicine for epilepsy or another seizure disorder, stopping this medicine suddenly may cause seizures.

For patients taking this medicine *for epilepsy or another seizure disorder:*

- Your doctor may want you to carry a medical identification card or bracelet stating that you are taking this medicine.

This medicine will add to the effects of alcohol and other CNS depressants (medicines that slow down the nervous system, possibly causing drowsiness). Some examples of CNS depressants are antihistamines or medicine for hay fever, other allergies, or colds; sedatives, tranquilizers, or sleeping medicine; prescription pain medicine or narcotics; barbiturates; medicine for seizures; muscle relaxants; or anesthetics, including some dental anesthetics. This effect may last for a few days after you stop taking this medicine. *Check with your doctor before taking any of the above while you are taking this medicine.*

*If you think you or someone else may have taken an overdose of this medicine, get emergency help at once.* Taking an overdose of a benzodiazepine or taking alcohol or other CNS depressants with the benzodiazepine may lead to unconsciousness and possibly death. Some signs of an overdose are continuing slurred speech or confusion, severe drowsiness, severe weakness, and staggering.

Before you have any medical tests, tell the medical doctor in charge that you are taking this medicine. The results of the metyrapone test may be affected by chlordiazepoxide.

If you develop any unusual and strange thoughts or behavior while you are taking this medicine, be sure to discuss it with your doctor. Some changes that have occurred in people taking this medicine are like those seen in people who drink alcohol and then act in a manner that is not normal. Other changes may be more unusual and extreme, such as confusion, agitation, and hallucinations (seeing, hearing, or feeling things that are not there).

This medicine may cause some people, especially older persons, to become drowsy, dizzy, lightheaded, clumsy or unsteady, or less alert than they are normally. Even if taken at bedtime, it may cause some people to feel drowsy or less alert on arising. *Make sure you know how you react to this medicine before you drive, use machines, or do anything else that could be dangerous if you are dizzy or are not alert.*

If you have been taking this medicine for insomnia, you may have difficulty sleeping (rebound insomnia) for the first few nights after you stop taking the medicine.

## Side Effects of This Medicine

Along with its needed effects, a medicine may cause some unwanted effects. Although not all of these side effects may occur, if they do occur they may need medical attention.

Check with your doctor as soon as possible if any of the following side effects occur:

*Less common or rare*

Behavior problems, including difficulty in concentrating and outbursts of anger; confusion or mental depression; convulsions (seizures); hallucinations (seeing, hearing, or feeling things that are not there); hypotension (low blood pressure); impaired memory—may be more common with triazolam; muscle weakness; skin rash or itching; sore throat, fever, and chills; trouble in sleeping; ulcers or sores in mouth or throat (continuing); uncontrolled movements of body, including the eyes; unusual bleeding or bruising; unusual excitement, nervousness, or irritability; unusual tiredness or weakness (severe); yellow eyes or skin

*Symptoms of overdose*

Confusion (continuing); drowsiness (severe); shakiness; slow heartbeat, shortness of breath, or troubled breathing; slow reflexes; slurred speech (continuing); staggering; weakness (severe)

Other side effects may occur that usually do not need medical attention. These side effects may go away during treatment as your body adjusts to the medicine. However, check with your doctor if any of the following side effects continue or are bothersome:

*More common*

Clumsiness or unsteadiness; dizziness or lightheadedness; drowsiness; slurred speech

*Less common or rare*

Abdominal or stomach cramps or pain; blurred vision or other changes in vision; changes in sexual drive or performance; constipation; diarrhea; dryness of mouth or increased thirst; false sense of well-being; fast or pounding heartbeat; headache; increased bronchial secretions or watering of mouth; muscle spasm; nausea or vomiting; problems with urination; trembling; unusual tiredness or weakness

Not all of the side effects listed above have been reported for each of these medicines, but they have been reported for at least one of them. All of the benzodiazepines are similar, so any of the above side effects may occur with any of these medicines.

For patients having *chlordiazepoxide, diazepam, or lorazepam injected:*

- Check with your doctor if there is redness, swelling, or pain at the place of injection.

After you stop using this medicine, your body may need time to adjust. If you took this medicine in high doses or for a long time, this may take up to 3 weeks. During this period of time check with your doctor if you notice any of the following side effects:

*More common*

Irritability; nervousness; trouble in sleeping

*Less common*

Abdominal or stomach cramps; confusion; fast or pounding heartbeat; increased sense of hearing; increased sensitivity to touch and pain; increased sweating; loss of sense of reality; mental depression; muscle cramps; nausea or vomiting; sensitivity of eyes to light; tingling, burning, or prickly sensations; trembling

*Rare*

Confusion as to time, place, or person; convulsions (seizures); feelings of suspicion or distrust; hallucinations (seeing, hearing, or feeling things that are not there)

Other side effects not listed above may also occur in some patients. If you notice any other effects, check with your doctor.

## Additional Information

Once a medicine has been approved for marketing for a certain use, experience may show that it is also useful for other medical problems. Although these uses are not included in product labeling, some of the benzodiazepines are used in certain patients with the following medical conditions:

- Nausea and vomiting caused by cancer chemotherapy
- Tension headache
- Tremors

Other than the above information, there is no additional information relating to proper use, precautions, or side effects for these uses.

Revised: 08/04/92
Interim revision: 08/17/94

# BENZONATATE    Systemic

A commonly used brand name in the U.S. and Canada is Tessalon. Generic name product may also be available in the U.S.

## Description

Benzonatate (ben-ZOE-na-tate) is used to relieve coughs due to colds or influenza (flu). It is not to be used for chronic cough that occurs with smoking, asthma, or emphysema or when there is an unusually large amount of mucus or phlegm (pronounced flem) with the cough.

Benzonatate relieves cough by acting directly on the lungs and the breathing passages. It may also act on the cough center in the brain.

This medicine is available only with your doctor's prescription, in the following dosage form:

*Oral*

- Capsules (U.S. and Canada)

## Before Using this Medicine

In deciding to use a medicine, the risks of taking the medicine must be weighed against the good it will do. This is a decision you and your doctor will make. For benzonatate, the following should be considered:

**Allergies**—Tell your doctor if you have ever had any unusual or allergic reaction to benzonatate or to tetracaine or other local anesthetics. Also tell your health care professional if you are allergic to any other substances, such as foods, preservatives, or dyes.

**Pregnancy**—Studies on effects in pregnancy have not been done in either humans or animals.

**Breast-feeding**—It is not known whether benzonatate passes into breast milk. Although most medicines pass into breast milk in small amounts, many of them may be used safely while breast-feeding. Mothers who are taking this medicine and who wish to breast-feed should discuss this with their doctor.

**Children**—Children may tend to chew the capsule before swallowing it. This may cause numbness (loss of feeling) in the mouth and throat, and choking may occur.

**Older adults**—Many medicines have not been studied specifically in older people. Therefore, it may not be known whether they work exactly the same way they do in younger adults or if they cause different side effects or problems in older people. There is no specific information comparing use of benzonatate in the elderly with use in other age groups.

**Other medicines**—Although certain medicines should not be used together at all, in other cases 2 different medicines may be used together even if an interaction might occur. In these cases, your doctor may want to change the dose, or other precautions may be necessary. Tell your health care professional if you are taking any other prescription or nonprescription (over-the-counter [OTC]) medicine.

**Other medical problems**—The presence of other medical problems may affect the use of benzonatate. Make sure you tell your doctor if you have any other medical problems, especially:

- Mucus or phlegm with cough—Since benzonatate decreases coughing, it makes it difficult to get rid of the mucus that may collect in the lungs and airways with some diseases

## Proper Use of This Medicine

Do not chew the capsules before swallowing them. If the benzonatate contained in the capsules comes in contact with the mouth, it may cause the mouth and throat to become numb (loss of feeling) and choking may occur.

**Dosing**—The dose of benzonatate will be different for different patients. *Follow your doctor's orders or the directions on the label.* The following information includes only the average doses of benzonatate. *If your dose is different, do not change it* unless your doctor tells you to do so.

- For *oral* dosage form (capsules):
  —For cough:
  - Adults—100 milligrams (mg) three times a day as needed.
  - Children—
    Up to 10 years of age: Use is not recommended.
    10 years of age and older: 100 mg three times a day as needed.

**Missed dose**—If you must take this medicine regularly and you miss a dose, take it as soon as possible. However, if it is almost time for your next dose, skip the missed dose and go back to your regular dosing schedule. Do not double doses.

**Storage**—To store this medicine:
- Store away from heat and direct light.
- Keep out of the reach of children.
- Do not store this medicine in the bathroom, near the kitchen sink, or in other damp places. Heat or moisture may cause the medicine to break down.

- Do not keep outdated medicine or medicine no longer needed. Be sure that any discarded medicine is out of the reach of children.

## Precautions While Using This Medicine

If your cough has not become better after 7 days or if you have a high fever, skin rash, or continuing headache with the cough, check with your doctor. These signs may mean that you have other medical problems.

## Side Effects of This Medicine

Along with its needed effects, a medicine may cause some unwanted effects. Although not all of these side effects may occur, if they do occur they may need medical attention.

Check with your doctor as soon as possible if any of the following side effects occur:

*Symptoms of overdose*
  Convulsions (seizures); restlessness; trembling

Other side effects may occur that usually do not need medical attention. These side effects may go away during treatment as your body adjusts to the medicine. However, check with your health care professional if any of the following side effects continue or are bothersome:

*Less common or rare*
  Constipation; dizziness (mild); drowsiness (mild); nausea or vomiting; skin rash; stuffy nose

Other side effects not listed above may also occur in some patients. If you notice any other effects, check with your doctor.

Revised: 02/23/94

# BENZOYL PEROXIDE Topical

Some commonly used brand names are:

In the U.S.—

| | |
|---|---|
| Acne Aid 10 Cream | Benzac W 2½ Gel |
| Acne-5 Lotion | Benzac W 5 Gel |
| Acne-10 Lotion | Benzac W 10 Gel |
| Ben-Aqua-2½ Gel | Benzac W Wash 5 |
| Ben-Aqua-5 Gel | Benzac W Wash 10 |
| Ben-Aqua-10 Gel | BenzaShave 5 Cream |
| Ben-Aqua-5 Lotion | BenzaShave 10 Cream |
| Ben-Aqua-10 Lotion | Brevoxyl 4 Gel |
| Ben-Aqua Masque 5 | Clearasil Maximum Strength |
| Benoxyl 5 Lotion | Medicated Anti-Acne 10 |
| Benoxyl 10 Lotion | Tinted Cream |
| Benzac Ac 2½ Gel | Clearasil Maximum Strength |
| Benzac Ac 5 Gel | Medicated Anti-Acne 10 |
| Benzac Ac 10 Gel | Vanishing Cream |
| Benzac 5 Gel | Clearasil Maximum Strength |
| Benzac 10 Gel | Medicated Anti-Acne 10 |
| | Vanishing Lotion |

| | |
|---|---|
| Clear By Design 2.5 Gel | Dryox 20 Gel |
| Cuticura Acne 5 Cream | Dryox Wash 5 |
| Del-Aqua-5 Gel | Dryox Wash 10 |
| Del-Aqua-10 Gel | Fostex 10 Bar |
| Desquam-E 2.5 Gel | Fostex 10 Cream |
| Desquam-E 5 Gel | Fostex 5 Gel |
| Desquam-E 10 Gel | Fostex 10 Gel |
| Desquam-X 10 Bar | Fostex 10 Wash |
| Desquam-X 2.5 Gel | Loroxide 5.5 Lotion |
| Desquam-X 5 Gel | Neutrogena Acne Mask 5 |
| Desquam-X 10 Gel | Noxzema Clear-ups Maximum |
| Desquam-X 5 Wash | Strength 10 Lotion |
| Desquam-X 10 Wash | Noxzema Clear-ups On-The- |
| Dry and Clear Double | Spot 10 Lotion |
| Strength 10 Cream | Oxy 10 Daily Face Wash |
| Dry and Clear 5 Lotion | Oxy 5 Tinted Lotion |
| Dryox 5 Gel | Oxy 10 Tinted Lotion |
| Dryox 10 Gel | Oxy 5 Vanishing Lotion |

Oxy 10 Vanishing Lotion
PanOxyl AQ 2½ Gel
PanOxyl AQ 5 Gel
PanOxyl AQ 10 Gel
PanOxyl 5 Bar
PanOxyl 10 Bar
PanOxyl 5 Gel
PanOxyl 10 Gel
Persa-Gel 5
Persa-Gel 10
Persa-Gel W 5
Persa-Gel W 10
pHisoAc BP 10 Cream
Propa P.H. 10 Acne Cover
    Stick

Propa P.H. 10 Liquid Acne
    Soap
Stri-Dex Maximum Strength
    Treatment 10 Cream
Theroxide 5 Lotion
Theroxide 10 Lotion
Theroxide 10 Wash
Topex 10 Lotion
Vanoxide 5 Lotion
Xerac BP 5 Gel
Xerac BP 10 Gel
Zeroxin-5 Gel
Zeroxin-10 Gel

Generic name product may also be available.

**In Canada—**

Acetoxyl 2.5 Gel
Acetoxyl 5 Gel
Acetoxyl 10 Gel
Acetoxyl 20 Gel
Acnomel B.P. 5 Lotion
Benoxyl 5 Lotion
Benoxyl 10 Lotion
Benoxyl 20 Lotion
Benoxyl 5 Wash
Benoxyl 10 Wash
Benzac W 5 Gel
Benzac W 10 Gel
Benzagel 5 Acne Lotion
Benzagel 5 Acne Wash
Benzagel 5 Gel
Benzagel 10 Gel
Clearasil BP Plus 5 Cream
Clearasil BP Plus 5 Lotion
Dermoxyl Aqua 5 Gel
Dermoxyl 2.5 Gel
Dermoxyl 5 Gel
Dermoxyl 10 Gel
Dermoxyl 20 Gel

Desquam-X 5 Bar
Desquam-X 5 Gel
Desquam-X 10 Gel
Desquam-X 5 Wash
Desquam-X 10 Wash
H₂Oxyl 2.5 Gel
H₂Oxyl 5 Gel
H₂Oxyl 10 Gel
H₂Oxyl 20 Gel
Loroxide 5 Lotion with Flesh-
    Tinted Base
Oxyderm 5 Lotion
Oxyderm 10 Lotion
Oxyderm 20 Lotion
Oxy 5 Vanishing Formula
    Lotion
PanOxyl 5 Bar
PanOxyl 10 Bar
PanOxyl 5 Gel
PanOxyl 10 Gel
PanOxyl 15 Gel
PanOxyl 20 Gel
Topex 5 Lotion

## Description

Benzoyl peroxide (BEN-zoe-ill per-OX-ide) is used to treat acne. It may also be used for other conditions as determined by your doctor.

Some of these preparations are available only with your doctor's prescription. Others are available without a prescription; however, your doctor may have special instructions on the proper use of benzoyl peroxide for your medical condition.

Benzoyl peroxide is available in the following dosage forms:

*Topical*
- Cleansing bar (U.S. and Canada)
- Cream (U.S. and Canada)
- Gel (U.S. and Canada)
- Lotion (U.S. and Canada)
- Cleansing lotion (U.S. and Canada)
- Facial mask (U.S.)
- Stick (U.S.)

## Before Using This Medicine

If you are using this medicine without a prescription, carefully read and follow any precautions on the label. For benzoyl peroxide, the following should be considered:

**Allergies**—Tell your doctor if you have ever had any unusual or allergic reaction to benzoyl peroxide. Also tell your health care professional if you are allergic to any other substances, such as preservatives or dyes.

**Pregnancy**—Studies on effects in pregnancy have not been done in either humans or animals. However, benzoyl peroxide may be absorbed through the skin.

**Breast-feeding**—Benzoyl peroxide may be absorbed through the mother's skin. It is not known whether it passes into the breast milk. However, this medicine has not been reported to cause problems in nursing babies.

**Children**—For children up to 12 years of age: Studies on this medicine have been done only in adult patients, and there is no specific information comparing use of benzoyl peroxide with use in other age groups. For children 12 years of age and older: Although there is no specific information comparing use of benzoyl peroxide in children with use in other age groups, this medicine is not expected to cause different side effects or problems in children 12 years of age and older than it does in adults.

**Older adults**—Many medicines have not been studied specifically in older people. Therefore, it may not be known whether they work exactly the same way they do in younger adults. Although there is no specific information comparing use of benzoyl peroxide in the elderly with use in other age groups, this medicine is not expected to cause different side effects or problems in older people than it does in younger adults.

**Other medicines**—Although certain medicines should not be used together at all, in other cases two different medicines may be used together even if an interaction might occur. In these cases, your doctor may want to change the dose, or other precautions may be necessary. Tell your health care professional if you are using any other topical prescription or nonprescription (over-the-counter [OTC]) medicine that is to be applied to the same area of the skin.

**Other medical problems**—The presence of other medical problems may affect the use of benzoyl peroxide. Make sure you tell your doctor if you have any other medical problems, especially:
- Red or raw skin—Irritation will occur if benzoyl peroxide is used on red or raw skin

## Proper Use of This Medicine

To use the *cream, gel, lotion, or stick form* of benzoyl peroxide:
- Before applying, wash the affected area with non-medicated soap and water or with a degreasing cleanser and then gently pat dry with a towel.
- Apply enough medicine to cover the affected areas, and rub in gently.

To use the *shave cream form* of benzoyl peroxide:
- Wet the area to be shaved.
- Apply a small amount of the shave cream and gently rub over entire area.
- Shave.
- Rinse the area and pat dry.

- After-shave lotions or other drying face products should not be used without checking with your doctor first.

To use the *cleansing bar, cleansing lotion, or soap form* of benzoyl peroxide:
- Use to wash the affected areas as directed.

To use the *facial mask form* of benzoyl peroxide:
- Before applying, wash the affected area with a non-medicated cleanser. Then rinse and pat dry.
- Using a circular motion, apply a thin layer of the mask evenly over the affected area.
- Allow the mask to dry for 15 to 25 minutes.
- Then rinse thoroughly with warm water and pat dry.

*Use benzoyl peroxide only as directed.* Do not use more of it and do not use it more often than recommended on the label, unless otherwise directed by your doctor.

*Keep this medicine away from the eyes, other mucous membranes, such as the mouth, lips, and inside of the nose, and sensitive areas of the neck.*

*Do not apply benzoyl peroxide to raw or irritated skin.*

**Dosing**—The dose of benzoyl peroxide will be different for different patients. *Follow your doctor's orders or the directions on the label.* The following information includes only the average doses of benzoyl peroxide. *If your dose is different, do not change it* unless your doctor tells you to do so.
- For acne:
  —For *cleansing bar* dosage form:
  - Adults and children 12 years of age and over—Use two or three times a day, or as directed by your doctor.
  - Children up to 12 years of age—Use and dose must be determined by your doctor.
  —For *cleansing lotion, cream,* or *gel* dosage forms:
  - Adults and children 12 years of age and over—Use on the affected area(s) of the skin one or two times a day.
  - Children up to 12 years of age—Use and dose must be determined by your doctor.
  —For *lotion* dosage form:
  - Adults and children 12 years of age and over—Use on the affected area(s) of the skin one to four times a day.
  - Children up to 12 years of age—Use and dose must be determined by your doctor.
  —For *facial mask* dosage form:
  - Adults and children 12 years of age and over—Use one time a week or as directed by your doctor.
  - Children up to 12 years of age—Use and dose must be determined by your doctor.

  —For *stick* dosage form:
  - Adults and children 12 years of age and over—Use on the affected area(s) of the skin one to three times a day.
  - Children up to 12 years of age—Use and dose must be determined by your doctor.

**Missed dose**—If you miss a dose of this medicine, apply or use it as soon as possible. Then go back to your regular dosing schedule.

**Storage**—To store this medicine:
- Keep out of the reach of children.
- Store away from heat and direct light.
- Keep the cream, gel, or liquid form of this medicine from freezing.
- Do not keep outdated medicine or medicine no longer needed. Be sure that any discarded medicine is out of the reach of children.

## Precautions While Using This Medicine

If your skin problem has not improved within 4 to 6 weeks, check with your doctor.

If this medicine causes too much redness, peeling, or dryness of your skin, check with your doctor. It may be necessary for you to reduce the number of times a day that you use the medicine and/or use a weaker strength of the medicine.

*When using benzoyl peroxide, do not use any of the following preparations on the same affected area as this medicine,* unless otherwise directed by your doctor:
  Abrasive soaps or cleansers
  Alcohol-containing preparations
  Any other topical acne preparation or preparation containing a peeling agent (for example, resorcinol, salicylic acid, sulfur, or tretinoin [vitamin A acid])
  Cosmetics or soaps that dry the skin
  Medicated cosmetics
  Other topical medicine for the skin

To use any of the above preparations on the same affected area as benzoyl peroxide may cause severe irritation of the skin.

*This medicine may bleach hair or colored fabrics.*

## Side Effects of This Medicine

Along with its needed effects, a medicine may cause some unwanted effects. Although not all of these side effects may occur, if they do occur they may need medical attention.

Check with your doctor as soon as possible if any of the following side effects occur:
*Less common or rare*
  Painful irritation of skin, including burning, blistering, crusting, itching, severe redness, or swelling; skin rash
*Symptoms of overdose*
  Burning, itching, scaling, redness, or swelling of skin (severe)

Other side effects may occur that usually do not need medical attention. These side effects may go away during treatment as your body adjusts to the medicine. However, check with your health care professional if any of the following side effects continue or are bothersome:

*Less common*
　　Dryness or peeling of skin (may occur after a few days); feeling of warmth, mild stinging, and redness of skin

Other side effects not listed above may also occur in some patients. If you notice any other effects, check with your health care professional.

## Additional Information

Once a medicine has been approved for marketing for a certain use, experience may show that it is also useful for other medical problems. Although these uses are not included in product labeling, benzoyl peroxide is used in certain patients with the following medical conditions:

- Decubital ulcer (bed sores)
- Stasis ulcer (a certain type of ulcer)

Other than the above information, there is no additional information relating to proper use, precautions, or side effects for these uses.

Annual revision: 01/15/92
Interim revision: 05/20/94

# BENZYL BENZOATE　Topical*†

A commonly used brand name is Ascabiol.

*Not commercially available in the U.S.
†Not commercially available in Canada.

## Description

Benzyl benzoate (ben-ZILL ben-ZOE-ate) is used to treat lice and scabies infestations. This medicine is believed to be absorbed by the lice and mites and to destroy them by acting on their nervous system.

This medicine is available without a prescription; however, your doctor may have special instructions on the proper use of this medicine for your medical condition.

Benzyl benzoate is available in the following dosage form:

*Topical*
- Emulsion (United Kingdom)

## Before Using This Medicine

If you are using this medicine without a prescription, carefully read and follow any precautions on the label. For topical benzyl benzoate, the following should be considered:

**Allergies**—Tell your doctor if you have ever had any unusual or allergic reaction to benzyl benzoate.

**Pregnancy**—Benzyl benzoate has not been reported to cause birth defects or other problems in humans. However, the manufacturer recommends that this medicine should be used by pregnant women only if it is necessary. Before taking this medicine, make sure your doctor knows if you are pregnant or if you may become pregnant.

**Breast-feeding**—Benzyl benzoate has not been reported to cause problems in nursing babies. However, the manufacturer recommends that breast-feeding be suspended during treatment.

**Children**—Although there is no specific information comparing use of benzyl benzoate in children with use in other age groups, this medicine is not expected to cause different side effects or problems in children than it does in adults.

**Older adults**—Many medicines have not been studied specifically in older people. Therefore, it may not be known whether they work exactly the same way they do in younger adults or if they cause different side effects or problems in older people. There is no specific information comparing use of benzyl benzoate in the elderly with use in other age groups. However, older people may have dry skin and the medicine may make the condition worse.

**Other medical problems**—The presence of other medical problems may affect the use of benzyl benzoate. Make sure you tell your doctor if you have any other medical problems, especially:

- Inflammation of the skin (severe)—Use of benzyl benzoate may make the condition worse

## Proper Use of This Medicine

Benzyl benzoate usually comes with patient directions. Read them carefully before using this medicine.

*Use this medicine only as directed. Do not use more of it and do not use it more often than recommended on the label.* To do so may increase the chance of absorption through the skin and the chance of side effects.

*Keep this medicine away from the eyes and other mucous membranes, such as the inside of the nose, because it may cause irritation.* If you accidentally get some in your eyes, flush them thoroughly with water at once.

*Do not use benzyl benzoate on open wounds, such as cuts or sores on the skin or scalp.* To do so may increase the amount of absorption, which may increase the chance of side effects.

Your sexual partner or partners, especially, and all members of your household may need to be treated also, since the infestation may spread to persons in close contact. If these persons have not been examined for infestation or if you have any questions about this, check with your doctor.

To use this medicine for *lice:*
- If your hair has any cream, lotion, ointment, or oil-based product on it, shampoo, rinse, and dry your hair and scalp well before applying benzyl benzoate.
- Apply enough medicine to thoroughly wet the dry hair and scalp or skin.
- Allow the medicine to remain on the affected areas for 24 hours.
- Then, thoroughly wash the affected areas with warm water and soap or regular shampoo.
- Rinse thoroughly and dry with a clean towel.
- After rinsing and drying, use a fine-toothed comb (less than 0.3 mm between the teeth) to remove any remaining nits (eggs) or nit shells from your hair, or, if you have fine hair, you may use a tweezer or your fingernails to pick nits out.

To use this medicine for *scabies:*
- If your skin has any cream, lotion, ointment, or oil on it, wash, rinse, and dry your skin well before applying benzyl benzoate.
- If you take a bath or shower before using benzyl benzoate, dry the skin well before applying the medicine.
- Apply enough medicine to cover the entire skin surface from the neck down, including the soles of your feet, and rub in well.
- Allow the medicine to remain on the body for 24 hours.
- Then, thoroughly wash the body with warm water and soap.
- Rinse thoroughly and dry with a clean towel.

Immediately after using benzyl benzoate, wash your hands to remove any medicine that may be on them.

Treatment may need to be repeated for severe infestation.

**Dosing**—The dose of benzyl benzoate will be different for different patients. *Follow your doctor's orders or the directions on the label.* The following information includes only the average doses of benzyl benzoate. *If your dose is different, do not change it* unless your doctor tells you to do so.

*The number of doses that you use each day, the time allowed between doses, and the length of time you use the medicine depend on the medical problem for which you are using benzyl benzoate.*
- For *topical* dosage form (emulsion):
  —For lice infestation:
    - Adults—Use just one time. For severe cases, treatment may be repeated two or three times after twenty-four hours.

- Children—
  For infants: Use mixed with three parts of water, just one time.
  For older children: Use mixed with an equal quantity of water, just one time.
—For scabies infestation:
- Adults—Use just one time. For severe cases, treatment may be repeated after twenty-four hours one time anytime within five days.
- Children—
  For infants: Use mixed with three parts of water, just one time.
  For older children: Use mixed with an equal quantity of water, just one time.

**Storage**—To store this medicine:
- Keep out of the reach of children.
- Store away from heat and direct light.
- Keep the medicine from freezing. Do not refrigerate.
- Do not keep outdated medicine or medicine no longer needed. Be sure that any discarded medicine is out of the reach of children.

## Precautions While Using This Medicine

To prevent reinfection or spreading of the infection to other people, good health habits are required. These include the following:
- For *lice infestation:*
  —Disinfecting or washing combs, curlers, and brushes in very hot water (65 °C or 150 °F) for about 10 minutes immediately after using.
  —Washing in very hot water all recently worn clothing and used bed linens and towels, and drying them in a hot dryer for at least 20 minutes. Articles that cannot be washed may be dry-cleaned, pressed with a hot iron, or just placed in a hot dryer.
  —Sealing stuffed toys and other non-washable articles in a plastic bag for 2 weeks, or placing these items in the freezer (in sealed plastic bags) for 12 to 24 hours.
  —Vacuuming all rugs, mattresses, pillows, furniture, and car seats to get rid of fallen hairs with lice.
- For *scabies infestation:* Washing all recently worn clothing such as underwear and pajamas, and used sheets, pillowcases, and towels in very hot water or dry-cleaning.

## Side Effects of This Medicine

Along with its needed effects, a medicine may cause some unwanted effects. Although not all of these side effects may occur, if they do occur they may need medical attention.

Check with your doctor as soon as possible if any of the following side effects occur:
*Symptoms of overdose*
  Blister formation, crusting, itching, oozing, reddening, or scaling of skin; difficulty in urinating (dribbling); jerking movements; sudden loss of consciousness

Other side effects may occur that usually do not need medical attention. These side effects may go away during treatment as your body adjusts to the medicine. However, check with your doctor if any of the following side effects continue or are bothersome:

*Less common or rare*
  Burning or itching of skin

Other side effects not listed above may also occur in some patients. If you notice any other effects, check with your doctor.

Developed: 01/21/94

---

# BETA-ADRENERGIC BLOCKING AGENTS    Ophthalmic

Some commonly used brand names are:

**In the U.S.—**
| | |
|---|---|
| Betagan C Cap B.I.D.[3] | Ocupress[2] |
| Betagan C Cap Q.D.[3] | OptiPranolol[4] |
| Betagan Standard Cap[3] | Timoptic[5] |
| Betoptic[1] | Timoptic in Ocudose[5] |
| Betoptic S[1] | |

**In Canada—**
| | |
|---|---|
| Apo-Timop[5] | Betoptic[1] |
| Betagan C Cap B.I.D.[3] | Gen-Timolol[5] |
| Betagan Standard Cap[3] | Timoptic[5] |

Note: For quick reference, the following beta-adrenergic blocking agents are numbered to match the corresponding brand names.

This information applies to the following medicines:
1. Betaxolol (be-TAX-oh-lol)
2. Carteolol (KAR-tee-oh-lole)†
3. Levobunolol (lee-voe-BYOO-noe-lole)
4. Metipranolol (met-i-PRAN-oh-lol)†
5. Timolol (TYE-moe-lole)

†Not commercially available in Canada.

## Description

Betaxolol, carteolol, levobunolol, metipranolol, and timolol are used to treat certain types of glaucoma. They appear to work by reducing the production of fluid in the eye. This lowers the pressure in the eye.

These medicines are available only with your doctor's prescription, in the following dosage forms:

*Ophthalmic*
  Betaxolol
  • Ophthalmic solution (eye drops) (U.S. and Canada)
  • Ophthalmic suspension (eye drops) (U.S.)
  Carteolol
  • Ophthalmic solution (eye drops) (U.S.)
  Levobunolol
  • Ophthalmic solution (eye drops) (U.S. and Canada)
  Metipranolol
  • Ophthalmic solution (eye drops) (U.S.)
  Timolol
  • Ophthalmic solution (eye drops) (U.S. and Canada)

## Before Using This Medicine

In deciding to use a medicine, the risks of taking the medicine must be weighed against the good it will do. This is a decision you and your doctor will make. For ophthalmic beta-adrenergic blocking agents, the following should be considered:

**Allergies**—Tell your doctor if you have ever had any unusual or allergic reaction to any of the beta-adrenergic blocking agents, either ophthalmic or systemic, such as acebutolol, atenolol, betaxolol, bisoprolol, carteolol, labetalol, levobunolol, metipranolol, metoprolol, nadolol, oxprenolol, penbutolol, pindolol, propranolol, sotalol, or timolol. Also tell your health care professional if you are allergic to any other substances, such as sulfites or preservatives.

**Pregnancy**—Ophthalmic beta-adrenergic blocking agents may be absorbed into the body. These medicines have not been studied in pregnant women. Studies in animals have not shown that betaxolol, levobunolol, metipranolol, or timolol causes birth defects. However, very large doses of carteolol given by mouth to pregnant rats have been shown to cause wavy ribs in rat babies. In addition, some studies in animals have shown that beta-adrenergic blocking agents increase the chance of death in the animal fetus. Before using ophthalmic beta-adrenergic blocking agents, make sure your doctor knows if you are pregnant or if you may become pregnant.

**Breast-feeding**—Betaxolol and timolol, and maybe other beta-adrenergic blocking agents, when taken by mouth, may pass into the breast milk. Since ophthalmic beta-adrenergic blocking agents may be absorbed into the body, they, too, may pass into the breast milk. However, it is not known whether ophthalmic beta-adrenergic blocking agents pass into the breast milk, and these medicines have not been reported to cause problems in nursing babies.

**Children**—Infants may be especially sensitive to the effects of ophthalmic beta-adrenergic blocking agents. This may increase the chance of side effects during treatment.

**Older adults**—Elderly people are especially sensitive to the effects of ophthalmic beta-adrenergic blocking agents. If too much medicine is absorbed into the body, the chance of side effects during treatment may be increased.

**Other medicines**—Although certain medicines should not be used together at all, in other cases two different medicines may be used together even if an interaction might occur. In these cases, your doctor may want to change the dose, or other precautions may be necessary. Tell your health care professional if you are using any other prescription or nonprescription (over-the-counter [OTC]) medicine.

**Other medical problems**—The presence of other medical problems may affect the use of ophthalmic beta-adrenergic blocking agents. Make sure you tell your doctor if you have any other medical problems, especially:

- Asthma (or history of), chronic bronchitis, emphysema, or other lung disease—Severe breathing problems, including death due to bronchospasm (spasm of the bronchial tubes), have been reported in patients with asthma following use of some ophthalmic beta-adrenergic blocking agents (carteolol, levobunolol, metipranolol, and timolol). Although most often not a problem, the possibility of wheezing or troubled breathing also exists with betaxolol
- Diabetes mellitus (sugar diabetes) or
- Hypoglycemia (low blood sugar)—Ophthalmic beta-adrenergic blocking agents may cover up some signs and symptoms of hypoglycemia (low blood sugar), such as fast heartbeat and trembling, although they do not cover up other signs, such as dizziness or sweating
- Heart or blood vessel disease—Ophthalmic beta-adrenergic blocking agents may decrease heart activity
- Overactive thyroid—Ophthalmic beta-adrenergic blocking agents may cover up certain signs and symptoms of hyperthyroidism (overactive thyroid). Suddenly stopping the use of ophthalmic beta-adrenergic blocking agents may cause a sudden and dangerous increase in thyroid symptoms

## Proper Use of This Medicine

To use:
- First, wash your hands. With the middle finger, apply pressure to the inside corner of the eye (and continue to apply pressure for 1 or 2 minutes after the medicine has been placed in the eye). *This is especially important if the ophthalmic beta-adrenergic blocking agent is used to treat infants and children.* Tilt the head back and with the index finger of the same hand, pull the lower eyelid away from the eye to form a pouch. Drop the medicine into the pouch and gently close the eyes. Do not blink. Keep the eyes closed for 1 or 2 minutes to allow the medicine to be absorbed.
- Immediately after using the eye drops, wash your hands to remove any medicine that may be on them.
- To keep the medicine as germ-free as possible, do not touch the applicator tip to any surface (including the eye). Also, keep the container tightly closed.
- If you are using the medication with the compliance cap (C Cap):
  —Before using the eye drops for the first time, make sure the number 1 or the correct day of the week appears in the window on the cap.
  —Remove the cap and use the eye drops as directed.
  —Replace the cap. Holding the cap between your thumb and forefinger, rotate the bottle until the cap clicks to the next position. This will tell you the time of your next dose.

  —After every dose, rotate the bottle until the cap clicks to the position that tells you the time of your next dose.

*Use this medicine only as directed.* Do not use more of it and do not use it more often than your doctor ordered. To do so may increase the chance of too much medicine being absorbed into the body and the chance of side effects.

**Dosing**—The dose of betaxolol, carteolol, levobunolol, metipranolol, or timolol will be different for different patients. *Follow your doctor's orders or the directions on the label.* The following information includes only the average doses. *If your dose is different, do not change it* unless your doctor tells you to do so.

*The number of doses of medicine that you use also depends on the strength of the medicine.*
*For betaxolol, carteolol, or metipranolol*
- For *ophthalmic drops* dosage forms:
  —For glaucoma:
    • Adults and older children—Topical, to the conjunctiva, 1 drop two times a day.
    • Infants and younger children—Dose must be determined by the doctor.
*For levobunolol or timolol*
- For *ophthalmic drops* dosage forms:
  —For glaucoma:
    • Adults and older children—Topical, to the conjunctiva, 1 drop one or two times a day.
    • Infants and younger children—Dose must be determined by the doctor.

**Missed dose**—If you miss a dose of this medicine and your dosing schedule is:
- One dose a day—Use the missed dose as soon as possible. However, if you do not remember the missed dose until the next day, skip the missed dose and go back to your regular dosing schedule. Do not double doses.
- More than one dose a day—Use the missed dose as soon as possible. However, if it is almost time for your next dose, skip the missed dose and go back to your regular dosing schedule. Do not double doses.

If you have any questions about this, check with your doctor.

**Storage**—To store this medicine:
- Keep out of the reach of children.
- Store away from heat and direct light.
- Keep this medicine from freezing.
- Do not keep outdated medicine or medicine no longer needed. Be sure that any discarded medicine is out of the reach of children.

## Precautions While Using This Medicine

Your doctor should check your eye pressure at regular visits to make certain that your glaucoma is being controlled.

*Before you have any kind of surgery, dental treatment, or emergency treatment, tell the medical doctor or dentist in charge that you are using this medicine.* Using an ophthalmic beta-adrenergic blocking agent during this time may cause an increased risk of side effects.

*For diabetic patients:*

- *Ophthalmic beta-adrenergic blocking agents may affect blood sugar levels. They may also cover up some signs of hypoglycemia (low blood sugar),* such as trembling or increase in pulse rate or blood pressure. However, other signs of low blood sugar, such as dizziness or sweating, are not affected. If you notice a change in the results of your blood or urine sugar tests or if you have any questions, check with your doctor.

Some ophthalmic beta-adrenergic blocking agents (betaxolol, carteolol, and metipranolol) may cause your eyes to become more sensitive to light than they are normally. Wearing sunglasses and avoiding too much exposure to bright light may help lessen the discomfort.

---

## Side Effects of This Medicine

Along with its needed effects, a medicine may cause some unwanted effects. Although not all of these side effects may occur, if they do occur they may need medical attention.

Check with your doctor as soon as possible if any of the following side effects occur:

*More common*

Redness of eyes or inside of eyelids

*Less common or rare*

Blurred vision or other change in vision; different size pupils of the eyes; discoloration of the eyeball; droopy upper eyelid; eye pain; redness or irritation of the tongue; seeing double; swelling, irritation or inflammation of eye or eyelid (severe)

*Symptoms of too much medicine being absorbed into the body*

Anxiety or nervousness; burning or prickling feeling on body; change in taste; chest pain; clumsiness or unsteadiness; confusion or mental depression; coughing, wheezing, or troubled breathing; decreased sexual ability; diarrhea; dizziness or feeling faint; drowsiness; hair loss; hallucinations (seeing, hearing, or feeling things that are not there); headache; irregular, slow, or pounding heartbeat; muscle or joint aches or pain; nausea or vomiting; raw or red areas of the skin; runny, stuffy, or bleeding nose; skin rash, hives, or itching; swelling of feet, ankles, or lower legs; trouble in sleeping; unusual tiredness or weakness

Other side effects may occur that usually do not need medical attention. These side effects may go away during treatment as your body adjusts to the medicine. However, check with your doctor if any of the following side effects continue or are bothersome:

*More common*

Decreased night vision; stinging of eye or other eye irritation (when medicine is applied)

*Less common or rare*

Browache; crusting of eyelashes; dryness of eye; increased sensitivity of eye to light; redness, itching, stinging, burning, or watering of eye or other eye irritation

Other side effects not listed above may also occur in some patients. If you notice any other effects, check with your doctor.

---

Revised: 05/12/93

---

# BETA-ADRENERGIC BLOCKING AGENTS    Systemic

Some commonly used brand names are:

**In the U.S.—**

| | |
|---|---|
| Betapace[13] | Lopressor[7] |
| Blocadren[14] | Normodyne[6] |
| Cartrol[5] | Sectral[1] |
| Corgard[8] | Tenormin[2] |
| Inderal[12] | Toprol-XL[7] |
| Inderal LA[12] | Trandate[6] |
| Kerlone[3] | Visken[11] |
| Levatol[10] | Zebeta[4] |

**In the Canada—**

| | |
|---|---|
| Apo-Atenolol[2] | Inderal[12] |
| Apo-Metoprolol[7] | Inderal LA[12] |
| Apo-Metoprolol (Type L)[7] | Lopresor[7] |
| Apo-Propranolol[12] | Lopresor SR[7] |
| Apo-Timol[14] | Monitan[1] |
| Betaloc[7] | Novo-Atenol[2] |
| Betaloc Durules[7] | Novometoprol[7] |
| Blocadren[14] | Novo-Pindol[11] |
| Corgard[8] | Novo-Timol[14] |
| Detensol[12] | Novopranol[12] |

| | |
|---|---|
| pms Propranolol[12] | Syn-Pindolol[11] |
| Sectral[1] | Tenormin[2] |
| Slow-Trasicor[9] | Trandate[6] |
| Sotacor[13] | Trasicor[9] |
| Syn-Nadolol[8] | Visken[11] |

Note: For quick reference, the following beta-adrenergic blocking agents are numbered to match the corresponding brand names.

This information applies to the following medicines:

1. Acebutolol (a-se-BYOO-toe-lole)
2. Atenolol (a-TEN-oh-lole)‡
3. Betaxolol (be-TAX-oh-lol)†
4. Bisoprolol (bis-OH-proe-lol)†
5. Carteolol (KAR-tee-oh-lole)†
6. Labetalol (la-BET-a-lole)
7. Metoprolol (me-TOE-proe-lole)§
8. Nadolol (NAY-doe-lole)§
9. Oxprenolol (ox-PREN-oh-lole)*
10. Penbutolol (pen-BYOO-toe-lole)†
11. Pindolol (PIN-doe-lole)
12. Propranolol (proe-PRAN-oh-lole)‡§

13. Sotalol (SOE-ta-lole)
14. Timolol (TIM-oh-lole)‡

---

*Not commercially available in the U.S.
†Not commercially available in Canada.
‡Generic name product may also be available in the U.S.
§Generic name product may also be available in Canada.

---

# Description

This group of medicines is known as beta-adrenergic blocking agents, beta-blocking agents, or, more commonly, beta-blockers. Beta-blockers are used in the treatment of high blood pressure (hypertension). Some beta-blockers are also used to relieve angina (chest pain) and in heart attack patients to help prevent additional heart attacks. Beta-blockers are also used to correct irregular heartbeat, prevent migraine headaches, and treat tremors. They may also be used for other conditions as determined by your doctor.

Beta-blockers work by affecting the response to some nerve impulses in certain parts of the body. As a result, they decrease the heart's need for blood and oxygen by reducing its workload. They also help the heart to beat more regularly.

Beta-adrenergic blocking agents are available only with your doctor's prescription, in the following dosage forms:

*Oral*

Acebutolol
• Capsules (U.S.)
• Tablets (Canada)
Atenolol
• Tablets (U.S. and Canada)
Betaxolol
• Tablets (U.S.)
Bisoprolol
• Tablets (U.S.)
Carteolol
• Tablets (U.S.)
Labetalol
• Tablets (U.S. and Canada)
Metoprolol
• Tablets (U.S. and Canada)
• Extended-release tablets (U.S. and Canada)
Nadolol
• Tablets (U.S. and Canada)
Oxprenolol
• Tablets (Canada)
• Extended-release tablets (Canada)
Penbutolol
• Tablets (U.S.)
Pindolol
• Tablets (U.S. and Canada)
Propranolol
• Extended-release capsules (U.S. and Canada)
• Oral solution (U.S.)
• Tablets (U.S. and Canada)
Sotalol
• Tablets (U.S. and Canada)
Timolol
• Tablets (U.S. and Canada)

*Parenteral*

Atenolol
• Injection (U.S.)
Labetalol
• Injection (U.S. and Canada)
Metoprolol
• Injection (U.S. and Canada)
Propranolol
• Injection (U.S. and Canada)

---

# Before Using This Medicine

In deciding to use a medicine, the risks of taking the medicine must be weighed against the good it will do. This is a decision you and your doctor will make. For the beta-blockers, the following should be considered:

**Allergies**—Tell your doctor if you have ever had any unusual or allergic reaction to the beta-blocker medicine prescribed. Also tell your health care professional if you are allergic to any other substances, such as foods, preservatives, or dyes.

**Pregnancy**—Use of some beta-blockers during pregnancy has been associated with low blood sugar, breathing problems, a lower heart rate, and low blood pressure in the newborn infant. Other reports have not shown unwanted effects on the newborn infant. Animal studies have shown some beta-blockers to cause problems in pregnancy when used in doses many times the usual human dose. Before taking any of these medicines, make sure your doctor knows if you are pregnant or if you may become pregnant.

**Breast-feeding**—It is not known whether bisoprolol, carteolol, or penbutolol passes into breast milk. All other beta-blockers pass into breast milk. Problems such as slow heartbeat, low blood pressure, and trouble in breathing have been reported in nursing babies. Mothers who are taking beta-blockers and who wish to breast-feed should discuss this with their doctor.

**Children**—Some of these medicines have been used in children and, in effective doses, have not been shown to cause different side effects or problems in children than they do in adults.

**Older adults**—Some side effects are more likely to occur in the elderly, who are usually more sensitive to the effects of beta-blockers. Also, beta-blockers may reduce tolerance to cold temperatures in elderly patients.

**Other medicines**—Although certain medicines should not be used together at all, in other cases 2 different medicines may be used together even if an interaction might occur. In these cases, your doctor may want to change the dose, or other precautions may be necessary. When you are taking or receiving a beta-blocker it is especially important that your health care professional know if you are taking any of the following:
• Allergen immunotherapy (allergy shots) or
• Allergen extracts for skin testing—Beta-blockers may increase the risk of serious allergic reaction to these medicines
• Aminophylline (e.g., Somophyllin) or
• Caffeine (e.g., NoDoz) or
• Dyphylline (e.g., Lufyllin) or

- Oxtriphylline (e.g., Choledyl) or
- Theophylline (e.g., Somophyllin-T)—The effects of both these medicines and beta-blockers may be blocked; in addition, theophylline levels in the body may be increased, especially in patients who smoke
- Antidiabetics, oral (diabetes medicine you take by mouth) or
- Insulin—There is an increased risk of hyperglycemia (high blood sugar); beta-blockers may cover up certain symptoms of hypoglycemia (low blood sugar) such as increases in pulse rate and blood pressure, and may make the hypoglycemia last longer
- Calcium channel blockers (bepridil [e.g., Bepadin], diltiazem [e.g., Cardizem], felodipine [e.g., Plendil], flunarizine [e.g., Sibelium], isradipine [e.g., DynaCirc], nicardipine [e.g., Cardene], nifedipine [e.g., Procardia], nimodipine [e.g., Nimotop], verapamil [e.g., Calan]) or
- Clonidine (e.g., Catapres) or
- Guanabenz (e.g., Wytensin)—Effects on blood pressure may be increased. In addition, unwanted effects may occur if clonidine, guanabenz, or a beta-blocker is stopped suddenly after use together. Unwanted effects on the heart may occur when beta-blockers are used with calcium channel blockers
- Cocaine—Cocaine may block the effects of beta-blockers; in addition, there is an increased risk of high blood pressure, fast heartbeat, and possibly heart problems if you use cocaine while taking a beta-blocker
- Monoamine oxidase (MAO) inhibitors (furazolidone [e.g., Furoxone], isocarboxazid [e.g., Marplan], phenelzine [e.g., Nardil], procarbazine [e.g., Matulane], selegiline [e.g., Eldepryl], tranylcypromine [e.g., Parnate])—Taking beta-blockers while you are taking or within 2 weeks of taking monoamine oxidase (MAO) inhibitors may cause severe high blood pressure

**Other medical problems**—The presence of other medical problems may affect the use of the beta blockers. Make sure you tell your doctor if you have any other medical problems, especially:

- Allergy, history of (asthma, eczema, hay fever, hives), or
- Bronchitis or
- Emphysema—Severity and duration of allergic reactions to other substances may be increased; in addition, beta-blockers can increase trouble in breathing
- Bradycardia (unusually slow heartbeat) or
- Heart or blood vessel disease—There is a risk of further decreased heart function; also, if treatment is stopped suddenly, unwanted effects may occur
- Diabetes mellitus (sugar diabetes)—Beta-blockers may cause hyperglycemia (high blood sugar) and circulation problems; in addition, if your diabetes medicine causes your blood sugar to be too low, beta-blockers may cover up some of the symptoms (fast heartbeat), although they will not cover up other symptoms such as dizziness or sweating
- Kidney disease or
- Liver disease—Effects of beta-blockers may be increased because of slower removal from the body
- Mental depression (or history of)—May be increased by beta-blockers
- Myasthenia gravis or
- Psoriasis—Beta-blockers may make these conditions worse

- Overactive thyroid—Stopping beta-blockers suddenly may increase symptoms; beta-blockers may cover up fast heartbeat, which is a sign of overactive thyroid

## Proper Use of This Medicine

For patients taking the *extended-release capsule or tablet* form of this medicine:

- Swallow the capsule or tablet whole.
- Do not crush, break (except metoprolol succinate extended-release tablets, which may be broken in half), or chew before swallowing.

For patients taking the *concentrated oral solution* form of *propranolol:*

- This medicine is to be taken by mouth even though it comes in a dropper bottle. The amount you should take is to be measured only with the specially marked dropper.
- Mix the medicine with some water, juice, or a carbonated drink. After drinking all the liquid containing the medicine, rinse the glass with a little more liquid and drink that also, to make sure you get all the medicine.

  If you prefer, you may mix this medicine with applesauce or pudding instead.

- Mix the medicine immediately before you are going to take it. Throw away any mixed medicine that you do not take immediately. Do not save medicine that has been mixed.

Ask your doctor about checking your pulse rate before and after taking beta-blocking agents. Then, while you are taking this medicine, check your pulse regularly. If it is much slower than your usual rate (or less than 50 beats per minute), check with your doctor. A pulse rate that is too slow may cause circulation problems.

To help you remember to take your medicine, try to get into the habit of taking it at the same time each day.

For patients taking this medicine *for high blood pressure:*

- In addition to the use of the medicine your doctor has prescribed, treatment for your high blood pressure may include weight control and care in the types of foods you eat, especially foods high in sodium. Your doctor will tell you which of these are most important for you. You should check with your doctor before changing your diet.
- Many patients who have high blood pressure will not notice any signs of the problem. In fact, many may feel normal. However, if high blood pressure is not treated, it can cause serious problems such as heart failure, blood vessel disease, stroke, or kidney disease.
- Remember that this medicine will not cure your high blood pressure but it does help control it. It is very important that you *take your medicine exactly as directed*, even if you feel well. You must continue to take it as directed if you expect to lower your blood pressure and keep it down. *You may have to take high blood pressure medicine for the rest of*

*your life.* Also, it is very important to keep your appointments with your doctor, even if you feel well.

**Dosing**—The dose of beta-blocker will be different for different patients. *Follow your doctor's orders or the directions on the label.* The following information includes only the average doses. *If your dose is different, do not change it* unless your doctor tells you to do so.

The number of capsules or tablets or teaspoonfuls of solution that you take depends on the strength of the medicine. Also, *the number of doses you take each day, the time allowed between doses, and the length of time you take the medicine depend on the medical problem for which you are taking the beta-blocker.*

*For acebutolol*
- For *oral* dosage forms (capsules and tablets):
  —For angina (chest pain) or irregular heartbeat:
   - Adults—200 milligrams (mg) two times a day. The dose may be increased up to a total of 1200 mg a day.
   - Children—Dose must be determined by your doctor.
  —For high blood pressure:
   - Adults—200 to 800 mg a day as a single dose or divided into two daily doses.
   - Children—Dose must be determined by your doctor.

*For atenolol*
- For *oral* dosage form (tablets):
  —For angina (chest pain):
   - Adults—50 to 100 mg once a day.
  —For high blood pressure:
   - Adults—25 to 100 mg once a day.
   - Children—Dose must be determined by your doctor.
  —For treatment after a heart attack:
   - Adults—50 mg ten minutes after the last intravenous dose, followed by another 50 mg twelve hours later. Then 100 mg once a day or 50 mg two times a day for six to nine days or until discharge from hospital.
- For *injection* dosage form:
  —For treatment of heart attacks:
   - Adults—5 mg given over 5 minutes. The dose is repeated ten minutes later.

*For betaxolol*
- For *oral* dosage form (tablets):
  —For high blood pressure:
   - Adults—10 mg once a day. Your doctor may double your dose after seven to fourteen days.
   - Children—Dose must be determined by your doctor.

*For bisoprolol*
- For *oral* dosage form (tablets):
  —For high blood pressure:
   - Adults—5 to 10 mg once a day.
   - Children—Dose must be determined by your doctor.

*For carteolol*
- For *oral* dosage form (tablets):
  —For high blood pressure:
   - Adults—2.5 to 10 mg once a day.
   - Children—Dose must be determined by your doctor.

*For labetalol*
- For *oral* dosage form (tablets):
  —For high blood pressure:
   - Adults—100 to 400 mg two times a day.
   - Children—Dose must be determined by your doctor.
- For *injection* dosage form:
  —For high blood pressure:
   - Adults—20 mg injected slowly over two minutes with additional injections of 40 and 80 mg given every ten minutes if needed, up to a total of 300 mg; may be given instead as an infusion at a rate of 2 mg per minute to a total dose of 50 to 300 mg.
   - Children—Dose must be determined by your doctor.

*For metoprolol*
- For *regular (short-acting) oral* dosage form (tablets):
  —For high blood pressure or angina (chest pain):
   - Adults—100 to 450 mg a day, taken as a single dose or in divided doses.
   - Children—Dose must be determined by your doctor.
  —For treatment after a heart attack:
   - Adults—50 mg every six hours starting fifteen minutes after last intravenous dose. Then 100 mg two times a day for three months to 1 year.
- For *long-acting oral* dosage forms (extended-release tablets):
  —For high blood pressure or angina (chest pain):
   - Adults—Up to 400 mg once a day.
   - Children—Dose must be determined by your doctor.
- For *injection* dosage form:
  —For treatment of a heart attack:
   - Adults—5 mg every two minutes for three doses.

*For nadolol*
- For *oral* dosage form (tablets):
  —For angina (chest pain):
   - Adults—40 to 240 mg once a day.
  —For high blood pressure:
   - Adults—40 to 320 mg once a day.
   - Children—Dose must be determined by your doctor.

*For oxprenolol*
- For *regular (short-acting) oral* dosage form (tablets):
  —For high blood pressure:
    - Adults—20 mg three times a day. Your doctor may increase your dose up to 480 mg a day.
    - Children—Dose must be determined by your doctor.
- For *long-acting oral* dosage form (extended-release tablets):
  —For high blood pressure:
    - Adults—80 to 160 mg once a day.
    - Children—Dose must be determined by your doctor.

*For penbutolol*
- For *oral* dosage form (tablets):
  —For high blood pressure:
    - Adults—20 mg once a day.
    - Children—Dose must be determined by your doctor.

*For pindolol*
- For *oral* dosage form (tablets):
  —For high blood pressure:
    - Adults—5 mg two times a day. Your doctor may increase your dose up to 60 mg a day.
    - Children—Dose must be determined by your doctor.

*For propranolol*
- For *regular (short-acting) oral* dosage forms (tablets and oral solution):
  —For angina (chest pain):
    - Adults—80 to 320 mg a day taken in two, three, or four divided doses.
  —For irregular heartbeat:
    - Adults—10 to 30 mg three or four times a day.
    - Children—500 micrograms (0.5 mg) to 4 mg per kilogram of body weight a day taken in divided doses.
  —For high blood pressure:
    - Adults—40 mg two times a day. Your doctor may increase your dose up to 640 mg a day.
    - Children—500 micrograms (0.5 mg) to 4 mg per kilogram of body weight a day taken in divided doses.
  —For diseased heart muscle (cardiomyopathy):
    - Adults—20 to 40 mg three or four times a day.
  —For treatment after a heart attack:
    - Adults—180 to 240 mg a day taken in divided doses.
  —For treating pheochromocytoma:
    - Adults—30 to 160 mg a day taken in divided doses.

—For preventing migraine headaches:
  - Adults—20 mg four times a day. Your doctor may increase your dose up to 240 mg a day.
—For trembling:
  - Adults—40 mg two times a day. Your doctor may increase your dose up to 320 mg a day.
- For *long-acting oral* dosage form (extended-release capsules):
  —For high blood pressure:
    - Adults—80 to 160 mg once a day. Doses up to 640 mg once a day may be needed in some patients.
  —For angina (chest pain):
    - Adults—80 to 320 mg once a day.
  —For preventing migraine headaches:
    - Adults—80 to 240 mg once a day.
- For *injection* dosage form:
  —For irregular heartbeat:
    - Adults—1 to 3 mg given at a rate not greater than 1 mg per minute. Dose may be repeated after two minutes and again after four hours if needed.
    - Children—10 to 100 micrograms (0.01 to 0.1 mg) per kilogram of body weight given intravenously every six to eight hours.

*For sotalol*
- For *oral* dosage form (tablets):
  —For irregular heartbeat:
    - Adults—80 mg two times a day. Your doctor may increase your dose up to 320 mg per day taken in two or three divided doses.
    - Children—Dose must be determined by your doctor.

*For timolol*
- For *oral* dosage form (tablets):
  —For high blood pressure:
    - Adults—10 mg two times a day. Your doctor may increase your dose up 60 mg per day taken as a single dose or in divided doses.
    - Children—Dose must be determined by your doctor.
  —For treatment after a heart attack:
    - Adults—10 mg two times a day.
  —For preventing migraine headaches:
    - Adults—10 mg two times a day. Your doctor may increase your dose up to 30 mg once a day or in divided doses.

**Missed dose**—Do not miss any doses. This is especially important when you are taking only one dose per day. Some conditions may become worse if this medicine is not taken regularly.

If you do miss a dose of this medicine, take it as soon as possible. However, if it is within 4 hours of your next dose (8 hours when using atenolol, betaxolol, bisoprolol, carteolol, labetalol, nadolol, penbutolol, sotalol, or extended-release [long-acting] metoprolol, oxprenolol, or propranolol), skip the missed dose and go back to your regular dosing schedule. Do not double doses.

**Storage**—To store this medicine:
- Keep out of the reach of children.
- Store away from heat and direct light.
- Do not store in the bathroom, near the kitchen sink, or in other damp places. Heat or moisture may cause the medicine to break down.
- Do not keep outdated medicine or medicine no longer needed. Be sure that any discarded medicine is out of the reach of children.

## Precautions While Using This Medicine

It is important that your doctor check your progress at regular visits. This is to make sure the medicine is working for you and to allow the dosage to be changed if needed.

*Do not stop taking this medicine without first checking with your doctor.* Your doctor may want you to reduce gradually the amount you are taking before stopping completely. Some conditions may become worse when the medicine is stopped suddenly, and the danger of heart attack is increased in some patients.

Make sure that you have enough medicine on hand to last through weekends, holidays, or vacations. You may want to carry an extra written prescription in your billfold or purse in case of an emergency. You can then have it filled if you run out of medicine while you are away from home.

Your doctor may want you to carry medical identification stating that you are taking this medicine.

*Before having any kind of surgery (including dental surgery) or emergency treatment, tell the medical doctor or dentist in charge that you are taking this medicine.*

For *diabetic patients:*
- *This medicine may cause your blood sugar levels to rise.* Also, *this medicine may cover up signs of hypoglycemia (low blood sugar),* such as change in pulse rate.

This medicine may cause some people to become dizzy, drowsy, or lightheaded. *Make sure you know how you react to this medicine before you drive, use machines, or do anything else that could be dangerous if you are dizzy or are not alert.* If the problem continues or gets worse, check with your doctor.

Beta-blockers may make you more sensitive to cold temperatures, especially if you have blood circulation problems. Beta-blockers tend to decrease blood circulation in the skin, fingers, and toes. Dress warmly during cold weather and be careful during prolonged exposure to cold, such as in winter sports.

Chest pain resulting from exercise or physical exertion is usually reduced or prevented by this medicine. This may tempt a patient to be overly active. *Make sure you discuss with your doctor a safe amount of exercise for your medical problem.*

Before you have any medical tests, tell the doctor in charge that you are taking this medicine. The results of some tests may be affected by this medicine.

Before you have any allergy shots, tell the doctor in charge that you are taking a beta-blocker. Beta-blockers may cause you to have a serious reaction to the allergy shot.

For patients with *allergies to foods, medicines, or insect stings:*
- There is a chance that this medicine will cause allergic reactions to be worse and harder to treat. If you have a severe allergic reaction while you are being treated with this medicine, check with a doctor right away so that it can be treated. Be sure to tell the doctor that you are taking a beta-blocker.

For patients taking this medicine *for high blood pressure:*
- *Do not take other medicines unless they have been discussed with your doctor.* This especially includes over-the-counter (nonprescription) medicines for appetite control, asthma, colds, cough, hay fever, or sinus problems since they may tend to increase your blood pressure.

For patients taking *labetalol by mouth:*
- *Dizziness, lightheadedness, or fainting may occur, especially when you get up from a lying or sitting position.* This is more likely to occur when you first start taking labetalol or when the dose is increased. *Getting up slowly may help.* When you get up from lying down, sit on the edge of the bed with your feet dangling for 1 to 2 minutes. Then stand up slowly. If the problem continues or gets worse, check with your doctor.
- The dizziness, lightheadedness, or fainting is also more likely to occur if you drink alcohol, stand for long periods of time, or exercise, or if the weather is hot. *While you are taking this medicine, be careful to limit the amount of alcohol you drink. Also, use extra care during exercise or hot weather or if you must stand for long periods of time.*

For patients receiving *labetalol by injection:*
- It is very important that you lie down flat while receiving labetalol and for up to 3 hours afterward. If you try to get up too soon, you may become dizzy or faint. *Do not try to sit or stand until your doctor or nurse tells you to do so.*

## Side Effects of This Medicine

Along with its needed effects, a medicine may cause some unwanted effects. Although not all of these side effects may occur, if they do occur they may need medical attention.

Check with your doctor as soon as possible if any of the following side effects occur:

*Less common*

Breathing difficulty and/or wheezing; cold hands and feet; mental depression; shortness of breath; slow heartbeat (especially less than 50 beats per minute); swelling of ankles, feet, and/or lower legs

*Rare*

Back pain or joint pain; chest pain; confusion (especially in elderly); dark urine—for acebutolol, bisoprolol, or labetalol; dizziness or lightheadedness when getting up from a lying or sitting position; fever and sore throat; hallucinations (seeing, hearing, or feeling things that are not there); irregular heartbeat; red, scaling, or crusted skin; skin rash; unusual bleeding and bruising; yellow eyes or skin—for acebutolol, bisoprolol, or labetalol

*Signs and symptoms of overdose (in the order in which they may occur)*

Slow heartbeat; dizziness (severe) or fainting; fast or irregular heartbeat; difficulty in breathing; bluish-colored fingernails or palms of hands; convulsions (seizures)

Other side effects may occur that usually do not need medical attention. These side effects may go away during treatment as your body adjusts to the medicine. However, check with your doctor if any of the following side effects continue or are bothersome:

*More common*

Decreased sexual ability; dizziness or lightheadedness; drowsiness (slight); trouble in sleeping; unusual tiredness or weakness

*Less common or rare*

Anxiety and/or nervousness; changes in taste—for labetalol only; constipation; diarrhea; dry, sore eyes; frequent urination—for acebutolol and carteolol only; itching of skin; nausea or vomiting; nightmares and vivid dreams; numbness and/or tingling of fingers and/or toes; numbness and/or tingling of skin, especially on scalp—for labetalol only; stomach discomfort; stuffy nose

Although not all of the side effects listed above have been reported for all of these medicines, they have been reported for at least one of them. Since all of the beta-adrenergic blocking agents are very similar, any of the above side effects may occur with any of these medicines. However, they may be more or less common with some agents than with others.

After you have been taking a beta-blocker for a while, it may cause unpleasant or even harmful effects if you stop taking it too suddenly. After you stop taking this medicine or while you are gradually reducing the amount you are taking, check with your doctor right away if any of the following occur:

Chest pain; fast or irregular heartbeat; general feeling of discomfort or illness or weakness; headache; shortness of breath (sudden); sweating; trembling

For patients taking *labetalol:*

• You may notice a tingling feeling on your scalp when you first begin to take labetalol. This is to be expected and usually goes away after you have been taking labetalol for a while.

Other side effects not listed above may also occur in some patients. If you notice any other effects, check with your doctor.

## Additional Information

Once a medicine has been approved for marketing for a certain use, experience may show that it is also useful for other medical problems. Although these uses are not included in product labeling, some beta-blockers are used in certain patients with the following medical conditions:

• Glaucoma
• Neuroleptic-induced akathisia (restlessness or the need to keep moving caused by some medicines used to treat nervousness or mental and emotional disorders)

Other than the above information, there is no additional information relating to proper use, precautions, or side effects for these uses.

Revised: 05/13/93

# BETA-ADRENERGIC BLOCKING AGENTS AND THIAZIDE DIURETICS   Systemic

Some commonly used brand names are:

**In the U.S.—**

| | |
|---|---|
| Corzide[4] | Tenoretic[1] |
| Inderide[6] | Timolide[7] |
| Inderide LA[6] | Ziac[2] |
| Lopressor HCT[3] | |

**In Canada—**

| | |
|---|---|
| Corzide[4] | Timolide[7] |
| Inderide[6] | Viskazide[5] |
| Tenoretic[1] | |

Note: For quick reference, the following beta-adrenergic blocking agents and thiazide diuretics are numbered to match the corresponding brand names.

This information applies to the following medicines:

1. Atenolol (a-TEN-oh-lole) and Chlorthalidone (klor-THAL-i-doan)‡
2. Bisoprolol (bis-OH-proe-lol) and Hydrochlorothiazide (hye-droe-klor-oh-THYE-a-zide)†
3. Metoprolol (me-TOE-proe-lole) and Hydrochlorothiazide†
4. Nadolol (NAY-doe-lole) and Bendroflumethiazide (ben-droe-floo-meth-EYE-a-zide)

5. Pindolol (PIN-doe-lole) and Hydrochlorothiazide*
6. Propranolol (proe-PRAN-oh-lole) and Hydrochlorothiazide‡
7. Timolol (TIM-oh-lole) and Hydrochlorothiazide

*Not commercially available in the U.S.
†Not commercially available in Canada.
‡Generic name product may also be available in the U.S.

## Description

Beta-adrenergic blocking agent (more commonly, beta-blockers) and thiazide diuretic combinations belong to the group of medicines known as antihypertensives (high blood pressure medicine). Both ingredients of the combination control high blood pressure, but they work in different ways. Beta-blockers (atenolol, bisoprolol, metoprolol, nadolol, pindolol, propranolol, and timolol) reduce the work load on the heart as well as having other effects. Thiazide diuretics (bendroflumethiazide, chlorthalidone, and hydrochlorothiazide) reduce the amount of fluid pressure in the body by increasing the flow of urine.

High blood pressure adds to the work load of the heart and arteries. If it continues for a long time, the heart and arteries may not function properly. This can damage the blood vessels of the brain, heart, and kidneys, resulting in a stroke, heart failure, or kidney failure. High blood pressure may also increase the risk of heart attacks. These problems may be less likely to occur if blood pressure is controlled.

Beta-blocker and thiazide diuretic combinations are available only with your doctor's prescription, in the following dosage forms:

*Oral*
    Atenolol and chlorthalidone
      • Tablets (U.S. and Canada)
    Bisoprolol and hydrochlorothiazide
      • Tablets (U.S.)
    Metoprolol and hydrochlorothiazide
      • Tablets (U.S.)
    Nadolol and bendroflumethiazide
      • Tablets (U.S. and Canada)
    Pindolol and hydrochlorothiazide
      • Tablets (Canada)
    Propranolol and hydrochlorothiazide
      • Extended-release capsules (U.S.)
      • Tablets (U.S. and Canada)
    Timolol and hydrochlorothiazide
      • Tablets (U.S. and Canada)

## Before Using This Medicine

In deciding to use a medicine, the risks of taking the medicine must be weighed against the good it will do. This is a decision you and your doctor will make. For the beta-blocker and thiazide diuretic combinations, the following should be considered:

**Allergies**—Tell your doctor if you have ever had any unusual or allergic reaction to beta-blockers, sulfonamides (sulfa drugs), bumetanide, furosemide, acetazolamide, dichlorphenamide, methazolamide, or any of the thiazide diuretics. Also tell your health care professional if you are allergic to any other substances, such as foods, preservatives, or dyes.

**Pregnancy**—Use of some beta-blockers during pregnancy has been associated with low blood sugar, breathing problems, a slower heart rate, and low blood pressure in the newborn infant. Other reports have not shown unwanted effects in the newborn infant. Animal studies have shown some beta-blockers to cause problems in pregnancy when used in doses many times the usual human dose.

Studies with thiazide diuretics have not been done in pregnant women. However, use of thiazide diuretics during pregnancy may cause side effects such as jaundice, blood problems, and low potassium in the newborn infant. Animal studies have not shown thiazide diuretic medicines to cause birth defects even when used in doses several times the usual human dose.

Before taking a beta-blocker and thiazide diuretic combination, make sure your doctor knows if you are pregnant or if you may become pregnant.

**Breast-feeding**—Atenolol, metoprolol, nadolol, propranolol, pindolol, timolol, and thiazide diuretics pass into breast milk. It is not known whether bisoprolol passes into breast milk. Thiazide diuretics may decrease the flow of breast milk.

**Children**—Although there is no specific information comparing use of this combination medicine in children with use in other age groups, this medicine is not expected to cause different side effects or problems in children than it does in adults. However, extra caution may be necessary in infants with jaundice, because these medicines can make the condition worse.

**Older adults**—Some side effects, especially dizziness or lightheadedness and signs and symptoms of too much potassium loss, may be more likely to occur in the elderly, who are usually more sensitive to the effects of this medicine. Also, beta-blockers may reduce tolerance to cold temperatures in elderly patients.

**Other medicines**—Although certain medicines should not be used together at all, in other cases 2 different medicines may be used together even if an interaction might occur. In these cases, your doctor may want to change the dose, or other precautions may be necessary. When you are taking beta-blocker and thiazide diuretic combinations, it is especially important that your health care professional know if you are taking any of the following:

• Allergy shots or
• Allergy skin tests—The beta-blocker contained in this medicine may increase the risk of a serious allergic reaction to these medicines
• Aminophylline (e.g., Somophyllin) or
• Caffeine (e.g., NoDoz) or
• Dyphylline (e.g., Lufylline) or
• Oxtriphylline (e.g., Choledyl) or
• Theophylline (e.g., Somophyllin-T)—The effects of these medicines and beta-blockers may be blocked; in addition, theophylline levels in the body may be increased, especially in patients who smoke

       

- Antidiabetics, oral (diabetes medicine you take by mouth) or
- Insulin—There is an increased risk of hyperglycemia (high blood sugar); the beta-blocker contained in this medicine may also cover up certain symptoms of hypoglycemia (low blood sugar), such as increases in pulse rate and blood pressure, and may make the hypoglycemia last longer
- Calcium channel blockers (amlodipine [e.g., Norvasc], bepridil [e.g., Bepadin], diltiazem [e.g., Cardizem], felodipine [e.g., Plendil], flunarizine [e.g., Sibelium], isradipine [e.g., DynaCirc], nicardipine [e.g., Cardene], nifedipine [e.g., Procardia], nimodipine [e.g., Nimotop], verapamil [e.g., Calan]) or
- Clonidine (e.g., Catapres) or
- Guanabenz (e.g., Wytensin) Effects on blood pressure may be increased. In addition, unwanted effects may occur if clonidine, guanabenz, or a beta-blocker are stopped suddenly after use together. Unwanted effects on the heart may occur when beta-blocker and thiazide diuretic combinations are used with calcium channel blockers
- Cocaine—Cocaine may block the effects of beta-blockers; in addition, there is an increased risk of high blood pressure, fast heartbeat, and possibly heart problems if you use cocaine while taking a beta-blocker and thiazide diuretic combination
- Digitalis glycosides (heart medicine)—Use with beta-blocker and thiazide diuretic combinations may cause high blood levels of digoxin, which may increase the chance of side effects
- Lithium—The thiazide diuretic contained in this combination may cause high blood levels of lithium, which may increase the chance of side effects
- Monoamine oxidase (MAO) inhibitors (furazolidone [e.g., Furoxone], isocarboxazid [e.g., Marplan], phenelzine [e.g., Nardil], procarbazine [e.g., Matulane], selegiline [e.g., Eldepryl], tranylcypromine [e.g., Parnate])—Taking a beta-blocker and thiazide diuretic combination while you are taking or within 2 weeks of taking monoamine oxidase (MAO) inhibitors may cause severe high blood pressure

**Other medical problems**—The presence of other medical problems may affect the use of the beta-blockers and thiazide diuretics. Make sure you tell your doctor if you have any other medical problems, especially:

- Allergy, history of (asthma, eczema, hay fever, hives), or
- Bronchitis or
- Emphysema—This combination medicine may make allergic reactions to other substances more severe or make the reaction last longer; in addition, the beta-blocker contained in this combination can increase trouble in breathing
- Bradycardia (unusually slow heartbeat) or
- Heart or blood vessel disease—This combination medicine may make these heart problems worse; also, if treatment is stopped suddenly, unwanted effects may occur
- Diabetes mellitus (sugar diabetes)—The beta-blocker contained in this medicine may cause hyperglycemia (high blood sugar) and circulation problems; in addition, if your diabetes medicine causes your blood sugar to be too low, beta-blockers may cover up some of the symptoms (fast heartbeat), although they will not cover up other symptoms such as dizziness or sweating; the thiazide diuretic contained in this medicine may increase the amount of sugar in the blood

- Gout (history of) or
- Lupus erythematosus (history of) or
- Pancreatitis (inflammation of the pancreas)—The thiazide diuretic contained in this medicine may make these conditions worse
- Kidney disease or
- Liver disease—Effects of this medicine may be increased because of slower removal from the body
- Mental depression (or history of) or
- Myasthenia gravis or
- Pheochromocytoma or
- Psoriasis or
- Raynaud's syndrome—The beta-blocker contained in this medicine may make these conditions worse
- Overactive thyroid—Stopping this medicine suddenly may increase symptoms of overactive thyroid; the beta-blocker contained in this medicine may cover up fast heartbeat, which is a sign of overactive thyroid

## Proper Use of This Medicine

In addition to the use of the medicine your doctor has prescribed, treatment for your high blood pressure may include weight control and care in the types of foods you eat, especially foods high in sodium. Your doctor will tell you which of these are most important for you. You should check with your doctor before changing your diet.

Many patients who have high blood pressure will not notice any signs of the problem. In fact, many may feel normal. It is very important that you *take your medicine exactly as directed* and that you keep your appointments with your doctor even if you feel well.

Remember that this medicine will not cure your high blood pressure but it does help control it. Therefore, you must continue to take it as directed if you expect to lower your blood pressure and keep it down. *You may have to take high blood pressure medicine for the rest of your life.* If high blood pressure is not treated, it can cause serious problems such as heart failure, blood vessel disease, stroke, or kidney disease.

For patients taking the *extended-release tablet* form of this medicine:

- Swallow the tablet whole.
- Do not crush, break, or chew before swallowing.

To help you remember to take your medicine, try to get into the habit of taking it at the same time each day.

Ask your doctor about checking your pulse rate before and after taking beta-blocking agents. Then, while you are taking this medicine, check your pulse regularly. If it is much slower than your usual rate (or less than 50 beats per minute), check with your doctor. A pulse rate that is too slow may cause circulation problems.

The thiazide diuretic (e.g., bendroflumethiazide, chlorthalidone, or hydrochlorothiazide) contained in this combination medicine may cause you to have an unusual feeling of tiredness when you begin to take it. You may also notice an increase in the amount of urine or in your frequency of urination. After you take the medicine for a while, these effects should lessen. To keep the increase in urine from affecting your sleep:

- If you are to take a single dose a day, take it in the morning after breakfast.
- If you are to take more than one dose a day, take the last dose no later than 6 p.m., unless otherwise directed by your doctor.

However, it is best to plan your dose or doses according to a schedule that will least affect your personal activities and sleep. Ask your health care professional to help you plan the best time to take this medicine.

*Do not miss any doses.* This is especially important when you are taking only one dose per day. Some conditions may become worse when this medicine is not taken regularly.

**Dosing**—The dose of beta-blocker and thiazide diuretic combinations will be different for different patients. *Follow your doctor's orders or the directions on the label.* The following information includes only the average doses of beta-blocker and thiazide diuretic combinations. *If your dose is different, do not change it* unless your doctor tells you to do so.

The number of capsules or tablets that you take depends on the strength of the medicine.

*For atenolol and chlorthalidone combination*
- For *oral* dosage form (tablets):
  —For high blood pressure:
  - Adults—1 or 2 tablets once a day.
  - Children—Dose must be determined by your doctor.

*For bisoprolol and hydrochlorothiazide combination*
- For *oral* dosage form (tablets):
  —For high blood pressure:
  - Adults—1 or 2 tablets once a day.
  - Children—Dose must be determined by your doctor.

*For metoprolol and hydrochlorothiazide combination*
- For *oral* dosage form (tablets):
  —For high blood pressure:
  - Adults—1 or 2 tablets a day.
  - Children—Dose must be determined by your doctor.

*For nadolol and bendroflumethiazide combination*
- For *oral* dosage form (tablets):
  —For high blood pressure:
  - Adults—1 tablet once a day.
  - Children—Dose must be determined by your doctor.

*For pindolol and hydrochlorothiazide combination*
- For *oral* dosage form (tablets):
  —For high blood pressure:
  - Adults—1 or 2 tablets once a day.
  - Children—Dose must be determined by your doctor.

*For propranolol and hydrochlorothiazide combination*
- For *regular (short-acting) oral* dosage form (tablets):
  —For high blood pressure:
  - Adults—1 or 2 tablets two times a day.
  - Children—Dose must be determined by your doctor.
- For *long-acting oral* dosage form (capsules):
  —For high blood pressure:
  - Adults—1 capsule a day.
  - Children—Dose must be determined by your doctor.

*For timolol and hydrochlorothiazide combination*
- For *oral* dosage form (tablets):
  —For high blood pressure:
  - Adults—1 tablet two times a day or 2 tablets once a day.
  - Children—Dose must be determined by your doctor.

**Missed dose**—If you miss a dose of this medicine, take it as soon as possible. However, if it is within 4 hours of your next dose (8 hours if you are using atenolol and chlorthalidone, bisoprolol and hydrochlorothiazide, nadolol and bendroflumethiazide, or extended-release propranolol and hydrochlorothiazide), skip the missed dose and go back to your regular dosing schedule. Do not double doses.

**Storage**—To store this medicine:
- Keep out of the reach of children.
- Store away from heat and direct light.
- Do not store in the bathroom, near the kitchen sink, or in other damp places. Heat or moisture may cause the medicine to break down.
- Do not keep outdated medicine or medicine no longer needed. Be sure that any discarded medicine is out of the reach of children.

## Precautions While Using This Medicine

It is important that your doctor check your progress at regular visits. This is to make sure the medicine is properly controlling your blood pressure and to allow the dosage to be changed if needed.

*Do not stop taking this medicine without first checking with your doctor.* Your doctor may want you to reduce gradually the amount you are taking before stopping completely. Some conditions may become worse when the medicine is stopped suddenly, and the risk of heart attack is increased in some patients.

Make sure that you have enough medicine on hand to last through weekends, holidays, or vacations. You may want to carry an extra written prescription in your billfold or purse in case of an emergency. You can then have it filled if you run out of medicine while you are away from home.

Your doctor may want you to carry medical identification stating that you are taking this medicine.

*Do not take other medicines unless they have been discussed with your doctor.* This especially includes over-the-counter (nonprescription) medicines for appetite control, asthma, colds, cough, hay fever, or sinus problems since they may increase your blood pressure.

*Before having any kind of surgery (including dental surgery) or emergency treatment, tell the medical doctor or dentist in charge that you are taking this medicine.*

For *diabetic patients*:
- *This medicine may increase your blood sugar levels.* Also, *this medicine may cover up signs of hypoglycemia (low blood sugar),* such as change in pulse rate. While you are taking this medicine, be especially careful in testing for sugar in your urine. If you have any questions about this, check with your doctor.

*The thiazide diuretic contained in this medicine may cause a loss of potassium from your body.*

- To help prevent this, your doctor may want you to:
  —eat or drink foods that have a high potassium content (for example, orange or other citrus fruit juices), or
  —take a potassium supplement, or
  —take another medicine to help prevent the loss of the potassium in the first place.
- It is very important to follow these directions. Also, it is important not to change your diet on your own. This is more important if you are already on a special diet (as for diabetes), or if you are taking a potassium supplement or a medicine to reduce potassium loss. Extra potassium may not be necessary and, in some cases, too much potassium could be harmful.

Check with your doctor if you become sick and have severe or continuing vomiting or diarrhea. These problems may cause you to lose additional water and potassium.

This medicine may cause some people to become dizzy, drowsy, lightheaded, or less alert than they are normally. *Make sure you know how you react to this medicine before you drive, use machines, or do anything else that could be dangerous if you are dizzy or are not alert.* If the problem continues or gets worse, check with your doctor.

The beta-blocker (atenolol, bisoprolol, metoprolol, nadolol, pindolol, propranolol, or timolol) contained in this medicine may make you more sensitive to cold temperatures, especially if you have blood circulation problems. Beta-blockers tend to decrease blood circulation in the skin, fingers, and toes. Dress warmly during cold weather and be careful during prolonged exposure to cold, such as in winter sports.

This medicine may cause your skin to be more sensitive to sunlight than it is normally. Exposure to sunlight, even for brief periods of time, may cause a skin rash, itching, redness or other discoloration of the skin, or a severe sunburn. When you begin taking this medicine:
- Stay out of direct sunlight, especially between the hours of 10:00 a.m. and 3:00 p.m., if possible.
- Wear protective clothing, including a hat. Also, wear sunglasses.
- Apply a sun block product that has a skin protection factor (SPF) of at least 15. Some patients may require a product with a higher SPF number, especially if they have a fair complexion. If you have any questions about this, check with your health care professional.
- Apply a sun block lipstick that has an SPF of at least 15 to protect your lips.
- Do not use a sunlamp or tanning bed or booth.

*If you have a severe reaction from the sun, check with your doctor.*

Before you have any medical tests, tell the doctor in charge that you are taking this medicine. The results of some tests may be affected by this medicine.

For patients with allergies to foods, medicines, or insect stings:
- There is a chance that this medicine will make allergic reactions worse and harder to treat. If you have a severe allergic reaction while you are being treated with this medicine, check with a doctor right away so that it can be treated.

## Side Effects of This Medicine

Along with its needed effects, a medicine may cause some unwanted effects. Although not all of these side effects may occur, if they do occur they may need medical attention.

Check with your doctor as soon as possible if any of the following side effects occur:

*Less common*
  Breathing difficulty and/or wheezing; cold hands and feet; mental depression; slow heartbeat (especially less than 50 beats per minute); swelling of ankles, feet, and/or lower legs

*Rare*
  Black, tarry stools; blood in urine or stools; chest pain; dark urine; fever, chills, cough, or sore throat; hallucinations (seeing, hearing, or feeling things that are not there); joint pain; lower back or side pain; pinpoint red spots on skin; red, scaling, or crusted skin; skin rash or hives; stomach pain (severe) with nausea and vomiting; unusual bleeding or bruising; or yellow eyes or skin

*Signs and symptoms of too much potassium or sodium loss*
  Confusion; convulsions (seizures); dryness of mouth; increased thirst; irregular heartbeats; irritability, mood or mental changes; muscle cramps or pain; nausea or vomiting, unusual tiredness or weakness; weak pulse

*Signs and symptoms of overdose (in the order in which they may occur)*

Slow heartbeat; dizziness (severe) or fainting; difficulty in breathing; bluish-colored fingernails or palms of hands; convulsions (seizures)

Other side effects may occur that usually do not need medical attention. These side effects may go away during treatment as your body adjusts to the medicine. However, check with your doctor if any of the following side effects continue or are bothersome:

*More common*

Decreased sexual ability; dizziness or lightheadedness; drowsiness (mild); trouble in sleeping

*Less common*

Anxiety or nervousness; constipation; diarrhea; increased sensitivity of skin to sunlight (skin rash, itching, redness or other discoloration of skin, or severe sunburn); loss of appetite; numbness or tingling of fingers and toes; stomach discomfort or upset; stuffy nose

*Rare*

Changes in taste; dry, sore eyes; itching of skin; nightmares and vivid dreams

Although not all of the above side effects have been reported for all of these medicines, they have been reported for at least one of the beta-blockers or thiazide diuretics. Since all of the beta-blockers are very similar and the thiazide diuretics are also very similar, any of the above side effects may occur with any of these medicines. However, they may be more common with some combinations than with others.

After you have been taking this medicine for a while, it may cause unpleasant or even harmful effects if you stop taking it too suddenly. After you stop taking this medicine or while you are gradually reducing the amount you are taking, check with your doctor right away if any of the following occur:

Chest pain; fast or irregular heartbeat; general feeling of discomfort, illness, or weakness; headache; shortness of breath (sudden); sweating; trembling

Other side effects not listed above may also occur in some patients. If you notice any other effects, check with your doctor.

Revised: 08/23/94

# BETA-CAROTENE—For Dietary Supplement    (Vitamin)    Systemic

Some commonly used brand names are:

**In the U.S.—**
Max-Caro            Solatene
Provatene
Generic name product is also available.

**In Canada—**
Generic name product is available.

## Description

Vitamins (VYE-ta-mins) are compounds that you *must* have for growth and health. They are needed in small amounts only and are usually available in the foods that you eat. Beta-carotene (bay-ta-KARE-oh-teen) is converted in the body to vitamin A, which is necessary for normal growth and health and for healthy eyes and skin.

In the absence of a dietary source of vitamin A, a lack of beta-carotene may also lead to a deficiency of vitamin A, which may cause a rare condition called night blindness (problems seeing in the dark). It may also cause dry eyes, eye infections, skin problems, and slowed growth. Your doctor may treat these problems by prescribing beta-carotene or vitamin A for you.

Beta-carotene or vitamin A supplements may be needed in patients with the following conditions:
- Cystic fibrosis
- Diarrhea, continuing
- Illness, long-term
- Injury, serious
- Liver disease
- Malabsorption problems
- Pancreas disease

If any of these conditions apply to you, you should take beta-carotene only on the advice of your doctor after need has been established.

Claims that beta-carotene is effective as a sunscreen have not been proven. Although beta-carotene is being studied for its ability to prevent certain types of cancer, there is not enough information to show that this treatment is effective.

Beta-carotene is available without a prescription. However, it may be a good idea to check with your doctor before taking beta-carotene on your own.

Beta-carotene is available in the following dosage forms:
*Oral*
- Capsules (U.S. and Canada)
- Tablets (U.S. and Canada)
- Chewable tablets (Canada)

## Importance of Diet

Vitamin supplements should be taken only if you cannot get enough vitamins in your diet; however, some diets may not contain all of the vitamins you need. This may occur with rapid weight loss, unusual diets (such as some reducing diets in which choice of foods is very limited), prolonged intravenous feeding, or malnutrition. A balanced diet should provide all the vitamins you normally need.

In order to get enough vitamins and minerals in your diet, it is important that you eat a balanced and varied diet. Follow carefully any diet program your doctor may recommend. For specific vitamin and/or mineral needs, ask your doctor or dietitian for a list of appropriate foods.

Beta-carotene is found in carrots; dark-green leafy vegetables, such as spinach, green leaf lettuce; tomatoes; sweet potatoes; broccoli; cantaloupe; and winter squash. The body converts beta-carotene into vitamin A. Ordinary cooking does not destroy beta-carotene.

Vitamins alone will not take the place of a good diet and will not provide energy. Your body needs other substances found in food, such as protein, minerals, carbohydrates, and fat. Vitamins themselves often cannot work without the presence of other foods. For example, some fat is needed so that beta-carotene can be absorbed into the body.

In some cases, it may not be possible for you to get enough food to supply you with the proper vitamins. In other cases, the amount of vitamins you need may be increased above normal. Therefore, a vitamin supplement may be needed.

## Before Using This Dietary Supplement

If you are taking this dietary supplement without a prescription, carefully read and follow any precautions on the label. For beta-carotene, the following should be considered:

**Allergies**—Tell your doctor if you have ever had any unusual or allergic reaction to beta-carotene. Also tell your health care professional if you are allergic to any other substances, such as foods, preservatives, or dyes.

**Pregnancy**—It is especially important that you are receiving enough vitamins when you become pregnant and that you continue to receive the right amount of vitamins throughout your pregnancy. The healthy growth and development of the fetus depend on a steady supply of nutrients from the mother.

Beta-carotene has not been studied in pregnant women. However, no problems with fertility or pregnancy have been reported in women taking up to 30 milligrams (mg) of beta-carotene a day. The effects of taking more than 30 mg a day are not known.

**Breast-feeding**—It is especially important that you receive the right amounts of vitamins so that your baby will also get the vitamins needed to grow properly. However, taking large amounts of a dietary supplement while breast-feeding may be harmful to the mother and/or baby and should be avoided.

**Children**—Normal daily requirements vary according to age. It is especially important that children receive enough vitamins in their diet for healthy growth and development.

**Older adults**—It is important that older people continue to receive enough vitamins in their diet for good health.

**Medicines or other dietary supplements**—Although certain medicines or dietary supplements should not be used together at all, in other cases they may be used together even if an interaction might occur. In these cases, your doctor may want to change the dose, or other precautions may be necessary. Tell your health care professional if you are taking any other dietary supplement or any prescription or nonprescription (over-the-counter [OTC]) medicine.

**Other medical problems**—The presence of other medical problems may affect the use of beta-carotene. Make sure you tell your doctor if you have any other medical problems, especially:
- Kidney disease or
- Liver disease—These conditions may cause high blood levels of beta-carotene, which may increase the chance of side effects

## Proper Use of This Dietary Supplement

Beta-carotene is safer than vitamin A (retinol) because vitamin A can be harmful in high doses. If you have high blood levels of vitamin A, then your body will convert less beta-carotene to vitamin A. However, you should take large doses of beta-carotene only under the direction of your doctor after need has been identified.

**Dosing**—For use as a nutritional supplement:
—For *oral* dosage forms (capsules or tablets):
- Adults and teenagers—6 to 15 milligrams (mg) of beta-carotene (the equivalent of 10,000 to 25,000 Units of vitamin A activity) a day.
- Children—3 to 6 mg of beta-carotene (the equivalent of 5000 to 10,000 Units of vitamin A activity) a day.

**Missed dose**—If you miss taking a vitamin for one or more days there is no cause for concern, since it takes some time for your body to become seriously low in vitamins. However, if your doctor has recommended that you take this vitamin, try to remember to take it as directed every day.

**Storage**—To store this dietary supplement:
- Keep out of the reach of children.
- Store away from heat and direct light.
- Do not store in the bathroom, near the kitchen sink, or in other damp places. Heat or moisture may cause the dietary supplement to break down.
- Keep the dietary supplement from freezing. Do not refrigerate.
- Do not keep outdated dietary supplements or those no longer needed. Be sure that any discarded dietary supplement is out of the reach of children.

## Side Effects of This Dietary Supplement

Along with its needed effects, a dietary supplement may cause some unwanted effects. The following side effects may go away during treatment as your body adjusts to the dietary supplement. However, check with your doctor if any of the following side effects continue or are bothersome:

*More common*
Yellowing of palms, hand, or soles of feet, and to a lesser extent the face (this may be a sign that your dose of beta-carotene as a nutritional supplement is too high)

*Rare*
Diarrhea; dizziness; joint pain; unusual bleeding or bruising

Other side effects not listed above may also occur in some patients. If you notice any other effects, check with your doctor.

Revised: 11/27/91
Interim revision(s): 05/11/92; 08/15/94

---

# BETA-CAROTENE—For Photosensitivity    Systemic

Some commonly used brand names are:
**In the U.S.—**
Max-Caro                    Solatene
Provatene
Generic name product is also available.
**In Canada—**
Generic name product is available.

## Description

Beta-carotene (bay-ta-KARE-oh-teen) is used to prevent or treat a sun reaction (photosensitivity) in patients with a disease called erythropoietic protoporphyria.

It may also be used to treat other conditions as determined by your doctor. However, beta-carotene has not been shown to be effective as a sunscreen.

Beta-carotene is available without a prescription. However, it may be a good idea to check with your doctor before taking it on your own.

Beta-carotene is available in the following dosage forms:
*Oral*
- Capsules (U.S. and Canada)
- Tablets (U.S. and Canada)
- Chewable tablets (Canada)

## Before Using This Medicine

If you are taking this medicine without a prescription, carefully read and follow any precautions on the label. For beta-carotene, the following should be considered:

**Allergies**—Tell your doctor if you have ever had any unusual or allergic reaction to beta-carotene. Also tell your health care professional if you are allergic to any other substances, such as foods, preservatives, or dyes.

**Pregnancy**—Beta-carotene has not been studied in pregnant women. However, no problems with fertility or pregnancy have been reported in women taking up to 30 milligrams (mg) of beta-carotene a day. The effects of taking more than 30 mg a day are not known.

**Breast-feeding**—Beta-carotene has not been reported to cause problems in nursing babies.

**Children**—This medicine has been tested in children and, in effective doses, has not been shown to cause different side effects or problems in children than it does in adults.

**Older adults**—Many medicines have not been studied specifically in older people. Therefore, it may not be known whether they work exactly the same way they do in younger adults. Although there is no specific information comparing use of beta-carotene in the elderly with use in other age groups, it is not expected to cause different side effects or problems in older people than it does in younger adults.

**Other medicines**—Although certain medicines should not be used together at all, in other cases two different medicines may be used together even if an interaction might occur. In these cases, your doctor may want to change the dose, or other precautions may be necessary. Tell your health care professional if you are taking any other prescription or nonprescription (over-the-counter [OTC]) medicine.

**Other medical problems**—The presence of other medical problems may affect the use of beta-carotene. Make sure you tell your doctor if you have any other medical problems, especially:
- Kidney disease or
- Liver disease—These conditions may cause high blood levels of beta-carotene, which may increase the chance of side effects

## Proper Use of This Medicine

**Dosing**—The dose of beta-carotene will be different for different patients. *Follow your doctor's orders or the directions on the label.* The following information includes only the average doses of beta-carotene. *If your dose is different, do not change it* unless your doctor tells you to do so.
- To treat or prevent a sun reaction in patients with erythropoietic protoporphyria:
  —For *oral* dosage forms (capsules or tablets):
  - Adults and teenagers—30 to 300 milligrams (mg) of beta-carotene (the equivalent of 50,000 to 500,000 Units of vitamin A activity) a day.

- Children—30 to 150 mg of beta-carotene (the equivalent of 50,000 to 250,000 Units of vitamin A activity) a day.

**Missed dose**—If you miss a dose of this medicine, take it as soon as possible. However, if it is almost time for your next dose, skip the missed dose and go back to your regular dosing schedule. Do not double doses.

**Storage**—To store this medicine:
- Keep out of the reach of children.
- Store away from heat and direct light.
- Do not store in the bathroom, near the kitchen sink, or in other damp places. Heat or moisture may cause the medicine to break down.
- Keep the medicine from freezing. Do not refrigerate.
- Do not keep outdated medicine or medicine no longer needed. Be sure that any discarded medicine is out of the reach of children.

## Side Effects of This Medicine

Along with its needed effects, a medicine may cause some unwanted effects. The following side effects may go away during treatment as your body adjusts to the medicine. However, check with your doctor if any of the following side effects continue or are bothersome:

*More common*
Yellowing of palms, hands, or soles of feet, and to a lesser extent the face

*Rare*
Diarrhea; dizziness; joint pain; unusual bleeding or bruising

Other side effects not listed above may also occur in some patients. If you notice any other effects, check with your doctor.

## Additional Information

Once a medicine has been approved for marketing for a certain use, experience may show that it is also useful for other medical problems. Although this use is not included in product labeling, beta-carotene is used in certain patients with the following medical condition:
- Polymorphous light eruption (a type of sun reaction)

Other than the above information, there is no additional information relating to proper use, precautions, or side effects for this use.

Revised: 11/27/91
Interim revision: 08/15/94

# BETHANECHOL   Systemic

Some commonly used brand names are:
**In the U.S.—**
Duvoid                        Urecholine
Urabeth
Generic name product may also be available.
**In Canada—**
Duvoid                        Urecholine

## Description

Bethanechol (be-THAN-e-kole) is taken to treat certain disorders of the urinary tract or bladder. It helps to cause urination and emptying of the bladder. Bethanechol may also be used for other conditions as determined by your doctor.

Bethanechol is available only with your doctor's prescription in the following dosage forms:
*Oral*
- Tablets (U.S. and Canada)
*Parenteral*
- Injection (U.S. and Canada)

## Before Using This Medicine

In deciding to use a medicine, the risks of taking the medicine must be weighed against the good it will do.

This is a decision you and your doctor will make. For bethanechol, the following should be considered:

**Allergies**—Tell your doctor if you have ever had any unusual or allergic reaction to bethanechol. Also tell your health care professional if you are allergic to any other substances, such as foods, preservatives, or dyes.

**Pregnancy**—Studies on effects in pregnancy have not been done in either humans or animals.

**Breast-feeding**—It is not known whether bethanechol passes into the breast milk.

**Children**—Although there is no specific information comparing use of bethanechol in children with use in other age groups, this medicine is not expected to cause different side effects or problems in children than it does in adults.

**Older adults**—Many medicines have not been studied specifically in older people. Therefore, it may not be known whether they work exactly the same way they do in younger adults. Although there is no specific information comparing use of bethanechol in the elderly with use in other age groups, it is not expected to cause different side effects or problems in older people than it does in younger adults.

**Other medicines**—Although certain medicines should not be used together at all, in other cases two different medicines may be used together even if an interaction might occur. In these cases, your doctor may want to change the dose, or other precautions may be necessary. Tell your health care professional if you are taking any other prescription or nonprescription (over-the-counter [OTC]) medicine.

**Other medical problems**—The presence of other medical problems may affect the use of bethanechol. Make sure you tell your doctor if you have any other medical problems, especially:

- Asthma or
- Epilepsy or
- Heart or blood vessel disease or
- Intestinal blockage or
- Low blood pressure or
- Parkinson's disease or
- Recent bladder or intestinal surgery or
- Stomach ulcer or other stomach problems or
- Urinary tract blockage or difficult urination—Bethanechol may make these conditions worse
- High blood pressure—Bethanechol may cause a rapid fall in blood pressure
- Overactive thyroid—Bethanechol may further increase the chance of heart problems

## Proper Use of This Medicine

*Take this medicine on an empty stomach* (either 1 hour before or 2 hours after meals) to lessen the possibility of nausea and vomiting, unless otherwise directed by your doctor.

*Take this medicine only as directed.* Do not take more of it, do not take it more often, and do not take it for a longer time than your doctor ordered. To do so may increase the chance of side effects.

**Dosing**—The dose of bethanechol will be different for different patients. *Follow your doctor's orders or the directions on the label.* The following information includes only the average doses of bethanechol. *If your dose is different, do not change it* unless your doctor tells you to do so.

- To empty the bladder:
  —For *oral* dosage form (tablets):
  - Adults—25 to 50 milligrams (mg) three or four times a day.
  - Children—Dose is based on body weight and must be determined by your doctor. The usual dose is 0.6 mg per kilogram (kg) (0.27 mg per pound) of body weight a day. This dose is divided into smaller doses and taken three or four times a day.
  —For *injection* dosage form:
  - Adults—5 mg injected under the skin three or four times a day.
  - Children—Dose is based on body weight and must be determined by your doctor. The usual dose is 0.2 mg per kg (0.09 mg per pound) of body weight a day. This dose is divided into smaller doses, which are injected under the skin three or four times a day.

**Missed dose**—If you miss a dose of this medicine and you remember within an hour or so of the missed dose, take it right away. However, if you do not remember until 2 or more hours after, skip the missed dose and go back to your regular dosing schedule. Do not double doses.

**Storage**—To store this medicine:
- Keep out of the reach of children.
- Store away from heat and direct light.
- Do not store the tablet form of this medicine in the bathroom, near the kitchen sink, or in other damp places. Heat or moisture may cause the medicine to break down.
- Do not keep outdated medicine or medicine no longer needed. Be sure that any discarded medicine is out of the reach of children.

## Precautions While Using This Medicine

Dizziness, lightheadedness, or fainting may occur, especially when you get up from a lying or sitting position. Getting up slowly may help lessen this problem.

## Side Effects of This Medicine

Along with its needed effects, a medicine may cause some unwanted effects. Although not all of these side effects may occur, if they do occur they may need medical attention.

Check with your doctor as soon as possible if any of the following side effects occur:
*Rare—more common with the injection*
    Shortness of breath, wheezing, or tightness in chest

Other side effects may occur that usually do not need medical attention. These side effects may go away during treatment as your body adjusts to the medicine. However, check with your doctor if any of the following side effects continue or are bothersome:
*Less common or rare—more common with the injection*
    Belching; blurred vision or change in near or distance vision; diarrhea; dizziness or lightheadedness; feeling faint; frequent urge to urinate; headache; increased watering of mouth or sweating; nausea or vomiting; redness or flushing of skin or feeling of warmth; seizures; sleeplessness, nervousness, or jitters; stomach discomfort or pain

Other side effects not listed above may also occur in some patients. If you notice any other effects, check with your doctor.

## Additional Information

Once a medicine has been approved for marketing for a certain use, experience may show that it is also useful for other medical problems. Although these uses are not

included in product labeling, bethanechol is used in certain patients with the following medical conditions:

- Certain stomach problems
- Gastroesophageal reflux (caused by acid in the stomach washing back up into the esophagus)
- Megacolon (an abnormally large or dilated colon)

Other than the above information, there is no additional information relating to proper use, precautions, or side effects for these uses.

Revised: 05/12/93
Interim revision: 06/27/94

# BIOTIN    Systemic

A commonly used brand name in the U.S. is Bio-Tn.
Generic name product is available in the U.S. and Canada.

Other commonly used names are vitamin H, coenzyme R, or vitamin Bw.

## Description

Vitamins (VYE-ta-mins) are compounds that you must have for growth and health. They are needed in only small amounts and are usually available in the foods that you eat. Biotin (BYE-oh-tin) is necessary for normal metabolism.

A lack of biotin is rare. However, if it occurs it may lead to skin rash, loss of hair, high blood levels of cholesterol, and heart problems.

Patients with the following conditions may be more likely to have a deficiency of biotin:

- Genetic disorder of biotin deficiency
- Seborrheic determatitis in infants
- Surgical removal of the stomach

If any of these conditions apply to you, you should take biotin supplements only on the advice of your doctor after need has been established.

Claims that biotin supplements are effective in the treatment of acne, eczema (a type of skin disorder), or hair loss have not been proven.

Some preparations are available only with your doctor's prescription. Others are available without a prescription; however, your doctor may have special instructions on the proper use and dose for your condition.

Biotin supplements are available in the following dosage forms:

*Oral*
- Capsules (U.S.)
- Tablets (U.S. and Canada)

*It is very important that you read and understand the following information.* If any of it causes you special concern, check with your doctor. Also, *if you have any questions* or if you want more information about this dietary supplement or your medical problem, *ask your doctor, nurse, or dietitian.*

## Importance of Diet

Many nutritionists recommend that, if possible, people should get all the biotin they need from foods. Some people may need more biotin than normal. For such people a supplement is important.

In order to get enough vitamins and minerals in your diet, it is important that you eat a balanced and varied diet. Follow carefully any diet program your doctor may recommend. For your specific vitamin and/or mineral needs, ask your doctor or dietitian for a list of appropriate foods.

Biotin is found in various foods, including liver, cauliflower, salmon, carrots, bananas, soy flour, cereals, and yeast. Biotin content of food is reduced by cooking and preserving.

Experts have developed a list of recommended dietary allowances (RDA) for most vitamins and some minerals. The RDA are not an exact number but a general idea of how much you need. They do not cover amounts needed for problems caused by a serious lack of vitamins and minerals. Because lack of biotin is rare, there are no RDA for it. The following intakes are thought to be plenty for most individuals:

Infants and children—
Birth to 6 months of age: 10 micrograms (mcg) a day.
6 months to 1 year of age: 15 mcg a day.
1 to 3 years of age: 20 mcg a day.
4 to 6 years of age: 25 mcg a day.
7 to 10 years of age: 30 mcg a day.
Adolescents and adults—30 to 100 mcg a day.

## Before Using This Dietary Supplement

If you are taking this dietary supplement without a prescription, carefully read and follow any precautions on the label. For biotin, the following should be considered:

**Pregnancy**—It is especially important that you are receiving enough vitamins and minerals when you become pregnant and that you continue to receive the right amount of vitamins and minerals throughout your pregnancy. The healthy growth and development of the fetus depend on a steady supply of nutrients from the mother. However, taking large amounts of a dietary supplement in pregnancy may be harmful to the mother and/or fetus and should be avoided.

**Children**—It is especially important that children receive enough biotin in their diet for healthy growth and development. Although there is no specific information comparing the use of biotin in children with use in other age groups, this medicine is not expected to cause different side effects or problems in children than in adults.

**Older adults**—It is important that older people continue to receive enough biotin in their daily diets.

## Proper Use of This Dietary Supplement

Some people believe that taking very large doses of a vitamin or mineral (called megadoses) is useful for treating certain medical problems. Studies have not proven this. Large doses should be taken only under the direction of your doctor after need has been identified.

**Dosing**—The dose of biotin for prevention of biotin deficiency is based on daily recommended intake. See the *Importance of Diet* section for the daily recommended intake for biotin.

**Missed dose**—If you miss taking biotin supplements for one or more days there is no cause for concern, since it takes some time for your body to become seriously low in biotin. However, if your doctor has recommended that you take biotin, try to remember to take it as directed every day.

**Storage**—To store this dietary supplement:
- Keep out of the reach of children.
- Store away from heat and direct light.
- Do not store in the bathroom, near the kitchen sink, or in other damp places. Heat or moisture may cause the dietary supplement to break down.
- Keep the dietary supplement from freezing. Do not refrigerate.
- Do not keep outdated dietary supplements or those no longer needed. Be sure that any discarded dietary supplement is out of the reach of children.

## Side Effects of This Dietary Supplement

No side effects have been reported for biotin, However, check with your doctor if you notice any unusual effects while you are taking it.

Revised: 09/26/91
Interim revision: 06/02/92; 07/28/94

# BISMUTH SUBSALICYLATE   Oral

Some commonly used brand names are:
**In the U.S.—**
Bismatrol
Bismatrol Extra Strength
Pepto-Bismol
Pepto-Bismol Easy-to-Swallow Caplets
Pepto-Bismol Maximum Strength

Generic name product may also be available.

**In Canada—**
Bismed
Pepto-Bismol
PMS-Bismuth Subsalicylate

## Description

Bismuth subsalicylate (BIS-muth sub-sa-LIS-a-late) is used to treat diarrhea. It is also used to relieve the symptoms of an upset stomach, such as heartburn, indigestion, and nausea.

This medicine is available without a prescription; however, your doctor may have special instructions on the proper use and dose for your medical problem. Bismuth subsalicylate is available in the following dosage forms:

*Oral*
- Oral suspension (U.S. and Canada)
- Tablets (U.S.)
- Chewable tablets (U.S. and Canada)

## Before Using This Medicine

If you are taking this medicine without a prescription, carefully read and follow any precautions on the label. For bismuth subsalicylate, the following should be considered:

**Allergies**—Tell your doctor if you have ever had any unusual or allergic reaction to bismuth subsalicylate or to other salicylates, such as aspirin, including methyl salicylate (oil of wintergreen), or to any of the following medicines:
- Carprofen (e.g., Rimadyl)
- Diclofenac (e.g., Voltaren)
- Diflunisal (e.g., Dolobid)
- Fenoprofen (e.g., Nalfon)
- Floctafenine (e.g., Idarac)
- Flurbiprofen taken by mouth (e.g., Ansaid)
- Ibuprofen (e.g., Motrin)
- Indomethacin (e.g., Indocin)
- Ketoprofen (e.g., Orudis)
- Ketorolac (e.g., Toradol)
- Meclofenamate (e.g., Meclomen)
- Mefenamic acid (e.g., Ponstel)
- Naproxen (e.g., Naprosyn)
- Oxyphenbutazone (e.g., Tandearil)
- Phenylbutazone (e.g., Butazolidin)
- Piroxicam (e.g., Feldene)
- Sulindac (e.g., Clinoril)
- Suprofen (e.g., Suprol)

- Tiaprofenic acid (e.g., Surgam)
- Tolmetin (e.g., Tolectin)
- Zomepirac (e.g., Zomax)

Also tell your health care professional if you are allergic to any other substances, such as certain foods, sulfites or other preservatives, or dyes.

**Diet**—Make certain your health care professional knows if you are on any special diet, such as a low-sodium or low-sugar diet.

**Pregnancy**—The occasional use of bismuth subsalicylate is not likely to cause problems in the fetus or in the newborn baby. However, based on what is known about the use of other salicylates, especially at high doses and for long periods of time, the following information may also apply for bismuth subsalicylate.

Salicylates have not been shown to cause birth defects in humans. However, studies in animals have shown that salicylates may cause birth defects.

There is a chance that regular use of salicylates late in pregnancy may cause unwanted effects on the heart or blood flow in the fetus or in the newborn infant.

Use of salicylates during the last 2 weeks of pregnancy may cause bleeding problems in the fetus before or during delivery or in the newborn infant. Also, too much use of salicylates during the last 3 months of pregnancy may increase the length of pregnancy, prolong labor, cause other problems during delivery, or cause severe bleeding in the mother before, during, or after delivery.

**Breast-feeding**—Salicylates pass into the breast milk. Although they have not been shown to cause problems in nursing babies, it is possible that problems may occur if large amounts of salicylates are taken regularly.

**Children**—The fluid loss caused by diarrhea may result in a severe condition. For this reason, medicine for diarrhea must not be given to young children (under 3 years of age) without first checking with their doctor. In older children with diarrhea, medicine for diarrhea may be used, but it is also very important that a sufficient amount of liquids be given to replace the fluid lost by the body. If you have any questions about this, check with your health care professional.

Also, children are usually more sensitive to the effects of salicylates, especially if they have a fever or have lost large amounts of body fluid because of vomiting, diarrhea, or sweating.

The bismuth in this medicine may cause severe constipation in children.

In addition, do not use this medicine to treat nausea or vomiting in children or teenagers who have or are recovering from the flu or chickenpox. If nausea or vomiting is present, check with the child's doctor because this could be an early sign of Reye's syndrome.

**Older adults**—The fluid loss caused by diarrhea may result in a severe condition. For this reason, elderly persons with diarrhea should not take this medicine without first checking with their doctor. It is also very important that a sufficient amount of liquids be taken to replace the fluid lost by the body. If you have any questions about this, check with your health care professional.

Also, the elderly may be more sensitive to the effects of salicylates. This may increase the chance of side effects during treatment. In addition, the bismuth in this medicine may cause severe constipation in the elderly.

**Other medicines**—Although certain medicines should not be used together at all, in other cases two different medicines may be used together even if an interaction might occur. In these cases, your doctor may want to change the dose, or other precautions may be necessary. When taking bismuth subsalicylate it is especially important that your health care professional know if you are taking any of the following:

- Anticoagulants (blood thinners) or
- Heparin—The salicylate in this medicine may increase the chance of bleeding
- Antidiabetics, oral (diabetes medicine you take by mouth)—This medicine may make the levels of sugar in the blood become too low
- Medicine for pain and/or inflammation (except narcotics)—If these medicines contain salicylates, use of bismuth subsalicylate (which also contains salicylate) may lead to increased side effects and overdose
- Probenecid (e.g., Benemid) or
- Sulfinpyrazone (e.g., Anturane)—Bismuth subsalicylate may make these medicines less effective for treating gout
- Tetracyclines by mouth (medicine for infection)—The tablet form of bismuth subsalicylate should be taken at least 1 to 3 hours before or after tetracyclines; otherwise it may decrease the effectiveness of the tetracycline

**Other medical problems**—The presence of other medical problems may affect the use of bismuth subsalicylate. Make sure you tell your doctor if you have any other medical problems, especially:

- Dysentery—This condition may get worse; a different kind of treatment may be needed
- Gout—The salicylate in this medicine may worsen the gout and make the medicines taken for gout less effective
- Hemophilia or other bleeding problems—The salicylate in this medicine may increase the chance of bleeding
- Kidney disease—There is a greater chance of side effects because the body may be unable to get rid of the bismuth subsalicylate
- Stomach ulcer—Use of this medicine may make the ulcer worse

## Proper Use of This Medicine

For safe and effective use of this medicine:

- Follow your doctor's instructions if this medicine was prescribed.
- Follow the manufacturer's package directions if you are treating yourself.

For patients using this medicine to treat diarrhea:

- *It is very important that the fluid lost by the body be replaced and that a proper diet be followed.* For the first 24 hours you should drink plenty of clear liquids, such as ginger ale, decaffeinated cola, decaffeinated tea, broth, and gelatin. During the next 24 hours you may eat bland foods, such as cooked cereals, bread, crackers, and applesauce. Fruits, vegetables, fried or spicy foods, bran, candy, and caffeine and alcoholic beverages may make the diarrhea worse.

- If too much fluid has been lost by the body due to the diarrhea a serious condition may develop. Check with your doctor as soon as possible if any of the following signs of too much fluid loss occur:

  Decreased urination
  Dizziness and lightheadedness
  Dryness of mouth
  Increased thirst
  Wrinkled skin

**Dosing**—The dose of bismuth subsalicylate will be different for different patients. *Follow your doctor's orders or the directions on the label.* The following information includes only the average doses of bismuth subsalicylate. *If your dose is different, do not change it* unless your doctor tells you to do so.

The number of tablets or tablespoonfuls or teaspoonfuls of suspension that you take depends on the strength of the medicine.

- For *oral* dosage form (suspension):
  —For diarrhea or upset stomach:
  - Adults and teenagers—The usual dose is 2 tablespoonfuls every half-hour to one hour if needed. You should not take more than 16 tablespoonfuls of the regular-strength suspension or 8 tablespoonfuls of the concentrate in twenty-four hours.
  - Children 9 to 12 years of age—The usual dose is 1 tablespoonful every half-hour to one hour. You should not take more than 8 tablespoonfuls of the regular-strength suspension or 4 tablespoonfuls of the concentrate in twenty-four hours.
  - Children 6 to 9 years of age—The usual dose is 2 teaspoonfuls every half-hour to one hour. You should not take more than 16 teaspoonfuls of the regular-strength suspension or 8 teaspoonfuls of the concentrate in twenty-four hours.
  - Children 3 to 6 years of age—The usual dose is 1 teaspoonful every half-hour to one hour. You should not take more than 8 teaspoonfuls of the regular-strength suspension or 4 teaspoonfuls of the concentrate in twenty-four hours.
  - Children up to 3 years of age—Dose is based on body weight:
    —For children weighing 6.4 to 8 kilograms (kg) (14 to 18 pounds): The usual dose is ½ teaspoonful of the regular-strength suspension or ¼ teaspoonful of the concentrate.
    —For children weighing over 13 kg (29 pounds): The usual dose is 1 teaspoonful of the regular-strength suspension or ½ teaspoonful of the concentrate.

- For *oral* dosage forms (tablets or chewable tablets):
  —For diarrhea or upset stomach:
  - Adults and teenagers—The usual dose is 2 tablets every half-hour to one hour. You should not take more than 16 tablets in twenty-four hours.
  - Children 9 to 12 years of age—The usual dose is 1 tablet every half-hour to one hour. You should not take more than 8 tablets in twenty-four hours.
  - Children up to 9 years of age—The oral suspension is the preferred dosage form for this age group.

**Missed dose**—If your doctor has ordered you to take this medicine according to a regular schedule and you miss a dose, take it as soon as you remember. However, if it is almost time for your next dose, skip the missed dose and go back to your regular dosing schedule. Do not double doses.

**Storage**—To store this medicine:

- Keep out of the reach of children. Overdose is very dangerous in young children.
- Store away from heat and direct light.
- Do not store the tablet form of this medicine in the bathroom, near the kitchen sink, or in other damp places. Heat or moisture may cause the medicine to break down.
- Keep the liquid form of this medicine from freezing.
- Do not keep outdated medicine or medicine no longer needed. Be sure that any discarded medicine is out of the reach of children.

## Precautions While Using This Medicine

*Check the labels of all over-the-counter (OTC), nonprescription, and prescription medicines you now take.* If any contain aspirin or other salicylates, be especially careful. Using other salicylate-containing products while taking this medicine may lead to overdose. If you have any questions about this, check with your health care professional.

For diabetic patients:

- False urine sugar test results may occur if you are regularly taking large amounts of bismuth subsalicylate or other salicylates.
- Smaller doses or occasional use of bismuth subsalicylate usually will not affect urine sugar tests. However, check with your health care professional (especially if your diabetes is not well-controlled) if:
  —you are not sure how much salicylate you are taking every day.
  —you notice any change in your urine sugar test results.
  —you have any other questions about this possible problem.

*If you think that you or anyone else may have taken an overdose, get emergency help at once.* Taking an overdose of this medicine may cause unconsciousness or death.

Signs of overdose include convulsions (seizures), hearing loss, confusion, ringing or buzzing in the ears, severe drowsiness or tiredness, severe excitement or nervousness, and fast or deep breathing.

If you are taking this medicine for diarrhea, check with your doctor:

- if your symptoms do not improve within 2 days or if they become worse.
- if you also have a high fever.

## Side Effects of This Medicine

Along with its needed effects, a medicine may cause some unwanted effects. Although not all of these side effects may occur, if they do occur they may need medical attention.

*When this medicine is used occasionally or for short periods of time at low doses, side effects usually are rare. However, check with your doctor immediately* if any of the following side effects occur, since they may indicate that too much medicine is being taken:

Anxiety; any loss of hearing; confusion; constipation (severe); diarrhea (severe or continuing); difficulty in speaking or slurred speech; dizziness or lightheadedness; drowsiness (severe); fast or deep breathing; headache (severe or continuing); increased sweating; increased thirst; mental depression; muscle spasms (especially of face, neck, and back); muscle weakness; nausea or vomiting (severe or continuing); ringing or buzzing in ears (continuing); stomach pain (severe or continuing); trembling; uncontrollable flapping movements of the hands (especially in elderly patients) or other uncontrolled body movements; vision problems

In some patients bismuth subsalicylate may cause dark tongue and/or grayish black stools. This is only temporary and will go away when you stop taking this medicine.

Other side effects not listed above may also occur in some patients. If you notice any other effects, check with your doctor.

---

Revised: 02/03/92
Interim revision: 09/01/94

---

# BLEOMYCIN   Systemic

A commonly used brand name in the U.S. and Canada is Blenoxane.

## Description

Bleomycin (blee-oh-MYE-sin) belongs to the general group of medicines called antineoplastics. It is used to treat some kinds of cancer.

Bleomycin seems to act by interfering with the growth of cancer cells, which are eventually destroyed. Since the growth of normal body cells may also be affected by bleomycin, other effects will also occur. Some of these may be serious and must be reported to your doctor. Other effects, like darkening of skin or hair loss, may not be serious but may cause concern. Some effects may not occur for months or years after the medicine is used.

This medicine may also be used for other conditions, as determined by your doctor.

Before you begin treatment with bleomycin, you and your doctor should talk about the good this medicine will do as well as the risks of using it.

Bleomycin is to be administered only by or under the immediate supervision of your doctor. It is available in the following dosage form:

*Parenteral*
- Injection (U.S. and Canada)

## Before Using This Medicine

In deciding to use a medicine, the risks of taking the medicine must be weighed against the good it will do. This is a decision you and your doctor will make. For bleomycin, the following should be considered:

**Allergies**—Tell your doctor if you have ever had any unusual or allergic reaction to bleomycin.

**Pregnancy**—Studies have not been done in pregnant women. However, there is a chance that this medicine may cause birth defects if either the male or female is receiving it at the time of conception or if it is used during pregnancy. Studies in mice given large doses of bleomycin have shown that it causes birth defects. In addition, many cancer medicines may cause sterility which could be permanent. Although sterility has not been reported with this medicine, the possibility should be kept in mind.

Be sure that you have discussed this with your doctor before receiving this medicine. It is best to use some kind of birth control while you are receiving bleomycin. Tell your doctor right away if you think you have become pregnant while receiving bleomycin.

**Breast-feeding**—Because bleomycin may cause serious side effects, breast-feeding is generally not recommended while you are receiving it.

**Children**—Although there is no specific information comparing use of bleomycin in children with use in other age groups, this medicine is not expected to cause different side effects or problems in children than it does in adults.

**Older adults**—Lung problems are more likely to occur in elderly patients (over 70 years of age), who are usually more sensitive to the effects of bleomycin.

**Other medical problems**—The presence of other medical problems may affect the use of bleomycin. Make sure you tell your doctor if you have any other medical problems, especially:

- Kidney disease—Effects of bleomycin may be increased because of slower removal from the body
- Liver disease—Bleomycin can cause liver problems
- Lung disease—Bleomycin may worsen the condition

**Smoking**—Tell your doctor if you smoke. The risk of lung problems is increased in people who smoke.

## Proper Use of This Medicine

Bleomycin is sometimes given together with certain other medicines. If you are using a combination of medicines, it is important that you receive each medicine at the proper time. If you are taking some of these medicines by mouth, ask your health care professional to help you plan a way to take them at the right times.

Bleomycin often causes nausea, vomiting, and loss of appetite. However, it is very important that you continue to receive the medicine, even if you begin to feel ill. Ask your health care professional for ways to lessen these effects.

**Dosing**—The dose of bleomycin will be different for different patients. The dose that is used may depend on a number of things, including what the medicine is being used for, the patient's weight, and whether or not other medicines are also being taken. *If you are receiving bleomycin at home, follow your doctor's orders or the directions on the label.* If you have any questions about the proper dose of bleomycin, ask your doctor.

## Precautions While Using This Medicine

*It is very important that your doctor check your progress at regular visits* to make sure that this medicine is working properly and to check for unwanted effects.

Before having any kind of surgery (including dental surgery) or emergency treatment, *tell the medical doctor or dentist in charge that you are receiving or have received this medicine.*

## Side Effects of This Medicine

Along with its needed effects, a medicine may cause some unwanted effects. Although not all of these side effects may occur, if they do occur they may need medical attention.

Also, because of the way these medicines act on the body, there is a chance that they might cause other unwanted effects that may not occur until months or years after the medicine is used. These delayed effects may include certain types of cancer, such as leukemia. Discuss these possible effects with your doctor.

*Check with your doctor or nurse immediately* if the following side effects occur:

*More common*
Fever and chills (occurring within 3 to 6 hours after a dose)

*Less common*
Confusion; faintness; wheezing

*Rare*
Chest pain (sudden severe); weakness in arms or legs (sudden)

Check with your health care professional as soon as possible if any of the following side effects occur:

*More common*
Cough; shortness of breath; sores in mouth and on lips

Other side effects may occur that usually do not need medical attention. These side effects may go away during treatment as your body adjusts to the medicine. Also, your health care professional may be able to tell you about ways to prevent or reduce some of these side effects. Check with your health care professional if any of the following side effects continue or are bothersome or if you have any questions about them:

*More common*
Darkening or thickening of skin; dark stripes on skin; itching of skin; skin rash or colored bumps on fingertips, elbows, or palms; skin redness or tenderness; swelling of fingers; vomiting and loss of appetite

*Less common*
Changes in fingernails or toenails; weight loss

Bleomycin may cause a temporary loss of hair in some people. After treatment has ended, normal hair growth should return, although it may take several months.

Side effects that affect your lungs (for example, cough and shortness of breath) may be more likely to occur if you smoke.

After you stop receiving bleomycin, it may still produce some side effects that need attention. During this period of time, check with your health care professional *immediately* if you notice either of the following:

Cough; shortness of breath

Other side effects not listed above may also occur in some patients. If you notice any other effects, check with your health care professional.

## Additional Information

Once a medicine has been approved for marketing for a certain use, experience may show that it is also useful for other medical problems. Although this use is not included in product labeling, bleomycin is used in certain patients with the following medical condition:

- Verruca vulgaris (warts)

For patients being treated with bleomycin for warts:

- Bleomycin is used to treat severe cases of warts when other treatments have not worked.
- Before using bleomycin, tell your doctor if you have problems with circulation. Bleomycin can cause paleness or coldness in fingers treated for warts.
- Bleomycin is injected directly into the wart. Because it is not absorbed into the body, it does not cause loss of hair, lung problems, or other unwanted effects described above. However, it may cause burning or pain at the place of injection. Skin rash or itching, nail loss, and pain or coldness in the finger where bleomycin was injected have also been reported.

Other than the above information, there is no additional information relating to proper use, precautions, or side effects for these uses.

Revised: 07/11/94

# BOTULINUM TOXIN TYPE A    Parenteral-Local

A commonly used brand name in the U.S. and Canada is Botox.

## Description

Botulinum toxin type A (BOT-yoo-lye-num) is used to treat certain eye conditions, such as:

- Blepharospasm—A condition in which the eyelid will not stay open, because of a spasm of a muscle of the eye.
- Strabismus—A condition in which the eyes do not line up properly.

Botulinum toxin type A is injected into the surrounding muscle or tissue of the eye, but not into the eye itself. Depending on your condition, more than one treatment may be required.

This medicine is to be administered only by, or under the immediate supervision of, your doctor. It is available in the following dosage form:

*Parenteral-Local*
- Injection (U.S. and Canada)

## Before Receiving This Medicine

In deciding to receive a medicine, the risks of receiving the medicine must be weighed against the good it will do. This is a decision you and your doctor will make. For botulinum toxin type A, the following should be considered:

**Allergies**—Tell your doctor if you have ever had any unusual or allergic reaction to botulinum toxin type A. Also tell your health care professional if you are allergic to any other substances.

**Pregnancy**—Studies on effects in pregnancy have not been done in either humans or animals.

**Breast-feeding**—It is not known whether botulinum toxin type A passes into the breast milk. However, this medicine has not been reported to cause problems in nursing babies.

**Children**—Studies on this medicine have been done only in adult patients, and there is no specific information comparing use of botulinum toxin type A in children up to 12 years of age with use in other age groups.

**Older adults**—Many medicines have not been studied specifically in older people. Therefore, it may not be known whether they work exactly the same way they do in younger adults. Although there is no specific information comparing use of botulinum toxin type A in the elderly with use in other age groups, this medicine is not expected to cause different side effects or problems in older people than it does in younger adults.

**Other medicines**—Although certain medicines should not be used together at all, in other cases two different medicines may be used together even if an interaction might occur. In these cases, your doctor may want to change the dose, or other precautions may be necessary. Tell your health care professional if you are using any other ophthalmic prescription or nonprescription (over-the-counter [OTC]) medicine.

**Other medical problems**—The presence of other medical problems may affect the use of botulinum toxin type A. Make sure you tell your doctor if you have any other medical problems, especially:

- Heart problems or other medical conditions that may worsen with rapidly increasing activity—Treatment with botulinum toxin type A may give you better vision and the desire to become more active in your daily life; this may put a strain on your heart and body
- Infection with *Clostridium botulinum* toxin (botulism poisoning), history of—Persons with a history of infection with *Clostridium botulinum* toxin (botulism poisoning) may have produced antibodies that may interfere with botulinum toxin type A therapy and make it less effective

## Proper Use of This Medicine

**Dosing**—The dose of botulinum toxin type A will be different for different patients. The following information includes only the average doses of botulinum toxin type A.

- For *injection* dosage form:
  —For certain eye conditions:
  - Adults and children 12 years of age and older—One or more injections into the muscles around the eyes one or more times, depending on the condition being treated.
  - Children up to 12 years of age—Use and dose must be determined by your doctor.

## Precautions After Receiving This Medicine

After you have received this medicine and your vision is better, you may find that you are a lot more active than you were before. You should increase your activities slowly and carefully to allow your heart and body time to get stronger. Also, before you start any exercise program, check with your doctor.

## Side Effects of This Medicine

Along with its needed effects, a medicine may cause some unwanted effects. Although not all of these side effects may occur, if they do occur they may need medical attention.

*Check with your doctor as soon as possible if any of the following side effects occur:*

*More common*

Dryness of the eye; inability to close the eyelid completely

*Less common or rare*

Decreased blinking; irritation of the cornea (colored portion) of the eye; turning outward or inward of the edge of the eyelid

Other side effects may occur that usually do not need medical attention. These side effects may go away as your body adjusts to the medicine. However, check with your doctor if any of the following side effects continue or are bothersome:

*More common*

Blue or purplish bruise on eyelid; drooping of the upper eyelid; eye pointing upward or downward instead of straight ahead; irritation or watering of the eye; sensitivity of the eye to light

*Less common or rare*

Difficulty finding the location of objects; double vision; skin rash; swelling of the eyelid skin

Other side effects not listed above may also occur in some patients. If you notice any other effects, check with your doctor.

## Additional Information

Once a medicine has been approved for marketing for a certain use, experience may show that it is also useful for other medical problems. Although these uses are not included in product labeling, botulinum toxin type A is used in certain patients with the following medical conditions:

- Spasms of the face
- Spasms of the neck

Revised: 01/09/92
Interim revision: 10/28/93

# BROMOCRIPTINE  Systemic

A commonly used brand name in the U.S. and Canada is Parlodel.

## Description

Bromocriptine (broe-moe-KRIP-teen) belongs to the group of medicines known as ergot alkaloids. It is used to treat certain menstrual problems or as a fertility medicine in some women who are unable to become pregnant. It is also used to stop milk production in some women who have abnormal milk leakage. Bromocriptine blocks release of a hormone called prolactin from the pituitary gland. Prolactin affects the menstrual cycle and milk production.

Bromocriptine is also used to treat some people who have Parkinson's disease. It works by stimulating certain parts of the brain and nervous system that are involved in this disease.

Bromocriptine is also used to treat acromegaly (overproduction of growth hormone) and pituitary prolactinomas (tumors of the pituitary gland).

Bromocriptine may be used to stop milk production after abortion or after the delivery of a baby in women who should not breast-feed for medical reasons or in women who do not wish to breast-feed. However, some serious side effects have occurred during the use of bromocriptine to stop milk flow after pregnancy or abortion. These side effects have included strokes, seizures (convulsions), and heart attacks. Some deaths have also occurred. You should discuss with your doctor the good that this medicine will do as well as the risks of using it.

Bromocriptine may also be used for other conditions as determined by your doctor.

Bromocriptine is available only with your doctor's prescription, in the following dosage forms:

*Oral*

- Capsules (U.S. and Canada)
- Tablets (U.S. and Canada)

## Before Using This Medicine

In deciding to use a medicine, the risks of taking the medicine must be weighed against the good it will do. This is a decision you and your doctor will make. For bromocriptine, the following should be considered:

**Allergies**—Tell your doctor if you have ever had any unusual or allergic reaction to bromocriptine or other ergot medicines such as ergotamine. Also tell your health care professional if you are allergic to any other substances, such as foods, preservatives, or dyes.

**Pregnancy**—Bromocriptine is not generally recommended for use during pregnancy. However, bromocriptine can be used during pregnancy in certain patients who are closely monitored by their doctor.

**Breast-feeding**—This medicine stops milk from being produced.

**Teenagers**—This medicine has been tested in teenagers and, in effective doses, has not been shown to cause different side effects or problems than it does in adults.

**Older adults**—Side effects such as confusion, hallucinations, or uncontrolled body movements may be more likely to occur in older patients.

**Other medicines**—Although certain medicines should not be used together at all, in other cases two different medicines may be used together even if an interaction might occur. In these cases, your doctor may want to change the dose, or other precautions may be necessary. When you are taking bromocriptine, it is especially important that your health care professional know if you are taking any of the following:

- Ergot alkaloids (dihydroergotamine [e.g., D.H.E. 45], ergoloid mesylates [e.g., Hydergine], ergonovine [e.g., Ergotrate], ergotamine [e.g., Gynergen], methylergonovine [e.g., Methergine], methysergide [e.g., Sansert])—Severe cases of high blood pressure have occurred with the use of bromocriptine. This may be made worse with the use of ergot alkaloids
- Estrogens (female hormones) or
- Oral contraceptives (birth control pills) or
- Progestins (hydroxyprogesterone [e.g., Delalutin], medroxyprogesterone [e.g., Provera], megestrol [e.g., Megace], norethindrone [e.g., Norlutin], norethindrone acetate [e.g., Norlutate], norgestrel [e.g., Ovrette], progesterone [e.g., Lipo-Lutin])—These medicines may interfere with the effects of bromocriptine when it is used to treat amenorrhea (abnormal stoppage of menstrual periods) or galactorrhea (milk flow that occurs abnormally, without nursing)

**Other medical problems**—The presence of other medical problems may affect the use of bromocriptine. Make sure you tell your doctor if you have any other medical problems, especially:

- High blood pressure (history of) or
- Pregnancy-induced high blood pressure (history of)—Rarely, bromocriptine can make the high blood pressure worse
- Liver disease—Toxic effects of bromocriptine may occur in patients with liver disease because the body is not able

to get the bromocriptine out of the bloodstream as it normally would
- Mental problems (history of)—Bromocriptine may make certain mental problems worse

## Proper Use of This Medicine

If bromocriptine upsets your stomach, it may be taken with meals or milk. Also, taking the dose at bedtime may help to lessen nausea if it occurs. If stomach upset continues, check with your doctor. Your doctor may recommend that you take the first dose vaginally.

**Dosing**—The dose of bromocriptine will be different for different patients. *Follow your doctor's orders or the directions on the label.* The following information includes only the average doses of bromocriptine. *If your dose is different, do not change it* unless your doctor tells you to do so.

The number of capsules or tablets that you take depends on the strength of the medicine. Also, *the number of doses you take each day, the time allowed between doses, and the length of time you take the medicine depend on the medical problem for which you are taking bromocriptine.*

- For *oral* dosage forms (capsules and tablets):
- —Adults and teenagers:
  - For acromegaly: 1.25 to 100 milligrams a day.
  - For female infertility: 1.25 to 7.5 milligrams a day, taken one to three times a day.
  - For menstrual cycle irregularity: 1.25 to 7.5 milligrams a day, taken one to three times a day.
  - For Parkinson's disease: 1.25 to 300 milligrams a day.
  - For pituitary tumors: 1.25 to 20 milligrams a day.
  - For unexpected breast milk production: 1.25 to 7.5 milligrams a day, taken one to three times a day.

**Missed dose**—If you miss a dose of this medicine and remember it within 4 hours, take the missed dose when you remember it. However, if a longer time has passed, skip the missed dose and go back to your regular dosing schedule. Do not double doses.

**Storage**—To store this medicine:
- Keep out of the reach of children.
- Store away from heat and direct light.
- Do not store in the bathroom, near the kitchen sink, or in other damp places. Heat or moisture may cause the medicine to break down.
- Do not keep outdated medicine or medicine no longer needed. Be sure that any discarded medicine is out of the reach of children.

## Precautions While Using This Medicine

It is important that your doctor check your progress at regular visits, to make sure that this medicine is working and to check for unwanted effects.

This medicine may cause some people to become drowsy, dizzy, or less alert than they are normally. *Make sure you know how you react to this medicine before you drive, use machines, or do anything else that could be dangerous if you are dizzy or are not alert.*

Dizziness is more likely to occur after the first dose of bromocriptine. It may be helpful if you get up slowly from a lying or sitting position. Taking the first dose at bedtime or when you are able to lie down may also lessen problems. Your doctor may also recommend that you take the first dose vaginally.

Bromocriptine may cause dryness of the mouth. For temporary relief, use sugarless candy or gum, melt bits of ice in your mouth, or use a saliva substitute. However, if dry mouth continues for more than 2 weeks, check with your medical doctor or dentist. Continuing dryness of the mouth may increase the chance of dental disease, including tooth decay, gum disease, and fungus infections.

It may take several weeks for bromocriptine to work. Do not stop taking this medicine or reduce the amount you are taking without first checking with your doctor.

Drinking alcohol while you are taking bromocriptine may cause you to have a certain reaction. *Avoid alcoholic beverages until you have discussed this with your doctor.* Some of the symptoms you may have if you drink any alcohol while you are taking this medicine are:

Blurred vision
Chest pain
Confusion
Fast or pounding heartbeat
Flushing or redness of face
Nausea
Sweating
Throbbing headache
Vomiting
Weakness (severe)

For females who are able to bear children and who are *taking this medicine for menstrual problems, to stop milk production, for acromegaly, or for pituitary tumors:*

- It is best to use some type of birth control while you are taking bromocriptine. However, do not use oral contraceptives ("the Pill") since they may prevent this medicine from working. If you wish to become pregnant, you and your doctor should decide on the best time for you to stop using birth control. Tell your doctor right away if you think you have become pregnant while taking this medicine. You and your doctor should discuss whether or not you should continue to take bromocriptine during pregnancy.
- *Check with your doctor right away* if you get blurred vision, a sudden headache, or severe nausea and vomiting.

For females *taking bromocriptine for infertility:*

- In general, it is best to use some type of birth control when you start taking bromocriptine. However, do not use oral contraceptives ("the Pill") since they may prevent this medicine from working. When your

normal menstrual cycle returns, you and your doctor can decide on the best time for you to stop using birth control. Tell your doctor right away if you think you have become pregnant while taking this medicine. You and your doctor should discuss whether or not you should continue to take bromocriptine during pregnancy.

- *Check with your doctor right away* if you get blurred vision, a sudden headache, or severe nausea and vomiting.

## Side Effects of This Medicine

Along with its needed effects, a medicine may cause some unwanted effects. Although not all of these side effects may occur, if they do occur they may need medical attention.

Some serious side effects have occurred during the use of bromocriptine to stop milk flow after pregnancy or abortion. These side effects have included strokes, seizures (convulsions), and heart attacks. Some deaths have also occurred. You should discuss with your doctor the good that this medicine will do as well as the risks of using it.

*Check with your doctor immediately* if any of the following side effects occur:

*Rare*

Black, tarry stools; bloody vomit; chest pain (severe); convulsions (seizures); fainting; fast heartbeat; headache (unusual); increased sweating; nausea and vomiting (continuing or severe); nervousness; shortness of breath (unexplained); vision changes (such as blurred vision or temporary blindness); weakness (sudden)

Check with your doctor as soon as possible if any of the following side effects occur:

*Less common—reported more often in patients with Parkinson's disease*

Confusion; hallucinations (seeing, hearing, or feeling things that are not there); uncontrolled movements of the body, such as the face, tongue, arms, hands, head, and upper body

*Rare—reported more often in patients taking large doses*

Abdominal or stomach pain (continuing or severe); increased frequency of urination; loss of appetite (continuing); lower back pain; runny nose (continuing); weakness

Other side effects may occur that usually do not need medical attention. These side effects may go away during treatment as your body adjusts to the medicine. However, check with your doctor if any of the following side effects continue or are bothersome:

*More common*

Dizziness or lightheadedness, especially when getting up from a lying or sitting position; nausea

*Less common*

Constipation; diarrhea; drowsiness or tiredness; dry mouth; leg cramps at night; loss of appetite; mental depression; stomach pain; stuffy nose; tingling or pain in fingers and toes when exposed to cold; vomiting

Some side effects may be more likely to occur in patients who are taking bromocriptine for Parkinson's disease, acromegaly, or pituitary tumors since they may be taking larger doses.

Other side effects not listed above may also occur in some patients. If you notice any other effects, check with your doctor.

---

## Additional Information

Once a medicine has been approved for marketing for a certain use, experience may show that it is also useful for other medical problems. Although these uses are not included in product labeling, bromocriptine is used in certain patients with the following medical conditions:

- Male infertility caused by excess prolactin (a hormone) in the blood
- Neuroleptic malignant syndrome

Other than the above information, there is no additional information relating to proper use, precautions, or side effects for these uses.

---

Revised: 06/04/93

---

# BRONCHODILATORS, ADRENERGIC     Inhalation

Some commonly used brand names are:

**In the U.S.—**

| | |
|---|---|
| Adrenalin Chloride[3] | Maxair[8] |
| Airet[1] | Medihaler-Epi[3] |
| Alupent[7] | Medihaler-Iso[6] |
| Arm-a-Med Isoetharine[5] | Metaprel[7] |
| Arm-a-Med Metaproterenol[7] | microNefrin[10] |
| AsthmaHaler Mist[3] | Nephron[10] |
| AsthmaNefrin[10] | Primatene Mist[3] |
| Brethaire[11] | Primatene Mist Suspension[3] |
| Bronitin Mist[3] | Proventil[1] |
| Bronkaid Mist[3] | S-2[10] |
| Bronkometer[5] | Tornalate[2] |
| Bronkosol[5] | Vaponefrin[10] |
| Dey-Lute Isoetharine S/F[5] | Ventolin[1] |
| Dey-Lute Metaproterenol[7] | Ventolin Nebules[1] |
| Isuprel[6] | Ventolin Rotacaps[1] |
| Isuprel Mistometer[6] | |

**In Canada—**

| | |
|---|---|
| Alupent[7] | Novo-Salmol[1] |
| Berotec[4] | Pro-Air[9] |
| Bricanyl[11] | Vaponefrin[10] |
| Bronkaid Mistometer[3] | Ventodisk[1] |
| Gen-Salbutamol[1] | Ventolin[1] |
| Isuprel[6] | Ventolin Nebules P.F.[1] |
| Isuprel Mistometer[6] | Ventolin Rotacaps[1] |
| Medihaler-Epi[3] | |

Other commonly used names are:
Salbutamol[1]
Orciprenaline[7]

Note: For quick reference, the following adrenergic bronchodilators are numbered to match the corresponding brand names.

This information applies to the following medicines:

1. Albuterol (al-BYOO-ter-ole)‡§
2. Bitolterol (bye-TOLE-ter-ole)†
3. Epinephrine (ep-i-NEF-rin)‡
4. Fenoterol (fen-OH-ter-ole)*
5. Isoetharine (eye-soe-ETH-a-reen)†‡
6. Isoproterenol (eye-soe-proe-TER-e-nole)‡
7. Metaproterenol (met-a-proe-TER-e-nole)‡
8. Pirbuterol (peer-BYOO-ter-ole)†
9. Procaterol (proe-KAY-ter-ole)*
10. Racepinephrine (race-ep-i-NEF-rin)
11. Terbutaline (ter-BYOO-ta-leen)

---

*Not commercially available in the U.S.
†Not commercially available in Canada.
‡Generic name product may also be available in the U.S.
§Generic name product may also be available in Canada.

## Description

Adrenergic bronchodilators are medicines that open up the bronchial tubes (air passages) of the lungs. They are taken by oral inhalation to treat the symptoms of bronchial asthma, chronic bronchitis, emphysema, and other lung diseases. They relieve cough, wheezing, shortness of breath, and troubled breathing by increasing the flow of air through the bronchial tubes.

Some of these medicines are also taken by oral inhalation to prevent bronchospasm (wheezing or difficulty in breathing) caused by exercise. In addition, some of these medicines are taken by oral inhalation to prevent attacks of bronchial asthma and bronchospasm. Also, racepinephrine may be used in the treatment of croup.

All of these medicines, except some epinephrine preparations, are available only with your doctor's prescription. Although some of the epinephrine preparations are available without a prescription, your doctor may have special instructions on the proper dose of epinephrine for your medical condition.

These medicines are available in the following dosage forms:

*Inhalation*

Albuterol
- Capsules for inhalation (U.S. and Canada)
- Inhalation aerosol (U.S. and Canada)
- Inhalation solution (U.S. and Canada)

Bitolterol
- Inhalation aerosol (U.S.)

Epinephrine
- Inhalation aerosol (U.S. and Canada)
- Inhalation solution (U.S.)

Fenoterol
- Inhalation aerosol (Canada)
- Inhalation solution (Canada)

Isoetharine
- Inhalation aerosol (U.S.)
- Inhalation solution (U.S.)

Isoproterenol
  • Inhalation aerosol (U.S. and Canada)
  • Inhalation solution (U.S. and Canada)
Metaproterenol
  • Inhalation aerosol (U.S. and Canada)
  • Inhalation solution (U.S. and Canada)
Pirbuterol
  • Inhalation aerosol (U.S.)
Procaterol
  • Inhalation aerosol (Canada)
Racepinephrine
  • Inhalation solution (U.S. and Canada)
Terbutaline
  • Inhalation aerosol (U.S. and Canada)

## Before Using This Medicine

In deciding to use a medicine, the risks of taking the medicine must be weighed against the good it will do. This is a decision you and your doctor will make. For inhalation adrenergic bronchodilators, the following should be considered:

**Allergies**—Tell your doctor if you have ever had any unusual or allergic reaction to albuterol, bitolterol, epinephrine, fenoterol, isoetharine, isoproterenol, metaproterenol, pirbuterol, procaterol, racepinephrine, terbutaline, or other inhalation medicines. Also tell your health care professional if you are allergic to any other substances, such as foods, preservatives, or dyes.

**Pregnancy**—
  • *For albuterol, bitolterol, and metaproterenol:* Albuterol, bitolterol, and metaproterenol have not been studied in pregnant women. However, studies in animals have shown that albuterol, bitolterol, and metaproterenol cause birth defects when given in doses many times the usual human inhalation dose.
  • *For epinephrine and racepinephrine:* Epinephrine and racepinephrine have not been studied in pregnant women. However, studies in animals have shown that epinephrine causes birth defects when given in doses many times the usual human inhalation dose. Use of epinephrine or racepinephrine during pregnancy may decrease the supply of oxygen to the fetus.
  • *For fenoterol:* Fenoterol has not been shown to cause birth defects or other problems in humans.
  • *For isoetharine and isoproterenol:* Studies on birth defects with isoetharine or isoproterenol have not been done in either humans or animals.
  • *For pirbuterol:* Pirbuterol has not been studied in pregnant women. However, in some animal studies, pirbuterol has been shown to cause miscarriage and death of the animal fetus when given in doses many times the usual human inhalation dose.
  • *For procaterol:* Procaterol has not been studied in pregnant women.
  • *For terbutaline:* Terbutaline has not been studied in pregnant women. It has not been shown to cause birth defects in animal studies when given in doses many times the human inhalation dose. However, terbutaline may delay labor.

**Breast-feeding**—
  • *For albuterol, bitolterol, fenoterol, isoetharine, isoproterenol, metaproterenol, pirbuterol, and procaterol:* It is not known whether albuterol, bitolterol, fenoterol, isoetharine, isoproterenol, metaproterenol, pirbuterol, or procaterol passes into the breast milk. Although most medicines pass into breast milk in small amounts, many of them may be used safely while breast-feeding. Mothers who are taking this medicine and who wish to breast-feed should discuss this with their doctor.
  • *For epinephrine and racepinephrine:* Epinephrine passes into the breast milk. Epinephrine and racepinephrine may cause unwanted side effects in babies of mothers using epinephrine or racepinephrine.
  • *For terbutaline:* Terbutaline passes into the breast milk. Although most medicines pass into breast milk in small amounts, many of them may be used safely while breast-feeding. Mothers who are taking this medicine and who wish to breast-feed should discuss this with their doctor.

**Children**—Although there is no specific information comparing use of albuterol, bitolterol, fenoterol, isoetharine, isoproterenol, metaproterenol, pirbuterol, procaterol, racepinephrine, or terbutaline in children with use in other age groups, these medicines are not expected to cause different side effects or problems in children than they do in adults.

Infants and children may be especially sensitive to the effects of epinephrine. Fainting has occurred after epinephrine was given to children with asthma.

**Older adults**—Many medicines have not been studied specifically in older people. Therefore, it may not be known whether they work exactly the same way they do in younger adults or if they cause different side effects or problems in older people. There is no specific information comparing use of inhalation adrenergic bronchodilators in the elderly.

**Other medicines**—Although certain medicines should not be used together at all, in other cases two different medicines may be used together even if an interaction might occur. In these cases, your doctor may want to change the dose, or other precautions may be necessary. When you are using inhalation adrenergic bronchodilators, it is especially important that your health care professional know if you are taking any of the following:
  • Beta-blockers (acebutolol [e.g., Sectral], atenolol [e.g., Tenormin], betaxolol [e.g., Betoptic, Kerlone], bisoprolol [e.g., Zebeta], carteolol [e.g., Cartrol], labetalol [e.g., Normodyne], levobunolol [e.g., Betagan], metoprolol [e.g., Lopressor], nadolol [e.g., Corgard], oxprenolol [e.g., Trasicor], penbutolol [e.g., Levatol], pindolol [e.g., Visken], propranolol [e.g., Inderal], sotalol [e.g., Sotacor], timolol [e.g., Blocadren, Timoptic])—These medicines may prevent the adrenergic bronchodilators from working properly
  • Cocaine or
  • Ergoloid mesylates (e.g., Hydergine) or
  • Ergotamine (e.g., Gynergen) or

- Maprotiline (e.g., Ludiomil) or
- Tricyclic antidepressants (medicine for depression)—The effects of these medicines on the heart and blood vessels may be increased
- Digitalis glycosides (heart medicine)—The chance of irregular heartbeat may be increased
- Monoamine oxidase (MAO) inhibitors (furazolidone [e.g., Furoxone], isocarboxazid [e.g., Marplan], phenelzine [e.g., Nardil], procarbazine [e.g., Matulane], tranylcypromine [e.g., Parnate])—Using adrenergic bronchodilators while you are taking or within 2 weeks of taking monoamine oxidase (MAO) inhibitors may increase the effects of MAO inhibitors

**Other medical problems**—The presence of other medical problems may affect the use of inhalation adrenergic bronchodilators. Make sure you tell your doctor if you have any other medical problems, especially:

- Brain damage
- Convulsions (seizures) (or history of)
- Diabetes mellitus (sugar diabetes)—Adrenergic bronchodilators may make the condition worse; your doctor may need to change the dose of your diabetes medicine
- Heart or blood vessel disease or
- High blood pressure—Adrenergic bronchodilators may make the condition worse
- Mental disease—Epinephrine may make the condition worse
- Overactive thyroid—The chance of side effects may be increased
- Parkinson's disease—Epinephrine may temporarily increase certain symptoms of Parkinson's disease, such as rigidity and tremor

## Proper Use of This Medicine

For patients using *epinephrine, isoetharine, isoproterenol, or racepinephrine:*

- Do not use if the solution turns pinkish to brownish in color or if it becomes cloudy.

Some epinephrine preparations are available without a doctor's prescription. However, *do not use this medicine without a doctor's prescription, unless your medical problem has been diagnosed as asthma by a doctor.*

Some of these preparations may come with patient directions. Read them carefully before using this medicine.

If you are using this medicine in a nebulizer or in a combination nebulizer and respirator, make sure you understand exactly how to use it. If you have any questions about this, check with your health care professional.

For patients using the *inhalation aerosol* form of this medicine:

- *Keep spray away from the eyes because it may cause irritation.*
- *Do not take more than 2 inhalations of this medicine at any one time,* unless otherwise directed by your doctor. Allow 1 to 2 minutes after the first inhalation to make certain that a second inhalation is necessary.
- Save your applicator. Refill units of this medicine may be available.

*Use this medicine only as directed. Do not use more of it and do not use it more often than recommended on the label, unless otherwise directed by your doctor.* To do so may increase the chance of serious side effects. Inhalation aerosol medicines have been reported to cause death when too much of the medicine was used.

**Dosing**—The dose of these medicines will be different for different patients. *Follow your doctor's orders or the directions on the label.* The following information includes only the average doses of these medicines. *If your dose is different, do not change it* unless your doctor tells you to do so.

The number of inhalations or the amount of medicine that you use depends on the strength of the medicine. Also, *the number of doses you take each day, the time allowed between doses, and the length of time you take the medicine depend on the medical problem for which you are taking the adrenergic bronchodilator.*

*For albuterol*

- For *inhalation aerosol* dosage form:
  —For symptoms of bronchial asthma, chronic bronchitis, emphysema, or other lung disease:
  - Adults and children 12 years of age and older—180 or 200 micrograms (mcg) (2 puffs) every four to six hours.
  - Children up to 12 years of age—Dose must be determined by your doctor.
  —For prevention of bronchospasm (wheezing or difficulty in breathing) caused by exercise:
  - Adults and children 12 years of age and older—180 or 200 mcg (2 puffs) fifteen minutes before exercise.
  - Children up to 12 years of age—Dose must be determined by your doctor.
- For *inhalation solution* dosage form:
  —For symptoms of bronchial asthma, chronic bronchitis, emphysema, or other lung disease:
  - Adults and children 12 years of age and older—1.25 to 5 milligrams (mg) of albuterol in 2 to 5 milliliters (mL) or more of sterile 0.9% sodium chloride solution or sterile water for inhalation, depending on the product. This medicine is usually used in a combination nebulizer and respirator and is taken by inhalation three or four times a day every four to six hours if needed. However, your doctor may use other inhalation methods to give you this medicine.
  - Children up to 12 years of age—Dose must be determined by your doctor.
- For *capsules for inhalation* dosage form:
  —For symptoms of bronchial asthma, chronic bronchitis, emphysema, or other lung disease:
  - Adults and children 12 years of age and older—200 or 400 mcg taken by inhalation every four to six hours.
  - Children up to 12 years of age—Dose must be determined by your doctor.

—For bronchospasm (wheezing or difficulty in breathing) caused by exercise:

- Adults and children 12 years of age and older—200 mcg taken by inhalation fifteen minutes before exercise.
- Children up to 12 years of age—Dose must be determined by your doctor.

*For bitolterol*
- For *inhalation aerosol* dosage form:
  —For prevention of symptoms of bronchial asthma, chronic bronchitis, emphysema, or other lung disease:
    - Adults and children 12 years of age and older—740 micrograms (mcg) (2 puffs) every eight hours.
    - Children up to 12 years of age—Dose must be determined by your doctor.
  —For treatment of symptoms of bronchial asthma, chronic bronchitis, emphysema, or other lung disease:
    - Adults and children 12 years of age and older—At first, 740 mcg (2 puffs), allowing one to three minutes between each puff. This dose may be followed by another dose of 370 mcg (1 puff), if needed. However, the dose taken each day should not be more than 740 mcg (2 puffs) every four hours or 1.11 milligrams (mg) (3 puffs) every six hours.
    - Children up to 12 years of age—Dose must be determined by your doctor.

*For epinephrine*
- For symptoms of bronchial asthma, chronic bronchitis, emphysema, or other lung disease:
  —For *inhalation aerosol* dosage form:
    - Adults and children 4 years of age and older—200 to 275 micrograms (mcg) (1 puff). The dose may be repeated after one to two minutes, if needed. Doses should be taken at least three hours apart.
    - Children up to 4 years of age—Dose must be determined by your doctor.
  —For *inhalation solution* dosage form:
    - Adults and children 6 years of age and older—This medicine should be used in a nebulizer as directed. The usual dose is 1 puff of a 1% solution. The dose may be repeated, if necessary, after one or two minutes as needed.
    - Children up to 6 years of age—Dose must be determined by your doctor.

*For epinephrine bitartrate*
- For *inhalation aerosol* dosage form:
  —For symptoms of bronchial asthma, chronic bronchitis, emphysema, or other lung disease:
    - Adults and children 4 years of age and older—160 micrograms (mcg) (1 puff) of epinephrine. The dose may be repeated after one minute, if needed. Doses should be taken at least three hours apart.
    - Children up to 4 years of age—Dose must be determined by your doctor.

*For fenoterol*
- For *inhalation aerosol* dosage form:
  —For symptoms of bronchial asthma, chronic bronchitis, emphysema, or other lung disease:
    - Adults and children 12 years of age and older—200 or 400 micrograms (mcg) (1 or 2 puffs), repeated up to four times a day if needed. This medicine should not be taken more often than every four hours.
    - Children up to 12 years of age—Dose must be determined by your doctor.
- For *inhalation solution* dosage form:
  —For symptoms of bronchial asthma, chronic bronchitis, emphysema, or other lung disease:
    - Adults and children 12 years of age and older—This medicine is usually used in a nebulizer and is taken by inhalation. However, your doctor may use other inhalation methods to give you this medicine. The usual dose is 500 mcg to 1 milligram (mg) as a 0.1% solution, diluted to 5 milliliters (mL) with 0.9% sodium chloride solution. The total amount of this solution should be inhaled over a period of ten to fifteen minutes. The dose may be repeated every six hours if needed.
    - Children up to 12 years of age—Dose must be determined by your doctor.

*For isoetharine*
- For *inhalation solution* dosage form:
  —For symptoms of bronchial asthma, chronic bronchitis, emphysema, or other lung disease:
    - Adults—This medicine is usually used in a nebulizer and is taken by inhalation. However, your doctor may use other inhalation methods to give you this medicine. The amount of medicine you use and whether it requires dilution depend on the product ordered by your doctor. This medicine usually should not be used more often than every four hours.
    - Children—Dose must be determined by your doctor.

*For isoetharine mesylate*
- For *inhalation aerosol* dosage form:
  —For symptoms of bronchial asthma, chronic bronchitis, emphysema, or other lung disease:
    - Adults—340 micrograms (mcg) (1 puff), repeated after one to two minutes if needed. This dose may be repeated every four hours as necessary.
    - Children—Dose must be determined by your doctor.

*For isoproterenol*
- For *inhalation solution* dosage form:
  —For symptoms of bronchial asthma, chronic bronchitis, emphysema, or other lung disease:
    • Adults and children—This medicine is usually used in a nebulizer and is taken by inhalation. However, your doctor may use other inhalation methods to give you this medicine. The usual dose is 6 to 12 puffs of a 0.25% solution, repeated every fifteen minutes, if needed, for three doses. No more than eight treatments should be taken in twenty-four hours. Or,
  —For severe bronchial asthma or asthma attack:
    • Adults—This medicine is usually used in a nebulizer and is taken by inhalation. However, your doctor may use other inhalation methods to give you this medicine. The usual dose is 5 to 15 deep puffs of a 0.5% solution or 3 to 7 deep puffs of a 1% solution, repeated once after five to ten minutes if needed. This dose may be taken up to five times a day if necessary.
    • Children—This medicine is usually used in a nebulizer and is taken by inhalation. However, your doctor may use other inhalation methods to give you this medicine. The usual dose is 5 to 15 deep puffs of a 0.5% solution, repeated once after five to ten minutes if needed. This dose may be taken up to five times a day if necessary.
  —For bronchospasm (wheezing or difficulty in breathing) in chronic lung disease:
    • Adults—This medicine is usually used in a nebulizer and is taken by inhalation. However, your doctor may use other inhalation methods to give you this medicine. The usual dose of this medicine when used in a nebulizer is 5 to 15 deep inhalations of a 0.5% solution or 3 to 7 deep inhalations of a 1% solution. This dose should not be taken more often than every three to four hours.
    • Children—This medicine is usually used in a nebulizer and is taken by inhalation. However, your doctor may use other inhalation methods to give you this medicine. The usual dose of this medicine when used in a nebulizer is 5 to 15 deep inhalations of a 0.5% solution. This dose should not be taken more often than every three to four hours.

*For isoproterenol hydrochloride*
- For *inhalation aerosol* dosage form:
  —For severe bronchial asthma or asthma attack:
    • Adults and children—120 to 131 micrograms (mcg) (1 puff), repeated after one to five minutes if needed. This dose is taken four to six times a day.

  —For symptoms of bronchial asthma, chronic bronchitis, emphysema, or other lung disease:
    • Adults and children—120 to 131 mcg (1 puff) taken not more often than once every three to four hours.

*For isoproterenol sulfate*
- For *inhalation aerosol* dosage form:
  —For symptoms of bronchial asthma, chronic bronchitis, emphysema, or other lung disease:
    • Adults and children—75 or 80 micrograms (mcg) (1 puff), repeated after two to five minutes if needed. This dose is taken four to six times a day.

*For metaproterenol*
- For *inhalation aerosol* dosage form:
  —For symptoms of bronchial asthma, chronic bronchitis, emphysema, or other lung disease:
    • Adults and children 12 years of age and older—1.3 to 2.25 milligrams (mg) (2 or 3 puffs) every three to four hours. The total dose should not be more than 9 mg (12 puffs) a day.
    • Children up to 12 years of age—Use is not recommended.
- For *inhalation solution* dosage form:
  —For attacks of bronchospasm (wheezing or difficulty in breathing):
    • Adults and children 12 years of age and older—This medicine is usually used in a nebulizer and is taken by inhalation. However, your doctor may use other inhalation methods to give you this medicine. The usual dose of this medicine when used in a nebulizer is 10 puffs of a 0.4 to 0.6% solution. This medicine should not be used more often than every four hours.
    • Children up to 12 years of age—Dose must be determined by your doctor.
  —For symptoms of bronchial asthma, chronic bronchitis, emphysema, or other lung disease:
    • Adults and children 12 years of age and older—This medicine is usually used in a nebulizer and is taken by inhalation. However, your doctor may use other inhalation methods to give you this medicine. The usual dose of this medicine when used in a nebulizer is 10 puffs of a 0.4 to 0.6% solution. This medicine should not be used more often than three or four times a day.
    • Children up to 12 years of age—Dose must be determined by your doctor.

*For pirbuterol*
- For *inhalation aerosol* dosage form:
  —For symptoms of bronchial asthma, chronic bronchitis, emphysema, or other lung disease:
    • Adults and children 12 years of age and older—200 or 400 micrograms (mcg) (1 or 2 puffs) every four to six hours. The total dose should not be more than 2.4 milligrams (mg) (12 puffs) a day.

- Children up to 12 years of age—Dose must be determined by your doctor.

*For procaterol*
- For *inhalation aerosol* dosage form:
   —For symptoms of bronchial asthma, chronic bronchitis, emphysema, or other lung disease:
      - Adults and children 12 years of age and older—20 micrograms (mcg) (2 puffs) three times a day.
      - Children up to 12 years of age—Dose must be determined by your doctor.
   —For bronchospasm (wheezing or difficulty in breathing) caused by exercise:
      - Adults and children 12 years of age and older—20 mcg (2 puffs) taken at least fifteen minutes before exercise.
      - Children up to 12 years of age—Dose must be determined by your doctor.

*For racepinephrine*
- For *inhalation solution* dosage form:
   —For symptoms of bronchial asthma, chronic bronchitis, emphysema, or other lung disease:
      - Adults and children 4 years of age and older—
         —For solution used in a nebulizer: 2 or 3 puffs of a 2.25% solution, followed in five minutes by 2 or 3 more puffs if needed. This dose may be taken four to six times a day.
         —For solution used in a combination nebulizer and respirator: 5 mL of a 0.1% solution used for a period of fifteen minutes every three to four hours.
      - Children up to 4 years of age—Dose must be determined by your doctor.

*For terbutaline*
- For *inhalation aerosol* dosage form:
   —For symptoms of bronchial asthma, chronic bronchitis, emphysema, or other lung disease:
      - Adults and children 12 years of age and older—200 to 500 micrograms (mcg) (1 or 2 puffs) every four to six hours. If 2 puffs are taken, allow sixty seconds between puffs.
      - Children up to 12 years of age—Dose must be determined by your doctor.

**Missed dose**—If you are using this medicine regularly and you miss a dose, use it as soon as possible. Then use any remaining doses for that day at regularly spaced intervals. Do not double doses.

**Storage**—To store this medicine:
- Keep out of the reach of children.
- Store away from heat.
- Store the solution form of this medicine away from direct light. Store the inhalation aerosol form of this medicine away from direct sunlight.
- Keep the medicine from freezing.
- Do not puncture, break, or burn the inhalation aerosol container, even if it is empty.
- Do not keep outdated medicine or medicine no longer needed. Be sure that any discarded medicine is out of the reach of children.

## Precautions While Using This Medicine

*If you still have trouble breathing after using this medicine, or if your condition becomes worse, check with your doctor at once.*

For *diabetic patients* using *epinephrine:*
- This medicine may cause your blood sugar levels to rise. If you notice a change in the results of your blood or urine sugar tests or if you have any questions, check with your doctor.

For patients using the *aerosol form* of this medicine:
- If you are also using the inhalation aerosol form of a corticosteroid (cortisone-like medicine, such as beclomethasone, dexamethasone, flunisolide, or triamcinolone) or ipratropium, *use the adrenergic bronchodilator inhalation aerosol first and then wait about 5 minutes before using the corticosteroid or ipratropium inhalation aerosol,* unless otherwise directed by your doctor. This will help the corticosteroid or ipratropium inhalation aerosol to reach the passages of the lungs (bronchioles) after the adrenergic bronchodilator inhalation aerosol opens them.

For patients using *albuterol inhalation aerosol:*
- If you use all of the medicine in one canister (container) in less than 2 weeks, check with your doctor. You may be using too much of the medicine.

Dryness of the mouth and throat may occur after use of this medicine. Rinsing the mouth with water after each dose may help prevent the dryness.

Some of these preparations may contain sulfites as a preservative. Sulfites may cause an allergic reaction in some people. *If you know that you are allergic to sulfites, do not use this medicine until you have carefully read the label or checked with your health care professional to make sure the medicine does not contain sulfites.* Signs of an allergic reaction to sulfites include bluish coloration of skin; severe dizziness or feeling faint; continuing flushing or redness of face or skin; increased wheezing or difficulty in breathing; skin rash, hives, or itching; or swelling of face, lips, or eyelids. *If any of these signs occur, check with your doctor immediately.*

## Side Effects of This Medicine

In some animal studies, albuterol and terbutaline were shown to increase the chance of benign (not cancerous) tumors. Terbutaline was also shown to increase the chance of ovarian cysts. The doses given were many times the inhalation dose of albuterol and the oral dose of terbutaline given to humans. It is not known if albuterol or terbutaline increases the chance of tumors in humans, or if terbutaline increases the chance of ovarian cysts in humans.

Along with its needed effects, a medicine may cause some unwanted effects. Although not all of these side effects may occur, if they do occur they may need medical attention.

*Check with your doctor immediately if any of the following side effects occur:*

Bluish coloration of skin; dizziness (severe) or feeling faint; flushing or redness of face or skin (continuing); increased wheezing or difficulty in breathing; skin rash, hives, or itching; swelling of face, lips, or eyelids

Check with your doctor as soon as possible if any of the following side effects occur:

*Rare*

Chest discomfort or pain; irregular heartbeat; numbness in hands or feet; unusual bruising

*With high doses*

Hallucinations (seeing, hearing, or feeling things that are not there)

*Symptoms of overdose*

Chest discomfort or pain (continuing or severe); chills or fever; convulsions (seizures); dizziness or lightheadedness (continuing or severe); fast or slow heartbeat (continuing); headache (continuing or severe); increase or decrease in blood pressure (severe); irregular or pounding heartbeat (continuing or severe); muscle cramps (severe); nausea or vomiting (continuing or severe); shortness of breath or troubled breathing (severe); trembling (severe); unusual anxiety, nervousness, or restlessness; unusually large pupils or blurred vision; unusual paleness and coldness of skin; weakness (severe)

Other side effects may occur that usually do not need medical attention. These side effects may go away during treatment as your body adjusts to the medicine. However, check with your doctor if any of the following side effects continue or are bothersome:

*More common*

Nervousness or restlessness; trembling

*Less common*

Coughing or other bronchial irritation; dizziness or light-headedness; drowsiness; dryness or irritation of mouth or throat; fast or pounding heartbeat; flushing or redness of face or skin; headache; increased sweating; increase in blood pressure; muscle cramps or twitching; nausea or vomiting; trouble in sleeping; unusual paleness; weakness

Not all of the side effects listed above have been reported for each of these medicines, but they have been reported for at least one of them. All of the adrenergic bronchodilators are similar, so any of the above side effects may occur with any of these medicines.

While you are using albuterol, bitolterol, fenoterol, metaproterenol, or terbutaline, you may notice an unusual or unpleasant taste. Also, pirbuterol may cause changes in smell or taste. These effects may be expected and will go away when you stop using the medicine.

Isoproterenol may cause the saliva to turn pinkish to red. This is to be expected while you are using this medicine.

Other side effects not listed above may also occur in some patients. If you notice any other effects, check with your doctor.

---

Revised: July 1990
Interim revision: 09/12/94

---

# BRONCHODILATORS, ADRENERGIC    Oral/Injection

Some commonly used brand names are:

**In the U.S.—**

| | |
|---|---|
| Adrenalin Chloride Solution[3] | Isuprel Glossets[6] |
| Alupent[7] | Metaprel[7] |
| Ana-Guard[3] | Prometa[7] |
| Brethine[8] | Proventil[1] |
| Bricanyl[8] | Proventil Repetabs[1] |
| Bronkephrine[4] | Sus-Phrine[3] |
| EpiPen Auto-Injector[3] | Ventolin[1] |
| EpiPen Jr. Auto-Injector[3] | Volmax[1] |
| Isuprel[6] | |

**In Canada—**

| | |
|---|---|
| Adrenalin[3] | EpiPen Jr. Auto-Injector[3] |
| Alupent[7] | Isuprel[6] |
| Berotec[5] | Novo-Salmol[1] |
| Bricanyl[8] | Ventolin[1] |
| EpiPen Auto-Injector[3] | Volmax[1] |

Other commonly used names are:
Salbutamol[1]
Orciprenaline[7]

Note: For quick reference the following adrenergic bronchodilators are numbered to match the corresponding brand names.

This information applies to the following medicines:
1. Albuterol (al-BYOO-ter-ole)‡
2. Ephedrine (e-FED-rin)‡§
3. Epinephrine (ep-i-NEF-rin)‡§
4. Ethylnorepinephrine (ETH-il-nor-ep-i-NEF-rin)†
5. Fenoterol (fen-OH-ter-ole)*
6. Isoproterenol (eye-soe-proe-TER-e-nole)‡
7. Metaproterenol (met-a-proe-TER-e-nole)‡
8. Terbutaline (ter-BYOO-ta-leen)

---

*Not commercially available in the U.S.
†Not commercially available in Canada.
‡Generic name product may also be available in the U.S.
§Generic name product may also be available in Canada.

---

## Description

Adrenergic bronchodilators are medicines that open up the bronchial tubes (air passages) of the lungs. They are used to treat the symptoms of bronchial asthma, chronic bronchitis, emphysema, and other lung diseases. They relieve cough, wheezing, shortness of breath, and troubled breathing by increasing the flow of air through the bronchial tubes.

Ephedrine may also be used for the relief of nasal congestion in hay fever or other allergies. In addition, ephedrine may be used in the treatment of narcolepsy (uncontrolled desire for sleep or sudden attacks of sleep) and certain types of mental depression.

Epinephrine injection (not including the auto-injector or the sterile suspension) may be used in eye surgery to stop bleeding, reduce congestion, and dilate the pupil. It may also be applied topically to the skin or mucous membranes to stop bleeding.

Epinephrine injection (including the auto-injector but not the sterile suspension) is used in the emergency treatment of allergic reactions to insect stings, medicines, foods, or other substances. It relieves skin rash, hives, and itching; wheezing; and swelling of the lips, eyelids, tongue, and inside of nose.

Adrenergic bronchodilators may be used for other conditions as determined by your doctor.

Ephedrine capsules are available without a prescription. However, your doctor may have special instructions on the proper dose of ephedrine for your medical condition.

All of the other adrenergic bronchodilators are available only with your doctor's prescription.

These medicines are available in the following dosage forms:

*Oral*
  Albuterol
  • Oral solution (Canada)
  • Syrup (U.S.)
  • Tablets (U.S. and Canada)
  • Extended-release tablets (U.S. and Canada)
  Ephedrine
  • Capsules (U.S.)
  Fenoterol
  • Tablets (Canada)
  Isoproterenol
  • Tablets (U.S.)
  Metaproterenol
  • Syrup (U.S. and Canada)
  • Tablets (U.S. and Canada)
  Terbutaline
  • Tablets (U.S. and Canada)
*Parenteral*
  Albuterol
  • Injection (Canada)
  Ephedrine
  • Injection (U.S. and Canada)
  Epinephrine
  • Injection (U.S. and Canada)
  Ethylnorepinephrine
  • Injection (U.S.)
  Isoproterenol
  • Injection (U.S. and Canada)
  Terbutaline
  • Injection (U.S.)

## Before Using This Medicine

In deciding to use a medicine, the risks of taking the medicine must be weighed against the good it will do. This is a decision you and your doctor will make. For adrenergic bronchodilators taken by mouth or given by injection, the following should be considered:

**Allergies**—Tell your doctor if you have ever had any unusual or allergic reaction to albuterol, ephedrine, epinephrine, ethylnorepinephrine, fenoterol, isoproterenol, metaproterenol, or terbutaline. Also tell your health care professional if you are allergic to any other substances, such as foods, preservatives, or dyes.

**Pregnancy**—
• *For albuterol:* Albuterol has not been studied in pregnant women. However, studies in animals have shown that albuterol causes birth defects when given in doses many times the usual human dose. In addition, although albuterol has been reported to delay preterm labor when taken by mouth, it has not been shown to stop preterm labor or prevent labor at term.
• *For ephedrine:* Studies on birth defects with ephedrine have not been done in either humans or animals. When ephedrine is used just before or during labor, its effects on the newborn infant or on the growth and development of the child are not known.
• *For epinephrine:* Epinephrine has not been studied in pregnant women. However, studies in animals have shown that epinephrine causes birth defects when given in doses many times the usual human dose. Also, use of epinephrine during pregnancy may decrease the supply of oxygen to the fetus. Epinephrine is not recommended for use during labor since it may delay the second stage of labor. In addition, high doses of epinephrine that decrease contractions of the uterus may result in excessive bleeding when used during labor and delivery.
• *For ethylnorepinephrine and isoproterenol:* Studies on birth defects with ethylnorepinephrine or isoproterenol have not been done in either humans or animals.
• *For fenoterol:* Fenoterol has not been shown to cause birth defects or other problems in humans.
• *For metaproterenol:* Metaproterenol has not been studied in pregnant women. However, studies in animals have shown that metaproterenol causes birth defects when given in doses many times the usual human dose. Also, studies in animals have shown that metaproterenol causes death of the animal fetus when given in doses many times the usual human dose.
• *For terbutaline:* Terbutaline has not been studied in pregnant women. It has not been shown to cause birth defects in animal studies when given in doses many times the usual human dose. However, terbutaline given by injection during pregnancy has been reported to cause an unusually fast heartbeat in the fetus. Although terbutaline is used to delay preterm labor, it may also delay labor at term.

**Breast-feeding—**

- *For albuterol, fenoterol, isoproterenol, and meta-proterenol:* It is not known whether albuterol, fenoterol, isoproterenol, or metaproterenol passes into the breast milk. Although most medicines pass into breast milk in small amounts, many of them may be used safely while breast-feeding. Mothers who are taking this medicine and who wish to breast-feed should discuss this with their doctor.
- *For ephedrine and epinephrine:* Ephedrine and epinephrine pass into the breast milk and may cause unwanted side effects in babies of mothers using ephedrine or epinephrine.
- *For terbutaline:* Terbutabline passes into the breast milk. Although most medicines pass into breast milk in small amounts, many of them may be used safely while breast-feeding. Mothers who are taking this medicine and who wish to breast-feed should discuss this with their doctor.

**Children—**Although there is no specific information comparing use of albuterol, ethylnorepinephrine, fenoterol, isoproterenol, metaproterenol, or terbutaline in children with use in other age groups, these medicines are not expected to cause different side effects or problems in children than they do in adults.

Infants may be especially sensitive to the effects of ephedrine.

Infants and children may be especially sensitive to the effects of epinephrine. Fainting has occurred after epinephrine was given to children with asthma.

**Older adults—**Many medicines have not been studied specifically in older people. Therefore, it may not be known whether they work exactly the same way they do in younger adults or if they cause different side effects or problems in older people. There is no specific information comparing use of adrenergic bronchodilators in the elderly with use in other age groups.

**Other medicines—**Although certain medicines should not be used together at all, in other cases two different medicines may be used together even if an interaction might occur. In these cases, your doctor may want to change the dose, or other precautions may be necessary. When you are taking adrenergic bronchodilators, it is especially important that your health care professional know if you are taking any of the following:

- Beta-blockers (acebutolol [e.g., Sectral], atenolol [e.g., Tenormin], betaxolol [e.g., Betoptic, Kerlone], bisoprolol [e.g., Zebeta], carteolol [e.g., Cartrol], labetalol [e.g., Normodyne], levobunolol [e.g., Betagan], metoprolol [e.g., Lopressor], nadolol [e.g., Corgard], oxprenolol [e.g., Trasicor], penbutolol [e.g., Levatol], pindolol [e.g., Visken], propranolol [e.g., Inderal], sotalol [e.g., Sotacor], timolol [e.g., Blocadren, Timoptic])—These medicines may prevent the adrenergic bronchodilators from working properly
- Cocaine or
- Ergoloid mesylates (e.g., Hydergine) or
- Ergotamine (e.g., Gynergen) or

- Maprotiline (e.g., Ludiomil) or
- Tricyclic antidepressants (medicine for depression)—The effects of these medicines on the heart and blood vessels may be increased
- Digitalis glycosides (heart medicine)—The chance of irregular heartbeat may be increased
- Monoamine oxidase (MAO) inhibitors (furazolidone [e.g., Furoxone], isocarboxazid [e.g., Marplan], phenelzine [e.g., Nardil], procarbazine [e.g., Matulane], tranylcypromine [e.g., Parnate])—Taking adrenergic bronchodilators while you are taking or within 2 weeks of taking monoamine oxidase (MAO) inhibitors may increase the effects of MAO inhibitors

**Other medical problems—**The presence of other medical problems may affect the use of adrenergic bronchodilators. Make sure you tell your doctor if you have any other medical problems, especially:

- Brain damage
- Convulsions (seizures) (history of)
- Diabetes mellitus (sugar diabetes)—Adrenergic bronchodilators may make the condition worse; your doctor may need to change the dose of your diabetes medicine
- Enlarged prostate—Ephedrine may make the condition worse
- Heart or blood vessel disease or
- High blood pressure—Adrenergic bronchodilators may make the condition worse
- Mental disease—Epinephrine may make the condition worse
- Overactive thyroid—The chance of side effects may be increased
- Parkinson's disease—Epinephrine may temporarily increase certain symptoms of Parkinson's disease, such as rigidity and tremor

## Proper Use of This Medicine

For patients taking *albuterol extended-release tablets:*
- Swallow the tablet whole.
- Do not crush, break, or chew before swallowing.

For patients taking *ephedrine:*
- Ephedrine may cause trouble in sleeping. To help prevent this, *take the last dose of ephedrine for each day a few hours before bedtime.* If you have any questions about this, check with your doctor.

For patients taking *isoproterenol sublingual tablets:*
- Do not chew or swallow the tablet. This medicine is meant to be absorbed through the lining of the mouth. Place the tablet under your tongue (sublingual) and let it slowly dissolve there. Do not swallow until the tablet has dissolved completely.

For patients using the *injection* form of this medicine:
- Do not use the epinephrine solution or suspension if it turns pinkish to brownish in color or if the solution becomes cloudy.
- *Use this medicine only for the conditions for which it was prescribed by your doctor.*

- Keep this medicine ready for use at all times. Also, keep the telephone numbers for your doctor and the nearest hospital emergency room readily available.
- Check the expiration date on the injection regularly. Replace the medicine before that date.
- This medicine is for injection only. If you will be giving yourself the injections, make sure you understand exactly how to give them. If you have any questions about this, check with your doctor.

For patients using *epinephrine injection* for an *allergic reaction emergency*:
- If an allergic reaction as described by your doctor occurs, *use the epinephrine injection immediately*.
- Notify your doctor immediately or go to the nearest hospital emergency room. If you have used the epinephrine injection, be sure to tell your doctor.
- If you have been stung by an insect, remove the insect's stinger with your fingernails, if possible. Be careful not to squeeze, pinch, or push it deeper into the skin. Ice packs or sodium bicarbonate (baking soda) soaks, if available, may then be applied to the area stung.
- If you are using the epinephrine auto-injector (automatic injection device):
  —It is important that you do not remove the safety cap on the auto-injector until you are ready to use it. This prevents accidental activation of the device during storage and handling.
  —Epinephrine auto-injector comes with patient directions. Read them carefully before you actually need to use this medicine. Then, when an emergency arises, you will know how to inject the epinephrine.
  —To use the epinephrine auto-injector:
    - Remove the gray safety cap.
    - Place the black tip on the thigh, at a right angle to the leg.
    - Press hard into the thigh until the auto-injector functions. Hold in place for several seconds. Then remove the auto-injector and discard.
    - Massage the injection area for 10 seconds.

*Use this medicine only as directed.* Do not use more of it and do not use it more often than your doctor ordered, or more than recommended on the label unless otherwise directed by your doctor. To do so may increase the chance of side effects.

**Dosing**—The dose of these medicines will be different for different patients. *Follow your doctor's orders or the directions on the label.* The following information includes only the average doses of these medicines. *If your dose is different, do not change it* unless your doctor tells you to do so.

The number of capsules or tablets, teaspoonfuls of solution or syrup, or amount of injection that you take depends on the strength of the medicine. Also, *the number of doses you take each day, the time allowed between*

*doses, and the length of time you take the medicine depend on the medical problem for which you are taking the adrenergic bronchodilator.*

*For albuterol*
- For symptoms of bronchial asthma, chronic bronchitis, emphysema, or other lung disease:
  —For *solution* dosage form:
    - Adults—2 to 4 milligrams (mg) of albuterol three or four times a day.
    - Children 6 to 12 years of age—2 mg of albuterol three or four times a day.
    - Children 2 to 6 years of age—Dose is based on body weight and must be determined by your doctor. The usual dose is 100 micrograms (mcg) of albuterol per kilogram (kg) (45 mcg per pound) of body weight three or four times a day.
    - Children up to 2 years of age—Dose must be determined by your doctor.
  —For *syrup* dosage form:
    - Adults and children 14 years of age and older—At first, 2 to 6 mg of albuterol three or four times a day. Then your doctor may increase your dose, if needed, up to 8 mg four times a day.
    - Children 6 to 14 years of age—At first, 2 mg of albuterol three or four times a day. Then your doctor may increase your dose, if needed, up to 24 mg a day taken in divided doses.
    - Children 2 to 6 years of age—Dose is based on body weight and must be determined by your doctor. At first, the usual dose is 100 mcg of albuterol per kg (45 mcg per pound) of body weight. Then your doctor may increase your dose, if needed, up to 200 mcg per kg (90 mcg per pound) of body weight. However, the dose should not be more than 4 mg three times a day.
    - Children up to 2 years of age—Dose must be determined by your doctor.
  —For *tablet* dosage form:
    - Older adults—At first, 2 mg of albuterol three or four times a day. Then your doctor may increase your dose, if needed, up to 8 mg three or four times a day.
    - Adults and children 12 years of age and older—At first, 2 to 6 mg of albuterol three or four times a day. Then your doctor may increase your dose, if needed, up to 8 mg four times a day.
    - Children 6 to 12 years of age—At first, 2 mg of albuterol three or four times a day. Then your doctor may increase your dose, if needed, up to 24 mg a day taken in divided doses.
    - Children up to 6 years of age—Dose must be determined by your doctor.
  —For *extended-release tablet* dosage form:
    - Adults and children 12 years of age and older—4 or 8 mg of albuterol every twelve hours.
    - Children up to 12 years of age—Dose must be determined by your doctor.

—For *injection* dosage form:
• Dose is usually based on body weight and must be determined by your doctor. Depending on your condition, this medicine is injected into either a muscle or vein or injected slowly into a vein over a period of time.
—Adults:
• The usual dose injected into a muscle is 8 mcg of albuterol per kg (3.6 mcg per pound) of body weight every four hours as needed, up to a total dose of 2 mg a day.
• The usual dose injected into a vein is 4 mcg per kg (1.8 mcg per pound) of body weight, given over a period of two to five minutes. The dose may be repeated after fifteen minutes, if needed, up to a total dose of 1 mg a day.
• When albuterol is injected slowly into a vein, it is given at a rate of 5 mcg per minute. Your doctor may increase the rate to 10 mcg per minute and then 20 mcg per minute every fifteen to thirty minutes, if needed.
—Children: Dose must be determined by your doctor.

*For ephedrine*
• For *capsule* dosage form:
—For nasal congestion, narcolepsy (uncontrolled desire for sleep), or symptoms of bronchial asthma, chronic bronchitis, emphysema, or other lung disease:
• Adults—25 or 50 milligrams (mg) every three or four hours, if needed.
• Children—Dose is based on body weight or size and must be determined by your doctor. The usual dose is 3 mg per kg (1.3 mg per pound) of body weight a day. This dose is divided into four to six doses.
• For *injection* dosage form:
—For symptoms of bronchial asthma, chronic bronchitis, emphysema, or other lung disease:
• Adults—12.5 to 25 mg injected into a muscle, a vein, or under the skin. Your doctor may give you another dose, if needed.
• Children—Dose is based on body weight and must be determined by your doctor. The usual dose is 3 mg per kg (1.3 mg per pound) of body weight a day. This dose is divided into four to six doses.

*For epinephrine*
• For *injection* dosage form:
—For symptoms of bronchial asthma, chronic bronchitis, emphysema, or other lung disease:
• Adults and teenagers—200 to 500 micrograms (mcg) injected under the skin. The dose may be repeated every twenty minutes to four hours as needed. Your doctor may increase your dose up to 1 mg a dose, if needed.

• Children—Dose is based on body weight or size and must be determined by your doctor. The usual dose is 10 mcg per kilogram (kg) (4.5 mcg per pound) of body weight, up to 500 mcg a dose. The dose may be repeated every fifteen minutes for two doses, then every four hours as needed.
—For allergic reactions:
• Adults—At first, 200 to 500 mcg injected into a muscle or under the skin. Then the dose may be repeated every ten to fifteen minutes as needed. Your doctor may increase your dose up to 1 mg a dose, if needed.
• Children—Dose is based on body weight or size and must be determined by your doctor. The usual dose is 10 mcg per kg (4.5 mcg per pound) of body weight, up to 500 mcg a dose. The dose may be repeated every fifteen minutes for two doses, then every four hours as needed.
• For *sterile suspension (injection)* dosage form:
—For symptoms of bronchial asthma, chronic bronchitis, emphysema, or other lung disease:
• Adults—At first, 500 mcg injected under the skin. Then 500 mcg to 1.5 milligrams (mg) injected no more often than every six hours as needed.
• Children—Dose is based on body weight or size and must be determined by your doctor. The usual dose is 25 mcg per kg (11 mcg per pound) of body weight. The dose may be repeated, if needed, but not more often than every six hours.

*For ethylnorepinephrine*
• For *injection* dosage form:
—For symptoms of bronchial asthma, chronic bronchitis, emphysema, or other lung disease:
• Adults—1 to 2 milligrams (mg) injected into a muscle or under the skin.
• Children—200 micrograms (mcg) to 1 mg injected into a muscle or under the skin.

*For fenoterol*
• For *tablet* dosage form:
—For symptoms of bronchial asthma, chronic bronchitis, emphysema, or other lung disease:
• Adults and children 12 years of age and older—At first, 2.5 milligrams (mg) two times a day. Then your doctor may increase your dose up to 5 mg three times a day, if needed. However, the medicine should not be taken more often than every six hours.
• Children up to 12 years of age—Dose must be determined by your doctor.

*For isoproterenol*
• For *tablet* dosage form:
—For symptoms of bronchial asthma, chronic bronchitis, emphysema, or other lung disease:
• Adults—10 to 15 milligrams (mg) dissolved under the tongue three or four times a day.

- Children—5 to 10 mg dissolved under the tongue three times a day.

*For metaproterenol*
- For *oral* dosage form (syrup or tablets):
  —For symptoms of bronchial asthma, chronic bronchitis, emphysema, or other lung disease:
  - Adults and children 9 years of age and older or weighing 27 kilograms (kg) (59 pounds) or more—20 milligrams (mg) three or four times a day.
  - Children 6 to 9 years of age and older or weighing up to 27 kg (59 pounds)—10 mg three or four times a day.
  - Children up to 6 years of age—Dose must be determined by your doctor.

*For terbutaline*
- For symptoms of bronchial asthma, chronic bronchitis, emphysema, or other lung disease:
  —For *tablet* dosage form:
  - Adults—2.5 to 5 milligrams (mg) three times a day, taken about every six hours.
  - Children 12 to 15 years of age—2.5 mg three times a day, taken about every six hours.
  - Children up to 12 years of age—Dose must be determined by your doctor.
  —For *injection* dosage form:
  - Adults—250 micrograms (mcg) injected under the skin. The dose may be repeated after fifteen to thirty minutes, if needed. However, not more than 500 mcg should be taken within a four-hour period.
  - Children up to 12 years of age—Dose must be determined by your doctor.

**Missed dose**—If you are using this medicine regularly and you miss a dose, use it as soon as possible. Then use any remaining doses for that day at regularly spaced intervals. Do not double doses.

**Storage**—To store this medicine:
- Keep out of the reach of children.
- Store away from heat and direct light.
- Do not store the capsule or tablet form of this medicine in the bathroom, near the kitchen sink, or in other damp places. Heat or moisture may cause the medicine to break down.
- Keep the injection or syrup form of this medicine from freezing.
- Store the suspension form of epinephrine injection in the refrigerator.
- Do not keep outdated medicine or medicine no longer needed. Be sure that any discarded medicine is out of the reach of children.

## Precautions While Using This Medicine

*If after using this medicine for asthma or other breathing problems you still have trouble breathing, or if your condition becomes worse, check with your doctor at once.*

For *diabetic patients* using *epinephrine:*
- This medicine may cause your blood sugar levels to rise. If you notice a change in the results of your blood or urine sugar tests or if you have any questions, check with your doctor.

For patients using *epinephrine injection* (including the auto-injector but not the sterile suspension) or *ethylnorepinephrine injection:*
- Some of the injection preparations may contain sulfites as a preservative. Sulfites may cause an allergic reaction in some people. If you know that you are allergic to sulfites, carefully read the label on the injection or check with your health care professional to find out if the injection contains sulfites.
- Although epinephrine injection may contain sulfites, it is still used to treat serious allergic reactions or other emergency conditions because other medicines may not work properly in a life-threatening situation.
- If you have any questions about when or whether you should use an epinephrine injection that contains sulfites, check with your doctor.
- Signs of an allergic reaction to sulfites include bluish coloration of skin; severe dizziness or feeling faint; continuing flushing or redness of face or skin; increased wheezing or difficulty in breathing; skin rash, hives, or itching; or swelling of face, lips, or eyelids. *If any of these signs occur, check with your doctor immediately.*

## Side Effects of This Medicine

In some animal studies, albuterol and terbutaline were shown to increase the chance of benign (not cancerous) tumors. Terbutaline was also shown to increase the chance of ovarian cysts. The doses given were many times the oral dose of albuterol or terbutaline given to humans. It is not known if albuterol or terbutaline increases the chance of tumors in humans, or if terbutaline increases the chance of ovarian cysts in humans.

Along with its needed effects, a medicine may cause some unwanted effects. Although not all of these side effects may occur, if they do occur they may need medical attention.

*Check with your doctor immediately if any of the following side effects occur:*

Bluish coloration of skin; dizziness (severe) or feeling faint; flushing or redness of face or skin (continuing); increased wheezing or difficulty in breathing; skin rash, hives, or itching; swelling of face, lips, or eyelids

Check with your doctor as soon as possible if any of the following side effects occur:

*Rare*

Chest discomfort or pain; irregular heartbeat

*With high doses*

Hallucinations (seeing, hearing, or feeling things that are not there); mood or mental changes (reported for ephedrine only)

*Symptoms of overdose*

> Bluish coloration of skin; chest discomfort or pain (continuing or severe); chills or fever; convulsions (seizures); dizziness or lightheadedness (continuing or severe); fast or slow heartbeat (continuing); headache (continuing or severe); increase or decrease in blood pressure (severe); irregular or pounding heartbeat (continuing or severe); muscle cramps (severe); nausea or vomiting (continuing or severe); shortness of breath or troubled breathing (severe); trembling (severe); unusual anxiety, nervousness, or restlessness; unusually large pupils or blurred vision; unusual paleness and coldness of skin; weakness (severe)

Other side effects may occur that usually do not need medical attention. These side effects may go away during treatment as your body adjusts to the medicine. However, check with your doctor if any of the following side effects continue or are bothersome:

*More common*

> Nervousness or restlessness; trembling

*Less common*

> Difficult or painful urination; dizziness or lightheadedness; drowsiness; fast or pounding heartbeat; flushing or redness of face or skin; headache; heartburn; increased sweating; increase in blood pressure; loss of appetite; muscle cramps or twitching; nausea or vomiting; trouble in sleeping; unusual paleness; weakness

Not all of the side effects listed above have been reported for each of these medicines, but they have been reported for at least one of them. All of the adrenergic bronchodilators are similar, so any of the above side effects may occur with any of these medicines.

While you are using albuterol, fenoterol, metaproterenol, or terbutaline, you may notice an unusual or unpleasant taste. This may be expected and will go away when you stop using the medicine.

Isoproterenol sublingual (under-the-tongue) tablets may cause the saliva to turn pinkish to red. This is to be expected while you are using this medicine.

Other side effects not listed above may also occur in some patients. If you notice any other effects, check with your doctor.

## Additional Information

Once a medicine has been approved for marketing for a certain use, experience may show that it is also useful for other medical problems. Although these uses are not included in product labeling, some of the adrenergic bronchodilators are used in certain patients with the following medical conditions:

- Premature labor (terbutaline)
- Urticaria (hives) (ephedrine)
- Hemorrhage (bleeding) of gums and teeth (epinephrine)
- Priapism (prolonged abnormal erection of penis) (epinephrine)

Other than the above information, there is no additional information relating to proper use, precautions, or side effects for these uses.

Revised: July 1990
Interim revision: 09/12/94

# BRONCHODILATORS, XANTHINE-DERIVATIVE    Systemic

Some commonly used brand names are:

**In the U.S.—**

| | |
|---|---|
| Aerolate III[4] | Solu-Phyllin[4] |
| Aerolate Jr.[4] | Theo-24[4] |
| Aerolate Sr.[4] | Theo 250[4] |
| Aquaphyllin[4] | Theobid Duracaps[4] |
| Asmalix[4] | Theobid Jr. Duracaps[4] |
| Bronkodyl[4] | Theochron[4] |
| Choledyl Delayed-release[3] | Theoclear-80[4] |
| Choledyl SA[3] | Theoclear L.A.-130[4] |
| Dilor[2] | Theoclear L.A.-260[4] |
| Dilor-400[2] | Theo-Dur[4] |
| Dyflex-200[2] | Theo-Dur Sprinkle[4] |
| Elixomin[4] | Theolair[4] |
| Elixophyllin[4] | Theolair-SR[4] |
| Elixophyllin SR[4] | Theomar[4] |
| Lanophyllin[4] | Theo-Sav[4] |
| Lufyllin[2] | Theospan-SR[4] |
| Lufyllin-400[2] | Theostat 80[4] |
| Neothylline[2] | Theo-Time[4] |
| Phyllocontin[1] | Theovent Long-Acting[4] |
| Quibron-T Dividose[4] | Theo-X[4] |
| Quibron-T/SR Dividose[4] | T-Phyl[4] |
| Respbid[4] | Truphylline[1] |
| Slo-bid Gyrocaps[4] | Truxophyllin[4] |
| Slo-Phyllin[4] | Uniphyl[4] |
| Slo-Phyllin Gyrocaps[4] | |

**In Canada—**

| | |
|---|---|
| Apo-Oxtriphylline[3] | Quibron-T/SR[4] |
| Choledyl[3] | Slo-Bid[4] |
| Choledyl SA[3] | Somophyllin-12[4] |
| Novotriphyl[3] | Theochron[4] |
| Phyllocontin[1] | Theo-Dur[4] |
| Phyllocontin-350[1] | Theolair[4] |
| PMS-Oxtriphylline[3] | Theolair-SR[4] |
| PMS Theophylline[4] | Theo-SR[4] |
| Pulmophylline[4] | Uniphyl[4] |

Note: For quick reference, the following bronchodilators, xanthine-derivatives are numbered to match the corresponding brand names.

This information applies to the following medicines:

1. Aminophylline (am-in-OFF-i-lin)‡§
2. Dyphylline (DYE-fi-lin)†‡
3. Oxtriphylline (ox-TRYE-fi-lin)‡
4. Theophylline (thee-OFF-i-lin)‡§

†Not commercially available in Canada.
‡Generic name product may also be available in the U.S.
§Generic name product may also be available in Canada.

## Description

Xanthine-derivative bronchodilators are used to treat and/or prevent the symptoms of bronchial asthma, chronic bronchitis, and emphysema. These medicines relieve cough, wheezing, shortness of breath, and troubled breathing. They work by opening up the bronchial tubes (air passages of the lungs) and increasing the flow of air through them.

Aminophylline and theophylline may also be used for other conditions as determined by your doctor.

The oral liquid, uncoated or chewable tablet, and capsule dosage forms of xanthine-derivative bronchodilators may be used for treatment of the acute attack and for chronic (long-term) treatment. The enteric-coated tablet and extended-release dosage forms are usually used only for chronic treatment. Sometimes, aminophylline rectal suppositories may be used but they generally are not recommended because of possible poor absorption.

These medicines are available only with your doctor's prescription, in the following dosage forms:

*Oral*
  Aminophylline
  • Oral solution (U.S.)
  • Tablets (U.S. and Canada)
  • Enteric-coated tablets (U.S.)
  • Extended-release tablets (U.S. and Canada)
  Dyphylline
  • Elixir (U.S.)
  • Tablets (U.S.)
  Oxtriphylline
  • Oral solution (U.S. and Canada)
  • Syrup (U.S. and Canada)
  • Tablets (U.S. and Canada)
  • Delayed-release tablets (U.S.)
  • Extended-release tablets (U.S. and Canada)
  Theophylline
  • Capsules (U.S.)
  • Extended-release capsules (U.S. and Canada)
  • Elixir (U.S. and Canada)
  • Oral solution (U.S. and Canada)
  • Syrup (U.S.)
  • Tablets (U.S. and Canada)
  • Extended-release tablets (U.S. and Canada)

*Parenteral*
  Aminophylline
  • Injection (U.S. and Canada)
  Aminophylline and Sodium Chloride
  • Injection (U.S.)
  Dyphylline
  • Injection (U.S.)
  Theophylline in Dextrose
  • Injection (U.S. and Canada)

*Rectal*
  Aminophylline
  • Suppositories (U.S.)

## Before Using This Medicine

In deciding to use a medicine, the risks of taking the medicine must be weighed against the good it will do. This is a decision you and your doctor will make. For xanthine-derivative bronchodilators, the following should be considered:

**Allergies**—Tell your doctor if you have ever had any unusual or allergic reaction to aminophylline, caffeine, dyphylline, ethylenediamine (contained in aminophylline), oxtriphylline, theobromine, or theophylline. Also tell your health care professional if you are allergic to any other substances, such as foods, preservatives, or dyes.

**Diet**—Make certain your health care professional knows if you are on any special diet, such as a low-sodium or low-sugar diet or a high-protein, low-carbohydrate or low-protein, high-carbohydrate diet.

Avoid eating or drinking large amounts of caffeine-containing foods or beverages, such as chocolate, cocoa, tea, coffee, and cola drinks, because they may increase the central nervous system (CNS) stimulant effects of the xanthine-derivative bronchodilators.

Also, eating charcoal broiled foods every day while taking aminophylline, oxtriphylline, or theophylline may keep these medicines from working properly.

**Pregnancy**—Studies on birth defects have not been done in humans. However, some studies in animals have shown that theophylline (including aminophylline and oxtriphylline) causes birth defects when given in doses many times the human dose. Also, use of aminophylline, oxtriphylline, or theophylline during pregnancy may cause unwanted effects such as fast heartbeat, jitteriness, irritability, gagging, vomiting, and breathing problems in the newborn infant. Studies on birth defects with dyphylline have not been done in either humans or animals.

**Breast-feeding**—Theophylline passes into the breast milk and may cause irritability, fretfulness, or trouble in sleeping in nursing babies of mothers taking aminophylline, oxtriphylline, or theophylline. Although dyphylline passes into the breast milk, it has not been reported to cause problems in nursing babies.

**Children**—The side effects of xanthine-derivative bronchodilators are more likely to occur in newborn infants, who are usually more sensitive to the effects of these medicines.

**Older adults**—The side effects of xanthine-derivative bronchodilators are more likely to occur in elderly patients, who are usually more sensitive than younger adults to the effects of these medicines.

**Other medicines**—Although certain medicines should not be used together at all, in other cases two different medicines may be used together even if an interaction might occur. In these cases, your doctor may want to change the dose, or other precautions may be necessary. When you are taking xanthine-derivative bronchodilators, it is especially important that your health care professional know if you are taking any of the following:

• Beta-blockers (acebutolol [e.g., Sectral], atenolol [e.g., Tenormin], betaxolol [e.g., Kerlone], bisoprolol [e.g., Zebeta], carteolol [e.g., Cartrol], labetalol [e.g., Normodyne], metoprolol [e.g., Lopressor], nadolol [e.g., Corgard], oxprenolol [e.g., Trasicor], penbutolol [e.g.,

Levatol], pindolol [e.g., Visken], propranolol [e.g., Inderal], sotalol [e.g., Sotacor], timolol [e.g., Blocadren])—Use of these medicines with xanthine-derivative bronchodilators may prevent either the beta-blocker or the bronchodilator from working properly

- Cimetidine (e.g., Tagamet) or
- Ciprofloxacin or
- Erythromycin (e.g., E-Mycin) or
- Nicotine chewing gum (e.g., Nicorette) or
- Norfloxacin or
- Ranitidine (e.g., Zantac) or
- Troleandomycin (e.g., TAO)—These medicines may increase the effects of aminophylline, oxtriphylline, or theophylline
- Corticosteroids (cortisone-like medicines)—Use of these medicines with aminophylline and sodium chloride injection may result in too much sodium in the blood
- Phenytoin (e.g., Dilantin)—The effects of phenytoin may be decreased by aminophylline, oxtriphylline, or theophylline
- Smoking tobacco or marijuana—If you smoke or have smoked tobacco or marijuana regularly within the last 2 years, the amount of medicine you need may vary, depending on how much and how recently you have smoked

**Other medical problems**—The presence of other medical problems may affect the use of xanthine-derivative bronchodilators. Make sure you tell your doctor if you have any other medical problems, especially:

- Alcohol abuse (or history of) or
- Fever or
- Liver disease or
- Respiratory infections, such as influenza (flu)—The effects of aminophylline, oxtriphylline, or theophylline may be increased
- Diarrhea—The absorption of xanthine-derivative bronchodilators, especially the extended-release dosage forms, may be decreased; therefore, the effects of these medicines may be decreased
- Enlarged prostate or
- Heart disease or
- High blood pressure or
- Stomach ulcer (or history of) or other stomach problems—Xanthine-derivative bronchodilators may make the condition worse
- Fibrocystic breast disease—Symptoms of this disease may be increased by xanthine-derivative bronchodilators
- Kidney disease—The effects of dyphylline may be increased
- Overactive thyroid—The effects of aminophylline, oxtriphylline, or theophylline may be decreased

## Proper Use of This Medicine

For patients *taking this medicine by mouth:*

- If you are taking the *capsule, tablet, liquid, or extended-release (not including the once-a-day capsule or tablet) form* of this medicine, *it works best when taken with a glass of water on an empty stomach* (either 30 minutes to 1 hour before meals or 2 hours after meals). That way the medicine will get into the blood sooner. However, in some cases your doctor may want you to take this medicine with meals or right after meals to lessen stomach upset. If you have

any questions about how you should be taking this medicine, check with your doctor.

- If you are taking the *once-a-day capsule or tablet form* of this medicine, *some products are to be taken each morning after fasting overnight and at least 1 hour before eating. However, other products are to be taken in the morning or evening with or without food. Be sure you understand exactly how to take the medicine prescribed for you.* Try to take the medicine about the same time each day.
- There are several different forms of xanthine-derivative bronchodilator capsules and tablets. If you are taking:
  —enteric-coated or delayed-release tablets, swallow the tablets whole. Do not crush, break, or chew before swallowing.
  —extended-release capsules, swallow the capsule whole. Do not crush, break, or chew before swallowing.
  —extended-release tablets, swallow the tablets whole. Do not break (unless tablet is scored for breaking), crush, or chew before swallowing.

*Use this medicine only as directed by your doctor.* Do not use more of it, do not use it more often, and do not use it for a longer time than your doctor ordered. To do so may increase the chance of serious side effects.

*In order for this medicine to help your medical problem, it must be taken every day in regularly spaced doses as ordered by your doctor.* This is necessary to keep a constant amount of this medicine in the blood. To help keep the amount constant, do not miss any doses.

**Dosing**—When you are taking aminophylline, dyphylline, oxtriphylline, or theophylline, it is very important that you get the exact amount of medicine that you need. The dose of these medicines will be different for different patients. Your doctor will determine the proper dose of the xanthine-derivative bronchodilator for you. *Follow your doctor's orders or the directions on the label.*

After you begin taking aminophylline, oxtriphylline, or theophylline, it is very important that your doctor check your blood level of theophylline at regular times to find out if your dose of aminophylline, oxtriphylline, or theophylline needs to be changed. *Do not change your dose of aminophylline, dyphylline, oxtriphylline, or theophylline* unless your doctor tells you to do so.

The number of capsules or tablets or teaspoonfuls of solution or syrup that you take depends on the strength of the medicine. Also, the number of doses you take each day and the time beween doses depend on whether you are taking a short-acting or a long-acting form of aminophylline, dyphylline, oxtriphylline, or theophylline.

**Missed dose**—If you miss a dose of this medicine, take it as soon as possible. However, if it is almost time for your next dose, skip the missed dose and go back to your regular dosing schedule. Do not double doses.

**Storage**—To store this medicine:
- Keep out of the reach of children.
- Store away from heat and direct light.
- Do not store the capsule or tablet form of this medicine in the bathroom, near the kitchen sink, or in other damp places. Heat or moisture may cause the medicine to break down.
- Keep the liquid form of this medicine from freezing.
- Do not keep outdated medicine or medicine no longer needed. Be sure that any discarded medicine is out of the reach of children.

## Precautions While Using This Medicine

Your doctor should check your progress at regular visits, especially for the first few weeks after you begin using this medicine. A blood test may be taken to help your doctor decide whether the dose of this medicine should be changed.

*Do not change brands or dosage forms of this medicine without first checking with your doctor.* Different products may not work the same way. If you refill your medicine and it looks different, check with your pharmacist.

This medicine may add to the central nervous system (CNS) stimulant effects of caffeine-containing foods or beverages such as chocolate, cocoa, tea, coffee, and cola drinks. *Avoid eating or drinking large amounts of these foods or beverages while using this medicine.* If you have any questions about this, check with your doctor.

For patients using *aminophylline, oxtriphylline, or theophylline*:
- Do not eat charcoal-broiled foods every day while using this medicine since these foods may keep the medicine from working properly.
- *Check with your doctor at once if you develop symptoms of influenza (flu) or a fever* since either of these may increase the chance of side effects with this medicine.
- Also, *check with your doctor if diarrhea occurs* because the dose of this medicine may need to be changed.

## Side Effects of This Medicine

Along with its needed effects, a medicine may cause some unwanted effects. Although not all of these side effects may occur, if they do occur they may need medical attention.

Check with your doctor as soon as possible if any of the following side effects occur:

*Less common*
    Heartburn and/or vomiting
*Rare*
    Skin rash or hives (with aminophylline only)
*Symptoms of overdose*
    Bloody or black, tarry stools; confusion or change in behavior; convulsions (seizures); diarrhea; dizziness or lightheadedness; fast breathing; fast, pounding, or irregular heartbeat; flushing or redness of face; headache; increased urination; irritability; loss of appetite; muscle twitching; nausea (continuing or severe) or vomiting; stomach cramps or pain; trembling; trouble in sleeping; unusual tiredness or weakness; vomiting blood or material that looks like coffee grounds

Other side effects may occur that usually do not need medical attention. These side effects may go away during treatment as your body adjusts to the medicine. However, check with your doctor if any of the following side effects continue or are bothersome:

*More common*
    Nausea; nervousness or restlessness

Other side effects not listed above may also occur in some patients. If you notice any other effects, check with your doctor.

## Additional Information

Once a medicine has been approved for marketing for a certain use, experience may show that it is also useful for other medical problems. Although this use is not included in product labeling, aminophylline and theophylline are used in certain patients with the following medical condition:
- Apnea (breathing problem) in newborns

Other than the above information, there is no additional information relating to proper use, precautions, or side effects for this use.

Revised: July 1990
Interim revision: 08/26/94

# BUPROPION   Systemic†

A commonly used brand name in the U.S. is Wellbutrin.
Another commonly used name is amfebutamone.

†Not commercially available in Canada.

## Description

Bupropion (byoo-PROE-pee-on) is used to relieve mental depression.

This medicine is available only with your doctor's prescription, in the following dosage form:

*Oral*
- Tablets (U.S.)

## Before Using This Medicine

In deciding to use a medicine, the risks of taking the medicine must be weighed against the good it will do. This is a decision you and your doctor will make. For bupropion, the following should be considered:

**Allergies**—Tell your doctor if you have ever had any unusual or allergic reaction to bupropion. Also tell your health care professional if you are allergic to any other substances, such as foods, preservatives, or dyes.

**Pregnancy**—Studies have not been done in pregnant women. However, bupropion has not been reported to cause birth defects or other problems in animal studies.

**Breast-feeding**—Bupropion passes into breast milk. Because it may cause unwanted effects in nursing babies, use of bupropion is not recommended during breast-feeding.

**Children**—Studies on this medicine have been done only in adult patients, and there is no specific information comparing use of bupropion in children with use in other age groups.

**Older adults**—This medicine has been tested in a limited number of patients 60 years of age and older and has not been shown to cause different side effects or problems in older people than it does in younger adults.

**Other medicines**—Although certain medicines should not be used together at all, in other cases two different medicines may be used together even if an interaction might occur. In these cases, your doctor may want to change the dose, or other precautions may be necessary. When you are taking bupropion, it is especially important that your health care professional know if you are taking any of the following:
- Alcohol or
- Antipsychotics (medicine for mental illness) or
- Fluoxetine (e.g., Prozac) or
- Lithium (e.g., Lithane) or
- Maprotiline (e.g., Ludiomil) or
- Trazodone (e.g., Desyrel) or

- Tricyclic antidepressants (amitriptyline [e.g., Elavil], amoxapine [e.g., Asendin], clomipramine [e.g., Anafranil], desipramine [e.g., Pertofrane], doxepin [e.g., Sinequan], imipramine [e.g., Tofranil], nortriptyline [e.g., Aventyl], protriptyline [e.g., Vivactil], trimipramine [e.g., Surmontil])—Using these medicines with bupropion may increase the risk of seizures
- Monoamine oxidase (MAO) inhibitors (furazolidone [e.g., Furoxone], isocarboxazid [e.g., Marplan], phenelzine [e.g., Nardil], procarbazine [e.g., Matulane], selegiline [e.g., Eldepryl], tranylcypromine [e.g., Parnate])—Taking bupropion while you are taking or within 2 weeks of taking MAO inhibitors may increase the chance of side effects; at least 14 days should be allowed between stopping treatment with one medicine and starting treatment with the other

**Other medical problems**—The presence of other medical problems may affect the use of bupropion. Make sure you tell your doctor if you have any other medical problems, especially:
- Anorexia nervosa or
- Brain tumor or
- Bulimia or
- Head injury, history of, or
- Seizure disorder—The risk of seizures may be increased when bupropion is taken by patients with these conditions
- Bipolar disorder (manic-depressive illness) or
- Other nervous, mental, or emotional conditions—Bupropion may make the condition worse
- Heart attack (recent) or heart disease—Bupropion may cause unwanted effects on the heart
- Kidney disease or
- Liver disease—Higher blood levels of bupropion may result, increasing the chance of side effects

## Proper Use of This Medicine

Use bupropion only as directed by your doctor. Do not use more of it, do not use it more often, and do not use it for a longer time than your doctor ordered. To do so may increase the chance of side effects.

To lessen stomach upset, this medicine may be taken with food, unless your doctor has told you to take it on an empty stomach.

Usually this medicine must be taken for several weeks before you feel better. Your doctor should check your progress at regular visits.

**Dosing**—The dose of bupropion will be different for different patients. *Follow your doctor's orders or the directions on the label.* The following information includes only the average doses of bupropion. *If your dose is different, do not change it* unless your doctor tells you to do so.

The number of tablets that you take depends on the strength of the medicine. Also, *the number of doses you take each day, the time allowed between doses, and the length of time you take the medicine depend on the medical problem for which you are taking bupropion.*

© 1994   The United States Pharmacopeial Convention, Inc.

- For *oral* dosage form (tablets):
  —For depression:
    - Adults—At first, 100 milligrams (mg) twice a day. Your doctor may increase your dose as needed. However, the dose is usually not more than 450 mg a day.
    - Children—Use and dose must be determined by your doctor.

**Missed dose**—If you miss a dose of this medicine, take it as soon as possible. However, if it is within 4 hours of your next dose, skip the missed dose and go back to your regular dosing schedule. Do not double doses.

**Storage**—To store this medicine:

- Keep out of the reach of children.
- Store away from heat and direct light.
- Do not store in the bathroom, near the kitchen sink, or in other damp places. Heat or moisture may cause the medicine to break down.
- Do not keep outdated medicine or medicine no longer needed. Be sure that any discarded medicine is out of the reach of children.

---

## Precautions While Using This Medicine

Your doctor should check your progress at regular visits, especially during the first few months of treatment with this medicine. The amount of bupropion you take may have to be changed often to meet the needs of your condition and to help avoid unwanted effects.

*If you have been taking this medicine regularly, do not stop taking it without first checking with your doctor.* Your doctor may want you to reduce gradually the amount you are taking before stopping completely. This will help reduce the possibility of side effects.

Drinking of alcoholic beverages should be limited or avoided, if possible, while taking bupropion. This will help prevent unwanted effects.

This medicine may cause some people to feel a false sense of well-being, or to become drowsy, dizzy, or less alert than they are normally. *Make sure you know how you react to this medicine before you drive, use machines, or do anything else that could be dangerous if you are dizzy or are not alert and clearheaded.*

---

## Side Effects of This Medicine

Along with its needed effects, a medicine may cause some unwanted effects. Although not all of these side effects may occur, if they do occur they may need medical attention.

*Check with your doctor as soon as possible if any of the following side effects occur:*

*More common*

Agitation or excitement; anxiety; confusion; fast or irregular heartbeat; headache (severe); restlessness; trouble in sleeping

*Less common*

Hallucinations; skin rash

*Rare*

Fainting; seizures (convulsions), especially with higher doses

Other side effects may occur that usually do not need medical attention. These side effects may go away during treatment as your body adjusts to the medicine. However, check with your doctor if any of the following side effects continue or are bothersome:

*More common*

Constipation; decrease in appetite; dizziness; dryness of mouth; increased sweating; nausea or vomiting; tremor; weight loss (unusual)

*Less common*

Blurred vision; difficulty concentrating; drowsiness; fever or chills; hostility or anger; tiredness; sleep disturbances; unusual feeling of well-being

Other side effects not listed above may also occur in some patients. If you notice any other effects, check with your doctor.

---

Revised: 07/29/94

---

# BUSERELIN   Systemic*

A commonly used brand name in Canada is Suprefact.

---

*Not commercially available in the U.S.

---

## Description

Buserelin (BYOO-se-rel-in) is used to treat cancer of the prostate gland.

It is similar to a hormone normally released from the hypothalamus gland. When given regularly, buserelin decreases testosterone levels. Reducing the amount of testosterone in the body is one way of treating cancer of the prostate.

Buserelin is available only with your doctor's prescription, in the following dosage forms:

*Nasal*

- Nasal solution (Canada)

---

© 1994   The United States Pharmacopeial Convention, Inc.

*Parenteral*
- Injection (Canada)

## Before Using This Medicine

In deciding to use a medicine, the risks of taking the medicine must be weighed against the good it will do. This is a decision you and your doctor will make. For buserelin, the following should be considered:

**Allergies**—Tell your doctor if you have ever had any unusual or allergic reaction to buserelin.

**Fertility**—Buserelin causes sterility which may be permanent. If you intend to have children, discuss this with your doctor before receiving this medicine.

**Older adults**—Many medicines have not been studied specifically in older people. Therefore, it may not be known whether they work exactly the same way they do in younger adults. Although there is no specific information comparing use of buserelin in the elderly to use in other age groups, it has been used mostly in elderly patients and is not expected to cause different side effects or problems in older people than it does in younger adults.

## Proper Use of This Medicine

*Buserelin comes with patient directions. Read these instructions carefully.*

For patients using the *injection* form of this medicine:
- Use the syringes provided in the kit. Other syringes may not provide the correct dose. These disposable syringes and needles are already sterilized and designed to be used one time only and then discarded. If you have any questions about the use of disposable syringes, check with your health care professional.
- After use, dispose of the syringes and needles in a safe manner. If a special container is not provided, ask your health care professional about the best way to dispose of syringes and needles.

For patients using the *nasal solution* form of this medicine:
- Use the nebulizer (spray pump) provided. Directions about how to use it are included. If you have any questions about the use of the nebulizer, check with your health care professional.

*Use this medicine only as directed by your doctor.* Do not use more or less of it, and do not use it more often than your doctor ordered. The exact amount of medicine you need has been carefully worked out. Using too much may increase the chance of side effects, while using too little may not improve your condition.

Buserelin sometimes causes unwanted effects such as hot flashes or decreased sexual ability. It may also cause a temporary increase in pain, trouble in urinating, or weakness in your legs when you begin to use it. However, it is very important that you continue to use the medicine, even after you begin to feel better. *Do not stop using this medicine without first checking with your doctor.*

**Dosing**—The dose of buserelin will be different for different patients. *Follow your doctor's orders or the directions on the label.* The following information includes only the average doses of buserelin. *If your dose is different, do not change it* unless your doctor tells you to do so.

*The number of doses you use each day, the time allowed between doses, and the length of time you use the medicine depend on the medical problem for which you are using buserelin.*

- For prostate cancer:
  —For *nasal* dosage forms:
  - Adults: 200 micrograms (mcg) (2 sprays) into each nostril every eight hours.
  —For *injection* dosage forms:
  - Adults: In the beginning, 500 mcg (0.5 milligrams [mg]) injected under the skin every eight hours. After a time, your doctor may lower your dose to 200 mcg (0.2 mg) once a day.

**Missed dose**—If you miss a dose of this medicine, use it as soon as possible. However, if it is almost time for the next dose, skip the missed dose and go back to your regular dosing schedule. Do not double doses.

**Storage**—To store this medicine:
- Keep out of the reach of children.
- Store away from heat and direct light.
- Keep the medicine from freezing.
- Do not keep outdated medicine or medicine no longer needed. Dispose of used syringes properly in the container provided. Be sure that any discarded medicine is out of the reach of children.

## Precautions While Using This Medicine

*It is very important that your doctor check your progress at regular visits* to make sure that this medicine is working properly and to check for unwanted effects.

## Side Effects of This Medicine

Along with its needed effects, a medicine may cause some unwanted effects. Although not all of these side effects may occur, if they do occur they may need medical attention.

The following side effects are symptoms of a flareup of your condition that may occur during the first few days of treatment. After a few days, these symptoms should lessen. However, they may require medical attention. Check with your doctor if any of the following side effects occur or get worse:

> Bone pain; numbness or tingling of hands or feet; trouble in urinating; weakness in legs

Other side effects may occur that usually do not need medical attention. These side effects may go away during treatment as your body adjusts to the medicine. However,

check with your doctor if any of the following side effects continue or are bothersome:

*More common*

Decrease in sexual desire; impotence; sudden sweating and feelings of warmth ("hot flashes")

*Less common*

Burning, itching, redness, or swelling at place of injection; diarrhea; dry or sore nose (with nasal solution); headache (with nasal solution); increased sweating (with nasal solution); loss of appetite; nausea or vomiting;

swelling and increased tenderness of breasts; swelling of feet or lower legs

Other side effects not listed above may also occur in some patients. If you notice any other effects, check with your doctor.

Revised: 07/11/94

# BUSPIRONE   Systemic

A commonly used brand name in the U.S. and Canada is BuSpar.

## Description

Buspirone (byoo-SPYE-rone) is used to treat certain anxiety disorders or to relieve the symptoms of anxiety. However, buspirone is usually not used for anxiety or tension caused by the stress of everyday life.

It is not known exactly how buspirone works to relieve the symptoms of anxiety.

Buspirone is available only with your doctor's prescription, in the following dosage form:

*Oral*

- Tablets (U.S. and Canada)

## Before Using This Medicine

In deciding to use a medicine, the risks of taking the medicine must be weighed against the good it will do. This is a decision you and your doctor will make. For buspirone, the following should be considered:

**Allergies**—Tell your doctor if you have ever had any unusual or allergic reaction to buspirone. Also tell your health care professional if you are allergic to any other substances, such as foods, preservatives, or dyes.

**Pregnancy**—Buspirone has not been studied in pregnant women. However, buspirone has not been shown to cause birth defects or other problems in animal studies.

**Breast-feeding**—It is not known whether buspirone passes into the breast milk of humans.

**Children**—Studies on this medicine have been done only in adult patients, and there is no specific information comparing use of buspirone in children up to 18 years of age with use in other age groups.

**Older adults**—This medicine has been tested and has not been shown to cause different side effects or problems in older people than it does in younger adults.

**Other medicines**—Although certain medicines should not be used together at all, in other cases 2 different medicines may be used together even if an interaction might

occur. In these cases, your doctor may want to change the dose, or other precautions may be necessary. When you are taking buspirone, it is especially important that your health care professional know if you are taking any of the following:

- Monoamine oxidase (MAO) inhibitors (furazolidone [e.g., Furoxone], isocarboxazid [e.g., Marplan], phenelzine [e.g., Nardil], procarbazine [e.g., Matulane], selegiline at doses more than 10 mg a day [e.g., Eldepryl], tranylcypromine [e.g., Parnate])—Taking buspirone while you are taking or within 2 weeks of taking monoamine oxidase (MAO) inhibitors may cause high blood pressure

**Other medical problems**—The presence of other medical problems may affect the use of buspirone. Make sure you tell your doctor if you have any other medical problems, especially:

- Drug abuse or dependence (history of)—There is a possibility that buspirone could become habit-forming, causing mental or physical dependence
- Kidney disease or
- Liver disease—The effects of buspirone may be increased, which may increase the chance of side effects

## Proper Use of This Medicine

*Take buspirone only as directed by your doctor.* Do not take more of it, do not take it more often, and do not take it for a longer time than your doctor ordered. To do so may increase the chance of unwanted effects.

After you begin taking buspirone, 1 to 2 weeks may pass before you feel the full effects of this medicine.

**Dosing**—The dose of buspirone will be different for different patients. *Follow your doctor's orders or the directions on the label.* The following information includes only the average doses of buspirone. *If your dose is different, do not change it* unless your doctor tells you to do so.

The number of tablets that you take depends on the strength of the medicine. Also, *the number of doses you take each day, the time allowed between doses, and the length of time you take the medicine depend on the medical problem for which you are taking buspirone.*

- For *oral* dosage forms (tablets):
  —Adults: To start, 5 milligrams three times a day. Your doctor may increase your dose by 5 milligrams a day every few days if needed. However, the dose is usually not more than 60 milligrams a day.
  —Children up to 18 years of age: Dose must be determined by the doctor.

**Missed dose**—If you are taking this medicine regularly and you miss a dose, take it as soon as possible. However, if it is almost time for your next dose, skip the missed dose and go back to your regular dosing schedule. Do not double doses.

**Storage**—To store this medicine:
- Keep out of the reach of children.
- Store away from heat and direct light.
- Do not store in the bathroom, near the kitchen sink, or in other damp places. Heat or moisture may cause the medicine to break down.
- Do not keep outdated medicine or medicine no longer needed. Be sure that any discarded medicine is out of the reach of children.

## Precautions While Using This Medicine

If you will be using buspirone regularly for a long time, your doctor should check your progress at regular visits to make sure the medicine does not cause unwanted effects.

Buspirone, when taken with alcohol or other CNS depressants (medicines that slow down the nervous system, possibly causing drowsiness), may increase the chance of drowsiness. Some examples of CNS depressants are antihistamines or medicine for hay fever, other allergies, or colds; sedatives, tranquilizers, or sleeping medicine; prescription pain medicine or narcotics; barbiturates; medicine for seizures; muscle relaxants; or anesthetics, including some dental anesthetics. Check with your doctor before taking any of the above while you are taking this medicine.

Buspirone may cause some people to become dizzy, lightheaded, drowsy, or less alert than they are normally. *Make sure you know how you react to this medicine before you drive, use machines, or do anything else that could be dangerous if you are dizzy or are not alert.*

*If you think you or someone else may have taken an overdose of buspirone, get emergency help at once.* Some symptoms of an overdose are severe dizziness or drowsiness; severe stomach upset, including nausea or vomiting; or unusually small pupils.

## Side Effects of This Medicine

Along with its needed effects, a medicine may cause some unwanted effects. Although not all of these side effects may occur, if they do occur they may need medical attention.

Check with your doctor as soon as possible if any of the following side effects occur:

*Rare*
Chest pain; confusion or mental depression; fast or pounding heartbeat; muscle weakness; numbness, tingling, pain, or weakness in hands or feet; sore throat or fever; uncontrolled movements of the body

*Symptoms of overdose*
Dizziness (severe); drowsiness (severe); stomach upset, including nausea or vomiting (severe); unusually small pupils

Other side effects may occur that usually do not need medical attention. These side effects may go away during treatment as your body adjusts to the medicine. However, check with your doctor if any of the following side effects continue or are bothersome:

*More common*
Dizziness or lightheadedness; headache; nausea; restlessness, nervousness, or unusual excitement

*Less common or rare*
Blurred vision; decreased concentration; drowsiness (more common with doses of more than 20 mg per day); dryness of mouth; muscle pain, spasms, cramps, or stiffness; ringing in the ears; stomach upset; trouble in sleeping, nightmares, or vivid dreams; unusual tiredness or weakness

Other side effects not listed above may also occur in some patients. If you notice any other effects, check with your doctor.

Revised: 03/09/93

# BUSULFAN  Systemic

A commonly used brand name in the U.S. and Canada is Myleran.

## Description

Busulfan (byoo-SUL-fan) belongs to the group of medicines known as alkylating agents. It is used to treat some kinds of cancer.

Busulfan seems to act by interfering with the function of the bone marrow. Since the growth of normal body cells may also be affected by busulfan, other effects will also occur. Some of these may be serious and must be reported to your doctor. Other effects may not be serious but may cause concern. Some effects may not occur for months or years after the medicine is used.

Before you begin treatment with busulfan, you and your doctor should talk about the good this medicine will do as well as the risks of using it.

Busulfan is available only with your doctor's prescription, in the following dosage form:
*Oral*
- Tablets (U.S. and Canada)

## Before Using This Medicine

In deciding to use a medicine, the risks of taking the medicine must be weighed against the good it will do. This is a decision you and your doctor will make. For busulfan, the following should be considered:

**Allergies**—Tell your doctor if you have ever had any unusual or allergic reaction to busulfan.

**Pregnancy**—Although only one case has been reported, there is a chance that this medicine may cause birth defects if either the male or the female is taking it at the time of conception or if it is taken during pregnancy. In addition, many cancer medicines may cause sterility which could be permanent. Sterility may occur with busulfan and the possibility should be kept in mind.

Be sure that you have discussed this with your doctor before taking this medicine. It is best to use some kind of birth control while you are taking busulfan. Tell your doctor right away if you think you have become pregnant while taking busulfan.

**Breast-feeding**—It is not known whether busulfan passes into breast milk. However, because this medicine may cause serious side effects, breast-feeding is generally not recommended while you are taking it.

**Children**—Although there is no specific information comparing use of busulfan in children with use in other age groups, this medicine is not expected to cause different side effects or problems in children than it does in adults.

**Older adults**—Many medicines have not been studied specifically in older people. Therefore, it may not be known whether they work exactly the same way they do in younger adults. Although there is no specific information comparing use of busulfan in the elderly with use in other age groups, this medicine is not expected to cause different side effects or problems in older people than it does in younger adults.

**Other medicines**—Although certain medicines should not be used together at all, in other cases two different medicines may be used together even if an interaction might occur. In these cases, your doctor may want to change the dose, or other precautions may be necessary. When taking busulfan it is especially important that your health care professional know if you are taking any of the following:
- Amphotericin B by injection (e.g., Fungizone) or
- Antithyroid agents (medicine for overactive thyroid) or
- Azathioprine (e.g., Imuran) or
- Chloramphenicol (e.g., Chloromycetin) or
- Colchicine or

- Flucytosine (e.g., Ancobon) or
- Ganciclovir (e.g., Cytovene) or
- Interferon (e.g., Intron A, Roferon-A) or
- Plicamycin (e.g., Mithracin) or
- Zidovudine (e.g., AZT, Retrovir) or
- If you have ever been treated with radiation or cancer medicines—Busulfan may increase the effects of these medicines or radiation therapy on the blood
- Probenecid (e.g., Benemid) or
- Sulfinpyrazone (e.g., Anturane)—Busulfan may raise the amount of uric acid in the blood. Since these medicines are used to lower uric acid levels, they may not be as effective in patients taking busulfan

**Other medical problems**—The presence of other medical problems may affect the use of busulfan. Make sure you tell your doctor if you have any other medical problems, especially:
- Chickenpox (including recent exposure) or
- Herpes zoster (shingles)—Risk of severe disease affecting other parts of the body
- Gout (history of) or
- Kidney stones (or history of)—Busulfan may increase levels of uric acid in the body, which can cause gout or kidney stones
- Head injury or
- Convulsions (history of)—Very high doses of busulfan can cause convulsions
- Infection—Busulfan may decrease your body's ability to fight infection

## Proper Use of This Medicine

*Take this medicine only as directed by your doctor.* Do not take more or less of it, and do not take it more often than your doctor ordered. The exact amount of medicine you need has been carefully worked out. Taking too much may increase the chance of side effects, while taking too little may not improve your condition.

Take each dose at the same time each day to make sure it has the best effect.

While you are taking this medicine, your doctor may want you to drink extra fluids so that you will pass more urine. This will help prevent kidney problems and keep your kidneys working well.

This medicine sometimes causes nausea and vomiting. However, it is very important that you continue to use the medicine, even if you begin to feel ill. *Do not stop taking this medicine without first checking with your doctor.* Ask your health care professional for ways to lessen these effects.

If you vomit shortly after taking a dose of busulfan, check with your doctor. You will be told whether to take the dose again or to wait until the next scheduled dose.

**Dosing**—The dose of busulfan will be different for different patients. The dose that is used may depend on a number of things, including what the medicine is being used for, the patient's weight, and whether or not other medicines are also being taken. *If you are taking busulfan at home, follow your doctor's orders or the directions on the label.* If you have any questions about the proper dose of busulfan, ask your doctor.

**Missed dose**—If you miss a dose of this medicine, skip the missed dose and go back to your regular dosing schedule. Do not double doses.

**Storage**—To store this medicine:

- Keep out of the reach of children.
- Store away from heat and direct light.
- Do not store in the bathroom, near the kitchen sink, or in other damp places. Heat or moisture may cause the medicine to break down.
- Do not keep outdated medicine or medicine no longer needed. Be sure that any discarded medicine is out of the reach of children.

---

## Precautions While Using This Medicine

*It is very important that your doctor check your progress at regular visits* to make sure that this medicine is working properly and to check for unwanted effects.

While you are being treated with busulfan, and after you stop treatment with it, *do not have any immunizations (vaccinations) without your doctor's approval.* Busulfan may lower your body's resistance and there is a chance you might get the infection the immunization is meant to prevent. In addition, other persons living in your household should not take oral polio vaccine since there is a chance they could pass the polio virus on to you. Also, avoid persons who have recently taken oral polio vaccine. Do not get close to them, and do not stay in the same room with them for very long. If you cannot take these precautions, you should consider wearing a protective face mask that covers the nose and mouth.

Busulfan can temporarily lower the number of white blood cells in your blood, increasing the chance of getting an infection. It can also lower the number of platelets, which are necessary for proper blood clotting. If this occurs, there are certain precautions you can take, especially when your blood count is low, to reduce the risk of infection or bleeding:

- If you can, avoid people with infections. *Check with your doctor immediately* if you think you are getting an infection or if you get a fever or chills, cough or hoarseness, lower back or side pain, or painful or difficult urination.
- *Check with your doctor immediately* if you notice any unusual bleeding or bruising; black, tarry stools; blood in urine or stools; or pinpoint red spots on your skin.
- Be careful when using a regular toothbrush, dental floss, or toothpick. Your medical doctor, dentist, or nurse may recommend other ways to clean your teeth and gums. Check with your medical doctor before having any dental work done.

- Do not touch your eyes or the inside of your nose unless you have just washed your hands and have not touched anything else in the meantime.
- Be careful not to cut yourself when you are using sharp objects such as a safety razor or fingernail or toenail cutters.
- Avoid contact sports or other situations where bruising or injury could occur.

Before you have any medical tests, tell the medical doctor in charge that you are taking this medicine. The results of some body tissue studies may be affected by this medicine.

---

## Side Effects of This Medicine

Along with its needed effects, a medicine may have some unwanted effects. Although not all of these side effects may occur, if they do occur they may need medical attention.

Also, because of the way these medicines act on the body, there is a chance that they might cause other unwanted effects that may not occur until months or years after the medicine is used. These delayed effects may include certain types of cancer, such as leukemia. Discuss these possible effects with your doctor.

*Check with your doctor or nurse immediately if any of the following side effects occur:*

*More common*
Black, tarry stools; blood in urine or stools; pinpoint red spots on skin; unusual bleeding or bruising

*Less common*
Cough or hoarseness; fever or chills; lower back or side pain; painful or difficult urination

Check with your doctor as soon as possible if any of the following side effects occur:

*Less common*
Joint pain; shortness of breath; sores in mouth and on lips; swelling of feet or lower legs

*Rare*
Blurred vision

Other side effects may occur that usually do not need medical attention. These side effects may go away during treatment as your body adjusts to the medicine. Also, your health care professional may be able to tell you about ways to prevent or reduce some of these side effects. Check with your health care professional if any of the following side effects continue or are bothersome or if you have any questions about them:

*More common*
Darkening of skin; missed or irregular menstrual periods
*Less common*
Confusion; diarrhea; dizziness; loss of appetite; nausea and vomiting; unusual tiredness or weakness; weight loss (sudden)

After you stop taking busulfan, it may still produce some side effects that need attention. During this period of

---

time, check with your doctor if you notice any of the following:

Black, tarry stools; blood in urine or stools; cough or hoarseness; fever or chills; lower back or side pain; painful or difficult urination; pinpoint red spots on skin; shortness of breath; unusual bleeding or bruising

Other side effects not listed above may also occur in some patients. If you notice any other effects, check with your doctor.

Revised: 06/12/92
Interim revision: 05/02/94

# BUTALBITAL AND ACETAMINOPHEN  Systemic†

Some commonly used brand names are:

**In the U.S.—**

| | |
|---|---|
| Amaphen[2] | Isocet[2] |
| Anolor-300[2] | Isopap[2] |
| Anoquan[2] | Medigesic[2] |
| Arcet[2] | Pacaps[2] |
| Bancap[1] | Pharmagesic[2] |
| Bucet[1] | Phrenilin[1] |
| Butace[2] | Phrenilin Forte[1] |
| Conten[1] | Repan[2] |
| Dolmar[2] | Sedapap[1] |
| Endolor[2] | Tencet[2] |
| Esgic[2] | Tencon[1] |
| Esgic-Plus[2] | Triad[2] |
| Ezol[2] | Triaprin[1] |
| Femcet[2] | Two-Dyne[2] |
| Fioricet[2] | |

Note: For quick reference, the following butalbital and acetaminophens are numbered to match the corresponding brand names.

This information applies to the following medicines:
1. Butalbital and Acetaminophen†‡
2. Butalbital, Acetaminophen, and Caffeine†‡

†Not commercially available in Canada.
‡Generic name product may also be available in the U.S.

## Description

Butalbital (byoo-TAL-bi-tal) and acetaminophen (a-seat-a-MIN-oh-fen) combination is a pain reliever and relaxant. It is used to treat tension headaches. Butalbital belongs to the group of medicines called barbiturates (bar-BI-tyoo-rates). Barbiturates act in the central nervous system (CNS) to produce their effects.

When you take butalbital for a long time, your body may get used to it so that larger amounts are needed to produce the same effects. This is called tolerance to the medicine. Also, butalbital may become habit-forming (causing mental or physical dependence) when it is used for a long time or in large doses. Physical dependence may lead to withdrawal side effects when you stop taking the medicine. In patients who get headaches, the first symptom of withdrawal may be new (rebound) headaches.

Some butalbital and acetaminophen combinations also contain caffeine (kaf-EEN). Caffeine may help to relieve headaches. However, caffeine can also cause physical dependence when it is used for a long time. This may lead to withdrawal (rebound) headaches when you stop taking it.

Butalbital and acetaminophen combination may also be used for other kinds of headaches or other kinds of pain as determined by your doctor.

Butalbital and acetaminophen combinations are available only with your doctor's prescription in the following dosage forms:

*Oral*
Butalbital and Acetaminophen
• Capsules (U.S.)
• Tablets (U.S.)
Butalbital, Acetaminophen, and Caffeine
• Capsules (U.S.)
• Tablets (U.S.)

## Before Using This Medicine

In deciding to use a medicine, the risks of taking the medicine must be weighed against the good it will do. This is a decision you and your doctor will make. For butalbital and acetaminophen combinations, the following should be considered:

**Allergies**—Tell your doctor if you have ever had any unusual or allergic reaction to butalbital or other barbiturates, or to acetaminophen, aspirin, or caffeine. Also tell your health care professional if you are allergic to any other substances, such as foods, preservatives, or dyes.

**Pregnancy—**

• *For butalbital:* Barbiturates such as butalbital have been shown to increase the chance of birth defects in humans. Also, one study in humans has suggested that barbiturates taken during pregnancy may increase the chance of brain tumors in the baby.
  Butalbital may cause breathing problems in the newborn baby if taken just before or during delivery.
• *For acetaminophen:* Although studies on birth defects with acetaminophen have not been done in pregnant women, it has not been reported to cause birth defects or other problems.
• *For caffeine:* Studies in humans have not shown that caffeine (contained in some of these combination medicines) causes birth defects. However, use of large amounts of caffeine during pregnancy may cause problems with the heart rhythm and the growth of the fetus. Also, studies in animals have shown that caffeine causes birth defects when given in very large

doses (amounts equal to those present in 12 to 24 cups of coffee a day).

**Breast-feeding—**

- *For butalbital:* Barbiturates such as butalbital pass into the breast milk and may cause drowsiness, unusually slow heartbeat, shortness of breath, or troubled breathing in nursing babies.
- *For acetaminophen:* Although acetaminophen has not been shown to cause problems in nursing babies, it passes into the breast milk in small amounts.
- *For caffeine:* Caffeine (present in some butalbital and acetaminophen combinations) passes into the breast milk in small amounts. Taking caffeine in the amounts present in these medicines has not been shown to cause problems in nursing babies. However, studies have shown that nursing babies may appear jittery and have trouble in sleeping when their mothers drink large amounts of caffeine-containing beverages. Therefore, breast-feeding mothers who use caffeine-containing medicines should probably limit the amount of caffeine they take in from other medicines or from beverages.

**Children—**

- *For butalbital:* Although barbiturates such as butalbital often cause drowsiness, some children become excited after taking them.
- *For acetaminophen:* Acetaminophen has been tested in children and, in effective doses, has not been shown to cause different side effects or problems than it does in adults.
- *For caffeine:* There is no specific information comparing use of caffeine in children up to 12 years of age with use in other age groups. However, caffeine is not expected to cause different side effects or problems in children than it does in adults.

**Older adults—**

- *For butalbital:* Certain side effects, such as confusion, excitement, or mental depression, may be especially likely to occur in elderly patients, who are usually more sensitive than younger adults to the effects of the butalbital in this combination medicine.
- *For acetaminophen:* Acetaminophen has been tested and has not been shown to cause different side effects or problems in older people than it does in younger adults.
- *For caffeine:* Many medicines have not been studied specifically in older people. Therefore, it may not be known whether they work exactly the same way they do in younger adults or if they cause different side effects or problems in older people. There is no specific information comparing use of caffeine in the elderly with use in other age groups.

**Other medicines—**Although certain medicines should not be used together at all, in other cases two different medicines may be used together even if an interaction might occur. In these cases, your doctor may want to change the dose, or other precautions may be necessary. When you are taking a butalbital and acetaminophen combination, it is especially important that your health care professional know if you are taking any of the following:

- Anticoagulants (blood thinners), or
- Carbamazepine (e.g., Tegretol) or
- Contraceptives, oral (birth control pills) containing estrogen, or
- Corticosteroids (cortisone-like medicines) or
- Corticotropin (e.g., ACTH)—Butalbital may make these medicines less effective
- Antidepressants, tricyclic (amitriptyline [e.g., Elavil], amoxapine [e.g., Asendin], clomipramine [e.g., Anafranil], desipramine [e.g., Pertofrane], doxepin [e.g., Sinequan], imipramine [e.g., Tofranil], nortriptyline [e.g., Aventyl], protriptyline [e.g., Vivactil], trimipramine [e.g., Surmontil]) or
- Central nervous system (CNS) depressants (medicines that often cause drowsiness)—These medicines may add to the effects of butalbital and increase the chance of drowsiness or other side effects
- Divalproex (e.g., Depakote) or
- Valproic acid (e.g., Depakene)—The chance of side effects may be increased

**Other medical problems—**The presence of other medical problems may affect the use of butalbital and acetaminophen combinations. Make sure you tell your doctor if you have any other medical problems, especially:

- Alcohol abuse (or history of) or
- Drug abuse or dependence (or history of)—Dependence on butalbital may develop; also, acetaminophen may cause liver damage in people who abuse alcohol
- Asthma (or history of), emphysema, or other chronic lung disease or
- Hepatitis or other liver disease or
- Hyperactivity (in children) or
- Kidney disease—The chance of serious side effects may be increased
- Diabetes mellitus (sugar diabetes) or
- Mental depression or
- Overactive thyroid or
- Porphyria (or history of)—Butalbital can make these conditions worse
- Heart disease (severe)—The caffeine in some butalbital and acetaminophen combinations can make some kinds of heart disease worse

## Proper Use of This Medicine

*Take this medicine only as directed by your doctor.* Do not take more of it, do not take it more often, and do not take it for a longer time than your doctor ordered. If butalbital and acetaminophen combination is taken regularly (for example, every day), it may become habit-forming (causing mental or physical dependence). The caffeine in some butalbital and acetaminophen combinations can also increase the chance of dependence. Dependence is especially likely to occur in patients who take these medicines to relieve frequent headaches. Taking too much of this medicine may also lead to liver damage or other medical problems.

This medicine will relieve a headache best if you *take it as soon as the headache begins*. If you get warning signs of a migraine, take this medicine as soon as you are sure that the migraine is coming. This may even stop the headache pain from occurring. *Lying down in a quiet, dark room for a while after taking the medicine also helps to relieve headaches.*

People who get a lot of headaches may need to take a different medicine to help prevent headaches. *It is important that you follow your doctor's directions about taking the other medicine, even if your headaches continue to occur.* Headache-preventing medicines may take several weeks to start working. Even after they do start working, your headaches may not go away completely. However, your headaches should occur less often, and they should be less severe and easier to relieve than before. This will reduce the amount of headache relievers that you need. If you do not notice any improvement after several weeks of headache-preventing treatment, check with your doctor.

**Dosing**—The dose of butalbital and acetaminophen combination medicines will be different for different patients. *Follow your doctor's orders or the directions on the label.* The following information includes only the average doses of these medicines. *If your dose is different, do not change it* unless your doctor tells you to do so.

The number of capsules or tablets that you take depends on the strength of the medicine.

- For *oral* dosage forms (capsules or tablets):
  —For tension headaches:
    - Adults—One or 2 capsules or tablets every four hours as needed. If your medicine contains 325 or 500 milligrams (mg) of acetaminophen in each capsule or tablet, you should not take more than six capsules or tablets a day. If your medicine contains 650 mg of acetaminophen in each capsule or tablet, you should not take more than four capsules or tablets a day.
    - Children—Dose must be determined by your doctor.

**Missed dose**—If your doctor has ordered you to take this medicine according to a regular schedule and you miss a dose, take it as soon as you remember. However, if it is almost time for your next dose, skip the missed dose and go back to your regular dosing schedule. *Do not double doses.*

**Storage**—To store this medicine:

- Keep out of the reach of children. Overdose is especially dangerous in young children.
- Store away from heat and direct light.
- Do not store this medicine in the bathroom, near the kitchen sink, or in other damp places. Heat or moisture may cause the medicine to break down.
- Do not keep outdated medicine or medicine no longer needed. Be sure that any discarded medicine is out of the reach of children.

## Precautions While Using This Medicine

*Check with your doctor:*

- If the medicine stops working as well as it did when you first started using it. This may mean that you are in danger of becoming dependent on the medicine. *Do not try to get better pain relief by increasing the dose.*
- *If you are having headaches more often than you did before you started taking this medicine.* This is especially important if a new headache occurs within 1 day after you took your last dose of this medicine, headaches begin to occur every day, or a headache continues for several days in a row. This may mean that you are dependent on the medicine. *Continuing to take this medicine will cause even more headaches later on.* Your doctor can give you advice on how to relieve the headaches.

*Check the labels of all nonprescription (over-the-counter [OTC]) or prescription medicines you now take. If any contain a barbiturate or acetaminophen, check with your health care professional.* Taking them together with this medicine may cause an overdose.

The butalbital in this medicine will add to the effects of alcohol and other CNS depressants (medicines that slow down the nervous system, possibly causing drowsiness). Some examples of CNS depressants are antihistamines or medicine for hay fever, other allergies, or colds; sedatives, tranquilizers, or sleeping medicine; other prescription pain medicine; narcotics; other barbiturates; medicine for seizures; muscle relaxants; or anesthetics, including some dental anesthetics. Also, drinking large amounts of alcoholic beverages regularly while taking this medicine may increase the chance of liver damage, especially if you take more of this medicine than your doctor ordered or if you take it regularly for a long time. *Therefore, do not drink alcoholic beverages, and check with your doctor before taking any of the medicines listed above, while you are using this medicine.*

This medicine may cause some people to become drowsy, dizzy, or lightheaded. *Make sure you know how you react to this medicine before you drive, use machines, or do anything else that could be dangerous if you are dizzy or are not alert and clearheaded.*

Before you have any medical tests, tell the person in charge that you are taking this medicine. Caffeine (present in some butalbital and acetaminophen combinations) interferes with the results of certain tests that use dipyridamole (e.g., Persantine) to help show how well blood is flowing to your heart. Caffeine should not be taken for 8 to 12 hours before the test. The results of other tests may also be affected by butalbital and acetaminophen combinations.

Before having any kind of surgery (including dental surgery) or emergency treatment, tell the medical doctor or dentist in charge that you are taking this medicine. Serious side effects can occur if your medical doctor or dentist gives you certain medicines without knowing that you have taken butalbital.

If you have been taking large amounts of this medicine, or if you have been taking it regularly for several weeks or more, *do not suddenly stop taking it without first checking with your doctor.* Your doctor may want you to reduce gradually the amount you are taking before stopping completely in order to lessen the chance of withdrawal side effects.

*If you think you or anyone else may have taken an overdose of this medicine, get emergency help at once.* Taking an overdose of this medicine or taking alcohol or CNS depressants with this medicine may lead to unconsciousness or possibly death. Signs of butalbital overdose include severe drowsiness, confusion, severe weakness, shortness of breath or unusually slow or troubled breathing, slurred speech, staggering, and unusually slow heartbeat. Signs of severe acetaminophen poisoning may not occur until 2 to 4 days after the overdose is taken, but treatment to prevent liver damage or death must be started within 24 hours or less after the overdose is taken.

## Side Effects of This Medicine

Along with its needed effects, a medicine may cause some unwanted effects. Although not all of these side effects may occur, if they do occur they may need medical attention.

*Check with your doctor immediately* if any of the following side effects occur, especially if several of them occur together:

*Rare*
Bleeding or crusting sores on lips; chest pain; fever with or without chills; hive-like swellings (large) on eyelids, face, lips, and/or tongue; muscle cramps or pain; red, thickened, or scaly skin; shortness of breath, troubled breathing, tightness in chest, or wheezing; skin rash, itching, or hives; sores, ulcers, or white spots in mouth (painful); sore throat

*Symptoms of overdose*
Anxiety, confusion, excitement, irritability, nervousness, restlessness, or trouble in sleeping (severe, especially

with products containing caffeine); convulsions (seizures) (for products containing caffeine); diarrhea, especially if occurring together with increased sweating, loss of appetite, and stomach cramps or pain; dizziness, lightheadedness, drowsiness, or weakness, (severe); frequent urination (for products containing caffeine); hallucinations (seeing, hearing, or feeling things that are not there); increased sensitivity to touch or pain (for products containing caffeine); muscle trembling or twitching (for products containing caffeine); nausea or vomiting, sometimes with blood; ringing or other sounds in ears (for products containing caffeine); seeing flashes of "zig-zag" lights (for products containing caffeine); shortness of breath or unusually slow or troubled breathing; slow, fast, or irregular heartbeat; slurred speech; staggering; swelling, pain, or tenderness in the upper abdomen or stomach area; unusual movements of the eyes

Also, check with your doctor as soon as possible if any of the following side effects occur:

*Less common*
Confusion (mild); mental depression; unusual excitement (mild)

*Rare*
Bloody or black, tarry stools; bloody urine; pinpoint red spots on skin; swollen or painful glands; unusual bleeding or bruising; unusual tiredness or weakness (mild)

Other side effects may occur that usually do not need medical attention. These side effects may go away during treatment as your body adjusts to the medicine. However, check with your doctor if any of the following side effects continue or are bothersome:

*More common*
Bloated or "gassy" feeling; dizziness or lightheadedness (mild); drowsiness (mild); nausea, vomiting, or stomach pain (occurring without other symptoms of overdose)

Other side effects not listed above may also occur in some patients. If you notice any other effects, check with your doctor.

Revised: 07/14/92
Interim revision: 07/15/94

# BUTALBITAL AND ASPIRIN    Systemic

Some commonly used brand names are:
**In the U.S.—**

| | |
|---|---|
| Axotal[1] | Isobutyl[2] |
| Butalgen[2] | Isolin[2] |
| Fiorgen[2] | Isollyl[2] |
| Fiorinal[2] | Laniroif[2] |
| Fiormor[2] | Lanorinal[2] |
| Fortabs[2] | Marnal[2] |
| Isobutal[2] | Vibutal[2] |

**In Canada—**

| | |
|---|---|
| Fiorinal[2] | Tecnal[2] |

Other commonly used names for the butalbital, aspirin, and caffeine combination medicine are butalbital-AC and butalbital compound.

Note: For quick reference, the following medicines are numbered to match the corresponding brand names.

This information applies to the following medicines:
1. For Butalbital and Aspirin†
2. For Butalbital, Aspirin#, and Caffeine‡

†Not commercially available in Canada.
‡Generic name product may also be available in the U.S.
#In Canada, *Aspirin* is a brand name. Acetylsalicylic acid is the generic name in Canada. ASA, a synonym for acetylsalicylic acid, is the term that commonly appears on Canadian product labels.

# Description

Butalbital (byoo-TAL-bi-tal) and aspirin (AS-pir-in) combination is a pain reliever and relaxant. It is used to treat tension headaches. Butalbital belongs to the group of medicines called barbiturates (bar-BI-tyoo-rates). Barbiturates act in the central nervous system (CNS) to produce their effects.

When you use butalbital for a long time, your body may get used to it so that larger amounts are needed to produce the same effects. This is called tolerance to the medicine. Also, butalbital may become habit-forming (causing mental or physical dependence) when it is used for a long time or in large doses. Physical dependence may lead to withdrawal side effects when you stop taking the medicine. In patients who get headaches, the first symptom of withdrawal may be new (rebound) headaches.

Some of these medicines also contain caffeine (kaf-EEN). Caffeine may help to relieve headaches. However, caffeine can also cause physical dependence when it is used for a long time. This may lead to withdrawal (rebound) headaches when you stop taking it.

Butalbital and aspirin combination is sometimes also used for other kinds of headaches or other kinds of pain, as determined by your doctor.

Butalbital and aspirin combination is available only with your doctor's prescription, in the following dosage forms:

*Oral*

Butalbital and Aspirin
* Tablets (U.S.)

Butalbital, Aspirin, and Caffeine
* Capsules (U.S. and Canada)
* Tablets (U.S. and Canada)

# Before Using This Medicine

In deciding to use a medicine, the risks of taking the medicine must be weighed against the good it will do. This is a decision you and your doctor will make. For butalbital and aspirin combinations, the following should be considered:

**Allergies**—Tell your doctor if you have ever had any unusual or allergic reaction to butalbital or other barbiturates; aspirin or other salicylates, including methyl salicylate (oil of wintergreen); caffeine; or any of the following medicines:

Diclofenac (e.g., Voltaren)
Diflunisal (e.g., Dolobid)
Etodolac (e.g., Lodine)
Fenoprofen (e.g., Nalfon)
Floctafenine (e.g., Idarac)
Flurbiprofen, oral (e.g., Ansaid)
Ibuprofen (e.g., Motrin)
Indomethacin (e.g., Indocin)
Ketoprofen (e.g., Orudis)
Ketorolac (e.g., Toradol)
Meclofenamate (e.g., Meclomen)
Mefenamic acid (e.g., Ponstel)
Nabumetone (e.g., Relafen)
Naproxen (e.g., Naprosyn)
Oxaprozin (e.g., Daypro)
Oxyphenbutazone (e.g., Tandearil)
Phenylbutazone (e.g., Butazolidin)
Piroxicam (e.g., Feldene)
Sulindac (e.g., Clinoril)
Suprofen (e.g., Suprol)
Tenoxicam (e.g., Mobiflex)
Tiaprofenic acid (e.g., Surgam)
Tolmetin (e.g., Tolectin)
Zomepirac (e.g., Zomax)

Also tell your health care professional if you are allergic to any other substances, such as foods, preservatives, or dyes.

**Pregnancy**—

* *For butalbital:* Barbiturates such as butalbital have been shown to increase the chance of birth defects in humans. Also, one study in humans has suggested that barbiturates taken during pregnancy may increase the chance of brain tumors in the baby. Butalbital may cause breathing problems in the newborn baby if taken just before or during delivery.

* *For aspirin:* Although studies in humans have not shown that aspirin causes birth defects, it has caused birth defects in animal studies.

*Do not take aspirin during the last 3 months of pregnancy unless it has been ordered by your doctor.* Some reports have suggested that use of aspirin late in pregnancy may cause a decrease in the newborn's weight and possible death of the fetus or newborn baby. However, the mothers in these reports had been taking much larger amounts of aspirin than are usually recommended. Studies of mothers taking aspirin in the doses that are usually recommended did not show these unwanted effects.

There is a chance that regular use of aspirin late in pregnancy may cause unwanted effects on the heart or blood flow in the fetus or in the newborn baby. Also, use of aspirin during the last 2 weeks of pregnancy may cause bleeding problems in the fetus before or during delivery or in the newborn baby. In addition, too much use of aspirin during the last 3 months of pregnancy may increase the length of pregnancy, prolong labor, cause other problems during delivery, or cause severe bleeding in the mother before, during, or after delivery.

* *For caffeine:* Studies in humans have not shown that caffeine causes birth defects. However, use of large amounts of caffeine during pregnancy may cause problems with the heart rhythm and the growth of the fetus. Also, studies in animals have shown that caffeine causes birth defects when given in very large doses (amounts equal to the amount in 12 to 24 cups of coffee a day).

**Breast-feeding**—Although this combination medicine has not been reported to cause problems, the chance always exists, especially if the medicine is taken for a long time or in large amounts.

- *For butalbital:* Barbiturates such as butalbital pass into the breast milk and may cause drowsiness, unusually slow heartbeat, shortness of breath, or troubled breathing in nursing babies.
- *For aspirin:* Aspirin passes into the breast milk. However, taking aspirin in the amounts present in these combination medicines has not been reported to cause problems in nursing babies.
- *For caffeine:* The caffeine in some of these combination medicines passes into the breast milk in small amounts. Taking caffeine in the amounts present in these medicines has not been reported to cause problems in nursing babies. However, studies have shown that nursing babies may appear jittery and have trouble in sleeping when their mothers drink large amounts of caffeine-containing beverages. Therefore, breast-feeding mothers who use caffeine-containing medicines should probably limit the amount of caffeine they take in from other medicines or from beverages.

**Children—**

- *For butalbital:* Although barbiturates such as butalbital often cause drowsiness, some children become excited after taking them.
- *For aspirin: Do not give a medicine containing aspirin to a child with fever or other symptoms of a virus infection, especially flu or chickenpox, without first discussing its use with your child's doctor.* This is very important because aspirin may cause a serious illness called Reye's syndrome in children with fever caused by a virus infection, especially flu or chickenpox. Children who do not have a virus infection may also be more sensitive to the effects of aspirin, especially if they have a fever or have lost large amounts of body fluid because of vomiting, diarrhea, or sweating. This may increase the chance of side effects during treatment.
- *For caffeine:* There is no specific information comparing use of caffeine in children up to 12 years of age with use in other age groups. However, caffeine is not expected to cause different side effects or problems in children than it does in adults.

**Teenagers—***Teenagers with fever or other symptoms of a virus infection, especially flu or chickenpox, should check with a doctor before taking this medicine.* The aspirin in this combination medicine may cause a serious illness called Reye's syndrome in teenagers with fever caused by a virus infection, especially flu or chickenpox.

**Older adults—**

- *For butalbital:* Confusion, depression, or excitement may be especially likely to occur in elderly patients, who are usually more sensitive than younger adults to the effects of butalbital.
- *For aspirin:* Elderly patients are more sensitive than younger adults to the effects of aspirin. This may increase the chance of side effects during treatment.
- *For caffeine:* Many medicines have not been studied specifically in older people. Therefore, it may not be

known whether they work exactly the same way they do in younger adults or if they cause different side effects or problems in older people. There is no specific information comparing use of caffeine in the elderly with use in other age groups.

**Other medicines—**Although certain medicines should not be used together at all, in other cases two different medicines may be used together even if an interaction might occur. In these cases, your doctor may want to change the dose, or other precautions may be necessary. When you are taking a butalbital and aspirin combination, it is especially important that your health care professional know if you are taking any of the following:

- Antacids, large amounts taken regularly, especially calcium- and/or magnesium-containing antacids or sodium bicarbonate (baking soda), or
- Urinary alkalizers (medicine that makes the urine less acid, such as acetazolamide [e.g., Diamox], dichlorphenamide [e.g., Daranide], methazolamide [e.g., Neptazane], potassium or sodium citrate and/or citric acid)—These medicines may cause aspirin to be removed from the body faster than usual, which may shorten the time that aspirin is effective; acetazolamide, dichlorphenamide, and methazolamide may also increase the chance of side effects when taken together with aspirin
- Anticoagulants (blood thinners) or
- Heparin—Use of these medicines together with aspirin may increase the chance of bleeding; also, butalbital may cause anticoagulants to be less effective
- Antidepressants, tricyclic (amitriptyline [e.g., Elavil], amoxapine [e.g., Asendin], clomipramine [e.g., Anafranil], desipramine [e.g., Pertofrane], doxepin [e.g., Sinequan], imipramine [e.g., Tofranil], nortriptyline [e.g., Aventyl], protriptyline [e.g., Vivactil], trimipramine [e.g., Surmontil]) or
- Central nervous system (CNS) depressants (medicines that often cause drowsiness)—These medicines may add to the effects of butalbital and increase the chance of drowsiness or other side effects
- Carbamazepine (e.g., Tegretol) or
- Contraceptives, oral (birth control pills), containing estrogen or
- Corticosteroids (cortisone-like medicines) or
- Corticotropin (e.g., ACTH)—Butalbital may make these medicines less effective
- Divalproex (e.g., Depakote) or
- Methotrexate (e.g., Folex, Mexate) or
- Valproic acid (e.g., Depakene) or
- Vancomycin (e.g., Vancocin)—The chance of serious side effects may be increased
- Probenecid (e.g., Benemid) or
- Sulfinpyrazone (e.g., Anturane)—Aspirin can keep these medicines from working properly for treating gout

**Other medical problems—**The presence of other medical problems may affect the use of butalbital and aspirin combinations. Make sure you tell your doctor if you have any other medical problems, especially:

- Alcohol abuse (or history of) or
- Drug abuse or dependence (or history of)—Dependence on butalbital may develop
- Asthma, especially if occurring together with other allergies and nasal polyps (or history of), or
- Emphysema or other chronic lung disease or

- Hyperactivity (in children) or
- Kidney disease or
- Liver disease—The chance of serious side effects may be increased
- Diabetes mellitus (sugar diabetes) or
- Mental depression or
- Overactive thyroid or
- Porphyria (or history of)—Butalbital may make these conditions worse
- Gout—Aspirin can make this condition worse and can also lessen the effects of some medicines used to treat gout
- Heart disease (severe)—The caffeine in some of these combination medicines can make some kinds of heart disease worse
- Hemophilia or other bleeding problems or
- Vitamin K deficiency—Aspirin increases the chance of serious bleeding
- Stomach ulcer, especially with a history of bleeding, or other stomach problems—Aspirin can make your condition worse

## Proper Use of This Medicine

*Take this medicine with food or a full glass (8 ounces) of water* to lessen stomach irritation.

*Do not take this medicine if it has a strong vinegar-like odor.* This odor means the aspirin in it is breaking down. If you have any questions about this, check with your health care professional.

*Take this medicine only as directed by your doctor.* Do not take more of it, do not take it more often, and do not take it for a longer time than your doctor ordered. If butalbital and aspirin combination is taken regularly (for example, every day), it may become habit-forming (causing mental or physical dependence). The caffeine in some butalbital and aspirin combinations can also increase the chance of dependence. Dependence is especially likely to occur in patients who take this medicine to relieve frequent headaches. Taking too much of this combination medicine can also lead to stomach problems or to other medical problems.

This medicine will relieve a headache best if you *take it as soon as the headache begins.* If you get warning signs of a migraine, take this medicine as soon as you are sure that the migraine is coming. This may even stop the headache pain from occurring. *Lying down in a quiet, dark room for a while after taking the medicine also helps to relieve headaches.*

People who get a lot of headaches may need to take a different medicine to help prevent headaches. *It is important that you follow your doctor's directions about taking the other medicine, even if your headaches continue to occur.* Headache-preventing medicines may take several weeks to start working. Even after they do start working, your headaches may not go away completely. However, your headaches should occur less often, and they should be less severe and easier to relieve than before. This will reduce the amount of headache relievers that you need. If you do not notice any improvement after

several weeks of headache-preventing treatment, check with your doctor.

**Dosing**—The dose of butalbital and aspirin combination medicines will be different for different patients. *Follow your doctor's orders or the directions on the label.* The following information includes only the average doses of the medicine. *If your dose is different, do not change it unless your doctor tells you to do so.*

*For Butalbital and Aspirin combination*

- For *oral* dosage form (tablets):
  —For tension headaches:
    - Adults—One tablet every four hours as needed. You should not take more than six tablets a day.
    - Children—Dose must be determined by your doctor.

*For Butalbital, Aspirin, and Caffeine combination*

- For *oral* dosage forms (capsules or tablets):
  —For tension headaches:
    - Adults—One or 2 capsules or tablets every four hours as needed. You should not take more than six capsules or tablets a day.
    - Children—Dose must be determined by your doctor.

**Missed dose**—If your doctor has ordered you to take this medicine according to a regular schedule and you miss a dose, take it as soon as you remember. However, if it is almost time for your next dose, skip the missed dose and go back to your regular dosing schedule. Do not double doses.

**Storage**—To store this medicine:

- Keep out of the reach of children. Overdose is especially dangerous in young children.
- Store away from heat and direct light.
- Do not store this medicine in the bathroom, near the kitchen sink, or in other damp places. Heat or moisture may cause the medicine to break down.
- Do not keep outdated medicine or medicine no longer needed. Be sure that any discarded medicine is out of the reach of children.

## Precautions While Using This Medicine

*Check with your doctor:*

- If the medicine stops working as well as it did when you first started using it. This may mean that you are in danger of becoming dependent on the medicine. *Do not try to get better pain relief by increasing the dose.*
- *If you are having headaches more often than you did before you started using this medicine.* This is especially important if a new headache occurs within 1 day after you took your last dose of headache medicine, headaches begin to occur every day, or a headache continues for several days in a row. This may mean that you are dependent on the headache medicine. *Continuing to take this medicine will cause*

*even more headaches later on.* Your doctor can give you advice on how to relieve the headaches.

*Check the labels of all nonprescription (over-the-counter [OTC]) and prescription medicines you now take. If any contain a barbiturate, aspirin, or other salicylates, including diflunisal, check with your health care professional.* Taking them together with this medicine may cause an overdose.

The butalbital in this medicine will add to the effects of alcohol and other CNS depressants (medicines that slow down the nervous system, possibly causing drowsiness). Some examples of CNS depressants are antihistamines or medicine for hay fever, other allergies, or colds; sedatives, tranquilizers, or sleeping medicine; other prescription pain medicine or narcotics; other barbiturates; medicine for seizures; muscle relaxants; or anesthetics, including some dental anesthetics. Also, stomach problems may be more likely to occur if you drink alcoholic beverages while you are taking aspirin. Therefore, *do not drink alcoholic beverages, and check with your doctor before taking any of the medicines listed above, while you are using this medicine.*

This medicine may cause some people to become drowsy, dizzy, or lightheaded. *Make sure you know how you react to this medicine before you drive, use machines, or do anything else that could be dangerous if you are dizzy or are not alert and clearheaded.*

Before having any kind of surgery (including dental surgery) or emergency treatment, tell the medical doctor or dentist in charge that you are taking this medicine. Serious side effects may occur if your medical doctor or dentist gives you certain other medicines without knowing that you have taken butalbital.

Do not take this medicine for 5 days before any planned surgery, including dental surgery, unless otherwise directed by your medical doctor or dentist. Taking aspirin during this time may cause bleeding problems.

Before you have any medical tests, tell the person in charge that you are taking this medicine. Caffeine (present in some butalbital and aspirin combinations) interferes with the results of certain tests that use dipyridamole (e.g., Persantine) to help show how well blood is flowing to your heart. Caffeine should not be taken for 8 to 12 hours before the test. The results of some other tests may also be affected by butalbital and aspirin combinations.

If you have been taking large amounts of this medicine, or if you have been taking it regularly for several weeks or more, *do not suddenly stop using it without first checking with your doctor.* Your doctor may want you to reduce gradually the amount you are taking before stopping completely, to lessen the chance of withdrawal side effects.

*If you think you or anyone else may have taken an overdose of this medicine, get emergency help at once.* Taking an overdose of this medicine or taking alcohol or CNS depressants with this medicine may lead to unconsciousness or death. Symptoms of overdose of this medicine include convulsions (seizures); hearing loss; confusion; ringing or buzzing in the ears; severe excitement, nervousness, or restlessness; severe dizziness; severe drowsiness; shortness of breath or troubled breathing; and severe weakness.

## Side Effects of This Medicine

Along with its needed effects, a medicine may cause some unwanted effects. Although not all of these side effects may occur, if they do occur they may need medical attention.

*The following side effects may mean that a serious allergic reaction is occurring. Check with your doctor or get emergency help immediately* if they occur, especially if several of them occur at the same time.

*Less common or rare*
Bluish discoloration or flushing or redness of skin (occurring together with other effects listed in this section); coughing, shortness of breath, troubled breathing, tightness in chest, or wheezing; difficulty in swallowing; dizziness or feeling faint (severe); hive-like swellings (large) on eyelids, face, lips, or tongue; skin rash, itching, or hives; stuffy nose (occurring together with other effects listed in this section)

*Also check with your doctor immediately* if any of the following side effects occur, especially if several of them occur together:

*Rare*
Bleeding or crusting sores on lips; chest pain; fever with or without chills; red, thickened, or scaly skin; sores, ulcers, or white spots in mouth (painful); sore throat (unexplained); tenderness, burning, or peeling of skin

*Symptoms of overdose*
Anxiety, confusion, excitement, irritability, nervousness, restlessness, or trouble in sleeping (severe, especially with products containing caffeine); convulsions (seizures, with products containing caffeine); diarrhea (severe or continuing); dizziness, lightheadedness, drowsiness, or weakness (severe); frequent urination (for products containing caffeine); hallucinations (seeing, hearing, or feeling things that are not there); increased sensitivity to touch or pain (for products containing caffeine); increased thirst; muscle trembling or twitching (for products containing caffeine); nausea or vomiting (severe or continuing), sometimes with blood; ringing or buzzing in ears (continuing) or hearing loss; seeing flashes of "zig-zag" lights (for products containing caffeine); slow, fast, or irregular heartbeat; slow, fast, irregular, or troubled breathing; slurred speech; staggering; stomach pain (severe); uncontrollable flapping movements of the hands, especially in elderly patients; unusual movements of the eyes; vision problems

Also, check with your doctor as soon as possible if any of the following side effects occur:

*Less common or rare*
Bloody or black, tarry stools; bloody urine; confusion or mental depression; muscle cramps or pain; pinpoint

red spots on skin; swollen or painful glands; unusual bleeding or bruising; unusual excitement (mild)

Other side effects may occur that usually do not need medical attention. These side effects may go away during treatment as your body adjusts to the medicine. However, check with your doctor if any of the following side effects continue or are bothersome:

*More common*

Bloated or "gassy" feeling; dizziness or lightheadedness (mild); drowsiness (mild); heartburn or indigestion; nausea, vomiting, or stomach pain (occurring without other symptoms of overdose)

Other side effects not listed above may also occur in some patients. If you notice any other effects, check with your doctor.

---

Revised: 07/14/92
Interim revision: 07/12/94

# CAFFEINE  Systemic

Some commonly used brand names are:

**In the U.S.—**

Caffedrine[1]
Caffedrine Caplets[1]
Dexitac[1]
Enerjets[1]
Keep Alert[1]
NoDoz[1]

NoDoz Maximum Strength
    Caplets[1]
Pep-Back[1]
Quick Pep[1]
Ultra Pep-Back[1]
Vivarin[1]

**In Canada—**

Caffedrine[1]
Wake-Up[1]

Note:  For quick reference, the following caffeine are numbered to match the corresponding brand names.

This information applies to the following medicines:
1. Caffeine (kaf-FEEN)
2. Citrated Caffeine (SIH-tray-ted)‡
3. Caffeine and Sodium Benzoate (SOE-dee-um BEN-zo-ate)†‡

†Not commercially available in Canada.
‡Generic name product may also be available in the U.S.

## Description

Caffeine (kaf-FEEN) belongs to the group of medicines called central nervous system (CNS) stimulants. It is used to help restore mental alertness when unusual tiredness or weakness or drowsiness occurs. Caffeine's use as an alertness aid should be only occasional. It is not intended to replace sleep and should not be used regularly for this purpose.

Caffeine is also used in combination with ergotamine (for treatment of migraine and cluster headaches) or with certain pain relievers, such as aspirin or aspirin and acetaminophen. When used in this way, caffeine may increase the effectiveness of the other medicines. Caffeine is sometimes used in combination with an antihistamine to overcome the drowsiness caused by the antihistamine.

Caffeine may also be used for other conditions as determined by your doctor.

Caffeine is present in coffee, tea, soft drinks, cocoa, and chocolate.

As a medicine, it is available without a prescription; however, your health care professional may have special instructions on its proper use. Caffeine is available in the following dosage forms:

*Oral*

Caffeine
• Extended-release capsules (U.S.)
• Tablets (U.S. and Canada)
Citrated caffeine
• Tablets (U.S.)

## Before Using This Medicine

If you are taking this medicine without a prescription, carefully read and follow any precautions on the label. For caffeine, the following should be considered:

**Allergies**—Tell your doctor if you have ever had any unusual or allergic reaction to aminophylline, caffeine, dyphylline, oxtriphylline, theobromine (also found in cocoa or chocolate), or theophylline. Also tell your health care professional if you are allergic to any other substances, such as foods, preservatives, or dyes.

**Pregnancy**—Studies in humans have shown that caffeine may cause miscarriage or may slow the growth of a developing fetus when given in doses greater than 300 mg a day. In addition, use of large amounts of caffeine by the mother during pregnancy may cause problems with the heart rhythm of the fetus. Therefore, it is recommended that pregnant women consume less than 300 mg of caffeine (an amount equal to 3 cups of coffee) a day. Studies in animals have shown that caffeine causes birth defects when given in very large doses (amounts equal to 12 to 24 cups of coffee a day) and problems with bone growth when given in smaller doses.

**Breast-feeding**—Caffeine passes into breast milk in small amounts and may build up in the nursing baby. Studies have shown that babies may appear jittery and have trouble in sleeping when their mothers drink large amounts of caffeine-containing beverages.

**Children**—With the exception of infants, there is no specific information comparing use of caffeine in children with use in other age groups. However, this medicine is not expected to cause different side effects or problems in children than it does in adults.

**Older adults**—Many medicines have not been studied specifically in older people. Therefore, it may not be known whether they work exactly the same way they do in younger adults or if they cause different side effects or problems in older people. There is no specific information comparing use of caffeine in the elderly with use in other age groups.

**Other medicines**—Although certain medicines should not be used together at all, in other cases 2 different medicines may be used together even if an interaction might occur. In these cases, your doctor may want to change the dose, or other precautions may be necessary. When you are taking caffeine, it is especially important that your health care professional know if you are taking any of the following:
• Amantadine (e.g., Symmetrel) or
• Amphetamines (e.g., Desoxyn, Dexedrine) or
• Appetite suppressants (diet pills), except fenfluramine (e.g., Pondimin), or
• Chlophedianol (e.g., Ulone) or
• Cocaine or
• Medicine for asthma or other breathing problems or
• Medicine for colds, sinus problems, hay fever or other allergies (including nose drops or sprays) or
• Methylphenidate (e.g., Ritalin) or
• Nabilone (e.g., Cesamet) or
• Other medicines or beverages containing caffeine or
• Pemoline (e.g., Cylert)—Using these medicines with caffeine may increase the CNS-stimulant effects, such as nervousness, irritability, or trouble in sleeping, or possibly cause convulsions (seizures) or changes in the rhythm of your heart

- Monoamine oxidase (MAO) inhibitors (furazolidone [e.g., Furoxone], isocarboxazid [e.g., Marplan], phenelzine [e.g., Nardil], procarbazine [e.g., Matulane], selegiline [e.g., Eldepryl], tranylcypromine [e.g., Parnate])—Taking large amounts of caffeine while you are taking or within 2 weeks of taking monoamine oxidase (MAO) inhibitors may cause extremely high blood pressure or dangerous changes in the rhythm of your heart; taking small amounts of caffeine may cause mild high blood pressure and fast heartbeat

**Other medical problems**—The presence of other medical problems may affect the use of caffeine. Make sure you tell your doctor if you have any other medical problems, especially:

- Agoraphobia (fear of being in open places) or
- Anxiety or
- Heart disease or
- High blood pressure or
- Panic attacks or
- Trouble in sleeping—Caffeine may make the condition worse
- Liver disease—Higher blood levels of caffeine may result, increasing the chance of side effects

## Proper Use of This Medicine

For patients taking the *extended-release form* of this medicine:

- Swallow the capsule whole.
- Do not break, crush, or chew the capsule before swallowing.

*Take caffeine in capsule or tablet form only as directed.* Do not take more of it, do not take it more often, and do not take it for a longer time than directed. Taking too much may increase the chance of side effects. It may also become habit-forming.

If you think this medicine is not working properly after you have taken it for a long time, *do not increase the dose.* To do so may increase the chance of side effects.

**Dosing**—The dose of caffeine will be different for different patients. *Follow the directions on the label.*

- For unusual tiredness or weakness, or drowsiness:
  —For *long-acting* dosage forms (extended-release capsules):
    - Adults and children 12 years of age and older—The usual dose is 200 to 250 milligrams (mg) of caffeine every three or four hours. You should not take more than 1 gram in twenty-four hours.
    - Children up to 12 years of age—Use is not recommended.
  —For *regular* (short-acting) dosage forms (tablets):
    - Adults and children 12 years of age and older—The usual dose is 100 to 200 mg of caffeine every three or four hours. You should not take more than 1 gram in twenty-four hours.
    - Children up to 12 years of age—Use is not recommended.

—For citrated caffeine (tablets):
  - Adults and children 12 years of age and older—The usual dose is 65 to 325 mg of caffeine three times a day, as needed. You should not take more than 1 gram in twenty-four hours.
  - Children up to 12 years of age—Use is not recommended.

**Storage**—To store this medicine:

- Keep out of the reach of children.
- Store away from heat and direct light.
- Do not store in the bathroom, near the kitchen sink, or in other damp places. Heat or moisture may cause the medicine to break down.
- Do not keep outdated medicine or medicine no longer needed. Be sure that any discarded medicine is out of the reach of children.

## Precautions While Using This Medicine

*Capsules or tablets containing caffeine are for occasional use only. They are not intended to replace sleep and should not be used regularly for this purpose. If unusual tiredness or weakness or drowsiness continues or returns often, check with your doctor.*

The recommended dose of this medicine contains about the same amount of caffeine as a cup of coffee. Do not drink large amounts of caffeine-containing coffee, tea, or soft drinks while you are taking this medicine. Also, do not take large amounts of other medicines that contain caffeine. To do so may cause unwanted effects.

The amount of caffeine in some common foods and beverages is as follows:

- Coffee, brewed—40 to 180 milligrams (mg) per cup.
- Coffee, instant—30 to 120 mg per cup.
- Coffee, decaffeinated—3 to 5 mg per cup.
- Tea, brewed American—20 to 90 mg per cup.
- Tea, brewed imported—25 to 110 mg per cup.
- Tea, instant—28 mg per cup.
- Tea, canned iced—22 to 36 mg per 12 ounces.
- Cola and other soft drinks, caffeine-containing—36 to 90 mg per 12 ounces.
- Cola and other soft drinks, decaffeinated—0 mg per 12 ounces.
- Cocoa—4 mg per cup.
- Chocolate, milk—3 to 6 mg per ounce.
- Chocolate, bittersweet—25 mg per ounce.

*Caffeine may cause nervousness or irritability, trouble in sleeping, dizziness, or a fast or pounding heartbeat. If these effects occur, discontinue the use of caffeine-containing beverages or medicines, or large amounts of chocolate-containing products.*

To prevent trouble in sleeping, do not take caffeine-containing beverages or medicines too close to bedtime.

## Side Effects of This Medicine

Along with its needed effects, a medicine may cause some unwanted effects. Although not all of these side effects may occur, they may be more likely to occur if caffeine is taken in large doses or more often than recommended. If they do occur, they may need medical attention.

Check with your doctor as soon as possible if any of the following side effects occur:

*More common*
> Diarrhea; dizziness; fast heartbeat; irritability, nervousness, or severe jitters in newborn babies; nausea (severe); tremors; trouble in sleeping; vomiting

*Symptoms of overdose*
> Abdominal or stomach pain; agitation, anxiety, excitement, or restlessness; confusion or delirium; convulsions (seizures)—in acute overdose; fast or irregular heartbeat; fever; frequent urination; headache; increased sensitivity to touch or pain; irritability; muscle trembling or twitching; nausea and vomiting, sometimes with blood; painful, swollen abdomen or vomiting in newborn babies; ringing or other sounds in ears; seeing flashes of "zig-zag" lights; trouble in sleeping; whole-body tremors in newborn babies

Other side effects may occur that usually do not need medical attention. These side effects may go away during treatment as your body adjusts to the medicine. However, check with your doctor if any of the following side effects continue or are bothersome:

*More common*
> Nausea (mild); nervousness or jitters (mild)

After you stop using this medicine, your body may need time to adjust. The length of time this takes depends on the amount of medicine you were using and how long you used it. During this time check with your doctor if you notice any of the following side effects:

*More common*
> Anxiety; dizziness; headache; irritability; muscle tension; nausea; nervousness; stuffy nose; unusual tiredness

Other side effects not listed above may also occur in some patients. If you notice any other effects, check with your doctor.

## Additional Information

Once a medicine has been approved for marketing for a certain use, experience may show that it is also useful for other medical problems. Although these uses are not included in product labeling, caffeine is used in certain patients with the following medical conditions:

- Neonatal apnea (breathing problems in newborn babies)
- Postoperative infant apnea (breathing problems after surgery in young babies)
- Psychiatric disorders requiring electroconvulsive or shock therapy (ECT)

Other than the above information, there is no additional information relating to proper use, precautions, or side effects for these uses.

Revised: 07/12/94

# CALCITONIN    Systemic

Some commonly used brand names are:

**In the U.S.—**
Calcimar[2]                    Miacalcin[2]
Cibacalcin[1]

**In Canada—**
Calcimar[2]

Note: For quick reference, the following calcitonin are numbered to match the corresponding brand names.

This information applies to the following medicines:
1. Calcitonin-Human†
2. Calcitonin-Salmon

†Not commercially available in Canada.

## Description

Calcitonin (kal-si-TOE-nin) is used to treat Paget's disease of bone. It also may be used to prevent continuing bone loss in women with postmenopausal osteoporosis and to treat hypercalcemia (too much calcium in the blood). This medicine may be used to treat other conditions as determined by your doctor.

Calcitonin is available only with your doctor's prescription, in the following dosage forms:

*Parenteral*
Calcitonin-Human
- Injection (U.S.)
Calcitonin-Salmon
- Injection (U.S. and Canada)

## Before Using This Medicine

In deciding to use a medicine, the risks of taking the medicine must be weighed against the good it will do. This is a decision you and your doctor will make. For calcitonin, the following should be considered:

**Allergies**—Tell your doctor if you have ever had any unusual or allergic reaction to calcitonin or other proteins. Also tell your health care professional if you are allergic to any other substances, such as foods, preservatives, or dyes.

**Diet**—Make certain your health care professional knows if your diet includes large amounts of calcium-containing foods and/or vitamin D–containing foods, such as milk or other dairy products. Calcium and vitamin D may cause the calcitonin to be less effective in treating a high blood calcium. Also let your health care professional know if you are on any special diet, such as low-sodium or low-sugar diet.

**Pregnancy**—Calcitonin has not been studied in pregnant women. However, in animal studies, calcitonin has been shown to lower the birth weight of the baby when the mother was given a dose of calcitonin many times the human dose.

**Breast-feeding**—Calcitonin has not been reported to cause problems in nursing babies. However, studies in animals have shown that calcitonin may decrease the flow of breast milk.

**Children**—Studies on this medicine have been done only in adult patients, and there is no specific information comparing the use of calcitonin in children with use in other age groups. Therefore, be sure to discuss with your doctor the use of this medicine in children.

**Older adults**—Many medicines have not been studied specifically in older people. Therefore, it may not be known whether they work exactly the same way they do in younger adults. Although there is no specific information comparing the use of calcitonin in the elderly with use in other age groups, this medicine is not expected to cause different side effects or problems in older people than it does in younger adults. Calcitonin is often used in elderly patients.

**Other medicine**—Although certain medicines should not be used together at all, in other cases two different medicines may be used together even if an interaction might occur. In these cases, your doctor may want to change the dose, or other precautions may be necessary. Tell your health care professional if you are using any other prescription or nonprescription (over-the-counter [OTC]) medicine.

---

## Proper Use of This Medicine

This medicine is for injection only. If you will be giving yourself the injections, make sure you understand exactly how to give them, including how to fill the syringe before injection. If you have any questions about this, check with your doctor.

Use the calcitonin only when the contents of the syringe are clear and colorless. Do not use it if it looks grainy or discolored.

**Dosing**—The dose of calcitonin will be different for different patients. *Follow your doctor's orders or the directions on the label.* The following information includes only the average doses of calcitonin. *If your dose is different, do not change it* unless your doctor tells you to do so.

*The number of doses you receive, the time allowed between doses, and the length of time you receive the medicine depends on the medical problem for which you are receiving calcitonin.*

*For calcitonin-human*

- For *injection* dosage form:
  —For Paget's disease of bone:
    - Adults—To start, 500 micrograms (mcg) injected under the skin once a day. Your doctor may reduce your dose or increase the time between doses. Or, your doctor may give you a smaller dose to start and increase your dose over two weeks.
    - Children—Dose must be determined by your doctor.

*For calcitonin-salmon*

- For *injection* dosage form:
  —For Paget's disease of bone:
    - Adults—To start, 100 Units injected into a muscle or under the skin once a day, once every other day, or three times a week. Your doctor may reduce your dose or increase the time between doses.
    - Children—Dose must be determined by your doctor.
  —For hypercalcemia (too much calcium in the blood):
    - Adults—To start, 4 Units per kilogram (kg) (1.8 Units per pound) of body weight injected into a muscle or under the skin every twelve hours. Your doctor may increase your dose or increase the time between doses.
    - Children—Dose must be determined by your doctor.
  —For postmenopausal osteoporosis:
    - Adults—100 Units injected into a muscle or under the skin once a day, once every other day, or three times a week. Or, your doctor may give you a smaller dose to start and increase your dose over two weeks.
    - Children—Dose must be determined by your doctor.

**Missed dose**—If you miss a dose of this medicine and your dosing schedule is:

- Two doses a day—If you remember within 2 hours of the missed dose, give it right away. Then go back to your regular dosing schedule. But if you do not remember the missed dose until later, skip it and go back to your regular dosing schedule. Do not double doses.
- One dose a day—Give the missed dose as soon as possible. Then go back to your regular dosing schedule. If you do not remember the missed dose until the next day, skip it and go back to your regular dosing schedule. Do not double doses.
- One dose every other day—Give the missed dose as soon as possible if you remember it on the day it

should be given. Then go back to your regular dosing schedule. If you do not remember the missed dose until the next day, give it at that time. Then skip a day and start your dosing schedule again.
- One dose three times a week—Give the missed dose the next day. Then set each injection back a day for the rest of the week. Go back to your regular Monday-Wednesday-Friday schedule the following week. Do not double doses.

If you have any questions about this, check with your doctor.

**Storage**—To store this medicine:
- Keep out of the reach of children.
- Store away from heat and direct light.
- Store *calcitonin-human* at a temperature below 77 °F. Do not refrigerate. Use prepared solution within 6 hours.
- Store *calcitonin-salmon* in the refrigerator. However, keep it from freezing.
- Do not keep outdated medicine or medicine no longer needed. Be sure that any discarded medicine is out of the reach of children.

## Precautions While Using This Medicine

Your doctor should check your progress at regular visits to make sure that this medicine does not cause unwanted effects.

If you are using this medicine for hypercalcemia (too much calcium in the blood), your doctor may want you to follow a low-calcium diet. If you have any questions about this, check with your doctor.

## Side Effects of This Medicine

Along with its needed effects, a medicine may cause some unwanted effects. Although not all of these side effects may occur, if they do occur they may need medical attention.

Check with your doctor as soon as possible if either of the following side effects occurs:

*Rare*

Skin rash or hives

Other side effects may occur that usually do not need medical attention. These side effects may go away during treatment as your body adjusts to the medicine. However, check with your doctor if any of the following side effects continue or are bothersome:

*More common*

Diarrhea; flushing or redness of face, ears, hands, or feet; loss of appetite; nausea or vomiting; pain, redness, soreness, or swelling at place of injection; stomach pain

*Less common*

Increased frequency of urination

*Rare*

Chills; dizziness; headache; pressure in chest; stuffy nose; tenderness or tingling of hands or feet; trouble in breathing; weakness

Other side effects not listed above may also occur in some patients. If you notice any other effects, check with your doctor.

## Additional Information

Once a medicine has been approved for marketing for a certain use, experience may show that it is also useful for other medical problems. Although this use is not included in product labeling, calcitonin is used in certain patients with the following medical condition:
- Osteoporosis caused by hormone problems, certain drugs, and other causes

Other than the above information, there is no additional information relating to proper use, precautions, or side effects for this use.

Annual revision: 05/13/92
Interim revision: 06/27/94

# CALCIUM CHANNEL BLOCKING AGENTS   Systemic

Some commonly used brand names are:

**In the U.S.—**

| | |
|---|---|
| Adalat[7] | DynaCirc[5] |
| Adalat CC[7] | Isoptin[9] |
| Bepadin[1] | Isoptin SR[9] |
| Calan[9] | Nimotop[8] |
| Calan SR[9] | Plendil[3] |
| Cardene[6] | Procardia[7] |
| Cardizem[2] | Procardia XL[7] |
| Cardizem CD[2] | Vascor[1] |
| Cardizem SR | Verelan[9] |
| Dilacor-XR[2] | |

**In Canada—**

| | |
|---|---|
| Adalat[7] | Nimotop[8] |
| Adalat FT[7] | Novo-Diltazem[2] |
| Adalat P.A.[7] | Novo-Nifedin[7] |
| Apo-Diltiaz[2] | Novo-Veramil[9] |
| Apo-Nifed[7] | Nu-Diltiaz[2] |
| Apo-Verap[9] | Nu-Nifed[7] |
| Cardene[6] | Nu-Verap[9] |
| Cardizem[2] | Plendil[3] |
| Cardizem SR[2] | Renedil[3] |
| Isoptin[9] | Sibelium[4] |
| Isoptin SR[9] | Syn-Diltiazem[2] |

Note: For quick reference, the following calcium channel blocking agents are numbered to match the corresponding brand names.

This information applies to the following medicines:
1. Bepridil (BE-pri-dil)†
2. Diltiazem (dil-TYE-a-zem)§
3. Felodipine (fe-LOE-di-peen)
4. Flunarizine (floo-NAR-i-zeen)*
5. Isradipine (is-RA-di-peen)†
6. Nicardipine (nye-KAR-de-peen)
7. Nifedipine (nye-FED-i-peen)‡
8. Nimodipine (nye-MOE-di-peen)
9. Verapamil (ver-AP-a-mil)‡§

*Not commercially available in the U.S.
†Not commercially available in Canada.
‡Generic name product may also be available in the U.S.
§Generic name product may also be available in Canada.

## Description

Bepridil, diltiazem, felodipine, flunarizine, isradipine, nicardipine, nifedipine, nimodipine, and verapamil belong to the group of medicines called calcium channel blockers.

Calcium channel blocking agents affect the movement of calcium into the cells of the heart and blood vessels. As a result, they relax blood vessels and increase the supply of blood and oxygen to the heart while reducing its workload.

Some of the calcium channel blocking agents are used to relieve and control angina pectoris (chest pain).

Some are also used to treat high blood pressure (hypertension). High blood pressure adds to the workload of the heart and arteries. If it continues for a long time, the heart and arteries may not function properly. This can damage the blood vessels of the brain, heart, and kidneys, resulting in a stroke, heart failure, or kidney failure. High blood pressure may also increase the risk of heart attacks. These problems may be less likely to occur if blood pressure is controlled.

Flunarizine is used to prevent migraine headaches.

Nimodipine is used to prevent and treat problems caused by a burst blood vessel in the head (also known as a ruptured aneurysm or subarachnoid hemorrhage).

Other calcium channel blocking agents may also be used for these and other conditions as determined by your doctor.

These medicines are available only with your doctor's prescription, in the following dosage forms:

*Oral*
Bepridil
  • Tablets (U.S.)
Diltiazem
  • Extended-release capsules (U.S. and Canada)
  • Tablets (U.S. and Canada)
Felodipine
  • Extended-release tablets (U.S. and Canada)
Flunarizine
  • Capsules (Canada)
Isradipine
  • Capsules (U.S.)
Nicardipine
  • Capsules (U.S. and Canada)

Nifedipine
  • Capsules (U.S. and Canada)
  • Tablets (Canada)
  • Extended-release tablets (U.S. and Canada)
Nimodipine
  • Capsules (U.S. and Canada)
Verapamil
  • Extended-release capsules (U.S.)
  • Tablets (U.S. and Canada)
  • Extended-release tablets (U.S. and Canada)

*Parenteral*
Diltiazem
  • Injection (U.S.)
Verapamil
  • Injection (U.S. and Canada)

## Before Using This Medicine

In deciding to use a medicine, the risks of taking the medicine must be weighed against the good it will do. This is a decision you and your doctor will make. For the calcium channel blocking agents, the following should be considered:

**Allergies**—Tell your doctor if you have ever had any unusual or allergic reaction to bepridil, diltiazem, felodipine, flunarizine, isradipine, nicardipine, nifedipine, nimodipine, or verapamil. Also tell your health care professional if you are allergic to any other substances, such as foods, preservatives, or dyes.

**Pregnancy**—Calcium channel blockers have not been studied in pregnant women. However, studies in animals have shown that large doses of calcium channel blockers cause birth defects, prolonged pregnancy, poor bone development, and stillbirth.

**Breast-feeding**—Although bepridil, diltiazem, nifedipine, verapamil, and possibly other calcium channel blockers, pass into breast milk, they have not been reported to cause problems in nursing babies.

**Children**—Although there is no specific information comparing use of this medicine in children with use in other age groups, it is not expected to cause different side effects or problems in children than it does in adults.

**Older adults**—Elderly people may be especially sensitive to the effects of calcium channel blockers. This may increase the chance of side effects during treatment.

**Other medicines**—Although certain medicines should not be used together at all, in other cases two different medicines may be used together even if an interaction might occur. In these cases, your doctor may want to change the dose, or other precautions may be necessary. When taking calcium channel blockers it is especially important that your health care professional know if you are taking any of the following:
  • Acetazolamide (e.g., Diamox) or
  • Amphotericin B by injection (e.g., Fungizone) or
  • Corticosteroids (cortisone-like medicine) or
  • Dichlorphenamide (e.g., Daranide) or

- Diuretics (water pills) or
- Methazolamide (e.g., Naptazane)—These medicines can cause hypokalemia (low levels of potassium in the body), which can increase the unwanted effects of bepridil
- Beta-blockers (acebutolol [e.g., Sectral], atenolol [e.g., Tenormin], betaxolol [e.g., Kerlone], carteolol [e.g., Cartrol], labetalol [e.g., Normodyne], metoprolol [e.g., Lopressor], nadolol [e.g., Corgard], oxprenolol [e.g., Trasicor], penbutolol [e.g., Levatol], pindolol [e.g., Visken], propranolol [e.g., Inderal], sotalol [e.g., Sotacor], timolol [e.g., Blocadren])—Effects of both may be increased. In addition, unwanted effects may occur if a calcium channel blocker or a beta-blocker is stopped suddenly after use together
- Carbamazepine (e.g., Tegretol) or
- Cyclosporine (e.g., Sandimmune) or
- Procainamide (e.g., Pronestyl) or
- Quinidine (e.g., Quinidex)—Effects of these medicines may be increased if they are used with some calcium channel blockers
- Digitalis glycosides (heart medicine)—Effects of these medicines may be increased if they are used with some calcium channel blockers
- Disopyramide (e.g., Norpace)—Effects of some calcium channel blockers on the heart may be increased

Also, tell your health care professional if you are using any of the following medicines in the eye:
- Betaxolol (e.g., Betoptic) or
- Levobunolol (e.g., Betagan) or
- Metipranolol (e.g., OptiPranolol) or
- Timolol (e.g., Timoptic)—Effects on the heart and blood pressure may be increased

**Other medical problems**—The presence of other medical problems may affect the use of the calcium channel blockers. Make sure you tell your doctor if you have any other medical problems, especially:
- Heart rhythm problems (history of)—Bepridil can cause serious heart rhythm problems
- Kidney disease or
- Liver disease—Effects of the calcium channel blocker may be increased
- Mental depression (history of)—Flunarizine may cause mental depression
- Parkinson's disease or similar problems—Flunarizine can cause parkinsonian-like effects
- Other heart or blood vessel disorders—Calcium channel blockers may make some heart conditions worse

## Proper Use of This Medicine

*Take this medicine exactly as directed* even if you feel well and do not notice any signs of chest pain. Do not take more of this medicine and do not take it more often than your doctor ordered. Do not miss any doses.

For patients taking *bepridil:*
- If this medicine causes upset stomach, it can be taken with meals or at bedtime.

For patients taking *diltiazem extended-release capsules:*
- Swallow the capsule whole, without crushing or chewing it.

- *Do not change to another brand without checking with your physician.* Different brands have different doses. If you refill your medicine and it looks different, check with your pharmacist.

For patients taking *nifedipine or verapamil extended-release capsules:*
- Swallow the capsule whole, without crushing or chewing it.

For patients taking *regular nifedipine or extended-release felodipine or nifedipine tablets:*
- Swallow the tablet whole, without breaking, crushing, or chewing it.
- If you are taking *Procardia XL*, you may sometimes notice what looks like a tablet in your stool. That is just the empty shell that is left after the medicine has been absorbed into your body.

For patients taking *verapamil extended-release tablets:*
- Swallow the tablet whole, without crushing or chewing it. However, if your doctor tells you to, you may break the tablet in half.
- Take the medicine with food or milk.

For patients taking this medicine *for high blood pressure:*
- In addition to the use of the medicine your doctor has prescribed, appropriate treatment for your high blood pressure may include weight control and care in the types of food you eat, especially foods high in sodium (salt). Your doctor will tell you which factors are most important for you. You should check with your doctor before changing your diet.
- Many patients who have high blood pressure will not notice any signs of the problem. In fact, many may feel normal. It is very important that you *take your medicine exactly as directed* and that you keep your appointments with your doctor even if you feel well.
- Remember that this medicine will not cure your high blood pressure but it does help control it. Therefore, you must continue to take it as directed if you expect to lower your blood pressure and keep it down. *You may have to take high blood pressure medicine for the rest of your life.* If high blood pressure is not treated, it can cause serious problems such as heart failure, blood vessel disease, stroke, or kidney disease.

**Dosing**—The dose of these medicines will be different for different patients. *Follow your doctor's orders or the directions on the label.* The following information includes only the average doses of these medicines. *If your dose is different, do not change it* unless your doctor tells you to do so.

The number of capsules or tablets that you take depends on the strength of the medicine. Also, *the number of doses you take each day, the time allowed between doses, and the length of time you take the medicine depend on the medical problem for which you are taking calcium channel blocking agents.*

*For bepridil*
- For *oral* dosage form (tablets):
  —For angina (chest pain):
  - Adults—200 to 300 milligrams (mg) once a day.
  - Children—Use and dose must be determined by your doctor.

*For diltiazem*
- For *long-acting oral* dosage form (extended-release capsules):
  —For high blood pressure:
  - Adults and teenagers—
    —For *Cardizem CD* or *Dilacor-XR:* 180 to 240 milligrams (mg) once a day.
    —For *Cardizem SR:* 60 to 120 mg two times a day.
  - Children—Dose must be determined by your doctor.
- For *regular (short-acting) oral* dosage form (tablets):
  —For angina (chest pain):
  - Adults and teenagers—30 mg three or four times a day. Your doctor may gradually increase your dose as needed.
  - Children—Dose must be determined by your doctor.
- For *injection* dosage form:
  —For arrhythmias (irregular heartbeat):
  - Adults and teenagers—Dose is based on body weight and must be determined by your doctor.
  - Children—Use and dose must be determined by your doctor.

*For felodipine*
- For *long-acting oral* dosage form (extended-release tablets):
  —For high blood pressure:
  - Adults—5 to 10 milligrams (mg) once a day.
  - Children—Use and dose must be determined by your doctor.
  —For angina (chest pain):
  - Adults—10 mg once a day.
  - Children—Use and dose must be determined by your doctor.

*For flunarizine*
- For *oral* dosage form (capsules):
  —To prevent headaches:
  - Adults—10 milligrams (mg) once a day in the evening.
  - Children—Dose must be determined by your doctor.

*For isradipine*
- For *oral* dosage form (capsules):
  —For high blood pressure:
  - Adults—2.5 milligrams (mg) two times a day. Your doctor may increase your dose as needed.
  - Children—Use and dose must be determined by your doctor.

*For nicardipine*
- For *oral* dosage form (capsules):
  —For high blood pressure or angina (chest pain):
  - Adults and teenagers—20 milligrams (mg) three times a day.
  - Children—Dose must be determined by your doctor.

*For nifedipine*
- For *regular (short-acting) oral* dosage form (capsules or tablets):
  —For high blood pressure or angina (chest pain):
  - Adults and teenagers—10 milligrams (mg) three times a day. Your doctor may increase your dose as needed.
  - Children—Dose must be determined by your doctor.
- For *long-acting oral* dosage form (extended-release tablets):
  —For high blood pressure or angina (chest pain):
  - Adults and teenagers—
    —For *Adalat CC* or *Procardia XL:* 30 or 60 mg once a day. Your doctor may increase your dose as needed.
    —For *Adalat P.A.:* 20 mg two times a day. Your doctor may increase your dose as needed.
  - Children—Dose must be determined by your doctor.

*For nimodipine*
- For *oral* dosage form (capsules):
  —To treat a burst blood vessel in the head:
  - Adults—60 milligrams (mg) every four hours.
  - Children—Dose must be determined by your doctor.

*For verapamil*
- For *regular (short-acting) oral* dosage form (tablets):
  —For angina (chest pain), arrhythmias (irregular heartbeat), or high blood pressure:
  - Adults and teenagers—40 to 120 milligrams (mg) three times a day. Your doctor may increase your dose as needed.
  - Children—Dose is based on body weight and must be determined by your doctor. The usual dose is 4 to 8 mg per kilogram (kg) (1.82 to 3.64 mg per pound) of body weight a day. This is divided into smaller doses.
- For *long-acting oral* dosage form (extended-release capsules):
  —For high blood pressure:
  - Adults and teenagers—240 to 480 mg once a day.
  - Children—Dose must be determined by your doctor.

- For *long-acting oral* dosage form (extended-release tablets):
  —For high blood pressure:
  - Adults and teenagers—120 mg once a day to 240 mg every twelve hours.
  - Children—Dose must be determined by your doctor.
- For *injection* dosage form:
  —For arrhythmias (irregular heartbeat):
  - Adults—5 to 10 mg slowly injected into a vein. The dose may be repeated after thirty minutes.
  - Children—Dose is based on body weight and must be determined by your doctor.
    —Infants up to 1 year of age: 100 to 200 micrograms (mcg) per kg (45.5 to 90.9 mcg per pound) of body weight injected slowly into a vein. The dose may be repeated after thirty minutes.
    —Children 1 to 15 years of age: 100 to 300 mcg per kg (45.5 to 136.4 mcg per pound) of body weight injected slowly into a vein. The dose may be repeated after thirty minutes.

**Missed dose**—If you miss a dose of this medicine, take it as soon as possible. However, if it is almost time for your next dose, skip the missed dose and go back to your regular dosing schedule. Do not double doses.

**Storage**—To store this medicine:
- Keep out of the reach of children.
- Store away from heat and direct light.
- Do not store in the bathroom, near the kitchen sink, or in other damp places. Heat or moisture may cause the medicine to break down.
- Do not keep outdated medicine or medicine no longer needed. Be sure that any discarded medicine is out of the reach of children.

## Precautions While Using This Medicine

It is important that your doctor check your progress at regular visits. This will allow your doctor to make sure the medicine is working properly and to change the dosage if needed.

If you have been using this medicine regularly for several weeks, do not suddenly stop using it. Stopping suddenly may bring on your previous problem. Check with your doctor for the best way to reduce gradually the amount you are taking before stopping completely.

Chest pain resulting from exercise or physical exertion is usually reduced or prevented by this medicine. This may tempt you to be overly active. *Make sure you discuss with your doctor a safe amount of exercise for your medical problem.*

After taking a dose of this medicine you may get a headache that lasts for a short time. This effect is more common if you are taking felodipine, isradipine, or nifedipine. This should become less noticeable after you have taken this medicine for a while. If this effect continues or if the headaches are severe, check with your doctor.

In some patients, tenderness, swelling, or bleeding of the gums may appear soon after treatment with this medicine is started. Brushing and flossing your teeth carefully and regularly and massaging your gums may help prevent this. *See your dentist regularly to have your teeth cleaned. Check with your medical doctor or dentist if you have any questions about how to take care of your teeth and gums, or if you notice any tenderness, swelling, or bleeding of your gums.*

For patients taking *bepridil, diltiazem,* or *verapamil:*
- *Ask your doctor how to count your pulse rate. Then, while you are taking this medicine, check your pulse regularly.* If it is much slower than your usual rate, or less than 50 beats per minute, check with your doctor. A pulse rate that is too slow may cause circulation problems.

For patients taking *flunarizine:*
- This medicine may cause some people to become drowsy or less alert than they are normally. This is more likely to happen when you begin to take it or when you increase the amount of medicine you are taking. *Make sure you know how you react to this medicine before you drive, use machines, or do anything else that could be dangerous if you are not alert.*

For patients taking this medicine *for high blood pressure:*
- *Do not take other medicines unless they have been discussed with your doctor.* This especially includes over-the-counter (nonprescription) medicines for appetite control, asthma, colds, cough, hay fever, or sinus problems, since they may tend to increase your blood pressure.

## Side Effects of This Medicine

Along with its needed effects, a medicine may cause some unwanted effects. Although not all of these side effects may occur, if they do occur they may need medical attention.

Not all of the side effects listed below have been reported for each of these medicines, but they have been reported for at least one of them. Since many of the effects of calcium channel blockers are similar, some of these side effects may occur with any of these medicines. However, they may be more common with some of these medicines than with others.

Check with your doctor as soon as possible if any of the following side effects occur:

*Less common*
  Breathing difficulty, coughing, or wheezing; irregular or fast, pounding heartbeat; skin rash; slow heartbeat (less than 50 beats per minute—bepridil, diltiazem, and verapamil only); swelling of ankles, feet, or lower legs (more common with felodipine and nifedipine)

*For flunarizine only—less common*

  Loss of balance control; mask-like face; mental depression; shuffling walk; stiffness of arms or legs; trembling and shaking of hands and fingers; trouble in speaking or swallowing

*Rare*

  Bleeding, tender, or swollen gums; chest pain (may appear about 30 minutes after medicine is taken); fainting; painful, swollen joints (for nifedipine only); trouble in seeing (for nifedipine only)

*For flunarizine and verapamil only—rare*

  Unusual secretion of milk

Other side effects may occur that usually do not need medical attention. These side effects may go away during treatment as your body adjusts to the medicine. However, check with your doctor if any of the following side effects continue or are bothersome:

*More common*

  Drowsiness (for flunarizine only); increased appetite and/or weight gain (for flunarizine only)

*Less common*

  Constipation; diarrhea; dizziness or lightheadedness (more common with bepridil and nifedipine); dryness of mouth (for flunarizine only); flushing and feeling of warmth (more common with nicardipine and nifedipine); headache (more common with felodipine, isradipine, and nifedipine); nausea (more common with bepridil and nifedipine); unusual tiredness or weakness

Other side effects not listed above may also occur in some patients. If you notice any other effects, check with your doctor.

## Additional Information

Once a medicine has been approved for marketing for a certain use, experience may show that it is also useful for other medical problems. Although these uses are not included in product labeling, calcium channel blockers are used in certain patients with the following medical conditions:

  • Hypertrophic cardiomyopathy (a heart condition) (verapamil)
  • Raynaud's phenomenon (circulation problems) (nicardipine and nifedipine)

Other than the above information, there is no additional information relating to proper use, precautions, or side effects for these uses.

Revised: 08/21/92
Interim revision: 09/07/94

# CALCIUM SUPPLEMENTS    Systemic

Some commonly used brand names are:

**In the U.S.—**

| | |
|---|---|
| BioCal[1] | Mallamint[1] |
| Calcarb 600[1] | Neo-Calglucon[4] |
| Calci-Chew[1] | Nephro-Calci[1] |
| Calciday 667[1] | Os-Cal 500[1] |
| Calcilac[1] | Oysco[1] |
| Calcium 600[1] | Oysco 500 Chewable[1] |
| Calglycine[1] | Oyst-Cal 500[1] |
| Calphosan[7] | Oyst-Cal 500 Chewable[1] |
| Caltrate 600[1] | Oystercal 500[1] |
| Chooz[1] | Posture[11] |
| Citracal[3] | Rolaids Calcium Rich[1] |
| Citracal Liquitabs[3] | Super Calcium 1200[1] |
| Dicarbosil[1] | Titralac[1] |
| Gencalc[1] | Tums[1] |
| Kalcinate[6] | Tums E-X[1] |

**In Canada—**

| | |
|---|---|
| Apo-Cal[1] | Caltrate 300[1] |
| Calciject[2] | Caltrate 600[1] |
| Calcite 500[1] | Caltrate Chewable[1] |
| Calcium 500[1] | Gramcal[9] |
| Calcium-Sandoz[4] | Mega-Cal[1] |
| Calcium-Sandoz Forte[9] | Nu-Cal[1] |
| Calcium Stanley[5] | Os-Cal[1] |
| Calsan[1] | Os-Cal Chewable[1] |

Note: For quick reference, the following calcium supplements are numbered to match the corresponding brand names.

This information applies to the following medicines:

1. Calcium Carbonate (KAL-see-um KAR-boh-nate)‡§
2. Calcium Chloride (KLOR-ide)‡§
3. Calcium Citrate (SIH-trayt)†‡
4. Calcium Glubionate (gloo-BY-oh-nate)§
5. Calcium Gluceptate and Calcium Gluconate (GLOO-coh-nate)*
6. Calcium Gluconate‡§
7. Calcium Glycerophosphate (gliss-er-o-FOS-fate) and Calcium Lactate (LAK-tate)†
8. Calcium Lactate‡§
9. Calcium Lactate-Gluconate and Calcium Carbonate*
10. Dibasic (dy-BAY-sic) Calcium Phosphate (FOS-fate)†‡
11. Tribasic (try-BAY-sic) Calcium Phosphate†

Note: This information does *not* apply to calcium carbonate used as an antacid.

*Not commercially available in the U.S.
†Not commercially available in Canada.
‡Generic name product may also be available in the U.S.
§In Canada, calcium glubionate is known as calcium glucono-galacto gluconate.

## Description

Calcium supplements are taken by patients who are unable to get enough calcium in their regular diet or who have a need for more calcium. They are used to prevent or treat several conditions that may cause hypocalcemia (not enough calcium in the blood). The body needs calcium to make strong bones. Calcium is also needed for the heart, muscles, and nervous system to work properly.

The bones serve as a storage site for the body's calcium. They are continuously giving up calcium to the bloodstream and then replacing it as the body's need for calcium changes from day to day. When there is not enough calcium in the blood to be used by the heart and other organs, your body will take the needed calcium from the bones. When you eat foods rich in calcium, the calcium will be restored to the bones and the balance between your blood and bones will be maintained.

Pregnant women, nursing mothers, children, and adolescents may need more calcium than they normally get from eating calcium-rich foods. Adult women may take calcium supplements to help prevent a bone disease called osteoporosis. Osteoporosis, which causes thin, porous, easily broken bones, may occur in women after menopause, but may sometimes occur in elderly men also. Osteoporosis in women past menopause is thought to be caused by a reduced amount of ovarian estrogen (a female hormone). However, a diet low in calcium for many years, especially in the younger adult years, may add to the risk of developing it. Other bone diseases in children and adults are also treated with calcium supplements.

These medicines may also be used for other conditions as determined by your doctor.

Some of these preparations are available only with your doctor's prescription. Others are available without a prescription; however, your doctor may have special instructions on the proper use and dose for your medical problem.

Calcium supplements are available in the following dosage forms:

*Oral*
Calcium Carbonate
- Capsules (U.S. and Canada)
- Oral suspension (U.S.)
- Tablets (U.S. and Canada)
- Chewable tablets (U.S. and Canada)
Calcium Citrate
- Tablets (U.S.)
- Tablets for solution (U.S.)
Calcium Glubionate
- Syrup (U.S. and Canada)
Calcium Gluceptate and Calcium Gluconate
- Oral solution (Canada)
Calcium Gluconate
- Tablets (U.S. and Canada)
Calcium Lactate
- Tablets (U.S. and Canada)
Calcium Lactate-Gluconate and Calcium Carbonate
- Tablets for solution (Canada)
Dibasic Calcium Phosphate
- Tablets (U.S.)
Tribasic Calcium Phosphate
- Tablets (U.S.)

*Parenteral*
Calcium Chloride
- Injection (U.S. and Canada)
Calcium Glubionate
- Injection (Canada)
Calcium Gluceptate
- Injection (U.S.)
Calcium Gluconate
- Injection (U.S. and Canada)
Calcium Glycerophosphate and Calcium Lactate
- Injection (U.S.)

A calcium "salt" contains calcium along with another substance, such as carbonate or gluconate. Some calcium salts have more calcium (elemental calcium) than others. For example, the amount of calcium in calcium carbonate is greater than that in calcium gluconate. To give you an idea of how different calcium supplements vary in calcium content, the following chart explains how many tablets of each type of supplement will provide 1000 milligrams of elemental calcium. When you look for a calcium supplement, be sure the number of milligrams on the label refers to the amount of elemental calcium, and not to the strength of each tablet.

| Calcium supplement | Strength of each tablet (in milligrams) | Amount of elemental calcium per tablet (in milligrams) | Number of tablets to provide 1000 milligrams of calcium |
|---|---|---|---|
| Calcium carbonate | 625 | 250 | 4 |
| | 650 | 260 | 4 |
| | 750 | 300 | 4 |
| | 835 | 334 | 3 |
| | 1250 | 500 | 2 |
| | 1500 | 600 | 2 |
| Calcium citrate | 950 | 200 | 5 |
| Calcium gluconate | 500 | 45 | 22 |
| | 650 | 58 | 17 |
| | 1000 | 90 | 11 |
| Calcium lactate | 325 | 42 | 24 |
| | 650 | 84 | 12 |
| Calcium phosphate, dibasic | 500 | 115 | 9 |
| Calcium phosphate, tribasic | 800 | 304 | 4 |
| | 1600 | 608 | 2 |

## Importance of Diet

Many nutritionists recommend that, if possible, people should get all the calcium they need from foods. However, many people do not get enough calcium from food. For example, people on weight-loss diets may consume too little food to provide enough calcium. Others may not be able to tolerate milk products because their bodies lack an enzyme called lactase, which helps the body digest milk. Still others may need more calcium than normal. For such people, a calcium supplement is important.

In order to get enough vitamins and minerals in your diet, it is important that you eat a balanced and varied diet. Follow carefully any diet program your doctor may recommend. For your specific vitamin and/or mineral needs, ask your doctor or dietitian for a list of appropriate foods.

Experts have developed a list of Recommended Dietary Allowances (RDA) of calcium. The RDA is not an exact number but a general idea of how much you need every day. The RDA do not cover amounts needed for problems caused by a serious lack of calcium.

The RDA for calcium are as follows:
  Infants and children—
    Birth to 6 months of age: 400 milligrams (mg) a day.
    6 months to 1 year of age: 600 mg a day.
    1 to 10 years of age: 800 mg a day.
  Adolescent and adult males—
    11 to 24 years of age: 1200 mg a day.
    24 years of age and over: 800 mg a day.
  Adolescent and adult females—
    11 to 24 years of age: 1200 mg a day.
    24 years of age and over: 800 mg a day.
  Pregnant women—1200 mg a day.
  Breast-feeding women—1200 mg a day.

Getting the proper amount of calcium in the diet every day and participating in weight-bearing exercise (walking, dancing, bicycling, aerobics, jogging), especially during the early years of life (up to about 35 years of age) is most important in helping to build and maintain bones as dense as possible to prevent the development of osteoporosis in later life.

The following table includes some calcium-rich foods. The calcium content of these foods can supply the daily RDA for calcium if the foods are eaten regularly in sufficient amounts.

| Food (amount) | Milligrams of calcium |
|---|---|
| Nonfat dry milk, reconstituted (1 cup) | 375 |
| Lowfat, skim, or whole milk (1 cup) | 290 to 300 |
| Yogurt (1 cup) | 275 to 400 |
| Sardines with bones (3 ounces) | 370 |
| Ricotta cheese, part skim (½ cup) | 340 |
| Salmon, canned, with bones (3 ounces) | 285 |
| Cheese, Swiss (1 ounce) | 272 |
| Cheese, cheddar (1 ounce) | 204 |
| Cheese, American (1 ounce) | 174 |
| Cottage cheese, lowfat (1 cup) | 154 |
| Tofu (4 ounces) | 154 |
| Shrimp (1 cup) | 147 |
| Ice milk (¾ cup) | 132 |

Vitamin D helps prevent calcium loss from your bones. It is sometimes called "the sunshine vitamin" because it is made in your skin when you are exposed to sunlight. If you get outside in the sunlight every day for 15 to 30 minutes, you should get all the vitamin D you need. However, in northern locations in winter, the sunlight may be too weak to make vitamin D in the skin. Vitamin D may also be obtained from your diet or from multivitamin preparations. Most milk is fortified with vitamin D.

*Do not use bonemeal or dolomite as a source of calcium.* The Food and Drug Administration has issued warnings that bonemeal and dolomite could be dangerous because these products may contain lead.

Remember:
- The total amount of calcium that you get every day includes what you get from food *and* what you may take as a supplement. Read the labels of processed foods. Many foods now have added calcium.
- This total intake of calcium need not be greater than the recommended amounts, unless ordered by your doctor. In some cases, excessive amounts of calcium may be harmful by causing kidney stones or kidney impairment.

## Before Using This Dietary Supplement

If you are taking this dietary supplement without a prescription, carefully read and follow any precautions on the label. For calcium supplements, the following should be considered:

**Pregnancy**—It is especially important that you are receiving enough calcium when you become pregnant and that you continue to receive the right amount of calcium throughout your pregnancy. The healthy growth and development of the fetus depend on a steady supply of nutrients from the mother. However, taking large amounts of a dietary supplement during pregnancy may be harmful to the mother and/or fetus and should be avoided.

**Breast-feeding**—It is especially important that you receive the right amount of calcium so that your baby will also get the calcium needed to grow properly. However, taking large amounts of a dietary supplement while breast-feeding may be harmful to the mother and/or baby and should be avoided.

**Children**—It is especially important that children receive enough calcium in their diet for healthy growth and development. Although there is no specific information about the use of calcium in children in doses higher than the normal daily requirements, it is not expected to cause different side effects or problems in children than in adults. Injectable forms of calcium should not be given to children because of the risk of irritating the injection site.

**Older adults**—It is important that older people continue to receive enough calcium in their daily diets. However, some older people may need to take extra calcium or larger doses because they do not absorb calcium as well as younger people. Check with your doctor if you have any questions about the amount of calcium you should be taking in each day.

**Medicines or other dietary supplements**—Although certain medicines or dietary supplements should not be used together at all, in other cases they may be used together even if an interaction might occur. In these cases, your doctor may want to change the dose, or other precautions may be necessary. When you are taking calcium supplements, it is especially important that your health care professional know if you are taking any of the following:
- Calcium-containing medicines, other—Taking excess calcium may cause too much calcium in the blood or urine and lead to medical problems

- Cellulose sodium phosphate (e.g., Calcibind)—Use with calcium supplements may decrease the effects of cellulose sodium phosphate
- Digitalis glycosides (heart medicine)—Use with calcium supplements by injection may increase the chance of irregular heartbeat
- Etidronate (e.g., Didronel)—Use with calcium supplements may decrease the effects of etidronate; etidronate should not be taken within 2 hours of calcium supplements
- Gallium nitrate (e.g., Ganite)—Use with calcium supplements may cause gallium nitrate to not work properly
- Magnesium sulfate (for injection)—Use with calcium supplements may cause either medicine to be less effective
- Phenytoin (e.g., Dilantin)—Use with calcium supplements may decrease the effects of both medicines; calcium supplements should not be taken within 1 to 3 hours of phenytoin
- Tetracyclines (medicine for infection) taken by mouth—Use with calcium supplements may decrease the effects of tetracycline; calcium supplements should not be taken within 1 to 3 hours of tetracyclines

**Other medical problems**—The presence of other medical problems may affect the use of calcium supplements. Make sure you tell your doctor if you have any other medical problems, especially:

- Diarrhea or
- Stomach or intestinal problems—Extra calcium or specific calcium preparations may be necessary in these conditions
- Heart disease—Calcium by injection may increase the chance of irregular heartbeat
- Hypercalcemia or
- Hypercalciuria—Calcium supplements may make these conditions worse
- Hyperparathyroidism or
- Sarcoidosis—Calcium supplements may increase the chance of hypercalcemia (too much calcium in the blood)
- Hypoparathyroidism—Use of calcium phosphate may cause high blood levels of phosphorus which could increase the chance of side effects
- Kidney disease or stones—Too much calcium may increase the chance of kidney stones

## Proper Use of This Dietary Supplement

Drink a full glass (8 ounces) of water or juice when taking a calcium supplement. However, if you are taking calcium carbonate as a phosphate binder in kidney dialysis, it is not necessary to drink a glass of water.

*This dietary supplement is best taken 1 to 1½ hours after meals*, unless otherwise directed by your doctor. However, patients with a condition known as achlorhydria may not absorb calcium supplements on an empty stomach and should take them with meals.

For patients taking *the chewable tablet form* of this dietary supplement:

- Chew the tablets completely before swallowing.

For patients taking *the syrup form* of this dietary supplement:

- Take the syrup before meals. This will allow the dietary supplement to work faster.
- Mix in water or fruit juice for infants or children.

Take this dietary supplement only as directed. Do not take more of it and do not take it more often than recommended on the label. To do so may increase the chance of side effects.

**Dosing**—The dose of calcium for prevention of calcium deficiency is based on the Recommended Dietary Allowances (RDA). See the *Importance of Diet* section for the RDA for calcium.

**Missed dose**—If you are taking this dietary supplement on a regular schedule and you miss a dose, take it as soon as possible, then go back to your regular dosing schedule.

**Storage**—To store this dietary supplement:

- Keep out of the reach of children.
- Store away from heat and direct light.
- Do not store in the bathroom, near the kitchen sink, or in other damp places. Heat or moisture may cause the dietary supplement to break down.
- Keep the liquid form of this dietary supplement from freezing.
- Do not keep outdated dietary supplements or those no longer needed. Be sure that any discarded dietary supplement is out of the reach of children.

## Precautions While Using This Dietary Supplement

If this dietary supplement has been ordered for you by your doctor and you will be taking it in large doses or for a long time, your doctor should check your progress at regular visits. This is to make sure the medicine is working properly and does not cause unwanted effects.

*Do not take calcium supplements within 1 to 2 hours of taking other medicine by mouth.* To do so may keep the other medicine from working properly.

Unless you are otherwise directed by your doctor, to make sure that calcium is used properly by your body:

- *Do not take other medicines or dietary supplements containing large amounts of calcium, phosphates, magnesium, or vitamin D unless your doctor has told you to do so or approved.*
- *Do not take calcium supplements within 1 to 2 hours of eating large amounts of fiber-containing foods, such as bran and whole-grain cereals or breads, especially if you are being treated for hypocalcemia (not enough calcium in your blood).*
- *Do not drink large amounts of alcohol or caffeine-containing beverages (usually more than 8 cups of coffee a day), or use tobacco.*

Recently, some calcium carbonate tablets have been shown to break up too slowly in the stomach to be properly absorbed into the body. If the calcium carbonate tablets you purchase are not specifically labeled as being "USP," check with your pharmacist. He or she may be able to help you determine which tablets are best.

## Side Effects of This Dietary Supplement

Along with its needed effects, a dietary supplement may cause some unwanted effects. Although the following side effects occur very rarely when the calcium supplement is taken as recommended, they may be more likely to occur if:

- It is taken in large doses.
- It is taken for a long time.
- It is taken by patients with kidney disease.

Check with your doctor as soon as possible if any of the following side effects occur:

*More common (for injection form only)*

Dizziness; flushing and/or sensation of warmth or heat; irregular heartbeat; nausea or vomiting; skin redness, rash, pain, or burning at injection site; sweating; tingling sensation

*Rare*

Drowsiness; difficult or painful urination; nausea or vomiting (continuing); weakness

*Early signs of overdose*

Constipation (severe); dryness of mouth; headache (continuing); increased thirst; irritability; loss of appetite; mental depression; metallic taste; unusual tiredness or weakness

*Late signs of overdose*

Confusion; drowsiness (severe); high blood pressure; increased sensitivity of eyes or skin to light; irregular, fast, or slow heartbeat; unusually large amount of urine or increased frequency of urination

Other side effects not listed above may also occur in some patients. If you notice any other effects, check with your doctor.

## Additional Information

Once a medicine or dietary supplement has been approved for marketing for a certain use, experience may show that it is also useful for other medical problems. Although this use is not included in product labeling, calcium supplements are used in certain patients with the following medical condition:

- Hyperphosphatemia (too much phosphate in the blood)

Other than the above information, there is no additional information relating to proper use, precautions, or side effects for this use.

Revised: 06/10/92
Interim revision: 08/22/94

# CAPREOMYCIN    Systemic

A commonly used brand name in the U.S. and Canada is Capastat.

## Description

Capreomycin (kap-ree-oh-MYE-sin) is used to treat tuberculosis (TB). It is given with other medicines for TB.

*To help clear up your tuberculosis (TB) completely, you must keep taking this medicine for the full time of treatment, even if you begin to feel better. This is very important. It is also important that you do not miss any doses.*

Capreomycin is available only with your doctor's prescription, in the following dosage form:

*Parenteral*

- Injection (U.S. and Canada)

## Before Receiving This Medicine

In deciding to use a medicine, the risks of taking the medicine must be weighed against the good it will do. This is a decision you and your doctor will make. For capreomycin, the following should be considered:

**Allergies**—Tell your doctor if you have ever had any unusual or allergic reaction to capreomycin. Also tell your health care professional if you are allergic to any other substances, such as foods, preservatives, or dyes.

**Pregnancy**—Capreomycin has not been studied in pregnant women. However, studies in rats given 3½ times the human dose have shown that capreomycin may cause birth defects.

**Breast-feeding**—It is not known whether capreomycin passes into breast milk. Although most medicines pass into breast milk in small amounts, many of them may be used safely while breast-feeding. Mothers who are taking this medicine and who wish to breast-feed should discuss this with their doctor.

**Children**—Studies on this medicine have been done only in adult patients, and there is no specific information comparing use of capreomycin in children with use in other age groups.

**Older adults**—Many medicines have not been studied specifically in older people. Therefore, it may not be known whether they work exactly the same way they do in younger adults or if they cause different side effects or problems in older people. There is no specific information comparing use of capreomycin in the elderly with use in other age groups.

**Other medicines**—Although certain medicines should not be used together at all, in other cases two different medicines may be used together even if an interaction might occur. In these cases, your doctor may want to change the dose, or other precautions may be necessary. When you are receiving capreomycin, it is especially important that your health care professional know if you are taking any of the following:

- Aminoglycosides by injection (amikacin [e.g., Amikin], gentamicin [e.g., Garamycin], kanamycin [e.g., Kantrex], neomycin [e.g., Mycifradin], netilmicin [e.g., Netromycin], streptomycin, tobramycin [e.g., Nebcin]) or
- Anti-infectives by mouth or by injection (medicine for infection) or
- Carmustine (e.g., BiCNU) or
- Chloroquine (e.g., Aralen) or
- Cisplatin (e.g., Platinol) or
- Combination pain medicine containing acetaminophen and aspirin (e.g., Excedrin) or other salicylates (with large amounts taken regularly) or
- Cyclosporine (e.g., Sandimmune) or
- Deferoxamine (e.g., Desferal) (with long-term use) or
- Gold salts (medicine for arthritis) or
- Hydroxychloroquine (e.g., Plaquenil) or
- Inflammation or pain medicines, except narcotics, or
- Lithium (e.g., Lithane) or
- Methotrexate (e.g., Mexate) or
- Penicillamine (e.g., Cuprimine) or
- Plicamycin (e.g., Mithracin) or
- Quinine (e.g., Quinamm) or
- Streptozocin (e.g., Zanosar) or
- Tiopronin (e.g., Thiola)—Use of any of these medicines with capreomycin may increase the chance of hearing, balance, or kidney side effects

**Other medical problems**—The presence of other medical problems may affect the use of capreomycin. Make sure you tell your doctor if you have any other medical problems, especially:

- Eighth-cranial-nerve disease (loss of hearing and/or balance)—Capreomycin may cause hearing and balance side effects
- Kidney disease—Capreomycin may cause serious side effects affecting the kidneys
- Myasthenia gravis or
- Parkinson's disease—Capreomycin may cause muscular weakness

## Proper Use of This Medicine

To help clear up your infection completely, *it is very important that you keep taking this medicine for the full time of treatment*, even if you begin to feel better after a few weeks. You may have to use it every day for as long as 1 to 2 years or more. If you stop using this medicine too soon, your symptoms may return.

**Dosing**—The dose of capreomycin will be different for different patients. The following information includes only the average doses of capreomycin. Your dose may be different if you have kidney disease.

- For *injection* dosage form:
  —For treatment of tuberculosis (TB):
  - Adults and adolescents—1 gram of capreomycin injected into the muscle once a day for 60 to 120 days. After this time, 1 gram of capreomycin is injected into the muscle 2 or 3 times a week. This medicine must be given with other medicines to treat tuberculosis (TB).
  - Children—Dose has not been determined.

## Side Effects of This Medicine

Along with its needed effects, a medicine may cause some unwanted effects. Although not all of these side effects may occur, if they do occur they may need medical attention.

Check with your doctor as soon as possible if any of the following side effects occur:

*More common*
  Greatly increased or decreased frequency of urination or amount of urine; increased thirst; loss of appetite; nausea; vomiting

*Less common*
  Any loss of hearing; clumsiness or unsteadiness; difficulty in breathing; dizziness; drowsiness; fever; irregular heartbeat; itching; muscle cramps or pain; pain, redness, hardness, unusual bleeding, or a sore at the place of injection; ringing or buzzing or a feeling of fullness in the ears; skin rash; swelling; unusual tiredness or weakness

Other side effects not listed above may also occur in some patients. If you notice any other effects, check with your doctor.

Revised: 06/27/94

# CAPSAICIN   Topical

Some commonly used brand names are:
**In the U.S.—**
  Zostrix
  Zostrix–HP
**In Canada—**
  Axsain
  Zostrix

## Description

Capsaicin (cap-SAY-sin) is used to help relieve a certain type of pain known as neuralgia (new-RAL-ja). Capsaicin is also used to temporarily help relieve the pain from osteoarthritis (OS-te-o-ar-THRI-tis) or rheumatoid arthritis (ROO-ma-toid ar-THRI-tis). This medicine will not cure any of these conditions.

Neuralgia is a pain from the nerves near the surface of your skin. This pain may occur after an infection with herpes zoster (shingles). It may also occur if you have diabetic neuropathy (di-a-BET-ick new-ROP-a-thee). Diabetic neuropathy is a condition that occurs in some persons with diabetes. The condition causes tingling and pain in the feet and toes. Capsaicin will help relieve the pain of diabetic neuropathy, but it will not cure diabetic neuropathy or diabetes.

Capsaicin may also be used for neuralgias caused by other conditions as determined by your doctor.

Capsaicin is available without a prescription; however, your doctor may have special instructions on the proper use of this medicine.

*Topical*
• Cream (U.S. and Canada)

## Before Using This Medicine

If you are using this medicine without a prescription, carefully read and follow any precautions on the label. For capsaicin, the following should be considered:

**Allergies**—Tell your health care professional if you have ever had any unusual or allergic reaction to capsaicin or to the fruit of capsicum plants (for example, hot peppers). Also tell your health care professional if you are allergic to any other substances, such as foods, preservatives, or dyes.

**Pregnancy**—Capsaicin has not been reported to cause birth defects or other problems in humans.

**Breast-feeding**—Capsaicin has not been reported to cause problems in nursing babies.

**Children**—Use is not recommended for infants and children up to 2 years of age, except as directed by your doctor. In children 2 years of age and older, this medicine is not expected to cause different side effects or problems than it does in adults.

**Older adults**—Many medicines have not been studied specifically in older people. Therefore, it may not be known whether they work exactly the same way they do in younger adults. Although there is no specific information comparing use of capsaicin in the elderly with use in other age groups, this medicine is not expected to cause different side effects or problems in older people than it does in younger adults.

**Other medical problems**—The presence of other medical problems may affect the use of capsaicin. Make sure you tell your health care professional if you have any other medical problems, especially:
• Broken or irritated skin on area to be treated with capsaicin

## Proper Use of This Medicine

If you are using capsaicin for the treatment of neuralgia caused by herpes zoster, do not apply the medicine until the zoster sores have healed.

It is not necessary to wash the areas to be treated before you apply capsaicin, but doing so will not cause harm.

Apply a small amount of cream and use your fingers to rub it well into the affected area so that little or no cream is left on the surface of the skin afterwards.

Wash your hands with soap and water after applying capsaicin to avoid getting the medicine in your eyes or on other sensitive areas of the body. However, if you are using capsaicin for arthritis in your hands, do not wash your hands for at least 30 minutes after applying the cream.

If a bandage is being used on the treated area, it should not be applied tightly.

When you first begin to use capsaicin, a warm, stinging, or burning sensation (feeling) may occur. This sensation is related to the action of capsaicin on the skin, and is to be expected. Although this sensation usually disappears after the first several days of treatment, it may last 2 to 4 weeks or longer. Heat, humidity, clothing, bathing in warm water, or sweating may increase the sensation. However, the sensation usually occurs less often and is less severe the longer you use the medicine. Reducing the number of doses of capsaicin that you use each day will not lessen the sensation, and may lengthen the period of time that you get the sensation. Also, reducing the number of doses you use may reduce the amount of pain relief that you get.

Capsaicin must be used regularly every day as directed if it is to work properly. Even then, it may not relieve your pain right away. The length of time it takes to work depends on the type of pain you have. In persons with arthritis, pain relief usually begins within 1 to 2 weeks. In most persons with neuralgia, relief usually begins within 2 to 4 weeks, although with head and neck neuralgias, relief may take as long as 4 to 6 weeks.

Once capsaicin has begun to relieve pain, you must continue to use it regularly 3 or 4 times a day to keep the pain from returning. If you stop using capsaicin and your pain returns, you can begin using it again.

**Dosing**—The dose of capsaicin may be different for different patients. *Follow your doctor's orders or the directions on the label.* The following information includes only the average dose of capsaicin. *If your dose is different, do not change it* unless your doctor tells you to do so:
• Apply regularly 3 or 4 times a day and rub in well.

**Missed dose**—If you miss a dose of this medicine, use it as soon as possible. However, if it is almost time for your next dose, skip the missed dose and go back to your regular dosing schedule. Do not double doses.

**Storage**—To store this medicine:
- Keep out of the reach of children.
- Store away from heat and direct light.
- Keep the medicine from freezing. Do not refrigerate.
- Do not keep outdated medicine or medicine no longer needed. Be sure that any discarded medicine is out of the reach of children.

## Precautions While Using This Medicine

If capsaicin gets into your eyes or on other sensitive areas of the body, it will cause a burning sensation. If capsaicin gets into your eyes, flush your eyes with water. If capsaicin gets on other sensitive areas of your body, wash the areas with warm (not hot) soapy water.

If your condition gets worse, or does not improve after 1 month, stop using this medicine and check with your doctor.

## Side Effects of This Medicine

Along with its needed effects, a medicine may cause some unwanted effects. Although not all of these side effects may occur, if they do occur they may need medical attention. Some side effects may occur that usually do not need medical attention. These side effects may go away during treatment as your body adjusts to the medicine. However, check with your doctor if any of the following side effects continue or are bothersome:

*More common*
    Warm, stinging, or burning feeling at the place of treatment

Other side effects not listed above may also occur in some patients. If you notice any other effects, check with your doctor.

Revised: 07/14/92

# CARBACHOL   Ophthalmic

Some commonly used brand names in the U.S. and Canada are Isopto Carbachol and Miostat.
Another commonly used name is carbamylcholine.

## Description

Carbachol (KAR-ba-kole) is used in the eye to treat glaucoma. Sometimes it is also used in eye surgery.

This medicine is available only with your doctor's prescription, in the following dosage forms:

*Ophthalmic*
- Intraocular solution (U.S. and Canada)
- Ophthalmic solution (eye drops) (U.S. and Canada)

## Before Using This Medicine

In deciding to use a medicine, the risks of taking the medicine must be weighed against the good it will do. This is a decision you and your doctor will make. For carbachol, the following should be considered:

**Allergies**—Tell your doctor if you have ever had any unusual or allergic reaction to carbachol. Also tell your health care professional if you are allergic to any other substances, such as preservatives.

**Pregnancy**—Studies on effects in pregnancy have not been done in either humans or animals. However, carbachol may be absorbed into the body.

**Breast-feeding**—Carbachol may be absorbed into the mother's body. However, it is not known whether carbachol passes into breast milk. Although most medicines pass into breast milk in small amounts, many of them may be used safely while breast-feeding. Mothers who

are using this medicine and who wish to breast-feed should discuss this with their doctor.

**Children**—Although there is no specific information comparing use of carbachol in children with use in other age groups, this medicine is not expected to cause different side effects or problems in children than it does in adults.

**Older adults**—Many medicines have not been studied specifically in older people. Therefore, it may not be known whether they work exactly the same way they do in younger adults. Although there is no specific information comparing use of carbachol in the elderly with use in other age groups, this medicine is not expected to cause different side effects or problems in older people than it does in younger adults.

**Other medicines**—Although certain medicines should not be used together at all, in other cases two different medicines may be used together even if an interaction might occur. In these cases, your doctor may want to change the dose, or other precautions may be necessary. Tell your health care professional if you are using any other prescription or nonprescription (over-the-counter [OTC]) medicine.

**Other medical problems**—The presence of other medical problems may affect the use of carbachol. Make sure you tell your doctor if you have any other medical problems, especially:
- Asthma or
- Eye problems (other) or
- Heart disease or
- Overactive thyroid or
- Parkinson's disease or

- Stomach ulcer or other stomach problems or
- Urinary tract blockage—Carbachol may make the condition worse

## Proper Use of This Medicine

*Use this medicine only as directed.* Do not use more of it and do not use it more often than your doctor ordered. To do so may increase the chance of too much medicine being absorbed into the body and the chance of side effects.

To use:

- First, wash your hands. Tilt the head back and, pressing your finger gently on the skin just beneath the lower eyelid, pull the lower eyelid away from the eye to make a space. Drop the medicine into this space. Let go of the eyelid and gently close the eyes. Do not blink. Keep the eyes closed and apply pressure to the inner corner of the eye with your finger for 1 or 2 minutes to allow the medicine to be absorbed by the eye.
- Immediately after using the eye drops, wash your hands to remove any medicine that may be on them.
- To keep the medicine as germ-free as possible, do not touch the applicator tip to any surface (including the eye). Also, keep the container tightly closed.

**Dosing**—The dose of carbachol will be different for different patients. *Follow your doctor's orders or the directions on the label.* The following information includes only the average doses of carbachol. If your dose is different, do not change it unless your doctor tells you to do so.

- For glaucoma:
  —For *ophthalmic solution (eye drops)* dosage form:
  - Adults and children—Use one drop in the eye one to three times a day.
- For use during surgery:
  —For *intraocular solution* dosage form:
  - Adults and children—Up to 0.5 milliliter (mL), used in the eye during surgery.

**Missed dose**—If you miss a dose of this medicine, apply it as soon as possible. However, if it is almost time for your next dose, skip the missed dose and go back to your regular dosing schedule. Do not double doses.

**Storage**—To store this medicine:

- Keep out of the reach of children.
- Store away from heat and direct light.
- Keep the medicine from freezing.
- Do not keep outdated medicine or medicine no longer needed. Be sure that any discarded medicine is out of the reach of children.

## Precautions While Using This Medicine

Your doctor should check your eye pressure at regular visits.

After you apply this medicine to your eyes, your pupils may become unusually small. This may cause you to see less well at night or in dim light. *Be especially careful if you drive, use machines, or do anything else at night or in dim light that could be dangerous if you are not able to see well.*

Also, for a short time after you apply this medicine, your vision may be blurred or there may be a change in your near or distance vision. *Make sure your vision is clear before you drive, use machines, or do anything else that could be dangerous if you are not able to see well.*

## Side Effects of This Medicine

Along with its needed effects, a medicine may cause some unwanted effects. Although not all of these side effects may occur, if they do occur they may need medical attention.

Check with your doctor as soon as possible if any of the following side effects occur:

*Rare*

Veil or curtain appearing across part of vision

*Symptoms of too much medicine being absorbed into the body*

Diarrhea, stomach cramps or pain, or vomiting; fainting; flushing or redness of face; frequent urge to urinate; increased sweating; irregular heartbeat; shortness of breath, wheezing, or tightness in chest; unusual tiredness or weakness; watering of mouth

Other side effects may occur that usually do not need medical attention. These side effects may go away during treatment as your body adjusts to the medicine. However, check with your doctor if any of the following side effects continue or are bothersome:

*More common*

Blurred vision or change in near or distance vision; eye pain; stinging or burning of the eye

*Less common*

Headache; irritation or redness of eyes; twitching of eyelids

Other side effects not listed above may also occur in some patients. If you notice any other effects, check with your doctor.

Revised: 06/21/94

# CARBAMAZEPINE   Systemic

Some commonly used brand names are:

**In the U.S.—**
> Epitol
> Tegretol
> Generic name product may also be available.

**In Canada—**
> Apo-Carbamazepine          Tegetrol Chewtabs
> Novocarbamaz              Tegetrol CR
> Tegretol

## Description

Carbamazepine (kar-ba-MAZ-e-peen) is used to control some types of seizures in the treatment of epilepsy. It is also used to relieve pain due to trigeminal neuralgia (tic douloureux). It should not be used for other more common aches or pains.

Carbamazepine may also be used for other conditions as determined by your doctor.

This medicine is available only with your doctor's prescription, in the following dosage forms:

*Oral*
- Suspension (U.S.)
- Tablets (U.S. and Canada)
- Chewable tablets (U.S. and Canada)
- Extended-release tablets (Canada)

## Before Using This Medicine

In deciding to use a medicine, the risks of taking the medicine must be weighed against the good it will do. This is a decision you and your doctor will make. For carbamazepine, the following should be considered:

**Allergies**—Tell your doctor if you have ever had any unusual or allergic reaction to carbamazepine or to any of the tricyclic antidepressants, such as amitriptyline, amoxapine, clomipramine, desipramine, doxepin, imipramine, nortriptyline, protriptyline, or trimipramine. Also tell your health care professional if you are allergic to any other substances, such as foods, preservatives, or dyes.

**Pregnancy**—Carbamazepine has not been studied in pregnant women. However, there have been reports of babies having low birth weight, small head size, skull and facial defects, underdeveloped fingernails, and delays in growth when their mothers had taken carbamazepine in high doses during pregnancy. In addition, birth defects have been reported in some babies when the mothers took other medicines for epilepsy during pregnancy. Also, studies in animals have shown that carbamazepine causes birth defects when given in large doses. Therefore, the use of carbamazepine during pregnancy should be discussed with your doctor.

**Breast-feeding**—Carbamazepine passes into the breast milk, and in some cases the baby may receive enough of it to cause unwanted effects. In animal studies, carbamazepine has affected the growth and appearance of the nursing babies.

**Children**—Behavior changes are more likely to occur in children.

**Older adults**—Confusion; restlessness and nervousness; irregular, pounding, or unusually slow heartbeat; and chest pain may be especially likely to occur in elderly patients, who are usually more sensitive than younger adults to the effects of carbamazepine.

**Other medicines**—Although certain medicines should not be used together at all, in other cases two different medicines may be used together even if an interaction might occur. In these cases, your doctor may want to change the dose, or other precautions may be necessary. When you are taking carbamazepine, it is especially important that your health care professional know if you are taking any of the following:

- Anticoagulants (blood thinners)—The effects of anticoagulants may be decreased; monitoring of blood clotting time may be necessary during and after carbamazepine treatment
- Cimetidine (e.g., Tagamet)—Blood levels of carbamazepine may be increased, leading to an increase in serious side effects
- Clarithromycin (e.g., Biaxin)—Blood levels of carbamazepine may be increased, increasing the risk of unwanted effects
- Corticosteroids (cortisone-like medicine)—The effects of corticosteroids may be decreased
- Diltiazem (e.g., Cardizem) or
- Erythromycin (e.g., E-Mycin, Erythrocin, Ilosone) or
- Propoxyphene (e.g., Darvon) or
- Verapamil (e.g., Calan)—Blood levels of carbamazepine may be increased; these medicines should not be used with carbamazepine
- Estrogens (female hormones) or
- Quinidine or
- Oral contraceptives (birth control pills) containing estrogen—The effects of these medicines may be decreased; use of a nonhormonal method of birth control or an oral contraceptive containing only a progestin may be necessary
- Isoniazid (e.g., INH)—The risk of serious side effects may be increased
- Monoamine oxidase (MAO) inhibitors (furazolidone [e.g., Furoxone], isocarboxazid [e.g., Marplan], phenelzine [e.g., Nardil], procarbazine [e.g., Matulane], selegiline [e.g., Eldepryl], tranylcypromine [e.g., Parnate])—Taking carbamazepine while you are taking or within 2 weeks of taking monoamine oxidase (MAO) inhibitors may cause sudden high body temperature, extremely high blood pressure, and severe convulsions; at least 14 days should be allowed between stopping treatment with one medicine and starting treatment with the other
- Other anticonvulsants (seizure medicine)—The effects of these medicines may be decreased; in addition, if these medicines and carbamazepine are used together during pregnancy, the risk of birth defects may be increased
- Tricyclic antidepressants (amitriptyline [e.g., Elavil], amoxapine [e.g., Asendin], clomipramine [e.g., Anafranil], desipramine [e.g., Pertofrane], doxepin [e.g., Sinequan], imipramine [e.g., Tofranil], nortriptyline [e.g.,

Aventyl], protriptyline [e.g., Vivactil], trimipramine [e.g., Surmontil])—Central nervous system depressant effects of carbamazepine may be increased while the anticonvulsant effects of carbamazepine may be decreased; seizures may occur more frequently

**Other medical problems**—The presence of other medical problems may affect the use of carbamazepine. Make sure you tell your doctor if you have any other medical problems, especially:

- Alcohol abuse (or history of)—Drinking alcohol may decrease the effectiveness of carbamazepine
- Anemia or other blood problems or
- Behavioral problems or
- Glaucoma or
- Heart or blood vessel disease or
- Problems with urination—Carbamazepine may make the condition worse
- Diabetes mellitus (sugar diabetes)—Carbamazepine may cause increased urine glucose levels
- Kidney disease or
- Liver disease—Higher blood levels of carbamazepine may result, increasing the chance of side effects

## Proper Use of This Medicine

*Carbamazepine should be taken with meals* to lessen the chance of stomach upset (nausea and vomiting).

*It is very important that you take this medicine exactly as directed by your doctor* to obtain the best results and lessen the chance of serious side effects. Do not take more of it, do not take it more often, and do not take it for a longer time than your doctor ordered.

If you are taking this medicine for pain relief:

- Carbamazepine is *not* an ordinary pain reliever. It should be used only when a doctor prescribes it for certain kinds of pain. *Do not take carbamazepine for any other aches or pains.*

If you are taking this medicine for epilepsy:

- *Do not suddenly stop taking this medicine without first checking with your doctor.* To keep your seizures under control, it is usually best to gradually reduce the amount of carbamazepine you are taking before stopping completely.

**Dosing**—The dose of carbamazepine will be different for different patients. *Follow your doctor's orders or the directions on the label.* The following information includes only the average doses of carbamazepine. *If your dose is different, do not change it* unless your doctor tells you to do so.

The number of tablets or teaspoonfuls of suspension that you take depends on the strength of the medicine. Also, *the number of doses you take each day, the time allowed between doses, and the length of time you take the medicine depend on the medical problem for which you are taking carbamazepine.*

- For *oral* dosage form (suspension):
  - For epilepsy:
    - Adults and teenagers—At first, 100 milligrams (mg) taken up to four times a day. Your doctor may increase your dose if needed. However, the dose is usually not more than 1200 mg a day.
    - Children 6 to 12 years of age—At first, 50 mg taken four times a day. Your doctor may increase your dose if needed. However, the dose is usually not more than 1000 mg a day.
    - Children up to 6 years of age—Dose is based on weight and will be determined by your doctor.
  - For trigeminal neuralgia:
    - Adults and teenagers—At first, 50 mg four times a day. Your doctor may increase your dose if needed. However, the dose is usually not more than 1200 mg a day.
    - Children—Use and dose must be determined by your doctor.
- For *oral* dosage form (tablets and chewable tablets):
  - For epilepsy:
    - Adults and teenagers—At first, 200 mg taken two times a day. Your doctor may increase your dose if needed. However, the dose is usually not more than 1200 mg a day.
    - Children 6 to 12 years of age—At first, 100 mg taken two times a day. Your doctor may increase your dose if needed. However, the dose is usually not more than 1000 mg a day.
    - Children up to 6 years of age—Dose is based on weight and will be determined by your doctor.
  - For trigeminal neuralgia:
    - Adults and teenagers—At first, 100 mg taken two times a day. Your doctor may increase your dose if needed. However, the dose is usually not more than 1200 mg a day.
    - Children—Use and dose must be determined by your doctor.
- For *oral extended-release tablet* dosage form:
  - For epilepsy:
    - Adults and teenagers—At first, 100 to 200 mg taken one or two times a day with meals. Your doctor may increase your dose if needed. However, the dose is usually not more than 1200 mg a day.
    - Children 6 to 12 years of age—At first, 100 mg taken in smaller doses during the day. Your doctor may increase your dose if needed. However, the dose is usually not more than 1000 mg a day.
    - Children up to 6 years of age—Use and dose must be determined by your doctor.
  - For trigeminal neuralgia:
    - Adults and teenagers—At first, 100 mg taken two times a day. Your doctor may increase your dose if needed. However, the dose is usually not more than 1200 mg a day.

- Children—Use and dose must be determined by your doctor.

**Missed dose**—If you miss a dose of this medicine, take it as soon as possible. However, if it is almost time for your next dose, skip the missed dose and go back to your regular dosing schedule. Do not double doses. However, if you miss more than one dose a day, check with your doctor.

**Storage**—To store this medicine:
- Keep out of the reach of children.
- Store away from heat and direct light.
- *Do not store the tablet forms of carbamazepine in the bathroom, near the kitchen sink, or in other damp places. Heat or moisture may cause the medicine to break down and become less effective.*
- Keep the liquid form of this medicine from freezing.
- Do not keep outdated medicine or medicine no longer needed. Be sure that any discarded medicine is out of the reach of children.

## Precautions While Using This Medicine

*It is very important that your doctor check your progress at regular visits.* Your doctor may want to have certain tests done to see if you are receiving the right amount of medicine or if certain side effects may be occurring without your knowing it. Also, the amount of medicine you are taking may have to be changed often.

This medicine will add to the effects of alcohol and other CNS depressants (medicines that cause drowsiness). Some examples of CNS depressants are antihistamines or medicine for hay fever, other allergies, or colds; sedatives, tranquilizers, or sleeping medicine; prescription pain medicine or narcotics; barbiturates; medicine for seizures; muscle relaxants; or anesthetics, including some dental anesthetics. *Check with your doctor before taking any of the above while you are using this medicine.*

This medicine may cause some people to become drowsy, dizzy, lightheaded, or less alert than they are normally, especially when they are starting treatment or increasing the dose. It may also cause blurred or double vision, weakness, or loss of muscle control in some people. *Make sure you know how you react to this medicine before you drive, use machines, or do anything else that could be dangerous if you are not alert and well-coordinated or able to see well.*

Some people who take carbamazepine may become more sensitive to sunlight than they are normally. Exposure to sunlight, even for brief periods of time, may cause a skin rash, itching, redness or other discoloration of the skin, or a severe sunburn. When you begin taking this medicine:
- Stay out of direct sunlight, especially between the hours of 10:00 a.m. and 3:00 p.m., if possible.
- Wear protective clothing, including a hat. Also, wear sunglasses.

- Apply a sun block product that has a skin protection factor (SPF) of at least 15. Some patients may require a product with a higher SPF number, especially if they have a fair complexion. If you have any questions about this, check with your health care professional.
- Apply a sun block lipstick that has an SPF of at least 15 to protect your lips.
- Do not use a sunlamp or tanning bed or booth.

*If you have a severe reaction from the sun, check with your doctor.*

*Oral contraceptives (birth control pills) containing estrogen may not work properly if you take them while you are taking carbamazepine. Unplanned pregnancies may occur. You should use a different or additional means of birth control while you are taking carbamazepine. If you have any questions about this, check with your health care professional.*

For diabetic patients:
- Carbamazepine may affect urine sugar levels. While you are using this medicine, be especially careful when testing for sugar in your urine. If you notice a change in the results of your urine sugar tests or have any questions about this, check with your doctor.

Before having any medical tests, tell the medical doctor in charge that you are taking this medicine. The results of some pregnancy tests and the metyrapone test may be affected by this medicine.

*Before having any kind of surgery, dental treatment, or emergency treatment, tell the medical doctor or dentist in charge that you are taking this medicine.* Taking carbamazepine together with medicines that are used during surgery or dental or emergency treatments may increase the CNS depressant effects.

Your doctor may want you to carry a medical identification card or bracelet stating that you are taking this medicine.

## Side Effects of This Medicine

Along with its needed effects, a medicine may cause some unwanted effects. Although not all of these side effects may occur, if they do occur they may need medical attention.

*Check with your doctor immediately* if any of the following side effects occur:
*Rare*
Black, tarry stools; blood in urine or stools; bone or joint pain; cough or hoarseness; darkening of urine; lower back or side pain; nosebleeds or other unusual bleeding or bruising; painful or difficult urination; pain, tenderness, swelling, or bluish color in leg or foot; pale stools; pinpoint red spots on skin; shortness of breath or cough; sores, ulcers, or white spots on lips or in the mouth; sore throat, chills, and fever; swollen or painful

glands; unusual tiredness or weakness; wheezing, tightness in chest, or troubled breathing; yellow eyes or skin

*Symptoms of overdose*

Body spasm in which head and heels are bent backward and body is bowed forward; clumsiness or unsteadiness; convulsions (seizures)—especially in small children; dizziness (severe) or fainting; drowsiness (severe); fast or irregular heartbeat; high or low blood pressure (hypertension or hypotension); irregular, slow, or shallow breathing; large pupils; nausea or vomiting (severe); overactive reflexes followed by underactive reflexes; poor control in body movements (for example, when reaching or stepping); sudden decrease in amount of urine; trembling, twitching, or abnormal body movements

In addition, check with your doctor as soon as possible if any of the following side effects occur:

*More common*

Blurred vision or double vision; continuous back-and-forth eye movements

*Less common*

Behavioral changes (especially in children); confusion, agitation, or hostility (especially in the elderly); diarrhea (severe); headache (continuing); increase in seizures; nausea and vomiting (severe); skin rash, hives, or itching; unusual drowsiness

*Rare*

Chest pain; difficulty in speaking or slurred speech; fainting; frequent urination; irregular, pounding, or unusually slow heartbeat; mental depression with restlessness and nervousness or other mood or mental changes; muscle or stomach cramps; numbness, tingling, pain, or weakness in hands and feet; rapid weight gain; rigidity; ringing, buzzing, or other unexplained sounds in the ears; sudden decrease in amount of urine; swelling of face, hands, feet, or lower legs; trembling; uncontrolled body movements; visual hallucinations (seeing things that are not there)

Other side effects may occur that usually do not need medical attention. These side effects may go away during treatment as your body adjusts to the medicine. However, check with your doctor if any of the following side effects continue or are bothersome:

*More common*

Clumsiness or unsteadiness; dizziness (mild); drowsiness (mild); lightheadedness; nausea or vomiting (mild)

*Less common or rare*

Aching joints or muscles; constipation; diarrhea; dryness of mouth; headache; increased sensitivity of skin to sunlight (skin rash, itching, redness or other discoloration of skin, or severe sunburn); increased sweating; irritation or soreness of tongue or mouth; loss of appetite; loss of hair; muscle or abdominal cramps; sexual problems in males; stomach pain or discomfort

Other side effects not listed above may also occur in some patients. If you notice any other effects, check with your doctor.

## Additional Information

Once a medicine has been approved for marketing for a certain use, experience may show that it is also useful for other medical problems. Although these uses are not included in product labeling, carbamazepine is used in certain patients with the following medical conditions:

- Neurogenic pain (a type of continuing pain)
- Bipolar disorder (manic-depressive illness)
- Central partial diabetes insipidus (water diabetes)
- Alcohol withdrawal
- Psychotic disorders (severe mental illness)

Other than the above information, there is no additional information relating to proper use, precautions, or side effects for these uses.

Revised: 08/26/94

# CARBOHYDRATES AND ELECTROLYTES   Systemic

Some commonly used brand names are:

**In the U.S.—**

| | |
|---|---|
| Infalyte[3] | Rehydralyte[1] |
| Naturalyte[1] | Resol‡[1] |
| Pedialyte[1] | |

**In Canada—**

| | |
|---|---|
| Lytren[1] | Pedialyte[1] |
| Gastrolyte[2] | Rapolyte[2] |

Other commonly used names are oral rehydration salts, ORS-bicarbonate, and ORS-citrate.§

Note: For quick reference, the following (family name) are numbered to match the corresponding brand names.

This information applies to the following medicines:

1. Dextrose and Electrolytes
2. Oral Rehydration Salts*§
3. Rice Syrup Solids and Electrolytes†

*Not commercially available in the U.S.
†Not commercially available in Canada.
‡ Resol is available to hospitals only.
§Distributed by the World Health Organization (WHO).

## Description

Carbohydrate and electrolytes combination is used to treat or prevent dehydration (the loss of too much water from the body) that may occur with severe diarrhea, especially in babies and young children. Although this medicine does not immediately stop the diarrhea, it replaces the water and some important salts (electrolytes), such as sodium and potassium, that are lost from the body during diarrhea, and helps prevent more serious problems. Some carbohydrate and electrolytes solutions may also be used after surgery when food intake has been stopped.

This medicine is available without a prescription; however, your doctor may have special instructions on the proper use and dose for you or your child.

Carbohydrate and electrolytes combination is available in the following dosage forms:

*Oral*
- Solution (U.S. and Canada)
- Powder for oral solution (Canada)

## Before Using This Medicine

If you are taking this medicine without a prescription, carefully read and follow any precautions on the label. For carbohydrate and electrolytes solutions, the following should be considered:

**Allergies**—Tell your doctor if you have ever had any unusual or allergic reaction to medicines containing potassium, sodium, citrates, rice, or sugar. Also tell your health care professional if you are allergic to any other substances, such as foods, preservatives, or dyes.

**Pregnancy**—Carbohydrate and electrolytes solutions have not been shown to cause birth defects or other problems in humans.

**Breast-feeding**—This medicine has not been reported to cause problems in nursing babies. Breast-feeding should continue, if possible, during treatment with carbohydrate and electrolytes solution.

**Children**—This medicine has been tested in children and, in effective doses, appears to be safe and effective in children. This medicine has not been tested in premature infants.

**Older adults**—This medicine has been tested and has been shown to be well tolerated by older people.

**Other medicines**—Although certain medicines should not be used together at all, in other cases two different medicines may be used together even if an interaction might occur. In these cases, your doctor may want to change the dose, or other precautions may be necessary. Tell your health care professional if you are taking any other prescription or nonprescription (over-the-counter [OTC]) medicine.

**Other medical problems**—The presence of other medical problems may affect the use of carbohydrate and electrolytes solutions. Make sure you tell your doctor if you have any other medical problems, especially:
- Difficult urination—This condition may prevent the carbohydrate and electrolytes solution from working properly
- Inability to drink or
- Vomiting (severe and continuing)—Treatment by injection may need to be given to patients with these conditions

- Intestinal blockage—Carbohydrate and electrolytes solution may be harmful if given to patients with this condition

## Proper Use of This Medicine

For patients using the *commercial powder form* of this medicine:
- Add 7 ounces of boiled, cooled tap water to the entire contents of one powder packet. Shake or stir the container for 2 or 3 minutes until all the powder is dissolved.
- Do not add more water to the solution after it is mixed.
- Do not boil the solution.
- Make and use a fresh solution each day.

For patients using the *powder form* of this medicine *distributed by the World Health Organization (WHO)*:
- Add the entire contents of one powder packet to enough drinking water to make one quart (32 ounces) or liter of solution. Shake the container for 2 or 3 minutes until all the powder is dissolved.
- Do not add more water to the solution after it is mixed.
- Do not boil the solution.
- Make and use a fresh solution each day.

Babies and small children should be given the solution slowly, in small amounts, with a spoon, as often as possible, during the first 24 hours of diarrhea.

Take as directed. Do not take it for a longer time than your doctor has recommended. To do so may increase the chance of side effects.

**Dosing**—The dose of these combination medicines will be different for different patients. *Follow your doctor's orders or the directions on the label.* The following information includes only the average doses of these medicines. *If your dose is different, do not change it* unless your doctor tells you to do so.

*For dextrose and electrolytes and for rice syrup solids and electrolytes*:
- For rehydration (to replace the water and some important salts [electrolytes]):
  —For *oral* dosage form (solution):
    - Adults and children over 10 years of age— Dose is based on body weight and must be determined by your doctor. At first, the usual dose is 50 to 100 milliliters (mL) per kilogram (kg) (23 to 45 mL per pound) of body weight taken over four to six hours. Your doctor may change the dose depending on your thirst and your response to the treatment.
    - Children up to 2 years of age—The dose is based on body weight and must be determined by your doctor. At first, the usual dose is 75 mL per kg (34 mL per pound) of body weight during the first eight hours and 75 mL per kg (34 mL

per pound) of body weight during the next six-teen hours. Your doctor may change the dose depending on your thirst and your response to the treatment. However, the dose is usually not more than 100 mL in any 20-minute period.

• Children 2 to 10 years of age—Dose is based on body weight and must be determined by your doctor. At first, the usual dose is 50 mL per kg (23 mL per pound) of body weight taken over the first four to six hours. Then, the dose is 100 mL per kg (45 mL per pound) of body weight taken over the next eighteen to twenty-four hours. Your doctor may change the dose depending on your thirst and your response to the treatment. However, the dose is usually not more than 100 mL in any 20-minute period.

*For oral rehydration salts*

• For rehydration (to replace the water and some important salts [electrolytes]):

–For *oral* dosage form (solution):

• Adults and teenagers—Dose is based on body weight and must be determined by your doctor. At first, the usual dose is 50 to 100 milliliters (mL) of solution per kilogram (kg) (23 to 45 mL per pound) of body weight taken over four to six hours. Your doctor may change the dose depending on your thirst and your response to the treatment.

• Children—Dose is based on body weight and must be determined by your doctor. At first, the usual dose is 50 to 100 mL per kg (23 to 46 mL per pound) of body weight taken over the first four hours. Your doctor may change the dose depending on your thirst and your response to the treatment.

**Storage**—To store this medicine:

• Keep out of the reach of children.
• Store away from heat and direct light.
• Do not store the powder packets in the bathroom, near the kitchen sink, or in other damp places. Heat or moisture may cause the medicine to break down.
• Store the liquid in the refrigerator. However, keep the medicine from freezing.
• Make a fresh solution each day. Discard unused solution at the end of each day. Be sure that any discarded medicine is out of the reach of children.

## Precautions While Using This Medicine

Eat soft foods, if possible, such as rice cereal, bananas, cooked peas or beans, and potatoes to keep up nutrition

until the diarrhea stops and regular food and milk can be taken again. Breast-fed infants should be given breast milk between doses of the solution.

If your diarrhea does not improve in 1 or 2 days, or if it becomes worse, check with your doctor.

Also, *check with your doctor immediately* if your baby or child appears to have severe thirst, doughy skin, sunken eyes, dizziness or lightheadedness, tiredness or weakness, irritability, difficult urination, loss of weight, or convulsions (seizures). These signs may mean that too much water has been lost from the body.

For patients (except nursing babies) using the *powder form* of this medicine:

• Drink plain water whenever thirsty between doses of solution.

For patients taking the *premixed liquid form* of this medicine:

• Do not drink fruit juices or eat foods containing added salt until the diarrhea has stopped.

## Side Effects of This Medicine

Along with its needed effects, a medicine may cause some unwanted effects. Although not all of these side effects may occur, if they do occur they may need medical attention.

Check with your doctor as soon as possible if any of the following side effects occur:

*Symptoms of too much sodium (salt) in the body*
 Convulsions (seizures); dizziness; fast heartbeat; high blood pressure; irritability; muscle twitching; restlessness; swelling of feet or lower legs; weakness

*Symptoms of too much fluid in the body*
 Puffy eyelids

Other side effects may occur that usually do not need medical attention. These side effects may go away during treatment as your body adjusts to the medicine. However, check with your doctor if the following side effect continues or is bothersome:

*More common*
 Vomiting (mild)

Other side effects not listed above may also occur in some patients. If you notice any other effects, check with your doctor.

Revised: 12/02/92

# CARBOL-FUCHSIN   Topical

A commonly used brand name in the U.S. is Castel Plus.
Another commonly used name is Castellani Paint.
Generic name product may also be available.

## Description

Carbol-fuchsin (kar-bol-FOOK-sin) is used to treat fungus infections, including athlete's foot and ringworm of the nails. It may also be used as a drying agent in skin conditions where there is too much moisture. This medicine may also be used for other infections as determined by your doctor.

Some preparations containing carbol-fuchsin topical solution are available only with your doctor's prescription. Others are available without a prescription; however, your doctor may have special instructions on the use of topical carbol-fuchsin solutions for your medical condition.

Topical carbol-fuchsin is available in the following dosage form:

*Topical*
- Solution (U.S.)

## Before Using This Medicine

If you are using this medicine without a prescription, carefully read and follow any precautions on the label. For carbol-fuchsin, the following should be considered:

**Allergies**—Tell your doctor if you have ever had any unusual or allergic reaction to carbol-fuchsin. Also tell your health care professional if you are allergic to any other substances, such as preservatives or dyes.

**Pregnancy**—Studies in humans have not shown that carbol-fuchsin causes birth defects or other problems in humans.

**Breast-feeding**—Carbol-fuchsin has not been reported to cause problems in nursing babies.

**Children**—If you are treating an infant or child with eczema, do not use carbol-fushsin more than once a day. Although there is no specific information comparing use of carbol-fuchsin in children treated for other conditions with use in other age groups, this medicine is not expected to cause different side effects or problems in children than it does in adults.

**Older adults**—Many medicines have not been studied specifically in older people. Therefore, it may not be known whether they work exactly the same way they do in younger adults or if they cause different side effects or problems in older people. There is no specific information comparing use of carbol-fuchsin in the elderly with use in other age groups.

**Other medicines**—Although certain medicines should not be used together at all, in other cases two different medicines may be used together even if an interaction might occur. In these cases, your doctor may want to change the dose, or other precautions may be necessary. Tell your health care professional if you are using any other topical prescription or nonprescription (over-the-counter [OTC]) medicine that is to be applied to the same area of the skin.

## Proper Use of This Medicine

*Carbol-fuchsin is a poison if swallowed. Use only on the affected areas as directed. Do not swallow this medicine.*

Before applying this medicine, wash the affected areas with soap and water, and dry thoroughly.

Using an applicator or swab, apply this medicine only to the affected areas. Do not apply to large areas of the body, unless otherwise directed by your doctor.

When this medicine is applied to the fingers or toes, do not bandage them.

To help clear up your infection completely, *it is very important that you keep using this medicine for the full time of treatment,* even if your symptoms begin to clear up after a few days. Since fungus infections may be very slow to clear up, you may have to continue using this medicine every day for as long as several months or more. If you stop using this medicine too soon, your symptoms may return. *Do not miss any doses.*

**Dosing**—The dose of carbol-fuchsin will be different for different patients. *Follow your doctor's orders or the directions on the label.* The following information includes only the average doses of carbol-fuchsin. *If your dose is different, do not change it* unless your doctor tells you to do so.
- For *topical* dosage form (solution):
   —For fungal infections or as a drying agent:
      • Adults and children—Apply to the affected area(s) of the skin one to three times a day.

**Missed dose**—If you miss a dose of this medicine, apply it as soon as possible. However, if it is almost time for your next dose, skip the missed dose and go back to your regular dosing schedule.

**Storage**—To store this medicine:
- Keep out of the reach of children.
- Store away from heat and direct light.
- Keep the medicine from freezing.
- Do not keep outdated medicine or medicine no longer needed. Be sure that any discarded medicine is out of the reach of children.

## Precautions While Using This Medicine

If your skin problem does not improve within 1 week, or if it becomes worse, check with your doctor.

*This medicine will stain skin and clothing.* Avoid getting it on your clothes. The stain will slowly wear off from your skin.

---

## Side Effects of This Medicine

Along with its needed effects, a medicine may cause some unwanted effects. Although not all of these side effects may occur, if they do occur they may need medical attention.

Check with your doctor as soon as possible if the following side effect occurs:

Skin irritation not present before use of this medicine

Other side effects may occur that usually do not need medical attention. These side effects may go away during treatment as your body adjusts to the medicine. However, check with your doctor if the following side effect continues or is bothersome:

Mild, temporary stinging

Other side effects not listed above may also occur in some patients. If you notice any other effects, check with your doctor.

---

Revised: 02/10/92
Interim revision: 07/21/94

---

# CARBONIC ANHYDRASE INHIBITORS   Systemic

Some commonly used brand names are:

In the U.S.—

| | |
|---|---|
| Ak-Zol[1] | Diamox Sequels[1] |
| Daranide[2] | Neptazane[3] |
| Dazamide[1] | Storzolamide[1] |
| Diamox[1] | |

In Canada—

| | |
|---|---|
| Acetazolam[1] | Diamox Sequels[1] |
| Apo-Acetazolamide[1] | Neptazane[3] |
| Diamox[1] | |

Another commonly used name for dichlorphenamide is diclofenamide.

Note: For quick reference, the following carbonic anhydrase inhibitors are numbered to match the corresponding brand names.

This information applies to the following medicines:
1. Acetazolamide (a-set-a-ZOLE-a-mide)‡
2. Dichlorphenamide (dye-klor-FEN-a-mide)†
3. Methazolamide (meth-a-ZOLE-a-mide)‡

†Not commercially available in Canada.
‡Generic name product may also be available in U.S.

---

## Description

Carbonic anhydrase inhibitors are used to treat glaucoma. Acetazolamide is also used as an anticonvulsant to control certain seizures in the treatment of epilepsy. It is also sometimes used to prevent or lessen some effects in mountain climbers who climb to high altitudes, and to treat other conditions as determined by your doctor.

These medicines are available only with your doctor's prescription, in the following dosage forms:

*Oral*

Acetazolamide
- Extended-release capsules (U.S. and Canada)
- Tablets (U.S. and Canada)

Dichlorphenamide
- Tablets (U.S.)

Methazolamide
- Tablets (U.S. and Canada)

*Parenteral*

Acetazolamide
- Injection (U.S. and Canada)

## Before Using This Medicine

In deciding to use a medicine, the risks of taking the medicine must be weighed against the good it will do. This is a decision you and your doctor will make. For carbonic anhydrase inhibitors, the following should be considered:

**Allergies**—Tell your doctor if you have ever had any unusual or allergic reaction to carbonic anhydrase inhibitors, sulfonamides (sulfa drugs), or thiazide diuretics (a type of water pill). Also tell your health care professional if you are allergic to any other substances, such as foods, preservatives, or dyes.

**Pregnancy**—Carbonic anhydrase inhibitors have not been studied in pregnant women. However, studies in animals have shown that carbonic anhydrase inhibitors cause birth defects. Before taking this medicine, make sure your doctor knows if you are pregnant or if you may become pregnant.

**Breast-feeding**—Carbonic anhydrase inhibitors may pass into the breast milk. These medicines are not recommended during breast-feeding, because they may cause unwanted effects in nursing babies. It may be necessary for you to use another medicine or to stop breast-feeding during treatment. Be sure you have discussed this with your doctor.

**Children**—Although there is no specific information comparing use of carbonic anhydrase inhibitors in children with use in other age groups, these medicines are not expected to cause different side effects or problems in children than they do in adults.

**Older adults**—Many medicines have not been studies specifically in older people. Therefore, it may not be known whether they work exactly the same way they do in younger adults. Although there is no specific information comparing use of carbonic anhydrase inhibitors in the elderly with use in other age groups, these medicines are

---

not expected to cause different side effects or problems in older people than they do in younger adults.

**Other medicines**—Although certain medicines should not be used together at all, in other cases two different medicines may be used together even if an interaction might occur. In these cases, your doctor may want to change the dose, or other precautions may be necessary. When you are using carbonic anhydrase inhibitors, it is especially important that your health care professional know if you are using any of the following:

- Amphetamines or
- Mecamylamine (e.g., Inversine) or
- Quinidine (e.g., Quinidex)—Use of carbonic anhydrase inhibitors may increase the chance of side effects
- Methenamine (e.g., Mandelamine)—Use of carbonic anhydrase inhibitors may decrease the effectiveness of methenamine

**Other medical problems**—The presence of other medical problems may affect the use of carbonic anhydrase inhibitors. Make sure you tell your doctor if you have any other medical problems, especially:

- Diabetes mellitus (sugar diabetes)—Use of carbonic anhydrase inhibitors may increase the patient's blood and urine sugar concentrations
- Emphysema or other chronic lung disease—Use of carbonic anhydrase inhibitors may increase the risk of acidosis (shortness of breath, troubled breathing)
- Gout or
- Low blood levels of potassium or sodium—Use of carbonic anhydrase inhibitors may make the condition worse
- Kidney disease or stones—Higher blood levels of carbonic anhydrase inhibitors may result, which may increase the chance of side effects; also, these medicines may make the condition worse
- Liver disease—Use of carbonic anhydrase inhibitors may increase the risk of electrolyte imbalance and may make the condition worse
- Underactive adrenal gland (Addison's disease)—Use of carbonic anhydrase inhibitors may increase the risk of electrolyte imbalance

## Proper Use of This Medicine

*Take this medicine only as directed.* Do not take more of it and do not take it more often than your doctor ordered. To do so may increase the chance of side effects without increasing the effectiveness of this medicine.

This medicine may be taken with meals to lessen the chance of stomach upset. However, if stomach upset (nausea or vomiting) continues, check with your doctor.

This medicine may cause an increase in the amount of urine or in your frequency of urination. If you continue to take the medicine every day, these effects should lessen or stop. To keep the increase in urine from affecting your nighttime sleep:

- If you are to take a single dose a day, take it in the morning after breakfast.
- If you are to take more than one dose a day, take the last dose no later than 6 p.m., unless otherwise directed by your doctor.

However, it is best to plan your dose or doses according to a schedule that will least affect your personal activities and sleep. Ask your health care professional to help you plan the best time to take this medicine.

**Dosing**—The doses of carbonic anhydrase inhibitors will be different for different patients. *Follow your doctor's orders or the directions on the label.* The following information includes only the average doses of these medicines. *If your dose is different, do not change it* unless your doctor tells you to do so.

The number of capsules or tablets that you take depends on the strength of the medicine. Also, *the number of doses you take each day, the time allowed between doses, and the length of time you take the medicine depend on the medical problem for which you are taking the carbonic anhydrase inhibitor.*

*For acetazolamide*

- For *oral* dosage form (extended-release capsules):
  —For glaucoma:
    - Adults—500 milligrams (mg) two times a day, in the morning and evening.
    - Children—Use and dose must be determined by your doctor.
  —For altitude sickness:
    - Adults—500 mg one or two times a day.
    - Children—Use and dose must be determined by your doctor.
- For *oral* dosage form (tablets):
  —For glaucoma:
    - Adults—250 mg one to four times a day.
    - Children—Dose is based on body weight and must be determined by your doctor. The usual dose is 10 to 15 mg per kilogram (kg) (4.5 to 6.8 mg per pound) of body weight a day in divided doses.
  —For epilepsy:
    - Adults and children—Dose is based on body weight and must be determined by your doctor. The usual dose is 10 mg per kg (4.5 mg per pound) of body weight a day in divided doses.
  —For altitude sickness:
    - Adults—250 mg two to four times a day.
    - Children—Use and dose must be determined by your doctor.
- For *injection* dosage form:
  —For glaucoma:
    - Adults—500 mg, injected into a muscle or vein, for one dose.
    - Children—Dose is based on body weight and must be determined by your doctor. The usual dose is 5 to 10 mg per kg (2.3 to 4.5 mg per pound) of body weight every six hours, injected into a muscle or vein.

*For dichlorphenamide*
- For *oral* dosage form (tablets):
  —For glaucoma:
    - Adults—25 to 50 milligrams (mg) one to three times a day.
    - Children—Use and dose must be determined by your doctor.

*For methazolamide*
- For *oral* dosage form (tablets):
  —For glaucoma:
    - Adults—50 to 100 milligrams (mg) two or three times a day.
    - Children—Use and dose must be determined by your doctor.

**Missed dose**—If you miss a dose of this medicine, take it as soon as possible. However, if it is almost time for your next dose, skip the missed dose and go back to your regular dosing schedule. Do not double doses.

**Storage**—To store this medicine:
- Keep out of the reach of children.
- Store away from heat and direct light.
- Do not store the capsule or tablet form of this medicine in the bathroom, near the kitchen sink, or in other damp places. Heat or moisture may cause the medicine to break down.
- Do not keep outdated medicine or medicine no longer needed. Be sure that any discarded medicine is out of the reach of children.

## Precautions While Using This Medicine

This medicine may cause some people to feel drowsy, dizzy, lightheaded, or more tired than they are normally. *Make sure you know how you react to this medicine before you drive, use machines, or do anything else that could be dangerous if you are not alert.*

It is important that your doctor check your progress at regular visits. Your doctor may want to do certain tests to see if the medicine is working properly or to see if certain side effects may be occurring without your knowing it.

*This medicine may cause a loss of potassium from your body.* To help prevent this, your doctor may want you to eat or drink foods that have a high potassium content (for example, orange or other citrus fruit juices) or take a potassium supplement. It is very important to follow these directions. Also, it is important not to change your diet on your own. This is more important if you are already on a special diet (as for diabetes) or if you are taking a potassium supplement. Extra potassium may not be necessary and, in some cases, too much potassium could be harmful.

For *diabetic patients:*
- This medicine may raise blood and urine sugar levels. While you are using this medicine, be especially careful in testing for sugar in your blood or urine.

If you have any questions about this, check with your doctor.

Your doctor may want you to increase the amount of fluids you drink while you are taking this medicine. This is to prevent kidney stones. However, do not increase the amount of fluids you drink without first checking with your doctor.

For patients taking *acetazolamide as an anticonvulsant:*
- *If you have been taking acetazolamide regularly for several weeks or more, do not suddenly stop taking it.* Your doctor may want you to reduce gradually the amount you are taking before stopping completely.

## Side Effects of This Medicine

Along with its needed effects, a medicine may cause some unwanted effects. Although not all of these side effects may occur, if they do occur they may need medical attention.

*Check with your doctor immediately* if either of the following side effects occurs:

*Rare*
Shortness of breath or trouble in breathing

Also, check with your doctor as soon as possible if any of the following side effects occur:

*More common*
Unusual tiredness or weakness

*Less common*
Blood in urine; difficult urination; mental depression; pain in lower back; pain or burning while urinating; sudden decrease in amount of urine

*Rare*
Bloody or black, tarry stools; clumsiness or unsteadiness; confusion; convulsions (seizures); darkening of urine; fever; hives, itching of skin, skin rash, or sores; muscle weakness (severe); pale stools; ringing or buzzing in the ears; sore throat; trembling; unusual bruising or bleeding; yellow eyes or skin

*Symptoms of too much potassium loss*
Dryness of mouth; increased thirst; irregular heartbeats; mood or mental changes; muscle cramps or pain; nausea or vomiting; unusual tiredness or weakness; weak pulse

Also, check with your doctor if you have any changes in your vision (especially problems with seeing faraway objects) when you first begin taking this medicine.

Other side effects may occur that usually do not need medical attention. These side effects may go away during treatment as your body adjusts to the medicine. However, check with your doctor if any of the following side effects continue or are bothersome:

*More common*
Diarrhea; general feeling of discomfort or illness; increase in frequency of urination or amount of urine (rare with methazolamide); loss of appetite; metallic taste in mouth; nausea or vomiting; numbness, tingling, or

burning in hands, fingers, feet, toes, mouth, lips, tongue, or anus; weight loss

*Less common or rare*

Constipation; dizziness or lightheadedness; drowsiness; feeling of choking or lump in the throat; headache; increased sensitivity of eyes to sunlight; loss of taste and smell; nervousness or irritability

Other side effects not listed above may also occur in some patients. If you notice any other effects, check with your doctor.

Revised: 06/21/94

---

# CARBOPLATIN    Systemic

Some commonly used brand names are:

**In the U.S.—**
   Paraplatin

**In Canada—**
   Paraplatin
   Paraplatin-AQ

## Description

Carboplatin (KAR-boe-pla-tin) belongs to the group of medicines known as alkylating agents. It is used to treat some kinds of cancer.

Carboplatin interferes with the growth of cancer cells, which are eventually destroyed. Since the growth of normal body cells may also be affected by carboplatin, other effects will also occur. Some of these may be serious and must be reported to your doctor. Other effects may not be serious but may cause concern. Some effects may not occur for months or years after the medicine is used.

Before you begin treatment with carboplatin, you and your doctor should talk about the good this medicine will do as well as the risks of using it.

Carboplatin is to be administered only by or under the immediate supervision of your doctor. It is available in the following dosage form:

*Parenteral*

• Injection (U.S. and Canada)

## Before Using This Medicine

In deciding to use a medicine, the risks of taking the medicine must be weighed against the good it will do. This is a decision you and your doctor will make. For carboplatin, the following should be considered:

**Allergies**—Tell your doctor if you have ever had any unusual or allergic reaction to carboplatin, cisplatin, or any other platinum-containing substance.

**Pregnancy**—There is a chance that this medicine may cause birth defects if either the male or female is taking it at the time of conception or if it is taken during pregnancy. Carboplatin causes toxic or harmful effects and birth defects in rats. In addition, many cancer medicines may cause sterility which could be permanent. Although sterility has not been reported with this medicine, the possibility should be kept in mind.

Be sure that you have discussed these possible effects with your doctor before receiving this medicine. It is best to use some kind of birth control while you are receiving carboplatin. Tell your doctor right away if you think you have become pregnant while receiving carboplatin. Before receiving carboplatin, make sure your doctor knows if you are pregnant or if you may become pregnant.

**Breast-feeding**—Because carboplatin may cause serious side effects, breast-feeding is generally not recommended while you are receiving it.

**Children**—Studies on this medicine have been done only in adult patients and there is no specific information comparing use of carboplatin in children with use in other age groups.

**Older adults**—Some side effects of carboplatin (especially blood problems or numbness or tingling in fingers or toes) may be more likely to occur in the elderly.

**Other medicines**—Although certain medicines should not be used together at all, in other cases two different medicines may be used together even if an interaction might occur. In these cases, your doctor may want to change the dose, or other precautions may be necessary. When receiving carboplatin it is especially important that your health care professional know if you have every been treated with radiation or cancer medicines or if you are taking any of the following:

• Amphotericin B by injection (e.g., Fungizone) or
• Antithyroid agents (medicine for overactive thyroid) or
• Azathioprine (e.g., Imuran) or
• Chloramphenicol (e.g., Chloromycetin) or
• Colchicine or
• Flucytosine (e.g., Ancobon) or
• Ganciclovir (e.g., Cytovene) or
• Interferon (e.g., Intron A, Roferon-A) or
• Plicamycin (e.g., Mithracin) or
• Zidovudine (e.g., AZT, Retrovir)—Carboplatin may increase the effects of these medicines or radiation on the blood

**Other medical problems**—The presence of other medical problems may affect the use of carboplatin. Make sure you tell your doctor if you have any other medical problems, especially:

• Chickenpox (including recent exposure) or
• Herpes zoster (shingles)—Risk of severe disease affecting other parts of the body
• Hearing problems—May be worsened by carboplatin

- Infection—Carboplatin decreases your body's ability to fight infection
- Kidney disease—Effects may be increased because of slower removal from the body

## Proper Use of This Medicine

This medicine is sometimes given together with certain other medicines. If you are using a combination of medicines, it is important that you receive each one at the proper time. If you are taking some of these medicines by mouth, ask your health care professional to help you plan a way to take them at the right times.

This medicine usually causes nausea and vomiting that may sometimes be severe. However, it is very important that you continue to receive the medicine, even if you begin to feel ill. Ask your health care professional for ways to lessen these effects, especially if they are severe.

**Dosing**—The dose of carboplatin will be different for different patients. The dose that is used may depend on a number of things, including what the medicine is being used for, the patient's size, and whether or not other medicines are also being taken. *If you are receiving carboplatin at home, follow your doctor's orders or the directions on the label.* If you have any questions about the proper dose of carboplatin, ask your doctor.

## Precautions While Using This Medicine

*It is very important that your doctor check your progress at regular visits* to make sure that this medicine is working properly and to check for unwanted effects.

While you are being treated with carboplatin, and after you stop treatment with it, *do not have any immunizations (vaccinations) without your doctor's approval.* Carboplatin may lower your body's resistance and there is a chance you might get the infection the immunization is meant to prevent. In addition, other persons living in your household should not take oral polio vaccine since there is a chance they could pass the polio virus on to you. Also, avoid persons who have taken oral polio vaccine. Do not get close to them, and do not stay in the same room with them for very long. If you cannot take these precautions, you should consider wearing a protective face mask that covers the nose and mouth.

Carboplatin can temporarily lower the number of white blood cells in your blood, increasing the chance of getting an infection. It can also lower the number of platelets, which are necessary for proper blood clotting. If this occurs, there are certain precautions you can take, especially when your blood count is low, to reduce the risk of infection or bleeding:

- If you can, avoid people with infections. *Check with your doctor immediately* if you think you are getting an infection or if you get a fever or chills, cough or hoarseness, lower back or side pain, or painful or difficult urination.
- *Check with your doctor immediately* if you notice any unusual bleeding or bruising; black, tarry stools;

blood in urine or stools; or pinpoint red spots on your skin.
- Be careful when using a regular toothbrush, dental floss, or toothpick. Your medical doctor, dentist, or nurse may recommend other ways to clean your teeth and gums. Check with your health care professional before having any dental work done.
- Do not touch your eyes or the inside of your nose unless you have just washed your hands and have not touched anything else in the meantime.
- Be careful not to cut yourself when you are using sharp objects such as a safety razor or fingernail or toenail cutters.
- Avoid contact sports or other situations where bruising or injury could occur.

## Side Effects of This Medicine

Along with its needed effects, a medicine may cause some unwanted effects. Although not all of these side effects may occur, if they do occur they may need medical attention.

Also, because of the way these medicines act on the body, there is a chance that they might cause other unwanted effects that may not occur until months or years after the medicine is used. These delayed effects may include certain types of cancer, such as leukemia. Discuss these possible effects with your doctor.

*Check with your doctor or nurse immediately* if any of the following side effects occur:

*Less common*
Black, tarry stools; blood in urine or stools; cough or hoarseness; fever or chills; lower back or side pain; painful or difficult urination; pinpoint red spots on skin; skin rash or itching; unusual bleeding or bruising

*Rare*
Wheezing

Check with your doctor as soon as possible if any of the following side effects occur:

*More common*
Pain at place of injection

*Less common*
Numbness or tingling in fingers or toes

*Rare*
Blurred vision; ringing in ears; sores in mouth and on lips

Other side effects may occur that usually do not need medical attention. These side effects may go away during treatment as your body adjusts to the medicine. Also, your health care professional may be able to tell you about ways to prevent or reduce some of these side effects. Check with your health care professional if any of the following side effects continue or are bothersome or if you have any questions about them:

*More common*
Nausea and vomiting; unusual tiredness or weakness

*Less common*
    Constipation or diarrhea; loss of appetite

This medicine may cause a temporary loss of hair in some people. After treatment with carboplatin has ended, normal hair growth should return.

Other side effects not listed above may also occur in some patients. If you notice any other effects, check with your doctor.

Revised: 06/03/92
Interim revision: 05/02/94

# CARBOPROST  Systemic

Some commonly used brand names are:
**In the U.S.—**
    Hemabate
**In Canada—**
    Prostin/15M

## Description

Carboprost (KAR-boe-prost) is given by injection to cause abortion. It is an oxytocic, which means it acts by causing the uterus to contract the way it does during labor and also helps the cervix to dilate.

Carboprost may also be used for other purposes as determined by your doctor.

Carboprost is to be administered only by or under the immediate care of your doctor. It is available in the following dosage form:
*Parenteral*
* Injection (U.S. and Canada)

## Before Receiving This Medicine

In deciding to use a medicine, the risks of taking the medicine must be weighed against the good it will do. This is a decision you and your doctor will make. For carboprost, the following should be considered:

**Allergies**—Tell your doctor if you have ever had any unusual or allergic reaction to carboprost or other oxytocics (medicines that stimulate the uterus to contract). Also tell your health care professional if you are allergic to any other substances, such as foods, preservatives, or dyes.

**Other medicines**—Although certain medicines should not be used together at all, in other cases two different medicines may be used together even if an interaction might occur. In these cases, your doctor may want to change the dose, or other precautions may be necessary. Tell your doctor if you are taking any prescription or nonprescription (over-the-counter [OTC]) medicine.

**Other medical problems**—The presence of other medical problems may affect the use of carboprost. Make sure you tell your doctor if you have any other medical problems, especially:
* Adrenal gland disease (history of)—Carboprost stimulates the body to produce steroids

* Anemia—In some patients, abortion with carboprost may result in loss of blood that may require a transfusion
* Asthma (or history of) or
* Lung disease—Carboprost may cause narrowing of the blood vessels in the lungs or narrowing of the lung passages
* Diabetes mellitus (sugar diabetes) (history of)
* Epilepsy (or history of)—Rarely, seizures have occurred with use of carboprost
* Fibroid tumors of the uterus or
* Uterus surgery (history of)—There is an increased risk of rupture of the uterus
* Glaucoma—Rarely, the pressure within the eye has increased during use of carboprost
* Heart or blood vessel disease (or history of) or
* High blood pressure (or history of) or
* Low blood pressure (or history of)—Carboprost may cause changes in heart function or blood pressure changes
* Jaundice (history of)
* Kidney disease (or history of)
* Liver disease (or history of)—The body may not get carboprost out of the bloodstream at the usual rate, which may make the medicine work longer or cause toxic effects

## Proper Use of This Medicine

**Dosing**—The dose of carboprost will be different for different patients. Your doctor will give you the dose of this medicine and follow your care in a hospital or another health care setting. The following information includes only the average doses of carboprost.
* For *injection* dosage form:
    —For causing an abortion in the second trimester of pregnancy (13th to 24th week):
      * Adults—At first, 100 to 250 micrograms (mcg) injected deep into a muscle. Then, 250 to 500 mcg every one and one-half to three and one-half hours for up to two days.
    —For bleeding of the uterus after pregnancy:
      * Adults—250 mcg injected deep into a muscle. Your doctor may repeat this dose every fifteen to ninety minutes as needed.

## Side Effects of This Medicine

Along with its needed effects, a medicine may cause some unwanted effects. Although not all of these side effects

may occur, if they do occur they may need medical attention.

*Tell the health care professional immediately* if any of the following side effects occur:

*Less common or rare*
Fast or slow heartbeat; headache (severe and continuing); hives or skin rash; increased pain of the uterus; pale, cool, blotchy skin on arms or legs; pressing or painful feeling in chest; shortness of breath; swelling of face, inside the nose, and eyelids; tightness in chest; trouble in breathing; weak or absent pulse in arms or legs; wheezing

Check with the health care professional as soon as possible if any of the following side effects occur:
Constipation; pain or inflammation at place of injection; tender or mildly bloated abdomen or stomach

Other side effects may occur that usually do not need medical attention. These side effects usually go away after the medicine is stopped. However, let the health care professional know if any of the following side effects continue or are bothersome:

*More common*
Diarrhea; nausea; vomiting
*Less common or rare*
Chills or shivering; dizziness; fever (temporary); flushing or redness of face; headache; stomach cramps or pain

This procedure may result in some effects, which occur after the procedure is completed, that need medical attention. Check with your doctor if you notice any of the following:
Chills or shivering (continuing); fever (continuing); foul-smelling vaginal discharge; increase in uterus bleeding; pain in lower abdomen

Other side effects not listed above may also occur in some patients. If you notice any other effects, check with your health care professional.

Revised: 10/26/92
Interim revision: 06/08/94

# CARMUSTINE   Systemic

A commonly used brand name in the U.S. and Canada is BiCNU. Another commonly used name is BCNU.

## Description

Carmustine (kar-MUS-teen) belongs to the group of medicines known as alkylating agents. It is used to treat some kinds of cancer.

Carmustine interferes with the growth of cancer cells, which are eventually destroyed. Since the growth of normal body cells may also be affected by carmustine, other effects will also occur. Some of these may be serious and must be reported to your doctor. Other effects, like hair loss, may not be serious but may cause concern. Some effects may not occur for months or years after the medicine is used.

Before you begin treatment with carmustine, you and your doctor should talk about the good this medicine will do as well as the risks of using it.

Carmustine is to be administered only by or under the immediate supervision of your doctor. It is available in the following dosage form:

*Parenteral*
• Injection (U.S. and Canada)

## Before Using This Medicine

In deciding to use a medicine, the risks of taking the medicine must be weighed against the good it will do.

This is a decision you and your doctor will make. For carmustine, the following should be considered:

**Allergies**—Tell your doctor if you have ever had any unusual or allergic reaction to carmustine.

**Pregnancy**—There is a chance that this medicine may cause birth defects if either the male or female is taking it at the time of conception or if it is taken during pregnancy. Carmustine causes toxic or harmful effects in the fetus of rats and rabbits and causes birth defects in rats at doses about the same as the human dose. In addition, many cancer medicines may cause sterility which could be permanent. Although this has only been reported in animals with this medicine, the possibility should be kept in mind.

Be sure that you have discussed this with your doctor before receiving this medicine. It is best to use some kind of birth control while you are receiving carmustine. Tell your doctor right away if you think you have become pregnant while receiving carmustine.

**Breast-feeding**—Because carmustine may cause serious side effects, breast-feeding is generally not recommended while you are receiving it.

**Children**—Although there is no specific information comparing use of carmustine in children with use in other age groups, this medicine is not expected to cause different side effects or problems in children than it does in adults.

**Older adults**—Many medicines have not been studied specifically in older people. Therefore, it may not be known whether they work exactly the same way they do in younger adults or if they cause different side effects or problems in older people. There is no specific information comparing use of carmustine in the elderly with use in other age groups.

**Other medicines**—Although certain medicines should not be used together at all, in other cases two different medicines may be used together even if an interaction might occur. In these cases, your doctor may want to change the dose, or other precautions may be necessary. When you are receiving carmustine, it is especially important that your health care professional know if you are taking any of the following:

- Amphotericin B by injection (e.g., Fungizone) or
- Antithyroid agents (medicine for overactive thyroid) or
- Azathioprine (e.g., Imuran) or
- Chloramphenicol (e.g., Chloromycetin) or
- Colchicine or
- Flucytosine (e.g., Ancobon) or
- Ganciclovir (e.g., Cytovene) or
- Interferon (e.g., Intron A, Roferon-A) or
- Plicamycin (e.g., Mithramycin) or
- Zidovudine (e.g., AZT, Retrovir) or
- If you have ever been treated with radiation or cancer medicines—Carmustine may increase the effects of these medicines or radiation therapy on the blood

**Other medical problems**—The presence of other medical problems may affect the use of carmustine. Make sure you tell your doctor if you have any other medical problems, especially:

- Chickenpox (including recent exposure) or
- Herpes zoster (shingles)—Risk of severe disease affecting other parts of the body
- Infection—Carmustine decreases your body's ability to fight infection
- Kidney disease—Effects of carmustine may be increased because of slower removal from the body
- Liver disease—Carmustine may cause side effects to the liver
- Lung disease—Risk of lung problems caused by carmustine may be increased

**Smoking**—Increased risk of lung problems

## Proper Use of This Medicine

Carmustine is sometimes given together with certain other medicines. If you are using a combination of medicines, it is important that you receive each one at the proper time. If you are taking some of these medicines by mouth, ask your health care professional to help you plan a way to take them at the right times.

This medicine often causes nausea and vomiting, which usually last no longer than 4 to 6 hours. It is very important that you continue to receive the medicine, even if you begin to feel ill. Ask your health care professional for ways to lessen these effects.

**Dosing**—The dose of carmustine will be different for different patients. The dose that is used may depend on a number of things, including what the medicine is being used for, the patient's size, and whether or not other medicines are also being taken. *If you are receiving carmustine at home, follow your doctor's orders or the directions on the label.* If you have any questions about the proper dose of carmustine, ask your doctor.

## Precautions While Using This Medicine

*It is very important that your doctor check your progress at regular visits* to make sure that this medicine is working properly and to check for unwanted effects.

While you are being treated with carmustine, and after you stop treatment with it, *do not have any immunizations (vaccinations) without your doctor's approval.* Carmustine may lower your body's resistance and there is a chance you might get the infection the immunization is meant to prevent. In addition, other persons living in your household should not take oral polio vaccine since there is a chance they could pass the polio virus on to you. Also, avoid persons who have taken oral polio vaccine. Do not get close to them, and do not stay in the same room with them for very long. If you cannot take these precautions, you should consider wearing a protective face mask that covers the nose and mouth.

Carmustine can temporarily lower the number of white blood cells in your blood, increasing the chance of getting an infection. It can also lower the number of platelets, which are necessary for proper blood clotting. If this occurs, there are certain precautions you can take, especially when your blood count is low, to reduce the risk of infection or bleeding:

- If you can, avoid people with infections. *Check with your doctor immediately* if you think you are getting an infection or if you get a fever or chills, cough or hoarseness, lower back or side pain, or painful or difficult urination.
- *Check with your doctor immediately* if you notice any unusual bleeding or bruising; black, tarry stools; blood in urine or stools; or pinpoint red spots on your skin.
- Be careful when using a regular toothbrush, dental floss, or toothpick. Your medical doctor, dentist, or nurse may recommend other ways to clean your teeth and gums. Check with your medical doctor before having any dental work done.
- Do not touch your eyes or the inside of your nose unless you have just washed your hands and have not touched anything else in the meantime.
- Be careful not to cut yourself when you are using sharp objects such as a safety razor or fingernail or toenail cutters.
- Avoid contact sports or other situations where bruising or injury could occur.

If carmustine accidentally seeps out of the vein into which it is injected, it may damage some tissues and cause scarring. *Tell the doctor or nurse right away if you notice redness, pain, or swelling at the place of injection.*

## Side Effects of This Medicine

Along with its needed effects, a medicine may cause some unwanted effects. Some side effects will have signs or symptoms that you can see or feel. Your doctor may watch for others by doing certain tests. Some of the unwanted effects that may be caused by carmustine are listed below. Although not all of these effects may occur, if they do occur, they may need medical attention.

Also, because of the way these medicines act on the body, there is a chance that they might cause other unwanted effects that may not occur until months or years after the medicine is used. These delayed effects may include certain types of cancer, such as leukemia. Discuss these possible effects with your doctor.

*Check with your doctor or nurse immediately* if any of the following side effects occur:

*More common*

Pain or redness at place of injection

*Less common*

Black, tarry stools; blood in urine or stools; cough or hoarseness; fever or chills; lower back or side pain; painful or difficult urination; pinpoint red spots on skin; unusual bleeding or bruising

Check with your health care professional as soon as possible if any of the following side effects occur:

*More common*

Shortness of breath

*Less common*

Flushing of face; sores in mouth and on lips; unusual tiredness or weakness

*Rare*

Decrease in urination; swelling of feet or lower legs

This medicine may also cause the following side effects that your doctor will watch for:

*More common*

Low red blood cell count; low white blood cell count

*Rare*

Liver problems; lung problems

Other side effects may occur that usually do not need medical attention. These side effects may go away during treatment as your body adjusts to the medicine. Also, your health care professional may be able to tell you about ways to prevent or reduce some of these side effects. Check with your health care professional if any of the following side effects continue or are bothersome or if you have any questions about them:

*More common*

Nausea and vomiting (usually lasting no longer than 4 to 6 hours)

*Less common*

Diarrhea; discoloration of skin along vein of injection; dizziness; loss of appetite; skin rash and itching; trouble in swallowing; trouble in walking

This medicine may cause a temporary loss of hair in some people. After treatment with carmustine has ended, normal hair growth should return.

Side effects that affect your lungs (for example, cough and shortness of breath) may be more likely to occur if you smoke.

After you stop receiving carmustine, it may still produce some side effects that need attention. During this period of time check with your health care professional if you notice any of the following:

Black, tarry stools; blood in urine or stools; cough or hoarseness; fever or chills; lower back or side pain; painful or difficult urination; pinpoint red spots on skin; shortness of breath; unusual bleeding or bruising

Other side effects not listed above may also occur in some patients. If you notice any other effects, check with your health care professional.

Revised: 07/15/94

# CELLULOSE SODIUM PHOSPHATE    Systemic†

A commonly used brand name in the U.S. is Calcibind.

†Not commercially available in Canada.

## Description

Cellulose sodium phosphate (SELL-u-lose SO-dee-um FOS-fate) is used to prevent the formation of calcium-containing kidney stones. It is used in patients whose bodies absorb too much calcium from their food.

Cellulose sodium phosphate works by combining with the calcium and some other minerals in food. This prevents the calcium from reaching the kidneys where the stones are formed.

Cellulose sodium phosphate is available only with your doctor's prescription, in the following dosage form:

*Oral*

• Powder for oral suspension (U.S.)

## Before Using This Medicine

In deciding to use a medicine, the risks of taking the medicine must be weighed against the good it will do. This is a decision you and your doctor will make. For

cellulose sodium phosphate, the following should be considered:

**Allergies**—Tell your doctor if you have ever had any unusual or allergic reaction to cellulose sodium phosphate. Also tell your health care professional if you are allergic to any other substances, such as foods, preservatives, or dyes.

**Diet**—Make certain your health care professional knows if you are on any special diet, such as a low-sodium or low-sugar diet. Also tell your health care professional if your diet contains large amounts of milk or other dairy products, spinach (or other dark green leafy vegetables), chocolate, brewed tea, or rhubarb or if you are taking vitamin C or magnesium supplements.

**Pregnancy**—Studies have not been done in either humans or animals. However, pregnant women usually need more calcium in their diet, and should not take cellulose sodium phosphate unless it is clearly needed. Be sure you have discussed the risks and benefits with your doctor.

**Breast-feeding**—It is not known whether cellulose sodium phosphate passes into breast milk. However, this medicine has not been reported to cause problems in nursing babies.

**Children**—Although there is no specific information comparing use of cellulose sodium phosphate in children with use in any other age group, its use is not recommended in children up to 16 years of age because of the increased need for calcium in growing children.

**Older adults**—Many medicines have not been studied specifically in older people. Therefore, it may not be known whether they work exactly the same way they do in younger adults or if they cause different side effects or problems in older people. There is no specific information comparing use of cellulose sodium phosphate in the elderly with use in other age groups.

**Other medicines**—Although certain medicines should not be used together at all, in other cases two different medicines may be used together even if an interaction might occur. In these cases, your doctor may want to change the dose, or other precautions may be necessary. When you are taking cellulose sodium phosphate, it is especially important that your health care professional know if you are taking any of the following:

- Calcium supplements, or calcium containing antacids or laxatives—Use may lead to too much calcium in the body, preventing the cellulose sodium phosphate from working properly
- Magnesium supplements, or magnesium containing antacids or laxatives—Cellulose sodium phosphate and magnesium should not be taken within 1 hour of each other

**Other medical problems**—The presence of other medical problems may affect the use of cellulose sodium phosphate. Make sure you tell your doctor if you have any other medical problems, especially:

- Bone disease—Cellulose sodium phosphate may make the condition worse

- Edema or swelling or
- Heart disease—The high sodium content of cellulose sodium phosphate may cause the body to hold water
- Intestinal problems or
- Parathyroid disease or problems—Cellulose sodium phosphate may increase the risk of bone problems

## Proper Use of This Medicine

*Take this medicine mixed in a full glass (8 ounces) of water, soft drink, or fruit juice.* After drinking all the liquid containing the medicine, rinse the glass with a little more liquid. Drink that also to make sure you get all the medicine.

*It is very important that you take cellulose sodium phosphate with meals.* If this medicine is taken an hour or more after a meal, it will not work properly.

*Take cellulose sodium phosphate only as directed.* Do not take more of it, do not take it more often, and do not take it for a longer time than your doctor ordered. To do so may increase the chance of side effects.

*Drink at least a full glass (8 ounces) of water, a soft drink, or fruit juice every hour while you are awake, unless otherwise directed by your doctor.* This also will help prevent kidney stones while you are taking cellulose sodium phosphate.

**Dosing**—The dose of cellulose sodium phosphate will be different for different patients. *Follow your doctor's orders or the directions on the label.* The following information includes only the average doses of cellulose sodium phosphate. *If your dose is different, do not change it* unless your doctor tells you to do so.

- To prevent kidney stones:
  - —Adults: At first, 10 to 15 grams a day (3.3 to 5 grams three times a day with meals). Then, your doctor may reduce your dose.
  - —Children: Use is not recommended.

**Missed dose**—If you miss a dose of this medicine, skip the missed dose and go back to your regular dosing schedule. Do not double doses.

**Storage**—To store this medicine:

- Keep out of the reach of children.
- Store away from heat and direct light.
- Do not store in the bathroom, near the kitchen sink, or in other damp places. Heat or moisture may cause the medicine to break down.
- Do not keep outdated medicine or medicine no longer needed. Be sure that any discarded medicine is out of the reach of children.

## Precautions While Using This Medicine

*It is important that your doctor check your progress at regular visits.* This is to make sure cellulose sodium phosphate is working properly and does not cause unwanted effects.

If you are taking a magnesium supplement, take it at least one hour before or after you take cellulose sodium phosphate. Otherwise, the magnesium may combine with this medicine and keep it from working properly.

Do not take vitamin C, or eat spinach (or other dark green leafy vegetables), chocolate, brewed tea, or rhubarb while you are taking cellulose sodium phosphate. They may increase the chance of kidney stones.

Do not drink milk or eat milk products (for example, cheese, ice cream, and yogurt) while you are taking this medicine, because dairy products are high in calcium. Drinking milk or eating milk products may keep cellulose sodium phosphate from working properly.

While you are taking cellulose sodium phosphate, do not eat salty foods or use extra salt on foods. To do so may increase the chance of unwanted effects.

For patients on a low-sodium diet:
- This medicine contains sodium. If you have any questions about this, check with your health care professional.

## Side Effects of This Medicine

Along with its needed effects, a medicine may cause some unwanted effects. Although not all of these side effects may occur, if they do occur they may need medical attention.

Check with your doctor as soon as possible if any of the following side effects occur:

*With long-term use*
    Convulsions (seizures); drowsiness; loss of appetite; mood or mental changes; muscle spasms or twitching; nausea or vomiting; trembling; unusual tiredness or weakness

Other side effects may occur that usually do not need medical attention. These side effects may go away during treatment as your body adjusts to the medicine. However, check with your doctor if any of the following side effects continue or are bothersome:

*More common*
    Abdominal or stomach discomfort; loose bowel movements or diarrhea

Other side effects not listed above may also occur in some patients. If you notice any other effects, check with your doctor.

Revised: 12/02/92
Interim revision: 05/13/94

# CEPHALOSPORINS  Systemic

Some commonly used brand names are:

**In the U.S.—**

| | |
|---|---|
| Ancef[4] | Keftab[18] |
| Ceclor[1] | Kefurox[17] |
| Cefadyl[20] | Kefzol[4] |
| Cefanex[18] | Mandol[3] |
| Cefizox[15] | Mefoxin[11] |
| Cefobid[8] | Monocid[7] |
| Cefotan[10] | Rocephin[16] |
| Ceftin[17] | Suprax[5] |
| Cefzil[13] | Tazicef[14] |
| Ceptaz[14] | Tazidime[14] |
| Claforan[9] | Ultracef[2] |
| C-Lexin[18] | Vantin[12] |
| Duricef[2] | Velosef[21] |
| Fortaz[14] | Zefazone[6] |
| Keflex[18] | Zinacef[17] |
| Keflin[19] | Zolicef[4] |

**In Canada—**

| | |
|---|---|
| Ancef[4] | Keflin[19] |
| Apo-Cephalex[18] | Kefurox[17] |
| Ceclor[1] | Kefzol[4] |
| Cefizox[15] | Mandol[3] |
| Cefobid[8] | Mefoxin[11] |
| Cefotan[10] | Novo-Lexin[18] |
| Ceftin[17] | Nu-Cephalex[18] |
| Ceptaz[14] | Rocephin[16] |
| Claforan[9] | Suprax[5] |
| Duricef[2] | Tazidime[14] |
| Fortaz[14] | Velosef[21] |
| Gen-Cefazolin[4] | Zinacef[17] |
| Keflex[18] | |

Note: For quick reference, the following cephalosporins are numbered to match the corresponding brand names.

This information applies to the following medicines:
1. Cefaclor (SEF-a-klor)
2. Cefadroxil (sef-a-DROX-ill)‡
3. Cefamandole (sef-a-MAN-dole)
4. Cefazolin (sef-A-zoe-lin)‡
5. Cefixime (sef-IX-eem)
6. Cefmetazole (sef-MET-a-zole)†
7. Cefonicid (se-FON-i-sid)†
8. Cefoperazone (sef-oh-PER-a-zone)
9. Cefotaxime (sef-oh-TAKS-eem)
10. Cefotetan (sef-oh-TEE-tan)
11. Cefoxitin (se-FOX-i-tin)
12. Cefpodoxime (sef-pode-OX-eem)†
13. Cefprozil (sef-PROE-zil)†
14. Ceftazidime (sef-TAY-zi-deem)
15. Ceftizoxime (sef-ti-ZOX-eem)
16. Ceftriaxone (sef-try-AX-one)
17. Cefuroxime (se-fyoor-OX-eem)
18. Cephalexin (sef-a-LEX-in)‡
19. Cephalothin (sef-A-loe-thin)‡
20. Cephapirin (sef-a-PYE-rin)†‡
21. Cephradine (SEF-ra-deen)‡

†Not commercially available in Canada.
‡Generic name product may also be available in the U.S.

## Description

Cephalosporins (sef-a-loe-SPOR-ins) are used in the treatment of infections caused by bacteria. They work by killing bacteria or preventing their growth.

Cephalosporins are used to treat infections in many different parts of the body. They are sometimes given with other antibiotics. Some cephalosporins are also given by injection to prevent infections before, during, and after surgery. However, cephalosporins will not work for colds, flu, or other virus infections.

Cephalosporins are available only with your doctor's prescription, in the following dosage forms:

*Oral*
Cefaclor
- Capsules (U.S. and Canada)
- Oral suspension (U.S. and Canada)
Cefadroxil
- Capsules (U.S. and Canada)
- Oral suspension (U.S.)
- Tablets (U.S.)
Cefixime
- Oral suspension (U.S. and Canada)
- Tablets (U.S. and Canada)
Cefpodoxime
- Oral suspension (U.S.)
- Tablets (U.S.)
Cefprozil
- Oral suspension (U.S.)
- Tablets (U.S.)
Cefuroxime
- Tablets (U.S. and Canada)
Cephalexin
- Capsules (U.S. and Canada)
- Oral suspension (U.S. and Canada)
- Tablets (U.S. and Canada)
Cephradine
- Capsules (U.S. and Canada)
- Oral suspension (U.S.)

*Parenteral*
Cefamandole
- Injection (U.S. and Canada)
Cefazolin
- Injection (U.S. and Canada)
Cefmetazole
- Injection (U.S.)
Cefonicid
- Injection (U.S.)
Cefoperazone
- Injection (U.S. and Canada)
Cefotaxime
- Injection (U.S. and Canada)
Cefotetan
- Injection (U.S. and Canada)
Cefoxitin
- Injection (U.S. and Canada)
Ceftazidime
- Injection (U.S. and Canada)
Ceftizoxime
- Injection (U.S. and Canada)
Ceftriaxone
- Injection (U.S. and Canada)
Cefuroxime
- Injection (U.S. and Canada)
Cephalothin
- Injection (U.S. and Canada)
Cephapirin
- Injection (U.S.)
Cephradine
- Injection (U.S.)

# Before Using This Medicine

In deciding to use a medicine, the risks of taking the medicine must be weighed against the good it will do. This is a decision you and your doctor will make. For the cephalosporins, the following should be considered:

**Allergies**—Tell your doctor if you have ever had any unusual or allergic reaction to any of the cephalosporins, penicillins, penicillin-like medicines, or penicillamine. Also tell your health care professional if you are allergic to any other substances, such as foods, preservatives, or dyes.

**Pregnancy**—Studies have not been done in humans. However, most cephalosporins have not been reported to cause birth defects or other problems in animal studies. Studies in rabbits have shown that cefoxitin may increase the risk of miscarriages and cause other problems.

**Breast-feeding**—Most cephalosporins pass into human breast milk, usually in small amounts. However, cephalosporins have not been reported to cause problems in nursing babies.

**Children**—Many cephalosporins have been tested in children and, in effective doses, have not been shown to cause different side effects or problems than they do in adults. However, there are some cephalosporins that have not been tested in children up to 1 year of age.

**Older adults**—Cephalosporins have been used in the elderly, and they are not expected to cause different side effects or problems in older people than they do in younger adults.

**Other medicines**—Although certain medicines should not be used together at all, in other cases 2 different medicines may be used together even if an interaction might occur. In these cases, your doctor may want to change the dose, or other precautions may be necessary. When you are taking a cephalosporin, it is especially important that your health care professional know if you are taking any of the following:
- Alcohol and alcohol-containing medicine (cefamandole, cefmetazole, cefoperazone, and cefotetan only)—Using alcohol and these cephalosporins together may cause abdominal or stomach cramps, nausea, vomiting, headache, dizziness or lightheadedness, shortness of breath, sweating, or facial flushing; this reaction usually begins within 15 to 30 minutes after alcohol is consumed and usually goes away over several hours
- Anticoagulants (blood thinners) or
- Carbenicillin by injection (e.g., Geopen) or
- Dipyridamole (e.g., Persantine) or
- Divalproex (e.g., Depakote) or
- Heparin (e.g., Panheprin) or
- Pentoxifylline (e.g., Trental) or
- Plicamycin (e.g., Mithracin) or
- Sulfinpyrazone (e.g., Anturane) or
- Ticarcillin (e.g., Ticar) or
- Thrombolytic agents or
- Valproic acid (e.g., Depakene)—Any of these medicines may increase the chance of bleeding, especially when used with cefamandole, cefmetazole, cefoperazone, or cefotetan

- Probenecid (e.g., Benemid) (except cefoperazone, ceftazidime, or ceftriaxone)—Probenecid increases the blood level of many cephalosporins. Although probenecid may be given with a cephalosporin by your doctor purposely to increase the blood level to treat some infections, in other cases this effect may be unwanted and may increase the chance of side effects

**Other medical problems**—The presence of other medical problems may affect the use of cephalosporins. Make sure you tell your doctor if you have any other medical problems, especially:

- Bleeding problems, history of (cefamandole, cefmetazole, cefoperazone, and cefotetan only)—These medicines may increase the chance of bleeding
- Kidney disease—Some cephalosporins need to be given at a lower dose to people with kidney disease. Also, cephalothin, especially, may increase the chance of kidney damage
- Liver disease (cefoperazone only)—Cefoperazone needs to be given at a lower dose to people with liver and kidney disease
- Phenylketonuria—Cefprozil oral suspension contains phenylalanine
- Stomach or intestinal disease, history of (especially colitis, including colitis caused by antibiotics, or enteritis)—Cephalosporins may cause colitis in some patients

## Proper Use of This Medicine

Cephalosporins may be taken on a full or empty stomach. If this medicine upsets your stomach, it may help to take it with food.

Cefuroxime axetil tablets and cefpodoxime should be taken with food to increase absorption of the medicine.

For patients taking the *oral liquid* form of this medicine:

- This medicine is to be taken by mouth even if it comes in a dropper bottle. If this medicine does not come in a dropper bottle, use a specially marked measuring spoon or other device to measure each dose accurately. The average household teaspoon may not hold the right amount of liquid.
- Do not use after the expiration date on the label since the medicine may not work properly after that date. Check with your pharmacist if you have any questions about this.

For patients unable to swallow *cefuroxime axetil tablets* whole ask your doctor for suggestions.

To help clear up your infection completely, *keep taking this medicine for the full time of treatment*, even if you begin to feel better after a few days. *If you have a "strep" infection, you should keep taking this medicine for at least 10 days. This is especially important in "strep" infections since serious heart or kidney problems could develop later* if your infection is not cleared up completely. Also, if you stop taking this medicine too soon, your symptoms may return.

This medicine works best when there is a constant amount in the blood or urine. *To help keep the amount constant, do not miss any doses. Also, it is best to take the doses at evenly spaced times, day and night*. For example, if you are to take 4 doses a day, the doses should be spaced about 6 hours apart. If this interferes with your sleep or other daily activities, or if you need help in planning the best times to take your medicine, check with your health care professional.

**Dosing**—The dose of these medicines will be different for different patients. *Follow your doctor's orders or the directions on the label*. The following information includes only the average doses of these medicines. Your dose may be different if you have kidney disease. *If your dose is different, do not change it* unless your doctor tells you to do so.

The number of capsules or tablets or teaspoonfuls of suspension that you take depends on the strength of the medicine. Also, *the number of doses you take each day, the time allowed between doses, and the length of time you take the medicine depend on the medical problem for which you are taking a cephalosporin.*

*For cefaclor*
- For bacterial infections
  —For *oral* dosage form (capsules or oral suspension):
    - Adults and teenagers—250 to 500 milligrams (mg) every eight hours.
    - Infants and children 1 month of age and older—6.7 to 13.4 mg per kilogram (kg) (3 to 6 mg per pound) of body weight every eight hours, or 10 to 20 mg per kg (4.5 to 9 mg per pound) of body weight every twelve hours.

*For cefadroxil*
- For bacterial infections
  —For *oral* dosage form (capsules, tablets, or oral suspension):
    - Adults and teenagers—500 milligrams (mg) every twelve hours, or 1 to 2 grams once a day.
    - Children—15 mg per kilogram (kg) (6.8 mg per pound) of body weight every twelve hours, or 30 mg per kg (13.6 mg per pound) of body weight once a day.

*For cefamandole*
- For bacterial infections
  —For *injection* dosage form:
    - Adults and teenagers—500 milligrams (mg) to 2 grams every four to eight hours, injected into a muscle or vein.
    - Infants and children 1 month of age and older—8.3 to 33.3 mg per kilogram (kg) (3.8 to 15.1 mg per pound) of body weight every four to eight hours, injected into a muscle or vein.

*For cefazolin*
- For bacterial infections
  —For *injection* dosage form:
    - Adults and teenagers—250 milligrams (mg) to 1.5 grams every six to eight hours, injected into a vein.

• Infants and children 1 month of age and older—6.25 to 25 mg per kilogram (kg) (2.8 to 11.4 mg per pound) of body weight every six hours, or 8.3 to 33.3 mg per kg (3.8 to 15.1 mg per pound) of body weight every eight hours, injected into a vein.

*For cefixime*

• For bacterial infections

—For *oral* dosage form (tablets or oral suspension):

• Adults and teenagers—200 milligrams (mg) every twelve hours, or 400 mg once a day. Gonorrhea is treated with a single, oral dose of 400 mg.

• Children 6 months of age to 12 years of age—4 mg per kilogram (kg) (1.8 mg per pound) of body weight every twelve hours, or 8 mg per kg (3.6 mg per pound) of body weight once a day.

*For cefmetazole*

• For bacterial infections

—For *injection* dosage form:

• Adults and teenagers—2 grams every six to twelve hours, injected into a vein, for five to fourteen days. Gonorrhea is treated with a single dose of 1 gram, injected into the muscle, along with a single, oral 1 gram dose of probenecid.

• Children—Dose must be determined by your doctor.

*For cefonicid*

• For bacterial infections

—For *injection* dosage form:

• Adults and teenagers—500 milligrams (mg) to 1 gram every twenty-four hours, injected into a vein or muscle.

• Children—Dose must be determined by your doctor.

*For cefoperazone*

• For bacterial infections

—For *injection* dosage form:

• Adults and teenagers—1 to 6 grams every twelve hours, or 2 to 4 grams every eight hours, injected into a vein.

• Children—Dose must be determined by your doctor.

*For cefotaxime*

• For bacterial infections

—For *injection* dosage form:

• Adults and teenagers—1 to 2 grams every four to twelve hours. Gonorrhea is usually treated with a single dose of 250 milligrams (mg), injected into a muscle.

• Newborns up to 1 week of age—50 mg per kilogram (kg) (22.7 mg per pound) of body weight every twelve hours, injected into a vein.

• Newborns 1 to 4 weeks of age—50 mg per kg (22.7 mg per pound) of body weight every eight hours, injected into a vein.

• Infants and children up to 50 kg of body weight (110 pounds)—8.3 to 30 mg per kg (3.8 to 13.6 mg per pound) of body weight every four hours, or 12.5 to 45 mg per kg (5.7 to 20.4 mg per pound) of body weight every six hours, injected into a vein.

• Children over 50 kg of body weight (110 pounds)—1 to 2 grams every four to twelve hours.

*For cefotetan*

• For bacterial infections

—For *injection* dosage form:

• Adults and teenagers—1 to 3 grams every twelve hours, injected into a vein or muscle.

• Children—Dose must be determined by your doctor.

*For cefoxitin*

• For bacterial infections

—For *injection* dosage form:

• Adults and teenagers—1 to 3 grams every four to eight hours, injected into a vein. Gonorrhea is treated with a single dose of 2 grams, injected into a muscle, and given along with a single, oral 1 gram dose of probenecid.

• Infants and children 3 months of age and over—13.3 to 26.7 milligrams (mg) per kilogram (kg) (6 to 12 mg per pound) of body weight every four hours, or 20 to 40 mg per kg (9 to 18 mg per pound) of body weight every six hours.

*For cefpodoxime*

• For bacterial infections

—For *oral* dosage forms (tablets or oral suspension):

• Adults and teenagers—100 to 400 milligrams (mg) every twelve hours for seven to fourteen days. Gonorrhea is treated with a single, oral dose of 200 mg.

• Infants and children 6 months to 12 years of age—5 mg per kilogram (kg) (2.3 mg per pound) of body weight every twelve hours for ten days.

• Infants up to 6 months of age—Dose must be determined by your doctor.

*For cefprozil*

• For bacterial infections

—For *oral* dosage forms (tablets or oral suspension):

• Adults and teenagers—250 to 500 milligrams (mg) every twelve to twenty-four hours for ten days.

• Children 2 to 12 years of age—7.5 mg per kilogram (kg) (3.4 mg per pound) of body weight every twelve hours for ten days.

• Infants and children 6 months to 12 years of age—15 mg per kg (6.8 mg per pound) of body weight every twelve hours for ten days.

*For ceftazidime*
- For bacterial infections
  —For *injection* dosage form:
    - Adults and teenagers—500 milligrams (mg) to 2 grams every eight to twelve hours.
    - Newborns up to 4 weeks of age—30 mg per kilogram (kg) (13.6 mg per pound) of body weight every twelve hours, injected into a vein.
    - Infants and children 1 month to 12 years of age—30 mg to 50 mg per kg (13.6 to 22.7 mg per pound) of body weight every eight hours, injected into a vein.

*For ceftizoxime*
- For bacterial infections
  —For *injection* dosage form:
    - Adults and teenagers—1 to 4 grams every eight to twelve hours injected into a vein.
    - Infants and children 6 months of age and older—50 milligrams (mg) per kilogram (kg) (22.7 mg per pound) of body weight every six to eight hours, injected into a vein.

*For ceftriaxone*
- For bacterial infections
  —For *injection* dosage form:
    - Adults and teenagers—1 to 2 grams every twenty-four hours, or 500 milligrams (mg) to 1 gram every twelve hours, injected into a vein or muscle. Gonorrhea is treated with a single 250 mg dose injected into a muscle.
    - Infants and children—25 to 50 mg per kilogram (kg) (11.4 to 22.7 mg per pound) of body weight every twelve hours, or 50 to 75 mg per kg (22.7 to 34.1 mg per pound) of body weight once a day, injected into a vein. Meningitis is treated with an initial dose of 100 mg per kg, then, 100 mg per kg once a day injected into a vein.

*For cefuroxime*
- For bacterial infections
  —For *oral* dosage form (tablets):
    - Adults and teenagers—125 to 500 milligrams (mg) every twelve hours. Gonorrhea is treated with a single, oral 1 gram dose.
    - Children up to 12 years of age—125 mg every twelve hours.
  —For *injection* dosage form:
    - Adults and teenagers—750 mg to 1.5 grams every eight hours injected into a vein or a muscle. Gonorrhea is treated with a single dose of 1.5 grams, injected into a muscle; the total 1.5-gram dose is divided into two doses and injected into muscles at two separate places on the body, and given along with a single oral 1 gram dose of probenecid.
    - Newborns—10 to 33.3 mg per kilogram (kg) (4.5 to 15.1 mg per pound) of body weight every eight hours, or 15 to 50 mg per kg (6.8 to 22.7 mg

per pound) of body weight every twelve hours, injected into a muscle or a vein.
    - Infants and children 3 months of age and over—16.7 to 33.3 mg per kg (7.6 to 15.1 mg per pound) of body weight every eight hours, injected into a muscle or a vein.

*For cephalexin*
- For bacterial infections
  —For *oral* dosage form (capsules, oral suspension, or tablets):
    - Adults and teenagers—250 to 500 milligrams (mg) every six to twelve hours.
    - Children—6.25 to 25 mg per kilogram (kg) (1.6 to 11.4 mg per pound) of body weight every six hours, or 12.5 to 50 mg per kg (5.7 to 22.7 mg per pound) of body weight every twelve hours.

*For cephalothin*
- For bacterial infections
  —For *injection* dosage form:
    - Adults and teenagers—500 milligrams (mg) to 2 grams every four to six hours, injected into a vein.
    - Children—13.3 to 26.6 mg per kilogram (kg) (6 to 12 mg per pound) of body weight every four hours, or 20 to 40 mg per kg (9.1 to 18.2 mg per pound) of body weight every six hours, injected into a vein.

*For cephapirin*
- For bacterial infections
  —For *injection* dosage form:
    - Adults and teenagers—500 milligrams (mg) to 1 gram every four to six hours, injected into a muscle or a vein.
    - Infants and children 3 months of age and over—10 to 20 mg per kilogram (kg) (4.5 to 9.1 mg per pound) of body weight every six hours, injected into a muscle or a vein.

*For cephradine*
- For bacterial infections
  —For *oral* dosage forms (capsules or oral suspension):
    - Adults and teenagers—250 to 500 milligrams (mg) every six hours, or 500 mg to 1 gram every twelve hours.
    - Children—6.25 to 25 mg per kilogram (kg) (2.8 to 11.4 mg per pound) of body weight every six hours.
  —For *injection* dosage form:
    - Adults and teenagers—500 mg to 1 gram every six hours, injected into a muscle or a vein.
    - Children 1 year of age and over—12.5 to 25 mg per kg (5.7 to 11.4 mg per pound) of body weight every six hours, injected into a muscle or a vein.

**Missed dose**—If you miss a dose of this medicine, take it as soon as possible. This will help to keep a constant amount of medicine in the blood or urine. However, if it is almost time for your next dose, skip the missed dose and go back to your regular dosing schedule. Do not double doses.

**Storage**—To store this medicine:

- Keep out of the reach of children.
- Store away from heat and direct light.
- Do not store the capsule or tablet form of this medicine in the bathroom, near the kitchen sink, or in other damp places. Heat or moisture may cause the medicine to break down.
- Store the oral liquid form of most cephalosporins in the refrigerator because heat will cause this medicine to break down. However, keep the medicine from freezing. Follow the directions on the label. Cefixime oral suspension (Suprax) does not need to be refrigerated.
- Do not keep outdated medicine or medicine no longer needed. Be sure that any discarded medicine is out of the reach of children.

## Precautions While Using This Medicine

If your symptoms do not improve within a few days, or if they become worse, check with your doctor.

*For diabetic patients:*

- *This medicine may cause false test results with some urine sugar tests.* Check with your doctor before changing your diet or the dosage of your diabetes medicine.

*For patients with phenylketonuria (PKU):*

- Cefprozil oral suspension contains phenylalanine. Check with your doctor before taking this medicine.

In some patients, cephalosporins may cause diarrhea:

- Severe diarrhea may be a sign of a serious side effect. *Do not take any diarrhea medicine without first checking with your doctor.* Diarrhea medicines may make your diarrhea worse or make it last longer.
- For mild diarrhea, diarrhea medicine containing kaolin or attapulgite (e.g., Kaopectate tablets, Diasorb) may be taken. However, other kinds of diarrhea medicine should not be taken. They may make your diarrhea worse or make it last longer.
- If you have any questions about this or if mild diarrhea continues or gets worse, check with your health care professional.

For patients receiving *cefamandole, cefmetazole, cefoperazone, or cefotetan by injection:*

- Drinking alcoholic beverages or taking other alcohol-containing preparations (for example, elixirs, cough syrups, tonics, or injections of alcohol) while receiving these medicines may cause problems. The problems may occur if you consume alcohol even several days after you stop taking the cephalosporin. Drinking alcoholic beverages may result in increased side effects such as abdominal or stomach cramps, nausea, vomiting, headache, fainting, fast or irregular heartbeat, difficult breathing, sweating, or redness of the face or skin. These effects usually start within 15 to 30 minutes after you drink alcohol and may not go away for up to several hours. Therefore, *you should not drink alcoholic beverages or take other alcohol-containing preparations while you are receiving these medicines and for several days after stopping them.*

## Side Effects of This Medicine

Along with its needed effects, a medicine may cause some unwanted effects. Although not all of these side effects may occur, if they do occur they may need medical attention.

*Check with your doctor immediately* if any of the following side effects occur:

*Less common or rare*

Abdominal or stomach cramps and pain (severe); fever; watery and severe diarrhea, which may also be bloody; (these side effects may also occur up to several weeks after you stop taking this medicine); unusual bleeding or bruising (more common for cefamandole, cefmetazole, cefoperazone, and cefotetan)

*Rare*

Blistering, peeling, or loosening of skin; convulsions (seizures); decrease in urine output; dizziness or lightheadedness; joint pain; loss of appetite; pain, redness, and swelling at place of injection; skin rash, itching, redness, or swelling; trouble in breathing; unusual tiredness or weakness; yellowing of the eyes or skin

Other side effects may occur that usually do not need medical attention. These side effects may go away during treatment as your body adjusts to the medicine. However, check with your doctor if any of the following side effects continue or are bothersome:

*More common (less common with some cephalosporins)*

Diarrhea (mild); nausea and vomiting; sore mouth or tongue; stomach cramps (mild)

*Less common or rare*

Vaginal itching or discharge

Other side effects not listed above may also occur in some patients. If you notice any other effects, check with your doctor.

Revised: 02/28/94

# CHARCOAL, ACTIVATED   Oral

Some commonly used brand names are:

**In the U.S.—**

| | |
|---|---|
| Actidose-Aqua[1] | Insta-Char[1] |
| Actidose with Sorbitol[2] | Insta-Char Aqueous |
| Charcoaid[2] | Suspension[1] |
| Charcocaps[1] | Liqui-Char[1] |

**In Canada—**

| | |
|---|---|
| Aqueous Charcodote[1] | Charcodote TFS[2] |
| Charac-50[1] | Insta-Char Aqueous |
| Charac-tol 50[2] | Suspension[1] |
| Charcodote[2] | Pediatric Aqueous Charcodote[1] |
| | Pediatric Charcodote[2] |

Note: For quick reference, the following medicines are numbered to match the corresponding brand names.

This information applies to the following medicines:

1. Activated Charcoal (AK-ti-vay-ted CHAR-kole)‡§
2. Activated Charcoal and Sorbitol (SOR-bi-tole)

‡Generic name product may also be available in the U.S.
§Generic name product may also be available in Canada.

## Description

Activated charcoal is used in the emergency treatment of certain kinds of poisoning. It helps prevent the poison from being absorbed by the body. Ordinarily, this medicine should not be used in poisoning if corrosive agents such as alkalis (lye) and strong acids, iron, boric acid, lithium, petroleum products (e.g., kerosene, gasoline, coal oil, fuel oil, paint thinner, cleaning fluid), ethyl alcohol, or methyl alcohol have been swallowed, since it will not prevent these poisons from being absorbed into the body.

Some activated charcoal products contain sorbitol. Sorbitol is a sweetener. It also works as a laxative, for the elimination of the poison from the body. *Products that contain sorbitol should be given only under the direct supervision of a doctor because severe diarrhea and vomiting may result.*

Activated charcoal (without sorbitol) may also be used to relieve diarrhea and intestinal gas.

Activated charcoal is available without a doctor's prescription; however, before using this medicine for poisoning, call a poison control center, your doctor, or an emergency room for advice. Also, your doctor may have special instructions on the proper use of this medicine for diarrhea or intestinal gas. Activated charcoal is available in the following dosage forms:

*Oral*

Activated Charcoal
- Capsules (U.S. and Canada)
- Powder (U.S. and Canada)
- Oral suspension (U.S. and Canada)
- Tablets (U.S.)

Activated Charcoal and Sorbitol
- Oral suspension (U.S. and Canada)

## Before Using This Medicine

In deciding to use a medicine, the risks of taking the medicine must be weighed against the good it will do.

This is a decision you and your doctor will make. Before you use activated charcoal *for diarrhea or intestinal gas*, the following should be considered:

**Allergies**—Tell your doctor if you have ever had any unusual or allergic reaction to activated charcoal. Also tell your health care professional if you are allergic to any other substances, such as foods, preservatives, or dyes.

**Diet**—Make certain your health care professional knows if you are on a low-sodium, low-sugar, or any other special diet. Most medicines contain more than their active ingredient.

**Pregnancy**—Activated charcoal has not been reported to cause birth defects or other problems in humans.

**Breast-feeding**—Activated charcoal has not been reported to cause problems in nursing babies.

**Children**—In babies and children under 3 years of age, activated charcoal should not be used regularly to relieve diarrhea and gas, since it may affect the child's nutrition. Also, the fluid loss caused by diarrhea may result in a severe condition. For this reason, a medicine for diarrhea must not be given to children without first checking with their doctor. If medicine for diarrhea is used, it is also very important that a sufficient amount of liquids be given to replace the fluid lost by the body. If you have any questions about this, check with your health care professional.

**Older adults**—Many medicines have not been studied specifically in older people. Therefore, it may not be known whether they work exactly the same way they do in younger adults. Although there is no specific information comparing the use of activated charcoal in the elderly, this medicine is not expected to cause different side effects or problems in older people than it does in younger adults.

However, the fluid loss caused by diarrhea may result in a severe condition. For this reason, elderly persons with diarrhea, in addition to using a medicine for diarrhea, must receive a sufficient amount of liquids to replace the fluid lost by the body. If you have any questions about this, check with your health care professional.

**Other medicines**—Although certain medicines should not be used together at all, in other cases two different medicines may be used together even if an interaction might occur. In these cases, your doctor may want to change the dose, or other precautions may be necessary. Tell your health care professional if you are taking any other prescription or nonprescription (over-the-counter [OTC]) medicine.

**Other medical problems**—The presence of other medical problems may affect the use of activated charcoal to relieve diarrhea. Make sure you tell your doctor if you have any other medical problems, especially:

- Dysentery—This condition may get worse; a different kind of treatment may be needed

## Proper Use of This Medicine

*Do not take this medicine mixed with chocolate syrup, ice cream, or sherbet,* since it may prevent the medicine from working properly.

For patients taking this medicine *for poisoning*:

- *Before taking this medicine for the treatment of poisoning, call a poison control center, your doctor, or an emergency room for advice.* It is a good idea to have these telephone numbers readily available.
- *It is very important that you shake the liquid form of this medicine well before taking it, some might have settled in the bottom. Be sure to drink all the liquid to get the full dose of activated charcoal.*
- If you have been told to take both this medicine and ipecac syrup to treat the poisoning, *do not take this medicine until after you have taken the ipecac syrup to cause vomiting and the vomiting has stopped. This is usually about 30 minutes.*

For patients taking this medicine *for diarrhea or intestinal gas:*

- *If you are taking any other medicine, do not take it within 2 hours of the activated charcoal.* Taking other medicines together with activated charcoal may prevent the other medicine from being absorbed by your body. If you have any questions about this, check with your health care professional.

*Importance of diet and fluid intake while treating diarrhea:*

- *In addition to using medicine for diarrhea, it is very important that you replace the fluid lost by the body and follow a proper diet.* For the first 24 hours you should drink plenty of caffeine-free clear liquids, such as ginger ale, decaffeinated cola, decaffeinated tea, broth, or gelatin. During the next 24 hours you may eat bland foods, such as cooked cereals, bread, crackers, and applesauce. Fruits, vegetables, fried or spicy foods, bran, candy, caffeine, and alcoholic beverages may make the condition worse.
- If too much fluid has been lost by the body due to the diarrhea, a serious condition may develop. Check with your doctor as soon as possible if any of the following signs of too much fluid loss occur:

  Decreased urination
  Dizziness and lightheadedness
  Dryness of mouth
  Increased thirst
  Wrinkled skin

**Storage**—To store this medicine:

- Keep out of the reach of children.
- Store away from heat and direct light.
- Do not store the capsule, tablet, or powder form of this medicine in the bathroom, near the kitchen sink, or in other damp places. Heat or moisture may cause the medicine to break down.
- Keep the liquid form of this medicine from freezing.
- Do not keep outdated medicine or medicine no longer needed. Be sure that any discarded medicine is out of the reach of children.

## Precautions While Using This Medicine

For patients taking this medicine *for diarrhea or intestinal gas:*

- If you are taking this medicine for intestinal gas and your condition has not improved after 7 days, check with your doctor.
- If you are taking this medicine for diarrhea and your condition has not improved after 2 days or if you have fever with the diarrhea, check with your doctor.

## Side Effects of This Medicine

Along with its needed effects, a medicine may cause some unwanted effects. Although not all of these side effects may occur, if they do occur they may need medical attention.

Check with your doctor as soon as possible if the following side effect occurs:

*Rare*
　Swelling or pain in stomach

Other side effects may occur that usually do not need medical attention. These side effects may go away during treatment as your body adjusts to the medicine. However, check with your doctor if any of the following side effects continue:

*More common (for sorbitol-containing preparations only)*
　Diarrhea; vomiting

Activated charcoal will cause your stools to turn black. This is to be expected while you are taking this medicine.

There have not been any other side effects reported with this medicine. However, if you notice any other effects, check with your doctor.

Revised: 08/16/91

# CHENODIOL  Systemic*†

A commonly used name is chenodeoxycholic acid.

*Not commercially available in the U.S.
†Not commercially available in Canada.

## Description

Chenodiol (kee-noe-DYE-ole) is used in the treatment of gallstone disease. It is taken by mouth to dissolve the gallstones.

Chenodiol is used in patients who do not need to have their gallbladder removed or in those in whom surgery is best avoided because of other medical problems. However, chenodiol works only in those patients who have a working gallbladder and whose gallstones are made of cholesterol. Chenodiol works best when these stones are small and of the "floating" type.

Chenodiol is available only with your doctor's prescription, in the following dosage form:
*Oral*
  • Tablets

## Before Using This Medicine

In deciding to use a medicine, the risks of taking the medicine must be weighed against the good it will do. This is a decision you and your doctor will make. For chenodiol, the following should be considered:

**Allergies**—Tell your doctor if you have ever had any unusual or allergic reaction to chenodiol or to other bile acid products.

**Diet**—If you have gallstones, your doctor may prescribe chenodiol and a personal high-fiber diet for you. Some foods that are high in fiber are whole grain breads and cereals, bran, fruit, and green, leafy vegetables. It has been found that such a diet may help dissolve the stones faster and may keep new stones from forming.

It may also be important for you to go on a reducing diet. However, check with your doctor before going on any diet.

**Pregnancy**—Chenodiol is not recommended for use during pregnancy. It has been shown to cause liver and kidney problems in animals when given in doses many times the human dose. Be sure you have discussed this with your doctor.

**Breast-feeding**—It is not known whether chenodiol passes into breast milk. Although most medicines pass into breast milk in small amounts, many of them may be used safely while breast-feeding. Mothers who are taking this medicine and who wish to breast-feed should discuss this with their doctor.

**Children**—Studies on this medicine have been done only in adult patients, and there is no specific information comparing use of chenodiol in children with use in other age groups.

**Older adults**—Many medicines have not been studied specifically in older people. Therefore, it may not be known whether they work exactly the same way they do in younger adults. Although there is no specific information comparing use of chenodiol in the elderly with use in other age groups, this medicine is not expected to cause different side effects or problems in older people than it does in younger adults.

**Other medicines**—Although certain medicines should not be used together at all, in other cases two different medicines may be used together even if an interaction might occur. In these cases, your doctor may want to change the dose, or other precautions may be necessary. Tell your health care professional if you are taking any other prescription or nonprescription (over-the-counter [OTC]) medicine.

**Other medical problems**—The presence of other medical problems may affect the use of chenodiol. Make sure you tell your doctor if you have any other medical problems, especially:
  • Biliary tract problems or
  • Blood vessel disease or
  • Pancreatitis (inflammation of pancreas)—These conditions may make it necessary to have surgery since treatment with chenodiol would take too long
  • Liver disease—Liver disease may become worse with use of chenodiol

## Proper Use of This Medicine

Take chenodiol with food or milk for best results, unless otherwise directed by your doctor.

*Take chenodiol for the full time of treatment, even if you begin to feel better.* If you stop taking this medicine too soon, the gallstones may not dissolve as fast or may not dissolve at all.

**Dosing**—The dose of chenodiol will be different for different patients. *Follow your doctor's orders or the directions on the label.* The following information includes only the average doses of chenodiol. *If your dose is different, do not change it unless your doctor tells you to do so:*
  • For *oral* dosage forms (tablets):
    —For gallstone disease:
      • Adults and children 12 years of age and older—250 milligrams (mg) a day for the first two weeks of treatment. Your doctor may then increase the dose by 250 mg a day until the proper treatment dose is reached. The treatment dose is based on body weight. It is usually 13 to 16 mg per kilogram (6 to 7 mg per pound) of body weight a day, divided into two doses, taken in the morning and at night. Each dose should be taken with food or milk.
      • Children up to 12 years of age—Use and dose must be determined by your doctor.

**Missed dose**—If you miss a dose of this medicine, take it as soon as possible. However, if it is almost time for your next dose, skip the missed dose and go back to your regular dosing schedule. Do not double doses.

**Storage**—To store this medicine:
- Keep out of the reach of children.
- Store away from heat and direct light.
- Do not store in the bathroom, near the kitchen sink, or in other damp places. Heat or moisture may cause the medicine to break down.
- Do not keep outdated medicine or medicine no longer needed. Be sure that any discarded medicine is out of the reach of children.

## Precautions While Using This Medicine

Do not take aluminum-containing antacids (e.g., ALternaGel, Maalox) while taking chenodiol. To do so may keep the chenodiol from working properly.

*It is important that your doctor check your progress at regular visits. Laboratory tests will have to be done every few months* while you are taking this medicine to make sure that the gallstones are dissolving and your liver is working properly.

*Check with your doctor immediately if severe abdominal or stomach pain, especially toward the upper right side, and severe nausea and vomiting occur.* These symptoms may mean that you have other medical problems or that your gallstone condition needs your doctor's attention.

## Side Effects of This Medicine

Along with its needed effects, a medicine may cause some unwanted effects. Although not all of these side effects may occur, if they do occur they may need medical attention.

Check with your doctor as soon as possible if the following side effect occurs:
*Less common or rare*
Diarrhea (severe)

Other side effects may occur that usually do not need medical attention. These side effects may go away during treatment as your body adjusts to the medicine. However, check with your doctor if any of the following side effects continue or are bothersome:
*More common*
Diarrhea (mild)
*Less common or rare*
Constipation; frequent urge for bowel movement; gas or indigestion (usually disappears within 2 to 4 weeks after the beginning of treatment); loss of appetite; nausea or vomiting; stomach cramps or pain

Other side effects not listed above may also occur in some patients. If you notice any other effects, check with your doctor.

Revised: 04/27/94

---

# CHLOPHEDIANOL Systemic*

A commonly used brand name in Canada is Ulone.

*Not commercially available in the U.S.

## Description

Chlophedianol (kloe-fe-DYE-a-nole) is used to relieve dry, irritating coughs. This medicine should not be used when there is mucus or phlegm (pronounced flem) with the cough.

Chlophedianol relieves cough by acting on the cough center in the brain.

Chlophedianol is available without a doctor's prescription; however, your doctor may have special instructions on the proper use of this medicine. It is available in the following dosage form:
*Oral*
- Syrup (Canada)

## Before Using This Medicine

If you are taking this medicine without a prescription, carefully read and follow any precautions on the label. For chlophedianol, the following should be considered:

**Allergies**—Tell your doctor if you have ever had any unusual or allergic reaction to chlophedianol. Also tell your health care professional if you are allergic to any other substances, such as foods, preservatives, or dyes.

**Pregnancy**—Studies on effects in pregnancy have not been done in either humans or animals.

**Breast-feeding**—It is not known whether chlophedianol passes into breast milk. Although most medicines pass into breast milk in small amounts, many of them may be used safely while breast-feeding. Mothers who are taking this medicine and who wish to breast-feed should discuss this with their doctor.

**Children**—This medicine has been tested in children 2 years of age or older. In effective doses, the medicine has not been shown to cause different side effects or problems in children then it does in adults.

**Older adults**—Many medicines have not been studied specifically in older people. Therefore, it may not be known whether they work exactly the same way they do in younger adults or if they cause different side effects or problems in older people. There is no specific information

comparing use of chlophedianol in the elderly with use in other age groups.

**Other medicines**—Although certain medicines should not be used together at all, in other cases two different medicines may be used together even if an interaction might occur. In these cases, your doctor may want to change the dose, or other precautions may be necessary. Tell your health care professional if you are taking any other prescription or nonprescription (over-the-counter [OTC]) medicine.

**Other medical problems**—The presence of other medical problems may affect the use of chlophedianol. Make sure you tell your doctor if you have any other medical problems, especially:

- Mucus or phlegm with cough—Since chlophedianol decreases coughing, it makes it difficult to get rid of the mucus that may collect in the lungs and airways with some diseases

## Proper Use of This Medicine

Do not take liquids immediately after taking this medicine. To do so may decrease the soothing effect of the syrup.

*Take this medicine only as directed.* Do not take more of it and do not take it more often than your doctor ordered or the label directs you to take. To do so may increase the chance of side effects.

**Dosing**—The dose of chlophedianol will be different for different patients. *Follow your doctor's orders or the directions on the label.* The following information includes only the average doses of chlophedianol. *If your dose is different, do not change it* unless your doctor tells you to do so.

- For *oral* dosage form (syrup):
  - —For cough:
    - Adults and children 12 years of age and older— 25 milligrams (mg) every six to eight hours as needed.
    - Children—

      Up to 2 years of age: Use is not recommended.

      2 to 6 years of age: 12.5 mg every six to eight hours as needed.

      6 to 12 years of age: 12.5 to 25 mg every six to eight hours as needed.

**Missed dose**—If you are taking this medicine on a regular schedule and you miss a dose, take it as soon as possible. However, if it is almost time for your next dose, skip the missed dose and go back to your regular dosing schedule. Do not double doses.

**Storage**—To store this medicine:

- Keep out of the reach of children.
- Store away from heat and direct light.
- Keep the syrup from freezing.

- Do not keep outdated medicine or medicine no longer needed. Be sure that any discarded medicine is out of the reach of children.

## Precautions While Using This Medicine

If your cough has not improved after 7 days, or if you have a high fever, skin rash, or continuing headache with the cough, check with your doctor. These signs may mean that you have other medical problems.

This medicine will add to the effects of alcohol and other CNS depressants (medicines that slow down the nervous system, possibly causing drowsiness). Some examples of CNS depressants are antihistamines or medicine for hay fever, other allergies, or colds; sedatives, tranquilizers, or sleeping medicine; prescription pain medicine or narcotics; barbiturates; medicine for seizures; muscle relaxants; or anesthetics, including some dental anesthetics. *Check with your doctor before taking any of the above while you are taking this medicine.*

This medicine may also add to the effects of CNS stimulants, such as appetite suppressants and caffeine-containing beverages like tea, coffee, cocoa, and cola drinks. *Avoid drinking large amounts of these beverages while taking this medicine.* If you have any questions about this, check with your doctor.

This medicine may cause some people to become drowsy or less alert than they are normally. *Make sure you know how you react to this medicine before you drive, use machines, or do anything else that could be dangerous if you are not alert.*

## Side Effects of This Medicine

Along with its needed effects, a medicine may cause some unwanted effects. Although not all of these side effects may occur, if they do occur they may need medical attention.

Check with your doctor as soon as possible if any of the following side effects occur:

*Rare*

Hallucinations (seeing, hearing, or feeling things that are not there); nightmares; skin rash or hives; unusual excitement or irritability

*With large doses*

Blurred vision; drowsiness or dizziness; dryness of the mouth; nausea or vomiting

Other side effects not listed above may also occur in some patients. If you notice any other effects, check with your doctor.

Revised: 02/23/94

# CHLORAL HYDRATE    Systemic

**In the U.S.—**
    Aquachloral Supprettes
    Generic name product may also be available.
**In Canada—**
    Novo-Chlorhydrate
    PMS-Chloral Hydrate
    Generic name product may also be available.

## Description

Chloral hydrate (KLOR-al HYE-drate) belongs to the group of medicines called sedatives and hypnotics. It is sometimes used before surgery or certain procedures to relieve anxiety or tension or to produce sleep. If your child is to take this medicine before a dental or medical procedure, it should be given to the child only at the health care facility where the procedure is to be done. This will allow the health care professional to monitor your child.

Chloral hydrate has been used in the treatment of insomnia (trouble in sleeping) and to help calm or relax patients who are nervous or tense. However, this medicine has generally been replaced by other medicines for the treatment of insomnia and nervousness or tension.

Chloral hydrate has also been used with analgesics (pain medicine) for control of pain following surgery. However, this medicine has generally been replaced by other medicines for control of pain following surgery.

Chloral hydrate comes in different strengths. Serious problems, including deaths, have occurred when children were given the wrong strength. *Make sure your doctor has told your pharmacist both how many milligrams (mg) and how many capsules, teaspoonfuls, or suppositories should be used.* This information is needed to be sure the right amount is given.

This medicine is available only with your doctor's prescription, in the following dosage forms:

*Oral*
- Capsules (U.S. and Canada)
- Syrup (U.S. and Canada)

*Rectal*
- Suppositories (U.S.)

## Before Using This Medicine

In deciding to use a medicine, the risks of taking the medicine must be weighed against the good it will do. This is a decision you and your doctor will make. For chloral hydrate, the following should be considered:

**Allergies**—Tell your doctor if you have ever had any unusual or allergic reaction to chloral hydrate. Also tell your health care professional if you are allergic to any other substances, such as foods, preservatives, or dyes.

**Pregnancy**—Studies on birth defects have not been done in either humans or animals. Too much use of chloral hydrate during pregnancy may cause the baby to become dependent on the medicine. This may lead to withdrawal side effects after birth.

**Breast-feeding**—Chloral hydrate passes into the breast milk and may cause drowsiness in babies of mothers using this medicine.

**Children**—This medicine comes in different strengths. Serious problems, including deaths, have occurred when children were given the wrong strength. *Make sure your doctor has told your pharmacist both how many milligrams (mg) and how many capsules, teaspoonfuls, or suppositories your child should receive.* This information is needed to be sure the right amount is given. With proper use, this medicine is not expected to cause different side effects or problems in children than it does in adults.

**Older adults**—Many medicines have not been studied specifically in older people. Therefore, it may not be known whether they work exactly the same way they do in younger adults. Although there is no specific information comparing use of chloral hydrate in the elderly with use in other age groups, this medicine is not expected to cause different side effects or problems in older people than it does in younger adults.

**Other medicines**—Although certain medicines should not be used together at all, in other cases two different medicines may be used together even if an interaction might occur. In these cases, your doctor may want to change the dose, or other precautions may be necessary. When you are taking chloral hydrate, it is especially important that your health care professional know if you are taking any of the following:

- Anticoagulants (blood thinners)—Chloral hydrate may change the amount of anticoagulant you need to take
- Central nervous system (CNS) depressants (medicine that causes drowsiness) or
- Tricyclic antidepressants (medicine for depression)—Using these medicines and chloral hydrate together may increase the CNS and other depressant effects

**Other medical problems**—The presence of other medical problems may affect the use of chloral hydrate. Make sure you tell your doctor if you have any other medical problems, especially:

- Alcohol abuse or dependence (or history of) or
- Drug abuse or dependence (or history of)—Dependence on chloral hydrate may develop
- Colitis or
- Proctitis or inflammation of the rectum—Chloral hydrate used rectally may make the condition worse
- Esophagitis or inflammation of the esophagus, or
- Gastritis or inflammation of the stomach, or
- Stomach ulcers—Chloral hydrate taken by mouth may make the condition worse
- Heart disease—Chloral hydrate may make the condition worse

- Kidney disease or
- Liver disease—Higher blood levels of chloral hydrate may occur, increasing the chance of side effects
- Porphyria—Acute attacks may be set off by chloral hydrate

## Proper Use of This Medicine

*Use this medicine only as directed by your doctor.* Do not use more of it, do not use it more often, and do not use it for a longer time than your doctor ordered. If too much is used, it may become habit-forming.

For patients taking *chloral hydrate capsules:*
- Swallow the capsule whole. Do not chew since the medicine may cause an unpleasant taste.
- Take this medicine with a full glass (8 ounces) of water, fruit juice, or ginger ale to lessen stomach upset.

For patients taking *chloral hydrate syrup:*
- Take each dose of medicine mixed with up to ½ glass (4 ounces) of clear liquid, such as water, apple juice, or ginger ale. This will help to improve flavor and lessen stomach upset.

For patients using *chloral hydrate rectal suppositories:*
- If the suppository is too soft to insert, chill it in the refrigerator for 30 minutes or run cold water over it before removing the foil wrapper.
- To insert suppository–First remove the foil wrapper and moisten the suppository with cold water. Lie down on your side and use your finger to push the suppository well up into the rectum.

**Dosing**—The dose of chloral hydrate will be different for different patients. *Follow your doctor's orders or the directions on the label.* The following information includes only the average doses of chloral hydrate. *If your dose is different, do not change it* unless your doctor tells you to do so.

This medicine comes in different strengths. *Make sure your doctor has told your pharmacist both how many milligrams (mg) and how many capsules, teaspoonfuls, or suppositories should be used.* This information is needed to be sure the right amount is given.

The number of capsules or teaspoonfuls of syrup that you take, or suppositories that you use, depends on the strength of the medicine. Also, *the number of doses you use each day, the time allowed between doses, and the length of time you use the medicine depend on the medical problem for which you are using chloral hydrate.*
- For *oral* dosage form (capsules or syrup):
  —For trouble in sleeping or sedation before surgery:
  - Adults—500 to 1000 milligrams (mg) taken thirty minutes before bedtime or surgery.
  —For daytime sedation:
  - Adults—250 mg taken three times a day after meals.
  —For sedation before a dental or medical procedure:
  - Children—Dose is based on body weight and must be determined by your doctor. The dose is usually 50 mg per kilogram (kg) (23 mg per pound) of body weight.
  —For sedation before an EEG (electroencephalograph) test:
  - Children—Dose is based on body weight and must be determined by your doctor. The usual dose is 25 mg per kg (11 mg per pound) of body weight.
- For *rectal* dosage form (suppositories):
  —For trouble in sleeping:
  - Adults—500 to 1000 mg at bedtime.
  —For daytime sedation:
  - Adults—325 mg three times a day.
  —For sedation before a dental or medical procedure:
  - Children—Dose is based on body weight and must be determined by your doctor. The dose is usually 50 mg per kg (23 mg per pound) of body weight.
  —For sedation before an EEG (electroencephalograph) test:
  - Children—Dose is based on body weight and must be determined by your doctor. The dose is usually 25 mg per kg (11 mg per pound) of body weight.

**Missed dose**—If you miss a dose of this medicine, skip the missed dose and go back to your regular dosing schedule. Do not double doses.

**Storage**—To store this medicine:
- Keep out of the reach of children. Overdose of chloral hydrate is especially dangerous in children.
- Store away from heat and direct light.
- Do not store the capsule form of this medicine in the bathroom, near the kitchen sink, or in other damp places. Heat or moisture may cause the medicine to break down.
- Keep the syrup form of this medicine from freezing.
- Do not keep outdated medicine or medicine no longer needed. Be sure that any discarded medicine is out of the reach of children.

## Precautions While Using This Medicine

If you will be using this medicine regularly for a long time:
- Your doctor should check your progress at regular visits to make sure that this medicine does not cause unwanted effects.
- Do not stop using it without first checking with your doctor. Your doctor may want you to reduce gradually the amount you are using before stopping completely.

This medicine will add to the effects of alcohol and other CNS depressants (medicines that slow down the nervous system, possibly causing drowsiness). Some examples of CNS depressants are antihistamines or medicine for hay fever, other allergies, or colds; sedatives, tranquilizers, or sleeping medicine; prescription pain medicine or narcotics; barbiturates; medicine for seizures; muscle relaxants; or anesthetics, including some dental anesthetics. *Check with your doctor before taking any of the above while you are using this medicine.*

*If you think you or someone else may have taken an overdose of this medicine, get emergency help at once.* Taking an overdose of chloral hydrate or taking alcohol or other CNS depressants with chloral hydrate may lead to unconsciousness and possibly death. Some signs of an overdose are continuing confusion, difficulty in swallowing, convulsions (seizures), severe drowsiness, severe weakness, shortness of breath or troubled breathing, staggering, and slow or irregular heartbeat.

This medicine may cause some people to become dizzy, lightheaded, drowsy, or less alert than they are normally. Even if taken at bedtime, it may cause some people to feel drowsy or less alert on arising. *Make sure you know how you react to this medicine before you drive, use machines, or do anything else that could be dangerous if you are dizzy or are not alert.*

## Side Effects of This Medicine

Along with its needed effects, a medicine may cause some unwanted effects. Although not all of these side effects may occur, if they do occur they may need medical attention.

Check with your doctor as soon as possible if any of the following side effects occur:

*Less common*
  Skin rash or hives

*Rare*
  Confusion; hallucinations (seeing, hearing, or feeling things that are not there); unusual excitement

*Symptoms of overdose*
  Confusion (continuing); convulsions (seizures); difficulty in swallowing; drowsiness (severe); low body temperature; nausea, vomiting, or stomach pain (severe); shortness of breath or troubled breathing; slow or irregular heartbeat; slurred speech; staggering; weakness (severe)

Other side effects may occur that do not need medical attention. These side effects may go away during treatment as your body adjusts to the medicine. However, check with your doctor if any of the following side effects continue or are bothersome:

*More common*
  Nausea; stomach pain; vomiting

*Less common*
  Clumsiness or unsteadiness; diarrhea; dizziness or lightheadedness; drowsiness; "hangover" effect

After you stop using this medicine, your body may need time to adjust. The length of time this takes depends on the amount of medicine you were using and how long you used it. During this period of time, check with your doctor if you notice any of the following side effects:

  Confusion; hallucinations (seeing, hearing, or feeling things that are not there); nausea or vomiting; nervousness; restlessness; stomach pain; trembling; unusual excitement

Other side effects not listed above may also occur in some patients. If you notice any other effects, check with your doctor.

Revised: 08/02/94

# CHLORAMBUCIL   Systemic

A commonly used brand name in the U.S. and Canada is Leukeran.

## Description

Chlorambucil (klor-AM-byoo-sill) belongs to the group of medicines called alkylating agents. It is used to treat some kinds of cancer.

Chlorambucil interferes with the growth of cancer cells, which are eventually destroyed. Since the growth of normal body cells may also be affected by chlorambucil, other effects will also occur. Some of these may be serious and must be reported to your doctor. Other effects may not be serious but may cause concern. Some effects may not occur for months or years after the medicine is used.

Before you begin treatment with chlorambucil, you and your doctor should talk about the good this medicine will do as well as the risks of using it.

Chlorambucil may also be used for other conditions as determined by your doctor.

Chlorambucil is available only with your doctor's prescription, in the following dosage form:
  *Oral*
  • Tablets (U.S. and Canada)

## Before Using This Medicine

In deciding to use a medicine, the risks of taking the medicine must be weighed against the good it will do.

This is a decision you and your doctor will make. For chlorambucil, the following should be considered:

**Allergies**—Tell your doctor if you have ever had any unusual or allergic reaction to chlorambucil or other cancer medicines.

**Pregnancy**—This medicine may cause birth defects if either the male or female is taking it at the time of conception or if it is taken during pregnancy. In addition, many cancer medicines may cause sterility which could be permanent. Sterility has been reported with this medicine and the possibility should be kept in mind.

Be sure that you have discussed this with your doctor before taking this medicine. It is best to use some kind of birth control while you are taking chlorambucil. Tell your doctor right away if you think you have become pregnant while taking chlorambucil.

**Breast-feeding**—Because chlorambucil may cause serious side effects, breast-feeding is generally not recommended while you are taking it.

**Children**—In general, this medicine has not been shown to cause different side effects or problems in children than it does in adults. However, some children with nephrotic syndrome (a kidney disease) may be more likely to have convulsions (seizures).

**Older adults**—Many medicines have not been studied specifically in older people. Therefore, it may not be known whether they work exactly the same way they do in younger adults or if they cause different side effects or problems in older people. There is no specific information comparing use of chlorambucil in the elderly with use in other age groups.

**Other medicines**—Although certain medicines should not be used together at all, in other cases two different medicines may be used together even if an interaction might occur. In these cases, your doctor may want to change the dose, or other precautions may be necessary. When you are taking chlorambucil it is especially important that your health care professional know if you are taking any of the following:

- Amphotericin B by injection (e.g., Fungizone) or
- Antithyroid agents (medicine for overactive thyroid) or
- Chloramphenicol (e.g., Chloromycetin) or
- Colchicine or
- Flucytosine (e.g., Ancobon) or
- Ganciclovir (e.g., Cytovene) or
- Interferon (e.g., Intron A, Roferon-A) or
- Plicamycin (e.g., Mithracin) or
- Zidovudine (e.g., AZT, Retrovir) or
- If you have ever been treated with radiation or cancer medicines—Chlorambucil may increase the effects of these medicines or radiation therapy on the blood
- Azathioprine (e.g., Imuran) or
- Corticosteroids (cortisone-like medicine) or
- Cyclophosphamide (e.g., Cytoxan) or
- Cyclosporine (e.g., Sandimmune) or
- Cytarabine (e.g., Cytosar-U) or
- Mercaptopurine (e.g., Purinethol) or
- Muromonab-CD3 (monoclonal antibody) (e.g., Orthoclone OKT3) or

- Tacrolimus (e.g., Prograf)—There may be an increased risk of infection and development of cancer because chlorambucil decreases the body's ability to fight them
- Probenecid (e.g., Benemid) or
- Sulfinpyrazone (e.g., Anturane)—Chlorambucil may increase the amount of uric acid in the blood. Since these medicines are used to lower uric acid levels, they may not work as well in patients taking chlorambucil

**Other medical problems**—The presence of other medical problems may affect the use of chlorambucil. Make sure you tell your doctor if you have any other medical problems, especially:

- Chickenpox (including recent exposure) or
- Herpes zoster (shingles)—Risk of severe disease affecting other parts of the body
- Convulsions (seizures) (history of) or
- Head injury—Increased risk of seizures
- Gout or
- Kidney stones (history of)—Chlorambucil may increase levels of uric acid in the body, which can cause gout or kidney stones
- Infection—Chlorambucil decreases your body's ability to fight infection

## Proper Use of This Medicine

*Take this medicine only as directed by your doctor.* Do not take more or less of it, and do not take it more often than your doctor ordered. The exact amount of medicine you need has been carefully worked out. Taking too much may increase the chance of side effects, while taking too little may not improve your condition.

Chlorambucil is sometimes given together with certain other medicines. If you are using a combination of medicines, make sure that you take each one at the proper time and do not mix them. Ask your health care professional to help you plan a way to remember to take your medicines at the right times.

While you are using chlorambucil, your doctor may want you to drink extra fluids so that you will pass more urine. This will help prevent kidney problems and keep your kidneys working well.

This medicine sometimes causes nausea and vomiting. However, it is very important that you continue to use the medicine, even if you begin to feel ill. *Do not stop using this medicine without first checking with your doctor.* Ask your health care professional for ways to lessen these effects.

If you vomit shortly after taking a dose of chlorambucil, check with your doctor. You will be told whether to take the dose again or to wait until the next scheduled dose.

**Dosing**—The dose of chlorambucil will be different for different patients. The dose that is used may depend on a number of things, including what the medicine is being used for, the patient's weight, and whether or not other medicines are also being taken. *If you are taking chlorambucil at home, follow your doctor's orders or the directions on the label.* If you have any questions about the proper dose of chlorambucil, ask your doctor.

**Missed dose**—If you miss a dose of this medicine and your dosing schedule is:

- One dose a day—Take the missed dose as soon as possible. Then go back to your regular dosing schedule. However, if you do not remember the missed dose until the next day, do not take it at all. Instead, take your regularly scheduled dose. Do not double doses.
- More than one dose a day—Take the missed dose as soon as possible. Then go back to your regular dosing schedule. However, if it is almost time for your next dose, skip the missed dose and go back to your regular dosing schedule. Do not double doses.

**Storage**—To store this medicine:

- Keep out of the reach of children.
- Store away from heat and direct light.
- Do not store in the bathroom, near the kitchen sink, or in other damp places. Heat or moisture may cause the medicine to break down.
- Do not keep outdated medicine or medicine no longer needed. Be sure that any discarded medicine is out of the reach of children.

## Precautions While Using This Medicine

*It is very important that your doctor check your progress at regular visits* to make sure this medicine is working properly and to check for unwanted effects.

While you are being treated with chlorambucil, and after you stop treatment with it, *do not have any immunizations (vaccinations) without your doctor's approval.* Chlorambucil may lower your body's resistance and there is a chance you might get the infection the immunization is meant to prevent. In addition, other persons living in your household should not take oral polio vaccine since there is a chance they could pass the polio virus on to you. Also, avoid persons who have recently taken oral polio vaccine. Do not get close to them, and do not stay in the same room with them for very long. If you cannot take these precautions, you should consider wearing a protective face mask that covers the nose and mouth.

Chlorambucil can temporarily lower the number of white blood cells in your blood, increasing the chance of getting an infection. It can also lower the number of platelets, which are necessary for proper blood clotting. If this occurs, there are certain precautions you can take, especially when your blood count is low, to reduce the risk of infection or bleeding:

- If you can, avoid people with infections. *Check with your doctor immediately* if you think you are getting an infection or if you get a fever or chills, cough or hoarseness, lower back or side pain, or painful or difficult urination.
- *Check with your doctor immediately* if you notice any unusual bleeding or bruising; black, tarry stools; blood in urine or stools; or pinpoint red spots on your skin.

- Be careful when using a regular toothbrush, dental floss, or toothpick. Your medical doctor, dentist, or nurse may recommend other ways to clean your teeth and gums. Check with your medical doctor before having any dental work done.
- Do not touch your eyes or the inside of your nose unless you have just washed your hands and have not touched anything else in the meantime.
- Be careful not to cut yourself when you are using sharp objects such as a safety razor or fingernail or toenail cutters.
- Avoid contact sports or other situations where bruising or injury could occur.

## Side Effects of This Medicine

Along with its needed effects, a medicine may have some unwanted effects. Although not all of these side effects may occur, if they do occur they may need medical attention.

Also, because of the way these medicines act on the body, there is a chance that they might cause other unwanted effects that may not occur until months or years after the medicine is used. These delayed effects may include certain types of cancer, such as leukemia. Discuss these possible effects with your doctor.

*Check with your doctor or nurse immediately* if any of the following side effects occur:

*Less common*
    Black, tarry stools; blood in urine or stools; cough or hoarseness; fever or chills; lower back or side pain; painful or difficult urination; pinpoint red spots on skin; sores in mouth and on lips; unusual bleeding or bruising

Check with your doctor as soon as possible if any of the following side effects occur:

*Less common*
    Joint pain; skin rash; swelling of feet or lower legs
*Rare*
    Agitation; blisters on skin; confusion; convulsions (seizures); hallucinations (seeing, hearing, or feeling things that are not there); muscle twitching; peeling or scaling of skin; shortness of breath; skin rash (severe); tremors; trouble in walking; weakness (severe) or paralysis; yellow eyes or skin

*Symptoms of overdose (in the order of frequency)*
    Black, tarry stools; blood in urine or stools; cough or hoarseness; fever or chills; lower back or side pain; painful or difficult urination; pinpoint red spots on skin; unusual bleeding or bruising; agitation; convulsions (seizures); trouble in walking

Other side effects may occur that usually do not need medical attention. These side effects may go away during treatment as your body adjusts to the medicine. Also, your health care professional may be able to tell you about ways to prevent or reduce some of these side effects. Check with your health care professional if any of the following side effects continue or are bothersome or if you have any questions about them:

*Less common*
> Changes in menstrual period; itching of skin; nausea and vomiting

After you stop using chlorambucil, it may still produce some side effects that need attention. During this period of time, check with your doctor if you notice any of the following side effects:

> Black, tarry stools; blood in urine or stools; cough or hoarseness; fever or chills; lower back or side pain; painful or difficult urination; pinpoint red spots on skin; shortness of breath; unusual bleeding or bruising

Other side effects not listed above may also occur in some patients. If you notice any other effects, check with your doctor.

## Additional Information

Once a medicine has been approved for marketing for a certain use, experience may show that it is also useful for other medical problems. Although these uses are not included in product labeling, chlorambucil is used in certain patients with the following medical conditions:

- Polycythemia vera
- Nephrotic syndrome

Other than the above information, there is no additional information relating to proper use, precautions, or side effects for these uses.

Revised: 07/15/94

# CHLORAMPHENICOL   Ophthalmic

Some commonly used brand names are:

**In the U.S.—**

| | |
|---|---|
| Ak-Chlor Ophthalmic Ointment | Econochlor Ophthalmic Ointment |
| Ak-Chlor Ophthalmic Solution | Econochlor Ophthalmic Solution |
| Chloracol Ophthalmic Solution | I-Chlor Ophthalmic Solution |
| Chlorofair Ophthalmic Ointment | Ocu-Chlor Ophthalmic Ointment |
| Chlorofair Ophthalmic Solution | Ocu-Chlor Ophthalmic Solution |
| Chloromycetin Ophthalmic Ointment | Ophthochlor Ophthalmic Solution |
| Chloromycetin for Ophthalmic Solution | Spectro-Chlor Ophthalmic Ointment |
| Chloroptic Ophthalmic Solution | Spectro-Chlor Ophthalmic Solution |
| Chloroptic S.O.P. | |

**In Canada—**

| | |
|---|---|
| Ak-Chlor Ophthalmic Solution | Ophtho-Chloram Ophthalmic Solution |
| Chloromycetin Ophthalmic Ointment | Pentamycetin Ophthalmic Ointment |
| Chloromycetin for Ophthalmic Solution | Pentamycetin Ophthalmic Solution |
| Chloroptic Ophthalmic Solution | Sopamycetin Ophthalmic Ointment |
| Chloroptic S.O.P. | Sopamycetin Ophthalmic Solution |
| Fenicol Ophthalmic Ointment | |

## Description

Chloramphenicol (klor-am-FEN-i-kole) belongs to the family of medicines called antibiotics. Chloramphenicol ophthalmic preparations are used to treat infections of the eye. This medicine may be given alone or with other medicines that are taken by mouth for eye infections.

Chloramphenicol is available only with your doctor's prescription, in the following dosage forms:

*Ophthalmic*
- Ophthalmic ointment (eye ointment) (U.S. and Canada)
- Ophthalmic solution (eye drops) (U.S. and Canada)

## Before Using This Medicine

In deciding to use a medicine, the risks of taking the medicine must be weighed against the good it will do. This is a decision you and your doctor will make. For chloramphenicol, the following should be considered:

**Allergies**—Tell your doctor if you have ever had any unusual or allergic reaction to chloramphenicol. Also tell your health care professional if you are allergic to any other substances, such as preservatives.

**Pregnancy**—Chloramphenicol ophthalmic preparations have not been shown to cause birth defects or other problems in humans.

**Breast-feeding**—Chloramphenicol ophthalmic preparations have not been reported to cause problems in nursing babies.

**Children**—Studies on this medicine have been done only in adult patients, and there is no specific information comparing use of this medicine in children with use in other age groups.

**Older adults**—Many medicines have not been studied specifically in older people. Therefore, it may not be known whether they work exactly the same way they do in younger adults or if they cause different side effects or problems in older people. There is no specific information comparing use of this medicine in the elderly with use in other age groups.

**Other medicines**—Although certain medicines should not be used together at all, in other cases two different medicines may be used together even if an interaction might occur. In these cases, your doctor may want to change the dose, or other precautions may be necessary. Tell your health care professional if you are using any other prescription or nonprescription (over-the-counter [OTC]) medicine.

## Proper Use of This Medicine

For patients using the *eye drop form* of chloramphenicol:

- Although the bottle may not be full, it contains exactly the amount of medicine your doctor ordered.
- To use:

  —First, wash your hands. Tilt the head back and, pressing your finger gently on the skin just beneath the lower eyelid, pull the lower eyelid away from the eye to make a space. Drop the medicine into this space. Let go of the eyelid and gently close the eyes. Do not blink. Keep the eyes closed and apply pressure to the inner corner of the eye with your finger for 1 or 2 minutes to allow the medicine to come into contact with the infection.

  —If you think you did not get the drop of medicine into your eye properly, use another drop.

  —To keep the medicine as germ-free as possible, do not touch the applicator tip or dropper to any surface (including the eye). Also, keep the container tightly closed.

To use the *eye ointment form* of chloramphenicol:

- First, wash your hands. Tilt the head back and, pressing your finger gently on the skin just beneath the lower eyelid, pull the lower eyelid away from the eye to make a space. Squeeze a thin strip of ointment into this space. A 1-cm (approximately 1/3-inch) strip of ointment is usually enough, unless you have been told by your doctor to use a different amount. Let go of the eyelid and gently close the eyes. Keep the eyes closed for 1 or 2 minutes to allow the medicine to come into contact with the infection.
- To keep the medicine as germ-free as possible, do not touch the applicator tip to any surface (including the eye). After using chloramphenicol eye ointment, wipe the tip of the ointment tube with a clean tissue and keep the tube tightly closed.

To help clear up your infection completely, *keep using this medicine for the full time of treatment*, even if your symptoms begin to clear up after a few days. If you stop using this medicine too soon, your symptoms may return. *Do not miss any doses.*

**Dosing**—The dose of chloramphenicol will be different for different patients. *Follow your doctor's orders or the directions on the label.* The following information includes only the average doses of chloramphenicol. *If your dose is different, do not change it unless your doctor tells you to do so.*

- For eye infection:
  —For *ophthalmic ointment* dosage form:
  - Adults and children—Use every three hours.
  —For *ophthalmic solution (eye drops)* dosage form:
  - Adults and children—One drop every one to four hours.

**Missed dose**—If you miss a dose of this medicine, apply it as soon as possible. However, if it is almost time for your next dose, skip the missed dose and go back to your regular dosing schedule.

**Storage**—To store this medicine:

- Keep out of the reach of children.
- Store away from heat and direct light.
- Keep the medicine from freezing.
- Do not keep outdated medicine or medicine no longer needed. Be sure that any discarded medicine is out of the reach of children.

## Precautions While Using This Medicine

If your symptoms do not improve within a few days, or if they become worse, check with your doctor.

## Side Effects of This Medicine

Along with its needed effects, a medicine may cause some unwanted effects. Although not all of these side effects may occur, if they do occur they may need medical attention.

*Check with your doctor immediately* if any of the following side effects occur:

*Rare*

Pale skin; sore throat and fever; unusual bleeding or bruising; unusual tiredness or weakness (the above side effects may also occur weeks or months after you stop using this medicine)

Check with your doctor as soon as possible if any of the following side effects occur:

*Less common*

Itching, redness, skin rash, swelling, or other sign of irritation not present before use of this medicine

Other side effects may occur that usually do not need medical attention. These side effects may go away during treatment as your body adjusts to the medicine. However, check with your doctor if either of the following side effects continues or is bothersome:

*Less common*

Burning or stinging

After application, eye ointments may be expected to cause your vision to blur for a few minutes.

Other side effects not listed above may also occur in some patients. If you notice any other effects, check with your doctor.

Revised: 01/15/92
Interim revision(s): 09/30/93; 12/13/93

# CHLORAMPHENICOL  Otic

Some commonly used brand names are:
**In the U.S.—**
  Chloromycetin
  Generic name product may also be available.
**In Canada—**
  Chloromycetin
  Sopamycetin

## Description

Chloramphenicol (klor-am-FEN-i-kole) belongs to the family of medicines called antibiotics. Chloramphenicol otic drops are used to treat infections of the ear canal. This medicine may be used alone or with other medicines that are taken by mouth for ear canal infections.

Chloramphenicol is available only with your doctor's prescription, in the following dosage form:

*Otic*
  • Solution (U.S. and Canada)

## Before Using This Medicine

In deciding to use a medicine, the risks of using the medicine must be weighed against the good it will do. This is a decision you and your doctor will make. For chloramphenicol otic, the following should be considered:

**Allergies—**Tell your doctor if you have ever had any unusual or allergic reaction to chloramphenicol. Also tell your health care professional if you are allergic to any other substances, such as preservatives.

**Pregnancy—**Chloramphenicol otic drops have not been shown to cause birth defects or other problems in humans.

**Breast-feeding—**Chloramphenicol otic drops have not been reported to cause problems in nursing babies.

**Children—**Although there is no specific information comparing use of chloramphenicol otic drops in children with use in other age groups, this medicine is not expected to cause different side effects or problems in children than it does in adults.

**Older adults—**Many medicines have not been studied specifically in older people. Therefore, it may not be known whether they work exactly the same way they do in younger adults or if they cause different side effects or problems in older people. There is no specific information comparing use of this medicine in the elderly with use in other age groups.

**Other medicines—**Although certain medicines should not be used together at all, in other cases two different medicines may be used together even if an interaction might occur. In these cases, your doctor may want to change the dose, or other precautions may be necessary. Tell your health care professional if you are using any other prescription or nonprescription (over-the-counter [OTC]) medicine.

**Other medical problems—**The presence of other medical problems may affect the use of chloramphenicol ear drops. Make sure you tell your doctor if you have any other medical problems, especially:
  • Opening in your ear drum—This medicine may cause unwanted effects if it goes past the ear drum into the middle ear

## Proper Use of This Medicine

To use:
  • Lie down or tilt the head so that the infected ear faces up. Gently pull the earlobe up and back for adults (down and back for children) to straighten the ear canal. Drop the medicine into the ear canal. Keep the ear facing up for about 1 or 2 minutes to allow the medicine to come into contact with the infection. A sterile cotton plug may be gently inserted into the ear opening to prevent the medicine from leaking out.
  • To keep the medicine as germ-free as possible, do not touch the dropper to any surface (including the ear). Also, keep the container tightly closed.

To help clear up your infection completely, *keep using this medicine for the full time of treatment,* even if your symptoms begin to clear up after a few days. If you stop using this medicine too soon, your symptoms may return. *Do not miss any doses.*

**Dosing—**The dose of otic chloramphenicol will be different for different patients. *Follow your doctor's orders or the directions on the label.* The following information includes only the average doses of otic chloramphenicol. *If your dose is different, do not change it* unless your doctor tells you to do so.
  • For *otic solution (ear drops)* dosage form:
    —For infections of the ear canal:
      • Adults and children—Use two or three drops in the ear every six to eight hours.

**Missed dose—**If you miss a dose of this medicine, apply it as soon as possible. However, if it is almost time for your next dose, skip the missed dose and go back to your regular dosing schedule.

**Storage—**To store this medicine:
  • Keep out of the reach of children.
  • Store away from heat and direct light.
  • Keep the medicine from freezing.
  • Do not keep outdated medicine or medicine no longer needed. Be sure that any discarded medicine is out of the reach of children.

## Precautions While Using This Medicine

If your symptoms do not improve within a few days, or if they become worse, check with your doctor.

## Side Effects of This Medicine

Along with its needed effects, a medicine may cause some unwanted effects. Although not all of these side effects may occur, if they do occur they may need medical attention.

*Check with your doctor immediately* if any of the following side effects occur:

*Rare*
  Pale skin; sore throat and fever; unusual bleeding or bruising; unusual tiredness or weakness (the above side effects may also occur weeks or months after you stop using this medicine)

Check with your doctor as soon as possible if any of the following side effects occur:

*Less common*
  Burning, itching, redness, skin rash, swelling, or other sign of irritation not present before use of this medicine

Other side effects not listed above may also occur in some patients. If you notice any other effects, check with your doctor.

Revised: 02/10/92
Interim revision: 02/17/94

---

# CHLORAMPHENICOL   Systemic

Some commonly used brand names are:
**In the U.S.—**
  Chloromycetin
  Generic name product may also be available.
**In Canada—**
  Chloromycetin                     Novochlorocap

## Description

Chloramphenicol (klor-am-FEN-i-kole) is used in the treatment of infections caused by bacteria. It works by killing bacteria or preventing their growth.

Chloramphenicol is used to treat serious infections in different parts of the body. It is sometimes given with other antibiotics. However, chloramphenicol should not be used for colds, flu, other virus infections, sore throats or other minor infections, or to prevent infections.

Chloramphenicol should only be used for serious infections in which other medicines do not work. This medicine may cause some serious side effects, including blood problems and eye problems. Symptoms of the blood problems include pale skin, sore throat and fever, unusual bleeding or bruising, and unusual tiredness or weakness. *You and your doctor should talk about the good this medicine will do as well as the risks of taking it.*

Chloramphenicol is available only with your doctor's prescription, in the following dosage forms:

*Oral*
  • Capsules (U.S. and Canada)
  • Oral suspension (U.S.)
*Parenteral*
  • Injection (U.S. and Canada)

## Before Using This Medicine

In deciding to use a medicine, the risks of taking the medicine must be weighed against the good it will do.

This is a decision you and your doctor will make. For chloramphenicol, the following should be considered:

**Allergies**—Tell your doctor if you have ever had any unusual or allergic reaction to chloramphenicol. Also tell your health care professional if you are allergic to any other substances, such as foods, preservatives, or dyes.

**Pregnancy**—Chloramphenicol has not been shown to cause birth defects in humans. However, use is not recommended within a week or two of your delivery date. Chloramphenicol may cause gray skin color, low body temperature, bloated stomach, uneven breathing, drowsiness, pale skin, sore throat and fever, unusual bleeding or bruising, unusual tiredness or weakness, or other problems in the infant.

**Breast-feeding**—Chloramphenicol passes into the breast milk and has been shown to cause unwanted effects, such as pale skin, sore throat and fever, unusual bleeding or bruising, unusual tiredness or weakness, or other problems in nursing babies. It may be necessary for you to take another medicine or to stop breast-feeding during treatment. Be sure you have discussed the risks and benefits of the medicine with your doctor.

**Children**—Newborn infants are especially sensitive to the side effects of chloramphenicol because they cannot remove the medicine from their body as well as older children and adults.

**Older adults**—Many medicines have not been studied specifically in older people. Therefore, it may not be known whether they work exactly the same way they do in younger adults or if they cause different side effects or problems in older people. There is no specific information comparing use of chloramphenicol in the elderly with use in other age groups.

**Other medicines**—Although certain medicines should not be used together at all, in other cases two different medicines may be used together even if an interaction might occur. In these cases, your doctor may want to change

the dose, or other precautions may be necessary. When you are taking chloramphenicol, it is especially important that your health care professional know if you are taking any of the following:

- Alfentanil or
- Antidiabetics, oral (diabetes medicine you take by mouth) or
- Phenobarbital or
- Warfarin (e.g., Coumadin)—Use of chloramphenicol with these medicines may increase the chance of side effects of these medicines
- Amphotericin B by injection (e.g., Fungizone) or
- Antineoplastics (cancer medicine) or
- Antithyroid agents (medicine for overactive thyroid) or
- Azathioprine (e.g., Imuran) or
- Colchicine or
- Cyclophosphamide (e.g., Cytoxan) or
- Ethotoin (e.g., Peganone) or
- Flucytosine (e.g., Ancobon) or
- Ganciclovir (e.g., Cytovene) or
- Interferon (e.g., Intron A, Roferon-A) or
- Mephenytoin (e.g., Mesantoin) or
- Mercaptopurine (e.g., Purinethol) or
- Methotrexate (e.g., Mexate) or
- Phenytoin (e.g., Dilantin) or
- Plicamycin (e.g., Mithracin) or
- Zidovudine (e.g., AZT, Retrovir) or
- X-ray treatment—Use of chloramphenicol with any of these medicines or with x-ray treatment may increase the risk of blood problems
- Clindamycin (e.g., Cleocin) or
- Erythromycins (medicine for infection) or
- Lincomycin (e.g., Lincocin)—Use of chloramphenicol with any of these medicines may decrease the effectiveness of these medicines
- Phenytoin (e.g., Dilantin)—Use of chloramphenicol with phenytoin may increase the chance of blood problems or increase the side effects of phenytoin

**Other medical problems**—The presence of other medical problems may affect the use of chloramphenicol. Make sure you tell your doctor if you have any other medical problems, especially:

- Anemia, bleeding, or other blood problems—Chloramphenicol may cause blood problems
- Liver disease—Patients with liver disease may have an increased risk of side effects

## Proper Use of This Medicine

Chloramphenicol is best taken with a full glass (8 ounces) of water on an empty stomach (either 1 hour before or 2 hours after meals), unless otherwise directed by your doctor.

For patients taking the oral liquid form of this medicine:

- Use a specially marked measuring spoon or other device to measure each dose accurately. The average household teaspoon may not hold the right amount of liquid.

To help clear up your infection completely, *keep taking this medicine for the full time of treatment*, even if you begin to feel better after a few days. *Do not miss any doses.*

**Dosing**—The dose of chloramphenicol will be different for different patients. *Follow your doctor's orders or the directions on the label.* The following information includes only the average doses of chloramphenicol. *If your dose is different, do not change it* unless your doctor tells you to do so.

The number of capsules or teaspoonfuls of suspension that you take depends on the strength of the medicine. Also, *the number of doses you take each day, the time allowed between doses, and the length of time you take the medicine depend on the medical problem for which you are taking chloramphenicol.*

- For infections caused by bacteria:
  —For *oral* dosage forms (capsules and suspension):
  - Adults and teenagers—Dose is based on body weight. The usual dose is 12.5 milligrams (mg) per kilogram (kg) (5.7 mg per pound) of body weight every six hours.
  - Children—
    —Infants up to 2 weeks of age: Dose is based on body weight. The usual dose is 6.25 mg per kg (2.8 mg per pound) of body weight every six hours.
    —Infants 2 weeks of age and older: Dose is based on body weight. The usual dose is 12.5 mg per kg (5.7 mg per pound) of body weight every six hours; or 25 mg per kg (11.4 mg per pound) of body weight every twelve hours.
  —For *injection* dosage form:
  - Adults and teenagers—Dose is based on body weight. The usual dose is 12.5 mg per kg (5.7 mg per pound) of body weight every six hours.
  - Children—
    —Infants up to 2 weeks of age: Dose is based on body weight. The usual dose is 6.25 mg per kg (2.8 mg per pound) of body weight every six hours.
    —Infants 2 weeks of age and older: Dose is based on body weight. The usual dose is 12.5 mg per kg (5.7 mg per pound) of body weight every six hours; or 25 mg per kg (11.4 mg per pound) of body weight every twelve hours.

**Missed dose**—If you miss a dose of this medicine, take it as soon as possible. However, if it is almost time for your next dose, skip the missed dose and go back to your regular dosing schedule. Do not double doses.

**Storage**—To store this medicine:
- Keep out of the reach of children.
- Store away from heat and direct light.
- Do not store the capsule form of this medicine in the bathroom, near the kitchen sink, or in other damp places. Heat or moisture may cause the medicine to break down.
- Keep the oral liquid form of this medicine from freezing.

- Do not keep outdated medicine or medicine no longer needed. Be sure that any discarded medicine is out of the reach of children.

## Precautions While Using This Medicine

If your symptoms do not improve within a few days, or if they become worse, check with your doctor.

*It is very important that your doctor check you at regular visits* for any blood problems that may be caused by this medicine.

Chloramphenicol may cause blood problems. These problems may result in a greater chance of infection, slow healing, and bleeding of the gums. Therefore, you should be careful when using regular toothbrushes, dental floss, and toothpicks. Dental work, whenever possible, should be done before you begin taking this medicine or delayed until your blood counts have returned to normal. Check with your medical doctor or dentist if you have any questions about proper oral hygiene (mouth care) during treatment.

For diabetic patients:

- *This medicine may cause false test results with urine sugar tests.* Check with your doctor before changing your diet or the dosage of your diabetes medicine.

## Side Effects of This Medicine

Along with its needed effects, a medicine may cause some serious unwanted effects. Although not all of these side effects may occur, if they do occur they may need medical attention.

*Stop taking this medicine and get emergency help immediately* if any of the following side effects occur:
### Rare—in babies only
Bloated stomach; drowsiness; gray skin color; low body temperature; uneven breathing; unresponsiveness

Also, *check with your doctor immediately* if any of the following side effects occur:
### Less common
Pale skin; sore throat and fever; unusual bleeding or bruising; unusual tiredness or weakness (the above side effects may also occur up to weeks or months after you stop taking this medicine)
### Rare
Confusion, delirium, or headache; eye pain, blurred vision, or loss of vision; numbness, tingling, burning pain, or weakness in the hands or feet; skin rash, fever, or difficulty in breathing

Other side effects may occur that usually do not need medical attention. These side effects may go away during treatment as your body adjusts to the medicine. However, check with your doctor if any of the following side effects continue or are bothersome:
### Less common
Diarrhea; nausea or vomiting

Other side effects not listed above may also occur in some patients. If you notice any other effects, check with your doctor.

Revised: 05/13/92
Interim revision: 03/17/94

---

# CHLORAMPHENICOL  Topical

A commonly used brand name in the U.S. and Canada is Chloromycetin.

## Description

Chloramphenicol (klor-am-FEN-i-kole) belongs to the family of medicines called antibiotics. Chloramphenicol cream is used to treat infections of the skin. It may be used alone or with other medicines that are taken by mouth for skin infections.

Chloramphenicol is available only with your doctor's prescription, in the following dosage form:
### Topical
- Cream (U.S. and Canada)

## Before Using This Medicine

In deciding to use a medicine, the risks of using the medicine must be weighed against the good it will do.

This is a decision you and your doctor will make. For chloramphenicol, the following should be considered:

**Allergies**—Tell your doctor if you have ever had any unusual or allergic reaction to chloramphenicol. Also tell your health care professional if you are allergic to any other substances, such as preservatives or dyes.

**Pregnancy**—Topical chloramphenicol has not been shown to cause birth defects or other problems in humans.

**Breast-feeding**—Topical chloramphenicol has not been reported to cause problems in nursing babies.

**Children**—Although there is no specific information comparing use of topical chloramphenicol in children with use in other age groups, this medicine is not expected to cause different side effects or problems in children than it does in adults.

**Older adults**—Many medicines have not been studied specifically in older people. Therefore, it may not be known

whether they work exactly the same way they do in younger adults or if they cause different side effects or problems in older people. There is no specific information comparing use of this medicine in the elderly with use in other age groups.

**Other medicines**—Although certain medicines should not be used together at all, in other cases two different medicines may be used together even if an interaction might occur. In these cases, your doctor may want to change the dose, or other precautions may be necessary. Tell your health care professional if you are using any other prescription or nonprescription (over-the-counter [OTC]) medicine.

## Proper Use of This Medicine

Before applying this medicine, wash the affected area with soap and water, and dry thoroughly.

To help clear up your infection completely, *keep using this medicine for the full time of treatment,* even if your symptoms begin to clear up after a few days. If you stop using this medicine too soon, your symptoms may return. *Do not miss any doses.* However, *do not use this medicine more often or for a longer time than your doctor ordered.*

**Dosing**—The dose of topical chloramphenicol will be different for different patients. *Follow your doctor's orders or the directions on the label.* The following information includes only the average dose of topical chloramphenicol. *If your dose is different, do not change it* unless your doctor tells you to do so.

• For *topical* dosage form (cream):
  —For bacterial skin infections:
    • Adults and children—Apply to the affected area(s) of the skin three or four times a day.

**Missed dose**—If you miss a dose of this medicine, apply it as soon as possible. However, if it is almost time for your next dose, skip the missed dose and go back to your regular dosing schedule.

**Storage**—To store this medicine:
• Keep out of the reach of children.
• Store away from heat and direct light.
• Keep the medicine from freezing.
• Do not keep outdated medicine or medicine no longer needed. Be sure that any discarded medicine is out of the reach of children.

## Precautions While Using This Medicine

If your skin problem does not improve within 1 week, or if it becomes worse, check with your doctor.

## Side Effects of This Medicine

Along with its needed effects, a medicine may cause some unwanted effects. Although not all of these side effects may occur, if they do occur they may need medical attention.

*Check with your doctor immediately* if any of the following side effects occur:
    *Rare*
        Pale skin; sore throat and fever; unusual bleeding or bruising; unusual tiredness or weakness (the above side effects may also occur weeks or months after you stop using this medicine)

Check with your doctor as soon as possible if any of the following side effects occur:
    *More common*
        Burning, itching, redness, skin rash, swelling, or other signs of irritation not present before use of this medicine

Other side effects not listed above may also occur in some patients. If you notice any other effects, check with your doctor.

Revised: 02/10/92
Interim revision: 06/13/94

---

# CHLORDIAZEPOXIDE AND AMITRIPTYLINE  Systemic†

Some commonly used brand names in the U.S. are Limbitrol and Limbitrol DS.
Generic name product may also be available.

†Not commercially available in Canada.

## Description

Chlordiazepoxide (klor-dy-az-e-POX-ide) and amitriptyline (a-mee-TRIP-ti-leen) combination is used to treat mental depression that occurs with anxiety or nervous tension.

This medicine is available only with your doctor's prescription, in the following dosage form:
    *Oral*
    • Tablets (U.S.)

## Before Using This Medicine

In deciding to use a medicine, the risks of taking the medicine must be weighed against the good it will do. This is a decision you and your doctor will make. For

chlordiazepoxide and amitriptyline combination, the following should be considered:

**Allergies**—Tell your doctor if you have ever had any unusual or allergic reaction to chlordiazepoxide (e.g., Librium) or other benzodiazepines (such as alprazolam [e.g., Xanax], bromazepam [e.g., Lectopam], clonazepam [e.g., Klonopin], clorazepate [e.g., Tranxene], diazepam [e.g., Valium], estazolam [e.g., ProSom], flurazepam [e.g., Dalmane], halazepam [e.g., Paxipam], ketazolam [e.g., Loftran], lorazepam [e.g., Ativan], midazolam [e.g., Versed], nitrazepam [e.g., Mogadon], oxazepam [e.g., Serax], prazepam [e.g., Centrax], quazepam [e.g., Doral], temazepam [e.g., Restoril], triazolam [e.g., Halcion]) or to amitriptyline (e.g., Elavil) or other tricyclic antidepressants (such as amoxapine [e.g., Asendin], clomipramine [e.g., Anafranil], desipramine [e.g., Pertofrane], doxepin [e.g., Sinequan], imipramine [e.g., Tofranil], nortriptyline [e.g., Aventyl], protriptyline [e.g., Vivactil], trimipramine [e.g., Surmontil]).

Also tell your health care professional if you are allergic to any other substances, such as foods, preservatives, or dyes.

**Pregnancy**—
- *Chlordiazepoxide*: Chlordiazepoxide has been reported to increase the chance of birth defects when used during the first 3 months of pregnancy.

 In addition, overuse of chlordiazepoxide during pregnancy may cause the baby to become dependent on the medicine. This may lead to withdrawal side effects in the baby after birth.

 Use of chlordiazepoxide during pregnancy, especially during the last weeks, may cause drowsiness, slow heartbeat, shortness of breath, or troubled breathing in the newborn baby. Chlordiazepoxide given just before or during labor may cause weakness in the newborn baby.
- *Amitriptyline*: Studies with amitriptyline have not been done in pregnant women. However, studies in animals have shown amitriptyline to cause birth defects when used in doses many times the human dose. Also, there have been reports of newborns suffering from muscle spasms and heart, breathing, and urinary problems when their mothers had taken tricyclic antidepressants (such as amitriptyline) immediately before delivery.

**Breast-feeding**—Chlordiazepoxide may pass into the breast milk and cause drowsiness, slow heartbeat, shortness of breath, or troubled breathing in babies of mothers taking this medicine. Although amitriptyline has also been found in breast milk, it has not been reported to cause problems in nursing babies.

**Children**—Children may be especially sensitive to the effects of chlordiazepoxide and amitriptyline combination. This may increase the chance of side effects during treatment.

**Older adults**—Elderly people are especially sensitive to the effects of chlordiazepoxide and amitriptyline combination. This may increase the chance of side effects during treatment.

**Other medicines**—Although certain medicines should not be used together at all, in other cases 2 different medicines may be used together even if an interaction might occur. In these cases, your doctor may want to change the dose, or other precautions may be necessary. When you are taking chlordiazepoxide and amitriptyline combination, it is especially important that your health care professional know if you are taking any of the following:
- Alcohol or
- Central nervous system (CNS) depressants (medicines that cause drowsiness)—Using these medicines with chlordiazepoxide and amitriptyline combination may increase the CNS depressant effects
- Amphetamines or
- Appetite suppressants (diet pills) or
- Medicine for asthma or other breathing problems or
- Medicine for colds, sinus problems, or hay fever or other allergies (including nose drops or sprays)—Using these medicines with chlordiazepoxide and amitriptyline combination may increase the risk of serious effects on your heart
- Antacids—Taking these medicines with chlordiazepoxide and amitriptyline combination may delay the combination medicine's effects
- Antihypertensives (high blood pressure medicine)—Taking these medicines with chlordiazepoxide and amitriptyline combination may increase the chance of low blood pressure (hypotension)
- Antithyroid agents (medicine for overactive thyroid) or
- Cimetidine (e.g., Tagamet)—Taking these medicines with chlordiazepoxide and amitriptyline combination may increase the chance of serious side effects
- Monoamine oxidase (MAO) inhibitors (furazolidone [e.g., Furoxone], isocarboxazid [e.g., Marplan], phenelzine [e.g., Nardil], procarbazine [e.g., Matulane], selegiline [e.g., Eldepryl], tranylcypromine [e.g., Parnate])—Taking chlordiazepoxide and amitriptyline combination while you are taking or within 2 weeks of taking monoamine oxidase (MAO) inhibitors may cause sudden very high body temperature, extremely high blood pressure, and severe convulsions; however, sometimes certain of these medicines may be used with this combination medicine under close supervision by your doctor

**Other medical problems**—The presence of other medical problems may affect the use of chlordiazepoxide and amitriptyline combination. Make sure you tell your doctor if you have any other medical problems, especially:
- Alcohol abuse (or history of) or
- Drug abuse or dependence (or history of)—Dependence on this medicine may develop
- Bipolar disorder (manic-depressive illness) or
- Blood problems or
- Difficulty in urinating or
- Emphysema, asthma, bronchitis, or other chronic lung disease or
- Enlarged prostate or
- Glaucoma or increased eye pressure or
- Heart disease or
- Mental illness (severe) or

- Myasthenia gravis or
- Porphyria—Chlordiazepoxide and amitriptyline combination may make the condition worse
- Epilepsy or history of seizures—The risk of seizures may be increased
- Hyperactivity—Chlordiazepoxide and amitriptyline combination may cause unexpected effects
- Kidney disease or
- Liver disease—Higher blood levels of chlordiazepoxide and amitriptyline may occur, increasing the chance of side effects
- Overactive thyroid or
- Stomach or intestinal problems—Use of this combination medicine may result in more serious problems

## Proper Use of This Medicine

To reduce stomach upset, take this medicine immediately after meals or with food unless your doctor has told you to take it on an empty stomach.

*Sometimes this medicine must be taken for several weeks before you begin to feel better.* Your doctor should check your progress at regular visits.

*Take this medicine only as directed by your doctor.* Do not take more of it, do not take it more often, and do not take it for a longer period of time than your doctor ordered. If too much is taken, it may increase unwanted effects or become habit-forming (causing mental or physical dependence).

If you think this medicine is not working properly after you have taken it for a few weeks, *do not increase the dose.* Instead, check with your doctor.

**Dosing**—The dose of chlordiazepoxide and amitriptyline combination will be different for different patients. *Follow your doctor's orders or the directions on the label.* The following information includes only the average doses of chlordiazepoxide and amitriptyline combination. *If your dose is different, do not change it* unless your doctor tells you to do so.

The number of tablets that you take depends on the strength of the medicine. Also, *the number of doses you take each day, the time allowed between doses, and the length of time you take the medicine depend on the medical problem for which you are taking chlordiazepoxide and amitriptyline combination.*

- For *oral* dosage forms (tablets):
  —Adults and adolescents: To start, 5 milligrams of chlordiazepoxide and 12.5 milligrams of amitriptyline or 10 milligrams of chlordiazepoxide and 25 milligrams of amitriptyline, taken three or four times a day. The doctor may adjust your dose if needed. However, the dose is usually not greater than 10 milligrams of chlordiazepoxide and 25 milligrams of amitriptyline taken six times a day.
  —Children up to 12 years of age: Dose must be determined by the doctor.

**Missed dose**—If you miss a dose of this medicine, skip the missed dose and go back to your regular dosing schedule. Do not double doses.

**Storage**—To store this medicine:
- Keep out of the reach of children. Overdose of this medicine is very dangerous in young children.
- Store away from heat and direct light.
- Do not store in the bathroom, near the kitchen sink, or in other damp places. Heat or moisture may cause the medicine to break down.
- Do not keep outdated medicine or medicine no longer needed. Be sure that any discarded medicine is out of the reach of children.

## Precautions While Using This Medicine

It is very important that your doctor check your progress at regular visits to allow dose adjustments and help reduce side effects.

*Do not stop taking this medicine without first checking with your doctor.* Your doctor may want you to reduce gradually the amount you are using before stopping completely. This may help prevent a possible worsening of your condition and reduce the possibility of withdrawal symptoms such as headache, nausea, and/or an overall feeling of discomfort.

This medicine will add to the effects of alcohol and other CNS depressants (medicines that slow down the nervous system, possibly causing drowsiness). Some examples of CNS depressants are antihistamines or medicine for hay fever, other allergies, or colds; sedatives, tranquilizers, or sleeping medicine; prescription pain medicine or narcotics; barbiturates; medicine for seizures; muscle relaxants; or anesthetics, including some dental anesthetics. This effect may last for a few days after you stop taking this medicine. *Check with your doctor before taking any of the above while you are using this medicine.*

*For diabetic patients:*
- This medicine may affect blood sugar levels. If you notice a change in the results of your blood or urine sugar tests or if you have any questions, check with your doctor.

Before you have any medical tests, tell the medical doctor in charge that you are taking this medicine. The results of the metyrapone test may be affected by this medicine.

*Before having any surgery, any dental treatment, or emergency treatment, tell the medical doctor or dentist in charge that you are using this medicine.* Taking chlordiazepoxide and amitriptyline combination together with medicines that are used during surgery or dental or emergency treatments may increase the CNS depressant effects.

This medicine may cause some people to become dizzy, lightheaded, drowsy, or less alert than they are normally. Even if taken at bedtime, it may cause some people to feel drowsy or less alert on arising. *Make sure you know how you react to this medicine before you drive, use* machines, or do anything else that could be dangerous if you are dizzy or are not alert.

*Dizziness, lightheadedness, or fainting may occur when you get up from a lying or sitting position.* Getting up slowly may help. If this problem continues or gets worse, check with your doctor.

Chlordiazepoxide and amitriptyline combination may cause dryness of the mouth. For temporary relief, use sugarless candy or gum, melt bits of ice in your mouth, or use a saliva substitute. However, if your mouth continues to feel dry for more than 2 weeks, check with your medical doctor or dentist. Continuing dryness of the mouth may increase the chance of dental disease, including tooth decay, gum disease, and fungus infections.

Chlordiazepoxide and amitriptyline combination may cause your skin to be more sensitive to sunlight than it is normally. Exposure to sunlight, even for brief periods of time, may cause a skin rash, itching, redness or other discoloration of the skin, or a severe sunburn. When you begin taking this medicine:

- Stay out of direct sunlight, especially between the hours of 10:00 a.m. and 3:00 p.m., if possible.
- Wear protective clothing, including a hat. Also, wear sunglasses.
- Apply a sun block product that has a skin protection factor (SPF) of at least 15. Some patients may require a product with a higher SPF number, especially if they have a fair complexion. If you have any questions about this, check with your health care professional.
- Apply a sun block lipstick that has an SPF of at least 15 to protect your lips.
- Do not use a sunlamp or tanning bed or booth.

*If you have a severe reaction from the sun, check with your doctor.*

## Side Effects of This Medicine

Along with its needed effects, a medicine may cause some unwanted effects. Although not all of these side effects may occur, if they do occur they may need medical attention.

Check with your doctor as soon as possible if any of the following side effects occur:

*Less common*

Blurred vision or other changes in vision; confusion or hallucinations (seeing, hearing, or feeling things that are not there); constipation; difficulty in urinating; eye pain; fainting; irregular heartbeat; mental depression; shakiness; trouble in sleeping; unusual excitement, nervousness, or irritability

*Rare*

Convulsions (seizures); increased sensitivity to sunlight; skin rash and itching; sore throat and fever; yellow eyes or skin

*Symptoms of overdose*

Agitation; confusion; convulsions (seizures); dizziness or lightheadedness (severe); drowsiness (severe); enlarged pupils; fast or irregular heartbeat; fever; hallucinations; muscle stiffness or rigidity; vomiting (severe)

Other side effects may occur that usually do not need medical attention. These side effects may go away during treatment as your body adjusts to the medicine. However, check with your doctor if any of the following side effects continue or are bothersome:

*More common*

Bloating; clumsiness or unsteadiness; dizziness or lightheadedness; drowsiness; dryness of mouth or unpleasant taste; headache; weight gain

*Less common*

Diarrhea; nausea or vomiting; unusual tiredness or weakness

*After you stop using this medicine, your body may need time to adjust.* If you took this medicine in high doses or for a long time, this may take up to 2 weeks. *During this time check with your doctor if you notice any of the following side effects:*

Convulsions (seizures); headache; increased sweating; irritability or restlessness; muscle cramps; nausea or vomiting; stomach cramps; trembling; trouble in sleeping, with vivid dreams

Other side effects not listed above may also occur in some patients. If you notice any other effects, check with your doctor.

Revised: 03/19/93

# CHLORDIAZEPOXIDE AND CLIDINIUM  Systemic

Some commonly used brand names are:

**In the U.S.—**
Clindex
Clinoxide
Clipoxide
Librax

Lidox
Lidoxide
Zebrax

Generic name product may also be available.

**In Canada—**
Apo-Chlorax
Corium

Librax

## Description

Chlordiazepoxide (klor-dye-az-e-POX-ide) and clidinium (kli-DI-nee-um) is a combination of medicines used to relax the digestive system and to reduce stomach acid. It is used to treat stomach and intestinal problems such as ulcers and colitis.

Chlordiazepoxide belongs to the group of medicines known as benzodiazepines. It is a central nervous system (CNS) depressant (a medicine that slows down the nervous system).

Clidinium belongs to the group of medicines known as anticholinergics. It helps lessen the amount of acid formed in the stomach. Clidinium also helps relieve abdominal or stomach spasms or cramps.

This combination is available only with your doctor's prescription, in the following dosage form:

*Oral*
- Capsules (U.S. and Canada)

## Before Using This Medicine

In deciding to use a medicine, the risks of taking the medicine must be weighed against the good it will do. This is a decision you and your doctor will make. For chlordiazepoxide and clidinium, the following should be considered:

**Allergies**—Tell your doctor if you have ever had any unusual or allergic reaction to benzodiazepines such as alprazolam [e.g., Xanax], bromazepam [e.g., Lectopam], chlordiazepoxide [e.g., Librium], clonazepam [e.g., Klonopin], clorazepate [e.g., Tranxene], diazepam [e.g., Valium], flurazepam [e.g., Dalmane], halazepam [e.g., Paxipam], ketazolam [e.g., Loftran], lorazepam [e.g., Ativan], midazolam [e.g., Versed], nitrazepam [e.g., Mogadon], oxazepam [e.g., Serax], prazepam [e.g., Centrax], temazepam [e.g., Restoril], or triazolam [e.g., Halcion], or to clidinium or any of the belladonna alkaloids (atropine, belladonna, hyoscyamine, and scopolamine). Also tell your health care professional if you are allergic to any other substances, such as foods, preservatives, or dyes.

**Pregnancy**—Clidinium (contained in this combination) has not been studied in pregnant women. However, clidinium has not been shown to cause birth defects or other problems in animal studies. Chlordiazepoxide (contained also in this combination) may cause birth defects if taken during the first 3 months of pregnancy. In addition, too much use of this medicine during pregnancy may cause the baby to become dependent on the medicine. This may lead to withdrawal side effects after birth. Make sure your doctor knows if you are pregnant or if you may become pregnant before taking chlordiazepoxide and clidinium.

**Breast-feeding**—Chlordiazepoxide may pass into the breast milk and cause unwanted effects, such as excessive drowsiness, in nursing babies. Also, because clidinium tends to decrease the secretions of the body, it is possible that the flow of breast milk may be reduced in some patients.

**Children**—There is no specific information comparing use of chlordiazepoxide and clidinium in children with use in other age groups. However, children are especially sensitive to the effects of chlordiazepoxide and clidinium. Therefore, this may increase the chance of side effects during treatment.

**Older adults**—Confusion or memory loss; constipation; difficult urination; drowsiness; dryness of mouth, nose, throat, or skin; and unusual excitement or agitation may be more likely to occur in the elderly, who are usually more sensitive than younger adults to the effects of chlordiazepoxide and clidinium.

**Other medicines**—Although certain medicines should not be used together at all, in other cases 2 different medicines may be used together even if an interaction might occur. In these cases, your doctor may want to change the dose, or other precautions may be necessary. When you are taking chlordiazepoxide and clidinium it is especially important that your health care professional know if you are taking any of the following:

- Antacids or
- Diarrhea medicine containing kaolin or attapulgite—These medicines may reduce the blood levels of chlordiazepoxide and clidinium, which may decrease their effects; they should be taken at least 2 to 3 hours before or after the chlordiazepoxide and clidinium combination
- Central nervous system (CNS) depressants (medicines that cause drowsiness) or
- Other anticholinergics (medicines for abdominal or stomach spasms or cramps)—Use with chlordiazepoxide and clidinium may increase the side effects of either medicine
- Ketoconazole (e.g., Nizoral)—Chlordiazepoxide and clidinium may reduce the blood level of ketoconazole, which may decrease its effects; therefore, chlordiazepoxide and clidinium should be taken at least 2 hours after ketoconazole
- Potassium chloride (e.g., Kay Ciel)—Use of chlordiazepoxide and clidinium may worsen or cause sores of the stomach or intestine

**Other medical problems**—The presence of other medical problems may affect the use of chlordiazepoxide and clidinium. Make sure you tell your doctor if you have any other medical problems, especially:

- Difficult urination or
- Dryness of mouth (severe and continuing) or
- Emphysema, asthma, bronchitis, or other chronic lung disease or
- Enlarged prostate or
- Glaucoma or
- Hiatal hernia or
- High blood pressure (hypertension) or
- Intestinal blockage or
- Mental depression or
- Mental illness (severe) or
- Myasthenia gravis or
- Ulcerative colitis (severe)—Use of chlordiazepoxide and clidinium may make these conditions worse
- Drug abuse or dependence—Taking chlordiazepoxide (contained in this combination) may become habit-forming, causing mental or physical dependence
- Kidney disease or
- Liver disease—Higher blood levels of chlordiazepoxide and clidinium may result, possibly increasing the chance of side effects

• Overactive thyroid—Use of chlordiazepoxide and clidinium may further increase the heart rate

## Proper Use of This Medicine

Take this medicine about ½ to 1 hour before meals unless otherwise directed by your doctor.

*Take this medicine only as directed by your doctor.* Do not take more of it, do not take it more often, and do not take it for a longer time than your doctor ordered. If too much is taken, it may become habit-forming.

**Dosing**—The dose of chlordiazepoxide and clidinium combination will be different for different people. *Follow your doctor's orders or the directions on the label.* The following information includes only the average doses of this combination medicine. *If your dose is different, do not change it* unless your doctor tells you to do so.

• For *oral* dosage form (capsules)
  —To relax the digestive system and to reduce stomach acid:
    • Adults—1 or 2 capsules one to four times a day, thirty to sixty minutes before meals or food. Your doctor may change the dose if needed. However, most people usually will not take more than 8 capsules a day.
    • Children—Dose must be determined by your doctor.
    • Older adults—To start, 1 capsule two times a day. Your doctor may change the dose if needed.

**Missed dose**—If you miss a dose of this medicine, take it as soon as possible. However, if it is almost time for your next dose, skip the missed dose and go back to your regular dosing schedule. Do not double doses.

**Storage**—To store this medicine:
• Keep out of the reach of children.
• Store away from heat and direct light.
• Do not store the capsule form of this medicine in the bathroom, near the kitchen sink, or in other damp places. Heat or moisture may cause the medicine to break down.
• Do not keep outdated medicine or medicine no longer needed. Be sure that any discarded medicine is out of the reach of children.

## Precautions While Using This Medicine

If you will be taking this medicine regularly for a long time your doctor should check your progress at regular visits.

Do not take this medicine within an hour of taking medicine for diarrhea. Taking them too close together will make this medicine less effective.

This medicine may cause some people to have blurred vision or to become dizzy, lightheaded, drowsy, or less alert than they are normally. *Make sure you know how you react to this medicine before you drive, use machines, or do anything else that could be dangerous if you are dizzy or are not alert or able to see well.*

This medicine will add to the effects of alcohol and other CNS depressants (medicines that slow down the nervous system, possibly causing drowsiness). Some examples of CNS depressants are sedatives, tranquilizers, or sleeping medicine; prescription pain medicine or narcotics; barbiturates; medicine for seizures; muscle relaxants; or anesthetics, including some dental anesthetics. *Check with your doctor before taking any of the above while you are using this medicine and also for a few days after you stop taking it.*

This medicine will often make you sweat less, causing your body temperature to increase. *Use extra care not to become overheated during exercise or hot weather while you are taking this medicine* as this could possibly result in heat stroke. Also, hot baths or saunas may make you feel dizzy or faint while you are taking this medicine.

Your mouth, nose, and throat may feel very dry while you are taking this medicine. For temporary relief of mouth dryness, use sugarless candy or gum, melt bits of ice in your mouth, or use a saliva substitute. However, if your mouth continues to feel dry for more than 2 weeks, check with your dentist. Continuing dryness of the mouth may increase the chance of dental disease, including tooth decay, gum disease, and fungus infections.

*Check with your doctor if you develop intestinal problems such as constipation.* This is especially important if you are taking other medicine while you are taking chlordiazepoxide and clidinium. If these problems are not corrected, serious complications may result.

If you will be taking this medicine in large doses or for a long time, do not stop taking it without first checking with your doctor. Your doctor may want you to reduce gradually the amount you are taking before stopping completely.

## Side Effects of This Medicine

Along with its needed effects, a medicine may cause some unwanted effects. Although not all of these side effects may occur, if they do occur they may need medical attention.

Check with your doctor as soon as possible if any of the following side effects occur:

*Less common or rare*
  Constipation; eye pain; mental depression; skin rash or hives; slow heartbeat, shortness of breath, or troubled breathing; sore throat and fever; trouble in sleeping; unusual excitement, nervousness, or irritability; yellow eyes or skin

*Symptoms of overdose*
  Confusion; difficult urination; drowsiness (severe); dryness of mouth, nose, or throat (severe); fast heartbeat; unusual warmth, dryness, and flushing of skin

Other side effects may occur that usually do not need medical attention. These side effects may go away during treatment as your body adjusts to the medicine. However, check with your doctor if any of the following side effects continue or are bothersome:

*More common*
Bloated feeling; decreased sweating; dizziness; drowsiness; dryness of mouth; headache

*Less common*
Blurred vision; decreased sexual ability; loss of memory; nausea; unusual tiredness or weakness

After you stop using this medicine, your body may need time to adjust. The length of time this takes depends on the amount of medicine you were using and how long you used it. During this time check with your doctor if you notice any of the following side effects:

Convulsions (seizures); muscle cramps; nausea or vomiting; stomach cramps; trembling

Other side effects not listed above may also occur in some patients. If you notice any other effects, check with your doctor.

Revised: 01/29/92
Interim revision: 08/10/94

# CHLORHEXIDINE    Dental†

A commonly used brand name in the U.S. is Peridex.

†Not commercially available in Canada.

## Description

Chlorhexidine (klor-HEX-i-deen) is used to treat gingivitis. It helps to reduce the inflammation (redness) and swelling of your gums and to reduce gum bleeding.

Gingivitis is caused by the bacteria that grow in the coating (plaque) that forms on your teeth between tooth brushings. Chlorhexidine destroys the bacteria, thereby preventing the gingivitis from occurring. However, chlorhexidine does *not* prevent plaque and tartar from forming; proper tooth brushing and flossing are still necessary and important.

Chlorhexidine is available only with your dentist's or medical doctor's prescription, in the following dosage form:

*Dental*
• Oral rinse (U.S.)

## Before Using This Medicine

In deciding to use a medicine, the risks of using the medicine must be weighed against the good it will do. This is a decision you and your dentist or medical doctor will make. For chlorhexidine, the following should be considered:

**Allergies**—Tell your dentist or medical doctor if you have ever had any unusual or allergic reaction to this medicine or to skin disinfectants containing chlorhexidine. Also tell your dentist or medical doctor and pharmacist if you are allergic to any other substances, such as foods, preservatives, or dyes.

**Pregnancy**—Chlorhexidine has not been studied in pregnant women. However, chlorhexidine has not been shown to cause birth defects or other problems in animal studies.

**Breast-feeding**—It is not known whether chlorhexidine passes into the breast milk. Although most medicines pass into breast milk in small amounts, many of them may be used safely while breast-feeding. Mothers who are taking this medicine and who wish to breast-feed should discuss this with their dentist or medical doctor.

**Children**—Studies on this medicine have been done only in adult patients, and there is no specific information comparing use of this medicine in children with use in other age groups.

**Older adults**—Many medicines have not been studied specifically in older people. Therefore, it may not be known whether they work exactly the same way they do in younger adults or if they cause different side effects or problems in older people. There is no specific information comparing use of this medicine in the elderly with use in other age groups.

**Other medicines**—Although certain medicines should not be used together at all, in other cases two different medicines may be used together even if an interaction might occur. In these cases, your dentist or medical doctor may want to change the dose, or other precautions may be necessary. Tell your dentist or health care provider if you are using any other prescription or nonprescription (over-the-counter [OTC]) medicine that is to be used in the mouth.

**Other medical problems**—The presence of other medical problems may affect the use of chlorhexidine. Make sure you tell your dentist or medical doctor if you have any other medical problems, especially:
• Front-tooth fillings (especially those having rough surfaces)—Chlorhexidine may cause staining that, in some cases, may be impossible to remove and may require replacement of the filling
• Gum problems (other)—Use of chlorhexidine may make other gum problems, such as periodontitis, worse

## Proper Use of This Medicine

Chlorhexidine oral rinse should be used after you have brushed and flossed your teeth. Rinse the toothpaste completely from your mouth with water before using the oral rinse. Do not eat or drink for several hours after using the oral rinse.

The cap on the original container of chlorhexidine can be used to measure the 15 mL (½ fluid ounce) dose of this medicine. Fill the cap to the "fill line." If you do not receive the dental rinse in its original container, make sure you have a measuring device to measure out the correct dose. Your pharmacist can help you with this.

Swish chlorhexidine around in the mouth for 30 seconds. Then spit out. *Use the medicine full strength.* Do not mix with water before using. *Do not swallow the medicine.*

**Dosing**—The dose of chlorhexidine oral rinse will be different for different patients. *Follow your dentist's or medical doctor's orders or the directions on the label.* The following information includes only the average doses of chlorhexidine oral rinse. *If your dose is different, do not change it* unless your dentist or medical doctor tells you to do so.

- For *oral rinse* dosage form:
  —For gingivitis:
  - Adults—Use 15 milliliters (mL) as a mouth wash for 30 seconds two times a day.
  - Children up to 18 years of age—Use and dose must be determined by your dentist or medical doctor.

**Missed dose**—If you miss a dose of this medicine, use it as soon as possible. However, if it is almost time for your next dose, skip the missed dose and go back to your regular dosing schedule. Do not double doses.

**Storage**—To store this medicine:
- Keep out of the reach of children.
- Store away from heat and direct light.
- Keep the medicine from freezing.
- Do not keep outdated medicine or medicine that is no longer needed. Be sure any discarded medicine is out of the reach of children.

## Precautions While Using This Medicine

Chlorhexidine may have a bitter aftertaste. Do not rinse your mouth with water immediately after using chlorhexidine, since doing so will increase the bitterness. Rinsing may also decrease the effect of the medicine.

Chlorhexidine may change the way foods taste to you. Sometimes this effect may last up to 4 hours after you use the oral rinse. In most cases, this effect will become less noticeable as you continue to use the medicine. When you stop using chlorhexidine, your taste should return to normal.

Chlorhexidine may cause staining and an increase in tartar (calculus) on your teeth. Brushing with a tartar-control toothpaste and flossing your teeth daily may help reduce this tartar build-up and staining. In addition, you should visit your dentist at least every 6 months to have your teeth cleaned and your gums examined.

If you think that a child weighing 22 pounds (10 kilograms) or less has swallowed more than 4 ounces of the dental rinse, *get emergency help at once.* In addition, if a child of any age drinks the dental rinse and has symptoms of alcohol intoxication, such as slurred speech, sleepiness, or a staggering or stumbling walk, *get emergency help at once.*

## Side Effects of This Medicine

Along with its needed effects, a medicine may cause some unwanted effects. Although not all of these side effects may occur, if they do occur they may need medical attention.

*Check with your doctor immediately* if any of the following side effects occur:
*Rare*
> Signs of allergic reaction, such as nasal congestion; shortness of breath or troubled breathing; skin rash, hives, or itching; or swelling of face

Other side effects may occur that usually do not need medical attention. These side effects may go away during treatment as your body adjusts to the medicine. However, check with your dentist or medical doctor if any of the following side effects continue or are bothersome:
*More common*
> Change in taste; increase in tartar (calculus) on teeth; staining of teeth, mouth, tooth fillings, and dentures or other mouth appliances
*Less common or rare*
> Mouth irritation; swollen glands on side of face or neck; tongue tip irritation

Other side effects not listed above may also occur in some patients. If you notice any other effects, check with your dentist or medical doctor.

Revised: 05/16/94

# CHLORMEZANONE   Systemic†

A commonly used brand name in the U.S. is Trancopal Caplets.

†Not commercially available in Canada.

## Description

Chlormezanone (klor-MEZ-an-own) is used to relieve nervousness or tension. This medication should not be used for nervousness or tension caused by the stress of everyday life.

Chlormezanone is available only with your doctor's prescription, in the following dosage form:

Oral
  • Tablets (U.S.)

## Before Using This Medicine

In deciding to use a medicine, the risks of taking the medicine must be weighed against the good it will do. This is a decision you and your doctor will make. For chlormezanone, the following should be considered:

**Allergies**—Tell your doctor if you have ever had any unusual or allergic reaction to chlormezanone. Also tell your health care professional if you are allergic to any other substances, such as foods, preservatives, or dyes.

**Pregnancy**—Studies on effects in pregnancy have not been done in either humans or animals.

**Breast-feeding**—Chlormezanone has not been reported to cause problems in nursing babies.

**Children**—Although there is no specific information comparing use of chlormezanone in children with use in other age groups, this medicine is not expected to cause different side effects or problems in children than it does in adults.

**Older adults**—Many medicines have not been studied specifically in older people. Therefore, it may not be known whether they work exactly the same way they do in younger adults. Although there is no specific information comparing use of chlormezanone in the elderly with use in other age groups, this medicine is not expected to cause different side effects or problems in older people than it does in younger adults.

**Other medicines**—Although certain medicines should not be used together at all, in other cases two different medicines may be used together even if an interaction might occur. In these cases, your doctor may want to change the dose, or other precautions may be necessary. When you are taking chlormezanone, it is especially important that your health care professional know if you are taking any of the following:
  • Central nervous system (CNS) depressants (medicine that causes drowsiness) or
  • Tricyclic antidepressants (medicine for depression)—Concurrent use may increase the CNS depressant effects of either these medications or chlormezanone

**Other medical problems**—The presence of other medical problems may affect the use of chlormezanone. Make sure you tell your doctor if you have any other medical problems, especially:
  • Drug abuse or dependence (or history of)—Dependence on chlormezanone may develop
  • Kidney disease or
  • Liver disease—Higher blood levels of chlormezanone may occur, increasing the chance of side effects

## Proper Use of This Medicine

*Take this medicine only as directed by your doctor.* Do not take more of it, do not take it more often, and do not take it for a longer time than your doctor ordered. If too much chlormezanone is taken, it may become habit-forming. Also, taking too much of this medicine may increase the chance of side effects.

**Dosing**—The dose of chlormezanone will be different for different patients. *Follow your doctor's orders or the directions on the label.* The following information includes only the average doses of chlormezanone. *If your dose is different, do not change it* unless your doctor tells you to do so.

The number of tablets that you take depends on the strength of the medicine. Also, *the number of doses you take each day, the time allowed between doses, and the length of time you take the medicine depend on the medical problem for which you are taking chlormezanone.*
  • For *oral* dosage forms (tablets):
    —Adults and adolescents: 100 to 200 milligrams three or four times a day.
    —Children 5 to 12 years of age: 50 to 100 milligrams three or four times a day.
    —Children up to 5 years of age: Dose must be determined by the doctor.

**Missed dose**—If you miss a dose of this medicine and remember within an hour or so of the missed dose, take it right away. However, if you do not remember until later, skip the missed dose and go back to your regular dosing schedule. Do not double doses.

**Storage**—To store this medicine:
  • Keep out of the reach of children.
  • Store away from heat and direct light.
  • Do not store in the bathroom, near the kitchen sink, or in other damp places. Heat or moisture may cause the medicine to break down.
  • Do not keep outdated medicine or medicine no longer needed. Be sure that any discarded medicine is out of the reach of children.

## Precautions While Using This Medicine

If you will be taking chlormezanone regularly for a long time:
  • Your doctor should check your progress at regular visits.

• Check with your doctor at least every 4 months to make sure you need to continue taking this medicine.

If you will be taking this medicine in large doses or for a long time, do not stop taking it without first checking with your doctor. Your doctor may want you to reduce gradually the amount you are taking before stopping completely.

Chlormezanone will add to the effects of alcohol and other CNS depressants (medicines that slow down the nervous system, possibly causing drowsiness). Some examples of CNS depressants are antihistamines or medicine for hay fever, other allergies, or colds; sedatives, tranquilizers, or sleeping medicine; prescription pain medicine or narcotics; barbiturates; medicine for seizures; muscle relaxants; or anesthetics, including some dental anesthetics. *Check with your doctor before taking any of the above while you are using this medicine.*

*If you think you or someone else may have taken an overdose of this medicine, get emergency help at once.* Taking an overdose of chlormezanone or taking alcohol or other CNS depressants with chlormezanone may lead to unconsciousness and possibly death. Some signs of an overdose are severe confusion, severe drowsiness, loss of reflexes, and continuing unusual tiredness or weakness.

This medicine may cause some people to become dizzy, drowsy, or less alert than they are normally. Even if taken at bedtime, it may cause some people to feel drowsy or less alert on arising. *Make sure you know how you react to this medicine before you drive, use machines, or do anything else that could be dangerous if you are dizzy or are not alert.*

## Side Effects of This Medicine

Along with its needed effects, a medicine may cause some unwanted effects. Although not all of these side effects may occur, if they do occur they may need medical attention.

Check with your doctor as soon as possible if any of the following side effects occur:

*Less common*
Confusion; mental depression

*Rare*
Abdominal or stomach pains; aching muscles and joints; fever and chills; skin rash or itching (severe); swelling of feet or lower legs; yellow eyes or skin; unusual excitement

*Signs and/or symptoms of overdose*
Confusion (severe); drowsiness (severe); loss of reflexes; unusual tiredness or weakness (continuing)

Other side effects may occur that usually do not need medical attention. These side effects may go away during treatment as your body adjusts to the medicine. However, check with your doctor if any of the following side effects continue or are bothersome:

*More common*
Drowsiness

*Less common*
Clumsiness or unsteadiness; difficulty in urination; dizziness; flushing or redness of skin; headache; nausea; trembling; weakness

Other side effects not listed above may also occur in some patients. If you notice any other effects, check with your doctor.

Revised: 03/09/93

# CHLOROQUINE  Systemic

Some commonly used brand names are:
**In the U.S.—**
Aralen
Aralen HCl
Generic name product may also be available.
**In Canada—**
Aralen

## Description

Chloroquine (KLOR-oh-kwin) is a medicine used to prevent and treat malaria and to treat some conditions such as liver disease caused by protozoa. It is also used in the treatment of arthritis to help relieve inflammation, swelling, stiffness, and joint pain and to help control the symptoms of systemic lupus erythematosus (lupus; SLE).

This medicine may be given alone or with one or more other medicines. It may also be used for other conditions as determined by your doctor.

Chloroquine is available only with your doctor's prescription, in the following dosage forms:
*Oral*
• Tablets (U.S. and Canada)
*Parenteral*
• Injection (U.S.)

## Before Using This Medicine

In deciding to use a medicine, the risks of taking the medicine must be weighed against the good it will do.

This is a decision you and your doctor will make. For chloroquine, the following should be considered:

**Allergies**—Tell your doctor if you have ever had any unusual or allergic reaction to chloroquine or hydroxychloroquine. Also tell your health care professional if you are allergic to any other substances, such as foods, preservatives, or dyes.

**Pregnancy**—Unless you are taking it for malaria or liver disease caused by protozoa, use of this medicine is not recommended during pregnancy. In animal studies, chloroquine has been shown to cause damage to the central nervous system (brain and spinal cord) of the fetus, including damage to hearing, sense of balance, bleeding inside the eyes, and other eye problems. However, when given in low doses (once a week) to prevent malaria, this medicine has not been shown to cause birth defects or other problems in humans.

**Breast-feeding**—Chloroquine passes into the breast milk. Chloroquine has not been reported to cause problems in nursing babies to date. However, babies and children are especially sensitive to the effects of chloroquine.

**Children**—Children are especially sensitive to the effects of chloroquine. This may increase the chance of side effects during treatment. Overdose is especially dangerous in children. Taking as little as 1 tablet (300-mg strength) has resulted in the death of a small child.

**Older adults**—Many medicines have not been studied specifically in older people. Therefore, it may not be known whether they work exactly the same way they do in younger adults or if they cause different side effects or problems in older people. There is no specific information comparing use of chloroquine in the elderly with use in other age groups.

**Other medicines**—Although certain medicines should not be used together at all, in other cases 2 different medicines may be used together even if an interaction might occur. In these cases, your doctor may want to change the dose, or other precautions may be necessary. Tell your health care professional if you are taking any other prescription or nonprescription (over-the-counter [OTC]) medicine.

**Other medical problems**—The presence of other medical problems may affect the use of chloroquine. Make sure you tell your doctor if you have any other medical problems, especially:

- Blood disease (severe)—Chloroquine may cause blood disorders
- Eye or vision problems—Chloroquine may cause serious eye side effects, especially in high doses
- Glucose-6-phosphate dehydrogenase (G6PD) deficiency—Chloroquine may cause serious blood side effects in patients with this deficiency
- Liver disease—May decrease the removal of chloroquine from the blood, increasing the chance of side effects
- Nerve or brain disease (severe), including convulsions (seizures)—Chloroquine may cause muscle weakness and, in high doses, seizures

- Porphyria—Chloroquine may cause episodes of porphyria to occur more frequently
- Psoriasis—Chloroquine may bring on severe attacks of psoriasis
- Stomach or intestinal disease (severe)—Chloroquine may cause stomach or intestinal irritation

## Proper Use of This Medicine

*Take this medicine with meals or milk* to lessen possible stomach upset, unless otherwise directed by your doctor.

*Keep this medicine out of the reach of children. Children are especially sensitive to the effects of chloroquine and overdose is especially dangerous in children.* Taking as little as 1 tablet (300-mg strength) has resulted in the death of a small child.

It is very important that you *take this medicine only as directed.* Do not take more of it, do not take it more often, and do not take it for a longer time than your doctor ordered. To do so may increase the chance of serious side effects.

If you are taking this medicine to help keep you from getting malaria, *keep taking it for the full time of treatment.* If you already have malaria, you should still keep taking this medicine for the full time of treatment even if you begin to feel better after a few days. This will help to clear up your infection completely. If you stop taking this medicine too soon, your symptoms may return.

Chloroquine works best when you take it on a regular schedule. For example, if you are to take it once a week to prevent malaria, it is best to take it on the same day each week. Or if you are to take 2 doses a day, 1 dose may be taken with breakfast and the other with the evening meal. *Make sure that you do not miss any doses.* If you have any questions about this, check with your health care professional.

For patients taking chloroquine *to prevent malaria:*

- Your doctor may want you to start taking this medicine 1 to 2 weeks before you travel to an area where there is a chance of getting malaria. This will help you to see how you react to the medicine. Also, it will allow time for your doctor to change to another medicine if you have a reaction to this medicine.
- Also, you should keep taking this medicine while you are in the area and for 4 weeks after you leave the area. No medicine will protect you completely from malaria. However, to protect you as completely as possible, *it is important to keep taking this medicine for the full time your doctor ordered.* Also, if fever develops during your travels or within 2 months after you leave the area, *check with your doctor immediately.*

For patients taking chloroquine *for arthritis or lupus:*

- This medicine must be taken regularly as ordered by your doctor in order for it to help you. It may take up to several weeks before you begin to feel better. It may take up to 6 months before you feel the full benefit of this medicine.

**Dosing**—The dose of chloroquine will be different for different patients. *Follow your doctor's orders or the directions on the label.* The following information includes only the average doses of chloroquine. *If your dose is different, do not change it* unless your doctor tells you to do so.

The number of tablets that you take depends on the strength of the medicine. Also, *the number of doses you take each day, the time allowed between doses, and the length of time you take the medicine depend on the medical problem for which you are taking chloroquine.*

- For *oral* dosage form (tablets):
  —For prevention of malaria:
  - Adults—500 milligrams (mg) once every seven days.
  - Children—Dose is based on body weight and must be determined by your doctor. The usual dose is 8.3 mg per kilogram (kg) (3.7 mg per pound) of body weight once every seven days.
  —For treatment of malaria:
  - Adults—Start with 1 gram. Then, 500 mg six to eight hours after the first dose, and 500 mg once a day on the second and third days of treatment.
  - Children—Dose is based on body weight and must be determined by your doctor. The usual dose is 41.7 mg per kg (18.9 mg per pound) of body weight divided up over three days. This dose is given as follows: Start with 16.7 mg per kg (7.5 mg per pound) of body weight, then 8.3 mg per kg (3.7 mg per pound) six hours, twenty-four hours, and forty-eight hours after the first dose.
  —For treatment of liver disease caused by protozoa:
  - Adults—Start with 250 mg four times a day for two days. Then 250 mg two times a day for at least two to three weeks.
  - Children—Dose is based on body weight and must be determined by your doctor. The usual dose is 10 mg per kg (4.5 mg per pound) of body weight a day for three weeks.
- For *injection* dosage form:
  —For treatment of malaria:
  - Adults—200 to 250 mg injected into a muscle. This dose may be repeated in six hours if needed.
  - Children—Dose is based on body weight and must be determined by your doctor. The usual dose is 4.4 mg per kg (2 mg per pound) of body weight injected into a muscle or under the skin. This dose may be repeated in six hours if needed. Chloroquine may also be injected slowly into a vein. If the medicine is given in this way, the dose must be determined by your doctor.
  —For treatment of liver disease caused by protozoa:
  - Adults—200 to 250 mg a day injected into a muscle for ten to twelve days.

- Children—Dose is based on body weight and must be determined by your doctor. The usual dose is 7.5 mg per kg (3.4 mg per pound) of body weight a day for ten to twelve days.

**Missed dose**—If you miss a dose of this medicine and your dosing schedule is:
- One dose every seven days—Take the missed dose as soon as possible. Then go back to your regular dosing schedule.
- One dose a day—Take the missed dose as soon as possible. But if you do not remember until the next day, skip the missed dose and go back to your regular dosing schedule. Do not double doses.
- More than one dose a day—Take it right away if you remember within an hour or so of the missed dose. But if you do not remember until later, skip the missed dose and go back to your regular dosing schedule. Do not double doses.

If you have any questions about this, check with your doctor.

**Storage**—To store this medicine:
- Keep out of the reach of children. Overdose of chloroquine is very dangerous in children.
- Store away from heat and direct light.
- Do not store in the bathroom, near the kitchen sink, or in other damp places. Heat or moisture may cause the medicine to break down.
- Do not keep outdated medicine or medicine no longer needed. Be sure that any discarded medicine is out of the reach of children.

## Precautions While Using This Medicine

If you will be taking this medicine for a long time, *it is very important that your doctor check you at regular visits* for any blood problems or muscle weakness that may be caused by this medicine. In addition, *check with your doctor immediately if blurred vision, difficulty in reading, or any other change in vision occurs during or after treatment.* Your doctor may want you to have your eyes checked by an ophthalmologist (eye doctor).

If your symptoms do not improve within a few days (or a few weeks or months for arthritis), or if they become worse, check with your doctor.

Chloroquine may cause blurred vision, difficulty in reading, or other change in vision. It may also cause some people to become lightheaded. *Make sure you know how you react to this medicine before you drive, use machines, or do anything else that could be dangerous if you are not able to see well.* If these reactions are especially bothersome, check with your doctor.

Malaria is spread by mosquitoes. If you are living in, or will be traveling to, an area where there is a chance of getting malaria, the following mosquito-control measures will help to prevent infection:
- If possible, sleep under mosquito netting to avoid being bitten by malaria-carrying mosquitoes.

- Wear long-sleeved shirts or blouses and long trousers to protect your arms and legs, especially from dusk through dawn when mosquitoes are out.
- Apply mosquito repellent to uncovered areas of the skin from dusk through dawn when mosquitoes are out.

## Side Effects of This Medicine

Along with its needed effects, a medicine may cause some unwanted effects. Although not all of these side effects may occur, if they do occur they may need medical attention. When this medicine is used for short periods of time, side effects usually are rare. However, when it is used for a long time and/or in high doses, side effects are more likely to occur and may be serious.

*Check with your doctor immediately* if any of the following side effects occur:

*Less common*

Blurred vision or any other change in vision

Note: The above side effects may also occur or get worse after you stop taking this medicine.

*Rare*

Convulsions (seizures); fatigue; feeling faint or light-headed; increased muscle weakness; mood or other mental changes; ringing or buzzing in ears or any loss of hearing; sore throat and fever; unusual bleeding or bruising; weakness

*Symptoms of overdose*

Drowsiness; headache; increased excitability

Other side effects may occur that usually do not need medical attention. These side effects may go away during treatment as your body adjusts to the medicine. However, check with your doctor if any of the following side effects continue or are bothersome:

*More common*

Diarrhea; difficulty in seeing to read; headache; itching (more common in black patients); loss of appetite; nausea or vomiting; stomach cramps or pain

*Less common*

Bleaching of hair or increased hair loss; blue-black discoloration of skin, fingernails, or inside of mouth; skin rash

Other side effects not listed above may also occur in some patients. If you notice any other effects, check with your doctor.

## Additional Information

Once a medicine has been approved for marketing for a certain use, experience may show that it is also useful for other medical problems. Although these uses are not included in product labeling, chloroquine is used in certain patients with the following medical conditions:

- Arthritis in children
- High levels of calcium in the blood associated with sarcoidosis
- Various skin disorders

Other than the above information, there is no additional information relating to proper use, precautions, or side effects for these uses.

Revised: 07/06/92
Interim revision: 08/17/94

# CHLOROXINE   Topical†

A commonly used brand name in the U.S. is Capitrol.

†Not commercially available in Canada.

## Description

Chloroxine (klor-OX-een) is used in the treatment of dandruff and seborrheic dermatitis of the scalp.

This medicine is available only with your doctor's prescription, in the following dosage form:

*Topical*
- Lotion shampoo (U.S.)

## Before Using This Medicine

In deciding to use a medicine, the risks of using the medicine must be weighed against the good it will do. This is a decision you and your doctor will make. For chloroxine, the following should be considered:

**Allergies**—Tell your doctor if you have ever had any unusual or allergic reaction to chloroxine, clioquinol (iodochlorhydroxyquin), iodoquinol (diiodohydroxyquin), or edetate disodium. Also tell your health care professional if you are allergic to any other substances, such as preservatives or dyes.

**Pregnancy**—Studies on effects in pregnancy have not been done in either humans or animals.

**Breast-feeding**—It is not known whether chloroxine passes into the breast milk. However, this medicine has not been reported to cause problems in nursing babies.

**Children**—Studies on this medicine have been done only in adult patients, and there is no specific information comparing use of this medicine in children with use in other age groups.

**Older adults**—Many medicines have not been studied specifically in older people. Therefore, it may not be known whether they work exactly the same way they do in younger adults or if they cause different side effects or problems in older people. There is no specific information comparing use of this medicine in the elderly with use in other age groups.

**Other medicines**—Although certain medicines should not be used together at all, in other cases two different medicines may be used together even if an interaction might occur. In these cases, your doctor may want to change the dose, or other precautions may be necessary. Tell your health care professional if you are using any other topical prescription or nonprescription (over-the-counter [OTC]) medicine that is to be applied to the same area of the skin.

## Proper Use of This Medicine

*Do not use this medicine if blistered, raw, or oozing areas are present on your scalp,* unless otherwise directed by your doctor.

*Keep this medicine away from the eyes.* If you should accidentally get some in your eyes, flush them thoroughly with cool water. Check with your doctor if eye irritation continues or is bothersome.

To use:
- Wet the hair and scalp with lukewarm water. Apply enough chloroxine to the scalp to work up a lather, and rub in well. Allow the lather to remain on the scalp for about 3 minutes, then rinse. Apply the medicine again and rinse thoroughly. Use the medicine two times a week or as directed by your doctor.

**Dosing**—The dose of chloroxine will be different for different patients. *Follow your doctor's orders or the directions on the label.* The following information includes only the average doses of chloroxine. *If your dose is different, do not change it* unless your doctor tells you to do so.
- For *topical* dosage form (lotion shampoo):
  —For dandruff or seborrheic dermatitis of the scalp:
  - Adults—Use two times a week.

- Children—Use and dose must be determined by your doctor.

**Missed dose**—If you miss a dose of this medicine, apply it as soon as possible.

**Storage**—To store this medicine:
- Keep out of the reach of children.
- Store away from heat and direct light.
- Keep the medicine from freezing.
- Do not keep outdated medicine or medicine no longer needed. Be sure that any discarded medicine is out of the reach of children.

## Precautions While Using This Medicine

This medicine may slightly discolor light-colored hair (for example, bleached, blond, or gray).

## Side Effects of This Medicine

Along with its needed effects, a medicine may cause some unwanted effects. Although not all of these side effects may occur, if they do occur they may need medical attention.

Check with your doctor as soon as possible if any of the following side effects occur:
  Irritation or burning of scalp not present before use of this medicine; skin rash

Other side effects may occur that usually do not need medical attention. However, check with your doctor if either of the following side effects continues or is bothersome:
  Dryness or increased itching of scalp

Other side effects not listed above may also occur in some patients. If you notice any other effects, check with your doctor.

Revised: 01/21/94

# CHLORZOXAZONE AND ACETAMINOPHEN  Systemic*

A commonly used brand name in Canada is Parafon Forte.

Another commonly used name for this combination medicine is chlorzoxazone with APAP.

*Not commercially available in the U.S.

## Description

Chlorzoxazone (klor-ZOX-a-zone) and acetaminophen (a-seat-a-MIN-oh-fen) combination medicine is used to help relax certain muscles in your body and relieve the pain and discomfort caused by strains, sprains, or other injuries to your muscles. However, this medicine does not take the place of rest, exercise or physical therapy, or other treatment that your doctor may recommend for your medical problem.

Chlorzoxazone acts in the central nervous system (CNS) to produce its muscle relaxant effects. Its actions in the CNS may also produce some of its side effects.

In Canada, this medicine is available without a prescription.

This medicine is available in the following dosage forms:

*Oral*
- Tablets (Canada)

## Before Using This Medicine

If you are taking this medicine without a prescription, carefully read and follow any precautions on the label. For chlorzoxazone and acetaminophen combination, the following should be considered:

**Allergies**—Tell your doctor if you have ever had any unusual or allergic reaction to acetaminophen, chlorzoxazone, or aspirin. Also tell your health care professional if you are allergic to any other substances, such as foods, preservatives, or dyes.

**Pregnancy**—Although studies on birth defects with chlorzoxazone or acetaminophen have not been done in pregnant women, these medicines have not been reported to cause birth defects or other problems.

**Breast-feeding**—Chlorzoxazone and acetaminophen have not been shown to cause problems in nursing babies. However, acetaminophen passes into the breast milk in small amounts.

**Children**—Studies on this combination medicine have been done only in adult patients, and there is no specific information about its use in children. However, chlorzoxazone and acetaminophen have been tested separately in children. In effective doses, these medicines have not been shown to cause different side effects or problems in children than they do in adults.

**Older adults**—Many medicines have not been studied specifically in older people. Therefore, it may not be known whether they work exactly the same way they do in younger adults or if they cause different side effects or problems in older people. There is no specific information comparing use of chlorzoxazone and acetaminophen combination, or of chlorzoxazone alone, in the elderly with use in other age groups. However, acetaminophen has been tested and has not been shown to cause different side effects or problems in older people than it does in younger adults.

**Other medicines**—Although certain medicines should not be used together at all, in other cases two different medicines may be used together even if an interaction might occur. In these cases, your doctor may want to change the dose, or other precautions may be necessary. When you are taking chlorzoxazone and acetaminophen combination, it is especially important that your health care professional know if you are taking any of the following:
- Antidepressants, tricyclic (amitriptyline [e.g., Elavil], amoxapine [e.g., Asendin], clomipramine [e.g., Anafranil], desipramine [e.g., Pertofrane], doxepin [e.g., Sinequan], imipramine [e.g., Tofranil], nortriptyline [e.g., Aventyl], protriptyline [e.g., Vivactil], trimipramine [e.g., Surmontil]) or

- Central nervous system (CNS) depressants (medicines that often cause drowsiness)—These medicines may add to the effects of chlorzoxazone and increase the chance of drowsiness or other side effects

**Other medical problems**—The presence of other medical problems may affect the use of chlorzoxazone and acetaminophen combination. Make sure you tell your doctor if you have any other medical problems, especially:
- Alcohol abuse or
- Allergies (asthma, eczema, hay fever, hives) or
- Hepatitis or other liver disease or
- Kidney disease—The chance of side effects may be increased

## Proper Use of This Medicine

*Take this medicine only as directed.* Do not take more of it, do not take it more often, and do not take it for a longer time than directed on the package label or by your doctor. To do so may increase the chance of side effects. This medicine may cause liver damage if too much is taken.

**Dosing**—The dose of chlorzoxazone and acetaminophen combination will be different for different patients. *Follow your doctor's orders or the directions on the label.* The following information includes only the average doses of this medicine. *If your dose is different, do not change it* unless your doctor tells you to do so.
- For *oral* dosage form (tablets):
  —For relieving painful, stiff muscles:
    - Adults—Two tablets four times a day.
    - Children—Use and dose must be determined by your doctor.

**Missed dose**—If you miss a dose of this medicine, take it as soon as you remember. However, if it is almost time for your next dose, skip the missed dose and go back to your regular dosing schedule. Do not double doses.

**Storage**—To store this medicine:
- Keep out of the reach of children.
- Store away from heat and direct light.
- Do not store this medicine in the bathroom, near the kitchen sink, or in other damp places. Heat or moisture may cause the medicine to break down.
- Do not keep outdated medicine or medicine no longer needed. Be sure that any discarded medicine is out of the reach of children.

## Precautions While Using This Medicine

If you will be taking this medicine for a long time (for example, for several months at a time), your doctor should check your progress at regular visits.

*Check the labels of all nonprescription (over-the-counter [OTC]) and prescription medicines you now take. If any of them contain chlorzoxazone or acetaminophen, check with your doctor or pharmacist. Using any of them together with this medicine may cause an overdose.*

This medicine will add to the effects of alcohol and other CNS depressants (medicines that slow down the nervous system, possibly causing drowsiness). Some examples of CNS depressants are antihistamines or medicine for hay fever, other allergies, or colds; sedatives, tranquilizers, or sleeping medicine; prescription pain medicine or narcotics; barbiturates; medicine for seizures; or anesthetics, including some dental anesthetics. Also, the risk of liver damage from acetaminophen may be greater if you use large amounts of alcoholic beverages with acetaminophen. Therefore, *do not drink alcoholic beverages, and check with your doctor before taking any of the medicines listed above, while you are taking this medicine.*

Taking the acetaminophen in this combination medicine together with certain other medicines may increase the chance of unwanted effects. The risk will depend on how much of each medicine you take every day, and on how long you take the medicines together. If your medical doctor or dentist directs you to take these medicines together on a regular basis, follow his or her directions carefully. However, *do not take any of the following medicines together with chlorzoxazone and acetaminophen combination for more than a few days, unless your doctor has directed you to do so and is following your progress.*

> Aspirin or other salicylates
> Diclofenac (e.g., Voltaren)
> Diflunisal (e.g., Dolobid)
> Etodolac (e.g., Lodine)
> Fenoprofen (e.g., Nalfon)
> Floctafenine (e.g., Idarac)
> Flurbiprofen, oral (e.g., Ansaid)
> Ibuprofen (e.g., Motrin)
> Indomethacin (e.g., Indocin)
> Ketoprofen (e.g., Orudis)
> Ketorolac (e.g., Toradol)
> Meclofenamate (e.g., Meclomen)
> Mefenamic acid (e.g., Ponstel)
> Nabumetone (e.g., Relafen)
> Naproxen (e.g., Naprosyn)
> Oxaprozin (e.g., Daypro)
> Phenylbutazone (e.g., Butazolidin)
> Piroxicam (e.g., Feldene)
> Sulindac (e.g., Clinoril)
> Tenoxicam (e.g., Mobiflex)
> Tiaprofenic acid (e.g., Surgam)
> Tolmetin (e.g., Tolectin)

This medicine may cause some people to become drowsy, dizzy, or less alert than they are normally. *Make sure you know how you react to this medicine before you drive, use machines, or do anything else that could be dangerous if you are dizzy or are not alert.*

Acetaminophen may interfere with the results of some medical tests. Before you have any medical tests, tell the doctor in charge if you have taken acetaminophen within the past 3 or 4 days. If possible, it is best to check with

the doctor first, to find out whether this medicine may be taken during the 3 or 4 days before the test.

For *diabetic patients:*
- Acetaminophen may cause false results with some blood glucose (sugar) tests. If you notice any change in your test results, or if you have any questions about this possible problem, check with your health care professional. This is especially important if your diabetes is not well-controlled.

*If you think that you or anyone else may have taken an overdose of this medicine, get emergency help at once.* Signs of overdose of this medicine include fast or irregular breathing and severe muscle weakness. Signs of severe acetaminophen poisoning may not appear for 2 to 4 days after the overdose is taken, but treatment to prevent liver damage or death must be started within 24 hours or less after the overdose is taken.

---

## Side Effects of This Medicine

Along with its needed effects, a medicine may cause some unwanted effects. Although not all of these side effects may occur, if they do occur they may need medical attention.

*Check with your doctor immediately* if any of the following side effects occur:

*Rare*
> Hive-like swellings (large) on face, eyelids, mouth, lips, or tongue; sudden decrease in amount of urine

*Symptoms of overdose*
> Diarrhea; fast or irregular breathing; increased sweating; loss of appetite; muscle weakness (severe); nausea or vomiting; pain, tenderness, or swelling in upper abdomen or stomach area; stomach cramps or pain

Also, check with your doctor as soon as possible if any of the following side effects occur:

*Rare*
> Bloody or black, tarry stools; bloody or cloudy urine; pain in lower back and/or side (severe and/or sharp); pinpoint red spots on skin; skin rash, hives, itching, or redness; sore throat and fever; unusual bleeding or bruising; unusual tiredness or weakness; yellow eyes or skin

Other side effects may occur that usually do not need medical attention. These side effects may go away during treatment as your body adjusts to the medicine. However, check with your doctor if any of the following side effects continue or are bothersome:

*More common*
> Dizziness or lightheadedness; drowsiness

*Less common*
> Constipation; headache; heartburn; unusual excitement, nervousness, restlessness, or irritability

This medicine sometimes causes the urine to turn orange or reddish purple. This is not harmful and will go away when you stop taking the medicine. If you have any questions about this, check with your doctor.

Other side effects not listed above may also occur in some patients. If you notice any other effects, check with your doctor.

Revised: 08/29/94

---

# CHOLECYSTOGRAPHIC AGENTS, ORAL    Diagnostic

Some commonly used brand names are:

**In the U.S.—**

| | |
|---|---|
| Bilivist[3] | Oragrafin Calcium[3] |
| Bilopaque[4] | Oragrafin Sodium[3] |
| Cholebrine[1] | Telepaque[2] |

**In Canada—**

Bilopaque[4]
Telepaque[2]

**Other—**

| | |
|---|---|
| Biloptin[3] | Felombrine[2] |
| Cistobil[2] | Jopanonsyre[2] |
| Colebrin[1] | Lumopaque[4] |
| Colebrina[1] | Neocontrast[2] |
| Colegraf[2] | |

Other commonly used names are:

Ipodate sodium[3]         Sodium tyropanoate[4]

Note: For quick reference, the following oral cholecystographic agents are numbered to match the corresponding brand names.

This information applies to the following medicines:

1. Iocetamic Acid (eye-oh-se-TAM-ik)†
2. Iopanoic Acid (eye-oh-pa-NOE-ik)
3. Ipodate (EYE-poe-date)†
4. Tyropanoate (tye-roe-pa-NOE-ate)

†Not commercially available in Canada.

---

## Description

Oral cholecystographic (ko-le-sis-to-GRAF-ik) agents are radiopaque agents. Radiopaque agents are drugs used to help diagnose certain medical problems. These agents contain iodine, which absorbs x-rays. Depending on how the radiopaque agent is given, it builds up in certain areas of the body. When radiopaque agents are inside the body they will appear white on the x-ray film. This creates the needed distinction, or contrast, between one organ and other tissues. This will help the doctor see any special conditions that may exist in that organ or part of the body.

The oral cholecystographic agents are taken by mouth before x-ray tests to help check for problems of the gallbladder and the biliary tract. Ipodate may also be used for other conditions as determined by your doctor.

These radiopaque agents are to be given only by or under the direct supervision of a doctor. They are available in the following dosage forms:

*Oral*

Iocetamic acid
  • Tablets (U.S.)
Iopanoic acid
  • Tablets (U.S. and Canada)

Ipodate
  • Capsules (U.S.)
  • Oral suspension (U.S.)
Tyropanoate
  • Capsules (U.S. and Canada)

---

## Before Having This Test

In deciding to use a diagnostic test, any risks of the test must be weighed against the good it will do. This is a decision you and your doctor will make. Also, test results may be affected by other things. For cholecystographic agents, the following should be considered:

**Allergies**—Tell your doctor if you have ever had any unusual or allergic reaction to iodine, to products containing iodine (for example, iodine-containing foods, such as seafoods, cabbage, kale, rape [turnip-like vegetable], turnips, or iodized salt), or to other radiopaque agents. Also tell your doctor if you are allergic to any other substance, such as preservatives.

**Pregnancy**—Studies on effects in pregnancy have not been done in humans with any of these agents. Studies in animals have been done only with iocetamic acid, which has not been shown to cause birth defects or other problems. However, on rare occasions, other radiopaque agents containing iodine have caused hypothyroidism (underactive thyroid) in the baby when given in late pregnancy. Also, x-rays of the abdomen are usually not recommended during pregnancy. This is to avoid exposing the fetus to radiation. Be sure you have discussed this with your doctor.

**Breast-feeding**—Iocetamic acid, iopanoic acid, and tyropanoate pass into the breast milk, and the other agents may pass into the breast milk also. However, these radiopaque agents have not been reported to cause problems in nursing babies.

**Children**—Although there is no specific information comparing use of cholecystographic agents in children with use in other age groups, tests using iopanoic acid and ipodate in children have not shown that these agents cause different side effects or problems in children than they do in adults.

**Older adults**—Many medicines have not been studied specifically in older people. Therefore, it may not be known whether they work exactly the same way they do in younger adults. Although there is no specific information comparing use of cholecystographic agents in the elderly with use in other age groups, these agents are not expected to cause different side effects or problems in older people than they do in younger adults.

**Other medicines**—Although certain medicines should not be used together at all, in other cases two different medicines may be used together even if an interaction might occur. In these cases, your doctor may want to change the dose, or other precautions may be necessary. Tell your doctor if you are taking any other prescription or nonprescription (over-the-counter [OTC]) medicine.

**Other medical problems**—The presence of other medical problems may affect the use of cholecystographic agents. Make sure you tell your doctor if you have any other medical problems, especially:

- Asthma, hay fever, or other allergies (history of)—Patients with these conditions have a greater chance of having a reaction, such as an allergic reaction
- Heart disease—Other problems, such as low blood pressure or slow heartbeat, may occur
- Kidney disease or
- Liver disease (severe)—Serious kidney problems may result
- Overactive thyroid—A sudden increase in symptoms, such as fast heartbeat or palpitations, fatigue, nervousness, excessive sweating, and muscle weakness may occur

## Preparation For This Test

**Dosing**—Take this radiopaque agent with water after dinner the evening or evenings before the examination, following the directions of your doctor.

Do not eat or drink anything but water after taking the medicine. Also, avoid smoking or chewing gum.

Your doctor may order a special diet or use of a laxative or enema in preparation for your test, depending on the type of test. If you have not received such instructions or if you do not understand them, check with your doctor in advance.

## Precautions After Having This Test

Make sure your doctor knows if you are planning to have any future thyroid tests. The results of the thyroid test may be affected, even weeks or months later, by the iodine in this agent.

## Side Effects of This Medicine

Along with its needed effects, a medicine may cause some unwanted effects. Although not all of these side effects may occur, if they do occur they may need medical attention.

*Check with your health care professional immediately* if any of the following side effects occur:

*Rare*

Itching; skin rash or hives; swelling of skin; unusual bleeding or bruising (with iopanoic acid only)

*Symptoms of overdose*

Severe diarrhea; severe nausea and vomiting; problems with urination

Other side effects may occur that usually do not need medical attention. These side effects should go away as the effects of the radiopaque agent wear off. However, check with your doctor if any of the following side effects continue or are bothersome:

*More common*

Mild diarrhea; mild to moderate nausea and vomiting

*Less common*

Abdominal or stomach spasms or cramps; severe diarrhea; difficult or painful urination; dizziness; frequent urge to urinate; headache; heartburn; severe or continuing nausea and vomiting

Other side effects not listed above may also occur in some patients. If you notice any other effects, check with your doctor.

## Additional Information

Once a medicine has been approved for marketing for a certain use, experience may show that it is also useful for other medical problems. Although not specifically included in product labeling, ipodate is used in certain patients with the following medical condition:

- Graves' disease

In addition to the above information, for patients with Graves' disease taking ipodate:

- Ipodate is used in patients with Graves' disease, who have an overactive thyroid, to reduce the amount of thyroid hormone produced by the thyroid gland.
- *Use this medicine only as directed by your doctor.* Do not take more of it, do not take it more often, and do not take it for a longer period of time than your doctor ordered. To do so may increase the chance of side effects.
- In order for it to work properly, *ipodate must be taken every day, as ordered by your doctor.*
- The information given above in the section *Preparation For This Test* will not apply to you.

Other than the above information, there is no additional information relating to proper use, precautions, or side effects for these uses.

Revised: 07/27/92

# CHOLESTYRAMINE    Oral

Some commonly used brand names in the U.S. and Canada are Questran and Questran Light.

## Description

Cholestyramine (koe-less-TEAR-a-meen) is used to lower high cholesterol levels in the blood. This may help prevent medical problems caused by cholesterol clogging the blood vessels. Cholestyramine is also used to remove substances called bile acids from your body. With some liver problems, there is too much bile acid in your body and this can cause severe itching.

Cholestyramine works by attaching to certain substances in the intestine. Since cholestyramine is not absorbed into the body, these substances also pass out of the body without being absorbed.

Cholestyramine may also be used for other conditions as determined by your doctor.

Cholestyramine is available only with your doctor's prescription, in the following dosage form:

*Oral*
- Powder (U.S. and Canada)

## Before Using This Medicine

In deciding to use a medicine, the risks of taking the medicine must be weighed against the good it will do. This is a decision you and your doctor will make. For cholestyramine, the following should be considered:

**Allergies**—Tell your doctor if you have ever had any unusual or allergic reaction to cholestyramine. Also tell your health care professional if you are allergic to any other substances, such as foods, preservatives, or dyes.

**Pregnancy**—Cholestyramine is not absorbed into the body and is not likely to cause problems. However, it may reduce absorption of vitamins into the body. Ask your doctor whether you need to take extra vitamins.

**Breast-feeding**—Cholestyramine is not absorbed into the body and is not likely to cause problems. However, the reduced absorption of vitamins by the mother may affect the nursing infant.

**Children**—This medicine has been tested in a limited number of children. In effective doses, the medicine has not been shown to cause different side effects or problems than it does in adults.

**Older adults**—Side effects may be more likely to occur in patients over 60 years of age, who are usually more sensitive to the effects of cholestyramine.

**Other medicines**—Although certain medicines should not be used together at all, in other cases two different medicines may be used together even if an interaction might occur. In these cases, your doctor may want to change the dose, or other precautions may be necessary. When you are taking cholestyramine it is especially important that your health care professional know if you are taking any of the following:

- Anticoagulants (blood thinners)—The effects of the anticoagulant may be changed and this may increase the chance of bleeding.
- Digitalis glycosides (heart medicine) or
- Diuretics (water pills) or
- Penicillin G, taken by mouth or
- Phenylbutazone or
- Propranolol (e.g., Inderal) or
- Tetracyclines, taken by mouth (medicine for infection) or
- Thyroid hormones or
- Vancomycin, taken by mouth—Cholestyramine may prevent these medicines from working properly

**Other medical problems**—The presence of other medical problems may affect the use of cholestyramine. Make sure you tell your doctor if you have any other medical problems, especially:

- Bleeding problems or
- Constipation or
- Gallstones or
- Heart or blood vessel disease or
- Hemorrhoids or
- Stomach ulcer or other stomach problems or
- Underactive thyroid—Cholestyramine may make these conditions worse
- Kidney disease—There is an increased risk of developing electrolyte problems (problems in the blood)
- Phenylketonuria—Phenylalanine in aspartame is included in the sugar-free brand of cholestyramine and should be avoided. Aspartame can cause problems in people with phenylketonuria. Therefore, it is best if you avoid using the sugar-free product.

## Proper Use of This Medicine

Take this medicine exactly as directed by your doctor. Try not to miss any doses and do not take more medicine than your doctor ordered.

*This medicine should never be taken in its dry form, since it could cause you to choke.* Instead, always mix as follows:

- Place the medicine in 2 ounces of any beverage and mix thoroughly. Then add an additional 2 to 4 ounces of beverage and again mix thoroughly (it will not dissolve) before drinking. After drinking all the liquid containing the medicine, rinse the glass with a little more liquid and drink that also, to make sure you get all the medicine.
- You may also mix this medicine with milk in hot or regular breakfast cereals, or in thin soups such as tomato or chicken noodle soup. Or you may add it to some pulpy fruits such as crushed pineapple, pears, peaches, or fruit cocktail.

For patients taking this medicine *for high cholesterol:*

- Importance of diet—Before prescribing medicine for your condition, your doctor will probably try to control your condition by prescribing a personal diet for you. Such a diet may be low in fats, sugars, and/or cholesterol. Many people are able to control their condition by carefully following their doctor's orders for proper diet and exercise. Medicine is prescribed only when additional help is needed. *Follow carefully the special diet your doctor gave you,* since the medicine is effective only when a schedule of diet and exercise is properly followed.

- Also, this medicine is less effective if you are greatly overweight. It may be very important for you to go on a reducing diet. However, check with your doctor before going on any diet.
- Remember that this medicine will not cure your cholesterol problem but it will help control it. Therefore, you must continue to take it as directed if you expect to lower your cholesterol level.

**Dosing**—The dose of cholestyramine will be different for different patients. *Follow your doctor's orders or the directions on the label.* The following information includes only the average doses of cholestyramine. *If your dose is different, do not change it* unless your doctor tells you to do so.

- For *oral* dosage form (powder for oral suspension):
  —For high cholesterol or pruritis (itching) related to biliary obstruction:
    - Adults—At first, 4 grams one or two times a day before meals. Then, your doctor may increase your dose to 8 to 24 grams a day. This is divided into two to six doses.
    - Children—At first, 4 grams a day. This is divided into two doses and taken before meals. Then, your doctor may increase your dose to 8 to 24 grams a day. This is divided into two or more doses.

**Missed dose**—If you miss a dose of this medicine, take it as soon as possible. Then go back to your regular dosing schedule. However, if it is almost time for your next dose, skip the missed dose and go back to your regular dosing schedule. Do not double doses.

**Storage**—To store this medicine:
- Keep out of the reach of children.
- Store away from heat and direct light.
- Do not store in the bathroom, near the kitchen sink, or in other damp places. Heat or moisture may cause the medicine to break down.
- Do not keep outdated medicine or medicine no longer needed. Be sure that any discarded medicine is out of the reach of children.

## Precautions While Using This Medicine

*It is very important that your doctor check your progress at regular visits.* This will allow your doctor to see if the medicine is working properly and to decide if you should continue to take it.

*Do not take any other medicine unless prescribed by your doctor* since cholestyramine may change the effect of other medicines.

*Do not stop taking this medicine without first checking with your doctor.* When you stop taking this medicine, your blood cholesterol levels may increase again. Your doctor may want you to follow a special diet to help prevent this from happening.

## Side Effects of This Medicine

In some animal studies, cholestyramine was found to cause tumors. It is not known whether cholestyramine causes tumors in humans.

Along with its needed effects, a medicine may cause some unwanted effects. Although not all of these side effects may occur, if they do occur they may need medical attention.

*Check with your doctor immediately* if any of the following side effects occur:
  *Rare*
    Black, tarry stools; stomach pain (severe) with nausea and vomiting

Check with your doctor as soon as possible if any of the following side effects occur:
  *More common*
    Constipation
  *Rare*
    Loss of weight (sudden)

Other side effects may occur that usually do not need medical attention. These side effects may go away during treatment as your body adjusts to the medicine. However, check with your doctor if any of the following side effects continue or are bothersome:
  *More common*
    Heartburn or indigestion; nausea or vomiting; stomach pain
  *Less common*
    Belching; bloating; diarrhea; dizziness; headache

Other side effects not listed above may also occur in some patients. If you notice any other effects, check with your doctor.

## Additional Information

Once a medicine has been approved for marketing for a certain use, experience may show that it is also useful for other medical problems. Although these uses are not

## CHORIONIC GONADOTROPIN Systemic

included in product labeling, cholestyramine is used in certain patients with the following medical conditions:

- Digitalis glycoside overdose
- Excess oxalate in the urine

Other than the above information, there is no additional information relating to proper use, precautions, or side effects for these uses.

Revised: 08/02/94

# CHORIONIC GONADOTROPIN    Systemic

Some commonly used brand names are:

**In the U.S.—**
| | |
|---|---|
| A.P.L. | Profasi |
| Pregnyl | |

Generic name product may also be available.

**In Canada—**
| | |
|---|---|
| A.P.L. | Profasi HP |

Generic name product may also be available.

Another commonly used name is human chorionic gonadotropin (hCG).

## Description

Chorionic gonadotropin (kor-ee-ON-ik goe-NAD-oh-troe-pin) is a drug whose actions are almost the same as those of luteinizing (loo-te-in-eye-ZING) hormone (LH), which is produced by the pituitary gland. It is a hormone also normally produced by the placenta in pregnancy. Chorionic gonadotropin has different uses for females and males.

In females, chorionic gonadotropin is used to help conception occur. It is usually given in combination with other drugs such as menotropins and urofollitropin. Many women being treated with these drugs usually have already tried clomiphene alone (e.g., Serophene) and have not been able to conceive yet. Chorionic gonadotropin is also used in *in vitro* fertilization (IVF) programs.

In males, LH and chorionic gonadotropin stimulate the testes to produce male hormones such as testosterone. Testosterone causes the enlargement of the penis and testes and the growth of pubic and underarm hair. It also increases the production of sperm.

Although chorionic gonadotropin has been prescribed to help some patients lose weight, it should *never* be used this way. When used improperly, chorionic gonadotropin can cause serious problems.

Chorionic gonadotropin is to be administered only by or under the immediate supervision of your doctor. It is available in the following dosage form:

*Parenteral*
- Injection (U.S. and Canada)

## Before Using This Medicine

In deciding to use a medicine, the risks of taking the medicine must be weighed against the good it will do. This is a decision you and your doctor will make. For chorionic gonadotropin, the following should be considered:

**Allergies**—Tell your doctor if you have ever had any unusual or allergic reaction to chorionic gonadotropin. Also tell your health care professional if you are allergic to any other substances, such as foods, preservatives, or dyes.

**Pregnancy**—If you become pregnant as a result of using this medicine with menotropins (e.g., Pergonal) or urofollitropin (e.g., Metrodin), there is an increased chance of a multiple pregnancy (for example, twins, triplets).

**Children**—Chorionic gonadotropin, when used for treating cryptorchidism (a birth defect where the testes remain inside the body), has caused the sexual organs of some male children to develop too rapidly.

**Other medicines**—Although certain medicines should not be used together at all, in other cases two different medicines may be used together even if an interaction might occur. In these cases, your doctor may want to change the dose, or other precautions may be necessary. Tell your health care professional if you are taking any prescription or nonprescription (over-the-counter [OTC]) medicine.

**Other medical problems**—The presence of other medical problems may affect the use of chorionic gonadotropin. Make sure you tell your doctor if you have any other medical problems, especially:

- Cancer of the prostate—Increases in the amount of testosterone in the bloodstream may make this condition worse
- Cyst on ovary or
- Fibroid tumors of the uterus—Chorionic gonadotropin can cause further growth of cysts on the ovary or fibroid tumors of the uterus
- Pituitary gland enlargement or tumor—Chorionic gonadotropin can cause the pituitary gland or a pituitary tumor to increase in size
- Unusual vaginal bleeding—Irregular vaginal bleeding is a sign that the endometrium is growing too much, of endometrial cancer, or of other hormone imbalances; the increases in estrogen production caused by ovulation can aggravate these problems of the endometrium. If other hormone imbalances are present, they should be treated before beginning ovulation induction

## Proper Use of This Medicine

**Dosing**—The dose of chorionic gonadotropin will be different for different patients. *Follow your doctor's orders or the directions on the label.* The following information includes only the average doses for chorionic gonadotropin. *If your dose is different, do not change it* unless your doctor tells you to do so.

*The number of doses you receive each day, the time allowed between doses, and the length of time you receive the medicine depend on the medical problem for which you are receiving chorionic gonadotropin.*

- For *injection* dosage form:
  —For treating men with problems related to low levels of male hormones:
  - Adults—1000 to 4000 Units injected into the muscle two to three times a week. You may need to receive this medicine for several weeks, months, or longer. If you are being treated for a low sperm count and have been on this medicine for six months, your doctor may give you another hormone medicine (menotropin or urofollitropin injection). You may need to receive both of these medicines together for up to twelve more months.
  —To help pregnancy occur in women:
  - Adults—5000 to 10,000 Units injected into the muscle on a day chosen by your doctor. The dose and day will depend on your hormone levels and the other medicines that you have been using.
  —For the treatment of cryptorchidism (condition where testes do not develop properly):
  - Children—1000 to 5000 Units injected into the muscle two to three times a week for up to ten doses.

## Precautions While Using This Medicine

*It is very important that your doctor check your progress at regular visits* to make sure that the medicine is working and to check for unwanted effects.

For women *taking this medicine to become pregnant:*
- Record your basal body temperature every day if told to do so by your doctor, so that you will know if you have begun to ovulate. It is important that intercourse take place around the time of ovulation to give you the best chance of becoming pregnant. Your doctor will likely want to monitor the development of the ovarian follicle(s) by measuring the amount of estrogen in your bloodstream and by checking the size of the follicle(s) with ultrasound examinations.

## Side Effects of This Medicine

Along with its needed effects, a medicine may cause some other effects. Although not all of these side effects may occur, if they do occur they may need medical attention.

Check with your doctor as soon as possible if any of the following side effects occur:
*For females only*
  *More common*
    Bloating (mild); stomach or pelvic pain
  *Less common or rare*
    Abdominal or stomach pain (severe); bloating (moderate to severe); decreased amount of urine; feeling of indigestion; nausea, vomiting, or diarrhea (continuing or severe); pelvic pain (severe); shortness of breath; swelling of feet or lower legs; weight gain (rapid)
*For boys only*
  *Less common*
    Acne; enlargement of penis and testes; growth of pubic hair; increase in height (rapid)

Other side effects may occur that usually do not need medical attention. These side effects may go away during treatment as your body adjusts to the medicine. However, check with your doctor if any of the following side effects continue or are bothersome:
*Less common*
  Enlargement of breasts; headache; irritability; mental depression; pain at place of injection; tiredness

After you stop receiving this medicine, it may continue to cause some side effects which require medical attention. During this period of time check with your doctor if you notice either of the following side effects:
*For females only*
  *Less common or rare*
    Abdominal or stomach pain (severe); bloating (moderate to severe); decreased amount of urine; feeling of indigestion; nausea, vomiting, or diarrhea (continuing or severe); pelvic pain (severe); shortness of breath; weight gain (rapid)

Other side effects not listed above may also occur in some patients. If you notice any other effects, check with your doctor.

Revised: 07/26/92
Interim revision: 06/03/94

# CHROMIC PHOSPHATE P 32    Therapeutic

A commonly used brand name in the U.S. is Phosphocol P 32.

## Description

Chromic phosphate (KROME-ik FOS-fate) P 32 is a radiopharmaceutical (ray-dee-oh-far-ma-SOO-ti-kal). Radiopharmaceuticals are agents used to diagnose certain medical problems or treat certain diseases.

Chromic phosphate P 32 is used to treat cancer or related problems. It is put by catheter into the pleura (sac that contains the lungs) or into the peritoneum (sac that contains the liver, stomach, and intestines) to treat the leaking of fluid inside these areas that is caused by cancer. It may also be given by injection to treat cancer in certain organs such as the ovaries and prostate.

Chromic phosphate P 32 is to be given only by or under the direct supervision of a doctor with specialized training in nuclear medicine. It is available in the following dosage form:

*Parenteral*
- Suspension (U.S.)

## Before Using This Medicine

In deciding to use a medicine, the risks of taking the medicine must be weighed against the good it will do. This is a decision you and your doctor will make. For chromic phosphate P 32, the following should be considered:

**Pregnancy**—Radiopharmaceuticals are usually not recommended for use during pregnancy to avoid exposing the fetus to radiation. However, some treatment using radiopharmaceuticals may be required even during pregnancy. Be sure you have discussed this with your doctor.

**Breast-feeding**—Chromic phosphate P 32 passes into the breast milk. If you must receive this radiopharmaceutical, it may be necessary for you to stop breast-feeding during treatment. Be sure you have discussed this with your doctor.

**Children**—There is no specific information comparing use of chromic phosphate P 32 in children with use in other age groups.

**Older adults**—Many medicines have not been studied specifically in older people. Therefore, it may not be known whether they work exactly the same way they do in younger adults. Although there is no specific information comparing use of chromic phosphate P 32 in the elderly with use in other age groups, this medicine is not expected to cause different side effects or problems in older people than it does in younger adults.

## Preparation for This Treatment

Your doctor may have special instructions for you in preparation for your treatment. If you have not received such instructions or if you do not understand them, check with your doctor in advance.

## Side Effects of This Medicine

Along with its needed effects, a medicine may cause some unwanted effects. Although not all of these side effects may occur, if they do occur they may need medical attention.

*Check with your health care professional immediately* if any of the following side effects occur:

*Less common or rare*
Abdominal or stomach pain (severe); chest pain; chills and/or fever; dry cough; nausea and vomiting (severe); sore throat and fever; troubled breathing; unusual bleeding or bruising; unusual tiredness or weakness

Other side effects may occur that usually do not need medical attention. These side effects may go away during treatment as your body adjusts to the medicine. However, check with your doctor if any of the following side effects continue or are bothersome:

*More common*
Abdominal or stomach cramps; diarrhea; feeling of discomfort; loss of appetite; nausea and vomiting; weakness

Other side effects not listed above may also occur in some patients. If you notice any other effects, check with your doctor.

Revised: 05/18/92

# CHROMIUM SUPPLEMENTS    Systemic

This information applies to the following medicines:
1. Chromic Chloride (KROME-ik KLOR-ide)‡§
2. Chromium (KROH-mee-um)‡§

‡Generic name product may also be available in the U.S.
§Generic name product may also be available in Canada.

## Description

Chromium supplements are used to prevent or treat chromium deficiency.

The body needs chromium for normal growth and health. For patients who are unable to get enough chromium in their regular diet or who have a need for more chromium, chromium supplements may be necessary. They are generally taken by mouth but some patients may have to receive them by injection.

Lack of chromium may lead to nerve problems and may decrease the body's ability to use sugar properly.

There is not enough evidence to show that chromium supplements may improve the way your body uses sugar (glucose tolerance).

Some chromium preparations are available only with your doctor's prescription. Others are available without a prescription; however, your doctor may have special instructions on the proper use and dose for your condition.

Chromium supplements are available in the following dosage forms:

*Oral*
Chromium
 • Tablets (U.S. and Canada)

*Parenteral*
Chromic Chloride
 • Injection (U.S. and Canada)

## Importance of Diet

Many nutritionists recommend that, if possible, people should get all the chromium they need from foods. However, some people do not get enough chromium from their diet. For example, people on weight-loss diets may consume too little food to provide enough chromium. Others may need more chromium than normal. For such people, a chromium supplement is important.

In order to get enough vitamins and minerals in your regular diet, it is important that you eat a balanced and varied diet. Follow carefully any diet program your doctor may recommend. For your specific vitamin and/or mineral needs, ask your doctor or dietitian for a list of appropriate foods.

Chromium is found in various foods, including brewer's yeast, calf liver, American cheese, and wheat germ.

Experts have developed a list of recommended dietary allowances (RDA) for most vitamins and some minerals. The RDA are not an exact number but a general idea of how much you need. They do not cover amounts needed for problems caused by serious lack of vitamins and minerals.

Because a lack of chromium is rare, there are no RDA for it. The following intakes are thought to be plenty for most individuals:
Infants and children—
 Birth to 6 months of age: 10–40 micrograms (mcg) per day.
 6 months to 1 year of age: 20–60 mcg per day.

1 to 3 years of age: 20–80 mcg per day.
4 to 6 years of age: 30–120 mcg per day.
7 to 10 years of age: 50–200 mcg per day.
Adolescents and adults—50–200 mcg per day.

## Before Using This Dietary Supplement

If you are taking this dietary supplement without a prescription, carefully read and follow any precautions on the label. For chromium, the following should be considered:

**Allergies**—Tell your doctor if you have ever had any unusual or allergic reaction to chromium. Also tell your health care professional if you are allergic to any other substances, such as foods, preservatives, or dyes.

**Pregnancy**—It is especially important that you are receiving enough vitamins and minerals when you become pregnant and that you continue to receive the right amount of vitamins and minerals throughout your pregnancy. The healthy growth and development of the fetus depend on a steady supply of nutrients from the mother. However, taking large amounts of a dietary supplement during pregnancy may be harmful to the mother and/or fetus and should be avoided.

**Breast-feeding**—It is important that you receive the right amounts of vitamins and minerals so that your baby will also get the vitamins and minerals needed to grow properly. However, taking large amounts of a dietary supplement while breast-feeding may be harmful to the mother and/or baby and should be avoided.

**Children**—It is especially important that children receive enough chromium in their diet for healthy growth and development. Although there is no specific information about the use of chromium in children in doses higher than normal daily requirements, it is not expected to cause different side effects or problems in children than it does in adults.

**Older adults**—It is important that older people continue to receive enough vitamins in their diet for good health. This medicine has been tested and has not been shown to cause different side effects or problems in older people than it does in younger adults.

**Medicines or other dietary supplements**—Although certain medicines or dietary supplements should not be used together at all, in other cases they may be used together even if an interaction might occur. In these cases, your doctor may want to change the dose, or other precautions may be necessary. Tell your health care professional if you are using any other dietary supplement or any prescription or over-the-counter (OTC) medication.

**Other medical problems**—The presence of other medical problems may affect the use of chromium. Make sure you tell your doctor if you have any other medical problems, especially:
 • Diabetes mellitus (sugar diabetes)—Taking chromium supplements when you have a chromium deficiency may cause a change in the amount of insulin you need

## Proper Use of This Dietary Supplement

Some people believe that taking very large doses of a vitamin or mineral (called megadoses) is useful for treating certain medical problems. Studies have not proven this. Large doses should be taken only under the direction of your doctor after need has been identified.

**Dosing**—The dose of chromium for prevention of chromium deficiency is based on daily recommended intake. See the *Importance of Diet* section for daily recommended intake for chromium.

**Missed dose**—If you miss taking chromium supplements for one or more days there is no cause for concern, since it takes some time for your body to become seriously low in chromium. However, if your doctor has recommended that you take chromium, try to remember to take it as directed every day.

**Storage**—To store this dietary supplement:
• Keep out of the reach of children.
• Store away from heat and direct light.
• Do not store in the bathroom, near the kitchen sink, or in other damp places. Heat or moisture may cause the dietary supplement to break down.
• Keep the dietary supplement from freezing. Do not refrigerate.
• Do not keep outdated dietary supplements or those no longer needed. Be sure that any discarded dietary supplement is out of the reach of children.

## Side Effects of This Dietary Supplement

No side effects have been reported for chromium. However, check with your doctor if you notice any unusual effects while you are taking it.

Revised: 03/24/92
Interim revision: 08/01/95

# CHYMOPAPAIN   Parenteral-Local

A commonly used brand name in the U.S. and Canada is Chymodiactin.

## Description

Chymopapain (kye-mo-PA-pane) is injected directly into a herniated ("slipped") disk in the spine to dissolve part of the disk and relieve the pain and other problems caused by the disk pressing on a nerve. Before you receive chymopapain, you will be given an anesthetic (either a general anesthetic to put you to sleep or a local anesthetic).

Very rarely, use of chymopapain may cause serious side effects, including paralysis of the legs or death. Another dangerous side effect of chymopapain injection is a severe allergic reaction called anaphylaxis. This side effect occurs in less than 1% of the patients receiving the medicine, but it occurs more often in women than in men. Before receiving chymopapain, you should discuss its use, and the possibility of anaphylaxis or other serious side effects, with your doctor.

Chymopapain injections are given only in a hospital, usually in an operating room, by your surgeon. This medicine is available in the following dosage form:
*Parenteral*
• Injection (U.S. and Canada)

## Before Receiving This Medicine

In deciding to use a medicine, the risks of receiving the medicine must be weighed against the good it will do. This is a decision you and your doctor will make. For chymopapain, the following should be considered:

**Allergies**—Tell your doctor if you have ever had any unusual or allergic reaction to chymopapain, papaya, meat tenderizer, contact lens cleaning solutions, beer, or iodine. Also tell your doctor if you are allergic to any other substances, such as foods, preservatives, or dyes.

**Pregnancy**—Studies on effects of pregnancy have not been done in either humans or animals.

**Breast-feeding**—It is not known whether chymopapain passes into breast milk. Although most medicines pass into breast milk in small amounts, many of them may be used safely while breast-feeding. Mothers who are receiving this medicine and who wish to breast-feed should discuss this with their doctor.

**Children**—Studies on this medicine have been done only in adult patients, and there is no specific information comparing use of chymopapain in children with use in other age groups.

**Older adults**—Many medicines have not been studied specifically in older people. Therefore, it may not be known whether they work exactly the same way they do in younger adults or if they cause different side effects or problems in older people. There is no specific information comparing use of chymopapain in the elderly with use in other age groups.

**Other medicines**—Although certain medicines should not be used together at all, in other cases two different medicines may be used together even if an interaction might occur. In these cases, your doctor may want to change the dose, or other precautions may be necessary. Tell your doctor if you are taking any other prescription or non-prescription (over-the-counter [OTC]) medicine.

**Other medical problems**—The presence of other medical problems may affect the use of chymopapain. Make sure you tell your doctor if you have ever received an injection of chymopapain, if you have had back surgery, or if you have any other medical problems, especially:

- Allergies or
- Stroke or bleeding in the brain (or if any member of your family has ever had these problems) or
- High blood pressure (hypertension)—The chance of side effects may be increased

## Proper Use of This Medicine

**Dosing**—The dose of chymopapain will be different for different patients and must be determined by your doctor.

## Side Effects of This Medicine

Along with its needed effects, a medicine may cause some unwanted effects. Very rarely, use of chymopapain has caused serious side effects, including paralysis of the legs or death. Also, this medicine may cause dangerous allergic reactions, especially in women.

Although not all of the following side effects may occur, if they do occur they may need medical attention. Tell your health care professional if any of the following side effects occur:

*Rare*
    Abdominal or stomach cramps or pain; changes of skin color, hot skin, pain, tenderness, or swelling of leg or foot; constipation (severe); decreased or uncontrolled

urination; fast or irregular breathing; headache (sudden, severe, and continuing); puffiness or swelling of the eyelids or around the eyes; runny nose; shortness of breath, troubled breathing, tightness in chest, or wheezing; skin rash, redness, hives, or itching; swelling of abdomen or stomach; uncontrolled bowel movements; vomiting; weakness in legs (severe) or problems with moving legs

Other side effects may occur that usually do not need medical attention. Pain and muscle spasms in the lower back may last for several days after you have received this medicine. Stiffness or soreness in the back may last for several months. Other side effects may go away after a short time. However, check with your doctor if any of the following side effects continue or are bothersome:

*More common*
    Back pain, stiffness, or soreness; muscle spasms in lower back
*Less common or rare*
    Cramps, pain, or mild weakness in legs; dizziness; feeling of burning in lower back; headache; nausea; numbness or tingling in legs or toes

Some side effects may not appear until several days or weeks after you have received chymopapain. Check with your doctor as soon as possible if any of the following side effects occur within 1 month after you have received this medicine:

    Back pain or muscle weakness (sudden and severe); skin rash, hives, or itching

Other side effects not listed above may also occur in some patients. If you notice any other effects, check with your doctor.

Revised: 07/26/94

# CICLOPIROX Topical

A commonly used brand name in the U.S. and Canada is Loprox.

## Description

Ciclopirox (sye-kloe-PEER-ox) is used to treat infections caused by fungus. It works by killing the fungus or preventing its growth.

Ciclopirox is applied to the skin to treat:
- ringworm of the body (tinea corporis);
- ringworm of the foot (tinea pedis; athlete's foot);
- ringworm of the groin (tinea cruris; jock itch);
- "sun fungus" (tinea versicolor; pityriasis versicolor); and
- certain other fungus infections, such as Candida (Monilia) infections.

Ciclopirox is available only with your doctor's prescription, in the following dosage forms:
*Topical*
- Cream (U.S. and Canada)
- Lotion (U.S. and Canada)

## Before Using This Medicine

In deciding to use a medicine, the risks of taking the medicine must be weighed against the good it will do. This is a decision you and your doctor will make. For ciclopirox, the following should be considered:

**Allergies**—Tell your doctor if you have ever had any unusual or allergic reaction to ciclopirox. Also tell your health care professional if you are allergic to any other substances, such as preservatives or dyes.

**Pregnancy**—Ciclopirox has not been studied in pregnant women. However, this medication has not been shown to cause birth defects or other problems in animal studies.

**Breast-feeding**—It is not known whether ciclopirox passes into breast milk. Although most medicines pass into breast milk in small amounts, many of them may be used safely while breast-feeding. Mothers who are using this medicine and who wish to breast-feed should discuss this with their doctor.

**Children**—Studies on this medicine have been done only in adult patients, and there is no specific information comparing use of ciclopirox in children under the age of 10 with use in other age groups.

**Older adults**—Many medicines have not been studied specifically in older people. Therefore, it may not be known whether they work exactly the same way they do in younger adults. Although there is no specific information comparing use of ciclopirox in the elderly with use in other age groups, this medicine is not expected to cause different side effects or problems in older people than it does in younger adults.

**Other medicines**—Although certain medicines should not be used together at all, in other cases two different medicines may be used together even if an interaction might occur. In these cases, your doctor may want to change the dose, or other precautions may be necessary. Tell your health care professional if you are using any other topical prescription or nonprescription (over-the-counter [OTC]) medicine that is to be applied to the same area of the skin.

## Proper Use of This Medicine

Apply enough ciclopirox to cover the affected and surrounding skin areas and rub in gently.

*Keep this medicine away from the eyes.*

When ciclopirox is used to treat certain types of fungus infections of the skin, an occlusive dressing (airtight covering, such as kitchen plastic wrap) should *not* be applied over the medicine. To do so may irritate the skin. *Do not apply an airtight covering over this medicine unless you have been directed to do so by your doctor.*

To help clear up your infection completely, *it is very important that you keep using ciclopirox for the full time of treatment,* even if your symptoms begin to clear up after a few days. Since fungus infections may be very slow to clear up, you may have to continue using this medicine every day for several weeks or more. If you stop using this medicine too soon, your symptoms may return. *Do not miss any doses.*

**Dosing**—The dose of topical ciclopirox will be different for different patients. *Follow your doctor's orders or the directions on the label.* The following information includes only the average doses of topical ciclopirox. *If your dose is different, do not change it* unless your doctor tells you to do so.

- For *topical* dosage forms (cream and lotion):
  —Fungus infections (treatment):
  - Adults and children 10 years of age and over—Apply two times a day, morning and evening.
  - Children up to 10 years of age—Use and dose must be determined by your doctor.

**Missed dose**—If you miss a dose of this medicine, apply it as soon as possible. However, if it is almost time for your next dose, skip the missed dose and go back to your regular dosing schedule.

**Storage**—To store this medicine:
- Keep out of the reach of children.
- Store away from heat and direct light.
- Keep the medicine from freezing.
- Do not keep outdated medicine or medicine no longer needed. Be sure that any discarded medicine is out of the reach of children.

## Precautions While Using This Medicine

If your skin problem does not improve within 2 to 4 weeks, or if it becomes worse, check with your doctor.

*To help clear up your infection completely and to help make sure it does not return, good health habits are also required.* The following measures will help reduce chafing and irritation and will also help keep the area cool and dry.

- *For patients using ciclopirox for ringworm of the groin (tinea cruris):*
  —Avoid wearing underwear that is tight-fitting or made from synthetic materials (for example, rayon or nylon). Instead, wear loose-fitting, cotton underwear.
  —Use a bland, absorbent powder (for example, talcum powder) or an antifungal powder (for example, tolnaftate) on the skin. It is best to use the powder between applications of ciclopirox.
- *For patients using ciclopirox for ringworm of the foot (tinea pedis):*
  —Carefully dry the feet, especially between the toes, after bathing.
  —Avoid wearing socks made from wool or synthetic materials (for example, rayon or nylon). Instead, wear clean, cotton socks and change them daily or more often if the feet sweat freely.
  —Wear sandals or well-ventilated shoes (for example, shoes with holes on top or on the side).
  —Use a bland, absorbent powder (for example, talcum powder) or an antifungal powder (for example, tolnaftate) between the toes, on the feet, and in socks and shoes freely once or twice a day. It is best to use the powder between applications of ciclopirox.

If you have any questions about these measures, check with your health care professional.

## Side Effects of This Medicine

Along with its needed effects, a medicine may cause some unwanted effects. Although not all of these side effects may occur, if they do occur they may need medical attention.

Check with your doctor as soon as possible if any of the following side effects occur:

*Rare*

Burning, itching, redness, swelling, or other signs of irritation not present before use of this medicine

Other side effects not listed above may also occur in some patients. If you notice any other effects, check with your doctor.

Revised: 05/26/94

---

# CINOXACIN  Systemic†

A commonly used brand name in the U.S. is Cinobac.

†Not commercially available in Canada.

## Description

Cinoxacin (sin-OX-a-sin) is used to prevent and treat infections of the urinary tract. It will not work for other infections or for colds, flu, or other virus infections.

Cinoxacin is available only with your doctor's prescription, in the following dosage form:

*Oral*
- Capsules (U.S.)

## Before Using This Medicine

In deciding to use a medicine, the risks of taking the medicine must be weighed against the good it will do. This is a decision you and your doctor will make. For cinoxacin, the following should be considered:

**Allergies**—Tell your doctor if you have ever had any unusual or allergic reaction to cinoxacin or to any related medicines such as ciprofloxacin (e.g., Cipro), enoxacin (e.g. Penetrex), lomefloxacin (e.g. Maxaquin), nalidixic acid (e.g., NegGram), norfloxacin (e.g., Noroxin), or ofloxacin (e.g., Floxin). Also tell your health care professional if you are allergic to any other substances, such as foods, preservatives, or dyes.

**Pregnancy**—Studies have not been done in humans. However, use is not recommended during pregnancy since cinoxacin has been shown to cause bone development problems in young animals.

**Breast-feeding**—It is not known whether cinoxacin passes into the breast milk. However, other related medicines do pass into the breast milk. Since cinoxacin has been shown to cause bone development problems in young animals, use is not recommended in nursing mothers.

**Children**—Since this medicine has been shown to cause bone development problems in young animals, its use is not recommended in children.

**Older adults**—Many medicines have not been studied specifically in older people. Therefore, it may not be known whether they work exactly the same way they do in younger adults. Although there is no specific information comparing use of cinoxacin in the elderly with use in other age groups, this medicine is not expected to cause different side effects or problems in older people than it does in younger adults.

**Other medical problems**—The presence of other medical problems may affect the use of cinoxacin. Make sure you tell your doctor if you have any other medical problems, especially:
- Kidney disease—Patients with kidney disease may have an increased risk of side effects

## Proper Use of This Medicine

Cinoxacin may be taken with food, unless you are otherwise directed by your doctor.

*Do not give this medicine to infants or children under 12 years of age,* unless otherwise directed by your doctor. It has been shown to cause bone development problems in young animals.

To help clear up your infection completely, *keep taking this medicine for the full time of treatment,* even if you begin to feel better after a few days. If you stop taking this medicine too soon, your symptoms may return.

This medicine works best when there is a constant amount in the urine. *To help keep the amount constant, do not miss any doses. Also, it is best to take the doses at evenly spaced times, day and night.* For example, if you are to take 4 doses a day, the doses should be spaced about 6 hours apart. If this interferes with your sleep or other daily activities, or if you need help in planning the best times to take your medicine, check with your health care professional.

**Dosing**—The dose of cinoxacin will be different for different patients. *Follow your doctor's orders or the directions on the label.* The following information includes only the average doses of cinoxacin. Your dose may be different if you have kidney disease. *If your dose is different, do not change it* unless your doctor tells you to do so.

The number of capsules that you take depends on the strength of the medicine. Also, *the number of doses you take each day, the time allowed between doses, and the length of time you take the medicine depend on the medical problem for which you are taking cinoxacin.*

- For *capsule* dosage form:
  —For the *prevention* of urinary tract infections:
  - Adults: 250 milligrams (mg) at bedtime for up to five months.
  - Children up to 18 years of age—Use is generally not recommended because it may cause bone development problems.

  —For the *treatment* of urinary tract infections:
  - Adults—250 milligrams (mg) every six hours; or 500 mg every twelve hours for seven to fourteen days.
  - Children up to 18 years of age—Use is generally not recommended because it may cause bone development problems.

**Missed dose**—If you do miss a dose of this medicine, take it as soon as possible. This will help to keep a constant amount of medicine in the urine. However, if it is almost time for your next dose, skip the missed dose and go back to your regular dosing schedule. Do not double doses.

**Storage**—To store this medicine:
- Keep out of the reach of children.
- Store away from heat and direct light.
- Do not store in the bathroom, near the kitchen sink, or in other damp places. Heat or moisture may cause the medicine to break down.
- Do not keep outdated medicine or medicine no longer needed. Be sure that any discarded medicine is out of the reach of children.

## Precautions While Using This Medicine

If your symptoms do not improve within a few days, or if they become worse, check with your doctor.

This medicine may also cause some people to become dizzy. *Make sure you know how you react to this medicine before you drive, use machines, or do anything else that could be dangerous if you are dizzy.* If this reaction is especially bothersome, check with your doctor.

## Side Effects of This Medicine

Along with its needed effects, a medicine may cause some unwanted effects. Although not all of these side effects may occur, if they do occur they may need medical attention.

Check with your doctor as soon as possible if any of the following side effects occur:

*More common*
   Skin rash, itching, redness, or swelling
*Less common*
   Dizziness; headache

Other side effects may occur that usually do not need medical attention. These side effects may go away during treatment as your body adjusts to the medicine. However, check with your doctor if any of the following side effects continue or are bothersome:

*Less common*
   Diarrhea; loss of appetite; nausea; stomach cramps; vomiting

Other side effects not listed above may also occur in some patients. If you notice any other effects, check with your doctor.

Revised: 04/15/93

---

# CIPROFLOXACIN   Ophthalmic

A commonly used brand name in the U.S. and Canada is Ciloxan.

## Description

Ophthalmic ciprofloxacin (sip-roe-FLOX-a-sin) is used in the eye to treat bacterial infections of the eye and corneal ulcers of the eye. Ophthalmic ciprofloxacin works by killing bacteria.

Ciprofloxacin ophthalmic preparation is available only with your doctor's prescription, in the following dosage form:
   *Ophthalmic*
   - Ophthalmic solution (eye drops) (U.S. and Canada)

## Before Using This Medicine

In deciding to use a medicine, the risks of using the medicine must be weighed against the good it will do. This is a decision you and your doctor will make. For ophthalmic ciprofloxacin, the following should be considered:

**Allergies**—Tell your doctor if you have ever had any unusual or allergic reaction to ophthalmic or systemic ciprofloxacin (e.g., Cipro) or any related medicines, such as cinoxacin (e.g., Cinobac), norfloxacin (e.g., Chibroxin or Noroxin), ofloxacin (e.g., Floxin), or nalidixic acid (e.g., NegGram). Also tell your health care professional if you are allergic to any other substances, such as foods, preservatives, or dyes.

**Pregnancy**—Ciprofloxacin has not been studied in pregnant women. However, studies in animals have not shown that ciprofloxacin causes birth defects.

**Breast-feeding**—It is not known whether ophthalmic ciprofloxin passes into breast milk. However, ciprofloxacin given by mouth does pass into breast milk. Although most medicines pass into breast milk in small amounts, many of them may be used safely while breast-feeding. Mothers who are using this medicine and who wish to breast-feed should discuss this with their doctor.

**Children**—Use is not recommended in infants and children up to 12 years of age. In children 12 years of age and older, this medicine is not expected to cause different side effects or problems than it does in adults.

**Older adults**—Many medicines have not been studied specifically in older people. Therefore, it may not be known whether they work exactly the same way they do in younger adults or if they cause different side effects or problems in older people. There is no specific information comparing use of ophthalmic ciprofloxacin in the elderly with use in other age groups.

**Other medicines**—Although certain medicines should not be used together at all, in other cases two different medicines may be used together even if an interaction might occur. In these cases, your doctor may want to change the dose, or other precautions may be necessary. Tell your health care professional if you using any other prescription or nonprescription (over-the-counter [OTC]) medicine that is to be used in the eye.

---

## Proper Use of This Medicine

To use:

- First, wash your hands. Then tilt the head back and pull the lower eyelid away from the eye to form a pouch. Drop the medicine into the pouch and gently close the eyes. Do not blink. Keep the eyes closed for 1 or 2 minutes to allow the medicine to come into contact with the infection.
- If you think you did not get the drop of medicine into your eyes properly, use another drop.
- To keep the medicine as germ-free as possible, do not touch the applicator tip to any surface (including the eye). Also, keep the container tightly closed.

To help clear up your eye infection completely, *keep using ophthalmic ciprofloxacin for the full time of treatment*, even if your symptoms have disappeared. *Do not miss any doses.*

**Dosing**—The dose of ophthalmic ciprofloxacin will be different for different patients. *Follow your doctor's orders or the directions on the label.* The following information includes only the average doses of ophthalmic ciprofloxacin. *If your dose is different, do not change it* unless your doctor tells you to do so.

*The number of doses you use each day, the time allowed between doses, and the length of time you use the medicine depend on the medical problem for which you are using ophthalmic ciprofloxacin.*

- For *ophthalmic solution* dosage form:
  —For bacterial conjunctivitis:
  - Adults and children 12 years of age and older— Use 1 drop in each eye every two hours, while you are awake, for two days. Then use 1 drop in each eye every four hours, while you are awake, for the next five days.
  - Infants and children up to 12 years of age— Use and dose must be determined by your doctor.
  —For corneal ulcers:
  - Adults and children 12 years of age and older— On day one, use 1 drop in the affected eye every fifteen minutes for six hours, then 1 drop every thirty minutes for the rest of the day, while you are awake. On day two, use 1 drop every hour, while you are awake. On days three through fourteen, use 1 drop every four hours, while you are awake.
  - Infants and children up to 12 years of age— Use and dose must be determined by your doctor.

**Missed dose**—If you miss a dose of this medicine, use it as soon as possible. However, if it is almost time for your next dose, skip the missed dose and go back to your regular dosing schedule.

**Storage**—To store this medicine:
- Keep out of the reach of children.
- Store away from heat and direct light.
- Keep the medicine from freezing. Do not refrigerate.
- Do not keep outdated medicine or medicine no longer needed. Be sure that any discarded medicine is out of the reach of children.

---

## Precautions While Using This Medicine

If your eye infection does not improve within a few days, or if it becomes worse, check with your doctor.

This medicine may cause your eyes to become more sensitive to light than they are normally. Wearing sunglasses and avoiding too much exposure to bright light may help lessen the discomfort.

---

## Side Effects of This Medicine

Along with its needed effects, a medicine may cause some unwanted effects. Although not all of these side effects may occur, if they do occur they may need medical attention.

Check with your doctor as soon as possible if any of the following side effects occur:

*Rare*

Blurred vision or other change in vision; irritation (severe) or redness of eye; nausea; skin rash

---

Other side effects may occur that usually do not need medical attention. These side effects may go away during treatment as your body adjusts to the medicine. However, check with your doctor if any of the following side effects continue or are bothersome:

*More common*

Burning or other discomfort of eye; crusting or crystals in corner of eye

*Less common*

Bad taste following use in the eye; feeling of something in eye; itching of eye; redness of the lining of the eyelids

*Rare*

Increased sensitivity of eyes to light; swelling of eyelid; tearing of eye

Other side effects not listed above may also occur in some patients. If you notice any other effects, check with your doctor.

Revised: 07/29/93

# CISAPRIDE   Systemic

A commonly used brand name in the U.S. and Canada is Prepulsid.

## Description

Cisapride (SIS-a-pride) is a medicine that increases the movements or contractions of the stomach and intestines. It is used to treat symptoms such as heartburn caused by a backward flow of stomach acid into the esophagus.

Cisapride is available only with your doctor's prescription. It is available in the following dosage forms:

*Oral*

- Oral suspension (Canada)
- Tablets (U.S. and Canada)

## Before Using This Medicine

In deciding to use a medicine, the risks of taking the medicine must be weighed against the good it will do. This is a decision you and your doctor will make. For cisapride, the following should be considered:

**Allergies**—Tell your doctor if you have ever had any unusual or allergic reaction to cisapride. Also tell your health care professional if you are allergic to any other substances, such as foods, preservatives, or dyes.

**Pregnancy**—Cisapride has not been studied in pregnant women. However, studies in animals have shown that cisapride causes harm to the fetus. Before taking this medicine, make sure your doctor knows if you are pregnant or if you may become pregnant.

**Breast-feeding**—Although cisapride passes into the breast milk, it has not been shown to cause problems in nursing babies.

**Children**—This medicine has been tested in a limited number of children. In effective doses, the medicine has not been shown to cause different side effects or problems than it does in adults.

**Older adults**—Elderly people are especially sensitive to the effects of cisapride. Cisapride stays in the body longer so the dose may be different than in younger people.

**Other medicines**—Although certain medicines should not be used together at all, in other cases two different medicines may be used together even if an interaction might occur. In these cases, your doctor may want to change the dose, or other precautions may be necessary. When you are taking cisapride, it is especially important that your health care professional know if you are taking any of the following:

- Amantadine (e.g., Symmetrel) or
- Anticholinergics (medicine for abdominal or stomach spasms or cramps) or
- Antidepressants (medicine for depression) or
- Antidyskinetics (medicine for Parkinson's disease or other conditions affecting control of muscles) or
- Antihistamines or
- Antipsychotics (medicine for mental illness) or
- Buclizine (e.g., Bucladin) or
- Carbamazepine (e.g., Tegretol) or
- Cyclizine (e.g., Marezine) or
- Cyclobenzaprine (e.g., Flexeril) or
- Disopyramide (e.g., Norpace) or
- Flavoxate (e.g., Urispas) or
- Ipratropium (e.g., Atrovent) or
- Meclizine (e.g., Antivert) or
- Methylphenidate (e.g., Ritalin) or
- Orphenadrine (e.g., Norflex) or
- Oxybutynin (e.g., Ditropen) or
- Procainamide (e.g., Pronestyl) or
- Promethazine (e.g., Phenergan) or
- Quinidine (e.g., Quinidex) or
- Trimeprazine (e.g., Temaril)—Cisapride may decrease the absorption of these medicines and cause them to be less effective

**Other medical problems**—The presence of other medical problems may affect the use of cisapride. Make sure you tell your doctor if you have any other medical problems, especially:

- Abdominal or stomach bleeding or
- Intestinal blockage—Cisapride may make these conditions worse
- Epilepsy or history of seizures—Cisapride has been reported to cause seizures in patients with a history of seizures

- Kidney disease or
- Liver disease—Higher blood levels of cisapride may result and a smaller dose may be needed

## Proper Use of This Medicine

*Take this medicine 15 minutes before meals and at bedtime with a beverage,* unless otherwise directed by your doctor.

**Dosing**—The dose of cisapride will be different for different patients. *Follow your doctor's orders or the directions on the label.* The following information includes only the average doses of cisapride. *If your dose is different, do not change it* unless your doctor tells you to do so.

- For *tablets and solution* dosage forms:
  —For heartburn caused by gastroesophageal reflux:
  - Adults and children 12 years of age and older: 5 to 20 milligrams (mg) of cisapride two to four times a day. Cisapride should be taken fifteen minutes before meals and at bedtime.
  - Children up to 12 years of age: Dose is based on body weight. The dose is usually 0.15 to 0.3 mg of cisapride per kilogram (0.07 to 0.14 mg per pound) of body weight three to four times a day, fifteen minutes before meals.

**Missed dose**—If you miss a dose of this medicine, take it as soon as possible. However, if it is almost time for your next dose, skip the missed dose and go back to your regular dosing schedule. Do not double doses.

**Storage**—To store this medicine:

- Keep out of the reach of children.
- Store away from heat and direct light.
- Do not store in the bathroom, near the kitchen sink, or in other damp places. Heat or moisture may cause the medicine to break down.
- Keep the medicine from freezing. Do not refrigerate.
- Do not keep outdated medicine or medicine no longer needed. Be sure that any discarded medicine is out of the reach of children.

## Precautions While Using This Medicine

This medicine may cause your body to absorb alcohol more quickly than you normally would. Therefore, you may notice the effects sooner. *Check with your doctor before drinking alcohol while you are using this medicine.*

This medicine may cause some people to become drowsy or less alert than they are normally. *Make sure you know how you react to this medicine before you drive, use machines, or do anything else that could be dangerous if you are dizzy or are not alert.*

## Side Effects of This Medicine

Along with its needed effects, a medicine may cause some unwanted effects. Although not all of these side effects may occur, if they do occur they may need medical attention.

*Check with your doctor immediately* if the following side effect occurs:

*Rare*
  Seizures
  Note: Seizures have occurred only in patients with a history of seizures.

Other side effects may occur that usually do not need medical attention. These side effects may go away during treatment as your body adjusts to the medicine. However, check with your doctor if any of the following side effects continue or are bothersome:

*Less common*
  Abdominal cramping, constipation, diarrhea, drowsiness, headache, nausea, unusual tiredness or weakness

Other side effects not listed above may also occur in some patients. If you notice any other effects, check with your doctor.

## Additional Information

Once a medicine has been approved for marketing for a certain use, experience may show that it is also useful for other medical problems. Although this use is not included in product labeling, cisapride is used in certain patients with the following medical condition:

- Gastroparesis (stomach condition)

Other than the above information, there is no additional information relating to proper use, precautions, or side effects for this use.

Developed: 08/27/93

---

# CISPLATIN  Systemic

Some commonly used brand names are:

**In the U.S.—**
  Platinol
  Platinol-AQ

**In Canada—**
  Platinol
  Platinol-AQ
Generic name product may also be available.

## Description

Cisplatin (sis-PLA-tin) belongs to the group of medicines known as alkylating agents. It is used to treat some kinds of cancer.

Cisplatin interferes with the growth of cancer cells, which are eventually destroyed. Since the growth of normal body cells may also be affected by cisplatin, other effects will also occur. Some of these may be serious and must be reported to your doctor. Other effects may not be serious but may cause concern. Some effects may not occur for months or years after the medicine is used.

Before you begin treatment with cisplatin, you and your doctor should talk about the good this medicine will do as well as the risks of using it.

Cisplatin is to be administered only by or under the immediate supervision of your doctor. It is available in the following dosage form:

*Parenteral*
- Injection (U.S. and Canada)

## Before Using This Medicine

In deciding to use a medicine, the risks of taking the medicine must be weighed against the good it will do. This is a decision you and your doctor will make. For cisplatin, the following should be considered:

**Allergies**—Tell your doctor if you have ever had any unusual or allergic reaction to cisplatin.

**Pregnancy**—There is a chance that this medicine may cause birth defects if either the male or female is taking it at the time of conception or if it is taken during pregnancy. Cisplatin causes toxic or harmful effects in the fetus in humans and birth defects in mice. In addition, many cancer medicines may cause sterility which could be permanent. Although sterility has not been reported with this medicine, the possibility should be kept in mind.

Be sure that you have discussed this with your doctor before receiving this medicine. It is best to use some kind of birth control while you are receiving cisplatin. Tell your doctor right away if you think you have become pregnant while receiving cisplatin.

**Breast-feeding**—Because cisplatin may cause serious side effects, breast-feeding is generally not recommended while you are receiving it.

**Children**—Hearing problems and loss of balance are more likely to occur in children, who are usually more sensitive to the effects of cisplatin.

**Older adults**—Many medicines have not been studied specifically in older people. Therefore, it may not be known whether they work exactly the same way they do in younger adults or if they cause different side effects or problems in older people. There is no specific information comparing use of cisplatin in the elderly with use in other age groups.

**Other medicines**—Although certain medicines should not be used together at all, in other cases two different medicines may be used together even if an interaction might occur. In these cases, your doctor may want to change the dose, or other precautions may be necessary. When you are receiving cisplatin, it is especially important that your health care professional know if you are taking any of the following:

- Amphotericin B by injection (e.g., Fungizone) or
- Antithyroid agents (medicine for overactive thyroid) or
- Azathioprine (e.g., Imuran) or
- Chloramphenicol (e.g., Chloromycetin) or
- Colchicine or
- Flucytosine (e.g., Ancobon) or
- Ganciclovir (e.g., Cytovene) or
- Interferon (e.g., Introl A, Roferon-A) or
- Plicamycin (e.g., Mithracin) or
- Zidovudine (e.g., AZT, Retrovir) or
- If you have ever been treated with radiation or cancer medicines—Cisplatin may increase the effects of these medicines or radiation therapy on the blood
- Anti-infectives by mouth or by injection (medicine for infection) or
- Chloroquine (e.g., Aralen) or
- Combination pain medicine containing acetaminophen and aspirin (e.g., Excedrin) or other salicylates (with large amounts taken regularly) or
- Cyclosporine (e.g., Sandimmune) or
- Deferoxamine (e.g., Desferal) (with long-term use) or
- Gold salts (medicine for arthritis) or
- Hydroxychloroquine (e.g., Plaquenil) or
- Inflammation or pain medicine, except narcotics, or
- Lithium (e.g., Lithane) or
- Penicillamine (e.g., Cuprimine) or
- Plicamycin (e.g., Mithracin) or
- Quinine (e.g., Quinamm) or
- Tiopronin (e.g., Thiola)—Risk of ear and kidney problems caused by cisplatin is increased
- Probenecid (e.g., Benemid) or
- Sulfinpyrazone (e.g., Anturane)—Cisplatin may raise the amount of uric acid in the blood. Since these medicines are used to lower uric acid levels, they may not work as well in patients receiving cisplatin

**Other medical problems**—The presence of other medical problems may affect the use of cisplatin. Make sure you tell your doctor if you have any other medical problems, especially:

- Chickenpox (including recent exposure) or
- Herpes zoster (shingles)—Risk of severe disease affecting other parts of the body
- Gout (history of) or
- Kidney stones (history of)—Cisplatin may increase levels of uric acid in the body, which can cause gout or kidney stones
- Hearing problems—May be worsened by cisplatin
- Infection—Cisplatin decreases your body's ability to fight infection
- Kidney disease—Effects of cisplatin may be increased because of slower removal from the body

## Proper Use of This Medicine

This medicine is sometimes given together with certain other medicines. If you are using a combination of medicines, it is important that you receive each one at the proper time. If you are taking some of these medicines by mouth, ask your health care professional to help you plan a way to take them at the right times.

While you are receiving this medicine, your doctor may want you to drink extra fluids so that you will pass more urine. This will help prevent kidney problems and keep your kidneys working well.

This medicine usually causes nausea and vomiting that may be severe. However, it is very important that you continue to receive the medicine, even if you begin to feel ill. Ask your health care professional for ways to lessen these effects, especially if they are severe.

**Dosing**—The dose of cisplatin will be different for different patients. The dose that is used may depend on a number of things, including what the medicine is being used for, the patient's size, and whether or not other medicines are also being taken. *If you are receiving cisplatin at home, follow your doctor's orders or the directions on the label.* If you have any questions about the proper dose of cisplatin, ask your doctor.

## Precautions While Using This Medicine

*It is very important that your doctor check your progress at regular visits* to make sure that this medicine is working properly and to check for unwanted effects.

While you are being treated with cisplatin, and after you stop treatment with it, *do not have any immunizations (vaccinations) without your doctor's approval.* Cisplatin may lower your body's resistance and there is a chance you might get the infection the immunization is meant to prevent. In addition, other persons living in your household should not take oral polio vaccine since there is a chance they could pass the polio virus on to you. Also, avoid persons who have recently taken oral polio vaccine. Do not get close to them, and do not stay in the same room with them for very long. If you cannot take these precautions, you should consider wearing a protective face mask that covers the nose and mouth.

Cisplatin can temporarily lower the number of white blood cells in your blood, increasing the chance of getting an infection. It can also lower the number of platelets, which are necessary for proper blood clotting. If this occurs, there are certain precautions you can take, especially when your blood count is low, to reduce the risk of infection or bleeding:

- If you can, avoid people with infections. *Check with your doctor immediately* if you think you are getting an infection or if you get a fever or chills, cough or hoarseness, lower back or side pain, or painful or difficult urination.
- *Check with your doctor immediately* if you notice any unusual bleeding or bruising; black, tarry stools; blood in urine or stools; or pinpoint red spots on your skin.
- Be careful when using a regular toothbrush, dental floss, or toothpick. Your medical doctor, dentist, or nurse may recommend other ways to clean your teeth

and gums. Check with your medical doctor before having any dental work done.

- Do not touch your eyes or the inside of your nose unless you have just washed your hands and have not touched anything else in the meantime.
- Be careful not to cut yourself when you are using sharp objects such as a safety razor or fingernail or toenail cutters.
- Avoid contact sports or other situations where bruising or injury could occur.

If cisplatin accidentally seeps out of the vein into which it is injected, it may damage some tissues and cause scarring. *Tell the doctor or nurse right away if you notice redness, pain, or swelling at the place of injection.*

## Side Effects of This Medicine

Along with its needed effects, a medicine may cause unwanted effects. Although not all of these side effects may occur, if they do occur they may need medical attention.

Also, because of the way cancer medicines act on the body, there is a chance that they might cause other unwanted effects that may not occur until months or years after the medicine is used. These delayed effects may include certain types of cancer, such as leukemia. Discuss these possible effects with your doctor.

*Check with your doctor or nurse immediately* if any of the following side effects occur:

*Less common*

Black, tarry stools; blood in urine or stools; cough or hoarseness; dizziness or faintness (during or shortly after a dose); fast heartbeat (during or shortly after a dose); fever or chills; lower back or side pain; painful or difficult urination; pain or redness at place of injection; pinpoint red spots on skin; swelling of face (during or shortly after a dose); unusual bleeding or bruising; wheezing (during or shortly after a dose)

Check with your doctor as soon as possible if any of the following side effects occur:

*More common*

Joint pain; loss of balance; ringing in ears; swelling of feet or lower legs; trouble in hearing; unusual tiredness or weakness

*Less common*

Convulsions (seizures); loss of reflexes; loss of taste; numbness or tingling in fingers or toes; trouble in walking

*Rare*

Agitation or confusion; blurred vision; change in ability to see colors (especially blue or yellow); muscle cramps; sores in mouth and on lips

Other side effects may occur that usually do not need medical attention. These side effects may go away during treatment as your body adjusts to the medicine. Also, your health care professional may be able to tell you about ways to prevent or reduce some of these side effects. Check with your health care professional if any of the following side effects continue or are bothersome or if you have any questions about them:

*More common*

  Nausea and vomiting (severe)

*Less common*

  Loss of appetite

After you stop receiving cisplatin, it may still produce some side effects that need attention. During this period of time check with your doctor if you notice any of the following side effects:

  Black, tarry stools; blood in urine or stools; convulsions (seizures); cough or hoarseness; decrease in urination; fever or chills; loss of balance; loss of reflexes; loss of taste; lower back or side pain; numbness or tingling in fingers or toes; painful or difficult urination; pinpoint red spots on skin; ringing in ears; swelling of feet or lower legs; trouble in hearing; trouble in walking; unusual bleeding or bruising

Other side effects not listed above may also occur in some patients. If you notice any other effects, check with your doctor.

Revised: 08/12/94

---

# CITRATES   Systemic

Some commonly used brand names are:

**In the U.S.—**

| | |
|---|---|
| Bicitra[4] | Polycitra-K Crystals[2] |
| Citrolith[3] | Polycitra-LC[5] |
| Oracit[4] | Polycitra Syrup[5] |
| Polycitra-K[2] | Urocit-K[1] |

**In Canada—**

  Oracit[4]

Other commonly used names for sodium citrate and citric acid are Albright's solution and modified Shohl's solution.

Note: For quick reference, the following citrates are numbered to match the corresponding brand names.

This information applies to the following medicines:
1. Potassium Citrate (poe-TASS-ee-um SIH-trayt)
2. Potassium Citrate and Citric Acid (SIH-trik A-sid)
3. Potassium Citrate and Sodium (SOE-dee-um) Citrate
4. Sodium Citrate and Citric Acid
5. Tricitrates (Try-SIH-trayts)

---

## Description

Citrates (SIH-trayts) are used to make the urine more alkaline (less acid). This helps prevent certain kinds of kidney stones. Citrates are sometimes used with other medicines to help treat kidney stones that may occur with gout. They are also used to make the blood more alkaline in certain conditions.

Citrates are available only with your doctor's prescription, in the following dosage forms:

*Oral*

Potassium Citrate
- Tablets (U.S.)

Potassium Citrate and Citric Acid
- Oral solution (U.S.)
- Crystals for oral solution (U.S.)

Potassium Citrate and Sodium Citrate
- Tablets (U.S.)

Sodium Citrate and Citric Acid
- Oral solution (U.S. and Canada)

Tricitrates
- Oral solution (U.S.)

## Before Using This Medicine

In deciding to use a medicine, the risks of taking the medicine must be weighed against the good it will do. This is a decision you and your doctor will make. For citrates, the following should be considered:

**Allergies**—Tell your doctor if you have ever had any unusual or allergic reaction to potassium citrate or potassium. Also tell your health care professional if you are allergic to any other substances, such as foods, preservatives, or dyes.

**Pregnancy**—Studies on effects in pregnancy have not been done in either humans or animals.

**Breast-feeding**—Although it is not known whether citrates pass into the breast milk, this medicine has not been reported to cause problems in nursing babies.

**Children**—Although there is no specific information comparing use of citrates in children with use in other age groups, these medicines are not expected to cause different side effects or problems in children than they do in adults.

**Older adults**—Many medicines have not been studied specifically in older people. Therefore, it may not be known whether they work exactly the same way they do in younger adults or if they cause different side effects or problems in older people. There is no specific information comparing use of citrates in the elderly with use in other age groups.

**Other medicines**—Although certain medicines should not be used together at all, in other cases two different medicines may be used together even if an interaction might occur. In these cases, your doctor may want to change the dose, or other precautions may be necessary. When you are taking citrates, it is especially important that your health care professional know if you are taking any of the following:
- Amiloride (e.g., Midamor) or
- Benazepril (e.g., Lotensin) or
- Captopril (e.g., Capoten) or

- Digitalis glycosides (heart medicine) or
- Enalapril (e.g., Vasotec) or
- Fosinopril (e.g., Monotril) or
- Heparin (e.g., Panheprin) or
- Lisinopril (e.g., Prinivil; Zestril) or
- Medicines for inflammation or pain (except narcotics) or
- Potassium-containing medicines (other) or
- Quinapril (e.g., Accuprol) or
- Ramipril (e.g., Altase) or
- Salt substitutes, low-salt foods or milk or
- Spironolactone (e.g., Aldactone) or
- Triamterene (e.g., Dyrenium)—Use with potassium-containing citrates may further increase potassium blood levels, possibly leading to serious side effects
- Antacids, especially those containing aluminum or sodium bicarbonate—Use with citrates may increase the risk of kidney stones; also, citrates may increase the amount of aluminum in the blood and cause serious side effects, especially in patients with kidney problems
- Methenamine (e.g., Mandelamine)—Use with citrates may make the methenamine less effective
- Quinidine (e.g., Quinidex)—Use with citrates may cause quinidine to build up in the bloodstream, possibly leading to serious side effects

**Other medical problems**—The presence of other medical problems may affect the use of citrates. Make sure you tell your doctor if you have any other medical problems, especially:

- Addison's disease (underactive adrenal glands) or
- Diabetes mellitus (sugar diabetes) or
- Kidney disease—The potassium in potassium-containing citrates may worsen or cause heart problems in patients with these conditions
- Diarrhea (chronic)—Treatment with citrates may not be effective; a change in dose of citrate may be needed
- Edema (swelling of the feet or lower legs) or
- High blood pressure or
- Toxemia of pregnancy—The sodium in sodium-containing citrates may cause the body to retain (keep) water
- Heart disease—The sodium in sodium-containing citrates may cause the body to retain (keep) water; the potassium in potassium-containing citrates may make heart disease worse
- Intestinal or esophageal blockage—Potassium citrate tablets may cause irritation of the stomach or intestines
- Stomach ulcer or other stomach problems—Potassium citrate–containing products may make these conditions worse
- Urinary tract infection—Citrates may make conditions worse

## Proper Use of This Medicine

For patients taking the *tablet form of this medicine:*
- Swallow the tablets whole. Do not crush, chew, or suck the tablet.
- Take with a full glass (8 ounces) of water.
- *If you have trouble swallowing the tablets or they seem to stick in your throat, check with your doctor at once.* If this medicine is not completely swallowed and not properly dissolved, it can cause severe irritation.

For patients taking the *liquid form of this medicine:*
- Dilute with a full glass (6 ounces) of water or juice and drink; follow with additional water, if desired.
- Chill, but do *not* freeze, this medicine before taking it, for a better taste.

For patients taking the *crystals form of this medicine:*
- Add the contents of one packet to at least 6 ounces of cool water or juice.
- Stir well to make sure the crystals are completely dissolved.
- Drink all the mixture to be sure you are taking the correct dose. Follow with additional water or juice, if desired.

*Take each dose immediately after a meal or within 30 minutes after a meal or bedtime snack.* This helps prevent the medicine from causing stomach pain or a laxative effect.

*Drink at least a full glass (8 ounces) of water or other liquid (except milk) every hour during the day (about 3 quarts a day), unless otherwise directed by your doctor.* This will increase the flow of urine and help prevent kidney stones.

*Take this medicine only as directed by your doctor.* Do not take more of it, do not take it more often, and do not take it for a longer time than your doctor ordered. *This is especially important if you are also taking a diuretic (water pill) or digitalis medicine for your heart.*

**Dosing**—The dose of these single or combination medicines will be different for different patients. *Follow your doctor's orders or the directions on the label.* The following information includes only the average doses of these medicines. *If your dose is different, do not change it* unless your doctor tells you to do so.

The number of tablets that you take or of teaspoonfuls or ounces of solution that you drink depends on the strength of the single or combination medicine. *Also, the number of doses you take each day, the time allowed between doses, and the length of time you take the medicine depend on the medical problem for which you are taking this single or combination medicine.*

*For potassium citrate*
- For *oral* dosage form (tablets):
  —To make the urine more alkaline (less acidic) and to prevent kidney stones:
  • Adults—At first, 1.08 to 2.16 grams three times a day with meals. Some people may take 1.62 grams four times a day with meals or within thirty minutes after a meal or bedtime snack. Your doctor may change your dose if needed. However, most people usually will not take more than 10.8 grams a day.
  • Children—Dose must be determined by your doctor.

*For potassium citrate and citric acid*
- For *oral* dosage form (solution):
  —To make the urine or blood more alkaline (less acidic) and to prevent kidney stones:
    • Adults—At first, 2 to 3 teaspoonfuls of solution, mixed with water or juice, four times a day, after meals and at bedtime. Your doctor may change the dose if needed.
  —To make the urine more alkaline (less acidic):
    • Children—At first, 1 to 3 teaspoonfuls of solution, mixed with water or juice, four times a day after meals and at bedtime. Your doctor may change the dose if needed.
- For *oral* dosage form (crystals for solution):
  —To make the urine or blood more alkaline (less acidic) and to prevent kidney stones:
    • Adults—At first, 3.3 grams of potassium citrate, mixed with water or juice, four times a day, after meals and at bedtime. Your doctor may change the dose if needed.
    • Children—Use is not recommended.

*For potassium citrate and sodium citrate*
- For *oral* dosage form (tablets):
  —To make the urine more alkaline (less acidic) and to prevent kidney stones:
    • Adults—At first, 1 to 4 tablets after meals and at bedtime.
    • Children—Dose must be determined by your doctor.

*For sodium citrate and citric acid*
- For *oral* dosage form (solution):
  —To make the urine and blood more alkaline (less acidic) and to prevent kidney stones:
    • Adults—At first, 2 to 6 teaspoonfuls of solution four times a day, after meals and at bedtime. The solution should be mixed in one to three ounces of water. Your doctor may change the dose if needed. However, most people will usually not take more than five ounces a day.
  —To make the contents of the stomach less acidic before surgery:
    • Adults—1 to 2 tablespoonfuls as a single dose. You may mix it in one to two tablespoonfuls of water.
  —To make the blood more alkaline (less acidic):
    • Children—At first, 1 to 3 teaspoonfuls of solution four times a day, after meals and at bedtime. The solution should be mixed in one to three ounces of water. Your doctor may change the dose if needed.

*For tricitrates*
- *For oral* dosage form (solution):
  —To make the urine and blood more alkaline (less acidic) and to prevent kidney stones:
    • Adults—At first, 1 to 2 tablespoonfuls of solution four times a day, after meals and at bedtime. Your doctor may change the dose if needed.

—To make the contents of the stomach less acidic before surgery:
  • Adults—1 tablespoonful as a single dose. You should mix the solution in one tablespoonful of water.
—To make the urine or blood more alkaline (less acidic):
  • Children—At first, 5 to 10 mL four times a day after meals and at bedtime. Your doctor may change the dose if needed.

**Missed dose**—If you miss a dose of this medicine, take it as soon as possible if remembered within 2 hours. However, if it is almost time for your next dose, skip the missed dose and go back to your regular dosing schedule. Do not double doses.

**Storage**—To store this medicine:
- Keep out of the reach of children.
- Store away from heat and direct light.
- Do not store in the bathroom, near the kitchen sink, or in other damp places. Heat or moisture may cause the medicine to break down.
- Keep the liquid form of this medicine from freezing.
- Do not keep outdated medicine or medicine no longer needed. Be sure that any discarded medicine is out of the reach of children.

## Precautions While Using This Medicine

It is important that your doctor check your progress at regular visits. This is to make sure the medicine is working properly and to check for unwanted effects.

Do not eat salty foods or use extra table salt on your food while you are taking citrates. This will help prevent kidney stones and unwanted effects.

Check with your doctor before starting any strenuous physical exercise, especially if you are out of condition and are taking any other medication. Exercise and certain medications may increase the amount of potassium in the blood.

For patients taking *potassium citrate–containing medicines:*
- Do not use salt substitutes and low-salt milk unless told to do so by your doctor. They may contain potassium.
- *Check with your doctor at once if you are taking the tablet form and notice black, tarry stools or other signs of stomach or intestinal bleeding.*
- Do not be alarmed if you notice what appears to be a whole tablet in the stool after taking potassium citrate tablets. Your body has received the proper amount of medicine from the tablet and has expelled the tablet shell. However, it is a good idea to check with your doctor also.
- If you are on a potassium-rich or potassium-restricted diet, check with your health care professional. Potassium citrate–containing medicines contain a large amount of potassium.

For patients taking *sodium citrate–containing medicines:*
- If you are on a sodium-restricted diet, check with your health care professional. Sodium citrate–containing medicines contain a large amount of sodium.

## Side Effects of This Medicine

Along with its needed effects, a medicine may cause some unwanted effects. Although not all of these side effects may occur, if they do occur they may need medical attention.

*Stop taking this medicine and check with your doctor immediately if any of the following side effects occur:*

*Rare*

Abdominal or stomach pain or cramping (severe); black, tarry stools; vomiting (severe), sometimes with blood

Also, check with your doctor as soon as possible if any of the following side effects occur:

Confusion; convulsions (seizures); dizziness; high blood pressure; irregular or fast heartbeat; irritability; mood or mental changes; muscle pain or twitching; nervousness or restlessness; numbness or tingling in hands, feet, or lips; shortness of breath, difficult breathing, or slow breathing; swelling of feet or lower legs; unexplained anxiety; unpleasant taste; unusual tiredness or weakness; weakness or heaviness of legs

Other side effects may occur that usually do not need medical attention. These side effects may go away during treatment as your body adjusts to the medicine. However, check with your doctor if any of the following side effects continue or are bothersome:

*Less common*

Abdominal or stomach soreness or pain (mild); diarrhea or loose bowel movements; nausea or vomiting

Other side effects not listed above may also occur in some patients. If you notice any other effects, check with your doctor.

Revised: 01/18/93
Interim revision: 08/29/94

---

# CLADRIBINE    Systemic

A commonly used brand name in the U.S. and Canada is Leustatin. Other commonly used names are 2-chlorodeoxyadenosine and 2-CdA.

## Description

Cladribine (KLAD-ri-been) belongs to the group of medicines called antimetabolites. It is used to treat hairy cell leukemia. It is also sometimes used to treat other kinds of cancer, as determined by your doctor.

Cladribine interferes with the growth of cancer cells, which are eventually destroyed. Since the growth of normal body cells may also be affected by cladribine, other effects will also occur. Some of these may be serious and must be reported to your doctor. Other effects may not be serious but may cause concern. Some effects may not occur for months or years after the medicine is used.

Before you begin treatment with cladribine, you and your doctor should talk about the good this medicine will do as well as the risks of using it.

Cladribine is to be administered only by or under the immediate supervision of your doctor. It is available in the following dosage form:

*Parenteral*
- Injection (U.S. and Canada)

## Before Using This Medicine

In deciding to use a medicine, the risks of taking the medicine must be weighed against the good it will do.

This is a decision you and your doctor will make. For cladribine, the following should be considered:

**Allergies**—Tell your doctor if you have ever had any unusual or allergic reaction to cladribine.

**Pregnancy**—There is a chance that this medicine may cause birth defects if either the male or female is taking it at the time of conception or if it is taken during pregnancy. Cladribine has been shown to cause birth defects in mice and rabbits. In addition, many cancer medicines may cause sterility which could be permanent. Although sterility has not been reported with this medicine, fertility problems do occur in male monkeys and the possibility should be kept in mind.

Be sure that you have discussed this with your doctor before receiving this medicine. It is best to use some kind of birth control while you are receiving cladribine. Tell your doctor right away if you think you have become pregnant while receiving cladribine.

**Breast-feeding**—It is not known whether cladribine passes into breast milk. However, because this medicine may cause serious side effects, breast-feeding is generally not recommended while you are receiving it.

**Children**—There is no specific information comparing use of cladribine in children with use in other age groups.

**Older adults**—Many medicines have not been studied specifically in older people. Therefore, it may not be known whether they work exactly the same way they do in younger adults. Although there is no specific information comparing use of cladribine in the elderly with use in other age groups, it is not expected to cause different side effects or problems in older people than it does in younger adults.

**Other medicines**—Although certain medicines should not be used together at all, in other cases two different medicines may be used together even if an interaction might occur. In these cases, your doctor may want to change the dose, or other precautions may be necessary. When you are receiving cladribine it is especially important that your health care professional know if you are taking any of the following:

- Amphotericin B by injection (e.g., Fungizone) or
- Antithyroid agents (medicine for overactive thyroid) or
- Azathioprine (e.g., Imuran) or
- Chloramphenicol (e.g., Chloromycetin) or
- Colchicine or
- Flucytosine (e.g., Ancobon) or
- Ganciclovir (e.g., Cytovene) or
- Interferon (e.g., Intron A, Roferon-A) or
- Plicamycin (e.g., Mithracin) or
- Zidovudine (e.g., AZT, Retrovir) or
- If you have ever been treated with radiation or cancer medicines—Cladribine may increase the effects of these medicines or radiation therapy on the blood
- Probenecid (e.g., Benemid) or
- Sulfinpyrazone (e.g., Anturane)—Cladribine may raise the amount of uric acid in the blood. Since these medicines are used to lower uric acid levels, they may not be as effective in patients receiving cladribine

**Other medical problems**—The presence of other medical problems may affect the use of cladribine. Make sure you tell your doctor if you have any other medical problems, especially:

- Chickenpox (including recent exposure) or
- Herpes zoster (shingles)—Risk of severe disease affecting other parts of the body
- Gout (history of) or
- Kidney stones (history of)—Cladribine may increase levels of uric acid in the body, which can cause gout or kidney stones
- Infection—Cladribine may decrease your body's ability to fight infection

## Proper Use of This Medicine

This medicine may cause mild nausea and may also cause vomiting. However, it is very important that you continue to receive the medicine even if you begin to feel ill. Ask your health care professional for ways to lessen these effects.

**Dosing**—The dose of cladribine will be different for different patients. The dose that is used may depend on a number of things, including what the medicine is being used for, the patient's weight, and whether or not other medicines are also being taken. *If you are receiving cladribine at home, follow your doctor's orders or the directions on the label.* If you have any questions about the proper dose of cladribine, ask your doctor.

## Precautions While Using This Medicine

*It is very important that your doctor check your progress at regular visits* to make sure that this medicine is working properly and to check for unwanted effects.

While you are being treated with cladribine, and after you stop treatment with it, *do not have any immunizations (vaccinations) without your doctor's approval.* Cladribine may lower your body's resistance and there is a chance you might get the infection the immunization is meant to prevent. In addition, other persons living in your household should not take oral polio vaccine since there is a chance they could pass the polio virus on to you. Also, avoid persons who have taken oral polio vaccine. Do not get close to them and do not stay in the same room with them for very long. If you cannot take these precautions, you should consider wearing a protective face mask that covers the nose and mouth.

Cladribine can temporarily lower the number of white blood cells in your blood, increasing the chance of getting an infection. It can also lower the number of platelets, which are necessary for proper blood clotting. If this occurs, there are certain precautions you can take, especially when your blood count is low, to reduce the risk of infection or bleeding:

- If you can, avoid people with infections, colds, or flu. *Check with your doctor immediately* if you think you are getting an infection or if you get a fever or chills, cough or hoarseness, lower back or side pain, or painful or difficult urination.
- *Check with your doctor immediately* if you notice any unusual bleeding or bruising; black, tarry stools; blood in urine or stools; or pinpoint red spots on your skin.
- Be careful when using a regular toothbrush, dental floss, or toothpick. Your medical doctor, dentist, or nurse may recommend other ways to clean your teeth and gums. Check with your medical doctor before having any dental work done.
- Do not touch your eyes or the inside of your nose unless you have just washed your hands and have not touched anything else in the meantime.
- Be careful not to cut yourself when you are using sharp objects such as a safety razor or fingernail or toenail cutters.
- Avoid contact sports or other situations where bruising or injury could occur.

## Side Effects of This Medicine

Along with its needed effects, a medicine may cause some unwanted effects. Some side effects will have signs or symptoms that you can see or feel. Your doctor may watch for others by doing certain tests.

Also, because of the way cancer medicines act on the body, there is a chance that they might cause other unwanted effects that may not occur until months or years after the medicine is used. These delayed effects may include certain types of cancer. Discuss these possible effects with your doctor.

*Check with your doctor or nurse immediately* if any of the following side effects occur:

*More common*
Black, tarry stools; blood in urine; cough or hoarseness; chills; fever; lower back or side pain; painful or difficult urination; pinpoint red spots on skin; unusual bleeding or bruising

Check with your health care professional as soon as possible if any of the following side effects occur:

*More common*
Skin rash

*Less common*
Pain or redness at place of injection; shortness of breath; stomach pain; swelling of feet or lower legs; unusually fast heartbeat

This medicine may also cause the following side effects that your doctor will watch out for:

*More common*
Anemia; low white cell counts in blood

Other side effects may occur that usually do not need medical attention. These side effects may go away during treatment as your body adjusts to the medicine. Also, your health care professional may be able to tell you about ways to prevent or reduce some of these side effects. Check with your health care professional if any of the following side effects continue or are bothersome or if you have any questions about them:

*More common*
Headache; loss of appetite; nausea; unusual tiredness; vomiting

*Less common*
Constipation; diarrhea; dizziness; general feeling of discomfort or illness; itching; muscle or joint pain; sweating; trouble in sleeping; weakness

Other side effects not listed above may also occur in some patients. If you notice any other effects, check with your doctor.

Developed: 07/26/94
Interim revision: 08/15/94

# CLARITHROMYCIN  Systemic

A commonly used brand name in the U.S. and Canada is Biaxin.

## Description

Clarithromycin (kla-RITH-roe-mye-sin) is used to treat bacterial infections in many different parts of the body. It works by killing bacteria or preventing their growth. It is also used to treat *Mycobacterium avium* complex (MAC) infection. However, this medicine will not work for colds, flu, or other virus infections. Clarithromycin may be used for other problems as determined by your doctor.

Clarithromycin is available only with your doctor's prescription, in the following dosage forms:

*Oral*
• Oral suspension (U.S.)
• Tablets (U.S. and Canada)

## Before Using This Medicine

In deciding to use a medicine, the risks of taking the medicine must be weighed against the good it will do. This is a decision you and your doctor will make. For clarithromycin, the following should be considered:

**Allergies**—Tell your doctor if you have ever had any unusual or allergic reaction to clarithromycin or to any related medicines, such as erythromycin. Also tell your health care professional if you are allergic to any other substances, such as foods, preservatives, or dyes.

**Pregnancy**—Clarithromycin has not been studied in pregnant women. However, studies in animals have shown that clarithromycin causes birth defects and other problems. Before taking this medicine, make sure your doctor knows if you are pregnant or if you may become pregnant.

**Breast-feeding**—Clarithromycin passes into breast milk.

**Children**—Studies on this medicine have not been done in children up to 6 months of age. In effective doses, the medicine has not been shown to cause different side effects or problems in children over the age of 6 months than it does in adults.

**Older adults**—This medicine has been tested in a limited number of elderly patients and has not been shown to cause different side effects or problems in older people than it does in younger adults.

**Other medicines**—Although certain medicines should not be used together at all, in other cases two different medicines may be used together even if an interaction might occur. In these cases, your doctor may want to change the dose, or other precautions may be necessary. When you are taking clarithromycin, it is especially important that your health care professional know if you are taking any of the following:
• Carbamazepine (e.g., Tegretol) or
• Terfenadine (e.g., Seldane) or
• Theophylline (e.g., Theodur, Slo-Bid)—Clarithromycin may increase the chance of side effects of these medicines
• Rifabutin (e.g., Mycobutin)—Rifabutin may decrease the amount of clarithromycin in the blood

- Zidovudine (e.g., Retrovir)—Clarithromycin may decrease the amount of zidovudine in the blood

**Other medical problems**—The presence of other medical problems may affect the use of clarithromycin. Make sure you tell your doctor if you have any other medical problems, especially:

- Kidney disease—Patients with severe kidney disease may have an increased chance of side effects

## Proper Use of This Medicine

Clarithromycin may be taken with meals or milk or on an empty stomach.

To help clear up your infection completely, *keep taking clarithromycin for the full time of treatment,* even if you begin to feel better after a few days. If you stop taking this medicine too soon, your symptoms may return.

If you are using *clarithromycin oral suspension*, use a specially marked measuring spoon or other device to measure each dose accurately. The average household teaspoon may not hold the right amount of liquid.

**Dosing**—The dose of clarithromycin will be different for different patients. *Follow your doctor's orders or the directions on the label.* The following information includes only the average doses of clarithromycin. Your dose may be different if you have kidney disease. *If your dose is different, do not change it* unless your doctor tells you to do so:

The number of tablets or teaspoonfuls of suspension that you take depends on the strength of the medicine.

- For *oral* dosage forms (suspension and tablets):
  —For bacterial infections:
  - Adults and teenagers—250 to 500 milligrams (mg) every twelve hours for seven to fourteen days.
  - Children 6 months of age and older—Use and dose must be determined by your doctor. However, 7.5 mg per kilogram (kg) (3.4 mg per pound) of body weight every twelve hours has been used.
  —For treatment of *Mycobacterium avium* complex (MAC):
  - Adults and teenagers—500 mg every twelve hours.
  - Children 6 months of age and older—7.5 mg per kg (3.4 mg per pound) of body weight, up to 500 mg, every twelve hours.

**Missed dose**—If you miss a dose of this medicine, take it as soon as possible. However, if it is almost time for your next dose, skip the missed dose and go back to your regular dosing schedule. Do not double doses.

**Storage**—To store this medicine:
- Keep out of the reach of children.
- Store away from heat and direct light.
- Do not store in the bathroom, near the kitchen sink, or in other damp places. Heat or moisture may cause the medicine to break down.
- Do not keep outdated medicine or medicine no longer needed. Be sure that any discarded medicine is out of the reach of children.

## Precautions While Using This Medicine

If your symptoms do not improve within a few days, or if they become worse, check with your doctor.

## Side Effects of This Medicine

Along with its needed effects, a medicine may cause some unwanted effects. Although neither of these side effects may occur, if they do occur they may need medical attention. Check with your doctor as soon as possible if either of the following side effects occur:

*Rare*
Unusual bleeding or bruising

Other side effects may occur that usually do not need medical attention. These side effects may go away during treatment as your body adjusts to the medicine. However, check with your doctor if any of the following side effects continue or are bothersome:

*Less common*
Abnormal taste; diarrhea; headache; nausea; stomach pain or discomfort; vomiting

Other side effects not listed above may also occur in some patients. If you notice any other effects, check with your doctor.

## Additional Information

Once a medicine has been approved for marketing for a certain use, experience may show that it is also useful for other medical problems. Although this use is not included in product labeling, clarithromycin is used in certain patients with the following medical condition:

- Legionnaires' disease

Other than the above information, there is no additional information relating to proper use, precautions, or side effects for this use.

Revised: 06/27/94

# CLINDAMYCIN   Systemic

Some commonly used brand names are:

**In the U.S.**
Cleocin
Cleocin Pediatric
Generic name product may also be available.

**In Canada**
Dalacin C                    Dalacin C Phosphate
Dalacin C Palmitate

## Description

Clindamycin (klin-da-MYE-sin) is used to treat bacterial infections. It will not work for colds, flu, or other virus infections.

Clindamycin is available only with your doctor's prescription, in the following dosage forms:

*Oral*
- Capsules (U.S. and Canada)
- Oral solution (U.S. and Canada)

*Parenteral*
- Injection (U.S. and Canada)

## Before Using This Medicine

In deciding to use a medicine, the risks of taking the medicine must be weighed against the good it will do. This is a decision you and your doctor will make. For clindamycin, the following should be considered:

**Allergies**—Tell your doctor if you have ever had any unusual or allergic reaction to clindamycin, lincomycin, or doxorubicin. Also tell your health care professional if you are allergic to any other substances, such as foods, preservatives, or dyes.

**Pregnancy**—Clindamycin has not been reported to cause birth defects or other problems in humans.

**Breast-feeding**—Clindamycin passes into the breast milk. However, clindamycin has not been reported to cause problems in nursing babies.

**Children**—This medicine has been tested in children and, in effective doses, has not been reported to cause different side effects or problems than it does in adults.

**Older adults**—Many medicines have not been studied specifically in older people. Therefore, it may not be known whether they work exactly the same way they do in younger adults or if they cause different side effects or problems in older people. There is no specific information comparing use of clindamycin in the elderly with use in other age groups.

**Other medicines**—Although certain medicines should not be used together at all, in other cases two different medicines may be used together even if an interaction might occur. In these cases, your doctor may want to change the dose, or other precautions may be necessary. When you are taking clindamycin, it is especially important that

your health care professional know if you are taking any of the following:
- Chloramphenicol (e.g., Chloromycetin) or
- Diarrhea medicine containing kaolin or attapulgite or
- Erythromycins (medicine for infection)—Taking these medicines along with clindamycin may decrease the effects of clindamycin

**Other medical problems**—The presence of other medical problems may affect the use of clindamycin. Make sure you tell your doctor if you have any other medical problems, especially:
- Kidney disease (severe) or
- Liver disease (severe)—Severe kidney or liver disease may increase blood levels of this medicine, increasing the chance of side effects
- Stomach or intestinal disease, history of (especially colitis, including colitis caused by antibiotics, or enteritis)—Patients with a history of stomach or intestinal disease may have an increased chance of side effects

## Proper Use of This Medicine

For patients taking the *capsule form* of clindamycin:
- *The capsule form of clindamycin should be taken with a full glass (8 ounces) of water or with meals* to prevent irritation of the esophagus (tube between the throat and stomach).

For patients taking the *oral liquid form* of clindamycin:
- Use a specially marked measuring spoon or other device to measure each dose accurately. The average household teaspoon may not hold the right amount of liquid.
- Do not use after the expiration date on the label. The medicine may not work properly after this date. Check with your pharmacist if you have any questions about this.

To help clear up your infection completely, *keep taking this medicine for the full time of treatment,* even if you begin to feel better after a few days. *If you have a "strep" infection, you should keep taking this medicine for at least 10 days. This is especially important in "strep" infections. Serious heart problems could develop later* if your infection is not cleared up completely. Also, if you stop taking this medicine too soon, your symptoms may return.

This medicine works best when there is a constant amount in the blood. *To help keep the amount constant, do not miss any doses. Also, it is best to take each dose at evenly spaced times day and night.* For example, if you are to take 4 doses a day, doses should be spaced about 6 hours apart. If this interferes with your sleep or other daily activities, or if you need help in planning the best times to take your medicine, check with your health care professional.

**Dosing**—The dose of clindamycin will be different for different patients. *Follow your doctor's orders or the* *directions on the label.* The following information includes only the average doses of clindamycin. *If your dose is different, do not change it* unless your doctor tells you to do so.

The number of capsules or teaspoonfuls of solution that you take depends on the strength of the medicine. Also, *the number of doses you take each day, the time allowed between doses, and the length of time you take the medicine depend on the medical problem for which you are taking clindamycin.*

- For bacterial infection:
  —For *oral* dosage forms (capsules and solution):
  - Adults and teenagers—150 to 300 milligrams (mg) every six hours.
  - Children—
    —Infants up to 1 month of age: Use and dose must be determined by your doctor.
    —Infants and children 1 month of age and older: Dose is based on body weight. The usual dose is 2 to 5 mg per kilogram (kg) (0.9 to 2.3 mg per pound) of body weight every six hours; or 2.7 to 6.7 mg per kg (1.2 to 3.0 mg per pound) of body weight every eight hours.
  —For *injection* dosage form:
  - Adults and teenagers—300 to 600 mg every six to eight hours injected into a muscle or vein; or 900 mg every eight hours injected into a muscle or vein.
  - Children—
    —Infants up to 1 month of age: Dose is based on body weight. The usual dose is 3.75 to 5 mg per kg (1.7 to 2.3 mg per pound) of body weight every six hours injected into a muscle or vein; or 5 to 6.7 mg per kg (2.3 to 3.0 mg per pound) of body weight every eight hours injected into a muscle or vein.
    —Infants and children 1 month of age and older: Dose is based on body weight. The usual dose is 3.75 to 10 mg per kg (1.7 to 4.5 mg per pound) of body weight every six hours injected into a muscle or vein; or 5 to 13.3 mg per kg (2.3 to 6.0 mg per pound) of body weight every eight hours injected into a muscle or vein.

**Missed dose**—If you miss a dose of this medicine, take it as soon as possible. This will help to keep a constant amount of medicine in the blood. However, if it is almost time for your next dose, skip the missed dose and go back to your regular dosing schedule. Do not double doses.

**Storage**—To store this medicine:
- Keep out of the reach of children.
- Store away from heat and direct light.
- Do not store the capsule form of this medicine in the bathroom, near the kitchen sink, or in other damp places. Heat or moisture may cause the medicine to break down.

- Do not refrigerate the oral liquid form of clindamycin. If chilled, the liquid may thicken and be difficult to pour. Follow the directions on the label.
- Do not keep outdated medicine or medicine no longer needed. Be sure that any discarded medicine is out of the reach of children.

## Precautions While Using This Medicine

It is important that your doctor check your progress at regular visits.

If your symptoms do not improve within a few days, or if they become worse, check with your doctor.

In some patients, clindamycin may cause diarrhea.
- Severe diarrhea may be a sign of a serious side effect. *Do not take any diarrhea medicine without first checking with your doctor.* Diarrhea medicines, such as loperamide (Imodium A-D) or diphenoxylate and atropine (Lomotil), may make your diarrhea worse or make it last longer.
- For mild diarrhea, diarrhea medicine containing attapulgite (e.g., Kaopectate tablets, Diasorb) may be taken. However, attapulgite may keep clindamycin from being absorbed into the body. Therefore, these diarrhea medicines should be taken at least 2 hours before or 3 to 4 hours after you take clindamycin by mouth.
- If you have any questions about this or if mild diarrhea continues or gets worse, check with your health care professional.

Before having surgery (including dental surgery) with a general anesthetic, tell the medical doctor or dentist in charge that you are taking clindamycin.

## Side Effects of This Medicine

Along with its needed effects, a medicine may cause some unwanted effects. Although not all of these side effects may occur, if they do occur they may need medical attention.

*Check with your doctor immediately* if any of the following side effects occur:

*More common*
Abdominal or stomach cramps and pain (severe); abdominal tenderness; diarrhea (watery and severe), which may also be bloody; fever (the above side effects may also occur up to several weeks after you stop taking this medicine)

*Less common*
Sore throat and fever; skin rash, redness, and itching; unusual bleeding or bruising

Other side effects may occur that usually do not need medical attention. These side effects may go away during treatment as your body adjusts to the medicine. However, check with your doctor if any of the following side effects continue or are bothersome:

*More common*

Diarrhea (mild); nausea and vomiting; stomach pain

*Less common*

Itching of rectal, or genital (sex organ) areas

Other side effects not listed above may also occur in some patients. If you notice any other effects, check with your doctor.

Revised: 08/12/92
Interim revision: 03/18/94

# CLINDAMYCIN   Topical

Some commonly used brand names are:

**In the U.S.**

Cleocin T Gel                    Cleocin T Topical Solution
Cleocin T Lotion                 Clinda-Derm

Generic name product may also be available.

**In Canada**

Dalacin T Topical Solution

## Description

Clindamycin (klin-da-MYE-sin) belongs to the family of medicines called antibiotics. Topical clindamycin is used to help control acne. It may be used alone or with one or more other medicines that are used on the skin or taken by mouth for acne. Topical clindamycin may also be used for other problems as determined by your doctor.

Clindamycin is available only with your doctor's prescription, in the following dosage forms:

*Topical*

- Gel (U.S.)
- Solution (U.S. and Canada)
- Suspension (U.S.)

## Before Using This Medicine

In deciding to use a medicine, the risks of using the medicine must be weighed against the good it will do. This is a decision you and your doctor will make. For topical clindamycin, the following should be considered:

**Allergies**—Tell your doctor if you have ever had any unusual or allergic reaction to this medicine or any of the other clindamycins (by mouth or by injection) or to lincomycin. Also tell your health care professional if you are allergic to any other substances, such as preservatives or dyes.

**Pregnancy**—Clindamycin has not been studied in pregnant women. However, this medicine has not been shown to cause birth defects or other problems in animal studies.

**Breast-feeding**—Small amounts of topical clindamycin are absorbed through the skin. It is possible that small amounts of the medicine may pass into the breast milk. However, this medicine has not been reported to cause problems in nursing babies.

**Children**—Studies on this medicine have been done only in adult patients, and there is no specific information comparing use of this medicine in children up to 12 years of age with use in other age groups.

**Older adults**—Many medicines have not been studied specifically in older people. Therefore, it may not be known whether they work exactly the same way they do in younger adults. Although there is no specific information comparing use of this medicine in the elderly with use in other age groups, this medicine is not expected to cause different side effects or problems in older people than it does in younger adults.

**Other medicines**—Although certain medicines should not be used together at all, in other cases two different medicines may be used together even if an interaction might occur. In these cases, your doctor may want to change the dose, or other precautions may be necessary. Tell your health care professional if you are using any other prescription or nonprescription (over-the-counter [OTC]) medicine.

**Other medical problems**—The presence of other medical problems may affect the use of topical clindamycin. Make sure you tell your doctor if you have any other medical problems, especially:

- History of stomach or intestinal disease (especially colitis, including colitis caused by antibiotics, or enteritis)—These conditions may increase the chance of side effects that affect the stomach and intestines

## Proper Use of This Medicine

Before applying this medicine, thoroughly wash the affected areas with warm water and soap, rinse well, and pat dry.

When applying the medicine, use enough to cover the affected area lightly. *You should apply the medicine to the whole area usually affected by acne, not just to the pimples themselves.* This will help keep new pimples from breaking out.

You should avoid washing the acne-affected areas too often. This may dry your skin and make your acne worse. Washing with a mild, bland soap 2 or 3 times a day should be enough, unless you have oily skin. If you have any questions about this, check with your doctor.

Topical clindamycin will not cure your acne. However, to help keep your acne under control, *keep using this medicine for the full time of treatment,* even if your symptoms begin to clear up after a few days. You may have to continue using this medicine every day for months or even longer in some cases. If you stop using this medicine too soon, your symptoms may return. *It is important that you do not miss any doses.*

For patients using the *topical solution form* of clindamycin:

- After washing or shaving, it is best to wait 30 minutes before applying this medicine. The alcohol in it may irritate freshly washed or shaved skin.
- This medicine contains alcohol and is flammable. *Do not use near heat, near open flame, or while smoking.*
- To apply this medicine:
  —This medicine comes in a bottle with an applicator tip, which may be used to apply the medicine directly to the skin. Use the applicator with a dabbing motion instead of a rolling motion (not like a roll-on deodorant, for example). Tilt the bottle and press the tip firmly against your skin. If needed, you can make the medicine flow faster from the applicator tip by slightly increasing the pressure against the skin. If the medicine flows too fast, use less pressure. If the applicator tip becomes dry, turn the bottle upside down and press the tip several times to moisten it.
  —Since this medicine contains alcohol, it will sting or burn. In addition, it has an unpleasant taste if it gets on the mouth or lips. Therefore, *do not get this medicine in the eyes, nose, or mouth, or on other mucous membranes.* Spread the medicine away from these areas when applying. If this medicine does get in the eyes, wash them out immediately, but carefully, with large amounts of cool tap water. If your eyes still burn or are painful, check with your doctor.
- It is important that you do not use this medicine more often than your doctor ordered. It may cause your skin to become too dry or irritated.

For patients using the *topical suspension form* of clindamycin:

- *Shake well* before applying.

**Dosing**—The dose of topical clindamycin will be different for different patients. *Follow your doctor's orders or the directions on the label.* The following information includes only the average doses of topical clindamycin. *If your dose is different, do not change it* unless your doctor tells you to do so.

*The number of doses you use each day, the time allowed between doses, and the length of time you use the medicine depend on the medical problem for which you are using clindamycin.*

- For *topical* dosage forms (gel, solution, and suspension):
  —For acne:
  • Adults and children 12 years of age and over— Apply two times a day to areas affected by acne.

- Infants and children up to 12 years of age— Use and dose must be determined by your doctor.

**Missed dose**—If you miss a dose of this medicine, apply it as soon as possible. However, if it is almost time for your next dose, skip the missed dose and go back to your regular dosing schedule.

**Storage**—To store this medicine:

- Keep out of the reach of children.
- Store away from heat and direct light.
- Keep the medicine from freezing.
- Do not keep outdated medicine or medicine no longer needed. Be sure that any discarded medicine is out of the reach of children.

---

## Precautions While Using This Medicine

If your acne does not improve within about 6 weeks, or if it becomes worse, check with your health care professional. However, treatment of acne may take up to 8 to 12 weeks before full improvement is seen.

If your doctor has ordered another medicine to be applied to the skin along with this medicine, it is best to apply them at different times. This may help keep your skin from becoming too irritated. Also, if the medicines are used at or near the same time, they may not work properly.

For patients using the *topical solution form* of clindamycin:

- This medicine may cause the skin to become unusually dry, even with normal use. If this occurs, check with your doctor.

In some patients, clindamycin may cause diarrhea.

- Severe diarrhea may be a sign of a serious side effect. *Do not take any diarrhea medicine without first checking with your doctor.* Diarrhea medicines may make your diarrhea worse or make it last longer.
- For mild diarrhea, only diarrhea medicine containing attapulgite (e.g., Kaopectate, Diasorb) may be taken. Other kinds of diarrhea medicine (e.g., Imodium A.D. or Lomotil) should not be taken. They may make your condition worse or make it last longer.
- If you have any questions about this or if mild diarrhea continues or gets worse, check with your health care professional.

You may continue to use cosmetics (make-up) while you are using this medicine for acne. However, it is best to use only "water-base" cosmetics. Also, it is best not to use cosmetics too heavily or too often. They may make your acne worse. If you have any questions about this, check with your doctor.

---

## Side Effects of This Medicine

Along with its needed effects, a medicine may cause some unwanted effects. Although not all of these side effects

may occur, if they do occur they may need medical attention.

*Check with your doctor immediately* if any of the following side effects occur:

> *Rare*
>> Abdominal or stomach cramps, pain, and bloating (severe); diarrhea (watery and severe), which may also be bloody; fever; increased thirst; nausea or vomiting; unusual tiredness or weakness; weight loss (unusual)—these side effects may also occur up to several weeks after you stop using this medicine

Also, check with your doctor as soon as possible if any of the following side effects occur:

> *Less common*
>> Skin rash, itching, redness, swelling, or other sign of irritation not present before use of this medicine

Other side effects may occur that usually do not need medical attention. These side effects may go away during treatment as your body adjusts to the medicine. However, check with your doctor if any of the following side effects continue or are bothersome:

> *More common*
>> Dryness, scaliness, or peeling of skin (for the topical solution)
> *Less common*
>> Abdominal pain; diarrhea (mild); irritation or oiliness of skin; stinging or burning feeling of skin

Other side effects not listed above may also occur in some patients. If you notice any other effects, check with your doctor.

Revised: 02/22/94

---

# CLINDAMYCIN   Vaginal†

A commonly used brand name in the U.S. is Cleocin.

†Not commercially available in Canada.

## Description

Clindamycin (klin-da-MYE-sin) is used to treat certain vaginal infections. It works by killing the bacteria. This medicine will not work for vaginal fungus or yeast infections.

Clindamycin is available only with your doctor's prescription, in the following dosage form:

> *Vaginal*
> • Cream (U.S.)

## Before Using This Medicine

In deciding to use a medicine, the risks of taking the medicine must be weighed against the good it will do. This is a decision you and your doctor will make. For vaginal clindamycin, the following should be considered:

**Allergies**—Tell your doctor if you have ever had any unusual or allergic reaction to clindamycin or lincomycin (e.g., Lincocin). Also tell your health care professional if you are allergic to any other substances, such as foods, preservatives, or dyes.

**Pregnancy**—Vaginal clindamycin is used during all stages of pregnancy. It was found to cause birth defects in one strain of mouse, but has not caused problems in other animals. Vaginal clindamycin has not been reported to cause birth defects or other problems in humans.

**Breast-feeding**—It is not known whether clindamycin used vaginally passes into the breast milk. Clindamycin taken by mouth does pass into the breast milk and has not been

reported to cause problems in nursing babies. Although most medicines pass into the breast milk in small amounts, many of them may be used safely while breast-feeding. Mothers who are using this medicine and who wish to breast-feed should discuss this with their doctor.

**Children**—Studies on this medicine have been done only in adult patients, and there is no specific information comparing use of vaginal clindamycin in children with use in other age groups.

**Older adults**—Many medicines have not been studied specifically in older people. Therefore, it may not be known whether they work exactly the same way they do in younger adults or if they cause different side effects or problems in older people. There is no specific information comparing use of vaginal clindamycin in the elderly with use in other age groups.

**Other medicines**—Although certain medicines should not be used together at all, in other cases two different medicines may be used together even if an interaction might occur. In these cases, your doctor may want to change the dose, or other precautions may be necessary. Tell your health care professional if you are taking or using any other prescription or nonprescription (over-the-counter [OTC]) medicine.

**Other medical problems**—The presence of other medical problems may affect the use of vaginal clindamycin. Make sure you tell your doctor if you have any other medical problems, especially:

• Stomach or intestinal disease, history of (especially colitis, including colitis caused by antibiotics, or enteritis)—Patients with a history of stomach or intestinal disease may have an increased chance of side effects including diarrhea

## Proper Use of This Medicine

Wash your hands before and after using this medicine.

Avoid getting this medicine in your eyes. If this medicine does get into your eyes, rinse them immediately with large amounts of cool tap water. If your eyes still burn or are painful, check with your doctor.

Vaginal clindamycin usually comes with patient directions. Read them carefully before using this medicine.

Use clindamycin vaginal cream exactly as directed by your doctor.

- *To fill the applicator*
  —Remove cap from the tube.
  —Screw one of the applicators onto the tube. Always use a new applicator. Never use one that has been used before.
  —Squeeze the medicine into the applicator slowly until it is full.
  —Remove the applicator from the tube. Replace the cap on the tube.
- *To insert the vaginal cream using the applicator*
  —Relax while lying on your back with your knees bent.
  —Hold the full applicator in one hand. Insert it slowly into the vagina. Stop before it becomes uncomfortable.
  —Slowly press the plunger until it stops.
  —Withdraw the applicator. The medicine will be left behind in the vagina.
- *To care for the applicator*
  —Throw the applicator away after you use it.

To help clear up your infection completely, *it is very important that you keep using this medicine for the full time of treatment,* even if your symptoms begin to clear up after a few days. If you stop using this medicine too soon, your symptoms may return. *Do not miss any doses.* Also, *continue using this medicine even if your menstrual period starts during the time of treatment.*

**Dosing**—The dose of vaginal clindamycin will be different for different patients. The following information includes only the average dose of vaginal clindamycin. *If your dose is different, do not change it* unless your doctor tells you to do so.

- For *vaginal cream* dosage form:
  —For bacterial vaginosis:
    - Adults and teenagers—One applicatorful (100 milligrams [mg]) inserted into the vagina once a day, usually at bedtime, for seven days.
    - Children—Use and dose must be determined by your doctor.

**Missed dose**—If you miss a dose of this medicine, use it as soon as possible. However, if it is almost time for your next dose, skip the missed dose and go back to your regular dosing schedule. Do not double doses.

**Storage**—To store this medicine:
- Keep out of the reach of children.
- Store away from heat and direct light.
- Keep the medicine from freezing. Do not refrigerate.
- Do not keep outdated medicine or medicine no longer needed. Be sure that any discarded medicine is out of the reach of children.

## Precautions While Using This Medicine

If your symptoms do not improve within a few days, or if they become worse, check with your doctor.

It is important that you visit your doctor after you have used all your medicine to make sure that the infection is gone.

This medicine may cause some people to become dizzy. Make sure you know how you react to this medicine before you drive, use machines, or do anything else that could be dangerous if you are dizzy.

Vaginal medicines usually leak out of the vagina during treatment. To keep the medicine from getting on your clothing, wear a minipad or sanitary napkin. Do not use tampons since they may soak up the medicine.

*To help clear up your infection completely and make sure it does not return,* good health habits are also required.

- Wear cotton panties (or panties or pantyhose with cotton crotches) instead of synthetic (for example, nylon or rayon) panties.
- Wear only freshly washed panties daily.

*Do not have sexual intercourse while you are using this medicine.* Having sexual intercourse may reduce the strength of the medicine. This may cause the medicine to not work as well.

*Do not use latex (rubber) contraceptive products such as condoms, diaphragms, or cervical caps for 72 hours after stopping treatment with vaginal clindamycin cream.* The cream contains oils that weaken or harm the latex products, causing them to not work properly to prevent pregnancy. If you have any questions about this, check with your health care professional.

## Side Effects of This Medicine

Along with its needed effects, a medicine may cause some unwanted effects. Although not all of these side effects may occur, if they do occur they may need medical attention.

Check with your doctor as soon as possible if any of the following side effects occur:

*More common*
   Itching of the vagina or genital area; pain during sexual intercourse; thick, white vaginal discharge with no odor or with mild odor

*Less common*

Diarrhea; dizziness; headache; nausea or vomiting; stomach pain or cramps

*Rare*

Burning, itching, rash, redness, swelling or other signs of skin problems not present before use of this medicine

After you stop using this medicine, your body may need time to adjust. The length of time this takes depends on the amount of medicine you were using and how long you used it. During this period of time check with your doctor if you notice any of the following side effects:

Itching of the vagina or genital area; pain during sexual intercourse; thick, white vaginal discharge with no odor or with mild odor

Other side effects not listed above may also occur in some patients. If you notice any other effects, check with your doctor.

Developed: 06/29/94

# CLIOQUINOL   Topical

A commonly used brand name in the U.S. and Canada is Vioform. Another commonly used name is iodochlorhydroxyquin.

## Description

Clioquinol (klye-oh-KWIN-ole) belongs to the family of medicines called anti-infectives. Clioquinol topical preparations are used to treat skin infections.

Clioquinol is available without a prescription; however, your doctor may have special instructions on the proper use of this medicine for your medical problem. It is available in the following dosage forms:

*Topical*
- Cream (U.S. and Canada)
- Ointment (U.S. and Canada)

## Before Using This Medicine

If you are using this medicine without a prescription, carefully read and follow any precautions on the label. For clioquinol, the following should be considered:

**Allergies**—Tell your doctor if you have ever had any unusual or allergic reaction to clioquinol, chloroxine (e.g., capitrol), iodine, or iodine-containing preparations. Also tell your health care professional if you are allergic to any other substances, such as preservatives or dyes.

**Pregnancy**—Clioquinol topical preparations have not been shown to cause birth defects or other problems in humans.

**Breast-feeding**—Clioquinol topical preparations have not been reported to cause problems in nursing babies.

**Children**—Clioquinol is not recommended in children under 2 years of age. Although there is no specific information comparing use of this medicine in children 2 years of age and over with use in other age groups, this medicine is not expected to cause different side effects or problems in children than it does in adults.

**Older adults**—Many medicines have not been studied specifically in older people. Therefore, it may not be known whether they work exactly the same way they do in younger adults. Although there is no specific information comparing use of this medicine in the elderly with use in other age groups, this medicine is not expected to cause different side effects or problems in older people than it does in younger adults.

**Other medicines**—Although certain medicines should not be used together at all, in other cases two different medicines may be used together even if an interaction might occur. In these cases, your doctor may want to change the dose, or other precautions may be necessary. Tell your health care professional if you are using any other prescription or nonprescription (over-the-counter [OTC]) medicine.

## Proper Use of This Medicine

Before applying this medicine, wash the affected area with soap and water, and dry thoroughly.

*Do not use this medicine in or around the eyes.*

To use the *cream form* of this medicine:
- Apply a thin layer of cream to the affected area and rub in gently until the cream disappears.

To use the *ointment form* of this medicine:
- Apply a thin layer of ointment to the affected area and rub in gently.

To help clear up your infection completely, *keep using this medicine for the full time of treatment,* even if your symptoms have disappeared. *Do not miss any doses.*

**Dosing**—The dose of clioquinol will be different for different patients. *Follow your doctor's orders or the directions on the label.* The following information includes only the average dose of clioquinol. *If your dose is different, do not change it* unless your doctor tells you to do so.
- For *topical* dosage forms (cream or ointment):
  —For bacterial or fungus infections:
    - Adults and children 2 years of age and over— Apply to the affected area(s) of the skin two or three times a day.

• Children up to 2 years of age—Use is not recommended.

**Missed dose**—If you miss a dose of this medicine, apply it as soon as possible. However, if it is almost time for your next dose, skip the missed dose and go back to your regular dosing schedule.

**Storage**—To store this medicine:

• Keep out of the reach of children.
• Store away from heat and direct light.
• Keep the medicine from freezing.
• Do not keep outdated medicine or medicine no longer needed. Be sure that any discarded medicine is out of the reach of children.

## Precautions While Using This Medicine

If your skin problem does not improve within 1 to 2 weeks, or if it becomes worse, check with your doctor.

This medicine may stain clothing, skin, hair, and nails yellow. Avoid getting this medicine on your clothing since bleaching may not remove the stain.

Before you have any medical tests, tell the doctor in charge that you are using this medicine. The results of some tests may be affected by this medicine.

## Side Effects of This Medicine

Along with its needed effects, a medicine may cause some unwanted effects. Although not all of these side effects may occur, if they do occur they may need medical attention.

*Check with your doctor immediately* if any of the following side effects occur:

*Rare*

Itching, rash, redness, swelling, or other sign of skin irritation not present before use of this medicine

Other side effects not listed above may also occur in some patients. If you notice any other effects, check with your doctor.

Revised: 02/10/92
Interim revision: 06/03/94

# CLIOQUINOL AND HYDROCORTISONE   Topical

Some commonly used brand names are:
**In the U.S.—**
Vioform-Hydrocortisone Cream
Vioform-Hydrocortisone Lotion
Vioform-Hydrocortisone Mild Cream
Vioform-Hydrocortisone Mild Ointment
Vioform-Hydrocortisone Ointment
**In Canada—**
Vioform-Hydrocortisone Cream
Vioform-Hydrocortisone Mild Cream
Vioform-Hydrocortisone Ointment

Another commonly used name is iodochlorhyroxyquin and hydrocortisone.

## Description

Clioquinol (klye-oh-KWIN-ole) and hydrocortisone (hye-droe-KOR-ti-sone) is a combined anti-infective and cortisone-like medicine. Clioquinol and hydrocortisone topical preparations are used to treat infections of the skin and to help provide relief from the redness, itching, and discomfort of many skin problems.

Clioquinol and hydrocortisone combination is available only with your doctor's prescription, in the following dosage forms:
*Topical*
• Cream (U.S. and Canada)
• Lotion (U.S.)
• Ointment (U.S. and Canada)

## Before Using This Medicine

In deciding to use a medicine, the risks of taking the medicine must be weighed against the good it will do.

This is a decision you and your doctor will make. For clioquinol and hydrocortisone combination, the following should be considered:

**Allergies**—Tell your doctor if you have ever had any unusual or allergic reaction to clioquinol, hydrocortisone, chloroxine (e.g., Capitrol), iodine, or iodine-containing preparations. Also tell your health care professional if you are allergic to any other substances, such as preservatives or dyes.

**Pregnancy**—Clioquinol and hydrocortisone topical preparations may be absorbed through the mother's skin. This medicine has not been shown to cause birth defects or other problems in humans. However, studies in animals have shown that it causes birth defects. Use of large amounts on the skin or use for a long time is not recommended during pregnancy.

**Breast-feeding**—Clioquinol and hydrocortisone topical preparations have not been reported to cause problems in nursing babies.

**Children**—Clioquinol and hydrocortisone combination is not recommended in children up to 2 years of age. Although there is no specific information comparing use of clioquinol and hydrocortisone combination in children over 2 years of age with use in other age groups, this medicine is not expected to cause different side effects or problems in these children than it does in adults.

**Older adults**—Many medicines have not been studied specifically in older people. Therefore, it may not be known

whether they work exactly the same way they do in younger adults. Although there is no specific information comparing use of clioquinol and hydrocortisone combination in the elderly with use in other age groups, this medicine is not expected to cause different side effects or problems in older people than it does in younger adults.

**Other medicines**—Although certain medicines should not be used together at all, in other cases two different medicines may be used together even if an interaction might occur. In these cases, your doctor may want to change the dose, or other precautions may be necessary. Tell your health care professional if you are using any other prescription or nonprescription (over-the-counter [OTC]) medicine.

**Other medical problems**—The presence of other medical problems may affect the use of clioquinol and hydrocortisone topical preparations. Make sure you tell your doctor if you have any other medical problems, especially:
- Skin infection (other)—Use of clioquinol and hydrocortisone topical preparations may make the condition worse

## Proper Use of This Medicine
Before applying this medicine, wash the affected area with soap and water, and dry thoroughly.

*Do not use this medicine in or around the eyes or on infants and children up to 2 years of age.*

To use the *cream form* of this medicine:
- Apply a thin layer of cream to the affected area and rub in gently until cream disappears.

To use the *lotion form* of this medicine:
- Gently squeeze bottle and apply a few drops of lotion to the affected area. Rub in gently until lotion disappears.

To use the *ointment form* of this medicine:
- Apply a thin layer of ointment to the affected area and rub in gently.

*Do not bandage or otherwise wrap the area of the skin being treated unless directed to do so by your doctor.*

*Check with your doctor before using this medicine on any other skin problems.* It should not be used on certain kinds of bacterial, virus, or fungus skin infections.

To help clear up your infection completely, *keep using this medicine for the full time of treatment*, even if your symptoms have disappeared. *Do not miss any doses.* However, *do not use this medicine more often or for a longer time than your doctor ordered.* To do so may increase the chance of absorption through the skin and the chance of side effects. In addition, too much use, especially on thin skin areas (for example, face, armpits, groin), may result in thinning of the skin and stretch marks.

**Dosing**—The dose of clioquinol and hydrocortisone combination will be different for different patients. *Follow your doctor's orders or the directions on the label.* The following information includes only the average dose of clioquinol and hydrocortisone combination. *If your dose is different, do not change it* unless your doctor tells you to do so.
- For *topical* dosage forms (cream, lotion, or ointment):
  —For bacterial and fungus infections:
  - Adults, teenagers, and children 2 years of age and over—Apply to the affected area(s) of the skin three or four times a day.
  - Children up to 2 years of age—Use is not recommended.

**Missed dose**—If you miss a dose of this medicine, apply it as soon as possible. However, if it is almost time for your next dose, skip the missed dose and go back to your regular dosing schedule.

**Storage**—To store this medicine:
- Keep out of the reach of children.
- Store away from heat and direct light.
- Keep the medicine from freezing.
- Do not keep outdated medicine or medicine no longer needed. Be sure that any discarded medicine is out of the reach of children.

## Precautions While Using This Medicine
If your skin problem does not improve within 1 to 2 weeks, or if it becomes worse, check with your doctor.

This medicine may be absorbed through the skin, and too much use can affect growth. *Children who must use this medicine should be followed closely by their doctor.*

This medicine may stain clothing, skin, hair, and nails yellow. Avoid getting this medicine on your clothing. Bleaching may not remove the stain.

## Side Effects of This Medicine
Along with its needed effects, a medicine may cause some unwanted effects. Although not all of these side effects may occur, if they do occur they may need medical attention.

*Check with your doctor immediately* if any of the following side effects occur:
*Rare*
 Blistering, burning, itching, peeling, skin rash, redness, swelling, or other sign of irritation not present before use of this medicine
*With prolonged use*
 Thinning of skin with easy bruising

Other side effects not listed above may also occur in some patients. If you notice any other effects, check with your doctor.

Revised: 02/10/92
Interim revision: 07/14/94

# CLOFAZIMINE    Systemic†

A commonly used brand name in the U.S. is Lamprene.

---

†Not commercially available in Canada.

---

## Description

Clofazimine (kloe-FA-zi-meen) is taken to treat leprosy (Hansen's disease). It is sometimes given with other medicines for leprosy. When this medicine is used to treat "flare-ups" of leprosy, it may be given with a cortisone-like medicine. Clofazimine may also be used for other problems as determined by your doctor.

This medicine is available only with your doctor's prescription, in the following dosage form:

*Oral*
- Capsules (U.S.)

---

## Before Using This Medicine

In deciding to use a medicine, the risks of taking the medicine must be weighed against the good it will do. This is a decision you and your doctor will make. For clofazimine, the following should be considered:

**Allergies**—Tell your doctor if you have ever had any unusual or allergic reaction to clofazimine. Also tell your health care professional if you are allergic to any other substances, such as foods, preservatives, or dyes.

**Pregnancy**—Clofazimine has not been studied in pregnant women. Although the skin of babies born to mothers who took clofazimine during pregnancy was deeply discolored, this medicine has not been shown to cause birth defects or other problems in humans. A gradual fading of the discoloration may occur over a period of about a year. Some animal studies have not shown that clofazimine causes birth defects. However, studies in mice have shown that clofazimine may cause slow bone formation of the skull and a decrease in successful pregnancies. Before you take clofazimine, make sure your doctor knows if you are pregnant or if you may become pregnant.

**Breast-feeding**—Clofazimine passes into the breast milk. Use is not recommended in nursing mothers.

**Children**—Studies on this medicine have been done only in adult patients, and there is no specific information comparing use of clofazimine in children with use in other age groups.

**Older adults**—Many medicines have not been studied specifically in older people. Therefore, it may not be known whether they work exactly the same way they do in younger adults or if they cause different side effects or problems in older people. There is no specific information comparing use of clofazimine in the elderly with use in other age groups.

**Other medicines**—Although certain medicines should not be used together at all, in other cases two different medicines may be used together even if an interaction might occur. In these cases, your doctor may want to change the dose, or other precautions may be necessary. Tell your health care professional if you are taking any other prescription or nonprescription (over-the-counter [OTC]) medicine.

**Other medical problems**—The presence of other medical problems may affect the use of clofazimine. Make sure you tell your doctor if you have any other medical problems, especially:
- Liver disease—Clofazimine may on rare occasion cause hepatitis and liver disease
- Stomach or intestinal problems, history of—Clofazimine often causes some stomach upset, but on rare occasion may cause severe, sharp abdominal pain and burning, which may be a sign of a serious side effect

---

## Proper Use of This Medicine

Clofazimine should be taken with meals or milk.

To help clear up your leprosy completely, *it is very important that you keep taking clofazimine for the full time of treatment,* even if you begin to feel better after a few months. You may have to take it every day for as long as 2 years to life. If you stop taking this medicine too soon, your symptoms may return.

This medicine works best when there is a constant amount in the blood. *To help keep the amount constant, do not miss any doses. Also, it is best to take each dose at the same time every day.* If you need help in planning the best time to take your medicine, check with your health care professional.

**Dosing**—The dose of clofazimine will be different for different patients. *Follow your doctor's orders or the directions on the label.* The following information includes only the average doses of clofazimine. *If your dose is different, do not change it* unless your doctor tells you to do so.

The number of capsules that you take depends on the strength of the medicine. Also, *the number of doses you take each day, the time allowed between doses, and the length of time you take the medicine depend on the medical problem for which you are taking clofazimine.*
- For the *treatment of leprosy (Hansen's disease):*
  —Adults and teenagers: 50 to 100 milligrams once a day. This medicine must be taken with other medicines for the treatment of Hansen's disease.
  —Children: Dose must be determined by the doctor.

**Missed dose**—If you miss a dose of this medicine, take it as soon as possible. However, if it is almost time for your next dose, skip the missed dose and go back to your regular dosing schedule. Do not double doses.

---

**Storage**—To store this medicine:
- Keep out of the reach of children.
- Store away from heat and direct light.
- Do not store in the bathroom, near the kitchen sink, or in other damp places. Heat or moisture may cause the medicine to break down.
- Do not keep outdated medicine or medicine no longer needed. Be sure that any discarded medicine is out of the reach of children.

## Precautions While Using This Medicine

If your symptoms do not improve within 1 to 3 months, or if they become worse, check with your doctor. It may take up to 6 months before the full benefit of this medicine is seen.

Clofazimine may cause pink or red to brownish-black discoloration of the skin within a few weeks after you start taking it. Because of the skin discoloration, some patients may become depressed. The discoloration will go away when you stop taking this medicine. However, it may take several months or years for the skin to clear up completely. *If skin discoloration causes you to feel very depressed or to have thoughts of suicide, check with your doctor immediately.*

This medicine may cause some people to become dizzy, drowsy, or less alert than they are normally. *Make sure you know how you react to this medicine before you drive, use machines, or do anything else that could be dangerous if you are dizzy or are not alert or able to see well.* If these reactions are especially bothersome, check with your doctor.

Clofazimine may cause your skin to become more sensitive to sunlight than it is normally. Exposure to sunlight, even for brief periods of time, may cause a skin rash, itching, redness, or other discoloration of the skin, or a severe sunburn. When you begin taking this medicine:
- Stay out of direct sunlight, especially between the hours of 10:00 a.m. and 3:00 p.m., if possible.
- Wear protective clothing, including a hat. Also, wear sunglasses.
- Apply a sun block product that has a skin protection factor (SPF) of at least 15. Some patients may require a product with a higher SPF number, especially if they have a fair complexion. If you have any questions about this, check with your health care professional.

- Apply a sun block lipstick that has an SPF of at least 15 to protect your lips.
- Do not use a sunlamp or tanning bed or booth.

*If you have a severe reaction, check with your doctor.*

Clofazimine may also cause dry, rough, or scaly skin. A skin cream, lotion, or oil may help to treat this problem.

## Side Effects of This Medicine

Along with its needed effects, a medicine may cause some unwanted effects. Although not all of these side effects may occur, if they do occur they may need medical attention.

*Check with your doctor immediately* if any of the following side effects occur:
*Rare*
    Bloody or black, tarry stools; colicky or burning abdominal or stomach pain; mental depression; yellow eyes or skin—may be an orange color if already have a pink to brownish-black skin or eye discoloration

Other side effects may occur that usually do not need medical attention. These side effects may go away during treatment as your body adjusts to the medicine. However, check with your doctor if any of the following side effects continue or are bothersome:
*More common*
    Diarrhea; dry, rough, or scaly skin; loss of appetite; nausea or vomiting; pink or red to brownish-black discoloration of skin and eyes; skin rash and itching
*Less common or rare*
    Changes in taste; dryness, burning, itching, or irritation of the eyes; increased sensitivity of skin to sunlight

Clofazimine commonly causes discoloration of the feces, lining of the eyelids, sputum, sweat, tears, and urine. Usually this side effect does not require medical attention, but the discoloration may not go away. However, *clofazimine may also cause bloody or black, tarry stools. This side effect may be a symptom of serious bleeding problems that do require medical attention.*

Other side effects not listed above may also occur in some patients. If you notice any other effects, check with your doctor.

Revised: 02/23/93

# CLOFIBRATE    Systemic

Some commonly used brand names are:

**In the U.S.—**
Abitrate
Atromid-S
Generic name product may also be available.

**In Canada—**
Atromid-S                Novofibrate
Claripex

## Description

Clofibrate (kloe-FYE-brate) is used to lower cholesterol and triglyceride (fat-like substances) levels in the blood. This may help prevent medical problems caused by such substances clogging the blood vessels.

Clofibrate may also be used for other conditions as determined by your doctor.

Clofibrate is available only with your doctor's prescription, in the following dosage form:

*Oral*
- Capsules (U.S. and Canada)

## Before Using This Medicine

In addition to its helpful effects in treating your medical problem, this medicine may have some harmful effects.

You may have read or heard about a study called the World Health Organization (WHO) Study. This study compared the effects in patients who used clofibrate with effects in those who used a placebo (sugar pill). The results of this study suggested that clofibrate might increase the patient's risk of cancer, liver disease, and pancreatitis (inflammation of the pancreas), although it might also decrease the risk of heart attack. It may also increase the risk of gallstones and problems from gallbladder surgery. Other studies have not found all of these effects. Be sure you have discussed this with your doctor before taking this medicine.

In deciding to use a medicine, the risks of taking the medicine must be weighed against the good it will do. This is a decision you and your doctor will make. For clofibrate, the following should be considered:

**Allergies**—Tell your doctor if you have ever had any unusual or allergic reaction to clofibrate. Also tell your health care professional if you are allergic to any other substances, such as foods, preservatives, or dyes.

**Diet**—Before prescribing medicine for your condition, your doctor will probably try to control your condition by prescribing a personal diet for you. Such a diet may be low in fats, sugars, and/or cholesterol. Many people are able to control their condition by carefully following their doctors' orders for proper diet and exercise. *Medicine is prescribed only when additional help is needed* and is effective only when a schedule of diet and exercise is properly followed.

Also, this medicine is less effective if you are greatly overweight. It may be very important for you to go on a reducing diet. However, check with your doctor before going on any diet.

Make certain your health care professional knows if you are on a low-sodium, low-sugar, or any other special diet. Most medicines contain more than their active ingredient.

**Pregnancy**—Use of clofibrate is not recommended during pregnancy. Although studies have not been done in pregnant women, studies in rabbits have shown that the fetus may not be able to break down and get rid of this medicine as well as the mother. Because of this, it is possible that clofibrate may be harmful to the fetus if you take it while you are pregnant or for up to several months before you become pregnant. Be sure that you have discussed this with your doctor before taking this medicine, especially if you plan to become pregnant in the near future.

**Breast-feeding**—Clofibrate passes into breast milk. This medicine is not recommended during breast-feeding because it may cause unwanted effects in nursing babies.

**Children**—Studies on this medicine have been done only in adult patients, and there is no specific information comparing use of clofibrate in children with use in other age groups. However, use is not recommended in children under 2 years of age since cholesterol is needed for normal development.

**Older adults**—Many medicines have not been studied specifically in older people. Therefore, it may not be known whether they work exactly the same way they do in younger adults. Although there is no specific information comparing use of clofibrate in the elderly with use in other age groups, this medicine is not expected to cause different side effects or problems in older people than it does in younger adults.

**Other medicines**—Although certain medicines should not be used together at all, in other cases two different medicines may be used together even if an interaction might occur. In these cases, your doctor may want to change the dose, or other precautions may be necessary. When you are taking clofibrate, it is especially important that your health care professional knows if you are taking the following:
- Anticoagulants (blood thinners)—Use with clofibrate may increase the effects of the anticoagulant

**Other medical problems**—The presence of other medical problems may affect the use of clofibrate. Make sure you tell your doctor if you have any other medical problems, especially:
- Gallstones or
- Stomach or intestinal ulcer—May make these conditions worse
- Heart disease or
- Kidney disease or

- Liver disease—Higher blood levels may result and increase the risk of side effects
- Underactive thyroid—Clofibrate may cause or make muscle disease worse

## Proper Use of This Medicine

*Use this medicine only as directed by your doctor.* Do not use more or less of it, and do not use it more often or for a longer time than your doctor ordered.

*Follow carefully the special diet your doctor gave you.* This is the most important part of controlling your condition and is necessary if the medicine is to work properly.

Stomach upset may occur but usually lessens after a few doses. Take this medicine with food or immediately after meals to lessen possible stomach upset.

**Dosing**—The dose of clofibrate will be different for different patients. *Follow your doctor's orders or the directions on the label.* The following information includes only the average doses of clofibrate. *If your dose is different, do not change it* unless your doctor tells you to do so.

The number of capsules that you take depends on the strength of the medicine.
- For *oral* dosage form (capsules):
  —For high cholesterol:
    - Adults—1.5 to 2 grams a day. This is divided into two to four doses.
    - Children—Dose must be determined by your doctor.

**Missed dose**—If you miss a dose of this medicine, take it as soon as possible. However, if it is almost time for your next dose, skip the missed dose and go back to your regular dosing schedule. Do not double doses.

**Storage**—To store this medicine:
- Keep out of the reach of children.
- Store away from heat and direct light.
- Do not store in the bathroom, near the kitchen sink, or in other damp places. Heat or moisture may cause the medicine to break down.
- Do not keep outdated medicine or medicine no longer needed. Be sure that any discarded medicine is out of the reach of children.

## Precautions While Using This Medicine

*It is very important that your doctor check your progress at regular visits.* This will allow your doctor to see if the medicine is working properly to lower your cholesterol and triglyceride levels and to decide if you should continue to take it.

*Do not stop taking this medicine without first checking with your doctor.* When you stop taking this medicine, your blood fat levels may increase again. Your doctor may want you to follow a special diet to help prevent that.

## Side Effects of This Medicine

Along with its needed effects, a medicine may cause some unwanted effects. Although not all of these side effects may occur, if they do occur they may need medical attention.

*Check with your doctor immediately* if you think you have taken an overdose or if any of the following side effects occur:
  *Rare*
    Chest pain; irregular heartbeat; shortness of breath; stomach pain (severe) with nausea and vomiting

Check with your doctor as soon as possible if any of the following side effects occur:
  *Rare*
    Blood in urine; cough or hoarseness; decrease in urination; fever or chills; lower back or side pain; painful or difficult urination; swelling of feet or lower legs

Other side effects may occur that usually do not need medical attention. These side effects may go away during treatment as your body adjusts to the medicine. However, check with your doctor if any of the following side effects continue or are bothersome:
  *More common*
    Diarrhea; nausea
  *Less common or rare*
    Decreased sexual ability; headache; increased appetite or weight gain (slight); muscle aches or cramps; sores in mouth and on lips; stomach pain, gas, or heartburn; unusual tiredness or weakness; vomiting

Other side effects not listed above may also occur in some patients. If you notice any other effects, check with your doctor.

## Additional Information

Once a medicine has been approved for marketing for a certain use, experience may show that it is also useful for other medical problems. Although this use is not included in product labeling, clofibrate is used in certain patients with the following medical condition:
- Certain types of diabetes insipidus (water diabetes)

Other than the above information, there is no additional information relating to proper use, precautions, or side effects for this use.

Revised: 11/24/92
Interim revision: 04/14/94

# CLOMIPHENE  Systemic

Some commonly used brand names are:

**In the U.S.—**
  Clomid                               Serophene
  Milophene
**In Canada—**
  Clomid                               Serophene

Another commonly used name is clomifene.

## Description

Clomiphene (KLOE-mi-feen) is used as a fertility medicine in some women who are unable to become pregnant.

Clomiphene probably works by changing the hormone balance of the body. In women, this causes ovulation to occur and prepares the body for pregnancy.

Clomiphene may also be used for other conditions in both females and males as determined by your doctor.

*The following information applies only to female patients taking clomiphene.* Check with your doctor if you are a male and have any questions about the use of clomiphene.

Clomiphene is available only with your doctor's prescription, in the following dosage form:

*Oral*
  • Tablets (U.S. and Canada)

## Before Using This Medicine

In deciding to use a medicine, the risks of taking the medicine must be weighed against the good it will do. This is a decision you and your doctor will make. For clomiphene, the following should be considered:

**Allergies**—Tell your doctor if you have ever had any unusual or allergic reaction to clomiphene. Also tell your health care professional if you are allergic to any other substances, such as foods, preservatives, or dyes.

**Pregnancy**—There is a chance that clomiphene may cause birth defects if it is taken after you become pregnant. *Stop taking this medicine and tell your doctor immediately if you think you have become pregnant* while still taking clomiphene.

If you become pregnant as a result of using this medicine, there is a chance of a multiple birth (for example, twins, triplets) occurring.

**Other medicines**—Although certain medicines should not be used together at all, in other cases two different medicines may be used together even if an interaction might occur. In these cases, your doctor may want to change the dose, or other precautions may be necessary. When you are taking clomiphene, it is especially important that your health care professional know if you are taking any other prescription or nonprescription (over-the-counter [OTC]) medicine.

**Other medical problems**—The presence of other medical problems may affect the use of clomiphene. Make sure you tell your doctor if you have any other medical problems, especially:

  • Cyst on ovary—Clomiphene may cause the cyst to increase in size
  • Endometriosis—Inducing ovulation (including using clomiphene) may worsen endometriosis because the body estrogen level is increased; estrogen can cause growth of endometriosis implants
  • Fibroid tumors of the uterus—Clomiphene may cause fibroid tumors to increase in size
  • Inflamed veins due to blood clots
  • Liver disease (or history of)
  • Mental depression
  • Unusual vaginal bleeding—Some irregular vaginal bleeding is a sign that the lining of the uterus is growing too much or is a sign of cancer of the uterus lining; these problems must be ruled out before clomiphene is used because clomiphene can make these conditions worse

## Proper Use of This Medicine

*Take this medicine only as directed by your doctor.* If you are to begin on Day 5, count the first day of your menstrual period as Day 1. Beginning on Day 5, take the correct dose every day for as many days as your doctor ordered. To help you to remember to take your dose of medicine, take it at the same time every day.

**Dosing**—The dose of clomiphene will be different for different patients. *Follow your doctor's orders or the directions on the label.* The following information includes only the average doses of clomiphene. *If your dose is different, do not change it* unless your doctor tells you to do so.

  • For *oral* dosage form (tablets):
    —For treating infertility:
      • Adults—25 to 50 milligrams (mg) a day for five days of each menstrual cycle. The treatment is usually started on the fifth day of your menstrual period. If you do not have menstrual cycles, you can begin taking your medicine at any time. If you do not become pregnant, your doctor may increase your dose up to 250 mg a day. Your treatment may be repeated until you do become pregnant or for up to four treatment cycles.

**Missed dose**—If you miss a dose of this medicine, take it as soon as possible. If you do not remember until it is time for the next dose, take both doses together; then go back to your regular dosing schedule. If you miss more than one dose, check with your doctor.

**Storage**—To store this medicine:
  • Keep out of the reach of children.
  • Store away from heat and direct light.

- Do not store in the bathroom, near the kitchen sink, or in other damp places. Heat or moisture may cause the medicine to break down.
- Do not keep outdated medicine or medicine no longer needed. Be sure that any discarded medicine is out of the reach of children.

## Precautions While Using This Medicine

*It is very important that your doctor check your progress at regular visits* to make sure this medicine is working and to check for unwanted effects.

At certain times in your menstrual cycle, your doctor may want you to use an ovulation prediction test kit. *Follow your doctor's instructions carefully.* Ovulation is controlled by luteinizing hormone (LH). LH is present in the blood and urine in very small amounts during most of the menstrual cycle but rises suddenly for a short time in the middle of the menstrual cycle. This sharp rise, the LH surge, usually causes ovulation within about 30 hours. A woman is most likely to become pregnant if she has intercourse within the 24 hours after detecting the LH surge. Ovulation prediction test kits are used to test for this large amount of LH in the urine. This method is better for predicting ovulation than measuring daily basal body temperature. It is important that intercourse take place at the correct time to give you the best chance of becoming pregnant.

There is a chance that clomiphene may cause birth defects if it is taken after you become pregnant. *Stop taking this medicine and tell your doctor immediately if you think you have become pregnant* while still taking clomiphene.

This medicine may cause blurred vision, difficulty in reading, or other changes in vision. It may also cause some people to become dizzy or lightheaded. *Make sure you know how you react to this medicine before you drive, use machines, or do anything else that could be dangerous if you are not clear-headed or able to see well.* If these reactions are especially bothersome, check with your doctor.

## Side Effects of This Medicine

Along with its needed effects, a medicine may cause some unwanted effects. Although not all of these side effects may occur, if they do occur they may need medical attention.

When this medicine is used for a short time at low doses, serious side effects usually are rare. *However, check with your doctor immediately* if any of the following side effects occur:

*More common*
  Bloating; stomach or pelvic pain
*Less common or rare*
  Shortness of breath (sudden)

Check with your doctor as soon as possible if any of the following side effects occur:

*Less common or rare*
  Blurred vision; decreased or double vision or other vision problems; sensitivity of eyes to light; yellow eyes or skin

Other side effects may occur that usually do not need medical attention. These side effects may go away during treatment as your body adjusts to the medicine. However, check with your doctor if any of the following side effects continue or are bothersome:

*More common*
  Hot flashes
*Less common or rare*
  Breast discomfort; dizziness or lightheadedness; headache; heavy menstrual periods or bleeding between periods; mental depression; nausea or vomiting; nervousness; restlessness or trouble in sleeping; tiredness

Other side effects not listed above may also occur in some patients. If you notice any other effects, check with your doctor.

## Additional Information

Once a medicine has been approved for marketing for a certain use, experience may show that it is also useful for other medical problems. Although these uses are not included in product labeling, clomiphene is used in certain patients with the following medical conditions:

- Male infertility caused by low production of sperm
- Certain problems of the male sexual organs caused by pituitary or hypothalamus gland problems (diagnosis)

*For males taking this medicine for treatment of infertility* caused by low sperm production:

- To decide on the best treatment for your medical problem, your doctor should be told:
  —if you have ever had any unusual or allergic reaction to clomiphene.
  —if you have either of the following medical problems:
    Liver disease
    Mental depression
- If you miss a dose of this medicine, take it as soon as possible. If you do not remember until it is time for the next dose, take both doses together, then go back to your regular dosing schedule. If you miss more than one dose, check with your doctor.
- It is important that your doctor check your progress at regular visits to find out if clomiphene is working and to check for unwanted effects.
- This medicine may cause vision problems, dizziness, or lightheadedness. *Make sure you know how you react to this medicine before you drive, use machines, or do anything else that could be dangerous if you are dizzy or are not clear-headed or able to see well.*
- Along with its needed effects, a medicine may cause some unwanted effects. Although not all of these side effects may occur, if they do occur they may need medical attention. When this medicine is used

for short periods of time at low doses, serious side effects usually are rare. However, check with your doctor if any of the following side effects occur:

*Less common or rare*
> Blurred vision; decreased or double vision or other vision problems; sensitivity of eyes to light; yellow eyes or skin

- Other side effects may occur that usually do not need medical attention. These side effects may go away during treatment as your body adjusts to the medicine. However, check with your doctor if any of the following side effects continue or are bothersome:

*Less common or rare*
> Breast enlargement; dizziness or lightheadedness; headache; mental depression; nausea or vomiting; nervousness; restlessness; tiredness; trouble in sleeping

Other than the above information, there is no additional information relating to proper use, precautions, or side effects for these uses.

Revised: July 1990
Interim revision: 06/04/94

# CLONIDINE  Systemic

Some commonly used brand names are:

**In the U.S.—**
Catapres
Catapres-TTS
Generic name product may also be available.

**In Canada—**
Catapres
Dixarit

## Description

Clonidine (KLOE-ni-deen) belongs to the general class of medicines called antihypertensives. It is used to treat high blood pressure (hypertension).

High blood pressure adds to the workload of the heart and arteries. If it continues for a long time, the heart and arteries may not function properly. This can damage the blood vessels of the brain, heart, and kidneys, resulting in a stroke, heart failure, or kidney failure. Hypertension may also increase the risk of heart attacks. These problems may be less likely to occur if blood pressure is controlled.

Clonidine works by controlling nerve impulses along certain nerve pathways. As a result, it relaxes blood vessels so that blood passes through them more easily. This helps to lower blood pressure.

Clonidine may also be used for other conditions as determined by your doctor.

Clonidine is available only with your doctor's prescription, in the following dosage forms:

*Oral*
- Tablets (U.S. and Canada)

*Transdermal*
- Skin patch (U.S.)

## Before Using This Medicine

In deciding to use a medicine, the risks of taking the medicine must be weighed against the good it will do.

This is a decision you and your doctor will make. For clonidine, the following should be considered:

**Allergies**—Tell your doctor if you have ever had any unusual or allergic reaction to clonidine. Also tell your health care professional if you are allergic to any other substance, such as foods, preservatives, or dyes.

**Pregnancy**—Clonidine has not been studied in pregnant women. However, studies in animals have shown that clonidine causes harmful effects in the fetus, but not birth defects.

**Breast-feeding**—Although clonidine passes into breast milk, it has not been reported to cause problems in nursing babies.

**Children**—Children may be more sensitive than adults to clonidine. Clonidine overdose has been reported when children accidentally took this medicine.

**Older adults**—Dizziness or faintness may be more likely to occur in the elderly, who are more sensitive than younger adults to the effects of clonidine.

**Other medicines**—Although certain medicines should not be used together at all, in other cases two different medicines may be used together even if an interaction might occur. In these cases, your doctor may want to change the dose, or other precautions may be necessary. When you are taking clonidine, it is especially important that your health care professional know if you are taking any of the following:

- Beta-blockers (acebutolol [e.g., Sectral], atenolol [e.g., Tenormin], betaxolol [e.g., Kerlone], carteolol [e.g., Cartrol], labetalol [e.g., Normodyne], metoprolol [e.g., Lopressor], nadolol [e.g., Corgard], oxprenolol [e.g., Trasicor], penbutolol [e.g., Levatol], pindolol [e.g., Visken], propranolol [e.g., Inderal], sotalol [e.g., Sotacor], timolol [e.g., Blocadren])—These medicines may increase the risk of harmful effects when clonidine treatment is stopped suddenly

- Tricyclic antidepressants (amitriptyline [e.g., Elavil], amoxapine [e.g., Asendin], clomipramine [e.g., Anafranil], desipramine [e.g., Pertofrane], doxepin [e.g., Sinequan], imipramine [e.g., Tofranil], nortriptyline [e.g., Aventyl], protriptyline [e.g., Vivactil], trimipramine [e.g., Surmontil])—These medicines may decrease clonidine's effects on blood pressure

**Other medical problems**—The presence of other medical problems may affect the use of clonidine. Make sure you tell your doctor if you have any other medical problems, especially:

- Heart or blood vessel disease—Clonidine may make these conditions worse
- Irritated or scraped skin (with transdermal system [skin patch] only)—The effects of clonidine may be increased if the skin patch is placed on an area of scraped or irritated skin because more medicine is absorbed into the body
- Kidney disease—Effects of clonidine may be increased because of slower removal of clonidine from the body
- Mental depression (history of) or
- Raynaud's syndrome—Clonidine may make these conditions worse
- Polyarteritis nodosa or
- Scleroderma or
- Systemic lupus erythematosus (SLE)—with transdermal system (skin patch) only—Effects of clonidine may be decreased because absorption of this medicine into the body is blocked

## Proper Use of This Medicine

For patients taking this medicine *for high blood pressure:*

- In addition to the use of the medicine your doctor has prescribed, treatment for your high blood pressure may include weight control and care in the types of foods you eat, especially foods high in sodium. Your doctor will tell you which of these are most important for you. You should check with your doctor before changing your diet.
- Many patients who have high blood pressure will not notice any signs of the problem. In fact, many may feel normal. It is very important that you *take your medicine exactly as directed* and that you keep your appointments with your doctor even if you feel well.
- Remember that this medicine will not cure your high blood pressure but it does help control it. Therefore, you must continue to use it as directed if you expect to lower your blood pressure and keep it down. *You may have to take high blood pressure medicine for the rest of your life.* If high blood pressure is not treated, it can cause serious problems such as heart failure, blood vessel disease, stroke, or kidney disease.

For patients using the *transdermal system (skin patch):*

- *Use this medicine exactly as directed by your doctor.* It will work only if applied correctly. *This medicine usually comes with patient instructions. Read them carefully before using.*

- Do not try to trim or cut the adhesive patch to adjust the dosage. Check with your doctor if you think the medicine is not working as it should.
- Apply the patch to a clean, dry area of skin on your upper arm or chest. Choose an area with little or no hair and free of scars, cuts, or irritation.
- The system should stay in place even during showering, bathing, or swimming. If the patch becomes loose, cover it with the extra adhesive overlay provided. Apply a new patch if the first one becomes too loose or falls off.
- Each dose is best applied to a different area of skin to prevent skin problems or other irritation.
- After removing a used patch, fold the patch in half with the sticky sides together. Make sure to dispose of it out of the reach of children.

To help you remember to use your medicine, try to get into the habit of using it at regular times. If you are taking the tablets, take them at the same time each day. If you are using the transdermal system (skin patch), try to change it at the same time and day of the week.

**Dosing**—The dose of clonidine will be different for different patients. *Follow your doctor's orders or the directions on the label.* The following information includes only the average doses of clonidine used for the treatment of high blood pressure. *If your dose is different, do not change it* unless your doctor tells you to do so:

- For *oral* dosage form (tablets):
  —For high blood pressure:
    - Adults—100 mcg (0.1 mg) two times a day. Your doctor may increase your dose up to 200 mcg (0.2 mg) to 600 mcg (0.6 mg) a day taken in divided doses.
    - Children—Use and dose must be determined by your doctor.
- For *transdermal* dosage form (skin patch):
  —For high blood pressure:
    - Adults—One transdermal dosage system (skin patch) applied once a week.
    - Children—Use and dose must be determined by your doctor.

**Missed dose**—If you miss a dose of this medicine, take it or use it as soon as possible. Then go back to your regular dosing schedule. *If you miss 2 or more doses of the tablets in a row or if you miss changing the transdermal patch for 3 or more days, check with your doctor right away.* If your body goes without this medicine for too long, your blood pressure may go up to a dangerously high level and some unpleasant effects may occur.

**Storage**—To store this medicine:

- Keep out of the reach of children.
- Store away from heat and direct light.
- Do not store in the bathroom, near the kitchen sink, or in other damp places. Heat or moisture may cause the medicine to break down.

• Do not keep outdated medicine or medicine no longer needed. Be sure that any discarded medicine is out of the reach of children.

## Precautions While Using This Medicine

It is important that your doctor check your progress at regular visits to make sure that this medicine is working properly.

*Check with your doctor before you stop using this medicine.* Your doctor may want you to reduce gradually the amount you are using before stopping completely.

*Make sure that you have enough clonidine on hand to last through weekends, holidays, or vacations.* You should not miss any doses. You may want to ask your doctor for another written prescription for clonidine to carry in your wallet or purse. You can then have it filled if you run out of medicine when you are away from home.

For patients taking this medicine *for high blood pressure:*

• *Do not take other medicines unless they have been discussed with your doctor.* This especially includes over-the-counter (nonprescription) medicines for appetite control, asthma, colds, cough, hay fever, or sinus problems, since they may tend to increase your blood pressure.

Clonidine will add to the effects of alcohol and other CNS depressants (medicines that slow down the nervous system, possibly causing drowsiness). Some examples of CNS depressants are antihistamines or medicine for hay fever, other allergies, or colds; sedatives, tranquilizers, or sleeping medicine; prescription pain medicine or narcotics; barbiturates; medicine for seizures; muscle relaxants; or anesthetics, including some dental anesthetics. *Check with your doctor before taking any of the above while you are using this medicine.*

Clonidine may cause some people to become drowsy or less alert than they are normally. This is more likely to happen when you begin to take it or when you increase the amount of medicine you are taking. *Make sure you know how you react to this medicine before you drive, use machines, or do anything else that could be dangerous if you are not alert.*

Before having any kind of surgery (including dental surgery) or emergency treatment, *tell the medical doctor or dentist in charge that you are using this medicine.*

Dizziness, lightheadedness, or fainting may occur after you take this medicine, especially when you get up from a lying or sitting position. Getting up slowly may help, but if the problem continues or gets worse, check with your doctor.

The dizziness, lightheadedness, or fainting is also more likely to occur if you drink alcohol, stand for long periods of time, exercise, or if the weather is hot. While you are taking clonidine, be careful to limit the amount of alcohol you drink. Also, use extra care during exercise or hot weather or if you must stand for a long time.

Clonidine may cause dryness of the mouth. For temporary relief, use sugarless candy or gum, melt bits of ice in your mouth, or use a saliva substitute. However, if your mouth continues to feel dry for more than 2 weeks, check with your medical doctor or dentist. Continuing dryness of the mouth may increase the chance of dental disease, including tooth decay, gum disease, and fungus infections.

## Side Effects of This Medicine

Along with its needed effects, a medicine may cause some unwanted effects. Although not all of these side effects may occur, if they do occur they may need medical attention.

*Check with your doctor immediately* if any of the following side effects occur:

*Signs and symptoms of overdose*
　Difficulty in breathing; dizziness (extreme) or faintness; pinpoint pupils of eyes; slow heartbeat; unusual tiredness or weakness (extreme)

Check with your doctor as soon as possible if any of the following side effects occur:

*More common—with transdermal system (skin patch) only*
　Itching or redness of skin

*Less common*
　Mental depression; swelling of feet and lower legs

*Rare*
　Paleness or cold feeling in fingertips and toes; vivid dreams or nightmares

Other side effects may occur that usually do not need medical attention. These side effects may go away during treatment as your body adjusts to the medicine. However, check with your doctor if any of the following side effects continue or are bothersome:

*More common*
　Constipation; dizziness; drowsiness; dryness of mouth; unusual tiredness or weakness

*Less common*
　Darkening of skin—with transdermal system (skin patch) only; decreased sexual ability; dizziness, lightheadedness, or fainting, especially when getting up from a lying or sitting position; dry, itching, or burning eyes; loss of appetite; nausea or vomiting; nervousness

After you have been using this medicine for a while, it may cause unpleasant or even harmful effects if you stop taking it too suddenly. After you stop taking this medicine, *check with your doctor immediately* if any of the following occur:
　Anxiety or tenseness; chest pain; fast or pounding heartbeat; headache; increased salivation; nausea; nervousness; restlessness; shaking or trembling of hands and fingers; stomach cramps; sweating; trouble in sleeping; vomiting

Other side effects not listed above may also occur in some patients. If you notice any other effects, check with your doctor.

## Additional Information

Once a medicine has been approved for marketing for a certain use, experience may show that it is also useful for other medical problems. Although this use is not included in product labeling, clonidine is used in certain patients with the following medical conditions:

- Migraine headache
- Symptoms associated with menopause or menstrual discomfort

- Symptoms of withdrawal associated with alcohol, nicotine, or narcotics
- Gilles de la Tourette's syndrome

Other than the above information, there is no additional information relating to proper use, precautions, or side effects for these uses.

Revised: 05/17/93

# CLONIDINE AND CHLORTHALIDONE  Systemic

A commonly used brand name in the U.S. and Canada is Combipres. Generic name product may also be available in the U.S.

## Description

Clonidine (KLOE-ni-deen) and chlorthalidone (klor-THAL-i-done) combinations are used in the treatment of high blood pressure (hypertension).

High blood pressure adds to the work load of the heart and arteries. If it continues for a long time, the heart and arteries may not function properly. This can damage the blood vessels of the brain, heart, and kidneys resulting in a stroke, heart failure, or kidney failure. Hypertension may also increase the risk of heart attacks. These problems may be less likely to occur if blood pressure is controlled.

Clonidine works by controlling nerve impulses along certain body nerve pathways. As a result, it relaxes blood vessels so that blood passes through them more easily. The chlorthalidone in this combination is a diuretic (water pill) that helps reduce the amount of water in the body by increasing the flow of urine.

Clonidine and chlorthalidone combination is available only with your doctor's prescription, in the following dosage form:

*Oral*
- Tablets (U.S. and Canada)

## Before Using This Medicine

In deciding to use a medicine, the risks of taking the medicine must be weighed against the good it will do. This is a decision you and your doctor will make. For clonidine and chlorthalidone, the following should be considered:

**Allergies**—Tell your doctor if you have ever had any unusual or allergic reaction to clonidine, chlorthalidone, sulfonamides (sulfa drugs), or other thiazide diuretics (water pills). Also tell your health care professional if you are allergic to any other substance, such as foods, preservatives, or dyes.

**Pregnancy**—Clonidine has not been studied in pregnant women. However, studies in animals have shown that clonidine does not cause birth defects but does cause other harmful effects in the fetus. When chlorthalidone is used during pregnancy, it may cause side effects including jaundice, blood problems, and low potassium in the newborn infant. Be sure you have discussed this with your doctor before taking this medicine.

**Breast-feeding**—Both clonidine and chlorthalidone pass into breast milk. Chlorthalidone may decrease the flow of breast milk. Therefore, you should avoid use of clonidine and chlorthalidone combination during the first month of breast-feeding.

**Children**—Studies on this medicine have been done only in adult patients, and there is no specific information comparing use of clonidine and chlorthalidone combination in children with use in other age groups. However, children may be more sensitive than adults to clonidine. Clonidine overdose has been reported when children accidentally took this medicine.

**Older adults**—Dizziness or lightheadedness and signs of too much potassium loss may be more likely to occur in the elderly, who are more sensitive to the effects of clonidine and chlorthalidone.

**Other medicines**—Although certain medicines should not be used together at all, in other cases two different medicines may be used together even if an interaction might occur. In these cases, your doctor may want to change the dose, or other precautions may be necessary. When you are taking clonidine and chlorthalidone, it is especially important that your health care professional know if you are taking any of the following:

- Beta-blockers (acebutolol [e.g., Sectral], atenolol [e.g., Tenormin], betaxolol [Kerlone], bisoprolol [Zebeta], carteolol [e.g., Cartrol], labetalol [e.g., Normodyne], metoprolol [e.g., Lopressor], nadolol [e.g., Corgard], oxprenolol [e.g., Trasicor], penbutolol [e.g., Levatol], pindolol [e.g., Visken], propranolol [e.g., Inderal], sotalol [e.g., Sotacor], timolol [e.g., Blocadren])—These medicines may increase the risk of harmful effects when clonidine and chlorthalidone combination treatment is stopped suddenly

- Cholestyramine or
- Colestipol—Use with clonidine and chlorthalidone combination may prevent the chlorthalidone portion of the medicine from working properly; take clonidine and chlorthalidone combination at least 1 hour before or 4 hours after cholestyramine or colestipol
- Digitalis glycosides (heart medicine)—This medicine may cause low potassium in the blood, which may increase the chance of side effects of digitalis glycosides
- Lithium (e.g., Lithane)—Use with clonidine and chlorthalidone combination may cause high blood levels of lithium, which may increase the chance of side effects
- Tricyclic antidepressants (amitriptyline [e.g., Elavil], amoxapine [e.g., Asendin], clomipramine [e.g., Anafranil], desipramine [e.g., Pertofrane], doxepin [e.g., Sinequan], imipramine [e.g., Tofranil], nortriptyline [e.g., Aventyl], protriptyline [e.g., Vivactil], trimipramine [e.g., Surmontil])—These medicines may decrease the effects of clonidine and chlorthalidone combination on blood pressure

**Other medical problems**—The presence of other medical problems may affect the use of clonidine and chlorthalidone. Make sure you tell your doctor if you have any other medical problems, especially:

- Diabetes mellitus (sugar diabetes)—This medicine may change the amount of diabetes medicine needed
- Gout—This medicine may increase the amount of uric acid in the blood, which can lead to gout
- Heart or blood vessel disease or
- Lupus erythematosus (history of) or
- Mental depression (history of) or
- Pancreatitis (inflammation of the pancreas) or
- Raynaud's syndrome—This medicine may make these conditions worse
- Kidney disease—Effects of this medicine may be increased because of slower removal from the body. If severe, the chlorthalidone portion of this medicine may not work
- Liver disease—If this medicine causes loss of too much water from the body, liver disease can become much worse

## Proper Use of This Medicine

This medicine may cause you to have an unusual feeling of tiredness when you begin to take it. You may also notice an increase in the amount of urine or in your frequency of urination. After taking the medicine for a while, these effects should lessen. It is best to plan your doses according to a schedule that will least affect your personal activities and sleep. Ask your health care professional to help you plan the best time to take this medicine.

In addition to the use of the medicine your doctor has prescribed, appropriate treatment for your high blood pressure may include weight control and care in the types of foods you eat, especially foods high in sodium. Your doctor will tell you which factors are most important for you. You should check with your doctor before changing your diet.

Many patients who have high blood pressure will not notice any signs of the problem. In fact, many may feel normal. It is very important that you *take your medicine*

*exactly as directed* and that you keep your appointments with your doctor even if you feel well.

Remember that this medicine will not cure your high blood pressure but it does help control it. Therefore, you must continue to take it as directed if you expect to lower your blood pressure and keep it down. *You may have to take high blood pressure medicine for the rest of your life.* If high blood pressure is not treated, it can cause serious problems such as heart failure, blood vessel disease, stroke, or kidney disease.

To help you remember to take your medicine, try to get into the habit of taking it at the same time each day.

**Dosing**—The dose of clonidine and chlorthalidone combination will be different for different patients. *Follow your doctor's orders or the directions on the label.* The following information includes only the average doses of clonidine and chlorthalidone combination. *If your dose is different, do not change it* unless your doctor tells you to do so.

The number of tablets that you take depends on the strength of the medicine.

- For *oral* dosage form (tablets):
  —For high blood pressure:
    - Adults—1 or 2 tablets two to four times a day.
    - Children—Dose must be determined by your doctor.

**Missed dose**—If you miss a dose of this medicine, take it as soon as possible. Then go back to your regular dosing schedule. *If you miss two or more doses in a row, check with your doctor right away.* If your body goes without this medicine for too long, your blood pressure may go up to a dangerously high level and some unpleasant effects may occur.

**Storage**—To store this medicine:
- Keep out of the reach of children.
- Store away from heat and direct light.
- Do not store in the bathroom, near the kitchen sink, or in other damp places. Heat or moisture may cause the medicine to break down.
- Do not keep outdated medicine or medicine no longer needed. Be sure that any discarded medicine is out of the reach of children.

## Precautions While Using This Medicine

It is important that your doctor check your progress at regular visits to make sure that this medicine is working properly.

*Check with your doctor before you stop taking this medicine.* Your doctor may want you to reduce gradually the amount you are taking before stopping completely.

*Make sure that you have enough medicine on hand to last through weekends, holidays, or vacations.* You should not miss taking any doses. You may want to ask your doctor for another written prescription to carry in your wallet or purse. You can then have it filled if you run out of medicine when you are away from home.

Before having any kind of surgery (including dental surgery) or emergency treatment, *make sure the medical doctor or dentist in charge knows that you are taking this medicine.*

*Do not take other medicines unless they have been discussed with your doctor.* This especially includes over-the-counter (nonprescription) medicines for appetite control, asthma, colds, cough, hay fever, or sinus problems, since they may tend to increase your blood pressure.

This medicine will add to the effects of alcohol and other CNS depressants (medicines that slow down the nervous system, possibly causing drowsiness). Some examples of CNS depressants are antihistamines or medicine for hay fever, other allergies, or colds; sedatives, tranquilizers, or sleeping medicine; prescription pain medicine or narcotics; barbiturates; medicine for seizures; muscle relaxants; or anesthetics, including some dental anesthetics. *Check with your doctor before taking any of the above while you are using this medicine.*

This medicine may cause some people to become drowsy or less alert than they are normally. This is more likely to happen when you begin to take it or when you increase the amount of medicine you are taking. *Make sure you know how you react to this medicine before you drive, use machines, or do anything else that could be dangerous if you are not alert.*

Dizziness, lightheadedness, or fainting may occur, especially when you get up from a lying or sitting position. Getting up slowly may help, but if the problem continues or gets worse, check with your doctor.

The dizziness, lightheadedness, or fainting is also more likely to occur if you drink alcohol, stand for long periods of time, exercise, or if the weather is hot. Drinking alcoholic beverages may also make the drowsiness worse. While you are taking this medicine, be careful to limit the amount of alcohol you drink. Also, use extra care during exercise or hot weather or if you must stand for long periods of time.

*This medicine may cause a loss of potassium from your body.*

- To help prevent this, your doctor may want you to:
  - —eat or drink foods that have a high potassium content (for example, orange or other citrus fruit juices), or
  - —take a potassium supplement, or
  - —take another medicine to help prevent the loss of the potassium in the first place.
- It is very important to follow these directions. Also, it is important not to change your diet on your own. This is more important if you are already on a special diet (as for diabetes), or if you are taking a potassium supplement or a medicine to reduce potassium loss. Extra potassium may not be necessary and, in some cases, too much potassium could be harmful.

Check with your doctor if you become sick and have severe or continuing vomiting or diarrhea. These problems may cause you to lose additional water and potassium.

For *diabetic patients:*

- The chlorthalidone contained in this medicine may raise blood sugar levels. While you are using this medicine, be especially careful in testing for sugar in your urine.

This medicine may cause your skin to be more sensitive to sunlight than it is normally. Exposure to sunlight, even for brief periods of time, may cause a skin rash, itching, redness or other discoloration of the skin, or a severe sunburn. When you begin taking this medicine:

- Stay out of direct sunlight, especially between the hours of 10:00 a.m. and 3:00 p.m., if possible.
- Wear protective clothing, including a hat. Also, wear sunglasses.
- Apply a sun block product that has a skin protection factor (SPF) of at least 15. Some patients may require a product with a higher SPF number, especially if they have a fair complexion. If you have any questions about this, check with your health care professional.
- Apply a sun block lipstick that has an SPF of at least 15 to protect your lips.
- Do not use a sunlamp or tanning bed or booth.

*If you have a severe reaction from the sun, check with your doctor.*

This medicine may cause dryness of the mouth. For temporary relief, use sugarless candy or gum, melt bits of ice in your mouth, or use a saliva substitute. However, if your mouth continues to feel dry for more than 2 weeks, check with your medical doctor or dentist. Continuing dryness of the mouth may increase the chance of dental disease, including tooth decay, gum disease, and fungus infections.

## Side Effects of This Medicine

Along with its needed effects, a medicine may cause some unwanted effects. Although not all of these side effects may occur, if they do occur they may need medical attention.

*Check with your doctor immediately* if any of the following side effects occur:

*Signs and symptoms of overdose*

Difficulty in breathing; dizziness (extreme) or faintness; feeling cold; pinpoint pupils of eyes; slow heartbeat; unusual tiredness or weakness (extreme)

Check with your doctor as soon as possible if any of the following side effects occur:

*Signs and symptoms of too much potassium loss*

Dryness of mouth; increased thirst; irregular heartbeat; mood or mental changes; muscle cramps or pain; nausea or vomiting; weak pulse

*Signs and symptoms of too much sodium loss*
> Confusion; convulsions (seizures); decreased mental activity; irritability; muscle cramps; unusual tiredness or weakness

*Less common*
> Mental depression; swelling of feet and lower legs

*Rare*
> Black, tarry stools; blood in urine or stools; cough or hoarseness; fever or chills; joint pain; lower back or side pain; paleness or cold feeling in fingertips and toes; pinpoint red spots on skin; skin rash or hives; stomach pain (severe) with nausea and vomiting; unusual bleeding or bruising; vivid dreams or nightmares; yellow eyes or skin

Other side effects may occur that usually do not need medical attention. These side effects may go away during treatment as your body adjusts to the medicine. However, check with your doctor if any of the following side effects continue or are bothersome:

*More common*
> Constipation; dizziness; drowsiness; dryness of mouth; unusual tiredness or weakness

*Less common*
> Decreased sexual ability; diarrhea; dizziness or lightheadedness when getting up from a lying or sitting position; dry, itching, or burning eyes; increased sensitivity of skin to sunlight; loss of appetite; nausea or vomiting; nervousness; upset stomach

After you have been using this medicine for a while, it may cause unpleasant or even harmful effects if you stop taking it too suddenly. After you stop taking this medicine, check with your doctor if any of the following occur:

> Anxiety or tenseness; chest pain; fast or irregular heartbeat; headache; increased salivation; nausea; nervousness; restlessness; shaking or trembling of hands and fingers; stomach cramps; sweating; trouble in sleeping; vomiting

Other side effects not listed above may also occur in some patients. If you notice any other effects, check with your doctor.

Revised: 08/02/94

---

# CLOTRIMAZOLE    Oral†

A commonly used brand name in the U.S. is Mycelex Troches.

†Not commercially available in Canada.

## Description

Clotrimazole (kloe-TRIM-a-zole) lozenges are dissolved slowly in the mouth to prevent and treat thrush. Thrush, also called candidiasis or white mouth, is a fungus infection of the mouth and throat. This medicine may also be used for other problems as determined by your doctor.

Clotrimazole is available only with your doctor's prescription, in the following dosage form:

*Oral*
- Lozenges (U.S.)

## Before Using This Medicine

In deciding to use a medicine, the risks of taking the medicine must be weighed against the good it will do. This is a decision you and your doctor will make. For clotrimazole, the following should be considered:

**Allergies**—Tell your doctor if you have ever had any unusual or allergic reaction to clotrimazole. Also tell your health care professional if you are allergic to any other substances, such as foods, preservatives, or dyes.

**Pregnancy**—Studies have not been done in humans. Studies in mice, rats, and rabbits given very high doses have not shown that clotrimazole causes birth defects. However, studies in rats and mice given high doses have

shown that clotrimazole lozenges may cause other harmful effects in the fetus.

**Breast-feeding**—It is not known whether clotrimazole passes into breast milk. However, only small amounts of clotrimazole are absorbed into the mother's body. Clotrimazole has not been reported to cause problems in nursing babies.

**Children**—Although this medicine has not been shown to cause different side effects or problems in children than it does in adults, it should not be given to children under 5 years of age since they may be too young to use the lozenges safely.

**Older adults**—Many medicines have not been studied specifically in older people. Therefore, it may not be known whether they work exactly the same way they do in younger adults. Although there is no specific information comparing use of clotrimazole lozenges in the elderly with use in other age groups, this medicine is not expected to cause different side effects or problems in older people than it does in younger adults.

## Proper Use of This Medicine

Clotrimazole lozenges should be held in the mouth and allowed to dissolve slowly and completely, then swallowed. This may take 15 to 30 minutes. *Do not chew the lozenges or swallow them whole.*

*Do not give clotrimazole lozenges to infants or children under 5 years of age.* They may be too young to use the lozenges safely.

To help clear up your infection completely, *it is very important that you keep using clotrimazole for the full time of treatment,* even if your symptoms begin to clear up after a few days. Since fungus infections may be very slow to clear up, you may have to continue using this medicine every day for two weeks or more. If you stop using this medicine too soon, your symptoms may return. *Do not miss any doses.*

**Dosing**—The dose of clotrimazole lozenges will be different for different patients. *Follow your doctor's orders or the directions on the label.* The following information includes only the average doses of clotrimazole lozenges. *If your dose is different, do not change it* unless your doctor tells you to do so.

- For the *treatment of thrush*:

    —Adults and children 5 years of age and older: Dissolve one 10-milligram lozenge slowly and completely in your mouth; this dose should be taken five times a day for at least fourteen days.

    —Children up to 5 years of age: This medicine is not recommended in children under 5 years of age since they may be too young to use the lozenges safely.

- For the *prevention of thrush*:

    —Adults and children 5 years of age and older: Dissolve one 10-milligram lozenge slowly and completely in your mouth; this dose should be taken three times a day.

    —Children up to 5 years of age: This medicine is not recommended in children under 5 years of age since they may be too young to use the lozenges safely.

**Missed dose**—If you miss a dose of this medicine, take it as soon as possible. However, if it is almost time for your next dose, skip the missed dose and go back to your regular dosing schedule.

**Storage**—To store this medicine:

- Keep out of the reach of children.
- Store away from heat and direct light.
- Do not store in the bathroom, near the kitchen sink, or in other damp places. Heat or moisture may cause the medicine to break down.
- Do not keep outdated medicine or medicine no longer needed. Be sure that any discarded medicine is out of the reach of children.

## Precautions While Using This Medicine

If your symptoms do not improve within 1 week, or if they become worse, check with your doctor.

## Side Effects of This Medicine

Along with its needed effects, a medicine may cause some unwanted effects. The following side effects may go away during treatment as your body adjusts to the medicine. However, check with your doctor if any of these effects continue or are bothersome:

*More common—when swallowed*

Abdominal or stomach cramping or pain; diarrhea; nausea or vomiting

Other side effects not listed above may also occur in some patients. If you notice any other effects, check with your doctor.

Revised: 02/23/93

---

# CLOTRIMAZOLE    Topical

Some commonly used brand names are:

**In the U.S.—**

| | |
|---|---|
| Lotrimin AF Cream | Lotrimin Lotion |
| Lotrimin AF Lotion | Lotrimin Solution |
| Lotrimin AF Solution | Mycelex Cream |
| Lotrimin Cream | Mycelex Solution |

Generic name product may also be available.

**In Canada—**

| | |
|---|---|
| Canesten Cream | Myclo Cream |
| Canesten Solution | Myclo Solution |
| Canesten Solution with | Myclo Spray Solution |
| Atomizer | Neo-Zol Cream |
| Clotrimaderm Cream | |

## Description

Clotrimazole (kloe-TRIM-a-zole) topical preparations are used to treat fungus infections.

Some of these preparations are available only with your doctor's prescription. Others are available without a prescription; however, your doctor may have special instructions on the proper dose for your medical condition.

Clotrimazole is available in the following dosage forms:

*Topical*
- Cream (U.S. and Canada)
- Lotion (U.S.)
- Solution (U.S. and Canada)

## Before Using This Medicine

If you are using this medicine without a prescription, carefully read and follow any precautions on the label. For topical clotrimazole, the following should be considered:

**Allergies**—Tell your doctor if you have ever had any unusual or allergic reaction to clotrimazole. Also tell your health care professional if you are allergic to any other substances, such as preservatives or dyes.

**Pregnancy**—Clotrimazole has not been studied in pregnant women during the first trimester (3 months). However, clotrimazole used vaginally during the second and third trimesters has not been shown to cause birth defects or other problems in humans.

**Breast-feeding**—It is not known whether topical clotrimazole passes into the breast milk. Although most medicines pass into breast milk in small amounts, many of them may be used safely while breast-feeding. Mothers who are using this medicine and who wish to breast-feed should discuss this with their doctor.

**Children**—This medicine has been tested in children and, in effective doses, has not been shown to cause different side effects or problems than it does in adults.

**Older adults**—Many medicines have not been studied specifically in older people. Therefore, it may not be known whether they work exactly the same way they do in younger adults. Although there is no specific information comparing use of topical clotrimazole in the elderly with use in other age groups, this medicine is not expected to cause different side effects or problems in older people than it does in younger adults.

**Other medicines**—Although certain medicines should not be used together at all, in other cases two different medicines may be used together even if an interaction might occur. In these cases, your doctor may want to change the dose, or other precautions may be necessary. Tell your health care professional if you are using any other topical prescription or nonprescription (over-the-counter [OTC]) medicine that is to be applied to the same area of the skin.

## Proper Use of This Medicine

Apply enough clotrimazole to cover the affected and surrounding skin areas, and rub in gently.

*Keep this medicine away from the eyes.*

When clotrimazole is used to treat certain types of fungus infections of the skin, an occlusive dressing (airtight covering, such as kitchen plastic wrap) should *not* be applied over the medicine. To do so may cause irritation of the skin. *Do not apply an occlusive dressing over this medicine unless you have been directed to do so by your doctor.*

To help clear up your infection completely, *it is very important that you keep using this medicine for the full time of treatment,* even if your symptoms begin to clear up after a few days. Since fungus infections may be very slow to clear up, you may have to continue using this medicine every day for several weeks or more. If you stop using this medicine too soon, your symptoms may return. *Do not miss any doses.*

**Dosing**—The dose of topical clotrimazole will be different for different patients. *Follow your doctor's orders or the directions on the label.* The following information includes only the average doses of topical clotrimazole. *If your dose is different, do not change it* unless your doctor tells you to do so:

*The number of doses you use each day, the time allowed between doses, and the length of time you use the medicine depend on the medical problem for which you are using clotrimazole.*

- For *topical* dosage forms (cream, lotion, and solution):
  —Fungal infections (treatment):
  - Adults and children—Use two times a day, morning and evening.

**Missed dose**—If you miss a dose of this medicine, apply it as soon as possible. However, if it is almost time for your next dose, skip the missed dose and go back to your regular dosing schedule.

**Storage**—To store this medicine:
- Keep out of the reach of children.
- Store away from heat and direct light.
- Keep the medicine from freezing.
- Do not keep outdated medicine or medicine no longer needed. Be sure that any discarded medicine is out of the reach of children.

## Precautions While Using This Medicine

If your skin problem does not improve within 4 weeks, or if it becomes worse, check with your doctor.

## Side Effects of This Medicine

Along with its needed effects, a medicine may cause some unwanted effects. Although not all of these side effects may occur, if they do occur they may need medical attention.

Check with your doctor as soon as possible if any of the following side effects occur:

Skin rash, hives, blistering, burning, itching, peeling, redness, stinging, swelling, or other sign of skin irritation not present before use of this medicine

Other side effects not listed above may also occur in some patients. If you notice any other effects, check with your doctor.

Revised: 03/29/94

# CLOTRIMAZOLE AND BETAMETHASONE   Topical

Some commonly used brand names are:
**In the U.S.—**
    Lotrisone
**In Canada—**
    Lotriderm

## Description

Clotrimazole (kloe-TRIM-a-zole) and betamethasone (bay-ta-METH-a-sone) combination is used to treat fungus infections. Clotrimazole works by killing the fungus or preventing its growth. Betamethasone, a corticosteroid (cortisone-like medicine or steroid), is used to help relieve redness, swelling, itching, and other discomfort of fungus infections.

Clotrimazole and betamethasone cream is applied to the skin to treat:

- athlete's foot (ringworm of the foot; tinea pedis);
- jock itch (ringworm of the groin; tinea cruris); and
- ringworm of the body (tinea corporis).

This medicine may also be used for other fungus infections of the skin as determined by your doctor.

This medicine is available only with your doctor's prescription, in the following dosage form:
*Topical*
- Cream (U.S. and Canada)

## Before Using This Medicine

In deciding to use a medicine, the risks of using the medicine must be weighed against the good it will do. This is a decision you and your doctor will make. For clotrimazole and betamethasone combination, the following should be considered:

**Allergies**—Tell your doctor if you have ever had any unusual or allergic reaction to this medicine or to clotrimazole (e.g., Gyne-Lotrimin, Lotrimin), betamethasone (e.g., Valisone), butoconazole (e.g., Femstat), econazole (e.g., Ecostatin, Spectazole), ketoconazole (e.g., Nizoral), miconazole (e.g., Monistat, Monistat-Derm), terconazole (e.g., Terazol 7), or to any of the other corticosteroids. Also tell your health care professional if you are allergic to any other substances, such as preservatives or dyes.

**Pregnancy**—Clotrimazole and betamethasone combination has not been studied in pregnant women. However, for the individual medicines:

- *Clotrimazole*—Clotrimazole (e.g., Gyne-Lotrimin), used in the vagina, has not been shown to cause birth defects or other problems in studies in rats or humans. However, clotrimazole (e.g., Mycelex), given by mouth, has been shown to cause a decrease in successful pregnancies, but no birth defects, in rats and mice.
- *Betamethasone*—Studies in animals have shown that corticosteroids, given by mouth or by injection, may cause birth defects, even at low doses. Also, some

of the stronger corticosteroids have been shown to cause birth defects when applied to the skin of animals.

Therefore, this medicine should not be used on large areas of the skin, in large amounts, or for a long time in pregnant patients. Before using this medicine, make sure your doctor knows if you are pregnant or if you may become pregnant.

**Breast-feeding**—It is not known whether topical clotrimazole and betamethasone combination passes into the breast milk, but it has not been reported to cause problems in nursing babies. However, clotrimazole and betamethasone may be absorbed into the mother's body.

- *Betamethasone*—Corticosteroids, given by mouth or by injection, do pass into the breast milk. They may cause unwanted effects, such as slower growth rate of nursing babies.

**Children**—Clotrimazole and betamethasone combination may rarely cause serious side effects. Some of these side effects may be more likely to occur in children, who may absorb greater amounts of this medicine than adults do. Long-term use in children may affect growth and development as well. Therefore, it is especially important that you discuss with the child's doctor the good that this medicine may do, as well as the risks of using it.

**Older adults**—Many medicines have not been studied specifically in older people. Therefore, it may not be known whether they work exactly the same way they do in younger adults or if they cause different side effects or problems in older people. There is no specific information comparing use of clotrimazole and betamethasone combination in the elderly with use in other age groups.

**Other medicines**—Although certain medicines should not be used together at all, in other cases two different medicines may be used together even if an interaction might occur. In these cases, your doctor may want to change the dose, or other precautions may be necessary. Tell your health care professional if you are using any other prescription or nonprescription (over-the-counter [OTC]) medicine.

**Other medical problems**—The presence of other medical problems may affect the use of clotrimazole and betamethasone combination. Make sure you tell your doctor if you have any other medical problems, especially:

- Herpes or
- Vaccinia (cowpox) or
- Varicella (chickenpox) or
- Other virus infections of the skin—Betamethasone may speed up the spread of virus infections
- Tuberculosis (TB) of the skin—Betamethasone may make a TB infection worse

## Proper Use of This Medicine

Before applying this medicine, wash the affected area with soap and water, and dry thoroughly.

*Do not use this medicine in the eyes.*

To use:

- *Check with your doctor before using this medicine on any other skin problems.* It should not be used on bacterial or virus infections. Also, it should only be used on certain kinds of fungus infections of the skin.
- Apply a thin layer of this medicine to the affected area(s) and surrounding skin. Rub in gently and thoroughly.

The use of any kind of occlusive dressing (airtight covering, such as kitchen plastic wrap) over this medicine may increase absorption of the medicine and the chance of irritation and other side effects. Therefore, *do not bandage, wrap, or apply any occlusive dressing over this medicine* unless directed by your doctor. Also, wear loose-fitting clothing when using this medicine on the groin area. When using this medicine on the diaper area of children, *avoid tight-fitting diapers and plastic pants.*

To help clear up your skin infection completely, *keep using this medicine for the full time of treatment,* even if your symptoms have disappeared. *Do not miss any doses.* However, *do not use this medicine more often or for a longer time than your doctor ordered.* To do so may increase absorption through your skin and the chance of side effects. In addition, too much use, especially on thin skin areas (for example, face, armpits, genitals [sex organs], between the toes, groin), may result in thinning of the skin and stretch marks.

**Dosing**—*Follow your doctor's orders or the directions on the label.* The following information includes only the average dose of clotrimazole and betamethasone combination. *If your dose is different, do not change it* unless your doctor tells you to do so.

- For *topical cream* dosage form:
  —For fungus infections:
  - Adults and children 12 years of age and over—Apply to the affected area(s) of the skin two times a day, morning and evening.
  - Children up to 12 years of age—Use and dose must be determined by your doctor.

**Missed dose**—If you miss a dose of this medicine, apply it as soon as possible. However, if it is almost time for your next dose, skip the missed dose and go back to your regular dosing schedule.

**Storage**—To store this medicine:

- Keep out of the reach of children.
- Store away from heat and direct light.
- Keep the medicine from freezing.
- Do not keep outdated medicine or medicine no longer needed. Be sure that any discarded medicine is out of the reach of children.

## Precautions While Using This Medicine

If your skin infection does not improve within a few days, or if it becomes worse, check with your doctor.

*To help clear up your skin infection completely and to help make sure it does not return, the following good health habits are important:*

- For patients using this medicine *for athlete's foot:*
  —Carefully dry the feet, especially between the toes, after bathing.
  —Avoid wearing socks made from wool or synthetic materials (for example, rayon or nylon). Instead, wear clean, cotton socks and change them daily or more often if your feet sweat freely.
  —Wear well-ventilated shoes (for example, shoes with holes) or sandals.
  —Use a bland, absorbent powder (for example, talcum powder) or an antifungal powder freely between the toes, on the feet, and in socks and shoes once or twice a day. Be sure to use the powder after clotrimazole and betamethasone cream has been applied and has disappeared into the skin. Do not use the powder as the only treatment for your fungus infection.

These measures will help keep the feet cool and dry.

- For patients using this medicine *for jock itch:*
  —Carefully dry the groin area after bathing.
  —Avoid wearing underwear that is tight-fitting or made from synthetic materials (for example, rayon or nylon). Instead, wear loose-fitting, cotton underwear.
  —Use a bland, absorbent powder (for example, talcum powder) or an antifungal powder freely once or twice a day. Be sure to use the powder after clotrimazole and betamethasone cream has been applied and has disappeared into the skin. Do not use the powder as the only treatment for your fungus infection.

These measures will help reduce chafing and irritation and will also help keep the groin area cool and dry.

- For patients using this medicine *for ringworm of the body:*
  —Carefully dry yourself after bathing.
  —Avoid too much heat and humidity if possible. Try to keep moisture from building up on affected areas of the body.
  —Wear well-ventilated clothing.
  —Use a bland, absorbent powder (for example, talcum powder) or an antifungal powder freely once or twice a day. Be sure to use the powder after clotrimazole and betamethasone cream has been applied and has disappeared into the skin. Do not use the powder as the only treatment for your fungus infection.

These measures will help keep the affected areas cool and dry.

If you have any questions about this, check with your health care professional

For diabetic patients:

- *Rarely, the corticosteroid in this medicine may cause higher blood and urine sugar levels. This is more likely to occur if you have severe diabetes and are using large amounts of this medicine.* Check with your doctor before changing your diet or the dosage of your diabetes medicine.

## Side Effects of This Medicine

Along with its needed effects, a medicine may cause some unwanted effects. Although not all of these side effects may occur, if they do occur they may need medical attention.

*Check with your doctor immediately* if any of the following side effects occur:

*Less common*
Blistering, burning, itching, peeling, dryness, redness, or other sign of skin irritation not present before use of this medicine

Additional side effects may occur if you use this medicine for a long time. Check with your doctor as soon as possible if any of the following side effects occur:

Acne or oily skin; increased hair growth, especially on the face; increased loss of hair, especially on the scalp; reddish purple lines on arms, face, legs, trunk, or groin; thinning of skin with easy bruising

Other side effects not listed above may also occur in some patients. If you notice any other effects, check with your doctor.

Revised: 02/10/92
Interim revision: 07/01/94

---

# CLOZAPINE  Systemic

Some commonly used brand names are:
**In the U.S. and Canada—**
Clozaril
**Other—**
Leponex

## Description

Clozapine (KLOE-za-peen) is used to treat schizophrenia in patients who have not been helped by or are unable to take other medicines.

Clozapine is only available from pharmacies that agree to participate with your doctor in a plan to monitor your blood tests. You will need to have blood tests done every week, and you will receive a 7-day supply of clozapine only if the results of your blood tests show that it is safe for you to take this medicine.

Clozapine is available in the following dosage form:
*Oral*
• Tablets (U.S. and Canada)

## Before Using This Medicine

In deciding to use a medicine, the risks of taking the medicine must be weighed against the good it will do. This is a decision you and your doctor will make. For clozapine, the following should be considered:

**Allergies**—Tell your doctor if you have ever had any unusual or allergic reaction to clozapine. Also tell your health care professional if you are allergic to any other substance, such as foods, preservatives, or dyes.

**Pregnancy**—Clozapine has not been studied in pregnant women. However, clozapine has not been shown to cause birth defects or other problems in animal studies.

**Breast-feeding**—Clozapine may pass into breast milk and cause sedation, decreased suckling, restlessness or irritability, seizures, or heart or blood vessel problems in nursing babies.

**Children**—Studies on this medicine have been done only in adult patients, and there is no specific information comparing use of clozapine in children with use in other age groups.

**Older adults**—Many medicines have not been tested in older people. Therefore, it may not be known whether they work exactly the same way they do in younger adults. Clozapine may be more likely to cause side effects in the elderly, including dizziness and fainting, low blood pressure, and confusion or excitement.

**Other medicines**—Although certain medicines should not be used together at all, in other cases 2 different medicines may be used together even if an interaction might occur. In these cases, your doctor may want to change the dose, or other precautions may be necessary. When you are taking clozapine, it is especially important that your health care professional know if you are taking any of the following:

• Alcohol or
• Central nervous system (CNS) depressants (medicines that cause drowsiness) or
• Tricyclic antidepressants (medicine for depression)—Clozapine may cause an increase in sedation or effects on the heart, or increase the risk of seizures
• Amphotericin B by injection (e.g., Fungizone) or
• Antineoplastics (cancer medicine) or
• Antithyroid agents (medicine for overactive thyroid) or
• Azathioprine (e.g., Imuran) or
• Chlorambucil (e.g., Leukeran) or
• Chloramphenicol (e.g., Chloromycetin) or
• Colchicine or
• Cyclophosphamide (e.g., Cytoxan) or
• Flucytosine (e.g., Ancobon) or

- Interferon (e.g., Intron A, Roferon-A) or
- Mercaptopurine (e.g., Purinethol) or
- Methotrexate (e.g., Mexate) or
- Plicamycin (e.g., Mithracin) or
- Zidovudine (e.g., Retrovir)—Taking clozapine with any of these medicines may cause increased blood problems
- Lithium—Using clozapine with lithium may increase the risk of seizures, or cause confusion or body movement disorders

**Other medical problems**—The presence of other medical problems may affect the use of clozapine. Make sure you tell your doctor if you have any other medical problems, especially:

- Blood diseases or
- Enlarged prostate or difficult urination or
- Gastrointestinal problems or
- Heart or blood vessel problems—Clozapine may make the condition worse
- Epilepsy or other seizure disorder—Clozapine may increase the risk of seizures
- Kidney or liver disease—Higher blood levels of clozapine may occur, increasing the chance of side effects

## Proper Use of This Medicine

*Take this medicine exactly as directed.* Do not take more of this medicine and do not take it more often than your doctor ordered. Do not miss any doses.

*This medicine has been prescribed for your current medical problem only.* It must not be given to other people or used for other problems unless you are directed to do so by your doctor.

**Dosing**—The dose of clozapine will be different for different patients. *Follow your doctor's orders or the directions on the label.* The following information includes only the average doses of clozapine. *If your dose is different, do not change it* unless your doctor tells you to do so.

The number of tablets that you take depends on the strength of the medicine. Also, *the number of doses you take each day, the time allowed between doses, and the length of time you take the medicine depend on your special needs.*

- For *oral* dosage form (tablets):
  —For schizophrenia:
    - Adults—At first, 25 milligrams (mg) once or twice a day. Your doctor may increase your dose as needed. However, the dose is usually not more than 900 mg a day.
    - Children up to 16 years of age—Use and dose must be determined by your doctor.

**Missed dose**—If you miss a dose of this medicine, take it as soon as possible. However, if it is almost time for your next dose, skip the missed dose and go back to your regular dosing schedule. Do not double doses.

**Storage**—To store this medicine:

- Keep out of the reach of children.
- Store away from heat and direct light.

- Do not store in the bathroom, near the kitchen sink, or in other damp places. Heat or moisture may cause the medicine to break down.
- Do not keep outdated medicine or medicine no longer needed. Be sure that any discarded medicine is out of the reach of children.

## Precautions While Using This Medicine

*It is important that you have your blood tests done weekly and that your doctor check your progress at regular visits.* This will allow your doctor to make sure the medicine is working properly and to change the dosage if needed.

If you have been using this medicine regularly, do not stop taking it without first checking with your doctor. Your doctor may want you to reduce gradually the amount you are taking before stopping completely.

This medicine will add to the effects of alcohol and other CNS depressants (medicines that slow down the nervous system, possibly causing drowsiness). Some examples of CNS depressants are antihistamines or medicine for hay fever, other allergies, or colds; sedatives, tranquilizers, or sleeping medicine; prescription pain medicine or narcotics; barbiturates; medicine for seizures; muscle relaxants; or anesthetics, including some dental anesthetics. *Check with your doctor before taking any of the above while you are using this medicine.*

Clozapine may cause drowsiness, blurred vision or convulsions (seizures). *Do not drive, climb, swim, operate machines or do anything else that could be dangerous* while you are taking this medicine.

Dizziness, lightheadedness, or fainting may occur, especially when you get up from a lying or sitting position. Getting up slowly may help. If this problem continues or gets worse, check with your doctor.

In some patients, clozapine may cause increased watering of the mouth. Other patients, however, may get dryness of the mouth. For temporary relief of mouth dryness, use sugarless gum or candy, melt bits of ice in your mouth, or use a saliva substitute. However, if your mouth continues to feel dry for more than 2 weeks, check with your medical doctor or dentist. Continuing dryness of the mouth may increase the chance of dental disease, including tooth decay, gum disease, and fungus infections.

## Side Effects of This Medicine

Along with its needed effects, a medicine may cause some unwanted effects. Although not all of these side effects may occur, if they do occur they may need medical attention.

Check with your doctor immediately if any of the following side effects occur:

*More common*
   Fast or irregular heartbeat; fever; low blood pressure

*Less common*
   High blood pressure

*Rare*

Chills; convulsions (seizures); difficult or fast breathing; increased sweating; loss of bladder control; muscle stiffness (severe); sore throat; sores, ulcers, or white spots on lips or in mouth; unusual bleeding or bruising; unusual tiredness or weakness; unusually pale skin

Check with your doctor as soon as possible if any of the following side effects occur:

*More common*

Dizziness or fainting

*Less common*

Blurred vision; confusion; restlessness or need to keep moving; trembling; unusual anxiety, nervousness, or irritability

*Rare*

Absence of or decrease in movement; decreased sexual ability; difficulty in sleeping; difficulty in urinating; headache (severe or continuing); lip smacking or puckering; mental depression; puffing of cheeks; rapid or worm-like movements of tongue; uncontrolled chewing movements; uncontrolled movements of arms and legs

*Symptoms of overdose*

Dizziness or fainting; drowsiness (severe); fast, slow, or irregular heartbeat; hallucinations (seeing, hearing, or feeling things that are not there); increased watering of mouth (severe); slow, irregular, or troubled breathing; unusual excitement, nervousness, or restlessness

Other side effects may occur that usually do not need medical attention. These side effects may go away during treatment as your body adjusts to the medicine. However, check with your doctor if any of the following side effects continue or are bothersome:

*More common*

Constipation; dizziness or lightheadedness (mild); drowsiness; headache (mild); increased watering of mouth; nausea or vomiting; unusual weight gain

*Less common*

Abdominal discomfort or heartburn; dryness of mouth

Other side effects not listed above may also occur in some patients. If you notice any other effects, check with your doctor.

Revised: 07/17/91
Interim revision: 03/25/92; 06/08/94

---

# COAL TAR  Topical

Some commonly used brand names are:

**In the U.S.—**

Alphosyl
Aquatar
Balnetar Therapeutic Tar Bath
Cutar Water Dispersible Emollient Tar
Denorex Extra Strength Medicated Shampoo
Denorex Extra Strength Medicated Shampoo with Conditioners
Denorex Medicated Shampoo
Denorex Medicated Shampoo and Conditioner
Denorex Mountain Fresh Herbal Scent Medicated Shampoo
DHS Tar Gel Shampoo
DHS Tar Shampoo
Doak Oil Forte Therapeutic Bath Treatment
Doak Oil Therapeutic Bath Treatment For All-Over Body Care
Doak Tar Lotion
Doak Tar Shampoo
Doctar Hair & Scalp Shampoo and Conditioner
Doctar Shampoo
Estar
Fototar
Ionil T Plus
Lavatar
Medotar

Pentrax Anti-Dandruff Tar Shampoo
Psorigel
PsoriNail Topical Solution
Taraphilic
Tarbonis
Tarpaste 'Doak'
T/Derm Tar Emollient
Tegrin Lotion for Psoriasis
Tegrin Medicated Cream Shampoo
Tegrin Medicated Shampoo Concentrated Gel
Tegrin Medicated Shampoo Extra Conditioning Formula
Tegrin Medicated Shampoo Herbal Formula
Tegrin Medicated Shampoo Original Formula
Tegrin Medicated Soap for Psoriasis
Tegrin Skin Cream for Psoriasis
Tersa-Tar Soapless Tar Shampoo
T/Gel Therapeutic Conditioner
T/Gel Therapeutic Shampoo
Theraplex T Shampoo
Zetar Emulsion
Zetar Medicated Antiseborrheic Shampoo

**In Canada—**

Alphosyl
Balnetar
Denorex
Doak Oil
Doak Oil Forte
Estar
Lavatar
Liquor Carbonis Detergens
Pentrax Extra-Strength Therapeutic Tar Shampoo
Psorigel

Tar Doak
Tarpaste
Tersa-Tar Mild Therapeutic Shampoo with Protein and Conditioner
Tersa-Tar Therapeutic Shampoo
T-Gel
Zetar Emulsion
Zetar Shampoo

## Description

Coal tar is used to treat eczema, psoriasis, seborrheic dermatitis, and other skin disorders.

Some of these preparations are available only with your doctor's prescription. Others are available without a prescription; however, your doctor may have special instructions on the proper use of coal tar for your medical condition.

Coal tar is available in the following dosage forms:

*Topical*

• Cleansing bar (U.S.)
• Cream (U.S. and Canada)
• Gel (U.S. and Canada)
• Lotion (U.S. and Canada)
• Ointment (U.S. and Canada)
• Shampoo (U.S. and Canada)
• Topical solution (U.S. and Canada)
• Topical suspension (U.S. and Canada)

## Before Using This Medicine

If you are using this medicine without a prescription, carefully read and follow any precautions on the label. For coal tar, the following should be considered:

**Allergies**—Tell your doctor if you have ever had any unusual or allergic reaction to coal tar or to any other tar. Also tell your health care professional if you are allergic to any other substances, such as preservatives or dyes.

**Pregnancy**—Studies on effects in pregnancy have not been done in either humans or animals.

**Breast-feeding**—It is not known whether coal tar passes into the breast milk. However, this medicine has not been reported to cause problems in nursing babies.

**Children**—Coal tar products should not be used on infants, unless otherwise directed by your doctor. Studies on this medicine have been done only in adult patients, and there is no specific information comparing use of this medicine in children with use in other age groups.

**Older adults**—Many medicines have not been studied specifically in older people. Therefore, it may not be known whether they work exactly the same way they do in younger adults or if they cause different side effects or problems in older people. There is no specific information comparing use of this medicine in the elderly with use in other age groups.

**Other medicines**—Although certain medicines should not be used together at all, in other cases two different medicines may be used together even if an interaction might occur. In these cases, your doctor may want to change the dose, or other precautions may be necessary. Tell your health care professional if you are using any other topical prescription or nonprescription (over-the-counter [OTC]) medicine that is to be applied to the same area of the skin.

## Proper Use of This Medicine

*Use this medicine only as directed.* Do not use more of it and do not use it more often than recommended on the label, unless otherwise directed by your doctor. To do so may increase the chance of side effects.

After applying coal tar, *protect the treated area from direct sunlight and do not use a sunlamp for 72 hours,* unless otherwise directed by your doctor, since a severe reaction may occur. Also, make sure you have removed all the coal tar medicine from your skin before you go back into direct sunlight or use a sunlamp.

*Do not apply this medicine to infected, blistered, raw, or oozing areas of the skin.*

*Keep this medicine away from the eyes.* If you should accidentally get some in your eyes, flush them thoroughly with water at once.

To use the *cream or ointment form* of this medicine:
- Apply enough medicine to cover the affected area, and rub in gently.

To use the *gel form* of this medicine:
- Apply enough gel to cover the affected area, and rub in gently. Allow the gel to remain on the affected area for 5 minutes, then remove excess gel by patting with a clean tissue.

To use the *shampoo form* of this medicine:
- Wet the scalp and hair with lukewarm water. Apply a generous amount of shampoo and rub into the scalp, then rinse. Apply the shampoo again, working up a rich lather, and allow to remain on the scalp for 5 minutes. Then rinse thoroughly.

To use the *nonshampoo liquid form* of this medicine:
- Some of these preparations are to be applied directly to dry or wet skin, some are to be added to lukewarm bath water, and some may be applied directly to dry or wet skin or added to lukewarm bath water. Make sure you know exactly how you should use this medicine. If you have any questions about this, check with your health care professional.
- If this medicine is to be applied directly to the skin, apply enough to cover the affected area, and rub in gently.
- Some of these preparations contain alcohol and are flammable. Do not use near heat, near open flame, or while smoking.

**Dosing**—The dose of coal tar will be different for different patients. *Follow your doctor's orders or the directions on the label.* The following information includes only the average doses of coal tar. *If your dose is different, do not change it* unless your doctor tells you to do so.
- For eczema, psoriasis, seborrheic dermatitis, and other skin disorders:
  —For *cleansing bar* dosage form:
    - Adults—Use one or two times a day, or as directed by your doctor.
    - Children—Use and dose must be determined by your doctor.
  —For *cream* dosage form:
    - Adults—Apply to the affected area(s) of the skin up to four times a day.
    - Children—Use and dose must be determined by your doctor.
  —For *gel* dosage form:
    - Adults—Apply to the affected area(s) of the skin one or two times a day.
    - Children—Use and dose must be determined by your doctor.
  —For *lotion* dosage form:
    - Adults—Apply directly to the affected area(s) of the skin or use as a bath, hand or foot soak, or as a hair rinse, depending on the product.
    - Children—Use and dose must be determined by your doctor.

—For *ointment* dosage form:
- Adults—Apply to the affected area(s) of the skin two or three times a day.
- Children—Use and dose must be determined by your doctor.

—For *shampoo* dosage form:
- Adults—Use once a day to once a week or as directed by your doctor.
- Children—Use and dose must be determined by your doctor.

—For *topical solution* dosage form:
- Adults—Apply to wet the skin or scalp, or use as a bath, depending on the product.
- Children—Use and dose must be determined by your doctor.

—For *topical suspension* dosage form:
- Adults—Use as a bath.
- Children—Use and dose must be determined by your doctor.

**Missed dose**—If you miss a dose of this medicine, apply it as soon as possible. However, if it is almost time for your next dose, skip the missed dose and go back to your regular dosing schedule. Do not double doses.

**Storage**—To store this medicine:
- Keep out of the reach of children.
- Store away from heat and direct light.
- Keep the medicine from freezing.
- Do not keep outdated medicine or medicine no longer needed. Be sure that any discarded medicine is out of the reach of children.

## Precautions While Using This Medicine

If this medicine is used on the scalp, it may temporarily discolor blond, bleached, or tinted hair.

*Coal tar may stain the skin or clothing.* Avoid getting it on your clothing. The stain on the skin will wear off after you stop using the medicine.

## Side Effects of This Medicine

In animal studies, coal tar has been shown to increase the chance of skin cancer.

Along with its needed effects, a medicine may cause some unwanted effects. Although not all of these side effects may occur, if they do occur they may need medical attention.

Check with your doctor as soon as possible if either of the following side effects occurs:

*Rare*

Skin irritation not present before use of this medicine; skin rash

Other side effects may occur that usually do not need medical attention. These side effects may go away during treatment as your body adjusts to the medicine. However, check with your health care professional if the following side effect continues or is bothersome:

*More common*

Stinging (mild)—especially for gel and solution dosage forms

Other side effects not listed above may also occur in some patients. If you notice any other effects, check with your health care professional.

Revised: 03/04/92
Interim revision: 06/03/94

# COCAINE Mucosal-Local

## Description

Cocaine (KOE-kane) is a local anesthetic. It is applied to certain areas of the body (for example, the nose, mouth, or throat) to cause loss of feeling. This allows some kinds of examinations or surgery to be done without causing pain.

Cocaine can cause psychological dependence (a strong desire to continue using the medicine because of the "high" feeling it produces). This may lead to cocaine abuse (more frequent use and/or use of larger amounts of cocaine) and to an increased chance of serious side effects. Cocaine abuse has caused death from heart or breathing failure.

Use of cocaine as a local anesthetic for an examination or surgery is not likely to cause psychological dependence or other serious side effects. However, if cocaine is absorbed into the body too quickly, serious side effects can occur. Also, some people are especially sensitive to the effects of cocaine. Unwanted effects may occur in these people even

with small amounts of the medicine. Before receiving cocaine as a local anesthetic, you should discuss its use with your doctor.

Cocaine is applied only by or under the immediate supervision of your doctor. It is available in the following dosage forms:

*Mucosal-Local*
- Crystals (U.S. and Canada)
- Solution (U.S.)

## Before Receiving This Medicine

In deciding to use a medicine, the risks of taking the medicine must be weighed against the good it will do. This is a decision you and your doctor will make. For cocaine, the following should be considered:

**Allergies**—Tell your doctor if you have ever had any unusual or allergic reaction to cocaine. Also tell your health care professional if you are allergic to any other substances, such as foods, preservatives, or dyes.

**Pregnancy**—Studies on birth defects or other problems have not been done in pregnant women receiving cocaine as a local anesthetic. However, studies in women who abused cocaine during pregnancy have shown that cocaine may cause birth defects, decreased birth weight and size, and problems affecting the baby's nervous system. These studies have also shown that too much use of cocaine may cause the baby to be born too soon, sometimes too soon to survive. Cocaine has also been shown to cause birth defects and other unwanted effects in animal studies.

**Breast-feeding**—Cocaine passes into the breast milk and may cause unwanted effects such as convulsions (seizures), high blood pressure, fast heartbeat, breathing problems, trembling, and unusual irritability in nursing babies. Therefore, after receiving this medicine you should stop breast-feeding your baby for about 2 days.

**Children**—Cocaine can cause serious side effects in any patient. Therefore, it is especially important that you discuss with the child's doctor the good that this medicine may do as well as the risks of using it.

**Older adults**—Side effects, including dizziness or lightheadedness or fast or irregular heartbeat, may be especially likely to occur in elderly patients, who are usually more sensitive than younger adults to the effects of cocaine.

**Other medicines**—Although certain medicines should not be used together at all, in other cases two different medicines may be used together even if an interaction might occur. In these cases, your doctor may want to change the dose, or other precautions may be necessary. When you are receiving cocaine, it is especially important that your health care professional know if you are taking any of the following:

- Amantadine (e.g., Symmetrel) or
- Amphetamines or
- Antimyasthenics (ambenonium [e.g., Mytelase], neostigmine [e.g., Prostigmin], pyridostigmine [e.g., Mestinon]) or
- Appetite suppressants (diet pills), except fenfluramine (e.g., Pondimin), or
- Beta-blockers (acebutolol [e.g., Sectral], atenolol [e.g., Tenormin], betaxolol [e.g., Kerlone], carteolol [e.g., Cartrol], labetalol [e.g., Normodyne], metoprolol [e.g., Lopressor], nadolol [e.g., Corgard], oxprenolol [e.g., Trasicor], penbutolol [e.g., Levatol], pindolol [e.g., Visken], propranolol [e.g., Inderal], sotalol [e.g., Sotacor], timolol [e.g., Blocadren]) or
- Betaxolol (ophthalmic) (e.g., Betoptic) or
- Caffeine (e.g., NoDoz) or
- Chlophedianol (e.g., Ulone) or
- Cyclophosphamide (e.g., Cytoxan) or
- Demecarium (e.g., Humorsol) or
- Echothiophate (e.g., Phospholine Iodide) or
- Guanadrel (e.g., Hylorel) or
- Guanethidine (e.g., Ismelin) or
- Isoflurophate (e.g., Floropryl) or
- Levobunolol (e.g., Betagan) or
- Levodopa (e.g., Dopar) or

- Malathion (e.g., Prioderm) or
- Medicine for asthma or other breathing problems or
- Medicine for colds, sinus problems, or hay fever or other allergies (including nose drops or sprays) or
- Methyldopa (e.g., Aldomet) or
- Methylphenidate (e.g., Ritalin) or
- Metipranolol (e.g., OptiPranolol) or
- Nabilone (e.g., Cesamet) or
- Pemoline (e.g., Cylert) or
- Thiotepa or
- Timolol (ophthalmic) (e.g., Timoptic)—The chance of serious side effects may be increased
- Monoamine oxidase (MAO) inhibitors (furazolidone [e.g., Furoxone], isocarboxazid [e.g., Marplan], phenelzine [e.g., Nardil], procarbazine [e.g., Matulane], selegiline [e.g., Eldepryl], tranylcypromine [e.g., Parnate])—Receiving cocaine while you are taking or within 2 weeks after you have taken an MAO inhibitor may increase the chance of serious side effects.

Also tell your doctor if you have recently used an insecticide (insect killer) or if you have been in an area that was recently treated with an insecticide. Some insecticides can slow the breakdown of cocaine in your body. This increases the chance of serious side effects.

**Other medical problems**—The presence of other medical problems may affect the use of cocaine. Make sure you tell your doctor if you have any other medical problems, especially:

- Cancer or
- Chest pain, or history of, or
- Convulsions (seizures), history of, or
- Fast or irregular heartbeat or
- Heart or blood vessel disease or
- High blood pressure or
- Liver disease or
- Myocardial infarction ("heart attack"), history of, or
- Overactive thyroid—The chance of serious side effects may be increased
- Tourette's syndrome—Cocaine can make your condition worse

---

## Proper Use of This Medicine

**Dosing**—The dose of cocaine will be different for different patients. It will depend on the reason a local anesthetic is needed and on the size of the area to which it is being applied. Your doctor or nurse will apply the medicine.

- For *mucosal-local* dosage forms (crystals or solution):

  —For causing loss of feeling before examinations or surgery:

  - Adults and teenagers—Your doctor or nurse will apply the smallest amount of cocaine that will produce the needed effect. The largest amount that is usually used is 400 milligrams (mg).

  - Children up to 12 years of age—Use and dose must be determined by your doctor.

## Precautions After Receiving This Medicine

Cocaine and some of its metabolites (substances to which cocaine is broken down in the body) will appear in your blood and urine for several days after you have received the medicine. Tests for possible drug use will then be "positive" for cocaine. If you must have such a test within 5 days or so after receiving cocaine, be sure to tell the person in charge that you have recently received cocaine for medical reasons. It may be helpful to have written information from your doctor stating why the medicine was used, the date on which you received it, and the amount you received.

## Side Effects of This Medicine

Along with its needed effects, a medicine may cause some unwanted effects. Although not all of these side effects may occur, if they do occur they may need medical attention.

After cocaine has been applied, your doctor or nurse will closely follow its effects. However, *tell your doctor or nurse immediately* if any of the following side effects occur:

*Signs and symptoms of too much medicine being absorbed into the body*

Abdominal or stomach pain; chills; confusion; dizziness or lightheadedness; excitement, nervousness, restlessness, or any mood or mental changes; fast or irregular heartbeat; general feeling of discomfort or illness; hallucinations (seeing, hearing, or feeling things that are not there); headache (sudden); increased sweating; nausea

Other side effects may occur that usually do not need medical attention. However, check with your doctor if the following side effects continue or are bothersome:

*More common*

Loss of sense of taste or smell (after application to the nose or mouth)

Other side effects not listed above may also occur in some patients. If you notice any other effects, *tell your doctor or nurse immediately*.

Revised: 08/08/92
Interim revision: 07/14/94

---

# COLCHICINE  Systemic

## Description

Colchicine (KOL-chi-seen) is used to prevent or treat attacks of gout (also called gouty arthritis). People with gout have too much uric acid in their blood and joints. An attack of gout occurs when uric acid causes inflammation (pain, redness, swelling, and heat) in a joint. Colchicine does not cure gout or take the place of other medicines that lower the amount of uric acid in the body. It prevents or relieves gout attacks by reducing inflammation. Colchicine is not an ordinary pain reliever and will not relieve most kinds of pain.

Colchicine may also be used for other conditions as determined by your doctor.

Colchicine may be used in 2 ways. Most people take small amounts of it regularly for a long time (months or even years) to prevent severe attacks or other problems caused by inflammation. Other people take large amounts of colchicine during a short period of time (several hours) only when the medicine is needed to relieve an attack that is occurring. The chance of serious side effects is much lower with the first (preventive) kind of treatment.

Because some of colchicine's side effects can be very serious, you should discuss with your doctor the good that this medicine can do as well as the risks of using it. Make sure you understand exactly how you are to use it, and follow the instructions carefully, to lessen the chance of unwanted effects.

This medicine is available only with your doctor's prescription, in the following dosage forms:

*Oral*
- Tablets (U.S. and Canada)

*Parenteral*
- Injection (U.S.)

## Before Using This Medicine

In deciding to use a medicine, the risks of taking the medicine must be weighed against the good it will do. This is a decision you and your doctor will make. For colchicine, the following should be considered:

**Allergies**—Tell your doctor if you have ever had any unusual or allergic reaction to colchicine. Also tell your health care professional if you are allergic to any other substances, such as foods, preservatives, or dyes.

**Pregnancy**—Studies in humans taking large amounts of colchicine to relieve attacks have not been done. Fertility problems have occurred in some men taking small amounts of colchicine regularly (preventive treatment), but these problems went away after treatment was stopped. Many other men taking preventive amounts of colchicine have fathered children without stopping treatment. Also, many women receiving preventive treatment with colchicine have become pregnant and given birth to normal, healthy babies. Some women receive preventive amounts of colchicine regularly for a medical condition that can cause fertility problems or miscarriages. Treatment with colchicine does not increase, and may actually decrease, the occurrence of these problems in women with this condition.

Colchicine has caused birth defects and other problems in animal studies.

**Breast-feeding**—Colchicine passes into breast milk. When breast-feeding mothers receive preventive treatment with one 0.6-milligram (mg) tablet twice a day, the amount that appears in the breast milk is not likely to cause problems in nursing babies. There is no information about whether colchicine can cause problems in nursing babies when the mother takes larger amounts of it. Mothers who are taking this medicine and who wish to breast-feed should discuss this with their doctor.

**Children**—Studies on the effects of colchicine in patients with gout have been done only in adults. Gout is very rare in children. However, colchicine is used in children 3 years of age and older who need preventive treatment for other medical conditions. It has not been reported to cause different side effects or problems in these children than it does in adults.

**Older adults**—Elderly people are especially sensitive to the effects of colchicine. Also, colchicine may stay in the body longer in older patients than it does in younger adults. This may increase the chance of side effects during treatment.

**Other medicines**—Although certain medicines should not be used together at all, in other cases two different medicines may be used together even if an interaction might occur. In these cases, your doctor may want to change the dose, or other precautions may be necessary. When you are taking colchicine, it is especially important that your health care professional know if you are taking any of the following:

- Amphotericin B by injection (e.g., Fungizone) or
- Antineoplastics (cancer medicine) or
- Antithyroid agents (medicine for overactive thyroid) or
- Azathioprine (e.g., Imuran) or
- Chloramphenicol (e.g., Chloromycetin) or
- Cyclophosphamide (e.g., Cytoxan) or
- Flucytosine (e.g., Ancobon) or
- Ganciclovir (e.g., Cytovene) or
- Interferon (e.g., Intron A, Roferon-A) or
- Mercaptopurine (e.g., Purinethol) or
- Methotrexate (e.g., Mexate) or
- Phenylbutazone (e.g., Butazolidin) or
- Plicamycin (e.g., Mithracin) or
- Zidovudine (e.g., Retrovir)—The chance of serious side effects caused by a decrease in the numbers of certain blood cells may be increased

**Other medical problems**—The presence of other medical problems may affect the use of colchicine. Make sure you tell your doctor if you have any other medical problems, especially:

- Alcohol abuse or
- Intestinal disease or
- Stomach ulcer or other stomach problems—The chance of stomach upset may be increased. Also, colchicine can make some kinds of stomach or intestinal problems worse

- Heart disease or
- Kidney disease or
- Liver disease—The chance of serious side effects may be increased because these conditions can cause colchicine to build up in the body
- Low white blood cell count or
- Low platelet count—The chance of serious side effects may be increased because colchicine can make these conditions worse

## Proper Use of This Medicine

Colchicine can build up in the body and cause serious side effects if too much of it is taken or if it is taken too often. Therefore, *do not take more of this medicine, and do not take it more often, than directed by your doctor.* This is especially important for elderly patients, who are more likely than younger adults to have colchicine build up in the body and who are also more sensitive to its effects.

For patients *taking small amounts of colchicine regularly (preventive treatment):*

- Take this medicine regularly as directed by your doctor, even if you feel well. If you are taking colchicine to prevent gout attacks, and you are also taking another medicine to reduce the amount of uric acid in your body, you probably will be able to stop taking colchicine after a while. However, if you stop taking it too soon, your attacks may return or get worse. If you are taking colchicine for certain other medical conditions, you may need to keep taking it for the rest of your life.
- If you are taking colchicine to prevent gout attacks, ask your doctor to recommend other medicine to be taken if an attack occurs. Most people receiving preventive amounts of colchicine should not take extra colchicine to relieve an attack. However, some people cannot take the other medicines that are used for gout attacks and will have to take extra colchicine. If you are one of these people, ask your doctor to tell you the largest amount of colchicine you should take for an attack and how long you should wait before starting to take the smaller preventive amounts again. Be sure to follow these directions carefully.

For patients *taking large amounts of colchicine only when needed to relieve an attack:*

- Start taking this medicine at the first sign of the attack for best results.
- *Stop taking this medicine as soon as the pain is relieved or at the first sign of nausea, vomiting, stomach pain, or diarrhea.* Also, stop taking colchicine when you have taken the largest amount that your doctor ordered for each attack, even if the pain is not relieved or none of these side effects occurs.
- The first few times you take colchicine, keep a record of each dose as you take it. Then, whenever stomach upset (nausea, vomiting, stomach pain, or diarrhea) occurs, count the number of doses you have taken. The next time you need colchicine, stop taking it before that number of doses is reached. For example,

if diarrhea occurs after your fifth dose of medicine, take no more than four doses the next time. If taking fewer doses does not prevent stomach upset from occurring after a few treatments, check with your doctor.

- After taking colchicine tablets to treat an attack, *do not take any more colchicine for at least 3 days. Also, after receiving the medicine by injection for an attack, do not take any more colchicine (tablets or injection) for at least 7 days.* Elderly patients may have to wait even longer between treatments and should check with their doctor for directions.

- If you are taking colchicine for an attack of gout, and you are also taking other medicine to reduce the amount of uric acid in your body, *do not stop taking the other medicine.* Continue taking the other medicine as directed by your doctor.

**Dosing**—The dose of colchicine will be different for different patients. *Follow your doctor's orders or the directions on the label.* The following information includes only the average doses of colchicine. *If your dose is different, do not change it* unless your doctor tells you to do so.

*The number of doses you take each day, the time allowed between doses, and the length of time you take the medicine depend on how often your attacks occur and on whether you are taking the medicine to prevent or to relieve attacks. The amount of medicine you take will also depend on how you react to the medicine.*

- For *oral* dosage form (tablets):
  —Adults:
    - For *preventing gout attacks*—Most people start with one 0.5-milligram (mg) or 0.6-mg tablet a day. If gout attacks continue to occur, the doctor may direct you to increase the dose to one tablet two or even three times a day for a while. Some people with mild gout may need only one tablet every other day, or even less.
    - For *treating a gout attack that has already started*—Your doctor will probably recommend one of the following treatment plans:
      —One or two 0.5-mg or 0.6-mg tablets for the first dose, then one 0.5-mg or 0.6-mg tablet every one or two hours, or
      —Two 0.5-mg or 0.6-mg tablets or one 1-mg tablet every two hours.
      For both plans, *stop taking this medicine after you have taken the largest amount ordered by your doctor.* If your doctor has not told you the largest amount that you should take for one attack, *do not take more than 6 mg of this medicine* (a total of twelve 0.5-mg tablets, ten 0.6-mg tablets, or six 1-mg tablets, spread over a period of several hours).
  —Children: Use and dose must be determined by the doctor.

- For *parenteral* dosage form (injection):
  —Adults:
    - For *preventing gout attacks*—0.5 or 1 mg one or two times a day, injected into a vein.
    - For *treating an attack of gout that has already started*—1 or 2 mg for the first dose, then 0.5 mg or 1 mg every six to twelve hours, injected into a vein. *After a total of 4 mg has been given, no more colchicine (tablets or injections) should be given for at least seven days.*
  —Children: Use and dose must be determined by the doctor.

**Missed dose**—If you are taking colchicine regularly (for example, every day) and you miss a dose, take it as soon as possible. However, if it is almost time for your next dose, skip the missed dose and go back to your regular dosing schedule. Do not double doses.

**Storage**—To store this medicine:
- Keep out of the reach of children.
- Store away from heat and direct light.
- Do not store this medicine in the bathroom, near the kitchen sink, or in other damp places. Heat or moisture may cause the medicine to break down.
- Do not keep outdated medicine or medicine no longer needed. Be sure that any discarded medicine is out of the reach of children.

## Precautions While Using This Medicine

If you must take colchicine for a long time (preventive treatment), your doctor may want to check your progress at regular visits. He or she may also want to check for certain side effects. Finding these side effects early can help to keep them from becoming serious.

Stomach problems may be more likely to occur if you drink large amounts of alcoholic beverages while taking colchicine. Also, drinking too much alcohol may increase the amount of uric acid in your blood. This may lessen the effects of colchicine when it is used to prevent gout attacks. Therefore, people who take colchicine should be careful to limit the amount of alcohol they drink.

For patients taking *small amounts of colchicine regularly (preventive treatment):*

- Attacks of gout or other problems caused by inflammation may continue to occur during treatment. However, the attacks or other problems should occur less often, and they should not be as severe as they were before you started taking colchicine. Even if you think the colchicine is not working, *do not stop taking it and do not increase the dose.* Check with your doctor instead.

## Side Effects of This Medicine

Along with its needed effects, a medicine may cause some unwanted effects. Although not all of these side effects may occur, if they do occur they may need medical attention.

*Stop taking this medicine immediately* if any of the following side effects occur:

### More common
Diarrhea; nausea or vomiting; stomach pain

*If any of these side effects continue for 3 hours or longer after you have stopped taking colchicine, check with your doctor.*

Also, *check with your doctor immediately* if any of the following side effects occur:

### Rare
Black, tarry stools; blood in urine or stools; difficulty in breathing when exercising; fever with or without chills; headache; large, hive-like swellings on the face, eyelids, mouth, lips, and/or tongue; pinpoint red spots on skin; sores, ulcers, or white spots on lips or in mouth; sore throat; unusual bleeding or bruising; unusual tiredness or weakness

### Signs and symptoms of overdose
Burning feeling in the stomach, throat, or skin; diarrhea (severe or bloody); nausea, stomach pain, or vomiting (severe)

Note: These side effects are usually the first signs of an overdose of colchicine tablets. They are not likely to occur when too much colchicine has been given by injection. Other signs and symptoms that may occur after an overdose of either the tablets or the injection include bleeding; fast, shallow breathing; convulsions (seizures); fever; and very severe muscle weakness. An overdose of colchicine can cause damage to the blood, heart, intestines, kidneys, liver, lungs, and muscles.

The following side effects may occur after an injection of colchicine. Check with your doctor as soon as possible if any of the following occur at or near the place of injection:

### Rare
Burning, "crawling," or tingling feeling in the skin; pain; peeling of skin; redness; swelling; tenderness

Also, check with your doctor as soon as possible if any of the following side effects occur:

### Rare
Muscle weakness; numbness in fingers or toes (usually mild); skin rash or hives

Other side effects may occur that usually do not need medical attention. However, check with your doctor if either of the following side effects continues or is bothersome:

### Less common
Loss of appetite

### With long-term use
Loss of hair

Other side effects not listed above may also occur in some patients. If you notice any other effects, check with your doctor.

---

## Additional Information

Once a medicine has been approved for marketing for a certain use, experience may show that it is also useful for other medical problems. Although these uses are not included in product labeling, colchicine is used in certain patients with the following medical conditions:

- Amyloidosis
- Behçet's syndrome
- Calcium pyrophosphate deposition disease (pseudogout)
- Cirrhosis of the liver
- Familial Mediterranean fever
- Pericarditis
- Sarcoid arthritis

If you are taking colchicine for any of these conditions, the following information may apply:

- For all of these conditions, colchicine is usually given regularly in small amounts to reduce inflammation (preventive treatment). This usually decreases the occurrence of severe attacks or other problems caused by inflammation.
- Colchicine is not a cure for these conditions. It will help prevent problems caused by inflammation only as long as you continue to take it.
- Some patients with calcium pyrophosphate deposition disease (pseudogout) or familial Mediterranean fever may take larger amounts of colchicine only when an attack occurs, to relieve the attack.

For patients taking colchicine for *familial Mediterranean fever:*

- Preventive treatment with colchicine may be helping you even if it does not reduce the number of severe attacks. Colchicine helps prevent other serious problems, such as kidney disease, that can occur in people with this condition. Therefore, even if you think that the colchicine isn't working, *do not stop taking it.* Check with your doctor instead.

Other than the above information, there is no additional information relating to proper use, precautions, or side effects for these uses.

---

Revised: 01/31/94

---

# COLESTIPOL  Oral

A commonly used brand name is:
**In the U.S.—**
  Colestid
**In Canada—**
  Colestid

## Description

Colestipol (koe-LES-ti-pole) is used to lower high cholesterol levels in the blood. This may help prevent medical problems caused by cholesterol clogging the blood vessels.

Colestipol works by attaching to certain substances in the intestine. Since colestipol is not absorbed into the body, these substances also pass out of the body without being absorbed.

Colestipol may also be used for other conditions as determined by your doctor.

Colestipol is available only with your doctor's prescription, in the following dosage form:
*Oral*
  • Powder (U.S. and Canada)

## Before Using This Medicine

In deciding to use a medicine, the risks of taking the medicine must be weighed against the good it will do. This is a decision you and your doctor will make. For colestipol, the following should be considered:

**Allergies**—Tell your doctor if you have ever had any unusual or allergic reaction to colestipol. Also tell your health care professional if you are allergic to any substances, such as foods, preservatives, or dyes.

**Diet**—Before prescribing medicine for your condition, your doctor will probably try to control your condition by prescribing a personal diet for you. Such a diet may be low in fats, sugars, and/or cholesterol. Many people are able to control their condition by carefully following their doctor's orders for proper diet and exercise. Medicine is prescribed only when additional help is needed and is effective only when a schedule of diet and exercise is properly followed.

Also, this medicine is less effective if you are greatly overweight. It may be very important for you to go on a reducing diet. However, check with your doctor before going on any diet.

Make certain your health care professional knows if you are on a low-sodium, low-sugar, or any other special diet.

**Pregnancy**—Colestipol is not absorbed into the body and is not likely to cause problems. However, it may reduce absorption of vitamins into the body. Ask your doctor whether you need to take extra vitamins.

**Breast-feeding**—Colestipol is not absorbed into the body and is not likely to cause problems.

**Children**—There is no specific information comparing use of colestipol in children with use in other age groups. However, use is not recommended in children under 2 years of age since cholesterol is needed for normal development.

**Older adults**—Side effects may be more likely to occur in patients over 60 years of age, who are usually more sensitive to the effects of colestipol.

**Other medicines**—Although certain medicines should not be used together at all, in other cases two different medicines may be used together even if an interaction might occur. In these cases, your doctor may want to change the dose, or other precautions may be necessary. When you are taking colestipol it is especially important that your health care professional knows if you are taking any of the following:
  • Anticoagulants (blood thinners)—The effects of the anticoagulant may be altered
  • Digitalis glycosides (heart medicine) or
  • Diuretics (water pills) or
  • Penicillin G, taken by mouth, or
  • Propranolol, taken by mouth, or
  • Tetracyclines (medicine for infection), taken by mouth, or
  • Thyroid hormones or
  • Vancomycin, taken by mouth—Colestipol may cause these medicines to be less effective; these medicines should be taken 4 to 5 hours apart from colestipol

**Other medical problems**—The presence of other medical problems may affect the use of colestipol. Make sure you tell your doctor if you have any other medical problems, especially:
  • Bleeding problems or
  • Constipation or
  • Gallstones or
  • Heart or blood vessel disease or
  • Hemorrhoids or
  • Stomach ulcer or other stomach problems or
  • Underactive thyroid—Colestipol may make these conditions worse
  • Kidney disease—There is an increased risk of developing electrolyte problems
  • Liver disease—Cholesterol levels may be raised

## Proper Use of This Medicine

*Take this medicine exactly as directed by your doctor.* Try not to miss any doses and do not take more medicine than your doctor ordered.

*Follow carefully the special diet your doctor gave you.* This is the most important part of controlling your condition and is necessary if the medicine is to work properly.

*This medicine should never be taken in its dry form,* since it could cause you to choke. Instead, always mix as follows:
  • Add this medicine to 3 ounces or more of water, milk, flavored drink, or your favorite juice or carbonated drink. If you use a carbonated drink, slowly

mix in the powder in a large glass to prevent too much foaming. Stir until it is completely mixed (it will *not* dissolve) before drinking. After drinking all the liquid containing the medicine, rinse the glass with a little more liquid and drink that also, to make sure you get all the medicine.

• You may also mix this medicine with milk in hot or regular breakfast cereals, or in thin soups such as tomato or chicken noodle soup. Or you may add it to some pulpy fruits such as crushed pineapple, pears, peaches, or fruit cocktail.

**Dosing**—The dose of colestipol will be different for different patients. *Follow your doctor's orders or the directions on the label.* The following information includes only the average doses of colestipol. *If your dose is different, do not change it* unless your doctor tells you to do so.

• For *oral* dosage form (powder for oral suspension):
—For high cholesterol:
  • Adults—15 to 30 grams a day. This is divided into two to four doses and taken before meals.
  • Children—Use and dose must be determined by your doctor.

**Missed dose**—If you miss a dose of this medicine, take it as soon as possible. Then go back to your regular dosing schedule. However, if it is almost time for your next dose, skip the missed dose and go back to your regular dosing schedule. Do not double doses.

**Storage**—To store this medicine:
• Keep out of the reach of children.
• Store away from heat and direct light.
• Do not store in the bathroom, near the kitchen sink or in other damp places. Heat or moisture may cause the medicine to break down.
• Do not keep outdated medicine or medicine no longer needed. Be sure that any discarded medicine is out of the reach of children.

## Precautions While Using This Medicine

*It is very important that your doctor check your progress at regular visits.* This will allow your doctor to see if the medicine is working properly to lower your cholesterol levels and to decide if you should continue to take it.

*Do not stop taking this medicine without first checking with your doctor.* When you stop taking this medicine, your blood cholesterol levels may increase again. Your doctor may want you to follow a special diet to help prevent this from happening.

*Do not take any other medicine unless prescribed by your doctor* since colestipol may interfere with other medicines.

## Side Effects of This Medicine

Along with its needed effects, a medicine may cause some unwanted effects. Although not all of these side effects may occur, if they do occur they may need medical attention.

*Check with your doctor immediately* if either of the following side effects occurs:
  *Rare*
    Black, tarry stools; stomach pain (severe) with nausea and vomiting

Check with your doctor as soon as possible if either of the following side effects occurs:
  *More common*
    Constipation
  *Rare*
    Loss of weight (sudden)

Other side effects may occur that usually do not need medical attention. These side effects may go away during treatment as your body adjusts to the medicine. However, check with your doctor if any of the following side effects continue or are bothersome:
  *Less common*
    Belching; bloating; diarrhea; dizziness; headache; nausea or vomiting; stomach pain

Other side effects not listed above may also occur in some patients. If you notice any other effects, check with your doctor.

## Additional Information

Once a medicine has been approved for marketing for a certain use, experience may show that it is also useful for other medical problems. Although these uses are not included in product labeling, colestipol is used in certain patients with the following medical conditions:

• Diarrhea caused by bile acids
• Digitalis glycoside overdose
• Excess oxalate in the urine
• Itching (pruritus) associated with partial biliary obstruction

Other than the above information, there is no additional information relating to proper use, precautions, or side effects for these uses.

Revised: 10/21/92
Interim revision: 04/14/94

# COLISTIN, NEOMYCIN, AND HYDROCORTISONE   Otic

Some commonly used brand names are:
**In the U.S.**
   Coly-Mycin S Otic
**In Canada**
   Coly-Mycin Otic

## Description

Colistin (koe-LIS-tin), neomycin (nee-oh-MYE-sin), and hydrocortisone (hye-droe-KOR-ti-sone) combination contains two antibiotics and a cortisone-like medicine. It is used in the ear to treat infections of the ear canal and to help provide relief from redness, irritation, and discomfort of certain ear problems.

Colistin, neomycin, and hydrocortisone combination is available only with your doctor's prescription, in the following dosage form:

*Otic*
   • Suspension (U.S. and Canada)

## Before Using This Medicine

In deciding to use a medicine, the risks of taking the medicine must be weighed against the good it will do. This is a decision you and your doctor will make. For colistin, neomycin, and hydrocortisone combination, the following should be considered:

**Allergies**—Tell your doctor if you have ever had any unusual or allergic reaction to this medicine or to any related antibiotics such as amikacin (e.g., Amikin), colistin by mouth or by injection (e.g., Coly-Mycin), gentamicin (e.g., Garamycin), kanamycin (e.g., Kantrex), neomycin by mouth or by injection (e.g., Mycifradin), netilmicin (e.g., Netromycin), paromomycin (e.g., Humatin), polymyxin B (e.g., Aerosporin), streptomycin, or tobramycin (e.g., Nebcin). Also tell your health care professional if you are allergic to any other substances, such as thimerosal or other preservatives.

**Pregnancy**—Colistin, neomycin, and hydrocortisone otic drops have not been shown to cause birth defects or other problems in humans.

**Breast-feeding**—Colistin, neomycin, and hydrocortisone otic drops have not been reported to cause problems in nursing babies.

**Children**—Although there is no specific information comparing use of colistin, neomycin, and hydrocortisone combination in children with use in other age groups, this medicine is not expected to cause different side effects or problems in children than it does in adults.

**Older adults**—Many medicines have not been studied specifically in older people. Therefore, it may not be known whether they work exactly the same way they do in younger adults. Although there is no specific information comparing use of colistin, neomycin, and hydrocortisone combination in the elderly with use in other age groups, this medicine is not expected to cause different side effects or problems in older people than it does in younger adults.

**Other medicines**—Although certain medicines should not be used together at all, in other cases two different medicines may be used together even if an interaction might occur. In these cases, your doctor may want to change the dose, or other precautions may be necessary. Tell your health care professional if you are using any other prescription or nonprescription (over-the-counter [OTC]) medicine that is to be used in the ear.

**Other medical problems**—The presence of other medical problems may affect the use of colistin, neomycin, and hydrocortisone combination. Make sure you tell your doctor if you have any other medical problems, especially:
   • Other ear infection or problem, including punctured eardrum—Use of colistin, neomycin, and hydrocortisone combination may make the condition worse or may increase the chance of side effects
   • Herpes simplex—Use of hydrocortisone may make the condition worse

## Proper Use of This Medicine

Before applying this medicine, thoroughly clean the ear canal and dry it with a sterile cotton applicator.

You may warm the ear drops to body temperature (37 °C or 98.6 °F), but no higher, by holding the bottle in your hand for a few minutes before applying. If this medicine gets too warm, it may break down and not work properly.

To apply this medicine:
   • Lie down or tilt the head so that the infected ear faces up. Gently pull the earlobe up and back for adults (down and back for children) to straighten the ear canal. Drop the medicine into the ear canal. Keep the ear facing up for about 5 minutes to allow the medicine to come into contact with the infection. A sterile cotton plug may be gently inserted into the ear opening to prevent the medicine from leaking out. However, your doctor may want you to keep a sterile cotton plug moistened with this medicine in your ear for the full time of treatment. If you have any questions about this, check with your doctor.

To keep the medicine as germ-free as possible, do not touch the dropper to any surface (including the ear). Also, keep the container tightly closed.

*Do not use this medicine for more than 10 days* unless otherwise directed by your doctor.

To help clear up your infection completely, *keep using this medicine for the full time of treatment,* even if your symptoms begin to clear up after a few days. If you stop using this medicine too soon, your symptoms may return. *Do not miss any doses.*

**Dosing**—The dose of otic colistin, neomycin, and hydrocortisone combination will be different for different patients. *Follow your doctor's orders or the directions on the label.* The following information includes only the average doses of otic colistin, neomycin, and hydrocortisone combination. *If your dose is different, do not change it* unless your doctor tells you to do so.

- For *otic suspension (ear drops)* dosage form:
  —For infections of the ear canal:
    - Adults—Use four drops in the ear every six to eight hours.
    - Children—Use up to three drops in the ear every six to eight hours.

**Missed dose**—If you miss a dose of this medicine, apply it as soon as possible. However, if it is almost time for your next dose, skip the missed dose and go back to your regular dosing schedule.

**Storage**—To store this medicine:
- Keep out of the reach of children.
- Store away from heat and direct light.
- Keep the medicine from freezing
- Do not keep outdated medicine or medicine no longer needed. Be sure that any discarded medicine is out of the reach of children.

## Precautions While Using This Medicine

If your symptoms do not improve within 1 week, or if they become worse, check with your doctor immediately.

## Side Effects of This Medicine

Along with its needed effects, a medicine may cause some unwanted effects. Although not all of these side effects may occur, if they do occur they may need medical attention.

*Check with your doctor immediately* if any of the following side effects occur:

*More common*
Itching, skin rash, redness, swelling, or other sign of irritation not present before use of this medicine

Other side effects not listed above may also occur in some patients. If you notice any other effects, check with your doctor.

Revised: 02/10/92
Interim revision(s): 04/13/92; 02/17/94

# COLONY STIMULATING FACTORS    Systemic

Some commonly used brand names are:
**In the U.S.—**
  Neupogen[1]
  Leukine[2]
**In Canada—**
  Neupogen[1]
Other commonly used names are:
  Granulocyte colony stimulating
    factor (G-CSF)[1]
  Granulocyte-macrophage
    colony stimulating factor
    (GM-CSF)[2]
Note: For quick reference, the following colony stimulating factors are numbered to match the corresponding brand names.

This information applies to the following medicines:
1. Filgrastim (fil-GRA-stim)
2. Sargramostim (sar-GRAM-o-stim)†

  †Not commercially available in Canada.

## Description

Filgrastim and sargramostim are synthetic (man-made) versions of substances naturally produced in your body. These substances, called colony stimulating factors, help the bone marrow to make new white blood cells.

When certain cancer medicines fight your cancer cells, they also affect those white blood cells that fight infection. To help prevent infections when these cancer medicines are used, colony stimulating factors may also be given.

Colony stimulating factors are available only with your doctor's prescription, in the following dosage form:
*Parenteral*
  Filgrastim
    - Injection (U.S. and Canada)
  Sargramostim
    - Injection (U.S.)

## Before Using This Medicine

In deciding to use a medicine, the risks of taking the medicine must be weighed against the good it will do. This is a decision you and your doctor will make. For colony stimulating factors, the following should be considered:

**Allergies**—Tell your doctor if you have ever had any unusual or allergic reaction to the colony stimulating factor. Also tell your health care professional if you are allergic to any other substances, such as foods, preservatives, or dyes.

**Pregnancy**—Colony stimulating factors have not been studied in pregnant women.
- *Filgrastim*—In studies in rabbits, filgrastim did not cause birth defects but did cause internal defects, a decrease in average weight, and death of the fetus in high doses.

- *Sargramostim*—Studies on birth defects have not been done in animals.

**Breast-feeding**—It is not known whether colony stimulating factors pass into the breast milk. However, these medicines have not been reported to cause problems in nursing babies.

**Children**—Although there is no specific information comparing use of colony stimulating factors in children with use in other age groups, this medicine is not expected to cause different side effects or problems in children than it does in adults.

**Older adults**—Many medicines have not been studied specifically in older people. Therefore, it may not be known whether they work exactly the same way they do in younger adults. Although there is no specific information comparing use of colony stimulating factors in the elderly with use in other age groups, this medicine has been used in many elderly patients and is not expected to cause different side effects or problems in older people than it does in younger adults.

**Other medicines**—Although certain medicines should not be used together at all, in other cases two different medicines may be used together even if an interaction might occur. In these cases, your doctor may want to change the dose, or other precautions may be necessary. Tell your health care professional if you are taking any other prescription or nonprescription (over-the-counter [OTC]) medicine.

**Other medical problems**—The presence of other medical problems may affect the use of colony stimulating factors. Make sure you tell your doctor if you have any other medical problems, especially:

- Conditions caused by inflammation or immune system problems—There is a chance these may be worsened by colony stimulating factor
- Heart disease—Risk of some unwanted effects (heart rhythm problems, retaining water) may be increased
- Kidney disease or
- Liver disease—May sometimes be worsened by colony stimulating factor
- Lung disease—Colony stimulating factor may cause shortness of breath

## Proper Use of This Medicine

If you are injecting this medicine yourself, *use it exactly as directed by your doctor.* Do not use more or less of it, and do not use it more often than your doctor ordered. The exact amount of medicine you need has been carefully worked out. Using too much will increase the risk of side effects, while using too little may not improve your condition.

*If you are injecting this medicine yourself, each package of colony stimulating factor will contain a patient instruction sheet. Read this sheet carefully* and make sure you understand:

- How to prepare the injection.
- Proper use of disposable syringes.

- How to give the injection.
- How long the injection is stable.

If you have any questions about any of this, check with your health care professional.

**Dosing**—The dose of colony stimulating factors will be different for different patients. The dose that is used may depend on a number of things, including what the medicine is being used for, the patient's body weight or size, and whether or not other medicines are also being taken. *If you are receiving colony stimulating factors at home, follow your doctor's orders or the directions on the label.* If you have any questions about the proper dose of colony stimulating factors, ask your doctor.

**Missed dose**—If you miss a dose of this medicine, check with your doctor.

**Storage**—To store this medicine:

- Keep out of the reach of children.
- Store in the refrigerator.
- Keep the medicine from freezing.
- Do not keep outdated medicine or medicine no longer needed. Ask your health care professional how you should dispose of any medicine you do not use. Be sure that any discarded medicine is out of the reach of children.

## Precautions While Using This Medicine

*It is very important that your doctor check your progress at regular visits* to make sure that this medicine is working properly and to check for unwanted effects.

Colony stimulating factors are used to prevent or reduce the risk of infection while you are being treated with cancer medicines. Because your body's ability to fight infection is reduced, *it is very important that you call your doctor at the first sign of any infection* (for example, if you get a fever or chills) so you can start antibiotic treatment right away.

Colony stimulating factors commonly cause mild bone pain, usually in the lower back or pelvis, about the time the white blood cells start to come back in your bone marrow. The pain is usually mild and lasts only a few days. Your doctor will probably prescribe a mild analgesic (painkiller) for you to take during that time. If you find that the analgesic is not strong enough, talk with your doctor about using something that will make you more comfortable.

## Side Effects of This Medicine

Along with its needed effects, a medicine may cause some unwanted effects. Although not all of these side effects may occur, if they do occur they may need medical attention.

The side effects listed below include only those that might be caused by colony stimulating factors. To find out about other side effects that may be caused by the cancer medicines you are also receiving, look under the information about those specific medicines.

Check with your doctor as soon as possible if any of the following side effects occur:

*For filgrastim*
  *Less common*
     Redness or pain at the site of subcutaneous (under the skin) injection
  *Rare*
     Fever; rapid or irregular heartbeat; sores on skin; wheezing
*For sargramostim*
  *Less common*
     Fever; redness or pain at the site of subcutaneous (under the skin) injection; shortness of breath; swelling of feet or lower legs; weight gain (sudden)
  *Rare*
     Chest pain; rapid or irregular heartbeat; sores on skin; wheezing

Other side effects may occur that usually do not need medical attention. These side effects may go away during treatment as your body adjusts to the medicine. However, check with your doctor if any of the following side effects continue or are bothersome:

*For both filgrastim and sargramostim*
  *More common*
     Headache; pain in joints or muscles; pain in lower back or pelvis; skin rash or itching
  *Less common*
     Pain in arms or legs
*For sargramostin only (in addition to the above)*
  *Less common or rare*
     Dizziness or faintness after first dose of medicine; flushing of face after first dose of medicine; weakness

Other side effects not listed above may also occur in some patients. If you notice any other effects, check with your doctor.

Revised: 08/07/92
Interim revision: 04/22/93; 07/14/94

# CONDOMS

Some commonly used brand names are:

**In the U.S.—**

| | |
|---|---|
| Embrace[2] | Ramses NuFORM[2] |
| Excita Extra[3] | Ramses Sensitol Lubricated[2] |
| Excita Fiesta[2] | Saxon Ribbed Lubricated[2] |
| Fourex Natural Skins[1] | Saxon Spermicidal[3] |
| Gold Circle Coin[2] | Saxon Ultra Thin[2] |
| Kimono[2] | Saxon Wet Lubricated[2] |
| Kimono Plus[3] | Sheik Elite[2] |
| Koromex with Nonoxynol 9[3] | Sheik Fetherlite Snug-Fit[2] |
| Lady Protex with Spermicidal Lubricant[3] | Sheik Non-Lubricated Plain End[2] |
| Lady Protex Ultra-Thin[2] | Sheik Non-Lubricated Reservoir End[2] |
| LifeStyles Extra Strength with Spermicide[3] | Today with Spermicidal Lubricant[3] |
| LifeStyles Form Fitting[2] | Trojan-Enz[2] |
| LifeStyles Lubricated[2] | Trojan-Enz Large Lubricated[2] |
| LifeStyles Spermicidally Lubricated[3] | Trojan-Enz Large with Spermicidal Lubricant[3] |
| LifeStyles Ultra Sensitive[2] | Trojan-Enz Lubricated[2] |
| LifeStyles Vibra-Ribbed[2] | Trojan-Enz with Spermicidal Lubricant[3] |
| Magnum Lubricated[2] | Trojan Extra Strength Lubricated[2] |
| Magnum with Spermicidal Lubricant[3] | Trojan Kling-Tite Naturalamb[1] |
| MAXX[2] | Trojan Naturalube Ribbed[2] |
| MAXX Plus[3] | Trojan Plus[2] |
| Mentor Lubricated[2] | Trojan Plus 2[3] |
| Mentor Plus Spermicidal Lubricant[3] | Trojan Ribbed[2] |
| Protex Arouse[2] | Trojan Ribbed with Spermicidal Lubricant[3] |
| Protex Contracept Plus with Spermicidal Lubricant[3] | Trojans[2] |
| Protex Secure[2] | Trojan for Women[2] |
| Protex Touch[2] | Trojan for Women with Spermicidal Lubricant[3] |
| Ramses Extra with Spermicidal Lubricant[3] | |
| Ramses Non-Lubricated Reservoir End[2] | |

**In Canada—**

| | |
|---|---|
| Conceptrol Shields[2] | Saxon Ribbed Lubricated[2] |
| Conceptrol Supreme[2] | Saxon Spermicidal[3] |
| Embrace[2] | Saxon Ultra Thin[2] |
| Fourex Natural Skins[1] | Saxon Wet Lubricated[2] |
| Gold Circle Coin[2] | Sheik Denim[2] |
| LifeStyles Extra Strength with Spermicide[3] | Sheik Elite[3] |
| LifeStyles Form Fitting[2] | Sheik Excita[3] |
| LifeStyles Lubricated[2] | Sheik Non-Lubricated[2] |
| LifeStyles Spermicidally Lubricated[3] | Sheik Sensi-Creme[2] |
| LifeStyles Ultra Sensitive[2] | Trojan-Enz[2] |
| LifeStyles Vibra-Ribbed[2] | Trojan-Enz Large Lubricated[2] |
| Ramses Extra[3] | Trojan-Enz Large with Spermicidal Lubricant[3] |
| Ramses Extra-15[3] | Trojan-Enz Lubricated[2] |
| Ramses Non-lubricated[2] | Trojan-Enz with Spermicidal Lubricant[3] |
| Ramses NuForm[2] | Trojan Kling-Tite Naturalamb[1] |
| Ramses Ribbed[3] | Trojan Naturalube Ribbed[2] |
| Ramses Sensitol[2] | Trojan Plus 2[3] |
| Ramses Ultra[2] | Trojan Ribbed[2] |
| Ramses Ultra-15[3] | Trojans[2] |

Note: For quick reference, the following condoms are numbered to match the corresponding brand names.

This information applies to the following medicines:
1. Lamb Cecum
2. Latex
3. Latex and Nonoxynol 9

## Description

Condoms (KON-dums) are used by a male partner during sexual intercourse as a form of birth control. Latex rubber condoms are also used during anal, vaginal, or oral sex to help protect against sexually transmitted diseases such as AIDS (HIV infection), genital herpes (herpes simplex

II), gonorrhea, syphilis, chlamydia, genital warts, and hepatitis.

*Condoms can be a highly effective form of birth control when they are used properly. However, pregnancy usually occurs in 12 of each 100 women during the first year of condom use.* You can discuss with your doctor what your options are for birth control and the pros and cons of using each method.

Condoms work to protect against sexually transmitted diseases (STDs) and as a birth control method by acting as barrier (wall) to keep blood, semen, and other fluids from passing from one partner to the other. The germs that can cause STDs are present in these fluids. With the proper use of latex condoms, these fluids are trapped inside the condom, along with sperm and any germs that may be present.

*Latex rubber condoms are preferred for the prevention of STDs.* Even though lamb intestine condoms are as effective as latex condoms in preventing pregnancy, it is not known whether they are as effective as latex condoms in protecting against all of the STDs, especially AIDS. Therefore, lamb intestine condoms should be used to protect against STDs *only* if you (or your partner) are allergic or sensitive to latex rubber condoms.

The use of a spermicide along with a condom increases the condom's ability to prevent pregnancy. Also, *laboratory studies* have shown that the spermicide nonoxynol 9 kills or stops the growth of the AIDS virus (HIV) and herpes simplex I and II viruses. It was also shown to be effective against other types of germs that cause gonorrhea, chlamydia, syphilis, trichomoniasis, and other STDs. *Although this has not been proven in human studies, some scientists believe that spermicides put into the vagina or on the outside of a latex condom may kill these germs before they are able to come in contact with the vagina or rectum (lower bowel).* Spermicides also provide a back-up in case the condom breaks, slips, or leaks during sexual intercourse.

The most effective way to protect yourself against STDs (such as AIDS) is by abstinence (not having sexual intercourse) or by having only one partner and making sure that person is not already infected and is *not* going to get an STD. However, if any of these methods are not likely or possible, using latex rubber condoms with an extra spermicide product is the best way to protect yourself. This is especially important if you cannot be sure a partner does not have an STD.

The use of a condom is recommended even when you are using other methods of birth control, such as birth control pills (the Pill), the cervical cap, the contraceptive sponge, diaphragm, and the intrauterine device (IUD), since these methods do not offer any protection from STDs.

The safety of using condoms with spermicides in the rectum (lower bowel), anus, or rectal area is not known. No side effects have been reported that are different from those reported for use in the vagina. However, some studies have reported that latex condoms are more likely to break during anal intercourse.

Condoms are available without a prescription in the following product forms:
- Lamb intestine condoms (U.S. and Canada)
- Latex condoms (U.S. and Canada)
- Latex condoms and nonoxynol 9 (a spermicide) (U.S. and Canada)

## Before Using This Product

In deciding to use condoms as a method of birth control or to prevent STDs, you need to consider the pros and cons involved with their use. This is a decision you and your sexual partner will make. The following information may help you in making your decision. Ask your health care professional for more information if you have any questions.

**Allergies**—If you have ever had any unusual or allergic reaction to condoms or other rubber products, it is best to check with your doctor before using latex condoms. Also, it is a good idea to check with your doctor before using condoms with nonoxynol 9 if you have ever had an allergic or unusual reaction to spermicides.

**Adolescents**—These products are frequently used by teenagers and have not been shown to cause different problems than they do in adults. However, some younger or first time users may need extra counseling and information on the importance of using condoms exactly as they are supposed to be used so they will work properly.

## Proper Use of This Product

Some condoms have a dry or wet lubricant applied to them. Use of a lubricant may help prevent condoms from breaking or slipping and prevent irritation to the vagina, anus, or rectum. It may be especially important to use a lubricant during anal intercourse, since some studies have shown that latex condoms break more often during anal intercourse. This is because there is greater friction (rubbing force) during anal intercourse, as compared with vaginal or oral intercourse. *If you need an extra lubricant, make sure it is a water-based product safe for use with condoms, cervical caps, or diaphragms.* Spermicides, especially gels and jellies, also provide some lubrication during sexual intercourse. *Oil-based products such as hand, face, or body cream; petroleum jelly; cooking oils or shortenings; or mineral or baby oil should not be used because they weaken the latex rubber.* (Even some products that easily rinse away with water are oil-based and should not be used.) This increases the chances of the condom breaking during sexual intercourse.

To use:
- *Before any genital contact occurs:*
  —Open the condom wrapper carefully, making sure you do not damage it before use. Always handle the unwrapped condom carefully. If the wrapper was already open, do not use the condom because the

condom may be damaged or weakened.

—Look at the unrolled condom before it is placed on the penis, to check it for any damage or defects. Occasionally, a condom may be damaged from improper storage, opening, or manufacturing. If the condom feels sticky, brittle, dried out, or gummy, do not use it. Also, check the tip for tears or holes. However, do not unroll the condom to look at it before you are ready to use it. Also, do not fill it with water to check it for leaks. Both of these actions will weaken the condom. When handling the condom, be careful also not to tear it with sharp or jagged fingernails and sharp rings or jewelry. Use a different condom if you have any doubts about any condom's quality or condition.

—Place the unrolled condom over the tip of the erect (hard) penis. Check the condom to make sure the correct side is touching the penis. If you accidentally put on the unrolled condom with the wrong side out, it should not be used. There is a chance that germs or sperm could get on the tip of the condom. If you then reversed the condom and unrolled it correctly, your partner would be in contact with the germs or sperm.

—Pinch the end of the condom to leave a half-inch of space for the semen to collect in. If the condom has a reservoir, pinch this reservoir to get rid of any air. Leaving this extra space will keep semen and other fluids from spilling out during intercourse.

—While still pinching the tip of the condom, completely unroll the condom down the length of the penis to its base. If the penis is uncircumcised, the foreskin should be pulled back before the condom is unrolled. To be most effective in preventing STDs, the condom must cover the entire penis.

—If you are using extra spermicide or lubricant, carefully spread some on the outside of the condom. It is a good idea to check the rest of the condom for any defects or damage at this time. A female partner should also use a spermicide inside the vagina.

• *After genital contact occurs:*

—If a condom breaks during intercourse, immediately put on a new condom. Also, apply more spermicide or lubricant.

—Immediately after ejaculation and before the penis becomes soft, firmly grasp the ring of the condom at the base of the penis. Carefully withdraw the penis to avoid tearing the condom or spilling semen. Discard the used condom properly.

—You must use a new condom each time you repeat intercourse. *Condoms should never be reused.* Spermicide or lubricant should also be re-applied outside of the new condom. A female partner should also put more spermicide in the vagina each time she has intercourse.

*For females using condoms with extra spermicide:*

• Condoms do not have to be used with spermicides, but the spermicide may provide a back-up in case the condom leaks or breaks.

• It is very important that the spermicide be placed properly in the vagina. It should be put deep into the vagina, directly on the cervix (opening to the uterus). The written instructions about how the product container and the applicator work, how much spermicide to use each time, and how long each application remains effective may be different for each product. Make sure you carefully read and follow the instructions that come with each product.

• *Make sure the spermicide you choose is labeled as being safe for use with latex diaphragms, cervical caps, or condoms.* Otherwise, it may cause the condom to weaken and leak or even break during intercourse.

**Storage**—To store:

• Store in a dark, cool, dry place. Avoid extreme temperatures and direct light. If you carry a condom with you, keep it in a wallet, loose pocket, or purse for no more than a few hours at time.

• Do not store in the bathroom or in other damp places. Heat or moisture may weaken condoms.

• Keep the product from freezing.

• Do not use outdated condoms or condoms that are clearly old or that have no date on the package. Only latex condoms with a pre-applied spermicide have an expiration date. After this time, the maker cannot guarantee the spermicide potency. Other condoms should have the date that they were made on the box. It is best if you do not buy condoms long before you use them, in case the storage has not been ideal. The best way to make sure you are using fresh condoms is to buy them only a short time before they will be used. Older condoms are more likely to break during sexual intercourse. If you have any questions about the storage and expiration dating of condoms, ask your health care professional.

• Be sure that any discarded condoms are out of the reach of children. Used condoms should be wrapped in tissue or paper. Discard them in the trash so that others will not accidentally handle them.

---

## Side Effects of This Product

Condoms occasionally cause allergies or local irritation in some people. They may cause itching, burning, stinging, or a rash. These reactions could be due to the latex itself, the lubricant, or the spermicide. Changing to a different brand of condom may solve this problem. Also, using a weaker strength of vaginal spermicide (if you are using extra spermicide) may be necessary, although it will be less effective. If any of these effects continue after you have changed products, you may have an allergy to these products or an infection and should contact a doctor as soon as possible.

Very rarely, some people may have a severe allergic reaction to latex rubber. *Check with a doctor immediately* if any of the following effects occur:

*Rare*

*For latex condoms only*

Difficulty in breathing; hives; swelling of the face or inside of the throat

Also, check with a doctor as soon as possible if any of the following effects occur:

*Rare*
*For latex condoms only*
*For females and males*
Redness of the inside of the eyelids; skin rash, redness, swelling, irritation, local swelling, or itching that occurs each time a latex condom is used; stuffy nose after using latex condoms
*For females only*
Vaginal bleeding, irritation, redness, rash, dryness, or whitish discharge that occurs each time a latex condom is used (signs of vaginal allergy)
*For latex condoms containing spermicide only*
*For females only*
Bladder pain; cloudy or bloody urine; increased frequency of urination; pain on urination

Other side effects may occur that usually do not need medical attention. Using a different brand of condom may help to eliminate these effects. However, check with your doctor if any of the following side effects continue or are bothersome:

*Less common*
Burning, stinging, warmth, itching, or other irritation of the skin, penis, rectum, or vagina; vaginal dryness or odor

Other side effects not listed above may also occur in some people. If you notice any other effects, check with your doctor.

Revised: 03/04/93

# COPPER INTRAUTERINE DEVICES (IUDs)

Some commonly used brand names are:
**In U.S.—**
ParaGard-T 380A[3]
**In Canada—**
Gyne-T [1]          Nova-T[2]
Gyne-T 380 Slimline[4]
Note: For quick reference, the following copper intrauterine devices are numbered to match the corresponding brand names.
This information applies to the following devices:

1. Copper-T 200 IUD*
2. Copper-T 200Ag IUD*
3. Copper-T 380A IUD†
4. Copper-T 380S IUD*

*Not commercially available in the U.S.
†Not commercially available in Canada.

## Description

A copper intrauterine device (KOP-er IN-tra-YOU-ta-rin de-VICE) (also called an IUD) is inserted by a health care professional into a woman's uterus as a long-term contraceptive (birth control method).

The copper-T IUD works by causing changes in the uterus that make becoming pregnant (conception) harder. The fertilization of the woman's egg with her partner's sperm is less likely with an IUD in place, but it can occur. Even so, the IUD makes it harder for the fertilized egg to become attached to the uterus walls making it hard to become pregnant. Having copper on the IUD is believed to improve the effects of the device. After the IUD is removed, most women can become pregnant.

*Studies have shown that pregnancy can occur in up to 4 of each 100 women using copper-T IUDs during the first year of use.* Other birth control methods such as not having intercourse, taking birth control pills (the Pill), or having surgery to become sterile are as effective or more effective. Methods that do not work as well include using condoms, diaphragms, vaginal sponges, or spermicides. Discuss with your health care professional what your options are for birth control and the risks and benefits of each method.

*IUDs do not protect a woman from sexually transmitted diseases (STDs), including human immunodeficiency virus (HIV) or acquired immunodeficiency syndrome (AIDS). The use of latex (rubber) condoms or abstinence is recommended for protection from these diseases.*

*Your lifestyle will determine how safe and reliable the copper-T IUD will be for you.* Problems that may occur with use of an IUD are far less likely to occur in women who have a long-term relationship with one sexual partner. Also, it is important that your sexual partner not have any other sexual partners. If you or your partner has more than one sexual partner it increases *your* chance of getting an infection in the vagina. If an infection is present in the vagina or uterus when the IUD is in the uterus it may make an infection more serious. *If your lifestyle changes while you are using an IUD or you get or are exposed to an STD, call your health care professional.*

Copper-T IUDs are available only from your doctor or other authorized health care professional in the following forms:

• Copper-T 200 Intrauterine Device (Canada)
• Copper-T 200Ag Intrauterine Device (Canada)
• Copper-T 380A Intrauterine Device (U.S.)
• Copper-T 380S Intrauterine Device (Canada)

## Before Receiving This Device

In deciding whether to use a copper-T IUD as a method of birth control, you need to consider the risks of using it as well as the good it can do. This is a decision you, your sexual partner, and your health care professional will make. For copper-T IUDs, the following should be considered:

**Allergies**—Tell your health care professional if you have ever had any unusual or allergic reaction to copper.

**Pregnancy**—IUD use is not recommended during pregnancy or if you plan to become pregnant in the near future. It is also not recommended in women who have had a pregnancy develop outside of the uterus (ectopic pregnancy).

There is a rare chance that a woman can become pregnant with the IUD in the uterus. If this happens, it is recommended that the IUD be removed or that the pregnancy be ended within the first 3 months. If the pregnancy continues, removing the IUD decreases the chance of a problem developing. However, whether the IUD is removed or not, some problems can occur. Some of these problems include miscarriage, premature labor and delivery, infection, and, very rarely, death of the mother.

Your health care professional will help you decide on the proper time to begin using an IUD after delivering a baby. Sometimes problems can occur if you start using the IUD too soon after delivery. These problems include having the IUD move out of place or having it press into the walls of the uterus or the cervix (opening to the uterus). These problems may harm the cervix or uterus, causing pain or unusual vaginal bleeding. *Call your health care professional immediately* if you have any problems.

**Breast-feeding**—The copper from an IUD has not been shown to cause problems in nursing babies.

**Teenagers**—Sexually active teenagers may need to use a contraceptive method that protects them against sexually transmitted diseases (STDs).

Teenagers who have not had children usually have more side effects than teenagers or adults who have had children. In some of these women, the IUD may move out of place. This may harm the uterus or cervix. Abdominal pain and increased menstrual bleeding also are more common in teenagers than in women who are older and have had children.

**Other medical problems**—The presence of other medical problems may affect the use of copper-T IUDs. Make sure you tell your health care professional if you have any other medical problems, especially:

- Abnormal uterus—May decrease the IUD's ability to prevent pregnancy or may increase the chance of problems, such as the IUD moving out of the uterus or pressing through the cervix or uterus
- Acquired immunodeficiency syndrome (AIDS), autoimmune diseases, treatable cancer, suspected or known cancer of the uterus or cervix, or any other condition that may decrease the ability of the body to fight infection—These conditions may increase the chance of a vaginal infection occurring with the use of an IUD
- Anemia or
- Bleeding problems, especially heavy bleeding during periods or bleeding between periods—Use of an IUD can

make these conditions worse, and heavy vaginal bleeding may cause the IUD to move out of place
- Diabetes, insulin-dependent or
- Heart defect—If an infection occurs during use of an IUD, the infection may become worse and/or be harder to treat in these patients
- Ectopic pregnancy (pregnancy not in the uterus), history of—The chance of an ectopic pregnancy may be increased if contraception fails during IUD use
- Fainting (history of) or
- Slow heartbeat (history of)—The chance of problems may be increased when, or soon after, the IUD is inserted
- Infection in the vagina or uterus or
- Recent infected abortion or
- Sexually transmitted disease in the last 12 months—Use of an IUD may make an infection worse
- Surgery involving the uterus or fallopian tubes—Certain surgeries done on the uterus or the fallopian tubes may increase the chance of problems if an IUD is present in the uterus
- Wilson's disease—Use of a copper IUD can make this condition worse

## Proper Use of This Device

IUDs come with patient information. *You must understand this information.* You should keep a copy for reference. *Be sure you understand possible problems with the copper-T IUD, especially side effects, risks, and warning signs of trouble.*

Spermicides such as contraceptive foams or creams are not needed to prevent pregnancy with a properly placed copper-T IUD.

*It is important that you check for the IUD threads every month (if not more often) especially after each menstrual period.* Feeling the IUD threads near the cervix lets you know that the copper-T IUD is still in place.
*To check for the IUD threads:*

- Wash your hands thoroughly.
- Squat and, using your middle finger, find the cervix high in the vagina.
- The IUD threads should hang down from the cervix.
- *Do not pull on the threads.*

**Dosing**—The length of time that you will be using the copper-T IUD depends on the device that you are using. *Follow your health care professional's orders to schedule the proper time to remove and replace your copper-T IUD.* You and your health care professional may choose to replace it sooner or begin a new method of birth control.

- For preventing pregnancy:
    —For copper-T 200 dosage form:
      - Adults and teenagers—One device inserted into the vagina by a health care professional and replaced within 24 months of use.

—For copper-T 200Ag dosage form:
- Adults and teenagers—One device inserted into the vagina by a health care professional and replaced within 30 months of use.

—For copper-T 380A dosage form:
- Adults and teenagers—One device inserted into the vagina by a health care professional and replaced within 10 years of use.

—For copper-T 380S dosage form:
- Adults and teenagers—One device inserted into the vagina by a health care professional and replaced within 30 months of use.

## Precautions While Using This Device

*It is very important to keep all medical appointments with your health care professional during the first year of IUD use.* After the first year, your health care professional will probably want to check your progress once a year. This will allow the health care professional to make sure that the device is still in place and working properly.

*Check with your medical doctor if you plan to have surgery of the uterus or fallopian tubes.* Your doctor may remove your IUD before the surgery. *Also, tell your health care professional if you plan to get heat or radiation therapy.* Some types of therapy such as treatments used in sports medicine may heat the copper on the IUD. This may cause harm to the area directly around the IUD. Your doctor may take the IUD out or help you choose another type of treatment.

*Tell your doctor immediately if you think that the IUD has moved out of place. Do not try to put the IUD back into place inside the uterus. Do not try to remove the IUD.*

Although IUDs are very reliable, there is a rare chance that the IUD may fail to protect some people from becoming pregnant. Very rarely a pregnancy can occur outside of the uterus; this is called an ectopic pregnancy. It can be hard to tell if an ectopic pregnancy has occurred. Unlike a normal pregnancy in the uterus which stops the menstrual period, some people can still have a menstrual period with an ectopic pregnancy. These women may not think they are pregnant.

*Notify your doctor immediately if you feel many of the following changes that can occur with a pregnancy:* Enlarged or tender breasts, lack of menstrual period, lower abdominal pain or cramping (possibly severe), sore abdomen, unusual tiredness or weakness, unusual vaginal bleeding (in some cases, very heavy).

*If you think you are pregnant or if you miss a period while you are using the IUD, tell your health care professional.* Until your doctor is able to see you, use another birth control method, such as condoms, to prevent pregnancy just in case you are not pregnant.

*Also, notify your doctor and use another birth control method, such as condoms,* if:
- you have unusual vaginal bleeding
- you are exposed to or get a sexually transmitted disease (STD)
- you feel the tip of the IUD at the cervix or you or your partner feels pain during sexual intercourse
- you cannot find the threads from the IUD or think that the thread length is different
- you or your sexual partner's lifestyle changes and one or both of you have more than one sexual partner
- you have unusual or severe lower abdominal pain or cramping, possibly with a fever
- you develop vaginal discharge or sores in the vaginal area

You can use other products in the vagina, such as tampons or condoms, while you are using a copper-T IUD.

## Side Effects of This Device

Along with its needed effects, a device may cause some unwanted effects. Although not all of these side effects may occur, if any do occur they may need medical attention.

*Get emergency help immediately* if any of the following side effects occur:

*Rare*
Abdominal pain or cramping (severe); vaginal bleeding (unexpected, heavy)

*Check with your health care professional immediately* if any of the following side effects occur:

*More common*
Faintness, dizziness, or sharp pain at time of IUD insertion; increased amount of menstrual bleeding at regular monthly periods; normal menstrual bleeding occurring earlier or lasting longer than expected

*Less common*
Abnormal vaginal bleeding (mild to moderate) not associated with a menstrual period; abdominal pain (dull or aching), odorous vaginal discharge, pain on urination with increased urge to urinate, and unusual vaginal bleeding

*Rare*
Abdominal pain or cramping, fever, nausea, and vomiting; painful sexual intercourse; unusual tiredness or weakness, and increased menstrual bleeding

Other side effects may occur that usually do not need medical attention. These side effects may go away during treatment as your body adjusts to the device. However, check with your health care professional if the following side effect continues or is bothersome:

*More common*
Increased abdominal pain and cramping at menstrual periods

After you stop using this device, you may become pregnant. The contraceptive effect of copper-T IUDs is usually reversible. If you stop using an IUD and still do not want to become pregnant, you should begin using another contraceptive method immediately to prevent pregnancy.

Other side effects not listed above may also occur in some patients. If you notice any other effects, check with your health care professional.

Developed: 06/29/94

---

# COPPER SUPPLEMENTS    Systemic

Another commonly used name for copper sulfate is cupric sulfate.

Note: For quick reference, the following copper supplements are numbered to match the corresponding brand names.

This information applies to the following medicines:
1. Copper Gluconate (KOP-er GLOO-coh-nate)‡
2. Copper Sulfate (SUL-fate)‡§

†Not commercially available in Canada.
‡Generic name product may also be available in the U.S.
§Generic name product may also be available in Canada.

## Description

Copper supplements are used to prevent or treat copper deficiency.

The body needs copper for normal growth and health. For patients who are unable to get enough copper in their regular diet or who have a need for more copper, copper supplements may be necessary. They are generally taken by mouth but some patients may have to receive them by injection.

Lack of copper may lead to anemia and osteoporosis (weak bones).

Patients with the following conditions may be more likely to have a deficiency of copper:
- Burns
- Diarrhea
- Intestine disease
- Kidney disease
- Pancreas disease
- Stomach removal
- Stress, continuing

In addition, premature infants may need additional copper.

If any of the above apply to you, you should take copper supplements only on the advice of your physician after need has been established.

Claims that copper supplements are effective in the treatment of arthritis or skin conditions have not been proven.

Use of copper supplements to cause vomiting has caused death and should be avoided.

Some preparations are available only with your doctor's prescription. Others are available without a prescription; however, your doctor may have special instructions on the proper use and dose for your condition.

Copper supplements are available in the following dosage forms:
*Oral*
Copper Gluconate
- Tablets (U.S.)
*Parenteral*
Copper Sulfate
- Injection (U.S. and Canada)

## Importance of Diet

Nutritionists recommend that, if possible, people should get all the copper they need from foods. However, some people do not get enough copper from their diets. For example, people on weight-loss diets may consume too little food to provide enough copper. Others may need more copper than normal. For such people, a copper supplement is important.

In order to get enough vitamins and minerals in your diet, it is important that you eat a balanced and varied diet. Follow carefully any diet program your doctor may recommend. For your specific vitamin and/or mineral needs, ask your doctor or dietitian for a list of appropriate foods.

Copper is found in various foods, including organ meats (especially liver), seafoods, beans, nuts, and whole-grains. Additional copper can come from drinking water from copper pipes, using copper cookware, and eating farm products sprayed with copper-containing chemicals. Copper may be decreased in foods that have high acid content and are stored in tin cans for a long time.

Experts have developed a list of recommended dietary allowances (RDA) for most vitamins and some minerals. The RDA are not an exact number but a general idea of how much you need. They do not cover amounts needed for problems caused by a serious lack of vitamins and minerals. There are no RDA for copper. The following intakes are thought to be plenty for most individuals:

- Infants and children—
  Birth to 6 months of age: 0.4 to 0.6 mg per day.
  6 months to 1 year of age: 0.6 to 0.7 mg per day.
  1 to 3 years of age: 0.7 to 1 mg per day.
  4 to 6 years of age: 1 to 1.5 mg per day.
  7 to 10 years of age: 1 to 2 mg per day.
- Adolescent males and females—1.5 to 2.5 mg per day.
- Adult males and females—1.5 to 3 mg per day.

Remember:

- The total amount of copper that you get every day includes what you get from the foods that you eat and what you may take as supplement.
- This total amount should not be greater than the above recommendations, unless ordered by your doctor.

## Before Using This Dietary Supplement

If you are taking this dietary supplement without a prescription, carefully read and follow any precautions on the label. For copper supplements, the following should be considered:

**Allergies**—Tell your health care professional if you are allergic to any substances, such as foods, preservatives, or dyes.

**Pregnancy**—It is especially important that you are receiving enough vitamins and minerals when you become pregnant and that you continue to receive the right amount of vitamins and minerals throughout your pregnancy. The healthy growth and development of the fetus depend on a steady supply of nutrients from the mother. However, taking large amounts of a dietary supplement in pregnancy may be harmful to the mother and/or fetus and should be avoided.

**Breast-feeding**—It is important that you receive the right amounts of vitamins and minerals so that your baby will also get the vitamins and minerals needed to grow properly. However, taking large amounts of a dietary supplement while breast-feeding may be harmful to the mother and/or baby and should be avoided.

**Children**—It is especially important that children receive enough copper in their diet for healthy growth and development. Although there is no specific information comparing use of copper in children with use in other age groups, this medicine is not expected to cause different side effects or problems in children than in adults.

**Older adults**—It is important that older people continue to receive enough copper in their daily diets.

**Medicines or other dietary supplements**—Although certain medicines or dietary supplements should not be used together at all, in other cases they may be used together even if an interaction might occur. In these cases, your doctor may want to change the dose, or other precautions may be necessary. When you are taking copper supplements, it is especially important that your health care professional know if you are taking any of the following:

- Penicillamine or
- Trientine or
- Zinc supplements (taken by mouth)—Use with copper supplements may decrease the amount of copper that gets into the body; copper supplements should be taken at least 2 hours after penicillamine, trientine, or zinc supplements

**Other medical problems**—The presence of other medical problems may affect the use of copper supplements. Make sure you tell your doctor if you have any other medical problems, especially:

- Wilson's disease (too much copper in the body)—Copper supplements may make this condition worse

## Proper Use of This Dietary Supplement

Some people believe that taking very large doses of a vitamin or mineral (called megadoses) is useful for treating certain medical problems. Studies have not proven this. Large doses should be taken only under the direction of your doctor after need has been identified.

**Dosing**—The dose of copper for prevention of copper deficiency is based on daily recommended intake. See the *Importance of Diet* section for daily recommended intake for copper.

**Missed dose**—If you miss taking copper supplements for one or more days there is no cause for concern, since it takes some time for your body to become seriously low in copper. However, if your doctor has recommended that you take copper try to remember to take it as directed every day.

**Storage**—To store this dietary supplement:

- Keep out of the reach of children.
- Store away from heat and direct light.
- Do not store in the bathroom, near the kitchen sink, or in other damp places. Heat or moisture may cause the dietary supplement to break down.
- Keep the dietary supplement from freezing. Do not refrigerate.
- Do not keep outdated dietary supplements or those no longer needed. Be sure that any discarded dietary supplement is out of the reach of children.

## Precautions While Using This Dietary Supplement

Do not take copper supplements and zinc supplements at the same time. It is best to take your copper supplement 2 hours after zinc supplements, to get the full benefit of each medicine.

## Side Effects of This Dietary Supplement

Along with its needed effects, a dietary supplement may cause some unwanted effects. Although copper supplements have not been reported to cause any side effects, *check with your doctor immediately* if any of the following side effects occur as a result of an overdose:

*Symptoms of overdose*

Black or bloody vomit; blood in urine; coma; diarrhea; dizziness or fainting; headache (severe or continuing); heartburn; loss of appetite; lower back pain; metallic taste; nausea (severe or continuing); pain or burning while urinating; vomiting; yellow eyes or skin

Other side effects not listed above may also occur in some patients. If you notice any other effects, check with your doctor.

Revised: 09/01/91
Interim revisions: 06/25/92; 08/17/94

---

# CORTICOSTEROIDS   Dental

Some commonly used brand names are:

**In the U.S.—**

| | |
|---|---|
| Kenalog in Orabase[2] | Oracort[2] |
| Orabase-HCA[1] | Oralone[2] |

**In Canada—**

Kenalog in Orabase[2]

Another commonly used name for hydrocortisone is cortisol.

Note: For quick reference, the following corticosteroids are numbered to match the corresponding brand names.

This information applies to the following medicines:

1. Hydrocortisone (hye-droe-KOR-ti-sone)
2. Triamcinolone (trye-am-SIN-oh-lone)

## Description

Dental corticosteroids (kor-ti-ko-STER-oyds) are used to relieve the discomfort and redness of some mouth and gum problems. These medicines are like cortisone. They belong to the general family of medicines called steroids.

Dental corticosteroids are available only with your medical doctor's or dentist's prescription in the following dosage forms:

*Dental*

Hydrocortisone
• Paste (U.S.)
Triamcinolone
• Paste (U.S. and Canada)

## Before Using This Medicine

In deciding to use a medicine, the risks of taking the medicine must be weighed against the good it will do. This is a decision you and your doctor or dentist will make. For dental corticosteroids, the following should be considered:

**Allergies**—Tell your doctor if you have ever had any unusual or allergic reaction to corticosteroids. Also tell your health care professional if you are allergic to any other substances, such as foods, preservatives, or dyes.

**Pregnancy**—When used properly, these medicines have not been shown to cause problems in humans. Studies on birth defects with dental corticosteroids have not been done in humans. However, studies in animals have shown that topical corticosteroids, such as the hydrocortisone or triamcinolone in this medicine, when applied to the skin in large amounts or used for a long time, could cause birth defects. Studies with dental paste have not been done in animals.

**Breast-feeding**—When used properly, dental corticosteroids have not been reported to cause problems in nursing babies.

**Children**—Children and teenagers who must use this medicine should be checked often by their doctor. Dental corticosteroids may be absorbed through the lining of the mouth and, if used too often or for too long a time, may interfere with growth in children. Before using this medicine in children, you should discuss its use with your child's medical doctor or dentist.

**Older adults**—Although there is no specific information comparing use of dental corticosteroids in the elderly with use in other age groups, these medicines are not expected to cause different side effects or problems in older people than they do in younger adults.

**Other medicines**—Although certain medicines should not be used together at all, in many cases two different medicines may be used together even if an interaction might occur. In these cases, your doctor or dentist may want to change the dose, or other precautions may be necessary. Tell your doctor, dentist, and pharmacist if you are taking or using any other prescription or nonprescription (over-the-counter [OTC]) medicine.

**Other medical problems**—The presence of other medical problems may affect the use of dental corticosteroids. Make sure you tell your doctor or dentist if you have any other medical problems, especially:

• Diabetes mellitus (sugar diabetes)—Too much use of corticosteroids may cause a loss of control of diabetes by increasing blood and urine glucose. However, this is not likely to happen when dental corticosteroids are used for a short period of time
• Herpes sores or
• Infection or sores of the mouth or throat or
• Tuberculosis—Corticosteroids may make existing infections worse or cause new infections

## Proper Use of This Medicine

To use hydrocortisone or triamcinolone:

• Using a cotton swab, press (do not rub) a small amount of paste onto the area to be treated until the paste sticks and a smooth, slippery film forms. Do not try to spread the medicine because it will become crumbly and gritty. Apply the paste at bedtime so the medicine can work overnight. The other applications of the paste should be made following meals.

*Do not use corticosteroids more often or for a longer time than your medical doctor or dentist ordered.* To do so may increase the chance of absorption through the lining of the mouth and the chance of side effects.

*Do not use any leftover medicine for future mouth problems without first checking with your medical doctor or dentist.* This medicine should *not* be used on many kinds of bacterial, virus, or fungus infections.

**Missed dose**—If your medical doctor or dentist has ordered you to use this medicine according to a regular schedule and you miss a dose, use it as soon as you remember. However, if it is almost time for your next dose, skip the missed dose and go back to your regular dosing schedule.

**Storage**—To store this medicine:
- Keep out of the reach of children.
- Store away from heat and direct light.
- Keep the medicine from freezing.

- Do not keep outdated medicine or medicine no longer needed. Be sure that any discarded medicine is out of the reach of children.

## Precautions While Using This Medicine

*Check with your medical doctor or dentist:*
- if your symptoms do not improve within 1 week.
- if your condition gets worse.

## Side Effects of This Medicine

Along with its needed effects, a medicine may cause some unwanted effects. Although not all of these side effects may occur, if they do occur they may need medical attention.

Check with your medical doctor or dentist as soon as possible if the following side effects occur:

Signs of infection or irritation such as burning, itching, blistering, or peeling not present before use of this medicine

Other side effects not listed above may also occur in some patients. If you notice any other effects, check with your medical doctor or dentist.

Revised: 11/18/92

---

# CORTICOSTEROIDS   Inhalation

Some commonly used brand names are:

**In the U.S.—**

| | |
|---|---|
| AeroBid[4] | Beclovent[1] |
| AeroBid-M[4] | Decadron Respihaler[3] |
| Azmacort[5] | Vanceril[1] |

**In Canada—**

| | |
|---|---|
| Azmacort[5] | |
| Beclodisk[1] | Bronalide[4] |
| Becloforte[1] | Pulmicort Nebuamp[2] |
| Beclovent[1] | Pulmicort Turbuhaler[2] |
| Beclovent Rotacaps[1] | Vanceril[1] |

Other commonly used names are:
Beclomethasone dipropionate[1]    Beclometasone dipropionate[1]
Beclometasone[1]

Note: For quick reference, the following corticosteroids are numbered to match the corresponding brand names.

This information applies to the following medicines:
1. Beclomethasone (be-kloe-METH-a-sone)
2. Budesonide (byoo-DESS-oh-nide)*
3. Dexamethasone (dex-a-METH-a-sone)†
4. Flunisolide (floo-NISS-oh-lide)
5. Triamcinolone (trye-am-SIN-oh-lone)

*Not commercially available in the U.S.
†Not commercially available in Canada.

## Description

Inhalation corticosteroids (kor-ti-koe-STER-oids) are cortisone-like medicines. They are used to help prevent the symptoms of asthma. When used regularly every day, inhalation corticosteroids decrease the number and severity of asthma attacks. However, they will not relieve an asthma attack that has already started.

Inhaled corticosteroids work by preventing certain cells in the lungs and breathing passages from releasing substances that cause asthma symptoms.

This medicine may be used with other asthma medicines, such as bronchodilators (medicines that open up narrowed breathing passages) or other corticosteroids taken by mouth.

Inhalation corticosteroids are available only with your doctor's prescription, in the following dosage forms:

*Inhalation*
Beclomethasone
- Aerosol (U.S. and Canada)
- Capsules for inhalation (Canada)
- Powder for inhalation (Canada)
Budesonide
- Powder for inhalation (Canada)
- Suspension for inhalation (Canada)
Dexamethasone
- Aerosol (U.S.)
Flunisolide
- Aerosol (U.S. and Canada)

Triamcinolone
• Aerosol (U.S. and Canada)

## Before Using This Medicine

In deciding to use a medicine, the risks of taking the medicine must be weighed against the good it will do. This is a decision you and your doctor will make. For inhalation corticosteroids, the following should be considered:

**Pregnancy**—When used in regular daily doses during pregnancy to keep the mother's asthma under control, these medicines have not been reported to cause breathing problems or birth defects in the baby.

**Breast-feeding**—It is not known whether inhaled corticosteroids pass into breast milk. Although most medicines pass into breast milk in small amounts, many of them may be used safely while breast-feeding. Mothers who are using this medicine and who wish to breast-feed should discuss this with their doctor.

**Children**—Inhalation corticosteroids have been tested in children and, in low effective doses, have not been shown to cause different side effects or problems than they do in adults.

There have been a few reports of slowed growth or reduced adrenal gland function in some children using inhaled corticosteroids in recommended doses. However, poorly contolled asthma may cause slowed growth, especially when corticosteroids taken by mouth are needed often. Your doctor will want you to use the lowest possible dose of an inhaled corticosteroid that controls asthma. This will lessen the chance of an effect on growth or adrenal gland function.

Regular use of inhaled corticosteroids may allow some children to stop using or decrease the amount of corticosteroids taken by mouth. This also will reduce the risk of slowed growth or reduced adrenal function.

Children who are using inhaled corticosteroids in large doses should avoid exposure to chickenpox or measles. When a child is exposed or the disease develops, the doctor's directions should be followed carefully.

Before this medicine is given to a child, you and your child's doctor should talk about the good this medicine will do as well as the risks of using it. Follow the doctor's directions very carefully to lessen the chance that unwanted effects will occur.

**Older adults**—Many medicines have not been studied specifically in older people. Therefore, it may not be known whether they work exactly the same way they do in younger adults. Although there is no specific information comparing use of inhaled corticosteroids in the elderly with use in other age groups, this medicine is not expected to cause different side effects or problems in older people than it does in younger adults.

**Other medicines**—Although certain medicines should not be used together at all, in other cases two different medicines may be used together even if an interaction might

occur. In these cases, your doctor may want to change the dose, or other precautions may be necessary. Tell your health care professional if you are taking any other prescription or nonprescription (over-the-counter [OTC]) medicine.

**Other medical problems**—The presence of other medical problems may affect the use of inhaled corticosteroids. Make sure you tell your doctor if you have any other medical problems, especially:

• Osteoporosis (bone disease)—Inhaled corticosteroids in high doses may make this condition worse in women who are past menopause and who are not receiving an estrogen replacement
• Tuberculosis (history of)—Use of this medicine may cause a tuberculosis infection to occur again

## Proper Use of This Medicine

Inhaled corticosteroids will not relieve an asthma attack that has already started. However, your doctor may want you to continue taking this medicine at the usual time, even if you use another medicine to relieve the asthma attack.

Use this medicine only as directed. Do not use more of it and do not use it more often than your doctor ordered. To do so may increase the chance of side effects.

*In order for this medicine to help prevent asthma attacks, it must be used every day in regularly spaced doses, as ordered by your doctor.* Up to four weeks may pass before you begin to notice improvement in your condition. It may take several months before you feel the full effects of this medicine. This may not take as long if you have already been taking certain other medicines for your asthma.

Gargling and rinsing your mouth with water after each dose may help prevent hoarseness, throat irritation, and infection in the mouth. However, do not swallow the water after rinsing. Your doctor may also want you to use a spacer device to lessen these problems.

Inhaled corticosteroids are used with a special inhaler and usually come with patient directions. *Read the directions carefully before using this medicine.* If you do not understand the directions or you are not sure how to use the inhaler, ask your health care professional to show you what to do. Also, *ask your health care professional to check regularly how you use the inhaler to make sure you are using it properly.*

For patients using *beclomethasone, flunisolide, or triamcinolone inhalation aerosol:*

• When you use the inhaler for the first time, it may not deliver the right amount of medicine with the first puff. Therefore, before using the inhaler, test it to make sure it works properly.
• *To test the inhaler:*
  —Insert the metal canister firmly into the clean mouthpiece according to the manufacturer's instructions. Check to make sure the canister is placed properly into the mouthpiece.

—Take the cover off the mouthpiece and shake the inhaler three or four times.

—Hold the canister well away from you against a light background and press the top of the canister, spraying the medicine once into the air. If you see a fine mist, you will know the inhaler is working properly to provide the right amount of medicine when you use it. If you do not see a fine mist, try a second time.

- *To use the inhaler:*

—Using your thumb and one or two fingers, hold the inhaler upright with the mouthpiece end down and pointing toward you.

—Take the cover off the mouthpiece. Check the mouthpiece and remove any foreign objects. Then gently shake the inhaler three or four times.

—Hold the mouthpiece away from your mouth and breathe out slowly and completely.

—Use the inhalation method recommended by your doctor.

- Open-mouth method—Place the mouthpiece about 1 or 2 inches (2 fingerwidths) in front of your widely opened mouth. Make sure the inhaler is aimed into your mouth so that the spray does not hit the roof of your mouth or your tongue.
- Closed-mouth method—Place the mouthpiece in your mouth between your teeth and over your tongue with your lips closed tightly around it. Do not block the mouthpiece with your teeth or tongue.

—Tilt your head back a little. Start to breathe in slowly and deeply through your mouth and, at the same time, press the top of the canister one time to get one puff of medicine. Continue to breathe in slowly for 5 to 10 seconds. Count the seconds while inhaling. It is important to press the top of the canister and breathe in slowly at the same time so the medicine is pulled into your lungs. This step may be difficult at first. If you are using the closed-mouth method and you see a fine mist coming from your mouth or nose, the inhaler is not being used correctly.

—Hold your breath as long as you can up to 10 seconds. This gives the medicine time to settle in your airways and lungs.

—Take the mouthpiece away from your mouth and breathe out slowly.

—If your doctor has told you to inhale more than one puff of medicine at each dose, gently shake the inhaler again, and take the second puff following exactly the same steps you used for the first puff.

—When you are finished, wipe off the mouthpiece and replace the cover to keep the mouthpiece clean and free of foreign objects.

- Your doctor may want you to use a spacer device with the inhaler. A spacer makes the inhaler easier to use. With a spacer, more of the medicine is able to reach your lungs, and less of it stays in the mouth and throat.

—*To use a spacer device with the inhaler:*

- Attach the spacer to the inhaler according to the manufacturer's directions. There are different types of spacers available, but the method of breathing remains the same with most spacers.
- Gently shake the inhaler and spacer three or four times.
- Hold the mouthpiece of the spacer away from your mouth and breathe out slowly to the end of a normal breath.
- Place the mouthpiece into your mouth between your teeth and over your tongue with your lips closed around it.
- Press down on the canister top once to release one puff of medicine into the spacer. Within one or two seconds, start to breathe in slowly and deeply through your mouth for 5 to 10 seconds. Count the seconds while inhaling. Do not breathe in through your nose.
- Then hold your breath as long as you can up to 10 seconds.
- Breathe out slowly. Do not remove the mouthpiece from your mouth. Breathe in and out slowly two or three times to make sure the spacer device is emptied.
- If your doctor has told you to take more than one puff of medicine at each dose, gently shake the inhaler and spacer again and take the second puff, following exactly the same steps you used for the first puff. Do not spray more than one puff at a time into the spacer.
- When you are finished, remove the spacer device from the inhaler and replace the cover of the mouthpiece.

- Clean the inhaler, mouthpiece, and spacer at least twice a week to prevent build-up of medicine and blockage of the mouthpiece.

—*To clean the inhaler:*

- Remove the metal canister from the inhaler and set it aside.
- Wash the mouthpiece and cover, the plastic case, and spacer with soap and warm water. Rinse well with warm, running water.
- Shake off the excess water and let the inhaler parts air dry completely before replacing the metal canister and cover.

- Check with your pharmacist to see if you should save the inhaler piece that comes with this medicine after the medicine is used up. Refill units may be available at a lower cost. However, remember that the inhaler is meant to be used only for the medicine that comes with it. Do not use the inhaler for any other inhalation aerosol medicine, even if the cartridge fits.

For patients using *beclomethasone capsules for inhalation:*

- *Do not swallow the capsules. The medicine will not work if you swallow it.*
- *To load the inhaler:*
  —Make sure your hands are clean and dry.
  —Do not insert the capsule into the inhaler until just before you are ready to use this medicine.
  —Take the inhaler from its container. Hold the inhaler by the mouthpiece and twist the barrel in either direction until it stops.
  —Take a capsule from its container. Hold the inhaler upright with the mouthpiece pointing downward. Press the capsule, with the clear end first, firmly into the raised small hole.
  —Make sure the top of the capsule is even with the top of the hole. This will push the old used capsule shell, if there is one, into the inhaler.
  —Hold the inhaler on its side with the white dot facing up. Twist the barrel quickly until it stops. This will break the capsule into two halves so the powder can be inhaled.
- *To use the inhaler:*
  —Hold the inhaler away from your mouth and breathe out slowly to the end of a normal breath.
  —Keep the inhaler on its side and place the mouthpiece in your mouth. Close your lips around it, and tilt your head slightly back. Do not block the mouthpiece with your teeth or tongue.
  —Breathe in slowly through your mouth until you have taken a full deep breath.
  —Take the inhaler from your mouth and hold your breath as long as you can up to 10 seconds. This gives the medicine time to settle in your airways and lungs.
  —Hold the inhaler well away from your mouth and breathe out to the end of a normal breath.
  —If your doctor has told you to use a second capsule, follow the same steps you used for the first capsule.
  —When you have finished using the inhaler, pull the two halves of the inhaler apart and throw away the empty capsule shells. There is no need to remove the shell left in the small hole, except before cleaning.
  —Put the two halves of the inhaler back together again and place it into its container to keep it clean.
- *To clean the inhaler:*
  —Every two weeks, take the inhaler apart and wash the two halves of the inhaler in clean, warm water. Make sure the empty capsule shell is removed from the small raised hole.
  —Shake out the excess water.
  —Allow all parts of the inhaler to dry before you put it back together.
- The inhaler should be replaced every 6 months.

For patients using *beclomethasone powder for inhalation:*

- *To load the inhaler:*
  —Make sure your hands are clean and dry.
  —Do not insert the cartridge until just before you are ready to use this medicine.
  —Take off the dark brown mouthpiece cover and make sure the mouthpiece is clean.
  —Hold the white cartridge by the exposed corners and gently pull it out until you see the ribbed sides of the cartridge.
  —Squeeze the ribbed sides and take out the cartridge unit from the body of the inhaler.
  —Place the disk containing the medicine onto the white wheel with the numbers facing up. Allow the underside of the disk to fit into the holes of the wheel.
  —Slide the cartridge unit with wheel and disk back into the body of the inhaler. Gently push the cartridge in and pull it out again. The disk will turn.
  —Continue to turn the disk in this way until the number 8 appears in the side indicator window. Each disk has eight blisters containing the medicine. The window will display how many doses you have left after you use it each time, by counting down from 8. For example, when you see the number 1, you have one dose left.
  —To replace the empty disk with a full disk, follow the same steps you used to load the inhaler. Do not throw away the wheel when you discard the empty disk.
- *To use the inhaler:*
  —Hold the inhaler flat in your hand. Lift the rear edge of the lid until it is fully upright.
  —The plastic needle on the front of the lid will break the blister containing one inhalation of medicine. When the lid is raised as far as it will go, both the upper and the lower surfaces of the blister will be pierced. Do not lift the lid if the cartridge is not in the inhaler. Doing this will break the needle and you will need a new inhaler.
  —After the blister is broken open, close the lid. Keeping the inhaler flat and well away from your mouth, breathe out to the end of a normal breath.
  —Raise the inhaler to your mouth, and place the mouthpiece in your mouth.
  —Close your lips around the mouthpiece and tilt your head slightly back. Do not block the mouthpiece with your teeth or tongue. Do not cover the air holes on the side of the mouthpiece.
  —Breathe in through your mouth as fast as you can until you have taken a full deep breath.
  —Hold your breath and remove the mouthpiece from your mouth. Continue holding your breath as long as you can up to 10 seconds before breathing out. This gives the medicine time to settle in your airways and lungs.
  —Hold the inhaler well away from your mouth and breathe out to the end of a normal breath.

—Prepare the cartridge for your next inhalation. Pull the cartridge out once and push it in once. The disk will turn to the next numbered dose as seen in the indicator window. Do not pierce the blister until just before the inhalation.

- *To clean the inhaler:* Brush away the loose powder each day with the brush provided.

- The inhaler should be replaced every 6 months.

For patients using *budesonide powder for inhalation:*

- *To load the inhaler:*

    —Unscrew the cover of the inhaler and lift it off.

    —Hold the inhaler upright with the brown piece pointing downward. Turn the brown piece of the inhaler in one direction as far as it will go. Then twist it back until it clicks.

- *To use the inhaler:*

    —Hold the inhaler away from your mouth and breathe out slowly to the end of a normal breath.

    —Place the mouthpiece in your mouth and close your lips around it. Tilt your head slightly back. Do not block the mouthpiece with your teeth or tongue.

    —Breathe in quickly and evenly through your mouth until you have taken a full deep breath.

    —Hold your breath and remove the inhaler from your mouth. Continue holding your breath as long as you can up to 10 seconds before breathing out. This gives the medicine time to settle in your airways and lungs.

    —Hold the inhaler well away from your mouth and breathe out to the end of a normal breath.

    —Replace the cover on the mouthpiece to keep it clean.

- When the indicator window begins to show a red mark, there are about 20 doses left. When the red mark covers the window, the inhaler is empty.

For patients using *budesonide suspension for inhalation:*

- This medicine is to be used in a power-operated nebulizer equipped with a face mask or mouthpiece. Your doctor will advise you on which nebulizer to use. Make sure you understand how to use the nebulizer. If you have any questions about this, check with your doctor.

- Any opened ampul should be protected from light. The medicine in an open ampul must be used within 12 hours after the ampul is opened. Ampuls should be used within 3 months after the envelope containing them is opened.

- *To prepare the medicine for use in the nebulizer:*

    —Remove one ampul from the sheet of five units and shake it gently.

    —Hold the ampul upright. Open it by twisting off the wing.

    —Squeeze the contents of the ampul into the cup of the nebulizer. If you use only half of the contents of an ampul, add enough of the sodium chloride solution provided to dilute the solution.

—Gently shake the nebulizer. Then attach the face mask to the nebulizer and connect the nebulizer to the air pump.

- *To use the medicine in the nebulizer:*

    —This medicine should be inhaled over a period of 10 to 15 minutes.

    —Breathe slowly and evenly, in and out, until no more mist is left in the nebulizer cup.

    —Rinse your mouth when you are finished with the treatment. Wash your face if you used a face mask.

- *To clean the nebulizer:*

    —After each treatment, wash the cup of the nebulizer and the mask or mouthpiece in warm water with a mild detergent.

    —Allow the nebulizer parts to dry before putting them back together again.

**Dosing**—The dose of these medicines will be different for different patients. *Follow your doctor's orders or the directions on the label.* The following information includes only the average doses of these medicines. *If your dose is different, do not change it* unless your doctor tells you to do so.

*For beclomethasone*

- For inhalation *aerosol:*

    —For bronchial asthma:

    • Adults and children 12 years of age and older—84 to 100 micrograms (mcg) (2 puffs) three or four times a day, or 168 to 200 mcg (4 puffs) two times a day. In severe asthma, your doctor may want you to take a higher dose.

    • Children 6 to 12 years of age—42 to 100 mcg (1 or 2 puffs) three or four times a day, or 168 to 200 mcg (4 puffs) two times a day.

    • Children up to 6 years of age—Use and dose must be determined by the doctor.

- For *capsules* for inhalation or *powder* for inhalation:

    —For bronchial asthma:

    • Adults and teenagers 14 years of age and older—At first, 200 mcg three or four times a day. Then your doctor may reduce the dose, based on your condition.

    • Children 6 to 14 years of age—At first, 100 mcg two to four times a day. Then your doctor may reduce the dose, based on your condition.

    • Children up to 6 years of age—Use and dose must be determined by the doctor.

*For budesonide*

- For *powder* for inhalation:

    —For bronchial asthma:

    • Adults and children 12 years of age and older—At first, 400 to 2400 micrograms (mcg) a day, divided into two to four doses. The higher dose is usually used for treatment of severe asthma or when the dose of corticosteroids taken by mouth is being reduced or stopped. Later, your doctor may reduce the dose to 200 to 400 mcg two times a day.

  • Children 6 to 12 years of age—At first, 100 to 200 mcg two times a day. The higher dose is usually used for treatment of severe asthma or when the dose of corticosteroids taken by mouth is being reduced or stopped.

  • Children up to 6 years of age—Use and dose must be determined by the doctor.

• For *suspension* for inhalation:

—For bronchial asthma:

  • Adults and children 12 years of age and older—500 to 2000 micrograms (mcg) mixed with enough sterile sodium chloride solution for inhalation, if necessary, to make 2 to 4 milliliters (mL). This solution is used in a nebulizer for a period of ten to fifteen minutes. The medicine should be used two times a day.

  • Children 3 months to 12 years of age—250 to 1000 mcg mixed with enough sterile sodium chloride solution for inhalation, if necessary, to make 2 to 4 mL. This solution is used in a nebulizer for a period of ten to fifteen minutes. The medicine should be used two times a day.

  • Children up to 3 months of age—Use and dose must be determined by the doctor.

*For flunisolide*

• For inhalation *aerosol*:

—For bronchial asthma:

  • Adults and children 4 years of age and older—500 micrograms (mcg) (2 puffs) two times a day, morning and evening.

  • Children up to 4 years of age—Use and dose must be determined by the doctor.

*For triamcinolone*

• For inhalation *aerosol*:

—For bronchial asthma:

  • Adults and children 12 years of age and older—At first, 200 micrograms (mcg) (2 puffs) two to four times a day. Then your doctor may reduce the dose, based on your condition. In severe asthma, your doctor may want you to take a higher dose.

  • Children 6 to 12 years of age—At first, 100 to 200 mcg (1 or 2 puffs) three or four times a day. Then your doctor may adjust your dose, based on your condition.

  • Children up to 6 years of age—Use and dose must be determined by the doctor.

**Missed dose**—If you miss a dose of this medicine, use it as soon as possible. Then use any remaining doses for that day at regularly spaced times.

**Storage**—To store this medicine:

• Keep out of the reach of children.

• Store away from heat and direct light.

• Do not store the capsule form of this medicine in the bathroom, near the kitchen sink, or in other damp places. Heat or moisture may cause the medicine to break down.

• Keep the aerosol or suspension form of this medicine from getting too cold or freezing. This medicine may be less effective if the container is cold when you use it.

• Do not puncture, break, or burn the aerosol container, even after it is empty.

• Do not keep outdated medicine or medicine no longer needed. Be sure that any discarded medicine is out of the reach of children.

---

## Precautions While Using This Medicine

*Check with your doctor if:*

• *You go through a period of unusual stress to your body, such as surgery, injury, or infection.*

• *You have an asthma attack* that does not improve after you take a bronchodilator medicine.

• *Signs of mouth, throat, or lung infection occur.*

• *Your symptoms do not improve or if your condition gets worse.*

Your doctor may want you to carry a medical identification card stating that you are using this medicine and that you may need additional medicine during times of emergency, a severe asthma attack or other illness, or unusual stress.

*Before you have any kind of surgery (including dental surgery) or emergency treatment, tell the medical doctor or dentist in charge that you are using this medicine.*

For patients who are also regularly taking a corticosteroid by mouth in tablet or liquid form:

• *Do not stop taking the corticosteroid taken by mouth without your doctor's advice, even if your asthma seems better.* Your doctor may want you to reduce gradually the amount you are taking before stopping completely to lessen the chance of unwanted effects.

• When your doctor tells you to reduce the dose, or to stop taking the corticosteroid taken by mouth, follow the directions carefully. Your body may need time to adjust to the change. The length of time this takes may depend on the amount of medicine you were taking and how long you took it. *It is especially important that your doctor check your progress at regular visits during this time.* Ask your doctor if there are special directions you should follow if you have a severe asthma attack, if you need any other medical or surgical treatment, or if certain side effects occur. Be certain that you understand these directions, and follow them carefully.

---

## Side Effects of This Medicine

Along with its needed effects, a medicine may cause some unwanted effects. Although not all of these side effects

may occur, if they do occur they may need medical attention.

*Check with your doctor immediately* if any of the following side effects occur just after you use this medicine:

*Rare*

Troubled breathing, tightness in chest, or wheezing

Also, check with your doctor as soon as possible if any of the following side effects occur:

*Less common*

Creamy white, curd-like patches in the mouth or throat and/or pain when eating or swallowing

*Rare*

Behavior changes; mental depression; nervousness; restlessness; pain or burning in the chest

Other side effects may occur that usually do not need medical attention. These side effects may go away during treatment as your body adjusts to the medicine. However, check with your doctor if any of the following side effects continue or are bothersome:

*More common*

Cough; dry mouth; hoarseness or other voice changes; sore throat

*Less common or rare*

Dry throat; headache; nausea; skin bruising or thinning; unpleasant taste

Other side effects not listed above may also occur in some patients. If you notice any other effects, check with your doctor.

Revised: 09/02/94

# CORTICOSTEROIDS   Nasal

Some commonly used brand names are:

**In the U.S.—**

| | |
|---|---|
| Beconase[1] | Nasalide[4] |
| Beconase AQ[1] | Vancenase[1] |
| Decadron Turbinaire[3] | Vancenase AQ[1] |
| Nasacort[5] | |

**In Canada—**

| | |
|---|---|
| Beconase[1] | Rhinocort Aqua[2] |
| Beconase AQ[1] | Rhinocort Turbuhaler[2] |
| Nasacort[5] | Vancenase[1] |
| Rhinalar[4] | |

Another commonly used name for beclomethasone is beclometasone.

Note: For quick reference, the following corticosteroids are numbered to match the corresponding brand names.

This information applies to the following medicines:

1. Beclomethasone (be-kloe-METH-a-sone)§
2. Budesonide (byoo-DES-oh-nide)*
3. Dexamethasone (dex-a-METH-a-sone)†
4. Flunisolide (floo-NISS-oh-lide)
5. Triamcinolone (trye-am-SIN-oh-lone)

*Not commercially available in the U.S.
†Not commercially available in the Canada.
§Generic name product may also be available in Canada.

## Description

Nasal corticosteroids (kor-ti-ko-STER-oids) are cortisone-like medicines. They belong to the family of medicines called steroids. These medicines are sprayed or inhaled into the nose to help relieve the stuffy nose, irritation, and discomfort of hay fever, other allergies, and other nasal problems. These medicines are also used to prevent nasal polyps from growing back after they have been removed by surgery.

These medicines are available only with your doctor's prescription, in the following dosage forms:

*Nasal*
Beclomethasone
• Aerosol (U.S. and Canada)
• Solution (U.S. and Canada)
Budesonide
• Powder (Canada)
• Solution (Canada)
Dexamethasone
• Aerosol (U.S.)
Flunisolide
• Solution (U.S. and Canada)
Triamcinolone
• Aerosol (U.S. and Canada)

## Before Using This Medicine

In deciding to use a medicine, the risks of taking the medicine must be weighed against the good it will do. This is a decision you and your doctor will make. For corticosteroids, the following should be considered:

**Allergies**—Tell your doctor if you have ever had any unusual or allergic reaction to corticosteroids. Also tell your health care professional if you are allergic to any other substances, such as foods, preservatives, or dyes.

**Pregnancy**—In one human study, use of beclomethasone oral inhalation by pregnant women did not cause birth defects or other problems. Studies on birth defects with budesonide, dexamethasone, flunisolide, or triamcinolone have not been done in humans.

In animal studies, corticosteroids taken by mouth or injection during pregnancy were shown to cause birth defects. Also, too much use of corticosteroids during pregnancy may cause other unwanted effects in the infant, such as slower growth and reduced adrenal gland function.

If corticosteroids are medically necessary during pregnancy to control nasal problems, nasal corticosteroids are generally considered safer than corticosteroids taken by mouth or injection. Also, use of nasal corticosteroids may allow some patients to stop using or decrease the amount of corticosteroids taken by mouth or injection.

**Breast-feeding**—Use of dexamethasone is not recommended in nursing mothers, since dexamethasone passes into breast milk and may affect the infant's growth.

It is not known whether beclomethasone, budesonide, flunisolide, or triamcinolone passes into breast milk. Although most medicines pass into breast milk in small amounts, many of them may be used safely while breast-feeding. Mothers who are taking this medicine and who wish to breast-feed should discuss this with their doctor.

**Children**—Corticosteroids taken by mouth or injection have been shown to slow or stop growth in children and cause reduced adrenal gland function. If corticosteroids are medically necessary to control nasal problems in a child, nasal corticosteroids are generally considered to be safer than corticosteroids taken by mouth or injection. Most nasal corticosteroids have not been shown to affect growth. Also, use of most nasal corticosteroids may allow some children to stop using or decrease the amount of corticosteroids taken by mouth or injection.

Before this medicine is given to a child, you and your child's doctor should talk about the good this medicine will do as well as the risks of using it. Follow the doctor's directions very carefully to lessen the chance of unwanted effects.

**Older adults**—Although there is no specific information comparing use of nasal corticosteroids in the elderly with use in other age groups, they are not expected to cause different side effects or problems in older people than they do in younger adults.

**Other medicines**—Although certain medicines should not be used together at all, in other cases two different medicines may be used together even if an interaction might occur. In these cases, your doctor may want to change the dose, or other precautions may be necessary. Tell your health care professional if you are taking any prescription or nonprescription (over-the-counter [OTC]) medicines.

**Other medical problems**—The presence of other medical problems may affect the use of corticosteroids. Make sure you tell your doctor if you have any other medical problems, especially:

- Amebiasis—Nasal corticosteroids may make this condition worse
- Glaucoma—Long-term use of nasal corticosteroids may worsen glaucoma by increasing the pressure within the eye
- Herpes simplex (virus) infection of the eye or
- Infections (virus, bacteria, or fungus)—Nasal corticosteroids may cover up the signs of these conditions
- Injury to the nose (recent) or
- Nose surgery (recent) or
- Sores in the nose—Nasal corticosteroids may prevent proper healing of these conditions

- Liver disease
- Tuberculosis (active or history of)
- Underactive thyroid

## Proper Use of This Medicine

This medicine usually comes with patient directions. *Read them carefully before using the medicine.* Beclomethasone, budesonide, dexamethasone, and triamcinolone are used with a special inhaler. If you do not understand the directions, or if you are not sure how to use the inhaler, check with your health care professional.

Before using this medicine, clear the nasal passages by blowing your nose. Then, with the nosepiece inserted into the nostril, aim the spray towards the inner corner of the eye.

*In order for this medicine to help you, it must be used regularly as ordered by your doctor.* This medicine usually begins to work in about 1 week, but up to 3 weeks may pass before you feel its full effects.

*Use this medicine only as directed.* Do not use more of it and do not use it more often than your doctor ordered. To do so may increase the chance of absorption through the lining of the nose and the chance of unwanted effects.

*Check with your doctor before using this medicine for nasal problems other than the one for which it was prescribed,* since it should not be used on many bacterial, virus, or fungus nasal infections.

Save the inhaler that comes with beclomethasone or dexamethasone, since refill units may be available at lower cost.

**Dosing**—The dose of nasal corticosteroids will be different for different patients. *Follow your doctor's orders or the directions on the label.* The following information includes only the average doses of nasal corticosteroids. *If your dose is different, do not change it* unless your doctor tells you to do so.

*For beclomethasone*
- For allergies or other nasal conditions:
  —For *nasal aerosol* dosage form:
    - Adults and children 6 years of age and older—One spray in each nostril two to four times a day.
    - Children up to 6 years of age—Use and dose must be determined by your doctor.
  —For *nasal solution* dosage form:
    - Adults and children 6 years of age and older—One or two sprays in each nostril two times a day.
    - Children up to 6 years of age—Use and dose must be determined by your doctor.

*For budesonide*
- For allergies or other nasal conditions:
  —For *nasal powder* dosage form:
    - Adults and children 6 years of age and older—Two inhalations in each nostril once a day in the morning.

- Children up to 6 years of age—Use and dose must be determined by your doctor.
—For *nasal solution* dosage form:
  - Adults and children 6 years of age and older—One or two sprays in each nostril one or two times a day.
  - Children up to 6 years of age—Use and dose must be determined by your doctor.

*For dexamethasone*
- For allergies or other nasal conditions:
—For *nasal aerosol* dosage form:
  - Adults and children 6 years of age and older—One or two sprays in each nostril two or three times a day for up to two weeks.
  - Children up to 6 years of age—Use and dose must be determined by your doctor.

*For flunisolide*
- For allergies or other nasal conditions:
—For *nasal solution* dosage form:
  - Adults and children 6 years of age and older—One or two sprays in each nostril one to three times a day.
  - Children up to 6 years of age—Use and dose must be determined by your doctor.

*For triamcinolone*
- For allergies or other nasal conditions:
—For *nasal aerosol* dosage form:
  - Adults and children 12 years of age and older—Two sprays in each nostril once a day.
  - Children up to 12 years of age—Use and dose must be determined by your doctor.

**Missed dose**—If you miss a dose of this medicine and remember within an hour or so, use it right away. However, if you do not remember until later, skip the missed dose and go back to your regular dosing schedule. Do not double doses.

**Storage**—To store this medicine:
- Keep out of the reach of children.
- Store away from heat and direct light.
- Do not store budesonide powder in the bathroom, near the kitchen sink, or in other damp places, especially if the cap has not been tightly screwed back on. Moisture may cause the medicine to break down.
- Keep the medicine from getting too cold or freezing. This medicine may be less effective if it is too cold when you use it.
- Do not puncture, break, or burn the beclomethasone, dexamethasone, or triamcinolone aerosol container, even after it is empty.
- Do not keep outdated medicine or medicine no longer needed. Also, discard any unused flunisolide or beclomethasone solution 3 months after you open the package. Be sure that any discarded medicine is out of the reach of children.

## Precautions While Using This Medicine

If you will be using this medicine for more than a few weeks, your doctor should check your progress at regular visits.

*Check with your doctor:*
- *if signs of a nose, sinus, or throat infection occur.*
- *if your symptoms do not improve within 7 days (for dexamethasone) or within 3 weeks (for beclomethasone, budesonide, flunisolide, or triamcinolone).*
- *if your condition gets worse.*

## Side Effects of This Medicine

Along with its needed effects, a medicine may cause some unwanted effects. Although not all of these side effects may occur, if they do occur they may need medical attention.

Check with your doctor as soon as possible if any of the following side effects occur:

*Less common or rare*
Bad smell; bloody mucus or unexplained nosebleeds; burning or stinging after use of spray or irritation inside nose (continuing); crusting, white patches, or sores inside nose; eye pain; gradual loss of vision; headache; hives; lightheadedness or dizziness; loss of sense of taste or smell; nausea or vomiting; shortness of breath, troubled breathing, tightness in chest, or wheezing; skin rash; sore throat, cough, or hoarseness; stomach pains; stuffy, dry, or runny nose or watery eyes (continuing); swelling of eyelids, face, or lips; unusual tiredness or weakness; white patches in throat

*Symptoms of overdose*
Acne; fullness or rounding of the face; menstrual changes

Other side effects may occur that usually do not need medical attention. These side effects may go away during treatment as your body adjusts to the medicine. However, check with your doctor if any of the following side effects continue or are bothersome:

*More common*
Burning, dryness, or other irritation inside the nose (mild, lasting only a short time); increase in sneezing; irritation of throat

*Less common*
Throat discomfort or itching

Not all of the side effects listed above have been reported for each of these medicines, but they have been reported for at least one of them. All of the nasal corticosteroids are very similar, so any of the above side effects may occur with any of these medicines.

Other side effects not listed above may also occur in some patients. If you notice any other effects, check with your doctor.

Revised: 05/16/94

# CORTICOSTEROIDS   Ophthalmic

Some commonly used brand names are:

**In the U.S.—**

| | |
|---|---|
| AK-Dex[2] | Inflamase Forte[6] |
| AK-Pred[6] | Inflamase Mild[6] |
| AK-Tate[6] | I-Pred[6] |
| Baldex[2] | Lite Pred[6] |
| Decadron[2] | Maxidex[2] |
| Dexair[2] | Ocu-Dex[2] |
| Dexotic[2] | Ocu-Pred[6] |
| Econopred[6] | Ocu-Pred-A[6] |
| Econopred Plus[6] | Ocu-Pred Forte[6] |
| Flarex[3] | Predair[6] |
| Fluor-Op[3] | Predair A[6] |
| FML Forte[3] | Predair Forte[6] |
| FML Liquifilm[3] | Pred Forte[6] |
| FML S.O.P.[3] | Pred Mild[6] |
| HMS Liquifilm[5] | Storz-Dexa[2] |
| I-Methasone[2] | Ultra Pred[6] |

**In Canada—**

| | |
|---|---|
| AK-Dex[2] | HMS Liquifilm[5] |
| AK-Tate[6] | Inflamase Forte[6] |
| Betnesol[1] | Inflamase Mild[6] |
| Cortamed[4] | Maxidex[2] |
| Decadron[2] | Ophtho-Tate[6] |
| Flarex[3] | Pred Forte[6] |
| FML Forte[3] | Pred Mild[6] |
| FML Liquifilm[3] | |

Another commonly used name for hydrocortisone is cortisol.

Note: For quick reference, the following corticosteroids are numbered to match the corresponding brand names.

This information applies to the following medicines:
1. Betamethasone (bay-ta-METH-a-sone)*
2. Dexamethasone (dex-a-METH-a-sone)‡
3. Fluorometholone (flure-oh-METH-oh-lone)
4. Hydrocortisone (hye-droe-KOR-ti-sone)*
5. Medrysone (ME-dri-sone)
6. Prednisolone (pred-NISS-oh-lone)‡§

*Not commercially available in the U.S.
‡Generic name product may also be available in U.S.
§Generic name product may also be available in Canada.

## Description

Ophthalmic corticosteroids (kor-ti-ko-STER-oids) (cortisone-like medicines) are used to prevent permanent damage to the eye, which may occur with certain eye problems. They also provide relief from redness, irritation, and other discomfort.

Corticosteroids for use in the eye are available only with your doctor's prescription, in the following dosage forms:

*Ophthalmic*
Betamethasone
• Solution (eye drops) (Canada)
Dexamethasone
• Ointment (U.S. and Canada)
• Solution (eye drops) (U.S. and Canada)
• Suspension (eye drops) (U.S. and Canada)
Fluorometholone
• Ointment (U.S.)
• Suspension (eye drops) (U.S. and Canada)
Hydrocortisone
• Ointment (Canada)
Medrysone
• Suspension (eye drops) (U.S. and Canada)

Prednisolone
• Solution (eye drops) (U.S. and Canada)
• Suspension (eye drops) (U.S. and Canada)

## Before Using This Medicine

In deciding to use a medicine, the risks of taking the medicine must be weighed against the good it will do. This is a decision you and your doctor will make. For ophthalmic corticosteroids, the following should be considered:

**Allergies**—Tell your doctor if you have ever had any unusual or allergic reaction to corticosteroids. Also tell your health care professional if you are allergic to any other substances, such as foods, preservatives, or dyes.

**Pregnancy**—Although studies on birth defects with ophthalmic corticosteroids have not been done in humans, these medicines have not been reported to cause birth defects or other problems. However, in animal studies, dexamethasone, fluorometholone, hydrocortisone, and prednisolone caused birth defects when applied to the eyes of pregnant animals. Also, fluorometholone and medrysone caused other unwanted effects in the animal fetus.

**Breast-feeding**—Ophthalmic corticosteroids have not been reported to cause problems in nursing babies.

**Children**—Children less than 2 years of age may be especially sensitive to the effects of ophthalmic corticosteroids. This may increase the chance of side effects. If this medicine has been ordered for a young child, you should discuss its use with your child's doctor. Be sure you follow all of the doctor's instructions very carefully.

**Older adults**—Although there is no specific information about the use of ophthalmic corticosteroids in the elderly, they are not expected to cause different side effects or problems in older people than they do in younger adults.

**Other medicines**—Although certain medicines should not be used together at all, in other cases two different medicines may be used together even if an interaction might occur. In these cases, your doctor may want to change the dose, or other precautions may be necessary. Tell your health care professional if you are using any other prescription or nonprescription (over-the-counter [OTC]) ophthalmic medicine.

**Other medical problems**—The presence of other medical problems may affect the use of ophthalmic corticosteroids. Make sure you tell your doctor if you have any other medical problems, especially:
• Cataracts—Corticosteroids may cause cataracts or make them worse
• Diabetes mellitus (sugar diabetes)—Patients with diabetes may be more likely to develop cataracts or glaucoma with the use of corticosteroids
• Glaucoma (or family history of)—Corticosteroids may cause glaucoma or make it worse

- Herpes infection of the eye or
- Tuberculosis of the eye (active or history of) or
- Any other eye infection—Ophthalmic corticosteroids may make existing infections worse or cause new infections

## Proper Use of This Medicine

For patients who wear *contact lenses:*

- Use of ophthalmic corticosteroids while you are wearing contact lenses (either hard lenses or soft lenses) may increase the chance of infection. Therefore, do not apply this medicine while you are wearing contact lenses. Also, check with an ophthalmologist (eye doctor) for advice on how long to wait after applying this medicine before inserting your contact lenses. It is possible that you may be directed not to wear contact lenses at all during the entire time of treatment and for a day or two after treatment has been stopped.

For patients using an *ophthalmic solution or suspension (eye drop) form* of this medicine:

- If you are using a suspension form of this medicine, always shake the container very well just before applying the eye drops.
- To use:
  —First, wash your hands. Tilt the head back and with the index finger of one hand, press gently on the skin just beneath the lower eyelid and pull the lower eyelid away from the eye to make a space. Drop the medicine into this space. Let go of the eyelid and gently close the eyes. Do not blink. Keep the eyes closed and apply pressure to the inner corner of the eye with your finger for 1 or 2 minutes, to allow the medicine to come into contact with the irritation.
  —If you think you did not get the drop of medicine into your eye properly, use another drop.
  —Remove any excess solution around the eye with a clean tissue, being careful not to touch the eye.
  —Immediately after using the eye drops, wash your hands to remove any medicine that may be on them.
  —To keep the medicine as germ-free as possible, do not touch the dropper or the applicator tip to any surface (including the eye). Always keep the container tightly closed.

For patients using an *ointment form* of this medicine:

- To use:
  —First, wash your hands. Tilt the head back and with the index finger of one hand, press gently on the skin just beneath the lower eyelid and pull the lower eyelid away from the eye to make a space. Squeeze a thin strip of ointment into this space. A 1-cm (approximately ⅓ inch) strip of ointment is usually enough unless otherwise directed by your doctor. Let go of the eyelid and gently close the eyes and keep them closed for 1 or 2 minutes, to allow the medicine to come into contact with the irritation.

—To keep the medicine as germ-free as possible, do not touch the applicator tip to any surface (including the eye). After using the eye ointment, wipe the tip of the ointment tube with a clean tissue. Do not wash the tip with water. Always keep the tube tightly closed.

*Do not use corticosteroids more often or for a longer time than your doctor ordered*. To do so may increase the chance of side effects, especially in children 2 years of age or younger.

*Do not use any leftover medicine for future eye problems without first checking with your doctor*. This medicine should not be used if certain kinds of infections are present. To do so may make the infection worse and possibly lead to eye damage.

**Dosing**—The dose of ophthalmic corticosteroids will be different for different patients. *Follow your doctor's orders or the directions on the label*. The following information includes only the average doses of ophthalmic corticosteroids. *If your dose is different, do not change it* unless your doctor tells you to do so.

*For betamethasone*
- For eye disorders:
  —For *ophthalmic solution (eye drops)* dosage form:
    - Adults and children—Use one or two drops in the eye every one or two hours, then space the doses further apart as the eye gets better.

*For dexamethasone*
- For eye disorders:
  —For *ophthalmic ointment* dosage form:
    - Adults and children—Use the ointment in the eye three or four times a day, then space the doses further apart as the eye gets better.
  —For *ophthalmic solution (eye drops)* dosage form:
    - Adults and children—Use one or two drops in the eye up to six times a day.
  —For *ophthalmic suspension (eye drops)* dosage form:
    - Adults and children—Use one or two drops in the eye four to six times a day.

*For fluorometholone*
- For eye disorders:
  —For *ophthalmic ointment* dosage form:
    - Adults and children—Use the ointment in the eye one to three times a day.
  —For *ophthalmic suspension (eye drops)* dosage form:
    - Adults and children—Use one or two drops in the eye two to four times a day.

*For hydrocortisone*
- For eye disorders:
  —For *ophthalmic ointment* dosage form:
    - Adults and children—Use the ointment in the eye three or four times a day, then space the doses further apart as the eye gets better.

*For medrysone*
- For eye disorders:
  —For *ophthalmic suspension (eye drops)* dosage form:
    - Adults and children—Use one drop in the eye up to every four hours.

*For prednisolone*
- For eye disorders:
  —For *ophthalmic solution (eye drops)* dosage form:
    - Adults and children—Use one or two drops in the eye up to six times a day.
  —For *ophthalmic suspension (eye drops)* dosage form:
    - Adults and children—Use one or two drops in the eye two to four times a day.

**Missed dose**—If you miss a dose of this medicine, apply it as soon as possible. However, if it is almost time for your next dose, skip the missed dose and go back to your regular dosing schedule.

**Storage**—To store this medicine:
- Keep out of the reach of children.
- Store away from heat and direct light.
- Keep the medicine from freezing.
- Do not keep outdated medicine or medicine no longer needed. Be sure that any discarded medicine is out of the reach of children.

## Precautions While Using This Medicine

If you will be using this medicine for more than a few weeks, an ophthalmologist (eye doctor) should examine your eyes at regular visits to make sure it does not cause unwanted effects.

If your eye condition does not improve after 5 to 7 days, or if it becomes worse, check with your doctor.

## Side Effects of This Medicine

Along with its needed effects, a medicine may cause some unwanted effects. Although not all of these side effects may occur, if they do occur they may need medical attention. Check with your doctor as soon as possible if any of the following side effects occur:

*Less common or rare*
Decreased vision; eye infection; eye pain; gradual blurring or loss of vision; nausea; vomiting

Other side effects may occur that usually do not need medical attention. These side effects may go away during treatment as your body adjusts to the medicine. However, check with your doctor if any of the following side effects continue or are bothersome:

*More frequent*
Blurred vision (mild and temporary, occurs after use of ointments)

*Less common or rare*
Burning, stinging, redness, or watering of the eyes

Other side effects not listed may also occur in some patients. If you notice any other effects, check with your doctor.

Revised: 01/05/94
Interim revision: 05/16/94

# CORTICOSTEROIDS  Otic

Some commonly used brand names are:

**In the U.S.—**
AK-Dex[2]                    I-Methasone[2]
Decadron[2]

**In Canada—**
AK-Dex[2]                    Cortamed[3]
Betnesol[1]                  Decadron[2]

Another commonly used name for hydrocortisone is cortisol.

Note: For quick reference, the following corticosteroids are numbered to match the corresponding brand names.

This information applies to the following medicines:
1. Betamethasone (bay-ta-METH-a-sone)*
2. Dexamethasone (dex-a-METH-a-sone)
3. Hydrocortisone (hye-droe-KOR-ti-sone)*

*Not commercially available in the U.S.

## Description

Otic corticosteroids (kor-ti-koe-STE-roids) (cortisone-like medicines) are used in the ear to relieve the redness, itching, and swelling caused by certain ear problems.

Otic corticosteroids are available only with your doctor's prescription, in the following dosage forms:

*Otic*
Betamethasone
- Solution (Canada)
Dexamethasone
- Solution (U.S. and Canada)
Hydrocortisone
- Ointment (Canada)

## Before Using This Medicine

In deciding to use a medicine, the risks of taking the medicine must be weighed against the good it will do. This is a decision you and your doctor will make. For otic corticosteroids, the following should be considered:

**Allergies**—Tell your doctor if you have ever had any unusual or allergic reaction to corticosteroids. Also tell your health care professional if you are allergic to any other substances, such as certain preservatives or dyes.

**Pregnancy**—Otic corticosteroids have not been shown to cause birth defects or other problems in pregnant women.

**Breast-feeding**—Otic corticosteroids have not been reported to cause problems in nursing infants.

**Children**—Although there is no specific information about the use of otic corticosteroids in children, they are not expected to cause different side effects or problems in children than they do in adults.

**Older adults**—Although there is no specific information about the use of otic corticosteroids in the elderly, they are not expected to cause different side effects or problems in older people than they do in younger adults.

**Other medical problems**—The presence of other medical problems may affect the use of otic corticosteroids. Make sure you tell your doctor if you have any other medical problems, especially:

- Any other ear infection or condition (or history of)—Otic corticosteroids may worsen existing infections or cause new infections
- Punctured ear drum—Using otic corticosteroids with a punctured ear drum may damage the ear

## Proper Use of This Medicine

To use *ear drops:*

- Lie down or tilt the head so that the affected ear faces up. Gently pull the earlobe up and back for adults (down and back for children) to straighten the ear canal. Drop the medicine into the ear canal. Keep the ear facing up for several (about 5) minutes to allow the medicine to run to the bottom of the ear canal. A sterile cotton plug may be gently inserted into the ear opening to prevent the medicine from leaking out. At first, your doctor may want you to put more medicine on the cotton plug during the day to keep it moist.

To use *ear ointment:*

- Apply a small amount of ointment to the area just inside the ear canal, using a clean finger or a piece of sterile gauze. Do not use a cotton-tipped swab unless your doctor has directed you to do so and has explained exactly how to use it.

To keep the medicine as germ-free as possible, do not touch the dropper or applicator tip to any surface (including the ear). Also, keep the container tightly closed.

*Do not use corticosteroids more often or for a longer time than your doctor ordered.* To do so may increase the chance of side effects.

*Do not use any leftover medicine for future ear problems without first checking with your doctor.* This medicine should not be used if certain kinds of infections are present. To do so may make the infection worse.

**Dosing**—The dose of otic corticosteroids will be different for different patients. *Follow your doctor's orders or the directions on the label.* The following information includes only the average doses of otic corticosteroids. *If your dose is different, do not change it* unless your doctor tells you to do so.

*For betamethasone*
- For *otic solution (ear drops)* dosage form:
  —For redness, itching, and swelling:
    • Adults and children—Use two or three drops in the ear every two or three hours. After symptoms are relieved, your doctor may lower the dose.

*For dexamethasone*
- For *otic solution (ear drops)* dosage form:
  —For redness, itching, and swelling:
    • Adults and children—Use three or four drops in the ear two or three times a day. After symptoms are relieved, your doctor may lower the dose.

*For hydrocortisone*
- For *otic ointment (ear ointment)* dosage form:
  —For redness, itching, and swelling:
    • Adults and children 2 years of age and older—Use two or three times a day in the ear. After symptoms are relieved, your doctor may lower the dose.
    • Children up to 2 years of age—Use and dose must be determined by your doctor.

**Missed dose**—If you miss a dose of this medicine, use it as soon as you remember. However, if it is almost time for your next dose, skip the missed dose and go back to your regular dosing schedule. Do not double doses.

**Storage**—To store this medicine:
- Keep out of the reach of children.
- Store away from heat and direct light.
- Keep the medicine from freezing.
- Do not keep outdated medicine or medicine no longer needed. Be sure that any discarded medicine is out of the reach of children.

## Precautions While Using This Medicine

If your condition does not improve within 5 to 7 days, or if it becomes worse, check with your doctor.

## Side Effects of This Medicine

Along with its needed effects, a medicine may cause some unwanted effects. The following side effects usually do not need medical attention and may go away during treatment as your body adjusts to the medicine. However, check with your doctor if either of the following side effects continues or is bothersome:

*Less common*
    Burning or stinging of the ear

There have not been any other common or important side effects reported with this medicine. However, if you notice any unusual effects, check with your doctor.

---

Revised: 03/31/92
Interim revision: 02/17/94

---

# CORTICOSTEROIDS—Low Potency    Topical

Some commonly used brand names are:

**In the U.S.—**

| | |
|---|---|
| Aclovate[1] | Dermtex HC[7] |
| Acticort 100[7] | DesOwen[3] |
| Aeroseb-Dex[4] | Epifoam[8] |
| Aeroseb-HC[7] | FoilleCort[8] |
| Ala-Cort[7] | Gly-Cort[7] |
| Ala-Scalp HP[7] | Gynecort[8] |
| Allercort[7] | Gynecort 10[8] |
| Alphaderm[7] | Hi-Cor 1.0[7] |
| Bactine[7] | Hi-Cor 2.5[7] |
| Beta-HC[7] | Hydro-Tex[7] |
| CaldeCORT Anti-Itch[7,8] | Hytone[7] |
| CaldeCORT Light[8] | LactiCare-HC[7] |
| Carmol-HC[8] | Lanacort[8] |
| Cetacort[7] | Lanacort 10[8] |
| Cloderm[2] | Lemoderm[7] |
| Cortaid[7,8] | Maximum Strength Cortaid[7] |
| Cort-Dome[7] | MyCort[7] |
| Cortef Feminine Itch[8] | 9-1-1[8] |
| Corticaine[8] | Nutracort[7] |
| Cortifair[7] | Penecort[7] |
| Cortril[7] | Pentacort[7] |
| Decaderm[4] | Pharma-Cort[8] |
| Decadron[4] | Rederm[7] |
| Decaspray[4] | Rhulicort[8] |
| Delacort[7] | S-T Cort[7] |
| Dermacort[7] | Synacort[7] |
| Dermarest DriCort[7] | Texacort[7] |
| DermiCort[7] | Tridesilon[3] |

**In Canada—**

| | |
|---|---|
| Barriere-HC[7] | Hyderm[8] |
| Cortacet[8] | Locacorten[5] |
| Cortate[7] | Novohydrocort[8] |
| Cortef[7,8] | Prevex HC[7] |
| Corticreme[8] | Sarna HC 1.0%[7] |
| Cortoderm[8] | Sential[7] |
| Drenison-¼[6] | Tridesilon[3] |
| Emo-Cort[7] | Unicort[7] |
| Emo-Cort Scalp Solution[7] | |

Other commonly used names are:

| | |
|---|---|
| cortisol[7] | flumetasone[5] |

Note: For quick reference, the following low potency corticosteroids are numbered to match the corresponding brand names.

This information applies to the following medicines:

1. Alclometasone (al-kloe-MET-a-sone)†
2. Clocortolone (kloe-KOR-toe-lone)†
3. Desonide (DESS-oh-nide)‡
4. Dexamethasone (dex-a-METH-a-sone)†
5. Flumethasone (floo-METH-a-sone)*
6. Flurandrenolide (flure-an-DREN-oh-lide) (Drenison-¼ only)
7. Hydrocortisone (hye-droe-KOR-ti-sone)‡
8. Hydrocortisone acetate (hye-droe-KOR-ti-sone AS-a-tate)‡

---

*Not commercially available in the U.S.
†Not commercially available in Canada.
‡Generic name product may also be available in the U.S.

## Description

Topical corticosteroids (kor-ti-ko-STER-oyds) are used to help relieve redness, swelling, itching, and discomfort of many skin problems. These medicines are like cortisone. They belong to the general family of medicines called steroids.

Most corticosteroids are available only with your doctor's prescription. Some strengths of hydrocortisone are available without a prescription; however, your doctor may have special instructions on the proper use for your medical condition.

Topical corticosteroids are available in the following dosage forms:

*Topical*
    Alclometasone
        • Cream (U.S.)
        • Ointment (U.S.)
    Clocortolone
        • Cream (U.S.)
    Desonide
        • Cream (U.S. and Canada)
        • Lotion (U.S.)
        • Ointment (U.S. and Canada)
    Dexamethasone
        • Cream (U.S.)
        • Gel (U.S.)
        • Topical aerosol (U.S.)
    Flumethasone
        • Cream (Canada)
        • Ointment (Canada)
    Flurandrenolide
        • Cream 0.0125% (Canada)
        • Ointment 0.0125% (Canada)
    Hydrocortisone
        • Cream (U.S. and Canada)
        • Lotion (U.S. and Canada)
        • Ointment (U.S. and Canada)
        • Topical solution (U.S. and Canada)
    Hydrocortisone acetate
        • Cream (U.S. and Canada)
        • Topical aerosol foam (U.S.)
        • Lotion (U.S.)
        • Ointment (U.S. and Canada)

## Before Using This Medicine

In deciding to use a medicine, the risks of taking the medicine must be weighed against the good it will do.

---

This is a decision you and your doctor will make. For topical corticosteroids, the following should be considered:

**Allergies**—Tell your doctor if you have ever had any unusual or allergic reaction to corticosteroids. Also tell your health care professional if you are allergic to any other substances, such as foods, preservatives, or dyes.

**Pregnancy**—When used properly, these medicines have not been shown to cause problems in humans. Studies on birth defects have not been done in humans. However, studies in animals have shown that topical corticosteroids, when applied to the skin in large amounts or used for a long time, could cause birth defects.

**Breast-feeding**—Topical corticosteroids have not been reported to cause problems in nursing babies when used properly. However, corticosteroids should not be applied to the breasts just before nursing.

**Children**—Children and teenagers who must use this medicine for a long time should be checked often by their doctor. Other more potent corticosteroids are absorbed through the skin and can affect growth or cause other unwanted effects. Topical corticosteroids can also be absorbed if they are applied to large areas of skin. These effects are less likely to occur with the use of the lower potency corticosteroids. However, before using this medicine in children, you should discuss its use with your child's doctor.

**Older adults**—This medicine is not expected to cause different side effects or problems in older people than it does in younger adults.

**Other medical problems**—The presence of other medical problems may affect the use of topical corticosteroids. Make sure you tell your doctor if you have any other medical problems, especially:
- Diabetes mellitus (sugar diabetes)—Too much use of corticosteroids may cause a loss of control of diabetes by increasing blood and urine glucose. However, this is not likely to happen when topical corticosteroids are used for a short time
- Infection or sores at the place of treatment or
- Tuberculosis—Corticosteroids may make existing infections worse or cause new infections
- Skin conditions that cause thinning of skin with easy bruising—Corticosteroids may make thinning of the skin worse

## Proper Use of This Medicine

Be very careful not to get this medicine in your eyes. Wash your hands after using your finger to apply the medicine. If you accidentally get this medicine in your eyes, flush them with water.

*Do not bandage or otherwise wrap the skin being treated* unless directed to do so by your doctor.

If your doctor has ordered an occlusive dressing (airtight covering, such as kitchen plastic wrap or a special patch) to be applied over this medicine, make sure you know how to apply it. Since occlusive dressings increase the amount of medicine absorbed through your skin and the possibility of side effects, use them only as directed. If you have any questions about this, check with your doctor.

For patients using the *topical aerosol form* of this medicine:
- This medicine usually comes with patient directions. Read them carefully before using this medicine.
- It is important to avoid breathing in the vapors from the spray or getting them in your eyes. If you accidentally get this medicine in your eyes, flush them with water.
- Do not use near heat, near an open flame, or while smoking.

*Do not use this medicine more often or for a longer time than your doctor ordered or than recommended on the package label.* To do so may increase the chance of absorption through the skin and the chance of side effects.

If this medicine has been prescribed for you, it is meant to treat a specific skin problem. *Do not use it for other skin problems, and do not use nonprescription hydrocortisone for skin problems that are not listed on the package label, without first checking with your doctor.* Topical corticosteroids should not be used on many kinds of bacterial, virus, or fungus skin infections.

**Missed dose**—If your doctor has ordered you to use this medicine on a regular schedule and you miss a dose, apply it as soon as possible. But if it is almost time for your next dose, skip the missed dose and apply it at the next regularly scheduled time.

**Storage**—To store this medicine:
- Keep out of the reach of children.
- Store away from heat and direct light.
- Keep the medicine from freezing.
- Do not puncture, break, or burn aerosol containers, even after they are empty.
- Do not keep outdated medicine or medicine no longer needed. Be sure that any discarded medicine is out of the reach of children.

## Precautions While Using This Medicine

Avoid using tight-fitting diapers or plastic pants on a child if this medicine is being used on the child's diaper area. Plastic pants and tight-fitting diapers may increase the chance of absorption of the medicine through the skin and the chance of side effects.

## Side Effects of This Medicine

Along with its needed effects, a medicine may cause some unwanted effects. Although not all of these side effects may occur, if they do occur they may need medical attention.

Check with your doctor as soon as possible if any of the following side effects occur:

*Less common or rare*
> Lack of healing of skin condition; skin pain, redness, itching, or pus-containing blisters; severe burning and continued itching of skin

Some side effects may occur that usually do not need medical attention. These side effects may go away during treatment as your body adjusts to the medicine. However, check with your doctor if any of the following side effects continue or are bothersome:

*Less common or rare*
> Burning, dryness, irritation, itching, or redness of skin; increased redness or scaling of skin sores; skin rash

When the gel, solution, lotion, or aerosol form of this medicine is applied, a mild, temporary stinging may be expected.

Other side effects not listed above may also occur in some patients. If you notice any other effects, check with your doctor.

Revised: 11/18/92

# CORTICOSTEROIDS—Medium to Very High Potency    Topical

Some commonly used brand names or other names are:

**In the U.S.—**

| | |
|---|---|
| Alphatrex[3] | Kenalog[18] |
| Aristocort[18] | Kenalog-H[18] |
| Aristocort A[18] | Kenonel[18] |
| Betatrex[3] | Licon[10] |
| Beta-Val[3] | Lidex[10] |
| Bio-Syn[9] | Lidex-E[10] |
| Cordran[11] | Locoid[15] |
| Cordran SP[11] | Maxiflor[7] |
| Cutivate[12] | Maxivate[3] |
| Cyclocort[1] | Psorcon[7] |
| Delta-Tritex[18] | Synalar[9] |
| Dermabet[3] | Synalar-HP[9] |
| Diprolene[3] | Synemol[9] |
| Diprolene AF[3] | Teladar[3] |
| Diprosone[3] | Temovate[4] |
| Elocon[17] | Temovate Scalp Application[4] |
| Florone[7] | Topicort[6] |
| Florone E[7] | Topicort LP[6] |
| Fluocet[9] | Triacet[18] |
| Fluocin[10] | Triderm[18] |
| Fluonid[9] | Ultravate[14] |
| Flurosyn[9] | Uticort[3] |
| Flutex[18] | Valisone[3] |
| Halog[13] | Valisone Reduced Strength[3] |
| Halog-E[13] | Valnac[3] |
| Kenac[18] | Westcort[16] |

**In Canada—**

| | |
|---|---|
| Aristocort C[18] | Elocom[17] |
| Aristocort D[18] | Eumovate[5] |
| Aristocort R[18] | Florone[7] |
| Beben[3] | Fluoderm[9] |
| Betacort Scalp Lotion[3] | Fluolar[9] |
| Betaderm[3] | Fluonide[9] |
| Betaderm Scalp Lotion[3] | Halog[13] |
| Betnovate[3] | Kenalog[18] |
| Betnovate-½[3] | Lidemol[10] |
| Celestoderm-V[3] | Lidex[10] |
| Celestoderm-V/2[3] | Lyderm[10] |
| Cyclocort[1] | Metaderm Mild[3] |
| Dermovate[4] | Metaderm Regular[3] |
| Dermovate Scalp Lotion[4] | Nerisone[8] |
| Diprolene[3] | Nerisone Oily[8] |
| Diprosone[3] | Novobetamet[3] |
| Drenison[11] | Prevex B[3] |
| Ectosone Mild[3] | Propaderm[2] |
| Ectosone Regular[3] | Synalar[9] |
| Ectosone Scalp Lotion[3] | Synamol[9] |

| | |
|---|---|
| Topicort[6] | Triaderm[18] |
| Topicort Mild[6] | Trianide Mild[18] |
| Topilene[3] | Trianide Regular[18] |
| Topisone[3] | Valisone Scalp Lotion[3] |
| Topsyn[10] | Westcort[16] |

Other commonly used names are:
> beclometasone[2]    fludroxycortide[11]

Note: For quick reference, the following medium to very high potency corticosteroids are numbered to match the corresponding brand names.

This information applies to the following medicines:

1. Amcinonide (am-SIN-oh-nide)
2. Beclomethasone (be-kloe-METH-a-sone)*
3. Betamethasone (bay-ta-METH-a-sone)‡
4. Clobetasol (kloe-BAY-ta-sol)
5. Clobetasone (kloe-BAY-ta-sone)*
6. Desoximetasone (des-ox-i-MET-a-sone)‡
7. Diflorasone (dye-FLOR-a-sone)
8. Diflucortolone (di-floo-KOR-toe-lone)*
9. Fluocinolone (floo-oh-SIN-oh-lone)‡
10. Fluocinonide (floo-oh-SIN-oh-nide)‡
11. Flurandrenolide (flure-an-DREN-oh-lide) (except Drenison-¼)‡
12. Fluticasone (floo-TIK-a-sone)†
13. Halcinonide (hal-SIN-oh-nide)
14. Halobetasol (hal-oh-BAY-ta-sol)†
15. Hydrocortisone butyrate (hye-droe-KOR-ti-sone bue-TEAR-ate)
16. Hydrocortisone valerate (hye-droe-KOR-ti-sone val-AIR-ate)
17. Mometasone (moe-MET-a-sone)
18. Triamcinolone (trye-am-SIN-oh-lone)‡

*Not commercially available in the U.S.
†Not commercially available in Canada.
‡Generic name product may also be available in the U.S.

## Description

Topical corticosteroids (kor-ti-ko-STER-oyds) are used to help relieve redness, swelling, itching, and discomfort of many skin problems. These medicines are like cortisone. They belong to the general family of medicines called steroids.

These corticosteroids are available only with your doctor's prescription. Topical corticosteroids are available in the following dosage forms:

*Topical*

Amcinonide
- Cream (U.S. and Canada)
- Lotion (U.S. and Canada)
- Ointment (U.S. and Canada)

Beclomethasone
- Cream (Canada)
- Lotion (Canada)
- Ointment (Canada)

Betamethasone
- Cream (U.S. and Canada)
- Gel (U.S. and Canada)
- Lotion (U.S. and Canada)
- Ointment (U.S. and Canada)
- Topical aerosol (U.S.)

Clobetasol
- Cream (U.S. and Canada)
- Ointment (U.S. and Canada)
- Solution (U.S. and Canada)

Clobetasone
- Cream (Canada)
- Ointment (Canada)

Desoximetasone
- Cream (U.S. and Canada)
- Gel (U.S. and Canada)
- Ointment (U.S.)

Diflorasone
- Cream (U.S. and Canada)
- Ointment (U.S. and Canada)

Diflucortolone
- Cream (Canada)
- Ointment (Canada)

Fluocinolone
- Cream (U.S. and Canada)
- Ointment (U.S. and Canada)
- Topical solution (U.S. and Canada)

Fluocinonide
- Cream (U.S. and Canada)
- Gel (U.S. and Canada)
- Ointment (U.S. and Canada)
- Topical solution (U.S. and Canada)

Flurandrenolide
- Cream (U.S. and Canada)
- Lotion (U.S.)
- Ointment (U.S. and Canada)
- Tape (U.S. and Canada)

Fluticasone
- Cream (U.S.)
- Ointment (U.S.)

Halcinonide
- Cream (U.S. and Canada)
- Ointment (U.S. and Canada)
- Topical solution (U.S. and Canada)

Halobetasol
- Cream (U.S.)
- Ointment (U.S.)

Hydrocortisone butyrate
- Cream (U.S.)
- Ointment (U.S.)

Hydrocortisone valerate
- Cream (U.S. and Canada)
- Ointment (U.S. and Canada)

Mometasone
- Cream (U.S. and Canada)
- Lotion (U.S. and Canada)
- Ointment (U.S. and Canada)

Triamcinolone
- Cream (U.S. and Canada)
- Lotion (U.S.)
- Ointment (U.S. and Canada)
- Topical aerosol (U.S.)

## Before Using This Medicine

In deciding to use a medicine, the risks of taking the medicine must be weighed against the good it will do. This is a decision you and your doctor will make. For corticosteroids, the following should be considered:

**Allergies**—Tell your doctor if you have ever had any unusual or allergic reaction to corticosteroids. Also tell your health care professional if you are allergic to any other substances, such as foods, preservatives, or dyes.

**Pregnancy**—When used properly, these medicines have not been shown to cause problems in humans. Studies on birth defects have not been done in humans. However, studies in animals have shown that topical corticosteroids, when applied to the skin in large amounts or used for a long time, could cause birth defects.

**Breast-feeding**—Topical corticosteroids have not been reported to cause problems in nursing babies when used properly. However, corticosteroids should not be applied to the breasts before nursing.

**Children**—Children and teenagers who must use this medicine should be checked often by their doctor since this medicine may be absorbed through the skin and can affect growth or cause other unwanted effects.

**Older adults**—Certain side effects may be more likely to occur in elderly patients since the skin of older adults may be naturally thin. These unwanted effects may include tearing of the skin or blood-containing blisters on the skin.

**Other medicines**—Although certain medicines should not be used together at all, in other cases two different medicines may be used together even if an interaction might occur. In these cases, your doctor may want to change the dose, or other precautions may be necessary. Tell your health care professional if you are taking or using any other prescription or nonprescription (over-the-counter [OTC]) medicine.

**Other medical problems**—The presence of other medical problems may affect the use of topical corticosteroids. Make sure you tell your doctor if you have any other medical problems, especially:

- Cataracts or
- Glaucoma—Corticosteroids may make these medical problems worse, especially when stronger corticosteroids are used in the eye area
- Diabetes mellitus (sugar diabetes)—Too much use of corticosteroids may cause a loss of control of diabetes by increasing blood and urine glucose. However, this is not likely to happen when topical corticosteroids are used for a short time

- Infection or sores at the place of treatment (unless your doctor also prescribed medicine for the infection) or
- Tuberculosis—Corticosteroids may make existing infections worse or cause new infections

## Proper Use of This Medicine

Be very careful not to get this medicine in your eyes. Wash your hands after using your finger to apply the medicine. If you accidentally get this medicine in your eyes, flush them with water.

*Do not bandage or otherwise wrap the skin being treated* unless directed to do so by your doctor.

If your doctor has ordered an occlusive dressing (airtight covering, such as kitchen plastic wrap or a special patch) to be applied over this medicine, make sure you know how to apply it. Since occlusive dressings increase the amount of medicine absorbed through your skin and the possibility of side effects, use them only as directed. If you have any questions about this, check with your doctor.

For patients using the *topical aerosol form* of this medicine:

- This medicine usually comes with patient directions. Read them carefully before using this medicine.
- It is important to avoid breathing in the vapors from the spray or getting them in your eyes. If you accidentally get this medicine in your eyes, flush them with water.
- Do not use near heat, near an open flame, or while smoking.

For patients using *flurandrenolide tape:*

- This medicine usually comes with patient directions. Read them carefully before using this medicine.

*Do not use this medicine more often or for a longer time than your doctor ordered.* To do so may increase the chance of absorption through the skin and the chance of side effects. In addition, too much use, especially on areas with thinner skin (for example, face, armpits, groin), may result in thinning of the skin and stretch marks or other unwanted effects.

*Do not use any leftover medicine for other skin problems without first checking with your doctor.* Topical corticosteroids should not be used on many kinds of bacterial, virus, or fungus skin infections.

**Missed dose**—If your doctor has ordered you to use this medicine on a regular schedule and you miss a dose, apply it as soon as possible. However, if it is almost time for your next dose, skip the missed dose and apply it at the next regularly scheduled time.

**Storage**—To store this medicine:

- Keep out of the reach of children.
- Store away from heat and direct light.
- Keep the medicine from freezing.
- Do not puncture, break, or burn aerosol containers, even after they are empty.

- Do not keep outdated medicine or medicine no longer needed. Be sure that any discarded medicine is out of the reach of children.

## Precautions While Using This Medicine

Avoid using tight-fitting diapers or plastic pants on a child if this medicine is being used on the child's diaper area. Plastic pants or tight-fitting diapers may increase the chance of absorption of the medicine through the skin and the chance of side effects.

## Side Effects of This Medicine

Along with its needed effects, a medicine may cause some unwanted effects. Although not all of these side effects may occur, if they do occur they may need medical attention.

Check with your doctor as soon as possible if any of the following side effects occur:

*Less frequent or rare*
> Blood-containing blisters on skin; increased skin sensitivity (for some brands of betamethasone lotion); lack of healing of skin condition; loss of top skin layer (for tape dosage forms); numbness in fingers; raised, dark red, wart-like spots on skin; skin pain, redness, itching or pus-containing blisters; severe burning and continued itching of skin; thinning of skin with easy bruising

Additional side effects may occur if you use this medicine improperly or for a long time. Check with your doctor if any of the following side effects occur:

*Rare*
> Acne or oily skin; backache; blurring or loss of vision (occurs gradually if certain products have been used near the eye); burning and itching of skin with pinhead-sized red blisters; eye pain (if certain products have been used near the eye); filling or rounding out of the face; increased blood pressure; irregular heartbeat; irregular menstrual periods; irritability; irritation of skin around mouth; loss of appetite (continuing); mental depression; muscle cramps, pain, or weakness; nausea; rapid weight gain or loss; reddish purple lines (stretch marks) on arms, face, legs, trunk, or groin; skin color changes; softening of skin; stomach bloating, pain, cramping, or burning; swelling of feet or lower legs; tearing of the skin; unusual decrease in sexual desire or ability (in men); unusual increase in hair growth, especially on the face; unusual loss of hair, especially on the scalp; unusual tiredness or weakness; vomiting; weakness of the arms, legs, or trunk (severe); worsening of infections

Some side effects may occur that usually do not need medical attention. These side effects may go away during treatment as your body adjusts to the medicine. However, check with your doctor if any of the following side effects continue or are bothersome:

*Less frequent or rare*
    Burning, dryness, irritation, itching, or redness of skin; increased redness or scaling of skin sores; skin rash

When the gel, solution, lotion, or aerosol form of this medicine is applied, a mild, temporary stinging may be expected.

Other side effects not listed above may also occur in some patients. If you notice any other effects, check with your doctor.

Revised: 11/18/92

# CORTICOSTEROIDS AND ACETIC ACID    Otic

Some commonly used brand names are:
**In the U.S.—**
    Otic Tridesilon Solution[1]
    VōSol HC[2]
**In Canada—**
    VōSol HC[2]
Another commonly used name for hydrocortisone is cortisol.
Note: For quick reference, the following corticosteroids and acetic acid combinations are numbered to match the corresponding brand names.
This information applies to the following medicines:
  1. Desonide (DESS-oh-nide) and Acetic Acid (a-SEAT-ic AS-id)
  2. Hydrocortisone (hye-droe-KOR-ti-sone) and Acetic Acid

## Description
Corticosteroid (kor-ti-koe-STE-roid) and acetic acid combinations are used to treat certain problems of the ear canal. They also help relieve the redness, itching, and swelling that may accompany these conditions.

These medicines may also be used for other conditions as determined by your doctor.

Corticosteroid and acetic acid combinations are available only with your doctor's prescription, in the following dosage forms:
  *Otic*
    Desonide and Acetic Acid
      • Solution (U.S.)
    Hydrocortisone and Acetic Acid
      • Solution (U.S. and Canada)

## Before Using This Medicine
In deciding to use a medicine, the risks of using the medicine must be weighed against the good it will do. This is a decision you and your doctor will make. For otic corticosteroids with acetic acid, the following should be considered:

**Allergies**—Tell your doctor if you have ever had any unusual or allergic reaction to corticosteroids or acetic acid. Also tell your health care professional if you are allergic to any other substances, such as certain preservatives or dyes.

**Pregnancy**—Corticosteroid and acetic acid combinations used in the ear have not been shown to cause birth defects or other problems in humans.

**Breast-feeding**—Otic corticosteroid and acetic acid combinations have not been reported to cause problems in nursing babies.

**Children**—Although there is no specific information comparing the use of otic corticosteroids in children with use in other age groups, this combination medicine is not expected to cause different side effects or problems in children than it does in adults.

**Older adults**—Although there is no specific information comparing the use of otic corticosteroids in the elderly with use in other age groups, they are not expected to cause different side effects or problems in older people than they do in younger adults.

**Other medical problems**—The presence of other medical problems may affect the use of otic corticosteroids. Make sure you tell your doctor if you have any other medical problems, especially:
  • Any other ear infection or condition—Otic corticosteroids may worsen existing infections or cause new infections
  • Punctured ear drum—Using otic corticosteroids when you have a punctured ear drum may damage the ear

## Proper Use of This Medicine
To use:
  • Lie down or tilt the head so that the affected ear faces up. Gently pull the ear lobe up and back for adults (down and back for children) to straighten the ear canal. Drop the medicine into the ear canal. Keep the ear facing up for several (about 5) minutes to allow the medicine to run to the bottom of the ear canal. A sterile cotton plug may be gently inserted into the ear opening to prevent the medicine from leaking out. At first, your doctor may want you to put more medicine on the cotton plug during the day to keep it moist.

To keep the medicine as germ-free as possible, avoid touching the dropper or applicator tip to any surface as much as possible (including the ear). Also, always keep the container tightly closed.

For patients using *hydrocortisone and acetic acid ear drops:*
  • *Do not wash the dropper or applicator tip,* because water may get into the medicine and make it weaker.

If necessary, you may wipe the dropper or applicator tip with a clean tissue.

Do not use corticosteroids more often or for a longer time than your doctor ordered. To do so may increase the chance of side effects.

*Do not use any leftover medicine for future ear problems without first checking with your doctor.* This medicine should not be used if certain kinds of infections are present. To do so may make the infection worse.

**Dosing**—The dose of otic corticosteroid and acetic acid combination will be different for different patients. *Follow your doctor's orders or the directions on the label.* The following information includes only the average doses of otic corticosteroid and acetic acid combination. *If your dose is different, do not change it* unless your doctor tells you to do so.

*For desonide and acetic acid*
• For *ear drops* dosage form:
  —For ear infections:
    • Adults and children—Use three or four drops in the ear three or four times a day.

*For hydrocortisone and acetic acid*
• For *ear drops* dosage form:
  —For ear infections:
    • Adults and children—Use two to five drops in the ear three or four times a day.

**Missed dose**—If you miss a dose of this medicine, apply it as soon as possible. However, if it is almost time for your next dose, skip the missed dose and go back to your regular dosing schedule.

**Storage**—To store this medicine:
• Keep out of the reach of children.
• Store away from heat and direct light.
• Keep the medicine from freezing.
• Do not keep outdated medicine or medicine no longer needed. Be sure that any discarded medicine is out of the reach of children.

## Precautions While Using This Medicine

If your condition does not improve within 5 to 7 days, or if it becomes worse, check with your doctor.

## Side Effects of This Medicine

Along with its needed effects, a medicine may cause some unwanted effects. The following side effects usually do not need medical attention and may go away during treatment as your body adjusts to the medicine or your condition improves. However, check with your doctor if any of the following side effects continue or are bothersome:

*Less common*
  Stinging, itching, irritation or burning of the ear

There have not been any other side effects reported with this medicine. However, if you notice any other effects, check with your doctor.

Revised: 03/31/92
Interim revision: 04/01/94

# CORTICOSTEROIDS/CORTICOTROPIN—Glucocorticoid Effects    Systemic

Some commonly used brand names are:
**In the U.S.—**

| | | |
|---|---|---|
| Acthar[2] | Cortrophin-Zinc[2] | Dexacen LA-8[4] | Key-Pred 50[7] |
| A-hydroCort[5] | Dalalone[4] | Dexamethasone Intensol[4] | Key-Pred SP[7] |
| AK-Dex[4] | Dalalone D.P.[4] | Dexasone[4] | Liquid Pred[8] |
| Amcort[9] | Dalalone L.A.[4] | Dexasone-LA[4] | Medralone-40[6] |
| A-methaPred[6] | Decadrol[4] | Dexone[4] | Medralone-80[6] |
| Aristocort[9] | Decadron[4] | Dexone 0.5[4] | Medrol[6] |
| Aristocort Forte[9] | Decadron-LA[4] | Dexone 0.75[4] | Medrol Enpak[6] |
| Aristocort Intralesional[9] | Decadron Phosphate[4] | Dexone 1.5[4] | Meprolone[6] |
| Aristospan Intra-articular[9] | Decaject[4] | Dexone 4[4] | Meticorten[8] |
| Aristospan Intralesional[9] | Decaject-L.A.[4] | Dexone LA[4] | Mymethasone[4] |
| Articulose-50[7] | Delta-Cortef[7] | Duralone-40[6] | Nor-Pred T.B.A.[7] |
| Articulose-L.A.[9] | Deltasone[8] | Duralone-80[6] | Orasone 1[8] |
| Celestone[1] | depMedalone 40[6] | Hexadrol[4] | Orasone 5[8] |
| Celestone Phosphate[1] | depMedalone 80[6] | Hexadrol Phosphate[4] | Orasone 10[8] |
| Celestone Soluspan[1] | Depoject-40[6] | H.P. Acthar Gel[2] | Orasone 20[8] |
| Cenocort A-40[9] | Depoject-80[6] | Hydeltrasol[7] | Orasone 50[8] |
| Cenocort Forte[9] | Depo-Medrol[6] | Hydeltra-T.B.A.[7] | Pediapred[7] |
| Cinalone 40[9] | Depopred-40[6] | Hydrocortone[5] | Predaject-50[7] |
| Cinonide 40[9] | Depopred-80[6] | Hydrocortone Acetate[5] | Predalone 50[7] |
| Cortef[5] | Depo-Predate 40[6] | Hydrocortone Phosphate[5] | Predalone T.B.A.[7] |
| Cortenema[5] | Depo-Predate 80[6] | Kenacort[9] | Predate 50[7] |
| Cortifoam[5] | Deronil[4] | Kenacort Diacetate[9] | Predate S[7] |
| Cortone Acetate[3] | Dexacen-4[4] | Kenaject-40[9] | Predate TBA[7] |
| | | Kenalog-10[9] | Predcor-25[7] |
| | | Kenalog-40[9] | Predcor-50[7] |
| | | Key-Pred 25[7] | Predcor-TBA[7] |

Predicort-50[7]
Predicort-RP[7]
Prednicen-M[8]
Prednisone Intensol[8]
Prelone[7]
Rep-Pred 40[6]
Rep-Pred 80[6]
Selestoject[1]
Solu-Cortef[5]
Solu-Medrol[6]
Solurex[4]

Solurex-LA[4]
Sterapred[8]
Sterapred DS[8]
Tac-3[9]
Triam-A[9]
Triam-Forte[9]
Triamolone 40[9]
Triamonide 40[9]
Tri-Kort[9]
Trilog[9]
Trilone[9]
Tristoject[9]

**In Canada—**
Acthar[2]
Acthar Gel (H.P.)[2]
Apo-Prednisone[8]
Aristocort[9]
Aristocort Forte[9]
Aristocort Intralesional[9]
Aristospan Intra-articular[9]
Betnelan[1]
Betnesol[1]
Celestone[1]
Celestone Soluspan[1]
Cortef[5]
Cortenema[5]
Cortifoam[5]
Cortone[3]

Decadron[4]
Decadron Phosphate[4]
Deltasone[8]
Depo-Medrol[6]
Deronil[4]
Dexasone[4]
Hexadrol[4]
Kenacort[9]
Kenalog-10[9]
Kenalog-40[9]
Medrol[6]
Oradexon[4]
Solu-Cortef[5]
Solu-Medrol[6]
Winpred[8]

Other commonly used names are:
ACTH[2]
Cortisol[5]

Note: For quick reference, the following corticosteroids/corticotropins are numbered to match the corresponding brand names.

This information applies to the following medicines:

1. Betamethasone (bay-ta-METH-a-sone)‡
2. Corticotropin (kor-ti-koe-TROE-pin)‡
3. Cortisone (KOR-ti-sone)‡§
4. Dexamethasone (dex-a-METH-a-sone)‡§
5. Hydrocortisone (hye-droe-KOR-ti-sone)
6. Methylprednisolone (meth-ill-pred-NISS-oh-lone)‡
7. Prednisolone (pred-NISS-oh-lone)‡
8. Prednisone (PRED-ni-sone)‡§
9. Triamcinolone (trye-am-SIN-oh-lone)‡§

The following information does *not* apply to desoxycorticosterone or fludrocortisone.

‡Generic name product may also be available in the U.S.
§Generic name product may also be available in Canada.

## Description

Corticosteroids (kor-ti-koe-STER-oyds) (cortisone-like medicines) are used to provide relief for inflamed areas of the body. They lessen swelling, redness, itching, and allergic reactions. They are often used as part of the treatment for a number of different diseases, such as severe allergies or skin problems, asthma, or arthritis. Corticosteroids may also be used for other conditions as determined by your doctor.

Your body naturally produces certain cortisone-like hormones that are necessary to maintain good health. If your body does not produce enough, your doctor may have prescribed this medicine to help make up the difference.

Corticotropin is not a corticosteroid. It is a hormone that occurs naturally in the body. Corticotropin is known as an adrenocorticotropic hormone, which means it causes the adrenal glands to produce cortisone-like hormones. Corticotropin is used as a test to determine whether your adrenal glands are producing enough hormones. Also, it is sometimes used instead of corticosteroids to treat many of the same medical problems.

Corticosteroids and corticotropin are very strong medicines. In addition to their helpful effects in treating your medical problem, they have side effects that can be very serious. If your adrenal glands are not producing enough cortisone-like hormones, taking this medicine is not likely to cause problems unless you take too much of it. If you are taking this medicine to treat another medical problem, be sure that you discuss the risks and benefits of this medicine with your doctor.

These medicines are available only with your doctor's prescription, in the following dosage forms:

*Oral*
Betamethasone
• Syrup (U.S.)
• Tablets (U.S. and Canada)
• Effervescent tablets (Canada)
• Extended-release tablets (Canada)
Cortisone
• Tablets (U.S. and Canada)
Dexamethasone
• Elixir (U.S.)
• Oral solution (U.S.)
• Tablets (U.S. and Canada)
Hydrocortisone
• Oral suspension (U.S.)
• Tablets (U.S. and Canada)
Methylprednisolone
• Tablets (U.S. and Canada)
Prednisolone
• Oral solution (U.S.)
• Syrup (U.S.)
• Tablets (U.S.)
Prednisone
• Oral solution (U.S.)
• Syrup (U.S.)
• Tablets (U.S. and Canada)
Triamcinolone
• Syrup (U.S. and Canada)
• Tablets (U.S. and Canada)

*Parenteral*
Betamethasone
• Injection (U.S. and Canada)
Corticotropin
• Injection (U.S. and Canada)
Cortisone
• Injection (U.S. and Canada)
Dexamethasone
• Injection (U.S. and Canada)
Hydrocortisone
• Injection (U.S. and Canada)
Methylprednisolone
• Injection (U.S. and Canada)
Prednisolone
• Injection (U.S.)
Triamcinolone
• Injection (U.S. and Canada)

*Rectal*
Betamethasone
• Enema (Canada)

Hydrocortisone
- Aerosol foam (U.S. and Canada)
- Enema (U.S. and Canada)

Methylprednisolone
- Enema (U.S.)

## Before Using This Medicine

In deciding to use a medicine, the risks of taking the medicine must be weighed against the good it will do. This is a decision you and your doctor will make. For corticosteroids and corticotropin, the following should be considered:

**Allergies**—Tell your doctor if you have ever had any unusual or allergic reaction to corticosteroids or corticotropin. Also tell your health care professional if you are allergic to any other substances, such as foods, preservatives, or dyes.

**Diet**—If you will be using this medicine for a long time, your doctor may want you to:
- Follow a low-salt diet and/or a potassium-rich diet.
- Watch your calories to prevent weight gain.
- Add extra protein to your diet. Make certain your health care professional knows if you are already on any special diet, such as a low-sodium or low-sugar diet.

**Pregnancy**—Studies on birth defects with corticosteroids or with corticotropin have not been done in humans. However, too much use of corticosteroids during pregnancy may cause the baby to have problems after birth, such as slower growth. Also, studies in animals have shown that corticosteroids cause birth defects and that corticotropin may cause other unwanted effects in the fetus.

**Breast-feeding**—Corticosteroids pass into breast milk and may cause problems with growth or other unwanted effects in nursing babies. Depending on the amount of medicine you are taking every day, it may be necessary for you to take another medicine or to stop breast-feeding during treatment. Corticotropin has not been shown to cause problems in nursing babies.

**Children**—Corticosteroids or corticotropin may cause infections such as chickenpox or measles to be more serious in children who catch them. These medicines can also slow or stop growth in children and in growing teenagers, especially when they are used for a long time. Before this medicine is given to children or teenagers, you should discuss its use with your child's doctor and then carefully follow the doctor's instructions.

**Older adults**—Older patients may be more likely to develop high blood pressure or bone disease from corticosteroids. Women are especially at risk of developing bone disease.

**Other medicines**—Although certain medicines should not be used together at all, in other cases two different medicines may be used together even if an interaction might occur. In these cases, your doctor may want to change the dose, or other precautions may be necessary. When

you are taking corticosteroids or corticotropin, it is especially important that your health care professional know if you are taking any of the following:
- Aminoglutethimide or
- Antacids (in large amounts) or
- Barbiturates, except butalbital, or
- Carbamazepine (e.g., Tegretol) or
- Griseofulvin (e.g., Fulvicin) or
- Mitotane (e.g., Lysodren) or
- Phenylbutazone (e.g., Butazolidin) or
- Phenytoin (e.g., Dilantin) or
- Primidone (e.g., Mysoline) or
- Rifampin (e.g., Rifadin)—Use of these medicines may make corticotropin or certain corticosteroids less effective
- Amphotericin B by injection (e.g., Fungizone)—Corticosteroids and this medicine decrease the amount of potassium in the blood. Serious side effects could occur if the level of potassium gets too low
- Antidiabetics, oral (diabetes medicine taken by mouth) or
- Insulin—Corticosteroids may increase blood glucose (sugar) levels
- Digitalis glycosides (heart medicine)—Corticosteroids decrease the amount of potassium in the blood. Digitalis can cause an irregular heartbeat or other problems more commonly if the blood potassium gets too low
- Diuretics (water pills) or
- Medicine containing potassium—Using corticosteroids with diuretics may cause the diuretic to be less effective. Also, corticosteroids may increase the risk of low blood potassium, which is also a problem with certain diuretics. Potassium supplements or a different type of diuretic is used in treating high blood pressure in those people who have problems keeping their blood potassium at a normal level. Corticosteroids may make these medicines less able to do this
- Immunizations (vaccinations)—While you are being treated with this medicine, and even after you stop taking it, do not have any immunizations without your doctor's approval. Also, other people living in your home should not receive oral polio vaccine, since there is a chance they could pass the polio virus on to you. In addition, you should avoid close contact with other people at school or work who have recently taken oral polio vaccine
- Skin test injections—Corticosteroids may cause false results in skin tests
- Sodium-containing medicine—Corticosteroids and corticotropin cause the body to retain (keep) more salt and water. Too much sodium may cause high blood sodium, high blood pressure, and excess body water

**Other medical problems**—The presence of other medical problems may affect the use of corticosteroids and corticotropin. Make sure you tell your doctor if you have any other medical problems, especially:
- Bone disease—These medicines may worsen bone disease because they cause the body to lose more calcium
- Chickenpox (including recent exposure) or
- Measles (including recent exposure)—Risk of severe disease affecting other parts of the body
- Colitis or
- Diverticulitis or
- Stomach ulcer or other stomach or intestine problems—These medicines may cover up symptoms of a worsening stomach or intestinal condition. A patient would not know

if his/her condition was getting worse and would not get medical help when needed
- Diabetes mellitus (sugar diabetes)—Corticosteroids may cause a loss of control of diabetes by increasing blood glucose (sugar)
- Fungus infection or any other infection or
- Herpes simplex infection of the eye or
- Infection at the place of treatment or
- Recent surgery or serious injury or
- Tuberculosis (active TB, nonactive TB, or past history of)— These medicines can cause slower healing, worsen existing infections, or cause new infections
- Glaucoma—Corticosteroids may cause the pressure within the eye to increase
- Heart disease or
- High blood pressure or
- Kidney disease (especially if you are receiving dialysis) or
- Kidney stones—These medicines cause the body to retain (keep) more salt and water. These conditions may be made worse by this extra body water
- High cholesterol levels—Corticosteroids may increase blood cholesterol levels
- Liver disease or
- Overactive thyroid or
- Underactive thyroid—With these conditions, the body may not eliminate the corticosteroid at the usual rate, which may change the medicine's effect
- Myasthenia gravis—When these medicines are first started, muscle weakness may occur. Your doctor may want to take special precautions because this could cause problems with breathing
- Systemic lupus erythematosus (SLE)—This condition may cause certain side effects of corticosteroids to occur more easily

## Proper Use of This Medicine

For patients taking this medicine by mouth:
- *Take this medicine with food* to help prevent stomach upset. If stomach upset, burning, or pain continues, check with your doctor.
- Stomach problems may be more likely to occur if you drink alcoholic beverages while being treated with this medicine. You should not drink alcoholic beverages while taking this medicine, unless you have first checked with your doctor.

For patients using this medicine rectally:
- This medicine usually comes with patient directions. Read them carefully before using this medicine.
- For patients using hydrocortisone enema:
  —Each bottle contains a single dose. Use it all, unless otherwise directed by your doctor.
  —For best results, use this medicine right after a bowel movement. Lie down on your left side when giving the enema.
  —Insert the rectal tip of the enema applicator gently to prevent damage to the rectal wall.
  —Stay on your left side for at least 30 minutes after the enema is given so the medicine can work. If you can, keep the medicine inside the rectum all night.

- For patients using hydrocortisone acetate rectal aerosol foam:
  —This medicine is used with a special applicator. Do not insert any part of the aerosol container into the rectum.

- For patients using methylprednisolone acetate for enema:
  —Each bottle contains a single dose. Use it all, unless otherwise directed by your doctor.
  —Insert the rectal tip of the enema applicator gently to prevent damage to the rectal wall.
  —If you have been directed to use this enema slowly (not all at once), shake the bottle once in a while while you are giving the enema.
  —Save your applicator. Refill units of this medicine may be available at a lower cost.

*Use this medicine only as directed by your doctor.* Do not use more or less of it, do not use it more often, and do not use it for a longer time than your doctor ordered. To do so may increase the chance of side effects.

**Dosing**—The dose of these medicines will be different for different patients. *Follow your doctor's orders or the directions on the label.* The following information gives the range of doses of these medicines for all uses, which can vary widely. The dose that you are receiving may be very different. *If your dose is different, do not change it* unless your doctor tells you to do so.

The number of capsules, tablets, teaspoonfuls of liquid or amount of injection that you use depends on the strength of the medicine. Also, *the number of doses you take each day, the time allowed between doses, and the length of time you take the medicine depend on the medical problem for which you are taking the corticosteroid. In addition, your doctor may need to change the dose from time to time.*

*For betamethasone*
- For *oral* dosage forms:
  —Syrup, tablets, effervescent tablets:
    • Adults and teenagers—Dose may range from 0.6 milligrams (mg) to 7.2 mg a day.
    • Children—Dose is based on body weight or size and must be determined by your doctor.
  —Extended-release tablets:
    • Adults and teenagers—2 to 6 mg a day.
    • Children—Dose is based on body weight or size and must be determined by your doctor.
- For *injection* dosage form:
  —Adults and teenagers: Up to 9 mg (betamethasone) a day, injected into a muscle, vein, joint, or lesion.
  —Children: Dose is based on body weight or size and must be determined by your doctor.

- For *rectal* dosage form (enema):
  —Adults and teenagers: 5 mg (betamethasone), given as directed, each night.
  —Children: Dose must be determined by your doctor.

*For corticotropin*
- For *injection* dosage forms:
  —Regular:
    • Adults and teenagers—10 to 80 Units every twelve to twenty-four hours, injected into a vein or muscle or under the skin.
    • Children—Dose is based on body weight or size and must be determined by your doctor.
  —Long-acting:
    • Adults and teenagers—40 to 80 Units every one to three days, injected into a muscle or under the skin.
    • Children—Dose is based on body weight or size and must be determined by your doctor.

*For cortisone*
- For *oral* dosage form (tablets):
  —Adults and teenagers: 25 to 300 milligrams (mg) a day, as a single dose or divided into several doses.
  —Children: Dose is based on body weight or size and must be determined by your doctor.
- For *injection* dosage form:
  —Adults and teenagers: 20 to 300 mg a day, injected into a muscle.
  —Children: Dose is based on body weight or size and must be determined by your doctor.

*For dexamethasone*
- For *oral* dosage forms (elixir, solution, tablets):
  —Adults and teenagers: 0.5 to 9 milligrams (mg) a day, as a single dose or divided into several doses.
  —Children: Dose is based on body weight or size and must be determined by your doctor.
- For *injection* dosage form:
  —Adults and teenagers: 0.2 to 16 mg (dexamethasone or dexamethasone phosphate) every three days to three weeks as needed. It is injected into a muscle, joint, or lesion.
  —Children: Dose is based on body weight or size and must be determined by your doctor.

*For hydrocortisone*
- For *oral* dosage forms (tablets, suspension):
  —Adults and teenagers: 20 to 240 milligrams (mg) (hydrocortisone) a day, as a single dose or divided into several doses.
  —Children: Dose is based on body weight or size and must be determined by your doctor.
- For *injection* dosage form:
  —Adults and teenagers:
    • 15 to 240 mg a day, injected into a muscle; or
    • 5 to 75 mg every two to three weeks, injected into a joint or lesion; or

    • 100 to 500 mg (hydrocortisone) every two to six hours as needed, injected into a muscle or vein or under the skin.
  —Children: Dose is based on body weight or size and must be determined by your doctor.
- For *rectal* dosage forms (enema, aerosol foam):
  —Enema:
    • Adults and teenagers—100 mg, given as directed, every night.
    • Children—Dose must be determined by your doctor.
  —Aerosol foam:
    • Adults and teenagers—90 mg (one applicatorful) one or two times a day.
    • Children—Dose must be determined by your doctor.

*For methylprednisolone*
- For *oral* dosage form (tablets):
  —Adults and teenagers: 4 to 160 milligrams (mg) a day, as a single dose or divided into several doses.
  —Children: Dose is based on body weight or size and must be determined by your doctor.
- For *injection* dosage form:
  —Adults and teenagers:
    • 4 to 120 mg every one day to five weeks as needed, injected into a muscle, joint, or lesion; or
    • 10 to 160 mg (methylprednisolone) repeated as needed, injected into a muscle or vein.
  —Children: Dose is based on body weight or size and must be determined by your doctor.
- For *rectal* dosage form (enema):
  —Adults and teenagers: 40 mg, given as directed, three to seven times a week.
  —Children: Dose is based on body weight or size and must be determined by your doctor.

*For prednisolone*
- For *oral* dosage forms (solution, syrup, tablets):
  —Adults and teenagers: 5 to 200 milligrams (mg) (prednisolone) a day, as needed, as a single dose or divided into several doses.
  —Children: Dose is based on body weight or size and must be determined by your doctor.
- For *injection* dosage form:
  —Adults and teenagers: 2 to 100 mg (prednisolone or prednisolone phosphate) a day as needed, injected into a muscle, vein, joint, or lesion.
  —Children: Dose is based on body weight or size and must be determined by your doctor.

*For prednisone*
- For *oral* dosage forms (solution, syrup, tablets):
  —Adults and teenagers: 5 to 200 milligrams (mg) a day, as needed, as a single dose or divided into several doses.

—Children: Dose is usually based on body weight or size and must be determined by your doctor.

*For triamcinolone*

- For *oral* dosage forms (syrup, tablets):
  —Adults and teenagers: 4 to 60 milligrams (mg) (triamcinolone) a day, as needed, as a single dose or divided into several doses.
  —Children: Dose is based on body weight or size and must be determined by your doctor.
- For *injection* dosage form:
  —Adults and teenagers: 0.5 to 80 mg repeated as needed, injected into a muscle, joint, or lesion, or under the skin.
  —Children: Dose is usually based on body weight or size and must be determined by your doctor.

**Missed dose**—If you miss a dose of this medicine and your dosing schedule is:

- One dose every other day—Take the missed dose as soon as possible if you remember it the same morning, then go back to your regular dosing schedule. If you do not remember the missed dose until later, wait and take it the following morning. Then skip a day and start your regular dosing schedule again.
- One dose a day—Take the missed dose as soon as possible, then go back to your regular dosing schedule. If you do not remember until the next day, skip the missed dose and do not double the next one.
- Several doses a day—Take the missed dose as soon as possible, then go back to your regular dosing schedule. If you do not remember until your next dose is due, double the next dose.

If you have any questions about this, check with your health care professional.

**Storage**—To store this medicine:

- Keep out of the reach of children.
- Store away from heat and direct light.
- Do not store tablets in the bathroom, near the kitchen sink, or in other damp places. Heat or moisture may cause the medicine to break down.
- Keep the liquid dosage forms of this medicine, including enemas, and hydrocortisone rectal aerosol foam from freezing.
- Do not puncture, break, or burn the hydrocortisone rectal aerosol foam container, even when it is empty.
- Do not keep outdated medicine or medicine no longer needed. Be sure that any discarded medicine is out of the reach of children.

---

## Precautions While Using This Medicine

*Your doctor should check your progress at regular visits.* Also, your progress may have to be checked after you have stopped using this medicine, since some of the effects may continue.

*Do not stop using this medicine without first checking with your doctor.* Your doctor may want you to reduce gradually the amount you are using before stopping completely.

Check with your doctor if your condition reappears or worsens after the dose has been reduced or treatment with this medicine is stopped.

If you will be using corticosteroids or corticotropin for a long time:

- *Your doctor may want you to follow a low-salt diet and/or a potassium-rich diet.*
- Your doctor may want you to watch your calories to prevent weight gain.
- Your doctor may want you to add extra protein to your diet.
- Your doctor may want you to have your eyes examined by an ophthalmologist (eye doctor) before and also sometime later during treatment.
- Your doctor may want you to carry a medical identification card stating that you are using this medicine.

Tell the doctor in charge that you are using this medicine:

- *Before having skin tests.*
- *Before having any kind of surgery (including dental surgery) or emergency treatment.*
- *If you get a serious infection or injury.*

*Avoid close contact with anyone who has chickenpox or measles.* This is especially important for children. *Tell your doctor right away if you think you have been exposed to chickenpox or measles.*

While you are being treated with this medicine, and after you stop taking it, *do not have any immunizations without your doctor's approval.* Also, other people living in your home should not receive oral polio vaccine, since there is a chance they could pass the polio virus on to you. In addition, you should avoid close contact with other people at school or work who have recently taken oral polio vaccine.

For *diabetic patients:*

- This medicine may affect blood sugar levels. If you notice a change in the results of your blood or urine sugar tests or if you have any questions, check with your doctor.

For patients having this medicine *injected into their joints:*

- If this medicine is injected into one of your joints, you should be careful not to put too much stress or strain on that joint for a while, even if it begins to feel better. Make sure your doctor has told you how much you are allowed to move this joint while it is healing.
- If redness or swelling occurs at the place of injection, and continues or gets worse, check with your doctor.

For patients using this medicine *rectally:*

- Check with your doctor if you notice rectal bleeding, pain, burning, itching, blistering, or any other sign of irritation not present before you started using this medicine, or if signs of infection occur.

## Side Effects of This Medicine

Corticosteroids or corticotropin may lower your resistance to infections. Also, any infection you get may be harder to treat. Always check with your doctor as soon as possible if you notice any signs of a possible infection, such as sore throat, fever, sneezing, or coughing.

Along with its needed effects, a medicine may cause some unwanted effects. Although not all of these side effects may occur, if they do occur they may need medical attention. When this medicine is used for short periods of time, side effects usually are rare. However, check with your doctor as soon as possible if any of the following side effects occur:

*Less common*
   Decreased or blurred vision; frequent urination; increased thirst; rectal bleeding, blistering, burning, itching, or pain not present before use of this medicine (when used rectally)

*Rare*
   Blindness (sudden, when injected in the head or neck area); confusion; excitement; false sense of well-being; hallucinations (seeing, hearing, or feeling things that are not there); mental depression; mood swings (sudden and wide); mistaken feelings of self-importance or being mistreated; redness, swelling, pain, or other sign of allergy or infection at place of injection; restlessness

Additional side effects may occur if you take this medicine for a long time. Check with your doctor if any of the following side effects occur:
   Abdominal or stomach pain or burning (continuing); acne or other skin problems; bloody or black, tarry stools; filling or rounding out of the face; irregular heartbeat; menstrual problems; muscle cramps or pain; muscle weakness; nausea; pain in back, hips, ribs, arms, shoulders, or legs; pitting, scarring, or depression of skin at place of injection; reddish purple lines on arms, face, legs, trunk, or

groin; swelling of feet or lower legs; thin, shiny skin; unusual bruising; unusual tiredness or weakness; vomiting; weight gain (rapid); wounds that will not heal

Other side effects may occur that usually do not need medical attention. These side effects may go away during treatment as your body adjusts to the medicine. However, check with your doctor if any of the following side effects continue or are bothersome:

*More common*
   Increased appetite; indigestion; loss of appetite (for triamcinolone only); nervousness or restlessness; trouble in sleeping

*Less common or rare*
   Darkening or lightening of skin color; dizziness; flushing of face or cheeks (after injection into the nose); headache; increased joint pain (after injection into a joint); increased sweating; lightheadedness; nosebleeds (after injection into the nose); unusual increase in hair growth on body or face

*After you stop using this medicine, your body may need time to adjust.* The length of time this takes depends on the amount of medicine you were using and how long you used it. If you have taken large doses of this medicine for a long time, your body may need one year to adjust. During this time, *check with your doctor immediately if any of the following side effects occur:*
   Abdominal, stomach, or back pain; dizziness; fainting; fever; loss of appetite (continuing); muscle or joint pain; nausea; reappearance of disease symptoms; shortness of breath; unexplained headaches (frequent or continuing); unusual tiredness or weakness; vomiting; weight loss (rapid)

Other side effects not listed above may also occur in some patients. If you notice any other effects, check with your doctor.

Revised: 04/14/92
Interim revision: 08/09/94

# COUGH/COLD COMBINATIONS　Systemic

Some commonly used brand names are:

**In the U.S.—**

Actagen-C Cough[41]
Actifed with Codeine Cough[41]
Adatuss D.C. Expectorant[97]
Alamine-C Liquid[28]
Alamine Expectorant[113]
Alka-Seltzer Plus Cold and Cough[49]
Alka-Seltzer Plus Night-Time Cold[42a]
Allerfrin with Codeine[41]
All-Nite Cold Formula[51]
Ambay Cough[1]
Ambenyl Cough[1]
Ambenyl-D Decongestant Cough Formula[114]
Ambophen Expectorant[9]
Amgenal Cough[1]
Ami-Tex LA[121]
Anamine HD[23]
Anaplex HD[23]
Anatuss[74]
Anatuss with Codeine[75]
Anatuss DM[114]
Anatuss LA[122]
Anti-Tuss DM Expectorant[94]
Aprodine with Codeine[41]
Banex[120]
Banex-LA[121]
Banex Liquid[120]
Bayaminic Expectorant[121]
Bayaminicol[27]
Baycodan[89]
Baycomine[103]
Baycomine Pediatric[103]
BayCotussend Liquid[106]
Baydec DM Drops[20]
Bayer Select Chest Cold Caplets[88a]
Bayer Select Flu Relief Caplets[50]
Bayer Select Head and Chest Cold Caplets[117]
Bayer Select Night Time Cold Caplets[54b]
Bayhistine DH[28]
Bayhistine Expectorant[113]
Baytussin AC[91]
Baytussin DM[94]
Benylin Expectorant Cough Formula[94]
Biphetane DC Cough[19]
Brexin[81]
Bromanate DC Cough[19]
Bromanyl[1]
Bromarest DX Cough[19b]

Bromatane DX Cough[19b]
Bromfed-DM[19b]
Bromotuss with Codeine[1]
Bromphen DC with Codeine Cough[19]
Bromphen DX Cough[19b]
Broncholate[118]
Bronkotuss Expectorant[82]
Brotane DX Cough[19b]
Calcidrine[90]
Carbinoxamine Compound[20]
Carbinoxamine Compound-Drops[20]
Carbodec DM Drops[20]
Cardec DM[20]
Cardec DM Drops[20]
Cardec DM Pediatric[20]
Cerose-DM[22]
Cheracol[91]
Cheracol D Cough[94]
Cheracol Plus[27]
Children's Formula Cough[94]
Children's Tylenol Cold Multi Symptom Plus Cough[50]
Children's Vicks NyQuil Cold/Cough Relief[29]
Chlorgest-HD[23]
Citra Forte[15 44]
Co-Apap[50]
Codamine[103]
Codamine Pediatric[103]
Codan[89]
Codegest Expectorant[111]
Codehist DH[28]
Codiclear DH[97]
Codimal DH[40]
Codimal DM[39]
Codimal Expectorant[121]
Codimal PH[38]
Codistan No. 1[94]
Comtrex Cough Formula[117]
Comtrex Daytime Caplets[108]
Comtrex Daytime Maximum Strength Cold, Cough, and Flu Relief[108]
Comtrex Daytime Maximum Strength Cold and Flu Relief[108]
Comtrex Hot Flu Relief[50]
Comtrex Maximum Strength Liqui-Gels[48]
Comtrex Multi-Symptom Cold Reliever[48]
Comtrex Multi-Symptom Non-Drowsy Caplets[108]

Comtrex Nighttime[50]
Comtrex Nighttime Maximum Strength Cold, Cough, and Flu Relief[50]
Comtrex Nighttime Maximum Strength Cold and Flu Relief[50]
Concentrin[114]
Conex[121]
Conex with Codeine Liquid[111]
Congess JR[122]
Congess SR[122]
Congestac Caplets[122]
Contac Cough & Chest Cold[117]
Contac Cough and Sore Throat[88a]
Contac Day Caplets[108]
Contac Jr. Children's Cold Medicine[107]
Contac Night Caplets[50b]
Contac Severe Cold and Flu Formula Caplets[48]
Contac Severe Cold Formula[50]
Contac Severe Cold Formula Night Strength[51]
Contuss[120]
Cophene-S[26]
Cophene-X[109a]
Cophene XP[115]
Cophene-XP[64]
Co-Tuss V[97]
CoTylenol Cold Medication[50]
C-Tussin Expectorant[113]
DayQuil Multi-Symptom Cold/Flu LiquiCaps[117]
DayQuil Non-Drowsy Cold/Flu[117]
DayQuil Sinus Pressure and Congestion Relief Caplets[117]
Decohistine DH[28]
Deconsal II[122]
Deconsal Pediatric[113]
Deconsal Sprinkle[120a]
Deproist Expectorant with Codeine[113]
Despec[120]
De-Tuss[106]
Detussin Expectorant[115]
Detussin Liquid[106]
Dexafed Cough[109]
Diabetic Tussin DM[94]
Dihistine DH[28]
Dihistine Expectorant[113]
Dilaudid Cough[99]
Dimacol Caplets[114]
Dimetane-DC Cough[19]
Dimetane-DX Cough[19b]
Dimetapp DM[19a]

Dimetapp DM Cold and Cough[19a]
Donatussin[62]
Donatussin DC[110]
Donatussin Drops[83]
Dondril[22]
Dorcol Children's Cough[114]
Dristan Cold and Flu[50]
Dristan Juice Mix-in Cold, Flu, and Cough[108]
Dura-Gest[120]
Duratuss[122]
Duratuss HD[115]
Dura-Vent[121]
ED-TLC[23]
ED Tuss HC[23]
Effective Strength Cough Formula[3]
Effective Strength Cough Formula with Decongestant[105]
Efficol Cough Whip (Cough Suppressant/Decongestant)[102]
Efficol Cough Whip (Cough Suppressant/Decongestant/Antihistamine)[27]
Efficol Cough Whip (Cough Suppressant/Expectorant)[94]
Endagen-HD[23]
Endal[120a]
Endal Expectorant[111]
Endal-HD[23]
Endal-HD Plus[23]
Enomine[120]
Entex[120]
Entex LA[121]
Entex Liquid[120]
Entex PSE[122]
Entuss-D[106 115]
Entuss Expectorant[97 98]
Entuss Pediatric Expectorant[115]
Eudal-SR[122]
Exgest LA[121]
Extra Action Cough[94]
Father John's Medicine Plus[63]
Fendol[123]
2/G-DM Cough[94]
Genatuss DM[94]
Genite[51]
Glycofed[122]
Glycotuss-dM[94]
Glydeine Cough[91]
GP-500[122]
Guaifed[122]
Guaifed-PD[122]
GuaiMAX-D[122]
Guaipax[121]
Guaitab[122]
GuiaCough CF[112]
GuiaCough PE[122]
Guiamid D.M. Liquid[94]
Guiatuss A.C.[91]
Guiatuss CF[112]

Guiatuss DAC[113]
Guiatuss-DM[94]
Guiatussin with Codeine Liquid[91]
Guiatussin DAC[113]
Guiatussin w/Dextromethorphan[94]
Guiatuss PE[122]
Halotussin-DM Expectorant[94]
Histafed C[41]
Histalet X[122]
Histatuss Pediatric[21]
Histine DM[19a]
Histussin HC[23]
Humibid DM[94]
Humibid DM Sprinkle[94]
Hycodan[89]
Hycomine[103]
Hycomine Compound[47]
Hycomine Pediatric[103]
Hycotuss Expectorant[97]
Hydromet[89]
Hydromine[103]
Hydromine Pediatric[103]
Hydropane[89]
Hydrophen[103]
Improved Sino-Tuss[46]
Iophen-C Liquid[92]
Iophen DM[95]
Ipsatol Cough Formula for Children[112]
Kiddy Koff[112]
KIE[119]
Kolephrin/DM Caplets[49,50a]
Kolephrin GG/DM[94]
Kolephrin NN Liquid[54]
Kophane[65]
Kophane Cough and Cold Formula[27]
Kwelcof Liquid[97]
Lanatuss Expectorant[85]
Mapap Cold Formula[50]
Marcof Expectorant[98]
Meda Syrup Forte[62]
Medi-Flu[50]
Medi-Flu Caplets[50]
Mediquell Decongestant Formula[105]
Midahist DH[28]
Mycotussin[106]
Myhistine DH[28]
Myhistine Expectorant[113]
Myhydromine[103]
Myhydromine Pediatric[103]
Myminic Expectorant[121]
Myminicol[27]
Myphetane DC Cough[19]
Myphetane DX Cough[19b]
Mytussin AC[91]

Mytussin DAC[113]
Mytussin DM[94]
Naldecon-CX Adult Liquid[111]
Naldecon-DX Adult Liquid[112]
Naldecon-DX Children's Syrup[112]
Naldecon-DX Pediatric Drops[112]
Naldecon-EX[121]
Naldecon-EX Pediatric Drops[121]
Naldecon Senior DX[94]
Naldelate DX Adult[112]
Nasatab LA[122]
Nolex LA[121]
Noratuss II Liquid[114]
Normatane DC[19]
Nortuss with Codeine[91]
Novagest Expectorant w/Codeine[113]
Novahistine DH Liquid[28]
Novahistine DMX Liquid[114]
Novahistine Expectorant[113]
Nucochem[104]
Nucochem Expectorant[113]
Nucochem Pediatric Expectorant[113]
Nucofed[104]
Nucofed Expectorant[113]
Nucofed Pediatric Expectorant[113]
Nucotuss Expectorant[113]
Nucotuss Pediatric Expectorant[113]
Nytcold Medicine[51]
Nytime Cold Medicine Liquid[51]
Omnicol[43]
Ordrine AT[101]
Ornex Severe Cold No Drowsiness Caplets[108]
Orthoxicol Cough[27]
Para-Hist HD[23]
Partuss LA[121]
PediaCare Children's Cough-Cold[29]
PediaCare Cough-Cold[29]
PediaCare Night Rest Cough-Cold Liquid[29]
Pediacof Cough[61]
Pedituss Cough[61]
Pentazine VC w/Codeine[5]
Pertussin All Night CS[94]
Pertussin All Night PM[51]
Phanadex[72a]
Phanatuss[94]
Phenameth DM[6]

　　*All rights reserved*

Phenameth VC with Codeine[37]
Phenergan with Codeine[5]
Phenergan with Dextromethorphan[6]
Phenergan VC with Codeine[37]
Phenhist DH w/ Codeine[28]
Phenhist Expectorant[113]
Phenylfenesin L.A.[121]
Pherazine w/Codeine[5]
Pherazine DM[6]
Pherazine VC with Codeine[37]
Pneumotussin HC[97]
Polaramine Expectorant[87]
Poly-Histine-CS[19]
Poly-Histine-DM[19a]
Primatuss Cough Mixture 4[3]
Primatuss Cough Mixture 4D[114]
Promethazine DM[6]
Promethazine VC w/ Codeine[37]
Prometh w/ Dextromethorphan[6]
Promethist w/ Codeine[37]
Prometh VC with Codeine[37]
Prominatuss Expectorant[121]
Prominicol Cough[69]
Promist HD Liquid[30]
Pseudo-Car DM[20]
Pseudodine C Cough[41]
P-V-Tussin[13 30]
Quelidrine Cough[57]
Remcol-C[8]

Rentamine Pediatric[21]
Rescaps-D S.R.[101]
Rescon-DM[29]
Rescon-GG[120a]
Respaire-60 SR[122]
Respaire-120 SR[122]
Rhinosyn-DM[29]
Rhinosyn-DMX Expectorant[94]
Rhinosyn-X[114]
Robafen AC Cough[91]
Robafen CF[112]
Robafen DAC[113]
Robafen DM[94]
Robitussin A-C[91]
Robitussin-CF[112]
Robitussin Cold and Cough Liqui-Gels[114]
Robitussin-DAC[113]
Robitussin-DM[94]
Robitussin Maximum Strength Cough and Cold[105]
Robitussin Night Relief[54a]
Robitussin Night Relief Colds Formula Liquid[53]
Robitussin-PE[122]
Robitussin Pediatric Cough & Cold[105]
Robitussin Severe Congestion Liqui-Gels[122]
Rolatuss Expectorant[60]
Rolatuss w/ Hydrocodone[34]
Rondamine-DM Drops[20]
Rondec-DM[20]
Rondec-DM Drops[20]

Ru-Tuss DE[122]
Ru-Tuss Expectorant[114]
Ru-Tuss with Hydrocodone Liquid[34]
Rymed[122]
Rymed Liquid[122]
Rymed-TR Caplets[122]
Ryna-C Liquid[28]
Ryna-CX Liquid[113]
Rynatuss[21]
Rynatuss Pediatric[21]
Safe Tussin 30[94]
Saleto-CF[107]
Scot-Tussin DM[3]
Silexin Cough[94]
Sinufed Timecelles[122]
Sinupan[120a]
SINUvent[121]
Snaplets-DM[102]
Snaplets-EX[121]
Snaplets-Multi[27]
SRC Expectorant[115]
Stamoist E[122]
Stamoist LA[121]
Statuss Green[34]
S-T Forte[71a]
S-T Forte 2[3a]
Sudafed Cold & Cough Liquid Caps[117]
Sudafed Cough[114]
Sudafed Severe Cold Formula Caplets[108]
Syracol Liquid[102]
TheraFlu/Flu, Cold and Cough Medicine[50]
TheraFlu Maximum Strength Non-Drowsy Formula Flu, Cold and Cough Medicine[108]

TheraFlu Nighttime Maximum Strength[50]
Threamine DM[27]
Threamine Expectorant[121]
T-Koff[24]
Tolu-Sed Cough[91]
Tolu-Sed DM[94]
Touro LA Caplets[122]
Triacin C Cough[41]
Triafed w/Codeine[41]
Triaminic-DM Cough Formula[102]
Triaminic Expectorant[121]
Triaminic Expectorant with Codeine[111]
Triaminic Expectorant DH[71]
Triaminic Nite Light[29]
Triaminicol Multi-Symptom Relief[27]
Triaminicol Multi-Symptom Relief Colds with Coughs[27]
Triaminic Sore Throat Formula[108]
Tricodene Cough & Cold[7]
Tricodene Forte[27]
Tricodene NN[27]
Tricodene Pediatric[102]
Tricodene Sugar Free[3]
Trifed-C Cough[41]
Triminol Cough[27]
Trinex[86]
Triphenyl Expectorant[121]
Tri-Tannate Plus Pediatric[21]
Tusquelin[25]

Tuss-Ade[101]
Tussafed[20]
Tussafed Drops[20]
Tussafin Expectorant[115]
Tuss Allergine Modified T.D.[101]
Tussanil DH[23 116]
Tussar-2[113]
Tussar DM[29]
Tussar SF[113]
Tuss-DM[94]
Tussex Cough[109]
Tussgen[106]
Tuss-Genade Modified[101]
Tussigon[89]
Tussionex[3a 4]
Tussi-Organidin DM Liquid[95]
Tussi-Organidin Liquid[92]
Tussirex with Codeine Liquid[78]
Tuss-LA[122]
Tusso-DM[95]
Tussogest[101]
Ty-Cold Cold Formula[50]
Tylenol Cold and Flu[50]
Tylenol Cold and Flu No Drowsiness Powder[108]
Tylenol Cold Medication[50]
Tylenol Cold Medication, Non-Drowsy[108]
Tylenol Cold Night Time[50a]
Tylenol Cough with Decongestant Maximum Strength[108]
Tylenol Maximum Strength Cough[88a]

Tylenol Maximum Strength Flu Gelcaps[108]
Tyrodone[106]
ULR-LA[121]
Uni-tussin DM[94]
Unproco[94]
Utex-S.R.[121]
Vanex Expectorant[115]
Vanex-HD[23]
Vanex-LA[121]
V-Dec-M[122]
Versacaps[122]
Vicks 44 Cough and Cold Relief Liqui-Caps[105]
Vicks 44D Dry Hacking Cough and Head Congestion[105]
Vicks 44M Cough, Cold and Flu Relief[50]
Vicks 44M Cough, Cold and Flu Relief LiquiCaps[50]
Vicks NyQuil Multi-Symptom Cold/Flu Relief[51]
Vicks NyQuil Multi-Symptom Liqui-Caps[51]
Vicks Pediatric Formula 44D Cough & Decongestant[105]
Vicks Pediatric Formula 44E[94]
Vicks Pediatric Formula 44M Multi-Symptom Cough & Cold[29]
Vicodin Tuss[97]
Viro-Med[50]
Zephrex[122]
Zephrex-LA[122]

**In Canada—**

Actifed DM[42]
Benylin with Codeine[113]
Caldomine-DH Forte[36]
Caldomine-DH Pediatric[36]
Calmylin with Codeine[11]
CoActifed[41]
CoActifed Expectorant[73]

Coristex-DH[100a]
Coristine-DH[100a]
Dimetane Expectorant[80]
Dimetane Expectorant-C[55]
Dimetane Expectorant-DC[56]
Dimetapp-DM[18]
Dorcol DM[112]
Entex LA[121]

Hycomine[72]
Hycomine-S Pediatric[72]
Novahistex C[100]
Novahistex DH[100a]
Novahistex DH Expectorant[110]
Novahistex DM[32]
Novahistine DH[33]
Novahistine DH Expectorant[68]

Omni-Tuss[67]
Ornade-DM 10[27]
Ornade-DM 15[27]
Ornade-DM 30[27]
Ornade Expectorant[84]
Robitussin A-C[14]
Robitussin-CF[112]
Robitussin with Codeine[14]
Robitussin-DM
Sudafed DM[105]

Sudafed Expectorant[122]
Triaminic-DM Expectorant[70]
Triaminic Expectorant[88]
Triaminic Expectorant DH[71]
Triaminicin with Codeine[52]
Triaminicol DM[35]
Tussaminic C[34a]

Tussaminic C Pediatric[34a]
Tussaminic DH[36]
Tussaminic Pediatric[36]
Tussionex[4]
Tuss-Ornade Spansules[26a]
Tylenol Cold Medication[50]
Tylenol Cold Medication, Non-Drowsy[108]

Note: For quick reference the following cough/cold combinations are numbered to match the preceding corresponding brand names.

**Antihistamine and antitussive combinations—**
1. Bromodiphenhydramine (broe-moe-dye-fen-HYE-dra-meen) and Codeine (KOE-deen)
2. No product available
3. Chlorpheniramine (klor-fen-EER-a-meen) and Dextromethorphan (dex-troe-meth-OR-fan)
3a. Chlorpheniramine and Hydrocodone (hye-droe-KOE-done)
4. Phenyltoloxamine (fen-ill-tole-OX-a-meen) and Hydrocodone
5. Promethazine (proe-METH-a-zeen) and Codeine†
6. Promethazine and Dextromethorphan
7. Pyrilamine and Codeine

**Antihistamine, antitussive, and analgesic combinations—**
8. Chlorpheniramine, Dextromethorphan (dex-troe-meth-OR-fan), and Acetaminophen (a-seat-a-MIN-oh-fen)

**Antihistamine, antitussive, and expectorant combinations—**
9. Bromodiphenhydramine (broe-moe-dye-fen-HYE-dra-meen), Diphenhydramine (dye-fen-HYE-dra-meen), Codeine (KOE-deen), Ammonium Chloride (a-MOE-nee-um KLOR-ide), and Potassium Guaiacolsulfonate (poe-TAS-ee-um gwye-a-kol-SUL-fon-ate)
10. No product available
11. Diphenhydramine, Codeine, and Ammonium Chloride
12. No product available
13. Phenindamine (fen-IN-da-meen), Hydrocodone (hye-droe-KOE-done), and Guaifenesin

14. Pheniramine (fen-EER-a-meen), Codeine, and Guaifenesin
15. Pheniramine, Pyrilamine (peer-ILL-a-meen), Hydrocodone, Potassium Citrate (poe-TAS-ee-um SI-trate), and Ascorbic Acid
16. No product available

**Antihistamine, decongestant, and antitussive combinations—**
17. No product available
18. Brompheniramine, Phenylephrine, Phenylpropanolamine, and Dextromethorphan (dex-troe-meth-OR-fan)
19. Brompheniramine, Phenylpropanolamine, and Codeine
19a. Brompheniramine, Phenylpropanolamine, and Dextromethorphan
19b. Brompheniramine, Pseudoephedrine (soo-doe-e-FED-rin), and Dextromethorphan
20. Carbinoxamine (kar-bi-NOX-a-meen), Pseudoephedrine, and Dextromethorphan
21. Chlorpheniramine (klor-fen-EER-a-meen), Ephedrine (e-FED-rin), Phenylephrine, and Carbetapentane (kar-bay-ta-PEN-tane)
22. Chlorpheniramine, Phenylephrine, and Dextromethorphan
23. Chlorpheniramine, Phenylephrine, and Hydrocodone (hye-droe-KOE-done)
24. Chlorpheniramine, Phenylephrine, Phenylpropanolamine, and Codeine
25. Chlorpheniramine, Phenylephrine, Phenylpropanolamine, and Dextromethorphan
26. Chlorpheniramine, Phenylephrine, Phenylpropanolamine, and Dihydrocodeine (dye-hye-droe-KOE-deen)
26a. Chlorpheniramine, Phenylpropanolamine, and Caramiphen (kar-AM-i-fen)
27. Chlorpheniramine, Phenylpropanolamine, and Dextromethorphan
28. Chlorpheniramine, Pseudoephedrine, and Codeine
29. Chlorpheniramine, Pseudoephedrine, and Dextromethorphan
30. Chlorpheniramine, Pseudoephedrine, and Hydrocodone
31. No product available
32. Diphenylpyraline, Phenylephrine, and Dextromethorphan
33. Diphenylpyraline, Phenylephrine, and Hydrocodone
34. Pheniramine (fen-EER-a-meen), Pyrilamine (peer-ILL-a-meen), Phenylephrine, Phenylpropanolamine, and Hydrocodone
34a. Pheniramine, Pyrilamine, Phenylpropanolamine, and Codeine
35. Pheniramine, Pyrilamine, Phenylpropanolamine, and Dextromethorphan
36. Pheniramine, Pyrilamine, Phenylpropanolamine, and Hydrocodone
37. Promethazine (proe-METH-a-zeen), Phenylephrine, and Codeine
38. Pyrilamine, Phenylephrine, and Codeine
39. Pyrilamine, Phenylephrine, and Dextromethorphan
40. Pyrilamine, Phenylephrine, and Hydrocodone
41. Triprolidine (trye-PROE-li-deen), Pseudoephedrine, and Codeine
42. Triprolidine, Pseudoephedrine, and Dextromethorphan

**Antihistamine, decongestant, antitussive, and analgesic combinations—**
42a. Brompheniramine (brome-fen-EER-a-meen), Phenylpropanolamine (fen-ill-proe-pa-NOLE-a-meen), Dextromethorphan (dex-troe-meth-OR-fan), and Aspirin
43. Chlorpheniramine (klor-fen-EER-a-meen), Phenindamine (fen-IN-da-meen), Phenylephrine (fen-ill-EF-rin), Dextromethorphan, Acetaminophen (a-seat-a-MIN-oh-fen), Salicylamide (sal-i-SILL-a-mide), Caffeine (kaf-EEN), and Ascorbic (a-SKOR-bik) Acid
44. Chlorpheniramine, Pheniramine (fen-EER-a-meen), Pyrilamine (peer-ILL-a-meen), Phenylephrine, Hydrocodone (hye-droe-KOE-done), Salicylamide, Caffeine, and Ascorbic Acid
45. No product available
46. Chlorpheniramine, Phenylephrine, Dextromethorphan, Acetaminophen, and Salicylamide
47. Chlorpheniramine, Phenylephrine, Hydrocodone (hye-droe-KOE-done), Acetaminophen, and Caffeine
48. Chlorpheniramine, Phenylpropanolamine (fen-ill-proe-pa-NOLE-a-meen), Dextromethorphan, and Acetaminophen
49. Chlorpheniramine, Phenylpropanolamine, Dextromethorphan, and Aspirin
50. Chlorpheniramine, Pseudoephedrine (soo-doe-e-FED-rin), Dextromethorphan, and Acetaminophen
50a. Chlorpheniramine, Pseudoephedrine, Dextromethorphan, Acetaminophen, and Caffeine
50b. Diphenhydramine (dye-fen-HYE-dra-meen), Pseudoephedrine, Dextromethorphan, and Acetaminophen
51. Doxylamine (dox-ILL-a-meen), Pseudoephedrine, Dextromethorphan, and Acetaminophen
52. Pheniramine, Pyrilamine, Phenylpropanolamine, Codeine, Acetaminophen, and Caffeine
53. Pyrilamine, Phenylephrine, Dextromethorphan, and Acetaminophen
54. Pyrilamine, Phenylpropanolamine, Dextromethorphan, and Sodium Salicylate (sa-LI-si-late)
54a. Pyrilamine, Pseudoephedrine, Dextromethorphan, and Acetaminophen
54b. Triprolidine, Pseudoephedrine, Dextromethorphan, and Acetaminophen

**Antihistamine, decongestant, antitussive, and expectorant combinations—**
55. Brompheniramine (brome-fen-EER-a-meen), Phenylephrine (fen-ill-EF-rin), Phenylpropanolamine (fen-ill-proe-pa-NOLE-a-meen), Codeine (KOE-deen), and Guaifenesin (gwye-FEN-e-sin)
56. Brompheniramine, Phenylephrine, Phenylpropanolamine, Hydrocodone (hye-droe-KOE-done), and Guaifenesin
57. Chlorpheniramine, Ephedrine, Phenylephrine, Dextromethorphan (dex-troe-meth-OR-fan), Ammonium Chloride, and Ipecac (IP-e-kak)
58. No product available
59. No product available
60. Chlorpheniramine, Phenylephrine, Codeine and Ammonium Chloride
61. Chlorpheniramine, Phenylephrine, Codeine, and Potassium Iodide (EYE-oh-dyed)
62. Chlorpheniramine, Phenylephrine, Dextromethorphan, and Guaifenesin
63. Chlorpheniramine, Phenylephrine, Dextromethorphan, Guaifenesin, and Ammonium Chloride

64. Chlorpheniramine, Phenylephrine, Phenylpropanolamine, Carbetapentane (kar-bay-ta-PEN-tane), and Potassium (poe-TAS-see-um) Guaiacolsulfonate (gwye-a-kol-SUL-fon-ate)
65. Chlorpheniramine, Phenylpropanolamine, Dextromethorphan, and Ammonium Chloride
66. No product available
67. Chlorpheniramine, Phenyltoloxamine (fen-ill-tole-OX-a-meen), Ephedrine, Codeine, and Guaiacol Carbonate (GYWE-a-kole KAR-bone-ate)
68. Diphenylpyraline (dye-fen-il-PEER-a-leen), Phenylephrine, Hydrocodone, and Guaifenesin
69. Pheniramine (fen-EER-a-meen), Pyrilamine, Phenylpropanolamine, Dextromethorphan, and Ammonium Chloride
70. Pheniramine, Pyrilamine, Phenylpropanolamine, Dextromethorphan, and Guaifenesin
71. Pheniramine, Pyrilamine, Phenylpropanolamine, Hydrocodone, and Guaifenesin
71a. Pheniramine, Phenylephrine, Phenylpropanolamine, Hydrocodone, and Guaifenesin
72. Pyrilamine, Phenylephrine, Hydrocodone, and Ammonium Chloride
72a. Pyrilamine, Phenylpropanolamine, Dextromethorphan, Guaifenesin, Potassium Citrate, and Citric Acid
73. Triprolidine (trye-PROE-li-deen), Pseudoephedrine (soo-doe-e-FED-rin), Codeine, and Guaifenesin

**Antihistamine, decongestant, antitussive, expectorant, and analgesic combinations—**

74. Chlorpheniramine (klor-fen-EER-a-meen), Phenylephrine (fen-ill-EF-rin), Phenylpropanolamine (fen-ill-proe-pa-NOLE-a-meen), Dextromethorphan (dex-troe-meth-OR-fan), Guaifenesin (gwye-FEN-e-sin), and Acetaminophen (a-seat-a-MIN-oh-fen)
75. Chlorpheniramine, Phenylpropanolamine, Codeine (KOE-deen), Guaifenesin, and Acetaminophen
76. No product available
77. No product available
78. Pheniramine (fen-EER-a-meen), Phenylephrine, Codeine, Sodium Citrate (SOE-dee-um SI-trate), Sodium Salicylate (sa-LI-sill-ate), and Caffeine (kaf-EEN)
79. No product available

**Antihistamine, decongestant, and expectorant combinations—**

80. Brompheniramine (brome-fen-EER-a-meen), Phenylephrine (fen-ill-EF-rin), Phenylpropanolamine (fen-ill-proe-pa-NOLE-a-meen), and Guaifenesin (gwye-FEN-e-sin)
81. Carbinoxamine (kar-bi-NOX-a-meen), Pseudoephedrine (soo-doe-e-FED-rin), and Guaifenesin
82. Chlorpheniramine (klor-fen-EER-a-meen), Ephedrine (e-FED-rin), and Guaifenesin
83. Chlorpheniramine, Phenylephrine, and Guaifenesin
84. Chlorpheniramine, Phenylpropanolamine, and Guaifenesin
85. Chlorpheniramine, Phenylpropanolamine, Guaifenesin, Sodium Citrate (SOE-dee-um SI-trate), and Citric (SI-trik) Acid
86. Chlorpheniramine, Pseudoephedrine, and Guaifenesin
87. Dexchlorpheniramine (dex-klor-fen-EER-a-meen), Pseudoephedrine, and Guaifenesin
88. Pheniramine (fen-EER-a-meen), Pyrilamine (peer-ILL-a-meen), Phenylpropanolamine, and Guaifenesin

**Antitussive and analgesic combination—**

88a. Dextromethorphan (dex-troe-meth-OR-fan) and Acetaminophen (a-seat-a-MIN-oh-fen)

**Antitussive and anticholinergic combination—**

89. Hydrocodone (hye-droe-KOE-done) and Homatropine (hoe-MA-troe-peen)†

**Antitussive and expectorant combinations—**

90. Codeine (KOE-deen) and Calcium Iodide (KAL-see-um EYE-oh-dyed)
91. Codeine and Guaifenesin (gwye-FEN-e-sin)
92. Codeine and Iodinated Glycerol (EYE-oh-di-nay-ted GLI-ser-ole)
93. No product available
94. Dextromethorphan and Guaifenesin
95. Dextromethorphan and Iodinated Glycerol
96. No product available
97. Hydrocodone (hye-droe-KOE-done) and Guaifenesin
98. Hydrocodone and Potassium Guaiacolsulfonate
99. Hydromorphone (hye-droe-MOR-fone) and Guaifenesin

**Decongestant and antitussive combinations—**

100. Phenylephrine (fen-ill-EF-rin) and Codeine (KOE-deen)
100a. Phenylephrine and Hydrocodone (hye-droe-KOE-done)
101. Phenylpropanolamine (fen-ill-proe-pa-NOLE-a-meen) and Caramiphen (kar-AM-i-fen)
102. Phenylpropanolamine and Dextromethorphan
103. Phenylpropanolamine and Hydrocodone (hye-droe-KOE-done)
104. Pseudoephedrine (soo-doe-e-FED-rin) and Codeine
105. Pseudoephedrine and Dextromethorphan
106. Pseudoephedrine and Hydrocodone

**Decongestant, antitussive, and analgesic combinations—**

107. Phenylpropanolamine (fen-ill-proe-pa-NOLE-a-meen), Dextromethorphan (dex-troe-meth-OR-fan), and Acetaminophen (a-seat-a-MIN-oh-fen)
108. Pseudoephedrine (soo-doe-e-FED-rin), Dextromethorphan, and Acetaminophen

**Decongestant, antitussive, and expectorant combinations—**

109. Phenylephrine (fen-ill-EF-rin), Dextromethorphan (dex-troe-meth-OR-fan), and Guaifenesin (gwye-FEN-e-sin)
109a. Phenylephrine, Phenylpropanolamine, Carbetapentane (kar-bay-ta-PEN-tane), and Potassium Guaiacolsulfonate (poe-TAS-see-um gwye-a-kol-SUL-fon-ate)
110. Phenylephrine, Hydrocodone (hye-droe-KOE-done), and Guaifenesin
111. Phenylpropanolamine (fen-ill-proe-pa-NOLE-a-meen), Codeine (KOE-deen), and Guaifenesin
112. Phenylpropanolamine, Dextromethorphan, and Guaifenesin
113. Pseudoephedrine (soo-doe-e-FED-rin), Codeine, and Guaifenesin
114. Pseudoephedrine, Dextromethorphan, and Guaifenesin
115. Pseudoephedrine, Hydrocodone, and Guaifenesin

**Decongestant, antitussive, expectorant, and analgesic combinations—**

116. Phenylpropanolamine (fen-ill-proe-pa-NOLE-a-meen), Hydrocodone (hye-droe-KOE-done), Guaifenesin (gwye-FEN-e-sin), and Salicylamide (sal-i-SILL-a-mide)

117. Pseudoephedrine (soo-doe-e-FED-rin), Dextromethorphan, Guaifenesin, and Acetaminophen

**Decongestant and expectorant combinations—**
118. Ephedrine (e-FED-rin) and Guaifenesin (gwye-FEN-e-sin)
119. Ephedrine and Potassium Iodide (poe-TAS-ee-um EYE-oh-dyed)
120. Phenylephrine (fen-ill-EF-rin), Phenylpropanolamine (fen-ill-proe-pa-NOLE-a-meen), and Guaifenesin
120a. Phenylephrine and Guaifenesin
121. Phenylpropanolamine and Guaifenesin
122. Pseudoephedrine (soo-doe-e-FED-rin) and Guaifenesin

**Decongestant, expectorant, and analgesic combination—**
123. Phenylephrine (fen-ill-EF-rin), Guaifenesin (gwye-FEN-e-sin), Acetaminophen (a-seat-a-MIN-oh-fen), Salicylamide and Caffeine

†Generic name product available in the U.S.

# Description

Cough/cold combinations are used mainly to relieve the cough due to colds, influenza, or hay fever. They are not to be used for the chronic cough that occurs with smoking, asthma, or emphysema or when there is an unusually large amount of mucus or phlegm (pronounced flem) with the cough.

Cough/cold combination products contain more than one ingredient. For example, some products may contain an antihistamine, a decongestant, and an analgesic, in addition to a medicine for coughing. If you are treating yourself, it is important to select a product that is best for your symptoms. Also, in general, it is best to buy a product that includes only those medicines you really need. If you have questions about which product to buy, check with your pharmacist.

Since different products contain ingredients that will have different precautions and side effects, it is important that you know the ingredients of the medicine you are taking. The different kinds of ingredients that may be found in cough/cold combinations include:

**Antihistamines—**Antihistamines are used to relieve or prevent the symptoms of hay fever and other types of allergy. They also help relieve some symptoms of the common cold, such as sneezing and runny nose. They work by preventing the effects of a substance called histamine, which is produced by the body. Some examples of antihistamines contained in these combinations are: chlorpheniramine, diphenhydramine, pheniramine, promethazine, and triprolidine.

**Decongestants—**Decongestants, such as ephedrine, phenylephrine, phenylpropanolamine (also known as PPA), and pseudoephedrine, produce a narrowing of blood vessels. This leads to clearing of nasal congestion. However, this effect may also increase blood pressure in patients who have high blood pressure.

**Antitussives—**To help relieve coughing these combinations contain either a narcotic (codeine, dihydrocodeine,

hydrocodone or hydromorphone) or a non-narcotic (carbetapentane, dextromethorphan, or noscapine) antitussive. These antitussives act directly on the cough center in the brain. Narcotics may become habit-forming, causing mental or physical dependence, if used for a long time. Physical dependence may lead to withdrawal side effects when you stop taking the medicine.

**Expectorants—**Guaifenesin works by loosening the mucus or phlegm in the lungs. Other ingredients added as expectorants (for example, ammonium chloride, calcium iodide, iodinated glycerol, ipecac, potassium guaiacolsulfonate, potassium iodide, and sodium citrate) have not been proven to be effective. In general, the best thing you can do to loosen mucus or phlegm is to drink plenty of water.

**Analgesics—**Analgesics, such as acetaminophen, aspirin, and other salicylates (such as salicylamide and sodium salicylate), are used in these combination medicines to help relieve the aches and pain that may occur with the common cold.

The use of too much acetaminophen and salicylates at the same time may cause kidney damage or cancer of the kidney or urinary bladder. This may occur if large amounts of both medicines are taken together for a long time. However, taking the recommended amounts of combination medicines that contain both acetaminophen and a salicylate for short periods of time has not been shown to cause these unwanted effects.

**Anticholinergics—**Anticholinergics such as homatropine may help produce a drying effect in the nose and chest.

Some of these combinations are available only with your doctor's prescription. Others are available without a prescription; however, your doctor or pharmacist may have special instructions on the proper dose of the medicine for your medical condition.

Cough/cold combinations are available in the following dosage forms:

**Antihistamine and antitussive combinations—**
*Oral*
  Bromodiphenhydramine and Codeine
  • Syrup (U.S.)
  Chlorpheniramine and Dextromethorphan
  • Oral solution (U.S.)
  Chlorpheniramine and Hydrocodone
  • Oral suspension (U.S.)
  Phenyltoloxamine and Hydrocodone
  • Capsules (Canada)
  • Oral suspension (U.S. and Canada)
  Promethazine and Codeine
  • Syrup (U.S.)
  Promethazine and Dextromethorphan
  • Syrup (U.S.)
  Pyrilamine and Codeine
  • Oral solution (U.S.)

**Antihistamine, antitussive, and analgesic combinations—**
*Oral*
  Chlorpheniramine, Dextromethorphan, and Acetaminophen
  • Capsules (U.S.)

**Antihistamine, antitussive, and expectorant combinations—**
*Oral*

Bromodiphenhydramine, Diphenhydramine, Codeine, Ammonium Chloride, and Potassium Guaiacolsulfonate
- Oral solution (U.S.)

Diphenhydramine, Codeine, and Ammonium Chloride
- Syrup (Canada)

Phenindamine, Hydrocodone, and Guaifenesin
- Tablets (U.S.)

Pheniramine, Codeine, and Guaifenesin
- Syrup (Canada)

Pheniramine, Pyrilamine, Hydrocodone, and Potassium Citrate
- Syrup (U.S.)

**Antihistamine, decongestant, and antitussive combinations—**
*Oral*

Brompheniramine, Phenylephrine, Phenylpropanolamine, and Dextromethorphan
- Elixir (Canada)
- Tablets (Canada)

Brompheniramine, Phenylpropanolamine, and Codeine
- Syrup (U.S.)

Brompheniramine, Phenylpropanolamine, and Dextromethorphan
- Syrup (U.S.)

Brompheniramine, Pseudoephedrine, and Dextromethorphan
- Syrup (U.S.)

Carbinoxamine, Pseudoephedrine, and Dextromethorphan
- Oral solution (U.S.)
- Syrup (U.S.)

Chlorpheniramine, Ephedrine, Phenylephrine, and Carbetapentane
- Oral suspension (U.S.)
- Tablets (U.S.)

Chlorpheniramine, Phenylephrine, and Dextromethorphan
- Oral solution (U.S.)
- Tablets (U.S.)

Chlorpheniramine, Phenylephrine, and Hydrocodone
- Syrup (U.S.)

Chlorpheniramine, Phenylephrine, Phenylpropanolamine, and Codeine
- Syrup (U.S.)

Chlorpheniramine, Phenylephrine, Phenylpropanolamine, and Dextromethorphan
- Syrup (U.S.)

Chlorpheniramine, Phenylephrine, Phenylpropanolamine, and Dihydrocodeine
- Syrup (U.S.)

Chlorpheniramine, Phenylpropanolamine, and Caramiphen
- Extended-release capsules (Canada)

Chlorpheniramine, Phenylpropanolamine, and Dextromethorphan
- Granules (U.S.)
- Oral gel (U.S.)
- Oral solution (U.S. and Canada)
- Syrup (U.S.)
- Tablets (U.S.)

Chlorpheniramine, Pseudoephedrine, and Codeine
- Elixir (U.S.)
- Oral solution (U.S.)
- Syrup (U.S.)

Chlorpheniramine, Pseudoephedrine, and Dextromethorphan
- Oral solution (U.S.)
- Syrup (U.S.)

Chlorpheniramine, Pseudoephedrine, and Hydrocodone
- Oral solution (U.S.)

Diphenylpyraline, Phenylephrine, and Dextromethorphan
- Syrup (Canada)

Diphenylpyraline, Phenylephrine, and Hydrocodone
- Oral solution (Canada)
- Syrup (Canada)

Pheniramine, Pyrilamine, Phenylephrine, Phenylpropanolamine, and Hydrocodone
- Oral solution (U.S.)

Pheniramine, Pyrilamine, Phenylpropanolamine, and Codeine
- Syrup (Canada)

Pheniramine, Pyrilamine, Phenylpropanolamine, and Dextromethorphan
- Syrup (Canada)

Pheniramine, Pyrilamine, Phenylpropanolamine, and Hydrocodone
- Oral solution (Canada)

Promethazine, Phenylephrine, and Codeine
- Syrup (U.S.)

Pyrilamine, Phenylephrine, and Codeine
- Syrup (U.S.)

Pyrilamine, Phenylephrine, and Dextromethorphan
- Oral solution (U.S.)

Pyrilamine, Phenylephrine, and Hydrocodone
- Syrup (U.S.)

Triprolidine, Pseudoephedrine, and Codeine
- Syrup (U.S. and Canada)
- Tablets (Canada)

Triprolidine, Pseudoephedrine, and Dextromethorphan
- Oral solution (Canada)

**Antihistamine, decongestant, antitussive, and analgesic combinations—**
*Oral*

Brompheniramine, Phenylpropanolamine, Dextromethorphan, and Aspirin
- Tablets (U.S.)

Chlorpheniramine, Phenindamine, Phenylephrine, Dextromethorphan, Acetaminophen, Salicylamide, Caffeine, and Ascorbic Acid
- Tablets (U.S.)

Chlorpheniramine, Pheniramine, Pyrilamine, Phenylephrine, Hydrocodone, Salicylamide, Caffeine, and Ascorbic Acid
- Capsules (U.S.)

Chlorpheniramine, Phenylephrine, Dextromethorphan, Acetaminophen, and Salicylamide
- Tablets (U.S.)

Chlorpheniramine, Phenylephrine, Hydrocodone, Acetaminophen, and Caffeine
- Tablets (U.S.)

Chlorpheniramine, Phenylpropanolamine, Dextromethorphan, and Acetaminophen
- Capsules (U.S.)
- Oral solution (U.S.)
- Tablets (U.S.)

Chlorpheniramine, Phenylpropanolamine, Dextromethorphan, and Aspirin
- Tablets (U.S.)

Chlorpheniramine, Pseudoephedrine, Dextromethorphan, and Acetaminophen
- Capsules (U.S.)
- Oral solution (U.S.)
- Tablets (U.S./Canada)

Chlorpheniramine, Pseudoephedrine, Dextromethorphan, Acetaminophen, and Caffeine
- Tablets (U.S.)

Diphenhydramine, Pseudoephedrine, Dextromethorphan, and Acetaminophen
- Capsules (U.S.)
- Oral solution (U.S.)

Doxylamine, Pseudoephedrine, Dextromethorphan, and Acetaminophen
- Oral solution (U.S.)

Pheniramine, Pyrilamine, Phenylpropanolamine, Codeine, Acetaminophen, and Caffeine
- Tablets (Canada)

Pyrilamine, Phenylephrine, Dextromethorphan, and Acetaminophen
- Oral solution (U.S.)

Pyrilamine, Phenylpropanolamine, Dextromethorphan, and Sodium Salicylate
- Oral solution (U.S.)

Pyrilamine, Pseudoephedrine, Dextromethorphan, and Acetaminophen
- Oral solution (U.S.)

Triprolidine, Psuedoephedrine, Dextromethorphan, and Acetaminophen
- Tablets (U.S.)

**Antihistamine, decongestant, antitussive, and expectorant combinations—**
*Oral*

Brompheniramine, Phenylephrine, Phenylpropanolamine, Codeine, and Guaifenesin
- Syrup (Canada)

Brompheniramine, Phenylephrine, Phenylpropanolamine, Hydrocodone, and Guaifenesin
- Oral solution (Canada)

Chlorpheniramine, Ephedrine, Phenylephrine, Dextromethorphan, Ammonium Chloride, and Ipecac
- Syrup (U.S.)

Chlorpheniramine, Phenylephrine, Codeine, and Ammonium Chloride
- Oral solution (U.S.)

Chlorpheniramine, Phenylephrine, Codeine, and Potassium Iodide
- Syrup (U.S.)

Chlorpheniramine, Phenylephrine, Dextromethorphan, and Guaifenesin
- Syrup (U.S.)

Chlorpheniramine, Phenylephrine, Dextromethorphan, Guaifenesin, and Ammonium Chloride
- Oral solution (U.S.)

Chlorpheniramine, Phenylephrine, Phenylpropanolamine, Carbetapentane, and Potassium Guaiacolsulfonate
- Capsules (U.S.)
- Syrup (U.S.)

Chlorpheniramine, Phenylpropanolamine, Dextromethorphan, and Ammonium Chloride
- Syrup (U.S.)

Chlorpheniramine, Phenyltoloxamine, Ephedrine, Codeine, and Guaiacol Carbonate
- Oral suspension (Canada)

Diphenylpyraline, Phenylephrine, Hydrocodone, and Guaifenesin
- Oral solution (Canada)

Pheniramine, Pyrilamine, Phenylpropanolamine, Dextromethorphan, and Ammonium Chloride
- Syrup (U.S.)

Pheniramine, Pyrilamine, Phenylpropanolamine, Dextromethorphan, and Guaifenesin
- Oral solution (Canada)

Pheniramine, Pyrilamine, Phenylpropanolamine, Hydrocodone, and Guaifenesin
- Oral solution (U.S.)

Pheniramine, Phenylephrine, Phenylpropanolamine, Hydrocodone, and Guaifenesin
- Oral solution (U.S.)

Pyrilamine, Phenylephrine, Hydrocodone, and Ammonium Chloride
- Syrup (Canada)

Pyrilamine, Phenylpropanolamine, Dextromethorphan, Guaifenesin, Potassium Citrate, and Citric Acid
- Syrup (U.S.)

Triprolidine, Pseudoephedrine, Codeine, and Guaifenesin
- Oral solution (Canada)

**Antihistamine, decongestant, antitussive, expectorant, and analgesic combinations—**
*Oral*

Chlorpheniramine, Phenylephrine, Phenylpropanolamine, Dextromethorphan, Guaifenesin, and Acetaminophen
- Syrup (U.S.)
- Tablets (U.S.)

Chlorpheniramine, Phenylpropanolamine, Codeine, Guaifenesin, and Acetaminophen
- Syrup (U.S.)
- Tablets (U.S.)

Pheniramine, Phenylephrine, Codeine, Sodium Citrate, Sodium Salicylate, and Caffeine
- Syrup (U.S.)

**Antihistamine, decongestant, and expectorant combinations—**
*Oral*

Brompheniramine, Phenylephrine, Phenylpropanolamine, and Guaifenesin
- Syrup (Canada)

Carbinoxamine, Pseudoephedrine, and Guaifenesin
- Capsules (U.S.)
- Oral solution (U.S.)

Chlorpheniramine, Ephedrine, and Guaifenesin
- Oral solution (U.S.)

Chlorpheniramine, Phenylephrine, and Guaifenesin
- Oral solution (U.S.)

Chlorpheniramine, Phenylpropanolamine, and Guaifenesin
- Oral solution (Canada)

Chlorpheniramine, Phenylpropanolamine, Guaifenesin, Sodium Citrate, and Citric Acid
- Oral solution (U.S.)

Chlorpheniramine, Pseudoephedrine, and Guaifenesin
- Extended-release tablets (U.S.)

Dexchlorpheniramine, Pseudoephedrine, and Guaifenesin
- Oral solution (U.S.)

Pheniramine, Pyrilamine, Phenylpropanolamine, and Guaifenesin
- Oral solution (Canada)

## Antitussive and anticholinergic combination—
*Oral*

Hydrocodone and Homatropine
- Syrup (U.S.)
- Tablets (U.S.)

## Antitussive and expectorant combinations—
*Oral*

Codeine and Calcium Iodide
- Syrup (U.S.)
Codeine and Guaifenesin
- Oral solution (U.S.)
- Syrup (U.S.)
Codeine and Iodinated Glycerol
- Oral solution (U.S.)
Dextromethorphan and Guaifenesin
- Capsules (U.S.)
- Extended-release capsules (U.S.)
- Oral gel (U.S.)
- Lozenges (U.S.)
- Oral solution (U.S.)
- Syrup (U.S.)
- Tablets (U.S.)
- Extended-release tablets (U.S.)
Dextromethorphan and Iodinated Glycerol
- Oral solution (U.S.)
Hydrocodone and Guaifenesin
- Oral solution (U.S.)
- Syrup (U.S.)
- Tablets (U.S.)
Hydrocodone and Potassium Guaiacolsulfonate
- Syrup (U.S.)
Hydromorphone and Guaifenesin
- Syrup (U.S.)

## Decongestant and antitussive combinations—
*Oral*

Phenylephrine and Codeine
- Oral solution (Canada)
Phenylephrine and Hydrocodone
- Oral solution (Canada)
Phenylpropanolamine and Caramiphen
- Extended-release capsules (U.S.)
- Oral solution (U.S.)
Phenylpropanolamine and Dextromethorphan
- Oral gel (U.S.)
- Granules (U.S.)
- Lozenges (U.S.)
- Oral solution (U.S.)
- Syrup (U.S.)
Phenylpropanolamine and Hydrocodone
- Oral solution (U.S.)
- Syrup (U.S.)
Pseudoephedrine and Codeine
- Capsules (U.S.)
- Syrup (U.S.)
Pseudoephedrine and Dextromethorphan
- Oral solution (Canada)
- Chewable tablets (U.S.)
Pseudoephedrine and Hydrocodone
- Oral solution (U.S.)
- Syrup (U.S.)

## Decongestant, antitussive, and analgesic combinations—
*Oral*

Phenylpropanolamine, Dextromethorphan, and Acetaminophen
- Oral solution (U.S.)
- Tablets (U.S.)
Pseudoephedrine, Dextromethorphan, and Acetaminophen
- Oral solution (U.S.)
- Tablets (U.S./Canada)

## Decongestant, antitussive, and expectorant combinations—
*Oral*

Phenylephrine, Dextromethorphan, and Guaifenesin
- Syrup (U.S.)
Phenylephrine, Phenylpropanolamine, Carbetapentane and Potassium Guaiacolsulfonate
- Capsules (U.S.)
Phenylephrine, Hydrocodone, and Guaifenesin
- Syrup (U.S.)
Phenylpropanolamine, Codeine, and Guaifenesin
- Oral solution (U.S.)
- Oral suspension (U.S.)
- Syrup (U.S.)
Phenylpropanolamine, Dextromethorphan, and Guaifenesin
- Oral solution (U.S.)
- Syrup (U.S.)
Pseudoephedrine, Codeine, and Guaifenesin
- Oral solution (U.S.)
- Syrup (U.S.)
Pseudoephedrine, Dextromethorphan, and Guaifenesin
- Capsules (U.S.)
- Oral solution (U.S.)
- Syrup (U.S.)
Pseudoephedrine, Hydrocodone, and Guaifenesin
- Oral solution (U.S.)
- Tablets (U.S.)

## Decongestant, antitussive, expectorant, and analgesic combinations—
*Oral*

Phenylpropanolamine, Hydrocodone, Guaifenesin, and Salicylamide
- Tablets (U.S.)
Pseudoephedrine, Dextromethorphan, Guaifenesin, and Acetaminophen
- Oral solution (U.S.)
- Tablets (U.S.)

## Decongestant and expectorant combinations—
*Oral*

Ephedrine and Guaifenesin
- Capsules (U.S.)
- Syrup (U.S.)
Ephedrine and Potassium Iodide
- Syrup (U.S.)
Phenylephrine, Phenylpropanolamine, and Guaifenesin
- Capsules (U.S.)
- Oral solution (U.S.)
- Tablets (U.S.)
Phenylephrine and Guaifenesin
- Extended-release capsules (U.S.)

Phenylpropanolamine and Guaifenesin
• Oral solution (U.S.)
• Syrup (U.S.)
• Extended-release tablets (U.S. and Canada)
Pseudoephedrine and Guaifenesin
• Extended-release capsules (U.S.)
• Oral solution (U.S.)
• Syrup (U.S.)
• Tablets (U.S.)
• Extended-release tablets (U.S.)

**Decongestant, expectorant, and analgesic combination—**
*Oral*

Phenylephrine, Guaifenesin, Acetaminophen, Salicylamide and Caffeine
• Tablets (U.S.)

## Before Using This Medicine

If you are taking this medicine without a prescription, carefully read and follow any precautions on the label. For cough/cold combinations, the following should be considered:

**Allergies**—Tell your doctor if you have ever had any unusual or allergic reaction to any of the ingredients contained in this medicine. Also tell your health care professional if you are allergic to any other substances, such as foods, preservatives, or dyes. In addition, if this medicine contains *aspirin or other salicylates*, before taking it, check with your doctor if you have ever had any unusual or allergic reaction to any of the following medicines:

Aspirin or other salicylates
Diclofenac (e.g., Voltaren)
Diflunisal (e.g., Dolobid)
Fenoprofen (e.g., Nalfon)
Floctafenine
Flurbiprofen, by mouth (e.g., Ansaid)
Ibuprofen (e.g., Motrin)
Indomethacin (e.g., Indocin)
Ketoprofen (e.g., Orudis)
Ketorolac (e.g., Toradol)
Meclofenamate (e.g., Meclomen)
Mefenamic acid (e.g., Ponstel)
Methyl salicylate (oil of wintergreen)
Naproxen (e.g., Naprosyn)
Oxyphenbutazone (e.g., Tandearil)
Phenylbutazone (e.g., Butazolidin)
Piroxicam (e.g., Feldene)
Sulindac (e.g., Clinoril)
Suprofen (e.g., Suprol)
Tiaprofenic acid (e.g., Surgam)
Tolmetin (e.g., Tolectin)
Zomepirac (e.g., Zomax)

**Diet**—Make certain your health care professional knows if you are on any special diet, such as a low-sodium or low-sugar diet.

**Pregnancy**—The occasional use of a cough/cold combination is not likely to cause problems in the fetus or in the newborn baby. However, when these medicines are used at higher doses and/or for a long time, the chance that problems might occur may increase. For the individual ingredients of these combinations, the following information should be considered before you decide to use a particular cough/cold combination:

• *Acetaminophen*—Studies on birth defects have not been done in humans. However, acetaminophen has not been shown to cause birth defects or other problems in humans.
• *Alcohol*—Some of these combination medicines contain a large amount of alcohol. Too much use of alcohol during pregnancy may cause birth defects.
• *Antihistamines*—Antihistamines have not been shown to cause problems in humans.
• *Caffeine*—Studies in humans have not shown that caffeine causes birth defects. However, studies in animals have shown that caffeine causes birth defects when given in very large doses (amounts equal to the amount of caffeine contained in 12 to 24 cups of coffee a day).
• *Codeine*—Although studies on birth defects with codeine have not been done in humans, it has not been reported to cause birth defects in humans. Codeine has not been shown to cause birth defects in animal studies, but it caused other unwanted effects. Also, regular use of narcotics during pregnancy may cause the baby to become dependent on the medicine. This may lead to withdrawal side effects after birth. In addition, narcotics may cause breathing problems in the newborn baby if taken by the mother just before delivery.
• *Hydrocodone*—Although studies on birth defects with hydrocodone have not been done in humans, it has not been reported to cause birth defects in humans. However, hydrocodone has been shown to cause birth defects in animals when given in very large doses. Also, regular use of narcotics during pregnancy may cause the baby to become dependent on the medicine. This may lead to withdrawal side effects after birth. In addition, narcotics may cause breathing problems in the newborn baby if taken by the mother just before delivery.
• *Iodides (e.g., calcium iodide and iodinated glycerol)*—Not recommended during pregnancy. Iodides have caused enlargement of the thyroid gland in the fetus and resulted in breathing problems in newborn babies whose mothers took iodides in large doses for a long period of time.
• *Phenylephrine*—Studies on birth defects with phenylephrine have not been done in either humans or animals.
• *Phenylpropanolamine*—Studies on birth defects with phenylpropanolamine have not been done in either humans or animals. However, it seems that women who take phenylpropanolamine in the weeks following delivery are more likely to suffer mental or mood changes.
• *Pseudoephedrine*—Studies on birth defects with pseudoephedrine have not been done in humans. In animal studies pseudoephedrine did not cause birth defects but did cause a decrease in average weight,

length, and rate of bone formation in the animal fetus when given in high doses.

- *Salicylates (e.g., aspirin)*—Studies on birth defects in humans have been done with aspirin, but not with salicylamide or sodium salicylate. Salicylates have not been shown to cause birth defects in humans. However, salicylates have been shown to cause birth defects in animals.

Some reports have suggested that too much use of aspirin late in pregnancy may cause a decrease in the newborn's weight and possible death of the fetus or newborn infant. However, the mothers in these reports had been taking much larger amounts of aspirin than are usually recommended. Studies of mothers taking aspirin in the doses that are usually recommended did not show these unwanted effects. However, there is a chance that regular use of salicylates late in pregnancy may cause unwanted effects on the heart or blood flow in the fetus or newborn baby.

Use of salicylates, especially aspirin, during the last 2 weeks of pregnancy may cause bleeding problems in the fetus before or during delivery, or in the newborn baby. Also, too much use of salicylates during the last 3 months of pregnancy may increase the length of pregnancy, prolong labor, cause other problems during delivery, or cause severe bleeding in the mother before, during, or after delivery. *Do not take aspirin during the last 3 months of pregnancy unless it has been ordered by your doctor.*

**Breast-feeding**—If you are breast-feeding, the chance that problems might occur depends on the ingredients of the combination. For the individual ingredients of these combinations, the following apply:

- *Acetaminophen*—Acetaminophen passes into the breast milk. However, it has not been reported to cause problems in nursing babies.
- *Alcohol*—Alcohol passes into the breast milk. However, the amount of alcohol in recommended doses of this medicine does not usually cause problems in nursing babies.
- *Antihistamines*—Small amounts of antihistamines pass into the breast milk. Antihistamine-containing medicine is not recommended for use while breast-feeding since most antihistamines are especially likely to cause side effects, such as unusual excitement or irritability, in the baby. Also, since antihistamines tend to decrease the secretions of the body, the flow of breast milk may be reduced in some patients.
- *Caffeine*—Small amounts of caffeine pass into the breast milk and may build up in the nursing baby. However, the amount of caffeine in recommended doses of this medicine does not usually cause problems in nursing babies.
- *Decongestants (e.g., ephedrine, phenylephrine, phenylpropanolamine, pseudoephedrine)*—Phenylephrine and phenylpropanolamine have not been reported to cause problems in nursing babies. Ephedrine and pseudoephedrine pass into the breast milk

and may cause unwanted effects in nursing babies (especially newborn and premature babies).

- *Iodides (e.g., calcium iodide and iodinated glycerol)*—These medicines pass into the breast milk and may cause unwanted effects, such as underactive thyroid, in the baby.
- *Narcotic antitussives (e.g., codeine, dihydrocodeine, hydrocodone, and hydromorphone)*—Small amounts of codeine have been shown to pass into the breast milk. However, the amount of codeine or other narcotic antitussives in recommended doses of this medicine has not been reported to cause problems in nursing babies.
- *Salicylates (e.g., aspirin)*—Salicylates pass into the breast milk. Although salicylates have not been reported to cause problems in nursing babies, it is possible that problems may occur if large amounts are taken regularly.

**Children**—Very young children are usually more sensitive to the effects of this medicine. *Before giving any of these combination medicines to a child, check the package label very carefully. Some of these medicines are too strong for use in children.* If you are not certain whether a specific product can be given to a child, or if you have any questions about the amount to give, check with your health care professional, especially if it contains:

- *Antihistamines*—Nightmares, unusual excitement, nervousness, restlessness, or irritability may be more likely to occur in children taking antihistamines.
- *Decongestants (e.g., ephedrine, phenylephrine, phenylpropanolamine, pseudoephedrine)*—Increases in blood pressure may be more likely to occur in children taking decongestants. Also, mental changes may be more likely to occur in young children taking phenylpropanolamine-containing combinations.
- *Narcotic antitussives (e.g., codeine, hydrocodeine, hydrocodone, and hydromorphone)*—Breathing problems may be especially likely to occur in children younger than 2 years of age taking narcotic antitussives. Also, unusual excitement or restlessness may be more likely to occur in children receiving these medicines.
- *Salicylates (e.g., aspirin)*—*Do not give medicines containing aspirin or other salicylates to a child with a fever or other symptoms of a virus infection, especially flu or chickenpox, without first discussing its use with your child's doctor.* This is very important because salicylates may cause a serious illness called Reye's syndrome in children with fever caused by a virus infection, especially flu or chickenpox. Also, children may be more sensitive to the aspirin or other salicylates contained in some of these medicines, especially if they have a fever or have lost large amounts of body fluid because of vomiting, diarrhea, or sweating.

**Teenagers**—*Do not give medicines containing aspirin or other salicylates to a teenager with a fever or other symptoms of a virus infection, especially flu or chickenpox,* *without first discussing its use with your child's doctor.* This is very important because salicylates may cause a serious illness called Reye's syndrome in teenagers with fever caused by a virus infection, especially flu or chickenpox.

**Older adults**—The elderly are usually more sensitive to the effects of this medicine, especially if it contains:

- *Antihistamines*—Confusion, difficult or painful urination, dizziness, drowsiness, feeling faint, or dryness of mouth, nose, or throat may be more likely to occur in elderly patients. Also, nightmares or unusual excitement, nervousness, restlessness, or irritability may be more likely to occur in the elderly taking antihistamines.
- *Decongestants (e.g., ephedrine, phenylephrine, phenylpropanolamine, pseudoephedrine)*—Confusion, hallucinations, drowsiness, or convulsions (seizures) may be more likely to occur in the elderly, who are usually more sensitive to the effects of this medicine. Also, increases in blood pressure may be more likely to occur in elderly persons taking decongestants.

**Other medicines**—Although certain medicines should not be used together at all, in other cases two different medicines may be used together even if an interaction might occur. In these cases, your doctor may want to change the dose, or other precautions may be necessary. Tell your health care professional if you are taking *any* other prescription or nonprescription (over-the-counter [OTC]) medicine, for example, aspirin or other medicine for allergies. Some medicines may change the way this medicine affects your body. Also, the effect of other medicines may be increased or reduced by some of the ingredients in this medicine. Check with your health care professional about which medicines you should not take with this medicine.

**Other medical problems**—The presence of other medical problems may affect the use of the cough/cold combination medicine. Make sure you tell your doctor if you have any other medical problems, especially:

- Alcohol abuse (or history of)—Acetaminophen-containing medicines increase the chance of liver damage; also, some of the liquid medicines contain a large amount of alcohol
- Anemia or
- Gout or
- Hemophilia or other bleeding problems or
- Stomach ulcer or other stomach problems—These conditions may become worse if you are taking a combination medicine containing aspirin or another salicylate
- Brain disease or injury or
- Colitis or
- Convulsions (seizures) (history of) or
- Diarrhea or
- Gallbladder disease or gallstones—These conditions may become worse if you are taking a combination medicine containing codeine, dihydrocodeine, hydrocodone, or hydromorphone
- Cystic fibrosis (in children)—Side effects of iodinated glycerol may be more likely in children with cystic fibrosis

- Diabetes mellitus (sugar diabetes)—Decongestants may put diabetic patients at greater risk of having heart or blood vessel disease
- Emphysema, asthma, or chronic lung disease (especially in children)—Salicylate-containing medicine may cause an allergic reaction in which breathing becomes difficult
- Enlarged prostate or
- Urinary tract blockage or difficult urination—Some of the effects of anticholinergics (e.g., homatropine) or antihistamines may make urinary problems worse
- Glaucoma—A slight increase in inner eye pressure may occur with the use of anticholinergics (e.g., homatropine) or antihistamines, which may make the condition worse
- Heart or blood vessel disease or
- High blood pressure—Decongestant-containing medicine may increase the blood pressure and speed up the heart rate; also, caffeine-containing medicine, if taken in large amounts, may speed up the heart rate
- Kidney disease—This condition may increase the chance of side effects of this medicine because the medicine may build up in the body
- Liver disease—Liver disease increases the chance of side effects because the medicine may build up in the body; also, if liver disease is severe, there is a greater chance that aspirin-containing medicine may cause bleeding
- Thyroid disease—If an overactive thyroid has caused a fast heart rate, the decongestant in this medicine may cause the heart rate to speed up further; also, if the medicine contains narcotic antitussives (e.g., codeine), iodides (e.g., iodinated glycerol), or salicylates, the thyroid problem may become worse

## Proper Use of This Medicine

To help loosen mucus or phlegm in the lungs, *drink a glass of water after each dose of this medicine*, unless otherwise directed by your doctor.

*Take this medicine only as directed.* Do not take more of it and do not take it more often than recommended on the label, unless otherwise directed by your doctor. To do so may increase the chance of side effects.

For patients *taking the extended-release capsule or tablet form of this medicine:*

- Swallow the capsule or tablet whole.
- Do not crush, break, or chew before swallowing.
- If the capsule is too large to swallow, you may mix the contents of the capsule with applesauce, jelly, honey, or syrup and swallow without chewing.

For patients *taking a combination medicine containing an antihistamine and/or aspirin or other salicylate:*

- Take with food or a glass of water or milk to lessen stomach irritation, if necessary.

*If a combination medicine containing aspirin has a strong vinegar-like odor, do not use it.* This odor means the medicine is breaking down. If you have any questions about this, check with your pharmacist.

**Missed dose**—If you must take this medicine regularly and you miss a dose, take it as soon as possible. However, if it is almost time for your next dose, skip the missed dose and go back to your regular dosing schedule. Do not double doses.

**Storage**—To store this medicine:

- Keep this medicine out of the reach of children. Overdose is very dangerous in young children.
- Store away from heat and direct light.
- Do not store the capsule or tablet form of this medicine in the bathroom, near the kitchen sink, or in other damp places. Heat or moisture may cause the medicine to break down.
- Keep the liquid form of this medicine from freezing. Do not refrigerate the syrup.
- Do not keep outdated medicine or medicine no longer needed. Be sure that any discarded medicine is out of the reach of children.

---

## Precautions While Using This Medicine

If your cough has not improved after 7 days or if you have a high fever, skin rash, continuing headache, or sore throat with the cough, check with your doctor. These signs may mean that you have other medical problems.

For patients *taking antihistamine-containing medicine:*

- Before you have any skin tests for allergies, tell the doctor in charge that you are taking this medicine. The results of the test may be affected by the antihistamine in this medicine.
- This medicine will add to the effects of alcohol and other CNS depressants (medicines that slow down the nervous system, possibly causing drowsiness). Some examples of CNS depressants are antihistamines or medicine for hay fever, other allergies, or colds; sedatives, tranquilizers, or sleeping medicine; prescription pain medicine or narcotics; barbiturates; medicine for seizures; muscle relaxants; or anesthetics, including some dental anesthetics. *Check with your doctor before taking any of the above while you are taking this medicine.*
- This medicine may cause some people to become drowsy, dizzy, or less alert than they are normally. *Make sure you know how you react to this medicine before you drive, use machines, or do anything else that could be dangerous if you are dizzy or are not alert.*
- When taking antihistamines on a regular basis, make sure your doctor knows if you are taking large amounts of aspirin at the same time (as in arthritis or rheumatism). Effects of too much aspirin, such as ringing in the ears, may be covered up by the antihistamine.
- Antihistamines may cause dryness of the mouth. For temporary relief, use sugarless candy or gum, melt bits of ice in your mouth, or use a saliva substitute. However, if your mouth continues to feel dry for more than 2 weeks, check with your medical doctor or dentist. Continuing dryness of the mouth may increase the chance of dental disease, including tooth decay, gum disease, and fungus infections.

For patients *taking decongestant-containing medicine:*

- This medicine may add to the central nervous system (CNS) stimulant and other effects of phenylpropanolamine (PPA)-containing diet aids. *Do not use medicines for diet or appetite control while taking this medicine unless you have checked with your doctor.*
- This medicine may cause some people to be nervous or restless or to have trouble in sleeping. If you have trouble in sleeping, *take the last dose of this medicine for each day a few hours before bedtime.* If you have any questions about this, check with your doctor.
- Before having any kind of surgery (including dental surgery) or emergency treatment, tell the medical doctor or dentist in charge that you are taking this medicine.

For patients *taking narcotic antitussive (codeine, dihydrocodeine, hydrocodone, or hydromorphone)–containing medicine:*

- This medicine will add to the effects of alcohol and other CNS depressants (medicines that slow down the nervous system, possibly causing drowsiness). Some examples of CNS depressants are antihistamines or medicine for hay fever, other allergies, or colds; sedatives, tranquilizers, or sleeping medicine; prescription pain medicine or narcotics; barbiturates; medicine for seizures; muscle relaxants; or anesthetics, including some dental anesthetics. *Check with your doctor before taking any of the above while you are taking this medicine.*
- This medicine may cause some people to become drowsy, dizzy, less alert than they are normally, or to feel a false sense of well-being. *Make sure you know how you react to this medicine before you drive, use machines, or do anything else that could be dangerous if you are dizzy or are not alert and clearheaded.*
- Nausea or vomiting may occur after taking a narcotic antitussive. This effect may go away if you lie down for a while. However, if nausea or vomiting continues, check with your doctor.
- Dizziness, lightheadedness, or fainting may be especially likely to occur when you get up suddenly from a lying or sitting position. Getting up slowly may help lessen this problem.
- Before having any kind of surgery (including dental surgery) or emergency treatment, tell the medical doctor or dentist in charge that you are taking this medicine.

For patients *taking iodide (calcium iodide, iodinated glycerol, or potassium iodide)-containing medicine:*

- Make sure your doctor knows if you are planning to have any future thyroid tests. The results of the thyroid test may be affected by the iodine in this medicine.

For patients *taking analgesic-containing medicine:*

- *Check the label of all nonprescription (over-the-counter [OTC]), and prescription medicines you now take.* If any contain acetaminophen or aspirin or other salicylates, including diflunisal or bismuth subsalicylate, be especially careful. Taking them while taking a cough/cold combination medicine that already contains them may lead to overdose. If you have any questions about this, check with your health care professional.
- Do not take aspirin-containing medicine for 5 days before any surgery, including dental surgery, unless otherwise directed by your medical doctor or dentist. Taking aspirin during this time may cause bleeding problems.

For *diabetic patients taking aspirin- or sodium salicylate–containing medicine:*

- False urine sugar test results may occur:

  —If you take 8 or more 325-mg (5-grain) doses of aspirin every day for several days in a row.

  —If you take 8 or more 325-mg (5-grain), or 4 or more 500-mg (10-grain) doses of sodium salicylate.

- Smaller doses or occasional use of aspirin or sodium salicylate usually will not affect urine sugar tests. If you have any questions about this, check with your health care professional, especially if your diabetes is not well controlled.

For patients *taking homatropine-containing medicine:*

- This medicine may make you sweat less, causing your body temperature to increase. *Use extra care not to become overheated during exercise or hot weather while you are taking this medicine,* since overheating may result in heat stroke. Also, hot baths or saunas may make you feel dizzy or faint while you are taking this medicine.

## Side Effects of This Medicine

Along with its needed effects, a medicine may cause some unwanted effects. Although serious side effects occur rarely when this medicine is taken as recommended, they may be more likely to occur if:

- too much medicine is taken.
- it is taken in large doses.
- it is taken for a long period of time.

*Get emergency help immediately if any of the following symptoms of overdose occur:*

*For narcotic antitussive (codeine, dihydrocodeine, hydrocodone, or hydromorphone)–containing*

Cold, clammy skin; confusion (severe); convulsions (seizures); drowsiness or dizziness (severe); nervousness or restlessness (severe); pinpoint pupils of eyes; slow heartbeat; slow or troubled breathing; weakness (severe)

*For acetaminophen-containing*

Diarrhea; increased sweating; loss of appetite; nausea or vomiting; stomach cramps or pain; swelling or tenderness in the upper abdomen or stomach area

*For salicylate-containing*

Any loss of hearing; bloody urine; confusion; convulsions (seizures); diarrhea (severe or continuing); dizziness or lightheadedness; drowsiness (severe); excitement or nervousness (severe); fast or deep breathing; fever; hallucinations (seeing, hearing, or feeling things that are not there); increased sweating; nausea or vomiting (severe or continuing); shortness of breath or troubled breathing (for salicylamide only); stomach pain (severe or continuing); uncontrollable flapping movements of the hands, especially in elderly patients; unusual thirst; vision problems

*For decongestant-containing*

Fast, pounding, or irregular heartbeat; headache (continuing and severe); nausea or vomiting (severe); nervousness or restlessness (severe); shortness of breath or troubled breathing (severe or continuing)

Also, check with your doctor as soon as possible if any of the following side effects occur:

*For all combinations*

Skin rash, hives, and/or itching

*For antihistamine- or anticholinergic-containing*

Clumsiness or unsteadiness; convulsions (seizures); drowsiness (severe); dryness of mouth, nose, or throat (severe); flushing or redness of face; hallucinations (seeing, hearing, or feeling things that are not there); restlessness (severe); shortness of breath or troubled breathing; slow or fast heartbeat

*For iodine-containing*

Headache (continuing); increased watering of mouth; loss of appetite; metallic taste; skin rash, hives, or redness; sore throat; swelling of face, lips, or eyelids

*For acetaminophen-containing*

Unexplained sore throat and fever; unusual tiredness or weakness; yellow eyes or skin

Other side effects may occur that usually do not need medical attention. These side effects may go away during treatment as your body adjusts to the medicine. However, check with your doctor if any of the following side effects continue or are bothersome:

Constipation; decreased sweating; difficult or painful urination; dizziness or lightheadedness; drowsiness; dryness of mouth, nose, or throat; false sense of well-being; increased sensitivity of skin to sun; nausea or vomiting; nightmares; stomach pain; thickening of mucus; trouble in sleeping; unusual excitement, nervousness, restlessness, or irritability; unusual tiredness or weakness

Not all of the side effects listed above have been reported for each of these medicines, but they have been reported for at least one of them. There are some similarities among these combination medicines, so many of the above side effects may occur with any of these medicines.

Other side effects not listed above may also occur in some patients. If you notice any other effects, check with your doctor.

Annual revision: 09/03/92

---

# CROMOLYN   Inhalation

A commonly used brand name in the U.S. and Canada is Intal. Another commonly used name is sodium cromoglycate.

## Description

Cromolyn (KROE-moe-lin) is used to prevent the symptoms of asthma. When it is used regularly, cromolyn lessens the number and severity of asthma attacks by reducing inflammation in the lungs. Cromolyn is also used just before exposure to conditions or substances (for example, allergens, chemicals, cold air, or air pollutants) that cause bronchospasm (wheezing or difficulty in breathing). In addition, this medicine is used to prevent bronchospasm following exercise. Cromolyn will not help an asthma or bronchospasm attack that has already started.

Cromolyn may be used alone or with other asthma medicines, such as bronchodilators (medicines that open up narrowed breathing passages) or corticosteroids (cortisone-like medicines).

Cromolyn inhalation works by acting on certain inflammatory cells in the lungs to prevent them from releasing substances that cause asthma symptoms or bronchospasm.

This medicine is available only with your doctor's prescription, in the following dosage forms:

   *Inhalation*
   • Capsules for inhalation (U.S. and Canada)
   • Inhalation aerosol (U.S. and Canada)
   • Inhalation solution (U.S. and Canada)

## Before Using This Medicine

In deciding to use a medicine, the risks of using the medicine must be weighed against the good it will do. This is a decision you and your doctor will make. For cromolyn inhalation, the following should be considered:

**Allergies**—Tell your doctor if you have ever had any unusual or allergic reaction to cromolyn or to any other inhalation aerosol medicine.

**Pregnancy**—Cromolyn has not been studied in pregnant women. However, when taken during pregnancy to control the mother's asthma, cromolyn has not been shown to cause problems in the baby. Studies in animals have shown that cromolyn causes a decrease in successful pregnancies and a decrease in the weight of the animal fetus only when given by injection in very large amounts.

**Breast-feeding**—It is not known whether cromolyn passes into the breast milk. However, this medicine has not been reported to cause problems in nursing babies. Although most medicines pass into breast milk in small amounts, many of them may be used safely while breast-feeding. Mothers who are using this medicine and who wish to breast-feed should discuss this with their doctor.

**Children**—Although there is no specific information comparing use of cromolyn inhalation in children 2 years of age and older with use in other age groups, this medicine is not expected to cause different side effects or problems in children than it does in adults.

**Older adults**—Many medicines have not been studied specifically in older people. Therefore, it may not be known whether they work exactly the same way they do in younger adults. Although there is no specific information comparing the use of cromolyn inhalation in the elderly with use in other age groups, this medicine is not expected to cause different side effects or problems in older people than it does in younger adults.

## Proper Use of This Medicine

*Cromolyn oral inhalation is used to help prevent symptoms of asthma or bronchospasm (wheezing or difficulty in breathing). Cromolyn will not relieve an asthma or a bronchospasm attack that has already started.*

*Use cromolyn inhalation only as directed.* Do not use more of it and do not use it more often than your doctor ordered. To do so may increase the chance of side effects.

Cromolyn inhalation usually comes with patient directions. Read them carefully before using this medicine. If you do not understand the directions that come with the inhaler or if you are not sure how to use the inhaler, ask your health care professional to show you how to use it. Also, ask your health care professional to check regularly how you use the inhaler to make sure you are using it properly.

For patients using *cromolyn inhalation aerosol:*
   • The cromolyn aerosol canister provides about 112 or 200 inhalations, depending on the size of the canister

your doctor ordered. You should try to keep a record of the number of inhalations you use so you will know when the canister is almost empty. This canister, unlike some other aerosol canisters, cannot be floated in water to test its fullness.

- When you use the inhaler for the first time, or if you have not used it for several days, the inhaler may not deliver the right amount of medicine with the first puff. Therefore, before using the inhaler, test it to make sure it works properly.

- *To test the inhaler:*

—Insert the metal canister firmly into the clean mouthpiece according to the manufacturer's instructions. Check to make sure the canister is placed properly into the mouthpiece.

—Take the cover off the mouthpiece and shake the inhaler well.

—Hold the canister well away from you against a light background and press the top of the canister, spraying the medicine one time into the air. If you see a fine mist, you will know the inhaler is working properly to provide the right amount of medicine when you use it. If you do not see a fine mist, try a second time.

- *To use the inhaler:*

—Using your thumb and one or two fingers, hold the inhaler upright with the mouthpiece end down and pointing toward you.

—Take the cover off the mouthpiece. Check the mouthpiece for any foreign objects. Do not use the inhaler with any other mouthpieces.

—Gently shake the inhaler three or four times.

—Hold the mouthpiece away from your mouth and breathe out slowly and completely to the end of a normal breath.

—Use the inhalation method recommended by your doctor.

- Open-mouth method: Place the mouthpiece about 1 to 2 inches (2 fingerwidths) in front of your widely opened mouth. Make sure the inhaler is aimed into your mouth so the spray does not hit the roof of your mouth or your tongue.

- Closed-mouth method: Place the mouthpiece in your mouth between your teeth and over your tongue with your lips closed tightly around it. Make sure your tongue or teeth are not blocking the opening.

—Tilt your head back a little. Start to breathe in slowly and deeply through your mouth and, at the same time, press the top of the canister once to get one puff of medicine. Continue to breathe in slowly for 3 to 4 seconds until you have taken a full deep breath. It is important to press down on the canister and breathe in slowly at the same time so the medicine is pulled into your lungs. This step may be difficult at first. If you are using the closed-mouth method and you see a fine mist coming from your

mouth or nose, the inhaler is not being used correctly.

—Hold your breath as long as you can up to 10 seconds (count slowly to ten). This gives the medicine time to get into your airways and lungs.

—Take the mouthpiece away from your mouth and breathe out slowly.

—Wait 1 minute between puffs. Then, gently shake the inhaler again, and take the second puff following exactly the same steps you used for the first puff. Breathe in only one puff at a time.

—If your doctor has told you to use an inhaled bronchodilator before using cromolyn, you should wait at least 2 minutes after using the bronchodilator before using cromolyn. This allows the cromolyn to get deeper into your lungs.

—When you are finished using the inhaler, wipe off the mouthpiece and replace the cover to keep the mouthpiece clean and free of foreign objects.

Your doctor may want you to use a spacer device with the inhaler. A spacer makes the inhaler easier to use. It allows more of the medicine to reach your lungs, rather than staying in your mouth and throat.

- *To use a spacer device with the inhaler:*

—Attach the spacer to the inhaler according to the manufacturer's directions. There are different types of spacers available, but the method of breathing remains the same with most spacers.

—Gently shake the inhaler and spacer well.

—Hold the mouthpiece of the spacer away from your mouth and breathe out slowly and completely.

—Place the mouthpiece of the spacer into your mouth between your teeth and over your tongue with your lips closed around it.

—Press down on the canister top once to release one puff of medicine into the spacer. Then, within one or two seconds, begin to breathe in slowly and deeply through your mouth for 5 to 10 seconds. Count the seconds while inhaling.

—Hold your breath as long as you can up to 10 seconds (count slowly to 10).

—Breathe out slowly. Do not remove the mouthpiece from your mouth. Breathe in and out slowly two or three times to make sure the spacer is emptied.

—Wait a minute between puffs. Then, gently shake the inhaler and spacer again and take the second puff, following exactly the same steps you used for the first puff. Do not spray more than one puff at a time into the spacer.

—When you are finished using the inhaler, remove the spacer device from the inhaler and replace the cover of the mouthpiece.

Clean the inhaler, mouthpiece, and spacer at least two times a week to prevent build-up of medicine and blockage of the mouthpiece.

- *To clean the inhaler:*
  - —Remove the metal canister from the inhaler and set the canister aside. Do not get the canister wet.
  - —Wash the mouthpiece and cover, the plastic case, and the spacer in warm soapy water. Rinse well with warm, running water.
  - —Shake off the excess water and let the inhaler parts air dry completely before putting the inhaler back together.

For patients using *cromolyn capsules for inhalation:*
- *Do not swallow the capsules. The medicine will not work if you swallow it.*
- This medicine is used with a special inhaler, either the *Spinhaler* or the *Halermatic*. If you do not understand the directions that come with the inhaler or if you are not sure how to use the inhaler, ask your health care professional to show you how to use it. Also, ask your health care professional to check regularly how you use the inhaler to make sure you are using it properly.
- If you are using *cromolyn capsules for inhalation* with the *Spinhaler:*
  - —To load the Spinhaler:
    - Make sure your hands are clean and dry.
    - Insert the capsule into the inhaler just before using this medicine.
    - Hold the inhaler upright with the mouthpiece pointing downward. Unscrew the body of the inhaler from the mouthpiece.
    - Keep the mouthpiece pointing downward and the propeller on the spindle. Remove the foil from the capsule and insert the colored end of the cromolyn capsule firmly into the cup of the propeller. Avoid too much handling of the capsule, because moisture from your hands may make the capsule soft.
    - Make sure the propeller moves freely.
    - Screw the body of the inhaler back into the mouthpiece and make certain that it is fastened well.
    - While keeping the inhaler upright with the mouthpiece pointing downward, slide the grey outer sleeve down firmly until it stops. This will puncture the capsule. Then slide the sleeve up as far as it will go. This step may be repeated a second time to make sure the capsule is punctured.
  - —To use the Spinhaler:
    - Check to make sure the mouthpiece is properly attached to the body of the inhaler.
    - Hold the inhaler away from your mouth and breathe out slowly to the end of a normal breath.
    - Place the mouthpiece in your mouth, close your lips around it, and tilt your head back. Do not block the mouthpiece with your teeth or tongue.

- Take a deep and rapid breath. You should hear and feel the vibrations of the rotating propeller as you breathe in.
- Take the inhaler from your mouth and hold your breath for a few seconds or as long as possible.
- Hold the inhaler away from your mouth and breathe out slowly and completely to the end of a normal breath. Do not breathe out through the inhaler because this may prevent the inhaler from working properly.
- Keep taking inhalations of this medicine until all the powder from the capsule is inhaled. A light dusting of powder remaining in the capsule is normal and is not a sign that the inhaler is not working properly.
- Throw away the empty capsule. Then return the inhaler to the container and replace the lid on the container.
- —To clean the Spinhaler:
  - At least once a week, brush off any powder left sticking to the propeller.
  - Take the inhaler apart and wash the parts of the inhaler with clean, warm water.
  - Wash the inside of the propeller shaft by moving the propeller on and off the steel spindle under water.
  - Shake out the excess water.
  - Allow all parts of the inhaler to dry completely before putting it back together.
  - The Spinhaler should be replaced after 6 months.
- If you are using *cromolyn capsules for inhalation* with the *Halermatic:*
  - —To load the Halermatic:
    - Make sure your hands are clean and dry.
    - Insert the capsule cartridge into the inhaler just before using this medicine.
    - Remove the mouthpiece cover. Then pull off the mouthpiece.
    - Push a cromolyn capsule cartridge firmly down to the bottom of the slot.
    - Slide the mouthpiece back on the body of the inhaler. Push down slowly as far as the mouthpiece will go. This punctures the capsule cartridge and lifts it into the rotation chamber. Do not repeat this step because the capsule cartridge needs to be punctured only once.
  - —To use the Halermatic:
    - Hold the inhaler away from your mouth and breathe out slowly to the end of a normal breath.
    - Place the mouthpiece in your mouth, close your lips around it, and tilt your head back. Do not block the flow of medicine into the lungs with your teeth or tongue.
    - Breathe in quickly and steadily through the mouthpiece.

- Hold your breath for a few seconds to keep the medicine in the lungs as long as possible. Then take the inhaler away from your mouth.
- Hold the inhaler well away from your mouth and breathe out to the end of a normal breath. Do not breathe out through the inhaler because this may prevent the inhaler from working properly.
- Keep taking inhalations of this medicine until all the powder from the capsule is inhaled. A light dusting of powder remaining in the capsule is normal and is not a sign that the inhaler is not working properly.
- Throw away the empty capsule cartridge.

—*To clean the Halermatic:*

- Brush away powder deposits each day with a brush.
- When powder deposits build up, wipe them away with a slightly damp cloth.
- The mouthpiece may be washed separately if necessary. However, do not wet the blue-based body of the inhaler. Be sure the mouthpiece grid is dry before putting the inhaler back together.
- The Halermatic should be replaced every 6 months.

For patients using *cromolyn inhalation solution:*

- Cromolyn inhalation solution comes in a small glass container called an ampul. The ampul must be broken gently to empty the contents. If you do not understand the manufacturer's directions, ask your health care professional to show you what to do.
- Do not use the solution in the ampul if it is cloudy or contains particles.
- *To break and empty the ampul:*
  —The glass ampul is weak at each end so the ends can be broken easily by hand.
  —Hold the ampul away from the nebulizer and your face when you break it. Hold the ampul at an angle and carefully break off the lower end. No solution will come out.
  —Turn the ampul over so the open end faces upward. Place a forefinger carefully over the open end.
  —Keep your finger firmly in place and break off the lower end of the ampul.
  —To empty the ampul, hold it over the bowl of the nebulizer unit and remove your finger to let the solution flow out.
  —Throw away any solution left in the nebulizer after you have taken your treatment.
- Use this medicine only in a power-operated nebulizer that has an adequate flow rate and is equipped with a face mask or mouthpiece. Your doctor will advise you on which nebulizer to use. Make sure you understand exactly how to use it. Hand-squeezed bulb nebulizers cannot be used with this medicine. If you

have any questions about this, check with your doctor.

For patients using *cromolyn oral inhalation* regularly (for example, every day):

- *In order for cromolyn to work properly, it must be inhaled every day in regularly spaced doses as ordered by your doctor.* Up to 4 weeks may pass before you feel the full effects of the medicine.

**Dosing**—The dose of cromolyn will be different for different patients. *Follow your doctor's orders or the directions on the label.* The following information includes only the average doses of cromolyn inhalation. *If your dose is different, do not change it* unless your doctor tells you to do so.

The number of doses you take each day, the time allowed between doses, and the length of time you take the medicine depend on the medical problem for which you are taking cromolyn inhalation.

- For *inhalation aerosol* dosage form:
  —For prevention of asthma symptoms:
    - Adults and children 5 years of age or older—1.6 or 2 milligrams (mg) (2 puffs) taken four times a day with doses spaced four to six hours apart.
    - Children up to 5 years of age—Use and dose must be determined by your doctor.
  —For prevention of bronchospasm caused by exercise or a condition or substance:
    - Adults and children 5 years of age or older—1.6 or 2 milligrams (mg) (2 puffs) taken at least ten to fifteen (but not more than sixty) minutes before exercise or exposure to any condition or substance that may cause an attack.
    - Children up to 5 years of age—Use and dose must be determined by your doctor.
- For *capsule for inhalation* dosage form:
  —For prevention of asthma symptoms:
    - Adults and children 2 years of age or older—20 mg (contents of 1 capsule) taken four times a day with doses spaced four to six hours apart.
    - Children up to 2 years of age—Use and dose must be determined by your doctor.
  —For prevention of bronchospasm caused by exercise or a condition or substance:
    - Adults and children 2 years of age or older—20 mg (contents of 1 capsule) taken at least ten to fifteen (but not more than sixty) minutes before exercise or exposure to any condition or substance that may cause an attack.
    - Children up to 2 years of age—Use and dose must be determined by your doctor.
- For *inhalation solution* dosage form:
  —For prevention of asthma symptoms:
    - Adults and children 2 years of age or older—20 mg (contents of 1 ampul) used in a nebulizer. This medicine should be used four times a day

with doses spaced four to six hours apart. Use a new ampul of solution for each dose.

- Children up to 2 years of age—Use and dose must be determined by your doctor.

—For prevention of bronchospasm caused by exercise or a condition or substance:

- Adults and children 2 years of age or older—20 mg (contents of 1 ampul) used in a nebulizer. This medicine should be used at least ten to fifteen (but not more than sixty) minutes before exercise or exposure to any condition or substance that may cause an attack. Use a new ampul of solution for each dose.
- Children up to 2 years of age—Use and dose must be determined by your doctor.

**Missed dose**—If you are using cromolyn regularly and you miss a dose, use it as soon as possible. Then use any remaining doses for that day at regularly spaced times.

**Storage**—To store this medicine:

- Keep out of the reach of children.
- Store the aerosol or solution form of this medicine at room temperature away from heat or cold. Keep this medicine from freezing.
- Store the capsule or solution form of this medicine away from direct light. Store the aerosol form of this medicine away from direct sunlight.
- Do not store the capsule form of this medicine in the bathroom, near the kitchen sink, or in other damp places. Heat or moisture may cause the medicine to break down.
- Do not puncture, break, or burn the aerosol container, even if it is empty.
- Do not keep outdated medicine or medicine no longer needed. Be sure that any discarded medicine is out of the reach of children.

## Precautions While Using This Medicine

*If your symptoms do not improve within 4 weeks or if your condition becomes worse after you begin using cromolyn, check with your doctor.*

*If you are also taking a corticosteroid or a bronchodilator for your asthma along with this medicine, do not stop taking the corticosteroid or bronchodilator even if*

*your asthma seems better, unless you are told to do so by your doctor.*

Dryness of the mouth or throat, throat irritation, and hoarseness may occur after you use this medicine. Gargling and rinsing your mouth or taking a drink of water after each dose may help prevent these effects.

## Side Effects of This Medicine

Along with its needed effects, a medicine may cause some unwanted effects. Although not all of these side effects may occur, if they do occur they may need medical attention.

Check with your doctor as soon as possible if any of the following side effects occur:

*Less common*
Increased wheezing, tightness in chest, or difficulty in breathing

*Rare*
Chest pain; chills; difficult or painful urination; difficulty in swallowing; dizziness; frequent urge to urinate; headache (severe or continuing); joint pain or swelling; muscle pain or weakness; skin rash, hives, or itching; sweating; swelling of the face, lips, eyelids, hands, feet, or inside of mouth

Other side effects may occur that usually do not need medical attention. These side effects may go away during treatment as your body adjusts to the medicine. However, check with your doctor if any of the following side effects continue or are bothersome:

*More common*
Cough; dryness of the mouth or throat; nausea; stuffy nose; throat irritation

*Less common*
Hoarseness; watering of the eyes

If you are using the cromolyn inhalation aerosol, you may notice an unpleasant taste. This may be expected and will go away when you stop using the medicine.

Other side effects not listed above may also occur in some patients. If you notice any other effects, check with your doctor.

Revised: 08/09/94

---

# CROMOLYN    Nasal

Some commonly used brand names are:

**In the U.S.—**
Nasalcrom

**In Canada—**
Rynacrom

Another commonly used name is sodium cromoglycate.

## Description

Cromolyn (KROE-moe-lin) nasal solution is used to help prevent or treat the symptoms (sneezing, wheezing, runny nose, itching) of seasonal (short-term) or chronic (long-term) allergic rhinitis. Cromolyn powder for nasal inhalation is used to help prevent seasonal (short-term) allergic rhinitis.

This medicine works by acting on certain cells in the body, called mast cells, to prevent them from releasing substances that cause the allergic reaction.

When cromolyn is used to treat chronic (long-term) allergic rhinitis, an antihistamine and/or a nasal decongestant may be used with this medicine, especially during the first few weeks of treatment.

Nasal cromolyn is available only with your doctor's prescription, in the following dosage forms:

*Nasal*
- Nasal insufflation (powder for nasal inhalation) (Canada)
- Nasal solution (U.S. and Canada)

## Before Using This Medicine

In deciding to use a medicine, the risks of using the medicine must be weighed against the good it will do. This is a decision you and your doctor will make. For nasal cromolyn, the following should be considered:

**Allergies**—Tell your doctor if you have ever had any unusual or allergic reaction to cromolyn. Also tell your health care professional if you are allergic to any other substances, such as foods, preservatives, or dyes.

**Pregnancy**—Nasal cromolyn has not been shown to cause birth defects in humans. However, studies in animals have shown that cromolyn, when given by injection in very large amounts, causes a decrease in successful pregnancies and a decrease in the weight of the animal fetus. Before using this medicine, make sure your doctor knows if you are pregnant or if you may become pregnant.

**Breast-feeding**—It is not known whether cromolyn passes into the breast milk. Although most medicines pass into breast milk in small amounts, many of them may be used safely while breast-feeding. Mothers who are using this medicine and who wish to breast-feed should discuss this with their doctor.

**Children**—Studies on this medicine have been done only in adult patients, and there is no specific information comparing use of nasal cromolyn in children up to 6 years of age (in Canada, up to 5 years of age) with use in other age groups. In older children, this medicine is not expected to cause different side effects or problems than it does in adults.

**Older adults**—Many medicines have not been studied specifically in older people. Therefore, it may not be known whether they work exactly the same way they do in younger adults. Although there is no specific information comparing use of nasal cromolyn in the elderly with use in other age groups, this medicine is not expected to cause different side effects or problems in older people than it does in younger adults.

**Other medical problems**—The presence of other medical problems may affect the use of nasal cromolyn. Make sure you tell your doctor if you have any other medical problems, especially:
- Polyps or growths inside the nose—Cromolyn may not work if nasal passages are blocked

## Proper Use of This Medicine

This medicine usually comes with patient directions. Read them carefully before using the medicine.

Before using this medicine, clear the nasal passages by blowing your nose.

For patients using *cromolyn nasal solution:*
- Cromolyn nasal solution is used with a special spray device.
- To keep clean, wipe the nosepiece with a clean tissue and replace the dust cap after use.

For patients using *cromolyn powder for nasal inhalation:*
- This medicine is used with a special inhaler. Be sure you understand exactly how to use it.
- To keep clean, wipe the nosepiece with a clean tissue and replace the dust cap after use. Only the nosepiece may be washed in warm water, but must be dried thoroughly. *The bulb unit should not be washed or dampened inside.*

*Use this medicine only as directed.* Do not use more of it and do not use it more often than your doctor ordered. To do so may increase the chance of side effects.

*In order for this medicine to work properly, it must be used every day in regularly spaced doses as ordered by your doctor:*
- For patients using cromolyn for *seasonal (short-term) allergic rhinitis,* up to 1 week may pass before you begin to feel better.
- For patients using cromolyn for *chronic (long-term) allergic rhinitis,* up to 4 weeks may pass before you feel the full effects of this medicine, although you may begin to feel better after 1 week.

**Dosing**—The dose of nasal cromolyn will be different for different patients. *Follow your doctor's orders or the directions on the label.* The following information includes only the average doses of nasal cromolyn. *If your dose is different, do not change it* unless your doctor tells you to do so.
- For *nasal solution* dosage form:
  —For allergic rhinitis:
    - Adults and children 6 years of age (in Canada, 5 years of age) and older—One spray into each nostril three to six times a day.
    - Children up to 6 years of age (in Canada, up to 5 years of age)—Use and dose must be determined by your doctor.
- For *powder for nasal inhalation* dosage form:
  —For allergic rhinitis:
    - Adults and children 5 years of age and older—One inhalation into each nostril four times a day

until condition is better; then, one inhalation into each nostril two or three times a day.
• Children up to 5 years of age—Use and dose must be determined by your doctor.

**Missed dose**—If you miss a dose of this medicine, use it as soon as possible. Then use any remaining doses for that day at regularly spaced intervals. Do not double doses.

**Storage**—To store this medicine:
• Keep out of the reach of children.
• Store away from heat and direct light.
• Store the powder form of this medicine in a dry place. Do not store it in the bathroom, near the kitchen sink, or in other damp places. Heat or moisture may cause the medicine to break down.
• Keep the solution form of this medicine from freezing.
• Do not keep outdated medicine or medicine no longer needed. Be sure that any discarded medicine is out of the reach of children.

## Precautions While Using This Medicine

*If your symptoms do not improve or if your condition becomes worse, check with your doctor.*

## Side Effects of This Medicine

Along with its needed effects, a medicine may cause some unwanted effects. Although not all of these side effects may occur, if they do occur they may need medical attention.

Check with your doctor as soon as possible if any of the following side effects occur:
*Rare*
Allergic reaction (coughing; difficulty in swallowing; hives or itching; swelling of face, lips, or eyelids; wheezing or difficulty in breathing); nosebleeds; skin rash

Other side effects may occur that usually do not need medical attention. These side effects may go away during treatment as your body adjusts to the medicine. However, check with your doctor if any of the following side effects continue or are bothersome:
*More common*
Burning, stinging, or irritation inside of nose; increase in sneezing
*Less common*
Cough; headache; postnasal drip; unpleasant taste

Other side effects not listed above may also occur in some patients. If you notice any other effects, check with your doctor.

Revised: 04/20/94

# CROMOLYN    Ophthalmic*

Some commonly used brand names in Canada are Opticrom and Vistacrom.
Other commonly used names are cromoglicic acid, cromoglycic acid, and sodium cromoglycate.

*Not commercially available at the present time in the U.S.

## Description

Cromolyn (KROE-moe-lin) ophthalmic solution is used in the eye to treat certain disorders of the eye caused by allergies. It works by acting on certain cells, called mast cells, to prevent them from releasing substances that cause the allergic reaction.

Cromolyn is available only with your doctor's prescription, in the following dosage form:
*Ophthalmic*
• Ophthalmic solution (eye drops) (Canada)

## Before Using This Medicine

In deciding to use a medicine, the risks of using the medicine must be weighed against the good it will do.

This is a decision you and your doctor will make. For ophthalmic cromolyn, the following should be considered:

**Allergies**—Tell your doctor if you have ever had any unusual or allergic reaction to cromolyn. Also tell your health care professional if you are allergic to any other substances, such as foods, preservatives, or dyes.

**Pregnancy**—Cromolyn has not been studied in pregnant women. Studies in animals have shown that cromolyn causes a decrease in successful pregnancies and a decrease in the weight of the animal fetus when given by injection in very large amounts. However, it is unlikely that ophthalmic cromolyn will cause problems in humans when used in the eye as directed.

**Breast-feeding**—It is not known whether cromolyn passes into the breast milk. Although most medicines pass into breast milk in small amounts, many of them may be used safely while breast-feeding. Mothers who are taking this medicine and who wish to breast-feed should discuss this with their doctor.

**Children**—Studies on this medicine have been done only in adult patients, and there is no specific information

comparing use of cromolyn in children up to 4 years of age with use in other age groups. For older children, this medicine is not expected to cause different side effects or problems than it does in adults.

**Older adults**—Many medicines have not been studied specifically in older people. Therefore, it may not be known whether they work exactly the same way they do in younger adults. Although there is no specific information comparing use of ophthalmic cromolyn in the elderly with use in other age groups, this medicine is not expected to cause different side effects or problems in older people than it does in younger adults.

## Proper Use of This Medicine

To use the *eye drops:*
- First, wash your hands. Tilt the head back and, pressing your finger gently on the skin just beneath the lower eyelid, pull the lower eyelid away from the eye to make a space. Drop the medicine into this space. Let go of the eyelid and gently close the eyes. Do not blink. Keep the eyes closed for 1 or 2 minutes to allow the medicine to be absorbed by the eye.
- If you think you did not get the drop of medicine into your eye properly, use another drop.
- To keep the medicine as germ-free as possible, do not touch the applicator tip to any surface (including the eye). Also, keep the container tightly closed.

*Use cromolyn eye drops only as directed.* Do not use more of this medicine and do not use it more often than your doctor ordered. To do so may increase the chance of side effects.

*In order for this medicine to work properly, it must be used every day in regularly spaced doses as ordered by your doctor.* A few days may pass before you begin to feel better. However, in some conditions, it may take several weeks before you begin to feel better.

**Dosing**—The dose of ophthalmic cromolyn will be different for different patients. *Follow your doctor's orders or the directions on the label.* The following information includes only the average doses of ophthalmic cromolyn. *If your dose is different, do not change it* unless your doctor tells you to do so.
- For *ophthalmic solution (eye drops)* dosage form:
  —For eye allergies:
    - Adults and children 4 years of age and older— Use one drop four to six times a day in regularly spaced doses.

- Children up to 4 years of age—Use and dose must be determined by your doctor.

**Missed dose**—If you miss a dose of this medicine, use it as soon as possible. Then go back to your regular dosing schedule.

**Storage**—To store this medicine:
- Keep out of the reach of children.
- Store away from heat and direct light.
- Keep the medicine from freezing.
- Do not keep outdated medicine or medicine no longer needed. Be sure that any discarded medicine is out of the reach of children.

## Precautions While Using This Medicine

*If your symptoms do not improve or if your condition becomes worse, check with your doctor.*

## Side Effects of This Medicine

Along with its needed effects, a medicine may cause some unwanted effects. Although not all of these side effects may occur, if they do occur they may need medical attention.

Check with your doctor as soon as possible if any of the following side effects occur:

*Rare*
Rash or redness around the eyes; swelling of the membrane covering the white part of the eye, redness of the white part of the eye, styes, or other eye irritation not present before therapy

Other side effects may occur that usually do not need medical attention. These side effects may go away during treatment as your body adjusts to the medicine. However, check with your doctor if any of the following side effects continue or are bothersome:

*More common*
Burning or stinging of eye (mild and temporary)

*Less common or rare*
Dryness or puffiness around the eye; watering or itching of eye (increased)

Other side effects not listed above may also occur in some patients. If you notice any other effects, check with your doctor.

Revised: 04/19/94

# CROMOLYN   Oral

Some commonly used brand names are:
**In the U.S.—**
     Gastrocrom
**In Canada—**
     Nalcrom
Another commonly used name is sodium cromoglycate.

## Description

Cromolyn (KROE-moe-lin) is used to treat the symptoms of mastocytosis. Mastocytosis is a rare condition caused by too many mast cells in the body. These mast cells release substances that cause the symptoms of the disease, such as abdominal pain, nausea, vomiting, diarrhea, headache, flushing or itching of skin, or hives.

Cromolyn works by acting on the mast cells in the body to prevent them from releasing substances that cause the symptoms of mastocytosis.

Cromolyn is available only with your doctor's prescription, in the following dosage form:

*Oral*
  • Capsules (U.S. and Canada)

## Before Using This Medicine

In deciding to use a medicine, the risks of taking the medicine must be weighed against the good it will do. This is a decision you and your doctor will make. For oral cromolyn, the following should be considered:

**Allergies**—Tell your doctor if you have ever had any unusual or allergic reaction to cromolyn. Also tell your health care professional if you are allergic to any other substances, such as foods, preservatives, or dyes.

**Diet**—Make certain your health care professional knows if you are on any special diet, such as a low-sodium diet. This medicine contains sodium.

**Pregnancy**—Cromolyn has not been studied in pregnant women. However, studies in animals have shown that cromolyn, when given by injection in very large amounts, causes a decrease in successful pregnancies and a decrease in the weight of the animal fetus. Before using this medicine, make sure your doctor knows if you are pregnant or if you may become pregnant.

**Breast-feeding**—It is not known whether cromolyn passes into the breast milk. Although most medicines pass into breast milk in small amounts, many of them may be used safely while breast-feeding. Mothers who are taking this medicine and who wish to breast-feed should discuss this with their doctor.

**Children**—Although there is no specific information comparing use of oral cromolyn in children with use in other age groups, this medicine is not expected to cause different side effects or problems in children than it does in adults.

**Older adults**—Many medicines have not been studied specifically in older people. Therefore, it may not be known whether they work exactly the same way they do in younger adults. Although there is no specific information comparing use of oral cromolyn in the elderly with use in other age groups, this medicine is not expected to cause different side effects or problems in older people than it does in younger adults.

**Other medicines**—Although certain medicines should not be used together at all, in other cases two different medicines may be used together even if an interaction might occur. In these cases, your doctor may want to change the dose, or other precautions may be necessary. Tell your health care professional if you are taking any other prescription or nonprescription (over-the-counter [OTC]) medicine.

**Other medical problems**—The presence of other medical problems may affect the use of oral cromolyn. Make sure you tell your doctor if you have any other medical problems, especially:
  • Kidney disease or
  • Liver disease—The effects of cromolyn may be increased, which may increase the chance of side effects

## Proper Use of This Medicine

Unless otherwise directed by your doctor, it is best to take oral cromolyn as follows:
  • Open the cromolyn capsule(s) and pour all of the powder into one-half glass (4 ounces) of hot water. Stir the solution until the powder is completely dissolved and the solution is clear. Then add an equal amount (one-half glass) of cold water to the solution while stirring.
  • Be sure to drink all of the liquid to get the full dose of medicine.
  • Do not mix this medicine with fruit juice, milk, or food because they may keep the medicine from working properly.

*Take cromolyn only as directed*. Do not take more of it and do not take it more often than your doctor ordered. To do so may increase the chance of side effects.

**Dosing**—The dose of cromolyn will be different for different patients. *Follow your doctor's orders or the directions on the label*. The following information includes only the average doses of cromolyn. *If your dose is different, do not change it* unless your doctor tells you to do so.
  • For *oral* dosage form (capsules):
    —For symptoms of mastocytosis:
      • Adults—200 milligrams (mg) dissolved in water and taken four times a day, thirty minutes before meals and at bedtime.
      • Children 2 to 12 years of age—100 mg dissolved in water and taken four times a day, thirty

minutes before meals and at bedtime. Your doctor may increase the dose if your symptoms are not under control within two to three weeks after you begin taking this medicine.

• Infants and children up to 2 years of age—Dose is based on body weight and must be determined by your doctor. The dose is usually 20 mg per kilogram (kg) (9.1 mg per pound) of body weight a day. This dose is divided into four doses. Your doctor may increase the dose if your symptoms are not under control within two to three weeks after you begin taking this medicine.

• Premature infants—Use is not recommended.

**Missed dose**—If you miss a dose of this medicine, take it as soon as possible. Then take any remaining doses for that day at regularly spaced times.

**Storage**—To store this medicine:
• Keep out of the reach of children.
• Store away from heat, in a tightly closed container.
• Do not store the capsule form of this medicine in the bathroom, near the kitchen sink, or in other damp places. Heat or moisture may cause the medicine to break down.
• Do not keep outdated medicine or medicine no longer needed. Be sure that any discarded medicine is out of the reach of children.

## Precautions While Using This Medicine

*If your symptoms do not improve or if your condition becomes worse, check with your doctor.*

## Side Effects of This Medicine

Along with its needed effects, a medicine may cause some unwanted effects. Although not all of these side effects may occur, if they do occur they may need medical attention.

*Check with your doctor immediately* if any of the following side effects occur:

*Rare*
Coughing; difficulty in swallowing; hives or itching of skin; swelling of face, lips, or eyelids; wheezing or difficulty in breathing

Also, check with your doctor as soon as possible if the following side effect occurs:

*Less common*
Skin rash

Other side effects may occur that usually do not need medical attention. These side effects may go away during treatment as your body adjusts to the medicine. However, check with your doctor if any of the following side effects continue or are bothersome:

*More common*
Diarrhea; headache

*Less common*
Abdominal pain; irritability; joint pain; nausea; trouble in sleeping

Note: If the above side effects occur in patients with mastocytosis, they are usually only temporary and could be symptoms of the disease.

Other side effects not listed above may also occur in some patients. If you notice any other effects, check with your doctor.

Revised: 09/06/94

---

# CROTAMITON   Topical

Some commonly used brand names are:

**In the U.S.—**
Eurax Cream
Eurax Lotion

**In Canada—**
Eurax Cream

## Description

Crotamiton (kroe-TAM-i-tonn) is used to treat scabies infection. It is also used to relieve the itching of certain skin conditions.

This medicine is available only with your doctor's prescription, in the following dosage forms:

*Topical*
• Cream (U.S. and Canada)
• Lotion (U.S.)

## Before Using This Medicine

In deciding to use a medicine, the risks of using the medicine must be weighed against the good it will do. This is a decision you and your doctor will make. For crotamiton, the following should be considered:

**Allergies**—Tell your doctor if you have ever had any unusual or allergic reaction to crotamiton. Also tell your health care professional if you are allergic to any other substances, such as preservatives or dyes.

**Pregnancy**—Studies on effects in pregnancy have not been done in either humans or animals.

**Breast-feeding**—Topical crotamiton has not been reported to cause problems in nursing babies.

**Children**—Studies on this medicine have been done only in adult patients, and there is no specific information

comparing use of this medicine in children with use in other age groups.

**Older adults**—Many medicines have not been studied specifically in older people. Therefore, it may not be known whether they work exactly the same way they do in younger adults or if they cause different side effects or problems in older people. There is no specific information comparing use of crotamiton in the elderly with use in other age groups.

**Other medicines**—Although certain medicines should not be used together at all, in other cases two different medicines may be used together even if an interaction might occur. In these cases, your doctor may want to change the dose, or other precautions may be necessary. Tell your health care professional if you are using any other topical prescription or nonprescription (over-the-counter [OTC]) medicine that is to be applied to the same area of the skin.

**Other medical problems**—The presence of other medical problems may affect the use of crotamiton. Make sure you tell your doctor if you have any other medical problems, especially:

- Severely inflamed skin or raw oozing areas of the skin—Use of crotamiton on these areas may make the condition worse

## Proper Use of This Medicine

*Keep crotamiton away from the mouth. It may be harmful if swallowed.*

*Use this medicine only as directed.* Do not use it more often than your doctor ordered. To do so may increase the chance of side effects.

*Keep crotamiton away from the eyes and other mucous membranes,* such as the inside of the nose. It may cause irritation. If you should accidentally get some in your eyes, flush them thoroughly with water at once.

This medicine usually comes with patient directions. Read them carefully before using.

If you take a bath or shower before using this medicine, dry the skin well before applying crotamiton.

For patients using this medicine *for scabies:*

- Apply enough medicine to cover the entire skin surface from the chin down, and rub in well. This applies especially to folds and creases in the skin and to the hands, feet (including the soles), between fingers and toes, and moist areas (such as underarms and groin).
- Do not wash off the first coat of this medicine.
- Apply a second coat of this medicine 24 hours after the first one.
- The next day, put on freshly washed or dry-cleaned clothing and change bedding in order to prevent reinfection.

- Then, 48 hours after the second application of this medicine, take a cleansing bath to remove the medicine.
- Your sexual partners, especially, and all members of your household may need to be treated also, since the infection may spread to persons in close contact. If these persons are not being treated or if you have any questions about this, check with your doctor.

**Dosing**—The dose of crotamiton will be different for different patients. *Follow your doctor's orders or the directions on the label.* The following information includes only the average doses of crotamiton. *If your dose is different, do not change it* unless your doctor tells you to do so.

- For *topical* dosage forms (cream and lotion):
  —For scabies:
  - Adults—Use two times. Apply one time the first day, and one time the second day. For severe cases, treatment may be repeated one time after one week.
  - Children—Use and dose must be determined by your doctor.
  —For pruritus:
  - Adults—Use when necessary according to the directions on the label or your doctor's instructions.
  - Children—Use and dose must be determined by your doctor.

**Storage**—To store this medicine:

- Keep out of the reach of children.
- Store away from heat and direct light.
- Keep the medicine from freezing.
- Do not keep outdated medicine or medicine no longer needed. Be sure that any discarded medicine is out of the reach of children.

## Precautions While Using This Medicine

*If your condition does not improve or if it becomes worse, check with your doctor.*

For patients using this medicine *for scabies:*

- To prevent reinfection or spreading of the infection to other people, good health habits are also required. These include machine washing all underwear, pajamas, sheets, pillowcases, towels, and washcloths in very hot water and drying them using the hot cycle of a dryer. Clothing or bedding that cannot be washed in this way should be dry cleaned.

## Side Effects of This Medicine

Along with its needed effects, a medicine may cause some unwanted effects. Although not all of these side effects may occur, if they do occur they may need medical attention.

Check with your doctor as soon as possible if either of the following side effects occur:

*Rare*
  Skin irritation or rash not present before use of this medicine

Other side effects not listed above may also occur in some patients. If you notice any other effects, check with your doctor.

Revised: 04/22/94

# CYCLANDELATE  Systemic

A commonly used brand name is Cyclospasmol.
Generic name product may also be available in the U.S.

## Description

Cyclandelate (sye-KLAN-de-late) belongs to the group of medicines commonly called vasodilators. These medicines increase the size of blood vessels. Cyclandelate is used to treat problems resulting from poor blood circulation.

In the U.S., cyclandelate is available only with your doctor's prescription. It is available in the following dosage forms:

*Oral*
  • Capsules (U.S.)
  • Tablets (Canada)

## Before Using This Medicine

In deciding to use a medicine, the risks of taking the medicine must be weighed against the good it will do. This is a decision you and your doctor will make. For cyclandelate, the following should be considered:

**Allergies**—Tell your doctor if you have ever had any unusual or allergic reaction to cyclandelate. Also tell your health care professional if you are allergic to any other substances, such as foods, preservatives, or dyes.

**Pregnancy**—Studies on effects in pregnancy have not been done in either humans or animals.

**Breast-feeding**—It is not known whether cyclandelate passes into breast milk. However, cyclandelate has not been reported to cause problems in nursing babies.

**Children**—Studies on this medicine have been done only in adult patients, and there is no specific information comparing use of cyclandelate in children with use in other age groups.

**Older adults**—Many medicines have not been studied specifically in older people. Therefore, it may not be known whether they work exactly the same way they do in younger adults. Although there is no specific information comparing use of cyclandelate in the elderly with use in other age groups, this medicine is not expected to cause different side effects or problems in older people than in younger adults.

**Other medicines**—Although certain medicines should not be used together at all, in other cases two different medicines may be used together even if an interaction might occur. In these cases, your doctor may want to change the dose, or other precautions may be necessary. Tell your health care professional if you are taking any other prescription or nonprescription (over-the-counter [OTC]) medicine, or if you smoke.

**Other medical problems**—The presence of other medical problems may affect the use of cyclandelate. Make sure you tell your doctor if you have any other medical problems, especially:
  • Angina (chest pain) or
  • Bleeding problems or
  • Glaucoma or
  • Hardening of the arteries or
  • Heart attack (recent) or
  • Stroke (recent)—The chance of unwanted effects may be increased

## Proper Use of This Medicine

*If this medicine upsets your stomach, it may be taken with meals, milk, or antacids.*

**Dosing**—The dose of cyclandelate will be different for different patients. *Follow your doctor's orders or the directions on the label.* The following information includes only the average doses of cyclandelate. *If your dose is different, do not change it* unless your doctor tells you to do so.

The number of capsules or tablets that you take depends on the strength of the medicine.
  • For *oral* dosage form (capsules or tablets):
    —For treating poor circulation:
      • Adults—At first, 1.2 to 1.6 grams a day. This is taken in divided doses before meals and at bedtime. Then, your doctor will gradually lower your dose to 400 to 800 milligrams (mg) a day. This is divided into two to four doses.
      • Children—Use and dose must be determined by your doctor.

**Missed dose**—If you miss a dose of this medicine, take it as soon as you remember. Then go back to your regular dosing schedule. However, if it is almost time for your next dose, skip the missed dose and go back to your regular dosing schedule. Do not double doses.

**Storage**—To store this medicine:
- Keep out of the reach of children.
- Store away from heat and direct light.
- Do not store in the bathroom, near the kitchen sink, or in other damp places. Heat or moisture may cause the medicine to break down.
- Do not keep outdated medicine or medicine no longer needed. Be sure that any discarded medicine is out of the reach of children.

---

## Precautions While Using This Medicine

It may take some time for this medicine to work. If you feel that the medicine is not working, do not stop taking it on your own. Instead, check with your doctor.

The helpful effects of this medicine may be decreased if you smoke.

*Dizziness may occur, especially when you get up from a lying or sitting position or climb stairs. Getting up*

*slowly may help.* If this problem continues or gets worse, check with your doctor.

---

## Side Effects of This Medicine

Along with its needed effects, a medicine may cause some unwanted effects. The following side effects may go away during treatment as your body adjusts to the medicine. However, check with your doctor if any of these effects continue or are bothersome:

*Less common*
> Belching, heartburn, nausea, or stomach pain; dizziness; fast heartbeat; flushing of face; headache; sweating; tingling sensation in face, fingers, or toes; weakness

Other side effects not listed above may also occur in some patients. If you notice any other effects, check with your doctor.

---

Revised: 10/15/92
Interim revision: 04/14/94

---

# CYCLOBENZAPRINE   Systemic

Some commonly used brand names are:

**In the U.S.—**
Cycoflex                    Flexeril
Generic name product may also be available.

**In Canada—**
Flexeril

---

## Description

Cyclobenzaprine (sye-kloe-BEN-za-preen) is used to help relax certain muscles in your body. It helps relieve the pain, stiffness, and discomfort caused by strains, sprains, or injuries to your muscles. However, this medicine does not take the place of rest, exercise or physical therapy, or other treatment that your doctor may recommend for your medical problem. Cyclobenzaprine acts on the central nervous system (CNS) to produce its muscle relaxant effects. Its actions on the CNS may also cause some of this medicine's side effects.

Cyclobenzaprine may also be used for other conditions as determined by your doctor.

Cyclobenzaprine is available only with your doctor's prescription, in the following dosage form:
*Oral*
- Tablets (U.S. and Canada)

---

## Before Using This Medicine

In deciding to use a medicine, the risks of taking the medicine must be weighed against the good it will do.

This is a decision you and your doctor will make. For cyclobenzaprine, the following should be considered:

**Allergies**—Tell your doctor if you have ever had any unusual or allergic reaction to cyclobenzaprine. Also tell your health care professional if you are allergic to any other substances, such as foods, preservatives, or dyes.

**Pregnancy**—Studies on birth defects with cyclobenzaprine have not been done in humans. However, cyclobenzaprine has not been shown to cause birth defects or other problems in animal studies.

**Breast-feeding**—It is not known whether cyclobenzaprine passes into breast milk. Although most medicines pass into the breast milk in small amounts, many of them may be used safely while breast-feeding. Mothers who are taking this medicine and who wish to breast-feed should discuss this with their doctor.

**Children**—Studies on this medicine have been done only in adult patients, and there is no specific information comparing use of cyclobenzaprine in children with use in other age groups.

**Teenagers**—Studies on this medicine have been done only in adult patients, and there is no specific information comparing use of cyclobenzaprine in teenagers up to 15 years of age with use in other age groups.

**Older adults**—Many medicines have not been studied specifically in older people. Therefore, it may not be known whether they work exactly the same way they do in younger adults or if they cause different side effects or

---

problems in older people. There is no specific information comparing use of cyclobenzaprine in the elderly with use in other age groups.

**Other medicines**—Although certain medicines should not be used together at all, in other cases two different medicines may be used together even if an interaction might occur. In these cases, your doctor may want to change the dose, or other precautions may be necessary. When you are taking cyclobenzaprine, it is especially important that your health care professional know if you are taking any of the following:

- Alcohol or
- Central nervous system (CNS) depressants or
- Tricyclic antidepressants (amitriptyline [e.g., Elavil], amoxapine [e.g., Asendin], clomipramine [e.g., Anafranil], desipramine [e.g., Pertofrane], doxepin [e.g., Sinequan], imipramine [e.g., Tofranil], nortriptyline [e.g., Aventyl], protriptyline [e.g., Vivactil], trimipramine [e.g., Surmontil])—The chance of side effects may be increased
- Monoamine oxidase (MAO) inhibitors (furazolidone [e.g., Furoxone], isocarboxazid [e.g., Marplan], phenelzine [e.g., Nardil], procarbazine [e.g., Matulane], selegiline (e.g., Eldepryl), tranylcypromine [e.g., Parnate])—Taking cyclobenzaprine while you are taking or within 2 weeks of taking monoamine oxidase (MAO) inhibitors may increase the chance of side effects

**Other medical problems**—The presence of other medical problems may affect the use of cyclobenzaprine. Make sure you tell your doctor if you have any other medical problems, especially:

- Glaucoma or
- Problems with urination—Cyclobenzaprine can make your condition worse
- Heart or blood vessel disease or
- Overactive thyroid—The chance of side effects may be increased

## Proper Use of This Medicine

Take this medicine only as directed by your doctor. Do not take more of it and do not take it more often than your doctor ordered. To do so may increase the chance of serious side effects.

**Dosing**—The dose of cyclobenzaprine will be different for different people. *Follow your doctor's orders or the directions on the label.* The following information includes only the average doses of cyclobenzaprine. *If your dose is different, do not change it* unless your doctor tells you to do so.

- For the *oral* dosage form (tablets):
  - —For relaxing stiff muscles:
    - Adults and teenagers 15 years of age and older—The usual dose is 10 milligrams (mg) three times a day. The largest amount should be no more than 60 mg (six 10-mg tablets) a day.
    - Children and teenagers up to 15 years of age—Dose must be determined by your doctor.

**Missed dose**—If you miss a dose of this medicine and remember within an hour or so of the missed dose, take it right away. Then go back to your regular dosing schedule. But if you do not remember until later, skip the missed dose and go back to your regular dosing schedule. Do not double doses.

**Storage**—To store this medicine:

- Keep out of the reach of children.
- Store away from heat and direct light.
- Do not store this medicine in the bathroom, near the kitchen sink, or in other damp places. Heat or moisture may cause the medicine to break down.
- Do not keep outdated medicine or medicine no longer needed. Be sure that any discarded medicine is out of the reach of children.

## Precautions While Using This Medicine

This medicine will add to the effects of alcohol and other CNS depressants (medicines that slow down the nervous system, possibly causing drowsiness). Some examples of CNS depressants are antihistamines or medicine for hay fever, other allergies, or colds; sedatives, tranquilizers, or sleeping medicine; prescription pain medicine or narcotics; barbiturates; medicine for seizures; other muscle relaxants; or anesthetics, including some dental anesthetics. *Check with your doctor before taking any of the above while you are using this medicine.*

This medicine may cause some people to have blurred vision or to become drowsy, dizzy, or less alert than they are normally. *Make sure you know how you react to this medicine before you drive, use machines, or do anything else that could be dangerous if you are dizzy or are not alert and able to see well.*

Cyclobenzaprine may cause dryness of the mouth. For temporary relief, use sugarless candy or gum, melt bits of ice in your mouth, or use a saliva substitute. However, if your mouth continues to feel dry for more than 2 weeks, check with your medical doctor or dentist. Continuing dryness of the mouth may increase the chance of dental disease, including tooth decay, gum disease, and fungus infections.

## Side Effects of This Medicine

Along with its needed effects, a medicine may cause some unwanted effects. Although not all of these side effects may occur, if they do occur they may need medical attention.

The following side effects may mean that you are having a serious allergic reaction to the medicine. *Get emergency help right away if any of them occurs:*

*Rare*

Changes in the skin color of the face; fast or irregular breathing; large swellings that look like hives on the face, eyelids, mouth, lips, and/or tongue; puffiness or swelling of the eyelids or the area around the eyes; shortness of breath, troubled breathing, tightness in chest, and/or wheezing; skin rash, hives, or itching

Also, check with your doctor immediately if any of the following side effects occur:

*Rare*

Fainting

*Symptoms of overdose*

Convulsions (seizures); drowsiness (severe); dry, hot, flushed skin; fast or irregular heartbeat; hallucinations (seeing, hearing, or feeling things that are not there); increase or decrease in body temperature; troubled breathing; unexplained muscle stiffness; unusual nervousness or restlessness (severe); vomiting (occurring together with other symptoms of overdose)

Also, check with your doctor as soon as possible if any of the following side effects occur:

*Rare*

Clumsiness or unsteadiness; confusion; mental depression or other mood or mental changes; problems in urinating; ringing or buzzing in the ears; skin rash, hives, or itching occurring without other symptoms of an allergic reaction listed above; unusual thoughts or dreams; yellow eyes or skin

Other side effects may occur that usually do not need medical attention. These side effects may go away during treatment as your body adjusts to the medicine. However, check with your doctor if any of the following side effects continue or are bothersome:

*More common*

Dizziness or lightheadedness; drowsiness; dryness of mouth

*Less common or rare*

Bloated feeling or gas, indigestion, nausea or vomiting, or stomach cramps or pain; blurred vision; constipation; decrease in blood pressure; diarrhea; excitement or nervousness; frequent urination; general feeling of discomfort or illness; headache; muscle twitching; numbness, tingling, pain, or weakness in hands or feet; pounding heartbeat; problems in speaking; trembling; trouble in sleeping; unpleasant taste or other taste changes; unusual muscle weakness; unusual tiredness

Other side effects not listed above may also occur in some patients. If you notice any other effects, check with your doctor.

## Additional Information

Once a medicine has been approved for marketing for a certain use, experience may show that it is also useful for other medical problems. Although this use is not included in product labeling, cyclobenzaprine is used in certain patients with fibromyalgia syndrome (also called fibrositis or fibrositis syndrome).

There is no additional information relating to proper use, precautions, or side effects for this use of cyclobenzaprine.

Revised: 07/28/94

# CYCLOPENTOLATE  Ophthalmic

Some commonly used brand names are:

**In the U.S.—**

| | |
|---|---|
| Ak-Pentolate | Ocu-Pentolate |
| Cyclogyl | Pentolair |
| I-Pentolate | Spectro-Pentolate |

Generic name product may also be available.

**In Canada**

| | |
|---|---|
| Ak-Pentolate | Minims Cyclopentolate |
| Cyclogyl | |

## Description

Cyclopentolate (sye-kloe-PEN-toe-late) is used to dilate (enlarge) the pupil. It is used before eye examinations (such as cycloplegic refraction or ophthalmoscopy), before or after certain eye surgery, and to treat certain eye conditions.

This medicine is available only with your doctor's prescription, in the following dosage form:

*Ophthalmic*

• Ophthalmic solution (eye drops) (U.S. and Canada)

## Before Using This Medicine

In deciding to use a medicine, the risks of using the medicine must be weighed against the good it will do.

This is a decision you and your doctor will make. For cyclopentolate, the following should be considered:

**Allergies**—Tell your doctor if you have ever had any unusual or allergic reaction to cyclopentolate. Also tell your health care professional if you are allergic to any other substances, such as preservatives.

**Pregnancy**—Cyclopentolate may be absorbed into the body. However, studies on effects in pregnancy have not been done in either humans or animals.

**Breast-feeding**—Cyclopentolate may be absorbed into the mother's body. It is not known whether cyclopentolate passes into the breast milk. However, cyclopentolate has not been reported to cause problems in nursing babies.

**Children**—Infants and young children and children with blond hair or blue eyes may be especially sensitive to the effects of cyclopentolate. This may increase the chance of side effects during treatment.

**Older adults**—Elderly people are especially sensitive to the effects of cyclopentolate. This may increase the chance of side effects during treatment.

**Other medicines**—Although certain medicines should not be used together at all, in other cases two different medicines may be used together even if an interaction might occur. In these cases, your doctor may want to change the dose, or other precautions may be necessary. Tell your health care professional if you are using any other prescription or nonprescription (over-the-counter [OTC]) medicine.

**Other medical problems**—The presence of other medical problems may affect the use of cyclopentolate. Make sure you tell your doctor if you have any other medical problems, especially:
- Brain damage (in children) or
- Down's syndrome (mongolism) (in children and adults) or
- Glaucoma or
- Spastic paralysis (in children)—Cyclopentolate may make the condition worse

## Proper Use of This Medicine

To use:
- First, wash your hands. Tilt the head back and with the index finger of one hand, press gently on the skin just beneath the lower eyelid and pull the lower eyelid away from the eye to make a space. Drop the medicine into this space. Let go of the eyelid and gently close the eyes. Do not blink. Keep the eyes closed and apply pressure to the inner corner of the eye with your finger for 2 or 3 minutes, to allow the medicine to be absorbed. *This is especially important in infants.*
- Immediately after using the eye drops, wash your hands to remove any medicine that may be on them. If you are using the eye drops for an infant or child, be sure to wash the infant's or child's hands also, and do not let any of the medicine get in the infant's or child's mouth.
- To keep the medicine as germ-free as possible, do not touch the applicator tip to any surface (including the eye). Also, keep the container tightly closed.

*Use this medicine only as directed.* Do not use more of it and do not use it more often than your doctor ordered. To do so may increase the chance of too much medicine being absorbed into the body and the chance of side effects.

**Dosing**—The dose of cyclopentolate will be different for different patients. *Follow your doctor's orders or the directions on the label.* The following information includes only the average doses of cyclopentolate. *If your dose is different, do not change it unless your doctor tells you to do so.*
- For *ophthalmic solution (eye drops)* dosage form:
  —For eye examinations:
    - Adults—One drop 40 to 50 minutes before the exam. Dose may be repeated in five to ten minutes.

- Children—One drop 40 to 50 minutes before the exam. After five to ten minutes, another drop may be used.
- Babies—One drop of 0.5% solution.

**Missed dose**—If you miss a dose of this medicine, apply it as soon as possible. However, if it is almost time for your next dose, skip the missed dose and go back to your regular dosing schedule. Do not double doses.

**Storage**—To store this medicine:
- Keep out of the reach of children. Overdose of this medicine is very dangerous for infants and children.
- Store away from heat and direct light.
- Keep the medicine from freezing.
- Do not keep outdated medicine or medicine no longer needed. Be sure that any discarded medicine is out of the reach of children.

## Precautions While Using This Medicine

After you apply this medicine to your eyes:
- Your pupils will become unusually large and you will have blurring of vision, especially for close objects. *Make sure your vision is clear before you drive, use machines, or do anything else that could be dangerous if you are not able to see well.*
- Your eyes will become more sensitive to light than they are normally. When you go out during the daylight hours, even on cloudy days, *wear sunglasses that block ultraviolet (UV) light to protect your eyes from sunlight and other bright lights.* Ordinary sunglasses may not protect your eyes. If you have any questions about the kind of sunglasses to wear, check with your doctor.

If these side effects continue for longer than 36 hours after you have stopped using this medicine, check with your doctor.

## Side Effects of This Medicine

Along with its needed effects, a medicine may cause some unwanted effects. Although not all of these side effects may occur, if they do occur they may need medical attention.

Check with your doctor as soon as possible if any of the following side effects occur:

*Symptoms of too much medicine being absorbed into the body*

Clumsiness or unsteadiness; confusion; fast or irregular heartbeat; fever; flushing or redness of face; hallucinations (seeing, hearing, or feeling things that are not there); skin rash; slurred speech; swollen stomach in infants; thirst or dryness of mouth; unusual behavior, especially in children; unusual drowsiness, tiredness, or weakness

Other side effects may occur that usually do not need medical attention. These side effects may go away during treatment as your body adjusts to the medicine. However,

check with your doctor if any of the following side effects continue or are bothersome:

> Blurred vision; burning of eye; eye irritation not present before therapy; increased sensitivity of eyes to light

Other side effects not listed above may also occur in some patients. If you notice any other effects, check with your doctor.

## Additional Information

Once a medicine has been approved for marketing for a certain use, experience may show that it is also useful for other medical problems. Although this use is not included in product labeling, cyclopentolate is used in certain patients with the following medical conditions:

- Posterior synechiae
- Uveitis

Other than the above information, there is no additional information relating to proper use, precautions, or side effects for these uses.

Revised: 03/04/92
Interim revision: 08/30/93

# CYCLOPHOSPHAMIDE    Systemic

Some commonly used brand names are:

**In the U.S.—**
Cytoxan                    Neosar
Generic name product may also be available.

**In Canada—**
Cytoxan                    Procytox

## Description

Cyclophosphamide (sye-kloe-FOSS-fa-mide) belongs to the group of medicines called alkylating agents. It is used to treat some kinds of cancer.

Cyclophosphamide interferes with the growth of cancer cells, which are eventually destroyed. Since the growth of normal body cells may also be affected by cyclophosphamide, other effects will also occur. Some of these may be serious and must be reported to your doctor. Other effects, like hair loss, may not be serious but may cause concern. Some effects may not occur for months or years after the medicine is used.

Cyclophosphamide is also used for treatment of some kinds of kidney disease.

Cyclophosphamide may also be used for other conditions as determined by your doctor.

Before you begin treatment with cyclophosphamide, you and your doctor should talk about the good this medicine will do as well as the risks of using it.

Cyclophosphamide is available only with your doctor's prescription, in the following dosage forms:

*Oral*
- Oral solution (U.S. and Canada)
- Tablets (U.S. and Canada)

*Parenteral*
- Injection (U.S. and Canada)

## Before Using This Medicine

In deciding to use a medicine, the risks of taking the medicine must be weighed against the good it will do.

This is a decision you and your doctor will make. For cyclophosphamide, the following should be considered:

**Allergies**—Tell your doctor if you have ever had any unusual or allergic reaction to cyclophosphamide.

**Pregnancy**—This medicine may cause several different birth defects if either the male or female is taking it at the time of conception or if it is taken during pregnancy. In addition, many cancer medicines may cause sterility. Although sterility occurs commonly with cyclophosphamide, it is usually only temporary.

Be sure that you have discussed this with your doctor before taking this medicine. It is best to use some kind of birth control while you are taking cyclophosphamide. Tell your doctor right away if you think you have become pregnant while taking cyclophosphamide.

**Breast-feeding**—Cyclophosphamide passes into the breast milk. Because this medicine may cause serious side effects, breast-feeding is generally not recommended while you are taking it.

**Children**—This medicine has been tested in children and has not been shown to cause different side effects or problems than it does in adults.

**Older adults**—Many medicines have not been studied specifically in older people. Therefore, it may not be known whether they work exactly the same way they do in younger adults. Although there is no specific information comparing use of cyclophosphamide in the elderly with use in other age groups, it is not expected to cause different side effects or problems in older people than it does in younger adults.

**Other medicines**—Although certain medicines should not be used together at all, in other cases two different medicines may be used together even if an interaction might occur. In these cases, your doctor may want to change the dose, or other precautions may be necessary. When

you are taking or receiving cyclophosphamide, it is especially important that your health care professional know if you are taking any of the following:

- Amphotericin B by injection (e.g., Fungizone) or
- Antithyroid agents (medicine for overactive thyroid) or
- Chloramphenicol (e.g., Chloromycetin) or
- Colchicine or
- Flucytosine (e.g., Ancobon) or
- Ganciclovir (e.g., Cytovene) or
- Interferon (e.g., Intron A, Roferon-A) or
- Plicamycin (e.g., Mithracin) or
- Zidovudine (e.g., AZT, Retrovir) or
- If you have ever been treated with radiation or cancer medicines—Cyclophosphamide may increase the effects of these medicines or radiation therapy on the blood
- Azathioprine (e.g., Imuran) or
- Chlorambucil (e.g., Leukeran) or
- Corticosteroids (cortisone-like medicine) or
- Cyclosporine (e.g., Sandimmune) or
- Mercaptopurine (e.g., Purinethol) or
- Muromonab-CD3 (monoclonal antibody) (e.g., Orthoclone OKT3)—There may be an increased risk of infection and development of cancer because cyclophosphamide reduces the body's ability to fight them
- Probenecid (e.g., Benemid) or
- Sulfinpyrazone (e.g., Anturane)—Cyclophosphamide may increase the amount of uric acid in the blood. Since these medicines are used to lower uric acid levels, they may not work as well in patients taking cyclophosphamide

**Other medical problems**—The presence of other medical problems may affect the use of cyclophosphamide. Make sure you tell your doctor if you have any other medical problems, especially:

- Chickenpox (including recent exposure) or
- Herpes zoster (shingles)—Risk of severe disease affecting other parts of the body
- Gout (history of) or
- Kidney stones—(history of)—Cyclophosphamide may increase levels of uric acid in the body, which can cause gout or kidney stones
- Infection—Cyclophosphamide can decrease your body's ability to fight infection
- Kidney disease—Effects of cyclophosphamide may be increased because of slower removal from the body
- Liver disease—The effect of cyclophosphamide may be decreased

## Proper Use of This Medicine

*Take this medicine only as directed by your doctor.* Do not take more or less of it, and do not take it more often than your doctor ordered. The exact amount of medicine you need has been carefully worked out. Taking too much may increase the chance of side effects, while taking too little may not improve your condition.

Cyclophosphamide is sometimes given together with certain other medicines. If you are using a combination of medicines, make sure that you take each one at the proper time and do not mix them. Ask your health care professional to help you plan a way to remember to take your medicines at the right times.

*While you are using cyclophosphamide, it is important that you drink extra fluids so that you will pass more urine.* Also, empty your bladder frequently, including at least once during the night. This will help prevent kidney and bladder problems and keep your kidneys working well. Cyclophosphamide passes from the body in the urine. If too much of it appears in the urine or if the urine stays in the bladder too long, it can cause dangerous irritation. *Follow your doctor's instructions carefully about how much fluid to drink every day.* Some patients may have to drink up to 7 to 12 cups (3 quarts) of fluid a day.

Usually it is best to take cyclophosphamide first thing in the morning, to reduce the risk of bladder problems. However, your doctor may want you to take it with food in smaller doses over the day, to lessen stomach upset or help the medicine work better. Follow your doctor's instructions carefully about when to take cyclophosphamide.

Cyclophosphamide often causes nausea, vomiting, and loss of appetite. However, it is very important that you continue to use the medicine even if you begin to feel ill. *Do not stop taking this medicine without first checking with your doctor.* Ask your health care professional for ways to lessen these effects.

If you vomit shortly after taking a dose of cyclophosphamide, check with your doctor. You will be told whether to take the dose again or to wait until the next scheduled dose.

**Dosing**—The dose of cyclophosphamide will be different for different patients. The dose that is used may depend on a number of things, including what the medicine is being used for, the patient's weight, whether the medicine is being given by mouth or by injection, and whether or not other medicines are also being taken. *If you are taking or receiving cyclophosphamide at home, follow your doctor's orders or the directions on the label.* If you have any questions about the proper dose of cyclophosphamide, ask your doctor.

**Missed dose**—If you miss a dose of this medicine, do not take the missed dose at all and do not double the next one. Instead, go back to your regular dosing schedule and check with your doctor.

**Storage**—To store this medicine:
- Keep out of the reach of children.
- Store away from heat and direct light.
- Do not store in the bathroom, near the kitchen sink, or in other damp places. Heat or moisture may cause the medicine to break down.
- Store the oral solution form of this medicine in the refrigerator. Keep it from freezing.
- Do not keep outdated medicine or medicine no longer needed. Be sure that any discarded medicine is out of the reach of children.

## Precautions While Using This Medicine

*It is very important that your doctor check your progress at regular visits* to make sure that this medicine is working properly and to check for unwanted effects.

While you are being treated with cyclophosphamide, and after you stop treatment with it, *do not have any immunizations (vaccinations) without your doctor's approval.* Cyclophosphamide may lower your body's resistance and there is a chance you might get the infection the immunization is meant to prevent. In addition, other persons living in your house should not take oral polio vaccine since there is a chance they could pass the polio virus on to you. Also, avoid persons who have recently taken oral polio vaccine. Do not get close to them, and do not stay in the same room with them for very long. If you cannot take these precautions, you should consider wearing a protective face mask that covers the nose and mouth.

Before having any kind of surgery, including dental surgery, or emergency treatment, make sure the medical doctor or dentist in charge knows that you are taking this medicine, especially if you have taken it within the last 10 days.

Cyclophosphamide can temporarily lower the number of white blood cells in your blood, increasing the chance of getting an infection. It can also lower the number of platelets, which are necessary for proper blood clotting. If this occurs, there are certain precautions you can take, especially when your blood count is low, to reduce the risk of infection or bleeding:

- If you can, avoid people with infections. *Check with your doctor immediately* if you think you are getting an infection or if you get a fever or chills, cough or hoarseness, lower back or side pain, or painful or difficult urination.
- *Check with your doctor immediately* if you notice any unusual bleeding or bruising; black, tarry stools; blood in urine or stools; or pinpoint red spots on your skin.
- Be careful when using a regular toothbrush, dental floss, or toothpick. Your medical doctor, dentist, or nurse may recommend other ways to clean your teeth and gums. Check with your medical doctor before having any dental work done.
- Do not touch your eyes or the inside of your nose unless you have just washed your hands and have not touched anything else in the meantime.
- Be careful not to cut yourself when you are using sharp objects such as a safety razor or fingernail or toenail cutters.
- Avoid contact sports or other situations where bruising or injury could occur.

Before you have any medical tests, tell the medical doctor in charge that you are taking this medicine. The results of some tests may be affected by this medicine.

## Side Effects of This Medicine

Along with its needed effects, a medicine may cause some unwanted effects. Although not all of these side effects may occur, if they do occur they may need medical attention.

Also, because of the way these medicines act on the body, there is a chance that they might cause other unwanted effects that may not occur until months or years after the medicine is used. These may include certain types of cancer, such as leukemia or bladder cancer. Discuss these possible effects with your doctor.

*Stop taking this medicine and check with your doctor immediately* if the following side effects occur:

*With high doses and/or long-term treatment*
  Blood in urine; painful urination

*Check with your doctor or nurse immediately* if any of the following side effects occur:

*Less common*
  Cough or hoarseness; fever or chills; lower back or side pain; painful or difficult urination

*Rare*
  Black, tarry stools; blood in urine or stools; pinpoint red spots on skin; shortness of breath (sudden); unusual bleeding or bruising

Check with your doctor as soon as possible if any of the following side effects occur:

*More common*
  Dizziness, confusion, or agitation; missing menstrual periods; unusual tiredness or weakness

*Less common*
  Fast heartbeat; joint pain; shortness of breath; swelling of feet or lower legs

*Rare*
  Frequent urination; redness, swelling, or pain at place of injection; sores in mouth and on lips; unusual thirst; yellow eyes or skin

Other side effects may occur that usually do not need medical attention. These side effects may go away during treatment as your body adjusts to the medicine. Also, your health care professional may be able to tell you about ways to prevent or reduce some of these side effects. Check with your health care professional if any of the following side effects continue or are bothersome or if you have any questions about them:

*More common*
  Darkening of skin and fingernails; loss of appetite; nausea or vomiting

*Less common*
  Diarrhea or stomach pain; flushing or redness of face; headache; increased sweating; skin rash, hives, or itching; swollen lips

Cyclophosphamide may cause a temporary loss of hair in some people. After treatment has ended, normal hair growth should return, although the new hair may be a slightly different color or texture.

After you stop using cyclophosphamide, it may still produce some side effects that need attention. During this period of time, *check with your doctor immediately* if you notice the following side effect:

Blood in urine

Other side effects not listed above may also occur in some patients. If you notice any other effects, check with your doctor.

## Additional Information

Once a medicine has been approved for marketing for a certain use, experience may show that it is also useful for other medical problems. Although these uses are not included in product labeling, cyclophosphamide is used in certain patients with the following medical conditions:

- Organ transplant rejection (prevention)
- Rheumatoid arthritis
- Wegener's granulomatosis
- Systemic lupus erythematosus
- Systemic dermatomyositis or
- Multiple sclerosis

Other than the above information, there is no additional information relating to proper use, precautions, or side effects for these uses.

Revised: 07/11/94

# CYCLOSERINE   Systemic†

A commonly used brand name is Seromycin.

†Not commercially available in Canada.

## Description

Cycloserine (sye-kloe-SER-een) belongs to the family of medicines called antibiotics. It is used to treat tuberculosis (TB). When cycloserine is used for TB, it is given with other medicines for TB. Cycloserine may also be used for other conditions as determined by your doctor.

*To help clear up your tuberculosis (TB) completely, you must keep taking this medicine for the full time of treatment, even if you begin to feel better. This is very important. It is also important that you do not miss any doses.*

Cycloserine is available only with your doctor's prescription, in the following dosage form:

*Oral*
- Capsules (U.S.)

## Before Using This Medicine

In deciding to use a medicine, the risks of taking the medicine must be weighed against the good it will do. This is a decision you and your doctor will make. For cycloserine, the following should be considered:

**Allergies**—Tell your doctor if you have ever had any unusual or allergic reaction to cycloserine. Also, tell your health care professional if you are allergic to any other substances, such as foods, preservatives, or dyes.

**Pregnancy**—Cycloserine has not been shown to cause birth defects or other problems in humans.

**Breast-feeding**—Cycloserine passes into the breast milk. However, cycloserine has not been reported to cause problems in nursing babies.

**Children**—Although there is no specific information comparing use of cycloserine in children with use in other age groups, this medicine is not expected to cause different side effects or problems in children than it does in adults.

**Older adults**—Many medicines have not been studied specifically in older people. Therefore, it may not be known whether they work exactly the same way they do in younger adults. Although there is no specific information comparing use of cycloserine in the elderly with use in other age groups, this medicine is not expected to cause different side effects or problems in older people than it does in younger adults.

**Other medicines**—Although certain medicines should not be used together at all, in other cases two different medicines may be used together even if an interaction might occur. In these cases, your doctor may want to change the dose, or other precautions may be necessary. When you are taking cycloserine, it is especially important that your health care professional know if you are taking the following:

- Ethionamide (e.g., Trecator-SC)—Ethionamide may increase the risk of nervous system side effects, especially seizures

**Other medical problems**—The presence of other medical problems may affect the use of cycloserine. Make sure you tell your doctor if you have any other medical problems, especially:

- Alcohol abuse (or history of) or
- Convulsive disorders such as seizures or epilepsy—Cycloserine may increase the risk of seizures in patients who drink alcohol or have a history of seizures
- Kidney disease—Cycloserine is removed from the body through the kidneys, and patients with kidney disease may need an adjustment in dose or the medicine may need to be discontinued

- Mental disorders such as mental depression, psychosis, or severe anxiety—Cycloserine may cause anxiety, mental depression, or psychosis

## Proper Use of This Medicine

Cycloserine may be taken after meals if it upsets your stomach.

To help clear up your infection completely, *it is very important that you keep taking this medicine for the full time of treatment,* even if you begin to feel better after a few weeks. If you are taking this medicine for TB, you may have to take it every day for as long as 1 to 2 years or more. If you stop taking this medicine too soon, your symptoms may return.

This medicine works best when there is a constant amount in the blood or urine. *To help keep the amount constant, do not miss any doses. Also, it is best to take the doses at evenly spaced times day and night.* For example, if you are to take 2 doses a day, the doses should be spaced about 12 hours apart. If this interferes with your sleep or other daily activities, or if you need help in planning the best times to take your medicine, check with your health care professional.

**Dosing**—The dose of cycloserine will be different for different patients. *Follow your doctor's orders or the directions on the label.* The following information includes only the average doses of cycloserine. *If your dose is different, do not change it* unless your doctor tells you to do so.

- For the *oral* dosage form (capsules):
  —For treatment of tuberculosis:
    - Adults and teenagers—250 milligrams (mg) two times a day to start. Your doctor may slowly increase your dose up to 250 mg three or four times a day. This medicine must be taken along with other medicines to treat tuberculosis.
    - Children—Use and dose must be determined by your doctor. Doses of 10 to 20 mg per kilogram (4.5 to 9.1 mg per pound) of body weight per day have been used. This medicine must be taken along with other medicines to treat tuberculosis.

**Missed dose**—If you do miss a dose of this medicine, take it as soon as possible. This will help to keep a constant amount of medicine in the blood or urine. However, if it is almost time for your next dose, skip the missed dose and go back to your regular dosing schedule. Do not double doses.

**Storage**—To store this medicine:
- Keep out of the reach of children.
- Store away from heat and direct light.
- Do not store in the bathroom, near the kitchen sink, or in other damp places. Heat or moisture may cause the medicine to break down.

- Do not keep outdated medicine or medicine no longer needed. Be sure that any discarded medicine is out of the reach of children.

## Precautions While Using This Medicine

It is very important that your doctor check your progress at regular visits.

If your symptoms do not improve within 2 to 3 weeks, or if they become worse, check with your doctor.

*If cycloserine causes you to feel very depressed or to have thoughts of suicide, check with your doctor immediately.* Your doctor will probably want to change your medicine.

This medicine may cause some people to become dizzy, drowsy, or less alert than they are normally. *Make sure you know how you react to this medicine before you drive, use machines, or do anything else that could be dangerous if you are dizzy or are not alert.* If these reactions are especially bothersome, check with your doctor.

Some of cycloserine's side effects (for example, convulsions [seizures]) may be more likely to occur if you drink alcoholic beverages regularly while you are taking this medicine. Therefore, *you should not drink alcoholic beverages while you are taking this medicine.*

## Side Effects of This Medicine

Along with its needed effects, a medicine may cause some unwanted effects. Although not all of these side effects may occur, if they do occur they may need medical attention.

*Check with your doctor immediately* if any of the following side effects occur:

*More common*
    Anxiety; confusion; dizziness; drowsiness; increased irritability; increased restlessness; mental depression; muscle twitching or trembling; nervousness; nightmares; other mood or mental changes; speech problems; thoughts of suicide

*Less common*
    Convulsions (seizures); numbness, tingling, burning pain, or weakness in the hands or feet; skin rash

Other side effects may occur that usually do not need medical attention. These side effects may go away during treatment as your body adjusts to the medicine. However, check with your doctor if the following side effect continues or is bothersome:

*More common*
    Headache

Other side effects not listed above may also occur in some patients. If you notice any other effects, check with your doctor.

## Additional Information

Once a medicine has been approved for marketing for a certain use, experience may show that it is also useful for other medical problems. Although this use is not included in product labeling, ethambutol is used in certain patients with the following medical condition:

- Atypical mycobacterial infections, such as *Mycobacterium avium* complex (MAC)

Other than the above information, there is no additional information relating to proper use, precautions, or side effects for this use.

---

Revised: 05/02/94

---

# CYCLOSPORINE   Systemic

A commonly used brand name in the U.S. and Canada is Sandimmune. Some other commonly used names are ciclosporin and cyclosporin A.

## Description

Cyclosporine (SYE-kloe-spor-een) belongs to the group of medicines known as immunosuppressive agents. It is used to reduce the body's natural immunity in patients who receive organ (for example, kidney, liver, and heart) transplants.

When a patient receives an organ transplant, the body's white blood cells will try to get rid of (reject) the transplanted organ. Cyclosporine works by preventing the white blood cells from doing this.

Cyclosporine may also be used for other conditions, as determined by your doctor.

Cyclosporine is a very strong medicine. It may cause side effects that could be very serious, such as high blood pressure and kidney and liver problems. It may also reduce the body's ability to fight infections. You and your doctor should talk about the good this medicine will do as well as the risks of using it.

Cyclosporine is available only with your doctor's prescription, in the following dosage forms:

*Oral*
- Capsules (U.S. and Canada)
- Oral solution (U.S. and Canada)

*Parenteral*
- Injection (U.S. and Canada)

## Before Using This Medicine

In deciding to use a medicine, the risks of taking the medicine must be weighed against the good it will do. This is a decision you and your doctor will make. For cyclosporine, the following should be considered:

**Allergies**—Tell your doctor if you have ever had any unusual or allergic reaction to cyclosporine.

**Pregnancy**—Studies have not been done in humans. However, studies in rats and rabbits have shown that cyclosporine at toxic doses (2 to 5 times the human dose) causes birth defects or death of the fetus.

**Breast-feeding**—Cyclosporine passes into breast milk. There is a chance that it could cause the same side effects in the baby that it does in people taking it. It may be necessary for you to stop breast-feeding during treatment. Be sure you have discussed the risks and benefits of the medicine with your doctor.

**Children**—This medicine has been tested in children and, in effective doses, has not been shown to cause different side effects or problems than it does in adults.

**Older adults**—Many medicines have not been studied specifically in older people. Therefore, it may not be known whether they work exactly the same way they do in younger adults. Although there is no specific information comparing use of cyclosporine in the elderly with use in other age groups, this medicine is not expected to cause different side effects or problems in older people than it does in younger adults.

**Other medicines**—Although certain medicines should not be used together at all, in other cases two different medicines may be used together even if an interaction might occur. In these cases, your doctor may want to change the dose, or other precautions may be necessary. When you are taking cyclosporine, it is especially important that your health care professional knows if you are taking any of the following:

- Amiloride or
- Spironolactone (e.g., Aldactone) or
- Triamterene (e.g., Dyrenium)—Since both cyclosporine and these medicines increase the amount of potassium in the body, potassium levels could become too high
- Androgens (male hormones) or
- Cimetidine (e.g., Tagamet) or
- Danazol (e.g., Danocrine) or
- Diltiazem (e.g., Cardizem) or
- Erythromycins (medicine for infection) or
- Estrogens (female hormones) or
- Ketoconazole (e.g., Nizoral)—May increase effects of cyclosporine by increasing the amount of this medicine in the body
- Azathioprine (e.g., Imuran) or
- Chlorambucil (e.g., Leukeran) or
- Corticosteroids (cortisone-like medicine) or
- Cyclophosphamide (e.g., Cytoxan) or
- Mercaptopurine (e.g., Purinethol) or
- Muromonab-CD3 (monoclonal antibody) (e.g., Orthoclone OKT3)—There may be an increased risk of infection and

cancer because both cyclosporine and these medicines decrease the body's ability to fight them
- Lovastatin (e.g., Mevacor)—May increase the risk of kidney problems

**Other medical problems**—The presence of other medical problems may affect the use of cyclosporine. Make sure you tell your doctor if you have any other medical problems, especially:
- Chickenpox (including recent exposure) or
- Herpes zoster (shingles)—Risk of severe disease affecting other parts of the body
- Infection—Cyclosporine decreases the body's ability to fight infection
- Intestine problems—Effects may be decreased because cyclosporine cannot be absorbed into the body
- Kidney disease—Cyclosporine can have harmful effects on the kidney when it is taken for long periods of time
- Liver disease—Effects of cyclosporine may be increased because of slower removal from the body

## Proper Use of This Medicine

*Take this medicine only as directed by your doctor.* Do not take more or less of it and do not take it more often than your doctor ordered. The exact amount of medicine you need has been carefully worked out. Taking too much may increase the chance of side effects, while taking too little may not improve your condition.

To help you remember to take your medicine, try to get into the habit of taking it at the same time each day. This will also help cyclosporine work better by keeping a constant amount in the blood.

This medicine is to be taken by mouth even if it comes in a dropper bottle. The amount you should take is to be measured only with the specially marked dropper provided with your prescription. The dropper should be wiped with a clean towel after it is used, and stored in its container. If the dropper needs to be cleaned, make sure it is completely dry before using it again.

To make cyclosporine taste better, mix it in a glass container with milk, chocolate milk, or orange juice (preferably at room temperature). Do not use a wax-lined or plastic disposable container. Stir it well, then drink it immediately. After drinking all the liquid containing the medicine, rinse the glass with a little more liquid and drink that also, to make sure you get all the medicine. Dry the dropper used to measure the cyclosporine, but do not rinse it with water.

If this medicine upsets your stomach, your doctor may recommend that you take it with meals. However, check with your doctor before you decide to do this on your own.

*Do not stop taking this medicine without first checking with your doctor.* You may have to take medicine for the rest of your life to prevent your body from rejecting the transplant.

**Dosing**—The dose of cyclosporine will be different for different patients. *Follow your doctor's orders or the*
directions on the label. The following information includes only the average doses of cyclosporine. *If your dose is different, do not change it* unless your doctor tells you to do so.

The number of capsules or teaspoonfuls of oral solution that you take depends on the strength of the medicine. Also, *the number of doses you take each day, the time allowed between doses, and the length of time you take the medicine depend on the medical problem for which you are taking cyclosporine.*
- For *oral* dosage forms (capsules, oral solution):
  —For transplant rejection:
    • Adults, teenagers, or children: Dose is based on body weight. The usual dose in the beginning is 12 to 15 milligrams (mg) per kilogram (kg) (5.5 to 6.8 mg per pound) a day. After a period of time, the dose may be decreased to 5 to 10 mg per kg (2.3 to 4.5 mg per pound) a day.
- For *injection* dosage form:
  —For transplant rejection:
    • Adults, teenagers, or children: Dose is based on body weight. The usual dose is 2 to 6 mg per kg (0.9 to 2.7 mg per pound) a day.

**Missed dose**—If you miss a dose of cyclosporine and remember it within 12 hours, take the missed dose as soon as you remember. However, if it is almost time for the next dose, skip the missed dose, go back to your regular dosing schedule, and check with your doctor. Do not double doses.

**Storage**—To store this medicine:
- Keep out of the reach of children.
- Store away from heat and direct light.
- Do not store in the bathroom, near the kitchen sink, or in other damp places. Heat or moisture may cause the medicine to break down.
- Do not store the oral solution in the refrigerator.
- Do not keep outdated medicine or medicine no longer needed. Be sure that any discarded medicine is out of the reach of children.

## Precautions While Using This Medicine

*It is very important that your doctor check your progress at regular visits.* Your doctor will want to do laboratory tests to make sure that cyclosporine is working properly and to check for unwanted effects.

While you are being treated with cyclosporine, and after you stop treatment with it, *do not have any immunizations (vaccinations) without your doctor's approval.* Cyclosporine lowers your body's resistance and there is a chance you might get the infection the immunization is meant to prevent. In addition, other persons living in your house should not take oral polio vaccine since there is a chance they could pass the polio virus on to you. Also, avoid persons who have recently taken oral polio vaccine. Do not get close to them, and do not stay in the same room with them for very long. If you cannot take these precautions, you should consider wearing a protective face mask that covers the nose and mouth.

In some patients (usually younger patients), tenderness, swelling, or bleeding of the gums may appear soon after treatment with cyclosporine is started. Brushing and flossing your teeth carefully and regularly and massaging your gums may help prevent this. *See your dentist regularly to have your teeth cleaned. Check with your medical doctor or dentist if you have any questions about how to take care of your teeth and gums, or if you notice any tenderness, swelling, or bleeding of your gums.*

## Side Effects of This Medicine

Along with its needed effects, a medicine may cause some unwanted effects. Some side effects will have signs or symptoms that you can see or feel. Your doctor will watch for others by doing certain tests.

Also, because of the way that cyclosporine acts on the body, there is a chance that it may cause effects that may not occur until years after the medicine is used. These delayed effects may include certain types of cancer, such as lymphomas or skin cancers. You and your doctor should discuss the good this medicine will do as well as the risks of using it.

*Check with your doctor or nurse immediately* if any of the following side effects occur:

*Less common*
Fever or chills; frequent urge to urinate

*Rare*
Blood in urine; flushing of face and neck (for injection only); wheezing or shortness of breath (for injection only)

Check with your doctor as soon as possible if any of the following side effects occur:

*More common*
Bleeding, tender, or enlarged gums

*Less common*
Convulsions (seizures)

*Rare*
Confusion; irregular heartbeat; numbness or tingling in hands, feet, or lips; shortness of breath or difficult breathing; stomach pain (severe) with nausea and vomiting; unexplained nervousness; unusual tiredness or weakness; weakness or heaviness of legs

This medicine may also cause the following side effects that your doctor will watch for:

*More common*
High blood pressure; kidney problems

*Less common*
Liver problems

Other side effects may occur that usually do not need medical attention. These side effects may go away during treatment as your body adjusts to the medicine. However, check with your doctor if any of the following side effects continue or are bothersome:

*More common*
Increase in hair growth; trembling and shaking of hands

*Less common*
Acne or oily skin; headache; leg cramps; nausea or vomiting

Other side effects not listed above may also occur in some patients. If you notice any other effects, check with your doctor.

Revised: 06/09/93
Interim revision: 05/12/94

# CYTARABINE  Systemic

Some commonly used brand names are:
**In the U.S.**
Cytosar-U
Generic name product may also be available.
**In Canada**
Cytosar
Other commonly used names are ara-C and cytosine arabinoside.

## Description

Cytarabine (sye-TARE-a-been) belongs to the group of medicines called antimetabolites. It is used to treat some kinds of cancer.

Cytarabine interferes with the growth of cancer cells, which are eventually destroyed. Since the growth of normal body cells may also be affected by cytarabine, other effects will also occur. Some of these may be serious and must be reported to your doctor. Other effects, like hair loss, may not be serious but may cause concern. Some effects may not occur for months or years after the medicine is used.

Before you begin treatment with cytarabine, you and your doctor should talk about the good this medicine will do as well as the risks of using it.

Cytarabine is to be administered only by or under the immediate supervision of your doctor. It is available in the following dosage form:

*Parenteral*
• Injection (U.S. and Canada)

## Before Using This Medicine

In deciding to use a medicine, the risks of taking the medicine must be weighed against the good it will do. This is a decision you and your doctor will make. For cytarabine, the following should be considered:

**Allergies**—Tell your doctor if you have ever had any unusual or allergic reaction to cytarabine.

**Pregnancy**—This medicine may cause birth defects (such as defects of the arms, legs, or ears, which occurred in two babies) if either the male or female is taking it at the time of conception or if it is taken during pregnancy. In addition, many cancer medicines may cause sterility. Although sterility has been reported with this medicine, it is usually only temporary.

Be sure that you have discussed this with your doctor before taking this medicine. It is best to use some kind of birth control while you are receiving cytarabine. Tell your doctor right away if you think you have become pregnant while receiving cytarabine.

**Breast-feeding**—Because cytarabine may cause serious side effects, breast-feeding is generally not recommended while you are receiving it.

**Children**—Although there is no specific information comparing use of cytarabine in children with use in other age groups, this medicine is not expected to cause different side effects or problems in children than it does in adults.

**Older adults**—Many medicines have not been studied specifically in older people. Therefore, it may not be known whether they work exactly the same way they do in younger adults. Although there is no specific information comparing use of cytarabine in the elderly with use in other age groups, this medicine is not expected to cause different side effects or problems in older people than it does in younger adults.

**Other medicines**—Although certain medicines should not be used together at all, in other cases two different medicines may be used together even if an interaction might occur. In these cases, your doctor may want to change the dose, or other precautions may be necessary. When you are receiving cytarabine, it is especially important that your health care professional know if you are taking any of the following:

- Amphotericin B by injection (e.g., Fungizone) or
- Antithyroid agents (medicine for overactive thyroid) or
- Azathioprine (e.g., Imuran) or
- Chloramphenicol (e.g., Chloromycetin) or
- Colchicine or
- Flucytosine (e.g., Ancobon) or
- Ganciclovir (e.g., Cytovene) or
- Interferon (e.g., Intron A, Roferon-A) or
- Plicamycin (e.g., Mithracin) or
- Zidovudine (e.g., AZT, Retrovir) or
- If you have ever been treated with radiation or cancer medicines—Cytarabine may increase the effects of these medicines or radiation therapy on the blood
- Azathioprine (e.g., Imuran) or
- Chlorambucil (e.g., Leukeran) or
- Corticosteroids (cortisone-like medicine) or

- Cyclosporine (e.g., Sandimmune) or
- Mercaptopurine (e.g., Purinethol) or
- Muromonab-CD3 (monoclonal antibody) (e.g., Orthoclone OKT3) or
- Tacrolimus (e.g., Prograf)—There may be an increased risk of infection because cytarabine decreases your body's ability to fight it
- Probenecid (e.g., Benemid) or
- Sulfinpyrazone (e.g., Anturane)—Cytarabine may raise the concentration of uric acid in the blood. Since these medicines are used to lower uric acid levels, they may not work as well in patients receiving cytarabine

**Other medical problems**—The presence of other medical problems may affect the use of cytarabine. Make sure you tell your doctor if you have any other medical problems, especially:

- Chickenpox (including recent exposure) or
- Herpes zoster (shingles)—Risk of severe disease affecting other parts of the body
- Gout (history of) or
- Kidney stones (history of)—Cytarabine may increase levels of uric acid in the body, which can cause gout or kidney stones
- Infection—Cytarabine can decrease your body's ability to fight infection
- Kidney disease or
- Liver disease—Effects of cytarabine may be increased because of slower removal from the body

## Proper Use of This Medicine

This medicine is sometimes given together with certain other medicines. If you are using a combination of medicines, it is important that you receive each one at the proper time. If you are taking some of these medicines by mouth, ask your health care professional to help you plan a way to take them at the right times.

While you are receiving this medicine, your doctor may want you to drink extra fluids so that you will pass more urine. This will help prevent kidney problems and keep your kidneys working well.

This medicine often causes nausea and vomiting. However, it is very important that you continue to receive the medicine even if you begin to feel ill. Ask your health care professional for ways to lessen these effects.

**Dosing**—The dose of cytarabine will be different for different patients. The dose that is used may depend on a number of things, including what the medicine is being used for, the patient's weight, and whether or not other medicines are also being taken. *If you are receiving cytarabine at home, follow your doctor's orders or the directions on the label.* If you have any questions about the proper dose of cytarabine, ask your doctor.

## Precautions While Using This Medicine

*It is very important that your doctor check your progress at regular visits* to make sure that this medicine is working properly and to check for unwanted effects.

While you are being treated with cytarabine, and after you stop treatment with it, *do not have any immunizations (vaccinations) without your doctor's approval.* Cytarabine may lower your body's resistance and there is a chance you might get the infection the immunization is meant to prevent. In addition, other persons living in your household should not take oral polio vaccine since there is a chance they could pass the polio virus on to you. Also, avoid persons who have taken oral polio vaccine. Do not get close to them and do not stay in the same room with them for very long. If you cannot take these precautions, you should consider wearing a protective face mask that covers the nose and mouth.

Cytarabine can temporarily lower the number of white blood cells in your blood, increasing the chance of getting an infection. It can also lower the number of platelets, which are necessary for proper blood clotting. If this occurs, there are certain precautions you can take, especially when your blood count is low, to reduce the risk of infection or bleeding:

- If you can, avoid people with infections. *Check with your doctor immediately* if you think you are getting an infection or if you get a fever or chills, cough or hoarseness, lower back or side pain, or painful or difficult urination.
- *Check with your doctor immediately* if you notice any unusual bleeding or bruising; black, tarry stools; blood in urine or stools; or pinpoint red spots on your skin.
- Be careful when using a regular toothbrush, dental floss, or toothpick. Your medical doctor, dentist, or nurse may recommend other ways to clean your teeth and gums. Check with your medical doctor before having any dental work done.
- Do not touch your eyes or the inside of your nose unless you have just washed your hands and have not touched anything else in the meantime.
- Be careful not to cut yourself when you are using sharp objects such as a safety razor or fingernail or toenail cutters.
- Avoid contact sports or other situations where bruising or injury could occur.

## Side Effects of This Medicine

Along with its needed effects, a medicine may cause some unwanted effects. Although not all of these side effects may occur, if they do occur they may need medical attention.

Also, because of the way these medicines act on the body, there is a chance that they might cause other unwanted effects that may not occur until months or years after the medicine is used. These delayed effects may include certain types of cancer, such as leukemia. Discuss these possible effects with your doctor.

*Check with your doctor or nurse immediately* if any of the following side effects occur:

*Less common*

Black, tarry stools; blood in urine; cough or hoarseness; fever or chills; lower back or side pain; painful or difficult urination; pinpoint red spots on skin; unusual bleeding or bruising

Check with your health care professional as soon as possible if any of the following side effects occur:

*More common*

Sores in mouth and on lips

*Less common*

Joint pain; numbness or tingling in fingers, toes, or face; swelling of feet or lower legs; unusual tiredness

*Rare*

Bone or muscle pain; chest pain; decrease in urination; difficulty in swallowing; fainting spells; general feeling of discomfort or illness or weakness; heartburn; irregular heartbeat; pain at place of injection; reddened eyes; shortness of breath; skin rash; weakness; yellow eyes or skin

Other side effects may occur that usually do not need medical attention. These side effects may go away during treatment as your body adjusts to the medicine. Also, your health care professional may be able to tell you about ways to prevent or reduce some of these side effects. Check with your health care professional if any of the following side effects continue or are bothersome or if you have any questions about them:

*More common*

Loss of appetite; nausea and vomiting

*Less common or rare*

Diarrhea; dizziness; headache; itching of skin; skin freckling

This medicine may cause a temporary loss of hair in some people. After treatment with cytarabine has ended, normal hair growth should return.

After you stop receiving cytarabine, it may still produce some side effects that need attention. During this period of time check with your doctor if you notice any of the following:

Black, tarry stools; blood in urine or stools; cough or hoarseness; fever or chills; lower back or side pain; painful or difficult urination; pinpoint red spots on skin; unusual bleeding or bruising

Other side effects not listed above may also occur in some patients. If you notice any other effects, check with your doctor.

Revised: 07/15/94

# DACARBAZINE  Systemic

## Description

Dacarbazine (da-KAR-ba-zeen) belongs to the group of medicines called alkylating agents. It is used to treat some kinds of cancer.

Dacarbazine interferes with the growth of cancer cells, which are eventually destroyed. Since the growth of normal body cells may also be affected by dacarbazine, other effects will also occur. Some of these may be serious and must be reported to your doctor. Other effects, like hair loss, may not be serious but may cause concern. Some effects may not occur for months or years after the medicine is used.

Before you begin treatment with dacarbazine, you and your doctor should talk about the good this medicine will do as well as the risks of using it.

Dacarbazine is to be administered only by or under the immediate supervision of your doctor. It is available in the following dosage form:

*Parenteral*
  • Injection (U.S. and Canada)

## Before Using This Medicine

In deciding to use a medicine, the risks of taking the medicine must be weighed against the good it will do. This is a decision you and your doctor will make. For dacarbazine, the following should be considered:

**Allergies**—Tell your doctor if you have ever had any unusual or allergic reaction to dacarbazine.

**Pregnancy**—There is a chance that this medicine may cause birth defects if either the male or female is taking it at the time of conception or if it is taken during pregnancy. In addition, many cancer medicines may cause sterility, which could be permanent. Although sterility has not been reported with this medicine, the possibility should be kept in mind. Dacarbazine has caused birth defects and a decrease in successful pregnancies in animal studies involving rats and rabbits given doses several times the usual human adult dose.

Be sure that you have discussed this with your doctor before taking this medicine. It is best to use some kind of birth control while you are receiving dacarbazine. Tell your doctor right away if you think you have become pregnant while receiving dacarbazine.

**Breast-feeding**—It is not known whether dacarbazine passes into breast milk. However, because this medicine may cause serious side effects, breast-feeding is generally not recommended while you are receiving it.

**Children**—Studies on this medicine have been done only in adult patients and there is no specific information comparing use of dacarbazine in children with use in other age groups.

**Older adults**—Many medicines have not been studied specifically in older people. Therefore, it may not be known whether they work exactly the same way they do in younger adults or if they cause different side effects or problems in older people. There is no specific information about the use of dacarbazine in the elderly.

**Other medicines**—Although certain medicines should not be used together at all, in other cases two different medicines may be used together even if an interaction might occur. In these cases, your doctor may want to change the dose, or other precautions may be necessary. When receiving dacarbazine it is especially important that your health care professional know if you are taking any of the following:

  • Amphotericin B by injection (e.g., Fungizone) or
  • Antithyroid agents (medicine for overactive thyroid) or
  • Azathioprine (e.g., Imuran) or
  • Chloramphenicol (e.g., Chloromycetin) or
  • Colchicine or
  • Flucytosine (e.g., Ancobon) or
  • Ganciclovir (e.g., Cytovene) or
  • Interferon (e.g., Intron A, Roferon-A) or
  • Plicamycin (e.g., Mithracin) or
  • Zidovudine (e.g., AZT, Retrovir) or
  • If you have ever been treated with radiation or cancer medicines—Dacarbazine may increase the effects of these medicines or radiation therapy on the blood

**Other medical problems**—The presence of other medical problems may affect the use of dacarbazine. Make sure you tell your doctor if you have any other medical problems, especially:

  • Chickenpox (including recent exposure) or
  • Herpes zoster (shingles)—Risk of severe disease affecting other parts of the body
  • Infection—Dacarbazine can decrease your body's ability to fight infection
  • Kidney disease or
  • Liver disease—Effects of dacarbazine may be increased because of slower removal from the body

## Proper Use of This Medicine

Dacarbazine is sometimes given together with certain other medicines. If you are using a combination of medicines, it is important that you receive each one at the proper time. If you are taking some of these medicines by mouth, ask your health care professional to help you plan a way to remember to take them at the right times.

This medicine often causes nausea, vomiting, and loss of appetite. The injection may also cause a feeling of burning or pain. However, it is very important that you continue to receive the medicine, even if you have discomfort or begin to feel ill. After 1 or 2 days, your stomach upset should lessen. Ask your health care professional for ways to lessen these effects.

**Dosing**—The dose of dacarbazine will be different for different patients. The dose that is used may depend on a number of things, including what the medicine is being used for, the patient's weight, and whether or not other medicines are also being taken. *If you are receiving dacarbazine at home, follow your doctor's orders or the directions on the label.* If you have any questions about the proper dose of dacarbazine, ask your doctor.

## Precautions While Using This Medicine

*It is very important that your doctor check your progress at regular visits* to make sure that this medicine is working properly and to check for unwanted effects.

While you are being treated with dacarbazine, and after you stop treatment with it, *do not have any immunizations (vaccinations) without your doctor's approval.* Dacarbazine may lower your body's resistance and there is a chance you might get the infection the immunization is meant to prevent. In addition, other persons living in your household should not take oral polio vaccine since there is a chance they could pass the polio virus on to you. Also, avoid persons who have taken oral polio vaccine. Do not get close to them, and do not stay in the same room with them for very long. If you cannot take these precautions, you should consider wearing a protective face mask that covers the nose and mouth.

Dacarbazine can temporarily lower the number of white blood cells in your blood, increasing the chance of getting an infection. It can also lower the number of platelets, which are necessary for proper blood clotting. If this occurs, there are certain precautions you can take, especially when your blood count is low, to reduce the risk of infection or bleeding:

- If you can, avoid people with infections. *Check with your doctor immediately* if you think you are getting an infection or if you get a fever or chills, cough or hoarseness, lower back or side pain, or painful or difficult urination.
- *Check with your doctor immediately* if you notice any unusual bleeding or bruising; black, tarry stools; blood in urine or stools; or pinpoint red spots on your skin.
- Be careful when using a regular toothbrush, dental floss, or toothpick. Your medical doctor, dentist, or nurse may recommend other ways to clean your teeth and gums. Check with your medical doctor before having any dental work done.
- Do not touch your eyes or the inside of your nose unless you have just washed your hands and have not touched anything else in the meantime.

- Be careful not to cut yourself when you are using sharp objects such as a safety razor or fingernail or toenail cutters.
- Avoid contact sports or other situations where bruising or injury could occur.

If dacarbazine accidentally seeps out of the vein into which it is injected, it may damage some tissues and cause scarring. *Tell the doctor or nurse right away if you notice redness, pain, or swelling at the place of injection.*

## Side Effects of This Medicine

Along with its needed effects, a medicine may cause some unwanted effects. Although not all of these side effects may occur, if they do occur they may need medical attention.

Also, because of the way these medicines act on the body, there is a chance that they might cause other unwanted effects that may not occur until months or years after the medicine is used. These delayed effects may include certain types of cancer, such as leukemia. Discuss these possible effects with your doctor.

*Check with your doctor or nurse immediately* if any of the following side effects occur:

*More common*
   Redness, pain, or swelling at place of injection

*Less common*
   Black, tarry stools; blood in urine or stools; cough or hoarseness; fever or chills; lower back or side pain; painful or difficult urination; pinpoint red spots on skin; unusual bleeding or bruising

*Rare*
   Shortness of breath; stomach pain; swelling of face; yellow eyes or skin

Check with your health care professional as soon as possible if the following side effect occurs:

*Rare*
   Sores in mouth and on lips

Other side effects may occur that usually do not need medical attention. These side effects may go away during treatment as your body adjusts to the medicine. Also, your health care professional may be able to tell you about ways to prevent or reduce some of these side effects. Check with your health care professional if any of the following side effects continue or are bothersome or if you have any questions about them:

*More common*
   Loss of appetite; nausea or vomiting (should lessen after 1 or 2 days)

*Less common*
   Feelings of uneasiness; flushing of face; muscle pain; numbness of face

This medicine may cause a temporary loss of hair in some people. After treatment with dacarbazine has ended, normal hair growth should return.

After you stop receiving dacarbazine, it may still produce some side effects that need attention. During this period of time check with your doctor if you notice any of the following:

  Black, tarry stools; blood in urine or stools; cough or hoarseness; fever or chills; lower back or side pain; painful or difficult urination; pinpoint red spots on skin; unusual bleeding or bruising

Other side effects not listed above may also occur in some patients. If you notice any other effects, check with your doctor.

Revised: 07/11/94

---

# DACTINOMYCIN   Systemic

A commonly used brand name in the U.S. and Canada is Cosmegen. Another commonly used name is actinomycin-D.

## Description

Dactinomycin (dak-ti-noe-MYE-sin) belongs to the group of medicines known as antineoplastics. It is used to treat some kinds of cancer.

Dactinomycin interferes with the growth of cancer cells, which are eventually destroyed. Since the growth of normal body cells may also be affected by dactinomycin, other effects will also occur. Some of these may be serious and must be reported to your doctor. Other effects, like hair loss, may not be serious but may cause concern. Some effects may not occur for months or years after the medicine is used.

Before you begin treatment with dactinomycin, you and your doctor should talk about the good this medicine will do as well as the risks of using it.

Dactinomycin is to be administered only by or under the immediate supervision of your doctor. It is available in the following dosage form:

*Parenteral*
  • Injection (U.S. and Canada)

## Before Using This Medicine

In deciding to use a medicine, the risks of taking the medicine must be weighed against the good it will do. This is a decision you and your doctor will make. For dactinomycin, the following should be considered:

**Allergies**—Tell your doctor if you have ever had any unusual or allergic reaction to dactinomycin.

**Pregnancy**—There is a chance that this medicine may cause birth defects if either the male or female is receiving it at the time of conception or if it is taken during pregnancy. Studies have shown that dactinomycin causes birth defects in animals. In addition, many cancer medicines may cause sterility which could be permanent. Although sterility has not been reported with this medicine, the possibility should be kept in mind.

Be sure that you have discussed this with your doctor before receiving this medicine. It is best to use some kind of birth control while you are receiving dactinomycin.

Tell your doctor right away if you think you have become pregnant while receiving dactinomycin.

**Breast-feeding**—It is not known whether dactinomycin passes into breast milk. However, because this medicine may cause serious side effects, breast-feeding is generally not recommended while you are receiving it.

**Children**—Because of increased toxicity, use of dactinomycin in infants less than 6 to 12 months of age is not recommended.

**Older adults**—Many medicines have not been studied specifically in older people. Therefore, it may not be known whether they work exactly the same way they do in younger adults or if they cause different side effects or problems in older people. There is no specific information about the use of dactinomycin in the elderly.

**Other medicines**—Although certain medicines should not be used together at all, in other cases two different medicines may be used together even if an interaction might occur. In these cases, your doctor may want to change the dose, or other precautions may be necessary. When receiving dactinomycin it is especially important that your health care professional know if you are taking any of the following:

  • Amphotericin B by injection (e.g., Fungizone) or
  • Antithyroid agents (medicine for overactive thyroid) or
  • Azathioprine (e.g., Imuran) or
  • Chloramphenicol (e.g., Chloromycetin) or
  • Flucytosine (e.g., Ancobon) or
  • Ganciclovir (e.g., Cytovene) or
  • Interferon (e.g., Intron A, Roferon-A) or
  • Plicamycin (e.g., Mithramycin) or
  • Zidovudine (e.g., AZT, Retrovir) or
  • If you have ever been treated with radiation or cancer medicine—Dactinomycin may increase the effects of these medicines or radiation therapy on the blood
  • Probenecid (e.g., Benemid) or
  • Sulfinpyrazone (e.g., Anturane)—Dactinomycin may increase concentrations of uric acid in the blood. Since these medicines are used to lower uric acid levels, they may not be as effective in patients receiving dactinomycin

**Other medical problems**—The presence of other medical problems may affect the use of dactinomycin. Make sure

you tell your doctor if you have any other medical problems, especially:

- Chickenpox (including recent exposure) or
- Herpes zoster (shingles)—Risk of severe disease affecting other parts of the body
- Gout (or history of) or
- Kidney stones—Dactinomycin may increase levels of uric acid in the body, which can cause gout or kidney stones
- Infection—Dactinomycin can decrease your body's ability to fight infection
- Liver disease—Effects of dactinomycin may be increased

## Proper Use of This Medicine

Dactinomycin is sometimes given together with certain other medicines. If you are receiving a combination of medicines, it is important that you receive each one at the proper time. If you are taking some of these medicines by mouth, ask your health care professional to help you plan a way to remember to take them at the right times.

This medicine often causes nausea and vomiting. However, it is very important that you continue to receive the medicine, even if you begin to feel ill. Ask your health care professional for ways to lessen these effects.

**Dosing**—The dose of dactinomycin will be different for different patients. The dose that is used may depend on a number of things, including what the medicine is being used for, the patient's weight, and whether or not other medicines are also being taken. *If you are receiving dactinomycin at home, follow your doctor's orders or the directions on the label.* If you have any questions about the proper dose of dactinomycin, ask your doctor.

## Precautions While Using This Medicine

*It is very important that your doctor check your progress at regular visits* to make sure that this medicine is working properly and to check for unwanted effects.

While you are being treated with dactinomycin, and after you stop treatment with it, *do not have any immunizations (vaccinations) without your doctor's approval*. Dactinomycin may lower your body's resistance, and there is a chance you might get the infection the immunization is meant to prevent. In addition, other persons living in your household should not take oral polio vaccine since there is a chance they could pass the polio virus on to you. Also, avoid persons who have taken oral polio vaccine. Do not get close to them, and do not stay in the same room with them for very long. If you cannot take these precautions, you should consider wearing a protective face mask that covers the nose and mouth.

Dactinomycin can temporarily lower the number of white blood cells in your blood increasing the chance of getting an infection. It can also lower the number of platelets, which are necessary for proper blood clotting. If this occurs, there are certain precautions you can take, especially when your blood count is low, to reduce the risk of infection or bleeding:

- If you can, avoid people with infections. *Check with your doctor immediately* if you think you are getting

an infection or if you get a fever or chills, cough or hoarseness, lower back or side pain, or painful or difficult urination.

- *Check with your doctor immediately* if you notice any unusual bleeding or bruising; black, tarry stools; blood in urine or stools; or pinpoint red spots on your skin.
- Be careful when using a regular toothbrush, dental floss, or toothpick. Your medical doctor, dentist, or nurse may recommend other ways to clean your teeth and gums. Check with your medical doctor before having any dental work done.
- Do not touch your eyes or the inside of your nose unless you have just washed your hands and have not touched anything else in the meantime.
- Be careful not to cut yourself when you are using sharp objects such as a safety razor or fingernail or toenail cutters.
- Avoid contact sports or other situations where bruising or injury could occur.

If dactinomycin accidentally seeps out of the vein into which it is injected, it may severely damage some tissues and cause scarring. *Tell the health care professional right away if you notice redness, pain, or swelling at the place of injection.*

## Side Effects of This Medicine

Along with its needed effects, a medicine may cause some unwanted effects. Although not all of these side effects may occur, if they do occur they may need medical attention.

Also, because of the way these medicines act on the body, there is a chance that they might cause other unwanted effects that may not occur until months or years after the medicine is used. These delayed effects may include certain types of cancer, such as leukemia. Discuss these possible effects with your doctor.

*Check with your doctor or nurse immediately* if any of the following side effects occur:

*Less common*
Black, tarry stools; blood in urine or stools; cough or hoarseness; fever or chills; lower back or side pain; painful or difficult urination; pinpoint red spots on skin; unusual bleeding or bruising

*Rare*
Pain at place of injection; wheezing

Check with your health care professional as soon as possible if any of the following side effects occur:

*More common*
Diarrhea (continuing); difficulty in swallowing; heartburn; sores in mouth and on lips; stomach pain (continuing)

*Rare*
Joint pain; swelling of feet or lower legs; yellow eyes or skin

Other side effects may occur that usually do not need medical attention. These side effects may go away during treatment as your body adjusts to the medicine. Also, your health care professional may be able to tell you about ways to prevent or reduce some of these side effects. Check with your health care professional if any of the following side effects continue or are bothersome or if you have any questions about them:

*More common*

Darkening of skin; nausea and vomiting; redness of skin; skin rash or acne; unusual tiredness

This medicine often causes a temporary loss of hair, sometimes including the eyebrows. After treatment with dactinomycin has ended, normal hair growth should return.

After you stop receiving dactinomycin, it may still produce some side effects that need attention. During this period of time check with your doctor if you notice any of the following:

Black, tarry stools; blood in urine or stools; cough or hoarseness; diarrhea; fever or chills; lower back or side pain; painful or difficult urination; pinpoint red spots on skin; sores in mouth and on lips; stomach pain; unusual bleeding or bruising; yellow eyes or skin

Other side effects not listed above may also occur in some patients. If you notice any other effects, check with your doctor.

Revised: 07/11/94

# DANAZOL Systemic

Some commonly used brand names are:
**In the U.S.—**
Danocrine
Generic name product may also be available.
**In Canada—**
Cyclomen

## Description

Danazol (DA-na-zole) may be used for a number of different medical problems. These include treatment of:

- pain and/or infertility due to endometriosis;
- a tendency for females to develop cysts in the breasts (fibrocystic breast disease); or
- hereditary angioedema, which causes swelling of the face, arms, legs, throat, windpipe, bowels, or sexual organs.

Danazol may also be used for other conditions as determined by your doctor.

This medicine is available only with your doctor's prescription, in the following dosage form:
*Oral*
- Capsules (U.S. and Canada)

## Before Using This Medicine

In deciding to use a medicine, the risks of taking the medicine must be weighed against the good it will do. This is a decision you and your doctor will make. For danazol, the following should be considered:

**Allergies**—Tell your doctor if you have ever had any unusual or allergic reaction to danazol, androgens (male hormones), or anabolic steroids. Also tell your health care professional if you are allergic to any other substances, such as foods, preservatives, or dyes.

**Pregnancy**—Danazol is not recommended for use during pregnancy, since it may cause a female baby to develop certain male characteristics.

**Breast-feeding**—Breast-feeding is not recommended while you are taking this medicine because it may cause unwanted effects in the baby.

**Children**—Danazol may cause male-like changes in female children and cause premature sexual development in male children. It may also slow or stop growth in any child.

**Older adults**—Many medicines have not been studied specifically in older people. Therefore, it may not be known whether they work exactly the same way they do in younger adults. Although there is no specific information comparing use of danazol in the elderly with use in other age groups, danazol has effects similar to androgens (male hormones). Androgens used in older males may increase the risk of developing prostate enlargement or cancer.

**Other medicines**—Although certain medicines should not be used together at all, in other cases two different medicines may be used together even if an interaction might occur. In these cases, your doctor may want to change the dose, or other precautions may be necessary. When you are taking danazol, it is especially important that your health care professional know if you are taking any of the following:

- Anticoagulants (blood thinners)—Danazol may increase the effects of these medicines and possibly increase the risk of severe bleeding

**Other medical problems**—The presence of other medical problems may affect the use of danazol. Make sure you tell your doctor if you have any other medical problems, especially:

- Diabetes mellitus (sugar diabetes)—Danazol may increase blood glucose levels

- Epilepsy or
- Heart disease or
- Kidney disease or
- Migraine headaches—These conditions can be made worse by the fluid retention (keeping too much body water) that can be caused by danazol
- Liver disease

## Proper Use of This Medicine

In order for danazol to help you, *it must be taken regularly for the full time of treatment* as ordered by your doctor.

**Dosing**—The dose of danazol will be different for different patients. *Follow your doctor's orders or the directions on the label.* The following information includes only the average doses of danazol. *If your dose is different, do not change it* unless your doctor tells you to do so.

The number of capsules that you take depends on the strength of the medicine. Also, *the number of doses you take each day, the time allowed between doses, and the length of time you take the medicine depend on the medical problems for which you are taking danazol.*

- For *capsules* dosage forms:
  —Adults:
  - For treatment of endometriosis: 100 to 400 milligrams two times a day.
  - For treatment of fibrocystic breast disease: 50 to 200 milligrams two times a day.
  - For prevention of attacks of hereditary angioedema: 200 milligrams two or three times a day. The dose may be lowered, depending upon your condition.

**Missed dose**—If you miss a dose of this medicine, take it as soon as possible. However, if it is almost time for your next dose, skip the missed dose and go back to your regular dosing schedule. Do not double doses.

**Storage**—To store this medicine:
- Keep out of the reach of children.
- Store away from heat and direct light.
- Do not store in the bathroom, near the kitchen sink, or in other damp places. Heat or moisture may cause the medicine to break down.
- Do not keep outdated medicine or medicine no longer needed. Be sure that any discarded medicine is out of the reach of children.

## Precautions While Using This Medicine

Your doctor should check your progress at regular visits to make sure that this medicine does not cause unwanted effects.

*For diabetic patients:*
- This medicine may affect blood glucose levels. If you notice a change in the results of your blood or urine glucose test or if you have any questions about this, check with your doctor.

*If you are taking danazol for endometriosis or fibrocystic breast disease:*
- During the time you are taking danazol, your menstrual period may not be regular or you may not have a menstrual period at all. This is to be expected when you are taking this medicine. If regular menstruation does not begin within 60 to 90 days after you stop taking this medicine, check with your doctor.
- During the time you are taking danazol, you should use birth control methods that do not contain hormones. If you have any questions about this, check with your health care professional.
- *If you suspect that you may have become pregnant, stop taking this medicine and check with your doctor.* Continued use of danazol during pregnancy may cause male-like changes in female babies.

Danazol may cause your skin to be more sensitive to sunlight than it is normally. Exposure to sunlight, even for brief periods of time, may cause a skin rash, itching, redness, or other discoloration of the skin, or a severe sunburn. When you begin taking this medicine:
- Stay out of direct sunlight, especially between the hours of 10:00 a.m. and 3:00 p.m., if possible.
- Wear protective clothing, including a hat. Also, wear sunglasses.
- Apply a sun block product that has a skin protection factor (SPF) of a least 15. Some patients may require a product with a higher SPF number, especially if they have a fair complexion. If you have questions about this, check with your health care professional.
- Apply a sun block lipstick that has an SPF of at least 15 to protect your lips.
- Do not use a sunlamp or tanning bed or booth.

*If you have a severe reaction from the sun, check with your doctor.*

## Side Effects of This Medicine

Along with its needed effects, a medicine may cause some unwanted effects. Although not all of these side effects may occur, if they do occur they may need medical attention.

Check with your doctor as soon as possible if any of the following side effects occur:

*For both females and males*
  *Less common*
    Acne or increased oiliness of skin or hair; muscle cramps or spasms; swelling of feet or lower legs; unusual tiredness or weakness; weight gain (rapid)

  *Rare*
    Bleeding gums; bloating, pain or tenderness of abdomen or stomach; blood in urine; changes in vision; chest pain; chills; cough; dark-colored urine; diarrhea; discharge from nipple; eye pain; fast heartbeat; fever; headache; hives or other skin rashes; joint pain; light-colored stools; loss of appetite (continuing); more frequent nosebleeds; muscle aches; nausea; pain, numbness, tingling, or burning in all

fingers except the smallest finger; purple- or red-colored, or other spots on body or inside the mouth or nose; sore throat; tingling, numbness, or weakness in legs, which may move upward to arms, trunk, or face; unusual bruising or bleeding; unusual tiredness, weakness, or general feeling of illness; vomiting; yellow eyes or skin

*For females only*

**More common**

Decrease in breast size; irregular menstrual periods; weight gain

**Rare**

Enlarged clitoris; hoarseness or deepening of voice; unnatural hair growth

*For males only*

**Rare**

Decrease in size of testicles

Other side effects may occur that usually do not need medical attention. These side effects may go away during treatment as your body adjusts to the medicine. However, check with your doctor if any of the following side effects continue or are bothersome:

*For both females and males*

**Less common**

Flushing or redness of skin; mood or mental changes; nervousness; sweating

**Rare**

Increased sensitivity of skin to sunlight

*For females only*

**Less common**

Burning, dryness, or itching of vagina or vaginal bleeding

Other side effects not listed above may also occur in some patients. If you notice any other effects, check with your doctor.

## Additional Information

Once a medicine has been approved for marketing for a certain use, experience may show that it is also useful for other medical problems. Although these uses are not included in product labeling, danazol is used in certain patients with the following medical conditions:

- Gynecomastia (excess breast development in males)
- Menorrhagia (excessively long menstrual periods)
- Precocious puberty in females (premature sexual development)

Other than the above information, there is no additional information relating to proper use, precautions, or side effects for these uses.

Revised: 02/19/93

# DANTROLENE   Systemic

Some commonly used brand names in the U.S. and Canada are Dantrium and Dantrium Intravenous.

## Description

Dantrolene (DAN-troe-leen) is used to help relax certain muscles in your body. It relieves the spasms, cramping, and tightness of muscles caused by certain medical problems such as multiple sclerosis (MS), cerebral palsy, stroke, or injury to the spine. Dantrolene does not cure these problems, but it may allow other treatment, such as physical therapy, to be more helpful in improving your condition. Dantrolene acts directly on the muscles to produce its relaxant effects.

Dantrolene is also used to prevent or treat a medical problem called malignant hyperthermia that may occur in some people during or following surgery or anesthesia. Malignant hyperthermia consists of a group of symptoms including very high fever, fast and irregular heartbeat, and breathing problems. It is believed that the tendency to develop malignant hyperthermia is inherited.

Dantrolene has been shown to cause cancer and noncancerous tumors in some animals (but not in others) when given in large doses for a long time. It is not known whether long-term use of dantrolene causes cancer or tumors in humans. Before taking this medicine, be sure that you have discussed this with your doctor.

This medicine is available only with your doctor's prescription, in the following dosage forms:

*Oral*

- Capsules (U.S. and Canada)

*Parenteral*

- Injection (U.S. and Canada)

## Before Using This Medicine

In deciding to use a medicine, the risks of taking the medicine must be weighed against the good it will do. This is a decision you and your doctor will make. For dantrolene, the following should be considered:

**Allergies**—Tell your doctor if you have ever had any unusual or allergic reaction to dantrolene. Also tell your health care professional if you are allergic to any other substances, such as foods, preservatives, or dyes.

**Pregnancy**—Dantrolene has not been shown to cause birth defects or other problems in humans.

**Breast-feeding**—Use of dantrolene is not recommended during breast-feeding.

**Children**—This medicine has been tested in children 5 years of age and older and has not been shown to cause different side effects or problems than it does in adults.

**Older adults**—Many medicines have not been studied specifically in older people. Therefore, it may not be known whether they work exactly the same way they do in younger adults or if they cause different side effects or problems in older people. There is no specific information comparing use of dantrolene in the elderly with use in other age groups.

**Other medicines**—Although certain medicines should not be used together at all, in other cases two different medicines may be used together even if an interaction might occur. In these cases, your doctor may want to change the dose, or other precautions may be necessary. When you are taking dantrolene, it is especially important that your health care professional know if you are taking any of the following:

- Acetaminophen (e.g., Tylenol) (with long-term, high-dose use) or
- Amiodarone (e.g., Cordarone) or
- Anabolic steroids (dromostanolone [e.g., Drolban], ethylestrenol [e.g., Maxibolin], nandrolone [e.g., Anabolin], oxandrolone [e.g., Anavar], oxymetholone [e.g., Anadrol], stanozolol [e.g., Winstrol]) or
- Androgens (male hormones) or
- Anti-infectives by mouth or by injection (medicine for infection) or
- Antithyroid agents (medicine for overactive thyroid) or
- Carbamazepine (e.g., Tegretol) or
- Carmustine (e.g., BiCNU) or
- Central nervous system (CNS) depressants (medicine that causes drowsiness) or
- Chloroquine (e.g., Aralen) or
- Daunorubicin (e.g., Cerubidine) or
- Disulfiram (e.g., Antabuse) or
- Divalproex (e.g., Depakote) or
- Estrogens (female hormones) or
- Etretinate (e.g., Tegison) or
- Gold salts (medicine for arthritis) or
- Hydroxychloroquine (e.g., Plaquenil) or
- Mercaptopurine (e.g., Purinethol) or
- Methotrexate (e.g., Mexate) or
- Methyldopa (e.g., Aldomet) or
- Naltrexone (e.g., Trexan) (with long-term, high-dose use) or
- Oral contraceptives (birth control pills) containing estrogen or
- Phenothiazines (acetophenazine [e.g., Tindal], chlorpromazine [e.g., Thorazine], fluphenazine [e.g., Prolixin], mesoridazine [e.g., Serentil], perphenazine [e.g., Trilafon], prochlorperazine [e.g., Compazine], promazine [e.g., Sparine], promethazine [e.g., Phenergan], thioridazine [e.g., Mellaril], trifluoperazine [e.g., Stelazine], triflupromazine [e.g., Vesprin], trimeprazine [e.g., Temaril]) or
- Phenytoin (e.g., Dilantin) or
- Plicamycin (e.g., Mithracin) or
- Tricyclic antidepressants (medicine for depression) (amitriptyline [e.g., Elavil], amoxapine [e.g., Asendin], clomipramine [e.g., Anafranil], desipramine [e.g., Pertofrane], doxepin [e.g., Sinequan], imipramine [e.g., Tofranil], nortriptyline [e.g., Aventyl], protriptyline [e.g., Vivactil], trimipramine [e.g., Surmontil]) or
- Valproic acid (e.g., Depakene)—The chance of side effects may be increased

**Other medical problems**—The presence of other medical problems may affect the use of dantrolene. Make sure you tell your doctor if you have any other medical problems, especially:

- Emphysema, asthma, bronchitis, or other chronic lung disease or
- Heart disease or
- Liver disease, such as hepatitis or cirrhosis (or history of)—The chance of serious side effects may be increased

## Proper Use of This Medicine

If you are unable to swallow the capsules, you may empty the number of capsules needed for one dose into a small amount of fruit juice or other liquid. Stir gently to mix the powder with the liquid before drinking. Drink the medicine right away. Rinse the glass with a little more liquid and drink that also to make sure that you have taken all of the medicine.

Dantrolene may be taken with or without food or on a full or empty stomach. However, if your doctor tells you to take the medicine a certain way, take it exactly as directed.

*Take this medicine only as directed by your doctor.* Do not take more of it and do not take it more often than your doctor ordered. Dantrolene may cause liver damage or other unwanted effects if too much is taken.

**Dosing**—The dose of dantrolene will be different for different patients. *Follow your doctor's orders or the directions on the label.* The following information includes only the average doses of dantrolene. *If your dose is different, do not change it* unless your doctor tells you to do so:

The number of capsules that you take depends on the strength of the medicine. Also, the number of doses you take each day, the time allowed between doses, and the length of time you take the medicine depend on the medical problem for which you are taking dantrolene.

- For *oral* dosage form (capsules):

  —For prevention or treatment of a malignant hyperthermic crisis:

  - Adults—Dose is based on body weight and must be determined by your doctor. The usual dose is 4 to 8 milligrams (mg) per kilogram (kg) (1.8 to 3.6 mg per pound) of body weight. The doctor will instruct you exactly when and how often to take your medicine.

  —To relieve spasms:

  - Adults—To start, 25 mg once a day. The doctor may increase your dose as needed and tolerated. However, the dose is usually not more than 100 mg four times a day.

  - Children—Dose is based on body weight and must be determined by your doctor. To start, the dose is usually 0.5 mg per kg (0.23 mg per pound) of body weight twice a day. The doctor may increase the dose as needed and tolerated. However, the dose is usually not more than 3 mg per kg or 100 mg four times a day.

- For *injection* dosage form:
  —For prevention or treatment of a malignant hyperthermia crisis:
    • Adults, teenagers, and children—Dose is based on body weight and must be determined by your doctor.

**Missed dose**—If you miss a dose of this medicine and remember within an hour or so of the missed dose, take it right away. Then go back to your regular dosing schedule. But if you do not remember until later, skip the missed dose and go back to your regular dosing schedule. Do not double doses.

**Storage**—To store this medicine:
- Keep out of the reach of children.
- Store away from heat and direct light.
- Do not store this medicine in the bathroom, near the kitchen sink, or in other damp places. Heat or moisture may cause the medicine to break down.
- Do not keep outdated medicine or medicine no longer needed. Be sure that any discarded medicine is out of the reach of children.

## Precautions While Using This Medicine

If you will be taking dantrolene for a long time (for example, for several months at a time), your doctor should check your progress at regular visits. It may be necessary to have certain blood tests to check for unwanted effects while you are taking dantrolene.

This medicine will add to the effects of alcohol and other CNS depressants (medicines that slow down the nervous system, possibly causing drowsiness). Some examples of CNS depressants are antihistamines or medicine for hay fever, other allergies, or colds; sedatives, tranquilizers, or sleeping medicine; prescription pain medicine or narcotics; barbiturates; medicine for seizures; other muscle relaxants; or anesthetics, including some dental anesthetics. Therefore, *do not drink alcoholic beverages, and check with your doctor before taking any of the medicines listed above, while you are using this medicine.*

This medicine may cause drowsiness, dizziness or lightheadedness, vision problems, or muscle weakness in some people. *Make sure you know how you react to this medicine before you drive, use machines, or do anything else that could be dangerous if you are dizzy or are not alert, well-coordinated, and able to see well.*

## Side Effects of This Medicine

Along with its needed effects, a medicine may cause some unwanted effects. Although not all of these side effects may occur, if they do occur they may need medical attention. Serious side effects are very rare when dantrolene is taken for a short time (for example, when it is used for a few days before, during, or after surgery or anesthesia to prevent or treat malignant hyperthermia). However, serious side effects may occur, especially when the medicine is taken for a long time.

*Check with your doctor immediately* if any of the following side effects occur:

*Less common*
Convulsions (seizures); pain, tenderness, changes in skin color, or swelling of foot or leg; shortness of breath or slow or troubled breathing

Also, check with your doctor as soon as possible if any of the following side effects occur:

*Less common*
Bloody or dark urine; chest pain; confusion; constipation (severe); diarrhea (severe); difficult urination; mental depression; skin rash, hives, or itching; yellow eyes or skin

Other side effects may occur that usually do not need medical attention. These side effects may go away during treatment as your body adjusts to the medicine. However, check with your doctor if any of the following side effects continue or are bothersome:

*More common*
Diarrhea (mild); dizziness or lightheadedness; drowsiness; general feeling of discomfort or illness; muscle weakness; nausea or vomiting; unusual tiredness

*Less common*
Abdominal or stomach cramps or discomfort; blurred or double vision or any change in vision; chills and fever; constipation (mild); difficulty in swallowing; frequent urge to urinate or uncontrolled urination; headache; loss of appetite; slurring of speech or other speech problems; sudden decrease in amount of urine; trouble in sleeping; unusual nervousness

Other side effects not listed above may also occur in some patients. If you notice any other effects, check with your doctor.

Revised: 05/10/93

# DAPIPRAZOLE    Ophthalmic

A commonly used brand name in the U.S. and Canada is Rev-Eyes.

## Description

Dapiprazole (da-PI-pray-zole) is used in the eye to reduce the size of the pupil after certain kinds of eye examinations.

Some eye examinations are best done when your pupil (the black center of the colored part of your eye) is very large, so the doctor can see into your eye better. This medicine helps to reduce the size of your pupil back to its normal size after the eye examination.

Dapiprazole is available in the following dosage form:

*Ophthalmic*
- Ophthalmic solution (eye drops) (U.S. and Canada)

## Before Using This Medicine

In deciding to use a medicine, the risks of using the medicine must be weighed against the good it will do. This is a decision you and your doctor will make. For dapiprazole, the following should be considered:

**Allergies**—Tell your doctor if you have ever had any unusual or allergic reaction to dapiprazole. Also tell your health care professional if you are allergic to any other substances, such as foods, preservatives, or dyes.

**Pregnancy**—Dapiprazole has not been studied in pregnant women. However, dapiprazole has not been shown to cause birth defects or other problems in animal studies.

**Breast-feeding**—It is not known whether dapiprazole passes into the breast milk. However, this medicine has not been reported to cause problems in nursing babies.

**Children**—Studies on this medicine have been done only in adult patients, and there is no specific information comparing use of dapiprazole in children with use in other age groups.

**Older adults**—Many medicines have not been studied specifically in older people. Therefore, it may not be known whether they work exactly the same way they do in younger adults. Although there is no specific information comparing use of dapiprazole in the elderly with use in other age groups, this medicine is not expected to cause different side effects or problems in older people than it does in younger adults.

**Other medicines**—Although certain medicines should not be used together at all, in other cases two different medicines may be used together even if an interaction might occur. In these cases, your doctor may want to change the dose, or other precautions may be necessary. Tell your health care professional if you are using any other ophthalmic (eye) prescription or nonprescription (over-the-counter [OTC]) medicine.

**Other medical problems**—The presence of other medical problems may affect the use of dapiprazole. Make sure you tell your doctor if you have any other medical problems, especially:
- Eye problems, other—Use of dapiprazole may make the condition worse

## Proper Use of This Medicine

**Dosing**—The dose of dapiprazole will be different for different patients. *Follow your doctor's orders or the directions on the label.* The following information includes only the average doses of dapiprazole. *If your dose is different, do not change it* unless your doctor tells you to do so.

- For *ophthalmic solution (eye drops)* dosage form:
  —For reduction of size of pupil of eye:
    - Adults—One drop, then one drop in five minutes, following eye examination.
    - Children—Use and dose must be determined by your doctor.

## Precautions While Using This Medicine

Even after using this medicine, you may have blurred vision or other vision problems. If any of these occur, *do not drive, use machines, or do anything else that could be dangerous if you are not able to see well.*

This medicine may cause your eyes to become more sensitive to light than they are normally. Wearing sunglasses and avoiding too much exposure to bright light may help lessen the discomfort.

## Side Effects of This Medicine

Along with its needed effects, a medicine may cause some unwanted effects. Although not all of these side effects may occur, if they do occur they may need medical attention.

*Check with your doctor as soon as possible if any of the following side effects occur:*

*Less common*
   Irritation (severe) or swelling of the clear part of the eye

Other side effects may occur that usually do not need medical attention. These side effects may go away during treatment as your body adjusts to the medicine. However, check with your doctor if any of the following side effects continue or are bothersome:

*More common*
   Burning of eye when medicine is applied; redness of the white part of the eye

*Less common*

Blurring of vision; browache; drooping of upper eyelid; dryness of eye; headache; increased sensitivity of eye to light; itching of eye; redness of eyelid; swelling of eyelid; swelling of the membrane covering the white part of the eye; tearing of eye

Other side effects not listed above may also occur in some patients. If you notice any other effects, check with your doctor.

Annual revision: 04/13/92
Interim revision: 08/16/93

# DAPSONE   Systemic

A commonly used brand name in Canada is Avlosulfon.
Another commonly used name is DDS.

## Description

Dapsone (DAP-sone), a sulfone, belongs to the family of medicines called anti-infectives.

Dapsone is used to treat leprosy (Hansen's disease) and to help control dermatitis herpetiformis, a skin problem. When it is used to treat leprosy, dapsone may be given with one or more other medicines. Dapsone may also be used for other conditions as determined by your doctor.

Dapsone is available only with your doctor's prescription, in the following dosage form:

*Oral*
• Tablets (U.S. and Canada)

## Before Using This Medicine

In deciding to use a medicine, the risks of taking the medicine must be weighed against the good it will do. This is a decision you and your doctor will make. For dapsone, the following should be considered:

**Allergies**—Tell your doctor if you have ever had any unusual or allergic reaction to dapsone or sulfonamides. Also tell your health care professional if you are allergic to any other substances, such as foods, preservatives, or dyes.

**Pregnancy**—Studies have not been done in humans or animals. However, reports on the use of dapsone in humans have not shown that this medicine causes birth defects or other problems.

**Breast-feeding**—Dapsone passes into the breast milk. Dapsone may cause blood problems in nursing babies with glucose-6-phosphate dehydrogenase (G6PD) deficiency. Breast-feeding may need to be stopped because of the risks to the baby.

**Children**—Although there is no specific information comparing use of dapsone in children with use in other age groups, this medicine is not expected to cause different side effects or problems in children than it does in adults.

**Older adults**—Many medicines have not been studied specifically in older people. Therefore, it may not be known whether they work exactly the same way they do in younger adults or if they cause different side effects or problems in older people. There is no specific information comparing use of dapsone in the elderly with use in other age groups.

**Other medicines**—Although certain medicines should not be used together at all, in other cases two different medicines may be used together even if an interaction might occur. In these cases, your doctor may want to change the dose, or other precautions may be necessary. When you are taking dapsone, it is especially important that your health care professional knows if you are taking any of the following:
• Acetohydroxamic acid (e.g., Lithostat) or
• Antidiabetics, oral (diabetes medicine you take by mouth) or
• Furazolidone (e.g., Furoxone) or
• Methyldopa (e.g., Aldomet) or
• Nitrofurantoin (e.g., Furadantin) or
• Primaquine or
• Procainamide (e.g., Pronestyl) or
• Quinidine (e.g., Quinidex) or
• Quinine (e.g., Quinamm) or
• Sulfonamides (sulfa medicine) or
• Vitamin K (e.g., AquaMEPHYTON, Synkayvite)—Use of dapsone with these medicines may increase the chance of side effects affecting the blood
• Dideoxyinosine (e.g., ddI, Videx)—Use of dideoxyinosine with dapsone may decrease the effectiveness of dapsone

**Other medical problems**—The presence of other medical problems may affect the use of dapsone. Make sure you tell your doctor if you have any other medical problems, especially:
• Anemia (severe) or
• Glucose-6-phosphate dehydrogenase (G6PD) deficiency or
• Methemoglobin reductase deficiency—There is an increased risk of severe blood disorders and a decrease in red blood cell survival
• Liver disease—Dapsone may on rare occasion cause liver damage

## Proper Use of This Medicine

For patients taking dapsone for leprosy:
• To help clear up your leprosy completely or to keep it from coming back, *it is very important that you keep taking this medicine for the full time of treatment,* even if you begin to feel better after a few weeks or months. You may have to take it every day

for as long as 3 years or more, or for life. If you stop taking this medicine too soon, your symptoms may return.

- This medicine works best when there is a constant amount in the blood. *To help keep the amount constant, do not miss any doses. Also, it is best to take each dose at the same time every day.* If you need help in planning the best time to take your medicine, check with your health care professional.

For patients taking dapsone for dermatitis herpetiformis:
- Your doctor may want you to follow a gluten-free diet. If you have any questions about this, check with your doctor.

**Dosing**—The dose of dapsone will be different for different patients. *Follow your doctor's orders or the directions on the label.* The following information includes only the average doses of dapsone. *If your dose is different, do not change it* unless your doctor tells you to do so.

The number of tablets that you take depends on the strength of the medicine. Also, *the number of doses you take each day, the time allowed between doses, and the length of time you take the medicine depend on the medical problem for which you are taking dapsone.*

- *For oral* dosage form (tablets):
  —For Hansen's disease (leprosy):
    - Adults and teenagers—50 to 100 milligrams (mg) once a day; or 1.4 mg per kilogram (kg) (0.6 mg per pound) of body weight once a day. Dapsone should be taken with other medicines to treat Hansen's disease.
    - Children—Dose is based on body weight. The usual dose is 1.4 mg per kg (0.6 mg per pound) of body weight once a day. Dapsone should be taken with other medicines to treat Hansen's disease.
  —For dermatitis herpetiformis:
    - Adults and teenagers—50 mg once a day to start. Your doctor will increase your dose, up to 300 mg once a day, until your symptoms are controlled. Then your dose will be decreased to the lowest dose that will still control your symptoms.
    - Children—Dose is based on body weight. The usual dose is 2 mg per kg (0.9 mg per pound) of body weight once a day to start. Your doctor will increase your dose until your symptoms are controlled. Then your dose will be decreased to the lowest dose that will still control your symptoms.

**Missed dose**—You may skip a missed dose if it does not make your symptoms come back or get worse. If your symptoms do come back or get worse, take the missed dose as soon as possible. Then go back to your regular dosing schedule.

**Storage**—To store this medicine:
- Keep out of the reach of children.
- Store away from heat and direct light.
- Do not store in the bathroom, near the kitchen sink, or in other damp places. Heat or moisture may cause the medicine to break down.
- Do not keep outdated medicine or medicine no longer needed. Be sure that any discarded medicine is out of the reach of children.

## Precautions While Using This Medicine

It is very important that your doctor check your progress at regular visits.

If your symptoms do not improve within 2 to 3 months (for leprosy), or within a few days (for dermatitis herpetiformis), or if they become worse, check with your doctor.

## Side Effects of This Medicine

Along with its needed effects, a medicine may cause some unwanted effects. Although not all of these side effects may occur, if they do occur they may need medical attention.

*Check with your doctor immediately* if any of the following side effects occur:

*More common*
> Back, leg, or stomach pains; bluish fingernails, lips, or skin; difficult breathing; fever; loss of appetite; pale skin; skin rash; unusual tiredness or weakness

*Rare*
> Itching, dryness, redness, scaling, or peeling of the skin, or loss of hair; mood or other mental changes; numbness, tingling, pain, burning, or weakness in hands or feet; sore throat; unusual bleeding or bruising; yellow eyes or skin

Other side effects may occur that usually do not need medical attention. These side effects may go away during treatment as your body adjusts to the medicine. However, check with your doctor if any of the following side effects continue or are bothersome:

*Rare*
> Headache; loss of appetite; nausea or vomiting; nervousness; trouble in sleeping

Other side effects not listed above may also occur in some patients. If you notice any other effects, check with your doctor.

## Additional Information

Once a medicine has been approved for marketing for a certain use, experience may show that it is also useful for other medical problems. Although these uses are not specifically included in product labeling, dapsone is used in certain patients with the following medical conditions:
- Actinomycotic mycetoma
- Granuloma annulare
- Malaria (prevention of)
- Pemphigoid

---

© 1994   The United States Pharmacopeial Convention, Inc.

- *Pneumocystis carinii* pneumonia
- Pyoderma gangrenosum
- Relapsing polychondritis
- Subcorneal pustular dermatosis
- Systemic lupus erythematosus

For patients taking this medicine for *Pneumocystis carinii* pneumonia (PCP):

- To help clear up PCP completely or to keep it from coming back, *it is very important that you keep taking this medicine for the full time of treatment.*
- If you miss a dose of this medicine, take it as soon as possible. This will help keep a constant amount of medicine in the blood. However, if it is almost time for your next dose, skip the missed dose and go back to your regular dosing schedule. Do not double doses.
- If your symptoms do not improve within 1 week, or if they become worse, check with your doctor.

Other than the above information, there is no additional information relating to proper use, precautions, or side effects for these uses.

Revised: 06/26/92
Interim revision: 03/17/94

# DAUNORUBICIN  Systemic

A commonly used brand name in the U.S. and Canada is Cerubidine.

## Description

Daunorubicin (daw-noe-ROO-bi-sin) belongs to the general group of medicines known as antineoplastics. It is used to treat some kinds of cancer.

Daunorubicin seems to interfere with the growth of cancer cells, which are eventually destroyed. Since the growth of normal body cells may also be affected by daunorubicin, other effects will also occur. Some of these may be serious and must be reported to your doctor. Other effects, like hair loss, may not be serious but may cause concern. Some effects may not occur for months or years after the medicine is used.

Before you begin treatment with daunorubicin, you and your doctor should talk about the good this medicine will do as well as the risks of using it.

Daunorubicin is to be administered only by or under the immediate supervision of your doctor. It is available in the following dosage form:

*Parenteral*
- Injection (U.S. and Canada)

## Before Using This Medicine

In deciding to use a medicine, the risks of taking the medicine must be weighed against the good it will do. This is a decision you and your doctor will make. For daunorubicin, the following should be considered:

**Allergies**—Tell your doctor if you have ever had any unusual or allergic reaction to daunorubicin.

**Pregnancy**—This medicine may cause birth defects if either the male or female is receiving it at the time of conception or if it is taken during pregnancy. In addition, many cancer medicines may cause sterility which could be permanent. Although sterility has been reported only in male dogs with this medicine, the possibility of an effect in human males should be kept in mind.

Be sure that you have discussed this with your doctor before receiving this medicine. It is best to use some kind of birth control while you are receiving daunorubicin. Tell your doctor right away if you think you have become pregnant while receiving daunorubicin.

**Breast-feeding**—Because daunorubicin may cause serious side effects, breast-feeding is generally not recommended while you are receiving it.

**Children**—Although daunorubicin is used in children, there is no specific information comparing use in children with use in other age groups.

**Older adults**—Heart problems are more likely to occur in the elderly, who are usually more sensitive to the effects of daunorubicin. The elderly may also be more likely to have blood problems.

**Other medicines**—Although certain medicines should not be used together at all, in other cases two different medicines may be used together even if an interaction might occur. In these cases, your doctor may want to change the dose, or other precautions may be necessary. When receiving daunorubicin it is especially important that your health care professional know if you are taking any of the following:

- Amphotericin B by injection (e.g., Fungizone) or
- Antithyroid agents (medicine for overactive thyroid) or
- Azathioprine (e.g., Imuran) or
- Chloramphenicol (e.g., Chloromycetin) or
- Colchicine or
- Flucytosine (e.g., Ancobon) or
- Ganciclovir (e.g., Cytovene) or
- Interferon (e.g., Intron A, Roferon-A) or
- Plicamycin (e.g., Mithracin) or
- Zidovudine (e.g., AZT, Retrovir) or
- If you have ever been treated with radiation or cancer medicines—Daunorubicin may increase the effects of these medicines or radiation therapy on the blood

- Probenecid (e.g., Benemid) or
- Sulfinpyrazone (e.g., Anturane)—Daunorubicin may raise the concentration of uric acid in the blood. Since these medicines are used to lower uric acid levels, they may not be as effective in patients receiving daunorubicin

**Other medical problems**—The presence of other medical problems may affect the use of daunorubicin. Make sure you tell your doctor if you have any other medical problems, especially:

- Chickenpox (including recent exposure) or
- Herpes zoster (shingles)—Risk of severe disease affecting other parts of the body
- Gout (history of) or
- Kidney stones—Daunorubicin may increase uric acid in the body, which can cause gout or kidney stones
- Heart disease—Risk of heart problems caused by daunorubicin may be increased
- Infection—Daunorubicin can decrease your body's ability to fight infection
- Kidney disease or
- Liver disease—Effects of daunorubicin may be increased because of slower removal from the body

## Proper Use of This Medicine

Daunorubicin is sometimes given together with certain other medicines. If you are using a combination of medicines, it is important that you receive each one at the proper time. If you are taking some of these medicines by mouth, ask your health care professional to help you plan a way to take them at the right times.

While you are receiving daunorubicin, your doctor may want you to drink extra fluids so that you will pass more urine. This will help prevent kidney problems and keep your kidneys working well.

This medicine often causes nausea and vomiting. However, it is very important that you continue to receive it, even if you begin to feel ill. Ask your health care professional for ways to lessen these effects.

**Dosing**—The dose of daunorubicin will be different for different patients. The dose that is used may depend on a number of things, including what the medicine is being used for, the patient's size, and whether or not other medicines are also being taken. *If you are receiving daunorubicin at home, follow your doctor's orders or the directions on the label.* If you have any questions about the proper dose of daunorubicin, ask your doctor.

## Precautions While Using This Medicine

*It is very important that your doctor check your progress at regular visits* to make sure that this medicine is working properly and to check for unwanted effects.

While you are being treated with daunorubicin, and after you stop treatment with it, *do not have any immunizations (vaccinations) without your doctor's approval.* Daunorubicin may lower your body's resistance and there is a chance you might get the infection the immunization is meant to prevent. In addition, other persons living in your household should not take oral polio vaccine since there is a chance they could pass the polio virus on to you. Also, avoid persons who have taken oral polio vaccine. Do not get close to them, and do not stay in the same room with them for very long. If you cannot take these precautions, you should consider wearing a protective face mask that covers the nose and mouth.

Daunorubicin can temporarily lower the number of white blood cells in your blood, increasing the chance of getting an infection. It can also lower the number of platelets, which are necessary for proper blood clotting. If this occurs, there are certain precautions you can take, especially when your blood count is low, to reduce the risk of infection or bleeding:

- If you can, avoid people with infections. *Check with your doctor immediately* if you think you are getting an infection or if you get a fever or chills, cough or hoarseness, lower back or side pain, or painful or difficult urination.
- *Check with your doctor immediately* if you notice any unusual bleeding or bruising; black, tarry stools; blood in urine or stools; or pinpoint red spots on your skin.
- Be careful when using a regular toothbrush, dental floss, or toothpick. Your medical doctor, dentist, or nurse may recommend other ways to clean your teeth and gums. Check with your medical doctor before having any dental work done.
- Do not touch your eyes or the inside of your nose unless you have just washed your hands and have not touched anything else in the meantime.
- Be careful not to cut yourself when you are using sharp objects such as a safety razor or fingernail or toenail cutters.
- Avoid contact sports or other situations where bruising or injury could occur.

If daunorubicin accidentally seeps out of the vein into which it is injected, it may damage some tissues and cause scarring. *Tell the doctor or nurse right away if you notice redness, pain, or swelling at the place of injection.*

## Side Effects of This Medicine

Along with its needed effects, a medicine may cause some unwanted effects. Although not all of these side effects may occur, if they do occur they may need medical attention.

Also, because of the way these medicines act on the body, there is a chance that they might cause other unwanted effects that may not occur until months or years after the medicine is used. These delayed effects may include certain types of cancer, such as leukemia. Discuss these possible effects with your doctor.

*Check with your doctor or nurse immediately* if any of the following side effects occur:

*Less common*

Cough or hoarseness; fever or chills; irregular heartbeat; lower back or side pain; pain at place of injection;

painful or difficult urination; shortness of breath; swelling of feet and lower legs

*Rare*

Black, tarry stools; blood in urine or stools; pinpoint red spots on skin; unusual bleeding or bruising

Check with your health care professional as soon as possible if any of the following side effects occur:

*More common*

Sores in mouth and on lips

*Less common*

Joint pain

*Rare*

Skin rash or itching

Other side effects may occur that usually do not need medical attention. These side effects may go away during treatment as your body adjusts to the medicine. Also, your health care professional may be able to tell you about ways to prevent or reduce some of these side effects. Check with your health care professional if any of the following side effects continue or are bothersome or if you have any questions about them:

*More common*

Nausea and vomiting

*Less common or rare*

Darkening or redness of skin; diarrhea

Daunorubicin causes the urine to turn reddish in color, which may stain clothes. This is not blood. It is perfectly normal and lasts for only 1 or 2 days after each dose is given.

This medicine often causes a temporary and total loss of hair. After treatment with daunorubicin has ended, normal hair growth should return.

After you stop receiving daunorubicin, it may still produce some side effects that need attention. During this period of time *check with your doctor immediately* if you notice any of the following side effects:

Irregular heartbeat; shortness of breath; swelling of feet and lower legs

Other side effects not listed above may also occur in some patients. If you notice any other effects, check with your health care professional.

Revised: 07/11/94

# DECONGESTANTS AND ANALGESICS    Systemic

Some commonly used brand names are:

**In the U.S.—**

Advil Cold and Sinus Caplets[8]
Allerest No-Drowsiness[6]
Bayer Select Head Cold Caplets[6]
Bayer Select Maximum Strength Sinus Pain Relief Caplets[6]
BC Cold Powder Non-Drowsy Formula[5]
CoAdvil Caplets[8]
Coldrine[6]
Congespirin for Children Cold Tablets[1]
Congespirin for Children Liquid Cold Medicine[2]
Contac Allergy/Sinus Day Caplets[6]
Contac Maximum Strength Sinus Caplets[6]
Contac Non-Drowsy Formula Sinus Caplets[6]
DayQuil Non-Drowsy Sinus Pressure and Pain Relief Caplets[6]
Dimetapp Sinus Caplets[8]
Dristan Cold Caplets[6]
Dristan Sinus Caplets[8]
Genex[2]
Motrin IB Sinus[8]
Motrin IB Sinus Caplets[8]
Naldegesic[6]
Ornex Maximum Strength Caplets[6]
Ornex No Drowsiness Caplets[6]
PhenAPAP No. 2[2]
Rhinocaps[3]

Saleto D[4]
Sinarest No-Drowsiness[6]
Sine-Aid[6]
Sine-Aid IB Caplets[8]
Sine-Aid Maximum Strength[6]
Sine-Aid Maximum Strength Caplets[6]
Sine-Aid Maximum Strength Gelcaps[6]
Sine-Off Maximum Strength No Drowsiness Formula Caplets[6]
Sinus Excedrin Extra Strength[6]
Sinus Excedrin Extra Strength Caplets[6]
Sinus-Relief[6]
Sinutab II Maximum Strength[6]
Sinutab Maximum Strength Without Drowsiness[6]
Sinutab Maximum Strength Without Drowsiness Caplets[6]
St. Joseph Cold Tablets for Children[2]
Sudafed Sinus Maximum Strength[6]
Sudafed Sinus Maximum Strength Caplets[6]
Tylenol Sinus Maximum Strength[6]
Tylenol Sinus Maximum Strength Caplets[6]
Tylenol Sinus Maximum Strength Gelcaps[6]
Ursinus Inlay[7]

**In Canada—**

Neo Citran Extra Strength Sinus[1]
Sinutab Without Drowsiness[6]
Sinutab Without Drowsiness Extra Strength[6]
Tylenol Sinus Medication[6]
Tylenol Sinus Medication Extra Strength[6]

Note: For quick reference, the following decongestants and analogs are numbered to match the corresponding brand names.

This information applies to the following medicines:

1. Phenylephrine (fen-ill-EF-rin) and Acetaminophen (a-seat-a-MIN-oh-fen)
2. Phenylpropanolamine (fen-ill-proe-pa-NOLE-a-meen) and Acetaminophen†
3. Phenylpropanolamine, Acetaminophen, and Aspirin (AS-pir-in)†
4. Phenylpropanolamine, Acetaminophen, Salicylamide (sal-i-SILL-a-mide), and Caffeine (kaf-EEN)†
5. Phenylpropanolamine and Aspirin†
6. Pseudoephedrine (soo-doe-e-FED-rin) and Acetaminophen
7. Pseudoephedrine and Aspirin†
8. Pseudoephedrine and Ibuprofen (eye-byoo-PRO-fen)†

†Not commercially available in Canada.

## Description

Decongestant and analgesic combinations are taken by mouth to relieve sinus and nasal congestion (stuffy nose) and headache of colds, allergy, and hay fever.

Decongestants, such as phenylephrine, phenylpropanolamine (also known as PPA), and pseudoephedrine produce a narrowing of blood vessels. This leads to clearing of nasal congestion, but it may also cause an increase in blood pressure in patients who have high blood pressure.

Analgesics, such as acetaminophen, ibuprofen, and salicylates (e.g., aspirin, salicylamide), are used in these combination medicines to help relieve headache and sinus pain.

Acetaminophen and salicylates may cause kidney damage or cancer of the kidney or urinary bladder if large amounts of both medicines are taken together for a long time. However, taking the recommended amounts of combination medicines that contain both acetaminophen and a salicylate for short periods of time has not been shown to cause these unwanted effects.

These medicines are available without a prescription. However, your doctor may have special instructions on the proper dose of these medicines for your medical condition. They are available in the following dosage forms:

*Oral*

Phenylephrine and Acetaminophen
- For oral solution (Canada)
- Chewable tablets (U.S.)

Phenylpropanolamine and Acetaminophen
- Capsules (U.S.)
- Oral solution (U.S.)
- Tablets (U.S.)
- Chewable tablets (U.S.)

Phenylpropanolamine, Acetaminophen, and Aspirin
- Capsules (U.S.)

Phenylpropanolamine, Acetaminophen, Salicylamide, and Caffeine
- Capsules (U.S.)

Phenylpropanolamine and Aspirin
- For oral solution (U.S.)

Pseudoephedrine and Acetaminophen
- Capsules (U.S.)
- Tablets (U.S. and Canada)

Pseudoephedrine and Aspirin
- Tablets (U.S.)

Pseudoephedrine and Ibuprofen
- Tablets (U.S.)

---

## Before Using This Medicine

If you are taking this medicine without a prescription, carefully read and follow any precautions on the label. For decongestant and analgesic combinations, the following should be considered:

**Allergies**—Tell your doctor if you have ever had any unusual or allergic reaction to any of the ingredients contained in this medicine.

If this medicine contains *aspirin, salicylamide,* or *ibuprofen,* before taking it check with your doctor if you have ever had any unusual or allergic reaction to any of the following medicines:

Aspirin or other salicylates
Diclofenac (e.g., Voltaren)
Diflunisal (e.g., Dolobid)
Etodolac (e.g., Lodine)
Fenoprofen (e.g., Nalfon)
Floctafenine (e.g., Idarac)
Flurbiprofen, by mouth (e.g., Ansaid)

Ibuprofen (e.g., Motrin)
Indomethacin (e.g., Indocin)
Ketoprofen (e.g., Orudis)
Ketorolac (e.g., Toradol)
Meclofenamate (e.g., Meclomen)
Mefenamic acid (e.g., Ponstel)
Methyl salicylate (oil of wintergreen)
Nabumetone (e.g., Relafen)
Naproxen (e.g., Naprosyn)
Oxaprozin (e.g., Daypro)
Oxyphenbutazone (e.g., Tandearil)
Phenylbutazone (e.g., Butazolidin)
Piroxicam (e.g., Feldene)
Sulindac (e.g., Clinoril)
Suprofen (e.g., Suprol)
Tenoxicam (e.g., Mobiflex)
Tiaprofenic acid (e.g., Surgam)
Tolmetin (e.g., Tolectin)
Zomepirac (e.g., Zomax)

Also tell your health care professional if you are allergic to any other substances, such as foods, preservatives, or dyes.

**Pregnancy**—The occasional use of decongestant and analgesic combinations at the doses recommended on the label is not likely to cause problems in the fetus or in the newborn baby. However, for the individual ingredients of these combinations, the following information applies:

- *Alcohol*—Some of these combination medicines contain large amounts of alcohol. Too much use of alcohol during pregnancy may cause birth defects.

- *Caffeine*—Studies in humans have not shown that caffeine causes birth defects. However, studies in animals have shown that caffeine causes birth defects when given in very large doses (amounts equal to the amount of caffeine contained in 12 to 24 cups of coffee a day).

- *Ibuprofen*—Studies on birth defects have not been done in humans. However, there is a chance that ibuprofen may cause unwanted effects on the heart or blood flow of the fetus or newborn baby if it is taken regularly during the last few months of pregnancy.

- *Phenylephrine*—Studies on birth defects have not been done in either humans or animals with phenylephrine.

- *Phenylpropanolamine*—Studies on birth defects have not been done in either humans or animals with phenylpropanolamine. However, it seems that women who take phenylpropanolamine in the weeks following delivery are more likely to suffer mental or mood changes.

- *Pseudoephedrine*—Studies on birth defects with pseudoephedrine have not been done in humans. In animal studies pseudoephedrine did not cause birth defects. However, when given to animals in high doses, pseudoephedrine did cause a decrease in average weight, length, and rate of bone formation in the animal fetus.

- *Salicylates (e.g., aspirin)*—Studies on birth defects in humans have been done with aspirin, but not with salicylamide. Although salicylates have been shown to cause birth defects in animals, they have not been shown to cause birth defects in humans.

Regular use of salicylates late in pregnancy may cause unwanted effects on the heart or blood flow in the fetus or newborn baby. Use of salicylates during the last 2 weeks of pregnancy may cause bleeding problems in the fetus before or during delivery, or in the newborn baby. Also, too much use of salicylates during the last 3 months of pregnancy may increase the length of pregnancy, prolong labor and cause other problems during delivery, or cause severe bleeding in the mother before, during, or after delivery. *Do not take aspirin during the last 3 months of pregnancy unless it has been ordered by your doctor.*

**Breast-feeding**—If you are breast-feeding the chance that problems might occur depends on the ingredients of the combination. For the individual ingredients of these combinations, the following apply:

- *Acetaminophen*—Acetaminophen passes into the breast milk. However, it has not been reported to cause problems in nursing babies.
- *Alcohol*—Alcohol passes into the breast milk. However, the amount of alcohol in recommended doses of this medicine does not usually cause problems in nursing babies.
- *Caffeine*—Small amounts of caffeine pass into the breast milk and may build up in the nursing baby. However, the amount of caffeine in recommended doses of this medicine does not usually cause problems in nursing babies.
- *Decongestants (e.g., phenylephrine, phenylpropanolamine, pseudoephedrine)*—Decongestants may pass into the breast milk and may cause unwanted effects in nursing babies of mothers taking this medicine.
- *Salicylates (e.g., aspirin, salicylamide)*—Salicylates pass into the breast milk. Although salicylates have not been reported to cause problems in nursing babies, it is possible that problems may occur if large amounts are taken regularly.

**Children**—Very young children are usually more sensitive to the effects of this medicine. *Before giving any of these combination medicines to a child, check the package label very carefully. Some of these medicines are too strong for use in children.* If you are not certain whether a specific product can be given to a child, or if you have any questions about the amount to give, check with your health care professional, especially if it contains:

- *Decongestants (e.g., phenylephrine, phenylpropanolamine, pseudoephedrine)*—Increases in blood pressure may be more likely to occur in children taking decongestants. Also, mental changes may be more likely to occur in young children taking phenylpropanolamine-containing combinations.
- *Salicylates (e.g., aspirin)*—*Do not give aspirin or other salicylates to a child with a fever or other symptoms of a virus infection, especially flu or chickenpox, without first discussing its use with your child's doctor.* This is very important because salicylates may cause a serious illness called Reye's syndrome in these children. Also, children may be more sensitive to the aspirin or other salicylates contained in some of these medicines, especially if they have a fever or have lost large amounts of body fluid because of vomiting, diarrhea, or sweating.

**Teenagers**—*Do not give aspirin or other salicylates to a teenager with a fever or other symptoms of a virus infection, especially flu or chickenpox, without first discussing its use with your child's doctor.* This is very important because salicylates may cause a serious illness called Reye's syndrome in these individuals.

**Older adults**—The elderly are usually more sensitive to the effects of this medicine.

**Other medicines**—Although certain medicines should not be used together at all, in other cases two different medicines may be used together even if an interaction might occur. In these cases, your doctor may want to change the dose, or other precautions may be necessary. Tell your health care professional if you are taking *any* other prescription or nonprescription (over-the-counter [OTC]) medicine, for example, aspirin or other medicine for allergies. Some medicines may change the way this medicine affects your body. Also, the effect of other medicines may be increased or reduced by some of the ingredients in this medicine. Check with your health care professional about which medicines you should not take together with this medicine.

**Other medical problems**—The presence of other medical problems may affect the use of decongestant and analgesic combinations. Make sure you tell your doctor if you have any other medical problems, especially:

- Alcohol abuse—Acetaminophen-containing medicine increases the chance of liver damage
- Anemia—Taking aspirin-, salicylamide-, or ibuprofen-containing medicine may make the anemia worse
- Asthma, allergies, and nasal polyps, history of—Taking salicylate- or ibuprofen-containing medicine may cause an allergic reaction in which breathing becomes difficult
- Diabetes mellitus (sugar diabetes)—The decongestant in this medicine may put the patient with diabetes at a greater risk of having heart or blood vessel disease
- Gout—Aspirin-containing medicine may make the gout worse and reduce the benefit of the medicines used for gout
- Hepatitis or other liver disease—Liver disease increases the chance of side effects because the medicine is not broken down and may build up in the body; also, if liver disease is severe there is a greater chance that aspirin-containing medicine may cause bleeding, and that ibuprofen-containing medicine may cause serious kidney damage
- Heart or blood vessel disease or
- High blood pressure—The decongestant in this medicine may cause the blood pressure to increase and may also speed up the heart rate; also, caffeine-containing medicine if taken in large amounts may increase the heart rate; ibuprofen-containing medicine may cause the blood pressure to increase

- Hemophilia or other bleeding problems—Aspirin- or ibuprofen-containing medicine increases the chance of bleeding
- Kidney disease—The kidneys may be affected, especially if too much of this medicine is taken for a long time
- Mental illness (history of)—The decongestant in this medicine may increase the chance of mental side effects
- Overactive thyroid—If an overactive thyroid has caused a fast heart rate, the decongestant in this medicine may cause the heart rate to speed up further
- Stomach ulcer or other stomach problems—Salicylate- or ibuprofen-containing medicine may make the ulcer worse or cause bleeding of the stomach
- Systemic lupus erythematosus (SLE)—Ibuprofen-containing medicine may put the patient with SLE at a greater risk of having unwanted effects on the central nervous system and/or kidneys
- Ulcers, sores, or white spots in the mouth—This may be a sign of a serious side effect of ibuprofen-containing medicine; if you already have ulcers or sores in the mouth you and your doctor may not be able to tell when this side effect occurs

## Proper Use of This Medicine

*Take this medicine only as directed.* Do not take more of it and do not take it more often than recommended on the label, unless otherwise directed by your doctor. To do so may increase the chance of side effects.

For *aspirin- or salicylamide-containing medicines:*
- If this medicine irritates your stomach, you may take it with food or a glass of water or milk to lessen the irritation.
- *If a combination medicine containing aspirin has a strong vinegar-like odor, do not use it.* This odor means the medicine is breaking down. If you have any questions about this, check with your pharmacist.

For *ibuprofen-containing medicines:*
- To lessen stomach upset, these medicines may be taken with food or an antacid.
- Take with a full glass (8 ounces) of water. Also, do not lie down for about 15 to 30 minutes after taking the medicine. Doing so may cause irritation that may lead to trouble in swallowing.

**Dosing**—The dose of these combination medicines will be different for different products. *Follow the the directions on the box if you are buying this medicine without a prescription. Or, follow your doctor's orders if this medicine was prescribed.* The following information includes only the average doses for these combinations.

The number of capsules or tablets or teaspoonfuls of liquid that you take depends on the strengths of the medicines.

There is a large variety of decongestant and analgesic combination products on the market. Some products are for use in adults only, while others may be used in children. If you have any questions about this, check with your health care professional.

- For *oral* dosage forms (capsules, liquid, or tablets):
  —For sinus pain and congestion:
  - Adults and children 12 years of age and older: 1 to 2 capsules or tablets every four to six hours.
  - Children up to 6 years of age: Use and dose must be determined by your doctor.
  - Children 6 to 12 years of age: 1 tablet, 4 to 6 chewable tablets, or 1 to 2 teaspoonfuls of liquid every four hours.

**Missed dose**—If you must take this medicine regularly and you miss a dose, take it as soon as possible. However, if it is almost time for your next dose, skip the missed dose and go back to your regular dosing schedule. Do not double doses.

**Storage**—To store this medicine:
- Keep this medicine out of the reach of children. Overdose is very dangerous in young children.
- Store away from heat and direct light.
- Do not store the capsule or tablet form of this medicine in the bathroom, near the kitchen sink, or in other damp places. Heat or moisture may cause the medicine to break down.
- Keep the liquid form of this medicine from freezing.
- Do not keep outdated medicine or medicine no longer needed. Be sure that any discarded medicine is out of the reach of children.

## Precautions While Using This Medicine

Check with your doctor if your symptoms do not improve or become worse, or if you have a high fever.

This medicine may add to the central nervous system (CNS) stimulant and other effects of phenylpropanolamine (PPA)-containing diet aids. *Do not use medicines for diet or appetite control while taking this medicine unless you have checked with your doctor.*

This medicine may cause some people to become nervous or restless or to have trouble in sleeping. If you have trouble in sleeping, *take the last dose of this medicine for each day a few hours before bedtime.* If you have any questions about this, check with your doctor.

Before having any kind of surgery (including dental surgery) or emergency treatment, tell the medical doctor or dentist in charge that you are taking this medicine.

*Check the label of all over-the-counter (OTC), nonprescription, and prescription medicines you now take.* If any of them contain acetaminophen, aspirin, other salicylates such as bismuth subsalicylate (e.g., Pepto Bismol) or magnesium salicylate (e.g., Nuprin Backache Caplets), or salicylic acid (present in some shampoos and skin products), *check with your health care professional. Using any of them together with this medicine may cause an overdose.*

*Do not drink alcoholic beverages while taking this medicine.* Stomach problems may be more likely to occur if you drink alcoholic beverages while you are taking aspirin or ibuprofen. Also, liver damage may be more likely to occur if you drink large amounts of alcoholic beverages while you are taking acetaminophen.

*If you think that you or anyone else may have taken an overdose of this medicine, get emergency help at once.* Taking an overdose of a salicylate may cause unconsciousness or death. The first sign of an aspirin overdose may be ringing or buzzing in the ears. Other signs include convulsions (seizures), hearing loss, confusion, severe drowsiness or tiredness, severe excitement or nervousness, and unusually fast or deep breathing. Signs of severe acetaminophen overdose may not appear until 2 to 4 days after the overdose is taken, but treatment to prevent liver damage or death must be started within 24 hours or less after the overdose is taken.

For patients *taking aspirin-containing medicine:*
- Do not take aspirin-containing medicine for 5 days before any surgery, including dental surgery, unless otherwise directed by your medical doctor or dentist. Taking aspirin during this time may cause bleeding problems.

For diabetic patients *taking salicylate-containing medicine:*
- False urine sugar test results may occur if you take 8 or more 325-mg (5-grain) doses of aspirin every day for several days in a row. Smaller doses or occasional use of aspirin usually will not affect urine sugar tests. If you have any questions about this, check with your health care professional, especially if your diabetes is not well controlled.

For patients *taking ibuprofen-containing medicine:*
- This medicine may cause some people to become confused, drowsy, dizzy, lightheaded, or less alert than they are normally. It may also cause blurred vision or other vision problems in some people. *Make sure you know how you react to this medicine before you drive, use machines, or do anything else that could be dangerous if you are dizzy or are not alert and able to see well.*

## Side Effects of This Medicine

Along with its needed effects, a medicine may cause some unwanted effects. Although serious side effects occur rarely when this medicine is taken as recommended, they may be more likely to occur if:
- too much medicine is taken.
- it is taken in large doses.
- it is taken for a long period of time.

*Get emergency help immediately if any of the following symptoms of overdose occur:*
*For all combinations*
Convulsions (seizures); dizziness or lightheadedness (severe); fast, slow, or irregular heartbeat; hallucinations (seeing, hearing, or feeling things that are not there); headache (continuing and severe); increased sweating; mood or mental changes; nausea or vomiting (severe or continuing); nervousness or restlessness (severe); shortness of breath or troubled breathing; stomach cramps or pain (severe or continuing); swelling or tenderness in the upper abdomen or stomach area; trouble in sleeping
*For acetaminophen-containing only*
Diarrhea; loss of appetite
*For aspirin- or salicylamide-containing only*
Any loss of hearing; changes in behavior (in children); confusion; diarrhea (severe or continuing); drowsiness or tiredness (severe, especially in children); fast or deep breathing (especially in children); ringing or buzzing in ears (continuing); uncontrollable flapping movements of the hands, (especially in elderly patients); unexplained fever; unusual thirst; vision problems

Also, check with your doctor as soon as possible if any of the following side effects occur:
*More common*
Nausea, vomiting, or stomach pain (mild—for combinations containing aspirin or ibuprofen)

*Less common or rare*
Bloody or black, tarry stools; bloody or cloudy urine; blurred vision or any changes in vision or eyes; changes in facial skin color; changes in hearing; changes or problems with urination; difficult or painful urination; fever; headache, severe, with fever and stiff neck; increased blood pressure; muscle cramps or pain; skin rash, hives, or itching; sores, ulcers, or white spots on lips or in mouth; swelling of face, fingers, feet, or lower legs; swollen and/or painful glands; unexplained sore throat and fever; unusual bleeding or bruising; unusual tiredness or weakness; vomiting of blood or material that looks like coffee grounds; weight gain (unusual); yellow eyes or skin

Other side effects may occur that usually do not need medical attention. These side effects may go away during treatment as your body adjusts to the medicine. However, check with your doctor if any of the following side effects continue or are bothersome:
*More common*
Heartburn or indigestion (for medicines containing salicylate or ibuprofen); nervousness or restlessness
*Less common*
Drowsiness (for medicines containing salicylamide)

Not all of the side effects listed above have been reported for each of these medicines, but they have been reported for at least one of them. There are some similarities among these combination medicines, so many of the above side effects may occur with any of these medicines.

Other side effects not listed above may also occur in some patients. If you notice any other effects, check with your doctor.

Revised: 09/07/94

# DEFEROXAMINE   Systemic

A commonly used brand name in the U.S. and Canada is Desferal. Another commonly used name is desferrioxamine.

## Description

Deferoxamine (dee-fer-OX-a-meen) is used to remove excess iron from the body. This may be necessary in certain patients with anemia who must receive many blood transfusions. It is also used to treat acute iron poisoning, especially in small children.

Deferoxamine combines with iron in the bloodstream. The combination of iron and deferoxamine is then removed from the body by the kidneys. By removing the excess iron, the medicine lessens damage to various organs and tissues of the body. This medicine may be used for other conditions as determined by your doctor.

Deferoxamine is to be administered only by or under the immediate supervision of your doctor. It is available in the following dosage form:

*Parenteral*
- Injection (U.S. and Canada)

## Before Receiving This Medicine

In deciding to use a medicine, the risks of taking the medicine must be weighed against the good it will do. This is a decision you and your doctor will make. For deferoxamine, the following should be considered:

**Allergies**—Tell your doctor if you have ever had any unusual or allergic reaction to deferoxamine. Also tell your health care professional if you are allergic to any other substances, such as foods, preservatives, or dyes.

**Pregnancy**—Deferoxamine has not been shown to cause birth defects or other problems in humans. However, in animal studies this medicine caused birth defects when given in doses just above the recommended human dose. In general, deferoxamine is not recommended for women who may become pregnant or for use during early pregnancy, unless the woman's life is in danger from too much iron.

**Breast-feeding**—It is not known whether deferoxamine passes into breast milk. Although most medicines pass into breast milk in small amounts, many of them may be used safely while breast-feeding. Mothers who are taking this medicine and who wish to breast-feed should discuss this with their doctor.

**Children**—Deferoxamine is not used for long-term treatment of children up to 3 years of age. Also, younger patients are more likely to develop hearing and vision problems with the use of deferoxamine in high doses for a long time.

**Older adults**—The combination of deferoxamine and vitamin C should be used with caution in older patients, since this combination may be more likely to cause heart problems in these patients than in younger adults.

**Other medicines**—Although certain medicines should not be used together at all, in other cases two different medicines may be used together even if an interaction might occur. In these cases, your doctor may want to change the dose, or other precautions may be necessary. When you are receiving deferoxamine, it is especially important that your health care professional know if you are taking the following:

- Ascorbic acid (vitamin C)—Use with deferoxamine may be harmful to body tissues, especially in the elderly

**Other medical problems**—The presence of other medical problems may affect the use of deferoxamine. Make sure you tell your doctor if you have any other medical problems, especially:

- Kidney disease—Patients with kidney disease may be more likely to have side effects

## Proper Use of This Medicine

Deferoxamine may sometimes be given at home to patients who do not need to be in the hospital. If you are receiving this medicine at home, *make sure you clearly understand and carefully follow your doctor's instructions.*

**Dosing**—The dose of deferoxamine will be different for different patients. *Follow your doctor's orders or the directions on the label.* The following information includes only the average doses of deferoxamine. *If your dose is different, do not change it* unless your doctor tells you to do so.

- For *injection* dosage form:
  —For acute iron toxicity:
  - Adults and children over 3 years of age—Dose is based on body weight and must be determined by your doctor. The usual dose is 90 milligrams (mg) per kilogram (kg) (41 mg per pound) of body weight, followed by 45 mg per kg (20 mg per pound) of body weight, injected into a muscle every four to twelve hours. If it is injected into a vein, the usual dose is 15 mg per kg (7 mg per pound) of body weight per hour every eight hours.
  - Children up to 3 years of age—The usual dose is 15 mg per kg (7 mg per pound) of body weight per hour, injected into a vein.
  —For chronic iron toxicity:
  - Adults and children over 3 years of age—The usual dose is 500 mg to 1 gram a day, injected into a muscle. Or, the medicine may be injected under the skin by an infusion pump. The usual dose is 1 to 2 grams (20 to 40 mg per kg [9 to 18 mg per pound] of body weight) a day, injected under the skin, over a period of eight to twenty-four hours. If you are receiving blood transfusions, the usual dose is 500 mg to 1 gram a day, injected into a muscle. An extra 2 grams of the medicine is injected into a vein with each unit

of blood at a rate of 15 mg per kg of body weight per hour.

- Children up to 3 years of age—Use and dose must be determined by your doctor. The usual dose is 10 mg per kg (5 mg per pound) of body weight a day, injected under the skin.

**Storage**—To store this medicine:

- Keep out of the reach of children.
- Store away from heat and direct light.
- Store the mixed medicine at room temperature for no longer than recommended by your doctor or the manufacturer. Do not refrigerate.
- Do not keep outdated medicine or medicine that is no longer needed. Be sure any discarded medicine is out of the reach of children.

---

## Precautions While Receiving This Medicine

*It is important that your doctor check your progress at regular visits* to make sure that this medicine is working properly and to prevent unwanted effects. Certain blood and urine tests must be done regularly to check for the need for dosage changes.

Deferoxamine may cause some people, especially younger patients, to have hearing and vision problems within a few weeks after they start taking it. *If you notice any problems with your vision, such as blurred vision, difficulty in seeing at night, or difficulty in seeing colors, or difficulty with your hearing, check with your doctor as soon as possible.* The dose of deferoxamine may need to be adjusted.

Do not take vitamin C unless your doctor has told you to do so.

---

## Side Effects of This Medicine

Along with its needed effects, a medicine may cause some unwanted effects. Although not all of these side effects may occur, if they do occur they may need medical attention.

Check with your doctor as soon as possible if any of the following side effects occur:

*More common*

Bluish fingernails, lips, or skin; blurred vision or other problems with vision; convulsions (seizures); difficulty in breathing (wheezing), or fast breathing; fast heartbeat; hearing problems; pain or swelling at place of injection; redness or flushing of skin; skin rash, hives, or itching

*Less common*

Diarrhea; difficult urination; fever; leg cramps; stomach and muscle cramps; stomach discomfort; unusual bleeding or bruising

Hearing and vision problems are more likely to occur in younger patients taking high doses and on long-term treatment.

Deferoxamine may cause the urine to turn orange-rose in color. This is to be expected while you are using this medicine.

Other side effects not listed above may also occur in some patients. If you notice any other effects, check with your doctor.

---

## Additional Information

Once a medicine has been approved for marketing for a certain use, experience may show that it is also useful for other medical problems. Although this use is not included in product labeling, deferoxamine is used in certain patients with the following medical condition:

- Aluminum toxicity (too much aluminum in the body)

Other than the above information, there is no additional information relating to proper use, precautions, or side effects for this use.

---

Revised: 05/27/94

---

# DESFLURANE   Inhalation-Systemic†

A commonly used brand name in the U.S. is Suprane.

---

†Not commercially available in Canada.

---

## Description

Desflurane (DES-flure-ane) belongs to the group of medicines known as general anesthetics (an-ess-THET-iks). Desflurane is used to cause general anesthesia (loss of consciousness) before and during surgery. It is breathed in (inhaled). Although desflurane can be used by itself, combinations of anesthetics are often used together. This helps produce more effective anesthesia in some patients.

*General anesthetics are given only by or under the immediate supervision of a medical doctor trained to use them.* If you will be receiving a general anesthetic during surgery, your doctor will give you the medicine and closely follow your progress.

Desflurane is available in the following dosage form:

- Inhalation (U.S.)

---

## Before Receiving This Medicine

In deciding to use a medicine, the risks of using the medicine must be weighed against the good it will do. For desflurane, the following should be considered:

---

© 1994  The United States Pharmacopeial Convention, Inc.

**Allergies**—Tell your doctor if you have ever had any unusual or allergic reaction to an anesthetic. Also tell your doctor if you are allergic to any other substances, such as foods, preservatives, or dyes.

**Pregnancy**—Desflurane has not been studied in pregnant women. It did not cause birth defects in animal studies. However, desflurane caused other unwanted effects in the animal fetus when given for many days in a row in amounts that were large enough to cause harmful effects in the mother.

**Breast-feeding**—Small amounts of desflurane may pass into the breast milk. Your doctor may want you to stop breast-feeding for about 24 hours after receiving the medicine.

**Children**—Desflurane has been tested in children. It is not used to start anesthesia in children who are awake because it causes irritation and other unwanted effects. However, when it is used to continue general anesthesia that has been started with another anesthetic, desflurane does not cause different side effects or problems in children than it does in adults.

**Older adults**—Desflurane has been tested and has not been shown to cause different side effects or problems in older people than it does in younger adults. However, older people usually need smaller amounts of an anesthetic than younger people. Your doctor will take your age into account when deciding on the right amount of desflurane for you.

**Other medicines**—Although certain medicines should not be used together at all, in other cases 2 different medicines may be used together even if an interaction might occur. In these cases, your doctor may want to change the dose, or other precautions may be necessary. When you are receiving a general anesthetic, it is especially important that your doctor know if you are taking **any** other prescription or nonprescription (over-the-counter [OTC]) medicine or any of the following:

- "Street" drugs, such as amphetamines ("uppers"), barbiturates ("downers"), cocaine, marijuana, phencyclidine (PCP or "angel dust"), and heroin or other narcotics—Serious, possibly fatal, side effects may occur if your doctor gives you an anesthetic without knowing that you have taken another medicine

**Other medical problems**—The presence of other medical problems may affect the use of desflurane. Make sure you tell your doctor if you have **any** other medical problems, especially:

- Diseases that can cause muscle weakness, such as familial periodic paralysis, muscular dystrophy, myasthenia gravis, or Eaton-Lambert syndrome, or
- Heart or blood vessel disease—The chance of side effects may be increased, but serious problems can be prevented if your doctor knows that these conditions are present before giving you an anesthetic
- Malignant hyperthermia, during or shortly after receiving an anesthetic (history of, or family history of). Signs of malignant hyperthermia include very high fever, fast and irregular heartbeat, muscle spasms or tightness, and breathing problems—This side effect may occur again

## Proper Use of This Medicine

**Dosing**—The dose of desflurane will be different for different patients. Your doctor will decide on the right amount for you, depending on:

- Your age.
- Your general physical condition.
- The kind of surgery being performed.
- Other medicines you are taking or will receive before and during surgery.

## Precautions After Receiving This Medicine

For patients going home within 24 hours after receiving a general anesthetic:

- General anesthetics may cause some people to feel drowsy, tired, or weak for a while after they have been given. They may also cause problems with coordination and one's ability to think. Therefore, for about 24 hours (or longer if necessary) after receiving a general anesthetic, *do not drive, use machines, or do anything else that could be dangerous if you are not alert.*
- Unless otherwise directed by your doctor or dentist, *do not drink alcoholic beverages or take other CNS depressants (medicines that slow down the nervous system, possibly causing drowsiness) for about 24 hours after you have received a general anesthetic.* To do so may add to the effects of the anesthetic. Some examples of CNS depressants are antihistamines or medicine for hay fever, other allergies, or colds; other sedatives, tranquilizers, or sleeping medicine; prescription pain medicine or narcotics; barbiturates; medicine for seizures; and muscle relaxants.

## Side Effects of This Medicine

Along with its needed effects, a medicine may cause some unwanted effects. Although not all of these side effects may occur, if they do occur they may need medical attention. While you are receiving and recovering from a general anesthetic, your health care professional will closely follow its effects. However, some effects may not be noticed until later.

The following side effects should go away as the effects of the anesthetic wear off. However, check with your doctor if any of them continue or are bothersome:

*More common*
    Coughing; nausea or vomiting

*Less common or rare*
    Dizziness; headache; irritated or red eyes; nervousness and restlessness; sore throat

Other side effects not listed above may also occur in some patients. If you notice any other effects, check with your doctor.

Developed: 12/21/93

# DESMOPRESSIN  Systemic

Some commonly used brand names are:

**In the U.S.—**
DDAVP
DDAVP Nasal Spray
DDAVP Rhinal Tube
Stimate

**In Canada—**
DDAVP
DDAVP Nasal Spray
DDAVP Rhinyle Drops

## Description

Desmopressin (des-moe-PRESS-in) is a hormone taken through the nose or given by injection to prevent or control the frequent urination, increased thirst, and loss of water associated with diabetes insipidus (water diabetes). It is used also to control frequent urination and increased thirst associated with certain types of brain injuries or brain surgery or bed-wetting. Desmopressin works by acting on the kidneys to reduce the flow of urine.

Desmopressin is also given by injection to treat some patients with certain bleeding problems such as hemophilia or von Willebrand's disease.

Desmopressin is available only with your doctor's prescription, in the following dosage forms:

*Nasal*
• Nasal solution (U.S. and Canada)
*Parenteral*
• Injection (U.S. and Canada)

## Before Using This Medicine

In deciding to use a medicine, the risks of taking the medicine must be weighed against the good it will do. This is a decision you and your doctor will make. For desmopressin, the following should be considered:

**Allergies**—Tell your doctor if you have ever had any unusual or allergic reaction to desmopressin. Also tell your health care professional if you are allergic to any other substances, such as foods, preservatives, or dyes.

**Pregnancy**—Studies have not been done in pregnant women. Desmopressin has been used before and during pregnancy to treat diabetes insipidus and has not been shown to cause birth defects.

**Breast-feeding**—Desmopressin passes into breast milk in very small amounts. However, it has not been reported to cause problems in nursing babies.

**Children**—Infants may be more sensitive to the effects of this medicine.

**Older adults**—Some side effects (confusion, drowsiness, continuing headache, problem with urination, weight gain) may be especially likely to occur in elderly patients, who are usually more sensitive than younger adults to the effects of desmopressin.

**Other medicines**—Although certain medicines should not be used together at all, in other cases two different medicines may be used together even if an interaction might

occur. In these cases, your doctor may want to change the dose, or other precautions may be necessary. Tell your health care professional if you are taking any other prescription or nonprescription (over-the-counter [OTC]) medicine.

**Other medical problems**—The presence of other medical problems may affect the use of desmopressin. Make sure you tell your doctor if you have any other medical problems, especially:

• Cystic fibrosis—Excess water retention and serious side effects may be more likely to occur in patients with this condition
• Heart or blood vessel disease or
• High blood pressure—Large doses of desmopressin can cause an increase in blood pressure
• Stuffy nose caused by cold or allergy—May prevent nasal desmopressin from being absorbed through the lining of the nose into the bloodstream

## Proper Use of This Medicine

For patients using the *nasal solution form* of this medicine:

• *Use this medicine only as directed.* Do not use more of it and do not use it more often than your doctor ordered. To do so may increase the chance of side effects.
• This medicine usually comes with patient directions. Read them carefully before using this medicine.

**Dosing**—When you are using desmopressin, it is very important that you get the exact amount of medicine that you need. The dose of desmopressin will be different for different patients. Your doctor will determine the proper dose of desmopressin for you.

*The number of doses you use each day, the time allowed between doses, and the length of time you use the medicine depend on the medical problem for which you are using desmopressin.*

• For *nasal* dosage form (nasal solution):
  —For preventing or controlling diabetes insipidus (water diabetes):
    • Adults and teenagers—At first, 10 micrograms (mcg) inhaled in a nostril at bedtime. Your doctor may increase the dose gradually each night if needed. Then, your doctor may want you to use 10 to 40 mcg. The dose may be used as a single dose or it may be divided into two or three doses a day.
    • Children up to 3 months of age—Dose must be determined by your doctor.
    • Children 3 months to 12 years of age—At first, 5 mcg (0.05 mL) inhaled in a nostril at bedtime. Your doctor may increase the dose gradually each night if needed. Then, your doctor may change the dose based on your body weight. The usual dose is 2 to 4 mcg per kilogram (kg) (0.91 to

1.82 mcg per pound) of body weight a day. The dose may used as a single dose or it may be divided into two doses a day.

—For controlling bed-wetting:

• Adults, teenagers, and children over 6 years of age—At first, 10 mcg inhaled into each nostril at bedtime. Then, your doctor may change the dose to 10 to 40 mcg a day.

• Children up to 6 years of age—Dose must be determined by your doctor.

• For *parenteral* dosage form (injection):

—For preventing or controlling frequent urination:

• Adults and teenagers—2 to 4 mcg injected into a vein or under the skin a day. This dose is usually divided into two doses.

—For treating some bleeding problems such as hemophilia or von Willebrand's disease:

• Adults and teenagers—0.3 mcg per kg (0.14 mcg per pound) of body weight mixed in fifty mL of 0.9% sodium chloride. This solution is injected into a vein slowly over fifteen to thirty minutes. Your doctor may repeat this treatment if needed.

• Children up to 3 months of age—Use is not recommended.

• Children 3 months of age or older—The dose is based on body weight and must be determined by your doctor:

—For children weighing 10 kg (22 pounds) or less—0.3 mcg per kg (0.135 mcg per pound) of body weight mixed in ten mL of 0.9% sodium chloride and injected over fifteen or thirty minutes into a vein by your doctor. Your doctor may repeat this treatment if needed.

—For children weighing more than 10 kg (22 pounds)—0.3 mcg per kg (0.14 mcg per pound) of body weight mixed in fifty mL of 0.9% sodium chloride and injected into a vein slowly over fifteen to thirty minutes by your doctor. Your doctor may repeat this treatment if needed.

**Missed dose**—*For nasal solution form of this medicine:* If you miss a dose of this medicine and your dosing schedule is—

• One dose a day—Use the missed dose as soon as possible. Then go back to your regular dosing schedule. However, if you do not remember the missed

dose until the next day, skip the missed dose and go back to your regular dosing schedule. Do not double doses.

• More than one dose a day—Use the missed dose as soon as possible. Then go back to your regular dosing schedule. However, if it is almost time for your next dose, skip the missed dose and go back to your regular dosing schedule. Do not double doses.

**Storage**—To store this medicine:

• Keep out of the reach of children.

• Store in the refrigerator. However, keep the medicine from freezing.

• Do not keep outdated medicine or medicine no longer needed. Be sure that any discarded medicine is out of the reach of children.

## Side Effects of This Medicine

Along with its needed effects, a medicine may cause some unwanted effects. Although not all of these effects may occur, if they do occur they may need medical attention.

*Check with your doctor immediately* if any of the following side effects occur:

Confusion; convulsions (seizures); drowsiness; headache (continuing); decreased urination; weight gain (rapid)

Other side effects may occur that usually do not need medical attention. These side effects may go away during treatment as your body adjusts to the medicine. However, check with your doctor if any of the following side effects continue or are bothersome:

*Less common or rare*

Abdominal or stomach cramps; flushing or redness of skin; headache; nausea; pain in the vulva (genital area outside of the vagina)

*With intranasal (through the nose) use*

Runny or stuffy nose

*With intravenous use*

Pain, redness, or swelling at place of injection

Other side effects not listed above may also occur in some patients. If you notice any other effects, check with your doctor.

Revised: 10/26/92
Interim revision: 06/02/94

# DEXTROMETHORPHAN    Systemic

Some commonly used brand names are:

**In the U.S.—**

| | |
|---|---|
| Benylin DM | Robitussin Cough Calmers |
| Children's Hold | Robitussin Maximum Strength |
| Cough-X | Cough Suppressant |
| Creo-Terpin | Robitussin Pediatric |
| Delsym | St. Joseph Cough Suppressant |
| Drixoral Cough Liquid Caps | for Children |
| Hold | Sucrets Cough Control |
| Mediquell | Formula |
| Pertussin Cough Suppressant | Trocal |
| Pertussin CS | Vicks Formula 44 Pediatric |
| Pertussin ES | Formula |

**In Canada—**

| | |
|---|---|
| Balminil D.M. | Ornex•DM 15 |
| Broncho-Grippol-DM | Ornex•DM 30 |
| Delsym | Robidex |
| DM Syrup | Robitussin Pediatric |
| Koffex | Sedatuss |
| Neo-DM | |

## Description

Dextromethorphan (dex-troe-meth-OR-fan) is used to relieve coughs due to colds or influenza (flu). It should not be used for chronic cough that occurs with smoking, asthma, or emphysema or when there is an unusually large amount of mucus or phlegm (flem) with the cough.

Dextromethorphan relieves cough by acting directly on the cough center in the brain.

This medicine is available without a prescription; however, your doctor may have special instructions on the proper use of this medicine for your medical condition. It is available in the following dosage forms:

*Oral*

- Capsules (U.S. and Canada)
- Lozenges (U.S.)
- Extended-release oral suspension (U.S. and Canada)
- Syrup (U.S. and Canada)
- Chewable tablets (U.S.)

## Before Using this Medicine

If you are taking this medicine without a prescription, carefully read and follow any precautions on the label. For dextromethorphan, the following should be considered:

**Allergies**—Tell your doctor if you have ever had any unusual or allergic reaction to dextromethorphan. Also tell your health care professional if you are allergic to any other substances, such as foods, preservatives, or dyes.

**Diet**—Make certain your health care professional knows if you are on a low-sodium, low-sugar, or any other special diet. Most medicines contain more than their active ingredient, and many liquid medicines contain alcohol.

**Pregnancy**—Dextromethorphan has not been shown to cause birth defects or other problems in humans.

**Breast-feeding**—Dextromethorphan has not been reported to cause problems in nursing babies.

**Children**—Although there is no specific information comparing use of dextromethorphan in children with use in other age groups, this medicine is not expected to cause different side effects or problems in children than it does in adults.

**Older adults**—Many medicines have not been studied specifically in older people. Therefore, it may not be known whether they work exactly the same way they do in younger adults or if they cause different side effects or problems in older people. There is no specific information comparing use of dextromethorphan in the elderly with use in other age groups.

**Other medicines**—Although certain medicines should not be used together at all, in other cases 2 different medicines may be used together even if an interaction might occur. In these cases, your doctor may want to change the dose, or other precautions may be necessary. When you are taking dextromethorphan it is especially important that your health care professional know if you are taking any of the following:

- Central nervous system (CNS) depressants (medicines that cause drowsiness)—The CNS depressant effects of either these medicines or dextromethorphan may be increased
- Monoamine oxidase (MAO) inhibitors (furazolidone [e.g., Furoxone], isocarboxazid [e.g., Marplan], phenelzine [e.g., Nardil], procarbazine [e.g., Matulane], tranylcypromine [e.g., Parnate])—Taking dextromethorphan if you are taking MAO inhibitors or have taken them within the past 2 weeks may cause coma, dizziness, excited or unusual behavior, fever, high blood pressure, nausea, sluggishness, spasms, and tremors

**Other medical problems**—The presence of other medical problems may affect the use of dextromethorphan. Make sure you tell your doctor if you have any other medical problems, especially:

- Asthma—Since dextromethorphan decreases coughing, it makes it difficult to get rid of the mucus that collects in the lungs and airways during asthma
- Liver disease—Dextromethorphan may build up in the body and cause unwanted effects
- Mucus or phlegm with cough—Since dextromethorphan decreases coughing, it makes it difficult to get rid of the mucus that may collect in the lungs and airways with some diseases

## Proper Use of This Medicine

*Use this medicine only as directed by your doctor or the directions on the label.* Do not use more of it, do not use it more often, and do not use it for a longer time than your doctor or the label says. Although this effect has happened only rarely, dextromethorphan has become habit-forming (causing mental or physical dependence) in some persons who used too much for a long time.

**Dosing**—The dose of dextromethrophan will be different for different patients. *Follow your doctor's orders or the* *directions on the label.* The following information includes only the average doses of dextromethrophan. *If your dose is different, do not change it* unless your doctor tells you to do so.

The number of capsules or tablets or teaspoonfuls of suspension or syrup that you take depends on the strength of the medicine.

- For *regular (short-acting) oral* dosage form (capsules, lozenges, syrup, or tablets):
  - —For cough:
    - Adults—10 to 20 milligrams (mg) every four hours or 30 mg every six to eight hours, as needed.
    - Children younger than 2 years of age—Use and dose must be determined by your doctor.
    - Children 2 to 6 years of age—2.5 to 5 mg every four hours or 7.5 mg every six to eight hours, as needed.
    - Children 6 to 12 years of age—5 to 10 mg every four hours or 15 mg every six to eight hours, as needed.
- For *long-acting oral* dosage form (extended-release oral suspension):
  - —For cough:
    - Adults—60 mg every twelve hours, as needed.
    - Children younger than 2 years of age—Use and dose must be determined by your doctor.
    - Children 2 to 6 years of age—15 mg every twelve hours, as needed.
    - Children 6 to 12 years of age—30 mg every twelve hours, as needed.

**Missed dose**—If you must take this medicine regularly and you miss a dose, take it as soon as possible. However, if it is almost time for your next dose, skip the missed dose and go back to your regular dosing schedule. Do not double doses.

**Storage**—To store this medicine:
- Store away from heat and direct light.
- Keep out of the reach of children.
- Do not store the tablet form of this medicine in the bathroom, near the kitchen sink, or in other damp places. Heat or moisture may cause the medicine to break down.
- Keep the liquid form of this medicine from freezing.
- Do not keep outdated medicine or medicine no longer needed. Be sure that any discarded medicine is out of the reach of children.

## Precautions While Using This Medicine

If your cough has not improved after 7 days or if you have a high fever, skin rash, or continuing headache with the cough, check with your doctor. These signs may mean that you have other medical problems.

## Side Effects of This Medicine

Along with its needed effects, a medicine may cause some unwanted effects. Although not all of these side effects may occur, if they do occur they may need medical attention.

Check with your doctor as soon as possible if any of the following side effects occur:

*Symptoms of overdose*
> Confusion; drowsiness or dizziness; nausea or vomiting (severe); unusual excitement, nervousness, restlessness, or irritability (severe)

Other side effects may occur that usually do not need medical attention. These side effects may go away during treatment as your body adjusts to the medicine. However, check with your health care professional if any of the following side effects continue or are bothersome:

*Less common or rare*
> Dizziness (mild); drowsiness (mild); nausea or vomiting; stomach pain

Other side effects not listed above may also occur in some patients. If you notice any other effects, check with your doctor.

Revised: 06/23/94

---

# DEXTROTHYROXINE   Systemic

Some commonly used brand names are:
**In the U.S.—**
  Choloxin
**In Canada—**
  Choloxin
**Other—**

| | |
|---|---|
| Biotirmone | Dynothel |
| Debetrol | Eulipos |
| Dethyrona | Lisolipin |
| Dethyrone | Nadrothyron-D |

## Description

Dextrothyroxine (dex-troe-thye-ROX-een) is used to lower high cholesterol levels in the blood. However, it has generally been replaced by safer medicines for the treatment of high cholesterol.

Dextrothyroxine is available only with your doctor's prescription, in the following dosage form:
*Oral*
- Tablets (U.S. and Canada)

## Before Using This Medicine

In deciding to use a medicine, the risks of taking the medicine must be weighed against the good it will do. This is a decision you and your doctor will make. For dextrothyroxine, the following should be considered:

**Allergies**—Tell your doctor if you have ever had any unusual or allergic reaction to dextrothyroxine. Also tell your health care professional if you are allergic to any other substances, such as foods, preservatives, or dyes.

**Diet**—Before prescribing medicine for your condition, your doctor will probably try to control your condition by prescribing a personal diet for you. Such a diet may be low in fats, sugars, and/or cholesterol. Many people are able to control their condition by carefully following their doctor's orders for proper diet and exercise. *Medicine is prescribed only when additional help is needed* and is effective only when a schedule of diet and exercise is properly followed.

Also, this medicine is less effective if you are greatly overweight. It may be very important for you to go on a reducing diet. However, check with your doctor before going on any diet.

Make certain your health care professional knows if you are on any special diet, such as a low-sodium or low-sugar diet.

**Pregnancy**—Dextrothyroxine has not been studied in pregnant women. However, studies in animals have not shown that dextrothyroxine causes birth defects or other problems. Before taking this medicine, make sure your doctor knows if you are pregnant or if you may become pregnant.

**Breast-feeding**—It is not known whether dextrothyroxine passes into breast milk. Although most medicines pass into breast milk in small amounts, many of them may be used safely while breast-feeding. Mothers who are taking this medicine and who wish to breast-feed should discuss this with their doctor.

**Children**—There is no specific information comparing use of dextrothyroxine in children to use in other age groups. However, use is not recommended in children under 2 years of age since cholesterol is needed for normal development.

**Older adults**—Side effects are more likely to occur in the elderly, who are usually more sensitive to the effects of dextrothyroxine.

**Other medicines**—Although certain medicines should not be used together at all, in other cases two different medicines may be used together even if an interaction might occur. In these cases, your doctor may want to change the dose, or other precautions may be necessary. When you are taking dextrothyroxine, it is especially important that your health care professional know if you are taking any of the following:

- Anticoagulants (blood thinners)—The effects of the anticoagulant may be altered; a change in dosage of the anticoagulant may be necessary

- Cholestyramine (e.g., Questran) or
- Colestipol (e.g., Colestid)—The effects of dextrothyroxine may decrease; these two medicines should be taken at least 4 to 5 hours before or after dextrothyroxine

**Other medical problems**—The presence of other medical problems may affect the use of dextrothyroxine. Make sure you tell your doctor if you have any other medical problems, especially:

- Diabetes mellitus (sugar diabetes)—Blood sugar levels may be increased
- Heart or blood vessel disease or
- High blood pressure or
- Overactive thyroid—Dextrothyroxine may make these conditions worse
- Kidney disease—Higher blood levels of dextrothyroxine may result and increase the chance of side effects
- Liver disease—May lead to an increase in cholesterol blood levels
- Underactive thyroid—There may be an increased sensitivity to the effects of dextrothyroxine

## Proper Use of This Medicine

*Take this medicine exactly as directed by your doctor.* Try not to miss any doses and do not take more medicine than your doctor ordered.

Remember that this medicine will not cure your cholesterol problem but it does help control it. Therefore, you must continue to take it as directed if you expect to lower your cholesterol level.

*Follow carefully the special diet your doctor gave you.* This is the most important part of controlling your condition, and is necessary if the medicine is to work properly.

**Dosing**—The dose of dextrothyroxine will be different for different patients. *Follow your doctor's orders or the directions on the label.* The following information includes only the average doses of dextrothyroxine. *If your dose is different, do not change it* unless your doctor tells you to do so:

The number of tablets that you take depends on the strength of the medicine.

- For *oral* dosage form (tablets):
  —For treatment of high cholesterol:
    - Adults—1 to 8 milligrams (mg) a day.
    - Children up to two years of age—Use is not recommended.
    - Children two years of age and older—50 to 100 micrograms (0.05 to 0.1 mg) per kilogram of body weight a day.

**Missed dose**—If you miss a dose of this medicine, take it as soon as possible. However, if it is almost time for your next dose, skip the missed dose and go back to your regular dosing schedule. Do not double doses.

**Storage**—To store this medicine:

- Keep out of the reach of children.
- Store away from heat and direct light.

- Do not store in the bathroom, near the kitchen sink, or in other damp places. Heat or moisture may cause the medicine to break down.
- Do not keep outdated medicine or medicine no longer needed. Be sure that any discarded medicine is out of the reach of children.

## Precautions While Using This Medicine

*It is very important that your doctor check your progress at regular visits.* This will allow your doctor to see if the medicine is working properly to lower your cholesterol levels and if you should continue to take it.

*Do not stop taking this medicine without first checking with your doctor.* When you stop taking this medicine, your blood cholesterol levels may increase again. Your doctor may want you to follow a special diet to help prevent this from happening.

Before having any kind of surgery (including dental surgery) or emergency treatment, *tell the medical doctor or dentist in charge that you are taking this medicine.*

## Side Effects of This Medicine

Along with its needed effects, a medicine may cause some unwanted effects. Although not all of these side effects may occur, if they do occur they may need medical attention.

*Check with your doctor immediately* if any of the following side effects occur:
   *Rare*
      Chest pain; fast or irregular heartbeat; stomach pain (severe) with nausea and vomiting

Check with your doctor as soon as possible if the following side effects occur, since they may indicate too much medicine is being taken:
   *Rare*
      Changes in appetite; changes in menstrual periods; diarrhea; fast or irregular heartbeat; fever; hand tremors; headache; increase in urination; irritability, nervousness, or trouble in sleeping; leg cramps; shortness of breath; skin rash or itching; sweating, flushing, or increased sensitivity to heat; unusual weight loss; vomiting

Other side effects not listed above may also occur in some patients. If you notice any other effects, check with your doctor.

Revised: 04/22/93

---

# DEZOCINE   Systemic†

A commonly used brand name in the U.S. is Dalgan.

   †Not commercially available in Canada.

## Description

Dezocine (DEZ-oh-seen) belongs to the group of medicines known as narcotic analgesics (nar-KOT-ik an-al-JEE-zicks). Narcotic analgesics act in the central nervous system (CNS) to relieve pain. Some of their side effects are also caused by actions in the CNS.

Dezocine is available only with your doctor's prescription. It is available in the following dosage form:
   *Parenteral*
   - Injection (U.S.)

## Before Using This Medicine

In deciding to use a medicine, the risks of using the medicine must be weighed against the good it will do. This is a decision you and your doctor will make. For dezocine, the following should be considered:

**Allergies**—Tell your doctor if you have ever had any unusual or allergic reaction to dezocine. Also tell your health care professional if you are allergic to any other substances, such as foods, preservatives, or dyes.

**Pregnancy**—Studies on birth defects with dezocine have not been done in pregnant women. Dezocine did not cause birth defects in animal studies. However, the birth weights of the newborn animals were lower than normal, probably because the pregnant animals ate less than usual.

Too much use of a narcotic during pregnancy may cause the baby to become dependent on the medicine. This may lead to withdrawal side effects after birth. Also, narcotics may cause breathing problems in the newborn infant if taken just before delivery.

**Breast-feeding**—It is not known whether dezocine passes into the breast milk. However, it has not been reported to cause problems in nursing babies.

**Children**—Studies on this medicine have been done only in adult patients, and there is no specific information comparing use of dezocine in patients up to 18 years of age with use in other age groups.

**Older adults**—Elderly people are especially sensitive to the effects of narcotic analgesics such as dezocine. This may increase the chance of side effects, especially breathing problems, during treatment.

**Other medicines**—Although certain medicines should not be used together at all, in other cases two different medicines may be used together even if an interaction might occur. In these cases, your doctor may want to change

the dose, or other precautions may be necessary. When you are using dezocine, it is especially important that your health care professional know if you are taking any of the following:

- Central nervous system (CNS) depressants, including other narcotics, or
- Tricyclic antidepressants (amitriptyline [e.g., Elavil], amoxapine [e.g., Asendin], clomipramine [e.g., Anafranil], desipramine [e.g., Pertofrane], doxepin [e.g., Sinequan], imipramine [e.g., Tofranil], nortriptyline [e.g., Aventyl], protriptyline [e.g., Vivactil], trimipramine [e.g., Surmontil])—The chance of side effects may be increased
- Naltrexone (e.g., Trexan)—Dezocine may not be effective in people taking naltrexone

**Other medical problems**—The presence of other medical problems may affect the use of dezocine. Make sure you tell your doctor if you have any other medical problems, especially:

- Alcohol abuse, or history of, or
- Drug dependence, especially narcotic abuse, or history of, or
- Emotional problems—The chance of side effects may be increased; also, withdrawal symptoms may occur if a narcotic you are dependent on is replaced by dezocine
- Brain disease or head injury or
- Colitis or other intestinal disease or
- Diarrhea or
- Emphysema, asthma, or other chronic lung disease or
- Enlarged prostate or problems with urination—Some of the side effects of narcotic analgesics can be dangerous if these conditions are present
- Heart or blood vessel disease, severe, or
- Gallbladder disease or gallstones or
- Kidney disease or
- Liver disease or
- Underactive thyroid—The chance of side effects may be increased

## Proper Use of This Medicine

Some narcotic analgesics given by injection may be used at home by patients who do not need to be in the hospital. If you are using dezocine at home, *make sure you clearly understand and carefully follow your doctor's directions.*

*Take this medicine only as directed by your doctor.* Do not use more of it, do not use it more often, and do not use it for a longer time than your doctor ordered. This is especially important for elderly patients, who are more sensitive than younger adults to the effects of narcotic analgesics. If too much is taken, the medicine may become habit-forming (causing mental or physical dependence) or lead to medical problems because of an overdose.

**Dosing**—The dose of dezocine will be different for different patients. *Follow your doctor's orders or the directions on the label.* The following information includes only the average doses of dezocine. *If your dose is different, do not change it* unless your doctor tells you to do so.

The number of milliliters (mL) of injection that you use for each dose depends on the strength of the medicine.

- For *parenteral* dosage form (injection):
  —For pain:
    - Adults—The usual dose is 10 milligrams (mg), injected into a muscle every three to six hours as needed. Some people may need only 5 mg and others may need 15 or 20 mg. The medicine may also be injected into a vein in a dose of 2.5 to 10 mg every two to four hours as needed. The total amount used in twenty-four hours should not be more than 120 mg. Elderly people, people who are very ill, and people with breathing problems may have to use lower doses than other adults.
    - Children and teenagers up to 18 years of age— Use and dose must be determined by your doctor.

**Missed dose**—If your doctor has ordered you to use dezocine according to a regular schedule and you miss a dose, use it as soon as you remember. However, if it is almost time for your next dose, skip the missed dose and go back to your regular dosing schedule. *Do not double doses.*

**Storage**—To store this medicine:

- Keep out of the reach of children. Overdose is very dangerous in young children.
- Store away from heat and direct light.
- Keep the medicine from freezing.
- Do not keep outdated medicine or medicine no longer needed. Be sure that any discarded medicine is out of the reach of children.

## Precautions While Using This Medicine

Dezocine will add to the effects of alcohol and other CNS depressants (medicines that slow down the nervous system, possibly causing drowsiness). Some examples of CNS depressants are antihistamines or medicine for hay fever, other allergies, or colds; sedatives, tranquilizers, or sleeping medicine; other prescription pain medicines including other narcotics; barbiturates; medicine for seizures; muscle relaxants; or anesthetics, including some dental anesthetics. *Do not drink alcoholic beverages, and check with your doctor before taking any of the medicines listed above, while you are using this medicine.*

This medicine may cause some people to become drowsy, dizzy, or lightheaded. *Make sure you know how you react to this medicine before you drive, use machines, or do anything else that could be dangerous if you are dizzy or are not alert.*

Dizziness, lightheadedness, or fainting may occur, especially when you get up suddenly from a lying or sitting position. Getting up slowly may help lessen this problem. Also, lying down for a while may help relieve these effects.

Nausea or vomiting may occur, especially after the first couple of doses. This effect may go away if you lie down for a while. However, if nausea or vomiting continues, check with your doctor.

Before having any kind of surgery (including dental surgery) or emergency treatment, tell the health care professional in charge that you are taking this medicine. Serious side effects may occur if your health care professional gives you certain medicines without knowing that you are using dezocine.

*If you think you or someone else may have taken an overdose, get emergency help at once.* Taking an overdose of this medicine or taking alcohol or CNS depressants with it may lead to unconsciousness or death. Signs of overdose of narcotic analgesics include convulsions (seizures), confusion, severe nervousness or restlessness, severe dizziness, severe drowsiness, slow or troubled breathing, and severe weakness.

## Side Effects of This Medicine

Along with its needed effects, a medicine may cause some unwanted effects. Although not all of these side effects may occur, if they do occur they may need medical attention.

*Get emergency help immediately if any of the following symptoms of overdose occur:*

Cold, clammy skin; confusion, nervousness, or restlessness (severe); convulsions (seizures); dizziness (severe); drowsiness (severe); low blood pressure; pinpoint pupils of eyes; slow heartbeat; slow or troubled breathing; weakness (severe)

Also, check with your doctor as soon as possible if any of the following side effects occur:

*Rare*

Chest pain; coughing occurring together with breathing problems; difficult, decreased, or frequent urination; difficult, slow, or shallow breathing; increase or decrease in blood pressure; irregular heartbeat; mental depression or other mood or mental changes; skin rash or itching; swelling of face, fingers, lower legs, or feet; weight gain

Other side effects may occur that usually do not need medical attention. These side effects may go away during treatment as your body adjusts to the medicine. However, check with your doctor if any of the following side effects continue or are bothersome:

*More common*

Drowsiness; nausea or vomiting

*Less common or rare*

Abdominal or stomach pain; anxiety or crying; blurred or double vision; confusion; constipation; diarrhea; dizziness or lightheadedness; flushing or redness of skin; slurred speech

After you stop using this medicine, your body may need time to adjust. The length of time this takes depends on the amount of medicine you were using and how long you used it. During this period of time check with your doctor if you notice any of the following side effects:

Body aches; diarrhea; fast heartbeat; fever, runny nose, or sneezing; gooseflesh; increased sweating; increased yawning; loss of appetite; nausea or vomiting; nervousness, restlessness, or irritability; shivering or trembling; stomach cramps; trouble in sleeping; unusually large pupils of eyes; weakness

Other side effects not listed above may also occur in some patients. If you notice any other effects, check with your doctor.

Revised: 08/29/94

# DIAZOXIDE   Oral

A commonly used brand name in the U.S. and Canada is Proglycem.

## Description

Diazoxide (dye-az-OX-ide) when taken by mouth is used in the treatment of hypoglycemia (low blood sugar). It works by preventing release of insulin from the pancreas.

Diazoxide is available only with your doctor's prescription, in the following dosage forms:

*Oral*

- Capsules (U.S. and Canada)
- Suspension (U.S. and Canada)

## Before Using This Medicine

In deciding to use a medicine, the risks of taking the medicine must be weighed against the good it will do.

This is a decision you and your doctor will make. For diazoxide, the following should be considered:

**Allergies**—Tell your doctor if you have ever had any unusual or allergic reaction to diazoxide, sulfonamides (sulfa medicine), or thiazide diuretics (certain types of water pills). Also tell your health care professional if you are allergic to any other substances, such as foods, preservatives, or dyes.

**Pregnancy**—Studies have not been done in pregnant women. However, too much use of diazoxide during pregnancy may cause unwanted effects (high blood sugar, loss of hair or increased hair growth, blood problems) in the baby. Studies in animals have shown that diazoxide causes some birth defects (in the skeleton, heart, and pancreas) and other problems (delayed birth, decrease in successful pregnancies).

**Breast-feeding**—It is not known whether diazoxide passes into breast milk. However, this medicine has not been reported to cause problems in nursing babies.

**Children**—Infants are more likely to retain (keep) body water because of diazoxide. In some infants, this may lead to certain types of heart problems. Also, a few children who received diazoxide for prolonged periods (longer than 4 years) developed changes in their facial structure.

**Older adults**—Many medicines have not been tested in older people. Therefore, it may not be known whether they work exactly the same way they do in younger adults or if they cause different side effects or problems in older people. There is no specific information comparing use of oral diazoxide in the elderly with use in other age groups.

**Other medicines**—Although certain medicines should not be used together at all, in other cases two different medicines may be used together even if an interaction might occur. In these cases, your doctor may want to change the dose, or other precautions may be necessary. When you are taking diazoxide, it is especially important that your health care professional know if you are taking any of the following:
- Amantadine (e.g., Symmetrel) or
- Antidepressants (medicine for depression) or
- Antihypertensives (high blood pressure medicine) or
- Antipsychotics (medicines for mental illness) or
- Bromocriptine (e.g., Parlodel) or
- Cyclandelate (e.g., Cyclospasmol) or
- Deferoxamine (e.g., Desferal) or
- Diuretics (water pills) or
- Hydralazine (e.g., Apresoline) or
- Isoxsuprine (e.g., Vasodilan) or
- Levobunolol (e.g., Betagan) (use in the eye) or
- Levodopa (e.g., Dopar) or
- Medicine for heart disease or
- Metipranolol (e.g., OptiPranolol) or
- Nabilone (e.g., Cesamet) (with high doses) or
- Narcotic pain medicine or
- Nicotinyl alcohol (e.g., Roniacol) or
- Nimodipine (e.g., Nimotop) or
- Nylidrin (e.g., Arlidin) or
- Papaverine (e.g., Pavabid) or
- Pentamidine (e.g., Pentam) or
- Pimozide (e.g., Orap) or
- Promethazine (e.g., Phenergan) or
- Timolol (e.g., Timoptic) (use in the eye) or
- Trimeprazine (e.g., Temaril)—Use of any of these medicines with diazoxide may cause low blood pressure
- Ethotoin (e.g., Peganone) or
- Mephenytoin (e.g., Mesantoin) or
- Phenytoin (e.g., Dilantin)—Any of these medicines and diazoxide may be less effective is they are taken at the same time

**Other medical problems**—The presence of other medical problems may affect the use of diazoxide. Make sure you tell your doctor if you have any other medical problems, especially:
- Angina (chest pain)
- Gout—Diazoxide may make this condition worse
- Heart attack (recent)
- Heart or blood vessel disease
- Kidney disease—The effects of diazoxide may last longer because the kidney may not be able to get the medicine out of the bloodstream as it normally would
- Liver disease
- Stroke (recent)

## Proper Use of This Medicine

*Take this medicine only as directed by your doctor.* Do not take more or less of it than your doctor ordered, and take it at the same time each day.

*Follow carefully the special diet your doctor gave you.* This is an important part of controlling your condition, and is necessary if the medicine is to work properly.

*Test for sugar in your urine or blood with a diabetic urine or blood test kit as directed by your doctor.* This is a convenient way to make sure your condition is being controlled, and it provides an early warning when it is not. Your doctor may also want you to test your urine for acetone.

**Dosing**—The dose of diazoxide will be different for different patients. *Follow your doctor's orders or the directions on the label.* The following information includes only the average doses of diazoxide. *If your dose is different, do not change it* unless your doctor tells you to do so.

The number of capsules that you take depends on the strength of the medicine.
- For *oral* dosage forms (capsules or suspension):
  —For treating hypoglycemia (low blood sugar):
    - Adults, teenagers, and children—Dose is based on body weight and must be determined by your doctor. At first, the usual dose is 1 milligram (mg) per kilogram (kg) (0.45 mg per pound) of body weight every eight hours. Then, your doctor may increase your dose to 3 to 8 mg per kg (1.4 to 3.6 mg per pound) of body weight a day. This dose may be divided into two or three doses.
    - Newborn babies and infants—Dose is based on body weight and must be determined by your doctor. At first, the usual dose is 3.3 mg per kg (1.5 mg per pound) of body weight every eight hours. Then, your doctor may increase the dose to 8 to 15 mg per kg (3.6 to 6.8 mg per pound) of body weight a day. This dose may be divided into two or three doses.

**Missed dose**—If you miss a dose of this medicine, take it as soon as possible. However, if it is almost time for your next dose, skip the missed dose and go back to your regular dosing schedule. Do not double doses.

**Storage**—To store this medicine:
- Keep out of the reach of children.
- Store away from heat and direct light.
- Do not store in the bathroom, near the kitchen sink, or in other damp places. Heat or moisture may cause the medicine to break down.

- Keep the oral liquid form of this medicine from freezing.
- Do not keep outdated medicine or medicine no longer needed. Be sure that any discarded medicine is out of the reach of children.

## Precautions While Using This Medicine

*It is very important that your doctor check your progress at regular visits,* especially during the first few weeks of treatment, to make sure that this medicine is working properly.

Before you have any kind of surgery, dental treatment, or emergency treatment, *tell the medical doctor or dentist in charge that you are using this medicine.*

*Do not take any other medicine, unless prescribed or approved by your doctor,* since some may interfere with this medicine's effects. This especially includes over-the-counter (OTC) or nonprescription medicine such as that for colds, cough, asthma, hay fever, or appetite control.

*Check with your doctor right away if symptoms of high blood sugar (hyperglycemia) occur.* These symptoms usually include:

Drowsiness
Flushed, dry skin
Fruit-like breath odor
Increased urination
Loss of appetite (continuing)
Unusual thirst

These symptoms may occur if the dose of the medicine is too high, or if you have a fever or infection or are experiencing unusual stress.

Check with your doctor as soon as possible also if these symptoms of low blood sugar (hypoglycemia) occur:

Anxiety
Chills
Cold sweats
Cool pale skin
Drowsiness
Excessive hunger
Fast pulse
Headache
Nausea
Nervousness
Shakiness
Unusual tiredness or weakness

Symptoms of both low blood sugar and high blood sugar must be corrected before they progress to a more serious condition. In either situation, you should check with your doctor immediately.

## Side Effects of This Medicine

Along with its needed effects, a medicine may cause some unwanted effects. Although not all of these side effects may occur, if they do occur they may need medical attention.

*Stop taking this medicine and get emergency help immediately if any of the following side effects occur:*

*Rare*

Chest pain caused by exercise or activity; confusion; numbness of the hands; shortness of breath (unexplained)

Check with your doctor as soon as possible if any of the following side effects occur:

*More common*

Decreased urination; swelling of feet or lower legs; weight gain (rapid)

*Less common*

Fast heartbeat

*Rare*

Fever; skin rash; stiffness of arms or legs; trembling and shaking of hands and fingers; unusual bleeding or bruising

Other side effects may occur that usually do not need medical attention. These side effects may go away during treatment as your body adjusts to the medicine. However, check with your doctor if any of the following side effects continue or are bothersome:

*Less common*

Changes in ability to taste; constipation; increased hair growth on forehead, back, arms, and legs; loss of appetite; nausea and vomiting; stomach pain

This medicine may cause a temporary increase in hair growth in some people when it is used for a long time. After treatment with diazoxide has ended, normal hair growth should return.

Other side effects not listed above may also occur in some patients. If you notice any other effects, check with your doctor.

---

Revised: 12/15/92
Interim revision: 05/24/94

---

# DIDANOSINE Systemic

A commonly used brand name in the U.S. and Canada is Videx. Another commonly used name is ddI.

## Description

Didanosine (di-DAN-oe-seen) (also known as ddI) is used in the treatment of the infection caused by the human immunodeficiency virus (HIV). HIV is the virus responsible for acquired immune deficiency syndrome (AIDS).

Didanosine (ddI) will not cure or prevent HIV infection or AIDS; however, it helps keep HIV from reproducing and appears to slow down the destruction of the immune system. This may help delay the development of problems usually related to AIDS or HIV disease. Didanosine will not keep you from spreading HIV to other people. People who receive this medicine may continue to have the problems usually related to AIDS or HIV disease.

Didanosine may cause some serious side effects, including pancreatitis (inflammation of the pancreas). Symptoms of pancreatitis include stomach pain, and nausea and vomiting. Didanosine may also cause peripheral neuropathy. Symptoms of peripheral neuropathy include tingling, burning, numbness, and pain in the hands or feet. *Check with your doctor if any new health problems or symptoms occur while you are taking didanosine.*

Didanosine is available only with your doctor's prescription, in the following dosage forms:

*Oral*
- Oral solution (U.S.)
- Oral suspension (U.S. and Canada)
- Tablets (U.S. and Canada)

## Before Using This Medicine

In deciding to use a medicine, the risks of taking the medicine must be weighed against the good it will do. This is a decision you and your doctor will make. For didanosine, the following should be considered:

**Allergies**—Tell your doctor if you have ever had any unusual or allergic reaction to didanosine. Also tell your health care professional if you are allergic to any other substances, such as foods, preservatives, or dyes.

**Diet**—Make certain your health care professional knows if you are on any special diet, such as a low-sodium (low-salt) diet. Didanosine chewable tablets and the oral solution packets contain a large amount of sodium. Also, didanosine tablets contain phenylalanine, which must be restricted in patients with phenylketonuria.

**Pregnancy**—Didanosine crosses the placenta. Studies in pregnant women have not been done. However, didanosine has not been shown to cause birth defects or other problems in animal studies. Also, it is not known whether didanosine reduces the chances that a baby born to an HIV-infected mother will also be infected.

**Breast-feeding**—It is not known whether didanosine passes into the breast milk. However, if your baby does not already have the AIDS virus, there is a chance that you could pass it to your baby by breast-feeding. Talk to your doctor first if you are thinking about breast-feeding your baby.

**Children**—Didanosine can cause serious side effects in any patient. Therefore, it is especially important that you discuss with your child's doctor the good that this medicine may do as well as the risks of using it. Your child must be carefully followed, and frequently seen, by the doctor while taking didanosine.

**Older adults**—Many medicines have not been studied specifically in older people. Therefore, it may not be known whether they work exactly the same way they do in younger adults or if they cause different side effects or problems in older people. There is no specific information comparing use of didanosine in the elderly with use in other age groups.

**Other medicines**—Although certain medicines should not be used together at all, in other cases 2 different medicines may be used together even if an interaction might occur. In these cases, your doctor may want to change the dose, or other precautions may be necessary. When you are taking didanosine, it is especially important that your health care professional know if you are taking any of the following:
- Alcohol or
- Asparaginase (e.g., Elspar) or
- Azathioprine (e.g., Imuran) or
- Estrogens (female hormones) or
- Furosemide (e.g., Lasix) or
- Methyldopa (e.g., Aldomet) or
- Pentamidine (e.g., Pentam, Pentacarinat) or
- Sulfonamides (e.g., Bactrim, Septra) or
- Sulindac (e.g., Clinoril) or
- Thiazide diuretics (e.g., Diuril, Hydrodiuril) or
- Valproic acid (e.g., Depakote)—Use of these medicines with didanosine may increase the chance of pancreatitis (inflammation of the pancreas)
- Chloramphenicol (e.g., Chloromycetin) or
- Cisplatin (e.g., Platinol) or
- Ethambutol (e.g., Myambutol) or
- Ethionamide (e.g., Trecator-SC) or
- Hydralazine (e.g., Apresoline) or
- Isoniazid (e.g., Nydrazid) or
- Lithium (e.g., Eskalith, Lithobid) or
- Metronidazole (e.g., Flagyl) or
- Nitrous oxide or
- Phenytoin (e.g., Dilantin) or
- Stavudine (e.g., D4T) or
- Vincristine (e.g., Oncovin) or
- Zalcitabine (e.g., HIVID)—Use of these medicines with didanosine may increase the chance of peripheral neuropathy (tingling, burning, numbness, or pain in your hands or feet)
- Ciprofloxacin (e.g., Cipro) or
- Enoxacin (e.g., Penetrex) or
- Itraconazole (e.g., Sporanox) or

- Ketoconazole (e.g., Nizoral) or
- Lomefloxacin (e.g., Maxaquin) or
- Norfloxacin (e.g., Noroxin) or
- Ofloxacin (e.g., Floxin) or
- Trimethoprim (e.g., Proloprim, Trimpex)—Use of these medicines with didanosine may keep these medicines from working properly; these medicines should be taken at least 2 hours before or 2 hours after taking didanosine
- Dapsone (e.g., Avlosulfon)—Use of dapsone with didanosine may increase the chance of peripheral neuropathy (tingling, burning, numbness, or pain in your hands or feet); it may also keep dapsone from working properly; dapsone should be taken at least 2 hours before or 2 hours after taking didanosine
- Nitrofurantoin (e.g., Macrodantin)—Use of nitrofurantoin with didanosine may increase the chance of pancreatitis (inflammation of the pancreas) and peripheral neuropathy (tingling, burning, numbness, or pain in your hands or feet)
- Tetracyclines (e.g., Achromycin, Minocin)—Use of tetracyclines with didanosine may increase the chance of pancreatitis (inflammation of the pancreas); it may also keep the tetracycline from working properly; tetracyclines should be taken at least 2 hours before or 2 hours after taking didanosine

**Other medical problems**—The presence of other medical problems may affect the use of didanosine. Make sure you tell your doctor if you have any other medical problems, especially:
- Alcoholism, active, or
- Increased blood triglycerides (substance formed in the body from fats in foods) or
- Pancreatitis (or a history of)—Patients with these medical problems may be at increased risk of pancreatitis (inflammation of the pancreas)
- Edema or
- Heart disease or
- High blood pressure or
- Kidney disease or
- Liver disease or
- Toxemia of pregnancy—The salt contained in the didanosine tablets and the oral solution packets may make these conditions worse
- Gouty arthritis—Didanosine may cause an attack or worsen gout
- Peripheral neuropathy—Didanosine may make this condition worse
- Phenylketonuria (PKU)—Didanosine tablets contain phenylalanine, which must be restricted in patients with PKU

## Proper Use of This Medicine

*Take this medicine exactly as directed by your doctor.* Do not take more of it, do not take it more often, and do not take it for a longer time than your doctor ordered. Also, do not stop taking this medicine without checking with your doctor first. However, stop taking didanosine and call your doctor right away if you get severe nausea, vomiting, and stomach pain.

*Otherwise, keep taking didanosine for the full time of treatment,* even if you begin to feel better.

For patients taking *didanosine pediatric oral suspension:*
- Use a specially marked measuring spoon or other device to measure each dose accurately. The average household teaspoon may not hold the right amount of liquid.

For patients taking *didanosine for oral solution:*
- Open the foil packet and pour its contents into approximately 1/2 glass (4 ounces) of water. *Do not mix with fruit juice* or other acid-containing drinks.
- Stir for approximately 2 to 3 minutes until the powder is dissolved.
- Drink at once.

For patients taking *didanosine tablets:*
- Tablets should be thoroughly chewed or crushed or mixed in at least 1 ounce of water before swallowing. The tablets are hard and some people may find them difficult to chew. If the tablets are mixed in water, stir well until a uniform suspension is formed and take at once.
- *Two tablets must be taken together by patients over 1 year of age.* These tablets contain a special buffer to keep didanosine from being destroyed in the stomach. In order to get the correct amount of buffer, 2 tablets always need to be taken together. Infants from 6 to 12 months of age will get enough buffer from just 1 tablet.

*Didanosine should be taken on an empty stomach* since food may decrease the absorption in the stomach and keep it from working properly. Didanosine should be taken at least 2 hours before or 2 hours after you eat.

This medicine works best when there is a constant amount in the blood. *To help keep the amount constant, do not miss any doses.* If you need help in planning the best times to take your medicine, check with your health care professional.

**Dosing**—The dose of didanosine will be different for different patients. *Follow your doctor's orders or the directions on the label.* The following information includes only the average doses of didanosine. *If your dose is different, do not change it* unless your doctor tells you to do so.

The number of tablets or teaspoonfuls of solution or suspension that you take depends on the strength of the medicine.
- For the treatment of advanced HIV infection or AIDS:
  —For *oral* dosage form (solution):
  - Adults and teenagers—Dose is based on body weight.
    —For patients weighing less than 60 kilograms (kg) (132 pounds): 167 milligrams (mg) every twelve hours.
    —For patients weighing 60 kg (132 pounds) or more: 250 mg every twelve hours.
  - Children—The oral solution is usually not used for small children.

—For *oral* dosage form (pediatric suspension):
  • Adults and teenagers—The pediatric oral suspension is usually not used in adults and teenagers.
  • Children—Dose is based on body size and must be determined by your doctor. The dose usually ranges from 31 to 125 mg every eight to twelve hours.
—For *oral* dosage form (tablets):
  • Adults and teenagers—Dose is based on body weight.
    —For patients weighing less than 60 kg (132 pounds): 125 mg every twelve hours.
    —For patients weighing 60 kg (132 pounds) or more: 200 mg every twelve hours.
  • Children—Dose is based on body size and must be determined by your doctor. The dose usually ranges from 25 to 100 mg every eight to twelve hours.

**Missed dose**—If you do miss a dose of this medicine, take it as soon as possible. However, if it is almost time for your next dose, skip the missed dose and go back to your regular dosing schedule. Do not double doses.

Only take medicine that your doctor has prescribed specifically for you. Do not share your medicine with others.

**Storage**—To store this medicine:
  • Keep out of the reach of children.
  • Store away from heat and direct light.
  • Do not store in the bathroom, near the kitchen sink, or in other damp places. Heat or moisture may cause the medicine to break down.
  • Do not keep outdated medicine or medicine no longer needed. Be sure that any discarded medicine is out of the reach of children.

## Precautions While Using This Medicine

*It is very important that your doctor check your progress at regular visits.*

*Do not take any other medicines without checking with your doctor first.* To do so may increase the chance of side effects from didanosine.

HIV may be acquired from or spread to other people through infected body fluids, including blood, vaginal fluid, or semen. *If you are infected, it is best to avoid any sexual activity involving an exchange of body fluids with other people. If you do have sex, always wear (or have your partner wear) a condom ("rubber").* Only use condoms made of latex, and *use them every time you have vaginal, anal, or oral sex.* The use of a spermicide (such as nonoxynol-9) may also help prevent transmission of HIV if it is not irritating to the vagina, rectum, or mouth. Spermicides have been shown to kill HIV in lab tests. Do not use oil-based jelly, cold cream, baby oil, or shortening as a lubricant—these products can cause the condom to break. Lubricants without oil, such as *K-Y jelly*, are recommended. Women may wish to carry their own condoms. Birth control pills and diaphragms will help protect against pregnancy, but they will not prevent someone from giving or getting the AIDS virus. *If you inject drugs*, get help to stop. *Do not share needles or equipment with anyone.* In some cities, more than half of the drug users are infected and sharing even 1 needle or syringe can spread the virus. If you have any questions about this, check with your health care professional.

## Side Effects of This Medicine

Along with its needed effects, a medicine may cause some unwanted effects. Although not all of these side effects may occur, if they do occur they may need medical attention.

*Check with your doctor immediately* if any of the following side effects occur:
  *Less common*
    Nausea and vomiting; stomach pain; tingling, burning, numbness, and pain in the hands or feet
  *Rare*
    Convulsions (seizures); fever and chills; shortness of breath; skin rash and itching; sore throat; swelling of feet or lower legs; unusual bleeding and bruising; unusual tiredness and weakness; yellow skin and eyes

Other side effects may occur that usually do not need medical attention. These side effects may go away during treatment as your body adjusts to the medicine. However, check with your doctor if any of the following side effects continue or are bothersome:
  *More common*
    Anxiety; diarrhea; difficulty in sleeping; dryness of mouth; headache; irritability; restlessness

Other side effects not listed above may also occur in some patients. If you notice any other effects, check with your doctor.

Revised: 06/22/94

# DIETHYLCARBAMAZINE    Systemic

A commonly used brand name in Canada is Hetrazan.
A generic name product may be available in the U.S.

## Description

Diethylcarbamazine (dye-eth-il-kar-BAM-a-zeen) is used in the treatment of certain worm infections. It is used to treat:

- Bancroft's filariasis;
- Eosinophilic lung (tropical pulmonary eosinophilia; tropical eosinophilia);
- Loiasis; and
- River blindness (onchocerciasis).

It will not work for other kinds of worm infections (for example, pinworms or tapeworms).

Diethylcarbamazine is available only with your doctor's prescription, in the following dosage form:

*Oral*
- Tablets (U.S. and Canada)

## Before Using This Medicine

In deciding to use a medicine, the risks of taking the medicine must be weighed against the good it will do. This is a decision you and your doctor will make. For diethylcarbamazine, the following should be considered:

**Allergies**—Tell your doctor if you have ever had any unusual or allergic reaction to diethylcarbamazine. Also tell your health care professional if you are allergic to any other substances, such as foods, preservatives, or dyes.

**Pregnancy**—Treatment of pregnant patients with diethylcarbamazine should be delayed until after delivery. However, diethylcarbamazine has not been shown to cause birth defects or other problems in humans.

**Breast-feeding**—Diethylcarbamazine has not been reported to cause problems in nursing babies.

**Children**—There is no specific information comparing use of diethylcarbamazine in children with use in other age groups.

**Older adults**—Many medicines have not been studied specifically in older people. Therefore, it may not be known whether they work exactly the same way they do in younger adults or if they cause different side effects or problems in older people. There is no specific information comparing use of diethylcarbamazine in the elderly with use in other age groups.

**Other medicines**—Although certain medicines should not be used together at all, in other cases two different medicines may be used together even if an interaction might occur. In these cases, your doctor may want to change the dose, or other precautions may be necessary. Tell your health care professional if you are taking any other prescription or nonprescription (over-the-counter [OTC]) medicine.

**Other medical problems**—The presence of other medical problems may affect the use of diethylcarbamazine. Make sure you tell your doctor if you have any other medical problems, especially:

- River blindness involving the eyes—Diethylcarbamazine may worsen the eye problems associated with river blindness

## Proper Use of This Medicine

Diethylcarbamazine should be taken immediately after meals.

To help clear up your infection completely, *keep taking this medicine for the full time of treatment,* even if your symptoms begin to clear up after a few days. In some patients, a second course of this medicine may be required to clear up the infection completely. If you stop taking this medicine too soon, your infection may return. *Do not miss any doses.*

**Dosing**—The dose of diethylcarbamazine will be different for different patients. *Follow your doctor's orders or the directions on the label.* The following information includes only the average doses of diethylcarbamazine. *If your dose is different, do not change it* unless your doctor tells you to do so.

The number of tablets that you take depends on the strength of the medicine. Also, *the number of doses you take each day, the time allowed between doses, and the length of time you take the medicine depend on the medical problem for which you are taking diethylcarbamazine.*

- For *oral* dosage form (tablets):
  - —For Bancroft's filariasis, loiasis, and river blindness:
    - Adults—Dose is based on body weight and must be determined by your doctor. The usual dose is 2 to 3 milligrams (mg) per kilogram (kg) (0.9 to 1.3 mg per pound) of body weight three times a day.
    - Children—Use and dose must be determined by your doctor.
  - —For eosinophilic lung:
    - Adults—Dose is based on body weight and must be determined by your doctor. The usual dose is 6 mg per kg (2.7 mg per pound) of body weight a day. This is taken for four to seven days.
    - Children—Use and dose must be determined by your doctor.

**Missed dose**—If you miss a dose of this medicine, take it as soon as possible. However, if it is almost time for your next dose, skip the missed dose and go back to your regular dosing schedule. Do not double doses.

**Storage**—To store this medicine:

- Keep out of the reach of children.
- Store away from heat and direct light.
- Do not store in the bathroom, near the kitchen sink, or in other damp places. Heat or moisture may cause the medicine to break down.
- Do not keep outdated medicine or medicine no longer needed. Be sure that any discarded medicine is out of the reach of children.

## Precautions While Using This Medicine

If your symptoms do not improve within a few days, or if they become worse, check with your doctor.

For patients taking diethylcarbamazine for river blindness:

- It is important that your doctor check your progress at regular visits. This is to help make sure that the infection is cleared up completely. Also, your doctor may want you to have your eyes checked by an ophthalmologist (eye doctor).
- Diethylcarbamazine may cause loss of vision, night blindness, or tunnel vision with prolonged use. This medicine may also cause some people to become dizzy. *Make sure you know how you react to this medicine before you drive, use machines, or do anything else that could be dangerous if you are dizzy or are not alert or able to see well.* If these reactions are especially bothersome, check with your doctor.

## Side Effects of This Medicine

Along with its needed effects, a medicine may cause some unwanted effects. Although not all of these side effects may occur, if they do occur they may need medical attention.

*Check with your doctor immediately* if any of the following side effects occur:

*More common*
Itching and swelling of face, especially eyes

*Less common*
Fever; painful and tender glands in neck, armpits, or groin; skin rash

Additional side effects may occur if you use this medicine for a long time in the treatment of river blindness. Check with your doctor as soon as possible if any of the following side effects occur:

Loss of vision; night blindness; tunnel vision

Other side effects may occur that usually do not need medical attention. These side effects may go away during treatment as your body adjusts to the medicine. However, check with your doctor if any of the following side effects continue or are bothersome:

*More common*
Dizziness; headache; joint pain; unusual tiredness or weakness

*Less common*
Nausea or vomiting

Other side effects not listed above may also occur in some patients. If you notice any other effects, check with your doctor.

## Additional Information

In addition to the above information, for patients taking diethylcarbamazine for river blindness:

- Doctors may also prescribe a corticosteroid (a cortisone-like medicine) for certain patients with river blindness, especially those with severe symptoms. This is to help reduce the inflammation caused by the death of the worms. If your doctor prescribes these two medicines together, it is important to take the corticosteroid along with diethylcarbamazine. Take them exactly as directed by your doctor. Do not miss any doses.

Revised: 07/22/92
Interim revision: 05/17/94

# DIFENOXIN AND ATROPINE Systemic†

A commonly used brand name in the U.S. is Motofen.

†Not commercially available in Canada.

## Description

Difenoxin (dye-fen-OX-in) and atropine (A-troe-peen) combination medicine is used along with other measures to treat severe diarrhea in adults. Difenoxin helps stop diarrhea by slowing down the movements of the intestines.

Since difenoxin is chemically related to some narcotics, it may be habit-forming if taken in doses that are larger than prescribed. To help prevent possible abuse, atropine (an anticholinergic) has been added. If higher-than-normal doses of the combination are taken, the atropine will cause unpleasant effects, making it unlikely that such doses will be taken again.

Difenoxin and atropine combination medicine should not be used in children. Children with diarrhea should be given solutions of carbohydrates (sugars) and electrolytes (important salts) to replace the water and important salts that are lost from the body during diarrhea.

This medicine is available only with your doctor's prescription, in the following dosage form:

*Oral*
- Tablets (U.S.)

## Before Using This Medicine

In deciding to use a medicine, the risks of taking the medicine must be weighed against the good it will do. This is a decision you and your doctor will make. For difenoxin and atropine, the following should be considered:

**Allergies**—Tell your doctor if you have ever had any unusual or allergic reaction to difenoxin or atropine. Also tell your health care professional if you are allergic to any other substances, such as foods, preservatives, or dyes.

**Pregnancy**—Difenoxin and atropine combination has not been studied in pregnant women. However, studies in rats have shown that difenoxin and atropine combination, when given in doses many times the human dose, increases the delivery time and the chance of death of the newborn.

**Breast-feeding**—Both difenoxin and atropine pass into the breast milk. Although it is not known how much of these drugs pass into the breast milk, difenoxin and atropine combination could cause serious effects in the nursing baby. Be sure you have discussed the risks and benefits of this medicine with your doctor.

**Children**—This medicine should not be used in children. Children, especially very young children, are very sensitive to the effects of difenoxin and atropine. This may increase the chance of side effects during treatment. Also, the fluid loss caused by diarrhea may result in a severe condition. For this reason, it is very important that a sufficient amount of liquids be given to replace the fluid lost by the body. If you have any questions about this, check with your health care professional.

**Older adults**—Shortness of breath or difficulty in breathing may be more likely to occur in elderly patients, who are usually more sensitive than younger adults to the effects of difenoxin. Also, the fluid loss caused by diarrhea may result in a severe condition. For this reason, elderly persons should not take this medicine without first checking with their doctor. It is also very important that a sufficient amount of liquids be taken to replace the fluid lost by the body. If you have any questions about this, check with your health care professional.

**Other medicines**—Although certain medicines should not be used together at all, in other cases two different medicines may be used together even if an interaction might occur. In these cases, your doctor may want to change the dose, or other precautions may be necessary. When you are taking difenoxin and atropine, it is especially important that your health care professional know if you are taking any of the following:

- Antibiotics, such as cephalosporins (e.g., Ceftin, Keflex), clindamycin (e.g., Cleocin), erythromycins (e.g., E.E.S., PCE), tetracyclines (e.g., Achromycin, Doryx)—These antibiotics may cause diarrhea. Difenoxin and atropine may make the diarrhea caused by antibiotics worse or make it last longer
- Central nervous system (CNS) depressants (medicines that cause drowsiness)—Effects, such as drowsiness, of CNS depressants or of difenoxin and atropine may become greater
- Monoamine oxidase (MAO) inhibitors (furazolidone [e.g., Furoxone], isocarboxazid [e.g., Marplan], phenelzine [e.g., Nardil], procarbazine [e.g., Matulane], tranylcypromine [e.g., Parnate])—Taking difenoxin and atropine while you are taking or within 2 weeks of taking MAO inhibitors may cause severe side effects; these medicines should not be used together
- Naltrexone (e.g., Trexan)—Withdrawal side effects may occur in patients who have become addicted to the difenoxin in this combination medicine; also, naltrexone will make this medicine less effective against diarrhea
- Other anticholinergics (medicine to help reduce stomach acid and abdominal or stomach spasms or cramps)—Use of other anticholinergics with this combination medicine may increase the effects of the atropine in this combination; however, this is not likely to happen with the usual doses of difenoxin and atropine

**Other medical problems**—The presence of other medical problems may affect the use of difenoxin and atropine. Make sure you tell your doctor if you have any other medical problems, especially:

- Alcohol abuse (or history of) or
- Drug abuse (history of)—There is a greater chance that this medicine may become habit-forming
- Colitis (severe)—A more serious problem of the colon may develop if you use this medicine
- Down's syndrome (mongolism)—Side effects may be more likely and severe in these patients
- Dysentery—This condition may get worse; a different kind of treatment may be needed
- Emphysema, asthma, bronchitis, or other chronic lung disease—There is a greater chance that this medicine may cause breathing problems in patients who have any of these conditions
- Enlarged prostate or
- Urinary tract blockage or difficult urination—Problems with urination may develop with the use of this medicine
- Gallbladder disease or gallstones—Use of this medicine may cause spasms of the biliary tract and make the condition worse
- Glaucoma—Severe pain in the eye may occur with the use of this medicine; however, the chance of this happening is low
- Heart disease—This medicine may have some effects on the heart, which may make the condition worse
- Hiatal hernia—The atropine in this medicine may make this condition worse; however, the chance of this happening is low
- High blood pressure (hypertension)—The atropine in this medicine may cause an increase in blood pressure; however, the chance of this happening is low

- Intestinal blockage—This medicine may make the condition worse
- Kidney disease—The atropine in this medicine may build up in the body and cause side effects
- Liver disease—The chance of central nervous system (CNS) side effects, including coma, may be greater in patients who have this condition
- Myasthenia gravis—This medicine may make the condition worse
- Overactive or underactive thyroid—Unwanted effects on breathing and heart rate may occur
- Overflow incontinence—This medicine may make the condition worse

## Proper Use of This Medicine

If this medicine upsets your stomach, your doctor may want you to take it with food.

*Take this medicine only as directed by your doctor.* Do not take more of it, do not take it more often, and do not take it for a longer time than your doctor ordered. If too much is taken, it may become habit-forming.

*Importance of diet and fluids while treating diarrhea:*

- *In addition to using medicine for diarrhea, it is very important that you replace the fluid lost by the body and follow a proper diet.* For the first 24 hours you should eat gelatin and drink plenty of caffeine-free clear liquids, such as ginger ale, decaffeinated cola, decaffeinated tea, and broth. During the next 24 hours you may eat bland foods, such as cooked cereals, bread, crackers, and applesauce. Fruits, vegetables, fried or spicy foods, bran, candy, caffeine, and alcoholic beverages may make the condition worse.
- If too much fluid has been lost by the body due to the diarrhea a serious condition may develop. Check with your doctor as soon as possible if any of the following symptoms of too much fluid loss occur:

  Decreased urination
  Dizziness and lightheadedness
  Dryness of mouth
  Increased thirst
  Wrinkled skin

**Dosing**—The dose of difenoxin and atropine combination medicine will be different for different patients. *Follow your doctor's orders or the directions on the label.* The following information includes only the average doses of difenoxin and atropine combination. *If your dose is different, do not change it* unless your doctor tells you to do so.

- For *oral* dosage form (tablets):
  —For severe diarrhea:
    - Adults and teenagers—The first dose is usually 2 milligrams (mg). After that, the dose is 1 mg taken after each loose stool or every three or four hours as needed. *Do not take more than 8 mg in any twenty-four-hour period.*
    - Children—Use is not recommended.

**Missed dose**—If you are taking this medicine on a regular schedule and you miss a dose, take it as soon as possible. However, if it is almost time for your next dose, skip the missed dose and go back to your regular dosing schedule. Do not double doses.

**Storage**—To store this medicine:

- Keep out of the reach of children. Overdose is especially dangerous in children, and even part of an adult's pill can cause serious problems in children.
- Store away from heat and direct light.
- Do not store in the bathroom, near the kitchen sink, or in other damp places. Heat or moisture may cause the medicine to break down.
- Do not keep outdated medicine or medicine no longer needed. Be sure that any discarded medicine is out of the reach of children.

## Precautions While Using This Medicine

Your doctor should check your progress at regular visits if you will be taking this medicine regularly for a long time.

*Check with your doctor if your diarrhea does not stop after 2 days or if you develop a fever.*

This medicine will add to the effects of alcohol and other CNS depressants (medicines that slow down the nervous system, possibly causing drowsiness). Some examples of CNS depressants are antihistamines or medicine for hay fever, other allergies, or colds; sedatives, tranquilizers, or sleeping medicine; prescription pain medicine or narcotics; barbiturates; medicine for seizures; muscle relaxants; or anesthetics, including some dental anesthetics. *Check with your doctor before taking any of the above while you are taking this medicine.*

*If you think you or someone else in your home may have taken an overdose of this medicine, get emergency help at once.* Taking an overdose of this medicine may lead to unconsciousness and possibly death. Symptoms of overdose include severe drowsiness; fast heartbeat; shortness of breath or troubled breathing; and unusual warmth, dryness, and flushing of skin.

Before having any kind of surgery (including dental surgery) or emergency treatment, tell the medical doctor or dentist in charge that you are using this medicine.

This medicine may cause some people to become dizzy, drowsy, or less alert than they are normally. Even if taken at bedtime, it may cause some people to feel drowsy or less alert on arising. *Make sure you know how you react to this medicine before you drive, use machines, or do anything else that could be dangerous if you are dizzy or are not alert.*

## Side Effects of This Medicine

Along with its needed effects, a medicine may cause some unwanted effects. Although not all of these side effects may occur, if they do occur they may need medical attention.

*When this medicine is used for short periods of time at low doses, side effects usually are rare. However, check with your doctor immediately* if any of the following side effects are severe and occur suddenly, since they may be signs of a more severe and dangerous problem with your bowels:

> Bloating; constipation; loss of appetite; stomach pain (severe) with nausea and vomiting

Check with your doctor also if any of the following effects occur, since they may be signs of an overdose of this medicine:

> Blurred vision (continuing) or changes in near vision; drowsiness (severe); dryness of mouth, nose, and throat (severe); fast heartbeat; shortness of breath or troubled breathing (severe); unusual excitement, nervousness, restlessness, or irritability; unusual warmth, dryness, and flushing of skin

Other side effects may occur that usually do not need medical attention. These side effects may go away during treatment as your body adjusts to the medicine. However, check with your doctor if any of the following side effects continue, worsen, or are bothersome:

> *Less common or rare*
>
> Blurred vision; confusion; difficult urination; dizziness or lightheadedness; drowsiness; dryness of skin and mouth; fever; headache; trouble in sleeping; unusual tiredness or weakness

After you stop using this medicine, your body may need time to adjust. The length of time this takes depends on the amount of medicine you were using and how long you used it. During this period of time check with your doctor if you notice any of the following side effects:

> Increased sweating; muscle cramps; nausea or vomiting; shivering or trembling; stomach cramps

Other side effects not listed above may also occur in some patients. If you notice any other effects, check with your doctor.

Revised: 07/15/94

# DIGITALIS MEDICINES    Systemic

Some commonly used brand names are:

**In the U.S.—**
Crystodigin[1]
Lanoxicaps[2]
Lanoxin[2]

**In Canada—**
Digitaline[1]
Lanoxin[2]
Novodigoxin[2]

Note: For quick reference, the following digitalis medicines are numbered to match the corresponding brand names.

This information applies to the following medicines:
1. Digitoxin (di-ji-TOX-in)§
2. Digoxin (di-JOX-in)‡§

---

‡Generic name product may also be available in U.S.
§Generic name product may also be available in Canada

## Description

Digitalis medicines are used to improve the strength and efficiency of the heart, or to control the rate and rhythm of the heartbeat. This leads to better blood circulation and reduced swelling of hands and ankles in patients with heart problems.

Although digitalis has been prescribed to help some patients lose weight, it should *never* be used in this way. When used improperly, digitalis can cause serious problems.

Digitalis medicines are available only with your doctor's prescription, in the following dosage forms:

*Oral*
Digitoxin
• Tablets (U.S. and Canada)
Digoxin
• Capsules (U.S.)
• Elixir (U.S. and Canada)
• Tablets (U.S. and Canada)

*Parenteral*
Digoxin
• Injection (U.S. and Canada)

## Before Using This Medicine

In deciding to use a medicine, the risks of taking the medicine must be weighed against the good it will do. This is a decision you and your doctor will make. For digitalis medicines, the following should be considered:

**Allergies**—Tell your doctor if you have ever had any unusual or allergic reaction to digitalis medicines. Also tell your health care professional if you are allergic to any other substances, such as foods, preservatives, or dyes.

**Pregnancy**—Digitalis medicines pass from the mother to the fetus. However, studies on effects in pregnancy have not been done in either humans or animals. Make sure your doctor knows if you are pregnant or if you may become pregnant before taking digitalis medicines.

**Breast-feeding**—Although small amounts of digitalis medicines pass into breast milk, they have not been reported to cause problems in nursing babies.

**Children**—This medicine has been tested in children and, in effective doses, has not been shown to cause different side effects or problems than it does in adults. However, the dose is very different for babies and children, and it is important to follow your doctor's instructions exactly.

**Older adults**—Signs and symptoms of overdose may be especially likely to occur in elderly patients, who are usually more sensitive than younger adults to the effects of digitalis medicines.

**Other medicines**—Although certain medicines should not be used together at all, in other cases 2 different medicines may be used together even if an interaction might occur. In these cases, your doctor may want to change the dose, or other precautions may be necessary. When you are taking or receiving digitalis medicines it is especially important that your health care professional know if you are taking any of the following:

- Amiodarone (e.g., Cordarone)—May cause levels of digitalis medicines in the body to be higher than usual, which could lead to signs or symptoms of overdose
- Amphetamines or
- Appetite suppressants (diet pills) or
- Digitalis medicines (other) or other heart medicine or
- Medicine for asthma or other breathing problems or
- Medicine for colds, sinus problems, or hay fever or other allergies (including nose drops or sprays)—May increase the risk of heart rhythm problems
- Calcium channel blocking agents (bepridil [e.g., Bepadin, Vascor], diltiazem [e.g., Cardizem, Cardizem CD, Cardizem SR], felodipine [e.g., Plendil], flunarizine [e.g., Sibelium], isradipine [e.g., DynaCirc], nicardipine [e.g., Cardene], nifedipine [e.g., Adalat, Procardia, Procardia XL], nimodipine [e.g., Nimotop], verapamil [e.g., Calan, Calan SR, Isoptin, Isoptin SR, Verelan] or
- Propafenone—May cause levels of digitalis medicines in the body to be higher than usual, which could lead to signs or symptoms of overdose
- Cholestyramine (e.g., Questran) or
- Colestipol (e.g., Colestid) or
- Diarrhea medicine or
- Sucralfate or
- If your diet contains large amounts of fiber, such as bran—May decrease effects of digitalis medicines by keeping them from being absorbed into the body; digitalis medicines should be taken several hours apart from these
- Diuretics (water pills) or
- Other medicines that decrease the amount of potassium in the body (corticosteroids [cortisone-like medicines], alcohol, capreomycin, corticotropin, insulin, laxatives, salicylates [aspirin], vitamin $B_{12}$, vitamin D [high doses])—These medicines can cause hypokalemia (low levels of potassium in the body), which can increase the unwanted effects of digitalis medicines
- Potassium-containing medicines or supplements—If levels of potassium in the body become too high, there is a serious risk of heart rhythm problems being caused by digitalis medicines
- Quinidine (e.g., Quinidex)—May cause levels of digitalis medicines in the body to be higher than usual, which could lead to signs or symptoms of overdose

**Other medical problems**—The presence of other medical problems may affect the use of digitalis medicines. Make sure you tell your doctor if you have any other medical problems, especially:

- Heart disease or
- Lung disease (severe)—The heart may be more sensitive to the effects of digitalis medicines
- Heart rhythm problems—Digitalis glycosides may make certain heart rhythm problems worse
- Kidney disease or
- Liver disease—Effects may be increased because of slower removal of digitalis medicines from the body
- Thyroid disease—Patients with low or high thyroid gland activity may be more or less sensitive to the effects of digitalis glycosides

---

## Proper Use of This Medicine

To keep your heart working properly, *take this medicine exactly as directed even though you may feel well.* Do not take more of it than your doctor ordered and do not miss any doses.

For patients taking the *liquid form of digoxin:*

- This medicine is to be taken by mouth even if it comes in a dropper bottle. The amount you should take is to be measured only with the specially marked dropper.

To help you remember to take your dose of medicine, try to take it at the same time every day.

Ask your doctor about checking your pulse rate. Then, while you are taking this medicine, check your pulse regularly. If it is much slower, or faster, than your usual rate (or less than 60 beats per minute), or if it changes in rhythm or force, check with your doctor. Such changes may mean that side effects are developing.

**Dosing**—When you are taking digitalis medicines, it is very important that you get the exact amount of medicine that you need. The dose of digitalis medicine will be different for different patients. Your doctor will determine the proper dose of digitalis medicine for you. *Follow your doctor's orders or the directions on the label.*

After you begin taking digitalis medicines, your doctor may sometimes check your blood level of digitalis medicine to find out if your dose needs to be changed. *Do not change your dose of digitalis medicine* unless your doctor tells you to do so.

The number of capsules or tablets or teaspoonfuls of solution that you take depends on the strength of the medicine.

**Missed dose**—If you do miss a dose of this medicine, and you remember it within 12 hours, take it as soon as you remember. However, if you do not remember until later, do not take the missed dose at all and do not double the next one. Instead, go back to your regular dosing schedule. If you have any questions about this or if you miss doses for 2 or more days in a row, check with your doctor.

**Storage**—To store this medicine:

- Keep out of the reach of children.
- Store away from heat and direct light.
- Do not store in the bathroom, near the kitchen sink, or in other damp places. Heat or moisture may cause the medicine to break down.
- Keep the oral liquid form of this medicine from freezing.

• Do not keep outdated medicine or medicine no longer needed. Be sure that any discarded medicine is out of the reach of children.

## Precautions While Using This Medicine

It is important that your doctor check your progress at regular visits to make sure the medicine is working properly. This will allow your doctor to make any changes in directions for taking it, if necessary.

*Do not stop taking this medicine without first checking with your doctor.* Stopping suddenly may cause a serious change in heart function.

*Keep this medicine out of the reach of children.* Digitalis medicines are a major cause of accidental poisoning in children.

*Watch for signs and symptoms of overdose* while you are taking digitalis medicine. Follow your doctor's directions carefully. The amount of this medicine needed to help most people is very close to the amount that could cause serious problems from overdose. Some early warning signs of overdose are loss of appetite, nausea, vomiting, diarrhea, or extremely slow heartbeat. In infants and small children, the earliest signs of overdose are changes in the rate and rhythm of the heartbeat. Children may not show the other symptoms as soon as adults.

*Before having any kind of surgery (including dental surgery) or emergency treatment, tell the medical doctor or dentist in charge that you are using this medicine.*

Your doctor may want you to carry a medical identification card or bracelet stating that you are taking this medicine.

*Do not take any other medicine unless ordered by your doctor.* Many over-the-counter (OTC) or nonprescription medicines contain ingredients that interfere with digitalis medicines or that may make your condition worse. These medicines include antacids; laxatives; asthma remedies; cold, cough, or sinus preparations; medicine for diarrhea; and reducing or diet medicines.

For patients taking the *tablet or capsule* form of this medicine:

• This medicine may look like other tablets or capsules you now take. It is very important that you do not get the medicines mixed up since this may have serious results. Ask your pharmacist for ways to avoid mix-ups with medicines that look alike.

## Side Effects of This Medicine

Along with its needed effects, a medicine may cause some unwanted effects. Although not all of these side effects may occur, if they do occur they may need medical attention.

Check with your doctor as soon as possible if any of the following side effects or symptoms of overdose occur:

*Rare*
    Skin rash or hives
*Signs and symptoms of overdose (in the order in which they may occur)*
    Loss of appetite; nausea or vomiting; lower stomach pain; diarrhea;. unusual tiredness or weakness (extreme); slow or irregular heartbeat (may be fast heartbeat in children); blurred vision or "yellow, green, or white vision" (yellow, green, or white halo seen around objects); drowsiness; confusion or mental depression; headache; fainting

Note: Overdose symptoms in infants and small children may occur at first only as changes in the heartbeat rate or rhythm, while in adults and older children the first symptoms may be mostly stomach upset, stomach pain, loss of appetite, or unusually slow heartbeat.

Other side effects not listed above may also occur in some patients. If you notice any other effects, check with your doctor.

Revised: 03/10/93

---

# DILOXANIDE    Systemic*†

Some commonly used brand names in other countries are Entamide and Furamide.

---

*Not commercially available in the U.S.
†Not commercially available in Canada.

---

## Description

Diloxanide (dye-LOKS-a-nide) is used to treat an infection called amebiasis, which is caused by protozoa (tiny, one-celled animals). It works by killing the protozoa.

Diloxanide is available only with your doctor's prescription in the following dosage form.

*Oral*
• Tablets (United Kingdom)

---

## Before Using This Medicine

In deciding to use a medicine, the risks of taking the medicine must be weighed against the good it will do. This is a decision you and your doctor will make. For diloxanide, the following should be considered:

**Allergies**—Tell your doctor if you have ever had any unusual or allergic reaction to diloxanide. Also tell your

health care professional if you are allergic to any other substances, such as foods, preservatives, or dyes.

**Pregnancy**—Diloxanide has not been studied in pregnant women. However, diloxanide has not been shown to cause birth defects or other problems in animal studies.

**Breast-feeding**—It is not known whether diloxanide passes into breast milk. Although most medicines pass into breast milk in small amounts, many of them may be used safely while breast-feeding. Mothers who are taking this medicine and who wish to breast-feed should discuss this with their doctor.

**Children**—Although there is no specific information comparing use of diloxanide in children with use in other age groups, this medicine is not expected to cause different side effects or problems in children than it does in adults.

**Older adults**—Many medicines have not been studied specifically in older people. Therefore, it may not be known whether they work exactly the same way they do in younger adults. Although there is no specific information comparing use of diloxanide in the elderly with use in other age groups, this medicine is not expected to cause different side effects or problems in older people than it does in younger adults.

**Other medicines**—Although certain medicines should not be used together at all, in other cases two different medicines may be used together even if an interaction might occur. In these cases, your doctor may want to change the dose, or other precautions may be necessary. Tell your health care professional if you are taking any other prescription or nonprescription (over-the-counter [OTC]) medicine.

## Proper Use of This Medicine

*Take this medicine after meals* to lessen possible stomach upset, unless otherwise directed by your doctor.

To help clear up your infection completely, *take this medicine for the full time of treatment. Do not miss any doses.*

**Dosing**—The dose of diloxanide will be different for different patients. *Follow your doctor's orders or the directions on the label.* The following information includes only the average doses of diloxanide. *If your dose is different, do not change it* unless your doctor tells you to do so.

- For *oral* dosage form (tablets):
  —For amebiasis:
    - Adults and children 12 years of age and older— Oral, 500 milligrams (mg) three times a day for ten days.
    - Children up to 12 years of age—Dose is based on body weight and must be determined by

your doctor. The usual dose is 20 mg per kilogram (kg) (9 mg per pound) of body weight per day given in three divided doses for ten days.

**Missed dose**—If you miss a dose of this medicine, take it as soon as possible. However, if it is almost time for your next dose, skip the missed dose and go back to your regular dosing schedule. Do not double doses.

**Storage**—To store this medicine:
- Keep out of the reach of children.
- Store away from heat and direct light.
- Do not store in the bathroom, near the kitchen sink, or in other damp places. Heat or moisture may cause the medicine to break down.
- Keep the medicine from freezing. Do not refrigerate.
- Do not keep outdated medicine or medicine no longer needed. Be sure that any discarded medicine is out of the reach of children.

## Precautions While Using This Medicine

It is important that your doctor check your progress after treatment. This is to make sure that the infection is cleared up completely, and to allow your doctor to check for any unwanted effects.

## Side Effects of This Medicine

Along with its needed effects, a medicine may cause some unwanted effects. Although not all of these side effects may occur, if they do occur they may need medical attention.

Check with your doctor as soon as possible if any of the following side effects occur:

*Rare*
  Skin rash

Other side effects may occur that usually do not need medical attention. These side effects may go away during treatment as your body adjusts to the medicine. However, check with your doctor if any of the following side effects continue or are bothersome:

*More common*
  Full feeling or passing gas; nausea
*Less common*
  Diarrhea; loss of appetite; stomach pain

Other side effects not listed above may also occur in some patients. If you notice any other effects, check with your doctor.

Developed: 08/15/94

# DIMETHYL SULFOXIDE    Mucosal

A commonly used brand name in the U.S. and Canada is Rimso-50.
Another commonly used name is DMSO.
Generic name product may also be available in the U.S.

## Description

Dimethyl sulfoxide (dye-METH-il sul-FOX-ide) is a purified preparation used in the bladder to relieve the symptoms of the bladder condition called interstitial cystitis. A catheter (tube) or syringe is used to put the solution into the bladder where it is allowed to remain for about 15 minutes. Then, the solution is expelled by urinating.

Interstitial cystitis is the only human use for dimethyl sulfoxide that is approved by the U.S. Food and Drug Administration (FDA).

Claims that dimethyl sulfoxide is effective for treating various types of arthritis, ulcers in scleroderma, muscle sprains and strains, bruises, infections of the skin, burns, wounds, and mental conditions have not been proven.

Although other preparations of dimethyl sulfoxide are available for industrial and veterinary (animal) use, they must not be used by humans, because of their unknown purity. Impurities in these preparations may cause serious unwanted effects in humans. Even if dimethyl sulfoxide is applied to the skin, it is absorbed into the body through the skin and mucous membranes.

This medicine is available only with your doctor's prescription, in the following dosage form:

Topical
- Bladder irrigation (U.S. and Canada)

## Before Using This Medicine

In deciding to use a medicine, the risks of taking the medicine must be weighed against the good it will do. This is a decision you and your doctor will make. For dimethyl sulfoxide, the following should be considered:

**Allergies**—Tell your doctor if you have ever had any unusual or allergic reaction to dimethyl sulfoxide. Also tell your health care professional if you are allergic to any other substances, such as preservatives.

**Pregnancy**—Dimethyl sulfoxide has not been studied in pregnant women. However, some studies in animals have shown that dimethyl sulfoxide causes birth defects when used on the skin and when given in high doses by injection. Before using this medicine, make sure your doctor knows if you are pregnant or if you may become pregnant.

**Breast-feeding**—Dimethyl sulfoxide is absorbed into the body. It is not known whether dimethyl sulfoxide passes into the breast milk. However, this medicine has not been reported to cause problems in nursing babies.

**Children**—Studies on this medicine have been done only in adult patients, and there is no specific information comparing use of this medicine in children with use in other age groups.

**Older adults**—Many medicines have not been studied specifically in older people. Therefore, it may not be known whether they work exactly the same way they do in younger adults or if they cause different side effects or problems in older people. There is no specific information comparing use of this medicine in the elderly with use in other age groups.

**Other medicines**—Although certain medicines should not be used together at all, in other cases two different medicines may be used together even if an interaction might occur. In these cases, your doctor may want to change the dose, or other precautions may be necessary. Tell your health care professional if you are using any other prescription or nonprescription (over-the-counter [OTC]) medicine.

## Proper Use of This Medicine

**Dosing**—The dose of dimethyl sulfoxide will be different for different patients. The following information includes only the average doses of dimethyl sulfoxide. *Your dose may be different.*

- For *bladder irrigation* dosage form:
  —For interstitial cystitis of bladder:
    - Adults—50 mL (milliliters) of a 50% solution is instilled into the bladder and left there for fifteen minutes. The treatment is repeated every two weeks until relief is obtained; then the treatment is repeated less often.
    - Children—Use and dose must be determined by your doctor.

## Side Effects of This Medicine

Along with its needed effects, a medicine may cause some unwanted effects. Although not all of these side effects may occur, if they do occur they may need medical attention.

*Check with your doctor immediately* if any of the following side effects occur:
Nasal congestion; shortness of breath or troubled breathing; skin rash, hives, or itching; swelling of face

Some patients may have some discomfort during the time this medicine is being put into the bladder. However, the discomfort usually becomes less each time the medicine is used.

Dimethyl sulfoxide may cause you to have a garlic-like taste within a few minutes after the medicine is put into the bladder. This effect may last for several hours. It may also cause your breath and skin to have a garlic-like odor, which may last up to 72 hours.

Other side effects not listed above may also occur in some patients. If you notice any other effects, check with your doctor.

Revised: 03/04/92
Interim revision: 03/28/94

# DINOPROST    Intra-amniotic*

A commonly used brand name in Canada is Prostin F₂ Alpha.

*Not commercially available in the U.S.

## Description

Dinoprost (DYE-noe-prost) is used to cause abortion during the second trimester of pregnancy. It may also be used for other purposes as determined by your doctor.

Dinoprost is to be administered only by or under the immediate care of your doctor. It is available in the following dosage form:

*Parenteral*
• Injection (Canada)

## Before Receiving This Medicine

In deciding to use a medicine, the risks of taking the medicine must be weighed against the good it will do. This is a decision you and your doctor will make. For dinoprost, the following should be considered:

**Allergies**—Tell your doctor if you have ever had any unusual or allergic reaction to dinoprost or other oxytocics (medicines that stimulate the uterus to contract). Also tell your health care professional if you are allergic to any other substances, such as foods, preservatives, or dyes.

**Other medicines**—Although certain medicines should not be used together at all, in other cases two different medicines may be used together even if an interaction might occur. In these cases, your doctor may want to change the dose, or other precautions may be necessary. Tell your doctor if you are taking any prescription or nonprescription (over-the-counter [OTC]) medicine.

**Other medical problems**—The presence of other medical problems may affect the use of dinoprost. Make sure you tell your doctor if you have any other medical problems, especially:
• Anemia (history of)—In some patients, abortion with dinoprost may result in loss of blood that may require a transfusion
• Asthma (or history of) or
• Lung disease—Dinoprost may cause narrowing of the blood vessels in the lungs or narrowing of the lung passages
• Diabetes mellitus (sugar diabetes) (history of)
• Epilepsy (or history of)—Rarely, dinoprost has been reported to cause seizures in patients who have epilepsy

• Fibroid tumors of the uterus or
• Uterus surgery (history of)—There is an increased risk of rupture of the uterus
• Glaucoma—Rarely the pressure within the eye has increased and constriction of the pupils has occurred during the use of dinoprost
• Heart or blood vessel disease (or history of) or
• High blood pressure (history of) or
• Low blood pressure (history of)—Dinoprost may cause changes in heart function or blood pressure changes
• Jaundice (history of)
• Kidney disease (or history of)
• Liver disease (or history of)—The body may not get dinoprost out of the bloodstream at the usual rate, which may make the medicine work longer or cause toxic effects

## Proper Use of This Medicine

**Dosing**—The dose of dinoprost will be different for different patients. Your doctor will give you the dose of this medicine and follow your care in a hospital or another health care setting.

• For *injection* dosage form:
—For aborting a pregnancy:
• Adults—Your doctor will slowly inject 40 milligrams (mg) into the amniotic sac (bag that surrounds the fetus). If needed, your doctor may give you another dose in twenty–four hours to complete the abortion.
—For inducing labor:
• Adults—Your doctor will slowly inject 1 to 4 mg a day into a vein.

## Side Effects of This Medicine

Along with its needed effects, a medicine may cause some unwanted effects. Although not all of these side effects may occur, if they do occur they may need medical attention.

*Tell the health care professional immediately* if any of the following side effects occur:

*Less common or rare*
Chest pain; coughing (sudden); cramping of the uterus (continuing and severe); fast heartbeat; hives; numbness in legs or other body parts; pale, cool, or blotchy skin on arms or legs; pressing or painful feeling in chest; redness and itching of skin; shortness of breath;

slow or irregular heartbeat; swelling of eyelids, face, or inside of nose; tightness in chest; trouble in breathing; weak or absent pulse in arms or legs; wheezing

Also, check with the health care professional as soon as possible if any of the following side effects occur:

*Less common or rare*
Abdominal or stomach pain (severe or continuing); blood in urine; constipation; decreased frequency of urination; difficult or painful urination; double vision or burning eyes; pain in legs, back, or shoulder; tender or mildly bloated abdomen

Other side effects may occur that usually do not need medical attention. These side effects usually go away after the medicine is stopped. However, let the health care professional know if any of the following side effects continue or are bothersome:

*More common*
Diarrhea; nausea; stomach cramps or pain; vomiting

*Less common*
Anxiety; breast fullness or tenderness; burning feeling in breasts; chills or shivering; cough (continuing); dizziness; drowsiness; fever (temporary); flushing or redness of face; headache; hiccups; increased sweating; inflammation and pain at place of injection; unusual thirst

After the procedure has been completed, this procedure may still produce some side effects that need medical attention. Check with your doctor if you notice any of the following side effects:

Chills or shivering (continuing); fever (continuing); foul-smelling vaginal discharge; pain in lower abdomen; unusual increase in uterus bleeding

Other side effects not listed above may also occur in some patients. If you notice any other effects, check with your health care professional.

## Additional Information

Once a medicine has been approved for marketing for a certain use, experience may show that it is also useful for other medical problems. Although these uses are not specifically included in product labeling, dinoprost is used in certain patients for the following medical procedures:

• Angiography (x-ray pictures of the blood vessels)
• Inducing labor

Other than the above information, there is no additional information relating to proper use, precautions, or side effects for these uses.

Revised: 10/26/92
Interim revision: 05/16/94

---

# DINOPROSTONE    Cervical/Vaginal

Some commonly used brand names are:
**In the U.S.—**
Prostin E$_2$
**In Canada—**
Prepidil

## Description

Dinoprostone (dye-noe-PROST-one) is an oxytocic, which means it acts by causing the cervix to dilate (open) and the uterus to contract (cramp) the way it does during labor.

Dinoprostone may also be used for other purposes as determined by your doctor.

Dinoprostone is to be administered only by or under the immediate care of your doctor. It is available in the following dosage forms:

*Cervical*
• Gel (Canada)

*Vaginal*
• Gel (Canada)
• Suppositories (U.S.)

## Before Receiving This Medicine

In deciding to use a medicine, the risks of taking the medicine must be weighed against the good it will do. This is a decision you and your doctor will make. For dinoprostone, the following should be considered:

**Allergies**—Tell your doctor if you have ever had any unusual or allergic reaction to dinoprostone or other oxytocics (drugs that stimulate the uterus to contract).

**Other medicines**—Although certain medicines should not be used together at all, in other cases two different medicines may be used together even if an interaction might occur. In these cases, your doctor may want to change the dose, or other precautions may be necessary. When you are receiving dinoprostone, it is especially important that your doctor knows if you are using any other vaginal prescription or nonprescription (over-the-counter [OTC]) medicine.

**Other medical problems**—The presence of other medical problems may affect the use of dinoprostone. Make sure you tell your doctor if you have any other medical problems, especially:

• Anemia (or history of)—Abortion with dinoprostone may result in loss of blood in some patients that may require a transfusion

- Asthma (or history of) or
- Lung disease—Dinoprostone may cause narrowing of the blood vessels in the lungs or narrowing of the lung passages
- Epilepsy (or history of)—Rarely, seizures have occurred with the use of dinoprostone
- Fibroid tumors of the uterus or
- Uterus surgery (history of)—There is an increased risk of rupture of the uterus
- Glaucoma—Rarely, the pressure within the eye has increased and constriction of the pupils has occurred during the use of dinoprostone
- Heart or blood vessel disease (or history of) or
- High blood pressure (or history of) or
- Low blood pressure (history of)—Dinoprostone may cause changes in heart function or blood pressure changes; 2 cases of a heart attack have occurred during the use of dinoprostone in patients with a history of heart disease
- Kidney disease (or history of) or
- Liver disease (or history of)—The body may not get dinoprostone out of the blood stream at the usual rate, which may make the dinoprostone work longer or cause an increased chance of side effects

## Proper Use of This Medicine

*After the suppository, cervical gel, or vaginal gel is inserted into the vagina, you will need to lie down* so that the medicine can be absorbed. The length of time you must remain lying down will depend on what form of the drug you are using.

**Dosing**—The dose of dinoprostone will be different for different patients. The following information includes only the average doses for dinoprostone. Your doctor will give you the dose of this medicine and follow your care in a hospital or other health care setting.

- For *cervical* dosage form (gel):
  —To widen the opening of the cervix just before labor:
  - Adults and teenagers—Your doctor will insert 0.5 milligram (mg) (one applicatorful) of dinoprostone into the canal of your cervix.
- For *vaginal* dosage form (gel):
  —To cause the uterus to contract for labor:
  - Adults and teenagers—Your doctor will insert 1 milligram (mg) (one applicatorful) of dinoprostone into your vagina. You may need another dose of 1 to 2 mg six hours after the first dose.

- For *cervical* dosage form (suppositories):
  —To cause the uterus to contract to abort a pregnancy:
  - Adults and teenagers—Your doctor will insert 20 milligrams (mg) (one suppository) into your vagina every three to five hours as needed.

## Side Effects of This Medicine

Along with its needed effects, a medicine may cause some unwanted effects. Although not all of these side effects may occur, if they do occur they may need medical attention.

*Tell the health care professional immediately* if any of the following side effects occur:
*Less common or rare*
Fast or slow heartbeat; hives; increased pain of the uterus; pale, cool, blotchy skin on arms or legs; pressing or painful feeling in chest; shortness of breath; swelling of face, inside the nose, and eyelids; tightness in chest; trouble in breathing; weak or absent pulse in arms or legs; wheezing

Other side effects may occur that usually do not need medical attention. These side effects usually go away after the medicine is stopped. However, let the health care professional know if any of the following side effects continue or are bothersome:
*More common*
Abdominal or stomach cramps; diarrhea; fever; nausea; vomiting
*Less common or rare*
Chills or shivering; constipation; flushing; headache; swelling of the vulva; tender or mildly bloated abdomen or stomach

This procedure may still result in some effects, which occur after the procedure is completed, that need medical attention. Check with your doctor if any of the following side effects occur:
Chills or shivering (continuing); fever (continuing); foul-smelling vaginal discharge; pain in lower abdomen; unusual increase in bleeding of the uterus

Other side effects not listed above may also occur in some patients. If you notice any other effects, check with your health care professional.

Revised: 10/26/92
Interim revision: 06/03/94

# DIPHENIDOL  Systemic†

A commonly used brand name in the U.S. is Vontrol.
Another commonly used name is difenidol.

†Not commercially available in Canada.

## Description

Diphenidol (dye-FEN-i-dole) is used to relieve or prevent nausea, vomiting, and dizziness caused by certain medical problems.

Diphenidol is available only with your doctor's prescription in the following dosage form:

*Oral*
- Tablets (U.S.)

## Before Using This Medicine

In deciding to use a medicine, the risks of taking the medicine must be weighed against the good it will do. This is a decision you and your doctor will make. For diphenidol, the following should be considered:

**Allergies**—Tell your doctor if you have ever had any unusual or allergic reaction to diphenidol. Also tell your health care professional if you are allergic to any other substances, such as foods, preservatives, or dyes.

**Pregnancy**—Diphenidol has not been shown to cause birth defects or other problems in human or animal studies.

**Breast-feeding**—Diphenidol has not been reported to cause problems in nursing babies.

**Children**—There is no specific information comparing use of diphenidol for dizziness in children with use in other age groups. Also, there is no specific information about the use of diphenidol for nausea and vomiting in children who weigh less than 22.8 kg (50 lbs).

**Older adults**—Many medicines have not been studied specifically in older people. Therefore, it may not be known whether they work exactly the same way they do in younger adults or if they cause different side effects or problems in older people. There is no specific information comparing use of diphenidol in the elderly with use in other age groups.

**Other medicines**—Although certain medicines should not be used together at all, in other cases 2 different medicines may be used together even if an interaction might occur. In these cases, your doctor may want to change the dose, or other precautions may be necessary. When you are taking diphenidol, it is especially important that your health care professional know if you are taking any of the following:
- Central nervous system (CNS) depressants (medicine that causes drowsiness) or
- Tricyclic antidepressants (medicine for depression)—Using these medicines with diphenidol may increase the CNS depressant effects

**Other medical problems**—The presence of other medical problems may affect the use of diphenidol. Make sure you tell your doctor if you have any other medical problems, especially:
- Enlarged prostate or
- Glaucoma or
- Intestinal blockage or
- Low blood pressure or
- Stomach ulcer—Diphenidol may make the condition worse
- Kidney disease or
- Urinary tract blockage—Higher blood levels of diphenidol may occur, increasing the chance of side effects

## Proper Use of This Medicine

If you are taking diphenidol to prevent nausea and vomiting, it may be taken with food or a glass of water or milk to lessen stomach irritation, unless otherwise directed by your doctor. However, if you are already suffering from nausea and vomiting, it is best to keep the stomach empty, and this medicine should be taken only with a small amount of water.

*Take this medicine only as directed.* Do not take more of it and do not take it more often than directed by your doctor. To do so may increase the chance of side effects.

**Dosing**—The dose of diphenidol will be different for different patients. *Follow your doctor's orders or the directions on the label.* The following information includes only the average doses of diphenidol. *If your dose is different, do not change it* unless your doctor tells you to do so.

The number of tablets that you take depends on the strength of the medicine. Also, *the number of doses you take each day, the time allowed between doses, and the length of time you take the medicine depend on the medical problem for which you are taking diphenidol.*
- For *oral* dosage form (tablets):
  —Adults: 25 to 50 milligrams (mg) every four hours as needed.
  —Children: The dose is based on body weight and must be determined by the doctor.

**Missed dose**—If your doctor has ordered you to take this medicine on a regular schedule and you miss a dose, take it as soon as possible. However, if it is almost time for your next dose, skip the missed dose and go back to your regular dosing schedule. Do not double doses.

**Storage**—To store this medicine:
- Keep out of the reach of children.
- Store away from heat and direct light.
- Do not store the tablet form of this medicine in the bathroom, near the kitchen sink, or in other damp places. Heat or moisture may cause the medicine to break down.
- Do not keep outdated medicine or medicine no longer needed. Be sure that any discarded medicine is out of the reach of children.

## Precautions While Using This Medicine

This medicine will add to the effects of alcohol and other CNS depressants (medicines that slow down the nervous system, possibly causing drowsiness). Some examples of CNS depressants are antihistamines or medicine for hay fever, other allergies, or colds; sedatives, tranquilizers, or sleeping medicine; prescription pain medicine or narcotics; barbiturates; medicine for seizures; muscle relaxants; or anesthetics, including some dental anesthetics. *Check with your doctor before taking any of the above while you are using this medicine.*

This medicine may cause some people to have blurred vision or to become dizzy, drowsy or less alert than they are normally. *Make sure you know how you react to this medicine before you drive, use machines, or do anything else that could be dangerous if you are dizzy or are not alert or able to see well.*

## Side Effects of This Medicine

Along with its needed effects, a medicine may cause some unwanted effects. Although not all of these side effects may occur, if they do occur they may need medical attention.

Check with your doctor as soon as possible if any of the following side effects occur:

*Rare*
Confusion; hallucinations (seeing, hearing, or feeling things that are not there)

*Symptoms of overdose*
Drowsiness (severe); shortness of breath or troubled breathing; unusual tiredness or weakness (severe)

Other side effects may occur that usually do not need medical attention. These side effects may go away during treatment as your body adjusts to the medicine. However, check with your doctor if any of the following side effects continue or are bothersome:

*More common*
Drowsiness

*Less common or rare*
Blurred vision; dizziness; dryness of mouth; headache; heartburn; nervousness, restlessness, or trouble in sleeping; skin rash; stomach upset or pain; unusual tiredness or weakness

Other side effects not listed above may also occur in some patients. If you notice any other effects, check with your doctor.

Revised: 04/16/93

# DIPHENOXYLATE AND ATROPINE    Systemic

Some commonly used brand names are:

**In the U.S.—**
Lofene        Lomotil
Logen         Lonox
Lomocot       Vi-Atro
Generic name product may also be available.

**In Canada—**
Lomotil

## Description

Diphenoxylate (dye-fen-OX-i-late) and atropine (A-troe-peen) is a combination medicine used along with other measures to treat severe diarrhea in adults. Diphenoxylate helps stop diarrhea by slowing down the movements of the intestines.

Since diphenoxylate is chemically related to some narcotics, it may be habit-forming if taken in doses that are larger than prescribed. To help prevent possible abuse, atropine (an anticholinergic) has been added. If higher than normal doses of the combination are taken, the atropine will cause unpleasant effects, making it unlikely that such doses will be taken again.

Diphenoxylate and atropine combination medicine should not be used in children. Children with diarrhea should be given solutions of carbohydrates (sugars) and important salts (electrolytes) to replace the water, sugars, and important salts that are lost from the body during diarrhea. For more information on these solutions, see the *Carbohydrates and Electrolytes (Systemic)* monograph.

This medicine is available only with your doctor's prescription in the following dosage forms:

*Oral*
- Oral solution (U.S.)
- Tablets (U.S. and Canada)

## Before Using This Medicine

In deciding to use a medicine, the risks of taking the medicine must be weighed against the good it will do. This is a decision you and your doctor will make. For diphenoxylate and atropine, the following should be considered:

**Allergies**—Tell your doctor if you have ever had any unusual or allergic reaction to diphenoxylate or atropine. Also tell your health care professional if you are allergic to any other substances, such as foods, preservatives, or dyes.

**Pregnancy**—Studies have not been done in humans. In animal studies this medicine given in larger doses than the usual human dose has not been shown to cause birth defects. However, some studies in rats have shown that this medicine reduces the weight gain of the pregnant rat and lessens the chance of conceiving or becoming pregnant when given in doses many times the usual human dose.

**Breast-feeding**—Although both diphenoxylate and atropine pass into the breast milk, this medicine has not been shown to cause problems in nursing babies.

**Children**—This medicine should not be used in children. Children, especially very young children, are very sensitive to the effects of diphenoxylate and atropine. This may increase the chance of side effects during treatment. Also, the fluid loss caused by diarrhea may result in a severe condition. For this reason, it is very important that a sufficient amount of liquids be given to replace the fluid lost by the body. If you have any questions about this, check with your health care professional.

**Older adults**—Shortness of breath or difficulty in breathing may be especially likely to occur in elderly patients, who are usually more sensitive than younger adults to the effects of diphenoxylate. Also, the fluid loss caused by diarrhea may result in a severe condition. For this reason, elderly persons should not take this medicine without first checking with their doctor. It is also very important that a sufficient amount of liquids be taken to replace the fluid lost by the body. If you have any questions about this, check with your health care professional.

**Other medicines**—Although certain medicines should not be used together at all, in other cases two different medicines may be used together even if an interaction might occur. In these cases, your doctor may want to change the dose, or other precautions may be necessary. When you are taking diphenoxylate and atropine, it is especially important that your health care professional know if you are taking any of the following:

- Antibiotics, such as cephalosporins (e.g., Ceftin, Keflex), clindamycin (e.g., Cleocin), erythromycins (e.g., E.E.S., PCE), tetracyclines (e.g., Achromycin, Doryx)—These antibiotics may cause diarrhea. Diphenoxylate and atropine may make the diarrhea caused by antibiotics worse or make it last longer
- Central nervous system (CNS) depressants (medicines that cause drowsiness)—Effects, such as drowsiness, of CNS depressants or of diphenoxylate and atropine may become greater
- Monoamine oxidase (MAO) inhibitors (furazolidone [e.g., Furoxone], isocarboxazid [e.g., Marplan], phenelzine [e.g., Nardil], procarbazine [e.g., Matulane], selegiline [e.g., Eldepryl], tranylcypromine [e.g., Parnate])—Taking diphenoxylate and atropine while you are taking or within 2 weeks of taking MAO inhibitors may cause severe side effects; these medicines should not be used together
- Naltrexone (e.g., Trexan)—Withdrawal side effects may occur in patients who have become addicted to the diphenoxylate in this combination medicine; also, naltrexone will make this medicine less effective against diarrhea
- Other anticholinergics (medicine to help reduce stomach acid and abdominal or stomach spasms or cramps)—Use of other anticholinergics with this combination medicine may increase the effects of the atropine in this combination; however, this is not likely to happen with the usual doses of diphenoxylate and atropine

**Other medical problems**—The presence of other medical problems may affect the use of diphenoxylate and atropine. Make sure you tell your doctor if you have any other medical problems, especially:

- Alcohol abuse (or history of) or
- Drug abuse (history of)—There is a greater chance that this medicine will become habit-forming

- Colitis (severe)—A more serious problem of the colon may develop if you use this medicine
- Down's syndrome (mongolism)—Side effects may be more likely and severe in these patients
- Dysentery—This condition may get worse; a different kind of treatment may be needed
- Emphysema, asthma, bronchitis, or other chronic lung disease—There is a greater chance that this medicine may cause serious breathing problems in patients who have any of these conditions
- Enlarged prostate or
- Urinary tract blockage or difficult urination—Severe problems with urination may develop with the use of this medicine
- Gallbladder disease or gallstones—Use of this medicine may cause spasms of the biliary tract and make the condition worse
- Glaucoma—Severe pain in the eye may occur with the use of this medicine; however, the chance of this happening is small
- Heart disease—This medicine may have some effects on the heart, which may make the condition worse
- Hiatal hernia—The atropine in this medicine may make this condition worse; however, the chance of this happening is small
- High blood pressure (hypertension)—The atropine in this medicine may cause an increase in blood pressure; however, the chance of this happening is small
- Intestinal blockage—This medicine may make the condition worse
- Kidney disease—The atropine in this medicine may build up in the body and cause side effects
- Liver disease—The chance of central nervous system (CNS) side effects, including coma, may be greater in patients who have this condition
- Myasthenia gravis—This medicine may make the condition worse
- Overactive or underactive thyroid—Unwanted effects on breathing and heart rate may occur
- Overflow incontinence—This medicine may make the condition worse

## Proper Use of This Medicine

If this medicine upsets your stomach, your doctor may want you to take it with food.

*Take this medicine only as directed by your doctor.* Do not take more of it, do not take it more often, and do not take it for a longer time than your doctor ordered. If too much is taken, it may become habit-forming.

For patients taking the liquid form of this medicine:

- This medicine is to be taken by mouth even if it comes in a dropper bottle. The amount to be taken is to be measured with the specially marked dropper.

*Importance of diet and fluids while treating diarrhea:*

- *In addition to using medicine for diarrhea, it is very important that you replace the fluid lost by the body and follow a proper diet.* For the first 24 hours you should eat gelatin and drink plenty of caffeine-free clear liquids, such as ginger ale, decaffeinated cola, decaffeinated tea, and broth. During the next

24 hours you may eat bland foods, such as cooked cereals, bread, crackers, and applesauce. Fruits, vegetables, fried or spicy foods, bran, candy, caffeine, and alcoholic beverages may make the condition worse.

- If too much fluid has been lost by the body due to the diarrhea a serious condition may develop. Check with your doctor as soon as possible if any of the following signs or symptoms of too much fluid loss occur:

  Decreased urination
  Dizziness and lightheadedness
  Dryness of mouth
  Increased thirst
  Wrinkled skin

**Dosing**—The dose of diphenoxylate and atropine combination medicine will be different for different patients. *Follow your doctor's orders or the directions on the label.* The following information includes only the average doses of diphenoxylate and atropine combination. *If your dose is different, do not change it* unless your doctor tells you to do so.

- For severe diarrhea:
  —For *oral* dosage form (oral solution):
    - Adults and teenagers—At first, the dose is 5 milligrams (mg) (2 teaspoonfuls) three or four times a day. Then, the dose is usually 5 mg (2 teaspoonfuls) once a day, as needed.
    - Children up to 12 years of age—Use is not recommended.
  —For *oral* dosage form (tablets):
    - Adults and teenagers—At first, the dose is 5 mg (2 tablets) three or four times a day. Then, the dose is usually 5 mg (2 tablets) once a day, as needed.
    - Children up to 12 years of age—Use is not recommended.

**Missed dose**—If you are taking this medicine on a regular schedule and you miss a dose, take it as soon as possible. However, if it is almost time for your next dose, skip the missed dose and go back to your regular dosing schedule. Do not double doses.

**Storage**—To store this medicine:

- Keep out of the reach of children since overdose is especially dangerous in children.
- Store away from heat and direct light.
- Do not store the tablet form of this medicine in the bathroom, near the kitchen sink, or in other damp places. Heat or moisture may cause the medicine to break down.
- Keep the liquid form of this medicine from freezing.
- Do not keep outdated medicine or medicine no longer needed. Be sure that any discarded medicine is out of the reach of children.

## Precautions While Using This Medicine

Your doctor should check your progress at regular visits if you will be taking this medicine regularly for a long time.

*Check with your doctor if your diarrhea does not stop after two days or if you develop a fever.*

This medicine will add to the effects of alcohol and other CNS depressants (medicines that slow down the nervous system, possibly causing drowsiness). Some examples of CNS depressants are antihistamines or medicine for hay fever, other allergies, or colds; sedatives, tranquilizers, or sleeping medicine; prescription pain medicine or narcotics; barbiturates; medicine for seizures; muscle relaxants; or anesthetics, including some dental anesthetics. *Check with your doctor before taking any of the above while you are taking this medicine.*

*If you think you or anyone else may have taken an overdose, get emergency help at once.* Taking an overdose of this medicine may lead to unconsciousness and possibly death. Signs or symptoms of overdose include severe drowsiness; shortness of breath or troubled breathing; fast heartbeat; and unusual warmth, dryness, and flushing of the skin.

Before having any kind of surgery (including dental surgery) or emergency treatment, tell the medical doctor or dentist in charge that you are taking this medicine.

This medicine may cause some people to become dizzy, drowsy, or less alert than they are normally. Even if taken at bedtime, it may cause some people to feel drowsy or less alert on arising. *Make sure you know how you react to this medicine before you drive, use machines, or do anything else that could be dangerous if you are dizzy or are not alert.*

## Side Effects of This Medicine

Along with its needed effects, a medicine may cause some unwanted effects. Although not all of these side effects may occur, if they do occur they may need medical attention.

*When this medicine is used for short periods of time at low doses, side effects usually are rare. However, check with your doctor immediately* if any of the following side effects are severe and occur suddenly, since they may be signs of a more severe and dangerous problem with your bowels:

Bloating; constipation; loss of appetite; stomach pain (severe) with nausea and vomiting

Check with your doctor immediately also if the following effects occur, since they may be signs of an overdose of this medicine:

Blurred vision (continuing) or changes in near vision; drowsiness (severe); dryness of mouth, nose, and throat (severe); fast heartbeat; shortness of breath or troubled breathing (severe); unusual excitement, nervousness, restlessness, or irritability; unusual warmth, dryness, and flushing of the skin

Other side effects may occur that usually do not need medical attention. These side effects may go away during treatment as your body adjusts to the medicine. However, check with your doctor if any of the following side effects continue, worsen, or are bothersome:

*Less common or rare*
> Blurred vision; confusion; difficult urination; dizziness or lightheadedness; drowsiness; dryness of skin and mouth; fever; headache; mental depression; numbness of hands or feet; skin rash or itching; swelling of the gums

After you stop using this medicine, your body may need time to adjust. The length of time this takes depends on the amount of medicine you were using and how long you used it. During this time check with your doctor if you notice any of the following side effects:

*Rare*
> Increased sweating; muscle cramps; nausea or vomiting; shivering or trembling; stomach cramps

Other side effects not listed above may also occur in some patients. If you notice any other effects, check with your doctor.

Revised: 08/22/94

# DIPHTHERIA AND TETANUS TOXOIDS AND PERTUSSIS VACCINE ADSORBED   Systemic

Some commonly used brand names in the U.S. are Acel-Imune, Tri-Immunol, and Tripedia.

Other commonly used names are acellular DTP, DTaP, DTP, DTwP, and whole-cell DTP.

Generic name product may also be available in the U.S. and Canada.

## Description

Diphtheria (dif-THEER-ee-a) and Tetanus (TET-n-us) Toxoids and Pertussis (per-TUSS-iss) Vaccine (also known as DTP) is a combination immunizing agent given by injection to prevent diphtheria, tetanus, and pertussis.

Diphtheria is a serious illness that can cause breathing difficulties, heart problems, nerve damage, pneumonia, and possibly death. The risk of serious complications and death is greater in very young children and in the elderly.

Tetanus (also known as lockjaw) is a serious illness that causes convulsions (seizures) and severe muscle spasms that can be strong enough to cause bone fractures of the spine. Tetanus causes death in 30 to 40 percent of cases.

Pertussis (also known as whooping cough) is a serious disease that causes severe spells of coughing that can interfere with breathing. Pertussis can also cause pneumonia, long-lasting bronchitis, seizures, brain damage, and death.

Immunization against diphtheria, tetanus, and pertussis is recommended for all infants and children from 6 or 8 weeks of age up until their 7th birthday. Children 7 years of age and older and adults should receive immunizing agents that contain only diphtheria and tetanus toxoids and not pertussis vaccine. Persons should receive the diphtheria and tetanus injections every 10 years for the rest of their lives.

Diphtheria, tetanus, and pertussis are serious diseases that can cause life-threatening illnesses. Although some serious side effects can occur after a dose of DTP (usually from the pertussis vaccine in DTP), this rarely happens. The chance of your child catching one of these diseases and being permanently injured or dying as a result is much greater than the chance of your child getting a serious side effect from the DTP vaccine.

DTP is available in the following dosage form:

*Parenteral*
- Injection (U.S. and Canada)

## Before Receiving This Vaccine

In deciding to use a medicine, the risks of taking the medicine must be weighed against the good it will do. This is a decision you and your doctor will make. For DTP, the following should be considered:

**Allergies**—Tell your doctor if your child has ever had any unusual or allergic reaction to diphtheria toxoid, tetanus toxoid, pertussis vaccine, or DTP. Also tell your health care professional if your child is allergic to any other substances, such as preservatives.

**Other medical problems**—The presence of other medical problems may affect the use of DTP. Make sure you tell your doctor if your child has any other medical problems, especially:
- Brain disease or
- Central nervous system (CNS) disease or
- Epilepsy or
- Fever or
- Spasms or
- Seizures (convulsions)—Use of DTP may make the condition worse or may increase the chance of side effects

## Proper Use of This Vaccine

**Dosing**—The dose of DTP will be different for different patients. The following information includes only the average doses of DTP.

- For *injection* dosage form:
  —For prevention of diphtheria, tetanus, and pertussis:
    - Adults and children 7 years of age and older—Use is not recommended.
    - Children 2 months to 7 years of age—One dose every four to eight weeks for a total of three doses, then a fourth dose six to twelve months after the third dose. A booster dose should be given at four to six years of age. (The booster dose is given only if the fourth dose was given before the child's fourth birthday.)

## Precautions After Receiving This Vaccine

At the time of the DTP injection, your doctor may give your child a dose of acetaminophen (or another medicine that helps prevent fever). This is to help prevent some of the side effects of DTP. Your doctor may also want your child to take this medicine every 4 hours for 24 hours after your child receives the DTP injection. Check with your doctor if you have any questions.

## Side Effects of This Vaccine

Along with its needed effects, a vaccine may cause some unwanted effects. Although not all of these side effects may occur, if they do occur they may need medical attention. *It is very important that you tell your doctor about any side effect that occurs after a dose of DTP, even though the side effect may have gone away without treatment.* Some types of side effects may mean that your child should not receive any more doses of DTP.

*Get emergency help immediately if any of the following side effects occur:*

*Rare*

Collapse; confusion; convulsions (seizures); crying for three or more hours; difficulty in breathing or swallowing; fever of 40.5 °C (105 °F) or more; headache (severe or continuing); hives; irritability (unusual); itching, especially of feet or hands; periods of unconsciousness or lack of awareness; reddening of skin, especially around ears; sleepiness (unusual and continuing); swelling of eyes, face, or inside of nose; unusual tiredness, weakness, or limpness (sudden and severe); vomiting (severe or continuing)

Other side effects may occur that usually do not need medical attention. These side effects may go away as your child's body adjusts to the vaccine. However, check with your doctor if any of the following side effects continue or are bothersome:

*More common*

Fever between 38 and 39 °C (100.4 and 102.2 °F) (may occur with fretfulness, drowsiness, vomiting, and loss of appetite); lump at place of injection (may be present for a few weeks after injection); redness, swelling, tenderness, or pain at place of injection

*Less common*

Fever between 39 and 40 °C (102.2 and 104 °F) (may occur with fretfulness, drowsiness, vomiting, and loss of appetite)

*Rare*

Fever between 40 and 40.5 °C (104 and 105 °F) (may occur with fretfulness, drowsiness, vomiting, and loss of appetite); skin rash; swollen glands on side of neck (following DTP injection into arm)

Other side effects not listed above may also occur in some patients. If you notice any other effects, check with your doctor.

Revised: 06/09/93
Interim revision: 03/29/94

# DIPIVEFRIN Ophthalmic

Some commonly used brand names are:
**In the U.S.—**
Propine C Cap B.I.D.
Generic name product may also be available.
**In Canada—**
Ophtho-Dipivefrin
Propine C Cap B.I.D.
Generic name product may also be available.
Another commonly used name is dipivefrine.

## Description

Dipivefrin (dye-PI-ve-frin) is used to treat certain types of glaucoma.

This medicine is available only with your doctor's prescription, in the following dosage form:
*Ophthalmic*
- Ophthalmic solution (eye drops) (U.S. and Canada)

## Before Using This Medicine

In deciding to use a medicine, the risks of taking the medicine must be weighed against the good it will do. This is a decision you and your doctor will make. For dipivefrin, the following should be considered:

**Allergies**—Tell your doctor if you have ever had any unusual or allergic reaction to dipivefrin or epinephrine. Also tell your health care professional if you are allergic to any other substances, such as preservatives.

**Pregnancy**—Dipivefrin has not been studied in pregnant women. However, this medication has not been shown to cause birth defects or other problems in animal studies.

**Breast-feeding**—Dipivefrin may be absorbed into the body, but it is not known whether dipivefrin passes into the breast milk.

**Children**—Although there is no specific information comparing use of this medicine in children with use in other age groups, this medicine is not expected to cause different side effects or problems in children than it does in adults.

**Older adults**—Many medicines have not been studied specifically in older people. Therefore, it may not be known whether they work exactly the same way they do in younger adults. Although there is no specific information comparing use of this medicine in the elderly with use in other age groups, this medicine is not expected to cause different side effects or problems in older people than it does in younger adults.

**Other medicines**—Although certain medicines should not be used together at all, in other cases two different medicines may be used together even if an interaction might occur. In these cases, your doctor may want to change the dose, or other precautions may be necessary. Tell your health care professional if you are using any other prescription or nonprescription (over-the-counter [OTC]) medicine.

**Other medical problems**—The presence of other medical problems may affect the use of dipivefrin. Make sure you tell your doctor if you have any other medical problems, especially:

- Eye disease or problems (other)—Dipivefrin may make the condition worse

## Proper Use of This Medicine

*Use this medicine only as directed*. Do not use more of it and do not use it more often than your doctor ordered. To do so may increase the chance of too much medicine being absorbed into the body and the chance of side effects.

To use:

- First, wash your hands. Tilt the head back and, pressing your finger gently on the skin just beneath the lower eyelid, pull the lower eyelid away from the eye to make a space. Drop the medicine into this space. Let go of the eyelid and gently close the eyes. Do not blink. Keep the eyes closed and apply pressure to the inner corner of the eye with your finger for 1 or 2 minutes to allow the medicine to be absorbed by the eye.
- Immediately after using the eye drops, wash your hands to remove any medicine that may be on them.
- To keep the medicine as germ-free as possible, do not touch the applicator tip to any surface (including the eye). Also, keep the container tightly closed.

- If you are using the medicine with the compliance cap (C Cap):
  —Before using the eye drops for the first time, make sure the number 1 or the correct day of the week appears in the window on the cap.
  —Remove the cap and use the eye drops as directed.
  —Replace the cap. Holding the cap between your thumb and forefinger, rotate the bottle until the cap clicks to the next station. This will tell you your next dose.
  —After every dose, rotate the bottle until the cap clicks to the position that tells you your next dose.

**Dosing**—The dose of dipivefrin will be different for different patients. *Follow your doctor's orders or the directions on the label.* The following information includes only the average doses of dipivefrin. *If your dose is different, do not change it* unless your doctor tells you to do so.

- For *ophthalmic solution* (eye drops) dosage form:
  —For glaucoma:
    • Adults and children—One drop every twelve hours.

**Missed dose**—If you miss a dose of this medicine, apply the missed dose as soon as possible. However, if it is almost time for your next dose, skip the missed dose and go back to your regular dosing schedule. Do not double doses.

**Storage**—To store this medicine:
- Keep out of the reach of children.
- Store away from heat and direct light.
- Keep the medicine from freezing.
- Do not keep outdated medicine or medicine no longer needed. Be sure that any discarded medicine is out of the reach of children.

## Precautions While Using This Medicine

Your doctor should check your eye pressure at regular visits.

## Side Effects of This Medicine

Along with its needed effects, a medicine may cause some unwanted effects. Although not all of these side effects may occur, if they do occur they may need medical attention.

Check with your doctor as soon as possible if either of the following side effects occurs:

*Rare—Signs and symptoms of too much medicine being absorbed into the body*
    Fast or irregular heartbeat; increase in blood pressure

Other side effects may occur that usually do not need medical attention. These side effects may go away during treatment as your body adjusts to the medicine. However,

check with your doctor if any of the following side effects continue or are bothersome:

*Less common*

Burning, stinging, or other eye irritation; increased sensitivity of eyes to light

Other side effects not listed above may also occur in some patients. If you notice any other effects, check with your doctor.

Revised: 05/14/92
Interim revision(s): 08/16/93; 10/19/93; 12/14/93

# DIPYRIDAMOLE  Diagnostic

Some commonly used brand names are:

**In the U.S.—**
Dipridacot                Persantine
I.V. Persantine
Generic name product may also be available.

**In Canada—**
Apo-Dipyridamole          Persantine
Novodipiradol

## Description

Dipyridamole (dye-peer-ID-a-mole) is used as part of a medical test that shows how well blood is flowing to your heart. The test can show your doctor whether any of the blood vessels that bring blood to the heart are blocked or in danger of becoming blocked. Your doctor can then decide on the best treatment for you. Exercise (for example, walking on a treadmill) is usually used to give your doctor this information. Dipyridamole is used instead of exercise for people who are not able to exercise at all, or cannot exercise hard enough.

The dose of dipyridamole that is used to test how well blood is flowing to your heart will be different for different patients and depends on your body weight.

For information on other uses of dipyridamole, see Dipyridamole (Therapeutic).

Dipyridamole is available only with your doctor's prescription, in the following dosage forms:

*Oral*
• Tablets (U.S. and Canada)

*Parenteral*
• Injection (U.S. and Canada)

## Before Having This Test

In deciding to use a diagnostic test, any risks of the test must be weighed against the good it will do. This is a decision you and your doctor will make. Also, test results may be affected by other things. For dipyridamole, the following should be considered:

**Allergies**—Tell your doctor if you have ever had any unusual or allergic reaction to dipyridamole. Also tell your health care professional if you are allergic to any other substances, such as foods, preservatives, or dyes.

**Pregnancy**—Although studies have not been done in pregnant women, dipyridamole has not been reported to cause birth defects or other problems. Also, dipyridamole has not been shown to cause birth defects or other problems in mice, rats, or rabbits given many times the maximum human dose.

**Breast-feeding**—Although dipyridamole passes into breast milk, it has not been reported to cause problems in nursing babies.

**Children**—This medicine has been tested only in adults, and there is no specific information comparing use of dipyridamole in children with use in other age groups.

**Older adults**—Dipyridamole for diagnostic use has been tested in older people. It has not been shown to cause different side effects or problems in older people than it does in younger adults.

**Other medicines**—Although certain medicines should not be used together at all, in other cases two different medicines may be used together even if an interaction might occur. In these cases, your doctor may want to change the dose, or other precautions may be necessary. Before you receive dipyridamole, it is especially important that your doctor knows if you are taking any of the following:

• Aminophylline (e.g., Somophyllin) or
• Caffeine (e.g., NoDoz) or
• Dyphylline (e.g., Lufyllin) or
• Oxtriphylline (e.g., Choledyl) or
• Theophylline (e.g., Somophyllin-T)—These medicines will interfere with the results of this test. Caffeine should not be taken for 8 to 12 hours before the test. It is present in many medicines (for example, stay-awake products, pain relievers, and medicines for relieving migraine headaches) and foods or beverages (for example, coffee, tea, colas or other soft drinks, cocoa, and chocolate). If you are not sure whether any medicine you are taking contains caffeine, check with your pharmacist

The other medicines listed here are used to treat asthma or other lung or breathing problems. They should not be taken for about 36 hours before the test. However, *do not stop taking the medicine on your own.* Instead, at least 3 or 4 days before the test, tell the doctor in charge of giving the test that you are taking the medicine. He or she can call the doctor who ordered the medicine for you, and together they will decide whether you should stop taking the medicine for a while

• Anticoagulants (blood thinners) or
• Aspirin or
• Carbenicillin by injection (e.g., Geopen) or
• Cefamandole (e.g., Mandol) or
• Cefoperazone (e.g., Cefobid) or

- Cefotetan (e.g., Cefotan) or
- Divalproex (e.g., Depakote) or
- Heparin or
- Inflammation or pain medicine, except narcotics, or
- Pentoxifylline (e.g., Trental) or
- Plicamycin (e.g., Mithracin) or
- Sulfinpyrazone (e.g., Anturane) or
- Ticarcillin (e.g., Ticar) or
- Ticlopidine (e.g., Ticlid) or
- Valproic acid (e.g., Depakene)—The chance of bleeding may be increased

**Other medical problems**—The presence of other medical problems may affect the use of dipyridamole. Make sure you tell your doctor if you have any other medical problems, especially:

- Asthma or history of or
- Chest pain—The chance of side effects may be increased
- Low blood pressure—Large amounts of dipyridamole can make your condition worse

## Side Effects of This Medicine

Along with its needed effects, a medicine may cause some unwanted effects. Although not all of these side effects may occur, if they do occur they may need medical attention.

While you are receiving dipyridamole, and for a while after you have received it, your doctor will closely follow its effects. If necessary, your doctor can give you a medicine that will stop any unwanted effects. *Tell your doctor right away if you notice any of the following side effects:*

*More common*

  Chest pain

*Less common or rare*

  Headache (severe and throbbing); shortness of breath, troubled breathing, tightness in chest, or wheezing

Other side effects may occur that usually do not need medical attention. These side effects may go away in a little while. However, check with your doctor if they continue or are bothersome:

*More common*

  Dizziness or lightheadedness; headache

*Less common*

  Flushing; nausea or vomiting

Other side effects not listed above may also occur in some patients. If you notice any other effects, check with your doctor.

Revised: 01/30/92
Interim revision: 08/17/94

# DIPYRIDAMOLE    Therapeutic

Some commonly used brand names are:

**In the U.S.—**

  Dipridacot                    Persantine
  Generic name product may also be available.

**In Canada—**

  Apo-Dipyridamole              Persantine
  Novodipiradol

## Description

Dipyridamole (dye-peer-ID-a-mole) is used to lessen the chance of stroke or other serious medical problems that may occur when a blood vessel is blocked by blood clots. It is given only when there is a larger-than-usual chance that these problems may occur. For example, it is given to people who have had diseased heart valves replaced by mechanical valves, because dangerous blood clots are especially likely to occur in these patients. Dipyridamole works by helping to prevent dangerous blood clots from forming.

Dipyridamole may also be used for other heart and blood conditions as determined by your doctor.

Dipyridamole is also sometimes used as part of a medical test that shows how well blood is flowing to your heart. For information on this use of dipyridamole, see Dipyridamole (Diagnostic).

Dipyridamole is available only with your doctor's prescription, in the following dosage forms:

*Oral*

- Tablets (U.S. and Canada)

*Parenteral*

- Injection (Canada)

## Before Using This Medicine

In deciding to use a medicine, the risks of taking the medicine must be weighed against the good it will do. This is a decision you and your doctor will make. For dipyridamole, the following should be considered:

**Allergies**—Tell your doctor if you have ever had any unusual or allergic reaction to dipyridamole. Also tell your health care professional if you are allergic to any other substances, such as foods, preservatives, or dyes.

**Pregnancy**—Although studies have not been done in pregnant women, dipyridamole has not been reported to cause birth defects or other problems. Also, dipyridamole has not been shown to cause birth defects or other problems in mice, rats, or rabbits given many times the maximum human dose.

**Breast-feeding**—Although dipyridamole passes into breast milk, it has not been reported to cause problems in nursing babies.

**Children**—This medicine has been tested only in adults, and there is no specific information comparing use of dipyridamole in children with use in other age groups.

**Older adults**—Dipyridamole has not been studied specifically in older people taking the medicine regularly to prevent blood clots from forming. Although there is no specific information comparing this use of dipyridamole in the elderly with use in other age groups, it is not expected to cause different side effects or problems in older people than it does in younger adults.

**Other medicines**—Although certain medicines should not be used together at all, in other cases two different medicines may be used together even if an interaction might occur. In these cases, your doctor may want to change the dose, or other precautions may be necessary. When you are taking dipyridamole, it is especially important that your health care professional know if you are taking any of the following:

- Anticoagulants (blood thinners) or
- Aspirin or
- Carbenicillin by injection (e.g., Geopen) or
- Cefamandole (e.g., Mandol) or
- Cefoperazone (e.g., Cefobid) or
- Cefotetan (e.g., Cefotan) or
- Divalproex (e.g., Depakote) or
- Heparin or
- Inflammation or pain medicine, except narcotics, or
- Pentoxifylline (e.g., Trental) or
- Plicamycin (e.g., Mithracin) or
- Sulfinpyrazone (e.g., Anturane) or
- Ticarcillin (e.g., Ticar) or
- Ticlopidine (e.g., Ticlid) or
- Valproic acid (e.g., Depakene)—The chance of bleeding may be increased

**Other medical problems**—The presence of other medical problems may affect the use of dipyridamole. Make sure you tell your doctor if you have any other medical problems, especially:

- Chest pain—The chance of side effects may be increased
- Low blood pressure—Large amounts of dipyridamole can make your condition worse

## Proper Use of This Medicine

This medicine works best when there is a constant amount in the blood. To help keep the amount constant, *dipyridamole must be taken in regularly spaced doses,* as ordered by your doctor.

This medicine works best when taken with a full glass (8 ounces) of water at least 1 hour before or 2 hours after meals. However, to lessen stomach upset, your doctor may want you to take the medicine with food or milk.

**Dosing**—The dose of dipyridamole will be different for different patients. *Follow your doctor's orders or the directions on the label.* The following information includes only the average doses of dipyridamole. *If your dose is different, do not change it* unless your doctor tells you to do so.

- For preventing blood clots:
  —For *oral* dosage form (tablets):
    - Adults—The usual dose is 75 to 100 milligrams (mg) four times a day taken together with an anticoagulant (blood-thinning) medicine.
    - Children—Use and dose must be determined by your doctor.

**Missed dose**—If you miss a dose of this medicine, take it as soon as possble. However, if it is within 4 hours of your next scheduled dose, skip the missed dose and go back to your regular dosing schedule. Do not double doses.

**Storage**—To store this medicine:

- Keep out of the reach of children.
- Store away from heat and direct light.
- Do not store in the bathroom, near the kitchen sink, or in other damp places. Heat or moisture may cause the medicine to break down.
- Do not keep outdated medicine or medicine no longer needed. Be sure that any discarded medicine is out of the reach of children.

## Precautions While Using This Medicine

Dipyridamole is sometimes used together with an anticoagulant (blood thinner) or aspirin. The combination of medicines may provide better protection against the formation of blood clots than any of the medicines used alone. However, the risk of bleeding may also be increased. To reduce the risk of bleeding:

- *Do not take aspirin, or any combination medicine containing aspirin, unless the same doctor who directed you to take dipyridamole also directs you to take aspirin.* This is especially important if you are taking an anticoagulant together with dipyridamole.
- If you have been directed to take aspirin together with dipyridamole, *take only the amount of aspirin ordered by your doctor.* If you need a medicine to relieve pain or a fever, your doctor may not want you to take extra aspirin. It is a good idea to discuss this with your doctor, so that you will know ahead of time what medicine to take.
- Your doctor should check your progress at regular visits.

*Tell all medical doctors and dentists you go to that you are taking dipyridamole, and whether or not you are taking an anticoagulant (blood thinner) or aspirin together with it.*

*Dizziness, lightheadedness, or fainting may occur,* especially when you get up from a lying or sitting position. Getting up slowly may help. If this problem continues or gets worse, check with your doctor.

## Side Effects of This Medicine

Along with its needed effects, a medicine may cause some unwanted effects. Although not all of these side effects

may occur, if they do occur they may need medical attention.

Check with your doctor as soon as possible if the following side effect occurs shortly after you start taking this medicine:

*Less common*
　Skin rash or itching

*Rare*
　Chest pain or tightness in chest

Other side effects may occur that usually do not need medical attention. These side effects may go away during treatment as your body adjusts to the medicine. However, check with your doctor if they continue or are bothersome:

*More common*
　Dizziness

*Less common*
　Flushing; headache; nausea or vomiting; stomach cramping; weakness

Other side effects not listed above may also occur in some patients. If you notice any other effects, check with your doctor.

Revised: 01/30/92
Interim revision: 08/17/94

---

# DISOPYRAMIDE    Systemic

Some commonly used brand names are:

**In the U.S.—**
　Norpace
　Norpace CR
　Generic name product may also be available.

**In Canada—**
　Norpace                        Rythmodan
　Norpace CR                  Rythmodan-LA

## Description

Disopyramide (dye-soe-PEER-a-mide) is used to correct irregular heartbeats to a normal rhythm and to slow an overactive heart. This allows the heart to work more efficiently.

Disopyramide is available only with your doctor's prescription, in the following dosage forms:

*Oral*
　• Capsules (U.S. and Canada)
　• Extended-release capsules (U.S.)
　• Extended-release tablets (Canada)

*Parenteral*
　• Injection (Canada)

## Before Using This Medicine

In deciding to use a medicine, the risks of taking the medicine must be weighed against the good it will do. This is a decision you and your doctor will make. For disopyramide, the following should be considered:

**Allergies**—Tell your doctor if you have ever had any unusual or allergic reaction to disopyramide. Also tell your health care professional if you are allergic to any other substance, such as foods, preservatives, or dyes.

**Pregnancy**—Disopyramide has not been studied in pregnant women. However, use of disopyramide in a small number of pregnant women seems to show that this medicine may cause contractions of the uterus. Studies in animals have shown that disopyramide increases the risk of miscarriages. Before taking this medicine, make sure your doctor knows if you are pregnant or if you may become pregnant.

**Breast-feeding**—Disopyramide passes into breast milk.

**Children**—This medicine has been tested in children and has not been shown to cause different side effects or problems than it does in adults.

**Older adults**—Some side effects, such as difficult urination and dry mouth, may be especially likely to occur in elderly patients, who are usually more sensitive than younger adults to the effects of disopyramide.

**Other medicines**—Although certain medicines should not be used together at all, in other cases two different medicines may be used together even if an interaction might occur. In these cases, your doctor may want to change the dose, or other precautions may be necessary. When you are taking disopyramide, it is especially important that your health care professional know if you are taking any of the following:

　• Other heart medicine—Effects on the heart may be increased
　• Pimozide (e.g., Orap)—Risk of heart rhythm problems may be increased

**Other medical problems**—The presence of other medical problems may affect the use of disopyramide. Make sure you tell your doctor if you have any other medical problems, especially:

　• Diabetes mellitus (sugar diabetes)—Disopyramide may cause low blood sugar
　• Difficult urination or
　• Enlarged prostate—Disopyramide may cause difficult urination
　• Glaucoma (history of) or
　• Myasthenia gravis—Disopyramide may make these conditions worse

- Kidney disease or
- Liver disease—Effects may be increased because of slower removal of disopyramide from the body

## Proper Use of This Medicine

*Take disopyramide exactly as directed by your doctor* even though you may feel well. Do not take more medicine than ordered.

For patients taking the *extended-release capsules:*
- Swallow the capsule whole without breaking, crushing, or chewing.

For patients taking the *extended-release tablets:*
- Do not crush or chew the tablet.

This medicine works best when there is a constant amount in the blood. *To help keep the amount constant, do not miss any doses. Also, it is best to take the doses at evenly spaced times day and night.* For example, if you are to take 4 doses a day, the doses should be spaced about 6 hours apart. If this interferes with your sleep or other daily activities, or if you need help in planning the best times to take your medicine, check with your health care professional.

**Dosing**—The dose of disopyramide will be different for different patients. *Follow your doctor's orders or the directions on the label.* The following information includes only the average doses of disopyramide. *If your dose is different, do not change it* unless your doctor tells you to do so:

The number of tablets or capsules that you take depends on the strength of the medicine.
- For *treatment* of arrhythmias:
  —For *short-acting oral* dosage forms (capsules):
  - Adults—300 milligrams (mg) for the first dose. Then 100 to 150 mg taken every six to eight hours.
  - Children—Dose is based on body weight and age. It must be determined by your doctor. The dose is usually 6 to 30 mg per kilogram (kg) of body weight (2.73 to 13.64 mg per pound) per day. This dose is evenly divided and taken every six hours.
  —For *long-acting oral* dosage forms (extended-release capsules or tablets):
  - Adults—200 or 300 mg every twelve hours.
  - Children—Use is not recommended.
  —For *injection* dosage form:
  - Adults—
    —*First few doses:* Dose is based on body weight and must be determined by your doctor. It is usually 2 mg per kg of body weight (0.91 mg per pound) injected in three divided doses, or, 2 mg per kg of body weight (0.91 mg per pound) infused over fifteen minutes.
    —*Dose following first few doses:* Dose is based on body weight and must be determined by your doctor. It is usually 0.4 mg per kg of

body weight (0.18 mg per pound) per hour given for up to twenty-four hours.
- Children—Use is not recommended.

**Missed dose**—*If you do miss a dose of this medicine, take it as soon as possible unless the next scheduled dose is in less than 4 hours.* If you do not remember until later, skip the missed dose and go back to your regular dosing schedule. Do not double doses.

**Storage**—To store this medicine:
- Keep out of the reach of children.
- Store away from heat and direct light.
- Do not store in the bathroom, near the kitchen sink, or in other damp places. Heat or moisture may cause the medicine to break down.
- Do not keep outdated medicine or medicine no longer needed. Be sure that any discarded medicine is out of the reach of children.

## Precautions While Using This Medicine

*Your doctor should check your progress at regular visits* to make sure the medicine is working properly.

*Do not stop taking this medicine without first checking with your doctor. Stopping suddenly may cause a serious change in heart function.*

*Dizziness, lightheadedness, or fainting may occur, especially when you get up from a lying or sitting position.* This is due to lowered blood pressure. Getting up slowly may help. This effect does not occur often at doses of disopyramide usually used; however, *make sure you know how you react to this medicine before you drive, use machines, or do anything else that could be dangerous if you are not alert.* If the problem continues or gets worse, check with your doctor.

*Avoid alcoholic beverages until you have discussed their use with your doctor.* Alcohol may make the low blood sugar effect worse and/or increase the possibility of dizziness or fainting.

*Disopyramide may cause hypoglycemia (low blood sugar) in some people. Patients with congestive heart disease or diabetes especially should be aware of the signs of hypoglycemia. (See Side Effects of This Medicine.) If these signs appear, eat or drink a food containing sugar and call your doctor right away.*

This medicine may cause blurred vision or other vision problems. If any of these occur, *do not drive, use machines, or do anything else that could be dangerous if you are not able to see well.*

Disopyramide may cause dryness of the mouth, nose, and throat. For temporary relief of mouth dryness, use sugarless candy or gum, melt bits of ice in your mouth, or use a saliva substitute. However, if dry mouth continues for more than 2 weeks, check with your medical doctor or dentist. Continuing dryness of the mouth may increase the chance of dental disease, including tooth decay, gum disease, and fungus infections.

This medicine will often make you sweat less, allowing your body temperature to increase. *Use extra care not to become overheated during exercise or hot weather while you are taking this medicine*, since overheating could possibly result in heat stroke.

## Side Effects of This Medicine

Along with its needed effects, a medicine may cause some unwanted effects. Although not all of these side effects may occur, if they do occur they may need medical attention.

Check with your doctor as soon as possible if any of the following side effects occur:

*More common*
>Difficult urination

*Less common*
>Chest pains; dizziness, lightheadedness, or fainting; fast or slow heartbeat; muscle weakness; shortness of breath (unexplained); swelling of feet or lower legs; weight gain (rapid)

*Rare*
>Eye pain; mental depression; sore throat and fever; yellow eyes or skin

*Signs and symptoms of hypoglycemia (low blood sugar)*
>Anxious feeling; chills; cold sweats; confusion; cool, pale skin; drowsiness; fast heartbeat; headache; hunger (excessive); nausea; nervousness; shakiness; unsteady walk; unusual tiredness or weakness

Other side effects may occur that usually do not need medical attention. These side effects may go away during treatment as your body adjusts to the medicine. However, check with your health care professional if any of the following side effects continue or are bothersome:

*More common*
>Dryness of mouth and throat

*Less common*
>Bloating or stomach pain; blurred vision; constipation; decreased sexual ability; dry eyes and nose; frequent urge to urinate; loss of appetite

Other side effects not listed above may also occur in some patients. If you notice any other effects, check with your doctor.

Revised: 05/14/93

# DISULFIRAM   Systemic

A commonly used brand name in the U.S. and Canada is Antabuse. Generic name product may also be available in the U.S.

## Description

Disulfiram (dye-SUL-fi-ram) is used to help overcome your drinking problem. It is not a cure for alcoholism, but rather will discourage you from drinking.

Disulfiram is available only with your doctor's prescription, in the following dosage form:

*Oral*
>• Tablets (U.S. and Canada)

## Before Using This Medicine

In deciding to use a medicine, the risks of taking the medicine must be weighed against the good it will do. This is a decision you and your doctor will make. For disulfiram, the following should be considered:

**Allergies**—Tell your doctor if you have had any unusual or allergic reactions to disulfiram, rubber, pesticides, or fungicides.

**Diet**—In addition to beverages, alcohol is found in many other products. Reading the list of ingredients on foods and other products before using them will help you to avoid alcohol. Do not use alcohol-containing foods such as sauces and vinegars.

**Pregnancy**—Disulfiram has not been studied in pregnant women. However, there have been a few reports of birth defects in infants whose mothers took disulfiram during pregnancy. Before taking this medicine, make sure your doctor knows if you are pregnant or if you may become pregnant.

**Breast-feeding**—Disulfiram has not been reported to cause problems in nursing babies.

**Children**—Studies on this medicine have been done only in adult patients, and there is no specific information comparing use of disulfiram in children with use in other age groups.

**Older adults**—Many medicines have not been studied specifically in older people. Therefore, it may not be known whether they work exactly the same way they do in younger adults or if they cause different side effects or problems in older people. There is no specific information comparing use of disulfiram in the elderly with use in other age groups.

**Other medicines**—Although certain medicines should not be used together at all, in other cases 2 different medicines may be used together even if an interaction might occur. In these cases, your doctor may want to change the dose, or other precautions may be necessary. When you are taking disulfiram, it is especially important that

your health care professional know if you are taking any of the following:

- Anticoagulants (blood thinners)—Taking disulfiram may increase the effects of anticoagulants, changing the amount you need to take
- Ethotoin (e.g., Peganone) or
- Mephenytoin (e.g., Mesantoin) or
- Phenytoin (e.g., Dilantin)—Taking these medicines with disulfiram may change the amount of anticonvulsant medicine you need to take
- Isoniazid (e.g., INH, Nydrazid)—Disulfiram may increase central nervous system (CNS) effects, such as dizziness, clumsiness, irritability, or trouble in sleeping
- Metronidazole (e.g., Flagyl) or
- Paraldehyde (e.g., Paral)—These medicines should not be taken with or within several days of disulfiram because serious side effects may occur

*Ethylene dibromide or organic solvents* (such as chemicals which may contain alcohol, acetaldehyde, paraldehyde, or other related chemicals used in factories and in hobbies [e.g., paint thinner])—Make sure you tell your doctor if you will come in contact with or breathe the fumes of ethylene dibromide or organic solvents while you are taking disulfiram.

**Other medical problems**—The presence of other medical problems may affect the use of disulfiram. Make sure you tell your doctor if you have any other medical problems, especially:

- Asthma or other lung disease, severe, or
- Diabetes mellitus (sugar diabetes) or
- Epilepsy or other seizure disorder or
- Heart or blood vessel disease or
- Kidney disease or
- Liver disease or cirrhosis of the liver or
- Underactive thyroid—A disulfiram-alcohol reaction may make the condition worse
- Depression or
- Severe mental illness—Disulfiram may make the condition worse
- Skin allergy—Disulfiram may cause an allergic reaction

## Proper Use of This Medicine

Before you take the first dose of this medicine, *make sure you have not taken any alcoholic beverage or alcohol-containing product or medicine* (for example, tonics, elixirs, and cough syrups) *during the past 12 hours.* If you are not sure about the alcohol content of medicines you may have taken, check with your health care professional.

*Take this medicine every day as directed by your doctor.* The medicine is usually taken each morning. However, if it makes you drowsy, ask your doctor if you may take it at bedtime instead.

**Dosing**—The dose of disulfiram will be different for different patients. *Follow your doctor's orders or the directions on the label.* The following information includes only the average doses of disulfiram. *If your dose is different, do not change it* unless your doctor tells you to do so.

- For *oral* dosage form (tablets):
  - —To help overcome drinking problems:
    - Adults and teenagers—At first, the dose is 500 milligrams (mg) or less, once a day for one or two weeks. Then, your doctor may lower your dose to 125 to 500 mg (usually to 250 mg) once a day.
    - Children—Use and dose must be determined by your doctor.

**Storage**—To store this medicine:
- Keep out of the reach of children.
- Store away from heat and direct light.
- Do not store in the bathroom, near the kitchen sink, or in other damp places. Heat or moisture may cause the medicine to break down.
- Do not keep outdated medicine or medicine no longer needed. Be sure that any discarded medicine is out of the reach of children.

## Precautions While Using This Medicine

*Do not drink any alcohol, even small amounts, while you are taking this medicine and for 14 days after you stop taking it,* because the alcohol may make you very sick. In addition to beverages, alcohol is found in many other products. Reading the list of ingredients on foods and other products before using them will help you to avoid alcohol. You can also avoid alcohol if you:

- Do not use alcohol-containing foods, products, or medicines, such as elixirs, tonics, sauces, vinegars, cough syrups, mouth washes, or gargles.
- *Do not come in contact with or breathe in the fumes of chemicals that may contain alcohol, acetaldehyde, paraldehyde, or other related chemicals,* such as paint thinner, paint, varnish, or shellac.
- *Use caution when using alcohol-containing products that are applied to the skin,* such as some transdermal (stick-on patch) medicines or rubbing alcohol, back rubs, after-shave lotions, colognes, perfumes, toilet waters, or after-bath preparations. Using such products while you are taking disulfiram may cause headache, nausea, or local redness or itching because the alcohol in these products may be absorbed into your body. Before using alcohol-containing products on your skin, first test the product by applying some to a small area of your skin. Allow the product to remain on your skin for 1 or 2 hours. If no redness, itching, or other unwanted effects occur, you should be able to use the product.
- *Do not use any alcohol-containing products on raw skin or open wounds.*

Check with your doctor if you have any questions.

Some of the symptoms you may experience if you use any alcohol while taking this medicine are:
Blurred vision
Chest pain
Confusion
Dizziness or fainting
Fast or pounding heartbeat

Flushing or redness of face
Increased sweating
Nausea and vomiting
Throbbing headache
Troubled breathing
Weakness

These symptoms will last as long as there is any alcohol left in your system, from 30 minutes to several hours. On rare occasions, if you have a severe reaction or have taken a large enough amount of alcohol, a heart attack, unconsciousness, convulsions (seizures), and death may occur.

Your doctor may want you to carry an identification card stating that you are using this medicine. This card should list the symptoms most likely to occur if alcohol is taken, and the doctor, clinic, or hospital to be contacted in case of an emergency. These cards may be available from the manufacturer. Ask your health care professional if you have any questions about this.

If you will be taking this medicine for a long period of time (for example, for several months at a time), your doctor should check your progress at regular visits.

*Before buying or using any liquid prescription or nonprescription medicine, check with your pharmacist to see if it contains any alcohol.*

This medicine may cause some people to become drowsy or less alert than they are normally. If this occurs, *do not drive, use machines, or do anything else that could be dangerous if you are not alert.*

Disulfiram will add to the effects of other CNS depressants (medicines that slow down the nervous system, possibly causing drowsiness). Some examples of CNS depressants are antihistamines or medicine for hay fever, other allergies, or colds; sedatives, tranquilizers, or sleeping medicine; prescription pain medicine or narcotics; barbiturates; medicine for seizures; muscle relaxants; or anesthetics, including some dental anesthetics. *Check with your doctor before taking any of the above while you are using this medicine.*

## Side Effects of This Medicine

Along with its needed effects, a medicine may cause some unwanted effects. Although not all of these side effects may occur, if they do occur they may need medical attention.

Check with your doctor as soon as possible if any of the following side effects occur:

*Less common*
Eye pain or tenderness or any change in vision; mood or mental changes; numbness, tingling, pain, or weakness in hands or feet

*Rare*
Darkening of urine; light gray–colored stools; severe stomach pain; yellow eyes or skin

Other side effects may occur that usually do not need medical attention. These side effects may go away during treatment as your body adjusts to the medicine. However, check with your doctor if any of the following side effects continue or are bothersome:

*More common*
Drowsiness

*Less common or rare*
Decreased sexual ability in males; headache; metallic or garlic-like taste in mouth; skin rash; unusual tiredness

Other side effects not listed above may also occur in some patients. If you notice any other effects, check with your doctor.

Revised: 01/27/92
Interim revision: 07/20/94

# DIURETICS, LOOP   Systemic

Some commonly used brand names are:
**In the U.S.—**
Bumex[1]                          Lasix[3]
Edecrin[2]                        Myrosemide[3]

**In Canada—**
Apo-Furosemide[3]                 Lasix Special[3]
Edecrin[2]                        Novosemide[3]
Furoside[3]                       Uritol[3]
Lasix[3]

Note: For quick reference, the following loop diuretics are numbered to match the corresponding brand names.

This information applies to the following medicines:
1. Bumetanide (byoo-MET-a-nide)†
2. Ethacrynic Acid (eth-a-KRIN-ik AS-id)
3. Furosemide (fur-OH-se-mide)‡§

†Not commercially available in Canada.
‡Generic name product may also be available in the U.S.
§Generic name product may also be available in Canada.

## Description

Loop diuretics are given to help reduce the amount of water in the body. They work by acting on the kidneys to increase the flow of urine.

Furosemide is also used to treat high blood pressure (hypertension) in those patients who are not helped by other medicines or in those patients who have kidney problems.

High blood pressure adds to the work load of the heart and arteries. If it continues for a long time, the heart and arteries may not function properly. This can damage the blood vessels of the brain, heart, and kidneys, resulting in a stroke, heart failure, or kidney failure. High blood pressure may also increase the risk of heart attacks. These problems may be less likely to occur if blood pressure is controlled.

Loop diuretics may also be used for other conditions as determined by your doctor.

This medicine is available only with your doctor's prescription, in the following dosage forms:

*Oral*
Bumetanide
• Tablets (U.S.)
Ethacrynic Acid
• Oral solution (U.S. and Canada)
• Tablets (U.S. and Canada)
Furosemide
• Oral solution (U.S. and Canada)
• Tablets (U.S. and Canada)

*Parenteral*
Bumetanide
• Injection (U.S.)
Ethacrynic Acid
• Injection (U.S. and Canada)
Furosemide
• Injection (U.S. and Canada)

## Before Using This Medicine

In deciding to use a medicine, the risks of taking the medicine must be weighed against the good it will do. This is a decision you and your doctor will make. For loop diuretics, the following should be considered:

**Allergies**—Tell your doctor if you have ever had any unusual or allergic reaction to bumetanide, ethacrynic acid, furosemide, sulfonamides (sulfa drugs), or thiazide diuretics (water pills). Also tell your health care professional if you are allergic to any other substances, such as foods, preservatives, or dyes.

**Pregnancy**—Studies have not been done in pregnant women. However, studies in animals have shown this medicine to cause harmful effects.

In general, diuretics are not useful for normal swelling of feet and hands that occurs during pregnancy. Diuretics should not be taken during pregnancy unless recommended by your doctor.

**Breast-feeding**—These medicines have not been reported to cause problems in nursing babies. Furosemide passes into breast milk; it is not known whether bumetanide or ethacrynic acid passes into breast milk.

**Children**—Although there is no specific information comparing the use of loop diuretics in children with use in any other age group, these medicines are not expected to cause different side effects in children than they do in adults.

**Older adults**—Dizziness, lightheadedness, or signs of too much potassium loss may be more likely to occur in the elderly, who are more sensitive to the effects of this medicine. Elderly patients may also be more likely to develop blood clots.

**Other medicines**—Although certain medicines should not be used together at all, in other cases two different medicines may be used together even if an interaction might occur. In these cases, your doctor may want to change the dose, or other precautions may be necessary. When you are taking loop diuretics, it is especially important that your health care professional know if you are taking *any* other medicines.

**Other medical problems**—The presence of other medical problems may affect the use of loop diuretics. Make sure you tell your doctor if you have any other medical problems, especially:
• Diabetes mellitus (sugar diabetes)—Loop diuretics may increase the amount of sugar in the blood
• Gout or
• Hearing problems or
• Pancreatitis (inflammation of the pancreas)—Loop diuretics may make these conditions worse
• Heart attack, recent—Use of loop diuretics after a recent heart attack may increase the chance of side effects
• Kidney disease (severe) or
• Liver disease—Higher blood levels of the loop diuretic may occur, which may increase the chance of side effects
• Lupus erythematosus (history of)—Ethacrynic acid and furosemide may make this condition worse

## Proper Use of This Medicine

This medicine may cause you to have an unusual feeling of tiredness when you begin to take it. You may also notice an increase in the amount of urine or in your frequency of urination. After you have taken the medicine for a while, these effects should lessen. In general, to keep the increase in urine from affecting your sleep:
• If you are to take a single dose a day, take it in the morning after breakfast.
• If you are to take more than one dose a day, take the last dose no later than 6 p.m., unless otherwise directed by your doctor.

However, it is best to plan your dose or doses according to a schedule that will least affect your personal activities and sleep. Ask your health care professional to help you plan the best time to take this medicine.

To help you remember to take your medicine, try to get into the habit of taking it at the same time each day.

For patients taking the *oral liquid form* of furosemide:
• This medicine is to be taken by mouth even if it comes in a dropper bottle. If this medicine does not come in a dropper bottle, use a specially marked measuring spoon or other device to measure each dose accurately, since the average household teaspoon may not hold the right amount of liquid.

For patients taking this medicine for *high blood pressure:*
• In addition to the use of the medicine your doctor has prescribed, appropriate treatment for your high blood pressure may include weight control and care in the types of foods you eat, especially foods high in sodium. Your doctor will tell you which factors

are most important for you. You should check with your doctor before changing your diet.

- Many patients who have high blood pressure will not notice any signs of the problem. In fact, many may feel normal. It is very important that you *take your medicine exactly as directed* and that you keep your appointments with your doctor even if you feel well.
- Remember that this medicine will not cure your high blood pressure but it does help control it. Therefore, you must continue to take it as directed if you expect to lower your blood pressure and keep it down. *You may have to take high blood pressure medicine for the rest of your life.* If high blood pressure is not treated, it can cause serious problems such as heart failure, blood vessel disease, stroke, or kidney disease.

If this medicine upsets your stomach, it may be taken with meals or milk. If stomach upset (nausea, vomiting, or stomach pain) continues or gets worse, or if you suddenly get severe diarrhea, check with your doctor.

**Dosing**—The dose of loop diuretics will be different for different patients. *Follow your doctor's orders or the directions on the label.* The following information includes only the average doses of loop diuretics. *If your dose is different, do not change it* unless your doctor tells you to do so.

The number of tablets or teaspoonfuls of solution that you take depends on the strength of the medicine. Also, *the number of doses you take each day, the time allowed between doses, and the length of time you take the medicine depend on the medical problem for which you are taking loop diuretics.*

*For bumetanide*
- For *oral* dosage form (tablets):
  —To lower the amount of water in the body:
  - Adults—0.5 to 2 milligrams (mg) once a day. Your doctor may increase your dose if needed.
  - Children—Dose must be determined by your doctor.
- For *injection* dosage form:
  —To lower the amount of water in the body:
  - Adults—0.5 to 1 mg injected into a muscle or a vein every two to three hours as needed.
  - Children—Dose must be determined by your doctor.

*For ethacrynic acid*
- For *oral* dosage form (oral solution or tablets):
  —To lower the amount of water in the body:
  - Adults—50 to 200 milligrams (mg) a day. This may be taken as a single dose or divided into smaller doses.
  - Children—At first, 25 mg a day. Your doctor may increase your dose as needed.

- For *injection* dosage form:
  —To lower the amount of water in the body:
  - Adults—50 mg injected into a vein every two to six hours as needed.
  - Children—Dose is based on body weight and must be determined by your doctor. The usual dose is 1 mg per kilogram (kg) (0.45 mg per pound) of body weight injected into a vein.

*For furosemide*
- For *oral* dosage form (oral solution or tablets):
  —To lower the amount of water in the body:
  - Adults—At first, 20 to 80 milligrams (mg) once a day. Then, your doctor may increase your dose as needed. Your doctor may tell you to take a dose once a day, two or three times a day, or every other day.
  - Children—Dose is based on body weight and must be determined by your doctor. The usual dose is 2 mg per kilogram (kg) (0.91 mg per pound) of body weight for one dose. Then, your doctor may increase your dose every six to eight hours as needed.
  —For high blood pressure:
  - Adults—40 mg two times a day. Your doctor may increase your dose.
- For *injection* dosage form:
  —To lower the amount of water in the body:
  - Adults—At first, 20 to 40 mg injected into a muscle or a vein for one dose. Then, your doctor may increase your dose every two hours as needed. Once the medicine is working, the dose is injected into a muscle or a vein one or two times a day.
  - Children—Dose is based on body weight and must be determined by your doctor. The usual dose is 1 mg per kg (0.45 mg per pound) of body weight injected into a muscle or a vein for one dose. Your doctor may increase your dose every two hours as needed.
  —For very high blood pressure:
  - Adults—40 to 200 mg injected into a vein.

**Missed dose**—If you miss a dose of this medicine, take it as soon as possible. However, if it is almost time for your next dose, skip the missed dose and go back to your regular dosing schedule. Do not double doses.

**Storage**—To store this medicine:
- Keep out of the reach of children.
- Store away from heat and direct light.
- Do not store in the bathroom, near the kitchen sink, or in other damp places. Heat or moisture may cause the medicine to break down.
- Keep the oral liquid form of this medicine from freezing.
- Do not keep outdated medicine or medicine no longer needed. Be sure that any discarded medicine is out of the reach of children.

## Precautions While Using This Medicine

It is important that your doctor check your progress at regular visits to make sure that this medicine is working properly.

*This medicine may cause a loss of potassium from your body:*

- To help prevent this, your doctor may want you to:
  —eat or drink foods that have a high potassium content (for example, orange or other citrus fruit juices), or
  —take a potassium supplement, or
  —take another medicine to help prevent the loss of the potassium in the first place.
- It is very important to follow these directions. Also, it is important not to change your diet on your own. This is more important if you are already on a special diet (as for diabetes), or if you are taking a potassium supplement or a medicine to reduce potassium loss. Extra potassium may not be necessary and, in some cases, too much potassium could be harmful.

To prevent the loss of too much water and potassium, tell your doctor if you become sick, especially with severe or continuing nausea and vomiting or diarrhea.

Before having any kind of surgery (including dental surgery) or emergency treatment, make sure the medical doctor or dentist in charge knows that you are taking this medicine.

*Dizziness, lightheadedness, or fainting may occur, especially when you get up from a lying or sitting position.* This is more likely to occur in the morning. *Getting up slowly may help.* When you get up from lying down, sit on the edge of the bed with your feet dangling for 1 or 2 minutes. Then stand up slowly. If the problem continues or gets worse, check with your doctor.

The dizziness, lightheadedness, or fainting is also more likely to occur if you drink alcohol, stand for long periods of time, exercise, or if the weather is hot. *While you are taking this medicine, be careful to limit the amount of alcohol you drink. Also, use extra care during exercise or hot weather or if you must stand for long periods of time.*

For *diabetic patients:*

- This medicine may affect blood sugar levels. While you are using this medicine, be especially careful in testing for sugar in your blood or urine.

For patients taking this medicine for *high blood pressure:*

- *Do not take other medicines unless they have been discussed with your doctor.* This especially includes over-the-counter (nonprescription) medicines for appetite control, asthma, colds, cough, hay fever, or sinus problems, since they may tend to increase your blood pressure.

For patients taking *furosemide:*

- Furosemide may cause your skin to be more sensitive to sunlight than it is normally. Exposure to sunlight, even for brief periods of time, may cause a skin rash, itching, redness or other discoloration of the skin, or a severe sunburn. When you begin taking this medicine:
  —Stay out of direct sunlight, especially between the hours of 10:00 a.m. and 3:00 p.m., if possible.
  —Wear protective clothing, including a hat. Also, wear sunglasses.
  —Apply a sun block product that has a skin protection factor (SPF) of at least 15. Some patients may require a product with a higher SPF number, especially if they have a fair complexion. If you have any questions about this, check with your health care professional.
  —Apply a sun block lipstick that has an SPF of at least 15 to protect your lips.
  —Do not use a sunlamp or tanning bed or booth.

*If you have a severe reaction from the sun, check with your doctor.*

## Side Effects of This Medicine

Along with its needed effects, a medicine may cause some unwanted effects. Although not all of these side effects may occur, if they do occur they may need medical attention.

Check with your doctor as soon as possible if any of the following side effects occur:

*Rare*

Black, tarry stools; blood in urine or stools; cough or hoarseness; fever or chills; joint pain; lower back or side pain; painful or difficult urination; pinpoint red spots on skin; ringing or buzzing in ears or any loss of hearing—more common with ethacrynic acid; skin rash or hives; stomach pain (severe) with nausea and vomiting; unusual bleeding or bruising; yellow eyes or skin; yellow vision—for furosemide only

*Signs and symptoms of too much potassium loss*

Dryness of mouth; increased thirst; irregular heartbeat; mood or mental changes; muscle cramps or pain; nausea or vomiting; unusual tiredness or weakness; weak pulse

Other side effects may occur that usually do not need medical attention. These side effects may go away during treatment as your body adjusts to the medicine. However, check with your doctor if any of the following side effects continue or are bothersome:

*More common*

Dizziness or lightheadedness when getting up from a lying or sitting position

*Less common or rare*

Blurred vision; chest pain—with bumetanide only; confusion—with ethacrynic acid only; diarrhea—more common with ethacrynic acid; headache; increased sensitivity of skin to sunlight—with furosemide only; loss of appetite—more common with ethacrynic acid; nervousness—with ethacrynic acid only; premature ejaculation or difficulty in keeping an erection—with bumetanide only; redness or pain at place of injection; stomach cramps or pain

Other side effects not listed above may also occur in some patients. If you notice any other effects, check with your doctor.

---

## Additional Information

Once a medicine has been approved for marketing for a certain use, experience may show that it is also useful for other medical problems. Although these uses are not included in product labeling, loop diuretics are used in certain patients with the following medical conditions:

- Hypercalcemia (too much calcium in the blood)
- Diagnostic aid for kidney disease

Other than the above information, there is no additional information relating to proper use, precautions, or side effects for these uses.

---

Revised: 08/02/94

---

# DIURETICS, POTASSIUM-SPARING  Systemic

Some commonly used brand names are:

**In the U.S.—**
| | |
|---|---|
| Aldactone[2] | Midamor[1] |
| Dyrenium[3] | |

**In Canada—**
| | |
|---|---|
| Aldactone[2] | Midamor[1] |
| Dyrenium[3] | Novospiroton[2] |

Note: For quick reference, the following potassium-sparing diuretics are numbered to match the corresponding brand names.

This information applies to the following medicines:

1. Amiloride (a-MILL-oh-ride)‡
2. Spironolactone (speer-on-oh-LAK-tone)‡
3. Triamterene (trye-AM-ter-een)

‡Generic name product may also be available in the U.S.

---

## Description

Potassium-sparing diuretics are commonly used to help reduce the amount of water in the body. Unlike some other diuretics, these medicines do not cause your body to lose potassium.

Amiloride and spironolactone are also used to treat high blood pressure (hypertension). High blood pressure adds to the workload of the heart and arteries. If the condition continues for a long time, the heart and arteries may not function properly. This can damage the blood vessels of the brain, heart, and kidneys, resulting in a stroke, heart failure, or kidney failure. High blood pressure may also increase the risk of heart attacks. These problems may be less likely to occur if blood pressure is controlled.

Spironolactone is also used to help increase the amount of potassium in the body when it is getting too low.

Potassium-sparing diuretics help to reduce the amount of water in the body by acting on the kidneys to increase the flow of urine. This also helps to lower blood pressure.

These medicines can also be used for other conditions as determined by your doctor.

Potassium-sparing diuretics are available only with your doctor's prescription, in the following dosage forms:

*Oral*
Amiloride
- Tablets (U.S. and Canada)

Spironolactone
- Tablets (U.S. and Canada)
Triamterene
- Capsules (U.S.)
- Tablets (Canada)

---

## Before Using This Medicine

In deciding to use a medicine, the risks of taking the medicine must be weighed against the good it will do. This is a decision you and your doctor will make. For potassium-sparing diuretics, the following should be considered:

**Allergies**—Tell your doctor if you have ever had any unusual or allergic reaction to amiloride, spironolactone, or triamterene. Also tell your health care professional if you are allergic to any other substances, such as foods, preservatives, or dyes.

**Pregnancy**—Studies have not been done in pregnant women. However, this medicine has not been shown to cause birth defects or other problems in animals.

In general, diuretics are not useful for normal swelling of feet and hands that occurs during pregnancy. Diuretics should not be taken during pregnancy unless recommended by your doctor.

**Breast-feeding**—Although amiloride, spironolactone, and triamterene may pass into breast milk, these medicines have not been reported to cause problems in nursing babies.

**Children**—This medicine has been tested in children and, in effective doses, has not been shown to cause different side effects or problems in children than it does in adults.

**Older adults**—Signs and symptoms of too much potassium are more likely to occur in the elderly, who are more sensitive than younger adults to the effects of this medicine.

**Other medicines**—Although certain medicines should not be used together at all, in other cases two different medicines may be used together even if an interaction might

---

occur. In these cases, your doctor may want to change the dose, or other precautions may be necessary. When you are taking potassium-sparing diuretics, it is especially important that your health care professional know if you are taking any of the following:

- Angiotensin-converting enzyme (ACE) inhibitors (benazepril [e.g., Lotensin], captopril [e.g., Capoten], enalapril [e.g., Vasotec], fosinopril [e.g., Monopril], lisinopril [e.g., Prinivil, Zestril], quinapril [e.g., Accupril], ramipril [e.g., Altace]) or
- Cyclosporine (e.g., Sandimmune) or
- Potassium-containing medicines or supplements—Use with potassium-sparing diuretics may cause high blood levels of potassium, which may increase the chance of side effects
- Digoxin—Use with spironolactone may cause high blood levels of digoxin, which may increase the chance of side effects
- Lithium (e.g., Lithane)—Use with potassium-sparing diuretics may cause high blood levels of lithium, which may increase the chance of side effects

**Other medical problems**—The presence of other medical problems may affect the use of potassium-sparing diuretics. Make sure you tell your doctor if you have any other medical problems, especially:

- Diabetes mellitus (sugar diabetes) or
- Kidney disease or
- Liver disease—Higher blood levels of potassium may occur, which may increase the chance of side effects
- Gout or
- Kidney stones (history of)—Triamterene may make these conditions worse
- Menstrual problems or breast enlargement—Spironolactone may make these conditions worse

## Proper Use of This Medicine

This medicine may cause you to have an unusual feeling of tiredness when you begin to take it. You may also notice an increase in the amount of urine or in your frequency of urination. After you have taken the medicine for a while, these effects should lessen. In general, to keep the increase in urine from affecting your sleep:

- If you are to take a single dose a day, take it in the morning after breakfast.
- If you are to take more than one dose a day, take the last dose no later than 6 p.m., unless otherwise directed by your doctor.

However, it is best to plan your dose or doses according to a schedule that will least affect your personal activities and sleep. Ask your health care professional to help you plan the best time to take this medicine.

To help you remember to take your medicine, try to get into the habit of taking it at the same time each day.

If this medicine upsets your stomach, it may be taken with meals or milk. If stomach upset (nausea, vomiting, stomach pain or cramps) continues, check with your doctor.

For patients taking this medicine for *high blood pressure:*

- In addition to the use of the medicine your doctor has prescribed, treatment for your high blood pressure may include weight control and care in the types of foods you eat, especially foods high in sodium. Your doctor will tell you which of these are most important for you. You should check with your doctor before changing your diet.
- Many patients who have high blood pressure will not notice any signs of the problem. In fact, many may feel normal. It is very important that you *take your medicine exactly as directed* and that you keep your appointments with your doctor even if you feel well.
- Remember that this medicine will not cure your high blood pressure but it does help control it. Therefore, you must continue to take it as directed if you expect to lower your blood pressure and keep it down. *You may have to take high blood pressure medicine for the rest of your life.* If high blood pressure is not treated, it can cause serious problems such as heart failure, blood vessel disease, stroke, or kidney disease.

**Dosing**—The dose of potassium-sparing diuretics will be different for different patients. *Follow your doctor's orders or the directions on the label.* The following information includes only the average doses of potassium-sparing diuretics. *If your dose is different, do not change it* unless your doctor tells you to do so.

The number of capsules or tablets that you take depends on the strength of the medicine. Also, *the number of doses you take each day, the time allowed between doses, and the length of time you take the medicine depend on the medical problem for which you are taking potassium-sparing diuretics.*

*For amiloride*
- For *oral* dosage form (tablets):
  —For high blood pressure or to lower the amount of water in the body:
  - Adults—5 to 10 milligrams (mg) once a day.
  - Children—Dose must be determined by your doctor.

*For spironolactone*
- For *oral* dosage form (tablets):
  —To lower the amount of water in the body:
  - Adults—At first, 25 to 200 milligrams (mg) a day. This is divided into two to four doses. Your doctor may increase your dose to 75 to 400 mg a day.
  - Children—Dose is based on body weight and must be determined by your doctor. The usual dose is 1 to 3 mg per kilogram (kg) (0.45 to 1.36 mg per pound) of body weight a day. The dose may be taken as a single dose or divided into two to four doses. Your doctor may increase your dose as needed.

—For high blood pressure:
• Adults—At first, 50 to 100 milligrams (mg) a day. This may be taken as a single dose or divided into two to four doses. Your doctor may gradually increase your dose up to 200 mg a day.
• Children—Dose is based on body weight and must be determined by your doctor. The usual dose is 1 to 3 mg per kg (0.45 to 1.36 mg per pound) of body weight a day. The dose may be taken as a single dose or divided into two to four doses. Your doctor may increase your dose as needed.
—To treat high aldosterone levels in the body:
• Adults—100 to 400 mg a day. This is divided into two to four doses and taken until you have surgery. If you are not having surgery, your doses may be smaller.
—For detecting high aldosterone levels in the body:
• Adults—400 mg a day, taken in two to four divided doses. Your doctor may want you to take this dose for as little as four days or as long as three to four weeks. Follow your doctor's instructions.
—To treat low potassium levels in the blood:
• Adults—25 to 100 mg a day. This may be taken as a single dose or divided into two to four doses.

*For triamterene*
• For *oral* dosage form (capsules or tablets):
—To lower the amount of water in the body:
• Adults—25 to 100 milligrams (mg) a day. Your doctor may gradually increase your dose.
• Children—Dose is based on body weight and must be determined by your doctor. To start, the usual dose is 2 to 4 mg per kilogram (kg) (0.9 to 1.82 mg per pound) of body weight a day or every other day. This is divided into smaller doses. Your doctor may increase your dose as needed.

**Missed dose**—If you miss a dose of this medicine, take it as soon as possible. However, if it is almost time for your next dose, skip the missed dose and go back to your regular dosing schedule. Do not double doses.

**Storage**—To store this medicine:
• Keep out of the reach of children.
• Store away from heat and direct light.
• Do not store in the bathroom, near the kitchen sink, or in other damp places. Heat or moisture may cause the medicine to break down.
• Do not keep outdated medicine or medicine no longer needed. Be sure that any discarded medicine is out of the reach of children.

## Precautions While Using This Medicine

It is important that your doctor check your progress at regular visits to make sure that this medicine is working properly.

This medicine does not cause a loss of potassium from your body as some other diuretics (water pills) do. Therefore, it is not necessary for you to get extra potassium in your diet, and too much potassium could even be harmful. Since salt substitutes and low-sodium milk may contain potassium, do not use them unless told to do so by your doctor.

Check with your doctor if you become sick and have severe or continuing nausea, vomiting, or diarrhea. These problems may cause you to lose additional water, which could be harmful, or to lose potassium, which could lessen the medicine's helpful effects.

Before having any kind of surgery (including dental surgery) or emergency treatment, tell the medical doctor or dentist in charge that you are taking this medicine.

Before you have any medical tests, tell the doctor in charge that you are taking this medicine. The results of some tests may be affected by this medicine.

For patients taking this medicine for *high blood pressure:*
• *Do not take other medicines unless they have been discussed with your doctor.* This especially includes over-the-counter (nonprescription) medicines for appetite control, asthma, colds, cough, hay fever, or sinus problems, since these medicines may tend to increase your blood pressure.

For patients taking *triamterene:*
• This medicine may cause your skin to be more sensitive to sunlight than it is normally. Exposure to sunlight, even for brief periods of time, may cause a skin rash, itching, redness or other discoloration of the skin, or a severe sunburn. When you begin taking this medicine:
—Stay out of direct sunlight, especially between the hours of 10:00 a.m. and 3:00 p.m., if possible.
—Wear protective clothing, including a hat. Also, wear sunglasses.
—Apply a sun block product that has a skin protection factor (SPF) of at least 15. Some patients may require a product with a higher SPF number, especially if they have a fair complexion. If you have any questions about this, check with your health care professional.
—Apply a sun block lipstick that has an SPF of at least 15 to protect your lips.
—Do not use a sunlamp or tanning bed or booth.
—If you have a severe reaction from the sun, check with your doctor.

## Side Effects of This Medicine

In rats, spironolactone has been found to increase the risk of tumors. It is not known if spironolactone increases the chance of tumors in humans.

Along with its needed effects, a medicine may cause some unwanted effects. Although not all of these side effects may occur, if they do occur they may need medical attention.

Check with your doctor as soon as possible if any of the following side effects occur:

*Rare*

*For amiloride, spironolactone, and triamterene*

Skin rash or itching; shortness of breath

*For spironolactone and triamterene only (in addition to effects listed above)*

Cough or hoarseness; fever or chills; lower back or side pain; painful or difficult urination

*For triamterene only (in addition to effects listed above)*

Black, tarry stools; blood in urine or stools; bright red tongue; burning, inflamed feeling in tongue; cracked corners of mouth; lower back pain (severe); pinpoint red spots on skin; unusual bleeding or bruising; weakness

*Signs and symptoms of too much potassium*

Confusion; irregular heartbeat; nervousness; numbness or tingling in hands, feet, or lips; shortness of breath or difficult breathing; unusual tiredness or weakness; weakness or heaviness of legs

Other side effects may occur that usually do not need medical attention. These side effects may go away during treatment as your body adjusts to the medicine. However, check with your doctor if any of the following side effects continue or are bothersome:

*More common (less common with amiloride and triamterene)*

Nausea and vomiting; stomach cramps and diarrhea

*Less common*

*For amiloride, spironolactone, and triamterene*

Dizziness; headache

*For amiloride and spironolactone only (in addition to effects listed above)*

Decreased sexual ability

*For amiloride only (in addition to effects listed above)*

Constipation; muscle cramps

*For spironolactone only (in addition to effects listed above for spironolactone)*

Breast tenderness in females; clumsiness; deepening of voice in females; enlargement of breasts in males; inability to have or keep an erection; increased hair growth in females; irregular menstrual periods; sweating

*For triamterene only (in addition to effects listed above for triamterene)*

Increased sensitivity of skin to sunlight

*Signs and symptoms of too little sodium*

Drowsiness; dryness of mouth; increased thirst; lack of energy

For *male patients:*

- Spironolactone sometimes causes enlarged breasts in males, especially when they take large doses of it for a long time. Breasts usually decrease in size gradually over several months after this medicine is stopped. If you have any questions about this, check with your doctor.

Other side effects not listed above may also occur in some patients. If you notice any other effects, check with your doctor.

## Additional Information

Once a medicine has been approved for marketing for a certain use, experience may show that it is also useful for other medical problems. Although these uses are not included in product labeling, spironolactone is used in certain patients with the following medical conditions:

- Polycystic ovary syndrome
- Hirsutism, female (increased hair growth)

Other than the above information, there is no additional information relating to proper use, precautions, or side effects for this use.

Revised: 10/15/92
Interim revision: 05/18/94

# DIURETICS, POTASSIUM-SPARING, AND HYDROCHLOROTHIAZIDE    Systemic

Some commonly used brand names are:

**In the U.S.—**

| | |
|---|---|
| Aldactazide[2] | Moduretic[1] |
| Dyazide[3] | Spirozide[2] |
| Maxzide[3] | |

Generic name product may also be available.

**In Canada—**

| | |
|---|---|
| Aldactazide[2] | Moduret[1] |
| Apo-Triazide[3] | Novo-Spirozine[2] |
| Dyazide[3] | Novo-Triamzide[3] |

Note: For quick reference, the following diuretics, potassium-sparing, and hydrochlorothiazides are numbered to match the corresponding brand names.

This information applies to the following medicines:

1. Amiloride (a-MILL-oh-ride) and Hydrochlorothiazide (hye-droe-klor-oh-THYE-a-zide)‡
2. Spironolactone (speer-on-oh-LAK-tone) and Hydrochlorothiazide‡
3. Triamterene (trye-AM-ter-een) and Hydrochlorothiazide‡

‡Generic name product may also be available in the U.S.

## Description

This medicine is a combination of two diuretics (water pills). It is commonly used to help reduce the amount of water in the body.

This combination is also used to treat high blood pressure (hypertension). High blood pressure adds to the work load of the heart and arteries. If it continues for a long time, the heart and arteries may not function properly. This can damage the blood vessels of the brain, heart, and kidneys, resulting in a stroke, heart failure, or kidney failure. High blood pressure may also increase the risk of heart attacks. These problems may be less likely to occur if blood pressure is controlled.

Diuretics help to reduce the amount of water in the body by acting on the kidneys to increase the flow of urine. This also helps to lower blood pressure.

This combination is also used to treat problems caused by too little potassium in the body.

This medicine is available only with your doctor's prescription, in the following dosage forms:

*Oral*

Amiloride and Hydrochlorothiazide
- Tablets (U.S. and Canada)

Spironolactone and Hydrochlorothiazide
- Tablets (U.S. and Canada)

Triamterene and Hydrochlorothiazide
- Capsules (U.S.)
- Tablets (U.S. and Canada)

## Before Using This Medicine

In deciding to use a medicine, the risks of taking the medicine must be weighed against the good it will do. This is a decision you and your doctor will make. For potassium-sparing diuretics and hydrochlorothiazide, the following should be considered:

**Allergies**—Tell your doctor if you have ever had any unusual or allergic reaction to amiloride, spironolactone, triamterene, sulfonamides (sulfa drugs), bumetanide, furosemide, acetazolamide, dichlorphenamide, methazolamide, or to hydrochlorothiazide or any of the other thiazide diuretics. Also tell your health care professional if you are allergic to any other substances, such as foods, preservatives, or dyes.

**Pregnancy**—In general, diuretics are not useful for normal swelling of feet and hands that occurs during pregnancy. They should not be taken during pregnancy unless recommended by your doctor.

**Breast-feeding**—Hydrochlorothiazide and spironolactone pass into breast milk. It is not known whether amiloride or triamterene passes into breast milk. Hydrochlorothiazide may also decrease the flow of breast milk. Therefore, you should avoid use of potassium-sparing diuretic and hydrochlorothiazide combinations during the first month of breast-feeding.

**Children**—Studies on this combination medicine have been done only in adult patients, and there is no specific information comparing use of potassium-sparing diuretic and hydrochlorothiazide combinations in children with use in other age groups.

**Older adults**—Dizziness or lightheadedness and signs and symptoms of too much potassium in the body or too little potassium in the body may be more likely to occur in the elderly, who are more sensitive than younger adults to the effects of this medicine.

**Other medicines**—Although certain medicines should not be used together at all, in other cases two different medicines may be used together even if an interaction might occur. In these cases, your doctor may want to change the dose, or other precautions may be necessary. When you are taking potassium-sparing diuretics and hydrochlorothiazide, it is especially important that your health care professional know if you are taking any of the following:

- Angiotensin-converting enzyme (ACE) inhibitors (benazepril [e.g., Lotensin], captopril [e.g., Capoten], enalapril [e.g., Vasotec], fosinopril [e.g., Monopril], lisinopril [e.g., Prinivil, Zestril], quinapril [e.g., Accupril], ramipril [e.g., Altace]) or
- Cyclosporine (e.g., Sandimmune) or
- Potassium-containing medicines or supplements—Use with potassium-sparing diuretic and hydrochlorothiazide combinations may cause high blood levels of potassium, which may increase the chance of side effects
- Cholestyramine or
- Colestipol—Use with potassium-sparing diuretic and hydrochlorothiazide combinations may prevent the diuretic from working properly; take the diuretic at least 1 hour before or 4 hours after cholestyramine or colestipol
- Digitalis glycosides (heart medicine)—Use with diuretics may cause high blood levels of digoxin, which may increase the chance of side effects
- Lithium (e.g., Lithane)—Use with diuretics may cause high blood levels of lithium, which may increase the chance of side effects

**Other medical problems**—The presence of other medical problems may affect the use of potassium-sparing diuretics and hydrochlorothiazde. Make sure you tell your doctor if you have any other medical problems, especially:

- Diabetes mellitus (sugar diabetes) or
- Kidney disease or
- Liver disease—Higher blood levels of potassium may occur, which may increase the chance of side effects
- Gout (history of) or
- Kidney stones (history of)—Triamterene and hydrochlorothiazide combination may make these conditions worse
- Heart or blood vessel disease—These medicines may cause high cholesterol levels or high triglyceride levels
- Lupus erythematosus (history of) or
- Pancreatitis (inflammation of pancreas)—Potassium-sparing diuretic and hydrochlorothiazide combinations may make these conditions worse
- Menstrual problems in women or breast enlargement in men—Spironolactone and hydrochlorothiazide combination may make these conditions worse

## Proper Use of This Medicine

This medicine may cause you to have an unusual feeling of tiredness when you begin to take it. You may also notice an increase in the amount of urine or in your frequency of urination. After you have taken the medicine for a while, these effects should lessen. In general, to keep the increase in urine from affecting your sleep:

- If you are to take a single dose a day, take it in the morning after breakfast.
- If you are to take more than one dose a day, take the last dose no later than 6 p.m., unless otherwise directed by your doctor.

However, it is best to plan your dose or doses according to a schedule that will least affect your personal activities and sleep. Ask your health care professional to help you plan the best time to take this medicine.

To help you remember to take your medicine, try to get into the habit of taking it at the same time each day.

If this medicine upsets your stomach, it may be taken with meals or milk. If stomach upset (nausea, vomiting, stomach pain, or cramps) continues, check with your doctor.

For patients taking this medicine for *high blood pressure:*

- In addition to the use of the medicine your doctor has prescribed, treatment for your high blood pressure may include weight control and care in the types of foods you eat, especially foods high in sodium. Your doctor will tell you which of these are most important for you. You should check with your doctor before changing your diet.
- Many patients who have high blood pressure will not notice any signs of the problem. In fact, many may feel normal. It is very important that you *take your medicine exactly as directed* and that you keep your appointments with your doctor even if you feel well.
- Remember that this medicine will not cure your high blood pressure but it does help control it. Therefore, you must continue to take it as directed if you expect to lower your blood pressure and keep it down. *You may have to take high blood pressure medicine for the rest of your life.* If high blood pressure is not treated, it can cause serious problems such as heart failure, blood vessel disease, stroke, or kidney disease.

**Dosing**—The dose of potassium-sparing diuretic and hydrochlorothiazide combinations will be different for different patients. *Follow your doctor's orders or the directions on the label.* The following information includes only the average doses of potassium-sparing diuretic and hydrochlorothiazide combinations. *If your dose is different, do not change it* unless your doctor tells you to do so.

The number of capsules or tablets that you take depends on the strength of the medicine. Also, *the number of doses you take each day depends on the strength of the medicine and the medical problem for which you are taking potassium-sparing diuretic and hydrochlorothiazide combinations.*

*For amiloride and hydrochlorothiazide combination*

- For *oral* dosage form (tablets):
  —For high blood pressure or lowering the amount of water in the body:
  - Adults—1 or 2 tablets a day.

- Children—Dose must be determined by your doctor.

*For spironolactone and hydrochlorothiazide combination*

- For *oral* dosage form (tablets):
  —For high blood pressure or lowering the amount of water in the body:
  - Adults—1 to 4 tablets a day.
  - Children—Dose is based on body weight and must be determined by your doctor.

*For triamterene and hydrochlorothiazide combination*

- For *oral* dosage form (capsules):
  —For high blood pressure or lowering the amount of water in the body:
  - Adults—1 or 2 capsules once a day.
  - Children—Dose must be determined by your doctor.
- For *oral* dosage form (tablets):
  —For high blood pressure or lowering the amount of water in the body:
  - Adults—1 to 4 tablets a day, depending on the strength of your tablet.
  - Children—Dose must be determined by your doctor.

**Missed dose**—If you miss a dose of this medicine, take it as soon as possible. However, if it is almost time for your next dose, skip the missed dose and go back to your regular dosing schedule. Do not double doses.

**Storage**—To store this medicine:

- Keep out of the reach of children.
- Store away from heat and direct light.
- Do not store in the bathroom, near the kitchen sink, or in other damp places. Heat or moisture may cause the medicine to break down.
- Do not keep outdated medicine or medicine no longer needed. Be sure that any discarded medicine is out of the reach of children.

## Precautions While Using This Medicine

It is important that your doctor check your progress at regular visits to make sure that this medicine is working properly.

*This medicine may cause a loss or increase of potassium in your body. Your doctor may have special instructions about whether or not you need to eat or drink foods or beverages that have a high potassium content (for example, orange or other citrus fruit juices), taking a potassium supplement, or using salt substitutes.* Since too much potassium can be harmful, it is important not to change your diet on your own. Tell your doctor if you are already on a special diet (as for diabetes). Since salt substitutes and low-sodium milk may contain potassium, do not use them unless told to do so by your doctor. Check with your health care professional if you need a list of foods that are high in potassium or if you have any questions.

Check with your doctor if you become sick and have severe or continuing vomiting or diarrhea. These problems may cause you to lose additional water and potassium and lead to low blood pressure.

For *diabetic patients:*

- Hydrochlorothiazide (contained in this combination medicine) may raise blood sugar levels. While you are taking this medicine, be especially careful in testing for sugar in your blood or urine.

Potassium-sparing diuretics and hydrochlorothiazide may cause your skin to be more sensitive to sunlight than it is normally. Exposure to sunlight, even for brief periods of time, may cause a skin rash, itching, redness or other discoloration of the skin, or a severe sunburn. When you begin taking this medicine:

- Stay out of direct sunlight, especially between the hours of 10:00 a.m. and 3:00 p.m., if possible.
- Wear protective clothing, including a hat. Also, wear sunglasses.
- Apply a sun block product that has a skin protection factor (SPF) of at least 15. Some patients may require a product with a higher SPF number, especially if they have a fair complexion. If you have any questions about this, check with your health care professional.
- Apply a sun block lipstick that has an SPF of at least 15 to protect your lips.
- Do not use a sunlamp or tanning bed or booth.

If you have a severe reaction from the sun, check with your doctor.

Before having any kind of surgery (including dental surgery) or emergency treatment, tell the medical doctor or dentist in charge that you are taking this medicine.

For patients taking *triamterene and hydrochlorothiazide combination:*

- Do not change brands of triamterene and hydrochlorothiazide without first checking with your doctor. Different products may not work the same way. If you refill your medicine and it looks different, check with your pharmacist.

For patients taking this medicine for *high blood pressure:*

- *Do not take other medicines unless they have been discussed with your doctor.* This especially includes over-the-counter (nonprescription) medicines for appetite control, asthma, colds, cough, hay fever, or sinus problems, since they may tend to increase your blood pressure.

Tell the doctor in charge that you are taking this medicine before you have any medical tests. The results of some tests may be affected by this medicine.

## Side Effects of This Medicine

In rats, spironolactone has been found to increase the risk of development of tumors. However, the doses given were many times the dose of spironolactone given to humans. It is not known whether spironolactone causes tumors in humans.

Along with its needed effects, a medicine may cause some unwanted effects. Although not all of these side effects may occur, if they do occur they may need medical attention.

Check with your doctor as soon as possible if any of the following side effects occur:

*Rare*

   Black, tarry stools; blood in urine or stools; cough or hoarseness; fever or chills; joint pain; lower back or side pain; painful or difficult urination; pinpoint red spots on skin; skin rash or hives; stomach pain (severe) with nausea and vomiting; unusual bleeding or bruising; yellow eyes or skin

*Signs and symptoms of changes in potassium*

   Confusion; dryness of mouth; increased thirst; irregular heartbeat; mood or mental changes; muscle cramps or pain; numbness or tingling in hands, feet, or lips; shortness of breath or difficulty breathing; unusual tiredness or weakness; weak pulse; weakness or heaviness of legs

*Reported for triamterene only (rare)*

   Bright red tongue; burning, inflamed feeling in tongue; cracked corners of mouth

Other side effects may occur that usually do not need medical attention. These side effects may go away during treatment as your body adjusts to the medicine. However, check with your doctor if any of the following side effects continue or are bothersome:

*More common (less common with triamterene)*

   Loss of appetite; nausea and vomiting; stomach cramps and diarrhea; upset stomach

*Less common*

   Decreased sexual ability; dizziness or lightheadedness when getting up from a lying or sitting position; headache; increased sensitivity of skin to sunlight

*Reported for amiloride only (less common)*

   Constipation

*Reported for spironolactone only (less common)*

   Breast tenderness in females; deepening of voice in females; enlargement of breasts in males; increased hair growth in females; irregular menstrual periods; sweating

Spironolactone sometimes causes enlarged breasts in males, especially when they take large doses of it for a long time. Breasts usually decrease in size gradually over several months after this medicine is stopped. If you have any questions about this, check with your doctor.

Other side effects not listed above may also occur in some patients. If you notice any other effects, check with your doctor.

Revised: 08/03/94

# DIURETICS, THIAZIDE   Systemic

Some commonly used brand names are:

**In the U.S.—**

| | |
|---|---|
| Anhydron[5] | Hydromox[11] |
| Aquatensen[8] | Hygroton[4] |
| Diucardin[7] | Metahydrin[12] |
| Diulo[9] | Mykrox[9] |
| Diuril[3] | Naqua[12] |
| Enduron[8] | Naturetin[1] |
| Esidrix[6] | Oretic[6] |
| Exna[2] | Renese[10] |
| Hydrex[2] | Saluron[7] |
| Hydro-chlor[6] | Thalitone[4] |
| Hydro-D[6] | Trichlorex[12] |
| HydroDIURIL[6] | Zaroxolyn[9] |

**In Canada—**

| | |
|---|---|
| Apo-Chlorthalidone[4] | Neo-Codema[6] |
| Apo-Hydro[6] | Novo-Hydrazide[6] |
| Diuchlor H[6] | Novo-Thalidone[4] |
| Duretic[8] | Uridon[4] |
| HydroDIURIL[6] | Urozide[6] |
| Hygroton[4] | Zaroxolyn[9] |
| Naturetin[1] | |

Note: For quick reference, the following diuretics, thiazide are numbered to match the corresponding brand names.

This information applies to the following medicines:

1. Bendroflumethiazide (ben-droe-floo-meth-EYE-a-zide)
2. Benzthiazide (benz-THYE-a-zide)†‡
3. Chlorothiazide (klor-oh-THYE-a-zide)†‡
4. Chlorthalidone (klor-THAL-i-doan)‡§
5. Cyclothiazide (sye-kloe-THYE-a-zide)†
6. Hydrochlorothiazide (hye-droe-klor-oh-THYE-a-zide)‡§
7. Hydroflumethiazide (hye-droe-floo-meth-EYE-a-zide)†‡
8. Methyclothiazide (meth-ee-kloe-THYE-a-zide)‡
9. Metolazone (me-TOLE-a-zone)
10. Polythiazide (pol-i-THYE-a-zide)†
11. Quinethazone (kwin-ETH-a-zone)†
12. Trichlormethiazide (trye-klor-meth-EYE-a-zide)†‡

†Not commercially available in Canada.
‡Generic name product may also be available in the U.S.
§Generic name product may also be available in Canada.

Thiazide diuretics are also used to help reduce the amount of water in the body by increasing the flow of urine. They may also be used for other conditions as determined by your doctor.

Thiazide diuretics are available only with your doctor's prescription, in the following dosage forms:

*Oral*

Bendroflumethiazide
- Tablets (U.S. and Canada)

Benzthiazide
- Tablets (U.S.)

Chlorothiazide
- Oral suspension (U.S.)
- Tablets (U.S.)

Chlorthalidone
- Tablets (U.S. and Canada)

Cyclothiazide
- Tablets (U.S.)

Hydrochlorothiazide
- Oral solution (U.S.)
- Tablets (U.S. and Canada)

Hydroflumethiazide
- Tablets (U.S.)

Methyclothiazide
- Tablets (U.S. and Canada)

Metolazone
- Tablets (U.S. and Canada)

Polythiazide
- Tablets (U.S.)

Quinethazone
- Tablets (U.S.)

Trichlormethiazide
- Tablets (U.S.)

*Parenteral*

Chlorothiazide
- Injection (U.S.)

## Description

Thiazide or thiazide-like diuretics are commonly used to treat high blood pressure (hypertension). High blood pressure adds to the workload of the heart and arteries. If it continues for a long time, the heart and arteries may not function properly. This can damage the blood vessels of the brain, heart, and kidneys, resulting in a stroke, heart failure, or kidney failure. High blood pressure may also increase the risk of heart attacks. These problems may be less likely to occur if blood pressure is controlled.

## Before Using This Medicine

In deciding to use a medicine, the risks of taking the medicine must be weighed against the good it will do. This is a decision you and your doctor will make. For thiazide diuretics, the following should be considered:

**Allergies**—Tell your doctor if you have ever had any unusual or allergic reaction to sulfonamides (sulfa drugs), bumetanide, furosemide, acetazolamide, dichlorphenamide, methazolamide, or to any of the thiazide diuretics. Also tell your health care professional if you are allergic to any other substances, such as foods, preservatives, or dyes.

**Pregnancy**—When this medicine is used during pregnancy, it may cause side effects including jaundice, blood problems, and low potassium in the newborn infant. In addition, although this medicine has not been shown to cause birth defects or other problems in animals, studies have not been done in humans.

In general, diuretics are not useful for normal swelling of feet and hands that occurs during pregnancy. They should not be taken during pregnancy unless recommended by your doctor.

**Breast-feeding**—Thiazide diuretics pass into breast milk. These medicines also may decrease the flow of breast milk. Therefore, you should avoid use of thiazide diuretics during the first month of breast-feeding.

**Children**—Although there is no specific information comparing the use of thiazide diuretics in children with use in other age groups, these medicines are not expected to cause different side effects or problems in children than they do in adults. However, extra caution may be necessary in infants with jaundice, because these medicines can make the condition worse.

**Older adults**—Dizziness or lightheadedness and signs of too much potassium loss may be more likely to occur in the elderly, who are more sensitive than younger adults to the effects of thiazide diuretics.

**Other medicines**—Although certain medicines should not be used together at all, in other cases two different medicines may be used together even if an interaction might occur. In these cases, your doctor may want to change the dose, or other precautions may be necessary. When you are taking thiazide diuretics, it is especially important that your health care professional know if you are taking any of the following:
- Cholestyramine or
- Colestipol—Use with thiazide diuretics may prevent the diuretic from working properly; take the diuretic at least 1 hour before or 4 hours after cholestyramine or colestipol
- Digitalis glycosides (heart medicine)—Use with thiazide diuretics may cause high blood levels of digoxin, which may increase the chance of side effects
- Lithium (e.g., Lithane)—Use with thiazide diuretics may cause high blood levels of lithium, which may increase the chance of side effects

**Other medical problems**—The presence of other medical problems may affect the use of thiazide diuretics. Make sure you tell your doctor if you have any other medical problems, especially:
- Diabetes mellitus (sugar diabetes)—Thiazide diuretics may increase the amount of sugar in the blood
- Gout (history of) or
- Lupus erythematosus (history of) or
- Pancreatitis (inflammation of the pancreas)—Thiazide diuretics may make these conditions worse
- Heart or blood vessel disease—Thiazide diuretics may cause high cholesterol levels or high triglyceride levels

- Liver disease or
- Kidney disease (severe)—Higher blood levels of the thiazide diuretic may occur, which may prevent the thiazide diuretic from working properly

## Proper Use of This Medicine

This medicine may cause you to have an unusual feeling of tiredness when you begin to take it. You may also notice an increase in the amount of urine or in your frequency of urination. After you have taken the medicine for a while, these effects should lessen. In general, to keep the increase in urine from affecting your sleep:
- If you are to take a single dose a day, take it in the morning after breakfast.
- If you are to take more than one dose a day, take the last dose no later than 6 p.m., unless otherwise directed by your doctor.

However, it is best to plan your dose or doses according to a schedule that will least affect your personal activities and sleep. Ask your health care professional to help you plan the best time to take this medicine.

To help you remember to take your medicine, try to get into the habit of taking it at the same time each day.

For patients taking this medicine for *high blood pressure:*
- In addition to the use of the medicine your doctor has prescribed, appropriate treatment for your high blood pressure may include weight control and care in the types of foods you eat, especially foods high in sodium. Your doctor will tell you which factors are most important for you. You should check with your doctor before changing your diet.
- Many patients who have high blood pressure will not notice any signs of the problem. In fact, many may feel normal. It is very important that you *take your medicine exactly as directed* and that you keep your appointments with your doctor even if you feel well.
- Remember that this medicine will not cure your high blood pressure but it does help control it. Therefore, you must continue to take it as directed if you expect to lower your blood pressure and keep it down. *You may have to take high blood pressure medicine for the rest of your life*. If high blood pressure is not treated, it can cause serious problems such as heart failure, blood vessel disease, stroke, or kidney disease.

For patients taking the *oral liquid form of hydrochlorothiazide,* which comes in a dropper bottle:
- This medicine is to be taken by mouth. The amount you should take is to be measured only with the specially marked dropper.

**Dosing**—The dose of these medicines will be different for different patients. *Follow your doctor's orders or the directions on the label*. The following information includes only the average doses of these medicines. *If your dose is different, do not change it* unless your doctor tells you to do so.

The number of tablets or teaspoonfuls of solution or suspension that you take depends on the strength of the medicine. Also, *the number of doses you take each day, the time allowed between doses, and the length of time you take the medicine depend on the medical problem for which you are taking thiazide diuretics.*

*For bendroflumethiazide*
- For *oral* dosage form (tablets):
  —To lower the amount of water in the body:
  - Adults—At first, 2.5 to 10 milligrams (mg) one or two times a day. Then, your doctor may lower your dose to 2.5 to 5 mg once a day. Or, your doctor may want you to take this dose once every other day or once a day for only three to five days out of the week.
  - Children—Dose is based on body weight and must be determined by your doctor. The usual dose is 50 to 100 micrograms (mcg) per kilogram (kg) (22.7 to 45.4 mcg per pound) of body weight once a day.
  —For high blood pressure:
  - Adults—2.5 to 20 mg a day. This may be taken as a single dose or divided into two doses.
  - Children—Dose is based on body weight and must be determined by your doctor. The usual dose is 50 to 400 mcg per kg (22.7 to 181.8 mcg per pound) of body weight a day. This may be taken as a single dose or divided into two doses.

*For benzthiazide*
- For *oral* dosage form (tablets):
  —To lower the amount of water in the body:
  - Adults—25 to 100 milligrams (mg) two times a day. Or, your doctor may want you to take this dose once every other day or once a day for only three to five days out of the week.
  - Children—Dose is based on body weight and must be determined by your doctor.
  —For high blood pressure:
  - Adults—50 to 100 mg a day. This may be taken as a single dose or divided into two doses.
  - Children—Dose is based on body weight and must be determined by your doctor.

*For chlorothiazide*
- For *oral* dosage forms (oral suspension or tablets):
  —To lower the amount of water in the body:
  - Adults—250 milligrams (mg) every six to twelve hours.
  - Children—Dose is based on body weight and must be determined by your doctor.
  —For high blood pressure:
  - Adults—250 to 1000 mg a day. This may be taken as a single dose or divided into smaller doses.
  - Children—Dose is based on body weight and must be determined by your doctor.

- For *injection* dosage form:
  —To lower the amount of water in the body:
  - Adults—250 mg injected into a vein every six to twelve hours.
  - Children—Use and dose must be determined by your doctor.
  —For high blood pressure:
  - Adults—500 to 1000 mg a day, injected into a vein. This dose may be given as a single dose or divided into two doses.
  - Children—Use and dose must be determined by your doctor.

*For chlorthalidone*
- For *oral* dosage form (tablets):
  —To lower the amount of water in the body:
  - Adults—25 to 100 milligrams (mg) once a day. Or, 100 to 200 mg taken once every other day or once a day for three days out of the week.
  - Children—Dose is based on body weight and must be determined by your doctor.
  —For high blood pressure:
  - Adults—25 to 100 mg once a day.
  - Children—Dose is based on body weight and must be determined by your doctor.

*For cyclothiazide*
- For *oral* dosage form (tablets):
  —To lower the amount of water in the body:
  - Adults—1 to 2 milligrams (mg) once a day. Or, your doctor may want you to take this dose once every other day or once a day for only two or three days out of the week.
  - Children—Dose is based on body weight and must be determined by your doctor.
  —For high blood pressure:
  - Adults—2 mg once a day.
  - Children—Dose is based on body weight and must be determined by your doctor.

*For hydrochlorothiazide*
- For *oral* dosage forms (oral solution or tablets):
  —To lower the amount of water in the body:
  - Adults—25 to 100 milligrams (mg) one or two times a day. Or, your doctor may want you to take this dose once every other day or once a day for three to five days out of the week.
  - Children—Dose is based on body weight and must be determined by your doctor.
  —For high blood pressure:
  - Adults—25 to 100 mg a day. This may be taken as a single dose or divided into two doses.
  - Children—Dose is based on body weight and must be determined by your doctor.

*For hydroflumethiazide*
- For *oral* dosage form (tablets):
  —To lower the amount of water in the body:
    - Adults—25 to 100 milligrams (mg) one or two times a day. Or, your doctor may want you to take this dose once every other day or once a day for three to five days out of the week.
    - Children—Dose is based on body weight and must be determined by your doctor.
  —For high blood pressure:
    - Adults—50 to 100 mg a day. This may be taken as a single dose or divided into two doses.
    - Children—Dose is based on body weight and must be determined by your doctor.

*For methyclothiazide*
- For *oral* dosage form (tablets):
  —To lower the amount of water in the body:
    - Adults—2.5 to 10 milligrams (mg) once a day. Or, your doctor may want you to take this dose once every other day or once a day for three to five days out of the week.
    - Children—Dose is based on body weight and must be determined by your doctor.
  —For high blood pressure:
    - Adults—2.5 to 5 mg once a day.
    - Children—Dose is based on body weight and must be determined by your doctor.

*For metolazone*
- For *oral* dosage form (*extended* metolazone tablets):
  —To lower the amount of water in the body:
    - Adults—5 to 20 milligrams (mg) once a day.
    - Children—Dose must be determined by your doctor.
  —For high blood pressure:
    - Adults—2.5 to 5 mg once a day.
    - Children—Dose must be determined by your doctor.
- For *oral* dosage form (*prompt* metolazone tablets):
  —For high blood pressure:
    - Adults—At first, 500 micrograms (mcg) once a day. Then, 500 to 1000 mcg once a day.
    - Children—Dose must be determined by your doctor.

*For polythiazide*
- For *oral* dosage form (tablets):
  —To lower the amount of water in the body:
    - Adults—1 to 4 milligrams (mg) once a day. Or, your doctor may want you to take this dose once every other day or once a day for three to five days out of the week.
    - Children—Dose is based on body weight and must be determined by your doctor.
  —For high blood pressure:
    - Adults—2 to 4 mg once a day.

- Children—Dose is based on body weight and must be determined by your doctor.

*For quinethazone*
- For *oral* dosage form (tablets):
  —To lower the amount of water in the body or for high blood pressure:
    - Adults—50 to 200 milligrams (mg) a day. This may be taken as a single dose or divided into two doses.
    - Children—Dose must be determined by your doctor.

*For trichlormethiazide*
- For *oral* dosage form (tablets):
  —To lower the amount of water in the body:
    - Adults—1 to 4 milligrams (mg) once a day. Or, your doctor may want you to take this dose once every other day or once a day for three to five days out of the week.
    - Children—Dose is based on body weight and must be determined by your doctor.
  —For high blood pressure:
    - Adults—2 to 4 mg once a day.
    - Children—Dose is based on body weight and must be determined by your doctor.

**Missed dose**—If you miss a dose of this medicine, take it as soon as possible. However, if it is almost time for your next dose, skip the missed dose and go back to your regular dosing schedule. Do not double doses.

**Storage**—To store this medicine:
- Keep out of the reach of children.
- Store away from heat and direct light.
- Do not store in the bathroom, near the kitchen sink, or in other damp places. Heat or moisture may cause the medicine to break down.
- Keep the oral liquid form of this medicine from freezing.
- Do not keep outdated medicine or medicine no longer needed. Be sure that any discarded medicine is out of the reach of children.

## Precautions While Using This Medicine

It is important that your doctor check your progress at regular visits to make sure that this medicine is working properly.

*This medicine may cause a loss of potassium from your body:*
- To help prevent this, your doctor may want you to:
  —eat or drink foods that have a high potassium content (for example, orange or other citrus fruit juices), or
  —take a potassium supplement, or
  —take another medicine to help prevent the loss of the potassium in the first place.
- It is very important to follow these directions. Also, it is important not to change your diet on your own.

This is more important if you are already on a special diet (as for diabetes), or if you are taking a potassium supplement or a medicine to reduce potassium loss. Extra potassium may not be necessary and, in some cases, too much potassium could be harmful.

Check with your doctor if you become sick and have severe or continuing vomiting or diarrhea. These problems may cause you to lose additional water and potassium.

For *diabetic patients:*
- Thiazide diuretics may raise blood sugar levels. While you are using this medicine, be especially careful in testing for sugar in your blood or urine.

Thiazide diuretics may cause your skin to be more sensitive to sunlight than it is normally. Exposure to sunlight, even for brief periods of time, may cause a skin rash, itching, redness or other discoloration of the skin, or a severe sunburn. When you begin taking this medicine:
- Stay out of direct sunlight, especially between the hours of 10:00 a.m. and 3:00 p.m., if possible.
- Wear protective clothing, including a hat. Also, wear sunglasses.
- Apply a sun block product that has a skin protection factor (SPF) of at least 15. Some patients may require a product with a higher SPF number, especially if they have a fair complexion. If you have any questions about this, check with your health care professional.
- Apply a sun block lipstick that has an SPF of at least 15 to protect your lips.
- Do not use a sunlamp or tanning bed or booth.

If you have a severe reaction from the sun, check with your doctor.

For patients taking this medicine for *high blood pressure:*
- *Do not take other medicines unless they have been discussed with your doctor.* This especially includes over-the-counter (nonprescription) medicines for appetite control, asthma, colds, cough, hay fever, or sinus problems, since they may tend to increase your blood pressure.

## Side Effects of This Medicine

Along with its needed effects, a medicine may cause some unwanted effects. Although not all of these side effects may occur, if they do occur they may need medical attention.

Check with your doctor as soon as possible if any of the following side effects occur:
*Rare*
  Black, tarry stools; blood in urine or stools; cough or hoarseness; fever or chills; joint pain; lower back or side pain; painful or difficult urination; pinpoint red spots on skin; skin rash or hives; stomach pain (severe) with nausea and vomiting; unusual bleeding or bruising; yellow eyes or skin
*Signs and symptoms of too much potassium loss*
  Dryness of mouth; increased thirst; irregular heartbeat; mood or mental changes; muscle cramps or pain; nausea or vomiting; unusual tiredness or weakness; weak pulse
*Signs and symptoms of too much sodium loss*
  Confusion; convulsions; decreased mental activity; irritability; muscle cramps; unusual tiredness or weakness

Other side effects may occur that usually do not need medical attention. These side effects may go away during treatment as your body adjusts to the medicine. However, check with your doctor if any of the following side effects continue or are bothersome:
*Less common*
  Decreased sexual ability; diarrhea; dizziness or lightheadedness when getting up from a lying or sitting position; increased sensitivity of skin to sunlight; loss of appetite; upset stomach

Other side effects not listed above may also occur in some patients. If you notice any other effects, check with your doctor.

## Additional Information

Once a medicine has been approved for marketing for a certain use, experience may show that it is also useful for other medical problems. Although these uses are not specifically included in product labeling, thiazide diuretics are used in certain patients with the following medical conditions:
- Diabetes insipidus (water diabetes)
- Kidney stones (calcium-containing)

For patients taking this medicine for *diabetes insipidus (water diabetes):*
- Some thiazide diuretics are used in the treatment of diabetes insipidus (water diabetes). In patients with water diabetes, this medicine causes a decrease in the flow of urine and helps the body hold water. Thus, the information given above about increased urine flow will not apply to you.

Other than the above information, there is no additional information relating to proper use, precautions, or side effects for these uses.

Revised: 06/07/92
Interim revision: 06/30/94

# DORNASE ALFA   Inhalation

A commonly used brand name in the U.S. and Canada is Pulmozyme. Other commonly used names are: rhDNase and DNase I.

## Description

Dornase alfa (DOR-nayse AL-fa) is used in the treatment of cystic fibrosis. It is used with other cystic fibrosis medicines, especially antibiotics, bronchodilators (medicines that open up narrowed breathing passages), and corticosteroids (cortisone-like medicines).

Cystic fibrosis is a condition in which thick mucus is formed in the lungs and breathing passages. The mucus blocks the airways and increases the chance of lung infections. The infections then cause the mucus to become even thicker, making it more difficult to breathe.

Dornase alfa will not cure cystic fibrosis. However, when it is used every day, it helps make breathing easier and reduces the number of serious lung infections that require treatment with antibiotics.

Dornase alfa is available only with your doctor's prescription, in the following dosage form:

*Inhalation*
- Solution for inhalation (U.S. and Canada)

## Before Using This Medicine

In deciding to use a medicine, the risks of taking the medicine must be weighed against the good it will do. This is a decision you and your doctor will make. For dornase alfa, the following should be considered:

**Allergies**—Tell your doctor if you have ever had any unusual or allergic reaction to dornase alfa. Also tell your health care professional if you are allergic to any other substances, such as foods, preservatives, or dyes.

**Pregnancy**—Dornase alfa has not been studied in pregnant women. However, this medicine has not been shown to cause birth defects or other problems in animal studies.

**Breast-feeding**—It is not known whether dornase alfa passes into breast milk. Although most medicines pass into breast milk in small amounts, many of them may be used safely while breast-feeding. Mothers who are taking this medicine and who wish to breast-feed should discuss this with their doctor.

**Children**—This medicine has been tested in children 5 years of age and older and, in effective doses, has not been shown to cause different side effects or problems than it does in adults. Dornase alfa has not been tested in children up to 5 years of age.

**Older adults**—Many medicines have not been studied specifically in older people. Therefore, it may not be known whether they work exactly the same way they do in younger adults. Although there is no specific information comparing use of dornase alfa in the elderly with use in other age groups, this medicine is not expected to cause

different side effects or problems in older people than it does in younger adults.

**Other medicines**—Although certain medicines should not be used together at all, in other cases two different medicines may be used together even if an interaction might occur. In these cases, your doctor may want to change the dose, or other precautions may be necessary. Tell your health care professional if you are taking any other prescription or nonprescription (over-the-counter [OTC]) medicine.

## Proper Use of This Medicine

Dornase alfa usually comes with patient instructions. Read them carefully before using this medicine.

Dornase alfa is packaged in small plastic containers called ampuls. Each ampul contains one full dose of dornase alfa. Do not use an ampul that has already been opened. Also, do not use an ampul of this medicine after the expiration date printed on the package.

*Do not use dornase alfa solution if it is cloudy or discolored.*

*Dornase alfa must be used in a nebulizer with a compressor.* Only the following nebulizers and compressors should be used with this medicine:

- Hudson T Up-draft II disposable jet nebulizer used with the Pulmo-Aide compressor
- Marquest Acorn II disposable jet nebulizer used with the Pulmo-Aide compressor
- Reusable PARI LC Jet+ nebulizer used with the PARI PRONEB compressor

Your health care professional will help you decide which nebulizer and compressor to use.

It is very important that you *use dornase alfa only as directed.* Use the mouthpiece provided with the nebulizer. Do not use a face mask with the nebulizer because less medicine will get into your lungs. *Make sure you understand exactly how to use this medicine in the nebulizer.*

In order to receive the full effects of this medicine, *you must use it every day as ordered by your doctor.* If possible, dornase alfa should be used at about the same time each day. You may notice some improvement in your condition within the first week of treatment. However, some patients may not feel the full effects of this medicine for weeks or months.

If you are taking any other medicines for cystic fibrosis, keep taking them as you did before you started using dornase alfa, unless otherwise directed by your doctor. However, *do not put any other inhaled medicine in the nebulizer at the same time that you use dornase alfa.* Other inhaled medicines may be taken in a clean nebulizer before or after your treatment with dornase alfa.

*To prepare the nebulizer for use:*
- Wash your hands well with soap and water before putting the nebulizer together and preparing the medicine. This will help prevent infection.
- Put the nebulizer together only on a clean surface. If dirt or germs get on the nebulizer or in the medicine, they may cause infection.
- After you put the nebulizer together, test the compressor (following the manufacturer's directions) to make sure it works properly. If you have any questions about this, ask your health care professional.

*To prepare the medicine for use in the nebulizer:*
- Remove one ampul of dornase alfa from the refrigerator. Hold the tab at the base of the ampul firmly. Twist off the top of the ampul, but do not squeeze the body of the ampul while doing so.
- Take the cap off the nebulizer cup. Turn the opened ampul upside down over the cup. Squeeze the ampul gently until all the contents are emptied into the cup. *It is very important that you use the full dose of this medicine.*
- Replace the cap on the nebulizer cup. Connect the nebulizer and compressor, following the manufacturer's directions.
- Turn on the compressor. Make sure there is mist coming from the nebulizer.

*To use the medicine in the nebulizer:*
- Place the mouthpiece between your teeth and on top of your tongue. Close your lips around the mouthpiece. Be sure that you do not block the airflow with your tongue or teeth.
- Breathe normally, in and out, through your mouth. *Do not breathe through your nose.* If you have trouble breathing only through your mouth, use a nose clip.
- During treatment, moisture may collect in the long connecting tube of the nebulizer. This should be expected. However, if you notice a leak or feel moisture coming from the nebulizer during the treatment, turn off the compressor. Then check to make sure the nebulizer cap is sealed correctly before you continue the treatment.
- When the nebulizer begins "spitting," gently tap the nebulizer cup. Continue breathing until the cup is empty or no more mist comes from the nebulizer.
- If you have to stop the treatment for some reason or if you start coughing during the treatment, turn off the compressor. To begin the treatment again, turn on the compressor and continue as before.
- The complete treatment usually takes 10 to 15 minutes. *Be sure to inhale the full dose of dornase alfa.*

*After using dornase alfa:*
- Turn off the compressor. Then take apart the nebulizer system.
- Follow the manufacturer's directions for care and cleaning of your nebulizer and compressor.

**Dosing**—The dose of dornase alfa will be different for different patients. *Follow your doctor's orders or the directions on the label.* The following information includes only the average doses of dornase alfa. *If your dose is different, do not change it* unless your doctor tells you to do so.
- For *inhalation* dosage form (inhalation solution):
  —For cystic fibrosis:
    • Adults and children 5 years of age and older—The usual dose is 2.5 milligrams (mg) (1 ampul), used in a nebulizer once a day for about 10 to 15 minutes. However, your doctor may want you to use this medicine two times a day at regularly spaced times.
    • Children up to 5 years of age—Use and dose must be determined by your doctor.

**Missed dose**—If you miss a dose of this medicine, take it as soon as possible. However, if it is almost time for your next dose, skip the missed dose and go back to your regular dosing schedule.

**Storage**—To store this medicine:
- Keep out of the reach of children
- Store away from heat and light.
- Store the medicine in the refrigerator in the foil pouches. However, keep the medicine from freezing. Do not leave this medicine out of the refrigerator for longer than a total of 24 hours. If an ampul of medicine is left out for longer than this, it should be thrown away and a new ampul used.
- Do not keep outdated medicine or medicine no longer needed. Be sure that any discarded medicine is out of the reach of children.

## Precautions While Using This Medicine

If your condition becomes worse, check with your doctor.

## Side Effects of This Medicine

Along with its needed effects, a medicine may cause some unwanted effects. The following side effects may go away during treatment as your body adjusts to the medicine. However, check with your doctor if any of the following side effects continue or are bothersome:

*More common*
   Chest pain or discomfort; sore throat; voice changes
*Less common*
   Hoarseness; redness, itching, pain, swelling, or other irritation of eyes; skin rash

Other side effects not listed above may also occur in some patients. If you notice any other effects, check with your doctor.

Developed: 09/02/94

# DOXAZOSIN   Systemic

A commonly used brand name in the U.S. and Canada is Cardura.

## Description

Doxazosin (dox-AY-zoe-sin) belongs to the general class of medicines called antihypertensives. It is used to treat high blood pressure (hypertension).

High blood pressure adds to the workload of the heart and arteries. If it continues for a long time, the heart and arteries may not function properly. This can damage the blood vessels of the brain, heart, and kidneys, resulting in a stroke, heart failure, or kidney failure. High blood pressure may also increase the risk of heart attacks. These problems may be less likely to occur if blood pressure is controlled.

Doxazosin works by relaxing blood vessels so that blood passes through them more easily. This helps to lower blood pressure.

Doxazosin may also be used for other conditions as determined by your doctor.

Doxazosin is available only with your doctor's prescription, in the following dosage form:

*Oral*
- Tablets (U.S. and Canada)

## Before Using This Medicine

In deciding to use a medicine, the risks of taking the medicine must be weighed against the good it will do. This is a decision you and your doctor will make. For doxazosin, the following should be considered:

**Allergies**—Tell your doctor if you have ever had any unusual or allergic reaction to doxazosin, prazosin, or terazosin. Also tell your health care professional if you are allergic to any other substances, such as foods, preservatives, or dyes.

**Pregnancy**—Doxazosin has not been studied in pregnant women. However, studies in rabbits have shown that doxazosin given at very high doses may cause death of the fetus. Before taking this medicine, make sure your doctor knows if you are pregnant or if you may become pregnant.

**Breast-feeding**—It is not known whether doxazosin passes into breast milk. However, doxazosin passes into the milk of rats. Although most medicines pass into breast milk in small amounts, many of them may be used safely while breast-feeding. Mothers who are taking this medicine and who wish to breast-feed should discuss this with their doctor.

**Children**—Studies on this medicine have been done only in adult patients, and there is no specific information comparing use of doxazosin in children with use in other age groups.

**Older adults**—Dizziness, lightheadedness, or fainting may be especially likely to occur in elderly patients, who are usually more sensitive than younger adults to the effects of doxazosin.

**Other medicines**—Although certain medicines should not be used together at all, in other cases two different medicines may be used together even if an interaction might occur. In these cases, your doctor may want to change the dose, or other precautions may be necessary. Tell your health care professional if you are using any other prescription or nonprescription (over-the-counter [OTC]) medicine.

**Other medical problems**—The presence of other medical problems may affect the use of doxazosin. Make sure you tell your doctor if you have any other medical problems, especially:
- Kidney disease—Possible increased sensitivity to the effects of doxazosin
- Liver disease—The effects of doxazosin may be increased, which may increase the chance of side effects

## Proper Use of This Medicine

For patients *taking this medicine for high blood pressure:*
- In addition to the use of the medicine your doctor has prescribed, treatment for your high blood pressure may include weight control and care in the types of foods you eat, especially foods high in sodium. Your doctor will tell you which of these are most important for you. You should check with your doctor before changing your diet.
- Many patients who have high blood pressure will not notice any signs of the problem. In fact, many may feel normal. It is very important that you *take your medicine exactly as directed* and that you keep your appointments with your doctor even if you feel well.
- Remember that doxazosin will not cure your high blood pressure but it does help control it. Therefore, you must continue to take it as directed if you expect to lower your blood pressure and keep it down. *You may have to take high blood pressure medicine for the rest of your life.* If high blood pressure is not treated, it can cause serious problems such as heart failure, blood vessel disease, stroke, or kidney disease.

To help you remember to take your medicine, try to get into the habit of taking it at the same time each day.

**Dosing**—The dose of doxazosin will be different for different patients. *Follow your doctor's orders or the directions on the label.* The following information includes only the average doses of doxazosin. *If your dose is different, do not change it* unless your doctor tells you to do so.

The number of tablets that you take depends on the strength of the medicine.

- For *oral* dosage form (tablets):
  —For high blood pressure:
  - Adults—1 milligram (mg) once a day to start. Your doctor may increase your dose slowly to as much as 16 mg once a day.
  - Children—Use and dose must be determined by your doctor.

**Missed dose**—If you miss a dose of this medicine, take it as soon as possible. However, if it is almost time for your next dose, skip the missed dose and go back to your regular dosing schedule. Do not double doses.

**Storage**—To store this medicine:
- Keep out of the reach of children.
- Store away from heat and direct light.
- Do not store in the bathroom, near the kitchen sink, or in other damp places. Heat or moisture may cause the medicine to break down.
- Do not keep outdated medicine or medicine no longer needed. Be sure that any discarded medicine is out of the reach of children.

## Precautions While Using This Medicine

It is important that your doctor check your progress at regular visits to make sure that this medicine is working properly. This is especially important for elderly patients, who may be more sensitive to the effects of this medicine.

*Do not take other medicines unless they have been discussed with your doctor.* This especially includes over-the-counter (nonprescription) medicines for appetite control, asthma, colds, cough, hay fever, or sinus problems, since they may tend to increase your blood pressure.

Dizziness, lightheadedness, or sudden fainting may occur after you take this medicine, especially when you get up from a lying or sitting position. These effects are more likely to occur when you take the first dose of this medicine. Taking the first dose at bedtime may prevent problems. However, *be especially careful if you need to get up during the night.* These effects may also occur with any doses you take after the first dose. Getting up slowly may help lessen this problem. *If you feel dizzy, lie down so that you do not faint.* Then sit for a few moments before standing to prevent the dizziness from returning.

The dizziness, lightheadedness, or sudden fainting is more likely to occur if you drink alcohol, stand for a long time, exercise, or if the weather is hot. *While you are taking this medicine, be careful to limit the amount of alcohol you drink. Also, use extra care during exercise or hot weather or if you must stand for a long time.*

Doxazosin may cause some people to become drowsy or less alert than they are normally. *Make sure you know how you react to this medicine before you drive, use machines, or do anything else that could be dangerous if you are dizzy, drowsy, or are not alert.* After you have taken several doses of this medicine, these effects should lessen.

## Side Effects of This Medicine

Along with its needed effects, a medicine may cause some unwanted effects. Although not all of these side effects may occur, if they do occur they may need medical attention.

Check with your doctor as soon as possible if any of the following side effects occur:
*More common*
  Dizziness or lightheadedness
*Less common*
  Dizziness or lightheadedness when getting up from a lying or sitting position; fainting (sudden); fast and pounding heartbeat; irregular heartbeat; shortness of breath; swelling of feet or lower legs

Other side effects may occur that usually do not need medical attention. These side effects may go away during treatment as your body adjusts to the medicine. However, check with your doctor if any of the following side effects continue or are bothersome:
*More common*
  Headache; unusual tiredness
*Less common*
  Nausea; nervousness, restlessness, unusual irritability; runny nose; sleepiness or drowsiness

Other side effects not listed above may also occur in some patients. If you notice any other effects, check with your doctor.

## Additional Information

Once a medicine has been approved for marketing for a certain use, experience may show that it is also useful for other medical problems. Although this use is not included in product labeling, doxazosin is used in certain patients with the following medical condition:
- Benign enlargement of the prostate

For patients taking this medicine for *benign enlargement of the prostate*:
- Doxazosin will not shrink the size of your prostate, but it does help to relieve the symptoms.

Other than the above information, there is no additional information relating to proper use, precautions, or side effects for this use.

Revised: 08/02/94

# DOXORUBICIN    Systemic

Some commonly used brand names are:

**In the U.S.—**
    Adriamycin PFS
    Adriamycin RDF
    Rubex
    Generic name product may also be available.

**In Canada—**
    Adriamycin PFS
    Adriamycin RDF

## Description

Doxorubicin (dox-oh-ROO-bi-sin) belongs to the general group of medicines known as antineoplastics. It is used to treat some kinds of cancer.

Doxorubicin seems to interfere with the growth of cancer cells, which are eventually destroyed. Since the growth of normal body cells may also be affected by doxorubicin, other effects will also occur. Some of these may be serious and must be reported to your doctor. Other effects, like hair loss, may not be serious but may cause concern. Some effects may not occur for months or years after the medicine is used.

Before you begin treatment with doxorubicin, you and your doctor should talk about the good this medicine will do as well as the risks of using it.

Doxorubicin is to be administered only by or under the supervision of your doctor. It is available in the following dosage form:

*Parenteral*
- Injection (U.S. and Canada)

## Before Using This Medicine

In deciding to use a medicine, the risks of taking the medicine must be weighed against the good it will do. This is a decision you and your doctor will make. For doxorubicin, the following should be considered:

**Allergies**—Tell your doctor if you have ever had any unusual or allergic reaction to doxorubicin or lincomycin.

**Pregnancy**—There is a chance that this medicine may cause birth defects if either the male or female is receiving it at the time of conception or if it is taken during pregnancy. Studies in rats and rabbits have shown that doxorubicin causes birth defects in the fetus and other problems (including miscarriage). In addition, many cancer medicines may cause sterility which could be permanent. Although sterility has been reported in animals and humans with this medicine, the effect is weaker in humans than in animals.

Be sure that you have discussed these possible effects with your doctor before receiving this medicine. It is best to use some kind of birth control while you are receiving doxorubicin. Tell your doctor right away if you think you

have become pregnant while receiving doxorubicin. Before receiving doxorubicin make sure your doctor knows if you are pregnant or if you may become pregnant.

**Breast-feeding**—Because doxorubicin may cause serious side effects, breast-feeding is generally not recommended while you are receiving it.

**Children**—Heart problems are more likely to occur in children under 2 years of age, who are usually more sensitive to the effects of doxorubicin.

**Older adults**—Heart problems are more likely to occur in the elderly, who are usually more sensitive to the effects of doxorubicin. The elderly may also be more likely to have blood problems.

**Other medicines**—Although certain medicines should not be used together at all, in other cases two different medicines may be used together even if an interaction might occur. In these cases, your doctor may want to change the dose, or other precautions may be necessary. When receiving doxorubicin it is especially important that your health care professional know if you are taking any of the following:

- Amphotericin B by injection (e.g., Fungizone) or
- Antithyroid agents (medicine for overactive thyroid) or
- Azathioprine (e.g., Imuran) or
- Chloramphenicol (e.g., Chloromycetin) or
- Colchicine or
- Flucytosine (e.g., Ancobon) or
- Ganciclovir (e.g., Cytovene) or
- Interferon (e.g., Intron A, Roferon-A) or
- Plicamycin (e.g., Mithracin) or
- Zidovudine (e.g., AZT, Retrovir) or
- If you have ever been treated with radiation or cancer medicines—Doxorubicin may increase the effects of these medicines or radiation therapy on the blood
- Probenecid (e.g., Benemid) or
- Sulfinpyrazone (e.g., Anturane)—Doxorubicin may raise the concentration of uric acid in the blood. Since these medicines are used to lower uric acid levels, they may not work as well in patients receiving doxorubicin

**Other medical problems**—The presence of other medical problems may affect the use of doxorubicin. Make sure you tell your doctor if you have any other medical problems, especially:

- Chickenpox (including recent exposure) or
- Herpes zoster (shingles)—Risk of severe disease affecting other parts of the body
- Gout or
- Kidney stones—Doxorubicin may increase levels of uric acid in the body, which can cause gout or kidney stones
- Heart disease—Risk of heart problems caused by doxorubicin may be increased
- Liver disease—Effects of doxorubicin may be increased because of slower removal from the body

## Proper Use of This Medicine

Doxorubicin is sometimes given together with certain other medicines. If you are receiving a combination of medicines, it is important that you receive each one at the proper time. If you are taking some of these medicines by mouth, ask your health care professional to help you plan a way to take them at the right times.

While you are using this medicine, your doctor may want you to drink extra fluids so that you will pass more urine. This will help prevent kidney problems and keep your kidneys working well.

Doxorubicin often causes nausea and vomiting. However, it is very important that you continue to receive it, even if you begin to feel ill. Ask your health care professional for ways to lessen these effects.

**Dosing**—The dose of doxorubicin will be different for different patients. The dose that is used may depend on a number of things, including what the medicine is being used for, the patient's body size, and whether or not other medicines are also being taken. *If you are receiving doxorubicin at home, follow your doctor's orders or the directions on the label.* If you have any questions about the proper dose of doxorubicin, ask your doctor.

## Precautions While Using This Medicine

*It is very important that your doctor check your progress at regular visits* to make sure that this medicine is working properly and to check for unwanted effects.

While you are being treated with doxorubicin, and after you stop treatment with it, *do not have any immunizations (vaccinations) without your doctor's approval.* Doxorubicin may lower your body's resistance, and there is a chance you might get the infection the immunization is meant to prevent. In addition, other persons living in your household should not take oral polio vaccine since there is a chance they could pass the polio virus on to you. Also, avoid persons who have taken oral polio vaccine. Do not get close to them, and do not stay in the same room with them for very long. If you cannot take these precautions, you should consider wearing a protective face mask that covers the nose and mouth.

Doxorubicin can temporarily lower the number of white blood cells in your blood, increasing the chance of getting an infection. It can also lower the number of platelets, which are necessary for proper blood clotting. If this occurs, there are certain precautions you can take, especially when your blood count is low, to reduce the risk of infection or bleeding:

- If you can, avoid people with infections. *Check with your doctor immediately* if you think you are getting an infection or if you get a fever or chills, cough or hoarseness, lower back or side pain, or painful or difficult urination.
- *Check with your doctor immediately* if you notice any unusual bleeding or bruising; black, tarry stools; blood in urine or stools; or pinpoint red spots on your skin.
- Be careful when using a regular toothbrush, dental floss, or toothpick. Your medical doctor, dentist, or nurse may recommend other ways to clean your teeth

and gums. Check with your medical doctor before having any dental work done.
- Do not touch your eyes or the inside of your nose unless you have just washed your hands and have not touched anything else in the meantime.
- Be careful not to cut yourself when you are using sharp objects such as a safety razor or fingernail or toenail cutters.
- Avoid contact sports or other situations where bruising or injury could occur.

If doxorubicin accidentally seeps out of the vein into which it is injected, it may damage some tissues and cause scarring. *Tell the doctor or nurse right away if you notice redness, pain, or swelling at the place of injection.*

## Side Effects of This Medicine

Along with its needed effects, a medicine may cause some unwanted effects. Although not all of these side effects may occur, if they do occur they may need medical attention.

Also, because of the way these medicines act on the body, there is a chance that they might cause other unwanted effects that may not occur until months or years after the medicine is used. These delayed effects may include certain types of cancer, such as leukemia. Discuss these possible effects with your doctor.

*Check with your doctor or nurse immediately* if any of the following side effects occur:

*Less common*
    Cough or hoarseness; fast or irregular heartbeat; fever or chills; lower back or side pain; pain at place of injection; painful or difficult urination; shortness of breath; swelling of feet and lower legs

*Rare*
    Black, tarry stools; blood in urine; pinpoint red spots on skin; unusual bleeding or bruising; wheezing

Check with your health care professional as soon as possible if any of the following side effects occur:

*More common*
    Sores in mouth and on lips
*Less common*
    Darkening or redness of skin (after x-ray treatment); joint pain; red streaks along injected vein
*Rare*
    Skin rash or itching

Other side effects may occur that usually do not need medical attention. These side effects may go away during treatment as your body adjusts to the medicine. Also, your health care professional may be able to tell you about ways to prevent or reduce some of these side effects. Check with your health care professional if any of the following side effects continue or are bothersome or if you have any questions about them:

*More common*
    Nausea and vomiting

*Less common*
> Darkening of soles, palms, or nails; diarrhea

Doxorubicin causes the urine to turn reddish in color, which may stain clothes. This is not blood. It is to be expected and only lasts for 1 or 2 days after each dose is given.

This medicine often causes a temporary and total loss of hair. After treatment with doxorubicin has ended, normal hair growth should return.

After you stop receiving doxorubicin, it may still produce some side effects that need attention. During this period

of time, *check with your doctor or nurse immediately* if you notice any of the following side effects:
> Fast or irregular heartbeat; shortness of breath; swelling of feet and lower legs

Other side effects not listed above may also occur in some patients. If you notice any other effects, check with your health care professional.

Revised: 07/11/94

# DRONABINOL   Systemic

A commonly used brand name in the U.S. and Canada is Marinol. Another commonly used name is delta-9-tetrahydrocannabinol (THC).

## Description

Dronabinol (droe-NAB-i-nol) is used to prevent the nausea and vomiting that may occur after treatment with cancer medicines. It is used only when other kinds of medicine for nausea and vomiting do not work. Dronabinol is also used to increase appetite in patients with acquired immunodeficiency syndrome (AIDS).

Dronabinol is available only with your doctor's prescription. Prescriptions cannot be refilled, and you must obtain a new prescription from your doctor each time you need this medicine. It is available in the following dosage form:

*Oral*
- Capsules (U.S. and Canada)

## Before Using This Medicine

In deciding to use a medicine, the risks of taking the medicine must be weighed against the good it will do. This is a decision you and your doctor will make. For dronabinol, the following should be considered:

**Allergies**—Tell your doctor if you have ever had any unusual or allergic reaction to dronabinol, marijuana products, or sesame oil. Also tell your health care professional if you are allergic to any other substances, such as foods, preservatives, or dyes.

**Pregnancy**—Studies have not been done in pregnant women. However, studies in animals have shown that dronabinol, given in doses many times the usual human dose, increases the risk of death of the fetus and decreases the number of live babies born.

**Breast-feeding**—Dronabinol passes into the breast milk. There is a possibility that the baby may become dependent on this medicine.

**Children**—Although there is no specific information comparing use of dronabinol in children with use in other age

groups, the effects that this medicine may have on the mind may be of special concern in children. Children should be watched closely while they are taking this medicine.

**Older adults**—This medicine has been tested in a limited number of patients up to 82 years of age and has not been shown to cause different side effects or problems in older people than it does in younger adults. However, the effects this medicine may have on the mind may be of special concern in the elderly. Therefore, older people should be watched closely while they are taking this medicine.

**Other medicines**—Although certain medicines should not be used together at all, in other cases 2 different medicines may be used together even if an interaction might occur. In these cases, your doctor may want to change the dose, or other precautions may be necessary. When you are taking dronabinol, it is especially important that your health care professional know if you are taking any of the following:

- Central nervous system (CNS) depressants (medicine that causes drowsiness) or
- Tricyclic antidepressants (medicine for depression)—Taking these medicines with dronabinol may increase the CNS depressant effects

**Other medical problems**—The presence of other medical problems may affect the use of dronabinol. Make sure you tell your doctor if you have any other medical problems, especially:

- Alcohol abuse (or history of) or
- Drug abuse or dependence (or history of)—Dependence on dronabinol may develop
- Heart disease or
- High blood pressure (hypertension) or
- Manic depression or
- Schizophrenia—Dronabinol may make the condition worse

## Proper Use of This Medicine

*Take this medicine only as directed by your physician.* Do not take more of it, do not take it more often, and do not take it for a longer time than your doctor ordered. If too much is taken, it may lead to medical problems because of an overdose.

**Dosing**—The dose of dronabinol will be different for different patients. *Follow your doctor's orders or the directions on the label.* The following information includes only the average doses of dronabinol. *If your dose is different, do not change it* unless your doctor tells you to do so.

The number of capsules that you take depends on the strength of the medicine. Also, *the number of doses you take each day, the time allowed between doses, and the length of time you take the medicine depend on the medical problem for which you are taking dronabinol.*

- For *oral* dosage form (capsules):
  —For nausea and vomiting caused by cancer medicines:
  - Adults and teenagers—Dose is based on body surface area. Your doctor will tell you how much medicine to take and when to take it.
  - Children—Use and dose must be determined by your doctor.
  —For increasing appetite in patients with AIDS:
  - Adults and teenagers—To start, 2.5 milligrams (mg) two times a day, taken before lunch and supper. Your doctor may change your dose depending on your condition. However, the dose is usually not more than 20 mg a day.
  - Children—Use and dose must be determined by your doctor.

**Missed dose**—If you miss a dose of this medicine, take it as soon as you remember. However, if it is almost time for your next dose, skip the missed dose and go back to your regular dosing schedule. *Do not double doses.*

**Storage**—To store this medicine:
- Keep out of the reach of children. Overdose is very dangerous in young children.
- Store away from heat and direct light.
- Do not store this medicine in the bathroom, near the kitchen sink, or in other damp places. Heat or moisture may cause the medicine to break down.
- Keep this medicine in the refrigerator but keep it from freezing.
- Do not keep outdated medicine or medicine no longer needed. Be sure that any discarded medicine is out of the reach of children.

## Precautions While Using This Medicine

Dronabinol will add to the effects of alcohol and other CNS depressants (medicines that slow down the nervous system, possibly causing drowsiness). Some examples of CNS depressants are antihistamines or medicine for hay fever, other allergies, or colds; sedatives, tranquilizers, or sleeping medicine; prescription pain medicines including

other narcotics; barbiturates; medicine for seizures; muscle relaxants; or anesthetics, including some dental anesthetics. *Check with your doctor before taking any of the above while you are taking this medicine.*

This medicine may cause some people to become drowsy, dizzy, or lightheaded, or to feel a false sense of well-being. *Make sure you know how you react to this medicine before you drive, use machines, or do anything else that could be dangerous if you are dizzy or are not alert and clearheaded.*

Dizziness, lightheadedness, or fainting may occur, especially when you get up suddenly from a lying or sitting position. Getting up slowly may help lessen this problem.

*If you think you or someone else may have taken an overdose of dronabinol, get emergency help at once.* Taking an overdose of this medicine or taking alcohol or CNS depressants with this medicine may lead to severe mental effects. Signs of overdose include changes in mood, confusion, hallucinations, mental depression, nervousness or anxiety, and fast or pounding heartbeat.

## Side Effects of This Medicine

Along with its needed effects, a medicine may cause some unwanted effects. Although not all of these side effects may occur, if they do occur they may need medical attention.

*Check with your health care professional immediately if any of the following side effects occur:*

*Less common (may also be signs of overdose)*
Changes in mood; confusion; fast or pounding heartbeat; hallucinations (seeing, hearing, or feeling things that are not there); mental depression; nervousness or anxiety

*Symptoms of overdose*
Being forgetful; change in your sense of smell, taste, sight, sound, or touch; change in how fast you think time is passing; constipation; problems in urinating; redness of eyes; slurred speech

Other side effects may occur that usually do not need medical attention. These side effects may go away during treatment as your body adjusts to the medicine. However, check with your doctor if any of the following side effects continue or are bothersome:

*More common*
Clumsiness or unsteadiness; dizziness; drowsiness; trouble thinking

*Less common or rare*
Blurred vision or any changes in vision; dryness of mouth; feeling faint or lightheaded; restlessness; unusual tiredness or weakness

Other side effects not listed above may also occur in some patients. If you notice any other effects, check with your doctor.

Revised: 06/07/93

# ECONAZOLE   Topical

Some commonly used brand names are:
**In the U.S.—**
    Spectazole
**In Canada—**
    Ecostatin

## Description

Econazole (e-KONE-a-zole) belongs to the family of medicines called antifungals, which are used to treat infections caused by a fungus. They work by killing the fungus or preventing its growth.

Econazole cream is applied to the skin to treat fungus infections. These include:

- ringworm of the body (tinea corporis);
- ringworm of the foot (tinea pedis; athlete's foot);
- ringworm of the groin (tinea cruris; jock itch);
- tinea versicolor (sometimes called "sun fungus"); and
- certain other fungus infections, such as Candida (Monilia) infections.

Econazole is available only with your doctor's prescription, in the following dosage form:

*Topical*
- Cream (U.S. and Canada)

## Before Using This Medicine

In deciding to use a medicine, the risks of using the medicine must be weighed against the good it will do. This is a decision you and your doctor will make. For topical econazole, the following should be considered:

**Allergies**—Tell your doctor if you have ever had any unusual or allergic reaction to econazole. Also tell your health care professional if you are allergic to any other substances, such as preservatives or dyes.

**Pregnancy**—Topical econazole has not been studied in pregnant women. Oral econazole has not been shown to cause birth defects in animal studies; however, it has been shown to cause other problems. Before using this medicine, make sure your doctor knows if you are pregnant or if you may become pregnant.

**Breast-feeding**—It is not known whether topical econazole passes into the breast milk. This medicine has not been reported to cause problems in nursing babies. However, econazole, when given by mouth, does pass into the milk of rats and has caused problems in the young.

**Children**—Although there is no specific information comparing use of this medicine in children with use in other age groups, this medicine is not expected to cause different side effects or problems in children than it does in adults.

**Older adults**—Many medicines have not been studied specifically in older people. Therefore, it may not be known whether they work exactly the same way they do in younger adults. Although there is no specific information comparing use of econazole in the elderly with use in other age groups, this medicine is not expected to cause different side effects or problems in older people than it does in younger adults.

## Proper Use of This Medicine

Apply enough econazole to cover the affected and surrounding skin areas, and rub in gently.

*Keep this medicine away from the eyes.*

When econazole is used to treat certain types of fungus infections of the skin, an occlusive dressing (airtight covering, such as kitchen plastic wrap) should *not* be applied over the medicine. To do so may cause irritation of the skin. *Do not apply an airtight covering over this medicine unless you have been directed to do so by your doctor.*

To help clear up your infection completely, *it is very important that you keep using econazole for the full time of treatment,* even if your symptoms begin to clear up after a few days. Since fungus infections may be very slow to clear up, you may have to continue using this medicine every day for several weeks or more. If you stop using this medicine too soon, your symptoms may return. *Do not miss any doses.*

**Dosing**—The dose of topical econazole will be different for different patients. *Follow your doctor's orders or the directions on the label.* The following information includes only the average dose of topical econazole. *If your dose is different, do not change it* unless your doctor tells you to do so.

- For *topical* dosage form (cream):
    —For fungus infections:
    - Adults and children—Apply to the affected area(s) of the skin one or two times a day. If you have to use the cream two times a day, apply it in the morning and evening.

**Missed dose**—If you miss a dose of this medicine, apply it as soon as possible. However, if it is almost time for your next dose, skip the missed dose and go back to your regular dosing schedule.

**Storage**—To store this medicine:
- Keep out of the reach of children.
- Store away from heat and direct light.
- Keep the medicine from freezing.
- Do not keep outdated medicine or medicine no longer needed. Be sure that any discarded medicine is out of the reach of children.

## Precautions While Using This Medicine

If your skin problem does not improve within 2 weeks or more, or if it becomes worse, check with your doctor.

*To help clear up your infection completely and to help make sure it does not return, good health habits are also required.*

- For patients using econazole for ringworm of the groin (tinea cruris; jock itch):
  —Avoid wearing underwear that is tight-fitting or made from synthetic materials (for example, rayon or nylon). Instead, wear loose-fitting, cotton underwear.
  —Use a bland, absorbent powder (for example, talcum powder) or an antifungal powder (for example, tolnaftate) on the skin. It is best not to use econazole cream or any other antifungal cream at the same time that you use the powder.

These measures will help reduce chafing and irritation and will also help keep the groin area cool and dry.

- For patients using econazole for ringworm of the foot (tinea pedis; athlete's foot):
  —Carefully dry the feet, especially between the toes, after bathing.
  —Avoid wearing socks made from wool or synthetic materials (for example, rayon or nylon). Instead, wear clean, cotton socks and change them daily or more often if the feet sweat freely.
  —Wear well-ventilated shoes (for example, shoes with holes) or sandals.
  —Use a bland, absorbent powder (for example, talcum powder) or an antifungal powder (for example, tolnaftate) between the toes, on the feet, and in socks and shoes freely once or twice a day. It is best not to use econazole cream or any other antifungal cream at the same time that you use the powder.

These measures will help keep the feet cool and dry.

If you have any questions about this, check with your health care professional.

## Side Effects of This Medicine

Along with its needed effects, a medicine may cause some unwanted effects. Although not all of these side effects may occur, if they do occur they may need medical attention.

Check with your doctor as soon as possible if any of the following side effects occur:

*Less common*
> Burning, itching, stinging, redness, or other sign of irritation not present before use of this medicine

Other side effects not listed above may also occur in some patients. If you notice any other effects, check with your doctor.

Revised: 04/14/92
Interim revision: 06/06/94

# EFLORNITHINE    Systemic†

A commonly used brand name in the U.S. is Ornidyl.

†Not commercially available in Canada.

## Description

Eflornithine (ee-FLOR-ni-theen) is used to treat African sleeping sickness, a disease caused by parasites.

Eflornithine is available only with your doctor's prescription, in the following dosage form:

*Parenteral*
- Injection (U.S.)

## Before Receiving This Medicine

In deciding to use a medicine, the risks of taking the medicine must be weighed against the good it will do. This is a decision you and your doctor will make. For eflornithine, the following should be considered:

**Allergies**—Tell your doctor if you have ever had any unusual or allergic reaction to eflornithine. Also tell your health care professional if you are allergic to any other substances, such as foods, preservatives, or dyes.

**Pregnancy**—Studies have not been done in humans. However, studies in animals have shown that eflornithine causes fetal death and birth defects. Before taking this medicine, make sure your doctor knows if you are pregnant or if you may become pregnant.

**Breast-feeding**—It is not known whether eflornithine passes into breast milk. Be sure you have discussed the risks and benefits of the medicine if you are thinking of breast-feeding your baby.

**Children**—Studies on this medicine have been done only in adult patients, and there is no specific information comparing use of eflornithine in children with use in other age groups.

**Older adults**—Many medicines have not been studied specifically in older people. Therefore, it may not be known whether they work exactly the same way they do in younger adults or if they cause different side effects or problems in older people. There is no specific information comparing use of eflornithine in the elderly with use in other age groups.

Other medicines—Although certain medicines should not be used together at all, in other cases two different medicines may be used together even if an interaction might occur. In these cases, your doctor may want to change the dose, or other precautions may be necessary. When you are receiving eflornithine, it is especially important that your health care professional know if you are taking any of the following:

- Amphotericin B by injection (e.g., Fungizone) or
- Antineoplastics (cancer medicine) or
- Antithyroid agents (medicine for overactive thyroid) or
- Azathioprine (e.g., Imuran) or
- Chloramphenicol (e.g., Chloromycetin) or
- Colchicine or
- Cyclophosphamide (e.g., Cytoxan) or
- Flucytosine (e.g., Ancobon) or
- Ganciclovir (e.g., Cytovene) or
- Interferon (e.g., Intron A, Roferon-A) or
- Mercaptopurine (e.g., Purinethol) or
- Methotrexate (e.g., Mexate) or
- Plicamycin (e.g., Mithracin) or
- Zidovudine (e.g., AZT, Retrovir)—Caution should be used if these medicines and eflornithine are used together; receiving eflornithine while you are using these medicines may make anemia and other blood problems worse
- Anti-infectives by mouth or by injection (medicine for infection) or
- Chloroquine (e.g., Aralen) or
- Cisplatin (e.g., Platinol) or
- Deferoxamine (e.g., Desferal) (with long-term use) or
- Hydroxychloroquine (e.g., Plaquenil) or
- Inflammation or pain medicine, except narcotics or
- Quinine (e.g., Quinamm)—Use of any of these medicines with eflornithine may increase the chance of hearing loss

Other medical problems—The presence of other medical problems may affect the use of eflornithine. Make sure you tell your doctor if you have any other medical problems, especially:

- Anemia or other blood problems—Eflornithine may cause blood problems, making the problems you already have worse
- Hearing loss—Long-term treatment with eflornithine may increase your chance of hearing loss
- Kidney disease—Patients with kidney disease may have an increased chance of side effects

## Proper Use of This Medicine

To ensure the best response, eflornithine must be given for the full time of treatment. Also, this medicine works best when there is a constant amount in the blood. To help keep the amount constant, eflornithine must be given on a regular schedule.

Dosing—The dose of eflornithine will be different for different patients. The following information includes only the average dose of eflornithine.

- For *injection* dosage form:
  - —For the treatment of African sleeping sickness:
    - Adults—Dose is based on body weight and must be determined by your doctor. The usual dose is 100 milligrams (mg) per kilogram (kg) (45 mg per pound) of body weight injected slowly into a vein over a period of at least forty-five minutes. This dose is given every six hours for fourteen days.
    - Children—Use and dose must be determined by your doctor.

## Precautions After Receiving This Medicine

Eflornithine can lower the number of white blood cells in your blood, increasing the chance of getting an infection. It can also lower the number of platelets, which are necessary for proper blood clotting. If this occurs, there are certain precautions you can take to reduce the risk of infection or bleeding:

- *Check with your doctor immediately* if you think you are getting an infection or if you get a fever or chills.
- *Check with your doctor immediately* if you notice any unusual bleeding or bruising; black, tarry stools; blood in urine or stools; or pinpoint red spots on your skin.
- Be careful when using a regular toothbrush, dental floss, or toothpick. Your medical doctor, dentist, or nurse may recommend other ways to clean your teeth and gums. Check with your medical doctor before having any dental work done.
- Be careful not to cut yourself when you are using sharp objects such as a safety razor or fingernail or toenail cutters.

*It is very important that your doctor check your progress at regular visits.* This medicine may cause blood problems.

## Side Effects of This Medicine

Along with its needed effects, a medicine may cause some unwanted effects. Although not all of these side effects may occur, if they do occur they may need medical attention.

*Check with your doctor immediately* if any of the following side effects occur:

*More common*
Sore throat and fever; unusual bleeding or bruising; unusual tiredness and weakness
*Rare*
Convulsions (seizures); loss of hearing

Other side effects may occur that usually do not need medical attention. These side effects may go away during

treatment as your body adjusts to the medicine. However, check with your doctor if any of the following side effects continue or are bothersome:

*More common*

Diarrhea; nausea; stomach pain; vomiting

*Rare*

Hair loss; headache

Other side effects not listed above may also occur in some patients. If you notice any other effects, check with your doctor.

Revised: 02/19/92
Interim revision: 08/16/94

# ENCAINIDE   Systemic*†

A commonly used brand name is Enkaid.

*Not commercially available in the U.S.
†Not commercially available in Canada.

## Description

Encainide (en-KAY-nide) belongs to the group of medicines known as antiarrhythmics. It is used to correct irregular heartbeats to a normal rhythm.

Encainide produces its helpful effects by slowing nerve impulses in the heart and making the heart tissue less sensitive.

There is a chance that encainide may cause new heart rhythm problems when it is used. Since it has been shown to cause severe problems in some patients, it is only used to treat serious heart rhythm problems. Discuss this possible effect with your doctor.

This medicine is available only with your doctor's prescription, in the following dosage form:

*Oral*

• Capsules

## Before Using This Medicine

In deciding to use a medicine, the risks of taking the medicine must be weighed against the good it will do. This is a decision you and your doctor will make. For encainide, the following should be considered:

**Allergies**—Tell your doctor if you have ever had any unusual or allergic reaction to encainide. Also tell your health care professional if you are allergic to any other substances, such as foods, preservatives, or dyes.

**Pregnancy**—Encainide has not been studied in pregnant women. However, this medicine has not been shown to cause birth defects or other problems in animal studies, but has been shown to reduce fertility in rats. Before taking encainide, make sure your doctor knows if you are pregnant or if you may become pregnant.

**Breast-feeding**—Encainide passes into the milk of some animals and may also pass into the milk of humans. However, this medicine has not been reported to cause problems in nursing babies.

**Children**—Studies on this medicine have been done only in adult patients. Therefore, be sure to discuss with your doctor the use of this medicine in children.

**Older adults**—Many medicines have not been tested in older people. Therefore, it may not be known whether they work exactly the same way they do in younger adults or if they cause different side effects or problems in older people. There is no specific information about the use of encainide in the elderly.

**Other medical problems**—The presence of other medical problems may affect the use of encainide. Make sure you tell your doctor if you have any other medical problems, especially:

• Diabetes mellitus—Encainide may raise blood sugar levels
• Kidney disease—Effects of encainide may be increased because of slower removal from the body
• Liver disease—Effects of encainide may be changed
• Recent heart attack—Risk of irregular heartbeats may be increased
• If you have a pacemaker—Encainide may interfere with the pacemaker and require more careful follow-up by the doctor

## Proper Use of This Medicine

*Take encainide exactly as directed by your doctor,* even though you may feel well. Do not take more or less of it than your doctor ordered.

This medicine works best when there is a constant amount in the blood. *To help keep the amount constant, do not miss any doses. Also, it is best to take each dose at evenly spaced times day and night.* For example, if you are to take 3 doses a day, doses should be spaced about 8 hours apart. If you need help in planning the best times to take your medicine, check with your health care professional.

**Dosing**—The dose of encainide will be different for different patients. *Follow your doctor's orders or the directions on the label.* The following information includes only the average doses of encainide. *If your dose is different, do not change it* unless your doctor tells you to do so:

• For *oral* dosage form (capsules):
—For irregular heartbeat:
• Adults—25 to 50 milligrams (mg) every eight hours.

- Children—Use and dose must be determined by your doctor.

**Missed dose**—If you do miss a dose of encainide and remember within 4 hours, take it as soon as possible. However, if you do not remember until later, skip the missed dose and go back to your regular dosing schedule. Do not double doses.

**Storage**—To store this medicine:
- Keep out of the reach of children.
- Store away from heat and direct light.
- Do not store in the bathroom, near the kitchen sink, or in other damp places. Heat or moisture may cause the medicine to break down.
- Do not keep outdated medicine or medicine no longer needed. Be sure that any discarded medicine is out of the reach of children.

## Precautions While Using This Medicine

It is important that your doctor check your progress at regular visits to make sure the medicine is working properly. This will allow changes to be made in the amount of medicine you are taking, if necessary.

Your doctor may want you to carry a medical identification card or bracelet stating that you are using this medicine.

*Before having any kind of surgery (including dental surgery) or emergency treatment, tell the medical doctor or dentist in charge that you are taking this medicine.*

Encainide may cause some people to become dizzy or light-headed. Make sure you know how you react to this medicine before you drive, use machines, or do anything else that could be dangerous if you are dizzy.

## Side Effects of This Medicine

Along with its needed effects, a medicine may cause some unwanted effects. Although not all of these side effects may occur, if they do occur they may need medical attention.

Check with your doctor as soon as possible if any of the following side effects occur:

*More common*
Chest pain; fast or irregular heartbeat

*Rare*
Shortness of breath; swelling of feet or lower legs; trembling or shaking

Other side effects may occur that usually do not need medical attention. These side effects may go away during treatment as your body adjusts to the medicine. However, check with your doctor if any of the following side effects continue or are bothersome:

*Less common*
Blurred or double vision; dizziness; headache; nausea; pain in arms or legs; skin rash; unusual tiredness or weakness

Other side effects not listed above may also occur in some patients. If you notice any other effects, check with your doctor.

Revised: 06/08/93

# ENOXAPARIN   Systemic

A commonly used brand name in the U.S. and Canada is Lovenox.

## Description

Enoxaparin (e-nox-a-PA-rin) is used to prevent deep venous thrombosis, a condition in which harmful blood clots form in the blood vessels of the legs. This medicine is used for several days after hip or knee replacement surgery, while you are unable to walk. It is during this time that blood clots are most likely to form. Enoxaparin also may be used for other conditions as determined by your doctor.

Enoxaparin is available only with your doctor's prescription, in the following dosage form:
*Parenteral*
- Injection (U.S. and Canada)

## Before Using This Medicine

In deciding to use a medicine, the risks of taking the medicine must be weighed against the good it will do.

This is a decision you and your doctor will make. For enoxaparin, the following should be considered:

**Allergies**—Tell your doctor if you have ever had any unusual or allergic reaction to enoxaparin or to heparin. Also tell your health care professional if you are allergic to any other substances, such as foods, especially pork or pork products, preservatives, or dyes.

**Pregnancy**—Enoxaparin has not been studied in pregnant women. However, it has not been shown to cause birth defects or other problems in animal studies.

**Breast-feeding**—It is not known whether this medicine passes into breast milk. Although most medicines pass into breast milk in small amounts, many of them may be used safely while breast-feeding. Mothers who are using this medicine and who wish to breast-feed should discuss this with their doctor.

**Children**—Studies on this medicine have been done only in adult patients, and there is no specific information

comparing use of enoxaparin in children with use in other age groups.

**Older adults**—This medicine has been tested and has not been shown to cause different side effects or problems in older people than it does in younger adults.

**Other medicines**—Although certain medicines should not be used together at all, in other cases two different medicines may be used together even if an interaction might occur. In these cases, your doctor may want to change the dose, or other precautions may be necessary. When you are using enoxaparin, it is especially important that your health care professional know if you are taking any of the following:

- Aspirin or
- Divalproex (e.g., Depakote) or
- Inflammation or pain medicine, except narcotics, or
- Plicamycin (e.g., Mithracin) or
- Sulfinpyrazone (e.g., Anturane) or
- Thrombolytic agents or
- Ticlopidine (e.g., Ticlid) or
- Valproic acid (e.g., Depakene)—Using any of these medicines together with enoxaparin may increase the risk of bleeding

**Other medical problems**—The presence of other medical problems may affect the use of enoxaparin. Make sure you tell your doctor if you have any other medical problems, especially:

- Blood disease or bleeding problems or
- Blood vessel problems or
- Heart infection or
- High blood pressure (hypertension) or
- Kidney disease or
- Liver disease or
- Stomach ulcer (active) or
- Threatened miscarriage—The risk of bleeding may be increased

Also, tell your doctor if you have received enoxaparin or heparin before and had a reaction to either of them called thrombocytopenia, or if new blood clots formed while you were receiving the medicine.

In addition, *tell your doctor if you have recently given birth, fallen or suffered a blow to the body or head, or had medical or dental surgery*. These events may increase the risk of serious bleeding when you are taking enoxaparin.

## Proper Use of This Medicine

If you are using enoxaparin at home, your health care professional will teach you how to inject yourself with the medicine. *Be sure to follow the directions carefully. Check with your health care professional if you have any problems using the medicine.*

*Put used syringes in a puncture-resistant, disposable container*, or dispose of them as directed by your health care professional.

**Dosing**—The dose of enoxaparin will be different for different patients. *Follow your doctor's orders or the directions on the label*. The following information includes only the average doses of enoxaparin. *If your dose is different, do not change it* unless your doctor tells you to do so.

- For *injection* dosage form:
    - —For prevention of deep venous thrombosis:
        - Adults—30 milligrams (mg) every twelve hours for seven to ten days.
        - Children—Use and dose must be determined by your doctor.

**Missed dose**—If you miss a dose of this medicine, use it as soon as possible. However, if it is almost time for your next dose, skip the missed dose and go back to your regular dosing schedule. Do not double doses.

**Storage**—To store this medicine:

- Keep out of the reach of children.
- Store away from heat and direct light.
- Keep the medicine from freezing. Do not refrigerate.
- Do not keep outdated medicine or medicine no longer needed. Be sure that any discarded medicine is out of the reach of children.

## Precautions While Using This Medicine

*Tell all your medical doctors and dentists that you are using this medicine.*

## Side Effects of This Medicine

Along with its needed effects, a medicine may cause some unwanted effects. Although not all of these side effects may occur, if they do occur they may need medical attention.

*Stop using this medicine and check with your doctor immediately* if any of the following side effects occur:

*Less common*

Blood in urine; bloody or black, tarry stools; bruising; chest discomfort; collection of blood under the skin; confusion; continuing bleeding or oozing from the nose and/or mouth, or surgical wound; convulsions; coughing up blood; fever; headache; irritability; lightheadedness; moderate to severe pain or numbness in the arms, legs, hands, feet; nosebleed; shortness of breath; swelling of hands and/or feet; unusual bleeding; unusual tiredness or weakness; vomiting of blood or material that looks like coffee grounds

*Rare*

Chest pain; dizziness or lightheadedness when getting up from a lying or sitting position; fast or irregular heartbeat; skin rash or hives; sudden fainting; swelling of the face, genitals, mouth, or tongue

Other side effects may occur that usually do not need medical attention. These side effects may go away during treatment as your body adjusts to the medicine. However,

check with your doctor if any of the following side effects continue or are bothersome:

*Less common*

Increased menstrual bleeding; irritation, pain, or redness at place of injection; nausea; vomiting

Other side effects not listed above may also occur in some patients. If you notice any other effects, check with your doctor.

Developed: 11/22/93

---

# ENTERAL NUTRITION FORMULAS    Systemic

Some commonly used brand names are:

**In the U.S.—**

| | |
|---|---|
| Accupep HPF[6] | Nutren 2.0[7] |
| Alitraq[6] | Nutren 1.0 with Fiber[3] |
| Amin-Aid[2] | NutriHep[2] |
| Attain[7] | Nutrilan Flavored |
| Carnation Instant Breakfast[4] | Supplements[7] |
| Carnation Instant Breakfast | NutriSource[3] |
| No Sugar Added[4] | NutriSource HN[3] |
| Casec[5] | NutriVent[2] |
| CitriSource[7] | Osmolite[7] |
| Citrotein[7] | Osmolite HN[7] |
| Compleat Modified[1] | Pediasure[7] |
| Compleat Regular[1] | Pediasure with Fiber[3] |
| Comply[7] | Peptamen[6] |
| Criticare HN[6] | Perative[2] |
| Elementra[5] | Polycose[5] |
| Ensure[7] | Pre-Attain[7] |
| Ensure with Fiber[3] | Precision HN[7] |
| Ensure HN[7] | Precision Isotonic Diet[7] |
| Ensure Plus[7] | Precision Low Residue[7] |
| Ensure Plus HN[7] | Profiber[3] |
| Entrition Half-Strength[7] | ProMod[5] |
| Entrition HN[7] | Promote[7] |
| Fiberlan[3] | Propac[5] |
| Fibersource[3] | Protain XL[2] |
| Fibersource HN[3] | Pulmocare[2] |
| Glucerna[2] | Reabilan[6] |
| Great Shake[4] | Reabilan HN[6] |
| Hepatic-Aid II[2] | Replete[7] |
| Immun-Aid[2] | Replete with Fiber[3] |
| Impact[2] | Resource[7] |
| Impact with Fiber[2,3] | Resource Plus[7] |
| Introlan[7] | Stresstein[2] |
| Introlite[7] | Sumacal[5] |
| Isocal[7] | Suplena[2] |
| Isocal HCN[7] | Sustacal[7] |
| Isocal HN[7] | Sustacal 8.8[7] |
| Isolan[7] | Sustacal with Fiber[3] |
| Isosource[7] | Sustacal HC[7] |
| Isosource HN[7] | Sustagen[4] |
| Isotein HN[7] | Tasty Shake[4] |
| Jevity[3] | Tolerex[6] |
| Lipisorb[2] | TraumaCal[2] |
| Lonalac[4] | Traum-Aid HBC[2] |
| Magnacal[7] | Travasorb Hepatic Diet[2] |
| MCT Oil[5] | Travasorb HN[6] |
| Menu Magic Instant | Travasorb Renal Diet[2] |
| Breakfast[4] | Travasorb STD[6] |
| Menu Magic Milk Shake[4] | TwoCal HN[7] |
| Meritene[4] | Ultracal[3] |
| Microlipid[5] | Ultralan[7] |
| Moducal[5] | Vital High Nitrogen[6] |
| Nepro[2] | Vitaneed[1] |
| Nutren 1.0[7] | Vivonex T.E.N.[6] |
| Nutren 1.5[7] | |

**In Canada—**

| | |
|---|---|
| CitriSource[7] | Nepro[2] |
| Citrotein[2] | NutriSource[3] |
| Compleat Modified[1] | NutriSource HN[3] |
| Enercal[7] | Osmolite HN[7] |
| Ensure[7] | Pediasure[7] |
| Ensure with Fiber[3] | Polycose[5] |
| Ensure High Protein[7] | ProMod[5] |
| Ensure Plus[7] | Pulmocare[2] |
| Glucerna[2] | Resource[7] |
| Impact[2] | Resource Plus[7] |
| Isosource[7] | Suplena[2] |
| Isosource HN[7] | Sustagen[4] |
| Jevity[3] | Tolerex[6] |
| MCT Oil[5] | Vital High Nitrogen[6] |
| Meritene[4] | Vivonex T.E.N.[6] |

Note: For quick reference, the following enteral nutrition formulas are numbered to match the corresponding brand names.

This information applies to the following enteral nutrition formulas:

1. Enteral nutrition formulas, blenderized
2. Enteral nutrition formulas, disease-specific
3. Enteral nutrition formulas, fiber-containing
4. Enteral nutrition formulas, milk-based
5. Enteral nutrition formulas, modular
6. Enteral nutrition formulas, monomeric (elemental)
7. Enteral nutrition formulas, polymeric

---

## Description

Enteral nutrition formulas are used as nutritional replacements for patients who are unable to get enough nutrients in their diet. These formulas are taken by mouth or through a feeding tube and are used by the body for energy and to form substances needed for normal body functions.

Patients with the following conditions may be more likely to need enteral feedings:

- Acquired immunodeficiency syndrome (AIDS)
- Burns
- Cancer
- Infections, prolonged
- Kidney problems
- Liver problems
- Lung problems
- Pancreas problems
- Stomach problems
- Surgery
- Trauma
- Vomiting, prolonged

Enteral nutrition formulas are available without a prescription. However, they should only be used under medical supervision.

The benefits of enteral formulas in healthy people have not been proven.

Enteral nutrition formulas are available in the following dosage forms:

*Oral*
  Blenderized Enteral Nutrition
  • Oral solution (U.S. and Canada)
  Disease-specific Enteral Nutrition
  • Oral solution (U.S. and Canada)
  • Powder for solution (U.S. and Canada)
  Fiber-containing Enteral Nutrition
  • Oral solution (U.S. and Canada)
  Milk-based Enteral Nutrition
  • Oral solution (U.S.)
  • Powder for solution (U.S. and Canada)
  Modular Enteral Nutrition
  • Oil (U.S. and Canada)
  • Oral solution (U.S. and Canada)
  • Oral powder (U.S. and Canada)
  Monomeric Enteral Nutrition
  • Oral solution (U.S. and Canada)
  • Powder for solution (U.S.)
  Polymeric Enteral Nutrition
  • Oral solution (U.S. and Canada)
  • Powder for solution (U.S.)

## Before Using This Enteral Nutrition Formula

If you are taking any of these enteral nutrition formulas without a prescription, carefully read and follow any precautions on the label. For enteral nutrition formulas, the following should be considered:

**Allergies**—Tell your doctor if you have ever had any unusual or allergic reaction to any of the ingredients listed for your enteral nutrition formula. Also tell your health care professional if you are allergic to any other substances, such as foods, preservatives, or dyes.

**Pregnancy**—Studies on effects in pregnancy have not been done in either humans or animals.

**Breast-feeding**—This enteral nutrition formula has not been reported to cause problems in nursing babies.

**Children**—Caution should be used when giving enteral feedings to children less than one year of age. Very young children may not be able to eliminate the feeding from the body. Although there is no specific information about the use of enteral feedings in older children, it is not expected to cause different side effects or problems in these children than it does in adults.

**Older adults**—Older adults may be at risk of developing problems related to the use of a nasogastric tube (tube going through the nose into the stomach), such as aspiration (sucking fluid into the lungs) or removing the nasogastric tube. The enteral feeding itself has not been shown to cause different side effects or problems in older people than it does in younger adults.

**Medicines**—Although certain medications and enteral nutrition formulas should not be used together at all, in other cases they may be used together even if an interaction might occur. In these cases, your doctor may want to change the dose, or other precautions may be necessary. Tell your health care professional if you are taking any prescription or nonprescription (over-the-counter [OTC]) medicine.

**Other medical problems**—The presence of other medical problems may affect the use of enteral feedings. Make sure you tell your doctor if you have any other medical problems, especially:

• Breathing problems or
• Dehydration or
• Diabetes mellitus (sugar diabetes) or
• Diarrhea or
• Heart problems or
• Hyperglycemia (high levels of sugar in the blood) or
• Hyperlipidemia or
• Lactose intolerance or
• Liver problems or
• Pancreas problems—Enteral feedings may make these conditions worse; your doctor may recommend a special formula for your condition
• Intestine problems or
• Stomach problems—These problems may prevent enteral formulas from being absorbed properly
• Kidney problems—Higher blood levels of certain ingredients of the enteral feeding may result, and a smaller amount of enteral feeding may be needed.
• Malnutrition, severe—Heart and nerve problems have been reported when feeding a patient who is severely malnourished; enteral formula may need to be used in smaller amounts

## Proper Use of This Enteral Nutrition Formula

Your enteral feeding may be given by mouth or by a feeding tube. Use the amount recommended by your doctor.

For patients taking the *oral liquid* form of enteral nutrition:

• This preparation is in ready-to-use form. No dilution is needed unless directed by your physician.
• Shake the preparation well before opening. Refrigerate after opening, out of the reach of children. Most formulas can be kept in the refrigerator for 1 to 2 days. Check the label of your product.

For patients using the *powder* form of this preparation:

• For mixing or other use, follow carefully the instructions on the package.
• Any unused solution should be kept in the refrigerator, out of the reach of children. Most formulas can be kept in the refrigerator for 1 to 2 days. Check the label of your product.

**Storage**—To store the unopened container:

• Keep out of the reach of children.
• Store away from heat and direct light.

- Do not store in the bathroom, near the kitchen sink, or in other damp places. Heat or moisture may cause the enteral nutrition formula to break down.
- Keep the enteral nutrition formula from freezing. Do not refrigerate, unless the product has been opened or mixed.
- Do not keep outdated enteral nutrition formulas or those no longer needed. Be sure that any discarded enteral nutrition formula is out of the reach of children.

## Precautions While Using This Enteral Nutrition Formula

Enteral feedings must be handled properly to protect them from bacteria. Enteral feedings should be used for no more than 12 hours at room temperature and then should be discarded.

If you are taking your enteral feeding through a tube, enteral formulas that are too thick may clog the feeding tube. If this happens, check with your doctor, nurse, dietitian, or pharmacist.

## Side Effects of This Enteral Nutrition Formula

Some problems may result from improper use of an enteral formula or use of the incorrect formula in your condition. Check with your doctor if any of the following problems occur:

*More common*

Confusion; convulsions (seizures); decrease in urine volume; dryness of mouth; frequent urination; increased thirst; irregular heartbeat; mood or mental changes; muscle cramps or pain; numbness or tingling in hands, feet, or lips; respiratory distress, shortness of breath or difficulty breathing; unexplained nervousness; unusual tiredness or weakness; weakness or heaviness of legs; weak pulse

Other problems may occur that usually do not need medical attention. They may go away during treatment as your body adjusts to the enteral nutrition formula. However, check with your doctor if any of the following side effects continue or are bothersome:

*More common*

Constipation; diarrhea; nausea or vomiting

Other side effects not listed above may also occur in some patients. If you notice any other effects, check with your doctor.

Developed: 08/31/93

# EPINEPHRINE  Ophthalmic

Some commonly used brand names are:

**In the U.S.—**
Epifrin[1]　　　　　　Glaucon[1]
Epinal[2]　　　　　　L-Epinephrine[1]
Eppy/N[2]

**In Canada—**
Epifrin[1]　　　　　　Eppy/N[2]
Epinal[2]　　　　　　Glaucon[1]

Note: For quick reference, the following medicines are numbered to match the corresponding brand names.

This information applies to the following medicines:
1. Epinephrine (ep-i-NEF-rin)‡
2. Epinephryl Borate (ep-i-NEF-rill BOR-ate)

‡Generic name product may also be available in the U.S.

## Description

Ophthalmic epinephrine is used to treat certain types of glaucoma. It may also be used in eye surgery.

This medicine is available only with your doctor's prescription, in the following dosage forms:

*Ophthalmic*

Epinephrine
- Ophthalmic solution (eye drops) (U.S. and Canada)

Epinephryl Borate
- Ophthalmic solution (eye drops) (U.S. and Canada)

## Before Using This Medicine

In deciding to use a medicine, the risks of taking the medicine must be weighed against the good it will do. This is a decision you and your doctor will make. For epinephrine, the following should be considered:

**Allergies**—Tell your doctor if you have ever had any unusual or allergic reaction to epinephrine. Also tell your health care professional if you are allergic to any other substances, such as preservatives.

**Pregnancy**—Ophthalmic epinephrine may be absorbed into the body. However, studies on effects in pregnancy have not been done in either humans or animals.

**Breast-feeding**—Ophthalmic epinephrine may be absorbed into the body. However, it is not known whether epinephrine passes into the breast milk.

**Children**—Studies on this medicine have been done only in adult patients, and there is no specific information comparing use of this medicine in children with use in other age groups.

**Older adults**—Many medicines have not been studied specifically in older people. Therefore, it may not be known whether they work exactly the same way they do in younger adults. Although there is no specific information comparing use of this medicine in the elderly with use in other age groups, this medicine is not expected to cause different side effects or problems in older people than it does in younger adults.

**Other medicines**—Although certain medicines should not be used together at all, in other cases two different medicines may be used together even if an interaction might occur. In these cases, your doctor may want to change the dose, or other precautions may be necessary. Tell your health care professional if you are using any other prescription or nonprescription (over-the-counter [OTC]) medicine.

**Other medical problems**—The presence of other medical problems may affect the use of epinephrine. Make sure you tell your doctor if you have any other medical problems, especially:

- Bronchial asthma or
- Diabetes mellitus (sugar diabetes) or
- Eye disease (other) or
- Heart or blood vessel disease or
- High blood pressure or
- Overactive thyroid—Epinephrine may make the condition worse
- Dental surgery on gums—Dental surgery may include the use of epinephrine in topical or injection form. Use of ophthalmic epinephrine during this time may increase blood levels of the medicine and increase the chance of side effects

## Proper Use of This Medicine

*Use this medicine only as directed.* Do not use more of it and do not use it more often than your doctor ordered. To do so may increase the chance of too much medicine being absorbed into the body and the chance of side effects.

To use:

- First, wash your hands. Tilt the head back and with the index finger of one hand, press gently on the skin just beneath the lower eyelid and pull the lower eyelid away from the eye to make a space. Drop the medicine into this space. Let go of the eyelid and gently close the eyes. Do not blink. Keep the eyes closed and apply pressure to the inner corner of the eye with your finger for 1 or 2 minutes, to allow the medicine to be absorbed.
- Immediately after using the eye drops, wash your hands to remove any medicine that may be on them.
- To keep the medicine as germ-free as possible, do not touch the applicator tip to any surface (including the eye). Also, keep the container tightly closed.

For patients using *epinephrine ophthalmic solution:*

- Do not use if the solution turns pinkish or brownish in color, or if it becomes cloudy.

For patients using *epinephryl borate ophthalmic solution:*

- The color of this solution may vary from colorless to amber yellow. Do not use if the solution turns dark brown or becomes cloudy.

**Dosing**—The dose of ophthalmic epinephrine will be different for different patients. *Follow your doctor's orders or the directions on the label.* The following information includes only the average doses of ophthalmic epinephrine. *If your dose is different, do not change it* unless your doctor tells you to do so.

*For epinephrine and epinephryl borate*

- For *ophthalmic solution (eye drops)* dosage forms:
  —For glaucoma:
    - Adults—One drop one or two times a day.
    - Children—Use and dose must be determined by your doctor.

**Missed dose**—If you miss a dose of this medicine, apply the missed dose as soon as possible. However, if it is almost time for your next dose, skip the missed dose and go back to your regular dosing schedule. Do not double doses.

**Storage**—To store this medicine:

- Keep out of the reach of children.
- Store away from heat and direct light.
- Keep the medicine from freezing.
- Do not keep outdated medicine or medicine no longer needed. Be sure that any discarded medicine is out of the reach of children.

## Precautions While Using This Medicine

Your doctor should check your eye pressure at regular visits.

## Side Effects of This Medicine

Along with its needed effects, a medicine may cause some unwanted effects. Although not all of these side effects may occur, if they do occur they may need medical attention.

Check with your doctor as soon as possible if any of the following side effects occur:

*Less common*

Blurred or decreased vision

*Symptoms of too much medicine being absorbed into the body*

Fast, irregular, or pounding heartbeat; feeling faint; increased sweating; paleness; trembling

Other side effects may occur that usually do not need medical attention. These side effects may go away during treatment as your body adjusts to the medicine. However, check with your doctor if any of the following side effects continue or are bothersome:

*More common*
    Headache or browache; stinging, burning, redness, or other eye irritation; watering of eyes

*Less common*
    Eye pain or ache

Other side effects not listed above may also occur in some patients. If you notice any other effects, check with your doctor.

Revised: 05/14/92
Interim revision: 08/17/93

# EPOETIN   Systemic

Some commonly used brand names are:

**In the U.S.—**
    Epogen
    Procrit

**In Canada—**
    Eprex

Other commonly used names are human erythropoietin, recombinant; EPO; and r-HuEPO.

## Description

Epoetin (eh-POH-ee-tin) is a man-made version of human erythropoietin (EPO). EPO is produced naturally in the body, mostly by the kidneys. It stimulates the bone marrow to produce red blood cells. If the body does not produce enough EPO, severe anemia can occur. This often occurs in people whose kidneys are not working properly. Epoetin is used to treat severe anemia in these people.

Epoetin may also be used to prevent or treat anemia caused by other conditions, as determined by your doctor.

Epoetin is given by injection. It is available only with your doctor's prescription and is available in the following dosage form:

*Parenteral*
- Injection (U.S. and Canada)

## Before Using This Medicine

In deciding to use a medicine, the risks of taking the medicine must be weighed against the good it will do. This is a decision you and your doctor will make. For epoetin, the following should be considered:

**Allergies**—Tell your doctor if you have ever had any unusual or allergic reaction to epoetin or to human albumin. Also tell your health care professional if you are allergic to any other substances, such as foods, preservatives, or dyes.

**Pregnancy**—Epoetin has not been reported to cause birth defects or other problems in humans. However, it did cause problems, including unwanted effects on the bones and spine, in some animal studies.

**Breast-feeding**—It is not known whether epoetin passes into the breast milk. However, it has not been reported to cause problems in nursing babies.

**Children**—There is no specific information about the use of epoetin in children up to 12 years of age.

**Older adults**—Epoetin has been given to elderly people. However, there is no specific information about whether epoetin works the same way it does in younger adults or whether it causes different side effects or problems in older people.

**Other medicines**—Although certain medicines should not be used together at all, in other cases two different medicines may be used together even if an interaction might occur. In these cases, your doctor may want to change the dose, or other precautions may be necessary. When you are taking epoetin, it is important that your health care professional know if you are taking any other prescription or nonprescription (over-the-counter [OTC]) medicine.

**Other medical problems**—The presence of other medical problems may affect the use of epoetin. Make sure you tell your doctor if you have any other medical problems, especially:
- Blood clots (history of) or other problems with the blood or
- Heart or blood vessel disease or
- High blood pressure—The chance of side effects may be increased
- Bone problems or
- Sickle cell anemia—Epoetin may not work properly
- Seizures (history of)—The chance of seizures may be increased

## Proper Use of This Medicine

Epoetin is usually given by a health care professional after a dialysis treatment. However, medicines given by injection are sometimes used at home. If you will be using epoetin at home, your health care professional will teach you how the injections are to be given. You will also have a chance to practice giving them. *Be certain that you understand exactly how the medicine is to be injected.*

**Dosing**—The dose of epoetin will be different for different patients. *Follow your doctor's orders or the directions on the label.* The following information includes only the average doses of epoetin. *If your dose is different, do not change it* unless your doctor tells you to do so.

- For *injection* dosage form:
  —For severe anemia:
    • Adults and teenagers—Dose is based on body weight and must be determined by your doctor. The usual dose is 50 to 100 Units per kilogram (kg) (23 to 45 Units per pound) of body weight three times a week, injected into a vein or under the skin. Your doctor may then gradually decrease the dose by 25 Units per kg (11 Units per pound) of body weight every four weeks or more until the lowest effective dose is reached.
    • Children up to 12 years of age—Dose must be determined by your doctor.

**Missed dose**—If you miss a dose of this medicine, use it as soon as possible. However, if it is almost time for your next dose, skip the missed dose and go back to your regular dosing schedule. Do not double doses.

**Storage**—To store this medicine:
- Keep out of the reach of children.
- Store in the refrigerator. However, keep the medicine from freezing.
- Do not keep outdated medicine or medicine no longer needed. Be sure that any discarded medicine is out of the reach of children.

## Precautions While Using This Medicine

Epoetin sometimes causes convulsions (seizures), especially during the first 90 days of treatment. During this time, it is best to avoid driving, operating heavy machinery, or other activities that could cause a serious injury if a seizure occurs while you are performing them.

People with severe anemia usually feel very tired and sick. When epoetin begins to work, usually in about 6 weeks, most people start to feel better. Some people are able to be more active. However, epoetin only corrects anemia. It has no effect on kidney disease or any other medical problem that needs regular medical attention. Therefore, even if you are feeling much better, *it is very important that you do not miss any appointments with your doctor or any dialysis treatments*.

Many people with kidney problems need to be on a special diet. Also, people with high blood pressure (which may be caused by kidney disease or by epoetin treatment) may need to be on a special diet and/or to take medicine to keep their blood pressure under control. After their anemia has been corrected, some people feel so much better that they want to eat more than before. To keep your kidney disease or your high blood pressure from getting worse, *it is very important that you follow your special diet and take your medicines regularly,* even if you are feeling better.

In addition to epoetin, your body needs iron to make red blood cells. Your doctor may direct you to take iron supplements. He or she may also direct you to take certain vitamins that help the iron work better. *Be sure to follow your doctor's orders carefully,* because epoetin will not work properly if there is not enough iron in your body.

## Side Effects of This Medicine

Along with its needed effects, a medicine may cause some unwanted effects. Although not all of these side effects may occur, if they do occur they may need medical attention.

*Check with your doctor immediately if any of the following side effects occur:*

*More common*
   Chest pain

*Less common*
   Convulsions (seizures); shortness of breath

Also, check with your doctor as soon as possible if any of the following side effects occur:

*More common*
   Fast heartbeat; headache; increased blood pressure; swelling of face, fingers, ankles, feet, or lower legs; vision problems; weight gain

*Rare*
   Skin rash or hives

Other side effects may occur that usually do not need medical attention. These side effects may go away during treatment as your body adjusts to the medicine. Epoetin sometimes causes an influenza-like reaction, with symptoms such as muscle aches, bone pain, chills, shivering, and sweating, occurring about 1 or 2 hours after an injection. These symptoms usually go away within 12 hours. However, check with your doctor if this influenza-like reaction or any of the following side effects continue or are bothersome:

*More common*
   Bone pain; diarrhea; muscle weakness (severe); nausea or vomiting; tiredness

Other side effects not listed above may also occur in some patients. If you notice any other effects, check with your doctor.

## Additional Information

For patients receiving epoetin who do not have anemia caused by kidney disease:

- The information about the importance of keeping dialysis appointments and following a special diet for people with kidney problems does not apply to you. However, your doctor may have other special directions for you to follow. Be sure to follow these directions carefully, even if you feel much better after receiving epoetin for a while.

Revised: 07/07/92
Interim revision(s): 05/02/94

# ERGOLOID MESYLATES　Systemic

Some commonly used brand names are:

**In the U.S.—**
　Gerimal　　　　　　　　　Hydergine LC
　Hydergine
　Generic name product may also be available.

**In Canada—**
　Hydergine
Another commonly used name is dihydrogenated ergot alkaloids.

## Description

Ergoloid mesylates (ER-goe-loid MESS-i-lates) belongs to the group of medicines known as ergot alkaloids. It is used to treat some mood, behavior, or other problems that may be due to changes in the brain from Alzheimer's disease or multiple small strokes.

This medicine is different from other ergot alkaloids such as ergotamine and methysergide. It is not useful for treating migraine headache. The exact way ergoloid mesylates acts on the body is not known.

This medicine is available only with your doctor's prescription, in the following dosage forms:

　*Oral*
　　• Capsules (U.S.)
　　• Oral solution (U.S.)
　　• Tablets (U.S. and Canada)
　*Sublingual (under-the-tongue)*
　　• Tablets (U.S.)

## Before Using This Medicine

In deciding to use a medicine, the risks of taking the medicine must be weighed against the good it will do. This is a decision you and your doctor will make. For ergoloid mesylates, the following should be considered:

**Allergies**—Tell your doctor if you have ever had any unusual or allergic reaction to ergot alkaloids. Also tell your health care professional if you are allergic to any other substances, such as foods, preservatives, or dyes.

**Other medicines**—Although certain medicines should not be used together at all, in other cases 2 different medicines may be used together even if an interaction might occur. In these cases, your doctor may want to change the dose, or other precautions may be necessary. Tell your health care professional if you are taking any other prescription or nonprescription (over-the-counter [OTC]) medicine.

**Other medical problems**—The presence of other medical problems may affect the use of ergoloid mesylates. Make sure you tell your doctor if you have any other medical problems, especially:
　• Liver disease—Higher blood levels of ergoloid mesylates may occur, increasing the chance of side effects

　• Low blood pressure or
　• Other mental problems or
　• Slow heartbeat—Ergoloid mesylates may make the condition worse

## Proper Use of This Medicine

*Take this medicine only as directed by your doctor.* Do not take more or less of it, and do not take it more often or for a longer period of time than your doctor ordered. To do so may increase the chance of unwanted effects.

For patients taking the *sublingual (under-the-tongue) tablets:*
　• Dissolve the tablet under your tongue. The sublingual tablet should not be chewed or swallowed, since it works much faster when absorbed through the lining of the mouth. Do not eat, drink, or smoke while a tablet is dissolving.

**Dosing**—The dose of ergoloid mesylates will be different for different patients. *Follow your doctor's orders or the directions on the label.* The following information includes only the average doses of ergoloid mesylates. *If your dose is different, do not change it* unless your doctor tells you to do so.

The number of tablets or milliliters of oral solution that you take depends on the strength of the medicine. Also, *the number of doses you take each day, the time allowed between doses, and the length of time you take the medicine depend on the medical problem for which you are taking ergoloid mesylates.*
　• For *oral* dosage forms (capsules, tablets, sublingual tablets, or oral solution):
　　—Adults: 1 to 2 milligrams (mg) three times a day.

**Missed dose**—If you miss a dose of this medicine, skip the missed dose and go back to your regular dosing schedule. Do not double doses. If you have any questions about this, or if you miss two or more doses in a row, check with your doctor.

**Storage**—To store this medicine:
　• Keep out of the reach of children.
　• Store away from heat and direct light.
　• Do not store in the bathroom, near the kitchen sink, or in other damp places. Heat or moisture may cause the medicine to break down.
　• Keep the oral solution from freezing.
　• Do not keep outdated medicine or medicine no longer needed. Be sure that any discarded medicine is out of the reach of children.

## Precautions While Using This Medicine

It is important that your doctor check your progress at regular visits to make sure this medicine is working and to check for unwanted effects.

It may take several weeks for this medicine to work. *However, do not stop taking this medicine without first checking with your doctor.*

## Side Effects of This Medicine

Along with its needed effects, a medicine may cause some unwanted effects. Although not all of these side effects may occur, if they do occur they may need medical attention.

Check with your doctor as soon as possible if any of the following side effects occur:

*Less common or rare*
  Dizziness or lightheadedness when getting up from a lying or sitting position; drowsiness; skin rash; slow pulse

*Signs and symptoms of overdose*
  Blurred vision; dizziness; fainting; flushing; headache; loss of appetite; nausea or vomiting; stomach cramps; stuffy nose

Other side effects may occur that usually do not need medical attention. These side effects may go away during treatment as your body adjusts to the medicine. However, check with your doctor if any of the following side effects continue or are bothersome:

*Less common or rare*
  Soreness under tongue (with sublingual use)

Other side effects not listed above may also occur in some patients. If you notice any other effects, check with your doctor.

Revised: 04/16/93

# ERGONOVINE/METHYLERGONOVINE  Systemic

Some commonly used brand names are:

**In the U.S.—**
  Ergotrate[1]
  Methergine[2]

**In Canada—**
  Ergotrate Maleate[1]

Other commonly used names are:
  Ergometrine[1]                    Methylergometrine[2]

Note: For quick reference, the following medicines are numbered to match the corresponding brand names.

This information applies to the following medicines:
  1. Ergonovine (er-goe-NOE-veen)§
  2. Methylergonovine (meth-ill-er-goe-NOE-veen)†

  †Not commercially available in Canada.
  §Generic name product may also be available in Canada.

## Description

Ergonovine and methylergonovine belong to the group of medicines known as ergot alkaloids. These medicines are usually given to stop excessive bleeding that sometimes occurs after abortion or a baby is delivered. They work by causing the muscle of the uterus to contract.

Ergonovine and methylergonovine may also be used for other conditions as determined by your doctor.

These medicines are available only on prescription and are to be administered only by or under the supervision of your doctor. They are available in the following dosage forms:

*Oral*
  Ergonovine
   • Tablets (U.S. and Canada)
  Methylergonovine
   • Tablets (U.S.)

*Parenteral*
  Ergonovine
   • Injection (U.S. and Canada)
  Methylergonovine
   • Injection (U.S.)

## Before Using This Medicine

In deciding to use a medicine, the risks of taking the medicine must be weighed against the good it will do. This is a decision you and your doctor will make. For ergonovine and methylergonovine, the following should be considered:

**Allergies**—Tell your doctor if you have ever had any unusual or allergic reaction to ergonovine, methylergonovine, or other ergot medicines. Also tell your health care professional if you are allergic to any other substances, such as foods, preservatives, or dyes.

**Breast-feeding**—This medicine passes into the breast milk and may cause unwanted effects, such as vomiting; decreased circulation in the hands, lower legs, and feet; diarrhea; weak pulse; unstable blood pressure; or convulsions (seizures) in infants of mothers taking large doses.

**Children**—Although there is no specific information comparing use of ergonovine or methylergonovine in children with use in other age groups, these medicines are not expected to cause different problems in children than they do in adults.

**Older adults**—Many medicines have not been studied specifically in older people. Therefore, it may not be known whether they work exactly the same way they do in younger adults or if they cause different side effects or problems in older people. There is no specific information

comparing use of ergonovine or methylergonovine in the elderly with use in other age groups.

**Other medicines**—Although certain medicines should not be used together at all, in other cases two different medicines may be used together even if an interaction might occur. In these cases, your doctor may want to change the dose, or other precautions may be necessary. When you are taking ergonovine or methylergonovine it is especially important that your health care professional know if you are taking any of the following:

- Bromocriptine (e.g., Parlodel) or
- Other ergot alkaloids (dihydroergotamine [e.g., D.H.E. 45], ergoloid mesylates [e.g., Hydergine], ergotamine [e.g., Gynergen], methysergide [e.g., Sansert])—Use of these medicines with ergonovine or methylergonovine may increase the chance of side effects of these medicines.
- Nitrates or
- Other medicines for angina—Use of these medicines with ergonovine or methylergonovine may keep these medicines from working properly

**Other medical problems**—The presence of other medical problems may affect the use of ergonovine or methylergonovine. Make sure you tell your doctor if you have any other medical problems, especially:

- Angina (chest pain) or other heart problems or
- Blood vessel disease or
- High blood pressure (or history of) or
- Stroke (history of)—These medicines may cause changes in how the heart works or blood pressure changes
- Infection—Infections may cause an increased sensitivity to the effect of these medicines
- Kidney disease
- Liver disease—The body may not remove these medicines from the bloodstream at the usual rate, which may make the medicine work longer or increase the chance for side effects
- Raynaud's phenomenon—Use of these medicines may cause worsening of the blood vessel narrowing that occurs with this disease

## Proper Use of This Medicine

*Take this medicine only as directed by your doctor.* Do not take more of it, do not take it more often, and do not take it for a longer time than your doctor ordered. If too much is taken or if it is taken for a longer time than your doctor ordered, it may cause serious effects.

**Dosing**—The dose of ergonovine or methylergonovine will be different for different patients. *Follow your doctor's orders or the directions on the label.* The following information includes only the average doses of ergonovine and methylergonovine. *If your dose is different, do not change it* unless your doctor tells you to do so.

*For ergonovine*

- For *oral* dosage forms (tablets):
  —For treatment of excessive uterine bleeding:
    - Adults—0.2 to 0.4 milligram, swallowed or placed under the tongue every six to twelve hours. Usually this medicine is taken for forty-eight hours or less.

- For *injection* dosage form:
  —For treatment of excessive uterine bleeding:
    - Adults—0.2 milligram, injected into a muscle or vein. This dose can be repeated up to five times if needed, with a two- to four-hour wait between doses.

*For methylergonovine*

- For *oral* dosage forms (tablets):
  —For treatment of excessive uterine bleeding:
    - Adults—0.2 to 0.4 milligram, taken every six to twelve hours. Usually this medicine is taken for forty-eight hours or less.
- For *injection* dosage form:
  —For treatment of excessive uterine bleeding:
    - Adults—0.2 milligram, injected into a muscle or vein. This dose can be repeated up to five times if needed, with a two- to four-hour wait between doses.

**Missed dose**—If you miss a dose of this medicine, do not take the missed dose at all and do not double the next one. Instead, go back to your regular dosing schedule. If you have any questions about this, check with your doctor.

**Storage**—To store this medicine:

- Keep out of the reach of children.
- Store away from heat and direct light.
- Do not store in the bathroom, near the kitchen sink, or in other damp places. Heat or moisture may cause the medicine to break down.
- Do not keep outdated medicine or medicine no longer needed. Be sure that any discarded medicine is out of the reach of children.

## Precautions While Using This Medicine

If you have an infection or illness of any kind, check with your doctor before taking this medicine, since you may be more sensitive to its effects.

## Side Effects of This Medicine

Along with its needed effects, a medicine may cause some unwanted effects. Although not all of these side effects may occur, if they do occur they may need medical attention.

*Check with the health care professional immediately* if any of the following side effects occur:

*Less common*
    Chest pain
*Rare*
    Blurred vision; convulsions (seizures); crushing chest pain; headache (sudden and severe); irregular heartbeat; unexplained shortness of breath

Check with your doctor as soon as possible if any of the following side effects occur:

*Less common*
  Slow heartbeat

*Rare*
  Itching of skin; pain in arms, legs, or lower back; pale or cold hands or feet; weakness in legs

*Symptoms of overdose*
  Bluish color of skin or inside of nose or mouth; chest pain; cool, pale, or numb arms or legs; confusion; cramping of the uterus (severe); decreased breathing rate; drowsiness; heartbeat changes; muscle pain; small pupils; tingling, itching, and cool skin; trouble in breathing; unconsciousness; unusual thirst; weak or absent pulse in arms or legs; weak pulse

*With long-term use*
  Dry, shriveled-looking skin on hands, lower legs, or feet; false feeling of insects crawling on the skin; pain and redness in an arm or leg; paralysis of one side of the body

Other side effects may occur that usually do not need medical attention. These side effects may go away during treatment as your body adjusts to the medicine. However, check with your doctor if any of the following side effects continue or are bothersome:

*More common*
  Cramping of the uterus; nausea; vomiting

*Less common*
  Abdominal or stomach pain; diarrhea; dizziness; headache (mild and temporary); ringing in the ears; stuffy nose; sweating; unpleasant taste

Other side effects not listed above may also occur in some patients. If you notice any other effects, check with your doctor.

Revised: 06/07/93

# ERGOTAMINE, BELLADONNA ALKALOIDS, AND PHENOBARBITAL   Systemic

Some commonly used brand names are:

**In the U.S.—**
  Bellergal-S

**In Canada—**
  Bellergal
  Bellergal Spacetabs

## Description

Ergotamine (er-GOT-a-meen), belladonna alkaloids (bell-a-DON-a AL-ka-loids), and phenobarbital (feen-oh-BAR-bi-tal) combination is used to treat some symptoms of menopause (such as hot flashes, sweating, restlessness, and trouble in sleeping). However, it is not effective against other problems that may occur after menopause, such as osteoporosis. This medicine is also used to prevent migraine or cluster headaches in people who get these headaches often. It is not used to treat a headache that has already started. This combination medicine may also be used for other problems as determined by your doctor.

The phenobarbital in this combination medicine belongs to the group of medicines known as barbiturates.

This medicine is available only with your doctor's prescription, in the following dosage forms:

*Oral*
  • Tablets (Canada)
  • Extended-release tablets (U.S. and Canada)

## Before Using This Medicine

In deciding to use a medicine, the risks of taking the medicine must be weighed against the good it will do.

This is a decision you and your doctor will make. For ergotamine, belladonna alkaloids, and phenobarbital combination, the following should be considered:

**Allergies**—Tell your doctor if you have ever had any unusual or allergic reaction to ergotamine or other ergot medicines, atropine, belladonna, or barbiturates. Also tell your health care professional if you are allergic to any other substances, such as foods, preservatives, or dyes.

**Pregnancy**—
  • *For ergotamine*—Ergotamine is not recommended for use during pregnancy since it has been shown to increase the chance of early labor, which could result in a miscarriage.
  • *For belladonna alkaloids*—Belladonna alkaloids have not been shown to cause problems in humans.
  • *For phenobarbital*—Barbiturates such as phenobarbital have been shown to increase the chance of birth defects. Also, when taken during pregnancy, barbiturates may cause bleeding problems in the newborn baby. Be sure that you have discussed these problems with your doctor before taking this medicine.

**Breast-feeding**—
  • *For ergotamine*—Ergotamine passes into the breast milk and may cause unwanted effects, such as vomiting, diarrhea, weak pulse, unstable blood pressure, or convulsions (seizures), in nursing babies whose mothers take large amounts of the medicine. Large amounts of ergotamine may also decrease the flow of breast milk.

- *For belladonna alkaloids*—Although belladonna alkaloids pass into the breast milk, the amount of belladonna alkaloids in this combination medicine has not been shown to cause problems in nursing babies. However, because the belladonna alkaloids tend to decrease the secretions of the body, it is possible that the flow of breast milk may be reduced in some patients.
- *For phenobarbital*—Phenobarbital passes into the breast milk. Taking this combination medicine two or three times a day is not likely to cause problems in nursing babies. However, larger amounts of the medicine may cause drowsiness, unusually slow heartbeat, shortness of breath, or troubled breathing in nursing babies.

Be sure that you discuss these possible problems with your doctor before taking this medicine.

**Children**—Children may be especially sensitive to the effects of the belladonna alkaloids and the phenobarbital in this combination medicine. This may increase the chance of side effects during treatment. Although there is no specific information about the use of ergotamine in children, it is not expected to cause different side effects or problems in children than it does in adults.

**Older adults**—Elderly people are especially sensitive to the effects of ergotamine, belladonna alkaloids, and barbiturates such as phenobarbital. This may increase the chance of side effects during treatment.

**Other medicines**—Although certain medicines should not be used together at all, in other cases two different medicines may be used together even if an interaction might occur. In these cases, your doctor may want to change the dose, or other precautions may be necessary. When you are taking this combination medicine, it is especially important that your health care professional know if you are taking any of the following:

- Antacids or
- Diarrhea medicine containing kaolin or attapulgite—These medicines may decrease the effects of the belladonna alkaloids and the phenobarbital in this combination medicine; to prevent this, take the 2 medicines at least 1 hour apart
- Anticoagulants (blood thinners)—The phenobarbital in this combination medicine may decrease the effects of anticoagulants; a change in the dose of anticoagulant may be needed
- Anticholinergics (medicine for abdominal or stomach spasms or cramps) or
- Carbamazepine (e.g., Tegretol) or
- Central nervous system (CNS) depressants (medicine that causes drowsiness) or
- Cocaine or
- Contraceptives, oral, (birth control pills) containing estrogens or progestins or
- Digitalis glycosides (heart medicine) or
- Monoamine oxidase (MAO) inhibitors (furazolidone [e.g., Furoxone], isocarboxazid [e.g., Marplan], phenelzine [e.g., Nardil], procarbazine [e.g., Matulane], selegiline [e.g., Eldepryl], tranylcypromine [e.g., Parnate] (taken currently or within the past 2 weeks) or

- Other ergot medicines (dihydroergotamine [e.g., D.H.E. 45], ergoloid mesylates [e.g., Hydergine], ergonovine [e.g., Ergotrate], methylergonovine [e.g., Methergine], methysergide [e.g., Sansert]) or
- Other medicines for migraine that contain ergotamine in combination with other ingredients, such as ergotamine and caffeine (e.g., Cafergot), or
- Potassium chloride (e.g., Kay Ciel) or
- Tricyclic antidepressants (amitriptyline [e.g., Elavil], amoxapine [e.g., Asendin], clomipramine [e.g., Anafranil], desipramine [e.g., Pertofrane], doxepin [e.g., Sinequan], imipramine [e.g., Tofranil], nortriptyline [e.g., Aventyl], protriptyline [e.g., Vivactil], trimipramine [e.g., Surmontil])—The chance of serious side effects may be increased
- Ketoconazole (e.g., Nizoral)—The belladonna alkaloids in this combination medicine may reduce the effects of ketoconazole; to prevent this, take the ergotamine, belladonna alkaloids, and phenobarbital combination at least 2 hours after taking ketoconazole

**Other medical problems**—The presence of other medical problems may affect the use of this combination medicine. Make sure you tell your doctor if you have any other medical problems, especially:

- Asthma (or history of), emphysema, or other chronic lung disease or
- Brain damage (in children) or
- Difficult urination or
- Down's syndrome (mongolism) or
- Dry mouth (severe and continuing) or
- Enlarged prostate or
- Heart or blood vessel disease or
- High blood pressure (severe) or
- Hyperactivity (in children) or
- Infection or
- Intestinal blockage or other intestinal problems or
- Itching (severe) or
- Kidney disease or
- Liver disease or
- Overactive thyroid or
- Porphyria or
- Spastic paralysis (in children) or
- Urinary tract blockage—The chance of side effects may be increased
- Glaucoma—The belladonna alkaloids in this combination medicine may make your condition worse

Also tell your doctor if you have recently had an angioplasty (a procedure done to improve the flow of blood in a blocked blood vessel) or surgery on a blood vessel, because the chance of side effects caused by the ergotamine in this combination medicine may be increased.

## Proper Use of This Medicine

*Take this medicine only as directed by your doctor.* If the amount you are to take does not seem to work, do not take more than your doctor ordered. Instead, check with your doctor. Taking too much of this medicine or taking it too often may cause serious effects such as nausea and vomiting; cold, painful hands or feet; or even gangrene. Also, if too much is used, it may become habit-forming.

To take the *extended-release tablet* form of this medicine:
- Swallow the tablet whole.
- Do not crush, break, or chew the tablet before swallowing it.

**Dosing**—The dose of this combination medicine will be different for different patients. *Follow your doctor's orders or the directions on the label.* The following information includes only the average doses of this medicine. *If your dose is different, do not change it* unless your doctor tells you to do so.
- For *oral tablet* dosage form:
  —For relieving symptoms of menopause and for preventing headaches:
    - Adults—One tablet in the morning, one tablet at noon, and two tablets at bedtime.
    - Children—Use and dose must be determined by your doctor.
- For *oral extended-release tablet* dosage form:
  —For relieving symptoms of menopause and for preventing headaches:
    - Adults—One tablet in the morning and one tablet in the evening.
    - Children—Use and dose must be determined by your doctor.

**Missed dose**—If you miss a dose of this medicine, skip the missed dose and go back to your regular dosing schedule. Do not double doses.

**Storage**—To store this medicine:
- Keep out of the reach of children since overdose is especially dangerous in children.
- Store away from heat and direct light.
- Do not store in the bathroom, near the kitchen sink, or in other damp places. Heat and moisture may cause the medicine to break down.
- Do not keep outdated medicine or medicine no longer needed. Be sure that any discarded medicine is out of the reach of children.

## Precautions While Using This Medicine

If you have been taking this medicine regularly, *do not stop taking it without first checking with your doctor.* Your doctor may want you to reduce gradually the amount you are using before stopping completely.

Do not take antacids or medicine for diarrhea within 1 hour of taking this medicine. Taking them too close together will make the belladonna alkaloids less effective.

This medicine will add to the effects of alcohol and other CNS depressants (medicines that slow down the nervous system, possibly causing drowsiness). Some examples of CNS depressants are antihistamines or medicine for hay fever, other allergies, or colds; sedatives, tranquilizers, or sleeping medicine; prescription pain medicine or narcotics; other barbiturates; medicine for seizures; muscle relaxants; or anesthetics, including some dental anesthetics. *Check with your doctor before taking any of the above*

*while you are taking this medicine.* Also, alcohol may make headaches worse, so it is best to avoid alcoholic beverages if you are taking this medicine to prevent headaches.

This medicine may cause some people to have blurred vision or to become drowsy, dizzy, lightheaded, or less alert than they are normally. *Make sure you know how you react to this medicine before you drive, use machines, or do anything else that could be dangerous if you are dizzy or are not alert and able to see well.*

Since smoking may increase some of the harmful effects of this medicine, it is best to avoid smoking while you are using it. If you have any questions about this, check with your doctor.

This medicine may make you more sensitive to cold temperatures, especially if you have blood circulation problems. It tends to decrease blood circulation in the skin, fingers, and toes. Dress warmly during cold weather and be careful during prolonged exposure to cold, such as in winter sports. This is especially important for elderly people, who are more likely than younger adults to already have problems with their circulation.

Belladonna alkaloids (contained in this combination medicine) will often make you sweat less, causing your body temperature to increase. *Use extra care not to become overheated during exercise or hot weather while you are taking this medicine,* as overheating may result in a heat stroke. Also, hot baths or saunas may make you feel dizzy or faint while you are taking this medicine. This is especially important in children taking this medicine.

This medicine may cause your eyes to become more sensitive to light than they are normally. Wearing sunglasses may help lessen the discomfort from bright light.

If you have a serious infection or illness of any kind, check with your doctor before taking this medicine, since you may be more sensitive to its effects.

This medicine may cause dryness of the mouth, nose and throat. For temporary relief of mouth dryness, use sugarless candy or gum, melt bits of ice in your mouth, or use a saliva substitute. However, if dry mouth continues for more than 2 weeks, check with your medical doctor or dentist. Continuing dryness of the mouth may increase the chance of dental disease, including tooth decay, gum disease, and fungus infections.

## Side Effects of This Medicine

Along with its needed effects, a medicine may cause some unwanted effects. Although not all of these side effects may occur, if they do occur they may need medical attention.

*Check with your doctor immediately* if the following side effects occur, because they may mean that you are developing a problem with blood circulation:
*Less common or rare*
  Anxiety or confusion (severe); change in vision; chest pain; increase in blood pressure; pain in arms, legs, or lower

back, especially if pain occurs in your calves or heels while you are walking; pale, bluish-colored, or cold hands or feet (not caused by cold temperatures and occurring together with other side effects listed in this section); red or violet-colored blisters on the skin of the hands or feet

*Also check with your doctor immediately* if any of the following side effects occur since they may be symptoms of an overdose:

Convulsions (seizures); diarrhea, nausea, vomiting, or stomach pain or bloating (severe) occurring together with other signs of overdose or of problems with blood circulation; dizziness, drowsiness, or weakness (severe), occurring together with other signs of overdose or of problems with blood circulation; fast or slow heartbeat; shortness of breath; unusual excitement

Also check with your doctor as soon as possible if any of the following side effects occur:

*More common*

Swelling of face, fingers, feet, and/or lower legs

*Less common or rare*

Skin rash, hives, or itching; sore throat and fever; unusual bleeding or bruising; weakness in legs; yellow eyes or skin

Other side effects may occur that usually do not need medical attention. These side effects may go away during treatment as your body adjusts to the medicine. However, check with your doctor if any of the following side effects continue or are bothersome:

*More common*

Constipation; decreased sweating; dizziness or lightheadedness; drowsiness; dryness of mouth, nose, throat, or skin

*Less common or rare*

Blurred vision, diarrhea, nausea, or vomiting (occurring without other signs of overdose or blood circulation problems); difficult urination (especially in older men); difficulty in swallowing; increased sensitivity of eyes to sunlight; loss of memory; reduced sweating; unusual excitement (especially in older adults); unusual tiredness or weakness

After you stop taking this medicine, your body may need time to adjust. The length of time this takes depends on the amount of medicine you were taking and how long you took it. During this time check with your doctor if your headaches or other symptoms begin again or worsen.

Other side effects not listed above may also occur in some patients. If you notice any other effects, check with your doctor.

---

Revised: 08/30/94

# ERYTHROMYCIN  Ophthalmic

A commonly used brand name in the U.S. and Canada is Ilotycin. Generic name product may also be available in the U.S.

## Description

Erythromycin (eh-rith-roe-MYE-sin) belongs to the family of medicines called antibiotics. Erythromycin ophthalmic preparations are used to treat infections of the eye. They also may be used to prevent certain eye infections of newborn babies, such as neonatal conjunctivitis and ophthalmia neonatorum. They may be used with other medicines for some eye infections.

Erythromycin is available only with your doctor's prescription, in the following dosage form:

*Ophthalmic*
• Ophthalmic ointment (U.S. and Canada)

## Before Using This Medicine

In deciding to use a medicine, the risks of taking the medicine must be weighed against the good it will do. This is a decision you and your doctor will make. For ophthalmic erythromycin, the following should be considered:

**Allergies**—Tell your doctor if you have ever had any unusual or allergic reaction to this or any of the other erythromycins. Also tell your health care professional if you are allergic to any other substances, such as preservatives.

**Pregnancy**—Ophthalmic erythromycin has not been shown to cause birth defects or other problems in humans.

**Breast-feeding**—Ophthalmic erythromycin has not been reported to cause problems in nursing babies.

**Children**—Studies on this medicine have been done only in adult patients, and there is no specific information comparing use of this medicine in children with use in other age groups.

**Older adults**—Many medicines have not been studied specifically in older people. Therefore, it may not be known whether they work exactly the same way they do in younger adults or if they cause different side effects or problems in older people. There is no specific information comparing use of this medicine in the elderly with use in other age groups.

## Proper Use of This Medicine

To use:
• First, wash your hands. Tilt the head back and with the index finger of one hand, press gently on the skin just beneath the lower eyelid and pull the lower eye lid away from the eye to make a space. Squeeze a thin strip of ointment into this space. A 1-cm (approximately 1/3-inch) strip of ointment is usually

enough unless otherwise directed by your doctor. Let go of the eyelid and gently close the eyes and keep them closed for 1 or 2 minutes, to allow the medicine to come into contact with the infection.

- To keep the medicine as germ-free as possible, do not touch the applicator tip to any surface (including the eye). After using erythromycin eye ointment, wipe the tip of the ointment tube with a clean tissue and keep the tube tightly closed.

To help clear up your infection completely, *keep using this medicine for the full time of treatment,* even if your symptoms begin to clear up after a few days. If you stop using this medicine too soon, your symptoms may return. *Do not miss any doses.*

**Dosing**—The dose of ophthalmic erythromycin will be different for different patients. *Follow your doctor's orders or the directions on the label.* The following information includes only the average doses of ophthalmic erythromycin. *If your dose is different, do not change it* unless your doctor tells you to do so.

- For *ophthalmic ointment* dosage form:
  —For treatment of eye infections:
  - Adults and children—Use once a day or more often as directed by your doctor.
  —For prevention of neonatal conjunctivitis and ophthalmia neonatorum:
  - Newborn babies—Use once at birth.

**Missed dose**—If you do miss a dose of this medicine, apply it as soon as possible. However, if it is almost time for your next dose, skip the missed dose and go back to your regular dosing schedule.

**Storage**—To store this medicine:
- Keep out of the reach of children.
- Store away from heat and direct light.
- Keep the medicine from freezing.
- Do not keep outdated medicine or medicine no longer needed. Be sure that any discarded medicine is out of the reach of children.

## Precautions While Using This Medicine

If your symptoms do not improve within a few days, or if they become worse, check with your doctor.

After application, eye ointments usually cause your vision to blur for a few minutes.

## Side Effects of This Medicine

Along with its needed effects, a medicine may cause some unwanted effects.

Check with your doctor as soon as possible if the following side effect occurs:
*Rare*
  Eye irritation not present before therapy

Other side effects not listed above may also occur in some patients. If you notice any other effects, check with your doctor.

Revised: 06/30/92
Interim revision: 08/17/93

# ERYTHROMYCIN    Topical

Some commonly used brand names are:
**In the U.S.—**

| | |
|---|---|
| Akne-Mycin | Erymax |
| A/T/S | Ery-Sol |
| Erycette | ETS |
| EryDerm | Staticin |
| Erygel | T-Stat |

Generic name product may also be available.
**In Canada—**
Sans-Acne
Staticin

## Description

Erythromycin (eh-rith-roe-MYE-sin) belongs to the family of medicines called antibiotics. Erythromycin topical preparations are used on the skin to help control acne. They may be used alone or with one or more other medicines that are applied to the skin or taken by mouth for acne. They may also be used for other problems, such as skin infections, as determined by your doctor.

Erythromycin is available only with your doctor's prescription, in the following dosage forms:

*Topical*
- Gel (U.S.)
- Ointment (U.S.)
- Pledgets (U.S.)
- Solution (U.S. and Canada)

## Before Using This Medicine

In deciding to use a medicine, the risks of taking the medicine must be weighed against the good it will do. This is a decision you and your doctor will make. For topical erythromycin, the following should be considered:

**Allergies**—Tell your doctor if you have ever had any unusual or allergic reaction to this or any of the other erythromycins. Also tell your health care professional if you are allergic to any other substances, such as preservatives or dyes.

**Pregnancy**—Topical erythromycin has not been studied in pregnant women. However, this medication has not been shown to cause birth defects or other problems in animal studies.

**Breast-feeding**—It is not known whether topical erythromycin passes into the breast milk. Erythromycin, given by mouth or by injection, does pass into the breast milk. However, erythromycin topical preparations have not been reported to cause problems in nursing babies.

**Children**—Erythromycin topical solution has been tested in children 12 years of age and older and, in effective doses, has not been shown to cause different side effects or problems than it does in adults.

**Older adults**—Many medicines have not been studied specifically in older people. Therefore, it may not be known whether they work exactly the same way they do in younger adults. Although there is no specific information comparing use of topical erythromycin in the elderly with use in other age groups, this medicine is not expected to cause different side effects or problems in older people than it does in younger adults.

**Other medicines**—Although certain medicines should not be used together at all, in other cases two different medicines may be used together even if an interaction might occur. In these cases, your doctor may want to change the dose, or other precautions may be necessary. Tell your health care professional if you are using any other topical prescription or nonprescription (over-the-counter [OTC]) medicine that is to be applied to the same area of the skin.

## Proper Use of This Medicine

Before applying this medicine, thoroughly wash the affected area with warm water and soap, rinse well, and pat dry. After washing or shaving, it is best to wait 30 minutes before applying the pledget (swab), topical gel, or topical liquid form. The alcohol in them may irritate freshly washed or shaved skin.

This medicine will not cure your acne. However, to help keep your acne under control, *keep using this medicine for the full time of treatment,* even if your symptoms begin to clear up after a few days. You may have to continue using this medicine every day for months or even longer in some cases. If you stop using this medicine too soon, your symptoms may return. *It is important that you do not miss any doses.*

**Dosing**—The dose of topical erythromycin will be different for different patients. *Follow your doctor's orders or the directions on the label.* The following information includes only the average doses of topical erythromycin. *If your dose is different, do not change it unless* your doctor tells you to do so.

- For acne:
  —For *gel* dosage form:
    • Adults—Apply to the affected area(s) of the skin two times a day, morning and evening.
    • Children—Dose must be determined by your doctor.
  —For *ointment* dosage form:
    • Adults, teenagers, and children—Apply to the affected area(s) of the skin two times a day, morning and evening.
  —For *pledgets* dosage form:
    • Adults, teenagers, and children—Apply to the affected area(s) of the skin two times a day.
  —For *topical solution* dosage form:
    • Adults, teenagers, and children 12 years of age and over—Apply to the affected area(s) of the skin two times a day, morning and evening.
    • Children up to 12 years of age—Dose must be determined by your doctor.

**Missed dose**—If you miss a dose of this medicine, apply it as soon as possible. However, if it is almost time for your next dose, skip the missed dose and go back to your regular dosing schedule.

For patients using the pledget (swab), topical gel, or topical liquid form of erythromycin:

- These forms contain alcohol and are flammable. *Do not use near heat, near open flame, or while smoking.*
- It is important that you do not use this medicine more often than your doctor ordered. It may cause your skin to become too dry or irritated.
- Also, you should avoid washing the acne-affected areas too often. This may dry your skin and make your acne worse. Washing with a mild, bland soap 2 or 3 times a day should be enough, unless you have oily skin. If you have any questions about this, check with your doctor.
- To use:
  —The topical liquid form of this medicine may come in a bottle with an applicator tip, which may be used to apply the medicine directly to the skin. Use the applicator with a dabbing motion instead of a rolling motion (not like a roll-on deodorant, for example). If the medicine does not come in an applicator bottle, you may moisten a pad with the medicine and then rub the pad over the whole affected area. Or you may also apply this medicine with your fingertips. Be sure to wash the medicine off your hands afterward.
  —Apply a thin film of medicine, using enough to cover the affected area lightly. *You should apply the medicine to the whole area usually affected by acne, not just to the pimples themselves.* This will help keep new pimples from breaking out.
  —The pledget (swab) form should be rubbed over the whole affected area. You may use extra pledgets (swabs), if needed, to cover larger areas.
  —Since these medicines contain alcohol, they may sting or burn. Therefore, *do not get these medicines in the eyes, nose, mouth, or on other mucous membranes.* Spread the medicine away from these areas when applying. If these medicines do get in the eyes,

wash them out immediately, but carefully, with large amounts of cool tap water. If your eyes still burn or are painful, check with your doctor.

**Storage**—To store this medicine:
- Keep out of the reach of children.
- Store away from heat and direct light.
- Keep the medicine from freezing.
- Do not keep outdated medicine or medicine no longer needed. Be sure that any discarded medicine is out of the reach of children.

## Precautions While Using This Medicine

If your acne does not improve within 3 to 4 weeks, or if it becomes worse, check with your health care professional. However, treatment of acne may take up to 8 to 12 weeks before you see full improvement.

For patients using the pledget (swab), topical gel, or topical liquid form of erythromycin:
- If your doctor has ordered another medicine to be applied to the skin along with this medicine, it is best to wait at least 1 hour before you apply the second medicine. This may help keep your skin from becoming too irritated. Also, if the medicines are used too close together, they may not work properly.
- After application of this medicine to the skin, mild stinging or burning may be expected and may last up to a few minutes or more.
- This medicine may also cause the skin to become unusually dry, even with normal use. If this occurs, check with your doctor.

- You may continue to use cosmetics (make-up) while you are using this medicine for acne. However, it is best to use only "water-base" cosmetics. Also, it is best not to use cosmetics too heavily or too often. They may make your acne worse. If you have any questions about this, check with your doctor.

## Side Effects of This Medicine

Along with its needed effects, a medicine may cause some unwanted effects. The following side effects may go away during treatment as your body adjusts to the medicine. However, check with your doctor if any of the following side effects continue or are bothersome:

*For erythromycin ointment*
*Less common*
   Peeling; redness
*For erythromycin pledget (swab), topical gel, or topical liquid form*
*More common*
   Dry or scaly skin; irritation; itching; stinging or burning feeling
*Less common*
   Peeling; redness

Other side effects not listed above may also occur in some patients. If you notice any other effects, check with your doctor.

Revised: 06/23/92
Interim revision: 06/07/94

# ERYTHROMYCIN AND BENZOYL PEROXIDE   Topical†

A commonly used brand name in the U.S. is Benzamycin.

†Not commercially available in Canada.

## Description

Erythromycin (eh-rith-roe-MYE-sin) and benzoyl peroxide (BEN-zoe-ill per-OX-ide) combination is used to help control acne.

This medicine is applied to the skin. It may be used alone or with other medicines that are applied to the skin or taken by mouth for acne.

Erythromycin and benzoyl peroxide combination is available only with your doctor's prescription, in the following dosage form:
*Topical*
- Topical gel (U.S.)

## Before Using This Medicine

In deciding to use a medicine, the risks of using the medicine must be weighed against the good it will do.

This is a decision you and your doctor will make. For erythromycin and benzoyl peroxide combination, the following should be considered:

**Allergies**—Tell your doctor if you have ever had any unusual or allergic reaction to this medicine, to any of the other erythromycins, or to benzoyl peroxide (e.g., PanOxyl). Also tell your health care professional if you are allergic to any other substances, such as preservatives or dyes.

**Pregnancy**—Studies on effects in pregnancy have not been done in either humans or animals. However, the benzoyl peroxide in this medicine may be absorbed into the body. Before using this medicine, make sure your doctor knows if you are pregnant or if you may become pregnant.

**Breast-feeding**—It is not known whether topical erythromycin or topical benzoyl peroxide passes into the breast milk. Erythromycin (e.g., E-Mycin), given by mouth or by injection, does pass into the breast milk. In addition, the benzoyl peroxide in this medicine may be absorbed into the mother's body. However, erythromycin and benzoyl peroxide combination has not been reported to cause problems in nursing babies.

**Children**—Studies on this medicine have been done only in adult patients, and there is no specific information comparing use of this medicine in children up to 12 years of age with use in other age groups.

**Older adults**—Many medicines have not been studied specifically in older people. Therefore, it may not be known whether they work exactly the same way they do in younger adults or if they cause different side effects or problems in older people. There is no specific information comparing use of this medicine in the elderly with use in other age groups.

**Other medicines**—Although certain medicines should not be used together at all, in other cases two different medicines may be used together even if an interaction might occur. In these cases, your doctor may want to change the dose, or other precautions may be necessary. Tell your health care professional if you are using any other topical prescription or nonprescription (over-the-counter [OTC]) medicine that is to be applied to the same area of the skin.

---

## Proper Use of This Medicine

*Do not use this medicine on raw or irritated skin.*

Before applying this medicine, thoroughly wash the affected area(s) with warm water and soap, rinse well, and gently pat dry. After washing or shaving, it is best to wait 30 minutes before applying the medicine. The alcohol in it may irritate freshly washed or shaved skin.

Avoid washing the acne-affected area(s) too often. This may dry your skin and make your acne worse. Washing with a mild, bland soap 2 or 3 times a day should be enough, unless you have oily skin. If you have any questions about this, check with your doctor.

To use:
- *Use this medicine only as directed.* Do not use more of it and do not use it more often than your doctor ordered. To do so may cause your skin to become too dry or irritated.
- After washing the affected area(s), you may apply this medicine with your fingertips. However, be sure to wash the medicine off your hands afterward.
- Apply and rub in a thin film of medicine, using enough to cover the affected area(s) lightly. *You should apply the medicine to the whole area usually affected by acne, not just to the pimples themselves.*
- Since this medicine contains alcohol, it may sting or burn. Therefore, *do not get this medicine in or around your eyes, nose, or mouth, or on other mucous membranes.* Spread the medicine away from these areas when applying. If this medicine does get in your eyes, wash them out immediately, but carefully, with large amounts of cool tap water. If your eyes still burn or are painful, check with your doctor.

Do not use this medicine after the expiration date on the label. The medicine may not work properly. Get a fresh supply from your pharmacist. Check with your pharmacist if you have any questions about this.

To help keep your acne under control, *keep using this medicine for the full time of treatment.* You may have to continue using this medicine every day for months or even longer in some cases.

**Dosing**—The dose of erythromycin and benzoyl peroxide combination will be different for different patients. *Follow your doctor's orders or the directions on the label.* The following information includes only the average dose of erythromycin and benzoyl peroxide combination. *If your dose is different, do not change it unless your doctor tells you to do so.*
- For *gel* dosage form:
  —For acne:
    - Adults and children 12 years of age and over—Apply to the affected area(s) of the skin two times a day, morning and evening, or as directed by your doctor.
    - Children up to 12 years of age—Dose must be determined by your doctor.

**Missed dose**—If you miss a dose of this medicine, apply it as soon as possible. However, if it is almost time for your next dose, skip the missed dose and go back to your regular dosing schedule.

**Storage**—To store this medicine:
- Keep out of the reach of children.
- Store in the refrigerator. Heat will cause this medicine to break down. However, keep the medicine from freezing. Follow the directions on the label.
- Do not keep outdated medicine or medicine no longer needed. Be sure that any discarded medicine is out of the reach of children.

---

## Precautions While Using This Medicine

If your acne does not improve within 3 to 4 weeks, or if it becomes worse, check with your health care professional. However, treatment of acne may take up to 8 to 12 weeks before you see full improvement.

If your doctor has ordered another medicine to be applied to the skin along with this medicine, it is best to apply the second medicine at least 1 hour after you apply the first medicine. This may help keep your skin from becoming too irritated. Also, if the medicines are used too close together, they may not work properly.

Mild stinging or burning of the skin may be expected after this medicine is applied. These effects may last up to a few minutes or more. If irritation continues, check with your doctor. You may have to use the medicine less often. Follow your doctor's directions.

This medicine may also cause the skin to become unusually dry, even with normal use. If this occurs, check with your doctor.

*This medicine may bleach hair or colored fabrics.*

You may continue to use cosmetics (make-up) while you are using this medicine for acne. However, it is best to use only "oil-free" cosmetics. Also, it is best not to use cosmetics too heavily or too often. They may make your acne worse. If you have any questions about this, check with your doctor.

## Side Effects of This Medicine

Along with its needed effects, a medicine may cause some unwanted effects. Although not all of these side effects may occur, if they do occur they may need medical attention.

Check with your doctor as soon as possible if any of the following side effects occur:

*Less common or rare*
> Burning, blistering, crusting, itching, severe redness, or swelling of the skin; painful irritation of the skin; skin rash

*Symptoms of topical overdose*
> Burning, itching, scaling, redness, or swelling of the skin (severe)

Other side effects may occur that usually do not need medical attention. These side effects may go away during treatment as your body adjusts to the medicine. However, check with your doctor if any of the following side effects continue or are bothersome:

*Less common*
> Dryness or peeling of the skin; feeling of warmth, mild stinging, or redness of the skin

Other side effects not listed above may also occur in some patients. If you notice any other effects, check with your doctor.

Revised: 06/26/92
Interim revision: 07/06/94

# ERYTHROMYCINS   Systemic

Some commonly used brand names are:

**In the U.S.—**

| | |
|---|---|
| E-Base[1] | Erythrocin[5, 6] |
| E-Mycin[1] | Erythrocot[6] |
| ERYC[1] | Ilotycin[1, 4] |
| Ery-Tab | Ilosone[2] |
| E.E.S.[3] | My-E[6] |
| EryPed[3] | PCE[1] |
| Erythro[3] | Wintrocin[6] |

**In Canada—**

| | |
|---|---|
| Apo-Erythro[1] | ERYC-333[1] |
| Apo-Erythro E-C[1] | Erythrocin[5, 6] |
| Apo-Erythro-ES[3] | Erythromid[1] |
| Apo-Erythro-S[6] | Ilosone[2] |
| E-Mycin[1] | Ilotycin[4] |
| E.E.S.[3] | Novo-rythro[2, 6] |
| Erybid[1] | Novo-rythro Encap[1] |
| EryPed[3] | PCE[1] |
| ERYC-250[1] | |

Note: For quick reference, the following erythromycins are numbered to match the corresponding brand names.

This information applies to the following medicines:

1. Erythromycin Base (er-ith-roe-MYE-sin)‡§
2. Erythromycin Estolate (ESS-toe-layt)‡
3. Erythromycin Ethylsuccinate (eth-ill-SUK-sin-ayt)‡
4. Erythromycin Gluceptate (gloo-SEP-tayt)
5. Erythromycin Lactobionate (lak-toe-BYE-oh-nayt)‡
6. Erythromycin Stearate (STEER-ate)‡

‡Generic name product may also be available in the U.S.
§Generic name product may also be available in Canada.

## Description

Erythromycins (eh-rith-roe-MYE-sins) are used to treat many kinds of infections. Erythromycins are also used to prevent "strep" infections in patients with a history of rheumatic heart disease who may be allergic to penicillin.

These medicines may also be used to treat Legionnaires' disease and for other problems as determined by your doctor. They will not work for colds, flu, or other virus infections.

Erythromycins are available only with your doctor's prescription, in the following dosage forms:

*Oral*

Erythromycin Base
- Delayed-release capsules (U.S. and Canada)
- Delayed-release tablets (U.S. and Canada)
- Tablets (U.S. and Canada)

Erythromycin Estolate
- Capsules (U.S. and Canada)
- Oral suspension (U.S. and Canada)
- Tablets (U.S. and Canada)

Erythromycin Ethylsuccinate
- Chewable tablets (U.S. and Canada)
- Oral suspension (U.S. and Canada)
- Tablets (U.S. and Canada)

Erythromycin Stearate
- Oral suspension (Canada)
- Tablets (U.S. and Canada)

*Parenteral*

Erythromycin Gluceptate
- Injection (U.S. and Canada)

Erythromycin Lactobionate
- Injection (U.S. and Canada)

## Before Using This Medicine

In deciding to use a medicine, the risks of taking the medicine must be weighed against the good it will do.

This is a decision you and your doctor will make. For erythromycins, the following should be considered:

**Allergies**—Tell your doctor if you have ever had any unusual or allergic reaction to erythromycins, or any related medicines, such as azithromycin or clarithromycin. Also tell your health care professional if you are allergic to any other substances, such as foods, preservatives, or dyes.

**Pregnancy**—Erythromycin estolate has caused side effects involving the liver in some pregnant women. However, none of the erythromycins has been shown to cause birth defects or other problems in human babies.

**Breast-feeding**—Erythromycins pass into the breast milk. However, erythromycins have not been shown to cause problems in nursing babies.

**Children**—This medicine has been tested in children and, in effective doses, has not been shown to cause different side effects or problems in children than it does in adults.

**Older adults**—This medicine has been tested and has not been shown to cause different side effects or problems in older people than it does in younger adults. However, older adults may be at increased risk of hearing loss, especially if they are taking high doses of erythromycin and/or have kidney or liver disease.

**Other medicines**—Although certain medicines should not be used together at all, in other cases two different medicines may be used together even if an interaction might occur. In these cases, your doctor may want to change the dose, or other precautions may be necessary. When you are taking or receiving erythromycins, it is especially important that your health care professional know if you are taking any of the following:
- Acetaminophen (e.g., Tylenol) (with long-term, high-dose use) or
- Amiodarone (e.g., Cordarone) or
- Anabolic steroids (nandrolone [e.g., Anabolin], oxandrolone [e.g., Anavar], oxymetholone [e.g., Anadrol], stanozolol [e.g., Winstrol]) or
- Androgens (male hormones) or
- Antithyroid agents (medicine for overactive thyroid) or
- Carmustine (e.g., BiCNU) or
- Chloroquine (e.g., Aralen) or
- Dantrolene (e.g., Dantrium) or
- Daunorubicin (e.g., Cerubidine) or
- Disulfiram (e.g., Antabuse) or
- Divalproex (e.g., Depakote) or
- Estrogens (female hormones) or
- Etretinate (e.g., Tegison) or
- Gold salts (medicine for arthritis) or
- Hydroxychloroquine (e.g., Plaquenil) or
- Mercaptopurine (e.g., Purinethol) or
- Methotrexate (e.g., Mexate) or
- Methyldopa (e.g., Aldomet) or
- Naltrexone (e.g., Trexan) (with long-term, high-dose use) or
- Oral contraceptives (birth control pills) containing estrogen or
- Other anti-infectives by mouth or by injection (medicine for infection) or
- Phenothiazines (acetophenazine [e.g., Tindal], chlorpromazine [e.g., Thorazine], fluphenazine [e.g., Prolixin],

mesoridazine [e.g., Serentil], perphenazine [e.g., Trilafon], prochlorperazine [e.g., Compazine], promazine [e.g., Sparine], promethazine [e.g., Phenergan], thioridazine [e.g., Mellaril], trifluoperazine [e.g., Stelazine], triflupromazine [e.g., Vesprin], trimeprazine [e.g., Temaril]) or
- Phenytoin (e.g., Dilantin) or
- Plicamycin (e.g., Mithracin) or
- Valproic acid (e.g., Depakene)—Use of these medicines with erythromycins, especially erythromycin estolate, may increase the chance of liver problems
- Aminophylline (e.g., Somophyllin) or
- Caffeine (e.g., NoDoz) or
- Oxtriphylline (e.g., Choledyl) or
- Theophylline (e.g., Somophyllin-T, Theo-Dur)—Use of these medicines with erythromycins may increase the chance of side effects from aminophylline, caffeine, oxtriphylline, or theophylline
- Astemizole (e.g., Hismanal) or
- Terfenadine (e.g., Seldane)—Use of astemizole or terfenadine with erythromycins may cause heart problems, such as an irregular heartbeat; these medicines should not be used together
- Carbamazepine (e.g., Tegretol)—Use of carbamazepine with erythromycin may increase the side effects of carbamazepine or increase the chance of liver problems
- Chloramphenicol (e.g., Chloromycetin) or
- Clindamycin (e.g., Cleocin) or
- Lincomycin (e.g., Lincocin)—Use of these medicines with erythromycins may decrease the effectiveness of these other antibiotics
- Cyclosporine (e.g., Sandimmune) or
- Warfarin (e.g., Coumadin)—Use of any of these medicines with erythromycins may increase the side effects of these medicines

**Other medical problems**—The presence of other medical problems may affect the use of erythromycins. Make sure you tell your doctor if you have any other medical problems, especially:
- Heart disease—High doses of erythromycin may increase the chance of side effects in patients with a history of an irregular heartbeat
- Liver disease—Erythromycins, especially erythromycin estolate, may increase the chance of side effects involving the liver
- Loss of hearing—High doses of erythromycins may, on rare occasion, cause hearing loss, especially if you have kidney or liver disease

## Proper Use of This Medicine

Generally, erythromycins are best taken with a full glass (8 ounces) of water on an empty stomach (at least 1 hour before or 2 hours after meals). If stomach upset occurs, these medicines may be taken with food. If you have questions about the erythromycin medicine you are taking, check with your health care professional.

For patients taking the *oral liquid form* of this medicine:
- This medicine is to be taken by mouth even if it comes in a dropper bottle. If this medicine does not come in a dropper bottle, use a specially marked measuring spoon or other device to measure each

dose accurately. The average household teaspoon may not hold the right amount of liquid.

- Do not use after the expiration date on the label. The medicine may not work properly after that date. Check with your pharmacist if you have any questions about this.

For patients taking the *chewable tablet form* of this medicine:

- Tablets must be chewed or crushed before they are swallowed.

For patients taking the *delayed-release capsule form (with enteric-coated pellets) or the delayed-release tablet form* of this medicine:

- Swallow capsules or tablets whole. Do not break or crush. If you are not sure about which type of capsule or tablet you are taking, check with your pharmacist.

To help clear up your infection completely, *keep taking this medicine for the full time of treatment,* even if you begin to feel better after a few days. *If you have a "strep" infection, you should keep taking this medicine for at least 10 days. This is especially important in "strep" infections. Serious heart problems could develop later* if your infection is not cleared up completely. Also, if you stop taking this medicine too soon, your symptoms may return.

This medicine works best when there is a constant amount in the blood. *To help keep the amount constant, do not miss any doses. Also, it is best to take the doses at evenly spaced times day and night.* For example, if you are to take 4 doses a day, the doses should be spaced about 6 hours apart. If this interferes with your sleep or other daily activities, or if you need help in planning the best times to take your medicine, check with your health care professional.

**Dosing**—The dose of erythromycin will be different for different patients. *Follow your doctor's orders or the directions on the label.* The following information includes only the average doses of erythromycin. *If your dose is different, do not change it* unless your doctor tells you to do so.

The number of capsules or tablets or teaspoonfuls of suspension that you take depends on the strength of the medicine. Also, *the number of doses you take each day, the time allowed between doses, and the length of time you take the medicine depend on the medical problem for which you are taking erythromycin.*

*For erythromycin base*

- For *oral* dosage forms (capsules, tablets):
  - —For treatment of infections:
    - Adults and teenagers—250 to 500 milligrams (mg) two to four times a day.
    - Children—Dose is based on body weight. The usual dose is 7.5 to 12.5 mg per kilogram (kg) (3.4 to 5.6 mg per pound) of body weight four

times a day, or 15 to 25 mg per kg (6.8 to 11.4 mg per pound) of body weight two times a day.
  - —For prevention of heart infections:
    - Adults and teenagers—Take 1 gram two hours before your dental appointment or surgery, then 500 mg six hours after taking the first dose.
    - Children—Dose is based on body weight. The usual dose is 20 mg per kg (9.1 mg per pound) of body weight two hours before the dental appointment or surgery, then 10 mg per kg (4.5 mg per pound) of body weight six hours after taking the first dose.

*For erythromycin estolate*

- For *oral* dosage forms (capsules, oral suspension, tablets):
  - —For treatment of infections:
    - Adults and teenagers—250 to 500 milligrams (mg) two to four times a day.
    - Children—Dose is based on body weight. The usual dose is 7.5 to 12.5 mg per kilogram (kg) (3.4 to 5.6 mg per pound) of body weight four times a day, or 15 to 25 mg per kg (6.8 to 11.4 mg per pound) of body weight two times a day.
  - —For prevention of heart infections:
    - Adults and teenagers—Take 1 gram two hours before your dental appointment or surgery, then 500 mg six hours after taking the first dose.
    - Children—Dose is based on body weight. The usual dose is 20 mg per kg (9.1 mg per pound) of body weight two hours before the dental appointment or surgery, then 10 mg per kg (4.5 mg per pound) of body weight six hours after taking the first dose.

*For erythromycin ethylsuccinate*

- For *oral* dosage forms (oral suspension, tablets):
  - —For treatment of infections:
    - Adults and teenagers—400 to 800 milligrams (mg) two to four times a day.
    - Children—Dose is based on body weight. The usual dose is 7.5 to 12.5 mg per kilogram (kg) (3.4 to 5.6 mg per pound) of body weight four times a day, or 15 to 25 mg per kg (6.8 to 11.4 mg per pound) of body weight two times a day.
  - —For prevention of heart infections:
    - Adults and teenagers—Take 1.6 grams two hours before your dental appointment or surgery, then 800 mg six hours after taking the first dose.
    - Children—Dose is based on body weight. The usual dose is 20 mg per kg (9.1 mg per pound) of body weight two hours before the dental appointment or surgery, then 10 mg per kg (4.5 mg per pound) of body weight six hours after taking the first dose.

*For erythromycin gluceptate*
- For *injection* dosage forms:
  - —For treatment of infections:
    - Adults and teenagers—250 to 500 milligrams (mg) injected into a vein every six hours; or 3.75 to 5 mg per kilogram (kg) (1.7 to 2.3 mg per pound) of body weight injected into a vein every six hours.
    - Children—Dose is based on body weight. The usual dose is 3.75 to 5 mg per kg (1.7 to 2.3 mg per pound) of body weight injected into a vein every six hours.

*For erythromycin lactobionate*
- For *injection* dosage forms:
  - —For treatment of infections:
    - Adults and teenagers—250 to 500 milligrams (mg) injected into a vein every six hours; or 3.75 to 5 mg per kilogram (kg) (1.7 to 2.3 mg per pound) of body weight injected into a vein every six hours.
    - Children—Dose is based on body weight. The usual dose is 3.75 to 5 mg per kg (1.7 to 2.3 mg per pound) of body weight injected into a vein every six hours.

*For erythromycin stearate*
- For *oral* dosage forms (oral suspension, tablets):
  - —For treatment of infections:
    - Adults and teenagers—250 to 500 milligrams (mg) two to four times a day.
    - Children—Dose is based on body weight. The usual dose is 7.5 to 12.5 mg per kilogram (kg) (3.4 to 5.6 mg per pound) of body weight four times a day; or 15 to 25 mg per kg (6.8 to 11.4 mg per pound) of body weight two times a day.
  - —For prevention of heart infections:
    - Adults and teenagers—Take 1 gram two hours before your dental appointment or surgery, then 500 mg six hours after taking the first dose.
    - Children—Dose is based on body weight. The usual dose is 20 mg per kg (9.1 mg per pound) of body weight two hours before the dental appointment or surgery, then 10 mg per kg (4.5 mg per pound) of body weight six hours after taking the first dose.

**Missed dose**—If you miss a dose of this medicine, take it as soon as possible. This will help to keep a constant amount of medicine in the blood. However, if it is almost time for your next dose, skip the missed dose and go back to your regular dosing schedule. Do not double doses.

**Storage**—To store this medicine:
- Keep out of the reach of children.
- Store away from heat and direct light.
- Do not store the capsule or tablet form of erythromycins in the bathroom, near the kitchen sink, or in other damp places. Heat or moisture may cause the medicine to break down.
- Store the oral liquid form of some erythromycins in the refrigerator because heat will cause this medicine to break down. However, keep the medicine from freezing. Follow the directions on the label.
- Do not keep outdated medicine or medicine no longer needed. Be sure that any discarded medicine is out of the reach of children.

## Precautions While Using This Medicine

If your symptoms do not improve within a few days, or if they become worse, check with your doctor.

## Side Effects of This Medicine

Along with its needed effects, a medicine may cause some unwanted effects. Although not all of these side effects may occur, if they do occur they may need medical attention.

*Check with your doctor immediately* if any of the following side effects occur:

*Less common*
  Fever; nausea; skin rash, redness, or itching; stomach pain (severe); unusual tiredness or weakness; vomiting; yellow eyes or skin–with erythromycin estolate (rare with other erythromycins)

*Less common–with erythromycin injection only*
  Pain, swelling, or redness at place of injection

*Rare*
  Fainting (repeated); irregular or slow heartbeat; loss of hearing (temporary)

Other side effects may occur that usually do not need medical attention. These side effects may go away during treatment as your body adjusts to the medicine. However, check with your doctor if any of the following side effects continue or are bothersome:

*More common*
  Abdominal or stomach cramping and discomfort; diarrhea; nausea or vomiting

*Less common*
  Sore mouth or tongue; vaginal itching and discharge

Other side effects not listed above may also occur in some patients. If you notice any other effects, check with your doctor.

## Additional Information

Once a medicine has been approved for marketing for a certain use, experience may show that it is also useful for other medical problems. Although these uses are not included in product labeling, erythromycins are used in certain patients with the following medical conditions:
- Acne
- Actinomycosis

- Anthrax
- Chancroid
- Gastroparesis
- Lyme disease
- Lymphogranuloma venereum
- Relapsing fever

Other than the above information, there is no additional information relating to proper use, precautions, or side effects for these uses.

Revised: 07/22/94

# ERYTHROMYCIN AND SULFISOXAZOLE    Systemic

Some commonly used brand names are:

**In the U.S.—**
Eryzole                Sulfimycin
Pediazole
Generic name product may also be available.

**In Canada—**
Pediazole

## Description

Erythromycin (eh-rith-roe-MYE-sin) and sulfisoxazole (sul-fi-SOX-a-zole) is a combination antibiotic used to treat ear infections in children. It may also be used for other problems as determined by your doctor. It will not work for colds, flu, or other virus infections.

Erythromycin and sulfisoxazole combination is available only with your doctor's prescription, in the following dosage form:

*Oral*
- Suspension (U.S. and Canada)

## Before Using This Medicine

In deciding to use a medicine, the risks of taking the medicine must be weighed against the good it will do. This is a decision you and your doctor will make. For erythromycin and sulfisoxazole, the following should be considered:

**Allergies**—Tell your doctor if you have ever had any unusual or allergic reaction to the erythromycins or sulfa medicines, furosemide (e.g., Lasix) or thiazide diuretics (water pills), oral antidiabetics (diabetes medicine you take by mouth), or glaucoma medicine you take by mouth (for example, acetazolamide [e.g., Diamox], dichlorphenamide [e.g., Daranide], methazolamide [e.g., Neptazane]). Also tell your health care professional if you are allergic to any other substances, such as foods, preservatives, or dyes.

**Pregnancy**—Studies have not been done in humans with either erythromycins or sulfa medicines. In addition, erythromycins have not been shown to cause birth defects or other problems in humans. However, studies in mice, rats, and rabbits have shown that some sulfa medicines cause birth defects, including cleft palate and bone problems.

**Breast-feeding**—Erythromycins and sulfa medicines pass into the breast milk. This medicine is not recommended for use during breast-feeding. It may cause liver problems, anemia, and other unwanted effects in nursing babies, especially those with glucose-6-phosphate dehydrogenase (G6PD) deficiency.

**Children**—This medicine has been tested in children over the age of 2 months and has not been shown to cause different side effects or problems than it does in adults.

**Older adults**—This medicine is intended for use in children and is not generally used in adult patients.

**Other medicines**—Although certain medicines should not be used together at all, in other cases two different medicines may be used together even if an interaction might occur. In these cases, your doctor may want to change the dose, or other precautions may be necessary. When you are taking erythromycin and sulfisoxazole, it is especially important that your health care professional know if you are taking any of the following:

- Acetaminophen (e.g., Tylenol) (with long-term, high-dose use) or
- Amiodarone (e.g., Cordarone) or
- Anabolic steroids (nandrolone [e.g., Anabolin], oxandrolone [e.g., Anavar], oxymetholone [e.g., Anadrol], stanozolol [e.g., Winstrol]) or
- Androgens (male hormones) or
- Antithyroid agents (medicine for overactive thyroid) or
- Carbamazepine (e.g., Tegretol) or
- Carmustine (e.g., BiCNU) or
- Chloroquine (e.g., Aralen) or
- Dantrolene (e.g., Dantrium) or
- Daunorubicin (e.g., Cerubidine) or
- Disulfiram (e.g., Antabuse) or
- Divalproex (e.g., Depakote) or
- Estrogens (female hormones) or
- Etretinate (e.g., Tegison) or
- Gold salts (medicine for arthritis) or
- Hydroxychloroquine (e.g., Plaquenil) or
- Mercaptopurine (e.g., Purinethol) or
- Methotrexate (e.g., Mexate) or
- Methyldopa (e.g., Aldomet) or
- Naltrexone (e.g., Trexan) (with long-term, high-dose use) or
- Oral contraceptives (birth control pills) containing estrogen or
- Other anti-infectives by mouth or by injection (medicine for infection) or
- Phenothiazines (acetophenazine [e.g., Tindal], chlorpromazine [e.g., Thorazine], fluphenazine [e.g., Prolixin],

mesoridazine [e.g., Serentil], perphenazine [e.g., Trilafon], prochlorperazine [e.g., Compazine], promazine [e.g., Sparine], promethazine [e.g., Phenergan], thioridazine [e.g. Mellaril], trifluoperazine [e.g., Stelazine], triflupromazine [e.g., Vesprin], trimeprazine [e.g., Temaril]) or
• Phenytoin (e.g., Dilantin) or
• Plicamycin (e.g., Mithracin) or
• Valproic acid (e.g., Depakene)—Use of erythromycin and sulfisoxazole with any of these medicines may increase the chance of side effects affecting the liver
• Acetohydroxamic acid (e.g., Lithostat) or
• Dapsone or
• Furazolidone (e.g., Furoxone) or
• Nitrofurantion (e.g., Furadantin) or
• Primaquine or
• Procainamide (e.g., Pronestyl) or
• Quinidine (e.g., Quinidex) or
• Quinine (e.g., Quinamm) or
• Sulfoxone (e.g., Diasone)—Use of erythromycin and sulfisoxazole with these medicines may increase the chance of side effects
• Alfentanil—Long-term use of erythromycin and sulfisoxazole may increase the action of alfentanil and increase the chance of side effects
• Aminophylline (e.g., Somophyllin) or
• Caffeine (e.g., NoDoz) or
• Oxtriphylline (e.g., Choledyl) or
• Theophylline (e.g., Slo-Phyllin, Somophyllin-T, Theodur)—Use of erythromycin and sulfisoxazole with these medicines may increase the side effects of these medicines
• Anticoagulants (blood thinners) or
• Antidiabetics, oral (diabetes medicine you take by mouth) or
• Ethotoin (e.g., Peganone) or
• Mephenytoin (e.g., Mesantoin)—Use of erythromycin and sulfisoxazole with these medicines may increase the effects of these medicines, thereby increasing the chance of side effects
• Chloramphenicol or
• Lincomycins—Use of erythromycin and sulfisoxazole with these medicines may decrease the effectiveness of these medicines
• Methenamine (e.g., Mandelamine)—Use of erythromycin and sulfisoxazole with this medicine may, on rare occasion, increase the chance of side effects affecting the kidneys
• Oral contraceptives (birth control pills) containing estrogen—Use of erythromycin and sulfisoxazole with oral contraceptives may decrease the effectiveness of oral contraceptives, increasing the chance of breakthrough bleeding and pregnancy
• Vitamin K (e.g., AquaMEPHYTON, Synkayvite)—Patients taking erythromycin and sulfisoxazole may have an increased need for vitamin K

**Other medical problems**—The presence of other medical problems may affect the use of erythromycin and sulfisoxazole. Make sure you tell your doctor if you have any other medical problems, especially:
• Anemia or other blood problems or
• Glucose-6-phosphate dehydrogenase (G6PD) deficiency—Erythromycin and sulfisoxazole may increase the chance of blood problems

• Kidney disease or
• Liver disease—Patients with liver or kidney disease may have an increased chance of side effects
• Loss of hearing—High doses of erythromycin and sulfisoxazole may increase the chance for hearing loss in some patients
• Porphyria—Erythromycin and sulfisoxazole may increase the chance of a porphyria attack

## Proper Use of This Medicine

*Erythromycin and sulfisoxazole combination is best taken with extra amounts of water* and may be taken with food. *Additional amounts of water should be taken several times every day,* unless otherwise directed by your doctor. Drinking extra water will help to prevent some unwanted effects (e.g., kidney stones) of sulfa medicines.

*Do not give this medicine to infants under 2 months of age,* unless otherwise directed by your doctor. Sulfa medicines may cause liver problems in these infants.

Use a specially marked measuring spoon or other device to measure each dose accurately. The average household teaspoon may not hold the right amount of liquid.

Do not use after the expiration date on the label. The medicine may not work properly after that date. Check with your pharmacist if you have any questions about this.

To help clear up your infection completely, *keep taking this medicine for the full time of treatment,* even if you begin to feel better after a few days. If you stop taking this medicine too soon, your symptoms may return.

This medicine works best when there is a constant amount in the blood. *To help keep the amount constant, do not miss any doses. Also, it is best to take the doses at evenly spaced times day and night.* For example, if you are to take 4 doses a day, the doses should be spaced about 6 hours apart. If this interferes with your sleep or other daily activities, or if you need help in planning the best times to take your medicine, check with your health care professional.

**Dosing**—The dose of erythromycin and sulfisoxazole combination will be different for different patients. *Follow your doctor's orders or the directions on the label.* The following information includes only the average doses of erythromycin and sulfisoxazole combination. *If your dose is different, do not change it* unless your doctor tells you to do so.
• For *oral* dosage form (suspension):
  —For infections caused by bacteria:
    • Adults and teenagers—This medicine is used only in children.
    • Children—This medicine is usually not used in children younger than 2 months of age. For children 2 months of age and older, the dose is based on body weight:
      —Children weighing less than 8 kilograms (kg) (under 18 pounds): Dose must be determined by your doctor.

—Children weighing 8 to 16 kg (18 to 35 pounds): 1/2 teaspoonful (2.5 milliliter [mL]) every six hours for ten days.
—Children weighing 16 to 24 kg (35 to 53 pounds): 1 teaspoonful (5 mL) every six hours for ten days.
—Children weighing 24 to 45 kg (53 to 100 pounds): 1 1/2 teaspoonfuls (7.5 mL) every six hours for ten days.
—Children weighing more than 45 kg (over 100 pounds): 2 teaspoonfuls (10 mL) every six hours for ten days.

**Missed dose**—If you miss a dose of this medicine, take it as soon as possible. This will help to keep a constant amount of medicine in the blood. However, if it is almost time for your next dose, skip the missed dose and go back to your regular dosing schedule. Do not double the dose.

**Storage**—To store this medicine:
- Keep out of the reach of children.
- Store away from heat and direct light.
- Store in the refrigerator because heat will cause this medicine to break down. However, keep the medicine from freezing. Follow the directions on the label.
- Do not keep outdated medicine or medicine no longer needed. Be sure that any discarded medicine is out of the reach of children.

## Precautions While Using This Medicine

*It is very important that your doctor check you at regular visits* for any blood problems that may be caused by this medicine, especially if you will be taking this medicine for a long time.

If your symptoms do not improve within a few days, or if they become worse, check with your doctor.

Erythromycin and sulfisoxazole may cause your skin to be more sensitive to sunlight than it is normally. Exposure to sunlight, even for brief periods of time, may cause a skin rash, itching, redness or other discoloration of the skin, or a severe sunburn. When you begin taking this medicine:
- Stay out of direct sunlight, especially between the hours of 10:00 a.m. and 3:00 p.m., if possible.
- Wear protective clothing, including a hat. Also, wear sunglasses.
- Apply a sun block product that has a skin protection factor (SPF) of at least 15. Some patients may require a product with a higher SPF number, especially if they have a fair complexion. If you have any questions about this, check with your health care professional.
- Apply a sun block lipstick that has an SPF of at least 15 to protect your lips.
- Do not use a sunlamp or tanning bed or booth.

*If you have a severe reaction from the sun, check with your doctor.*

Erythromycin and sulfisoxazole combination may cause blood problems. These problems may result in a greater chance of infection, slow healing, and bleeding of the gums. Therefore, you should be careful when using regular toothbrushes, dental floss, and toothpicks. Dental work should be delayed until your blood counts have returned to normal. Check with your medical doctor or dentist if you have any questions about proper oral hygiene (mouth care) during treatment.

## Side Effects of This Medicine

Along with its needed effects, a medicine may cause some unwanted effects. Although not all of these side effects may occur, if they do occur they may need medical attention.

*Check with your doctor immediately* if any of the following side effects occur:

*More common*
Itching; skin rash

*Less common*
Aching of joints and muscles; difficulty in swallowing; pale skin; redness, blistering, peeling, or loosening of skin; sore throat and fever; unusual bleeding or bruising; unusual tiredness or weakness; yellow eyes or skin

*Rare*
Blood in urine; dark or amber urine; temporary loss of hearing (with kidney disease and high doses); lower back pain; pain or burning while urinating; pale stools; severe stomach pain; swelling of front part of neck

In addition to the side effects listed above, check with your doctor as soon as possible if the following side effect occurs:

*More common*
Increased sensitivity to sunlight

Other side effects may occur that usually do not need medical attention. These side effects may go away during treatment as your body adjusts to the medicine. However, check with your doctor if any of the following side effects continue or are bothersome:

*More common*
Abdominal or stomach cramping and discomfort; diarrhea; headache; loss of appetite; nausea or vomiting

*Less common*
Sore mouth or tongue

Other side effects not listed above may also occur in some patients. If you notice any other effects, check with your doctor.

## Additional Information

Once a medicine has been approved for marketing for a certain use, experience may show that it is also useful for other medical problems. Although this use is not specifically included in product labeling, erythromycin and sulfisoxazole combination is used in certain patients with the following medical condition:

- Sinusitis (sinus infection)

Other than the above information, there is no additional information relating to proper use, precautions, or side effects for this use.

---

Revised: 08/27/92
Interim revision: 03/18/94

---

# ESTRAMUSTINE   Systemic

Some commonly used brand names are:
**In the U.S.—**
  Emcyt
**In Canada—**
  Emcyt
**Other—**
  Estracyt

## Description

Estramustine (ess-tra-MUSS-teen) belongs to the general group of medicines called antineoplastics. It is used to treat some cases of prostate cancer.

Estramustine is a combination of two medicines, an estrogen and mechlorethamine. The way that estramustine works against cancer is not completely understood. However, it seems to interfere with the growth of cancer cells, which are eventually destroyed.

Estramustine is available only with your doctor's prescription, in the following dosage form:

*Oral*
- Capsules (U.S. and Canada)

## Before Using This Medicine

In deciding to use a medicine, the risks of taking the medicine must be weighed against the good it will do. This is a decision you and your doctor will make. For estramustine, the following should be considered:

**Allergies**—Tell your doctor if you have ever had any unusual or allergic reaction to estramustine, estrogens, or mechlorethamine.

**Pregnancy**—There is a chance that this medicine may cause birth defects if the male is taking it at the time of conception. It may also cause permanent sterility after it has been taken for a while. Be sure that you have discussed this with your doctor before taking this medicine. Before taking estramustine, make sure your doctor knows if you intend to have children.

**Older adults**—Many medicines have not been studied specifically in older people. Therefore, it may not be known whether they work exactly the same way they do in younger adults or if they cause different side effects or problems in older people. There is no specific information comparing use of estramustine in the elderly with use in other age groups.

**Other medicines**—Although certain medicines should not be used together at all, in other cases two different medicines may be used together even if an interaction might occur. In these cases, your doctor may want to change the dose, or other precautions may be necessary. When you are taking estramustine, it is especially important that your health care professional know if you are taking any of the following:

- Acetaminophen (e.g., Tylenol) (with long-term, high-dose use) or
- Amiodarone (e.g., Cordarone) or
- Anabolic steroids (nandrolone [e.g., Anabolin], oxandrolone [e.g., Anavar], oxymetholone [e.g., Anadrol], stanozolol [e.g., Winstrol]) or
- Androgens (male hormones) or
- Anti-infectives by mouth or by injection (medicine for infection) or
- Antithyroid agents (medicine for overactive thyroid) or
- Carbamazepine (e.g., Tegretol) or
- Carmustine (e.g., BiCNU) or
- Chloroquine (e.g., Aralen) or
- Dantrolene (e.g., Dantrium) or
- Disulfiram (e.g., Antabuse) or
- Divalproex (e.g., Depakote) or
- Estrogens (female hormones) or
- Etretinate (e.g., Tegison) or
- Gold salts (medicine for arthritis) or
- Hydroxychloroquine (e.g., Plaquenil) or
- Mercaptopurine (e.g., Purinethol) or
- Methotrexate (e.g., Mexate) or
- Methyldopa (e.g., Aldomet) or
- Naltrexone (e.g., Trexan) (with long-term, high-dose use) or
- Oral contraceptives (birth control pills) containing estrogen or
- Phenothiazines (acetophenazine [e.g., Tindal], chlorpromazine [e.g., Thorazine], fluphenazine [e.g., Prolixin], mesoridazine [e.g., Serentil], perphenazine [e.g., Trilafon], prochlorperazine [e.g., Compazine], promazine [e.g., Sparine], promethazine [e.g., Phenergan], thioridazine [e.g., Mellaril], trifluoperazine [e.g., Stelazine], triflupromazine [e.g., Vesprin], trimeprazine [e.g., Temaril]) or
- Phenytoin (e.g., Dilantin) or
- Plicamycin (e.g., Mithracin) or
- Valproic acid (e.g., Depakene)—May increase the risk of liver problems

**Other medical problems**—The presence of other medical problems may affect the use of estramustine. Make sure

you tell your doctor if you have any other medical problems, especially:
- Asthma or
- Epilepsy or
- Mental depression (or history of) or
- Migraine headaches or
- Kidney disease—Fluid retention sometimes caused by estramustine may worsen these conditions
- Blood clots (or history of) or
- Stroke (or history of) or
- Recent heart attack or stroke—May be worsened because of blood vessel problems caused by estramustine
- Chickenpox (including recent exposure) or
- Herpes zoster (shingles)—Risk of severe disease affecting other parts of the body
- Diabetes mellitus (sugar diabetes)—Estramustine may change the amount of antidiabetic medicine needed
- Gallbladder disease (or history of)—May be worsened by estramustine
- Heart or blood vessel disease—Estramustine can cause circulation problems
- Jaundice or hepatitis (or history of) or other liver disease—Effects, including liver problems, may be increased
- Stomach ulcer—May be aggravated by estramustine

**Smoking**—Because smoking causes narrowing of blood vessels, it can increase the risk of serious circulation problems, which can lead to stroke or heart attack.

## Proper Use of This Medicine

*Use this medicine only as directed by your doctor*. Do not use more or less of it, and do not use it more often than your doctor ordered. The exact amount of medicine you need has been carefully worked out. Taking too much may increase the chance of side effects, while taking too little may not improve your condition.

Do not take estramustine within 1 hour before or 2 hours after meals or after the time you take milk, milk formulas, or other dairy products, since they may keep the medicine from working properly.

This medicine commonly causes nausea and sometimes causes vomiting. However, it may have to be taken for several weeks to months to be effective. Even if you begin to feel ill, *do not stop using this medicine without first checking with your doctor*. Ask your health care professional for ways to lessen these effects.

If you vomit shortly after taking a dose of estramustine, check with your doctor. You will be told whether to take the dose again or to wait until the next scheduled dose.

**Dosing**—The dose of estramustine will be different for different patients. The dose that is used may depend on a number of things, including what the medicine is being used for, the patient's size, and whether or not other medicines are also being taken. *If you are taking estramustine at home, follow your doctor's orders or the directions on the label*. If you have any questions about the proper dose of estramustine, ask your doctor.

**Missed dose**—If you miss a dose of this medicine, skip the missed dose and go back to your regular dosing schedule. Do not double doses.

**Storage**—To store this medicine:
- Keep out of the reach of children.
- Store in the refrigerator, away from direct light.
- Do not store in the bathroom, near the kitchen sink, or in other damp places. Heat or moisture may cause the medicine to break down.
- Do not keep outdated medicine or medicine no longer needed. Be sure that any discarded medicine is out of the reach of children.

## Precautions While Using This Medicine

*It is very important that your doctor check your progress at regular visits* to make sure that the medicine is working properly and does not cause unwanted effects.

While you are being treated with estramustine, and after you stop treatment with it, *do not have any immunizations (vaccinations) without your doctor's approval*. Estramustine may lower your body's resistance and there is a chance you might get the infection the immunization is meant to prevent. In addition, other persons living in your household should not take oral polio vaccine since there is a chance they could pass the polio virus on to you. Also, avoid persons who have recently taken oral polio vaccine. Do not get close to them and do not stay in the same room with them for very long. If you cannot take these precautions, you should consider wearing a protective face mask that covers the nose and mouth.

## Side Effects of This Medicine

Along with its needed effects, a medicine may cause some unwanted effects. Although not all of these side effects may occur, if they do occur they may need medical attention.

*Check with your doctor immediately* if any of the following side effects occur. If your doctor is not available, go to the nearest hospital emergency room.
  *Rare*
    Black, tarry stools; blood in urine or stools; cough or hoarseness; fever or chills; headaches (severe or sudden); loss of coordination (sudden); lower back or side pain; painful or difficult urination; pains in chest, groin, or leg (especially calf of leg); pinpoint red spots on skin; shortness of breath (sudden, for no apparent reason); slurred speech (sudden); unusual bleeding or bruising; vision changes (sudden); weakness or numbness in arm or leg

Check with your doctor as soon as possible if any of the following side effects occur:
  *More common*
    Swelling of feet or lower legs
  *Rare*
    Skin rash or fever; unusual tiredness or weakness

Other side effects may occur that usually do not need medical attention. These side effects may go away during

treatment as your body adjusts to the medicine. However, check with your doctor if any of the following side effects continue or are bothersome or if you have any questions about them:

*More common*
Breast tenderness or enlargement; decreased interest in sex; diarrhea; nausea

*Less common*
Trouble in sleeping; vomiting

Other side effects not listed above may also occur in some patients. If you notice any other effects, check with your doctor.

Revised: 07/11/94

# ESTROGENS   Systemic

Some commonly used brand names are:

**In the U.S.—**

| | |
|---|---|
| Aquest[6] | Estroject-LA[3] |
| Clinagen LA 40[3] | Estro-L.A.[3] |
| Deladiol-40[3] | Estrone '5'[6] |
| Delestrogen[3] | Estro-Span[3] |
| depGynogen[3] | Estrovis[9] |
| Depo-Estradiol[3] | Gynogen L.A. 20[3] |
| Depogen[3] | Gynogen L.A. 40[3] |
| Dioval 40[3] | Kestrone-5[6] |
| Dioval XX[3] | Menaval-20[3] |
| Dura-Estrin[3] | Menest[5] |
| Duragen-20[3] | Ogen .625[7] |
| Duragen-40[3] | Ogen 1.25[7] |
| E-Cypionate[3] | Ogen 2.5[7] |
| Estinyl[8] | Ortho-Est[7] |
| Estrace[3] | Premarin[4] |
| Estraderm[3] | Premarin Intravenous[4] |
| Estragyn 5[6] | Stilphostrol[2] |
| Estragyn LA 5[3] | TACE[1] |
| Estra-L 40[3] | Valergen-10[3] |
| Estratab[5] | Valergen-20[3] |
| Estro-A[6] | Valergen-40[3] |
| Estro-Cyp[3] | Wehgen[6] |
| Estrofem[3] | |

**In Canada—**

| | |
|---|---|
| C.E.S.[4] | Femogex[3] |
| Congest[4] | Honvol[2] |
| Delestrogen[3] | Neo-Estrone[5] |
| Estinyl[8] | Ogen[7] |
| Estrace[3] | Premarin[4] |
| Estraderm[3] | Premarin Intravenous[4] |

Other commonly used names are:

| | |
|---|---|
| DES[2] | Piperazine Estrone Sulfate[7] |

Note: For quick reference, the following estrogens are numbered to match the corresponding brand names.

This information applies to the following medicines:

1. Chlorotrianisene (klor-oh-trye-AN-i-seen)†
2. Diethylstilbestrol (dye-eth-il-stil-BESS-trole)‡
3. Estradiol (ess-tra-DYE-ole)‡
4. Estrogens, Conjugated (ESS-troe-jenz, CON-ju-gate-ed)§
5. Estrogens, Esterified (ess-TAIR-i-fyed)
6. Estrone (ESS-trone)†‡
7. Estropipate (ess-troe-PI-pate)‡
8. Ethinyl Estradiol (ETH-in-il ess-tra-DYE-ole)
9. Quinestrol (quin-ESS-trole)†

†Not commercially available in Canada.
‡Generic name product may also be available in the U.S.
§Generic name product may also be available in Canada.

## Description

Estrogens (ESS-troe-jenz) are female hormones. They are produced by the body and are necessary for the normal sexual development of the female and for the regulation of the menstrual cycle during the childbearing years.

The ovaries begin to produce less estrogen after menopause (the change of life). This medicine is prescribed to make up for the lower amount of estrogen. This should relieve signs of menopause, such as hot flashes and unusual sweating, chills, faintness, or dizziness.

Estrogens are prescribed for several reasons:

- to provide additional hormone when the body does not produce enough of its own, as during the menopause or following certain kinds of surgery.
- in the treatment of selected cases of breast cancer in men and women.
- in the treatment of men with certain kinds of cancer of the prostate.
- to help prevent weakening of bones (osteoporosis) in women past menopause.

Estrogens may also be used for other conditions as determined by your doctor.

There is *no* medical evidence to support the belief that the use of estrogens will keep the patient feeling young, keep the skin soft, or delay the appearance of wrinkles. Nor has it been proven that the use of estrogens during the menopause will relieve emotional and nervous symptoms, unless these symptoms are caused by other menopausal symptoms, such as hot flashes or hot flushes.

Estrogens are very useful medicines. However, in addition to their helpful effects in treating your medical problem, they sometimes have side effects that could be very serious. *A paper called "Information for the Patient" should be given to you with your prescription. Read this carefully.* Also, before you use an estrogen, you and your doctor should discuss the good that it will do as well as the risks of using it.

Estrogens are available only with your doctor's prescription, in the following dosage forms:

*Oral*
Chlorotrianisene
- Capsules (U.S.)

Diethylstilbestrol
- Tablets (U.S. and Canada)

Estradiol
- Tablets (U.S. and Canada)

Estrogens, Conjugated
- Tablets (U.S. and Canada)

Estrogens, Esterified
- Tablets (U.S. and Canada)

Estropipate
- Tablets (U.S. and Canada)

Ethinyl Estradiol
- Tablets (U.S. and Canada)

Quinestrol
- Tablets (U.S.)

*Parenteral*

Diethylstilbestrol
- Injection (U.S. and Canada)

Estradiol
- Injection (U.S. and Canada)

Estrogens, Conjugated
- Injection (U.S. and Canada)

Estrone
- Injection (U.S.)

*Topical*

Estradiol
- Transdermal system (stick-on patch) (U.S. and Canada)

## Before Using This Medicine

In deciding to use a medicine, the risks of taking the medicine must be weighed against the good it will do. This is a decision you and your doctor will make. For estrogens, the following should be considered:

**Allergies**—Tell your doctor if you have ever had any unusual or allergic reaction to estrogens. Also tell your health care professional if you are allergic to any other substances, such as foods, preservatives, or dyes.

**Pregnancy**—Estrogens are not recommended for use during pregnancy, since some have been shown to cause serious birth defects in humans and animals. Some daughters of women who took diethylstilbestrol (DES) during pregnancy have developed reproductive (genital) tract problems and, rarely, cancer of the vagina or cervix (opening to the uterus) when they reached childbearing age. Some sons of women who took DES during pregnancy have developed urinary-genital tract problems.

**Breast-feeding**—Use of this medicine is not recommended in nursing mothers. Estrogens pass into the breast milk and their possible effect on the baby is not known.

**Older adults**—This medicine has been tested and has not been shown to cause different side effects or problems in older women than it does in younger women.

**Other medicines**—Although certain medicines should not be used together at all, in other cases two different medicines may be used together even if an interaction might occur. In these cases, your doctor may want to change the dose, or other precautions may be necessary. When you are taking estrogens, it is especially important that

your health care professional know if you are taking any of the following:

- Acetaminophen (e.g., Tylenol) (with long-term, high-dose use) or
- Amiodarone (e.g., Cordarone) or
- Anabolic steroids (nandrolone [e.g., Anabolin], oxandrolone [e.g., Anavar], oxymetholone [e.g., Anadrol], stanozolol [e.g., Winstrol]) or
- Androgens (male hormones) or
- Anti-infectives by mouth or by injection (medicine for infection) or
- Antithyroid agents (medicine for overactive thyroid) or
- Carbamazepine (e.g., Tegretol) or
- Carmustine (e.g., BiCNU) or
- Chloroquine (e.g., Aralen) or
- Dantrolene (e.g., Dantrium) or
- Daunorubicin (e.g., Cerubidine) or
- Disulfiram (e.g., Antabuse) or
- Divalproex (e.g., Depakote) or
- Etretinate (e.g., Tegison) or
- Gold salts (medicine for arthritis) or
- Hydroxychloroquine (e.g., Plaquenil) or
- Mercaptopurine (e.g., Purinethol) or
- Methotrexate (e.g., Mexate) or
- Methyldopa (e.g., Aldomet) or
- Naltrexone (e.g., Trexan) (with long-term, high-dose use) or
- Oral contraceptives (birth control pills) containing estrogen or
- Phenothiazines (acetophenazine [e.g., Tindal], chlorpromazine [e.g., Thorazine], fluphenazine [e.g., Prolixin], mesoridazine [e.g., Serentil], perphenazine [e.g., Trilafon], prochlorperazine [e.g., Compazine], promazine [e.g., Sparine], promethazine [e.g., Phenergan], thioridazine [e.g., Mellaril], trifluoperazine [e.g., Stelazine], triflupromazine [e.g., Vesprin], trimeprazine [e.g., Temaril]) or
- Phenytoin (e.g., Dilantin) or
- Plicamycin (e.g., Mithracin) or
- Valproic acid (e.g., Depakene)—Estrogens and all of these medicines can cause liver damage. Your doctor may want you to have extra blood tests that tell about your liver, if you must take any of these medicines with estrogens
- Bromocriptine (e.g., Parlodel)—Estrogens may interfere with the effects of bromocriptine
- Cyclosporine (e.g., Sandimmune)—Estrogens can increase the chance of toxic effects to the kidney or liver from cyclosporine because estrogens can interfere with the body's ability to get the cyclosporine out of the bloodstream as it normally would

**Other medical problems**—The presence of other medical problems may affect the use of estrogens. Make sure you tell your doctor if you have any other medical problems, especially:

*For all patients*
- Blood clots (or history of during previous estrogen therapy)—Estrogens may worsen blood clots or cause new clots to form
- Breast cancer (active or suspected)—Estrogens may cause growth of the tumor in some cases
- Changes in vaginal bleeding of unknown causes—Some irregular vaginal bleeding is a sign that the lining of the uterus is growing too much or is a sign of cancer of the uterus lining; estrogens may make these conditions worse

- Endometriosis—Estrogens may worsen endometriosis by causing growth of endometriosis implants
- Fibroid tumors of the uterus—Estrogens may cause fibroid tumors to increase in size
- Gallbladder disease or gallstones (or history of)—Estrogens may possibly increase the risk of gallbladder disease or gallstones
- Jaundice (or history of during pregnancy)—Estrogens may worsen or cause jaundice in these patients
- Liver disease—Toxic drug effects may occur in patients with liver disease because the body is not able to get this medicine out of the bloodstream as it normally would
- Porphyria—Estrogens can make porphyria worse

*For males treated for breast or prostate cancer*
- Blood clots or
- Heart or circulation disease or
- Stroke—Males with these medical problems may be more likely to have clotting problems while taking estrogens; the doses of estrogens used to treat male breast or prostate cancer have been shown to increase the chances of heart attack, phlebitis (inflamed veins) caused by a blood clot, or blood clots in the lungs

## Proper Use of This Medicine

For patients taking any of the estrogens by mouth:

- *Take this medicine only as directed by your doctor. Do not take more of it and do not take it for a longer time than your doctor ordered.* Try to take the medicine at the same time each day to reduce the possibility of side effects and to allow it to work better.
- Nausea may occur during the first few weeks after you start taking estrogens. This effect usually disappears with continued use. If the nausea is bothersome, it can usually be prevented or reduced by taking each dose with food or immediately after food.

For patients using the transdermal (stick-on patch) form of estradiol:

- This medicine comes with patient directions. Read them carefully before using this medicine.
- Wash and dry your hands thoroughly before and after handling.
- Apply the patch to a clean, dry, non-oily skin area of your abdomen (stomach) or buttocks that has little or no hair and is free of cuts or irritation.
- *Do not apply to the breasts.* Also, do not apply to the waistline or anywhere else where tight clothes may rub the patch loose.
- Press the patch firmly in place with the palm of your hand for about 10 seconds. Make sure there is good contact, especially around the edges.
- If a patch becomes loose or falls off, you may reapply it or discard it and apply a new patch.
- Each dose is best applied to a different area of skin on your abdomen so that at least 1 week goes by before the same area is used again. This will help prevent skin irritation.

**Dosing**—The dose of these medicines will be different for different patients. *Follow your doctor's orders or the directions on the label.* The following information includes only the average doses of these medicines. *If your dose is different, do not change it* unless your doctor tells you to do so.

The number of capsules or tablets that you take or the amount of injection you use depends on the strength of the medicine. Also, *the number of doses you take or use each day, the time allowed between doses, and the length of time you take or use the medicine depend on the medical problem for which you are taking or using estrogen.*

*For chlorotrianisene*
- For *oral* dosage form (capsules):
  —For treating a genital skin condition (vulvar squamous hyperplasia), inflammation of the vagina (atrophic vaginitis), ovary disorders (female hypogonadism), or symptoms of menopause:
    - Adults—12 to 25 milligrams (mg) a day. Your doctor may want you to take this medicine every day or only on certain days each month.
  —For treating prostate cancer:
    - Adults—12 to 25 mg a day.

*For conjugated estrogens*
- For *oral* dosage form (tablets):
  —For treating a genital skin condition (vulvar squamous hyperplasia), inflammation of the vagina (atrophic vaginitis), or to prevent loss of bone (osteoporosis):
    - Adults—0.3 to 1.25 milligrams (mg) a day. Your doctor may want you to take the medicine each day or only on certain days of the month.
  —For treating ovary problems (female hypogonadism):
    - Adults—2.5 to 7.5 mg a day. This dose is divided up and taken in smaller doses. Your doctor may want you to take the medicine only on certain days of the month.
  —For treating symptoms of menopause:
    - Adults—0.625 to 1.25 mg a day. Your doctor may want you to take the medicine each day or only on certain days of the month.
  —For treating ovary problems (failure or removal of the ovary):
    - Adults—1.25 mg a day. Your doctor may want you to take the medicine each day or only on certain days of the month.
  —For treating breast cancer in women after menopause and in men:
    - Adults—10 mg three times a day for at least three months.
  —For treating prostate cancer:
    - Adults—1.25 to 2.5 mg three times a day.

- For *injection* dosage form:
  - —For controlling abnormal bleeding of the uterus:
    - Adults—25 mg injected into a muscle or vein. This may be repeated in six to twelve hours if needed.

### For diethylstilbestrol

- For *oral* dosage forms (tablets and enteric-coated tablets):
  - —For treating breast cancer in women after menopause and in men:
    - Adults—15 milligrams (mg) a day.
  - —For treating prostate cancer:
    - Adults—At first, 1 to 3 mg a day. Later, your doctor may decrease your dose to 1 mg a day.

### For diethylstilbestrol diphosphate

- For *oral* dosage form (tablets):
  - —For treating prostate cancer:
    - Adults—50 to 200 milligrams (mg) three times a day.
- For *injection* dosage form:
  - —For treating prostate cancer:
    - Adults—At first, 500 mg mixed in solution with sodium chloride or dextrose injection and injected slowly into a vein. Your doctor may increase your dose to 1 gram a day for five or more straight days as needed. Then, your doctor may lower your dose to 250 to 500 mg one or two times a week.

### For esterified estrogens

- For *oral* dosage form (tablets):
  - —For treating a genital skin condition (vulvar squamous hyperplasia) or inflammation of the vagina (atrophic vaginitis):
    - Adults—0.3 to 1.25 milligrams (mg) a day. Your doctor may want you to take the medicine each day or only on certain days of the month.
  - —For treating ovary problems (female hypogonadism):
    - Adults—2.5 to 7.5 mg a day. This dose may be divided up and taken in smaller doses. Your doctor may want you to take the medicine each day or only on certain days of the month.
  - —For treating symptoms of menopause:
    - Adults—0.625 to 1.25 mg a day. Your doctor may want you to take the medicine each day or only on certain days of the month.
  - —For treating ovary problems (failure or removal of the ovary):
    - Adults—1.25 mg a day. Your doctor may want you to take the medicine each day or only on certain days of the month.
  - —For treating breast cancer in women after menopause and in men:
    - Adults—10 mg three times a day for at least three months.

- —For treating prostate cancer:
  - Adults—1.25 to 2.5 mg three times a day.

### For estradiol

- For *oral* dosage form (tablets):
  - —For treating a genital skin condition (vulvar squamous hyperplasia), inflammation of the vagina (atrophic vaginitis), ovary problems (female hypogonadism or failure or removal of the ovary), or symptoms of menopause:
    - Adults—0.5 to 2 milligrams (mg) a day. Your doctor may want you to take the medicine each day or only on certain days of the month.
  - —For treating breast cancer in women after menopause and in men:
    - Adults—10 mg three times a day for at least three months.
  - —For treating prostate cancer:
    - Adults—1 to 2 mg three times a day.
  - —For preventing bone loss (osteoporosis):
    - Adults—0.5 mg a day. Your doctor may want you to take the medicine each day or only on certain days of the month.
- For *transdermal* dosage form (patches):
  - —For treating a genital skin condition (vulvar squamous hyperplasia), inflammation of the vagina (atrophic vaginitis), symptoms of menopause, ovary problems (female hypogonadism or failure or removal of the ovary), or to prevent bone loss (osteoporosis):
    - Adults—0.05 or 0.1 milligram (mg) (one patch) applied to the skin and worn for one-half of a week. Then, remove that patch and apply a new patch. A new patch should be applied two times a week.

### For estradiol cypionate

- For *injectable* dosage form:
  - —For treating ovary problems (female hypogonadism):
    - Adults—1.5 to 2 milligrams (mg) injected into a muscle once a month.
  - —For treating symptoms of menopause:
    - Adults—1 to 5 mg injected into a muscle every three to four weeks.

### For estradiol valerate

- For *injection* dosage form:
  - —For treating a genital skin condition (vulvar squamous hyperplasia), inflammation of the vagina (atrophic vaginitis), symptoms of menopause, or ovary problems (female hypogonadism or failure or removal of the ovary):
    - Adults—10 to 20 milligrams (mg) injected into a muscle every four weeks as needed.
  - —For treating prostate cancer:
    - Adults—30 mg injected into a muscle every one or two weeks.

*For estrone*
- For *injection* dosage form:
  - —For controlling abnormal bleeding of the uterus:
    - Adults—2 to 5 milligrams (mg) a day, injected into a muscle for several days.
  - —For treating ovary problems (female hypogonadism, failure or removal of the ovary):
    - Adults—0.1 to 2 mg a week. This is injected into a muscle as a single dose or divided into more than one dose. Your doctor may want you to receive the medicine each week or only during certain weeks of the month.
  - —For treating a genital skin condition (vulvar squamous hyperplasia), inflammation of the vagina (atrophic vaginitis), or symptoms of menopause:
    - Adults—0.1 to 0.5 mg injected into a muscle two or three times a week. Your doctor may want you to receive the medicine each week or only during certain weeks of the month.
  - —For treating prostate cancer:
    - Adults—2 to 4 mg injected into a muscle two or three times a week.

*For estropipate*
- For oral dosage form (tablets):
  - —For treating a genital skin condition (vulvar squamous hyperplasia), inflammation of the vagina (atrophic vaginitis), or symptoms of menopause:
    - Adults—0.75 to 6 milligrams (mg) a day. Your doctor may want you to take the medicine each day or only on certain days of the month.
  - —For treating ovary problems (female hypogonadism, failure or removal of the ovary):
    - Adults—1.5 to 9 mg a day. Your doctor may want you to take the medicine each day or only on certain days of the month.

*For ethinyl estradiol*
- For *oral* dosage form (tablets):
  - —For treating ovary problems (female hypogonadism):
    - Adults—0.05 milligrams (mg) one to three times a day for three to six months. Your doctor may want you to take the medicine each day or only on certain days of the month.
  - —For treating symptoms of menopause:
    - Adults—0.02 to 0.05 mg a day. Your doctor may want you to take the medicine each day or only on certain days of the month.
  - —For treating breast cancer in women after menopause:
    - Adults—1 mg three times a day.
  - —For treating prostate cancer:
    - Adults—0.15 to 3 mg a day.

*For quinestrol*
- For *oral* dosage form (tablets):
  - —For treating a genital skin condition (vulvar squamous hyperplasia), inflammation of the vagina (atrophic vaginitis), symptoms of menopause, or ovary problems (female hypogonadism, failure or removal of the ovary):
    - Adults—At first, 100 micrograms (mcg) a day for seven days. Then, no medicine is taken for seven days. After that, your doctor will lower your dose to 100 to 200 mcg taken once a week.

**Missed dose—**
- For patients taking any of the estrogens by mouth: If you miss a dose of this medicine, take it as soon as possible. However, if it is almost time for your next dose, skip the missed dose and go back to your regular dosing schedule. Do not double doses.
- For patients using the transdermal (stick-on patch) form of estradiol: If you forget to apply a new patch when you are supposed to, apply it as soon as possible. However, if it is almost time for the next patch, skip the missed one and go back to your regular schedule. Do not apply more than one patch at a time.

**Storage**—To store this medicine:
- Keep out of the reach of children.
- Store away from heat and direct light.
- Do not store in the bathroom medicine cabinet because the heat or moisture may cause the medicine to break down.
- Keep the injectable form of this medicine from freezing.
- Do not keep outdated medicine or medicine no longer needed. Be sure that any discarded medicine is out of the reach of children.

---

## Precautions While Using This Medicine

*It is very important that your doctor check your progress at regular visits to make sure this medicine does not cause unwanted effects.* These visits will usually be every year, but some doctors require them more often.

It is not yet known whether the use of estrogens increases the risk of breast cancer in women. Therefore, it is very important that you regularly check your breasts for any unusual lumps or discharge. You should also have a mammogram (x-ray pictures of the breasts) done if your doctor recommends it. Because breast cancer has occurred in men taking estrogens, regular self-breast exams and exams by your doctor for any unusual lumps or discharge should be done.

In some patients using estrogens, tenderness, swelling, or bleeding of the gums may occur. Brushing and flossing your teeth carefully and regularly and massaging your gums may help prevent this. See your dentist regularly to have your teeth cleaned. Check with your medical doctor or dentist if you have any questions about how to take care of your teeth and gums, or if you notice any tenderness, swelling, or bleeding of your gums.

*If you think that you may be pregnant, stop using the medicine immediately and check with your doctor.* Continued use of some estrogens during pregnancy may cause birth defects in the child. DES may also increase the risk of vaginal cancer developing in daughters when they reach childbearing age.

Do not give this medicine to anyone else. Your doctor has prescribed it only for you after studying your health record and the results of your physical examination. Estrogens may be dangerous for other people because of differences in their health and body make-up.

## Side Effects of This Medicine

Discuss these possible effects with your doctor:

• The prolonged use of estrogens has been reported to increase the risk of endometrial cancer (cancer of the lining of the uterus) in women after the menopause. This risk seems to increase as the dose and the length of use increase. When estrogens are used in low doses for less than 1 year, there is less risk. The risk is also reduced if a progestin (another female hormone) is added to, or replaces part of, your estrogen dose. If the uterus has been removed by surgery (total hysterectomy), there is no risk of endometrial cancer.

• It is not yet known whether the use of estrogens increases the risk of breast cancer in women. Although some large studies show an increased risk, most studies and information gathered to date do not support this idea. Breast cancer has been reported in men taking estrogens.

• In studies with oral contraceptives (birth control pills) containing estrogens, cigarette smoking was shown to cause an increased risk of serious side effects affecting the heart or blood circulation, such as dangerous blood clots, heart attack, or stroke. The risk increased as the amount of smoking and the age of the smoker increased. Women aged 35 and over were at greatest risk when they smoked while using oral contraceptives containing estrogens. It is not known if this risk exists with the use of estrogens for symptoms of menopause. However, smoking may make estrogens less effective.

The following side effects may be caused by blood clots, which could lead to stroke, heart attack, or death. These side effects rarely occur, and, when they do occur, they occur in men treated for cancer using high doses of estrogens. *Get emergency help immediately* if any of the following side effects occur:

*Rare—For males being treated for breast or prostate cancer only*

Headache (sudden or severe); loss of coordination (sudden); loss of vision or change of vision (sudden); pains in chest, groin, or leg, especially in calf of leg; shortness of breath (sudden and unexplained); slurring of speech (sudden); weakness or numbness in arm or leg

Also, check with your doctor as soon as possible if any of the following side effects occur:

*More common*

Breast pain (in females and males); increased breast size (in females and males); swelling of feet and lower legs; weight gain (rapid)

*Less common or rare*

Changes in vaginal bleeding (spotting, breakthrough bleeding, prolonged or heavier bleeding, or complete stoppage of bleeding); lumps in, or discharge from, breast (in females and males); pains in stomach, side, or abdomen; uncontrolled jerky muscle movements; yellow eyes or skin

Other side effects may occur that usually do not need medical attention. These side effects may go away during treatment as your body adjusts to the medicine. However, check with your doctor if any of the following side effects continue or are bothersome:

*More common*

Bloating of stomach; cramps of lower stomach; loss of appetite; nausea; skin irritation or redness where skin patch was worn

*Less common*

Diarrhea (mild); dizziness (mild); headaches (mild); migraine headaches; problems in wearing contact lenses; unusual decrease in sexual desire (in males); unusual increase in sexual desire (in females); vomiting (usually with high doses)

Also, many women who are taking estrogens with a progestin (another female hormone) will start having monthly vaginal bleeding, similar to menstrual periods again. This effect will continue for as long as the medicine is taken. However, monthly bleeding will not occur in women who have had the uterus removed by surgery (total hysterectomy).

Other side effects not listed above may also occur in some patients. If you notice any other effects, check with your doctor.

Revised: 06/18/93
Interim revision: 06/30/94

# ESTROGENS Vaginal

Some commonly used brand names are:

**In the U.S.—**
Estrace[2]          Ortho Dienestrol[1]
Ogen[5]            Premarin[3]

**In Canada—**
Oestrilin[4]        Premarin[3]
Ortho Dienestrol[1]

Another commonly used name for estropipate is piperazine estrone sulfate.

Note: For quick reference, the following estrogens are numbered to match the corresponding brand names.

This information applies to the following medicines:
1. Dienestrol (dye-en-ESS-trole)‡
2. Estradiol (ess-tra-DYE-ole)
3. Conjugated Estrogens (CON-ju-gate-ed ESS-troe-jenz)
4. Estrone (ESS-trone)*
5. Estropipate (ess-troe-PI-pate)†‡

*Not commercially available in the U.S.
†Not commercially available in Canada.
‡Generic name product may also be available in the U.S.

## Description

Estrogens (ESS-troe-jenz) are female hormones. They are produced by the body and are necessary for the normal sexual development of the female and for the regulation of the menstrual cycle during the childbearing years.

Uncomfortable changes may occur in vaginal tissues when the body does not produce enough estrogens, as during the menopause or following certain kinds of surgery. In order to relieve such uncomfortable conditions, estrogens are prescribed for vaginal use in the form of special creams or suppositories.

When used vaginally or on the skin, most estrogens are absorbed into the bloodstream and produce many of the same effects in the body as when they are taken by mouth or given by injection.

Estrogens are very useful medicines. However, in addition to their helpful effects in treating your medical problem, they sometimes have side effects that could be very serious. *A paper called "Information for the Patient" is given to you with your prescription. Read this carefully.* Also, you should discuss with your doctor the good that this medicine will do as well as the risks of using it.

Estrogens for vaginal use are available only with your doctor's prescription, in the following dosage forms:

*Vaginal*
Dienestrol
• Cream (U.S. and Canada)
Estradiol
• Cream (U.S.)
Conjugated Estrogens
• Cream (U.S. and Canada)
Estrone
• Cream (Canada)
• Suppositories (Canada)
Estropipate
• Cream (U.S.)

## Before Using This Medicine

In deciding to use a medicine, the risks of using the medicine must be weighed against the good it will do. This is a decision you and your doctor will make. For vaginal estrogens, the following should be considered:

**Allergies**—Tell your doctor if you have ever had any unusual or allergic reaction to estrogens. Also tell your health care professional if you are allergic to any other substances, such as foods, preservatives, or dyes.

**Pregnancy**—Estrogens are not recommended for use during pregnancy, since some have been shown to cause serious birth defects in humans and animals.

**Breast-feeding**—Use of this medicine is not recommended in nursing mothers. Estrogens pass into the breast milk and their possible effect on the baby is not known.

**Older adults**—This medicine has been tested and has not been shown to cause different side effects or problems in older people than it does in younger adults.

**Other medicines**—Although certain medicines should not be used together at all, in other cases two different medicines may be used together even if an interaction might occur. In these cases, your doctor may want to change the dose, or other precautions may be necessary. When you are using vaginal estrogens, it is especially important that your health care professional know if you are taking any of the following:

• Acetaminophen (e.g., Tylenol) (with long-term, high-dose use) or
• Amiodarone (e.g., Cordarone) or
• Anabolic steroids (nandrolone [e.g., Anabolin], oxandrolone [e.g., Anavar], oxymetholone [e.g., Anadrol], stanozolol [e.g., Winstrol]) or
• Androgens (male hormones) or
• Anti-infectives by mouth or by injection (medicine for infection) or
• Antithyroid agents (medicine for overactive thyroid) or
• Carbamazepine (e.g., Tegretol) or
• Carmustine (e.g., BiCNU) or
• Chloroquine (e.g., Aralen) or
• Dantrolene (e.g., Dantrium) or
• Daunorubicin (e.g., Cerubidine) or
• Disulfiram (e.g., Antabuse) or
• Divalproex (e.g., Depakote) or
• Etretinate (e.g., Tegison) or
• Gold salts (medicine for arthritis) or
• Hydroxychloroquine (e.g., Plaquenil) or
• Mercaptopurine (e.g., Purinethol) or
• Methotrexate (e.g., Mexate) or
• Methyldopa (e.g., Aldomet) or
• Naltrexone (e.g., Trexan) (with long-term, high-dose use) or
• Oral contraceptives (birth control pills) containing estrogen or
• Phenothiazines (acetophenazine [e.g., Tindal], chlorpromazine [e.g., Thorazine], fluphenazine [e.g., Prolixin], mesoridazine [e.g., Serentil], perphenazine [e.g., Trilafon], prochlorperazine [e.g., Compazine], promazine [e.g., Sparine], promethazine [e.g., Phenergan], thioridazine

[e.g., Mellaril], trifluoperazine [e.g., Stelazine], triflu-promazine [e.g., Vesprin], trimeprazine [e.g., Temaril]) or
- Phenytoin (e.g., Dilantin) or
- Plicamycin (e.g., Mithracin) or
- Valproic acid (e.g., Depakene)—Estrogens and all of these medicines can cause liver damage. Your doctor may want you to have extra blood tests that tell about your liver, if you must take any of these medicines with estrogens
- Bromocriptine (e.g., Parlodel)—Estrogens may interfere with the effects of bromocriptine
- Cyclosporine (e.g., Sandimmune)—Estrogens can increase the chance of toxic effects to the kidney or liver from cyclosporine because estrogens can interfere with the body's ability to get the cyclosporine out of the bloodstream as it normally would

**Other medical problems**—The presence of other medical problems may affect the use of estrogens. Make sure you tell your doctor if you have any other medical problems, especially:
- Blood clots (or history of during previous estrogen therapy)—Estrogens may worsen blood clots or cause new clots to form
- Breast cancer (active or suspected)—Estrogens may cause growth of the tumor in some cases
- Changes in vaginal bleeding of unknown causes—Some irregular vaginal bleeding is a sign that the lining of the uterus is growing too much or is a sign of cancer of the uterus lining; estrogens may make these conditions worse
- Endometriosis—Estrogens may worsen endometriosis by causing growth of endometriosis implants
- Fibroid tumors of the uterus—Estrogens may cause fibroid tumors to increase in size
- Gallbladder disease or gallstones (or history of)—Estrogens may possibly increase the risk of gallbladder disease or gallstones
- Jaundice (or history of during pregnancy)—Estrogens may worsen or cause jaundice in these patients
- Liver disease—Toxic drug effects may occur in patients with liver disease because the body is not able to get this medicine out of the bloodstream as it normally would
- Porphyria—Estrogens can worsen porphyria

## Proper Use of This Medicine

*Use this medicine only as directed. Do not use more of it and do not use it for a longer time than your doctor ordered.*

This medicine is often used at bedtime to increase effectiveness through better absorption. To protect your clothing while using this medicine, you may find sanitary napkins helpful.

Vaginal creams and some vaginal suppositories are inserted with a plastic dose applicator. Directions for using the applicator are included with your medicine. If you do not receive the directions or do not understand them, ask your health care professional for information or additional explanation.

**Dosing**—The dose of vaginal estrogens will be different for different women. *Follow your doctor's orders or the directions on the label.* The following information includes only the average doses of these medicines. *If your dose is different, do not change it* unless your doctor tells you to do so.

*For dienestrol*
- For *vaginal* dosage form (cream):
  —Adults: At first, one applicatorful of cream inserted into the vagina one to two times a day, for one to two weeks. The dosage and how often you use the medicine will likely be reduced after your condition improves. Then, usually your doctor will want you to use this medicine for three weeks of each month, with one week of no medicine between each three weeks of medicine.

*For estradiol*
- For *vaginal* dosage form (cream):
  —Adults: At first, 200 to 400 micrograms (0.2 to 0.4 milligrams) of estradiol inserted into the vagina once a day, for one to two weeks. The dosage and how often you use the medicine will likely be reduced after your condition improves. Then, usually your doctor will want you to use this medicine for three weeks of each month, with one week of no medicine between each three weeks of medicine.

*For conjugated estrogens*
- For *vaginal* dosage form (cream):
  —Adults: 1.25 to 2.5 milligrams of conjugated estrogens inserted into the vagina once a day. Usually your doctor will want you to use this medicine for three weeks of each month, with one week of no medicine between each three weeks of medicine.

*For estrone*
- For *vaginal* dosage form (cream):
  —Adults: 2 to 4 milligrams of estrone inserted into the vagina once a day.
- For *vaginal* dosage form (suppository):
  —Adults: 0.25 to 0.5 milligrams of estrone inserted into the vagina once a day.

*For estropipate*
- For *vaginal* dosage form (cream):
  —Adults: 3 to 6 milligrams of estropipate inserted into the vagina once a day. Usually your doctor will want you to use this medicine for three weeks of each month, with one week of no medicine between each three weeks of medicine.

**Missed dose**—If you miss a dose of this medicine and do not remember it until the next day, do not use the missed dose at all. Instead, go back to your regular dosing schedule.

**Storage**—To store this medicine:
- Keep out of the reach of children.
- Store away from heat and direct light.
- Keep the medicine from freezing.

- Do not keep outdated medicine or medicine no longer needed. Be sure that any discarded medicine is out of the reach of children.

## Precautions While Using This Medicine

*It is very important that your doctor check your progress at regular visits to make sure this medicine does not cause unwanted effects.* These visits will usually be every year, but some doctors require them more often.

It is not yet known whether the use of estrogens increases the risk of breast cancer in women. Therefore, it is very important that you regularly check your breasts for any unusual lumps or discharge. You should also have a mammogram (x-ray pictures of the breasts) done if your doctor recommends it.

In some patients using estrogens, tenderness, swelling, or bleeding of the gums may occur. Brushing and flossing your teeth carefully and regularly and massaging your gums may help prevent this. See your dentist regularly to have your teeth cleaned. Check with your medical doctor or dentist if you have any questions about how to take care of your teeth and gums, or if you notice any tenderness, swelling, or bleeding of your gums.

*If you think that you may be pregnant, stop using the medicine immediately and check with your doctor.* Continued use of some estrogens during pregnancy may cause birth defects in the child.

Do not give this medicine to anyone else. Your doctor has prescribed it only for you after studying your health record and the results of your physical examination. Estrogens may be dangerous for other people because of differences in their health and body make-up.

Certain brands of vaginal estrogen products contain oils in the cream bases. Oils can weaken latex rubber condoms, diaphragms, or cervical caps. This increases the chances of a condom breaking during sexual intercourse. The rubber in cervical caps or diaphragms may break down faster and wear out sooner. Check with your health care professional to make sure the vaginal estrogen product you are using can be used with latex rubber birth control devices.

## Side Effects of This Medicine

Discuss these possible effects with your doctor:

- The prolonged use of estrogens has been reported to increase the risk of endometrial cancer (cancer of the lining of the uterus) in women after the menopause. This risk seems to increase as the dose and the length of use increase. When estrogens are used in low doses for less than 1 year, there is less risk. The risk is also reduced if a progestin (another female hormone) is added to, or replaces part of, your estrogen dose. If the uterus has been removed by surgery (total hysterectomy), there is no risk of endometrial cancer.

- It is not yet known whether the use of estrogens increases the risk of breast cancer in women. Although some large studies show an increased risk, most studies and information gathered to date do not support this idea.

- In studies with oral contraceptives (birth control pills) containing estrogens, cigarette smoking was shown to cause an increased risk of serious side effects affecting the heart or blood circulation, such as dangerous blood clots, heart attack, or stroke. The risk increased as the amount of smoking and the age of the smoker increased. Women aged 35 and over were at greatest risk when they smoked while using oral contraceptives containing estrogens. It is not known if this risk exists with the use of estrogens for symptoms of menopause. However, smoking may make estrogens less effective.

Check with your doctor as soon as possible if any of the following side effects occur:

*More common*

Pain, tenderness, or enlargement of breasts; swelling of feet and lower legs; weight gain (rapid)

*Less common or rare*

Changes in vaginal bleeding (spotting, breakthrough bleeding, prolonged or heavier bleeding, or complete stoppage of bleeding); lumps in, or discharge from, breast; pains in stomach, side, or abdomen; swelling, redness, or itching around vaginal area; uncontrolled jerky muscle movements; yellow eyes or skin

Other side effects may occur that usually do not need medical attention. These side effects may go away during treatment as your body adjusts to the medicine. However, check with your doctor if any of the following side effects continue or are bothersome:

*More common*

Bloating of stomach; cramps of lower stomach; loss of appetite

*Less common*

Diarrhea (mild); dizziness (mild); headaches (mild); migraine headaches; problems in wearing contact lenses; unusual increase in sexual desire

Also, many women who are using estrogens with a progestin (another female hormone) will start having monthly vaginal bleeding, similar to menstrual periods again. This effect will continue for as long as the medicine is taken. However, monthly bleeding will not occur in women who have had the uterus removed by surgery (total hysterectomy).

Other side effects not listed above may also occur in some patients. If you notice any other effects, check with your doctor.

Revised: 06/16/93

---

# ESTROGENS AND PROGESTINS   Oral Contraceptives   Systemic

Some commonly used brand names are:

**In the U.S.—**

| | |
|---|---|
| Brevicon[5] | Nelova 1/50M[6] |
| Demulen 1/35[2] | Nelulen 1/35E[2] |
| Demulen 1/50[2] | Nelulen 1/50E[2] |
| Desogen[1] | Nordette[3] |
| GenCept 0.5/35[5] | Norethin 1/35E[5] |
| GenCept 1/35[5] | Norethin 1/50M[6] |
| GenCept 10/11[5] | Norinyl 1+50[6] |
| Genora 0.5/35[5] | Norinyl 1+35[5] |
| Genora 1/35[5] | Ortho-Cept[1] |
| Genora 1/50[6] | Ortho-Cyclen[7] |
| Jenest[5] | Ortho-Novum 1/35[5] |
| Levlen[3] | Ortho-Novum 7/7/7[5] |
| Loestrin 1/20[4] | Ortho-Novum 10/11[5] |
| Loestrin 1.5/30[4] | Ortho-Novum 1/50[6] |
| Lo/Ovral[8] | Ortho Tri-Cyclen[7] |
| ModiCon[5] | Ovcon-35[5] |
| N.E.E. 1/35[5] | Ovcon-50[5] |
| N.E.E. 1/50[5] | Ovral[8] |
| Nelova 0.5/35E[5] | Tri-Levlen[3] |
| Nelova 1/35E[5] | Tri-Norinyl[5] |
| Nelova 10/11[5] | Triphasil[3] |

**In Canada—**

| | |
|---|---|
| Brevicon 0.5/35[5] | Ortho 7/7/7[5] |
| Brevicon 1/35[5] | Ortho 10/11[5] |
| Cyclen[7] | Ortho-Cept[1] |
| Demulen 30[2] | Ortho-Novum 0.5[6] |
| Demulen 50[2] | Ortho-Novum 1/50[6] |
| Loestrin 1.5/30[4] | Ortho-Novum 1/80[6] |
| Marvelon[1] | Ortho-Novum 2[6] |
| Minestrin 1/20[4] | Ovral[8] |
| Min-Ovral[3] | Synphasic[5] |
| Norinyl 1/50[6] | Tri-Cyclen[7] |
| Ortho 0.5/35[5] | Triphasil[3] |
| Ortho 1/35[5] | Triquilar[3] |

Note: For quick reference, the following estrogens and progestins are numbered to match the corresponding brand names.

This information applies to the following medicines:

1. Desogestrel (des-oh-JES-trel) and Ethinyl Estradiol (ETH-in-il ess-tra-DYE-ole)
2. Ethynodiol (e-thye-noe-DYE-ole) Diacetate and Ethinyl Estradiol
3. Levonorgestrel (LEE-voe-nor-jess-trel) and Ethinyl Estradiol
4. Norethindrone (nor-eth-IN-drone) Acetate and Ethinyl Estradiol
5. Norethindrone and Ethinyl Estradiol
6. Norethindrone and Mestranol
7. Norgestimate (nor-JES-ti-mate) and Ethinyl Estradiol
8. Norgestrel (nor-JESS-trel) and Ethinyl Estradiol

For information about Norethindrone (e.g., Micronor) or Norgestrel (e.g., Ovrette) when used as single-ingredient oral contraceptives, see *Progestins (Systemic)*.

## Description

Oral contraceptives are known also as the Pill, OC's, BC's, BC tablets, or birth control pills. They usually contain two types of female hormones, estrogens (ESS-troe-jenz) and progestins (proe-JESS-tins). When taken by mouth on a regular schedule, they change the hormone balance of the body, which prevents pregnancy.

Sometimes these preparations can be used in the treatment of conditions that are helped by added hormones. Oral contraceptives do not prevent or cure venereal diseases (VD), however.

Before you take an oral contraceptive, you and your doctor should discuss the benefits and risks of using these medicines. Besides surgery or not having intercourse, these medicines are the most effective method of preventing pregnancy. However, oral contraceptives sometimes have side effects that could be very serious.

To make the use of oral contraceptives as safe and reliable as possible, you should understand how and when to take them and what effects may be expected. *A paper with information for the patient will be given to you with your filled prescription, and will provide many details concerning the use of oral contraceptives. Read this paper carefully* and ask your health care professional if you need additional information or explanation.

Oral contraceptives are available only with your doctor's prescription, in the following dosage forms:

*Oral*
Desogestrel and Ethinyl Estradiol
  • Tablets (U.S. and Canada)
Ethynodiol Diacetate and Ethinyl Estradiol
  • Tablets (U.S. and Canada)
Levonorgestrel and Ethinyl Estradiol
  • Tablets (U.S. and Canada)
Norethindrone Acetate and Ethinyl Estradiol
  • Tablets (U.S. and Canada)
Norethindrone and Ethinyl Estradiol
  • Tablets (U.S. and Canada)
Norethindrone and Mestranol
  • Tablets (U.S. and Canada)
Norgestimate and Ethinyl Estradiol
  • Tablets (U.S. and Canada)
Norgestrel and Ethinyl Estradiol
  • Tablets (U.S. and Canada)

## Before Using This Medicine

In deciding to use a medicine, the risks of taking the medicine must be weighed against the good it will do. This is a decision you and your doctor will make. For estrogen and progestin birth control pills, the following should be considered:

**Allergies**—Tell your doctor if you have ever had any unusual or allergic reaction to estrogens or progestins. Also tell your health care professional if you are allergic to any other substances, such as foods, preservatives, or dyes.

**Pregnancy**—Oral contraceptives are not recommended for use during pregnancy.

**Breast-feeding**—The estrogens in oral contraceptives pass into the breast milk. It is not known what effect oral contraceptives may have on the infant. Studies have shown oral contraceptives to cause tumors in humans and animals. Use of "high-dose" birth control medicines is not recommended during breast-feeding. It may be necessary for you to use another method of birth control or to stop breast-feeding while taking oral contraceptives. However, your doctor may allow you to begin using one of the "low-dose" oral contraceptives after you have been breast-feeding for a while.

**Children**—This medicine is frequently used for birth control in teenage females and has not been shown to cause different side effects or problems than it does in adults. However, some teenagers may need extra information on the importance of taking this medication exactly as prescribed in order for it to work.

**Other medicines**—Although certain medicines should not be used together at all, in other cases two different medicines may be used together even if an interaction might occur. In these cases, your doctor may want to change the dose, or other precautions may be necessary. When you are taking estrogen and progestin birth control pills, it is especially important that your health care professional know if you are taking any of the following:

- Acetaminophen (e.g., Tylenol) (with long-term, high-dose use)
- Adrenocorticoids (cortisone-like medicine)
- Amiodarone (e.g., Cordarone)
- Anabolic steroids (nandrolone [e.g., Anabolin], oxandrolone [e.g., Anavar], oxymetholone [e.g., Anadrol], stanozolol [e.g., Winstrol])
- Androgens (male hormones)
- Anticoagulants (blood thinners)
- Anti-infectives by mouth or by injection (medicine for infection)
- Antithyroid agents (medicine for overactive thyroid)
- Barbiturates
- Bromocriptine (e.g., Parlodel)
- Carbamazepine (e.g., Tegretol)
- Carmustine (e.g., BiCNU)
- Chloroquine (e.g., Aralen)
- Dantrolene (e.g., Dantrium)
- Daunorubicin (e.g., Cerubidine)
- Disulfiram (e.g., Antabuse)
- Divalproex (e.g., Depakote)
- Estrogens (female hormones)
- Etretinate (e.g., Tegison)
- Gold salts (medicine for arthritis)
- Griseofulvin (e.g., Fulvicin)
- Hydroxychloroquine (e.g., Plaquenil)
- Mercaptopurine (e.g., Purinethol)
- Methotrexate (e.g., Mexate)
- Methyldopa (e.g., Aldomet)
- Naltrexone (e.g., Trexan) (with long-term, high-dose use)
- Phenothiazines (acetophenazine [e.g., Tindal], chlorpromazine [e.g., Thorazine], fluphenazine [e.g., Prolixin], mesoridazine [e.g., Serentil], perphenazine [e.g., Trilafon], prochlorperazine [e.g., Compazine], promazine [e.g., Sparine], promethazine [e.g., Phenergan], thioridazine [e.g., Mellaril], trifluoperazine [e.g., Stelazine], triflupromazine [e.g., Vesprin], trimeprazine [e.g., Temaril])
- Phenylbutazone (e.g., Butazolidin)
- Phenytoin (e.g., Dilantin)
- Plicamycin (e.g., Mithracin)
- Primidone (e.g., Mysoline)
- Rifampin (e.g., Rifadin)

- Tricyclic antidepressants (amitriptyline [e.g., Elavil], amoxapine [e.g., Asendin], clomipramine [e.g., Anafranil], desipramine [e.g., Pertofrane], doxepin [e.g., Sinequan], imipramine [e.g., Tofranil], nortriptyline [e.g., Aventyl], protriptyline [e.g., Vivactil], trimipramine [e.g., Surmontil])
- Valproic acid (e.g., Depakene)

**Other medical problems**—The presence of other medical problems may affect the use of estrogen and progestin birth control pills. Make sure you tell your doctor if you have any other medical problems, especially:

- Angina pectoris (chest pains on exertion)
- Asthma
- Blood clots (or history of)
- Bone disease
- Breast disease (not cancerous, such as fibrocystic disease [breast cysts], breast lumps, or abnormal mammograms [x-ray pictures of the breast])
- Cancer (or history of or family history of breast cancer)
- Changes in vaginal bleeding
- Diabetes mellitus (sugar diabetes)
- Endometriosis
- Epilepsy
- Fibroid tumors of the uterus
- Gallbladder disease or gallstones (or history of)
- Heart or circulation disease
- High blood cholesterol
- High blood pressure (hypertension)
- Jaundice (or history of, including jaundice during pregnancy)
- Kidney disease
- Liver disease (such as jaundice or porphyria)
- Lumps in breasts
- Mental depression (or history of)
- Migraine headaches
- Scanty or irregular menstrual periods
- Stroke (history of)
- Too much calcium in the blood
- Tuberculosis
- Varicose veins

## Proper Use of This Medicine

*Take this medicine only as directed by your doctor. This medicine must be taken exactly on schedule to prevent pregnancy.* Try to take the medicine at the same time each day, not more than 24 hours apart, to reduce the possibility of side effects and to provide the best protection.

Nausea may occur during the first few weeks after you start taking this medicine. This effect usually disappears with continued use. If the nausea is bothersome, it can usually be prevented or reduced by taking each dose with food or immediately after food.

Since one of the most important factors in the proper use of oral contraceptives is taking every dose exactly on schedule, you should never let your tablet supply run out. Always keep 1 extra month's supply of tablets on hand.

To keep the extra month's supply from becoming too old, use it next, after the pills now being used, and replace the extra supply each month on a regular schedule. The tablets will keep well when kept dry and at room temperature (light will fade some tablet colors but will not change the medicine's effect).

Keep the tablets in the container in which you received them. Most containers aid you in keeping track of your dosage schedule.

It is very important that you take the tablets in the same order that they appear in the container. Tablets of different colors in the same package are also different in strength. *Taking the tablets out of order may reduce the effectiveness of the medicine.*

- *Monophasic (one-phase) cycle* dosing schedule: Most available dosing schedules are of the monophasic type. If you are taking tablets of one strength (color) for 20 or 21 days, you are using a monophasic schedule. For the 28-day monophasic cycle you will also take an additional 7 inactive tablets, which are of another color.
- *Biphasic (two-phase) cycle* dosing schedule:
  —If you are using a biphasic 21-day schedule, you are taking tablets of one strength (color) for 7 to 10 days (the 1st phase). You then take tablets of a second strength (color) for the next 11 to 14 days (the 2nd phase). For the 28-day biphasic cycle you will also take an additional 7 inactive tablets, which are of a third color.
  —If you are using a biphasic 24-day schedule, you are taking tablets of one strength (color) for 17 days (the 1st phase). You then take tablets of a second strength (color) for the next 7 days (the 2nd phase).
- *Triphasic (three-phase) cycle* dosing schedule: If you are using a triphasic 21-day schedule, you are taking tablets of one strength (color) for 6 or 7 days depending on the medicine prescribed (the 1st phase). You then take tablets of a second strength (color) for the next 5 to 9 days depending on the medicine prescribed (the 2nd phase). After that, you take tablets of a third strength (color) for the next 5 to 10 days depending on the medicine prescribed (the 3rd phase). At this point, you will have taken a total of 21 tablets. For the 28-day triphasic cycle you will also take an additional 7 inactive tablets, which are of a fourth color.

**Dosing—**Your health care professional may begin your dose on the first day of your menstrual period (called day-1 start), on the fifth day of your menstrual period (called day-5 start), or on Sunday (called Sunday start). *When you begin on a certain day it is important that you follow that schedule, even when you miss a dose. Do not change your schedule on your own.* If the schedule that you have been put on is not convenient, check with your health care professional about changing schedules.

- For *oral* dosage forms (monophasic, biphasic, or triphasic tablets):
  —For contraception:
  • Adults and teenagers—
    For 21-day cycle: Take one tablet a day for twenty-one days. Skip seven days. Then repeat the cycle.
    For 28-day cycle: Take one tablet a day for twenty-eight days. Then repeat the cycle.

**Missed dose—***Follow your doctor's orders or the directions on the label* if you miss a dose of this medicine. The following information includes only some of the ways to handle missed doses. Your health care professional may want you to stop taking the medicine and use other birth control methods for the rest of the month until you have your menstrual period. Then your health care professional can help you begin your medicine again.

*For monophasic, biphasic, or triphasic cycles:*

- If you miss the first tablet of a new cycle—Take the missed tablet as soon as you remember and take the next tablet at the usual time. You may take 2 tablets in one day. Then continue your regular dosing schedule. Also, use another birth control method until you have taken seven days of your tablets after the last missed dose.
- If you miss 1 tablet during the cycle—Take the missed tablet as soon as you remember. Take the next tablet at the usual time. You may take 2 tablets in one day. Then continue your regular dosing schedule.
- If you miss 2 tablets in a row in the first or second week—Take 2 tablets on the day that you remember and 2 tablets the next day. Continue taking 1 tablet a day. Also, use another birth control method until you begin a new cycle.
- If you miss 2 tablets in a row in the third week; or
- If you miss 3 or more tablets in a row at any time during the cycle—

  Using a day-1 start: Throw out your current cycle and begin taking a new cycle. Also, use another birth control method until you have taken seven days of your tablets after the last missed dose. You may not have a menstrual period this month. But if you miss two menstrual periods in a row, call your health care professional.

  Using a day-5 start: Keep taking one tablet a day from your current pack until the end of the cycle. Use another birth control method until you begin a new cycle. You should have a menstrual period this month. If you do not, call your health care professional.

  Using a Sunday start: Keep taking one tablet a day from your current pack until Sunday. Then, on Sunday, throw out your old pack and begin a new pack. Also, use another birth control method until you have taken seven days of your tablets after the last missed dose. You may not have a menstrual period this month. But if you miss two menstrual periods in a row, call your health care professional.

If you miss any of the last 7 (inactive) tablets of a 28-day cycle, there is no danger of pregnancy. However, the first tablet (active) of the next month's cycle must be taken on the regularly scheduled day, in spite of any missed doses, if pregnancy is to be avoided. The active and inactive tablets are colored differently for your convenience.

**Storage**—To store this medicine:
- Keep out of the reach of children.
- Store away from heat and direct light.
- Do not store in the bathroom, near the kitchen sink, or in other damp places. Heat and moisture may cause the medicine to break down.
- Do not keep outdated medicine or medicine no longer needed. Be sure that any discarded medicine is out of the reach of children.

## Precautions While Using This Medicine

*It is very important that your doctor check your progress at regular visits* to make sure this medicine does not cause unwanted effects. These visits will usually be every 6 to 12 months, but some doctors require them more often.

*When you begin to use oral contraceptives,* your body will require at least 7 days to adjust before pregnancy will be prevented; therefore, you should *use a second method of birth control for the first cycle (or 3 weeks)* to ensure full protection.

*Tell the medical doctor or dentist in charge that you are taking this medicine before any kind of surgery (including dental surgery) or emergency treatment,* since this medicine may cause serious blood clots, heart attack, or stroke.

The following medicines may reduce the effectiveness of oral contraceptives. *You should use a second method of birth control during each cycle in which any of the following medicines are used:*

Ampicillin
Adrenocorticoids (cortisone-like medicine)
Bacampicillin
Barbiturates
Carbamazepine (e.g., Tegretol)
Chloramphenicol (e.g., Chloromycetin)
Dihydroergotamine (e.g., D.H.E. 45)
Griseofulvin (e.g., Fulvicin)
Mineral oil
Neomycin, oral
Penicillin V
Phenylbutazone (e.g., Butazolidin)
Phenytoin (e.g., Dilantin)
Primidone (e.g., Mysoline)
Rifampin (e.g., Rifadin)
Sulfonamides (sulfa medicine)
Tetracyclines (medicine for infection)
Tranquilizers
Valproic acid (e.g., Depakene)

Check with your doctor if you have any questions about this.

Vaginal bleeding of various amounts may occur between your regular menstrual periods during the first 3 months of use. This is sometimes called spotting when slight, or breakthrough bleeding when heavier. If this should occur:
- Continue on your regular dosing schedule.
- The bleeding usually stops within 1 week.
- Check with your doctor if the bleeding continues for more than 1 week.
- After you have been taking oral contraceptives on schedule and for more than 3 months, check with your doctor.

Missed menstrual periods may occur:
- if you have not taken the medicine exactly as scheduled. Pregnancy must be considered a possibility.
- if the medicine is not properly adjusted for your needs.
- if you have taken oral contraceptives for a long time, usually 2 or more years, and stop their use.

Check with your doctor if you miss any menstrual periods so that the cause may be determined.

In some patients using estrogen-containing oral contraceptives, tenderness, swelling, or bleeding of the gums may occur. Brushing and flossing your teeth carefully and regularly and massaging your gums may help prevent this. See your dentist regularly to have your teeth cleaned. Check with your medical doctor or dentist if you have any questions about how to take care of your teeth and gums, or if you notice any tenderness, swelling, or bleeding of your gums. Also, it has been shown that estrogen-containing oral contraceptives may cause a healing problem called dry socket after a tooth has been removed. If you are going to have a tooth removed, tell your dentist or oral surgeon that you are taking oral contraceptives.

Some people who take oral contraceptives may become more sensitive to sunlight than they are normally. When you begin taking this medicine, avoid too much sun and do not use a sunlamp until you see how you react to the sun, especially if you tend to burn easily. If you have a severe reaction, check with your doctor. Some people may develop brown, blotchy spots on exposed areas. These spots usually disappear gradually when the medicine is stopped.

If you wear contact lenses and notice a change in vision or are not able to wear them, check with your doctor.

*If you suspect that you may have become pregnant, stop taking this medicine immediately and check with your doctor.*

If you are scheduled for any laboratory tests, tell your doctor that you are taking birth control pills.

Do not give this medicine to anyone else. Your doctor has prescribed it only for you after studying your health record and the results of your physical examination. Oral contraceptives may be dangerous for other people because of differences in their health and body make-up.

Check with your doctor before taking any leftover oral contraceptives from an old prescription, especially after a pregnancy. Your old prescription may be dangerous to you now or may allow you to become pregnant if your health has changed since your last physical examination.

## Side Effects of This Medicine

Discuss these possible effects with your doctor:

- Along with their needed effects, birth control tablets sometimes cause some unwanted effects such as benign (not cancerous) liver tumors, liver cancer, blood clots, heart attack, and stroke, and problems of the gallbladder, liver, and uterus. Although these effects are rare, they can be very serious and may cause death.
- *Cigarette smoking* during the use of oral contraceptives has been found to increase the risk of serious side effects affecting the heart and/or blood circulation, such as dangerous blood clots, heart attack, or stroke. The risk increases as the age of the patient and the amount of smoking increase. This risk is greater in women age 35 and over. *To reduce the risk of serious side effects, do not smoke cigarettes while using oral contraceptives.*

The following side effects may be caused by blood clots, which could lead to stroke, heart attack, or death. Although these side effects rarely occur, they require immediate medical attention. *Get emergency help immediately* if any of the following side effects occur:

Abdominal or stomach pain (sudden, severe, or continuing); coughing up blood; headache (severe or sudden); loss of coordination (sudden); loss of vision or change in vision (sudden); pains in chest, groin, or leg (especially in calf of leg); shortness of breath (sudden or unexplained); slurring of speech (sudden); weakness, numbness, or pain in arm or leg (unexplained)

Check with your doctor as soon as possible if any of the following side effects occur:

*Less common or rare*

Bulging eyes; changes in vaginal bleeding (spotting, breakthrough bleeding, prolonged bleeding, or complete stoppage of bleeding); double vision; fainting; frequent urge to urinate or painful urination; increased blood pressure; loss of vision (gradual, partial, or complete); lumps in, or discharge from, breast; mental depression; pains in stomach, side, or abdomen; skin rash, redness, or other skin irritation; swelling, pain, or tenderness in upper abdomen (stomach) area; unusual or dark-colored mole; vaginal discharge (thick, white, or curd-like); vaginal itching or irritation; yellow eyes or skin

Other side effects may occur that usually do not need medical attention. These side effects may go away during treatment as your body adjusts to the medicine. However, check with your doctor if any of the following side effects continue or are bothersome:

*More common*

Acne (usually less common after first 3 months); bloating of stomach; cramps of lower stomach; increase or decrease in appetite; nausea; swelling of ankles and feet; swelling and increased tenderness of breasts; unusual tiredness or weakness; unusual weight gain

*Less common or rare*

Brown, blotchy spots on exposed skin;. diarrhea (mild); dizziness; headaches or migraine headaches; increased body and facial hair; increased sensitivity to contact lenses; increased skin sensitivity to sun; irritability; some loss of scalp hair; unusual decrease or increase in sexual desire; vomiting; weight loss

Other side effects not listed above may also occur in some patients. If you notice any other effects, check with your doctor.

Revised: August 1990
Interim revision: 06/08/93; 07/12/94

# ETHAMBUTOL   Systemic

Some commonly used brand names are:
**In the U.S.—**
    Myambutol
**In Canada—**
    Etibi
    Myambutol

## Description

Ethambutol (e-THAM-byoo-tole) is used to treat tuberculosis (TB). It is used with other medicines for TB. This medicine may also be used for other problems as determined by your doctor.

*To help clear up your tuberculosis (TB) completely, you must keep taking this medicine for the full time of treatment, even if you begin to feel better. This is very important. It is also important that you do not miss any doses.*

Ethambutol is available only with your doctor's prescription, in the following dosage form:

*Oral*
- Tablets (U.S. and Canada)

## Before Using This Medicine

In deciding to use a medicine, the risks of taking the medicine must be weighed against the good it will do.

This is a decision you and your doctor will make. For ethambutol, the following should be considered:

**Allergies**—Tell your doctor if you have ever had any unusual or allergic reaction to ethambutol. Also tell your health care professional if you are allergic to any other substances, such as foods, preservatives, or dyes.

**Pregnancy**—Pregnant women with tuberculosis (TB) should be treated with TB medicines, including ethambutol. Ethambutol has not been shown to cause birth defects or other problems in humans. However, studies in animals have shown that ethambutol causes cleft palate, skull and spine defects, absence of one eye, and hare lip.

**Breast-feeding**—Ethambutol passes into breast milk. However, ethambutol has not been shown to cause problems in nursing babies.

**Children**—This medicine has been tested in children 13 years of age or older and has not been shown to cause different side effects or problems than it does in adults. Ethambutol may be used for children with TB when other medicines cannot be used. However, ethambutol is usually not used in children younger than 6 years of age because it may be hard to tell if they are having side effects affecting their eyes.

**Older adults**—Many medicines have not been studied specifically in older people. Therefore, it may not be known whether they work exactly the same way they do in younger adults. Although there is no specific information comparing use of ethambutol in the elderly with use in other age groups, this medicine is not expected to cause different side effects or problems in older people than it does in younger adults.

**Other medicines**—Although certain medicines should not be used together at all, in other cases two different medicines may be used together even if an interaction might occur. In these cases, your doctor may want to change the dose, or other precautions may be necessary. Tell your health care professional if you are taking any other prescription or nonprescription (over-the-counter [OTC]) medicine.

**Other medical problems**—The presence of other medical problems may affect the use of ethambutol. Make sure you tell your doctor if you have any other medical problems, especially:
- Gouty arthritis—Ethambutol may cause or worsen attacks of gout
- Kidney disease—Patients with kidney disease may be more likely to have side effects
- Optic neuritis (eye nerve damage)—Ethambutol may cause or worsen eye disease

## Proper Use of This Medicine

Ethambutol may be taken with food if this medicine upsets your stomach.

To help clear up your tuberculosis (TB) completely, *it is very important that you keep taking this medicine for*

*the full time of treatment,* even if you begin to feel better after a few weeks. You may have to take it every day for as long as 1 to 2 years or more. *It is important that you do not miss any doses.*

**Dosing**—The dose of ethambutol will be different for different patients. *Follow your doctor's orders or the directions on the label.* The following information includes only the average doses of ethambutol. *If your dose is different, do not change it* unless your doctor tells you to do so.

The number of tablets that you take depends on the strength of the medicine.
- For *oral* dosage form (tablets):
  —For the treatment of tuberculosis (TB):
    - Adults and children 13 years of age and older—15 to 25 milligrams (mg) per kilogram (kg) (6.8 to 11.4 mg per pound) of body weight once a day. Instead, your doctor may tell you to take 50 mg per kg (22.8 mg per pound) of body weight, up to a total of 2.5 grams, two times a week. Another dose that your doctor may tell you to take is 25 to 30 mg per kg (11.4 to 13.6 mg per pound) of body weight, up to a total of 2.5 grams, three times a week. Ethambutol must be taken with other medicines to treat tuberculosis.
    - Infants and children up to 13 years of age—Use and dose must be determined by your doctor.

**Missed dose**—If you miss a dose of this medicine, take it as soon as possible. However, if it is almost time for your next dose, skip the missed dose and go back to your regular dosing schedule. Do not double doses.

**Storage**—To store this medicine:
- Keep out of the reach of children.
- Store away from heat and direct light.
- Do not store in the bathroom, near the kitchen sink, or in other damp places. Heat or moisture may cause the medicine to break down.
- Do not keep outdated medicine or medicine no longer needed. Be sure that any discarded medicine is out of the reach of children.

## Precautions While Using This Medicine

If your symptoms do not improve within 2 to 3 weeks, or if they become worse, check with your doctor.

It is very important that your doctor check your progress at regular visits.

*Check with your doctor immediately if blurred vision, eye pain, red-green color blindness, or loss of vision occurs during treatment.* Your doctor may want you to have your eyes checked by an ophthalmologist (eye doctor). *Also, make sure you know how you react to this medicine before you drive, use machines, or do anything else that could be dangerous if you are not alert or able to see well.*

## Side Effects of This Medicine

Along with its needed effects, a medicine may cause some unwanted effects. Although not all of these side effects may occur, if they do occur they may need medical attention.

*Check with your doctor immediately* if any of the following side effects occur:

*Less common*
Chills; pain and swelling of joints, especially big toe, ankle, or knee; tense, hot skin over affected joints

*Rare*
Blurred vision, eye pain, red-green color blindness, or any loss of vision (more common with high doses); fever; joint pain; numbness, tingling, burning pain, or weakness in hands or feet; skin rash

Other side effects may occur that usually do not need medical attention. These side effects may go away during treatment as your body adjusts to the medicine. However, check with your doctor if any of the following side effects continue or are bothersome:

*Less common*
Confusion; headache; loss of appetite; nausea and vomiting; stomach pain

Other side effects not listed above may also occur in some patients. If you notice any other effects, check with your doctor.

## Additional Information

Once a medicine has been approved for marketing for a certain use, experience may show that it is also useful for other medical problems. Although this use is not included in product labeling, ethambutol is used in certain patients with the following medical condition:

• Atypical mycobacterial infections, such as *Mycobacterium avium* complex (MAC)

Other than the above information, there is no additional information relating to proper use, precautions, or side effects for this use.

Revised: 06/22/94

# ETHCHLORVYNOL   Systemic

A commonly used brand name in the U.S. and Canada is Placidyl. Generic name product may also be available in the U.S.

## Description

Ethchlorvynol (eth-klor-VI-nole) is used to treat insomnia (trouble in sleeping). However, it has generally been replaced by other medicines for the treatment of insomnia. If ethchlorvynol is used regularly (for example, every day) to help produce sleep, it is usually not effective for more than 1 week.

This medicine is available only with your doctor's prescription, in the following dosage form:

*Oral*
• Capsules (U.S. and Canada)

## Before Using This Medicine

In deciding to use a medicine, the risks of taking the medicine must be weighed against the good it will do. This is a decision you and your doctor will make. For ethchlorvynol, the following should be considered:

**Allergies**—Tell your doctor if you have ever had any unusual or allergic reaction to ethchlorvynol. Also tell your health care professional if you are allergic to any other substances, such as foods, preservatives, or dyes.

**Pregnancy**—Ethchlorvynol has not been studied in pregnant women. However, use of ethchlorvynol during the first 6 months of pregnancy is not recommended because studies in animals have shown that high doses of ethchlorvynol increase the chance of stillbirths and decrease the chance of the newborn surviving. Taking ethchlorvynol during the last 3 months of pregnancy may cause slow heartbeat, shortness of breath, troubled breathing, or withdrawal side effects in the newborn baby.

**Breast-feeding**—It is not known whether ethchlorvynol passes into the breast milk.

**Children**—Studies on this medicine have been done only in adult patients and there is no specific information comparing use of ethchlorvynol in children with use in other age groups.

**Older adults**—Elderly people may be especially sensitive to the effects of ethchlorvynol. This may increase the chance of side effects during treatment.

**Other medicines**—Although certain medicines should not be used together at all, in other cases 2 different medicines may be used together even if an interaction might occur. In these cases, your doctor may want to change the dose, or other precautions may be necessary. When you are taking ethchlorvynol, it is especially important that your health care professional know if you are taking any of the following:

• Anticoagulants (blood thinners)—Ethchlorvynol may change the amount of anticoagulant you need to take

- Central nervous system (CNS) depressants (medicine that causes drowsiness) or
- Tricyclic antidepressants (medicine for depression)—Using these medicines together with ethchlorvynol may increase the CNS and other depressant effects

**Other medical problems**—The presence of other medical problems may affect the use of ethchlorvynol. Make sure you tell your doctor if you have any other medical problems, especially:

- Alcohol abuse (or history of) or
- Drug abuse or dependence (or history of)—Dependence on ethchlorvynol may develop
- Kidney disease or
- Liver disease—Higher blood levels of ethchlorvynol may result and increase the chance of side effects
- Mental depression or
- Porphyria—Ethchlorvynol may make the condition worse

## Proper Use of This Medicine

*Ethchlorvynol is best taken with food or a glass of milk* to lessen the possibility of dizziness, clumsiness, or unsteadiness, which may occur shortly after you take this medicine.

*Take this medicine only as directed by your doctor.* Do not take more of it, do not take it more often, and do not take it for a longer time than your doctor ordered. If too much is taken, it may become habit-forming.

**Dosing**—The dose of ethchlorvynol will be different for different patients. *Follow your doctor's orders or the directions on the label.* The following information includes only the average doses of ethchlorvynol. *If your dose is different, do not change it* unless your doctor tells you to do so.

- For *oral* dosage forms (capsules):
  —Adults: 500 to 1000 milligrams at bedtime.
  —Children: Dose must be determined by the doctor.

**Storage**—To store this medicine:

- Keep out of the reach of children. Overdose of ethchlorvynol is especially dangerous in children.
- Store away from heat and direct light.
- Do not store in the bathroom, near the kitchen sink, or in other damp places. Heat or moisture may cause the medicine to break down.
- Do not keep outdated medicine or medicine no longer needed. Be sure that any discarded medicine is out of the reach of children.

## Precautions While Using This Medicine

If you will be taking this medicine regularly for a long time:

- Your doctor should check your progress at regular visits.
- Do not stop taking it without first checking with your doctor. Your doctor may want you to reduce gradually the amount you are taking before stopping completely.

This medicine will add to the effects of alcohol and other CNS depressants (medicines that slow down the nervous system, possibly causing drowsiness). Some examples of CNS depressants are antihistamines or medicine for hay fever, other allergies, or colds; sedatives, tranquilizers, or sleeping medicine; prescription pain medicine or narcotics; barbiturates; medicine for seizures; muscle relaxants; or anesthetics, including some dental anesthetics. *Check with your doctor before taking any of the above while you are taking this medicine.*

*If you think you or someone else may have taken an overdose of this medicine, get emergency help at once.* Taking an overdose of ethchlorvynol or taking alcohol or other CNS depressants with ethchlorvynol may lead to unconsciousness and possibly death. Some signs of an overdose are continuing confusion, severe weakness, shortness of breath or slow or troubled breathing, slurred speech, staggering, and slow heartbeat.

This medicine may cause some people to become dizzy, lightheaded, drowsy, or less alert than they are normally. Even if taken at bedtime, it may cause some people to feel drowsy or less alert on arising. *Make sure you know how you react to this medicine before you drive, use machines, or do anything else that could be dangerous if you are dizzy or are not alert.*

## Side Effects of This Medicine

Along with its needed effects, a medicine may cause some unwanted effects. Although not all of these side effects may occur, if they do occur they may need medical attention.

Check with your doctor as soon as possible if any of the following side effects occur:

*Less common*
Skin rash or hives; unusual bleeding or bruising; unusual excitement, nervousness, or restlessness

*Rare*
Darkening of urine; itching; pale stools; yellow eyes or skin

*Symptoms of overdose*
Confusion (continuing); double vision; low body temperature; numbness, tingling, pain, or weakness in hands or feet; shortness of breath or slow or troubled breathing; slow heartbeat; slurred speech; staggering; trembling; unusual movements of the eyes; weakness (severe)

Other side effects may occur that usually do not need medical attention. These side effects may go away during treatment as your body adjusts to the medicine. However, check with your doctor if any of the following side effects continue or are bothersome:

*More common*
Blurred vision; dizziness or lightheadedness; indigestion; nausea or vomiting; numbness of face; stomach pain; unpleasant aftertaste; unusual tiredness or weakness

*Less common*
Clumsiness or unsteadiness; confusion; drowsiness (daytime)

After you stop using this medicine, your body may need time to adjust. If you took this medicine in high doses or for a long time, this may take up to 2 weeks. During this period of time check with your doctor if you notice any of the following side effects:

Convulsions (seizures); hallucinations (seeing, hearing, or feeling things that are not there); muscle twitching; nausea or vomiting; restlessness, nervousness, or irritability; sweating; trembling; trouble in sleeping; weakness

Other side effects not listed above may also occur in some patients. If you notice any other effects, check with your doctor.

Revised: 03/09/90

# ETHIONAMIDE    Systemic†

A commonly used brand name in the U.S. is Trecator-SC.

†Not commercially available in Canada.

## Description

Ethionamide (e-thye-ON-am-ide) is used with other medicines to treat tuberculosis (TB). Ethionamide may also be used for other problems as determined by your doctor.

*To help clear up your tuberculosis (TB) completely, you must keep taking this medicine for the full time of treatment, even if you begin to feel better. This is very important. It is also important that you do not miss any doses.*

Ethionamide is available only with your doctor's prescription, in the following dosage form:
*Oral*
- Tablets (U.S.)

## Before Using This Medicine

In deciding to use a medicine, the risks of taking the medicine must be weighed against the good it will do. This is a decision you and your doctor will make. For ethionamide, the following should be considered:

**Allergies**—Tell your doctor if you have ever had any unusual or allergic reaction to ethionamide, isoniazid (e.g., INH; Nydrazid), pyrazinamide, or niacin (e.g., Nicobid; nicotinic acid). Also tell your health care professional if you are allergic to any other substances, such as foods, preservatives, or dyes.

**Pregnancy**—Ethionamide causes birth defects in rats and rabbits given doses greater than the usual human dose. However, women with tuberculosis (TB) should be treated with medicines to treat TB. If you have any concerns, talk to your doctor.

**Breast-feeding**—It is not known whether ethionamide passes into breast milk. Although most medicines pass into breast milk in small amounts, many of them may be used safely while breast-feeding. Mothers who are taking this medicine and who wish to breast-feed should discuss this with their doctor.

**Children**—Although there is no specific information comparing use of ethionamide in children with use in other age groups, this medicine is not expected to cause different side effects or problems in children than it does in adults.

**Older adults**—Many medicines have not been studied specifically in older people. Therefore, it may not be known whether they work exactly the same way they do in younger adults or if they cause different side effects or problems in older people. There is no specific information comparing use of ethionamide in the elderly with use in other age groups.

**Other medicines**—Although certain medicines should not be used together at all, in other cases two different medicines may be used together even if an interaction might occur. In these cases, your doctor may want to change the dose, or other precautions may be necessary. When you are taking ethionamide, it is especially important that your health care professional know if you are taking any of the following:
- Cycloserine—Use of ethionamide with cycloserine may increase the chance for nervous system side effects, such as convulsions (seizures)

**Other medical problems**—The presence of other medical problems may affect the use of ethionamide. Make sure you tell your doctor if you have any other medical problems, especially:
- Diabetes mellitus (sugar diabetes)—Diabetes may be harder to control in patients taking ethionamide
- Liver disease (severe)—Patients with severe liver disease may have an increased chance of side effects

## Proper Use of This Medicine

Ethionamide may be taken with or after meals if it upsets your stomach.

To help clear up your tuberculosis (TB) completely, *it is very important that you keep taking this medicine for the full time of treatment,* even if you begin to feel better after a few weeks. You may have to take it every day for 1 to 2 years or more. *It is important that you do not miss any doses.*

Your doctor may also want you to take pyridoxine (e.g., Hexa-Betalin; vitamin $B_6$) every day to help prevent or lessen some of the side effects of ethionamide. If so, *it is very important to take pyridoxine every day along with this medicine. Do not miss any doses.*

**Dosing**—The dose of ethionamide will be different for different patients. *Follow your doctor's orders or the directions on the label.* The following information includes only the average doses of ethionamide. *If your dose is different, do not change it* unless your doctor tells you to do so.

- For *oral* dosage form (tablets):
  —For the treatment of tuberculosis (TB):
  - Adults and teenagers—250 milligrams (mg) every eight to twelve hours. Ethionamide must be taken with other medicines to treat tuberculosis.
  - Children—Dose is based on body weight. The usual dose is 4 to 5 mg per kilogram of body weight every eight hours. Ethionamide must be taken with other medicines to treat tuberculosis.

**Missed dose**—If you do miss a dose of either of these medicines, take it as soon as possible. However, if it is almost time for your next dose, skip the missed dose and go back to your regular dosing schedule. Do not double doses.

**Storage**—To store this medicine:

- Keep out of the reach of children.
- Store away from heat and direct light.
- Do not store in the bathroom, near the kitchen sink, or in other damp places. Heat or moisture may cause the medicine to break down.
- Do not keep outdated medicine or medicine no longer needed. Be sure that any discarded medicine is out of the reach of children.

## Precautions While Using This Medicine

If your symptoms do not improve within 2 to 3 weeks, or if they become worse, check with your doctor.

It is very important that your doctor check your progress at regular visits. Also, *check with your doctor immediately if blurred vision or any loss of vision, with or without eye pain, occurs during treatment.* Your doctor may want you to have your eyes checked by an ophthalmologist (eye doctor).

Since this medicine may cause blurred vision or loss of vision, *make sure you know how you react to this medicine before you drive, use machines, or do anything else that could be dangerous if you are not able to see well.*

*If this medicine causes clumsiness; unsteadiness; or numbness, tingling, burning, or pain in the hands and feet, check with your doctor immediately.* These may be early warning symptoms of more serious nerve problems that could develop later.

## Side Effects of This Medicine

Along with its needed effects, a medicine may cause some unwanted effects. Although not all of these side effects may occur, if they do occur they may need medical attention.

*Check with your doctor immediately* if any of the following side effects occur:

*Less common*
Clumsiness or unsteadiness; confusion; mental depression; mood or other mental changes; numbness, tingling, burning, or pain in hands and feet; yellow eyes or skin

*Rare*
Blurred vision or loss of vision, with or without eye pain; changes in menstrual periods; coldness; decreased sexual ability (in males); difficulty in concentrating; dry, puffy skin; faster heartbeat; increased hunger; nervousness; shakiness; skin rash; swelling of front part of neck; weight gain

Other side effects may occur that usually do not need medical attention. These side effects may go away during treatment as your body adjusts to the medicine. However, check with your doctor if any of the following side effects continue or are bothersome:

*More common*
Dizziness (especially when getting up from a lying or sitting position); loss of appetite; metallic taste; nausea or vomiting; sore mouth

*Less common or rare*
Enlargement of the breasts (in males)

Other side effects not listed above may also occur in some patients. If you notice any other effects, check with your doctor.

## Additional Information

Once a medicine has been approved for marketing for a certain use, experience may show that it is also useful for other medical problems. Although these uses are not included in product labeling, ethionamide is used in certain patients with the following medical conditions:

- Atypical mycobacterial infections, such as *Mycobacterium avium* complex (MAC)
- Leprosy (Hansen's disease)

Other than the above information, there is no additional information relating to proper use, precautions, or side effects for these uses.

Revised: 06/22/94

# ETIDRONATE  Systemic

A commonly used brand name in the U.S. and Canada is Didronel. Another commonly used name is EHDP.

## Description

Etidronate (eh-tih-DROE-nate) is used to treat Paget's disease of bone. It may also be used to treat or prevent a certain type of bone problem that may occur after hip replacement surgery or spinal injury.

Etidronate is also used to treat hypercalcemia (too much calcium in the blood) that may occur with some types of cancer.

This medicine is available only with your doctor's prescription, in the following dosage forms:

*Oral*
- Tablets (U.S. and Canada)

*Parenteral*
- Injection (U.S.)

## Before Using This Medicine

In deciding to use a medicine, the risks of taking the medicine must be weighed against the good it will do. This is a decision you and your doctor will make. For etidronate, the following should be considered:

**Allergies**—Tell your doctor if you have ever had any unusual or allergic reaction to etidronate. Also tell your health care professional if you are allergic to any other substances, such as foods, preservatives, or dyes.

**Diet**—Make certain your health care professional knows if your diet includes large amounts of calcium, such as milk or other dairy products, or if you are on any special diet, such as a low-sodium or low-sugar diet. Calcium in the diet may prevent the absorption of oral etidronate.

**Pregnancy**—Studies have not been done in humans. However, studies in rats injected with large doses of etidronate have shown that etidronate causes deformed bones in the fetus.

**Breast-feeding**—It is not known if etidronate passes into breast milk. However, this medicine has not been reported to cause problems in nursing babies.

**Children**—Some changes in bone growth may occur in children, but will usually go away when the medicine is stopped.

**Older adults**—When etidronate is given by injection along with a large amount of fluids, older people tend to retain (keep) the excess fluid.

**Other medicines**—Although certain medicines should not be used together at all, in other cases two different medicines may be used together even if an interaction might occur. In these cases, your doctor may want to change the dose, or other precautions may be necessary. When you are taking etidronate, it is especially important that

your health care professional know if you are taking any of the following:

- Antacids containing calcium, magnesium, or aluminum or
- Mineral supplements or other medicines containing calcium, iron, magnesium, or aluminum—These medicines may decrease the effects of etidronate, and should be taken at least 2 hours before or after taking etidronate

**Other medical problems**—The presence of other medical problems may affect the use of etidronate. Make sure you tell your doctor if you have any other medical problems, especially:

- Bone fracture, especially of arm or leg—Etidronate may increase the risk of bone fractures
- Intestinal or bowel disease—Etidronate may increase the risk of diarrhea
- Kidney disease—High blood levels of etidronate may result causing cause serious side effects

## Proper Use of This Medicine

*Take etidronate with water on an empty stomach* at least 2 hours before or after food (midmorning is best) or at bedtime. Food may decrease the amount of etidronate absorbed by your body.

*Take etidronate only as directed.* Do not take more of it, do not take it more often, and do not take it for a longer time than your doctor ordered. To do so may increase the chance of side effects.

In some patients, etidronate takes up to 3 months to work. If you feel that the medicine is not working, do not stop taking it on your own. Instead, check with your doctor.

It is important that you eat a well-balanced diet with an adequate amount of calcium and vitamin D (found in milk or other dairy products). Too much or too little of either may increase the chance of side effects while you are taking etidronate. Your doctor can help you choose the meal plan that is best for you. *However, do not take any food, especially milk, milk formulas, or other dairy products, or antacids, mineral supplements, or other medicines that are high in calcium or iron (high amounts of these minerals may also be in some vitamin preparations), magnesium, or aluminum* within 2 hours of taking etidronate. To do so may keep this medicine from working properly.

**Dosing**—The dose of etidronate will be different for different patients. *Follow your doctor's order or the directions on the label.* The following information includes only the average doses of etidronate. *If your dose is different, do not change it* unless your doctor tells you to do so.

- For *oral* dosage form (tablets):
  —For treating Paget's disease of bone:
    - Adults—Dose is based on body weight and must be determined by your doctor. The dose to start is 5 milligrams (mg) per kilogram (kg) (2.3 mg per pound) of body weight a day, usually as a

single dose, for not more than six months. Some people may need 6 to 10 mg per kg (2.7 to 4.6 mg per pound) of body weight a day for not more than six months. Others may need 11 to 20 mg per kg (5 to 9.1 mg per pound) of body weight a day for not more than three months. Your doctor may change your dose depending on your response to treatment.

- Children—Dose must be determined by your doctor.

—For treating or preventing a certain type of bone problem that may occur after hip replacement:

- Adults—Dose is based on body weight and must be determined by your doctor. The usual dose is 20 mg per kg (9.1 mg per pound) of body weight a day for one month before surgery, and for three months after surgery.
- Children—Dose must be determined by your doctor.

—For treating or preventing a certain type of bone problem that may occur after spinal injury:

- Adults—Dose is based on body weight and must be determined by your doctor. The usual dose is 20 mg per kg (9.1 mg per pound) of body weight a day for two weeks, beginning as soon as possible after your injury. Your doctor may then decrease your dose to 10 mg per kg (4.5 mg per pound) of body weight for an additional ten weeks.
- Children—Dose must be determined by your doctor.

—For treating hypercalcemia (too much calcium in the blood):

- Adults—Dose is based on body weight and must be determined by your doctor. The usual dose is 20 mg per kg (9.1 mg per pound) of body weight a day for thirty days. Treatment usually does not continue beyond ninety days.
- Children—Dose must be determined by your doctor.

- For *injection* dosage form:

—For treating hypercalcemia (too much calcium in the blood):

- Adults—Dose is based on body weight and must be determined by your doctor. The usual dose is 7.5 mg per kg (3.4 mg per pound) of body weight, injected slowly into your vein over 2 hours. This dose is repeated for two more days. Your doctor may repeat the treatment after at least seven days.
- Children—Dose must be determined by your doctor.

**Missed dose**—If you miss a dose of this medicine, take it as soon as possible. However, if it is almost time for your next dose, skip the missed dose and go back to your regular dosing schedule. Do not double doses.

**Storage**—To store this medicine:

- Keep out of the reach of children.
- Store away from heat and direct light.
- Do not store in the bathroom, near the kitchen sink, or in other damp places. Heat or moisture may cause the medicine to break down.
- Do not keep outdated medicine or medicine no longer needed. Be sure that any discarded medicine is out of the reach of children.

## Precautions While Using This Medicine

*It is important that your doctor check your progress at regular visits* even if you are between treatments and are not taking this medicine. If your condition has improved and your doctor has told you to stop taking etidronate, your progress must still be checked. The results of laboratory tests or the occurrence of certain symptoms will tell your doctor if more medicine must be taken. Your doctor may want you to begin another course of treatment after you have been off the medicine for at least 3 months.

If this medicine causes you to have nausea or diarrhea and it continues, check with your doctor. The dose may need to be changed.

If bone pain occurs or worsens during treatment, check with your doctor.

## Side Effects of This Medicine

Along with its needed effects, a medicine may cause some unwanted effects. Although not all of these side effects may occur, if they do occur they may need medical attention.

Check with your doctor as soon as possible if any of the following side effects occur:

*More common*
Bone pain or tenderness (increased, continuing, or returning—in patients with Paget's disease)

*Less common*
Bone fractures, especially of the thigh bone

*Rare*
Hives; skin rash or itching; swelling of the arms, legs, face, lips, tongue, and/or throat

Other side effects may occur that usually do not need medical attention. These side effects may go away during treatment as your body adjusts to the medicine. However, check with your doctor if any of the following side effects continue or are bothersome:

*More common—at higher doses*
    Diarrhea; nausea
*Less common—with injection*
    Loss of taste or metallic or altered taste

Other side effects not listed above may also occur in some patients. If you notice any other effects, check with your doctor.

Revised: 08/19/92
Interim revision: 08/10/94

# ETOPOSIDE   Systemic

A commonly used brand name is:
**In the U.S.—**
    VePesid
**In Canada—**
    VePesid
    Generic name product may also be available.
Another commonly used name is VP-16.

## Description

Etoposide (e-TOE-poe-side) belongs to the group of medicines known as antineoplastic agents. It is used to treat cancer of the testicles and certain types of lung cancer. It is also sometimes used to treat some other kinds of cancer in both males and females.

The exact way that etoposide acts against cancer is not known. However, it seems to interfere with the growth of the cancer cells, which are eventually destroyed. Since the growth of normal body cells may also be affected by etoposide, other effects will also occur. Some of these may be serious and must be reported to your doctor. Other effects, like hair loss, may not be serious but may cause concern. Some effects may not occur for months or years after the medicine is used.

Before you begin treatment with etoposide, you and your doctor should talk about the good this medicine will do as well as the risks of using it.

This medicine is available only with your doctor's prescription, in the following dosage forms:
*Oral*
    • Capsules (U.S. and Canada)
*Parenteral*
    • Injection (U.S. and Canada)

## Before Using This Medicine

In deciding to use a medicine, the risks of taking the medicine must be weighed against the good it will do. This is a decision you and your doctor will make. For etoposide, the following should be considered:

**Allergies**—Tell your doctor if you have ever had any unusual or allergic reaction to etoposide.

**Pregnancy**—There is a good chance that this medicine will cause birth defects if it is being used at the time of conception or during pregnancy. In addition, many cancer medicines may cause sterility which could be permanent. Although sterility has not been reported with etoposide, the possibility should be kept in mind.

Be sure that you have discussed this with your doctor before receiving this medicine. It is best to use some kind of birth control while you are taking etoposide. Tell your doctor right away if you think you have become pregnant while taking etoposide. Before taking etoposide make sure your doctor knows if you are pregnant or if you may become pregnant.

**Breast-feeding**—Because etoposide may cause serious side effects, breast-feeding is generally not recommended while you are receiving it.

**Children**—Although this medicine has been used in children, there is no specific information comparing use of etoposide in children with use in other age groups.

**Older adults**—Many medicines have not been studied specifically in older people. Therefore, it may not be known whether they work exactly the same way they do in younger adults or if they cause different side effects or problems in older people. There is no specific information comparing use of etoposide in the elderly with use in other age groups.

**Other medicines**—Although certain medicines should not be used together at all, in other cases two different medicines may be used together even if an interaction might occur. In these cases, your doctor may want to change the dose, or other precautions may be necessary. When you are taking or receiving etoposide, it is especially important that your health care professional know if you are taking any of the following:
    • Amphotericin B by injection (e.g., Fungizone) or
    • Antithyroid agents (medicine for overactive thyroid) or
    • Azathioprine (e.g., Imuran) or
    • Chloramphenicol (e.g., Chloromycetin) or
    • Colchicine or
    • Flucytosine (e.g., Ancobon) or
    • Ganciclovir (e.g., Cytovene) or
    • Interferon (e.g., Intron A, Roferon-A) or
    • Plicamycin (e.g., Mithracin) or
    • Zidovudine (e.g., AZT, Retrovir)
    • If you have ever been treated with radiation or cancer medicines—Etoposide may increase the effects of these medicines or radiation therapy on the blood

**Other medical problems**—The presence of other medical problems may affect the use of etoposide. Make sure you tell your doctor if you have any other medical problems, especially:
- Chickenpox (including recent exposure) or
- Herpes zoster (shingles)—Risk of severe disease affecting other parts of the body
- Infection—Etoposide can decrease your body's ability to fight infection
- Kidney disease or
- Liver disease—Effects of etoposide may be increased because of slower removal from the body

## Proper Use of This Medicine

*Take etoposide only as directed by your doctor.* Do not use more or less of it, and do not use it more often than your doctor ordered. The exact amount of medicine you need has been carefully worked out. Taking too much may increase the chance of side effects, while taking too little may not improve your condition.

Etoposide is sometimes given together with certain other medicines. If you are using a combination of medicines, make sure that you take each one at the proper time and do not mix them. If you are taking some of these medicines by mouth, ask your health care professional to help you plan a way to remember to take your medicines at the right times.

Etoposide often causes nausea, vomiting, and loss of appetite, which may be severe. However, it is very important that you continue to receive the medicine, even if you begin to feel ill. Ask your health care professional for ways to lessen these effects.

If you vomit shortly after taking a dose of etoposide, check with your doctor. You will be told whether to take the dose again or to wait until the next dose.

**Dosing**—The dose of etoposide will be different for different patients. The dose that is used may depend on a number of things, including what the medicine is being used for, the patient's size, whether the medicine is being given by mouth or by injection, and whether or not other medicines are also being taken. *If you are taking or receiving etoposide at home, follow your doctor's orders or the directions on the label.* If you have any questions about the proper dose of etoposide, ask your doctor.

**Missed dose**—If you miss a dose of this medicine, do not take the missed dose at all and do not double the next one. Instead, go back to your regular dosing schedule and check with your doctor.

**Storage**—To store this medicine:
- Keep out of the reach of children.
- Store in the refrigerator.
- Do not store in the bathroom, near the kitchen sink, or in other damp places. Heat or moisture may cause the medicine to break down.
- Do not keep outdated medicine or medicine no longer needed. Be sure that any discarded medicine is out of the reach of children.

## Precautions While Using This Medicine

*It is very important that your doctor check your progress at regular visits* to make sure that etoposide is working properly and to check for unwanted effects.

While you are being treated with etoposide, and after you stop treatment with it, *do not have any immunizations (vaccinations) without your doctor's approval.* Etoposide may lower your body's resistance and there is a chance you might get the infection the immunization is meant to prevent. In addition, other persons living in your household should not take oral polio vaccine since there is a chance they could pass the polio virus on to you. Also, avoid persons who have recently taken oral polio vaccine. Do not get close to them and do not stay in the same room with them for very long. If you cannot take these precautions, you should consider wearing a protective face mask that covers the nose and mouth.

Etoposide can temporarily lower the number of white blood cells in your blood, increasing the chance of getting an infection. It can also lower the number of platelets, which are necessary for proper blood clotting. If this occurs, there are certain precautions you can take, especially when your blood count is low, to reduce the risk of infection or bleeding:
- If you can, avoid people with infections. *Check with your doctor immediately* if you think you are getting an infection or if you get a fever or chills, cough or hoarseness, lower back or side pain, or painful or difficult urination.
- *Check with your doctor immediately* if you notice any unusual bleeding or bruising; black, tarry stools; blood in urine or stools; or pinpoint red spots on your skin.
- Be careful when using a regular toothbrush, dental floss, or toothpick. Your medical doctor, dentist, or nurse may recommend other ways to clean your teeth and gums. Check with your medical doctor before having any dental work done.
- Do not touch your eyes or the inside of your nose unless you have just washed your hands and have not touched anything else in the meantime.
- Be careful not to cut yourself when you are using sharp objects such as a safety razor or fingernail or toenail cutters.
- Avoid contact sports or other situations where bruising or injury could occur.

## Side Effects of This Medicine

Along with its needed effects, a medicine may cause some unwanted effects. Although not all of these side effects may occur, if they do occur they may need medical attention.

Also, because of the way these medicines act on the body, there is a chance that they might cause other unwanted effects that may not occur until months or years after the medicine is used. These delayed effects may include certain types of cancer, such as leukemia. Discuss these possible effects with your doctor.

*Check with your doctor or nurse immediately* if any of the following side effects occur:

   *Less common*
      Black, tarry stools; blood in urine or stools; cough or hoarseness; fever or chills; lower back or side pain; painful or difficult urination; pinpoint red spots on skin; unusual bleeding or bruising

Check with your health care professional as soon as possible if any of the following side effects occur:

   *Less common*
      Fast heartbeat; shortness of breath or wheezing; sores in mouth or on lips
   *Rare*
      Back pain; difficulty in walking; numbness or tingling in fingers and toes; pain at place of injection; skin rash or itching; sweating; swelling of face or tongue; tightness in throat; weakness

Other side effects may occur that usually do not need medical attention. These side effects may go away during treatment as your body adjusts to the medicine. Also, your health care professional may be able to tell you about ways to prevent or reduce some of these side effects. Check with your health care professional if any of the following side effects continue or are bothersome or if you have any questions about them:

   *More common*
      Loss of appetite; nausea and vomiting
   *Less common*
      Diarrhea; unusual tiredness

This medicine often causes a temporary loss of hair. After treatment with etoposide has ended, normal hair growth should return.

Other side effects not listed above may also occur in some patients. If you notice any other effects, check with your doctor or nurse.

Revised: 08/09/92
Interim revision: 08/08/94

# ETRETINATE   Systemic

A commonly used brand name in the U.S. and Canada is Tegison.

## Description

Etretinate (e-TRET-i-nate) is used to treat severe psoriasis. It is usually used only after other medicines have been tried and have failed to help the psoriasis.

*Etretinate must not be used to treat women who are able to bear children unless other forms of treatment have been tried first and have failed. Etretinate must not be taken during pregnancy, because it causes birth defects in humans. In addition, if you take etretinate, you must plan on never having children in the future. If you are able to bear children, it is very important that you read, understand, and follow the pregnancy warnings for etretinate.*

It is also recommended that etretinate not be used to treat children unless all other forms of treatment have been tried first and have failed. Etretinate may interfere with bone growth. In addition, children may be more sensitive to the side effects of the medicine.

This medicine is available only with your doctor's prescription, in the following dosage form:

   *Oral*
   • Capsules (U.S. and Canada)

## Before Using This Medicine

In deciding to use a medicine, the risks of taking the medicine must be weighed against the good it will do. This is a decision you and your doctor will make. For etretinate, the following should be considered:

**Allergies**—Tell your doctor if you have ever had any unusual or allergic reaction to etretinate, isotretinoin, tretinoin, or vitamin A–like preparations. Also tell your health care professional if you are allergic to any other substances, such as foods, preservatives, or dyes.

**Pregnancy**—*Etretinate must not be taken during pregnancy, because it causes birth defects in humans. In addition, since it is not known how long pregnancy should be avoided after treatment stops, you must plan on never having children if you are treated with etretinate. If you are able to bear children, you must have a pregnancy test within 2 weeks before beginning treatment with etretinate to make sure you are not pregnant. Therapy with etretinate will then be started on the second or third day of your next normal menstrual period. Also, etretinate must not be taken unless an effective form of contraception (birth control) is used for at least 1 month before beginning treatment. Contraception must be continued during treatment and for as long as you are able to become pregnant after etretinate is stopped. Be sure you have discussed this information with your doctor.*

**Breast-feeding**—It is not known whether etretinate passes into the breast milk. However, etretinate is not recommended during breast-feeding or if you plan to breast-feed in the future, because it may cause unwanted effects in nursing babies.

**Children**—It is recommended that etretinate not be used to treat children, unless all other forms of treatment have been tried first and have failed. Etretinate may interfere with bone growth. In addition, children may be more sensitive to the side effects of the medicine.

**Older adults**—Many medicines have not been studied specifically in older people. Therefore, it may not be known whether they work exactly the same way they do in younger adults or if they cause different side effects or problems in older people. There is no specific information comparing use of etretinate in the elderly with use in other age groups.

**Other medicines**—Although certain medicines should not be used together at all, in other cases two different medicines may be used together even if an interaction might occur. In these cases, your doctor may want to change the dose, or other precautions may be necessary. When you are using etretinate, it is especially important that your health care professional know if you are using any of the following:

- Abrasive or medicated soaps or cleansers or
- Cosmetics or soaps that dry the skin or
- Medicated cosmetics or "cover-ups" or
- Topical acne preparation or preparation containing a peeling agent, such as benzoyl peroxide, resorcinol, salicylic acid, sulfur, or tretinoin (vitamin A acid), or
- Topical alcohol-containing preparation, such as after-shave lotion, astringent, cologne, perfume, or shaving cream or lotion, or
- Topical medicine for the skin, other—Use of etretinate with these products will increase the chance of dryness and other irritation of the skin
- Isotretinoin (e.g., Accutane) or
- Methotrexate (e.g., Mexate) or
- Tretinoin (vitamin A acid) (e.g., Retin-A) or
- Vitamin A or any preparation containing vitamin A (e.g., Alphalin)—Use of etretinate with these products will cause an increase in side effects
- Tetracyclines (medicine for infection)—Use of etretinate may increase the chance of the side effect called pseudotumor cerebri, which is a swelling of the brain

**Other medical problems**—The presence of other medical problems may affect the use of etretinate. Make sure you tell your doctor if you have any other medical problems, especially:

- Alcoholism or excess use of alcohol (or history of) or
- Diabetes mellitus (sugar diabetes) (or a family history of) or
- Heart or blood vessel disease (or history of increased risk of or family history of) or
- High triglyceride (a fat-like substance) levels in the blood (history of or a family history of) or
- Severe weight problems—Use of etretinate may increase blood levels of triglyceride (a fat-like substance), which may increase the chance of heart or blood vessel problems in patients who have a family history of high triglycerides, are greatly overweight, are diabetic, or use a lot of alcohol. For persons with diabetes mellitus, use of etretinate may also change blood sugar levels
- Liver disease (or history of or family history of)—Use of etretinate may make the condition worse

## Proper Use of This Medicine

*Take each dose of etretinate with milk or a fatty food.* This is important because taking fats with etretinate will help your body absorb the medicine better. *However, you should follow a low-fat diet during the rest of the day* because eating a high-fat diet while you are taking this medicine may cause high triglyceride (fat-like substance) levels in the blood. This may increase the chance of heart and blood vessel disease.

*It is very important that you take etretinate only as directed.* Do not take more of it, do not take it more often, and do not take it for a longer period of time than your doctor ordered. To do so may increase the chance of side effects.

**Dosing**—The dose of etretinate will be different for different patients. *Follow your doctor's orders or the directions on the label.* The following information includes only the average doses of etretinate. *If your dose is different, do not change it* unless your doctor tells you to do so.

The number of capsules that you take depends on the strength of the medicine. Also, *the number of doses you take each day, the time allowed between doses, and the length of time you take the medicine depend on the medical problem for which you are taking etretinate.*

- For *oral* dosage form (capsules):
  —For psoriasis:
    - Adults and teenagers—Dose is based on body weight and must be determined by your doctor. The usual dose is 0.75 to 1 milligram (mg) per kilogram (kg) (0.34 to 0.45 mg per pound) of body weight a day, divided into several doses.
    - Children—Use is usually not recommended.

**Missed dose**—If you miss a dose of this medicine, take it as soon as possible with milk or a fatty food. However, if it is almost time for your next dose, skip the missed dose and go back to your regular dosing schedule. Do not double doses.

**Storage**—To store this medicine:
- Keep out of the reach of children.
- Store away from heat and direct light.
- Do not store in the bathroom, near the kitchen sink, or in other damp places. Heat or moisture may cause the medicine to break down.
- Do not keep outdated medicine or medicine no longer needed. Be sure that any discarded medicine is out of the reach of children.

## Precautions While Using This Medicine

*Your doctor should check your progress at regular visits* to make sure this medicine does not cause unwanted effects.

*Etretinate causes birth defects in humans if taken during pregnancy. In addition, it is not known how long pregnancy should be avoided after treatment stops, to prevent* birth defects. *Therefore, you must plan on never having children if you are treated with etretinate. For as long as you are able to become pregnant, you must use a reliable form of birth control. In addition, you must not change your birth control method unless you have checked with your doctor first. If you suspect that you may have become pregnant while taking etretinate, stop taking the medicine immediately and check with your doctor. Also, if you become pregnant at any time after you have stopped taking this medicine, check with your doctor as soon as possible. In either case, you should talk to your doctor about the risks of continuing the pregnancy.*

It is not known how long etretinate stays in the blood. *Therefore, to prevent the possibility of a pregnant patient receiving your blood, you must plan on never donating blood to a blood bank if you are being treated with etretinate or if you have ever been treated with etretinate.*

*Do not take vitamin A or any vitamin supplement containing vitamin A while you are taking this medicine.* To do so may increase the chance of side effects.

Drinking too much alcohol while you are taking this medicine may cause high triglyceride (fat-like substance) levels in the blood. This may increase the chance of heart and blood vessel disease. Therefore, *while taking this medicine, do not drink alcoholic beverages or, at least, reduce the amount you usually drink.* If you have any questions about this, check with your doctor.

For *diabetic patients*:

- This medicine may affect blood sugar levels. If you notice a change in the results of your blood or urine sugar tests or if you have any questions, check with your doctor.

In some patients, etretinate may cause a decrease in night vision. This decrease may occur suddenly. If it does occur, *do not drive, use machines, or do anything else that could be dangerous if you are not able to see well.* Also, check with your doctor.

Etretinate may cause dryness of the eyes. Therefore, if you wear contact lenses, your eyes may be more sensitive to them while you are taking etretinate and for several weeks or longer after you stop taking it. To help relieve dryness of the eyes, check with your doctor about using an eye lubricating solution, such as artificial tears. If your eyes become inflamed, check with your doctor.

Some people who take this medicine may become more sensitive to sunlight than they are normally. When you begin taking this medicine:

- Stay out of direct sunlight, especially between the hours of 10:00 a.m. and 3:00 p.m., if possible.
- Wear protective clothing, including a hat and sunglasses.
- Apply a sun block product that has a skin protection factor (SPF) of at least 15. Some patients may require a product with a higher SPF number, especially if they have a fair complexion. If you have

any questions about this, check with your health care professional.

- Do not use a sunlamp or tanning bed or booth.

*If you have a severe reaction, check with your doctor.*

This medicine may cause dryness of the mouth and nose. For temporary relief of mouth dryness, use sugarless candy or gum, melt bits of ice in your mouth, or use a saliva substitute. However, if dry mouth continues for more than 2 weeks, check with your medical doctor or dentist. Continuing dryness of the mouth may increase the chance of dental disease, including tooth decay, gum disease, and fungus infections.

During the first month of treatment with etretinate, your psoriasis may seem to get worse before it gets better. There may be more redness or itching, but this usually goes away during treatment. It may take 2 or 3 months before the full effects of etretinate are seen. If irritation or other symptoms of your condition become severe, check with your doctor.

## Side Effects of This Medicine

Along with its needed effects, a medicine may cause some unwanted effects. Although not all of these side effects may occur, if they do occur they may need medical attention.

*Stop taking this medicine and check with your doctor immediately* if any of the following side effects occur:

*Less common*

Blurred or double vision or other changes in vision; dark-colored urine; flu-like symptoms; yellow eyes or skin

*Rare*

Headache (severe or continuing); nausea and vomiting

Check with your doctor as soon as possible if any of the following side effects occur:

*More common*

Bone or joint pain, tenderness, or stiffness; burning, redness, itching, feeling of dryness, pain, tenderness, excessive tearing (continuing), or other sign of inflammation or irritation of eyes; cramps or pain in upper abdomen or stomach area; muscle cramps; unusual bruising

*Less common*

Change in hearing, earache or pain in ear, or drainage from ear

*Rare*

Bleeding or inflammation of gums; confusion; mental depression; mood or mental changes

Other side effects may occur that usually do not need medical attention. These side effects may go away during treatment as your body adjusts to the medicine. However, check with your doctor if any of the following side effects continue or are bothersome:

*More common*

Changes in appetite; chapped lips; dryness of nose or nosebleeds; dryness, redness, scaling, itching, rash, or other sign of inflammation or irritation of the skin; headache (mild); increased sensitivity to contact lenses (may occur during and after treatment); increased sensitivity of skin to sunlight; peeling of skin on fingertips, palms of hands, or soles of feet; thinning of hair; unusual thirst; unusual tiredness

*Less common*

Dizziness; dryness of mouth; fever; nausea (mild); redness or soreness around fingernails; loosening of the fingernails; soreness of tongue; soreness, cracking, swelling, or unusual redness of lips

Other side effects not listed above may also occur in some patients. If you notice any other effects, check with your doctor.

Revised: June 1990
Interim revision: 06/17/94

# FACTOR IX    Systemic

Some commonly used brand names are:

**In the U.S.—**

| | |
|---|---|
| AlphaNine | Mononine |
| AlphaNine SD | Profilnine Heat-Treated |
| Bebulin VH | Proplex T |
| Konÿne 80 | |

**In Canada—**

AlphaNine
Bebulin VH

Other commonly used names are Christmas factor, plasma thrombo-plastin component (PTC), and prothrombin complex concentrate (PCC).

## Description

Factor IX is a protein produced naturally in the body. It helps the blood form clots to stop bleeding. Injections of factor IX are used to treat hemophilia B, which is sometimes called Christmas disease. This is a condition in which the body does not make enough factor IX. If you do not have enough factor IX and you become injured, your blood will not form clots as it should, and you may bleed into and damage your muscles and joints.

Injections of one form of factor IX, called factor IX complex, also are used to treat certain people with hemophilia A. In hemophilia A, sometimes called classical hemophilia, the body does not make enough factor VIII, and, just as in hemophilia B, the blood cannot form clots as it should. Injections of factor IX complex may be used in patients in whom the medicine used to treat hemophilia A is no longer effective. Injections of factor IX complex also may be used for other conditions as determined by your doctor.

The factor IX product that your doctor will give you is obtained naturally from human blood. It has been treated and is not likely to contain harmful viruses such as hepatitis B virus, hepatitis C (non-A, non-B) virus, or human immunodeficiency virus (HIV), the virus that causes acquired immunodeficiency syndrome (AIDS).

Factor IX is available only with your doctor's prescription, in the following dosage form:

*Parenteral*
- Injection (U.S. and Canada)

## Before Using This Medicine

In deciding to use a medicine, the risks of using the medicine must be weighed against the good it will do. This is a decision you and your doctor will make. For factor IX, the following should be considered:

**Allergies**—Tell your doctor if you have ever had any unusual or allergic reaction to injections of factor IX or mouse protein. Also tell your health care professional if you are allergic to any other substances, such as foods, preservatives, or dyes.

**Pregnancy**—Studies on effects in pregnancy have not been done in either humans or animals.

**Breast-feeding**—It is not known whether the ingredients in factor IX products pass into breast milk. Although most medicines pass into breast milk in small amounts, many of them may be used safely while breast-feeding. Mothers who are using this medicine and who wish to breast-feed should discuss this with their doctor.

**Children**—Blood clots may be especially likely to occur in premature and newborn babies, who are usually more sensitive than adults to the effects of injections of factor IX.

**Older adults**—This medicine has been tested and has not been shown to cause different side effects or problems in older people than it does in younger adults.

**Other medicines**—Although certain medicines should not be used together at all, in other cases two different medicines may be used together even if an interaction might occur. In these cases, your doctor may want to change the dose, or other precautions may be necessary. Tell your health care professional if you are using any other prescription or nonprescription (over-the-counter [OTC]) medicine.

**Other medical problems**—The presence of other medical problems may affect the use of factor IX products. Make sure you tell your doctor if you have any other medical problems, especially:

- Liver disease—Risk of bleeding or developing blood clots may be increased

## Proper Use of This Medicine

Some medicines given by injection may sometimes be given at home to patients who do not need to be in the hospital. If you are using this medicine at home, your health care professional will teach you how to prepare and inject the medicine. You will have a chance to practice preparing and injecting it. *Be sure that you understand exactly how the medicine is to be prepared and injected.*

To prepare this medicine:

- Take the dry medicine and the liquid (diluent) out of the refrigerator and *bring them to room temperature*, as directed by your doctor.
- When injecting the liquid (diluent) into the dry medicine, *aim the stream of liquid (diluent) against the wall of the container of dry medicine* to prevent foaming.
- *Swirl the container gently to dissolve the medicine. Do not shake the container.*

*Use this medicine right away*. It should not be kept longer than 3 hours after it has been prepared.

*A plastic disposable syringe and filter needle must be used with this medicine.* The medicine may stick to the inside of a glass syringe, and you may not receive a full dose.

*Do not reuse syringes and needles. Put used syringes and needles in a puncture-resistant disposable container,* or dispose of them as directed by your health care professional.

**Dosing**—The dose of factor IX will be different for different patients. The dose you receive will be based on:

- The condition for which you are using this medicine.
- Your body weight.
- The amount of factor IX your body is able to make.
- How much, how often, and where in your body you are bleeding.
- Whether or not your body has built up a defense (antibody) against this medicine.

Your dose of this medicine may even be different at different times. It is important that you *follow your doctor's orders.*

**Missed dose**—If you miss a dose of this medicine, check with your doctor as soon as possible for instructions.

**Storage**—To store this medicine:

- Keep out of the reach of children.
- Some factor IX products must be stored in the refrigerator, and some may be kept at room temperature for short periods of time. Store this medicine as directed by your doctor or the manufacturer.
- Do not keep outdated medicine or medicine no longer needed. Be sure that any discarded medicine is out of the reach of children.

## Precautions While Using This Medicine

If you were recently diagnosed with hemophilia B, you should receive a hepatitis B vaccine to reduce even further your risk of getting hepatitis B from factor IX products.

After a while, your body may build up a defense (antibody) against this medicine. *Tell your doctor if this medicine seems to be less effective than usual.*

*It is recommended that you carry identification stating that you have hemophilia A or hemophilia B.* If you have any questions about what kind of identification to carry, check with your health care professional.

## Side Effects of This Medicine

Along with its needed effects, a medicine may cause some unwanted effects. Although not all of these side effects may occur, if they do occur they may need medical attention.

*Check with your doctor immediately* if any of the following side effects occur, because they may mean that you are having a serious allergic reaction to the medicine:

*Less common or rare*

Changes in facial skin color; fast or irregular breathing; puffiness or swelling of the eyelids or around the eyes; shortness of breath, troubled breathing, tightness in chest, and/or wheezing; skin rash, hives, and/or itching

*Also, check with your doctor immediately* if any of the following side effects occur, because they may mean that you are developing a problem with blood clotting:

*More common*

Bluish coloring (especially of the hands and feet); convulsions; dizziness or lightheadedness when getting up from a lying or sitting position; increased heart rate; large blue or purplish patches in the skin (at places of injection); nausea or vomiting; pains in chest, groin, or legs (especially calves); persistent bleeding from puncture sites, gums, inner linings of the nose and/or mouth, or blood in the stool or urine; severe pain or pressure in the chest and/or the neck, back, or left arm; severe, sudden headache; shortness of breath or fast breathing; sudden loss of coordination; sudden and unexplained slurred speech, vision changes, and/or weakness or numbness in arm or leg

*Also, check with your doctor immediately* if any of the following side effects occur, because they may mean that your medicine is being given too fast:

*Less common*

Burning or stinging at place of injection; changes in blood pressure or pulse rate; chills; drowsiness; fever; headache; nausea or vomiting; redness of face; shortness of breath

Other side effects not listed above may also occur in some patients. If you notice any other effects, check with your doctor.

Revised: 08/27/93

# FAT EMULSIONS   Systemic

Some commonly used brand names are:
**In the U.S.—**
Intralipid                      Liposyn III
Liposyn II
**In Canada—**
Intralipid
Liposyn II

## Description

Fat emulsions are used as dietary supplements for patients who are unable to get enough fat in their diet, usually because of certain illnesses or recent surgery. Fats are used by the body for energy and to form substances needed for normal body functions.

Fat emulsions are available by injection only with your doctor's prescription, in the following dosage form:

*Parenteral*
- Injection (U.S. and Canada)

## Before Using This Medicine

In deciding to use a medicine, the risks of using the medicine must be weighed against the good it will do. This is a decision you and your doctor will make. For fat emulsions, the following should be considered:

**Allgeries**—Tell your doctor if you have ever had any unusual or allergic reaction to eggs, soybeans, beans, peas, or fat emulsions. Also tell your health care professional if you are allergic to any other substances, such as foods, preservatives, or dyes.

**Pregnancy**—Studies on effects in pregnancy have not been done in either animals or humans.

**Breast-feeding**—It is not known whether fat emulsions pass into the breast milk. However, this medicine has not been reported to cause problems in nursing babies.

**Children**—Fat emulsions may cause or worsen lung problems or jaundice if given to premature infants. Although there is no specific information comparing use of fat emulsions in older children with use in other age groups, it is not expected to cause different side effects or problems in older children than it does in adults.

**Older adults**—Many medicines have not been studied specifically in older people. Therefore, it may not be known whether they work exactly the same way they do in younger adults or if they cause different side effects or problems in older people. Although there is no specific information comparing use of fat emulsions in the elderly with use in other age groups, this medicine is not expected to cause different side effects or problems in older people than it does in younger adults.

**Other medicines**—Although certain medicines should not be used together at all, in other cases two different medicines may be used together even if an interaction might occur. In these cases, your doctor may want to change the dose, or other precautions may be necessary. Tell your health care professional if you are using any other prescription or nonprescription (over-the-counter [OTC]) medicine.

**Other medical problems**—The presence of other medical problems may affect the use of fat emulsions. Make sure you tell your doctor if you have any other medical problems, especially:
- Blood problems or
- Diabetes mellitus (sugar diabetes) or
- High cholesterol levels or
- Infection or
- Jaundice or
- Kidney disease or
- Liver disease or
- Lung disease or
- Pancreas disease—Fat emulsions may make these conditions worse

## Proper Use of This Medicine

**Dosing**—The amount of fat emulsions to be used will be different for different patients. *Follow your doctor's orders or the directions on the label.* The following information includes only the average dose of fat emulsions. *If your dose is different, do not change it* unless your doctor tells you to do so.

The amount of fat emulsions that is infused into your vein depends on the strength of the fat emulsions used.
- For *injection* dosage form:
  —For nutritional supplement:
    - Adults and teenagers—At first, the dose is 0.5 to 1 milliliter (mL) per minute injected slowly into a vein over a period of fifteen to thirty minutes. Your doctor may increase the rate of the injection until up to 250 to 500 mL have been injected over four to six hours.
    - Children—At first, the dose is 0.1 mL per minute injected slowly into a vein over a period of fifteen minutes. Your doctor may increase the rate of the injection up to 50 to 100 mL per hour.

**Storage**—To store this medicine:
- Keep out of the reach of children.
- Store away from heat and direct light.
- Do not store in the bathroom, near the kitchen sink, or in other damp places. Heat or moisture may cause the medicine to break down.
- Keep the medicine from freezing. Do not refrigerate.
- Do not keep outdated medicine or medicine no longer needed. Be sure that any discarded medicine is out of the reach of children.

## Precautions While Using This Medicine

It is very important that your doctor check your progress weekly while you are receiving fat emulsions to make sure that this medicine does not cause unwanted effects.

Fat emulsions can lower your ability to fight infection. If you think you are getting an infection, check with your doctor.

## Side Effects of This Medicine

Along with its needed effects, a medicine may cause some unwanted effects. Although not all of these side effects may occur, if they do occur they may need medical attention.

Check with your doctor as soon as possible if any of the following side effects occur:

*More common*
    Chills; fever; sore throat
*Rare*
    Bluish color of skin; chest or back pain; difficulty in breathing; headache; hives; unusual bleeding or bruising; unusual irritability; unusual tiredness or weakness; yellow eyes or skin

Other side effects may occur that usually do not need medical attention. These side effects may go away during treatment as your body adjusts to the medicine. However, check with your doctor if any of the following side effects continue or are bothersome:

*More common*
    Redness, swelling, or pain at place of injection
*Less common*
    Diarrhea; dizziness; flushing; nausea and vomiting

Other side effects not listed above may also occur in some patients. If you notice any other effects, check with your doctor.

Revised: 05/12/93
Interim revision: 06/27/94

# FECAL OCCULT BLOOD TEST KITS

Some commonly used brand names are:
**In the U.S.—**

| | |
|---|---|
| ColoCare[2] | Hematest[2] |
| ColoScreen[1][2] | HemaWipe[2] |
| ColoScreen III[2] | HemeSelect[2] |
| ColoScreen Self-Test[2] | Hemoccult[1][2] |
| DigiWipe[1] | Hemoccult II[2] |
| EZ Detect[2] | Hemoccult SENSA[1][2] |
| HemaChek[2] | Hemoccult II SENSA[2] |

**In Canada—**
Colo-Rectal Test[2]          Hematest[2]

Note: For quick reference, the following fecal occult blood test kits are numbered to match the corresponding brand names.

This information applies to the following medicines:
1. Fecal Occult Blood Test Kits for Clinic Use†
2. Fecal Occult Blood Test Kits for Home Use

†Not commercially available in Canada.

## Description

Fecal occult blood tests are designed to detect small, hidden amounts of blood in the bowel movement (feces). These tests are usually used to detect the small amounts of bleeding that come painlessly from cancers of the colon or rectum. These cancers may bleed without symptoms. They are frequently fatal if allowed to grow until the patient has symptoms of abdominal pain, anemia, or changes in bowel habits. Colon or rectal cancers are more likely to be cured if found in early stages.

A positive fecal occult blood test does not always mean that you have colon or rectal cancer. Rather, it means that more tests are needed to find the cause of the bleeding. Blood may come from many sources in the digestive tract, such as ulcers, diarrhea, or hemorrhoids. Other blood sources which may react include menstrual blood or blood in the urine. Some physicians will, in fact, use

a fecal occult blood test to help find bleeding problems other than cancer.

Most test kits are given out when a physical examination is done. Others may be bought without a prescription in a pharmacy. Most kits also provide a toll-free number for advice on using the kits.

## Before Using This Test Kit

It is important to get the best results possible from fecal occult blood test kits. Therefore, the following should be considered before you use these test kits:

**Diet**—Most kits recommend following a special diet. Red meats that are not completely cooked (for example, rare) may contain hemoglobin, the substance with which the test reacts. In addition, some fruits and vegetables, such as horseradish, broccoli, carrots, cauliflower, radishes, turnips, mushrooms, cucumbers, cantaloupes, and grapefruit, contain peroxidase, another chemical the test may react with. Large quantities of these foods should be avoided for 2 days before beginning testing and during the test period.

**Medicines**—Certain medicines may affect the results of the fecal occult blood test. Check with your doctor if you are taking any medicines, especially:

• Aspirin or other salicylates or
• Corticosteroids (cortisone-like medicine) or
• Medicine for pain and/or inflammation, except narcotics, or
• Reserpine—These medicines irritate the digestive tract and may cause bleeding that will give a positive test

- Ascorbic acid (vitamin C)—Large amounts may block a positive test reaction
- Rectal medicines—Use of rectal medicines may affect test results

**Medical conditions**—The presence of other medical conditions may affect the results of the fecal occult blood test. Make sure you tell your doctor if you have any other medical conditions, especially:

- Colitis or
- Constipation or
- Diarrhea or
- Diverticulitis or
- Hemorrhoids or
- Irritation of throat (severe) or
- Menstrual period or
- Nosebleeds or
- Stomach ulcer—These conditions may also cause blood to appear in the stool, resulting in a positive test

## Proper Use of This Test

Check the expiration date printed on the package before purchasing. Do not use an outdated test kit. Outdated test kits will not work properly.

Read test instructions carefully. Proceed only after you understand the instructions. Most test kits include a toll-free number for consumer questions, or you may ask questions of your health care professional.

Stop collection/testing in the presence of diarrhea, constipation, or hemorrhoid problems, or during menstrual periods.

For bowl tests:

- Remove bowl cleanser by repeated flushing (at least 3 times) and then flush urine before bowel movement. If a continuous-cleaning product is being used, remove it from the tank system and flush several times to clear away the chemicals.
- Follow test instructions carefully for timing of reactions and watching for color changes. Use a watch or clock with a second hand. Have another person observe for color changes if you have trouble seeing.
- Complete the "control" tests as the kit directs.
- Record results with the materials provided in the kit, to be discussed with your medical doctor.

For card tests:
- Samples should be collected from 2 different areas of the feces for 3 separate bowel movements.
- Samples should be sent to the physician as soon as collected. They should not be stored for more than 5 days (14 days for *HemeSelect, Hemoccult,* and *Hemoccult SENSA*).

For wipe tests:
- Samples should be sent to the physician as soon as collected. They should not be stored for more than 5 days (14 days for *HemaWipe*).

For patients mailing test cards/slides to doctor's office or clinic:
- U.S. postal regulations prohibit mailing completed cards/slides in standard paper envelopes. Approved mailing pouches must be used.

**Storage**—To store this product:
- Keep out of the reach of children.
- Do not store in warm, humid conditions or in direct sunlight.

## About Your Test Results

In most cases the tests are returned to the clinic or doctor's office for final development, and you will be notified if any of the tests are positive or if further testing is necessary.

A positive result means that there was some blood found in the feces. Further testing may be necessary to find the cause. It does not necessarily mean you have cancer. Only 5 to 10 percent of persons with positive fecal occult blood tests are found to have cancer.

A negative result means that no blood was found in the feces. It shows that you were not bleeding from your digestive system during the test period. However, a cancer may bleed off and on, and be missed by the test. Although it is unlikely that you have colon or rectal cancer, you should continue to watch for cancer warning signals such as changes in bowel habits or blood in the feces. You should also have a cancer check-up at regular intervals, as recommended by your health care professional.

Revised: 06/18/92

# FELBAMATE   Systemic†

A commonly used brand name in the U.S. is Felbatol.
Another commonly used name is FBM.

---

†Not commercially available in Canada.

---

## Description

Felbamate (FEL-ba-mate) is used to control some types
of seizures in the treatment of epilepsy. Felbamate acts
on the central nervous system (CNS) to make it more
difficult for seizures to start or to continue. This medicine
cannot cure epilepsy and will only work to control seizures
for as long as you continue to use it.

Felbamate is available only with your doctor's prescription, in the following dosage forms:

*Oral*
- Suspension (U.S.)
- Tablets (U.S.)

## Before Using This Medicine

In deciding to use a medicine, the risks of taking the
medicine must be weighed against the good it will do.
This is a decision you and your doctor will make. For
felbamate, the following should be considered:

**Allergies**—Tell your doctor if you have ever had any unusual or allergic reaction to felbamate or to medicines
like felbamate such as carbromal, carisoprodol (Soma,
Rela), mebutamate, meprobamate (Equanil, Miltown), or
tybamate (Tybatran). Also tell your health care professional if you are allergic to any other substances, such as
foods, preservatives, or dyes.

**Pregnancy**—Felbamate has not been studied in pregnant
women. However, studies in pregnant animals have shown
that felbamate may cause lowered birth weight and lowered survival of offspring when given to the mother in
doses more than one and one-half times the usual human
dose. Before taking this medicine, make sure your doctor
knows if you are pregnant or if you may become pregnant.

**Breast-feeding**—Felbamate passes into breast milk. However, it is not known whether this medicine causes problems in nursing babies.

**Children**—This medicine has been tested in children and,
in effective doses, has not been shown to cause different
side effects or problems than it does in adults.

**Older adults**—Many medicines have not been studied specifically in older people. Therefore, it may not be known
whether they work exactly the same way they do in
younger adults or if they cause different side effects or
problems in older people. There is no specific information
comparing use of felbamate in the elderly with use in
other age groups. However, older people are more likely
to have other illnesses and to use other medicines that
may affect the way felbamate works. Your doctor may
start with a lower felbamate dose or may increase the
dose more slowly.

**Other medicines**—Although certain medicines should not
be used together at all, in other cases two different medicines may be used together even if an interaction might
occur. In these cases, your doctor may want to change
the dose, or other precautions may be necessary. When
you are taking felbamate, it is especially important that
your health care professional know if you are taking any
of the following:
- Carbamazepine (e.g., Tegretol) or
- Phenytoin (e.g., Dilantin) or
- Valproic acid (e.g., Depakene)—Higher or lower blood levels of these medicines or felbamate may occur, which
  may increase the chance of unwanted effects; your doctor
  may need to change the dose of either these medicines
  or felbamate

**Other medical problems**—The presence of other medical
problems may affect the use of felbamate. Make sure
you tell your doctor if you have any other medical problems, especially:
- Anemia or other blood problems (or history of) or
- Liver problems (or history of)—Felbamate may make the
  condition worse

---

## Proper Use of This Medicine

*Take this medicine only as directed by your doctor,* to
benefit your condition as much as possible. Do not take
more of it, do not take it more often, and do not take it
for a longer time than your doctor ordered.

For patients taking the *oral liquid form* of this medicine:
- Shake the bottle well before measuring the dose.
- Use a specially marked measuring spoon, a plastic syringe,
  or a small marked measuring cup to measure each dose
  accurately. The average household teaspoon may not hold
  the right amount of liquid.

To lessen stomach upset, felbamate may be taken with
food, unless your doctor has told you to take it on an
empty stomach.

**Dosing**—The dose of felbamate will be different for different patients. *Follow your doctor's orders or the directions on the label.* The following information includes
only the average doses of felbamate. *If your dose is different, do not change it* unless your doctor tells you to
do so.

The number of tablets or teaspoonfuls of suspension that
you take depends on the strength of the medicine.
- For *oral* dosage forms (suspension or tablets):
  —For epilepsy:
    - Adults and teenagers 14 years of age and
      older—At first, usually 1200 milligrams (mg) a
      day, divided into three or four smaller doses.
      Your doctor may increase the dose gradually over
      several weeks if needed. However, the dose is
      usually not more than 3600 mg a day.
    - Children 2 to 14 years of age—At first, usually
      15 mg per kilogram (kg) [6.8 mg per pound] of

---

body weight per day, divided into smaller doses that are given three or four times during the day. Your doctor may increase the dose gradually over a few weeks if needed. However, the dose is usually not more than 45 mg per kg [20.5 mg per pound] per day or 3600 mg, whichever is less.

**Missed dose**—If you miss a dose of this medicine, take it as soon as possible. However, if it is almost time for your next dose, skip the missed dose and go back to your regular dosing schedule. Do not double doses.

**Storage**—To store this medicine:

• Keep out of the reach of children.
• Store away from heat and direct sunlight.
• Do not store in the bathroom, near the kitchen sink, or in other damp places. Heat or moisture may cause the medicine to break down.
• Do not keep outdated medicine or medicine no longer needed. Be sure that any discarded medicine is out of the reach of children.

## Precautions While Using This Medicine

*It is important that your doctor check your progress at regular visits.* This is necessary to allow dose adjustments and to test for serious unwanted effects.

*Do not stop taking felbamate without first checking with your doctor.* Your doctor may want you to gradually reduce the amount you are taking before stopping completely. Stopping the medicine suddenly may cause your seizures to return or to occur more often.

Felbamate may cause blurred vision, double vision, or other changes in vision. It may also cause some people to become dizzy or drowsy. *Make sure you know how you react to this medicine before you drive, use machines, or do anything else that could be dangerous if you are not alert or able to see well.* If these reactions are especially bothersome, check with your doctor.

## Side Effects of This Medicine

Felbamate may cause some serious side effects, including blood problems and liver problems. *You and your doctor should discuss the good this medicine will do as well as the risks of receiving it.*

Along with its needed effects, a medicine may cause some unwanted effects. Some side effects will have signs or symptoms that you can see or feel. Your doctor may watch for others by doing certain tests. Although not all of these side effects may occur, if they do occur they may need medical attention.

*Check with your doctor immediately* if any of the following side effects occur:
*More common*
Fever; purple or red spots on skin
*Rare*
Black or tarry stools; blood in urine or stools; chills; continuing abdominal pain; continuing headache; continuing vomiting; dark-colored urine; general feeling of tiredness or weakness; light-colored stools; nosebleeds or other unusual bruising or bleeding; shortness of breath, trouble in breathing, wheezing, or tightness in chest; sore throat; sores, ulcers, or white spots on lips or in mouth; swelling of face; swollen or painful glands; yellow eyes or skin

*Check with your doctor as soon as possible* if any of the following side effects occur:
*More common*
Walking in unusual manner
*Less common*
Agitation, aggression, or other mood or mental changes; clumsiness or unsteadiness; skin rash; tremor
*Rare*
Chest pain; hives or itching; muscle cramps; nasal congestion; pain; sensitivity of skin to sunlight; swollen lymph nodes

Other side effects may occur that usually do not need medical attention. These side effects may go away during treatment as your body adjusts to the medicine. However, check with your doctor if any of the following side effects continue or are bothersome:
*More common*
Abdominal pain; change in your sense of taste; constipation; difficulty in sleeping; dizziness; headache; indigestion; loss of appetite; nausea; vomiting
*Less common*
Blurred or double vision; coughing; diarrhea; drowsiness; ear congestion or pain; runny nose; sneezing; weight loss

This medicine may also cause the following side effects that you doctor will watch for:
*Rare*
Blood problems

Other side effects not listed above may also occur in some patients. If you notice any other effects, check with your doctor.

Developed: 08/30/94
Interim revision: 10/06/94

# FENFLURAMINE   Systemic

**In the U.S.—**
Pondimin

**In Canada—**
Ponderal                          Pondimin
Ponderal Pacaps

## Description

Fenfluramine (fen-FLURE-a-meen) is an appetite suppressant used in the short-term treatment of obesity. For a few weeks, fenfluramine, in combination with dieting, exercise, and changes in eating habits, can help obese patients lose weight. However, since fenfluramine's appetite-reducing effect may be temporary, it may be useful only for the first few weeks of dieting until new habits are established.

Fenfluramine may also be used for other conditions as determined by your doctor.

This medicine is available only with your doctor's prescription, in the following dosage forms:

*Oral*
- Extended-release capsules (Canada)
- Tablets (U.S. and Canada)

## Before Using This Medicine

In deciding to use a medicine, the risks of taking the medicine must be weighed against the good it will do. This is a decision you and your doctor will make. For fenfluramine, the following should be considered:

**Allergies**—Tell your doctor if you have ever had any unusual or allergic reaction to this medicine or amphetamine, dextroamphetamine, ephedrine, epinephrine, isoproterenol, metaproterenol, methamphetamine, norepinephrine, phenylephrine, phenylpropanolamine, pseudoephedrine, terbutaline, or other appetite suppressants. Also tell your health care professional if you are allergic to any other substances, such as foods, preservatives, or dyes.

**Pregnancy**—Studies have not been done in pregnant women. However, animal studies have shown that fenfluramine, when given at many times the human dose, reduces fertility and may have toxic or harmful effects on the fetus.

**Breast-feeding**—It is not known if fenfluramine passes into breast milk. However, this medicine has not been reported to cause problems in nursing babies.

**Children**—Fenfluramine should not be used as an appetite suppressant by children under 12 years of age.

**Older adults**—Many medicines have not been studied specifically in older people. Therefore, it may not be known whether they work exactly the same way they do in younger adults or if they cause different side effects or problems in older people. There is no specific information comparing use of fenfluramine in the elderly to use in other age groups.

**Other medicines**—Although certain medicines should not be used together at all, in other cases two different medicines may be used together even if an interaction might occur. In these cases, your doctor may want to change the dose, or other precautions may be necessary. When you are taking fenfluramine, it is especially important that your health care professional know if you are taking any of the following:

- Central nervous system (CNS) depressants (medicine that causes drowsiness) or
- Tricyclic antidepressants (medicine for depression)—Using these medicines with fenfluramine may increase the CNS depressant effects
- Monoamine oxidase (MAO) inhibitors (furazolidone [e.g., Furoxone], isocarboxazid [e.g., Marplan], phenelzine [e.g., Nardil], procarbazine [e.g., Matulane], selegiline [e.g., Eldepryl], tranylcypromine [e.g., Parnate])—Taking fenfluramine while you are taking or within 2 weeks of taking monoamine oxidase (MAO) inhibitors may cause sudden extremely high blood pressure; at least 14 days should be allowed between stopping treatment with one medicine and starting treatment with the other

**Other medical problems**—The presence of other medical problems may affect the use of appetite suppressants. Make sure you tell your doctor if you have any other medical problems, especially:

- Alcohol abuse (or history of) or
- Drug abuse or dependence (or history of)—Dependence on fenfluramine may develop
- Diabetes mellitus (sugar diabetes)—The amount of insulin or oral antidiabetic medicine that you need to take may change
- Glaucoma or
- Heart or blood vessel disease or
- High blood pressure or
- Mental depression or
- Mental illness (severe)—Fenfluramine may make the condition worse

## Proper Use of This Medicine

*Take fenfluramine only as directed by your doctor*. Do not take more of it, do not take it more often, and do not take it for a longer time than your doctor ordered. If too much is taken, it may become habit-forming.

If you think this medicine is not working properly after you have taken it for a few weeks, *do not increase the dose*. Instead, check with your doctor.

For patients taking the *long-acting form* of this medicine:
- These capsules or tablets are to be swallowed whole. Do not break, crush, or chew before swallowing.

**Dosing**—The dose of fenfluramine will be different for different patients. *Follow your doctor's orders or the directions on the label*. The following information includes only the average doses of fenfluramine. *If your*

dose is different, do not change it unless your doctor tells you to do so.
- For *oral extended-release capsule* dosage form:
  —For appetite suppression:
  • Adults—At first, 60 milligrams (mg) once a day. Your doctor may need to adjust your dose.
  • Children—Use is not recommended.
- For *oral tablet* dosage form:
  —For appetite suppression:
  • Adults—At first, 20 mg three times a day, taken thirty to sixty minutes before meals. Your doctor may need to adjust your dose.
  • Children—Use is not recommended.

**Storage**—To store this medicine:
- Keep out of the reach of children.
- Store away from heat and direct light.
- Do not store in the bathroom, near the kitchen sink, or in other damp places. Heat or moisture may cause the medicine to break down.
- Do not keep outdated medicine or medicine no longer needed. Be sure that any discarded medicine is out of the reach of children.

## Precautions While Using This Medicine

Your doctor should check your progress at regular visits in order to make sure that this medicine does not cause unwanted effects.

Fenfluramine will add to the effects of alcohol and other CNS depressants (medicines that cause drowsiness). Some examples of CNS depressants are antihistamines or medicine for hay fever, other allergies, or colds; sedatives, tranquilizers, or sleeping medicine; prescription pain medicine or narcotics; barbiturates; medicine for seizures; muscle relaxants; or anesthetics, including some dental anesthetics. *Check with your medical doctor or dentist before taking any such depressants while you are using this medicine.*

This medicine may cause some people to have a false sense of well-being or to become dizzy, lightheaded, drowsy, or less alert than they are normally. *Make sure you know how you react to this medicine before you drive, use machines, or do anything else that could be dangerous if you are dizzy or are not alert.*

*Before having any kind of surgery, dental treatment, or emergency treatment, tell the medical doctor or dentist in charge that you are using this medicine.* Taking fenfluramine together with medicines that are used during surgery or dental or emergency treatments may increase the CNS depressant effects.

If you have been taking fenfluramine for a long time or in large doses and *you think you may have become mentally or physically dependent on it, check with your doctor.*

- Some signs of dependence on fenfluramine are:
  —a strong desire or need to continue taking the medicine.
  —a need to increase the dose to receive the effects of the medicine.
  —withdrawal side effects (for example, mental depression, trouble in sleeping, or nightmares when you stop taking the medicine).

For *diabetic patients:*
- This medicine may affect blood sugar levels. If you notice a change in the results of your urine or blood sugar test or if you have any questions, check with your doctor.

If you will be taking fenfluramine in large doses for a long time, *do not stop taking it without first checking with your doctor.* Your doctor may want you to reduce gradually the amount you are taking before stopping completely.

## Side Effects of This Medicine

Along with its needed effects, a medicine may cause some unwanted effects. Although not all of these side effects may occur, if they do occur they may need medical attention.

Check with your doctor as soon as possible if any of the following side effects occur:
*Less common*
 Confusion or mental depression; skin rash or hives
*Rare*
 Difficult or troubled breathing brought on by physical effort; increased blood pressure
*Symptoms of overdose*
 Abdominal or stomach cramps; fast breathing; fever; nausea or vomiting (severe); tremor

Other side effects may occur that usually do not need medical attention. These side effects may go away during treatment as your body adjusts to the medicine. However, check with your doctor if any of the following side effects continue or are bothersome:
*More common*
 Diarrhea; drowsiness; dryness of mouth
*Less common*
 Blurred vision; changes in sexual desire or decreased sexual ability; clumsiness or unsteadiness; constipation; difficult or painful urination; difficulty in talking; dizziness or lightheadedness; false sense of well-being; frequent urge to urinate or increased urination; headache; increased sweating; irritability; nausea or vomiting; nervousness or restlessness; nightmares; pounding heartbeat; stomach cramps or pain; trouble in sleeping or nightmares; unpleasant taste; unusual tiredness or weakness

After you stop using this medicine, your body may need time to adjust. The length of time this takes depends on the amount of medicine you were using and how long you used it. During this time check with your doctor if you notice any of the following side effects:

Mental depression; trouble in sleeping or nightmares

Other side effects not listed above may also occur in some patients. If you notice any other effects, check with your doctor.

## Additional Information

Once a medicine has been approved for marketing for a certain use, experience may show that it is also useful for other medical problems. Although this use is not included in product labeling, fenfluramine is used in certain patients with the following medical condition:

• Infantile autism

Other than the above information, there is no additional information relating to proper use, precautions, or side effects for these uses.

Revised: 08/29/94

# FENTANYL    Transdermal-Systemic

A commonly used brand name in the U.S. and Canada is Duragesic.

## Description

Fentanyl (FEN-ta-nil) belongs to the group of medicines called narcotic analgesics (nar-KOT-ik an-al-GEE-ziks). Narcotic analgesics are used to relieve pain. The transdermal system (skin patch) form of fentanyl is used to treat chronic pain (pain that continues for a long time).

Fentanyl acts in the central nervous system (CNS) to relieve pain. Some of its side effects are also caused by actions in the CNS.

When a narcotic is used for a long time, it may become habit-forming (causing mental or physical dependence). However, *people who have continuing pain should not let the fear of dependence keep them from using narcotics to relieve their pain.* Mental dependence (addiction) is not likely to occur when narcotics are used for this purpose. Physical dependence may lead to withdrawal side effects if treatment is stopped suddenly. However, severe withdrawal side effects can usually be prevented by reducing the dose gradually over a period of time before treatment is stopped completely.

This medicine is available only with your doctor's prescription. Prescriptions for transdermal fentanyl cannot be refilled. You will need to obtain a new prescription from your doctor each time you need the medicine. This medicine is available in the following dosage form:

*Transdermal*
• Transdermal system (stick-on skin patch) (U.S. and Canada)

## Before Using This Medicine

In deciding to use a medicine, the risks of using the medicine must be weighed against the good it will do. This is a decision you and your health care professional will make. For fentanyl, the following should be considered:

**Allergies**—Tell your health care professional if you have ever had any unusual or allergic reaction to fentanyl, alfentanil (e.g., Alfenta), or sufentanil (e.g., Sufenta). Also tell your health care professional if you are allergic to any other substances, including the adhesives that keep stick-on bandages in place.

**Pregnancy**—Although studies on birth defects with fentanyl have not been done in pregnant women, it has not been reported to cause birth defects. However, using any narcotic regularly during pregnancy may cause physical dependence in the fetus. This may lead to withdrawal side effects after birth. Also, use of this medicine near the end of pregnancy may cause drowsiness and breathing problems in newborn babies.

**Breast-feeding**—Fentanyl passes into the breast milk. Nursing babies whose mothers are using this medicine regularly may receive enough of it to cause unwanted effects such as drowsiness, breathing problems, and physical dependence. Similar effects may also occur with some other narcotics if they are taken regularly in large amounts. A mother who wishes to breast-feed and who needs treatment for continuing pain should discuss the risks and benefits of different pain treatments with her health care professional.

**Children**—Studies with the fentanyl skin patch have been done only in adult patients, and there is no specific information comparing the use of this medicine in children with use in other age groups.

**Teenagers**—Studies with the fentanyl skin patch have been done only in patients 18 years of age and older. There is no specific information comparing the use of this medicine in teenagers with use in other age groups.

**Older adults**—Elderly people are especially sensitive to the effects of narcotic analgesics. This may increase the chance of side effects, especially breathing problems, during treatment. Your health care professional will take this into consideration when deciding on the amount of transdermal fentanyl you should receive.

**Other medicines**—Although certain medicines should not be used together at all, in other cases two different medicines may be used together even if an interaction might occur. In these cases, your health care professional may want to change the dose, or other precautions may be necessary. When you are using fentanyl, it is especially important that your health care professional know if you are taking any of the following:

- Buprenorphine (e.g., Buprenex) or
- Dezocine (e.g., Dalgan) or
- Nalbuphine (e.g., Nubain) or
- Pentazocine (e.g., Talwin)—Like all narcotic analgesics, these medicines may add to the effects of fentanyl, which may increase the chance of side effects or overdose. However, buprenorphine, dezocine, nalbuphine, and pentazocine sometimes decrease the effects of fentanyl, so that fentanyl might be less effective in relieving pain. Also, these medicines can cause withdrawal side effects if they are given to someone who is physically dependent on fentanyl
- Central nervous system (CNS) depressants (medicines that cause drowsiness), including other narcotics, or
- Tricyclic antidepressants—These medicines may add to the effects of fentanyl. This may increase the chance of serious side effects
- Naltrexone (e.g., Trexan)—Fentanyl will not be effective in people taking naltrexone

**Other medical problems**—The presence of other medical problems may affect the use of fentanyl. Make sure you tell your health care professional if you have any other medical problems, especially:

- Alcohol abuse, or history of, or
- Drug dependence, especially narcotic abuse or dependence, or history of, or
- Emotional problems or
- Kidney disease or
- Liver disease or
- Underactive thyroid—The chance of side effects may be increased
- Brain tumor or
- Diarrhea caused by antibiotic treatment or poisoning or
- Emphysema, asthma, or other chronic lung disease or
- Enlarged prostate or problems with urination or
- Gallbladder disease or gallstones or
- Intestinal problems such as colitis or Crohn's disease— Some of the side effects of fentanyl can cause serious problems in people who have these medical problems
- Slow heartbeat—Fentanyl can make this condition worse

## Proper Use of This Medicine

*Transdermal fentanyl comes with patient instructions. Read them carefully before using the product.* If you do not receive any printed instructions with the medicine, check with your pharmacist.

To use:

- *Use this medicine exactly as directed by your doctor.* It will work only if it has been applied correctly.
- Fentanyl skin patches are packaged in sealed pouches. *Do not remove the patch from the sealed pouch until you are ready to apply it.*
- When handling the skin patch, *be careful not to touch the adhesive (sticky) surface with your hand.* The adhesive part of the system contains some fentanyl, which can be absorbed into your body too fast through the skin of your hand. If any of the medicine

does get on your hand, *rinse the area right away with a lot of clear water. Do not use soap or other cleansers.*

- *Be careful not to tear the patch or make any holes in it.* Damage to a patch may allow fentanyl to pass into your skin too quickly. This can cause an overdose.
- Apply the patch to a dry, flat skin area on your upper arm, chest, or back. *Choose a place where the skin is not very oily and is free of scars, cuts, burns, or any other skin irritations. Also, do not apply this medicine to areas that have received radiation (x-ray) treatment.*
- The patch will stay in place better if it is applied to an area with little or no hair. If you need to apply the patch to a hairy area, you may first clip the hair with scissors, *but do not shave it off.*
- If you need to clean the area before applying the medicine, *use only plain water. Do not use soaps, other cleansers, lotions, or anything that contains oils or alcohol.* Be sure that the skin is completely dry before applying the medicine.
- Remove the liner covering the sticky side of the skin patch. Then press the patch firmly in place, using the palm of your hand, for about 30 seconds. Make sure that the entire adhesive surface is attached to your skin, especially around the edges.
- If you need to apply more than 1 patch at a time, *place the patches far enough apart so that the edges do not touch or overlap each other.*
- Wash your hands with a lot of clear water after applying the medicine. Do not use soap or other cleansers.
- Remove the patch after 72 hours (3 days). *Choose a different place on your skin to apply the next patch.* If possible, use a place on the other side of your body. *Wait at least 3 days before using the first area again.*

After a patch is applied, the fentanyl it contains passes into the skin a little at a time. A certain amount of the medicine must build up in the skin before it is absorbed into the body. Therefore, up to a day may pass before the first dose begins to work. Your health care professional may need to change the dose during the first several applications (each kept in place for 3 days) before finding the amount that works best for you. Even if you feel that the medicine is not working, *do not increase the amount of transdermal fentanyl that you apply.* Instead, check with your health care professional.

You will probably need to take a faster-acting narcotic to relieve pain during the first few days of transdermal fentanyl treatment. You may continue to need another narcotic while your dose of fentanyl is being adjusted, and also to relieve any "break through" pain that occurs later on. *Be sure that you do not take more of the other narcotic, and do not take it more often, than directed. Taking other narcotics together with fentanyl can increase the chance of an overdose.*

**Dosing**—The dose of transdermal fentanyl will be different for different patients. *Follow your doctor's orders or the directions on the label.* The following information includes only the average doses of this medicine. *If your dose is different, do not change it* unless your doctor tells you to do so.

- For *transdermal* dosage form (stick-on patch):
  —For relief of severe, continuing pain:
    - Adults—If you have not already been using other narcotics regularly, your first dose will probably be one patch that releases 25 micrograms (mcg) of fentanyl every hour. If you have already been using other narcotics regularly, your first dose will depend on the amount of other narcotic you have been taking every day. If necessary, your health care professional will change the dose after 3 days, when the first patch is replaced. The size of the new dose will depend on how well the medicine is working and on whether you had any side effects during the first 3-day application. Other changes in dose may be needed later on. Some people may need to use more than one patch at a time.
    - Children—Use and dose must be determined by the doctor.

**Missed dose**—If you miss a dose of this medicine, apply it as soon as possible. Remove the new patch 3 days after applying it.

**Storage**—To store this medicine:
- Keep out of the reach of children.
- Store away from heat and direct light.
- Do not keep outdated medicine or medicine no longer needed. To dispose of this medicine, first fold the patch in half, with the sticky side inside. If the patch has not been used, take it out of the pouch and remove the liner that covers the sticky side of the patch before folding it in half. Then flush it down the toilet right away.

## Precautions While Using This Medicine

Check with your health care professional at regular times while using fentanyl. Be sure to report any side effects.

After you have been using this medicine for a while, "break through" pain may occur more often than usual, and it may not be relieved by your regular dose of medicine. If this occurs, *do not increase the amount of transdermal fentanyl or other narcotic that you are taking without first checking with your health care professional.*

This medicine will add to the effects of alcohol and other CNS depressants (medicines that can make you drowsy or less alert). Some examples of CNS depressants are antihistamines or medicine for hay fever, other allergies, or colds; sedatives, tranquilizers, or sleeping medicine;

other prescription pain medicine or narcotics; barbiturates; medicine for seizures; muscle relaxants; or anesthetics, including some dental anesthetics. You will probably be directed to take other pain relievers if you still have pain while using transdermal fentanyl. However, *check with your health care professional before taking any of the other medicines listed above while you are using this medicine.*

Fentanyl may cause some people to become drowsy, dizzy, or lightheaded, or to feel a false sense of well-being. *Make sure you know how you react to this medicine before you drive, use machines, or do anything else that could be dangerous if you are dizzy or not alert and clearheaded.* These effects usually go away after a few days of treatment, when your body gets used to the medicine. However, *check with your health care professional if drowsiness that is severe enough to interfere with your activities continues for more than a few days.*

Dizziness, lightheadedness, or even fainting may occur when you get up suddenly from a lying or sitting position. *Getting up slowly may help lessen this problem.* Also, lying down for a while may relieve dizziness or lightheadedness.

Nausea or vomiting may occur, especially during the first several days of treatment. Lying down for a while may relieve these effects. However, if they are especially bothersome or if they continue for more than a few days, check with your health care professional. You may be able to take another medicine to help prevent these problems.

Using narcotics for a long time can cause severe constipation. To prevent this, your health care professional may direct you to take laxatives, drink a lot of fluids, or increase the amount of fiber in your diet. *Be sure to follow the directions carefully,* because continuing constipation can lead to more serious problems.

Heat can cause the fentanyl in the patch to be absorbed into your body faster. This may increase the chance of serious side effects or an overdose. While you are using this medicine, *do not use a heating pad, a sunlamp, or a heated water bed, and do not take sunbaths or long baths or showers in hot water.* Also, *check with your health care professional if you get a fever.*

*Before having any kind of surgery (including dental surgery) or emergency treatment, tell the medical doctor or dentist in charge that you are using this medicine.* Serious side effects can occur if your medical doctor or dentist gives you certain other medicines without knowing that you are using fentanyl.

You may bathe, shower, or swim while wearing a fentanyl skin patch. However, be careful to wash and dry the area around the patch gently. Rubbing may cause the patch to get loose or come off. If this does occur, throw away the patch and apply a new one in a different place. Make sure the area is completely dry before applying the new patch.

If you have been using this medicine regularly for several weeks or more, *do not suddenly stop using it without first checking with your health care professional.* You may be directed to reduce gradually the amount you are using before stopping treatment completely, or to take another narcotic for a while, to lessen the chance of withdrawal side effects.

*Using too much transdermal fentanyl, or taking too much of another narcotic while using transdermal fentanyl, may cause an overdose. If this occurs, get emergency help right away.* An overdose can cause severe breathing problems (breathing may even stop), unconsciousness, and death. Serious signs of an overdose include very slow breathing (fewer than 8 breaths a minute) and drowsiness that is so severe that you are not able to answer when spoken to or, if asleep, cannot be awakened. Other signs of an overdose may include cold, clammy skin; low blood pressure; pinpoint pupils of eyes; and slow heartbeat. *It may be best to have a family member or a friend check on you several times a day when you start using a narcotic regularly, and whenever your dose is increased,* so that he or she can get help for you if you cannot do so yourself.

## Side Effects of This Medicine

Along with its needed effects, a medicine may cause some unwanted effects. Although not all of these side effects may occur, if they do occur they may need medical attention.

*Get emergency help immediately if the following signs of overdose occur:*

Cold, clammy skin; convulsions (seizures); drowsiness that is so severe that you are not able to answer when spoken to or, if asleep, cannot be awakened; low blood pressure; pinpoint pupils of eyes; slow heartbeat; very slow (fewer than 8 breaths a minute) or troubled breathing

Also, check with your doctor as soon as possible if any of the following side effects occur:

*More common*

Decrease in amount of urine or in the frequency of urination; hallucinations (seeing, hearing, or feeling things that are not there)

*Less common*

Chest pain; difficulty in speaking; fainting; irregular heartbeat; mood or mental changes; problems with walking; redness, swelling, itching, or bumps on the skin at place of application; spitting blood

*Rare*

Any change in vision; bladder pain; difficulty in speaking; fever with or without chills; fluid-filled blisters on skin; frequent urge to urinate; noisy breathing, shortness of breath, tightness in chest, or wheezing; red, thickened, or scaly skin; swelling of abdomen or stomach area; swollen and/or painful glands; unusual bruising

Other side effects may occur that usually do not need medical attention. These side effects may go away during treatment as your body adjusts to the medicine. However, check with your doctor if any of the following side effects continue or are bothersome:

*More common*

Abdominal or stomach pain that was not present before treatment; confusion; constipation; diarrhea; dizziness, drowsiness, or lightheadedness; false sense of well-being; feeling anxious; headache; indigestion; loss of appetite; nausea or vomiting; nervousness; sweating; weakness

*Less common*

Bloated feeling or gas; feeling anxious and restless at the same time; feeling of crawling, tingling, or burning of the skin; memory loss; unusual dreams

After you stop using this medicine, your body may need time to adjust. The length of time this takes depends on the amount of medicine you were using and how long you used it. During this period of time check with your doctor if you notice any of the following side effects:

Body aches; diarrhea; fast heartbeat; fever, runny nose, or sneezing; gooseflesh; increased sweating; increased yawning; loss of appetite; nausea or vomiting; nervousness, restlessness, or irritability; shivering or trembling; stomach cramps; trouble in sleeping; unusually large pupils of eyes; weakness

Other side effects not listed above may also occur in some patients. If you notice any other effects, check with your doctor.

Developed: 07/27/94

# FINASTERIDE   Systemic

A commonly used brand name in the in the U.S. and Canada is Proscar.

## Description

Finasteride (fi-NAS-teer-ide) belongs to the group of medicines called enzyme inhibitors. It is used to treat enlargement of the prostate (benign prostatic hyperplasia or BPH), a condition that causes urinary problems in men.

Finasteride blocks an enzyme called 5-alpha-reductase, which is necessary to change testosterone to another hormone that causes the prostate to grow. As a result, the size of the prostate is decreased. The effect of finasteride on the prostate lasts only as long as the medicine is taken. If it is stopped, the prostate begins to grow again.

*Oral*
- Tablets (U.S. and Canada)

## Before Using This Medicine

In deciding to use a medicine, the risks of taking the medicine must be weighed against the good it will do. This is a decision you and your doctor will make. For finasteride, the following should be considered:

**Allergies**—Tell your doctor if you have ever had any unusual or allergic reaction to finasteride. Also tell your health care professional if you are allergic to any other substances, such as foods, preservatives, or dyes.

**Pregnancy**—Women who are or may become pregnant should not be exposed to finasteride, because it can cause changes in the genitals (sex organs) of male infants. Therefore, you should use a condom to prevent contact of your semen with your sexual partner while you are taking finasteride. Discuss with your doctor the need to stop taking finasteride if your partner wishes to become pregnant.

While you are taking finasteride, you may notice a decrease in the amount of semen when you ejaculate. This should not affect your sexual performance and is not a sign of any change in fertility.

**Older adults**—This medicine has been tested and has not been shown to cause different side effects or problems in older people than it does in younger adults.

**Other medicines**—Although certain medicines should not be used together at all, in other cases two different medicines may be used together even if an interaction might occur. In these cases, your doctor may want to change the dose, or other precautions may be necessary. When you are taking finasteride, it is especially important that your health care professional know if you are taking any of the following:
- Amantadine (e.g., Symmetrel) or
- Amphetamines or
- Anticholinergics (medicine for abdominal or stomach spasms or cramps) or
- Antidepressants (medicine for depression) or
- Antidyskinetics (medicine for Parkinson's disease or other conditions affecting control of muscles or
- Antihistamines or
- Antipsychotics (medicine for mental illness) or
- Appetite suppressants (diet pills) or
- Buclizine (e.g., Bucladin) or
- Carbamazepine (e.g., Tegretol) or
- Cyclizine (e.g., Marezine) or
- Cyclobenzaprine (e.g., Flexeril) or
- Disopyramide (e.g., Norpace) or
- Flavoxate (e.g., Urispas) or
- Ipratropium (e.g., Atrovent) or
- Meclizine (e.g., Antivert) or
- Medicine for asthma or other breathing problems or
- Medicine for colds, sinus problems, or hay fever or other allergies (including nose drops or sprays) or
- Methylphenidate (e.g., Ritalin) or

- Orphenadrine (e.g., Norflex) or
- Oxybutynin (e.g., Ditropan)
- Procainamide (e.g., Pronestyl) or
- Promethazine (e.g., Phenergan) or
- Quinidine (e.g., Quinidex) or
- Trimeprazine (e.g., Temaril)—These medicines can cause problems with urination, which could reduce the effects of finasteride

**Other medical problems**—The presence of other medical problems may affect the use of finasteride. Make sure you tell your doctor if you have any other medical problems, especially:
- Liver disease—Effects of finasteride may be increased because of slower removal from the body

## Proper Use of This Medicine

To help you remember to take your medicine, try to get into the habit of taking it at the same time each day.

Remember that this medicine does not cure BPH but it does help reduce the size of the prostate. Therefore, you must continue to take it if you expect to keep the size of your prostate down. *You may have to take medicine for the rest of your life.* Do not stop taking this medicine without first discussing it with your doctor.

Finasteride tablets may be crushed to make them easier to swallow.

This medicine helps to reduce urinary problems in men with BPH. In general, it is best to avoid drinking fluids, especially coffee or alcohol, in the evening. Then your sleep will not be disturbed by your needing to urinate during the night.

**Dosing**—The dose of finasteride will be different for different patients. *Follow your doctor's orders or the directions on the label.* The following information includes only the average dose of finasteride. *If your dose is different, do not change it* unless your doctor tells you to do so:
- Adults: 5 mg (one tablet) once a day.

**Missed dose**—If you miss a dose of this medicine, take it as soon as possible. However, if it is almost time for your next dose, skip the missed dose and go back to your regular dosing schedule. Do not double doses.

**Storage**—To store this medicine:
- Keep out of the reach of children.
- Store away from heat and direct light.
- Do not store in the bathroom, near the kitchen sink, or in other damp places. Heat or moisture may cause the medicine to break down.
- Do not keep outdated medicine or medicine no longer needed. Be sure that any discarded medicine is out of the reach of children.

## Precautions While Using This Medicine

*Do not take other medicines unless they have been discussed with your doctor.* This especially includes over-the-counter (nonprescription) medicines for appetite control, asthma, colds, cough, hay fever, or sinus problems.

These medicines may cause problems with urination and could reduce the effects of finasteride.

Women who are or who may become pregnant should not handle crushed finasteride tablets because of the risk that it could be absorbed into the body and harm the infant.

## Side Effects of This Medicine

Along with its needed effects, a medicine may cause some unwanted effects. The following side effects may go away during treatment as your body adjusts to the medicine.

However, check with your doctor if any of the following side effects continue or are bothersome:

*Less common or rare*
> Decreased libido (decreased interest in sex); decreased volume of ejaculate (amount of semen); impotence (inability to have or keep an erection)

Other side effects not listed above may also occur in some patients. If you notice any other effects, check with your doctor.

Revised: 03/03/93

---

# FLAVOXATE    Systemic

A commonly used brand name in the U.S. and Canada is Urispas.

## Description

Flavoxate (fla-VOX-ate) belongs to the group of medicines called antispasmodics. It is taken by mouth to help decrease muscle spasms of the bladder and relieve difficult urination.

Flavoxate is available only with your doctor's prescription, in the following dosage form:

*Oral*
- Tablets (U.S. and Canada)

## Before Using This Medicine

In deciding to use a medicine, the risks of taking the medicine must be weighed against the good it will do. This is a decision you and your doctor will make. For flavoxate, the following should be considered:

**Allergies**—Tell your doctor if you have ever had any unusual or allergic reaction to flavoxate. Also tell your health care professional if you are allergic to any other substances, such as foods, preservatives, or dyes.

**Pregnancy**—Flavoxate has not been studied in pregnant women. However, flavoxate has not been shown to cause birth defects or other problems in animal studies.

**Breast-feeding**—Flavoxate has not been reported to cause problems in nursing babies.

**Children**—Although there is no specific information comparing the use of flavoxate in children with use in other age groups, this medicine is not expected to cause different side effects or problems in children than it does in adults.

**Older adults**—Confusion may be especially likely to occur in elderly patients, who are usually more sensitive than younger adults to the effects of flavoxate.

**Other medicines**—Although certain medicines should not be used together at all in other cases two different medicines may be used together even if an interaction might occur. In these cases, your doctor may want to change the dose, or other precautions may be necessary. Tell your health care professional if you are taking any other prescription or nonprescription (over-the-counter [OTC]) medicine.

**Other medical problems**—The presence of other medical problems may affect the use of flavoxate. Make sure you tell your doctor if you have any other medical problems, especially:
- Bleeding (severe) or
- Glaucoma or
- Intestinal blockage or other intestinal or stomach problems or
- Urinary tract blockage—Use of flavoxate may make these conditions worse
- Enlarged prostate—Use of flavoxate may cause difficult urination

## Proper Use of This Medicine

This medicine is usually taken with water on an empty stomach. However, your doctor may want you to take it with food or milk to lessen stomach upset.

*Take this medicine only as directed.* Do not take more of it, do not take it more often, and do not take it for a longer time than your doctor ordered. To do so may increase the chance of side effects.

**Dosing**—The dose of flavoxate will be different for different patients. *Follow your doctor's orders or the directions on the label.* The following information includes only the average dose of flavoxate. *If your dose is different, do not change it* unless your doctor tells you to do so. The number of tablets that you take depends on the strength of the medicine.
- Adults and children 12 years of age and older: 100 to 200 milligrams three or four times a day.

- Children up to 12 years of age: Dose must be determined by the doctor.

**Missed dose**—If you miss a dose of this medicine, take it as soon as possible. However, if it is almost time for your next dose, skip the missed dose and go back to your regular dosing schedule. Do not double doses.

**Storage**—To store this medicine:
- Keep out of the reach of children.
- Store away from heat and direct light.
- Do not store in the bathroom, near the kitchen sink, or in other damp places. Heat or moisture may cause the medicine to break down.
- Do not keep outdated medicine or medicine no longer needed. Be sure that any discarded medicine is out of the reach of children.

## Precautions While Using This Medicine

This medicine may cause your eyes to become more sensitive to light than they are normally. Wearing sunglasses may help lessen the discomfort from bright light.

This medicine may cause some people to become drowsy or have blurred vision. *Make sure you know how you react to this medicine before you drive, use machines, or do anything else that could be dangerous if you are not alert or able to see well.*

Flavoxate may make you sweat less, causing your body temperature to increase. *Use extra care not to become overheated during exercise or hot weather while you are taking this medicine,* since overheating may result in heat stroke. Also, hot baths or saunas may make you feel dizzy or faint while you are taking this medicine.

Your mouth and throat may feel very dry while you are taking this medicine. For temporary relief of mouth dryness, use sugarless candy or gum, melt bits of ice in your mouth, or use a saliva substitute. However, if your mouth continues to feel dry for more than 2 weeks, check with your medical doctor or dentist. Continuing dryness of the mouth may increase the chance of dental disease, including tooth decay, gum disease, and fungus infections.

## Side Effects of This Medicine

Along with its needed effects, a medicine may cause some unwanted effects. Although not all of these side effects may occur, if they do occur they may need medical attention.

Check with your doctor as soon as possible if any of the following side effects occur:
*Rare*
Confusion; eye pain; skin rash or hives; sore throat and fever
*Symptoms of overdose*
Clumsiness or unsteadiness; dizziness (severe); drowsiness (severe); fever; flushing or redness of face; hallucinations (seeing, hearing, or feeling things that are not there); shortness of breath or troubled breathing; unusual excitement, nervousness, restlessness, or irritability

Other side effects may occur that usually do not need medical attention. These side effects may go away during treatment as your body adjusts to the medicine. However, check with your doctor if any of the following side effects continue or are bothersome:
*More common*
Drowsiness; dryness of mouth and throat
*Less common or rare*
Blurred vision; constipation; difficult urination; difficulty concentrating; dizziness; fast heartbeat; headache; increased sensitivity of eyes to light; increased sweating; nausea or vomiting; nervousness; stomach pain

Other side effects not listed above may also occur in some patients. If you notice any other effects, check with your doctor.

Revised: 01/18/93

# FLECAINIDE   Systemic

A commonly used brand name in the U.S. and Canada is Tambocor.

## Description

Flecainide (FLEK-a-nide) belongs to the group of medicines known as antiarrhythmics. It is used to correct irregular heartbeats to a normal rhythm.

Flecainide produces its helpful effects by slowing nerve impulses in the heart and making the heart tissue less sensitive.

There is a chance that flecainide may cause new or make worse existing heart rhythm problems when it is used. Since it has been shown to cause severe problems in some patients, it is only used to treat serious heart rhythm problems. Discuss this possible effect with your doctor.

This medicine is available only with your doctor's prescription, in the following dosage form:
*Oral*
- Tablets (U.S. and Canada)

## Before Using This Medicine

In deciding to use a medicine, the risks of taking the medicine must be weighed against the good it will do. This is a decision you and your doctor will make. For flecainide, the following should be considered:

**Allergies**—Tell your doctor if you have ever had any unusual or allergic reaction to flecainide, lidocaine, tocainide, or anesthetics. Also tell your health care professional if you are allergic to any other substances, such as foods, preservatives, or dyes.

**Pregnancy**—Flecainide has not been studied in pregnant women. However, studies in one kind of rabbit given about 4 times the usual human dose have shown that flecainide causes birth defects. Before taking flecainide, make sure your doctor knows if you are pregnant or if you may become pregnant.

**Breast-feeding**—Flecainide passes into breast milk. However, this medicine has not been shown to cause problems in nursing babies.

**Children**—Studies on this medicine have been done only in adult patients, and there is no specific information comparing use of flecainide in children with use in other age groups.

**Older adults**—Elderly people are especially sensitive to the effects of flecainide. Flecainide may be more likely to cause irregular heartbeat in the elderly.

**Other medicines**—Although certain medicines should not be used together at all, in other cases two different medicines may be used together even if an interaction might occur. In these cases, your doctor may want to change the dose, or other precautions may be necessary. When you are taking flecainide it is especially important that your health care professional knows if you are taking any of the following:
- Other medicine for heart rhythm problems—Both wanted and unwanted effects on the heart may increase

**Other medical problems**—The presence of other medical problems may affect the use of flecainide. Make sure you tell your doctor if you have any other medical problems, especially:
- Congestive heart failure—Flecainide may make this condition worse
- Kidney disease or
- Liver disease—Effects of flecainide may be increased because of slower removal from the body
- Recent heart attack—Risk of irregular heartbeats may be increased
- If you have a pacemaker—Flecainide may interfere with the pacemaker and require more careful follow-up by the doctor

## Proper Use of This Medicine

*Take flecainide exactly as directed by your doctor*, even though you may feel well. Do not take more medicine than ordered.

This medicine works best when there is a constant amount in the blood. *To help keep this amount constant, do not miss any doses. Also, it is best to take the doses 12 hours apart, in the morning and at night*, unless otherwise directed by your doctor. If you need help in planning the best times to take your medicine, check with your health care professional.

**Dosing**—The dose of flecainide will be different for different patients. *Follow your doctor's orders or the directions on the label.* The following information includes only the average doses of flecainide. *If your dose is different, do not change it* unless your doctor tells you to do so.

The number of tablets that you take depends on the strength of the medicine.
- For *oral* dosage form (tablets):
  —For correcting irregular heartbeat:
  - Adults—50 to 150 milligrams (mg) every twelve hours.
  - Children—Use and dose must be determined by your doctor.

**Missed dose**—If you miss a dose of flecainide and remember within 6 hours, take it as soon as possible. However, if you do not remember until later, skip the missed dose and go back to your regular dosing schedule. Do not double doses.

**Storage**—To store this medicine:
- Keep out of the reach of children.
- Store away from heat and direct light.
- Do not store in the bathroom, near the kitchen sink, or in other damp places. Heat or moisture may cause the medicine to break down.
- Do not keep outdated medicine or medicine no longer needed. Be sure that any discarded medicine is out of the reach of children.

## Precautions While Using This Medicine

It is important that your doctor check your progress at regular visits to make sure the medicine is working properly. This will allow for changes to be made in the amount of medicine you are taking, if necessary.

Your doctor may want you to carry a medical identification card or bracelet stating that you are using this medicine.

*Before having any kind of surgery (including dental surgery) or emergency treatment, tell the medical doctor or dentist in charge that you are taking this medicine.*

Flecainide may cause some people to become dizzy, lightheaded, or less alert than they are normally. *Make sure you know how you react to this medicine before you drive, use machines, or do anything else that could be dangerous if you are dizzy or are not alert.*

If you have been using this medicine regularly for several weeks, do not suddenly stop using it. Check with your doctor for the best way to reduce gradually the amount you are taking before stopping completely.

## Side Effects of This Medicine

Along with its needed effects, a medicine may cause some unwanted effects. Although not all of these side effects may occur, if they do occur they may need medical attention.

Check with your doctor as soon as possible if any of the following side effects occur:

*Less common*
Chest pain; irregular heartbeat; shortness of breath; swelling of feet or lower legs; trembling or shaking

*Rare*
Yellow eyes or skin

Other side effects may occur that usually do not need medical attention. These side effects may go away during treatment as your body adjusts to the medicine. However, check with your doctor if any of the following side effects continue or are bothersome:

*More common*
Blurred vision or seeing spots; dizziness or lightheadedness

*Less common*
Anxiety or mental depression; constipation; headache; nausea or vomiting; skin rash; stomach pain or loss of appetite; unusual tiredness or weakness

Other side effects not listed above may also occur in some patients. If you notice any other effects, check with your doctor.

Revised: 09/24/92
Interim revision: 04/29/94

# FLOXURIDINE   Systemic†

A commonly used brand name in the U.S. is FUDR.
Generic name product may also be available in the U.S.

†Not commercially available in Canada.

## Description

Floxuridine (flox-YOOR-i-deen) belongs to the group of medicines known as antimetabolites. It is used to treat some kinds of cancer.

Floxuridine interferes with the growth of cancer cells, which are eventually destroyed. Since the growth of normal body cells may also be affected by floxuridine, other effects will also occur. Some of these may be serious and must be reported to your doctor. Other effects, like hair loss, may not be serious but may cause concern. Some effects may not occur for months or years after the medicine is used.

Before you begin treatment with floxuridine, you and your doctor should talk about the good this medicine will do as well as the risks of using it.

Floxuridine is to be administered only by or under the immediate supervision of your doctor. It is available in the following dosage form:

*Parenteral*
• Injection (U.S.)

## Before Using This Medicine

In deciding to use a medicine, the risks of taking the medicine must be weighed against the good it will do.

This is a decision you and your doctor will make. For floxuridine, the following should be considered:

**Allergies**—Tell your doctor if you have ever had any unusual or allergic reaction to floxuridine.

**Pregnancy**—There is a chance that this medicine may cause birth defects if either the male or female is receiving it at the time of conception or if it is taken during pregnancy. Floxuridine has been shown to cause birth defects in mice and rats. In addition, many cancer medicines may cause sterility which could be permanent. Although sterility has not been reported with this medicine, the possibility should be kept in mind.

Be sure that you have discussed this with your doctor before receiving this medicine. It is best to use some kind of birth control while you are receiving floxuridine. Tell your doctor right away if you think you have become pregnant while receiving floxuridine.

**Breast-feeding**—Tell your doctor if you are breast-feeding or if you intend to breast-feed during treatment with this medicine. Because floxuridine may cause serious side effects, breast-feeding is generally not recommended while you are receiving it.

**Children**—There is no specific information comparing use of floxuridine in children with use in other age groups.

**Older adults**—Many medicines have not been studied specifically in older people. Therefore, it may not be known whether they work exactly the same way they do in younger adults or if they cause different side effects or problems in older people. Although there is no specific information comparing use of floxuridine in the elderly with use in other age groups, this medicine is not expected to cause different side effects or problems in older people than it does in younger adults.

**Other medicines**—Although certain medicines should not be used together at all, in other cases two different medicines may be used together even if an interaction might occur. In these cases, your doctor may want to change the dose, or other precautions may be necessary. When you are receiving floxuridine, it is especially important that your health care professional know if you are taking any of the following:

- Amphotericin B by injection (e.g., Fungizone) or
- Antithyroid agents (medicine for overactive thyroid) or
- Azathioprine (e.g., Imuran) or
- Chloramphenicol (e.g., Chloromycetin) or
- Colchicine or
- Flucytosine (e.g., Ancobon) or
- Ganciclovir (e.g., Cytovene) or
- Interferon (Intron A, Roferon-A) or
- Plicamycin (e.g., Mithracin) or
- Zidovudine (e.g., AZT, Retrovir) or
- If you have ever been treated with radiation or cancer medicines—Floxuridine may increase the effects of these medicines or radiation on the blood

**Other medical problems**—The presence of other medical problems may affect the use of floxuridine. Make sure you tell your doctor if you have any other medical problems, especially:

- Chickenpox (including recent exposure) or
- Herpes zoster (shingles)—Risk of severe disease affecting other parts of the body
- Hepatitis (history of)—Increased risk of hepatitis
- Kidney disease or
- Liver disease (other)—Effects of floxuridine may be increased because of slower removal from the body
- Infection—Floxuridine can decrease your body's ability to fight infection

## Proper Use of This Medicine

Floxuridine sometimes causes nausea and vomiting. *Tell your doctor if this occurs, especially if you have stomach pain.*

**Dosing**—The dose of floxuridine will be different for different patients. The dose that is used may depend on a number of things, including what the medicine is being used for, the patient's weight, and whether or not other medicines are also being taken. *If you are receiving floxuridine at home, follow your doctor's orders or the directions on the label.* If you have any questions about the proper dose of floxuridine, ask your doctor.

## Precautions While Using This Medicine

*It is very important that your doctor check your progress at regular visits* to make sure that this medicine is working properly and to check for unwanted effects.

While you are being treated with floxuridine, and after you stop treatment with it, *do not have any immunizations (vaccinations) without your doctor's approval.* Floxuridine may lower your body's resistance and there is a chance you might get the infection the immunization is

meant to prevent. In addition, other persons living in your household should not take oral polio vaccine since there is a chance they could pass the polio virus on to you. Also, avoid persons who have recently taken oral polio vaccine. Do not get close to them and do not stay in the same room with them for very long. If you cannot take these precautions, you should consider wearing a protective face mask that covers the nose and mouth.

## Side Effects of This Medicine

Along with its needed effects, a medicine may cause some unwanted effects. Although not all of these side effects may occur, if they do occur they may need medical attention.

Also, because of the way these medicines act on the body, there is a chance that they might cause other unwanted effects that may not occur until months or years after the medicine is used. These delayed effects may include certain types of cancer, such as leukemia. Discuss these possible effects with your doctor.

*Check with your doctor or nurse immediately* if any of the following side effects occur:

*More common*

Diarrhea; sores in mouth and on lips; stomach pain or cramps

*Less common*

Black, tarry stools; heartburn; nausea and vomiting; scaling or redness of hands or feet; swelling or soreness of the tongue

*Rare*

Blood in urine or stools; cough or hoarseness; fever or chills; lower back or side pain; painful or difficult urination; pinpoint red spots on skin; trouble in walking; unusual bleeding or bruising; yellow eyes or skin

Other side effects may occur that usually do not need medical attention. These side effects may go away during treatment as your body adjusts to the medicine. Also, your health care professional may be able to tell you about ways to prevent or reduce some of these side effects. Check with your health care professional if any of the following side effects continue or are bothersome or if you have any questions about them:

*Less common or rare*

Loss of appetite; skin rash or itching

This medicine sometimes causes temporary thinning of hair. After treatment with floxuridine has ended, normal hair growth should return.

Other side effects not listed above may also occur in some patients. If you notice any other effects, check with your health care professional.

Revised: 07/26/94

# FLUCYTOSINE  Systemic

Some commonly used brand names are:
**In the U.S.—**
Ancobon
**In Canada**
Ancotil
Other commonly used names are 5-fluorocytosine and 5-FC.

## Description

Flucytosine (floo-SYE-toe-seen) belongs to the group of medicines called antifungals. It is used to treat certain fungus infections.

Flucytosine is available only with your doctor's prescription, in the following dosage form:
*Oral*
• Capsules (U.S. and Canada)

## Before Using This Medicine

In deciding to use a medicine, the risks of taking the medicine must be weighed against the good it will do. This is a decision you and your doctor will make. For flucytosine, the following should be considered:

**Allergies**—Tell your doctor if you have ever had any unusual or allergic reaction to flucytosine. Also tell your health care professional if you are allergic to any other substances, such as foods, preservatives, or dyes.

**Pregnancy**—Flucytosine has not been reported to cause birth defects or other problems in humans. However, studies in rats have shown that flucytosine causes birth defects.

**Breast-feeding**—Flucytosine has not been reported to cause problems in nursing babies.

**Children**—Although there is no specific information comparing use of flucytosine in children with use in other age groups, this medicine is not expected to cause different side effects or problems in children than it does in adults.

**Older adults**—Many medicines have not been studied specifically in older people. Therefore, it may not be known whether they work exactly the same way they do in younger adults. Although there is no specific information comparing use of flucytosine in the elderly with use in other age groups, this medicine is not expected to cause different side effects or problems in older people than it does in younger adults.

**Other medicines**—Although certain medicines should not be used together at all, in other cases two different medicines may be used together even if an interaction might occur. In these cases, your doctor may want to change the dose, or other precautions may be necessary. When you are taking flucytosine, it is especially important that your health care professional knows if you are taking any of the following:
• Amphotericin B by injection (e.g., Fungizone) or
• Antineoplastics (cancer medicine) or

• Antithyroid agents (medicine for overactive thyroid) or
• Azathioprine (e.g., Imuran) or
• Chloramphenicol (e.g., Chloromycetin) or
• Colchicine or
• Cyclophosphamide (e.g., Cytoxan) or
• Ganciclovir (e.g., Cytovene) or
• Interferon (e.g., Intron A, Roferon-A) or
• Mercaptopurine (e.g., Purinethol) or
• Methotrexate (e.g., Mexate) or
• Plicamycin (e.g., Mithracin) or
• Zidovudine (e.g., AZT, Retrovir) or
• X-ray treatment—Use of flucytosine with any of these medicines may increase the chance for side effects of the blood

**Other medical problems**—The presence of other medical problems may affect the use of flucytosine. Make sure you tell your doctor if you have any other medical problems, especially:
• Blood disease—Flucytosine may cause blood problems
• Kidney disease—Patients with kidney disease may have an increased chance of side effects
• Liver disease—Flucytosine may cause liver side effects

## Proper Use of This Medicine

In some patients this medicine may cause nausea or vomiting. If you are taking more than 1 capsule for each dose, you may space them out over a period of 15 minutes to help lessen the nausea or vomiting. If this does not help or if you have any questions, check with your doctor.

To help clear up your infection completely, *keep taking this medicine for the full time of treatment,* even if you begin to feel better after a few days. *Do not miss any doses.*

**Dosing**—The dose of flucytosine will be different for different patients. *Follow your doctor's orders or the directions on the label.* The following information includes only the average doses of flucytosine. *If your dose is different, do not change it* unless your doctor tells you to do so.
• For *oral* dosage form (capsules):
—For fungus infections:
• Adults and children—Dose is based on body weight. The usual dose is 12.5 to 37.5 milligrams (mg) per kilogram (kg) (5.7 to 17 mg per pound) of body weight every six hours.

**Missed dose**—If you miss a dose of this medicine, take it as soon as possible. However, if it is almost time for your next dose, skip the missed dose and go back to your regular dosing schedule. Do not double doses.

**Storage**—To store this medicine:
• Keep out of the reach of children.
• Store away from heat and direct light.
• Do not store in the bathroom, near the kitchen sink, or in other damp places. Heat or moisture may cause the medicine to break down.

- Do not keep outdated medicine or medicine no longer needed. Be sure that any discarded medicine is out of the reach of children.

## Precautions While Using This Medicine

Your doctor should check your progress at regular visits to make sure that this medicine does not cause unwanted effects.

Flucytosine may cause blood problems. These problems may result in a greater chance of infection, slow healing, and bleeding of the gums. Therefore, you should be careful when using regular toothbrushes, dental floss, and toothpicks. Dental work, whenever possible, should be done before you begin taking this medicine or delayed until your blood counts have returned to normal. Check with your medical doctor or dentist if you have any questions about proper oral hygiene (mouth care) during treatment.

Flucytosine may cause your skin to be more sensitive to sunlight than it is normally. Exposure to sunlight, even for brief periods of time, may cause skin rash, itching, redness, or other discoloration of the skin, or a severe sunburn. When you begin taking this medicine:

- Stay out of direct sunlight, especially between the hours of 10:00 a.m. and 3:00 p.m., if possible.
- Wear protective clothing, including a hat. Also, wear sunglasses.
- Apply a sun block product that has a skin protection factor (SPF) of at least 15. Some patients may require a product with a higher SPF number, especially if they have a fair complexion. If you have any questions about this, check with your health care professional.
- Apply a sun block lipstick that has an SPF of at least 15 to protect your lips.
- Do not use a sunlamp or tanning bed or booth.

*If you have a severe reaction from the sun, check with your doctor.*

This medicine may also cause some people to become dizzy, lightheaded, drowsy, or less alert than they are normally. *Make sure you know how you react to this medicine before you drive, use machines, or do anything else that could be dangerous if you are dizzy or are not alert.* If these reactions are especially bothersome, check with your doctor.

## Side Effects of This Medicine

Along with its needed effects, a medicine may cause some unwanted effects. Although not all of these side effects may occur, if they do occur they may need medical attention.

*Check with your doctor immediately* if any of the following side effects occur:

*More common*

Skin rash, redness, or itching; sore throat and fever; unusual bleeding or bruising; unusual tiredness or weakness; yellow eyes or skin

*Less common*

Confusion; hallucinations (seeing, hearing, or feeling things that are not there); increased sensitivity of skin to sunlight

Other side effects may occur that usually do not need medical attention. These side effects may go away during treatment as your body adjusts to the medicine. However, check with your doctor if any of the following side effects continue or are bothersome:

*More common*

Abdominal pain; diarrhea; loss of appetite; nausea or vomiting

*Less common*

Dizziness or lightheadedness; drowsiness; headache

Other side effects not listed above may also occur in some patients. If you notice any other effects, check with your doctor.

Revised: 07/24/92
Interim revision: 03/17/94

# FLUDARABINE   Systemic

A commonly used brand name in the U.S. and Canada is Fludara.

## Description

Fludarabine (floo-DARE-a-been) belongs to the group of medicines called antimetabolites. It is used to treat chronic lymphocytic leukemia (CLL), a type of cancer.

Fludarabine interferes with the growth of cancer cells, which are eventually destroyed. Since the growth of normal body cells may also be affected by fludarabine, other effects will also occur. Some of these may be serious and must be reported to your doctor. Other effects may not be serious but may cause concern. Some effects may not occur for months or years after the medicine is used.

Before you begin treatment with fludarabine, you and your doctor should talk about the good this medicine will do as well as the risks of using it.

Fludarabine is to be administered only by or under the immediate supervision of your doctor. It is available in the following dosage form:

*Parenteral*

- Injection (U.S. and Canada)

## Before Using This Medicine

In deciding to use a medicine, the risks of taking the medicine must be weighed against the good it will do. This is a decision you and your doctor will make. For fludarabine, the following should be considered:

**Allergies**—Tell your doctor if you have ever had any unusual or allergic reaction to fludarabine.

**Pregnancy**—There is a chance that this medicine may cause birth defects if either the male or female is taking it at the time of conception or if it is taken during pregnancy. Fludarabine has been shown to cause birth defects in rats and rabbits. In addition, many cancer medicines may cause sterility which could be permanent. Although sterility has not been reported with this medicine, it does occur in animals and the possibility should be kept in mind.

Be sure that you have discussed this with your doctor before taking this medicine. It is best to use some kind of birth control while you are receiving fludarabine. Tell your doctor right away if you think you have become pregnant while receiving fludarabine.

**Breast-feeding**—It is not known whether fludarabine passes into breast milk. However, because this medicine may cause serious side effects, breast-feeding is generally not recommended while you are receiving it.

**Children**—There is no specific information comparing use of fludarabine in children with use in other age groups.

**Older adults**—Many medicines have not been studied specifically in older people. Therefore, it may not be known whether they work exactly the same way they do in younger adults. Although there is no specific information comparing use of fludarabine in the elderly with use in other age groups, it is not expected to cause different side effects or problems in older people than it does in younger adults.

**Other medicines**—Although certain medicines should not be used together at all, in other cases two different medicines may be used together even if an interaction might occur. In these cases, your doctor may want to change the dose, or other precautions may be necessary. When receiving fludarabine it is especially important that your health care professional know if you are taking any of the following:

- Amphotericin B by injection (e.g., Fungizone) or
- Antithyroid agents (medicine for overactive thyroid) or
- Azathioprine (e.g., Imuran) or
- Chloramphenicol (e.g., Chloromycetin) or
- Colchicine or
- Flucytosine (e.g., Ancobon) or
- Ganciclovir (e.g., Cytovene) or
- Interferon (e.g., Intron A, Roferon-A) or
- Plicamycin (e.g., Mithracin) or
- Zidovudine (e.g., AZT, Retrovir) or
- If you have ever been treated with radiation or cancer medicines—Fludarabine may increase the effects of these medicines or radiation therapy on the blood

- Probenecid (e.g., Benemid) or
- Sulfinpyrazone (e.g., Anturane)—Fludarabine may raise the amount of uric acid in the blood. Since these medicines are used to lower uric acid levels, they may not be as effective in patients receiving fludarabine

**Other medical problems**—The presence of other medical problems may affect the use of fludarabine. Make sure you tell your doctor if you have any other medical problems, especially:

- Chickenpox (including recent exposure) or
- Herpes zoster (shingles)—Risk of severe disease affecting other parts of the body
- Gout (history of) or
- Kidney stones (history of)—Fludarabine may increase levels of uric acid in the body, which can cause gout or kidney stones
- Infection—Fludarabine may decrease your body's ability to fight infection
- Kidney disease—Effects of fludarabine may be increased because of slower removal from the body

## Proper Use of This Medicine

This medicine may cause nausea and vomiting. However, it is very important that you continue to receive the medicine even if you begin to feel ill. Ask your health care professional for ways to lessen these effects.

**Dosing**—The dose of fludarabine will be different for different patients. The dose that is used may depend on a number of things, including what the medicine is being used for, the patient's size, and whether or not other medicines are also being taken. *If you are receiving fludarabine at home, follow your doctor's orders or the directions on the label.* If you have any questions about the proper dose of fludarabine, ask your doctor.

## Precautions While Using This Medicine

*It is very important that your doctor check your progress at regular visits* to make sure that this medicine is working properly and to check for unwanted effects.

While you are being treated with fludarabine, and after you stop treatment with it, *do not have any immunizations (vaccinations) without your doctor's approval*. Fludarabine may lower your body's resistance and there is a chance you might get the infection the immunization is meant to prevent. In addition, other persons living in your household should not take oral polio vaccine since there is a chance they could pass the polio virus on to you. Also, avoid persons who have recently taken oral polio vaccine. Do not get close to them and do not stay in the same room with them for very long. If you cannot take these precautions, you should consider wearing a protective face mask that covers the nose and mouth.

Fludarabine can temporarily lower the number of white blood cells in your blood, increasing the chance of getting an infection. It can also lower the number of platelets, which are necessary for proper blood clotting. If this occurs, there are certain precautions you can take, especially when your blood count is low, to reduce the risk of infection or bleeding:

- If you can, avoid people with infections. *Check with your doctor immediately* if you think you are getting an infection or if you get a fever or chills, cough or hoarseness, lower back or side pain, or painful or difficult urination.
- *Check with your doctor immediately* if you notice any unusual bleeding or bruising; black, tarry stools; blood in urine or stools; or pinpoint red spots on your skin.
- Be careful when using a regular toothbrush, dental floss, or toothpick. Your medical doctor, dentist, or nurse may recommend other ways to clean your teeth and gums. Check with your medical doctor before having any dental work done.
- Do not touch your eyes or the inside of your nose unless you have just washed your hands and have not touched anything else in the meantime.
- Be careful not to cut yourself when you are using sharp objects such as a safety razor or fingernail or toenail cutters.
- Avoid contact sports or other situations where bruising or injury could occur.

## Side Effects of This Medicine

Along with its needed effects, a medicine may cause some unwanted effects. Although not all of these side effects may occur, if they do occur they may need medical attention.

Also, because of the way cancer medicines act on the body, there is a chance that they might cause other unwanted effects that may not occur until months or years after the medicine is used. These delayed effects may include certain types of cancer. Discuss these possible effects with your doctor.

*Check with your doctor or nurse immediately* if any of the following side effects occur:

*More common*

Cough or hoarseness; fever or chills; lower back or side pain; painful or difficult urination; shortness of breath

*Less common*

Black, tarry stools; blood in urine; pinpoint red spots on skin; unusual bleeding or bruising

Check with your health care professional as soon as possible if any of the following side effects occur:

*More common*

Pain

*Less common*

Agitation or confusion; blurred vision; loss of hearing; numbness or tingling in fingers, toes, or face; sores in mouth and on lips; swelling of feet or lower legs; unusual tiredness or weakness

Other side effects may occur that usually do not need medical attention. These side effects may go away during treatment as your body adjusts to the medicine. Also, your health care professional may be able to tell you about ways to prevent or reduce some of these side effects. Check with your health care professional if any of the following side effects continue or are bothersome or if you have any questions about them:

*More common*

Diarrhea; nausea or vomiting; skin rash

*Less common*

Aching muscles; general feeling of discomfort or illness; headache; loss of appetite

This medicine may rarely cause a temporary loss of hair in some people. After treatment with fludarabine has ended, normal hair growth should return.

After you stop treatment with fludarabine, it may still produce some side effects that need attention. During this period of time, check with your doctor if you notice the following:

*Rare*

Cough or hoarseness; fever or chills; loss of vision; lower back or side pain; painful or difficult urination

Other side effects not listed above may also occur in some patients. If you notice any other effects, check with your doctor.

Revised: 08/02/94

# FLUDROCORTISONE   Systemic

A commonly used brand name in the U.S. and Canada is Florinef.

## Description

Fludrocortisone (floo-droe-KOR-tis-sone) is a corticosteroid (kor-ti-koe-STE-roid) (cortisone-like medicine). It belongs to the family of medicines called steroids. Your body naturally produces similar corticosteroids, which are necessary to maintain the balance of certain minerals and water for good health. If your body does not produce enough corticosteroids, your doctor may have prescribed this medicine to help make up the difference.

Fludrocortisone may also be used to treat other medical conditions as determined by your doctor.

Fludrocortisone is available only with your doctor's prescription, in the following dosage form:

*Oral*
- Tablets (U.S. and Canada)

## Before Using This Medicine

In deciding to use a medicine, the risks of taking the medicine must be weighed against the good it will do. This is a decision you and your doctor will make. For fludrocortisone, the following should be considered:

**Allergies**—Tell your doctor if you have ever had any unusual or allergic reaction to fludrocortisone. Also tell your health care professional if you are allergic to any other substances, such as foods, preservatives, or dyes.

**Diet**—Your doctor may want you to control the amount of sodium in your diet. When fludrocortisone is used to treat certain types of kidney diseases, too much sodium may cause high blood sodium, high blood pressure, and excess body water.

**Pregnancy**—Studies on birth defects in humans or animals have not been done with fludrocortisone. However, it is possible that too much use of this medicine during pregnancy may cause the baby to have an underactive adrenal gland after birth.

**Breast-feeding**—Fludrocortisone passes into the breast milk and may cause problems with growth or other unwanted effects in the nursing baby.

**Children**—Fludrocortisone may slow or stop growth in children or growing adolescents when used for a long time. The natural production of corticosteroids by the body may also be decreased by the use of this medicine. Before this medicine is given to a child or adolescent, you and your child's doctor should talk about the good this medicine will do as well as the risks of using it. Follow the doctor's directions very carefully to lessen the chance that these unwanted effects will occur.

**Older adults**—Many medicines have not been studied specifically in older people. Therefore, it may not be known whether they work exactly the same way they do in younger adults or if they cause different side effects or problems in older people. There is no specific information comparing the use of fludrocortisone in the elderly with its use in other age groups.

**Other medicines**—Although certain medicines should not be used together at all, in other cases two different medicines may be used together even if an interaction might occur. In these cases, your doctor may want to change the dose, or other precautions may be necessary. When you are taking fludrocortisone, it is especially important that your health care professional know if you are taking any of the following:
- Acetazolamide (e.g., Diamox) or
- Amphotericin B by injection (e.g., Fungizone) or
- Azlocillin (e.g., Azlin) or
- Capreomycin (e.g., Capastat) or
- Carbenicillin by injection (e.g., Geopen) or
- Corticotropin (ACTH) or

- Dichlorphenamide (e.g., Daranide) or
- Diuretics (water pills) or
- Insulin or
- Laxatives (with overdose or chronic misuse) or
- Methazolamide (e.g., Neptazane) or
- Mezlocillin (e.g., Mezlin) or
- Piperacillin (e.g., Pipracil) or
- Salicylates or
- Sodium bicarbonate (e.g., baking soda) or
- Ticarcillin (e.g., Ticar) or
- Ticarcillin and clavulanate (e.g., Timentin) or
- Vitamin $B_{12}$ (e.g., AlphaRedisol, Rubramin-PC) (when used in megaloblastic anemia) or
- Vitamin D—Fludrocortisone and these medicines decrease the amount of potassium in the blood, which may increase the chance of severe low blood potassium
- Alcohol—Alcohol and fludrocortisone decrease the amount of potassium in the blood, which may increase the chance of severe low blood potassium; alcohol may also make fludrocortisone less effective by causing the body to get rid of it faster
- Barbiturates or
- Carbamazepine (e.g., Tegretol) or
- Griseofulvin (e.g., Fulvicin) or
- Phenylbutazone (e.g., Butazolidin) or
- Phenytoin (e.g., Dilantin) or
- Primidone (e.g., Mysoline) or
- Rifampin (e.g., Rifadin)—Using these medicines may make fludrocortisone less effective because they cause the body to get rid of it faster
- Digitalis glycosides (heart medicine)—Fludrocortisone decreases the amount of potassium in the blood, which may increase the chance of irregular heartbeat
- Other corticosteroids (cortisone-like medicine)—Using any corticosteroid medicine with fludrocortisone will cause the body to get rid of both medicines faster. This may make either or both medicines less effective. Also, fludrocortisone and other corticosteroids decrease the amount of potassium in the blood, which may increase the chance of severe low blood potassium
- Sodium-containing medicine—When using fludrocortisone to treat certain types of kidney diseases, too much sodium may cause high blood sodium, high blood pressure, and excess body water

**Other medical problems**—The presence of other medical problems may affect the use of fludrocortisone. Make sure you tell your doctor if you have any other medical problems, especially:
- Bone disease—Fludrocortisone may make bone disease worse because it causes more calcium to pass into the urine
- Edema (swelling of feet or lower legs) or
- Heart disease or
- High blood pressure or
- Kidney disease—Fludrocortisone causes the body to retain (keep) more salt and water. These conditions may be made worse by this extra body water
- Liver disease or
- Thyroid disease—The body may not get fludrocortisone out of the bloodstream at the usual rate, which may increase the effect of fludrocortisone or cause more side effects

## Proper Use of This Medicine

*Take this medicine only as directed by your doctor.* Do not take more or less of it, do not take it more often, and do not take it for a longer time than your doctor ordered. To do so may increase the chance of side effects.

**Dosing**—The dose of fludrocortisone will be different for different patients. *Follow your doctor's orders or the directions on the label.* The following information includes only the average doses of fludrocortisone. *If your dose is different, do not change it* unless your doctor tells you to do so.

- For *oral* dosage forms (tablets):
  —Adults
  - For adrenal gland deficiency: 50 to 200 micrograms a day.
  - For adrenogenital syndrome: 100 to 200 micrograms a day.
  —Children: For adrenal gland deficiency: 50 to 100 micrograms a day.

**Missed dose**—If you miss a dose of this medicine, take it as soon as you remember. However, if it is almost time for your next dose, skip the missed dose and go back to your regular dosing schedule. Do not double doses.

**Storage**—To store this medicine:
- Keep out of the reach of children.
- Store away from heat and direct light.
- Do not store in the bathroom, near the kitchen sink, or in other damp places. Heat or moisture may cause the medicine to break down.
- Do not keep outdated medicine or medicine no longer needed. Be sure that any discarded medicine is out of the reach of children.

## Precautions While Using This Medicine

*Your doctor should check your progress at regular visits* to make sure this medicine does not cause unwanted effects.

If you will be using this medicine for a long time, your doctor may want you to carry a medical identification card stating that you are using this medicine.

While you are taking fludrocortisone, be careful to limit the amount of alcohol you drink.

## Side Effects of This Medicine

Along with its needed effects, a medicine may cause some unwanted effects. Although not all of these side effects may occur, if they do occur they may need medical attention.

*Check with your doctor immediately* if any of the following side effects occur:

*Less common or rare*
  Cough; difficulty swallowing; hives; irregular breathing or shortness of breath; irregular heartbeat; redness and itching of skin; redness of eyes; swelling of nasal passages, face, or eyelids; swollen neck veins; unusual tiredness or weakness

Check with your doctor as soon as possible if any of the following side effects occur:

*Less common or rare*
  Dizziness; headache (severe or continuing); loss of appetite; muscle cramps or pain; nausea; swelling of feet or lower legs; weakness in arms, legs, or trunk (severe); weight gain (rapid); vomiting

Other side effects not listed above may also occur in some patients. If you notice any other effects, check with your doctor.

## Additional Information

Once a medicine has been approved for marketing for a certain use, experience may show that it is also useful for other medical problems. Although these uses are not included in product labeling, fludrocortisone is used in certain patients with the following medical conditions:

- Idiopathic orthostatic hypotension (a certain type of low blood pressure)
- Too much acid in the blood, caused by kidney disease

Other than the above information, there is no additional information relating to proper use, precautions, or side effects for these uses.

Revised: 06/15/93

# FLUOROQUINOLONES   Systemic

Some commonly used brand names are:

**In the U.S.—**
| | |
|---|---|
| Cipro[1] | Maxaquin[3] |
| Cipro IV[1] | Noroxin[4] |
| Floxin[5] | Penetrex[2] |
| Floxin IV[5] | |

**In Canada—**
| | |
|---|---|
| Cipro[1] | Maxaquin[3] |
| Floxin[5] | Penetrex[2] |

Note: For quick reference, the following fluoroquinolones are numbered to match the corresponding brand names.

This information applies to the following medicines:
1. Ciprofloxacin (sip-roe-FLOX-a-sin)
2. Enoxacin (en-OX-a-sin)
3. Lomefloxacin (loe-me-FLOX-a-sin)
4. Norfloxacin (nor-FLOX-a-sin)
5. Ofloxacin (oe-FLOX-a-sin)

## Description

Fluoroquinolones (flu-roe-KWIN-a-lones) are used to treat bacterial infections in many different parts of the body. They work by killing bacteria or preventing their growth. However, these medicines will not work for colds, flu, or other virus infections. Fluoroquinolones may be used for other problems as determined by your doctor.

Fluoroquinolones are available only with your doctor's prescription, in the following dosage forms:

*Oral*

Ciprofloxacin
  • Tablets (U.S. and Canada)
Enoxacin
  • Tablets (U.S. and Canada)
Lomefloxacin
  • Tablets (U.S. and Canada)
Norfloxacin
  • Tablets (U.S. and Canada)
Ofloxacin
  • Tablets (U.S. and Canada)

*Parenteral*

Ciprofloxacin
  • Injection (U.S. and Canada)
Ofloxacin
  • Injection (U.S.)

## Before Using This Medicine

In deciding to use a medicine, the risks of taking the medicine must be weighed against the good it will do. This is a decision you and your doctor will make. For the fluoroquinolones, the following should be considered:

**Allergies**—Tell your doctor if you have ever had any unusual or allergic reaction to any of the fluoroquinolones or to any related medicines such as cinoxacin (e.g., Cinobac) or nalidixic acid (e.g., NegGram). Also tell your health care professional if you are allergic to any other substances, such as foods, preservatives, or dyes.

**Pregnancy**—Studies have not been done in humans. However, use is not recommended during pregnancy since fluoroquinolones have been reported to cause bone development problems in young animals.

**Breast-feeding**—Some of the fluoroquinolones are known to pass into human breast milk. Since fluoroquinolones have been reported to cause bone development problems in young animals, breast-feeding is not recommended during treatment with these medicines.

**Children**—Use is not recommended for infants or children since fluoroquinolones have been shown to cause bone development problems in young animals. However, your doctor may choose to use one of these medicines if other medicines cannot be used.

**Teenagers**—Use is not recommended for teenagers up to 18 years of age since fluoroquinolones have been shown to cause bone development problems in young animals. However, your doctor may choose to use one of these medicines if other medicines cannot be used.

**Older adults**—These medicines have been tested and, in effective doses, have not been shown to cause different side effects or problems in older people than they do in younger adults.

**Other medicines**—Although certain medicines should not be used together at all, in other cases two different medicines may be used together even if an interaction might occur. In these cases, your doctor may want to change the dose, or other precautions may be necessary. When you are taking a fluoroquinolone, it is especially important that your health care professional know if you are taking any of the following:

  • Aminophylline or
  • Oxtriphylline (e.g., Choledyl) or
  • Theophylline (e.g., Somophyllin-T, Theodur, Elixophyllin)—Enoxacin, ciprofloxacin, and norfloxacin may increase the chance of side effects of aminophylline, oxtriphylline, or theophylline
  • Antacids, aluminum-, calcium-, or magnesium-containing, or
  • Iron supplements or
  • Sucralfate—Antacids, iron, or sucralfate may keep any of the fluoroquinolones from working properly
  • Caffeine—Enoxacin, ciprofloxacin, and norfloxacin may increase the chance of side effects of caffeine
  • Didanosine (e.g., Videx, ddI)—Didanosine may keep any of the fluoroquinolones from working properly
  • Warfarin (e.g., Coumadin)—Enoxacin, ciprofloxacin, and norfloxacin may increase the effect of warfarin, increasing the chance of bleeding

**Other medical problems**—The presence of other medical problems may affect the use of fluoroquinolones. Make sure you tell your doctor if you have any other medical problems, especially:

  • Brain or spinal cord disease, including hardening of the arteries in the brain or epilepsy or other seizures—Fluoroquinolones may cause nervous system side effects
  • Kidney disease or
  • Kidney disease and liver disease—Patients with kidney disease (alone) or kidney disease and liver disease (together) may have an increased chance of side effects

## Proper Use of This Medicine

*Do not take fluoroquinolones if you are pregnant. Do not give fluoroquinolones to infants, children, or teenagers* unless otherwise directed by your doctor. These medicines have been shown to cause bone development problems in young animals.

*Fluoroquinolones are best taken with a full glass (8 ounces) of water. Several additional glasses of water should be taken every day,* unless you are otherwise directed by your doctor. Drinking extra water will help to prevent some unwanted effects of ciprofloxacin and norfloxacin.

Ciprofloxacin and lomefloxacin may be taken with meals or on an empty stomach.

Enoxacin, norfloxacin, and ofloxacin should be taken on an empty stomach.

To help clear up your infection completely, *keep taking your medicine for the full time of treatment,* even if you begin to feel better after a few days. If you stop taking this medicine too soon, your symptoms may return.

This medicine works best when there is a constant amount in the blood or urine. *To help keep the amount constant, do not miss any doses. Also, it is best to take the doses at evenly spaced times, day and night.* For example, if you are to take 2 doses a day, the doses should be spaced about 12 hours apart. If this interferes with your sleep or other daily activities, or if you need help in planning the best times to take your medicine, check with your health care professional.

**Dosing**—The dose of fluoroquinolones will be different for different patients. *Follow your doctor's orders or the directions on the label.* The following information includes only the average doses of fluoroquinolones. Your dose may be different if you have kidney disease. *If your dose is different, do not change it* unless your doctor tells you to do so.

The number of tablets that you take depends on the strength of the medicine. Also, *the number of doses you take each day, the time allowed between doses, and the length of time you take the medicine depend on the medical problem for which you are using a fluoroquinolone.*

*For ciprofloxacin*
- For *oral* dosage form (tablets):
  —Adults: 250 to 750 milligrams (mg) every twelve hours for five to fourteen days, depending on the medical problem being treated.
  —Children up to 18 years of age: This medicine is not recommended in infants, children, or teenagers.
- For *injection* dosage form:
  —Adults: 200 to 400 mg every twelve hours.
  —Children up to 18 years of age: This medicine is not recommended in infants, children, or teenagers.

*For enoxacin*
- For *oral* dosage form (tablets):
  —Adults: 200 to 400 mg every twelve hours for seven to fourteen days, depending on the medical problem being treated. Gonorrhea is usually treated with a single, oral dose of 400 mg.
  —Children up to 18 years of age: This medicine is not recommended in infants, children, or teenagers.

*For lomefloxacin*
- For *oral* dosage form (tablets):
  —Adults: 400 mg once a day for ten to fourteen days, depending on the medical problem being treated.
  —Children up to 18 years of age: This medicine is not recommended in infants, children, or teenagers.

*For norfloxacin*
- For *oral* dosage form (tablets):
  —Adults: 400 mg every twelve hours for three to twenty-one days, depending on the medical problem

being treated. Gonorrhea is usually treated with a single, oral dose of 800 mg.
  —Children up to 18 years of age: This medicine is not recommended in infants, children, or teenagers.

*For ofloxacin*
- For *oral* dosage form (tablets):
  —Adults: 200 to 400 mg every twelve hours for three to ten days, depending on the medical problem being treated. Gonorrhea is usually treated with a single, oral dose of 400 mg.
  —Children up to 18 years of age: This medicine is not recommended in infants, children, or teenagers.
- For *injection* dosage form:
  —Adults: 200 to 400 mg every twelve hours for three to ten days, depending on the medical problem being treated. Gonorrhea is usually treated with a single, oral dose of 400 mg.
  —Children up to 18 years of age: This medicine is not recommended in infants, children, or teenagers.

**Missed dose**—If you miss a dose of this medicine, take it as soon as possible. This will help to keep a constant amount of medicine in the blood or urine. However, if it is almost time for your next dose, skip the missed dose and go back to your regular dosing schedule. Do not double doses.

**Storage**—To store this medicine:
- Keep out of the reach of children.
- Store away from heat and direct light.
- Do not store in the bathroom, near the kitchen sink, or in other damp places. Heat or moisture may cause the medicine to break down.
- Do not keep outdated medicine or medicine no longer needed. Be sure that any discarded medicine is out of the reach of children.

## Precautions While Using This Medicine

If your symptoms do not improve within a few days, or if they become worse, check with your doctor.

*If you are taking aluminum- or magnesium-containing antacids, or sucralfate do not take them at the same time that you take this medicine.* It is best to take these medicines at least 2 hours before or 2 hours after taking norfloxacin or ofloxacin, at least 4 hours before or 2 hours after taking ciprofloxacin or lomefloxacin, and at least 8 hours before or 2 hours after taking enoxacin. These medicines may keep fluoroquinolones from working properly.

Some people who take fluoroquinolones may become more sensitive to sunlight than they are normally. Exposure to sunlight, even for brief periods of time, may cause severe sunburn; skin rash, redness, itching, or discoloration; or vision changes. When you begin taking this medicine:
- Stay out of direct sunlight, especially between the hours of 10:00 a.m. and 3:00 p.m., if possible.
- Wear protective clothing, including a hat and sunglasses.

- Apply a sun block product that has a skin protection factor (SPF) of at least 15. Some patients may require a product with a higher SPF number, especially if they have a fair complexion. If you have any questions about this, check with your health care professional.
- Do not use a sunlamp or tanning bed or booth.

*If you have a severe reaction from the sun, check with your doctor.*

Fluoroquinolones may also cause some people to become dizzy, lightheaded, drowsy, or less alert than they are normally. *Make sure you know how you react to this medicine before you drive, use machines, or do anything else that could be dangerous if you are dizzy or are not alert.* If these reactions are especially bothersome, check with your doctor.

---

## Side Effects of This Medicine

Along with its needed effects, a medicine may cause some unwanted effects. Although not all of these side effects may occur, if they do occur they may need medical attention.

*Check with your doctor immediately* if any of the following side effects occur:

*Rare*

Agitation; confusion; fever; hallucinations (seeing, hearing, or feeling things that are not there); pain at site of injection; peeling of the skin; shakiness or tremors; shortness of breath; skin rash, itching, or redness; swelling of face or neck

Other side effects may occur that usually do not need medical attention. These side effects may go away during treatment as your body adjusts to the medicine. However, check with your doctor if any of the following side effects continue or are bothersome:

*More common*

Abdominal or stomach pain or discomfort; diarrhea; dizziness; drowsiness; headache; lightheadedness; nausea or vomiting; nervousness; trouble in sleeping

*Less frequent or rare*

Increased sensitivity of skin to sunlight

Other side effects not listed above may also occur in some patients. If you notice any other effects, check with your doctor.

---

Revised: 05/20/93

---

# FLUOROURACIL   Systemic

A commonly used brand name in the U.S. and Canada is Adrucil. Generic name product may also be available in the U.S. and Canada. Another commonly used name is 5-FU.

---

## Description

Fluorouracil (flure-oh-YOOR-a-sill) belongs to the group of medicines known as antimetabolites. It is used to treat some kinds of cancer.

Fluorouracil interferes with the growth of cancer cells, which are eventually destroyed. Since the growth of normal body cells may also be affected by fluorouracil, other effects will also occur. Some of these may be serious and must be reported to your doctor. Other effects, like hair loss, may not be serious but may cause concern. Some effects may not occur for months or years after the medicine is used.

Before you begin treatment with fluorouracil, you and your doctor should talk about the good this medicine will do as well as the risks of using it.

Fluorouracil is to be administered only by or under the immediate supervision of your doctor. It is available in the following dosage form:

*Parenteral*

- Injection (U.S. and Canada)

## Before Using This Medicine

In deciding to use a medicine, the risks of taking the medicine must be weighed against the good it will do. This is a decision you and your doctor will make. For fluorouracil, the following should be considered:

**Allergies**—Tell your doctor if you have ever had any unusual or allergic reaction to fluorouracil.

**Pregnancy**—Tell your doctor if you are pregnant or if you intend to have children. There is a chance that this medicine may cause birth defects if either the male or female is receiving it at the time of conception or if it is taken during pregnancy. Fluorouracil has been reported to cause birth defects in mice given doses slightly higher than the human dose. Also, there has been one case of a baby born with several birth defects after the mother received fluorouracil. In addition, many cancer medicines may cause sterility. Although sterility has been reported with this medicine, it is usually only temporary; the possibility should be kept in mind.

Be sure that you have discussed this with your doctor before receiving this medicine. It is best to use some kind of birth control while you are receiving fluorouracil. Tell your doctor right away if you think you have become pregnant while receiving fluorouracil.

**Breast-feeding**—Tell your doctor if you are breast-feeding or if you intend to breast-feed during treatment with this medicine. It is not known whether fluorouracil passes into breast milk. However, because fluorouracil may cause serious side effects, breast-feeding is generally not recommended while you are receiving it.

**Children**—Although there is no specific information comparing use of fluorouracil in children with use in other age groups, it is not expected to cause different side effects or problems in children than it does in adults.

**Older adults**—Many medicines have not been studied specifically in older people. Therefore, it may not be known whether they work exactly the same way they do in younger adults. Although there is no specific information comparing use of fluorouracil in the elderly with use in other age groups, it is not expected to cause different side effects or problems in older people than it does in younger adults.

**Other medicines**—Although certain medicines should not be used together at all, in other cases two different medicines may be used together even if an interaction might occur. In these cases, your doctor may want to change the dose, or other precautions may be necessary. When you are receiving fluorouracil, it is especially important that your health care professional know if you are taking any of the following:

- Amphotericin B by injection (e.g., Fungizone) or
- Antithyroid agents (medicine for overactive thyroid) or
- Azathioprine (e.g., Imuran) or
- Chloramphenicol (e.g., Chloromycetin) or
- Colchicine or
- Flucytosine (e.g., Ancobon) or
- Ganciclovir (e.g., Cytovene) or
- Interferon (e.g., Intron A, Roferon-A) or
- Plicamycin (e.g., Mithracin) or
- Zidovudine (e.g., AZT, Retrovir) or
- If you have ever been treated with radiation or cancer medicines—Fluorouracil may increase the effects of these medicines or radiation on the blood

**Other medical problems**—The presence of other medical problems may affect the use of fluorouracil. Make sure you tell your doctor if you have any other medical problems, especially:

- Chickenpox (including recent exposure) or
- Herpes zoster (shingles)—Risk of severe disease affecting other parts of the body
- Infection—Fluorouracil can decrease your body's ability to fight infection
- Kidney disease or
- Liver disease—Effects of fluorouracil may be increased because of slower removal from the body

## Proper Use of This Medicine

This medicine is sometimes given together with certain other medicines. If you are using a combination of medicines, it is important that you receive each one at the proper time. If you are taking some of these medicines by mouth, ask your health care professional to help you plan a way to remember to take them at the right times.

Fluorouracil often causes nausea and vomiting. However, it is very important that you continue to receive the medicine, even if your stomach is upset. Ask your health care professional for ways to lessen these effects.

**Dosing**—The dosing of fluorouracil will be different for different patients. The dose that is used may depend on a number of things, including what the medicine is being used for, the patient's weight, and whether or not other medicines are also being taken. *If you are receiving fluorouracil at home, follow your doctor's orders or the directions on the label.* If you have any questions about the proper dose of fluorouracil, ask your doctor.

## Precautions While Using This Medicine

*It is very important that your doctor check your progress at regular visits* to make sure that this medicine is working properly and to check for unwanted effects.

While you are being treated with fluorouracil, and after you stop treatment with it, *do not have any immunizations (vaccinations) without your doctor's approval.* Fluorouracil may lower your body's resistance and there is a chance you might get the infection the immunization is meant to prevent. In addition, other persons living in your household should not take oral polio vaccine since there is a chance they could pass the polio virus on to you. Also, avoid persons who have recently taken oral polio vaccine. Do not get close to them and do not stay in the same room with them for very long. If you cannot take these precautions, you should consider wearing a protective face mask that covers the nose and mouth.

Fluorouracil can temporarily lower the number of white blood cells in your blood, increasing the chance of getting an infection. It can also lower the number of platelets, which are necessary for proper blood clotting. If this occurs, there are certain precautions you can take, especially when your blood count is low, to reduce the risk of infection or bleeding:

- If you can, avoid people with infections. *Check with your doctor immediately* if you think you are getting an infection or if you get a fever or chills, cough or hoarseness, lower back or side pain, or painful or difficult urination.
- *Check with your doctor immediately* if you notice any unusual bleeding or bruising; black, tarry stools; blood in urine or stools; or pinpoint red spots on your skin.
- Be careful when using a regular toothbrush, dental floss, or toothpick. Your medical doctor, dentist, or nurse may recommend other ways to clean your teeth and gums. Check with your medical doctor before having any dental work done.
- Do not touch your eyes or the inside of your nose unless you have just washed your hands and have not touched anything else in the meantime.
- Be careful not to cut yourself when you are using sharp objects such as a safety razor or fingernail or toenail cutters.

- Avoid contact sports or other situations where bruising or injury could occur.

## Side Effects of This Medicine

Along with its needed effects, a medicine may cause some unwanted effects. Although not all of these side effects may occur, if they do occur they may need medical attention.

Also, because of the way these medicines act on the body, there is a chance that they might cause other unwanted effects that may not occur until months or years after the medicine is used. These delayed effects may include certain types of cancer, such as leukemia. Discuss these possible effects with your doctor.

*Check with your doctor or nurse immediately* if any of the following side effects occur:

*More common*
Diarrhea; heartburn; sores in mouth and on lips

*Less common*
Black, tarry stools; cough or hoarseness; fever or chills; lower back or side pain; nausea and vomiting (severe); painful or difficult urination; stomach cramps

*Rare*
Blood in urine or stools; pinpoint red spots on skin; unusual bleeding or bruising

Check with your health care professional as soon as possible if any of the following side effects occur:

*Rare*
Chest pain; shortness of breath; tingling of hands and feet, followed by pain, redness, and swelling; trouble with balance

Other side effects may occur that usually do not need medical attention. These side effects may go away during treatment as your body adjusts to the medicine. Also, your health care professional may be able to tell you about ways to prevent or reduce some of these side effects. Check with your health care professional if any of the following side effects continue or are bothersome or if you have any questions about them:

*More common*
Loss of appetite; nausea and vomiting; skin rash and itching; weakness

*Less common*
Dry or cracked skin

This medicine often causes a temporary loss of hair. After treatment with fluorouracil has ended, normal hair growth should return.

After you stop receiving fluorouracil, it may still produce some side effects that need attention. During this period of time, *check with your doctor or nurse immediately* if you notice any of the following:

Black, tarry stools; blood in urine or stools; cough or hoarseness; fever or chills; lower back or side pain; painful or difficult urination; pinpoint red spots on skin; unusual bleeding or bruising

Other side effects not listed above may also occur in some patients. If you notice any other effects, check with your health care professional.

Revised: 07/26/94

# FLUOROURACIL Topical

Some commonly used brand names are:
**In the U.S.—**
Efudex
Fluoroplex
**In Canada—**
Efudex
Fluoroplex
Another commonly used name is 5-FU.

## Description

Fluorouracil (flure-oh-YOOR-a-sill) belongs to the group of medicines known as antimetabolites. When applied to the skin, it is used to treat certain skin problems, including cancer or conditions that could become cancerous if not treated.

Fluorouracil interferes with the growth of abnormal cells, which are eventually destroyed.

Fluorouracil is available only with your doctor's prescription, in the following dosage forms:
*Topical*
- Cream (U.S. and Canada)
- Topical solution (U.S. and Canada)

## Before Using This Medicine

In deciding to use a medicine, the risks of using the medicine must be weighed against the good it will do. This is a decision you and your doctor will make. For topical fluorouracil, the following should be considered:

**Allergies**—Tell your doctor if you have ever had any unusual or allergic reaction to fluorouracil.

**Pregnancy**—Tell your doctor if you are pregnant or if you intend to become pregnant. Although fluorouracil applied to the skin has not been shown to cause problems in humans, some of it is absorbed through the skin and there is a chance that it could cause birth defects. Be sure that you have discussed this with your doctor before using this medicine.

**Breast-feeding**—Although fluorouracil applied to the skin has not been shown to cause problems in nursing babies, some of it is absorbed through the skin.

**Children**—There is no specific information comparing use of fluorouracil on the skin in children with use in other age groups.

**Older adults**—Many medicines have not been studied specifically in older people. Therefore, it may not be known whether they work exactly the same way they do in younger adults or if they cause different side effects or problems in older people. Although there is no specific information comparing use of fluorouracil on the skin in the elderly with use in other age groups, this medicine is not expected to cause different side effects or problems in older people than it does in younger adults.

**Other medical problems**—The presence of other medical problems may affect the use of fluorouracil on the skin. Make sure you tell your doctor if you have any other medical problems, especially:

- Other skin problems—May be aggravated

## Proper Use of This Medicine

Keep using this medicine for the full time of treatment. However, *do not use this medicine more often or for a longer time than your doctor ordered.* Apply enough medicine each time to cover the entire affected area with a thin layer.

After washing the area with soap and water and drying carefully, use a cotton-tipped applicator or your fingertips to apply the medicine in a thin layer to your skin.

If you apply this medicine with your fingertips, make sure you *wash your hands immediately afterwards,* to prevent any of the medicine from accidentally getting in your eyes or mouth.

Fluorouracil may cause redness, soreness, scaling, and peeling of affected skin after 1 or 2 weeks of use. This effect may last for several weeks after you stop using the medicine and is to be expected. Sometimes a pink, smooth area is left when the skin treated with this medicine heals. This area will usually fade after 1 to 2 months. Do not stop using this medicine without first checking with your doctor. If the reaction is very uncomfortable, check with your doctor.

**Dosing**—The dose of fluorouracil will be different for different patients. *Follow your doctor's orders or the directions on the label.* The following information includes only the average doses of fluorouracil. *If your dose is different, do not change it* unless your doctor tells you to do so.

- For *cream* dosage form:
  —For precancerous skin condition caused by the sun:
    - Adults—Use the 1% cream on the affected areas of skin one or two times a day. The 5% cream is sometimes used on the hands.

- Children—Use and dose must be determined by your doctor.
  —For skin cancer:
    - Adults—Use the 5% cream on the affected areas of skin two times a day. Treatment may continue for several weeks.
    - Children—Use and dose must be determined by your doctor.

- For *topical solution* dosage form:
  —For precancerous skin condition caused by the sun:
    - Adults—Use the 1% solution on the affected areas of skin one or two times a day. The 2% or 5% solution is sometimes used on the hands.
    - Children—Use and dose must be determined by your doctor.
  —For skin cancer:
    - Adults—Use the 5% solution on the affected areas of skin two times a day. Treatment may continue for several weeks.
    - Children—Use and dose must be determined by your doctor.

**Missed dose**—If you miss a dose of this medicine, apply it as soon as you remember. However, if more than a few hours have passed, skip the missed dose and go back to your regular dosing schedule. If you miss more than one dose, check with your doctor.

**Storage**—To store this medicine:

- Keep out of the reach of children.
- Store away from heat and direct light.
- Do not store in the bathroom, near the kitchen sink, or in other damp places. Heat or moisture may cause the medicine to break down.
- Protect the solution from freezing.
- Do not keep outdated medicine or medicine no longer needed. Be sure that any discarded medicine is out of the reach of children.

## Precautions While Using This Medicine

*It is very important that your doctor check your progress at regular visits* to make sure that this medicine is working properly and to check for unwanted effects.

*Apply this medicine very carefully when using it on your face. Avoid getting any in your eyes, nose, or mouth.*

While using this medicine, and for 1 or 2 months after you stop using it, your skin may become more sensitive to sunlight than usual and too much sunlight may increase the effect of the drug. *During this period of time:*

- Stay out of direct sunlight, especially between the hours of 10:00 a.m. and 3:00 p.m., if possible.
- Wear protective clothing, including a hat and sunglasses.

- Apply a sun block product that has a skin protection factor (SPF) of at least 15. Some patients may require a product with a higher SPF number, especially if they have a fair complexion. If you have any questions about this, check with your health care professional.
- Do not use a sunlamp or tanning bed or booth.

*If you have a severe reaction from the sun, check with your doctor.*

## Side Effects of This Medicine

Along with its needed effects, a medicine may cause some unwanted effects. Although not all of these side effects may occur, if they do occur they may need medical attention.

*Check with your doctor immediately* if the following side effects occur:
  Redness and swelling of normal skin

Other side effects may occur that usually do not need medical attention. These side effects may go away during treatment as your body adjusts to the medicine. However, check with your doctor if any of the following side effects continue, worsen, or are bothersome:

*More common*
  Burning feeling where medicine is applied; increased sensitivity of skin to sunlight; itching; oozing; skin rash; soreness or tenderness of skin

*Less common or rare*
  Darkening of skin; scaling; watery eyes

Other side effects not listed above may also occur in some patients. If you notice any other effects, check with your doctor.

Revised: 06/09/93
Interim revision: 05/02/94

# FLUOXETINE   Systemic

A commonly used brand name in the U.S. and Canada is Prozac.

## Description

Fluoxetine (floo-OX-uh-teen) is used to treat mental depression. It is also used to treat obsessive-compulsive disorder.

This medicine is available only with your doctor's prescription, in the following dosage form:
*Oral*
- Capsules (U.S. and Canada)
- Oral Solution (U.S. and Canada)

## Before Using This Medicine

There have been recent suggestions that the use of fluoxetine may be related to increased thoughts about suicide in a very small number of patients. More study is needed to determine if the medicine caused this effect. Be sure you discuss this, and any possible precautions you should take, with your doctor before taking fluoxetine.

In deciding to use a medicine, the risks of taking the medicine must be weighed against the good it will do. This is a decision you and your doctor will make. For fluoxetine, the following should be considered:

**Allergies**—Tell your doctor if you have ever had any unusual or allergic reaction to fluoxetine. Also tell your health care professional if you are allergic to any other substances, such as foods, preservatives, or dyes.

**Pregnancy**—Studies have not been done in pregnant women. However, fluoxetine has not been shown to cause birth defects or other problems in animal studies.

**Breast-feeding**—Fluoxetine passes into breast milk and may cause unwanted effects, such as vomiting, watery stools, crying, and sleep problems in nursing babies. It may be necessary for you to take another medicine or to stop breast-feeding during treatment. Be sure you have discussed the risks and benefits of the medicine with your doctor.

**Children**—Studies on this medicine have been done only in adult patients, and there is no specific information comparing use of fluoxetine in children with use in other age groups.

**Older adults**—Many medicines have not been tested in older people. Therefore, it may not be known whether they work exactly the same way they do in younger adults or if they cause different side effects or problems in older people. In studies done to date that included elderly people, fluoxetine did not cause different side effects or problems in older people than it did in younger adults.

**Other medicines**—Although certain medicines should not be used together at all, in other cases two different medicines may be used together even if an interaction might occur. In these cases, your doctor may want to change the dose, or other precautions may be necessary. When you are taking fluoxetine, it is especially important that your health care professional know if you are taking any of the following:
- Anticoagulants (blood thinners) or
- Digitalis glycosides (heart medicine)—Higher or lower blood levels of these medicines or fluoxetine may occur; your doctor may need to change the dose of either medicine
- Central nervous system (CNS) depressants (medicines that cause drowsiness)—The CNS depressant effects may be increased

- Monoamine oxidase (MAO) inhibitors (furazolidone [e.g., Furoxone], isocarboxazid [e.g., Marplan], pargyline [e.g., Eutonyl], phenelzine [e.g., Nardil], procarbazine [e.g., Matulane], tranylcypromine [e.g., Parnate])—Taking fluoxetine while you are taking or within 2 weeks of taking MAO inhibitors may cause confusion, agitation, restlessness, stomach or intestinal symptoms, sudden high body temperature, extremely high blood pressure, and severe convulsions; at least 14 days should be allowed between stopping treatment with an MAO inhibitor and starting treatment with fluoxetine; if you have been taking fluoxetine, at least 5 weeks should be allowed before starting treatment with an MAO inhibitor
- Phenytoin—Taking this medicine with fluoxetine may result in higher blood levels of phenytoin, which increases the chance of serious side effects.
- Tryptophan—Taking this medicine with fluoxetine may result in increased agitation or restlessness, and stomach or intestinal problems

**Other medical problems**—The presence of other medical problems may affect the use of fluoxetine. Make sure you tell your doctor if you have any other medical problems, especially:

- Diabetes—The amount of insulin or oral antidiabetic medicine that you need to take may change
- Kidney disease or
- Liver disease—Higher blood levels of fluoxetine may occur, increasing the chance of side effects
- Seizure disorders (history of)—The risk of seizures may be increased

## Proper Use of This Medicine

*Take this medicine only as directed by your doctor,* to benefit your condition as much as possible. Do not take more of it, do not take it more often, and do not take it for a longer time than your doctor ordered.

If this medicine upsets your stomach, it may be taken with food.

*Sometimes fluoxetine must be taken for up to 4 weeks or longer before you begin to feel better. Your doctor should check your progress at regular visits during this time.*

**Dosing**—The dose of fluoxetine will be different for different patients. *Follow your doctor's orders or the directions on the label.* The following information includes only the average doses of fluoxetine. *If your dose is different, do not change it* unless your doctor tells you to do so:

The number of capsules or teaspoonfuls of solution that you take depends on the strength of the medicine. Also, *the number of doses you take each day, the time allowed between doses, and the length of time you take the medicine depend on the medical problem for which you are taking fluoxetine.*

- For *oral* dosage forms (capsules or solution):
  —For depression or obsessive-compulsive disorder:
    - Adults—At first, usually 20 milligrams (mg) a day, taken as a single dose in the morning.

- Children—Use and dose must be determined by your doctor.

**Missed dose**—If you miss a dose of this medicine, it is not necessary to make up the missed dose. Skip the missed dose and continue with your next scheduled dose. Do not double doses.

**Storage**—To store this medicine:
- Keep out of the reach of children.
- Store away from heat and direct light.
- Do not store in the bathroom, near the kitchen sink, or in other damp places. Heat or moisture may cause the medicine to break down.
- Do not keep outdated medicine or medicine no longer needed. Be sure that any discarded medicine is out of the reach of children.

## Precautions While Using This Medicine

It is important that your doctor check your progress at regular visits, to allow dosage adjustments and help reduce any side effects.

This medicine will add to the effects of alcohol and other CNS depressants (medicines that slow down the nervous system, possibly causing drowsiness). Some examples of CNS depressants are antihistamines or medicine for hay fever, other allergies, or colds; sedatives, tranquilizers, or sleeping medicine; prescription pain medicine or narcotics; barbiturates; medicine for seizures; muscle relaxants; or anesthetics, including some dental anesthetics. *Check with your doctor before taking any of the above while you are using this medicine.*

*If you develop a skin rash or hives, stop taking fluoxetine and check with your doctor as soon as possible.*

*For diabetic patients*:
- This medicine may affect blood sugar levels. If you notice a change in the results of your blood or urine sugar tests or if you have any questions, check with your doctor.

This medicine may cause some people to become drowsy. *Make sure you know how you react to fluoxetine before you drive, use machines, or do anything else that could be dangerous if you are not alert.*

*Dizziness, lightheadedness, or fainting may occur,* especially when you get up from a lying or sitting position. Getting up slowly may help. If this problem continues or gets worse, check with your doctor.

*This medicine may cause dryness of the mouth. For temporary relief, use sugarless gum or candy, melt bits of ice in your mouth, or use a saliva substitute.* However, if your mouth continues to feel dry for more than 2 weeks, check with your medical doctor or dentist. Continuing dryness of the mouth may increase the chance of dental disease, including tooth decay, gum disease, and fungus infections.

## Side Effects of This Medicine

Along with its needed effects, a medicine may cause some unwanted effects. Although not all of these side effects may occur, if they do occur they may need medical attention.

*Check with your doctor as soon as possible if any of the following side effects occur:*

### Less common

Chills or fever; joint or muscle pain; skin rash, hives, or itching; trouble in breathing

### Rare

Convulsions (seizures); signs of hypoglycemia (low blood sugar); including anxiety or nervousness, chills, cold sweats, confusion, cool, pale skin, difficulty in concentration, drowsiness, excessive hunger, fast heartbeat, headache, shakiness or unsteady walk, or unusual tiredness or weakness; skin rash or hives that may occur with burning or tingling in fingers, hands, or arms, chills or fever, joint or muscle pain, swelling of feet or lower legs, swollen glands, or trouble in breathing

### Symptoms of overdose

Agitation and restlessness; convulsions (seizures); nausea and vomiting (severe); unusual excitement

Other side effects may occur that usually do not need medical attention. These side effects may go away during treatment as your body adjusts to the medicine. However, check with your doctor if any of the following side effects continue or are bothersome:

### More common

Anxiety and nervousness; diarrhea; drowsiness; headache; increased sweating; nausea; trouble in sleeping

### Less common

Abnormal dreams; change in taste; changes in vision; chest pain; constipation; cough; decreased appetite or weight loss; decreased sexual drive or ability; decrease in concentration; dizziness or lightheadedness; dryness of mouth; fast or irregular heartbeat; feeling of warmth or heat; flushing or redness of skin, especially on face and neck; frequent urination; increased appetite; menstrual pain; stomach cramps, gas, or pain; stuffy nose; tiredness or weakness; tremor; vomiting

Other side effects not listed above may also occur in some patients. If you notice any other effects, check with your doctor.

Revised: 08/04/92
Interim revision(s): 04/29/94

---

# FLUTAMIDE  Systemic

Some commonly used brand names are:
**In the U.S.—**
Eulexin
**In Canada—**
Euflex

## Description

Flutamide (FLOO-ta-mide) is used to treat cancer of the prostate gland.

Flutamide belongs to the group of medicines known as antiandrogens. It blocks the effect of testosterone in the body. Giving flutamide with another medicine that decreases testosterone levels is one way of treating cancer of the prostate.

Flutamide is available only with your doctor's prescription, in the following dosage forms:

### Oral

- Capsules (U.S.)
- Tablets (Canada)

## Before Using This Medicine

In deciding to use a medicine, the risks of taking the medicine must be weighed against the good it will do.

This is a decision you and your doctor will make. For flutamide, the following should be considered:

**Allergies**—Tell your doctor if you have ever had any unusual or allergic reaction to flutamide.

**Pregnancy**—This medicine causes low sperm count and the medicine it is used with causes sterility which may be permanent. If you intend to have children, be sure that you have discussed this with your doctor before taking this medicine.

**Older adults**—Many medicines have not been studied specifically in older people. Therefore, it may not be known whether they work exactly the same way they do in younger adults or if they cause different side effects or problems in older people. The effects of a dose of flutamide may last a little longer in elderly patients. However, the dose that is prescribed has that taken into account. Flutamide is not expected to cause different side effects or problems in older people than in younger adults.

## Proper Use of This Medicine

*Take this medicine exactly as directed by your doctor.* Do not use more or less of it, and do not use it more often than your doctor ordered. The exact amount of medicine you need has been carefully worked out. Taking too much may increase the chance of side effects, while taking too little may not improve your condition.

Flutamide is usually taken with another medicine. *It is very important that the two medicines be used as directed. Follow your doctor's instructions very carefully about when to use these medicines.*

Flutamide in combination therapy sometimes causes unwanted effects such as hot flashes or decreased sexual ability. It may also cause difficulty in urinating when you begin to take it. However, it is very important that you continue to take the medicine, even after you begin to feel better. *Do not stop taking this medicine without first checking with your doctor.*

If you vomit shortly after taking a dose of flutamide, check with your doctor. You will be told whether to take the dose again or to wait until the next scheduled dose.

**Dosing**—The dose of flutamide may be different for different patients. *Follow your doctor's orders or the directions on the label.* The following information includes only the average doses of flutamide. *If your dose is different, do not change it* unless your doctor tells you to do so.

- For *oral* dosage forms (capsules or tablets):
  —For prostate cancer:
    - Adults—250 milligrams (mg) every eight hours. This is usually taken in combination with another medicine that decreases testosterone levels.

**Missed dose**—If you miss a dose of this medicine, take it as soon as possible. However, if it is almost time for your next dose, skip the missed dose and go back to your regular dosing schedule. Do not double doses.

**Storage**—To store this medicine:
- Keep out of the reach of children.
- Store away from heat and direct light.
- Do not store in the bathroom, near the kitchen sink, or in other damp places. Heat or moisture may cause the medicine to break down.
- Do not keep outdated medicine or medicine no longer needed. Be sure that any discarded medicine is out of the reach of children.

## Precautions While Using This Medicine

*It is very important that your doctor check your progress at regular visits* to make sure that this medicine is working properly and to check for unwanted effects.

## Side Effects of This Medicine

Along with its needed effects, a medicine may cause some unwanted effects. Although not all of these side effects may occur, if they do occur they may need medical attention.

*Check with your doctor immediately* if any of the following side effects occur:

*Rare*

Bluish-colored lips, fingernails, or palms of hands; dark urine; dizziness (extreme) or fainting; feeling of extreme pressure in head; itching; loss of appetite; nausea or vomiting; pain in right side; shortness of breath; weak and fast heartbeat; yellow eyes or skin

This medicine may also cause the following side effects that your doctor will watch out for:

*Rare*

High blood pressure; liver problems; methemoglobinemia (a blood problem)

Other side effects may occur that usually do not need medical attention. The side effects listed below are for flutamide used together with the medicine that decreases testosterone. These side effects may go away during treatment as your body adjusts to the medicine. However, check with your health care professional if any of the following side effects continue or are bothersome:

*More common*

Diarrhea; impotence or decrease in sexual desire; sweating and feelings of warmth (sudden)

*Less common*

Loss of appetite; numbness or tingling of hands or feet; swelling and increased tenderness of breasts; swelling of feet or lower legs

Other side effects not listed above may also occur in some patients. If you notice any other effects, check with your doctor.

Revised: 08/03/94

---

# FOLIC ACID    Vitamin B$_9$    Systemic

Some commonly used brand names are:
**In the U.S.—**
 Folvite
 Generic name product may also be available.
**In Canada—**
 Apo-Folic                    Novo-Folacid
 Folvite
 Generic name product may also be available.
Another commonly used name is Vitamin B$_9$.

## Description

Vitamins (VYE-ta-mins) are compounds that you *must* have for growth and health. They are needed in small amounts only and are usually available in the foods that you eat. Folic (FOE-lik) acid (vitamin B$_9$) is necessary for strong blood.

Lack of folic acid may lead to anemia (weak blood). Your doctor may treat this by prescribing folic acid for you.

Patients with the following conditions may be more likely to have a deficiency of folic acid:

- Alcoholism
- Anemia, hemolytic
- Diarrhea (continuing)
- Fever (prolonged)
- Hemodialysis
- Illness (prolonged)
- Intestinal diseases
- Liver disease
- Stress (continuing)
- Surgical removal of stomach

In addition, infants smaller than normal, breast-fed infants, or those receiving unfortified formulas (such as evaporated milk or goat's milk) may need additional folic acid.

If any of the above apply to you, you should take folic acid supplements only on the advice of your doctor after need has been established.

Some studies have found that folic acid taken by women before they become pregnant and during early pregnancy may reduce the chances of certain birth defects (neural tube defects).

Claims that folic acid and other B vitamins are effective for preventing mental problems have not been proven. Many of these treatments involve large and expensive amounts of vitamins.

Some strengths of folic acid are available only with your doctor's prescription. Others are available without a prescription. However, it may be a good idea to check with your doctor before taking folic acid on your own.

Folic acid is available in the following dosage forms:

*Oral*
- Tablets (U.S. and Canada)

*Parenteral*
- Injection (U.S. and Canada)

---

## Importance of Diet

Vitamin supplements should be taken only if you cannot get enough vitamins in your diet; however, some diets may not contain all of the vitamins you need. This may occur with rapid weight loss, unusual diets (such as some reducing diets in which choice of foods is limited), prolonged intravenous feeding, or malnutrition. A balanced diet should provide all the vitamins you normally need.

In order to get enough vitamins and minerals in your diet, it is important that you eat a balanced and varied diet. Follow carefully any diet program your doctor may recommend. For your specific vitamin and/or mineral needs, ask your doctor for a list of appropriate foods.

Folic acid is found in various foods, including vegetables, especially green vegetables; potatoes; cereal and cereal products; fruits; and organ meats (for example, liver or kidney). It is best to eat fresh fruits and vegetables whenever possible since they contain the most vitamins. Food processing may destroy some of the vitamins. For example, heat may reduce the amount of folic acid in foods.

Vitamins alone will not take the place of a good diet and will not provide energy. Your body also needs other substances found in food such as protein, minerals, carbohydrates, and fat. Vitamins themselves often cannot work without the presence of other foods.

In some cases, it may not be possible for you to get enough food to supply you with the proper vitamins. In other cases, the amount of vitamins you need may be increased above normal. Therefore, a vitamin supplement may be needed.

Experts have developed a list of recommended dietary allowances (RDA) for most of the vitamins. The RDA are not an exact number but a general idea of how much you need. They do not cover amounts needed for problems caused by a serious lack of vitamins.

The RDA for folic acid are:

- Infants and children—
  Birth to 6 months of age: 25 micrograms (mcg) per day.
  6 months to 1 year of age: 35 mcg per day.
  1 to 3 years of age: 50 mcg per day.
  4 to 6 years of age: 75 mcg per day.
  7 to 10 years of age: 100 mcg per day.
- Adolescent and adult males—
  11 to 14 years of age: 150 mcg per day.
  15 years of age and over: 200 mcg per day.
- Adolescent and adult females—
  11 to 14 years of age: 200 mcg per day.
  15 years of age and over: 180 mcg per day.
- Pregnant females—400 mcg per day.
- Breast-feeding females—
  First 6 months: 280 mcg per day.
  Second 6 months: 260 mcg per day.

Remember:
- The total amount of each vitamin that you get every day includes what you get from the foods that you eat *and* what you may take as a supplement.

- This total amount should not be greater than the RDA, unless ordered by your doctor.

## Before Using This Dietary Supplement

In deciding to use a medicine, the risks of taking the medicine must be weighed against the good it will do. This is a decision you and your doctor will make. For folic acid, the following should be considered:

**Allergies**—Tell your doctor if you have ever had any unusual or allergic reaction to folic acid. Also tell your health care professional if you are allergic to any other substances, such as foods, preservatives, or dyes.

**Pregnancy**—It is especially important that you are receiving enough vitamins when you become pregnant and that you continue to receive the right amount of vitamins, especially folic acid, throughout your pregnancy. The healthy growth and development of the fetus depend on a steady supply of nutrients from the mother. However, taking large amounts of a dietary supplement in pregnancy may be harmful to the mother and/or fetus and should be avoided.

Your doctor may recommend that you take folic acid alone or as part of a multivitamin supplement before you become pregnant and during early pregnancy. Folic acid may reduce the chances of your baby being born with a certain type of birth defect (neural tube defects).

**Breast-feeding**—It is especially important that you receive the right amounts of vitamins so that your baby will also get the vitamins needed to grow properly. However, taking large amounts of a dietary supplement while breast-feeding may be harmful to the mother and/or baby and should be avoided.

**Children**—Normal daily requirements vary according to age. It is especially important that children receive enough vitamins in their diet for healthy growth and development. Although there is no specific information about the use of folic acid in children in doses higher than the normal daily requirements, it is not expected to cause different side effects or problems in children than in adults.

**Older adults**—It is important that older people continue to receive enough vitamins in their diet for good health. Although there is no specific information about the use of folic acid in older people in doses higher than the normal daily requirements, it is not expected to cause different side effects or problems in older people than in younger adults.

**Medicines or other dietary supplements**—Although certain dietary supplements should not be used together at all, in other cases they may be used together even if an interaction might occur. In these cases, your doctor may want to change the dose, or other precautions may be necessary. Tell your health care professional if you are taking any other dietary supplement or any prescription or nonprescription (over-the-counter [OTC]) medicine.

**Other medical problems**—The presence of other medical problems may affect the use of folic acid. Make sure you tell your doctor if you have any other medical problems, especially:

- Pernicious anemia (a type of blood problem)—Taking folic acid while you have pernicious anemia may cause serious side effects. You should be sure that you do not have pernicious anemia before beginning folic acid supplementation

## Proper Use of This Dietary Supplement

Some people believe that taking very large doses of vitamins (called megadoses or megavitamin therapy) is useful for treating certain medical problems. Studies have not proven this. Large doses should be taken only under the direction of your doctor after need has been identified.

**Dosing**—The dose of folic acid for prevention of folic acid deficiency is based on the Recommended Dietary Allowances (RDA). See the *Importance of Diet* section for the RDA for folic acid.

**Missed dose**—If you miss taking a vitamin for one or more days there is no cause for concern, since it takes some time for your body to become seriously low in vitamins. However, if your doctor has recommended that you take this vitamin, try to remember to take it as directed every day.

**Storage**—To store this dietary supplement:

- Keep out of the reach of children.
- Store away from heat and direct light.
- Do not store in the bathroom, near the kitchen sink, or in other damp places. Heat or moisture may cause the dietary supplement to break down.
- Do not keep outdated dietary supplements or those no longer needed. Be sure that any discarded dietary supplement is out of the reach of children.

## Side Effects of This Dietary Supplement

Along with its needed effects, a dietary supplement may cause some unwanted effects. Although folic acid does not usually cause any side effects, check with your doctor as soon as possible if any of the following side effects occur:

*Rare*

Fever; reddened skin; shortness of breath; skin rash or itching; tightness in chest; troubled breathing; wheezing

Other side effects not listed above may also occur in some patients. If you notice any other effects, check with your doctor.

Revised: 05/20/92
Interim revision: 08/17/94

# FOSCARNET   Systemic†

A commonly used brand name in the U.S. is Foscavir.
Other commonly used names are phosphonoformic acid and PFA.

---

†Not commercially available in Canada.

---

## Description

Foscarnet (foss-KAR-net) is used to treat the symptoms of cytomegalovirus (CMV) infection of the eyes in patients with acquired immune deficiency syndrome (AIDS). Foscarnet will not cure this eye infection, but it may help to control worsening of the symptoms. Foscarnet may also be used for other serious viral infections as determined by your doctor. However, it does not work in treating certain viruses, such as the common cold or the flu.

Foscarnet is administered only by or under the supervision of your doctor. It is available in the following dosage form:

*Parenteral*
- Injection (U.S.)

## Before Receiving This Medicine

In deciding to use a medicine, the risks of taking the medicine must be weighed against the good it will do. This is a decision you and your doctor will make. For foscarnet, the following should be considered:

**Allergies**—Tell your doctor if you have ever had any unusual or allergic reaction to foscarnet. Also tell your health care professional if you are allergic to any other substances, such as foods, preservatives, or dyes.

**Pregnancy**—Foscarnet has not been studied in pregnant women. However, studies in animals have shown that foscarnet causes birth defects. Before taking this medicine, make sure your doctor knows if you are pregnant or if you may become pregnant.

**Breast-feeding**—It is not known whether foscarnet passes into the breast milk. Although most medicines pass into breast milk in small amounts, many of them may be used safely while breast-feeding. Mothers who are taking this medicine and who wish to breast-feed should discuss this with their doctor.

**Children**—There is no specific information comparing use of foscarnet in children with use in other age groups. Foscarnet can cause serious side effects in any patient. Therefore, it is especially important that you discuss with the child's doctor the good that this medicine may do as well as the risks of using it.

**Older adults**—Many medicines have not been studied specifically in older people. Therefore, it may not be known whether they work exactly the same way they do in younger adults or if they cause different side effects or problems in older people. There is no specific information comparing use of foscarnet in the elderly with use in other age groups.

**Other medicines**—Although certain medicines should not be used together at all, in other cases 2 different medicines may be used together even if an interaction might occur. In these cases, your doctor may want to change the dose, or other precautions may be necessary. When you are taking foscarnet, it is especially important that your health care professional know if you are taking any of the following:
- Carmustine (e.g., BiCNU) or
- Cisplatin (e.g., Platinol) or
- Combination pain medicine containing acetaminophen and aspirin (e.g., Excedrin) or other salicylates (with large amounts taken regularly) or
- Cyclosporine (e.g., Sandimmune) or
- Deferoxamine (e.g., Desferal) (with long-term use) or
- Gold salts (medicine for arthritis) or
- Inflammation or pain medicine, except narcotics, or
- Lithium (e.g., Lithane) or
- Methotrexate (e.g., Mexate) or
- Other anti-infectives (e.g., amphotericin B) or
- Penicillamine (e.g., Cuprimine) or
- Plicamycin (e.g., Mithracin) or
- Streptozocin (e.g., Zanosar) or
- Tiopronin (e.g., Thiola)—Use of these medicines may increase the chance of side effects affecting the kidneys
- Pentamidine (e.g., Pentam)—Use of pentamidine injection with foscarnet may lower the level of important minerals (calcium and magnesium) in the blood; it may also increase the chance of side effects affecting the kidneys

**Other medical problems**—The presence of other medical problems may affect the use of foscarnet. Make sure you tell your doctor if you have any other medical problems, especially:
- Anemia—Foscarnet may cause or worsen anemia
- Dehydration or
- Kidney disease—Patients who are dehydrated or have kidney disease may have an increased chance of side effects

---

## Proper Use of This Medicine

To ensure the best response, foscarnet must be given for the full time of treatment. Also, this medicine works best when there is a constant amount in the blood. To help keep the amount constant, foscarnet must be given on a regular schedule.

*Several glasses of water should be taken every day, unless otherwise directed by your doctor. Drinking extra water will help to prevent some unwanted effects foscarnet has on the kidneys.*

This medicine may cause sores on the genitals (sex organs). Washing your genitals after urination may decrease the chance of your developing this problem.

**Dosing**—The dose of foscarnet will be different for different patients. *Follow your doctor's orders or the directions on the label.* The following information includes only the average doses of foscarnet. *If your dose is different, do not change it* unless your doctor tells you to do so.

---

- For *injection* dosage form:
  —For cytomegalovirus (CMV) retinitis induction (first stage of dosing):
    - Adults and children—The usual dose is 60 milligrams (mg) per kilogram (kg) (27.3 mg per pound) of body weight every eight hours for fourteen to twenty-one days. Each dose is injected slowly into a vein by an infusion pump over at least one hour.
  —For CMV retinitis maintenance (second stage of dosing):
    - Adults and children—The usual dose is 90 to 120 mg per kg (41 to 54.5 mg per pound) of body weight once a day. This dose is injected slowly into a vein by an infusion pump over at least two hours.

## Precautions After Receiving This Medicine

It is very important that your doctor check your progress at regular visits. This will allow your doctor to check for possible unwanted effects.

It is also *very important that your ophthalmologist (eye doctor) check your eyes* at regular visits since you may have some loss of eyesight due to retinitis even while you are receiving foscarnet.

## Side Effects of This Medicine

Along with their needed effects, medicines like foscarnet can sometimes cause serious side effects such as kidney problems; these are described below. Foscarnet may also decrease the amount of calcium in your blood, causing you to have a tingling sensation around your mouth, and pain or numbness in your hands and feet. If this occurs, especially while you are receiving the medicine, notify your health care professional immediately.

Along with its needed effects, a medicine may cause some unwanted effects. Although not all of these side effects may occur, if they do occur they may need medical attention.

*Check with your doctor immediately* if any of the following side effects occur:

*More common*
  Increased or decreased frequency of urination or amount of urine; increased thirst

*Less common*
  Convulsions (seizures); fever, chills, and sore throat; muscle twitching; pain at place of injection; pain or numbness in hands or feet; tingling sensation around mouth; tremor; unusual tiredness and weakness

*Rare*
  Sores or ulcers on the mouth or throat, penis, or vulva

Other side effects may occur that usually do not need medical attention. These side effects may go away during treatment as your body adjusts to the medicine. However, check with your doctor if any of the following side effects continue or are bothersome:

*More common*
  Abdominal or stomach pain; anxious feeling; confusion; dizziness; headache; loss of appetite; nausea and vomiting; unusual tiredness or weakness

Other side effects not listed above may also occur in some patients. If you notice any other effects, check with your doctor.

## Additional Information

Once a medicine has been approved for marketing for a certain use, experience may show that it is also useful for other medical problems. Although these uses are not included in product labeling, foscarnet is used in certain patients with the following medical conditions:

- Cytomegalovirus infections in places other than the eyes, such as the lungs, esophagus, or intestines
- Herpes simplex infections of the lips and mouth that do not respond to treatment with acyclovir in patients with HIV infection
- Varicella-zoster infection (shingles) that does not respond to treatment with acyclovir in patients with HIV infection

Other than the above information, there is no additional information relating to proper use, precautions, or side effects for these uses.

Revised: 07/22/94

# FRUCTOSE, DEXTROSE, AND PHOSPHORIC ACID    Oral

A commonly used brand name in the U.S. and Canada is Emetrol.

## Description

Fructose (FRUK-tose), dextrose (DEX-trose), and phosphoric (fos-FOR-ik) acid combination is used to treat nausea and vomiting. However, this combination has not been proven to be effective.

This medicine is available without a prescription; however, your doctor may have special instructions on the proper use and dose for your medical problem. Fructose, dextrose, and phosphoric acid combination is available in the following dosage form:

*Oral*
  - Oral solution (U.S. and Canada)

## Before Using This Medicine

If you are taking this medicine without a prescription, carefully read and follow any precautions on the label. For fructose, dextrose, and phosphoric acid combination, the following should be considered:

**Allergies**—Tell your doctor if you have ever had any unusual or allergic reaction to fructose, dextrose, or phosphoric acid.

**Pregnancy**—Studies on effects in pregnancy have not been done in either humans or animals.

**Breast-feeding**—This medicine has not been reported to cause problems in nursing babies.

**Children**—The fluid loss caused by vomiting may result in a severe condition, especially in children under 3 years of age. Do not give medicine for vomiting to children without first checking with their doctor.

**Older adults**—The fluid loss caused by vomiting may result in a severe condition. Elderly persons should not take any medicine for vomiting without first checking with their doctor.

**Other medical problems**—The presence of other medical problems may affect the use of fructose, dextrose, and phosphoric acid. Make sure you tell your doctor if you have any other medical problems, especially:

- Appendicitis, symptoms of, or
- Inflamed bowel, symptoms of—Make sure nausea and vomiting are not due to appendicitis or inflamed bowel before using this product. These conditions may become more severe if they are not treated by your doctor
- Diabetes mellitus—The sugars contained in this medicine may cause problems in diabetics
- Fructose intolerance, hereditary—The fructose in this medicine may cause severe side effects in patients with this condition

## Proper Use of This Medicine

For safe use of this medicine:

- Follow your doctor's instructions if this medicine was prescribed.
- Follow the manufacturer's package directions if you are treating yourself.

Do not dilute this medicine with other liquids. Also, do not drink any other liquids immediately before or after taking this medicine. To do so may keep this medicine from working properly.

**Dosing**—The dose of this combination product will be different for different patients. *Follow your doctor's orders or the directions on the label.* The following information includes only the average doses. *If your dose is different, do not change it* unless your doctor tells you to do so.

- For *oral* dosage form (oral solution):
  —For morning sickness:
    • Pregnant women: One or two tablespoonfuls upon arising and every three hours as needed.

—For nausea:
  • Adults: One or two tablespoonfuls. Dose may be repeated every fifteen minutes until nausea stops. You should not take this product for more than one hour (5 doses) without checking with your doctor.
  • Children over 3 years of age: One or two teaspoonfuls. Dose may be repeated every fifteen minutes until nausea stops. This product should not be taken for more than one hour (5 doses) without checking with your doctor.
  • Children under 3 years of age: Use is not recommended.

**Storage**—To store this medicine:
- Keep out of the reach of children.
- Store away from heat and direct light.
- Keep the medicine from freezing.
- Do not keep outdated medicine or medicine no longer needed. Be sure that any discarded medicine is out of the reach of children.

## Precautions While Using This Medicine

*Check with your doctor if your nausea and vomiting continue or become worse after you have taken this medicine.*

*Do not take this medicine if you have any signs of appendicitis or inflamed bowel* (such as stomach or lower abdominal pain, cramping, bloating, soreness, or continuing or severe nausea or vomiting). Instead, check with your doctor as soon as possible.

## Side Effects of This Medicine

Along with its needed effects, a medicine may cause some unwanted effects. Although not all of these side effects may occur, if they do occur they may need medical attention.

Stop using this medicine and check with your doctor as soon as possible if any of the following side effects occur:
  *Signs of fructose intolerance*
    Fainting; swelling of face, arms, and legs; unusual bleeding; vomiting; weight loss; yellow eyes or skin

Other side effects may occur that usually do not need medical attention. These side effects may go away during treatment as your body adjusts to the medicine. However, check with your doctor if any of the following side effects continue or are bothersome:
  *Less common—more common with large doses*
    Diarrhea; stomach or abdominal pain

Other side effects not listed above may also occur in some patients. If you notice any other effects, check with your doctor.

Revised: 05/12/93

# FURAZOLIDONE Oral†

Some commonly used brand names in the U.S. are Furoxone and Furoxone Liquid.

†Not commercially available in Canada.

## Description

Furazolidone (fyoor-a-ZOE-li-done) is used to treat bacterial and protozoal (proe-toe-ZOE-al) infections. It works by killing bacteria and protozoa (tiny, one-celled animals). Some protozoa are parasites that can cause many different kinds of infections in the body.

Furazolidone is taken by mouth. It works inside the intestinal tract to treat cholera, colitis and/or diarrhea caused by bacteria, and giardiasis (jee-ar-DYE-a-siss). This medicine is sometimes given with other medicines for bacterial infections.

*Furazolidone may cause some serious side effects when taken with certain foods, beverages, or other medicines.* Check with your health care professional for a list of products that should be avoided.

Furazolidone is available only with your doctor's prescription, in the following dosage forms:

*Oral*
- Oral suspension (U.S.)
- Tablets (U.S.)

## Before Using This Medicine

In deciding to use a medicine, the risks of taking the medicine must be weighed against the good it will do. This is a decision you and your doctor will make. For furazolidone, the following should be considered:

**Allergies**—Tell your doctor if you have ever had any unusual or allergic reaction to furazolidone or to any related medicines such as nitrofurantoin (e.g., Furadantin) or nitrofurazone (e.g., Furacin). Also tell your health care professional if you are allergic to any other substances, such as foods, preservatives, or dyes.

**Pregnancy**—Studies have not been done in humans. However, furazolidone has not been shown to cause birth defects or other problems in humans or in animals given high doses for a long time.

**Breast-feeding**—It is not known whether furazolidone passes into breast milk. However, breast-feeding is not recommended for nursing babies up to 1 month of age because furazolidone may cause anemia.

**Children**—Because furazolidone may cause anemia, use in infants up to 1 month of age is not recommended.

**Older adults**—Many medicines have not been studied specifically in older people. Therefore, it may not be known whether they work exactly the same way they do in younger adults or if they cause different side effects or problems in older people. There is no specific information

comparing use of furazolidone in the elderly with use in other age groups.

**Other medicines**—Although certain medicines should not be used together at all, in other cases two different medicines may be used together even if an interaction might occur. In these cases, your doctor may want to change the dose, or other precautions may be necessary. When you are taking furazolidone, it is especially important that your health care professional know if you are taking any of the following:
- Amphetamines or
- Appetite suppressants (diet pills) or
- Ephedrine (e.g., Primatene) or
- Isocarboxazid (e.g., Marplan) or
- Phenelzine (e.g., Nardil) or
- Phenylephrine (e.g., Neo-Synephrine) or
- Phenylpropanolamine (e.g., Dexatrim) or
- Procarbazine (e.g., Matulane) or
- Pseudoephedrine (e.g., Sudafed) or
- Selegiline (e.g., Eldepryl) or
- Tranylcypromine (e.g., Parnate) or
- Tricyclic antidepressants (amitriptyline [e.g., Elavil], amoxapine [e.g., Asendin], clomipramine [e.g., Anafranil], desipramine [e.g., Pertofrane], doxepin [e.g., Sinequan], imipramine [e.g., Tofranil], nortriptyline [e.g., Aventyl], protriptyline [e.g., Vivactil], trimipramine [e.g., Surmontil])—The use of furazolidone with any of these medicines may result in a severe increase in blood pressure

**Other medical problems**—The presence of other medical problems may affect the use of furazolidone. Make sure you tell your doctor if you have any other medical problems, especially:
- Glucose-6-phosphate dehydrogenase deficiency (lack of G6PD enzyme)—Patients with G6PD-deficiency may develop mild anemia while taking furazolidone

## Proper Use of This Medicine

*Do not give furazolidone to infants up to 1 month of age,* unless otherwise directed by your doctor. This medicine may cause anemia in these patients.

Furazolidone may be taken with food.

To use the *oral suspension*:
- Use a specially marked measuring spoon or other device to measure each dose accurately. The average household teaspoon may not hold the right amount of liquid.

To help clear up your infection completely, *keep taking furazolidone for the full time of treatment,* even if you begin to feel better after a few days. If you stop taking this medicine too soon, your symptoms may return. *Do not miss any doses.*

**Dosing**—The dose of furazolidone will be different for different patients. *Follow your doctor's orders or the directions on the label.* The following information includes only the average doses of furazolidone. *If your* *dose is different, do not change it* unless your doctor tells you to do so.

The number of tablets or teaspoonfuls of suspension that you take depends on the strength of the medicine. Also, *the number of doses you take each day, the time allowed between doses, and the length of time you take the medicine depend on the medical problem for which you are taking furazolidone.*

- For *oral* dosage forms (oral suspension or tablets):
    —For cholera or diarrhea caused by bacteria:
    - Adults—100 milligrams (mg) taken four times a day for five to seven days.
    - Children up to 1 month of age—Use is not recommended.
    - Children 1 month of age and over—Dose is based on body weight and must be determined by your doctor. The usual dose is 1.25 mg per kilogram (kg) (0.56 mg per pound) of body weight taken four times a day for five to seven days.
    —For giardiasis:
    - Adults—100 mg taken four times a day for seven to ten days.
    - Children up to 1 month of age—Use is not recommended.
    - Children 1 month of age and over—Dose is based on body weight and must be determined by your doctor. The usual dose is 1.25 mg to 2 mg per kg (0.56 to 0.90 mg per pound) of body weight taken four times a day for seven to ten days.

**Missed dose**—If you miss a dose of this medicine, take it as soon as possible. However, if it is almost time for your next dose, skip the missed dose and go back to your regular dosing schedule. Do not double doses.

**Storage**—To store this medicine:
- Keep out of the reach of children.
- Store away from heat and direct light.
- Do not store the tablet form of this medicine in the bathroom, near the kitchen sink, or in other damp places. Heat or moisture may cause the medicine to break down.
- Keep the oral suspension form of this medicine from freezing.
- Do not keep outdated medicine or medicine no longer needed. Be sure that any discarded medicine is out of the reach of children.

---

## Precautions While Using This Medicine

It is important that your doctor check your progress at regular visits. This is to check whether or not the infection is cleared up completely.

If your symptoms do not improve within a week, or if they become worse, check with your doctor.

Drinking alcoholic beverages or taking other alcohol-containing preparations (for example, elixirs, cough syrups, tonics, or injections of alcohol) while taking furazolidone may rarely cause problems. These problems include increased side effects such as redness of the face, difficult breathing, fainting, and a feeling of tightness in the chest. These side effects usually go away within 24 hours without treatment. However, these effects may occur if you drink for up to 4 days after you stop taking furazolidone. Therefore, *you should not drink alcoholic beverages or take other alcohol-containing preparations while you are taking furazolidone and for 4 days after stopping it.*

Certain foods, drinks, or other medicines may cause very dangerous reactions, such as severe high blood pressure, when taken with furazolidone. Aged or fermented foods and drinks commonly contain tyramine or other substances that increase blood pressure. To avoid such reactions, the following measures are recommended:

- *Do not eat foods that have a high tyramine content (most common in foods that are aged or fermented to increase their flavor), such as cheeses; yeast or meat extracts; fava or broad bean pods; smoked or pickled meat, poultry, or fish; fermented sausage (bologna, pepperoni, salami, summer sausage) or other fermented meat; or any overripe fruit. If a list of these foods is not given to you, ask your health care professional to provide one.*
- *Do not drink alcoholic beverages or alcohol-free or reduced-alcohol beer and wine.*
- Do not eat or drink large amounts of caffeine-containing food or beverages such as chocolate, coffee, tea, or cola.
- *Do not take any other medicines unless approved or prescribed by your doctor.* This includes nonprescription (over-the-counter [OTC]) appetite suppressants (diet pills) or medicine for colds, sinus problems, or hay fever or other allergies.
- *Do not take any of the above-listed foods, drinks, or medicine for at least 2 weeks after you stop taking furazolidone.* They may continue to react with this medicine during that time.
- Other foods may also contain tyramine or other substances that increase blood pressure. However, these products generally do not cause serious problems when taken with furazolidone, especially if eaten when fresh and in small amounts. These include yogurt, sour cream, cream cheese, cottage cheese, chocolate, and soy sauce. If you have any questions about this, ask your health care professional. Also ask for a list of foods, beverages, or medicines that may cause serious problems when taken with furazolidone.

---

## Side Effects of This Medicine

Along with its needed effects, a medicine may cause some unwanted effects. Although not all of these side effects may occur, if they do occur they may need medical attention.

*Check with your doctor immediately* if any of the following side effects occur:

> *Rare*
>> Fever; itching; joint pain; skin rash or redness; sore throat

Other side effects may occur that usually do not need medical attention. These side effects may go away during treatment as your body adjusts to the medicine. However, check with your doctor if any of the following side effects continue or are bothersome:

> *Less common*
>> Abdominal or stomach pain; diarrhea; headache; nausea or vomiting

This medicine commonly causes dark yellow to brown discoloration of urine. This side effect does not usually need medical attention.

Other side effects not listed above may also occur in some patients. If you notice any other effects, check with your doctor.

Annual revision: 10/06/92
Interim revision: 08/08/94

# GALLIUM NITRATE   Systemic†

A commonly used brand name in the U.S. is Ganite.

†Not commercially available in Canada; however it is available by emergency drug release from the Health Protection Branch.

## Description

Gallium nitrate (GAL-ee-um NYE-trate) is used to treat hypercalcemia (too much calcium in the blood) that may occur with some types of cancer.

This medicine is available only with your doctor's prescription in the following dosage form:

*Parenteral*
- Injection (U.S.)

## Before Receiving This Medicine

In deciding to use a medicine, the risks of taking the medicine must be weighed against the good it will do. This is a decision you and your doctor will make. For gallium nitrate the following should be considered:

**Allergies**—Tell your doctor if you have ever had any unusual or allergic reaction to gallium nitrate. Also tell your health care professional if you are allergic to any other substances, such as foods, preservatives, or dyes.

**Diet**—Make certain your health care professional knows if your diet includes large amounts of calcium-containing foods and/or vitamin D, such as milk or other dairy products. Calcium and vitamin D may cause the gallium nitrate to be less effective in treating high blood calcium. Also let your health care professional know if you are on any special diet, such as a low-sodium or a low-sugar diet.

**Pregnancy**—Gallium nitrate has not been studied in pregnant women.

**Breast-feeding**—It is not known whether gallium nitrate passes into breast milk. However, this medicine is not recommended during breast-feeding, because it may cause unwanted effects in nursing babies.

**Children**—Studies on this medicine have been done only in adult patients, and there is no specific information comparing use of gallium nitrate in children with use in other age groups.

**Older adults**—Many medicines have not been studied specifically in older people. Therefore, it may not be known whether they work exactly the same way they do in younger adults or if they cause different side effects or problems in older people. There is no specific information comparing use of gallium nitrate in the elderly with use in other age groups.

**Other medicines**—Although certain medicines should not be used together at all, in other cases two different medicines may be used together even if an interaction might occur. In these cases, your doctor may want to change the dose, or other precautions may be necessary. When you are taking gallium nitrate, it is especially important that your health care professional know if you are taking any of the following:
- Anti-infectives by mouth or by injection (medicine for infection) or
- Carmustine (e.g., BiCNU) or
- Cisplatin (e.g., Platinol) or
- Combination pain medicine containing acetaminophen and aspirin (e.g., Excedrin) or other salicylates (with large amounts taken regularly) or
- Cyclosporine (e.g., Sandimmune) or
- Deferoxamine (e.g., Desferal) (with long-term use) or
- Gold salts (medicine for arthritis) or
- Inflammation or pain medicine, except narcotics or
- Lithium (e.g., Lithane) or
- Methotrexate (e.g., Mexate) or
- Penicillamine (e.g., Cuprimine) or
- Plicamycin (e.g., Mithracin) or
- Streptozocin (e.g., Zanosar) or
- Tiopronin (e.g., Thiola)—Use with gallium nitrate may cause or worsen kidney problems
- Calcium-containing preparations or
- Vitamin D–containing preparations—Use with gallium nitrate may prevent gallium nitrate from working properly

**Other medical problems**—The presence of other medical problems may affect the use of gallium nitrate. Make sure you tell your doctor if you have any other medical problems, especially:
- Kidney disease—Gallium nitrate may make this condition worse

## Proper Use of This Medicine

**Dosing**—The dose of gallium nitrate will be different for different patients. *Follow your doctor's orders.*
- For *injection* dosage form:
  - For treatment of too much calcium in the blood:
    - Adults and children 12 years of age and older—The dose is based on body surface and must be determined by your doctor. Gallium nitrate is injected slowly into a vein over 24 hours, for five days. The dose may be repeated in three to four weeks.
    - Children up to 12 years of age—Use and dose have not been determined.

**Storage**—To store this medicine:
- Keep out of the reach of children.
- Store away from heat and direct light.
- Do not store in the bathroom, near the kitchen sink, or in other damp places. Heat or moisture may cause the medicine to break down.
- Keep the medicine from freezing. Do not refrigerate.
- Do not keep outdated medicine or medicine no longer needed. Be sure that any discarded medicine is out of the reach of children.

## Precautions While Receiving This Medicine

*It is important that your doctor check your progress at regular visits* while you are receiving this medicine. If your condition has improved and you are no longer receiving gallium nitrate, your progress must still be checked. The results of laboratory tests or the occurrence of certain symptoms will tell your doctor if your condition is coming back.

Your doctor may want you to follow a low-calcium diet while you are receiving this medicine. If you have any questions about this, check with your doctor.

## Side Effects of This Medicine

Along with its needed effects, a medicine may cause some unwanted effects. Although not all of these side effects may occur, if they do occur they may need medical attention.

*More common*
Blood in urine; bone pain; greatly increased or decreased frequency of urination or amount of urine; increased

thirst; loss of appetite; muscle weakness; nausea or vomiting

*Less common*
Abdominal cramps; confusion; muscle spasms

*Rare*
Unusual tiredness or weakness

Other side effects may occur that usually do not need medical attention. These side effects may go away during treatment as your body adjusts to the medicine. However, check with your doctor if any of the following side effects continue or are bothersome:

*More common*
Diarrhea; metallic taste

Other side effects not listed above may also occur in some patients. If you notice any other effects, check with your doctor.

Revised: 06/15/93

# GANCICLOVIR   Systemic

A commonly used brand name in the U.S. and Canada is Cytovene. Another commonly used name is DHPG.

## Description

Ganciclovir (gan-SYE-kloe-vir) is an antiviral. It is used to treat infections caused by viruses.

Ganciclovir is used to treat the symptoms of cytomegalovirus (CMV) infection of the eyes in people whose immune system is not working fully. This includes patients with acquired immune deficiency syndrome (AIDS). Ganciclovir will not cure this eye infection, but it may help to control worsening of the symptoms. It is also used to help prevent CMV infection in patients who receive organ or bone marrow transplants. Ganciclovir may also be used for other serious CMV infections as determined by your doctor. However, it does not work in treating certain viruses, such as the common cold or the flu.

This medicine may cause some serious side effects, including anemia and other blood problems. Before you begin treatment with ganciclovir, you and your doctor should talk about the good this medicine will do as well as the risks of using it.

Ganciclovir is to be administered by or under the supervision of your doctor. It is available in the following dosage form:

*Parenteral*
• Injection (U.S. and Canada)

## Before Receiving This Medicine

In deciding to use a medicine, the risks of taking the medicine must be weighed against the good it will do. This is a decision you and your doctor will make. For ganciclovir, the following should be considered:

**Allergies**—Tell your doctor if you have ever had any unusual or allergic reaction to acyclovir or ganciclovir. Also tell your doctor and pharmacist if you are allergic to any other substances, such as foods, preservatives, or dyes.

**Pregnancy**—Use of ganciclovir during pregnancy should be avoided whenever possible since ganciclovir has caused cancer and birth defects in animal studies. The use of birth control is recommended during ganciclovir therapy. Your partner should use a condom if he is receiving ganciclovir. Animal studies have shown that ganciclovir causes a decrease in fertility.

**Breast-feeding**—Breast-feeding should be stopped during treatment with this medicine because ganciclovir may cause serious unwanted effects in nursing babies.

**Children**—Ganciclovir can cause serious side effects in any patient. Therefore, it is especially important that you discuss with the child's doctor the good that this medicine may do as well as the risks of using it.

**Older adults**—Many medicines have not been studied specifically in older people. Therefore, it may not be known whether they work exactly the same way they do in younger adults or if they cause different side effects or problems in older people. There is no specific information

comparing use of ganciclovir in the elderly with use in other age groups.

**Other medicines**—Although certain medicines should not be used together at all, in other cases 2 different medicines may be used together even if an interaction might occur. In these cases, your doctor may want to change the dose, or other precautions may be necessary. When you are taking ganciclovir, it is especially important that your doctor and pharmacist know if you are taking any of the following:

- Amphotericin B by injection (e.g., Fungizone) or
- Antineoplastics (cancer medicine) or
- Antithyroid agents (medicine for overactive thyroid) or
- Azathioprine (e.g., Imuran) or
- Chloramphenicol (e.g., Chloromycetin) or
- Colchicine or
- Cyclophosphamide (e.g., Cytoxan) or
- Flucytosine (e.g., Ancobon) or
- Interferon (e.g., Intron A, Roferon-A) or
- Mercaptopurine (e.g., Purinethol) or
- Methotrexate (e.g., Mexate) or
- Plicamycin (e.g., Mithracin) or
- Zidovudine (e.g., AZT, Retrovir)—Caution should be used if these medicines and ganciclovir are used together; receiving ganciclovir while you are using these medicines may make anemia and other blood problems worse

**Other medical problems**—The presence of other medical problems may affect the use of ganciclovir. Make sure you tell your doctor if you have any other medical problems, especially:

- Kidney disease—Ganciclovir may build up in the blood in patients with kidney disease, increasing the chance of side effects

## Proper Use of This Medicine

To get the best results, *ganciclovir must be given for the full time of treatment.* Also, this medicine works best when there is a constant amount in the blood. To help keep the amount constant, ganciclovir must be given on a regular schedule.

**Dosing**—The dose of ganciclovir will be different for different patients. *Follow your doctor's orders or the directions on the label.* The following information includes only the average doses of ganciclovir. *If your dose is different, do not change it* unless your doctor tells you to do so.

- For *injection* dosage form:
  —For treatment of CMV retinitis:
  - Adults and teenagers—Dose is based on body weight. At first, 5 milligrams (mg) per kilogram (11 mg per pound) of body weight is injected into a vein every twelve hours for fourteen to twenty-one days. Then, 5 mg per kilogram of body weight is injected into a vein once a day for seven days of the week; or 6 mg per kilogram of body weight is injected into a vein once a day for five days of the week.
  - Children—Use and dose must be determined by your doctor.

  —For prevention of CMV in transplant patients:
  - Adults and teenagers—Dose is based on body weight. At first, 5 mg per kilogram (11 mg per pound) of body weight is injected into a vein every twelve hours for seven to fourteen days. Then the dose is reduced to 5 mg per kilogram of body weight once a day for seven days of the week; or 6 mg per kilogram of body weight once a day for five days of the week.
  - Children—Use and dose must be determined by your doctor.

## Precautions After Receiving This Medicine

Ganciclovir can lower the number of white blood cells in your blood, increasing the chance of getting an infection. It can also lower the number of platelets, which are necessary for proper blood clotting. If this occurs, there are certain precautions you can take to reduce the risk of infection or bleeding:

- *Check with your doctor immediately* if you think you are getting an infection or if you get a fever or chills.
- *Check with your doctor immediately* if you notice any unusual bleeding or bruising; black, tarry stools; blood in urine or stools; or pinpoint red spots on your skin.
- Be careful when using a regular toothbrush, dental floss, or toothpick. Your medical doctor, dentist, or nurse may recommend other ways to clean your teeth and gums. Check with your medical doctor before having any dental work done.
- Be careful not to cut yourself when you are using sharp objects such as a safety razor or fingernail or toenail cutters.

The *use of birth control is recommended for both men and women.* Women should use effective birth control methods while receiving this medicine. Men should use a condom during treatment with this medicine and for at least 90 days after treatment has been completed.

*It is very important that your doctor check you at regular visits* for any blood problems that may be caused by this medicine.

It is also *very important that your ophthalmologist (eye doctor) check your eyes* at regular visits since it is still possible that you may have some loss of eyesight during ganciclovir treatment.

## Side Effects of This Medicine

Along with their needed effects, medicines like ganciclovir can sometimes cause serious side effects such as blood problems; these are described below. Discuss these possible effects with your doctor.

Along with its needed effects, a medicine may cause some unwanted effects. Although not all of these side effects may occur, if they do occur they may need medical attention.

*Check with your doctor immediately* if any of the following side effects occur:

*More common*
*For injection into the vein only*
Sore throat and fever; unusual bleeding or bruising

*Less common*
*For injection into the vein only*
Mood or other mental changes; nervousness; pain at place of injection; skin rash; tremor; unusual tiredness and weakness

*For injection into the eye only*
Decreased vision or any change in vision

Other side effects may occur that usually do not need medical attention. These side effects may go away during treatment as your body adjusts to the medicine. However, check with your doctor if any of the following side effects continue or are bothersome:

*Less common*
Abdominal or stomach pain; loss of appetite; nausea and vomiting

Other side effects not listed above may also occur in some patients. If you notice any other effects, check with your doctor.

---

Annual revision: 08/20/93

---

# GEMFIBROZIL    Systemic

A commonly used brand name in the U.S. and Canada is Lopid.

## Description

Gemfibrozil (gem-FI-broe-zil) is used to lower cholesterol and triglyceride (fat-like substances) levels in the blood. This may help prevent medical problems caused by such substances clogging the blood vessels.

Gemfibrozil is available only with your doctor's prescription, in the following dosage forms:

*Oral*
- Capsules (Canada)
- Tablets (U.S. and Canada)

## Before Using This Medicine

In addition to its helpful effects in treating your medical problem, this type of medicine may have some harmful effects.

Results of a large study using gemfibrozil seem to show that it may cause a higher rate of some cancers in humans. In addition, the action of gemfibrozil is similar to that of another medicine called clofibrate. Studies with clofibrate have suggested that it may increase the patient's risk of cancer, liver disease, pancreatitis (inflammation of the pancreas), gallstones and problems from gallbladder surgery, although it may also decrease the risk of heart attacks. Other studies have not found all of these effects.

Studies with gemfibrozil in rats found an increased risk of liver tumors when doses up to 10 times the human dose were given for a long time.

Be sure you have discussed this with your doctor before taking this medicine.

In deciding to use a medicine, the risks of taking the medicine must be weighed against the good it will do.

This is a decision you and your doctor will make. For gemfibrozil, the following should be considered:

**Allergies**—Tell your doctor if you have ever had any unusual or allergic reaction to gemfibrozil. Also tell your health care professional if you are allergic to any other substances, such as foods, preservatives, or dyes.

**Diet**—Before prescribing medicine for your condition, your doctor will probably try to control your condition by prescribing a personal diet for you. Such a diet may be low in fats, sugars, and/or cholesterol. Many people are able to control their condition by carefully following their doctor's orders for proper diet and exercise. *Medicine is prescribed only when additional help is needed* and is effective only when a schedule of diet and exercise is properly followed.

Also, this medicine is less effective if you are greatly overweight. It may be very important for you to go on a reducing diet. However, check with your doctor before going on any diet.

Make certain your health care professional knows if you are on a low-sodium, low-sugar, or any other special diet. Most medicines contain more than their active ingredient.

**Pregnancy**—Gemfibrozil has not been studied in pregnant women. However, studies in animals have shown that high doses of gemfibrozil may increase the number of fetal deaths, decrease birth weight, or cause some skeletal defects. Before taking this medicine, make sure your doctor knows if you are pregnant or if you may become pregnant.

**Breast-feeding**—It is not known whether gemfibrozil passes into breast milk. However, studies in animals have shown that high doses of gemfibrozil may increase the risk of some kinds of tumors. Therefore, you should consider this when deciding whether to breast-feed your baby while taking this medicine.

**Children**—There is no specific information about the use of gemfibrozil in children. However, use is not recommended in children under 2 years of age since cholesterol is needed for normal development.

**Older adults**—Many medicines have not been studied specifically in older people. Therefore, it may not be known whether they work exactly the same way they do in younger adults or if they cause different side effects or problems in older people. There is no specific information comparing use of gemfibrozil in the elderly with use in other age groups.

**Other medicines**—Although certain medicines should not be used together at all, in other cases two different medicines may be used together even if an interaction might occur. In these cases, your doctor may want to change the dose, or other precautions may be necessary. When you are taking gemfibrozil it is especially important that your health care professional know if you are taking any of the following:

• Anticoagulants (blood thinners)—Use with gemfibrozil may increase the effect of the anticoagulant
• Lovastatin—Use with gemfibrozil may cause muscle or kidney problems or make them worse

**Other medical problems**—The presence of other medical problems may affect the use of gemfibrozil. Make sure you tell your doctor if you have any other medical problems, especially:

• Gallbladder disease or
• Gallstones—Gemfibrozil may make these conditions worse
• Kidney disease or
• Liver disease—Higher blood levels of gemfibrozil may result, which may increase the chance of side effects; a decrease in the dose of gemfibrozil may be needed

## Proper Use of This Medicine

*Use this medicine only as directed by your doctor.* Do not use more or less of it, and do not use it more often or for a longer time than your doctor ordered.

This medicine is usually taken twice a day. If you are taking 2 doses a day, it is best to take the medicine 30 minutes before your breakfast and evening meal.

*Follow carefully the special diet your doctor gave you.* This is the most important part of controlling your condition and is necessary if the medicine is to work properly.

**Dosing**—The dose of gemfibrozil will be different for different patients. *Follow your doctor's orders or the directions on the label.* The following information includes only the average doses of gemfibrozil. *If your dose is different, do not change it* unless your doctor tells you to do so:

• For *oral* dosage forms (tablets):
  —Adults: 600 milligrams two times a day to be taken thirty minutes before the morning and evening meals.

**Missed dose**—If you miss a dose of this medicine, take it as soon as possible. However, if it is almost time for

your next dose, skip the missed dose and go back to your regular dosing schedule. Do not double doses.

**Storage**—To store this medicine:

• Keep out of the reach of children.
• Store away from heat and direct light.
• Do not store in the bathroom, near the kitchen sink, or in other damp places. Heat or moisture may cause the medicine to break down.
• Do not keep outdated medicine or medicine no longer needed. Be sure that any discarded medicine is out of the reach of children.

## Precautions While Using This Medicine

*It is very important that your doctor check your progress at regular visits.* This will allow your doctor to see if the medicine is working properly to lower your cholesterol and triglyceride levels and to decide if you should continue to take it.

*Do not stop taking this medication without first checking with your doctor.* When you stop taking this medicine, your blood cholesterol levels may increase again. Your doctor may want you to follow a special diet to help prevent this from happening.

## Side Effects of This Medicine

Along with its needed effects, a medicine may cause some unwanted effects. Although not all of these side effects may occur, if they do occur they may need medical attention.

*Check with your doctor immediately* if any of the following side effects occur:

*Rare*
Cough or hoarseness; fever or chills; lower back or side pain; painful or difficult urination; stomach pain (severe) with nausea and vomiting

Check with your doctor as soon as possible if either of the following side effects occurs:

*Rare*
Muscle pain; unusual tiredness or weakness

Other side effects may occur that usually do not need medical attention. These side effects may go away during treatment as your body adjusts to the medicine. However, check with your doctor if any of the following side effects continue or are bothersome:

*More common*
Stomach pain, gas, or heartburn
*Less common*
Diarrhea; nausea or vomiting; skin rash

Other side effects not listed above may also occur in some patients. If you notice any other effects, check with your doctor.

Revised: 05/24/93

# GENTAMICIN   Ophthalmic

Some commonly used brand names are:

**In the U.S.—**

| | |
|---|---|
| Garamycin | Gentak |
| Genoptic Liquifilm | Gentrasul |
| Genoptic S.O.P. | Ocu-Mycin |
| Gentacidin | Spectro-Genta |
| Gentafair | |

Generic name product may also be available.

**In Canada—**

| | |
|---|---|
| Alcomicin | Gentrasul |
| Garamycin | |

Another commonly used name is gentamycin.

## Description

Gentamicin (jen-ta-MYE-sin) belongs to the family of medicines called antibiotics. Gentamicin ophthalmic preparations are used to treat infections of the eye.

Gentamicin is available only with your doctor's prescription, in the following dosage forms:

*Ophthalmic*
- Ophthalmic ointment (U.S. and Canada)
- Ophthalmic solution (eye drops) (U.S. and Canada)

## Before Using This Medicine

In deciding to use a medicine, the risks of using the medicine must be weighed against the good it will do. This is a decision you and your doctor will make. For ophthalmic gentamicin, the following should be considered:

**Allergies**—Tell your doctor if you have ever had any unusual or allergic reaction to this medicine or to any related antibiotic, such as amikacin (e.g., Amikin), gentamicin by injection (e.g., Garamycin), kanamycin (e.g., Kantrex), neomycin (e.g., Mycifradin), netilmicin (e.g., Netromycin), streptomycin, or tobramycin (e.g., Nebcin). Also tell your health care professional if you are allergic to any other substances, such as preservatives.

**Pregnancy**—Gentamicin ophthalmic preparations have not been shown to cause birth defects or other problems in humans.

**Breast-feeding**—Gentamicin ophthalmic preparations have not been reported to cause problems in nursing babies.

**Children**—Studies on this medicine have been done only in adult patients, and there is no specific information comparing use of this medicine in children with use in other age groups.

**Older adults**—Many medicines have not been studied specifically in older people. Therefore, it may not be known whether they work exactly the same way they do in younger adults or if they cause different side effects or problems in older people. There is no specific information comparing use of this medicine in the elderly with use in other age groups.

## Proper Use of This Medicine

For patients using the *eye drop form* of this medicine:
- The bottle is only partially full to provide proper drop control.
- To use:
  —First, wash your hands. Tilt the head back and with the index finger of one hand, press gently on the skin just beneath the lower eyelid and pull the lower eyelid away from the eye to make a space. Drop the medicine into this space. Let go of the eyelid and gently close the eyes. Do not blink. Keep the eyes closed for 1 or 2 minutes, to allow the medicine to come into contact with the infection.
- If you think you did not get the drop of medicine into your eye properly, use another drop.
- To keep the medicine as germ-free as possible, do not touch the applicator tip to any surface (including the eye). Also, keep the container tightly closed.

For patients using the *eye ointment form* of this medicine:
- First, wash your hands. Tilt the head back and with the index finger of one hand, press gently on the skin just beneath the lower eyelid and pull the lower eyelid away from the eye to make a space. Squeeze a thin strip of ointment into this space. A 1-cm (approximately ⅓-inch) strip of ointment is usually enough unless otherwise directed by your doctor. Let go of the eyelid and gently close the eyes and keep them closed for 1 or 2 minutes, to allow the medicine to come into contact with the infection.
- To keep the medicine as germ-free as possible, do not touch the applicator tip to any surface (including the eye). After using gentamicin eye ointment, wipe the tip of the ointment tube with a clean tissue and keep the tube tightly closed.

To help clear up your infection completely, *keep using this medicine for the full time of treatment,* even if your symptoms have disappeared. *Do not miss any doses.*

**Dosing**—The dose of ophthalmic gentamicin will be different for different patients. *Follow your doctor's orders or the directions on the label.* The following information includes only the average doses of ophthalmic gentamicin. *If your dose is different, do not change it* unless your doctor tells you to do so.
- For *ophthalmic ointment* dosage form:
  —For eye infections:
    - Adults and children—Use every eight to twelve hours.
- For *ophthalmic solution (eye drops)* dosage form:
  —For mild to moderate eye infections:
    - Adults and children—One drop every four hours.
  —For severe eye infections:
    - Adults and children—One drop every hour.

---

---

**Missed dose**—If you do miss a dose of this medicine, apply it as soon as possible. However, if it is almost time for your next dose, skip the missed dose and go back to your regular dosing schedule.

**Storage**—To store this medicine:
- Keep out of the reach of children.
- Store away from heat and direct light.
- Keep the medicine from freezing.
- Do not keep outdated medicine or medicine no longer needed. Be sure that any discarded medicine is out of the reach of children.

## Precautions While Using This Medicine

If your symptoms do not improve within a few days, or if they become worse, check with your doctor.

## Side Effects of This Medicine

Along with its needed effects, a medicine may cause some unwanted effects. Although not all of these side effects may occur, if they do occur they may need medical attention.

*Check with your doctor immediately* if any of the following side effects occur:

*Less common*
Itching, redness, swelling, or other sign of irritation not present before use of this medicine

Other side effects may occur that usually do not need medical attention. These side effects may go away during treatment as your body adjusts to the medicine. However, check with your doctor if either of the following side effects continues or is bothersome:

*Less common*
Burning or stinging

After application, eye ointments usually cause your vision to blur for a few minutes.

Other side effects not listed above may also occur in some patients. If you notice any other effects, check with your doctor.

Revised: 6/23/92
Interim revision: 8/30/93

# GENTAMICIN  Otic*

A commonly used brand name in Canada is Garamycin Otic Solution*.

*Not commercially available in the U.S.

## Description

Gentamicin (jen-ta-MYE-sin) belongs to the family of medicines called antibiotics. Gentamicin otic preparations are used to treat infections of the ear canal.

Gentamicin is available only with your doctor's prescription, in the following dosage form:

*Otic*
- Solution (Canada)

## Before Using This Medicine

In deciding to use a medicine, the risks of using the medicine must be weighed against the good it will do. This is a decision you and your doctor will make. For gentamicin otic preparations, the following should be considered:

**Allergies**—Tell your doctor if you have ever had any unusual or allergic reaction to this medicine or to any related antibiotics such as amikacin (e.g., Amikin), gentamicin by injection (e.g., Garamycin), kanamycin (e.g., Kantrex), neomycin (e.g., Mycifradin), netilmicin (e.g., Netromycin), streptomycin, or tobramycin (e.g., Nebcin). Also tell your health care professional if you are allergic to any other substances, such as preservatives.

**Pregnancy**—Gentamicin otic preparations have not been shown to cause birth defects or other problems in humans.

**Breast-feeding**—Gentamicin otic preparations have not been reported to cause problems in nursing babies.

**Children**—Although there is no specific information comparing use of this medicine in children with use in other age groups, this medicine is not expected to cause different side effects or problems in children than it does in adults.

**Older adults**—Many medicines have not been studied specifically in older people. Therefore, it may not be known whether they work exactly the same way they do in younger adults. Although there is no specific information comparing use of this medicine in the elderly with use in other age groups, this medicine is not expected to cause different side effects or problems in older people than it does in younger adults.

**Other medical problems**—The presence of other medical problems may affect the use of gentamicin otic preparations. Make sure you tell your doctor if you have any other medical problems, especially:
- Any other ear infection or problem (including punctured eardrum)—Use of gentamicin otic preparations in persons with this condition may lead to systemic absorption, and increase the chance of side effects

## Proper Use of This Medicine

To use:

- Lie down or tilt the head so that the infected ear faces up. Gently pull the earlobe up and back for adults (down and back for children) to straighten the ear canal. Drop the medicine into the ear canal. Keep the ear facing up for about 1 or 2 minutes to allow the medicine to come into contact with the infection. A sterile cotton plug may be gently inserted into the ear opening to prevent the medicine from leaking out.
- To keep the medicine as germ-free as possible, do not touch the applicator tip to any surface (including the ear). Also, keep the container tightly closed.

To help clear up your infection completely, *keep using this medicine for the full time of treatment,* even if your symptoms have disappeared. *Do not miss any doses.* .

**Dosing**—The dose of gentamicin otic will be different for different patients. *Follow your doctor's orders or the directions on the label.* The following information includes only the average doses of gentamicin otic. *If your dose is different, do not change it* unless your doctor tells you to do so.

- For *ear drops* dosage form:
  - —For ear infections:
    - Adults and children—Place three or four drops in the ear three times a day.

**Missed dose**—If you miss a dose of this medicine, apply it as soon as possible. However, if it is almost time for your next dose, skip the missed dose and go back to your regular dosing schedule.

**Storage**—To store this medicine:

- Keep out of the reach of children.
- Store away from heat and direct light.
- Keep the medicine from freezing.
- Do not keep outdated medicine or medicine no longer needed. Be sure that any discarded medicine is out of the reach of children.

## Precautions While Using This Medicine

If your symptoms do not improve within a few days, or if they become worse, check with your doctor.

## Side Effects of This Medicine

Along with its needed effects, a medicine may cause some unwanted effects. Although not all of these side effects may occur, if they do occur they may need medical attention.

*Check with your doctor immediately* if any of the following side effects occur:

*Less common*
> Itching, redness, swelling, or other sign of irritation not present before use of this medicine

Other side effects may occur that usually do not need medical attention. These side effects may go away during treatment as your body adjusts to the medicine. However, check with your doctor if either of the following side effects continues or is bothersome:

*Less common*
> Burning or stinging

Other side effects not listed above may also occur in some patients. If you notice any other effects, check with your doctor.

---

Revised: 08/12/92
Interim revision: 04/11/94

---

# GENTAMICIN   Topical

Some commonly used brand names are:

**In the U.S.—**
Garamycin                    G-Myticin
Gentamar
Generic name product may also be available.

**In Canada—**
Garamycin

## Description

Gentamicin (jen-ta-MYE-sin) belongs to the family of medicines called antibiotics. Gentamicin topical preparations are used to treat infections of the skin.

Gentamicin is available only with your doctor's prescription, in the following dosage forms:

*Topical*
- Cream (U.S. and Canada)
- Ointment (U.S. and Canada)

## Before Using This Medicine

In deciding to use a medicine, the risks of using the medicine must be weighed against the good it will do. This is a decision you and your doctor will make. For topical gentamicin, the following should be considered:

**Allergies**—Tell your doctor if you have ever had any unusual or allergic reaction to this medicine or any related antibiotics, such as amikacin (e.g., Amikin), gentamicin by injection (e.g., Garamycin), kanamycin (e.g., Kantrex), neomycin (e.g., Mycifradin), netilmicin (e.g., Netromycin), streptomycin, or tobramycin (e.g., Nebcin). Also tell your health care professional if you are allergic to any other substances, such as preservatives or dyes.

**Pregnancy**—Gentamicin topical preparations have not been shown to cause birth defects or other problems in humans.

**Breast-feeding**—Gentamicin topical preparations have not been reported to cause problems in nursing babies.

**Children**—This medicine has been tested in children over 1 year of age and, in effective doses, has not been shown to cause different side effects or problems than it does in adults.

**Older adults**—Many medicine have not been studied specifically in older people. Therefore, it may not be known whether they work exactly the same way they do in younger adults. Although there is no specific information comparing use of this medicine in the elderly with use in other age groups, this medicine is not expected to cause different side effects or problems in older people than it does in younger adults.

**Other medicines**—Although certain medicines should not be used together at all, in other cases two different medicines may be used together even if an interaction might occur. In these cases, your doctor may want to change the dose, or other precautions may be necessary. Tell your health care professional if you are using any other topical prescription or nonprescription (over-the-counter [OTC]) medicine that is to be applied to the same area of the skin.

## Proper Use of This Medicine

Before applying this medicine, wash the affected area with soap and water, and dry thoroughly. Apply a small amount to the affected area and rub in gently.

After this medicine is applied, the treated area may be covered with a gauze dressing if desired.

To help clear up your infection completely, *keep using this medicine for the full time of treatment,* even though your symptoms may have disappeared. *Do not miss any doses.*

**Dosing**—The dose of topical gentamicin will be different for different patients. *Follow your doctor's orders or the directions on the label.* The following information includes only the average dose of topical gentamicin. *If your dose is different, do not change it* unless your doctor tells you to do so.

- For *topical* dosage forms (cream or ointment):
  —For bacterial infections:
    - Adults and children 1 year of age and over— Apply to affected area(s) of the skin three or four times a day.

**Missed dose**—If you miss a dose of this medicine, apply it as soon as possible. However, if it is almost time for your next dose, skip the missed dose and go back to your regular dosing schedule.

**Storage**—To store this medicine:
- Keep out of the reach of children.
- Store away from heat and direct light.
- Keep the medicine from freezing.
- Do not keep outdated medicine or medicine no longer needed. Be sure that any discarded medicine is out of the reach of children.

## Precautions While Using This Medicine

If your skin problem does not improve within 1 week, or if it becomes worse, check with your doctor.

## Side Effects of This Medicine

Along with its needed effects, a medicine may cause some unwanted effects. Although not all of these side effects may occur, if they do occur they may need medical attention.

*Check with your doctor immediately* if any of the following side effects occur:

*Less common*
    Itching, redness, swelling, or other sign of irritation not present before use of this medicine

Other side effects not listed above may also occur in some patients. If you notice any other effects, check with your doctor.

Revised: 06/23/92
Interim revision: 06/08/94

# GENTIAN VIOLET    Topical†

†Not commercially available in Canada.

## Description

Gentian violet (JEN-shun VYE-oh-let) belongs to the group of medicines called antifungals. Topical gentian violet is used to treat some types of fungus infections inside the mouth (thrush) and of the skin.

Gentian violet is available without a prescription; however, your doctor may have special instructions on the proper use of gentian violet for your medical condition.

Gentian violet is available in the following dosage form:
*Topical*
- Solution (U.S.)

## Before Using This Medicine

If you are using this medicine without a prescription, carefully read and follow any precautions on the label. For gentian violet, the following should be considered:

**Allergies**—Tell your doctor if you have ever had any unusual or allergic reaction to gentian violet. Also tell your health care professional if you are allergic to any other substances, such as preservatives or dyes.

**Pregnancy**—Gentian violet topical solution has not been shown to cause birth defects or other problems in humans.

**Breast-feeding**—Gentian violet topical solution has not been reported to cause problems in nursing babies.

**Children**—Although there is no specific information comparing use of this medicine in children with use in other age groups, this medicine is not expected to cause different side effects or problems in children than it does in adults.

**Older adults**—Many medicines have not been studied specifically in older people. Therefore, it may not be known whether they work exactly the same way they do in younger adults. Although there is no specific information comparing use of this medicine in the elderly with use in other age groups, this medicine is not expected to cause different side effects or problems in older people than it does in younger adults.

**Other medical problems**—The presence of other medical problems may affect the use of gentian violet. Make sure you tell your doctor if you have any other medical problems, especially:
- Ulcerative skin condition on the face—Use of gentian violet may cause tattooing of the area

## Proper Use of This Medicine

Using a cotton swab, apply enough gentian violet to cover only the affected area.

If you are applying this medicine to affected areas in the mouth, avoid swallowing any of the medicine.

If you are using this medicine in a child's mouth, make sure you understand exactly how to apply it so that it is not swallowed. If you have any questions about this, check with your health care professional.

*Do not apply an occlusive dressing (airtight covering, such as kitchen plastic wrap) over this medicine.* It may cause irritation of the skin.

To help clear up your infection completely, *keep using this medicine for the full time of treatment,* even if your condition has improved. *Do not miss any doses.*

**Dosing**—The dose of gentian violet will be different for different patients. *Follow your doctor's orders or the directions on the label.* The following information includes only the average dose of gentian violet. *If your dose is different, do not change it* unless your doctor tells you to do so.
- For *topical solution* dosage form:
  —For fungus infections:
    - Adults and children—Apply to the affected area(s) of the skin two or three times a day for three days.

**Missed dose**—If you miss a dose of this medicine, apply it as soon as possible. However, if it is almost time for your next dose, skip the missed dose and go back to your regular dosing schedule.

**Storage**—To store this medicine:
- Keep out of the reach of children.
- Store away from heat and direct light.
- Keep the medicine from freezing.
- Do not keep outdated medicine or medicine no longer needed. Be sure that any discarded medicine is out of the reach of children.

## Precautions While Using This Medicine

*Gentian violet will stain the skin and clothing.* Avoid getting the medicine on your clothes.

## Side Effects of This Medicine

Along with its needed effects, a medicine may cause some unwanted effects. Although not all of these side effects may occur, if they do occur they may need medical attention.

Check with your doctor as soon as possible if the following side effect occurs:

Skin irritation not present before use of this medicine

Other side effects not listed above may also occur in some patients. If you notice any other effects, check with your doctor.

Revised: 06/23/92
Interim revision: 06/22/94

# GENTIAN VIOLET   Vaginal

A commonly used brand name in the U.S. is Genapax.

## Description

Vaginal gentian violet (JEN-shun VYE-oh-let) is used to treat fungus (yeast) infections.

Vaginal gentian violet is available only with your doctor's prescription, in the following dosage form:

*Vaginal*
- Tampons (U.S.)

## Before Using This Medicine

In deciding to use a medicine, the risks of using the medicine must be weighed against the good it will do. This is a decision you and your doctor will make. For gentian violet, the following should be considered:

**Allergies**—Tell your doctor if you have ever had any unusual or allergic reaction to gentian violet. Also tell your health care professional if you are allergic to any other substances, such as foods, preservatives, or dyes.

**Pregnancy**—Studies on effects in pregnancy have not been done in either humans or animals.

**Breast-feeding**—It is not known whether gentian violet, applied to the vagina, is absorbed into the body and passes into the breast milk. However, gentian violet tampons have not been reported to cause problems in nursing babies.

**Children**—Studies on this medicine have been done only in adult patients, and there is no specific information comparing use of vaginal gentian violet in children with use in other age groups.

**Older adults**—Many medicines have not been studied specifically in older people. Therefore, it may not be known whether they work exactly the same way they do in younger adults. Although there is no specific information comparing use of vaginal gentian violet in the elderly with use in other age groups, this medicine is not expected to cause different side effects or problems in older people than it does in younger adults.

**Other medicines**—Although certain medicines should not be used together at all, in other cases two different medicines may be used together even if an interaction might occur. In these cases, your doctor may want to change the dose, or other precautions may be necessary. Tell your health care professional if you are using any other vaginal prescription or nonprescription (over-the-counter [OTC]) medicine.

## Proper Use of This Medicine

Gentian violet usually comes with patient directions. Read them carefully before using this medicine.

After insertion, remove the tampon from the vagina after 3 to 4 hours unless otherwise directed by your doctor.

To help clear up your infection completely, *keep using this medicine for the full time of treatment,* even though your condition may have improved. *Do not miss any doses.*

While you are using gentian violet tampons, the use of regular (non-medicated) tampons is not recommended. They will soak up the medicine that stays in the vagina after the gentian violet tampon is taken out. During your menstrual period you should wear a minipad or sanitary napkin instead.

**Dosing**—The dose of gentian violet will be different for different patients. *Follow your doctor's orders or the directions on the label.* The following information includes only the average doses of gentian violet. *If your dose is different, do not change it* unless your doctor tells you to do so.

- For *vaginal* dosage form (tampons):
  —For treating a vaginal fungus (yeast) infection:
    • Adults and teenagers—5 milligrams (one tampon) inserted into your vagina one or two times a day for twelve days in a row. The tampon should be left in your vagina for three to four hours.

**Missed dose**—If you miss a dose of this medicine, insert it as soon as possible. However, if it is almost time for your next dose, skip the missed dose and go back to your regular dosing schedule.

**Storage**—To store this medicine:
- Keep out of the reach of children.
- Store away from heat and direct light.
- Do not keep outdated medicine or medicine no longer needed. Be sure that any discarded medicine is out of the reach of children.

## Precautions While Using This Medicine

If your symptoms do not improve within a few days, or if they become worse, check with your doctor.

Gentian violet will stain the skin and clothing. Vaginal medicines usually will come out of the vagina during treatment. To keep the medicine from getting on your clothing, wear a minipad or sanitary napkin.

*To help clear up your infection completely and to help make sure it does not return, good health habits are also needed.*

- Wear cotton panties (or panties or pantyhose with cotton crotches) instead of synthetic (for example, nylon or rayon) panties.
- Wear only clean panties.

If you have any questions about this, check with your health care professional.

Many vaginal infections are spread by having sex. A male sexual partner may carry the germs on or in his penis. While you are using this medicine, it may be a good idea for your partner to wear a condom during sex to avoid re-infection. Also, your partner may need to be treated. *Do not stop using this medicine if you have sex during treatment.*

Some women may want to use a douche before putting each dose in the vagina. Some doctors will allow the use of a vinegar and water douche or other douche. However, others do not allow any douching. If you do use a douche, *do not overfill the vagina.* To do so may push the douche up into the uterus and possibly cause inflammation or infection. Also, *do not douche if you are pregnant since this may harm the fetus.* If you have any questions about this, check with your health care professional.

## Side Effects of This Medicine

Along with its needed effects, a medicine may cause some unwanted effects. Although not all of these side effects

may occur, if they do occur they may need medical attention.

Check with your doctor as soon as possible if any of the following side effects occur:

> Vaginal burning, itching, pain, or other sign of irritation not present before use of this medicine

Other side effects not listed above may also occur in some patients. If you notice any other effects, check with your doctor.

Revised: 10/26/92
Interim revision: 06/04/94

# GLUCAGON   Systemic

A commonly used brand name in the U.S. and Canada is Glucagon Emergency Kit.

## Description

Glucagon (GLOO-ka-gon) belongs to the group of medicines called hormones. It is an emergency medicine used to treat severe hypoglycemia (low blood sugar) in patients with diabetes who have passed out or cannot take some form of sugar by mouth.

Glucagon is also used during x-ray tests of the stomach and bowels. Glucagon helps to improve test results by relaxing the muscles of the stomach and bowels. This also makes the testing more comfortable for the patient.

Glucagon may also be used for other conditions as determined by your doctor.

Glucagon is available only with your doctor's prescription, in the following dosage form:

*Parenteral*
- Injection (U.S. and Canada)

## Before Using This Medicine

In deciding to use a medicine, the risks of taking the medicine must be weighed against the good it will do. This is a decision you and your doctor will make. For glucagon, the following should be considered:

**Allergies**—Tell your doctor if you have ever had any unusual or allergic reaction to glucagon or other proteins. Also, tell your health care professional if you are allergic to any other substances, such as foods, preservatives, or dyes.

**Pregnancy**—Glucagon has not been studied in pregnant women. However, glucagon has not been shown to cause birth defects or other problems in animal studies.

**Breast-feeding**—It is not known whether glucagon passes into breast milk. However, this medicine has not been reported to cause problems in nursing babies.

**Children**—This medicine has been tested in children and, in effective doses, has not been shown to cause different side effects or problems than it does in adults.

**Older adults**—Many medicines have not been studied specifically in older people. Therefore, it may not be known whether they work exactly the same way they do in younger adults. Although there is no specific information comparing use of glucagon in the elderly with use in other age groups, it is not expected to cause different side effects or problems in older people than it does in younger adults.

**Other medicines**—Although certain medicines should not be used together at all, in other cases two different medicines may be used together even if an interaction might occur. In these cases, your doctor may want to change the doses or other precautions may be necessary. Tell your health care professional if you are using any other prescription or nonprescription (over-the-counter [OTC]) medicine.

**Other medical problems**—The presence of other medical problems may affect the use of glucagon. Make sure you tell your doctor if you have any other medical problems, especially:

- Diabetes mellitus—When glucagon is used for test or x-ray procedures in diabetes that is well-controlled, too high blood sugar may occur; otherwise, glucagon is an important part of the management of diabetes because it is used to treat hypoglycemia (low blood sugar)
- Insulinoma (tumors of the pancreas gland that make too much insulin) (or history of)—Blood sugar concentrations may decrease
- Pheochromocytoma—Glucagon can cause high blood pressure

## Proper Use of This Medicine

**Dosing**—The dose of glucagon will be different for different patients. *Follow your doctor's orders or the directions on the label.* The following information includes only the average doses of glucagon. *If your dose is different, do not change it* unless your doctor tells you to do so.

- As an *emergency treatment for hypoglycemia:*
  —Adults and adolescents: 0.5 to 1 milligram. The dose may be repeated in 20 minutes if necessary.
  —Children: Dose is based on body weight (25 micrograms of glucagon per kilogram [11.4 micrograms per pound] of body weight). The dose may be repeated in 20 minutes if necessary.

Glucagon is an emergency medicine and must be used only as directed by your doctor. *Make sure that you and your family or a friend understand exactly when and how to use this medicine before it must be used.*

Some brands of glucagon come in a kit of 2 vials (one powder containing the medicine and one liquid to mix the medicine with). The contents of these 2 vials must be mixed before use. Other brands of glucagon are packaged in a kit with a vial of powder containing the medicine and a syringe filled with liquid to mix the medicine with. *Directions for mixing and injecting are in the package. Read them carefully* and ask your health care professional for additional explanation, if necessary.

If your glucagon kit does not already have a syringe in it, your doctor may want you to inject glucagon with the type of syringe you normally use to inject your insulin. Other patients may be told to use a different type of syringe that will allow a deeper injection. If you have any questions about the type of syringe you should be using, check with your health care professional. Also, you should *regularly check to see if you have a sterile syringe and needles always available* to be used for the glucagon. It is a good idea to keep a sterile syringe taped to the glucagon carton.

Glucagon is usually mixed when an emergency occurs. However, it may be mixed ahead of time and kept in the refrigerator, ready for use. The date of mixing should then be written on the package. Mixed glucagon kept more than 48 hours (2 full days) (even if it is refrigerated) should be discarded and replaced by a fresh preparation.

Glucagon should not be mixed after the expiration date printed on the kit and on one vial. *Check the date regularly and replace the medicine before it expires.* The printed expiration date does not apply after mixing.

**Storage**—To store this medicine:
- Keep out of the reach of children.
- Store away from heat and direct light.
- Store the unmixed medication at room temperature.
- Do not store the unmixed or mixed medication in the bathroom, near the kitchen sink, or in other damp places. Heat or moisture may cause the medicine to break down.
- Store the mixed solution in the refrigerator for no longer than 48 hours. Do not allow it to freeze.
- Do not keep outdated medicine or medicine no longer needed. Be sure that any discarded medicine is out of the reach of children.

## Precautions While Using This Medicine

*Diabetic patients should be aware of the symptoms of hypoglycemia (low blood sugar). These symptoms may develop in a very short time and may result from:*
- using too much insulin ("insulin reaction") or as a side effect from oral antidiabetes medicines.
- delaying or missing a scheduled snack or meal.
- sickness (especially with vomiting).
- exercising more than usual.

*Unless corrected, hypoglycemia will lead to unconsciousness, convulsions (seizures), and possibly death. Early symptoms of hypoglycemia include:*
Abdominal or stomach pain (mild)
Anxious feeling
Chills (continuing)
Cold sweats
Confusion
Cool pale skin
Difficulty in concentrating
Drowsiness
Excessive hunger
Fast heartbeat
Headache (continuing)
Nausea or vomiting (continuing)
Nervousness
Shakiness
Unsteady walk
Unusual tiredness or weakness
Vision changes

- Symptoms of hypoglycemia can differ from person to person. It is important that you learn your own signs of low blood sugar so that you can treat it quickly. It is a good idea also to check your blood sugar to confirm that it is low.
- *Eat or drink something containing sugar and check with your doctor right away if mild symptoms of low blood sugar (hypoglycemia) appear.* Doing this when symptoms of hypoglycemia first appear will usually prevent them from getting worse, and will probably make the use of glucagon unnecessary. Good sources of sugar include glucose tablets or gel, fruit juice, corn syrup, honey, nondiet soft drinks, or sugar cubes or table sugar (dissolved in water).
- *Tell someone to take you to your doctor or to a hospital right away if the symptoms do not improve after eating or drinking a sweet food. Do not try to drive yourself.*
- Even if you correct these symptoms by eating sugar, it is very important to call your doctor or hospital emergency service right away. Then, eat some food (such as crackers and cheese, half a sandwich, or milk) to keep your blood sugar from going down again.

- Check your blood sugar again to make sure it is not still too low.
- *If severe symptoms such as convulsions (seizures) or unconsciousness occur, diabetics should not eat or drink anything.* There is a chance that they could choke from not swallowing correctly. Emergency medical help should be obtained immediately.

*If it becomes necessary to inject glucagon in an unconscious patient, a family member or friend should know the following:*

- *After injection, turn the unconscious patient on his or her side.* Glucagon may cause some patients to vomit and this position will reduce the possibility of choking.
- *Call the patient's doctor at once.*
- The patient should become conscious in less than 15 minutes after glucagon is injected into the muscle, but if not, a second dose may be given. *Get the patient to a doctor or to hospital emergency care as soon as possible,* since being unconscious too long can be harmful.
- *When the patient is conscious and can swallow, give some form of sugar.* Glucagon is not effective for much longer than 1½ hours and is *used only until the patient is able to swallow.* Fruit juice, corn syrup, honey, and sugar cubes or table sugar (dissolved in water) all work quickly. Then, if a snack or meal is not scheduled for an hour or more, the patient should also eat some crackers and cheese or half a sandwich, or drink a glass of milk. This will prevent hypoglycemia from occurring again before the next meal or snack.
- The patient or care-giver should continue to monitor the patient's blood sugar. For about 3 to 4 hours after the patient is conscious, check his or her blood sugar every hour.
- *If nausea prevents a patient from swallowing some form of sugar for an hour after glucagon is given, medical help should be obtained.*

*Keep your doctor informed of any hypoglycemic episodes or use of glucagon even if the symptoms are successfully controlled and there seem to be no continuing problems.* Complete information is necessary to provide the best possible treatment of any condition.

*Replace your supply* of glucagon as soon as possible, in case another hypoglycemic episode occurs.

You should wear a medical I.D. bracelet or chain at all times. In addition, you should carry an identification card that lists your medical conditions and medications.

## Side Effects of This Medicine

Along with its needed effects, a medicine may cause some unwanted effects. Although not all of these side effects may occur, if they do occur they may need medical attention.

*Get emergency help immediately* if any of the following side effects occur:

*Less common*
Dizziness; lightheadedness; trouble in breathing

*Symptoms of overdose*
Irregular heartbeat; loss of appetite; muscle cramps or pain; nausea (continuing); vomiting (continuing); weakness of arms, legs, and trunk (severe)

Check with your doctor as soon as possible if any of the following side effects occur:

*Less common*
Skin rash or hives

Other side effects may occur that usually do not need medical attention. These side effects may go away during treatment as your body adjusts to the medicine. However, check with your doctor if any of the following side effects continue or are bothersome:

Nausea; vomiting

Other side effects not listed above may also occur in some patients. If you notice any other effects, check with your doctor.

## Additional Information

Once a medicine has been approved for marketing for a certain use, experience may show that it is also useful for other medical problems. Although these uses are not included in product labeling, glucagon is used in certain patients with the following medical conditions or undergoing certain medical procedures:

- Overdose of beta-blocker medicines
- Overdose of calcium channel blockers
- Removing food or an object stuck in the esophagus
- Hysterosalpingography (x-ray examination of the uterus and fallopian tubes)

Other than the above information, there is no additional information relating to proper use, precautions, or side effects for these uses.

Revised: 01/13/93

# GLUTETHIMIDE   Systemic†

Generic name product may be available in the U.S.

†Not commercially available in Canada.

## Description

Glutethimide (gloo-TETH-i-mide) is used to treat insomnia (trouble in sleeping). However, it has generally been replaced by safer and more effective medicines for the treatment of insomnia. If glutethimide is used regularly (for example, every day) to help produce sleep, it is usually not effective for more than 7 days.

This medicine is available only with your doctor's prescription, in the following dosage forms:

*Oral*
- Capsules (U.S.)
- Tablets (U.S.)

## Before Using This Medicine

In deciding to use a medicine, the risks of taking the medicine must be weighed against the good it will do. This is a decision you and your doctor will make. For glutethimide the following should be considered:

**Allergies**—Tell your doctor if you have ever had any unusual or allergic reaction to glutethimide. Also tell your health care professional if you are allergic to any other substances, such as foods, preservatives, or dyes.

**Pregnancy**—Studies of effects in pregnancy have not been done in either humans or animals. However, too much use of glutethimide during pregnancy may cause the baby to become dependent on the medicine. This may lead to withdrawal side effects after birth.

**Breast-feeding**—Glutethimide passes into the breast milk and may cause drowsiness in nursing babies.

**Children**—Studies on this medicine have been done only in adult patients and there is no specific information comparing use of glutethimide in children with use in other age groups.

**Older adults**—Elderly people may be especially sensitive to the effects of glutethimide. This may increase the chance of side effects during treatment.

**Other medicines**—Although certain medicines should not be used together at all, in other cases 2 different medicines may be used together even if an interaction might occur. In these cases, your doctor may want to change the dose, or other precautions may be necessary. When you are taking glutethimide it is especially important that your health care professional know if you are taking any of the following:
- Anticoagulants (blood thinners)—Glutethimide may change the amount of anticoagulant you need to take
- Central nervous system (CNS) depressants, other (medicine that causes drowsiness) or

- Tricyclic antidepressants (medicine for depression)—Using these medicines together with glutethimide may increase the CNS and other depressant effects

**Other medical problems**—The presence of other medical problems may affect the use of glutethimide. Make sure you tell your doctor if you have any other medical problems, especially:
- Enlarged prostate or
- Intestinal blockage or
- Irregular heartbeat or
- Porphyria or
- Stomach ulcer or
- Urinary tract blockage—Glutethimide may make the condition worse
- Kidney disease—Higher blood levels of glutethimide may result and increase the chance of side effects

## Proper Use of This Medicine

*Take this medicine only as directed by your doctor.* Do not take more of it, do not take it more often, and do not take it for a longer time than your doctor ordered. If too much is taken, it may become habit-forming.

**Dosing**—The dose of glutethimide will be different for different patients. *Follow your doctor's orders or the directions on the label.* The following information includes only the average doses of glutethimide. *If your dose is different, do not change it* unless your doctor tells you to do so.
- For *oral* dosage forms (capsules or tablets):
  —Adults: 500 milligrams (1 capsule or tablet) at bedtime.
  —Children: Dose must be determined by the doctor.

**Storage**—To store this medicine:
- Keep out of the reach of children since overdose is especially dangerous in children.
- Store away from heat and direct light.
- Do not store in the bathroom, near the kitchen sink, or in other damp places. Heat or moisture may cause the medicine to break down.
- Do not keep outdated medicine or medicine no longer needed. Be sure that any discarded medicine is out of the reach of children.

## Precautions While Using This Medicine

If you will be taking this medicine regularly for a long time:
- Your doctor should check your progress at regular visits.
- Do not stop taking it without first checking with your doctor. Your doctor may want you to reduce gradually the amount you are taking before stopping completely.

This medicine will add to the effects of alcohol and other CNS depressants (medicines that slow down the nervous system, possibly causing drowsiness). Some examples of CNS depressants are antihistamines or medicine for hay fever, other allergies, or colds; sedatives, tranquilizers, or sleeping medicine; prescription pain medicine or narcotics; barbiturates; medicine for seizures; muscle relaxants; or anesthetics, including some dental anesthetics. *Check with your doctor before taking any of the above while you are using this medicine.*

Before you have any medical tests, tell the doctor in charge that you are taking this medicine. The results of the metyrapone test may be affected by this medicine.

*If you think you or someone else may have taken an overdose of this medicine, get emergency help at once.* Taking an overdose of glutethimide or taking alcohol or other CNS depressants with glutethimide may lead to unconsciousness and possibly death. Some signs of an overdose are continuing confusion, severe weakness, shortness of breath or slow or troubled breathing, convulsions (seizures), slurred speech, staggering, and slow heartbeat.

This medicine may cause some people to become dizzy, drowsy, or less alert than they are normally. Even if taken at bedtime, it may cause some people to feel drowsy or less alert on arising. *Make sure you know how you react to this medicine before you drive, use machines, or do anything else that could be dangerous if you are dizzy or are not alert.*

## Side Effects of This Medicine

Along with its needed effects, a medicine may cause some unwanted effects. Although not all of these side effects may occur, if they do occur they may need medical attention.

Check with your doctor as soon as possible if any of the following side effects occur:

*Less common*
    Skin rash

*Rare*
    Sore throat and fever; unusual bleeding or bruising; unusual excitement; unusual tiredness or weakness

*Symptoms of overdose*
    Bluish coloration of skin; confusion (continuing); convulsions (seizures); fever; low body temperature; memory problems; muscle spasms or twitching; shortness of breath or slow or troubled breathing; slow heartbeat; slowness or loss of reflexes; slurred speech; staggering; trembling; trouble in concentrating; weakness (severe)

Other side effects may occur that usually do not need medical attention. These side effects may go away during treatment as your body adjusts to the medicine. However, check with your doctor if any of the following side effects continue or are bothersome:

*More common*
    Drowsiness (daytime)

*Less common*
    Blurred vision; clumsiness or unsteadiness; confusion; dizziness; "hangover" effect; headache; nausea; vomiting

After you stop using this medicine, your body may need time to adjust. The length of time this takes depends on the amount of medicine you were using and how long you used it. During this period of time check with your doctor if you notice any of the following side effects:

    Convulsions (seizures); fast heartbeat; hallucinations (seeing, hearing, or feeling things that are not there); increased dreaming; muscle cramps or spasms; nausea or vomiting; nightmares; stomach cramps or pain; trembling; trouble in sleeping

Other side effects not listed above may also occur in some patients. If you notice any other effects, check with your doctor.

Revised: 05/12/93

---

# GLYCERIN   Systemic

Some commonly used brand names in the U.S. are Glyrol and Osmoglyn.
Generic name product may also be available in the U.S.

## Description

Glycerin (GLI-ser-in), when taken by mouth, is used to treat certain conditions in which there is increased eye pressure, such as glaucoma. It may also be used before eye surgery to reduce pressure in the eye.

Glycerin may also be used for other conditions as determined by your doctor.

This medicine is available only with your doctor's prescription, in the following dosage form:
*Oral*
    • Oral solution (U.S.)

## Before Using This Medicine

In deciding to use a medicine, the risks of taking the medicine must be weighed against the good it will do. This is a decision you and your doctor will make. For glycerin, the following should be considered:

**Allergies**—Tell your doctor if you have ever had any unusual or allergic reaction to glycerin. Also tell your health care professional if you are allergic to any other substances, such as foods, preservatives, or dyes.

**Pregnancy**—Studies on effects in pregnancy have not been done in either humans or animals.

**Breast-feeding**—It is not known whether glycerin passes into breast milk. This medicine has not been reported to cause problems in nursing babies.

**Children**—Although there is no specific information comparing use of glycerin in children with use in other age groups, this medicine is not expected to cause different side effects or problems in children than it does in adults.

**Older adults**—Glycerin reduces water in the body, and there may be an increased risk that elderly patients taking it could become dehydrated.

**Other medicines**—Although certain medicines should not be used together at all, in other cases two different medicines may be used together even if an interaction might occur. In these cases, your doctor may want to change the dose, or other precautions may be necessary. Tell your health care professional if you are taking any other prescription or nonprescription (over-the-counter [OTC]) medicine.

**Other medical problems**—The presence of other medical problems may affect the use of glycerin. Make sure you tell your doctor if you have any other medical problems, especially:
- Diabetes mellitus (sugar diabetes)—Use of glycerin may increase the chance of dehydration (loss of too much body water)
- Confused mental states or
- Heart disease or
- Kidney disease—Glycerin may make these conditions worse

## Proper Use of This Medicine

*It is very important that you take this medicine only as directed.* Do not take more of it and do not take it more often than your doctor ordered.

To improve the taste of this medicine, mix it with a small amount of unsweetened lemon, lime, or orange juice, pour over cracked ice, and sip through a straw.

**Dosing**—The dose of glycerin will be different for different patients. *Follow your doctor's orders or the directions on the label.* The following information includes only the average doses of glycerin. *If your dose is different, do not change it* unless your doctor tells you to do so.
- For *oral* dosage form (oral solution):
  —To lower pressure in the eye:
    - Adults—Dose is based on body weight and must be determined by your doctor. The usual dose is 1 to 2 grams per kilogram (kg) (0.45 to 0.91 grams per pound) of body weight taken one time. Then, additional doses of 500 milligrams (mg) per kg (227 mg per pound) of body weight every six hours may be taken if needed.
    - Children—Dose is based on body weight and must be determined by your doctor. The usual dose is 1 to 1.5 grams per kg (0.45 to 0.68 grams per pound) of body weight taken one time. The dose may be repeated in four to eight hours if needed.

**Missed dose**—If you miss a dose of this medicine, take it as soon as possible. However, if it is almost time for your next dose, skip the missed dose and go back to your regular dosing schedule. Do not double doses.

**Storage**—To store this medicine:
- Keep out of the reach of children.
- Store away from heat and direct light.
- Do not store in the bathroom, near the kitchen sink, or in other damp places. Heat or moisture may cause the medicine to break down.
- Keep the medicine from freezing.
- Do not keep outdated medicine or medicine no longer needed. Be sure that any discarded medicine is out of the reach of children.

## Precautions While Using This Medicine

Your doctor should check your progress at regular visits to make sure that this medicine is working properly.

In some patients, headaches may occur when this medicine is taken. To help prevent or relieve the headache, lie down while you are taking this medicine and for a short time after taking it. If headaches become severe or continue, check with your doctor.

## Side Effects of This Medicine

Along with its needed effects, a medicine may cause some unwanted effects. Although not all of these side effects may occur, if they do occur they may need medical attention.

Check with your doctor as soon as possible if either of the following side effects occurs:

*Less common*
Confusion
*Rare*
Irregular heartbeat

Other side effects may occur that usually do not need medical attention. These side effects may go away during treatment as your body adjusts to the medicine. However, check with your doctor if any of the following side effects continue or are bothersome:

*More common*
Headache; nausea or vomiting
*Less common*
Diarrhea; dizziness; dryness of mouth or increased thirst

Other side effects not listed above may also occur in some patients. If you notice any other effects, check with your doctor.

## Additional Information

Once a medicine has been approved for marketing for a certain use, experience may show that it is also useful for other medical problems. Although this use is not included in product labeling, glycerin is used in certain patients with the following medical conditions:

- Cerebral edema (swelling of the brain)

Other than the above information, there is no additional information relating to proper use, precautions, or side effects for these uses.

---

Revised: 08/03/94

---

# GOLD COMPOUNDS    Systemic

Some commonly used brand names are:

**In the U.S.—**

Myochrysine[3]          Solganal[2]
Ridaura[1]

**In Canada—**

Myochrysine[3]          Ridaura[1]

Note: For quick reference, the following gold compounds are numbered to match the corresponding brand names.

This information applies to the following medicines:

1. Auranofin (au-RANE-oh-fin)
2. Aurothioglucose (aur-oh-thye-oh-GLOO-kose)
3. Gold Sodium Thiomalate (gold SO-dee-um thye-oh-MAH-late)‡

---

‡Generic name product may also be available in the U.S.

---

## Description

The gold compounds are used in the treatment of rheumatoid arthritis. They may also be used for other conditions as determined by your doctor.

In addition to the helpful effects of this medicine in treating your medical problem, it has side effects that can be very serious. Before you take this medicine, you should discuss with your doctor the good that this medicine will do as well as the risks of using it.

Auranofin is available only with your doctor's prescription. The other gold compounds are given by your health care professional.

These medicines are available in the following dosage forms:

*Oral*

Auranofin
- Capsules (U.S. and Canada)

*Parenteral*

Aurothioglucose
- Injection (U.S.)
Gold sodium thiomalate
- Injection (U.S. and Canada)

## Before Using This Medicine

In deciding to use a medicine, the risks of taking the medicine must be weighed against the good it will do.

This is a decision you and your doctor will make. For gold compounds, the following should be considered:

**Allergies**—Tell your doctor if you have ever had any unusual or allergic reaction to gold or other metals, if you have received a gold compound before and developed serious side effects from it, or if any medicine you have taken has caused an allergy or a reaction that affected your blood. Also tell your health care professional if you are allergic to any other substances, such as foods, preservatives, or dyes.

**Pregnancy**—Studies on birth defects with gold compounds have not been done in humans. However, studies in animals have shown that gold compounds may cause birth defects.

**Breast-feeding**—Aurothioglucose and gold sodium thiomalate pass into the breast milk and may cause unwanted effects in nursing babies. It is not known whether auranofin passes into the breast milk.

**Children**—Auranofin has been tested only in adult patients and there is no specific information about its use in children. However, aurothioglucose and gold sodium thiomalate have been tested in children and have not been shown to cause different side effects or problems than they do in adults.

**Older adults**—These medicines have been tested and have not been shown to cause different side effects or problems in older people than they do in younger adults.

**Other medicines**—Although certain medicines should not be used together at all, in other cases two different medicines may be used together even if an interaction might occur. In these cases, your doctor may want to change the dose, or other precautions may be necessary. When you are taking a gold compound, it is important that your health care professional know if you are taking *any* other prescription or nonprescription (over-the-counter [OTC]) medicine, especially:

- Penicillamine (e.g., Cuprimine)—The chance of side effects may be increased.

**Other medical problems**—The presence of other medical problems may affect the use of gold compounds. Make sure you tell your doctor if you have any other medical problems, especially:

- Blood or blood vessel disease or
- Colitis or
- Kidney disease (or history of) or
- Lupus erythematosus or
- Sjögren's syndrome or
- Skin disease—The chance of unwanted effects may be increased

## Proper Use of This Medicine

In order for this medicine to work, it must be taken regularly as ordered by your doctor. Continue receiving the injections or taking auranofin even if you think the medicine is not working. You may not notice the effects of this medicine until after three to six months of regular use.

For patients taking *auranofin:*

- *Do not take more of this medicine than ordered by your doctor.* Taking too much auranofin may increase the chance of serious unwanted effects.

If you have any questions about this, check with your doctor.

**Dosing**—The dose of these medicines will be different for different patients. *Follow your doctor's orders or the directions on the label.* The following information includes only the average doses of these medicines. *If your dose is different, do not change it* unless your doctor tells you to do so.

*For auranofin*

- For *oral* dosage form (capsules):
  —For arthritis:
    - Adults—6 milligrams (mg) once a day or 3 mg twice a day. After six months, your doctor may increase the dose to 3 mg three times a day.
    - Children—Dose must be determined by your doctor.

*For aurothioglucose*

- For *injection* dosage form:
  —For arthritis:
    - Adults and teenagers—10 milligrams (mg) for the first dose, then 25 mg once a week for the next two weeks, then 25 or 50 mg once a week. The medicine is injected into a muscle. After several months, the injections may be given less often (25 or 50 mg every two weeks for a while, then every three or four weeks).
    - Children 6 to 12 years of age—2.5 mg for the first dose, then 6.25 mg once a week for the next two weeks, then 12.5 mg once a week. The medicine is injected into a muscle. After several months, the injections may be given less often (6.25 or 12.5 mg every three or four weeks).
    - Children younger than 6 years of age—Dose must be determined by your doctor.

*For gold sodium thiomalate*

- For *injection* dosage form:
  —For arthritis:
    - Adults and teenagers—10 milligrams (mg) for the first dose, then 25 mg a week later, then 25 or 50 mg once a week. The medicine is injected into a muscle. After several months, the injections may be given less often (25 or 50 mg every two weeks for a while, then every three or four weeks).
    - Children—10 mg for the first dose, then 1 mg per kilogram (about 0.45 mg per pound) of body weight, but not more than a total of 50 mg, once a week. The medicine is injected into a muscle. After several months, the same dose may be given less often (every two weeks for a while, then every three or four weeks).

**Missed dose**—For patients taking *auranofin:* If you miss a dose of this medicine, and your dosing schedule is—

- One dose a day—Take the missed dose as soon as possible. However, if you do not remember until the next day, skip the missed dose and go back to your regular dosing schedule. Do not double doses.
- More than one dose a day—Take the missed dose as soon as possible. However, if it is almost time for your next dose, skip the missed dose and go back to your regular dosing schedule. Do not double doses.

**Storage**—To store this medicine:

- Keep out of the reach of children.
- Store away from heat and direct light.
- Do not store this medicine in the bathroom, near the kitchen sink, or in other damp places. Heat or moisture may cause the medicine to break down.
- Do not keep outdated medicine or medicine no longer needed. Be sure that any discarded medicine is out of the reach of children.

## Precautions While Using This Medicine

Gold compounds may cause some people to become more sensitive to sunlight than they are normally. These people may break out in a rash after being in the sun, or a skin rash that is already present may become worse. To protect yourself, it is best to:

- Stay out of direct sunlight, especially between the hours of 10:00 a.m. and 3:00 p.m., if possible.
- Wear protective clothing.
- Ask your doctor if you may apply a sun block product. Products that have a skin protection factor (SPF) of at least 15 work best, but some patients may require a product with a higher SPF number, especially if they have a fair complexion.
- Do not use a sunlamp or tanning bed or booth.

If you have a severe reaction from the sun, check with your doctor.

For patients taking *auranofin:*

- Your doctor should check your progress at regular visits. Blood and urine tests may be needed to make certain that this medicine is not causing unwanted effects.

For patients receiving *gold injections:*

- Immediately following an injection of this medicine, side effects such as dizziness, feeling faint, flushing or redness of the face, nausea or vomiting, increased sweating, or unusual weakness may occur. These will usually go away after you lie down for a few minutes. If any of these effects continue or become worse, or if you notice any other effects within 10 minutes or so after receiving an injection, tell your health care professional right away.
- Joint pain may occur for 1 or 2 days after you receive an injection of this medicine. This effect usually disappears after the first few injections. However, if this continues or is bothersome, check with your doctor.

## Side Effects of This Medicine

Gold compounds have been shown to cause tumors and cancer of the kidney when given to animals in large amounts for a long time. However, these effects have not been reported in humans receiving gold compounds for arthritis. If you have any questions about this, check with your doctor.

Along with its needed effects, a medicine may cause some unwanted effects. Although not all of these side effects may occur, side effects may occur at any time during treatment with this medicine *and up to many months after treatment has ended,* and they may need medical attention.

Check with your doctor as soon as possible if any of the following side effects occur:

*More common*

Irritation or soreness of tongue—less common with auranofin; metallic taste—less common with auranofin; skin rash or itching; redness, soreness, swelling, or bleeding of gums—rare with auranofin; ulcers, sores, or white spots on lips or in mouth or throat

*Less common*

Bloody or cloudy urine; hives

*Rare*

Abdominal or stomach pain, cramping, or burning (severe); bloody or black, tarry stools; confusion; convulsions (seizures); coughing, hoarseness, difficulty in breathing, shortness of breath, tightness in chest, or wheezing; dark urine; decreased urination; decreased vision; difficulty in swallowing; feeling of something in the eye; fever; hair loss; hallucinations (hearing, seeing, or feeling things that are not there); irritation of nose, throat, or upper chest area, possibly with hoarseness or coughing; irritation of vagina; nausea, vomiting, or heartburn (severe and/or continuing); numbness, tingling, pain, or weakness, especially in the face, hands, arms, or feet; pale stools; painful or difficult urination; pain in lower back, side, or lower abdomen (stomach) area; pain, redness, itching, or tearing of eyes; pinpoint red spots on skin; problems with muscle coordination; red, thickened, or scaly skin; sore throat and fever with or without chills; swelling of face, fingers, ankles, lower legs, or feet; swellings (large) on face, eyelids, mouth, lips, and/or tongue; swollen and/or painful glands; unusual bleeding or bruising; unusual tiredness or weakness; vomiting of blood or material that looks like coffee grounds; yellow eyes or skin

Other side effects may occur that usually do not need medical attention. These side effects may go away during treatment as your body adjusts to the medicine. However, check with your doctor if the following side effects continue or are bothersome:

*More common with auranofin; rare with injections*

Abdominal or stomach cramps or pain (mild or moderate); bloated feeling, gas, or indigestion (mild or moderate); decrease or loss of appetite; diarrhea or loose stools; nausea or vomiting (mild or moderate)

*Less common*

Constipation—with auranofin; joint pain—with injections

Some patients receiving auranofin have noticed changes in the taste of certain foods. If you notice a metallic taste while receiving any gold compound, check with your doctor as soon as possible. If you notice any other taste changes while you are taking auranofin, it is not necessary to check with your doctor unless you find this effect especially bothersome.

Other side effects not listed above may also occur in some patients. If you notice any other effects, check with your doctor.

Revised: June 1990
Interim revision: 08/22/94

# GONADORELIN  Systemic

A commonly used brand name in the U.S. and Canada is Factrel.

Other commonly used names are gonadotropin-releasing hormone, GnRH, and LHRH.

## Description

Gonadorelin (goe-nad-oh-RELL-in) is a medicine that is the same as gonadotropin-releasing hormone (GnRH) that is naturally released from the hypothalamus gland. GnRH causes the pituitary gland to release other hormones (luteinizing hormone [LH] and follicle-stimulating hormone [FSH]). These other hormones control development in children and fertility in adults.

Gonadorelin is used to test how well the hypothalamus and the pituitary glands are working. It is also used to cause ovulation (release of an egg from the ovary) in women who do not have regular ovulation and menstrual periods because the hypothalamus gland does not release enough GnRH.

Gonadorelin may also be used for other conditions as determined by your doctor.

Gonadorelin is available in the following dosage form:

*Parenteral*
- Injection (U.S. and Canada)

## Before Using This Medicine

In deciding to use a medicine, the risks of using the medicine must be weighed against the good it will do. This is a decision you and your doctor will make. For gonadorelin, the following should be considered:

**Allergies**—Tell your doctor if you have ever had any unusual or allergic reaction to gonadorelin. Also tell your health care professional if you are allergic to any other substances, such as foods, preservatives, or dyes.

**Pregnancy**—Gonadorelin has not been studied in pregnant women. However, it has not been shown to cause birth defects or other problems in animal studies.

**Breast-feeding**—Gonadorelin has not been reported to cause problems in nursing babies.

**Children**—This medicine has been tested and used in children and, in effective doses, has not been shown to cause different side effects or problems in children than it does in adults.

**Other medicines**—Although certain medicines should not be used together at all, in other cases two different medicines may be used together even if an interaction might occur. In these cases, your doctor may want to change the dose, or other precautions may be necessary. When you are using gonadorelin, it is especially important that your health care professional know if you are taking any other prescription or nonprescription (over-the-counter [OTC]) medicine.

## Proper Use of This Medicine

If you are having a test done with gonadorelin, one or more samples of your blood will be taken. Then gonadorelin is given by an intravenous (into a vein) or a subcutaneous (under the skin) injection. At regular times after it is given, more blood samples will be taken. Then the results of the test will be studied.

**Dosing**—The dose of gonadorelin will be different for different patients. *Follow your doctor's orders.* The following information includes only the average doses of gonadorelin.

- For *injectable* dosage form:
  —For testing the hypothalamus and pituitary glands:
    - Adults—0.1 milligram (mg) injected once under the skin or into a vein.
    - Children 12 years of age and older—0.1 mg injected once under the skin or into a vein.

## Side Effects of This Medicine

Along with its needed effects, a medicine may cause some unwanted effects. Although the following side effects usually occur rarely with the use of repeated injections, they require immediate medical attention. *Get emergency help immediately* if any of the following side effects occur:

  Difficulty in breathing; flushing (continuing)

Check with your doctor as soon as possible if any of the following side effects occur:

*With repeated doses*
  Hardening of skin around place of injection; hives; skin rash (at place of injection or over entire body)

Other side effects may occur that usually do not need medical attention. These side effects may go away during treatment as your body adjusts to the medicine. However, check with your doctor if any of the following side effects continue or are bothersome:

*Less common*
  Abdominal or stomach discomfort; flushing (lasting only a short time); headaches; itching, pain, or swelling at place of injection; lightheadedness; nausea

Other side effects not listed above may also occur in some patients. If you notice any other effects, check with your doctor.

## Additional Information

Once a medicine has been approved for marketing for a certain use, experience may show that it is also useful for other medical problems. Although not specifically included in product labeling, gonadorelin is used in certain patients with the following medical conditions:

- Delayed puberty
- Infertility in males

Other than the above information, there is no additional information relating to proper use, precautions, or side effects for these uses.

Revised: August 1990
Interim revision: 05/16/94

# GOSERELIN   Systemic

A commonly used brand name in the U.S. and Canada is Zoladex.

## Description

Goserelin (GOE-se-rel-in) is used to treat cancer of the prostate gland. It is usually given once a month.

Goserelin is similar to a hormone normally released from the hypothalamus gland. When given regularly, it decreases testosterone levels. Reducing the amount of testosterone in the body is one way of treating cancer of the prostate.

Goserelin is to be given only by or under the supervision of your doctor. It is injected under the skin and is available in the following dosage form:

*Parenteral*
- Implants (U.S. and Canada)

## Before Using This Medicine

In deciding to use a medicine, the risks of taking the medicine must be weighed against the good it will do. This is a decision you and your doctor will make. For goserelin, the following should be considered:

**Allergies**—Tell your doctor if you have ever had any unusual or allergic reaction to goserelin.

**Fertility**—Goserelin causes sterility which may be permanent. If you intend to have children, discuss this with your doctor before receiving this medicine.

**Older adults**—Many medicines have not been tested in older people. Therefore, it may not be known whether they work exactly the same way they do in younger adults. Although there is no specific information comparing use of goserelin in the elderly to use in other age groups, it has been used mostly in elderly patients and is not expected to cause different side effects or problems in older people than it does in younger adults.

## Proper Use of This Medicine

Goserelin sometimes causes unwanted effects such as hot flashes or decreased sexual ability. It may also cause a temporary increase in pain, numbness or tingling of hands or feet, trouble in urinating, or weakness in your legs when you begin treatment with it. However, it is very important that you continue to receive the medicine, even

after you begin to feel better. *Do not stop treatment with this medicine without first checking with your doctor.*

**Dosing**—The dose of goserelin may be different for different patients. Goserelin implants are usually given by a doctor in the office or hospital. The following information includes only the average dose of goserelin:

- For *implant* dosage form:
  —For prostate cancer:
    - Adults—3.6 milligrams (mg) (one implant) injected under the skin every twenty-eight days.

**Missed dose**—If you miss getting a dose of this medicine, get it as soon as possible.

## Precautions While Using This Medicine

*It is very important that your doctor check your progress at regular visits* to make sure that this medicine is working properly and to check for unwanted effects.

## Side Effects of This Medicine

Along with its needed effects, a medicine may cause some unwanted effects. Although not all of these side effects may occur, if they do occur they may need medical attention.

The following side effects are symptoms of a flareup of your condition that may occur during the first few days of treatment. After a few days, these symptoms should lessen. However, they may need medical attention. Check with your doctor if any of the following side effects occur or get worse:

Bone pain; numbness or tingling of hands or feet; trouble in urinating; weakness in legs

Also check with your doctor as soon as possible if any of the following side effects occur:

*Less common*
Chest pain; irregular heartbeat; joint pain; painful or cold hands or feet; shortness of breath; skin rash; weakness (sudden)

Other side effects may occur that usually do not need medical attention. These side effects may go away during treatment as your body adjusts to the medicine. However,

check with your doctor if any of the following side effects continue or are bothersome:

*More common*

Decrease in sexual desire; impotence; sudden sweating and feelings of warmth ("hot flashes")

*Less common*

Anxiety or mental depression; constipation; diarrhea; dizziness; headache; loss of appetite; nausea or vomiting; swelling and increased tenderness of breasts; swelling of feet or lower legs; trouble in sleeping; unusual tiredness or weakness; weight gain

Other side effects not listed above may also occur in some patients. If you notice any other effects, check with your doctor.

Revised: 07/90
Interim revision: 07/08/94

# GRISEOFULVIN    Systemic

Some commonly used brand names are:

**In the U.S.—**
| | |
|---|---|
| Fulvicin P/G | Grisactin |
| Fulvicin-U/F | Grisactin Ultra |
| Grifulvin V | Gris-PEG |

**In Canada—**
| | |
|---|---|
| Fulvicin P/G | Grisovin-FP |
| Fulvicin U/F | |

## Description

Griseofulvin (gri-see-oh-FUL-vin) belongs to the group of medicines called antifungals. It is used to treat fungus infections of the skin, hair, fingernails, and toenails. This medicine may be taken alone or used along with medicines that are applied to the skin for fungus infections.

Griseofulvin is available only with your doctor's prescription, in the following dosage forms:

*Oral*
- Capsules (U.S.)
- Suspension (U.S.)
- Tablets (U.S. and Canada)

## Before Using This Medicine

In deciding to use a medicine, the risks of taking the medicine must be weighed against the good it will do. This is a decision you and your doctor will make. For griseofulvin, the following should be considered:

**Allergies**—Tell your doctor if you have ever had any unusual or allergic reaction to penicillins, penicillamine (e.g., Cuprimine), or griseofulvin. Also tell your health care professional if you are allergic to any other substances, such as foods, preservatives, or dyes.

**Diet**—Griseofulvin is absorbed best when it is taken with a high fat meal, such as a cheeseburger, whole milk, or ice cream. Tell your doctor if you are on a low-fat diet.

**Pregnancy**—Griseofulvin should not be used during pregnancy. The birth of twins that were joined together has been reported, although rarely, in women who took griseofulvin during the first 3 months of pregnancy. In addition, studies in rats and dogs have shown that griseofulvin causes birth defects and other problems.

**Breast-feeding**—It is not known if griseofulvin is excreted in breast milk. However, griseofulvin has not been reported to cause problems in nursing babies.

**Children**—This medicine has been tested in a limited number of children 2 years of age or older. In effective doses, the medicine has not been shown to cause different side effects or problems than it does in adults.

**Older adults**—Many medicines have not been studied specifically in older people. Therefore, it may not be known whether they work exactly the same way they do in younger adults. Although there is no specific information comparing use of griseofulvin in the elderly with use in other age groups, this medicine is not expected to cause different side effects or problems in older people than it does in younger adults.

**Other medicines**—Although certain medicines should not be used together at all, in other cases two different medicines may be used together even if an interaction might occur. In these cases, your doctor may want to change the dose, or other precautions may be necessary. When you are taking griseofulvin, it is especially important that your health care professional knows if you are taking any of the following:

- Anticoagulants (blood thinners)—Griseofulvin may decrease the effectiveness of anticoagulants in some patients
- Oral contraceptives (birth control pills) containing estrogen—Griseofulvin may decrease the effectiveness of birth control pills, which may result in breakthrough bleeding and unwanted pregnancies

**Other medical problems**—The presence of other medical problems may affect the use of griseofulvin. Make sure you tell your doctor if you have any other medical problems, especially:

- Liver disease—Griseofulvin may on rare occasion cause side effects affecting the liver
- Lupus erythematosus or lupus-like diseases—Griseofulvin may worsen lupus symptoms in patients who have lupus erythematosus or lupus-like diseases
- Porphyria—Griseofulvin may increase attacks of porphyria in patients with acute intermittent porphyria

## Proper Use of This Medicine

*Griseofulvin is best taken with or after meals, especially fatty ones (for example, whole milk or ice cream).* This lessens possible stomach upset and helps to clear up the infection by helping your body absorb the medicine better. *However, if you are on a low-fat diet, check with your doctor.*

For patients taking the *oral liquid form of griseofulvin:*

- Use a specially marked measuring spoon or other device to measure each dose accurately. The average household teaspoon may not hold the right amount of liquid.

To help clear up your infection completely, *keep taking this medicine for the full time of treatment,* even if you begin to feel better after a few days. *Do not miss any doses.*

**Dosing**—The dose of griseofulvin will be different for different patients. *Follow your doctor's orders or the directions on the label.* The following information includes only the average doses of griseofulvin. *If your dose is different, do not change it* unless your doctor tells you to do so.

The number of capsules or tablets or teaspoonfuls of suspension that you take depends on the strength of the medicine. Also, *the number of doses you take each day, the time allowed between doses, and the length of time you take the medicine depend on the medical problem for which you are taking griseofulvin.*

- For microsize capsules, tablets, and suspension:
  - —Adults and teenagers:
    - Treatment of fungus infections of the feet and nails—500 milligrams (mg) every twelve hours.
    - Treatment of fungus infections of the scalp, skin, and groin—250 mg every twelve hours; or 500 mg once a day.
  - —Children:
    - Treatment of fungus infections—Dose is based on body weight. The usual dose is 5 mg per kilogram (kg) (2.3 mg per pound) of body weight every twelve hours; or 10 mg per kg (4.6 mg per pound) of body weight once a day.
- For ultramicrosize tablets:
  - —Adults and teenagers:
    - Treatment of fungus infections of the feet and nails—250 to 375 mg every twelve hours.
    - Treatment of fungus infections of the scalp, skin, and groin—125 to 187.5 mg every twelve hours; or 250 to 375 mg once a day.
  - —Infants and children up to 2 years of age:
    - Treatment of fungus infections—Use and dose must be determined by your doctor.
  - —Children 2 years of age and over:
    - Treatment of fungus infections—Dose is based on body weight. The usual dose is 2.75 to 3.65 mg per kg (1.25 to 1.7 mg per pound) of body weight every twelve hours; or 5.5 to 7.3 mg per kg (2.5 to 3.3 mg per pound) of body weight once a day.

**Missed dose**—If you miss a dose of this medicine, take it as soon as possible. However, if it is almost time for your next dose, skip the missed dose and go back to your regular dosing schedule. Do not double doses.

**Storage**—To store this medicine:

- Keep out of the reach of children.
- Store away from heat and direct light.
- Do not store the capsule or tablet form of this medicine in the bathroom, near the kitchen sink, or in other damp places. Heat or moisture may cause the medicine to break down.
- Keep the oral liquid form of this medicine from freezing.
- Do not keep outdated medicine or medicine no longer needed. Be sure that any discarded medicine is out of the reach of children.

## Precautions While Using This Medicine

Your doctor should check your progress at regular visits to make sure that griseofulvin does not cause unwanted effects.

*Oral contraceptives (birth control pills) containing estrogen may not work properly if you take them while you are taking griseofulvin. Unplanned pregnancies may occur. You should use a different or additional means of birth control while you are taking griseofulvin and for one month after stopping griseofulvin.* If you have any questions about this, check with your health care professional.

Griseofulvin may increase the effects of alcohol. If taken with alcohol it may also cause fast heartbeat, flushing, increased sweating, or redness of the face. Therefore, if you have this reaction, do not drink alcoholic beverages while you are taking this medicine, unless you have first checked with your doctor.

This medicine may cause some people to become dizzy or less alert than they are normally. *Make sure you know how you react to this medicine before you drive, use machines, or do other things that could be dangerous if you are dizzy or are not alert.* If these reactions are especially bothersome, check with your doctor.

Griseofulvin may cause your skin to be more sensitive to sunlight than it is normally. Exposure to sunlight, even for brief periods of time, may cause a skin rash, itching, redness or other discoloration of the skin, or a severe sunburn. When you begin taking this medicine:

- Stay out of direct sunlight, especially between the hours of 10:00 a.m. and 3:00 p.m., if possible.
- Wear protective clothing, including a hat. Also, wear sunglasses.
- Apply a sun block product that has a skin protection factor (SPF) of at least 15. Some patients may require a product with a higher SPF number, especially if they have a fair complexion. If you have

any questions about this, check with your health care professional.

- Apply a sun block lipstick that has an SPF of at least 15 to protect your lips.
- Do not use a sunlamp or tanning bed or booth.

*If you have a severe reaction from the sun, check with your doctor.*

## Side Effects of This Medicine

Griseofulvin has been shown to cause liver and thyroid tumors in some animals. *You and your doctor should discuss the good this medicine will do, as well as the risks of taking it.*

Along with its needed effects, a medicine may cause some unwanted effects. Although not all of these side effects may occur, if they do occur they may need medical attention.

Check with your doctor as soon as possible if any of the following side effects occur:

*Less common*
Confusion; increased sensitivity of skin to sunlight; skin rash, hives, or itching; soreness or irritation of mouth or tongue

*Rare*
Numbness, tingling, pain, or weakness in hands or feet; sore throat and fever; yellow eyes or skin

Other side effects may occur that usually do not need medical attention. These side effects may go away during treatment as your body adjusts to the medicine. However, check with your doctor if any of the following side effects continue or are bothersome:

*More common*
Headache

*Less common*
Diarrhea; dizziness; nausea or vomiting; stomach pain; trouble in sleeping; unusual tiredness

Other side effects not listed above may also occur in some patients. If you notice any other effects, check with your doctor.

Revised: 09/06/92
Interim revision: 03/17/94

---

# GROWTH HORMONE   Systemic

Some commonly used brand names are:

**In the U.S.—**
Humatrope[2]
Protropin[1]

**In Canada—**
Humatrope[2]
Protropin[1]

Note: For quick reference, the following growth hormone are numbered to match the corresponding brand names.

This information applies to the following medicines:
1. Somatrem (SOE-ma-trem)
2. Somatropin (soe-ma-TROE-pin)

Other commonly used names are GH and human growth hormone (hGH).

## Description

Somatrem and somatropin are man-made versions of human growth hormone. Growth hormone is naturally produced by the pituitary gland and is necessary to stimulate growth in children. If a child fails to grow normally because his or her body is not producing enough growth hormone, this medicine may be used to stimulate growth.

This medicine is available only with your doctor's prescription, in the following dosage forms:

*Parenteral*
Somatrem
- Injection (U.S. and Canada)
Somatropin
- Injection (U.S. and Canada)

## Before Using This Medicine

In deciding to use a medicine, the risks of taking the medicine must be weighed against the good it will do. This is a decision you and your doctor will make. For growth hormone, the following should be considered:

**Allergies**—Tell your doctor if you have ever had any unusual or allergic reaction to growth hormone. Also tell your health care professional if you are allergic to any other substances, such as foods, preservatives, or dyes.

**Other medicines**—Although certain medicines should not be used together at all, in other cases two different medicines may be used together even if an interaction might occur. In these cases, your doctor may want to change the dose, or other precautions may be necessary. When you are taking growth hormone, it is especially important that your health care professional know if you are taking any of the following:

- Corticosteroids (cortisone-like medicines)—These medicines can interfere with the effects of growth hormone

**Other medical problems**—The presence of other medical problems may affect the use of growth hormone. Make sure you tell your doctor if you have any other medical problems, especially:

- Underactive thyroid—This condition can interfere with the effects of growth hormone

## Proper Use of This Medicine

**Dosing**—The dose of these medicines will be different for different patients. *Follow your doctor's orders or the directions on the label.* The following information includes only the average doses of these medicines. *If your dose is different, do not change it* unless your doctor tells you to do so.

*For somatrem and somatropin*

- For *injection* dosage form:
  —For stimulating growth:
    - Children—Dose is based on body weight and must be determined by your doctor. The usual dose is 0.025 to 0.05 milligram (mg) per kilogram (kg) (0.01 to 0.02 mg per pound) of body weight. This is injected into a muscle or under the skin every other day or three times a week.

## Precautions While Using This Medicine

*It is important that your doctor check your progress at regular visits.*

## Side Effects of This Medicine

Leukemia has been reported in a few patients after treatment with growth hormone. However, it is not definitely known whether the leukemia was caused by the growth hormone. Leukemia has also been reported in patients whose bodies do not make enough growth hormone and who have not yet been treated with man-made growth hormone. However, discuss this possible effect with your doctor.

If hGH is given to children or adults with normal growth, who do not need growth hormone, serious unwanted effects may occur because levels in the body become too high. These effects include the development of diabetes, abnormal growth of bones and internal organs such as the heart, kidneys, and liver, atherosclerosis (hardening of the arteries), and hypertension (high blood pressure).

Along with its needed effects, a medicine may cause some unwanted effects. Although not all of these side effects may occur, if they do occur they may need medical attention. When growth hormone is used to promote growth in children who have a lack of naturally produced human growth hormone, serious side effects do not usually occur. However, check with your doctor as soon as possible if any of the following side effects occur:

*Rare*

Limp; pain and swelling at place of injection; pain in hip or knee; skin rash or itching

Other side effects not listed above may also occur in some patients. If you notice any other effects, check with your doctor.

Revised: 11/18/92
Interim revision: 06/30/94

---

# GUAIFENESIN   Systemic

Some commonly used brand names are:

**In the U.S.—**

| | |
|---|---|
| Amonidrin | Humibid Sprinkle |
| Anti-Tuss | Hytuss |
| Breonesin | Hytuss-2X |
| Diabetic Tussin EX | Malotuss |
| Fenesin | Mytussin |
| Gee-Gee | Naldecon Senior EX |
| Genatuss | Nortussin |
| GG-CEN | Pneumomist |
| Glyate | Robitussin |
| Glycotuss | Scot-tussin |
| Glytuss | Sinumist-SR |
| Guiatuss | Touro Ex |
| Halotussin | Uni-tussin |
| Humibid L.A. | |

Generic name product may also be available.

**In Canada—**

| | |
|---|---|
| Balminil Expectorant | Resyl |
| Benylin-E | Robitussin |

Another commonly used name is glyceryl guaiacolate.

## Description

Guaifenesin (gwye-FEN-e-sin) is used to relieve coughs due to colds or influenza (flu). Guaifenesin works by loosening the mucus or phlegm (pronounced flem) in the lungs.

Guaifenesin is available without a prescription; however, your doctor may have special instructions on the proper dose of this medicine for your medical condition. It is available in the following dosage forms:

*Oral*

- Capsules (U.S.)
- Extended-release capsules (U.S.)
- Oral solution (U.S.)
- Syrup (U.S. and Canada)
- Tablets (U.S. and Canada)
- Extended-release tablets (U.S.)

## Before Using This Medicine

If you are taking this medicine without a prescription, carefully read and follow any precautions on the label. For guaifenesin, the following should be considered:

**Allergies**—Tell your doctor if you have ever had any unusual or allergic reaction to guaifenesin. Also tell your health care professional if you are allergic to any other substances, such as foods, preservatives, or dyes.

**Pregnancy**—Studies have not been done in either humans or animals.

---

**Breast-feeding**—It is not known whether guaifenesin passes into breast milk. However, guaifenesin has not been reported to cause problems in nursing babies.

**Children**—Although there is no specific information comparing use of guaifenesin in children with use in other age groups, this medicine is not expected to cause different side effects or problems in children than it does in adults. However, check with your doctor before using this medicine in children who have a chronic cough, such as occurs with asthma, or who have an unusually large amount of mucus or phlegm with the cough. Children with these conditions may need a different kind of medicine.

**Older adults**—Many medicines have not been studied specifically in older people. Therefore, it may not be known whether they work exactly the same way they do in younger adults. Although there is no specific information comparing use of guaifenesin in the elderly with use in other age groups, this medicine is not expected to cause different side effects or problems in older people than it does in younger adults.

## Proper Use of This Medicine

To help loosen mucus or phlegm in the lungs, *drink a glass of water after each dose of this medicine,* unless otherwise directed by your doctor.

For patients taking the *extended-release tablet* form of this medicine:

- Swallow the tablet whole. Do not crush, break, or chew before swallowing.

**Dosing**—The dose of guaifenesin will be different for different patients. *Follow your doctor's orders or the directions on the label.* The following information includes only the average doses of guaifenesin. *If your dose is different, do not change it* unless your doctor tells you to do so.

- For *regular (short-acting) oral* dosage forms (capsules, oral solution, syrup, or tablets):
  —For cough:
  - Adults—200 to 400 milligrams (mg) every four hours.
  - Children younger than 2 years of age—Use and dose must be determined by your doctor.
  - Children 2 to 6 years of age—50 to 100 mg every four hours.
  - Children 6 to 12 years of age—100 to 200 mg every four hours.

- For *long-acting oral* dosage forms (extended-release capsules or tablets):
  —For cough:
  - Adults—600 to 1200 mg every twelve hours.
  - Children younger than 2 years of age—Use is not recommended.
  - Children 2 to 6 years of age—300 mg every twelve hours.
  - Children 6 to 12 years of age—600 mg every twelve hours.

**Missed dose**—If you must take this medicine regularly and you miss a dose, take it as soon as possible. However, if it is almost time for your next dose, skip the missed dose and go back to your regular dosing schedule. Do not double doses.

**Storage**—To store this medicine:

- Keep out of the reach of children.
- Store away from heat and direct light.
- Do not store the capsule or tablet form of this medicine in the bathroom, near the kitchen sink, or in other damp places. Heat or moisture may cause the medicine to break down.
- Do not refrigerate the syrup form of this medicine.
- Do not keep outdated medicine or medicine no longer needed. Be sure that any discarded medicine is out of the reach of children.

## Precautions While Using This Medicine

If your cough has not improved after 7 days or if you have a high fever, skin rash, continuing headache, or sore throat with the cough, check with your doctor. These signs may mean that you have other medical problems.

## Side Effects of This Medicine

Along with its needed effects, a medicine may cause some unwanted effects. Although not all of these side effects may occur, if they do occur they may need medical attention. Some side effects may occur that usually do not need medical attention. These side effects may go away during treatment as your body adjusts to the medicine. However, check with your doctor if any of the following side effects continue or are bothersome:

*Less common or rare*
  Diarrhea; drowsiness; nausea or vomiting; stomach pain

Other side effects not listed above may also occur in some patients. If you notice any other effects, check with your doctor.

Revised: 06/23/94

# GUANABENZ Systemic†

## Description

Guanabenz (GWAHN-a-benz) belongs to the general class of medicines called antihypertensives. It is used to treat high blood pressure (hypertension).

High blood pressure adds to the work load of the heart and arteries. If it continues for a long time, the heart and arteries may not function properly. This can damage the blood vessels of the brain, heart, and kidneys, resulting in a stroke, heart failure, or kidney failure. High blood pressure may also increase the risk of heart attacks. These problems may be less likely to occur if blood pressure is controlled.

Guanabenz works by controlling nerve impulses along certain nerve pathways. As a result, it relaxes blood vessels so that blood passes through them more easily. This helps to lower blood pressure.

Guanabenz is available only with your doctor's prescription, in the following dosage form:

*Oral*
- Tablets (U.S.)

## Before Using This Medicine

In deciding to use a medicine, the risks of taking the medicine must be weighed against the good it will do. This is a decision you and your doctor will make. For guanabenz, the following should be considered:

**Allergies**—Tell your doctor if you have ever had any unusual or allergic reaction to guanabenz. Also tell your health care professional if you are allergic to any other substance, such as foods, preservatives, or dyes.

**Pregnancy**—Guanabenz has not been studied in pregnant women. However, studies in rats have shown that guanabenz given in doses 9 to 10 times the maximum human dose caused a decrease in fertility. In addition, 3 to 6 times the maximum human dose caused birth defects (in the skeleton) in mice, and 6 to 9 times the maximum human dose caused death of the fetus in rats. Before taking this medicine, make sure your doctor knows if you are pregnant or if you may become pregnant.

**Breast-feeding**—It is not known whether guanabenz passes into the breast milk. However, this medicine has not been reported to cause problems in nursing babies.

**Children**—Studies on this medicine have been done only in adult patients, and there is no specific information comparing use of guanabenz in children with use in other age groups.

**Older adults**—Many medicines have not been studied specifically in older people. Therefore, it may not be known whether they work exactly the same way they do in younger adults or if they cause different side effects or problems in older people. There is no specific information comparing use of guanabenz in the elderly with use in other age groups. However, dizziness, faintness, or drowsiness may be more likely to occur in the elderly, who are usually more sensitive to the effects of guanabenz.

**Other medicines**—Although certain medicines should not be used together at all, in other cases two different medicines may be used together even if an interaction might occur. In these cases, your doctor may want to change the dose, or other precautions may be necessary. When you are taking guanabenz, it is especially important that your health care professional know if you are taking any of the following:

- Beta-blockers (acebutolol [e.g., Sectral], atenolol [e.g., Tenormin], betaxolol [Kerlone], carteolol [e.g., Cartrol], labetalol [e.g., Normodyne], metoprolol [e.g., Lopressor], nadolol [e.g., Corgard], oxprenolol [e.g., Trasicor], penbutolol [e.g., Levatol], pindolol [e.g., Visken], propranolol [e.g., Inderal], sotalol [e.g., Sotacor], timolol [e.g., Blocadren])—Effects on blood pressure may be increased. Also, the risk of unwanted effects when guanabenz treatment is stopped suddenly may be increased

**Other medical problems**—The presence of other medical problems may affect the use of guanabenz. Make sure you tell your doctor if you have any other medical problems, especially:

- Heart or blood vessel disease—Lowering blood pressure may make some conditions worse
- Kidney disease or
- Liver disease—Effects of guanabenz may be increased because of slower removal of guanabenz from the body

## Proper Use of This Medicine

In addition to the use of the medicine your doctor has prescribed, treatment for your high blood pressure may include weight control and care in the types of foods you eat, especially foods high in sodium. Your doctor will tell you which of these are most important for you. You should check with your doctor before changing your diet.

Many patients who have high blood pressure will not notice any signs of the problem. In fact, many may feel normal. It is very important that you *take your medicine exactly as directed* and that you keep your appointments with your doctor even if you feel well.

Remember that this medicine will not cure your high blood pressure but it does help control it. Therefore, you must continue to take it as directed if you expect to lower your blood pressure and keep it down. *You may have to take high blood pressure medicine for the rest of your life.* If high blood pressure is not treated, it can cause serious problems such as heart failure, blood vessel disease, stroke, or kidney disease.

To help you remember to take your medicine, try to get into the habit of taking it at the same time each day.

**Dosing**—The dose of guanabenz will be different for different patients. *Follow your doctor's orders or the directions on the label.* The following information includes only the average doses of guanabenz. *If your dose is different, do not change it* unless your doctor tells you to do so.

The number of tablets that you take depends on the strength of the medicine.

- For *oral* dosage form (tablets):
  —For high blood pressure:
    - Adults—At first, 4 milligrams (mg) two times a day. Then, your doctor may gradually increase your dose.
    - Children—Use and dose must be determined by your doctor.

**Missed dose**—

- If you miss a dose of this medicine, take it as soon as possible. However, if it is almost time for your next dose, skip the missed dose and go back to your regular dosing schedule. Do not double doses.
- If you miss two or more doses in a row, check with your doctor. If your body suddenly goes without this medicine, some unpleasant effects may occur. If you have any questions about this, check with your doctor.

**Storage**—To store this medicine:

- Keep out of the reach of children.
- Store away from heat and direct light.
- Do not store in the bathroom, near the kitchen sink, or in other damp places. Heat or moisture may cause the medicine to break down.
- Do not keep outdated medicine or medicine no longer needed. Be sure that any discarded medicine is out of the reach of children.

## Precautions While Using This Medicine

It is important that your doctor check your progress at regular visits to make sure that this medicine is working properly.

Check with your doctor before you stop taking guanabenz. Your doctor may want you to reduce gradually the amount you are taking before stopping completely.

Before having any kind of surgery (including dental surgery) or emergency treatment, tell the medical doctor or dentist in charge that you are using this medicine.

*Do not take other medicines unless they have been discussed with your doctor.* This especially includes over-the-counter (nonprescription) medicines for appetite control, asthma, colds, cough, hay fever, or sinus problems, since they may tend to increase your blood pressure.

Guanabenz will add to the effects of alcohol and other CNS depressants (medicines that slow down the nervous system, possibly causing drowsiness). Some examples of CNS depressants are antihistamines or medicine for hay fever, other allergies, or colds; sedatives, tranquilizers, or sleeping medicine; prescription pain medicine or narcotics; barbiturates; medicine for seizures; muscle relaxants; or anesthetics, including some dental anesthetics. *Check with your doctor before taking any of the above while you are using this medicine.*

Guanabenz may cause some people to become dizzy, drowsy, or less alert than they are normally. *Make sure you know how you react to this medicine before you drive, use machines, or do anything else that could be dangerous if you are dizzy or are not alert.*

Guanabenz may cause dryness of the mouth, nose, and throat. For temporary relief of mouth dryness, use sugarless candy or gum, melt bits of ice in your mouth, or use a saliva substitute. However, if your mouth continues to feel dry for more than 2 weeks, check with your medical doctor or dentist. Continuing dryness of the mouth may increase the chance of dental disease, including tooth decay, gum disease, and fungus infections.

## Side Effects of This Medicine

Along with its needed effects, a medicine may cause some unwanted effects. Although not all of these side effects may occur, if they do occur they may need medical attention.

Check with your doctor as soon as possible if any of the following side effects occur:

*Signs and symptoms of overdose*
  Dizziness (severe); faintness; irritability; nervousness; pinpoint pupils; slow heartbeat; unusual tiredness or weakness

Other side effects may occur that usually do not need medical attention. These side effects may go away during treatment as your body adjusts to the medicine. However, check with your doctor if any of the following side effects continue or are bothersome:

*More common*
  Dizziness; drowsiness; dryness of mouth; weakness

*Less common or rare*
  Decreased sexual ability; headache; nausea

After you have been using this medicine for a while, unpleasant effects may occur if you stop taking it too suddenly. After you stop taking this medicine, check with your doctor if any of the following effects occur:
  Anxiety or tenseness; chest pain; fast or irregular heartbeat; headache; increased salivation; increase in sweating; nausea or vomiting; nervousness or restlessness; shaking or trembling of hands or fingers; stomach cramps; trouble in sleeping

Other side effects not listed above may also occur in some patients. If you notice any other effects, check with your doctor.

Revised: 10/15/92
Interim revision: 04/14/94

# GUANADREL  Systemic†

A commonly used brand name in the U.S. is Hylorel.

†Not commercially available in Canada.

## Description

Guanadrel (GWAHN-a-drel) belongs to the general class of medicines called antihypertensives. It is used to treat high blood pressure (hypertension).

High blood pressure adds to the work load of the heart and arteries. If it continues for a long time, the heart and arteries may not function properly. This can damage the blood vessels of the brain, heart, and kidneys resulting in a stroke, heart failure, or kidney failure. High blood pressure may also increase the risk of heart attacks. These problems may be less likely to occur if blood pressure is controlled.

Guanadrel works by controlling nerve impulses along certain nerve pathways. As a result, it relaxes the blood vessels so that blood passes through them more easily. This helps to lower blood pressure.

Guanadrel is available only with your doctor's prescription, in the following dosage form:

*Oral*
- Tablets (U.S.)

## Before Using This Medicine

In deciding to use a medicine, the risks of taking the medicine must be weighed against the good it will do. This is a decision you and your doctor will make. For guanadrel, the following should be considered:

**Allergies**—Tell your doctor if you have ever had any unusual or allergic reaction to guanadrel. Also tell your health care professional if you are allergic to any other substance, such as foods, preservatives, or dyes.

**Pregnancy**—Guanadrel has not been studied in pregnant women. However, guanadrel has not been shown to cause birth defects or other problems in animal studies.

**Breast-feeding**—It is not known whether guanadrel passes into breast milk. However, it has not been reported to cause problems in nursing babies.

**Children**—Studies on this medicine have been done only in adult patients, and there is no specific information comparing use of guanadrel in children with use in other age groups.

**Older adults**—Dizziness or faintness may be more likely to occur in the elderly, who are usually more sensitive to the effects of guanadrel.

**Other medicines**—Although certain medicines should not be used together at all, in other cases two different medicines may be used together even if an interaction might occur. In these cases, your doctor may want to change the dose, or other precautions may be necessary. When you are taking guanadrel, it is especially important that your health care professional know if you are taking any of the following:

- Chlorprothixene (e.g., Taractan) or
- Loxapine (e.g., Loxitane) or
- Thiothixene (e.g., Navane) or
- Tricyclic antidepressants (amitriptyline [e.g., Elavil], amoxapine [e.g., Asendin], clomipramine [e.g., Anafranil], desipramine [e.g., Pertofrane], doxepin [e.g., Sinequan], imipramine [e.g., Tofranil], nortriptyline [e.g., Aventyl], protriptyline [e.g., Vivactil], trimipramine [e.g., Surmontil]) or
- Trimeprazine (e.g., Temaril)—May decrease the effects of guanadrel on blood pressure
- Monoamine oxidase (MAO) inhibitors (furazolidone [e.g., Furoxone], isocarboxazid [e.g., Marplan], phenelzine [e.g., Nardil], procarbazine [e.g., Matulane], selegiline [e.g., Eldepryl], tranylcypromine [e.g., Parnate])—Taking guanadrel while you are taking or within 2 weeks of taking MAO inhibitors may cause a severe increase in blood pressure

**Other medical problems**—The presence of other medical problems may affect the use of guanadrel. Make sure you tell your doctor if you have any other medical problems, especially:

- Asthma (history of) or
- Diarrhea or
- Pheochromocytoma or
- Stomach ulcer (history of)—May be worsened by guanadrel
- Fever—Effects of guanadrel may be increased
- Heart or blood vessel disease or
- Heart attack or stroke (recent)—Lowering blood pressure may make problems resulting from these conditions worse

## Proper Use of This Medicine

In addition to the use of the medicine your doctor has prescribed, treatment for your high blood pressure may include weight control and care in the types of foods you eat, especially foods high in sodium. Your doctor will tell you which of these are most important for you. You should check with your doctor before changing your diet.

Many patients who have high blood pressure will not notice any signs of the problem. In fact, many may feel normal. It is very important that you *take your medicine exactly as directed* and that you keep your appointments with your doctor even if you feel well.

Remember that guanadrel will not cure your high blood pressure but it does help control it. Therefore, you must continue to take it as directed if you expect to lower your blood pressure and keep it down. *You may have to take high blood pressure medicine for the rest of your life.* If high blood pressure is not treated, it can cause serious problems such as heart failure, blood vessel disease, stroke, or kidney disease.

To help you remember to take your medicine, try to get into the habit of taking it at the same time each day.

**Dosing**—The dose of guanadrel will be different for different patients. *Follow your doctor's orders or the directions on the label.* The following information includes only the average doses of guanadrel. *If your dose is different, do not change it* unless your doctor tells you to do so.

The number of tablets that you take depends on the strength of the medicine.

- For *oral* dosage form (tablets):
  —For high blood pressure:
    - Adults—At first, 5 milligrams (mg) two times a day. Then, your doctor may increase your dose to 20 to 75 mg a day, divided into two to four doses.
    - Children—Use and dose must be determined by your doctor.

**Missed dose**—If you miss a dose of guanadrel, take it as soon as possible. However, if it is almost time for your next dose, skip the missed dose and go back to your regular dosing schedule. Do not double doses.

**Storage**—To store this medicine:

- Keep out of the reach of children.
- Store away from heat and direct light.
- Do not store in the bathroom, near the kitchen sink, or in other damp places. Heat or moisture may cause the medicine to break down.
- Do not keep outdated medicine or medicine no longer needed. Be sure that any discarded medicine is out of the reach of children.

## Precautions While Using This Medicine

It is important that your doctor check your progress at regular visits to make sure that this medicine is working properly.

*Dizziness, lightheadedness, or fainting may occur, especially when you get up from a lying or sitting position.* This may be more likely to occur in the morning. *Getting up slowly may help.* If you feel dizzy, sit or lie down. When you get up from lying down, sit on the edge of the bed with your feet dangling for 1 or 2 minutes. Then stand up slowly. If the problem continues or gets worse, check with your doctor.

The dizziness, lightheadedness, or fainting is also more likely to occur if you drink alcohol, stand for long periods of time, exercise, or if the weather is hot. *While you are taking guanadrel, be careful to limit the amount of alcohol you drink. Also, use extra care during exercise or hot weather or if you must stand for long periods of time.*

*Do not take other medicines unless they have been discussed with your doctor.* This especially includes over-the-counter (nonprescription) medicines for appetite control, asthma, colds, cough, hay fever, or sinus problems, since they may tend to increase your blood pressure.

Before having any kind of surgery (including dental surgery) or emergency treatment, tell the medical doctor or dentist in charge that you are taking guanadrel.

Tell your doctor if you get a fever since that may change the amount of medicine you have to take.

## Side Effects of This Medicine

Along with its needed effects, a medicine may cause some unwanted effects. Although not all of these side effects may occur, if they do occur they may need medical attention.

*Check with your doctor immediately* if either of the following side effects occurs since they may be symptoms of an overdose:

*Rare*
Blurred vision; dizziness or faintness (severe)

Check with your doctor as soon as possible if any of the following side effects occur:

*More common*
Swelling of feet or lower legs

*Less common or rare*
Chest pain; shortness of breath

Other side effects may occur that usually do not need medical attention. These side effects may go away during treatment as your body adjusts to the medicine. However, check with your doctor if any of the following side effects continue or are bothersome:

*More common*
Difficulty in ejaculating; dizziness, lightheadedness, or fainting, especially when getting up from a lying or sitting position; drowsiness or tiredness

*Less common or rare*
Diarrhea or increase in bowel movements; dryness of mouth; headache; muscle pain or tremors; nighttime urination

Other side effects not listed above may also occur in some patients. If you notice any other effects, check with your doctor.

Revised: 10/21/92
Interim revision: 04/14/94

# GUANETHIDINE   Systemic

**In the U.S.—**
    Ismelin
  Generic name product may also be available.
**In Canada—**
    Apo-Guanethidine
    Ismelin

## Description

Guanethidine (gwahn-ETH-i-deen) belongs to the general class of medicines called antihypertensives. It is used to treat high blood pressure (hypertension).

High blood pressure adds to the work load of the heart and arteries. If it continues for a long time, the heart and arteries may not function properly. This can damage the blood vessels of the brain, heart, and kidneys, resulting in a stroke, heart failure, or kidney failure. High blood pressure may also increase the risk of heart attacks. These problems may be less likely to occur if blood pressure is controlled.

Guanethidine works by controlling nerve impulses along certain nerve pathways. As a result, it relaxes the blood vessels so that blood passes through them more easily. This helps to lower blood pressure.

Guanethidine is available only with your doctor's prescription, in the following dosage form:
    *Oral*
      • Tablets (U.S. and Canada)

## Before Using This Medicine

In deciding to use a medicine, the risks of taking the medicine must be weighed against the good it will do. This is a decision you and your doctor will make. For guanethidine, the following should be considered:

**Allergies**—Tell your doctor if you have ever had any unusual or allergic reaction to guanethidine. Also tell your health care professional if you are allergic to any other substance, such as foods, preservatives, or dyes.

**Pregnancy**—Studies on effects in pregnancy have not been done in either humans or animals.

**Breast-feeding**—Small amounts of guanethidine pass into breast milk. However, this medicine has not been reported to cause problems in nursing babies.

**Children**—Although there is no specific information comparing use of guanethidine in children with use in other age groups, this medicine is not expected to cause different side effects or problems in children than it does in adults.

**Older adults**—Many medicines have not been studied specifically in older people. Therefore, it may not be known whether they work exactly the same way they do in younger adults. Although there is no specific information comparing use of guanethidine in the elderly with use in other age groups, dizziness, lightheadedness, or fainting may be more likely to occur in the elderly, who are more sensitive to the effects of guanethidine.

**Other medicines**—Although certain medicines should not be used together at all, in other cases two different medicines may be used together even if an interaction might occur. In these cases, your doctor may want to change the dose, or other precautions may be necessary. When you are taking guanethidine, it is especially important that your health care professional knows if you are taking any of the following:

- Antidiabetics, oral (diabetes medicine you take by mouth)—Effects may be increased by guanethidine
- Loxapine (e.g., Loxitane) or
- Thioxanthenes (chlorprothixene [e.g., Taractan], thiothixene [e.g., Navane]) or
- Tricyclic antidepressants (amitriptyline [e.g., Elavil], amoxapine [e.g., Asendin], clomipramine [e.g., Anafranil], desipramine [e.g., Pertofrane], doxepin [e.g., Sinequan], imipramine [e.g., Tofranil], nortriptyline [e.g., Aventyl], protriptyline [e.g., Vivactil], trimipramine [e.g., Surmontil]) or
- Trimeprazine (e.g., Temaril)—May decrease the effects of guanethidine on blood pressure
- Minoxidil (e.g., Loniten)—Effects on blood pressure may be greatly increased
- Monoamine oxidase (MAO) inhibitors (furazolidone [e.g., Furoxone], isocarboxazid [e.g., Marplan], phenelzine [e.g., Nardil], procarbazine [e.g., Matulane], selegiline [e.g., Eldepryl], tranylcypromine [e.g., Parnate])—Taking guanethidine while you are taking or within 2 weeks of taking MAO inhibitors may cause a severe increase in blood pressure

**Other medical problems**—The presence of other medical problems may affect the use of guanethidine. Make sure you tell your doctor if you have any other medical problems, especially:

- Asthma (history of) or
- Diarrhea or
- Pheochromocytoma or
- Stomach ulcer (history of)—May be worsened by guanethidine
- Diabetes mellitus (sugar diabetes)—Effects of medicine used to treat this may be increased by guanethidine
- Fever—Effects of guanethidine may be increased
- Heart or blood vessel disease or
- Heart attack or stroke (recent)—Lowering blood pressure may make problems resulting from these conditions worse
- Kidney disease—May be worsened. Also, effects of guanethidine may be increased because of slower removal of this medicine from the body
- Liver disease—Effects of guanethidine may be increased because of slower removal from the body

## Proper Use of This Medicine

In addition to the use of the medicine your doctor has prescribed, treatment for your high blood pressure may include weight control and care in the types of foods you eat, especially foods high in sodium. Your doctor will tell you which of these are most important for you. You should check with your doctor before changing your diet.

Many patients who have high blood pressure will not notice any signs of the problem. In fact, many may feel normal. It is very important that you *take your medicine exactly as directed* and that you keep your appointments with your doctor even if you feel well.

Remember that guanethidine will not cure your high blood pressure but it does help control it. Therefore, you must continue to take it as directed if you expect to lower your blood pressure and keep it down. *You may have to take high blood pressure medicine for the rest of your life.* If high blood pressure is not treated, it can cause serious problems such as heart failure, blood vessel disease, stroke, or kidney disease.

To help you remember to take your medicine, try to get into the habit of taking it at the same time each day.

**Dosing**—The dose of guanethidine will be different for different patients. *Follow your doctor's orders or the directions on the label.* The following information includes only the average doses of guanethidine. *If your dose is different, do not change it* unless your doctor tells you to do so.

The number of tablets that you take depends on the strength of the medicine.

- For *oral* dosage form (tablets):
  —For high blood pressure:
  - Adults—At first, 10 or 12.5 milligrams (mg) once a day. Then, your doctor may increase your dose to 25 to 50 mg once a day.
  - Children—The dose is based on body weight. The usual dose is 200 micrograms (mcg) per kilogram (kg) (90.9 mcg per pound) of body weight a day. Then, your doctor may increase your dose as needed.

**Missed dose**—If you miss a dose of guanethidine, take it as soon as possible. However, if it is almost time for your next dose, skip the missed dose and go back to your regular dosing schedule. Do not double doses.

**Storage**—To store this medicine:
- Keep out of the reach of children.
- Store away from heat and direct light.
- Do not store in the bathroom, near the kitchen sink, or in other damp places. Heat or moisture may cause the medicine to break down.
- Do not keep outdated medicine or medicine no longer needed. Be sure that any discarded medicine is out of the reach of children.

## Precautions While Using This Medicine

It is important that your doctor check your progress at regular visits to make sure that this medicine is working properly.

*Dizziness, lightheadedness, or fainting may occur, especially when you get up from a lying or sitting position.* This is more likely to occur in the morning. *Getting up slowly may help.* When you get up from lying down, sit on the edge of the bed with your feet dangling for 1 or 2 minutes. Then stand up slowly. If the problem continues or gets worse, check with your doctor.

The dizziness, lightheadedness, or fainting is also more likely to occur if you drink alcohol, stand for long periods of time, exercise, or if the weather is hot. *While you are taking this medicine, be careful in the amount of alcohol you drink. Also, use extra care during exercise or hot weather or if you must stand for long periods of time.*

*Do not take other medicines unless they have been discussed with your doctor.* This especially includes over-the-counter (nonprescription) medicines for appetite control, asthma, colds, cough, hay fever, or sinus problems, since they may tend to increase your blood pressure.

Before having any kind of surgery (including dental surgery) or emergency treatment, tell the medical doctor or dentist in charge that you are taking this medicine.

Tell your doctor if you get a fever since that may change the amount of medicine you have to take.

## Side Effects of This Medicine

Along with its needed effects, a medicine may cause some unwanted effects. Although not all of these side effects may occur, if they do occur they may need medical attention.

Check with your doctor as soon as possible if any of the following side effects occur:

*More common*
　Swelling of feet or lower legs
*Less common or rare*
　Chest pain; shortness of breath

Other side effects may occur that usually do not need medical attention. These side effects may go away during treatment as your body adjusts to the medicine. However, check with your doctor if any of the following side effects continue or are bothersome:

*More common*
　Diarrhea or increase in bowel movements; dizziness, light-headedness, or fainting, especially when getting up from a lying or sitting position; sexual problems in males; slow heartbeat; stuffy nose; unusual tiredness or weakness

*Less common or rare*
> Blurred vision; drooping eyelids; dryness of mouth; headache; loss of hair on scalp; muscle pain or tremors; nausea or vomiting; nighttime urination; skin rash

Other side effects not listed above may also occur in some patients. If you notice any other effects, check with your doctor.

Revised: 08/05/92
Interim revision: 04/25/94

# GUANETHIDINE AND HYDROCHLOROTHIAZIDE    Systemic

Some commonly used brand names are:
**In the U.S.—**
  Esimil
**In Canada—**
  Ismelin-Esidrix

## Description

Guanethidine (gwahn-ETH-i-deen) and hydrochlorothiazide (hye-droe-klor-oh-THYE-a-zide) combination is used to treat high blood pressure (hypertension).

High blood pressure adds to the work load of the heart and arteries. If it continues for a long time, the heart and arteries may not function properly. This can damage the blood vessels of the brain, heart, and kidneys, resulting in a stroke, heart failure, or kidney failure. High blood pressure may also increase the risk of heart attacks. These problems may be less likely to occur if blood pressure is controlled.

Guanethidine works by controlling nerve impulses along certain nerve pathways. As a result, it relaxes the blood vessels so that blood passes through them more easily. The hydrochlorothiazide in this combination is a thiazide diuretic (water pill) that helps reduce the amount of water in the body by increasing the flow of urine.

Guanethidine and hydrochlorothiazide combination is available only with your doctor's prescription, in the following dosage form:
*Oral*
  • Tablets (U.S. and Canada)

## Before Using This Medicine

In deciding to use a medicine, the risks of taking the medicine must be weighed against the good it will do. This is a decision you and your doctor will make. For guanethidine and hydrochlorothiazide, the following should be considered:

**Allergies**—Tell your doctor if you have ever had any unusual or allergic reaction to guanethidine, sulfonamides (sulfa drugs), hydrochlorothiazide, bumetanide, furosemide, acetazolamide, dichlorphenamide, methazolamide, or to other thiazide diuretics (water pills). Also tell your health care professional if you are allergic to any other substance, such as foods, preservatives, or dyes.

**Pregnancy**—When hydrochlorothiazide is used during pregnancy, it may cause side effects including jaundice, blood problems, and low potassium in the newborn infant. However, this medicine has not been shown to cause birth defects.

**Breast-feeding**—Guanethidine and hydrochlorothiazide pass into breast milk. However, this medicine has not been reported to cause problems in nursing babies.

**Children**—Although there is no specific information about the use of this medicine in children, it is not expected to cause different side effects or problems in children than it does in adults. However, extra caution may be necessary in infants with jaundice, because thiazide diuretics can make the condition worse.

**Older adults**—Dizziness, lightheadedness, fainting, or signs and symptoms of too much potassium loss may be more likely to occur in the elderly, who are more sensitive to the effects of guanethidine and hydrochlorothiazide.

**Other medicines**—Although certain medicines should not be used together at all, in other cases two different medicines may be used together even if an interaction might occur. In these cases, your doctor may want to change the dose, or other precautions may be necessary. When you are taking guanethidine and hydrochlorothiazide, it is especially important that your health care professional know if you are taking any of the following:
  • Antidiabetics, oral (diabetes medicine you take by mouth)—Effects may be increased by guanethidine
  • Cholestyramine or
  • Colestipol—Use with thiazide diuretics may prevent the diuretic from working properly; take the diuretic at least 1 hour before or 4 hours after cholestyramine or colestipol
  • Digitalis glycosides (heart medicine)—Hydrochlorothiazide may cause low potassium in the blood, which can lead to symptoms of digitalis toxicity
  • Lithium (e.g., Lithane)—Risk of lithium overdose, even at usual doses, may be increased
  • Loxapine (e.g., Loxitane) or
  • Thioxanthenes (chlorprothixene [e.g., Taractan], thiothixene [e.g., Navane]) or
  • Tricyclic antidepressants (amitriptyline [e.g., Elavil], amoxapine [e.g., Asendin], clomipramine [e.g., Anafranil], desipramine [e.g., Pertofrane], doxepin [e.g., Sinequan], imipramine [e.g., Tofranil], nortriptyline [e.g., Aventyl], protriptyline [e.g., Vivactil], trimipramine [e.g., Surmontil]) or

- Trimeprazine (e.g., Temaril)—May decrease the effects of guanethidine on blood pressure
- Monoamine oxidase (MAO) inhibitors (furazolidone [e.g., Furoxone], isocarboxazid [e.g., Marplan], phenelzine [e.g., Nardil], procarbazine [e.g., Matulane], selegiline [e.g., Eldepryl], tranylcypromine [e.g., Parnate])—Taking guanethidine while you are taking or within 2 weeks of taking MAO inhibitors may cause a severe increase in blood pressure

**Other medical problems**—The presence of other medical problems may affect the use of guanethidine and hydrochlorothiazide. Make sure you tell your doctor if you have any other medical problems, especially:

- Asthma (history of) or
- Diarrhea or
- Pheochromocytoma or
- Stomach ulcer (history of)—May be worsened by guanethidine
- Diabetes mellitus (sugar diabetes)—Effects of medicine used to treat this may be increased by guanethidine. Hydrochlorothiazide may change the amount of diabetes medicine needed
- Fever—Effects of guanethidine may be increased
- Gout (history of)—Hydrochlorothiazide may increase the amount of uric acid in the blood, which can lead to gout
- Heart or blood vessel disease or
- Heart attack or stroke (recent)—Lowering blood pressure may make problems resulting from these conditions worse
- Kidney disease—May be worsened. Also, effects may be increased because of slower removal of guanethidine from the body
- Liver disease—Effects may be increased because of slower removal of guanethidine from the body
- Lupus erythematosus (history of)—Hydrochlorothiazide may worsen the condition
- Pancreatitis (inflammation of the pancreas)

## Proper Use of This Medicine

This medicine may cause you to have an unusual feeling of tiredness when you begin to take it. You may also notice an increase in the amount of urine or in your frequency of urination. After taking the medicine for a while, these effects should lessen. In general, in order to keep the increase in urine from affecting your sleep:

- If you are to take a single dose a day, take it in the morning after breakfast.
- If you are to take more than one dose a day, take the last dose no later than 6 p.m., unless otherwise directed by your doctor.

However, it is best to plan your dose or doses according to a schedule that will least affect your personal activities and sleep. Ask your health care professional to help you plan the best time to take this medicine.

In addition to the use of the medicine your doctor has prescribed, treatment for your high blood pressure may include weight control and care in the types of foods you eat, especially foods high in sodium. Your doctor will tell you which of these are most important for you. You should check with your doctor before changing your diet.

Many patients who have high blood pressure will not notice any signs of the problem. In fact, many may feel normal. It is very important that you *take your medicine exactly as directed* and that you keep your appointments with your doctor even if you feel well.

Remember that this medicine will not cure your high blood pressure but it does help control it. Therefore, you must continue to take it as directed if you expect to lower your blood pressure and keep it down. *You may have to take high blood pressure medicine for the rest of your life.* If high blood pressure is not treated, it can cause serious problems such as heart failure, blood vessel disease, stroke, or kidney disease.

To help you remember to take your medicine, try to get into the habit of taking it at the same time each day.

**Dosing**—The dose of guanethidine and hydrochlorothiazide combination will be different for different patients. *Follow your doctor's orders or the directions on the label.* The following information includes only the average dose of guanethidine and hydrochlorothiazide combination. *If your dose is different, do not change it* unless your doctor tells you to do so.

- For *oral* dosage form (tablets):
  —For high blood pressure:
  - Adults—2 tablets a day.
  - Children—Dose must be determined by your doctor.

**Missed dose**—If you miss a dose of this medicine, take it as soon as possible. However, if it is almost time for your next dose, skip the missed dose and go back to your regular dosing schedule. Do not double doses.

**Storage**—To store this medicine:
- Keep out of the reach of children.
- Store away from heat and direct light.
- Do not store in the bathroom, near the kitchen sink, or in other damp places. Heat or moisture may cause the medicine to break down.
- Do not keep outdated medicine or medicine no longer needed. Be sure that any discarded medicine is out of the reach of children.

## Precautions While Using This Medicine

It is important that your doctor check your progress at regular visits to make sure that this medicine is working properly.

*Do not take other medicines unless they have been discussed with your doctor.* This especially includes over-the-counter (nonprescription) medicines for appetite control, asthma, colds, cough, hay fever, or sinus problems, since they may tend to increase your blood pressure.

This medicine may cause a loss of potassium from your body.
- To help prevent this, your doctor may want you to:
  —eat or drink foods that have a high potassium content (for example, orange or other citrus fruit juices), or

—take a potassium supplement, or

—take another medicine to help prevent the loss of the potassium in the first place.

- It is very important to follow these directions. Also, it is important not to change your diet on your own. This is more important if you are already on a special diet (as for diabetes), or if you are taking a potassium supplement or a medicine to reduce potassium loss. Extra potassium may not be necessary and, in some cases, too much potassium could be harmful.

Check with your doctor if you become sick and have severe or continuing vomiting or diarrhea. These problems may cause you to lose additional water and potassium.

*Dizziness, lightheadedness, or fainting may occur, especially when you get up from a lying or sitting position.* This is more likely to occur in the morning. *Getting up slowly* may help. When you get up from lying down, sit on the edge of the bed with your feet dangling for 1 or 2 minutes. Then stand up slowly. If the problem continues or gets worse, check with your doctor.

The dizziness, lightheadedness, or fainting is also more likely to occur if you drink alcohol, stand for long periods of time or exercise, or if the weather is hot. *While you are taking this medicine, be careful in the amount of alcohol you drink. Also, use extra care during exercise or hot weather or if you must stand for long periods of time.*

For *diabetic patients*:

- This medicine may raise blood sugar levels. While you are using this medicine, be especially careful in testing for sugar in your blood or urine. If you have any questions about this, check with your doctor.

Some people who take this medicine may become more sensitive to sunlight than they are normally. Exposure to sunlight, even for brief periods of time, may cause severe sunburn; skin rash, redness, itching, or discoloration; or vision changes. When you begin taking this medicine:

- Stay out of direct sunlight, especially between the hours of 10:00 a.m. and 3:00 p.m., if possible.
- Wear protective clothing, including a hat and sunglasses.
- Apply a sun block product that has a skin protection factor (SPF) of at least 15. Some patients may require a product with a higher SPF number, especially if they have a fair complexion. If you have any questions about this, check with your health care professional.
- Do not use a sunlamp or tanning bed or booth.

If you have a severe reaction from the sun, check with your doctor.

Tell your doctor if you get a fever since that may change the amount of medicine you have to take.

Before having any kind of surgery (including dental surgery) or emergency treatment, tell the medical doctor or dentist in charge that you are taking this medicine.

## Side Effects of This Medicine

Along with its needed effects, a medicine may cause some unwanted effects. Although not all of these side effects may occur, if they do occur they may need medical attention.

Check with your doctor as soon as possible if any of the following side effects occur, especially since some of them may mean that your body is losing too much potassium:

*Signs and symptoms of too much potassium loss*

Dryness of mouth; increased thirst; irregular heartbeats; mood or mental changes; muscle cramps or pain; nausea or vomiting; unusual tiredness or weakness; weak pulse

*Signs and symptoms of too much sodium loss*

Confusion; convulsions; decreased mental activity; irritability; muscle cramps; unusual tiredness or weakness

*Less common*

Chest pain

*Rare*

Black, tarry stools; blood in urine or stools; cough or hoarseness; fever or chills; joint pain; lower back or side pain; painful or difficult urination; pinpoint red spots on skin; skin rash or hives; sore throat and fever; stomach pain (severe) with nausea and vomiting; unusual bleeding or bruising; yellow eyes or skin

Other side effects may occur that usually do not need medical attention. These side effects may go away during treatment as your body adjusts to the medicine. However, check with your doctor if any of the following side effects continue or are bothersome:

*More common*

Diarrhea or increase in bowel movements; dizziness, lightheadedness, or fainting, especially when getting up from a lying or sitting position; sexual problems in males; slow heartbeat; stuffy nose

*Less common or rare*

Blurred vision; drooping eyelids; headache; increased sensitivity of skin to sunlight; loss of appetite; loss of hair; nighttime urination

Other side effects not listed above may also occur in some patients. If you notice any other effects, check with your doctor.

Revised: 07/14/92
Interim revision: 04/29/94

# GUANFACINE  Systemic†

A commonly used brand name in the U.S. is Tenex.

†Not commercially available in Canada.

## Description

Guanfacine (GWAHN-fa-seen) belongs to the general class of medicines called antihypertensives. It is used to treat high blood pressure (hypertension).

High blood pressure adds to the workload of the heart and arteries. If it continues for a long time, the heart and arteries may not function properly. This can damage the blood vessels of the brain, heart, and kidneys, resulting in a stroke, heart failure, or kidney failure. High blood pressure may also increase the risk of heart attacks. These problems may be less likely to occur if blood pressure is controlled.

Guanfacine works by controlling nerve impulses along certain nerve pathways. As a result, it relaxes blood vessels so that blood passes through them more easily. This helps to lower blood pressure.

Guanfacine is available only with your doctor's prescription, in the following dosage form:

*Oral*
- Tablets (U.S.)

## Before Using This Medicine

In deciding to use a medicine, the risks of taking the medicine must be weighed against the good it will do. This is a decision you and your doctor will make. For guanfacine, the following should be considered:

**Allergies**—Tell your doctor if you have ever had any unusual or allergic reaction to guanfacine. Also tell your health care professional if you are allergic to any other substance, such as foods, preservatives, or dyes.

**Pregnancy**—Guanfacine has not been studied in pregnant women. However, guanfacine has not been shown to cause birth defects or other problems in rats or rabbits given many times the human dose. In rats and rabbits given extremely high doses (up to 200 times the human dose), there was an increase in deaths of the animal fetus.

**Breast-feeding**—It is not known whether guanfacine passes into breast milk. However, this medicine has not been reported to cause problems in nursing babies.

**Children**—Studies on this medicine have been done only in adult patients, and there is no specific information comparing use of guanfacine in children with use in other age groups.

**Older adults**—Dizziness, drowsiness, or faintness may be more likely to occur in the elderly, who are more sensitive to the effects of guanfacine.

**Other medicines**—Although certain medicines should not be used together at all, in other cases two different medicines may be used together even if an interaction might occur. In these cases, your doctor may want to change the dose, or other precautions may be necessary. Tell your health care professional if you are taking any other prescription or nonprescription (over-the-counter [OTC]) medicine.

**Other medical problems**—The presence of other medical problems may affect the use of guanfacine. Make sure you tell your doctor if you have any other medical problems, especially:
- Heart disease or
- Heart attack or stroke (recent)—Lowering blood pressure may make problems resulting from these conditions worse
- Liver disease—Effects may be increased because of slower removal of guanfacine from the body
- Mental depression—Guanfacine may cause mental depression

## Proper Use of This Medicine

In addition to the use of the medicine your doctor has prescribed, treatment for your high blood pressure may include weight control and care in the types of foods you eat, especially foods high in sodium. Your doctor will tell you which of these are most important for you. You should check with your doctor before changing your diet.

Many patients who have high blood pressure will not notice any signs of the problem. In fact, many may feel normal. It is very important that you *take your medicine exactly as directed* and that you keep your appointments with your doctor even if you feel well.

Remember that this medicine will not cure your high blood pressure but it does help control it. Therefore, you must continue to use it as directed if you expect to lower your blood pressure and keep it down. *You may have to take high blood pressure medicine for the rest of your life.* If high blood pressure is not treated, it can cause serious problems such as heart failure, blood vessel disease, stroke, or kidney disease.

Take your daily dose of guanfacine at bedtime. (If you are taking more than one dose a day, take your last dose at bedtime). Taking it this way will help lessen daytime drowsiness.

**Dosing**—The dose of guanfacine will be different for different patients. *Follow your doctor's orders or the directions on the label.* The following information includes only the average doses of guanfacine. *If your dose is different, do not change it* unless your doctor tells you to do so.

The number of tablets that you take depends on the strength of the medicine.

- For *oral* dosage form (tablets):
  —For high blood pressure:
    - Adults—At first, 1 milligram (mg) once a day at bedtime. Then, your doctor may gradually increase your dose up to 3 mg a day, if needed.
    - Children—Dose must be determined by your doctor.

**Missed dose**—If you miss a dose of this medicine, take it as soon as possible. However, if it is almost time for your next dose, skip the missed dose and go back to your regular dosing schedule. Do not double doses. *If you miss taking guanfacine for two or more days in a row, check with your doctor.* If your body suddenly goes without this medicine, some unwanted effects may occur. If you have any questions about this, check with your doctor.

**Storage**—To store this medicine:
- Keep out of the reach of children.
- Store away from heat and direct light.
- Do not store in the bathroom, near the kitchen sink, or in other damp places. Heat or moisture may cause the medicine to break down.
- Do not keep outdated medicine or medicine no longer needed. Be sure any discarded medicine is out of the reach of children.

## Precautions While Using This Medicine

It is important that your doctor check your progress at regular visits to make sure this medicine is working properly.

Check with your doctor before you stop taking guanfacine. Your doctor may want you to reduce gradually the amount you are taking before stopping completely.

Make sure that you have enough guanfacine on hand to last through weekends, holidays, and vacations. You should not miss any doses. You may want to ask your doctor for another written prescription for guanfacine to carry in your wallet or purse. You can then have it filled if you run out when you are away from home.

Before having any kind of surgery (including dental surgery) or emergency treatment, tell the medical doctor or dentist in charge that you are using this medicine.

*Do not take other medicines unless they have been discussed with your doctor.* This especially includes over-the-counter (nonprescription) medicines for appetite control, asthma, colds, cough, hay fever, or sinus problems, since they may tend to increase your blood pressure.

Guanfacine will add to the effects of alcohol and other CNS depressants (medicines that slow down the nervous system, possibly causing drowsiness). Some examples of CNS depressants are antihistamines or medicine for hay fever, other allergies, or colds; sedatives, tranquilizers, or sleeping medicine; prescription pain medicine or narcotics; barbiturates; medicine for seizures; muscle relaxants; or anesthetics, including some dental anesthetics. *Check with your doctor before taking any of the above while you are using this medicine.*

Guanfacine may cause some people to become dizzy, drowsy, or less alert than they are normally. *Make sure you know how you react to this medicine before you drive, use machines, or do anything else that could be dangerous if you are dizzy or are not alert.*

Guanfacine may cause dryness of the mouth, nose, and throat. For temporary relief of mouth dryness, use sugarless candy or gum, melt bits of ice in your mouth, or use a saliva substitute. However, if dry mouth continues for more than 2 weeks, check with your physician or dentist. Continuing dryness of the mouth may increase the chance of dental disease, including tooth decay, gum disease, and fungus infections.

## Side Effects of This Medicine

Along with its needed effects, a medicine may cause some unwanted effects. Although not all of these side effects may occur, if they do occur they may need medical attention.

Check with your doctor as soon as possible if any of the following side effects occur:

*Less common*
    Confusion; mental depression
*Signs and symptoms of overdose*
    Difficulty in breathing; dizziness (extreme) or faintness; slow heartbeat; unusual tiredness or weakness (severe)

Other side effects may occur that usually do not need medical attention. These side effects may go away during treatment as your body adjusts to the medicine. However, check with your doctor if any of the following side effects continue or are bothersome:

*More common*
    Constipation; dizziness; drowsiness; dryness of mouth
*Less common*
    Decreased sexual ability; dry, itching, or burning eyes; headache; nausea or vomiting; trouble in sleeping; unusual tiredness or weakness

After you have been using this medicine for a while, unwanted effects may occur if you stop taking it too suddenly. After you stop taking this medicine, check with your doctor if any of the following side effects occur:

    Anxiety or tenseness; chest pain; fast or irregular heartbeat; headache; increased salivation; nausea or vomiting; nervousness or restlessness; shaking or trembling of hands and fingers; stomach cramps; sweating; trouble in sleeping

Other side effects not listed above may also occur in some patients. If you notice any other effects, check with your doctor.

Revised: 10/21/92
Interim revision: 07/05/94

# HAEMOPHILUS B CONJUGATE VACCINE    Systemic

Some commonly used brand names are:

**In the U.S.—**

| | |
|---|---|
| Act-Hib | Pedvaxhib |
| Hibtiter | Prohibit |

**In Canada—**

| | |
|---|---|
| Act-Hib | Pedvaxhib |
| Hibtiter | Prohibit |

Other commonly used names are: HbOC, PRP-D, PRP-OMP, and PRP-T.

## Description

Haemophilus b conjugate (hem-OFF-fil-us BEE KON-ja-gat) vaccine is an active immunizing agent used to prevent infection by *Haemophilus influenzae* type b (Hib) bacteria. The vaccine works by causing your body to produce its own protection (antibodies) against the disease.

Haemophilus b conjugate vaccine is an haemophilus b vaccine that has been prepared by adding a diphtheria-, meningococcal-, or tetanus-related substance. However, this vaccine does *not* take the place of the regular diphtheria or tetanus toxoid injections (for example, DTP, DT, or T) that children should receive, the regular tetanus toxoid or diphtheria and tetanus toxoid injections (for example T or Td) that adults should receive, or the meningococcal vaccine injection that some children and adults should receive.

Infection by *Haemophilus influenzae* type b (Hib) bacteria can cause life-threatening illnesses, such as meningitis, which affects the brain; epiglottitis, which can cause death by suffocation; pericarditis, which affects the heart; pneumonia, which affects the lungs; and septic arthritis, which affects the bones and joints. Hib meningitis causes death in 5 to 10% of children who are infected. Also, approximately 30% of children who survive Hib meningitis are left with some type of serious permanent damage, such as mental retardation, deafness, epilepsy, or partial blindness.

Immunization against Hib is recommended for all children 2 months up to 5 years of age (i.e., up to the 5th birthday).

Immunization against Hib may also be recommended for adults and children over 5 years of age with certain medical problems.

This vaccine is to be administered only by or under the supervision of your doctor or other authorized health care professional. It is available in the following dosage form:

*Parenteral*
- Injection (U.S. and Canada)

## Before Receiving This Vaccine

In deciding to use a medicine, the risks of taking the medicine must be weighed against the good it will do. This is a decision you and your doctor will make. For haemophilus b conjugate vaccine, the following should be considered:

**Allergies**—Tell your doctor if you have ever had any unusual or allergic reaction to haemophilus b conjugate vaccine, haemophilus b polysaccharide vaccine, diphtheria or tetanus toxoid, or meningococcal vaccine. Also tell your health care professional if you are allergic to any other substances, such as preservatives.

**Pregnancy**—Studies on effects in pregnancy have not been done in either humans or animals.

**Breast-feeding**—This vaccine has not been reported to cause problems in nursing babies.

**Children**—This vaccine is not recommended for children less than 2 months of age.

**Older adults**—Many medicines have not been studied specifically in older people. Therefore, it may not be known whether they work exactly the same way they do in younger adults. Although there is no specific information comparing use of this vaccine in the elderly with use in other age groups, this vaccine is not expected to cause different side effects or problems in older people than it does in younger adults.

**Other medicines**—Although certain medicines should not be used together at all, in other cases two different medicines may be used together even if an interaction might occur. In these cases, your doctor may want to change the dose, or other precautions may be necessary. Tell your health care professional if you are using any other prescription or nonprescription (over-the-counter [OTC]) medicine.

**Other medical problems**—The presence of other medical problems may affect the use of haemophilus b conjugate vaccine. Make sure you tell your doctor if you have any other medical problems, especially:

- Fever or
- Serious illness—The symptoms of the condition may be confused with some of the possible side effects of the vaccine

## Proper Use of This Vaccine

**Dosing**—Haemophilus b conjugate vaccine is an haemophilus b vaccine that has been prepared by adding a diphtheria-, meningococcal-, or tetanus-related substance to it. If the vaccine was prepared using a diphtheria-related substance, it is called either HbOC or PRP-D. If the vaccine was prepared using a meningococcal-related substance, it is called PRP-OMP. If the vaccine was prepared using a tetanus-related substance, it is called PRP-T. *All of these subtypes of haemophilus b conjugate vaccine work the same way*, but may be given at different ages or times.

The dose of haemophilus b conjugate vaccine will be different for different patients. The following information includes only the average doses of haemophilus b conjugate vaccine.

- For prevention of *Haemophilus influenzae* type b infection:

    —For *HbOC or PRP-T injection* dosage form:
    - Adults and children 5 years of age and older— Use and dose must be determined by your doctor.
    - Infants 2 to 6 months of age at the first dose— Three doses, two months apart, then a booster dose at fifteen months of age. The doses are injected into a muscle.
    - Children 7 to 11 months of age at the first dose—Two doses, two months apart, then a booster dose at fifteen months of age. The doses are injected into a muscle.
    - Children 12 to 14 months of age at the first dose—One dose, then a booster dose at fifteen months of age. The doses are injected into a muscle.
    - Children 15 to 59 months of age at the first dose—One dose injected into a muscle.

    —For *PRP-D injection* dosage form:
    - Adults and children 5 years of age and older— Use and dose must be determined by your doctor.
    - Infants and children up to 15 months of age— Use is not recommended.
    - Children 15 to 59 months of age at the first dose—One dose injected into a muscle.

    —For *PRP-OMP injection* dosage form:
    - Adults and children 5 years of age and older— Use and dose must be determined by your doctor.
    - Infants 2 to 6 months of age at the first dose— Two doses, two months apart, then a booster dose at twelve months of age. The doses are injected into a muscle.
    - Children 7 to 11 months of age at the first dose—Two doses, two months apart, then a booster dose at fifteen months of age. The doses are injected into a muscle.
    - Children 12 to 14 months of age at the first dose—One dose, then a booster dose at fifteen months of age. The doses are injected into a muscle.

- Children 15 to 59 months of age at the first dose—One dose injected into a muscle.

## After Receiving This Vaccine

This vaccine may interfere with laboratory tests that check for Hib disease. Make sure your doctor knows that you have received Hib vaccine if you are treated for a severe infection during the 2 weeks after you receive this vaccine.

## Side Effects of This Vaccine

Along with its needed effects, a vaccine may cause some unwanted effects. Although not all of these side effects may occur, if they do occur they may need medical attention.

*Get emergency help immediately* if any of the following side effects occur:

*Symptoms of allergic reactions*
> Difficulty in breathing or swallowing; hives; itching (especially of feet or hands); reddening of skin (especially around ears); swelling of eyes, face, or inside of nose; unusual tiredness or weakness (sudden and severe)

*Check with your doctor immediately* if the following side effect occurs:

*Rare*
> Convulsions (seizures)

Other side effects may occur that usually do not need medical attention. However, check with your doctor if any of the following side effects continue or are bothersome:

*More common*
> Fever of up to 102 °F (39 °C) (usually lasts less than 48 hours); irritability; loss of appetite; lack of interest; redness at place of injection; reduced physical activity; tenderness at place of injection; tiredness

*Less common*
> Diarrhea; fever over 102 °F (39 °C) (usually lasts less than 48 hours); hard lump, swelling, or warm feeling at place of injection; skin rash; vomiting

Other side effects not listed above may also occur in some patients. If you notice any other effects, check with your doctor.

Revised: 06/21/93
Interim revision: 03/29/94

# HAEMOPHILUS B POLYSACCHARIDE VACCINE   Systemic*†

Commonly used names are:

| | |
|---|---|
| Haemophilus influenzae type b polysaccharide vaccine | Hib CPS |
| | Hib polysaccharide vaccine |
| HbPV | PRP |

*Not commercially available in the U.S.
†Not commercially available in Canada.

## Description

Haemophilus b polysaccharide (hem-OFF-fil-us BEE pol-i-SAK-ka-ryd) vaccine is an active immunizing agent used to prevent infection by *Haemophilus influenzae* type b (Hib) bacteria. The vaccine works by causing your body to produce its own protection (antibodies) against the disease.

The following information applies only to the Haemophilus b polysaccharide vaccine.

Infection by *Haemophilus influenzae* type b (Hib) bacteria can cause life-threatening illnesses, such as meningitis, which affects the brain; epiglottitis, which can cause death by suffocation; pericarditis, which affects the heart; pneumonia, which affects the lungs; and septic arthritis, which affects the bones and joints. Hib meningitis causes death in 5 to 10% of children who are infected. Also, approximately 30% of children who survive Hib meningitis are left with some type of serious permanent damage, such as mental retardation, deafness, epilepsy, or partial blindness.

Immunization against Hib is recommended for all children 24 months up to 5 years of age (i.e., up to the 5th birthday). In addition, immunization is recommended for children 18 to 24 months of age, especially:

- Children attending day-care facilities.
- Children with chronic illnesses associated with increased risk of Hib disease. These illnesses include asplenia, sickle cell disease, antibody deficiency syndromes, immunosuppression, and Hodgkin's disease.
- Children 18 to 24 months of age who have already had Hib disease. These children may get the disease again if they are not immunized. Children who developed Hib disease when 24 months of age or older do not need to be immunized, since most children in this age group will develop antibodies against the disease.
- Children with human immunodeficiency virus (HIV) infection or acquired immunodeficiency syndrome (AIDS).
- Children of certain racial groups, such as American Indian and Alaskan Eskimo. Children in these groups seem to be at increased risk of Hib disease.
- Children living close together with groups of other persons. Close living conditions increase a child's risk of being exposed to persons who have Hib infection or who carry the bacteria.

It is recommended that children immunized when they were 18 to 24 months of age receive a second dose of vaccine, since these children may not produce enough antibodies to fully protect them from Hib disease. Children who were first immunized when they were 24 months of age or older do not need to be reimmunized.

This vaccine is available only from your doctor or other authorized health care professional, in the following dosage form:

*Parenteral*
- Injection

## Before Receiving This Vaccine

In deciding to use a medicine, the risks of taking the medicine must be weighed against the good it will do. This is a decision you and your doctor will make. For haemophilus b polysaccharide vaccine, the following should be considered:

**Allergies**—Tell your doctor if you have ever had any unusual or allergic reaction to haemophilus b polysaccharide vaccine or haemophilus b conjugate vaccine. Also tell your health care professional if you are allergic to any other substances, such as preservatives.

**Children**—This vaccine is not recommended for children less than 18 months of age.

**Other medicines**—Although certain medicines should not be used together at all, in other cases two different medicines may be used together even if an interaction might occur. In these cases, your doctor may want to change the dose, or other precautions may be necessary. Tell your health care professional if you are using any other prescription or nonprescription (over-the-counter [OTC]) medicine.

**Other medical problems**—The presence of other medical problems may affect the use of haemophilus b polysaccharide vaccine. Make sure you tell your doctor if you have any other medical problems, especially:

- Fever or
- Serious illness—The symptoms of the condition may be confused with the possible side effects of the vaccine

## Proper Use of This Vaccine

**Dosing**—The dose of haemophilus b polysaccharide vaccine will be different for different patients. The following information includes only the average doses of haemophilus b polysaccharide vaccine.

- For *injection* dosage form:
  - —For prevention of *Haemophilus influenzae* type b infection:
    - Adults and children 5 years of age and older—Use is not recommended.
    - Children up to 18 months of age—Use is not recommended.

• Children 18 to 24 months of age—Use and dose must be determined by your doctor.
• Children 24 months to 5 years of age—One dose injected under the skin or into a muscle.

## Side Effects of This Vaccine

Along with its needed effects, a vaccine may cause some unwanted effects. Although not all of these side effects may occur, if they do occur they may need medical attention.

*Get emergency help immediately* if any of the following side effects occur:

*Symptoms of allergic reaction*
Difficulty in breathing or swallowing; hives; itching (especially of feet or hands); reddening of skin (especially around ears); swelling of eyes, face, or inside of nose; unusual tiredness or weakness (sudden and severe)

*Check with your doctor immediately* if the following side effect occurs:

*Rare*
Convulsions (seizures)

Other side effects may occur that usually do not need medical attention. However, check with your doctor if any of the following side effects continue or are bothersome:

*More common*
Diarrhea; fever up to 102 °F (39 °C) (usually lasts less than 48 hours); irritability; lack of appetite; lack of interest; redness at place of injection; reduced physical activity; tenderness at place of injection

*Less common*
Fever over 102 °F (39 °C) (usually lasts less than 48 hours); hard lump at place of injection; itching; joint aches or pains; skin rash; swelling at place of injection; trouble in sleeping; vomiting

Other side effects not listed above may also occur in some patients. If you notice any other effects, check with your doctor.

Revised: 06/21/93
Interim revision: 03/29/94

# HALOFANTRINE    Systemic*†

A commonly used brand name is Halfan.

*Not commercially available in the U.S.
†Not commercially available in Canada.

## Description

Halofantrine (ha-loe-FAN-trin) is used to treat certain types of malaria infection. It works by killing the malaria parasites (tiny one-celled animals).

Halofantrine is available only with your doctor's prescription, in the following dosage forms:

*Oral*
• Oral suspension (United Kingdom)
• Tablets (United Kingdom)

## Before Using This Medicine

In deciding to use a medicine, the risks of taking the medicine must be weighed against the good it will do. This is a decision you and your doctor will make. For halofantrine, the following should be considered:

**Allergies**—Tell your doctor if you have ever had any unusual or allergic reaction to halofantrine. Also tell your health care professional if you are allergic to any other substances, such as foods, preservatives, or dyes.

**Pregnancy**—Halofantrine has not been studied in pregnant women. However, it has been found to cause unwanted effects, including death of the fetus, in animals. Before taking this medicine, make sure your doctor knows if you are pregnant or if you may become pregnant.

**Breast-feeding**—Halofantrine may pass into breast milk and cause unwanted effects in nursing babies. It may be necessary for you to take another medicine or to stop breast-feeding while taking halofantrine. Be sure you have discussed the risks and benefits of the medicine with your doctor.

**Children**—Although there is no specific information comparing use of halofantrine in children with use in other age groups, this medicine is not expected to cause different side effects or problems in children than it does in adults.

**Older adults**—Many medicines have not been studied specifically in older people. Therefore, it may not be known whether they work exactly the same way they do in younger adults or if they cause different side effects or problems in older people. There is no specific information comparing use of halofantrine in the elderly with use in other age groups.

**Other medicines**—Although certain medicines should not be used together at all, in other cases two different medicines may be used together even if an interaction might occur. In these cases, your doctor may want to change the dose, or other precautions may be necessary. When you are taking halofantrine, it is especially important that your health care professional know if you are taking any of the following:
• Mefloquine (e.g., Lariam)—Recent use of mefloquine or use of mefloquine with halofantrine may cause fast and irregular heartbeat

**Other medical problems**—The presence of other medical problems may affect the use of halofantrine. Make sure you tell your doctor if you have any other medical problems, especially:

- Heart problems especially abnormal heartbeat or
- Thiamine deficiency or
- Unexplained sudden fainting—These conditions increase the chance of side effects affecting the heart, including fast irregular heartbeat

## Proper Use of This Medicine

Halofantrine is best taken on an empty stomach to decrease the chance of side effects.

To help clear up your infection completely, *take this medicine exactly as directed by your doctor for the full time of treatment.* Your symptoms may come back if you stop your treatment too early. Your doctor may also instruct you to take a second course of treatment after one week.

**Dosing**—The dose of halofantrine will be different for different patients. *Follow your doctor's orders or the directions on the label.* The following information includes only the average doses of halofantrine. *If your dose is different, do not change it* unless your doctor tells you to do so.

The number of tablets or teaspoonfuls of suspension that you take depends on the strength of the medicine. Also, *the number of doses you take each day, the time allowed between doses, and the length of time you take the medicine depend on the medical problem for which you are taking halofantrine.*

- For malaria:
  —For *oral* dosage form (oral suspension):
  - Adults and children over 12 years of age—500 milligrams (mg), taken on an empty stomach every six hours three times a day for one day. Treatment may need to be repeated after one week.
  - Children—Dose is based on age and/or body weight. Treatment may need to be repeated after one week.
    —1 to 2 years of age: 100 mg, taken on an empty stomach every six hours three times a day for one day.
    —2 to 5 years of age: 150 mg, taken on an empty stomach every six hours three times a day for one day.
    —5 to 8 years of age: 200 mg, taken on an empty stomach every six hours three times a day for one day.
    —8 to 10 years of age: 250 mg, taken on an empty stomach every six hours three times a day for one day.
    —10 to 12 years of age: 300 mg, taken on an empty stomach every six hours three times a day for one day.

  —For *oral* dosage form (tablets):
  - Adults and children over 37 kilograms (81.4 pounds) of body weight—500 mg, taken on an empty stomach every six hours three times a day for one day. Treatment may need to be repeated after one week.
  - Children—Dose is based on body weight and must be determined by your doctor. Treatment may need to be repeated after one week.
    —Up to 23 kilograms (50.6 pounds) of body weight: Dosage has not been established.
    —23 to 31 kilograms (50.6 to 68.2 pounds) of body weight: 250 mg, taken on an empty stomach every six hours three times a day for one day.
    —32 to 37 kilograms (70.4 to 81.4 pounds) of body weight: 375 mg, taken on an empty stomach every six hours three times a day for one day.

**Missed dose**—If you miss a dose of this medicine, take it as soon as possible. However, if it is almost time for your next dose, skip the missed dose and go back to your regular dosing schedule. Do not double doses.

**Storage**—To store this medicine:
- Keep out of the reach of children.
- Store away from heat and direct light.
- Do not store in the bathroom, near the kitchen sink, or in other damp places. Heat or moisture may cause the medicine to break down.
- Keep the liquid form of this medicine from freezing.
- Do not keep outdated medicine or medicine no longer needed. Be sure that any discarded medicine is out of the reach of children.

## Precautions While Using This Medicine

It is important that your doctor check your progress after treatment. This is to make sure that the infection is cleared up completely, and to allow your doctor to check for any unwanted effects.

If your symptoms do not improve after you have taken this medicine for the full course of treatment, or if they become worse, check with your doctor.

Malaria is spread by the bites of certain kinds of infected female mosquitoes. If you are living in, or will be traveling to, an area where there is a chance of getting malaria, the following mosquito-control measures will help to prevent infection:

- If possible, avoid going out between dusk and dawn because it is at these times when mosquitoes most commonly bite.
- Wear long-sleeved shirts and long trousers to protect your arms and legs, especially from dusk through dawn when mosquitoes are out.
- Apply insect repellant, preferably one containing DEET, to uncovered areas of the skin from dusk through dawn when mosquitoes are out.

- If possible, sleep in a screened or air-conditioned room or under mosquito netting sprayed with insecticide to avoid being bitten by malaria-carrying mosquitoes.
- Use mosquito coils or sprays to kill mosquitoes in living and sleeping quarters during evening and night-time hours.

## Side Effects of This Medicine

Along with its needed effects, a medicine may cause some unwanted effects. Although not all of these side effects may occur, if they do occur they may need medical attention.

*Check with your doctor immediately* if any of the following side effects occur:

*Rare*

Anxiety; black or decreased amount of urine; chest or lower back pain; fast and irregular heartbeat; feeling restless; flushing of the whole body; rapid breathing

Other side effects may occur that usually do not need medical attention. These side effects may go away during treatment as your body adjusts to the medicine. However, check with your doctor if any of the following side effects continue or are bothersome:

*Less common*

Abdominal or stomach pain; diarrhea; nausea; skin itching or rash; vomiting

Other side effects not listed above may also occur in some patients. If you notice any other effects, check with your doctor.

Revised: 8/31/93

# HALOPERIDOL   Systemic

Some commonly used brand names are:

**In the U.S.—**
Haldol
Haldol Decanoate
Generic name product may also be available.

**In Canada—**
Apo-Haloperidol          Novo-Peridol
Haldol                   Peridol
Haldol LA                PMS Haloperidol
Generic name product may also be available.

## Description

Haloperidol (ha-loe-PER-i-dole) is used to treat nervous, mental, and emotional conditions. It is also used to control the symptoms of Tourette's disorder. Haloperidol may also be used for other conditions as determined by your doctor.

Haloperidol is available only with your doctor's prescription, in the following dosage forms:

*Oral*
- Solution (U.S. and Canada)
- Tablets (U.S. and Canada)

*Parenteral*
- Injection (U.S. and Canada)

## Before Using This Medicine

In deciding to use a medicine, the risks of taking the medicine must be weighed against the good it will do. This is a decision you and your doctor will make. For haloperidol, the following should be considered:

**Allergies**—Tell your doctor if you have ever had any unusual or allergic reaction to haloperidol. Also tell your health care professional if you are allergic to any other substances, such as foods, preservatives, or dyes.

**Pregnancy**—Haloperidol has not been studied in pregnant women. However, studies in animals given 2 to 20 times the usual maximum human dose of haloperidol have shown reduced fertility, delayed delivery, cleft palate, and an increase in the number of stillbirths and newborn deaths.

**Breast-feeding**—Haloperidol passes into breast milk. Animal studies have shown that haloperidol in breast milk causes drowsiness and unusual muscle movements in the nursing offspring. Breast-feeding is not recommended during treatment with haloperidol.

**Children**—Side effects, especially muscle spasms of the neck and back, twisting movements of the body, trembling of fingers and hands, and inability to move the eyes are more likely to occur in children, who usually are more sensitive than adults to the effects of haloperidol.

**Older adults**—Constipation, dizziness or fainting, drowsiness, dryness of mouth, trembling of the hands and fingers, and symptoms of tardive dyskinesia (such as rapid, worm-like movements of the tongue or any other uncontrolled movements of the mouth, tongue, or jaw, and/or arms and legs) are especially likely to occur in elderly patients, who are usually more sensitive than younger adults to the effects of haloperidol.

**Other medicines**—Although certain medicines should not be used together at all, in other cases 2 different medicines may be used together even if an interaction might occur. In these cases, your doctor may want to change the dose, or other precautions may be necessary. When you are taking haloperidol, it is especially important that

your health care professional know if you are taking any of the following:

- Amoxapine (e.g., Ascendin) or
- Metoclopramide (e.g., Reglan) or
- Metyrosine (e.g., Demser) or
- Other antipsychotics (medicine for mental illness) or
- Pemoline (e.g., Cylert) or
- Pimozide (e.g., Orap) or
- Promethazine (e.g., Phenergan) or
- Rauwolfia alkaloids (alseroxylon [e.g., Rauwiloid], deserpidine [e.g., Harmonyl], rauwolfia serpentina [e.g., Raudixin], reserpine [e.g., Serpasil]) or
- Trimeprazine (e.g., Temaril)—Taking these medicines with haloperidol may increase the frequency and severity of certain side effects
- Central nervous system (CNS) depressants (medicine that causes drowsiness) or
- Tricyclic antidepressants (medicine for depression)—Taking these medicines with haloperidol may result in increased CNS and other depressant effects, and in an increased chance of low blood pressure (hypotension)
- Epinephrine (e.g., Adrenalin)—Severe low blood pressure or irregular heartbeat may occur
- Levodopa (e.g., Dopar, Larodopa)—Haloperidol may interfere with the effects of this medicine
- Lithium (e.g., Eskalith, Lithane)—Although lithium and haloperidol are sometimes used together, their use must be closely monitored by your doctor, who may change the amount of medicine you need to take

**Other medical problems**—The presence of other medical problems may affect the use of haloperidol. Make sure you tell your doctor if you have any other medical problems, especially:

- Alcohol abuse—The risk of heat stroke may be increased
- Difficult urination or
- Glaucoma or
- Heart or blood vessel disease or
- Lung disease or
- Parkinson's disease—Haloperidol may make the condition worse
- Epilepsy—The risk of seizures may be increased
- Kidney disease or
- Liver disease—Higher blood levels of haloperidol may occur, increasing the chance of side effects
- Overactive thyroid—Serious unwanted effects may occur

## Proper Use of This Medicine

If this medicine upsets your stomach, it may be taken with food or milk to lessen stomach irritation.

For patients taking the *liquid form of this medicine*:

- This medicine is to be taken by mouth even if it comes in a dropper bottle. Each dose is to be measured with the specially marked dropper provided with your prescription. Do not use other droppers since they may not deliver the correct amount of medicine.
- This medicine is best taken alone. However, if necessary, it may be mixed with water. If this is done, the mixture should be taken immediately after mixing. Haloperidol should not be taken in tea or coffee,

since they cause the medicine to separate out of solution.

*Take this medicine only as directed by your doctor.* Do not take more of it, do not take it more often, and do not take it for a longer time than your doctor ordered. This is particularly important for children or elderly patients, since they may react very strongly to this medicine.

Continue taking this medicine for the full time of treatment. *Sometimes haloperidol must be taken for several days to several weeks before its full effect is reached.*

**Dosing**—The dose of haloperidol will be different for different patients. *Follow your doctor's orders or the directions on the label.* The following information includes only the average doses of haloperidol. *If your dose is different, do not change it* unless your doctor tells you to do so.

The number of tablets or teaspoonfuls of solution that you take or injections that you receive depends on the strength of the medicine. Also, *the number of doses you take each day, the time allowed between doses, and the length of time you take the medicine depend on the medical problem for which you are using haloperidol.*

- For *oral* dosage forms (solution and tablets):
  —Adults and adolescents: To start, 500 micrograms to 5 milligrams two or three times a day. Your doctor may increase your dose if needed. However, the dose is usually not more than 100 milligrams a day.
  —Children 3 to 12 years of age or weighing 15 to 40 kilograms (33 to 88 pounds): Dose is based on body weight. The usual dose is 25 to 150 micrograms per kilogram (11 to 68 micrograms per pound) a day, taken in smaller doses two or three times a day.
  —Children up to 3 years of age: Dose must be determined by the doctor.
  —Older adults: To start, 500 micrograms to 2 milligrams two or three times a day. The doctor may increase your dose if needed.
- For *short-acting injection* dosage form:
  —Adults and adolescents: To start, 2 to 5 milligrams, usually injected into a muscle. The dose may be repeated every one to eight hours, depending on your condition.
  —Children: Dose must be determined by the doctor.
- For *long-acting or depot injection* dosage form:
  —Adults and adolescents: To start, the dose is usually 10 to 15 times the daily oral dose you were taking, injected into a muscle once a month. The doctor may adjust how much of this medicine you need and how often you will need it, depending on your condition.
  —Children: Dose must be determined by the doctor.

**Missed dose**—If you miss a dose of this medicine, take it as soon as possible. Then take any remaining doses for that day at regularly spaced intervals. Do not double doses.

**Storage**—To store this medicine:
- Keep out of the reach of children.
- Store away from heat and direct light.
- Do not store the tablet form of this medicine in the bathroom, near the kitchen sink, or in other damp places. Heat or moisture may cause the medicine to break down.
- Keep the liquid form of this medicine from freezing.
- Do not keep outdated medicine or medicine no longer needed. Be sure that any discarded medicine is out of the reach of children.

## Precautions While Using This Medicine

Your doctor should check your progress at regular visits, especially during the first few months of treatment with this medicine. The amount of haloperidol you take may be changed often to meet the needs of your condition. This also helps prevent side effects.

*Do not stop taking this medicine without first checking with your doctor.* Your doctor may want you to reduce gradually the amount you are taking before stopping completely. This will allow your body time to adjust and help avoid a worsening of your medical condition.

This medicine will add to the effects of alcohol and other CNS depressants (medicines that slow down the nervous system, possibly causing drowsiness). Some examples of CNS depressants are antihistamines or medicine for hay fever, other allergies, or colds; sedatives, tranquilizers, or sleeping medicine; prescription pain medicine or narcotics; barbiturates; medicine for seizures; muscle relaxants; or anesthetics, including some dental anesthetics. *Check with your doctor before taking any of the above while you are taking this medicine.*

This medicine may cause some people to become dizzy, drowsy, or less alert than they are normally, especially as the amount of medicine is increased. Even if you take haloperidol at bedtime, you may feel drowsy or less alert on arising. *Make sure you know how you react to this medicine before you drive, use machines, or do anything else that could be dangerous if you are dizzy or are not alert.*

Although not a problem for many patients, dizziness, lightheadedness, or fainting may occur, especially when you get up from a lying or sitting position. Getting up slowly may help. However, if the problem continues or gets worse, check with your doctor.

This medicine will often make you sweat less, causing your body temperature to increase. *Use extra care not to become overheated during exercise or hot weather while you are taking this medicine, since overheating may result in heat stroke.* Also, hot baths or saunas may make you feel dizzy or faint while you are taking this medicine.

Before using any prescription or over-the-counter (OTC) medicine for colds or allergies, check with your doctor. These medicines may increase the chance of heat stroke or other unwanted effects, such as dizziness, dry mouth, blurred vision, and constipation, while you are taking haloperidol.

*Before having any kind of surgery, dental treatment, or emergency treatment, tell the medical doctor or dentist in charge that you are using this medicine.* Taking haloperidol together with medicines that are used during surgery or dental or emergency treatments may increase the CNS depressant effects.

Haloperidol may cause your skin to be more sensitive to sunlight than it is normally. Exposure to sunlight, even for brief periods of time, may cause a skin rash, itching, redness or other discoloration of the skin, or a severe sunburn. When you begin taking this medicine:
- Stay out of direct sunlight, especially between the hours of 10:00 a.m. and 3:00 p.m., if possible.
- Wear protective clothing, including a hat. Also, wear sunglasses.
- Apply a sun block product that has a skin protection factor (SPF) of at least 15. Some patients may require a product with a higher SPF number, especially if they have a fair complexion. If you have any questions about this, check with your health care professional.
- Apply a sun block lipstick that has an SPF of at least 15 to protect your lips.
- Do not use a sunlamp or tanning bed or booth.

*If you have a severe reaction from the sun, check with your doctor.*

Haloperidol may cause dryness of the mouth. For temporary relief, use sugarless candy or gum, melt bits of ice in your mouth, or use a saliva substitute. However, if your mouth continues to feel dry for more than 2 weeks, check with your medical doctor or dentist. Continuing dryness of the mouth may increase the chance of dental disease, including tooth decay, gum disease, and fungus infections.

If you are *receiving this medicine by injection:*
- The effects of the long-acting injection form of this medicine may last for up to 6 weeks. *The precautions and side effects information for this medicine applies during this time.*

## Side Effects of This Medicine

Along with its needed effects, haloperidol can sometimes cause serious side effects. Tardive dyskinesia (a movement disorder) may occur and may not go away after you stop using the medicine. Signs of tardive dyskinesia include fine, worm-like movements of the tongue, or other uncontrolled movements of the mouth, tongue, cheeks, jaw, or arms and legs. Other serious but rare side effects may also occur. These include severe muscle stiffness, fever, unusual tiredness or weakness, fast heartbeat, difficult breathing, increased sweating, loss of bladder control, and seizures (neuroleptic malignant syndrome). *You and your doctor should discuss the good this medicine will do as well as the risks of taking it.*

*Stop taking haloperidol and get emergency help immediately* if any of the following side effects occur:

*Rare*

Convulsions (seizures); difficult or fast breathing; fast heartbeat or irregular pulse; fever (high); high or low blood pressure; increased sweating; loss of bladder control; muscle stiffness (severe); unusually pale skin; unusual tiredness or weakness

Check with your doctor as soon as possible if any of the following side effects occur:

*More common*

Difficulty in speaking or swallowing; inability to move eyes; loss of balance control; mask-like face; muscle spasms, especially of the neck and back; restlessness or need to keep moving (severe); shuffling walk; stiffness of arms and legs; trembling and shaking of fingers and hands; twisting movements of body; weakness of arms and legs

*Less common*

Decreased thirst; difficulty in urination; dizziness, light-headedness, or fainting; hallucinations (seeing or hearing things that are not there); lip smacking or puckering; puffing of cheeks; rapid or worm-like movements of tongue; skin rash; uncontrolled chewing movements; uncontrolled movements of arms and legs

*Rare*

Confusion; hot, dry skin, or lack of sweating; increased blinking or spasms of eyelid; muscle weakness; sore throat and fever; uncontrolled twisting movements of neck, trunk, arms, or legs; unusual bleeding or bruising; unusual facial expressions or body positions; yellow eyes or skin

*Symptoms of overdose*

Difficulty in breathing (severe); dizziness (severe); drowsiness (severe); muscle trembling, jerking, stiffness, or uncontrolled movements (severe); unusual tiredness or weakness (severe)

Other side effects may occur that usually do not need medical attention. These side effects may go away during treatment as your body adjusts to the medicine. However, check with your doctor if any of the following side effects continue or are bothersome:

*More common*

Blurred vision; changes in menstrual period; constipation; dryness of mouth; swelling or pain in breasts (in females); unusual secretion of milk; weight gain

*Less common*

Decreased sexual ability; drowsiness; increased sensitivity of skin to sun (skin rash, itching, redness or other discoloration of skin, or severe sunburn); nausea or vomiting

Some side effects, such as trembling of fingers and hands, or uncontrolled movements of the mouth, tongue, and jaw, may occur after you have stopped taking this medicine. If you notice any of these effects, check with your doctor as soon as possible.

Other side effects not listed above may also occur in some patients. If you notice any other effects, check with your doctor.

## Additional Information

Once a medicine has been approved for marketing for a certain use, experience may show that it is also useful for other medical problems. Although these uses are not included in product labeling, haloperidol is used in certain patients with the following medical conditions:

- Huntington's chorea (an hereditary movement disorder)
- Infantile autism
- Nausea and vomiting caused by cancer chemotherapy

Other than the above information, there is no additional information relating to proper use, precautions, or side effects for these uses.

Revised: 03/19/93

# HALOPROGIN    Topical

A commonly used brand name in the U.S. and Canada is Halotex.

## Description

Haloprogin (ha-loe-PROE-jin) belongs to the group of medicines called antifungals. It is used to treat some types of fungus infections.

Haloprogin is available only with your doctor's prescription, in the following dosage forms:

*Topical*

- Cream (U.S. and Canada)
- Solution (U.S. and Canada)

## Before Using This Medicine

In deciding to use a medicine, the risks of using the medicine must be weighed against the good it will do. This is a decision you and your doctor will make. For haloprogin, the following should be considered:

**Allergies**—Tell your doctor if you have ever had any unusual or allergic reaction to haloprogin. Also tell your health care professional if you are allergic to any other substances, such as preservatives or dyes.

**Pregnancy**—Haloprogin has not been studied in pregnant women. However, this medicine has not been shown to cause birth defects or other problems in animal studies.

**Breast-feeding**—It is not known whether topical haloprogin is absorbed into the body and passes into the breast milk. Although most medicines pass into breast milk in small amounts, many of them may be used safely while breast-feeding. Mothers who are using this medicine and who wish to breast-feed should discuss this with their doctor.

**Children**—Studies on this medicine have been done only in adult patients, and there is no specific information comparing use of haloprogin in children with use in other age groups.

**Older adults**—Many medicines have not been studied specifically in older people. Therefore, it may not be known whether they work exactly the same way they do in younger adults. Although there is no specific information comparing use of this medicine in the elderly with use in other age groups, this medicine is not expected to cause different side effects or problems in older people than it does in younger adults.

## Proper Use of This Medicine

Apply enough haloprogin to cover the affected area, and rub in gently.

*Keep this medicine away from the eyes.*

To help clear up your infection completely, *keep using this medicine for the full time of treatment,* even if your condition has improved. *Do not miss any doses.*

**Dosing**—The dose of topical haloprogin will be different for different patients. *Follow your doctor's orders or the directions on the label.* The following information includes only the average doses of topical haloprogin. *If your dose is different, do not change it* unless your doctor tells you to do so.

*The number of doses you use each day, the time allowed between doses, and the length of time you use the medicine depend on the medical problem for which you are using topical haloprogin.*
- For *cream* or *topical solution* dosage forms:
  —For treatment of fungus infections:
    - Adults—Use 2 times a day for 2 to 4 weeks.

- Children—Use and dose must be determined by your doctor.

**Missed dose**—If you miss a dose of this medicine, apply it as soon as possible. However, if it is almost time for your next dose, skip the missed dose and go back to your regular dosing schedule.

**Storage**—To store this medicine:
- Keep out of the reach of children.
- Store away from heat and direct light.
- Keep the medicine from freezing.
- Do not keep outdated medicine or medicine no longer needed. Be sure that any discarded medicine is out of the reach of children.

## Precautions While Using This Medicine

If your skin problem does not improve within 4 weeks, or if it becomes worse, check with your doctor.

## Side Effects of This Medicine

Along with its needed effects, a medicine may cause some unwanted effects. Although not all of these side effects may occur, if they do occur they may need medical attention.

Check with your doctor as soon as possible if any of the following side effects occur:
   Blistering, burning, itching, or other sign of skin irritation not present before use of this medicine

When you apply the solution form of this medicine, a mild temporary stinging may be expected.

Other side effects not listed above may also occur in some patients. If you notice any other effects, check with your doctor.

Revised: 06/21/93

# HEADACHE MEDICINES, ERGOT DERIVATIVE–CONTAINING    Systemic

Some commonly used brand names are:
**In the U.S.—**
Cafergot[3]            Ergomar[2]
Cafertine[3]          Ergostat[2]
Cafetrate[3]          Gotamine[3]
D.H.E. 45[1]          Migergot[3]
Ercaf[3]              Wigraine[3]
Ergo-Caff[3]

**In Canada—**
Cafergot[3]                      Gravergol[7]
Cafergot-PB[5]                   Gynergen[2]
Dihydroergotamine-Sandoz[1]      Medihaler Ergotamine[2]
Ergodryl[8]                      Megral[6]
Ergomar[2]                       Wigraine[4]

Note: For quick reference, the following ergot derivative–containing headache medicines are numbered to match the corresponding brand names.

This information applies to the following medicines:

1. Dihydroergotamine (dye-hye-droe-er-GOT-a-meen)
2. Ergotamine (er-GOT-a-meen)
3. Ergotamine and Caffeine (kaf-EEN)‡
4. Ergotamine, Caffeine, and Belladonna Alkaloids (bell-a-DON-a AL-ka-loids)*
5. Ergotamine, Caffeine, Belladonna Alkaloids, and Pentobarbital (pen-toe-BAR-bi-tal)*
6. Ergotamine, Caffeine, and Cyclizine (SYE-kli-zeen)*
7. Ergotamine, Caffeine, and Dimenhydrinate (dye-men-HYE-dri-nate)*
8. Ergotamine, Caffeine, and Diphenhydramine (dye-fen-HYE-dra-mine)*

---

*Not commercially available in the U.S.
‡Generic name product may also be available in the U.S.

---

# Description

Dihydroergotamine and ergotamine belong to the group of medicines known as ergot alkaloids. They are used to treat severe, throbbing headaches, such as migraine and cluster headaches. Dihydroergotamine and ergotamine are not ordinary pain relievers. They will not relieve any kind of pain other than throbbing headaches. Because these medicines can cause serious side effects, they are usually used for patients whose headaches are not relieved by acetaminophen, aspirin, or other pain relievers.

Dihydroergotamine and ergotamine may cause blood vessels in the body to constrict (become narrower). This effect can lead to serious side effects that are caused by a decrease in the flow of blood (blood circulation) to many parts of the body.

The caffeine present in many ergotamine-containing combinations helps ergotamine work better and faster by causing more of it to be quickly absorbed into the body. The belladonna alkaloids, cyclizine, dimenhydrinate, and diphenhydramine in some combinations help to relieve nausea and vomiting, which often occur together with the headaches. Cyclizine, dimenhydinate, diphenhydramine, and pentobarbital also help the patient relax and even sleep. This also helps relieve headaches.

Dihydroergotamine is also used for other conditions, as determined by your doctor.

These medicines are available only with your doctor's prescription, in the following dosage forms:

*Oral*
  Ergotamine
    • Inhalation aerosol (Canada)
    • Sublingual tablets (U.S. and Canada)
    • Tablets (Canada)
  Ergotamine and Caffeine
    • Tablets (U.S. and Canada)
  Ergotamine, Caffeine, and Belladonna Alkaloids
    • Tablets (Canada)
  Ergotamine, Caffeine, Belladonna Alkaloids, and Pentobarbital
    • Tablets (Canada)
  Ergotamine, Caffeine, and Cyclizine
    • Tablets (Canada)
  Ergotamine, Caffeine, and Dimenhydrinate
    • Capsules (Canada)
  Ergotamine, Caffeine, and Diphenhydramine
    • Capsules (Canada)
*Parenteral*
  Dihydroergotamine
    • Injection (U.S. and Canada)
*Rectal*
  Ergotamine and Caffeine
    • Suppositories (U.S. and Canada)
  Ergotamine, Caffeine, and Belladonna Alkaloids
    • Suppositories (Canada)
  Ergotamine, Caffeine, Belladonna Alkaloids, and Pentobarbital
    • Suppositories (Canada)

---

# Before Using This Medicine

In deciding to use a medicine, the risks of taking the medicine must be weighed against the good it will do. This is a decision you and your doctor will make. For these headache medicines, the following should be considered:

**Allergies**—Tell your doctor if you have ever had any unusual or allergic reaction to atropine, belladonna, pentobarbital or other barbiturates, caffeine, cyclizine, dimenhydrinate, diphenhydramine, or an ergot medicine. Also tell your health care professional if you are allergic to any other substances, such as foods, preservatives, or dyes.

**Pregnancy**—Use of dihydroergotamine or ergotamine by pregnant women may cause serious harm, including death of the fetus and miscarriage. Therefore, *these medicines should not be used during pregnancy*.

**Breast-feeding**—

- *For dihydroergotamine and ergotamine:* These medicines pass into the breast milk and may cause unwanted effects, such as vomiting, diarrhea, weak pulse, changes in blood pressure, or convulsions (seizures) in nursing babies. Large amounts of these medicines may also decrease the flow of breast milk.

- *For caffeine:* Caffeine passes into the breast milk. Large amounts of it may cause the baby to appear jittery or to have trouble in sleeping.

- *For belladonna alkaloids, cyclizine, dimenhydrinate, and diphenhydramine:* These medicines have drying effects. Therefore, it is possible that they may reduce the amount of breast milk in some people. Dimenhydrinate passes into the breast milk. Cylizine may also pass into the breast milk.

- *For pentobarbital:* Pentobarbital passes into the breast milk. Large amounts of it may cause unwanted effects such as drowsiness in nursing babies.

Be sure that you discuss these possible problems with your doctor before taking any of these medicines.

**Children**—

- *For dihydroergotamine and ergotamine:* These medicines are used to relieve severe, throbbing headaches in children 6 years of age or older. They have not been shown to cause different side effects or problems in children than they do in adults. However, these medicines can cause serious side effects in any patient. Therefore, it is especially important that you discuss with the child's doctor the good that this medicine may do as well as the risks of using it.

- *For belladonna alkaloids:* Young children, especially children with spastic paralysis or brain damage, may be especially sensitive to the effects of belladonna alkaloids. This may increase the chance of side effects during treatment.
- *For cyclizine, dimenhydrinate, diphenhydramine, and pentobarbital:* Although these medicines often cause drowsiness, some children become excited after taking them.

**Older adults—**
- *For dihydroergotamine and ergotamine:* The chance of serious side effects caused by decreases in blood flow is increased in elderly people receiving these medicines.
- *For belladonna alkaloids, cyclizine, dimenhydrinate, diphenhydramine, and pentobarbital:* Elderly people are more sensitive than younger adults to the effects of these medicines. This may increase the chance of side effects such as excitement, depression, dizziness, drowsiness, and confusion.

**Other medicines—**Although certain medicines should not be used together at all, in other cases two different medicines may be used together even if an interaction might occur. In these cases, your doctor may want to change the dose, or other precautions may be necessary. Many medicines can add to or decrease the effects of the belladonna alkaloids, caffeine, cyclizine, dimenhydrinate, diphenhydramine, or pentobarbital present in some of these headache medicines. Therefore, you should tell your health care professional if you are taking *any* other prescription or nonprescription (over-the-counter [OTC]) medicine. This is especially important if any medicine you take causes excitement, trouble in sleeping, dryness of the mouth, dizziness, or drowsiness.

When you are taking dihydroergotamine or ergotamine, it is especially important that your health care professional know if you are taking any of the following:
- Cocaine or
- Epinephrine by injection [e.g., Epi-Pen] or
- Other ergot medicines (ergoloid mesylates [e.g., Hydergine], ergonovine [e.g., Ergotrate], methylergonovine [e.g., Methergine], methysergide [e.g., Sansert])—The chance of serious side effects caused by dihydroergotamine or ergotamine may be increased

**Other medical problems—**The presence of other medical problems may affect the use of these headache medicines. Make sure you tell your doctor if you have any other medical problems, especially:
- Agoraphobia (fear of open or public places) or
- Panic attacks or
- Stomach ulcer or
- Trouble in sleeping (insomnia)—Caffeine can make your condition worse
- Diarrhea—Rectal dosage forms (suppositories) will not be effective if you have diarrhea
- Difficult urination or
- Enlarged prostate or
- Glaucoma (not well controlled) or
- Heart or blood vessel disease or
- High blood pressure (not well controlled) or
- Infection or
- Intestinal blockage or other intestinal problems or
- Itching (severe) or
- Kidney disease or
- Liver disease or
- Mental depression or
- Overactive thyroid or
- Urinary tract blockage—The chance of side effects may be increased

Also, tell your doctor if you need, or if you have recently had, an angioplasty (a procedure done to improve the flow of blood in a blocked blood vessel) or surgery on a blood vessel. The chance of serious side effects caused by dihydroergotamine or ergotamine may be increased.

## Proper Use of This Medicine

*Use this medicine only as directed by your doctor. Do not use more of it, and do not use it more often, than directed.* If the amount you are to use does not relieve your headache, check with your doctor. Taking too much dihydroergotamine or ergotamine, or taking it too often, may cause serious effects, especially in elderly patients. Also, if a headache medicine (especially ergotamine) is used too often for migraines, it may lose its effectiveness or even cause a type of physical dependence. If this occurs, your headaches may actually get worse.

This medicine works best if you:
- *Use it at the first sign of headache or migraine attack. If you get warning signals of a coming migraine, take it before the headache actually starts.*
- *Lie down in a quiet, dark room until you are feeling better.*

Your doctor may direct you to take another medicine to help prevent headaches. *It is important that you follow your doctor's directions, even if your headaches continue to occur.* Headache-preventing medicines may take several weeks to start working. Even after they do start working, your headaches may not go away completely. However, your headaches should occur less often, and they should be less severe and easier to relieve. This can reduce the amount of dihydroergotamine, ergotamine, or pain relievers that you need. If you do not notice any improvement after several weeks of headache-preventing treatment, check with your doctor.

For patients using *dihydroergotamine:*
- Dihydroergotamine is given only by injection. Your health care professional will teach you how to inject yourself with the medicine. Be sure to follow the directions carefully. Check with your health care

professional if you have any problems using the medicine.

For patients using *ergotamine inhalation* [e.g., Medihaler Ergotamine]:

- This medicine comes with patient directions. Read them carefully before using the medicine, and check with your health care professional if you have any questions.
- To use the inhaler—Remove the cap, then shake the container well. After breathing out, place the mouthpiece of the inhaler in your mouth. Aim it at the back of the throat. Breathe in; at the same time, press the vial down into the adapter. After inhaling the medicine, hold your breath as long as you can.

For patients using the *sublingual (under-the-tongue) tablets of ergotamine:*

- To use—Place the tablet under your tongue and let it remain there until it disappears. The sublingual tablet should not be chewed or swallowed, because it works faster when it is absorbed into the body through the lining of the mouth. Do not eat, drink, or smoke while the tablet is under your tongue.

For patients using *rectal suppository forms of a headache medicine:*

- If the suppository is too soft to use, chill it in the refrigerator for 30 minutes or run cold water over it before removing the foil wrapper.
- If you have been directed to use part of a suppository, you should divide the suppository into pieces that all contain the same amount of medicine. To do this, use a sharp knife and carefully cut the suppository lengthwise (from top to bottom) into pieces that are the same size. The suppository will be easier to cut if it has been kept in the refrigerator.
- To insert the suppository—First remove the foil wrapper and moisten the suppository with cold water. Lie down on your side and use your finger to push the suppository well up into the rectum.

**Dosing**—The dose of these headache medicines will be different for different patients. *Follow your doctor's orders or the directions on the label.* The following information includes only the average doses of these medicines. *If your dose is different, do not change it* unless your doctor tells you to do so.

*For dihydroergotamine*

- Adults: For relieving a migraine or cluster headache—1 mg. If your headache is not better, and no side effects are occurring, a second 1-mg dose may be used at least one hour later.
- Children 6 years of age and older: For relieving a migraine headache—It is not likely that a child will be receiving dihydrogergotamine at home. If a child needs the medicine, the dose will have to be determined by the doctor.

*For ergotamine*

- Some headache medicines contain only ergotamine. Some of them contain other medicines along with the ergotamine. The number of tablets, capsules, or suppositories that you need for each dose depends on the amount of ergotamine in them. The size of each dose, and the number of doses that you take, also depends on the reason you are taking the medicine and on how you react to the medicine.
- For *oral* (capsule or tablet) and *sublingual* (under-the-tongue tablet) dosage forms:
  —Adults:
    - For relieving a migraine or cluster headache—1 or 2 mg of ergotamine. If your headache is not better, and no side effects are occurring, a second dose and even a third dose may be taken; however the doses should be taken at least 30 minutes apart. People who usually need more than one dose of the medicine, and who do not get side effects from it, may be able to take a larger first dose of not more than 3 mg of ergotamine. This may provide better relief of the headache with only one dose. *The medicine should not be taken more often 2 times a week, at least five days apart.*
    - For preventing cluster headaches—The dose of ergotamine, and the number of doses you need every day, will depend on how many headaches you usually get each day. For some people, 1 or 2 mg of ergotamine once a day may be enough. Other people may need to take 1 or 2 mg of ergotamine 2 or 3 times a day.
    - For all uses—*Do not take more than 6 mg of ergotamine a day in the form of capsules or tablets.*
  —Children 6 years of age and older: For relieving migraine headaches—1 mg of ergotamine. If the headache is not better, and no side effects are occurring, a second dose and even a third dose may be taken; however, the doses should be taken at least 30 minutes apart. *Children should not take more than 3 mg of ergotamine a day in the form of capsules or tablets. Also, this medicine should not be taken more often than 2 times a week, at least five days apart.*
- For *rectal suppository* dosage forms:
  —Adults: For relieving migraine or cluster headaches—Usually 1 mg of ergotamine, but the dose may range from half of this amount to up to 2 mg. If your headache is not better, and no side effects are occurring, a second dose and even a third dose may be used; however the doses should be taken at least 30 minutes apart. People who usually need more than one dose of the medicine, and who do not get side effects from it, may be able to use a larger first dose of not more than 3 mg. This may provide better relief of the headache with only one dose. *Adults should not use more than 4 mg of ergotamine a day in suppository form. Also, this*

*medicine should not be used more often than 2 times a week, at least five days apart.*

—Children 6 years of age and older: For relieving migraine headaches—One-half or 1 mg of ergotamine. *Children should not receive more than 1 mg a day of ergotamine in suppository form. Also, this medicine should not be used more often than 2 times a week, at least five days apart.*

- For the *oral inhalation* dosage form:
  —Adults: For relieving a migraine or cluster headache—1 spray (1 inhalation). Another inhalation may be used at least 5 minutes later, if needed. Up to a total of 6 inhalations a day may be used, at least 5 minutes apart. *This medicine should not be used more often than 2 times a week, at least five days apart.*
  —Children: To be determined by the doctor.

**Storage**—To store this medicine:

- Keep out of the reach of children since overdose is especially dangerous in children.
- Store away from heat and direct light.
- Do not store in the bathroom, near the kitchen sink, or in other damp places. Heat or moisture may cause the medicine to break down.
- Suppositories should be stored in a cool place, but not allowed to freeze. Some manufacturers recommend keeping them in a refrigerator; others do not. Follow the directions on the package. However, cutting the suppository into smaller pieces, if you need to do so, will be easier if the suppository is kept in the refrigerator.
- Do not puncture, break, or burn the ergotamine inhalation aerosol container, even after it is empty.
- Do not keep outdated medicine or medicine no longer needed. Be sure that any discarded medicine is out of the reach of children.

---

## Precautions While Using This Medicine

*Check with your doctor:*

- If your migraine headaches are worse than they were before you started using this medicine, or your headache medicine stops working as well as it did when you first started using it. This may mean that you are in danger of becoming dependent on the headache medicine. *Do not try to get better relief by increasing the dose.*
- If your migraine headaches are occurring more often than they did before you started using this medicine. This is especially important if a new headache occurs within 1 day after you took your last dose of headache medicine, or if you are having headaches every day. This may mean that you are dependent on the headache medicine. *Continuing to take this medicine will cause even more headaches later on.* Your doctor can give you advice on how to relieve the headaches.

Drinking alcoholic beverages can make headaches worse or cause new headaches to occur. People who suffer from severe headaches should probably avoid alcoholic beverages, especially during a headache.

Smoking may increase some of the harmful effects of dihydroergotamine or ergotamine. It is best to avoid smoking for several hours after taking these medicines.

Dihydroergotamine and ergotamine may make you more sensitive to cold temperatures, especially if you have blood circulation problems. They tend to decrease blood flow in the skin, fingers, and toes. Dress warmly during cold weather and be careful during prolonged exposure to cold temperatures. This is especially important for older patients, who are more likely than younger adults to already have problems with their circulation.

If you have a serious infection or illness of any kind, check with your doctor before using this medicine, since you may be more sensitive to its effects.

For patients using *ergotamine inhalation* [e.g., Medihaler Ergotamine]:

- Cough, hoarseness, or throat irritation may occur. Gargling and rinsing your mouth after each dose may help prevent the hoarseness and irritation. However, check with your doctor if these or any other side effects continue or are bothersome.

For patients taking one of the combination medicines that contains *caffeine:*

- Caffeine may interfere with the results of a test that uses dipyridamole (e.g., Persantine) to help find out how well your blood is flowing through certain blood vessels. You should not have any caffeine for at least 12 hours before the test.
- Caffeine may also interfere with some other laboratory tests. Before having any other laboratory tests, tell the person in charge if you have taken a medicine that contains caffeine.

For patients taking one of the combination medicines that contains *belladonna alkaloids, cyclizine, dimenhydrinate, diphenhydramine, or pentobarbital:*

- These medicines may cause some people to have blurred vision or to become drowsy, dizzy, lightheaded, or less alert than they are normally. These effects may be especially severe if you also take CNS depressants (medicines that slow down the nervous system, possibly causing drowsiness) together with one of these combination medicines. Some examples of CNS depressants are antihistamines or medicine for hay fever, other allergies, or colds; sedatives, tranquilizers, or sleeping medicine; prescription pain medicine or narcotics; barbiturates; medicine for seizures; muscle relaxants; and antiemetics (medicines that prevent or relieve nausea or vomiting). If you are not able to lie down for a while, *make sure you know how you react to this medicine or combination of medicines before you drive, use machines, or do anything else that could be dangerous if you are dizzy or are not alert and able to see well.*

- Belladonna alkaloids, cyclizine, dimenhydrinate, and diphenhydramine may cause dryness of the mouth, nose, and throat. For temporary relief of mouth dryness, use sugarless candy or gum, melt bits of ice in your mouth, or use a saliva substitute.
- Belladonna alkaloids may interfere with certain laboratory tests that check the amount of acid in your stomach. They should not be taken for 24 hours before the test.
- Cyclizine, dimenhydrinate, and diphenhydramine may interfere with skin tests that show whether you are allergic to certain substances. They should not be taken for 3 days before the test.

## Side Effects of This Medicine

Along with its needed effects, a medicine may cause some unwanted effects. Although not all of these side effects may occur, if they do occur they may need medical attention.

*Check with your doctor immediately* if the following side effects occur, because they may mean that you are developing a problem with blood circulation:

*Less common or rare*

Anxiety or confusion (severe); change in vision; chest pain; increase in blood pressure; pain in arms, legs, or lower back, especially if pain occurs in your calves or heels while you are walking; pale, bluish-colored, or cold hands or feet (not caused by cold temperatures and occurring together with other side effects listed in this section); red or violet-colored blisters on the skin of the hands or feet

*Also check with your doctor immediately* if any of the following side effects occur, because they may mean that you have taken an overdose of the medicine:

*Less common or rare*

Convulsions (seizures); diarrhea, nausea, vomiting, or stomach pain or bloating (severe) occurring together with other signs of overdose or of problems with blood circulation; dizziness, drowsiness, or weakness (severe), occurring together with other signs of overdose or of problems with blood circulation; fast or slow heartbeat; diarrhea; headaches, more often and/or more severe than before; problems with moving bowels, occurring together with pain or discomfort in the rectum (with rectal suppositories only); shortness of breath; unusual excitement

The following side effects may go away after a little while. *Do not take any more medicine while they are present.* If any of them occur together with other signs of problems with blood circulation, *check with your doctor right away.* Even if any of the following side effects occur without other signs of problems with blood circulation, *check with your doctor if any of them continue for more than one hour:*

*More common*

Itching of skin; coldness, numbness, or tingling in fingers, toes, or face; weakness in legs

Also, check with your doctor as soon as possible if you notice any of the following side effects:

*More common*

Swelling of face, fingers, feet, or lower legs

Other side effects may occur that usually do not need medical attention. These side effects may go away after a little while. However, check with your doctor if any of the following side effects continue or are bothersome:

*More common*

Diarrhea, nausea, or vomiting (occurring without other signs of overdose or problems with blood circulation); dizziness or drowsiness (occurring without other signs of overdose or problems with blood circulation, especially with combinations containing cyclizine, dimenhydrinate, diphenhydramine, or pentobarbital); nervousness or restlessness; dryness of mouth (especially with combinations containing belladonna alkaloids, cyclizine, dimenhydrinate, or diphenhydramine)

After you stop taking this medicine, your body may need time to adjust. The length of time this takes depends on the amount of medicine you were taking and how long you took it. During this time check with your doctor if your headaches begin again or worsen.

Other side effects not listed above may also occur in some patients. If you notice any other effects, check with your doctor.

## Additional Information

Once a medicine has been approved for marketing for a certain use, experience may show that it is also useful for other medical problems. Although this use is not specifically included in product labeling, dihydroergotamine is sometimes used together with another medicine (heparin) to help prevent blood clots that may occur after certain kinds of surgery. It is also used to prevent or treat low blood pressure in some patients.

For patients receiving this medicine for *preventing blood clots:*

- You may need to receive this medicine two or three times a day for several days in a row. This may increase the chance of problems caused by decreased blood flow. Your health care professional will be following your progress, to make sure that this medicine is not causing problems with blood circulation.

For patients using this medicine to *prevent or treat low blood pressure:*

- Take this medicine every day as directed by your doctor.
- The dose of dihydroergotamine will depend on whether the medicine is going to be injected under the skin or into a muscle, and, sometimes, on the weight of the patient. For these reasons, the dose will have to be determined by your doctor.
- Your doctor will need to check your progress at regular visits, to make sure that the medicine is working properly without causing side effects.

- This medicine is less likely to cause problems with blood circulation in patients with low blood pressure than it is in patients with normal or high blood pressure.
- In patients being treated for low blood pressure, an increase in blood pressure is the wanted effect, not a side effect that may need medical attention.

Other than the above information, there is no additional information relating to proper use, precautions, or side effects for these uses.

Revised: 09/08/92

# HEPARIN   Systemic

Some commonly used brand names are:
**In the U.S.**
    Calciparine                 Liquaemin
    Generic name product may also be available.
**In Canada**
    Calcilean                 Hepalean
    Calciparine            Heparin Leo
    Generic name product may also be available.

## Description

Heparin (HEP-a-rin) is an anticoagulant. It is used to decrease the clotting ability of the blood and help prevent harmful clots from forming in the blood vessels. This medicine is sometimes called a blood thinner, although it does not actually thin the blood. Heparin will not dissolve blood clots that have already formed, but it may prevent the clots from becoming larger and causing more serious problems.

Heparin is often used as a treatment for certain blood vessel, heart, and lung conditions. Heparin is also used to prevent blood clotting during open-heart surgery, bypass surgery, and dialysis. It is also used in low doses to prevent the formation of blood clots in certain patients, especially those who must have certain types of surgery or who must remain in bed for a long time.

Heparin is available only with your doctor's prescription, in the following dosage form:

*Parenteral*
- Injection (U.S. and Canada)

## Before Using This Medicine

In deciding to use a medicine, the risks of taking the medicine must be weighed against the good it will do. This is a decision you and your doctor will make. For heparin, the following should be considered:

**Allergies**—Tell your doctor if you have ever had any unusual or allergic reaction to heparin, to beef, or to pork. Also tell your health care professional if you are allergic to any other substances, such as foods, preservatives, or dyes.

**Pregnancy**—Heparin has not been shown to cause birth defects or bleeding problems in the baby. However, use during the last 3 months of pregnancy or during the month following the baby's delivery may cause bleeding problems in the mother.

**Breast-feeding**—Heparin does not pass into the breast milk. However, heparin can rarely cause bone problems in the nursing mother. This effect has been reported to occur when heparin is used for 2 weeks or more. Be sure to discuss this with your doctor.

**Children**—Heparin has been tested in children and, in effective doses, has not been shown to cause different side effects or problems than it does in adults.

**Older adults**—Bleeding problems may be more likely to occur in elderly patients, especially women, who are usually more sensitive than younger adults to the effects of heparin.

**Other medicines**—Although certain medicines should not be used together at all, in other cases two different medicines may be used together even if an interaction might occur. In these cases, your doctor may want to change the dose, or other precautions may be necessary. When you are taking heparin, it is especially important that your health care professional know if you are taking any of the following:

- Aspirin or
- Carbenicillin by injection (e.g., Geopen) or
- Cefamandole (e.g., Mandol) or
- Cefoperazone (e.g., Cefobid) or
- Cefotetan (e.g., Cefotan) or
- Dipyridamole (e.g., Persantine) or
- Divalproex (e.g., Depakote) or
- Medicine for inflammation or pain, except narcotics, or
- Medicine for overactive thyroid or
- Pentoxifylline (e.g., Trental) or
- Plicamycin (e.g., Mithracin) or
- Probenecid (e.g., Benemid) or
- Sulfinpyrazone (e.g., Anturane) or
- Ticarcillin (e.g., Ticar) or
- Valproic acid (e.g., Depakene)—Using any of these medicines together with heparin may increase the risk of bleeding

Also, tell your doctor if you are now receiving any kind of medicine by intramuscular (IM) injection.

**Other medical problems**—The presence of other medical problems may affect the use of heparin. Make sure you tell your doctor if you have any other medical problems, especially:

- Allergies or asthma (history of)—The risk of an allergic reaction to heparin may be increased
- Blood disease or bleeding problems or
- Colitis or stomach ulcer (or history of) or
- Diabetes mellitus (sugar diabetes) (severe) or
- High blood pressure (hypertension) or
- Kidney disease or
- Liver disease or
- Tuberculosis (active)—The risk of bleeding may be increased

Also, tell your doctor if you have received heparin before and had a reaction to it called thrombocytopenia, or if new blood clots formed while you were receiving the medicine.

In addition, it is important that you tell your doctor if you have recently had any of the following conditions or medical procedures:

- Childbirth or
- Falls or blows to the body or head or
- Heavy or unusual menstrual bleeding or
- Insertion of intrauterine device (IUD) or
- Medical or dental surgery or
- Spinal anesthesia or
- X-ray (radiation) treatment—The risk of serious bleeding may be increased

## Proper Use of This Medicine

*If you are using these injections at home, make sure your doctor has explained exactly how this medicine is to be given.*

To obtain the best results without causing serious bleeding, *use this medicine exactly as directed by your doctor. Be certain that you are using the right amount of heparin, and that you use it according to schedule.* Be especially careful that you do not use more of it, do not use it more often, and do not use it for a longer time than your doctor ordered.

*Your doctor should check your progress at regular visits.* A blood test must be taken regularly to see how fast your blood is clotting so that your doctor can decide on the proper amount of heparin you should be receiving each day.

**Dosing**—The dose of heparin will be different for different patients and must be determined by your doctor. The dose you receive will be based on the type of heparin you receive, the condition for which you are receiving heparin, and your body weight.

**Missed dose**—If you miss a dose of this medicine, use it as soon as possible. However, if it is almost time for your next dose, do not use the missed dose at all and do not double the next one. *Doubling the dose may cause bleeding.* Instead, go back to your regular dosing schedule. It is best to keep a record of each dose as you use it to avoid mistakes. Be sure to give your doctor a record of any doses you miss. If you have any questions about this, check with your doctor.

**Storage**—To store this medicine:

- Keep out of the reach of children.
- Store away from heat and direct light.
- Keep the medicine from freezing.
- Do not keep outdated medicine or medicine no longer needed. Be sure that any discarded medicine is out of the reach of children.

## Precautions While Using This Medicine

*Do not take aspirin while using this medicine.* Many nonprescription (over-the-counter [OTC]) medicines and some prescription medicines contain aspirin. Check the labels of all medicines you take. Also, do not take ibuprofen unless it has been ordered by your doctor. In addition, there are many other medicines that may change the way heparin works or increase the chance of bleeding if they are used together with heparin. It is best to check with your health care professional before taking any other medicine while you are using heparin.

*Tell all medical doctors and dentists you visit that you are using this medicine.*

It is recommended that you carry identification stating that you are using heparin. If you have any questions about what kind of identification to carry, check with your health care professional.

While you are using this medicine, it is very important that you avoid sports and other activities that may cause you to be injured. Report to your doctor any falls, blows to the body or head, or other injuries, since serious bleeding inside the body may occur without your knowing about it.

Take special care in brushing your teeth and in shaving. Use a soft toothbrush and floss gently. Also, it is best to use an electric shaver rather than a blade.

## Side Effects of This Medicine

Since many things can affect the way your body reacts to this medicine, you should always watch for signs of unusual bleeding. Unusual bleeding may mean that your body is getting more heparin than it needs.

Along with its needed effects, a medicine may cause some unwanted effects. Although not all of these side effects may occur, if they do occur they may need medical attention.

*Check with your doctor immediately* if any of the following signs and symptoms of bleeding inside the body occur:

Abdominal or stomach pain or swelling; back pain or backaches; blood in urine; bloody or black, tarry stools; constipation; coughing up blood; dizziness; headaches (severe or continuing); joint pain, stiffness, or swelling; vomiting of blood or material that looks like coffee grounds

Also, *check with your doctor immediately* if any of the following side effects occur, since they may mean that you are having a serious allergic reaction to the medicine:

> Changes in the skin color of the face; fast or irregular breathing; puffiness or swelling of the eyelids or around the eyes; shortness of breath, troubled breathing, tightness in chest, and/or wheezing; skin rash, hives, and/or itching

Also, check with your doctor as soon as possible if any of the following occur:

> Bleeding from gums when brushing teeth; heavy bleeding or oozing from cuts or wounds; unexplained bruising or purplish areas on skin; unexplained nosebleeds; unusually heavy or unexpected menstrual bleeding

Other side effects that may need medical attention may occur while you are using this medicine. Check with your doctor as soon as possible if any of the following side effects occur:

*Less common or rare*

> Back or rib pain (with long-term use only); change in skin color, especially near the place of injection or in the fingers, toes, arms, or legs; chest pain; chills and/or fever; collection of blood under skin (blood blister) at place of injection; decrease in height (with long-term use only); frequent or persistent erection; irritation, pain, redness, or ulcers at place of injection; itching and burning feeling, especially on the bottom of the feet; nausea and/or vomiting; numbness or tingling in hands or feet; pain, coldness, or blue color of skin of arms or legs; peeling of skin; runny nose; tearing of eyes; unusual hair loss (with long-term use only)

Other side effects not listed above may also occur in some patients. If you notice any other effects, check with your doctor.

Revised: August 1990
Interim revision: 08/23/94

---

# HEPATITIS B VACCINE RECOMBINANT    Systemic

Some commonly used brand names are:

**In the U.S.—**
> Engerix-B
> Recombivax HB
> Recombivax HB Dialysis Formulation

**In Canada—**
> Engerix-B
> Recombivax HB
> Recombivax HB Dialysis Formulation

Another commonly used name is HB vaccine.

## Description

Hepatitis (hep-ah-TY-tiss) B vaccine recombinant is an active immunizing agent used to prevent infection by the hepatitis B virus. The vaccine works by causing your body to produce its own protection (antibodies) against the disease.

Hepatitis B vaccine recombinant is made without any human blood or blood products or any other substances of human origin and cannot give the hepatitis B virus (HBV) or the human immunodeficiency virus (HIV) to you.

HBV infection is a major cause of serious liver diseases, such as virus hepatitis and cirrhosis, and a type of liver cancer called primary hepatocellular carcinoma.

Pregnant women who have hepatitis B infection or are carriers of hepatitis B virus can give the disease to their babies when they are born. These babies often suffer serious long-term illnesses from the disease.

Immunization against hepatitis B disease is recommended for all newborn babies, infants, children, and adolescents up to 20 years old. It is also recommended for adults who live in areas that have a high rate of hepatitis B disease or who may be at increased risk of infection from hepatitis B virus. These adults include:

- Sexually active homosexual and bisexual males, including those with HIV infection.
- Sexually active heterosexual persons with multiple partners.
- Persons who may be exposed to the virus by means of blood, blood products, or human bites, such as health care workers, employees in medical facilities, patients and staff of live-in facilities and day-care programs for the mentally retarded, morticians and embalmers, police and fire department personnel, and military personnel.
- Persons who have kidney disease or who undergo blood dialysis for kidney disease.
- Persons with blood clotting disorders who receive transfusions of clotting-factor concentrates.
- Household and sexual contacts of HBV carriers.
- Persons in areas with high risk of HBV infection, such as Alaskan Eskimos, Pacific Islanders, and refugees from areas that have a high rate of hepatitis B disease; persons accepting orphans or adoptees from these areas; and travelers to these areas.
- Persons who use illegal injectable drugs and inmates of prisons.

This vaccine is available only from your doctor or other authorized health care professional, in the following dosage form:

*Parenteral*
- Injection (U.S. and Canada)

---

© 1994   The United States Pharmacopeial Convention, Inc.

## Before Receiving This Vaccine

In deciding to use a medicine, the risks of using the medicine must be weighed against the good it will do. This is a decision you and your doctor will make. For hepatitis B recombinant vaccine, the following should be considered:

**Allergies**—Tell your doctor if you have ever had any unusual or allergic reaction to this vaccine or to the hepatitis B vaccine made from human plasma. Also tell your health care professional if you are allergic to any other substances, such as foods (especially baker's yeast). The vaccine is made by using baker's yeast; persons allergic to baker's yeast may also be allergic to the vaccine.

**Pregnancy**—Studies on effects in pregnancy have not been done in either humans or animals. However, since the vaccine does not contain contagious particles, it is not expected to cause problems during pregnancy.

**Breast-feeding**—It is not known whether hepatitis B vaccine passes into the breast milk. However, since the vaccine does not contain contagious particles, it is not expected to cause problems in nursing babies.

**Children**—Hepatitis B vaccine has been tested in newborns, infants, and children and, in effective doses, has not been shown to cause different side effects or problems than it does in adults. The vaccine strength for use in dialysis patients has been studied only in adult patients, and there is no specific information about its use in children receiving dialysis.

**Older adults**—This vaccine is not expected to cause different side effects or problems in older people than it does in younger adults. However, persons over 50 years of age may not become as immune to the virus as do younger adults.

**Other medicines**—Although certain medicines should not be used together at all, in other cases two different medicines may be used together even if an interaction might occur. In these cases, your doctor may want to change the dose, or other precautions may be necessary. Before you receive hepatitis B vaccine, it is especially important that your health care professional know if you are using any other prescription or nonprescription (over-the-counter [OTC]) medicine.

**Other medical problems**—The presence of other medical problems may affect the use of hepatitis B vaccine. Make sure you tell your doctor if you have any other medical problems, especially:

- Heart disease (severe) or
- Lung disease (severe)—Some of the side effects of the vaccine may make the condition worse
- Immune deficiency condition—The condition may decrease the useful effects of hepatitis B vaccine. The dose of the vaccine may need to be increased
- Moderate or severe illness with or without fever—The symptoms of the condition may be confused with the possible side effects of the vaccine

## Proper Use of This Vaccine

**Dosing**—The dose of hepatitis B vaccine will be different for different patients. *Follow your doctor's orders.* The following information includes only the average doses of hepatitis B vaccine.

- For *injection* dosage form:
  - For prevention of hepatitis B infection:
    - Adults, adolescents, and older children—2.5 to 20 micrograms (mcg) injected into the arm muscle at the first office visit, then one month and six months after the first dose, for a total of three doses.
    - Adults who also receive or will receive blood dialysis—40 mcg injected into the arm muscle at the first office visit, then one month and six months after the first dose, for a total of three doses; or 40 mcg injected into the arm muscle at the first office visit, then one month, two months, and six months after the first dose, for a total of four doses.
    - Infants and young children—2.5 to 20 mcg injected into the thigh muscle at the first office visit, then one month and six months after the first dose, for a total of three doses.
    - Newborn babies—2.5 to 20 mcg injected into the thigh muscle at birth or within seven days of birth, then one month and six months after the first dose, for a total of three doses; or 10 or 20 mcg injected into the thigh muscle at birth or within seven days of birth, then one month, two months, and twelve months after the first dose, for a total of four doses.

## Side Effects of This Vaccine

Along with its needed effects, a vaccine may cause some unwanted effects. Although not all of these side effects may occur, if they do occur they may need medical attention.

*Get emergency help immediately* if any of the following side effects occur:

*Symptoms of allergic reaction—Rare*
> Difficulty in breathing or swallowing; hives; itching, especially of feet or hands; reddening of skin, especially around ears; swelling of eyes, face, or inside of nose; unusual tiredness or weakness (sudden and severe)

Check with your doctor as soon as possible if any of the following side effects occur:

*Rare*
> Aches or pain in joints, fever, or skin rash or welts (may occur days to weeks following the vaccine); blurred vision or other vision changes; muscle weakness or numbness or tingling of limbs

Other side effects may occur that usually do not need medical attention. However, check with your doctor if any of the following side effects continue or are bothersome:

*More common*

Soreness at the place of injection

*Less common*

Dizziness; fever of 37.7 °C (100 °F) or over; hard lump, redness, swelling, pain, itching, purple spot, tenderness, or warmth at place of injection; headache; unusual tiredness or weakness

*Rare*

Aches or pain in muscles; back pain or stiffness or pain in neck or shoulder; chills; diarrhea or stomach cramps

or pain; feeling of bodily discomfort; increased sweating; headache (mild), sore throat, runny nose, or fever (mild); itching; lack of appetite or decreased appetite; nausea or vomiting; sudden redness of skin; swelling of glands in armpit or neck; trouble in sleeping

Other side effects not listed above may also occur in some patients. If you notice any other effects, check with your doctor.

Revised: 02/23/94

---

# HISTAMINE   Diagnostic*

* Not commercially available in the U.S.

## Description

Histamine (HISS-ta-meen) is used to help diagnose problems or disease of the stomach. This test determines how much acid your stomach produces.

How the stomach test is done: Before this medicine is given, the stomach contents are emptied through a tube. Then the dose of histamine, which is based on body weight, is injected under the skin. Five minutes later, the stomach contents are emptied and tested for acidity. This procedure may be repeated several times. An antihistamine medicine may be given before the histamine is injected to prevent a possible unwanted effect.

Histamine is to be used only under the supervision of a doctor. It is available in the following dosage form:

*Parenteral*

• Injection (Canada)

## Before Having This Test

In deciding to use a diagnostic test, any risks of the test must be weighed against the good it will do. This is a decision you and your doctor will make. Also, test results may be affected by other things. For histamine, the following should be considered:

**Allergies**—Tell your health care professional if you are allergic to any substances, such as foods, preservatives, or dyes.

**Pregnancy**—Studies have not been done in either humans or animals.

**Breast-feeding**—It is not known whether histamine passes into the breast milk. However, histamine has not been reported to cause problems in nursing babies.

**Children**—There is no specific information comparing the use of histamine in children with use in other age groups.

**Older adults**—Many medicines have not been studied specifically in older people. Therefore, it may not be known whether they work exactly the same way they do in younger adults or if they cause different side effects or problems in older people. There is no specific information comparing use of histamine in the elderly with use in other age groups.

**Other medicines**—Although certain medicines should not be used together at all, in other cases two different medicines may be used together even if an interaction might occur. In these cases, your doctor may want to change the dose, or other precautions may be necessary. When you are receiving histamine, it is especially important that your health care professional know if you are taking any of the following:

• Antacids or
• Anticholinergics (medicine for abdominal or stomach spasms or cramps) or
• Cimetidine (e.g., Tagamet) or
• Famotidine (e.g., Pepcid) or
• Nizatidine (e.g., Axid) or
• Omeprazole (e.g., Prilosec) or
• Ranitidine (e.g., Zantac)—These medicines decrease the effect that histamine has on the production of stomach acid, and the test may not work

**Other medical problems**—The presence of other medical problems may affect the use of histamine. Make sure you tell your doctor if you have any other medical problems, especially:

• Heart disease—Histamine's effect on the heart may make the condition worse
• High blood pressure (severe) or
• Low blood pressure—Histamine may increase the high blood pressure further or lower an already low blood pressure
• Kidney disease (severe)—The histamine may build up in the body and cause side effects
• Lung disease (especially asthma)—There is a chance that this test may make the condition worse; for example, an asthma attack may occur

• Pheochromocytoma—Histamine may cause serious damage to the brain and blood vessels.

## Preparation For This Test

Your doctor may ask you to avoid certain medicines before the histamine test is done. *Follow your doctor's instructions carefully.* Otherwise, this test may not work and may have to be done again.

*Do not eat anything for twelve hours before the test,* unless otherwise directed by your doctor. Having food in the stomach may affect the interpretation of the test results.

## Precautions During This Test

Do not swallow saliva during the test. The saliva may affect the results of the test.

## Side Effects of This Medicine

Along with its needed effects, histamine may cause some unwanted effects. Although not all of these side effects may occur, if they do occur they may need medical attention.

*Check with your doctor or nurse immediately* if any of the following side effects occur:

*More common*

Dizziness, lightheadedness, or fainting; fast or pounding heartbeat; headache (continuing or severe); nervousness

*Less common or rare*

Convulsions (seizures); difficulty in breathing; flushing or redness of face

*With large doses*

Bluish coloration of face; blurred vision; chest discomfort or pain; decrease in blood pressure (sudden); diarrhea (severe); difficulty in breathing (severe); nausea and vomiting (severe)

Other side effects may occur that usually do not need medical attention. These side effects should go away as the effects of the medicine wear off. However, check with your doctor if any of the following side effects continue or are bothersome:

*More common*

Abdominal or stomach spasms or cramps; diarrhea; metallic taste; nausea or vomiting; stomach pain; swelling or redness at place of injection

Other side effects not listed above may also occur in some patients. If you notice any other effects, check with your doctor.

Revised: 06/02/93

---

# HISTAMINE H$_2$-RECEPTOR ANTAGONISTS   Systemic

Some commonly used brand names are:

**In the U.S.—**

| | |
|---|---|
| Axid[3] | Tagamet[1] |
| Pepcid[2] | Zantac[4] |
| Pepcid I.V.[2] | |

**In Canada—**

| | |
|---|---|
| Apo-Cimetidine[1] | Pepcid I.V.[2] |
| Apo-Ranitidine[4] | Peptol[1] |
| Axid[3] | Tagamet[1] |
| Novocimetine[1] | Zantac[4] |
| Pepcid[2] | Zantac-C[4] |

Note: For quick reference, the following histamine H$_2$-receptor antagonists are numbered to match the corresponding brand names.

This information applies to the following medicines:

1. Cimetidine (sye-MET-i-deen)§
2. Famotidine (fa-MOE-ti-deen)
3. Nizatidine (ni-ZA-ti-deen)
4. Ranitidine (ra-NIT-ti-deen)

§Generic name product may also be available in Canada.

## Description

Histamine H$_2$-receptor antagonists, also known as H$_2$-blockers, are used to treat duodenal ulcers and prevent their return. They are also used to treat gastric ulcers and in some conditions, such as Zollinger-Ellison disease, in which the stomach produces too much acid. H$_2$-blockers may also be used for other conditions as determined by your doctor.

H$_2$-blockers work by decreasing the amount of acid produced by the stomach.

They are available only with your doctor's prescription, in the following dosage forms:

*Oral*

Cimetidine
• Oral solution (U.S. and Canada)
• Tablets (U.S. and Canada)
Famotidine
• Oral suspension (U.S.)
• Tablets (U.S. and Canada)
Nizatidine
• Capsules (U.S. and Canada)
Ranitidine
• Capsules (U.S. and Canada)
• Syrup (U.S. and Canada)
• Tablets (U.S. and Canada)

*Parenteral*

Cimetidine
• Injection (U.S. and Canada)
Famotidine
• Injection (U.S. and Canada)

Ranitidine
  • Injection (U.S. and Canada)

## Before Using This Medicine

In deciding to use a medicine, the risks of taking the medicine must be weighed against the good it will do. This is a decision you and your doctor will make. For $H_2$-blockers, the following should be considered:

**Allergies**—Tell your doctor if you have ever had any unusual or allergic reaction to cimetidine, famotidine, nizatidine, or ranitidine.

**Pregnancy**—$H_2$-blockers have not been studied in pregnant women. In animal studies, famotidine and ranitidine have not been shown to cause birth defects or other problems. However, one study in rats suggested that cimetidine may affect male sexual development. More studies are needed to confirm this. Also, studies in rabbits with very high doses have shown that nizatidine causes miscarriages and low birth weights. Make sure your doctor knows if you are pregnant or if you may become pregnant before taking $H_2$-blockers.

**Breast-feeding**—Cimetidine, famotidine, nizatidine, and ranitidine pass into the breast milk and may cause unwanted effects, such as decreased amount of stomach acid and increased excitement, in the nursing baby. It may be necessary for you to take another medicine or to stop breast-feeding during treatment. Be sure you have discussed the risks and benefits of the medicine with your doctor.

**Children**—This medicine has been tested in children and, in effective doses, has not been shown to cause different side effects or problems than it does in adults when used for short periods of time.

**Older adults**—Confusion and dizziness may be especially likely to occur in elderly patients, who are usually more sensitive than younger adults to the effects of $H_2$-blockers.

**Other medicines**—Although certain medicines should not be used together at all, in other cases two different medicines may be used together even if an interaction might occur. In these cases, your doctor may want to change the dose, or other precautions may be necessary. When you are taking or receiving $H_2$-blockers it is especially important that your health care professional know if you are taking any of the following:
  • Aminophylline (e.g., Somophyllin) or
  • Anticoagulants (blood thinners) or
  • Caffeine (e.g., NoDoz) or
  • Metoprolol (e.g., Lopressor) or
  • Oxtriphylline (e.g., Choledyl) or
  • Phenytoin (e.g., Dilantin) or
  • Propranolol (e.g., Inderal) or
  • Theophylline (e.g., Somophyllin-T) or
  • Tricyclic antidepressants (amitriptyline [e.g., Elavil], amoxapine [e.g., Asendin], clomipramine [e.g., Anafranil], desipramine [e.g., Pertofrane], doxepin [e.g., Sinequan], imipramine [e.g., Tofranil], nortriptyline [e.g., Aventyl], protriptyline [e.g., Vivactil], trimipramine [e.g.,

Surmontil])—Use of these medicines with cimetidine has been shown to increase the effects of cimetidine. This is less of a problem with ranitidine and has not been reported for famotidine or nizatidine. However, all of the $H_2$-blockers are similar, so drug interactions may occur with any of them
  • Ketoconazole—$H_2$-blockers may decrease the effects of ketoconazole; $H_2$-blockers should be taken at least 2 hours after ketoconazole

**Other medical problems**—The presence of other medical problems may affect the use of $H_2$-blockers. Make sure you tell your doctor if you have any other medical problems, especially:
  • Kidney disease or
  • Liver disease—The $H_2$-blocker may build up in the bloodstream, which may increase the risk of side effects

## Proper Use of This Medicine

For patients taking:
  • One dose a day—Take it at bedtime, unless otherwise directed.
  • Two doses a day—Take one in the morning and one at bedtime.
  • Several doses a day—Take them with meals and at bedtime for best results.

It may take several days before this medicine begins to relieve stomach pain. To help relieve this pain, antacids may be taken with the $H_2$-blocker, unless your doctor has told you not to use them. However, you should wait one-half to one hour between taking the antacid and the $H_2$-blocker.

*Take this medicine for the full time of treatment, even if you begin to feel better.* Also, it is important that you keep your appointments with your doctor for check-ups so that your doctor will be better able to tell you when to stop taking this medicine.

**Dosing**—The dose of histamine $H_2$-receptor antagonists (also called $H_2$-blockers) will be different for different patients. *Follow your doctor's orders or the directions on the label.* The following information includes only the average doses of these medicines. *If your dose is different, do not change it unless your doctor tells you to do so.*

*The number of capsules or tablets or teaspoonfuls of solution, suspension, or syrup that you take depends on the strength of the medicine. Also, the number of doses you take each day, the time allowed between doses, and the length of time you take the medicine depend on the medical problem for which you are taking the $H_2$-receptor antagonist.*

*For cimetidine*
  • For *oral* dosage forms (solution and tablets):
    —To treat duodenal or gastric ulcers:
      • Older adults, adults, and teenagers—300 milligrams (mg) four times a day, with meals and at bedtime. Some people may take 400 or 600

mg two times a day, on waking up and at bedtime. Others may take 800 mg at bedtime.
- Children—20 to 40 mg per kilogram (kg) (9.1 to 18.2 mg per pound) of body weight a day, divided into four doses, taken with meals and at bedtime.

—To prevent duodenal ulcers:
- Older adults, adults, and teenagers—300 mg two times a day, on waking up and at bedtime. Instead some people may take 400 mg at bedtime.
- Children—Dose must be determined by your doctor.

—To treat conditions in which the stomach produces too much acid:
- Adults—300 mg four times a day, with meals and at bedtime. Your doctor may change the dose if needed.
- Children—Dose must be determined by your doctor.

—To treat gastroesophageal reflux disease:
- Adults—800 to 1600 mg a day, divided into smaller doses. Treatment usually lasts for 12 weeks.
- Children—Dose must be determined by your doctor.

- For *injectable* dosage form:
—To treat duodenal ulcers, gastric ulcers or conditions in which the stomach produces too much acid:
- Older adults, adults, and teenagers—300 mg injected into muscle, every six to eight hours. Or, 300 mg injected slowly into a vein every six to eight hours. Instead, 900 mg may be injected slowly into a vein around the clock at the rate of 37.5 mg per hour. Some people may need 150 mg at first, before beginning the around-the-clock treatment.
- Children—5 to 10 mg per kg (2.3 to 4.5 mg per pound) of body weight injected into a vein or muscle, every six to eight hours. Or, 5 to 10 mg per kg (2.3 to 4.6 mg per pound) of body weight injected slowly into a vein every six to eight hours.

—To prevent stress-related bleeding:
- Older adults, adults, and teenagers—50 mg per hour injected slowly around the clock for up to 7 days.
- Children—Dose must be determined by your doctor.

## For famotidine

- For *oral* dosage forms (solution and tablets):
—To treat duodenal ulcers:
Older adults, adults, and teenagers—40 milligrams (mg) once a day at bedtime. Some people may take 20 mg two times day.
- Children—Dose must be determined by your doctor.

—To prevent duodenal ulcers:
- Older adults, adults, and teenagers—20 mg once a day at bedtime.
- Children—Dose must be determined by your doctor.

—To treat gastric ulcers:
- Older adults, adults, and teenagers—40 mg once a day at bedtime.
- Children—Dose must be determined by your doctor.

—To treat conditions in which the stomach produces too much acid:
- Older adults, adults, and children—20 mg every six hours. Your doctor may change the dose if needed.
- Children—Dose must be determined by your doctor.

—To treat gastroesophageal reflux disease:
- Older adults, adults, and teenagers—20 mg two times a day, usually for up to 6 weeks.
- Children weighing more than 10 kg (4.5 pounds): 1 to 2 mg per kilogram (kg) (0.5 to 0.9 mg per pound) of body weight a day divided into two doses.
- Children weighing less than 10 kg (4.5 pounds): 1 to 2 mg per kg (0.5 to 0.9 mg per pound) of body weight a day, divided into three doses.

- For *injectable* dosage form:
—To treat duodenal ulcers, gastric ulcers, or conditions in which the stomach produces too much acid:
- Older adults, adults, and teenagers—20 mg injected into a vein, every twelve hours. Or, 20 mg injected slowly into a vein every twelve hours.
- Children—Dose must be determined by your doctor.

## For nizatidine

- For *oral* dosage form (capsules):
—To treat duodenal or gastric ulcers:
- Older adults, adults, and teenagers—300 milligrams (mg) once a day at bedtime. Some people may take 150 mg two times a day.
- Children—Dose must be determined by your doctor.

—To prevent duodenal ulcers:
- Adults and teenagers—150 mg once a day at bedtime.
- Children—Dose must be determined by your doctor.

—To treat gastroesophageal reflux disease:
- Adults and teenagers—150 mg two times a day.
- Children—Dose must be determined by your doctor.

*For ranitidine*

- For *oral* dosage form (capsules, syrup, or tablets):
  - —To treat duodenal ulcers:
    - Older adults, adults, teenagers—150 milligrams (mg) two times a day. Some people may take 300 mg once a day at bedtime.
    - Children—2 to 4 mg per kilogram (kg) (1 to 2 mg per pound) of body weight two times a day. However, your dose will not be more than 300 mg a day.
  - —To prevent duodenal ulcers:
    - Older adults, adults, teenagers—150 mg at bedtime.
    - Children—Dose must be detemined by your doctor.
  - —To treat gastric ulcers:
    - Older adults, adults, teenagers—150 mg two times a day.
    - Children—2 to 4 mg per kg (1 to 2 mg per pound) of body weight two times a day. However, your dose will not be more than 300 mg a day.
  - —To treat some conditions in which the stomach produces too much acid:
    - Older adults, adults, teenagers—150 mg two times a day. Your doctor may change the dose if needed.
    - Children—Dose must be determined by your doctor.
  - —To treat gastroesophageal reflux disease:
    - Older adults, adults, and teenagers—150 mg two times a day. Your dose may be increased if needed.
    - Children—2 to 8 mg per kg (1 to 3.6 mg per pound) of body weight a day, three times a day. However, most children will usually take not more than 300 mg a day.
- For *injectable* dosage form:
  - —To treat duodenal ulcers, gastric ulcers, or conditions in which the stomach produces too much acid:
    - Older adults, adults, and teenagers—50 mg injected into a muscle every six to eight hours. Or, 50 mg injected slowly into a vein every six to eight hours. Instead, you may receive 6.25 mg per hour injected slowly around the clock. However, most people will usually not need more than 400 mg a day.
  - —To treat duodenal or gastric ulcers:
    - Children—2 to 4 mg per kg (1 to 2 mg per pound) of body weight a day, injected slowly into a vein.

**Missed dose**—If you miss a dose of this medicine, take it as soon as possible. However, if it is almost time for your next dose, skip the missed dose and go back to your regular dosing schedule. Do not double doses.

**Storage**—To store this medicine:

- Keep out of the reach of children.
- Store away from heat and direct light.
- Do not store the tablet form of this medicine in the bathroom, near the kitchen sink, or in other damp places. Heat or moisture may cause the medicine to break down.
- Keep the liquid form of this medicine from freezing.
- Do not keep outdated medicine or medicine no longer needed. Be sure that any discarded medicine is out of the reach of children.

## Precautions While Using This Medicine

Some tests may be affected by this medicine. Tell the doctor in charge that you are taking this medicine before:

- You have any skin tests for allergies.
- You have any tests to determine how much acid your stomach produces.

Remember that certain medicines, such as aspirin, and certain foods and drinks (e.g., citrus products, carbonated drinks, etc.) irritate the stomach and may make your problem worse.

Cigarette smoking tends to decrease the effect of H$_2$-blockers by increasing the amount of acid produced by the stomach. This is more likely to affect the stomach's nighttime production of acid. While taking H$_2$-blockers, stop smoking completely, or at least do not smoke after taking the last dose of the day.

Drinking alcoholic beverages while taking an H$_2$-receptor antagonist has been reported to increase the blood levels of alcohol. You should consult your health care professional for guidance.

Check with your doctor if your ulcer pain continues or gets worse.

## Side Effects of This Medicine

Along with its needed effects, a medicine may cause some unwanted effects. Although not all of these side effects may occur, if they do occur they may need medical attention.

Check with your doctor as soon as possible if any of the following side effects occur:

*Rare*

  Burning, itching, redness, skin rash; confusion; fast, pounding, or irregular heartbeat; fever; slow heartbeat; sore throat and fever; swelling; tightness in chest; unusual bleeding or bruising; unusual tiredness or weakness

Other side effects may occur that usually do not need medical attention. These side effects may go away during treatment as your body adjusts to the medicine. However,

check with your doctor if any of the following side effects continue or are bothersome:

*Less common or rare*

Blurred vision; constipation; decreased sexual ability (especially in patients with Zollinger-Ellison disease who have received high doses of cimetidine for at least 1 year); decrease in sexual desire; diarrhea; dizziness; drowsiness; dryness of mouth or skin; headache; increased sweating; joint or muscle pain; loss of appetite; loss of hair (temporary); nausea or vomiting; ringing or buzzing in ears; skin rash; swelling of breasts or breast soreness in females and males

Not all of the side effects listed above have been reported for each of these medicines, but they have been reported for at least one of them. All of the H₂-blockers are similar, so any of the above side effects may occur with any of these medicines.

Other side effects not listed above may also occur in some patients. If you notice any other effects, check with your doctor.

## Additional Information

Once a medicine has been approved for marketing for a certain use, experience may show that it is also useful for other medical problems. Although these uses are not included in product labeling, H₂-blockers are used in certain patients with the following medical conditions:

- Damage to the stomach and/or intestines due to stress or trauma
- Hives
- Pancreatic problems
- Stomach or intestinal ulcers (sores) resulting from damage caused by medication used to treat rheumatoid arthritis

Other than the above information, there is no additional information relating to proper use, precautions, or side effects for these uses.

Revised: 09/29/92
Interim revision: 08/31/94

---

# HMG-CoA REDUCTASE INHIBITORS    Systemic

Some commonly used brand names are:

**In the U.S.—**

| | |
|---|---|
| Mevacor[1] | Zocor[3] |
| Pravachol[2] | |

**In Canada—**

| | |
|---|---|
| Mevacor[1] | Zocor[3] |
| Pravachol[2] | |

Other commonly used names are:

| | |
|---|---|
| Epistatin[3] | Mevinolin[1] |
| Eptastatin[2] | Synvinolin[3] |

Note: For quick reference, the following HMG-CoA reductase inhibitors are numbered to match the corresponding brand names.

This information applies to the following medicines:

1. Lovastatin (LOE-va-sta-tin)
2. Pravastatin (PRA-va-stat-in)
3. Simvastatin (SIM-va-stat-in)

## Description

Lovastatin, pravastatin, and simvastatin are used to lower levels of cholesterol and other fats in the blood. This may help prevent medical problems caused by cholesterol clogging the blood vessels.

These medicines belong to the group of medicines called 3-hydroxy-3-methylglutaryl coenzyme A (HMG-CoA) reductase inhibitors. They work by blocking an enzyme that is needed by the body to make cholesterol. Thus, less cholesterol is made.

HMG-CoA reductase inhibitors are available only with your doctor's prescription, in the following dosage form:

*Oral*

Lovastatin
- Tablets (U.S. and Canada)

Pravastatin
- Tablets (U.S. and Canada)

Simvastatin
- Tablets (U.S and Canada)

## Before Using This Medicine

In deciding to use a medicine, the risks of taking the medicine must be weighed against the good it will do. This is a decision you and your doctor will make. For HMG-CoA reductase inhibitors, the following should be considered:

**Allergies**—Tell your doctor if you have ever had any unusual or allergic reaction to HMG-CoA reductase inhibitors. Also tell your health care professional if you are allergic to any other substances, such as foods, preservatives, or dyes.

**Diet**—Before prescribing medicines to lower your cholesterol, your doctor will probably try to control your condition by prescribing a personal diet for you. Such a diet may be low in fats, sugars, and/or cholesterol. Many people are able to control their condition by carefully following their doctor's orders for proper diet and exercise. *Medicine is prescribed only when additional help is needed* and is effective only when a schedule of diet and exercise is properly followed.

Also, this medicine is less effective if you are greatly overweight. It may be very important for you to go on a reducing diet. However, check with your doctor before going on any diet.

**Pregnancy**—Use of an HMG-CoA reductase inhibitor is not recommended during pregnancy or in a woman who plans to become pregnant in the near future. These medicines block formation of cholesterol, which is necessary for the fetus to develop properly. In addition, lovastatin has been shown to cause birth defects in animals given very high doses. Be sure you have discussed this with your doctor.

**Breast-feeding**—These medicines are not recommended for use during breast-feeding because they may cause unwanted effects in nursing babies.

**Children**—Studies on this medicine have been done only in adult patients, and there is no specific information comparing use of HMG-CoA reductase inhibitors in children with use in other age groups.

**Older adults**—Many medicines have not been studied specifically in older people. Therefore, it may not be known whether they work exactly the same way they do in younger adults or if they cause different side effects or problems in older people. There is no specific information comparing the use of HMG-CoA reductase inhibitors in the elderly with use in other age groups.

**Other medicines**—Although certain medicines should not be used together at all, in other cases two different medicines may be used together even if an interaction might occur. In these cases, your doctor may want to change the dose, or other precautions may be necessary. When you are taking HMG-CoA reductase inhibitors, it is especially important that your health care professional know if you are taking any of the following:

- Cyclosporine (e.g., Sandimmune) or
- Gemfibrozil (e.g., Lopid) or
- Niacin—Use of these medicines with an HMG-CoA reductase inhibitor may increase the risk of developing muscle problems and kidney failure

**Other medical problems**—The presence of other medical problems may affect the use of HMG-CoA reductase inhibitors. Make sure you tell your doctor if you have any other medical problems, especially:

- Alcohol abuse (or history of) or
- Liver disease—Use of this medicine may make liver problems worse
- Convulsions (seizures), not well-controlled, or
- Organ transplant with immunosuppressant therapy or
- If you have recently had major surgery—Patients with these conditions may be at risk of developing problems that may lead to kidney failure

## Proper Use of This Medicine

*Use this medicine only as directed by your doctor.* Do not use more or less of it, and do not use it more often or for a longer time than your doctor ordered.

Remember that this medicine will not cure your condition but it does help control it. Therefore, you must continue to take it as directed if you expect to keep your cholesterol levels down.

*Follow carefully the special diet your doctor gave you.* This is the most important part of controlling your condition, and is necessary if the medicine is to work properly.

For patients taking *lovastatin:*

- This medicine works better when it is taken with food. If you are taking this medicine once a day, take it with the evening meal. If you are taking more than one dose a day, take each dose with a meal or snack.

**Dosing**—The dose of lovastatin, pravastatin, or simvastatin will be different for different patients. *Follow your doctor's orders or the directions on the label.* The following information includes only the average doses. *If your dose is different, do not change it* unless your doctor tells you to do so:

The number of tablets that you take depends on the strength of the medicine.

*For lovastatin*
- For *oral* dosage form (tablets):
  —For high cholesterol:
    - Adults—20 to 80 milligrams (mg) a day taken as a single dose or in divided doses. Take with meals.
    - Children—Use is not recommended.

*For pravastatin*
- For *oral* dosage form (tablets):
  —For high cholesterol:
    - Adults—10 to 40 mg once a day at bedtime.
    - Children—Use is not recommended.

*For simvastatin*
- For *oral* dosage form (tablets):
  —For high cholesterol:
    - Adults—5 to 40 mg once a day in the evening.
    - Children—Use is not recommended.

**Missed dose**—If you miss a dose of this medicine, take it as soon as possible. However, if it is almost time for your next dose, skip the missed dose and go back to your regular dosing schedule. Do not double doses.

**Storage**—To store this medicine:
- Keep out of the reach of children.
- Store away from heat and direct light.
- Do not store in the bathroom, near the kitchen sink, or in other damp places. Heat or moisture may cause the medicine to break down.
- Keep the medicine from freezing. Do not refrigerate.
- Do not keep outdated medicine or medicine no longer needed. Be sure that any discarded medicine is out of the reach of children.

## Precautions While Using This Medicine

*It is very important that your doctor check your progress at regular visits.* This will allow your doctor to see if the medicine is working properly to lower your cholesterol levels and that it does not cause unwanted effects.

*Do not stop taking this medicine without first checking with your doctor.* When you stop taking this medicine, your blood cholesterol levels may increase again. Your doctor may want you to follow a special diet to help prevent this from happening.

*Before having any kind of surgery (including dental surgery) or emergency treatment, tell the medical doctor or dentist in charge that you are taking this medicine.*

## Side Effects of This Medicine

Along with its needed effects, a medicine may cause some unwanted effects. Although not all of these side effects may occur, if they do occur they may need medical attention.

Check with your doctor as soon as possible if any of the following side effects occur:

*Less common*
*For lovastatin, pravastatin, and simvastatin*
Fever; muscle aches or cramps; unusual tiredness or weakness
*For lovastatin only (in addition to those listed above)*
Blurred vision

Other side effects may occur that usually do not need medical attention. These side effects may go away during treatment as your body adjusts to the medicine. However, check with your doctor if any of the following side effects continue or are bothersome:

*Less common*
*For lovastatin, pravastatin, and simvastatin*
Constipation; diarrhea; dizziness; gas; heartburn; headache; nausea; skin rash; stomach pain
*For lovastatin only (in addition to those listed above)*
Decreased sexual ability; trouble in sleeping

Other side effects not listed above may also occur in some patients. If you notice any other effects, check with your doctor.

Revised: 06/18/93

---

# HYDRALAZINE    Systemic

Some commonly used brand names are:
**In the U.S.—**
Apresoline
Generic name product may also be available.
**In Canada—**
Apresoline
Novo-Hylazin

*Parenteral*
• Injection (U.S. and Canada)

## Description

Hydralazine (hye-DRAL-a-zeen) belongs to the general class of medicines called antihypertensives. It is used to treat high blood pressure (hypertension).

High blood pressure adds to the work load of the heart and arteries. If it continues for a long time, the heart and arteries may not function properly. This can damage the blood vessels of the brain, heart, and kidneys, resulting in a stroke, heart failure, or kidney failure. High blood pressure may also increase the risk of heart attacks. These problems may be less likely to occur if blood pressure is controlled.

Hydralazine works by relaxing blood vessels and increasing the supply of blood and oxygen to the heart while reducing its work load.

Hydralazine may also be used for other conditions as determined by your doctor.

Hydralazine is available only with your doctor's prescription, in the following dosage forms:
*Oral*
• Tablets (U.S. and Canada)

## Before Using This Medicine

In deciding to use a medicine, the risks of taking the medicine must be weighed against the good it will do. This is a decision you and your doctor will make. For hydralazine, the following should be considered:

**Allergies**—Tell your doctor if you have ever had any unusual or allergic reaction to hydralazine. Also tell your health care professional if you are allergic to any other substance, such as foods, preservatives, or dyes.

**Pregnancy**—Hydralazine has not been studied in pregnant women. However, blood problems have been reported in infants of mothers who took hydralazine during pregnancy. In addition, studies in mice have shown that hydralazine causes birth defects (cleft palate, defects in head and face bones). These birth defects may also occur in rabbits, but do not occur in rats. Before taking this medicine, make sure your doctor knows if you are pregnant or if you may become pregnant.

**Breast-feeding**—It is not known whether hydralazine passes into breast milk.

**Children**—Although there is no specific information comparing use of hydralazine in children with use in other age groups, this medicine is not expected to cause different side effects or problems in children than it does in adults.

**Older adults**—Many medicines have not been studied specifically in older people. Therefore, it may not be known whether they work exactly the same way they do in younger adults. Although there is no specific information comparing use of hydralazine in the elderly with use in other age groups, this medicine is not expected to cause different side effects or problems in older people than it does in younger adults. However, dizziness or lightheadedness may be more likely to occur in the elderly, who are more sensitive to the effects of hydralazine.

**Other medicines**—Although certain medicines should not be used together at all, in other cases two different medicines may be used together even if an interaction might occur. In these cases, your doctor may want to change the dose, or other precautions may be necessary. When you are taking hydralazine, it is especially important that your health care professional know if you are taking the following:

- Diazoxide (e.g., Proglycem)—Effect on blood pressure may be increased

**Other medical problems**—The presence of other medical problems may affect the use of hydralazine. Make sure you tell your doctor if you have any other medical problems, especially:

- Heart or blood vessel disease or
- Stroke—Lowering blood pressure may make problems resulting from these conditions worse
- Kidney disease—Effects may be increased because of slower removal of hydralazine from the body

## Proper Use of This Medicine

For patients taking this medicine *for high blood pressure:*

- In addition to the use of the medicine your doctor has prescribed, treatment for your high blood pressure may include weight control and care in the types of foods you eat, especially foods high in sodium. Your doctor will tell you which of these are most important for you. You should check with your doctor before changing your diet.
- Many patients who have high blood pressure will not notice any signs of the problem. In fact, many may feel normal. It is very important that you *take your medicine exactly as directed* and that you keep your appointments with your doctor even if you feel well.
- Remember that hydralazine will not cure your high blood pressure but it does help control it. Therefore, you must continue to take it as directed if you expect to lower your blood pressure and keep it down. *You may have to take high blood pressure medicine for the rest of your life.* If high blood pressure is not treated, it can cause serious problems such as heart failure, blood vessel disease, stroke, or kidney disease.

To help you remember to take your medicine, try to get into the habit of taking it at the same time each day.

**Dosing**—The dose of hydralazine will be different for different patients. *Follow your doctor's orders or the directions on the label.* The following information includes only the average doses of hydralazine. *If your dose is different, do not change it* unless your doctor tells you to do so.

The number of tablets that you take depends on the strength of the medicine.

- For *oral* dosage form (tablets):
  —For high blood pressure:
  - Adults—10 to 50 milligrams (mg) four times a day.
  - Children—Dose is based on body weight or size. The usual dose is 0.75 to 7.5 mg per kilogram (kg) (0.34 to 3.4 mg per pound) of body weight a day. This is divided into two to four doses.
- For *injection* dosage form:
  —For high blood pressure:
  - Adults—10 to 40 mg injected into a muscle or a vein. Your doctor may repeat the dose as needed.
  - Children—Dose is based on body weight or size. The usual dose is 1.7 to 3.5 mg per kg (0.77 to 1.6 mg per pound) of body weight a day. This is divided into four to six doses and injected into a muscle or a vein.

**Missed dose**—If you miss a dose of this medicine, take it as soon as possible. However, if it is almost time for your next dose, skip the missed dose and go back to your regular dosing schedule. Do not double doses.

**Storage**—To store this medicine:

- Keep out of the reach of children.
- Store away from heat and direct light.
- Do not store in the bathroom, near the kitchen sink, or in other damp places. Heat or moisture may cause the medicine to break down.
- Do not keep outdated medicine or medicine no longer needed. Be sure that any discarded medicine is out of the reach of children.

## Precautions While Using This Medicine

It is important that your doctor check your progress at regular visits to make sure that this medicine is working properly.

For patients taking this medicine *for high blood pressure:*

- *Do not take other medicines unless they have been discussed with your doctor.* This especially includes over-the-counter (nonprescription) medicines for appetite control, asthma, colds, cough, hay fever, or sinus, since they may tend to increase your blood pressure.

Hydralazine may cause some people to have headaches or to feel dizzy. *Make sure you know how you react to this medicine before you drive, use machines, or do anything else that could be dangerous if you are dizzy or are not alert.*

## Side Effects of This Medicine

Along with its needed effects, a medicine may cause some unwanted effects. Although not all of these side effects may occur, if they do occur they may need medical attention.

In general, side effects with hydralazine are rare at lower doses. However, check with your doctor as soon as possible if any of the following occur:

*Less common*
> Blisters on skin; chest pain; general feeling of discomfort or illness or weakness; joint pain; numbness, tingling, pain, or weakness in hands or feet; skin rash or itching; sore throat and fever; swelling of feet or lower legs; swelling of the lymph glands

Other side effects may occur that usually do not need medical attention. These side effects may go away during treatment as your body adjusts to the medicine. However, check with your doctor if any of the following side effects continue or are bothersome:

*More common*
> Diarrhea; fast or irregular heartbeat; headache; loss of appetite; nausea or vomiting; pounding heartbeat

*Less common*
> Constipation; dizziness or lightheadedness; redness or flushing of face; shortness of breath; stuffy nose; watering or irritated eyes

Other side effects not listed above may also occur in some patients. If you notice any other effects, check with your doctor.

## Additional Information

Once a medicine has been approved for marketing for a certain use, experience may show that it is also useful for other medical problems. Although this use is not specifically included in product labeling, hydralazine is used in certain patients with the following medical condition:
- Congestive heart failure

Other than the above information, there is no additional information relating to proper use, precautions, or side effects for this use.

Revised: 06/09/92
Interim revision: 04/29/94

# HYDRALAZINE AND HYDROCHLOROTHIAZIDE   Systemic†

Some commonly used brand names are:
**In the U.S.—**
| | |
|---|---|
| Apresazide | Aprozide |
| Apresoline-Esidrix | Hydra-zide |

Generic name product may also be available.

†Not commercially available in Canada.

## Description

Hydralazine (hye-DRAL-a-zeen) and hydrochlorothiazide (hye-droe-klor-oh-THYE-a-zide) combination is used to treat high blood pressure (hypertension).

High blood pressure adds to the work load of the heart and arteries. If it continues for a long time, the heart and arteries may not function properly. This can damage the blood vessels of the brain, heart, and kidneys, resulting in a stroke, heart failure, or kidney failure. High blood pressure may also increase the risk of heart attacks. These problems may be less likely to occur if blood pressure is controlled.

Hydralazine works by relaxing blood vessels and increasing the supply of blood and oxygen to the heart while reducing its work load. The hydrochlorothiazide in this combination helps reduce the amount of water in the body by acting on the kidneys to increase the flow of urine.

This medicine is available only with your doctor's prescription, in the following dosage forms:

*Oral*
- Capsules (U.S.)
- Tablets (U.S.)

## Before Using This Medicine

In deciding to use a medicine, the risks of taking the medicine must be weighed against the good it will do. This is a decision you and your doctor will make. For hydralazine and hydrochlorothiazide, the following should be considered:

**Allergies**—Tell your doctor if you have ever had any unusual or allergic reaction to hydralazine, sulfonamides (sulfa drugs), indapamide, or any of the thiazide diuretics (water pills). Also tell your health care professional if you are allergic to any other substance, such as foods, preservatives, or dyes.

**Pregnancy**—When hydrochlorothiazide is used during pregnancy, it may cause side effects including jaundice, blood problems, and low potassium in the newborn infant.
Studies with hydralazine have not been done in humans. However, blood problems have been reported in infants of mothers who took hydralazine during pregnancy. In addition, studies in mice have shown that hydralazine causes birth defects (cleft palate, defects in head and face bones); these birth defects may also occur in rabbits, but do not occur in rats.

**Breast-feeding**—Hydrochlorothiazide passes into breast milk. However, neither hydralazine nor hydrochlorothiazide has been reported to cause problems in nursing babies.

**Children**—Although there is no specific information comparing use of this medicine in children with use in other age groups, this medicine is not expected to cause different side effects or problems in children than it does in adults. However, extra caution may be necessary in infants with jaundice, because thiazide diuretics can make this condition worse.

**Older adults**—Many medicines have not been studied specifically in older people. Therefore, it may not be known whether they work exactly the same way they do in younger adults. Although there is no specific information comparing use of hydralazine and hydrochlorothiazide combination in the elderly with use in other age groups, this medicine is not expected to cause different side effects or problems in older people than it does in younger adults. However, dizziness or lightheadedness or symptoms of too much potassium loss may be more likely to occur in the elderly, who are usually more sensitive to the effects of this medicine. Also, this medicine may reduce tolerance to cold temperatures in elderly patients.

**Other medicines**—Although certain medicines should not be used together at all, in other cases two different medicines may be used together even if an interaction might occur. In these cases, your doctor may want to change the dose, or other precautions may be necessary. When you are taking hydralazine and hydrochlorothiazide, it is especially important that your health care professional know if you are taking any of the following:
- Cholestyramine or
- Colestipol—Use with thiazide diuretics may prevent the diuretic from working properly; take the diuretic at least 1 hour before or 4 hours after cholestyramine or colestipol
- Diazoxide (e.g., Proglycem)—Effect on blood pressure may be increased
- Digitalis glycosides (heart medicine)—Hydrochlorothiazide may cause low potassium in the blood, which can lead to symptoms of digitalis toxicity
- Lithium (e.g., Lithane)—Risk of lithium overdose, even at usual doses, may be increased

**Other medical problems**—The presence of other medical problems may affect the use of hydralazine and hydrochlorothiazide. Make sure you tell your doctor if you have any other medical problems, especially:
- Diabetes mellitus (sugar diabetes)—Hydrochlorothiazide may change the amount of diabetes medicine needed
- Gout (history of)—Hydrochlorothiazide may increase the amount of uric acid in the blood, which can lead to gout
- Heart or blood vessel disease or
- Stroke (recent)—Lowering blood pressure may make problems resulting from these conditions worse
- Kidney disease—Hydrochlorothiazide may worsen this condition. Also, the blood pressure lowering effects may be increased because of slower removal of hydralazine from the body
- Liver disease—If hydrochlorothiazide causes loss of too much water from the body, liver disease can become much worse
- Lupus erythematosus (history of)—Hydrochlorothiazide may worsen the condition
- Pancreatitis (inflammation of the pancreas)

# Proper Use of This Medicine

This medicine may cause you to have an unusual feeling of tiredness when you begin to take it. You may also notice an increase in the amount of urine or in your frequency of urination. After taking the medicine for a while, these effects should lessen. To keep the increase in urine from affecting your sleep:
- If you are to take a single dose a day, take it in the morning after breakfast.
- If you are to take more than one dose a day, take the last dose no later than 6 p.m., unless otherwise directed by your doctor.

However, it is best to plan your dose or doses according to a schedule that will least affect your personal activities and sleep. Ask your health care professional to help you plan the best time to take this medicine.

In addition to the use of the medicine your doctor has prescribed, treatment for your high blood pressure may include weight control and care in the types of foods you eat, especially foods high in sodium. Your doctor will tell you which of these are most important for you. You should check with your doctor before changing your diet.

Many patients who have high blood pressure will not notice any signs of the problem. In fact, many may feel normal. It is very important that you *take your medicine exactly as directed* and that you keep your appointments with your doctor even if you feel well.

Remember that this medicine will not cure your high blood pressure but it does help control it. Therefore, you must continue to take it as directed if you expect to lower your blood pressure and keep it down. *You may have to take high blood pressure medicine for the rest of your life.* If high blood pressure is not treated, it can cause serious problems such as heart failure, blood vessel disease, stroke, or kidney disease.

To help you remember to take your medicine, try to get into the habit of taking it at the same time each day.

**Dosing**—The dose of hydralazine and hydrochlorothiazide combination will be different for different patients. *Follow your doctor's orders or the directions on the label.* The following information includes only the average dose of hydralazine and hydrochlorothiazide combination. *If your dose is different, do not change it* unless your doctor tells you to do so.

The number of capsules or tablets that you take depends on the strength of the medicine.
- For *oral* dosage forms (capsules or tablets):
  —For high blood pressure:
    - Adults—1 capsule or tablet two times a day.
    - Children—Dose must be determined by your doctor.

**Missed dose**—If you miss a dose of this medicine, take it as soon as possible. However, if it is almost time for your next dose, skip the missed dose and go back to your regular dosing schedule. Do not double doses.

**Storage**—To store this medicine:
- Keep out of the reach of children.
- Store away from heat and direct light.
- Do not store in the bathroom, near the kitchen sink, or in other damp places. Heat or moisture may cause the medicine to break down.
- Do not keep outdated medicine or medicine no longer needed. Be sure that any discarded medicine is out of the reach of children.

## Precautions While Using This Medicine

It is important that your doctor check your progress at regular visits to make sure that this medicine is working properly.

*Do not take other medicines unless they have been discussed with your doctor.* This especially includes over-the-counter (nonprescription) medicines for appetite control, asthma, colds, cough, hay fever, or sinus problems, since they may tend to increase your blood pressure.

This medicine may cause some people to have headaches or to feel dizzy. *Make sure you know how you react to this medicine before you drive, use machines, or do anything else that could be dangerous if you are dizzy or are not alert.*

*Dizziness, lightheadedness, or fainting may occur, especially when you get up from a lying or sitting position.* This is more likely to occur in the morning. *Getting up slowly may help.* When you get up from lying down, sit on the edge of the bed with your feet dangling for 1 or 2 minutes. Then stand up slowly. If the problem continues or gets worse, check with your doctor.

The dizziness, lightheadedness, or fainting is also more likely to occur if you drink alcohol, stand for a long time, exercise, or if the weather is hot. *While you are taking this medicine, be careful in the amount of alcohol you drink. Also, use extra care during exercise or hot weather or if you must stand for a long time.*

*This medicine may cause a loss of potassium from your body.*
- To help prevent this, your doctor may want you to:
  —eat or drink foods that have a high potassium content (for example, orange or other citrus fruit juices), or
  —take a potassium supplement, or
  —take another medicine to help prevent the loss of the potassium in the first place.
- It is very important to follow these directions. Also, it is important not to change your diet on your own. This is more important if you are already on a special diet (as for diabetes), or if you are taking a potassium supplement or a medicine to reduce potassium loss. Extra potassium may not be necessary and, in some cases, too much potassium could be harmful.

Check with your doctor if you become sick and have severe or continuing nausea, vomiting, or diarrhea. These problems may cause you to lose additional water and potassium.

For *diabetic patients*:
- Thiazide diuretics may raise blood sugar levels. While you are using this medicine, be especially careful in testing for sugar in your blood or urine. If you have any questions about this, check with your doctor.

Some people who take this medicine may become more sensitive to sunlight than they are normally. Exposure to sunlight, even for brief periods of time, may cause severe sunburn; skin rash, redness, itching, or discoloration; or vision changes. When you begin taking this medicine:
- Stay out of direct sunlight, especially between the hours of 10:00 a.m. and 3:00 p.m., if possible.
- Wear protective clothing, including a hat and sunglasses.
- Apply a sun block product that has a skin protection factor (SPF) of at least 15. Some patients may require a product with a higher SPF number, especially if they have a fair complexion. If you have any questions about this, check with your health care professional.
- Do not use a sunlamp or tanning bed or booth.

If you have a severe reaction from the sun, check with your doctor.

## Side Effects of This Medicine

Along with its needed effects, a medicine may cause some unwanted effects. Although not all of these side effects may occur, if they do occur they may need medical attention.

Check with your doctor as soon as possible if any of the following side effects occur:

*Signs and symptoms of too much potassium loss*
  Dryness of mouth; increased thirst; irregular heartbeats; mood or mental changes; muscle cramps or pain; weak pulse

*Signs and symptoms of too much sodium loss*
  Confusion; convulsions; decreased mental activity; irritability; muscle cramps; unusual tiredness or weakness

*Less common*
  Blisters on skin; chest pain; general feeling of discomfort or illness or weakness; joint pain; numbness, tingling, pain, or weakness in hands or feet; skin rash or itching; sore throat and fever; swelling of the lymph glands

*Rare*
  Lower back or side pain; severe stomach pain with nausea and vomiting; unusual bleeding or bruising; yellow eyes or skin

Other side effects may occur that usually do not need medical attention. These side effects may go away during treatment as your body adjusts to the medicine. However, check with your doctor if any of the following side effects continue or are bothersome:

*More common*
  Diarrhea; fast or irregular heartbeat; headache; loss of appetite; nausea or vomiting

*A'*

*Less common*
> Constipation; decreased sexual ability; dizziness or light-headedness, especially when getting up from a lying or sitting position; increased sensitivity of skin to sunlight; redness or flushing of face; shortness of breath with exercise or work; stuffy nose; watering or irritated eyes

Other side effects not listed above may also occur in some patients. If you notice any other effects, check with your doctor.

---

Revised: 08/24/92
Interim revision: 04/29/94

---

# HYDROCORTISONE   Rectal

Some commonly used brand names are:

**In the U.S.—**

| | |
|---|---|
| Anucort-HC | Corticaine |
| Anusol-HC | Hemril-HC |
| Cort-Dome High Potency | Proctocort |

Generic name product may also be available.

**In Canada**

| | |
|---|---|
| Cortiment-10 | Rectocort |
| Cortiment-40 | |

Another commonly used name is cortisol.

## Description

Rectal hydrocortisone (hye-droe-KOR-ti-sone) is used to help relieve swelling, itching, and discomfort of some rectal problems. Rectal hydrocortisone may also be applied to the area around the anus or rectum to relieve itching and discomfort. Hydrocortisone is a corticosteroid (kor-ti-ko-STER-oyd), which is a cortisone-like medicine. Hydrocortisone belongs to the general family of medicines called steroids.

Some hydrocortisone products for rectal use are available without a prescription; however, your doctor may have special instructions on the proper dose for your medical condition. Other hydrocortisone products for rectal use are available only with your doctor's prescription.

Rectal hydrocortisone is available in the following dosage forms:

*Rectal*
- Cream (U.S.)
- Ointment (Canada)
- Suppositories (U.S. and Canada)

## Before Using This Medicine

In deciding to use rectal hydrocortisone, the risks of using it must be weighed against the good it will do. This is a decision you and possibly your doctor will make. The following information may help you in making your decision:

**Allergies**—If you have ever had any unusual or allergic reaction to hydrocortisone or other corticosteroids, it is best to check with your doctor before using rectal hydrocortisone.

**Pregnancy**—When used properly, this medicine has not been shown to cause problems in humans. Studies on birth defects with rectal hydrocortisone have not been done in humans. However, studies in animals have shown that topical corticosteroids, such as the hydrocortisone contained in this medicine, when used in large amounts or for a long time, may be absorbed through the skin and could cause birth defects.

**Breast-feeding**—When used properly, rectal hydrocortisone has not been reported to cause problems in nursing babies.

**Children**—Children and teenagers who must use this medicine should be checked often by their doctor. Hydrocortisone may be absorbed through the lining of the rectum and, rarely, may affect growth, especially if used in large amounts or for a long time. Before using this medicine in children, you should discuss its use with your child's doctor.

**Older adults**—Although there is no specific information comparing use of rectal hydrocortisone in the elderly with use in other age groups, this medicine is not expected to cause different side effects or problems in older people than it does in younger adults.

**Other medical problems**—The presence of other medical problems may affect the use of rectal hydrocortisone. Since in some cases rectal hydrocortisone should not be used, check with your doctor if you have any of the following:
- Diabetes mellitus (sugar diabetes)—Too much use of hydrocortisone may cause a loss of control of diabetes by increasing blood and urine glucose. However, this is not likely to happen when hydrocortisone is used for a short period of time
- Infection or sores at the place of treatment or
- Tuberculosis—Corticosteroids may make existing infections worse or cause new infections
- Skin conditions that cause thinning of skin with easy bruising—Corticosteroids may make thinning of the skin worse

## Proper Use of This Medicine

For patients using *hydrocortisone rectal cream or ointment:*
- If you are applying this medicine to the outer rectal area, first bathe and dry the rectal area. Then apply a small amount and rub it in gently.

- If you have been directed to insert this medicine into the rectum, first attach the plastic applicator tip onto the opened tube. Insert the applicator tip into the rectum and gently squeeze the tube to deliver the medicine. Remove the applicator tip from the tube and wash it with hot, soapy water. Replace the cap of the tube after use.

For patients using *hydrocortisone suppositories:*
- If the suppository is too soft to insert, chill it in the refrigerator for 30 minutes or run cold water over it before removing the foil wrapper.
- To insert suppository: First remove the foil wrapper and moisten the suppository with cold water. Lie down on your side and use your finger to push the suppository well up into the rectum.

*Do not use rectal hydrocortisone in larger amounts, more often, or for a longer time than your doctor ordered or the package label directs.* To do so may increase the chance of absorption through the lining of the rectum and the chance of side effects.

*If this medicine was ordered by your doctor, do not use any leftover medicine for future rectal problems without first checking with your doctor. Also, if you are treating yourself, check with your doctor before using rectal hydrocortisone for problems other than those stated on the package, or if you suspect that an infection may be present.* The medicine should not be used if many kinds of bacterial, virus, or fungus infections are present.

**Missed dose**—If your doctor has ordered you to use this medicine according to a regular schedule and you miss a dose, use it as soon as you remember. However, if it is almost time for your next dose, skip the missed dose and go back to your regular dosing schedule. Do not double doses.

**Storage**—To store this medicine:
- Keep out of the reach of children.
- Store away from heat and direct light.

- Do not store hydrocortisone suppositories in the bathroom medicine cabinet because the heat or moisture may cause the medicine to break down.
- Keep the medicine from freezing.
- Do not keep outdated medicine or medicine no longer needed. Be sure that any discarded medicine is out of the reach of children.

## Precautions While Using This Medicine
Avoid using tight-fitting diapers or plastic pants on children using this medicine. Plastic pants and tight-fitting diapers may increase the chance of absorption of the medicine through the skin and the chance of side effects.

## Side Effects of This Medicine
Along with its needed effects, a medicine may cause some unwanted effects. Although not all of these side effects may occur, if they do occur they may need medical attention.

Check with your doctor as soon as possible if any of the following side effects occur:
 Signs of irritation or infection such as rectal bleeding, pain, burning, itching, or blistering not present before use of this medicine

Additional side effects may occur if you use this medicine for a long time. Check with your doctor as soon as possible if any of the following side effects occur:
 Reddish-purple lines (stretch marks) on treated areas; thinning of skin with easy bruising

Other side effects not listed above may also occur in some patients. If you notice any other effects, check with your doctor.

Revised: 11/18/92

# HYDROXYCHLOROQUINE  Systemic

A commonly used brand name in the U.S. and Canada is Plaquenil.

## Description
Hydroxychloroquine (hye-drox-ee-KLOR-oh-kwin) belongs to the family of medicines called antiprotozoals. Protozoa are tiny, one-celled animals. Some are parasites that can cause many different kinds of infections in the body.

This medicine is used to prevent and to treat malaria and to treat some conditions such as liver disease caused by protozoa. It is also used in the treatment of arthritis to help relieve inflammation, swelling, stiffness, and joint pain and to help control the symptoms of lupus erythematosus (lupus; SLE).

This medicine may be given alone or with one or more other medicines. It may also be used for other conditions as determined by your doctor.

Hydroxychloroquine is available only with your doctor's prescription, in the following dosage form:
*Oral*
- Tablets (U.S. and Canada)

## Before Using This Medicine

In deciding to use a medicine, the risks of taking the medicine must be weighed against the good it will do. This is a decision you and your doctor will make. For hydroxychloroquine, the following should be considered:

**Allergies**—Tell your doctor if you have ever had any unusual or allergic reaction to hydroxychloroquine or chloroquine. Also tell your health care professional if you are allergic to any other substances, such as foods, preservatives, or dyes.

**Pregnancy**—Unless you are taking it for malaria or liver disease caused by protozoa, use of this medicine is not recommended during pregnancy. In animal studies, hydroxychloroquine has been shown to cause damage to the central nervous system (brain and spinal cord) of the fetus, including damage to hearing, sense of balance, bleeding inside the eyes, and other eye problems. However, when given in low doses (once a week) to prevent malaria, this medicine has not been shown to cause birth defects or other problems in pregnant women.

**Breast-feeding**—A very small amount of hydroxychloroquine passes into the breast milk. It has not been reported to cause problems in nursing babies to date. However, babies and children are especially sensitive to the effects of hydroxychloroquine.

**Children**—Children are especially sensitive to the effects of hydroxychloroquine. This may increase the chance of side effects during treatment. Overdose is especially dangerous in children. Taking as few as 3 or 4 tablets (250-mg strength) of chloroquine has resulted in death in small children. Because hydroxychloroquine is so similar to chloroquine, it is probably just as toxic.

**Older adults**—Many medicines have not been studied specifically in older people. Therefore, it may not be known whether they work exactly the same way they do in younger adults or if they cause different side effects or problems in older people. There is no specific information comparing use of hydroxychloroquine in the elderly with use in other age groups.

**Other medicines**—Although certain medicines should not be used together at all, in other cases 2 different medicines may be used together even if an interaction might occur. In these cases, your doctor may want to change the dose, or other precautions may be necessary. Tell your health care professional if you are taking any other prescription or nonprescription (over-the-counter [OTC]) medicine.

**Other medical problems**—The presence of other medical problems may affect the use of hydroxychloroquine. Make sure you tell your doctor if you have any other medical problems, especially:

- Blood disease (severe)—Hydroxychloroquine may cause blood disorders
- Eye or vision problems—Hydroxychloroquine may cause serious eye side effects, especially in high doses
- Glucose-6-phosphate dehydrogenase (G6PD) deficiency—Hydroxychloroquine may cause serious blood side effects in patients with this deficiency
- Liver disease—May decrease the removal of hydroxychloroquine from the blood, increasing the chance of side effects
- Nerve or brain disease (severe), including convulsions (seizures)—Hydroxychloroquine may cause muscle weakness and, in high doses, seizures
- Porphyria—Hydroxychloroquine may worsen the symptoms of porphyria
- Psoriasis—Hydroxychloroquine may bring on severe attacks of psoriasis
- Stomach or intestinal disease (severe)—Hydroxychloroquine may cause stomach irritation

## Proper Use of This Medicine

*Take this medicine with meals or milk* to lessen possible stomach upset, unless otherwise directed by your doctor.

*Keep this medicine out of the reach of children. Children are especially sensitive to the effects of hydroxychloroquine and overdose is especially dangerous in children.* Taking as few as 3 or 4 tablets (250-mg strength) of chloroquine has resulted in death in small children. Hydroxychloroquine is probably just as dangerous.

It is very important that you *take this medicine only as directed.* Do not take more of it, do not take it more often, and do not take it for a longer time than your doctor ordered. To do so may increase the chance of serious side effects.

If you are taking this medicine to help keep you from getting malaria, *keep taking it for the full time of treatment.* If you already have malaria, you should still keep taking this medicine for the full time of treatment even if you begin to feel better after a few days. This will help to clear up your infection completely. If you stop taking this medicine too soon, your symptoms may return.

Hydroxychloroquine works best when you take it on a regular schedule. For example, if you are to take it once a week to prevent malaria, it is best to take it on the same day each week. Or if you are to take 2 doses a day, 1 dose may be taken with breakfast and the other with the evening meal. *Make sure that you do not miss any doses.* If you have any questions about this, check with your health care professional.

**Dosing**—The dose of hydroxychloroquine will be different for different patients. *Follow your doctor's orders or the directions on the label.* The following information includes only the average doses of hydroxychloroquine. *If your dose is different, do not change it* unless your doctor tells you to do so.

*The number of doses you take each day, the time allowed between doses, and the length of time you take the medicine depend on the medical problem for which you are taking hydroxychloroquine.*

- For *tablets* dosage form:
  —For prevention of malaria:
  - Adults—400 milligrams (mg) taken once every seven days.
  - Children—Dose is based on body weight and must be determined by your doctor. The usual dose is 6.4 mg per kilogram (kg) (2.9 mg per pound) of body weight taken once every seven days.
  —For treatment of malaria:
  - Adults—800 mg taken as a single dose. This may sometimes be followed by a dose of 400 mg taken six to eight hours after the first dose, then 400 mg once a day on the second and third days.
  - Children—Dose is based on body weight and must be determined by your doctor. The usual dose is 32 mg per kg (14.5 mg per pound) of body weight taken over a period of three days.
  —For treatment of arthritis:
  - Adults—Dose is based on body weight and must be determined by your doctor. The usual dose is 6.5 mg per kg (2.9 mg per pound) of body weight per day.

**Missed dose**—If you miss a dose of this medicine, take it as soon as possible. However, if it is almost time for your next dose, skip the missed dose and go back to your regular dosing schedule. Do not double doses.

For patients taking hydroxychloroquine *to prevent malaria:*

- Your doctor may want you to start taking this medicine 1 to 2 weeks before you travel to an area where there is a chance of getting malaria. This will help you to see how you react to the medicine. Also, it will allow time for your doctor to change to another medicine if you have a reaction to this medicine.
- Also, you should keep taking this medicine while you are in the area and for 4 to 6 weeks after you leave the area. No medicine will protect you completely from malaria. However, to protect you as completely as possible, *it is important to keep taking this medicine for the full time your doctor ordered.* Also, if fever develops during your travels or within 2 months after you leave the area, *check with your doctor immediately.*

For patients taking hydroxychloroquine *for arthritis or lupus:*

- This medicine must be taken regularly as ordered by your doctor in order for it to help you. It may take up to several weeks before you begin to feel better. It may take up to 6 months before you feel the full benefit of this medicine.

For patients *unable to swallow hydroxychloroquine tablets:*

- Your pharmacist can crush the tablets and put each dose in a capsule. Contents of the capsules may then be mixed with a teaspoonful of jam, jelly, or jello.

Be sure you take all the food in order to get the full dose of medicine.

**Storage**—To store this medicine:

- Keep out of the reach of children. Overdose of hydroxychloroquine is very dangerous in children.
- Store away from heat and direct light.
- Do not store in the bathroom, near the kitchen sink, or in other damp places. Heat or moisture may cause the medicine to break down.
- Do not keep outdated medicine or medicine no longer needed. Be sure that any discarded medicine is out of the reach of children.

## Precautions While Using This Medicine

If you will be taking this medicine for a long time, *it is very important that your doctor check you at regular visits* for any blood problems or muscle weakness that may be caused by this medicine. In addition, *check with your doctor immediately if blurred vision, difficulty in reading, or any other change in vision occurs during or after treatment.* Your doctor may want you to have your eyes checked by an ophthalmologist (eye doctor).

If your symptoms do not improve within a few days (or a few weeks or months for arthritis), or if they become worse, check with your doctor.

Hydroxychloroquine may cause blurred vision, difficulty in reading, or other change in vision. It may also cause some people to become dizzy or lightheaded. *Make sure you know how you react to this medicine before you drive, use machines, or do anything else that could be dangerous if you are dizzy or are not alert or able to see well.* If these reactions are especially bothersome, check with your doctor.

Malaria is spread by mosquitoes. If you are living in, or will be traveling to, an area where there is a chance of getting malaria, the following mosquito-control measures will help to prevent infection:

- If possible, sleep under mosquito netting to avoid being bitten by malaria-carrying mosquitoes.
- Wear long-sleeved shirts or blouses and long trousers to protect your arms and legs, especially from dusk through dawn when mosquitoes are out.
- Apply mosquito repellent to uncovered areas of the skin from dusk through dawn when mosquitoes are out.

## Side Effects of This Medicine

Along with its needed effects, a medicine may cause some unwanted effects. Although not all of these side effects may occur, if they do occur they may need medical attention. When this medicine is used for short periods of time, side effects usually are rare. However, when it is used for a long time and/or in high doses, side effects are more likely to occur and may be serious.

*Check with your doctor immediately* if any of the following side effects occur:

*Less common*

Blurred vision or any other change in vision—this side effect may also occur or get worse after you stop taking this medicine

*Rare*

Convulsions (seizures); unusual tiredness; increased muscle weakness; mood or other mental changes; ringing or buzzing in ears or any loss of hearing; sore throat and fever; unusual bleeding or bruising; weakness

*Symptoms of overdose*

Drowsiness; headache; increased excitability

Other side effects may occur that usually do not need medical attention. These side effects may go away during treatment as your body adjusts to the medicine. However, check with your doctor if any of the following side effects continue or are bothersome:

*More common*

Diarrhea; difficulty in seeing to read; headache; itching (more common in black patients); loss of appetite; nausea or vomiting; stomach cramps or pain

*Less common*

Bleaching of hair or increased hair loss; blue-black discoloration of skin, fingernails, or inside of mouth; dizziness or lightheadedness; nervousness or restlessness; skin rash

Other side effects not listed above may also occur in some patients. If you notice any other effects, check with your doctor.

## Additional Information

Once a medicine has been approved for marketing for a certain use, experience may show that it is also useful for other medical problems. Although these uses are not included in product labeling, hydroxychloroquine is used in certain patients with the following medical conditions:

- Arthritis, juvenile
- Hypercalcemia, sarcoid-associated
- Polymorphous light eruption
- Porphyria cutanea tarda
- Urticaria, solar
- Vasculitis, chronic cutaneous

Other than the above information, there is no additional information relating to proper use, precautions, or side effects for these uses.

Revised: 10/06/92
Interim revision: 05/19/94

# HYDROXYPROPYL CELLULOSE   Ophthalmic

A commonly used brand name in the U.S. and Canada is Lacrisert.

## Description

Hydroxypropyl cellulose (hye-drox-ee-PROE-pil SELL-yoo-lose) belongs to the group of medicines known as artificial tears. It is inserted in the eye to relieve dryness and irritation caused by reduced tear flow that occurs in certain eye diseases.

This medicine is available only with your doctor's prescription, in the following dosage form:

*Ophthalmic*

- Ocular system (eye system) (U.S. and Canada)

## Before Using This Medicine

In deciding to use a medicine, the risks of using the medicine must be weighed against the good it will do. This is a decision you and your doctor will make. For hydroxypropyl cellulose, the following should be considered:

**Allergies**—Tell your doctor if you have ever had any unusual or allergic reaction to hydroxypropyl cellulose. Also tell your health care professional if you are allergic to any other substances, such as preservatives.

**Pregnancy**—Hydroxypropyl cellulose has not been shown to cause birth defects or other problems in humans.

**Breast-feeding**—Hydroxypropyl cellulose has not been reported to cause problems in nursing babies.

**Children**—Although there is no specific information comparing use of this medicine in children with use in other age groups, this medicine is not expected to cause different side effects or problems in children than it does in adults.

**Older adults**—Many medicines have not been studied specifically in older people. Therefore, it may not be known whether they work exactly the same way they do in younger adults. Although there is no specific information comparing use of this medicine in the elderly with use in other age groups, this medicine is not expected to cause different side effects or problems in older people than it does in younger adults.

## Proper Use of This Medicine

To use:

- This medicine usually comes with patient directions. Read them carefully before using this medicine. It is very important that you understand how to insert this eye system properly. If you have any questions about this, check with your doctor.

- Before opening the package containing this medicine, wash your hands thoroughly with soap and water.
- If the eye system accidentally comes out of your eye, as sometimes occurs when the eye is rubbed, do not put it back in the eye, since it may be contaminated. Instead, insert another eye system if needed.
- You may have to use this medicine for several weeks before your eye symptoms get better.

**Dosing**—The dose of hydroxypropyl cellulose will be different for different patients. *Follow your doctor's orders or the directions on the label.* The following information includes only the average doses of hydroxypropyl cellulose. *If your dose is different, do not change it* unless your doctor tells you to do so.

*The number of doses you use, the time allowed between doses, and the length of time you use the medicine depend on the medical problem for which you are using hydroxypropyl cellulose.*

- For *eye system* dosage form:
  —For dry eyes or eye irritation:
    • Adults and children—Place one insert in the eye each day.

**Missed dose**—If you forget to insert an eye system at the proper time, insert it as soon as possible. Then go back to your regular dosing schedule.

**Storage**—To store this medicine:
- Keep out of the reach of children.
- Store away from heat and direct light.
- Do not keep outdated medicine or medicine no longer needed. Be sure that any discarded medicine is out of the reach of children.

## Precautions While Using This Medicine

This medicine may cause blurred vision for a short time after each dose is applied. *Make sure your vision is clear before you drive, use machines, or do anything else that could be dangerous if you are not able to see well.*

This medicine may also cause your eyes to become more sensitive to light than they are normally. Wearing sunglasses and avoiding too much exposure to bright light may help lessen the discomfort.

If your eye symptoms get worse or if you get new eye symptoms, remove the eye system and check with your doctor as soon as possible.

## Side Effects of This Medicine

Along with its needed effects, a medicine may cause some unwanted effects. The following side effects may go away during treatment as your body adjusts to the medicine. However, check with your doctor if any of these effects continue or are bothersome:

*Less common*
> Blurred vision; eye redness or discomfort or other irritation not present before use of this medicine; increased sensitivity of eyes to light; matting or stickiness of eyelashes; swelling of eyelids; watering of eyes

Other side effects not listed above may also occur in some patients. If you notice any other effects, check with your doctor.

Revised: 06/21/93

# HYDROXYPROPYL METHYLCELLULOSE    Ophthalmic

Some commonly used brand names are:

**In the U.S.—**

| | |
|---|---|
| Gonak | Lacril |
| Goniosol | Moisture Drops |
| Isopto Alkaline | Tearisol |
| Isopto Plain | Tears Naturale II |
| Isopto Tears | Tears Renewed |
| Just Tears | Ultra Tears |

**In Canada—**

| | |
|---|---|
| Isopto Tears | Tears Naturale |
| Moisture Drops | |

Another commonly used name is hypromellose.

## Description

Hydroxypropyl methylcellulose (hye-drox-ee-PROE-pil meth-ill-SELL-yoo-lose) belongs to the group of medicines known as artificial tears. It is used to relieve dryness and irritation caused by reduced tear flow. It helps prevent damage to the eye in certain eye diseases. Hydroxypropyl methylcellulose may also be used to moisten hard contact lenses and artificial eyes. In addition, it may be used in certain eye examinations.

Some of these preparations are available only with your doctor's prescription. Others are available without a prescription; however, your doctor may have special instructions on the proper use of this medicine for your medical problem.

Hydroxypropyl methylcellulose is available in the following dosage form:

*Ophthalmic*
- Ophthalmic solution (eye drops) (U.S. and Canada)

## Before Using This Medicine

If you are using this medicine without a prescription, carefully read and follow any precautions on the label. For hydroxypropyl methylcellulose, the following should be considered:

**Allergies**—Tell your doctor if you have ever had any unusual or allergic reaction to hydroxypropyl methylcellulose. Also tell your health care professional if you are allergic to any other substances, such as preservatives.

**Pregnancy**—Hydroxypropyl methylcellulose has not been shown to cause birth defects or other problems in humans.

**Breast-feeding**—Hydroxypropyl methylcellulose has not been reported to cause problems in nursing babies.

**Children**—Although there is no specific information comparing use of hydroxypropyl methylcellulose in children with use in other age groups, this medicine is not expected to cause different side effects or problems in children than it does in adults.

**Older adults**—Many medicine have not been studied specifically in older people. Therefore, it may not be known whether they work exactly the same way they do in younger adults. Although there is no specific information comparing use of hydroxypropyl methylcellulose in the elderly with use in other age groups, this medicine is not expected to cause different side effects or problems in older people than it does in younger adults.

## Proper Use of This Medicine

To use:

- First, wash your hands. Then tilt the head back and pull the lower eyelid away from the eye to form a pouch. Drop the medicine into the pouch and gently close the eyes. Do not blink. Keep the eyes closed for 1 or 2 minutes to allow the medicine to be absorbed.
- To keep the medicine as germ-free as possible, do not touch the applicator tip to any surface (including the eye). Also, keep the container tightly closed.

*Do not use this medicine for more than 3 days,* unless otherwise directed by your doctor. To do so may increase the chance of side effects.

For patients *wearing hard contact lenses*:

- Take care not to float the lens from your eye when applying this medicine. If you have any questions about this, check with your health care professional.

**Dosing**—The dose of hydroxypropyl methylcellulose will be different for different patients. *Follow your doctor's orders or the directions on the label.* The following information includes only the average doses of hydroxypropyl methylcellulose. *If your dose is different, do not change it* unless your doctor tells you to do so.

*The number of doses you use each day, the time allowed between doses, and the length of time you use the medicine depend on the medical problem for which you are using hydroxypropyl methylcellulose.*

- For dry eyes:
  —For *ophthalmic solution (eye drops)* dosage form:
  - Adults and children—Use 1 drop three or four times a day.

**Storage**—To store this medicine:

- Keep out of the reach of children.
- Store away from heat and direct light.
- Keep the medicine from freezing.
- Do not keep outdated medicine or medicine no longer needed. Be sure that any discarded medicine is out of the reach of children.

## Precautions While Using This Medicine

*If you experience eye pain, changes in vision, continued redness or irritation of the eye, or if your symptoms continue or become worse, check with your doctor.*

## Side Effects of This Medicine

Along with its needed effects, a medicine may cause some unwanted effects. Although not all of these side effects may occur, if they do occur they may need medical attention.

Check with your doctor as soon as possible if the following side effect occurs:

Eye irritation not present before use of this medicine

Other side effects may occur that usually do not need medical attention. These side effects may go away during treatment as your body adjusts to the medicine. However, check with your health care professional if any of the following side effects continue or are bothersome:

*Less common—more common with 1% solution*
Blurred vision; matting or stickiness of eyelashes

Other side effects not listed above may also occur in some patients. If you notice any other effects, check with your health care professional.

Revised: 06/21/93

# HYDROXYUREA    Systemic

A commonly used brand name in the U.S. and Canada is Hydrea.

## Description

Hydroxyurea (hye-DROX-ee-yoo-REE-ah) belongs to the group of medicines called antimetabolites. It is used to treat some kinds of cancer.

Hydroxyurea seems to interfere with the growth of cancer cells, which are eventually destroyed. Since the growth of normal body cells may also be affected by hydroxyurea, other effects will also occur. Some of these may be serious and must be reported to your doctor. Other effects may not be serious but may cause concern. Some effects may not occur for months or years after the medicine is used.

Before you begin treatment with hydroxyurea, you and your doctor should talk about the good this medicine will do as well as the risks of using it.

Hydroxyurea is available only with your doctor's prescription, in the following dosage form:
*Oral*
- Capsules (U.S. and Canada)

## Before Using This Medicine

In deciding to use a medicine, the risks of taking the medicine must be weighed against the good it will do. This is a decision you and your doctor will make. For hydroxyurea, the following should be considered:

**Allergies**—Tell your doctor if you have ever had any unusual or allergic reaction to hydroxyurea.

**Pregnancy**—Tell your doctor if you are pregnant or if you intend to have children. There is a chance that this medicine may cause birth defects if either the male or female is taking it at the time of conception or if it is taken during pregnancy. Studies have shown that hydroxyurea causes birth defects in animals. In addition, many cancer medicines may cause sterility. Although sterility seems to be only temporary with this medicine, the possibility should be kept in mind.

Be sure that you have discussed this with your doctor before taking this medicine. It is best to use some kind of birth control while you are taking hydroxyurea. Tell your doctor right away if you think you have become pregnant while taking hydroxyurea.

**Breast-feeding**—Tell your doctor if you are breast-feeding or if you intend to breast-feed during treatment with this medicine. Because hydroxyurea may cause serious side effects, breast-feeding is generally not recommended while you are taking it.

**Children**—Side effects may be likely to occur in children, who may be more sensitive to the effects of hydroxyurea.

**Older adults**—Side effects may be more likely to occur in the elderly, who may be more sensitive to the effects of hydroxyurea.

**Other medicines**—Although certain medicines should not be used together at all, in other cases two different medicines may be used together even if an interaction might occur. In these cases, your doctor may want to change the dose, or other precautions may be necessary. When you are taking hydroxyurea, it is especially important that your health care professional know if you are taking any of the following:
- Amphotericin B by injection (e.g., Fungizone) or
- Antithyroid agents (medicine for overactive thyroid) or
- Azathioprine (e.g., Imuran) or
- Chloramphenicol (e.g., Chloromycetin) or
- Colchicine or
- Flucytosine (e.g., Ancobon) or
- Ganciclovir (e.g., Cytovene) or
- Interferon (e.g., Intron A, Roferon-A) or
- Plicamycin (e.g., Mithracin) or
- Zidovudine (e.g., AZT, Retrovir) or
- If you have ever been treated with x-rays or cancer medicines—Hydroxyurea may increase the effects of these medicines or radiation therapy on the blood
- Probenecid (e.g., Benemid) or
- Sulfinpyrazone (e.g., Anturane)—Hydroxyurea may increase the amount of uric acid in the blood. Since these medicines are used to lower uric acid levels, they may not be as effective in patients taking hydroxyurea

**Other medical problems**—The presence of other medical problems may affect the use of hydroxyurea. Make sure you tell your doctor if you have any other medical problems, especially:
- Anemia—May be worsened
- Chickenpox (including recent exposure) or
- Herpes zoster (shingles)—Risk of severe disease affecting other parts of the body
- Gout or
- Kidney stones—Hydroxyurea may increase levels of uric acid in the body, which can cause gout or kidney stones
- Infection—Hydroxyurea may decrease your body's ability to fight infection
- Kidney disease—Effects may be increased because of slower removal of hydroxyurea from the body

## Proper Use of This Medicine

*Take hydroxyurea only as directed by your doctor.* Do not use more or less of it, and do not use it more often than your doctor ordered. The exact amount of medicine you need has been carefully worked out. Taking too much may increase the chance of side effects, while taking too little may not improve your condition.

For patients who *cannot swallow the capsules:*
- The contents of the capsule may be emptied into a glass of water and then taken immediately. Some powder may float on the surface of the water, but that is just filler from the capsule.

This medicine is sometimes given together with certain other medicines. If you are using a combination of medicines, make sure that you take each one at the right time and do not mix them. Ask your health care professional to help you plan a way to take your medicine at the right times.

While you are using this medicine, your doctor may want you to drink extra fluids so that you will pass more urine. This will help prevent kidney problems and keep your kidneys working well.

This medicine commonly causes nausea, vomiting, and diarrhea. However, it is very important that you continue to use the medicine, even if you begin to feel ill. Ask your health care professional for ways to lessen these effects.

If you vomit shortly after taking a dose of hydroxyurea, check with your doctor. You will be told whether to take the dose again or to wait until the next scheduled dose.

**Dosing**—The dose of hydroxyurea will be different for different patients. The dose that is used may depend on a number of things, including what the medicine is being used for, the patient's weight, and whether or not other medicines are also being taken. *If you are taking hydroxyurea at home, follow your doctor's orders or the directions on the label.* If you have any questions about the proper dose of hydroxyurea, ask your doctor.

**Missed dose**—If you miss a dose of this medicine, do not take the missed dose at all and do not double the next one. Instead, go back to your regular dosing schedule and check with your doctor.

**Storage**—To store this medicine:
- Keep out of the reach of children.
- Store away from heat and direct light.
- Do not store in the bathroom, near the kitchen sink, or in other damp places. Heat or moisture may cause the medicine to break down.
- Do not keep outdated medicine or medicine no longer needed. Be sure that any discarded medicine is out of the reach of children.

## Precautions While Using This Medicine

*It is very important that your doctor check your progress at regular visits* to make sure that this medicine is working properly and to check for unwanted effects.

While you are being treated with hydroxyurea, and after you stop treatment with it, *do not have any immunizations (vaccinations) without your doctor's approval.* Hydroxyurea may lower your body's resistance and there is a chance you might get the infection the immunization is meant to prevent. In addition, other persons living in your household should not take oral polio vaccine since there is a chance they could pass the polio virus on to you. Also, avoid persons who have recently taken oral polio vaccine. Do not get close to them and do not stay in the same room with them for very long. If you cannot

take these precautions, you should consider wearing a protective face mask that covers the nose and mouth.

Hydroxyurea can temporarily lower the number of white blood cells in your blood, increasing the chance of getting an infection. It can also lower the number of platelets, which are necessary for proper blood clotting. If this occurs, there are certain precautions you can take, especially when your blood count is low, to reduce the risk of infection or bleeding:

- If you can, avoid people with infections. *Check with your doctor immediately* if you think you are getting an infection or if you get a fever or chills, cough or hoarseness, lower back or side pain, or painful or difficult urination.
- *Check with your doctor immediately* if you notice any unusual bleeding or bruising; black, tarry stools; blood in urine or stools; or pinpoint red spots on your skin.
- Be careful when using a regular toothbrush, dental floss, or toothpick. Your medical doctor, dentist, or nurse may recommend other ways to clean your teeth and gums. Check with your medical doctor before having any dental work done.
- Do not touch your eyes or the inside of your nose unless you have just washed your hands and have not touched anything else in the meantime.
- Be careful not to cut yourself when you are using sharp objects such as a safety razor or fingernail or toenail cutters.
- Avoid contact sports or other situations where bruising or injury could occur.

## Side Effects of This Medicine

Along with their needed effects, medicines like hydroxyurea can sometimes cause unwanted effects such as blood problems and other side effects. These and others are described below. Also, because of the way these medicines act on the body, there is a chance that they might cause other unwanted effects that may not occur until months or years after the medicine is used. These delayed effects may include certain types of cancer, such as leukemia. Ask your health care professional for ways to lessen these effects.

Although not all of these side effects may occur, if they do occur they may need medical attention.

*Check with your doctor or nurse immediately* if any of the following side effects occur:

*Less common*
Cough or hoarseness; fever or chills; lower back or side pain; painful or difficult urination

*Rare*
Black, tarry stools; blood in urine or stools; pinpoint red spots on skin; unusual bleeding or bruising

Check with your doctor as soon as possible if any of the following side effects occur:

*Less common*
Sores in mouth and on lips

*Rare*

Confusion; convulsions (seizures); dizziness; hallucinations (seeing, hearing, or feeling things that are not there); headache; joint pain; swelling of feet or lower legs

Other side effects may occur that usually do not need medical attention. These side effects may go away during treatment as your body adjusts to the medicine. Also, your health care professional may be able to tell you about ways to prevent or reduce some of these side effects. Check with your health care professional if any of the following side effects continue or are bothersome or if you have any questions about them:

*More common*

Diarrhea; drowsiness; loss of appetite; nausea or vomiting

*Less common*

Constipation; redness of skin; skin rash and itching

After you stop taking hydroxyurea, your body may need time to adjust. The length of time this takes depends on the amount of medicine you were using and how long you used it. During this period of time check with your doctor if you notice any of the following side effects:

Black, tarry stools; blood in urine or stools; cough or hoarseness; fever or chills; lower back or side pain; painful or difficult urination; pinpoint red spots on skin; unusual bleeding or bruising

Other side effects not listed above may also occur in some patients. If you notice any other effects, check with your doctor.

Revised: 06/16/92
Interim revision: 06/21/94

# IDARUBICIN Systemic

A commonly used brand name in the U.S. and Canada is Idamycin.

## Description

Idarubicin (eye-da-RUE-bi-sin) belongs to the general group of medicines known as antineoplastics. It is used to treat some kinds of cancer, including leukemia.

Idarubicin seems to interfere with the growth of cancer cells, which are eventually destroyed. Since the growth of normal body cells may also be affected by idarubicin, other effects will also occur. Some of these may be serious and must be reported to your doctor. Other effects, like hair loss, may not be serious but may cause concern. Some effects may not occur for months or years after the medicine is used.

Before you begin treatment with idarubicin, you and your doctor should talk about the good this medicine will do as well as the risks of using it.

Idarubicin is to be administered only by or under the supervision of your doctor. It is available in the following dosage form:

*Parenteral*
- Injection (U.S. and Canada)

## Before Using This Medicine

In deciding to use a medicine, the risks of taking the medicine must be weighed against the good it will do. This is a decision you and your doctor will make. For idarubicin, the following should be considered:

**Allergies**—Tell your doctor if you have ever had any unusual or allergic reaction to idarubicin.

**Pregnancy**—There is a chance that this medicine may cause birth defects if either the male or female is receiving it at the time of conception or if it is taken during pregnancy. Studies in rats and rabbits have shown that idarubicin causes birth defects in the fetus and other problems (including miscarriage). In addition, many cancer medicines may cause sterility which could be permanent. Although sterility has been reported only in male dogs with this medicine, the possibility of an effect in human males should be kept in mind.

Be sure that you have discussed these possible effects with your doctor before receiving this medicine. It is best to use some kind of birth control while you are receiving idarubicin. Tell your doctor right away if you think you have become pregnant while receiving idarubicin. Before receiving idarubicin make sure your doctor knows if you are pregnant or if you may become pregnant.

**Breast-feeding**—Because idarubicin may cause serious side effects, breast-feeding is generally not recommended while you are receiving it.

**Children**—There is no specific information comparing use of idarubicin in children with use in other age groups.

**Older adults**—Heart problems are more likely to occur in the elderly, who are usually more sensitive to the effects of idarubicin.

**Other medicines**—Although certain medicines should not be used together at all, in other cases two different medicines may be used together even if an interaction might occur. In these cases, your doctor may want to change the dose, or other precautions may be necessary. When you are receiving idarubicin, it is especially important that your health care professional know if you have ever been treated with x-rays or cancer medicines or if you are taking any of the following:

- Amphotericin B by injection (e.g., Fungizone) or
- Antithyroid agents (medicine for overactive thyroid) or
- Azathioprine (e.g., Imuran) or
- Chloramphenicol (e.g., Chloromycetin) or
- Colchicine or
- Flucytosine (e.g., Ancobon) or
- Ganciclovir (e.g., Cytovene) or
- Interferon (e.g., Intron A, Roferon-A) or
- Plicamycin (e.g., Mithracin) or
- Zidovudine (e.g., AZT, Retrovir)—Idarubicin may increase the effects of these medicines or radiation therapy on the blood
- Probenecid (e.g., Benemid) or
- Sulfinpyrazone (e.g., Anturane)—Idarubicin may raise the concentration of uric acid in the blood, which these medicines are used to lower

**Other medical problems**—The presence of other medical problems may affect the use of idarubicin. Make sure you tell your doctor if you have any other medical problems, especially:

- Chickenpox (including recent exposure) or
- Herpes zoster (shingles)—Risk of severe disease affecting other parts of the body
- Gout or
- Kidney stones—Idarubicin may increase levels of a chemical called uric acid in the body, which can cause gout or kidney stones
- Heart disease—Risk of heart problems caused by idarubicin may be increased
- Kidney disease or
- Liver disease—Effects may be increased because of slower removal of idarubicin from the body

## Proper Use of This Medicine

Idarubicin is sometimes given together with certain other medicines. If you are receiving a combination of medicines, it is important that you receive each one at the proper time. If you are taking some of these medicines by mouth, ask your health care professional to help you plan a way to take them at the right times.

While you are receiving this medicine, your doctor may want you to drink extra fluids so that you will pass more urine. This will help prevent kidney problems and keep your kidneys working well.

Idarubicin often causes nausea and vomiting. However, it is very important that you continue to receive it, even if you begin to feel ill. Ask your health care professional for ways to lessen these effects.

**Dosing**—The dose of idarubicin will be different for different patients. The dose that is used may depend on a number of things, including what the medicine is being used for, the patient's size, and whether or not other medicines are also being taken. *If you are receiving idarubicin at home, follow your doctor's orders or the directions on the label.* If you have any questions about the proper dose of idarubicin, ask your doctor.

## Precautions While Using This Medicine

*It is very important that your doctor check your progress at regular visits* to make sure that this medicine is working properly and to check for unwanted effects.

While you are being treated with idarubicin, and after you stop treatment with it, *do not have any immunizations (vaccinations) without your doctor's approval.* Idarubicin may lower your body's resistance, and there is a chance you might get the infection the immunization is meant to prevent. In addition, other persons living in your household should not take or should not have recently taken oral polio vaccine since there is a chance they could pass the polio virus on to you. Also, avoid other persons who have taken oral polio vaccine. Do not get close to them, and do not stay in the same room with them for very long. If you cannot take these precautions, you should consider wearing a protective face mask that covers the nose and mouth.

Idarubicin can lower the number of white blood cells in your blood temporarily, increasing the chance of getting an infection. It can also lower the number of platelets, which are necessary for proper blood clotting. If this occurs, there are certain precautions you can take, especially when your blood count is low, to reduce the risk of infection or bleeding:

- If you can, avoid people with infections. *Check with your doctor immediately* if you think you are getting an infection or if you get a fever or chills, cough or hoarseness, lower back or side pain, or painful or difficult urination.
- *Check with your doctor immediately* if you notice any unusual bleeding or bruising; black, tarry stools; blood in urine or stools; or pinpoint red spots on your skin.
- Be careful when using a regular toothbrush, dental floss, or toothpick. Your medical doctor, dentist, or nurse may recommend other ways to clean your teeth and gums. Check with your medical doctor before having any dental work done.
- Do not touch your eyes or the inside of your nose unless you have just washed your hands and have not touched anything else in the meantime.
- Be careful not to cut yourself when you are using sharp objects such as a safety razor or fingernail or toenail cutters.

- Avoid contact sports or other situations where bruising or injury could occur.

If idarubicin accidentally seeps out of the vein into which it is injected, it may damage some tissues and cause scarring. *Tell the health care professional right away if you notice redness, pain, or swelling at the place of injection.*

## Side Effects of This Medicine

Along with their needed effects, medicines like idarubicin can sometimes cause unwanted effects such as heart problems, blood problems, loss of hair, and other side effects. These and others are described below. Also, because of the way these medicines act on the body, there is a chance that they might cause other unwanted effects that may not occur until months or years after the medicine is used. These delayed effects may include certain types of cancer, such as leukemia. Discuss these possible effects with your doctor.

Although not all of these side effects may occur, if they do occur they may need medical attention.

*Check with your health care professional immediately* if any of the following side effects occur:

*More common*
  Black, tarry stools; blood in urine or stools; cough or hoarseness; fever or chills; lower back or side pain; painful or difficult urination; pinpoint red spots on skin; unusual bleeding or bruising

*Less common*
  Fast or irregular heartbeat; pain at place of injection; shortness of breath; swelling of feet and lower legs

*Rare*
  Stomach pain (severe)

Check with your health care professional as soon as possible if any of the following side effects occur:

*More common*
  Sores in mouth and on lips

*Less common*
  Joint pain

*Rare*
  Skin rash or hives

Other side effects may occur that usually do not need medical attention. These side effects may go away during treatment as your body adjusts to the medicine. Also, your health care professional may be able to tell you about ways to prevent or reduce some of these side effects. Check with your health care professional if any of the following side effects continue or are bothersome or if you have any questions about them:

*More common*
  Diarrhea or stomach cramps; headache; nausea and vomiting

*Less common*
  Darkening or redness of skin (after x-ray treatment); numbness or tingling of fingers, toes, or face

Idarubicin causes the urine to turn reddish in color, which may stain clothes. This is not blood. It is perfectly normal and lasts for only a day or two after each dose is given.

This medicine often causes a temporary and total loss of hair. After treatment with idarubicin has ended, normal hair growth should return.

After you stop receiving idarubicin, it may still produce some side effects that need attention. During this period of time, *check with your health care professional immediately* if you notice any of the following side effects:

> Fast or irregular heartbeat; shortness of breath; swelling of feet and lower legs

Other side effects not listed above may also occur in some patients. If you notice any other effects, check with your health care professional.

Revised: 06/18/93
Interim revision: 06/21/94

# IDOXURIDINE   Ophthalmic

Some commonly used brand names in the U.S. and Canada are Herplex Liquifilm and Stoxil.

## Description

Idoxuridine (eye-dox-YOOR-i-deen) belongs to the family of medicines called antivirals. Idoxuridine is used to treat virus infections of the eye.

Idoxuridine is available only with your doctor's prescription, in the following dosage forms:

*Ophthalmic*
- Ophthalmic ointment (U.S. and Canada)
- Ophthalmic solution (eye drops) (U.S. and Canada)

## Before Using This Medicine

In deciding to use a medicine, the risks of using the medicine must be weighed against the good it will do. This is a decision you and your doctor will make. For idoxuridine, the following should be considered:

**Allergies**—Tell your doctor if you have ever had any unusual or allergic reaction to idoxuridine or to iodine or iodine-containing preparations. Also tell your health care professional if you are allergic to any other substances, such as preservatives.

**Pregnancy**—Idoxuridine ophthalmic preparations have not been shown to cause birth defects or other problems in humans. However, studies in animals have shown that idoxuridine causes protruding eyes (eyes that stick out too far) and deformed front legs in rabbits. Before using this medicine, make sure your doctor knows if you are pregnant or if you may become pregnant.

**Breast-feeding**—It is not known whether idoxuridine passes into the breast milk. Although most medicines pass into breast milk in small amounts, many of them may be used safely while breast-feeding. Mothers who are using this medicine and who wish to breast-feed should discuss this with their doctor.

**Children**—Studies on this medicine have been done only in adult patients, and there is no specific information comparing use of this medicine in children with use in other age groups.

**Older adults**—Many medicines have not been studied specifically in older people. Therefore, it may not be known whether they work exactly the same way they do in younger adults or if they cause different side effects or problems in older people. There is no specific information comparing use of idoxuridine in the elderly with use in other age groups.

**Other medicines**—Although certain medicines should not be used together at all, in other cases two different medicines may be used together even if an interaction might occur. In these cases, your doctor may want to change the dose, or other precautions may be necessary. When you are using idoxuridine, it is especially important that your health care professional know if you are using the following:

- Eye product containing boric acid—Boric acid may interact with the idoxuridine preparation causing a gritty substance to form or may interact with the preservative in the idoxuridine preparation causing a toxic effect in the eye

## Proper Use of This Medicine

For patients using the *eye drop form* of idoxuridine:
- The bottle is only partially full to provide proper drop control.
- To use:
  —First, wash your hands. Then tilt the head back and pull the lower eyelid away from the eye to form a pouch. Drop the medicine into the pouch and gently close the eyes. Do not blink. Keep the eyes closed for 1 or 2 minutes to allow the medicine to come into contact with the infection.
  —If you think you did not get the drop of medicine into your eye properly, use another drop.
  —To keep the medicine as germ-free as possible, do not touch the applicator tip to any surface (including the eye). Also, keep the container tightly closed.

For patients using the *eye ointment form* of idoxuridine:
- To use:

   —First, wash your hands. Then pull the lower eyelid away from the eye to form a pouch. Squeeze a thin strip of ointment into the pouch. A 1-cm (approximately ⅓-inch) strip of ointment is usually enough unless otherwise directed by your doctor. Gently close the eyes and keep them closed for 1 or 2 minutes to allow the medicine to come into contact with the infection.

   —To keep the medicine as germ-free as possible, do not touch the applicator tip to any surface (including the eye). After using idoxuridine eye ointment, wipe the tip of the ointment tube with a clean tissue and keep the tube tightly closed.

*Do not use this medicine more often or for a longer time than your doctor ordered.* To do so may cause problems in the eyes. If you have any questions about this, check with your doctor.

To help clear up your infection completely, *keep using this medicine for the full time of treatment,* even though your symptoms may have disappeared. *Do not miss any doses.*

**Dosing**—The dose of idoxuridine will be different for different patients. *Follow your doctor's orders or the directions on the label.* The following information includes only the average doses of idoxuridine. *If your dose is different, do not change it* unless your doctor tells you to do so.

*The number of doses you use each day, the time allowed between doses, and the length of time you use the medicine depend on the medical problem for which you are using idoxuridine.*
- For virus infections of the eye:
   —For *eye ointment* dosage form:
      • Adults and children—Use every four hours during the day (five times a day).
   —For *eye solution (eye drops)* dosage form:
      • Adults and children—Use every hour during the day and every two hours during the night. After the eye condition gets better, use every two hours during the day and every four hours during the night.

**Missed dose**—If you miss a dose of this medicine, apply it as soon as possible. However, if it is almost time for your next dose, skip the missed dose and go back to your regular dosing schedule.

**Storage**—To store this medicine:
- Keep out of the reach of children.
- Store in the refrigerator or in a cool place because heat will cause this medicine to break down. How-ever, keep the medicine from freezing. Follow the directions on the label.
- Do not keep outdated medicine or medicine no longer needed. Be sure that any discarded medicine is out of the reach of children.

## Precautions While Using This Medicine

It is very important that your doctor check your progress at regular visits.

If your symptoms do not improve within a week, or if they become worse, check with your doctor.

This medicine may cause your eyes to become more sensitive to light than they are normally. Wearing sunglasses and avoiding too much exposure to bright light may help lessen the discomfort.

## Side Effects of This Medicine

Along with its needed effects, a medicine may cause some unwanted effects. Although not all of these side effects may occur, if they do occur they may need medical attention.

Check with your doctor as soon as possible if any of the following side effects occur:

*Less common*
   Increased sensitivity of eyes to light; itching, redness, swelling, pain, or other sign of irritation not present before use of this medicine

*Rare*
   Blurring, dimming, or haziness of vision

Other side effects may occur that usually do not need medical attention. These side effects may go away during treatment as your body adjusts to the medicine. However, check with your doctor if the following side effect continues or is bothersome:

*Less common*
   Excess flow of tears

After application, eye ointments usually cause your vision to blur for a few minutes.

Other side effects not listed above may also occur in some patients. If you notice any other effects, check with your doctor.

Revised: 06/21/93

# IFOSFAMIDE  Systemic

A commonly used brand name in the U.S. and Canada is IFEX.

## Description

Ifosfamide (eye-FOSS-fa-mide) belongs to the group of medicines called alkylating agents. It is used to treat cancer of the testicles as well as some other kinds of cancer. Another medicine, called mesna, is usually given along with ifosfamide to prevent bladder problems that can be caused by ifosfamide.

Ifosfamide interferes with the growth of cancer cells, which are eventually destroyed. Since the growth of normal body cells may also be affected by ifosfamide, other effects will also occur. Some of these may be serious and must be reported to your doctor. Other effects, like hair loss, may not be serious but may cause concern. Some effects may not occur for months or years after the medicine is used.

Before you begin treatment with ifosfamide, you and your doctor should talk about the good this medicine will do as well as the risks of using it.

Ifosfamide is to be administered only by or under the immediate supervision of your doctor. It is available in the following dosage form:

*Parenteral*
  Injection (U.S. and Canada)

## Before Using This Medicine

In deciding to use a medicine, the risks of taking the medicine must be weighed against the good it will do. This is a decision you and your doctor will make. For ifosfamide, the following should be considered:

**Allergies**—Tell your doctor if you have ever had any unusual or allergic reaction to ifosfamide.

**Pregnancy**—Tell your doctor if you are pregnant or if you intend to have children. There is a chance that this medicine may cause birth defects if either the male or female is taking it at the time of conception or if it is taken during pregnancy. Ifosfamide causes birth defects in animals. In addition, many cancer medicines may cause sterility which could be permanent. Although sterility has not been reported with this medicine, the possibility should be kept in mind.

Be sure that you have discussed this with your doctor before taking this medicine. It is best to use some kind of birth control while you are receiving ifosfamide. Tell your doctor right away if you think you have become pregnant while receiving ifosfamide.

**Breast-feeding**—Tell your doctor if you are breast-feeding or if you intend to breast-feed during treatment with this medicine. Because ifosfamide may cause serious side effects, breast-feeding is generally not recommended while you are receiving it.

**Children**—Although there is no specific information comparing use of ifosfamide in children with use in other age groups, this medicine is not expected to cause different side effects or problems in children than it does in adults.

**Older adults**—Many medicines have not been studied specifically in older people. Therefore, it may not be known whether they work exactly the same way they do in younger adults or if they cause different side effects or problems in older people. There is no specific information comparing use of ifosfamide in the elderly with use in other age groups.

**Other medicines**—Although certain medicines should not be used together at all, in other cases two different medicines may be used together even if an interaction might occur. In these cases, your doctor may want to change the dose, or other precautions may be necessary. When you are taking ifosfamide, it is especially important that your doctor and pharmacist know if you are taking any of the following:
- Amphotericin B by injection (e.g., Fungizone) or
- Antithyroid agents (medicine for overactive thyroid) or
- Azathioprine (e.g., Imuran) or
- Chloramphenicol (e.g., Chloromycetin) or
- Colchicine or
- Flucytosine (e.g., Ancobon) or
- Ganciclovir (e.g., Cytovene) or
- Interferon (e.g., Intron A, Roferon-A) or
- Plicamycin (e.g., Mithracin) or
- Zidovudine (e.g., AZT, Retrovir) or
- If you have ever been treated with x-rays or cancer medicines—Ifosfamide may increase the effects of these medicines or radiation therapy on the blood

**Other medical problems**—The presence of other medical problems may affect the use of ifosfamide. Make sure you tell your doctor if you have any other medical problems, especially:
- Chickenpox (including recent exposure) or
- Herpes zoster (shingles)—Risk of severe disease affecting other parts of the body
- Infection—Ifosfamide can decrease your body's ability to fight infection
- Kidney disease—Effects may be increased because of slower removal of ifosamide from the body
- Liver disease—Effects may be increased or decreased because the liver both makes ifosfamide work and removes it from the body

## Proper Use of This Medicine

Ifosfamide is sometimes given together with certain other medicines. If you are using a combination of medicines, make sure that you take each one at the proper time and do not mix them. Ask your doctor, nurse, or pharmacist to help you plan a way to remember to take your medicines at the right times.

While you are receiving ifosfamide, it is important that you drink extra fluids so that you will pass more urine. Also, empty your bladder frequently, including at least once during the night. This will help prevent kidney and bladder problems and keep your kidneys working well. Ifosfamide passes from the body in the urine. If too much of it appears in the urine or if the urine stays in the bladder too long, it can cause dangerous irritation. Follow your doctor's instructions carefully about how much fluid to drink every day. Some patients may have to drink up to 7 to 12 cups (3 quarts) of fluid a day.

Ifosfamide often causes nausea and vomiting. However, it is very important that you continue to receive the medicine even if you begin to feel ill. Ask your health care professional for ways to lessen these effects.

**Dosing**—The dose of ifosfamide will be different for different patients. The dose that is used may depend on a number of things, including what the medicine is being used for, the patient's size, and whether or not other medicines are also being taken. *If you are receiving ifosfamide at home, follow your doctor's orders or the directions on the label.* If you have any questions about the proper dose of ifosfamide, ask your doctor.

## Precautions While Using This Medicine

*It is very important that your doctor check your progress at regular visits* to make sure that this medicine is working properly and to check for unwanted effects.

While you are being treated with ifosfamide, and after you stop treatment with it, *do not have any immunizations (vaccinations) without your doctor's approval.* Ifosfamide may lower your body's resistance and there is a chance you might get the infection the immunization is meant to prevent. In addition, other persons living in your house should not take oral polio vaccine since there is a chance they could pass the polio virus on to you. Also, avoid persons who have recently taken oral polio vaccine. Do not get close to them, and do not stay in the same room with them for very long. If you cannot take these precautions, you should consider wearing a protective face mask that covers the nose and mouth.

Ifosfamide can temporarily lower the number of white blood cells in your blood, increasing the chance of getting an infection. It can also lower the number of platelets, which are necessary for proper blood clotting. If this occurs, there are certain precautions you can take to reduce the risk of infection or bleeding:

- If you can, avoid people with infections. *Check with your doctor immediately* if you think you are getting an infection or if you get a fever or chills, cough or hoarseness, lower back or side pain, or painful or difficult urination.
- *Check with your doctor immediately* if you notice any unusual bleeding or bruising; black, tarry stools; blood in urine or stools; or pinpoint red spots on your skin.
- Be careful when using a regular toothbrush, dental floss, or toothpick. Your medical doctor, dentist, or nurse may recommend other ways to clean your teeth and gums. Check with your medical doctor before having any dental work done.

- Do not touch your eyes or the inside of your nose unless you have just washed your hands and have not touched anything else in the meantime.
- Be careful not to cut yourself when you are using sharp objects such as a safety razor or fingernail or toenail cutters.
- Avoid contact sports or other situations where bruising or injury could occur.

## Side Effects of This Medicine

Along with their needed effects, medicines like ifosfamide can sometimes cause unwanted effects such as blood problems, loss of hair, and problems with the bladder. These and others are described below. Also, because of the way these medicines act on the body, there is a chance that they might cause other unwanted effects that may not occur until months or years after the medicine is used. These may include certain types of cancer, such as leukemia. Discuss these possible effects with your doctor.

Although not all of these side effects may occur, if they do occur they may need medical attention.

*Check with your doctor immediately* if any of the following side effects occur:

*More common*

Blood in urine; frequent urination; painful urination

*Less common*

Cough or hoarseness; fever or chills; lower back or side pain

*Rare*

Black, tarry stools; blood in stools; pinpoint red spots on skin; unusual bleeding or bruising

Check with your doctor as soon as possible if any of the following side effects occur:

*More common*

Agitation; confusion; hallucinations (seeing, hearing, or feeling things that are not there); unusual tiredness

*Less common*

Dizziness; redness, swelling, or pain at place of injection

*Rare*

Cough or shortness of breath; convulsions (seizures); sores in mouth and on lips

Other side effects may occur that usually do not need medical attention. These side effects may go away during treatment as your body adjusts to the medicine. Also, your health care professional may be able to tell you about ways to prevent or reduce some of these side effects. Check with your doctor if any of the following side effects continue or are bothersome or if you have any questions about them:

*More common*

Nausea and vomiting

Ifosfamide often causes a temporary loss of hair. After treatment has ended, normal hair growth should return.

After you stop receiving ifosfamide, it may still produce some side effects that need attention. During this period of time, *check with your doctor immediately* if you notice the following side effect:

Blood in urine

Other side effects not listed above may also occur in some patients. If you notice any other effects, check with your doctor.

Revised: 09/09/92
Interim revision: 06/21/94

# IMIPENEM AND CILASTATIN   Systemic

Some commonly used brand names are:

**In the U.S.—**
Primaxin IM
Primaxin IV

**In Canada—**
Primaxin

## Description

Imipenem (i-mi-PEN-em) and cilastatin (sye-la-STAT-in) combination is used in the treatment of infections caused by bacteria. It works by killing bacteria or preventing their growth. This medicine will not work for colds, flu, or other virus infections.

Imipenem and cilastatin combination is used to treat infections in many different parts of the body. It is sometimes given with other antibiotics.

This medicine is available only with your doctor's prescription, in the following dosage form:

*Parenteral*
• Injection (U.S. and Canada)

## Before Receiving This Medicine

In deciding to use a medicine, the risks of taking the medicine must be weighed against the good it will do. This is a decision you and your doctor will make. For imipenem and cilastatin, the following should be considered:

**Allergies**—Tell your doctor if you have ever had any unusual or allergic reaction to imipenem and cilastatin, penicillins or cephalosporins. Also tell your health care professional if you are allergic to any other substances, such as foods, preservatives, or dyes.

**Pregnancy**—Studies have not been done in humans. However, imipenem and cilastatin combination has not been reported to cause birth defects or other problems in animal studies.

**Breast-feeding**—It is not known whether imipenem or cilastatin passes into the breast milk. However, this medicine has not been reported to cause problems in nursing babies.

**Children**—This medicine has been tested in a limited number of children 12 years of age and older and, in effective doses, has not been reported to cause different side effects or problems in children than it does in adults.

**Older adults**—Many medicines have not been studied specifically in older people. Therefore, it may not be known whether they work exactly the same way they do in younger adults. Although there is no specific information comparing use of imipenem and cilastatin in the elderly with use in other age groups, this medicine is not expected to cause different side effects or problems in older people than it does in younger adults.

**Other medicines**—Although certain medicines should not be used together at all, in other cases two different medicines may be used together even if an interaction might occur. In these cases, your doctor may want to change the dose, or other precautions may be necessary. Tell your health care professional if you are taking any other prescription or nonprescription (over-the-counter [OTC]) medicine.

**Other medical problems**—The presence of other medical problems may affect the use of imipenem and cilastatin. Make sure you tell your doctor if you have any other medical problems, especially:

• Central nervous system (CNS) disorders (for example, brain disease or history of seizures)—Patients with nervous system disorders, including seizures, may be more likely to have side effects
• Kidney disease—Patients with kidney disease may be more likely to have side effects

## Proper Use of This Medicine

To help clear up your infection completely, *imipenem and cilastatin combination must be given for the full time of treatment,* even if you begin to feel better after a few days. Also, this medicine works best when there is a constant amount in the blood or urine. To help keep the amount constant, it must be given on a regular schedule.

**Dosing**—The dose of imipenem and cilastatin combination will be different for different patients. *Follow your doctor's orders or the directions on the label.* The following information includes only the average doses of imipenem and cilastatin combination. *If your dose is different, do not change it* unless your doctor tells you to do so.

• For *injection* dosage form:
  —For bacterial infections:
    • Adults and children 12 years of age and over— 250 milligrams (mg) to 1 gram injected into a

vein every six to eight hours; or 500 to 750 mg injected into a muscle every twelve hours, depending on how severe your infection is.
- Children up to 12 years of age—Use and dose must be determined by your doctor.

## Precautions While Using This Medicine

*Some patients may develop tremors or seizures while receiving this medicine. If you already have a history of seizures and you are taking anticonvulsants, you should continue to take them* unless otherwise directed by your doctor.

In some patients, imipenem and cilastatin combination may cause diarrhea.
- Severe diarrhea may be a sign of a serious side effect. *Do not take any diarrhea medicine without first checking with your doctor.* Diarrhea medicines may make your diarrhea worse or make it last longer.
- For mild diarrhea, diarrhea medicine containing kaolin (e.g., Kaopectate liquid) or attapulgite (e.g., Kaopectate tablets, Diasorb) may be taken. However, other kinds of diarrhea medicine should not be taken. They may make your diarrhea worse or make it last longer.
- If you have any questions about this or if mild diarrhea continues or gets worse, check with your health care professional.

## Side Effects of This Medicine

Along with its needed effects, a medicine may cause some unwanted effects. Although not all of these side effects may occur, if they do occur they may need medical attention.

*Check with your health care professional immediately* if any of the following side effects occur:

*More common*

Confusion; convulsions (seizures); dizziness; pain at place of injection; skin rash, hives, itching, fever, or wheezing; tremors

*Less common*

Dizziness; increased sweating; nausea or vomiting; unusual tiredness or weakness

*Rare*

Fever; severe abdominal or stomach cramps and pain; watery and severe diarrhea, which may also be bloody (these side effects may also occur up to several weeks after you stop receiving this medicine)

Other side effects may occur that usually do not need medical attention. These side effects may go away during treatment as your body adjusts to the medicine. However, check with your doctor if the following side effects continue or are bothersome:

*More common*

Diarrhea; nausea and vomiting

Other side effects not listed above may also occur in some patients. If you notice any other effects, check with your doctor.

Revised: 09/08/92
Interim revision: 04/01/94

# IMMUNE GLOBULIN INTRAVENOUS (HUMAN)   Systemic

Some commonly used brand names are:

**In the U.S.—**

| | |
|---|---|
| Gamimune N | Polygam |
| Gammagard | Sandoglobulin |
| Gammar–IV | Venoglobulin–I |
| Iveegam | |

**In Canada—**

Gamimune N
Iveegam

Other commonly used names are IGIV and IVIG.

## Description

Immune globulin intravenous (IGIV) belongs to a group of medicines known as immunizing agents. IGIV is used to prevent or treat some illnesses that can occur when your body does not produce enough of its own immunity to prevent those diseases.

IGIV is manufactured from plasma that comes from blood that has been donated by many people. The immunity to diseases that is in the donated blood is used by your own body to increase your immunity.

IGIV is also used to treat a disorder known as idiopathic thrombocytopenic purpura (ITP). When a person has ITP, there is an increase in the breakdown of a part of the blood known as platelets. Low platelet levels in the blood increase a person's chance of bleeding or hemorrhaging. IGIV is used to increase the number of platelets in the blood to prevent this bleeding.

IGIV does not contain harmful products of hepatitis B virus, human immunodeficiency virus (HIV), acquired immunodeficiency syndrome (AIDS), or AIDS-related complex (ARC).

IGIV is available in the following dosage form:

*Parenteral*

- Injection (U.S. and Canada)

## Before Using This Medicine

In deciding to use a medicine, the risks of taking the medicine must be weighed against the good it will do. This is a decision you and your doctor will make. For

immune globulin intravenous (IGIV), the following should be considered:

**Allergies**—Tell your doctor if you have ever had any unusual or allergic reaction to intramuscular or intravenous immune globulins. Also tell your health care professional if you are allergic to any other substances, such as foods, preservatives, or dyes.

**Diet**—Make certain your health care professional knows if you are on any special diet, such as a low-sodium or low-sugar diet.

**Pregnancy**—Studies on effects in pregnancy have not been done in either humans or animals.

**Breast-feeding**—It is not known whether IGIV passes into the breast milk. Although most medicines pass into breast milk in small amounts, many of them may be used safely while breast-feeding. Mothers who are using this medicine and who wish to breast-feed should discuss this with their doctor.

**Children**—Although there is no specific information comparing use of IGIV in children with use in other age groups, this medicine is not expected to cause different side effects or problems in children than it does in adults.

**Older adults**—Many medicines have not been studied specifically in older people. Therefore, it may not be known whether they work exactly the same way they do in younger adults. Although there is no specific information comparing use of IGIV in the elderly with use in other age groups, this medicine is not expected to cause different side effects or problems in older people than it does in younger adults.

**Other medicines**—Although certain medicines should not be used together at all, in other cases two different medicines may be used together even if an interaction might occur. In these cases, your doctor may want to change the dose, or other precautions may be necessary. Tell your health care professional if you are using any other prescription or nonprescription (over-the-counter [OTC]) medicine.

**Other medical problems**—The presence of other medical problems may affect the use of IGIV. Make sure you tell your doctor if you have any other medical problems, especially:

- Agammaglobulinemia or
- Hypogammaglobulinemia—Patients with these conditions who have never received immune globulin substitution therapy or who were last treated more than 8 weeks ago may have more side effects to IGIV
- Heart problems or
- Immunoglobulin A (IgA) deficiencies—IGIV may make the conditions worse

## Proper Use of This Medicine

**Dosing**—The dose of IGIV will be different for different patients. Doses are based on body weight and the condition for which you are being treated. The following information includes only the average doses of IGIV. *If your dose is different, do not change it* unless your doctor tells you to do so.

- For *injection* dosage form:
  —For immunodeficiency:
    - Adults and children—200 to 800 milligrams per kilogram (mg/kg) (90 to 360 milligrams per pound) of body weight per month, injected into a vein.
  —For idiopathic thrombocytopenic purpura (ITP):
    - Adults and children—Either 400 milligrams per kilogram (mg/kg) (180 milligrams per pound) of body weight per day for 2 to 5 days or 1 gram per kilogram (450 milligrams per pound) of body weight per day for 1 or 2 days, injected into a vein. Doses are usually repeated every 10 to 21 days.
  —For bacterial infection secondary to B-cell chronic lymphocytic leukemia (CLL):
    - Adults and children—400 milligrams per kilogram (mg/kg) (180 milligrams per pound) of body weight, given once every 3 or 4 weeks, injected into a vein.
  —For any other condition: The dose will be determined by your doctor.

## Side Effects of This Medicine

Along with its needed effects, a medicine may cause some unwanted effects. Although not all of these side effects may occur, if they do occur they may need medical attention.

*Check with your doctor immediately* if any of the following side effects occur:

*Symptoms of overdose*
  Chest tightness; chills; dizziness; fever; nausea; redness of face; sweating; unusual tiredness or weakness; vomiting

Check with your doctor as soon as possible if any of the following side effects occur:

*More common*
  Fast or pounding heartbeat; troubled breathing

*Less common*
  Bluish coloring of lips or nailbeds; burning sensation in head; faintness or lightheadedness; unusual tiredness or weakness; wheezing

Other side effects may occur that usually do not need medical attention. These side effects may go away during treatment as your body adjusts to the medicine. However, check with your doctor if any of the following side effects continue or are bothersome:

*More common*

　　Backache; general feeling of discomfort or illness; head-ache; joint pain; muscle pain

*Less common*

　　Chest, back, or hip pain; hives; leg cramps; redness, rash, or pain at place of injection

Other side effects not listed above may also occur in some patients. If you notice any other effects, check with your doctor.

---

Revised: 06/21/93
Interim revision: 02/23/94

---

# INDAPAMIDE    Systemic

Some commonly used brand names are:

**In the U.S.—**
　　Lozol

**In Canada—**
　　Lozide

---

## Description

Indapamide (in-DAP-a-mide) belongs to the group of medicines known as diuretics. It is commonly used to treat high blood pressure (hypertension).

High blood pressure adds to the workload of the heart and arteries. If it continues for a long time, the heart and arteries may not function properly. This can damage the blood vessels of the brain, heart, and kidneys resulting in a stroke, heart failure, or kidney failure. High blood pressure may also increase the risk of heart attacks. These problems may be less likely to occur if blood pressure is controlled.

Indapamide is also used to help reduce the amount of water in the body by increasing the flow of urine.

Indapamide is available only with your doctor's prescription, in the following dosage form:

*Oral*
　　• Tablets (U.S. and Canada)

---

## Before Using This Medicine

In deciding to use a medicine, the risks of taking the medicine must be weighed against the good it will do. This is a decision you and your doctor will make. For indapamide, the following should be considered:

**Allergies**—Tell your doctor if you have ever had any unusual or allergic reaction to indapamide or other sulfonamide-type medicines. Also tell your health care professional if you are allergic to any other substances, such as foods, preservatives, or dyes.

**Pregnancy**—Indapamide has not been studied in pregnant women. However, indapamide has not been shown to cause birth defects or other problems in animal studies.

In general, diuretics are not useful for normal swelling of feet and hands that occurs during pregnancy. Diuretics should not be taken during pregnancy unless recommended by your doctor.

**Breast-feeding**—It is not known whether indapamide passes into breast milk. However, this medicine has not been reported to cause problems in nursing babies.

**Children**—Studies on this medicine have been done only in adult patients, and there is no specific information comparing use of indapamide in children with use in other age groups.

**Older adults**—Dizziness or lightheadedness and signs and symptoms of too much potassium loss are more likely to occur in the elderly, who are usually more sensitive than younger adults to the effects of indapamide.

**Other medicines**—Although certain medicines should not be used together at all, in other cases two different medicines may be used together even if an interaction might occur. In these cases, your doctor may want to change the dose, or other precautions may be necessary. When you are taking indapamide, it is especially important that your health care professional know if you are taking any of the following:

　　• Digitalis glycosides (heart medicine)—Use with indapamide may increase the chance of side effects of digitalis glycosides
　　• Lithium (e.g., Lithane)—Use with indapamide may cause high blood levels of lithium, which may increase the chance of side effects

**Other medical problems**—The presence of other medical problems may affect the use of indapamide. Make sure you tell your doctor if you have any other medical problems, especially:

　　• Diabetes mellitus (sugar diabetes) or
　　• Gout (history of)—Indapamide may make these conditions worse
　　• Kidney disease—May prevent indapamide from working properly
　　• Liver disease—Higher blood levels of indapamide may occur, which may increase the chance of side effects

---

## Proper Use of This Medicine

Indapamide may cause you to have an unusual feeling of tiredness when you begin to take it. You may also notice an increase in the amount of urine or in your frequency of urination. After taking the medicine for a while,

---

these effects should lessen. In general, to keep the increase in urine from affecting your sleep:

- If you are to take a single dose a day, take it in the morning after breakfast.
- If you are to take more than one dose a day, take the last dose no later than 6 p.m., unless otherwise directed by your doctor.

However, it is best to plan your dose or doses according to a schedule that will least affect your personal activities and sleep. Ask your health care professional to help you plan the best time to take this medicine.

To help you remember to take indapamide, try to get into the habit of taking it at the same time each day.

For patients taking indapamide for *high blood pressure:*

- In addition to the use of the medicine your doctor has prescribed, treatment for your high blood pressure may include weight control and care in the types of foods you eat, especially foods high in sodium. Your doctor will tell you which of these are most important for you. You should check with your doctor before changing your diet.
- Many patients who have high blood pressure will not notice any signs of the problem. In fact, many may feel normal. It is very important that you *take your medicine exactly as directed* and that you keep your appointments with your doctor even if you feel well.
- Remember that this medicine will not cure your high blood pressure but it does help control it. Therefore, you must continue to take it as directed if you expect to lower your blood pressure and keep it down. *You may have to take high blood pressure medicine for the rest of your life.* If high blood pressure is not treated, it can cause serious problems such as heart failure, blood vessel disease, stroke, or kidney disease.

**Dosing**—The dose of indapamide will be different for different patients. *Follow your doctor's orders or the directions on the label.* The following information includes only the average doses of indapamide. *If your dose is different, do not change it* unless your doctor tells you to do so:

- For *oral* dosage forms (tablets):
  —Adults: 2.5 to 5 milligrams once a day.

**Missed dose**—If you miss a dose of this medicine, take it as soon as possible. However, if it is almost time for your next dose, skip the missed dose and go back to your regular dosing schedule. Do not double doses.

**Storage**—To store this medicine:

- Keep out of the reach of children.
- Store away from heat and direct light.
- Do not store in the bathroom, near the kitchen sink, or in other damp places. Heat or moisture may cause the medicine to break down.

- Do not keep outdated medicine or medicine no longer needed. Be sure that any discarded medicine is out of the reach of children.

## Precautions While Using This Medicine

It is important that your doctor check your progress at regular visits to make sure that indapamide is working properly.

*This medicine may cause a loss of potassium from your body:*

- To help prevent this, your doctor may want you to:
  —eat or drink foods that have a high potassium content (for example, orange or other citrus fruit juices), or
  —take a potassium supplement, or
  —take another medication to help prevent the loss of the potassium in the first place.
- It is very important to follow these directions. Also, it is important not to change your diet on your own. This is more important if you are already on a special diet (as for diabetes), or if you are taking a potassium supplement or a medicine to reduce potassium loss. Extra potassium may not be necessary and, in some cases, too much potassium could be harmful.

Check with your doctor if you become sick and have severe or continuing vomiting or diarrhea. These problems may cause you to lose additional water and potassium.

For patients taking this medicine for *high blood pressure:*

- *Do not take other medicines unless they have been discussed with your doctor.* This especially includes over-the-counter (nonprescription) medicines for appetite control, asthma, colds, hay fever, or sinus problems, since they may tend to increase your blood pressure.

## Side Effects of This Medicine

Along with its needed effects, a medicine may cause some unwanted effects. Although not all of these side effects may occur, if they do occur they may need medical attention.

Check with your doctor as soon as possible if any of the following side effects occur:

Dryness of mouth; increased thirst; irregular heartbeat; mood or mental changes; muscle cramps or pain; nausea or vomiting; unusual tiredness or weakness; weak pulse

*Rare*

Skin rash, itching, or hives

Other side effects may occur that usually do not need medical attention. These side effects may go away during treatment as your body adjusts to the medicine. However,

check with your doctor if any of the following side effects continue or are bothersome:

*Less common or rare*
> Diarrhea; dizziness or lightheadedness, especially when getting up from a lying or sitting position; headache; loss of appetite; trouble in sleeping; stomach upset

Other side effects not listed above may also occur in some patients. If you notice any other effects, check with your doctor.

Revised: 01/20/93

# INFANT FORMULAS   Systemic

Some commonly used brand names are:

**In the U.S.—**

| | |
|---|---|
| Alimentum[1] | RCF[3] |
| Carnation Follow-Up Formula[2] | Similac 13[2] |
| Carnation Good Start[2] | Similac 20[2] |
| Enfamil[2] | Similac 24[2] |
| Enfamil Human Milk Fortifier[2] | Similac 27[2] |
| Enfamil with Iron[2] | Similac with Iron 20[2] |
| Enfamil Premature Formula[2] | Similac with Iron 24[2] |
| Enfamil Premature Formula with Iron[2] | Similac Natural Care Human Milk Fortifier[2] |
| Gerber Baby Formula[2] | Similac PM 60/40[2] |
| Gerber Soy Formula[3] | Similac Special Care 20[2] |
| Isomil[3] | Similac Special Care 24[2] |
| Isomil SF[3] | Similac Special Care with Iron 24[2] |
| I-Soyalac[3] | SMA 13[2] |
| Lactofree[2] | SMA 20[2] |
| Nursoy[3] | SMA 24[2] |
| Nutramigen[1] | SMA 27[2] |
| Preemie SMA 20[2] | SMA Lo-Iron 13[2] |
| Preemie SMA 24[2] | SMA Lo-Iron 20[2] |
| Pregestimil[1] | SMA Lo-Iron 24[2] |
| ProSobee[3] | Soyalac[3] |

**In Canada—**

| | |
|---|---|
| Alimentum[1] | Similac 27[2] |
| Isomil[3] | Similac PM 60/40[2] |
| Nursoy[3] | Similac Special Care 20[2] |
| Nutramigen[1] | Similac Special Care 24[2] |
| Preemie SMA 20[2] | SMA 13[2] |
| Preemie SMA 24[2] | SMA 20[2] |
| Pregestimil[1] | SMA 24[2] |
| ProSobee[3] | SMA 27[2] |
| RCF[3] | SMA Lo-Iron 13[2] |
| Similac 13[2] | SMA Lo-Iron 20[2] |
| Similac 20[2] | SMA Lo-Iron 24[2] |
| Similac 24[2] | |

Note: For quick reference, the following infant formulas are numbered to match the corresponding brand names.

This monograph includes information on the following:
1. Infant Formulas, Hypoallergenic
2. Infant Formulas, Milk-based
3. Infant Formulas, Soy-based

## Description

Infant formulas are used to supply all or part of the nutrients infants need for growth and development. These formulas are used by the body for energy and to form substances for normal body functions.

The amount and type of nutrients contained in infant formulas are regulated by the Food and Drug Administration (FDA). The FDA also regulates the manufacturing process, labeling, and recall procedure for infant formulas.

Infant formulas are available without a prescription. However, they should only be used under medical supervision. They are available in the following forms:

*Oral*
> Infant Formulas, Hypoallergenic (for infants allergic to milk)
> • Oral concentrate (U.S. and Canada)
> • Oral solution (U.S. and Canada)
> • Powder for oral solution (U.S. and Canada)

> Infant Formulas, Milk-based (for infants not allergic to milk)
> • Oral concentrate (U.S.)
> • Oral powder (U.S.)
> • Oral solution (U.S. and Canada)
> • Powder for oral solution (U.S. and Canada)

> Infant Formulas, Soy-based (for infants allergic to milk but not to soy)
> • Oral concentrate (U.S. and Canada)
> • Oral solution (U.S. and Canada)
> • Powder for oral solution (U.S. and Canada)

## Before Using This Infant Formula

If you are giving your infant this infant formula, carefully read and follow any precautions on the label. For infant formulas, the following should be considered:

**Allergies**—Tell your doctor if your infant has ever had any unusual or allergic reaction to infant formulas. Also tell your health care professional if your infant is allergic to any other substances, such as foods, preservatives, or dyes.

**Children**—Problems may occur if the infant formula is not mixed properly or is not used under medical care.

**Medicines, dietary supplements, or infant formulas**—Although certain medicines, dietary supplements, or infant formulas should not be used together at all, in other cases they may be used together even if an interaction might occur. In these cases, your doctor may want to change the feeding schedule, or other precautions may be necessary. When you are giving your infant an infant formula, it is especially important that your health care professional know if you are giving your infant any dietary supplements or any prescription or nonprescription (over-the-counter [OTC]) medicine.

**Other medical problems**—The presence of other medical problems may affect the use of infant formulas. Make sure you tell your doctor if your infant has any medical problems, especially:

- Breathing problems or
- Dehydration or
- Diabetes mellitus (sugar diabetes) or
- Diarrhea or
- Heart problems or
- Hyperglycemia (high levels of sugar in the blood) or
- Liver problems or
- Pancreas problems—Infant formulas may make these conditions worse
- Intestine problems or
- Stomach problems—These problems may prevent infant formulas from being absorbed properly
- Kidney problems—Higher blood levels of certain ingredients of the infant formula may result, and a smaller amount of infant formula may be needed
- Phenylketonuria—Infant formulas contain phenylalanine, which may make the condition worse

## Proper Use of This Infant Formula

Infant formulas may be given by mouth or, in some cases, by a tube feeding. Use the amount of infant formula and the feeding schedule recommended by your doctor.

For infants receiving the *concentrate or powder for oral solution* form of this preparation:

- For mixing or other use, follow carefully the instructions on the package.
- Any unused solution should be kept in the refrigerator. Most formulas can be kept in the refrigerator for 1 to 2 days. Check the label of your product.

For infants receiving the *oral liquid* form of this preparation:

- This preparation is in ready-to-use form. No dilution is needed unless directed by your doctor.
- Shake the preparation well before opening. Refrigerate after opening. Most formulas can be kept in the refrigerator for 1 to 2 days. Check the label of your product.

For infants receiving *Enfamil Human Milk Fortifier*:

- This powder should be added to mother's breast milk. For mixing or other use, follow carefully the instructions on the package.
- Any unused solution should be kept in the refrigerator for up to 1 day.

For infants receiving *Similac Natural Care*:

- This liquid should be added to the mother's breast milk. It may also be fed alternating with breast milk to low-birth-weight infants as directed by the infant's doctor. For mixing or other use, follow carefully the instructions on the package.
- Any unused solution should be kept in the refrigerator for up to 1 day.

**Feeding**—The amount of an infant formula to be given will be different for different infants. *Follow your doctor's orders*.

**Storage**—To store the unopened container:

- Keep out of the reach of children.
- Store away from heat and direct light.
- Do not store in the bathroom, near the kitchen sink, or in other damp places. Heat or moisture may cause the infant formula to break down.
- Keep the infant formula from freezing. Do not refrigerate until after the product has been opened or mixed.
- Do not keep outdated infant formulas or those no longer needed. Be sure that any discarded infant formula is out of the reach of children.

## Side Effects of This Infant Formula

Along with its needed effects, an infant formula may cause some unwanted effects. Although not all of these side effects may occur, if they do occur they may need medical attention.

*More common*

Diarrhea; unusual thirst; unusual tiredness or weakness

Note: Diarrhea can lead to severe fluid loss in your infant very quickly. Diarrhea can be caused by improper infant formula preparation. Make sure that you are following the directions for mixing on the container of your product.

*Less common*

Signs of milk allergy (hives, wheezing); signs of milk intolerance (abdominal bloating, diarrhea, stomach cramps, vomiting)

Developed: 09/23/93

# INFLUENZA VIRUS VACCINE  Systemic

Some commonly used brand names are:

**In the U.S.—**
Flu-Imune
Fluogen
FluShield
Fluzone
Generic name product may also be available.

**In Canada—**
Fluviral
Fluzone
Another commonly used name is flu vaccine.

# Description

Influenza (in-floo-EN-za) Virus Vaccine is an active immunizing agent given by injection each year. It is also known as a "Flu shot." The vaccine helps to prevent infection by influenza viruses.

There are many kinds of influenza viruses, but not all will cause problems in any given year. Therefore, before the influenza vaccine for each year is produced, the World Health Organization (WHO) and the U.S. and Canadian Public Health Services decide which influenza viruses will be most likely to cause influenza infection that year. Then they include the antigens to these viruses in the influenza vaccine made available. Usually, both the U.S. and Canada use the same influenza vaccine; however, they are not required to do so.

It is necessary to receive an influenza vaccine injection each year, since influenza infections are usually caused by viruses with different antigens each year and because the immunity gained by the vaccine lasts less than a year.

Influenza is a virus infection of the throat, bronchial tubes, and lungs. Influenza infection causes fever, chills, cough, headache, and muscle aches and pains in your back, arms, and legs. In addition, adults and children weakened by other diseases or medical conditions and persons 65 years of age and over, even if they are healthy, may get a much more serious illness and may have to be treated in a hospital. Each year thousands of persons die as a result of an influenza infection.

The best way to help prevent influenza infection is to get an influenza vaccination each year, usually in early November. Immunization against influenza is recommended for everyone, including infants 6 months of age and over, all children, and all adults.

This vaccine is to be administered only by or under the supervision of your doctor or other health care professional. It is available in the following dosage form:

*Parenteral*
- Injection (U.S. and Canada)

# Before Receiving This Vaccine

In deciding to use a medicine, the risks of taking the medicine must be weighed against the good it will do. This is a decision you and your doctor will make. For influenza vaccine, the following should be considered:

**Allergies**—Tell your doctor if you have ever had any unusual or allergic reaction to influenza vaccine or to antibiotics, such as gentamicin sulfate, streptomycin sulfate, or other aminoglycosides. Influenza vaccine available in the U.S. or Canada may contain these antibiotics. Also tell your health care professional if you are allergic to any other substances, such as foods (especially eggs) or preservatives (especially sodium bisulfite or thimerosal). Influenza vaccine is grown in the fluids of chick embryos.

**Pregnancy**—Influenza vaccine has not been shown to cause birth defects or other problems in humans.

**Breast-feeding**—Influenza vaccine has not been reported to cause problems in nursing babies.

**Children**—Use is not recommended for infants up to 6 months of age. In addition, only the split-virus vaccine should be given to children 6 months up to 13 years of age. Also, some side effects of the vaccine, such as fever, unusual tiredness or weakness, or aches or pains in muscles, are more likely to occur in infants and children, who are usually more sensitive than adults to the effects of influenza vaccine.

**Older adults**—This vaccine is not expected to cause different side effects or problems in older persons than it does in younger adults. However, elderly persons may not become as immune to head and upper chest influenza infections as younger adults, although the vaccine may still be effective in preventing lower chest influenza infections and other complications of influenza.

**Other medicines**—Although certain medicines should not be used together at all, in other cases two different medicines may be used together even if an interaction might occur. In these cases, your doctor may want to change the dose, or other precautions may be necessary. Tell your health care professional if you are using any other prescription or nonprescription (over-the-counter [OTC]) medicine.

**Other medical problems**—The presence of other medical problems may affect the use of influenza vaccine. Make sure you tell your doctor if you have any other medical problems, especially:

- Bronchitis, pneumonia, or other illness involving lungs or bronchial tubes—Use of influenza vaccine may make the condition worse
- Convulsions (seizures) caused by fever (history of)—Fever, a possible side effect of the vaccine, may cause the condition to occur again
- Guillain-Barré syndrome (GBS) (history of)—Use of influenza vaccine may reactivate the condition
- Severe illness with fever—The symptoms of the condition may be confused with the possible side effects of the vaccine

# Proper Use of This Vaccine

**Dosing**—The dose of influenza vaccine will be different for different patients. *Follow your doctor's orders.* The following information includes only the average dose of influenza vaccine.

- For *injection* dosage form:
  —To help prevent influenza infection:
    - Adults and children 6 months of age and older—One injection each year.

# Side Effects of This Vaccine

In 1976, a number of persons who received the "swine flu" influenza vaccine developed Guillain-Barré syndrome (GBS). Most of these persons were over 25 years of age. Although only 10 out of one million persons receiving the vaccine actually developed GBS, this number was 6 times more than would normally have been expected. Most of the persons who got GBS recovered completely from the paralysis it caused.

It is assumed that the "swine flu" virus included in the 1976 vaccine caused the problem, but this has not been proven. Since that time, the "swine flu" virus has not been used in influenza vaccines, and there has been no recurrence of GBS associated with influenza vaccinations.

Along with its needed effects, a vaccine may cause some unwanted effects. Although not all of these side effects may occur, if they do occur they may need medical attention.

**Get emergency help immediately** if any of the following side effects occur:

*Symptoms of allergic reaction*

Difficulty in breathing or swallowing; hives; itching, especially of feet or hands; reddening of skin, especially

around ears; swelling of eyes, face, or inside of nose; unusual tiredness or weakness (sudden and severe)

Other side effects may occur that usually do not need medical attention. These side effects generally do not last for more than 1 or 2 days. However, check with your doctor if any of the following side effects continue or are bothersome:

*More common*

Tenderness, redness, or hard lump at place of injection

*Less common*

Fever, general feeling of discomfort or illness, or aches or pains in muscles

Other side effects not listed above may also occur in some patients. If you notice any other effects, check with your doctor.

Revised: 07/12/94

# INSULIN   Systemic

Some commonly used brand names are:

**In the U.S.—**

| | |
|---|---|
| Humulin 50/50[7] | Novolin R[2] |
| Humulin 70/30[7] | NPH Iletin I[4] |
| Humulin L[9] | NPH Iletin II[4] |
| Humulin N[5] | NPH Insulin[4] |
| Humulin R[2] | NPH-N[4] |
| Humulin U Ultralente[11] | Regular (Concentrated) |
| Lente Iletin I[8] | Iletin II, U-500[1] |
| Lente Iletin II[8] | Regular Iletin I[1] |
| Lente Insulin[8] | Regular Iletin II[1] |
| Lente L[8] | Regular Insulin[1] |
| Novolin 70/30[7] | Ultralente U[10] |
| Novolin L[9] | Velosulin Human[2] |
| Novolin N[5] | |

**In Canada—**

| | |
|---|---|
| Humulin 10/90[7] | Novolin ge 30/70[7] |
| Humulin 20/80[7] | Novolin ge 40/60[7] |
| Humulin 30/70[7] | Novolin ge 50/50[7] |
| Humulin 40/60[7] | Novolin ge Lente[9] |
| Humulin 50/50[7] | Novolin ge NPH[5] |
| Humulin-L[9] | Novolin ge Toronto[2] |
| Humulin-N[5] | Novolin ge Ultralente[11] |
| Humulin-R[2] | NPH Iletin[4] |
| Humulin-U[11] | NPH Iletin II[4] |
| Insulin-Toronto[1] | NPH Insulin[4] |
| Lente Iletin[8] | Regular Iletin[1] |
| Lente Iletin II[8] | Regular Iletin II[1] |
| Lente Insulin[8] | Semilente Insulin[12] |
| Novolin ge 10/90[7] | Ultralente Insulin[10] |
| Novolin ge 20/80[7] | Velosulin Human[2] |

Other commonly used names are:

| | |
|---|---|
| lente insulin[8] | regular insulin[1] |
| NPH insulin[4] | semilente insulin[12] |
| PZI insulin [13] | ultralente insulin[10] |

Note: For quick reference, the following insulins are numbered to match the corresponding brand names.

This information applies to the following medicines:

1. Insulin (IN-su-lin)
2. Insulin Human
3. Buffered Insulin Human*†
4. Isophane (EYE-so-fayn) Insulin
5. Isophane Insulin, Human
6. Isophane Insulin and Insulin*†
7. Isophane Insulin, Human and Insulin Human
8. Insulin Zinc
9. Insulin Zinc, Human
10. Extended Insulin Zinc
11. Extended Insulin Zinc, Human
12. Prompt Insulin Zinc*
13. Protamine Zinc Insulin*†

*Not commercially available in the U.S.
†Not commercially available in Canada.

## Description

Insulin (IN-su-lin) is a hormone that helps the body turn the food we eat into energy. This occurs whether we make our own insulin in the pancreas gland or take it by injection.

Diabetes mellitus (sugar diabetes) is a condition where the body does not make enough insulin to meet its needs or does not properly use the insulin it makes.

Insulin can be obtained from beef or pork pancreas glands or from new processes that produce human insulin. All types of insulin must be injected because, if taken by mouth, insulin is destroyed by chemical reactions in the stomach.

One or more injections of insulin a day may be needed to control your diabetes. Insulin is usually injected before meals or at bedtime. Your doctor will discuss the number of injections you will need, the kind of insulin to use, the correct dose, and the right time to take it.

A prescription is not necessary to purchase most insulin. However, your doctor must first determine your insulin needs and provide you with special instructions for control of your diabetes. Insulin is available in the following dosage forms:

*Parenteral*

Insulin
- Injection (U.S. and Canada)

Insulin Human
- Injection (U.S. and Canada)

Buffered Insulin Human
- Injection

Isophane Insulin
- Injection (U.S. and Canada)

Isophane Insulin and Insulin
- Injection

Isophane Insulin, Human
- Injection (U.S. and Canada)

Isophane Insulin, Human, and Insulin Human
- Injection (U.S. and Canada)

Insulin Zinc
- Injection (U.S. and Canada)

Insulin Zinc, Human
- Injection (U.S. and Canada)

Extended Insulin Zinc
- Injection (U.S. and Canada)

Extended Insulin Zinc, Human
- Injection (U.S. and Canada)

Prompt Insulin Zinc
- Injection (Canada)

Protamine Zinc Insulin
- Injection

## Before Using This Medicine

In deciding to use a medicine, the risks of taking the medicine must be weighed against the good it will do. This is a decision you and your doctor will make. For insulin, the following should be considered:

**Allergies**—Tell your doctor if you have ever had any unusual or allergic reaction to insulin. Also tell your health care professional if you are allergic to any other substances, such as foods, preservatives, or dyes.

**Diet**—If you have insulin-dependent diabetes (type I), your doctor will prescribe both insulin and a personalized meal plan for you. Such a diet is low in fat and simple sugars such as table sugar, and sweet foods and beverages. This meal plan is also high in complex carbohydrates (starchy foods) such as cereals, grains, bread, pasta or noodles, starchy vegetables, and dried beans, peas, or lentils. The daily number of calories in this meal plan should be adjusted by your doctor or a registered dietitian to help you reach and maintain a healthy body weight. In addition, meals and snacks are arranged to meet the energy needs of your body at different times of the day. *It is very important that you carefully follow your meal plan.*

**Pregnancy**—Your requirements for insulin change during pregnancy. Because it is especially important for the health of both you and the baby that your blood sugar be closely controlled, be sure to tell your doctor if you suspect you are pregnant or if you are planning to become pregnant.

**Breast-feeding**—Insulin does not pass into breast milk and will not affect the nursing infant.

**Other medicines**—Although certain medicines should not be used together at all, in other cases two different medicines may be used together even if an interaction might occur. In these cases, your doctor may want to change the dose, or other precautions may be necessary. When using insulin, it is especially important that your health care professional know if you are taking any of the following:

- Beta-blockers—Beta-blockers may increase the risk of developing either high or low blood sugar levels. Also, they can mask symptoms of low blood sugar (such as rapid pulse). Because of this, a person with diabetes might not recognize low blood sugar and might not take immediate steps to treat it. Beta-blockers can also cause a low blood sugar level to last longer than it would have normally
- Corticosteroids (e.g., prednisone or other cortisone-like medicines)—Your dose of either medicine may need to be adjusted because the corticosteroids may interfere with insulin and thus increase your blood sugar

**Other medical problems**—The presence of other medical problems may affect the dose of insulin you need. Be sure to tell your doctor if you have any other medical problems, especially:

- Infections or
- Kidney disease or
- Liver disease or
- Thyroid disease—These conditions may change your daily insulin dose

## Proper Use of This Medicine

Make sure you have the type and strength of insulin that your doctor ordered for you. You may find that keeping an insulin label with you is helpful when buying insulin supplies. The concentration (strength) of insulin is measured by units, and is sometimes expressed in terms such as U-100 insulin.

Insulin doses are measured and given with specially marked insulin syringes. These syringes come in 3 sizes: 30 units, 50 units, and 100 units. Your insulin syringe will allow you to measure the units of insulin that have been prescribed for you, and allow you to easily read the measuring scale.

There are several important steps that will help you successfully prepare your insulin injection. To draw the insulin up into the syringe correctly, you need to follow these steps:

- Wash your hands.
- If your insulin is the intermediate- or long-acting kind (cloudy), be sure that it is completely mixed. Mix the insulin by slowly rolling the bottle between your hands or gently tipping the bottle over a few times.
- Never shake the bottle vigorously (hard).
- Do not use the insulin if it looks lumpy or grainy, seems unusually thick, sticks to the bottle, or seems to be even a little discolored. Do not use the insulin if it contains crystals or if the bottle looks frosted.

Regular insulin (short-acting) should be used only if it is clear and colorless.

- Remove the colored protective cap on the bottle. Do *not* remove the rubber stopper.
- Wipe the top of the bottle with an alcohol swab.
- Remove the needle cover of the insulin syringe.
- Draw air into the syringe by pulling back on the plunger. The amount of air should be equal to your insulin dose.
- Gently push the needle through the top of the rubber stopper.
- Push plunger in all the way, to inject air into the bottle.
- Turn the bottle with syringe upside down in one hand. Be sure the tip of the needle is covered by the insulin. With your other hand, draw the plunger back slowly to draw the correct dose of insulin into the syringe.
- Check the insulin in the syringe for air bubbles. To remove air bubbles, push the insulin slowly back into the bottle and draw up your dose again.
- Check your dose again.
- Remove the needle from the bottle and re-cover the needle.

If you are mixing more than 1 type of insulin in the same syringe, you also need to know about the following:

- When mixing regular insulin with another type of insulin, *always* draw the regular insulin into the syringe first. When mixing 2 types of insulins other than regular insulin, it does not matter in what order you draw them.
- After you decide on a certain order for drawing up your insulin, you should use the same order each time.
- Some mixtures of insulins have to be injected immediately. Others may be stable for longer periods of time, which means that you can wait before you inject the mixture. Check with your health care professional to find out which type you have.
- If your mixture is stable and you mixed it ahead of time, gently turn the filled syringe back and forth to remix the insulins before you inject them. Do not shake the syringe.

After you have your syringe prepared, you are ready to inject the insulin into your body. To do this:

- Clean the site where the injection is to be made with an alcohol swab, and let the area dry.
- Inject the insulin into fatty tissue. Injection sites include your thighs, abdomen (stomach area), upper arms, or buttocks. Generally, insulin is absorbed into the bloodstream most evenly from the abdomen. If you are either thin or greatly overweight, you may be given special instructions for giving yourself insulin injections.
- Pinch up a large area of skin and hold it firmly. With your other hand, hold the syringe like a pencil. Push the needle straight into the pinched-up skin at a 90-degree angle. Be sure the needle is all the way

in. Drawing back on the syringe each time to check for blood (also called routine aspiration) is not necessary.

- Push the plunger all the way down, using less than 5 seconds to inject the dose. Hold an alcohol swab near the needle and pull the needle straight out of the skin.
- Press the swab against the injection site for several seconds. Do not rub.

For patients using *disposable syringes:*

- Manufacturers of disposable syringes recommend that they be used only once, because the sterility of a reused syringe cannot be guaranteed. However, some patients prefer to reuse a syringe until its needle becomes dull. Most insulins have chemicals added that keep them from growing the bacteria that are usually found on the skin. Because of this, some patients may decide to reuse a disposable syringe. However, the syringe should be thrown away when the needle becomes dull, has been bent, or has come into contact with any surface other than the cleaned and swabbed area of skin. Also, if you plan to reuse a syringe, the needle must be recapped after each use. Check with your health care professional to find out the best way to reuse syringes.
- Laws in some states require that used insulin syringes and needles be destroyed. Be careful when you recap, bend, or break a needle, because these actions increase the chances of a needle-stick injury. It is best to put used syringes and needles in a disposable container that is puncture-resistant or to use a needle-clipping device. The chances of a syringe being reused by someone else is lower if the plunger is taken out of the barrel and broken in half when you dispose of a syringe.

For patients using *a glass syringe and metal needle:*

- This type of syringe and needle may be used repeatedly if it is sterilized each time. You should get an instruction sheet that tells you how to do this. If you need more information on this, ask your health care professional.

For patients using *an insulin-infusion pump:*

- Regular insulin is the only insulin product that should be used with insulin infusion pumps.
- Do not use the insulin injection if it looks lumpy, cloudy, unusually thick, or even slightly discolored, or if it contains crystals. Use the insulin only if it is clear and colorless.
- Do not mix the buffered regular insulin injection with any other insulin. If you do, crystals may form that will block the pump catheter. Also, the potency of the insulin may change.
- It is important to follow the pump manufacturer's directions on how to load the syringe and/or pump reservoir. Your correct insulin dose may not be given if loading is not done correctly.

- Check the infusion tubing and infusion-site dressing often for improper insulin infusion, as your health care professional recommends.

**Dosing**—The dose of these medicines will be different for different patients. *Follow your doctor's orders or the directions on the label.* The following information applies to the average doses of these medicines. *If your dose is different, do not change it* unless your doctor tells you to do so.

The number of injections that you receive depends on the strength or type of the medicine. Also, *the number of doses you receive each day, the time allowed between doses, and the length of time you receive the medicine depend on the amount of sugar in your blood or urine.*

*For regular insulin (R)—crystalline zinc, human buffered, and human regular insulins*

- For *injection* dosage form:
  —For treating sugar diabetes (diabetes mellitus):
  - Adults and teenagers—The dose is based on your blood sugar and must be determined by your doctor. The medicine is injected under the skin fifteen or thirty minutes before meals up to four times a day.
  - Children—Dose is based on your blood sugar and body size, and must be determined by your doctor.
  —For treating uncontrolled diabetes (diabetic ketoacidosis):
  - Adults—The dose is based on your blood sugar and body weight, and must be determined by your doctor. The usual dose is 0.1 USP Units per kilogram (kg) (0.05 USP Units per pound) of body weight injected slowly into a vein each hour.
  - Children—The dose is based on your blood sugar and body size, and must be determined by your doctor.

*For isophane insulin (NPH)—isophane and human isophane insulins*

- For *injection* dosage form:
  —For treating sugar diabetes (diabetes mellitus):
  - Adults and teenagers—The dose is based on your blood sugar and must be determined by your doctor. The medicine is injected under the skin thirty to sixty minutes before breakfast. You may need a dose before another meal or at bedtime.
  - Children—Dose is based on your blood sugar and body size, and must be determined by your doctor.

*For isophane insulin/insulin (NPH/R)—human isophane/regular insulin*

- For *injection* dosage form:
  —For treating sugar diabetes (diabetes mellitus):
  - Adults and teenagers—The dose is based on your blood sugar and must be determined by

your doctor. The medicine is injected under the skin fifteen to thirty minutes before breakfast.
  - Children—Dose is based on your blood sugar and body size, and must be determined by your doctor.

*For insulin zinc (L)—lente and human lente insulins*

- For *injection* dosage form:
  —For treating sugar diabetes (diabetes mellitus):
  - Adults and teenagers—The dose is based on your blood sugar and must be determined by your doctor. The medicine is injected under the skin thirty to sixty minutes before breakfast. You may need a dose before another meal or at bedtime.
  - Children—Dose is based on your blood sugar and body size, and must be determined by your doctor.

*For insulin zinc extended (U)—ultralente and human ultralente insulins*

- For *injection* dosage form:
  —For treating sugar diabetes (diabetes mellitus):
  - Adults and teenagers—The dose is based on your blood sugar and must be determined by your doctor. The medicine is injected under the skin thirty to sixty minutes before breakfast.
  - Children—Dose is based on your blood sugar and body size, and must be determined by your doctor.

*For prompt insulin zinc (S)—semilente and human semilente insulins*

- For *injection* dosage form:
  —For treating sugar diabetes (diabetes mellitus):
  - Adults and teenagers—The dose is based on your blood sugar and must be determined by your doctor. The medicine is injected under the skin thirty to sixty minutes before breakfast. You may need a dose thirty minutes before another meal or at bedtime.
  - Children—Dose is based on your blood sugar and body size, and must be determined by your doctor.

*For protamine zinc insulin (PZI)—protamine zinc insulin*

- For *injection* dosage form:
  —For treating sugar diabetes (diabetes mellitus):
  - Adults and teenagers—The dose is based on your blood sugar and must be determined by your doctor. The medicine is injected under the skin thirty to sixty minutes before breakfast.
  - Children—Dose is based on your blood sugar and body size, and must be determined by your doctor.

**Storage**—Storage and expiration date:

- When buying insulin, always check the package expiration date to make sure the insulin will be used before it expires.

- This expiration date applies *only* when the insulin has been stored in the refrigerator. Expiration is much shorter if the insulin is left unrefrigerated. Do not use insulin after the expiration date stated on the label even if the bottle has never been opened. Check with your pharmacist about a possible exchange of bottles.

- An unopened bottle of insulin should be refrigerated until needed. It should never be frozen. Remove the insulin from the refrigerator and allow it to reach room temperature before injecting.

- An insulin bottle in use may be kept at room temperature for up to 1 month. Insulin that has been kept at room temperature for longer than a month should be thrown away.

- Do not expose insulin to extremely hot temperatures or to sunlight. Do not leave insulin in the hot summer sun or in a hot closed car. Extreme heat will cause insulin to become less effective much more quickly.

## Precautions While Using This Medicine

*It is very important that your doctor check your progress at regular visits,* especially during the first few weeks of insulin treatment.

*It is very important to follow carefully any instructions from your health care team about:*

- Alcohol—Drinking alcohol may cause severe low blood sugar. Discuss this with your health care team.

- Tobacco—If you have been smoking for a long time and suddenly stop, your dosage of insulin may need to be reduced. If you decide to quit, tell your doctor first.

- Meal plan—To be successful in your treatment, you must closely follow the diet your doctor or dietitian prescribed for you. Do not miss or delay your meals.

- Exercise—Ask your doctor what kind of exercise to do, the best time to do it, and how much you should do daily.

- Blood tests—This is the best way to tell whether your diabetes is being controlled properly. Blood sugar testing is a useful guide to help you and your health care team adjust your insulin dose, meal plan, and exercise schedule.

- Urine ketone tests—You will also be asked at certain times to test for acetone, which is an acid that may be released from your bloodstream into your urine when your blood glucose is too high.

- Injection sites—If you carefully select and rotate the sites where you give your insulin injections, you may be able to prevent skin problems. Also, the insulin may be better absorbed into the bloodstream.

- Other medicines—Do not take other medicines unless they have been discussed with your doctor. This especially includes nonprescription medicines such as aspirin, and those for appetite control, asthma, colds, cough, hay fever, or sinus problems.

*Insulin can cause low blood sugar (also called insulin reaction or hypoglycemia). Symptoms of low blood sugar are:*

Anxious feeling
Cold sweats
Confusion
Cool pale skin
Difficulty in concentration
Drowsiness
Excessive hunger
Headache
Nausea
Nervousness
Rapid pulse
Shakiness
Unusual tiredness or weakness
Vision changes

- Different people may feel different symptoms of low blood sugar (hypoglycemia). It is important that you learn the symptoms of low blood sugar that you usually have so that you can treat it quickly.

- The symptoms of hypoglycemia (low blood sugar) may develop quickly and may result from:
  —delaying or missing a scheduled meal or snack.
  —exercising more than usual.
  —drinking a significant amount of alcohol.
  —taking certain medicines.
  —using too much insulin.
  —sickness (especially with vomiting or diarrhea).

- Eating some form of quick-acting sugar when symptoms of hypoglycemia first appear will usually prevent them from getting worse. Good sources of sugar include:
  Glucose tablets or gel that you can buy
  A restaurant sugar packet
  Fruit juice (4 to 6 ounces or one-half cup)
  Corn syrup (1 tablespoon)
  Honey (1 tablespoon)
  Regular (non-diet) soft drinks (4 to 6 ounces or one-half cup)
  Sugar cubes (6 one-half-inch sized) or table sugar (dissolved in water)

- Do not use chocolate because its fat slows down the sugar entering into the bloodstream.

- If a snack is not scheduled for an hour or more you should also eat some crackers and cheese, or a half a sandwich, or ice cream, or a peanut butter cookie, or drink an 8 ounce glass of milk.

- Symptoms of low blood sugar must be treated before they lead to unconsciousness (passing out). Glucagon is also used in emergency situations such as unconsciousness. Have a glucagon kit available, along with a syringe and needle, and know how to prepare and use it. Members of your household should know how and when to use it, also. Check the expiration date of the glucagon and remind yourself when to buy a new kit. If your kit has expired, ask your pharmacist to exchange it for a new one.

*Hyperglycemia (high blood sugar) is another problem related to uncontrolled diabetes.* If you have any symptoms of high blood sugar, you need to contact your health care team right away. If it is not treated, severe hyperglycemia can lead to ketoacidosis (diabetic coma) and death. The symptoms of hyperglycemia appear more slowly than those of low blood sugar and usually include:

Increased urination
Unusual thirst
Dry mouth
Drowsiness
Flushed, dry skin
Fruit-like breath odor
Loss of appetite
Stomach ache, nausea, or vomiting
Tiredness
Troubled breathing (rapid and deep)
Increased blood sugar level

- Symptoms of ketoacidosis (diabetic coma) that need immediate hospitalization include:

  Flushed, dry skin
  Fruit-like breath odor
  Stomach ache, nausea, or vomiting
  Troubled breathing (rapid and deep)

- Hyperglycemia (high blood sugar) symptoms may occur if you:
  —have a fever, diarrhea, or infection.
  —do not take enough insulin.
  —skip a dose of insulin.
  —do not exercise as much as usual.
  —overeat or do not follow your meal plan.

- Your doctor may recommend changes in your insulin dose or meal plan to avoid hyperglycemia. Symptoms of high blood sugar must be corrected before they progress to more serious conditions. Check with your doctor often to make sure you are controlling your blood sugar.

*In case of emergency*—There may be a time when you need emergency help for a problem caused by your diabetes. You need to be prepared for these emergencies. It is a good idea to:

- Wear a medical identification (I.D.) bracelet or neck chain at all times. Also, carry an I.D. card in your wallet or purse that says that you have diabetes and lists all of your medicines.
- Keep an extra supply of insulin and syringes with needles on hand.
- Have a glucagon kit and a syringe and needle available and know how to prepare and use it if severe hypoglycemia (low blood sugar) occurs.
- Keep some kind of quick-acting sugar handy to treat hypoglycemia (low blood sugar) symptoms.

*In case of illness:*

- When you become ill with a cold, fever, or the flu, you need to take your usual insulin dose, even if you feel too sick to eat. This is especially true if you have

nausea, vomiting, or diarrhea. Infection usually increases your need for insulin. Call your doctor for specific instructions.

- Continue taking your insulin and try to stay on your regular meal plan. However, if you have trouble eating solid food, drink fruit juices, non-diet soft drinks, or clear soups, or eat small amounts of bland foods. A dietitian or your doctor can give you a list of foods and the amounts to use for sick days.
- Test your blood sugar level at least every 4 hours while you are awake and check your urine for acetone. If acetone is present, call your doctor at once. If you have severe or prolonged vomiting, check with your doctor. Even when you start feeling better, let your doctor know how you are doing.

*Travel*—If you take a few special precautions when you travel, you are less likely to have problems related to your diabetes during trips away from home. It is a good idea to:

- Carry a recent prescription from your doctor for your diabetes medicine and also for the type of syringe and needles you use.
- Do not make major changes in your meal plan or medicine schedule without advice from your health care team.
- Carry your diabetic supplies on your person or in a purse or briefcase to reduce the possibility of loss.
- Carry snack foods with you in case of delays between meals.
- Make allowances for changing time zones and keep your meal times as close to usual as possible.
- In hot climates, use an insulated container for your insulin.
- When traveling to foreign countries, it is advisable to pack enough diabetic supplies to last until you return home and to have extra or reserve supplies kept separate from your main supplies.
- Carry a letter from your doctor with all the details of your diabetes and medicines you need, including your need for syringes.
- When carrying a large quantity of diabetic supplies, divide them throughout your hand-carried luggage to avoid problems if something is lost, and to avoid possible freezing in airplane storage areas.

Revised: September 1990
Interim revision: 06/28/93; 07/12/94

# INTERFERON, GAMMA    Systemic†

A commonly used brand name in the U.S. is Actimmune.

†Not commercially available in Canada.

## Description

Gamma interferon (in-ter-FEER-on) is a synthetic (man-made) version of a substance naturally produced by cells in the body to help fight infections and tumors. Gamma interferon is used to treat chronic granulomatous disease.

Gamma interferon is available only with your doctor's prescription, in the following dosage form:

*Parenteral*
- Injection (U.S.)

## Before Using This Medicine

In deciding to use a medicine, the risks of taking the medicine must be weighed against the good it will do. This is a decision you and your doctor will make. For gamma interferon, the following should be considered:

**Allergies**—Tell your doctor if you have ever had any unusual or allergic reaction to gamma interferon.

**Pregnancy**—Gamma interferon has not been studied in pregnant women. However, in monkeys given 100 times the human dose of gamma interferon and in mice, there was an increase in deaths of the fetus. Also, in mice, toxic doses of gamma interferon caused bleeding of the uterus.

**Breast-feeding**—It is not known whether gamma interferon passes into the breast milk. However, because this medicine may cause serious side effects, breast-feeding may not be recommended while you are receiving it. Discuss with your doctor whether or not you should breast-feed while you are receiving gamma interferon.

**Children**—Studies on this medicine have been done mostly in children and it is not expected to cause different side effects or problems than it does in adults.

**Older adults**—Many medicines have not been studied specifically in older people. Therefore, it may not be known whether they work exactly the same way they do in younger adults or if they cause different side effects or problems in older people. There is no specific information comparing use of gamma interferon in the elderly with use in other age groups.

**Other medicines**—Although certain medicines should not be used together at all, in other cases two different medicines may be used together even if an interaction might occur. In these cases, your doctor may want to change the dose, or other precautions may be necessary. Tell your health care professional if you are taking any other prescription or nonprescription (over-the-counter [OTC]) medicine.

**Other medical problems**—The presence of other medical problems may affect the use of gamma interferon. Make sure you tell your doctor if you have any other medical problems, especially:
- Convulsions (seizures) or
- Mental problems (or history of)—Risk of problems affecting the central nervous system may be increased
- Heart disease or
- Multiple sclerosis or
- Systemic lupus erythematosus—May be worsened by gamma interferon

## Proper Use of This Medicine

If you are injecting this medicine yourself, *use it exactly as directed by your doctor.* Do not use more or less of it, and do not use it more often than your doctor ordered. The exact amount of medicine you need has been carefully worked out. Using too much will increase the risk of side effects, while using too little may not improve your condition.

*Each package of gamma interferon contains a patient instruction sheet. Read this sheet carefully* and make sure you understand:
- How to prepare the injection.
- Proper use of disposable syringes.
- How to give the injection.
- How long the injection is stable.

If you have any questions about any of this, check with your health care professional.

While you are using gamma interferon, your doctor may want you to drink extra fluids. This will help prevent low blood pressure due to loss of too much water.

Gamma interferon often causes flu-like symptoms, which can be severe. This effect is less likely to cause problems if you inject your gamma interferon at bedtime.

**Dosing**—The dose of gamma interferon will be different for different patients. The dose that is used may depend on a number of things, including the patient's body size. *If you are receiving gamma interferon at home, follow your doctor's orders or the directions on the label.* If you have any questions about the proper dose of gamma interferon, ask your doctor.

**Missed dose**—If you miss a dose of this medicine, do not give the missed dose at all and do not double the next one. Check with your doctor for further instructions.

**Storage**—To store this medicine:
- Keep out of the reach of children.
- Store in the refrigerator.
- Keep the medicine from freezing.
- Do not keep outdated medicine or medicine no longer needed. Ask your health care professional how you should dispose of any medicine you do not use. Be sure that any discarded medicine is out of the reach of children.

## Precautions While Using This Medicine

*It is very important that your doctor check your progress at regular visits* to make sure that this medicine is working properly and to check for unwanted effects.

This medicine commonly causes a flu-like reaction, with aching muscles, fever and chills, and headache. To prevent problems from your temperature going too high, your doctor may ask you to take acetaminophen before each dose of gamma interferon. You may also need to take it after a dose to bring your temperature down. *Follow your doctor's instructions carefully about taking your temperature, and how much and when to take the acetaminophen.*

## Side Effects of This Medicine

Along with its needed effects, a medicine may cause some unwanted effects. Although not all of these side effects may occur, if they do occur they may need medical attention.

Check with your doctor as soon as possible if any of the following side effects occur:

*Rare*

Black, tarry stools; blood in urine or stools; confusion; cough or hoarseness; loss of balance control; lower back or side pain; mask-like face; painful or difficult urination; pinpoint red spots on skin; shuffling walk; stiffness of arms or legs; trembling and shaking of hands and fingers; trouble in speaking or swallowing; trouble in thinking or concentrating; trouble in walking; unusual bleeding or bruising

Other side effects may occur that usually do not need medical attention. These side effects may go away during treatment as your body adjusts to the medicine. However, check with your doctor if any of the following side effects continue or are bothersome:

*More common*

Aching muscles; diarrhea; fever and chills; general feeling of discomfort or illness; headache; nausea or vomiting; skin rash; unusual tiredness

*Less common*

Back pain; dizziness; joint pain; loss of appetite; weight loss

Other side effects not listed above may also occur in some patients. If you notice any other effects, check with your doctor.

Revised: 06/04/92
Interim revision: 07/05/94

# INTERFERONS, ALPHA  Systemic

Some commonly used brand names are:

**In the U.S.—**
Alferon N[4]
Roferon-A[1]
Intron A[2]

**In Canada—**
Roferon-A
Intron A[2]
Wellferon[3]

Note: For quick reference, the following alpha interferons are numbered to match the corresponding brand names.

This information applies to the following medicines:
1. Interferon Alfa-2a, Recombinant
2. Interferon Alfa-2b, Recombinant
3. Interferon Alfa-n1 (lns)*
4. Interferon Alfa-n3†

*Not commercially available in the U.S.
†Not commercially available in Canada.

## Description

Interferons (in-ter-FEER-ons) are substances naturally produced by cells in the body to help fight infections and tumors. They may also be synthetic (man-made) versions of these substances. Alpha interferons are used to treat hairy cell leukemia and AIDS-related Kaposi's sarcoma. They are also used to treat laryngeal papillomatosis (growths in the respiratory tract) in children, genital warts, and some kinds of hepatitis.

Alpha interferons may also be used for other conditions as determined by your doctor.

Alpha interferons are available only with your doctor's prescription, in the following dosage form:

*Parenteral*

Interferon Alfa-2a, Recombinant
• Injection (U.S. and Canada)
Interferon Alfa-2b, Recombinant
• Injection (U.S. and Canada)
Interferon Alfa-n1 (lns)
• Injection (Canada)
Interferon Alfa-n3
• Injection (U.S.)

## Before Using This Medicine

In deciding to use a medicine, the risks of taking the medicine must be weighed against the good it will do. This is a decision you and your doctor will make. For interferons, the following should be considered:

**Allergies**—Tell your doctor if you have ever had any unusual or allergic reaction to alpha interferon.

**Pregnancy**—Alpha interferons have not been shown to cause birth defects or other problems in humans. However, in monkeys given 20 to 500 times the human dose of recombinant interferon alfa-2a or 90 to 180 times the usual dose of recombinant interferon alfa-2b there was an increase in deaths of the fetus.

**Breast-feeding**—It is not known whether alpha interferons pass into the breast milk. However, because this medicine may cause serious side effects, breast-feeding may not be recommended while you are receiving it. Discuss with your doctor whether or not you should breast-feed while you are are receiving alpha interferon.

**Children**—There is no specific information comparing use of alpha interferon for cancer or genital warts in children with use in other age groups.

**Teenagers**—Alpha interferons may cause changes in the menstrual cycle. Discuss this possible effect with your doctor.

**Older adults**—Some side effects of alpha interferons (chest pain, irregular heartbeat, unusual tiredness, confusion, mental depression, trouble in thinking or concentrating) may be more likely to occur in the elderly, who are usually more sensitive to the effects of alpha interferons.

**Other medicines**—Although certain medicines should not be used together at all, in other cases two different medicines may be used together even if an interaction might occur. In these cases, your doctor may want to change the dose, or other precautions may be necessary. Tell your health care professional if you are taking any other prescription or nonprescription (over-the-counter [OTC]) medicine.

**Other medical problems**—The presence of other medical problems may affect the use of alpha interferons. Make sure you tell your doctor if you have any other medical problems, especially:

- Bleeding problems—May be worsened by recombinant interferon alfa-2b
- Chickenpox (including recent exposure) or
- Herpes zoster (shingles)—Risk of severe disease affecting other parts of the body
- Convulsions (seizures) or
- Mental problems (or history of)—Risk of problems affecting the central nervous system may be increased
- Diabetes mellitus (sugar diabetes) or
- Heart attack (recent) or
- Heart disease or
- Kidney disease or
- Liver disease or
- Lung disease—May be worsened by alpha interferons
- Problems with overactive immune system—Alpha interferons make the immune system even more active
- Thyroid disease—Recombinant interferon alfa-2b can cause thyroid problems when it is used to treat hepatitis

## Proper Use of This Medicine

If you are injecting this medicine yourself, *use it exactly as directed by your doctor.* Do not use more or less of it, and do not use it more often than your doctor ordered. The exact amount of medicine you need has been carefully worked out. Using too much will increase the risk of side effects, while using too little may not improve your condition.

*Each package of alpha interferon contains a patient instruction sheet. Read this sheet carefully* and make sure you understand:

- How to prepare the injection.
- Proper use of disposable syringes.
- How to give the injection.
- How long the injection is stable.

If you have any questions about any of this, check with your health care professional.

While you are using alpha interferon, your doctor may want you to drink extra fluids. This will help prevent low blood pressure due to loss of too much water.

Alpha interferons often cause unusual tiredness, which can be severe. This effect is less likely to cause problems if you inject your interferon at bedtime.

**Dosing**—The dose of alpha interferons will be different for different patients. The dose that is used may depend on a number of things, including what the medicine is being used for, the patient's size, and whether or not other medicines are also being taken. *If you are receiving alpha interferons at home, follow your doctor's orders or the directions on the label.* If you have any questions about the proper dose of alpha interferons, ask your doctor.

**Missed dose**—If you miss a dose of this medicine, do not give the missed dose at all and do not double the next one. Check with your doctor for further instructions.

**Storage**—To store this medicine:

- Keep out of the reach of children.
- Store in the refrigerator.
- Keep the medicine from freezing.
- Do not keep outdated medicine or medicine no longer needed. Ask your health care professional how you should dispose of any medicine you do not use. Be sure that any discarded medicine is out of the reach of children.

## Precautions While Using This Medicine

*It is very important that your doctor check your progress at regular visits* to make sure that this medicine is working properly and to check for unwanted effects.

*Do not change to another brand of alpha interferon without checking with your physician.* Different kinds of alpha interferon have different doses. If you refill your medicine and it looks different, check with your pharmacist.

This medicine will add to the effects of alcohol and other CNS depressants (medicines that slow down the nervous system, possibly causing drowsiness). Some examples of CNS depressants are antihistamines or medicine for hay fever, other allergies, or colds; sedatives, tranquilizers, or sleeping medicine; prescription pain medicine or narcotics; barbiturates; medicine for seizures; muscle relaxants; or anesthetics, including some dental anesthetics. *Check with your doctor before taking any of the above while you are using this medicine.*

Alpha interferon may cause some people to become unusually tired or dizzy, or less alert than they are normally. *Make sure you know how you react to this medicine before you drive, use machines, or do anything else that could be dangerous if you are dizzy or if you are not alert.*

This medicine commonly causes a flu-like reaction, with aching muscles, fever and chills, and headache. To prevent problems from your temperature going too high, your doctor may ask you to take acetaminophen before each dose of interferon. You may also need to take it after a dose to bring your temperature down. *Follow your doctor's instructions carefully about taking your temperature, and how much and when to take the acetaminophen.*

Alpha interferon can lower the number of white blood cells in your blood temporarily, increasing the chance of getting an infection. It can also lower the number of platelets, which are necessary for proper blood clotting. If this occurs, there are certain precautions you can take, especially when your blood count is low, to reduce the risk of infection or bleeding:

- If you can, avoid people with infections. *Check with your doctor immediately* if you think you are getting an infection or if you get a fever or chills, cough or hoarseness, lower back or side pain, or painful or difficult urination.

- *Check with your doctor immediately* if you notice any unusual bleeding or bruising; black, tarry stools; blood in urine or stools; or pinpoint red spots on your skin.

- Be careful when using a regular toothbrush, dental floss, or toothpick. Your medical doctor, dentist, or nurse may recommend other ways to clean your teeth and gums. Check with your medical doctor before having any dental work done.

- Do not touch your eyes or the inside of your nose unless you have just washed your hands and have not touched anything else in the meantime.

- Be careful not to cut yourself when you are using sharp objects such as a safety razor or fingernail or toenail cutters.

- Avoid contact sports or other situations where bruising or injury could occur.

## Side Effects of This Medicine

Along with its needed effects, a medicine may cause some unwanted effects. Although not all of these side effects may occur, if they do occur they may need medical attention.

Because this medicine is used for many different conditions and in many different doses, the actual frequency of side effects may vary. In general, side effects are less common with low doses than with high doses. Also, when alpha interferon is used for genital warts, very little of it gets into the rest of the body, so side effects are generally less common than in other conditions.

Check with your doctor as soon as possible if any of the following side effects occur:

*Less common*

Confusion; mental depression; nervousness; numbness or tingling of fingers, toes, and face; trouble in sleeping; trouble in thinking or concentrating

*Rare*

Black, tarry stools; blood in urine or stools; chest pain; cough or hoarseness; fever or chills (beginning after 3 weeks of treatment); irregular heartbeat; lower back or side pain; painful or difficult urination; pinpoint red spots on skin; unusual bleeding or bruising

Other side effects may occur that usually do not need medical attention. These side effects may go away during treatment as your body adjusts to the medicine. However, check with your doctor if any of the following side effects continue or are bothersome:

*More common*

Aching muscles; change in taste or metallic taste; fever and chills (should lessen after the first 1 or 2 weeks of treatment); general feeling of discomfort or illness; headache; loss of appetite; nausea and vomiting; skin rash; unusual tiredness

*Less common or rare*

Back pain; blurred vision; diarrhea; dizziness; dryness of mouth; dry skin or itching; increased sweating; joint pain; leg cramps; sores in mouth and on lips; weight loss

Alpha interferon may cause a temporary loss of some hair. After treatment has ended, normal hair growth should return.

Other side effects not listed above may also occur in some patients. If you notice any other effects, check with your doctor.

## Additional Information

Once a medicine has been approved for marketing for a certain use, experience may show that it is also useful for other medical problems. Although these uses are not included in product labeling, alpha interferons are used in certain patients with the following medical conditions:

- Bladder cancer
- Cervical cancer

- Chronic myelocytic leukemia
- Kidney cancer
- Laryngeal papillomatosis (growths on larynx)
- Lymphomas, non-Hodgkin's
- Malignant melanoma
- Multiple myeloma
- Mycosis fungoides

Other than the above information, there is no additional information relating to proper use, precautions, or side effects for these uses.

Revised: 01/16/92
Interim revision(s): 04/17/93; 07/05/94

# INULIN    Diagnostic†

Generic name product available in the U.S.

†Not commercially available in Canada.

## Description

Inulin (IN-yoo-lin) is used as a test to help diagnose problems or disease of the kidneys. This test determines how well your kidneys are working.

Inulin passes out of the body entirely in the urine. Measuring the amount of inulin in the blood after it has been given can help the doctor determine if the kidneys are working properly.

How test is done: Inulin is given through an intravenous infusion (run into a vein). The dose of inulin will be different for different patients. The doctor will determine your dose according to your weight and size. Several times during the test, blood and sometimes urine samples are taken. A tube called a catheter may be placed in your bladder to help take the urine samples. The amount of inulin in your blood or urine is measured. Then the results of the test are studied.

Inulin is to be used only under the supervision of a doctor. It is available in the following dosage form:

*Parenteral*
- Injection (U.S.)

## Before Having This Test

In deciding to use a diagnostic test, the risks of the test must be weighed against the good it will do. This is a decision you and your doctor will make. Also, test results may be affected by other things. For inulin, the following should be considered:

**Allergies**—Tell your doctor if you have ever had any unusual or allergic reaction to inulin. Also tell your doctor if you are allergic to any other substances, such as foods, preservatives, or dyes.

**Pregnancy**—Inulin has not been shown to cause birth defects or other problems in humans.

**Breast-feeding**—Inulin has not been reported to cause problems in nursing babies.

**Children**—This medicine has been used in children. In effective doses, inulin has not been shown to cause different side effects or problems than it does in adults.

**Older adults**—Many medicines have not been studied specifically in older people. Therefore, it may not be known whether they work exactly the same way they do in younger adults. Although there is no specific information comparing the use of inulin in the elderly with use in other age groups, this medicine is not expected to cause different side effects or problems in older people than it does in younger adults.

**Other medical problems**—The presence of other medical problems may affect the use of inulin. Make sure you tell your doctor if you have any other medical problems, especially:

- Heart disease or
- Liver disease or
- Underactive adrenal gland or
- Underactive thyroid—These conditions may affect the inulin test results by reducing the amount of inulin that is cleared from the blood

## Preparation for This Test

Your doctor may ask you to drink a certain amount of water before and during the test. *Follow your doctor's instructions carefully.* Otherwise, this test may not work and may have to be done again.

## Side Effects of This Medicine

Along with its needed effects, a medicine may cause some unwanted effects. Although inulin does not usually cause any side effects, check with your doctor if you notice any unusual effects.

Revised: 06/23/94

# IOBENGUANE, RADIOIODINATED    Therapeutic*†

A commonly used name for iobenguane is meta-iodobenzylguanidine or mIBG.

*Not commercially available in the U.S.
†Not commercially available in Canada.

## Description

Radioiodinated iobenguane is a radiopharmaceutical (ray-dee-oh-far-ma-SOO-ti-kal). Radiopharmaceuticals are radioactive agents, which may be used to find and treat certain diseases or to study the function of the body's organs.

Radioiodinated iobenguane is used to treat certain kinds of cancer of the adrenal glands.

When very small doses of radioiodinated iobenguane are given, the radioactivity taken up by the adrenal gland helps find tumors of the adrenal glands. An image of the gland on film or on a computer screen can be provided to help with the diagnosis.

*The information that follows applies only to the use of radioiodinated iobenguane in treating cancer of the adrenal gland.*

Radioiodinated iobenguane is to be given only by or under the direct supervision of a doctor with specialized training in nuclear medicine. Radioiodinated iobenguane is available in the following dosage form:

*Parenteral*
- Injection

## Before Using This Medicine

In deciding to use a medicine, the risks of taking the medicine must be weighed against the good it will do. This is a decision you and your doctor will make. For radioiodinated iobenguane, the following should be considered:

**Pregnancy**—This radiopharmaceutical is not recommended for use during pregnancy. This is to avoid exposing the fetus to harmful levels of radiation.

**Breast-feeding**—Some radiopharmaceuticals pass into the breast milk and may expose the baby to radiation. If you must receive radioiodinated iobenguane, it may be necessary for you to stop breast-feeding after receiving it. Be sure you have discussed this with your doctor.

**Children and adolescents**—Children and adolescents are especially sensitive to the effects of radiation. This may increase the chance of side effects during and after treatment. Be sure you have discussed this with your doctor.

**Older adults**—Radioiodinated iobenguane has been used in older people and has not been shown to cause different side effects or problems in older people than it does in younger adults.

**Other medicines**—Although certain medicines should not be used together at all, in other cases two different medicines may be used together even if an interaction might occur. In these cases, your doctor may want to change the dose, or other precautions may be necessary. When you are receiving radioiodinated iobenguane, it is especially important that your doctor knows if you are taking any of the following:

- Amphetamines or
- Appetite suppressants (diet pills) or
- Calcium channel blocking agents (diltiazem [e.g., Cardizem], nicardipine [e.g., Cardene], nifedipine [e.g., Procardia], verapamil [e.g., Calan]) or
- Cocaine or
- Guanethidine (e.g., Ismelin) or
- Haloperidol (e.g., Haldol) or
- Labetalol (e.g., Normodyne) or
- Loxapine (e.g., Loxitane) or
- Medicines for colds, sinus problems, or hay fever or other allergies (including nose drops or sprays) or
- Phenothiazines (acetophenazine [e.g., Tindal], chlorpromazine [e.g., Thorazine], fluphenazine [e.g., Prolixin], mesoridazine [e.g., Serentil], perphenazine [e.g., Trilafon], prochlorperazine [e.g., Compazine], promazine [e.g., Sparine], promethazine [e.g., Phenergan], thioridazine [e.g., Mellaril], trifluoperazine [e.g., Stelazine], triflupromazine [e.g., Vesprin], trimeprazine [e.g., Temaril]) or
- Reserpine (e.g., Serpasil) or
- Thiothixene (e.g., Navane) or
- Tricyclic antidepressants (amitriptyline [e.g., Elavil], amoxapine [e.g., Asendin], clomipramine [e.g., Anafranil], desipramine [e.g., Pertofrane], doxepin [e.g., Sinequan], imipramine [e.g., Tofranil], nortriptyline [e.g., Aventyl], protriptyline [e.g., Vivactil], trimipramine [e.g., Surmontil])—These medicines may keep the affected organ or tissue from getting the amount of radioiodinated iobenguane it needs to fight the disease

**Other medical problems**—The presence of other medical problems may affect the use of radioiodinated iobenguane. Make sure you tell your doctor if you have any other medical problems.

## Preparation for This Treatment

Your doctor may have special instructions for you in preparation for your treatment. If you have not received such instructions or you do not understand them, check with your doctor in advance.

This radiopharmaceutical contains radioactive iodine, which may be taken up in your thyroid. To protect your thyroid, your doctor will prescribe a medicine (e.g., potassium iodide or SSKI) that contains non-radioactive iodine. You must take this medicine before starting treatment with radioiodinated iobenguane and continue taking it after treatment for as long as your doctor tells you.

## Side Effects of This Medicine

Along with its needed effects, a medicine may cause some unwanted effects. Although not all of these side effects

may occur, if they do occur they may need medical attention.

*Check with your doctor as soon as possible* if any of the following side effects occur after treatment for tumors of the adrenal gland:

*Rare*

Pale skin; sore throat and fever; unusual bleeding or bruising; unusual tiredness or weakness

Other side effects may occur that usually do not need medical attention. These side effects may go away during treatment as your body adjusts to the medicine. However,

check with your doctor if the following side effects continue or are bothersome:

*Less common or rare*

Flushing of skin; nausea; slight and temporary increase in blood pressure

Other side effects not listed above may also occur in some patients. If you notice any other effects, check with your doctor.

Revised: 05/05/93

# IODINATED GLYCEROL   Systemic*†

## Description

Iodinated glycerol (EYE-oh-di-nay-ted GLI-ser-ole) is used to thin and loosen mucus secretions. It is used in the treatment of respiratory tract conditions such as asthma, bronchitis, emphysema, sinusitis, and cystic fibrosis.

Iodinated glycerol is available only with your doctor's prescription. This medicine may be available in the following dosage forms:

*Oral*

- Elixir
- Oral solution
- Tablets

## Before Using This Medicine

In deciding to use a medicine, the risks of taking the medicine must be weighed against the good it will do. This is a decision you and your doctor will make. For iodinated glycerol, the following should be considered:

**Allergies**—Tell your doctor if you have ever had any unusual or allergic reaction to iodinated glycerol, iodine, or iodine-containing preparations. Also tell your health care professional if you are allergic to any other substances, such as foods, preservatives, or dyes.

**Pregnancy**—Iodinated glycerol is not recommended for use during pregnancy because it may cause enlargement of the thyroid gland in the fetus and result in breathing problems.

**Breast-feeding**—Iodinated glycerol is not recommended for use in nursing mothers because it may cause skin rash and thyroid problems in the baby.

**Children**—Swelling of the neck (goiter or enlarged thyroid gland) may be especially likely to occur in children with cystic fibrosis. These patients are usually more sensitive than adults to this effect of iodinated glycerol.

**Older adults**—Many medicines have not been studied specifically in older people. Therefore, it may not be known whether they work exactly the same way they do in younger adults. Although there is no specific information comparing use of iodinated glycerol in the elderly with use in other age groups, this medicine is not expected to cause different side effects or problems in older people than it does in younger adults.

**Other medicines**—Although certain medicines should not be used together at all, in other cases two different medicines may be used together even if an interaction might occur. In these cases, your doctor may want to change the dose, or other precautions may be necessary. When you are taking iodinated glycerol, it is especially important that your health care professional know if you are taking any of the following:

- Antithyroid agents (medicine for overactive thyroid) or
- Lithium (e.g., Lithane)—Taking these medicines with iodinated glycerol may increase the chance of goiter or an underactive thyroid

**Other medical problems**—The presence of other medical problems may affect the use of iodinated glycerol. Make sure you tell your doctor if you have any other medical problems, especially:

- Acne (teenage)—Iodinated glycerol may make the condition worse
- Cystic fibrosis (in children)—Iodinated glycerol may increase the chance of goiter in these patients
- Thyroid disease (or history of)—Iodinated glycerol may increase the chance of goiter in patients with an overactive thyroid; also, prolonged use of iodinated glycerol may result in an underactive thyroid

## Proper Use of This Medicine

For patients taking the *oral solution form of iodinated glycerol*:

- This medicine is to be taken by mouth even if it comes in a dropper bottle.

- Take this medicine mixed in water or another liquid. Be sure to drink all of the liquid to get the full dose of medicine.

To help thin and loosen mucus in the lungs, *drink a glass of water after each dose of this medicine* unless otherwise directed by your doctor.

*Take iodinated glycerol only as directed.* Do not take more of it, do not take it more often, and do not take it for a longer time than your doctor ordered. To do so may increase the chance of side effects.

**Dosing**—The dose of iodinated glycerol will be different for different patients. *Follow your doctor's orders or the directions on the label.* The following information includes only the average doses of iodinated glycerol. *If your dose is different, do not change it* unless your doctor tells you to do so.

The number of tablets or teaspoonfuls of elixir or solution that you take depends on the strength of the medicine. Also, *the number of doses you take each day, the time allowed between doses, and the length of time you take the medicine depend on the medical problem for which you are taking iodinated glycerol.*

- For *oral* dosage form (elixir, solution, or tablets):
  —To thin and loosen mucus in the lungs:
  - Adults—60 milligrams (mg) four times a day.
  - Children—Dose is based on body weight and must be determined by your doctor. However, the usual dose is 30 mg four times a day.

**Missed dose**—If you miss a dose of this medicine, take it as soon as possible. However, if it is almost time for your next dose, skip the missed dose and go back to your regular dosing schedule. Do not double doses.

**Storage**—To store this medicine:
- Keep out of the reach of children.
- Store away from heat and direct light.
- Do not store the tablet form of this medicine in the bathroom, near the kitchen sink, or in other damp places. Heat or moisture may cause the medicine to break down.
- Keep the liquid form of this medicine from freezing.

- Do not keep outdated medicine or medicine no longer needed. Be sure that any discarded medicine is out of the reach of children.

## Precautions While Using This Medicine

Your doctor should check your progress at regular visits to make sure this medicine is working properly and does not cause unwanted effects.

## Side Effects of This Medicine

Along with its needed effects, a medicine may cause some unwanted effects. Although not all of these side effects may occur, if they do occur they may need medical attention.

Check with your doctor as soon as possible if any of the following side effects occur:

*Rare*
> Chills or fever; headache (continuing); joint pain; loss of appetite; pain on chewing or swallowing; skin rash, hives, or redness; sore throat; swelling of face, lips, or eyelids; tenderness or swelling below or in front of ear

*With long-term use*
> Burning of mouth and throat; dry skin; headache (severe); increased watering of the mouth; irritation of eyes; metallic taste; runny nose, sneezing, and other symptoms of head cold; soreness of teeth and gums; swelling around the eyes; swelling of neck; unusual sensitivity to cold; unusual tiredness or weakness; unusual weight gain

Other side effects may occur that usually do not need medical attention. These side effects may go away during treatment as your body adjusts to the medicine. However, check with your doctor if any of the following side effects continue or are bothersome:

*More common*
> Diarrhea; nausea or vomiting; stomach pain

Other side effects not listed above may also occur in some patients. If you notice any other effects, check with your doctor.

Revised: 08/30/94

# IODINE Topical†

Generic name product is available in the U.S.

†Not commercially available in Canada.

## Description

Topical iodine (EYE -oh-din) is used to prevent and treat infections that may occur in minor scrapes and cuts. It works by killing bacteria that can cause infections.

This medicine is available in the following dosage form:
*Topical*
- Tincture (U.S.)

## Before Using This Medicine

If you are using this medicine without a prescription, carefully read and follow any precautions on the label. For topical iodine, the following should be considered:

**Allergies**—Tell your doctor if you have ever had any unusual or allergic reaction to iodine. Also tell your health care professional if you are allergic to any other substances, such as foods, preservatives, or dyes.

**Pregnancy**—Use of topical iodine is not recommended during pregnancy because it has been shown to cause thyroid problems in the newborn infant. Before using this medicine, make sure your doctor knows if you are pregnant or you may become pregnant.

**Breast-feeding**—Topical iodine passes into the breast milk and has been shown to cause unwanted effects, such as thyroid problems in nursing babies. It may be necessary for you to use another medicine or to stop breast-feeding during treatment. Be sure you have discussed the risks and benefits of the medicine with your doctor.

**Children**—Use of topical iodine is not recommended for newborn infants because it may cause skin and thyroid problems.

**Older adults**—Many medicines have not been studied specifically in older people. Therefore, it may not be known whether they work exactly the same way they do in younger adults. Although there is no specific information comparing use of topical iodine in the elderly with use in other age groups, this medicine is not expected to cause different side effects or problems in older people than it does in younger adults.

**Other medicines**—Although certain medicines should not be used together at all, in other cases two different medicines may be used together even if an interaction might occur. In these cases, your doctor may want to change the dose, or other precautions may be necessary. Tell your health care professional if you are using any other topical prescription or nonprescription (over-the-counter [OTC]) medicine that is to be applied to the same area of the skin.

**Other medical problems**—The presence of other medical problems may affect the use of topical iodine. Make sure you tell your doctor if you have any other medical problems, especially:
- Animal bites or
- Deep wounds or
- Serious burns—The chance of side effects may be increased

## Proper Use of This Medicine

Use this medicine only as directed.

This medicine is for external use only. Do not swallow it.

*Keep this medicine away from the eyes because it may cause irritation.* If you should accidentally get some in your eyes, wash it away with water immediately.

*Do not use topical iodine on deep, puncture wounds, animal bites, or serious burns.* To do so may increase the chance of side effects.

Do not cover the wound to which you have applied topical iodine with a tight dressing or bandage since this may increase the chance of side effects.

**Dosing**—*Follow your doctor's orders or the directions on the label before using this medicine.* The following information includes only the average doses of iodine. *If your dose is different, do not change it* unless your doctor tells you to do so.
- For *topical* dosage form (tincture):
  —For minor bacterial skin infections:
    - Adults and children 1 month of age and over—Use when necessary, according to the directions on the label or your doctor's instructions. Do not use for more than ten days.
    - Infants and children under 1 month of age—Use is not recommended.

To help clear up your infection completely, it *is very important that you keep using topical iodine for the full time of treatment. Do not miss any doses.*

**Missed dose**—If you miss a dose of this medicine, apply it as soon as possible. However, if it is almost time for your next dose, skip the missed dose and go back to your regular dosing schedule.

**Storage**—To store this medicine:
- Keep out of the reach of children.
- Store away from heat and direct light.
- Keep the medicine from freezing. Do not refrigerate.
- Do not keep outdated medicine or medicine no longer needed. Be sure that any discarded medicine is out of the reach of children.

## Precautions While Using This Medicine

Check with your doctor if the skin problem for which you are using topical iodine becomes worse, or if you develop a constant irritation such as itching or burning that was not present before you started using this medicine.

This medicine can stain your skin and clothing. Alcohol may be used to remove iodine stain on the skin. Stains on clothing can be removed by washing and rinsing them in ammonia diluted with water. Stains on starched linens can be removed by washing them in soap and water.

## Side Effects of This Medicine

Along with its needed effects, a medicine may cause some unwanted effects. Although not all of these side effects may occur, if they do occur they may need medical attention.

Check with your doctor as soon as possible if any of the following side effects occur:

*Rare*
  Blistering, crusting, irritation, itching, or reddening of skin

*Symptoms of overdose (when swallowed)*
  Abdominal or stomach pain; diarrhea; fever; nausea; not being able to pass urine; thirst, severe; vomiting

Other side effects not listed above may also occur in some patients. If you notice any other effects, check with your doctor.

Developed: 02/22/94

# IODINE, STRONG   Systemic

Another commonly used name in the U.S. and Canada is Lugol's solution.

## Description

Strong iodine (EYE-oh-dine) is used to treat overactive thyroid, iodine deficiency, and to protect the thyroid gland from the effects of radiation from radioactive forms of iodine. It may be used before and after administration of a radioactive medicine containing radioactive iodine or after accidental exposure to radiation (for example, from nuclear power plant accidents). It may also be used for other conditions as determined by your doctor.

Strong iodine is available only with your doctor's prescription, in the following dosage form:

*Oral*
  • Oral solution (U.S. and Canada)

## Before Using This Medicine

In deciding to use a medicine, the risks of taking the medicine must be weighed against the good it will do. This is a decision you and your doctor will make. For strong iodine, the following should be considered:

**Allergies**—Tell your doctor if you have ever had any unusual or allergic reaction to iodine or potassium iodide. Also tell your health care professional if you are allergic to any substances, such as foods, preservatives, or dyes.

**Pregnancy**—Taking strong iodine during pregnancy may cause thyroid problems or goiter in the newborn infant.

**Breast-feeding**—Strong iodine may cause skin rash and thyroid problems in nursing babies.

**Children**—Strong iodine may cause skin rash and thyroid problems in infants.

**Older adults**—Many medicines have not been studied specifically in older people. Therefore, it may not be known whether they work exactly the same way they do in younger adults. Although there is no specific information comparing use of strong iodine in the elderly with use in other age groups, this medicine is not expected to cause different side effects or problems in older people than it does in younger adults.

**Other medicines**—Although certain medicines should not be used together at all, in other cases two different medicines may be used together even if an interaction might occur. In these cases, your doctor may want to change the dose, or other precautions may be necessary. When you are taking strong iodine, it is especially important that your health care professional know if you are taking any of the following:

  • Amiloride (e.g., Midamor) or
  • Spironolactone (e.g., Aldactone) or
  • Triamterene (e.g., Dyrenium)—Use of these medicines with strong iodine may increase the amount of potassium in the blood and increase the chance of side effects
  • Antithyroid agents (medicine for overactive thyroid) or
  • Lithium (e.g., Lithane)—Use of these medicines with strong iodine may increase the chance of side effects

**Other medical problems**—The presence of other medical problems may affect the use of strong iodine. Make sure you tell your doctor if you have any other medical problems, especially:

  • Bronchitis or
  • Other lung conditions—Use of strong iodine may make this condition worse
  • Hyperkalemia (too much potassium in the blood) or
  • Kidney disease—Use of strong iodine may increase the amount of potassium in the blood and increase the chance of side effects

## Proper Use of This Medicine

For patients taking this medicine for *radiation exposure:*

  • Take this medicine only when directed to do so by state or local public health authorities.
  • Take this medicine once a day for 10 days, unless otherwise directed by public health authorities. *Do not take more of it and do not take it more often than directed.* Taking more of the medicine will not protect you better and may result in a greater chance of side effects.

If strong iodine upsets your stomach, *take it after meals or with food or milk* unless otherwise directed by your doctor. If stomach upset (nausea, vomiting, stomach pain, or diarrhea) continues, check with your doctor.

This medicine is to be taken by mouth even if it comes in a dropper bottle.

Do not use this solution if it turns brownish yellow.

Take strong iodine in a full glass (8 ounces) of water or in fruit juice, milk, or broth to improve the taste and lessen stomach upset. Be sure to drink all of the liquid to get the full dose of medicine.

If crystals form in strong iodine solution, they may be dissolved by warming the closed container of solution in warm water and then gently shaking the container.

**Dosing**—The dose of strong iodine will be different for different patients. *Follow your doctor's orders or the directions on the label.* The following information includes only the average doses of strong iodine. *If your dose is different, do not change it* unless your doctor tells you to do so.

- For *oral* dosage form (solution):
  —To treat overactive thyroid (hyperthyroid):
  - Adults and teenagers—One milliliter (mL) three times a day. The first dose is taken at least one hour after the first dose of your antithyroid medicine.
  - Children—Use and dose must be determined by your doctor.
  —To prepare for surgery to remove thyroid gland:
  - Adults, teenagers, and children—3 to 5 drops (approximately 0.1 to 0.3 mL) three times a day for ten days before surgery. This medicine is usually given along with your antithyroid medicine.
  —To protect the thyroid gland against radiation exposure:
  - Adults and teenagers—130 mg once a day for ten days.
  - Children—65 mg once a day for ten days.
  —To treat iodine deficiency:
  - Adults and teenagers—0.3 to 1 mL three to four times a day.
  - Children—Use and dose must be determined by your doctor.

**Missed dose**—If you miss a dose of this medicine, take it as soon as possible. However, if it is almost time for your next dose, skip the missed dose and go back to your regular dosing schedule. Do not double doses.

**Storage**—To store this medicine:
- Keep out of the reach of children.
- Store away from heat and direct light.
- Do not store in the bathroom, near the kitchen sink, or in other damp places.

- Keep the medicine from freezing. Do not refrigerate.
- Do not keep outdated medicine or medicine no longer needed. Be sure that any discarded medicine is out of the reach of children.

## Precautions While Using This Medicine

Your doctor should check your progress at regular visits to make sure that this medicine does not cause unwanted effects.

For patients on a low-potassium diet:
- *This medicine contains potassium.* Check with your health care professional before you take this medicine.

## Side Effects of This Medicine

Along with its needed effects, a medicine may cause some unwanted effects. Although not all of these side effects may occur, if they do occur they may need medical attention. When this medicine is used for a short time at low doses, side effects usually are rare.

Check with your doctor as soon as possible if any of the following side effects occur:

*Less common*
Hives; joint pain; swelling of the arms, face, legs, lips, tongue, and/or throat; swelling of the lymph glands

*With long-term use*
Burning of mouth or throat; confusion; headache (severe); increased watering of mouth; irregular heartbeat; metallic taste; numbness, tingling, pain, or weakness in hands or feet; soreness of teeth and gums; stomach upset; symptoms of head cold; unusual tiredness; weakness or heaviness of legs

Other side effects may occur that usually do not need medical attention. These side effects may go away during treatment as your body adjusts to the medicine. However, check with your doctor if any of the following side effects continue or are bothersome:

*Less common*
Diarrhea; nausea or vomiting; stomach pain

Other side effects not listed above may also occur in some patients. If you notice any other effects, check with your doctor.

Revised: 04/15/92
Interim revision: 08/10/94

# IODOQUINOL   Oral

Some commonly used brand names are:

**In the U.S.—**
Diquinol                              Yodoxin
Yodoquinol
Generic name product may also be available.

**In Canada—**
Diodoquin                             Yodoxin
Another commonly used name is diiodohydroxyquin.

## Description

Iodoquinol (eye-oh-doe-KWIN-ole) belongs to the group of medicines called antiprotozoals. Although sometimes used to treat other types of infection, it is used most often in the treatment of intestinal infections such as amebiasis.

Iodoquinol is available only with your doctor's prescription, in the following dosage form:

*Oral*
- Tablets (U.S. and Canada)

## Before Using This Medicine

In deciding to use a medicine, the risks of taking the medicine must be weighed against the good it will do. This is a decision you and your doctor will make. For iodoquinol, the following should be considered:

**Allergies**—Tell your doctor if you have ever had any unusual or allergic reaction to iodoquinol, chloroxine (e.g., Capitrol), clioquinol (e.g., Vioform), iodine, pamaquine, pentaquine, or primaquine. Also tell your health care professional if you are allergic to any other substances, such as foods, preservatives, or dyes.

**Pregnancy**—Iodoquinol has not been reported to cause birth defects or other problems in humans.

**Breast-feeding**—Iodoquinol has not been reported to cause problems in nursing babies.

**Children**—Children may be more likely to develop side effects, especially if given high doses for a long time.

**Older adults**—Many medicines have not been studied specifically in older people. Therefore, it may not be known whether they work exactly the same way they do in younger adults or if they cause different side effects or problems in older people. There is no specific information comparing use of iodoquinol in the elderly with use in other age groups.

**Other medicines**—Although certain medicines should not be used together at all, in other cases two different medicines may be used together even if an interaction might occur. In these cases, your doctor may want to change the dose, or other precautions may be necessary. Tell your health care professional if you are taking any other prescription or nonprescription (over-the-counter [OTC]) medicine.

**Other medical problems**—The presence of other medical problems may affect the use of iodoquinol. Make sure you tell your doctor if you have any other medical problems, especially:
- Eye disease—Iodoquinol may cause side effects affecting the eye or make eye disease worse
- Kidney disease or
- Liver disease or
- Thyroid disease—Patients with kidney disease, liver disease, or thyroid disease may have an increased chance of side effects

## Proper Use of This Medicine

*Take this medicine after meals* to lessen possible stomach upset, unless otherwise directed by your doctor.

If these tablets are too large to swallow whole, they may be crushed and mixed with a small amount of applesauce or chocolate syrup.

To help clear up your infection completely, *keep taking this medicine for the full time of treatment,* even if you begin to feel better after a few days. *Do not miss any doses.*

**Dosing**—The dose of iodoquinol will be different for different patients. *Follow your doctor's orders or the directions on the label.* The following information includes only the average doses of iodoquinol. *If your dose is different, do not change it* unless your doctor tells you to do so.

The number of tablets that you take depends on the strength of the medicine.
- For *oral* dosage form (tablets):
  —For amebiasis:
    - Adults—630 or 650 milligrams (mg) taken three times a day for twenty days.
    - Children—Dose is based on body weight and must be determined by your doctor. The usual dose is 10 to 13.3 mg per kilogram (kg) (4.5 to 6 mg per pound) of body weight taken three times a day for twenty days.

**Missed dose**—If you miss a dose of this medicine, take it as soon as possible. However, if it is almost time for your next dose, skip the missed dose and go back to your regular dosing schedule. Do not double doses.

**Storage**—To store this medicine:
- Keep out of the reach of children.
- Store away from heat and direct light.
- Do not store in the bathroom, near the kitchen sink, or in other damp places. Heat or moisture may cause the medicine to break down.
- Do not keep outdated medicine or medicine no longer needed. Be sure that any discarded medicine is out of the reach of children.

## Precautions While Using This Medicine

This medicine may cause blurred vision or loss of vision. *Make sure you know how you react to this medicine before you drive, use machines, or do anything else that could be dangerous if you are not able to see well.* If these reactions are especially bothersome, check with your doctor.

*If you must have thyroid function tests, make sure the doctor knows that you are taking this medicine or have taken it within the past 6 months.*

## Side Effects of This Medicine

Along with its needed effects, a medicine may cause some unwanted effects. Although not all of these side effects may occur, if they do occur they may need medical attention.

*Check with your doctor immediately* if any of the following side effects occur:

*Less common*

Fever or chills; skin rash, hives, or itching; swelling of neck

*With long-term use of high doses—especially in children*

Blurred vision or any change in vision; clumsiness or unsteadiness; decreased vision or eye pain; increased weakness; muscle pain; numbness, tingling, pain, or weakness in hands or feet

Other side effects may occur that usually do not need medical attention. These side effects may go away during treatment as your body adjusts to the medicine. However, check with your doctor if any of the following side effects continue or are bothersome:

*More common*

Diarrhea; nausea or vomiting; stomach pain

*Less common*

Headache; itching of the rectal area

Blurred vision or any change in vision; decreased vision; eye pain; or numbness, tingling, pain, or weakness in hands or feet may be more likely to occur in children, especially with long-term use of high doses.

Other side effects not listed above may also occur in some patients. If you notice any other effects, check with your doctor.

Revised: 10/06/92
Interim revision: 06/06/94

---

# IPECAC    Oral

Available in the U.S. and Canada as generic name product.

## Description

Ipecac (IP-e-kak) is used in the emergency treatment of certain kinds of poisoning. It is used to cause vomiting of the poison.

Only the syrup form of ipecac should be used. A bottle of ipecac labeled as being Ipecac Fluidextract or Ipecac Tincture should not be used. These dosage forms are too strong and may cause serious side effects or death. Only ipecac syrup contains the proper strength of ipecac for treating poisonings.

Ordinarily, this medicine should not be used if strychnine, corrosives such as alkalies (lye) and strong acids, or petroleum distillates such as kerosene, gasoline, coal oil, fuel oil, paint thinner, or cleaning fluid have been swallowed. It may cause seizures, additional injury to the throat, or pneumonia.

*Ipecac should not be used to cause vomiting as a means of losing weight.* If used regularly for this purpose, serious heart problems or even death may occur.

This medicine in amounts of more than 1 ounce is available only with your doctor's prescription. It is available in ½- and 1-ounce bottles without a prescription. However, before using ipecac syrup, call a poison control center, your doctor, or an emergency room for advice.

*Oral*

• Syrup (U.S. and Canada)

## Before Using This Medicine

*Before using this medicine to cause vomiting in poisoning, call a poison control center, your doctor, or an emergency room for advice.* It is a good idea to have these telephone numbers readily available. In addition, before you use ipecac, the following should be considered:

**Pregnancy**—Studies on effects in pregnancy have not been done in either humans or animals.

**Children**—Infants and very young children are at a greater risk of choking with their own vomit (or getting vomit in their lungs). Therefore, it is especially important to call a poison control center, your doctor, or an emergency room for instructions before giving ipecac to an infant or young child.

**Older adults**—This medicine has been tested and has not been shown to cause different side effects or problems in older people than it does in younger adults.

**Other medical problems**—The presence of other medical problems may affect the use of ipecac. Make sure you tell your doctor or the person you talk to at the poison control center or the emergency room if you have any other medical problems, especially:

• Heart disease—There is an increased risk of heart problems, such as unusually fast heartbeat, if the ipecac is not vomited

## Proper Use of This Medicine

*It is very important that you take this medicine only as directed.* Do not take more of it and do not take it more often than recommended on the label, unless otherwise directed. When too much ipecac is used, it can cause damage to the heart and other muscles, and may even cause death.

*Do not give this medicine to unconscious or very drowsy persons,* since the vomited material may enter the lungs and cause pneumonia.

To help this medicine cause vomiting of the poison, adults should drink 1 full glass (8 ounces) of water and children should drink ½ to 1 full glass (4 to 8 ounces) of water immediately after taking this medicine. Water may be given first in the case of a small or scared child.

*Do not take this medicine with milk, milk products, or with carbonated beverages.* Milk or milk products may prevent this medicine from working properly, and carbonated beverages may cause swelling of the stomach.

If vomiting does not occur within 20 to 30 minutes after you have taken the first dose of this medicine, take a second dose. If vomiting does not occur after you have taken the second dose, you must immediately see your doctor or go to an emergency room.

If you have been told to take both this medicine and activated charcoal to treat the poisoning, *do not take the activated charcoal until after you have taken this medicine to cause vomiting and vomiting has stopped. This takes usually about 30 minutes.*

**Dosing**—The dose of ipecac will be different for different patients. *Follow your doctor's orders or the directions on the label.* The following information includes only the average doses of ipecac. *If your dose is different, do not change it* unless your doctor tells you to do so.

- For *oral* dosage form (syrup):
  —For treatment of poisoning:
    - Adults and teenagers—The usual dose is 15 to 30 milliliters (mL) (1 to 2 tablespoonfuls), followed immediately by one full glass (240 mL) of water. The dose may be repeated one time after twenty to thirty minutes if vomiting does not occur.
    - Children 1 to 12 years of age—The usual dose is 15 mL (1 tablespoonful). One-half to one full glass (120 to 240 mL) of water should be taken right before or right after the dose. The dose

may be repeated one time after twenty to thirty minutes if vomiting does not occur.
    - Children 6 months to 1 year of age—The usual dose is 5 to 10 mL (1 to 2 teaspoonfuls). One-half to one full glass (120 to 240 mL) of water should be taken right before or right after the dose. The dose may be repeated one time after twenty to thirty minutes if vomiting does not occur.
    - Children up to 6 months of age—Ipecac must be given only under the direction of your doctor.

**Storage**—To store this medicine:
- Keep out of the reach of children since overdose is very dangerous in children.
- Store away from heat and direct light.
- Keep the syrup from freezing.
- Do not keep outdated medicine or medicine no longer needed. Be sure that any discarded medicine is out of the reach of children.
- Do not keep a bottle of ipecac that has been opened. Ipecac may evaporate over a period of time. It is best to replace it with a new one.

## Side Effects of This Medicine

Along with its needed effects, a medicine may cause some unwanted effects. Although side effects usually do not occur with recommended doses of ipecac, if they do occur they may need medical attention.

Check with your doctor as soon as possible if any of the following side effects occur:

*Symptoms of overdose (may also occur if ipecac is taken regularly)*
Diarrhea; fast or irregular heartbeat; nausea or vomiting (continuing more than 30 minutes); stomach cramps or pain; troubled breathing; unusual tiredness or weakness; weakness, aching, and stiffness of muscles, especially those of the neck, arms, and legs

Other side effects not listed above may also occur in some patients. If you notice any other effects, check with your doctor.

Revised: 08/04/94

# IPRATROPIUM    Inhalation

A commonly used brand name in the U.S. and Canada is Atrovent.

## Description

Ipratropium is a bronchodilator (medicine that opens up narrowed breathing passages). It is taken by inhalation to help control the symptoms of lung diseases, such as

bronchial asthma, chronic bronchitis, and emphysema. When ipratropium is used regularly every day, it may be used alone or with other bronchodilators to help decrease coughing, wheezing, shortness of breath, and troubled breathing by increasing the flow of air into the lungs.

When ipratropium inhalation is used to treat acute attacks of asthma, it is used only in a nebulizer and must be used in combination with other bronchodilators.

Ipratropium is available only with your doctor's prescription, in the following dosage forms:

*Inhalation*
- Inhalation aerosol (U.S. and Canada)
- Inhalation solution (U.S. and Canada)

## Before Using This Medicine

In deciding to use a medicine, the risks of using the medicine must be weighed against the good it will do. This is a decision you and your doctor will make. For ipratropium, the following should be considered:

**Allergies**—Tell your doctor if you have ever had any unusual or allergic reaction to ipratropium, atropine, belladonna, hyoscyamine, or scopolamine, or to other inhalation aerosol medicines.

**Pregnancy**—Ipratropium has not been studied in pregnant women. However, it has not been shown to cause birth defects or other problems in animal studies.

**Breast-feeding**—It is not known whether ipratropium passes into the breast milk. Although most medicines pass into breast milk in small amounts, many of them may be used safely while breast-feeding. Mothers who are using this medicine and who wish to breast-feed should discuss this with their doctor.

**Children**—Although there is no specific information comparing the use of ipratropium in children up to 5 years of age with other age groups, this medicine is not expected to cause different side effects or problems in children than it does in adults.

**Older adults**—Ipratropium inhalation has been tested in a small number of patients 65 years of age or older. This medicine is not expected to cause different side effects or problems in older people than it does in younger adults.

**Other medicines**—Although certain medicines should not be used together at all, in other cases two different medicines may be used together even if an interaction might occur. In these cases, your doctor may want to change the dose, or other precautions may be necessary. When you are taking ipratropium, it is especially important that your health care professional know if you are taking any other prescription or nonprescription (over-the-counter [OTC]) medicine.

**Other medical problems**—The presence of other medical problems may affect the use of ipratropium. Make sure you tell your doctor if you have any other medical problem, especially:
- Difficult urination—Ipratropium may make the condition worse
- Glaucoma—Ipratropium may make the condition worse if it gets into the eyes

## Proper Use of This Medicine

*Ipratropium is used to help control the symptoms of lung diseases, such as chronic bronchitis, emphysema, and asthma. However, for treatment of bronchospasm or asthma attacks that have already started, ipratropium inhalation solution is used only in a nebulizer and in combination with other bronchodilators.*

*It is very important that you use ipratropium only as directed. Do not use more of it and do not use it more often than your doctor ordered.* To do so may increase the chance of side effects.

*Keep the spray or solution away from the eyes* because this medicine may cause irritation or blurred vision. Closing your eyes while you are inhaling ipratropium may help keep the medicine out of your eyes. Rinsing your eyes with cool water may help if any medicine does get into your eyes.

Ipratropium usually comes with patient directions. Read them carefully before using this medicine.

For patients using *ipratropium inhalation aerosol:*
- If you do not understand the directions or you are not sure how to use the inhaler, ask your health care professional to show you how to use it. Also, ask your health care professional to check regularly how you use the inhaler to make sure you are using it properly.
- When you use the inhaler for the first time, or if you have not used it for a while, the inhaler may not deliver the right amount of medicine with the first puff. Therefore, before using the inhaler, test it to make sure it works properly.

- *To test the inhaler:*
  —Insert the metal canister firmly into the clean mouthpiece according to the manufacturer's instructions. Check to make sure it is placed properly into the mouthpiece.
  —Take the cover off the mouthpiece and shake the inhaler three or four times.
  —Hold the inhaler well away from you against a light background and press the top of the canister, spraying the medicine into the air. If you see a fine mist, you will know the inhaler is working properly to provide the right amount of medicine when you use it. If you do not see a fine mist, try a second time.

- *To use the inhaler:*
  —Using your thumb and one or two fingers, hold the inhaler upright, with the mouthpiece end down and pointing toward you.
  —Take off the cover off the mouthpiece. Check the mouthpiece for any foreign object. Then, gently shake the inhaler and canister three or four times.
  —Hold the mouthpiece away from your mouth and breathe out slowly and completely.

—Use the inhalation method recommended by your doctor.

- Open-mouth method—Place the mouthpiece about 1 or 2 inches (2 fingerwidths) in front of your widely opened mouth. Make sure the inhaler is aimed into your mouth so the spray does not hit the roof of your mouth or your tongue.

- Closed-mouth method—Place the mouthpiece in your mouth between your teeth and over your tongue with your lips closed tightly around it. Make sure your tongue or teeth are not blocking the opening.

—Tilt your head back a little. Start to breathe in slowly and deeply through your mouth and, at the same time, press the top of the canister once to get one puff of medicine. Continue to breathe in slowly until you have taken a full breath. Try to inhale for 3 to 4 seconds. It is important to press down on the top of the canister and breathe in at the same time so the medicine is pulled into your lungs. This step may be difficult at first. If you are using the closed-mouth method and you see a fine mist coming from your mouth or nose, the inhaler is not being used correctly.

—After inhaling the spray into your lungs, hold your breath as long as you can up to 10 seconds. This gives the medicine time to settle into your airways and lungs.

—Take the mouthpiece away from your mouth and breathe out slowly.

—If your doctor has told you to inhale more than one puff of medicine at each dose, gently shake the inhaler again, and take the second puff following exactly the same steps you used for the first puff.

—When you are finished, wipe off the mouthpiece and replace the cover to keep the mouthpiece clean and free of foreign objects.

Your doctor may want you to use a spacer device with the inhaler. A spacer makes the inhaler easier to use. With a spacer, more of the medicine is able to reach your lungs and less of it stays in the mouth and throat.

- *To use a spacer device with the inhaler:*
  —Attach the spacer to the inhaler according to the manufacturer's directions. There are different types of spacers available, but the method of breathing remains the same with most spacers.
  —Gently shake the inhaler and spacer three or four times.
  —Hold the mouthpiece of the spacer away from your mouth and breathe out slowly to the end of a normal breath.
  —Place the mouthpiece into your mouth between your teeth and over your tongue with your lips closed around it.
  —Press down on the canister top once to release one puff of medicine into the spacer. Within one

or two seconds, start to breathe in slowly and deeply through your mouth for 5 to 10 seconds. Count the seconds while inhaling. Do not breathe in through your nose.

—Then hold your breath as long as you can up to 10 seconds.

—Breathe out slowly. Do not remove the mouthpiece from your mouth. Breathe in and out slowly three or four times to be sure the spacer device is emptied.

—If your doctor has told you to take more than one puff of medicine at each dose, gently shake the inhaler and spacer again and take the second puff, following exactly the same steps you used for the first puff.

—When you are finished, remove the spacer device from the inhaler and replace the cover of the mouthpiece.

Clean the inhaler, mouthpiece, and spacer at least twice a week to prevent build-up of medicine and blockage of the mouthpiece.

- *To clean the inhaler:*
  —Remove the metal canister from the inhaler and set aside.
  —Wash the mouthpiece and cover, the plastic case, and the spacer with soap and hot water. Rinse well with warm, running water.
  —Shake off the excess water and let the inhaler parts air dry completely before replacing the metal canister and cover.
  —The metal canister stem may get dirty or blocked. While the canister is out of the mouthpiece, check the two small holes in the stem of the canister.
  —If the holes seem blocked, rinse them with clear, lukewarm water.
  —Let the canister dry completely before you put it back into the dry mouthpiece.
  —Replace the cover to keep the mouthpiece clean.

- *To check how full the canister is:*
  —Place only the canister in a container of water.
  —If the canister floats at the top of the water, it is empty and needs replacing. If it sinks to the bottom of the water, it is full. When the canister stands upright in the water, it is about one-half full.
  —Take the canister out of the water and let it dry completely before putting it back into the dry mouthpiece.

For patients using *ipratropium inhalation solution:*
- Use this medicine only in a power-operated nebulizer with an adequate flow rate and equipped with a face mask or mouthpiece. Your doctor will tell you which nebulizer to use. Make sure you understand exactly how to use it. If you have any questions about this, check with your doctor.

- *To prepare the medicine for use in the nebulizer:*
  —*If you are using the single-dose vial of ipratropium:*
  - Break away one vial by pulling it firmly from the strip.
  - Twist off the top to open the vial. Use the contents of the vial as soon as possible after opening it.
  - Squeeze the contents of the vial into the cup of the nebulizer. If your doctor has told you to use less than a full vial of solution, use a syringe to withdraw the correct amount of solution from the vial and add it to the nebulizer cup. Be sure to throw away the syringe after one use.
  —*If you are using the multiple-dose bottle of ipratropium:*
  - Use a syringe to withdraw the correct amount of solution from the bottle and add it to the nebulizer cup. Do not use the same syringe more than once.
- If you have been told to dilute the ipratropium inhalation solution in the nebulizer cup with the sodium chloride solution provided, use a new syringe to add the sodium chloride solution to the cup as directed by your health care professional.
- If your doctor told you to use another inhalation solution with the ipratropium inhalation solution, add that solution also to the nebulizer cup.
- *To use the nebulizer:*
  —Gently shake the nebulizer cup to mix the solutions well.
  —Connect the nebulizer tube to the air or oxygen pump and begin the treatment. Adjust the mask, if you are using one, to prevent mist from getting into your eyes.
  —Use the method of breathing your doctor told you to use to take the treatment. One way is to breathe slowly and deeply through the mask or mouthpiece. Another way is to breathe in and out normally with the mouthpiece in your mouth, taking a deep breath every one or two minutes. Continue to breathe in the medicine as instructed until no more mist is formed in the nebulizer cup or until you hear a sputtering (spitting or popping) sound.
  —When you have finished, replace the caps on the solutions. Store the bottles in the refrigerator until the next treatment.
  —Clean the nebulizer according to the manufacturer's directions.

For patients using *ipratropium* regularly (for example, every day):

- *In order for ipratropium to work properly, it must be inhaled every day in regularly spaced doses as ordered by your doctor.*

**Dosing**—The dose of ipratropium will be different for different patients. *Follow your doctor's orders or the directions on the label.* The following information includes only the average doses of ipratropium. *If your dose is different, do not change it* unless your doctor tells you to do so.

- For symptoms of lung diseases, such as bronchial asthma, chronic bronchitis, or emphysema:
  —For *inhalation aerosol* dosage form:
  - Adults and children 12 years of age and older—18 to 40 micrograms (mcg) (1 to 2 puffs) three or four times a day, at regularly spaced times.
  - Children up to 12 years of age—Use and dose must be determined by your doctor.
  —For *inhalation solution* dosage form:
  - Adults and children 12 years of age and older—250 to 500 mcg mixed, if necessary, with the sodium chloride solution provided with this medicine, to make 3 to 5 milliliters (mL) of solution. This mixture is used in a nebulizer three or four times a day, every six to eight hours.
  - Children 5 to 12 years of age—125 to 250 mcg mixed, if necessary, with the sodium chloride solution provided with this medicine, to make 3 to 5 milliliters (mL) of solution. This mixture is used in a nebulizer three or four times a day, every four to six hours as needed.
  - Children up to 5 years of age—Use and dose must be determined by your doctor.

**Missed dose**—If you use ipratropium inhalation regularly and you miss a dose of this medicine, use it as soon as possible. Then use any remaining doses for that day at regularly spaced times.

**Storage**—To store this medicine:

- Keep out of the reach of children.
- Store away from heat.
- Store the solution form of this medicine away from direct light. Store the aerosol form of this medicine away from direct sunlight.
- Keep the medicine from freezing.
- Store any opened bottles of the solution form of this medicine in the refrigerator.
- Do not puncture, break, or burn the aerosol container, even if it is empty.
- Do not keep outdated medicine or medicine no longer needed. Be sure that any discarded medicine is out of the reach of children.

## Precautions While Using This Medicine

*Check with your doctor at once if your symptoms do not improve within 30 minutes after using a dose of this medicine or if your condition gets worse.*

For patients using *ipratropium inhalation solution:*

- *If you are also using cromolyn inhalation solution, do not mix that solution with the ipratropium inhalation solution from the 20-mL multiple-dose vial for use in a nebulizer. To do so will cause the solution to become cloudy and prevent the cromolyn from* working properly. However, if your condition requires you to use cromolyn inhalation solution with ipratropium inhalation solution, it may be mixed with ipratropium inhalation solution from the 2-mL single-dose vial.

Ipratropium may cause dryness of the mouth or throat. For temporary relief of mouth dryness, use sugarless candy or gum, melt bits of ice in your mouth, or use a saliva substitute. However, if your mouth continues to feel dry for more than 2 weeks, check with your medical doctor or dentist. Continuing dryness of the mouth may increase the chance of dental disease, including tooth decay, gum disease, and fungus infections.

## Side Effects of This Medicine

Along with its needed effects, a medicine may cause some unwanted effects. Although not all of these side effects may occur, if they do occur they may require medical attention.

Check with your doctor as soon as possible if any of the following side effects occur:

*Less common*
> Increased wheezing, tightness in chest, or difficulty in breathing

*Rare*
> Difficulty in swallowing; severe eye pain; skin rash or hives; swelling of tongue or lips; ulcers or sores in mouth and on lips

Other side effects may occur that usually do not need medical attention. These side effects may go away during treatment as your body adjusts to the medicine. However, check with your doctor if any of the following side effects continue or are bothersome:

*More common*
> Cough or dryness of mouth or throat; headache or dizziness; nervousness; stomach upset or nausea

*Less common or rare*
> Blurred vision or other changes in vision; constipation (continuing); difficult urination; metallic or unpleasant taste; pounding heartbeat; stuffy nose; trembling; trouble in sleeping; unusual tiredness or weakness

Other side effects not listed above may also occur in some patients. If you notice any other effects, check with your doctor.

Revised: 08/29/94

# IPRATROPIUM   Nasal*

A commonly used brand name in Canada is Atrovent.

*Not commercially available in the U.S.

## Description

Ipratropium (i-pra-TROE-pee-um) nasal aerosol is used to relieve runny nose caused by continuing nasal inflammation.

When this medicine is sprayed into your nose, it works by preventing the glands in your nose from producing large amounts of fluid.

Ipratropium is available only with your doctor's prescription, in the following dosage form:

*Nasal*
• Nasal aerosol (Canada)

## Before Using This Medicine

In deciding to use a medicine, the risks of using the medicine must be weighed against the good it will do. This is a decision you and your doctor will make. For ipratropium nasal aerosol, the following should be considered:

**Allergies**—Tell your doctor if you have ever had any unusual or allergic reaction to ipratropium, atropine, belladonna, hyoscyamine, or scopolamine, or to other nasal aerosol medicines.

**Pregnancy**—Ipratropium has not been studied in pregnant women. However, it has not been shown to cause birth defects in animal studies.

**Breast-feeding**—It is not known whether ipratropium nasal aerosol passes into the breast milk. Although most medicines pass into breast milk in small amounts, many of them may be used safely while breast-feeding. Mothers who are using this medicine and who wish to breast-feed should discuss this with their doctor.

**Children**—Although there is no specific information comparing the use of ipratropium nasal aerosol in children with use in other age groups, this medicine is not expected to cause different side effects or problems in children than it does in adults.

**Older adults**—Many medicines have not been studied specifically in older people. Therefore, it may not be known whether they work exactly the same way they do in younger adults. Although there is no specific information comparing the use of ipratropium nasal aerosol in the elderly with use in other age groups, this medicine is not expected to cause different side effects in older people than it does in younger adults.

**Other medicines**—Although certain medicines should not be used together at all, in other cases two different medicines may be used together even if an interaction might occur. In these cases, your doctor may want to change the dose, or other precautions may be necessary. Tell your health care professional if you are taking any other prescription or nonprescription (over-the-counter [OTC]) medicine.

**Other medical problems**—The presence of other medical problems may affect the use of ipratropium nasal aerosol. Make sure you tell your doctor if you have any other medical problem, especially:

- Glaucoma—If ipratropium nasal aerosol is sprayed into the eyes, it may make the condition worse

## Proper Use of This Medicine

*It is very important that you use ipratropium nasal aerosol only as directed.* Do not use more of it and do not use it more often than your doctor ordered. To do so may increase the chance of side effects.

*Keep the aerosol spray away from the eyes.* If the spray accidently gets in your eyes, it may cause irritation and blurred vision. Rinsing your eyes with cool water may help if any medicine does get into your eyes.

Ipratropium nasal aerosol usually comes with patient directions. Read them carefully before using this medicine.

If you do not understand the directions or if you are not sure how to use the ipratropium nasal aerosol, ask your health care professional to show you how to use it.

When you use the nasal aerosol for the first time or if you have not used it for a while, the spray device may not deliver the right amount of medicine with the first spray. Therefore, before using the aerosol, test the device to make sure it works properly.

*To test the aerosol spray device:*
- Insert the canister firmly into the clean nosepiece according to the manufacturer's instructions. Check to make sure it is placed properly into the nosepiece.
- Take the cover off the nosepiece and shake the aerosol container well.
- Hold the aerosol container against a light background and press the top of the canister once or twice, spraying the medicine away from yourself, into the air. If you see a fine mist of medicine, you will know that the spray device is working properly and that you will get the right amount of medicine when you use it.

*To use the nasal aerosol:*
- Gently blow your nose, making sure your nostrils are clear.
- Hold the aerosol container upright between your thumb and forefinger, with the nosepiece down and pointing toward you.
- Take off the nosepiece cover and gently shake the aerosol container well.
- Insert the nosepiece into one nostril. Point it slightly toward the outside nostril wall. Hold your other nostril closed with one finger.
- Tilt your head back a little. Press down on the top of the canister to release one spray. Do not breathe

in at the same time you are spraying the medicine. If the spray tends to drip out, you may sniff gently to keep the spray in your nose.
- If your doctor has told you to use more than one spray in the same nostril, slightly change the direction of the nosepiece in your nostril and spray again.
- Remove the nosepiece from your nostril.
- Gently shake the container well. Place the nosepiece into the second nostril.
- Repeat the same steps for spraying the medicine into the second nostril that you used for the first nostril.
- Remove the nosepiece from your nostril.
- When you have finished, replace the cover on the nosepiece to keep it clean.
- Do not blow your nose for the next 15 minutes.

Clean the aerosol spray device often to prevent the medicine from building up and blocking the nosepiece.

*To clean the aerosol spray device:*
- After each use—Wipe off the nosepiece.
- At least once a week:
  —Remove the canister from the nosepiece.
  —Wash the nosepiece well in lukewarm water.
  —If you use soap or detergent, rinse the nosepiece well in clear water.
  —Shake off the excess water and let the nosepiece air dry completely.
  —The canister stem may get dirty or blocked. While the canister is out of the nosepiece, check the two small holes in the stem of the canister.
  —If the holes seem blocked, rinse them with clear, lukewarm water.
  —Let the canister air dry completely before you put it back into the dry nosepiece.
  —Replace the cover to keep the nosepiece clean.

**Dosing**—The dose of ipratropium nasal aerosol will be different for different patients. *Follow your doctor's orders or the directions on the label.* The following information includes only the average doses of ipratropium nasal aerosol. *If your dose is different, do not change it* unless your doctor tells you to do so:
- For *nasal* aerosol:
  —For runny nose:
    • Adults and children 12 years of age and older—40 micrograms (mcg) (2 sprays) into each nostril two to four times a day. Do not use more often than every 6 hours. Do not use more than 16 sprays in twenty-four hours.
    • Children up to 12 years of age—Use is not recommended.

**Missed dose**—If you are using ipratropium nasal aerosol regularly and you miss a dose of this medicine, use it as soon as possible. Then use any remaining doses for that day at regularly spaced times.

**Storage**—To store this medicine:
- Keep out of the reach of children.
- Store away from heat and direct sunlight.
- Keep the medicine from freezing.
- Do not puncture, break, or burn the container, even if it is empty.
- Do not keep outdated medicine or medicine no longer needed. Be sure that any discarded medicine is out of the reach of children.

## Precautions While Using This Medicine

*If your symptoms do not improve within one or two weeks or if your condition becomes worse, check with your doctor.*

Ipratropium nasal aerosol may cause dryness of the mouth or throat. For temporary relief, use sugarless candy or gum, melt bits of ice in your mouth, or use a saliva substitute. However, if your mouth continues to feel dry for more than 2 weeks, check with your medical doctor or dentist. Continuing dryness of the mouth may increase the chance of dental disease, including tooth decay, gum disease, and fungus infections.

## Side Effects of This Medicine

Along with its needed effects, a medicine may cause some unwanted effects. Although not all of these side effects may occur, if they do occur they may require medical attention.

Check with your doctor as soon as possible if any of the following side effects occur:

*Rare*

Blurred vision or other changes in vision; difficult or painful urination; difficulty in swallowing; eye pain; fast or irregular heartbeat; skin rash or hives; swelling of tongue or lips; sores in mouth and on lips; wheezing, tightness in chest, or difficulty in breathing

Other side effects may occur that usually do not need medical attention. These side effects may go away during treatment as your body adjusts to the medicine. However, check with your doctor if any of the following side effects continue or are bothersome:

*More common*

Dryness of nose or mouth; headache; irritation and crusting in nose

*Less common or rare*

Bleeding or burning in nose; diarrhea or constipation; dryness of throat; nausea; nervousness; stomach pain; stuffy nose

Other side effects not listed above may occur in some patients. If you notice any other effects, check with your doctor.

Developed: 08/09/94

---

# IRON SUPPLEMENTS    Systemic

Some commonly used brand names are:

**In the U.S.—**

| | |
|---|---|
| Femiron[1] | Fumerin[1] |
| Feostat[1] | Hemocyte[1] |
| Feostat Drops[1] | Hytinic[5] |
| Feosol[3] | InFeD[4] |
| Fergon[2] | Ircon[1] |
| Fer-In-Sol[3] | Mol-Iron[3] |
| Fer-In-Sol Drops[3] | Niferex[5] |
| Fer-In-Sol Syrup[3] | Niferex-150[5] |
| Fer-Iron Drops[3] | Nu-Iron[5] |
| Fero-Gradumet[3] | Nu-Iron 150[5] |
| Ferospace[3] | Palmiron[1] |
| Ferralet[2] | Simron[2] |
| Ferralyn Lanacaps[3] | Slow Fe[3] |
| Ferra-TD[3] | Span-FF[1] |
| Fumasorb[1] | |

**In Canada**

| | |
|---|---|
| Apo-Ferrous Gluconate[2] | Neo-Fer[1] |
| Apo-Ferrous Sulfate[3] | Novoferrogluc[2] |
| Fer-In-Sol Drops[3] | Novoferrosulfa[3] |
| Fer-In-Sol Syrup[3] | Novofumar[1] |
| Fero-Grad[3] | Palafer[1] |
| Fertinic[2] | Palafer Pediatric Drops[1] |
| Imferon[4] | PMS Ferrous Sulfate[3] |
| Jectofer[6] | Slow Fe[3] |

Note: For quick reference, the following iron supplements are numbered to match the corresponding brand names.

This information applies to the following medicines:
1. Ferrous Fumarate (FER-us FYOO-ma-rate)‡
2. Ferrous Gluconate (FER-us GLOO-koe-nate)‡§
3. Ferrous Sulfate (FER-us SUL-fate)‡§
4. Iron Dextran (DEX-tran)
5. Iron-Polysaccharide (pol-i-SAK-a-ride)†
6. Iron Sorbitol (SOR-bi-tole)*

*Not commercially available in the U.S.
†Not commercially available in Canada.
‡Generic name product may also be available in the U.S.
§Generic name product may also be available in Canada.

---

## Description

Iron is a mineral that the body needs to produce red blood cells. When the body does not get enough iron, it cannot produce the number of normal red blood cells needed to keep you in good health. This condition is called iron deficiency (iron shortage) or iron deficiency anemia.

Although many people in the U.S. get enough iron from their diet, some must take additional amounts to meet their needs. For example, iron is sometimes lost with slow or small amounts of bleeding in the body that you would not be aware of and which can only be detected by your doctor. Your doctor can determine if you have an iron deficiency, what is causing the deficiency, and if an iron supplement is necessary.

Lack of iron may lead to unusual tiredness, shortness of breath, a decrease in physical performance, learning problems in children, and may increase your chance of getting an infection.

Patients with the following conditions may be more likely to have a deficiency of iron:
- Bleeding problems
- Burns
- Hemodialysis
- Intestinal diseases
- Stomach removal

In addition, premature infants and those receiving unfortified formulas may need additional iron.

If any of the above apply to you, you should take iron supplements only on the advice of your doctor after need has been established.

Some iron preparations are available only with your doctor's prescription. Others are available without a prescription; however, your doctor may have special instructions on the proper use and dose for your condition.

Iron supplements are available in the following dosage forms:

*Oral*

Ferrous Fumarate
- Capsules (Canada)
- Extended-release capsules (U.S.)
- Solution (U.S. and Canada)
- Suspension (U.S. and Canada)
- Tablets (U.S. and Canada)
- Chewable tablets (U.S.)

Ferrous Gluconate
- Capsules (U.S.)
- Elixir (U.S.)
- Syrup (Canada)
- Tablets (U.S. and Canada)

Ferrous Sulfate
- Capsules (U.S.)
- Extended-release capsules (U.S. and Canada)
- Elixir (U.S.)
- Solution (U.S. and Canada)
- Tablets (U.S. and Canada)
- Enteric-coated tablets (U.S. and Canada)
- Extended-release tablets (U.S. and Canada)

Iron-Polysaccharide
- Capsules (U.S.)
- Elixir (U.S.)
- Tablets (U.S.)

*Parenteral*

Iron Dextran
- Injection (U.S. and Canada)

Iron Sorbitol
- Injection (Canada)

## Importance of Diet

Many nutritionists recommend that, if possible, people should get all the iron they need from foods. However, many people do not get enough iron from food. For example, people on weight-loss diets may consume too little food to provide enough iron. Others may need more iron than normal. For such people, an iron supplement is important.

In order to get enough vitamins and minerals in your diet, it is important that you eat a balanced and varied diet. Follow carefully any diet program your doctor may recommend. For your specific vitamin and/or mineral needs, ask your doctor or dietitian for a list of appropriate foods.

Experts have developed a list of Recommended Dietary Allowances (RDA) of iron. The RDA are not an exact number but a general idea of how much you need every day. The RDA do not cover amounts needed for problems caused by a serious lack of iron.

The daily RDA for iron are as follows (Note that the RDA are expressed as an actual amount of iron. The drug form [e.g., ferrous fumarate, ferrous gluconate, ferrous sulfate] has a different strength):
- Infants and children—
  Birth to 6 months of age: 6 milligrams (mg) per day.
  6 months to 10 years of age: 10 mg per day.
- Adolescent and adult males—
  11 to 18 years of age: 12 mg per day.
  19 years of age and over: 10 mg per day.
- Adolescent and adult females—
  11 to 50 years of age: 15 mg per day.
  51 years of age and over: 10 mg per day.
- Pregnant females—30 mg per day.
- Breast-feeding females—15 mg per day.

Iron is found in the diet in two forms—heme iron, which is well absorbed and nonheme iron, which is poorly absorbed. The best dietary source of absorbable iron (heme iron) is lean red meat. Chicken, turkey, and fish are also sources of iron, but they contain less than red meat. Foods rich in vitamin C (e.g., citrus fruits and fresh vegetables) eaten with small amounts of heme iron-containing foods, such as meat, may increase the amount of iron absorbed from cereals, beans, and other vegetables, which contain poorly absorbed iron (nonheme iron). Some foods (e.g., milk, eggs, spinach, fiber, coffee, tea) may decrease the amount of nonheme iron absorbed from foods. Additional iron may be added to food from cooking in iron pots.

## Before Using This Dietary Supplement

If you are taking this dietary supplement without a prescription, carefully read and follow any precautions on the label. For iron supplements, the following should be considered:

**Allergies**—Tell your doctor if you have ever had any unusual or allergic reaction to iron medicine. Also tell your health care professional if you are allergic to any other substances, such as foods, preservatives, or dyes.

**Pregnancy**—During the first 3 months of pregnancy, a proper diet usually provides enough iron. However, during the last 6 months, in order to meet the increased needs of the developing baby, an iron supplement may be recommended by your doctor. However, taking large amounts of a dietary supplement in pregnancy may be harmful to the mother and/or fetus and should be avoided.

**Breast-feeding**—Iron normally is present in breast milk in small amounts. When prescribed by a doctor, iron preparations are not known to cause problems during breast-feeding. However, nursing mothers are advised to check with their doctor before taking iron supplements or any other medication. Taking large amounts of a dietary supplement while breast-feeding may be harmful to the mother and/or infant and should be avoided.

**Children**—Iron supplements, when prescribed by your doctor, are not expected to cause different side effects in children than they do in adults. However, it is important to follow the directions carefully, since iron overdose in children is especially dangerous.

**Older adults**—Elderly people sometimes do not absorb iron as easily as younger adults and may need a larger dose. If you think you need to take an iron supplement, check with your doctor first. Only your doctor can decide if you need an iron supplement and how much you should take.

**Medicines or other dietary supplements**—Although certain medicines or dietary supplements should not be used together at all, in other cases they may be used together even if an interaction might occur. In these cases, your doctor may want to change the dose, or other precautions may be necessary. When you are taking iron supplements, it is especially important that your health care professional know if you are taking any of the following:

- Acetohydroxamic acid (e.g., Lithostat)—Use with iron supplements may cause either medicine to be less effective
- Dimercaprol—Iron supplements and dimercaprol may combine in the body to form a harmful chemical
- Etidronate or
- Tetracyclines (taken by mouth) (medicine for infection)—Use with iron supplements may make these medicines less effective; iron supplements should be taken 2 hours after etidronate or tetracycline

**Other medical problems**—The presence of other medical problems may affect the use of iron supplements. Make sure you tell your doctor if you have any other medical problems, especially:

- Arthritis (rheumatoid) or
- Asthma or allergies—The injected form of iron may make these conditions worse

- Blood disease (other than iron-deficiency anemia) or
- Colitis or other intestinal problems or
- Stomach ulcer—Iron supplements may make these conditions worse
- Kidney infection or
- Liver disease—Higher blood levels of the iron supplement may occur, which may increase the chance of side effects

## Proper Use of This Dietary Supplement

After you start using this dietary supplement, continue to return to your doctor to see if you are benefiting from the iron. Some blood tests may be necessary for this.

Iron is best taken on an empty stomach, with water or fruit juice (adults: full glass or 8 ounces; children: ½ glass or 4 ounces), about 1 hour before or 2 hours after meals. However, to lessen the possibility of stomach upset, iron may be taken with food or immediately after meals.

For safe and effective use of iron supplements:

- Follow your doctor's instructions if this dietary supplement was prescribed.
- Follow the manufacturer's package directions if you are treating yourself. If you think you still need iron after taking it for 1 or 2 months, check with your doctor.

*Liquid forms of iron supplement* tend to stain the teeth. To prevent, reduce, or remove these stains:

- Mix each dose in water, fruit juice, or tomato juice. You may use a drinking tube or straw to help keep the iron supplement from getting on the teeth.
- When doses of liquid iron supplement are to be given by dropper, the dose may be placed well back on the tongue and followed with water or juice.
- Iron stains on teeth can usually be removed by brushing with baking soda (sodium bicarbonate) or medicinal peroxide (hydrogen peroxide 3%).

**Dosing**—The dose of iron for prevention of iron deficiency is based on the Recommended Dietary Allowances (RDA). See the *Importance of Diet* section for the RDA for iron.

**Missed dose**—If you miss a dose of this dietary supplement, skip the missed dose and go back to your regular dosing schedule. Do not double doses.

**Storage**—To store this dietary supplement:

- Keep out of the reach of children because iron overdose is especially dangerous in children. As few as 3 or 4 adult iron tablets can cause serious poisoning in small children. Vitamin-iron products for use during pregnancy and flavored vitamins with iron often cause iron overdose in small children.
- Store away from heat and direct light.
- Do not store in the bathroom, near the kitchen sink, or in other damp places. Heat or moisture may cause the dietary supplement to break down.
- Keep the liquid form of this dietary supplement from freezing.

- Do not keep outdated dietary supplements or those no longer needed. Be sure that any discarded dietary supplement is out of the reach of children.

## Precautions While Using This Dietary Supplement

When iron is combined with certain foods it may lose much of its value. If you are taking iron, the following foods should be avoided or only taken in very small amounts for at least 1 hour before or 2 hours after you take iron:

Cheese and yogurt
Eggs
Milk
Spinach
Tea or coffee
Whole-grain breads and cereals and bran

Do not take iron supplements and antacids or calcium supplements at the same time. It is best to space doses of these 2 products 1 to 2 hours apart, to get the full benefit from each medicine or dietary supplement.

If you are taking iron supplement *without a doctor's prescription:*

- Do not take iron supplements by mouth if you are receiving iron injections. To do so may result in iron poisoning.
- Do not regularly take large amounts of iron for longer than 6 months without checking with your doctor. People differ in their need for iron, and those with certain medical conditions can gradually become poisoned by taking too much iron over a period of time. Also, unabsorbed iron can mask the presence of blood in the stool, which may delay discovery of a serious condition.
- Your total daily intake of iron must be considered, not just the amount contained in iron supplements. Iron-fortified bread, cereals, and other foods must be added for the total amount.

If you have been taking a long-acting or coated iron tablet and your stools have *not* become black, check with your doctor. The tablets may not be breaking down properly in your stomach, and you may not be receiving enough iron.

It is important to keep iron preparations out of the reach of children. Keep a 1-ounce bottle of *syrup* of ipecac available at home to be taken in case of an iron overdose emergency when a doctor, poison control center, or emergency room orders its use.

*If you think you or anyone else has taken an overdose of iron medicine:*

- *Immediate medical attention is very important.*
- *Call your doctor, a poison control center, or the nearest hospital emergency room at once.* Always keep these phone numbers readily available.
- *Follow any instructions given to you.* If syrup of ipecac has been ordered and given, do not delay going to the emergency room while waiting for the ipecac syrup to empty the stomach, since it may require 20 to 30 minutes to show results.
- *Go to the emergency room without delay.*
- *Take the container of iron medicine with you.*

Early signs of iron overdose may not appear for up to 60 minutes or more. Do not delay going to the emergency room while waiting for signs to appear.

## Side Effects of This Dietary Supplement

Along with its needed effects, a dietary supplement may cause some unwanted effects. Although not all of these effects may occur, if they do occur they may need medical attention.

Check with your doctor if any of the following side effects occur:

*More common—with the injection only*

Backache or muscle pain; chills; dizziness; fever with increased sweating; headache; metallic taste; nausea or vomiting; numbness, pain, or tingling of hands or feet; pain or redness at injection site; skin rash or hives; troubled breathing

*More common—when taken by mouth only*

Abdominal or stomach pain, cramping, or soreness (continuing)

*Less common or rare—when taken by mouth only*

Chest or throat pain, especially when swallowing; stools with signs of blood (red or black color)

*Early symptoms of iron overdose*

Diarrhea (may contain blood); nausea; stomach pain or cramping (sharp); vomiting, severe (may contain blood)

Note: Symptoms of iron overdose may not occur for up to 60 minutes or more after the overdose was taken. By this time you should have had emergency room treatment. Do not delay going to emergency room while waiting for signs to appear.

*Late symptoms of iron overdose*

Bluish-colored lips, fingernails, and palms of hands; convulsions (seizures); drowsiness; pale, clammy skin; unusual tiredness or weakness; weak and fast heartbeat

Other side effects may occur that usually do not need medical attention. These side effects may go away during treatment as your body adjusts to the dietary supplement. However, check with your doctor if any of the following side effects continue or are bothersome:

*More common*

Constipation; diarrhea; nausea; vomiting

*Less common*

Darkened urine; heartburn

Stools commonly become dark green or black when iron preparations are taken by mouth. This is caused by unabsorbed iron and is harmless. However, in rare cases, black stools of a sticky consistency may occur along with other side effects such as red streaks in the stool, cramping, soreness, or sharp pains in the stomach or abdominal area. Check with your doctor immediately if these side effects appear.

If you have been receiving injections of iron, you may notice a brown discoloration of your skin. This color usually fades within several weeks or months.

Other side effects not listed above may also occur in some patients. If you notice any other effects, check with your doctor.

Revised: 04/16/92
Interim revision(s): 06/29/92; 08/22/94

# ISOMETHEPTENE, DICHLORALPHENAZONE, AND ACETAMINOPHEN   Systemic

Some commonly used brand names are:

**In the U.S.—**

| | |
|---|---|
| Amidrine | Migquin |
| I.D.A. | Migratine |
| Iso-Acetazone | Migrazone |
| Isocom | Migrend |
| Midchlor | Migrex |
| Midrin | Mitride |
| Migrapap | |

## Description

Isometheptene (eye-soe-meth-EP-teen), dichloralphenazone (dye-klor-al-FEN-a-zone), and acetaminophen (a-seat-a-MIN-oh-fen) combination is used to treat certain kinds of headaches, such as "tension" headaches and migraine headaches. This combination is not used regularly (for example, every day) to prevent headaches. It should be taken only after headache pain begins, or after a warning sign that a migraine is coming appears. Isometheptene helps to relieve throbbing headaches, but it is not an ordinary pain reliever. Dichloralphenazone helps you to relax, and acetaminophen relieves pain.

This medicine is available only with your doctor's prescription, in the following dosage form:

*Oral*
- Capsules (U.S.)

## Before Using This Medicine

In deciding to use a medicine, the risks of taking the medicine must be weighed against the good it will do. This is a decision you and your doctor will make. For this combination medicine, the following should be considered:

**Allergies**—Tell your doctor if you have ever had any unusual or allergic reaction to acetaminophen or to this combination medicine. Also tell your health care professional if you are allergic to any other substances, such as foods, preservatives, or dyes.

**Pregnancy**—Studies with this combination medicine have not been done in either humans or animals.

**Breast-feeding**—Acetaminophen passes into the breast milk in small amounts. However, this medicine has not been shown to cause problems in nursing babies.

**Children**—Studies with this medicine have been done only in adult patients, and there is no specific information about its use in children.

**Older adults**—Many medicines have not been tested in older people. Therefore, it may not be known whether they work exactly the same way they do in younger adults or if they cause different side effects or problems in older people. There is no specific information comparing use of this combination medicine in the elderly with use in other age groups.

**Other medicines**—Although certain medicines should not be used together at all, in other cases two different medicines may be used together even if an interaction might occur. In these cases, your doctor may want to change the dose, or other precautions may be necessary. When you are taking this combination medicine, it is especially important that your health care professional know if you are taking any of the following:

- Monoamine oxidase (MAO) inhibitors (furazolidone [e.g., Furoxone], isocarboxazid [e.g., Marplan], phenelzine [e.g., Nardil], procarbazine [e.g., Matulane], selegiline [e.g., Eldepryl], tranylcypromine [e.g., Parnate])—Taking this combination medicine while you are taking or within 2 weeks of taking a monoamine oxidase (MAO) inhibitor may increase the chance of side effects

**Other medical problems**—The presence of other medical problems may affect the use of this medicine. Make sure you tell your doctor if you have any other medical problems, especially:

- Alcohol abuse or
- Heart attack (recent) or
- Heart or blood vessel disease or
- Kidney disease or
- Liver disease or
- Stroke (recent) or
- Virus infection of the liver (viral hepatitis)—The chance of side effects may be increased
- Glaucoma, not well controlled, or
- High blood pressure (hypertension), not well controlled—The isometheptene in this combination medicine may make these conditions worse

## Proper Use of This Medicine

*Take this medicine only as directed by your doctor.* Do not take more of it, do not take it more often than directed, and do not take it every day for several days in a row. If the amount you are to take does not relieve your headache, check with your doctor. If a headache medicine is used too often, it may lose its effectiveness or even cause a type of physical dependence. If this occurs, your headaches may actually get worse. Also, taking too much acetaminophen can cause liver damage.

This medicine works best if you:

- *Take it as soon as the headache begins.* If you get warning signals of a migraine, take this medicine as soon as you are sure that the migraine is coming. This may even stop the headache pain from occurring.
- *Lie down in a quiet, dark room until you are feeling better.*

People who get a lot of headaches may need to take a different medicine to help prevent headaches. *It is important that you follow your doctor's directions, even if your headaches continue to occur.* Headache-preventing medicines may take several weeks to start working. Even after they do start working, your headaches may not go away completely. However, your headaches should occur less often, and they should be less severe and easier to relieve, than before. This will reduce the amount of headache relievers that you need. If you do not notice any improvement after several weeks of headache-preventing treatment, check with your doctor.

**Dosing**—The dose of this combination medicine will be different for different patients. *Follow your doctor's orders or the directions on the label.* The following information includes only the average doses of this medicine. *If your dose is different, do not change it unless your doctor tells you to do so.*

- *For "tension" headaches:*
  —Adults: 1 or 2 capsules every 4 hours, as needed. Not more than 8 capsules a day.
  —Children: Dose must be determined by the doctor.
- *For migraine headaches:*
  —Adults: 2 capsules for the first dose, then 1 capsule every hour, as needed. Not more than 5 capsules in 12 hours.
  —Children: Dose must be determined by the doctor.

**Storage**—To store this medicine:

- Keep out of the reach of children.
- Store away from heat and direct light.
- Do not store in the bathroom, near the kitchen sink, or in other damp places. Heat and moisture may cause the medicine to break down.
- Do not keep outdated medicine or medicine no longer needed. Be sure that any discarded medicine is out of the reach of children.

## Precautions While Using This Medicine

*Check with your doctor:*

- *If the medicine stops working as well as it did when you first started using it.* This may mean that you

are in danger of becoming dependent on the medicine. *Do not try to get better relief by increasing the dose.*

- *If you are having headaches more often than you did before you started using this medicine.* This is especially important if a new headache occurs within 1 day after you took your last dose of headache medicine, headaches begin to occur every day, or a headache continues for several days in a row. This may mean that you are dependent on the medicine. *Continuing to take this medicine will cause even more headaches later on.* Your doctor can give you advice on how to relieve the headaches.

*Check the labels of all nonprescription (over-the-counter [OTC]) and prescription medicines you now take.* Taking other medicines that contain acetaminophen together with this medicine may lead to an overdose. If you have any questions about this, check with your health care professional.

This medicine may cause some people to become drowsy, dizzy, or less alert than they are normally. These effects may be especially severe if you also take CNS depressants (medicines that slow down the nervous system, possibly causing drowsiness) together with this medicine. Some examples of CNS depressants are antihistamines or medicine for hay fever, other allergies, or colds; sedatives, tranquilizers, or sleeping medicine; prescription pain medicine or narcotics; barbiturates; medicine for seizures; muscle relaxants; antiemetics (medicines that prevent or relieve nausea or vomiting), and anesthetics. If you are not able to lie down for a while, *make sure you know how you react to this medicine or combination of medicines before you drive, use machines, or do anything else that could be dangerous if you are drowsy or dizzy or are not alert.*

*Do not drink alcoholic beverages while taking this medicine.* To do so may increase the chance of liver damage caused by acetaminophen, especially if you drink large amounts of alcoholic beverages regularly. Also, because drinking alcoholic beverages may make your headaches worse or cause new headaches to occur, people who often get headaches should probably avoid alcohol.

## Side Effects of This Medicine

Along with its needed effects, a medicine may cause some unwanted effects. Although not all of these side effects may occur, if they do occur they may need medical attention.

Check with your doctor as soon as possible if any of the following side effects occur:

*Less common*
  Unusual tiredness or weakness
*Rare*
  Black, tarry stools; blood in urine or stools; pinpoint red spots on skin; skin rash, hives, or itching; sore throat and fever; unusual bleeding or bruising; yellow eyes or skin

*Symptoms of dependence on this medicine*
> Headaches, more severe and/or more frequent than before

*Symptoms of acetaminophen overdose*
> Diarrhea; increased sweating; loss of appetite; nausea or vomiting; pain, tenderness, and/or swelling in the upper abdominal (stomach) area; stomach cramps or pain

Other side effects may occur that usually do not need medical attention. These side effects may go away during treatment as your body adjusts to the medicine. However,

check with your doctor if any of the following side effects continue or are bothersome:

*More common*
> Drowsiness

*Rare*
> Dizziness; fast or irregular heartbeat

Other side effects not listed above may also occur in some patients. If you notice any other effects, check with your doctor.

Revised: 08/18/92

# ISONIAZID  Systemic

Some commonly used brand names are:
**In the U.S.—**
  Laniazid                     Nydrazid
  Generic name product may also be available.
**In Canada—**
  Isotamine                    PMS Isoniazid
Another commonly used name is INH.

## Description

Isoniazid (eye-soe-NYE-a-zid) is used to prevent or treat tuberculosis (TB). It may be given alone to prevent, or, in combination with other medicines, to treat TB. This medicine may also be used for other problems as determined by your doctor.

This medicine may cause some serious side effects, including damage to the liver. Liver damage is more likely to occur in patients over 50 years of age. *You and your doctor should talk about the good this medicine will do, as well as the risks of taking it.*

*If you are being treated for active tuberculosis (TB): To help clear up your TB completely, you must keep taking this medicine for the full time of treatment, even if you begin to feel better. This is very important. It is also important that you do not miss any doses.*

Isoniazid is available only with your doctor's prescription, in the following dosage forms:
*Oral*
  • Syrup (U.S. and Canada)
  • Tablets (U.S. and Canada)
*Parenteral*
  • Injection (U.S.)

## Before Using This Medicine

In deciding to use a medicine, the risks of taking the medicine must be weighed against the good it will do.

This is a decision you and your doctor will make. For isoniazid, the following should be considered:

**Allergies**—Tell your doctor if you have ever had any unusual or allergic reaction to isoniazid, ethionamide (e.g., Trecator-SC), pyrazinamide, or niacin (e.g., Nicobid, nicotinic acid). Also tell your health care professional if you are allergic to any other substances, such as foods, preservatives, or dyes.

**Diet**—Make certain your health care professional knows if you are on a low-sodium, low-sugar, or any other special diet. Most medicines contain more than just the active ingredient, and many liquid medicines contain alcohol.

**Pregnancy**—Isoniazid has not been shown to cause birth defects or other problems in humans or animals. Studies in rats and rabbits have shown that isoniazid may increase the risk of fetal death. However, tuberculosis is a very serious disease and many women have been treated with isoniazid during pregnancy with no problems to their babies.

**Breast-feeding**—Isoniazid passes into the breast milk. However, isoniazid has not been reported to cause problems in nursing babies. Also, there is not enough isoniazid in breast milk to protect or treat babies that have been exposed to tuberculosis.

**Children**—Isoniazid can cause serious side effects in any patient. Therefore, it is especially important that you discuss with the child's doctor the good that this medicine may do as well as the risks of using it.

**Older adults**—Hepatitis may be especially likely to occur in older patients, who are usually more sensitive than younger adults to the effects of isoniazid.

**Other medicines**—Although certain medicines should not be used together at all, in other cases two different medicines may be used together even if an interaction might occur. In these cases, your doctor may want to change the dose, or other precautions may be necessary. When

you are taking or receiving isoniazid it is especially important that your health care professional know if you are taking any of the following:

- Acetaminophen (e.g., Tylenol) (with long-term, high-dose use) or
- Amiodarone (e.g., Cordarone) or
- Anabolic steroids (nandrolone [e.g., Anabolin], oxandrolone [e.g., Anavar], oxymetholone [e.g., Anadrol], stanozolol [e.g., Winstrol]) or
- Androgens (male hormones) or
- Antithyroid agents (medicine for overactive thyroid) or
- Carmustine (e.g., BiCNU) or
- Chloroquine (e.g., Aralen) or
- Dantrolene (e.g., Dantrium) or
- Daunorubicin (e.g., Cerubidine) or
- Disulfiram (e.g., Antabuse) or
- Divalproex (e.g., Depakote) or
- Estrogens (female hormones) or
- Etretinate (e.g., Tegison) or
- Gold salts (medicine for arthritis) or
- Hydroxychloroquine (e.g., Plaquenil) or
- Mercaptopurine (e.g., Purinethol) or
- Methotrexate (e.g., Mexate) or
- Methyldopa (e.g., Aldomet) or
- Naltrexone (e.g., Trexan) (with long-term, high-dose use) or
- Oral contraceptives (birth control pills) containing estrogen or
- Other anti-infectives by mouth or by injection (medicine for infection) or
- Phenothiazines (acetophenazine [e.g., Tindal], chlorpromazine [e.g., Thorazine], fluphenazine [e.g., Prolixin], mesoridazine [e.g., Serentil], perphenazine [e.g., Trilafon], prochlorperazine [e.g., Compazine], promazine [e.g., Sparine], promethazine [e.g., Phenergan], thioridazine [e.g., Mellaril], trifluoperazine [e.g., Stelazine], triflupromazine [e.g., Vesprin], trimeprazine [e.g., Temaril]) or
- Plicamycin (e.g., Mithracin) or
- Valproic acid (e.g., Depakene)—These medicines may increase the chance of liver damage if taken with isoniazid
- Carbamazepine (e.g., Tegretol) or
- Phenytoin (e.g., Dilantin)—These medicines may increase the chance of liver damage if taken with isoniazid. There may also be an increased chance of side effects of carbamazepine and phenytoin
- Disulfiram (e.g., Antabuse)—This medicine may increase the chance of liver damage and side effects, such as dizziness, lack of coordination, irritability, and trouble in sleeping
- Ketoconazole (e.g., Nizoral) or
- Rifampin (e.g., Rifadin)—Use of these medicines with isoniazid can lower the blood levels of ketoconazole or rifampin, decreasing their effects

**Other medical problems**—The presence of other medical problems may affect the use of isoniazid. Make sure you tell your doctor if you have any other medical problems, especially:

- Alcohol abuse (or history of) or
- Liver disease—There may be an increased chance of hepatitis with daily drinking of alcohol or in patients with liver disease
- Kidney disease (severe)—There may be an increased chance of side effects in patients with severe kidney disease

- Seizure disorders such as epilepsy—There may be an increased chance of seizures (convulsions) in some patients

## Proper Use of This Medicine

If you are taking isoniazid by mouth and it upsets your stomach, take it with food. Antacids may also help. However, do not take aluminum-containing antacids within 1 hour of taking isoniazid. They may keep this medicine from working properly.

For patients taking the *oral liquid form* of isoniazid:

- Use a specially marked measuring spoon or other device to measure each dose accurately. The average household teaspoon may not hold the right amount of liquid.

To help clear up your tuberculosis (TB) completely, *it is very important that you keep taking this medicine for the full time of treatment,* even if you begin to feel better after a few weeks. You may have to take it every day for as long as 6 months to 2 years. *It is important that you do not miss any doses.*

Your doctor may also want you to take pyridoxine (e.g., Hexa-Betalin, vitamin B$_6$) every day to help prevent or lessen some of the side effects of isoniazid. This is not usually needed in children, who receive enough pyridoxine in their diet. If it is needed, *it is very important to take pyridoxine every day along with this medicine. Do not miss any doses.*

**Dosing**—The dose of isoniazid will be different for different patients. *Follow your doctor's orders or the directions on the label.* The following information includes only the average doses of isoniazid. *If your dose is different, do not change it* unless your doctor tells you to do so.

The number of tablets or teaspoonfuls of syrup that you take depends on the strength of the medicine.

- For *oral dosage forms* (tablets, syrup):
  —For prevention of tuberculosis:
  - Adults and teenagers—300 milligrams (mg) once a day.
  - Children—Dose is based on body weight. The usual dose is 10 mg per kilogram (kg) (4.5 mg per pound) of body weight, up to 300 mg, once a day.
  —For treatment of tuberculosis:
  - Adults and teenagers—300 mg once a day; or 15 mg per kg (6.8 mg per pound) of body weight, up to 900 mg, two times a week or three times a week, depending on the schedule your doctor chooses for you.
  - Children—Dose is based on body weight. The usual dose is 10 to 20 mg per kg (4.5 to 9.1 mg per pound) of body weight, up to 300 mg, once a day; or 20 to 40 mg per kg (9.1 to 18.2 mg per pound) of body weight, up to 900 mg, two times a week or three times a week, depending on the schedule your doctor chooses for you.

- For *injection* dosage form:
  —For prevention of tuberculosis:
  - Adults and teenagers—300 mg once a day.
  - Children—Dose is based on body weight. The usual dose is 10 mg per kg (4.5 mg per pound) of body weight, up to 300 mg, once a day.
  —For treatment of tuberculosis:
  - Adults and teenagers—300 mg once a day; or 15 mg per kg (6.8 mg per pound) of body weight, up to 900 mg, two times a week or three times a week, depending on the schedule your doctor chooses for you.
  - Children—Dose is based on body weight. The usual dose is 10 to 20 mg per kg (4.5 to 9.1 mg per pound) of body weight, up to 300 mg, once a day; or 20 to 40 mg per kg (9.1 to 18.2 mg per pound) of body weight, up to 900 mg, two times a week or three times a week, depending on the schedule your doctor chooses for you.

**Missed dose**—If you miss a dose of this medicine, take it as soon as possible. However, if it is almost time for your next dose, skip the missed dose and go back to your regular dosing schedule. Do not double doses.

**Storage**—To store this medicine:
- Keep out of the reach of children.
- Store away from heat and direct light.
- Do not store the tablet form of this medicine in the bathroom, near the kitchen sink, or in other damp places. Heat or moisture may cause the medicine to break down.
- Keep the oral liquid form of this medicine from freezing.
- Do not keep outdated medicine or medicine no longer needed. Be sure that any discarded medicine is out of the reach of children.

## Precautions While Using This Medicine

It is very important that your doctor check your progress at regular visits. Also, *check with your doctor immediately if blurred vision or loss of vision, with or without eye pain, occurs during treatment.* Your doctor may want you to have your eyes checked by an ophthalmologist (eye doctor).

If your symptoms do not improve within 2 to 3 weeks, or if they become worse, check with your doctor.

Certain foods such as cheese (Swiss or Cheshire) or fish (tuna, skipjack, or Sardinella) may rarely cause reactions in some patients taking isoniazid. Check with your doctor if redness or itching of the skin, hot feeling, fast or pounding heartbeat, sweating, chills or clammy feeling, headache, or lightheadedness occurs while you are taking this medicine.

Liver problems may be more likely to occur if you drink alcoholic beverages regularly while you are taking this medicine. Also, the regular use of alcohol may keep this medicine from working properly. Therefore, *you should strictly limit the amount of alcoholic beverages you drink while you are taking this medicine.*

*If this medicine causes you to feel very tired or very weak; or causes clumsiness; unsteadiness; a loss of appetite; nausea; numbness, tingling, burning, or pain in the hands and feet; or vomiting, check with your doctor immediately.* These may be early warning signs of more serious liver or nerve problems that could develop later.

*For diabetic patients:*
- *This medicine may cause false test results with some urine sugar tests.* Check with your doctor before changing your diet or the dosage of your diabetes medicine.

## Side Effects of This Medicine

Along with its needed effects, a medicine may cause some unwanted effects. Although not all of these side effects may occur, if they do occur they may need medical attention.

*Check with your doctor immediately* if any of the following side effects occur:

*More common*
 Clumsiness or unsteadiness; dark urine; loss of appetite; nausea or vomiting; numbness, tingling, burning, or pain in hands and feet; unusual tiredness or weakness; yellow eyes or skin

*Rare*
 Blurred vision or loss of vision, with or without eye pain; convulsions (seizures); fever and sore throat; joint pain; mental depression; mood or other mental changes; skin rash; unusual bleeding or bruising

Other side effects may occur that usually do not need medical attention. These side effects may go away during treatment as your body adjusts to the medicine. However, check with your doctor if any of the following side effects continue or are bothersome:

*More common*
 Diarrhea; stomach pain
*For injection form*
 Irritation at the place of injection

Dark urine and yellowing of the eyes or skin (signs of liver problems) are more likely to occur in patients over 50 years of age.

Other side effects not listed above may also occur in some patients. If you notice any other effects, check with your doctor.

Revised: 06/22/94

# ISOPROTERENOL AND PHENYLEPHRINE  Systemic

Some commonly used brand names are:

**In the U.S.—**
 Duo-Medihaler
**In Canada—**
 Duo-Medihaler

## Description

Isoproterenol (eye-soe-proe-TER-e-nole) and phenylephrine (fen-ill-EF-rin) combination medicine is used to treat bronchial asthma, bronchitis, emphysema, and other lung diseases. It relieves wheezing, shortness of breath, and troubled breathing.

This medicine is available only with your doctor's prescription, in the following dosage form:

*Inhalation*
 • Inhalation aerosol (U.S. and Canada)

## Before Using This Medicine

In deciding to use a medicine, the risks of taking the medicine must be weighed against the good it will do. This is a decision you and your doctor will make. For isoproterenol and phenylephrine combination, the following should be considered:

**Allergies**—Tell your doctor if you have ever had any unusual or allergic reaction to isoproterenol and phenylephrine or to medicines like them, such as amphetamines, ephedrine, epinephrine, metaproterenol, norepinephrine, phenylpropanolamine, pseudoephedrine, or terbutaline, or to other inhalation aerosol medicines. Also tell your health care professional if you are allergic to any other substances, such as foods, preservatives, or dyes.

**Pregnancy**—Studies on effects in pregnancy with isoproterenol and phenylephrine have not been done in either humans or animals. However, use of phenylephrine during late pregnancy or during labor may cause a lack of oxygen and slow heartbeat in the fetus.

**Breast-feeding**—It is not known whether isoproterenol and phenylephrine pass into the breast milk. Although most medicines pass into breast milk in small amounts, many of them may be used safely while breast-feeding. Mothers who are using this medicine and who wish to breast-feed should discuss this with their doctor.

**Children**—Studies on isoproterenol and phenylephrine combination have been done only in adult patients, and there is no specific information comparing use of isoproterenol and phenylephrine combination in children with use in other age groups.

**Older adults**—Many medicines have not been studied specifically in older people. Therefore, it may not be known whether they work exactly the same way they do in younger adults or if they cause different side effects or problems in older people. There is no specific information comparing use of isoproterenol and phenylephrine combination in the elderly with use in other age groups.

**Other medicines**—Although certain medicines should not be used together at all, in other cases two different medicines may be used together even if an interaction might occur. In these cases, your doctor may want to change the dose, or other precautions may be necessary. When you are taking isoproterenol and phenylephrine combination, it is especially important that your health care professional know if you are taking any of the following:

 • Beta-blockers (acebutolol [e.g., Sectral], atenolol [e.g., Tenormin], betaxolol [e.g., Kerlone], bisoprolol [e.g., Zebeta], carteolol [e.g., Cartrol], labetalol [e.g., Normodyne], metoprolol [e.g., Lopressor], nadolol [e.g., Corgard], oxprenolol [e.g., Trasicor], penbutolol [e.g., Levatol], pindolol [e.g., Visken], propranolol [e.g., Inderal], sotalol [e.g., Sotacor], timolol [e.g., Blocadren])—Taking these medicines with isoproterenol and phenylephrine combination may prevent either medicine from working properly
 • Cocaine—The effects of phenylephrine (contained in this combination medicine) may be increased
 • Digitalis glycosides (heart medicine)—Taking these medicines with isoproterenol and phenylephrine combination may increase the chance of irregular heartbeat
 • Ergoloid mesylates (e.g., Hydergine) or
 • Ergotamine (e.g., Cafergot, Gynergen)—The effects of either these medicines or phenylephrine (contained in this combination medicine) may be increased
 • Maprotiline (e.g., Ludiomil) or
 • Tricyclic antidepressants (amitriptyline [e.g., Elavil], amoxapine [e.g., Asendin], clomipramine (e.g., Anafranil), desipramine [e.g., Pertofrane], doxepin [e.g., Sinequan], imipramine [e.g., Tofranil], nortriptyline [e.g., Aventyl], protriptyline [e.g., Vivactil], trimipramine [e.g., Surmontil])—Taking isoproterenol and phenylephrine combination with these medicines may increase the effects on the heart, possibly resulting in fast or irregular heartbeat, severe high blood pressure, or fever
 • Methyldopa (e.g., Aldomet)—The effects of methyldopa may be decreased; also, the effects of phenylephrine (contained in this combination medicine) may be increased
 • Monoamine oxidase (MAO) inhibitors (furazolidone [e.g., Furoxone], isocarboxazid [e.g., Marplan], phenelzine [e.g., Nardil], procarbazine [e.g., Matulane], tranylcypromine [e.g., Parnate])—Taking phenylephrine (contained in this combination medicine) while you are taking or within 2 weeks of taking monoamine oxidase (MAO) inhibitors may increase the effects of phenylephrine, possibly resulting in serious side effects

**Other medical problems**—The presence of other medical problems may affect the use of isoproterenol and phenylephrine combination. Make sure you tell your doctor if you have any other medical problems, especially:

 • Diabetes mellitus (sugar diabetes)
 • Heart or blood vessel disease or
 • High blood pressure—The condition may become worse
 • Overactive thyroid—The chance of side effects may be increased

## Proper Use of This Medicine

This medicine usually comes with patient directions. Read them carefully before using this medicine.

Keep spray away from the eyes.

*Do not take more than 2 inhalations of this medicine at any one time,* unless otherwise directed by your doctor. Allow 1 to 5 minutes after the first inhalation to make certain that a second inhalation is necessary.

Save your applicator. Refill units of this medicine may be available.

*Use this medicine only as directed.* Do not use more of it and do not use it more often than your doctor ordered. To do so may increase the chance of serious side effects. Isoproterenol inhalation preparations have been reported to cause death when too much of the medicine was used.

**Dosing**—The dose of isoproterenol and phenylephrine combination will be different for different patients. *Follow your doctor's orders or the directions on the label.* The following information includes only the average doses of isoproterenol and phenylephrine combination. *If your dose is different, do not change it* unless your doctor tells you to do so.

* For *inhalation aerosol* dosage form:
  —For symptoms of bronchial asthma, bronchitis, emphysema, or other lung disease:
    * Adults and children 12 years of age and older— One inhalation (puff), repeated after two to five minutes if necessary, four to six times a day.
    * Children up to 12 years of age—Dose must be determined by your doctor.

**Storage**—To store this medicine:
* Keep out of the reach of children.
* Store away from heat and direct sunlight.
* Keep the medicine from freezing.
* Do not puncture, break, or burn container, even if it is empty.
* Do not keep outdated medicine or medicine no longer needed. Be sure that any discarded medicine is out of the reach of children.

## Precautions While Using This Medicine

*If you still have trouble breathing after using this medicine, or if your condition becomes worse, check with your doctor at once.*

If you are also using the inhalation aerosol form of a corticosteroid (cortisone-like medicine, such as beclomethasone, dexamethasone, flunisolide, or triamcinolone) or ipratropium, *use the isoproterenol and phenylephrine inhalation aerosol first and then wait about 5 minutes before using the corticosteroid or ipratropium inhalation aerosol,* unless otherwise directed by your doctor. This will allow the corticosteroid or ipratropium inhalation aerosol to better reach the passages of the lungs (bronchioles) after isoproterenol and phenylephrine inhalation aerosol opens them.

## Side Effects of This Medicine

Along with its needed effects, a medicine may cause some unwanted effects. Although not all of these side effects may occur, if they do occur they may need medical attention.

Check with your doctor as soon as possible if any of the following side effects occur:
*Rare*
    Chest pain; irregular heartbeat
*Symptoms of overdose*
    Chest pain (continuing or severe); dizziness or lightheadedness (continuing or severe); fast, slow, or pounding heartbeat (continuing); headache (continuing or severe); increase in blood pressure; irregular heartbeat (continuing or severe); nausea or vomiting (continuing or severe); sensation of fullness in head; tingling in hands or feet; trembling (severe); unusual anxiety, nervousness, or restlessness; weakness (severe)

Other side effects may occur that usually do not need medical attention. These side effects may go away during treatment as your body adjusts to the medicine. However, check with your doctor if any of the following side effects continue or are bothersome:
*More common*
    Nervousness; restlessness; trouble in sleeping
*Less common*
    Dizziness or lightheadedness; fast or pounding heartbeat; flushing or redness of face or skin; headache; increased sweating; nausea or vomiting; trembling; weakness

This medicine may cause the saliva to turn pinkish to red in color. This is to be expected while you are using this medicine.

Other side effects not listed above may also occur in some patients. If you notice any other effects, check with your doctor.

Revised: August 1990
Interim revision: 09/02/94

# ISOTRETINOIN    Systemic

Some commonly used brand names are:

**In the U.S.—**
Accutane

**In Canada—**
Accutane Roche

## Description

Isotretinoin (eye-soe-TRET-i-noyn) is used to treat severe, disfiguring nodular acne. It should be used only after other acne medicines have been tried and have failed to help the acne. Isotretinoin may also be used to treat other skin diseases as determined by your doctor.

*Isotretinoin must not be used to treat women who are able to bear children unless other forms of treatment have been tried first and have failed. Isotretinoin must not be taken during pregnancy, because it causes birth defects in humans. If you are able to bear children, it is very important that you read, understand, and follow the pregnancy warnings for isotretinoin.*

This medicine is available only with your doctor's prescription and should be prescribed only by a doctor who has special knowledge in the diagnosis and treatment of severe, uncontrollable cystic acne.

Isotretinoin is available in the following dosage form:

*Oral*
- Capsules (U.S. and Canada)

## Before Using This Medicine

*Isotretinoin comes with patient information. It is very important that you read and understand this information. Be sure to ask your doctor about anything you do not understand.*

In deciding to use a medicine, the risks of taking the medicine must be weighed against the good it will do. This is a decision you and your doctor will make. For isotretinoin, the following should be considered:

**Allergies**—Tell your doctor if you have ever had any unusual or allergic reaction to isotretinoin, etretinate, tretinoin, or vitamin A preparations. Also tell your health care professional if you are allergic to any other substances, such as foods, preservatives, or dyes.

**Pregnancy**—*Isotretinoin must not be taken during pregnancy, because it causes birth defects in humans. In addition, isotretinoin must not be taken if there is a chance that you may become pregnant during treatment or within one month following treatment.* Women who are able to have children must have a pregnancy blood test within 2 weeks before beginning treatment with isotretinoin to make sure they are not pregnant. Treatment with isotretinoin will then be started on the second or third day of the woman's next normal menstrual period. In addition, you must have a pregnancy blood test each month while you are taking this medicine and one month after treatment is completed. Also, *isotretinoin must not be*

*taken unless an effective form of contraception (birth control) has been used for at least 1 month before the beginning of treatment. Contraception must be continued during the period of treatment, which is up to 20 weeks, and for 1 month after isotretinoin is stopped. Be sure you have discussed this information with your doctor. In addition, you will be asked to sign an informed consent form stating that you understand the above information.*

**Breast-feeding**—It is not known whether isotretinoin passes into the breast milk. However, isotretinoin is not recommended during breast-feeding, because it may cause unwanted effects in nursing babies.

**Children**—Children may be especially sensitive to the effects of isotretinoin. This may increase the chance of side effects during treatment.

**Older adults**—Many medicines have not been studied specifically in older people. Therefore, it may not be known whether they work exactly the same way they do in younger adults or if they cause different side effects or problems in older people. There is no specific information comparing use of isotretinoin in the elderly with use in other age groups.

**Other medicines**—Although certain medicines should not be used together at all, in other cases two different medicines may be used together even if an interaction might occur. In these cases, your doctor may want to change the dose, or other precautions may be necessary. When you are using isotretinoin, it is especially important that your health care professional know if you are using any of the following:

- Etretinate (e.g., Tegison) or
- Tretinoin (vitamin A acid) (e.g., Retin-A) or
- Vitamin A or any preparation containing vitamin A—Use of isotretinoin with these medicines will result in an increase in side effects
- Tetracyclines (medicine for infection)—Use of isotretinoin with these medicines may increase the chance of a side effect called pseudotumor cerebri, which is a swelling of the brain

**Other medical problems**—The presence of other medical problems may affect the use of isotretinoin. Make sure you tell your doctor if you have any other medical problems, especially:

- Alcoholism or excess use of alcohol (or history of) or
- Diabetes mellitus (sugar diabetes) (or a family history of) or
- Family history of high triglyceride (a fat-like substance) levels in the blood or
- Severe weight problems—Use of isotretinoin may increase blood levels of triglyceride (a fat-like substance), which may increase the chance of heart or blood vessel problems in patients who have a family history of high triglycerides, are greatly overweight, are diabetic, or use a lot of alcohol. For persons with diabetes mellitus, use of isotretinoin may also change blood sugar levels

## Proper Use of This Medicine

*It is very important that you take isotretinoin only as directed.* Do not take more of it, do not take it more often, and do not take it for a longer time than your doctor ordered. To do so may increase the chance of side effects.

**Dosing**—The dose of isotretinoin will be different for different patients. *Follow your doctor's orders or the directions on the label.* The following information includes only the average doses of isotretinoin. *If your dose is different, do not change it* unless your doctor tells you to do so.

The number of capsules that you take depends on the strength of the medicine. Also, *the number of doses you take each day, the time allowed between doses, and the length of time you take the medicine depend on the medical problem for which you are taking isotretinoin.*

- For *oral* dosage form (capsules):
  —For acne:
    - Adults and teenagers—Dose is based on body weight and must be determined by your doctor. The usual dose is 0.5 to 1 milligram (mg) per kilogram (kg) (0.23 to 0.45 mg per pound) of body weight a day, divided into two doses.
    - Children—Use is usually not recommended.

**Missed dose**—If you miss a dose of this medicine, take it as soon as possible. However, if it is almost time for your next dose, skip the missed dose and go back to your regular dosing schedule. Do not double doses.

**Storage**—To store this medicine:
- Keep out of the reach of children.
- Store away from heat and direct light.
- Do not store in the bathroom, near the kitchen sink, or in other damp places. Heat or moisture may cause the medicine to break down.
- Do not keep outdated medicine or medicine no longer needed. Be sure that any discarded medicine is out of the reach of children.

## Precautions While Using This Medicine

Your doctor should check your progress at regular visits to make sure this medicine does not cause unwanted effects.

*Isotretinoin causes birth defects in humans if taken during pregnancy. Therefore, if you suspect that you may have become pregnant, stop taking this medicine immediately and check with your doctor.*

*Do not donate blood to a blood bank while you are taking isotretinoin or for 30 days after you stop taking it.* This is to prevent the possibility of a pregnant patient receiving the blood.

*Do not take vitamin A or any vitamin supplement containing vitamin A while taking this medicine,* unless otherwise directed by your doctor. To do so may increase the chance of side effects.

Drinking too much alcohol while taking this medicine may cause high triglyceride (fat-like substance) levels in the blood and possibly increase the chance of unwanted effects on the heart and blood vessels. Therefore, *while taking this medicine, it is best that you do not drink alcoholic beverages or that you at least reduce the amount you usually drink.* If you have any questions about this, check with your doctor.

For diabetic patients:
- This medicine may affect blood sugar levels. If you notice a change in the results of your blood or urine sugar tests or if you have any questions, check with your doctor.

In some patients, isotretinoin may cause a decrease in night vision. This decrease may occur suddenly. If it does occur, *do not drive, use machines, or do anything else that could be dangerous if you are not able to see well.* Also, check with your doctor.

Isotretinoin may cause dryness of the eyes. Therefore, if you wear contact lenses, your eyes may be more sensitive to them during the time you are taking isotretinoin and for up to about 2 weeks after you stop taking it. To help relieve dryness of the eyes, check with your doctor about using an eye lubricating solution, such as artificial tears. If eye inflammation occurs, check with your doctor.

Some people who take this medicine may become more sensitive to sunlight than they are normally. When you first begin taking this medicine, avoid too much sun and do not use a sunlamp until you see how you react to the sun, especially if you tend to burn easily. If you have a severe reaction, check with your doctor.

Isotretinoin may cause dryness of the mouth and nose. For temporary relief of mouth dryness, use sugarless candy or gum, melt bits of ice in your mouth, or use a saliva substitute. However, if dry mouth continues for more than 2 weeks, check with your medical doctor or dentist. Continuing dryness of the mouth may increase the chance of dental disease, including tooth decay, gum disease, and fungus infections.

For patients taking isotretinoin for acne:
- When you begin taking isotretinoin, your acne may seem to get worse before it gets better. If irritation or other symptoms of your condition become severe, check with your doctor.

## Side Effects of This Medicine

Along with its needed effects, a medicine may cause some unwanted effects. Although not all of these side effects may occur, if they do occur they may need medical attention.

Check with your doctor as soon as possible if any of the following side effects occur:
*More common*
  Burning, redness, itching, or other sign of eye inflammation; nosebleeds; scaling, redness, burning, pain, or other sign of inflammation of lips

*Less common*

Mental depression; skin infection or rash

*Rare*

Abdominal or stomach pain (severe); bleeding or inflammation of gums; blurred vision or other changes in vision; diarrhea (severe); headache (severe or continuing); mood changes; nausea and vomiting; pain or tenderness of eyes; rectal bleeding; yellow eyes or skin

Other side effects may occur that usually do not need medical attention. These side effects may go away during treatment as your body adjusts to the medicine. However, check with your doctor if any of the following side effects continue or are bothersome:

*More common*

Dryness of mouth or nose; dryness or itching of skin

*Less common*

Dryness of eyes; headache (mild); increased sensitivity of skin to sunlight; pain, tenderness, or stiffness in muscles, bones, or joints; peeling of skin on palms of hands or soles of feet; stomach upset; thinning of hair; unusual tiredness

Other side effects not listed above may also occur in some patients. If you notice any other effects, check with your doctor.

Revised: June 1990
Interim revision: 07/14/94

---

# ISOXSUPRINE   Systemic

A commonly used brand name in the U.S. and Canada is Vasodilan.

Generic name product may also be available in the U.S.

## Description

Isoxsuprine (eye-SOX-syoo-preen) belongs to the group of medicines called vasodilators. Vasodilators increase the size of blood vessels. Isoxsuprine is used to treat problems resulting from poor blood circulation.

It may also be used for other conditions as determined by your doctor.

Isoxsuprine is available only with your doctor's prescription, in the following dosage forms:

*Oral*

• Tablets (U.S. and Canada)

*Parenteral*

• Injection (Canada)

## Before Using This Medicine

In deciding to use a medicine, the risks of taking the medicine must be weighed against the good it will do. This is a decision you and your doctor will make. For isoxsuprine, the following should be considered:

**Allergies**—Tell your doctor if you have ever had any unusual or allergic reaction to isoxsuprine. Also tell your health care professional if you are allergic to any other substances, such as foods, preservatives, or dyes.

**Pregnancy**—Isoxsuprine has not been shown to cause birth defects in humans. However, isoxsuprine given shortly before delivery may cause fast heartbeat and other problems (low blood sugar, bowel problems, low blood pressure) in the newborn.

**Breast-feeding**—Isoxsuprine has not been reported to cause problems in nursing babies.

**Older adults**—Many medicines have not been studied specifically in older people. Therefore, it may not be known whether they work exactly the same way they do in younger adults or if they cause different side effects or problems in older people. There is no specific informaiton comparing use of isoxsuprine in the elderly with use in other age groups. However, isoxsuprine may reduce tolerance to cold temperatures in elderly patients.

**Other medicines**—Although certain medicines should not be used together at all, in other cases two different medicines may be used together even if an interaction might occur. In these cases, your doctor may want to change the dose, or other precautions may be necessary. Tell your health care professional if you are taking any other prescription or nonprescription (over-the-counter [OTC]) medicine, or if you smoke.

**Other medical problems**—The presence of other medical problems may affect the use of isoxsuprine. Make sure you tell your doctor if you have any other medical problems, especially:

• Angina (chest pain) or
• Bleeding problems or
• Glaucoma or
• Hardening of the arteries or
• Heart attack (recent) or
• Stroke (recent)—The chance of side effects may be increased

## Proper Use of This Medicine

*If this medicine upsets your stomach, it may be taken with meals, milk, or antacids.*

**Dosing**—The dose of isoxsuprine will be different for different patients. *Follow your doctor's orders or the directions on the label.* The following information includes only the average doses of isoxsuprine. *If your dose is different, do not change it* unless your doctor tells you to do so.

The number of tablets that you take depends on the strength of the medicine.

- For *oral* dosage form (tablets):
  —For poor blood circulation:
    - Adults—10 to 20 milligrams (mg) three or four times a day.

**Missed dose**—If you miss a dose of this medicine, take it as soon as possible. However, if it is almost time for your next dose, skip the missed dose and go back to your regular dosing schedule. Do not double doses.

**Storage**—To store this medicine:

- Keep out of the reach of children.
- Store away from heat and direct light.
- Do not store in the bathroom, near the kitchen sink, or in other damp places. Heat or moisture may cause the medicine to break down.
- Do not keep outdated medicine or medicine no longer needed. Be sure that any discarded medicine is out of the reach of children.

---

## Precautions While Using This Medicine

It may take some time for this medicine to work. If you feel that the medicine is not working, do not stop taking it on your own. Instead, check with your doctor.

The helpful effects of this medicine may be decreased if you smoke. If you have any questions about this, check with your doctor.

*Dizziness may occur, especially when you get up from a lying or sitting position or climb stairs. Getting up slowly may help.* If this problem continues or gets worse, check with your doctor.

---

## Side Effects of This Medicine

Along with its needed effects, a medicine may cause some unwanted effects. Although not all of these side effects may occur, if they do occur they may need medical attention.

Check with your doctor as soon as possible if any of the following side effects occur:

*Rare*

Chest pain; dizziness or faintness (more common for injection); fast heartbeat (more common for injection); shortness of breath; skin rash

Other side effects may occur that usually do not need medical attention. These side effects may go away during treatment as your body adjusts to the medicine. However, check with your doctor if the following side effects continue or are bothersome:

*Less common*

Nausea or vomiting (more common for injection)

Other side effects not listed above may also occur in some patients. If you notice any other effects, check with your doctor.

---

## Additional Information

Although this use is not included in U.S. product labeling, isoxsuprine is used in certain women to stop premature labor.

*In addition to the above information, the following information applies when this medicine is used to stop premature labor:*

- Before you begin treatment with this medicine, tell your doctor if you have any of the following medical problems:
  Asthma
  Diabetes mellitus (sugar diabetes)
  Heart disease
  High blood pressure
  Overactive thyroid
- *Check with your doctor immediately:*
  —if your contractions begin again or your water breaks.
  —if you notice chest pain or shortness of breath while taking isoxsuprine.

---

Revised: 07/06/92
Interim revision: 07/15/94

---

# JAPANESE ENCEPHALITIS VIRUS VACCINE    Systemic†

A commonly used brand name in the U.S. is Je-Vax.

†Not commercially available in Canada.

## Description

Japanese encephalitis (in-cef-a-LY-tis) virus vaccine is an immunizing agent used to help prevent infection by the Japanese encephalitis virus. Japanese encephalitis is caused by the bite of a mosquito that lives in certain parts of Asia. The vaccine works by causing your body to produce its own protection (antibodies) against the virus.

This vaccine is available only from your doctor or other authorized health care professional, in the following dosage form:

*Parenteral*
- Injection (U.S.)

## Before Receiving This Vaccine

In deciding to use a medicine, the risks of receiving the medicine must be weighed against the good it will do. This is a decision you and your doctor will make. For Japanese encephalitis virus vaccine, the following should be considered:

**Allergies**—Tell your doctor if you have ever had any unusual or allergic reaction to thimerosal, formaldehyde, gelatin, or rodent protein or brain products. Also tell your health care professional if you are allergic to any other substances, such as foods, preservatives, or dyes.

**Pregnancy**—Studies on effects in pregnancy have not been done in either humans or animals.

**Breast-feeding**—It is not known whether this vaccine passes into breast milk. Although most medicines pass into breast milk in small amounts, many of them may be used safely while breast-feeding. Mothers who are receiving this vaccine and who wish to breast-feed should discuss this with their doctor.

**Children**—Studies on this vaccine have been done only in adults and children 1 year of age and older. There is no specific information comparing use of this vaccine in infants under 1 year of age with use in other age groups.

**Older adults**—Many medicines have not been studied specifically in older people. Therefore, it may not be known whether they work exactly the same way they do in younger adults. Although there is no specific information comparing use of Japanese encephalitis virus vaccine in the elderly with use in other age groups, this vaccine is not expected to cause different side effects or problems in older people than it does in younger adults. In addition, immunization may be especially useful for the elderly, since older persons may have a higher risk of illness following infection with the Japanese encephalitis virus.

**Other medical problems**—The presence of other medical problems may affect the use of this vaccine. Make sure you tell your doctor if you have any other medical problems, especially:
- Hives (history of)—May increase the chance of side effects of the vaccine

## Proper Use of This Vaccine

*It is important that you receive 3 doses of the vaccine.* If there is not enough time for you to get all 3 doses, you may get 2 doses of the vaccine. However, *2 doses of the vaccine will not protect you as well as 3 doses.*

*It is important that you receive all 3 doses of the vaccine at least 10 days before you plan on traveling out of the country.* There is a chance of side effects that do not show up right away, and, if they do occur, they may need medical attention. In addition, the 10 days will give your body time to produce antibodies against the Japanese encephalitis virus.

**Dosing**—The number of doses you receive and the time allowed between doses of Japanese encephalitis virus vaccine will be different for different patients.
- For help preventing Japanese encephalitis:
  —For *injection* dosage form:
    - Adults and children 1 year of age and older— One dose injected under the skin on days zero, seven, and thirty, for a total of three doses.
    - Children up to 1 year of age—Use and dose must be determined by your doctor.

## Precautions After Receiving This Vaccine

Since the vaccine may not protect everyone completely, *it is very important that you still use precautions to reduce your chance of mosquito bites.* These include using insect repellents and mosquito netting, wearing protective clothing, and staying indoors during twilight and after dark.

## Side Effects of This Vaccine

Along with its needed effects, a medicine may cause some unwanted effects. Although not all of these side effects may occur, if they do occur they may need medical attention. *It is very important that you tell your doctor about any side effect that occurs after a dose of the vaccine,* even if the side effect goes away without treatment. Some types of side effects may mean that you should not receive any more doses of the vaccine.

*Get emergency help immediately* if the following side effect occurs:
*Rare*
    Swelling of face, lips, eyelids, throat, tongue, hands, or feet

*Check with your doctor immediately* if any of the following side effects occur:

### Rare
Hives; tiredness or weakness (severe or unusual); wheezing or troubled breathing

Although the following side effects usually do not need medical attention and may go away on their own, *their presence may also mean that more serious side effects are about to occur*. Therefore, check with your doctor as soon as possible if any of the following side effects occur:

### More common
Tenderness, soreness, redness, or swelling at place of injection

### Less common
Abdominal pain; aches or pains in muscles; chills or fever; dizziness; general feeling of discomfort or illness; headache; itching or skin rash; nausea or vomiting

### Rare
Joint swelling

Other side effects not listed above may also occur in some patients. If you notice any other effects, check with your doctor.

Revised: 06/21/93

# KANAMYCIN Oral†

†Not commercially available in Canada.

## Description

Oral kanamycin (kan-a-MYE-sin) belongs to the family of medicines called antibiotics. It is used before surgery affecting the bowel to help prevent infection during surgery.

Kanamycin is available only with your doctor's prescription, in the following dosage form:

*Oral*
- Capsules (U.S.)

## Before Using This Medicine

In deciding to use a medicine, the risks of taking the medicine must be weighed against the good it will do. This is a decision you and your doctor will make. For oral kanamycin, the following should be considered:

**Allergies**—Tell your doctor if you have ever had any unusual or allergic reaction to oral kanamycin or to any related antibiotics such as amikacin (e.g., Amikin), gentamicin (e.g., Garamycin), kanamycin by injection (e.g., Kantrex), neomycin (e.g., Mycifradin), netilmicin (e.g., Netromycin), streptomycin, or tobramycin (e.g., Nebcin). Also tell your health care professional if you are allergic to any other substances, such as foods, preservatives, or dyes.

**Pregnancy**—Oral kanamycin has not been reported to cause birth defects or other problems in humans.

**Breast-feeding**—Oral kanamycin has not been reported to cause problems in nursing babies.

**Children**—Although there is no specific information comparing use of oral kanamycin in children with use in other age groups, this medicine is not expected to cause different side effects or problems in children than it does in adults.

**Older adults**—Many medicines have not been studied specifically in older people. Therefore, it may not be known whether they work exactly the same way they do in younger adults or if they cause different side effects or problems in older people. There is no specific information comparing use of oral kanamycin in the elderly with use in other age groups.

**Other medicines**—Although certain medicines should not be used together at all, in other cases two different medicines may be used together even if an interaction might occur. In these cases, your doctor may want to change the dose, or other precautions may be necessary. Tell your health care professional if you are taking any other prescription or nonprescription (over-the-counter [OTC]) medicine.

**Other medical problems**—The presence of other medical problems may affect the use of oral kanamycin. Make sure you tell your doctor if you have any other medical problems, especially:
- Blockage of the bowel—Oral kanamycin should never be used in patients who have a blockage of the bowel
- Eighth-cranial-nerve disease (loss of hearing and/or balance)—Use of oral kanamycin may increase problems related to hearing and/or balance
- Kidney disease or
- Ulcers of the bowel—Use of kanamycin in patients with either condition may cause an increase in side effects

## Proper Use of This Medicine

This medicine may be taken on a full or empty stomach.

*Keep taking this medicine for the full time of treatment. Do not miss any doses.*

**Dosing**—The dose of oral kanamycin will be different for different patients. *Follow your doctor's orders or the directions on the label.* The following information includes only the average doses of oral kanamycin. *If your dose is different, do not change it* unless your doctor tells you to do so.
- For *oral* dosage form (capsule):
  —For patients in a coma from liver disease:
    - Adults and children—2 to 3 grams every six hours.
  —For cleaning the bowel before surgery:
    - Adults and children—1 gram every hour for four hours; then, 1 gram every six hours for thirty-six to seventy-two hours.

**Missed dose**—For patients taking *oral kanamycin before any surgery affecting the bowel:*
- If you miss a dose of this medicine, take it as soon as possible. However, if it is almost time for your next dose, skip the missed dose and go back to your regular dosing schedule. Do not double doses.

**Storage**—To store this medicine:
- Keep out of the reach of children.
- Store away from heat and direct light.
- Do not store in the bathroom, near the kitchen sink, or in other damp places. Heat and moisture may cause the medicine to break down.
- Do not keep outdated medicine or medicine no longer needed. Be sure that any discarded medicine is out of the reach of children.

## Side Effects of This Medicine

Along with its needed effects, a medicine may cause some unwanted effects. Although not all of these side effects may occur, if they do occur they may need medical attention.

*Check with your doctor immediately* if any of the following side effects occur:

*Rare—with long-term use and high doses*
> Any loss of hearing; clumsiness; dizziness; greatly decreased frequency of urination or amount of urine; increased thirst; ringing or buzzing or a feeling of fullness in the ears; unsteadiness

Other side effects may occur that usually do not need medical attention. These side effects may go away during treatment as your body adjusts to the medicine. However, check with your doctor if any of the following side effects continue or are bothersome:

*More common*
> Diarrhea; nausea or vomiting

*Rare—with prolonged treatment*
> Increased amount of gas; light-colored, frothy, fatty-appearing stools

Other side effects not listed above may also occur in some patients. If you notice any other effects, check with your doctor.

Revised: 09/08/92
Interim revision: 03/17/94

# KAOLIN AND PECTIN    Oral

Some commonly used brand names are:
**In the U.S.—**
Kao-Spen                     K-P
Kapectolin
Generic product may also be available.
**In Canada—**
Donnagel-MB

## Description

Kaolin (KAY-oh-lin) and pectin (PEK-tin) combination medicine is used to treat diarrhea.

Kaolin is a clay-like powder believed to work by attracting and holding onto the bacteria or germ that may be causing the diarrhea.

This medicine is available without a prescription; however, the product's directions and warnings should be carefully followed. In addition, your doctor may have special instructions on the proper dose or use of kaolin and pectin combination medicine for your medical condition. Kaolin and pectin combination is available in the following dosage form:

*Oral*
> • Oral suspension (U.S. and Canada)

## Before Using This Medicine

If you are taking this medicine without a prescription, carefully read and follow any precautions on the label. For kaolin and pectin combination, the following should be considered:

**Pregnancy**—This medicine is not absorbed into the body and is not likely to cause problems.

**Breast-feeding**—This medicine is not absorbed into the body and is not likely to cause problems.

**Children**—The fluid loss caused by diarrhea may result in a severe condition. For this reason, antidiarrheals must not be given to young children (under 3 years of age) without first checking with their doctor. In older children with diarrhea, antidiarrheals may be used, but it is also very important that a sufficient amount of liquids be given to replace the fluid lost by the body. If you have any questions about this, check with your health care professional.

**Older adults**—The fluid loss caused by diarrhea may result in a severe condition. For this reason, elderly persons with diarrhea, in addition to using an antidiarrheal, must receive a sufficient amount of liquids to replace the fluid lost by the body. If you have any questions about this, check with your health care professional.

**Other medicines**—Although certain medicines should not be used together at all, in other cases two different medicines may be used together even if an interaction might occur. In these cases, your doctor may want to change the dose, or other precautions may be necessary. Tell your health care professional if you are taking any other prescription or nonprescription (over-the-counter [OTC]) medicine.

**Other medical problems**—The presence of other medical problems may affect the use of kaolin and pectin. Make sure you tell your doctor if you have any other medical problems, especially:
> • Dysentery—This condition may get worse; a different kind of treatment may be needed

## Proper Use of This Medicine

*Do not use kaolin and pectin combination to treat your diarrhea if you have a fever or if there is blood or mucus in your stools.* Contact your doctor.

Take this medicine, following the directions in the product package, after each loose bowel movement until the diarrhea is controlled, unless otherwise directed by your doctor.

*Importance of diet and fluid intake while treating diarrhea:*

- *In addition to using medicine for diarrhea, it is very important that you replace the fluid lost by the body and follow a proper diet.* For the first 24 hours you should eat gelatin and drink plenty of clear liquids, such as ginger ale, decaffeinated cola, decaffeinated tea, and broth. During the next 24 hours you may eat bland foods, such as cooked cereals, bread, crackers, and applesauce. Fruits, vegetables, fried or spicy foods, bran, candy, and caffeine and alcoholic beverages may make the condition worse.

- If too much fluid has been lost by the body due to the diarrhea, a serious condition may develop. Check with your doctor as soon as possible if any of the following signs or symptoms of too much fluid loss occur:

    Decreased urination
    Dizziness and lightheadedness
    Dryness of mouth
    Increased thirst
    Wrinkled skin

**Dosing**—The dose of kaolin and pectin combination will be different for different patients. *Follow your doctor's orders or the directions on the label.* The following information includes only the average doses of kaolin and pectin.

The number of tablespoonfuls of suspension that you take depends on the strength of the medicine.

- For diarrhea:
    —For *oral* dosage form (suspension):
    - Adults—The usual dose is 4 to 8 tablespoonfuls (60 to 120 milliliters [mL]) taken after each loose bowel movement.
    - Children 12 years of age and over—The usual dose is 3 to 4 tablespoonfuls (45 to 60 mL) taken after each loose bowel movement.
    - Children 6 to 12 years of age—The usual dose is 2 to 4 tablespoonfuls (30 to 60 mL) taken after each loose bowel movement.
    - Children 3 to 6 years of age—The usual dose is 1 to 2 tablespoonfuls (15 to 30 mL) taken after each loose bowel movement.
    - Children up to 3 years of age—Use and dose must be determined by your doctor.

**Storage**—To store this medicine:
- Keep out of the reach of children.
- Store away from heat and direct light.
- Keep this medicine from freezing.
- Do not keep outdated medicine or medicine no longer needed. Be sure that any discarded medicine is out of the reach of children.

## Precautions While Using This Medicine

*Check with your doctor if your diarrhea does not stop after 1 or 2 days or if you develop a fever.*

*If you are taking any other medicine, do not take it within 2 to 3 hours of taking kaolin and pectin.* Taking the medicines together may prevent the other medicine from being absorbed by your body. If you have any questions about this, check with your health care professional.

## Side Effects of This Medicine

Along with its needed effects, a medicine may cause some unwanted effects. No serious side effects have been reported for this medicine. However, this medicine may cause constipation in some patients, especially if they take a lot of it. Check with your doctor as soon as possible if constipation continues or is bothersome.

Other side effects not listed above may also occur in some patients. If you notice any other effects, check with your doctor.

Revised: 08/04/94

# KAOLIN, PECTIN, BELLADONNA ALKALOIDS, AND OPIUM   Systemic†

Some commonly used brand names are:
**In the U.S.—**
Amogel PG              Kapectolin PG
Donnagel-PG            Quiagel PG
Donnapectolin-PG

†Not commercially available in Canada.

## Description

Kaolin (KAY-oh-lin), pectin (PEK-tin), belladonna alkaloids (bell-a-DON-a AL-ka-loyds), and opium (OH-pee-um) combination medicine is used to treat diarrhea.

In some states, this medicine is available without a prescription. However, the product's directions and warnings should be carefully followed. In addition, your doctor may have special instructions on the proper dose or use of this medicine for your medical condition. This medicine is available in the following dosage form:

*Oral*
- Oral suspension (U.S.)

## Before Using This Medicine

If you are taking this medicine without a prescription, carefully read and follow any precautions on the label.

For kaolin, pectin, belladonna alkaloids, and opium, the following should be considered:

**Allergies**—Tell your doctor if you have ever had any unusual or allergic reaction to any of the belladonna alkaloids (atropine, hyoscyamine, scopolamine) or medicines like morphine, codeine, or papaverine. Also, tell your health care professional if you are allergic to any other substances, such as foods, preservatives, or dyes.

**Pregnancy**—This medicine has not been shown to cause problems in humans. However, too much use of opium (contained in this combination medicine) during pregnancy may cause the baby to become dependent on the medicine. This may lead to withdrawal side effects after birth.

**Breast-feeding**—This medicine has not been reported to cause problems in nursing babies.

**Children**—Children are especially sensitive to the effects of belladonna alkaloids and opium (contained in this combination medicine). This may increase the chance of side effects during treatment. Also, the fluid loss caused by the diarrhea may result in a severe condition. For these reasons, do not give this medicine for diarrhea to young children (under 6 years of age) without first checking with their doctor. In older children with diarrhea, medicine for diarrhea may be used, but it is also very important that a sufficient amount of liquids be given to replace the fluid lost by the body. If you have any questions about this, check with your health care professional.

**Older adults**—Elderly people are especially sensitive to the effects of belladonna alkaloids and opium (contained in this combination medicine). This may increase the chance of side effects during treatment. Also, the fluid loss caused by the diarrhea may result in a severe condition. For this reason, elderly persons should not take this medicine without first checking with their doctor. It is also very important that a sufficient amount of liquids be taken to replace the fluid lost by the body. If you have any questions about this, check with your health care professional.

**Other medicines**—Although certain medicines should not be used together at all, in other cases two different medicines may be used together even if an interaction might occur. In these cases, your doctor may want to change the dose, or other precautions may be necessary. When you are taking belladonna alkaloids and opium (contained in this combination medicine), it is especially important that your health care professional know if you are taking any of the following:

- Central nervous system (CNS) depressants—Effects, such as drowsiness, of CNS depressants or of belladonna alkaloids and opium may become greater
- Ketoconazole [e.g., Nizoral]—Use of this medicine with ketoconazole may decrease the effectiveness of ketoconazole
- Monoamine oxidase (MAO) inhibitors (furazolidone [e.g., Furoxone], isocarboxazid [e.g., Marplan], phenelzine [e.g., Nardil], procarbazine [e.g., Matulane], tranylcypromine [e.g., Parnate])—Taking belladonna alkaloids while you

are taking or within 2 weeks of taking MAO inhibitors may cause an increase in the effects of belladonna alkaloids
- Naltrexone (e.g., Trexan)—Withdrawal side effects may occur in patients who have become addicted to the opium in this combination medicine; also, naltrexone will make this medicine less effective against diarrhea
- Potassium chloride (e.g., Kay Ciel)—Use with belladonna alkaloids may worsen stomach and intestinal problems caused by potassium

**Other medical problems**—The presence of other medical problems may affect the use of this medicine. Make sure you tell your doctor if you have any other medical problems, especially:

- Alcohol or drug abuse or dependence (history of)—There is a greater chance that this medicine may become habit-forming
- Brain damage (children) or
- Down's syndrome (mongolism) or
- Spastic paralysis (children)—The effects of belladonna alkaloids may be increased
- Colitis or other intestinal disease—A more serious condition may develop with the use of this medicine
- Difficult urination or
- Dryness of the mouth (severe and continuing) or
- Emphysema, asthma, bronchitis, or other chronic lung disease or
- Enlarged prostate or
- Gallbladder disease or gallstones or
- Glaucoma or
- Heart disease or
- Hiatal hernia or
- Irregular heartbeat—The belladonna alkaloids contained in this medicine may make these conditions worse
- Dysentery—This condition may get worse; a different kind of treatment may be needed
- Kidney disease or
- Liver disease—Higher blood levels of the belladonna alkaloids and opium may result, increasing the chance of side effects
- Underactive thyroid—This medicine may cause central nervous system (CNS) depression and breathing problems in patients with this condition

## Proper Use of This Medicine

If this medicine upsets your stomach, you may take it with food.

*Take this medicine only as directed on the label or as ordered by your doctor.* Do not take more of it, do not take it more often, and do not take it for a long time. If too much is taken, it may become habit-forming.

*Importance of diet and fluids while treating diarrhea:*
- *In addition to using medicine for diarrhea, it is very important that you replace the fluid lost by the body and follow a proper diet.* For the first 24 hours you should eat gelatin and drink plenty of caffeine-free clear liquids, such as ginger ale, decaffeinated cola, decaffeinated tea, and broth. During the next 24 hours you may eat bland foods, such as cooked cereals, bread, crackers, and applesauce. Fruits, vegetables, fried or spicy foods, bran, candy, caffeine,

and alcoholic beverages may make the condition worse.

- If too much fluid has been lost by the body due to the diarrhea, a serious condition may develop. Check with your doctor as soon as possible if any of the following signs of too much fluid loss occur:

    Decreased urination
    Dizziness and lightheadedness
    Dryness of mouth
    Increased thirst
    Wrinkled skin

**Dosing**—The dose of kaolin, pectin, belladonna alkaloids, and opium combination medicine will be different for different patients. *Follow your doctor's orders or the directions on the label.* The following information includes only the average doses of kaolin, pectin, belladonna alkaloids, and opium combination medicine. *If your dose is different, do not change it* unless your doctor tells you to do so.

- For *oral* dosage form (suspension):
    —For diarrhea:
    - Adults and teenagers—At first, the dose is 2 tablespoonfuls (30 milliliters [mL]). Then the dose is 1 tablespoonful (15 mL) every three hours as needed. You should not take more than four doses in twenty-four hours.
    - Children over 6 years of age—At first, the dose is 2 teaspoonfuls (10 mL). Then the dose is 1 or 2 teaspoonfuls (5 or 10 mL) every three hours as needed. You should not take more than four doses in twenty-four hours.
    - Children up to 6 years of age—Dose must be determined by your doctor.

**Storage**—To store this medicine:

- Keep out of the reach of children since overdose is especially dangerous in children.
- Store away from heat and direct light.
- Keep this medicine from freezing.
- Do not keep outdated medicine or medicine no longer needed. Be sure that any discarded medicine is out of the reach of children.

## Precautions While Using This Medicine

*Check with your doctor if your diarrhea does not stop after 1 or 2 days or if you develop a fever.*

This medicine will add to the effects of alcohol and other CNS depressants (medicines that slow down the nervous system, possibly causing drowsiness). Some examples of CNS depressants are antihistamines or medicine for hay fever, other allergies, or colds; sedatives, tranquilizers, or sleeping medicine; prescription pain medicine or narcotics; barbiturates; medicine for seizures; muscle relaxants; or anesthetics, including some dental anesthetics. *Check*

*with your doctor before taking any of the above while you are taking this medicine.*

This medicine may cause some people to become dizzy, drowsy, or less alert than they are normally. Even if taken at bedtime, it may cause some people to feel drowsy or less alert on arising. *Make sure you know how you react to this medicine before you drive, use machines, or do anything else that could be dangerous if you are dizzy or are not alert.*

This medicine may cause your eyes to become more sensitive to light than they are normally. Wearing sunglasses and avoiding too much exposure to bright light may help lessen the discomfort.

This medicine may make you sweat less, causing your body temperature to increase. *Use extra care not to become overheated during exercise or hot weather while you are taking this medicine,* since overheating may result in heat stroke. Also, hot baths or saunas may make you feel dizzy or faint while you are taking this medicine.

This medicine may cause dryness of the mouth, nose, and throat. For temporary relief, use sugarless candy or gum, melt bits of ice in your mouth, or use a saliva substitute. However, if your mouth continues to feel dry for more than 2 weeks, check with your medical doctor or dentist. Continuing dryness of the mouth may increase the chance of dental disease, including tooth decay, gum disease, and fungus infections.

## Side Effects of This Medicine

Along with its needed effects, a medicine may cause some unwanted effects. Although not all of these side effects appear very often, when they do occur they may need medical attention.

*Check with your doctor immediately* if any of the following side effects are severe and occur suddenly since they may be signs of a more severe and dangerous problem with your bowels:

*Rare*
    Bloating; constipation; loss of appetite; stomach pain (severe) with nausea and vomiting

Also, check with your doctor as soon as possible if the following effects occur:

*Rare*
    Eye pain; hallucinations (seeing, hearing, or feeling things that are not there); shortness of breath; skin rash or itching; slow heartbeat; troubled breathing

Other side effects may occur that usually do not need medical attention. These side effects may go away during treatment as your body adjusts to the medicine. However, check with your doctor if any of the following side effects continue or are bothersome:

*More common with large doses*
    Confusion; constipation; decreased sweating; difficult urination; dizziness; drowsiness; dryness of mouth, nose,

throat, or skin; faintness; fast heartbeat; headache; increased sweating; lightheadedness; redness or flushing of face; unusual tiredness or weakness

*Less common*

Blurred vision; decreased sexual ability; increased sensitivity of eyes to sunlight; loss of memory (especially in the elderly); nervousness; reduced sense of taste

Other side effects not listed above may also occur in some patients. If you notice any other effects, check with your doctor.

Revised: 05/15/91
Interim revision: 08/17/94

---

# KAOLIN, PECTIN, AND PAREGORIC    Systemic

Some commonly used brand names are:

**In the U.S.—**
Kapectolin with Paregoric        Parepectolin

**In Canada—**
Donnagel-PG

## Description

Kaolin (KAY-oh-lin), pectin (PEK-tin), and paregoric (par-e-GOR-ik) combination medicine is used to treat diarrhea.

In some states, this medicine is available without a prescription; however, the product's directions and warnings should be carefully followed. In addition, your doctor may have special instructions on the proper dose or use of this medicine for your medical condition. It is available in the following dosage form:

*Oral*

• Oral suspension (U.S. and Canada)

## Before Using This Medicine

If you are taking this medicine without a prescription, carefully read and follow any precautions on the label. For kaolin, pectin, and paregoric, the following should be considered:

**Allergies**—If you have ever had an unusual or allergic reaction to morphine, codeine, or papaverine. Also, tell your health care professional if you are allergic to any other substances, such as foods, preservatives, or dyes.

**Pregnancy**—This medicine has not been shown to cause problems in humans. However, too much use of opium preparations such as paregoric (contained in this combination medicine) during pregnancy may cause the baby to become dependent on the medicine. This may lead to withdrawal side effects after birth.

**Breast-feeding**—Although the paregoric in this medicine passes into breast milk, it has not been reported to cause problems in nursing babies.

**Children**—Children are especially sensitive to the effects of paregoric (contained in this combination medicine). This may increase the chance of side effects during treatment. Also, the fluid loss caused by the diarrhea may result in a severe condition. For this reason, antidiarrheals must not be given to young children (under 3 years of age) without first checking with their doctor. In older children with diarrhea, antidiarrheals may be used, but it is also very important that a sufficient amount of liquids be given to replace the fluid lost by the body. If you have any questions about this, check with your health care professional.

**Older adults**—Elderly people are especially sensitive to the effects of paregoric (contained in this combination medicine). This may increase the chance of side effects during treatment. Also, the fluid loss caused by the diarrhea may result in a severe condition. For this reason, elderly persons should not take this medicine without first checking with their doctor. It is also very important that a sufficient amount of liquids be taken to replace the fluid lost by the body. If you have any questions about this, check with your health care professional.

**Other medicines**—Although certain medicines should not be used together at all, in other cases two different medicines may be used together even if an interaction might occur. In these cases, your doctor may want to change the dose, or other precautions may be necessary. When you are taking this medicine, it is especially important that your health care professional know if you are taking any of the following:

• Central nervous system (CNS) depressants—Effects, such as drowsiness, of CNS depressants or of paregoric may become greater

**Other medical problems**—The presence of other medical problems may affect the use of this medicine. Make sure you tell your doctor if you have any other medical problems, especially:

• Alcohol or drug abuse or dependence (history of)—There is a greater chance that this medicine may become habit-forming
• Colitis or other intestinal disease—A more serious condition may develop with the use of this medicine
• Diarrhea caused by antibiotics—This medicine may make the diarrhea caused by antibiotics worse or make it last longer
• Difficult urination or
• Emphysema, asthma, bronchitis, or other chronic lung disease, or
• Enlarged prostate or
• Gallbladder disease or gallstones or
• Heart disease or
• Irregular heartbeat—The paregoric contained in this medicine may make these conditions worse

- Dysentery—This condition may get worse; a different kind of treatment may be needed
- Kidney disease or
- Liver disease—In patients with kidney or liver disease, paregoric may accumulate in the body; smaller doses of this medicine may be needed
- Underactive thyroid—This medicine may cause central nervous system (CNS) depression and breathing problems in patients with this condition

## Proper Use of This Medicine

If this medicine upsets your stomach, you may take it with food.

*Take this medicine only as directed on the label or as ordered by your doctor.* Do not take more of it, do not take it more often, and do not take it for a long time. If too much is taken, it may become habit-forming.

*Importance of diet and fluid intake while treating diarrhea:*

- *In addition to using medicine for diarrhea, it is very important that you replace the fluid lost by the body and follow a proper diet.* For the first 24 hours you should eat gelatin and drink plenty of clear liquids, such as ginger ale, decaffeinated cola, decaffeinated tea, and broth. During the next 24 hours you may eat bland foods, such as cooked cereals, bread, crackers, and applesauce. Fruits, vegetables, fried or spicy foods, bran, candy, and caffeine and alcoholic beverages may make the condition worse.
- If too much fluid has been lost by the body due to the diarrhea a serious condition may develop. Check with your doctor as soon as possible if any of the following signs of too much fluid loss occur:
  Decreased urination
  Dizziness and lightheadedness
  Dryness of mouth
  Increased thirst
  Wrinkled skin

**Dosing**—The dose of kaolin, pectin, and paregoric combination medicine will be different for different patients. *Follow your doctor's orders or the directions on the label.* The following information includes only the average doses of kaolin, pectin, and paregoric combination medicine. *If your dose is different, do not change it* unless your doctor tells you to do so.

- For *oral* dosage form (suspension):
  —For diarrhea:
  - Adults and teenagers—The usual dose is 1 or 2 tablespoonfuls (15 or 30 milliliters [mL]) after each loose bowel movement. You should not take more than 4 doses in twelve hours.
  - Children 6 years of age and over—The usual dose is 2 teaspoonfuls (10 mL) after each loose bowel movement. You should not take more than 4 doses in twelve hours.
  - Children 3 to 6 years of age—The usual dose is 1½ teaspoonfuls (7.5 mL) after each loose

bowel movement. You should not take more than 4 doses in twelve hours.
  - Children 1 to 3 years of age—The usual dose is ½ teaspoonful (2.5 mL) after each loose bowel movement. You should not take more than 4 doses in twelve hours.
  - Children up to 1 year of age—Dose must be determined by your doctor.

**Storage**—To store this medicine:
- Keep out of the reach of children since overdose is especially dangerous in children.
- Store away from heat and direct light.
- Do not store this medicine in the refrigerator. If it does get cold and you notice any solid particles in it, throw it away.
- Keep this medicine from freezing.
- Keep the container for this medicine tightly closed to prevent the alcohol from evaporating and the medicine from becoming stronger.
- Do not keep outdated medicine or medicine no longer needed. Be sure that any discarded medicine is out of the reach of children.

## Precautions While Using This Medicine

*Check with your doctor if your diarrhea does not stop after 1 or 2 days or if you develop a fever.*

This medicine will add to the effects of alcohol and other CNS depressants (medicines that slow down the nervous system, possibly causing drowsiness). Some examples of CNS depressants are antihistamines or medicine for hay fever, other allergies, or colds; sedatives, tranquilizers, or sleeping medicine; prescription pain medicine or narcotics; barbiturates; medicine for seizures; muscle relaxants; or anesthetics, including some dental anesthetics. *Check with your doctor before taking any of the above while you are taking this medicine.*

This medicine may cause some people to become dizzy, drowsy, or less alert than they are normally. Even if taken at bedtime, it may cause some people to feel drowsy or less alert on arising. *Make sure you know how you react to this medicine before you drive, use machines, or do anything else that could be dangerous if you are dizzy or are not alert.*

## Side Effects of This Medicine

Along with its needed effects, a medicine may cause some unwanted effects. Although not all of these side effects appear very often, when they do occur they may require medical attention. *Check with your doctor immediately if any of the following side effects are severe and occur suddenly since they may indicate a more severe and dangerous problem with your bowels:*

*Rare*
  Bloating; constipation (severe); loss of appetite; stomach pain (severe) with nausea and vomiting

Also, check with your doctor as soon as possible if the following effects occur:

*Rare*

Decreased blood pressure; fast heartbeat; increased sweating; mental depression; redness or flushing of face; shortness of breath, wheezing, or troubled breathing; skin rash, hives, or itching

Other side effects may occur that usually do not need medical attention. These side effects may go away during treatment as your body adjusts to the medicine. However, check with your doctor if any of the following side effects continue or are bothersome:

*More common with large doses*

Constipation; difficult or painful urination or frequent urge to urinate; dizziness, feeling faint, lightheadedness, unusual tiredness or weakness; drowsiness; nervousness or restlessness

Other side effects not listed above may also occur in some patients. If you notice any other effects, check with your doctor.

Revised: 06/12/91
Interim revision: 08/10/94

# KETOCONAZOLE   Topical

Some commonly used brand names in the U.S. and Canada are Nizoral Cream and Nizoral Shampoo.

## Description

Ketoconazole (kee-toe-KOE-na-zole) is used to treat infections caused by a fungus or yeast. It works by killing the fungus or yeast or preventing its growth.

Ketoconazole cream is used to treat:

- Athlete's foot (tinea pedis; ringworm of the foot);
- Ringworm of the body (tinea corporis);
- Ringworm of the groin (tinea cruris; jock itch);
- Seborrheic dermatitis;
- "Sun fungus" (tinea versicolor; pityriasis versicolor); and
- Yeast infection of the skin (cutaneous candidiasis).

Ketoconazole shampoo is used to treat dandruff.

This medicine may also be used for other fungus infections of the skin as determined by your doctor.

Ketoconazole is available only with your doctor's prescription, in the following dosage forms:

*Topical*
- Cream (U.S. and Canada)
- Shampoo (U.S. and Canada)

## Before Using This Medicine

In deciding to use a medicine, the risks of using the medicine must be weighed against the good it will do. This is a decision you and your doctor will make. For topical ketoconazole, the following should be considered:

**Allergies**—Tell your doctor if you have ever had any unusual or allergic reaction to ketoconazole, miconazole or other imidazoles, or sulfites. The cream form of ketoconazole contains sulfites. Also tell your health care professional if you are allergic to any other substances, such as preservatives or dyes.

**Pregnancy**—Ketoconazole has not been studied in pregnant women. However, studies in animals have shown that ketoconazole causes birth defects or other problems. Before using this medicine, make sure your doctor knows if you are pregnant or if you may become pregnant.

**Breast-feeding**—It is not known whether topical ketoconazole, used on a regular basis, is absorbed into the mother's body enough to pass into the breast milk. However, this medicine was not absorbed through the skin after a single dose. Therefore, it is unlikely to cause problems in nursing babies.

**Children**—Studies on this medicine have been done only in adult patients, and there is no specific information comparing use of this medicine in children with use in other age groups.

**Older adults**—Many medicines have not been studied specifically in older people. Therefore, it may not be known whether they work exactly the same way they do in younger adults or if they cause different side effects or problems in older people. There is no specific information comparing use of topical ketoconazole in the elderly with use in other age groups.

**Other medicines**—Although certain medicines should not be used together at all, in other cases two different medicines may be used together even if an interaction might occur. In these cases, your doctor may want to change the dose, or other precautions may be necessary. Tell your health care professional if you are using any other prescription or nonprescription (over-the-counter [OTC]) medicine.

## Proper Use of This Medicine

*Keep this medicine away from the eyes.*

For patients using the *cream form* of this medicine:
- Apply enough ketoconazole cream to cover the affected and surrounding skin areas, and rub in gently.
- To help clear up your infection completely, *it is very important that you keep using ketoconazole cream*

*for the full time of treatment,* even if your symptoms begin to clear up after a few days. Since fungus or yeast infections may be very slow to clear up, you may have to continue using this medicine every day for up to several weeks. If you stop using this medicine too soon, your symptoms may return. *Do not miss any doses.*

For patients using the *shampoo form* of this medicine:

- Wet your hair and scalp well with water.
- Apply enough shampoo to work up a good lather and gently massage it over your entire scalp for about 1 minute.
- Rinse your hair and scalp with warm water.
- Repeat application, then leave the shampoo on your scalp for 3 minutes more.
- Rinse your hair and scalp well with warm water, and dry your hair.

**Dosing**—The dose of topical ketoconazole will be different for different patients. *Follow your doctor's orders or the directions on the label.* The following information includes only the average doses of topical ketoconazole. *If your dose is different, do not change it* unless your doctor tells you to do so.

*The number of doses you use each day, the time allowed between doses, and the length of time you use the medicine depend on the medical problem for which you are using topical ketoconazole.*

- For *cream* dosage form:
  —For cutaneous candidiasis, tinea corporis, tinea cruris, tinea pedis, or pityriasis versicolor:
  - Adults—Apply once a day to the affected skin and surrounding area.
  - Children—Use and dose must be determined by your doctor.
  —For seborrheic dermatitis:
  - Adults—Apply two times a day to the affected skin and surrounding area.
  - Children—Use and dose must be determined by your doctor.
- For *shampoo* dosage form:
  —For dandruff:
  - Adults—Use every 4 days for 4 weeks. Then use once every 1 or 2 weeks to keep dandruff under control.
  - Children—Use and dose must be determined by your doctor.

**Missed dose**—If you miss a dose of this medicine, apply it as soon as possible. However, if it is almost time for your next dose, skip the missed dose and go back to your regular dosing schedule.

**Storage**—To store this medicine:

- Keep out of the reach of children.
- Store away from heat and direct light.
- Keep the medicine from freezing.
- Do not keep outdated medicine or medicine no longer needed. Be sure that any discarded medicine is out of the reach of children.

## Precautions While Using This Medicine

For patients using the *cream form* of this medicine:

- If your skin problem does not improve within 2 to 4 weeks, or if it becomes worse, check with your doctor.
- *To help clear up your infection completely and to help make sure it does not return, good health habits are also required.*
- For patients using ketoconazole cream for *athlete's foot* (tinea pedis; ringworm of the foot), the following instructions will help keep the feet cool and dry.
  —Avoid wearing socks made from wool or synthetic materials (for example, rayon or nylon). Instead, wear clean, cotton socks and change them daily or more often if your feet sweat a lot.
  —Wear sandals or well-ventilated shoes (for examples, shoes with holes).
  —Use a bland, absorbent powder (for example, talcum powder) or an antifungal powder between the toes, on the feet, and in socks and shoes one or two times a day. It is best to use the powder between the times you use ketoconazole cream.
  If you have any questions about these instructions, check with your health care professional.
- For patients using ketoconazole cream for *ringworm of the groin* (tinea cruris; jock itch), the following instructions will help reduce chafing and irritation and will also help keep the groin area cool and dry.
  —Avoid wearing underwear that is tight-fitting or made from synthetic materials (for example, rayon or nylon). Instead, wear loose-fitting, cotton underwear.
  —Use a bland, absorbent powder (for example, talcum powder) or an antifungal powder on the skin. It is best to use the powder between the times you use ketoconazole cream.
  If you have any questions about these instructions, check with your health care professional.

## Side Effects of This Medicine

Along with its needed effects, a medicine may cause some unwanted effects. Although not all of these side effects may occur, if they do occur they may need medical attention.

Check with your doctor as soon as possible if any of the following side effects occur:

*More common*
 Itching, stinging, or irritation not present before use of this medicine

Other side effects not listed above may also occur in some patients. If you notice any other effects, check with your doctor.

Revised: 06/21/93

---

# KETOROLAC    Ophthalmic

A commonly used brand name in the U.S. and Canada is Acular.

## Description

Ophthalmic ketorolac (kee-toe-ROLE-ak) is an anti-inflammatory medicine. It is used in the eye to treat itching caused by seasonal allergic conjunctivitis (an allergy that occurs at only certain times of the year).

This medicine may also be used to prevent or treat other conditions, as determined by your ophthalmologist (eye doctor).

*Ophthalmic*
 • Ophthalmic solution (eye drops) (U.S. and Canada)

## Before Using This Medicine

In deciding to use a medicine, the risks of using the medicine must be weighed against the good it will do. This is a decision you and your doctor will make. For ophthalmic ketorolac, the following should be considered:

**Allergies**—Tell your doctor if you have ever had any unusual or allergic reaction to aspirin or other salicylates, ophthalmic ketorolac, systemic ketorolac (e.g., Toradol), diclofenac (e.g., Voltaren), or any of the other ophthalmic or systemic anti-inflammatory medicines.

Also tell your health care professional if you are allergic to any other substances, such as preservatives.

**Pregnancy**—Ophthalmic ketorolac has not been studied in pregnant women. However, studies in some animals have shown that ophthalmic ketorolac causes birth defects. Before using this medicine, make sure your doctor knows if you are pregnant or if you may become pregnant.

**Breast-feeding**—Ophthalmic ketorolac has not been reported to cause problems in nursing babies.

**Children**—Studies on this medicine have been done only in adult patients, and there is no specific information comparing use of ophthalmic ketorolac in children with use in other age groups.

**Older adults**—Many medicines have not been studied specifically in older people. Therefore, it may not be known whether they work exactly the same way they do in younger adults. Although there is no specific information comparing use of ophthalmic ketorolac in the elderly with use in other age groups, this medicine is not expected to cause different side effects or problems in older people than it does in younger adults.

**Other medicines**—Although certain medicines should not be used together at all, in other cases two different medicines may be used together even if an interaction might occur. In these cases, your doctor may want to change the dose, or other precautions may be necessary. Tell your health care professional if you are using any other ophthalmic prescription or non-prescription (over-the-counter [OTC]) medicine.

## Proper Use of This Medicine

To use:
 • First, wash your hands. Tilt the head back and, pressing your finger gently on the skin just beneath the lower eyelid, pull the lower eyelid away from the eye to make a space. Drop the medicine into this space. Let go of the eyelid and gently close the eyes. Do not blink. Keep the eyes closed for 1 or 2 minutes to allow the medicine to be absorbed by the eye.
 • If you think you did not get the drop of medicine into your eye properly, use another drop.
 • To keep the medicine as germ-free as possible, do not touch the applicator tip to any surface (including the eye). Also, keep the container tightly closed.

**Dosing**—The dose of ophthalmic ketorolac will be different for different patients. *Follow your doctor's orders or the directions on the label.* The following information includes only the average dose of ophthalmic ketorolac. *If your dose is different, do not change it* unless your doctor tells you to do so.
 • For *ophthalmic solution (eye drops)* dosage form:
  —For itching of the eye
   • Adults—Use one drop in each eye four times a day for up to one week or as directed by your doctor.
   • Children—Use and dose must be determined by your doctor.

**Missed dose**—If you miss a dose of this medicine, use it as soon as possible. However, if it is almost time for your next dose, skip the missed dose and go back to your regular dosing schedule. Do not double doses.

**Storage**—To store this medicine:
- Keep out of the reach of children.
- Store away from heat and direct light.
- Keep the medicine from freezing. Do not refrigerate.
- Do not keep outdated medicine or medicine no longer needed. Be sure that any discarded medicine is out of the reach of children.

## Precautions While Using This Medicine

If your symptoms do not improve within a few days, or if they become worse, check with your doctor.

While applying this medicine, your eyes will probably sting or burn for a short time. This is to be expected.

## Side Effects of This Medicine

Along with its needed effects, a medicine may cause some unwanted effects. Although not all of these side effects may occur, if they do occur they may need medical attention.

Check with your doctor as soon as possible if any of the following side effects occur:

*Less common or rare*
  Burning, itching, redness, swelling, tearing, or other sign of eye irritation not present before therapy or becoming worse during therapy; skin rash around eye

Other side effects may occur that usually do not need medical attention. These side effects may go away during treatment as your body adjusts to the medicine. However, check with your doctor if any of the following side effects continue or are bothersome:

*More common*
  Stinging or burning of eye when medicine is applied

Other side effects not listed above may also occur in some patients. If you notice any other effects, check with your doctor.

## Additional Information

Once a medicine has been approved for marketing for a certain use, experience may show that it is also useful for other medical problems. Although this use is not included in product labeling, ophthalmic ketorolac is used in certain patients with the following medical condition:
- Inflammation, ocular (redness of the eye that occurs after eye surgery in patients having cataracts removed from their eyes)

For patients using this medicine for *ocular inflammation after eye surgery:*
- Make sure you tell your doctor if you have hemophilia or other bleeding problems, since the possibility of bleeding may be increased during eye surgery.

Other than the above information, there is no additional information relating to proper use, precautions, or side effects for this use.

Developed: 08/11/94

---

# KETOROLAC    Systemic

Some commonly used brand names are:

**In the U.S.—**
  Toradol<sup>IM</sup>          Toradol<sup>ORAL</sup>
**In Canada—**
  Toradol          Toradol<sup>IM</sup>

## Description

Ketorolac (kee-TOE-role-ak) is used to relieve pain. It belongs to the group of medicines called anti-inflammatory analgesics. Ketorolac is not a narcotic and is not habit-forming. It will not cause physical or mental dependence, as narcotics can. However, ketorolac is sometimes used together with a narcotic to provide better pain relief than either medicine used alone.

Ketorolac is available only with your doctor's prescription, in the following dosage forms:

*Oral*
- Tablets (U.S. and Canada)

*Parenteral*
- Injection (U.S. and Canada)

## Before Using This Medicine

In deciding to use a medicine, the risks of taking the medicine must be weighed against the good it will do. This is a decision you and your doctor will make. For ketorolac, the following should be considered:

**Allergies**—Tell your doctor if you have ever had any unusual or allergic reaction to ketorolac or to any of the following medicines:
  Aspirin or other salicylates
  Diclofenac (e.g., Voltaren)
  Diflunisal (e.g., Dolobid)
  Etodolac (e.g., Lodine)
  Fenoprofen (e.g., Nalfon)
  Floctafenine (e.g., Idarac)
  Flurbiprofen, oral (e.g., Ansaid)
  Ibuprofen (e.g., Motrin)
  Indomethacin (e.g., Indocin)
  Ketoprofen (e.g., Orudis)
  Meclofenamate (e.g., Meclomen)
  Mefenamic acid (e.g., Ponstel)
  Nabumetone (e.g., Relafen)

Naproxen (e.g., Naprosyn)
Oxaprozin (e.g., Daypro)
Oxyphenbutazone (e.g., Tandearil)
Phenylbutazone (e.g., Butazolidin)
Piroxicam (e.g., Feldene)
Sulindac (e.g., Clinoril)
Suprofen (e.g., Suprol)
Tenoxicam (e.g., Mobiflex)
Tiaprofenic acid (e.g., Surgam)
Tolmetin (e.g., Tolectin)
Zomepirac (e.g., Zomax)

Also tell your health care professional if you are allergic to any other substances, such as foods, preservatives, or dyes.

**Pregnancy**—Studies on birth defects with ketorolac have not been done in pregnant women. However, it crosses the placenta. There is a chance that regular use of ketorolac during the last few months of pregnancy may cause unwanted effects on the heart or blood flow of the fetus or newborn baby. Ketorolac has not been shown to cause birth defects in animal studies. However, animal studies have shown that, if taken late in pregnancy, ketorolac may increase the length of pregnancy, prolong labor, or cause other problems during delivery.

**Breast-feeding**—Small amounts of ketorolac pass into the breast milk. Mothers who are taking this medicine and who wish to breast-feed should discuss this with their doctor.

**Children**—Studies on this medicine have been done only in adult patients, and there is no specific information comparing use of ketorolac in children with use in other age groups.

**Older adults**—Stomach or intestinal problems, swelling of the face, feet, or lower legs, or sudden decrease in the amount of urine, may be especially likely to occur in elderly patients, who are usually more sensitive than younger adults to the effects of anti-inflammatory analgesics such as ketorolac. Also, elderly people are more likely than younger adults to get very sick if the medicine causes stomach problems. Studies in older adults have shown that ketorolac stays in the body longer than it does in younger people. Your doctor will consider this when deciding on how much ketorolac should be given for each dose and how often it should be given.

**Other medicines**—Although certain medicines should not be used together at all, in other cases two different medicines may be used together even if an interaction might occur. In these cases, your doctor may want to change the dose, or other precautions may be necessary. When you are using ketorolac, it is especially important that your health care professional know if you are taking any of the following:

- Anticoagulants (blood thinners) or
- Cefamandole (e.g., Mandol) or
- Cefoperazone (e.g., Cefobid) or
- Cefotetan (e.g., Cefotan) or
- Heparin or
- Moxalactam (e.g., Moxam) or
- Plicamycin (e.g., Mithracin) or

- Valproic acid (e.g., Depakene)—Use of any of these medicines together with ketorolac may increase the chance of bleeding
- Aspirin or other salicylates or
- Other medicine for inflammation or pain, except narcotics—The chance of serious side effects may be increased
- Lithium (e.g., Lithane) or
- Methotrexate (e.g., Mexate)—Higher blood levels of lithium or methotrexate and an increased chance of side effects may occur
- Probenecid (e.g., Benemid)—Higher blood levels of ketorolac and an increased chance of side effects may occur

**Other medical problems**—The presence of other medical problems may affect the use of ketorolac. Make sure you tell your doctor if you smoke tobacco or if you have any other medical problems, especially:

- Alcohol abuse or
- Diabetes mellitus (sugar diabetes) or
- Edema (swelling of face, fingers, feet or lower legs caused by too much fluid in the body) or
- Kidney disease or
- Liver disease (severe) or
- Systemic lupus erythematosus (SLE)—The chance of serious side effects may be increased
- Asthma or
- Colitis, stomach ulcer, or other stomach problems or
- Heart disease or
- High blood pressure—Ketorolac may make your condition worse
- Hemophilia or other bleeding problems—Ketorolac may increase the chance of serious bleeding

## Proper Use of This Medicine

For patients taking *ketorolac tablets:*

- To lessen stomach upset, ketorolac tablets should be taken with food (a meal or a snack) or with an antacid. However, your doctor may want you to take the first few doses 30 minutes before meals or 2 hours after meals. This helps the medicine work a little faster when you first begin to take it.
- Take this medicine with a full glass of water. Also, do not lie down for about 15 to 30 minutes after taking it. This helps to prevent irritation that may lead to trouble in swallowing.

For patients using *ketorolac injection*:

- Medicines given by injection are sometimes used at home. If you will be using ketorolac at home, your health care professional will teach you how the injections are to be given. You will also have a chance to practice giving injections. *Be certain that you understand exactly how the medicine is to be injected.*

*For safe and effective use of this medicine, do not use more of it, do not use it more often, and do not use it for a longer time than ordered by your doctor.* Using too much of this medicine increases the chance of unwanted effects, especially in elderly patients.

**Dosing**—The dose of ketorolac will be different for different patients. *Follow your doctor's orders or the directions on the label.* The following information includes only the average doses of ketorolac. *If your dose is different, do not change it* unless your doctor tells you to do so.

- For *oral* dosage form (tablets):
  —For pain:
  - Adults—One 10-milligram (mg) tablet four times a day, four to six hours apart. Your doctor may want you to take two tablets for the first dose only. This helps the medicine start working a little faster.
  - Children—Use and dose must be determined by your doctor.
- For *injection* dosage form:
  —For pain:
  - Adults—15 or 30 mg four times a day, at least 4 to 6 hours apart. This amount of medicine may be contained in 1 mL or in one-half (0.5) mL of the injection, depending on the strength. Sometimes, larger amounts are used for the first dose only. This helps the medicine start working a little faster.
  - Children—Use and dose must be determined by your doctor.

**Missed dose**—If you have been directed to use this medicine according to a regular schedule, and you miss a dose, use it as soon as possible. However, if it is almost time for your next dose, skip the missed dose and go back to your regular dosing schedule. Do not double doses.

**Storage**—To store this medicine:
- Keep out of the reach of children.
- Store away from heat and direct light.
- Do not store ketorolac tablets in the bathroom, near the kitchen sink, or in other damp places. Heat or moisture may cause the medicine to break down.
- Keep the injection form of ketorolac from freezing. Do not store it in the refrigerator.
- Do not keep outdated medicine or medicine no longer needed. Be sure that any discarded medicine is out of the reach of children.

## Precautions While Using This Medicine

Taking certain other medicines together with ketorolac may increase the chance of unwanted effects. The risk will depend on how much of each medicine you take every day, and on how long you take the medicines together. Therefore, do not take acetaminophen (e.g., Tylenol) or aspirin or other salicylates together with ketorolac for more than a few days, unless otherwise directed by your medical doctor or dentist. Also, *do not take any of the following medicines together with ketorolac, unless your medical doctor or dentist has directed you to do so and is following your progress*:

Diclofenac (e.g., Voltaren)
Diflunisal (e.g., Dolobid)

Etodolac (e.g., Lodine)
Fenoprofen (e.g., Nalfon)
Floctafenine (e.g., Idarac)
Flurbiprofen, oral (e.g., Ansaid)
Ibuprofen (e.g., Motrin)
Indomethacin (e.g., Indocin)
Ketoprofen (e.g., Orudis)
Meclofenamate (e.g., Meclomen)
Mefenamic acid (e.g., Ponstel)
Nabumetone (e.g., Relafen)
Naproxen (e.g., Naprosyn)
Oxaprozin (e.g., Daypro)
Phenylbutazone (e.g., Butazolidin)
Piroxicam (e.g., Feldene)
Sulindac (e.g., Clinoril)
Tenoxicam (e.g., Mobiflex)
Tiaprofenic acid (e.g., Surgam)
Tolmetin (e.g., Tolectin)

Ketorolac may cause some people to become dizzy or drowsy. If either of these side effects occurs, *do not drive, use machines, or do anything else that could be dangerous if you are not alert.*

## Side Effects of This Medicine

Along with its needed effects, a medicine may cause some unwanted effects. Although not all of these side effects may occur, if they do occur they may need medical attention.

*Stop using this medicine and check with your doctor immediately if any of the following side effects occur:*
  *Rare*
  Bleeding or crusting sores on lips; blue lips and fingernails; chest pain; convulsions; fainting; shortness of breath, fast, irregular, noisy or troubled breathing, tightness in chest, and/or wheezing; vomiting of blood or material that looks like coffee grounds

Also, check with your doctor as soon as possible if any of the following side effects occur:
  *Less common*
  Swelling of face, fingers, lower legs, ankles, and/or feet; weight gain (unusual)
  *Rare*
  Abdominal or stomach pain, cramping, or burning (severe); bleeding from rectum or bloody or black, tarry stools; bloody or cloudy urine; bruising (not at place of injection) or small red spots on skin; burning, red, tender, thick, scaly, or peeling skin; decrease in amount of urine (sudden); fever with or without chills or sore throat; hallucinations (seeing, hearing, or feeling things that are not there); hives or itching of skin; increased blood pressure; increased sweating; muscle cramps or pain; nausea, heartburn, and/or indigestion (severe and continuing); nosebleeds; pain in lower back and/or side; puffiness or swelling of the eyelids or around the eyes; skin rash; sores, ulcers, or white spots on lips or in mouth; swollen and/or painful glands; swollen tongue; thirst (continuing); unusual tiredness or weakness

Other side effects may occur that usually do not need medical attention. These side effects may go away during treatment as your body adjusts to the medicine. However, check with your doctor if any of the following side effects continue or are bothersome:

*More common*

Abdominal or stomach pain (mild or moderate); bruising at place of injection; drowsiness; indigestion; nausea

*Less common or rare*

Bloating or gas; burning or pain at place of injection; constipation; diarrhea; dizziness; feeling of fullness in abdominal or stomach area; headache; increased sweating; vomiting

Other side effects not listed above may also occur in some patients. If you notice any other effects, check with your doctor.

---

Revised: 05/14/93

---

# LAXATIVES   Oral

Some commonly used brand names and other names are:

**In the U.S.—**

Afko-Lube[43]
Afko-Lube Lax[37]
Agoral[24]
Agoral
  Marshmallow[24]
Agoral Plain[22]
Agoral Raspberry[24]
Alaxin[44]
Alophen[33]
Alphamul[31]
Bilagog[17]
Bilax[39]
Bisac-Evac[26]
Black-Draught[27]
Black-Draught
  Lax-Senna[34]
Caroid Laxative[30]
Carter's Little
  Pills[26]
Cholac[13]
Cholan-HMB[32]
Chronulac[13]
Cillium[5]
Citrate of
  magnesia[14]
Citroma[14]
Citro-Nesia[14]
Citrucel Orange
  Flavor[6]
Citrucel Sugar-Free
  Orange Flavor[3]
Colace[43]
Colax[41]
Cologel[3]
Constilac[13]
Constulose[13]
Correctol[41]
Correctol Extra
  Gentle[43]
Dacodyl[26]
Decholin[32]
Deficol[26]
Dialose[43]
Dialose Plus[41]
Diocto[43]
Diocto-C[37]
Diocto-K[43]
Diocto-K Plus[37]
Dioctyl sodium
  sulfosuccinate[43]
Dioeze[43]
Diosuccin[43]
Dio-Sul[43]
Diothron[37]
Disanthrol[37]
Disolan[41]
Disolan Forte[11]
Disonate[43]
Disoplex[12]
Di-Sosul[43]
Di-Sosul Forte[37]
Docucal-P[41]
Docu-K Plus[37]
Doss[43]
Doxidan[41]
Doxinate[43]
DSMC Plus[37]
D-S-S[43]
D-S-S plus[37]

Dulcolax[26]
Duosol[43]
Duphalac[13]
Effer-syllium[6]
Emulsoil[31]
Enulose[13]
Epsom salts[17]
Equalactin[4]
Espotabs[33]
Evac-U-Gen[33]
Evac-U-Lax[33]
Ex-Lax[33]
Ex-Lax Maximum
  Relief Formula[33]
Ex-Lax Pills[33]
Extra Gentle Ex-Lax[41]
Feen-a-Mint[41]
Feen-a-Mint Gum[33]
Feen-a-Mint Pills[41]
Fiberall[6]
Fibercon[4]
FiberNorm[4]
Fleet Flavored Castor
  Oil[31]
Fleet Laxative[26]
Fleet Phospho-Soda[18]
Fletcher's Castoria[34]
Generlac[13]
Gentlax S[42]
Gentle Nature[35]
Haley's M-O[19]
Hepahydrin[32]
Hydrocil Instant[6]
Kasof[3]
Kellogg's Castor Oil[31]
Kondremul Plain[22]
Kondremul with
  Cascara[23]
Kondremul with
  Phenolphthalein[24]
Konsyl[5]
Konsyl-D[6]
Konsyl-Orange[6]
Laxinate 100[43]
Liqui-Doss[22]
Liquid petrolatum[22]
Mag-Ox 400[16]
Maltsupex[1]
Maox[16]
Medilax[33]
Metamucil[6]
Metamucil Apple
  Crisp Fiber
  Wafers[6]
Metamucil Cinnamon
  Spice Fiber Wafers[6]
Metamucil Orange
  Flavor[6]
Metamucil
  Sugar-Free,
  Lemon-Lime
  Flavor[6]
Metamucil
  Sugar-Free,
  Orange Flavor[6]
Metamucil Sunrise
  Smooth,
  Citrus Flavor[6]

Metamucil Sunrise
  Smooth,
  Orange Flavor[6]
Metamucil Sunrise
  Smooth Sugar-Free,
  Citrus Flavor[6]
Metamucil Sunrise
  Smooth Sugar-Free,
  Orange Flavor[6]
Metamucil Sunrise
  Smooth Sugar-Free,
  Regular Flavor[6]
Milkinol[22]
Mitrolan[4]
Modane[33]
Modane Bulk[6]
Modane Soft[43]
Molatoc[43]
Molatoc-CST[37]
Naturacil[5]
Nature's Remedy[29]
Neo-Cultol[22]
Neolax[39]
Neoloid[31]
Nujol[22]
Nytilax[35]
Perdiem[8]
Perdiem Plain[5]
Peri-Colace[37]
Petrogalar Plain[22]
Phenolax[33]
Phenolphthalein
  Petrogalar[24]
Phillips' Gelcaps[41]
Phillips' LaxCaps[41]
Phillips' Milk of
  Magnesia[15]
Poloxalkol[44]
Portalac[13]
Pro-Cal-Sof[43]
Pro-Lax[6]
Prompt[10]
Pro-Sof[43]
Pro-Sof Liquid
  Concentrate[43]
Pro-Sof Plus[37]
Purge[31]
Regulace[37]
Regulax SS[43]
Reguloid Natural[6]
Reguloid Orange[6]
Regutol[43]
Sal hepatica[18]
Senexon[34]
Senokot[34]
Senokot-S[42]
Senolax[34]
Serutan[6]
Serutan Toasted
  Granules[7]
Siblin[5]
Stulex[43]
Surfak[43]
Syllact[5]
Syllamalt[2]
Trilax[40]
Versabran[6]
V-Lax[6]
X-Prep Liquid[34]
Zymenol[22]

**In Canada—**

Agarol[21]
Bisacolax[26]
Chronulac[13]
Citro-Mag[14]
Colace[43]
Doss[38]
Doxidan[41]
Dulcodos[36]
Dulcolax[26]
Ex-Lax[33]
Ex-Lax Pills[33]
Extra Gentle
  Ex-Lax[41]
Fibrepur[6]
Glysennid[35]
Karacil[6]

Kondremul[22]
Lactulax[13]
Lansoÿl[22]
Laxit[26]
Magnolax[20]
Metamucil[6]
Metamucil Instant
  Mix, Orange
  Flavor[6]
Metamucil Orange
  Flavor[6]
Metamucil Sugar
  Free[6]
Metamucil
  Sugar-Free,
  Orange Flavor[6]

Mitrolan[4]
Peri-Colace[37]
Phillips' Magnesia
  Tablets[15]
Phillips' Milk of
  Magnesia[15]
Prodiem[9]
Prodiem Plain[6]
Regulex[43]
Regulex-D[38]
Senokot[34]
Senokot-S[42]
Siblin[5]

Note: For quick reference the following laxatives are numbered to match the corresponding brand names.

**Bulk-forming laxatives—**
1. Malt Soup Extract
2. Malt Soup Extract and Psyllium (SILL-i-yum)
3. Methylcellulose (meth-ill-SELL-yoo-lose)‡
4. Polycarbophil (pol-i-KAR-boe-fil)
5. Psyllium
6. Psyllium Hydrophilic Mucilloid (hye-droe-FILL-ik MYOO-sill-oid)
7. Psyllium Hydrophilic Mucilloid and Carboxymethyl-cellulose (kar-box-ee-meth-ill-SELL-yoo-lose)

**Bulk-forming and stimulant combinations—**
8. Psyllium and Senna
9. Psyllium Hydrophilic Mucilloid and Senna
10. Psyllium Hydrophilic Mucilloid and Sennosides

**Bulk-forming, stimulant, and stool softener (emollient) combinations—**
11. Carboxymethylcellulose, Casanthranol (ka-SAN-thra-nole), and Docusate (DOK-yoo-sate)

**Bulk-forming and stool softener (emollient) combinations—**
12. Carboxymethylcellulose and Docusate

**Hyperosmotic laxatives—Lactulose:**
13. Lactulose

**Hyperosmotic laxatives—Saline:**
14. Magnesium Citrate (mag-NEE-zhum SI-trate)‡
15. Magnesium Hydroxide‡
16. Magnesium Oxide
17. Magnesium Sulfate (SUL-fate)‡
18. Sodium Phosphate (SOE-dee-um FOS-fate)‡

**Hyperosmotic and lubricant combinations—**
19. Milk of Magnesia and Mineral Oil
20. Milk of Magnesia, Mineral Oil, and Glycerin

**Hyperosmotic, lubricant, and stimulant combinations—**
21. Mineral Oil, Glycerin, and Phenolphthalein (fee-nole-THAY-leen)

**Lubricant laxatives—**
22. Mineral Oil‡

**Lubricant and stimulant combinations—**
23. Mineral Oil and Cascara (kas-KAR-a) Sagrada
24. Mineral Oil and Phenolphthalein
25. Product not available

**Stimulant laxatives—**
26. Bisacodyl (bis-a-KOE-dill)‡
27. Casanthranol
28. Cascara Sagrada‡

29. Cascara Sagrada and Aloe
30. Cascara Sagrada and Phenolphthalein
31. Castor (KAS-tor) Oil‡
32. Dehydrocholic (dee-hye-droe-KOE-lik) Acid‡
33. Phenolphthalein
34. Senna
35. Sennosides

**Stimulant and stool softener (emollient) combinations—**
36. Bisacodyl and Docusate
37. Casanthranol and Docusate‡
38. Danthron and Docusate
39. Dehydrocholic Acid and Docusate
40. Dehydrocholic Acid, Docusate, and Phenolphthalein
41. Docusate and Phenolphthalein
42. Senna and Docusate

**Stool softener (emollient) laxatives—**
43. Docusate‡
44. Poloxamer 188 (pol-OX-a-mer)

‡Generic name product may also be available.

# Description

Oral laxatives are medicines taken by mouth to encourage bowel movements to relieve constipation.

There are several different types of oral laxatives and they work in different ways. Since directions for use are different for each type, it is important to know which one you are taking. The different types of oral laxatives include:

**Bulk-formers—**Bulk-forming laxatives are not digested but absorb liquid in the intestines and swell to form a soft, bulky stool. The bowel is then stimulated normally by the presence of the bulky mass. Some bulk-forming laxatives, like psyllium and polycarbophil, may be prescribed by your doctor to treat diarrhea.

**Hyperosmotics—**Hyperosmotic laxatives encourage bowel movements by drawing water into the bowel from surrounding body tissues. This provides a soft stool mass and increased bowel action.

There are two types of hyperosmotic laxatives taken by mouth—the saline and the lactulose types. The *saline type* is often called "salts." They are used for rapid emptying of the lower intestine and bowel. They are not used for long-term or repeated correction of constipation. With smaller doses than those used for the laxative effect, some saline laxatives are used as antacids. The information that follows applies only to their use as laxatives. Sodium phosphate may also be prescribed for other conditions as determined by your doctor.

The *lactulose type* is a special sugar-like laxative that works the same way as the saline type. However, it produces results much more slowly and is often used for long-term treatment of chronic constipation. Lactulose may sometimes be used in the treatment of certain medical conditions to reduce the amount of ammonia in the blood. It is available only with your doctor's prescription.

**Lubricants—**Lubricant laxatives, such as mineral oil, taken by mouth encourage bowel movements by coating the bowel and the stool mass with a waterproof film. This keeps moisture in the stool. The stool remains soft and its passage is made easier.

**Stimulants—**Stimulant laxatives, also known as contact laxatives, encourage bowel movements by acting on the intestinal wall. They increase the muscle contractions that move along the stool mass. Stimulant laxatives are a popular type of laxative for self-treatment. However, they also are more likely to cause side effects. One of the stimulant laxatives, dehydrocholic acid, may also be used for treating certain conditions of the biliary tract.

**Stool softeners (emollients)—**Stool softeners encourage bowel movements by helping liquids mix into the stool and prevent dry, hard stool masses. This type of laxative has been said not to *cause* a bowel movement but instead *allows* the patient to have a bowel movement without straining.

**Combinations—**There are many products that you can buy for constipation that contain more than one type of laxative. For example, a product may contain both a stool softener and a stimulant laxative. In general, combination products may be more likely to cause side effects because of the multiple ingredients. In addition, they may not offer any advantage over products containing only one type of laxative. *If you are taking a combination laxative, make certain you know the proper use and precautions for each of the different ingredients.*

Most laxatives (except saline laxatives) may be used to provide relief:
- during pregnancy.
- for a few days after giving birth.
- during preparation for examination or surgery.
- for constipation of bedfast patients.
- for constipation caused by other medicines.
- following surgery when straining should be avoided.
- following a period of poor eating habits or a lack of physical exercise in order to develop normal bowel function (bulk-forming laxatives only).
- for some medical conditions that may be made worse by straining, for example:
    Heart disease
    Hemorrhoids
    Hernia (rupture)
    High blood pressure (hypertension)
    History of stroke

Saline laxatives have more limited uses and may be used to provide rapid results:
- during preparation for examination or surgery.
- for elimination of food or drugs from the body in cases of poisoning or overdose.
- for simple constipation that happens on occasion (although another type of laxative may be preferred).
- in supplying a fresh stool sample for diagnosis.

Most laxatives are available without a prescription; however, your doctor may have special instructions for the proper use and dose for your medical condition. They are available in the following dosage forms:

*Oral*

**Bulk-forming laxatives—**
Malt Soup Extract
- Powder (U.S.)
- Oral solution (U.S.)
- Tablets (U.S.)

Malt Soup Extract and Psyllium
- Powder (U.S.)

Methylcellulose
- Capsules (U.S.)
- Granules (U.S.)
- Powder (U.S.)
- Oral solution (U.S.)
- Tablets (U.S.)

Polycarbophil
- Tablets (U.S.)
- Chewable tablets (U.S. and Canada)

Psyllium
- Caramels (U.S.)
- Granules (U.S. and Canada)
- Powder (U.S.)

Psyllium Hydrophilic Mucilloid
- Granules (Canada)
- Powder (U.S. and Canada)
- Effervescent powder (U.S. and Canada)
- Wafers (U.S.)

Psyllium Hydrophilic Mucilloid and Carboxymethylcellulose
- Granules (U.S.)

**Bulk-forming and stimulant combinations—**
Psyllium and Senna
- Granules (U.S.)

Psyllium Hydrophilic Mucilloid and Senna
- Granules (Canada)

Psyllium Hydrophilic Mucilloid and Sennosides
- Powder (U.S.)

**Bulk-forming, stimulant, and stool softener (emollient) combination—**
Carboxymethylcellulose, Casanthranol, and Docusate
- Capsules (U.S.)

**Bulk-forming and stool softener (emollient) combination—**
Carboxymethylcellulose and Docusate
- Capsules (U.S.)

**Hyperosmotic laxative—Lactulose:**
Lactulose
- Solution (U.S. and Canada)

**Hyperosmotic laxatives—Saline:**
Magnesium Citrate
- Oral solution (U.S. and Canada)

Magnesium Hydroxide
- Milk of magnesia (U.S. and Canada)
- Tablets (U.S. and Canada)

Magnesium Oxide
- Tablets (U.S.)

Magnesium Sulfate
- Crystals (U.S.)
- Tablets (U.S.)

Sodium Phosphate
- Effervescent powder (U.S.)
- Oral solution (U.S.)

**Hyperosmotic and lubricant combinations—**
Milk of Magnesia and Mineral Oil
- Emulsion (U.S.)

Milk of Magnesia, Mineral Oil, and Glycerin
- Emulsion (Canada)

**Hyperosmotic, lubricant, and stimulant combination—**
Mineral Oil, Glycerin, and Phenolphthalein
- Emulsion (Canada)

**Lubricant laxatives—**
Mineral Oil
- Oil (U.S. and Canada)
- Emulsion (U.S. and Canada)
- Gel (U.S. and Canada)
- Oral suspension (U.S.)

**Lubricant and stimulant combinations—**
Mineral Oil and Cascara Sagrada
- Emulsion (U.S.)

Mineral Oil and Phenolphthalein
- Emulsion (U.S.)
- Oral suspension (U.S.)

**Stimulant laxatives—**
Bisacodyl
- Tablets (U.S. and Canada)

Casanthranol
- Syrup (U.S.)

Cascara Sagrada
- Fluidextract (U.S.)
- Tablets (U.S.)

Cascara Sagrada and Aloe
- Tablets (U.S.)

Cascara Sagrada and Phenolphthalein
- Tablets (U.S.)

Castor Oil
- Oil (U.S. and Canada)
- Emulsion (U.S.)

Dehydrocholic Acid
- Tablets (U.S.)

Phenolphthalein
- Chewing gum (U.S.)
- Tablets (U.S. and Canada)
- Chewable tablets (U.S. and Canada)
- Wafers (U.S.)

Senna
- Granules (U.S. and Canada)
- Oral solution (U.S.)
- Syrup (U.S. and Canada)
- Tablets (U.S. and Canada)

Sennosides
- Tablets (U.S. and Canada)

**Stimulant and stool softener (emollient) combinations—**
Bisacodyl and Docusate
- Tablets (Canada)

Casanthranol and Docusate
- Capsules (U.S. and Canada)
- Syrup (U.S.)
- Tablets (U.S.)

Danthron and Docusate
- Capsules (Canada)
- Tablets (Canada)

Dehydrocholic Acid and Docusate
- Capsules (U.S.)
- Tablets (U.S.)

Dehydrocholic Acid, Docusate, and Phenolphthalein
- Capsules (U.S.)

Docusate and Phenolphthalein
- Capsules (U.S. and Canada)
- Tablets (U.S. and Canada)
- Chewable tablets (U.S.)

Senna and Docusate
- Tablets (U.S. and Canada)

**Stool softener (emollient) laxatives—**
Docusate
- Capsules (U.S. and Canada)
- Oral solution (U.S. and Canada)
- Syrup (U.S. and Canada)
- Tablets (U.S.)
Poloxamer 188 (pol-OX-a-mer)
- Capsules (U.S.)

## Before Using This Medicine

**Importance of diet, fluids, and exercise to prevent constipation**—Laxatives are to be used to provide short-term relief only, unless otherwise directed by a doctor. A proper diet containing roughage (whole grain breads and cereals, bran, fruit, and green, leafy vegetables), with 6 to 8 full glasses (8 ounces each) of liquids each day, and daily exercise are most important in maintaining healthy bowel function. Also, for individuals who have problems with constipation, foods such as pastries, puddings, sugar, candy, cake, and cheese may make the constipation worse.

If you are taking this medicine without a prescription, carefully read and follow any precautions on the label. For oral laxatives, the following should be considered:

**Allergies**—Tell your doctor if you have ever had any unusual or allergic reaction to laxatives. Also tell your health care professional if you are allergic to any other substances, such as foods, preservatives, or dyes.

**Diet**—Make certain your health care professional knows if you are on any special diet, such as a low-sodium or low-sugar diet. Some laxatives have large amonts of sodium or sugars in them.

**Pregnancy**—Although laxatives are often used during pregnancy, some types are better than others. Stool softeners (emollient) laxatives and bulk-forming laxatives are probably used most often. If you are using a laxative during pregnancy, remember that:
- Some laxatives (in particular, the bulk-formers) contain a large amount of sodium or sugars, which may have possible unwanted effects such as increasing blood pressure or causing water to be held in the body.
- Saline laxatives containing magnesium, potassium, or phosphates may have to be avoided if your kidney function is not normal.
- Mineral oil is usually not used during pregnancy because of possible unwanted effects on the mother or infant. Mineral oil may interfere with the absorption of nutrients and vitamins in the mother. Also, if taken for a long time during pregnancy, mineral oil may cause severe bleeding in the newborn infant.
- Stimulant laxatives may cause unwanted effects in the expectant mother if improperly used. Castor oil in particular should not be used as it may cause contractions of the womb.

**Breast-feeding**—Laxatives containing cascara, danthron, and phenolphthalein may pass into the breast milk. Although the amount of laxative in the milk is generally thought to be too small to cause problems in the baby, your doctor should be told if you plan to use such laxatives. Some reports claim that diarrhea has been caused in the infant.

**Children**—*Laxatives should not be given to young children (up to 6 years of age) unless prescribed by their doctor.* Since children usually cannot describe their symptoms very well, they should be checked by a doctor before being given a laxative. The child may have a condition that needs other treatment. If so, laxatives will not help, and may even cause unwanted effects or make the condition worse.

Mineral oil should not be given to young children (up to 6 years of age) because a form of pneumonia may be caused by the inhalation of oil droplets into the lungs.

Also, bisacodyl tablets should not be given to children up to 6 years of age because if chewed they may cause stomach irritation.

**Older adults**—Mineral oil should not be taken by bedridden elderly persons because a form of pneumonia may be caused by the inhalation of oil droplets into the lungs. Also, stimulant laxatives (e.g., bisacodyl, casanthranol, or phenolphthalein), if taken too often, may worsen weakness, lack of coordination, or dizziness and lightheadedness.

**Other medicines**—Although certain medicines should not be used together at all, in other cases two different medicines may be used together even if an interaction might occur. In these cases, your doctor may want to change the dose, or other precautions may be necessary. When you are taking oral laxatives, it is especially important that your health care professional know if you are taking any of the following:
- Anticoagulants, oral (blood thinners you take by mouth) or
- Digitalis glycosides (heart medicine)—The use of magnesium-containing laxatives may reduce the effects of these medicines
- Ciprofloxacin (e.g., Cipro) or
- Etidronate (e.g., Didronel) or
- Sodium polysterene sulfonate—Use of magnesium-containing laxatives will keep these medicines from working
- Tetracyclines taken by mouth (medicine for infection)—Use of bulk-forming or magnesium-containing laxatives will keep the tetracycline medicine from working

**Other medical problems**—The presence of other medical problems may affect the use of oral laxatives. Make sure you tell your doctor if you have any other medical problems, especially:
- Appendicitis (or signs of) or
- Rectal bleeding of unknown cause—These conditions need immediate attention by a doctor
- Colostomy or
- Intestinal blockage or
- Ileostomy—The use of laxatives may create other problems if these conditions are present

- Diabetes mellitus (sugar diabetes)—Diabetic patients should be careful since some laxatives contain large amounts of sugars, such as dextrose, galactose, and/or sucrose
- Heart disease or
- High blood pressure—Some laxatives contain large amounts of sodium, which may make these conditions worse
- Kidney disease—Magnesium and potassium (contained in some laxatives) may build up in the body if kidney disease is present; a serious condition may develop
- Swallowing difficulty—Mineral oil should not be used since it may get into the lungs by accident and cause pneumonia; also, bulk-forming laxatives may get lodged in the esophagus of patients who have difficulty in swallowing

## Proper Use of This Medicine

For safe and effective use of your laxative:
- Follow your doctor's instructions if this laxative was prescribed.
- Follow the manufacturer's package directions if you are treating yourself.

With all kinds of laxatives, at least 6 to 8 glasses (8 ounces each) of liquids should be taken each day. This will help make the stool softer.

For *patients taking laxatives containing a bulk-forming ingredient:*
- Do not try to swallow in the dry form. Take with liquid.
- To allow bulk-forming laxatives to work properly and to prevent intestinal blockage, it is necessary to drink plenty of fluids during their use. Each dose should be taken in or with a full glass (8 ounces) or more of cold water or fruit juice. This will provide enough liquid for the laxative to work properly. A second glass of water or juice by itself is often recommended with each dose for best effect and to avoid side effects.
- When taking a product that contains only a bulk-forming ingredient, results often may be obtained in 12 hours. However, this may not occur for some individuals until after 2 or 3 days.

For *patients taking laxatives containing a stool softener (emollient):*
- Liquid forms may be taken in milk or fruit juice to improve flavor.
- When taking a product that contains only a stool softener, results usually occur 1 to 2 days after the first dose. However, this may not occur for some individuals until after 3 to 5 days.

For *patients taking laxatives containing a hyperosmotic ingredient:*
- Each dose should be taken in or with a full glass (8 ounces) or more of cold water or fruit juice. This will provide enough liquid for the laxative to work properly. A second glass of water or juice by itself is often recommended with each dose for best effect and, in the case of saline laxatives, to prevent you from becoming dehydrated.

- The unpleasant taste produced by some hyperosmotic laxatives may be improved by following each dose with citrus fruit juice or citrus-flavored carbonated beverage.
- Lactulose may not produce laxative results for 24 to 48 hours.
- Saline laxatives usually produce results within ½ to 3 hours following a dose. When a larger dose is taken on an empty stomach, the results are quicker. When a smaller dose is taken with food, the results are delayed. Therefore, large doses of saline laxatives are usually not taken late in the day on an empty stomach.

For *patients taking laxatives containing mineral oil:*
- Mineral oil should not be taken within 2 hours of meals because of possible interference with food digestion and absorption of nutrients and vitamins.
- Mineral oil is usually taken at bedtime (but not while lying down) for convenience and because it requires about 6 to 8 hours to produce results.

For *patients taking laxatives containing a stimulant ingredient:*
- Stimulant laxatives are usually taken on an empty stomach for rapid effect. Results are slowed if taken with food.
- Many stimulant laxatives (but not castor oil) are often taken at bedtime to produce results the next morning (although some may require 24 hours or more).
- *Castor oil* is not usually taken late in the day because its results occur within 2 to 6 hours.
- The unpleasant taste of *castor oil* may be improved by chilling in the refrigerator for at least an hour and then stirring the dose into a full glass of cold orange juice just before it is taken. Also, flavored preparations of castor oil are available.
- *Bisacodyl tablets* are specially coated to allow them to work properly without causing irritation and/or nausea. To protect this coating, do not chew, crush, or take the tablets within an hour of milk or antacids.
- Because of the way *phenolphthalein* works in the body, a single dose may cause a laxative effect in some people for up to 3 days.

**Dosing**—There are a large variety of laxative products on the market. The dose of laxatives will be different for different products. The number of capsules or tablets or teaspoonfuls of crystals, gel, granules, liquid, or powder that you use; the number of caramels or wafers that you eat; or the number of pieces of gum that you chew depends on the strength of the medicine. *Follow your doctor's orders if this medicine was prescribed, or follow the directions on the box if you are buying this medicine without a prescription.*

**Storage**—To store this medicine:
- Keep out of the reach of children.
- Store away from heat and direct light.

- Do not store the capsule, tablet, granules, or powder form of this medicine in the bathroom, near the kitchen sink, or in other damp places. Heat or moisture may cause the medicine to break down.
- Keep the liquid form of this medicine from freezing.
- Do not keep outdated medicine or medicine no longer needed. Be sure that any discarded medicine is out of the reach of children.

## Precautions While Using This Medicine

*Do not take any type of laxative:*
- *if you have signs of appendicitis or inflamed bowel* (such as stomach or lower abdominal pain, cramping, bloating, soreness, nausea, or vomiting). Instead, check with your doctor as soon as possible.
- *for more than 1 week* unless your doctor has prescribed or ordered a special schedule for you. This is true even when you have had no results from the laxative.
- *within 2 hours of taking other medicine* because the desired effect of the other medicine may be reduced.
- *if you do not need it,* as for the common cold, "to clean out your system," or as a "tonic to make you feel better."
- *if you miss a bowel movement for a day or two.*
- *if you develop a skin rash* while taking a laxative or if you had a rash the last time you took it. Instead, check with your doctor.

*If you notice a sudden change in bowel habits or function that lasts longer than 2 weeks,* or that keeps returning off and on, check with your doctor before using a laxative. This will allow the cause of your problem to be determined before it may become more serious.

The "laxative habit"—Laxative products are overused by many people. Such a practice often leads to dependence on the laxative action to produce a bowel movement. In severe cases, overuse of some laxatives has caused damage to the nerves, muscles, and tissues of the intestines and bowel. If you have any questions about the use of laxatives, check with your health care professional.

Many laxatives often contain large amounts of sugars, carbohydrates, and sodium. If you are on a low-sugar, low-caloric, or low-sodium diet, check with your health care professional before using a laxative.

For *patients taking laxatives containing mineral oil:*
- Mineral oil should not be taken often or for long periods of time because:
  —gradual build-up in body tissues may create additional problems.
  —the use of mineral oil may interfere with the body's ability to absorb certain food nutrients and vitamins A, D, E, and K.
- Large doses of mineral oil may cause some leakage from the rectum. The use of absorbent pads or a decrease in dose may be necessary to prevent the soiling of clothing.

- Do not take mineral oil within 2 hours of a stool softener (emollient laxative). The stool softener may increase the amount of mineral oil absorbed.

For *patients taking laxatives containing a stimulant ingredient:*
- Stimulant laxatives are most often associated with:
  —overuse and the laxative habit.
  —skin rashes.
  —intestinal cramping after dosing (especially if taken on an empty stomach).
  —potassium loss.

## Side Effects of This Medicine

Along with its needed effects, a medicine may cause some unwanted effects. Although not all of these side effects may occur, if they do occur they may need medical attention.

Check with your doctor as soon as possible if any of the following side effects occur:
*For bulk-forming–containing*
   Difficulty in breathing; intestinal blockage; skin rash or itching; swallowing difficulty (feeling of lump in throat)
*For hyperosmotic–containing*
   Confusion; dizziness or lightheadedness; irregular heartbeat; muscle cramps; unusual tiredness or weakness
*For stimulant–containing*
   Confusion; irregular heartbeat; muscle cramps; pink to red coloration of alkaline urine and stools (for phenolphthalein only); pink to red, red to violet, or red to brown coloration of alkaline urine (for cascara, danthron, and/or senna only); skin rash; unusual tiredness or weakness; yellow to brown coloration of acid urine (for cascara, phenolphthalein, and/or senna only)
*For stool softener (emollient)–containing*
   Skin rash

Other side effects may occur that usually do not need medical attention. These side effects are less common and may go away during treatment as your body adjusts to the medicine. However, check with your doctor if any of the following side effects continue or are bothersome:
*For hyperosmotic–containing*
   Cramping; diarrhea; gas; increased thirst
*For lubricant–containing*
   Skin irritation surrounding rectal area
*For stimulant–containing*
   Belching; cramping; diarrhea; nausea
*For stool softener (emollient)-containing*
   Stomach and/or intestinal cramping; throat irritation (liquid forms only)

Other side effects not listed above may also occur in some patients. If you notice any other effects, check with your doctor.

## Additional Information

Once a medicine has been approved for marketing for a certain use, experience may show that it is also useful for other medical problems. Although this use is not included in product labeling, psyllium hydrophilic mucilloid is used in certain patients with high cholesterol (hypercholesterolemia).

For patients taking psyllium hydrophilic mucilloid for *high cholesterol*:

- Importance of diet—Before prescribing medicine for your condition, your doctor will probably try to control your condition by prescribing a personal diet for you. Such a diet may be low in fats, sugars, and/or cholesterol. Many people are able to control their condition by carefully following their doctor's orders for proper diet and exercise. Medicine is prescribed only when additional help is needed. *Follow carefully the special diet your doctor gave you,* since the medicine is effective only when a schedule of diet and exercise is properly followed.
- Do not try to swallow the powder form of this medicine in the dry form. Mix with liquid following the directions in the package.
- Remember that this medicine will not cure your cholesterol problem but it will help control it. Therefore, you must continue to take it as directed by your doctor if you expect to lower your cholesterol level.

Other than the above information, there is no additional information relating to proper use, precautions, or side effects for this use.

Revised: 06/25/93
Interim revision: 06/28/94

# LAXATIVES   Rectal

Some commonly used brand names are:

**In the U.S.—**

| | |
|---|---|
| Bisco-Lax[1] | Fleet Enema[7] |
| Ceo-Two[5] | Fleet Enema Mineral Oil[4] |
| Clysodrast[1] | Fleet Laxative[1] |
| Dacodyl[1] | Sani-Supp[3] |
| Deficol[1] | Senokot[6] |
| Dulcolax[1] | Theralax[1] |
| Fleet Babylax[3] | Therevac Plus[2] |
| Fleet Bisacodyl[1] | Therevac-SB[2] |
| Fleet Bisacodyl Prep[1] | |

**In Canada**

| | |
|---|---|
| Bisacolax[1] | Fleet Enema Mineral Oil[4] |
| Dulcolax[1] | Laxit[1] |
| Fleet Enema[7] | Senokot[6] |

Note: For quick reference, the following laxatives are numbered to match the corresponding brand names.

This information applies to the following medicines:
1. Bisacodyl (bis-a-KOE-dill)‡§
2. Docusate (DOK-yoo-sate)
3. Glycerin (GLI-ser-in)‡§
4. Mineral Oil
5. Potassium Bitartrate and Sodium Bicarbonate (SOE-dee-um Bye-KAR-boe-nate)
6. Senna
7. Sodium Phosphates (soe-dee-um FOS-fates)

‡Generic product may also be available in the U.S.
§Generic name product may also be available in Canada.

## Description

Rectal laxatives are used as enemas or suppositories to produce bowel movements in a short time.

There are several different types of rectal laxatives and they work in different ways. Since directions for use are different for each type, it is important to know which one you are taking. The different types of rectal laxatives include:

**Carbon dioxide–releasing**—Carbon dioxide–releasing laxatives (e.g., potassium bitartrate and sodium bicarbonate) are suppositories that encourage bowel movements by forming carbon dioxide, a gas. This gas pushes against the intestinal wall, causing contractions that move along the stool mass.

**Hyperosmotic**—Hyperosmotic laxatives (e.g., glyceria; sodium phosphates) draw water into the bowel from surrounding body tissues. This provides a soft stool mass and increased bowel action.

**Lubricant**—Mineral oil coats the bowel and the stool mass with a waterproof film. This keeps moisture in the stool. The stool remains soft and its passage is made easier.

**Stimulants**—Stimulant laxatives (e.g., bisacodyl; senna), also known as contact laxatives, act on the intestinal wall. They increase the muscle contractions that move along the stool mass.

**Stool softeners (emollients)**—Stool softeners (emollient laxatives—e.g., docusate) encourage bowel movements by helping liquids mix into the stool and prevent dry, hard stool masses. This type of laxative has been said not to *cause* a bowel movement but instead *allows* the patient to have a bowel movement without straining.

Rectal laxatives may provide relief in a number of situations such as:
- before giving birth.
- for a few days after giving birth.
- preparation for examination or surgery.

- to aid in developing normal bowel function following a period of poor eating habits or a lack of physical exercise (glycerin suppositories only).
- following surgery when straining should be avoided.
- constipation caused by other medicines.

Some of these laxatives are available only with your doctor's prescription. Others are available without a prescription; however, your doctor may have special instructions for the proper use and dose for your medical condition. They are available in the following dosage forms:

*Rectal*

Bisacodyl
- Enema (U.S. and Canada)
- Suppositories (U.S. and Canada)
- Powder for enema (U.S.)

Docusate
- Enema (U.S.)

Glycerin
- Enema (U.S.)
- Suppositories (U.S. and Canada)

Mineral Oil
- Enema (U.S. and Canada)

Potassium Bitartrate and Sodium Bicarbonate
- Suppositories (U.S.)

Senna
- Suppositories (U.S. and Canada)

Sodium Phosphates
- Enema (U.S. and Canada)

## Before Using This Medicine

**Importance of diet, fluids, and exercise to prevent constipation**—Laxatives are to be used to provide short-term relief only, unless otherwise directed by your doctor. A proper diet containing roughage (whole grain breads and cereals, bran, fruit, and green, leafy vegetables), with 6 to 8 full glasses (8 ounces each) of liquids each day, and daily exercise are most important in maintaining healthy bowel function. Also, for individuals who have problems with constipation, foods such as pastries, puddings, sugar, candy, cake, and cheese may make the constipation worse.

If you are using this medicine without a prescription, carefully read and follow any precautions on the label. For rectal laxatives, the following should be considered:

**Allergies**—Tell your doctor if you have ever had any unusual or allergic reaction to rectal laxatives. Also tell your health care professional if you are allergic to any other substances, such as preservatives or dyes.

**Children**—*Laxatives should not be given to young children (up to 6 years of age) unless prescribed by their doctor.* Since children cannot usually describe their symptoms very well, they should be checked by a doctor before being given a laxative. The child may have a condition that needs other treatment. If so, laxatives will not help and may even cause unwanted effects or make the condition worse.

Also, weakness, increased sweating, and convulsions (seizures) may be especially likely to occur in children receiving enemas or rectal solutions, since they may be more sensitive than adults to their effects.

**Older adults**—Weakness, increased sweating, and convulsions (seizures) may be especially likely to occur in elderly patients, since they may be more sensitive than younger adults to the effects of rectal laxatives.

**Other medical problems**—The presence of other medical problems may affect the use of rectal laxatives. Make sure you tell your doctor if you have any other medical problems, especially:

- Appendicitis (or signs of) or
- Rectal bleeding of unknown cause—These conditions need immediate attention by a doctor
- Intestinal blockage—The use of laxatives may create other problems if this condition is present

## Proper Use of This Medicine

For safe and effective use of laxatives:
- Follow your doctor's orders if this laxative was prescribed.
- Follow the manufacturer's package directions if you are treating yourself.

For patients using *the enema form* of this medicine:
- This medicine usually comes with patient directions. Read them carefully before using this medicine.
- Lubricate anus with petroleum jelly before inserting the enema applicator.
- Gently insert the rectal tip of the enema applicator to prevent damage to the rectal wall.
- Results often may be obtained with:
  —bisacodyl enema in 15 minutes to 1 hour.
  —docusate enema in 2 to 15 minutes.
  —glycerin enema in 15 minutes to 1 hour.
  —mineral oil enema in 2 to 15 minutes.
  —senna enema in 30 minutes, but may not occur for some individuals for up to 2 hours.
  —sodium phosphates enema in 2 to 5 minutes.

For patients using *the suppository form* of this medicine:
- If the suppository is too soft to insert, chill the suppository in the refrigerator for 30 minutes or run cold water over it, before removing the foil wrapper.
- To insert suppository: First remove the foil wrapper and moisten the suppository with cold water. Lie down on your side and use your finger to push the suppository well up into the rectum.
- Results often may be obtained with:
  —bisacodyl suppositories in 15 minutes to 1 hour.
  —carbon dioxide–releasing suppositories in 5 to 30 minutes.
  —glycerin suppositories in 15 minutes to 1 hour.
  —senna suppositories in 30 minutes, but may not occur for some individuals for up to 2 hours.

**Dosing**—There are a large variety of laxative products on the market. The dose of laxatives will be different for different products. The amount of enema or the number of suppositories that you use depends on the strength of the medicine. *Follow your doctor's orders if this medicine was prescribed, or follow the directions on the box if you are buying this medicine without a prescription.*

**Storage**—To store this medicine:

- Keep out of the reach of children.
- Store away from heat and direct light.
- Do not store in the bathroom, near the kitchen sink, or in other damp places. Heat or moisture may cause the medicine to break down.
- Do not keep outdated medicine or medicine no longer needed. Be sure that any discarded medicine is out of the reach of children.

## Precautions While Using This Medicine

*Do not use any type of laxative:*

- *if you have signs of appendicitis or inflamed bowel* (such as stomach or lower abdominal pain, cramping, bloating, soreness, nausea, or vomiting). Instead, check with your doctor as soon as possible.
- *more often than your doctor prescribed. This is true even when you have had no results from the laxative.*
- *if you do not need it,* as for the common cold, "to clean out your system," or as a "tonic to make you feel better."
- *if you miss a bowel movement for a day or two.*

*If you notice a sudden change in bowel habits or function that lasts longer than 2 weeks,* or keeps returning off and on, check with your doctor before using a laxative. This will allow the cause of your problem to be determined before it becomes more serious.

The "laxative habit"—Laxative products are overused by many people. Such a practice often leads to dependence on the laxative action to produce a bowel movement. In severe cases, overuse of some laxatives has caused damage to the nerves, muscles, and tissues of the intestines and bowel. If you have any questions about the use of laxatives, check with your health care professional.

For patients using *the enema form* of this medicine:

- *Check with your doctor if you notice rectal bleeding, blistering, pain, burning, itching, or other sign of irritation not present before you started using this medicine.*

For patients using *the suppository form* of this medicine:

- Do not lubricate the suppository with mineral oil or petroleum jelly before inserting into the rectum. To do so may affect the way the suppository works. Moisten only with water.

## Side Effects of This Medicine

Along with its needed effects, a medicine may cause some unwanted effects. Although not all of these side effects may occur, if they do occur they may need medical attention.

Check with your doctor as soon as possible if any of the following side effects occur:

*Less common*
    Rectal bleeding, blistering, burning, itching, or pain (with enemas only)

Other side effects may occur that usually do not need medical attention. These side effects may go away during treatment as your body adjusts to the medicine. However, check with your doctor if the following side effect continues or is bothersome:

*Less common*
    Skin irritation surrounding rectal area

Other side effects not listed above may also occur in some patients. If you notice any other effects, check with your doctor.

Revised: 06/25/93
Interim revision(s): 06/28/94

# LEUCOVORIN   Systemic

A commonly used brand name in the U.S. is Wellcovorin.
Generic name product may also be available in the U.S. and Canada.
Other commonly used names are citrovorum factor and folinic acid.

## Description

Leucovorin (loo-koe-VOR-in) is used as an antidote to the harmful effects of methotrexate (a cancer medicine) that is given in high doses. It is used also to prevent or treat certain kinds of anemia. Leucovorin acts the same way in the body as folic acid, which may be low in these patients.

Leucovorin is also used along with fluorouracil (a cancer medicine) to treat cancer of the colon (bowel).

Leucovorin is available only with a prescription and is to be given only by or under the supervision of your doctor. It is available in the following dosage forms:

*Oral*
- Tablets (U.S. and Canada)
*Parenteral*
- Injection (U.S. and Canada)

## Before Using This Medicine

In deciding to use a medicine, the risks of taking the medicine must be weighed against the good it will do. This is a decision you and your doctor will make. For leucovorin, the following should be considered:

**Allergies**—Tell your doctor if you have ever had any unusual or allergic reaction to leucovorin. Also tell your health care professional if you are allergic to any other substance, such as foods, sulfites or other preservatives, or dyes.

**Pregnancy**—Studies on effects in pregnancy have not been done in either humans or animals.

**Breast-feeding**—It is not known whether leucovorin passes into the breast milk. However, it has not been reported to cause problems in nursing babies.

**Children**—In children with seizures, leucovorin may increase the number of seizures that occur.

**Older adults**—Many medicines have not been studied specifically in older people. Therefore, it may not be known whether they work exactly the same way they do in younger adults or if they cause different side effects or problems in older people. There is no specific information comparing use of leucovorin in the elderly with use in other age groups.

**Other medicines**—Although certain medicines should not be used together at all, in other cases two different medicines may be used together even if an interaction might occur. In these cases, your doctor may want to change the dose, or other precautions may be necessary. Tell your health care professional if you are taking any other prescription or nonprescription (over-the-counter [OTC]) medicine.

**Other medical problems**—The presence of other medical problems may affect the use of leucovorin. If you are taking leucovorin as an antidote to methotrexate, make sure you tell your doctor if you have any other medical problems, especially:

- Kidney disease—Levels of methotrexate may be increased because of its slower removal from the body, so the dose of leucovorin may not be enough to block the unwanted effects of methotrexate
- Nausea and vomiting—Not enough leucovorin may be absorbed into the body to block the unwanted effects of methotrexate

## Proper Use of This Medicine

It is very important that you *take leucovorin exactly as directed,* especially when it is being taken to counteract the harmful effects of cancer medicine. *Do not miss any doses. Also, it is best to take the doses at evenly spaced times day and night.* For example, if you are to take 4 doses a day, the doses should be spaced about 6 hours apart. If this interferes with your sleep or other daily activities, or if you need help in planning the best times to take your medicine, check with your health care professional.

*Do not stop taking leucovorin without checking with your doctor.* It is very important that you get exactly the right amount.

**Dosing**—The dose of leucovorin will be different for different patients. *Follow your doctor's orders or the directions on the label.* The following information includes only the average doses of leucovorin. *If your dose is different, do not change it* unless your doctor tells you to do so.

The number of tablets or doses of injection that you take depends on the strength of the medicine. Also, *the number of doses you take each day, the time allowed between doses, and the length of time you take the medicine depend on the medical problem for which you are taking leucovorin.*

- For use as an antidote to methotrexate:
  —For *oral* (tablets) or *injection* dosage forms:
  - Adults, teenagers, and children—Dose is based on body size and must be determined by your doctor.
- For use as an antidote to other medicines:
  —For *oral* (tablets) or *injection* dosage forms:
  - Adults, teenagers, and children—Dose may range from 0.4 milligrams (mg) to 15 mg a day and must be determined by your doctor.
- For certain kinds of anemia:
  —For *oral* (tablets) or *injection* dosage forms:
  - Adults, teenagers, and children—Up to 1 mg a day.
- For colon cancer:
  —For *injection* dosage forms:
  - Adults and teenagers—Dose is based on body size and must be determined by your doctor.
  - Children—Dose must be determined by your doctor.

**Missed dose**—If you miss a dose of leucovorin or if you vomit shortly after taking a dose, *check with your doctor right away.* Your doctor may want you to take extra leucovorin to make up for what you missed. Do not take more medicine on your own, however, since it is very important that you receive just the right dose at the right time.

**Storage**—To store this medicine:

- Keep out of the reach of children.
- Store away from heat and direct light.
- Do not store in the bathroom, near the kitchen sink, or in other damp places. Heat or moisture may cause the medicine to break down.
- Do not keep outdated medicine or medicine no longer needed. Be sure that any discarded medicine is out of the reach of children.

## Side Effects of This Medicine

Along with its needed effects, a medicine may cause some unwanted effects. Leucovorin usually does not cause any side effects. However, *check with your doctor immediately* if any of the following side effects occur shortly after you receive this medicine:

  Skin rash, hives, or itching; wheezing

Other side effects not listed above may also occur in some patients. If you notice any other effects, check with your doctor.

---

Revised: 07/23/92
Interim revision: 07/05/94

---

# LEUPROLIDE  Systemic

Some commonly used brand names in the U.S. and Canada are Lupron and Lupron Depot.
Another commonly used name is leuprorelin.

---

## Description

Leuprolide (loo-PROE-lide) may be used for a number of different medical problems. These include treatment of:

  • cancer of the prostate gland in men;
  • pain and/or infertility due to endometriosis in women.

Leuprolide is similar to a hormone normally released from the hypothalamus gland.

When given regularly to men, leuprolide decreases testosterone levels. Reducing the amount of testosterone in the body is one way of treating cancer of the prostate.

When given regularly to women, leuprolide decreases estrogen levels. Reducing the amount of estrogen in the body is one way of treating endometriosis.

Leuprolide is available only with your doctor's prescription, in the following dosage form:

  *Parenteral*
  • Injection (U.S. and Canada)

---

## Before Using This Medicine

In deciding to use a medicine, the risks of taking the medicine must be weighed against the good it will do. This is a decision you and your doctor will make. For leuprolide, the following should be considered:

**Allergies**—Tell your doctor if you have ever had any unusual or allergic reaction to leuprolide, buserelin, gonadorelin, histrelin, or nafarelin.

**Pregnancy**—Tell your doctor if you intend to have children.

  • For men: Leuprolide may cause sterility which probably is only temporary. Be sure that you have discussed this with your doctor before receiving this medicine.
  • For women: There is a chance that leuprolide may cause birth defects if it is taken after you become pregnant. It could also cause a miscarriage if taken during pregnancy. *Stop using this medicine and tell your doctor immediately if you think you have become pregnant* while receiving this medicine.

**Older adults**—Many medicines have not been studied specifically in older people. Therefore, it may not be known whether they work exactly the same way they do in younger adults. Although there is no specific information comparing use of leuprolide in the elderly to use in other age groups, it is not expected to cause different side effects or problems in older people than it does in younger adults.

**Other medical problems**—The presence of other medical problems may affect the use of leuprolide. Make sure you tell your doctor if you have any other medical problems, especially:

  • Bleeding from the vagina with unknown cause (for use in endometriosis)
  • Problems in passing urine (for use for cancer of the prostate)—May get worse for a short time after leuprolide treatment is started

---

## Proper Use of This Medicine

*Leuprolide comes with patient directions. Read these instructions carefully.*

Use the syringes provided in the kit. Other syringes may not provide the correct dose. These disposable syringes and needles are already sterilized and designed to be used one time only and then discarded. If you have any questions about the use of disposable syringes, check with your health care professional.

*Use this medicine only as directed by your doctor.* Do not use more or less of it, and do not use it more often than your doctor ordered. The exact amount of medicine you need has been carefully worked out. Using too much may increase the chance of side effects, while using too little may not improve your condition.

For patients receiving leuprolide for *endometriosis*:

  • Leuprolide sometimes causes unwanted effects such as hot flashes or decreased interest in sex. It may also cause a temporary increase in pain when you first begin to use it. However, it is very important that you continue to use the medicine, even after you begin to feel better. *Do not stop using this medicine without first checking with your doctor.*

For patients receiving leuprolide for *cancer of the prostate:*

- Leuprolide sometimes causes unwanted effects such as hot flashes or decreased sexual ability. It may also cause a temporary increase in pain or difficulty in urinating, as well as temporary numbness or tingling of hands or feet or weakness when you first begin to use it. However, it is very important that you continue to use the medicine, even after you begin to feel better. *Do not stop using this medicine without first checking with your doctor.*

**Dosing**—The dose of leuprolide will be different for different patients. *Follow your doctor's orders or the directions on the label.* The following information includes only the average doses of leuprolide. *If your dose is different, do not change it* unless your doctor tells you to do so:

- For injection dosage form:
  —For *endometriosis:*
  - Adults—3.75 milligrams (mg) injected into the muscle once a month.
  —For *cancer of the prostate:*
  - Adults—
    1 mg injected under the skin once a day or 7.5 mg injected into the muscle once a month.

**Missed dose**—If you are using this medicine every day and you miss a dose, give it as soon as possible. However, if you do not remember until the next day, skip the missed dose and go back to your regular dosing schedule. Do not double doses.

**Storage**—To store this medicine:

- Keep out of the reach of children.
- Store away from heat and direct light.
- Keep the medicine from freezing.
- Do not keep outdated medicine or medicine no longer needed. Dispose of used syringes properly in the container provided. Be sure that any discarded medicine is out of the reach of children.

## Precautions While Using This Medicine

*It is very important that your doctor check your progress at regular visits* to make sure that this medicine is working properly and to check for unwanted effects.

For patients receiving leuprolide for *endometriosis:*

- During the time you are receiving leuprolide, your menstrual period may not be regular or you may not have a menstrual period at all. This is to be expected when being treated with this medicine. If regular menstruation does not begin within 60 to 90 days after you stop receiving this medicine, check with your doctor.
- During the time you are receiving leuprolide, you should use birth control methods which do not contain hormones. If you have any questions about this, check with your health care professional.

- *If you suspect you may have become pregnant, stop using this medicine and check with your doctor.* There is a chance that continued use of leuprolide during pregnancy could cause birth defects or a miscarriage.

## Side Effects of This Medicine

Along with its needed effects, a medicine may cause some unwanted effects. Some side effects will have signs or symptoms that you can see or feel. Your doctor may watch for others by doing certain tests.

The following side effects may be caused by blood clots but occur only rarely. However, they require immediate medical attention. *Get emergency help immediately* if any of the following side effects occur:

*For males only*
  *Rare*
    Pains in groin or legs (especially in calves of legs); shortness of breath (sudden)

Check with your doctor as soon as possible if any of the following side effects occur:

*For both females and males*
  *Less common*
    Fast or irregular heartbeat
*For females only*
  *Less common*
    Deepening of voice; increased hair growth
*For males only*
  *Less common*
    Chest pain

Other side effects may occur that usually do not need medical attention. These side effects may go away during treatment as your body adjusts to the medicine. However, check with your doctor if any of the following side effects continue or are bothersome:

*For both females and males*
  *More common*
    Sudden sweating and feelings of warmth ("hot flashes")
  *Less common*
    Blurred vision; burning, itching, redness, or swelling at place of injection; dizziness; headache; nausea or vomiting; numbness or tingling of hands or feet; swelling of feet or lower legs; trouble in sleeping; weight gain
*For females only*
  *More common*
    Light, irregular vaginal bleeding; stopping of menstrual periods
  *Less common*
    Burning, dryness, or itching of vagina; decreased interest in sex; increased tenderness of breasts; mood changes; pelvic pain

---

*For males only*
*Less common*
Bone pain; constipation; decreased size of testicles; impotence or decreased interest in sex; loss of appetite; swelling and increased tenderness of breasts

Other side effects not listed above may also occur in some patients. If you notice any other effects, check with your doctor.

Revised: 06/25/93

# LEVAMISOLE   Systemic

A commonly used brand name in the U.S. and Canada is Ergamisol.

## Description

Levamisole (lee-VAM-i-sole) is used with another cancer medicine (fluorouracil) to help make it work better against cancer of the colon.

Levamisole is available only with your doctor's prescription in the following dosage form:
*Oral*
• Tablets (U.S. and Canada)

## Before Using This Medicine

In deciding to use a medicine, the risks of taking the medicine must be weighed against the good it will do. This is a decision you and your doctor will make. For levamisole, the following should be considered:

**Allergies**—Tell your doctor if you have ever had any unusual or allergic reaction to levamisole or to any other medicines.

**Pregnancy**—Levamisole has not been studied in pregnant women. However, studies in rats and rabbits have not shown that levamisole causes birth defects or other problems.

**Breast-feeding**—It is not known whether levamisole passes into the breast milk in humans, although it passes into cows' milk. However, this medicine has not been reported to cause problems in nursing babies.

**Children**—Studies on this medicine have been done only in adult patients, and there is no specific information comparing use of levamisole in children with use in other age groups.

**Older adults**—Many medicines have not been studied specifically in older people. Therefore, it may not be known whether they work exactly the same way they do in younger adults or if they cause different side effects or problems in older people. Although there is no specific information comparing use of levamisole in the elderly with use in other age groups, this medicine has been used in elderly patients and is not expected to cause different side effects or problems in older people than it does in younger adults.

**Other medicines**—Although certain medicines should not be used together at all, in other cases two different medicines may be used together even if an interaction might occur. In these cases, your doctor may want to change the dose, or other precautions may be necessary. Tell your health care professional if you are taking any other prescription or nonprescription (over-the-counter [OTC]) medicine.

**Other medical problems**—The presence of other medical problems may affect the use of levamisole. Make sure you tell your doctor if you have any other medical problems, especially:
• Infection—Levamisole may decrease your body's ability to fight infection

## Proper Use of This Medicine

*Take this medicine only as directed by your doctor.* Do not take more or less of it, and do not take it more often than your doctor ordered. The exact amount of medicine you need has been carefully worked out. Taking too much may increase the chance of side effects, while taking too little may not improve your condition.

If you vomit shortly after taking a dose of levamisole, check with your doctor. You will be told whether to take the dose again or to wait until the next scheduled dose.

**Dosing**—The dose of levamisole will be different for different patients. The dose that is used may depend on a number of things, including what the medicine is being used for and whether or not other medicines are also being taken. *If you are taking levamisole at home, follow your doctor's orders or the directions on the label.* If you have any questions about the proper dose of levamisole, ask your doctor.

**Missed dose**—If you miss a dose of this medicine, do not take the missed dose at all and do not double the next one. Instead, go back to your regular dosing schedule and check with your doctor.

**Storage**—To store this medicine:
• Keep out of the reach of children.
• Store away from heat and direct light.
• Do not store in the bathroom, near the kitchen sink, or in other damp places. Heat or moisture may cause the medicine to break down.

- Do not keep outdated medicine or medicine no longer needed. Be sure that any discarded medicine is out of the reach of children.

## Precautions While Using This Medicine

*It is very important that your doctor check your progress at regular visits* to make sure that this medicine is working properly and to check for unwanted effects.

## Side Effects of This Medicine

Along with its needed effects, a medicine may cause some unwanted effects. Although not all of these side effects may occur, if they do occur they may need medical attention.

*Check with your doctor immediately* if any of the following side effects occur:

*Less common*
> Fever or chills; unusual feeling of discomfort or weakness

*Rare*
> Black, tarry stools; blood in urine or stools; cough or hoarseness; lower back or side pain; painful or difficult urination; pinpoint red spots on skin; unusual bleeding or bruising

Check with your doctor as soon as possible if the following side effects occur:

*Less common*
> Sores in mouth and on lips

*Rare*
> Blurred vision; confusion; convulsions (seizures); lip smacking or puffing; numbness, tingling, or pain in face, hands, or feet; paranoia (feelings of persecution); puffing of cheeks; rapid or worm-like movements of tongue; trembling or shaking; trouble in walking; uncontrolled movements of arms and legs

Other side effects may occur that usually do not need medical attention. These side effects may go away during treatment as your body adjusts to the medicine. Also, your health care professional may be able to tell you about ways to prevent or reduce some of these side effects. However, check with your doctor if any of the following side effects continue or are bothersome:

*More common*
> Diarrhea; metallic taste; nausea

*Less common*
> Anxiety or nervousness; dizziness; headache; mental depression; nightmares; pain in joints or muscles; skin rash or itching; trouble in sleeping; unusual tiredness or sleepiness; vomiting

Levamisole may cause a temporary loss of hair in some people. After treatment has ended, normal hair growth should return.

Other side effects not listed above may also occur in some patients. If you notice any other effects, check with your doctor.

Revised: 08/12/92
Interim revisin: 07/08/94

# LEVOCABASTINE    Ophthalmic

A commonly used brand name in the U.S. and Canada is Livostin.

## Description

Levocabastine (lee-voe-KAB-as-teen) is used to treat certain disorders of the eye caused by allergies. It works by preventing the effects of a substance called histamine, which is produced in certain cells in your eyes and which causes the allergic reaction.

Levocabastine is available only with your doctor's prescription, in the following dosage form:

*Ophthalmic*
- Ophthalmic suspension (eye drops) (U.S. and Canada)

## Before Using This Medicine

In deciding to use a medicine, the risks of using the medicine must be weighed against the good it will do. This is a decision you and your doctor will make. For levocabastine, the following should be considered:

**Allergies**—Tell your doctor if you have ever had any unusual or allergic reaction to levocabastine. Also tell your health care professional if you are allergic to any other substances, such as preservatives.

**Pregnancy**—Levocabastine has not been studied in pregnant women. However, studies in animals have shown that levocabastine, when given in very high doses, causes birth defects. Before using this medicine, make sure your doctor knows if you are pregnant or if you may become pregnant.

**Breast-feeding**—Although levocabastine passes into the breast milk, it has not been reported to cause problems in nursing babies. However, be sure you have discussed the risks and benefits of the medicine with your doctor.

**Children**—Studies on this medicine have been done only in adult patients and there is no specific information comparing use of levocabastine in children up to 12 years of age with use in other age groups.

**Older adults**—Many medicines have not been studied specifically in older people. Therefore, it may not be known whether they work exactly the same way they do in younger adults or if they cause different side effects or problems in older people. There is no specific information comparing use of levocabastine in the elderly with use in other age groups.

**Other medicines**—Although certain medicines should not be used together at all, in other cases two different medicines may be used together even if an interaction might occur. In these cases, your doctor may want to change the dose, or other precautions may be necessary. Tell your health care professional if you are using any other prescription or nonprescription (over the-counter [OTC]) medicine.

## Proper Use of This Medicine

To use the *eye drops:*

- First, wash your hands. Tilt the head back and, pressing your finger gently on the skin just beneath the lower eyelid, pull the lower eyelid away from the eye to make a space. Drop the medicine into this space. Let go of the eyelid and gently close the eyes. Do not blink. Keep the eyes closed for 1 or 2 minutes to allow the medicine to be absorbed by the eye.
- If you think you did not get the drop of medicine into your eye properly, use another drop.
- To keep the medicine as germ-free as possible, do not touch the applicator tip to any surface (including the eye). Also, keep the container tightly closed.

*In order for this medicine to work properly, it must be used every day in regularly spaced doses as ordered by your doctor.* A few days may pass before you begin to feel better.

**Dosing**—The dose of levocabastine will be different for different patients. *Follow your doctor's orders or the directions on the label.* The following information includes only the average dose of levocabastine. *If your dose is different, do not change it* unless your doctor tells you to do so.

- For *ophthalmic suspension (eye drops)* dosage form:
  —For eye allergy:
    - Adults and children over 12 years of age—Use one drop in each eye four times a day for up to two weeks.
    - Children up to 12 years of age—Use and dose must be determined by your doctor.

**Missed dose**—If you miss a dose of this medicine, use it as soon as possible. Then go back to your regular dosing schedule.

**Storage**—To store this medicine:

- Keep out of the reach of children.
- Store away from heat and direct light.
- Keep the medicine from freezing. Do not refrigerate.
- Do not keep outdated medicine or medicine no longer needed. Be sure that any discarded medicine is out of the reach of children.

## Precautions While Using This Medicine

*If your symptoms do not improve within 3 days or if your condition becomes worse, check with your doctor.*

After application of this medicine to the eye, occasional stinging or burning may occur.

## Side Effects of This Medicine

Along with its needed effects, a medicine may cause some unwanted effects. Although not all of these side effects may occur, if they do occur they may need medical attention.

Check with your doctor as soon as possible if any of the following side effects occur:

*Less common*
 Headache
*Rare*
 Change in vision or trouble in seeing; cough; eye pain; nausea; redness, tearing, discharge, or other eye irritation not present before therapy or becoming worse during therapy; skin rash; sore throat; swelling of eyelids; troubled breathing; unusual tiredness or weakness

Other side effects may occur that usually do not need medical attention. These side effects may go away during treatment as your body adjusts to the medicine. However, check with your doctor if any of the following side effects continue or are bothersome:

*More common*
 Burning or stinging when medicine is applied
*Less common*
 Dry eyes; dry mouth; feeling sleepy

Other side effects not listed above may also occur in some patients. If you notice any other effects, check with your doctor.

Developed: 08/11/94

# LEVOCARNITINE   Systemic†

Some commonly used brand names in the U.S. are Carnitor and VitaCarn.
Generic name product may also be available in the U.S.
Another commonly used name is L-Carnitine.

†Not commercially available in Canada.

## Description

Levocarnitine (lee-voe-KAR-ni-teen) is a substance that helps the cells use fat to produce energy needed by the body. It is needed in small amounts only and is usually available in the foods that you eat. Lack of carnitine can lead to liver, heart, and muscle problems. Your doctor may treat lack of carnitine by prescribing levocarnitine for you.

Carnitine comes in two forms. Levocarnitine (L-Carnitine) should not be confused with the D,L-carnitine form (labeled as "vitamin $B_T$"). Only the L-form of carnitine is used by the body. The D,L-form does not help the body use fat and can actually interfere with and cause a lack of levocarnitine.

Certain levocarnitine products have been specifically approved by the U.S. Food and Drug Administration for medical use and are available only with your doctor's prescription. Other levocarnitine products are sold without a prescription as food supplements.

Levocarnitine is available in the following dosage forms:

*Oral*
- Capsules (U.S.)
- Solution (U.S.)
- Tablets (U.S.)

*Parenteral*
- Injection (U.S.)

## Before Using This Dietary Supplement

If you are taking this dietary supplement without a prescription, carefully read and follow any precautions on the label. For levocarnitine, the following should be considered:

**Allergies**—Tell your health care professional if you are allergic to any substances, such as foods, preservatives, or dyes.

**Pregnancy**—Studies have not been done in humans. However, levocarnitine has not been shown to cause birth defects or other problems in animal studies. Normal healthy fetal growth and development may depend on a steady supply of nutrients such as levocarnitine from mother to fetus.

**Breast-feeding**—Levocarnitine has not been shown to cause problems in nursing babies. It normally is present in breast milk, even in women not taking supplements of it, because it is obtained from the diet.

**Children**—Although there is no specific information comparing use of levocarnitine in children with use in other age groups, this dietary supplement is not expected to cause different side effects or problems in children than it does in adults.

**Older adults**—Many dietary supplements have not been studied specifically in older people. Therefore, it may not be known whether they work exactly the same way they do in younger adults. Although there is no specific information comparing use of levocarnitine in the elderly with use in other age groups, this medicine is not expected to cause different side effects or problems in older people than it does in younger adults.

**Medicines or other dietary supplements**—Although certain medicines or dietary supplements should not be used together at all, in other cases they may be used together even if an interaction might occur. In these cases, your doctor may want to change the dose, or other precautions may be necessary. Tell your health care professional if you are taking any other dietary supplement or any prescription or nonprescription (over-the-counter [OTC]) medicine.

## Proper Use of This Dietary Supplement

Take levocarnitine with or just after meals. Also, if you are taking it in liquid form, drink it slowly. It will be less likely to upset your stomach if you take it this way.

This dietary supplement is also less likely to cause unwanted effects when there is a constant amount in the blood. If you are taking more than one dose a day, take the doses at evenly spaced times throughout the day. Doses should be spaced at least 3 to 4 hours apart. If you need help in planning the best times to take your dietary supplement, check with your health care professional.

**Dosing**—The dose of levocarnitine will be different for different patients. *Follow your doctor's orders or the directions on the label.* The following information includes only the average doses of levocarnitine. *If your dose is different, do not change it* unless your doctor tells you to do so.

The number of capsules or tablets or of teaspoonfuls of solution that you take or the number of injections you receive depends on the strength of the medicine. Also, *the number of doses you take each day, the time allowed between doses, and the length of time you take the medicine depend on the medical problem for which you are taking levocarnitine.*

*Do NOT change brands or dosage forms of levocarnitine without first checking with your doctor. Different products may not work in the same way. If you refill your dietary supplement and it looks different, check with your pharmacist.*

- For *oral* dosage form (capsules):
  —To prevent carnitine deficiency:
    - Adults and teenagers—1 gram taken two or three times a day with meals.
    - Children—The dose is based on body weight and must be determined by your doctor. The usual dose at first is 50 milligrams (mg) per kilogram (kg) (22.7 mg per pound) of body weight a day, divided into smaller amounts with meals. Your doctor may change the dose if needed.
- For *oral* dosage form (solution):
  —To prevent or treat carnitine deficiency:
    - Adults and teenagers—At first, 1 gram taken once a day with food. Your doctor may change the dose if needed.
    - Children—The dose is based on body weight and must be determined by your doctor. The usual dose at first is 50 mg per kg (22.7 mg per pound) of body weight a day, divided into smaller amounts with meals. Your doctor may change the dose if needed.
- For *oral* dosage form (tablets):
  —To prevent or treat carnitine deficiency:
    - Adults and teenagers—1 gram taken two or three times a day with meals.
    - Children—The dose is based on body weight and must be determined by your doctor. The usual dose at first is 50 mg per kg (22.7 mg per pound) of body weight a day, divided into smaller amounts with meals. Your doctor may change the dose if needed.
- For *injection* dosage form:
  —To treat carnitine deficiency:
    - Adults and children—The dose is based on body weight and must be determined by your doctor. The usual dose is 50 mg per kg (22.7 mg per pound) of body weight a day injected into a vein. Your doctor may change the dose if needed.

**Missed dose**—If you miss a dose of this dietary supplement, skip the missed dose and go back to your regular dosing schedule. Do not double doses. Taking doses too close together may increase stomach upset.

**Storage**—To store this dietary supplement:
- Keep out of the reach of children.
- Store away from heat and direct light.
- Do not store in the bathroom, near the kitchen sink, or in other damp places. Heat or moisture may cause the dietary supplement to break down.
- Keep the oral solution form of this dietary supplement from freezing. Do not refrigerate.
- Do not keep outdated dietary supplements or those no longer needed. Be sure that any discarded dietary supplement is out of the reach of children.

## Precautions While Using This Dietary Supplement

Do *not* change brands or dosage forms of levocarnitine without first checking with your doctor. Different products may not work in the same way. If you refill your dietary supplement and it looks different, check with your pharmacist.

## Side Effects of This Dietary Supplement

Along with its needed effects, a dietary supplement may cause some unwanted effects. The following side effects may go away during treatment as your body adjusts to the medicine. However, check with your doctor if any of these effects continue or are bothersome:

*More common*
  Body odor; diarrhea or stomach cramps; nausea or vomiting

Other side effects not listed above may also occur in some patients. If you notice any other effects, check with your doctor.

## Additional Information

Once a medicine or dietary supplement has been approved for marketing for a certain use, experience may show that it is also useful for other medical problems. Although this use is not included in product labeling, levocarnitine is used in certain patients with the following medical condition:

- Carnitine deficiency that results from treatment with valproic acid

Other than the above information, there is no additional information relating to proper use, precautions, or side effects for this use.

Revised: 03/04/92
Interim revision(s): 08/10/92; 08/29/94

# LEVODOPA  Systemic

Some commonly used brand names are:

**In the U.S.—**
Dopar[2]            Sinemet[1]
Larodopa[2]         Sinemet CR[1]

**In Canada—**
Larodopa[2]
Sinemet[1]
Sinemet CR[1]

Note: For quick reference, the following levodopa are numbered to match the corresponding brand names.
This information applies to the following medicines:
  1. Carbidopa and Levodopa (KAR-bi-doe-pa and LEE-voe-doe-pa)
  2. Levodopa

# Description

Levodopa is used alone or in combination with carbidopa to treat Parkinson's disease, sometimes referred to as shaking palsy or paralysis agitans. Some patients require the combination of medicine, while others benefit from levodopa alone. By improving muscle control, this medicine allows more normal movements of the body.

Levodopa alone or in combination is available only with your doctor's prescription. It is available in the following dosage forms:

*Oral*

Carbidopa and Levodopa
- Tablets (U.S. and Canada)
- Extended-release tablets (U.S. and Canada)

Levodopa
- Capsules (U.S.)
- Tablets (U.S. and Canada)

# Before Using This Medicine

In deciding to use a medicine, the risks of taking the medicine must be weighed against the good it will do. This is a decision you and your doctor will make. For levodopa and for carbidopa and levodopa combination, the following should be considered:

**Allergies**—Tell your doctor if you have ever had any unusual or allergic reaction to levodopa alone or in combination with carbidopa. Also tell your health care professional if you are allergic to any other substances, such as foods, preservatives, or dyes.

**Diet**—Since protein may interfere with the body's response to levodopa, high protein diets should be avoided. Intake of normal amounts of protein should be spaced equally throughout the day.

For patients taking levodopa by itself:
- Pyridoxine (vitamin $B_6$) has been found to reduce the effects of levodopa when levodopa is taken by itself. This does not happen with the combination of carbidopa and levodopa. *If you are taking levodopa by itself, do not take vitamin products containing vitamin $B_6$ during treatment, unless prescribed by your doctor.*
- Large amounts of pyridoxine are also contained in some foods such as avocado, bacon, beans, beef liver, dry skim milk, oatmeal, peas, pork, sweet potato, tuna, and certain health foods. Check with your doctor about how much of these foods you may have in your diet while you are taking levodopa. Also, ask your health care professional for help when selecting vitamin products.

**Pregnancy**—Studies have not been done in pregnant women. However, studies in animals have shown that levodopa affects the baby's growth both before and after birth if given during pregnancy in doses many times the human dose. Also, studies in rabbits have shown that levodopa, alone or in combination with carbidopa, causes birth defects.

**Breast-feeding**—Levodopa and carbidopa pass into the breast milk and may cause unwanted side effects in the nursing baby. Also, levodopa may reduce the flow of breast milk.

**Children**—Studies on this medicine have been done only in adult patients, and there is no specific information comparing use of levodopa or carbidopa in children with use in other age groups.

**Older adults**—Elderly people are especially sensitive to the effects of levodopa. This may increase the chance of side effects during treatment.

**Other medicines**—Although certain medicines should not be used together at all, in other cases 2 different medicines may be used together even if an interaction might occur. In these cases, your doctor may want to change the dose, or other precautions may be necessary. When you are taking levodopa or carbidopa and levodopa combination, it is especially important that your health care professional know if you are taking any of the following:
- Cocaine—Cocaine use by individuals taking levodopa, alone or in combination with carbidopa, may cause an irregular heartbeat
- Ethotoin (e.g., Peganone) or
- Haloperidol (e.g., Haldol) or
- Mephenytoin (e.g., Mesantoin) or
- Phenothiazines (acetophenazine [e.g., Tindal], chlorpromazine [e.g., Thorazine], fluphenazine [e.g., Prolixin], mesoridazine [e.g., Serentil], perphenazine [e.g., Trilafon], prochlorperazine [e.g., Compazine], promazine [e.g., Sparine], promethazine [e.g., Phenergan], thioridazine [e.g., Mellaril], trifluoperazine [e.g., Stelazine], triflupromazine [e.g., Vesprin], trimeprazine [e.g., Temaril]) or
- Phenytoin (e.g., Dilantin)—Taking these medicines with levodopa may lessen the effects of levodopa
- Monoamine oxidase (MAO) inhibitors (furazolidone [e.g., Furoxone], isocarboxazid [e.g., Marplan], phenelzine [e.g., Nardil], procarbazine [e.g., Matulane], tranylcypromine [e.g., Parnate])—Taking levodopa while you are taking or within 2 weeks of taking monoamine oxidase (MAO) inhibitors may cause sudden extremely high blood pressure; at least 14 days should be allowed between stopping treatment with one medicine and starting treatment with the other medicine
- Pyridoxine (vitamin $B_6$, e.g., Hexa-Betalin), present in some foods and vitamin formulas (for levodopa used alone)—Pyridoxine reverses the effects of levodopa
- Selegiline—Dosage of levodopa or carbidopa and levodopa combination may need to be decreased

**Other medical problems**—The presence of other medical problems may affect the use of levodopa. Make sure you tell your doctor if you have any other medical problems, especially:
- Diabetes mellitus (sugar diabetes)—The amount of insulin or antidiabetic medicine that you need to take may change
- Emphysema, asthma, bronchitis, or other chronic lung disease or
- Glaucoma or
- Heart or blood vessel disease or
- Hormone problems or

- Melanoma (a type of skin cancer) (or history of) or
- Mental illness—Levodopa may make the condition worse
- Kidney disease or
- Liver disease—Higher blood levels of levodopa may occur, increasing the chance of side effects
- Seizure disorders, such as epilepsy (history of)—The risk of seizures may be increased
- Stomach ulcer (history of)—The ulcer may occur again

## Proper Use of This Medicine

It is best not to take this medicine with or after food, especially high-protein food, since food may decrease levodopa's effect. However, *to lessen possible stomach upset, your doctor may want you to take food shortly after taking this medicine (about 15 minutes after)*. If stomach upset is severe or continues, check with your doctor.

*Take this medicine only as directed.* Do not take more or less of it, and do not take it more often than your doctor ordered.

For patients taking *carbidopa and levodopa extended-release tablets*:

- Swallow the tablet whole without crushing or chewing, unless your doctor tells you not to. If your doctor tells you to, you may break the tablet in half.

Some people must take this medicine for several weeks or months before full benefit is received. *Do not stop taking it even if you do not think it is working.* Instead, check with your doctor.

**Dosing**—The dose of levodopa or carbidopa and levodopa combination will be different for different patients. *Follow your doctor's orders or the directions on the label.* The following information includes only the average doses of levodopa or carbidopa and levodopa combination. *If your dose is different, do not change it* unless your doctor tells you to do so.

The number of capsules or tablets that you take depends on the strength of the medicine. Also, *the number of doses you take each day, the time allowed between doses, and the length of time you take the medicine depend on your special needs.*

*For levodopa*

- For Parkinson's disease:
  —For *oral* dosage form (capsules and tablets):
    - Adults and teenagers—At first, 250 milligrams (mg) two to four times a day. Your doctor may increase your dose if needed. However, the dose is usually not more than 8000 mg a day.
    - Children up to 12 years of age—Use and dose must be determined by your doctor.

*For levodopa and carbidopa combination*

- For Parkinson's disease:
  —For *oral tablet* dosage form:
    - Adults—At first, 1 tablet three or four times a day. Your doctor may need to change your dose, depending on how you respond to this combination medicine.

- Children and teenagers—Use and dose must be determined by your doctor.
  —For *oral extended-release tablet* dosage form:
    - Adults—At first, 1 tablet two times a day. However, you may need to take more than this. Your doctor will decide the right dose for you, depending on your condition and the other medicines you may be taking for Parkinson's disease.
    - Children and teenagers—Use and dose must be determined by your doctor.

**Missed dose**—If you miss a dose of this medicine, take it as soon as possible. However, if your next scheduled dose is within 2 hours, skip the missed dose and go back to your regular dosing schedule. Do not double doses.

**Storage**—To store this medicine:

- Keep out of the reach of children.
- Store away from heat and direct light.
- Do not store in the bathroom, near the kitchen sink, or in other damp places. Heat or moisture may cause the medicine to break down.
- Do not keep outdated medicine or medicine no longer needed. Be sure that any discarded medicine is out of the reach of children.

## Precautions While Using This Medicine

Before having any kind of surgery (including dental surgery) or emergency treatment, tell the medical doctor or dentist in charge that you are taking this medicine.

For *diabetic patients*:

- This medicine may cause test results for urine sugar or ketones to be wrong. Check with your doctor before depending on home tests using the paper-strip or tablet method.

This medicine may cause some people to become drowsy or less alert than they are normally. *Make sure you know how you react to this medicine before you drive, use machines, or do anything else that could be dangerous if you are not alert.*

*Dizziness, lightheadedness, or fainting may occur, especially when you get up from a lying or sitting position.* Getting up slowly may help. If the problem continues or gets worse, check with your doctor.

For patients taking levodopa by itself:

- Pyridoxine (vitamin B$_6$) has been found to reduce the effects of levodopa when levodopa is taken by itself. This does not happen with the combination of carbidopa and levodopa. *If you are taking levodopa by itself, do not take vitamin products containing vitamin B$_6$ during treatment, unless prescribed by your doctor.*
- Large amounts of pyridoxine are also contained in some foods such as avocado, bacon, beans, beef liver, dry skim milk, oatmeal, peas, pork, sweet potato, tuna, and certain health foods. Check with your doctor about how much of these foods you may have in

your diet while you are taking levodopa. Also, ask your health care professional for help when selecting vitamin products.

As your condition improves and your body movements become easier, *be careful not to overdo physical activities. Injuries resulting from falls may occur.* Physical activities must be increased gradually to allow your body to adjust to changing balance, circulation, and coordination. *This is especially important in the elderly.*

After taking this medicine for long periods of time, such as a year or more, some patients suddenly lose the ability to move. Their muscles do not seem to work. This loss of movement may last from a few minutes to several hours. The patient then is able to move as before. This condition may unexpectedly occur again and again. If you should have this problem, sometimes called the "on-off" effect, check with your doctor.

## Side Effects of This Medicine

Along with its needed effects, a medicine may cause some unwanted effects. Although not all of these side effects may occur, if they do occur they may need medical attention.

Check with your doctor as soon as possible if any of the following side effects occur:

*More common*
   Mental depression; mood or mental changes (such as aggressive behavior); unusual and uncontrolled movements of the body

*Less common—more common when levodopa is used alone*
   Difficult urination; dizziness or lightheadedness when getting up from a lying or sitting position; irregular heartbeat; nausea or vomiting (severe or continuing);

spasm or closing of eyelids (not more common when levodopa is used alone)

*Rare*
   High blood pressure; stomach pain; unusual tiredness or weakness

Other side effects may occur that usually do not need medical attention. These side effects may go away during treatment as your body adjusts to the medicine. However, check with your doctor if any of the following side effects continue or are bothersome:

*More common*
   Anxiety, confusion, or nervousness (especially in elderly patients receiving other medicine for Parkinson's disease)

*Less common*
   Constipation (more common when levodopa is used alone); diarrhea; dryness of mouth; flushing of skin; headache; loss of appetite; muscle twitching; nightmares (more common when levodopa is used alone); trouble in sleeping

This medicine may sometimes cause the urine and sweat to be darker in color than usual. The urine may at first be reddish, then turn to nearly black after being exposed to air. Some bathroom cleaning products will produce a similar effect when in contact with urine containing this medicine. This is to be expected during treatment with this medicine.

Other side effects not listed above may also occur in some patients. If you notice any other effects, check with your doctor.

Revised: 08/18/92
Interim revision: 08/17/94

# LIDOCAINE—For Self-Injection   Systemic†

A commonly used brand name in the U.S. is LidoPen.
This information does *not* apply to any other dosage forms or brand names of lidocaine.

†Not commercially available in Canada.

## Description

Lidocaine (LYE-doe-kane) belongs to the group of medicines called antiarrhythmics. It is used to change an abnormal rhythm in the heart back to normal. Lidocaine produces its helpful effects by slowing abnormal nerve impulses in the heart and reducing irritability of heart tissues.

Lidocaine is usually given by a health care professional when a rapid effect is needed. However, this dosage form has been prescribed by your doctor as part of the early management of a heart attack when certain abnormal

heart rhythms occur. It is designed to be used by the patient under instructions from a doctor.

This form of lidocaine is available only with your doctor's prescription and *is to be administered only under direct orders from your doctor.* It is available in the following dosage form:

*Parenteral*
   • Injection (U.S.)

## Before Using This Medicine

In deciding to use a medicine, the risks of taking the medicine must be weighed against the good it will do. This is a decision you and your doctor will make. For lidocaine, the following should be considered:

**Allergies**—Tell your doctor if you have ever had any unusual or allergic reaction to lidocaine, flecainide, tocainide, or anesthetics.

**Pregnancy**—Lidocaine has not been studied in pregnant women. However, this medicine may reduce the blood supply to the unborn baby.

**Breast-feeding**—It is not known whether lidocaine passes into breast milk. However, this medicine has not been reported to cause problems in nursing babies.

**Children**—Although there is no specific information comparing use of lidocaine in children with use in other age groups, this medicine is not expected to cause different side effects or problems in children than it does in adults.

**Older adults**—Elderly people are especially sensitive to the effects of lidocaine. This may increase the chance of side effects during treatment.

**Other medicines**—Although certain medicines should not be used together at all, in other cases two different medicines may be used together even if an interaction might occur. In these cases, your doctor may want to change the dose, or other precautions may be necessary. When you are receiving lidocaine it is especially important that your health care professional know if you are taking any of the following:

- Ethotoin (e.g., Peganone) or
- Mephenytoin (e.g., Mesantoin) or
- Phenytoin (e.g., Dilantin)—Risk of slow heartbeat may be increased. Other effects of lidocaine may be decreased because these medicines may cause it to be removed from the body more quickly

**Other medical problems**—The presence of other medical problems may affect the use of lidocaine. Make sure you tell your doctor if you have any other medical problems, especially:

- Congestive heart failure or
- Kidney disease or
- Liver disease—Effects may be increased because of slower removal of lidocaine from the body

## Proper Use of This Medicine

This medicine should be kept within easy reach, along with your doctor's telephone number. Check the expiration date on the lidocaine regularly. Replace the medicine before it expires.

Be familiar with possible symptoms of a heart attack and how to recognize them. If they occur, *telephone your doctor immediately.* The special device your doctor gave you will transmit your electrocardiogram (ECG or EKG) over the telephone. Your doctor will look at your ECG and tell you whether you need to use this medicine.

*Lidocaine comes with patient directions. Read them carefully before you actually need to use this medicine.* Then, when an emergency arises, you will know how to inject the lidocaine.

To use the lidocaine self-injector:

- Remove the gray safety cap.
- Place the black end of the self-injector on the thickest part of your thigh and press hard until the injector functions. You should feel a needle prick.
- Hold the device firmly in place for 10 seconds, then remove it. Massage the injection area for 10 seconds.

**Dosing**—The dose of lidocaine will be different for different patients. *Follow your doctor's orders or the directions on the label.* The following information includes only the average doses of lidocaine. *If your dose is different, do not change it* unless your doctor tells you to do so.

- For *injection* dosage form:
  —For arrhythmia (abnormal heart rhythm):
  - Adults—4.3 milligrams (mg) per kilogram (kg) (1.95 mg per pound) of body weight injected into the muscle. The dose may be repeated after sixty to ninety minutes if needed.
  - Children—Dose must be determined by your doctor. Use is not recommended in children weighing less than 50 kg (23 pounds).

**Storage**—To store this medicine:

- Keep out of the reach of children.
- Store away from heat and direct light.
- Keep the medicine from freezing.

## Precautions While Using This Medicine

*Do not administer this injection unless instructed to do so by your doctor.* Your doctor is trained to read the electrocardiogram and decide whether an abnormal heart rhythm is occurring.

Unless it is absolutely necessary, *do not attempt to drive after using this medicine.* Follow your doctor's instructions about what to do next, including going to the doctor's office or hospital emergency room, if necessary.

## Side Effects of This Medicine

Along with its needed effects, a medicine may cause some unwanted effects. Although not all of these side effects may occur, if they do occur they may need medical attention.

*Check with your doctor immediately* if any of the following side effects occur:

*Rare*

Convulsions (seizures); difficulty in breathing; itching; skin rash; swelling of skin

Check with your doctor as soon as possible if any of the following side effects occur:

*Signs and symptoms of overdose*

Blurred or double vision; dizziness (severe) or fainting; nausea or vomiting; ringing in ears; slow heartbeat; tremors or twitching

Other side effects may occur that usually do not need medical attention. However, check with your doctor if the following side effects continue or are bothersome:

*Less common or rare*

Anxiety or nervousness; dizziness; drowsiness; feelings of coldness, heat, or numbness; pain at place of injection

Other side effects not listed above may also occur in some patients. If you notice any other effects, check with your doctor.

Revised: 10/21/92
Interim revision: 10/27/93

---

# LIDOCAINE AND PRILOCAINE    Topical

A commonly used brand name in the U.S. and Canada is EMLA.

Another commonly used name for lidocaine is lignocaine.

## Description

This medicine contains a mixture of 2 local anesthetics (an-ess-THET-iks), lidocaine (LYE-doe-kane) and prilocaine (PRIL-oh-kane). It is used to produce numbness or loss of feeling before certain painful procedures, such as injections, drawing blood from a vein, or removing small growths (warts, for example) from the skin.

This medicine deadens the nerve endings in the skin. It does not cause unconsciousness as general anesthetics used for surgery do.

In the U.S., this medicine is available only with your doctor's prescription. In Canada, it is available without a prescription. However, your doctor may have special instructions on the proper use and dose, depending on the reason you are using this medicine.

*Topical*
• Cream (U.S. and Canada)

## Before Using This Medicine

In deciding to use a medicine, the risks of using the medicine must be weighed against the good it will do. This is a decision you and your doctor will make. For this medicine, the following should be considered:

**Allergies**—Tell your doctor if you have ever had any unusual or allergic reaction to lidocaine, prilocaine, or other local anesthetics given by injection or applied to any part of the body as a liquid, cream, ointment, or spray. Also tell your health care professional if you are allergic to any other substances, such as foods, preservatives, or dyes.

**Pregnancy**—This mixture of lidocaine and prilocaine has not been studied in pregnant women. However, lidocaine and prilocaine (separately) have been given to pregnant women and have not been reported to cause birth defects or other problems.

**Breast-feeding**—Small amounts of lidocaine, and probably of prilocaine also, pass into breast milk. Many medicines that pass into breast milk in small amounts may be used safely while breast-feeding. Mothers who are breast-feeding and who wish to use this medicine should discuss this with their doctor.

**Children**—This medicine has been tested in children. Very young children (less than 1 year of age) may be especially sensitive to the effects of lidocaine and prilocaine. This may increase the chance of side effects. However, in effective doses, this medicine has not been shown to cause different side effects or problems in children older than 1 year of age than it does in adults.

Young children are often frightened when they receive injections or have other painful procedures done. This medicine helps prevent pain, but it will not calm a frightened child. Parents can help by staying calm and by comforting and reassuring the child.

**Older adults**—This medicine has not been studied specifically in older people. However, it is possible that the chance of some side effects may be increased in elderly people. Experience with local anesthetics given by injection or applied to other areas of the body (for example, the throat or the inside of the mouth) has shown that elderly people are usually more sensitive than younger adults to the effects of local anesthetics.

**Other medicines**—Although certain medicines should not be used together at all, in other cases two different medicines may be used together even if an interaction might occur. In these cases, your doctor may want to change the dose, or other precautions may be necessary. Before using this medicine, tell your health care professional if you are taking any other prescription or nonprescription (over-the-counter [OTC]) medicine, especially:

• Sulfonamides (sulfa medicine)—The chance of a side effect (methemoglobinemia) may be increased, especially in infants.

**Other medical problems**—The presence of other medical problems may affect the use of this medicine. Make sure you tell your doctor if you have any other medical problems, especially:

• Broken or inflamed skin, burns, or open wounds at place of application or
• Atopic dermatitis or
• Eczema—More of this medicine can be absorbed into the body quickly, which increases the chance of side effects
• Glucose-6-phosphate dehydrogenase (G6PD) deficiency—A possible side effect of this medicine (methemoglobinemia) may be more likely to occur

• Liver disease (severe)—The chance of side effects may be increased if large amounts of this medicine are absorbed into the body quickly
• Methemoglobinemia—This medicine may make your condition worse

## Proper Use of This Medicine

For safe and effective use of this medicine:
• Use this medicine only when directed to do so by your health care professional. *Do not use it for any other reason without first checking with your doctor.* This medicine may be more likely than other topical anesthetics to cause unwanted effects if it is used too much, because more of it is absorbed into the body through the skin.
• Unless otherwise directed by your health care professional, *do not apply this medicine to open wounds, burns, or broken or inflamed skin.*
• *Be careful not to get any of this medicine in your eyes,* because it can cause severe eye irritation. If any of the medicine does get into your eye, *do not rub or wipe the eye, even if it hurts. Instead, check with your doctor right away.*
• Be careful not to get any of this medicine on your lips or in your mouth.
• *Follow carefully any directions given to you by your health care professional about how this medicine should be used.* If you have not received other instructions about how to apply this medicine, *follow the patient directions that come with the medicine.*
• *Check with your health care professional if you have any questions* about how to apply this medicine, where to apply it, or what time to apply it.

To use:
• Apply a thick layer of medicine to the area or areas where local anesthesia (numbness or loss of feeling) is needed. *Do not spread out the medicine.*
• This medicine is used together with a special bandage (called an occlusive dressing). *Check with your health care professional if you did not receive any bandages with the medicine.* Cover the medicine with the bandage. *Seal the edges of the bandage tightly, making sure that none of the medicine leaks out.* Do not lift the bandage or otherwise disturb it. Keeping the medicine tightly covered helps it work properly.
• If your health care professional has directed you to remove the bandage and wipe off the medicine after a certain amount of time, follow the directions carefully. Then clean the area with the antiseptic solution recommended by your health care professional. *If your health care professional has not directed you to remove the bandage and the medicine, keep them in place until your health care professional removes them.*

**Dosing**—The dose of this medicine will be different for different patients. *Follow your doctor's orders or the directions that come with the medicine.* The following

information includes only the average doses of this medicine. *If your dose is different, do not change it* unless your doctor tells you to do so.
• For *topical* dosage form (cream):
—For preventing pain caused by injections or drawing blood from a vein:
• Adults and children—Apply 2.5 grams of cream (one-half of the amount in a 5-gram tube) in a thick layer to an area about two inches by two inches (twenty to twenty-five square centimeters) in size. Your health care professional may direct you to apply the medicine in two places. The medicine should remain in place, covered by the bandage that comes with it, for at least one hour.
—For preventing pain caused by certain procedures:
• Adults—The size of the area to be covered by a thick layer of this medicine and the amount of time that the medicine must be kept in place depend on the procedure that is being done. The medicine sometimes needs to be kept in place, covered with the bandage, for two hours or more.
• Children—The size of the area to be covered by a thick layer of this medicine and the amount of time that the medicine must be kept in place depend on the procedure being done. However, the largest area that may be covered by this medicine depends on the child's weight and must be determined by your doctor. The medicine sometimes needs to be kept in place, covered with the bandage, for two hours or more.

**Storage**—To store this medicine:
• Keep out of the reach of children.
• Store away from heat and direct light.
• Keep the medicine from freezing.
• Do not keep outdated medicine or medicine no longer needed. Be sure that any discarded medicine is out of the reach of children.

## Precautions After Using This Medicine

After applying this medicine to the skin of a child, *watch the child carefully to make sure that he or she does not loosen or remove the bandage. Also, keep the child from getting any of the medicine into his or her mouth.* This medicine can cause serious side effects, especially in children, if any of it gets into the mouth or is swallowed.

During the time that the area to which the medicine was applied feels numb, serious injury can occur without your knowing about it. *Be especially careful to avoid injury until the anesthetic wears off or feeling returns to the area.* For example, do not scratch or rub the area or allow very hot or very cold objects to touch it.

## Side Effects of This Medicine

Along with its needed effects, a medicine may cause some unwanted effects. Although not all of these side effects

may occur, if they do occur they may need medical attention.

*The following side effects may mean that a serious allergic reaction is occurring. Check with your doctor or get emergency help immediately* if they occur, especially if several of them occur at the same time.

*Rare*

Coughing, shortness of breath, troubled breathing, tightness in chest, or wheezing; difficulty in swallowing; large, hive-like swellings on eyelids, face, lips, or tongue; severe dizziness or feeling faint; skin rash, itching, or hives; stuffy nose

*Also check with your health care professional, or get emergency help right away*, if any of the following side effects occur:

*Signs of too much medicine being absorbed into the body*

Blue or blue-purple color of lips, fingernails, or skin; blurred or double vision; dark urine; dizziness or drowsiness; feeling hot, cold, or numb; headache; irregular or fast heartbeat; muscle twitching or trembling; nausea or vomiting; ringing or buzzing in the ears; shortness of breath or troubled breathing; unusual excitement, nervousness, or restlessness; unusual tiredness or weakness

Note: The above side effects are not likely to occur when usual amounts of this medicine are used properly. However, they may occur if the medicine is used too often, applied to broken skin (for example, cuts or scrapes), applied to very large areas, or kept on the skin too long.

Other side effects may occur that usually do not need medical attention. However, check with your doctor if any of the following side effects continue or are bothersome:

*More common*

Burning feeling, swelling, itching, or skin rash at place of application (without other signs of an allergic reaction listed above); white or red skin at place of application

Other side effects not listed above may also occur in some patients. If you notice any other effects, check with your doctor.

## Additional Information

Once a medicine has been approved for marketing for a certain use, experience may show that it is also useful for other uses. Although this use is not included in product labeling, this medicine is used to produce loss of feeling in the genital area of adults before certain kinds of procedures are done. When used for this purpose, the medicine will be applied and removed by your doctor.

Other than the above information, there is no additional information relating to precautions or side effects for this use.

Revised: 08/18/93

# LINCOMYCIN    Systemic

A commonly used brand name is:
**In the U.S.—**
    Lincocin               Lincorex
**In Canada—**
    Lincocin

## Description

Lincomycin belongs to the family of medicines called antibiotics. These medicines are used to treat infections. They will not work for colds, flu, or other virus infections.

Lincomycin is available only with your doctor's prescription, in the following dosage forms:

*Oral*
- Capsules (U.S. and Canada)

*Parenteral*
- Injection (U.S. and Canada)

## Before Using This Medicine

In deciding to use a medicine, the risks of taking the medicine must be weighed against the good it will do.

This is a decision you and your doctor will make. For lincomycin, the following should be considered:

**Allergies**—Tell your doctor if you have ever had any unusual or allergic reaction to lincomycin, clindamycin, or doxorubicin. Also tell your health care professional if you are allergic to any other substances, such as foods, preservatives, or dyes.

**Pregnancy**—Lincomycin has not been reported to cause birth defects or other problems in humans.

**Breast-feeding**—Lincomycin passes into the breast milk. However, lincomycin has not been reported to cause problems in nursing babies.

**Children**—Lincomycin has been used in children 1 month of age or older and has not been reported to cause different side effects or problems than it does in adults.

**Older adults**—Many medicines have not been studied specifically in older people. Therefore, it may not be known whether they work exactly the same way they do in younger adults or if they cause different side effects or problems in older people. There is no specific information comparing use of lincomycin in the elderly with use in other age groups.

**Other medicines**—Although certain medicines should not be used together at all, in other cases two different medicines may be used together even if an interaction might occur. In these cases, your doctor may want to change the dose, or other precautions may be necessary. When you are taking lincomycin, it is especially important that your health care professional know if you are taking any of the following:

- Chloramphenicol (e.g., Chloromycetin) or
- Diarrhea medicine containing kaolin or attapulgite or
- Erythromycins (medicine for infection)—Taking these medicines along with lincomycin may decrease the effects of lincomycin
- Diarrhea medicine, such as loperamide (Imodium A-D)—Patients who take diarrhea medicine, such as loperamide (Imodium A-D) or diphenoxylate and atropine (Lomotil), may worsen diarrhea that is a side effect of lincomycin

**Other medical problems**—The presence of other medical problems may affect the use of lincomycin. Make sure you tell your doctor if you have any other medical problems, especially:

- Kidney disease (severe) or
- Liver disease (severe)—Severe kidney or liver disease may increase blood levels of this medicine, increasing the chance of side effects
- Stomach or intestinal disease, history of (especially colitis, including colitis caused by antibiotics, or enteritis)—Patients with a history of stomach or intestinal disease may have an increased chance of side effects

## Proper Use of This Medicine

Lincomycin is best taken with a full glass (8 ounces) of water on an empty stomach (either 1 hour before or 2 hours after meals), unless otherwise directed by your doctor.

To help clear up your infection completely, *keep taking this medicine for the full time of treatment,* even if you begin to feel better after a few days. *If you have a "strep" infection, you should keep taking this medicine for at least 10 days. This is especially important in "strep" infections. Serious heart problems could develop later* if your infection is not cleared up completely. Also, if you stop taking this medicine too soon, your symptoms may return.

This medicine works best when there is a constant amount in the blood. *To help keep the amount constant, do not miss any doses. Also, it is best to take each dose at evenly spaced times day and night.* For example, if you are to take 4 doses a day, doses should be spaced about 6 hours apart. If this interferes with your sleep or other daily activities, or if you need help in planning the best times to take your medicine, check with your health care professional.

**Dosing**—The dose of lincomycin will be different for different patients. *Follow your doctor's orders or the directions on the label.* The following information includes only the average doses of lincomycin. *If your dose is different, do not change it* unless your doctor tells you to do so.

- For infections caused by bacteria:
  —For *oral* dosage form (capsules):
  - Adults and teenagers—500 milligrams (mg) every six to eight hours.
  - Infants up to 1 month of age—Use and dose must be determined by your doctor.
  - Children 1 month of age and older—Dose is based on body weight. The usual dose is 7.5 to 15 mg per kilogram (kg) (3.4 to 6.8 mg per pound) of body weight every six hours; or 10 to 20 mg per kg (4.5 to 9.1 mg per pound) of body weight every eight hours.
  —For *injection* dosage form:
  - Adults and teenagers—600 mg to 1 gram injected into a vein over at least one hour, every eight to twelve hours; or 600 mg injected into a muscle every twelve to twenty-four hours.
  - Infants up to 1 month of age—Use and dose must be determined by your doctor.
  - Children 1 month of age and older—Dose is based on body weight. The usual dose is 10 mg per kg (4.5 mg per pound) of body weight injected into a muscle every twelve to twenty-four hours; or 3.3 to 6.7 mg per kg (1.5 to 3 mg per pound) of body weight injected into a vein every eight hours; or 5 to 10 mg per kg (2.3 to 4.5 mg per pound) of body weight injected into a vein every twelve hours.

**Missed dose**—If you miss a dose of this medicine, take it as soon as possible. This will help to keep a constant amount of medicine in the blood. However, if it is almost time for your next dose, skip the missed dose and go back to your regular dosing schedule. Do not double doses.

**Storage**—To store this medicine:

- Keep out of the reach of children.
- Store away from heat and direct light.
- Do not store the capsule form of this medicine in the bathroom, near the kitchen sink, or in other damp places. Heat or moisture may cause the medicine to break down.
- Do not keep outdated medicine or medicine no longer needed. Be sure that any discarded medicine is out of the reach of children.

## Precautions While Using This Medicine

It is important that your doctor check your progress at regular visits.

If your symptoms do not improve within a few days, or if they become worse, check with your doctor.

In some patients, lincomycin may cause diarrhea.

- Severe diarrhea may be a sign of a serious side effect. *Do not take any diarrhea medicine without first checking with your doctor.* Diarrhea medicines may make your diarrhea worse or make it last longer.
- For mild diarrhea, diarrhea medicine containing attapulgite (e.g., Kaopectate tablets, Diasorb) may be

taken. However, kaolin or attapulgite may keep lincomycin from being absorbed into the body. Therefore, these diarrhea medicines should be taken at least 2 hours before or 3 to 4 hours after you take lincomycin by mouth. Other kinds of diarrhea medicine should not be taken. They may make your diarrhea worse or make it last longer.

- If you have any questions about this or if mild diarrhea continues or gets worse, check with your health care professional.

Before having surgery (including dental surgery) with a general anesthetic, tell the medical doctor or dentist in charge that you are taking lincomycin.

## Side Effects of This Medicine

Along with its needed effects, a medicine may cause some unwanted effects. Although not all of these side effects may occur, if they do occur they may need medical attention.

*Check with your doctor immediately* if any of the following side effects occur:

*More common*
> Abdominal or stomach cramps and pain (severe); abdominal tenderness; diarrhea (watery and severe), which may also be bloody; fever

> Note: The above side effects may also occur up to several weeks after you stop taking this medicine.

*Less common*
> Skin rash, redness, and itching; sore throat and fever; unusual bleeding and bruising

Other side effects may occur that usually do not need medical attention. These side effects may go away during treatment as your body adjusts to the medicine. However, check with your doctor if any of the following side effects continue or are bothersome:

*More common*
> Diarrhea (mild); nausea and vomiting; stomach pain

*Less common*
> Itching of rectal or genital (sex organ) areas

Other side effects not listed above may also occur in some patients. If you notice any other effects, check with your doctor.

Revised: 10/06/92
Interim revision: 03/24/94

# LINDANE    Topical

Some commonly used brand names are:

**In the U.S.—**

| | |
|---|---|
| Bio-Well | Kwell |
| GBH | Kwildane |
| G-well | Scabene |
| Kildane | Thionex |

Generic name product may also be available.

**In Canada—**

| | |
|---|---|
| GBH | Kwellada |
| Hexit | PMS Lindane |

Generic name product may also be available.

Another commonly used name for lindane is gamma benzene hexachloride.

## Description

Lindane (LIN-dane), formerly known as gamma benzene hexachloride, is an insecticide and is used to treat scabies and lice infestations.

Lindane cream and lotion are usually used to treat only scabies infestation. Lindane shampoo is used to treat only lice infestations.

Lindane is available only with your doctor's prescription, in the following dosage forms:

*Topical*
- Cream (U.S. and Canada)
- Lotion (U.S. and Canada)
- Shampoo (U.S. and Canada)

## Before Using This Medicine

In deciding to use a medicine, the risks of using the medicine must be weighed against the good it will do. This is a decision you and your doctor will make. For lindane, the following should be considered:

**Allergies**—Tell your doctor if you have ever had any unusual or allergic reaction to lindane. Also tell your health care professional if you are allergic to any other substances, such as preservatives or dyes.

**Pregnancy**—Lindane is absorbed through the skin and could possibly cause toxic effects in the central nervous system (CNS) of the unborn baby. *Use lindane only as directed by your doctor. Do not use more of it, do not use it more often, and do not use it for a longer time than your doctor ordered. In addition, you should not be treated with lindane more than twice during your pregnancy.*

**Breast-feeding**—Lindane is absorbed through the mother's skin and is present in breast milk. Even though lindane has not been reported to cause problems in nursing babies, you should use another method of feeding your baby for 2 days after you use lindane. Be sure you have discussed this with your doctor.

**Children**—Infants and children are especially sensitive to the effects of lindane. This may increase the chance of side effects during treatment. In addition, use of lindane is not recommended in premature infants.

**Older adults**—Absorption of lindane may be increased in the elderly. This may increase the chance of problems during treatment with this medicine.

**Other medicines**—Although certain medicines should not be used together at all, in other cases two different medicines may be used together even if an interaction might occur. In these cases, your doctor may want to change the dose, or other precautions may be necessary. When you are using lindane, it is especially important that your health care professional know if you are using any other prescription or nonprescription (over-the-counter [OTC]) medicine.

**Other medical problems**—The presence of other medical problems may affect the use of lindane. Make sure you tell your doctor if you have any other medical problems, especially:

- Seizure disorder—Use of lindane may make the condition worse
- Skin rash or raw or broken skin—Condition may increase the absorption of lindane and the chance of side effects

## Proper Use of This Medicine

*Lindane is poisonous. Keep it away from the mouth because it is harmful and may be fatal if swallowed.*

*Use lindane only as directed by your doctor. Do not use more of it, do not use it more often, and do not use it for a longer time than your doctor ordered. To do so may increase the chance of absorption through the skin and the chance of lindane poisoning.*

*Keep lindane away from the eyes.* If you should accidentally get some in your eyes, flush them thoroughly with water at once and contact your doctor.

*Do not use lindane on open wounds, such as cuts or sores on the skin or scalp.* To do so may increase the chance of lindane poisoning.

*When applying lindane to another person, you should wear plastic disposable or rubber gloves, especially if you are pregnant or are breast-feeding.* This will prevent lindane from being absorbed through your skin. If you have any questions about this, check with your doctor.

Lindane usually comes with patient directions. Read them carefully before using lindane.

Your sexual partner or partners, especially, and all members of your household may need to be treated also, since the infestation may spread to persons in close contact. If these persons have not been checked for an infestation or if you have any questions about this, check with your doctor.

To use the *cream or lotion form of lindane for scabies:*
- If your skin has any cream, lotion, ointment, or oil on it, wash, rinse, and dry your skin well before applying lindane.

- If you take a warm bath or shower before using lindane, dry the skin well before applying it.
- Apply enough lindane to your dry skin to cover the entire skin surface from the neck down, including the soles of your feet, and rub in well.
- Leave lindane on for no more than 8 hours, then remove by washing thoroughly.

To use the *shampoo form of lindane for lice:*
- If your hair has any cream, lotion, ointment, or oil-based product on it, shampoo, rinse, and dry your hair and scalp well before applying lindane.
- If you apply this shampoo in the shower or in the bathtub, make sure the shampoo is not allowed to run down on other parts of your body. Also, do not apply this shampoo in a bathtub where the shampoo may run into the bath water in which you are sitting. To do so may increase the chance of absorption through the skin. When you rinse out the shampoo, be sure to thoroughly rinse your entire body also to remove any shampoo that may have gotten on it.
- Apply enough shampoo to your dry hair (1 ounce or less for short hair, 1½ ounces for medium length hair, and 2 ounces or less for long hair) to thoroughly wet the hair and skin or scalp of the affected and surrounding hairy areas.
- Thoroughly rub the shampoo into the hair and skin or scalp and allow to remain in place for 4 minutes. Then, use just enough water to work up a good lather.
- Rinse thoroughly and dry with a clean towel.
- When the hair is dry, comb with a fine-toothed comb to remove any remaining nits (eggs) or nit shells.
- *Do not use as a regular shampoo.*

**Dosing**—*Follow your doctor's orders or the directions on the label.* The following information includes only the average doses of lindane. *If your dose is different, do not change it* unless your doctor tells you to do so.
- For cream and lotion dosage forms:
  —For scabies:
    - Adults and children—Apply to the affected area(s) of the skin one time.
    - Premature infants—Use is not recommended.
- For shampoo dosage form:
  —For lice:
    - Adults and children—Apply to the scalp or the affected area(s) of the skin one time. Treatment may be repeated after seven days if necessary.
    - Premature infants—Use is not recommended.

**Storage**—To store this medicine:
- Keep out of the reach of children.
- Store away from heat and direct light.
- Keep lindane from freezing.
- Do not keep outdated lindane or lindane no longer needed. Be sure that any discarded lindane is out of the reach of children.

## Precautions While Using This Medicine

To help prevent reinfestation or spreading of the infestation to other persons:

- For scabies—All recently worn underwear and pajamas and used sheets, pillowcases, and towels should be washed in very hot water or dry-cleaned.
- For lice—All recently worn clothing and used bed linens and towels should be washed in very hot water or dry-cleaned.

## Side Effects of This Medicine

In infants and children, the risk of lindane being absorbed through the skin and causing unwanted side effects is greater than in adults. In premature newborn infants, use of lindane is not recommended, because lindane may be more likely to be absorbed through their skin than through the skin of older infants. You should discuss these possible effects with your doctor.

Along with its needed effects, a medicine may cause some unwanted effects. Although not all of these side effects may occur, if they do occur they may need medical attention.

Check with your doctor as soon as possible if any of the following side effects occur:
> *Rare*
>> Skin irritation not present before use of lindane; skin rash
> *Symptoms of lindane poisoning*
>> Convulsions (seizures); dizziness, clumsiness, or unsteadiness; fast heartbeat; muscle cramps; nervousness, restlessness, or irritability; vomiting

After you stop using lindane, itching may occur and continue for 1 to several weeks. If this continues longer or is bothersome, check with your doctor.

Other side effects not listed above may also occur in some patients. If you notice any other effects, check with your doctor.

Revised: 08/15/94

---

# LITHIUM   Systemic

Some commonly used brand names are:

**In the U.S.—**

| | |
|---|---|
| Cibalith-S | Lithobid |
| Eskalith | Lithonate |
| Eskalith CR | Lithotabs |
| Lithane | |

Generic name product may also be available.

**In Canada—**

| | |
|---|---|
| Carbolith | Lithane |
| Duralith | Lithizine |

## Description

Lithium (LITH-ee-um) is used to treat the manic stage of bipolar disorder (manic-depressive illness). Manic-depressive patients experience severe mood changes, ranging from an excited or manic state (for example, unusual anger or irritability or a false sense of well-being) to depression or sadness. Lithium is used to reduce the frequency and severity of manic states. Lithium may also reduce the frequency and severity of depression in bipolar disorder.

It is not known how lithium works to stabilize a person's mood. However, it does act on the central nervous system. It helps you to have more control over your emotions and helps you cope better with the problems of living.

It is important that you and your family understand all the effects of lithium. These effects depend on your individual condition and response and the amount of lithium you use. You also must know when to contact your doctor if there are problems with the medicine's use.

Lithium may also be used for other conditions as determined by your doctor.

This medicine is available only with your doctor's prescription, in the following dosage forms:
> *Oral*
> - Capsules (U.S. and Canada)
> - Slow-release capsules (Canada)
> - Syrup (U.S.)
> - Tablets (U.S. and Canada)
> - Extended-release tablets (U.S. and Canada)

## Before Using This Medicine

In deciding to use a medicine, the risks of taking the medicine must be weighed against the good it will do. This is a decision you and your doctor will make. For lithium, the following should be considered:

**Allergies**—Tell your doctor if you have ever had any unusual or allergic reaction to lithium. Also tell your health care professional if you are allergic to any other substances, such as foods, preservatives, or dyes.

**Diet**—Make certain your health care professional knows if you are on a low-sodium or low-salt diet. Too little salt in your diet could lead to serious side effects.

**Pregnancy**—Lithium is not recommended for use during pregnancy, especially during the first 3 months. Studies have shown that lithium may rarely cause thyroid problems and heart or blood vessel defects in the baby. It has also been shown to cause muscle weakness and severe drowsiness in newborn babies of mothers taking lithium near time of delivery.

**Breast-feeding**—Lithium passes into the breast milk. It has been reported to cause unwanted effects such as muscle weakness, lowered body temperature, and heart problems in nursing babies. Before taking this medicine, be sure you have discussed with your doctor the risks and benefits of breast-feeding.

**Children**—Lithium may cause weakened bones in children during treatment.

**Older adults**—Unusual thirst, an increase in amount of urine, diarrhea, drowsiness, loss of appetite, muscle weakness, trembling, slurred speech, nausea or vomiting, goiter, or symptoms of underactive thyroid are especially likely to occur in elderly patients, who are often more sensitive than younger adults to the effects of lithium.

**Other medicines**—Although certain medicines should not be used together at all, in other cases 2 different medicines may be used together even if an interaction might occur. In these cases, your doctor may want to change the dose, or other precautions may be necessary. When you are taking lithium, it is especially important that your health care professional know if you are taking any of the following:

- Antipsychotics (medicine for mental illness)—Blood levels of both medicines may change, increasing the chance of serious side effects
- Diuretics (water pills) or
- Inflammation or pain medicine, except narcotics—Higher blood levels of lithium may occur, increasing the chance of serious side effects
- Medicine for asthma, bronchitis, emphysema, sinusitis, or cystic fibrosis that contains the following:
    Calcium iodide or
    Iodinated glycerol or
    Potassium iodide—Unwanted effects on the thyroid gland may occur

**Other medical problems**—The presence of other medical problems may affect the use of lithium. Make sure you tell your doctor if you have any other medical problems, especially:

- Brain disease or
- Schizophrenia—You may be especially sensitive to lithium, and mental effects (such as increased confusion) may occur
- Diabetes mellitus (sugar diabetes)—Lithium may increase the blood levels of insulin; the dose of insulin you need to take may change
- Difficult urination or
- Infection (severe, occurring with fever, prolonged sweating, diarrhea, or vomiting) or
- Kidney disease—Higher blood levels of lithium may occur, increasing the chance of serious side effects
- Epilepsy or
- Goiter or other thyroid disease, or
- Heart disease or
- Parkinson's disease or
- Psoriasis—Lithium may make the condition worse
- Leukemia (history of)—Lithium may cause the leukemia to occur again

## Proper Use of This Medicine

Take this medicine after a meal or snack. Doing so will reduce stomach upset, tremors, or weakness and may also prevent a laxative effect.

For patients taking the *long-acting or slow-release form* of lithium:

- Swallow the tablet or capsule whole.
- Do not break, crush, or chew before swallowing.

For patients taking the *syrup form* of lithium:

- Dilute the syrup in fruit juice or another flavored beverage before taking.

*During treatment with lithium, drink 2 or 3 quarts of water or other fluids each day, and use a normal amount of salt in your food,* unless otherwise directed by your doctor.

*Take this medicine exactly as directed.* Do not take more or less of it, do not take it more or less often, and do not take it for a longer time than your doctor ordered. To do so may increase the chance of unwanted effects.

*Sometimes lithium must be taken for 1 to several weeks before you begin to feel better.*

*In order for lithium to work properly, it must be taken every day in regularly spaced doses as ordered by your doctor.* This is necessary to keep a constant amount of lithium in your blood. To help keep the amount constant, do not miss any doses and *do not stop taking the medicine even if you feel better.*

**Dosing**—The dose of lithium will be different for different patients. *Follow your doctor's orders or the directions on the label.* The following information includes only the average doses of lithium. *If your dose is different, do not change it* unless your doctor tells you to do so.

The number of capsules or tablets or teaspoonfuls of syrup that you take depends on the strength of the medicine. Also, *the number of doses you take each day, the time allowed between doses, and the length of time you take the medicine depend on the medical problem for which you are using lithium.*

- For *short-acting oral* dosage forms (capsules, tablets, syrup):
    —Adults and adolescents: To start, 300 to 600 milligrams three times a day.
    —Children up to 12 years of age: The dose is based on body weight. To start, the usual dose is 15 to 20 milligrams per kilogram of body weight (6.8 to 9 milligrams per pound) a day, given in smaller doses two or three times during the day.
- For *long-acting oral* dosage forms (slow-release capsules, extended-release tablets):
    —Adults and adolescents: 300 to 600 milligrams three times a day, or 450 to 900 milligrams two times a day.
    —Children up to 12 years of age: Dose must be determined by the doctor.

**Missed dose**—If you miss a dose of this medicine, take it as soon as possible. However, if it is within 4 hours (about 6 hours for extended-release tablets or slow-release capsules) of your next dose, skip the missed dose and go back to your regular dosing schedule. Do not double doses.

**Storage**—To store this medicine:

- Keep out of the reach of children.
- Store away from heat and direct light.
- Do not store in the bathroom, near the kitchen sink, or in other damp places. Heat or moisture may cause the medicine to break down.
- Keep the syrup form of this medicine from freezing.
- Do not keep outdated medicine or medicine no longer needed. Be sure that any discarded medicine is out of the reach of children.

## Precautions While Using This Medicine

*Your doctor should check your progress at regular visits* to make sure that the medicine is working properly and that possible side effects are avoided. Laboratory tests may be necessary.

Lithium may not work properly if you drink large amounts of caffeine-containing coffee, tea, or colas.

This medicine may cause some people to become dizzy, drowsy, or less alert than they are normally. *Make sure you know how you react to this medicine before you drive, use machines, or do anything else that could be dangerous if you are dizzy or are not alert.*

*Use extra care in hot weather and during activities that cause you to sweat heavily, such as hot baths, saunas, or exercising.* The loss of too much water and salt from your body could lead to serious side effects from this medicine.

*If you have an infection or illness that causes heavy sweating, vomiting, or diarrhea,* check with your doctor. The loss of too much water and salt from your body could lead to serious side effects from lithium.

*Do not go on a diet to lose weight and do not make a major change in your diet without first checking with your doctor.* Improper dieting could cause the loss of too much water and salt from your body and could lead to serious side effects from this medicine.

For patients taking the *slow-release capsules or the extended-release tablets:*

- Do not use this medicine interchangeably with other lithium products.

*It is important that you and your family know the early symptoms of lithium overdose or toxicity and when to call the doctor.*

## Side Effects of This Medicine

Along with its needed effects, a medicine may cause some unwanted effects. Although not all of these side effects may occur, if they do occur they may need medical attention.

*Check with your doctor immediately if any of the following side effects occur:*

> *Early symptoms of overdose or toxicity*
>> Diarrhea; drowsiness; loss of appetite; muscle weakness; nausea or vomiting; slurred speech; trembling

> *Late symptoms of overdose or toxicity*
>> Blurred vision; clumsiness or unsteadiness; confusion; convulsions (seizures); dizziness; increase in amount of urine; trembling (severe)

Check with your doctor as soon as possible if any of the following side effects occur:

> *Less common*
>> Fainting; fast or slow heartbeat; irregular pulse; troubled breathing (especially during hard work or exercise); unusual tiredness or weakness; weight gain

> *Rare*
>> Blue color and pain in fingers and toes; coldness of arms and legs; dizziness; eye pain; headache; noises in the ears; vision problems

> *Signs of low thyroid function*
>> Dry, rough skin; hair loss; hoarseness; mental depression; sensitivity to cold; swelling of feet or lower legs; swelling of neck; unusual excitement

Other side effects may occur that usually do not need medical attention. These side effects may go away during treatment as your body adjusts to the medicine. However, check with your doctor if any of the following side effects continue or are bothersome:

> *More common*
>> Increased frequency of urination or loss of bladder control—more common in women than in men, usually beginning 2 to 7 years after start of treatment; increased thirst; nausea (mild); trembling of hands (slight)

> *Less common*
>> Acne or skin rash; bloated feeling or pressure in the stomach; muscle twitching (slight)

Other side effects not listed above may also occur in some patients. If you notice any other effects, check with your doctor.

## Additional Information

Once a medicine has been approved for marketing for a certain use, experience may show that it is also useful for other medical problems. Although these uses are not

included in product labeling, lithium is used in certain patients with the following medical conditions:

- Cluster headaches
- Mental depression
- Neutropenia (a blood condition in which there is a decreased number of a certain type of white blood cells)

Other than the above information, there is no additional information relating to proper use, precautions, or side effects for these uses.

Revised: 03/09/93

# LODOXAMIDE Ophthalmic†

A commonly used brand name in the U.S. is Alomide.
Another commonly used name is lodoxamide trometamol.

†Not commercially available in Canada.

## Description

Lodoxamide (loe-DOX-a-mide) ophthalmic solution is used in the eye to treat certain disorders of the eye caused by allergies. It works by acting on certain cells, called mast cells, to prevent them from releasing substances that cause the allergic reaction.

Lodoxamide is available only with your doctor's prescription, in the following dosage form:

*Ophthalmic*
- Ophthalmic solution (eye drops) (U.S.)

## Before Using This Medicine

In deciding to use a medicine, the risks of using the medicine must be weighed against the good it will do. This is a decision you and your doctor will make. For lodoxamide, the following should be considered:

**Allergies**—Tell your doctor if you have ever had any unusual or allergic reaction to lodoxamide. Also tell your health care professional if you are allergic to any other substances, such as foods, preservatives, or dyes.

**Pregnancy**—Lodoxamide has not been studied in pregnant women. However, lodoxamide has not been shown to cause birth defects or other problems in animal studies.

**Breast-feeding**—It is not known whether lodoxamide passes into the breast milk. Although most medicines pass into breast milk in small amounts, many of them may be used safely while breast-feeding. Mothers who are using this medicine and who wish to breast-feed should discuss this with their doctor.

**Children**—Studies on this medicine have been done only in adult patients, and there is no specific information comparing use of lodoxamide in children up to 2 years of age with use in other age groups. For older children, this medicine is not expected to cause different side effects or problems than it does in adults.

**Older adults**—Many medicines have not been studied specifically in older people. Therefore, it may not be known whether they work exactly the same way they do in younger adults or if they cause different side effects or problems in older people. There is no specific information comparing use of lodoxamide in the elderly with use in other age groups.

## Proper Use of This Medicine

To use the *eye drops:*
- First, wash your hands. Tilt the head back and, pressing your finger gently on the skin just beneath the lower eyelid, pull the lower eyelid away from the eye to make a space. Drop the medicine into this space. Let go of the eyelid and gently close the eyes. Do not blink. Keep the eyes closed for 1 or 2 minutes to allow the medicine to be absorbed by the eye.
- If you think you did not get the drop of medicine into your eye properly, use another drop.
- To keep the medicine as germ-free as possible, do not touch the applicator tip to any surface (including the eye). Also, keep the container tightly closed.

*In order for this medicine to work properly, it should be used every day in regularly spaced doses as ordered by your doctor.*

**Dosing**—The dose of ophthalmic lodoxamide will be different for different patients. *Follow your doctor's orders or the directions on the label.* The following information includes only the average doses of ophthalmic lodoxamide. *If your dose is different, do not change it* unless your doctor tells you to do so.
- For *ophthalmic solution (eye drops)* dosage form:
  —For eye allergies:
    - Adults and children 2 years of age and older—Use one drop four times a day at regularly spaced times for up to three months.
    - Children up to 2 years of age—Use and dose must be determined by your doctor.

**Missed dose**—If you miss a dose of this medicine, use it as soon as possible. Then go back to your regular dosing schedule.

**Storage**—To store this medicine:
- Keep out of the reach of children.
- Store away from heat and direct light.
- Keep the medicine from freezing.

- Do not keep outdated medicine or medicine no longer needed. Be sure that any discarded medicine is out of the reach of children.

## Precautions While Using This Medicine

*If your symptoms do not improve or if your condition becomes worse, check with your doctor.*

## Side Effects of This Medicine

Along with its needed effects, a medicine may cause some unwanted effects. Although not all of these side effects may occur, if they do occur they may need medical attention.

Check with your doctor as soon as possible if any of the following side effects occur:

*Less common*
Blurred vision; feeling of something in eye, itching, discomfort, redness, tearing or discharge, or other eye or eyelid irritation (not present before you started using this medicine or becoming worse while you are using this medicine)

*Rare*
Dizziness; mucus from eye, eye pain, or swelling of eye or eyelid (not present before you started using this medicine or becoming worse while you are using this medicine); headache; sensitivity of eyes to light; skin rash

Other side effects may occur that usually do not need medical attention. These side effects may go away during treatment as your body adjusts to the medicine. However, check with your doctor if any of the following side effects continue or are bothersome:

*More common*
Burning or stinging (when medicine is applied)

*Less common or rare*
Aching eyes; crusting in corner of eye or on eyelid; drowsiness or sleepiness; dryness of nose or eyes; feeling of heat in eye; heat sensation on body; nausea or stomach discomfort; scales on eyelid or eyelash; sneezing; sticky feeling of eyes; tired eyes

Other side effects not listed above may also occur in some patients. If you notice any other effects, check with your doctor.

Developed: 03/29/94

# LOMUSTINE  Systemic

A commonly used brand name in the U.S. and Canada is CeeNU. Another commonly used name is CCNU.

## Description

Lomustine (loe-MUS-teen) belongs to the group of medicines known as alkylating agents. It is used to treat some kinds of cancer.

Lomustine interferes with the growth of cancer cells, which are eventually destroyed. Since the growth of normal body cells may also be affected by lomustine, other effects will also occur. Some of these may be serious and must be reported to your doctor. Other effects, like hair loss, may not be serious but may cause concern. Some effects may not occur for months or years after the medicine is used.

Before you begin treatment with lomustine, you and your doctor should talk about the good this medicine will do as well as the risks of using it.

Lomustine is available only with your doctor's prescription, in the following dosage form:
*Oral*
- Capsules (U.S. and Canada)

## Before Using This Medicine

In deciding to use a medicine, the risks of taking the medicine must be weighed against the good it will do.

This is a decision you and your doctor will make. For lomustine, the following should be considered:

**Allergies**—Tell your doctor if you have ever had any unusual or allergic reaction to lomustine.

**Pregnancy**—Tell your doctor if you are pregnant or if you intend to have children. There is a chance that this medicine may cause birth defects if either the male or female is taking it at the time of conception or if it is taken during pregnancy. Lomustine causes birth defects in rats and causes toxic or harmful effects in the fetus of rats and rabbits at doses about the same as the human dose. In addition, many cancer medicines may cause sterility which could be permanent. Sterility has been reported in animals and humans with this medicine.

Be sure that you have discussed this with your doctor before taking this medicine. It is best to use some kind of birth control while you are taking lomustine. Tell your doctor right away if you think you have become pregnant while taking lomustine.

**Breast-feeding**—Tell your doctor if you are breast-feeding or if you intend to breast-feed during treatment with this medicine. Because lomustine may cause serious side effects, breast-feeding is generally not recommended while you are receiving it.

**Children**—Although there is no specific information comparing use of lomustine in children with use in other age groups, this medicine is not expected to cause different side effects or problems in children than it does in adults.

**Older adults**—Many medicines have not been studied specifically in older people. Therefore, it may not be known whether they work exactly the same way they do in younger adults or if they cause different side effects or problems in older people. There is no specific information comparing use of lomustine in the elderly with use in other age groups.

**Other medicines**—Although certain medicines should not be used together at all, in other cases two different medicines may be used together even if an interaction might occur. In these cases, your doctor may want to change the dose, or other precautions may be necessary. When you are taking lomustine, it is especially important that your health care professional know if you have ever been treated with x-rays or cancer medicines or if you are taking any of the following:
- Amphotericin B by injection (e.g., Fungizone) or
- Antithyroid agents (medicine for overactive thyroid) or
- Azathioprine (e.g., Imuran) or
- Chloramphenicol (e.g., Chloromycetin) or
- Colchicine or
- Flucytosine (e.g., Ancobon) or
- Ganciclovir (e.g., Cytovene) or
- Interferon (e.g., Intron A, Roferon-A) or
- Plicamycin (e.g., Mithracin) or
- Zidovudine (e.g., AZT, Retrovir)—Lomustine may increase the effects of these medicines or radiation therapy on the blood

**Other medical problems**—The presence of other medical problems may affect the use of lomustine. Make sure you tell your doctor if you have any other medical problems, especially:
- Chickenpox (including recent exposure) or
- Herpes zoster (shingles)—Risk of severe disease affecting other parts of the body
- Infection—Lomustine can decrease your body's ability to fight infection
- Kidney disease—Effects of lomustine may be increased because of slower removal from the body
- Lung disease—Risk of lung problems caused by lomustine may be increased

## Proper Use of This Medicine

*Take this medicine only as directed by your doctor.* Do not take more or less of it than your doctor ordered. The exact amount of medicine you need has been carefully worked out. Taking too much may increase the chance of side effects, while taking too little may not improve your condition.

In order that you receive the proper dose of lomustine, there may be two or more different types of capsules in the container. This is not an error. It is important that you take all of the capsules in the container as one dose so that you receive the right dose of the medicine.

This medicine is sometimes given together with certain other medicines. If you are using a combination of medicines, make sure that you take each one at the right time

and do not mix them. Ask your health care professional to help you plan a way to remember to take your medicines at the right times.

Nausea and vomiting occur often after lomustine is taken, but usually last less than 24 hours. Loss of appetite may last for several days. This medicine is best taken on an empty stomach at bedtime so that it will cause less stomach upset. Ask your health care professional for other ways to lessen these effects.

If you vomit shortly after taking a dose of lomustine, check with your doctor. You may be told to take the dose again.

**Dosing**—The dose of lomustine will be different for different patients. The dose that is used may depend on a number of things, including what the medicine is being used for, the patient's size, and whether or not other medicines are also being taken. *If you are taking lomustine at home, follow your doctor's orders or the directions on the label.* If you have any questions about the proper dose of lomustine, ask your doctor.

## Precautions While Using This Medicine

*It is important that your doctor check your progress at regular visits* to make sure that this medicine is working properly and to check for unwanted effects.

While you are being treated with lomustine, and after you stop treatment with it, *do not have any immunizations (vaccinations) without your doctor's approval.* Lomustine may lower your body's resistance and there is a chance you might get the infection the immunization is meant to prevent. In addition, other persons living in your household should not take oral polio vaccine since there is a chance they could pass the polio virus on to you. Also, avoid persons who have recently taken oral polio vaccine. Do not get close to them, and do not stay in the same room with them for very long. If you cannot take these precautions, you should consider wearing a protective face mask that covers the nose and mouth.

Lomustine can temporarily lower the number of white blood cells in your blood, increasing the chance of getting an infection. It can also lower the number of platelets, which are necessary for proper blood clotting. If this occurs, there are certain precautions you can take, especially when your blood count is low, to reduce the risk of infection or bleeding:
- If you can, avoid people with infections. *Check with your doctor immediately* if you think you are getting an infection or if you get a fever or chills, cough or hoarseness, lower back or side pain, or painful or difficult urination.
- *Check with your doctor immediately* if you notice any unusual bleeding or bruising; black, tarry stools; blood in urine or stools; or pinpoint red spots on your skin.
- Be careful when using a regular toothbrush, dental floss, or toothpick. Your medical doctor, dentist, or nurse may recommend other ways to clean your teeth

and gums. Check with your medical doctor before having any dental work done.

- Do not touch your eyes or the inside of your nose unless you have just washed your hands and have not touched anything else in the meantime.
- Be careful not to cut yourself when you are using sharp objects such as a safety razor or fingernail or toenail cutters.
- Avoid contact sports or other situations where bruising or injury could occur.

## Side Effects of This Medicine

Along with their needed effects, medicines like lomustine can sometimes cause unwanted effects such as blood problems, loss of hair, and other side effects; these are described below. Also, because of the way these medicines act on the body, there is a chance that they might cause other unwanted effects that may not occur until months or years after the medicine is used. These delayed effects may include certain types of cancer, such as leukemia. Discuss these possible effects with your doctor.

Although not all of these side effects may occur, if they do occur they may need medical attention.

*Check with your doctor or nurse immediately* if any of the following side effects occur:

*Less common*
> Black, tarry stools; blood in urine or stools; cough or hoarseness; fever or chills; lower back or side pain; painful or difficult urination; pinpoint red spots on skin; unusual bleeding or bruising

Check with your doctor as soon as possible if any of the following side effects occur:

*Less common*
> Awkwardness; confusion; decrease in urination; slurred speech; sores in mouth and on lips; swelling of feet or lower legs; unusual tiredness or weakness

*Rare*
> Cough; shortness of breath

Other side effects may occur that usually do not need medical attention. These side effects may go away during treatment as your body adjusts to the medicine. Also, your health care professional may be able to tell you about ways to prevent or reduce some of these side effects. Check with your health care professional if any of the following side effects continue or are bothersome or if you have any questions about them:

*More common*
> Loss of appetite
> Nausea and vomiting (usually last less than 24 hours)

*Less common*
> Darkening of skin; diarrhea; skin rash and itching

This medicine may cause a temporary loss of hair in some people. After treatment with lomustine has ended, normal hair growth should return.

After you stop using this medicine, it may still produce some side effects that need attention. During this period of time, check with your doctor if you notice any of the following side effects:

> Black, tarry stools; blood in urine or stools; cough or hoarseness; fever or chills; lower back or side pain; painful or difficult urination; pinpoint red spots on skin; unusual bleeding or bruising

Other side effects not listed above may also occur in some patients. If you notice any other effects, check with your doctor.

Revised: 08/09/92
Interim revision: 06/21/94

# LOPERAMIDE    Oral

Some commonly used brand names are:

**In the U.S.—**
> Imodium
> Imodium A-D

Imodium A-D Caplets

**In Canada—**
> Imodium

## Description

Loperamide (loe-PER-a-mide) is a medicine used along with other measures to treat diarrhea. Loperamide helps stop diarrhea by slowing down the movements of the intestines.

In the U.S., loperamide capsules are available only with your doctor's prescription, while the liquid form and the tablet form are available without a prescription. In Canada, all the dosage forms are available without a prescription.

Loperamide is available in the following dosage forms:

*Oral*
- Capsules (U.S. and Canada)
- Oral solution (U.S. and Canada)
- Tablets (U.S. and Canada)

## Before Using This Medicine

If you are taking this medicine without a prescription, carefully read and follow any precautions on the label. For loperamide, the following should be considered:

**Allergies**—Tell your doctor if you have ever had any unusual or allergic reaction to loperamide. Also tell your

health care professional if you are allergic to any other substances, such as foods, preservatives, or dyes.

**Pregnancy**—Studies have not been done in humans. However, studies in animals have not shown that loperamide causes cancer or birth defects or lessens the chances of becoming pregnant when given in doses many times the human dose.

**Breast-feeding**—It is not known whether loperamide passes into the breast milk. However, this medicine has not been reported to cause problems in nursing babies.

**Children**—This medicine should not be used in children under 2 years of age. Children, especially very young children, are very sensitive to the effects of loperamide. This may increase the chance of side effects during treatment. Also, the fluid loss caused by diarrhea may result in a severe condition. For these reasons, do not give medicine for diarrhea to young children without first checking with their doctor. In older children with diarrhea, medicine for diarrhea may be used, but it is also very important that a sufficient amount of liquids be given to replace the fluid lost by the body. If you have any questions about this, check with your health care professional.

**Older adults**—The fluid loss caused by diarrhea may result in a severe condition. For this reason, elderly persons with diarrhea, in addition to using medicine for diarrhea, must receive a sufficient amount of liquids to replace the fluid lost by the body. If you have any questions about this, check with your health care professional.

**Other medicines**—Although certain medicines should not be used together at all, in other cases two different medicines may be used together even if an interaction might occur. In these cases, your doctor may want to change the dose, or other precautions may be necessary. When you are taking loperamide, it is especially important that your health care professional know if you are taking any of the following:

- Antibiotics such as cephalosporins (e.g., Ceftin, Keflex), clindamycin (e.g., Cleocin), erythromycins (e.g., E.E.S., PCE), tetracyclines (e.g., Achromycin, Doryx)—These antibiotics may cause diarrhea; loperamide may make the diarrhea caused by antibiotics worse or make it last longer
- Narcotic pain medicine—There is a greater chance that severe constipation may occur if loperamide is used together with narcotic pain medicine

**Other medical problems**—The presence of other medical problems may affect the use of loperamide. Make sure you tell your doctor if you have any other medical problems, especially:

- Colitis (severe)—A more serious problem of the colon may develop if you use this medicine
- Dysentery—This condition may get worse; a different kind of treatment may be needed
- Liver disease—The chance of severe central nervous system (CNS) side effects may be greater in patients with liver disease

## Proper Use of This Medicine

For safe and effective use of this medicine:

- *Follow your doctor's instructions if this medicine was prescribed.*
- Follow the manufacturer's package directions if you are treating yourself.

*Importance of diet and fluid intake while treating diarrhea:*

- *In addition to using medicine for diarrhea, it is very important that you replace the fluid lost by the body and follow a proper diet.* For the first 24 hours, you should drink plenty of caffeine-free clear liquids, such as ginger ale, decaffeinated cola, decaffeinated tea, broth, and gelatin. During the next 24 hours you may eat bland foods, such as cooked cereals, bread, crackers, and applesauce. Fruits, vegetables, fried or spicy foods, bran, candy, caffeine, and alcoholic beverages may make the condition worse.
- If too much fluid has been lost by the body due to the diarrhea, a serious condition may develop. Check with your doctor as soon as possible if any of the following signs of too much fluid loss occur:
  Decreased urination
  Dizziness and lightheadedness
  Dryness of mouth
  Increased thirst
  Wrinkled skin

**Missed dose**—If you must take this medicine regularly and you miss a dose, skip the missed dose and go back to your regular dosing schedule. Do not double doses.

**Storage**—To store this medicine:

- Keep out of the reach of children
- Store away from heat and direct light.
- Do not store the capsule or tablet form of this medicine in the bathroom, near the kitchen sink, or in other damp places. Heat or moisture may cause the medicine to break down.
- Keep the liquid form of this medicine from freezing.
- Do not keep outdated medicine or medicine no longer needed. Be sure that any discarded medicine is out of the reach of children.

## Precautions While Using This Medicine

Loperamide should not be used for more than 2 days, unless directed by your doctor. If you will be taking this medicine regularly for a long time, your doctor should check your progress at regular visits.

*Check with your doctor if your diarrhea does not stop after two days or if you develop a fever.*

## Side Effects of This Medicine

Along with its needed effects, a medicine may cause some unwanted effects. *When this medicine is used for short periods of time at low doses, side effects usually are rare.*

*However, check with your doctor immediately* if any of the following side effects are severe and occur suddenly since they may be signs of a more severe and dangerous problem with your bowels:

> *Rare*
>> Bloating; constipation; loss of appetite; stomach pain (severe) with nausea and vomiting

Also, check with your doctor as soon as possible if the following side effect occurs:

> *Rare*
>> Skin rash

Other side effects may occur that usually do not need medical attention. These side effects may go away during treatment as your body adjusts to the medicine. However, check with your doctor if any of the following side effects continue or are bothersome:

> *Rare*
>> Drowsiness or dizziness; dryness of mouth

Other side effects not listed above may also occur in some patients. If you notice any other effects, check with your doctor.

Revised: 05/15/91

# LORACARBEF    Systemic†

A commonly used brand name in the U.S. is Lorabid.

†Not commercially available in Canada.

## Description

Loracarbef (loe-ra-KAR-bef) is used to treat bacterial infections in many different parts of the body. It works by killing bacteria or preventing their growth. This medicine will not work for colds, flu, or other virus infections.

Loracarbef is available only with your doctor's prescription, in the following dosage forms:

*Oral*
- Capsules (U.S.)
- Oral suspension (U.S.)

## Before Using This Medicine

In deciding to use a medicine, the risks of taking the medicine must be weighed against the good it will do. This is a decision you and your doctor will make. For loracarbef, the following should be considered:

**Allergies**—Tell your doctor if you have ever had any unusual or allergic reaction to loracarbef or to any related medicines such as penicillins or cephalosporins. Also tell your health care professional if you are allergic to any other substances, such as foods, preservatives, or dyes.

**Pregnancy**—Loracarbef has not been studied in pregnant women. However, loracarbef has not been shown to cause birth defects or other problems in animal studies.

**Breast-feeding**—It is not known whether loracarbef passes into breast milk.

**Children**—This medicine has been tested in a limited number of children 6 months of age and older. In effective doses, the medicine has not been shown to cause different side effects or problems than it does in adults.

**Older adults**—This medicine has been tested in a limited number of elderly patients and has not been shown to cause different side effects or problems in older people than it does in younger adults.

**Other medicines**—Although certain medicines should not be used together at all, in other cases two different medicines may be used together even if an interaction might occur. In these cases, your doctor may want to change the dose, or other precautions may be necessary. When you are taking loracarbef, it is especially important that your health care professional know if you are taking any of the following:

- Probenecid (e.g., Benemid)—Probenecid increases the blood level of loracarbef, increasing the chance of side effects

**Other medical problems**—The presence of other medical problems may affect the use of loracarbef. Make sure you tell your doctor if you have any other medical problems, especially:

- Kidney disease—Kidney disease may increase the blood level of loracarbef, increasing the chance of side effects

## Proper Use of This Medicine

Loracarbef should be taken at least 1 hour before or at least 2 hours after meals.

To help clear up your infection completely, *keep taking loracarbef for the full time of treatment,* even if you begin to feel better after a few days. *If you have a "strep" infection, you should keep taking this medicine for at least 10 days. This is especially important in "strep" infections. Serious heart problems could develop later* if your infection is not cleared up completely. Also, if you stop taking this medicine too soon, your symptoms may return.

This medicine works best when there is a constant amount in the blood or urine. *To help keep the amount constant, do not miss any doses. Also, it is best to take the doses at evenly spaced times, day and night.* If this interferes with your sleep or other daily activities, or if you need help in planning the best times to take your medicine, check with your health care professional.

**Dosing**—The dose of loracarbef will be different for different patients. *Follow your doctor's orders or the directions on the label.* The following information includes only the average doses of loracarbef. Your dose may be different if you have kidney disease. *If your dose is different, do not change it* unless your doctor tells you to do so.

The number of capsules or teaspoonfuls of suspension that you take depends on the strength of the medicine. Also, *the number of doses you take each day, the time allowed between doses, and the length of time you take the medicine depend on the medical problem for which you are taking loracarbef.*

- For *oral* dosage forms (capsules or oral suspension):
  —For bronchitis:
    - Adults and children 13 years of age and older—200 to 400 milligrams (mg) every twelve hours for seven days.
    - Children 6 months to 12 years of age—Use and dose to be determined by your doctor.
  —For otitis media (ear infection):
    - Children 6 months to 12 years of age—Dose is based on body weight and must be determined by your doctor.
  —For pneumonia:
    - Adults and children 13 years of age and older—400 mg every twelve hours for fourteen days.
    - Children 6 months to 12 years of age—Use and dose to be determined by your doctor.
  —For sinusitis:
    - Adults and children 13 years of age and older—400 mg every twelve hours for ten days.
    - Children 6 months to 12 years of age—Use and dose to be determined by your doctor.
  —For skin and soft tissue infections:
    - Adults and children 13 years of age and older—200 mg every twelve hours for seven days.
    - Children 6 months to 12 years of age—Dose is based on body weight and must be determined by your doctor.
  —For streptococcal pharyngitis ("strep throat"):
    - Adults and children 13 years of age and older—200 mg every twelve hours for ten days.
    - Children 6 months to 12 years of age—Dose is based on body weight and must be determined by your doctor.
  —For urinary tract infections:
    - Adults and children 13 years of age and older—200 to 400 mg every twelve to twenty-four hours for seven to fourteen days.
    - Children 6 months to 12 years of age—Use and dose to be determined by your doctor.

**Missed dose**—If you do miss a dose of this medicine, take it as soon as possible. This will help to keep a constant amount of medicine in the blood or urine. However, if it is almost time for your next dose, skip the missed dose and go back to your regular dosing schedule. Do not double doses.

**Storage**—To store this medicine:
- Keep out of the reach of children.
- Store away from heat and direct light.
- Do not store the capsule form of this medicine in the bathroom, near the kitchen sink, or in other damp places. Heat or moisture may cause the medicine to break down.
- Do not keep outdated medicine or medicine no longer needed. Be sure that any discarded medicine is out of the reach of children.

## Precautions While Using This Medicine

If your symptoms do not improve within a few days, or if they become worse, check with your doctor.

In some patients, loracarbef may cause diarrhea.
- Severe diarrhea may be a sign of a serious side effect. *Do not take any diarrhea medicine without first checking with your doctor.* Diarrhea medicines may make your diarrhea worse or last longer.
- For mild diarrhea, diarrhea medicine containing kaolin or attapulgite (e.g., Kaopectate tablets, Diasorb) may be taken. However, other kinds of diarrhea medicine should not be taken. They may make your diarrhea worse or last longer.
- If you have any questions about this or if mild diarrhea continues or gets worse, check with your health care professional.

## Side Effects of This Medicine

Along with its needed effects, a medicine may cause some unwanted effects. Although not all of these side effects may occur, if they do occur they may need medical attention.

Check with your doctor as soon as possible if any of the following side effects occur:

*More common*
  Itching; skin rash

Other side effects may occur that usually do not need medical attention. These side effects may go away during treatment as your body adjusts to the medicine. However, check with your doctor if any of the following side effects continue or are bothersome:

*More common*
  Diarrhea; loss of appetite; nausea and vomiting; stomach pain

*Rare*

> Dizziness; drowsiness; headache; itching or discharge from the vagina; nervousness; trouble in sleeping

Other side effects not listed above may also occur in some patients. If you notice any other effects, check with your doctor.

Revised: 08/18/93

# LOXAPINE    Systemic

Some commonly used brand names are:

**In the U.S.—**
> Loxitane                           Loxitane IM
> Loxitane C

Generic name product may also be available.

**In Canada—**
> Loxapac

## Description

Loxapine (LOX-a-peen) is used to treat nervous, mental, and emotional conditions.

Loxapine is available only with your doctor's prescription, in the following dosage forms:

*Oral*
- Solution (U.S. and Canada)
- Capsules (U.S.)
- Tablets (Canada)

*Parenteral*
- Injection (U.S. and Canada)

## Before Using This Medicine

In deciding to use a medicine, the risks of taking the medicine must be weighed against the good it will do. This is a decision you and your doctor will make. For loxapine, the following should be considered:

**Allergies**—Tell your doctor if you have ever had any unusual or allergic reaction to loxapine or amoxapine. Also tell your health care professional if you are allergic to any other substances, such as foods, preservatives, or dyes.

**Pregnancy**—Loxapine has not been shown to cause birth defects or other problems in humans. However, animal studies have shown unwanted effects in the fetus.

**Breast-feeding**—It is not known if loxapine passes into breast milk.

**Children**—Studies on this medicine have been done only in adult patients, and there is no specific information comparing use of loxapine in children with use in other age groups.

**Older adults**—Elderly patients are usually more sensitive than younger adults to the effects of loxapine. Constipation, dizziness or fainting, drowsiness, dry mouth, trembling of the hands and fingers, and symptoms of tardive dyskinesia (such as rapid, worm-like movements of the

tongue or any other uncontrolled movements of the mouth, tongue, or jaw, and/or arms and legs) are especially likely to occur in elderly patients.

**Other medicines**—Although certain medicines should not be used together at all, in other cases 2 different medicines may be used together even if an interaction might occur. In these cases, your doctor may want to change the dose, or other precautions may be necessary. When you are taking loxapine, it is especially important that your health care professional know if you are taking any of the following:

- Amoxapine (e.g., Asendin) or
- Methyldopa (e.g., Aldomet) or
- Metoclopramide (e.g., Reglan) or
- Metyrosine (e.g., Demser) or
- Other antipsychotics (medicine for mental illness) or
- Pemoline (e.g., Cylert) or
- Pimozide (e.g., Orap) or
- Promethazine (e.g., Phenergan) or
- Rauwolfia alkaloids (alseroxylon [e.g., Rauwiloid], deserpidine [e.g., Harmonyl], rauwolfia serpentina [e.g., Raudixin], reserpine [e.g., Serpasil]) or
- Trimeprazine (e.g., Temaril)—Taking these medicines with loxapine may increase the chance and seriousness of some side effects
- Central nervous system (CNS) depressants (medicine that causes drowsiness) or
- Tricyclic antidepressants (medicine for depression)—Taking these medicines with loxapine may increase the CNS depressant effects
- Guanadrel (e.g., Hylorel) or
- Guanethidine (e.g., Ismelin)—Loxapine may decrease the effects of these medicines

**Other medical problems**—The presence of other medical problems may affect the use of loxapine. Make sure you tell your doctor if you have any other medical problems, especially:

- Alcohol abuse—CNS depressant effects may be increased
- Difficult urination
- Enlarged prostate or
- Glaucoma (or predisposition to) or
- Parkinson's disease—Loxapine may make the condition worse
- Heart or blood vessel disease—An increased risk of low blood pressure (hypotension) or changes in the rhythm of your heart may occur
- Liver disease—Higher blood levels of loxapine may occur, increasing the chance of side effects

- Seizure disorders—Loxapine may increase the risk of seizures

## Proper Use of This Medicine

This medicine may be taken with food or a full glass (8 ounces) of water or milk to reduce stomach irritation.

For patients taking the *oral solution*:

- Measure the solution only with the dropper provided by the manufacturer. This will give a more accurate dose.

The liquid medicine must be mixed with orange juice or grapefruit juice just before you take it to make it easier to take.

*Do not take more of this medicine, do not take it more often, and do not take it for a longer time than your doctor ordered.* To do so may increase the chance of unwanted effects.

**Dosing**—The dose of loxapine will be different for different patients. *Follow your doctor's orders or the directions on the label.* The following information includes only the average doses of loxapine. *If your dose is different, do not change it* unless your doctor tells you to do so.

The number of capsules or tablets or amount of solution that you take depends on the strength of the medicine. Also, *the number of doses you take each day, the time allowed between doses, and the length of time you take the medicine depend on the medical problem for which you are taking loxapine.*

- For *oral* dosage forms (capsules, oral solution, or tablets):
  —Adults: To start, 10 milligrams taken two times a day. Your doctor may increase your dose if needed.
  —Children up to 16 years of age: The dose must be determined by the doctor.
- For *injection* dosage form:
  —Adults: 12.5 to 50 milligrams every four to six hours, injected into a muscle.
  —Children up to 16 years of age: The dose must be determined by the doctor.

**Missed dose**—If you miss a dose of this medicine, take it as soon as possible. However, if it is within one hour of your next dose, skip the missed dose and go back to your regular dosing schedule. Do not double doses.

**Storage**—To store this medicine:

- Keep out of the reach of children.
- Store away from heat and direct light.
- Do not store the capsule or tablet form of this medicine in the bathroom, near the kitchen sink, or in other damp places. Heat or moisture may cause the medicine to break down.
- Keep the liquid form of this medicine from freezing.
- Do not keep outdated medicine or medicine no longer needed. Be sure that any discarded medicine is out of the reach of children.

## Precautions While Using This Medicine

Your doctor should check your progress at regular visits, especially during the first few months of treatment with this medicine. The amount of loxapine you take may be changed often to meet the needs of your condition and to help avoid side effects.

*Do not stop taking this medicine without first checking with your doctor.* Your doctor may want you to reduce gradually the amount you are taking before stopping completely. This will allow your body time to adjust and to keep your condition from becoming worse.

This medicine will add to the effects of alcohol and other CNS depressants (medicines that slow down the nervous system, possibly causing drowsiness). Some examples of CNS depressants are antihistamines or medicine for hay fever, other allergies, or colds; sedatives, tranquilizers, or sleeping medicine; prescription pain medicine or narcotics; barbiturates; medicine for seizures; or anesthetics, including some dental anesthetics. *Check with your doctor before taking any of the above while you are taking this medicine.*

Do not take this medicine within two hours of taking antacids or medicine for diarrhea. Taking loxapine and antacids or medicine for diarrhea too close together may make this medicine less effective.

This medicine may cause some people to become drowsy or less alert than they are normally, especially as the amount of medicine is increased. Even if you take this medicine at bedtime, you may feel drowsy or less alert on arising. *Make sure you know how you react to this medicine before you drive, use machines, or do anything else that could be dangerous if you are not alert.*

Although it is not a problem for most patients, dizziness, lightheadedness, or fainting may occur, especially when you get up from a lying or sitting position. Getting up slowly may help. However, if the problem continues or gets worse, check with your doctor.

Loxapine may cause your skin to be more sensitive to sunlight than it is normally. Exposure to sunlight, even for brief periods of time, may cause a skin rash, itching, redness or other discoloration of the skin, or a severe sunburn. When you begin taking this medicine:

- Stay out of direct sunlight, especially between the hours of 10:00 a.m. and 3:00 p.m., if possible.
- Wear protective clothing, including a hat. Also, wear sunglasses.
- Apply a sun block product that has a skin protection factor (SPF) of at least 15. Some patients may require a product with a higher SPF number, especially if they have a fair complexion. If you have any questions about this, check with your health care professional.
- Apply a sun block lipstick that has an SPF of at least 15 to protect your lips.
- Do not use a sunlamp or tanning bed or booth.

*If you have a severe reaction from the sun, check with your doctor.*

Loxapine may cause dryness of the mouth. For temporary relief, use sugarless candy or gum, melt bits of ice in your mouth, or use a saliva substitute. However, if your mouth continues to feel dry for more than 2 weeks, check with your medical doctor or dentist. Continuing dryness of the mouth may increase the chance of dental disease, including tooth decay, gum disease, and fungus infections.

*Before having any kind of surgery, dental treatment, or emergency treatment, tell the medical doctor or dentist in charge that you are taking this medicine.* Taking loxapine together with medicines that are used during surgery or dental or emergency treatments may increase the CNS depressant effects.

## Side Effects of This Medicine

Along with its needed effects, loxapine can sometimes cause serious side effects. Tardive dyskinesia (a movement disorder) may occur and may not go away after you stop using the medicine. Signs of tardive dyskinesia include fine, worm-like movements of the tongue, or other uncontrolled movements of the mouth, tongue, cheeks, jaw, or arms and legs. Other serious but rare side effects may also occur. These include severe muscle stiffness, fever, unusual tiredness or weakness, fast heartbeat, difficult breathing, increased sweating, loss of bladder control, and seizures (neuroleptic malignant syndrome). *You and your doctor should discuss the good this medicine will do as well as the risks of taking it.*

*Stop taking loxapine and get emergency help immediately* if any of the following side effects occur:

*Rare*

Convulsions (seizures); difficult or fast breathing; fast heartbeat or irregular pulse; fever (high); high or low blood pressure; increased sweating; loss of bladder control; muscle stiffness (severe); unusually pale skin; unusual tiredness or weakness

*Check with your doctor immediately* if any of the following side effects occur:

*More common*

Lip smacking or puckering; puffing of cheeks; rapid or fine, worm-like movements of tongue; uncontrolled chewing movements; uncontrolled movements of arms or legs

Also, check with your doctor as soon as possible if any of the following side effects occur:

*More common (occurring with increase of dosage)*

Difficulty in speaking or swallowing; loss of balance control; mask-like face; restlessness or desire to keep moving; shuffling walk; slowed movements; stiffness of arms and legs; trembling and shaking of fingers and hands

*Less common*

Constipation (severe); difficult urination; inability to move eyes; muscle spasms, especially of the neck and back; skin rash; twisting movements of the body

*Rare*

Sore throat and fever; increased blinking or spasms of eyelid; uncontrolled twisting movements of neck, trunk, arms, or legs; unusual bleeding or bruising; unusual facial expressions or body positions; yellow eyes or skin

*Symptoms of overdose*

Dizziness (severe); drowsiness (severe); muscle trembling, jerking, stiffness, or uncontrolled movements (severe); troubled breathing (severe); unusual tiredness or weakness (severe)

Other side effects may occur that usually do not need medical attention. These side effects may go away during treatment as your body adjusts to the medicine. However, check with your doctor if any of the following side effects continue or are bothersome:

*More common*

Blurred vision; confusion; dizziness, lightheadedness, or fainting; drowsiness; dryness of mouth

*Less common*

Constipation (mild); decreased sexual ability; enlargement of breasts (males and females); headache; increased sensitivity of skin to sun; missing menstrual periods; nausea or vomiting; trouble in sleeping; unusual secretion of milk; weight gain

Certain side effects of this medicine may occur after you have stopped taking it. Check with your doctor as soon as possible if you notice any of the following effects after you have stopped taking loxapine:

Dizziness; nausea and vomiting; rapid or worm-like movements of the tongue; stomach upset or pain; trembling of fingers and hands; uncontrolled chewing movements

Other side effects not listed above may also occur in some patients. If you notice any other effects, check with your doctor.

## Additional Information

Once a medicine has been approved for marketing for a certain use, experience may show that it is also useful for other medical problems. Although this use is not included in product labeling, loxapine is used in certain patients with the following medical condition:

• Anxiety associated with mental depression

Other than the above information, there is no additional information relating to proper use, precautions, or side effects for this use.

Revised: 01/29/93

# LYPRESSIN  Systemic

A commonly used brand name in the U.S. is Diapid.

## Description

Lypressin (lye-PRESS-in) is a hormone used to prevent or control the frequent urination, increased thirst, and loss of water associated with diabetes insipidus (water diabetes).

Lypressin is available only with your doctor's prescription, in the following dosage form:

*Nasal*
- Nasal spray (U.S.)

## Before Using This Medicine

In deciding to use a medicine, the risks of taking the medicine must be weighed against the good it will do. This is a decision you and your doctor will make. For lypressin, the following should be considered:

**Allergies**—Tell your doctor if you have ever had any unusual or allergic reaction to lypressin or vasopressin. Also tell your health care professional if you are allergic to any other substances, such as foods, preservatives, or dyes.

**Pregnancy**—Studies on the effects in pregnancy have not been done in either humans or animals.

**Breast-feeding**—It is not known whether lypressin passes into breast milk. However, this medicine has not been reported to cause problems in nursing babies.

**Children**—Although there is no specific information comparing use of lypressin in children with use in other age groups, this medicine is not expected to cause different side effects or problems in children than it does in adults.

**Older adults**—Many medicines have not been studied specifically in older people. Therefore, it may not be known whether they work exactly the same way they do in younger adults or if they cause different side effects or problems in older people. There is no specific information comparing use of lypressin in the elderly with use in other age groups.

**Other medicines**—Although certain medicines should not be used together at all, in other cases two different medicines may be used together even if an interaction might occur. In these cases, your doctor may want to change the dose, or other precautions may be necessary. Tell your health care professional if you are taking any other prescription or nonprescription (over-the-counter [OTC]) medicine.

**Other medical problems**—The presence of other medical problems may affect the use of lypressin. Make sure you tell your doctor if you have any other medical problems, especially:
- Hay fever or other allergies or
- Infection of ears, lungs, nose, or throat or

- Stuffy nose—May prevent nasal lypressin from being absorbed into the bloodstream, through the lining of the nose
- High blood pressure—Lypressin may increase blood pressure

## Proper Use of This Medicine

*Use this medicine only as directed.* Do not use more of it and do not use it more often than your doctor ordered. To do so may increase the chance of unwanted effects.

To use:
- Blow nose gently. Hold the bottle in an upright position. With head upright, spray the medicine into each nostril by squeezing the bottle quickly and firmly. Do not lie down when spraying this medicine.

Rinse the tip of the bottle with hot water, taking care not to suck water into the bottle, and dry with a clean tissue. Replace the cap right after use.

**Dosing**—The dose of lypressin will be different for different patients. *Follow your doctor's orders or the directions on the label.* The following information includes only the average doses of lypressin. *If your dose is different, do not change it* unless your doctor tells you to do so.
- For *nasal* dosage forms:
  —Adults: One or two sprays in each nostril four times a day.
  —Children six weeks of age and older: One or two sprays in each nostril four times a day.
  —Children less than six weeks of age: Use is generally not recommended.

**Missed dose**—If you miss a dose of this medicine, use it as soon as possible. However, if it is almost time for your next dose, skip the missed dose and go back to your regular dosing schedule. Do not double doses.

**Storage**—To store this medicine:
- Keep out of the reach of children.
- Store away from heat and direct light.
- Do not store in the bathroom, near the kitchen sink, or in other damp places. Heat or moisture may cause the medicine to break down.
- Keep the medicine from freezing.
- Do not keep outdated medicine or medicine no longer needed. Be sure that any discarded medicine is out of the reach of children.

## Side Effects of This Medicine

Along with its needed effects, a medicine may cause some unwanted effects. Although not all of these effects may occur, if they do occur they may need medical attention.

*Check with your doctor immediately* if any of the following side effects occur since they may be signs or symptoms of too much fluid in the body or overdose:

Coma; confusion; convulsions (seizures); drowsiness; headache (continuing); problems with urination; weight gain

Check with your doctor as soon as possible if any of the following side effects occur:

*Rare*

Cough (continuing); feeling of tightness in chest; shortness of breath or troubled breathing

Other side effects may occur that usually do not need medical attention. These side effects may go away during treatment as your body adjusts to the medicine. However, check with your doctor if any of the following side effects continue or are bothersome:

*Less common or rare*

Abdominal or stomach cramps; headache; heartburn; increased bowel movements; irritation or pain in the eye; itching, irritation, or sores inside nose; runny or stuffy nose

Other side effects not listed above may also occur in some patients. If you notice any other effects, check with your doctor.

Revised: 07/01/93

# MAFENIDE Topical†

A commonly used brand name in the U.S. is Sulfamylon.

†Not commercially available in Canada.

## Description

Mafenide (MA-fe-nide), a sulfa medicine, is used to prevent and treat bacterial or fungus infections. It works by preventing growth of the fungus or bacteria.

Mafenide cream is applied to the skin and/or burned area(s) to prevent and treat bacterial or fungus infections that may occur in burns.

Other medicines are used along with this medicine for burns. Patients with severe burns or burns over a large area of the body must be treated in a hospital.

This medicine is available only with your doctor's prescription, in the following dosage form:

*Topical*
- Cream (U.S.)

## Before Using This Medicine

In deciding to use a medicine, the risks of taking the medicine must be weighed against the good it will do. This is a decision you and your doctor will make. For mafenide, the following should be considered:

**Allergies**—Tell your doctor if you have ever had any unusual or allergic reaction to mafenide, acetazolamide (e.g., Diamox), oral antidiabetics (diabetes medicine you take by mouth), dichlorphenamide (e.g., Daranide), furosemide (e.g., Lasix), methazolamide (e.g., Neptazane), other sulfa medicines, or thiazide diuretics (water pills). Also tell your health care professional if you are allergic to any other substances, such as preservatives or dyes.

**Pregnancy**—Studies on effects in pregnancy have not been done in either humans or animals. However, use is not recommended in women during their child-bearing years unless the burn area covers more than 20% of the total body surface. In addition, sulfa medicines may increase the chance of liver problems in newborn infants and should not be used near the due date of the pregnancy.

**Breast-feeding**—Mafenide, when used on skin and/or burns, is absorbed into the mother's body. It is not known whether this medicine passes into breast milk. Sulfa medicines given by mouth do pass into the breast milk, and may cause liver problems, anemia (iron-poor blood), and other unwanted effects in nursing babies, especially those with glucose-6-phosphate dehydrogenase deficiency (lack of G6PD enzyme). Be sure you have discussed the risks and benefits of mafenide with your doctor.

**Children**—Use of mafenide is not recommended in premature or newborn infants up to 2 months of age. Sulfa medicines may cause liver problems in these infants.

**Older adults**—Many medicines have not been tested in older people. Therefore, it may not be known whether they work exactly the same way they do in younger adults or if they cause different side effects or problems in older people. There is no specific information comparing use of mafenide in the elderly with use in other age groups.

**Other medicines**—Although certain medicines should not be used together at all, in other cases two different medicines may be used together even if an interaction might occur. In these cases, your doctor may want to change the dose, or other precautions may be necessary. Tell your health care professional if you are using any other prescription or nonprescription (over-the-counter [OTC]) medicine.

**Other medical problems**—The presence of other medical problems may affect the use of mafenide. Make sure you tell your doctor if you have any other medical problems, especially:

- Blood problems—Use of mafenide may make the condition worse
- Glucose-6-phosphate dehydrogenase deficiency (lack of G6PD enzyme)—Use of mafenide in persons with this condition may result in hemolytic anemia
- Kidney problems or
- Lung problems or
- Metabolic acidosis—Use of mafenide in persons with any of these conditions may increase the risk of a side effect called metabolic acidosis

## Proper Use of This Medicine

To use:
- Before applying this medicine, cleanse the affected area(s). Remove dead or burned skin and other debris.
- Wear a sterile glove to apply this medicine. Apply a thin layer (about 1/16 inch) of mafenide to the affected area(s). Keep the affected area(s) covered with the medicine at all times.
- If this medicine is rubbed off the affected area(s) by moving around or if it is washed off during bathing, showering, or the use of a whirlpool bath, reapply the medicine.
- After this medicine has been applied, the treated area(s) may be covered with a dressing or left uncovered as desired.

To help clear up your skin and/or burn infection completely, *keep using mafenide for the full time of treatment.* You should keep using this medicine until the burn area has healed or is ready for skin grafting. *Do not miss any doses.*

**Dosing**—The dose of topical mafenide will be different for different patients. *Follow your doctor's orders or the directions on the label.* The following information includes only the average doses of topical mafenide. *If your* *dose is different, do not change it* unless your doctor tells you to do so.

- For *topical* dosage form (cream):
  —For bacterial or fungus infection:
    • Adults and children 2 months of age and over—Use one or two times a day.
    • Infants and children up to 2 months of age—Use is not recommended.

**Missed dose**—If you miss a dose of this medicine, apply it as soon as possible. However, if it is almost time for your next dose, skip the missed dose and go back to your regular dosing schedule.

**Storage**—To store this medicine:
- Keep out of the reach of children.
- Store away from heat and direct light.
- Keep the medicine from freezing.
- Do not keep outdated medicine or medicine no longer needed. Be sure that any discarded medicine is out of the reach of children.

## Precautions While Using This Medicine

It is important that your doctor check your progress at regular visits.

If your skin infection or burn does not improve within a few days or if your more serious burns or burns over larger areas do not improve within a few weeks, or if they become worse, check with your doctor.

## Side Effects of This Medicine

Along with its needed effects, a medicine may cause some unwanted effects. Although not all of these side effects may occur, if they do occur they may need medical attention.

*Check with your doctor immediately* if any of the following side effects occur:
  *Less common*
    Itching; skin rash or redness; swelling of face or skin; wheezing or troubled breathing
  *Rare*
    Bleeding or oozing of skin; drowsiness; fast, deep breathing; nausea

Other side effects may occur that usually do not need medical attention. These side effects may go away during treatment as your body adjusts to the medicine. However, check with your doctor if any of the following side effects continue or are bothersome:
  *More common*
    Pain or burning feeling on treated area(s)

Other side effects not listed above may also occur in some patients. If you notice any other effects, check with your doctor.

Revised: 04/22/94

# MAGNESIUM SUPPLEMENTS   Systemic

Some commonly used brand names are:

**In the U.S.—**

| | |
|---|---|
| Citroma[2] | Maox[7] |
| Citro-Nesia[2] | Phillips' Milk of Magnesia[5] |
| Concentrated Phillips' Milk of Magnesia[5] | Slow-Mag[1] |
| Mag-Ox[7] | Uro-Mag[7] |
| Mag-Tab SR[6] | |

**In Canada—**

| | |
|---|---|
| Citro-Mag[2] | Magnesium-Rougier[3] |
| Mag 2[8] | Phillips' Milk of Magnesia[5] |
| Maglucate[4] | |

Note: For quick reference, the following magnesium supplements are numbered to match the corresponding brand names.

This information applies to the following medicines:
1. Magnesium Chloride (mag-NEE-zhum KLOR-ide)†‡
2. Magnesium Citrate (SIH-trayt)#‡
3. Magnesium Gluceptate (gloo-SEP-tate)*
4. Magnesium Gluconate (GLOO-ko-nate)‡
5. Magnesium Hydroxide (hye-DROX-ide)+#‡§
6. Magnesium Lactate (LAK-tate)†‡
7. Magnesium Oxide (OX-ide)+#‡§

8. Magnesium Pidolate (PID-o-late)*
9. Magnesium Sulfate (SUL-fate)#**‡§

*Not commercially available in the U.S.
†Not commercially available in Canada.
+See *Antacids (Oral-Local)* for antacid use of magnesium hydroxide and magnesium oxide.
#See *Laxatives (Local)* for laxative use of magnesium citrate, magnesium hydroxide, and magnesium oxide and magnesium sulfate.
**See *Magnesium Sulfate (Systemic)* for use in seizures and uterine tetany.
‡Generic name product may also be available in the U.S.
§Generic name product may also be available in Canada.

## Description

Magnesium is used as a dietary supplement for patients who are deficient in magnesium. Although a balanced diet usually supplies all the magnesium a person needs, magnesium supplements may be needed by patients who have lost magnesium because of illness or treatment with certain medicines.

Lack of magnesium may lead to irritability, muscle weakness, and irregular heartbeat.

Some magnesium preparations are available only with your doctor's prescription. Others are available without a prescription; however, your doctor may have special instructions on the proper dose for your medical condition. You should take magnesium supplements only under the supervision of your doctor.

Magnesium supplements are available in the following dosage forms:

*Oral*

Magnesium Chloride
- Tablets (U.S.)

Magnesium Citrate
- Oral solution (U.S. and Canada)

Magnesium Gluceptate
- Oral solution (Canada)

Magnesium Gluconate
- Tablets (U.S. and Canada)

Magnesium Hydroxide
- Chewable tablets (U.S. and Canada)
- Oral solution (U.S. and Canada)

Magnesium Lactate
- Extended-release tablets (U.S.)

Magnesium Oxide
- Capsules (U.S.)
- Tablets (U.S. and Canada)

Magnesium Pidolate
- Powder for oral solution (Canada)

Magnesium Sulfate
- Crystals (U.S.)

*Parenteral*

Magnesium Chloride
- Injection (U.S.)

Magnesium Sulfate
- Injection (U.S. and Canada)

## Importance of Diet

Many nutritionists recommend that, if possible, people should get all the magnesium they need from foods. However, some people may not get enough magnesium from food. For example, people on weight-loss diets may consume too little food to provide enough magnesium. Others may lose magnesium from the body because of illness or treatment with certain medicines. For such people, a magnesium supplement, taken under a doctor's care, is important.

In order to get enough vitamins and minerals in your diet, it is important that you eat a balanced and varied diet. Follow carefully any diet program your doctor may recommend. For your specific vitamin and/or mineral needs, ask your doctor or dietitian for a list of appropriate foods.

The best dietary sources of magnesium include green leafy vegetables, nuts, peas, beans, and cereal grains in which the germ or outer layers have not been removed. Hard water has been found to contain more magnesium than soft water. A diet high in fat may cause less magnesium to be absorbed. Cooking may decrease the magnesium content of food.

Experts have developed Recommended Dietary Allowances (RDA) for vitamins and other nutrients, based on the amount you need for good health. RDA cover the needs of most healthy people. They do not cover the needs of those who require extra vitamins or nutrients because of disease or serious lack of good nutrition. RDA should not be thought of as the amount of vitamins or other nutrients you need every day. Instead, they are the amounts you should eat on an average over time.

The RDA for magnesium are:
- Infants and children—
  Birth to 6 months of age: 40 milligrams (mg) per day.
  6 months to 1 year of age: 60 mg per day.
  1 to 3 years of age: 80 mg per day.
  4 to 6 years of age: 120 mg per day.
  7 to 10 years of age: 170 mg per day.
- Adolescent and adult males—
  11 to 14 years of age: 270 mg per day.
  15 to 18 years of age: 400 mg per day.
  19 years of age and over: 350 mg per day.
- Adolescent and adult females—
  11 to 14 years of age: 280 mg per day.
  15 to 18 years of age: 300 mg per day.
  19 years of age and over: 280 mg per day.
- Pregnant females—320 mg per day.
- Breast-feeding females—
  First 6 months: 355 mg per day.
  Second 6 months: 340 mg per day.

Remember:
- The total amount of magnesium that you get every day includes what you get from food *and* what you may take as a supplement.
- The total intake of magnesium averaged over several days need not be greater than twice the RDA, unless ordered by your doctor. In some cases, excessive amounts of magnesium may be harmful.

## Before Using This Dietary Supplement

If you are taking this dietary supplement without a prescription, carefully read and follow any precautions on the label. For magnesium supplements, the following should be considered:

**Allergies**—Tell your doctor if you have ever had any unusual or allergic reaction to magnesium. Also tell your health care professional if you are allergic to any other substances, such as foods, preservatives, or dyes.

**Pregnancy**—It is especially important that you are receiving enough vitamins and minerals when you become pregnant and that you continue to receive the right amount of vitamins and minerals throughout your pregnancy. The healthy growth and development of the fetus depend on a steady supply of nutrients from the mother. However, taking large amounts of dietary supplements during pregnancy may be harmful to the mother and/or fetus and should be avoided.

**Breast-feeding**—It is especially important that you receive the right amount of vitamins and minerals so that your baby will also get the vitamins and minerals needed to grow properly. However, taking large amounts of a dietary supplement while breast-feeding may be harmful to the mother and/or baby and should be avoided.

**Children**—Although there is no specific information comparing use of oral magnesium in children with use in other age groups, dietary supplements are not expected to cause different side effects in children than they do in adults.

**Older adults**—Many dietary supplements have not been studied specifically in older people. Therefore, it may not be known whether they work exactly the same way they do in younger adults or if they cause different side effects, or problems in older people. There is no specific information comparing use of magnesium in the elderly with use in other age groups.

Studies have shown that older adults may have lower blood levels of magnesium than younger adults. Your doctor may recommend that you take a magnesium supplement.

**Medicines or other dietary supplements**—Although certain medicines or other dietary supplements should not be used together at all, in other cases they may be used together even if an interaction might occur. In these cases, your doctor may want to change the dose, or other precautions may be necessary. When you are taking magnesium, it is especially important that your health care professional know if you are taking any of the following:

- Cellulose sodium phosphate—Use with magnesium supplements may prevent cellulose sodium phosphate from working properly; magnesium supplements should be taken at least 1 hour before or after cellulose sodium phosphate
- Magnesium-containing medications, other, including magnesium enemas—Use with magnesium supplements may cause high blood levels of magnesium, which may increase the chance of side effects
- Sodium polystyrene sulfonate—Use with magnesium supplements may cause the magnesium supplement to be less effective
- Tetracyclines, oral—Use with magnesium supplements may prevent the tetracycline from working properly; magnesium supplements should be taken at least 1 to 3 hours before or after oral tetracycline

**Other medical problems**—The presence of other medical problems may affect the use of magnesium. Make sure you tell your doctor if you have any other medical problems, especially:

- Heart disease—Magnesium supplements may make this condition worse
- Kidney problems—Magnesium supplements may increase the risk of hypermagnesemia (too much magnesium in the blood), which could cause serious side effects; your doctor may need to change your dose.

## Proper Use of This Dietary Supplement

Magnesium supplements should be taken with meals. Taking magnesium supplements on an empty stomach may cause diarrhea.

For patients taking the *extended-release form* of this dietary supplement:
- Swallow the tablets whole. Do not chew or suck on the tablet.
- Some tablets may be broken or crushed and sprinkled on applesauce or other soft food. However, check with your health care professional first, since this should not be done for most tablets.

For patients taking the *powder form* of this dietary supplement:
- Pour powder into a glass.
- Add water and stir.

**Dosing**—The dose of magnesium for prevention of magnesium deficiency is based on the Recommended Dietary Allowances (RDA). See the *Importance of Diet* section for the RDA for magnesium.

**Missed dose**—If you miss taking your magnesium supplement for one or more days there is no cause for concern, since it takes some time for your body to become seriously low in magnesium. However, if your doctor has recommended that you take magnesium, try to remember to take it as directed every day.

**Storage**—To store this dietary supplement:
- Keep out of the reach of children.
- Store away from heat and direct light.
- Do not store in the bathroom, near the kitchen sink, or in other damp places. Heat or moisture may cause the dietary supplement to break down.
- Keep the dietary supplement from freezing. Do not refrigerate.
- Do not keep dietary supplements that are outdated or are no longer needed. Be sure that any discarded dietary supplement is out of the reach of children.

## Side Effects of This Dietary Supplement

Along with its needed effects, a dietary supplement may cause some unwanted effects. Although not all of these side effects may occur, if they do occur they may need medical attention.

*Check with your doctor immediately* if any of the following side effects occur:

*Rare (with injectable magnesium only)*
Dizziness or fainting; flushing; irritation and pain at injection site—for intramuscular administration only; muscle paralysis; troubled breathing

*Symptoms of overdose (rare in patients with normal kidney function)*

Blurred or double vision; coma; dizziness or fainting; drowsiness (severe); increased or decreased urination; slow heartbeat; troubled breathing

Other side effects may occur that usually do not need medical attention. These side effects may go away during treatment as your body adjusts to the medicine. However, check with your doctor if the following side effect continues or is bothersome:

*Less common (with oral magnesium)*

Diarrhea

Other side effects not listed above may also occur in some patients. If you notice any other effects, check with your doctor.

---

Revised: 12/03/92
Interim revision(s): 03/28/93; 08/23/94

---

# MALATHION　Topical

Some commonly used brand names are:

**In the U.S.—**
Ovide

**Other—**
Derbac-M
Suleo-M

## Description

Malathion (mal-a-THYE-on) belongs to the group of medicines known as pediculicides (medicines that kill lice).

Malathion is applied to the hair and scalp to treat head lice infections. It acts by killing both the lice and their eggs.

This medicine is available only with your doctor's prescription, in the following dosage form:

*Topical*
• Lotion (U.S.)

## Before Using This Medicine

In deciding to use a medicine, the risks of taking the medicine must be weighed against the good it will do. This is a decision you and your doctor will make. For malathion, the following should be considered:

**Allergies—**Tell your doctor if you have ever had any unusual or allergic reaction to malathion. Also tell your health care professional if you are allergic to any other substances, such as preservatives or dyes.

**Pregnancy—**Malathion may be absorbed through the skin. Although it has not been studied in pregnant women, malathion has not been shown to cause birth defects or other problems in animal studies.

**Breast-feeding—**Malathion may be absorbed through the mother's skin. It is not known whether malathion passes into the breast milk. Although most medicines pass into breast milk in small amounts, many of them may be used safely while breast-feeding. Mothers who are using this medicine and who wish to breast-feed should discuss this with their doctor.

**Children—**This medicine has been tested in children 2 years of age and older and, in effective doses, has not been shown to cause different side effects or problems than it does in adults. There is no specific information comparing use of malathion in children less than 2 years of age with use in other age groups.

**Older adults—**Many medicines have not been studied specifically in older people. Therefore, it may not be known whether they work exactly the same way they do in younger adults or if they cause different side effects or problems in older people. There is no specific information comparing use of malathion in the elderly with use in other age groups.

**Other medicines—**Although certain medicines should not be used together at all, in other cases two different medicines may be used together even if an interaction might occur. In these cases, your doctor may want to change the dose, or other precautions may be necessary. When you are using malathion, it is especially important that your health care professional know if you are using any of the following:

• Antimyasthenics (ambenonium, neostigmine, pyridostigmine) or
• Demecarium, echothiophate, or isoflurophate eye medicine—Use of malathion with these medicines may increase the chance of side effects

**Other medical problems—**The presence of other medical problems may affect the use of malathion. Make sure you tell your doctor if you have any other medical problems, especially:

• Anemia (severe) or
• Brain surgery, recent, or
• Liver disease or
• Malnutrition—These conditions may increase the chance of some side effects of malathion
• Asthma or
• Epilepsy or other seizure disorders or
• Heart disease or
• Myasthenia gravis or other nerve/muscle disease or
• Parkinson's disease or
• Stomach ulcer or other stomach or intestinal problems—Use of malathion may make the condition worse

## Proper Use of This Medicine

*Malathion is a poison.* Keep it away from the mouth because it is harmful if swallowed.

---

*Use this medicine only as directed by your doctor.* Do not use more of it, do not use it more often, and do not use it for a longer time than your doctor ordered. To do so may increase the chance of absorption through the skin and the chance of malathion poisoning.

To use:
- Apply malathion by sprinkling on dry hair and rubbing in until the hair and scalp are thoroughly moistened.
- Immediately after using this medicine, wash your hands to remove any medicine that may be on them.
- Allow the hair to dry naturally. Use no heat (as from a hair dryer) and leave the hair uncovered.
- After the medicine has been allowed to remain on the hair and scalp for 8 to 12 hours, *wash the hair with a nonmedicated shampoo and then rinse thoroughly.*
- After rinsing, use a fine-toothed comb to remove the dead lice and eggs from the hair.

*Keep this medicine away from the eyes.* If you should accidentally get some in your eyes, flush them thoroughly with water at once.

This medicine is flammable. Do not use near heat, near open flame, or while smoking.

Head lice can be easily transferred from one person to another by direct contact with clothing, hats, scarves, bedding, towels, washcloths, hairbrushes and combs, or hairs from infected persons. Therefore, *all household members of your family should be examined for head lice and receive treatment if they are found to be infected.* If you have any questions about this, check with your doctor.

**Dosing**—The dose of malathion will be different for different patients. *Follow your doctor's orders or the directions on the label.* The following information includes only the average doses of malathion. *If your dose is different, do not change it* unless your doctor tells your to do so.
- For *lotion* dosage form:
  —For head lice infestations:
    - Adults and children 2 years of age and older—Apply to the hair and scalp one time. Treatment may be repeated after seven to nine days if necessary.
    - Children up to 2 years of age—Use and dose must be determined by your doctor.

**Storage**—To store this medicine:
- Keep out of the reach of children.
- Store away from heat and direct light.
- Keep the medicine from freezing.
- Do not keep outdated medicine or medicine no longer needed. Be sure that any discarded medicine is out of the reach of children.

## Precautions While Using This Medicine

To prevent reinfection or the spreading of the infection to other people, good health habits are also required. These include the following:
- Wash all clothing, bedding, towels, and washcloths in very hot water or dry-clean them.
- Wash all hairbrushes and combs in very hot soapy water and do not share them with other people.
- Clean the house or room by thorough vacuuming.

If you have any questions about this, check with your doctor.

Breathing in even small amounts of carbamate- or organophosphate-type insecticides or pesticides (for example, carbaryl [Sevin], demeton [Systox], diazinon, malathion, parathion, ronnel [Trolene]) may add to the effects of this medicine. Farmers, gardeners, residents of communities undergoing insecticide or pesticide spraying or dusting, workers in plants manufacturing such products, or other persons exposed to such poisons should protect themselves by wearing a mask over the nose and mouth, changing clothes frequently, and washing hands often while using this medicine.

## Side Effects of This Medicine

Along with its needed effects, a medicine may cause some unwanted effects. Although not all of these side effects may occur, if they do occur they may need medical attention.

Check with your doctor as soon as possible if any of the following side effects occur:
*Rare*
  Skin rash

When malathion is applied to the skin in recommended doses, symptoms of poisoning have not been reported. However, the chance may exist, especially if the skin is broken. *Symptoms of malathion poisoning* include:
  Abdominal or stomach cramps; anxiety or restlessness; clumsiness or unsteadiness; confusion or mental depression; convulsions (seizures); diarrhea; difficult or labored breathing; dizziness; drowsiness; increased sweating; increased watering of mouth or eyes; loss of bowel or bladder control; muscle twitching of eyelids, face, and neck; pinpoint pupils; slow heartbeat; trembling; unusual weakness

Other side effects may occur that usually do not need medical attention. These side effects may go away during treatment as your body adjusts to the medicine. However,

check with your doctor if either of the following side effects continues or is bothersome:

*Less common or rare*
Stinging or irritation of scalp

Other side effects not listed above may also occur in some patients. If you notice any other effects, check with your doctor.

Revised: 07/25/94

# MANGANESE SUPPLEMENTS Systemic

Note: For quick reference, the following manganese supplements are numbered to match the corresponding brand names.
This information applies to the following medicines:
1. Manganese Gluconate (MAN-ga-nees GLOO-coh-nate)‡§
2. Manganese Sulfate (SUL-fate)†§

†Not commercially available in Canada.
‡Generic name product may also be available in the U.S.
§Generic name product may also be available in Canada.

## Description

Manganese supplements are used to prevent or treat manganese deficiency.

The body needs manganese for normal growth and health. For patients who are unable to get enough manganese in their regular diet or who have a need for more manganese, manganese supplements may be necessary.

Manganese deficiency has not been reported in humans. Lack of manganese in animals has been found to cause improper formation of bone and cartilage, may decrease the body's ability to use sugar properly, and may cause growth problems.

Some manganese preparations are available only with your doctor's prescription. Others are available without a prescription; however, your doctor may have special instructions on the proper use and dose for your condition.

Manganese supplements are available in the following dosage forms:
*Oral*
Manganese Gluconate
• Tablets (U.S. and Canada)
*Parenteral*
Manganese Sulfate
• Injection (U.S.)

## Importance of Diet

Many nutritionists recommend that, if possible, people should get all the manganese they need from foods. However, some people may not get enough manganese from their diet. For such people, a manganese supplement is important.

In order to get enough vitamins and minerals in your regular diet, it is important that you eat a balanced and varied diet. Follow carefully any diet program your doctor may recommend. For your specific vitamin and/or mineral needs, ask your doctor or dietitian for a list of appropriate foods.

Manganese is found in whole grains, cereal products, lettuce, dry beans, and peas.

Experts have developed a list of recommended dietary allowances (RDA) for most vitamins and some minerals. The RDA are not an exact number but a general idea of how much you need. They do not cover amounts needed for problems caused by serious lack of vitamins and minerals.

Because a lack of manganese is rare, there are no RDA for it. The following intakes are thought to be plenty for most individuals:
• Infants and children—
  Birth to 6 months of age: 0.3 to 0.6 milligrams (mg) per day.
  6 months to 1 year of age: 0.6 to 1 mg per day.
  1 to 3 years of age: 1 to 1.5 mg per day.
  4 to 6 years of age: 1.5 to 2 mg per day.
  7 to 10 years of age: 2 to 3 mg per day.
• Adolescents and adults—2 to 5 mg per day.

## Before Using This Dietary Supplement

If you are taking this dietary supplement without a prescription, carefully read and follow any precautions on the label. For manganese, the following should be considered:

**Allergies**—Tell your doctor if you have ever had any unusual or allergic reaction to manganese. Also tell your health care professional if you are allergic to any other substances, such as foods, preservatives, or dyes.

**Pregnancy**—It is especially important that you are receiving enough vitamins and minerals when you become pregnant and that you continue to receive the right amount of vitamins and minerals throughout your pregnancy. The healthy growth and development of the fetus depend on a steady supply of nutrients from the mother. However, taking large amounts of a dietary supplement in pregnancy may be harmful to the mother and/or fetus and should be avoided.

**Breast-feeding**—It is important that you receive the right amounts of vitamins and minerals so that your baby will also get the vitamins and minerals needed to grow properly. However, taking large amounts of a dietary supplement while breast-feeding may be harmful to the mother and/or baby and should be avoided.

**Children**—It is especially important that children receive enough manganese in their diet for healthy growth and development. Although there is no specific information about the use of manganese in children in doses higher than normal daily requirements, it is not expected to cause different side effects or problems in children than it does in adults.

**Older adults**—It is important that older people continue to receive enough vitamins and minerals in their diet for good health. Manganese has been tested and has not been shown to cause different side effects or problems in older people than it does in younger adults.

**Medicines or other dietary supplements**—Although certain medicines or dietary supplements should not be used together at all, in other cases they may be used together even if an interaction might occur. In these cases, your doctor may want to change the dose, or other precautions may be necessary. Tell your health care professional if you are taking any other dietary supplement or any prescription or nonprescription (over-the-counter [OTC]) medicines.

**Other medical problems**—The presence of other medical problems may affect the use of manganese. Make sure you tell your doctor if you have any other medical problems, especially:

- Biliary disease or
- Liver disease—Taking manganese supplements may cause high blood levels of manganese, and dosage of manganese may have to be changed

## Proper Use of This Dietary Supplement

Some people believe that taking very large doses of a vitamin or mineral (called megadoses) is useful for treating certain medical problems. Studies have not proven this. Large doses should be taken only under the direction of your doctor after need has been identified.

**Dosing**—The dose of manganese for prevention of manganese deficiency is based on the daily recommended intake. See the *Importance of Diet* section for the daily recommended intake for manganese.

**Missed dose**—If you miss taking manganese supplements for one or more days there is no cause for concern, since it takes some time for your body to become seriously low in manganese. However, if your doctor has recommended that you take manganese, try to remember to take it as directed every day.

**Storage**—To store this dietary supplement:

- Keep out of the reach of children.
- Store away from heat and direct light.
- Do not store in the bathroom, near the kitchen sink, or in other damp places. Heat or moisture may cause the dietary supplement to break down.
- Keep the dietary supplement from freezing. Do not refrigerate.
- Do not keep outdated dietary supplements or those no longer needed. Be sure that any discarded dietary supplement is out of the reach of children.

## Side Effects of This Dietary Supplement

No side effects have been reported for manganese. However, check with your doctor if you notice any unusual effects while you are taking it.

Revised: 02/01/92
Interim revisions: 08/07/92; 08/15/94

# MAPROTILINE    Systemic

A commonly used brand name in the U.S. and Canada is Ludiomil.
   Generic name product may also be available in the U.S.

## Description

Maprotiline (ma-PROE-ti-leen) is used to relieve mental depression, including anxiety that sometimes occurs with depression.

Maprotiline is available only with your doctor's prescription, in the following dosage form:

*Oral*
- Tablets (U.S. and Canada)

## Before Using This Medicine

In deciding to use a medicine, the risks of taking the medicine must be weighed against the good it will do. This is a decision you and your doctor will make. For maprotiline, the following should be considered:

**Allergies**—Tell your doctor if you have ever had any unusual or allergic reaction to maprotiline or tricyclic antidepressants. Also tell your health care professional if you are allergic to any other substances, such as foods, preservatives, or dyes.

**Pregnancy**—Maprotiline has not been studied in pregnant women. However, this medicine has not been shown to cause birth defects or other problems in animal studies.

**Breast-feeding**—Maprotiline passes into the breast milk. However, this medicine has not been reported to cause problems in nursing babies.

**Children**—Studies on this medicine have been done only in adult patients, and there is no specific information comparing use of maprotiline in children with use in other age groups.

**Older adults**—Drowsiness, dizziness or lightheadedness; confusion; vision problems; dryness of mouth; constipation; and difficulty in urinating may be especially likely to occur in elderly patients, who are usually more sensitive than younger adults to the effects of maprotiline.

**Other medicines**—Although certain medicines should not be used together at all, in other cases two different medicines may be used together even if an interaction might occur. In these cases, your doctor may want to change the dose, or other precautions may be necessary. When you are taking maprotiline, it is especially important that your health care professional know if you are taking any of the following:

- Amphetamines or
- Appetite suppressants (diet pills) or
- Medicine for asthma or other breathing problems or
- Medicine for colds, sinus problems, or hay fever or other allergies (including nose drops or sprays)—Using these medicines with maprotiline may cause serious unwanted effects on your heart and blood pressure
- Central nervous system (CNS) depressants (medicines that cause drowsiness)—Taking these medicines with maprotiline may increase the CNS depressant effects
- Monoamine oxidase (MAO) inhibitors (furazolidone [e.g., Furoxone], isocarboxazid [e.g., Marplan], phenelzine [e.g., Nardil], procarbazine [e.g., Matulane], selegiline [e.g., Eldepryl], tranylcypromine [e.g., Parnate])—Taking maprotiline while you are taking or within 2 weeks of taking monoamine oxidase (MAO) inhibitors may cause very serious side effects, such as sudden high body temperature, extremely high blood pressure, and severe convulsions; at least 14 days should be allowed between stopping treatment with one medicine and starting treatment with the other

**Other medical problems**—The presence of other medical problems may affect the use of maprotiline. Make sure you tell your doctor if you have any other medical problems, especially:

- Alcohol abuse or
- Seizure disorders (including epilepsy)—The risk of seizures may be increased
- Asthma or
- Difficult urination or
- Enlarged prostate or
- Glaucoma or
- Mental illness (severe) or
- Stomach or intestinal problems—Maprotiline may make the condition worse
- Heart or blood vessel disease or
- Overactive thyroid—Serious effects on your heart may occur

- Liver disease—Higher blood levels of maprotiline may occur, increasing the chance of side effects

## Proper Use of This Medicine

*Take this medicine only as directed by your doctor* to benefit your condition as much as possible. Do not take more of it, do not take it more often, and do not take it for a longer time than your doctor ordered.

*Sometimes this medicine must be taken for up to two or three weeks before you begin to feel better.* Your doctor should check your progress at regular visits.

**Dosing**—The dose of maprotiline will be different for different patients. *Follow your doctor's orders or the directions on the label.* The following information includes only the average doses of maprotiline. *If your dose is different, do not change it* unless your doctor tells you to do so.

The number of tablets that you take depends on the strength of the medicine. Also, *the number of doses you take each day, the time allowed between doses, and the length of time you take the medicine depend on the medical problem for which you are taking maprotiline.*

- For *oral* dosage form (tablets):
  —For depression:
  - Adults—At first, 25 milligrams (mg) taken one to three times a day. Your doctor may increase your dose as needed. However, the dose is usually not more than 150 mg a day, unless you are in the hospital. Some hospitalized patients may need higher doses.
  - Children—Use and dose must be determined by your doctor.

**Missed dose**—If you miss a dose of this medicine and your dosing schedule is:

- One dose a day at bedtime—Do not take the missed dose in the morning since it may cause disturbing side effects during waking hours. Instead, check with your doctor.
- More than one dose a day—Take the missed dose as soon as possible. Then go back to your regular dosing schedule. However, if it is almost time for your next dose, skip the missed dose and go back to your regular dosing schedule. Do not double doses. If you have any questions about this, check with your doctor.

**Storage**—To store this medicine:

- Keep out of the reach of children.
- Store away from heat and direct light.
- Do not store in the bathroom, near the kitchen sink, or in other damp places. Heat or moisture may cause the medicine to break down.
- Do not keep outdated medicine or medicine no longer needed. Be sure that any discarded medicine is out of the reach of children.

## Precautions While Using This Medicine

It is very important that your doctor check your progress at regular visits. This will allow your dosage to be changed if necessary and will help to reduce side effects.

This medicine will add to the effects of alcohol and other CNS depressants (medicines that slow down the nervous system, possibly causing drowsiness). Some examples of CNS depressants are antihistamines or medicine for hay fever, other allergies, or colds; sedatives, tranquilizers, or sleeping medicine; prescription pain medicine or narcotics; barbiturates; medicine for seizures; or anesthetics, including some dental anesthetics. *Check with your doctor before taking any of the above while you are using this medicine.*

This medicine may cause blurred vision, especially during the first few weeks of treatment. It may also cause some people to become drowsy or less alert than they are normally. *If these effects occur, do not drive, use machines, or do anything else that could be dangerous if you are not alert or able to see well.*

*Dizziness, lightheadedness, or fainting may occur,* especially when you get up from a lying or sitting position. Getting up slowly may help. If this problem continues or gets worse, check with your doctor.

Maprotiline may cause dryness of the mouth. For temporary relief, use sugarless gum or candy, melt bits of ice in your mouth, or use a saliva substitute. However, if your mouth continues to feel dry for more than 2 weeks, check with your medical doctor or dentist. Continuing dryness of the mouth may increase the chance of dental disease, including tooth decay, gum disease, and fungus infections.

*Before having any kind of surgery, dental treatment, or emergency treatment, tell the medical doctor or dentist in charge that you are using this medicine.* Taking maprotiline together with medicines that are used during surgery or dental or emergency treatments may increase the CNS depressant effects.

*Do not stop taking this medicine without first checking with your doctor.* Your doctor may want you to reduce gradually the amount you are taking before stopping completely. This will allow your body to adjust properly and will reduce the possibility of unwanted effects.

## Side Effects of This Medicine

Along with its needed effects, a medicine may cause some unwanted effects. Although not all of these side effects may occur, if they do occur they may need medical attention.

Check with your doctor as soon as possible if any of the following side effects occur:

*More common*
> Skin rash, redness, swelling, or itching

*Less common*
> Constipation (severe); nausea or vomiting; shakiness or trembling; seizures (convulsions); unusual excitement; weight loss

*Rare*
> Breast enlargement—in males and females; confusion (especially in the elderly); difficulty in urinating; fainting; hallucinations (seeing, hearing, or feeling things that are not there); inappropriate secretion of milk—in females; irregular heartbeat (pounding, racing, skipping); sore throat and fever; swelling of testicles; yellow eyes or skin

*Symptoms of overdose*
> Convulsions (seizures); dizziness (severe); drowsiness (severe); fast or irregular heartbeat; fever; muscle stiffness or weakness (severe); restlessness or agitation; trouble in breathing; vomiting

Other side effects may occur that usually do not need medical attention. These side effects may go away during treatment as your body adjusts to the medicine. However, check with your doctor if any of the following side effects continue or are bothersome:

*More common*
> Blurred vision; decreased sexual ability; dizziness or lightheadedness (especially in the elderly); drowsiness; dryness of mouth; headache; increased or decreased sexual drive; tiredness or weakness

*Less common*
> Constipation (mild); diarrhea; heartburn; increased appetite and weight gain; increased sensitivity of skin to sunlight; increased sweating; trouble in sleeping; weight loss

After you stop taking this medicine, your body will need time to adjust. This usually takes about 3 to 10 days. Continue to follow the precautions listed above during this period of time.

Other side effects not listed above may also occur in some patients. If you notice any other effects, check with your doctor.

## Additional Information

Once a medicine has been approved for marketing for a certain use, experience may show that it is also useful for other medical problems. Although this use in not included in product labeling, maprotiline is used in certain patients with the following medical condition:

- Chronic neurogenic pain (a certain type of pain that is continuing)

Other than the above information, there is no additional information relating to proper use, precautions, or side effects for these uses.

Revised: 08/29/94

# MEASLES VIRUS VACCINE LIVE   Systemic

A commonly used brand name in the U.S. is Attenuvax.
Generic name product may be available in Canada.

## Description

Measles (MEE-zills) Virus Vaccine Live is an immunizing agent used to prevent infection by the measles virus. It works by causing your body to produce its own protection (antibodies) against the virus. This vaccine does not protect you against German measles (Rubella). A separate immunization is needed for that type of measles.

The following information applies only to the vaccine made from the more attenuated line of Enders' attenuated Edmonston strain of measles virus. Different types of measles vaccine may be available in countries other than the U.S. and Canada.

Measles (also known as coughing measles, hard measles, morbilli, red measles, rubeola, and ten-day measles) is an infection that is easily spread from one person to another. Infection with measles can cause serious problems, such as pneumonia, ear infections, sinus problems, convulsions (seizures), brain damage, and possibly death. The risk of serious complications and death is greater for adults and infants than for children and teenagers.

Immunization against measles is recommended for everyone 15 months of age (in Canada, 12 months of age) up to persons born in 1957. In addition, there may be special reasons why children from 6 months of age up to 15 months of age (up to 12 months of age in Canada) may also require measles vaccine.

Immunization against measles is not usually recommended for infants younger than 12 months of age, unless the risk of their getting a measles infection is high. This is because antibodies they received from their mothers before birth may interfere with the effectiveness of the vaccine. Children who were immunized against measles before 12 months of age should be immunized twice again.

You can be considered to be immune to measles only if you received 2 doses of measles vaccine starting on or after your first birthday and have the medical record to prove it, if you have a doctor's diagnosis of a previous measles infection, or if you have had a blood test showing immunity to measles.

This vaccine is to be administered only by or under the supervision of your doctor or other health care professional. It is available in the following dosage form:

*Parenteral*
- Injection (U.S. and Canada)

## Before Receiving This Vaccine

In deciding to use a medicine, the risks of taking the medicine must be weighed against the good it will do.

This is a decision you and your doctor will make. For measles vaccine, the following should be considered:

**Allergies**—Tell your doctor if you have ever had any unusual or allergic reaction to measles vaccine or to any form of the antibiotic neomycin or streptomycin. Also tell your health care professional if you are allergic to any other substances, such as foods (especially eggs) or preservatives. The measles vaccine available in the U.S. and Canada is grown in a chick embryo cell culture.

**Pregnancy**—Although studies on effects in pregnancy have not been done in humans and problems have not been shown to occur, use of measles vaccine during pregnancy, or becoming pregnant within 3 months after receiving measles vaccine, is not recommended. Since the natural measles infection has been shown to increase the chance of birth defects and other problems, it is thought that the live virus vaccine might cause similar problems.

**Breast-feeding**—It is not known whether measles vaccine passes into breast milk. Although most medicines pass into breast milk in small amounts, many of them may be used safely while breast-feeding. Mothers who are receiving this vaccine and who wish to breast-feed should discuss this with their doctor.

**Children**—In the U.S., measles vaccine is usually not recommended for infants up to 15 months of age. In Canada, use is not recommended for infants up to 12 months of age. In special cases, such as children traveling outside the U.S. or children living in high-risk areas, measles vaccine may be given to children as young as 6 months of age.

**Other medicines**—Although certain medicines should not be used together at all, in other cases two different medicines may be used together even if an interaction might occur. In these cases, your doctor may want to change the dose, or other precautions may be necessary. Before you receive measles vaccine, it is especially important that your health care professional know if you have received any of the following:
- Treatment with x-rays or cancer medicines—Treatment may increase the action of the vaccine, causing an increase in vaccine side effects, or treatment may interfere with the useful effect of the vaccine

**Other medical problems**—The presence of other medical problems may affect the use of measles vaccine. Make sure you tell your doctor if you have any other medical problems, especially:
- Brain or head injury or
- Convulsions (seizures) due to fever (history of)—Fever, a side effect of measles vaccine, may make the condition worse
- Immune deficiency condition (or family history of)—Condition may increase the chance and severity of side effects of the vaccine and/or may decrease the useful effects of the vaccine

- Severe illness with fever—The symptoms of the condition may be confused with the possible side effects of the vaccine
- Tuberculosis—Use of measles vaccine may make the condition worse or may interfere with the tuberculin skin test

## Proper Use of This Vaccine

**Dosing**—The dose of measles vaccine will be different for different patients. The following information includes only the average doses of measles vaccine.

- For *injection* dosage form:
  —For prevention of measles:
    - Adults and children 12 years of age and older—One dose injected under the skin, followed by a second dose at least one month later.
    - Children up to 6 months of age—Use is not recommended.
    - Children 6 to 15 months of age—Use and dose must be determined by your doctor.
    - Children 15 months to 12 years of age—One dose injected under the skin, followed by a second dose when the child is between 4 to 12 years of age. The second dose must be given at least one month after the first dose.

## Precautions After Receiving This Vaccine

*Do not become pregnant for 3 months after receiving measles vaccine without first checking with your doctor.* There is a chance that this vaccine may cause birth defects.

Tell your doctor that you have received this vaccine:

- If you are to receive a tuberculin skin test within 6 weeks after receiving this vaccine. The results of the test may be affected by this vaccine.
- If you are to receive any other live virus vaccines within 1 month after receiving this vaccine.
- If you are to receive blood transfusions or other blood products within 2 weeks after receiving this vaccine.
- If you are to receive gamma globulin or other globulins within 2 weeks after receiving this vaccine.

## Side Effects of This Vaccine

Along with its needed effects, a vaccine may cause some unwanted effects. Although not all of these side effects may occur, if they do occur they may need medical attention.

*Get emergency help immediately* if any of the following side effects occur:
*Symptoms of allergic reaction*
  Difficulty in breathing or swallowing; hives; itching, especially of feet or hands; reddening of skin, especially around ears; swelling of eyes, face, or inside of nose; unusual tiredness or weakness (sudden and severe)

Check with your doctor as soon as possible if any of the following side effects occur:
*More common*
  Fever over 103 °F (39.4 °C)
*Rare*
  Bruising or purple spots on skin; confusion; convulsions (seizures); double vision; headache (severe or continuing); irritability; stiff neck; vomiting

Other side effects may occur that usually do not need medical attention. However, check with your doctor if any of the following side effects continue or are bothersome:

*More common*
  Burning or stinging at place of injection; fever of 100 °F (37.7 °C) or less
*Less common*
  Fever between 100 and 103 °F (37.7 and 39.4 °C); itching, swelling, redness, tenderness, or hard lump at place of injection; skin rash

Fever or skin rash may occur from 5 to 12 days after vaccination and usually lasts several days.

Some side effects, such as fever over 103 °F (39.4 °C), swelling of glands in neck, or swelling, blistering, or pain at place of injection, may be more frequent or more severe or may last longer in persons who received inactivated (killed) measles vaccine (available in the U.S. from 1963 to 1967 and in Canada until 1970). If any of these side effects occur, check with your doctor as soon as possible.

Other side effects not listed above may also occur in some patients. If you notice any other effects, check with your doctor.

Revised: 07/12/94

# MEBENDAZOLE    Systemic

Some commonly used brand names are:
**In the U.S.—**
  Vermox
**In Canada—**
  Vermox
**Other—**
  Mebendacin        Nemasole
  Mebutar

## Description

Mebendazole (me-BEN-da-zole) belongs to the family of medicines called anthelmintics (ant-hel-MIN-tiks). Anthelmintics are medicines used in the treatment of worm infections.

Mebendazole is used to treat:
- Common roundworms (ascariasis);
- Hookworm infections (uncinariasis);
- Pinworms (enterobiasis; oxyuriasis);
- Whipworms (trichuriasis); and
- More than one worm infection at a time.

This medicine may also be used for other worm infections as determined by your doctor.

Mebendazole works by keeping the worm from absorbing sugar (glucose). This gradually causes loss of energy and death of the worm.

Mebendazole is available only with your doctor's prescription, in the following dosage form:
*Oral*
- Chewable tablets (U.S. and Canada)

## Before Using This Medicine

In deciding to use a medicine, the risks of taking the medicine must be weighed against the good it will do. This is a decision you and your doctor will make. For mebendazole, the following should be considered:

**Allergies**—Tell your doctor if you have ever had any unusual or allergic reaction to mebendazole. Also tell your health care professional if you are allergic to any other substances, such as foods, preservatives, or dyes.

**Pregnancy**—Mebendazole is not recommended for use during pregnancy. It has been shown to cause birth defects and other problems in rats given a single dose, which was several times the usual human dose. However, mebendazole did not cause birth defects or other problems in women who took this medicine during the first 3 months of pregnancy. Be sure you have discussed this with your doctor.

**Breast-feeding**—It is not known whether mebendazole passes into the breast milk. However, this medicine has not been reported to cause problems in nursing babies.

**Children**—This medicine has been tested in a limited number of children 2 years of age or older and, in effective doses, has not been shown to cause different side effects or problems in children than it does in adults.

**Older adults**—Many medicines have not been studied specifically in older people. Therefore, it may not be known whether they work exactly the same way they do in younger adults or if they cause different side effects or problems in older people. There is no specific information comparing use of mebendazole in the elderly with use in other age groups.

**Other medicines**—Although certain medicines should not be used together at all, in other cases two different medicines may be used together even if an interaction might occur. In these cases, your doctor may want to change the dose, or other precautions may be necessary. Tell your health care professional if you are taking any prescription or nonprescription (over-the-counter [OTC]) medicine.

**Other medical problems**—The presence of other medical problems may affect the use of mebendazole. Make sure you tell your doctor if you have any other medical problems, especially:
- Crohn's disease or
- Liver disease or
- Ulcerative colitis—Patients with these diseases may have an increased chance of side effects from mebendazole

## Proper Use of This Medicine

Mebendazole usually comes with patient directions. Read them carefully before using this medicine.

No special preparations (for example, special diets, fasting, other medicines, laxatives, or enemas) are necessary before, during, or immediately after taking mebendazole.

Mebendazole tablets may be chewed, swallowed whole, or crushed and mixed with food.

For patients taking *mebendazole for hookworms, roundworms, or whipworms:*
- To help clear up your infection completely, *take this medicine exactly as directed by your doctor for the full time of treatment.* In some patients a second course of this medicine may be required to clear up the infection completely. *Do not miss any doses.*

For patients taking *mebendazole for pinworms:*
- To help clear up your infection completely, *take this medicine exactly as directed by your doctor.* A second course of this medicine is usually required to clear up the infection completely.
- Pinworms may be easily passed from one person to another, especially in a household. Therefore, all household members may have to be treated at the same time. This helps to prevent infection or reinfection of other household members. Also, all household members may have to be treated again in 2 to 3 weeks to clear up the infection completely.

For patients taking mebendazole for infections in which *high doses* are needed:
- *Mebendazole is best taken with meals, especially fatty ones (for example, meals that include whole milk or ice cream).* This helps to clear up the infection by helping your body absorb the medicine better. *However, if you are on a low-fat diet, check with your doctor.*

**Dosing**—The dose of mebendazole will be different for different patients. *Follow your doctor's orders or the directions on the label.* The following information includes only the average doses of mebendazole. *If your dose is different, do not change it* unless your doctor tells you to do so.

*The number of doses you take each day, the time allowed between doses, and the length of time you take the medicine depend on the medical problem for which you are taking mebendazole.*

- For *oral* dosage form (chewable tablets):
  —For common roundworms, hookworms, and whipworms:
    - Adults and children 2 years of age and over—100 milligrams (mg) two times a day, morning and evening, for three days. Treatment may need to be repeated in two to three weeks.
    - Children up to 2 years of age—Use and dose must be determined by your doctor.
  —For pinworms:
    - Adults and children 2 years of age and over—100 mg once a day for one day. Treatment may need to be repeated in two to three weeks.
    - Children up to 2 years of age—Use and dose must be determined by your doctor.
  —For more than one worm infection at a time:
    - Adults and children 2 years of age and over—100 mg two times a day, morning and evening, for three days.
    - Children up to 2 years of age—Use and dose must be determined by your doctor.

**Missed dose**—If you miss a dose of this medicine, take it as soon as possible. However, if it is almost time for your next dose, skip the missed dose and go back to your regular dosing schedule. Do not double doses.

**Storage**—To store this medicine:

- Keep out of the reach of children.
- Store away from heat and direct light.
- Do not store in the bathroom, near the kitchen sink, or in other damp places. Heat or moisture may cause the medicine to break down.
- Do not keep outdated medicine or medicine no longer needed. Be sure that any discarded medicine is out of the reach of children.

## Precautions While Using This Medicine

It is important that your doctor check your progress at regular visits, especially in infections in which high doses are needed. This is to make sure that the infection is cleared up completely and to allow your doctor to check for any unwanted effects.

If your symptoms do not improve within a few days, or if they become worse, check with your doctor.

For patients taking *mebendazole for pinworms:*

- In some patients, pinworms may return after treatment with mebendazole. Washing (not shaking) all bedding and nightclothes (pajamas) after treatment may help to prevent this.
- Some doctors may also recommend other measures to help keep your infection from returning. If you have any questions about this, check with your doctor.

For patients taking *mebendazole for hookworms or whipworms:*

- In hookworm and whipworm infections anemia may occur. Therefore, your doctor may want you to take iron supplements to help clear up the anemia. If so, it is important to take iron every day while you are being treated for hookworms or whipworms; do not miss any doses. Your doctor may also want you to keep taking iron supplements for up to 6 months after you stop taking mebendazole. If you have any questions about this, check with your doctor.

## Side Effects of This Medicine

Along with its needed effects, a medicine may cause some unwanted effects. Although not all of these side effects may occur, if they do occur they may need medical attention.

Check with your doctor as soon as possible if any of the following side effects occur:

*Rare*

Fever; skin rash or itching; sore throat and fever; unusual tiredness and weakness

Other side effects may occur that usually do not need medical attention. These side effects may go away during treatment as your body adjusts to the medicine. However, check with your doctor if any of the following side effects continue or are bothersome:

*Less common*

Abdominal or stomach pain or upset; diarrhea; nausea or vomiting

*Rare*

Dizziness; hair loss; headache

Other side effects not listed above may also occur in some patients. If you notice any other effects, check with your doctor.

Revised: 10/06/92
Interim revision: 06/06/94

# MECAMYLAMINE    Systemic†

A commonly used brand name in the U.S. is Inversine.

†Not commercially available in Canada.

## Description

Mecamylamine (mek-a-MILL-a-meen) belongs to the general class of medicines called antihypertensives. It is used to treat high blood pressure (hypertension).

High blood pressure adds to the workload of the heart and arteries. If it continues for a long time, the heart and arteries may not function properly. This can damage the blood vessels of the brain, heart, and kidneys, resulting in a stroke, heart failure, or kidney failure. High blood pressure may also increase the risk of heart attacks. These problems may be less likely to occur if blood pressure is controlled.

Mecamylamine works by controlling impulses along certain nerve pathways. As a result, it relaxes blood vessels so that blood passes through them more easily. This helps to lower blood pressure.

Mecamylamine is available only with your doctor's prescription, in the following dosage form:

*Oral*
- Tablets (U.S.)

## Before Using This Medicine

In deciding to use a medicine, the risks of taking the medicine must be weighed against the good it will do. This is a decision you and your doctor will make. For mecamylamine, the following should be considered:

**Allergies**—Tell your doctor if you have ever had any unusual or allergic reaction to mecamylamine. Also tell your health care professional if you are allergic to any other substances, such as foods, preservatives, or dyes.

**Pregnancy**—Studies on effects in pregnancy have not been done in either humans or animals. However, in general, use of this medicine during pregnancy is not recommended because pregnant women may be more sensitive to its effects. In addition, mecamylamine may cause bowel problems in the unborn baby.

**Breast-feeding**—It is not known whether mecamylamine passes into breast milk. However, this medicine has not been reported to cause problems in nursing babies.

**Children**—Studies on this medicine have been done only in adult patients, and there is no specific information comparing use of mecamylamine in children with use in other age groups.

**Older adults**—Dizziness or lightheadedness may be more likely to occur in the elderly, who are more sensitive to the effects of mecamylamine.

**Other medicines**—Although certain medicines should not be used together at all, in many cases two different medicines may be used together even if an interaction might occur. In these cases, changes in dose or other precautions may be necessary. When taking mecamylamine it is especially important that your health care professional know if you are taking any of the following:

- Antibiotics or
- Sulfonamides (sulfa medicine)—Patients with chronic pyelonephritis being treated with these medications should not be treated with mecamylamine
- Antimyasthenics (ambenonium [e.g., Mytelase], neostigmine [e.g., Prostigmin], pyridostigmine [e.g., Mestinon])—Effects of these medicines may be decreased by mecamylamine
- Urinary alkalizers (medicine that makes the urine less acid, such as acetazolamide [e.g., Diamox], calcium- and/or magnesium-containing antacids, dichlorphenamide [e.g., Daranide], methazolamide [e.g., Neptazane], potassium or sodium citrate and/or citric acid, sodium bicarbonate [baking soda])—Effects of mecamylamine may be increased because these medicines cause it to be removed more slowly from the body

**Other medical problems**—The presence of other medical problems may affect the use of mecamylamine. Make sure you tell your doctor if you have any other medical problems, especially:

- Bladder or prostate problems—Mecamylamine may interfere with urination
- Bowel problems—Patients with bowel problems who take mecamylamine may be at inceased risk for serious bowel side effects of mecamylamine
- Diarrhea or
- Fever or infection or
- Nausea or vomiting—Effects of mecamylamine on blood pressure may be increased
- Glaucoma—Mecamylamine may make this condition worse
- Heart or blood vessel disease or
- Heart attack or stroke (recent)—Lowering of blood pressure by mecamylamine may make problems resulting from these conditions worse
- Kidney disease—Effects of mecamylamine may be increased because of slower removal of mecamylamine from the body

## Proper Use of This Medicine

In addition to the use of the medicine your doctor has prescribed, treatment for your high blood pressure may include weight control and care in the types of foods you eat, especially foods high in sodium. Your doctor will tell you which of these are most important for you. You should check with your doctor before changing your diet.

Many patients who have high blood pressure will not notice any signs of the problem. In fact, many may feel normal. *It is very important that you take your medicine exactly as directed and that you keep your appointments with your doctor* even if you feel well.

Remember that this medicine will not cure your high blood pressure but it does help control it. Therefore, you must continue to take it as directed if you expect to lower your blood pressure and keep it down. *You may have to take high blood pressure medicine for the rest of your life.* If high blood pressure is not treated, it can cause serious problems such as heart failure, blood vessel disease, stroke, or kidney disease.

To help you remember to take your medicine, try to get into the habit of taking it at the same time each day.

**Dosing**—The dose of mecamylamine will be different for different patients. *Follow your doctor's orders or the directions on the label.* The following information includes only the average doses of mecamylamine. *If your dose is different, do not change it* unless your doctor tells you to do so:

- For *oral* dosage forms (tablets):
  —Adults: 2.5 milligrams two times a day to 25 milligrams three times a day.

**Missed dose**—If you miss a dose of this medicine, take it as soon as possible. Then go back to your regular dosing schedule. *If you miss two or more doses in a row, check with your doctor right away.* If your body goes without this medicine for too long, your blood pressure may go up to a dangerously high level.

**Storage**—To store this medicine:

- Keep out of the reach of children.
- Store away from heat and direct light.
- Do not store in the bathroom, near the kitchen sink, or in other damp places. Heat or moisture may cause the medicine to break down.
- Do not keep outdated medicine or medicine no longer needed. Be sure that any discarded medicine is out of the reach of children.

## Precautions While Using This Medicine

It is important that your doctor check your progress at regular visits to make sure that this medicine is working properly.

*Check with your doctor before you stop taking this medicine.* Your doctor may want you to reduce gradually the amount you are taking before stopping completely.

*Make sure that you have enough medicine on hand to last through weekends, holidays, or vacations.* You should not miss taking any doses. You may want to ask your doctor for another written prescription for mecamylamine to carry in your wallet or purse. You can then have it filled if you run out of medicine when you are away from home.

*Do not take other medicines unless they have been discussed with your doctor.* This especially includes over-the-counter (nonprescription) medicines for appetite control, asthma, colds, cough, hay fever, or sinus problems, since they may tend to increase your blood pressure.

*Dizziness, lightheadedness, or fainting may occur, especially when you get up from a lying or sitting position.* This is more likely to occur in the morning. *Getting up slowly may help.* When you get up from lying down, sit on the edge of the bed with your feet dangling for one or two minutes. Then stand up slowly. If you feel dizzy, sit or lie down. If the problem continues or gets worse, check with your doctor.

The dizziness, lightheadedness, or fainting is also more likely to occur if you drink alcohol, stand for a long time, exercise, or if the weather is hot. *While you are taking this medicine, be careful to limit the amount of alcohol you drink. Also, use extra care during exercise or hot weather or if you must stand for a long time.*

Sodium bicarbonate (commonly known as baking soda) may cause you to get a greater than normal effect from this medicine. To prevent problems, check with your health care professional before using an antacid or medicine for heartburn since some of these contain sodium bicarbonate.

Tell your doctor if you get a fever or infection since that may change the amount of medicine you have to take.

Mecamylamine may cause dryness of the mouth, nose, and throat. For temporary relief of mouth dryness, use sugarless candy or gum, melt bits of ice in your mouth, or use a saliva substitute. However, if your mouth continues to feel dry for more than 2 weeks, check with your medical doctor or dentist. Continuing dryness of the mouth may increase the chance of dental disease, including tooth decay, gum disease, and fungus infections.

Before having any kind of surgery (including dental surgery) or emergency treatment, tell the medical doctor or dentist in charge that you are taking this medicine.

## Side Effects of This Medicine

Along with its needed effects, a medicine may cause some unwanted effects. Although not all of these side effects may occur, if they do occur they may need medical attention.

Check with your doctor as soon as possible if any of the following side effects occur:

*More common*
    Dizziness or lightheadedness, especially when getting up from a lying or sitting position

*Less common*
    Difficult urination

*Rare*
    Bloating and frequent loose stools; confusion or excitement; constipation (severe); convulsions (seizures); mental depression; shortness of breath; trembling; uncontrolled movements of face, hands, arms, or legs

Other side effects may occur that usually do not need medical attention. These side effects may go away during treatment as your body adjusts to the medicine. However,

check with your doctor if any of the following side effects continue or are bothersome:

*More common*

Constipation; drowsiness; unusual tiredness

*Less common or rare*

Blurred vision; decreased sexual ability or interest in sex; dryness of mouth; enlarged pupils; loss of appetite; nausea and vomiting; weakness

Other side effects not listed above may also occur in some patients. If you notice any other effects, check with your doctor.

Revised: 01/20/93

# MECHLORETHAMINE   Systemic

A commonly used brand name in the U.S. and Canada is Mustargen. Other commonly used names are chlormethine and nitrogen mustard.

## Description

Mechlorethamine (me-klor-ETH-a-meen) belongs to the group of medicines called alkylating agents. It is used to treat some kinds of cancer as well as some noncancerous conditions.

Mechlorethamine interferes with the growth of cancer cells, which are eventually destroyed. Since the growth of normal body cells may also be affected by mechlorethamine, other effects will also occur. Some of these may be serious and must be reported to your doctor. Other effects, like hair loss, may not be serious but may cause concern. Some effects may not occur for months or years after the medicine is used.

Before you begin treatment with mechlorethamine, you and your doctor should talk about the good this medicine will do as well as the risks of using it.

Mechlorethamine is to be administered only by or under the immediate supervision of your doctor. It is available in the following dosage form:

*Parenteral*

• Injection (U.S. and Canada)

## Before Using This Medicine

In deciding to use a medicine, the risks of taking the medicine must be weighed against the good it will do. This is a decision you and your doctor will make. For mechlorethamine, the following should be considered:

**Allergies**—Tell your doctor if you have ever had any unusual or allergic reaction to mechlorethamine, including a reaction if it was applied to the skin.

**Pregnancy**—Tell your doctor if you are pregnant or if you intend to have children. This medicine may cause birth defects if either the male or female is receiving it at the time of conception or if it is used during pregnancy. In addition, many cancer medicines may cause sterility which could be permanent. Sterility has been reported with mechlorethamine and the possibility should be kept in mind.

Be sure that you have discussed this with your doctor before receiving this medicine. It is best to use some kind of birth control while you are receiving mechlorethamine. Tell your doctor right away if you think you have become pregnant while receiving mechlorethamine.

**Breast-feeding**—Tell your doctor if you are breast-feeding or if you intend to breast-feed during treatment with this medicine. Because mechlorethamine may cause serious side effects, breast-feeding is generally not recommended while you are receiving it.

**Children**—Although there is no specific information about the use of mechlorethamine in children, it is not expected to cause different side effects or problems in children than it does in adults.

**Older adults**—Many medicines have not been tested in older people. Therefore, it may not be known whether they work exactly the same way they do in younger adults or if they cause different side effects or problems in older people. There is no specific information about the use of mechlorethamine in the elderly.

**Other medicines**—Although certain medicines should not be used together at all, in other cases two different medicines may be used together even if an interaction might occur. In these cases, your doctor may want to change the dose, or other precautions may be necessary. When you are receiving mechlorethamine, it is especially important that your health care professional know if you are taking any of the following:

• Amphotericin B by injection (e.g., Fungizone) or
• Antithyroid agents (medicine for overactive thyroid) or
• Azathioprine (e.g., Imuran) or
• Chloramphenicol (e.g., Chloromycetin) or
• Colchicine or
• Flucytosine (e.g., Ancobon) or
• Interferon (e.g., Intron A, Roferon-A) or
• Plicamycin (e.g., Mithracin) or
• Zidovudine (e.g., Retrovir) or
• If you have ever been treated with x-rays or cancer medicines—Mechlorethamine may increase the effects of these medicines or radiation therapy on the blood
• Probenecid (e.g., Benemid) or
• Sulfinpyrazone (e.g., Anturane)—Mechlorethamine may raise the concentration of uric acid in the blood, which these medicines are used to lower

**Other medical problems**—The presence of other medical problems may affect the use of mechlorethamine. Make sure you tell your doctor if you have any other medical problems, especially:

- Chickenpox (including recent exposure) or
- Herpes zoster (shingles)—Risk of severe disease affecting other parts of the body
- Gout or
- Kidney stones—Mechlorethamine may increase levels of a chemical called uric acid in the body, which can cause gout and kidney stones
- Infection—Mechlorethamine can reduce immunity to infection

## Proper Use of This Medicine

Mechlorethamine is sometimes given together with certain other medicines. If you are using a combination of medicines, it is important that you receive each one at the proper time. If you are taking some of these medicines by mouth, ask your health care professional to help you plan a way to take them at the right times.

While you are using this medicine, your doctor may want you to drink extra fluids so that you will pass more urine. This will help prevent kidney problems and keep your kidneys working well.

Mechlorethamine often causes nausea and vomiting, which usually last only 8 to 24 hours. It is very important that you continue to receive the medicine, even if you begin to feel ill. Ask your health care professional for ways to lessen these effects.

**Dosing**—The dose of mechlorethamine will be different for different patients. The dose that is used may depend on a number of things, including what the medicine is being used for, the patient's weight, and whether or not other medicines are also being taken. *If you are receiving mechlorethamine at home, follow your doctor's orders or the directions on the label.* If you have any questions about the proper dose of mechlorethamine, ask your doctor.

## Precautions While Using This Medicine

*It is very important that your doctor check your progress at regular visits* to make sure that this medicine is working properly and to check for unwanted effects.

While you are being treated with mechlorethamine, and after you stop treatment with it, *do not have any immunizations (vaccinations) without your doctor's approval.* Mechlorethamine may lower your body's resistance and there is a chance you might get the infection the immunization is meant to prevent. In addition, other persons living in your household should not take or should not have recently taken oral polio vaccine since there is a chance they could pass the polio virus on to you. Also, avoid other persons who have taken oral polio vaccine. Do not get close to them, and do not stay in the same room with them for very long. If you cannot take these precautions, you should consider wearing a protective face mask that covers the nose and mouth.

Mechlorethamine can lower the number of white blood cells in your blood temporarily, increasing the chance of getting an infection. It can also lower the number of platelets, which are necessary for proper blood clotting. If this occurs, there are certain precautions you can take, especially when your blood count is low, to reduce the risk of infection or bleeding:

- If you can, avoid people with infections. *Check with your doctor immediately* if you think you are getting an infection or if you get a fever or chills, cough or hoarseness, lower back or side pain, or painful or difficult urination.
- *Check with your doctor immediately* if you notice any unusual bleeding or bruising; black, tarry stools; blood in urine or stools; or pinpoint red spots on your skin.
- Be careful when using a regular toothbrush, dental floss, or toothpick. Your medical doctor, dentist, or nurse may recommend other ways to clean your teeth and gums. Check with your medical doctor before having any dental work done.
- Do not touch your eyes or the inside of your nose unless you have just washed your hands and have not touched anything else in the meantime.
- Be careful not to cut yourself when you are using sharp objects such as a safety razor or fingernail or toenail cutters.
- Avoid contact sports or other situations where bruising or injury could occur.

If mechlorethamine accidentally seeps out of the vein into which it is injected, it may damage some tissues and cause scarring. *Tell the health care professional right away if you notice redness, pain, or swelling at the place of injection.*

## Side Effects of This Medicine

Along with their needed effects, medicines like mechlorethamine can sometimes cause blood problems, loss of hair, and other side effects. These and others are described below. Also, because of the way these medicines act on the body, there is a chance that they might cause other effects that may not occur until months or years after these medicine is used. These delayed effects may include certain types of cancer, such as leukemia. Discuss these possible effects with your doctor.

Although not all of these side effects may occur, if they do occur they may need medical attention.

*Check with your doctor or nurse immediately* if any of the following side effects occur:

*Less common*

Black, tarry stools; blood in urine or stools; cough or hoarseness; fever or chills; lower back or side pain; pain or redness at place of injection; painful or difficult urination; pinpoint red spots on skin; unusual bleeding or bruising

*Rare*
    Shortness of breath, itching, or wheezing

Check with your health care professional as soon as possible if any of the following side effects occur:

*More common*
    Missing menstrual periods; painful rash

*Less common*
    Dizziness; joint pain; loss of hearing; ringing in ears; swelling of feet or lower legs

*Rare*
    Numbness, tingling, or burning of fingers, toes, or face; sores in mouth and on lips; yellow eyes or skin

Other side effects may occur that usually do not need medical attention. These side effects may go away during treatment as your body adjusts to the medicine. Also, your health care professional may be able to tell you about ways to prevent or reduce some of these side effects. Check with your health care professional if any of the following side effects continue or are bothersome or if you have any questions about them:

*More common*
    Nausea and vomiting (usually lasts only 8 to 24 hours)

*Less common*
    Confusion; diarrhea; drowsiness; headache; loss of appetite; metallic taste; weakness

This medicine may cause a temporary loss of hair in some people. After treatment with mechlorethamine has ended, normal hair growth should return.

After you stop receiving mechlorethamine, it may still produce some side effects that need attention. During this period of time, check with your doctor if you notice any of the following side effects:

    Black, tarry stools; blood in urine or stools; cough or hoarseness; fever or chills; lower back or side pain; painful or difficult urination; pinpoint red spots on skin; unusual bleeding or bruising

Other side effects not listed above may also occur in some patients. If you notice any other effects, check with your doctor.

Revised: 8/90
Interim revision: 07/29/93; 06/21/94

---

# MECHLORETHAMINE    Topical*†

Other commonly used names are chlormethine and nitrogen mustard.

*Not commercially available in the U.S.
†Not commercially available in Canada.

## Description

Mechlorethamine (me-klor-ETH-a-meen) belongs to the group of medicines called alkylating agents. It is used to treat certain skin conditions that could turn to cancer if left untreated.

Mechlorethamine interferes with the growth of problem cells, which are eventually destroyed. However, there is also a chance that mechlorethamine can cause some kinds of skin cancer, especially after it has been used for several years.

Before you begin treatment with mechlorethamine, you and your doctor should talk about the good this medicine will do as well as the risks of using it.

Mechlorethamine is available only with your doctor's prescription, in the following dosage forms:

*Topical*
- Ointment (U.S. and Canada)
- Topical solution (U.S. and Canada)

## Before Using This Medicine

In deciding to use a medicine, the risks of taking the medicine must be weighed against the good it will do. This is a decision you and your doctor will make. For mechlorethamine applied to the skin, the following should be considered:

**Allergies**—Tell your doctor if you have ever had any unusual or allergic reaction to mechlorethamine.

**Pregnancy**—Although mechlorethamine applied to the skin has not been shown to cause problems in humans, some of it may be absorbed through the skin.

**Breast-feeding**—Although mechlorethamine applied to the skin has not been shown to cause problems in nursing babies, some of it may be absorbed through the skin. Because this medicine can cause serious side effects, breast-feeding is generally not recommended while you are using it.

**Children**—There is no specific information about use of mechlorethamine on the skin in children.

**Older adults**—Many medicines have not been tested in older people. Therefore, it may not be known whether they work exactly the same way they do in younger adults or if they cause different side effects or problems in older people. There is no specific information about the use of mechlorethamine on the skin in the elderly.

## Proper Use of This Medicine

Mechlorethamine may be used either as a solution or as an ointment. If you are using the solution, it must be mixed just before you use it since it breaks down quickly.

*Mix the solution carefully according to your doctor's or pharmacist's directions.*

When preparing the solution, remember:
- Do not use the mechlorethamine if the solution is discolored or if droplets of water appear in the vial.
- Avoid inhaling the powder or any vapors. If some of the powder or solution accidentally gets on your skin, *immediately* wash that area of skin. Use a large amount of water and continue to wash for at least 15 minutes. If eye contact occurs, use an eyewash recommended by your doctor. Keep this eyewash on hand. *Follow carefully any other instructions your doctor may have given you.*
- All equipment used must be specially cleaned, even if it is to be thrown away. *Follow carefully your doctor's instructions* for doing this, using the special solution recommended.

Take a shower and rinse carefully just before you apply mechlorethamine solution or ointment, unless otherwise directed by your doctor. Make sure your skin is completely dry before applying the ointment. Do not shower again until the next treatment.

Apply the solution or ointment all over the body, until the entire amount for a dose is used up. Wear rubber or plastic gloves if you are using your hands. To apply the solution, a 2-inch-wide soft brush or gauze may be used instead. Let the solution dry.

Mechlorethamine should be applied more lightly to the groin, armpits, inside the bends of the elbows, and behind the knees. These areas are more likely to get irritated.

Avoid contact with the eyes, nose, or mouth, unless otherwise directed by your doctor.

Mechlorethamine is usually applied once a day. However, follow your doctor's instructions. Continue to use the medicine as long as you are told to. This may be months or years. However, do not use this medicine more often or for a longer time than ordered. To do so may increase the chance of unwanted effects.

**Dosing**—The dose of mechlorethamine will be different for different patients. *Follow your doctor's orders or the directions on the label.* The following information includes only the average doses of mechlorethamine. *If your dose is different, do not change it* unless your doctor tells you to do so.
- For *topical* dosage forms (ointment or solution):
  - —For mycosis fungoides:
    - Adults—Apply to the entire skin surface once a day. Several months after this medicine has helped your problem, your doctor may decrease the treatments to several times a week.

- Children—Dose must be determined by your doctor.

**Missed dose**—If you miss a dose of this medicine, go back to your regular dosing schedule and check with your doctor. Do not change the amount you are using unless directed to do so by your doctor.

**Storage**—To store this medicine:
- Keep out of the reach of children.
- Store away from heat and direct light. This applies to either the ointment or the vials of mechlorethamine used to make the solution. The solution should not be stored but instead should be freshly made just before it is used.
- Do not store in the bathroom, near the kitchen sink, or in other damp places. Heat or moisture may cause the medicine to break down.
- Do not keep outdated medicine or medicine no longer needed. Be sure that any discarded medicine is out of the reach of children.

## Precautions While Using This Medicine

*It is very important that your doctor check your progress at regular visits* to make sure that mechlorethamine is working properly and to check for unwanted effects.

## Side Effects of This Medicine

Along with its needed effects, a medicine may cause some unwanted effects. When mechlorethamine is applied to the skin, it does not usually cause the same effects as when it is given by injection. *However, stop using this medicine and check with your doctor immediately* if the following side effects occur:

Hives; shortness of breath (sudden); skin rash or itching; sore, reddened skin

Check with your doctor also if you develop dry skin. There may be a lotion or ointment that you can use to help this. However, do not use anything else on your skin unless directed by your doctor.

Your skin color may darken after you have used this medicine for a while. The effect will go away after you have stopped using the medicine.

Other side effects not listed above may also occur in some patients. If you notice any other effects, check with your doctor.

Revised: 08/90
Interim revision: 07/12/94

# MECLIZINE/BUCLIZINE/CYCLIZINE   Systemic

Some commonly used brand names are:

**In the U.S.—**
| | |
|---|---|
| Antivert[3] | D-Vert 15[3] |
| Antivert/25[3] | D-Vert 30[3] |
| Antivert/50[3] | Marezine[2] |
| Bonine[3] | Meni-D[3] |
| Bucladin-S Softabs[1] | Ru-Vert M[3] |

**In Canada—**
| | |
|---|---|
| Bonamine[3] | Marzine[2] |

Note: For quick reference, the following medicines are numbered to match the corresponding brand names.

This information applies to the following medicines:
1. Buclizine (BYOO-kli-zeen)†
2. Cyclizine (SYE-kli-zeen)
3. Meclizine (MEK-li-zeen)‡

†Not commercially available in Canada.
‡Generic name product may also be available in the U.S.

## Description

Buclizine (BYOO-kli-zeen), cyclizine (SYE-kli-zeen), and meclizine (MEK-li-zeen) are used to prevent and treat nausea, vomiting, and dizziness associated with motion sickness, and dizziness caused by other medical problems.

Some of these preparations are available only with your doctor's prescription. Others are available without a prescription; however, your doctor may have special instructions on the proper dose of the medicine for your medical condition. They are available in the following dosage forms:

*Oral*
Buclizine
  • Chewable tablets (U.S.)
Cyclizine
  • Tablets (U.S.)
Meclizine
  • Capsules (U.S.)
  • Tablets (U.S. and Canada)
  • Chewable tablets (U.S.)

*Parenteral*
Cyclizine
  • Injection (U.S. and Canada)

## Before Using This Medicine

If you are taking this medicine without a prescription, carefully read and follow any precautions on the label. For buclizine, cyclizine, and meclizine, the following should be considered:

**Allergies**—Tell your doctor if you have ever had any unusual or allergic reaction to buclizine, cyclizine, or meclizine. Also tell your health care professional if you are allergic to any other substances, such as foods, preservatives, or dyes.

**Pregnancy**—These medicines have not been shown to cause birth defects or other problems in humans. However, studies in animals have shown that buclizine, cyclizine, and meclizine given in doses many times the usual human dose cause birth defects, such as cleft palate.

**Breast-feeding**—Although these medicines may pass into the breast milk, they have not been reported to cause problems in nursing babies. However, since these medicines tend to decrease the secretions of the body, it is possible that the flow of breast milk may be reduced in some patients.

**Children**—There is no specific information comparing use of buclizine, cyclizine, and meclizine in children with use in other age groups. However, children may be especially sensitive to the anticholinergic effects (e.g., dryness of mouth, nose, and throat) of these medicines.

**Older adults**—There is no specific information comparing use of buclizine, cyclizine, and meclizine in the elderly with use in other age groups. However, older people may be especially sensitive to the anticholinergic effects (e.g., dryness of mouth, nose, and throat) of these medicines.

**Other medicines**—Although certain medicines should not be used together at all, in other cases two different medicines may be used together even if an interaction might occur. In these cases, your doctor may want to change the dose, or other precautions may be necessary. When you are taking buclizine, cyclizine, or meclizine, it is especially important that your health care professional know if you are taking the following:
  • Alcohol or
  • Central nervous system (CNS) depressants, other (medicines that cause drowsiness)—Use with buclizine, cyclizine, or meclizine may increase the side effects of either medicine

**Other medical problems**—The presence of other medical problems may affect the use of buclizine, cyclizine, or meclizine. Make sure you tell your doctor if you have any other medical problems, especially:
  • Enlarged prostate or
  • Glaucoma or
  • Intestinal blockage or
  • Urinary tract blockage—Buclizine, cyclizine, or meclizine may make these conditions worse
  • Heart failure—Cyclizine may make the condition worse

## Proper Use of This Medicine

Take this medicine with food or a glass of water or milk to lessen stomach irritation, if necessary.

This medicine is used to relieve or prevent the symptoms of motion sickness or dizziness caused by other medical problems. Take it only as directed. Do not take more of it or take it more often than stated on the label or ordered by your doctor. To do so may increase the chance of side effects.

**Dosing**—The dose of buclizine, cyclizine, or meclizine will be different for different patients. *Follow your doctor's orders or the directions on the label.* The following information includes only the average doses of buclizine, cyclizine, or meclizine. *If your dose is different, do not change it* unless your doctor tells you to do so.

*For buclizine*

- For *oral* dosage form (chewable tablets):
  - —To prevent motion sickness:
    - Adults and teenagers—50 milligrams (mg) thirty minutes before travel. The dose may be repeated in four to six hours if needed. The dose is usually not more than 150 mg a day.
    - Children—Dose must be determined by your doctor.

*For cyclizine*

- For *oral* dosage form (tablets):
  - —To prevent and treat motion sickness:
    - Adults and teenagers—50 milligrams (mg) thirty minutes before travel. The dose may be repeated in four to six hours if needed. The dose is usually not more than 200 mg a day.
    - Children—Dose is based on body weight and must be determined by your doctor. The usual dose is 1 mg per kilogram (0.5 mg per pound) of body weight three times a day. Or, for children 6 to 12 years of age may take 25 mg thirty minutes before travel. The dose may be repeated in six to eight hours if needed. The dose is usually not more than 75 mg a day.
- For *injection* dosage form:
  - —To treat motion sickness:
    - Adults and teenagers—50 mg injected into a muscle every four to six hours as needed.
    - Children—Dose is based on body weight and must be determined by your doctor. The usual dose is 1 mg per kilogram (0.5 mg per pound) of body weight injected into a muscle three times a day if needed.

*For meclizine*

- For *oral* dosage forms (capsules, chewable tablets, tablets):
  - —To prevent and treat motion sickness:
    - Adults and teenagers—25 to 50 milligrams (mg) one hour before travel. The dose may be repeated every twenty-four hours as needed.
    - Children—Dose must be determined by your doctor.
  - —To prevent and treat dizziness:
    - Adults and teenagers—25 to 100 mg a day as needed, in divided doses.
    - Children—Dose must be determined by your doctor.

**Missed dose**—If you must take this medicine regularly and you miss a dose, take the missed dose as soon as possible. However, if it is almost time for your next dose, skip the missed dose and go back to your regular dosing schedule. Do not double doses.

**Storage**—To store this medicine:
- Keep out of the reach of children.
- Store away from heat and direct light.
- Do not store the tablets in the bathroom, near the kitchen sink, or in other damp places. Heat or moisture may cause the medicine to break down.
- Do not keep outdated medicine or medicine no longer needed. Be sure that any discarded medicine is out of the reach of children.

---

## Precautions While Using This Medicine

Tell the doctor in charge that you are taking this medicine before you have any skin tests for allergies. The results of the test may be affected by this medicine.

Buclizine, cyclizine, or meclizine will add to the effects of alcohol and other CNS depressants (medicines that slow down the nervous system, possibly causing drowsiness). Some examples of CNS depressants are antihistamines or medicine for hay fever, other allergies, or colds; sedatives, tranquilizers, or sleeping medicine; prescription pain medicine or narcotics; barbiturates; medicine for seizures; muscle relaxants; or anesthetics, including some dental anesthetics. *Check with your doctor before taking any of the above while you are using this medicine.*

This medicine may cause some people to become drowsy or less alert than they are normally. *Make sure you know how you react to this medicine before you drive, use machines, or do anything else that could be dangerous if you are not alert.*

Buclizine, cyclizine, and meclizine may cause dryness of the mouth. For temporary relief use sugarless candy or gum, melt bits of ice in your mouth, or use a saliva substitute. However, if your mouth continues to feel dry for more than 2 weeks, check with your medical doctor or dentist. Continuing dryness of the mouth may increase the chance of dental disease, including tooth decay, gum disease, and fungus infections.

---

## Side Effects of This Medicine

Along with its needed effects, a medicine may cause some unwanted effects. The following side effects may go away during treatment as your body adjusts to the medicine; however, check with your doctor if they continue or are bothersome:

*More common*

Drowsiness

*Less common or rare*

Blurred vision; constipation; difficult or painful urination; dizziness; dryness of mouth, nose, and throat; fast heartbeat; headache; loss of appetite; nervousness, restlessness, or trouble in sleeping; skin rash; upset stomach

Not all of the side effects listed above have been reported for each of these medicines, but they have been reported for at least one of them. Buclizine, cyclizine, and meclizine are similar, so any of the above side effects may occur with any of these medicines.

Other side effects not listed above may also occur in some patients. If you notice any other effects, check with your doctor.

Revised: 12/02/92
Interim revision: 05/13/94

# MEFLOQUINE    Systemic†

A commonly used brand name in the U.S. is Lariam.

†Not commercially available in Canada.

## Description

Mefloquine (ME-floe-kwin) is used to prevent or treat malaria. It works by killing malaria parasites (tiny, one-celled animals) or preventing their growth.

Mefloquine will not actually prevent you from becoming infected with malaria. However, it will prevent the development of symptoms of malaria in people who are living in, or will be traveling to, an area where there is a chance of getting malaria. This medicine may also be used to treat malaria in patients who have already developed symptoms of malaria. Mefloquine may be taken alone or with other medicines for malaria.

This medicine may cause some serious side effects. Therefore, it is usually used only to prevent the symptoms of malaria or to treat serious malaria infections in areas where it is known that other medicines may not work.

Mefloquine is available only with your doctor's prescription, in the following dosage form:

*Oral*
- Tablets (U.S.)

## Before Using This Medicine

In deciding to use a medicine, the risks of taking the medicine must be weighed against the good it will do. This is a decision you and your doctor will make. For mefloquine, the following should be considered:

**Allergies**—Tell your doctor if you have ever had any unusual or allergic reaction to mefloquine, quinidine (e.g., Quinidex), quinine (e.g., Quinamm), or any related medicines. Also tell your health care professional if you are allergic to any other substances, such as foods, preservatives, or dyes.

**Pregnancy**—Mefloquine has not been studied in pregnant women, and its use is not recommended during pregnancy. Studies in animals have shown that mefloquine may cause birth defects and other problems.

However, mefloquine has been used in some women in the second and third trimesters of pregnancy. It is important to prevent malaria since if a pregnant woman gets malaria, there is an increased chance of premature births, stillbirths, and abortion.

It is best if pregnant women can avoid traveling to areas where there is a chance of getting malaria. However, if travel is necessary and mefloquine is used, women who may become pregnant should use effective birth control measures while taking this medicine and for 2 months after taking the last dose.

**Breast-feeding**—Mefloquine passes into the breast milk in small amounts.

**Children**—Studies on mefloquine use in children have shown that this medicine causes side effects in children like those seen in adults, e.g., nausea, vomiting, and dizziness. Its use is not recommended in infants and children up to 2 years of age or those weighing up to 15 kg (33 pounds).

**Older adults**—Many medicines have not been studied specifically in older people. Therefore, it may not be known whether they work exactly the same way they do in younger adults or if they cause different side effects or problems in older people. There is no specific information comparing use of mefloquine in the elderly with use in other age groups.

**Other medicines**—Although certain medicines should not be used together at all, in other cases two different medicines may be used together even if an interaction might occur. In these cases, your doctor may want to change the dose, or other precautions may be necessary. When you are taking mefloquine, it is especially important that your health care professional know if you are taking any of the following:

- Bepridil (e.g., Vascor) or
- Beta-adrenergic blocking agents (acebutolol [e.g., Sectral], atenolol [e.g., Tenormin], betaxolol [e.g., Kerlone], carteolol [e.g., Cartrol], labetalol [e.g., Normodyne], metoprolol [e.g., Lopressor], nadolol [e.g., Corgard], oxprenolol [e.g., Trasicor], penbutolol [e.g., Levatol], pindolol [e.g., Visken], propranolol [e.g., Inderal], sotalol [e.g., Sotacor], timolol [e.g., Blocadren]) or
- Diltiazem (e.g., Cardizem) or
- Flunarizine (e.g., Sibelium) or
- Isradipine (e.g., DynaCirc) or
- Nicardipine (e.g., Cardene) or
- Nifedipine (e.g., Procardia) or
- Nimodipine (e.g., Nimotop) or
- Quinidine (e.g., Quinidex) or

- Quinine (e.g., Quinamm) or
- Verapamil (e.g., Calan)—Use of these medicines together with mefloquine may result in slow heartbeat and other heart problems; also, an increased chance of convulsions (seizures) may occur when quinine is taken together with mefloquine
- Chloroquine (e.g., Aralen)—Use of chloroquine with mefloquine may increase the chance of convulsions (seizures)
- Divalproex (e.g., Depakote) or
- Valproic acid (e.g., Depakene)—Use of these medicines together with mefloquine may result in low blood levels of valproic acid and an increased chance of convulsions (seizures)
- Typhoid vaccine, oral (e.g., Vivotif Vaccine)—Use of the oral typhoid vaccine with mefloquine may keep the vaccine from working properly

**Other medical problems**—The presence of other medical problems may affect the use of mefloquine. Make sure you tell your doctor if you have any other medical problems, especially:

- Convulsions (seizures) or
- Epilepsy or
- Heart block or
- Psychiatric (mental) disorders, history of—Mefloquine may make these conditions worse

## Proper Use of This Medicine

*Do not give this medicine to infants and children up to 2 years of age or to those weighing less than 15 kg (33 pounds).*

Mefloquine is best taken with a full glass (8 ounces) of water and with food, unless otherwise directed by your doctor.

For patients taking *mefloquine* to *prevent the symptoms of malaria:*

- Your doctor will want you to start taking this medicine 1 week before you travel to an area where there is a chance of getting malaria. This will help you to see how you react to the medicine. Also, it will allow time for your doctor to prescribe another medicine for you if you have a reaction to this medicine.
- Also, you should keep taking this medicine while you are in the area and for 4 weeks after you leave the area. No medicine will protect you completely from malaria. However, to protect you as completely as possible, *it is important that you keep taking this medicine for the full time your doctor ordered.* Also, if fever or "flu-like" symptoms develop during your travels or within 2 to 3 months after you leave the area, *check with your doctor immediately.*
- This medicine works best when you take it on a regular schedule. For example, if you are to take it once a week, it is best to take it on the same day each week. *Do not miss any doses.* If you have any questions about this, check with your health care professional.

For patients taking *mefloquine* to *treat malaria:*

- To help clear up your infection completely, *take this medicine exactly as directed by your doctor.*

**Dosing**—The dose of mefloquine will be different for different patients. *Follow your doctor's orders or the directions on the label.* The following information includes only the average doses of mefloquine. *If your dose is different, do not change it* unless your doctor tells you to do so.

*The number of doses you take each day, the time allowed between doses, and the length of time you take the medicine depend on whether you are using mefloquine to prevent or to treat malaria.*

- For *oral* dosage form (tablets):
  —For prevention of malaria:
    - Adults and children weighing over 45 kilograms (kg) (99 pounds)—250 milligrams (mg) (1 tablet) one week before traveling to an area where malaria occurs. Then 250 mg once a week while staying in the area and every week for four weeks after leaving the area.
    - Children—Dose is based on body weight and must be determined by your doctor.
      —Children weighing up to 15 kg (33 pounds): Use is not recommended.
      —Children weighing 15 to 19 kg (33 to 41.8 pounds): 62.5 mg (¼ tablet) one week before traveling to an area where malaria occurs. Then 62.5 mg once a week while staying in the area and every week for four weeks after leaving the area.
      —Children weighing 20 to 30 kg (44 to 66 pounds): 125 mg (½ tablet) one week before traveling to an area where malaria occurs. Then 125 mg once a week while staying in the area and every week for four weeks after leaving the area.
      —Children weighing 31 to 45 kg (68.2 to 99 pounds): 187.5 mg (¾ tablet) one week before traveling to an area where malaria occurs. Then 187.5 mg once a week while staying in the area and every week for four weeks after leaving the area.
  —For treatment of malaria:
    - Adults—1250 mg as a single dose.
    - Children—Dose is based on body weight and must be determined by your doctor. The usual dose is 16.5 mg per kg (7 mg per pound) of body weight as a single dose.

**Missed dose**—If you miss a dose of this medicine, take it as soon as possible. This will help to keep you taking your medicine on a regular schedule. However, if it is almost time for your next dose, skip the missed dose and go back to your regular dosing schedule. Do not double doses.

**Storage**—To store this medicine:
- Keep out of the reach of children.
- Store away from heat and direct light.
- Do not store in the bathroom, near the kitchen sink, or in other damp places. Heat or moisture may cause the medicine to break down.
- Do not keep outdated medicine or medicine no longer needed. Be sure that any discarded medicine is out of the reach of children.

## Precautions While Using This Medicine

Mefloquine may cause vision problems. It may also cause some people to become dizzy or lightheaded or to have hallucinations (seeing, hearing, or feeling things that are not there). *Make sure you know how you react to this medicine before you drive, use machines, or do anything else that could be dangerous if you are dizzy or are not alert or able to see well.* This is especially important for people whose jobs require fine coordination. If these reactions are especially bothersome, check with your doctor.

Malaria is spread by the bite of certain kinds of infected female mosquitoes. If you are living in, or will be traveling to, an area where there is a chance of getting malaria, the following mosquito-control measures will help to prevent infection:

- If possible, sleep under mosquito netting to avoid being bitten by malaria-carrying mosquitoes.
- Wear long-sleeved shirts or blouses and long trousers to protect your arms and legs, especially from dusk through dawn when mosquitoes are out.
- Apply mosquito repellant, preferably one containing DEET, to uncovered areas of the skin from dusk through dawn when mosquitoes are out.
- Using a pyrethrum-containing flying insect spray to kill mosquitoes in living and sleeping quarters during evening and nighttime hours.

*If you are taking quinidine (e.g., Quinidex) or quinine (e.g., Quinamm) talk to your doctor before you take mefloquine. While you are taking mefloquine, take mefloquine at least 12 hours after the last dose of quinidine or quinine.* Taking mefloquine and either of these medicines at the same time may result in a greater chance of serious side effects.

For patients taking *mefloquine* to *treat malaria:*
- If your symptoms do not improve within a few days, or if they become worse, check with your doctor.

## Side Effects of This Medicine

Along with its needed effects, a medicine may cause some unwanted effects. Although not all of these side effects may occur, if they do occur they may need medical attention.

*Check with your doctor immediately* if any of the following side effects occur:
  *Rare*
      Anxiety; confusion; convulsions (seizures); hallucinations (seeing, hearing, or feeling things that are not there); mental depression; mood or mental changes; restlessness; slow heartbeat

Other side effects may occur that usually do not need medical attention. These side effects may go away during treatment as your body adjusts to the medicine. However, check with your doctor if any of the following side effects continue or are bothersome:
  *More common*
      Abdominal or stomach pain; diarrhea; difficulty concentrating; dizziness; headache; lightheadedness; loss of appetite; nausea or vomiting; trouble in sleeping; visual changes

Other side effects not listed above may also occur in some patients. If you notice any other effects, check with your doctor.

Revised: 10/06/92
Interim revision(s): 08/26/94

# MELPHALAN   Systemic

A commonly used brand name in the U.S. and Canada is Alkeran. Other commonly used names are L-PAM and phenylalanine mustard.

## Description

Melphalan (MEL-fa-lan) belongs to the group of medicines called alkylating agents. It is used to treat some kinds of cancer.

Melphalan interferes with the growth of cancer cells, which are eventually destroyed. Since the growth of normal body cells may also be affected by melphalan, other effects will also occur. Some of these may be serious and must be reported to your doctor. Other effects may not be serious but may cause concern. Some effects may not occur for months or years after the medicine is used.

Before you begin treatment with melphalan, you and your doctor should talk about the good this medicine will do as well as the risks of using it.

Melphalan is available only with your doctor's prescription, in the following dosage form:
  *Oral*
- Tablets (U.S. and Canada)

## Before Using This Medicine

In deciding to use a medicine, the risks of taking the medicine must be weighed against the good it will do. This is a decision you and your doctor will make. For melphalan, the following should be considered:

**Allergies**—Tell your doctor if you have ever had any unusual or allergic reaction to melphalan or chlorambucil.

**Pregnancy**—Tell your doctor if you are pregnant or if you intend to have children. There is a chance that this medicine may cause birth defects if either the male or female is taking it at the time of conception or if it is taken during pregnancy. In addition, many cancer medicines may cause sterility which could be permanent. Sterility has been reported with melphalan and the possibility should be kept in mind.

Be sure that you have discussed this with your doctor before taking this medicine. It is best to use some kind of birth control while you are taking melphalan. Tell your doctor right away if you think you have become pregnant while taking melphalan.

**Breast-feeding**—Tell your doctor if you are breast-feeding or if you intend to breast-feed during treatment with this medicine. Because melphalan may cause serious side effects, breast-feeding is generally not recommended while you are taking it.

**Children**—There is no specific information about the use of melphalan in children.

**Older adults**—Many medicines have not been tested in older people. Therefore, it may not be known whether they work exactly the same way they do in younger adults or if they cause different side effects or problems in older people. There is no specific information about the use of melphalan in the elderly.

**Other medicines**—Although certain medicines should not be used together at all, in other cases two different medicines may be used together even if an interaction might occur. In these cases, your doctor may want to change the dose, or other precautions may be necessary. When you are taking melphalan, it is especially important that your health care professional know if you are taking any of the following:

- Amphotericin B by injection (e.g., Fungizone) or
- Antithyroid agents (medicine for overactive thyroid) or
- Azathioprine (e.g., Imuran) or
- Chloramphenicol (e.g., Chloromycetin) or
- Colchicine or
- Flucytosine (e.g., Ancobon) or
- Interferon (e.g., Intron A, Roferon-A) or
- Plicamycin (e.g., Mithracin) or
- Zidovudine (e.g., Retrovir) or
- If you have ever been treated with x-rays or cancer medicines—Melphalan may increase the effects of these medicines or radiation therapy on the blood
- Probenecid (e.g., Benemid) or
- Sulfinpyrazone (e.g., Anturane)—Melphalan may raise the concentration of uric acid in the blood, which these medicines are used to lower

**Other medical problems**—The presence of other medical problems may affect the use of melphalan. Make sure you tell your doctor if you have any other medical problems, especially:

- Chickenpox (including recent exposure) or
- Herpes zoster (shingles)—Risk of severe disease affecting other parts of the body
- Gout (history of) or
- Kidney stones (history of)—Melphalan may increase levels of a chemical called uric acid in the body, which can cause gout or kidney stones
- Infection—Melphalan can reduce immunity to infection
- Kidney disease

## Proper Use of This Medicine

*Take melphalan only as directed by your doctor.* Do not take more or less of it, do not take it more often, and do not take it for a longer time than your doctor ordered. The exact amount of medicine you need has been carefully worked out. Taking too much may increase the chance of side effects, while taking too little may not improve your condition.

This medicine is sometimes given together with certain other medicines. If you are using a combination of medicines, make sure that you take each one at the proper time and do not mix them. Ask your health care professional to help you plan a way to remember to take your medicine at the right times.

While you are using melphalan, your doctor may want you to drink extra fluids so that you will pass more urine. This will help prevent kidney problems and keep your kidneys working well.

This medicine often causes nausea, vomiting, and loss of appetite. However, it may have to be taken for several months to be effective. Even if you begin to feel ill, *do not stop using this medicine without first checking with your doctor.* Ask your health care professional for ways to lessen these effects.

If you vomit shortly after taking a dose of melphalan, check with your doctor. You will be told whether to take the dose again or to wait until the next scheduled dose.

**Dosing**—The dose of melphalan will be different for different patients. The dose that is used may depend on a number of things, including what the medicine is being used for, the patient's weight, whether the medicine is being given by mouth or by injection, and whether or not other medicines are also being taken. *If you are taking or receiving melphalan at home, follow your doctor's orders or the directions on the label.* If you have any questions about the proper dose of melphalan, ask your doctor.

**Missed dose**—If you miss a dose of this medicine, do not take the missed dose at all and do not double the next one. Instead, go back to your regular dosing schedule and check with your doctor.

**Storage**—To store this medicine:

- Keep out of the reach of children.
- Store in the original glass container away from heat and direct light.
- Do not store in the bathroom, near the kitchen sink, or in other damp places. Heat or moisture may cause the medicine to break down.
- Do not keep outdated medicine or medicine no longer needed. Be sure that any discarded medicine is out of the reach of children.

## Precautions While Using This Medicine

*It is very important that your doctor check your progress at regular visits* to make sure that this medicine is working properly and to check for unwanted effects.

While you are being treated with melphalan, and after you stop treatment with it, *do not have any immunizations (vaccinations) without your doctor's approval.* Melphalan may lower your body's resistance and there is a chance you might get the infection the immunization is meant to prevent. In addition, other persons living in your household should not take or should not have recently taken oral polio vaccine since there is a chance they could pass the polio virus on to you. Also, avoid other persons who have taken oral polio vaccine. Do not get close to them and do not stay in the same room with them for very long. If you cannot take these precautions, you should consider wearing a protective face mask that covers the nose and mouth.

Melphalan can lower the number of white blood cells in your blood temporarily, increasing the chance of getting an infection. It can also lower the number of platelets, which are necessary for proper blood clotting. If this occurs, there are certain precautions you can take, especially when your blood count is low, to reduce the risk of infection or bleeding:

- If you can, avoid people with infections. *Check with your doctor immediately* if you think you are getting an infection or if you get a fever or chills, cough or hoarseness, lower back or side pain, or painful or difficult urination.
- *Check with your doctor immediately* if you notice any unusual bleeding or bruising; black, tarry stools; blood in urine or stools; or pinpoint red spots on your skin.
- Be careful when using a regular toothbrush, dental floss, or toothpick. Your medical doctor, dentist, or nurse may recommend other ways to clean your teeth and gums. Check with your medical doctor before having any dental work done.
- Do not touch your eyes or the inside of your nose unless you have just washed your hands and have not touched anything else in the meantime.
- Be careful not to cut yourself when you are using sharp objects such as a safety razor or fingernail or toenail cutters.
- Avoid contact sports or other situations where bruising or injury could occur.

## Side Effects of This Medicine

Along with their needed effects, medicines like melphalan can sometimes cause unwanted effects such as blood problems and other side effects. These and others are described below. Also, because of the way these medicines act on the body, there is a chance that they might cause other unwanted effects that may not occur until months or years after the medicine is used. These delayed effects may include certain types of cancer, such as leukemia. Discuss these possible effects with your doctor.

Although not all of these side effects may occur, if they do occur they may need medical attention.

*Check with your doctor immediately* if any of the following side effects occur:

*Less common*
Black, tarry stools; blood in urine or stools; cough or hoarseness; fever or chills; lower back or side pain; painful or difficult urination; pinpoint red spots on skin; skin rash or itching (sudden); unusual bleeding or bruising

Check with your doctor as soon as possible if any of the following side effects occur:

*Less common or rare*
Joint pain; sores in mouth and on lips; swelling of feet or lower legs

Other side effects may occur that usually do not need medical attention. These side effects may go away during treatment as your body adjusts to the medicine. Also, your health care professional may be able to tell you about ways to prevent or reduce some of these side effects. Check with your health care professional if the following side effects continue or are bothersome or if you have any questions about them:

*Less common*
Nausea and vomiting

After you stop taking melphalan, it may still produce some side effects that need attention. During this period of time, check with your doctor if you notice any of the following side effects:

Black, tarry stools; blood in urine or stools; cough or hoarseness; fever or chills; lower back or side pain; painful or difficult urination; pinpoint red spots on skin; unusual bleeding or bruising

Other side effects not listed above may also occur in some patients. If you notice any other effects, check with your doctor.

Revised: 08/90
Interim revision: 07/29/93; 07/11/94

# MENINGOCOCCAL POLYSACCHARIDE VACCINE   Systemic

A commonly used brand name in the U.S. and Canada is Menomune.

## Description

Meningococcal polysaccharide (ma-nin-ja-KOK-kal pol-i-SAK-ka-ryd) vaccine is an active immunizing agent used to prevent infection by certain groups of meningococcal bacteria. The vaccine works by causing your body to produce its own protection (antibodies) against the disease.

The following information applies only to the meningococcal vaccine used for meningococcal bacteria Groups A, C, Y, and W-135. These groups cause approximately 50% of meningococcal meningitis cases in the U.S. The vaccine will not protect against infection caused by other meningococcal bacteria groups, such as Group B.

Meningococcal infection can cause life-threatening illnesses, such as meningococcal meningitis, which affects the brain, and meningococcemia, which affects the blood. Approximately 10% of persons with meningococcal meningitis and 30% of persons with meningococcemia die. These diseases are more likely to occur in young children and in persons with certain diseases or conditions that make them more susceptible to a meningococcal infection or more likely to develop serious problems from a meningococcal infection.

Immunization against meningococcal disease is recommended for persons 2 years of age or older who are at risk of getting the disease because:

- they have certain diseases or conditions that make them more susceptible to a meningococcal infection or more likely to develop serious problems from a meningococcal infection.
- they are living in, working in, or visiting an area where there is a high possibility of getting meningococcal disease.

Usually a person needs to receive meningococcal vaccine only once. However, additional injections may be needed for young children who remain at high risk of meningococcal disease.

Meningococcal polysaccharide vaccine is to be administered only by or under the supervision of your doctor or other health care professional. It is available in the following dosage form:

*Parenteral*
- Injection (U.S. and Canada)

## Before Receiving This Vaccine

In deciding to use a medicine, the risks of taking the medicine must be weighed against the good it will do. This is a decision you and your doctor will make. For meningococcal vaccine, the following should be considered:

**Allergies**—Tell your doctor if you have ever had any unusual or allergic reaction to meningococcal vaccine. Also tell your health care professional if you are allergic to any other substances, such as food (especially lactose) or preservatives (especially thimerosal). This vaccine contains lactose and thimerosal.

**Pregnancy**—Meningococcal vaccine has not been shown to cause birth defects or other problems in humans.

**Breast-feeding**—Meningococcal vaccine has not been reported to cause problems in nursing babies.

**Children**—Use of meningococcal vaccine is not recommended in infants and children younger than 2 years of age. This vaccine has been tested in older children and, in effective doses, has not been shown to cause different side effects or problems than it does in adults.

**Older adults**—Many medicines have not been studied specifically in older people. Therefore, it may not be known whether they work exactly the same way they do in younger adults. Although there is no specific information comparing use of this vaccine in the elderly with use in other age groups, this vaccine is not expected to cause different side effects or problems in older people than it does in younger adults.

**Other medicines**—Although certain medicines should not be used together at all, in other cases two different medicines may be used together even if an interaction might occur. In these cases, your doctor may want to change the dose, or other precautions may be necessary. Before you receive meningococcal vaccine, it is especially important that your health care professional know if you have received any of the following:

- Cancer medicines or
- Corticosteroids (e.g., cortisone-like medicines) or
- Radiation therapy—May reduce the useful effect of the vaccine

**Other medical problems**—The presence of other medical problems may affect the use of meningococcal vaccine. Make sure you tell your doctor if you have any other medical problems, especially:

- Severe illness with fever—The symptoms of the condition may be confused with the possible side effects of the vaccine

## Proper Use of This Vaccine

**Dosing**—The dose of meningococcal vaccine will be different for different patients. The following information includes only the average doses of meningococcal vaccine.

- For *injection* dosage form:
  —For prevention of meningococcal meningitis:
  - Adults and children 2 years of age and older—One dose injected under the skin.
  - Children up to 2 years of age—Use is not recommended.

## Side Effects of This Vaccine

Along with its needed effects, a vaccine may cause some unwanted effects. Although not all of these side effects may occur, if they do occur they may need medical attention.

*Get emergency help immediately* if any of the following side effects occur:

*Symptoms of allergic reactions*
Difficulty in breathing or swallowing; hives; itching, especially of feet or hands; reddening of skin, especially around ears; swelling of eyes, face, or inside of nose; unusual tiredness or weakness (sudden and severe)

Other side effects may occur that usually do not need medical attention. However, check with your doctor if any of the following side effects continue or are bothersome:

*More common*
Redness at place of injection—may last 1 or 2 days; tenderness, soreness, or pain at place of injection

*Less common*
Chills; fever over 100 °F (37.8 °C); general feeling of discomfort or illness; hard lump at place of injection; headache; tiredness or weakness

Other side effects not listed above may also occur in some patients. If you notice any other effects, check with your doctor.

Revised: 07/12/94

---

# MENOTROPINS   Systemic

A commonly used brand name in the U.S. and Canada is Pergonal. Another commonly used name is human menopausal gonadotropins (HMG).

## Description

Menotropins (men-oh-TROE-pins) are a mixture of follicle-stimulating hormone (FSH) and luteinizing hormone (LH) that are naturally produced by the pituitary gland.

*Use in females*:
FSH is primarily responsible for stimulating growth of the ovarian follicle, which includes the developing egg, the cells surrounding the egg that produce the hormones needed to support a pregnancy, and the fluid around the egg. As the follicle grows, an increasing amount of the hormone estrogen is produced by the cells in the follicle and released into the bloodstream. Estrogen causes the endometrium (lining of the uterus) to thicken before ovulation occurs. The higher blood levels of estrogen will also tell the hypothalamus and pituitary gland to slow the production and release of FSH.

LH also helps to increase the amount of estrogen produced by the follicle cells. However, its main function is to cause ovulation. The sharp rise in the blood level of LH that triggers ovulation is called the LH surge. After ovulation, the group of hormone-producing follicle cells become the corpus luteum, which will produce estrogen and large amounts of another hormone, progesterone. Progesterone causes the endometrium to mature so that it can support implantation of the fertilized egg or embryo. If implantation of a fertilized egg does not occur, the levels of estrogen and progesterone decrease, the endometrium sloughs off, and menstruation occurs.

Menotropins are usually given in combination with human chorionic gonadotropin (hCG). The actions of hCG are almost the same as those of LH. It is given to simulate the natural LH surge. This results in ovulation at an expected time.

Many women choosing treatment with menotropins have already tried clomiphene (e.g., Serophene) and have not been able to conceive yet. Menotropins may also be used to cause the ovary to produce several follicles, which can then be harvested for use in gamete intrafallopian transfer (GIFT) or *in vitro* fertilization (IVF).

*Use in males*:
Menotropins are used to stimulate the production of sperm in some forms of male infertility.

Menotropins are to be given only by or under the supervision of your doctor. It is available in the following dosage form:

*Parenteral*
- Injection (U.S. and Canada)

## Before Using This Medicine

In deciding to use a medicine, the risks of taking the medicine must be weighed against the good it will do. This is a decision you and your doctor will make. For menotropins, the following should be considered:

**Allergies**—Tell your doctor if you have ever had any unusual or allergic reaction to menotropins. Also tell your health care professional if you are allergic to any other substances, such as foods, preservatives, or dyes.

**Pregnancy**—If you become pregnant as a result of using this medicine, there is an increased chance of a multiple pregnancy.

**Other medicines**—Although certain medicines should not be used together at all, in other cases two different medicines may be used together even if an interaction might occur. In these cases, your doctor may want to change

the dose, or other precautions may be necessary. Tell your health care professional if you are taking any other prescription or nonprescription (over-the-counter [OTC]) medicine.

**Other medical problems**—The presence of other medical problems may affect the use of menotropins. Make sure you tell your doctor if you have any other medical problems, especially:

- Cyst on ovary—Menotropins can cause further growth of cysts on the ovary
- Unusual vaginal bleeding—Some irregular vaginal bleeding is a sign that the endometrium is growing too rapidly, possibly of endometrial cancer, or some hormone imbalances; the increases in estrogen production caused by menotropins can make these problems worse. If a hormonal imbalance is present, it should be treated before the beginning of menotropins therapy

## Proper Use of This Medicine

**Dosing**—The dose of menotropins will be different for different patients. *Follow your doctor's orders or the directions on the label.* The following information includes only the average doses of menotropins. *If your dose is different, do not change it* unless your doctor tells you to do so.

- For *injection* dosage form:
  —For causing ovulation to help in becoming pregnant:
    - Adults—75 Units of FSH and 75 Units of LH injected into a muscle once a day for seven or more days. Usually your doctor will give you another medicine called chorionic gonadotropin (hCG) the day after the last dose of menotropins.
  —For help in becoming pregnant while using other pregnancy methods (assisted reproductive technology [ART]):
    - Adults—150 Units of FSH and 150 Units of LH injected into a muscle once a day for seven or more days. Usually your doctor will give you another medicine called chorionic gonadotropin (hCG) the day after the last dose of menotropins.
  —For producing sperm:
    - Adults—75 Units of FSH and 75 Units of LH injected into a muscle three times a week for four or more months. Usually your doctor will give you another medicine called chorionic gonadotropin before and during treatment with menotropins. If needed, your doctor may increase your dose to 150 Units of FSH and 150 Units of LH three times a week after four months.

## Precautions While Using This Medicine

*It is very important that your doctor check your progress at regular visits* to make sure that the medicine is working properly and to check for unwanted effects. Your doctor will likely want to watch the development of the ovarian follicle(s) by measuring the amount of estrogen in your bloodstream and by checking the size of the follicle(s) with ultrasound examinations.

*For females only:*

- If your doctor has asked you to record your basal body temperatures (BBTs) daily, make sure that you do this every day. It is important that intercourse take place around the time of ovulation to give you the best chance of becoming pregnant. *Follow your doctor's instructions carefully.*

## Side Effects of This Medicine

Along with its needed effects, a medicine may cause some unwanted effects. Although not all of these side effects may occur, if they do occur they may need medical attention.

Check with your doctor as soon as possible if any of the following side effects occur:

*For females only*
  *More common*

    Bloating (mild); pain, swelling, or irritation at place of injection; rash at place of injection or on body; stomach or pelvic pain

  *Less common or rare*

    Abdominal or stomach pain (severe); bloating (moderate to severe); decreased amount of urine; feeling of indigestion; nausea, vomiting, or diarrhea (continuing or severe); pelvic pain (severe); shortness of breath; swelling of the lower legs; weight gain (rapid)

*For males only*
  *More common*

    Dizziness; fainting; headache; irregular heartbeat; loss of appetite; more frequent nosebleeds; shortness of breath

Other side effects may occur that usually do not need medical attention. These side effects may go away during treatment as your body adjusts to the medicine. However, check with your doctor if the following side effect continues or is bothersome:

*For males only*
  *Less common*
    Enlargement of breasts

After you stop using this medicine, your body may need time to adjust. The length of time this takes depends on the amount of medicine you were using and how long you used it. During this period of time check with your doctor if you notice any of the following side effects:

*For females only*
    Abdominal or stomach pain (severe); bloating (moderate to severe); decreased amount of urine; feeling of indigestion; nausea, vomiting, or diarrhea (continuing or severe); pelvic pain (severe); shortness of breath; weight gain (rapid)

Other side effects not listed above may also occur in some patients. If you notice any other effects, check with your doctor.

Annual revision: 07/07/92
Interim revision: 06/30/94

# MEPROBAMATE  Systemic

Some commonly used brand names are:
**In the U.S.—**

| | |
|---|---|
| Equanil | 'Miltown'-400 |
| Meprospan 200 | 'Miltown'-600 |
| Meprospan 400 | Probate |
| 'Miltown'-200 | Trancot |

Generic name product may also be available.

**In Canada—**

| | |
|---|---|
| Apo-Meprobamate | Meprospan-400 |
| Equanil | Miltown |

## Description

Meprobamate (me-proe-BA-mate) is used to relieve nervousness or tension. This medicine should not be used for nervousness or tension caused by the stress of everyday life.

Meprobamate is available only with your doctor's prescription, in the following dosage forms:

*Oral*
- Extended-release capsules (U.S. and Canada)
- Tablets (U.S. and Canada)

## Before Using This Medicine

In deciding to use a medicine, the risks of taking the medicine must be weighed against the good it will do. This is a decision you and your doctor will make. For meprobamate, the following should be considered:

**Allergies**—Tell your doctor if you have ever had any unusual or allergic reaction to meprobamate or to medicines like meprobamate such as carbromal, carisoprodol, mebutamate, or tybamate. Also tell your health care professional if you are allergic to any other substances, such as foods, preservatives, or dyes.

**Pregnancy**—Meprobamate has been reported to increase the chance of birth defects if taken during the first 3 months of pregnancy.

**Breast-feeding**—Meprobamate passes into the breast milk and may cause drowsiness in babies of mothers taking this medicine.

**Children**—Studies on this medicine have been done only in adult patients, and there is no specific information comparing use of meprobamate in children with use in other age groups.

**Older adults**—Elderly people may be especially sensitive to the effects of meprobamate. This may increase the chance of side effects during treatment.

**Other medicines**—Although certain medicines should not be used together at all, in other cases two different medicines may be used together even if an interaction might occur. In these cases, your doctor may want to change the dose, or other precautions may be necessary. When you are taking meprobamate, it is especially important that your health care professional know if you are taking any of the following:
- Central nervous system (CNS) depressants (medicines that cause drowsiness) or
- Tricyclic antidepressants (medicine for depression)—Taking these medicines with meprobamate may increase the CNS depressant effects

**Other medical problems**—The presence of other medical problems may affect the use of meprobamate. Make sure you tell your doctor if you have any other medical problems, especially:
- Alcohol abuse (or history of) or
- Drug abuse or dependence (or history of)—Dependence on meprobamate may develop
- Epilepsy—The risk of seizures may be increased
- Kidney disease or
- Liver disease—Higher blood levels of meprobamate may occur, increasing the chance of side effects
- Porphyria—Meprobamate may make the condition worse

## Proper Use of This Medicine

*Take this medicine only as directed by your doctor.* Do not take more of it, do not take it more often, and do not take it for a longer time than your doctor ordered. If too much is taken, it may become habit-forming.

**Dosing**—The dose of meprobamate will be different for different patients. *Follow your doctor's orders or the directions on the label.* The following information includes only the average doses of meprobamate. *If your dose is different, do not change it* unless your doctor tells you to do so:
- For *regular (short-acting)* tablets:
  - Adults and children 12 years of age and older: 400 milligrams three or four times a day, or 600 milligrams two times a day.

—Children 6 to 12 years of age: 100 to 200 milligrams two or three times a day.

—Children up to 6 years of age: Dose must be determined by the doctor.

• For *long-acting* dosage forms (extended-release tablets):

—Adults and children 12 years of age or older: 400 to 800 milligrams two times a day, in the morning and at bedtime.

—Children 6 to 12 years of age: 200 milligrams two times a day, in the morning and at bedtime.

—Children up to 6 years of age: Dose must be determined by the doctor.

**Missed dose**—If you miss a dose of this medicine and remember within an hour or so of the missed dose, take it right away. However, if you do not remember until later, skip the missed dose and go back to your regular dosing schedule. Do not double doses.

**Storage**—To store this medicine:

• Keep out of the reach of children. Overdose of meprobamate is very dangerous in children.

• Store away from heat and direct light.

• Do not store in the bathroom, near the kitchen sink, or in other damp places. Heat or moisture may cause the medicine to break down.

• Do not keep outdated medicine or medicine no longer needed. Be sure that any discarded medicine is out of the reach of children.

## Precautions While Using This Medicine

If you will be taking this medicine regularly for a long time:

• Your doctor should check your progress at regular visits.

• Check with your doctor at least every 4 months to make sure you need to continue taking this medicine.

If you will be taking this medicine in large doses or for a long time, do not stop taking it without first checking with your doctor. Your doctor may want you to reduce gradually the amount you are taking before stopping completely.

This medicine will add to the effects of alcohol and other CNS depressants (medicines that slow down the nervous system, possibly causing drowsiness). Some examples of CNS depressants are antihistamines or medicine for hay fever, other allergies, or colds; sedatives, tranquilizers, or sleeping medicine; prescription pain medicine or narcotics; barbiturates; medicine for seizures; muscle relaxants; or anesthetics, including some dental anesthetics. *Check with your doctor before taking any of the above while you are taking this medicine.*

Before you have any medical tests, tell the medical doctor in charge that you are taking this medicine. The results of some tests, such as the metyrapone test and the phentolamine test, may be affected by this medicine.

*If you think you or someone else may have taken an overdose of this medicine, get emergency help at once.* Taking an overdose of meprobamate or taking alcohol or other CNS depressants with meprobamate may lead to unconsciousness and possibly death. Some signs of an overdose are severe confusion, drowsiness, or weakness; shortness of breath or slow or troubled breathing; slurred speech; staggering; and slow heartbeat.

This medicine may cause some people to become dizzy, lightheaded, drowsy, or less alert than they are normally. Even if taken at bedtime, it may cause some people to feel drowsy or less alert on arising. *Make sure you know how you react to this medicine before you drive, use machines, or do anything else that could be dangerous if you are dizzy or are not alert.*

Meprobamate may cause dryness of the mouth. For temporary relief, use sugarless candy or gum, melt bits of ice in your mouth, or use a saliva substitute. However, if your mouth continues to feel dry for more than 2 weeks, check with your medical doctor or dentist. Continuing dryness of the mouth may increase the chance of dental disease, including tooth decay, gum disease, and fungus infections.

## Side Effects of This Medicine

Along with its needed effects, a medicine may cause some unwanted effects. Although not all of these side effects may occur, if they do occur they may need medical attention.

Check with your doctor as soon as possible if any of the following side effects occur:

*Less common*

Skin rash, hives, or itching

*Rare*

Confusion; fast, pounding, or irregular heartbeat; sore throat and fever; unusual bleeding or bruising; unusual excitement; wheezing, shortness of breath, or troubled breathing

*Symptoms of overdose*

Confusion (severe); dizziness or lightheadedness (continuing); drowsiness (severe); shortness of breath or slow or troubled breathing; slow heartbeat; slurred speech; staggering; weakness (severe)

Other side effects may occur that usually do not need medical attention. These side effects may go away during treatment as your body adjusts to the medicine. However, check with your doctor if any of the following side effects continue or are bothersome:

*More common*

Clumsiness or unsteadiness; drowsiness

*Less common*

Blurred vision or change in near or distant vision; diarrhea; dizziness or lightheadedness; false sense of wellbeing; headache; nausea or vomiting; unusual tiredness or weakness

After you stop using this medicine, your body may need time to adjust. If you took this medicine in high doses or for a long time, this may take about 2 days. During this period of time check with your doctor if you notice any of the following side effects:

> Clumsiness or unsteadiness; confusion; convulsions (seizures); hallucinations (seeing, hearing, or feeling things that are not there); increased dreaming; muscle twitching; nausea or vomiting; nervousness or restlessness; nightmares; trembling; trouble in sleeping

Other side effects not listed above may also occur in some patients. If you notice any other effects, check with your doctor.

---

Revised: 01/13/93

---

# MEPROBAMATE AND ASPIRIN  Systemic

Some commonly used brand names are:

**In the U.S.—**

| | |
|---|---|
| Epromate-M | Meprogesic |
| Equagesic | Meprogesic Q |
| Heptogesic | Micrainin |

Generic name product may also be available.

**In Canada—**
Equagesic‡

---

‡In Canada, Equagesic also contains ethoheptazine citrate.

---

## Description

Meprobamate (me-proe-BA-mate) and aspirin (AS-pir-in) combination is used to relieve pain, anxiety, and tension in certain disorders or diseases.

This medicine is available only with your doctor's prescription, in the following dosage form:

*Oral*
- Tablets (U.S. and Canada)

---

## Before Using This Medicine

In deciding to use a medicine, the risks of taking the medicine must be weighed against the good it will do. This is a decision you and your doctor will make. For meprobamate and aspirin combination, the following should be considered:

**Allergies**—Tell your doctor if you have ever had any unusual or allergic reaction to meprobamate or to medicines like meprobamate such as carbromal, carisoprodol, mebutamate, or tybamate, or to aspirin or other salicylates, including methyl salicylate (oil of wintergreen), or to any of the following medicines:

> Diclofenac (e.g., Voltaren)
> Diflunisal (e.g., Dolobid)
> Etodolac (e.g., Lodine)
> Fenoprofen (e.g., Nalfon)
> Floctafenine (e.g., Idarac)
> Flurbiprofen, oral (e.g., Ansaid)
> Ibuprofen (e.g., Motrin)
> Indomethacin (e.g., Indocin)
> Ketoprofen (e.g., Orudis)
> Ketorolac (e.g., Toradol)
> Meclofenamate (e.g., Meclomen)
> Mefenamic acid (e.g., Ponstel)
> Naproxen (e.g., Naprosyn)
> Oxyphenbutazone (e.g., Tandearil)
> Phenylbutazone (e.g., Butazolidin)

> Piroxicam (e.g., Feldene)
> Sulindac (e.g., Clinoril)
> Suprofen (e.g., Suprol)
> Tiaprofenic acid (e.g., Surgam)
> Tolmetin (e.g., Tolectin)
> Zomepirac (e.g., Zomax)

Also tell your health care professional if you are allergic to any other substances, such as foods, preservatives, or dyes.

**Pregnancy**—Meprobamate (contained in this combination medicine) has been reported to increase the chance of birth defects if taken during the first 3 months of pregnancy.

Studies in humans have not shown that aspirin (contained in this combination medicine) causes birth defects. However, studies in animals have shown that aspirin causes birth defects. Some reports have suggested that too much use of aspirin late in pregnancy may cause a decrease in the newborn's weight and possible death of the fetus or newborn infant. However, the mothers in these reports had been taking much larger amounts of aspirin than are usually recommended. Studies of mothers taking aspirin in the doses that are usually recommended did not show these unwanted effects. However, regular use of aspirin late in pregnancy may cause unwanted effects on the heart or blood flow in the fetus or in the newborn infant. Also, use of aspirin during the last 2 weeks of pregnancy may cause bleeding problems in the fetus before or during delivery or in the newborn infant. In addition, too much use of aspirin during the last 3 months of pregnancy may increase the length of pregnancy, prolong labor, cause other problems during delivery, or cause severe bleeding in the mother before, during, or after delivery.

**Breast-feeding**—Meprobamate (contained in this combination medicine) passes into the breast milk and may cause drowsiness in babies of mothers taking this medicine. Although aspirin (contained in this combination medicine) passes into the breast milk, it has not been shown to cause problems in nursing babies.

**Children**—*Do not give a medicine containing aspirin to a child with a fever or other symptoms of a virus infection, especially flu or chickenpox, without first discussing this with your child's doctor. This is very important because aspirin may cause a serious illness called Reye's* syndrome in children with fever caused by a virus infection, especially flu or chickenpox. Children who do not have a virus infection may also be more sensitive to the effects of aspirin (contained in this combination medicine), especially if they have a fever or have lost large amounts of body fluid because of vomiting, diarrhea, or sweating. This may increase the chance of side effects during treatment.

**Teenagers**—*Teenagers with fever or other symptoms of a virus infection, especially flu or chickenpox, should check with a doctor before taking this medicine.* The aspirin in this combination medicine may cause a serious illness called Reye's syndrome in teenagers with fever caused by a virus infection, especially flu or chickenpox.

**Older adults**—Elderly people may be especially sensitive to the effects of meprobamate and aspirin. This may increase the chance of side effects during treatment.

**Other medicines**—Although certain medicines should not be used together at all, in other cases two different medicines may be used together even if an interaction might occur. In these cases, your doctor may want to change the dose, or other precautions may be necessary. When you are taking meprobamate and aspirin combination, it is especially important that your health care professional know if you are taking any of the following:

- Anticoagulants (blood thinners) or
- Carbenicillin by injection (e.g., Geopen) or
- Cefamandole (e.g., Mandol) or
- Cefoperazone (e.g., Cefobid) or
- Cefotetan (e.g., Cefotan) or
- Dipyridamole (e.g., Persantine) or
- Divalproex (e.g., Depakote) or
- Heparin or
- Inflammation or pain medicine, except narcotics, or
- Moxalactam (e.g., Moxam) or
- Pentoxifylline (e.g., Trental) or
- Plicamycin (e.g., Mithracin) or
- Ticarcillin (e.g., Ticar) or
- Valproic acid (e.g., Depakene)—Taking these medicines together with aspirin may increase the chance of bleeding
- Antidiabetics, oral (diabetes medicine you take by mouth)—Aspirin may increase the effects of the antidiabetic medicine; a change in dose may be needed if meprobamate and aspirin combination is taken regularly
- Central nervous system (CNS) depressants (medicine that causes drowsiness) or
- Tricyclic antidepressants (medicine for depression)—Taking these medicines with meprobamate and aspirin combination may increase the CNS depressant effects
- Methotrexate (e.g., Mexate)—The chance of serious side effects may be increased
- Probenecid (e.g., Benemid)—Aspirin may keep probenecid from working properly in the treatment of gout
- Sulfinpyrazone (e.g., Anturane)—Aspirin may keep sulfinpyrazone from working properly in the treatment of gout; also, there may be an increased chance of bleeding
- Urinary alkalizers (medicine that makes the urine less acid, such as acetazolamide [e.g., Diamox], calcium- and/or magnesium-containing antacids, dichlorphenamide [e.g., Daranide], methazolamide [e.g., Neptazane], potassium or sodium citrate and/or citric acid, sodium bicarbonate [baking soda])—These medicines may make aspirin less

effective by causing it to be removed from the body more quickly
- Vancomycin (e.g., Vancocin)—Hearing loss may occur and may lead to deafness

**Other medical problems**—The presence of other medical problems may affect the use of meprobamate and aspirin combination. Make sure you tell your doctor if you have any other medical problems, especially:

- Alcohol abuse (or history of) or
- Drug abuse or dependence (or history of)—Dependence on meprobamate may develop
- Anemia or
- Stomach ulcer or other stomach problems—Aspirin may make your condition worse
- Asthma, allergies, and nasal polyps (history of) or
- Kidney disease or
- Liver disease—The chance of side effects may be increased.
- Epilepsy—The risk of seizures may be increased
- Gout—Aspirin may make this condition worse and may also lessen the effects of some medicines used to treat gout
- Hemophilia or other bleeding problems—The chance of bleeding may be increased by aspirin
- Porphyria—Meprobamate may make the condition worse

## Proper Use of This Medicine

*Take this medicine with food or a full glass (8 ounces) of water* to lessen stomach irritation.

*If this combination medicine containing aspirin has a strong vinegar-like odor, do not use it.* This odor means the medicine is breaking down. If you have any questions about this, check with your pharmacist.

*Take this medicine only as directed by your doctor.* Do not take more of it, do not take it more often, and do not take it for a longer time than your doctor ordered. If too much meprobamate is taken, it may become habit-forming. Also, taking too much aspirin may cause stomach problems or lead to medical problems because of an overdose.

**Dosing**—The dose of meprobamate and aspirin combination will be different for different patients. *Follow your doctor's orders or the directions on the label.* The following information includes only the average doses of meprobamate and aspirin combination. *If your dose is different, do not change it* unless your doctor tells you to do so:

- Adults—Oral, 1 or 2 tablets three or four times a day, as needed.
- Children up to 12 years of age: Use is not recommended.

**Storage**—To store this medicine:

- Keep this medicine out of the reach of children. Overdose of meprobamate is very dangerous in children.
- Store away from heat and direct light.

---

- Do not store in the bathroom, near the kitchen sink, or in other damp places. Heat or moisture may cause the medicine to break down.
- Do not keep outdated medicine or medicine no longer needed. Be sure that any discarded medicine is out of the reach of children.

## Precautions While Using This Medicine

If you will be taking this medicine regularly for a long time:

- Your doctor should check your progress at regular visits.
- Check with your doctor at least every 4 months to make sure you need to continue taking this medicine.

If you will be taking this medicine in large doses or for a long time, do not stop taking it without first checking with your doctor. Your doctor may want you to reduce gradually the amount you are taking before stopping completely.

*Check the labels of all nonprescription (over-the-counter [OTC]) and prescription medicines you now take.* If any contain aspirin or other salicylates (including bismuth subsalicylate [e.g., Pepto-Bismol]), be especially careful. Taking or using any of these medicines while taking this combination medicine containing aspirin may lead to overdose. If you have any questions about this, check with your health care professional.

This medicine will add to the effects of alcohol and other CNS depressants (medicines that slow down the nervous system, possibly causing drowsiness). Some examples of CNS depressants are antihistamines or medicine for hay fever, other allergies, or colds; sedatives, tranquilizers, or sleeping medicine; prescription pain medicine or narcotics; barbiturates; medicine for seizures; muscle relaxants; or anesthetics, including some dental anesthetics. *Check with your doctor before taking any of the above while you are taking this medicine.*

Stomach problems may be more likely to occur if you drink alcoholic beverages while being treated with this medicine, especially if you are taking the medicine in high doses or for a long time. Check with your doctor if you have any questions about this.

Too much use of this medicine together with certain other medicines may increase the chance of stomach problems. Therefore, do not regularly take this medicine together with any of the following medicines, unless directed to do so by your medical doctor or dentist:

Acetaminophen (e.g., Tylenol)
Diclofenac (e.g., Voltaren)
Diflunisal (e.g., Dolobid)
Etodolac (e.g., Lodine)
Fenoprofen (e.g., Nalfon)
Floctafenine (e.g., Idarac)
Flurbiprofen (oral) (e.g., Ansaid)
Ibuprofen (e.g., Motrin)
Indomethacin (e.g., Indocin)
Ketoprofen (e.g., Orudis)
Ketorolac (e.g., Toradol)

Meclofenamate (e.g., Meclomen)
Mefenamic acid (e.g., Ponstel)
Naproxen (e.g., Naprosyn)
Phenylbutazone (e.g., Butazolidin)
Piroxicam (e.g., Feldene)
Sulindac (e.g., Clinoril)
Tiaprofenic acid (e.g., Surgam)
Tolmetin (e.g., Tolectin)

If you are taking a laxative containing cellulose, do not take it within 2 hours of taking this medicine. Taking these medicines close together may make this medicine less effective by preventing the aspirin (contained in this combination medicine) from being absorbed by your body.

For diabetic patients:

- False urine sugar test results may occur if you take 8 or more 325-mg (5-grain) doses of aspirin (contained in this combination medicine) every day for several days in a row. Smaller doses or occasional use of aspirin usually will not affect urine sugar tests. If you have any questions about this, check with your doctor, especially if your diabetes is not well controlled.

Before you have any medical tests, tell the medical doctor in charge that you are taking this medicine. The results of some tests, such as the metyrapone test and the phentolamine test, may be affected by this medicine.

If you plan to have surgery, including dental surgery, do not take aspirin (contained in this combination medicine) for 5 days before the surgery, unless otherwise directed by your medical doctor or dentist. Taking aspirin during this time may cause bleeding problems.

*If you think you or someone else may have taken an overdose of this medicine, get emergency help at once.* Taking an overdose of this medicine or taking alcohol or other CNS depressants with it may lead to unconsciousness and possibly death. Some signs of an overdose are continuing ringing or buzzing in ears; any hearing loss; severe confusion, drowsiness, or weakness; shortness of breath or slow or troubled breathing; staggering; and slow heartbeat.

This medicine may cause some people to become dizzy, lightheaded, drowsy, or less alert than they are normally. *Make sure you know how you react to this medicine before you drive, use machines, or do anything else that could be dangerous if you are dizzy or are not alert.*

Meprobamate (contained in this combination medicine) may cause dryness of the mouth. For temporary relief, use sugarless candy or gum, melt bits of ice in your mouth, or use a saliva substitute. However, if your mouth continues to feel dry for more than 2 weeks, check with your medical doctor or dentist. Continuing dryness of the mouth may increase the chance of dental disease, including tooth decay, gum disease, and fungus infections.

## Side Effects of This Medicine

Along with its needed effects, a medicine may cause some unwanted effects. Although not all of these side effects

may occur, if they do occur they may need medical attention.

*Check with your doctor immediately* if any of the following side effects occur:

*Rare*

Wheezing, shortness of breath, troubled breathing, or tightness in chest

*Symptoms of overdose*

Any loss of hearing; bloody urine; confusion (severe); convulsions (seizures); diarrhea (severe or continuing); dizziness or lightheadedness (continuing); drowsiness (severe); fast or deep breathing; hallucinations (seeing, hearing, or feeling things that are not there); headache (severe or continuing); increased sweating; nausea or vomiting (continuing); nervousness or excitement (severe); ringing or buzzing in ears (continuing); slow heartbeat; slurred speech; staggering; stomach pain (severe or continuing); unexplained fever; unusual or uncontrolled flapping movements of the hands, especially in elderly patients; unusual thirst; vision problems; weakness (severe)

*Symptoms of overdose in children*

Changes in behavior; drowsiness or tiredness (severe); fast or deep breathing

Also, check with your doctor as soon as possible if any of the following side effects occur:

*Rare*

Bloody or black, tarry stools; confusion; skin rash, hives, or itching; sore throat and fever; unusual bleeding or bruising; unusual excitement; unusual tiredness or

weakness; vomiting of blood or material that looks like coffee grounds

Other side effects may occur that usually do not need medical attention. These side effects may go away during treatment as your body adjusts to the medicine. However, check with your doctor if any of the following side effects continue or are bothersome:

*More common*

Drowsiness; heartburn or indigestion; nausea with or without vomiting; stomach pain (mild)

*Less common*

Blurred vision or change in near or distant vision; dizziness or lightheadedness; headache

After you stop using this medicine, your body may need time to adjust. The length of time this takes depends on the amount of medicine you were using and how long you used it. During this period of time check with your doctor if you notice any of the following side effects:

Clumsiness or unsteadiness; confusion; convulsions (seizures); hallucinations (seeing, hearing, or feeling things that are not there); increased dreaming; muscle twitching; nausea or vomiting; nervousness or restlessness; nightmares; trembling; trouble in sleeping

Other side effects not listed above may also occur in some patients. If you notice any other effects, check with your doctor.

Revised: 01/13/93

# MERCAPTOPURINE   Systemic

A commonly used brand name in the U.S. and Canada is Purinethol. Another commonly used name is 6-MP.

## Description

Mercaptopurine (mer-kap-toe-PYOOR-een) belongs to the group of medicines known as antimetabolites. It is used to treat some kinds of cancer.

Mercaptopurine interferes with the growth of cancer cells, which are eventually destroyed. Since the growth of normal body cells may also be affected by mercaptopurine, other effects will also occur. Some of these may be serious and must be reported to your doctor. Other effects may not be serious but may cause concern. Some effects may not occur for months or years after the medicine is used.

Before you begin treatment with mercaptopurine, you and your doctor should talk about the good this medicine will do as well as the risks of using it.

Mercaptopurine may also be used for other conditions as determined by your doctor.

Mercaptopurine is available only with your doctor's prescription, in the following dosage form:

*Oral*

• Tablets (U.S. and Canada)

## Before Using This Medicine

In deciding to use a medicine, the risks of taking the medicine must be weighed against the good it will do. This is a decision you and your doctor will make. For mercaptopurine, the following should be considered:

**Allergies**—Tell your doctor if you have ever had any unusual or allergic reaction to mercaptopurine.

**Pregnancy**—Tell your doctor if you are pregnant or if you intend to have children. There is a chance that this medicine may cause birth defects if either the male or female is taking it at the time of conception or if it is taken during pregnancy. However, studies have not been done in humans. Mercaptopurine has been shown to cause damage to the fetus in rats and increases the risk of miscarriage or premature births in humans. In addition, many cancer medicines may cause sterility which could be permanent. Although this has not been reported with this medicine, the possibility should be kept in mind.

Be sure that you have discussed this with your doctor before taking this medicine. It is best to use some kind of birth control while you are taking mercaptopurine. Tell your doctor right away if you think you have become pregnant while taking mercaptopurine.

**Breast-feeding**—Tell your doctor if you are breast-feeding or if you intend to breast-feed during treatment with this medicine. Because mercaptopurine may cause serious side effects, breast-feeding is generally not recommended while you are taking it.

**Children**—Although there is no specific information about the use of mercaptopurine in children, it is not expected to cause different side effects or problems in children than it does in adults.

**Older adults**—Many medicines have not been tested in older people. Therefore, it may not be known whether they work exactly the same way they do in younger adults or if they cause different side effects or problems in older people. There is no specific information about the use of mercaptopurine in the elderly.

**Other medicines**—Although certain medicines should not be used together at all, in other cases two different medicines may be used together even if an interaction might occur. In these cases, your doctor may want to change the dose, or other precautions may be necessary. When you are taking mercaptopurine, it is especially important that your health care professional know if you are taking any of the following:

- Acetaminophen (e.g., Tylenol) (with long-term, high-dose use) or
- Amiodarone (e.g., Cordarone) or
- Anabolic steroids (dromostanolone [e.g., Drolban], ethylestrenol [e.g., Maxibolin], nandrolone [e.g., Anabolin], oxandrolone [e.g., Anavar], oxymetholone [e.g., Anadrol], stanozolol [e.g., Winstrol]) or
- Androgens (male hormones) or
- Anti-infectives by mouth or by injection (medicine for infection) or
- Carbamazepine (e.g., Tegretol) or
- Chloroquine (e.g., Aralen) or
- Dantrolene (e.g., Dantrium) or
- Disulfiram (e.g., Antabuse) or
- Divalproex (e.g., Depakote) or
- Estrogens (female hormones) or
- Etretinate (e.g., Tegison) or
- Gold salts or
- Hydroxychloroquine (e.g., Plaquenil) or
- Methyldopa (e.g., Aldomet) or
- Naltrexone (e.g., Trexan) (with long-term, high-dose use) or
- Oral contraceptives (birth control pills) containing estrogen or
- Phenothiazines (acetophenazine [e.g., Tindal], chlorpromazine [e.g., Thorazine], fluphenazine [e.g., Prolixin], mesoridazine [e.g., Serentil], perphenazine [e.g., Trilafon], prochlorperazine [e.g., Compazine], promazine [e.g., Sparine], promethazine [e.g., Phenergan], thioridazine

[e.g., Mellaril], trifluoperazine [e.g., Stelazine], triflupromazine [e.g., Vesprin], trimeprazine [e.g., Temaril]) or
- Phenytoin (e.g., Dilantin) or
- Valproic acid (e.g., Depakene)—Risk of unwanted effects on the liver may be increased
- Adrenocorticoids (cortisone-like medicine) or
- Cyclosporine (e.g., Sandimmune) or
- Muromonab-CD3 (monoclonal antibody) (e.g., Orthoclone OKT3)—There may be an increased risk of infection and development of cancer because mercaptopurine reduces the body's immunity
- Allopurinol (e.g., Zyloprim)—Effects of mercaptopurine may be increased because allopurinol blocks its removal from the body
- Amphotericin B by injection (e.g., Fungizone) or
- Antithyroid agents (medicine for overactive thyroid) or
- Azathioprine (e.g., Imuran) or
- Chloramphenicol (e.g., Chloromycetin) or
- Colchicine or
- Flucytosine (e.g., Ancobon) or
- Interferon (e.g., Intron A, Roferon-A) or
- Plicamycin (e.g., Mithracin) or
- Zidovudine (e.g., Retrovir) or
- If you have ever been treated with x-rays or cancer medicines—Mercaptopurine may increase the effects of these medicines or radiation therapy on the blood
- Probenecid (e.g., Benemid) or
- Sulfinpyrazone (e.g., Anturane)—Mercaptopurine may raise the concentration of uric acid in the blood, which these medicines are used to lower

**Other medical problems**—The presence of other medical problems may affect the use of mercaptopurine. Make sure you tell your doctor if you have any other medical problems, especially:

- Chickenpox (including recent exposure) or
- Herpes zoster (shingles)—Risk of severe disease affecting other parts of the body
- Gout (history of) or
- Kidney stones (history of)—Mercaptopurine may increase levels of a chemical called uric acid in the body, which can cause gout or kidney stones
- Infection—Mercaptopurine can reduce immunity to infection
- Kidney disease or
- Liver disease—Effects may be increased because of slower removal of mercaptopurine from the body

## Proper Use of This Medicine

*Use this medicine only as directed by your doctor.* Do not use more or less of it, and do not use it more often than your doctor ordered. The exact amount of medicine you need has been carefully worked out. Taking too much may increase the chance of side effects, while taking too little may not improve your condition.

Mercaptopurine is often given together with certain other medicines. If you are using a combination of medicines, make sure that you take each one at the right time and do not mix them. Ask your health care professional to help you plan a way to remember to take your medicines at the right times.

While you are using mercaptopurine, your doctor may want you to drink extra fluids so that you will pass more urine. This will help prevent kidney problems and keep your kidneys working well.

If you vomit shortly after taking a dose of mercaptopurine, check with your doctor. You will be told whether to take the dose again or to wait until the next scheduled dose.

**Dosing**—The dose of mercaptopurine will be different for different patients. The dose that is used may depend on a number of things, including what the medicine is being used for, the patient's weight, and whether or not other medicines are also being taken. *If you are taking mercaptopurine at home, follow your doctor's orders or the directions on the label.* If you have any questions about the proper dose of mercaptopurine, ask your doctor.

**Missed dose**—If you miss a dose of this medicine, do not take the missed dose at all and do not double the next one. Instead, go back to your regular dosing schedule and check with your doctor.

**Storage**—To store this medicine:
- Keep out of the reach of children.
- Store away from heat and direct light.
- Do not store in the bathroom, near the kitchen sink, or in other damp places. Heat or moisture may cause the medicine to break down.
- Do not keep outdated medicine or medicine no longer needed. Be sure that any discarded medicine is out of the reach of children.

---

## Precautions While Using This Medicine

*It is very important that your doctor check your progress at regular visits* to make sure that this medicine is working properly and to check for unwanted effects.

*Avoid alcoholic beverages until you have discussed their use with your doctor.* Alcohol may increase the harmful effects of this medicine.

While you are being treated with mercaptopurine, and after you stop treatment with it, *do not have any immunizations (vaccinations) without your doctor's approval.* Mercaptopurine may lower your body's resistance and there is a chance you might get the infection the immunization is meant to prevent. In addition, other persons living in your household should not take or should not have recently taken oral polio vaccine since there is a chance they could pass the polio virus on to you. Also, avoid other persons who have taken oral polio vaccine. Do not get close to them and do not stay in the same room with them for very long. If you cannot take these precautions, you should consider wearing a protective face mask that covers the nose and mouth.

Mercaptopurine can lower the number of white blood cells in your blood temporarily, increasing the chance of getting an infection. It can also lower the number of platelets, which are necessary for proper blood clotting. If this occurs, there are certain precautions you can take, especially when your blood count is low, to reduce the risk of infection or bleeding:

- If you can, avoid people with infections. *Check with your doctor immediately* if you think you are getting an infection or if you get a fever or chills, cough or hoarseness, lower back or side pain, or painful or difficult urination.
- *Check with your doctor immediately* if you notice any unusual bleeding or bruising; black, tarry stools; blood in urine or stools; or pinpoint red spots on your skin.
- Be careful when using a regular toothbrush, dental floss, or toothpick. Your medical doctor, dentist, or nurse may recommend other ways to clean your teeth and gums. Check with your medical doctor before having any dental work done.
- Do not touch your eyes or the inside of your nose unless you have just washed your hands and have not touched anything else in the meantime.
- Be careful not to cut yourself when you are using sharp objects such as a safety razor or fingernail or toenail cutters.
- Avoid contact sports or other situations where bruising or injury could occur.

Tell the doctor in charge that you are taking this medicine before you have any medical tests. The results of tests for the amount of sugar or uric acid in the blood measured by a machine called a sequential multiple analyzer (SMA) may be affected by this medicine.

---

## Side Effects of This Medicine

Along with their needed effects, medicines like mercaptopurine can sometimes cause unwanted effects such as blood problems, liver problems, and other side effects. These and others are described below. Also, because of the way these medicines act on the body, there is a chance that they might cause other unwanted effects that may not occur until months or years after the medicine is used. These delayed effects may include certain types of cancer, such as leukemia. Discuss these possible effects with your doctor.

Although not all of these side effects may occur, if they do occur they may need medical attention.

*Check with your doctor immediately* if any of the following side effects occur:

*Less common*
> Black, tarry stools; blood in urine or stools; cough or hoarseness; fever or chills; lower back or side pain; painful or difficult urination; pinpoint red spots on skin; unusual bleeding or bruising

Check with your doctor as soon as possible if any of the following side effects occur:

*More common*
> Unusual tiredness or weakness; yellow eyes or skin

*Less common*
> Joint pain; loss of appetite; nausea and vomiting; swelling of feet or lower legs

*Rare*

Sores in mouth and on lips

Other side effects may occur that usually do not need medical attention. These side effects may go away during treatment as your body adjusts to the medicine. Also, your health care professional may be able to tell you about ways to prevent or reduce some of these side effects. Check with your health care professional if any of the following side effects continue or are bothersome or if you have any questions about them:

*Less common*

Darkening of skin; diarrhea; headache; skin rash and itching; weakness

After you stop taking mercaptopurine, it may still produce some side effects that need attention. During this period of time, check with your doctor if you notice any of the following side effects:

Black, tarry stools; blood in urine or stools; cough or hoarseness; fever or chills; lower back or side pain; painful or difficult urination; pinpoint red spots on skin; unusual bleeding or bruising; yellow eyes or skin

Other side effects not listed above may also occur in some patients. If you notice any other effects, check with your doctor.

Revised: August 1990
Interim revision: 07/29/93; 06/21/94

---

# MESALAMINE  Rectal

Some commonly used brand names are:

**In the U.S.—**
Rowasa

**In Canada—**
Salofalk

Other commonly used names are 5-aminosalicylic acid, 5-ASA, and mesalazine.

## Description

Mesalamine (me-SAL-a-meen) is used to treat inflammatory bowel disease, such as ulcerative colitis. This medicine works inside the bowel by helping to reduce the inflammation and other symptoms.

Mesalamine is available only with your doctor's prescription. It is available in the following dosage forms:

*Rectal*
- Enema (U.S. and Canada)
- Suppositories (U.S. and Canada)

## Before Using This Medicine

In deciding to use a medicine, the risks of using the medicine must be weighed against the good it will do. This is a decision you and your doctor will make. For mesalamine, the following should be considered:

**Allergies**—Tell your doctor if you have ever had any unusual or allergic reaction to mesalamine, olsalazine, sulfasalazine, or salicylates (e.g., aspirin). Also tell your health care professional if you are allergic to any other substances, such as foods, preservatives, or dyes.

**Pregnancy**—Studies have not been done in humans. However, mesalamine has not been shown to cause birth defects or other problems in animal studies.

**Breast-feeding**—It is not known whether mesalamine passes into the breast milk.

**Children**—Studies on this medicine have been done only in adult patients, and there is no specific information comparing use of mesalamine in children with use in other age groups.

**Older adults**—Many medicines have not been studied specifically in older people. Therefore, it may not be known whether they work exactly the same way they do in younger adults or if they cause different side effects or problems in older people. There is no specific information comparing use of mesalamine in the elderly with use in other age groups.

**Other medicines**—Although certain medicines should not be used together at all, in other cases two different medicines may be used together even if an interaction might occur. In these cases, your doctor may want to change the dose, or other precautions may be necessary. Tell your health care professional if you are taking any other medicines.

**Other medical problems**—The presence of other medical problems may affect the use of mesalamine. Make sure you tell your doctor if you have any other medical problems, especially:
- Kidney disease—The use of mesalamine may cause further damage to the kidneys

## Proper Use of This Medicine

This medicine usually comes with patient directions. Read them carefully before using this medicine.

For best results, empty your bowel just before using this rectal enema.

*Keep using this medicine for the full time of treatment* even if you begin to feel better after a few days. *Do not miss any doses.*

**Dosing**—The dose of mesalamine may be different for different patients. *Follow your doctor's orders or the*

*directions on the label.* The following information includes only the average doses of mesalamine. *If your dose is different, do not change it* unless your doctor tells you to do so.

- For *enema* dosage form:
  - —For inflammatory bowel disease:
    - Adults—4 grams (1 unit), used as directed, every night. May have to be used for up to several weeks.
    - Children—Use and dose must be determined by your doctor.
- For *suppository* dosage form:
  - —For inflammatory bowel disease:
    - Adults—500 mg, inserted into your rectum, two or three times a day.
    - Children—Use and dose must be determined by your doctor.

**Missed dose**—If you miss a dose of this medicine, use it as soon as possible if you remember it that same night. However, if you do not remember it until the next morning, skip the missed dose and go back to your regular dosing schedule.

**Storage**—To store this medicine:
- Keep out of the reach of children.
- Store away from heat and direct light.
- Keep the enema from freezing.
- Keep the suppositories at room temperature.
- Do not keep outdated medicine or medicine no longer needed. Be sure that any discarded medicine is out of the reach of children.

---

## Precautions While Using This Medicine

It is important that your doctor check your progress at regular visits.

Check with your doctor if you notice rectal bleeding, blistering, pain, burning, itching, or other sign of irritation not present before you started using this medicine.

---

## Side Effects of This Medicine

Along with its needed effects, a medicine may cause some unwanted effects. Although not all of these side effects may occur, if they do occur they may need medical attention.

*Stop using this medicine and check with your doctor immediately* if any of the following side effects occur:

*Rare*

Abdominal or stomach cramps or pain (severe); bloody diarrhea; fever; headache (severe); skin rash

Also, check with your doctor as soon as possible if the following side effect occurs:

*Rare*

Rectal irritation

Other side effects may occur that usually do not need medical attention. These side effects may go away during treatment as your body adjusts to the medicine. However, check with your doctor if the following side effects continue or are bothersome:

*More common*

Abdominal or stomach cramps or pain (mild); gas or flatulence; headache (mild); nausea

*Less common or rare*

Loss of hair

Other side effects not listed above may also occur in some patients. If you notice any other effects, check with your doctor.

---

Revised: 06/28/91
Interim revision: 07/05/94

---

# MESNA    Systemic

Some commonly used brand names are:

**In the U.S.—**
MESNEX

**In Canada—**
Uromitexan

## Description

Mesna is used to reduce the harmful effects of some cancer medicines on the bladder.

Mesna is to be given only by or under the immediate supervision of your doctor. It is available in the following dosage form:

*Parenteral*
- Injection (U.S. and Canada)

## Before Using This Medicine

In deciding to use a medicine, the risks of taking the medicine must be weighed against the good it will do. This is a decision you and your doctor will make. For mesna, the following should be considered:

**Allergies**—Tell your doctor if you have ever had any unusual or allergic reaction to mesna.

**Pregnancy**—Mesna has not been shown to cause birth defects or other problems in humans.

**Breast-feeding**—It is not known whether mesna passes into the breast milk. However, this medicine has not been reported to cause problems in nursing babies.

**Children**—Although there is no specific information comparing use of mesna in children with use in other age groups, this medicine is not expected to cause different side effects or problems in children than it does in adults.

**Older adults**—Many medicines have not been studied specifically in older people. Therefore, it may not be known whether they work exactly the same way they do in younger adults or if they cause different side effects or problems in older people. There is no specific information comparing use of mesna in the elderly with use in other age groups.

---

## Proper Use of This Medicine

**Dosing**—The dose of mesna will be different for different patients and must be determined by your doctor. Mesna is usually given by a doctor or nurse in the hospital. If you have any questions about the proper dose of mesna, ask your doctor.

---

## Side Effects of This Medicine

Along with its needed effects, a medicine may cause some unwanted effects. Although not all of these side effects may occur, if they do occur they may need medical attention.

Check with your doctor as soon as possible if either of the following side effects occur:
*Rare*
　Skin rash or itching

Other side effects may occur that usually do not need medical attention. These side effects may go away during treatment as your body adjusts to the medicine. However, check with your doctor if any of the following side effects continue or are bothersome:
*Less common*
　Diarrhea; nausea or vomiting; unpleasant taste

Other side effects not listed above may also occur in some patients. If you notice any other effects, check with your doctor.

---

Annual revision: 08/09/92
Interim revision: 07/06/94

---

# METHACHOLINE　Inhalation†

A commonly used brand name in the U.S. is Provocholine.

---

†Not commercially available in Canada.

---

## Description

Methacholine (METH-a-koe-leen) is used to help find out whether a patient has asthma.

Before the test with methacholine inhalation is given, another test will be done to find out how well your lungs are working.

How test is done: Although there are 5 different strengths of methacholine solution that may be used in this test, not all of them may be necessary. It depends on how you react to each increasing strength of solution during the test. The weakest strength solution is used first. It is placed in a nebulizer and 5 inhalations are taken by mouth. After 3 to 5 minutes, a test will be done to determine what effect the medicine had on your lungs. Each time the test dose is repeated, a stronger solution will be used. During this test, wheezing and difficulty in breathing may occur. If these effects do occur, your doctor may give you a bronchodilator (medicine that opens up the bronchial tubes [air passages] of the lungs) by inhalation to relieve the discomfort.

Methacholine is to be used only by or under the immediate supervision of a doctor. It is available in the following dosage form:
*Inhalation*
• Inhalation solution (U.S.)

## Before Having This Test

In deciding to use a diagnostic test, any risks of the test must be weighed against the good it will do. This is a decision you and your doctor will make. Also, test results may be affected by other things. For methacholine, the following should be considered:

**Allergies**—Tell your doctor if you have ever had any unusual or allergic reaction to methacholine or to similar medicines, such as ambenonium, bethanechol, neostigmine, and pyridostigmine. Also tell your health care professional if you are allergic to any other substances, such as foods, preservatives, or dyes.

**Pregnancy**—Studies on birth defects have not been done in either humans or animals. However, if the test is necessary, women who are able to bear children should be given the test within 10 days after the beginning of the last menstrual period or within 2 weeks after a pregnancy test has shown they are not pregnant.

**Breast-feeding**—It is not known whether methacholine passes into the breast milk. Although most medicines pass into breast milk in small amounts, many of them may be used safely while breast-feeding. Mothers who are receiving the methacholine test and who wish to breast-feed should discuss this with their doctor.

**Children**—Although there is no specific information comparing use of methacholine in children less than 5 years old with use in other age groups, this medicine is not expected to cause different side effects or problems in these children than it does in adults.

**Older adults**—Many medicines have not been studied specifically in older people. Therefore, it may not be known whether they work exactly the same way they do in younger adults or if they cause different side effects or problems in older people. There is no specific information comparing use of methacholine in the elderly with use in other age groups.

**Other medicines**—Although certain medicines should not be used together at all, in other cases two different medicines may be used together even if an interaction might occur. In these cases, your doctor may want to change the dose, or other precautions may be necessary. When you are receiving the methacholine test, it is especially important that your health care professional know if you are taking or using any of the following:

- Anticholinergics (medicine for abdominal or stomach spasms or cramps) or
- Corticosteroids (cortisone-like medicines) or
- Cromolyn (e.g., Intal) or
- Medicine for breathing problems, colds, sinus problems, or hay fever or other allergies (including nose drops or sprays) or
- Smoking tobacco—These medicines or smoking tobacco may affect the results of this test
- Beta-blockers (acebutolol [e.g., Sectral], atenolol [e.g., Tenormin], betaxolol [e.g., Kerlone], bisoprolol [e.g., Zebeta], carteolol [e.g., Cartrol], labetalol [e.g., Normodyne], metoprolol [e.g., Lopressor], nadolol [e.g., Corgard], oxprenolol [e.g., Trasicor], penbutolol [e.g., Levatol], pindolol [e.g., Visken], propranolol [e.g., Inderal], sotalol [e.g., Sotacor], timolol [e.g., Blocadren])— These medicines may increase the reaction to the methacholine test

**Other medical problems**—The presence of other medical problems may affect the use of methacholine . Make sure you tell your doctor if you have any other medical problems, especially:

- Asthma (or if any member of your family has asthma), hay fever, allergic rhinitis, wheezing, chronic lung disease, or respiratory virus illness—Methacholine may cause severe difficulty in breathing
- Epilepsy or
- Heart or blood vessel disease or

- Stomach ulcer or
- Thyroid disease or
- Urinary tract blockage—Use of methacholine may make the condition worse

## Preparation for This Test

Unless otherwise directed by your doctor:

- *For 24 hours before the test, do not take any extended-release capsule or tablet form of aminophylline, oxtriphylline, or theophylline. For 12 hours before the test, do not use any other medicine,* especially anticholinergics (medicine for abdominal or stomach spasms or cramps) or medicine for breathing problems, sinus problems, or hay fever or other allergies (including nose drops or sprays). To do so may affect the results of this test.

## Side Effects of This Medicine

Along with its needed effects, a medicine may cause some unwanted effects. Although not all of these side effects may occur, if they do occur they may need medical attention.

*Check with your health care professional immediately* if any of the following side effects occur:

Wheezing, tightness in chest, or difficulty in breathing (continuing or severe)

Other side effects may occur that usually do not need medical attention. These side effects should go away as the effects of the medicine wear off. However, check with your doctor if any of the following side effects continue or are bothersome:

*Less common or rare*

Headache or lightheadedness; irritation of throat; itching

Other side effects not listed above may also occur in some patients. If you notice any other effects, check with your doctor.

Revised: 08/09/94

---

# METHENAMINE   Systemic

Some commonly used brand names are:

**In the U.S.—**

| | |
|---|---|
| Hiprex | Urex |
| Mandelamine | |

Generic name product may also be available.

**In Canada**

| | |
|---|---|
| Hip-Rex | Mandelamine |

## Description

Methenamine (meth-EN-a-meen) belongs to the family of medicines called anti-infectives. It is used to help prevent and treat infections of the urinary tract. Methenamine is available only with your doctor's prescription, in the following dosage forms:

*Oral*

- Enteric-coated tablets (U.S.)
- Granules for oral solution (U.S.)

---

- Oral suspension (U.S.)
- Tablets (U.S. and Canada)

## Before Using This Medicine

In deciding to use a medicine, the risks of taking the medicine must be weighed against the good it will do. This is a decision you and your doctor will make. For methenamine, the following should be considered:

**Allergies**—Tell your doctor if you have ever had any unusual or allergic reaction to methenamine. Also tell your health care professional if you are allergic to any other substances, such as foods, preservatives, or dyes.

**Pregnancy**—Methenamine has not been studied in either humans or animals. However, individual case reports on the use of methenamine during pregnancy have not shown that this medicine causes birth defects or other problems in humans.

**Breast-feeding**—Methenamine passes into the breast milk. However, methenamine has not been reported to cause problems in nursing babies.

**Children**—Although there is no special information comparing use of methenamine in children with use in other age groups, this medicine is not expected to cause different side effects or problems in children than it does in adults.

**Older adults**—Many medicines have not been studied specifically in older people. Therefore, it may not be known whether they work exactly the same way they do in younger adults or if they cause different side effects or problems in older people. There is no specific information comparing use of methenamine in the elderly with use in other age groups.

**Other medicines**—Although certain medicines should not be used together at all, in other cases two different medicines may be used together even if an interaction might occur. In these cases, your doctor may want to change the dose, or other precautions may be necessary. When you are taking methenamine, it is especially important that your health care professional knows if you are taking any of the following:

- Thiazide diuretics (water pills) or
- Urinary alkalizers (medicine that makes the urine less acid, such as acetazolamide [e.g., Diamox], calcium- and/or magnesium-containing antacids, dichlorphenamide [e.g., Daranide], methazolamide [e.g., Neptazane], potassium or sodium citrate and/or citric acid, sodium bicarbonate [baking soda])—Use of methenamine with any of these medicines may decrease the effectiveness of methenamine

**Other medical problems**—The presence of other medical problems may affect the use of methenamine. Make sure you tell your doctor if you have any other medical problems, especially:

- Dehydration (severe) or
- Kidney disease (severe)—Patients with severe kidney disease who take methenamine may have an increase in side effects that affect the kidneys

- Liver disease (severe)—Patients with severe liver disease who take methenamine may have an increase in symptoms of their liver disease

## Proper Use of This Medicine

Before you start taking this medicine, check your urine with phenaphthazine paper or another test to see if it is acid. *Your urine must be acidic (pH 5.5 or below) for this medicine to work properly.* If you have any questions about this, check with your health care professional.

The following changes in your diet may help make your urine more acid; however, check with your doctor first if you are on a special diet (for example, for diabetes). Avoid most fruits (especially citrus fruits and juices), milk and other dairy products, and other foods that make the urine less acid. Also, avoid antacids unless otherwise directed by your doctor. Eating more protein and foods such as cranberries (especially cranberry juice with vitamin C added), plums, or prunes may also help. If your urine is still not acid enough, check with your doctor.

If this medicine causes nausea or upset stomach, it may be taken after meals and at bedtime.

For patients taking the *dry granule form of this medicine:*

- Dissolve the contents of each packet in 2 to 4 ounces of cold water immediately before taking. Stir well. Be sure to drink all the liquid to get the full dose of medicine.

For patients taking the *oral liquid form of this medicine:*

- Use a specially marked measuring spoon or other device to measure each dose accurately. The average household teaspoon may not hold the right amount of liquid.

For patients taking the *enteric-coated tablet form of this medicine:*

- Swallow tablets whole. Do not break, crush, or take if chipped.

To help clear up your infection completely, *keep taking this medicine for the full time of treatment,* even if you begin to feel better after a few days. *Do not miss any doses.*

**Dosing**—The dose of methenamine will be different for different patients. *Follow your doctor's orders or the directions on the label.* The following information includes only the average doses of methenamine. *If your dose is different, do not change it* unless your doctor tells you to do so.

The number of tablets or teaspoonfuls of solution or suspension that you take depends on the strength of the medicine.

- For the treatment of urinary tract infections:
  —For *oral* dosage form (methenamine hippurate tablets):
    - Adults and children 12 years of age and over— 1 gram two times a day. Take in the morning and the evening.

- Children up to 6 years of age—Use and dose must be determined by your doctor.
- Children 6 to 12 years of age—500 milligrams (mg) to 1 gram two times a day. Take in the morning and the evening.

—For *oral* dosage form (methenamine mandelate enteric-coated tablets, regular tablets, solution, and suspension):

- Adults and children 12 years of age and over—1 gram four times a day. Take after meals and at bedtime.
- Children up to 6 years of age—Dose is based on body weight. The usual dose is 18.3 mg per kilogram (kg) (8.3 mg per pound) of body weight four times a day. Take after meals and at bedtime.
- Children 6 to 12 years of age—500 mg four times a day. Take after meals and at bedtime.

**Missed dose**—If you miss a dose of this medicine, take it as soon as possible. However, if it is almost time for your next dose, skip the missed dose and go back to your regular dosing schedule. Do not double doses.

**Storage**—To store this medicine:
- Keep out of the reach of children.
- Store away from heat and direct light.
- Do not store the dry granule or tablet form of this medicine in the bathroom, near the kitchen sink, or in other damp places. Heat or moisture may cause the medicine to break down.
- Keep the oral liquid form of this medicine from freezing.
- Do not keep outdated medicine or medicine no longer needed. Be sure that any discarded medicine is out of the reach of children.

## Precautions While Using This Medicine

If your symptoms do not improve within a few days, or if they become worse, check with your doctor.

## Side Effects of This Medicine

Along with its needed effects, a medicine may cause some unwanted effects. Although not all of these side effects may occur, if they do occur they may need medical attention.

*Check with your doctor immediately* if any of the following side effects occur:

*Less common*
  Skin rash
*Rare*
  Blood in urine; lower back pain; pain or burning while urinating

Other side effects may occur that usually do not need medical attention. These side effects may go away during treatment as your body adjusts to the medicine. However, check with your doctor if any of the following side effects continue or are bothersome:

*Less common*
  Nausea and vomiting

Other side effects not listed above may also occur in some patients. If you notice any other effects, check with your doctor.

Revised: 10/20/92
Interim revision: 03/17/94

# METHOTREXATE—For Cancer  Systemic

Some commonly used brand names are:
**In the U.S.—**
Folex                    Mexate
Folex PFS               Mexate-AQ
Generic name product may also be available in the U.S. and Canada.
Another commonly used name is amethopterin.

## Description

Methotrexate (meth-o-TREX-ate) belongs to the group of medicines known as antimetabolites. It is used to treat some kinds of cancer.

Methotrexate blocks an enzyme needed by the cell to live. This interferes with the growth of cancer cells, which are eventually destroyed. Since the growth of normal body cells may also be affected by methotrexate, other effects will also occur. Some of these may be serious and must be reported to your doctor. Other effects, like hair loss, may not be serious but may cause concern. Some effects may not occur for months or years after the medicine is used.

Before you begin treatment with methotrexate, you and your doctor should talk about the good this medicine will do as well as the risks of using it.

Methotrexate is available only with your doctor's prescription, in the following dosage forms:
*Oral*
- Tablets (U.S. and Canada)
*Parenteral*
- Injection (U.S. and Canada)

## Before Using This Medicine

In deciding to use a medicine, the risks of taking the medicine must be weighed against the good it will do.

This is a decision you and your doctor will make. For methotrexate, the following should be considered:

**Allergies**—Tell your doctor if you have ever had any unusual or allergic reaction to methotrexate.

**Pregnancy**—Tell your doctor if you are pregnant or if you intend to have children. There is a good chance that this medicine may cause birth defects if either the male or female is taking it at the time of conception or if it is taken during pregnancy. Methotrexate may cause harm or even death of the fetus. In addition, many cancer medicines may cause sterility which could be permanent. Although sterility is probably rare with this medicine, the possibility should be kept in mind.

Be sure that you have discussed this with your doctor before taking this medicine. It is best to use some kind of birth control while you are taking methotrexate. Tell your doctor right away if you think you have become pregnant while taking methotrexate.

**Breast-feeding**—Tell your doctor if you are breast-feeding or if you intend to breast-feed during treatment with this medicine. Because methotrexate may cause serious side effects, breast-feeding is generally not recommended while you are taking it.

**Children**—Newborns and other infants may be more sensitive to the effects of methotrexate. However, in other children it is not expected to cause different side effects or problems than it does in adults.

**Older adults**—Side effects may be more likely to occur in the elderly, who are usually more sensitive to the effects of methotrexate.

**Other medicines**—Although certain medicines should not be used together at all, in other cases two different medicines may be used together even if an interaction might occur. In these cases, your doctor may want to change the dose, or other precautions may be necessary. When you are taking methotrexate, it is especially important that your health care professional know if you are taking any other prescription or nonprescription (over-the-counter [OTC]) medicine. They should also be told if you have ever been treated with x-rays or cancer medicines or if you drink alcohol.

**Other medical problems**—The presence of other medical problems may affect the use of methotrexate. Make sure you tell your doctor if you have any other medical problems, especially:

- Alcohol abuse (or history of)—Increased risk of unwanted effects on the liver
- Chickenpox (including recent exposure) or
- Herpes zoster (shingles)—Risk of severe disease affecting other parts of the body
- Colitis
- Disease of the immune system
- Gout (history of) or
- Kidney stones (or history of)—Methotrexate may increase levels of a chemical called uric acid in the body, which can cause gout or kidney stones
- Infection—Methotrexate can reduce immunity to infection

- Intestine blockage or
- Kidney disease or
- Liver disease—Effects may be increased because of slower removal of methotrexate from the body
- Mouth sores or inflammation or
- Stomach ulcer—May be worsened

## Proper Use of This Medicine

*Take this medicine only as directed by your doctor.* Do not take more or less of it, and do not take it more often than your doctor ordered. The exact amount of medicine you need has been carefully worked out. Taking too much may increase the chance of side effects, while taking too little may not improve your condition.

Methotrexate is often given together with certain other medicines. If you are using a combination of medicines, make sure that you take each one at the proper time and do not mix them. Ask your health care professional to help you plan a way to remember to take your medicines at the right times.

While you are using methotrexate, your doctor may want you to drink extra fluids so that you will pass more urine. This will help the drug to pass from the body, and will prevent kidney problems and keep your kidneys working well.

Methotrexate commonly causes nausea and vomiting. Even if you begin to feel ill, *do not stop using this medicine without first checking with your doctor.* Ask your health care professional for ways to lessen these effects.

If you vomit shortly after taking a dose of methotrexate, check with your doctor. You will be told whether to take the dose again or to wait until the next scheduled dose.

**Dosing**—The dose of methotrexate will be different for different patients. The dose that is used may depend on a number of things, including what the medicine is being used for, the patient's size, whether the medicine is being given by mouth or by injection, and whether or not other medicines are also being taken. *If you are taking or receiving methotrexate at home, follow your doctor's orders or the directions on the label.* If you have any questions about the proper dose of methotrexate, ask your doctor.

**Missed dose**—If you miss a dose of this medicine, do not take the missed dose at all and do not double the next one. Instead, go back to your regular dosing schedule and check with your doctor.

**Storage**—To store this medicine:

- Keep out of the reach of children.
- Store away from heat and direct light.
- Do not store in the bathroom, near the kitchen sink, or in other damp places. Heat or moisture may cause the medicine to break down.
- Do not keep outdated medicine or medicine no longer needed. Be sure that any discarded medicine is out of the reach of children.

## Precautions While Using This Medicine

*It is very important that your doctor check your progress at regular visits* to make sure that this medicine is working properly and to check for unwanted effects.

*Do not drink alcohol while using this medicine.* Alcohol can increase the chance of liver problems.

Some patients who take methotrexate may become more sensitive to sunlight than they are normally. When you first begin taking methotrexate, avoid too much sun and do not use a sunlamp until you see how you react to the sun, especially if you tend to burn easily. In case of a severe burn, check with your doctor.

*Do not take medicine for inflammation or pain (aspirin or other salicylates, diclofenac, diflunisal, fenoprofen, ibuprofen, indomethacin, ketoprofen, meclofenamate, mefenamic acid, naproxen, phenylbutazone, piroxicam, sulindac, suprofen, tolmetin) without first checking with your doctor.* These medicines may increase the effects of methotrexate, which could be harmful.

While you are being treated with methotrexate, and after you stop treatment with it, *do not have any immunizations (vaccinations) without your doctor's approval.* Methotrexate may lower your body's resistance and there is a chance you might get the infection the immunization is meant to prevent. In addition, other persons living in your household should not take or should not have recently taken oral polio vaccine since there is a chance they could pass the polio virus on to you. Also, avoid other persons who have taken oral polio vaccine. Do not get close to them, and do not stay in the same room with them for very long. If you cannot take these precautions, you should consider wearing a protective face mask that covers the nose and mouth.

Methotrexate can lower the number of white blood cells in your blood temporarily, increasing the chance of getting an infection. It can also lower the number of platelets, which are necessary for proper blood clotting. If this occurs, there are certain precautions you can take, especially when your blood count is low, to reduce the risk of infection or bleeding:

- If you can, avoid people with infections. *Check with your doctor immediately* if you think you are getting an infection or if you get a fever or chills, cough or hoarseness, lower back or side pain, or painful or difficult urination.
- *Check with your doctor immediately* if you notice any unusual bleeding or bruising; black, tarry stools; blood in urine or stools; or pinpoint red spots on your skin.
- Be careful when using a regular toothbrush, dental floss, or toothpick. Your medical doctor, dentist, or nurse may recommend other ways to clean your teeth and gums. Check with your medical doctor before having any dental work done.
- Do not touch your eyes or the inside of your nose unless you have just washed your hands and have not touched anything else in the meantime.
- Be careful not to cut yourself when you are using sharp objects such as a safety razor or fingernail or toenail cutters.
- Avoid contact sports or other situations where bruising or injury could occur.

## Side Effects of This Medicine

Along with their needed effects, medicines like methotrexate can sometimes cause unwanted effects such as blood problems, kidney problems, stomach or liver problems, loss of hair, and other side effects. These and others are described below. Also, because of the way these medicines act on the body, there is a chance that they might cause other unwanted effects that may not occur until months or years after the medicine is used. These delayed effects may include certain types of cancer, such as leukemia. Discuss these possible effects with your doctor.

Although not all of these side effects may occur, if they do occur they may need medical attention.

*Check with your doctor immediately* if any of the following side effects occur:
  *More common*
    Black, tarry stools; bloody vomit; diarrhea; reddening of skin; sores in mouth and on lips; stomach pain
  *Less common*
    Blood in urine or stools; blurred vision; confusion; convulsions (seizures); cough or hoarseness; fever or chills; lower back or side pain; painful or difficult urination; pinpoint red spots on skin; shortness of breath; swelling of feet or lower legs; unusual bleeding or bruising

Check with your doctor as soon as possible if any of the following side effects occur:
  *Less common*
    Back pain; dark urine; dizziness; drowsiness; headache; joint pain; unusual tiredness or weakness; yellow eyes or skin

Other side effects may occur that usually do not need medical attention. These side effects may go away during treatment as your body adjusts to the medicine. Also, your health care professional may be able to tell you about ways to prevent or reduce some of these side effects. Check with your health care professional if any of the following side effects continue or are bothersome or if you have any questions about them:
  *More common*
    Loss of appetite; nausea or vomiting
  *Less common*
    Acne; boils; pale skin; skin rash or itching

This medicine may cause a temporary loss of hair in some people. After treatment with methotrexate has ended, normal hair growth should return.

After you stop using methotrexate, it may still produce some side effects that need attention. During this period of time, check with your doctor as soon as possible if you notice any of the following side effects:

Back pain; blurred vision; confusion; convulsions (seizures); dizziness; drowsiness; fever; headache; unusual tiredness or weakness

Other side effects not listed above may also occur in some patients. If you notice any other effects, check with your doctor.

Revised: 8/90
Interim revision: 06/21/94

# METHOTREXATE—For Noncancerous Conditions   Systemic

Some commonly used brand names are:

**In the U.S.—**
Folex
Folex PFS
Mexate

Mexate-AQ
Rheumatrex

**In Canada—**
Rheumatrex
Generic name product may also be available in the U.S. and Canada.
Another commonly used name is amethopterin.

## Description

Methotrexate (meth-o-TREX-ate) belongs to the group of medicines known as antimetabolites. It is used to treat psoriasis and rheumatoid arthritis. It may also be used for other conditions as determined by your doctor.

Methotrexate blocks an enzyme needed by the cell to live. This interferes with the growth of certain cells, such as skin cells in psoriasis that are growing rapidly. Since the growth of normal body cells may also be affected by methotrexate, other effects will also occur. Some of these may be serious and must be reported to your doctor. Other effects, like hair loss, may not be serious but may cause concern. Some effects may not occur for months or years after the medicine is used.

Before you begin treatment with methotrexate, you and your doctor should talk about the good this medicine will do as well as the risks of using it.

Methotrexate is available only with your doctor's prescription, in the following dosage forms:

*Oral*
• Tablets (U.S. and Canada)
*Parenteral*
• Injection (U.S. and Canada)

## Before Using This Medicine

In deciding to use a medicine, the risks of taking the medicine must be weighed against the good it will do. This is a decision you and your doctor will make. For methotrexate, the following should be considered:

**Allergies**—Tell your doctor if you have ever had any unusual or allergic reaction to methotrexate.

**Pregnancy**—There is a good chance that this medicine may cause birth defects if either the male or female is taking it at the time of conception or if it is taken during pregnancy. Methotrexate may cause harm or even death of the fetus. In addition, this medicine may rarely cause temporary sterility.

Methotrexate is not recommended during pregnancy. Be sure that you have discussed this with your doctor before taking this medicine. It is best to use some kind of birth control while you are taking methotrexate. Tell your doctor right away if you think you have become pregnant while taking methotrexate.

**Breast-feeding**—Tell your doctor if you are breast-feeding or if you intend to breast-feed during treatment with this medicine. Because methotrexate may cause serious side effects, breast-feeding is generally not recommended while you are taking it.

**Children**—Newborns and other infants may be more sensitive to the effects of methotrexate. However, in other children it is not expected to cause different side effects or problems than it does in adults.

**Older adults**—Side effects may be more likely to occur in the elderly, who are usually more sensitive to the effects of methotrexate.

**Other medicines**—Although certain medicines should not be used together at all, in other cases two different medicines may be used together even if an interaction might occur. In these cases, your doctor may want to change the dose, or other precautions may be necessary. When you are taking methotrexate, it is especially important that your health care professional know if you are taking any other prescription or nonprescription (over-the-counter [OTC]) medicine. They should also be told if you have ever been treated with x-rays or cancer medicines or if you drink alcohol.

**Other medical problems**—The presence of other medical problems may affect the use of methotrexate. Make sure you tell your doctor if you have any other medical problems, especially:
• Alcohol abuse (or history of)—Increased risk of unwanted effects on the liver
• Chickenpox (including recent exposure) or
• Herpes zoster (shingles)—Risk of severe disease affecting other parts of the body
• Colitis
• Disease of the immune system
• Infection—Methotrexate can reduce immunity to infection

- Intestine blockage or
- Kidney disease or
- Liver disease—Effects may be increased because of slower removal of methotrexate from the body
- Mouth sores or inflammation or
- Stomach ulcer—May be worsened

## Proper Use of This Medicine

*Take this medicine only as directed by your doctor.* Do not take more or less of it, and do not take it more often than your doctor ordered. The exact amount of medicine you need has been carefully worked out. Taking too much may increase the chance of side effects, while taking too little may not improve your condition.

Methotrexate may cause nausea. Even if you begin to feel ill, *do not stop using this medicine without first checking with your doctor.* Ask your health care professional for ways to lessen these effects. If you begin vomiting, check with your doctor.

If you vomit shortly after taking a dose of methotrexate, check with your doctor. You will be told whether to take the dose again or to wait until the next scheduled dose.

**Dosing**—The dose of methotrexate will be different for different patients. *Follow your doctor's orders or the directions on the label.* The following information includes only the average doses of methotrexate. *If your dose is different, do not change it* unless your doctor tells you to do so.

The number of tablets that you take or doses of injection that you use depends on the strength of the medicine. Also, *the number of doses you take each day, the time allowed between doses, and the length of time you take the medicine depend on the medical problem for which you are taking methotrexate.*

- For *oral* dosage form (tablets):
  - —For psoriasis or rheumatoid arthritis:
    - Adults—2.5 to 5 milligrams (mg) every twelve hours for three doses once a week, or 10 mg once a week. Your doctor may increase the dose as needed.
    - Children—Dose must be determined by your doctor.
- For *injection* dosage form:
  - —For psoriasis:
    - Adults—To start, 10 mg injected into a muscle or vein once a week. Your doctor may increase the dose as needed.
    - Children—Dose must be determined by your doctor.

**Missed dose**—If you miss a dose of this medicine, do not take the missed dose at all and do not double the next one. Instead, go back to your regular dosing schedule and check with your doctor.

**Storage**—To store this medicine:
- Keep out of the reach of children.
- Store away from heat and direct light.
- Do not store in the bathroom, near the kitchen sink, or in other damp places. Heat or moisture may cause the medicine to break down.
- Do not keep outdated medicine or medicine no longer needed. Be sure that any discarded medicine is out of the reach of children.

## Precautions While Using This Medicine

*It is very important that your doctor check your progress at regular visits* to make sure that this medicine is working properly and to check for unwanted effects.

*Do not drink alcohol while using this medicine.* Alcohol can increase the chance of liver problems.

Some patients who take methotrexate may become more sensitive to sunlight than they are normally. When you first begin taking methotrexate, avoid too much sun and do not use a sunlamp until you see how you react to the sun, especially if you tend to burn easily. In case of a severe burn, check with your doctor. This is especially important if you are taking this medicine for psoriasis because sunlight can make the psoriasis worse.

*Do not take medicine for inflammation or pain (aspirin or other salicylates, diclofenac, diflunisal, fenoprofen, ibuprofen, indomethacin, ketoprofen, meclofenamate, mefenamic acid, naproxen, phenylbutazone, piroxicam, sulindac, suprofen, tolmetin) without first checking with your doctor.* These medicines may increase the effects of methotrexate, which could be harmful.

While you are being treated with methotrexate, and after you stop treatment with it, *do not have any immunizations (vaccinations) without your doctor's approval.* Methotrexate may lower your body's resistance and there is a chance you might get the infection the immunization is meant to prevent. In addition, other persons living in your household should not take or should not have recently taken oral polio vaccine since there is a chance they could pass the polio virus on to you. Also, avoid other persons who have taken oral polio vaccine. Do not get close to them, and do not stay in the same room with them for very long. If you cannot take these precautions, you should consider wearing a protective face mask that covers the nose and mouth.

Methotrexate can lower the number of white blood cells in your blood temporarily, increasing the chance of getting an infection. It can also lower the number of platelets, which are necessary for proper blood clotting. If this occurs, there are certain precautions you can take, especially when your blood count is low, to reduce the risk of infection or bleeding:

- If you can, avoid people with infections. *Check with your doctor immediately* if you think you are getting an infection or if you get a fever or chills, cough or hoarseness, lower back or side pain, or painful or difficult urination.
- *Check with your doctor immediately* if you notice any unusual bleeding or bruising; black, tarry stools;

blood in urine or stools; or pinpoint red spots on your skin.

- Be careful when using a regular toothbrush, dental floss, or toothpick. Your medical doctor, dentist, or nurse may recommend other ways to clean your teeth and gums. Check with your medical doctor before having any dental work done.
- Do not touch your eyes or the inside of your nose unless you have just washed your hands and have not touched anything else in the meantime.
- Be careful not to cut yourself when you are using sharp objects such as a safety razor or fingernail or toenail cutters.
- Avoid contact sports or other situations where bruising or injury could occur.

## Side Effects of This Medicine

Along with their needed effects, medicines like methotrexate can sometimes cause unwanted effects such as blood problems, kidney problems, stomach or liver problems, loss of hair, and other side effects. These and others are described below. Also, because of the way these medicines act on the body, there is a chance that they might cause other unwanted effects that may not occur until months or years after the medicine is used. These delayed effects may include certain types of cancer, such as leukemia. Discuss these possible effects with your doctor.

Although not all of these side effects may occur, if they do occur they may need medical attention.

*Check with your doctor immediately* if any of the following side effects occur:

*Less common*
> Diarrhea; reddening of skin; sores in mouth and on lips; stomach pain

*Rare*
> Black, tarry stools; blood in urine or stools; blurred vision; convulsions (seizures); cough or hoarseness; fever or chills; lower back or side pain; painful or difficult urination; pinpoint red spots on skin; shortness of breath; unusual bleeding or bruising

Check with your doctor as soon as possible if any of the following side effects occur:

*Rare*
> Back pain; dark urine; dizziness; drowsiness; headache; unusual tiredness or weakness; yellow eyes or skin

Other side effects may occur that usually do not need medical attention. These side effects may go away during treatment as your body adjusts to the medicine. Also, your health care professional may be able to tell you about ways to prevent or reduce some of these side effects. Check with your health care professional if any of the following side effects continue or are bothersome or if you have any questions about them:

*Less common or rare*
> Acne; boils; loss of appetite; nausea or vomiting; pale skin; skin rash or itching

This medicine may cause a temporary loss of hair in some people. After treatment with methotrexate has ended, normal hair growth should return.

Other side effects not listed above may also occur in some patients. If you notice any other effects, check with your doctor.

## Additional Information

Once a medicine has been approved for marketing for a certain use, experience may show that it is also useful for other medical problems. Although these uses are not included in product labeling, methotrexate is used in certain patients with the following medical conditions:

- Psoriatic arthritis
- Systemic dermatomyositis

Other than the above information, there is no additional information relating to proper use, precautions, or side effects for these uses.

Revised: 08/90
Interim revision(s): 07/08/93; 07/05/94

# METHOXSALEN    Systemic

Some commonly used brand names are:

**In the U.S.—**
8-MOP
Oxsoralen-Ultra

**In Canada—**
Oxsoralen                    Ultra MOP

## Description

Methoxsalen (meth-OX-a-len) belongs to the group of medicines called psoralens. It is used along with ultraviolet light (found in sunlight and some special lamps) in a treatment called PUVA to treat vitiligo, a disease in which skin color is lost, and psoriasis, a skin condition associated with red and scaly patches.

Methoxsalen is also used with ultraviolet light in the treatment of white blood cells. This treatment is called photopheresis and is used to treat the skin problems associated with mycosis fungoides, which is a type of lymphoma.

Methoxsalen may also be used for other conditions as determined by your doctor.

This medicine is available only with your doctor's prescription, in the following dosage forms:

*Oral*
- Hard gelatin capsules (U.S. and Canada)
- Soft gelatin capsules (U.S. and Canada)

## Before Using This Medicine

Methoxsalen is a very strong medicine that increases the skin's sensitivity to sunlight. In addition to causing serious sunburns if not properly used, it has been reported to increase the chance of skin cancer and cataracts. Also, like too much sunlight, PUVA can cause premature aging of the skin. Therefore, methoxsalen should be used only as directed and it should *not* be used simply for suntanning. Before using this medicine, be sure that you have discussed its use with your doctor.

In deciding to use a medicine, the risks of using the medicine must be weighed against the good it will do. This is a decision you and your doctor will make. For methoxsalen, the following should be considered:

**Allergies**—Tell your doctor if you have ever had any unusual or allergic reaction to methoxsalen. Also tell your health care professional if you are allergic to any other substances, such as foods, preservatives, or dyes.

**Diet**—Eating certain foods while you are taking methoxsalen may increase your skin's sensitivity to sunlight. To help prevent this, avoid eating limes, figs, parsley, parsnips, mustard, carrots, and celery while you are being treated with this medicine.

**Pregnancy**—Studies on effects in pregnancy have not been done in either humans or animals.

**Breast-feeding**—It is not known whether methoxsalen passes into breast milk. Although most medicines pass into breast milk in small amounts, many of them may be used safely while breast-feeding. Mothers who are using this medicine and who wish to breast-feed should discuss this with their doctor.

**Children**—Some of the side effects are more likely to occur in children up to 12 years of age, since these children may be more sensitive to the effects of methoxsalen.

**Older adults**—Many medicines have not been studied specifically in older people. Therefore, it may not be known whether they work exactly the same way they do in younger adults or if they cause different side effects or problems in older people. There is no specific information comparing use of methoxsalen in the elderly with use in other age groups.

**Other medicines**—Although certain medicines should not be used together at all, in other cases two different medicines may be used together even if an interaction might occur. In these cases, your doctor may want to change the dose, or other precautions may be necessary. When you are using methoxsalen, it is especially important that

your health care professional know if you are using the following:
- Arsenicals or recent treatment with x-rays, or cancer medicines or plans to have x-rays in the near future—Arsenicals, x-rays and cancer medicines increase the chance of side effects from treatment with PUVA

**Other medical problems**—The presence of other medical problems may affect the use of methoxsalen. Make sure you tell your doctor if you have any other medical problems, especially:
- Allergy to sunlight (or family history of) or
- Infection or
- Lupus erythematosus or
- Porphyria or
- Skin cancer (history of) or
- Skin conditions (other) or
- Stomach problems—Use of PUVA may make the condition worse
- Eye problems, such as cataracts or loss of the lens of the eye—The light treatment may make the condition worse or may cause damage to the eye
- Heart or blood vessel disease (severe)—The heat or prolonged standing associated with each light treatment may make the condition worse
- Liver disease—Condition may cause increased blood levels of the medicine and cause an increase in side effects

## Proper Use of This Medicine

Methoxsalen usually comes with patient directions. Read them carefully before using this medicine.

This medicine may take 6 to 8 weeks to really help your condition. *Do not increase the amount of methoxsalen you are taking or spend extra time in the sunlight or under an ultraviolet lamp.* This will not make the medicine act any more quickly and may result in a serious burn.

If this medicine upsets your stomach:
- Patients taking the hard gelatin capsules may take them with food or milk.
- Patients taking the soft gelatin capsules may take them with low fat food or low fat milk.

**Dosing**—The dose of methoxsalen will be different for different patients. *Follow your doctor's orders or the directions on the label.* The following information includes only the average doses of methoxsalen. *If your dose is different, do not change it* unless your doctor tells you to do so.

The number of capsules that you take depends on the strength of the medicine. Also, *the number of doses you take each day, the time allowed between doses, and the length of time you take the medicine depend on the medical problem for which you are taking methoxsalen.*
- For *oral* dosage form (hard gelatin capsule):
  —For vitiligo:
    - Adults and children 12 years of age and over—20 milligrams (mg) per day taken two to four hours before ultraviolet light A (UVA) exposure. This treatment (methoxsalen and UVA)

is given two or three times a week with the treatment spaced at least forty-eight hours apart.

- Children up to 12 years of age—Use and dose must be determined by your doctor.

—For psoriasis:

- Adults and children 12 years of age and over—Dose is based on body weight and must be determined by your doctor. However, the usual dose is 0.6 mg per kilogram (kg) (0.27 mg per pound) of body weight taken two hours before UVA exposure. This treatment (methoxsalen and UVA) is given two or three times a week with the treatment spaced at least forty-eight hours apart.
- Children up to 12 years of age—Use and dose must be determined by your doctor.

- For *oral* dosage form (soft gelatin capsule):

—For psoriasis:

- Adults and children 12 years of age and over—Dose is based on body weight and must be determined by your doctor. The usual dose is 0.4 mg per kg (0.18 mg per pound) of body weight taken one and one-half to two hours before UVA exposure. This treatment (methoxsalen and UVA) is given two or three times a week, with the treatment spaced at least forty-eight hours apart.
- Children up to 12 years of age—Use and dose must be determined by your doctor.

**Missed dose**—If you are late in taking, or miss taking, a dose of this medicine, notify your doctor so your light treatment can be rescheduled. Remember that exposure to sunlight or ultraviolet light must take place a certain number of hours *after* you take the medicine or it will not work. For patients taking the hard gelatin capsules, this is 2 to 4 hours. For patients taking the soft gelatin capsules, this is 1½ to 2 hours. If you have any questions about this, check with your doctor.

**Storage**—To store this medicine:

- Keep out of the reach of children.
- Store away from heat and direct light.
- Do not store in the bathroom, near the kitchen sink, or in other damp places. Heat or moisture may cause the medicine to break down.
- Do not keep outdated medicine or medicine no longer needed. Be sure that any discarded medicine is out of the reach of children.

## Precautions While Using This Medicine

Your doctor should check your progress at regular visits to make sure this medicine is working and that it does not cause unwanted effects. Eye examinations should be included.

This medicine increases the sensitivity of your skin and lips to sunlight. Therefore, *exposure to the sun, even through window glass or on a cloudy day, could cause*

*a serious burn.* If you must go out during the daylight hours:

- *Before each treatment, cover your skin for at least 24 hours* by wearing protective clothing, such as long-sleeved shirts, full-length slacks, wide-brimmed hat, and gloves. In addition, *protect your lips with a special sun block lipstick that has a skin protection factor (SPF) of at least 15.* Check with your doctor before using sun block products on other parts of your body before a treatment, since sun block products should not be used on the areas of your skin that are to be treated.
- *After each treatment, cover your skin for at least 8 hours* by wearing protective clothing. In addition, use a sun block product that has a skin protection factor (SPF) of at least 15 on your lips and on those areas of your body that cannot be covered.

If you have any questions about this, check with your health care professional.

Your skin may continue to be sensitive to sunlight for some time after treatment with this medicine. Use extra caution for at least 48 hours following each treatment if you plan to spend any time in the sun. In addition, do not sunbathe anytime during your course of treatment with methoxsalen.

*For 24 hours after you take each dose of methoxsalen, your eyes should be protected during daylight hours with special wraparound sunglasses that totally block or absorb ultraviolet light* (ordinary sunglasses are not adequate). This is to prevent cataracts. Your doctor will tell you what kind of sunglasses to use. These glasses should be worn even in indirect light, such as light coming through window glass or on a cloudy day.

This medicine may cause your skin to become dry or itchy. *However, check with your doctor before applying anything to your skin to treat this problem.*

## Side Effects of This Medicine

Along with its needed effects, a medicine may cause some unwanted effects. Although not all of these side effects may occur, if they do occur they may need medical attention.

*Check with your doctor immediately* if you think you have taken an overdose or if any of the following side effects occur, since they may indicate a serious burn:

Blistering and peeling of skin; reddened, sore skin; swelling (especially of feet or lower legs)

Other side effects may occur that usually do not need medical attention. These side effects may go away during treatment as your body adjusts to the medicine. However, check with your doctor if any of the following side effects continue for more than 48 hours or are bothersome:

*More common*

Itching of skin; nausea

*Less common*

Dizziness; headache; mental depression; nervousness; trouble in sleeping

Treatment with this medicine usually causes a slight reddening of your skin 24 to 48 hours after the treatment. This is an expected effect and is no cause for concern. However, check with your doctor right away if your skin becomes sore and red or blistered.

There is an increased risk of developing skin cancer after use of methoxsalen. You should check your body regularly and show your doctor any skin sores that do not heal, new skin growths, and skin growths that have changed in the way they look or feel.

Premature aging of the skin may occur as a result of prolonged methoxsalen therapy. This effect is permanent and is similar to what happens when a person sunbathes for long periods of time.

Other side effects not listed above may also occur in some patients. If you notice any other effects, check with your doctor.

Revised: 06/24/94

# METHOXSALEN    Topical

Some commonly used brand names are:
**In the U.S.—**
 Oxsoralen Lotion
**In Canada—**
 Oxsoralen Lotion
 UltraMOP Lotion

## Description

Methoxsalen (meth-OX-a-len) belongs to the group of medicines called psoralens. It is used along with ultraviolet light (found in sunlight and some special lamps) in a treatment called psoralen plus ultraviolet light A (PUVA) to treat vitiligo, a disease in which skin color is lost. Methoxsalen may also be used for other conditions as determined by your doctor.

Methoxsalen is available only with a prescription and is to be administered by or under the direct supervision of your doctor, in the following dosage form:

*Topical*
 • Topical solution (U.S. and Canada)

## Before Using This Medicine

Methoxsalen is a very strong medicine that increases the skin's sensitivity to sunlight. In addition to causing serious sunburns if not properly used, it has been reported to increase the chance of skin cancer. Also, like too much sunlight, PUVA can cause premature aging of the skin. Therefore, methoxsalen should be used only as directed and should *not* be used simply for suntanning. Before using this medicine, be sure that you have discussed its use with your doctor.

In deciding to use a medicine, the risks of using the medicine must be weighed against the good it will do. This is a decision you and your doctor will make. For topical methoxsalen, the following should be considered:

**Allergies**—Tell your doctor if you have ever had any unusual or allergic reaction to methoxsalen. Also tell your health care professional if you are allergic to any other substances, such as foods, preservatives, or dyes.

**Diet**—Eating certain foods while you are using methoxsalen may increase your skin's sensitivity to sunlight. To help prevent this, avoid eating limes, figs, parsley, parsnips, mustard, carrots, and celery while you are being treated with this medicine.

**Pregnancy**—Studies on effects in pregnancy have not been done in either humans or animals.

**Breast-feeding**—It is not known whether methoxsalen passes into breast milk. Although most medicines pass into breast milk in small amounts, many of them may be used safely while breast-feeding. Mothers who are taking this medicine and who wish to breast-feed should discuss this with their doctor.

**Children**—Studies on this medicine have been done only in adult patients, and there is no specific information comparing use of methoxsalen in children up to 12 years of age with use in other age groups.

**Older adults**—Many medicines have not been studied specifically in older people. Therefore, it may not be known whether they work exactly the same way they do in younger adults or if they cause different side effects or problems in older people. There is no specific information comparing use of topical methoxsalen in the elderly with use in other age groups.

**Other medicines**—Although certain medicines should not be used together at all, in other cases two different medicines may be used together even if an interaction might occur. In these cases, your doctor may want to change the dose, or other precautions may be necessary. When you are using topical methoxsalen, it is especially important that your health care professional know if you are receiving the following:
 • Recent treatment with x-rays or cancer medicines or plans to have x-rays in the near future—Increases the chance of side effects from treatment with PUVA

**Other medical problems**—The presence of other medical problems may affect the use of topical methoxsalen. Make sure you tell your doctor if you have any other medical problems, especially:

- Allergy to sunlight (or family history of) or
- Infection or
- Lupus erythematosus or
- Porphyria or
- Skin cancer (history of) or
- Skin conditions (other)—Use of PUVA may make the condition worse
- Heart or blood vessel disease (severe)—The heat or prolonged standing associated with each light treatment may make the condition worse

## Proper Use of This Medicine

Use this medicine only under the direct supervision of your doctor.

After UVA exposure, wash the treated area of skin with soap and water. Then use a sunscreen or wear protective clothing to protect the area.

**Dosing**—Follow your doctor's directions in using this medicine. The following information includes only the average doses of methoxsalen. *If your dose is different, do not change it* unless your doctor tells you to do so.

- For *topical solution* dosage form:
  —For vitiligo:
    - Adults and children 12 years of age and over—Apply to the affected area of the skin and allow to dry for one to two minutes, then apply again within two to two and one-half hours before UVA exposure.
    - Children under 12 years of age—Use and dose must be determined by your doctor.

## Precautions While Using This Medicine

It is important that you visit your doctor as directed for treatments and to have your progress checked.

This medicine increases the sensitivity of the treated areas of your skin to sunlight. Therefore, *exposure to the sun, even through window glass or on a cloudy day, could cause a serious burn.* After each light treatment, thoroughly wash the treated areas of your skin. Also, if you must go out during daylight hours, cover the treated areas of your skin for at least 12 to 48 hours following treatment by wearing protective clothing or a sun block product that has a skin protection factor (SPF) of at least 15. Some patients may require a product with a higher SPF number, especially if they have a fair complexion. If you have any questions about this, check with your health care professional.

The treated areas of your skin may continue to be sensitive to sunlight for some time after treatment with this medicine. Use extra caution for at least 72 hours following each treatment if you plan to spend any time in the sun. In addition, do not sunbathe anytime during your course of treatment with methoxsalen.

This medicine may cause your skin to become dry or itchy. *However, check with your doctor before applying anything to your skin to treat this problem.*

## Side Effects of This Medicine

Along with its needed effects, a medicine may cause some unwanted effects. Although not all of these side effects may occur, if they do occur they may need medical attention.

*Check with your doctor immediately* if any of the following side effects occur, since they may indicate a serious burn:

Blistering and peeling of skin; reddened, sore skin; swelling, especially of the feet or lower legs

There is an increased risk of developing skin cancer after use of methoxsalen. You should check the treated areas of your body regularly and show your doctor any skin sores that do not heal, new skin growths, and skin growths that have changed in the way they look or feel.

Premature aging of the skin may occur as a result of prolonged methoxsalen therapy. This effect is permanent and is similar to the result of sunbathing for long periods of time.

Other side effects not listed above may also occur in some patients. If you notice any other effects, check with your doctor.

## Additional Information

Once a medicine has been approved for marketing for a certain use, experience may show that it is also useful for other medical problems. Although these uses are not included in product labeling, topical methoxsalen is used in certain patients with the following medical conditions:

- Alopecia areata
- Eczema
- Inflammatory dermatoses
- Lichen planus
- Mycosis fungoides
- Need to increase tolerance of skin to sunlight
- Psoriasis

Other than the above information, there is no additional information relating to proper use, precautions, or side effects for these uses.

Revised: 05/26/94

# METHYLDOPA   Systemic

Some commonly used brand names are:
**In the U.S.—**
Aldomet
Generic name product may also be available.

**In Canada—**
Aldomet           Dopamet
Apo-Methyldopa    Novomedopa
Generic name product may also be available.

© 1994   The United States Pharmacopeial Convention, Inc.          *All rights reserved*

# Description

Methyldopa (meth-ill-DOE-pa) belongs to the general class of medicines called antihypertensives. It is used to treat high blood pressure (hypertension).

High blood pressure adds to the work load of the heart and arteries. If it continues for a long time, the heart and arteries may not function properly. This can damage the blood vessels of the brain, heart, and kidneys, resulting in a stroke, heart failure, or kidney failure. High blood pressure may also increase the risk of heart attacks. These problems may be less likely to occur if blood pressure is controlled.

Methyldopa works by controlling impulses along certain nerve pathways. As a result, it relaxes blood vessels so that blood passes through them more easily. This helps to lower blood pressure.

Methyldopa is available only with your doctor's prescription, in the following dosage forms:

*Oral*
- Oral suspension (U.S.)
- Tablets (U.S. and Canada)

*Parenteral*
- Injection (U.S. and Canada)

# Before Using This Medicine

In deciding to use a medicine, the risks of taking the medicine must be weighed against the good it will do. This is a decision you and your doctor will make. For methyldopa, the following should be considered:

**Allergies**—Tell your doctor if you have ever had any unusual or allergic reaction to methyldopa. Also tell your health care professional if you are allergic to any other substances, such as foods, sulfites or other preservatives, or dyes. Some methyldopa products may contain sulfites. Your health care professional can help you avoid products that may cause a problem.

**Pregnancy**—Methyldopa has not been studied in pregnant women in the first and second trimesters (the first 6 months of pregnancy). However, studies in pregnant women during the third trimester (the last 3 months of pregnancy) have not shown that methyldopa causes birth defects or other problems.

**Breast-feeding**—Although methyldopa passes into breast milk, it has not been reported to cause problems in nursing babies.

**Children**—Although there is no specific information comparing use of methyldopa in children with use in other age groups, this medicine is not expected to cause different side effects or problems in children than it does in adults.

**Older adults**—Dizziness or lightheadedness and drowsiness may be more likely to occur in the elderly, who are more sensitive to the effects of methyldopa.

**Other medicines**—Although certain medicines should not be used together at all, in other cases two different medicines may be used together even if an interaction might occur. In these cases, your doctor may want to change the dose, or other precautions may be necessary. When you are taking methyldopa, it is especially important that your health care professional know if you are taking any of the following:

- Monoamine oxidase (MAO) inhibitors (furazolidone [e.g., Furoxone], isocarboxazid [e.g., Marplan], phenelzine [e.g., Nardil], procarbazine [e.g., Matulane], selegiline [e.g., Eldepryl], tranylcypromine [e.g., Parnate])—Taking methyldopa while you are taking or within 2 weeks of taking MAO inhibitors may cause nervousness in patients receiving MAO inhibitors; headache, severe high blood pressure, and hallucinations have been reported

**Other medical problems**—The presence of other medical problems may affect the use of methyldopa. Make sure you tell your doctor if you have any other medical problems, especially:

- Angina (chest pain)—Methyldopa may worsen the condition
- Kidney disease or
- Liver disease—Effects of methyldopa may be increased because of slower removal from the body
- Mental depression (history of)—Methyldopa can cause mental depression
- Parkinson's disease—Methyldopa may worsen condition
- Pheochromocytoma—Methyldopa may interfere with tests for the condition; in addition, there have been reports of increased blood pressure
- If you have taken methyldopa in the past and developed liver problems

# Proper Use of This Medicine

In addition to the use of the medicine your doctor has prescribed, treatment for your high blood pressure may include weight control and care in the types of foods you eat, especially foods high in sodium. Your doctor will tell you which of these are most important for you. You should check with your doctor before changing your diet.

Many patients who have high blood pressure will not notice any signs of the problem. In fact, many may feel normal. It is very important that you *take your medicine exactly as directed* and that you keep your appointments with your doctor even if you feel well.

Remember that methyldopa will not cure your high blood pressure but it does help control it. Therefore, you must continue to take it as directed if you expect to lower your blood pressure and keep it down. *You may have to take high blood pressure medicine for the rest of your life.* If high blood pressure is not treated, it can cause serious problems such as heart failure, blood vessel disease, stroke, or kidney disease.

To help you remember to take your medicine, try to get into the habit of taking it at the same time each day.

**Dosing**—The dose of methyldopa will be different for different patients. *Follow your doctor's orders or the* *directions on the label.* The following information includes only the average doses of methyldopa. *If your dose is different, do not change it* unless your doctor tells you to do so.

The number of tablets or teaspoonfuls of suspension that you take depends on the strength of the medicine.

- For *oral* dosage form (suspension or tablets):
  —For high blood pressure:
  - Adults—250 milligrams (mg) to 2 grams a day. This is divided into two to four doses.
  - Children—Dose is based on body weight or size and must be determined by your doctor. The usual dose is 10 mg per kilogram (kg) (4.5 mg per pound) of body weight a day. This is divided into two to four doses. Your doctor may increase the dose as needed.
- For *injection* dosage form:
  —For high blood pressure:
  - Adults—250 to 500 mg mixed in 100 milliliters (mL) of solution (5% dextrose) and slowly injected into a vein every six hours as needed.
  - Children—Dose is based on body weight and must be determined by your doctor. The usual dose is 5 to 10 mg per kg (2.3 to 4.5 mg per pound) of body weight. This is mixed in a solution (5% dextrose) and slowly injected into a vein every six hours as needed.

**Missed dose**—If you miss a dose of this medicine, take it as soon as possible. However, if it is almost time for your next dose, skip the missed dose and go back to your regular dosing schedule. Do not double doses.

**Storage**—To store this medicine:
- Keep out of the reach of children.
- Store away from heat and direct light.
- Do not store in the bathroom, near the kitchen sink, or in other damp places. Heat or moisture may cause the medicine to break down.
- Keep the oral liquid form of this medicine from freezing.
- Do not keep outdated medicine or medicine no longer needed. Be sure that any discarded medicine is out of the reach of children.

## Precautions While Using This Medicine

It is important that your doctor check your progress at regular visits to make sure that this medicine is working properly.

*Do not take other medicines unless they have been discussed with your doctor.* This especially includes over-the-counter (nonprescription) medicines for appetite control, asthma, colds, cough, hay fever, or sinus problems, since they may tend to increase your blood pressure.

*If you have a fever and there seems to be no reason for it, check with your doctor.* This is especially important

during the first few weeks you take methyldopa, since fever may be a sign of a serious reaction to this medicine.

Before having any kind of surgery (including dental surgery) or emergency treatment, make sure the medical doctor or dentist in charge knows that you are taking this medicine.

Methyldopa may cause some people to become drowsy or less alert than they are normally. This is more likely to happen when you begin to take it or when you increase the amount of medicine you are taking. *Make sure you know how you react to this medicine before you drive, use machines, or do anything else that could be dangerous if you are not alert.*

Dizziness, lightheadedness, or fainting may occur, especially when you get up from a lying or sitting position. Getting up slowly may help, but if the problem continues or gets worse, check with your doctor.

Methyldopa may cause dryness of the mouth. For temporary relief, use sugarless candy or gum, melt bits of ice in your mouth, or use a saliva substitute. However, if your mouth continues to feel dry for more than 2 weeks, check with your medical doctor or dentist. Continuing dryness of the mouth may increase the chance of dental disease, including tooth decay, gum disease, and fungus infections.

Tell the doctor in charge that you are taking this medicine before you have any medical tests. The results of some tests may be affected by this medicine.

## Side Effects of This Medicine

Along with its needed effects, a medicine may cause some unwanted effects. Although not all of these side effects may occur, if they do occur they may need medical attention.

*Check with your doctor immediately* if the following side effect occurs:
> *Less common*
>> Fever, shortly after starting to take this medicine

Check with your doctor as soon as possible if any of the following side effects occur:
> *More common*
>> Swelling of feet or lower legs
> *Less common*
>> Mental depression or anxiety; nightmares or unusually vivid dreams
> *Rare*
>> Dark or amber urine; diarrhea or stomach cramps (severe or continuing); fever, chills, troubled breathing, and fast heartbeat; general feeling of discomfort or illness or weakness; joint pain; pale stools; skin rash or itching; stomach pain (severe) with nausea and vomiting; tiredness or weakness after having taken this medicine for several weeks (continuing); yellow eyes or skin

Other side effects may occur that usually do not need medical attention. These side effects may go away during

treatment as your body adjusts to the medicine. However, check with your doctor if any of the following side effects continue or are bothersome:

*More common*

Drowsiness; dryness of mouth; headache

*Less common*

Decreased sexual ability or interest in sex; diarrhea; dizziness or lightheadedness when getting up from a lying or sitting position; nausea or vomiting; numbness, tingling, pain, or weakness in hands or feet; slow heartbeat; stuffy nose; swelling of breasts or unusual milk production

Other side effects not listed above may also occur in some patients. If you notice any other effects, check with your doctor.

Revised: 08/05/92
Interim revision: 04/29/94

---

# METHYLDOPA AND THIAZIDE DIURETICS    Systemic

Some commonly used brand names are:

**In the U.S.—**
Aldoclor[1]                           Aldoril[2]

**In Canada—**
Aldoril[2]                            PMS Dopazide[2]
Novodoparil[2]                        Supres[1]

Note: For quick reference, the following methyldopa and thiazide diuretics are numbered to match the corresponding brand names.

This information applies to the following medicines:

1. Methyldopa (meth-ill-DOE-pa) and Chlorothiazide (klor-oh-THYE-a-zide)‡
2. Methyldopa and Hydrochlorothiazide (hye-droe-klor-oh-THYE-a-zide)‡

‡Generic name product may also be available in the U.S.

## Description

Combinations of methyldopa and a thiazide diuretic (chlorothiazide or hydrochlorothiazide) are used to treat high blood pressure (hypertension).

High blood pressure adds to the workload of the heart and arteries. If it continues for a long time, the heart and arteries may not function properly. This can damage the blood vessels of the brain, heart, and kidneys, resulting in a stroke, heart failure, or kidney failure. High blood pressure may also increase the risk of heart attacks. These problems may be less likely to occur if blood pressure is controlled.

Methyldopa works by controlling nerve impulses along certain nerve pathways. As a result, it relaxes blood vessels so that blood passes through them more easily. Thiazide diuretics help reduce the amount of water in the body by increasing the flow of urine. These actions help to lower blood pressure.

This medicine is available only with your doctor's prescription, in the following dosage forms:

*Oral*

Methyldopa and Chlorothiazide
• Tablets (U.S. and Canada)
Methyldopa and Hydrochlorothiazide
• Tablets (U.S. and Canada)

## Before Using This Medicine

In deciding to use a medicine, the risks of taking the medicine must be weighed against the good it will do. This is a decision you and your doctor will make. For methyldopa and thiazide diuretics, the following should be considered:

**Allergies**—Tell your doctor if you have ever had any unusual or allergic reaction to methyldopa, sulfonamides (sulfa drugs), bumetanide, furosemide, indapamide, acetazolamide, dichlorphenamide, methazolamide, or thiazide diuretics (water pills). Also tell your health care professional if you are allergic to any other substances, such as foods, sulfites or other preservatives, or dyes.

**Pregnancy**—Studies in humans have not shown that methyldopa causes birth defects or other problems. However, when thiazide diuretics are used during pregnancy, they may cause side effects including jaundice, blood problems, and low potassium in the newborn infant. Thiazide diuretics have not been shown to cause birth defects.

**Breast-feeding**—This medicine passes into breast milk. Thiazide diuretics may decrease the flow of breast milk. Therefore, you should avoid use of thiazide diuretics during the first month of breast-feeding.

**Children**—Although there is no specific information comparing use of this medicine in children with use in other age groups, it is not expected to cause different side effects or problems in children than it does in adults.

**Older adults**—Dizziness or lightheadedness, drowsiness, or signs of too much potassium loss may be more likely to occur in the elderly, who are more sensitive to the effects of methyldopa and thiazide diuretics.

**Other medicines**—Although certain medicines should not be used together at all, in other cases two different medicines may be used together even if an interaction might occur. In these cases, your doctor may want to change the dose, or other precautions may be necessary. When you are taking methyldopa and thiazide diuretics, it is especially important that your health care professional know if you are taking any of the following:

- Digitalis glycosides (heart medicine)—Thiazide diuretics may cause low potassium in the blood, which can lead to symptoms of digitalis toxicity
- Lithium (e.g., Lithane)—Risk of lithium overdose, even at usual doses, may be increased
- Monoamine oxidase (MAO) inhibitors (furazolidone [e.g., Furoxone], isocarboxazid [e.g., Marplan], phenelzine [e.g., Nardil], procarbazine [e.g., Matulane], selegiline [e.g., Eldepryl], tranylcypromine [e.g., Parnate])—Taking methyldopa while you are taking or within 2 weeks of taking MAO inhibitors may cause nervousness; headache, severe high blood pressure, and hallucinations have been reported

**Other medical problems**—The presence of other medical problems may affect the use of methyldopa and thiazide diuretics. Make sure you tell your doctor if you have any other medical problems, especially:

- Angina (chest pain)—Methyldopa may worsen the condition
- Diabetes mellitus (sugar diabetes)—Thiazide diuretics may change the amount of diabetes medicine needed
- Gout (history of)—Thiazide diuretics may increase the amount of uric acid in the blood, which can lead to gout
- High cholesterol—Thiazide diuretics may raise cholesterol levels
- Kidney disease—Effects of methyldopa and thiazide diuretics may be increased because of slower removal from the body. If severe, thiazide diuretics may not work
- Liver disease—Effects of methyldopa may be increased because of slower removal from the body. If thiazide diuretics cause loss of too much water from the body, liver disease can become much worse
- Lupus erythematosus (history of)—Thiazide diuretics may worsen the condition
- Mental depression (history of)—Methyldopa can cause mental depression
- Pancreatitis (inflammation of the pancreas)
- Parkinson's disease—Methyldopa may worsen the condition
- Pheochromocytoma—Methyldopa may interfere with tests for the condition; in addition, there have been reports of increased blood pressure
- If you have taken methyldopa in the past and developed liver problems

## Proper Use of This Medicine

In addition to the use of the medicine your doctor has prescribed, appropriate treatment for your high blood pressure may include weight control and care in the types of foods you eat, especially foods high in sodium. Your doctor will tell you which factors are most important for you. You should check with your doctor before changing your diet.

Many patients who have high blood pressure will not notice any signs of the problem. In fact, many may feel normal. It is very important *that you take your medicine exactly as directed* and that you keep your appointments with your doctor even if you feel well.

Remember that this medicine will not cure your high blood pressure but it does help control it. Therefore, you must continue to take it as directed if you expect to lower your blood pressure and keep it down. *You may have to take high blood pressure medicine for the rest of your life.* If high blood pressure is not treated, it can cause serious problems such as heart failure, blood vessel disease, stroke, or kidney disease.

This medicine may cause you to have an unusual feeling of tiredness when you begin to take it. You may also notice an increase in the amount of urine or in your frequency of urination. After taking the medicine for a while, these effects should lessen. In general, to keep the increase in urine from affecting your sleep:

- If you are to take a single dose a day, take it in the morning after breakfast.
- If you are to take more than one dose a day, take the last dose no later than 6 p.m., unless otherwise directed by your doctor.

However, it is best to plan your dose or doses according to a schedule that will least affect your personal activities and sleep. Ask your health care professional to help you plan the best time to take this medicine.

To help you remember to take your medicine, try to get into the habit of taking it at the same time each day.

**Dosing**—The dose of methyldopa and thiazide diuretic combinations will be different for different patients. *Follow your doctor's orders or the directions on the label.* The following information includes only the average doses of methyldopa and thiazide diuretic combinations. *If your dose is different, do not change it* unless your doctor tells you to do so:

*For methyldopa and chlorothiazide*

- For *oral* dosage form (tablets):
  —Adults: Two to four tablets a day, taken as a single dose or in divided doses.
  —Children: Dose must be determined by your doctor.

*For methyldopa and hydrochlorothiazide*

- For *oral* dosage form (tablets):
  —Adults: Two to four tablets a day, taken as a single dose or in divided doses.
  —Children: Dose must be determined by your doctor.

**Missed dose**—If you miss a dose of this medicine, take it as soon as possible. However, if it is almost time for your next dose, skip the missed dose and go back to your regular dosing schedule. Do not double doses.

**Storage**—To store this medicine:

- Keep out of the reach of children.
- Store away from heat and direct light.
- Do not store in the bathroom, near the kitchen sink, or in other damp places. Heat or moisture may cause the medicine to break down.

• Do not keep outdated medicine or medicine no longer needed. Be sure that any discarded medicine is out of the reach of children.

## Precautions While Using This Medicine

It is important that your doctor check your progress at regular visits to make sure that this medicine is working properly.

*Do not take other medicines unless they have been discussed with your doctor.* This especially includes over-the-counter (nonprescription) medicines for appetite control, asthma, colds, cough, hay fever, or sinus problems, since they may tend to increase your blood pressure.

*This medicine may cause a loss of potassium from your body:*

• To help prevent this, your doctor may want you to:
  —eat or drink foods that have a high potassium content (for example, orange or other citrus fruit juices), or
  —take a potassium supplement, or
  —take another medicine to help prevent the loss of the potassium in the first place.
• It is very important to follow these directions. Also, it is important not to change your diet on your own. This is more important if you are already on a special diet (as for diabetes), or if you are taking a potassium supplement or a medicine to reduce potassium loss. Extra potassium may not be necessary and, in some cases, too much potassium could be harmful.

Check with your doctor if you become sick and have severe or continuing vomiting or diarrhea. These problems may cause you to lose additional water and potassium.

Before having any kind of surgery (including dental surgery) or emergency treatment, tell the medical doctor or dentist in charge that you are taking this medicine.

*If you have a fever and there seems to be no reason for it, check with your doctor.* This is especially important during the first few weeks you take this medicine since fever may be a sign of a serious reaction to methyldopa.

This medicine may cause some people to become drowsy or less alert than they are normally. This is more likely to happen when you begin to take it or when you increase the amount of medicine you are taking. *Make sure you know how you react to this medicine before you drive, use machines, or do anything else that could be dangerous if you are not alert.*

Dizziness, lightheadedness, or fainting may occur, especially when you get up from a lying or sitting position. Getting up slowly may help, but if the problem continues or gets worse, check with your doctor.

The dizziness, lightheadedness, or fainting is also more likely to occur if you drink alcohol, stand for long periods of time, exercise, or if the weather is hot. Drinking alcoholic beverages may also make the drowsiness worse.

*While you are taking this medicine, be careful in the amount of alcohol you drink.* Also, use extra care during exercise or hot weather or if you must stand for long periods of time.

For *diabetic patients*:

• This medicine may raise blood sugar levels. While you are using this medicine, be especially careful in testing for sugar in your urine. If you have any questions about this, check with your doctor.

This medicine may cause dryness of the mouth. For temporary relief, use sugarless candy or gum, melt bits of ice in your mouth, or use a saliva substitute. However, if your mouth continues to feel dry for more than 2 weeks, check with your medical doctor or dentist. Continuing dryness of the mouth may increase the chance of dental disease, including tooth decay, gum disease, and fungus infections.

Thiazide diuretics may cause your skin to be more sensitive to sunlight than it is normally. Exposure to sunlight, even for brief periods of time, may cause a skin rash, itching, redness or other discoloration of the skin, or a severe sunburn. When you begin taking this medicine:

• Stay out of direct sunlight, especially between the hours of 10:00 a.m. and 3:00 p.m., if possible.
• Wear protective clothing, including a hat. Also, wear sunglasses.
• Apply a sun block product that has a skin protection factor (SPF) of at least 15. Some patients may require a product with a higher SPF number, especially if they have a fair complexion. If you have any questions about this, check with your health care professional.
• Apply a sun block lipstick that has an SPF of at least 15 to protect your lips.
• Do not use a sunlamp or tanning bed or booth.

*If you have a severe reaction from the sun, check with your doctor.*

Before you have any medical tests, tell the doctor in charge that you are taking this medicine. The results of some tests may be affected by this medicine.

## Side Effects of This Medicine

Along with its needed effects, a medicine may cause some unwanted effects. Although not all of these side effects may occur, if they do occur they may need medical attention.

*Check with your doctor immediately* if the following side effect occurs:

*Rare*
Unexplained fever shortly after starting to take this medicine

*Check with your doctor as soon as possible if any of the following side effects occur, especially since some of them may mean that your body is losing too much potassium:*

*Signs and symptoms of too much potassium loss*
Dry mouth; increased thirst; irregular heartbeats; muscle cramps or pain; nausea or vomiting; unusual tiredness or weakness; weak pulse

*Less common*

Mental depression or anxiety; nightmares or unusually vivid dreams

*Rare*

Cough or hoarseness; dark or amber urine; diarrhea or stomach cramps (severe or continuing); fever, chills, troubled breathing, and fast heartbeat; general feeling of discomfort or illness or weakness; joint pain; lower back or side pain; painful or difficult urination; pale stools; skin rash, hives, or itching; stomach pain (severe) with nausea and vomiting; tiredness or weakness after having taken this medicine for several weeks (continuing); yellow eyes or skin

Other side effects may occur that usually do not need medical attention. These side effects may go away during treatment as your body adjusts to the medicine. However, check with your doctor if any of the following side effects continue or are bothersome:

*More common*

Dizziness or lightheadedness when getting up from a lying or sitting position; drowsiness; dryness of mouth; headache

*Less common*

Decreased sexual ability or interest in sex; diarrhea; increased sensitivity of skin to sunlight (skin rash, itching, redness or other discoloration of skin or severe sunburn after exposure to sunlight); loss of appetite; numbness, tingling, pain, or weakness in hands or feet; slow heartbeat; stuffy nose; swelling of breasts or unusual milk production

Other side effects not listed above may also occur in some patients. If you notice any other effects, check with your doctor.

Revised: 04/13/93

# METHYLENE BLUE    Systemic

A commonly used brand name in the U.S. is Urolene Blue.
Generic name product may also be available in the U.S. and Canada.
Other commonly used names are aniline violet, methylthionine chloride, and tetramethylthionine chloride.

## Description

Methylene (METH-i-leen) blue is used to treat a condition called methemoglobinemia. This condition occurs when the blood cannot deliver oxygen where it is needed in the body. Methylene blue is also used as a dye to stain certain parts of the body before or during surgery.

*Oral*
- Tablets (U.S.)

*Parenteral*
- Injection (U.S. and Canada)

## Before Using This Medicine

In deciding to use a medicine, the risks of taking the medicine must be weighed against the good it will do. This is a decision you and your doctor will make. For methylene blue, the following should be considered:

**Allergies**—Tell your doctor if you have ever had any unusual or allergic reaction to methylene blue. Also tell your health care professional if you are allergic to any other substances, such as foods, preservatives, or dyes.

**Pregnancy**—Studies on effects in pregnancy have not been done in either humans or animals.

**Breast-feeding**—It is not known whether methylene blue passes into breast milk. Although most medicines pass into breast milk in small amounts, many of them may be used safely while breast-feeding. Mothers who are taking this medicine and who wish to breast-feed should discuss this with their doctor.

**Children**—Babies are especially sensitive to the effects of methylene blue. This may increase the chance of side effects during treatment.

**Older adults**—Many medicines have not been studied specifically in older people. Therefore, it may not be known whether they work exactly the same way they do in younger adults. Although there is no specific information comparing the use of methylene blue in the elderly with use in other age groups, this medicine is not expected to cause different side effects or problems in older people than it does in younger adults.

**Other medicines**—Although certain medicines should not be used together at all, in other cases two different medicines may be used together even if an interaction might occur. In these cases, your doctor may want to change the dose, or other precautions may be necessary. Tell your health care professional if you are taking any other prescription or nonprescription (over-the-counter [OTC]) medicine.

**Other medical problems**—The presence of other medical problems may affect the use of methylene blue. Make sure you tell your doctor if you have any other medical problems, especially:
- Glucose-6-phosphate dehydrogenase (G6PD) deficiency—Methylene blue may cause anemia or make methemoglobinemia worse
- Kidney disease—In patients with kidney disease methylene blue may accumulate in the body; smaller doses of this medicine may be needed

• Methemoglobinemia to treat cyanide toxicity—Methylene blue may make cyanide toxicity worse by increasing the amount of cyanide in the blood

## Proper Use of This Medicine

For patients taking the *tablet* form of this medicine:
• Take tablets after meals with a full glass (8 ounces) of water.

*Take this medicine only as directed*. Do not take more of it and do not take it more often than recommended on the label unless directed by your doctor. To do so may increase the chance of side effects.

**Dosing**—The dose of methylene blue will be different for different patients. *Follow your doctor's orders or the directions on the label*. The following information includes only the average doses of methylene blue. *If your dose is different, do not change it* unless your doctor tells you to do so.

• For *oral* dosage form (tablets):
  —For methemoglobinemia:
    • Adults and children—100 to 300 milligrams (mg) a day.
• For *injection* dosage form:
  —For methemoglobinemia:
    • Adults and children—Dose is based on body weight or size and must be determined by your doctor. The dose is usually 1 to 2 mg per kilogram (kg) (0.45 to 0.9 mg per pound) of body weight, or 25 to 50 mg per square meter of body surface area, injected into a vein over a period of five minutes. A second dose may be given after one hour, if needed.

**Missed dose**—If you miss a dose of this medicine, take it as soon as possible. However, if it is almost time for your next dose, skip the missed dose and go back to your regular dosing schedule. Do not double doses.

**Storage**—To store this medicine:
• Keep out of the reach of children.
• Store away from heat and direct light.
• Do not store in the bathroom, near the kitchen sink, or in other damp places. Heat or moisture may cause the medicine to break down.

• Keep the medicine from freezing. Do not refrigerate.
• Do not keep outdated medicine or medicine no longer needed. Be sure that any discarded medicine is out of the reach of children.

## Precautions While Using This Medicine

Before you have any medical tests, tell the doctor in charge that you are taking this medicine. The results of some tests may be affected by this medicine.

## Side Effects of This Medicine

Along with its needed effects, a medicine may cause some unwanted effects. Although not all of these side effects may occur, if they do occur they may need medical attention.

*Check with your doctor immediately* if any of the following side effects occur:

*Symptoms of overdose*
  Anxiety; back pain; bluish fingernails, lips, or skin; chest pain; chills; confusion; difficulty in breathing; dizziness; headache; leg pain; nausea and vomiting; severe sweating; stomach pain; trembling; unusual tiredness or weakness

Other side effects may occur that usually do not need medical attention. These side effects may go away during treatment as your body adjusts to the medicine. However, check with your doctor if any of the following side effects continue or are bothersome:

*More common*
  Greenish blue to blue discoloration of urine and stools
*Less common*
  Diarrhea; nausea and vomiting; painful urination or increased need to urinate (with tablet form)

Other side effects not listed above may also occur in some patients. If you notice any other effects, check with your doctor.

Developed: 05/27/94

---

# METHYLPHENIDATE    Systemic

Some commonly used brand names are:
**In the U.S.—**
  Ritalin
  Ritalin-SR
  Generic name product may also be available.
**In Canada—**
  PMS-Methylphenidate
  Ritalin
  Ritalin SR

## Description

Methylphenidate (meth-ill-FEN-i-date) belongs to the group of medicines called central stimulants. It is used to treat children with attention-deficit hyperactivity disorder (ADHD).

Methylphenidate works by increasing attention and decreasing restlessness in children who are overactive, cannot concentrate for very long or are easily distracted, and are emotionally unstable. This medicine is used as part of a total treatment program that also includes social, educational, and psychological treatment.

Methylphenidate is also used in the treatment of narcolepsy (uncontrollable desire for sleep or sudden attacks of deep sleep).

This medicine is available only with a doctor's prescription. Prescriptions cannot be refilled. A new written prescription must be obtained from your doctor each time you or your child needs this medicine.

Methylphenidate is available in the following dosage forms:

*Oral*
- Tablets (U.S. and Canada)
- Extended-release tablets (U.S. and Canada)

## Before Using This Medicine

In deciding to use a medicine, the risks of taking the medicine must be weighed against the good it will do. This is a decision you and your doctor will make. For methylphenidate, the following should be considered:

**Allergies**—Tell your doctor if you have ever had any unusual or allergic reaction to methylphenidate. Also tell your health care professional if you are allergic to any other substances, such as foods, preservatives, or dyes.

**Pregnancy**—Studies on effects in pregnancy have not been done in either humans or animals.

**Breast-feeding**—It is not known whether methylphenidate passes into breast milk.

**Children**—Loss of appetite, trouble in sleeping, stomach pain, and weight loss, may be especially likely to occur in children, who are usually more sensitive than adults to the effects of methylphenidate. Also, there have been reports of children's growth rate being slowed when methylphenidate was used for a long time. Some doctors recommend drug-free periods during treatment with methylphenidate.

**Older adults**—Many medicines have not been studied specifically in older people. Therefore, it may not be known whether they work exactly the same way they do in younger adults or if they cause different side effects or problems in older people. There is no specific information comparing use of methylphenidate in the elderly with use in other age groups.

**Other medicines**—Although certain medicines should not be used together at all, in other cases 2 different medicines may be used together even if an interaction might occur. In these cases, your doctor may want to change the dose, or other precautions may be necessary. When you are taking methylphenidate, it is especially important

that your health care professional know if you are taking any of the following:
- Amantadine (e.g., Symmetrel) or
- Amphetamines or
- Appetite suppressants (diet pills), except fenfluramine (e.g., Pondimin) or
- Caffeine (e.g., NoDoz) or
- Chlophedianol (e.g., Ulone) or
- Cocaine or
- Medicine for asthma or other breathing problems or
- Medicine for colds, sinus problems, hay fever or other allergies (including nose drops or sprays) or
- Nabilone (e.g., Cesamet) or
- Pemoline (e.g., Cylert)—Using these medicines with methylphenidate may cause severe nervousness, irritability, trouble in sleeping, or possibly irregular heartbeat or seizures
- Monoamine oxidase (MAO) inhibitors (furazolidone [e.g., Furoxone], isocarboxazid [e.g., Marplan], phenelzine [e.g., Nardil], procarbazine [e.g., Matulane], selegiline at doses more than 10 milligrams a day [e.g., Eldepryl], tranylcypromine [e.g., Parnate])—Taking methylphenidate while you are taking or within 2 weeks of taking MAO inhibitors may cause sudden extremely high blood pressure and severe convulsions; at least 14 days should be allowed between stopping treatment with one medicine and starting treatment with the other
- Pimozide (e.g., Orap)—The cause of tics may be masked

**Other medical problems**—The presence of other medical problems may affect the use of methylphenidate. Make sure you tell your doctor if you have any other medical problems, especially:
- Alcohol abuse (or history of) or
- Drug abuse or dependence (or history of)—Dependence on methylphenidate may develop
- Epilepsy or other seizure disorders—The risk of convulsions (seizures) may be increased
- Gilles de la Tourette's disorder (or history of) or
- Glaucoma or
- High blood pressure or
- Psychosis or
- Severe anxiety, agitation, tension, or depression or
- Tics (other than Tourette's disorder)—Methylphenidate may make the condition worse

## Proper Use of This Medicine

*Take this medicine only as directed by your doctor.* Do not take more of it, do not take it more often, and do not take it for a longer time than your doctor ordered. If too much is taken, it may become habit-forming.

Take this medicine about 30 to 45 minutes before meals. To do so will help it to work better.

If you are taking the long-acting form of this medicine:
- These tablets are to be swallowed whole. Do not break, crush, or chew before swallowing.

To help prevent trouble in sleeping, take the last dose of this medicine for each day before 6 p.m., unless otherwise directed by your doctor.

If you think this medicine is not working properly after you have taken it for several weeks, *do not increase the dose*. Instead, check with your doctor.

**Dosing**—The dose of methylphenidate will be different for different patients. *Follow your doctor's orders or the directions on the label.* The following information includes only the average doses of methylphenidate. *If your dose is different, do not change it* unless your doctor tells you to do so.

The number of tablets that you take depends on the strength of the medicine. Also, *the number of doses you take each day, the time allowed between doses, and the length of time you take the medicine depend on the medical problem for which you are using methylphenidate.*

- For *short-acting oral* dosage forms (tablets):
  —Adults and adolescents: 5 to 20 milligrams two or three times a day, taken thirty to forty-five minutes before meals.
  —Children 6 years of age and over: To start, 5 milligrams two times a day, before breakfast and lunch. Your doctor may increase your dose if needed by 5 to 10 milligrams a week until symptoms improve or a maximum dose is reached.
  —Children up to 6 years of age: The dose must be determined by the doctor.
- For *long-acting oral* dosage forms (extended-release tablets):
  —Adults and adolescents: 20 milligrams one to three times a day, spaced eight hours apart, and taken on an empty stomach.
  —Children 6 years of age and over: 20 milligrams one to three times a day, spaced eight hours apart, and taken on an empty stomach.
  —Children up to 6 years of age: The dose must be determined by the doctor.

**Missed dose**—If you miss a dose of this medicine, take it as soon as possible. Then take any remaining doses for that day at regularly spaced intervals. Do not double doses.

**Storage**—To store this medicine:
- Keep out of the reach of children.
- Store away from heat and direct light.
- Do not store in the bathroom, near the kitchen sink, or in other damp places. Heat or moisture may cause the medicine to break down.
- Do not keep outdated medicine or medicine no longer needed. Be sure that any discarded medicine is out of the reach of children.

## Precautions While Using This Medicine

Your doctor should check your progress at regular visits to make sure that this medicine does not cause unwanted effects.

If you will be taking this medicine in large doses for a long time, *do not stop taking it without first checking with your doctor*. Your doctor may want you to reduce gradually the amount you are taking before stopping completely.

*If you have been using this medicine for a long time and you think you may have become mentally or physically dependent on it, check with your doctor.* Some signs of dependence on methylphenidate are:

- A strong desire or need to continue taking the medicine.
- A need to increase the dose to receive the effects of the medicine.
- Withdrawal side effects (for example, mental depression, unusual behavior, or unusual tiredness or weakness) occurring after the medicine is stopped.

## Side Effects of This Medicine

Along with its needed effects, a medicine may cause some unwanted effects. Although not all of these side effects may occur, if they do occur they may need medical attention.

Check with your doctor as soon as possible if any of the following side effects occur:

*More common*
Fast heartbeat

*Less common*
Bruising; chest pain; fever; joint pain; skin rash or hives; uncontrolled movements of the body

*Rare*
Blurred vision or any change in vision; convulsions (seizures); sore throat and fever; unusual tiredness or weakness

*With long-term use*
Mood or mental changes; weight loss

*Symptoms of overdose*
Agitation; confusion; convulsions (seizures); delirium or hallucinations; dryness of mouth; false sense of well-being; fast, pounding, or irregular heartbeat; fever and sweating; headache (severe); increased blood pressure; muscle twitching; trembling or tremors; vomiting

Other side effects may occur that usually do not need medical attention. These side effects may go away during treatment as your body adjusts to the medicine. However, check with your doctor if any of the following side effects continue or are bothersome:

*More common*
Loss of appetite; nervousness; trouble in sleeping

*Less common*
Dizziness; drowsiness; headache; nausea; stomach pain

After you stop using this medicine, your body may need time to adjust. The length of time this takes depends on the amount of medicine you were using and how long you used it. During this period of time check with your doctor if you notice any of the following side effects:

Mental depression (severe); unusual behavior; unusual tiredness or weakness

Other side effects not listed above may also occur in some patients. If you notice any other effects, check with your doctor.

Revised: 03/09/93

# METHYSERGIDE   Systemic

A commonly used brand name in the U.S. and Canada is Sansert.

## Description

Methysergide (meth-i-SER-jide) belongs to the group of medicines known as ergot alkaloids. It is used to prevent migraine headaches and some kinds of throbbing headaches. It is not used to treat an attack once it has started. The exact way methysergide acts on the body is not known.

This medicine is available only with your doctor's prescription, in the following dosage form:

*Oral*
- Tablets (U.S. and Canada)

## Before Using This Medicine

In deciding to use a medicine, the risks of taking the medicine must be weighed against the good it will do. This is a decision you and your doctor will make. For methysergide, the following should be considered:

**Allergies**—Tell your doctor if you have ever had any unusual or allergic reaction to methysergide or to other ergot medicines. Also tell your health care professional if you are allergic to any other substances, such as foods, preservatives, or dyes.

**Pregnancy**—Studies with methysergide have not been done in either humans or animals.

**Breast-feeding**—This medicine passes into the breast milk and may cause unwanted effects such as vomiting, diarrhea, weak pulse, unstable blood pressure, and convulsions (seizures) in nursing babies.

**Children**—Methysergide can cause serious side effects in any patient. Therefore, it is especially important that you discuss with the child's doctor the good that this medicine may do as well as the risks of using it.

**Older adults**—Elderly people are especially sensitive to the effects of methysergide. This may increase the chance of side effects during treatment.

**Other medicines**—Although certain medicines should not be used together at all, in other cases two different medicines may be used together even if an interaction might occur. In these cases, your doctor may want to change the dose, or other precautions may be necessary. When you are taking methysergide, it is important that your

health care professional know if you are using any other prescription or nonprescription (over-the-counter [OTC]) medicine, or if you smoke.

**Other medical problems**—The presence of other medical problems may affect the use of methysergide. Make sure you tell your doctor if you have any other medical problems, especially:

- Arthritis or
- Heart or blood vessel disease or
- Infection or
- Itching (severe) or
- Kidney disease or
- Liver disease or
- Lung disease—The chance of serious side effects may be increased
- High blood pressure or
- Stomach ulcer—Methysergide can make your condition worse

## Proper Use of This Medicine

*Take this medicine only as directed by your doctor.* If the amount you are to take does not prevent your headaches from occurring as often as before, do not take more than your doctor ordered. Instead, check with your doctor. Taking too much of this medicine or taking it too frequently may cause serious effects such as nausea and vomiting; cold, painful hands or feet; or even gangrene.

*If this medicine upsets your stomach, it may be taken with meals or milk.* If stomach upset continues or is severe, check with your doctor.

**Dosing**—The dose of methysergide will be different for different patients. *Follow your doctor's orders or the directions on the label.* The following information includes only the average doses of methysergide. *If your dose is different, do not change it* unless your doctor tells you to do so.

- For *oral* dosage form (tablets:)
  —For preventing migraine and other throbbing headaches:
    - Adults—2 milligrams (mg) (one tablet) two or three times a day.
    - Children—Use is not recommended.

**Missed dose**—If you miss a dose of this medicine, skip the missed dose and go back to your regular dosing schedule. Do not double doses.

**Storage**—To store this medicine:
- Keep out of the reach of children.
- Store away from heat and direct light.
- Do not store in the bathroom, near the kitchen sink, or in other damp places. Heat or moisture may cause the medicine to break down.
- Do not keep outdated medicine or medicine no longer needed. Be sure that any discarded medicine is out of the reach of children.

## Precautions While Using This Medicine

If you have been taking this medicine regularly, *do not stop taking it without first checking with your doctor.* Your doctor may want you to reduce gradually the amount you are using before stopping completely. If you stop taking it suddenly, your headaches may return or worsen.

Your doctor will tell you how long you should take this medicine. Usually it is not taken for longer than 6 months at a time. *If the doctor tells you to stop taking the medicine for a while, do not continue to take it.* If your body does not get a rest from the medicine, it can have harmful effects.

This medicine may cause some people to become dizzy, lightheaded, drowsy, or less alert than they are normally. Even if taken at bedtime, it may cause some people to feel drowsy or less alert on arising. *Make sure you know how you react to this medicine before you drive, use machines, or do anything else that could be dangerous if you are dizzy or are not alert.*

If dizziness occurs, get up slowly after lying or sitting down. If the problem continues or gets worse, check with your doctor.

Since drinking alcoholic beverages may make headaches worse, it is best to avoid alcohol while you are suffering from them. If you have any questions about this, check with your doctor.

Since smoking may increase some of the harmful effects of this medicine, it is best to avoid smoking while you are using it. If you have any questions about this, check with your doctor.

This medicine may make you more sensitive to cold temperatures, especially if you have blood circulation problems. It tends to decrease blood circulation in the skin, fingers, and toes. Dress warmly during cold weather and be careful during prolonged exposure to cold, such as in winter sports. This is especially important for elderly people, who are more likely than younger adults to already have problems with their circulation.

Check with your doctor if a serious infection or illness of any kind occurs while you are taking methysergide, since an infection may make you more sensitive to the medicine's effects.

## Side Effects of This Medicine

Along with its needed effects, a medicine may cause some unwanted effects. Although not all of these side effects may occur, if they do occur they may need medical attention.

*Check with your doctor immediately* if any of the following side effects occur:

Chest pain or tightness in chest; difficult or painful urination; dizziness (severe); fever or chills; increase or decrease (large) in the amount of urine; leg cramps; pain in arms, legs, groin, lower back, or side; pale or cold hands or feet; shortness of breath or difficult breathing; swelling of hands, ankles, feet, or lower legs

Check with your doctor as soon as possible if the following side effects occur:

*More common*

Abdominal or stomach pain; itching; numbness and tingling of fingers, toes, or face; weakness in the legs

*Less common or rare*

Changes in vision; clumsiness or unsteadiness; cough or hoarseness; excitement or difficulty in thinking; fast or slow heartbeat; feeling of being outside the body; hallucinations (seeing, hearing, or feeling things that are not there); loss of appetite or weight loss; mental depression; nightmares; raised red spots on skin; redness or flushing of face; skin rash

Other side effects may occur that usually do not need medical attention. These side effects may go away during treatment as your body adjusts to the medicine. However, check with your doctor if any of the following side effects continue or are bothersome:

*More common*

Diarrhea; dizziness or lightheadedness, especially when you get up from a lying or sitting position; drowsiness; nausea or vomiting

*Less common or rare*

Constipation; heartburn; trouble in sleeping

After you stop using this medicine, your body may need time to adjust. The length of time this takes depends on the amount of medicine you were using and how long you used it. During this time check with your doctor if your headaches begin again or worsen.

Other side effects not listed above may also occur in some patients. If you notice any other effects, check with your doctor.

Revised: July 1990
Interim revision: 08/17/94

# METOCLOPRAMIDE Systemic

Some commonly used brand names are:

**In the U.S.—**
| | |
|---|---|
| Clopra | Reclomide |
| Octamide | Reglan |
| Octamide PFS | |

Generic name product may also be available.

**In Canada—**
| | |
|---|---|
| Apo-Metoclop | Maxeran |
| Emex | Reglan |

## Description

Metoclopramide (met-oh-KLOE-pra-mide) is a medicine that increases the movements or contractions of the stomach and intestines. When given by injection it is used to help diagnose certain problems of the stomach and/or intestines. It is also used by injection to prevent the nausea and vomiting that may occur after treatment with anticancer medicines. Another medicine may be used with metoclopramide to prevent side effects that may occur when metoclopramide is used with anticancer medicines.

When taken by mouth, metoclopramide is used to treat the symptoms of a certain type of stomach problem called diabetic gastroparesis. It relieves symptoms such as nausea, vomiting, continued feeling of fullness after meals, and loss of appetite. Metoclopramide is also used, for a short time, to treat symptoms such as heartburn in patients who suffer esophageal injury from a backward flow of gastric acid into the esophagus.

Metoclopramide may also be used for other conditions as determined by your doctor.

Metoclopramide is available only with your doctor's prescription. It is available in the following dosage forms:

*Oral*
- Tablets (U.S. and Canada)
- Syrup (U.S. and Canada)

*Parenteral*
- Injection (U.S. and Canada)

## Before Using This Medicine

In deciding to use a medicine, the risks of taking the medicine must be weighed against the good it will do. This is a decision you and your doctor will make. For metoclopramide, the following should be considered:

**Allergies**—Tell your doctor if you have ever had any unusual or allergic reaction to metoclopramide, procaine, or procainamide. Also tell your health care professional if you are allergic to any other substances, such as foods, preservatives, or dyes.

**Pregnancy**—Not enough studies have been done in humans to determine metoclopramide's safety during pregnancy. However, metoclopramide has not been shown to cause birth defects or other problems in animal studies.

**Breast-feeding**—Although metoclopramide passes into the breast milk, it has not been shown to cause problems in nursing babies.

**Children**—Muscle spasms, especially of jaw, neck, and back, and tic-like (jerky) movements of head and face may be especially likely to occur in children, who are usually more sensitive than adults to the effects of metoclopramide. Premature and full-term infants may develop blood problems if given high doses of metoclopramide.

**Older adults**—Shuffling walk and trembling and shaking of hands may be especially likely to occur in elderly patients after they have taken metoclopramide over a long time.

**Other medicines**—Although certain medicines should not be used together at all, in other cases 2 different medicines may be used together even if an interaction might occur. In these cases, your doctor may want to change the dose, or other precautions may be necessary. When you are taking metoclopramide, it is especially important that your health care professional know if you are taking the following:
- Central nervous system (CNS) depressants (medicine that causes drowsiness)—Use with metoclopramide may cause severe drowsiness

**Other medical problems**—The presence of other medical problems may affect the use of metoclopramide. Make sure you tell your doctor if you have any other medical problems, especially:
- Abdominal or stomach bleeding or
- Asthma or
- High blood pressure or
- Intestinal blockage or
- Parkinson's disease—Metoclopramide may make these conditions worse
- Epilepsy—Metoclopramide may increase the risk of having a seizure
- Kidney disease (severe) or
- Liver disease (severe)—Higher blood levels of metoclopramide may result, possibly increasing the chance of side effects

## Proper Use of This Medicine

*Take this medicine 30 minutes before meals and at bedtime,* unless otherwise directed by your doctor.

*Take metoclopramide only as directed.* Do not take more of it, do not take it more often, and do not take it for a longer time than your doctor ordered. To do so may increase the chance of side effects.

**Dosing**—The dose of metoclopramide will be different for different patients. *Follow your doctor's orders or the directions on the label.* The following information includes only the average doses of metoclopramide. *If your dose is different, do not change it* unless your doctor tells you to do so.

The number of tablets or teaspoonfuls of syrup that you take depends on the strength of the medicine. Also, *the number of doses you take each day, the time allowed between doses, and the length of time you take the medicine depend on the medical problem for which you are taking metoclopramide.*

- For *oral* dosage forms (syrup or tablets):
  —To treat the symptoms of a stomach problem called diabetic gastroparesis:
    • Adults and teenagers—10 milligrams (mg) thirty minutes before symptoms are likely to begin or before each meal and at bedtime. The dose may be taken up to four times a day. However, most people usually will not take more than 500 micrograms (mcg) per kilogram (kg) (227 mcg per pound) of body weight a day.
    • Children—Dose must be determined by your doctor.
  —For heartburn:
    • Adults and teenagers—10 to 15 mg thirty minutes before symptoms are likely to begin or before each meal and at bedtime. The dose may be taken up to four times a day. However, most people usually will not take more than 500 mcg per kg (227 mcg per pound) of body weight a day.
    • Children—Dose must be determined by your doctor.
  —To increase movements or contractions of the stomach and intestines:
    • Children 5 to 14 years of age—2.5 to 5 mg three times a day, thirty minutes before meals. Some children may receive 100 to 200 mcg per kg (45.5 to 90.9 mcg per pound) of body weight, thirty minutes before meals and at bedtime.
- For *injection* dosage form:
  —To increase movements or contractions of the stomach and intestine:
    • Adults and teenagers—10 mg injected into a vein.
    • Children—Dose is based on body weight and must be determined by your doctor. The usual dose is 1 mg per kilogram (kg) (0.45 mg per pound) of body weight injected into a vein. Your doctor may repeat this dose after sixty minutes if needed.
  —To prevent nausea and vomiting caused by anticancer medicines:
    • Adults and teenagers—Dose is based on body weight and must be determined by your doctor. The usual dose is 1 to 2 mg per kg (0.45 to 0.9 mg per pound) of body weight, injected slowly into a vein, thirty minutes before you take your anticancer medicine. Your doctor may repeat this dose every two or three hours if needed. Some people may need a larger dose to start.
    • Children—1 mg per kg (0.45 mg per pound) of body weight injected into a vein. Your doctor may repeat this dose after sixty minutes if needed.
  —To prevent vomiting after surgery:
    • Adults and teenagers—10 to 20 mg injected into a muscle near the end of surgery.
    • Children—Dose must be determined by your doctor.

**Missed dose**—If you miss a dose of this medicine, take it as soon as possible. However, if it is almost time for your next dose, skip the missed dose and go back to your regular dosing schedule. Do not double doses.

**Storage**—To store this medicine:
- Keep out of the reach of children.
- Store away from heat and direct light.
- Do not store the tablet form of this medicine in the bathroom, near the kitchen sink, or in other damp places. Heat or moisture may cause the medicine to break down.
- Keep the syrup form of this medicine from freezing.
- Do not keep outdated medicine or medicine no longer needed. Be sure that any discarded medicine is out of the reach of children.

## Precautions While Using This Medicine

This medicine will add to the effects of alcohol and other CNS depressants (medicines that slow down the nervous system, possibly causing drowsiness). Some examples of CNS depressants are antihistamines or medicine for hay fever, other allergies, or colds; sedatives, tranquilizers, or sleeping medicine; prescription pain medicine or narcotics; barbiturates; medicine for seizures; muscle relaxants; or anesthetics, including some dental anesthetics. *Check with your doctor before taking any of the above while you are using this medicine.*

This medicine may cause some people to become dizzy, lightheaded, drowsy, or less alert than they are normally. *Make sure you know how you react to this medicine before you drive, use machines, or do anything else that could be dangerous if you are dizzy or are not alert.*

## Side Effects of This Medicine

Along with its needed effects, a medicine may cause some unwanted effects. Although not all of these side effects may occur, if they do occur they may need medical attention.

Check with your doctor as soon as possible if any of the following side effects occur:

*Rare*

Chills; difficulty in speaking or swallowing; dizziness or fainting; fast or irregular heartbeat; fever; general feeling of tiredness or weakness; headache (severe or continuing); increase in blood pressure; lip smacking or puckering; loss of balance control; mask-like face; rapid or worm-like movements of tongue; shuffling walk; sore throat; stiffness of arms or legs; trembling and shaking of hands and fingers; uncontrolled chewing movements; uncontrolled movements of arms and legs

*With high doses—may occur within minutes of receiving a dose of metoclopramide and last for 2 to 24 hours*

Aching or discomfort in lower legs; panic-like sensation; sensation of crawling in legs; unusual nervousness, restlessness, or irritability

*Symptoms of overdose—may also occur rarely with usual doses, especially in children and young adults, and with high doses used to treat the nausea and vomiting caused by anticancer medicines*

Confusion; drowsiness (severe)

Other side effects may occur that usually do not need medical attention. These side effects may go away during treatment as your body adjusts to the medicine. However, check with your doctor if any of the following side effects continue or are bothersome:

*More common*

Diarrhea—with high doses; drowsiness; restlessness

*Less common or rare*

Breast tenderness and swelling; changes in menstruation; constipation; depression; increased flow of breast milk; nausea; skin rash; trouble in sleeping; unusual dryness of mouth; unusual irritability

Other side effects not listed above may also occur in some patients. If you notice any other effects, check with your doctor.

---

## Additional Information

Once a medicine has been approved for marketing for a certain use, experience may show that it is also useful for other medical problems. Although these uses are not included in product labeling, metoclopramide is used in certain patients with the following medical conditions:

- Failure of the stomach to empty its contents
- Nausea and vomiting caused by other medicines
- Persistent hiccups
- Prevention of aspirating fluid into the lungs during surgery
- Vascular headaches

Other than the above information, there is no additional information relating to proper use, precautions, or side effects for these uses.

---

Revised: 05/20/92
Interim revision: 08/16/94

---

# METRONIDAZOLE   Systemic

Some commonly used brand names are:

**In the U.S.—**

| | |
|---|---|
| Flagyl | Metric 21 |
| Flagyl I.V. | Metro I.V. |
| Flagyl I.V. RTU | Protostat |

Generic name product may also be available.

**In Canada—**

| | |
|---|---|
| Apo-Metronidazole | Novonidazol |
| Flagyl | Trikacide |

Generic name product may also be available.

---

## Description

Metronidazole (me-troe-NI-da-zole) is used to treat infections. It may also be used for other problems as determined by your doctor. It will not work for colds, flu, or other virus infections.

Metronidazole is available only with your doctor's prescription, in the following dosage forms:

*Oral*
- Capsules (Canada)
- Tablets (U.S. and Canada)

*Parenteral*
- Injection (U.S. and Canada)

---

## Before Using This Medicine

In deciding to use a medicine, the risks of taking the medicine must be weighed against the good it will do.

This is a decision you and your doctor will make. For metronidazole, the following should be considered:

**Allergies**—Tell your doctor if you have ever had any unusual or allergic reaction to metronidazole. Also tell your health care professional if you are allergic to any other substances, such as foods, preservatives, or dyes.

**Pregnancy**—Studies have not been done in humans. Metronidazole has not been shown to cause birth defects in animal studies; however, use is not recommended during the first trimester of pregnancy.

**Breast-feeding**—Use is not recommended in nursing mothers since metronidazole passes into the breast milk and may cause unwanted effects in the baby. However, in some infections your doctor may want you to stop breast-feeding and take this medicine for a short time. During this time the breast milk should be squeezed out or sucked out with a breast pump and thrown away. One or two days after you finish taking this medicine, you may go back to breast-feeding.

**Children**—Metronidazole has been used in children and, in effective doses, has not been shown to cause different side effects or problems in children than it does in adults.

**Older adults**—Many medicines have not been studied specifically in older people. Therefore, it may not be known whether they work exactly the same way they do in younger adults or if they cause different side effects or problems in older people. There is no specific information comparing use of metronidazole in the elderly with use in other age groups.

**Other medicines**—Although certain medicines should not be used together at all, in other cases two different medicines may be used together even if an interaction might occur. In these cases, your doctor may want to change the dose, or other precautions may be necessary. When you are taking metronidazole, it is especially important that your health care professional knows if you are taking any of the following:

- Anticoagulants (blood thinners)—Patients taking anticoagulants with metronidazole may have an increased chance of bleeding
- Disulfiram (e.g., Antabuse)—Patients taking disulfiram with metronidazole may have an increase in side effects affecting the central nervous system

**Other medical problems**—The presence of other medical problems may affect the use of metronidazole. Make sure you tell your doctor if you have any other medical problems, especially:

- Blood disease or a history of blood disease—Metronidazole may make the condition worse
- Central nervous system (CNS) disease, including epilepsy—Metronidazole may increase the chance of seizures (convulsions) or other CNS side effects
- Heart disease—Metronidazole by injection may make heart disease worse
- Liver disease, severe—Patients with severe liver disease may have an increase in side effects

## Proper Use of This Medicine

If this medicine upsets your stomach, it may be taken with meals or a snack. If stomach upset (nausea, vomiting, stomach pain, or diarrhea) continues, check with your doctor.

To help clear up your infection completely, *keep taking this medicine for the full time of treatment,* even if you begin to feel better after a few days. If you stop taking this medicine too soon, your symptoms may return.

In some kinds of infections, this medicine works best when there is a constant amount in the blood. *To help keep the amount constant, do not miss any doses. Also, it is best to take the doses at evenly spaced times, day and night.* For example, if you are to take 4 doses a day, the doses should be spaced about 6 hours apart. If this interferes with your sleep or other daily activities, or if you need help in planning the best times to take your medicine, check with your health care professional.

**Dosing**—The dose of metronidazole will be different for different patients. *Follow your doctor's orders or the directions on the label.* The following information includes only the average doses of metronidazole. *If your dose is different, do not change it* unless your doctor tells you to do so.

The number of capsules or tablets that you take depends on the strength of the medicine. Also, *the number of doses you take each day, the time allowed between doses, and the length of time you take the medicine depend on the medical problem for which you are taking metronidazole.*

- *For oral* dosage forms (capsules, tablets):
  —For bacterial infections:
  - Adults and teenagers—Dose is based on body weight. The usual dose is 7.5 milligrams (mg) per kilogram (kg) (3.4 mg per pound) of body weight, up to a maximum dose of 1 gram, every six hours for at least seven days.
  - Children—Dose is based on body weight. The usual dose is 7.5 mg per kg (3.4 mg per pound) of body weight every six hours; or 10 mg per kg (4.5 mg per pound) every eight hours.
  —For amebiasis infections:
  - Adults and teenagers—500 to 750 mg three times a day for five to ten days.
  - Children—Dose is based on body weight. The usual dose is 11.6 to 16.7 mg per kg (5.3 to 7.6 mg per pound) of body weight three times a day for ten days.
  —For trichomoniasis infections:
  - Adults and teenagers—A single dose of 2 grams; or 1 gram two times a day for one day; or 250 mg three times a day for seven days.
  - Children—Dose is based on body weight. The usual dose is 5 mg per kg (2.3 mg per pound) of body weight three times a day for seven days.
- For *injection* dosage form:
  —For bacterial infections:
  - Adults and children over 1 week of age—Dose is based on body weight. The usual dose is 15 mg per kg (6.8 mg per pound) of body weight one time to start, then 7.5 mg per kg (3.4 mg per pound) of body weight injected into a vein every six hours for at least seven days.
  - Preterm infants—Dose is based on body weight. The usual dose is 15 mg per kg (6.8 mg per pound) of body weight one time to start, then 7.5 mg per kg (3.4 mg per pound) of body weight, injected into a vein, every twelve hours starting forty-eight hours after the first dose.
  - Full-term infants—Dose is based on body weight. The usual dose is 15 mg per kg (6.8 mg per pound) of body weight one time to start, then 7.5 mg per kg (3.4 mg per pound) of body weight, injected into a vein, every twelve hours starting twenty-four hours after the first dose.
  —For treatment before and during bowel surgery:
  - Adults and teenagers—Dose is based on body weight. The usual dose is 15 mg per kg (6.8 mg per pound), injected into a vein, one hour before surgery, then 7.5 mg per kg (3.4 mg per pound) of body weight, injected into a vein, six hours and twelve hours after the first dose.
  - Children—Use and dose must be determined by your doctor.

**Missed dose**—If you miss a dose of this medicine, take it as soon as possible. This will help to keep a constant amount of medicine in the blood. However, if it is almost time for your next dose, skip the missed dose and go back to your regular dosing schedule. Do not double doses.

**Storage**—To store this medicine:
- Keep out of the reach of children.
- Store away from heat and direct light.
- Do not store the capsule or tablet form of this medicine in the bathroom, near the kitchen sink, or in other damp places. Heat or moisture may cause the medicine to break down.
- Do not keep outdated medicine or medicine no longer needed. Be sure that any discarded medicine is out of the reach of children.

## Precautions While Using This Medicine

If your symptoms do not improve within a few days, or if they become worse, check with your doctor.

Drinking alcoholic beverages while taking this medicine may cause stomach pain, nausea, vomiting, headache, or flushing or redness of the face. Other alcohol-containing preparations (for example, elixirs, cough syrups, tonics) may also cause problems. These problems may last for at least a day after you stop taking metronidazole. Also, this medicine may cause alcoholic beverages to taste different. Therefore, *you should not drink alcoholic beverages or take other alcohol-containing preparations while you are taking this medicine and for at least a day after stopping it.*

Metronidazole may cause dryness of the mouth, an unpleasant or sharp metallic taste, and a change in taste sensation. For temporary relief of dry mouth, use sugarless candy or gum, melt bits of ice in your mouth, or use a saliva substitute. However, if your mouth continues to feel dry for more than 2 weeks, check with your medical doctor or dentist. Continuing dryness of the mouth may increase the chance of dental disease, including tooth decay, gum disease, and fungus infections.

This medicine may also cause some people to become dizzy or lightheaded. *Make sure you know how you react to this medicine before you drive, use machines, or do anything else that could be dangerous if you are dizzy or are not alert.* If these reactions are especially bothersome, check with your doctor.

If you are taking this medicine for trichomoniasis (an infection of the sex organs in males and females), your doctor may want to treat your sexual partner at the same time you are being treated, even if he or she has no symptoms. Also, it may be desirable to use a condom (prophylactic) during intercourse. These measures will help keep you from getting the infection back again from your partner. If you have any questions about this, check with your doctor.

## Side Effects of This Medicine

Along with its needed effects, a medicine may cause some unwanted effects. Although not all of these side effects may occur, if they do occur they may need medical attention.

*Check with your doctor immediately* if any of the following side effects occur:
> *Less common*
>> Numbness, tingling, pain, or weakness in hands or feet
> *Rare*
>> Convulsions (seizures)

Also, check with your doctor as soon as possible if any of the following side effects occur:
> *Less common*
>> Any vaginal irritation, discharge, or dryness not present before use of this medicine; clumsiness or unsteadiness; mood or other mental changes; skin rash, hives, redness, or itching; sore throat and fever; stomach and back pain (severe)
> *For injection form*
>> Pain, tenderness, redness, or swelling over vein in which the medicine is given

Other side effects may occur that usually do not need medical attention. These side effects may go away during treatment as your body adjusts to the medicine. However, check with your doctor if any of the following side effects continue or are bothersome:
> *More common*
>> Diarrhea; dizziness or lightheadedness; headache; loss of appetite; nausea or vomiting; stomach pain or cramps
> *Less common or rare*
>> Change in taste sensation; dryness of mouth; unpleasant or sharp metallic taste

In some patients metronidazole may cause dark urine. This is only temporary and will go away when you stop taking this medicine.

Other side effects not listed above may also occur in some patients. If you notice any other effects, check with your doctor.

## Additional Information

Once a medicine has been approved for marketing for a certain use, experience may show that it is also useful for other medical problems. Although these uses are not included in product labeling, metronidazole is used in certain patients with the following medical conditions:
- Antibiotic-associated colitis
- Bacterial vaginosis
- Balantidiasis
- Dental infections
- Gastritis or ulcer due to *Helicobacter pylori*
- Giardiasis
- Inflammatory bowel disease

For patients taking this medicine for *giardiasis*:
- After treatment, it is important that your doctor check whether or not the infection in your intestinal tract has been cleared up completely.

Other than the above information, there is no additional information relating to proper use, precautions, or side effects for this use.

---

Revised: 10/20/92
Interim revision: 03/24/94

---

# METRONIDAZOLE    Topical

A commonly used brand name in the U.S. and Canada is MetroGel.

## Description

Topical metronidazole (me-troe-NI-da-zole) is applied to the skin in adults to help control rosacea (roe-ZAY-she-ah), also known as acne rosacea and "adult acne." This medicine helps to reduce the redness of the skin and the number of pimples, usually found on the face, in patients with rosacea.

Topical metronidazole is available only with your doctor's prescription, in the following dosage form:

*Topical*
- Gel (U.S. and Canada)

## Before Using This Medicine

In deciding to use a medicine, the risks of taking the medicine must be weighed against the good it will do. This is a decision you and your doctor will make. For topical metronidazole, the following should be considered:

**Allergies**—Tell your doctor if you have ever had any unusual or allergic reaction to metronidazole. Also tell your health care professional if you are allergic to any other substances, such as preservatives or dyes.

**Pregnancy**—Topical metronidazole has not been studied in pregnant women. However, metronidazole given by mouth (e.g., Flagyl) has not been shown to cause birth defects or other problems in animal studies.

**Breast-feeding**—Topical metronidazole is absorbed into the mother's body only in small amounts. The small amounts of this medicine that are absorbed are unlikely to cause serious problems in nursing babies.

**Children**—Rosacea is usually considered an adult disease. Therefore, topical metronidazole is not generally used in children.

**Older adults**—Many medicines have not been studied specifically in older people. Therefore, it may not be known whether they work exactly the same way they do in younger adults or if they cause different side effects or problems in older people. There is no specific information comparing use of topical metronidazole in the elderly with use in other age groups.

**Other medicines**—Although certain medicines should not be used together at all, in other cases two different medicines may be used together even if an interaction might occur. In these cases, your doctor may want to change the dose, or other precautions may be necessary. Tell your health care professional if you are using any other topical prescription or nonprescription (over-the-counter [OTC]) medicine that is to be applied to the same area of the skin.

## Proper Use of This Medicine

*Do not use this medicine in or near the eyes.* Watering of the eyes may occur when the medicine is used too close to the eyes.

If this medicine does get into your eyes, wash them out immediately, but carefully, with large amounts of cool tap water. If your eyes still burn or are painful, check with your doctor.

Before applying this medicine, thoroughly wash the affected area(s) with a mild, nonirritating cleanser, rinse well, and gently pat dry.

To use:
- After washing the affected area(s), apply this medicine with your fingertips.
- Apply and rub in a thin film of medicine, using enough to cover the affected area(s) lightly. *You should apply the medicine to the whole area usually affected by rosacea, not just to the pimples themselves.*
- Wash the medicine off your hands.

To help keep your rosacea under control, *keep using this medicine for the full time of treatment*. You may have to continue using this medicine every day for 9 weeks or longer. *Do not miss any doses.*

**Dosing**—The dose of topical metronidazole will be different for different patients. *Follow your doctor's orders or the directions on the label.* The following information includes only the average doses of topical metronidazole. *If your dose is different, do not change it* unless your doctor tells you to do so.

- For *topical* dosage form (gel):
  —For rosacea:
    • Adults—Apply to the affected area(s) of skin two times a day, morning and evening, for nine weeks.
    • Children—Use and dose must be determined by your doctor.

**Missed dose**—If you miss a dose of this medicine, apply it as soon as possible. However, if it is almost time for your next dose, skip the missed dose and go back to your regular dosing schedule.

**Storage**—To store this medicine:
- Keep out of the reach of children.
- Store away from heat and direct light.
- Keep the medicine from freezing.
- Do not keep outdated medicine or medicine no longer needed. Be sure that any discarded medicine is out of the reach of children.

## Precautions While Using This Medicine

If your rosacea does not improve within 3 weeks, or if it becomes worse, check with your doctor. However, treatment of rosacea may take up to 9 weeks or longer before you see full improvement.

Stinging or burning of the skin may be expected after this medicine is applied. These effects may last up to a few minutes or more. If irritation continues, check with

your doctor. You may have to use the medicine less often or stop using it altogether. Follow your doctor's directions.

You may continue to use cosmetics (make-up) while you are using this medicine for rosacea. However, it is best to use only "oil-free" cosmetics. Also, it is best not to use cosmetics too heavily or too often. They may make your rosacea worse. If you have any questions about this, check with your doctor.

## Side Effects of This Medicine

Along with its needed effects, a medicine may cause some unwanted effects. The following side effects may go away during treatment as your body adjusts to the medicine. However, check with your doctor if any of these effects continue or are bothersome:

*Less common*
  Dry skin; redness or other signs of skin irritation not present before use of this medicine; stinging or burning of the skin; watering of eyes

Other side effects not listed above may also occur in some patients. If you notice any other effects, check with your doctor.

Revised: 06/24/94

# METRONIDAZOLE    Vaginal

Some commonly used brand names are:
**In the U.S.—**
  MetroGel-Vaginal
**In Canada—**
  Flagyl

## Description

Metronidazole (me-troe-NI-da-zole), is used to treat certain vaginal infections. It works by killing bacteria. This medicine will not work for vaginal fungus or yeast infections.

Metronidazole is available only with your doctor's prescription, in the following dosage forms:
*Vaginal*
- Cream (Canada)
- Gel (U.S.)
- Inserts (tablets) (Canada)

## Before Using This Medicine

In deciding whether to use a medicine, the risks of using the medicine must be weighed against the good it will do. This is a decision you and your doctor will make. For

vaginal metronidazole, the following should be considered:

**Allergies**—Tell your doctor if you have ever had any unusual or allergic reaction to metronidazole. Also tell your health care professional if you are allergic to any other substances, such as foods, preservatives, or dyes.

**Pregnancy**—Vaginal metronidazole has not been studied in pregnant women. Metronidazole given by mouth (e.g., Flagyl) has not been shown to cause birth defects. Before taking this medicine, make sure your doctor knows if you are pregnant or if you may become pregnant.

**Breast-feeding**—Use is not recommended in nursing mothers since metronidazole passes into breast milk and may cause unwanted effects in the baby. In addition, metronidazole may change the taste of your breast milk. Your doctor may want you to stop breast-feeding and use this medicine for a short time. During this time the breast milk should be pumped or drawn out with a breast pump and thrown away. Two days after you finish using this medicine, you may go back to breast-feeding.

**Children**—Studies on these medicines have been done only in adult patients, and there is no specific information comparing use of vaginal metronidazole in children with use in other age groups.

**Older adults**—Many medicines have not been studied specifically in older people. Therefore, it may not be known whether they work exactly the same way they do in younger adults or if they cause different side effects or problems in older people. There is no specific information comparing use of metronidazole in the elderly with use in other age groups.

**Other medicines**—Although certain medicines should not be used together at all, in other cases two different medicines may be used together even if an interaction might occur. In these cases, your doctor may want to change the dose, or other precautions may be necessary. When you are using vaginal metronidazole it is especially important that your health care professional knows if you are taking any of the following:

- Alcohol or alcohol-containing medicines (e.g., NyQuil, Geritol)—Metronidazole can cause serious side effects such as abdominal cramping, flushing, headache, nausea, or vomiting when it is used with alcohol
- Anticoagulants (blood thinners)—Taking metronidazole may increase the effects of anticoagulants, changing the amount you need to take
- Disulfiram (e.g., Antabuse)—Severe confusion or mental problems can occur if metronidazole is used together with disulfiram or if it is used up to 2 weeks after disulfiram treatment has been stopped

**Other medical problems**—The presence of other medical problems may affect the use of vaginal metronidazole. Make sure you tell your doctor if you have any other medical problems, especially:

- Central nervous system (CNS) disease, including epilepsy—Metronidazole may increase the chance of seizures (convulsions) or other side effects
- Liver disease, severe—Patients with severe liver disease may have an increase in side effects
- Low white blood cell count (or history of)—Metronidazole may make the condition worse

## Proper Use of This Medicine

*Wash your hands before and after using the medicine.* Also, keep the medicine out of your eyes.

If this medicine does get into your eyes, wash them out immediately, but carefully, with large amounts of tap water. If your eyes still burn or are painful, check with your doctor.

Vaginal metronidazole products usually come with patient directions. Read them carefully before using this medicine.

Use vaginal metronidazole exactly as directed by your doctor.

- *To fill the applicator*
  —For cream or gel dosage forms:
    - Break the metal seal at the opening of the tube by using the point on the top of the cap.
    - Screw the applicator onto the tube.
    - Squeeze the medicine into the applicator slowly until it is full.
    - Remove the applicator from the tube. Replace the cap on the tube.
  —For insert dosage form:
    - Place the insert into the applicator. Wet the insert with water for a few seconds.
- *To insert vaginal metronidazole using the applicator*
  —For all dosage forms:
    - Relax while lying on your back with your knees bent.
    - Hold the full applicator in one hand. Insert it slowly into the vagina. Stop before it becomes uncomfortable.
    - Slowly press the plunger until it stops.
    - Withdraw the applicator. The medicine will be left behind in the vagina.
- *To care for the applicator*
  —For all dosage forms:
    - Clean the applicator after use by pulling the plunger out of the applicator and washing both parts completely in warm soapy water.
    - Rinse well.
    - After drying the applicator, replace the plunger.

To help clear up your infection completely, *it is very important that you keep using this medicine for the full time of treatment,* even if your symptoms begin to clear up after a few days. If you stop using this medicine too soon, your symptoms may return. *Do not miss any doses.* Also, *continue using this medicine even if your menstrual period starts during the time of treatment.*

**Dosing**—The dose of vaginal metronidazole will be different for different patients. The following information includes only the average doses of vaginal metronidazole. *If your dose is different, do not change it* unless your doctor tells you to do so.

- *For vaginal cream* dosage form:
  —For bacterial vaginosis or trichomoniasis:
    - Adults and teenagers—One applicatorful (500 milligrams [mg]), inserted into the vagina. Use the medicine one or two times a day for ten or twenty days.
    - Children—Use and dose must be determined by your doctor.
- *For vaginal gel* dosage form:
  —For bacterial vaginosis:
    - Adults and teenagers—One applicatorful (37.5 mg), inserted into the vagina two times a

day. Use the medicine once in the morning and once in the evening for five days.
- Children—Use and dose must be determined by your doctor.

- *For vaginal inserts* dosage form:
  —For bacterial vaginosis or trichomoniasis:
    - Adults and teenagers—One 500-mg insert, inserted high into the vagina. Use the medicine once a day in the evening for ten or twenty days.
    - Children—Use and dose must be determined by your doctor.

**Missed dose**—If you miss a dose of this medicine, use it as soon as possible. However, if it is almost time for your next dose, skip the missed dose and go back to your regular dosing schedule.

**Storage**—To store this medicine:
- Keep out of the reach of children.
- Store away from heat and direct light.
- Do not store the vaginal inserts in the bathroom, near the kitchen sink, or in other damp places. Heat or moisture may cause the medicine to break down.
- Keep this medicine from freezing.
- Do not keep outdated medicine or medicine no longer needed. Be sure that any discarded medicine is out of the reach of children.

## Precautions While Using This Medicine

If your symptoms do not improve within a few days, or if they become worse, check with your doctor.

It is important that you visit your doctor after you have used all your medicine to make sure that the infection is gone.

Drinking alcoholic beverages while using this medicine may cause stomach pain, nausea, vomiting, headache, or flushing or redness of the face. Alcohol-containing medicines (for example, elixirs, cough syrups, tonics) may also cause problems. The chance of these problems occurring may continue for at least a day after you stop using metronidazole. Therefore, *you should not drink alcoholic beverages or take other alcohol-containing medicines while you are using this medicine and for at least a day after stopping it.*

This medicine may cause some people to become dizzy or lightheaded. *Make sure you know how you react to this medicine before you drive, use machines, or do anything else that could be dangerous if you are dizzy or are not alert.* If these reactions are especially bothersome, check with your doctor.

Vaginal medicines usually leak out of the vagina during treatment. To keep the medicine from getting on your clothing, wear a minipad or sanitary napkin. *Do not use tampons* (like those used for menstrual periods) since they may soak up the medicine.

*To help clear up your infection completely and to help make sure it does not return,* good health habits are also required.
- Wear cotton panties (or panties or pantyhose with cotton crotches) instead of synthetic (for example, nylon or rayon) panties.
- Wear only freshly washed panties daily.

*Do not have sexual intercourse while you are using this medicine.* Having sexual intercourse may reduce the strength of the medicine. This may cause the medicine to not work as well.

Many vaginal infections (for example, trichomoniasis) are spread by having sexual intercourse. You can give the infection to your sexual partner, and he can give the infection back to you later. Your partner may also need to be treated for some infections. *Until you are sure that the infection is completely cleared up after your treatment with this medicine, your partner should wear a condom during sexual intercourse.* If you have any questions about this, check with your health care professional.

## Side Effects of This Medicine

Along with its needed effects, a medicine may cause some unwanted effects. Although not all of these side effects may occur, if they do occur they may need medical attention.

Check with your doctor as soon as possible if any of the following side effects occur:
*More common*
Itching in the vagina; pain during sexual intercourse; thick, white vaginal discharge with no odor or with a mild odor

*Less common*
Abdominal or stomach cramping or pain; burning or irritation of penis of sexual partner; burning on urination or need to urinate more often; itching, stinging or redness of the genital area

Other side effects may occur that usually do not need medical attention. These side effects may go away during treatment as your body adjusts to the medicine. However, check with your doctor if any of the following side effects continue or are bothersome:
*Less common*
Diarrhea; dizziness or lightheadedness; dryness of mouth; headache; feeling of a furry tongue; loss of appetite; metallic taste or other change in taste sensation; nausea; vomiting

Metronidazole may cause your urine to become dark. This is harmless and will go away when you stop using this medicine.

After you stop using this medicine, your body may need time to adjust. The length of time this takes depends on the amount of medicine you were using and how long you used it. During this period of time check with your doctor if you notice any of the following side effects:

> Any vaginal or genital irritation or itching; pain during sexual intercouse; thick, white discharge not present before treatment, with no odor or with a mild odor

Other side effects not listed above may also occur in some patients. If you notice any other effects, check with your doctor.

---

Developed: 05/16/94

---

# METYRAPONE    Systemic

A commonly used brand name is:

**In the U.S.—**
Metopirone
**In Canada—**
Metopirone

---

## Description

Metyrapone (me-TEER-a-pone) is used in the diagnosis of certain problems of the adrenal glands. These glands are located near the kidneys. The adrenal glands produce a steroid chemical called cortisol (hydrocortisone) that helps the body respond to stress or illness. From the results of a metyrapone test, your doctor will be able to tell if your adrenal glands produce the correct amount of cortisol under stress or during illnesses.

How test is done: Metyrapone is taken by mouth in one or more doses the day before the testing is done. The next day, blood and/or urine samples are taken. A tube called a catheter may be placed in your bladder to help take the urine sample. The amount of hormones in your blood or urine is measured. Then the results of the test are studied.

Metyrapone may also be used for other conditions as determined by your doctor.

Metyrapone is available only with your doctor's prescription, in the following dosage form:

*Oral*
- Tablets (U.S. and Canada)

## Before Using This Medicine

In deciding to use a medicine, the risks of taking the medicine must be weighed against the good it will do. This is a decision you and your doctor will make. For metyrapone, the following should be considered:

**Allergies**—Tell your doctor if you have ever had any unusual or allergic reaction to metyrapone. Also, tell your health care professional if you are allergic to any other substances, such as foods, preservatives, or dyes.

**Pregnancy**—Metyrapone has not been fully studied in pregnant women. However, some small studies have shown that metyrapone can affect the production of chemicals by the pituitary and adrenal glands of the fetus. Also, the large amounts of estrogen produced by your body

during pregnancy may cause false results in metyrapone testing. Before you take metyrapone, make sure your doctor knows if you are pregnant or if you may become pregnant.

**Breast-feeding**—It is not known whether metyrapone passes into the breast milk. However, use of metyrapone is not recommended during breast-feeding because it may cause unwanted effects in nursing babies.

**Children**—This medicine has been tested in children and has not been shown to cause different side effects or problems in children than it does in adults.

**Older adults**—Although there is no specific information about the use of metyrapone in the elderly, it is not expected to cause different side effects or problems in older people than it does in younger adults.

**Other medicines**—Although certain medicines should not be used together at all, in other cases 2 different medicines may be used together even if an interaction might occur. In these cases, your doctor may want to change the dose, or other precautions may be necessary. When you are taking metyrapone, it is especially important that your health care professional know if you are also taking any other medicines, since many medicines can cause false results in metyrapone testing. This may result in a wrong diagnosis. It is especially important that your doctor know if you are taking any of the following:

- Alcohol (with chronic use)
- Barbiturates
- Carbamazepine (e.g., Tegretol)
- Corticosteroids (cortisone-like medicine)
- Estrogens (female hormones)
- Griseofulvin (e.g., Fulvicin)
- Oral contraceptives (birth control pills) containing estrogen
- Phenylbutazone (e.g., Butazolidin)
- Phenytoin (e.g., Dilantin)
- Primidone (e.g., Mysoline)
- Rifampin (e.g., Rifadin)

**Other medical problems**—The presence of other medical problems may affect the use of metyrapone. Make sure you tell your doctor if you have any other medical problems, especially:

- Breast cancer or
- Diabetes mellitus (sugar diabetes) or
- Heart disease or
- Liver disease or

- Low blood sugar or
- Thyroid disease—These conditions may cause false results in metyrapone testing and result in a wrong diagnosis
- Excessive body hair in females—Long-term use may increase growth of body hair
- Porphyria—Metyrapone may worsen active cases of porphyria
- Underactive adrenal or pituitary gland—Metyrapone may severely reduce the amount of certain hormones produced by the adrenal glands; these hormones are needed to respond to stress or illness

## Proper Use of This Medicine

Metyrapone may cause nausea and vomiting, especially if taken in larger doses. Taking each dose with food or milk or immediately after eating may lessen this effect.

Before you have any medical tests, tell the doctor in charge that you are taking this medicine. The results of some tests may be affected by this medicine.

**Dosing**—The dose of metyrapone will be different for different patients. *Follow your doctor's orders.* The dose will be given by your doctor. The following information includes only the average doses of metyrapone.

- For *tablet* dosage form:
  —For testing the adrenal glands:
  - Adults—750 milligrams (mg) (3 tablets) every four hours for six doses. Or, your doctor may want you to take 2000 to 3000 mg (8 to 12 tablets) as a single dose at eleven p.m.
  - Children—Dose is based on body weight and must be determined by your doctor. The usual dose is 15 mg per kilogram (kg) (6.8 mg per pound) of body weight every four hours for six doses.

**Missed dose**—If you are taking metyrapone every day to treat Cushing's syndrome and you miss a dose, take it as soon as possible. However, if it is almost time for your next dose, skip the missed dose and go back to your regular dosing schedule. Do not double doses. If you are taking metyrapone for a test procedure and you miss a dose, contact your physician. Missing doses or taking them on the wrong schedule may cause false test results.

**Storage**—To store this medicine:
- Keep out of the reach of children.
- Store away from heat and direct light.
- Do not store in the bathroom, near the kitchen sink, or in other damp places. Heat or moisture may cause the medicine to break down.
- Do not keep outdated medicine or medicine no longer needed. Be sure that any discarded medicine is out of the reach of children.

## Precautions While Using This Medicine

This medicine may cause some people to become dizzy, lightheaded, drowsy, or less alert than they are normally. Even if taken at bedtime, it may cause some people to feel drowsy or less alert on arising. *Make sure you know how you react to this medicine before you drive, use machines, or do anything else that could be dangerous if you are dizzy or are not alert.*

## Side Effects of This Medicine

Along with its needed effects, a medicine may cause some unwanted effects. Although not all of these side effects may occur, if they do occur they may need medical attention.

*Check with your doctor immediately* if any of the following side effects occur:
*Rare (with long-term use)*
  Irregular heartbeat

Check with your doctor as soon as possible if any of the following side effects occur:
*Less common*
  Skin rash
*Rare (usually with long-term use)*
  Enlargement of clitoris; muscle cramps or pain; sore throat or fever; swelling of feet or lower legs; unusual bleeding or bruising; unusual tiredness or weakness; weight gain (rapid)
*Symptoms of overdose*
  Abdominal or stomach pain (severe); confusion; decrease in consciousness; diarrhea (severe); nausea (severe); nervousness; unusual thirst; vomiting (severe); weakness (sudden)

Other side effects may occur that usually do not need medical attention. These side effects may go away during treatment as your body adjusts to the medicine. However, check with your doctor if any of the following side effects continue or are bothersome:
*More common*
  Dizziness; drowsiness; headache; lightheadedness; nausea
*Rare*
  Confusion or mental slowing; excessive hair growth; greater-than-normal loss of scalp hair; increased sweating; loss of appetite; upper abdominal or stomach pain; vomiting; worsening of acne

Other side effects not listed above may also occur in some patients. If you notice any other effects, check with your doctor.

## Additional Information

Once a medicine has been approved for marketing for a certain use, experience may show that it is also useful for other medical problems. Although this use is not included in product labeling, metyrapone is used in certain patients with the following medical condition:
- Cushing's syndrome (diagnosis and treatment)

Since treatment for Cushing's syndrome may require longer therapy, side effects are more likely to occur.

Revised: 07/08/92
Interim revision: 06/30/94

# METYROSINE    Systemic†

A commonly used brand name in the U.S. is Demser.

†Not commercially available in Canada.

## Description

Metyrosine (me-TYE-roe-seen) belongs to the general class of medicines called antihypertensives. It is used to treat high blood pressure (hypertension) caused by a disease called pheochromocytoma (a noncancerous tumor of the adrenal gland).

Metyrosine reduces the amount of certain chemicals in the body. When these chemicals are present in large amounts, they cause high blood pressure.

Metyrosine is available only with your doctor's prescription, in the following dosage form:

*Oral*
- Capsules (U.S.)

## Before Using This Medicine

In deciding to use a medicine, the risks of taking the medicine must be weighed against the good it will do. This is a decision you and your doctor will make. For metyrosine, the following should be considered:

**Allergies**—Tell your doctor if you have ever had any unusual or allergic reaction to metyrosine. Also tell your health care professional if you are allergic to any other substances, such as foods, sulfites or other preservatives, or dyes.

**Pregnancy**—Studies on effects in pregnancy have not been done in either humans or animals.

**Breast-feeding**—It is not known whether metyrosine passes into breast milk. However, this medicine has not been reported to cause problems in nursing babies.

**Children**—Studies on this medicine have been done only in adult patients, and there is no specific information comparing use of metyrosine in children with use in other age groups.

**Older adults**—Many medicines have not been studied specifically in older people. Therefore, it may not be known whether they work exactly the same way they do in younger adults or if they cause different side effects or problems in older people. There is no specific information comparing use of metyrosine in the elderly with use in other age groups.

**Other medicines**—Although certain medicines should not be used together at all, in other cases two different medicines may be used together even if an interaction might occur. In these cases, your doctor may want to change the dose, or other precautions may be necessary. Tell your health care professional if you are taking any other prescription or nonprescription (over-the-counter [OTC]) medicine.

**Other medical problems**—The presence of other medical problems may affect the use of metyrosine. Make sure you tell your doctor if you have any other medical problems, especially:
- Kidney disease or
- Liver disease—Effects of metyrosine may be increased because of slower removal from the body
- Mental depression (or history of) or
- Parkinson's disease—Metyrosine may make these conditions worse

## Proper Use of This Medicine

*Take this medicine only as directed by your doctor.* Do not take more or less of it than your doctor ordered.

To help you remember to take your medicine, try to get into the habit of taking it at the same times each day.

**Dosing**—The dose of metyrosine will be different for different patients. *Follow your doctor's orders or the directions on the label.* The following information includes only the average doses of metyrosine. *If your dose is different, do not change it* unless your doctor tells you to do so:
- For *oral* dosage forms (capsules):
  —Adults and children 12 years of age and older: 1000 milligrams to 3000 milligrams (1 to 3 grams) a day, divided into four doses.

**Missed dose**—If you miss a dose of this medicine, take it as soon as possible. However, if it is almost time for your next dose, skip the missed dose and go back to your regular dosing schedule. Do not double doses.

**Storage**—To store this medicine:
- Keep out of the reach of children.
- Store away from heat and direct light.
- Do not store in the bathroom, near the kitchen sink, or in other damp places. Heat or moisture may cause the medicine to break down.
- Do not keep outdated medicine or medicine no longer needed. Be sure that any discarded medicine is out of the reach of children.

## Precautions While Using This Medicine

It is important that your doctor check your progress at regular visits to make sure that this medicine is working properly and to check for unwanted effects.

*While taking this medicine, it is important that you drink plenty of fluids and urinate often.* This will help prevent kidney problems and keep your kidneys working well. If you have any questions about how much you should drink, check with your doctor.

This medicine will add to the effects of alcohol and other CNS depressants (medicines that slow down the nervous system, possibly causing drowsiness). Some examples of CNS depressants are antihistamines or medicine for hay fever, other allergies, or colds; sedatives, tranquilizers, or sleeping medicine; prescription pain medicine or narcotics; barbiturates; medicine for seizures; tricyclic antidepressants (medicine for depression); muscle relaxants; or anesthetics, including some dental anesthetics. *Check with your doctor before taking any of the above while you are taking this medicine.*

*Before having any kind of surgery (including dental surgery), tell the medical doctor or dentist in charge that you are taking this medicine.*

This medicine may cause most people to become drowsy or less alert than they are normally. *Make sure you know how you react to this medicine before you drive, use machines, or do anything else that could be dangerous if you are not alert.*

## Side Effects of This Medicine

Along with its needed effects, a medicine may cause some unwanted effects. Although not all of these side effects may occur, if they do occur they may need medical attention.

Check with your doctor as soon as possible if any of the following side effects occur:

*More common*
  Diarrhea; drooling; trembling and shaking of hands and fingers; trouble in speaking

*Less common*
  Anxiety; confusion; hallucinations (seeing, hearing, or feeling things that are not there); mental depression

*Rare*
  Black, tarry stools; blood in urine or stools; unusual bleeding or bruising; muscle spasms, especially of neck and back; painful urination; pinpoint red spots on skin; restlessness; shortness of breath; shuffling walk; skin rash and itching; swelling of feet or lower legs; tic-like (jerky) movements of head, face, mouth, and neck; unusual tiredness or weakness

Other side effects may occur that usually do not need medical attention. These side effects may go away during treatment as your body adjusts to the medicine. However, check with your doctor if any of the following side effects continue or are bothersome:

*More common*
  Drowsiness

*Less common*
  Decreased sexual ability in men; dryness of mouth; nausea, vomiting, or stomach pain; stuffy nose; swelling of breasts or unusual milk production

After you stop taking this medicine, it may still produce some side effects that need attention. During this period of time check with your doctor if you notice the following side effect:

  Diarrhea

Also, after you stop taking this medicine, you may have feelings of increased energy or you may have trouble sleeping. However, these effects should last only for two or three days.

Other side effects not listed above may also occur in some patients. If you notice any other effects, check with your doctor.

Revised: 01/20/93

# MEXILETINE  Systemic

A commonly used brand name in the U.S. and Canada is Mexitil.

## Description

Mexiletine (MEX-i-le-teen) belongs to the group of medicines known as antiarrhythmics. It is used to correct irregular heartbeats to a normal rhythm.

Mexiletine produces its helpful effects by slowing nerve impulses in the heart and making the heart tissue less sensitive.

Mexiletine is available only with your doctor's prescription, in the following dosage form:

*Oral*
  • Capsules (U.S. and Canada)

## Before Using This Medicine

In deciding to use a medicine, the risks of taking the medicine must be weighed against the good it will do. This is a decision you and your doctor will make. For mexiletine, the following should be considered:

**Allergies**—Tell your doctor if you have ever had any unusual or allergic reaction to mexiletine, lidocaine, or tocainide. Also tell your health care professional if you are allergic to any other substance, such as foods, preservatives, or dyes.

**Pregnancy**—Mexiletine has not been studied in pregnant women. However, studies in animals have shown that mexiletine causes a decrease in successful pregnancies but no birth defects. Before taking this medicine, make sure your doctor knows if you are pregnant or if you may become pregnant.

**Breast-feeding**—Mexiletine passes into breast milk. Because this medicine may cause serious side effects, breast-feeding is generally not recommended while you are receiving it. Be sure you have discussed this with your doctor before taking mexiletine.

**Children**—Studies on this medicine have been done only in adult patients, and there is no specific information comparing use of mexiletine in children with use in other age groups.

**Older adults**—Many medicines have not been studied specifically in older people. Therefore, it may not be known whether they work exactly the same way they do in younger adults or if they cause different side effects or problems in older people. There is no specific information comparing use of mexiletine in the elderly with use in other age groups.

**Other medicines**—Although certain medicines should not be used together at all, in other cases two different medicines may be used together even if an interaction might occur. In these cases, your doctor may want to change the dose, or other precautions may be necessary. Tell your health care professional if you are taking any other prescription or nonprescription (over-the-counter [OTC]) medicine.

**Smoking**—Smoking may decrease the effects of mexiletine.

**Other medical problems**—The presence of other medical problems may affect the use of mexiletine. Make sure you tell your doctor if you have any other medical problems, especially:

- Congestive heart failure or
- Low blood pressure—Mexiletine may make these conditions worse
- Heart attack (severe) or
- Liver disease—Effects may last longer because of slower removal of mexiletine from the body
- Seizures (history of)—Mexiletine can cause seizures

## Proper Use of This Medicine

*Take mexiletine exactly as directed by your doctor*, even though you may feel well. Do not take more medicine than ordered.

To lessen the possibility of stomach upset, mexiletine should be taken with food or immediately after meals or with milk or an antacid.

This medicine works best when there is a constant amount in the blood. *To help keep this amount constant, do not miss any doses. Also it is best to take the doses at evenly spaced times day and night.* For example, if you are to take 3 doses a day, the doses should be spaced about 8 hours apart. If this interferes with your sleep or other daily activities, or if you need help in planning the best times to take your medicine, check with your health care professional.

**Dosing**—The dose of mexiletine will be different for different patients. *Follow your doctor's orders or the directions on the label.* The following information includes only the average dose of mexiletine. *If your dose is different, do not change it* unless your doctor tells you to do so.

The number of capsules that you take depends on the strength of the medicine.

- For *oral* dosage form (capsules):
  —For irregular heartbeat (arrhythmias):
    - Adults—At first, 200 milligrams (mg) every eight hours. Then, your doctor may raise or lower your dose as needed.
    - Children—Use and dose must be determined by your doctor.

**Missed dose**—If you miss a dose of this medicine and remember within 4 hours, take it as soon as possible. Then go back to your regular dosing schedule. However, if you do not remember until later, skip the missed dose and go back to your regular dosing schedule. Do not double doses.

**Storage**—To store this medicine:

- Keep out of the reach of children.
- Store away from heat and direct light.
- Do not store in the bathroom, near the kitchen sink, or in other damp places. Heat or moisture may cause the medicine to break down.
- Do not keep outdated medicine or medicine no longer needed. Be sure that any discarded medicine is out of the reach of children.

## Precautions While Using This Medicine

It is important that your doctor check your progress at regular visits to make sure the medicine is working properly. This will allow for changes to be made in the amount of medicine you are taking, if necessary.

Your doctor may want you to carry a medical identification card or bracelet stating that you are using this medicine.

*Before having any kind of surgery (including dental surgery) or emergency treatment, tell the medical doctor or dentist in charge that you are taking this medicine.*

Mexiletine may cause some people to become dizzy, lightheaded, or less alert than they are normally. *Make sure you know how you react to this medicine before you drive, use machines, or do anything else that could be dangerous if you are dizzy or are not alert.*

## Side Effects of This Medicine

Along with its needed effects, a medicine may cause some unwanted effects. Although not all of these side effects may occur, if they do occur they may need medical attention.

Check with your doctor as soon as possible if any of the following side effects occur:

*Less common*
Chest pain; fast or irregular heartbeat; shortness of breath

*Rare*
Convulsions (seizures); fever or chills; unusual bleeding or bruising

Other side effects may occur that usually do not need medical attention. These side effects may go away during treatment as your body adjusts to the medicine. However, check with your doctor if any of the following side effects continue or are bothersome:

*More common*
Dizziness or lightheadedness; heartburn; nausea and vomiting; nervousness; trembling or shaking of the hands; unsteadiness or difficulty in walking

*Less common*
Blurred vision; confusion; constipation or diarrhea; headache; numbness or tingling of fingers and toes; ringing in the ears; skin rash; slurred speech; trouble in sleeping; unusual tiredness or weakness

Other side effects not listed above may also occur in some patients. If you notice any other effects, check with your doctor.

Revised: 10/06/92
Interim revision: 07/14/94

---

# MICONAZOLE    Topical

Some commonly used brand names are:

**In the U.S.—**
Micatin                          Zeasorb-AF
Monistat-Derm
Generic name product may also be available.

**In Canada—**
Micatin                          Monistat-Derm

## Description

Miconazole (mi-KON-a-zole) belongs to the group of medicines called antifungals. Topical miconazole is used to treat some types of fungus infections.

Some of these preparations may be available without a prescription; however, your doctor may have special instructions on the proper use of these medicines for your medical problem. Others are available only with your doctor's prescription.

Topical miconazole is available in the following dosage forms:

*Topical*
- Aerosol powder (U.S.)
- Aerosol solution (U.S.)
- Cream (U.S. and Canada)
- Lotion (U.S. and Canada)
- Powder (U.S.)

## Before Using This Medicine

If you are using this medicine without a prescription, carefully read and follow any precautions on the label. For miconazole, the following should be considered:

**Allergies**—Tell your doctor if you have ever had any unusual or allergic reaction to miconazole. Also, tell your health care professional if you are allergic to any other substances, such as preservatives or dyes.

**Pregnancy**—Miconazole topical preparations have not been shown to cause birth defects or other problems in humans.

**Breast-feeding**—Miconazole topical preparations have not been reported to cause problems in nursing babies.

**Children**—Although there is no specific information comparing use of topical miconazole in children with use in other age groups, this medicine is not expected to cause different side effects or problems in children than it does in adults.

**Older adults**—Many medicines have not been studied specifically in older people. Therefore, it may not be known whether they work exactly the same way they do in younger adults. Although there is no specific information comparing use of topical miconazole in the elderly with use in other age groups, this medicine is not expected to cause different side effects or problems in older people than it does in younger adults.

**Other medicines**—Although certain medicines should not be used together at all, in other cases two different medicines may be used together even if an interaction might occur. In these cases, your doctor may want to change the dose, or other precautions may be necessary. Tell your health care professional if you are using any other topical prescription or nonprescription (over-the-counter [OTC]) medicine that is to be applied to the same area of the skin.

## Proper Use of This Medicine

*Keep this medicine away from the eyes.*

Apply enough miconazole to cover the affected area, and rub in gently.

To use the *aerosol powder form* of miconazole:
- Shake well before using.
- From a distance of 6 to 10 inches, spray the powder on the affected areas. If it is used on the feet, spray it between the toes, on the feet, and in the socks and shoes.
- Do not inhale the powder.
- Do not use near heat, near open flame, or while smoking.

To use the *aerosol solution form* of miconazole:
- Shake well before using.
- From a distance of 4 to 6 inches, spray the solution on the affected areas. If it is used on the feet, spray it between the toes and on the feet.
- Do not inhale the vapors from the spray.
- Do not use near heat, near open flame, or while smoking.

To use the *powder form* of miconazole:
- If the powder is used on the feet, sprinkle it between the toes, on the feet, and in the socks and shoes.

When miconazole is used to treat certain types of fungus infections of the skin, an occlusive dressing (airtight covering, such as kitchen plastic wrap) should *not* be applied over this medicine. To do so may cause irritation of the skin. *Do not apply an occlusive dressing over this medicine unless you have been directed to do so by your doctor.*

To help clear up your infection completely, *keep using this medicine for the full time of treatment,* even if your condition has improved. *Do not miss any doses.*

**Dosing**—The dose of topical miconazole will be different for different patients. *Follow your doctor's orders or the directions on the label.* The following information includes only the average doses of topical miconazole. *If your dose is different, do not change it* unless your doctor tells you to do so.
- For *aerosol powder, aerosol solution, cream,* and *powder* dosage forms:
  —For fungus infections:
    - Adults and children—Apply to the affected area(s) of the skin two times a day, morning and evening.

- For *cream* and *lotion* dosage forms:
  —For sun fungus:
    - Adults and children—Apply to the affected area(s) of the skin once a day.

**Missed dose**—If you miss a dose of this medicine, apply it as soon as possible. However, if it is almost time for your next dose, skip the missed dose and go back to your regular dosing schedule.

**Storage**—To store this medicine:
- Keep out of the reach of children.
- Store away from heat and direct light.
- Do not store the powder form of this medicine in the bathroom, near the kitchen sink, or in other damp places. Heat or moisture may cause the medicine to break down.
- Keep the cream, lotion, and aerosol solution forms of this medicine from freezing.
- Do not puncture, break, or burn the aerosol powder or aerosol solution container.
- Do not keep outdated medicine or medicine no longer needed. Be sure that any discarded medicine is out of the reach of children.

## Precautions While Using This Medicine

If your skin problem does not improve within 4 weeks, or if it becomes worse, check with your health care professional.

## Side Effects of This Medicine

Along with its needed effects, a medicine may cause some unwanted effects. Although not all of these side effects may occur, if they do occur they may need medical attention.

Check with your doctor as soon as possible if any of the following side effects occur:

> Blistering, burning, redness, skin rash, or other sign of skin irritation not present before use of this medicine

Other side effects not listed above may also occur in some patients. If you notice any other effects, check with your doctor.

Revised: 07/25/94

# MIDAZOLAM   Systemic

A commonly used brand name in the U.S. and Canada is Versed.

## Description

Midazolam (mid-AY-zoe-lam) is used to produce sleepiness or drowsiness and to relieve anxiety before surgery or certain procedures. It is also used to produce loss of consciousness before and during surgery.

*Midazolam is given only by or under the immediate supervision of a doctor trained to use this medicine.* If you will be receiving midazolam during surgery, your doctor or anesthesiologist will give you the medicine and closely follow your progress.

Midazolam is available in the following dosage form:
*Parenteral*
- Injection (U.S. and Canada)

## Before Receiving This Medicine

In deciding to use a medicine, the risks of taking the medicine must be weighed against the good it will do. This is a decision you and your doctor will make. For midazolam, the following should be considered:

**Allergies**—Tell your doctor if you have ever had any unusual or allergic reaction to midazolam or other benzodiazepines (such as alprazolam [e.g., Xanax], bromazepam [e.g., Lectopam], chlordiazepoxide [e.g., Librium], clonazepam [e.g., Klonopin], diazepam [e.g., Valium], estazolam [e.g., ProSom], flurazepam [e.g., Dalmane], halazepam [e.g., Paxipam], ketazolam [e.g., Loftran], lorazepam [e.g., Ativan], nitrazepam [e.g., Mogadon], oxazepam [e.g., Serax], prazepam [e.g., Centrax], quazepam [e.g., Doral], temazepam [e.g., Restoril], triazolam [e.g., Halcion]). Also, tell your health care professional if you are allergic to any other substances, such as foods, preservatives, or dyes.

**Pregnancy**—Midazolam is not recommended for use during pregnancy because it may cause birth defects. Other benzodiazepines, such as chlordiazepoxide (e.g., Librium) and diazepam (e.g., Valium) that are related chemically and in action to midazolam, have been reported to increase the chance of birth defects when used during the first 3 months of pregnancy. Also, use of midazolam during pregnancy, especially during the last few days, may cause drowsiness, slow heartbeat, shortness of breath, or troubled breathing in the newborn infant. In addition, receiving midazolam just before or during labor may cause weakness in the newborn infant.

**Breast-feeding**—It is not known whether midazolam passes into the breast milk. However, this medicine has not been reported to cause problems in nursing babies.

**Children**—Although there is no specific information comparing use of midazolam in children with use in other age groups, this medicine is not expected to cause different side effects or problems in children than it does in adults.

**Older Adults**—Elderly people are especially sensitive to the effects of midazolam. This may increase the chance of side effects during the use of this medicine. Also, time to complete recovery after midazolam is given may be slower in the elderly than in younger adults.

**Other medicines**—Although certain medicines should not be used together at all, in other cases 2 different medicines may be used together even if an interaction might occur. In these cases, your doctor may want to change the dose, or other precautions may be necessary. When you are receiving midazolam, it is especially important

that your health care professional know if you are taking any of the following:
- Central nervous system (CNS) depressants (medicine that causes drowsiness)—The CNS depressant and other effects of either these medicines or midazolam may be increased; also, the effects of midazolam may be prolonged

**Other medical problems**—The presence of other medical problems may affect the use of midazolam. Make sure you tell your doctor if you have any other medical problems, especially:
- Heart disease or
- Kidney disease or
- Liver disease or
- Obesity (overweight)—The effects of midazolam may be prolonged
- Lung disease or
- Myasthenia gravis or other muscle and nerve disease—Midazolam may make the condition worse

## Proper Use of This Medicine

**Dosing**—The dose of midazolam will be different for different patients. Your doctor will decide on the right amount for you. The dose will depend on:
- Your age;
- Your weight;
- Your general physical condition;
- The kind of surgery or other procedure you are having; and
- Other medicines you are taking or will receive before and during the procedure.

## Precautions After Receiving This Medicine

For patients going home within 24 hours after receiving midazolam:
- Midazolam may cause some people to feel drowsy, tired, or weak for one or two days after it has been given. It may also cause problems with coordination and one's ability to think. Therefore, *do not drive, use machines, or do anything else that could be dangerous if you are not alert* until the effects of the medicine have disappeared or until the day after you receive midazolam, whichever period of time is longer.
- *Do not drink alcoholic beverages or take other CNS depressants (medicines that slow down the nervous system, possibly causing drowsiness) for about 24 hours after you have received midazolam, unless otherwise directed by your doctor.* To do so may add to the effects of the medicine. Some examples of CNS depressants are antihistamines or medicine for hay fever, other allergies, or colds; other sedatives, tranquilizers, or sleeping medicine; prescription pain medicine or narcotics; medicine for seizures; and muscle relaxants.

## Side Effects of This Medicine

Some side effects may occur that usually do not need medical attention. The following side effects may go away as the effects of midazolam wear off. However, check with your doctor if any of the following side effects continue or are bothersome:

*Less common or rare*

Blurred vision or other changes in vision; coughing; dizziness, lightheadedness, or feeling faint; drowsiness (prolonged); headache; hiccups; nausea or vomiting; numbness, tingling, pain, or weakness in hands or feet;

redness, pain, lump or hardness, or muscle stiffness at place of injection

Other side effects not listed above may also occur in some patients. If you notice any other effects, check with your doctor.

Revised: 11/11/91
Interim revision: 08/17/94

# MINOXIDIL   Systemic

A commonly used brand name in the U.S. and Canada is Loniten. Generic name product may also be available in the U.S.

## Description

Minoxidil (mi-NOX-i-dill) belongs to the general class of medicines called antihypertensives. It is used to treat high blood pressure (hypertension).

High blood pressure adds to the workload of the heart and arteries. If it continues for a long time, the heart and arteries may not function properly. This can damage the blood vessels of the brain, heart, and kidneys, resulting in a stroke, heart failure, or kidney failure. High blood pressure may also increase the risk of heart attacks. These problems may be less likely to occur if blood pressure is controlled.

Minoxidil works by relaxing blood vessels so that blood passes through them more easily. This helps to lower blood pressure.

Minoxidil has other effects that could be bothersome for some patients. These include increased hair growth, weight gain, fast heartbeat, and chest pain. Before you take this medicine, be sure that you have discussed the use of it with your doctor.

Minoxidil is being applied to the scalp in liquid form by some balding men to stimulate hair growth. However, improper use of liquids made from minoxidil tablets can result in minoxidil being absorbed into the body, where it may cause unwanted effects on the heart and blood vessels.

Minoxidil is available only with your doctor's prescription, in the following dosage form:

*Oral*

• Tablets (U.S. and Canada)

## Before Using This Medicine

In deciding to use a medicine, the risks of taking the medicine must be weighed against the good it will do. This is a decision you and your doctor will make. For minoxidil, the following should be considered:

**Allergies**—Tell your doctor if you have ever had any unusual or allergic reaction to minoxidil. Also tell your health care professional if you are allergic to any other substances, such as foods, preservatives, or dyes.

**Pregnancy**—Minoxidil has not been studied in pregnant women. However, there have been reports of babies born with extra thick or dark hair on their bodies after the mothers took minoxidil during pregnancy. Discuss this possible effect with your doctor.

Studies in rats found a decreased rate of conception, and studies in rabbits at 5 times the human dose have shown a decrease in successful pregnancies. Minoxidil did not cause birth defects in rats or rabbits.

**Breast-feeding**—Although minoxidil passes into breast milk, it has not been reported to cause problems in nursing babies.

**Children**—Although there is no specific information comparing use of minoxidil in children with use in other age groups, this medicine is not expected to cause different side effects or problems in children than it does in adults.

**Older adults**—Elderly patients may be more sensitive to the effects of minoxidil. In addition, minoxidil may reduce tolerance to cold temperatures in elderly patients.

**Other medicines**—Although certain medicines should not be used together at all, in other cases two different medicines may be used together even if an interaction might occur. In these cases, your doctor may want to change the dose, or other precautions may be necessary. When taking minoxidil it is especially important that your health care professional know if you are taking any of the following:

• Guanethidine (e.g., Ismelin) or
• Nitrates (medicine for angina)—Severe lowered blood pressure may occur

**Other medical problems**—The presence of other medical problems may affect the use of minoxidil. Make sure you tell your doctor if you have any other medical problems, especially:

• Angina (chest pain)—Minoxidil may make this condition worse
• Heart attack or stroke (recent)—Lowering blood pressure may make problems resulting from heart attack or stroke worse

- Heart or blood vessel disease—Minoxidil can cause fluid buildup, which can cause problems
- Kidney disease—Effects may be increased because of slower removal of minoxidil from the body
- Pheochromocytoma—Minoxidil may cause the tumor to be more active

## Proper Use of This Medicine

In addition to the use of the medicine your doctor has prescribed, treatment for your high blood pressure may include weight control and care in the types of foods you eat, especially foods high in sodium. Your doctor will tell you which of these are most important for you. You should check with your doctor before changing your diet.

Many patients who have high blood pressure will not notice any signs of the problem. In fact, many may feel normal. It is very important that you *take your medicine exactly as directed* and that you keep your appointments with your doctor even if you feel well.

Remember that minoxidil will not cure your high blood pressure but it does help control it. Therefore, you must continue to take it as directed if you expect to lower your blood pressure and keep it down. *You may have to take high blood pressure medicine for the rest of your life.* If high blood pressure is not treated, it can cause serious problems such as heart failure, blood vessel disease, stroke, or kidney disease.

To help you remember to take your medicine, try to get into the habit of taking it at the same time each day.

This medicine is usually given together with certain other medicines. If you are using a combination of drugs, make sure that you take each medicine at the proper time and do not mix them. Ask your health care professional to help you plan a way to remember to take your medicines at the right time.

**Dosing**—The dose of minoxidil will be different for different patients. *Follow your doctor's orders or the directions on the label.* The following information includes only the average doses of minoxidil. *If your dose is different, do not change it* unless your doctor tells you to do so:

- For *oral* dosage forms (tablets):
  —Adults and children over 12 years of age: 5 to 40 milligrams taken as a single dose or in divided doses.
  —Children up to 12 years of age: 200 micrograms to 1 milligram per kilogram of body weight a day to be taken as a single dose or in divided doses.

**Missed dose**—If you miss a dose of this medicine and remember it within a few hours, take it when you remember. However, if you do not remember until the next day, skip the missed dose and go back to your regular dosing schedule. Do not double doses.

**Storage**—To store this medicine:
- Keep out of the reach of children.
- Store away from heat and direct light.
- Do not store in the bathroom, near the kitchen sink, or in other damp places. Heat or moisture may cause the medicine to break down.
- Do not keep outdated medicine or medicine no longer needed. Be sure that any discarded medicine is out of the reach of children.

## Precautions While Using This Medicine

It is important that your doctor check your progress at regular visits to make sure that this medicine is working properly.

Ask your doctor about checking your pulse rate before and after taking minoxidil. Then, while you are taking this medicine, *check your pulse regularly while you are resting.* If it increases by 20 beats or more a minute, check with your doctor right away.

While you are taking minoxidil, *weigh yourself every day.* A weight gain of 2 to 3 pounds (about 1 kg) in an adult is normal and should be lost with continued treatment. However, if you suddenly gain 5 pounds (2 kg) or more (for a child, 2 pounds [1 kg] or more) or if you notice swelling of your feet or lower legs, check with your doctor right away.

*Do not take other medicines unless they have been discussed with your doctor.* This especially includes over-the-counter (nonprescription) medicines for appetite control, asthma, colds, cough, hay fever, or sinus problems, since they may tend to increase your blood pressure.

## Side Effects of This Medicine

Along with its needed effects, a medicine may cause some unwanted effects. Although not all of these side effects may occur, if they do occur they may need medical attention.

*Check with your doctor immediately* if any of the following side effects occur:
*More common*
  Fast or irregular heartbeat; weight gain (rapid) of more than 5 pounds (2 pounds in children)
*Less common*
  Chest pain; shortness of breath

Check with your doctor as soon as possible if any of the following side effects occur:
*More common*
  Bloating; flushing or redness of skin; swelling of feet or lower legs
*Less common*
  Numbness or tingling of hands, feet, or face
*Rare*
  Skin rash and itching

Other side effects may occur that usually do not need medical attention. These side effects may go away during treatment as your body adjusts to the medicine. However,

check with your doctor if any of the following side effects continue or are bothersome:

*More common*

Increase in hair growth, usually on face, arms, and back

*Less common or rare*

Breast tenderness in males and females; headache

This medicine causes a temporary increase in hair growth in most people. Hair may grow longer and darker in both men and women. This may first be noticed on the face several weeks after you start taking minoxidil. Later, new hair growth may be noticed on the back, arms, legs, and scalp. Talk to your doctor about shaving or using a hair remover during this time. After treatment with minoxidil has ended, the hair will stop growing, although it may take several months for the new hair growth to go away.

Other side effects not listed above may also occur in some patients. If you notice any other effects, check with your doctor.

Revised: 05/26/93

---

# MINOXIDIL    Topical

A commonly used brand name in the U.S. and Canada is Rogaine. Generic name product may also be available in Canada.

## Description

Minoxidil (mi-NOX-i-dill) applied to the scalp is used to stimulate hair growth in men and women with a certain type of baldness. The exact way that it works is not known.

If hair growth is going to occur with the use of minoxidil, it usually occurs after the medicine has been used for about 4 months and lasts only as long as the medicine continues to be used. The new hair will be lost within a few months after minoxidil treatment is stopped.

This medicine is available only with your doctor's prescription, in the following dosage form:

*Topical*

• Topical solution (U.S. and Canada)

## Before Using This Medicine

In deciding to use a medicine, the risks of using the medicine must be weighed against the good it will do. This is a decision you and your doctor will make. For topical minoxidil, the following should be considered:

**Allergies**—Tell your doctor if you have ever had any unusual or allergic reaction to minoxidil. Also tell your health care professional if you are allergic to any other substances, such as preservatives or dyes.

**Pregnancy**—Topical minoxidil has not been studied in pregnant women. However, some studies in animals have shown that minoxidil, when given by mouth, causes problems during pregnancy, although the studies have not shown that the medicine causes birth defects. Before using this medicine, make sure your doctor knows if you are pregnant or if you may become pregnant.

**Breast-feeding**—It is not known whether topical minoxidil passes into breast milk. However, minoxidil, taken by mouth, does pass into breast milk. Minoxidil is not recommended during breast-feeding, because it may cause problems in nursing babies.

**Older adults**—Many medicines have not been studied specifically in older people. Therefore, it may not be known whether they work exactly the same way they do in younger adults or if they cause different side effects or problems in older people. There is no specific information comparing use of minoxidil on the scalp in the elderly with use in other age groups.

**Other medicines**—Although certain medicines should not be used together at all, in other cases two different medicines may be used together even if an interaction might occur. In these cases, your doctor may want to change the dose, or other precautions may be necessary. When you are using topical minoxidil, it is especially important that your health care professional know if you are taking any other prescription or nonprescription (over-the-counter [OTC]) medicine or if you are using any of the following on your scalp:

• Corticosteroids (cortisone-like medicine) or
• Petrolatum (e.g., Vaseline) or
• Tretinoin (e.g., Retin A)—Use of these products on your scalp may cause too much topical minoxidil to be absorbed into the body and may increase the chance of side effects
• Minoxidil, systemic (e.g., Loniten)—Use of topical minoxidil with minoxidil taken by mouth for high blood pressure may increase the chance of side effects

**Other medical problems**—The presence of other medical problems may affect the use of topical minoxidil. Make sure you tell your doctor if you have any other medical problems, especially:

• Any other skin problems or an irritation or a sunburn on the scalp—The condition may cause too much topical minoxidil to be absorbed into the body and may increase the chance of side effects

• Heart disease or
• Hypertension (high blood pressure)—The condition may get worse if too much medicine is absorbed into the body

## Proper Use of This Medicine

This medicine usually comes with patient instructions. It is important that you read the instructions carefully.

*It is very important that you use this medicine only as directed.* Do not use more of it and do not use it more often than your doctor ordered. To do so may increase the chance of it being absorbed through the skin. For the same reason, do not apply minoxidil to other parts of your body. Absorption into the body may affect the heart and blood vessels and cause unwanted effects.

*Do not use any other skin products on the same skin area on which you use minoxidil.*

To apply minoxidil solution:

- Shampoo your hair each morning before applying minoxidil. Make sure your hair and scalp are completely dry before applying this medicine.
- Apply the amount prescribed to the area of the scalp being treated, beginning in the center of the area. Follow your doctor's instructions on how to apply the solution, using the applicator provided.
- Immediately after using this medicine, wash your hands to remove any medicine that may be on them.
- Do not use a hairdryer to dry the scalp after you apply minoxidil solution. Blowing with a hairdryer on the scalp may make the treatment less effective.
- If you are using this medicine at bedtime, do not go to bed until at least 30 minutes after you use it. That way, less of the medicine will rub off on the pillowcase.

If your scalp becomes abraded, irritated, or sunburned, check with your doctor before applying minoxidil.

*Keep this medicine away from the eyes, nose, and mouth.* If you should accidentally get some in your eyes, nose, or mouth, flush the area thoroughly with cool tap water. If you are using the pump spray, be careful not to breathe the spray in.

**Dosing**—The dose of topical minoxidil will be different for different patients. *Follow your doctor's orders or the directions on the label.* The following information includes only the average dose of topical minoxidil. *If your dose is different, do not change it* unless your doctor tells you to do so.

- For *topical solution* dosage form:
  —For hair growth:
    - Adults—Apply to the scalp two times a day.

**Missed dose**—If you miss a dose of this medicine, go back to your regular dosing schedule. Do not double doses.

**Storage**—To store this medicine:
- Keep out of the reach of children.
- Store away from heat and direct light.
- Keep the medicine from freezing.
- Do not keep outdated medicine or medicine no longer needed. Be sure that any discarded medicine is out of the reach of children.

## Precautions While Using This Medicine

It is important that your doctor check your progress at regular visits to make sure that this medicine is working properly and to check for unwanted effects.

Tell your doctor if you notice itching, redness, or burning of your scalp after you apply minoxidil. If the itching, redness, or burning is severe, wash the medicine off and check with your doctor before using it again.

## Side Effects of This Medicine

Along with its needed effects, a medicine may cause some unwanted effects. Although not all of these side effects may occur, if they do occur they may need medical attention.

Check with your doctor as soon as possible if any of the following side effects occur:

*Less common*
    Itching or skin rash
*Rare*
    Blurred vision or other change in vision; burning of scalp; decrease of sexual ability or desire; dizziness; increased hair loss; lightheadedness; soreness at root of hair; swelling of face
*Signs and symptoms of too much medicine being absorbed into the body—Rare*
    Chest pain; fast or irregular heartbeat; flushing; headache; numbness or tingling of hands, feet, or face; swelling of face, hands, feet, or lower legs; weight gain (rapid)

Other side effects may occur that usually do not need medical attention. These side effects may go away during treatment as your body adjusts to the medicine. However, check with your doctor if either of the following side effects continues or is bothersome:

*Less common*
    Dry or flaking skin; reddened skin

Other side effects not listed above may also occur in some patients. If you notice any other effects, check with your doctor.

Revised: 04/14/92
Interim revision: 07/14/94

# MISOPROSTOL   Systemic

A commonly used brand name in the U.S. and Canada is Cytotec.

## Description

Misoprostol (mye-soe-PROST-ole) is taken to prevent stomach ulcers in patients taking anti-inflammatory drugs, including aspirin. Misoprostol may also be used for other conditions as determined by your doctor.

Misoprostol helps the stomach protect itself against acid damage. It also decreases the amount of acid produced by the stomach.

This medicine is available only with your doctor's prescription, in the following dosage form:

*Oral*
   • Tablets (U.S. and Canada)

## Before Using This Medicine

In deciding to use a medicine, the risks of taking the medicine must be weighed against the good it will do. This is a decision you and your doctor will make. For misoprostol, the following should be considered:

**Allergies**—Tell your doctor if you have ever had any unusual or allergic reaction to misoprostol. Also tell your health care professional if you are allergic to any other substances, such as foods, preservatives, or dyes.

**Pregnancy**—*Misoprostol must not be used during pregnancy*. It has been shown to cause contractions and bleeding of the uterus. Misoprostol may also cause miscarriage.

Before starting to take this medicine you must have had a negative pregnancy test within the previous 2 weeks. Also, you must start taking misoprostol only on the second or third day of your next normal menstrual period. In addition, it will be necessary that you use an effective form of birth control while taking this medicine. Be sure that you have discussed this with your doctor before taking this medicine.

**Breast-feeding**—It is not known whether misoprostol passes into breast milk. However, misoprostol is not recommended for use during breast-feeding because it may cause diarrhea in nursing babies.

**Children**—Studies on this medicine have been done only in adult patients, and there is no specific information comparing use of misoprostol in children with use in other age groups.

**Older adults**—This medicine has been tested and has not been shown to cause different side effects or problems in older people than it does in younger adults.

**Other medicines**—Although certain medicines should not be used together at all, in other cases two different medicines may be used together even if an interaction might occur. In these cases, your doctor may want to change the dose, or other precautions may be necessary. Tell your

health care professional if you are taking any other prescription or nonprescription (over-the-counter [OTC]) medicine.

**Other medical problems**—The presence of other medical problems may affect the use of misoprostol. Make sure you tell your doctor if you have any other medical problems, especially:
   • Blood vessel disease—Medicines similar to misoprostol have been shown to make this condition worse
   • Epilepsy (uncontrolled)—Medicines similar to misoprostol have been shown to cause convulsions (seizures)

## Proper Use of This Medicine

Misoprostol is best taken with or after meals and at bedtime, unless otherwise directed by your doctor.

**Dosing**—The dose of misoprostol will be different for different patients. *Follow your doctor's orders or the directions on the label*. The following information includes only the average doses of misoprostol. *If your dose is different, do not change it* unless your doctor tells you to do so.
   • To prevent stomach ulcers in patients taking anti-inflammatory medicines including aspirin:
     —For *oral* dosage form (tablets):
       • Adults—200 micrograms (mcg) four times a day, with or after meals and at bedtime. Or, your dose may be 400 mcg two times day with the last dose taken at bedtime. Your doctor may reduce the dose to 100 mcg if you are sensitive to high doses.
       • Children and teenagers—Dose must be determined by your doctor.

**Missed dose**—If you miss a dose of this medicine, take it as soon as possible. However, if it is almost time for your next dose, skip the missed dose and go back to your regular dosing schedule. Do not double doses.

**Storage**—To store this medicine:
   • Keep out of the reach of children.
   • Store away from heat and direct light.
   • Do not store in the bathroom, near the kitchen sink, or in other damp places. Heat or moisture may cause the medicine to break down.
   • Do not keep outdated medicine or medicine no longer needed. Be sure that any discarded medicine is out of the reach of children.

## Precautions While Using This Medicine

*Misoprostol may cause miscarriage if taken during pregnancy. Therefore, if you suspect that you may have become pregnant, stop taking this medicine immediately and check with your doctor.*

This medicine may cause diarrhea in some people. The diarrhea will usually disappear within a few days as your body adjusts to the medicine. However, check with your doctor if the diarrhea is severe and/or does not stop after a week. Your doctor may have to lower the dose of misoprostol you are taking.

## Side Effects of This Medicine

Along with its needed effects, a medicine may cause some unwanted effects. Some side effects may occur that usually do not need medical attention. These side effects may go away during treatment as your body adjusts to the medicine. However, check with your doctor if any of the following side effects continue or are bothersome:

*More common*
Abdominal or stomach pain (mild); diarrhea

*Less common or rare*
Bleeding from vagina; constipation; cramps in lower abdomen or stomach area; gas; headache; nausea and/or vomiting

Other side effects not listed above may also occur in some patients. If you notice any other effects, check with your doctor.

## Additional Information

Once a medicine has been approved for marketing for a certain use, experience may show that it is also useful for other medical problems. Although this use is not included in product labeling, misoprostol is used in certain patients with the following medical condition:

- Duodenal ulcers

For patients taking this medicine for *duodenal ulcers*:

- Antacids may be taken with misoprostol, if needed, to help relieve stomach pain, unless you are otherwise directed by your doctor. However, do not take magnesium-containing antacids, since they may cause diarrhea or worsen the diarrhea that is sometimes caused by misoprostol.
- Take this medicine for the full time of treatment, even if you begin to feel better. Also, it is important that you keep your appointments with your doctor so that your doctor will be better able to tell you when to stop taking this medicine.
- *Misoprostol is not normally taken for more than 4 weeks when used to treat duodenal ulcers.* However, your doctor may order treatment for a second 4-week period if needed.

Other than the above information, there is no additional information relating to proper use, precautions, or side effects for these uses.

Revised: 04/14/92
Interim revision: 08/10/94

# MITOMYCIN   Systemic

A commonly used brand name in the U.S. and Canada is Mutamycin.

## Description

Mitomycin (mye-toe-MYE-sin) belongs to the group of medicines known as antineoplastics. It is used to treat some kinds of cancer.

Mitomycin interferes with the growth of cancer cells, which are eventually destroyed. Since the growth of normal body cells may also be affected by mitomycin, other effects will also occur. Some of these may be serious and must be reported to your doctor. Other effects, like hair loss, may not be serious but may cause concern. Some effects may not occur for months or years after the medicine is used.

Before you begin treatment with mitomycin, you and your doctor should talk about the good this medicine will do as well as the risks of using it.

Mitomycin is to be administered only by or under the immediate supervision of your doctor. It is available in the following dosage form:

*Parenteral*
- Injection (U.S. and Canada)

## Before Using This Medicine

In deciding to use a medicine, the risks of taking the medicine must be weighed against the good it will do. This is a decision you and your doctor will make. For mitomycin, the following should be considered:

**Allergies**—Tell your doctor if you have ever had any unusual or allergic reaction to mitomycin.

**Pregnancy**—Tell your doctor if you are pregnant or if you intend to have children. There is a chance that this medicine may cause birth defects if either the male or female is taking it at the time of conception or if it is taken during pregnancy. Studies have shown that mitomycin causes birth defects in animals. In addition, many cancer medicines may cause sterility which could be permanent. Although sterility has not been reported with this medicine, the possibility should be kept in mind.

Be sure that you have discussed this with your doctor before taking this medicine. It is best to use some kind of birth control while you are receiving mitomycin. Tell your doctor right away if you think you have become pregnant while receiving mitomycin.

**Breast-feeding**—Tell your doctor if you are breast-feeding or if you intend to breast-feed during treatment with this medicine. Because mitomycin may cause serious side effects, breast-feeding is generally not recommended while you are receiving it.

**Children**—Although there is no specific information about the use of mitomycin in children, it is not expected to cause different side effects or problems in children than it does in adults.

**Older adults**—Many medicines have not been tested in older people. Therefore, it may not be known whether they work exactly the same way they do in younger adults or if they cause different side effects or problems in older people. There is no specific information about the use of mitomycin in the elderly.

**Other medicines**—Although certain medicines should not be used together at all, in other cases two different medicines may be used together even if an interaction might occur. In these cases, your doctor may want to change the dose, or other precautions may be necessary. When you are receiving mitomycin, it is especially important that your health care professional know if you have ever been treated with x-rays or cancer medicines or if you are taking any of the following:

- Amphotericin B by injection (e.g., Fungizone) or
- Antithyroid agents (medicine for overactive thyroid) or
- Azathioprine (e.g., Imuran) or
- Chloramphenicol (e.g., Chloromycetin) or
- Colchicine or
- Flucytosine (e.g., Ancobon) or
- Interferon (e.g., Intron A, Roferon-A) or
- Plicamycin (e.g., Mithracin) or
- Zidovudine (e.g., Retrovir)—Mitomycin may increase the effects of these medicines or radiation therapy on the blood

**Other medical problems**—The presence of other medical problems may affect the use of mitomycin. Make sure you tell your doctor if you have any other medical problems, especially:

- Bleeding problems
- Chickenpox (including recent exposure) or
- Herpes zoster (shingles)—Risk of severe disease affecting other parts of the body
- Infection—Mitomycin can reduce immunity to infection
- Kidney disease—May be worsened

## Proper Use of This Medicine

Mitomycin is usually given together with certain other medicines. If you are using a combination of medicines, it is important that you receive each one at the proper time. If you are taking some of these medicines by mouth, ask your health care professional to help you plan a way to remember to take them at the right times.

This medicine often causes nausea, vomiting, and loss of appetite. However, it is very important that you continue to receive the medicine, even if you begin to feel ill. Ask your health care professional for ways to lessen these effects.

**Dosing**—The dose of mitomycin will be different for different patients. The dose that is used may depend on a number of things, including what the medicine is being used for, the patient's size, and whether or not other medicines are also being taken. *If you are receiving mitomycin at home, follow your doctor's orders or the directions on the label.* If you have any questions about the proper dose of mitomycin, ask your doctor.

## Precautions While Using This Medicine

*It is very important that your doctor check your progress at regular visits* to make sure that this medicine is working properly and to check for unwanted effects.

While you are being treated with mitomycin, and after you stop treatment with it, *do not have any immunizations (vaccinations) without your doctor's approval.* Mitomycin may lower your body's resistance and there is a chance you might get the infection the immunization is meant to prevent. In addition, other persons living in your household should not take or should not have recently taken oral polio vaccine since there is a chance they could pass the polio virus on to you. Also, avoid other persons who have taken oral polio vaccine. Do not get close to them, and do not stay in the same room with them for very long. If you cannot take these precautions, you should consider wearing a protective face mask that covers the nose and mouth.

Mitomycin can lower the number of white blood cells in your blood temporarily, increasing the chance of getting an infection. It can also lower the number of platelets, which are necessary for proper blood clotting. If this occurs, there are certain precautions you can take, especially when your blood count is low, to reduce the risk of infection or bleeding:

- If you can, avoid people with infections. *Check with your doctor immediately* if you think you are getting an infection or if you get a fever or chills, cough or hoarseness, lower back or side pain, or painful or difficult urination.
- *Check with your doctor immediately* if you notice any unusual bleeding or bruising; black, tarry stools; blood in urine or stools; or pinpoint red spots on your skin.
- Be careful when using a regular toothbrush, dental floss, or toothpick. Your medical doctor, dentist, or nurse may recommend other ways to clean your teeth and gums. Check with your medical doctor before having any dental work done.
- Do not touch your eyes or the inside of your nose unless you have just washed your hands and have not touched anything else in the meantime.
- Be careful not to cut yourself when you are using sharp objects such as a safety razor or fingernail or toenail cutters.
- Avoid contact sports or other situations where bruising or injury could occur.

If mitomycin accidentally seeps out of the vein into which it is injected, it may damage the skin and cause scarring.

In some patients, this may occur weeks or even months after this medicine is given. *Tell the doctor or nurse right away if you notice redness, pain, or swelling at the place of injection or anywhere else on your skin.*

## Side Effects of This Medicine

Along with their needed effects medicines like mitomycin can sometimes cause unwanted effects such as blood problems, loss of hair, and other side effects. These and others are described below. Also, because of the way these medicines act on the body, there is a chance that they might cause other unwanted effects that may not occur until months or years after the medicine is used. These delayed effects may include certain types of cancer, such as leukemia. Discuss these possible effects with your doctor.

Although not all of these side effects may occur, if they do occur they may need medical attention.

*Check with your doctor or nurse immediately* if any of the following side effects occur:

*Less common*
  Black, tarry stools; blood in urine or stools; cough or hoarseness; fever or chills; lower back or side pain; painful or difficult urination; pinpoint red spots on skin; unusual bleeding or bruising

*Rare*
  Redness or pain, especially at place of injection

Check with your doctor as soon as possible if any of the following side effects occur:

*Less common*
  Cough; decreased urination; shortness of breath; sores in mouth and on lips; swelling of feet or lower legs

*Rare*
  Bloody vomit

Other side effects may occur that usually do not need medical attention. These side effects may go away during treatment as your body adjusts to the medicine. Also, your health care professional may be able to tell you about ways to prevent or reduce some of these side effects. Check with your doctor if any of the following side effects continue or are bothersome or if you have any questions about them:

*More common*
  Loss of appetite; nausea and vomiting
*Less common*
  Numbness or tingling in fingers and toes; purple-colored bands on nails; skin rash; unusual tiredness or weakness

Mitomycin sometimes causes a temporary loss of hair. After treatment has ended, normal hair growth should return.

After you stop receiving mitomycin, it may still produce some side effects that need attention. During this period of time, *check with your doctor immediately* if you notice the following:

  Blood in urine

Also, check with your doctor if you notice any of the following:

  Black, tarry stools; blood in stools; cough or hoarseness; decreased urination; fever or chills; lower back or side pain; painful or difficult urination; pinpoint red spots on skin; red or painful skin; shortness of breath; swelling of feet or lower legs; unusual bleeding or bruising

Other side effects not listed above may also occur in some patients. If you notice any other effects, check with your doctor.

Annual revision: 06/90
Interim revision(s): 07/30/93; 07/05/94

---

# MITOTANE    Systemic

A commonly used brand name in the U.S. and Canada is Lysodren.

## Description

Mitotane (MYE-toe-tane) is a medicine that acts on a part of the body called the adrenal cortex. It is used to treat some kinds of cancer that affect the adrenal cortex. Also, it is sometimes used when the adrenal cortex is overactive without being cancerous.

Mitotane reduces the amounts of adrenocorticoids (cortisone-like hormones) produced by the adrenal cortex. These steroids are important for various functions of the body, including growth. However, too much of these steroids can cause problems.

Mitotane is available only with your doctor's prescription, in the following dosage form:

*Oral*
  • Tablets (U.S. and Canada)

## Before Using This Medicine

In deciding to use a medicine, the risks of taking the medicine must be weighed against the good it will do. This is a decision you and your doctor will make. For mitotane, the following should be considered:

**Allergies**—Tell your doctor if you have ever had any unusual or allergic reaction to mitotane. Also tell your health care professional if you are allergic to any other substance, such as foods, preservatives, or dyes.

**Pregnancy**—Mitotane has not been shown to cause problems in humans.

**Breast-feeding**—Although it is not known whether mitotane passes into the breast milk, it has not been reported to cause problems in nursing babies.

**Children**—Although there is no specific information about the use of mitotane in children, it is not expected to cause different side effects or problems in children than it does in adults.

**Older adults**—Many medicines have not been tested in older people. Therefore, it may not be known whether they work exactly the same way they do in younger adults or if they cause different side effects or problems in older people. There is no specific information about the use of mitotane in the elderly.

**Other medicines**—Although certain medicines should not be used together at all, in other cases two different medicines may be used together even if an interaction might occur. In these cases, your doctor may want to change the dose, or other precautions may be necessary. When you are taking mitotane, it is especially important that your health care professional know if you are taking any of the following:

- Central nervous system (CNS) depressants—CNS depressant effects may be increased

**Other medical problems**—The presence of other medical problems may affect the use of mitotane. Make sure you tell your doctor if you have any other medical problems, especially:

- Infection
- Liver disease—Effects may be increased because of slower removal of mitotane from the body

## Proper Use of This Medicine

*Take mitotane only as directed by your doctor.* Do not take more or less of it, and do not take it more often than your doctor ordered.

*Do not stop taking this medicine without first checking with your doctor.* To do so may increase the chance of unwanted effects.

**Dosing**—The dose of mitotane will be different for different patients. The dose that is used may depend on a number of things, including what the medicine is being used for and whether or not other medicines are also being taken. *If you are taking mitotane at home, follow your doctor's orders or the directions on the label.* If you have any questions about the proper dose of mitotane, ask your doctor.

**Missed dose**—If you miss a dose of this medicine, take the missed dose as soon as you remember it. However, if it is almost time for the next dose, skip the missed dose and do not double the next one. Instead, go back to your regular dosing schedule and check with your doctor.

**Storage**—To store this medicine:
- Keep out of the reach of children.

- Store away from heat and direct light.
- Do not store in the bathroom, near the kitchen sink, or in other damp places. Heat or moisture may cause the medicine to break down.
- Do not keep outdated medicine or medicine no longer needed. Be sure that any discarded medicine is out of the reach of children.

## Precautions While Using This Medicine

*It is very important that your doctor check your progress at regular visits* to make sure this medicine is working properly and to check for unwanted effects.

Your doctor may want you to carry an identification card stating that you are taking this medicine.

This medicine will add to the effects of alcohol and other CNS depressants (medicines that slow down the nervous system, possibly causing drowsiness). Some examples of CNS depressants are antihistamines or medicine for hay fever, other allergies, or colds; sedatives, tranquilizers, or sleeping medicine; prescription pain medicine or narcotics; barbiturates; medicine for seizures; tricyclic antidepressants (medicine for depression); muscle relaxants; or anesthetics, including some dental anesthetics. *Check with your doctor before taking any of the above while you are using this medicine.*

This medicine may cause some people to become dizzy, drowsy, or less alert than they are normally. *Make sure you know how you react to this medicine before you drive, use machines, or do anything else that could be dangerous if you are dizzy or are not alert.*

*Check with your doctor right away if you get an injury, infection, or illness of any kind.* This medicine may weaken your body's defenses against infection or inflammation.

## Side Effects of This Medicine

Along with its needed effects, a medicine may cause some unwanted effects. Although not all of these side effects may occur, if they do occur they may need medical attention.

Check with your doctor as soon as possible if any of the following side effects occur:

*More common*
  Darkening of skin; diarrhea; dizziness; drowsiness; loss of appetite; mental depression; nausea and vomiting; skin rash; unusual tiredness

*Less common*
  Blood in urine; blurred vision; double vision

*Rare*
  Shortness of breath; wheezing

Other side effects may occur that usually do not need medical attention. These side effects may go away during treatment as your body adjusts to the medicine. However, check with your health care professional if any of the following side effects continue or are bothersome:

*Less common*
   Aching muscles; dizziness or lightheadedness when getting up from a lying or sitting position; fever; flushing or redness of skin; muscle twitching

Other side effects not listed above may also occur in some patients. If you notice any other effects, check with your doctor.

Revised: 08/90
Interim revision: 06/30/94

# MITOXANTRONE   Systemic

A commonly used brand name in the U.S. and Canada is Novantrone.

## Description

Mitoxantrone (mye-toe-ZAN-trone) belongs to the general group of medicines known as antineoplastics. It is used to treat some kinds of cancer.

Mitoxantrone seems to interfere with the growth of cancer cells, which are eventually destroyed. Since the growth of normal body cells may also be affected by mitoxantrone, other effects will also occur. Some of these may be serious and must be reported to your doctor. Other effects, like hair loss, may not be serious but may cause concern. Some effects may not occur for months or years after the medicine is used.

Before you begin treatment with mitoxantrone, you and your doctor should talk about the good this medicine will do as well as the risks of using it.

Mitoxantrone is to be administered only by or under the immediate supervision of your doctor. It is available in the following dosage form:

*Parenteral*
   • Injection (U.S. and Canada)

## Before Using This Medicine

In deciding to use a medicine, the risks of taking the medicine must be weighed against the good it will do. This is a decision you and your doctor will make. For mitoxantrone, the following should be considered:

**Allergies**—Tell your doctor if you have ever had any unusual or allergic reaction to mitoxantrone.

**Pregnancy**—Tell your doctor if you are pregnant or if you intend to have children. There is a chance that this medicine may cause birth defects if either the male or female is receiving it at the time of conception or if it is taken during pregnancy. Mitoxantrone has been reported to cause low birth weight and slow growth of the kidney in rats and premature birth in rabbits. In addition, many cancer medicines may cause sterility which could be permanent. Although sterility has not been reported with this medicine, the possibility should be kept in mind.

Be sure that you have discussed this with your doctor before receiving this medicine. It is best to use some kind of birth control while you are receiving mitoxantrone. Tell your doctor right away if you think you have become pregnant while receiving mitoxantrone.

**Breast-feeding**—if you are breast-feeding or if you intend to breast-feed during treatment with this medicine. Because mitoxantrone may cause serious side effects, breast-feeding is generally not recommended while you are receiving it.

**Children**—There is no specific information about the use of mitoxantrone in children.

**Older adults**—Many medicines have not been tested in older people. Therefore, it may not be known whether they work exactly the same way they do in younger adults or if they cause different side effects or problems in older people. There is no specific information about the use of mitoxantrone in the elderly.

**Other medicines**—Although certain medicines should not be used together at all, in other cases two different medicines may be used together even if an interaction might occur. In these cases, your doctor may want to change the dose, or other precautions may be necessary. When you are receiving mitoxantrone, it is especially important that your health care professional know if you are taking any of the following:
   • Amphotericin B by injection (e.g., Fungizone) or
   • Antithyroid agents (medicine for overactive thyroid) or
   • Chloramphenicol (e.g., Chloromycetin) or
   • Colchicine or
   • Flucytosine (e.g., Ancobon) or
   • Interferon (e.g., Intron A, Roferon-A) or
   • Plicamycin (e.g., Mithracin) or
   • Zidovudine (e.g., Retrovir) or
   • If you have been treated with x-rays or cancer medicines—Mitoxantrone may increase the effects of these medicines or radiation therapy on the blood
   • Probenecid (e.g., Benemid) or
   • Sulfinpyrazone (e.g., Anturane)—Mitoxantrone may increase the concentration of uric acid in the blood, which these medicines are used to lower

**Other medical problems**—The presence of other medical problems may affect the use of mitoxantrone. Make sure you tell your doctor if you have any other medical problems, especially:
   • Chickenpox (including recent exposure) or
   • Herpes zoster (shingles)—Risk of severe disease affecting other parts of the body

- Gout (history of) or
- Kidney stones—Mitoxantrone may increase levels of a chemical called uric acid in the body, which can cause gout or kidney stones
- Heart disease—Risk of heart problems caused by mitoxantrone may be increased
- Infection—Mitoxantrone can reduce immunity to infection
- Liver disease—Effects may be increased because of slower removal of mitoxantrone from the body

---

## Proper Use of This Medicine

Mitoxantrone is sometimes given together with certain other medicines. If you are using a combination of medicines, it is important that you receive each one at the proper time. If you are taking some of these medicines by mouth, ask your health care professional to help you plan a way to take them at the right times.

While you are receiving mitoxantrone, your doctor may want you to drink extra fluids so that you will pass more urine. This will help prevent kidney problems and keep your kidneys working well.

Mitoxantrone often causes nausea and vomiting. However, it is very important that you continue to receive the medicine, even if your stomach is upset. Ask your health care professional for ways to lessen these effects.

**Dosing**—The dose of mitoxantrone will be different for different patients. The dose that is used may depend on a number of things, including what the medicine is being used for, the patient's size, and whether or not other medicines are also being taken. *If you are receiving mitoxantrone at home, follow your doctor's orders or the directions on the label.* If you have any questions about the proper dose of mitoxantrone, ask your doctor.

---

## Precautions While Using This Medicine

It is very important that your doctor check your progress at regular visits to make sure that this medicine is working properly and to check for unwanted effects.

While you are being treated with mitoxantrone, and after you stop treatment with it, *do not have any immunizations (vaccinations) without your doctor's approval.* Mitoxantrone may lower your body's resistance and there is a chance you might get the infection the immunization is meant to prevent. In addition, other persons living in your household should not take or should not have recently taken oral polio vaccine since there is a chance they could pass the polio virus on to you. Also, avoid other persons who have taken oral polio vaccine. Do not get close to them and do not stay in the same room with them for very long. If you cannot take these precautions, you should consider wearing a protective face mask that covers the nose and mouth.

*Tell your doctor right away if you think you have become pregnant while receiving mitoxantrone.* There is a chance that it may cause birth defects or other problems if it is used during pregnancy.

Mitoxantrone can lower the number of white blood cells in your blood temporarily, increasing the chance of getting an infection. It can also lower the number of platelets, which are necessary for proper blood clotting. If this occurs, there are certain precautions you can take, especially when your blood count is low, to reduce the risk of infection or bleeding:

- If you can, avoid people with infections. *Check with your doctor immediately* if you think you are getting an infection or if you get a fever or chills, cough or hoarseness, lower back or side pain, or painful or difficult urination.
- *Check with your doctor immediately* if you notice any unusual bleeding or bruising; black, tarry stools; blood in urine or stools; or pinpoint red spots on your skin.
- Be careful when using a regular toothbrush, dental floss, or toothpick. Your medical doctor, dentist, or nurse may recommend other ways to clean your teeth and gums. Check with your medical doctor before having any dental work done.
- Do not touch your eyes or the inside of your nose unless you have just washed your hands and have not touched anything else in the meantime.
- Be careful not to cut yourself when you are using sharp objects such as a safety razor or fingernail or toenail cutters.
- Avoid contact sports or other situations where bruising or injury could occur.

---

## Side Effects of This Medicine

Along with their needed effects, medicines like mitoxantrone can sometimes cause unwanted effects such as blood problems, loss of hair, and other side effects. These and others are described below. Also, because of the way these medicines act on the body, there is a chance that they might cause other unwanted effects that may not occur until months or years after the medicine is used. These delayed effects may include certain types of cancer, such as leukemia. Discuss these possible effects with your doctor.

Although not all of these side effects may occur, if they do occur they may need medical attention.

*Check with your doctor or nurse immediately* if any of the following side effects occur:

*More common*

Black, tarry stools; cough or shortness of breath

*Less common*

Blood in urine or stools; fast or irregular heartbeat; fever or chills; lower back or side pain; painful or difficult urination; pinpoint red spots on skin; swelling of feet and lower legs; unusual bleeding or bruising

Check with your health care professional as soon as possible if any of the following side effects occur:

*More common*

Sores in mouth and on lips; stomach pain

*Less common*

> Decrease in urination; seizures; sore, red eyes; yellow eyes or skin

*Rare*

> Blue skin at place of injection; pain or redness at place of injection; skin rash

Other side effects may occur that usually do not need medical attention. These side effects may go away during treatment as your body adjusts to the medicine. Also, your health care professional may be able to tell you about ways to prevent or reduce some of these side effects. Check with your health care professional if any of the following side effects continue or are bothersome:

*More common*

> Diarrhea; headache; nausea and vomiting

Mitoxantrone may cause the urine to turn a blue-green color. It may also cause the whites of the eyes to turn a blue color. These effects are normal and last for only 1 or 2 days after each dose is given.

This medicine often causes a temporary loss of hair. After treatment with mitoxantrone has ended, normal hair growth should return.

Other side effects not listed above may also occur in some patients. If you notice any other effects, check with your health care professional.

Revised: 06/02/92
Interim revision: 07/30/93; 06/30/94

# MOLINDONE   Systemic†

Some commonly used brand names in the U.S. are Moban and Moban Concentrate.

†Not commercially available in Canada.

## Description

Molindone (moe-LIN-done) is used to treat nervous, mental, and emotional conditions.

Molindone is available only with your doctor's prescription, in the following dosage forms:

*Oral*

- Solution (U.S.)
- Tablets (U.S.)

## Before Using This Medicine

In deciding to use a medicine, the risks of taking the medicine must be weighed against the good it will do. This is a decision you and your doctor will make. For molindone, the following should be considered:

**Allergies**—Tell your doctor if you have ever had any unusual or allergic reaction to molindone, phenothiazines, thioxanthenes, haloperidol, or loxapine. Also tell your health care professional if you are allergic to any other substances, such as foods, preservatives, or dyes.

**Pregnancy**—Molindone has not been shown to cause birth defects or other problems in humans. However, studies in mice have shown a slight decrease in successful pregnancies.

**Breast-feeding**—It is not known if molindone passes into breast milk.

**Children**—Studies on this medicine have been done only in adult patients, and there is no specific information comparing use of molindone in children with use in other age groups.

**Older adults**—Elderly patients are usually more sensitive than younger adults to the effects of molindone. Constipation, dizziness or lightheadedness, drowsiness, dryness of mouth, trembling of the hands and fingers, and symptoms of tardive dyskinesia (such as rapid, worm-like movements of the tongue or any other uncontrolled movements of the mouth, tongue, or jaw, and/or arms and legs) are especially likely to occur in elderly patients.

**Other medicines**—Although certain medicines should not be used together at all, in other cases 2 different medicines may be used together even if an interaction might occur. In these cases, your doctor may want to change the dose, or other precautions may be necessary. When you are taking molindone, it is especially important that your health care professional know if you are taking any of the following:

- Amoxapine (e.g., Asendin) or
- Methyldopa (e.g., Aldomet) or
- Metoclopramide (e.g., Reglan) or
- Metyrosine (e.g., Demser) or
- Other antipsychotics (medicine for mental illness) or
- Pemoline (e.g., Cylert) or
- Pimozide (e.g., Orap) or
- Promethazine (e.g., Phenergan) or
- Rauwolfia alkaloids (alseroxylon [e.g., Rauwiloid], deserpidine [e.g., Harmonyl], rauwolfia serpentina [e.g., Raudixin], reserpine [e.g., Serpasil]) or
- Trimeprazine (e.g., Temaril)—Taking these medicines with molindone may increase the chance and seriousness of some side effects
- Central nervous system (CNS) depressants (medicine that causes drowsiness) or
- Tricyclic antidepressants (medicine for depression)—Taking these medicines with molindone may increase the CNS depressant effects
- Lithium (e.g., Eskalith, Lithane)—The chance of serious side effects may be increased

**Other medical problems**—The presence of other medical problems may affect the use of molindone. Make sure

you tell your doctor if you have any other medical problems, especially:

- Brain tumor or
- Intestinal blockage—Molindone may interfere with the diagnosis of these conditions
- Difficult urination or
- Enlarged prostate or
- Glaucoma or
- Liver disease or
- Parkinson's disease—Molindone may make the condition worse

## Proper Use of This Medicine

Molindone should be taken with food or a full glass (8 ounces) of water or milk to reduce stomach irritation.

The liquid form of molindone may be taken undiluted or mixed with milk, water, fruit juice, or carbonated beverages.

*Take this medicine only as directed by your doctor.* Do not take more of it, do not take it more often, and do not take it for a longer time than your doctor ordered. To do so may increase the chance of side effects.

*Sometimes this medicine must be taken for several weeks before its full effect is reached in the treatment of certain mental and emotional conditions.*

**Dosing**—The dose of molindone will be different for different patients. *Follow your doctor's orders or the directions on the label.* The following information includes only the average doses of molindone. *If your dose is different, do not change it* unless your doctor tells you to do so.

The number of tablets or amount of solution that you take depends on the strength of the medicine. Also, *the number of doses you take each day, the time allowed between doses, and the length of time you take the medicine depend on the medical problem for which you are using molindone.*

- For *oral* dosage forms (solution or tablets):
  - —Adults: To start, 50 to 75 milligrams a day, taken in smaller doses three or four times during the day. For maintenance, the dose you take will depend on your condition and may be from 15 to 225 milligrams a day, taken in smaller doses three or four times during the day.
  - —Children up to 12 years of age: The dose must be determined by the doctor.

**Missed dose**—If you miss a dose of this medicine, take it as soon as possible. However, if it is within 2 hours of your next dose, skip the missed dose and go back to your regular dosing schedule. Do not double doses.

**Storage**—To store this medicine:

- Keep out of the reach of children.
- Store away from heat and direct light.
- Do not store the tablets in the bathroom, near the kitchen sink, or in other damp places. Heat or moisture may cause the medicine to break down.

- Keep the liquid form of this medicine from freezing
- Do not keep outdated medicine or medicine no longer needed. Be sure that any discarded medicine is out of the reach of children.

## Precautions While Using This Medicine

Your doctor should check your progress at regular visits. This will allow the dosage of the medicine to be adjusted when necessary and also will reduce the possibility of side effects.

*Do not stop taking this medicine without first checking with your doctor.* Your doctor may want you to reduce gradually the amount you are taking before stopping completely.

*Do not take molindone within 1 or 2 hours of taking antacids or medicine for diarrhea.* Taking them too close together may make molindone less effective.

This medicine will add to the effects of alcohol and other CNS depressants (medicines that slow down the nervous system, possibly causing drowsiness). Some examples of CNS depressants are antihistamines or medicine for hay fever, other allergies, or colds; sedatives, tranquilizers, or sleeping medicine; prescription pain medicine or narcotics; barbiturates; medicine for seizures; muscle relaxants; or anesthetics, including some dental anesthetics. *Check with your doctor before taking any of the above while you are using this medicine.*

Molindone may cause some people to become drowsy or less alert than they are normally, especially during the first few weeks the medicine is being taken. Even if you take this medicine only at bedtime, you may feel drowsy or less alert on arising. *Make sure you know how you react to this medicine before you drive, use machines, or do anything else that could be dangerous if you are not alert.*

*Dizziness or lightheadedness may occur,* especially when you get up from a lying or sitting position. Getting up slowly may help. If the problem continues or gets worse, check with your doctor.

These medicines may make you sweat less, causing your body temperature to increase. *Use extra care not to become overheated during exercise or hot weather while you are taking this medicine, since overheating may result in heat stroke.* Also, hot baths or saunas may make you feel dizzy or faint while you are taking this medicine.

Molindone may cause dryness of the mouth. For temporary relief, use sugarless candy or gum, melt bits of ice in your mouth, or use a saliva substitute. However, if your mouth continues to feel dry for more than 2 weeks, check with your medical doctor or dentist. Continuing dryness of the mouth may increase the chance of dental disease, including tooth decay, gum disease, and fungus infection.

## Side Effects of This Medicine

Along with its needed effects, molindone can sometimes cause serious side effects. Tardive dyskinesia (a movement disorder) may occur and may not go away after you stop using the medicine. Symptoms of tardive dyskinesia include fine, worm-like movements of the tongue, or other uncontrolled movements of the mouth, tongue, cheeks, jaw, or arms and legs. Other serious but rare side effects may also occur. These include severe muscle stiffness, fever, unusual tiredness or weakness, fast heartbeat, difficult breathing, increased sweating, loss of bladder control, and seizures (neuroleptic malignant syndrome). *You and your doctor should discuss the good this medicine will do as well as the risks of taking it.*

*Stop taking molindone and get emergency help immediately* if any of the following side effects occur:

*Rare*
> Convulsions (seizures); difficult or fast breathing; fast heartbeat or irregular pulse; fever (high); high or low (irregular) blood pressure; increased sweating; loss of bladder control; muscle stiffness (severe); unusually pale skin; unusual tiredness or weakness

Also, check with your doctor as soon as possible if any of the following side effects occur:

*More common*
> Difficulty in talking or swallowing; inability to move eyes; lip smacking or puckering; loss of balance control; mask-like face; muscle spasms, especially of the neck and back; puffing of cheeks; rapid or worm-like movements of tongue; restlessness or need to keep moving (severe); shuffling walk; stiffness of arms and legs; trembling and shaking of hands; twisting movements of body; uncontrolled movements of arms and legs; unusual chewing movements

*Less common*
> Mental depression
*Rare*
> Confusion; hot, dry skin, or lack of sweating; muscle weakness; skin rash; yellow eyes or skin

Other side effects may occur that usually do not need medical attention. These side effects may go away during treatment as your body adjusts to the medicine. However, check with your doctor if any of the following side effects continue or are bothersome:

*More common*
> Blurred vision; constipation; decreased sweating; difficult urination; dizziness or lightheadedness, especially when getting up suddenly from a lying or sitting position; drowsiness; dryness of mouth; headache; nausea; stuffy nose

*Less common*
> Changes in menstrual periods; decreased sexual ability; false sense of well-being; swelling of breasts; unusual secretion of milk

Some side effects may occur after you have stopped taking this medicine. Check with your doctor as soon as possible if you notice any of the following effects:

> Lip smacking or puckering; puffing of cheeks; rapid or worm-like movements of tongue; uncontrolled chewing movements; uncontrolled movements of arms and legs

Other side effects not listed above may also occur in some patients. If you notice any other effects, check with your doctor.

Revised: 03/19/93

---

# MOLYBDENUM SUPPLEMENTS Systemic†

A commonly used brand name in the U.S. is Molypen.
Generic name product may also be available.

†Not commercially available in Canada.

## Description

The body needs molybdenum for normal growth and health. For patients who are unable to get enough molybdenum in their regular diet or who have a need for more molybdenum, molybdenum supplements may be necessary. They are generally taken by mouth in multivitamin/mineral products but some patients may have to receive them by injection.

A deficiency of molybdenum is rare. However, if the body does not get enough molybdenum, certain enzymes needed by the body are affected. This may lead to a build up of unwanted substances in some people.

Injectable molybdenum is administered only by or under the supervision of your doctor. This medicine is available in the following dosage forms:

*Oral*
> Molybdenum is available orally as part of a multivitamin/mineral combination.

*Parenteral*
> • Injection (U.S.)

## Importance of Diet

Many nutritionists recommend that, if possible, people should get all the molybdenum they need from foods. However, some people do not get enough molybdenum from their diet. For example, people on weight-loss diets may consume too little food to provide enough molybdenum. Others may need more molybdenum than normal. For such people, a molybdenum supplement is important.

In order to get enough vitamins and minerals in your regular diet, it is important that you eat a balanced and varied diet. Follow carefully any diet program your doctor may recommend. For your specific vitamin and/or mineral needs, ask your doctor or dietitian for a list of appropriate foods.

The amount of molybdenum in foods depends on the soil in which the food is grown. Some soils have more molybdenum than others. Peas, beans, cereal products, leafy vegetables, and low-fat milk are good sources of molybdenum.

Experts have developed a list of recommended dietary allowances (RDA) for most vitamins and some minerals. The RDA are not an exact number but a general idea of how much you need. They do not cover amounts needed for problems caused by serious lack of vitamins and minerals.

Because a lack of molybdenum is rare, there are no RDA for it. The following intakes are thought to be plenty for most individuals:

Infants and children—

  Birth to 6 months of age: 15–30 micrograms (mcg) per day.

  6 months to 1 year of age: 20–40 mcg per day.

  1 to 3 years of age: 25–50 mcg per day.

  4 to 6 years of age: 30–75 mcg per day.

  7 to 10 years of age: 50–150 mcg per day.

Adolescents and adults—75–250 mcg per day.

## Before Using This Dietary Supplement

In deciding to use a dietary supplement, the risks of taking the dietary supplement must be weighed against the good it will do. This is a decision you and your doctor will make. For molybdenum, the following should be considered:

**Allergies**—Tell your doctor if you have ever had any unusual or allergic reaction to molybdenum. Also tell your health care professional if you are allergic to any other substances, such as foods, preservatives, or dyes.

**Pregnancy**—It is especially important that you are receiving enough vitamins and minerals when you become pregnant and that you continue to receive the right amount of vitamins and minerals throughout your pregnancy. The healthy growth and development of the fetus depend on a steady supply of nutrients from the mother. However, taking large amounts of a dietary supplement in pregnancy may be harmful to the mother and/or fetus and should be avoided.

**Breast-feeding**—It is important that you receive the right amounts of vitamins and minerals so that your baby will

also get the vitamins and minerals needed to grow properly. However, taking large amounts of a dietary supplement while breast-feeding may be harmful to the mother and/or baby and should be avoided.

**Children**—It is especially important that children receive enough molybdenum in their diet for healthy growth and development.

**Older adults**—It is important that older people continue to receive enough vitamins in their diet for good health.

**Medicines or other dietary supplements**—Although certain medicines or dietary supplements should not be used together at all, in other cases they may be used together even if an interaction might occur. In these cases, your doctor may want to change the dose, or other precautions may be necessary. Tell your health care professional if you are taking any other dietary supplement or any prescription or nonprescription (over-the-counter [OTC]) medicine.

**Other medical problems**—The presence of other medical problems may affect the use of molybdenum. Make sure you tell your doctor if you have any other medical problems, especially:

- Copper deficiency—Molybdenum may make this condition worse
- Kidney diease or
- Liver disease—These conditions may cause higher blood levels of molybdenum, which may increase the chance of unwanted effects

## Proper Use of This Dietary Supplement

Molybdenum is available orally only as part of a multivitamin/mineral product.

Some people believe that taking very large doses of a vitamin or mineral (called megadoses) is useful for treating certain medical problems. Studies have not proven this. Large doses should be taken only under the direction of your doctor after need has been identified.

**Dosing**—The dose of molybdenum for prevention of molybdenum deficiency is based on daily recommended intake. See the *Importance of Diet* section for daily recommended intake for molybdenum.

**Missed dose**—If you miss taking your multivitamin containing molybdenum for one or more days there is no cause for concern, since it takes some time for your body to become seriously low in molybdenum. However, if your doctor has recommended that you take molybdenum, try to remember to take it as directed every day.

**Storage**—To store this dietary supplement:

- Keep out of the reach of children.
- Store away from heat and direct light.
- Do not store in the bathroom, near the kitchen sink, or in other damp places. Heat or moisture may cause the dietary supplement to break down.
- Keep the dietary supplement from freezing. Do not refrigerate.

- Do not keep outdated dietary supplements or those no longer needed. Be sure that any discarded dietary supplement is out of the reach of children.

## Precautions While Using This Dietary Supplement

Large amounts of molybdenum may cause your body to lose copper. Your doctor may recommend that you take a copper supplement while on molybdenum therapy.

## Side Effects of This Dietary Supplement

Along with its needed effects, a dietary supplement may cause some unwanted effects. Although molybdenum has not been reported to cause any side effects, *check with your doctor immediately* if any of the following side effects occur as a result of a molybdenum overdose:

*Symptoms of overdose*
> Joint pain; side, lower back, or stomach pain; swelling of feet or lower legs

Other side effects not listed above may also occur in some patients. If you notice any other effects, check with your doctor.

Revised: 03/02/92
Interim revision: 07/31/92; 08/10/94

---

# MONOOCTANOIN  Local†

A commonly used brand name in the U.S. is Moctanin.

†Not commercially available in Canada.

## Description

Monooctanoin (mono-OCK-ta-noyn) is used to dissolve cholesterol gallstones. Gallstones, which are found in the gallbladder or bile duct, sometimes remain in the bile duct even after the gallbladder has been removed by surgery. These stones may be too large to pass out of the body on their own. A catheter or tube is used to put the solution of monooctanoin into the bile duct where it will come in contact with the gallstone or gallstones and dissolve them. This is done for a period of 1 to 3 weeks.

Monooctanoin is available only with your doctor's prescription. It is available in the following dosage form:

*Local*
- Irrigation (U.S.)

## Before Using This Medicine

In deciding to use a medicine, the risks of taking the medicine must be weighed against the good it will do. This is a decision you and your doctor will make. For monooctanoin, the following should be considered:

**Allergies**—Tell your doctor if you have ever had any unusual or allergic reaction to monooctanoin or any vegetable oils. Also, tell your doctor if you are allergic to any other substances, such as foods, preservatives, or dyes.

**Pregnancy**—Studies with this medicine have not been done in either humans or animals.

**Breast-feeding**—It is not known whether monooctanoin passes into the breast milk. However, this medicine has not been reported to cause problems in nursing babies.

**Children**—Studies on this medicine have been done only in adult patients, and there is no specific information comparing use of monooctanoin in children with use in other age groups.

**Older adults**—Many medicines have not been studied specifically in older people. Therefore, it may not be known whether they work exactly the same way they do in younger adults or if they cause different side effects or problems in older people. There is no specific information comparing use of monooctanoin in the elderly with use in other age groups.

**Other medical problems**—The presence of other medical problems may affect the use of monooctanoin. Make sure you tell your doctor if you have any other medical problems, especially:
- Biliary tract problems (other) or
- Jaundice or
- Pancreatitis (inflammation of the pancreas)—Monooctanoin may make these conditions worse
- Duodenal ulcer (recent) or
- Intestinal problems—Monooctanoin may make these conditions worse and may increase the chance of bleeding
- Liver disease (severe)—Unwanted effects may occur if the liver is not working properly

## Proper Use of This Medicine

**Dosing**—The dose of monooctanoin will be different for different patients. The following information includes only the average doses of monooctanoin.
- For *irrigation* dosage form:
  —For gallstone disease:
    - Adults and teenagers—The usual dose is 3 to 5 milliliters (mL) per hour given through a catheter or tube. The dose is given over a period of 7 to 21 days.
    - Children—Dose must be determined by your doctor.

## Side Effects of This Medicine

Along with its needed effects, a medicine may cause some unwanted effects. Although not all of these side effects appear very often, when they do occur they may require medical attention.

Check with your doctor as soon as possible if any of the following side effects occur:

*Less common or rare*
> Abdominal or stomach pain (severe); back pain (severe); drowsiness (severe); fever, chills, or sore throat; nausea (continuing); shortness of breath (severe)

Other side effects may occur that usually do not need medical attention. These side effects may go away during treatment as your body adjusts to the medicine. However, check with your doctor if any of the following side effects continue or are bothersome:

*More common*
> Abdominal or stomach pain (mild) or burning sensation

*Less common or rare*
> Back pain (mild); diarrhea; flushing or redness of face; loss of appetite; metallic taste; nausea or vomiting

Other side effects not listed above may also occur in some patients. If you notice any other effects, check with your doctor.

Revised: 08/16/91
Interim revision: 07/15/94

# MORICIZINE    Systemic†

A commonly used brand name in the U.S. is Ethmozine.

†Not commercially available in Canada.

## Description

Moricizine (mor-IH-siz-een) belongs to the group of medicines known as antiarrhythmics. It is used to correct irregular or rapid heartbeats to a normal rhythm by making the heart tissue less sensitive.

There is a chance that moricizine may cause new or make worse existing heart rhythm problems when it is used. Since other antiarrhythmic medicines have been shown to cause severe problems in some patients, moricizine is only used to treat serious heart rhythm problems. Discuss this possible effect with your doctor.

This medicine is available only with your doctor's prescription, in the following dosage form:

*Oral*
- Tablets (U.S.)

## Before Using This Medicine

In deciding to use a medicine, the risks of taking the medicine must be weighed against the good it will do. This is a decision you and your doctor will make. For moricizine, the following should be considered:

**Allergies**—Tell your doctor if you have ever had any unusual or allergic reaction to moricizine. Also tell your health care professional if you are allergic to any other substances, such as foods, preservatives, or dyes.

**Pregnancy**—Moricizine has not been studied in pregnant women. However, this medicine has not been shown to cause birth defects or other problems in animal studies, although it affected weight gain in some animals. Before taking moricizine, make sure your doctor knows if you are pregnant or if you may become pregnant.

**Breast-feeding**—Moricizine passes into the milk of some animals and may also pass into the milk of humans. However, this medicine has not been reported to cause problems in nursing babies.

**Children**—Studies on this medicine have been done only in adult patients, and there is no specific information comparing use of moricizine in children with use in other age groups.

**Older adults**—Many medicines have not been studied specifically in older people. Therefore, it may not be known whether they work exactly the same way they do in younger adults or if they cause different side effects or problems in older people. There is no specific information comparing use of moricizine in the elderly with use in other age groups, although the risk of some unwanted effects may be increased.

**Other medicines**—Although certain medicines should not be used together at all, in other cases two different medicines may be used together even if an interaction might occur. In these cases, your doctor may want to change the dose, or other precautions may be necessary. Tell your health care professional if you are taking any other prescription or nonprescription (over-the-counter [OTC]) medicine.

**Other medical problems**—The presence of other medical problems may affect the use of moricizine. Make sure you tell your doctor if you have any other medical problems, especially:

- Kidney disease or
- Liver disease—Effects may be increased because of slower removal of moricizine from the body
- Heart disease or
- Recent heart attack or
- If you have a pacemaker—Risk of irregular heartbeats may be increased

## Proper Use of This Medicine

*Take moricizine exactly as directed by your doctor,* even though you may feel well. Do not take more or less of it than your doctor ordered.

This medicine works best when there is a constant amount in the blood. *To help keep the amount constant, do not miss any doses. Also, it is best to take each dose at evenly spaced times day and night.* For example, if you are to take 3 doses a day, doses should be spaced about 8 hours apart. If you need help in planning the best times to take your medicine, check with your health care professional.

**Dosing**—The dose of moricizine will be different for different patients. *Follow your doctor's orders or the directions on the label.* The following information includes only the average doses of moricizine. *If your dose is different, do not change it* unless your doctor tells you to do so.

The number of tablets that you take depends on the strength of the medicine.

- For *oral* dosage form (tablets):
  —For irregular heartbeat (arrhythmias):
    - Adults—600 to 900 milligrams (mg) a day. This is divided into three doses and taken every eight hours.
    - Children—Use and dose must be determined by your doctor.

**Missed dose**—If you miss a dose of moricizine and remember within 4 hours, take it as soon as possible. However, if you do not remember until later, skip the missed dose and go back to your regular dosing schedule. Do not double doses.

**Storage**—To store this medicine:

- Keep out of the reach of children.
- Store away from heat and direct light.
- Do not store in the bathroom, near the kitchen sink, or in other damp places. Heat or moisture may cause the medicine to break down.
- Do not keep outdated medicine or medicine no longer needed. Be sure that any discarded medicine is out of the reach of children.

## Precautions While Using This Medicine

It is important that your doctor check your progress at regular visits to make sure the medicine is working properly. This will allow changes to be made in the amount of medicine you are taking, if necessary.

Your doctor may want you to carry a medical identification card or bracelet stating that you are using this medicine.

*Before having any kind of surgery (including dental surgery) or emergency treatment, tell the medical doctor or dentist in charge that you are taking this medicine.*

Moricizine may cause some people to become dizzy or lightheaded. Make sure you know how you react to this medicine before you drive, use machines, or do anything else that could be dangerous if you are dizzy.

## Side Effects of This Medicine

Along with its needed effects, a medicine may cause some unwanted effects. Although not all of these side effects may occur, if they do occur they may need medical attention.

Check with your doctor as soon as possible if any of the following side effects occur:

*Less common*

Chest pain; fast or irregular heartbeat; shortness of breath; swelling of feet or lower legs

*Rare*

Fever (sudden, high)

Other side effects may occur that usually do not need medical attention. These side effects may go away during treatment as your body adjusts to the medicine. However, check with your doctor if any of the following side effects continue or are bothersome:

*More common*

Dizziness

*Less common*

Blurred vision; diarrhea; dryness of mouth; headache; nausea or vomiting; nervousness; numbness or tingling in arms or legs or around mouth; pain in arms or legs; stomach pain; trouble in sleeping; unusual tiredness or weakness

Other side effects not listed above may also occur in some patients. If you notice any other effects, check with your doctor.

Revised: 09/27/92
Interim revision: 06/30/94

# MRI CONTRAST AGENTS    Diagnostic

This information applies to the following medicines:
1. Gadodiamide (gad-oh-DYE-a-mide)
2. Gadopentetate (gad-o-PEN-te-tate)†
3. Gadoteridol (gad-oh-TER-i-dol)†

†Not commercially available in Canada.

## Description

MRI (magnetic resonance imaging) contrast agents (also called paramagnetic agents) are used to help provide a clear picture during MRI. MRI is a special kind of diagnostic procedure. It uses magnets and computers to create images or "pictures" of certain areas inside the body. Unlike x-rays, it does not involve ionizing radiation.

MRI contrast agents are given by injection before or during MRI to help diagnose problems or diseases of the brain or the spine. In addition, gadopentetate is used to help diagnose problems in other parts of the body, such as the bones and joints, breast, liver, soft tissues, and uterus.

MRI contrast agents may also be used to diagnose other conditions as determined by your doctor.

MRI contrast agents are injected into a vein. The doses of these agents will be different for different patients depending on the weight of the person.

These agents are to be used only by or under the supervision of a doctor.

## Before Having This Test

In deciding to use a diagnostic test, any risks of the test must be weighed against the good it will do. This is a decision you and your doctor will make. Also, test results may be affected by other things. For MRI contrast agents, the following should be considered:

**Allergies**—Tell your doctor if you have ever had any unusual or allergic reaction to contrast agents such as gadodiamide, gadopentetate, or gadoteridol. Also, tell your doctor if you are allergic to any other substances, such as foods, preservatives, or dyes.

**Pregnancy**—Studies have not been done in pregnant women. However, in animal studies, MRI contrast agents caused a delay in development of the animal fetus, increased the risk of losing the fetus, and caused birth defects and other side effects in the offspring when these agents were given to the mother in doses many times the human dose. Also, it is not known yet what effect the magnetic field used in MRI might have on the development of the fetus. Be sure you have discussed this with your doctor.

**Breast-feeding**—It is not known what amount of MRI contrast agents passes into the breast milk. However, your doctor may want you to stop breast-feeding for some time after you receive an MRI contrast agent. Be sure you have discussed this with your doctor.

**Children**—Although there is no specific information comparing use of MRI contrast agents in children with use in other age groups, these agents are not expected to cause different side effects or problems in children than they do in adults.

**Older adults**—These contrast agents have been tested and have not been shown to cause different side effects or problems in older people than they do in younger adults.

**Other medical problems**—The presence of other medical problems may affect the use of MRI contrast agents. Make sure you tell your doctor if you have any other medical problems, especially:

- Allergies or asthma (history of)—If you have a history of allergies or asthma, you may be at greater risk of having an allergic reaction to the contrast agent
- Anemia or
- Low blood pressure—MRI contrast agents may make these conditions worse
- Epilepsy—There may be an increased chance of seizures
- Kidney disease (severe)—Kidney disease can cause the MRI agent to stay in the body longer than usual, which may increase the chance of side effects
- Sickle cell disease—There may be a greater risk of blockage of the blood vessels in patients with this condition

## Preparation for This Test

Your doctor may have special instructions for you to get ready for your test, depending on the type of test you are having. If you do not understand the instructions you receive or if you have not received any instructions, check with your doctor ahead of time.

## Side Effects of This Medicine

Along with their needed effects, MRI contrast agents may cause some unwanted effects. Although not all of these side effects may occur, if they do occur they may need medical attention.

*Less common or rare*

Convulsions (seizures); fast or irregular heartbeat; itching, watery eyes; skin rash or hives; swelling of face; thickening of tongue; unusual tiredness or weakness (severe); wheezing, tightness in chest, or troubled breathing

Other side effects may occur that usually do not need medical attention. These side effects may go away as your body adjusts to this agent. However, check with your doctor if any of the following side effects continue or are bothersome:

*More common*

Coldness at the place of injection; dizziness; headache; nausea

*Less common or rare*

Agitation; anxiety; changes in taste; chest pains; confusion; diarrhea; dryness of mouth; fever; increased watering of mouth; pain and/or burning sensation at place of injection; ringing or buzzing in ears; stomach pain; unusual warmth and flushing of skin; vomiting; weakness or tiredness

Not all of the side effects listed above have been reported for each of these agents, but they have been reported for at least one of them. There are some similarities among these agents, so many of the above side effects may occur with any of them.

Other side effects not listed above may also occur in some patients. If you notice any other effects, check with your doctor.

Revised: 08/19/94

---

# MUMPS VIRUS VACCINE LIVE    Systemic

A commonly used brand name in the U.S. and Canada is Mumpsvax.

## Description

Mumps Virus Vaccine Live is an active immunizing agent used to prevent infection by the mumps virus. It works by causing your body to produce its own protection (antibodies) against the virus.

The following information applies only to the Jeryl Lynn strain of mumps vaccine. Different types of mumps vaccines may be available in countries other than the U.S. and Canada.

Mumps is an infection that can cause serious problems, such as encephalitis and meningitis, which affect the brain. In addition, adolescent boys and men are very susceptible to a condition called orchitis, which causes pain and swelling in the testicles and scrotum and, in rare cases, sterility. Also, mumps infection can cause spontaneous abortion in women during the first three months of pregnancy.

Although immunization against mumps is recommended for everyone (children, adolescents, and adults) born in or after 1957, it is especially important for:

- persons born between 1967 and 1977.
- children 12 months of age and older, including school-age children, children in day-care centers, and children of pregnant women who have not yet received their own mumps vaccination.
- boys nearing the age of puberty, adolescent boys, and men.
- women of child-bearing age who are not pregnant.
- persons vaccinated during the years 1950 through 1978 (especially during the years 1950 through 1967) with either the inactivated (killed) mumps vaccine or with an unknown type of mumps vaccine.
- persons traveling outside the U.S.

Immunization against mumps is not recommended for infants younger than 12 months of age, because antibodies they received from their mothers before birth may interfere with the effectiveness of the vaccine. Children who were immunized against mumps before 12 months of age should be immunized again.

If the mumps vaccine is going to be given in a combination immunization that includes measles vaccine, the person to be immunized should be at least 15 months old to make sure the measles vaccine is effective.

You can be considered to be immune to mumps only if you:

- received mumps vaccine on or after your first birthday and have the medical record to prove it, or
- have a doctor's diagnosis of a previous mumps infection, or
- have had a laboratory test that shows that you are immune to mumps.

This vaccine is to be administered only by or under the supervision of your doctor or other health care professional. It is available in the following dosage form:

*Parenteral*
- Injection (U.S. and Canada)

## Before Receiving This Vaccine

In deciding to use a medicine, the risks of taking the medicine must be weighed against the good it will do. This is a decision you and your doctor will make. For mumps vaccine, the following should be considered:

**Allergies**—Tell your doctor if you have ever had any unusual or allergic reaction to mumps vaccine or to any form of the antibiotic neomycin. Also tell your health care professional if you are allergic to any other substances, such as foods (especially eggs) or preservatives. The mumps vaccine available in the U.S. and Canada is grown in a chick embryo cell culture.

**Pregnancy**—Tell your doctor if you are now pregnant or if you may become pregnant within 3 months after receiving this vaccine. Studies on effects in pregnancy have not been done in either humans or animals. However, use during pregnancy is not recommended, because mumps vaccine may infect the placenta, although the vaccine has not been shown to infect the fetus or to cause birth defects.

**Breast-feeding**—It is not known whether mumps vaccine passes into breast milk. Although most medicines pass into breast milk in small amounts, many of them may be used safely while breast-feeding. Mothers who are receiving this vaccine and who wish to breast-feed should discuss this with their doctor.

**Children**—Use is not recommended for infants up to 12 months of age.

**Other medicines**—Although certain medicines should not be used together at all, in other cases two different medicines may be used together even if an interaction might occur. In these cases, your doctor may want to change the dose, or other precautions may be necessary. Before receiving mumps vaccine, it is especially important that your health care professional know if you have received any of the following:

- Treatment with x-rays or cancer medicines—May decrease the useful effect of mumps vaccine

**Other medical problems**—The presence of other medical problems may affect the use of mumps vaccine. Make sure you tell your doctor if you have any other medical problems, especially:

- Immune deficiency condition (or family history of)—The condition may decrease the useful effect of the vaccine or may increase the risk and severity of side effects
- Serious illness with fever—The symptoms of the illness may be confused with the possible side effects of the vaccine
- Tuberculosis—Mumps vaccine will interfere with the results of the skin test for tuberculosis for 4 or more weeks

## Proper Use of This Vaccine

**Dosing**—The dose of mumps vaccine will be different for different patients. The following information includes only the average doses of mumps vaccine.

- For *injection* dosage form:
  —For prevention of mumps:
  - Adults and children 12 months of age and older—One dose injected under the skin.
  - Children up to 12 months of age—Use is not recommended.

## Precautions After Receiving This Vaccine

*Do not become pregnant for 3 months after receiving mumps vaccine without first checking with your doctor.* There is a chance that this vaccine may cause problems during pregnancy.

Tell your doctor that you have received this vaccine:

- if you are to receive a tuberculin skin test within 6 weeks after receiving this vaccine. The results of the test may be affected by this vaccine.
- if you are to receive any other live virus vaccines within 1 month after receiving this vaccine.
- if you are to receive blood transfusions or other blood products within 2 weeks after receiving this vaccine.
- if you are to receive gamma globulin or other globulins within 2 weeks after receiving this vaccine.

## Side Effects of This Vaccine

Along with its needed effects, a medicine may cause some unwanted effects. Although not all of these side effects may occur, if they do occur they may need medical attention.

*Get emergency help immediately* if any of the following side effects occur:

*Symptoms of allergic reaction*
Difficulty in breathing or swallowing; hives; itching, especially of feet or hands; reddening of skin, especially around ears; swelling of eyes, face, or inside of nose; unusual tiredness or weakness (sudden and severe)

Check with your doctor as soon as possible if any of the following side effects occur:

*Rare*
Bruising or purple spots on skin; confusion; convulsions (seizures); fever over 103 °F (39.4 °C); headache (severe or continuing); irritability; pain, tenderness, or swelling in testicles and scrotum (in adolescent boys and men); stiff neck; vomiting

Other side effects may occur that usually do not need medical attention. However, check with your doctor if any of the following side effects continue or are bothersome:

*More common*
Burning or stinging at place of injection

*Less common or rare*
Fever of 100 °F (37.7 °C) or less; itching, swelling, redness, tenderness, or hard lump at place of injection; skin rash; swollen glands on side of face or neck

Other side effects not listed above may also occur in some patients. If you notice any other effects, check with your doctor.

Revised: 07/12/94

# MUPIROCIN    Topical

A commonly used brand name in the U.S. and Canada is Bactroban. Another commonly used name is pseudomonic acid.

## Description

Mupirocin (myoo-PEER-oh-sin) is used to treat bacterial infections. It works by killing bacteria or preventing their growth.

Mupirocin ointment is applied to the skin to treat impetigo. It may also be used for other bacterial skin infections as determined by your doctor.

Mupirocin is available in the U.S. only with your doctor's prescription. It is available in Canada without a prescription; however, your doctor may have special instructions on the proper use of this medicine for your medical problem. Mupirocin is available in the following dosage form:

*Topical*
- Ointment (U.S. and Canada)

## Before Using This Medicine

In deciding to use a medicine, the risks of taking the medicine must be weighed against the good it will do. This is a decision you and your doctor will make. For topical mupirocin, the following should be considered:

**Allergies**—Tell your doctor if you have ever had any unusual or allergic reaction to mupirocin. Also tell your health care professional if you are allergic to any other substances, such as preservatives or dyes.

**Pregnancy**—Topical mupirocin has not been studied in pregnant women. However, this medication has not been shown to cause birth defects or other problems in animal studies.

**Breast-feeding**—It is not known whether topical mupirocin passes into the breast milk. However, this medicine is unlikely to pass into the breast milk in large amounts, since very little mupirocin is absorbed into the mother's body when applied to the skin.

**Children**—Studies on this medicine have been done only in adult patients, and there is no specific information comparing use of mupirocin in children with use in other age groups.

**Older adults**—Many medicines have not been studied specifically in older people. Therefore, it may not be known whether they work exactly the same way they do in younger adults or if they cause different side effects or problems in older people. There is no specific information comparing use of mupirocin in the elderly with use in other age groups.

**Other medicines**—Although certain medicines should not be used together at all, in other cases two different med-

icines may be used together even if an interaction might occur. In these cases, your doctor may want to change the dose, or other precautions may be necessary. Tell your health care professional if you are using any other prescription or nonprescription (over-the-counter [OTC]) medicine that is to be applied to the same area of skin.

## Proper Use of This Medicine

*Do not use this medicine in the eyes.*

To use:
- Before applying this medicine, wash the affected area(s) with soap and water, and dry thoroughly. Then apply a small amount to the affected area(s) and rub in gently.
- After applying this medicine, the treated area(s) may be covered with a gauze dressing if desired.

*To help clear up your skin infection completely, keep using mupirocin for the full time of treatment,* even if your symptoms have disappeared. *Do not miss any doses.*

**Dosing**—*Follow your doctor's orders or the directions on the label.* The following information includes only the average dose of mupirocin. *If your dose is different, do not change it* unless your doctor tells you to do so.
- For *ointment* dosage form:
  —Impetigo:
    - Adults and children—Apply three times a day.

**Missed dose**—If you miss a dose of this medicine, apply it as soon as possible. However, if it is almost time for your next dose, skip the missed dose and go back to your regular dosing schedule.

**Storage**—To store this medicine:
- Keep out of the reach of children.
- Store away from heat and direct light.
- Keep the medicine from freezing.
- Do not keep outdated medicine or medicine no longer needed. Be sure that any discarded medicine is out of the reach of children.

## Precautions While Using This Medicine

If your skin infection does not improve within 3 to 5 days, or if it becomes worse, check with your health care professional.

## Side Effects of This Medicine

Along with its needed effects, a medicine may cause some unwanted effects. The following side effects may go away during treatment as your body adjusts to the medicine. However, check with your doctor if any of these effects continue or are bothersome:

*Less common*
   Dry skin; skin burning, itching, pain, rash, redness, stinging, or swelling

Other side effects not listed above may also occur in some patients. If you notice any other effects, check with your doctor.

Revised: 06/24/94

---

# MUROMONAB-CD3    Systemic

A commonly used brand name in the U.S. and Canada is Orthoclone OKT3.

## Description

Muromonab (myoor-oh-MON-ab)-CD3 is a monoclonal antibody. It is used to reduce the body's natural immunity in patients who receive organ (for example, kidney) transplants.

When a patient receives an organ transplant, the body's white blood cells will try to get rid of (reject) the transplanted organ. Muromonab-CD3 works by preventing the white blood cells from doing this.

The effect of muromonab-CD3 on the white blood cells may also reduce the body's ability to fight infections. Before you begin treatment, you and your doctor should talk about the good this medicine will do as well as the risks of using it.

Muromonab-CD3 is to be administered only by or under the immediate supervision of your doctor. It is available in the following dosage form:

*Parenteral*
   • Injection (U.S. and Canada)

## Before Using This Medicine

In deciding to use a medicine, the risks of taking the medicine must be weighed against the good it will do. This is a decision you and your doctor will make. For muromonab-CD3, the following should be considered:

**Allergies**—Tell your doctor if you have ever had any unusual or allergic reaction to muromonab-CD3 or to rodents (such as mice or rats). Muromonab-CD3 is grown in a mouse cell culture. Also tell your health care professional if you are allergic to any other substance, such as preservatives.

**Pregnancy**—Studies have not been done in either humans or animals.

**Breast-feeding**—Muromonab-CD3 has not been reported to cause problems in nursing babies. However, it may be necessary for you to stop breast-feeding during treatment. Be sure you have discussed the risks and benefits of the medicine with your doctor.

**Children**—Although there is no specific information comparing use of muromonab-CD3 in children with use in other age groups, this medicine is not expected to cause different side effects or problems in children than it does in adults.

**Older adults**—Many medicines have not been studied specifically in older people. Therefore, it may not be known whether they work exactly the same way they do in younger adults or if they cause different side effects or problems in older people. There is no specific information comparing use of muromonab-CD3 in the elderly with use in other age groups.

**Other medicines**—Although certain medicines should not be used together at all, in other cases two different medicines may be used together even if an interaction might occur. In these cases, your doctor may want to change the dose, or other precautions may be necessary. When you are receiving muromonab-CD3, it is especially important that your health care professional know if you are taking any of the following:

   • Azathioprine (e.g., Imuran) or
   • Chlorambucil (e.g., Leukeran) or
   • Corticosteroids (cortisone-like medicine) or
   • Cyclophosphamide (e.g., Cytoxan) or
   • Cyclosporine (e.g., Sandimmune) or
   • Mercaptopurine (e.g., Purinethol)—There may be an increased risk of infection and development of cancer because muromonab-CD3 reduces the body's ability to fight them

**Other medical problems**—The presence of other medical problems may affect the use of muromonab-CD3. Make sure you tell your doctor if you have any other medical problems, especially:

   • Chickenpox (including recent exposure) or
   • Herpes zoster (shingles)—Risk of severe disease affecting other parts of the body
   • Infection—Muromonab-CD3 decreases your body's ability to fight infection

## Proper Use of This Medicine

**Dosing**—The dose of muromonab-CD3 may be different for different patients. Muromonab-CD3 is usually given

---

© 1994   The United States Pharmacopeial Convention, Inc.

by a doctor or nurse in the hospital. The following information includes only the average doses of muromonab-CD3:

- For *injection* dosage form:
  —To prevent organ transplant rejection:
  - Adults—5 milligrams (mg) injected into a vein once a day.
  - Children less than 12 years of age—Dose is based on body weight and must be determined by your doctor.

## Precautions While Using This Medicine

*It is very important that your doctor check your progress at regular visits* to make sure that this medicine is working properly and to check for unwanted effects.

While you are being treated with muromonab-CD3 and after you stop treatment with it, *do not have any immunizations (vaccinations) without your doctor's approval.* Muromonab-CD3 may lower your body's resistance and there is a chance you might get the infection the immunization is meant to prevent. In addition, other persons living in your house should not take oral polio vaccine since there is a chance they could pass the polio virus on to you. Also, avoid persons who have recently taken oral polio vaccine. Do not get close to them and do not stay in the same room with them for very long. If you cannot take these precautions, you should consider wearing a protective face mask that covers the nose and mouth.

Treatment with muromonab-CD3 may also increase the chance of getting other infections. If you can, avoid people with colds or other infections. If you think you are getting a cold or other infection, check with your doctor.

This medicine commonly causes chest pain, dizziness, fever and chills, shortness of breath, stomach upset, and trembling within a few hours after the first dose. These effects should be much less after the second dose and should not occur after that. However, *check with your health care professional immediately* if you have severe shortness of breath after the first dose or if the effects continue.

## Side Effects of This Medicine

Along with its needed effects, a medicine may cause some unwanted effects. Because of the way that muromonab-CD3 acts on the body, there is a chance that it may cause effects that may not occur until years after the medicine is used. These delayed effects may include certain types of cancer, such as lymphomas. Discuss these possible effects with your doctor.

Although not all of these side effects may occur, if they do occur, they may need medical attention.

*Check with your doctor or nurse immediately* if the following side effect occurs with the first dose of this medicine:

*Less common*
  Shortness of breath (severe)

Check with your doctor as soon as possible if any of the following side effects occur within the first 2 or 3 days after a dose:

*More common*
  Chest pain; diarrhea; dizziness or faintness; fever and chills; headache; nausea and vomiting; rapid or irregular heartbeat; shortness of breath or wheezing; trembling and shaking of hands

*Less common*
  Stiff neck; unusual sensitivity of eyes to light

*Rare*
  Confusion; convulsions (seizures); hallucinations (seeing, hearing, or feeling things that are not there); unusual tiredness

After you stop using this medicine, it may still produce some side effects that need medical attention. **During this period of time check with your doctor if you notice the following side effects:**

  Fever and chills

Other side effects not listed above may also occur in some patients. If you notice any other effects, **check with your doctor.**

Revised: 08/09/92
Interim revision: 07/05/94

# NABILONE Systemic*

A commonly used brand name in Canada is Cesamet.

*Not commercially available in the U.S.

## Description

Nabilone (NAB-i-lone) is chemically related to marijuana. It is used to prevent the nausea and vomiting that may occur after treatment with cancer medicines. It is used only when other kinds of medicine for nausea and vomiting do not work.

Nabilone is available only with your doctor's prescription. Prescriptions cannot be refilled and you must obtain a new prescription from your doctor each time you need this medicine. Nabilone is available in the following dosage form:

*Oral*
- Capsules (Canada)

## Before Using This Medicine

In deciding to use a medicine, the risks of taking the medicine must be weighed against the good it will do. This is a decision you and your doctor will make. For nabilone, the following should be considered:

**Allergies**—Tell your doctor if you have ever had any unusual or allergic reaction to nabilone or marijuana products. Also tell your health care professional if you are allergic to any other substances, such as foods, preservatives, or dyes.

**Pregnancy**—Studies have not been done in pregnant women. However, studies in animals have shown a decrease in successful pregnancies and a decrease in the number of live babies born, when nabilone was given in doses many times the usual human dose.

**Breast-feeding**—It is not known whether nabilone passes into the breast milk. However, nabilone is not recommended during breast-feeding because other medicines similar to nabilone that pass into the breast milk have been shown to cause unwanted effects in the nursing baby.

**Children**—Studies on this medicine have been done only in adult patients, and there is no specific information comparing use of nabilone in children with use in other age groups.

**Older adults**—Fast or pounding heartbeat, feeling faint or lightheaded, and unusual tiredness or weakness may be especially likely to occur in elderly patients, who are usually more sensitive than younger adults to the effects of nabilone. Also, the effects this medicine may have on the mind may be of special concern in the elderly. Therefore, older people should be watched closely while taking this medicine.

**Other medicines**—Although certain medicines should not be used together at all, in other cases 2 different medicines may be used together even if an interaction might occur. In these cases, your doctor may want to change the dose, or other precautions may be necessary. When you are taking nabilone, it is especially important that your health care professional know if you are taking any of the following:

- Central nervous system (CNS) depressants (medicine that causes drowsiness) or
- Tricyclic antidepressants (medicine for depression)—Taking these medicines with nabilone may increase the CNS depressant effects

**Other medical problems**—The presence of other medical problems may affect the use of nabilone. Make sure you tell your doctor if you have any other medical problems, especially:

- Alcohol abuse (or history of) or
- Drug abuse or dependence (or history of)—Dependence on nabilone may develop
- Heart disease or
- High blood pressure or
- Low blood pressure or
- Manic depression or
- Schizophrenia—Nabilone may make the condition worse
- Liver disease (severe)—Higher blood levels of nabilone may occur, increasing the chance of side effects

## Proper Use of This Medicine

*Take this medicine only as directed by your doctor.* Do not take more of it, do not take it more often, and do not take it for a longer time than your doctor ordered. If too much is taken, it may lead to other medical problems because of an overdose.

**Dosing**—The dose of nabilone will be different for different patients. *Follow your doctor's orders or the directions on the label.* The following information includes only the average doses of nabilone. *If your dose is different, do not change it* unless your doctor tells you to do so.

- For *oral* dosage forms (capsules):
  —For nausea and vomiting caused by cancer medicines:
    - Adults and teenagers—Usually 1 or 2 milligrams (mg) twice a day. Your doctor will tell you how and when to take this medicine while you are taking your cancer medicine.
    - Children—Use and dose must be determined by your doctor.

**Missed dose**—If you miss a dose of this medicine, take it as soon as you remember. However, if it is almost time for your next dose, skip the missed dose and go back to your regular dosing schedule. *Do not double doses.*

**Storage**—To store this medicine:
- Keep out of the reach of children.
- Store away from heat and direct light.

- Do not store this medicine in the bathroom, near the kitchen sink, or in other damp places. Heat or moisture may cause the medicine to break down.
- Do not keep outdated medicine or medicine no longer needed. Be sure that any discarded medicine is out of the reach of children.

## Precautions While Using This Medicine

Nabilone will add to the effects of alcohol and other central nervous system (CNS) depressants (medicines that slow down the nervous system, possibly causing drowsiness). Some examples of CNS depressants are antihistamines or medicine for hay fever, other allergies, or colds; sedatives, tranquilizers, or sleeping medicine; prescription pain medicines including other narcotics; barbiturates; medicine for seizures; muscle relaxants; or anesthetics, including some dental anesthetics. *Check with your doctor before taking any of the above while you are taking this medicine.*

*If you think you or someone else may have taken an overdose, get emergency help at once.* Taking an overdose of this medicine or taking alcohol or CNS depressants with this medicine may cause severe mental effects. Symptoms of overdose include changes in mood; confusion; difficulty in breathing; dizziness (severe) or fainting; hallucinations (seeing, hearing, or feeling things that are not there); increase in blood pressure; mental depression; nervousness or anxiety; fast, slow, irregular, or pounding heartbeat; and unusual tiredness or weakness (severe).

This medicine may cause some people to become drowsy, dizzy, or lightheaded, or to feel a false sense of well-being. *Make sure you know how you react to this medicine before you drive, use machines, or do anything else that could be dangerous if you are dizzy or are not alert and clearheaded.*

Dizziness, lightheadedness, or fainting may occur, especially when you get up suddenly from a lying or sitting position. Getting up slowly may help lessen this problem.

Nabilone may cause dryness of the mouth. For temporary relief, use sugarless candy or gum, melt bits of ice in your mouth, or use a saliva substitute. However, if your mouth continues to feel dry for more than 2 weeks, check with your medical doctor or dentist. Continuing dryness of the mouth may increase the chance of dental disease, including tooth decay, gum disease, and fungus infections.

## Side Effects of This Medicine

Along with its needed effects, a medicine may cause some unwanted effects. Although not all of these side effects may occur, if they do occur they may need medical attention.

*Check with your health care professional immediately if any of the following side effects occur:*

*Symptoms of overdose*

Changes in mood; confusion; difficulty in breathing; dizziness (severe) or fainting; fast, slow, irregular, or pounding heartbeat; hallucinations (seeing, hearing, or feeling things that are not there); increase in blood pressure; mental depression; nervousness or anxiety; unusual tiredness or weakness (severe)

Other side effects may occur that usually do not need medical attention. These side effects may go away during treatment as your body adjusts to the medicine. However, check with your doctor if any of the following side effects continue or are bothersome:

*More common*

Clumsiness or unsteadiness; difficulty concentrating; dizziness; drowsiness; dryness of mouth; false sense of well-being; headache

*Less common or rare*

Blurred vision or any changes in vision; dizziness or lightheadedness, especially when getting up from a lying or sitting position—more common with high doses; loss of appetite; muscle pain or weakness

Other side effects not listed above may also occur in some patients. If you notice any other effects, check with your doctor.

Revised: 06/17/93

---

# NAFARELIN    Systemic

## Description

Nafarelin (NAF-a-re-lin) is used to treat endometriosis. Endometriosis is a condition in which tissue similar to the lining of the uterus implants in other places in a woman's pelvis area. These growths increase in response to estrogen. Nafarelin works by stopping the production of estrogen by the ovaries.

Nafarelin is usually only used in those women who cannot or do not want to take danazol (e.g., Danocrine), oral contraceptives (birth control pills), or a progestin (another type of female hormone) or choose not to undergo surgery. Danazol and nafarelin work equally well for pain caused by endometriosis, but each has different types of side effects. Danazol is similar to testosterone. Because of this, it causes side effects such as acne, oily skin or hair, rapid weight gain, decreased breast size, enlarged

clitoris, hoarseness or deepening of the voice, and unnatural hair growth. Most of the side effects of nafarelin
are related to the lower amount of estrogen in the bloodstream. This includes a temporary thinning of the bones
that occurs with a continued shortage of estrogen. Because it is not yet known if repeating therapy with nafarelin can increase a woman's risk of osteoporosis (brittle
bones) and an increased risk of broken bones in later life,
nafarelin therapy is usually only used for short periods
of time (a few months) and is generally not repeated.

*Nasal*
- Spray solution (U.S. and Canada)

## Before Using This Medicine

In deciding to use a medicine, the risks of taking the
medicine must be weighed against the good it will do.
This is a decision you and your doctor will make. For
nafarelin, the following should be considered:

**Allergies**—Tell your doctor if you have ever had any unusual or allergic reaction to nafarelin. Also tell your health
care professional if you are allergic to any other substances, such as foods, preservatives, or dyes.

**Pregnancy**—Nafarelin is not recommended during pregnancy. Nafarelin has not been studied in pregnant women.
Some animal studies showed an increase in stillbirths and
decreases in fetal weight, which would be expected from
the changes in hormones caused by nafarelin. Because of
this, you and your partner should use a birth control
method that does not contain hormones, such as condoms,
a diaphragm, or a cervical cap, with a spermicide. If you
suspect that you may have become pregnant, stop taking
this medicine and check with your doctor.

**Breast-feeding**—It is not known whether nafarelin passes
into the breast milk.

**Other medicines**—Although certain medicines should not
be used together at all, in other cases two different medicines may be used together even if an interaction might
occur. In these cases, your doctor may want to change
the dose, or other precautions may be necessary. When
you are taking nafarelin, it is especially important that
your health care professional know if you are taking the
following:
- Nasal decongestant sprays—It is not known whether nasal
  decongestant sprays can decrease the amount of nafarelin
  that enters the bloodstream through the lining of the nose.
  For this reason, you should allow at least 30 minutes to
  pass before you use a nasal decongestant spray after using
  nafarelin

**Other medical problems**—The presence of other medical
problems may affect the use of nafarelin. Make sure you
tell your doctor if you have any other medical problems,
especially:
- Other conditions that increase the chances for osteoporosis
  (brittle bones)—Since nafarelin causes a temporary thinning of the bones, it is important that your doctor know
  if you already have an increased risk of osteoporosis. Some
  things that can increase your risk for having osteoporosis

include cigarette smoking, alcohol abuse, taking or drinking a lot of caffeine, and a family history of osteoporosis
or easily broken bones. Some medicines, such as adrenocorticoids (cortisone-like medicines) or anticonvulsants
(seizure medicine), can also cause thinning of the bones

## Proper Use of This Medicine

You will be given a fact sheet with your prescription for
nafarelin that explains how to use the pump spray bottle.
If you have any questions about using the pump spray,
ask your health care professional.

To use *nafarelin spray:*
- Before you use each new bottle of nafarelin, the spray
  pump needs to be started. To do this, point the bottle
  away from you and pump the bottle firmly about
  7 times. A spray should come out by the seventh
  time you pump the spray bottle. *This only needs to
  be done once for each new bottle of nafarelin.* Be
  careful not to breathe in this spray. You could inhale
  extra doses of nafarelin, since the medicine is dissolved in the spray.
- Before you take your daily doses of nafarelin, blow
  your nose gently. Hold your head forward a little.
  Put the spray tip into one nostril. Aim the tip toward
  the back and outside of your nostril. You do not need
  to put the tip too far into your nose.
- Close your other nostril off by pressing on the outside
  of your nose with a finger. Then, sniff in the spray
  as you pump the bottle once.
- Take the spray bottle out of your nose. Tilt your
  head back for a few seconds, to let the spray get
  onto the back of your nose.
- Repeat these steps for each dose of medicine.
- Each time you use the spray bottle, wipe off the tip
  with a clean tissue or cloth. Keep the blue safety
  clip and plastic cap on the bottle when you are not
  using it.
- Every 3 or 4 days you should clean the tip of the
  spray bottle. To do this, hold the bottle sideways.
  Rinse the tip with warm water, while wiping the tip
  with your finger or soft cloth for about 15 seconds.
  Dry the tip with a soft cloth or tissue. Replace the
  cap right after use. Be careful not to get water into
  the bottle, since this could dilute the medicine.

**Dosing**—The dose of nafarelin will be different for different patients. *Follow your doctor's orders or the directions on the label.* The following information includes
only the average dose of nafarelin. *If your dose is different, do not change it* unless your doctor tells you to
do so.
- For *nasal solution* dosage form:
  —For treating endometriosis:
    - Adults and teenagers—200 micrograms (mcg)
      (one spray) inhaled into one nostril in the morn-
      ing and one spray inhaled into the other nostril
      in the evening, for six months. Begin your treat-
      ment on Day 2, 3, or 4 of your menstrual period.

**Missed dose**—If you miss a dose of this medicine, take it as soon as possible. However, if it is almost time for your next dose, skip the missed dose and go back to your regular dosing schedule. Do not double doses.

**Storage**—To store this medicine:
- Keep out of the reach of children.
- The bottle should be stored standing upright, with the tip up.
- Store away from heat and direct light.
- Keep the medicine from freezing. Do not refrigerate.
- Do not keep outdated medicine or medicine no longer needed. Be sure that any discarded medicine is out of the reach of children.

## Precautions While Using This Medicine

Your doctor should check your progress at regular visits to make sure that this medicine is working properly and to check for unwanted effects.

Using nafarelin can cause dryness of the vagina. If this is uncomfortable, especially during sex, there are several water-based vaginal lubricant products that you can use. Using a lubricant may also help to prevent soreness or damage to the vagina from sex. If you decide to use a lubricant during sex and you are using condoms, a cervical cap, or a diaphragm, make sure the lubricant you choose will not damage the birth control device. Some products contain oils, which can break down latex rubber and cause any of these types of birth control devices to rip or tear.

## Side Effects of This Medicine

In some animal studies, nafarelin was shown to increase the chance of certain types of tumors. The doses given were higher and were used longer than those used in humans. These effects have not been found in humans using recommended doses.

Along with its needed effects, a medicine may cause some unwanted effects. Although not all of these side effects may occur, if they do occur they may need medical attention.

Check with your doctor as soon as possible if any of the following side effects occur:

*More common*
Light vaginal bleeding between regular menstrual periods, which does not need the use of a pad or tampon ("spotting"); longer or heavier menstrual periods; vaginal bleeding between regular menstrual periods, which may need the use of a pad or tampon ("breakthrough bleeding")

*Rare*
Allergic reaction (shortness of breath, chest pain, hives); joint pain; pelvic or lower abdomen bloating or tenderness (mild); unexpected or excess flow of milk

Other side effects may occur that usually do not need medical attention. Some of these side effects may go away during treatment as your body adjusts to the medicine. However, check with your doctor if any of the following side effects continue or are bothersome:

*More common*
Lower estrogen in the bloodstream (acne, decreased sex drive, dryness of the vagina, hot flashes, pain during sex, decreased breast size, palpitations, oily skin); stopping of menstrual periods

*Less common or rare*
Breast pain; headache (mild and transient); irritated or runny nose; mental depression (mild and transient); mood swings; skin rash; weight changes

Other side effects not listed above may also occur in some patients. If you notice any other effects, check with your doctor.

Revised: 10/26/92
Interim revision: 07/05/94

---

# NAFTIFINE    Topical

A commonly used brand name in the U.S. and Canada is Naftin.

## Description

Naftifine (NAF-ti-feen) is used to treat fungus infections. It works by killing the fungus or preventing its growth.

Naftifine is applied to the skin to treat:
- athlete's foot (ringworm of the foot; tinea pedis);
- jock itch (ringworm of the groin; tinea cruris); and
- ringworm of the body (tinea corporis).

This medicine may also be used for other fungus infections of the skin as determined by your doctor.

Naftifine is available with or without your doctor's prescription, in the following dosage forms:

*Topical*
- Cream (U.S. and Canada)
- Gel (U.S. and Canada)

## Before Using This Medicine

In deciding to use a medicine, the risks of taking the medicine must be weighed against the good it will do. This is a decision you and your doctor will make. For topical naftifine, the following should be considered:

**Allergies**—Tell your doctor if you have ever had any unusual or allergic reaction to naftifine. Also tell your health care professional if you are allergic to any other substances, such as preservatives or dyes.

**Pregnancy**—Topical naftifine has not been studied in pregnant women. However, naftifine, when given by mouth, has not been shown to cause birth defects or other problems in animal studies.

**Breast-feeding**—Topical naftifine is absorbed into the body. However, it is not known whether naftifine passes into the breast milk. In addition, this medicine has not been reported to cause problems in nursing babies. Mothers who are using this medicine and who wish to breast-feed should discuss this with their doctor.

**Children**—Studies on this medicine have been done only in adult patients, and there is no specific information comparing use of naftifine in children with use in other age groups.

**Older adults**—Many medicines have not been studied specifically in older people. Therefore, it may not be known whether they work exactly the same way they do in younger adults or if they cause different side effects or problems in older people. There is no specific information comparing use of naftifine in the elderly with use in other age groups.

**Other medicines**—Although certain medicines should not be used together at all, in other cases two different medicines may be used together even if an interaction might occur. In these cases, your doctor may want to change the dose, or other precautions may be necessary. Tell your health care professional if you are using any other prescription or non-prescription (over-the-counter [OTC]) medicine.

---

## Proper Use of This Medicine

*Keep this medicine away from the eyes and mucous membranes such as the inside of the nose, mouth, or vagina.*

The area to which you have applied naftifine should not be covered with an occlusive dressing (airtight covering such as plastic wrap or bandage) unless otherwise directed by your doctor.

To use:
- Apply enough naftifine to cover the affected skin and surrounding areas, and rub in gently.
- After applying naftifine, wash your hands to remove any medicine that may be on them.

To help clear up your skin infection completely, *keep using naftifine for the full time of treatment.* You should keep using this medicine for 1 to 2 weeks after your symptoms have disappeared. If you stop using this medicine too soon, your symptoms may return. *Do not miss any doses.*

**Dosing**—The dose of naftifine will be different for different patients. *Follow your doctor's orders or the directions on the label.* The following information includes only the average doses of naftifine. *If your dose is different, do not change it* unless your doctor tells you to do so.

- For fungus infections:
  —For *cream* dosage form:
  - Adults—Apply to the affected area(s) of the skin once a day.
  - Children—Use and dose must be determined by your doctor.
  —For *gel* dosage form:
  - Adults—Apply to the affected area(s) of the skin two times a day, morning and evening.
  - Children—Use and dose must be determined by your doctor.

**Missed dose**—If you miss a dose of this medicine, apply it as soon as possible. However, if it is almost time for your next dose, skip the missed dose and go back to your regular dosing schedule.

**Storage**—To store this medicine:
- Keep out of the reach of children.
- Store away from heat and direct light.
- Keep the medicine from freezing.
- Do not keep outdated medicine or medicine no longer needed. Be sure that any discarded medicine is out of the reach of children.

---

## Precautions While Using This Medicine

If your skin infection does not improve within 4 weeks, or if it becomes worse, check with your doctor.

*To help clear up your skin infection completely and to help make sure it does not return, the following good health habits are important:*

- *For patients using naftifine for athlete's foot*, these measures will help keep the feet cool and dry:
  —Carefully dry the feet, especially between the toes, after bathing.
  —Avoid wearing socks made from wool or synthetic materials (for example, rayon or nylon). Instead, wear clean, cotton socks and change them daily or more often if your feet sweat very much.
  —Wear well-ventilated shoes (for example, shoes with holes on top or on the side) or sandals.
  —Use a bland, absorbent powder (for example, talcum powder) or an antifungal powder freely between the toes, on the feet, and in socks and shoes once or twice a day. Be sure to use the powder after naftifine has been applied and has disappeared into the skin. Do not use the powder as the only treatment for your fungus infection.

- *For patients using naftifine for jock itch*, these measures will help reduce chafing and irritation and will also help keep the groin area cool and dry:
  —Carefully dry the groin area after bathing.
  —Avoid wearing underwear that is tight-fitting or made from synthetic materials (for example, rayon

or nylon). Instead, wear loose-fitting, cotton underwear.

—Use a bland, absorbent powder (for example, talcum powder) or an antifungal powder freely once or twice a day. Be sure to use the powder after naftifine has been applied and has disappeared into the skin. Do not use the powder as the only treatment for your fungus infection.

- *For patients using naftifine for ringworm of the body*, these measures will help keep the affected areas cool and dry:
  —Carefully dry yourself after bathing.
  —Avoid too much heat and humidity if possible. Try to keep moisture from building up on affected areas of the body.
  —Wear well-ventilated clothing.
  —Use a bland, absorbent powder (for example, talcum powder) or an antifungal powder freely once or twice a day. Be sure to use the powder after naftifine has been applied and has disappeared into the skin. Do not use the powder as the only treatment for your fungus infection.

If you have any questions about this, check with your health care professional.

## Side Effects of This Medicine

Along with its needed effects, a medicine may cause some unwanted effects. The following side effects may go away during treatment as your body adjusts to the medicine. However, check with your doctor if any of these effects continue or are bothersome:

*More common*

Burning or stinging feeling on treated area(s)

*Less common*

Dry skin; itching, redness, or other sign of skin irritation not present before use of this medicine

Other side effects not listed above may also occur in some patients. If you notice any other effects, check with your doctor.

Revised: 07/25/94

---

# NALIDIXIC ACID    Systemic

A commonly used brand name in the U.S. and Canada is NegGram.

## Description

Nalidixic (nal-i-DIX-ik) acid is used to treat infections of the urinary tract. It may be used for other problems as determined by your doctor.

Nalidixic acid is available only with your doctor's prescription, in the following dosage forms:

*Oral*
- Suspension (U.S.)
- Tablets (U.S. and Canada)

## Before Using This Medicine

In deciding to use a medicine, the risks of taking the medicine must be weighed against the good it will do. This is a decision you and your doctor will make. For nalidixic acid, the following should be considered:

**Allergies**—Tell your doctor if you have ever had any unusual or allergic reaction to nalidixic acid, or to any related medicines such as cinoxacin (e.g., Cinobac), ciprofloxacin (e.g., Cipro), enoxacin (e.g. Penetrex), lomefloxacin (e.g., Maxaquin), norfloxacin (e.g., Noroxin), or ofloxacin (e.g., Floxin). Also tell your health care professional if you are allergic to any other substances, such as foods, preservatives, or dyes.

**Pregnancy**—Studies have not been done in humans. However, use is not recommended during pregnancy since nalidixic acid has been shown to cause bone development problems in young animals.

**Breast-feeding**—Nalidixic acid passes into the breast milk. This medicine may cause blood problems in nursing babies with glucose-6-phosphate dehydrogenase (G6PD) deficiency. However, problems in other nursing babies have not been reported.

**Children**—This medicine is not recommended for use in infants up to 3 months of age since nalidixic acid has been shown to cause bone problems in young animals.

**Older adults**—This medicine has been studied in a limited number of elderly patients and has not been shown to cause different side effects or problems in older people than it does in younger adults.

**Other medicines**—Although certain medicines should not be used together at all, in other cases two different medicines may be used together even if an interaction might occur. In these cases, your doctor may want to change the dose, or other precautions may be necessary. When you are taking nalidixic acid, it is especially important that your health care professional know if you are taking any of the following:

- Anticoagulants (blood thinners)—Patients taking nalidixic acid with anticoagulants may have an increased chance of bleeding

**Other medical problems**—The presence of other medical problems may affect the use of nalidixic acid. Make sure

you tell your doctor if you have any other medical problems, especially:

- Convulsive disorders, history of (seizures, epilepsy) or
- Hardening of the arteries in the brain (severe)—Patients with these medical problems may have an increased chance of side effects affecting the nervous system
- Glucose-6-phosphate dehydrogenase (G6PD) deficiency—Patients with G6PD deficiency may have an increased chance of side effects affecting the blood
- Kidney disease (severe) or
- Liver disease—Patients with liver disease or severe kidney disease may have an increase in side effects

## Proper Use of This Medicine

*Do not give this medicine to infants or children* unless otherwise directed by your doctor. It has been shown to cause bone problems in young animals and may cause these problems in children.

Nalidixic acid is best taken with a full glass (8 ounces) of water on an empty stomach (either 1 hour before or 2 hours after meals). However, if this medicine causes nausea or upset stomach, it may be taken with food or milk.

For patients taking the *oral liquid form* of this medicine:

- Use a specially marked measuring spoon or other device to measure each dose accurately. The average household teaspoon may not hold the right amount of liquid.

To help clear up your infection completely, *keep taking this medicine for the full time of treatment,* even if you begin to feel better after a few days. *Do not miss any doses.*

**Dosing**—The dose of nalidixic acid will be different for different patients. *Follow your doctor's orders or the directions on the label.* The following information includes only the average doses of nalidixic acid. *If your dose is different, do not change it* unless your doctor tells you to do so.

The number of tablets or teaspoonfuls of suspension that you take depends on the strength of the medicine. Also, *the number of doses you take each day, the time allowed between doses, and the length of time you take the medicine depend on the medical problem for which you are taking nalidixic acid.*

- For *oral* dosage forms (oral suspension or tablets):
  —Adults and children 12 years of age and older: 1 gram (g) every six hours for one to two weeks to start; then, 500 milligrams (mg) every six hours.
  —Children 3 months to 12 years of age: The dose is based on body weight and must be determined by the doctor.
  —Infants up to 3 months of age: This medicine is not recommended in infants up to 3 months of age since nalidixic acid has been shown to cause bone problems in young animals.

**Missed dose**—If you do miss a dose of this medicine, take it as soon as possible. However, if it is almost time for your next dose, skip the missed dose and go back to your regular dosing schedule. Do not double doses.

**Storage**—To store this medicine:

- Keep out of the reach of children.
- Store away from heat and direct light.
- Do not store the tablet form of this medicine in the bathroom, near the kitchen sink, or in other damp places. Heat or moisture may cause the medicine to break down.
- Keep the oral liquid form of this medicine from freezing.
- Do not keep outdated medicine or medicine no longer needed. Be sure that any discarded medicine is out of the reach of children.

## Precautions While Using This Medicine

If you will be taking this medicine for more than 2 weeks, your doctor should check your progress at regular visits.

If your symptoms do not improve within 2 days, or if they become worse, check with your doctor.

This medicine may cause blurred vision or other vision problems. It may also cause some people to become dizzy, drowsy, or less alert than they are normally. *Make sure you know how you react to this medicine before you drive, use machines, or do anything else that could be dangerous if you are dizzy or are not alert or able to see well.* If these reactions are especially bothersome, check with your doctor.

Nalidixic acid may cause your skin to be more sensitive to sunlight than it is normally. Exposure to sunlight, even for brief periods of time, may cause a skin rash, itching, redness or other discoloration of the skin, or a severe sunburn. When you begin taking this medicine:

- Stay out of direct sunlight, especially between the hours of 10:00 a.m. and 3:00 p.m., if possible.
- Wear protective clothing, including a hat. Also, wear sunglasses.
- Apply a sun block product that has a skin protection factor (SPF) of at least 15. Some patients may require a product with a higher SPF number, especially if they have a fair complexion. If you have any questions about this, check with your health care professional.
- Apply a sun block lipstick that has an SPF of at least 15 to protect your lips.
- Do not use a sunlamp or tanning bed or booth.

*If you have a severe reaction from the sun, check with your doctor.*

For diabetic patients:

- *This medicine may cause false test results with some urine glucose (sugar) tests.* Check with your doctor before changing your diet or the dosage of your diabetes medicine.

## Side Effects of This Medicine

Along with its needed effects, a medicine may cause some unwanted effects. Although not all of these side effects may occur, if they do occur they may need medical attention.

*Check with your doctor immediately* if any of the following side effects occur:

*More common*
   Blurred or decreased vision; change in color vision; double vision; halos around lights; overbright appearance of lights

*Rare*
   Bulging of fontanel (soft spot) on top of head of an infant; convulsions (seizures); dark or amber urine; hallucinations (seeing, hearing, or feeling things that are not there); headache (severe); mood or other mental changes; pale skin; pale stools; skin rash and itching; sore throat and fever; stomach pain (severe); unusual bleeding or bruising; unusual tiredness or weakness; yellow eyes or skin

Other side effects may occur that usually do not need medical attention. These side effects may go away during treatment as your body adjusts to the medicine. However, check with your doctor if any of the following side effects continue or are bothersome:

*More common*
   Diarrhea; dizziness; drowsiness; headache; nausea or vomiting; stomach pain

*Less common*
   Increased sensitivity of skin to sunlight

Other side effects not listed above may also occur in some patients. If you notice any other effects, check with your doctor.

Revised: 05/14/93

# NALTREXONE    Systemic

A commonly used brand name in the U.S. is Trexan.

## Description

Naltrexone (nal-TREX-zone) is used to help narcotic addicts who have stopped taking narcotics to stay drug-free. The medicine is not a cure for addiction. It is used as part of an overall program that may include counseling, attending support group meetings, and other treatment recommended by your doctor.

Naltrexone is not a narcotic. It works by blocking the effects of narcotics, especially the "high" feeling that makes you want to use them. It will not produce any narcotic-like effects or cause mental or physical dependence.

Naltrexone will cause withdrawal symptoms in people who are physically dependent on narcotics. Therefore, naltrexone treatment is started after you are no longer dependent on narcotics. The length of time this takes may depend on which narcotic you took, the amount you took, and how long you took it. Before you start taking this medicine, be sure to tell your doctor if you think you are still having withdrawal symptoms.

Naltrexone is available only with your doctor's prescription, in the following dosage form:

*Oral*
   • Tablets (U.S.)

## Before Using This Medicine

In deciding to use a medicine, the risks of taking the medicine must be weighed against the good it will do.

This is a decision you and your doctor will make. For naltrexone, the following should be considered:

**Allergies**—Tell your doctor if you have ever had any unusual or allergic reaction to naltrexone. Also tell your health care professional if you are allergic to any other substances, such as foods, preservatives, or dyes.

**Pregnancy**—Studies on birth defects with naltrexone have not been done in humans. Studies in animals have shown that naltrexone causes unwanted effects when given in very large doses.

**Breast-feeding**—It is not known whether naltrexone passes into the breast milk. However, this medicine has not been reported to cause problems in nursing babies.

**Children**—Naltrexone has been tested only in adult patients and there is no specific information about its use in patients up to 18 years of age.

**Older adults**—Many medicines have not been tested in older people. Therefore, it may not be known whether they work exactly the same way they do in younger adults or if they cause different side effects or problems in older people. There is no specific information about the use of naltrexone in the elderly.

**Other medical problems**—The presence of other medical problems may affect the use of naltrexone. Make sure you tell your doctor if you have any other medical problems, especially:
   • Hepatitis or other liver disease—The chance of side effects may be increased

## Proper Use of This Medicine

*Take naltrexone regularly as ordered by your doctor.* It may be helpful to have someone else, such as a family member, doctor, or nurse, give you each dose as scheduled.

**Dosing**—The dose of naltrexone will be different for different patients. *Follow your doctor's orders or the directions on the label.* The following information includes only the average doses of naltrexone. *If your dose is different, do not change it* unless your doctor tells you to do so.

- For *oral* dosage form (tablets):
  —For treating narcotic addiction:
  - Adults—25 milligrams (mg) (one-half tablet) for the first dose, then another 25 mg one hour later. After that, the dose is 350 mg a week. Your doctor will direct you to divide up this weekly dose and take naltrexone according to one of the following schedules:
    —50 mg (one tablet) every day; or
    —50 mg a day during the week and 100 mg (two tablets) on Saturday; or
    —100 mg every other day; or
    —100 mg on Mondays and Wednesdays, and 150 mg (three tablets) on Fridays; or
    —150 mg every 3 days.
  - Children and teenagers up to 18 years of age— Dose must be determined by your doctor.

**Missed dose**—If you miss a dose of this medicine, and your regular dosing schedule is:

- One tablet every day:
  —Take the missed dose as soon as possible. However, if you do not remember until the next day, skip the missed dose and go back to your regular dosing schedule. Do not double the next day's dose.
- One tablet every weekday and two tablets on Saturday:
  —If you miss a weekday dose, follow the directions for one tablet every day.
  —If you miss the Saturday dose, take it as soon as possible. However, if you do not remember until Sunday, take one tablet on Sunday. Then go back to your regular dosing schedule on Monday.
- Two tablets every other day:
  —Take two tablets as soon as you remember, then skip a day, then go back to taking the medicine every other day; or
  —Take two tablets as soon as possible if you remember the same day. However, if you do not remember until the next day, take one tablet the next day. Then go back to your regular dosing schedule.
- Two tablets on Monday and Wednesday and three tablets on Friday:
  —If you miss one of the Monday or Wednesday doses, take it as soon as possible. However, if you do not remember until the next day, take one tablet

the next day. Then go back to your regular dosing schedule.
  —If you miss the Friday dose, take it as soon as possible if you remember the same day. However, if you do not remember until Saturday, take two tablets on Saturday. If you do not remember until Sunday, take one tablet on Sunday. Then go back to your regular dosing schedule on Monday.
- Three tablets every three days:
  —Take three tablets as soon you remember, then skip two days, then go back to taking the medicine every three days; or
  —Take three tablets as soon as possible if you remember the same day. However, if you do not remember until the next day, take two tablets, then skip a day and go back to your regular dosing schedule. If you do not remember until the second day, take one tablet. Then go back to your regular dosing schedule.

**Storage**—To store this medicine:
- Keep out of the reach of children.
- Store away from heat and direct light.
- Do not store this medicine in the bathroom, near the kitchen sink, or in other damp places. Heat or moisture may cause the medicine to break down.
- Do not keep outdated medicine.

## Precautions While Using This Medicine

*It is very important that your doctor check your progress at regular visits.* Your doctor may want to do certain blood tests to see if the medicine is causing unwanted effects.

Remember that use of naltrexone is only part of your treatment. *Be sure that you follow all of your doctor's orders, including seeing your therapist and/or attending support group meetings on a regular basis.*

*Do not try to overcome the effects of naltrexone by taking very large amounts of narcotics.* To do so may cause coma or death.

Naltrexone also blocks the useful effects of narcotics. *Always use a non-narcotic medicine to treat pain, diarrhea, or cough.* If you have any questions about the proper medicine to use, check with your health care professional.

*Never share this medicine with anyone else.* This is especially important if the other person is using narcotics because naltrexone will cause withdrawal symptoms.

*Tell all medical doctors, dentists, and pharmacists you go to that you are taking naltrexone.*

*It is recommended that you carry identification stating that you are taking naltrexone.* Identification cards may be available from your doctor.

## Side Effects of This Medicine

Along with its needed effects, a medicine may cause some unwanted effects. Although not all of these side effects

may occur, if they do occur they may need medical attention.

Check with your doctor as soon as possible if any of the following side effects occur:

*More common*
   Skin rash

*Rare*
   Abdominal or stomach pain (severe); blurred vision or aching, burning, or swollen eyes; confusion; discomfort while urinating and/or frequent urination; earache; fever; hallucinations (seeing, hearing, or feeling things that are not there); increased blood pressure; itching; mental depression or other mood or mental changes; nosebleeds (unexplained); pain, tenderness, or color changes in legs or feet; ringing or buzzing in ears; shortness of breath; swelling of face, feet, or lower legs; swollen glands; weight gain

Other side effects may occur that usually do not need medical attention. These side effects may go away during treatment as your body adjusts to the medicine. However, check with your doctor if any of the following side effects continue or are bothersome:

*More common*
   Abdominal or stomach cramping or pain (mild or moderate); anxiety, nervousness, restlessness, and/or trouble in sleeping; headache; joint or muscle pain; nausea or vomiting; unusual tiredness

*Less common or rare*
   Chills; constipation; cough, hoarseness, runny or stuffy nose, sinus problems, sneezing, and/or sore throat; diarrhea; dizziness; fast or pounding heartbeat; increased thirst; irritability; loss of appetite; sexual problems in males

Other side effects not listed above, possibly including withdrawal symptoms, may also occur in some patients. If you notice any other effects, check with your doctor.

---

Revised: June 1990
Interim revision: 08/16/94

---

# NAPHAZOLINE   Ophthalmic

Some commonly used brand names are:

**In the U.S.—**

| | |
|---|---|
| Ak-Con | Muro's Opcon |
| Albalon | Nafazair |
| Allerest | Naphcon |
| Allergy Drops | Naphcon Forte |
| Clear Eyes Lubricating Eye Redness Reliever | Ocu-Zoline Sterile Ophthalmic Solution |
| Comfort Eye Drops | VasoClear |
| Degest 2 | VasoClear A |
| Estivin II | Vasocon Regular |
| I-Naphline | |

Generic name product may also be available.

**In Canada—**

| | |
|---|---|
| Ak-Con | Naphcon Forte |
| Albalon Liquifilm | Vasocon |

## Description

Naphazoline (naf-AZ-oh-leen) is used to relieve redness due to minor eye irritations, such as those caused by colds, dust, wind, smog, pollen, swimming, or wearing contact lenses.

Some of these preparations are available only with your doctor's prescription. Others are available without a prescription; however, your doctor may have special instructions on the proper use of this medicine for your medical problem.

Naphazoline is available in the following dosage form:

*Ophthalmic*
   • Ophthalmic solution (eye drops) (U.S. and Canada)

## Before Using This Medicine

If you are using this medicine without a prescription, carefully read and follow any precautions on the label.

For ophthalmic naphazoline, the following should be considered:

**Allergies**—Tell your doctor if you have ever had any unusual or allergic reaction to naphazoline. Also tell your health care professional if you are allergic to any other substances, such as preservatives.

**Pregnancy**—This medicine may be absorbed into the body. However, studies on effects in pregnancy have not been done in either humans or animals.

**Breast-feeding**—Naphazoline may be absorbed into the mother's body. However, this medicine has not been reported to cause problems in nursing babies.

**Children**—Use by infants and children is not recommended, since they are especially sensitive to the effects of naphazoline.

**Older adults**—Many medicines have not been studied specifically in older people. Therefore, it may not be known whether they work exactly the same way they do in younger adults or if they cause different side effects or problems in older people. There is no specific information comparing use of naphazoline in the elderly with use in other age groups.

**Other medicines**—Although certain medicines should not be used together at all, in other cases two different medicines may be used together even if an interaction might occur. In these cases, your doctor may want to change the dose, or other precautions may be necessary. Tell your health care professional if you are using any other prescription or nonprescription (over-the-counter [OTC]) medicine.

**Other medical problems**—The presence of other medical problems may affect the use of ophthalmic naphazoline. Make sure you tell your doctor if you have any other medical problems, especially:

- Diabetes mellitus (sugar diabetes) or
- Heart disease or
- High blood pressure or
- Overactive thyroid—Use of ophthalmic naphazoline may make the condition worse
- Eye disease, infection, or injury—The symptoms of the condition may be confused with possible side effects of ophthalmic naphazoline

## Proper Use of This Medicine

Do not use naphazoline ophthalmic solution if it becomes cloudy or changes color.

*Naphazoline should not be used in infants and children.* It may cause severe slowing down of the central nervous system (CNS), which may lead to unconsciousness. It may also cause a severe decrease in body temperature.

*Use this medicine only as directed.* Do not use more of it, do not use it more often, and do not use it for more than 72 hours, unless otherwise directed by your doctor. To do so may make your eye redness and irritation worse and may also increase the chance of side effects.

To use:

- First, wash your hands. With the middle finger, apply pressure to the inside corner of the eye (and continue to apply pressure for 1 or 2 minutes after the medicine has been placed in the eye). Tilt the head back and with the index finger of the same hand, pull the lower eyelid away from the eye to form a pouch. Drop the medicine into the pouch and gently close the eyes. Do not blink. Keep the eyes closed for 1 or 2 minutes to allow the medicine to be absorbed.
- To keep the medicine as germ-free as possible, do not touch the applicator tip to any surface (including the eye). Also, keep the container tightly closed.

**Dosing**—The dose of ophthalmic naphazoline will be different for different patients. *Follow your doctor's orders or the directions on the label.* The following information includes only the average doses of ophthalmic naphazoline. *If your dose is different, do not change it* unless your doctor tells you to do so.

- For *ophthalmic solution (eye drop)* dosage form:
  —For eye redness:
    - Adults—Use one drop not more often than every four hours.
    - Children—Use is not recommended.

**Storage**—To store this medicine:

- Keep out of the reach of children.
- Store away from heat and direct light.
- Keep the medicine from freezing.
- Do not keep outdated medicine or medicine no longer needed. Be sure that any discarded medicine is out of the reach of children.

## Precautions While Using This Medicine

*If eye pain or change in vision occurs or if redness or irritation of the eye continues, gets worse, or lasts for more than 72 hours, stop using the medicine and check with your doctor.*

## Side Effects of This Medicine

Along with its needed effects, a medicine may cause some unwanted effects. Although not all of these side effects may occur, if they do occur they may need medical attention.

When this medicine is used for short periods of time at recommended doses, side effects usually are rare. However, check with your doctor as soon as possible if any of the following occur:

*With overuse or long-term use*
  Increase in eye irritation
*Symptoms of too much medicine being absorbed into the body*
  Dizziness; headache; increased sweating; nausea; nervousness; weakness
*Symptoms of overdose*
  Decrease in body temperature; drowsiness; slow heartbeat; weakness (severe)

Other side effects may occur that usually do not need medical attention. These side effects may go away during treatment as your body adjusts to the medicine. However, check with your health care professional if either of the following side effects continues or is bothersome:

*Less common or rare*
  Blurred vision; large pupils

Other side effects not listed above may also occur in some patients. If you notice any other effects, check with your health care professional.

Revised: 05/14/92
Interim revision: 02/24/94

# NARCOTIC ANALGESICS—For Pain Relief   Systemic

Some commonly used brand names are:

**In the U.S.—**

| | |
|---|---|
| Astramorph[9] | MSIR[9] |
| Astramorph PF[9] | Nubain[10] |
| Buprenex[1] | Numorphan[13] |
| Darvon[15] | Pantopon[11] |
| Darvon-N[15] | Profene[15] |
| Demerol[7] | Pro Pox[15] |
| Dilaudid[5] | Propoxycon[15] |
| Dilaudid-HP[5] | RMS Uniserts[9] |
| Dolene[15] | Roxanol[9] |
| Dolophine[8] | Roxanol 100[9] |
| Doraphen[15] | Roxanol SR[9] |
| Doxaphene[15] | Stadol[2] |
| Duramorph[9] | Roxicodone[12] |
| Levo-Dromoran[6] | Talwin[14] |
| Methadose[8] | Talwin-Nx[14] |
| M S Contin[9] | |

**In Canada—**

| | |
|---|---|
| Darvon-N[15] | Novopropoxyn[15] |
| Demerol[7] | Nubain[10] |
| Dilaudid[5] | Numorphan[13] |
| Dilaudid-HP[5] | Pantopon[11] |
| Epimorph[9] | Paveral[3] |
| Hycodan[4]# | Robidone[4] |
| Levo-Dromoran[6] | Roxanol[9] |
| Morphine H.P.[9] | 642[15] |
| Morphitec[9] | Stadol[2] |
| M.O.S.[9] | Statex[9] |
| M.O.S.-S.R.[9] | Supeudol[12] |
| M S Contin[9] | Talwin[14] |

Other commonly used names are:

| | |
|---|---|
| dextropropoxyphene[15] | papaveretum[11] |
| dihydromorphinone[5] | pethidine[7] |
| levorphan[6] | |

Note: For quick reference, the following narcotic analgesics are numbered to match the corresponding brand names.

This information applies to the following medicines:

1. Buprenorphine (byoo-pre-NOR-feen)
2. Butorphanol (byoo-TOR-fa-nole)
3. Codeine (KOE-deen)‡§
4. Hydrocodone (hye-droe-KOE-done)*
5. Hydromorphone (hye-droe-MOR-fone)‡
6. Levorphanol (lee-VOR-fa-nole)‡
7. Meperidine (me-PER-i-deen)‡§
8. Methadone (METH-a-done)‡**
9. Morphine (MOR-feen)‡§
10. Nalbuphine (NAL-byoo-feen)‡
11. Opium Injection (OH-pee-um)
12. Oxycodone (ox-i-KOE-done)
13. Oxymorphone (ox-i-MOR-fone)
14. Pentazocine (pen-TAZ-oh-seen)
15. Propoxyphene (proe-POX-i-feen)‡

This information does *not* apply to Opium Tincture or Paregoric.

---

*Not commercially available in the U.S.
‡Generic name product may also be available in the U.S.
§Generic name product may also be available in Canada.
#For Canadian product only. In the U.S., *Hycodan* also contains homatropine; in Canada, *Hycodan* contains only hydrocodone.
**In Canada, methadone is available only through doctors who have received special approval to prescribe it.

---

## Description

Narcotic (nar-KOT-ik) analgesics (an-al-JEE-zicks) are used to relieve pain. Some of these medicines are also used just before or during an operation to help the anesthetic work better. Codeine and hydrocodone are also used to relieve coughing. Methadone is also used to help some people control their dependence on heroin or other narcotics. Narcotic analgesics may also be used for other conditions as determined by your doctor.

Narcotic analgesics act in the central nervous system (CNS) to relieve pain. Some of their side effects are also caused by actions in the CNS.

If a narcotic is used for a long time, it may become habit-forming (causing mental or physical dependence). Physical dependence may lead to withdrawal side effects when you stop taking the medicine.

These medicines are available only with your medical doctor's or dentist's prescription. For some of them, prescriptions cannot be refilled and you must obtain a new prescription from your medical doctor or dentist each time you need the medicine. In addition, other rules and regulations may apply when methadone is used to treat narcotic dependence.

These medicines are available in the following dosage forms:

*Oral*

Codeine
  • Oral solution (U.S. and Canada)
  • Tablets (U.S. and Canada)
Hydrocodone
  • Syrup (Canada)
  • Tablets (Canada)
Hydromorphone
  • Tablets (U.S. and Canada)
Levorphanol
  • Tablets (U.S. and Canada)
Meperidine
  • Syrup (U.S.)
  • Tablets (U.S. and Canada)
Methadone
  • Oral concentrate (U.S.)
  • Oral solution (U.S.)
  • Tablets (U.S.)
  • Dispersible tablets (U.S.)
Morphine
  • Oral solution (U.S. and Canada)
  • Syrup (Canada)
  • Tablets (U.S. and Canada)
  • Extended-release tablets (U.S. and Canada)
Oxycodone
  • Oral solution (U.S.)
  • Tablets (U.S. and Canada)
Pentazocine
  • Tablets (Canada)
Pentazocine and Naloxone
  • Tablets (U.S.)
Propoxyphene
  • Capsules (U.S. and Canada)
  • Oral suspension (U.S.)
  • Tablets (U.S. and Canada)

*Parenteral*

Buprenorphine
  • Injection (U.S.)

Butorphanol
  • Injection (U.S. and Canada)
Codeine
  • Injection (U.S. and Canada)
Hydromorphone
  • Injection (U.S. and Canada)
Levorphanol
  • Injection (U.S. and Canada)
Meperidine
  • Injection (U.S. and Canada)
Methadone
  • Injection (U.S.)
Morphine
  • Injection (U.S. and Canada)
Nalbuphine
  • Injection (U.S. and Canada)
Opium
  • Injection (U.S. and Canada)
Oxymorphone
  • Injection (U.S. and Canada)
Pentazocine
  • Injection (U.S. and Canada)

*Rectal*
Hydromorphone
  • Suppositories (U.S. and Canada)
Morphine
  • Suppositories (U.S. and Canada)
Oxycodone
  • Suppositories (Canada)
Oxymorphone
  • Suppositories (U.S. and Canada)

## Before Using This Medicine

In deciding to use a medicine, the risks of taking the medicine must be weighed against the good it will do. This is a decision you and your doctor will make. For narcotic analgesics, the following should be considered:

**Allergies**—Tell your doctor if you have ever had any unusual or allergic reaction to any of the narcotic analgesics. Also tell your health care professional if you are allergic to any other substances, such as foods, preservatives, or dyes.

**Pregnancy**—Although studies on birth defects with narcotic analgesics have not been done in pregnant women, these medicines have not been reported to cause birth defects. However, hydrocodone, hydromorphone, and morphine caused birth defects in animals when given in very large doses. Buprenorphine and codeine did not cause birth defects in animal studies, but they caused other unwanted effects. Butorphanol, nalbuphine, pentazocine, and propoxyphene did not cause birth defects in animals. There is no information about whether other narcotic analgesics cause birth defects in animals.

Too much use of a narcotic during pregnancy may cause the baby to become dependent on the medicine. This may lead to withdrawal side effects after birth. Also, some of these medicines may cause breathing problems in the newborn infant if taken just before delivery.

**Breast-feeding**—Most narcotic analgesics have not been reported to cause problems in nursing babies. However, when the mother is taking large amounts of methadone (in a methadone maintenance program), the nursing baby may become dependent on the medicine. Also, butorphanol, codeine, meperidine, morphine, opium, and propoxyphene pass into the breast milk.

**Children**—Breathing problems may be especially likely to occur in children younger than 2 years of age. These children are usually more sensitive than adults to the effects of narcotic analgesics. Also, unusual excitement or restlessness may be more likely to occur in children receiving these medicines.

**Older adults**—Elderly people are especially sensitive to the effects of narcotic analgesics. This may increase the chance of side effects, especially breathing problems, during treatment.

**Other medicines**—Although certain medicines should not be used together at all, in other cases two different medicines may be used together even if an interaction might occur. In these cases, your doctor may want to change the dose, or other precautions may be necessary. When you are taking a narcotic analgesic, it is especially important that your health care professional know if you are taking any of the following:

  • Carbamazepine (e.g., Tegretol)—Propoxyphene may increase the blood levels of carbamazepine, which increases the chance of serious side effects
  • Central nervous system (CNS) depressants or
  • Monoamine oxidase (MAO) inhibitors (furazolidone [e.g., Furoxone], isocarboxazid [e.g., Marplan], pargyline [e.g., Eutonyl], phenelzine [e.g., Nardil], procarbazine [e.g., Matulane], tranylcypromine [e.g., Parnate] (taken currently or within the past 2 weeks) or
  • Tricyclic antidepressants (amitriptyline [e.g., Elavil], amoxapine [e.g., Asendin], clomipramine [e.g., Anafranil], desipramine [e.g., Pertofrane], doxepin [e.g., Sinequan], imipramine [e.g., Tofranil], nortriptyline [e.g., Aventyl], protriptyline [e.g., Vivactil], trimipramine [e.g., Surmontil])—The chance of side effects may be increased; the combination of meperidine (e.g., Demerol) and MAO inhibitors is especially dangerous
  • Naltrexone (e.g., Trexan)—Narcotics will not be effective in people taking naltrexone
  • Rifampin (e.g., Rifadin)—Rifampin decreases the effects of methadone and may cause withdrawal symptoms in people who are dependent on methadone
  • Zidovudine (e.g., AZT, Retrovir)—Morphine may increase the blood levels of zidovudine and increase the chance of serious side effects

**Other medical problems**—The presence of other medical problems may affect the use of narcotic analgesics. Make sure you tell your doctor if you have any other medical problems, especially:

  • Alcohol abuse, or history of, or
  • Drug dependence, especially narcotic abuse, or history of, or
  • Emotional problems—The chance of side effects may be increased; also, withdrawal symptoms may occur if a narcotic you are dependent on is replaced by buprenorphine, butorphanol, nalbuphine, or pentazocine
  • Brain disease or head injury or
  • Emphysema, asthma, or other chronic lung disease or

- Enlarged prostate or problems with urination or
- Gallbladder disease or gallstones—Some of the side effects of narcotic analgesics can be dangerous if these conditions are present
- Colitis or
- Heart disease or
- Kidney disease or
- Liver disease or
- Underactive thyroid—The chance of side effects may be increased
- Convulsions (seizures), history of—Some of the narcotic analgesics can cause convulsions

---

## Proper Use of This Medicine

Some narcotic analgesics given by injection may be given at home to patients who do not need to be in the hospital. If you are using an injection form of this medicine at home, *make sure you clearly understand and carefully follow your doctor's instructions.*

To take the *syrup form of meperidine:*

- Unless otherwise directed by your medical doctor or dentist, *take this medicine mixed with a half glass (4 ounces) of water* to lessen the numbing effect of the medicine on your mouth and throat.

To take the *oral liquid forms of methadone:*

- *This medicine may have to be mixed with water or another liquid before you take it.* Read the label carefully for directions. If you have any questions about this, check with your health care professional.

To take the *dispersible tablet form of methadone:*

- *These tablets must be stirred into water or fruit juice just before each dose is taken.* Read the label carefully for directions. If you have any questions about this, check with your health care professional.

To take *oral liquid forms of morphine:*

- This medicine may be mixed with a glass of fruit juice just before you take it, if desired, to improve the taste.

To take *long-acting morphine tablets:*

- *These tablets must be swallowed whole.* Do not break, crush, or chew them before swallowing.

To use *suppositories:*

- If the suppository is too soft to insert, chill it in the refrigerator for 30 minutes or run cold water over it before removing the foil wrapper.
- To insert the suppository: First remove the foil wrapper and moisten the suppository with cold water. Lie down on your side and use your finger to push the suppository well up into the rectum.

*Take this medicine only as directed by your medical doctor or dentist.* Do not take more of it, do not take it more often, and do not take it for a longer time than your medical doctor or dentist ordered. This is especially important for young children and elderly patients, who are especially sensitive to the effects of narcotic analgesics.

If too much is taken, the medicine may become habit-forming (causing mental or physical dependence) or lead to medical problems because of an overdose.

If you think this medicine is not working properly after you have been taking it for a few weeks, *do not increase the dose.* Instead, check with your doctor.

**Missed dose**—If your medical doctor or dentist has ordered you to take this medicine according to a regular schedule and you miss a dose, take it as soon as you remember. However, if it is almost time for your next dose, skip the missed dose and go back to your regular dosing schedule. *Do not double doses.*

**Storage**—To store this medicine:

- Keep out of the reach of children. Overdose is very dangerous in young children.
- Store away from heat and direct light.
- Do not store tablets or capsules in the bathroom, near the kitchen sink, or in other damp places. Heat or moisture may cause the medicine to break down.
- Store hydromorphone, oxycodone, or oxymorphone suppositories in the refrigerator.
- Keep liquid (including injections) and suppository forms of the medicine from freezing.
- Do not keep outdated medicine or medicine no longer needed. Be sure that any discarded medicine is out of the reach of children.

---

## Precautions While Using This Medicine

If you will be taking this medicine for a long time (for example, for several months at a time), your doctor should check your progress at regular visits.

Narcotic analgesics will add to the effects of alcohol and other CNS depressants (medicines that slow down the nervous system, possibly causing drowsiness). Some examples of CNS depressants are antihistamines or medicine for hay fever, other allergies, or colds; sedatives, tranquilizers, or sleeping medicine; other prescription pain medicines including other narcotics; barbiturates; medicine for seizures; muscle relaxants; or anesthetics, including some dental anesthetics. *Do not drink alcoholic beverages, and check with your medical doctor or dentist before taking any of the medicines listed above, while you are using this medicine.*

This medicine may cause some people to become drowsy, dizzy, or lightheaded, or to feel a false sense of well-being. *Make sure you know how you react to this medicine before you drive, use machines, or do anything else that could be dangerous if you are dizzy or are not alert and clearheaded.*

Dizziness, lightheadedness, or fainting may occur, especially when you get up suddenly from a lying or sitting position. Getting up slowly may help lessen this problem.

Nausea or vomiting may occur, especially after the first couple of doses. This effect may go away if you lie down for a while. However, if nausea or vomiting continues, check with your medical doctor or dentist. Lying down

---

© 1994   The United States Pharmacopeial Convention, Inc.

for a while may also help relieve some other side effects, such as dizziness or lightheadedness, that may occur.

Before having any kind of surgery (including dental surgery) or emergency treatment, tell the medical doctor or dentist in charge that you are taking this medicine.

Narcotic analgesics may cause dryness of the mouth. For temporary relief, use sugarless candy or gum, melt bits of ice in your mouth, or use a saliva substitute. However, if dry mouth continues for more than 2 weeks, check with your dentist. Continuing dryness of the mouth may increase the chance of dental disease, including tooth decay, gum disease, and fungus infections.

If you have been taking this medicine regularly for several weeks or more, *do not suddenly stop using it without first checking with your doctor.* Your doctor may want you to reduce gradually the amount you are taking before stopping completely, in order to lessen the chance of withdrawal side effects.

*If you think you or someone else may have taken an overdose, get emergency help at once.* Taking an overdose of this medicine or taking alcohol or CNS depressants with this medicine may lead to unconsciousness or death. Signs of overdose include convulsions (seizures), confusion, severe nervousness or restlessness, severe dizziness, severe drowsiness, slow or troubled breathing, and severe weakness.

## Side Effects of This Medicine

Along with its needed effects, a medicine may cause some unwanted effects. Although not all of these side effects may occur, if they do occur they may need medical attention.

*Get emergency help immediately if any of the following symptoms of overdose occur:*

Cold, clammy skin; confusion; convulsions (seizures); dizziness (severe); drowsiness (severe); low blood pressure; nervousness or restlessness (severe); pinpoint pupils of eyes; slow heartbeat; slow or troubled breathing; weakness (severe)

Also, check with your doctor as soon as possible if any of the following side effects occur:

*Less common or rare*

Dark urine (for propoxyphene only); fast, slow, or pounding heartbeat; feelings of unreality; hallucinations (seeing, hearing, or feeling things that are not there); hives, itching, or skin rash; increased sweating (more common with hydrocodone, meperidine, and methadone); irregular breathing; mental depression or other mood or mental changes; pale stools (for propoxyphene only); redness or flushing of face (more common with hydrocodone, meperidine, and methadone); ringing or buzzing in the ears; shortness of breath, wheezing, or troubled breathing; swelling of face; trembling or uncontrolled muscle movements; unusual excitement or restlessness (especially in children); yellow eyes or skin (for propoxyphene only)

Other side effects may occur that usually do not need medical attention. These side effects may go away during treatment as your body adjusts to the medicine. However, check with your doctor if any of the following side effects continue or are bothersome:

*More common*

Dizziness, lightheadedness, or feeling faint; drowsiness; nausea or vomiting

*Less common or rare*

Blurred or double vision or other changes in vision; constipation (more common with long-term use and with codeine); decrease in amount of urine; difficult or painful urination; dry mouth; false sense of well-being; frequent urge to urinate; general feeling of discomfort or illness; headache; loss of appetite; nervousness or restlessness; nightmares or unusual dreams; redness, swelling, pain, or burning at place of injection; stomach cramps or pain; trouble in sleeping; unusual tiredness or weakness

After you stop using this medicine, your body may need time to adjust. The length of time this takes depends on the amount of medicine you were using and how long you used it. During this period of time check with your doctor if you notice any of the following side effects:

Body aches; diarrhea; fast heartbeat; fever, runny nose, or sneezing; gooseflesh; increased sweating; increased yawning; loss of appetite; nausea or vomiting; nervousness, restlessness, or irritability; shivering or trembling; stomach cramps; trouble in sleeping; unusually large pupils of eyes; weakness

Other side effects not listed above may also occur in some patients. If you notice any other effects, check with your doctor.

Revised: July 1990

---

# NARCOTIC ANALGESICS—For Surgery and Obstetrics   Systemic

Some commonly used brand names are:

**In the U.S.—**

| | |
|---|---|
| Alfenta[1] | Duramorph[6] |
| Astramorph[6] | Nubain[7] |
| Astramorph PF[6] | Stadol[3] |
| Buprenex[2] | Sublimaze[4] |
| Demerol[5] | Sufenta[8] |

**In Canada—**

| | |
|---|---|
| Alfenta[1] | Stadol[3] |
| Demerol[5] | Sublimaze[4] |
| Epimorph[6] | Sufenta[8] |
| Nubain[7] | |

Another commonly used name for meperidine is pethidine.

Note: For quick reference, the following narcotic analgesics are numbered to match the corresponding brand names.

This information applies to the following medicines:
1. Alfentanil (al-FEN-ta-nil)
2. Buprenorphine (byoo-pre-NOR-feen)
3. Butorphanol (byoo-TOR-fa-nole)
4. Fentanyl (FEN-ta-nil)‡
5. Meperidine (me-PER-i-deen)‡§
6. Morphine (MOR-feen)‡§
7. Nalbuphine (NAL-byoo-feen)‡
8. Sufentanil (soo-FEN-ta-nil)

‡Generic name product may also be avilable in the U.S.
§Generic name product may also be available in Canada.

## Description

Narcotic analgesics (nar-KOT-ik an-al-JEE-zicks) are given to relieve pain before and during surgery (including dental surgery) or during labor and delivery. These medicines may also be given before or together with an anesthetic (either a general anesthetic or a local anesthetic), even when the patient is not in pain, to help the anesthetic work better.

When a narcotic analgesic is used for surgery or obstetrics (labor and delivery), it will be given by or under the immediate supervision of a medical doctor or dentist, or by a specially trained nurse, in the doctor's office or in a hospital.

The following information applies only to these special uses of narcotic analgesics. If you are taking or receiving a narcotic analgesic to relieve pain after surgery, or for any other reason, ask your health care professional for additional information about the medicine and its use.

These medicines are available in the following dosage forms:

*Parenteral*
Alfentanil
• Injection (U.S. and Canada)
Buprenorphine
• Injection (U.S.)
Butorphanol
• Injection (U.S. and Canada)
Fentanyl
• Injection (U.S. and Canada)
Meperidine
• Injection (U.S. and Canada)
Morphine
• Injection (U.S. and Canada)
Nalbuphine
• Injection (U.S. and Canada)
Sufentanil
• Injection (U.S. and Canada)

## Before Receiving This Medicine

In deciding to use a medicine, the risks of using the medicine must be weighed against the good it will do. This is a decision you and your doctor will make. For narcotic analgesics, the following should be considered:

**Allergies**—Tell your doctor if you have ever had any unusual or allergic reaction to a narcotic analgesic. Also tell your health care professional if you are allergic to any other substances, such as foods, preservatives, or dyes.

**Pregnancy**—Although studies on birth defects have not been done in pregnant women, these medicines have not been reported to cause birth defects. However, in animal studies, many narcotics have caused birth defects or other unwanted effects when they were given for a long time in amounts that were large enough to cause harmful effects in the mother.

Use of a narcotic during labor and delivery sometimes causes drowsiness or breathing problems in the newborn baby. If this happens, your health care professional can give the baby another medicine that will overcome these effects. Narcotics are usually not used during the delivery of a premature baby.

**Breast-feeding**—Some narcotics have been shown to pass into the breast milk. However, these medicines have not been reported to cause problems in nursing babies.

**Children**—Children younger than 2 years of age may be especially sensitive to the effects of narcotic analgesics. This may increase the chance of side effects.

**Older adults**—Elderly people are especially sensitive to the effects of narcotic analgesics. This may increase the chance of side effects.

**Other medicines**—Although certain medicines should not be used together at all, in other cases two different medicines may be used together even if an interaction might occur. In these cases, it may be necessary to change the dose, or other precautions may be necessary. It is very important that you tell the person in charge if you are taking:
• Any other medicine, prescription or nonprescription (over-the-counter [OTC]), or
• "Street" drugs, such as amphetamines ("uppers"), barbiturates ("downers"), cocaine (including "crack"), marijuana, phencyclidine (PCP, "angel dust"), and heroin or other narcotics—Serious side effects may occur if anyone gives you an anesthetic without knowing that you have taken another medicine

**Other medical problems**—The presence of other medical problems may affect the use of narcotic analgesics. Make sure you tell your doctor if you have *any* other medical problems.

## Precautions After Receiving This Medicine

For patients going home within a few hours after surgery:
• Narcotic analgesics and other medicines that may be given with them during surgery may cause some people to feel drowsy, tired, or weak for up to a few days after they have been given. Therefore, for at least 24 hours (or longer if necessary) after receiving this medicine, *do not drive, use machines, or do anything else that could be dangerous if you are dizzy or are not alert*.
• Unless otherwise directed by your medical doctor or dentist, *do not drink alcoholic beverages or take other CNS depressants (medicines that slow down the nervous system, possibly causing drowsiness) for*

*about 24 hours after you have received this medicine*. To do so may add to the effects of the narcotic analgesic. Some examples of CNS depressants are antihistamines or medicine for hay fever, other allergies, or colds; sedatives, tranquilizers, or sleeping medicine; prescription pain medicine or narcotics; barbiturates; medicine for seizures; and muscle relaxants.

## Side Effects of This Medicine

Along with its needed effects, a medicine may cause some unwanted effects. Before you leave the hospital or doctor's office, your health care professional will closely follow the effects of this medicine. However, some effects may continue, or may not be noticed until later.

The following side effects usually do not need medical attention. They will gradually go away as the effects of the medicine wear off. However, check with your medical doctor or dentist if any of the following side effects continue or are bothersome:

*More common*
> Dizziness, lightheadedness, or feeling faint; drowsiness; nausea or vomiting; unusual tiredness or weakness

*Less common or rare*
> Blurred or double vision or other vision problems; confusion; constipation; difficult or painful urination; dryness of mouth; general feeling of discomfort or illness; headache; mental depression or other mood or mental changes; nightmares or unusual dreams

Other side effects not listed above may also occur in some patients. If you notice any other effects, check with your doctor.

Revised: July 1990

---

# NARCOTIC ANALGESICS AND ACETAMINOPHEN   Systemic

Some commonly used brand names are:

**In the U.S.—**

| | |
|---|---|
| Acetaco[1] | Myapap with Codeine[1] |
| Aceta with Codeine[1] | Norcet[4] |
| Allay[4] | Norcet 7.5[4] |
| Amacodone[4] | Percocet[6] |
| Anexsia[4] | Phenaphen with Codeine |
| Anexsia 7.5[4] |    No.2[1]# |
| Anodynos DHC[4] | Phenaphen with Codeine |
| Anolor DH 5[4] |    No.3[1]# |
| Bancap-HC[4] | Phenaphen with Codeine |
| Capital with Codeine[1] |    No.4[1]# |
| Codalan No.1[2] | Phenaphen-650 with Codeine[1] |
| Codalan No.2[2] | Polygesic[4] |
| Codalan No.3[2] | Propacet 100[8] |
| Co-Gesic[4] | Propain-HC[4] |
| Compal[3] | Pro Pox with APAP[8] |
| Darvocet-N 50[8] | Proval[1] |
| Darvocet-N 100[8] | Pyregesic-C[1] |
| Demerol-APAP[5] | Rogesic No.3[4] |
| Dolacet[4] | Roxicet[6] |
| Dolene-AP-65[8] | Roxicet 5/500[6] |
| Doxapap-N[8] | Senefen III[4] |
| D-Rex 65[8] | Talacen[7] |
| Duocet[4] | Tylaprin with Codeine[1] |
| Duradyne DHC[4] | Tylenol with Codeine[1] |
| E-Lor[8] | Tylenol with Codeine No.1[1] |
| Genagesic[8] | Tylenol with Codeine No.2[1] |
| HY-5[4] | Tylenol with Codeine No.3[1] |
| Hycomed[4] | Tylenol with Codeine No.4[1] |
| Hycopap[4] | Tylox[6] |
| Hyco-Pap[4] | Ty-Pap with Codeine[1] |
| Hydrocet[4] | Ty-Tab with Codeine No.2[1] |
| Hydrogesic[4] | Ty-Tab with Codeine No.3[1] |
| HY-PHEN[4] | Ty-Tab with Codeine No.4[1] |
| Lorcet-HD[4] | Ultragesic[4] |
| Lorcet Plus[4] | Vapocet[4] |
| Lortab[4] | Vicodin[4] |
| Lortab 5[4] | Vicodin ES[4] |
| Lortab 7[4] | Wygesic[8] |
| Megagesic[4] | Zydone[4] |
| M-Gesic[1] | |

**In Canada—**

| | |
|---|---|
| Atasol-8[2] | Novogesic C8[2] |
| Atasol-15[2] | Novogesic C15[2] |
| Atasol-30[2] | Novogesic C30[2] |
| Codamin #2[2] | Oxycocet[6] |
| Codamin #3[2] | Percocet[6] |
| Codaminophen[2] | Percocet-Demi[6] |
| Empracet-30[1] | Rounox and Codeine 15[1] |
| Empracet-60[1] | Rounox and Codeine 30[1] |
| Emtec-30[1] | Rounox and Codeine 60[1] |
| Endocet[6] | Tylenol No.1[2] |
| Exdol-8[2] | Tylenol No.1 Forte[2] |
| Exdol-15[2] | Tylenol with Codeine[2] |
| Exdol-30[2] | Tylenol with Codeine No.2[2] |
| Lenoltec with Codeine No.1[2] | Tylenol with Codeine No.3[2] |
| Lenoltec with Codeine No.2[2] | Tylenol with Codeine No.4[1] |
| Lenoltec with Codeine No.3[2] | Veganin[2] |
| Lenoltec with Codeine No.4[1] | |

Other commonly used names are:

| | |
|---|---|
| APAP with codeine[1] | hydrocodone with APAP[4] |
| drocode, acetaminophen, and | oxycodone with APAP[6] |
|    caffeine[3] | propoxyphene with APAP[8] |

Note: For quick reference, the following narcotic analgesics and acetaminophen combinations are numbered to match the corresponding brand names.

This information applies to the following medicines:

1. Acetaminophen (a-seat-a-MIN-oh-fen) and Codeine (KOE-deen)‡
2. Acetaminophen, Codeine, and Caffeine (kaf-EEN)§
3. Dihydrocodeine (dye-hye-droe-KOE-deen), Acetaminophen, and Caffeine†
4. Hydrocodone (hye-droe-KOE-done) and Acetaminophen†‡
5. Meperidine (me-PER-i-deen) and Acetaminophen†
6. Oxycodone (ox-i-KOE-done) and Acetaminophen‡
7. Pentazocine (pen-TAZ-oh-seen) and Acetaminophen†
8. Propoxyphene (proe-POX-i-feen) and Acetaminophen†‡

---

†Not commercially available in Canada.
‡Generic name product may also be available in the U.S.
§Generic name product may also be available in Canada.
#In Canada, *Phenaphen with Codeine* is different from the product with that name in the U.S. The Canadian product contains phenobarbital, ASA, and codeine.

# Description

Combination medicines containing narcotic (nar-KOT-ik) analgesics (an-al-JEE-zicks) and acetaminophen are used to relieve pain. A narcotic analgesic and acetaminophen used together may provide better pain relief than either medicine used alone. In some cases, relief of pain may come at lower doses of each medicine.

Narcotic analgesics act in the central nervous system (CNS) to relieve pain. Many of their side effects are also caused by actions in the CNS. When narcotics are used for a long time, your body may get used to them so that larger amounts are needed to relieve pain. This is called tolerance to the medicine. Also, when narcotics are used for a long time or in large doses, they may become habit-forming (causing mental or physical dependence). Physical dependence may lead to withdrawal symptoms when you stop taking the medicine.

Acetaminophen does not become habit-forming when taken for a long time or in large doses, but it may cause other unwanted effects, including liver damage, if too much is taken.

In the U.S., these medicines are available only with your medical doctor's or dentist's prescription. In Canada, some acetaminophen, codeine, and caffeine combinations are available without a prescription.

These medicines are available in the following dosage forms:

*Oral*

Acetaminophen and Codeine
- Capsules (U.S.)
- Elixir (U.S. and Canada)
- Oral suspension (U.S.)
- Tablets (U.S. and Canada)

Acetaminophen, Codeine, and Caffeine
- Capsules (Canada)
- Tablets (U.S. and Canada)

Dihydrocodeine, Acetaminophen, and Caffeine
- Capsules (U.S.)

Hydrocodone and Acetaminophen
- Capsules (U.S.)
- Oral solution (U.S.)
- Tablets (U.S.)

Meperidine and Acetaminophen
- Tablets (U.S.)

Oxycodone and Acetaminophen
- Capsules (U.S.)
- Oral solution (U.S.)
- Tablets (U.S. and Canada)

Pentazocine and Acetaminophen
- Tablets (U.S.)

Propoxyphene and Acetaminophen
- Capsules (U.S.)
- Tablets (U.S.)

# Before Using This Medicine

In deciding to use a medicine, the risks of taking the medicine must be weighed against the good it will do. This is a decision you and your doctor will make. For narcotic analgesic and acetaminophen combinations, the following should be considered:

**Allergies**—Tell your doctor if you have ever had any unusual or allergic reaction to acetaminophen or to a narcotic analgesic. Also tell your health care professional if you are allergic to any other substances, such as foods, preservatives, or dyes.

**Pregnancy**—

- *For acetaminophen:* Although studies on birth defects with acetaminophen have not been done in pregnant women, it has not been reported to cause birth defects or other problems.
- *For narcotic analgesics:* Although studies on birth defects with narcotic analgesics have not been done in pregnant women, they have not been reported to cause birth defects. However, hydrocodone caused birth defects in animal studies when very large doses were used. Codeine did not cause birth defects in animals, but it caused slower development of bones and other toxic or harmful effects in the fetus. Pentazocine and propoxyphene did not cause birth defects in animals. There is no information about whether dihydrocodeine, meperidine, or oxycodone cause birth defects in animals.

Too much use of a narcotic during pregnancy may cause the fetus to become dependent on the medicine. This may lead to withdrawal side effects in the newborn baby. Also, some of these medicines may cause breathing problems in the newborn baby if taken just before or during delivery.

- *For caffeine:* Studies in humans have not shown that caffeine (contained in some of these combination medicines) causes birth defects. However, studies in animals have shown that caffeine causes birth defects when given in very large doses (amounts equal to those present in 12 to 24 cups of coffee a day).

**Breast-feeding**—Acetaminophen, codeine, meperidine, and propoxyphene pass into the breast milk. It is not known whether other narcotic analgesics pass into the breast milk. However, these medicines have not been reported to cause problems in nursing babies.

**Children**—Breathing problems may be especially likely to occur when narcotic analgesics are given to children younger than 2 years of age. These children are usually more sensitive than adults to the effects of narcotic analgesics. Also, unusual excitement or restlessness may be more likely to occur in children receiving these medicines.

Acetaminophen has been tested in children and has not been shown to cause different side effects or problems in children than it does in adults.

**Older adults**—Elderly people are especially sensitive to the effects of narcotic analgesics. This may increase the chance of side effects, especially breathing problems, during treatment.

Acetaminophen has been tested and has not been shown to cause different side effects or problems in older people than it does in younger adults.

**Other medicines**—Although certain medicines should not be used together at all, in other cases two different medicines may be used together even if an interaction might occur. In these cases, your doctor may want to change the dose, or other precautions may be necessary. When you are taking a narcotic analgesic and acetaminophen combination, it is especially important that your health care professional know if you are taking any of the following:

- Carbamazepine (e.g., Tegretol)—Propoxyphene may increase the blood levels of carbamazepine, which increases the chance of serious side effects
- Central nervous system (CNS) depressants or
- Monoamine oxidase (MAO) inhibitors (furazolidone [e.g., Furoxone], isocarboxazid [e.g., Marplan], pargyline [e.g., Eutonyl], phenelzine [e.g., Nardil], procarbazine [e.g., Matulane], tranylcypromine [e.g., Parnate]) (taken currently or within the past 2 weeks) or
- Tricyclic antidepressants (amitriptyline [e.g., Elavil], amoxapine [e.g., Asendin], clomipramine [e.g., Anafranil], desipramine [e.g., Pertofrane], doxepin [e.g., Sinequan], imipramine [e.g., Tofranil], nortriptyline [e.g., Aventyl], protriptyline [e.g., Vivactil], trimipramine [e.g., Surmontil])—Taking these medicines together with a narcotic analgesic may increase the chance of serious side effects
- Naltrexone (e.g., Trexan)—Naltrexone keeps narcotic analgesics from working to relieve pain; people taking naltrexone should take pain relievers that do not contain a narcotic
- Zidovudine (e.g., AZT, Retrovir)—Acetaminophen may increase the blood levels of zidovudine, which increases the chance of serious side effects

**Other medical problems**—The presence of other medical problems may affect the use of narcotic analgesic and acetaminophen combinations. Make sure you tell your doctor if you have any other medical problems, especially:

- Alcohol and/or other drug abuse, or history of, or
- Brain disease or head injury or
- Colitis or
- Convulsions (seizures), history of, or
- Emotional problems or mental illness or
- Emphysema, asthma, or other chronic lung disease or
- Hepatitis or other liver disease or
- Kidney disease or
- Underactive thyroid—The chance of serious side effects may be increased
- Enlarged prostate or problems with urination or
- Gallbladder disease or gallstones—Some of the effects of narcotic analgesics may be especially serious in people with these medical problems
- Heart disease—Caffeine (present in some of these combination medicines) can make some kinds of heart disease worse

## Proper Use of This Medicine

*Take this medicine only as directed by your medical doctor or dentist.* Do not take more of it, do not take it more often, and do not take it for a longer time than your medical doctor or dentist ordered. This is especially important for young children and elderly patients, who may be more sensitive than other people to the effects of narcotic analgesics. If too much of a narcotic analgesic is taken, it may become habit-forming (causing mental or physical dependence) or lead to medical problems because of an overdose. Taking too much acetaminophen may cause liver damage.

If you think that this medicine is not working properly after you have been taking it for a few weeks, *do not increase the dose.* Instead, check with your medical doctor or dentist.

**Missed dose**—If your medical doctor or dentist has ordered you to take this medicine according to a regular schedule and you miss a dose, take it as soon as you remember. However, if it is almost time for your next dose, skip the missed dose and go back to your regular dosing schedule. *Do not double doses.*

**Storage**—To store this medicine:

- Keep out of the reach of children. Overdose is very dangerous in young children.
- Store away from heat and direct light.
- Do not store tablets or capsules in the bathroom, near the kitchen sink, or in other damp places. Heat or moisture may cause the medicine to break down.
- Keep the liquid forms of this medicine from freezing.
- Do not keep outdated medicine or medicine no longer needed. Be sure that any discarded medicine is out of the reach of children.

## Precautions While Using This Medicine

If you will be taking this medicine for a long time (for example, for several months at a time), or in high doses, your doctor should check your progress at regular visits.

*Check the labels of all nonprescription (over-the-counter [OTC]) and prescription medicines you now take.* If any contain acetaminophen or a narcotic be especially careful, since taking them while taking this medicine may lead to overdose. If you have any questions about this, check with your medical doctor, dentist, or pharmacist.

The narcotic analgesic in this medicine will add to the effects of alcohol and other CNS depressants (medicines that slow down the nervous system, possibly causing drowsiness). Some examples of CNS depressants are antihistamines or medicine for hay fever, other allergies, or colds; sedatives, tranquilizers, or sleeping medicine; other prescription pain medicine or narcotics; barbiturates; medicine for seizures; muscle relaxants; or anesthetics, including some dental anesthetics. Also, there may be a greater risk of liver damage if large amounts of alcoholic beverages are used while you are taking acetaminophen. *Do not drink alcoholic beverages, and check with your medical doctor or dentist before taking any of the medicines listed above, while you are using this medicine.*

Too much use of the acetaminophen in this combination medicine together with certain other medicines may increase the chance of unwanted effects. The risk will depend on how much of each medicine you take every day, and on how long you take the medicines together. If your doctor directs you to take these medicines together on a regular basis, follow his or her directions carefully. However, do not take this medicine together with any of the following medicines for more than a few days, unless your doctor has directed you to do so and is following your progress:

Aspirin or other salicylates
Diclofenac (e.g., Voltaren)
Diflunisal (e.g., Dolobid)
Fenoprofen (e.g., Nalfon)
Floctafenine (e.g., Idarac)
Flurbiprofen, oral (e.g., Ansaid)
Ibuprofen (e.g., Motrin)
Indomethacin (e.g., Indocin)
Ketoprofen (e.g., Orudis)
Ketorolac (e.g., Toradol)
Meclofenamate (e.g., Meclomen)
Mefenamic acid (e.g., Ponstel)
Naproxen (e.g., Naprosyn)
Phenylbutazone (e.g., Butazolidin)
Piroxicam (e.g., Feldene)
Sulindac (e.g., Clinoril)
Tiaprofenic acid (e.g., Surgam)
Tolmetin (e.g., Tolectin)

This medicine may cause some people to become drowsy, dizzy, or lightheaded, or to feel a false sense of well-being. *Make sure you know how you react to this medicine before you drive, use machines, or do anything else that could be dangerous if you are dizzy or are not alert and clearheaded.*

Dizziness, lightheadedness, or fainting may occur, especially when you get up suddenly from a lying or sitting position. Getting up slowly may help lessen this problem.

Nausea or vomiting may occur, especially after the first couple of doses. This effect may go away if you lie down for a while. However, if nausea or vomiting continues, check with your medical doctor or dentist. Lying down for a while may also help relieve some other side effects, such as dizziness or lightheadedness, that may occur.

Before having any kind of surgery (including dental surgery) or emergency treatment, tell the medical doctor or dentist in charge that you are taking this medicine.

Narcotic analgesics may cause dryness of the mouth. For temporary relief, use sugarless candy or gum, melt bits of ice in your mouth, or use a saliva substitute. However, if dry mouth continues for more than 2 weeks, check with your dentist. Continuing dryness of the mouth may increase the chance of dental disease, including tooth decay, gum disease, and fungus infections.

If you have been taking this medicine regularly for several weeks or more, *do not suddenly stop taking it without first checking with your doctor.* Your doctor may want you to reduce gradually the amount you are taking before stopping completely, to lessen the chance of withdrawal side effects. This will depend on which of these medicines you have been taking, and the amount you have been taking every day.

*If you think you or someone else may have taken an overdose of this medicine, get emergency help at once.* Taking an overdose of this medicine or taking alcohol or CNS depressants with this medicine may lead to unconsciousness or death. Signs of overdose of narcotics include convulsions (seizures), confusion, severe nervousness or restlessness, severe dizziness, severe drowsiness, shortness of breath or troubled breathing, and severe weakness. Signs of severe acetaminophen overdose may not occur until several days after the overdose is taken.

## Side Effects of This Medicine

Along with its needed effects, a medicine may cause some unwanted effects. Although not all of these side effects may occur, if they do occur they may need medical attention.

*Get emergency help immediately if any of the following symptoms of overdose occur:*

Cold, clammy skin; confusion (severe); convulsions (seizures); diarrhea; dizziness (severe); drowsiness (severe); increased sweating; low blood pressure; nausea or vomiting (continuing); nervousness or restlessness (severe); pinpoint pupils of eyes; shortness of breath or unusually slow or troubled breathing; slow heartbeat; stomach cramps or pain; weakness (severe)

Also, check with your doctor as soon as possible if any of the following side effects occur:

*Less common or rare*

Black, tarry stools; bloody or cloudy urine; confusion; dark urine; difficult or painful urination; fast, slow, or pounding heartbeat; frequent urge to urinate; hallucinations (seeing, hearing, or feeling things that are not there); increased sweating; irregular breathing or wheezing; mental depression; pain in lower back and/or side (severe and/or sharp); pale stools; pinpoint red spots on skin; redness or flushing of face; ringing or buzzing in ears; skin rash, hives, or itching; sore throat and fever; sudden decrease in amount of urine; swelling of face; trembling or uncontrolled muscle movements; unusual bleeding or bruising; unusual excitement (especially in children); yellow eyes or skin

Other side effects may occur that usually do not need medical attention. These side effects may go away during treatment as your body adjusts to the medicine. However, check with your medical doctor or dentist if any of the following side effects continue or are bothersome:

*More common*

Dizziness, lightheadedness, or feeling faint; drowsiness; nausea or vomiting; unusual tiredness or weakness

*Less common or rare*

Blurred or double vision or other changes in vision; constipation (more common with long-term use and with codeine or meperidine); dry mouth; false sense of well-being; general feeling of discomfort or illness; headache; loss of appetite; nervousness or restlessness; nightmares or unusual dreams; trouble in sleeping

Although not all of the side effects listed above have been reported for all of these combination medicines, they have been reported for at least one of them. However, since all of the narcotic analgesics are very similar, any of the above side effects may occur with any of these medicines.

After you stop using this medicine, your body may need time to adjust. The length of time this takes depends on which of these medicines you were taking, the amount of medicine you were using, and how long you used it.

During this time check with your doctor if you notice any of the following side effects:

> Body aches; diarrhea; fast heartbeat; fever, runny nose, or sneezing; gooseflesh; increased sweating; increased yawning; loss of appetite; nausea or vomiting; nervousness, restlessness, or irritability; shivering or trembling; stomach cramps; trouble in sleeping; weakness

Other side effects not listed above may also occur in some patients. If you notice any other effects, check with your doctor.

Revised: July 1990

---

# NARCOTIC ANALGESICS AND ASPIRIN    Systemic

Some commonly used brand names are:

**In the U.S.—**

Azdone[5]
Bexophene[10]
Cotanal-65[10]
Damason-P[6]
Darvon Compound[10]
Darvon Compound-65[10]
Darvon with A.S.A.[9]
Darvon-N with A.S.A.[9]
Doraphen Compound-65[10]
Doxaphene Compound[10]
Emcodeine No.2[2]
Emcodeine No.3[2]

Emcodeine No.4[2]
Empirin with Codeine No.2[2]
Empirin with Codeine No.3[2]
Empirin with Codeine No.4[2]
Lortab ASA[5]
Margesic A-C[10]
Percodan[7]
Percodan-Demi[7]
Pro Pox Plus[10]
Roxiprin[7]
Synalgos-DC[1]
Talwin Compound[8]

**In Canada—**

A.C.&C[3]
Anacin with Codeine[3]
Ancasal 8[3]
Ancasal 15[3]
Ancasal 30[3]
C2 Buffered with Codeine[4]
C2 with Codeine[3]
Coryphen with Codeine[2]
Darvon-N Compound[10]
Darvon-N with A.S.A.[9]
Endodan[7]

Novopropoxyn Compound[10]
Oxycodan[7]
Percodan[7]
Percodan-Demi[7]
692[10]
222 Forte[3]
222[3]
282[3]
292[3]
293[3]

Other commonly used names are:

dihydrocodeine compound[1]
drocode and aspirin[1]

propoxyphene hydrochloride compound[10]

Note: For quick reference, the following narcotic analgesics and aspirin combinations are numbered to match the corresponding brand names.

This information applies to the following medicines:

1. Aspirin, Caffeine, and Dihydrocodeine (dye-hye-droe-KOE-deen)†‡
2. Aspirin (AS-pir-in) and Codeine (KOE-deen)‡#
3. Aspirin, Codeine, and Caffeine (kaf-EEN)*#
4. Aspirin, Codeine, and Caffeine, Buffered*#
5. Hydrocodone (hye-droe-KOE-done) and Aspirin†
6. Hydrocodone, Aspirin, and Caffeine†
7. Oxycodone (ox-i-KOE-done) and Aspirin‡#
8. Pentazocine (pen-TAZ-oh-seen) and Aspirin†
9. Propoxyphene (proe-POX-i-feen) and Aspirin#
10. Propoxyphene, Aspirin, and Caffeine‡#

---

*Not commercially available in the U.S.
†Not commercially available in Canada.
‡Generic name product may also be available in the U.S.
§Generic name product may also be available in Canada.
#In Canada, *Aspirin* is a brand name. Acetylsalicylic acid is the generic name in Canada. ASA, a synonym for acetylsalicylic acid, is the term that commonly appears on Canadian product labels.

## Description

Combination medicines containing narcotic (nar-KOT-ik) analgesics (an-al-JEE-zicks) and aspirin are used to relieve pain. A narcotic analgesic and aspirin used together may provide better pain relief than either medicine used alone. In some cases, relief of pain may come at lower doses of each medicine.

Narcotic analgesics act in the central nervous system (CNS) to relieve pain. Many of their side effects are also caused by actions in the CNS. When narcotics are used for a long time, your body may get used to them so that larger amounts are needed to relieve pain. This is called tolerance to the medicine. Also, when narcotics are used for a long time or in large doses, they may become habit-forming (causing mental or physical dependence). Physical dependence may lead to withdrawal symptoms when you stop taking the medicine.

Aspirin does not become habit-forming when taken for a long time or in large doses, but it may cause other unwanted effects if too much is taken.

In the U.S., these medicines are available only with your medical doctor's or dentist's prescription. In Canada, some strengths of aspirin, codeine, and caffeine combination are available without a prescription.

These medicines are available in the following dosage forms:

*Oral*

Aspirin, Caffeine, and Dihydrocodeine
• Capsules (U.S.)
Aspirin and Codeine
• Tablets (U.S. and Canada)
Aspirin, Codeine, and Caffeine
• Tablets (Canada)
Aspirin, Codeine, and Caffeine, Buffered
• Tablets (Canada)
Hydrocodone and Aspirin
• Tablets (U.S.)
Hydrocodone, Aspirin, and Caffeine
• Tablets (U.S.)

---

© 1994   The United States Pharmacopeial Convention, Inc.

Oxycodone and Aspirin
- Tablets (U.S. and Canada)

Pentazocine and Aspirin
- Tablets (U.S.)

Propoxyphene and Aspirin
- Capsules (U.S. and Canada)
- Tablets (U.S.)

Propoxyphene, Aspirin, and Caffeine
- Capsules (U.S. and Canada)
- Tablets (Canada)

## Before Using This Medicine

In deciding to use a medicine, the risks of taking the medicine must be weighed against the good it will do. This is a decision you and your doctor will make. For narcotic analgesic and aspirin combinations, the following should be considered:

**Allergies**—Tell your doctor if you have ever had any unusual or allergic reaction to a narcotic analgesic, aspirin or other salicylates, including methyl salicylate (oil of wintergreen), or any of the following medicines:

Diclofenac (e.g., Voltaren)
Diflunisal (e.g., Dolobid)
Fenoprofen (e.g., Nalfon)
Floctafenine (e.g., Idarac)
Flurbiprofen, oral (e.g., Ansaid)
Ibuprofen (e.g., Motrin)
Indomethacin (e.g., Indocin)
Ketoprofen (e.g., Orudis)
Ketorolac (e.g., Toradol)
Meclofenamate (e.g., Meclomen)
Mefenamic acid (e.g., Ponstel)
Naproxen (e.g., Naprosyn)
Oxyphenbutazone (e.g., Tandearil)
Phenylbutazone (e.g., Butazolidin)
Piroxicam (e.g., Feldene)
Sulindac (e.g., Clinoril)
Suprofen (e.g., Suprol)
Tiaprofenic acid (e.g., Surgam)
Tolmetin (e.g., Tolectin)
Zomepirac (e.g., Zomax)

Also tell your health care professional if you are allergic to any other substances, such as foods, preservatives, or dyes.

**Pregnancy**—

- *For aspirin:* Studies in humans have not shown that aspirin causes birth defects. However, studies in animals have shown that aspirin causes birth defects.

  Some reports have suggested that too much use of aspirin late in pregnancy may cause a decrease in the newborn's weight and possible death of the fetus or newborn baby. However, the mothers in these reports had been taking much larger amounts of aspirin than are usually recommended. Studies of mothers taking aspirin in the doses that are usually recommended did not show these effects. However, regular use of aspirin late in pregnancy may cause unwanted effects on the heart or blood flow in the fetus or in the newborn baby. Also, use of aspirin during the last 2 weeks of pregnancy may cause

bleeding problems in the fetus before or during delivery or in the newborn baby.

Too much use of aspirin during the last 3 months of pregnancy may increase the length of pregnancy, prolong labor, cause other problems during delivery, or cause severe bleeding in the mother before, during, or after delivery. *Do not take aspirin during the last 3 months of pregnancy unless it has been ordered by your doctor.*

- *For narcotic analgesics:* Although studies on birth defects with narcotic analgesics have not been done in pregnant women, they have not been reported to cause birth defects. However, hydrocodone caused birth defects in animal studies when given in very large doses. Codeine did not cause birth defects in animals, but it caused slower development of bones and other toxic or harmful effects on the fetus. Pentazocine and propoxyphene did not cause birth defects in animals. There is no information about whether dihydrocodeine or oxycodone causes birth defects in animals.

  Too much use of a narcotic during pregnancy may cause the fetus to become dependent on the medicine. This may lead to withdrawal side effects in the newborn baby. Also, some of these medicines may cause breathing problems in the newborn baby if taken just before or during delivery.

- *For caffeine:* Studies in humans have not shown that caffeine (contained in some of these combination medicines) causes birth defects. However, studies in animals have shown that caffeine causes birth defects when given in very large doses (amounts equal to those present in 12 to 24 cups of coffee a day).

**Breast-feeding**—These combination medicines have not been reported to cause problems in nursing babies. However, aspirin, caffeine, codeine, and propoxyphene pass into the breast milk. It is not known whether dihydrocodeine, hydrocodone, oxycodone, or pentazocine passes into the breast milk.

**Children**—*Do not give a medicine containing aspirin to a child or a teenager with a fever or other symptoms of a virus infection, especially flu or chickenpox, without first discussing its use with your child's doctor.* This is very important because aspirin may cause a serious illness called Reye's syndrome in children with fever caused by a virus infection, especially flu or chickenpox. Children who do not have a virus infection may also be more sensitive to the effects of aspirin, especially if they have a fever or have lost large amounts of body fluid because of vomiting, diarrhea, or sweating. This may increase the chance of side effects during treatment.

The narcotic analgesic in this combination medicine can cause breathing problems, especially in children younger than 2 years of age. These children are usually more sensitive than adults to the effects of narcotic analgesics. Also, unusual excitement or restlessness may be more likely to occur in children receiving these medicines.

**Older adults**—Elderly people are especially sensitive to the effects of aspirin and of narcotic analgesics. This may increase the chance of side effects, especially breathing problems caused by narcotic analgesics, during treatment.

**Other medicines**—Although certain medicines should not be used together at all, in other cases two different medicines may be used together even if an interaction might occur. In these cases, your doctor may want to change the dose, or other precautions may be necessary. When you are taking a narcotic analgesic and aspirin combination, it is especially important that your health care professional know if you are taking any of the following:

- Anticoagulants (blood thinners) or
- Carbenicillin by injection (e.g., Geopen) or
- Cefamandole (e.g., Mandol) or
- Cefoperazone (e.g., Cefobid) or
- Cefotetan (e.g., Cefotan) or
- Dipyridamole (e.g., Persantine) or
- Divalproex (e.g., Depakote) or
- Heparin or
- Medicine for inflammation or pain, except narcotics, or
- Moxalactam (e.g., Moxam) or
- Pentoxifylline (e.g., Trental) or
- Plicamycin (e.g., Mithracin) or
- Ticarcillin (e.g., Ticar) or
- Valproic acid (e.g., Depakene)—Taking these medicines together with aspirin may increase the chance of bleeding
- Antidiabetics, oral (diabetes medicine you take by mouth)—Aspirin may increase the effects of the antidiabetic medicine; a change in the dose of the antidiabetic medicine may be needed if aspirin is taken regularly
- Carbamazepine (e.g., Tegretol)—Propoxyphene can increase the blood levels of carbamazepine, which increases the chance of serious side effects
- Central nervous system (CNS) depressants or
- Diarrhea medicine or
- Methotrexate (e.g., Mexate) or
- Tricyclic antidepressants (amitriptyline [e.g., Elavil], amoxapine [e.g., Asendin], clomipramine [e.g., Anafranil], desipramine [e.g., Pertofrane], doxepin [e.g., Sinequan], imipramine [e.g., Tofranil], nortriptyline [e.g., Aventyl], protriptyline [e.g., Vivactil], trimipramine [e.g., Surmontil])—or
- Vancomycin (e.g., Vancocin)—The chance of side effects may be increased
- Naltrexone (e.g., Trexan)—Naltrexone keeps narcotic analgesics from working to relieve pain; people taking naltrexone should use pain relievers that do not contain a narcotic
- Probenecid (e.g., Benemid) or
- Sulfinpyrazone (e.g., Anturane)—Aspirin can keep these medicines from working as well for treating gout; also, use of sulfinpyrazone and aspirin together may increase the chance of bleeding
- Urinary alkalizers (medicine that makes the urine less acid, such as acetazolamide [e.g., Diamox], calcium- and/or magnesium-containing antacids, dichlorphenamide [e.g., Daranide], methazolamide [e.g., Neptazane], potassium or sodium citrate and/or citric acid, sodium bicarbonate [baking soda])—These medicines may make aspirin less effective by causing it to be removed from the body more quickly

- Zidovudine (e.g., AZT, Retrovir)—Higher blood levels of zidovudine and an increased chance of serious side effects may occur

**Other medical problems**—The presence of other medical problems may affect the use of narcotic analgesic and aspirin combinations. Make sure you tell your doctor if you have any other medical problems, especially:

- Alcohol and/or other drug abuse, or history of, or
- Asthma, allergies, and nasal polyps (history of) or
- Brain disease or head injury or
- Colitis or
- Convulsions (seizures), history of, or
- Emotional problems or mental illness or
- Emphysema or other chronic lung disease or
- Kidney disease or
- Liver disease or
- Underactive thyroid—The chance of serious side effects may be increased
- Anemia or
- Overactive thyroid or
- Stomach ulcer or other stomach problems—Aspirin may make these conditions worse
- Enlarged prostate or problems with urination or
- Gallbladder disease or gallstones—Narcotic analgesics have side effects that may be dangerous if these medical problems are present
- Gout—Aspirin can make this condition worse and can also lessen the effects of some medicines used to treat gout
- Heart disease—Large amounts of aspirin and caffeine (present in some of these combination medicines) can make some kinds of heart disease worse
- Hemophilia or other bleeding problems or
- Vitamin K deficiency—Aspirin increases the chance of serious bleeding

## Proper Use of This Medicine

*Take this medicine with food or a full glass (8 ounces) of water* to lessen stomach irritation.

*Do not take this medicine if it has a strong vinegar-like odor.* This odor means the aspirin in it is breaking down. If you have any questions about this, check with your health care professional.

*Take this medicine only as directed by your medical doctor or dentist.* Do not take more of it, do not take it more often, and do not take it for a longer time than your medical doctor or dentist ordered. This is especially important for children and elderly patients, who are usually more sensitive to the effects of these medicines. If too much of a narcotic analgesic is taken, it may become habit-forming (causing mental or physical dependence) or lead to medical problems because of an overdose. Also, taking too much aspirin may cause stomach problems or lead to medical problems because of an overdose.

If you think that this medicine is not working as well after you have been taking it for a few weeks, *do not increase the dose.* Instead, check with your medical doctor or dentist.

**Missed dose**—If your medical doctor or dentist has ordered you to take this medicine according to a regular schedule and you miss a dose, take it as soon as you remember. However, if it is almost time for your next dose, skip the missed dose and go back to your regular dosing schedule. *Do not double doses.*

**Storage**—To store this medicine:
- Keep out of the reach of children. Overdose is very dangerous in young children.
- Store away from heat and direct light.
- Do not store this medicine in the bathroom, near the kitchen sink, or in other damp places. Heat or moisture may cause the medicine to break down.
- Do not keep outdated medicine or medicine no longer needed. Be sure that any discarded medicine is out of the reach of children.

## Precautions While Using This Medicine

If you will be taking this medicine for a long time (for example, for several months at a time), your doctor should check your progress at regular visits.

*Check the labels of all nonprescription (over-the-counter [OTC]) and prescription medicines you now take.* If any contain a narcotic, aspirin, or other salicylates, be especially careful, since taking them while taking this medicine may lead to overdose. If you have any questions about this, check with your medical doctor, dentist, or pharmacist.

This medicine will add to the effects of alcohol and other CNS depressants (medicines that slow down the nervous system, possibly causing drowsiness). Some examples of CNS depressants are antihistamines or medicine for hay fever, other allergies, or colds; sedatives, tranquilizers, or sleeping medicine; other prescription pain medicine or narcotics; barbiturates; medicine for seizures; muscle relaxants; or anesthetics, including some dental anesthetics. Also, stomach problems may be more likely to occur if you drink alcoholic beverages while you are taking aspirin. *Do not drink alcoholic beverages, and check with your medical doctor or dentist before taking any of the medicines listed above, while you are using this medicine.*

Taking acetaminophen or certain other medicines together with the aspirin in this combination medicine may increase the chance of unwanted effects. The risk will depend on how much of each medicine you take every day, and on how long you take the medicines together. If your doctor directs you to take these medicines together on a regular basis, follow his or her directions carefully. However, do not take acetaminophen or any of the following medicines together with this combination medicine for more than a few days, unless your doctor has directed you to do so and is following your progress:

Diclofenac (e.g., Voltaren)
Diflunisal (e.g., Dolobid)
Fenoprofen (e.g., Nalfon)
Floctafenine (e.g., Idarac)
Flurbiprofen, oral (e.g., Ansaid)
Ibuprofen (e.g., Motrin)
Indomethacin (e.g., Indocin)
Ketoprofen (e.g., Orudis)
Ketorolac (e.g., Toradol)

Meclofenamate (e.g., Meclomen)
Mefenamic acid (e.g., Ponstel)
Naproxen (e.g., Naprosyn)
Phenylbutazone (e.g., Butazolidin)
Piroxicam (e.g., Feldene)
Sulindac (e.g., Clinoril)
Tiaprofenic acid (e.g., Surgam)
Tolmetin (e.g., Tolectin)

This medicine may cause some people to become drowsy, dizzy, or lightheaded, or to feel a false sense of well-being. *Make sure you know how you react to this medicine before you drive, use machines, or do anything else that could be dangerous if you are dizzy or are not alert and clearheaded.*

Dizziness, lightheadedness, or fainting may occur, especially when you get up suddenly from a lying or sitting position. Getting up slowly may help lessen this problem.

Nausea or vomiting may occur, especially after the first couple of doses. This effect may go away if you lie down for a while. However, if nausea or vomiting continues, check with your doctor. Lying down for a while may also help some other side effects, such as dizziness or lightheadedness.

Before having any kind of surgery (including dental surgery) or emergency treatment, tell the medical doctor or dentist in charge that you are taking this medicine.

Do not take this medicine for 5 days before any surgery, including dental surgery, unless otherwise directed by your medical doctor or dentist. Taking aspirin during this time may cause bleeding problems.

If you are taking one of the combination medicines containing buffered aspirin, and you are also taking a tetracycline antibiotic, do not take the two medicines within 3 to 4 hours of each other. Taking them too close together may prevent the tetracycline from being absorbed by your body. If you have any questions about this, check with your health care professional.

For *diabetic patients:*
- False urine sugar test results may occur if you are regularly taking 8 or more 325-mg (5-grain) or 5 or more 500-mg doses of aspirin a day. Smaller amounts or occasional use of aspirin usually will not affect urine sugar tests. If you have any questions about this, check with your health care professional, especially if your diabetes is not well controlled.

Narcotic analgesics may cause dryness of the mouth. For temporary relief, use sugarless candy or gum, melt bits of ice in your mouth, or use a saliva substitute. However, if dry mouth continues for more than 2 weeks, check with your dentist. Continuing dryness of the mouth may increase the chance of dental disease, including tooth decay, gum disease, and fungus infections.

If you have been taking this medicine regularly for several weeks or more, *do not suddenly stop using it without first checking with your doctor.* Depending on which of these medicines you have been taking, and the amount you have been taking every day, your doctor may want you to reduce gradually the amount you are taking before stopping completely, to lessen the chance of withdrawal side effects.

*If you think you or someone else may have taken an overdose of this medicine, get emergency help at once.* Taking an overdose of this medicine or taking alcohol or CNS depressants with this medicine may lead to unconsciousness or death. Signs of overdose of this medicine include convulsions (seizures); hearing loss; confusion; ringing or buzzing in the ears; severe excitement, nervousness, or restlessness; severe dizziness, severe drowsiness, shortness of breath or troubled breathing, and severe weakness.

## Side Effects of This Medicine

Along with its needed effects, a medicine may cause some unwanted effects. Although not all of these side effects may occur, if they do occur they may need medical attention.

*Get emergency help immediately if any of the following symptoms of overdose occur:*

Any loss of hearing; bloody urine; cold, clammy skin; confusion (severe); convulsions (seizures); diarrhea (severe or continuing); dizziness or lightheadedness (severe); drowsiness (severe); excitement, nervousness, or restlessness (severe); fever; hallucinations (seeing, hearing, or feeling things that are not there); headache (severe or continuing); increased sweating; increased thirst; low blood pressure; nausea or vomiting (severe or continuing); pinpoint pupils of eyes; ringing or buzzing in the ears; shortness of breath or unusually slow or troubled breathing; slow heartbeat; stomach pain (severe or continuing); uncontrollable flapping movements of the hands (especially in elderly patients); vision problems; weakness (severe)

Also, check with your doctor as soon as possible if any of the following side effects occur:

*Less common or rare*

Bloody or black, tarry stools; confusion; dark urine; fast, slow, or pounding heartbeat; increased sweating (more common with hydrocodone); irregular breathing; mental depression; pale stools; redness or flushing of face (more common with hydrocodone); skin rash, hives, or itching; stomach pain (severe); swelling of face; tightness in chest or wheezing; trembling or uncontrolled muscle movements; unusual excitement (especially in

children); unusual tiredness or weakness; vomiting of blood or material that looks like coffee grounds; yellow eyes or skin

Other side effects may occur that usually do not need medical attention. These side effects may go away during treatment as your body adjusts to the medicine. However, check with your doctor if any of the following side effects continue or are bothersome:

*More common*

Dizziness, lightheadedness, or feeling faint; drowsiness; heartburn or indigestion; nausea or vomiting; stomach pain (mild)

*Less common or rare*

Blurred or double vision or other changes in vision; constipation (more common with long-term use and with codeine); difficult, painful, or decreased urination; dryness of mouth; false sense of well-being; frequent urge to urinate; general feeling of discomfort or illness; headache; loss of appetite; nervousness or restlessness; nightmares or unusual dreams; trouble in sleeping; unusual tiredness; unusual weakness

Although not all of the side effects listed above have been reported for all of these medicines, they have been reported for at least one of them. However, since all of the narcotic analgesics are very similar, any of the above side effects may occur with any of these medicines.

After you stop using this medicine, your body may need time to adjust. The length of time this takes depends on which of these medicines you were taking, the amount of medicine you were using, and how long you used it. During this period of time check with your doctor if you notice any of the following side effects:

Body aches; diarrhea; fever, runny nose, or sneezing; gooseflesh; increased sweating; increased yawning; loss of appetite; nausea or vomiting; nervousness, restlessness, or irritability; shivering or trembling; stomach cramps; trouble in sleeping; weakness

Other side effects not listed above may also occur in some patients. If you notice any other effects, check with your medical doctor or dentist.

Revised: July 1990

---

# NATAMYCIN     Ophthalmic†

A commonly used brand name in the U.S. is Natacyn.
Another commonly used name is pimaricin.

   †Not commercially available in Canada.

## Description

Natamycin (na-ta-MYE-sin) belongs to the group of medicines called antifungals. It is used to treat some types of fungus infections of the eye.

Natamycin is available only with your doctor's prescription, in the following dosage form:

*Ophthalmic*
- Ophthalmic suspension (eye drops) (U.S.)

## Before Using This Medicine

In deciding to use a medicine, the risks of taking the medicine must be weighed against the good it will do. This is a decision you and your doctor will make. For ophthalmic natamycin, the following should be considered:

**Allergies**—Tell your doctor if you have ever had any unusual or allergic reaction to natamycin. Also tell your health care professional if you are allergic to any other substances, such as preservatives.

**Pregnancy**—Studies on effects in pregnancy have not been done in either humans or animals.

**Breast-feeding**—It is not known whether natamycin passes into breast milk. Although most medicines pass into breast milk in small amounts, many of them may be used safely while breast-feeding. Mothers who are using this medicine and who wish to breast-feed should discuss this with their doctor.

**Children**—Studies on this medicine have been done only in adult patients, and there is no specific information comparing use of natamycin in children with use in other age groups.

**Older adults**—Many medicines have not been studied specifically in older people. Therefore, it may not be known whether they work exactly the same way they do in younger adults. Although there is no specific information comparing use of natamycin in the elderly with use in other age groups, this medicine is not expected to cause different side effects or problems in older people than it does in younger adults.

## Proper Use of This Medicine

The bottle is only partially full to provide proper drop control.

To use:
- First, wash your hands. Tilt the head back and, pressing your finger gently on the skin just beneath the lower eyelid, pull the lower eyelid away from the eye to make a space. Drop the medicine into this space. Let go of the eyelid and gently close the eyes. Do not blink. Keep the eyes closed for 1 or 2 minutes to allow the medicine to come into contact with the infection.
- If you think you did not get the drop of medicine into your eye properly, use another drop.
- To keep the medicine as germ-free as possible, do not touch the applicator tip to any surface (including the eye). Also, keep the container tightly closed.

To help clear up your eye infection completely, *keep using this medicine for the full time of treatment*, even if your condition has improved. *Do not miss any doses.*

**Dosing**—The dose of ophthalmic natamycin will be different for different patients. *Follow your doctor's orders or the directions on the label*. The following information includes only the average doses of ophthalmic natamycin. *If your dose is different, do not change it* unless your doctor tells you to do so.

- For fungus infection of the eye:
  —For *eye drops* dosage form:
    - Adults—Use one drop in the eye every four to six hours. For more serious infections, your doctor may tell you to use one drop in the eye every one or two hours for three or four days, then one drop six to eight times a day thereafter.
    - Children—Use and dose must be determined by your doctor.

**Missed dose**—If you miss a dose of this medicine, apply it as soon as possible. Then go back to your regular dosing schedule.

**Storage**—To store this medicine:
- Keep out of the reach of children.
- Store away from heat and direct light.
- Keep the medicine from freezing.
- Do not keep outdated medicine or medicine no longer needed. Be sure that any discarded medicine is out of the reach of children.

## Precautions While Using This Medicine

Your doctor should check your progress at regular visits. For some eye infections, these visits may be as often as several times a week.

If your symptoms do not improve within 7 to 10 days, or if they become worse, check with your doctor.

## Side Effects of This Medicine

Along with its needed effects, a medicine may cause some unwanted effects. Although not all of these side effects may occur, if they do occur they may need medical attention.

Check with your doctor as soon as possible if any of the following side effects occur:

Eye irritation, redness, or swelling not present before use of this medicine

Other side effects not listed above may also occur in some patients. If you notice any other effects, check with your doctor.

Revised: 05/16/94

# NEDOCROMIL  Inhalation

A commonly used brand name in the U.S. and Canada is Tilade.

## Description

Nedocromil (ne-DOK-roe-mil) is used to prevent the symptoms of asthma. When it is used regularly, nedocromil lessens the number and severity of asthma attacks by reducing inflammation in the lungs. Nedocromil is also used just before exposure to conditions or substances (for example, allergens, chemicals, cold air, or air pollutants) that cause reactions, to prevent bronchospasm (wheezing or difficulty in breathing). In addition, nedocromil is used to prevent bronchospasm following exercise. This medicine will not help an asthma or bronchospasm attack that has already started.

Nedocromil may be used alone or with other asthma medicines, such as bronchodilators (medicines that open up narrowed breathing passages) and corticosteroids (cortisone-like medicines).

Nedocromil works by acting on certain inflammatory cells in the lungs to prevent them from releasing substances that cause asthma symptoms and/or bronchospasm.

This medicine is available only with your doctor's prescription, in the following dosage form:

*Inhalation*
 • Inhalation aerosol (U.S. and Canada)

## Before Using This Medicine

In deciding to use a medicine, the risks of using the medicine must be weighed against the good it will do. This is a decision you and your doctor will make. For nedocromil, the following should be considered:

**Allergies**—Tell your doctor if you have ever had any unusual or allergic reaction to nedocromil or to any other inhalation aerosol medicine.

**Pregnancy**—Nedocromil has not been studied in pregnant women. However, nedocromil has not been shown to cause birth defects or other problems in animal studies.

**Breast-feeding**—It is not known whether nedocromil passes into breast milk. Although most medicines pass into breast milk in small amounts, many of them may be used safely while breast-feeding. Mothers who are using this medicine and who wish to breast-feed should discuss this with their doctor.

**Children**—Nedocromil has been tested in a limited number of children 6 years of age and older. In effective doses, it is not expected to cause different side effects or problems in children than it does in adults.

**Older adults**—Many medicines have not been studied specifically in older people. Therefore, it may not be known whether they work the same way they do in younger adults. Although there is no specific information comparing use of nedocromil in the elderly with use in other age groups, it is not expected to cause different side effects or problems in older people than it does in younger adults.

## Proper Use of This Medicine

*Nedocromil is used to help prevent symptoms of asthma or bronchospasm (wheezing or difficulty in breathing).* When this medicine is used regularly, it decreases the number and severity of asthma attacks. Nedocromil will not relieve an asthma or bronchospasm attack that has already started.

Nedocromil inhalation aerosol usually comes with patient directions. Read them carefully before using this medicine. If you do not understand the directions or if you are not sure how to use the inhaler, ask your health care professional to show you what to do. Also, ask your health care professional to check regularly how you use the inhaler to make sure you are using it properly.

The nedocromil aerosol canister provides about 56 or 112 inhalations, depending on the size of the canister your doctor ordered. You should keep a record of the number of inhalations you use so you will know when the canister is almost empty. This canister, unlike other aerosol canisters, cannot be floated in water to test its fullness.

When you use the inhaler for the first time, or if you have not used it for several days, the inhaler may not deliver the right amount of medicine with the first puff. Therefore, before using the inhaler, test it to make sure it works properly.

*To test the inhaler:*
 • Insert the metal canister firmly into the clean mouthpiece according to the manufacturer's instructions. Check to make sure the canister is placed properly into the mouthpiece.
 • Take the cover off the mouthpiece and shake the inhaler well.
 • Hold the canister well away from you against a light background, and press the top of the canister, spraying the medicine one time into the air. If you see a fine mist, you will know the inhaler is working properly to provide the right amount of medicine when you use it. If you do not see a fine mist, try a second time.

*To use the inhaler:*
 • Using your thumb and one or two fingers, hold the inhaler upright with the mouthpiece end down and pointing toward you.
 • Take the cover off the mouthpiece. Check the mouthpiece for any foreign objects. Do not use the inhaler with any other mouthpieces.
 • Gently shake the inhaler three or four times.
 • Hold the mouthpiece away from your mouth and breathe out slowly and completely to the end of a normal breath.

- Use the inhalation method recommended by your doctor.
  - —Open-mouth method: Place the mouthpiece about 1 to 2 inches (2 fingerwidths) in front of your widely opened mouth. Make sure the inhaler is aimed into your mouth so the spray does not hit the roof of your mouth or your tongue. Close your eyes just before spraying to keep the spray out of your eyes.
  - —Closed-mouth method: Place the mouthpiece in your mouth between your teeth and over your tongue with your lips closed tightly around it. Make sure your tongue or teeth are not blocking the opening.
- Tilt your head back a little. Start to breathe in slowly and deeply through your mouth and, at the same time, press the top of the canister once to get one puff of medicine. Continue to breathe in slowly for 3 to 4 seconds until you have taken a full breath. It is important to press down on the canister and breathe in slowly at the same time so the medicine is pulled into your lungs. This step may be difficult at first. If you are using the closed-mouth method and you see a fine mist coming from your mouth or nose, the inhaler is not being used correctly.
- Hold your breath as long as you can for up to 10 seconds (count slowly to 10). This gives the medicine time to get into your airways and lungs.
- Take the mouthpiece away from your mouth and breathe out slowly.
- If your doctor has told you to inhale more than one puff of medicine at each dose, wait 1 minute between puffs. Then, gently shake the inhaler again, and take the second puff following exactly the same steps you used for the first puff. Breathe in only one puff at a time.
- If your doctor has told you to use an inhaled bronchodilator before using nedocromil, you should wait at least 2 minutes after using the bronchodilator before using nedocromil. This allows the nedocromil to get deeper into your lungs.
- When you are finished, wipe off the mouthpiece and replace the cover to keep the mouthpiece clean and free of foreign objects.

Your doctor may want you to use a spacer device with the inhaler. A spacer makes the inhaler easier to use. It allows more of the medicine to reach your lungs and helps make sure that less of it stays in your mouth and throat.

*To use a spacer device with the inhaler:*

- Attach the spacer to the inhaler according to the manufacturer's directions. There are different types of spacers available, but the method of breathing remains the same with most spacers.
- Gently shake the inhaler and spacer three or four times.
- Hold the mouthpiece of the spacer away from your mouth and breathe out slowly to the end of a normal breath.

- Place the mouthpiece into your mouth between your teeth and over your tongue with your lips closed around it.
- Press down on the canister top once to release one puff of medicine into the spacer. Then, within one or two seconds, begin to breathe in slowly and deeply through your mouth for 5 to 10 seconds. Count the seconds while inhaling. Do not breathe in through your nose.
- Hold your breath as long as you can for up to 10 seconds (count slowly to ten).
- Breathe out slowly. Do not remove the mouthpiece from your mouth. Breathe in and out slowly two or three times to make sure the spacer device is emptied.
- If your doctor has told you to take more than one puff of medicine at each dose, wait a minute between puffs. Then, gently shake the inhaler and spacer again and take the second puff, following exactly the same steps you used for the first puff.
- When you have finished, remove the spacer device from the inhaler and replace the cover of the mouthpiece.

*To clean the inhaler:*

- Clean the inhaler often to prevent build-up of medicine and blocking of the mouthpiece. The mouthpiece can be washed every day and should be washed at least twice a week.
- Remove the metal canister from the inhaler and set it aside. Do not get the canister wet.
- Wash the mouthpiece in hot water.
- Shake off the excess water and let the mouthpiece air dry completely before replacing the metal canister and cover.

For patients using nedocromil regularly (for example, every day):

- *In order for nedocromil to work properly, it must be inhaled every day in regularly spaced doses as ordered by your doctor.*
- Usually about 2 to 4 weeks may pass before you begin to feel the full effects of this medicine.

**Missed dose**—If you are using nedocromil regularly and you miss a dose of this medicine, take it as soon as possible. Then take any remaining doses for that day at regularly spaced times.

**Dosing**—The dose of nedocromil will be different for different patients. *Follow your doctor's orders or the directions on the label.* The following information includes only the average doses of nedocromil. *If your dose is different, do not change it* unless your doctor tells you to do so:

- For *inhalation* dosage form (inhalation aerosol):
  - —For prevention of asthma symptoms:
    - • Adults and children 12 years of age or older— 3.5 or 4 milligrams (mg) (2 puffs) two to four times a day at regularly spaced times.

- Children up to 12 years of age—Use and dose must be determined by the doctor.
—For prevention of bronchospasm caused by exercise or a substance:
  - Adults and children 12 years of age or older—4 mg (2 puffs) as a single dose up to thirty minutes before exercise or exposure to any condition or substance that may cause an attack.
  - Children up to 12 years of age—Use and dose must be determined by the doctor.

**Storage**—To store this medicine:
- Keep out of the reach of children.
- Store away from heat and direct sunlight.
- Keep the medicine from freezing.
- Do not puncture, break, or burn the aerosol container, even if it is empty.
- Do not keep outdated medicine or medicine no longer needed. Be sure that any discarded medicine is out of the reach of children.
- Always keep the dust cover on the mouthpiece when the inhaler is not in use.

## Precautions While Using This Medicine

*If your symptoms do not improve within 2 to 4 weeks, check with your doctor. Also, check with your doctor if your condition becomes worse.*

You may also be taking a corticosteroid or a bronchodilator for asthma along with this medicine. *Do not stop taking the corticosteroid or bronchodilator even if your asthma seems better, unless you are told to do so by your doctor.*

Throat irritation and/or an unpleasant taste may occur after you use this medicine. Gargling and rinsing the mouth after each dose may help prevent these effects.

## Side Effects of This Medicine

Along with its needed effects, a medicine may cause some unwanted effects. Although not all of these side effects may occur, if they do occur they may need medical attention.

Check with your doctor as soon as possible if any of the following side effects occur:

*Less common*
> Increased wheezing, tightness in chest, or difficulty in breathing

Other side effects may occur that usually do not need medical attention. These side effects may go away during treatment as your body adjusts to the medicine. However, check with your doctor if any of the following side effects continue or are bothersome:

*Less common*
> Cough; headache; nausea; runny or stuffy nose; throat irritation

After you use nedocromil inhalation aerosol, you may notice an unpleasant taste. This may be expected and will usually go away after a while.

Other side effects not listed above may also occur in some patients. If you notice any other effects, check with your doctor.

Revised: 08/09/94

---

# NEOMYCIN    Ophthalmic*†

## Description

Neomycin (nee-oh-MYE-sin) belongs to the family of medicines called antibiotics. Neomycin ophthalmic preparations are used to treat infections of the eye.

Neomycin is available only with your doctor's prescription, in the following dosage form:

*Ophthalmic*
- Ophthalmic ointment

## Before Using This Medicine

In deciding to use a medicine, the risks of taking the medicine must be weighed against the good it will do. This is a decision you and your doctor will make. For

neomycin ophthalmic preparations, the following should be considered:

**Allergies**—Tell your doctor if you have ever had any unusual or allergic reaction to this medicine or to any related antibiotic, such as amikacin (e.g., Amikin), gentamicin (e.g., Garamycin), kanamycin (e.g., Kantrex), netilmicin (e.g., Netromycin), streptomycin, or tobramycin (e.g., Nebcin). Also tell your health care professional if you are allergic to any other substances, such as preservatives.

**Pregnancy**—Neomycin ophthalmic preparations have not been shown to cause birth defects or other problems in humans.

**Breast-feeding**—Neomycin ophthalmic preparations have not been reported to cause problems in nursing babies.

**Children**—Studies on this medicine have been done only in adult patients, and there is no specific information

comparing use of neomycin in children with use in other age groups.

**Older adults**—Many medicines have not been studied specifically in older people. Therefore, it may not be known whether they work exactly the same way they do in younger adults or if they cause different side effects or problems in older people. There is no specific information comparing use of neomycin in the elderly with use in other age groups.

---

### Proper Use of This Medicine

To use:

- First, wash your hands. Tilt the head back and, pressing your finger gently on the skin just beneath the lower eyelid, pull the lower eyelid away from the eye to make a space. Squeeze a thin strip of ointment into this space. A 1-cm (approximately ⅓-inch) strip of ointment is usually enough, unless you have been told by your doctor to use a different amount. Let go of the eyelid and gently close the eyes. Keep the eyes closed for 1 or 2 minutes to allow the medicine to come into contact with the infection.

- To keep the medicine as germ-free as possible, do not touch the applicator tip to any surface (including the eye). After using neomycin eye ointment, wipe the tip of the ointment tube with a clean tissue and keep the tube tightly closed.

To help clear up your infection completely, *keep using this medicine for the full time of treatment,* even if your symptoms have disappeared. *Do not miss any doses.*

**Dosing**—The dose of ophthalmic neomycin will be different for different patients. *Follow your doctor's orders or the directions on the label.* The following information includes only the average doses of ophthalmic neomycin. *If your dose is different, do not change it* unless your doctor tells you to do so.

- For eye infection:
  - —For *eye ointment* dosage form:
    - Adults and children—Use in the eye every eight to twenty-four hours.

**Missed dose**—If you miss a dose of this medicine, apply it as soon as possible. However, if it is almost time for your next dose, skip the missed dose and go back to your regular dosing schedule.

**Storage**—To store this medicine:

- Keep out of the reach of children.
- Store away from heat and direct light.
- Keep the medicine from freezing.
- Do not keep outdated medicine or medicine no longer needed. Be sure that any discarded medicine is out of the reach of children.

---

### Precautions While Using This Medicine

If your symptoms do not improve within a few days, or if they become worse, check with your doctor.

---

### Side Effects of This Medicine

Along with its needed effects, a medicine may cause some unwanted effects. Although not all of these side effects may occur, if they do occur they may need medical attention.

*Check with your doctor immediately* if any of the following side effects occur:

*More common*
  Itching, rash, redness, swelling, or other sign of irritation not present before use of this medicine

Other side effects may occur that usually do not need medical attention. These side effects may go away during treatment as your body adjusts to the medicine. However, check with your doctor if either of the following side effects continues or is bothersome:

*Less common*
  Burning or stinging

After application, eye ointments may be expected to cause your vision to blur for a few minutes.

Other side effects not listed above may also occur in some patients. If you notice any other effects, check with your doctor.

---

Revised: 05/16/94

---

# NEOMYCIN    Oral

---

A commonly used brand name in the U.S. and Canada is Mycifradin. Generic name product may also be available in the U.S.

---

### Description

Oral neomycin (nee-oh-MYE-sin) is used to help lessen the symptoms of hepatic coma, a complication of liver disease. In addition, it may be used with another medicine before any surgery affecting the bowels to help prevent infection during surgery.

Neomycin is available only with your doctor's prescription, in the following dosage forms:

*Oral*
- Solution (U.S. and Canada)
- Tablets (U.S. and Canada)

---

## Before Using This Medicine

In deciding to use a medicine, the risks of taking the medicine must be weighed against the good it will do. This is a decision you and your doctor will make. For oral neomycin, the following should be considered:

**Allergies**—Tell your doctor if you have ever had any unusual or allergic reaction to oral neomycin, or to any related antibiotics such as amikacin (e.g., Amikin), gentamicin (e.g., Garamycin), kanamycin (e.g., Kantrex), neomycin by injection (e.g., Mycifradin), netilmicin (e.g., Netromycin), streptomycin, or tobramycin (e.g., Nebcin). Also tell your health care professional if you are allergic to any other substances, such as foods, preservatives, or dyes.

**Pregnancy**—Studies have shown that neomycin may damage the infant's kidneys. In addition, some reports have shown that related medicines, especially streptomycin and tobramycin (e.g., Nebcin), may damage the infant's hearing and sense of balance. Be sure you have discussed this with your doctor.

**Breast-feeding**—It is not known whether neomycin passes into the breast milk. However, neomycin has not been reported to cause problems in nursing babies.

**Children**—Damage to hearing, sense of balance, and kidneys is more likely to occur in premature infants and neonates, who are more sensitive than adults to the effects of neomycin.

**Older adults**—Serious side effects, such as damage to hearing, sense of balance, and kidneys may occur in elderly patients, who are usually more sensitive than younger adults to the effects of neomycin.

**Other medicines**—Although certain medicines should not be used together at all, in other cases two different medicines may be used together even if an interaction might occur. In these cases, your doctor may want to change the dose, or other precautions may be necessary. Tell your health care professional if you are taking any other prescription or nonprescription (over-the-counter [OTC]) medicine.

**Other medical problems**—The presence of other medical problems may affect the use of oral neomycin. Make sure you tell your doctor if you have any other medical problems, especially:

- Blockage of the bowel
- Eighth-cranial-nerve disease (loss of hearing and/or balance)—Oral neomycin may increase the chance of hearing loss and/or balance problems
- Kidney disease—Patients with kidney disease may have an increased chance of side effects
- Myasthenia gravis or
- Parkinson's disease—Patients with myasthenia gravis or Parkinson's disease may have an increased chance of developing muscular weakness
- Ulcers of the bowel—Patients with ulcers of the bowel may have an increased chance of side effects since more neomycin may be absorbed by the body

## Proper Use of This Medicine

This medicine may be taken on a full or empty stomach.

For patients taking the *oral liquid form* of neomycin:
- Use a specially marked measuring spoon or other device to measure each dose accurately. The average household teaspoon may not hold the right amount of liquid.

*Keep taking this medicine for the full time of treatment. Do not miss any doses.*

**Dosing**—The dose of oral neomycin will be different for different patients. *Follow your doctor's orders or the directions on the label.* The following information includes only the average doses of oral neomycin. *If your dose is different, do not change it* unless your doctor tells you to do so.

- For *oral* dosage forms (solution, tablets):
  —For patients in a coma from liver disease:
    - Adults and teenagers—1 to 3 grams every six hours for five or six days.
    - Children—Dose is based on body size (not weight) and must be determined by your doctor. That dose is given every six hours for five or six days.
  —For cleaning the bowel before surgery:
    - Adults and teenagers—1 gram every hour for four hours, then 1 gram every four hours for the rest of a twenty-four hour period; or 1 gram nineteen hours before surgery, 1 gram eighteen hours before surgery, and 1 gram nine hours before surgery.
    - Children—Dose is based on body weight. The usual dose is 14.7 milligrams (mg) per kilogram (kg) (6.7 mg per pound) of body weight every four hours for three days.

**Missed dose**—If you miss a dose of this medicine, take it as soon as possible. However, if it is almost time for your next dose, skip the missed dose and go back to your regular dosing schedule. Do not double doses.

**Storage**—To store this medicine:
- Keep out of the reach of children.
- Store away from heat and direct light.
- Do not store the tablet form of this medicine in the bathroom, near the kitchen sink, or in other damp places. Heat or moisture may cause the medicine to break down.
- Keep the oral liquid form of this medicine from freezing.
- Do not keep outdated medicine or medicine no longer needed. Be sure that any discarded medicine is out of the reach of children.

## Side Effects of This Medicine

Along with its needed effects, a medicine may cause some unwanted effects. Although not all of these side effects

may occur, if they do occur they may need medical attention.

*Check with your doctor immediately* if any of the following side effects occur:

   *Rare*
      Any loss of hearing; clumsiness; diarrhea; difficulty in breathing; dizziness; drowsiness; greatly decreased frequency of urination or amount of urine; increased amount of gas; increased thirst; light-colored, frothy, fatty-appearing stools; ringing or buzzing or a feeling of fullness in the ears; skin rash; unsteadiness; weakness

Other side effects may occur that usually do not need medical attention. These side effects may go away during treatment as your body adjusts to the medicine. However, check with your doctor if any of the following side effects continue or are bothersome:

   *More common*
      Irritation or soreness of the mouth or rectal area; nausea or vomiting

Other side effects not listed above may also occur in some patients. If you notice any other effects, check with your doctor.

Revised: 10/20/92
Interim revision: 03/17/94

# NEOMYCIN   Topical

A commonly used brand name in the U.S. and Canada is Myciguent. Generic name product may also be available in the U.S.

## Description

Neomycin (nee-oh-MYE-sin) belongs to the family of medicines called antibiotics. Neomycin topical preparations are used to help prevent infections of the skin. This medicine may be used for other problems as determined by your doctor.

Neomycin topical preparations are available without a prescription; however, your doctor may have special instructions on the proper use of topical neomycin for your medical problem.

Topical neomycin is available in the following dosage forms:

   *Topical*
   • Cream (U.S.)
   • Ointment (U.S. and Canada)

## Before Using This Medicine

In deciding to use a medicine, the risks of using the medicine must be weighed against the good it will do. This is a decision you and your doctor will make. For topical neomycin, the following should be considered:

**Allergies**—Tell your doctor if you have ever had any unusual or allergic reaction to this medicine or to any related antibiotic, such as amikacin (e.g., Amikin), gentamicin (e.g., Garamycin), kanamycin (e.g., Kantrex), neomycin by mouth or by injection (e.g., Mycifradin), netilmicin (e.g., Netromycin), streptomycin, or tobramycin (e.g., Nebcin). Also tell your health care professional if you are allergic to any other substances, such as preservatives or dyes.

**Pregnancy**—Neomycin topical preparations have not been shown to cause birth defects or other problems in humans.

**Breast-feeding**—Neomycin topical preparations have not been reported to cause problems in nursing babies.

**Children**—Studies on this medicine have been done only in adult patients, and there is no specific information comparing use of topical neomycin in children with use in other age groups.

**Older adults**—Many medicines have not been studied specifically in older people. Therefore, it may not be known whether they work exactly the same way they do in younger adults or if they cause different side effects or problems in older people. There is no specific information comparing use of topical neomycin in the elderly with use in other age groups.

**Other medicines**—Although certain medicines should not be used together at all, in other cases two different medicines may be used together even if an interaction might occur. In these cases, your doctor may want to change the dose, or other precautions may be necessary. Tell your health care professional if you are using any other topical prescription or nonprescription (over-the-counter [OTC]) medicine that is to be applied to the same area of the skin.

## Proper Use of This Medicine

If you are using this medicine without a prescription, do not use it to treat deep wounds, puncture wounds, serious burns, or raw areas without first checking with your health care professional.

Do not use this medicine in the eyes.

Before applying this medicine, wash the affected area with soap and water, and dry thoroughly.

For patients using the *cream form* of this medicine:
   • Apply a generous amount of cream to the affected area, and rub in gently until the cream disappears.

For patients using the *ointment form* of this medicine:
- Apply a generous amount of ointment to the affected area, and rub in gently.

After this medicine is applied, the treated area may be covered with a gauze dressing if desired.

To help clear up your infection completely, *keep using this medicine for the full time of treatment,* even if your symptoms have disappeared. *Do not miss any doses.*

**Dosing**—The dose of topical neomycin will be different for different patients. *Follow your doctor's orders or the directions on the label.* The following information includes only the average dose of topical neomycin. *If your dose is different, do not change it* unless your doctor tells you to do so.
- For *topical* dosage forms (cream or ointment):
  —For minor bacterial skin infections:
  - Adults and children—Apply to the affected area(s) of the skin one to three times a day.

**Missed dose**—If you miss a dose of this medicine, apply it as soon as possible. However, if it is almost time for your next dose, skip the missed dose and go back to your regular dosing schedule.

**Storage**—To store this medicine:
- Keep out of the reach of children.
- Store away from heat and direct light.
- Keep the medicine from freezing.
- Do not keep outdated medicine or medicine no longer needed. Be sure that any discarded medicine is out of the reach of children.

## Precautions While Using This Medicine

If your skin problem does not improve within 1 week, or if it becomes worse, check with your health care professional.

## Side Effects of This Medicine

Along with its needed effects, a medicine may cause some unwanted effects. Although not all of these side effects may occur, if they do occur they may need medical attention.

*Check with your doctor immediately* if any of the following side effects occur:
> *More common*
>> Itching, rash, redness, swelling, or other sign of skin irritation not present before use of this medicine
> *Rare*
>> Any loss of hearing

Other side effects not listed above may also occur in some patients. If you notice any other effects, check with your doctor.

Revised: 08/15/94

---

# NEOMYCIN AND POLYMYXIN B    Topical†

A commonly used brand name in the U.S. is Neosporin Cream‡.

†Not commercially available in Canada.
‡In Canada, Neosporin cream also contains gramicidin.

## Description

Neomycin (nee-oh-MYE-sin) and polymyxin (pol-i-MIX-in) B combination is used to prevent bacterial infections. It works by killing bacteria.

Neomycin and polymyxin B cream is applied to the skin to prevent minor bacterial skin infections. It may also be used for other problems as determined by your doctor.

This medicine is available without a prescription; however, your doctor may have special instructions on the proper use of this medicine for your medical problem.

Neomycin and polymyxin B combination is available in the following dosage form:
*Topical*
- Cream (U.S.)

## Before Using This Medicine

If you are using this medicine without a prescription, carefully read and follow any precautions on the label. For neomycin and polymyxin B topical preparations, the following should be considered:

**Allergies**—Tell your doctor if you have ever had any unusual or allergic reaction to neomycin and polymyxin B combination or to any related antibiotic: Amikacin (e.g., Amikin), colistimethate (e.g., Coly-Mycin M), colistin (e.g., Coly-Mycin S), gentamicin (e.g., Garamycin), kanamycin (e.g., Kantrex), neomycin by mouth or by injection (e.g., Mycifradin), netilmicin (e.g., Netromycin), paromomycin (e.g., Humatin), polymyxin B by injection (e.g., Aerosporin), streptomycin, or tobramycin (e.g., Nebcin). Also, tell your health care professional if you are allergic to any other substances, such as preservatives or dyes.

**Pregnancy**—Neomycin and polymyxin B topical preparations have not been shown to cause birth defects or other problems in humans.

**Breast-feeding**—Neomycin and polymyxin B topical preparations have not been reported to cause problems in nursing babies.

**Children**—Although there is no specific information comparing use of neomycin and polymyxin B combination in children with use in other age groups, this medicine is not expected to cause different side effects or problems in children than it does in adults.

**Older adults**—Many medicines have not been studied specifically in older people. Therefore, it may not be known whether they work exactly the same way they do in younger adults or if they cause different side effects or problems in older people. There is no specific information comparing use of neomycin and polymyxin B combination in the elderly with use in other age groups.

**Other medicines**—Although certain medicines should not be used together at all, in other cases two different medicines may be used together even if an interaction might occur. In these cases, your doctor may want to change the dose, or other precautions may be necessary. Tell your health care professional if you are using any other topical prescription or nonprescription (over-the-counter [OTC]) medicine that is to be applied to the same area of the skin.

## Proper Use of This Medicine

If you are using this medicine without a prescription, *do not use it to treat deep wounds, puncture wounds, animal bites, serious burns, or raw areas* without first checking with your health care professional.

*Do not use this medicine in the eyes.*

To use:

- Before applying this medicine, wash the affected area(s) with soap and water, and dry thoroughly.
- Apply a small amount of this medicine to the affected area(s) and rub in gently.
- After applying this medicine, the treated area(s) may be covered with a gauze dressing if desired.

*Do not use this medicine for longer than 1 week or on large areas of the skin,* unless otherwise directed by your doctor. To do so may increase the chance of side effects.

To help clear up your skin infection completely, *keep using this medicine for the full time of treatment,* even if your symptoms have disappeared. *Do not miss any doses.*

**Dosing**—The dose of neomycin and polymyxin B combination will be different for different patients. *Follow your doctor's orders or the directions on the label.* The following information includes only the average dose of neomycin and polymyxin B combination. *If your dose is different, do not change it* unless your doctor tells you to do so.

- For *topical* dosage form (cream):
  —For prevention of minor bacterial infections:
    - Adults and children 2 years of age and older— Apply to the affected area(s) of the skin one to three times a day.
    - Children up to 2 years of age—Use and dose must be determined by your doctor.

**Missed dose**—If you miss a dose of this medicine, apply it as soon as possible. However, if it is almost time for your next dose, skip the missed dose and go back to your regular dosing schedule.

**Storage**—To store this medicine:

- Keep out of the reach of children.
- Store away from heat and direct light.
- Keep the medicine from freezing.
- Do not keep outdated medicine or medicine no longer needed. Be sure that any discarded medicine is out of the reach of children.

## Precautions While Using This Medicine

If your skin infection does not improve within 1 week, or if it becomes worse, check with your health care professional.

## Side Effects of This Medicine

Along with its needed effects, a medicine may cause some unwanted effects. Although not all of these side effects may occur, if they do occur they may need medical attention.

*Check with your doctor immediately* if any of the following side effects occur:

*More common*
　Itching, pain, skin rash, swelling, redness, or other sign of skin irritation not present before use of this medicine

*Rare*
　Loss of hearing

Other side effects not listed above may also occur in some patients. If you notice any other effects, check with your doctor.

Revised: 06/09/94

# NEOMYCIN, POLYMYXIN B, AND BACITRACIN    Ophthalmic

Some commonly used brand names are:

**In the U.S.—**

Ak-Spore Ophthalmic
   Ointment
Neocidin Ophthalmic
   Ointment
Neosporin Ophthalmic
   Ointment
Neotal

Ocu-Spor-B
Ocusporin
Ocutricin Ophthalmic
   Ointment
Ophthalmic
Spectro-Sporin

Generic name product may also be available.

**In Canada—**

Neosporin Ophthalmic
   Ointment

## Description

Neomycin (nee-oh-MYE-sin), polymyxin (pol-i-MIX-in) B, and bacitracin (bass-i-TRAY-sin) combination antibiotic medicine is used to treat infections of the eye.

Neomycin, polymyxin B, and bacitracin combination is available only with your doctor's prescription, in the following dosage form:

*Ophthalmic*
- Ophthalmic ointment (U.S. and Canada)

## Before Using This Medicine

In deciding to use a medicine, the risks of using the medicine must be weighed against the good it will do. This is a decision you and your doctor will make. For neomycin, polymyxin B, and bacitracin ophthalmic combination, the following should be considered:

**Allergies**—Tell your doctor if you have ever had any unusual or allergic reaction to this medicine or to any related antibiotic, such as amikacin (e.g., Amikin), colistimethate (e.g., Coly-Mycin M), colistin (e.g., Coly-Mycin S), gentamicin (e.g., Garamycin), kanamycin (e.g., Kantrex), netilmicin (e.g., Netromycin), paromomycin (e.g., Humatin), streptomycin, or tobramycin (e.g., Nebcin). Also tell your health care professional if you are allergic to any other substances, such as preservatives or dyes.

**Pregnancy**—Neomycin, polymyxin B, and bacitracin ophthalmic combination has not been shown to cause birth defects or other problems in humans.

**Breast-feeding**—Neomycin, polymyxin B, and bacitracin ophthalmic combination has not been reported to cause problems in nursing babies.

**Children**—Studies on this medicine have been done only in adult patients, and there is no specific information comparing use of neomycin, polymyxin B, and bacitracin combination in children with use in other age groups.

**Older adults**—Many medicines have not been studied specifically in older people. Therefore, it may not be known whether they work exactly the same way they do in younger adults or if they cause different side effects or problems in older people. There is no specific information comparing use of neomycin, polymyxin B, and bacitracin combination in the elderly with use in other age groups.

## Proper Use of This Medicine

To use:
- First, wash your hands. Tilt the head back and, pressing your finger gently on the skin just beneath the lower eyelid, pull the lower eyelid away from the eye to make a space. Squeeze a thin strip of ointment into this space. A 1-cm (approximately ⅓-inch) strip of ointment is usually enough, unless you have been told by your doctor to use a different amount. Let go of the eyelid and gently close the eyes. Keep the eyes closed for 1 or 2 minutes to allow the medicine to come into contact with the infection.
- To keep the medicine as germ-free as possible, do not touch the applicator tip to any surface (including the eye). After using neomycin, polymyxin B, and bacitracin eye ointment, wipe the tip of the ointment tube with a clean tissue and keep the tube tightly closed.

To help clear up your infection completely, *keep using this medicine for the full time of treatment,* even if your symptoms have disappeared. *Do not miss any doses.*

**Dosing**—The dose of neomycin, polymyxin B, and bacitracin ophthalmic combination will be different for different patients. *Follow your doctor's orders or the directions on the label.* The following information includes only the average dose of neomycin, polymyxin B, and bacitracin ophthalmic combination. *If your dose is different, do not change it* unless your doctor tells you to do so.

- For eye infections:
  - —For *eye ointment* dosage forms:
    - Adults and children—Use a thin strip of ointment in the eyes every three or four hours for seven to ten days.

**Missed dose**—If you miss a dose of this medicine, apply it as soon as possible. However, if it is almost time for your next dose, skip the missed dose and go back to your regular dosing schedule.

**Storage**—To store this medicine:
- Keep out of the reach of children.
- Store away from heat and direct light.
- Keep the medicine from freezing.
- Do not keep outdated medicine or medicine no longer needed. Be sure that any discarded medicine is out of the reach of children.

## Precautions While Using This Medicine

If your symptoms do not improve within a few days, or if they become worse, check with your doctor.

## Side Effects of This Medicine

Along with its needed effects, a medicine may cause some unwanted effects. Although not all of these side effects may occur, if they do occur they may need medical attention.

*Check with your doctor immediately* if any of the following side effects occur:

*More common*

　　Itching, rash, redness, swelling, or other sign of irritation not present before use of this medicine

After application, eye ointments usually cause your vision to blur for a few minutes.

Other side effects not listed above may also occur in some patients. If you notice any other effects, check with your doctor.

Revised: 05/16/94

---

# NEOMYCIN, POLYMYXIN B, AND BACITRACIN    Topical

Some commonly used brand names are:

**In the U.S.—**

Bactine First Aid Antibiotic　　Neosporin Ointment
Foille　　Topisporin
Mycitracin
Neosporin Maximum Strength
　　Ointment

Generic name product may also be available in the U.S. and Canada.

## Description

Neomycin (nee-oh-MYE-sin), polymyxin (pol-i-MIX-in) B, and bacitracin (bass-i-TRAY-sin) is a combination antibiotic medicine used to help prevent infections of the skin.

Neomycin, polymyxin B, and bacitracin combination is available without a prescription; however, your doctor may have special instructions on the proper use of this medicine for your medical problem.

Topical neomycin, polymyxin B, and bacitracin combination is available in the following dosage form:

*Topical*

• Ointment (U.S. and Canada)

## Before Using This Medicine

If you are using this medicine without a prescription, carefully read and follow any precautions on the label. For topical neomycin, polymyxin B, and bacitracin combination, the following should be considered:

**Allergies**—Tell your doctor if you have ever had any unusual or allergic reaction to this medicine or to any related antibiotic, such as amikacin (e.g., Amikin), colistimethate (e.g., Coly-Mycin M), colistin (e.g., Coly-Mycin S), gentamicin (e.g., Garamycin), kanamycin (e.g., Kantrex), neomycin by mouth or by injection (e.g., Mycifradin), netilmicin (e.g., Netromycin), paromomycin (e.g., Humatin), polymyxin B by injection (e.g., Aerosporin), streptomycin, or tobramycin (e.g., Nebcin). Also tell your health care professional if you are allergic to any other substances, such as preservatives or dyes.

**Pregnancy**—Neomycin, polymyxin B, and bacitracin topical preparations have not been studied in pregnant women. However, this medicine has not been shown to cause birth defects or other problems in humans.

**Breast-feeding**—It is not known whether topical neomycin, polymyxin B, and bacitracin combination passes into breast milk. However, this medicine has not been reported to cause problems in nursing babies.

**Children**—Studies on this medicine have been done only in adult patients, and there is no specific information comparing use of topical neomycin, polymyxin B, and bacitracin combination in children with use in other age groups.

**Older adults**—Many medicines have not been studied specifically in older people. Therefore, it may not be known whether they work exactly the same way they do in younger adults or if they cause different side effects or problems in older people. There is no specific information comparing use of topical neomycin, polymyxin B, and bacitracin combination in the elderly with use in other age groups.

**Other medicines**—Although certain medicines should not be used together at all, in other cases two different medicines may be used together even if an interaction might occur. In these cases, your doctor may want to change the dose, or other precautions may be necessary. Tell your health care professional if you are using any other prescription or nonprescription (over-the-counter [OTC]) medicine.

## Proper Use of This Medicine

If you are using this medicine without a prescription, do not use it to treat deep wounds, puncture wounds, serious burns, or raw areas without first checking with your health care professional.

Do not use this medicine in the eyes.

Before applying this medicine, wash the affected area with soap and water, and dry thoroughly.

After applying this medicine, the treated area may be covered with a gauze dressing if desired.

To help clear up your infection completely, *keep using this medicine for the full time of treatment,* even if your symptoms have disappeared. *Do not miss any doses.*

**Dosing**—The dose of topical neomycin, polymyxin B, and bacitracin combination will be different for different patients. *Follow your doctor's orders or the directions on the label.* The following information includes only the average doses of topical neomycin, polymyxin B, and bacitracin combination. *If your dose is different, do not change it* unless your doctor tells you to do so.

- For *topical* dosage form (ointment):
  —For prevention of minor bacterial infections:
    - Adults and children—Apply to the affected area(s) of the skin two to five times a day.

**Missed dose**—If you miss a dose of this medicine, apply it as soon as possible. However, if it is almost time for your next dose, skip the missed dose and go back to your regular dosing schedule.

**Storage**—To store this medicine:
- Keep out of the reach of children.
- Store away from heat and direct light.
- Keep the medicine from freezing.
- Do not keep outdated medicine or medicine no longer needed. Be sure that any discarded medicine is out of the reach of children.

## Precautions While Using This Medicine

If your skin problem does not improve within 1 week, or if it becomes worse, check with your health care professional.

## Side Effects of This Medicine

Along with its needed effects, a medicine may cause some unwanted effects. Although not all of these side effects may occur, if they do occur they may need medical attention.

*Check with your doctor immediately* if any of the following side effects occur:

*More common*
> Itching, skin rash, redness, swelling, or other sign of irritation not present before use of this medicine

*Rare*
> Any loss of hearing

Other side effects not listed above may also occur in some patients. If you notice any other effects, check with your doctor.

Revised: 07/25/94

# NEOMYCIN, POLYMYXIN B, AND GRAMICIDIN   Ophthalmic

Some commonly used brand names are:
**In the U.S.—**
| | |
|---|---|
| Ak-Spore Ophthalmic Solution | Ocu-Spor-G |
| Neocidin Ophthalmic Solution | Ocutricin Ophthalmic Solution |
| Neosporin Ophthalmic Solution | P.N. Ophthalmic |
| | Tribiotic |
| | Tri-Ophthalmic |

Generic name product may also be available.
**In Canada—**
Neosporin Ophthalmic Solution

## Description

Neomycin (nee-oh-MYE-sin), polymyxin (pol-i-MIX-in) B, and gramicidin (gram-i-SYE-din) is a combination antibiotic medicine used to treat infections of the eye.

Neomycin, polymyxin B, and gramicidin combination is available only with your doctor's prescription, in the following dosage form:

*Ophthalmic*
- Ophthalmic solution (eye drops) (U.S. and Canada)

## Before Using This Medicine

In deciding to use a medicine, the risks of taking the medicine must be weighed against the good it will do. This is a decision you and your doctor will make. For neomycin, polymyxin B, and gramicidin ophthalmic drops, the following should be considered:

**Allergies**—Tell your doctor if you have ever had any unusual or allergic reaction to this medicine or to any related antibiotic, such as amikacin (e.g., Amikin), colistimethate (e.g., Coly-Mycin M), colistin (e.g., Coly-Mycin S), gentamicin (e.g., Garamycin), kanamycin (e.g., Kantrex), netilmicin (e.g., Netromycin), paromomycin (e.g., Humatin), streptomycin, or tobramycin (e.g., Nebcin). Also tell your health care professional if you are allergic to any other substances, such as preservatives.

**Pregnancy**—Neomycin, polymyxin B, and gramicidin combination has not been shown to cause birth defects or other problems in humans.

**Breast-feeding**—Neomycin, polymyxin B, and gramicidin combination has not been reported to cause problems in nursing babies.

**Children**—Studies on this medicine have been done only in adult patients, and there is no specific information comparing use of this combination in children with use in other age groups.

**Older adults**—Many medicines have not been studied specifically in older people. Therefore, it may not be known whether they work exactly the same way they do in younger adults or if they cause different side effects or problems in older people. There is no specific information comparing use of neomycin, polymyxin B, and gramicidin combination in the elderly with use in other age groups.

## Proper Use of This Medicine

The bottle is only partially full to provide proper drop control.

To use:

- First, wash your hands. Tilt the head back and, pressing your finger gently on the skin just beneath the lower eyelid, pull the lower eyelid away from the eye to make a space. Drop the medicine into this space. Let go of the eyelid and gently close the eyes. Do not blink. Keep the eyes closed for 1 or 2 minutes to allow the medicine to come into contact with the infection.
- If you think you did not get the drop of medicine into your eye properly, use another drop.
- To keep the medicine as germ-free as possible, do not touch the applicator tip or dropper to any surface (including the eye). Also, keep the container tightly closed.

To help clear up your infection completely, *keep using this medicine for the full time of treatment,* even if your symptoms have disappeared. *Do not miss any doses.*

**Dosing**—The dose of neomycin, polymyxin B, and gramicidin ophthalmic combination will be different for different patients. *Follow your doctor's orders or the directions on the label.* The following information includes only the average doses of neomycin, polymyxin B, and gramicidin ophthalmic combination. *If your dose is different, do not change it* unless your doctor tells you to do so.

- For eye infections:
  - —For *eye drops* dosage form:
    - Adults and children—Use one drop in the eye two to four times a day for seven to ten days. If you have a more serious infection, your doctor

may want you to use one drop in the eye every fifteen to thirty minutes at first. Then your doctor may have you use the medicine less often.

**Missed dose**—If you miss a dose of this medicine, apply it as soon as possible. However, if it is almost time for your next dose, skip the missed dose and go back to your regular dosing schedule.

**Storage**—To store this medicine:

- Keep out of the reach of children.
- Store away from heat and direct light.
- Keep the medicine from freezing.
- Do not keep outdated medicine or medicine no longer needed. Be sure that any discarded medicine is out of the reach of children.

## Precautions While Using This Medicine

If your symptoms do not improve within a few days, or if they become worse, check with your doctor.

## Side Effects of This Medicine

Along with its needed effects, a medicine may cause some unwanted effects. Although not all of these side effects may occur, if they do occur they may need medical attention.

*Check with your doctor immediately* if any of the following side effects occur:

*More common*

Itching, rash, redness, swelling, or other sign of irritation in or around the eye not present before use of this medicine

Other side effects may occur that usually do not need medical attention. These side effects may go away during treatment as your body adjusts to the medicine. However, check with your doctor if either of the following side effects continues or is bothersome:

*Less common*

Burning or stinging of the eye

Other side effects not listed above may also occur in some patients. If you notice any other effects, check with your doctor.

Revised: 06/21/94

# NEOMYCIN, POLYMYXIN B, AND HYDROCORTISONE    Ophthalmic

Some commonly used brand names are:

**In the U.S.—**

| | |
|---|---|
| Ak-Spore H.C. | Cortomycin |
| Bacticort | Hydromycin |
| Cobiron | I-Neocort |
| Cortisporin Ophthalmic | Ocutricin HC |
| Suspension | Triple-Gen |

Generic name product may also be available.

**In Canada—**

Cortisporin Ophthalmic
Suspension

## Description

Neomycin (nee-oh-MYE-sin), polymyxin (pol-i-MIX-in) B, and hydrocortisone (hye-droe-KOR-ti-sone) is a combination antibiotic and cortisone-like medicine. It is used to treat infections of the eye and to help provide relief from redness, irritation, and discomfort of certain eye problems.

Neomycin, polymyxin B, and hydrocortisone combination is available only with your doctor's prescription, in the following dosage form:

*Ophthalmic*
- Ophthalmic suspension (eye drops) (U.S. and Canada)

## Before Using This Medicine

In deciding to use a medicine, the risks of using the medicine must be weighed against the good it will do. This is a decision you and your doctor will make. For neomycin, polymyxin B, and hydrocortisone ophthalmic drops, the following should be considered:

**Allergies**—Tell your doctor if you have ever had any unusual or allergic reaction to this medicine or to any related antibiotic, such as amikacin (e.g., Amikin), colistimethate (e.g., Coly-Mycin M), colistin (e.g., Coly-Mycin S), gentamicin (e.g., Garamycin), kanamycin (e.g., Kantrex), netilmicin (e.g., Netromycin), paromomycin (e.g., Humatin), streptomycin, or tobramycin (e.g., Nebcin). Also tell your health care professional if you are allergic to any other substances, such as preservatives.

**Pregnancy**—Neomycin, polymyxin B, and hydrocortisone ophthalmic preparations have not been studied in pregnant women. However, studies in animals have shown that topical corticosteroids cause birth defects. Before using this medicine, make sure your doctor knows if you are pregnant or if you may become pregnant.

**Breast-feeding**—Neomycin, polymyxin B, and hydrocortisone ophthalmic drops have not been reported to cause problems in nursing babies.

**Children**—Studies on this medicine have been done only in adult patients, and there is no specific information comparing use in children with use in other age groups.

**Older adults**—Many medicines have not been studied specifically in older people. Therefore, it may not be known whether they work exactly the same way they do in younger adults or if they cause different side effects or problems in older people. There is no specific information comparing use of ophthalmic neomycin, polymyxin B, and hydrocortisone combination in the elderly with use in other age groups.

**Other medical problems**—The presence of other medical problems may affect the use of neomycin, polymyxin B, and hydrocortisone ophthalmic drops. Make sure you tell your doctor if you have any other medical problems, especially:
- Any other eye infection or condition—Use of neomycin, polymyxin B, and hydrocortisone ophthalmic drops may make the condition worse

## Proper Use of This Medicine

The bottle is only partially full to provide proper drop control.

To use:
- First, wash your hands. Then tilt the head back and pull the lower eyelid away from the eye to form a pouch. Drop the medicine into the pouch and gently close the eyes. Do not blink. Keep the eyes closed for 1 or 2 minutes to allow the medicine to come into contact with the infection.
- If you think you did not get the drop of medicine into your eye properly, use another drop.
- To keep the medicine as germ-free as possible, do not touch the applicator tip to any surface (including the eye). Also, keep the container tightly closed.

To help clear up your infection completely, *keep using this medicine for the full time of treatment,* even if your symptoms have disappeared. *Do not miss any doses.*

**Dosing**—The dose of ophthalmic neomycin, polymyxin B, and hyrdocortisone combination will be different for different patients. *Follow your doctor's orders or the directions on the label.* The following information includes only the average doses of ophthalmic neomycin, polymyxin B, and hydrocortisone combination. *If your dose is different, do not change it* unless your doctor tells you to do so.

*The number of doses you use each day, the time allowed between doses, and the length of time you use the medicine depend on the medical problem for which you are using ophthalmic neomycin, polymyxin B, and hydrocortisone combination.*
- For eye infection:
  —For *ophthalmic suspension* dosage forms:
    - Adults and children—One drop every three to four hours.

**Missed dose**—If you miss a dose of this medicine, apply it as soon as possible. However, if it is almost time for your next dose, skip the missed dose and go back to your regular dosing schedule.

*Do not use any leftover medicine for future eye problems without checking with your doctor first.* This medicine should not be used on many different kinds of infection.

**Storage**—To store this medicine:
- Keep out of the reach of children.
- Store away from heat and direct light.
- Keep the medicine from freezing.
- Do not keep outdated medicine or medicine no longer needed. Be sure that any discarded medicine is out of the reach of children.

## Precautions While Using This Medicine

If you will be using this medicine for a long time (for example, longer than 6 weeks), your doctor should check your eyes at regular visits.

If your symptoms do not improve within a few days, or if they become worse, check with your doctor.

## Side Effects of This Medicine

Along with its needed effects, a medicine may cause some unwanted effects. Although not all of these side effects may occur, if they do occur they may need medical attention.

*Check with your doctor immediately* if any of the following side effects occur:

*More common*
 Itching, rash, redness, swelling, or other sign of irritation not present before use of this medicine

Other side effects may occur that usually do not need medical attention. These side effects may go away during treatment as your body adjusts to the medicine. However, check with your doctor if either of the following side effects continues or is bothersome:

*Less common*
 Burning or stinging

Other side effects not listed above may also occur in some patients. If you notice any other effects, check with your doctor.

Revised: 07/01/93

# NEOMYCIN, POLYMYXIN B, AND HYDROCORTISONE   Otic

Some commonly used brand names are:

**In the U.S.—**

| | |
|---|---|
| AK-Spore HC Otic | Ortega Otic-M |
| Cortisporin | Otocort |
| LazerSporin-C | Otoreid-HC |
| Octicair | Pediotic |

**In Canada—**
 Cortisporin

## Description

Neomycin (nee-oh-MYE-sin), polymyxin (pol-i-MIX-in) B, and hydrocortisone (hye-droe-KOR-ti-sone) is a combination antibiotic and cortisone-like medicine. It is used to treat infections of the ear canal and to help provide relief from redness, irritation, and discomfort of certain ear problems.

Neomycin, polymyxin B, and hydrocortisone preparation is available only with your doctor's prescription, in the following dosage forms:

*Otic*
- Solution (U.S. and Canada)
- Suspension (U.S. and Canada)

## Before Using This Medicine

In deciding to use a medicine, the risks of using the medicine must be weighed against the good it will do. This is a decision you and your doctor will make. For neomycin, polymyxin B, and hydrocortisone otic preparations, the following should be considered:

**Allergies**—Tell your doctor if you have ever had any unusual or allergic reaction to this medicine or to any related antibiotic, such as amikacin (e.g., Amikin), colistimethate (e.g., Coly-Mycin M), colistin (e.g., Coly-Mycin S), gentamicin (e.g., Garamycin), kanamycin (e.g., Kantrex), neomycin by mouth or by injection (e.g., Mycifradin), netilmicin (e.g., Netromycin), paromomycin (e.g., Humatin), polymyxin B by injection (e.g., Aerosporin), streptomycin, or tobramycin (e.g., Nebcin). Also tell your health care professional if you are allergic to any other substances, such as preservatives or dyes.

**Pregnancy**—Neomycin, polymyxin B, and hydrocortisone otic preparations have not been studied in pregnant women. However, studies in animals have shown that topical corticosteroids (such as hydrocortisone) cause birth defects. Before using this medicine, make sure your doctor knows if you are pregnant or if you may become pregnant.

**Breast-feeding**—Neomycin, polymyxin B, and hydrocortisone otic preparations have not been reported to cause problems in nursing babies.

**Children**—Although there is no specific information comparing use of otic neomycin, polymyxin B, and hydrocortisone preparation in children with use in other age groups, this preparation is not expected to cause different side effects or problems in children than it does in adults.

**Older adults**—Many medicines have not been studied specifically in older people. Therefore, it may not be known whether they work exactly the same way they do in younger adults. Although there is no specific information comparing use of otic neomycin, polymyxin B, and hydrocortisone preparation in the elderly with use in other age groups, this preparation is not expected to cause different side effects or problems in older people than it does in younger adults.

**Other medicines**—Although certain medicines should not be used together at all, in other cases two different medicines may be used together even if an interaction might occur. In these cases, your doctor may want to change the dose, or other precautions may be necessary. Tell your health care professional if you are using any other otic (for the ear) prescription or nonprescription (over-the-counter [OTC] medicine).

**Other medical problems**—The presence of other medical problems may affect the use of neomycin, polymyxin B, and hydrocortisone otic preparations. Make sure you tell your doctor if you have any other medical problems, especially:

- Any other ear infection or condition (including punctured eardrum)—Use of neomycin, polymyxin B, and hydrocortisone otic preparations may make the condition worse

## Proper Use of This Medicine

You may warm the ear drops to body temperature (37 °C or 98.6 °F), but no higher, by holding the bottle in your hand for a few minutes before using the medicine. If the medicine gets too warm, it may break down and not work at all.

To use:

- Lie down or tilt the head so that the infected ear faces up. Gently pull the earlobe up and back for adults (down and back for children) to straighten the ear canal. Drop the medicine into the ear canal. Keep the ear facing up for about 5 minutes to allow the medicine to come into contact with the infection. A sterile cotton plug may be gently inserted into the ear opening to prevent the medicine from leaking out. However, your doctor may want you to keep a sterile cotton plug moistened with this medicine in your ear for the full time of treatment. If you have any questions about this, check with your doctor.
- To keep the medicine as germ-free as possible, do not touch the dropper to any surface (including the ear). Also, keep the container tightly closed.

To help clear up your infection completely, *keep using this medicine for the full time of treatment,* even if your symptoms have disappeared. *Do not miss any doses.*

**Dosing**—The dose of neomycin, polymyxin B, and hydrocortisone otic preparation will be different for different patients. *Follow your doctor's orders or the directions*

*on the label.* The following information includes only the average doses of neomycin, polymyxin B, and hydrocortisone otic preparation. *If your dose is different, do not change it* unless your doctor tells you to do so.

- For *otic (ear drops)* dosage forms:
  —For ear canal infection:
  - Adults—Use four drops in the ear three or four times a day.
  - Children—Use three drops in the ear three or four times a day.
  —For mastoid cavity infection:
  - Adults—Use four to ten drops in the ear every six to eight hours.
  - Children—Use four or five drops in the ear every six to eight hours.

**Missed dose**—If you miss a dose of this medicine, apply it as soon as possible. However, if it is almost time for your next dose, skip the missed dose and go back to your regular dosing schedule.

*Do not use this medicine for more than 10 days* unless otherwise directed by your doctor.

**Storage**—To store this medicine:

- Keep out of the reach of children.
- Store away from heat and direct light.
- Keep the medicine from freezing.
- Do not keep outdated medicine or medicine no longer needed. Be sure that any discarded medicine is out of the reach of children.

## Precautions While Using This Medicine

If your symptoms do not improve within 1 week, or if they become worse, check with your doctor.

## Side Effects of This Medicine

Along with its needed effects, a medicine may cause some unwanted effects. Although not all of these side effects may occur, if they do occur they may need medical attention.

*Check with your doctor immediately* if any of the following side effects occur:

*More common*

Itching, skin rash, redness, swelling, or other sign of irritation in or around the ear not present before use of this medicine

Other side effects not listed above may also occur in some patients. If you notice any other effects, check with your doctor.

Revised: 06/21/94

# NIACIN—For High Cholesterol    Systemic

Some commonly used brand names are:

**In the U.S.**

| | |
|---|---|
| Endur-Acin | Nico-400 |
| Nia-Bid | Nicobid Temples |
| Niac | Nicolar |
| Niacels | Nicotinex Elixir |
| Niacor | Slo-Niacin |

Generic name product may also be available.

**In Canada**

Novo-Niacin

Generic name product may also be available.

Other commonly used names are nicotinic acid or vitamin B$_3$.

## Description

Niacin (NYE-a-sin) is used to help lower high cholesterol and fat levels in the blood. This may help prevent medical problems caused by cholesterol and fat clogging the blood vessels.

Some strengths of niacin are available only with your doctor's prescription. Others are available without a prescription, since niacin is also a vitamin. However, it is best to take it only under your doctor's direction so that you can be sure you are taking the correct dose.

Niacin for use in the treatment of high cholesterol is available in the following dosage forms:

*Oral*
- Extended-release capsules (U.S.)
- Solution (U.S.)
- Tablets (U.S. and Canada)
- Extended-release tablets (U.S. and Canada)

## Before Using This Medicine

If you are taking this medicine without a prescription, carefully read and follow any precautions on the label. For niacin, the following should be considered:

**Allergies**—Tell your doctor if you have ever had any unusual or allergic reaction to niacin. Also tell your health care professional if you are allergic to any other substances, such as foods, preservatives, or dyes.

**Diet**—Before prescribing medicine for your condition, your doctor will probably try to control your condition by prescribing a personal diet for you. Such a diet may be low in fats, sugars, and/or cholesterol. Many people are able to control their condition by carefully following their doctor's orders for proper diet and exercise. *Medicine is prescribed only when additional help is needed* and is effective only when a schedule of diet and exercise is properly followed.

Also, this medicine is less effective if you are greatly overweight. It may be very important for you to go on a reducing diet. However, check with your doctor before going on any diet.

Make certain your health care professional know if you are on any special diet, such as a low-sodium or low-sugar diet.

**Pregnancy**—Studies have not been done in either humans or animals.

**Breast-feeding**—Niacin has not been reported to cause problems in nursing babies.

**Children**—There is no specific information comparing the use of niacin for high cholesterol in children with use in other age groups. However, use is not recommended in children under 2 years of age since cholesterol is needed for normal development.

**Older adults**—Many medicines have not been studied specifically in older people. Therefore, it may not be known whether they work exactly the same way they do in younger adults or if they cause different side effects or problems in older people. Although there is no specific information comparing the use of niacin for high cholesterol in the elderly with use in other age groups, it is not expected to cause different side effects or problems in older people than in younger adults.

**Other medicines**—Although certain medicines should not be used together at all, in other cases two different medicines may be used together even if an interaction might occur. In these cases, your doctor may want to change the dose, or other precautions may be necessary. Tell your health care professional if you are using any other prescription or nonprescription (over-the-counter [OTC]) medicine.

**Other medical problems**—The presence of other medical problems may affect the use of niacin. Make sure you tell your doctor if you have any other medical problems, especially:
- Bleeding problems or
- Diabetes mellitus (sugar diabetes) or
- Glaucoma or
- Gout or
- Liver disease or
- Low blood pressure or
- Stomach ulcer—Niacin may make these conditions worse

## Proper Use of This Medicine

*Use this medicine only as directed by your doctor.* Do not use more or less of it, do not use it more often, and do not use it for a longer time than your doctor ordered. To do so may increase the chance of unwanted effects.

Remember that niacin will not cure your condition but it does help control it. Therefore, you must continue to take it as directed if you expect to keep your cholesterol levels down.

*Follow carefully the special diet your doctor gave you.* This is the most important part of controlling your condition, and is necessary if the medicine is to work properly.

If this medicine upsets your stomach, it may be taken with meals or milk. If stomach upset (nausea or diarrhea) continues, check with your doctor.

For patients taking the *extended-release capsule form* of this medicine:

- Swallow the capsule whole. Do not crush, break, or chew before swallowing. However, if the capsule is too large to swallow, you may mix the contents of the capsule with jam or jelly and swallow without chewing.

For patients taking the *extended-release tablet form* of this medicine:

- Swallow the tablet whole. If the tablet is scored, it may be broken, but not crushed or chewed, before being swallowed.

**Dosing**—The dose of niacin will be different for different patients. *Follow your doctor's orders or the directions on the label.* The following information includes only the average doses of niacin. *If your dose is different, do not change it* unless your doctor tells you to do so.

The number of capsules or tablets or teaspoonfuls of solution that you take depends on the strength of the medicine.

- For *oral* dosage form (extended-release capsules, extended-release tablets, oral solution, or regular tablets):
  - —For treatment of high cholesterol:
    - Adults and teenagers—1 to 2 grams three times a day.
    - Children—Use and dose must be determined by your doctor.

**Missed dose**—If you miss a dose of this medicine, take it as soon as possible. However, if it is almost time for your next dose, skip the missed dose and go back to your regular dosing schedule. Do not double doses.

**Storage**—To store this medicine:

- Keep out of the reach of children.
- Store away from heat and direct light.
- Do not store in the bathroom, near the kitchen sink, or in other damp places. Heat or moisture may cause the medicine to break down.
- Keep the liquid form of this medicine from freezing.
- Do not keep outdated medicine or medicine no longer needed. Be sure that any discarded medicine is out of the reach of children.

## Precautions While Using This Medicine

*It is very important that your doctor check your progress at regular visits.* This will allow your doctor to see if the medicine is working properly to lower your cholesterol and triglyceride (fat) levels and if you should continue to take it.

*Do not stop taking niacin without first checking with your doctor.* When you stop taking this medicine, your blood cholesterol levels may increase again. Your doctor may want you to follow a special diet to help prevent this from happening.

This medicine may cause you to feel dizzy or faint, especially when you get up from a lying or sitting position. Getting up slowly may help. This effect should lessen after a week or two as your body gets used to the medicine. However, if the problem continues or gets worse, check with your doctor.

## Side Effects of This Medicine

Along with its needed effects, a medicine may cause some unwanted effects. Although not all of these side effects may occur, if they do occur they may need medical attention. *Check with your doctor immediately* if any of the following side effects occur:

*Less common*
  *With prolonged use of extended-release niacin*
    Darkening of urine; light gray-colored stools; loss of appetite; severe stomach pain; yellow eyes or skin

Other side effects may occur that usually do not need medical attention. These side effects may go away during treatment as your body adjusts to the medicine. However, check with your doctor if any of the following side effects continue or are bothersome:

*Less common*
    Feeling of warmth; flushing or redness of skin, especially on face and neck; headache
*With high doses*
    Diarrhea; dizziness or faintness; dryness of skin; fever; frequent urination; itching of skin; joint pain; muscle aching or cramping; nausea or vomiting; side, lower back, or stomach pain; swelling of feet or lower legs; unusual thirst; unusual tiredness or weakness; unusually fast, slow, or irregular heartbeat

Other side effects not listed above may also occur in some patients. If you notice any other effects, check with your health care professional.

Revised: 11/09/91
Interim revision: 08/10/94

# NIACIN   (Vitamin B₃)   Systemic

Some commonly used brand names are:

**In the U.S.**

| | |
|---|---|
| Endur-Acin | Nico-400 |
| Nia-Bid | Nicobid Tempules |
| Niac | Nicolar |
| Niacels | Nicotinex Elixir |
| Niacor | Slo-Niacin |

Generic name product may also be available.

**In Canada**

Novo-Niacin

Generic name product may also be available.

Other commonly used names are niacinamide (nye-a-SIN-a-mide), nicotinic acid, nicotinamide, or vitamin B₃.

## Description

Vitamins (VYE-ta-mins) are compounds that you *must* have for growth and health. They are needed in small amounts only and are usually available in the foods that you eat. Niacin (NYE-a-sin) is necessary for many normal functions of the body, including normal tissue metabolism. It may have other effects as well.

Lack of niacin may lead to a condition called pellagra, with diarrhea, stomach problems, skin problems, sores in the mouth, anemia (weak blood), and mental problems. Your doctor may treat this by prescribing niacin for you.

Patients with the following conditions may be more likely to have a lack of niacin:

- Cancer
- Diabetes mellitus (sugar diabetes)
- Diarrhea (prolonged)
- Fever (prolonged)
- Hartnup disease
- Infection (prolonged)
- Intestinal problems
- Liver disease
- Mouth or throat sores
- Overactive thyroid
- Pancreas disease
- Stomach ulcer
- Stress (prolonged)
- Surgical removal of stomach

If any of the above apply to you, you should take niacin supplements only on the advice of your physician after need has been established.

Claims that niacin is effective for treatment of acne, alcoholism, unwanted effects of drug abuse, leprosy, motion sickness, muscle problems, poor circulation, and mental problems, and for prevention of heart attacks, have not been proven. Many of these treatments involve large and expensive amounts of vitamins.

Some strengths of niacin are available only with your doctor's prescription. Others are available without a prescription. However, it may be a good idea to check with your health care professional before taking niacin on your own.

This medicine is available in the following dosage forms:

*Oral*

Niacin
- Extended-release capsules (U.S.)
- Solution (U.S.)
- Tablets (U.S. and Canada)
- Extended-release tablets (U.S. and Canada)

Niacinamide
- Tablets (U.S. and Canada)

*Parenteral*

Niacin
- Injection (U.S.)

Niacinamide
- Injection (U.S.)

## Importance of Diet

Vitamin supplements should be taken only if you cannot get enough vitamins in your diet; however, some diets may not contain all of the vitamins you need. This may occur with rapid weight loss, unusual diets (such as some reducing diets in which choice of foods is very limited), prolonged intravenous feeding, or malnutrition. A balanced diet should provide all the vitamins you normally need.

In order to get enough vitamins and minerals in your diet, it is important that you eat a balanced and varied diet. Follow carefully any diet program your doctor may recommend. For your specific vitamin and/or mineral needs, ask your doctor for a list of appropriate foods.

Niacin is found in meats, eggs, and milk and dairy products. Little niacin is lost from foods during ordinary cooking.

Vitamins alone will not take the place of a good diet and will not provide energy. Your body also needs other substances found in food such as protein, minerals, carbohydrates, and fat. Vitamins themselves often cannot work without the presence of other foods.

In some cases, it may not be possible for you to get enough food to supply you with the proper vitamins. In other cases, the amount of vitamins you need may be increased above normal. Therefore, a vitamin supplement may be needed.

Experts have developed a list of recommended dietary allowances (RDA) for most of the vitamins. The RDA are not an exact number but a general idea of how much you need. They do not cover amounts needed for problems caused by a serious lack of vitamins.

Niacin (Vitamin B₃) (Systemic)

The RDA for niacin are:
- Infants and children—
  Birth to 6 months of age: 5 mg per day.
  6 months to 1 year of age: 6 mg per day.
  1 to 3 years of age: 9 mg per day.
  4 to 6 years of age: 12 mg per day.
  7 to 10 years of age: 13 mg per day.
- Adolescent and adult males—
  11 to 14 years of age: 17 mg per day.
  15 to 18 years of age: 20 mg per day.
  19 to 50 years of age: 19 mg per day.
  50 years of age and over: 15 mg per day.
- Adolescent and adult females—
  11 to 50 years of age: 15 mg per day.
  50 years of age and over: 13 mg per day.
- Pregnant females—17 mg per day.
- Lactating females—20 mg per day.

Remember:
- The total amount of each vitamin that you get every day includes what you get from the foods that you eat *and* what you may take as a supplement.
- Your total amount should not be greater than the RDA, unless ordered by your doctor. Taking too much niacin over a period of time may cause unwanted effects such as high blood sugar, peptic ulcer, gout, heart problems, or liver problems.

---

## Before Using This Dietary Supplement

If you are taking this dietary supplement without a prescription, carefully read and follow any precautions on the label. For niacin or niacinamide, the following should be considered:

**Allergies**—Tell your doctor if you have ever had any unusual or allergic reaction to niacin or niacinamide. Also tell your health care professional if you are allergic to any other substances, such as foods, preservatives, or dyes.

**Pregnancy**—It is especially important that you are receiving enough vitamins when you become pregnant and that you continue to receive the right amount of vitamins throughout your pregnancy. The healthy growth and development of the fetus depend on a steady supply of nutrients from the mother. However, taking large amounts of a dietary supplement in pregnancy may be harmful to the mother and/or fetus and should be avoided.

**Breast-feeding**—It is especially important that you receive the right amounts of vitamins so that your baby will also get the vitamins needed to grow properly. However, taking large amounts of a dietary supplement while breast-feeding may be harmful to the mother and/or baby and should be avoided.

**Children**—Normal daily requirements vary according to age. It is especially important that children receive enough vitamins in their diet for healthy growth and development. Although there is no specific information about the use of niacin in children in doses higher than the normal daily requirements, it is not expected to cause different side effects or problems in children than in adults.

**Older adults**—It is important that older people continue to receive enough vitamins in their diet for good health.

**Medicines or other dietary supplements**—Although certain medicines or dietary supplements should not be used together at all, in other cases they may be used together even if an interaction might occur. In these cases, your doctor may want to change the dose, or other precautions may be necessary. Tell your health care professional if you are using any other dietary supplement or any prescription or nonprescription (over-the-counter [OTC]) medicine.

**Other medical problems**—The presence of other medical problems may affect the use of niacin or niacinamide. Make sure you tell your doctor if you have any other medical problems, especially:
- Bleeding problems or
- Diabetes mellitus (sugar diabetes) or
- Glaucoma or
- Gout or
- Liver disease or
- Low blood pressure or
- Stomach ulcer—Niacin or niacinamide may make these conditions worse

---

## Proper Use of This Dietary Supplement

Some people believe that taking very large doses of vitamins (called megadoses or megavitamin therapy) is useful for treating certain medical problems. Studies have not proven this. Large doses should be taken only under the direction of your doctor after need has been identified.

If this dietary supplement upsets your stomach, it may be taken with meals or milk. If stomach upset (nausea or diarrhea) continues, check with your doctor.

For patients taking the *extended-release capsule form* of this dietary supplement:
- Swallow the capsule whole. Do not crush, break, or chew before swallowing. However, if the capsule is too large to swallow, you may mix the contents of the capsule with jam or jelly and swallow without chewing.

For patients taking the *extended-release tablet form* of this dietary supplement:
- Swallow the tablet whole. If the tablet is scored, it may be broken, but not crushed or chewed, before being swallowed.

**Dosing**—The dose of niacin for prevention of niacin deficiency is based on the Recommended Dietary Allowances (RDA). See the *Importance of Diet* section for the RDA for niacin.

**Missed dose**—If you miss taking a vitamin for one or more days there is no cause for concern, since it takes some time for your body to become seriously low in vitamins. However, if your doctor has recommended that you take this vitamin, try to remember to take it as directed every day.

**Storage**—To store this dietary supplement:

- Keep out of the reach of children.
- Store away from heat and direct light.
- Do not store in the bathroom, near the kitchen sink, or in other damp places. Heat or moisture may cause the dietary supplement to break down.
- Keep the liquid form of this dietary supplement from freezing.
- Do not keep outdated dietary supplements or those no longer needed. Be sure that any discarded dietary supplement is out of the reach of children.

## Precautions While Using This Dietary Supplement

This dietary supplement may cause you to feel dizzy or faint, especially when you get up from a lying or sitting position. Getting up slowly may help. This effect should lessen after a week or two as your body gets used to the dietary supplement. However, if the problem continues or gets worse, check with your doctor.

## Side Effects of This Dietary Supplement

Along with its needed effects, a dietary supplement may cause some unwanted effects. Although not all of these side effects may occur, if they do occur they may need medical attention.

*Check with your doctor immediately* if any of the following side effects occur:

*With injection only*
Skin rash or itching; wheezing

*With prolonged use of extended-release niacin*
Darkening of urine; light gray-colored stools; loss of appetite; severe stomach pain; yellow eyes or skin

Other side effects may occur that usually do not need medical attention. These side effects may go away during treatment as your body adjusts to the dietary supplement. However, check with your health care professional if any of the following side effects continue or are bothersome:

*Less common—with niacin only*
Feeling of warmth; flushing or redness of skin, especially on face and neck; headache

*With high doses*
Diarrhea; dizziness or faintness; dryness of skin; fever; frequent urination; itching of skin; joint pain; muscle aching or cramping; nausea or vomiting; side, lower back, or stomach pain; swelling of feet or lower legs; unusual thirst; unusual tiredness or weakness; unusually fast, slow, or irregular heartbeat

Other side effects not listed above may also occur in some patients. If you notice any other effects, check with your health care professional.

Revised: 11/09/91
Interim revision: 08/10/94

# NICLOSAMIDE    Oral†

A commonly used brand name in the U.S. is Niclocide.

†Not commercially available in Canada.

## Description

Niclosamide (ni-KLOE-sa-mide) belongs to the family of medicines called anthelmintics (ant-hel-MIN-tiks). Anthelmintics are medicines used in the treatment of worm infections.

Niclosamide is used to treat broad or fish tapeworm, dwarf tapeworm, and beef tapeworm infections. Niclosamide may also be used for other tapeworm infections as determined by your doctor. It will not work for other types of worm infections (for example, pinworms or roundworms).

Niclosamide works by killing tapeworms on contact. The killed worms are then passed in the stool. However, you may not notice them since they are sometimes destroyed in the intestine.

Niclosamide is available only with your doctor's prescription, in the following dosage form:

*Oral*
- Chewable tablets (U.S.)

## Before Using This Medicine

In deciding to use a medicine, the risks of taking the medicine must be weighed against the good it will do. This is a decision you and your doctor will make. For niclosamide, the following should be considered:

**Allergies**—Tell your doctor if you have ever had any unusual or allergic reaction to niclosamide. Also tell your health care professional if you are allergic to any other substances, such as foods, preservatives, or dyes.

**Pregnancy**—Studies have not been done in pregnant women. However, niclosamide has not been shown to cause birth defects or other problems in rats and rabbits given 25 times the usual human dose or in mice given 12 times the usual human dose.

**Breast-feeding**—It is not known whether niclosamide passes into the breast milk. However, this medicine has not been reported to cause problems in nursing babies.

**Children**—This medicine has been tested in a limited number of children 2 years of age or older and, in effective doses, has not been reported to cause different side effects or problems in children than it does in adults.

**Older adults**—Many medicines have not been studied specifically in older people. Therefore, it may not be known whether they work exactly the same way they do in younger adults or if they cause different side effects or problems in older people. There is no specific information comparing use of niclosamide in the elderly with use in other age groups.

**Other medicines**—Although certain medicines should not be used together at all, in other cases two different medicines may be used together even if an interaction might occur. In these cases, your doctor may want to change the dose, or other precautions may be necessary. Tell your health care professional if you are taking any other prescription or nonprescription (over-the-counter [OTC]) medicine.

---

## Proper Use of This Medicine

No special preparations (for example, special diets, fasting, other medicines, laxatives, or enemas) are necessary before, during, or immediately after taking niclosamide.

Niclosamide may be taken on an empty stomach (either 1 hour before or 2 hours after a meal). However, to prevent stomach upset, it is best taken after a light meal (for example, breakfast).

Niclosamide tablets should be thoroughly chewed or crushed and then swallowed with a small amount of water. If this medicine is being given to a young child, the tablets should be crushed to a fine powder and mixed with a small amount of water to form a paste.

For patients taking this medicine for *beef tapeworms or broad or fish tapeworms:*

- To help clear up your infection completely, *take this medicine exactly as directed by your doctor*. Usually one dose is enough. However, in some patients a second dose of this medicine may be required to clear up the infection completely.

For patients taking this medicine for *dwarf tapeworms:*

- To help clear up your infection completely, *keep taking this medicine for the full time of treatment (usually 7 days)*, even if your symptoms begin to clear up after a few days. In some patients, a second course of this medicine may be required to clear up the infection completely. If you stop taking this medicine too soon, your infection may return. *Do not miss any doses*. Some patients with tapeworm infections may not notice any symptoms or may have only mild symptoms.

**Dosing**—The dose of niclosamide will be different for different patients. *Follow your doctor's orders or the directions on the label*. The following information includes only the average doses of niclosamide. *If your dose is different, do not change it* unless your doctor tells you to do so.

*The number of doses you take each day, the time allowed between doses, and the length of time you take the medicine depend on the medical problem for which you are taking niclosamide.*

- For *oral* dosage form (tablets):
  —For fish tapeworm or beef tapeworm:
    - Adults—2 grams as a single dose. Treatment may be repeated in seven days if needed.
    - Children—Dose is based on body weight and must be determined by your doctor.
      —For children weighing 11 to 34 kilograms (kg) (24.2 to 74.8 pounds): 1 gram as a single dose. Treatment may be repeated in seven days if needed.
      —For children weighing over 34 kg (74.8 pounds): 1.5 grams as a single dose. Treatment may be repeated in seven days if needed.
  —For dwarf tapeworm:
    - Adults—2 grams a day for seven days. Treatment may be repeated in seven to fourteen days if needed.
    - Children—Dose is based on body weight and must be determined by your doctor.
      —For children weighing 11 to 34 kg (24.2 to 74.8 pounds): 1 gram on the first day. Then 500 milligrams (mg) once a day for the next six days. Treatment may be repeated in seven to fourteen days if needed.
      —For children weighing over 34 kg (74.8 pounds): 1.5 grams on the first day. Then 1 gram once a day for the next six days. Treatment may be repeated in seven to fourteen days if needed.

**Missed dose**—If you miss a dose of this medicine, take it as soon as possible. However, if it is almost time for your next dose, skip the missed dose and go back to your regular dosing schedule. Do not double doses.

**Storage**—To store this medicine:
- Keep out of the reach of children.
- Store away from heat and direct light.
- Do not store in the bathroom, near the kitchen sink, or in other damp places. Heat or moisture may cause the medicine to break down.
- Do not keep outdated medicine or medicine no longer needed. Be sure that any discarded medicine is out of the reach of children.

---

## Precautions While Using This Medicine

It is important that your doctor check your progress at regular visits. This is to make sure that the infection is cleared up completely.

---

If your symptoms do not improve within a few days, or if they become worse, check with your doctor.

## Side Effects of This Medicine

Along with its needed effects, a medicine may cause some unwanted effects. The following side effects may go away during treatment as your body adjusts to the medicine. However, check with your doctor if any of the following side effects continue or are bothersome:

*Less common*
> Abdominal or stomach cramps or pain; diarrhea; loss of appetite; nausea or vomiting

*Rare*
> Unpleasant taste; dizziness or lightheadedness; drowsiness; itching of the rectal area; skin rash

Other side effects not listed above may also occur in some patients. If you notice any other effects, check with your doctor.

Revised: 10/20/92
Interim revision: 08/12/94

---

# NICOTINE    Systemic

Some commonly used brand names are:

**In the U.S.—**
| | |
|---|---|
| Habitrol | Nicorette DS |
| Nicoderm | Nicotrol |
| Nicorette | ProStep |

**In Canada—**
| | |
|---|---|
| Habitrol | Nicorette |
| Nicoderm | Nicotrol |

## Description

Nicotine (NIK-o-teen), in a flavored chewing gum or a skin patch, is used to help you stop smoking. It is used for up to 12 to 20 weeks as part of a supervised stop-smoking program. These programs may include education, counseling, and psychological support. Using nicotine replacement products without taking part in a supervised stop-smoking program has not been shown to be effective.

- As you chew nicotine gum, nicotine passes through the lining of your mouth and into your body.
- When you wear a nicotine patch, nicotine passes through your skin into your bloodstream.

This nicotine takes the place of nicotine that you would otherwise get from smoking. In this way, the withdrawal effects of not smoking are less severe. Then, as your body adjusts to not smoking, the use of the nicotine gum is decreased gradually, or the strength of the patches is decreased over a few weeks. Finally, use is stopped altogether.

Children, pregnant women, and nonsmokers should not use nicotine gum or patches because of unwanted effects.

Nicotine gum and patches are available only with your doctor's prescription, in the following dosage forms:

*Oral*
- Chewing gum tablets (U.S. and Canada)

*Topical*
- Transdermal (stick-on) skin patch (U.S. and Canada)

## Before Using This Medicine

In deciding to use a medicine, the risks of taking the medicine must be weighed against the good it will do. This is a decision you and your doctor will make. For nicotine gum, the following should be considered:

**Allergies—**Tell your doctor if you have ever had any unusual or allergic reaction to nicotine. Also tell your health care professional if you are allergic to any other substances, such as foods, preservatives, or dyes. If you plan to use the nicotine patches, tell your doctor if you have ever had a rash or irritation from adhesive tape or bandages.

**Pregnancy—**Nicotine, whether from smoking or from the gum or patches, is not recommended during pregnancy. Studies in humans show that miscarriages have occurred in pregnant women using nicotine replacement products. In addition, studies in animals have shown that nicotine can cause harmful effects in the fetus.

**Breast-feeding—**Nicotine passes into breast milk and may cause unwanted effects in the baby. It may be necessary for you to stop breast-feeding during treatment.

**Children—**Small amounts of nicotine can cause serious harm in children. Even used nicotine patches contain enough nicotine to cause problems in children.

**Older adults—**Nicotine gum and patches have been used in a limited number of patients 60 years of age or older, and have not been shown to cause different side effects or problems in older people than in younger adults.

**Other medicines—**Although certain medicines should not be used together at all, in other cases 2 different medicines may be used together even if an interaction might occur. In these cases, your doctor may want to change the dose, or other precautions may be necessary. When you are using nicotine gum or patches, it is especially important that your health care professional know if you are taking any of the following:

- Aminophylline (e.g., Somophyllin) or
- Insulin or
- Oxtriphylline (e.g., Choledyl) or
- Propoxyphene (e.g., Darvon) or
- Propranolol (e.g., Inderal) or
- Theophylline (e.g., Somophyllin-T)—Stopping smoking may increase the effects of these medicines; the amount of medicine you need to take may change

**Other medical problems**—The presence of other medical problems may affect the use of nicotine gum or patches. Make sure you tell your doctor if you have any other medical problems, especially:

- Dental problems (with gum only) or
- Diabetes mellitus (sugar diabetes) or
- Heart or blood vessel disease or
- High blood pressure or
- Inflammation of mouth or throat (with gum only) or
- Irritated skin (with patches only) or
- Overactive thyroid or
- Pheochromocytoma (PCC) or
- Stomach ulcer or
- Temporomandibular (jaw) joint disorder (TMJ) (with gum only)—Nicotine gum or patches may make the condition worse

## Proper Use of This Medicine

For patients using the *chewing gum tablets:*

- Nicotine gum usually comes with patient directions. *Read the directions carefully before using this medicine.*
- *When you feel the urge to smoke, chew one piece of gum very slowly* until you taste it or feel a slight tingling in your mouth. Stop chewing, and place ("park") the chewing gum tablet between your cheek and gum until the taste or tingling is almost gone. Then chew slowly until you taste it again. Continue chewing and stopping ("parking") in this way for about 30 minutes in order to get the full dose of nicotine.
- *Do not chew too fast,* do not chew more than one piece at a time, and do not chew a piece of gum too soon after another. To do so may cause unwanted side effects or an overdose. Also, slower chewing will reduce the possibility of belching.
- *Use nicotine gum exactly as directed by your doctor.* Remember that it is also important to participate in a stop-smoking program during treatment. This may make it easier for you to stop smoking.
- As your urge to smoke becomes less frequent, *gradually reduce the number of pieces of gum you chew each day* until you are chewing one or two pieces a day. This may be possible within 2 to 3 months.
- *Remember to carry nicotine gum with you at all times* in case you feel the sudden urge to smoke. One cigarette may be enough to start you on the smoking habit again.
- Using hard sugarless candy between doses of gum may help to relieve the discomfort in your mouth.

For patients using the *transdermal system (skin patch):*

- *Use this medicine exactly as directed by your doctor.* It will work only if applied correctly. *This medicine usually comes with patient instructions. Read them carefully before using this product.* Remember that it is also important to participate in a stop-smoking program during treatment. This may make it easier for you to stop smoking.
- Do not remove the patch from its sealed pouch until you are ready to put it on your skin. The patch may not work as well if it is unwrapped too soon.
- Do not try to trim or cut the adhesive patch to adjust the dosage. Check with your doctor if you think the medicine is not working as it should.
- Apply the patch to a clean, dry area of skin on your upper arm, chest, or back. Choose an area that is not very oily, has little or no hair, and is free of scars, cuts, burns, or any other skin irritations.
- Press the patch firmly in place with the palm of your hand for about 10 seconds. Make sure there is good contact with your skin, especially around the edges of the patch.
- The patch should stay in place even when you are showering, bathing, or swimming. Apply a new patch if one falls off.
- Rinse your hands with plain water after you have finished applying the patch to your skin. Nicotine on your hands could get into your eyes and nose and cause stinging, redness, or more serious problems. Using soap to wash your hands will increase the amount of nicotine that passes through your skin.
- After 16 or 24 hours, depending on which product you are using, remove the patch. Choose a different place on your skin to apply the next patch. Do not put a new patch in the same place for at least one week. Do not leave the patch on for more than 24 hours. It will not work as well after that time and it may irritate your skin.
- After removing a used patch, fold the patch in half with the sticky sides together. Place the folded, used patch in its protective pouch or in aluminum foil. Make sure to dispose of it out of the reach of children and pets.
- Try to change the patch at the same time each day. If you want to change the time when you put on your patch, just remove the patch you are wearing and put on a new patch. After that, apply a fresh patch at the new time each day.

**Dosing**—The dose of nicotine will be different for different patients. *Follow your doctor's orders or the directions on the label.* The following information includes only the average doses of nicotine. *If your dose is different, do not change it* unless your doctor tells you to do so.

- For the *oral* dosage form (chewing gum tablets):
  —To help you stop smoking:
    - Adults and older children—The usual dose is 20 to 24 milligrams (mg) a day. However, the

number of pieces of nicotine gum you chew each day depends on how often you have the urge to smoke, how fast you chew, and the strength of the gum. You should not chew more than 30 pieces of 2-mg strength gum or more than 15 pieces of 4-mg strength gum (a total of 60 mg) a day.

- Children up to 12 years of age—Use and dose must be determined by your doctor.

- For the *transdermal* (stick-on) skin patch:
  —To help you stop smoking:
    - Adults—The dose you receive will be based on your body weight, how often you have the urge to smoke, and the strength of the patch you use. This dose will be determined by your doctor.
    - Children—Use and dose must be determined by your doctor.

**Storage**—To store this medicine:

- Keep out of the reach of children because even small doses of nicotine can cause serious harm in children.
- Store away from heat and direct light.
- Do not store in the bathroom, near the kitchen sink, or in other damp places. Heat or moisture may cause the medicine to break down.
- Do not keep outdated medicine or medicine no longer needed. Be sure that any discarded medicine is out of the reach of children and pets.

## Precautions While Using This Medicine

*Your doctor should check your progress at regular visits* to make sure that the nicotine gum or patches are working properly and that possible side effects are avoided.

*Do not smoke during treatment with nicotine gum or patches* because of the risk of nicotine overdose.

*Nicotine should not be used in pregnancy.* If there is a possibility you might become pregnant, you may want to use some type of birth control. If you think you may have become pregnant, stop taking this medicine immediately and check with your doctor.

*Nicotine products must be kept out of the reach of children and pets.* Even used nicotine patches contain enough nicotine to cause problems in children. If a child chews or swallows one or more pieces of nicotine gum, contact your doctor or poison control center at once. If a child puts on a nicotine patch or plays with a patch that is out of the sealed pouch, take it away from the child and contact your doctor or poison control center at once.

For patients using the *chewing gum tablets:*

- *Do not chew more than 30 2-mg pieces, or 15 4-mg pieces of gum a day.* Chewing too many pieces may be harmful because of the risk of overdose.
- *Do not use nicotine gum for longer than 6 months.* To do so may result in physical dependence on the nicotine.

- *If the gum sticks to your dental work, stop using it and check with your medical doctor or dentist.* Dentures or other dental work may be damaged because nicotine gum is stickier and harder to chew than ordinary gum.

For patients using the *transdermal system (skin patch):*

- Mild itching, burning, or tingling may occur when the patch is first applied, and should go away within an hour. After a patch is removed, the skin underneath it may be somewhat red. It should not remain red for more than a day. *If you get a skin rash from the patch, or if the skin becomes swollen or very red, call your doctor.* Do not put on a new patch. If you become allergic to the nicotine in the patch, you could get sick from using cigarettes or other products that contain nicotine.

- *Do not use nicotine patches for longer than 12 to 20 weeks* (depending on the product) if you have stopped smoking, because continuing use of nicotine in any form can be harmful and addictive.

## Side Effects of This Medicine

Along with its needed effects, a medicine may cause some unwanted effects. Although not all of these side effects may occur, if they do occur they may need medical attention.

Check with your doctor as soon as possible if any of the following side effects occur:

*More common*
  Injury to mouth, teeth, or dental work—with chewing gum only
*Rare*
  Hives, itching, rash, redness, or swelling; irregular heartbeat
*Symptoms of overdose (may occur in the following order)*
  Nausea and/or vomiting; increased watering of mouth (severe); abdominal or stomach pain (severe); diarrhea (severe); cold sweat; headache (severe); dizziness (severe); drooling; disturbed hearing and vision; confusion; weakness (severe); fainting; low blood pressure; difficulty in breathing (severe); fast, weak, or irregular heartbeat; convulsions (seizures)

Other side effects may occur that usually do not need medical attention. These side effects may go away during treatment as your body adjusts to the medicine. However, check with your doctor if any of the following side effects continue or are bothersome:

*More common*
  Belching—with chewing gum only; fast heartbeat; headache (mild); increased appetite; increased watering of mouth (mild)—with chewing gum only; jaw muscle ache—with chewing gum only; redness, itching, and/or burning at site of application of patch—usually stops within an hour; sore mouth or throat—with chewing gum only

*Less common or rare*
- Constipation; coughing (increased); diarrhea; dizziness or lightheadedness (mild); drowsiness; dryness of mouth; hiccups—with chewing gum only; hoarseness—with chewing gum only; irritability or nervousness; loss of appetite; menstrual pain; muscle or joint pain; stomach upset or indigestion (mild); sweating (increased); trouble in sleeping or unusual dreams

Other side effects not listed above may also occur in some patients. If you notice any other effects, check with your doctor.

Revised: 09/08/92
Interim revision(s): 05/19/94

# NICOTINYL ALCOHOL    Systemic*

A commonly used brand name in Canada is Roniacol.

*Not commercially available in the U.S.

## Description

Nicotinyl (nik-oh-TIN-ill) alcohol belongs to the group of medicines called vasodilators. Vasodilators increase the size of blood vessels and are used to treat problems resulting from poor blood circulation.

Nicotinyl alcohol is available without a prescription, in the following dosage form:

*Oral*
- Extended-release tablets (Canada)

## Before Using This Medicine

If you are taking this medicine without a prescription, carefully read and follow any precautions on the label. For nicotinyl alcohol, the following should be considered:

**Allergies**—Tell your doctor if you have ever had any unusual or allergic reaction to nicotinyl alcohol. Also tell your health care professional if you are allergic to any other substances, such as foods, preservatives, or dyes.

**Pregnancy**—Studies on effects in pregnancy have not been done in either humans or animals.

**Breast-feeding**—It is not known whether nicotinyl alcohol passes into breast milk. However, this medicine has not been reported to cause problems in nursing babies.

**Older adults**—Many medicines have not been studied specifically in older people. Therefore, it may not be known whether they work exactly the same way they do in younger adults or if they cause different side effects or problems in older people. There is no specific information comparing use of nicotinyl alcohol in the elderly with use in other age groups. However, nicotinyl alcohol may reduce tolerance to cold temperatures in elderly patients.

**Other medicines**—Although certain medicines should not be used together at all, in other cases two different medicines may be used together even if an interaction might occur. In these cases, your doctor may want to change the dose, or other precautions may be necessary. Tell your

health care professional if you are taking any other prescription or nonprescription (over-the-counter [OTC]) medicine, or if you smoke.

**Other medical problems**—The presence of other medical problems may affect the use of nicotinyl alcohol. Make sure you tell your doctor if you have any other medical problems, especially:
- Angina (chest pain) or
- Diabetes mellitus (sugar diabetes) or
- Heart attack (recent) or
- Stomach ulcer
- Stroke (recent)—Nicotinyl alcohol can make your condition worse
- Glaucoma or
- High cholesterol levels—The chance of side effects may be increased

## Proper Use of This Medicine

Nicotinyl alcohol tablets should be swallowed whole. Do not break, crush, or chew the tablets before swallowing them.

**Dosing**—The dose of nicotinyl alcohol will be different for different patients. *Follow your doctor's orders or the directions on the label.* The following information includes only the average doses of nicotinyl alcohol. *If your dose is different, do not change it* unless your doctor tells you to do so:
- For *oral* dosage forms (tablets):
  —Adults: 150 to 300 milligrams two times a day, taken in the morning and evening.

**Missed dose**—If you miss a dose of this medicine, take it as soon as you remember. However, if it is almost time for your next dose, skip the missed dose and go back to your regular dosing schedule. Do not double doses.

**Storage**—To store this medicine:
- Keep out of the reach of children.
- Store away from heat and direct light.
- Do not store in the bathroom, near the kitchen sink, or in other damp places. Heat or moisture may cause the medicine to break down.
- Do not keep outdated medicine or medicine no longer needed. Be sure that any discarded medicine is out of the reach of children.

## Precautions While Using This Medicine

It may take some time for this medicine to work. If you feel that the medicine is not working, do not stop taking it on your own. Instead, check with your doctor.

The helpful effects of this medicine may be decreased if you smoke.

## Side Effects of This Medicine

Along with its needed effects, a medicine may cause some unwanted effects. Although not all of these side effects may occur, if they do occur they may need medical attention.

Check with your doctor as soon as possible if any of the following side effects occur:

*Rare*
Swelling of feet or lower legs; yellow eyes or skin

Other side effects may occur that usually do not need medical attention. These side effects may go away during treatment as your body adjusts to the medicine. However, check with your doctor if any of the following side effects continue or are bothersome:

*More common*
Flushing; warmth or tingling

*Less common or rare*
Diarrhea; dizziness or faintness; increased hair loss; nausea and vomiting; skin rash

Other side effects not listed above may also occur in some patients. If you notice any other effects, check with your doctor.

Revised: 04/06/93

---

# NITRATES—Lingual Aerosol  Systemic

This information applies to nitroglycerin oral spray.
A commonly used brand name in the U.S. and Canada is Nitrolingual.
Another commonly used name is glyceryl trinitrate.

## Description

Nitrates (NYE-trates) are used to treat the symptoms of angina (chest pain). Depending on the type of dosage form and how it is taken, nitrates are used to treat angina in three ways:

- to relieve an attack that is occurring by using the medicine when the attack begins;
- to prevent attacks from occurring by using the medicine just before an attack is expected to occur; or
- to reduce the number of attacks that occur by using the medicine regularly on a long-term basis.

When used as a lingual (in the mouth) spray, nitroglycerin is used either to relieve the pain of angina attacks or to prevent an expected angina attack.

Nitroglycerin works by relaxing blood vessels and increasing the supply of blood and oxygen to the heart while reducing its work load.

Nitroglycerin as discussed here is available only with your doctor's prescription, in the following dosage form:

*Oral*
- Lingual aerosol (U.S. and Canada)

## Before Using This Medicine

In deciding to use a medicine, the risks of taking the medicine must be weighed against the good it will do. This is a decision you and your doctor will make. For

nitroglycerin lingual aerosol, the following should be considered:

**Allergies**—Tell your doctor if you have ever had any unusual or allergic reaction to nitrates or nitrites. Also tell your health care professional if you are allergic to any other substances, such as certain foods, preservatives, or dyes.

**Pregnancy**—Studies on effects in pregnancy have not been done in either humans or animals.

**Breast-feeding**—It is not known whether this medicine passes into breast milk. Although most medicines pass into breast milk in small amounts, many of them may be used safely while breast-feeding. Mothers who are taking this medicine and who wish to breast-feed should discuss this with their doctor.

**Children**—Studies on this medicine have been done only in adult patients, and there is no specific information comparing use of nitroglycerin in children with use in other age groups.

**Older adults**—Dizziness or lightheadedness may be more likely to occur in the elderly, who may be more sensitive to the effects of nitrates.

**Other medicines**—Although certain medicines should not be used together at all, in other cases two different medicines may be used together even if an interaction might occur. In these cases, your doctor may want to change the dose, or other precautions may be necessary. When you are taking nitroglycerin, it is especially important that your health care professional know if you are taking any of the following:

- Antihypertensives (high blood pressure medicine) or
- Other heart medicine—May increase the effects of nitroglycerin on blood pressure

**Other medical problems**—The presence of other medical problems may affect the use of nitroglycerin. Make sure you tell your doctor if you have any other medical problems, especially:

- Anemia (severe)
- Glaucoma—May be worsened by nitroglycerin
- Head injury (recent) or
- Stroke (recent)—Nitroglycerin may increase pressure in the brain, which can make problems worse
- Heart attack (recent)—Nitroglycerin may lower blood pressure, which can aggravate problems associated with heart attack
- Kidney disease or
- Liver disease—Effects may be increased because of slower removal of nitroglycerin from the body
- Overactive thyroid

## Proper Use of This Medicine

*Use nitroglycerin spray exactly as directed by your doctor.* It will work only if used correctly.

*This medicine usually comes with patient instructions. Read them carefully before you actually need to use it.* Then, if you need the medicine quickly, you will know how to use it.

To use nitroglycerin lingual spray:

- Remove the plastic cover. *Do not shake the container.*
- Hold the container upright. With the container held close to your mouth, press the button to spray onto or under your tongue. *Do not inhale the spray.*
- Release the button and close your mouth. Avoid swallowing immediately after using the spray.

For patients using nitroglycerin oral spray *to relieve the pain of an angina attack*:

- *When you begin to feel an attack of angina starting (chest pains or a tightness or squeezing in the chest), sit down. Then use 1 or 2 sprays as directed by your doctor.* This medicine works best when you are standing or sitting. However, since you may become dizzy, lightheaded, or faint soon after using a spray, it is safer to sit rather than stand while the medicine is working. If you become dizzy or faint while sitting, take several deep breaths and bend forward with your head between your knees.
- Remain calm and you should feel better in a few minutes.
- *This medicine usually gives relief in less than 5 minutes.* However, if the pain is not relieved, use a second spray. If the pain continues for another 5 minutes, a third spray may be used. *If you still have the chest pains after a total of 3 sprays in a 15-minute period, contact your doctor or go to a hospital emergency room immediately.*

For patients using nitroglycerin oral spray *to prevent an expected angina attack*:

- You may prevent anginal chest pains for up to 1 hour by using a spray 5 to 10 minutes before expected emotional stress or physical exertion that in the past seemed to bring on an attack.

**Dosing**—The dose of nitroglycerin lingual spray will be different for different patients. *Follow your doctor's orders or the directions on the label.* The following information includes only the average doses of nitroglycerin lingual spray. *If your dose is different, do not change it unless your doctor tells you to do so.*

- For *oral* dosage form (lingual spray):
  —For chest pain:
  - Adults—One or two sprays on or under the tongue. The dose may be repeated every five minutes as needed. If the chest pain is not relieved after a total of three sprays in a fifteen-minute period, call your doctor or go to the emergency room right away.

**Storage**—To store this medicine:

- Keep out of the reach of children.
- Store away from heat and direct light.
- Keep the medicine from freezing.
- Do not puncture, break, or burn the aerosol container, even after it is empty.
- Do not keep outdated medicine or medicine no longer needed. Be sure that any discarded medicine is out of the reach of children.

## Precautions While Using This Medicine

*If you have been using this medicine regularly for several weeks, do not suddenly stop using it.* Stopping suddenly may bring on attacks of angina. Check with your doctor for the best way to reduce gradually the amount you are using before stopping completely.

*Dizziness, lightheadedness, or faintness may occur,* especially when you get up quickly from a lying or sitting position. Getting up slowly may help. If you feel dizzy, sit or lie down.

The dizziness, lightheadedness, or fainting is also more likely to occur if you drink alcohol, stand for long periods of time, exercise, or if the weather is hot. *While you are taking this medicine, be careful to limit the amount of alcohol you drink. Also, use extra care during exercise or hot weather or if you must stand for long periods of time.*

*After using a dose of this medicine you may get a headache that lasts for a short time. This is a common side effect,* which should become less noticeable after you have used the medicine for a while. If this effect continues or if the headaches are severe, check with your doctor.

## Side Effects of This Medicine

Along with its needed effects, a medicine may cause some unwanted effects. Although not all of these side effects

may occur, if they do occur they may need medical attention.

Check with your doctor as soon as possible if any of the following side effects occur:

*Rare*

Blurred vision; dryness of mouth; headache (severe or prolonged); skin rash

*Signs and symptoms of overdose (in the order in which they may occur)*

Bluish-colored lips, fingernails, or palms of hands; dizziness (extreme) or fainting; feeling of extreme pressure in head; shortness of breath; unusual tiredness or weakness; weak and fast heartbeat; fever; convulsions (seizures)

Other side effects may occur that usually do not need medical attention. These side effects may go away during treatment as your body adjusts to the medicine. However, check with your doctor if any of the following side effects continue or are bothersome:

*More common*

Dizziness or lightheadedness, especially when getting up from a lying or sitting position; fast pulse; flushing of face and neck; headache; nausea or vomiting; restlessness

Other side effects not listed above may also occur in some patients. If you notice any other effects, check with your doctor.

Revised: 10/06/93

---

# NITRATES—Oral   Systemic

Some commonly used brand names are:

**In the U.S.—**

| | |
|---|---|
| Cardilate[1] | Nitrocap[4] |
| Dilatrate-SR[2] | Nitrocap T.D.[4] |
| Duotrate[5] | Nitroglyn[4] |
| IMDUR[3] | Nitrolin[4] |
| ISMO[3] | Nitronet[4] |
| Iso-Bid[2] | Nitrong [4] |
| Isonate[2] | Nitrospan[4] |
| Isorbid[2] | Pentylan[5] |
| Isordil[2] | Peritrate[5] |
| Isotrate[2] | Peritrate SA[5] |
| Klavikordal[4] | Sorbitrate[2] |
| Monoket[3] | Sorbitrate SA[2] |
| Niong[4] | |

**In Canada—**

| | |
|---|---|
| Apo-ISDN[2] | Nitrong SR[4] |
| Cardilate[1] | Novosorbide[2] |
| Cedocard-SR[2] | Peritrate[5] |
| Coronex[2] | Peritrate Forte[5] |
| Isordil[2] | Peritrate SA[5] |

Other commonly used names are:

| | |
|---|---|
| Eritrityl tetranitrate[1] | Pentaerithrityl tetranitrate[5] |
| Erythritol tetranitrate[1] | P.E.T.N.[5] |
| Glyceryl trinitrate[4] | |

Note: For quick reference, the following nitrates are numbered to match the corresponding brand names.

This information applies to the following medicines:

1. Erythrityl Tetranitrate (e-RI-thri-till tet-ra-NYE-trate)
2. Isosorbide Dinitrate (eye-soe-SOR-bide dye-NYE-trate)‡
3. Isosorbide Mononitrate (eye-soe-SOR-bide mon-oh-NYE-trate)†
4. Nitroglycerin (nye-troe-GLI-ser-in)‡
5. Pentaerythritol Tetranitrate (pen-ta-er-ITH-ri-tole tet-ra-NYE-trate)‡

Note: This information does *not* apply to amyl nitrite or mannitol hexanitrate.

†Not commercially available in Canada.
‡Generic name product may also be available in the U.S.

## Description

Nitrates (NYE-trates) are used to treat the symptoms of angina (chest pain). Depending on the type of dosage form and how it is taken, nitrates are used to treat angina in three ways:

- to relieve an attack that is occurring by using the medicine when the attack begins;
- to prevent attacks from occurring by using the medicine just before an attack is expected to occur; or
- to reduce the number of attacks that occur by using the medicine regularly on a long-term basis.

When taken orally and swallowed, nitrates are used to reduce the number of angina attacks that occur. They do not act fast enough to relieve the pain of an angina attack.

Nitrates work by relaxing blood vessels and increasing the supply of blood and oxygen to the heart while reducing its work load.

Nitrates may also be used for other conditions as determined by your doctor.

The nitrates discussed here are available only with your doctor's prescription, in the following dosage forms:

*Oral*

Erythrityl tetranitrate
- Tablets (U.S. and Canada)

Isosorbide dinitrate
- Capsules (U.S.)
- Extended-release capsules (U.S.)
- Tablets (U.S. and Canada)
- Chewable tablets (U.S.)
- Extended-release tablets (U.S. and Canada)

Isosorbide mononitrate
- Extended-release tablets (U.S.)
- Tablets (U.S.)

Nitroglycerin
- Extended-release capsules (U.S.)
- Extended-release tablets (U.S. and Canada)

Pentaerythritol tetranitrate
- Extended-release capsules (U.S.)
- Tablets (U.S. and Canada)
- Extended-release tablets (U.S. and Canada)

---

## Before Using This Medicine

In deciding to use a medicine, the risks of taking the medicine must be weighed against the good it will do. This is a decision you and your doctor will make. For nitrates, the following should be considered:

**Allergies**—Tell your doctor if you have ever had any unusual or allergic reaction to nitrates or nitrites. Also tell your health care professional if you are allergic to any other substances, such as certain foods, preservatives, or dyes.

**Pregnancy**—Nitrates have not been studied in pregnant women. However, studies in rabbits given large doses of isosorbide dinitrate have shown adverse effects on the fetus. Before taking these medicines, make sure your doctor knows if you are pregnant or if you may become pregnant.

**Breast-feeding**—It is not known whether these medicines pass into breast milk. Although most medicines pass into breast milk in small amounts, many of them may be used safely while breast-feeding. Mothers who are taking these medicines and who wish to breast-feed should discuss this with their doctor.

**Children**—Studies on these medicines have been done only in adult patients, and there is no specific information comparing use of nitrates in children with use in other age groups.

**Older adults**—Dizziness or lightheadedness may be more likely to occur in the elderly, who may be more sensitive to the effects of nitrates.

**Other medicines**—Although certain medicines should not be used together at all, in other cases two different medicines may be used together even if an interaction might occur. In these cases, your doctor may want to change the dose, or other precautions may be necessary. When you are taking nitrates, it is especially important that your health care professional know if you are taking any of the following:

- Antihypertensives (high blood pressure medicine) or
- Other heart medicine—May increase the effects of nitrates on blood pressure

**Other medical problems**—The presence of other medical problems may affect the use of nitrates. Make sure you tell your doctor if you have any other medical problems, especially:

- Anemia (severe)
- Glaucoma—May be worsened by nitrates
- Head injury (recent) or
- Stroke (recent)—Nitrates may increase pressure in the brain, which can make problems worse
- Heart attack (recent)—Nitrates may lower blood pressure, which can aggravate problems associated with heart attack
- Kidney disease or
- Liver disease—Effects may be increased because of slower removal of nitroglycerin from the body
- Overactive thyroid

## Proper Use of This Medicine

*Take this medicine exactly as directed by your doctor.* It will work only if taken correctly.

*This form of nitrate is used to reduce the number of angina attacks. In most cases, it will not relieve an attack that has already started,* because it works too slowly (the extended-release form releases medicine gradually over a 6-hour period to provide its effect for 8 to 10 hours). Check with your doctor if you need a fast-acting medicine to relieve the pain of an angina attack.

*Take this medicine with a full glass (8 ounces) of water on an empty stomach.* If taken either 1 hour before or 2 hours after meals, it will start working sooner.

*Extended-release capsules and tablets are not to be broken, crushed, or chewed before they are swallowed.* If broken up, they will not release the medicine properly.

**Dosing**—The dose of nitrates will be different for different patients. *Follow your doctor's orders or the directions on the label.* The following information includes only the average doses of nitrates. *If your dose is different, do not change it* unless your doctor tells you to do so.

The number of capsules or tablets that you take depends on the strength of the medicine. Also, *the number of doses you take each day, the time allowed between doses, and the length of time you take the medicine depend on the medical problem for which you are taking nitrates.*

*For erythrityl tetranitrate*

- For angina (chest pain):
  —For *oral* dosage form (tablets):
  - Adults—5 to 10 milligrams (mg) three or four times a day.
  - Children—Dose must be determined by your doctor.

*For isosorbide dinitrate*

- For angina (chest pain):
  —For *regular (short-acting) oral* dosage forms (capsules or tablets):
  - Adults—5 to 40 mg four times a day.
  - Children—Dose must be determined by your doctor.
  —For *long-acting oral* dosage forms (extended-release capsules or tablets):
  - Adults—20 to 80 mg every eight to twelve hours.
  - Children—Dose must be determined by your doctor.

*For isosorbide mononitrate*

- For angina (chest pain):
  —For *regular (short-acting) oral* dosage form (tablets):
  - Adults—20 mg two times a day. The two doses should be taken seven hours apart.
  - Children—Use and dose must be determined by your doctor.

—For *long-acting oral* dosage forms (extended-release tablets):

- Adults—30 to 240 mg once a day.
- Children—Use and dose must be determined by your doctor.

*For nitroglycerin*

- For angina (chest pain):

—For *long-acting oral* dosage forms (capsules or tablets):

- Adults—1.3 to 9.0 mg every eight to twelve hours.
- Children—Dose must be determined by your doctor.

*For pentaerythritol tetranitrate*

- For angina (chest pain):

—For *regular (short-acting) oral* dosage forms (tablets):

- Adults—10 to 20 mg four times a day.
- Children—Dose must be determined by your doctor.

—For *long-acting oral* dosage forms (capsules or tablets):

- Adults—30 to 80 mg two times a day.
- Children—Dose must be determined by your doctor.

**Missed dose**—If you are taking this medicine regularly and you miss a dose, take it as soon as possible. However, if the next scheduled dose is within 2 hours (or within 6 hours for extended-release capsules or tablets), skip the missed dose and go back to your regular dosing schedule. Do not double doses.

**Storage**—To store this medicine:

- Keep out of the reach of children.
- Store away from heat and direct light.
- Do not store in the bathroom, near the kitchen sink, or in other damp places. Heat or moisture may cause the medicine to break down.
- Do not keep outdated medicine or medicine no longer needed. Be sure that any discarded medicine is out of the reach of children.

---

## Precautions While Using This Medicine

*If you have been taking this medicine regularly for several weeks or more, do not suddenly stop using it.* Stopping suddenly may bring on attacks of angina. Check with your doctor for the best way to reduce gradually the amount you are taking before stopping completely.

*Dizziness, lightheadedness, or faintness may occur,* especially when you get up quickly from a lying or sitting position. Getting up slowly may help. If you feel dizzy, sit or lie down.

The dizziness, lightheadedness, or fainting is also more likely to occur if you drink alcohol, stand for long periods of time, exercise, or if the weather is hot. *While you are taking this medicine, be careful to limit the amount of alcohol you*

drink. *Also, use extra care during exercise or hot weather or if you must stand for long periods of time.*

*After taking a dose of this medicine you may get a headache that lasts for a short time. This is a common side effect,* which should become less noticeable after you have taken the medicine for a while. If this effect continues, or if the headaches are severe, check with your doctor.

For patients taking the *extended-release dosage forms of isosorbide dinitrate or pentaerythritol tetranitrate*:

- Partially dissolved tablets have been found in the stools of a few patients taking the extended-release tablets. Be alert to this possibility, especially if you have frequent bowel movements, diarrhea, or digestive problems. Notify your doctor if any such tablets are discovered. The tablets must be properly digested to provide the correct dose of medicine.

---

## Side Effects of This Medicine

Along with its needed effects, a medicine may cause some unwanted effects. Although not all of these side effects may occur, if they do occur they may need medical attention.

Check with your doctor as soon as possible if any of the following side effects occur:

*Rare*

Blurred vision; dryness of mouth; headache (severe or prolonged); skin rash

*Signs and symptoms of overdose (in the order in which they may occur)*

Bluish-colored lips, fingernails, or palms of hands; dizziness (extreme) or fainting; feeling of extreme pressure in head; shortness of breath; unusual tiredness or weakness; weak and fast heartbeat; fever; convulsions (seizures)

Other side effects may occur that usually do not need medical attention. These side effects may go away during treatment as your body adjusts to the medicine. However, check with your doctor if any of the following side effects continue or are bothersome:

*More common*

Dizziness or lightheadedness, especially when getting up from a lying or sitting position; fast pulse; flushing of face and neck; headache; nausea or vomiting; restlessness

Other side effects not listed above may also occur in some patients. If you notice any other effects, check with your doctor.

---

Revised: 10/06/93
Interim revision: 02/22/94

# NITRATES—Sublingual, Chewable, or Buccal   Systemic

Some commonly used brand names are:

**In the U.S.—**

| | |
|---|---|
| Cardilate[1] | Nitrogard[3] |
| Isonate[2] | Nitrostat[3] |
| Isorbid[2] | Sorbitrate[2] |
| Isordil[2] | |

**In Canada—**

| | |
|---|---|
| Apo-ISDN[2] | Isordil[2] |
| Cardilate[1] | Nitrogard SR[3] |
| Coronex[2] | Nitrostat[3] |

Other commonly used names are:

| | |
|---|---|
| Eritrityl tetranitrate[1] | Glyceryl trinitrate[3] |
| Erythritol tetranitrate[1] | |

Note: For quick reference, the following nitrates are numbered to match the corresponding brand names.

This information applies to the following medicines:
1. Erythrityl Tetranitrate (e-RI-thri-till tet-ra-NYE-trate)
2. Isosorbide Dinitrate (eye-soe-SOR-bide dye-NYE-trate)‡
3. Nitroglycerin (nye-troe-GLI-ser-in)‡§

Note: This information does *not* apply to amyl nitrite or pentaerythritol tetranitrate.

‡Generic name product may also be available in the U.S.
§Generic name product may also be available in Canada.

## Description

Nitrates (NYE-trates) are used to treat the symptoms of angina (chest pain). Depending on the type of dosage form and how it is taken, nitrates are used to treat angina in three ways:

- to relieve an attack that is occurring by using the medicine when the attack begins;
- to prevent attacks from occurring by using the medicine just before an attack is expected to occur; or
- to reduce the number of attacks that occur by using the medicine regularly on a long-term basis.

Nitrates are available in different forms. Sublingual nitrates are generally placed under the tongue where they dissolve and are absorbed through the lining of the mouth. Some can also be used buccally, being placed under the lip or in the cheek. The chewable dosage forms, after being chewed and held in the mouth before swallowing, are absorbed in the same way. *It is important to remember that each dosage form is different and that the specific directions for each type must be followed if the medicine is to work properly.*

Nitrates that are used *to relieve the pain* of an angina attack include:

- sublingual nitroglycerin;
- buccal nitroglycerin;
- sublingual isosorbide dinitrate; and
- chewable isosorbide dinitrate.

Those that can be used *to prevent expected attacks* of angina include:

- sublingual nitroglycerin;
- buccal nitroglycerin;
- sublingual erythrityl tetranitrate;
- sublingual isosorbide dinitrate; and
- chewable isosorbide dinitrate.

Products that are used regularly on a long-term basis *to reduce the number of attacks* that occur include:

- buccal nitroglycerin;
- oral/sublingual erythrityl tetranitrate; and
- chewable isosorbide dinitrate; and
- sublingual isosorbide dinitrate.

Nitrates work by relaxing blood vessels and increasing the supply of blood and oxygen to the heart while reducing its work load.

Nitrates may also be used for other conditions as determined by your doctor.

The nitrates discussed here are available only with your doctor's prescription, in the following dosage forms:

*Buccal*
   Nitroglycerin
   - Extended-release tablets (U.S. and Canada)

*Chewable*
   Isosorbide dinitrate
   - Tablets (U.S.)

*Sublingual*
   Erythrityl tetranitrate
   - Tablets (U.S. and Canada)
   Isosorbide dinitrate
   - Tablets (U.S. and Canada)
   Nitroglycerin
   - Tablets (U.S. and Canada)

## Before Using This Medicine

In deciding to use a medicine, the risks of taking the medicine must be weighed against the good it will do. This is a decision you and your doctor will make. For nitrates, the following should be considered:

**Allergies**—Tell your doctor if you have ever had any unusual or allergic reaction to nitrates or nitrites. Also tell your health care professional if you are allergic to any other substances, such as certain foods, preservatives, or dyes.

**Pregnancy**—Nitrates have not been studied in pregnant women. However, studies in rabbits given large doses of isosorbide dinitrate have shown adverse effects on the fetus. Before taking these medicines, make sure your doctor knows if you are pregnant or if you may become pregnant.

**Breast-feeding**—It is not known whether these medicines pass into breast milk. Although most medicines pass into breast milk in small amounts, many of them may be used safely while breast-feeding. Mothers who are taking these medicines and who wish to breast-feed should discuss this with their doctor.

**Children**—Studies on these medicines have been done only in adult patients, and there is no specific information comparing use of nitrates in children with use in other age groups.

**Older adults**—Dizziness or lightheadedness may be more likely to occur in the elderly, who may be more sensitive to the effects of nitrates.

**Other medicines**—Although certain medicines should not be used together at all, in other cases two different medicines may be used together even if an interaction might occur. In these cases, your doctor may want to change the dose, or other precautions may be necessary. When you are taking nitrates, it is especially important that your health care professional know if you are taking any of the following:

- Antihypertensives (high blood pressure medicine) or
- Other heart medicine—May increase the effects of nitrates on blood pressure

**Other medical problems**—The presence of other medical problems may affect the use of nitroglycerin. Make sure you tell your doctor if you have any other medical problems, especially:

- Anemia (severe)
- Glaucoma—May be worsened by nitrates
- Head injury (recent) or
- Stroke (recent)—Nitrates may increase pressure in the brain, which can make problems worse
- Heart attack (recent)—Nitrates may lower blood pressure, which can aggravate problems associated with heart attack
- Kidney disease or
- Liver disease—Effects may be increased because of slower removal of nitroglycerin from the body
- Overactive thyroid

## Proper Use of This Medicine

*Take this medicine exactly as directed by your doctor.* It will work only if taken correctly.

*Sublingual tablets should not be chewed, crushed, or swallowed.* They work much faster when absorbed through the lining of the mouth. Place the tablet under the tongue, between the lip and gum, or between the cheek and gum and let it dissolve there. Do not eat, drink, smoke, or use chewing tobacco while a tablet is dissolving.

*Buccal extended-release tablets should not be chewed, crushed, or swallowed.* They are designed to release a dose of nitroglycerin over a period of hours, not all at once.

- Allow the tablet to dissolve slowly in place between the upper lip and gum (above the front teeth), or between the cheek and upper gum. If food or drink is to be taken during the 3 to 5 hours when the tablet is dissolving, place the tablet between the *upper* lip and gum, above the front teeth. If you have dentures, you may place the tablet anywhere between the cheek and gum.
- Touching the tablet with your tongue or drinking hot liquids may cause the tablet to dissolve faster.

- Do not go to sleep while a tablet is dissolving because it could slip down your throat and cause choking.
- If you accidentally swallow the tablet, replace it with another one.
- Do not use chewing tobacco while a tablet is in place.

*Chewable tablets must be chewed well and held in the mouth for about 2 minutes before you swallow them.* This will allow the medicine to be absorbed through the lining of the mouth.

For patients using *nitroglycerin or isosorbide dinitrate to relieve the pain of an angina attack*:

- *When you begin to feel an attack of angina starting (chest pains or a tightness or squeezing in the chest), sit down. Then place a tablet in your mouth, either sublingually or buccally, or chew a chewable tablet.* This medicine works best when you are standing or sitting. However, since you may become dizzy, lightheaded, or faint soon after using a tablet, it is safer to sit rather than stand while the medicine is working. If you become dizzy or faint while sitting, take several deep breaths and bend forward with your head between your knees.
- Remain calm and you should feel better in a few minutes.
- *This medicine usually gives relief in 1 to 5 minutes.* However, if the pain is not relieved, and you are using:

  —Sublingual tablets, either sublingually or buccally: Use a second tablet. If the pain continues for another 5 minutes, a third tablet may be used. *If you still have the chest pains after a total of 3 tablets in a 15-minute period, contact your doctor or go to a hospital emergency room immediately.*

  —Buccal extended-release tablets: *Use a sublingual (under the tongue) nitroglycerin tablet and check with your doctor.* Do not use another buccal tablet since the effects of a buccal tablet last for several hours.

For patients using *nitroglycerin, erythrityl tetranitrate, or isosorbide dinitrate to prevent an expected angina attack*:

- You may prevent anginal chest pains for up to 1 hour (6 hours for the extended-release nitroglycerin tablet) by using a buccal or sublingual tablet or chewing a chewable tablet 5 to 10 minutes before expected emotional stress or physical exertion that in the past seemed to bring on an attack.

For patients using *isosorbide dinitrate or extended-release buccal nitroglycerin regularly on a long-term basis to reduce the number of angina attacks that occur*:

- Chewable or sublingual isosorbide dinitrate and buccal extended-release nitroglycerin tablets can be used either to prevent angina attacks or to help relieve an attack that has already started.

**Dosing**—The dose of nitrates will be different for different patients. *Follow your doctor's orders or the directions on the label.* The following information includes only the average doses of nitrates. *If your dose is different, do not change it* unless your doctor tells you to do so.

*For erythrityl tetranitrate*
- For angina (chest pain):
  —For *buccal or sublingual* dosage form (tablets):
    - Adults—5 to 10 milligrams (mg) three or four times a day.
    - Children—Dose must be determined by your doctor.

*For isosorbide dinitrate*
- For angina (chest pain):
  —For *chewable* dosage form (tablets):
    - Adults—5 mg every two to three hours, chewed well and held in mouth for one or two minutes.
    - Children—Dose must be determined by your doctor.
  —For *buccal or sublingual* dosage form (tablets):
    - Adults—2.5 to 5 mg every two to three hours.
    - Children—Dose must be determined by your doctor.

*For nitroglycerin*
- For angina (chest pain):
  —For *buccal* dosage form (extended-release tablets):
    - Adults—1 mg every five hours while awake. Your doctor may increase your dose.
    - Children—Dose must be determined by your doctor.
  —For *sublingual* dosage form (tablets):
    - Adults—150 to 600 micrograms (mcg) (0.15 to 0.6 mg) every five minutes. If you still have chest pain after a total of three tablets in fifteen minutes, call your doctor or go to the emergency room right away.
    - Children—Dose must be determined by your doctor.

**Missed dose**—For patients using isosorbide dinitrate or extended-release buccal nitroglycerin regularly on a long-term basis to reduce the number of angina attacks that occur:
- If you miss a dose of this medicine, use it as soon as possible. However, if the next scheduled dose is within 2 hours, skip the missed dose and go back to your regular dosing schedule. Do not double doses.

**Stability and proper storage—**
*For sublingual nitroglycerin*
- Sublingual nitroglycerin tablets may lose some of their strength if they are exposed to air, heat, or moisture for long periods of time. However, if you screw the cap on tightly after each use and you properly store the bottle, the tablets should retain their strength until the expiration date on the bottle.

- Some people think they should test the strength of their sublingual nitroglycerin tablets by looking for a tingling or burning sensation, a feeling of warmth or flushing, or a headache after a tablet has been dissolved under the tongue. This kind of testing is not completely reliable since some patients may be unable to detect these effects. In addition, newer, stabilized sublingual nitroglycerin tablets are less likely to produce these detectable effects.
- To help keep the nitroglycerin tablets at full strength:
  —keep the medicine in the original glass, screw-cap bottle. For patients who wish to carry a small number of tablets with them for emergency use, a specially designed container is available. However, only containers specifically labeled as suitable for use with nitroglycerin sublingual tablets should be used.
  —remove the cotton plug that comes in the bottle and *do not* put it back.
  —*put the cap on the bottle quickly and tightly after each use.*
  —to select a tablet for use, pour several into the bottle cap, take one, and pour the others back into the bottle. Try not to hold them in the palm of your hand because they may pick up moisture and crumble.
  —do not keep other medicines in the same bottle with the nitroglycerin since they will weaken the nitroglycerin effect.
  —keep the medicine handy at all times but try not to carry the bottle close to the body. Medicine may lose strength because of body warmth. Instead, carry the tightly closed bottle in your purse or the pocket of a jacket or other loose-fitting clothing whenever possible.
  —store the bottle of nitroglycerin tablets in a cool, dry place. Storage at average room temperature away from direct heat or direct sunlight is best. Do not store in the refrigerator or in a bathroom medicine cabinet because the moisture usually present in these areas may cause the tablets to crumble if the container is not tightly closed. Do not keep the tablets in your automobile glove compartment.
- Keep out of the reach of children.
- Do not keep outdated medicine or medicine no longer needed. Be sure that any discarded medicine is out of the reach of children.

*For erythrityl tetranitrate, isosorbide dinitrate, and buccal extended-release nitroglycerin*
- These forms of nitrates are more stable than sublingual nitroglycerin.
- Keep out of the reach of children.
- Store away from heat and direct light.
- Do not store in the bathroom, near the kitchen sink, or in other damp places. Heat or moisture may cause the medicine to break down.

• Do not keep outdated medicine or medicine no longer needed. Be sure that any discarded medicine is out of the reach of children.

---

## Precautions While Using This Medicine

*If you have been taking this medicine regularly for several weeks, do not suddenly stop using it.* Stopping suddenly may bring on attacks of angina. Check with your doctor for the best way to reduce gradually the amount you are taking before stopping completely.

*Dizziness, lightheadedness, or faintness may occur,* especially when you get up quickly from a lying or sitting position. Getting up slowly may help. If you feel dizzy, sit or lie down.

The dizziness, lightheadedness, or fainting is also more likely to occur if you drink alcohol, stand for long periods of time, exercise, or if the weather is hot. *While you are taking this medicine, be careful to limit the amount of alcohol you drink. Also, use extra care during exercise or hot weather or if you must stand for long periods of time.*

*After taking a dose of this medicine you may get a headache that lasts for a short time. This is a common side effect,* which should become less noticeable after you have taken the medicine for a while. If this effect continues or if the headaches are severe, check with your doctor.

---

## Side Effects of This Medicine

Along with its needed effects, a medicine may cause some unwanted effects. Although not all of these side effects may occur, if they do occur they may need medical attention.

Check with your doctor as soon as possible if any of the following side effects occur:

*Rare*

Blurred vision; dryness of mouth; headache (severe or prolonged); skin rash

*Signs and symptoms of overdose (in the order in which they may occur)*

Bluish-colored lips, fingernails, or palms of hands; dizziness (extreme) or fainting; feeling of extreme pressure in head; shortness of breath; unusual tiredness or weakness; weak and fast heartbeat; fever; convulsions (seizures)

Other side effects may occur that usually do not need medical attention. These side effects may go away during treatment as your body adjusts to the medicine. However, check with your doctor if any of the following side effects continue or are bothersome:

*More common*

Dizziness or lightheadedness, especially when getting up from a lying or sitting position; fast pulse; flushing of face and neck; headache; nausea or vomiting; restlessness

Other side effects not listed above may also occur in some patients. If you notice any other effects, check with your doctor.

---

Revised: 10/06/93

---

# NITRATES—Topical    Systemic

Some commonly used brand names are:

**In the U.S.—**

| | |
|---|---|
| Deponit[2] | Nitrol[1] |
| Nitro-Bid[1] | Nitrong[1] |
| Nitrodisc[2] | Nitrostat[1] |
| Nitro-Dur[2] | NTS[2] |
| Nitro-Dur II[2] | Transderm-Nitro[2] |

**In Canada—**

| | |
|---|---|
| Nitro-Bid[1] | Nitrong[1] |
| Nitrol[1] | Transderm-Nitro[2] |

Another commonly used name for nitroglycerin is glyceryl trinitrate.

Note: For quick reference, the following nitrates are numbered to match the corresponding brand names.

This information applies to the following medicines:

1. Nitroglycerin Ointment‡
2. Nitroglycerin Transdermal Patches‡

‡Generic name product may also be available in the U.S.

## Description

Nitrates (NYE-trates) are used to treat the symptoms of angina (chest pain). Depending on the type of dosage form and how it is taken, nitrates are used to treat angina in three ways:

• to relieve an attack that is occurring by using the medicine when the attack begins;

• to prevent attacks from occurring by using the medicine just before an attack is expected to occur; or

• to reduce the number of attacks that occur by using the medicine regularly on a long-term basis.

When applied to the skin, nitrates are used to reduce the number of angina attacks that occur. The only nitrate available for this purpose is topical nitroglycerin (nye-troe-GLI-ser-in).

Topical nitroglycerin is absorbed through the skin. It works by relaxing blood vessels and increasing the supply of blood and oxygen to the heart while reducing its work

---

load. This helps prevent future angina attacks from occurring.

Topical nitroglycerin may also be used for other conditions as determined by your doctor.

Nitroglycerin as discussed here is available only with your doctor's prescription, in the following dosage forms:

*Topical*
- Ointment (U.S. and Canada)
- Transdermal (stick-on) patch (U.S. and Canada)

## Before Using This Medicine

In deciding to use a medicine, the risks of taking the medicine must be weighed against the good it will do. This is a decision you and your doctor will make. For nitroglycerin applied to the skin, the following should be considered:

**Allergies**—Tell your doctor if you have ever had any unusual or allergic reaction to nitrates or nitrites. Also tell your health care professional if you are allergic to any other substances, such as certain foods, preservatives, or dyes.

**Pregnancy**—Nitrates have not been studied in pregnant women. Before taking these medicines, make sure your doctor knows if you are pregnant or if you may become pregnant.

**Breast-feeding**—It is not known whether this medicine passes into breast milk. Although most medicines pass into breast milk in small amounts, many of them may be used safely while breast-feeding. Mothers who are taking these medicines and who wish to breast-feed should discuss this with their doctor.

**Children**—Studies on these medicines have been done only in adult patients, and there is no specific information comparing use of nitrates in children with use in other age groups.

**Older adults**—Dizziness or lightheadedness may be more likely to occur in the elderly, who may be more sensitive to the effects of nitrates.

**Other medicines**—Although certain medicines should not be used together at all, in other cases two different medicines may be used together even if an interaction might occur. In these cases, your doctor may want to change the dose, or other precautions may be necessary. When you are using nitroglycerin, it is especially important that your health care professional know if you are taking any of the following:
- Antihypertensives (high blood pressure medicine) or
- Other heart medicine—May increase the effects of nitroglycerin on blood pressure

**Other medical problems**—The presence of other medical problems may affect the use of nitroglycerin. Make sure you tell your doctor if you have any other medical problems, especially:
- Anemia (severe)
- Glaucoma—May be worsened by nitroglycerin

- Head injury (recent) or
- Stroke (recent)—Nitroglycerin may increase pressure in the brain, which can make problems worse
- Heart attack (recent)—Nitroglycerin may lower blood pressure, which can aggravate problems associated with heart attack
- Kidney disease or
- Liver disease—Effects may be increased because of slower removal of nitroglycerin from the body
- Overactive thyroid

## Proper Use of This Medicine

*Use nitroglycerin exactly as directed by your doctor.* It will work only if applied correctly.

*The ointment and transdermal forms of nitroglycerin are used to reduce the number of angina attacks. They will not relieve an attack that has already started* because they work too slowly. Check with your doctor if you need a fast-acting medicine to relieve the pain of an angina attack.

*This medicine usually comes with patient instructions. Read them carefully before using.*

For patients using the *ointment* form of this medicine:
- Before applying a new dose of ointment, remove any ointment remaining on the skin from a previous dose. This will allow the fresh ointment to release the nitroglycerin properly.
- This medicine comes with dose-measuring papers. Use them to measure the length of ointment squeezed from the tube and to apply the ointment to the skin. *Do not rub or massage the ointment into the skin; just spread in a thin, even layer, covering an area of the same size each time it is applied.*
- Apply the ointment to skin that has little or no hair.
- Apply each dose of ointment to a different area of skin to prevent irritation or other skin problems.
- If your doctor has ordered an occlusive dressing (airtight covering, such as kitchen plastic wrap) to be applied over this medicine, make sure you know how to apply it. Since occlusive dressings increase the amount of medicine absorbed through the skin and the possibility of side effects, use them only as directed. If you have any questions about this, check with your health care professional.

For patients using the *transdermal (stick-on patch) system:*
- Do not try to trim or cut the adhesive patch to adjust the dosage. Check with your doctor if you think the medicine is not working as it should.
- Apply the patch to a clean, dry skin area with little or no hair and free of scars, cuts, or irritation. Remove the previous patch before applying a new one.
- Apply a new patch if the first one becomes loose or falls off.
- Apply each dose to a different area of skin to prevent skin irritation or other problems.

**Dosing**—The dose of nitroglycerin will be different for different patients. *Follow your doctor's orders or the directions on the label.* The following information includes only the average doses of nitrates. *If your dose is different, do not change it* unless your doctor tells you to do so.

*For nitroglycerin*

- For angina (chest pain):
  —For *ointment* dosage form:
    - Adults—15 to 30 milligrams (mg) (about one to two inches of ointment squeezed from tube) every six to eight hours.
    - Children—Use and dose must be determined by your doctor.
  —For *transdermal system (skin patch)* dosage form:
    - Adults—Apply one transdermal dosage system (skin patch) to intact skin once a day. The patch is usually left on for 12 to 14 hours a day and then taken off. Follow your doctor's instructions for when to put on and take off the skin patch.
    - Children—Use and dose must be determined by your doctor.

**Missed dose**—

- For patients using the *ointment* form of this medicine: If you miss a dose of this medicine, apply it as soon as possible unless the next scheduled dose is within 2 hours. Then go back to your regular dosing schedule. Do not increase the amount used.
- For patients using the *transdermal (stick-on patch) system*: If you miss a dose of this medicine, apply it as soon as possible. Then go back to your regular dosing schedule.

**Storage**—

- To store the *ointment* form of this medicine:
  —Keep out of the reach of children.
  —Store the tube of nitroglycerin ointment in a cool place and keep it tightly closed.
  —Do not keep outdated medicine or medicine no longer needed. Be sure that any discarded medicine is out of the reach of children.
- To store the *transdermal (stick-on patch) system*:
  —Keep out of the reach of children.
  —Store away from heat and direct light.
  —Do not store in the bathroom, near the kitchen sink, or in other damp places. Heat or moisture may cause the medicine to break down.
  —Do not keep outdated medicine or medicine no longer needed. Be sure that any discarded medicine is out of the reach of children.

## Precautions While Using This Medicine

*If you have been using nitroglycerin regularly for several weeks or more, do not suddenly stop using it.* Stopping suddenly may bring on attacks of angina. Check with your doctor for the best way to reduce gradually the amount you are using before stopping completely.

*Dizziness, lightheadedness, or faintness may occur,* especially when you get up quickly from a lying or sitting position. Getting up slowly may help. If you feel dizzy, sit or lie down.

The dizziness, lightheadedness, or fainting is also more likely to occur if you drink alcohol, stand for long periods of time, exercise, or if the weather is hot. *While you are taking this medicine, be careful to limit the amount of alcohol you drink. Also, use extra care during exercise or hot weather or if you must stand for long periods of time.*

*After using a dose of this medicine you may get a headache that lasts for a short time. This is a common side effect,* which should become less noticeable after you have used the medicine for a while. If this effect continues, or if the headaches are severe, check with your doctor.

## Side Effects of This Medicine

Along with its needed effects, a medicine may cause some unwanted effects. Although not all of these side effects may occur, if they do occur they may need medical attention.

Check with your doctor as soon as possible if any of the following side effects occur:

*Rare*

Blurred vision; dryness of mouth; headache (severe or prolonged)

*Signs and symptoms of overdose (in the order in which they may occur)*

Bluish-colored lips, fingernails, or palms of hands; dizziness (extreme) or fainting; feeling of extreme pressure in head; shortness of breath; unusual tiredness or weakness; weak and fast heartbeat; fever; convulsions (seizures)

Other side effects may occur that usually do not need medical attention. These side effects may go away during treatment as your body adjusts to the medicine. However, check with your doctor if any of the following side effects continue or are bothersome:

*More common*

Dizziness or lightheadedness, especially when getting up from a lying or sitting position; fast pulse; flushing of face and neck; headache; nausea or vomiting; restlessness

*Less common*

Sore, reddened skin

Other side effects not listed above may also occur in some patients. If you notice any other effects, check with your doctor.

Revised: 10/06/93

# NITROFURANTOIN   Systemic

Some commonly used brand names are:

**In the U.S.—**

| | |
|---|---|
| Furadantin | Macrobid |
| Furalan | Macrodantin |
| Furatoin | Nitrofuracot |

Generic name product may also be available.

**In Canada—**

| | |
|---|---|
| Apo-Nitrofurantoin | Macrodantin |

## Description

Nitrofurantoin (nye-troe-fyoor-AN-toyn) belongs to the family of medicines called anti-infectives. It is used to treat infections of the urinary tract. It may also be used for other conditions as determined by your doctor.

Nitrofurantoin is available only with your doctor's prescription, in the following dosage forms:

*Oral*
- Capsules (U.S. and Canada)
- Extended-release Capsules (U.S.)
- Oral Suspension (U.S.)
- Tablets (U.S. and Canada)

## Before Using This Medicine

In deciding to use a medicine, the risks of taking the medicine must be weighed against the good it will do. This is a decision you and your doctor will make. For nitrofurantoin, the following should be considered:

**Allergies**—Tell your doctor if you have ever had any unusual or allergic reaction to nitrofurantoin or to any related medicines such as furazolidone (e.g., Furoxone) or nitrofurazone (e.g., Furacin). Also tell your health care professional if you are allergic to any other substances, such as foods, preservatives, or dyes.

**Pregnancy**—Nitrofurantoin should not be used if you are within a week or 2 of your delivery date or during labor and delivery. It may cause problems in the infant.

**Breast-feeding**—Nitrofurantoin passes into the breast milk in small amounts and may cause problems in nursing babies, especially those with glucose-6-phosphate dehydrogenase (G6PD) deficiency.

**Children**—Infants up to 1 month of age should not be given this medicine because they are especially sensitive to the effects of nitrofurantoin.

**Older adults**—Elderly people may be more sensitive to the effects of nitrofurantoin. This may increase the chance of side effects during treatment.

**Other medicines**—Although certain medicines should not be used together at all, in other cases two different medicines may be used together even if an interaction might occur. In these cases, your doctor may want to change the dose, or other precautions may be necessary. When you are taking nitrofurantoin, it is especially important that your health care professional know if you are taking any of the following:

- Acetohydroxamic acid (e.g., Lithostat) or
- Antidiabetics, oral (diabetes medicine you take by mouth) or
- Dapsone or
- Furazolidone (e.g., Furoxone) or
- Methyldopa (e.g., Aldomet) or
- Primaquine or
- Procainamide (e.g., Pronestyl) or
- Quinidine (e.g., Quinidex) or
- Sulfonamides (sulfa medicine) or
- Sulfoxone (e.g., Diasone) or
- Vitamin K (e.g., AquaMEPHYTON, Synkayvite)—Patients who take nitrofurantoin with any of these medicines may have an increase in side effects affecting the blood
- Carbamazepine (e.g., Tegretol) or
- Chloroquine (e.g., Aralen) or
- Cisplatin (e.g., Platinol) or
- Cytarabine (e.g., Cytosar-U) or
- Diphtheria, tetanus, and pertussis (DTP) vaccine or
- Disulfiram (e.g., Antabuse) or
- Ethotoin (e.g., Peganone) or
- Hydroxychloroquine (e.g., Plaquenil) or
- Lindane, topical (e.g., Kwell) or
- Lithium (e.g., Lithane) or
- Mephenytoin (e.g., Mesantoin) or
- Mexiletine (e.g., Mexitil) or
- Other anti-infectives by mouth or by injection (medicine for infection) or
- Pemoline (e.g., Cylert) or
- Phenytoin (e.g., Dilantin) or
- Pyridoxine (e.g., Hexa-Betalin) (with long-term, high-dose use) or
- Vincristine (e.g., Oncovin)—Patients who take nitrofurantoin with any of these medicines, or who have received a DTP vaccine within the last 30 days or are going to receive a DTP may have an increase in side effects affecting the nervous system
- Probenecid (e.g., Benemid) or
- Sulfinpyrazone (e.g., Anturane)—Patients who take nitrofurantoin with any of these medicines may have an increase in side effects
- Quinine (e.g., Quinamm)—Patients who take nitrofurantoin with quinine may have an increase in side effects affecting the blood and the nervous system

**Other medical problems**—The presence of other medical problems may affect the use of nitrofurantoin. Make sure you tell your doctor if you have any other medical problems, especially:

- Glucose-6-phosphate dehydrogenase (G6PD) deficiency—Nitrofurantoin may cause anemia in patients with G6PD deficiency
- Kidney disease (other than infection)—The chance of side effects of this medicine may be increased and the medicine may be less effective in patients with kidney disease
- Lung disease or
- Nerve damage—Patients with lung disease or nerve damage may have an increase in side effects when they take nitrofurantoin

## Proper Use of This Medicine

*Do not give this medicine to infants up to 1 month of age.*

Nitrofurantoin is best taken with food or milk. This may lessen stomach upset and help your body absorb the medicine better.

For patients taking the *oral liquid form of this medicine:*

- Shake the oral liquid forcefully before each dose to help make it pour more smoothly and to be sure the medicine is evenly mixed.

- Use a specially marked measuring spoon or other device to measure each dose accurately. The average household teaspoon may not hold the right amount of liquid.

- Nitrofurantoin may be mixed with water, milk, fruit juices, or infants' formulas. If it is mixed with other liquids, take the medicine immediately after mixing. Be sure to drink all the liquid in order to get the full dose of medicine.

For patients taking the *extended-release capsule* form of this medicine:

- Swallow the capsules whole.

- Do not open, crush, or chew the capsules before swallowing them.

To help clear up your infection completely, *keep taking this medicine for the full time of treatment,* even if you begin to feel better after a few days. *Do not miss any doses.*

**Dosing**—The dose of nitrofurantoin will be different for different patients. *Follow your doctor's orders or the directions on the label.* The following information includes only the average doses of nitrofurantoin. *If your dose is different, do not change it* unless your doctor tells you to do so.

- For the *capsule, oral suspension, and tablet* dosage forms:
  - —Adults and adolescents: 50 to 100 mg every six hours.
  - —Children 1 month of age and older: Dose is based on body weight and will be determined by your doctor.
  - —Children up to 1 month of age: Use is not recommended.

- For the *extended-release capsule* dosage form:
  - —Adults and children 12 years of age and older: 100 mg every twelve hours for seven days.
  - —Children up to 12 years of age: Dose must be determined by the doctor.

**Missed dose**—If you do miss a dose of this medicine, take it as soon as possible. However, if it is almost time for your next dose, skip the next dose and go back to your regular dosing schedule. Do not double doses.

**Storage**—To store this medicine:

- Keep out of the reach of children.

- Store away from heat and direct light.

- Do not store the capsule or tablet form of this medicine in the bathroom, near the kitchen sink, or in other damp places. Heat or moisture may cause the medicine to break down.

- Keep the oral liquid form of this medicine from freezing.

- Do not keep outdated medicine or medicine no longer needed. Be sure that any discarded medicine is out of the reach of children.

## Precautions While Using This Medicine

It is important that your doctor check your progress at regular visits if you will be taking this medicine for a long time.

If your symptoms do not improve within a few days, or if they become worse, check with your doctor.

For *diabetic patients:*

- *This medicine may cause false test results with some urine sugar tests.* Check with your doctor before changing your diet or the dosage of your diabetes medicine.

## Side Effects of This Medicine

Along with its needed effects, a medicine may cause some unwanted effects. Although not all of these side effects may occur, if they do occur they may need medical attention.

*Check with your doctor immediately* if any of the following side effects occur:

*More common*

Chest pain; chills; cough; fever; troubled breathing

*Less common*

Dizziness; drowsiness; headache; numbness, tingling, or burning of face or mouth; sore throat and fever; unusual muscle weakness; unusual tiredness or weakness

*Rare*

Itching; joint pain; pale skin; skin rash; yellow eyes or skin

Other side effects may occur that usually do not need medical attention. These side effects may go away during treatment as your body adjusts to the medicine. However, check with your doctor if any of the following side effects continue or are bothersome:

*More common*

Abdominal or stomach pain or upset; diarrhea; loss of appetite; nausea or vomiting

This medicine may cause the urine to become rust-yellow to brown. This side effect does not require medical attention.

Other side effects not listed above may also occur in some patients. If you notice any other effects, check with your doctor.

Revised: 01/19/93

# NONSTEROIDAL ANTI-INFLAMMATORY DRUGS   Systemic

Some commonly used brand names are:

**In the U.S.—**

| | |
|---|---|
| Advil[7] | Ibuprohm[7] |
| Advil Caplets[7] | Ibuprohm Caplets[7] |
| Advil, Children's[7] | Ibu-Tab[7] |
| Aleve[13] | Indocin[8] |
| Anaprox[13] | Indocin SR[8] |
| Anaprox DS[13] | Lodine[3] |
| Ansaid[6] | Meclomen[10] |
| Bayer Select Ibuprofen | Medipren[7] |
| Caplets[7] | Medipren Caplets[7] |
| Cataflam[1] | Midol IB[7] |
| Clinoril[17] | Motrin[7] |
| Cotylbutazone[15] | Motrin, Children's[7] |
| Cramp End[7] | Motrin-IB[7] |
| Daypro[14] | Motrin-IB Caplets[7] |
| Dolgesic[7] | Nalfon[7] |
| Dolobid[2] | Nalfon 200[4] |
| Excedrin IB[7] | Naprosyn[13] |
| Excedrin IB Caplets[7] | Nuprin[7] |
| Feldene[16] | Nuprin Caplets[7] |
| Genpril[7] | Orudis[9] |
| Genpril Caplets[7] | Oruvail[9] |
| Haltran[7] | Pamprin-IB[7] |
| Ibifon 600 Caplets[7] | Ponstel[11] |
| Ibren[7] | Relafen[12] |
| Ibu[7] | Rufen[7] |
| Ibu-200[7] | Tolectin 200[20] |
| Ibu-4[7] | Tolectin 400[20] |
| Ibu-6[7] | Tolectin 600[20] |
| Ibu-8[7] | Trendar[7] |
| Ibuprin[7] | Voltaren[1] |

**In Canada—**

| | |
|---|---|
| Actiprofen Caplets[7] | Froben SR[6] |
| Advil[7] | Idarac[5] |
| Advil Caplets[7] | Indocid[8] |
| Albert Tiafen[19] | Indocid SR[8] |
| Alka Butazolidin[15] | Medipren Caplets[7] |
| Anaprox[13] | Mobiflex[18] |
| Anaprox DS[13] | Motrin[7] |
| Ansaid[6] | Motrin-IB[7] |
| Apo-Diclo[1] | Nalfon[4] |
| Apo-Diflunisal[2] | Naprosyn[13] |
| Apo-Flurbiprofen[6] | Naprosyn-E[13] |
| Apo-Ibuprofen[7] | Naprosyn-SR[13] |
| Apo-Indomethacin[8] | Naxen[13] |
| Apo-Keto[9] | Novo-Difenac[1] |
| Apo-Keto-E[9] | Novo-Difenac SR[1] |
| Apo-Napro-Na[13] | Novo-Diflunisal[2] |
| Apo-Napro-Na DS[13] | Novo-Flurprofen[6] |
| Apo-Naproxen[13] | Novo-Keto-EC[9] |
| Apo-Phenylbutazone[15] | Novo-Methacin[8] |
| Apo-Piroxicam[16] | Novo-Naprox[13] |
| Apo-Sulin[17] | Novo-Naprox Sodium[13] |
| Butazolidin[15] | Novo-Naprox Sodium DS[13] |
| Clinoril[17] | Novo-Pirocam[16] |
| Dolobid[2] | Novo-Profen[7] |
| Feldene[16] | Novo-Sundac[17] |
| Froben[6] | Novo-Tolmetin[20] |

| | |
|---|---|
| Nu-Diclo[11] | Relafen[12] |
| Nu-Flurbiprofen[6] | Rhodis[9] |
| Nu-Ibuprofen[7] | Rhodis-EC[9] |
| Nu-Indo[8] | Surgam[19] |
| Nu-Naprox[13] | Surgam SR[19] |
| Nu-Pirox[16] | Synflex[13] |
| Nu-Sulindac[17] | Synflex DS[13] |
| Orudis[9] | Tolectin 200[20] |
| Orudis-E[9] | Tolectin 600[20] |
| Orudis-SR[9] | Tolectin DS[20] |
| Oruvail[9] | Voltaren[1] |
| Ponstan[11] | Voltaren Rapide[1] |
| | Voltaren SR[1] |

Other commonly used names are:

| | |
|---|---|
| Etodolic acid[3] | Meclofenamic acid[10] |
| Indometacin[8] | |

Note: For quick reference, the following (family name) are numbered to match the corresponding brand names.

This information applies to the following medicines:

1. Diclofenac (dye-KLOE-fen-ak)
2. Diflunisal (dye-FLOO-ni-sal)‡
3. Etodolac (ee-TOE-doe-lak)†
4. Fenoprofen (fen-oh-PROE-fen)‡
5. Floctafenine (flok-ta-FEN-een)*
6. Flurbiprofen (flure-BI-proe-fen)‡§
7. Ibuprofen (eye-byoo-PROE-fen)‡§
8. Indomethacin (in-doe-METH-a-sin)‡
9. Ketoprofen (kee-toe-PROE-fen)‡
10. Meclofenamate (me-kloe-FEN-am-ate)†‡
11. Mefenamic (me-fe-NAM-ik) Acid
12. Nabumetone (na-BYOO-me-tone)
13. Naproxen (na-PROX-en)‡
14. Oxaprozin (ox-a-PROE-zin)†
15. Phenylbutazone (fen-ill-BYOO-ta-zone)‡
16. Piroxicam (peer-OX-i-kam)‡
17. Sulindac (sul-IN-dak)‡
18. Tenoxicam (ten-OX-i-kam)*
19. Tiaprofenic (tie-a-pro-FEN-ik) Acid*
20. Tolmetin (TOLE-met-in)‡

This information does *not* apply to aspirin or other salicylates or to ketorolac (e.g., Toradol).

*Not commercially available in the U.S.
†Not commercially available in Canada.
‡Generic name product may also be available in the U.S.
§Generic name product may also be available in the Canada.

## Description

Nonsteroidal anti-inflammatory drugs (also called NSAIDs) are used to relieve some symptoms caused by arthritis (rheumatism), such as inflammation, swelling, stiffness, and joint pain. However, this medicine does not cure arthritis and will help you only as long as you continue to take it.

Some of these medicines are also used to relieve other kinds of pain or to treat other painful conditions, such as:

- gout attacks;
- bursitis;
- tendinitis;
- sprains, strains, or other injuries; or
- menstrual cramps.

Ibuprofen and naproxen are also used to reduce fever.

Meclofenamate is also used to reduce the amount of bleeding in some women who have very heavy menstrual periods.

Nonsteroidal anti-inflammatory drugs may also be used to treat other conditions as determined by your doctor.

Any nonsteroidal anti-inflammatory drug can cause side effects, especially when it is used for a long time or in large doses. Some of the side effects are painful or uncomfortable. Others can be more serious, resulting in the need for medical care and sometimes even death. If you will be taking this medicine for more than one or two months or in large amounts, you should discuss with your doctor the good that it can do as well as the risks of taking it. Also, it is a good idea to ask your doctor about other forms of treatment that might help to reduce the amount of this medicine that you take and/or the length of treatment.

One of the nonsteroidal anti-inflammatory drugs, phenylbutazone, is especially likely to cause very serious side effects. These serious side effects are more likely to occur in patients 40 years of age or older than in younger adults, and the risk becomes greater as the patient's age increases. Before you take phenylbutazone, be sure that you have discussed its use with your doctor. *Also, do not use phenylbutazone to treat any painful condition other than the one for which it was prescribed by your doctor.*

Although ibuprofen and naproxen may be used instead of aspirin to treat many of the same medical problems, they must not be used by people who are allergic to aspirin.

The 200-mg strength of ibuprofen and the 220-mg strength of naproxen are available without a prescription. However, your health care professional may have special instructions on the proper dose of these medicines for your medical condition.

Other nonsteroidal anti-inflammatory drugs and other strengths of ibuprofen and naproxen are available only with your medical doctor's or dentist's prescription. These medicines are available in the following dosage forms:

*Oral*

Diclofenac
- Tablets (U.S. and Canada)
- Delayed-release tablets (U.S. and Canada)
- Extended-release tablets (Canada)

Diflunisal
- Tablets (U.S. and Canada)

Etodolac
- Capsules (U.S.)
- Tablets (U.S.)

Fenoprofen
- Capsules (U.S. and Canada)
- Tablets (U.S. and Canada)

Floctafenine
- Tablets (Canada)

Flurbiprofen
- Extended-release capsules (Canada)
- Tablets (U.S. and Canada)

Ibuprofen
- Oral suspension (U.S.)
- Tablets (U.S. and Canada)

Indomethacin
- Capsules (U.S. and Canada)
- Extended-release capsules (U.S. and Canada)
- Oral suspension (U.S.)

Ketoprofen
- Capsules (U.S. and Canada)
- Extended-release capsules (U.S. and Canada)
- Delayed-release tablets (Canada)
- Extended-release tablets (Canada)

Meclofenamate
- Capsules (U.S.)

Mefenamic Acid
- Capsules (U.S. and Canada)

Nabumetone
- Tablets (U.S. and Canada)

Naproxen
- Oral suspension (U.S. and Canada)
- Tablets (U.S. and Canada)
- Delayed-release tablets (Canada)
- Extended-release tablets (Canada)

Oxaprozin
- Tablets (U.S.)

Phenylbutazone
- Capsules (U.S.)
- Tablets (U.S. and Canada)
- Buffered tablets (Canada)

Piroxicam
- Capsules (U.S. and Canada)

Sulindac
- Tablets (U.S. and Canada)

Tenoxicam
- Tablets (Canada)

Tiaprofenic Acid
- Extended-release capsules (Canada)
- Tablets (Canada)

Tolmetin
- Capsules (U.S. and Canada)
- Tablets (U.S. and Canada)

*Rectal*

Diclofenac
- Suppositories (Canada)

Indomethacin
- Suppositories (U.S. and Canada)

Ketoprofen
- Suppositories (Canada)

Naproxen
- Suppositories (Canada)

Piroxicam
- Suppositories (Canada)

## Before Using This Medicine

In deciding to use a medicine, the risks of taking the medicine must be weighed against the good it will do.

This is a decision you and your health care professional will make. For the nonsteroidal anti-inflammatory drugs, the following should be considered:

**Allergies**—Tell your health care professional if you have ever had any unusual or allergic reaction to any of the nonsteroidal anti-inflammatory drugs, or to any of the following medicines:

- Aspirin or other salicylates
- Ketorolac (e.g., Toradol)
- Oxyphenbutazone (e.g., Oxalid, Tandearil)
- Suprofen (e.g., Suprol)
- Zomepirac (e.g., Zomax)

Also tell your health care professional if you are allergic to any other substances, such as foods, preservatives, or dyes.

**Diet**—Make certain your health care professional knows if you are on any special diet, such as a low-sodium or low-sugar diet. Some of these medicines contain sodium or sugar.

**Pregnancy**—Studies on birth defects with these medicines have not been done in humans. However, there is a chance that these medicines may cause unwanted effects on the heart or blood flow of the fetus or newborn baby if they are taken regularly during the last few months of pregnancy. Also, studies in animals have shown that these medicines, if taken late in pregnancy, may increase the length of pregnancy, prolong labor, or cause other problems during delivery. If you are pregnant, do not take any of these medicines, including nonprescription (over-the-counter [OTC]) ibuprofen or naproxen, without first discussing its use with your doctor.

Studies in animals have not shown that fenoprofen, floctafenine, flurbiprofen, ibuprofen, ketoprofen, nabumetone, naproxen, phenylbutazone, piroxicam, tiaprofenic acid, or tolmetin causes birth defects. Diflunisal caused birth defects of the spine and ribs in rabbits, but not in mice or rats. Diclofenac and meclofenamate caused unwanted effects on the formation of bones in animals. Etodolac and oxaprozin caused birth defects in animals. Indomethacin caused slower development of bones and damage to nerves in animals. In some animal studies, sulindac caused unwanted effects on the development of bones and organs. Studies on birth defects with mefenamic acid have not been done in animals.

Even though most of these medicines did not cause birth defects in animals, many of them did cause other harmful or toxic effects on the fetus, usually when they were given in such large amounts that the pregnant animals became sick.

**Breast-feeding—**

- *For indomethacin:* Indomethacin passes into the breast milk and has been reported to cause unwanted effects in nursing babies.
- *For meclofenamate:* Use of meclofenamate by nursing mothers is not recommended because in animal studies it caused unwanted effects on the newborn's development.

- *For phenylbutazone:* Phenylbutazone passes into the breast milk and may cause unwanted effects, such as blood problems, in nursing babies.
- *For piroxicam:* Studies in animals have shown that piroxicam may decrease the amount of milk.

Although other anti-inflammatory analgesics have not been reported to cause problems in nursing babies, diclofenac, diflunisal, fenoprofen, flurbiprofen, meclofenamate, mefenamic acid, naproxen, piroxicam, and tolmetin pass into the breast milk. It is not known whether etodolac, floctafenine, ibuprofen, ketoprofen, nabumetone, oxaprozin, sulindac, or tiaprofenic acid passes into human breast milk.

**Children—**

- *For ibuprofen:* Ibuprofen has been tested in children 6 months of age and older. It has not been shown to cause different side effects or problems than it does in adults.
- *For indomethacin and for tolmetin:* Indomethacin and tolmetin have been tested in children 2 years of age and older and have not been shown to cause different side effects or problems than they do in adults.
- *For naproxen:* Studies with naproxen in children 2 years of age and older have shown that skin rash may be more likely to occur.
- *For oxaprozin:* Oxaprozin has been used in children with arthritis. However, there is no specific information comparing use of this medicine in children with use in other age groups.
- *For phenylbutazone:* Use of phenylbutazone in children up to 15 years of age is not recommended.
- *For other anti-inflammatory analgesics:* There is no specific information on the use of other anti-inflammatory analgesics in children.

Most of these medicines, especially indomethacin and phenylbutazone, can cause serious side effects in any patient. Therefore, it is especially important that you discuss with the child's doctor the good that this medicine may do as well as the risks of using it.

**Older adults**—Certain side effects, such as confusion, swelling of the face, feet, or lower legs, or sudden decrease in the amount of urine, may be especially likely to occur in elderly patients, who are usually more sensitive than younger adults to the effects of nonsteroidal anti-inflammatory drugs. Also, elderly people are more likely than younger adults to get very sick if these medicines cause stomach problems. With phenylbutazone, blood problems may also be more likely to occur in the elderly.

**Other medicines**—Although certain medicines should not be used together at all, in other cases two different medicines may be used together even if an interaction might occur. In these cases, your doctor may want to change the dose, or other precautions may be necessary. When you are taking a nonsteroidal anti-inflammatory drug, it is especially important that your health care professional know if you are taking any of the following:

- Anticoagulants (blood thinners) or
- Cefamandole (e.g., Mandol) or
- Cefoperazone (e.g., Cefobid) or
- Cefotetan (e.g., Cefotan) or
- Heparin or
- Plicamycin (e.g., Mithracin) or
- Valproic acid—The chance of bleeding may be increased
- Aspirin—The chance of serious side effects may be increased if aspirin is used together with a nonsteroidal anti-inflammatory drug on a regular basis
- Ciprofloxacin (e.g., Cipro) or
- Enoxacin (e.g., Penetrex) or
- Itraconazole (e.g., Sporanox) or
- Ketoconazole (e.g., Nizoral) or
- Lomefloxacin (e.g., Maxaquin) or
- Norfloxacin (e.g., Noroxin) or
- Ofloxacin (e.g., Floxin) or
- Tetracyclines, oral—The buffered form of phenylbutazone (e.g., Alka Butazolidin) may keep these medicines from working properly if the 2 medicines are taken too close together
- Cyclosporine (e.g., Sandimmune) or
- Digitalis glycosides (heart medicine) or
- Lithium (e.g., Lithane) or
- Methotrexate (e.g., Mexate) or
- Phenytoin (e.g., Dilantin)—Higher blood levels of these medicines and an increased chance of side effects may occur
- Penicillamine (e.g., Cuprimine)—The chance of serious side effects may be increased, especially with phenylbutazone (e.g., Cotylbutazone)
- Probenecid (e.g., Benemid)—Higher blood levels of the nonsteroidal anti-inflammatory drug and an increased chance of side effects may occur
- Triamterene (e.g., Dyrenium)—The chance of kidney problems may be increased, especially with indomethacin
- Zidovudine (e.g., AZT, Retrovir)—The chance of serious side effects may be increased, especially with indomethacin

**Other medical problems**—The presence of other medical problems may affect the use of nonsteroidal anti-inflammatory drugs. Make sure you tell your doctor if you have any other medical problems, especially:

- Alcohol abuse or
- Bleeding problems or
- Colitis, Crohn's disease, diverticulitis, stomach ulcer, or other stomach or intestinal problems or
- Diabetes mellitus (sugar diabetes) or
- Hemorrhoids or
- Hepatitis or other liver disease or
- Kidney disease (or history of) or
- Rectal irritation or bleeding, recent, or
- Systemic lupus erythematosus (SLE) or
- Tobacco use (or recent history of)—The chance of side effects may be increased
- Anemia or
- Asthma or
- Epilepsy or
- Fluid retention (swelling of feet or lower legs) or
- Heart disease or
- High blood pressure or
- Kidney stones (or history of) or

- Low platelet count or
- Low white blood cell count or
- Mental illness or
- Parkinson's disease or
- Polymyalgia rheumatica or
- Porphyria or
- Temporal arteritis—Some nonsteroidal anti-inflammatory drugs may make these conditions worse
- Ulcers, sores, or white spots in mouth—Ulcers, sores, or white spots in the mouth sometimes mean that the medicine is causing serious side effects; if these sores or spots are already present before you start taking the medicine, it will be harder for you and your doctor to recognize that these side effects might be occurring

## Proper Use of This Medicine

For patients taking *a capsule, tablet (including caplet), or liquid form* of this medicine:

- *Take tablet or capsule forms of these medicines with a full glass (8 ounces) of water.* Also, do not lie down for about 15 to 30 minutes after taking the medicine. This helps to prevent irritation that may lead to trouble in swallowing.
- To lessen stomach upset, these medicines should be taken with food or an antacid. This is especially important when you are taking indomethacin, mefenamic acid, phenylbutazone, or piroxicam, which should always be taken with food or an antacid. Taking the extended-release tablet dosage form of flurbiprofen or naproxen and taking nabumetone with food may also help the medicine be absorbed into your body more quickly. However, your doctor may want you to take the first 1 or 2 doses of other nonsteroidal anti-inflammatory drugs 30 minutes before meals or 2 hours after meals. This helps the medicine start working a little faster when you first begin to take it. However, after the first few doses, take the medicine with food or an antacid.
- It is not necessary to take delayed-release (enteric-coated) tablets with food or an antacid, because the enteric coating helps protect your stomach from the irritating effects of the medicine. Also, it is not necessary to take ketoprofen extended-release capsules (e.g., Oruvail) with food or an antacid, because the medicine inside the capsules is enteric coated.
- If you will be taking your medicine together with an antacid, one that contains magnesium and aluminum hydroxides (e.g., Maalox) may be the best kind of antacid to use, unless your doctor has directed you to use another antacid. However, do not mix the liquid form of ibuprofen, indomethacin, or naproxen together with an antacid, or any other liquid, before taking it. To do so may cause the medicine to break down. If stomach upset (indigestion, nausea, vomiting, stomach pain, or diarrhea) continues or if you have any questions about how you should be taking this medicine, check with your health care professional.
- Some of these medicines must be swallowed whole. Tablets should not be crushed, chewed, or broken, and capsules should not be emptied out, before you

take the medicine. These include delayed-release (enteric-coated) or extended-release tablets or capsules, diflunisal tablets (e.g., Dolobid), and phenylbutazone tablets (e.g., Butazolidin). If you are not sure whether you are taking a delayed-release or extended-release form of your medicine, check with your pharmacist.

For patients using *a suppository form* of this medicine:

- If the suppository is too soft to insert, chill it in the refrigerator for 30 minutes or run cold water over it before removing the foil wrapper.
- To insert the suppository: First remove the foil wrapper and moisten the suppository with cold water. Lie down on your side and use your finger to push the suppository well up into the rectum.
- Indomethacin suppositories should be kept inside the rectum for at least one hour so that all of the medicine can be absorbed by your body. This helps the medicine work better.

For patients taking *nonprescription (over-the-counter [OTC]) ibuprofen or naproxen:*

- This medicine comes with a patient information sheet. Read it carefully. If you have any questions about this information, check with your health care professional.

*For safe and effective use of this medicine, do not take more of it, do not take it more often, and do not take it for a longer time than ordered by your health care professional or directed on the nonprescription (over-the-counter [OTC]) package label.* Taking too much of any of these medicines may increase the chance of unwanted effects, especially in elderly patients.

*When used for severe or continuing arthritis, a nonsteroidal anti-inflammatory drug must be taken regularly as ordered by your doctor* in order for it to help you. These medicines usually begin to work within one week, but in severe cases up to two weeks or even longer may pass before you begin to feel better. Also, several weeks may pass before you feel the full effects of the medicine.

For patients taking *mefenamic acid:*

- *Always take mefenamic acid with food or antacids.*
- *Do not take mefenamic acid for more than 7 days at a time* unless otherwise directed by your doctor. To do so may increase the chance of side effects, especially in elderly patients.

For patients taking *phenylbutazone:*

- Phenylbutazone is intended to treat your current medical problem only. *Do not take it for any other aches or pains.* Also, phenylbutazone should be used for the shortest time possible because of the chance of serious side effects, especially in patients who are 40 years of age or older.

**Dosing**—The dose of these medicines will be different for different patients. *Follow your doctor's orders or the directions on the label.* The following information includes only the average doses of these medicines. *If your dose is different, do not change it* unless your doctor tells you to do so.

The number of capsules or tablets or teaspoonfuls of suspension that you take, or the number of suppositories that you use, depends on the strength of the medicine. Also, *the number of doses you take each day, the time allowed between doses, and the length of time you take the medicine depend on the medical problem for which you are taking the medicine.*

People with arthritis usually need to take more of a nonsteroidal anti-inflammatory drug during a "flare-up" than they do between "flare-ups" of arthritis symptoms. Therefore, your dose may need to be increased or decreased as your condition changes.

*For diclofenac*

- For *tablet* dosage form:
  —For relieving pain or menstrual cramps:
  - Adults—50 milligrams (mg) three times a day as needed. Your doctor may direct you to take 100 mg for the first dose only.
  - Children—Use and dose must be determined by your doctor.
  —For rheumatoid arthritis:
  - Adults—At first, 50 mg three or four times a day. Your doctor may increase the dose, if necessary, up to a total of 225 mg a day. After your condition improves your doctor may direct you to take a lower dose.
  - Children—Use and dose must be determined by your doctor.
  —For osteoarthritis:
  - Adults—At first, 50 mg two or three times a day. Usually, no more than a total of 150 mg a day should be taken. After your condition improves your doctor may direct you to take a lower dose.
  - Children—Use and dose must be determined by your doctor.
  —For spondylitis (lower back pain):
  - Adults—At first, 25 mg four or five times a day. After your condition improves your doctor may direct you to take a lower dose.
  - Children—Use and dose must be determined by your doctor.
- For *delayed-release tablet* dosage form:
  —For rheumatoid arthritis:
  - Adults—At first, 50 mg three or four times a day. Your doctor may increase the dose, if necessary, up to a total of 225 mg a day. After your condition improves your doctor may direct you to take a lower dose.
  - Children—Use and dose must be determined by your doctor.
  —For osteoarthritis:
  - Adults—At first, 50 mg two or three times a day. Usually, no more than a total of 150 mg a

day should be taken. After your condition improves your doctor may direct you to take a lower dose.

• Children—Use and dose must be determined by your doctor.

—For spondylitis (lower back pain):

• Adults—At first, 25 mg four or five times a day. After your condition improves your doctor may direct you to take a lower dose.

• Children—Use and dose must be determined by your doctor.

• For *extended-release tablet* dosage form:

—For rheumatoid arthritis, osteoarthritis, or spondylitis:

• Adults—Usually 75 or 100 mg once a day, in the morning or evening. Some people may need 75 mg twice a day, in the morning and evening. Take the medicine at the same time every day.

• Children—Use and dose must be determined by your doctor.

• For *rectal* dosage form (suppositories):

—For rheumatoid arthritis, osteoarthritis, or spondylitis:

• Adults—One 50-mg or 100-mg suppository, inserted into the rectum. The suppository is usually used only at night by people who take tablets during the day. Usually, no more than a total of 150 mg of diclofenac should be used in a day from all dosage forms combined.

• Children—Use and dose must be determined by your doctor.

### For diflunisal

• For *oral* dosage form (tablets):

—For pain:

• Adults—1000 milligrams (mg) for the first dose, then 500 mg every eight to twelve hours as needed. Some people may need only 500 mg for the first dose, then 250 mg every eight to twelve hours as needed. Usually, no more than a total of 1500 mg a day should be taken.

• Children—Dose must be determined by your doctor.

—For rheumatoid arthritis or osteoarthritis:

• Adults—At first, 250 or 500 mg twice a day. Your doctor may increase the dose, if necessary, up to a total of 1500 mg a day. After your condition improves your doctor may direct you to take a lower dose.

• Children—Dose must be determined by your doctor.

### For etodolac

• For *oral* dosage forms (capsules or tablets):

—For pain:

• Adults—400 milligrams (mg) for the first dose, then 200 to 400 mg every six to eight hours as needed. Usually, no more than a total of 1200 mg a day should be taken.

• Children—Use and dose must be determined by your doctor.

—For osteoarthritis:

• Adults—At first, 400 mg two or three times a day or 300 mg three or four times a day. Usually, no more than a total of 1200 mg a day should be taken. After your condition improves your doctor may direct you to take a lower dose.

• Children—Use and dose must be determined by your doctor.

### For fenoprofen

• For *oral* dosage forms (capsules or tablets):

—For pain:

• Adults—200 milligrams (mg) every four to six hours as needed.

• Children—Use and dose must be determined by your doctor.

—For arthritis:

• Adults—At first, 300 to 600 mg three or four times a day. Your doctor may increase the dose, if necessary, up to a total of 3200 mg a day. After your condition improves your doctor may direct you to take a lower dose.

• Children—Use and dose must be determined by your doctor.

### For floctafenine

• For *oral* dosage form (tablets):

—For pain:

• Adults—200 to 400 milligrams (mg) every six to eight hours, as needed. Usually, no more than 1200 mg a day should be taken.

• Children—Use is not recommended.

### For flurbiprofen

• For *oral tablet* dosage form:

—For menstrual cramps:

• Adults—50 milligrams (mg) four times a day.

• Children—Use and dose must be determined by your doctor.

—For bursitis, tendinitis, or athletic injuries:

• Adults—50 mg every four to six hours as needed.

• Children—Use and dose must be determined by your doctor.

—For rheumatoid arthritis or osteoarthritis:

• Adults—At first, 200 to 300 mg a day, divided into smaller amounts that are taken two to four times a day. Usually, no more than a total of 300 mg a day should be taken. After your condition improves your doctor may direct you to take a lower dose.

• Children—Use and dose must be determined by your doctor.

—For spondylitis (lower back pain):

• Adults—At first, 50 mg four times a day. Your doctor may increase the dose, if necessary, up to a total of 300 mg a day. After your condition

improves your doctor may direct you to take a lower dose.
- Children—Use and dose must be determined by your doctor.
- For *extended-release capsule* dosage form:
  —For arthritis:
    - Adults—200 mg once a day, in the evening. Take the medicine at the same time every day.
    - Children—Use and dose must be determined by your doctor.

*For ibuprofen*
- For *oral* dosage forms (tablets or oral suspension):
  —For pain or menstrual cramps:
    - Adults and teenagers—200 to 400 milligrams (mg) every four to six hours as needed. If you are taking the medicine without a prescription from your health care professional, do not take more than a total of 1200 mg (six 200-mg tablets) a day.
    - Children up to 12 years of age—Use and dose must be determined by your doctor.
  —For fever:
    - Adults and teenagers—200 to 400 mg every four to six hours as needed. If you are taking the medicine without a prescription from your health care professional, do not take more than a total of 1200 mg (six 200-mg tablets) a day.
    - Children 6 months to 12 years of age—The medicine should be used only with a prescription from your doctor. The dose is based on body weight and on the body temperature. For fevers lower than 102.5 °F (39.2 °C) the dose is 5 mg per kilogram (kg) (about 2.2 mg per pound) of body weight. For higher fevers the dose is 10 mg per kg (about 4.5 mg per pound) of body weight.
    - Infants younger than 6 months of age—Use and dose must be determined by your doctor.
  —For arthritis:
    - Adults and teenagers—At first, a total of 1200 to 3200 mg a day, divided into smaller amounts that are taken three or four times a day. After your condition improves your doctor may direct you to take a lower dose.
    - Children 6 months to 12 years of age—The dose is based on body weight. At first, a total of 30 to 40 mg per kg (about 13.6 to 18 mg per pound) of body weight a day, divided into smaller amounts that are taken three or four times a day. Your doctor may increase the dose, if necessary, up to a total of 50 mg per kg (about 21 mg per pound) of body weight a day. After your condition improves your doctor may direct you to take a lower dose.
    - Infants younger than 6 months of age—Use and dose must be determined by your doctor.

*For indomethacin*
- For *capsule or oral suspension* dosage forms:
  —For arthritis:
    - Adults—At first, 25 or 50 milligrams (mg) two to four times a day. Your doctor may increase the dose, if necessary, up to a total of 200 mg a day. After your condition improves your doctor may direct you to take a lower dose.
    - Children—The dose is based on body weight. At first, 1.5 to 2.5 mg per kilogram (kg) (about 0.7 to 1.1 mg per pound) of body weight a day, divided into smaller amounts that are taken three or four times a day. Your doctor may increase the dose, if necessary, up to a total of 4 mg per kg (about 1.8 mg per pound) of body weight or 200 mg a day, whichever is less. After your condition improves your doctor may direct you to take a lower dose.
  —For gout:
    - Adults—100 mg for the first dose, then 50 mg three times a day. After the pain is relieved, your doctor may direct you to take a lower dose for a while before stopping treatment completely.
    - Children—Use and dose must be determined by your doctor.
  —For bursitis or tendinitis:
    - Adults—25 mg three or four times a day or 50 mg three times a day.
    - Children—Use and dose must be determined by your doctor.
- For *extended-release capsule* dosage form:
  —For arthritis:
    - Adults—75 mg once a day, in the morning or evening. Some people may need to take 75 mg twice a day, in the morning and evening. Take the medicine at the same time each day.
    - Children—Dose must be determined by your doctor.
- For *rectal suppository* dosage form:
  —For arthritis, bursitis, tendinitis, or gout:
    - Adults—One 50-mg suppository, inserted into the rectum up to four times a day.
    - Children—One 50-mg suppository, inserted into the rectum up to four times a day. The suppository dosage form is too strong for small children. However, the suppositories may be used for large or heavy children if they need doses as large as 50 mg.

*For ketoprofen*
- For *capsule or delayed-release tablet* dosage forms:
  —For pain or menstrual cramps:
    - Adults—25 to 50 milligrams (mg) every six to eight hours as needed. Some people may need to take as much as 75 mg every six to eight hours. Doses larger than 75 mg are not likely to give better relief.

• Children—Use and dose must be determined by your doctor.

—For arthritis:

• Adults—At first, 50 mg four times a day or 75 mg three times a day. Your doctor may increase the dose, if necessary, up to a total of 300 mg a day. After your condition improves your doctor may direct you to take a lower dose.

• Children—Use and dose must be determined by your doctor.

• For *extended-release capsule or extended-release tablet* dosage forms:

—For arthritis:

• Adults—150 or 200 mg once a day, in the morning or evening. Take the medicine at the same time every day.

• Children—Use and dose must be determined by your doctor.

• For *rectal suppository* dosage form:

—For arthritis:

• Adults—50 or 100 mg twice a day, inserted into the rectum, in the morning and evening. Sometimes, the suppository is used only at night by people who take an oral dosage form (capsules or delayed-release tablets) during the day. Usually, no more than a total of 300 mg of ketoprofen should be used in a day from all dosage forms combined.

• Children—Use and dose must be determined by your doctor.

*For meclofenamate*

• For *oral* dosage form (capsules):

—For arthritis:

• Adults and teenagers 14 years of age and older—At first, 50 milligrams (mg) four times a day. Your doctor may increase the dose, if necessary, up to a total of 400 mg a day. After your condition improves your doctor may direct you to take a lower dose.

• Children up to 14 years of age—Use and dose must be determined by your doctor.

—For pain:

• Adults and teenagers 14 years of age and older—50 mg every four to six hours. Some people may need as much as 100 mg every four to six hours.

• Children up to 14 years of age—Use and dose must be determined by your doctor.

—For menstrual cramps and heavy menstrual bleeding:

• Adults and teenagers 14 years of age and older—100 mg three times a day for up to six days.

• Children up to 14 years of age—Use and dose must be determined by your doctor.

*For mefenamic acid*

• For *oral* dosage form (capsules):

—For pain and for menstrual cramps:

• Adults and teenagers 14 years of age and older—500 milligrams (mg) for the first dose, then 250 mg every six hours as needed for up to seven days.

• Children up to 14 years of age—Use and dose must be determined by your doctor.

*For nabumetone*

• For *oral* dosage form (tablets):

—For arthritis:

• Adults—At first, 1000 milligrams (mg) once a day, in the morning or evening, or 500 mg twice a day, in the morning and evening. Your doctor may increase the dose, if necessary, up to a total of 2000 mg a day. After your condition improves your doctor may direct you to take a lower dose.

• Children—Use and dose must be determined by your doctor.

*For naproxen*

• For *naproxen (e.g., Naprosyn) tablet, oral suspension, and delayed-release tablet* dosage forms:

—For arthritis:

• Adults—At first, 250, 375, or 500 milligrams (mg) two times a day, in the morning and evening. Your doctor may increase the dose, if necessary, up to a total of 1500 mg a day. After your condition improves your doctor may direct you to take a lower dose.

• Children—The dose is based on body weight. At first, 5 mg per kilogram (kg) (about 2.25 mg per pound) of body weight twice a day. After your condition improves your doctor may direct you to take a lower dose.

—For bursitis, tendinitis, menstrual cramps, and other kinds of pain:

• Adults—500 mg for the first dose, then 250 mg every six to eight hours as needed.

• Children—Use and dose must be determined by your doctor.

—For gout:

• Adults—750 mg for the first dose, then 250 mg every eight hours until the attack is relieved.

• Children—Use and dose must be determined by your doctor.

• For *naproxen extended-release tablet (e.g., Naprosyn-E)* dosage form:

—For arthritis:

• Adults—750 mg once a day, in the morning or evening.

• Children—The extended-release tablets are too strong for use in children.

- For *naproxen (e.g., Naprosyn) rectal suppository* dosage form:
  - —For arthritis:
    - Adults—One 500-mg suppository, inserted into the rectum at bedtime. The suppository is usually used only at night by people who take an oral dosage form (tablets, oral suspension, or delayed-release tablets) during the day. Usually, no more than a total of 1500 mg of naproxen should be used in a day from all dosage forms combined.
    - Children—The suppositories are too strong for use in children.
- For *naproxen sodium (e.g., Aleve, Anaprox) tablet* dosage form:
  - —For arthritis:
    - Adults—At first, 275 or 550 mg two times a day, in the morning and evening, or 275 mg in the morning and 550 mg in the evening. Your doctor may increase the dose, if necessary, up to a total of 1650 mg a day. After your condition improves your doctor may direct you to take a lower dose.
    - Children—Naproxen sodium tablets are too strong for most children. Naproxen (e.g., Naprosyn) tablets or oral suspension are usually used for children.
  - —For bursitis and tendinitis:
    - Adults—550 mg for the first dose, then 275 mg every six to eight hours as needed.
    - Children—Use and dose must be determined by your doctor. Naproxen sodium tablets are too strong for most children.
  - —For gout:
    - Adults—825 mg for the first dose, then 275 mg every eight hours until the attack is relieved.
    - Children—Use and dose must be determined by your doctor. Naproxen sodium tablets are too strong for most children.
  - —For pain, fever, and menstrual cramps:
    - Adults and children 12 years of age or older—For nonprescription (over-the-counter [OTC]) use: 220 mg (one tablet) every eight to twelve hours as needed. Some people may get better relief if they take 440 mg (two tablets) for the first dose, then 220 mg twelve hours later on the first day only. If you are taking this medicine without a prescription from your health care professional, do not take more than three 220-mg tablets a day. If you are older than 65 years of age, do not take more than two 220-mg tablets a day. Your health care professional may direct you to take larger doses.
    - Children up to 12 years of age—Use and dose must be determined by your doctor.

- For *oxaprozin*
  - For *oral* dosage form (tablets):
    - —For arthritis:
      - Adults—At first, 600 milligrams (mg) once or twice a day, or 1200 mg once a day. Some people may need a larger amount for the first dose only. Your doctor may increase the dose, if necessary, up to 1800 mg a day. This large dose should always be divided into smaller amounts that are taken two or three times a day. After your condition improves your doctor may direct you to take a lower dose.
      - Children—Use and dose must be determined by your doctor.
- For *phenylbutazone*
  - For *oral* dosage forms (capsules, tablets, and buffered tablets):
    - —For severe arthritis:
      - Adults and teenagers 15 years of age and older—At first, 100 milligrams (mg) three or four times a day. Some people may need a higher dose of 200 mg three times a day. After your condition improves your doctor may direct you to take a lower dose for a while before stopping treatment completely. This medicine should not be taken for longer than a few weeks.
      - Children up to 15 years of age—Use is not recommended.
    - —For gout:
      - Adults—400 mg for the first dose, then 100 mg every four hours for one week or less.
      - Children up to 15 years of age—Use is not recommended.
- For *piroxicam*
  - For *oral* dosage form (capsules):
    - —For arthritis:
      - Adults—20 milligrams (mg) once a day or 10 mg twice a day.
      - Children—Dose must be determined by your doctor.
    - —For menstrual cramps:
      - Adults—40 mg once a day for one day only, then 20 mg once a day if needed.
      - Children—Dose must be determined by your doctor.
  - For *rectal* dosage form (suppositories):
    - —For arthritis:
      - Adults—20 mg once a day or 10 mg twice a day.
      - Children—Dose must be determined by your doctor.
- For *sulindac*
  - For *oral* dosage form (tablets):
    - —For arthritis:
      - Adults—At first, 150 or 200 milligrams (mg) twice a day. After your condition improves, your doctor may direct you to take a lower dose.

- Children—Use and dose must be determined by your doctor.

—For gout, bursitis, or tendinitis:

- Adults—At first, 200 mg twice a day. After the pain is relieved, your doctor may direct you to take a lower dose for a while before treatment is stopped completely.
- Children—Use and dose must be determined by your doctor.

*For tenoxicam*
- For *oral* dosage form (tablets):
   —For arthritis:
   - Adults and teenagers 16 years of age and older—At first, 20 milligrams (mg) once a day, at the same time each day. For some people, a smaller dose of 10 mg (one-half tablet) a day may be enough.
   - Children and teenagers up to 16 years of age— Dose must be determined by your doctor.

*For tiaprofenic acid*
- For *oral tablet* dosage form:
   —For arthritis:
   - Adults—At first, 200 milligrams (mg) three times a day or 300 mg twice a day. After your condition improves, your doctor may direct you to take a lower dose.
   - Children—Use and dose must be determined by your doctor.
- For *extended-release capsule* dosage form:
   —For arthritis:
   - Adults—600 mg (two capsules) once a day, at the same time each day.
   - Children—Use and dose must be determined by your doctor.

*For tolmetin*
- For *oral* dosage forms (capsules or tablets):
   —For arthritis:
   - Adults—At first, 400 milligrams (mg) three times a day. Your doctor may increase the dose, if necessary, up to a total of 1800 mg a day. After your condition improves, your doctor may direct you to take a lower dose.
   - Children 2 years of age and older—The dose is based on body weight. At first, 20 mg per kilogram (kg) (about 9 mg per pound) of body weight a day, divided into smaller amounts that are taken three or four times a day. Your doctor may increase the dose, if necessary, up to 30 mg per kg (about 13.5 mg per pound) of body weight a day. After your condition improves, your doctor may direct you to take a lower dose.
   - Children up to 2 years of age—Dose must be determined by your doctor.

**Missed dose**—If your health care professional has ordered you to take this medicine according to a regular schedule, and you miss a dose, take it as soon as you remember. However, if it is almost time for your next dose, skip the missed dose and go back to your regular dosing schedule. (For long-acting medicines or extended-release dosage forms that are only taken once or twice a day, take the missed dose only if you remember within an hour or two after the dose should have been taken. If you do not remember until later, skip the missed dose and go back to your regular dosing schedule.) Do not double doses.

**Storage**—To store this medicine:
- Keep out of the reach of children.
- Store away from heat and direct light.
- Do not store tablets or capsules in the bathroom, near the kitchen sink, or in other damp places. Heat or moisture may cause the medicine to break down.
- Keep liquid and suppository forms of this medicine from freezing.
- Do not keep outdated medicine or medicine no longer needed. Be sure that any discarded medicine is out of the reach of children.

---

## Precautions While Using This Medicine

*If you will be taking this medicine for a long time, as for arthritis (rheumatism), your doctor should check your progress at regular visits.* Your doctor may want to do certain tests to find out if unwanted effects are occurring, especially if you are taking phenylbutazone. The tests are very important because serious side effects, including ulcers, bleeding, or blood problems, can occur without any warning.

Stomach problems may be more likely to occur if you drink alcoholic beverages while being treated with this medicine. Also, alcohol may add to the depressant side effects of phenylbutazone. Therefore, *do not regularly drink alcoholic beverages while taking this medicine,* unless otherwise directed by your doctor.

Taking two or more of the nonsteroidal anti-inflammatory drugs together on a regular basis may increase the chance of unwanted effects. Also, taking acetaminophen, aspirin or other salicylates, or ketorolac (e.g., Toradol) regularly while you are taking a nonsteroidal anti-inflammatory drug may increase the chance of unwanted effects. The risk will depend on how much of each medicine you take every day, and on how long you take the medicines together. If your health care professional directs you to take these medicines together on a regular basis, follow his or her directions carefully. However, *do not take acetaminophen or aspirin or other salicylates together with this medicine for more than a few days, and do not take any ketorolac (e.g., Toradol) while you are taking this medicine, unless your doctor has directed you to do so and is following your progress.*

Before having any kind of surgery (including dental surgery), tell the medical doctor or dentist in charge that you are taking this medicine. If possible, this should be done when your surgery is first being planned. Some of the nonsteroidal anti-inflammatory drugs can increase the chance of bleeding during and after surgery. It may be necessary for you to stop treatment for a while, or to change to a different nonsteroidal anti-inflammatory drug that is less likely to cause bleeding.

This medicine may cause some people to become confused, drowsy, dizzy, lightheaded, or less alert than they are normally. It may also cause blurred vision or other vision problems in some people. *Make sure you know how you react to this medicine before you drive, use machines, or do anything else that could be dangerous if you are confused, dizzy, or drowsy, or if you are not alert and able to see well.* If these reactions are especially bothersome, check with your doctor.

For patients taking *the buffered form of phenylbutazone (e.g., Alka-Butazolidin):*

- This medicine contains antacids that can keep other medicines from working properly if the 2 medicines are taken to close together. *Always take this medicine:*
  
  —*At least 6 hours before or 2 hours after taking ciprofloxacin (e.g., Cipro) or lomefloxacin (e.g., Maxaquin).*
  
  —*At least 8 hours before or 2 hours after taking enoxacin (e.g., Penetrex).*
  
  —*At least 2 hours after taking itraconazole (e.g., Sporanox).*
  
  —*At least 3 hours before or after taking ketoconazole (e.g., Nizoral).*
  
  —*At least 2 hours before or after taking norfloxacin (e.g., Noroxin) or ofloxacin (e.g., Floxin).*
  
  —*At least 1 to 3 hours before or after taking a tetracycline antibiotic by mouth.*
  
  —*At least 1 or 2 hours before or after taking any other medicine by mouth.*

For patients taking *mefenamic acid:*

- If diarrhea occurs while you are using this medicine, *stop taking it and check with your doctor immediately. Do not take it again without first checking with your doctor,* because severe diarrhea may occur each time you take it.

Some people who take nonsteroidal anti-inflammatory drugs may become more sensitive to sunlight than they are normally. Exposure to sunlight, even for brief periods of time, may cause severe sunburn; blisters on the skin; skin rash, redness, itching, or discoloration; or vision changes. When you begin taking this medicine:

- Stay out of direct sunlight, especially between the hours of 10:00 a.m. and 3:00 p.m., if possible.
- Wear protective clothing, including a hat and sunglasses.
- Apply a sun block product that has a skin protection factor (SPF) of at least 15. Some patients may require a product with a higher SPF number, especially if they have a fair complexion. If you have any questions about this, check with your health care professional.

- Do not use a sunlamp or tanning bed or booth.

If you have a severe reaction from the sun, check with your doctor.

Serious side effects, including ulcers or bleeding, can occur during treatment with this medicine. Sometimes serious side effects can occur without any warning. However, possible warning signs often occur, including severe abdominal or stomach cramps, pain, or burning; black, tarry stools; severe, continuing nausea, heartburn, or indigestion; and/or vomiting of blood or material that looks like coffee grounds. *Stop taking this medicine and check with your doctor immediately if you notice any of these warning signs.*

*Check with your doctor immediately if chills, fever, muscle aches or pains, or other influenza-like symptoms occur, especially if they occur shortly before, or together with, a skin rash.* Very rarely, these effects may be the first signs of a serious reaction to this medicine.

Nonsteroidal anti-inflammatory drugs may cause a serious type of allergic reaction called anaphylaxis. Although this is rare, it may occur more often in patients who are allergic to aspirin or to any of the nonsteroidal anti-inflammatory drugs. *Anaphylaxis requires immediate medical attention.* The most serious signs of this reaction are very fast or irregular breathing, gasping for breath, wheezing, or fainting. Other signs may include changes in color of the skin of the face; very fast but irregular heartbeat or pulse; hive-like swellings on the skin; and puffiness or swellings of the eyelids or around the eyes. If these effects occur, get emergency help at once. Ask someone to drive you to the nearest hospital emergency room. If this is not possible, do not try to drive yourself. Call an ambulance, lie down, cover yourself to keep warm, and prop your feet higher than your head. Stay in that position until help arrives.

For patients taking *ibuprofen* or *naproxen* without a prescription:

- Check with your medical doctor or dentist:
  
  —if your symptoms do not improve or if they get worse.
  
  —if you are using this medicine to bring down a fever and the fever lasts more than 3 days or returns.
  
  —if the painful area is red or swollen.

---

## Side Effects of This Medicine

Along with its needed effects, a medicine may cause some unwanted effects. Although not all of these side effects may occur, if they do occur they may need medical attention.

Stop taking this medicine and get emergency help right away if any of the following side effects occur:

*Rare—For all nonsteroidal anti-inflammatory drugs*

Fainting; fast or irregular breathing; fast, irregular heartbeat or pulse; hive-like swellings (large) on face, eyelids, mouth, lips, or tongue; puffiness or swelling of the eyelids or around the eyes; shortness of breath, troubled breathing, wheezing, or tightness in chest

*Also, stop taking this medicine and check with your doctor immediately* if any of the following side effects occur:

*More common—for mefenamic acid only*
Diarrhea

*More common—for phenylbutazone only*
Swelling of face, hands, feet, or lower legs; weight gain (rapid)

*Symptoms of phenylbutazone overdose*
Bluish color of fingernails, lips, or skin; headache (severe and continuing)

*Rare—for all nonsteroidal anti-inflammatory drugs*
Abdominal or stomach pain, cramping, or burning (severe); bloody or black, tarry stools; chest pain; convulsions (seizures); fever with or without chills; nausea, heartburn, and/or indigestion (severe and continuing); pinpoint red spots on skin; sores, ulcers, or white spots on lips or in mouth; spitting up blood; unexplained nosebleeds; unusual bleeding or bruising; vomiting of blood or material that looks like coffee grounds

Also, check with your doctor as soon as possible if any of the following side effects occur:

*More common*
Bleeding from rectum (with suppositories); headache (severe), especially in the morning (for indomethacin only); skin rash

*Less common or rare*
Bladder pain; bleeding from cuts or scratches that lasts longer than usual; bleeding or crusting sores on lips; bloody or cloudy urine or any problem with urination, such as difficult, burning, or painful urination; change in urine color or odor; frequent urge to urinate; sudden, large increase or decrease in the amount of urine; or loss of bladder control; blurred vision or any change in vision; burning feeling in throat, chest, or stomach; confusion, forgetfulness, mental depression, or other mood or mental changes; cough or hoarseness; decreased hearing, any other change in hearing, or ringing or buzzing in ears; difficulty in swallowing; eye pain, irritation, dryness, redness, and/or swelling; hallucinations (seeing, hearing, or feeling things that are not there); headache (severe), throbbing, or with stiff neck or back; hives, itching of skin, or any other skin problem, such as blisters, redness or other color change, tenderness, burning, peeling, thickening, or scaliness; increased blood pressure; irritated tongue; light-colored stools; loosening or splitting of fingernails; muscle cramps, pain, or weakness; numbness, tingling, pain, or weakness in hands or feet; pain in lower back and/or side (severe); swelling and/or tenderness in upper abdominal or stomach area; swelling of face, feet, or lower legs (if taking phenylbutazone, stop taking it and check with your doctor immediately); swelling of

lips or tongue; swollen and/or painful glands (especially in the neck or throat area); thirst (continuing); trouble in speaking; unexplained runny nose or sneezing; unexplained, unexpected, or unusually heavy vaginal bleeding; unusual tiredness or weakness; weight gain (rapid) (if taking phenylbutazone, stop taking it and check with your doctor immediately); yellow eyes or skin

Other side effects may occur that usually do not need medical attention. These side effects may go away during treatment as your body adjusts to the medicine. However, check with your doctor if any of the following side effects continue or are bothersome:

*More common*
Abdominal or stomach cramps, pain, or discomfort (mild to moderate); diarrhea (if taking mefenamic acid, stop taking it and check with your doctor immediately); dizziness, drowsiness, or lightheadedness; headache (mild to moderate); heartburn, indigestion, nausea, or vomiting

*Less common or rare*
Bitter taste or other taste change; bloated feeling, gas, or constipation; decreased appetite or loss of appetite; fast or pounding heartbeat; flushing or hot flashes; general feeling of discomfort or illness; increased sensitivity of eyes to light; increased sensitivity of skin to sunlight; increased sweating; irritation, dryness, or soreness of mouth; nervousness, anxiety, irritability, trembling, or twitching; rectal irritation (with suppositories); trouble in sleeping; unexplained weight loss; unusual tiredness or weakness without any other symptoms

Although not all of the side effects listed above have been reported for all of these medicines, they have been reported for at least one of them. However, since all anti-inflammatory analgesics are very similar, it is possible that any of the above side effects may occur with any of these medicines.

Some side effects may occur many days or weeks after you have stopped using phenylbutazone. During this time *check with your doctor immediately* if you notice any of the following side effects:

Sore throat and fever; ulcers, sores, or white spots in mouth; unusual bleeding or bruising; unusual tiredness or weakness

Other side effects not listed above may also occur in some patients. If you notice any other effects, check with your doctor.

---

Revised: 09/13/94

# NORFLOXACIN Ophthalmic

Some commonly used brand names are:

**In the U.S.—**
Chibroxin

**In Canada—**
Noroxin

## Description

Norfloxacin (nor-FLOX-a-sin) is an antibiotic. The ophthalmic preparation is used to treat infections of the eye.

Norfloxacin is available only with your doctor's prescription, in the following dosage form:

*Ophthalmic*
- Ophthalmic solution (eye drops) (U.S. and Canada)

## Before Using This Medicine

In deciding to use a medicine, the risks of taking the medicine must be weighed against the good it will do. This is a decision you and your doctor will make. For ophthalmic norfloxacin, the following should be considered:

**Allergies**—Tell your doctor if you have ever had any unusual or allergic reaction to norfloxacin or to any related medicines, such as cinoxacin (e.g., Cinobac), ciprofloxacin (e.g., Cipro or Ciloxan), enoxacin (e.g., Penetrax), lomefloxacin (e.g., Maxaquin), nalidixic acid (e.g., NegGram), or ofloxacin (e.g., Floxin or Ocuflox). Also tell your health care professional if you are allergic to any other substances, such as foods, preservatives, or dyes.

**Pregnancy**—Studies have not been done in humans. However, norfloxacin taken by mouth can cause bone problems in young animals. Since it is not known whether ophthalmic norfloxacin can cause bone problems in infants, use is not recommended during pregnancy.

**Breast-feeding**—It is not known whether ophthalmic norfloxacin passes into the breast milk. Low doses of norfloxacin taken by mouth do not pass into breast milk, but other related medicines do. Also, norfloxacin taken by mouth can cause bone problems in young animals. Since it is not known whether ophthalmic norfloxacin can cause bone problems in infants, use is not recommended in nursing mothers.

**Children**—Use is not recommended in infants and children up to 1 year of age. Norfloxacin taken by mouth has been shown to cause bone problems in young animals. It is not known whether ophthalmic norfloxacin can cause bone problems in infants. In children 1 year of age and older, this medicine is not expected to cause different side effects or problems than it does in adults.

**Older adults**—Many medicines have not been studied specifically in older people. Therefore, it may not be known whether they work exactly the same way they do in younger adults. Although there is no specific information comparing use of ophthalmic norfloxacin in the elderly with use in other age groups, this medicine is not expected to cause different side effects or problems in older people than it does in younger adults.

**Other medicines**—Although certain medicines should not be used together at all, in other cases two different medicines may be used together even if an interaction might occur. In these cases, your doctor may want to change the dose, or other precautions may be necessary. Tell your health care professional if you are taking or using any prescription or nonprescription (over -the-counter [OTC]) medicine.

## Proper Use of This Medicine

To use:
- First, wash your hands. Tilt the head back and with the index finger of one hand, press gently on the skin just beneath the lower eyelid and pull the lower eyelid away from the eye to make a space. Drop the medicine into this space. Let go of the eyelid and gently close the eyes. Do not blink. Keep the eyes closed for 1 or 2 minutes, to allow the medicine to come into contact with the infection.
- If you think you did not get the drop of medicine into your eye properly, use another drop.
- To keep the medicine as germ-free as possible, do not touch the applicator tip to any surface (including the eye). Also, keep the container tightly closed.

**Dosing**—The dose of ophthalmic norfloxacin will be different for different patients. *Follow your doctor's orders or the directions on the label.* The following information includes only the average doses of ophthalmic norfloxacin. *If your dose is different, do not change it* unless your doctor tells you to do so:
- For infants and children up to 1 year of age: Use is not recommended.
- For adults and children 1 year of age and over: Place 1 drop in each eye four times a day for 7 days.

To help clear up your infection completely, *keep using this medicine for the full time of treatment,* even if your symptoms begin to clear up after a few days. If you stop using this medicine too soon, your symptoms may return. *Do not miss any doses.*

**Missed dose**—If you do miss a dose of this medicine, apply it as soon as possible. However, if it is almost time for your next dose, skip the missed dose and go back to your regular dosing schedule.

**Storage**—To store this medicine:
- Keep out of the reach of children.
- Store away from heat and direct light.
- Keep the medicine from freezing.
- Do not keep outdated medicine or medicine no longer needed. Be sure that any discarded medicine is out of the reach of children.

## Precautions While Using This Medicine

If your symptoms do not improve within a few days, or if they become worse, check with your doctor.

This medicine may cause your eyes to become more sensitive to light than they are normally. Wearing sunglasses and avoiding too much exposure to bright light may help lessen the discomfort.

## Side Effects of This Medicine

Along with its needed effects, a medicine may cause some unwanted effects. Although not all of these side effects may occur, if they do occur they may need medical attention.

*Check with your doctor immediately* if any of the following side effects occur:

*Rare*
   Skin rash or other sign of allergic reaction

Other side effects may occur that usually do not need medical attention. These side effects may go away during treatment as your body adjusts to the medicine. However, check with your doctor if any of the following side effects continue or are bothersome:

*More common*
   Burning or other eye discomfort

*Less common*
   Bitter taste following use in the eye; increased sensitivity of eye to light; redness of the lining of the eyelids; swelling of the membrane covering the white part of the eye

Other side effects not listed above may also occur in some patients. If you notice any other effects, check with your doctor.

Revised: 12/22/93

---

# NYLIDRIN    Systemic*

Some commonly used brand names are:

**In Canada—**
   Arlidin                          PMS Nylidrin
   Arlidin Forte

*Not commercially available in the U.S.

## Description

Nylidrin (NYE-li-drin) belongs to the group of medicines called vasodilators. Vasodilators increase the size of blood vessels. Nylidrin is used to treat problems due to poor blood circulation.

Nylidrin is available only with your doctor's prescription, in the following dosage form:

*Oral*
   • Tablets (Canada)

## Before Using This Medicine

In deciding to use a medicine, the risks of taking the medicine must be weighed against the good it will do. This is a decision you and your doctor will make. For nylidrin, the following should be considered:

**Allergies**—Tell your doctor if you have ever had any unusual or allergic reaction to nylidrin. Also tell your health care professional if you are allergic to any other substances, such as foods, preservatives, or dyes.

**Pregnancy**—Studies on effects in pregnancy have have not been done in either humans or animals.

**Breast-feeding**—It is not known whether nylidrin passes into breast milk. Although most medicines pass into breast milk in small amounts, many of them may be used safely while breast-feeding. Mothers who are taking this medicine and who wish to breast-feed should discuss this with their doctor.

**Older adults**—Many medicines have not been studied specifically in older people. Therefore, it may not be known whether they work exactly the same way they do in younger adults or if they cause different side effects or problems in older people. There is no specific information comparing use of nylidrin in the elderly with use in other age groups. However, nylidrin may reduce tolerance to cold temperatures in elderly patients.

**Other medicines**—Although certain medicines should not be used together at all, in other cases two different medicines may be used together even if an interaction might occur. In these cases, your doctor may want to change the dose, or other precautions may be necessary. Tell your health care professional if you are taking any other prescription or nonprescription (over-the-counter [OTC]) medicine, or if you smoke.

**Other medical problems**—The presence of other medical problems may affect the use of nylidrin. Make sure you tell your doctor if you have any other medical problems, especially:

   • Angina (chest pain) or
   • Fast heartbeat or
   • Heart attack (recent) or other heart disease or
   • Overactive thyroid gland or
   • Stomach ulcer—Nylidrin may make these conditions worse

## Proper Use of This Medicine

Nylidrin may cause you to have a fast or pounding heartbeat. To keep this from affecting your sleep, do not take the last dose of the day at bedtime. Instead, it is best to plan your dose or doses according to a schedule that will least affect your sleep. Ask your health care professional to help you plan the best time to take this medicine.

**Dosing**—The dose of nylidrin will be different for different patients. *Follow your doctor's orders or the directions on the label.* The following information includes only the average doses of nylidrin. *If your dose is different, do not change it* unless your doctor tells you to do so:

- For *oral* dosage form (tablets):
  —Adults: 3 to 12 milligrams (mg) three or four times a day.

**Missed dose**—If you miss a dose of this medicine, take the missed dose as soon as you remember. However, if it is almost time for the next dose, skip the missed dose and go back to your regular dosing schedule. Do not double doses.

**Storage**—To store this medicine:

- Keep out of the reach of children.
- Store away from heat and direct light.
- Do not store in the bathroom, near the kitchen sink, or in other damp places. Heat or moisture may cause the medicine to break down.
- Do not keep outdated medicine or medicine no longer needed. Be sure that any discarded medicine is out of the reach of children.

---

## Precautions While Using This Medicine

It may take some time for this medicine to work. If you feel that the medicine is not working, do not stop taking it on your own. Instead, check with your doctor.

The helpful effects of this medicine may be decreased if you smoke. If you have any questions about this, check with your doctor.

---

## Side Effects of This Medicine

Along with its needed effects, a medicine may cause some unwanted effects. Although not all of these side effects may occur, if they do occur they may need medical attention.

Check with your doctor as soon as possible if any of the following side effects occur:

*Less common*
　Dizziness; fast or irregular heartbeat; weakness or tiredness (continuing)

*Signs and symptoms of overdose*
　Blurred vision; chest pain; decrease in urination or inability to urinate; fever; metallic taste

Other side effects may occur that usually do not need medical attention. These side effects may go away during treatment as your body adjusts to the medicine. However, check with your doctor if any of the following side effects continue or are bothersome:

*Less common*
　Chilliness; flushing or redness of face; headache; nausea and vomiting; nervousness; trembling

Other side effects not listed above may also occur in some patients. If you notice any other effects, check with your doctor.

---

Revised: 05/14/93

---

# NYSTATIN  Oral

Some commonly used brand names are:

**In the U.S.—**
　Mycostatin　　　　　　Nystex
　Nilstat
　Generic name product may also be available.

**In Canada—**
　Mycostatin　　　　　　Nilstat
　Nadostine　　　　　　PMS Nystatin

## Description

Nystatin (nye-STAT-in) belongs to the group of medicines called antifungals. The dry powder, lozenge (pastille), and liquid forms of this medicine are used to treat fungus infections in the mouth.

Nystatin is available only with your doctor's prescription, in the following dosage forms:

*Oral*

- Lozenges (Pastilles) (U.S.)
- Oral suspension (U.S. and Canada)
- Powder for oral suspension (U.S. and Canada)
- Tablets (U.S. and Canada)

## Before Using This Medicine

In deciding to use a medicine, the risks of taking the medicine must be weighed against the good it will do. This is a decision you and your doctor will make. For nystatin, the following should be considered:

**Allergies**—Tell your doctor if you have ever had any unusual or allergic reaction to nystatin. Also tell your health care professional if you are allergic to any other substances, such as foods, preservatives, or dyes.

**Pregnancy**—Studies in humans have not shown that oral nystatin causes birth defects or other problems.

**Breast-feeding**—Oral nystatin has not been reported to cause problems in nursing babies.

**Children**—This medicine has been tested in children and has not been reported to cause different side effects or problems in children than it does in adults. However, since children up to 5 years of age may be too young to use the lozenges (pastilles) or tablets safely, the oral suspension dosage form is best for this age group.

**Older adults**—Many medicines have not been studied specifically in older people. Therefore, it may not be known whether they work exactly the same way they do in younger adults or if they cause different side effects or problems in older people. There is no specific information comparing use of oral nystatin in the elderly with use in other age groups.

## Proper Use of This Medicine

For patients taking the *dry powder form of nystatin:*

- Add about ⅛ teaspoonful of dry powder to about 4 ounces of water immediately before taking. Stir well.
- After it is mixed, take this medicine by dividing the whole amount (4 ounces) into several portions. Hold each portion of the medicine in your mouth or swish it around in your mouth for as long as possible, gargle, and swallow. Be sure to use all the liquid to get the full dose of medicine.

For patients taking the *lozenge (pastille) form of nystatin:*

- Nystatin lozenges (pastilles) should be held in the mouth and allowed to dissolve slowly and completely. This may take 15 to 30 minutes. Also, the saliva should be swallowed during this time. *Do not chew or swallow the lozenges whole.*
- *Do not give nystatin lozenges (pastilles) to infants or children up to 5 years of age.* They may be too young to use the lozenges safely.

For patients taking the *oral liquid form of nystatin:*

- This medicine is to be taken by mouth even if it comes in a dropper bottle. If it does come in a dropper bottle, use the specially marked dropper to measure each dose accurately.
- Take this medicine by placing one-half of the dose in each side of your mouth. Hold the medicine in your mouth or swish it around in your mouth for as long as possible, then gargle and swallow.

Patients with full or partial dentures may need to soak their dentures nightly in nystatin for oral suspension to eliminate the fungus from the dentures. In rare cases when this does not eliminate the fungus, it may be necessary to have new dentures made.

To help clear up your infection completely, *keep taking this medicine for the full time of treatment,* even if your condition has improved. *Do not miss any doses.*

**Dosing**—The dose of nystatin will be different for different patients. *Follow your doctor's orders or the directions on the label.* The following information includes only the average doses of nystatin. *If your dose is different, do not change it* unless your doctor tells you to do so.

The number of lozenges, tablets, or milliliters (mL) of suspension that you take depends on the strength of the medicine. Also, *the number of doses you take each day, the time allowed between doses, and the length of time you take the medicine depend on the medical problem for which you are taking nystatin.*

- For the *lozenge (pastille) and tablet* dosage forms:
  —Adults and children 5 years of age and older: 1 or 2 lozenges or tablets three to five times a day for up to fourteen days.
  —Children up to 5 years of age: Children this young may not be able to use the lozenges or tablets safely. The oral suspension is better for this age group.

- For the *suspension* dosage form:
  —Adults and children 5 years of age and older: 4 to 6 milliliters (mL) (about 1 teaspoonful) four times a day.
  —For older infants: 2 mL four times a day.
  —For premature and low-birth-weight infants: 1 mL four times a day.

**Missed dose**—If you do miss a dose of this medicine, take it as soon as possible. However, if it is almost time for your next dose, skip the missed dose and go back to your regular dosing schedule. Do not double doses.

**Storage**—To store this medicine:

- Keep out of the reach of children.
- Store away from heat and direct light.
- Do not store the tablet or dry powder form of this medicine in the bathroom, near the kitchen sink, or in other damp places. Heat or moisture may cause the medicine to break down.
- Store the lozenge (pastille) form in the refrigerator. Heat will cause this medicine to break down.
- Keep the oral liquid form of this medicine from freezing.
- Do not keep outdated medicine or medicine no longer needed. Be sure that any discarded medicine is out of the reach of children.

## Side Effects of This Medicine

Along with its needed effects, a medicine may cause some unwanted effects. The following side effects may go away during treatment as your body adjusts to the medicine. However, check with your doctor if any of the following side effects continue or are bothersome:

*Less common*
    Diarrhea; nausea or vomiting; stomach pain

Other side effects not listed above may also occur in some patients. If you notice any other effects, check with your doctor.

## Additional Information

Once a medicine has been approved for marketing for a certain use, experience may show that it is also useful for other medical problems. Although this use is not included in product labeling, nystatin is used in certain patients with the following medical condition:

- Candidiasis, oral (fungus infection of the mouth) (prevention)

Other than the above information, there is no additional information relating to proper use, precautions, or side effects for this use.

Revised: 01/19/93

---

# NYSTATIN   Topical

Some commonly used brand names are:

**In the U.S.—**

| | |
|---|---|
| Mycostatin | Nystex |
| Nilstat | |

Generic name product may also be available.

**In Canada—**

| | |
|---|---|
| Mycostatin | Nilstat |
| Nadostine | Nyaderm |

## Description

Nystatin (nye-STAT-in) belongs to the group of medicines called antifungals. Topical nystatin is used to treat some types of fungus infections.

Nystatin is available only with your doctor's prescription, in the following dosage forms:

*Topical*
- Cream (U.S. and Canada)
- Ointment (U.S. and Canada)
- Topical powder (U.S. and Canada)

## Before Using This Medicine

In deciding to use a medicine, the risks of using the medicine must be weighed against the good it will do. This is a decision you and your doctor will make. For nystatin, the following should be considered:

**Allergies**—Tell your doctor if you have ever had any unusual or allergic reaction to nystatin. Also tell your health care professional if you are allergic to any other substances, such as preservatives or dyes.

**Pregnancy**—Nystatin topical preparations have not been shown to cause birth defects or other problems in humans.

**Breast-feeding**—It is not known whether nystatin passes into the breast milk. Although most medicines pass into breast milk in small amounts, many of them may be used safely while breast-feeding. Mothers who are using this medicine and who wish to breast-feed should discuss this with their doctor.

**Children**—Although there is no specific information comparing use of topical nystatin in children with use in other age groups, this medicine is not expected to cause different side effects or problems in children than it does in adults.

**Older adults**—Many medicines have not been studied specifically in older people. Therefore, it may not be known whether they work exactly the same way they do in younger adults or if they cause different side effects or problems in older people. There is no specific information comparing use of topical nystatin in the elderly with use in other age groups.

**Other medicines**—Although certain medicines should not be used together at all, in other cases two different medicines may be used together even if an interaction might occur. In these cases, your doctor may want to change the dose, or other precautions may be necessary. Tell your health care professional if you are using any other topical prescription or nonprescription (over-the-counter [OTC]) medicine that is to be applied to the same area of the skin.

## Proper Use of This Medicine

Topical nystatin should not be used in the eyes.

Apply enough nystatin to cover the affected area.

For patients using the *powder form* of this medicine on the feet:
- Sprinkle the powder between the toes, on the feet, and in socks and shoes.

The use of any kind of occlusive dressing (airtight covering, such as kitchen plastic wrap) over this medicine may increase the chance of irritation. Therefore, *do not bandage, wrap, or apply any occlusive dressing over this medicine* unless directed to do so by your doctor. When using this medicine on the diaper area of children, *avoid tight-fitting diapers and plastic pants.*

To help clear up your infection completely, *keep using this medicine for the full time of treatment,* even if your condition has improved. *Do not miss any doses.*

**Dosing**—The dose of topical nystatin will be different for different patients. *Follow your doctor's orders or the directions on the label.* The following information includes only the average dose of topical nystatin. *If your dose is different, do not change it* unless your doctor tells you to do so.

- For *topical* dosage forms (cream, ointment, or powder):
  —For fungus infections:
    - Adults and children—Apply to the affected area(s) of the skin two or three times a day.

**Missed dose**—If you miss a dose of this medicine, apply it as soon as possible. Then go back to your regular dosing schedule.

**Storage**—To store this medicine:
- Keep out of the reach of children.
- Store away from heat and direct light.
- Do not store the powder form of this medicine in the bathroom, near the kitchen sink, or in other damp places. Heat or moisture may cause the medicine to break down.
- Keep the cream and ointment forms of this medicine from freezing.

- Do not keep outdated medicine or medicine no longer needed. Be sure that any discarded medicine is out of the reach of children.

## Side Effects of This Medicine

Along with its needed effects, a medicine may cause some unwanted effects. Although not all of these side effects may occur, if they do occur they may need medical attention.

Check with your doctor as soon as possible if the following side effect occurs:

Skin irritation not present before use of this medicine

Other side effects not listed above may also occur in some patients. If you notice any other effects, check with your doctor.

Revised: 07/25/94

---

# NYSTATIN  Vaginal

Some commonly used brand names are:
**In the U.S.—**
Mycostatin                      Nilstat
Generic name product may also be available.

**In Canada—**
Mycostatin                      Nilstat
Nadostine                       Nyaderm

## Description
Nystatin (nye-STAT-in) belongs to the group of medicines called antifungals. Vaginal nystatin is used to treat fungus infections of the vagina. Nystatin vaginal cream or tablets may also be used for other problems as determined by your doctor.

Nystatin is available only with your doctor's prescription, in the following dosage forms:

*Vaginal*
- Cream (Canada)
- Tablets (U.S. and Canada)

## Before Using This Medicine
In deciding to use a medicine, the risks of taking the medicine must be weighed against the good it will do. This is a decision you and your doctor will make. For nystatin, the following should be considered:

**Allergies**—Tell your doctor if you have ever had any unusual or allergic reaction to nystatin. Also tell your health care professional if you are allergic to any other substances, such as foods, preservatives, or dyes.

**Pregnancy**—Studies have not been done in animals. However, nystatin vaginal tablets have not been shown to cause birth defects or other problems in humans.

**Breast-feeding**—It is not known whether nystatin passes into breast milk. However, this medicine has not been reported to cause problems in nursing babies.

**Children**—Studies on this medicine have been done only in adults, and there is no specific information comparing use of vaginal nystatin in children with use in other age groups.

**Older adults**—Many medicines have not been studied specifically in older people. Therefore, it may not be known whether they work exactly the same way they do in younger adults or if they cause different side effects or problems in older people. There is no specific information comparing the use of vaginal nystatin in the elderly with use in other age groups.

**Other medicines**—Although certain medicines should not be used together at all, in other cases two different medicines may be used together even if an interaction might occur. In these cases, your doctor may want to change the dose, or other precautions may be necessary. Tell your health care professional if you are using any other vaginal prescription or nonprescription (over-the-counter [OTC]) medicine.

## Proper Use of This Medicine
Nystatin usually comes with patient directions. Read them carefully before using this medicine.

This medicine is usually inserted into the vagina with an applicator. However, if you are pregnant, check with your doctor before using the applicator to insert the vaginal tablet.

To help clear up your infection completely, *keep using this medicine for the full time of treatment,* even if your condition has improved. Also, keep using this medicine even if you begin to menstruate during the time of treatment. *Do not miss any doses.*

**Dosing**—The dose of nystatin will be different for different patients. *Follow your doctor's orders or the directions on the label.* The following information includes only the average doses of nystatin. *If your dose is different, do not change it* unless your doctor tells you to do so.

- For treating fungus (yeast) infections:
  —For *vaginal cream* dosage form:
  - Adults and teenagers—One 100,000-Unit applicatorful inserted into the vagina one or two times a day for two weeks. Or, your doctor may want you to insert one 500,000-Unit applicatorful into the vagina once a day.
  - Children—Dose must be determined by your doctor.
  —For *vaginal tablet* dosage form:
  - Adults and teenagers—One 100,000-unit tablet inserted into the vagina one or two times a day for two weeks.
  - Children—Dose must be determined by your doctor.

**Missed dose**—If you do miss a dose of this medicine, insert it as soon as possible. However, if it is almost time for your next dose, skip the missed dose and go back to your regular dosing schedule.

**Storage**—To store this medicine:
- Keep out of the reach of children.
- Store away from heat and direct light.
- Do not store in the bathroom, near the kitchen sink, or in other damp places. Heat or moisture may cause the medicine to break down.

- Do not keep outdated medicine or medicine no longer needed. Be sure that any discarded medicine is out of the reach of children.

## Precautions While Using This Medicine

*To help cure the infection and to help prevent reinfection, good health habits are required.*
- Wear cotton panties (or panties or pantyhose with cotton crotches) instead of synthetic (for example, nylon, rayon) underclothes.
- Wear freshly laundered underclothes.

If you have any questions about this, check with your health care professional.

If you have any questions about douching or intercourse during the time of treatment with nystatin, check with your doctor.

Since there may be some vaginal drainage while you are using this medicine, a sanitary napkin may be worn to protect your clothing.

## Side Effects of This Medicine

Along with its needed effects, a medicine may cause some unwanted effects. Although not all of these side effects may occur, if they do occur they may need medical attention.

Check with your doctor as soon as possible if the following side effect occurs:

*Rare*
Vaginal irritation not present before use of this medicine

Other side effects not listed above may also occur in some patients. If you notice any other effects, check with your doctor.

Revised: 09/08/92
Interim revision: 06/30/94

---

# NYSTATIN AND TRIAMCINOLONE   Topical†

Some commonly used brand names are:

**In the U.S.—**

| | |
|---|---|
| Dermacomb | Myco-Triacet II |
| Myco II | Mykacet |
| Mycobiotic II | Mykacet II |
| Mycogen II | Mytrex |
| Mycolog II | Tristatin II |

Generic name product may also be available.

†Not commercially available in Canada.

## Description

Nystatin (nye-STAT-in) and triamcinolone (trye-am-SIN-oh-lone) combination contains an antifungal and a corticosteroid (kor-ti-co-STI-roid) (cortisone-like medicine).

Antifungals are used to treat infections caused by a fungus. They work by killing the fungus or preventing its growth. This medicine will not work for other kinds of infections. Corticosteroids belong to the family of medicines called steroids. They are used to help relieve redness, swelling, itching, and other discomfort of many skin problems.

This medicine is used to treat certain fungus infections, such as Candida (Monilia), and to help relieve the discomfort of the infection.

Topical corticosteroids may rarely cause some serious side effects. Some of the side effects may be more likely to occur in children. *Before using this medicine in children, be sure to talk to your doctor about these problems, as well as the good this medicine may do.*

Nystatin and triamcinolone combination is available only with your doctor's prescription, in the following dosage forms:

*Topical*
- Cream (U.S.)
- Ointment (U.S.)

## Before Using This Medicine

In deciding to use a medicine, the risks of using the medicine must be weighed against the good it will do. This is a decision you and your doctor will make. For nystatin and triamcinolone combination, the following should be considered:

**Allergies**—Tell your doctor if you have ever had any unusual or allergic reaction to nystatin or triamcinolone. Also tell your health care professional if you are allergic to any other substances, such as preservatives or dyes.

**Pregnancy**—Nystatin and triamcinolone combination has not been studied in pregnant women. However, studies in animals have shown that corticosteroids given by mouth or by injection may cause birth defects, even at low doses. Also, some of the stronger corticosteroids have been shown to cause birth defects when applied to the skin of animals. Therefore, this medicine should not be used on large areas of skin, in large amounts, or for a long time in pregnant patients. Before using this medicine, make sure your doctor knows if you are pregnant or if you may become pregnant.

**Breast-feeding**—It is not known whether nystatin or triamcinolone passes into the breast milk. Although this combination medicine has not been reported to cause problems in humans, topical corticosteroids may be absorbed into the body. Corticosteroids that are given by mouth or by injection do pass into the breast milk and may cause unwanted effects, such as interfering with nursing babies' growth.

**Children**—Children may be especially sensitive to the effects of topical nystatin and triamcinolone combination. This may increase the chance of side effects during treatment. Therefore, it is especially important that you discuss with your child's doctor the good that this medicine may do as well as the risks of using it.

**Older adults**—Many medicines have not been studied specifically in older people. Therefore, it may not be known

whether they work exactly the same way they do in younger adults. Although there is no specific information comparing use of topical nystatin and triamcinolone combination in the elderly with use in other age groups, this medicine is not expected to cause different side effects or problems in older people than it does in younger adults.

**Other medicines**—Although certain medicines should not be used together at all, in other cases two different medicines may be used together even if an interaction might occur. In these cases, your doctor may want to change the dose, or other precautions may be necessary. When you are using nystatin and triamcinolone combination, it is especially important that your health care professional know if you are using any other prescription or nonprescription (over-the-counter [OTC]) medicine.

**Other medical problems**—The presence of other medical problems may affect the use of nystatin and triamcinolone combination. Make sure you tell your doctor if you have any other medical problems, especially:

- Herpes
- Vaccinia (cowpox)
- Varicella (chickenpox)
- Other virus infections of the skin—Triamcinolone may speed up the spread of virus infections
- Tuberculosis (TB) of the skin—Triamcinolone may make a TB infection worse

## Proper Use of This Medicine

*Do not use this medicine in or around the eyes.*

*Check with your doctor before using this medicine on any other skin problems.* It should not be used on bacterial or virus infections. Also, it should only be used on certain fungus infections of the skin.

Apply a thin layer of this medicine to the affected area and rub in gently and thoroughly.

The use of any kind of airtight covering over this medicine may increase absorption of the medicine and the chance of irritation and other side effects. Therefore, *do not bandage, wrap, or apply any airtight covering or other occlusive dressing (for example, kitchen plastic wrap) over this medicine* unless directed to do so by your doctor. Also, wear loose-fitting clothing when using this medicine on the groin area. When using this medicine on the diaper area of children, *avoid tight-fitting diapers and plastic pants.*

To help clear up your infection completely, *keep using this medicine for the full time of treatment,* even if your symptoms have disappeared. *Do not miss any doses.* However, *do not use this medicine more often or for a longer time than your doctor ordered.* To do so may increase absorption through your skin and the chance of side effects. In addition, too much use, especially on thin skin areas (for example, face, armpits, groin), may result in thinning of the skin and stretch marks.

**Dosing**—The dose of topical nystatin and triamcinolone combination will be different for different patients. *Follow your doctor's orders or the directions on the label.*

The following information includes only the average doses of topical nystatin and triamcinolone combination. *If your dose is different, do not change it* unless your doctor tells you to do so.

- For fungus infections:
  —For cream dosage form:
  - Adults and children—Apply to the affected area(s) of the skin two times a day, morning and evening
  —For ointment dosage form:
  - Adults and children—Apply to the affected area(s) of the skin two or three times a day.

**Missed dose**—If you miss a dose of this medicine, apply it as soon as possible. However, if it is almost time for your next dose, skip the missed dose and go back to your regular dosing schedule.

**Storage**—To store this medicine:
- Keep out of the reach of children.
- Store away from heat and direct light.
- Keep the medicine from freezing.
- Do not keep outdated medicine or medicine no longer needed. Be sure that any discarded medicine is out of the reach of children.

## Precautions While Using This Medicine

*To help clear up your infection completely and to help make sure it does not return, good health habits are also required.* Keep the affected area as cool and dry as possible.

If your skin problem does not improve within 2 or 3 weeks, or if it becomes worse, check with your doctor.

The corticosteroid in this medicine may be absorbed through the skin and may be more likely to cause side effects in children. Long-term use may affect growth and development as well. *Children who must use this medicine should be followed closely by their doctor.*

For diabetic patients:
- *Although rare, the corticosteroid in this medicine may cause higher blood and urine sugar levels, especially if you have severe diabetes and are using large amounts of this medicine.* Check with your doctor before changing your diet or the dosage of your diabetes medicine.

## Side Effects of This Medicine

Along with its needed effects, a medicine may cause some unwanted effects. Although not all of these side effects may occur, if they do occur they may need medical attention.

*Check with your doctor immediately* if any of the following side effects occur:

*Rare*
Blistering, burning, dryness, itching, peeling, or other sign of irritation not present before use of this medicine

Additional side effects may occur if you use this medicine for a long time. Check with your doctor as soon as possible if any of the following side effects occur:

Acne or oily skin; increased hair growth, especially on the face; increased loss of hair, especially on the scalp; reddish purple lines on arms, face, legs, trunk, or groin; thinning of skin with easy bruising

Many of the above side effects are more likely to occur in children, who may absorb greater amounts of this medicine.

Other side effects not listed above may also occur in some patients. If you notice any other effects, check with your doctor.

Revised: 08/15/94

# OCTREOTIDE Systemic

A commonly used brand name in the U.S. and Canada is Sandostatin.

## Description

Octreotide (oak-TREE-oh-tide) is used to treat the severe diarrhea and other symptoms that occur with certain intestinal tumors. It does not cure the tumor but it helps the patient live a more normal life. Octreotide may also be used for other medical conditions as determined by your doctor.

Octreotide is available only with your doctor's prescription, in the following dosage form:

*Parenteral*
- Injection (U.S. and Canada)

## Before Using This Medicine

In deciding to use a medicine, the risks of using the medicine must be weighed against the good it will do. This is a decision you and your doctor will make. For octreotide, the following should be considered:

**Allergies**—Tell your doctor if you have ever had any unusual or allergic reaction to octreotide. Also tell your health care professional if you are allergic to any other substances, such as foods, preservatives, or dyes.

**Pregnancy**—Studies have not been done in humans. However, studies in rats and rabbits have not shown that octreotide causes birth defects or other problems, even when given in doses many times the human dose.

**Breast-feeding**—It is not known whether octreotide passes into the breast milk. However, octreotide has not been reported to cause problems in nursing babies.

**Children**—This medicine has been tested in a limited number of children as young as 1 month of age and has not been shown to cause different side effects or problems than it does in adults.

**Older adults**—This medicine has been used in persons up to 83 years of age and has not been shown to cause different side effects or problems in older people than it does in younger adults.

**Other medicines**—Although certain medicines should not be used together at all, in other cases two different medicines may be used together even if an interaction might occur. In these cases, your doctor may want to change the dose, or other precautions may be necessary. When you are taking octreotide, it is especially important that your health care professional know if you are taking any of the following:
- Antidiabetics, oral (diabetes medicine you take by mouth) or
- Glucagon or
- Insulin—Octreotide may cause high or low blood sugar; your doctor may need to change the dose of your diabetes medicine

- Growth hormone—Octreotide may cause high or low blood sugar; your doctor may need to change the dose of this medicine

**Other medical problems**—The presence of other medical problems may affect the use of octreotide. Make sure you tell your doctor if you have any other medical problems, especially:
- Diabetes mellitus (sugar diabetes)—Octreotide may cause high or low blood sugar; your doctor may need to change the dose of your diabetes medicine
- Gallbladder disease or gallstones (or history of)—This medicine may increase the chance of having gallstones
- Kidney disease (severe)—If you have this condition, octreotide may remain longer in the body; your doctor may need to change the dose of your medicine

## Proper Use Of This Medicine

To control the symptoms of your medical problem, this medicine must be taken daily in evenly spaced doses as ordered by your doctor. He or she will tell you how much octreotide you need to take each day and how to divide the doses through the day. *Make sure that you understand exactly how to use this medicine.*

Octreotide is packaged in a kit containing an ampul opener, alcohol swabs, and ampuls of the medicine. *Directions on how to use the medicine are in the package. Read them carefully* and ask your health care professional for additional explanation, if necessary.

**Dosing**—The dose of octreotide will be different for different patients. *Follow your doctor's orders or the directions on the label.* The following information includes only the average doses of octreotide. *If your dose is different, do not change it* unless your doctor tells you to do so.
- For *injection* dosage form:
  —For treating the severe diarrhea that occurs with intestinal tumors:
    - Adults and teenagers—At first, 0.05 milligrams (mg) injected under the skin, one or two times a day. Then, the dose is slowly increased. Some people may need doses as high as 0.1 to 0.6 mg a day for the first two weeks. However, the dose is usually not more than 0.75 mg a day.
    - Children—The dose is based on body weight and must be determined by your doctor. The usual dose is 0.001 to 0.01 mg per kilogram (kg) (0.0005 to 0.005 mg per pound) of body weight a day, injected under the skin.

**Missed dose**—If you miss a dose of this medicine, use it as soon as you remember it. However, if it is almost time for the next dose, skip the missed dose and go back to your regular dosing schedule. Do not double doses. Although you will not be harmed by forgetting a dose, the symptoms that you are trying to control (for example, diarrhea) may reappear. To be able to control your symptoms, your doses should be evenly spaced over a period of 24 hours. If you have any questions about this, check with your health care professional.

**Storage**—To store this medicine:

- Keep out of the reach of children.
- Store the ampuls of octreotide in the refrigerator until they are to be used. Remove the ampul that is going to be used from the refrigerator and allow it to reach room temperature before using it. Using octreotide at room temperature will help lessen the burning sensation that some people feel when injecting octreotide. Ampuls may be kept at room temperature for the day they will be used; however, they should not be kept at room temperature for longer than 24 hours.
- Do not keep outdated medicine or medicine no longer needed. Be sure that any discarded medicine and syringes are out of the reach of children.

## Precautions While Using This Medicine

*It is very important that your doctor check your progress at regular visits* to make sure that this medicine is working properly and to check for unwanted effects.

*It is very important to follow any instructions from your doctor about the careful selection and rotation of injection sites on your body.* This will help prevent skin problems, such as irritation.

## Side Effects of This Medicine

Along with its needed effects, a medicine may cause some unwanted effects. Although these problems are rare, patients using octreotide may develop symptoms of high blood sugar (hyperglycemia) or low blood sugar (hypoglycemia). *If any of the following symptoms of hyperglycemia or hypoglycemia occur, stop using octreotide and check with your doctor right away:*

*Symptoms of hyperglycemia usually include:*
> Drowsiness; dry mouth; flushed, dry skin; fruit-like breath odor; increased urination; loss of appetite; stomach-ache, nausea, or vomiting; troubled breathing (rapid

and deep); unusual thirst; unusual tiredness; weight loss (rapid)

*Early symptoms of hypoglycemia include:*
> Anxious feeling; chills; cool pale skin; difficulty in concentrating; headache; hunger; nausea; nervousness; shakiness; sweating; unusual tiredness; weakness

Other side effects may occur that usually do not need medical attention. These side effects may go away during treatment as your body adjusts to the medicine. However, check with your doctor if any of the following side effects continue or are bothersome:

*More common*
> Abdominal or stomach pain or discomfort; diarrhea; nausea and vomiting; pain, stinging, tingling, or burning sensation at place of injection, with redness and swelling

*Less common or rare*
> Dizziness or lightheadedness; unusual tiredness or weakness; headache; redness or flushing of face; swelling of feet and lower legs

Other side effects not listed above may also occur in some patients. If you notice any other effects, check with your doctor.

## Additional Information

Once a medicine has been approved for marketing for a certain use, experience may show that it is also useful for other medical problems. Although this use is not included in product labeling, octreotide is used in certain patients with the following medical conditions:

- Acromegaly (enlargement of the face, hands, and feet because of too much growth hormone)
- Acquired immune deficiency syndrome (AIDS)–related diarrhea
- Insulin-producing tumors of the pancreas

Other than the above information, there is no additional information relating to proper use, precautions, or side effects for these uses.

Revised: 12/15/92
Interim revision: 06/30/94

# OFLOXACIN    Ophthalmic†

A commonly used brand name in the U.S. is Ocuflox.

†Not commercially available in Canada.

## Description

Ofloxacin (oh-FLOKS-a-sin) is an antibiotic used to treat bacterial infections of the eye.

Ofloxacin is available only with your doctor's prescription, in the following dosage form:

*Ophthalmic*
- Ophthalmic solution (eye drops) (U.S.)

## Before Using This Medicine

In deciding to use a medicine, the risks of using the medicine must be weighed against the good it will do.

This is a decision you and your doctor will make. For ophthalmic ofloxacin, the following should be considered:

**Allergies**—Tell your doctor if you have ever had any unusual or allergic reaction to ophthalmic or systemic ofloxacin (e.g., Floxin) or any related medicines, such as cinoxacin (e.g., Cinobac), ciprofloxacin (e.g., Ciloxan or Cipro), enoxacin (e.g., Penetrex), lomefloxacin (e.g., Maxaquin), nalidixic acid (e.g., NegGram), or norfloxacin (e.g., Chibroxin or Noroxin). Also tell your health care professional if you are allergic to any other substances, such as foods, preservatives, or dyes.

**Pregnancy**—Ophthalmic ofloxacin has not been studied in pregnant women. However, studies in animals that were given very high doses of ofloxacin by mouth have shown that ofloxacin can cause birth defects or other problems. Before taking this medicine, make sure your doctor knows if you are pregnant or if you may become pregnant.

**Breast-feeding**—It is not known whether ophthalmic ofloxacin passes into breast milk. However, ofloxacin given by mouth does pass into breast milk. Although most medicines pass into breast milk in small amounts, many of them may be used safely while breast-feeding. Mothers who are using this medicine and who wish to breast-feed should discuss this with their doctor.

**Children**—Use is not recommended in infants up to 1 year of age. In children 1 year of age and older, this medicine is not expected to cause different side effects or problems than it does in adults.

**Older adults**—Many medicines have not been studied specifically in older people. Therefore, it may not be known whether they work exactly the same way they do in younger adults or if they cause different side effects or problems in older people. There is no specific information comparing use of ophthalmic ofloxacin in the elderly with use in other age groups.

**Other medicines**—Although certain medicines should not be used together at all, in other cases two different medicines may be used together even if an interaction might occur. In these cases, your doctor may want to change the dose, or other precautions may be necessary. Tell your health care professional if you're using any other prescription or nonprescription (over-the-counter [OTC]) medicine that is to be used in the eye.

## Proper Use of This Medicine

To use:

- First, wash your hands. Tilt the head back and with the index finger of one hand, press gently on the skin just beneath the lower eyelid and pull the lower eyelid away from the eye to make a space. Drop the medicine into this space. Let go of the eyelid and gently close the eyes. Do not blink. Keep the eyes closed for 1 to 2 minutes, to allow the medicine to come into contact with the infection.
- If you think you did not get the drop of medicine into your eyes properly, use another drop.

- To keep the medicine as germ-free as possible, do not touch the applicator tip to any surface (including the eye). Also, keep the container tightly closed.

To help clear up your eye infection completely, *keep using ophthalmic ofloxacin for the full time of treatment,* even if your symptoms have disappeared. *Do not miss any doses.*

**Dosing**—The dose of ophthalmic ofloxacin will be different for different patients. *Follow your doctor's orders or the directions on the label.* The following information includes only the average doses of ophthalmic ofloxacin. *If your dose is different, do not change it* unless your doctor tells you to do so.

- For *ophthalmic (eye drops)* dosage form:
  —For eye infection:
    - Adults and children 1 year of age and older— Use 1 drop in each eye every two to four hours, while you are awake, for two days. Then, use 1 drop in each eye four times a day for up to five more days.
    - Infants up to 1 year of age—Use and dose must be determined by your doctor.

**Missed dose**—If you miss a dose of this medicine, use it as soon as possible. However, if it is almost time for your next dose, skip the missed dose and go back to your regular dosing schedule.

**Storage**—To store this medicine:
- Keep out of the reach of children.
- Store away from heat and direct light.
- Keep the medicine from freezing. Do not refrigerate.
- Do not keep outdated medicine or medicine no longer needed. Be sure that any discarded medicine is out of the reach of children.

## Precautions While Using This Medicine

If your eye infection does not improve within 7 days, or if it becomes worse, check with your doctor.

This medicine may cause your eyes to become more sensitive to light than they are normally. Wearing sunglasses and avoiding too much exposure to bright light may help lessen the discomfort.

## Side Effects of This Medicine

Along with its needed effects, a medicine may cause some unwanted effects. Although not all of these side effects may occur, if they do occur they may need medical attention.

Check with your doctor as soon as possible if the following side effect occurs:

*Rare*
Dizziness

Other side effects may occur that usually do not need medical attention. These side effects may go away during treatment as your body adjusts to the medicine. However,

check with your doctor if any of the following side effects continue or are bothersome:

*More common*

Burning of eye

*Less common*

Increased sensitivity of eye to light; stinging, redness, itching, tearing, or dryness of eye

Other side effects not listed above may also occur in some patients. If you notice any other effects, check with your doctor.

Developed: 12/21/93

---

# OLSALAZINE    Oral

A commonly used brand name in the U.S. and Canada is Dipentum. Other commonly used names are sodium azodisalicylate and azodisal sodium.

## Description

Olsalazine (ole-SAL-a-zeen) is used in patients who have had ulcerative colitis to prevent the condition from occurring again. It works inside the bowel by helping to reduce the inflammation and other symptoms of the disease.

Olsalazine is available only with your doctor's prescription, in the following dosage form:

*Oral*

• Capsules (U.S. and Canada)

## Before Using This Medicine

In deciding to use a medicine, the risks of taking the medicine must be weighed against the good it will do. This is a decision you and your doctor will make. For olsalazine, the following should be considered:

**Allergies**—Tell your doctor if you have ever had any unusual or allergic reaction to olsalazine, mesalamine, or any salicylates (for example, aspirin). Also tell your health care professional if you are allergic to any other substances, such as foods, preservatives, or dyes.

**Pregnancy**—Studies have not been done in humans. However, studies in rats have shown that olsalazine causes birth defects and other problems at doses 5 to 20 times the human dose. Before taking this medicine, make sure your doctor knows if you are pregnant or if you may become pregnant.

**Breast-feeding**—It is not known whether olsalazine passes into the breast milk.

**Children**—Studies on this medicine have been done only in adult patients, and there is no specific information comparing use of olsalazine in children with use in other age groups.

**Older adults**—Many medicines have not been studied specifically in older people. Therefore, it may not be known whether they work exactly the same way they do in younger adults. Although there is no specific information comparing use of olsalazine in the elderly with use in

other age groups, this medicine is not expected to cause different side effects or problems in older people than it does in younger adults.

**Other medicines**—Although certain medicines should not be used together at all, in other cases two different medicines may be used together even if an interaction might occur. In these cases, your doctor may want to change the dose, or other precautions may be necessary. When you are using olsalazine, it is especially important that your health care professional know if you are taking any other medicines.

**Other medical problems**—The presence of other medical problems may affect the use of olsalazine. Make sure you tell your doctor if you have any other medical problems, especially:

• Kidney disease—The use of olsalazine may cause further damage to the kidneys

## Proper Use of This Medicine

Olsalazine is best taken with food, to lessen stomach upset and diarrhea. If stomach or intestinal problems continue or are bothersome, check with your doctor.

*Keep taking this medicine for the full time of treatment,* even if you begin to feel better after a few days. *Do not miss any doses.*

**Dosing**—The dose of olsalazine will be different for different patients. *Follow your doctor's orders or the directions on the label.* The following information includes only the average doses of olsalazine. *If your dose is different, do not change it* unless your doctor tells you to do so.

• For *oral* dosage form (capsules):

—To prevent ulcerative colitis from occurring again:

• Adults and teenagers—500 milligrams (mg) two times a day.

• Children—Use and dose must be determined by your doctor.

**Missed dose**—If you miss a dose of this medicine, take it as soon as possible. However, if it is almost time for your next dose, skip the missed dose and go back to your regular dosing schedule. Do not double doses.

**Storage**—To store this medicine:

- Keep out of the reach of children.
- Store away from heat and direct light.
- Do not store this medicine in the bathroom, near the kitchen sink, or in other damp places. Heat or moisture may cause the medicine to break down.
- Do not keep outdated medicine or medicine no longer needed. Be sure that any discarded medicine is out of the reach of children.

---

## Precautions While Using This Medicine

*It is very important that your doctor check your progress at regular visits*, especially if you will be taking it for a long time. Olsalazine may cause blood problems.

---

## Side Effects of This Medicine

Along with its needed effects, a medicine may cause some unwanted effects. Although not all of these side effects may occur, if they do occur they may need medical attention.

*Check with your doctor as soon as possible if any of the following side effects occur:*

> *Rare*
>> Bloody diarrhea; fever; pale skin; skin rash; sore throat; unusual bleeding or bruising; unusual tiredness or weakness; yellow eyes or skin

Other side effects may occur that usually do not need medical attention. These side effects may go away during treatment as your body adjusts to the medicine. However, check with your doctor if any of the following side effects continue or are bothersome:

> *More common*
>> Abdominal or stomach pain or upset; diarrhea; loss of appetite; nausea or vomiting
> *Less common*
>> Aching joints and muscles; acne; anxiety or depression, drowsiness or dizziness; headache; insomnia

Other side effects not listed above may also occur in some patients. If you notice any other effects, check with your doctor.

---

Revised: 05/13/91
Interim revision: 07/05/94

---

# OMEPRAZOLE  Systemic

Some commonly used brand names are:

**In the U.S.—**
  Prilosec
**In Canada—**
  Losec

## Description

Omeprazole (o-MEP-ra-zole) is used to treat certain conditions in which there is too much acid in the stomach. It is used to treat duodenal ulcers and gastroesophageal reflux disease, a condition in which the acid in the stomach washes back up into the esophagus. Omeprazole is also used to treat Zollinger-Ellison disease, a condition in which the stomach produces too much acid. It may also be used for other conditions as determined by your doctor.

Omeprazole works by decreasing the amount of acid produced by the stomach.

This medicine is available only with your doctor's prescription.

> *Oral*
> - Delayed-release capsules (U.S. and Canada)

## Before Using This Medicine

In deciding to use a medicine, the risks of taking the medicine must be weighed against the good it will do.

This is a decision you and your doctor will make. For omeprazole, the following should be considered:

**Allergies**—Tell your doctor if you have ever had any unusual or allergic reaction to omeprazole. Also tell your health care professional if you are allergic to any other substances, such as foods, preservatives, or dyes.

**Pregnancy**—Studies have not been done in humans. However, studies in animals have shown that omeprazole may cause harm to the fetus.

**Breast-feeding**—Omeprazole may pass into the breast milk. Since this medicine has been shown to cause unwanted effects, such as tumors and cancer in animals, it may be necessary for you to take another medicine or to stop breast-feeding during treatment. Be sure you have discussed the risks and benefits of the medicine with your doctor.

**Children**—There is no specific information comparing the use of omeprazole in children with use in other age groups.

**Older adults**—Many medicines have not been studied specifically in older people. Therefore, it may not be known whether they work exactly the same way they do in younger adults or if they cause different side effects or problems in older people. There is no specific information comparing use of omeprazole in the elderly with use in other age groups.

**Other medicines**—Although certain medicines should not be used together at all, in other cases two different medicines may be used together even if an interaction might occur. In these cases, your doctor may want to change the dose, or other precautions may be necessary. When you are taking omeprazole, it is especially important that your health care professional know if you are taking any of the following:

- Anticoagulants (blood thinners) or
- Diazepam (e.g., Valium) or
- Phenytoin (e.g., Dilantin)—Use with omeprazole may cause high blood levels of these medicines, which may increase the chance of side effects

**Other medical problems**—The presence of other medical problems may affect the use of omeprazole. Make sure you tell your doctor if you have any other medical problems, especially:

- Liver disease or a history of liver disease—This condition may cause omeprazole to build up in the body

## Proper Use of This Medicine

Take omeprazole immediately before a meal, preferably in the morning.

It may take several days before this medicine begins to relieve stomach pain. To help relieve this pain, antacids may be taken with omeprazole, unless your doctor has told you not to use them.

Swallow the capsule whole. Do not crush, break, chew, or open the capsule.

*Take this medicine for the full time of treatment, even if you begin to feel better.* Also, keep your appointments with your doctor for check-ups so that your doctor will be better able to tell you when to stop taking this medicine.

**Dosing**—The dose of omeprazole will be different for different patients. *Follow your doctor's orders or the directions on the label.* The following information includes only the average doses of omeprazole. *If your dose is different, do not change it* unless your doctor tells you to do so.

- For *oral* dosage form (capsules):
  —To treat gastroesophageal reflux disease:
  - Adults—20 milligrams (mg) taken once a day for four to eight weeks. Or, your doctor may tell you to take 40 mg a day for certain conditions.
  - Children—Dose must be determined by your doctor.
  —To treat conditions in which the stomach produces too much acid:
  - Adults—60 milligrams (mg) taken once a day. Your doctor may change the dose as needed. Your treatment may be continued for as long as it is needed.
  - Children—Dose must be determined by your doctor.

—To treat duodenal ulcers:
- Adults—20 mg taken once a day. Or, your doctor may tell you to take 40 mg a day for certain conditions.
- Children—Dose must be determined by your doctor.

**Missed dose**—If you miss a dose of this medicine, take it as soon as possible. However, if it is almost time for your next dose, skip the missed dose and go back to your regular dosing schedule. Do not double doses.

**Storage**—To store this medicine:
- Keep out of the reach of children.
- Store away from heat and direct light.
- Do not store in the bathroom, near the kitchen sink, or in other damp places. Heat or moisture may cause the medicine to break down.
- Do not keep outdated medicine or medicine no longer needed. Be sure that any discarded medicine is out of the reach of children.

## Precautions While Using This Medicine

If your condition does not improve, or if it becomes worse, check with your doctor.

## Side Effects of This Medicine

Along with its needed effects, a medicine may cause some unwanted effects. Although not all of these side effects may occur, if they do occur they may need medical attention.

Check with your doctor as soon as possible if any of the following side effects occur:

*Rare*

Bloody or cloudy urine; continuing ulcers or sores in mouth; difficult, burning, or painful urination; frequent urge to urinate; sore throat and fever; unusual bleeding or bruising; unusual tiredness or weakness

Other side effects may occur that usually do not need medical attention. These side effects may go away during treatment as your body adjusts to the medicine. However, check with your doctor if any of the following side effects continue or are bothersome:

*More common*

Abdominal or stomach pain

*Less common*

Chest pain; constipation; diarrhea or loose stools; dizziness; gas; headache; heartburn; muscle pain; nausea and vomiting; skin rash or itching; unusual drowsiness; unusual tiredness

Other side effects not listed above may also occur in some patients. If you notice any other effects, check with your doctor.

## Additional Information

Once a medicine has been approved for marketing for a certain use, experience may show that it is also useful for other medical problems. Although this use is not included in product labeling, omeprazole is used in certain patients with the following medical condition:

• Gastric ulcer

Other than the above information, there is no additional information relating to proper use, precautions, or side effects for these uses.

---

Revised: 02/25/92
Interim revision: 07/28/94

# ONDANSETRON  Systemic

A commonly used brand name in the U.S. and Canada is Zofran.

## Description

Ondansetron (on-DAN-se-tron) is used to prevent the nausea and vomiting that may occur after treatment with anti-cancer medicines.

Ondansetron is to be given only by or under the immediate supervision of your doctor. It is available in the following dosage form:

*Parenteral*
• Injection (U.S. and Canada)

## Before Using This Medicine

In deciding to use a medicine, the risks of taking the medicine must be weighed against the good it will do. This is a decision you and your doctor will make. For ondansetron, the following should be considered:

**Allergies**—Tell your doctor if you have ever had any unusual or allergic reaction to ondansetron. Also tell your health care professional if you are allergic to any other substances, such as foods, preservatives, or dyes.

**Pregnancy**—Ondansetron has not been studied in pregnant women. However, this medicine has not been shown to cause birth defects or other problems in animal studies.

**Breast-feeding**—It is not known whether ondansetron passes into the breast milk.

**Children**—This medicine has been tested in a limited number of children 4 years of age or older. In effective doses, the medicine has not been shown to cause different side effects or problems than it does in adults.

**Older adults**—This medicine has been tested in a limited number of patients 65 years of age or older and has not been shown to cause different side effects or problems in older people than it does in younger adults.

**Other medicines**—Although certain medicines should not be used together at all, in other cases two different medicines may be used together even if an interaction might occur. In these cases, your doctor may want to change the dose, or other precautions may be necessary. Tell your health care professional if you are taking any other prescription or nonprescription (over-the-counter [OTC]) medicine.

## Proper Use of This Medicine

**Dosing**—The dose of ondansetron will be different for different patients. *Follow your doctor's orders or the directions on the label.* The following information includes only the average dose of ondansetron. *If your dose is different, do not change it* unless your doctor tells you to do so.

• For *injection* dosage form:
—For prevention of nausea and vomiting:
• Adults and children 4 years of age and older—The dose is based on body weight and must be determined by your doctor. It is usually 150 micrograms (mcg) per kilogram (kg) (68 mcg per pound) of body weight. It is injected into a vein over a period of fifteen minutes, beginning thirty minutes before the cancer medicine is given. The dose of ondansetron is repeated four and eight hours following the first dose.
• Children up to 4 years of age—Dose must be determined by your doctor.

## Side Effects of This Medicine

Along with its needed effects, a medicine may cause some unwanted effects. Although not all of these side effects may occur, if they do occur they may need medical attention.

*Check with your health care professional immediately* if any of the following side effects occur:
*Rare*
Shortness of breath; tightness in chest; troubled breathing; wheezing

Other side effects may occur that usually do not need medical attention. These side effects may go away during treatment as your body adjusts to the medicine. However, check with your doctor if any of the following side effects continue or are bothersome:
*More common*
Constipation; diarrhea; fever and/or chills; headache

*Less common*

Abdominal pain or stomach cramps; dizziness or light-headedness; drowsiness; dryness of mouth; skin rash; unusual tiredness or weakness

Other side effects not listed above may also occur in some patients. If you notice any other effects, check with your doctor.

Revised: 07/16/91
Interim revision: 07/15/94

# OPIUM PREPARATIONS    Systemic

Some commonly used names are:

**In the U.S.—**
Camphorated Opium Tincture[2]
Laudanum[1]

**In Canada—**
Camphorated Opium Tincture[2]
Laudanum[1]

Note: For quick reference, the following opium preparations are numbered to match the corresponding brand names.

This information applies to the following medicines:

1. Opium Tincture (OH-pee-um)
2. Paregoric (par-e-GOR-ik)

## Description

Opium preparations are used along with other measures to treat severe diarrhea. These medicines belong to the group of medicines called narcotics. If too much of a narcotic is taken, it may become habit-forming, causing mental or physical dependence. Physical dependence may lead to withdrawal side effects when you stop taking the medicine.

Opium preparations are available only with your doctor's prescription, in the following dosage forms:

*Oral*

Opium Tincture
• Oral liquid (U.S. and Canada)
Paregoric
• Oral liquid (U.S. and Canada)

## Before Using This Medicine

In deciding to use a medicine, the risks of taking the medicine must be weighed against the good it will do. This is a decision you and your doctor will make. For opium preparations, the following should be considered:

**Allergies**—Tell your doctor if you have ever had any unusual or allergic reaction to morphine, codeine, or papaverine. Also tell your health care professional if you are allergic to any other substances, such as foods, preservatives, or dyes.

**Pregnancy**—Opium preparations have not been studied in pregnant women. However, morphine (contained in these medicines) has caused birth defects in animals when given in very large doses.

Regular use of opium preparations during pregnancy may cause the fetus to become dependent on the medicine.

This may lead to withdrawal side effects in the newborn baby. Also, these medicines may cause breathing problems in the newborn baby, especially if they are taken just before delivery.

**Breast-feeding**—Opium preparations have not been reported to cause problems in nursing babies.

**Children**—Breathing problems may be especially likely to occur in children up to 2 years of age, who are usually more sensitive than adults to the effects of opium preparations.

**Older adults**—Breathing problems may be especially likely to occur in elderly patients, who are usually more sensitive than younger adults to the effects of opium preparations.

**Other medicines**—Although certain medicines should not be used together at all, in other cases two different medicines may be used together even if an interaction might occur. In these cases, your doctor may want to change the dose, or other precautions may be necessary. When you are taking an opium preparation, it is especially important that your health care professional know if you are taking any of the following:

• Anticholinergics (medicine for abdominal or stomach spasms or cramps) or
• Central nervous system (CNS) depressants, especially other narcotics, or
• Other diarrhea medicine or
• Tricyclic antidepressants (amitriptyline [e.g., Elavil], amoxapine [e.g., Asendin], clomipramine [e.g., Anafranil], desipramine [e.g., Pertofrane], doxepin [e.g., Sinequan], imipramine [e.g., Tofranil], nortriptyline [e.g., Aventyl], protriptyline [e.g., Vivactil], trimipramine [e.g., Surmontil])—The chance of side effects is increased
• Naltrexone (e.g., Trexan)—Naltrexone blocks the effects of opium preparations and makes them less effective in treating diarrhea

**Other medical problems**—The presence of other medical problems may affect the use of opium preparations. Make sure you tell your doctor if you have any other medical problems, especially:

• Alcohol or other drug abuse (or history of) or
• Colitis or
• Heart disease or
• Kidney disease or

- Liver disease or
- Underactive thyroid—The chance of side effects may be increased
- Brain disease or head injury or
- Emphysema, asthma, bronchitis, or other chronic lung disease or
- Enlarged prostate or problems with urination or
- Gallbladder disease or gallstones—Some of the side effects of opium preparations can be dangerous if these conditions are present
- Convulsions (seizures), history of—Opium can rarely cause convulsions

## Proper Use of This Medicine

This medicine is to be taken by mouth even if it comes in a dropper bottle. The amount you should take is to be measured with the special dropper provided with your prescription and diluted with water just before you take each dose. This will cause the medicine to turn milky in color, but it will still work.

If your prescription does not come in a dropper bottle and the directions on the bottle say to take it by the teaspoonful, it is not necessary to dilute it before using.

If this medicine upsets your stomach, your doctor may want you to take it with food.

*Take this medicine only as directed by your doctor.* Do not take more of it, do not take it more often, and do not take it for a longer time than your doctor ordered. This is especially important for young children and for elderly patients, who are especially sensitive to the effects of opium preparations. If too much is taken, this medicine may become habit-forming (causing mental or physical dependence) or lead to problems because of an overdose.

**Dosing**—The dose of these medicines will be different for different patients. *Follow your doctor's orders or the directions on the label.* The following information includes only the average doses of these medicines. *If your dose is different, do not change it* unless your doctor tells you to do so.

*For opium tincture (laudanum)*
- For *oral liquid* dosage form (drops):
  —For diarrhea:
    - Adults—5 to 16 drops of liquid, measured with the dropper in the bottle and mixed with a little water, four times a day until diarrhea is controlled.
    - Children—Dose must be determined by your doctor.

*For paregoric*
- For *oral liquid* dosage form:
  —For diarrhea:
    - Adults—1 or 2 teaspoonfuls one to four times a day until diarrhea is controlled. Use a measuring spoon to measure the dose. An ordinary household teaspoon that is used at the table may not hold the right amount of medicine.

- Children 2 years of age and older—0.25 to 0.5 milliliters (mL) (4 to 8 drops), mixed with a little water, one to four times a day until diarrhea is controlled. This amount of medicine must be measured with a dropper or a special measuring device that can be used for very small amounts of liquid. If you did not receive a dropper or measuring device with the medicine, check with your pharmacist.

**Missed dose**—If you miss a dose of this medicine, take it as soon as you remember. However, if it is almost time for your next dose, skip the missed dose and go back to your regular dosing schedule. *Do not double doses.*

**Storage**—To store this medicine:
- Keep out of the reach of children. Overdose is very dangerous in young children.
- Store away from heat and direct light.
- Keep the container for this medicine tightly closed to prevent the alcohol from evaporating and the medicine from becoming stronger.
- Do not store this medicine in the refrigerator or allow the medicine to freeze. If it does get cold and you notice any solid particles in it, throw it away.
- Do not keep outdated medicine or medicine no longer needed. Be sure that any discarded medicine is out of the reach of children.

## Precautions While Using This Medicine

*Check with your doctor if your diarrhea does not stop after 1 or 2 days or if you develop a fever.*

This medicine will add to the effects of alcohol and other CNS depressants (medicines that slow down the nervous system, possibly causing drowsiness). Some examples of CNS depressants are antihistamines or medicine for hay fever, other allergies, or colds; sedatives, tranquilizers, or sleeping medicine; prescription pain medicine or other narcotics; barbiturates; medicine for seizures; muscle relaxants; or anesthetics, including some dental anesthetics. *Do not drink alcoholic beverages, and check with your doctor before taking any of the medicines listed above, while you are taking this medicine.*

This medicine may cause some people to become drowsy, dizzy, lightheaded, or less alert than they are normally. Even if taken at bedtime, it may cause some people to feel drowsy or less alert on arising. *Make sure you know how you react to this medicine before you drive, use machines, or do anything else that could be dangerous if you are dizzy or are not alert.*

Dizziness, lightheadedness, or fainting may be especially likely to occur when you get up suddenly from a lying or sitting position. Getting up slowly may help lessen this problem. If you feel very dizzy, lightheaded, or faint after taking this medicine, lying down for a while may help.

If you have been taking this medicine regularly for several weeks or more, *do not stop using it without first checking with your doctor.* Your doctor may want you to reduce gradually the amount you are using before stopping completely, to lessen the chance of withdrawal side effects.

*If you think you or someone else may have taken an overdose, get emergency help at once.* Taking an overdose of this medicine or taking alcohol or other CNS depressants with this medicine may lead to unconsciousness and possibly death. Signs of overdose include convulsions (seizures), confusion, severe nervousness or restlessness, severe dizziness, severe drowsiness, slow or irregular breathing, and severe weakness.

---

## Side Effects of This Medicine

Along with its needed effects, a medicine may cause some unwanted effects. Although not all of these side effects may occur, if they do occur they may need medical attention.

*Get emergency help immediately if any of the following symptoms of overdose occur:*

> Cold, clammy skin; confusion; convulsions (seizures); dizziness (severe); drowsiness (severe); low blood pressure; nervousness or restlessness (severe); pinpoint pupils of eyes; slow heartbeat; slow or irregular breathing; weakness (severe)

Also, *check with your doctor immediately* if any of the following side effects are severe and occur suddenly since they may indicate a more severe and dangerous problem with your bowels:

> *Rare*
> Bloating; constipation; loss of appetite; nausea or vomiting; stomach cramps or pain

In addition, check with your doctor as soon as possible if any of the following side effects occur:

> *Rare*
> Fast heartbeat; increased sweating; mental depression; redness or flushing of face; shortness of breath, wheezing, or troubled breathing; skin rash, hives, or itching; slow heartbeat

Other side effects may occur that usually do not need medical attention. These side effects may go away during treatment as your body adjusts to the medicine. However, check with your doctor if any of the following side effects continue or are bothersome:

> *More common with large doses*
> Difficult or painful urination; dizziness, lightheadedness, or feeling faint; drowsiness; frequent urge to urinate; nervousness or restlessness; unusual decrease in amount of urine; unusual tiredness or weakness

After you stop using this medicine, your body may need time to adjust. The length of time this takes depends on the amount of medicine you were using and how long you used it. During this period of time check with your doctor if you notice any of the following side effects:

> Body aches; diarrhea; fever, runny nose, or sneezing; gooseflesh; increased sweating; increased yawning; loss of appetite; nausea or vomiting; nervousness, restlessness, or irritability; shivering or trembling; stomach cramps; trouble in sleeping; unusually large pupils of eyes; weakness (severe)

Other side effects not listed above may also occur in some patients. If you notice any other effects, check with your doctor.

Revised: 10/05/92
Interim revision: 09/08/94

---

# ORPHENADRINE   Systemic

Some commonly used brand names are:

**In the U.S.—**

| | |
|---|---|
| Banflex | Myotrol |
| Blanex | Neocyten |
| Disipal | Noradex |
| Flexagin | Norflex |
| Flexain | O-Flex |
| Flexoject | Orflagen |
| Flexon | Orfro |
| K-Flex | Orphenate |
| Marflex | Tega-Flex |
| Myolin | |

Generic name product may also be available.

**In Canada—**

| | |
|---|---|
| Disipal | Norflex |

---

## Description

Orphenadrine (or-FEN-a-dreen) is used to help relax certain muscles in your body and relieve the pain and discomfort caused by strains, sprains, or other injury to your muscles. One form of orphenadrine is also used to relieve trembling caused by Parkinson's disease. However, this medicine does not take the place of rest, exercise or physical therapy, or other treatment that your doctor may recommend for your medical problem.

Orphenadrine acts in the central nervous system (CNS) to produce its muscle relaxant effects. Orphenadrine also has other actions (anticholinergic) that produce its helpful effects in Parkinson's disease. Orphenadrine's CNS and anticholinergic actions may also be responsible for some of its side effects.

In the U.S., this medicine is available only with your doctor's prescription. In Canada, it may be available without a prescription. It is available in the following dosage forms:

> *Oral*
> • Tablets (U.S. and Canada)
> • Extended-release tablets (U.S. and Canada)

*Parenteral*
* Injection (U.S. and Canada)

## Before Using This Medicine

In deciding to use a medicine, the risks of taking the medicine must be weighed against the good it will do. This is a decision you and your doctor will make. For orphenadrine, the following should be considered:

**Allergies**—Tell your doctor if you have ever had any unusual or allergic reaction to orphenadrine. Also tell your health care professional if you are allergic to any other substances, such as foods, preservatives, or dyes.

**Pregnancy**—Orphenadrine has not been reported to cause birth defects or other problems in humans.

**Breast-feeding**—It is not known whether orphenadrine passes into the breast milk. However, orphenadrine has not been reported to cause problems in nursing babies.

**Children**—Studies on this medicine have been done only in adult patients, and there is no specific information about its use in children.

**Older adults**—Many medicines have not been tested in older people. Therefore, it may not be known whether they work exactly the same way they do in younger adults or if they cause different side effects or problems in older people. There is no specific information about the use of orphenadrine in the elderly.

**Other medicines**—Although certain medicines should not be used together at all, in other cases two different medicines may be used together even if an interaction might occur. In these cases, your doctor may want to change the dose, or other precautions may be necessary. When you are taking orphenadrine, it is especially important that your health care professional know if you are taking any of the following:
* Central nervous system (CNS) depressants
* Tricyclic antidepressants (amitriptyline [e.g., Elavil], amoxapine [e.g., Asendin], clomipramine [e.g., Anafranil], desipramine [e.g., Pertofrane], doxepin [e.g., Sinequan], imipramine [e.g., Tofranil], nortriptyline [e.g., Aventyl], protriptyline [e.g., Vivactil], trimipramine [e.g., Surmontil])—The chance of side effects may be increased

**Other medical problems**—The presence of other medical problems may affect the use of orphenadrine. Make sure you tell your doctor if you have any other medical problems, especially:
* Disease of the digestive tract, especially esophagus disease, stomach ulcer, or intestinal blockage, or
* Enlarged prostate or
* Fast or irregular heartbeat or
* Glaucoma or
* Myasthenia gravis or
* Urinary tract blockage—Orphenadrine has side effects that may be harmful to people with these conditions
* Heart disease or
* Kidney disease or
* Liver disease—The chance of side effects may be increased

## Proper Use of This Medicine

**Missed dose**—If you miss a dose of this medicine and remember within an hour or so of the missed dose, take it right away. But if you do not remember until later, skip the missed dose and go back to your regular dosing schedule. Do not double doses.

**Storage**—To store this medicine:
* Keep out of the reach of children.
* Store away from heat and direct light.
* Do not store this medicine in the bathroom, near the kitchen sink, or in other damp places. Heat or moisture may cause the medicine to break down.
* Do not keep outdated medicine or medicine no longer needed. Be sure that any discarded medicine is out of the reach of children.

## Precautions While Using This Medicine

If you will be taking this medicine for a long time (for example, more than a few weeks), your doctor should check your progress at regular visits.

This medicine may add to the effects of alcohol and other CNS depressants (medicines that slow down the nervous system, possibly causing drowsiness). Some examples of CNS depressants are antihistamines or medicine for hay fever, other allergies, or colds; sedatives, tranquilizers, or sleeping medicine; prescription pain medicine or narcotics; barbiturates; medicine for seizures; other muscle relaxants; or anesthetics, including some dental anesthetics. *Do not drink alcoholic beverages, and check with your doctor before taking any of the medicines listed above, while you are using this medicine.*

This medicine may cause some people to have blurred vision or to become drowsy, dizzy, lightheaded, faint, or less alert than they are normally. It may also cause muscle weakness in some people. *Make sure you know how you react to this medicine before you drive, use machines, or do anything else that could be dangerous if you are dizzy or are not alert and able to see well.*

Orphenadrine may cause dryness of the mouth. For temporary relief, use sugarless candy or gum, melt bits of ice in your mouth, or use a saliva substitute. However, if dry mouth continues for more than 2 weeks, check with your dentist. Continuing dryness of the mouth may increase the chance of dental disease, including tooth decay, gum disease, and fungus infections.

## Side Effects of This Medicine

Along with its needed effects, a medicine may cause some unwanted effects. Although not all of these side effects may occur, if they do occur they may need medical attention.

Check with your doctor as soon as possible if any of the following side effects occur:
*Less common*
> Decreased urination; eye pain; fainting; fast or pounding heartbeat

*Rare*

Hallucinations (seeing, hearing, or feeling things that are not there); shortness of breath, troubled breathing, tightness in chest, and/or wheezing; skin rash, hives, itching, or redness; sores, ulcers, or white spots on lips or in mouth; swollen and/or painful glands; unusual bruising or bleeding; unusual tiredness or weakness

Other side effects may occur that usually do not need medical attention. These side effects may go away during treatment as your body adjusts to the medicine. However, check with your doctor if any of the following side effects continue or are bothersome:

*More common*

Dryness of mouth

*Less common or rare*

Abdominal or stomach cramps or pain; blurred or double vision or other vision problems; confusion; constipation; difficult urination; dizziness or lightheadedness; drowsiness; excitement, irritability, nervousness, or restlessness; headache; muscle weakness; nausea or vomiting; trembling; unusually large pupils of eyes

Other side effects not listed above may also occur in some patients. If you notice any other effects, check with your doctor.

Revised: August 1990

---

# ORPHENADRINE AND ASPIRIN    Systemic

Some commonly used brand names are:

**In the U.S.—**

| | |
|---|---|
| Norgesic | N3 Gesic |
| Norgesic Forte | N3 Gesic Forte |
| Norphadrine | Orphenagesic |
| Norphadrine Forte | Orphenagesic Forte |

**In Canada—‡**

| | |
|---|---|
| Norgesic | Norgesic Forte |

‡In Canada, *Aspirin* is a brand name. Acetylsalicylic acid is the generic name in Canada. ASA, a synonym for acetylsalicylic acid, is the term that commonly appears on Canadian product labels.

---

## Description

Orphenadrine (or-FEN-a-dreen) and aspirin (AS-pir-in) combination is used to help relax certain muscles in your body and relieve the pain and discomfort caused by strains, sprains, or other injury to your muscles. However, this medicine does not take the place of rest, exercise, or other treatment that your doctor may recommend for your medical problem.

Orphenadrine acts in the central nervous system (CNS) to produce its muscle relaxant effects. Actions in the CNS may also be responsible for some of its side effects. Orphenadrine also has other actions (antimuscarinic) that may be responsible for some of its side effects.

This combination medicine also contains caffeine (kaf-EEN).

In the U.S., this combination medicine is available only with your doctor's prescription. In Canada, it is available without a prescription.

These medicines are available in the following dosage forms:

*Oral*

• Tablets (U.S. and Canada)

## Before Using This Medicine

In deciding to use a medicine, the risks of taking the medicine must be weighed against the good it will do. This is a decision you and your doctor will make. For orphenadrine and aspirin combination, the following should be considered:

**Allergies**—Tell your doctor if you have ever had any unusual or allergic reaction to orphenadrine, caffeine, aspirin or other salicylates including methyl salicylate (oil of wintergreen), or to any of the following medicines:

Diclofenac (e.g., Voltaren)
Diflunisal (e.g., Dolobid)
Etodolac (e.g., Lodine)
Fenoprofen (e.g., Nalfon)
Floctafenine (e.g., Idarac)
Flurbiprofen, oral (e.g., Ansaid)
Ibuprofen (e.g., Motrin)
Indomethacin (e.g., Indocin)
Ketoprofen (e.g., Orudis)
Ketorolac (e.g., Toradol)
Meclofenamate (e.g., Meclomen)
Mefenamic acid (e.g., Ponstel)
Nabumetone (e.g., Relafen)
Naproxen (e.g., Naprosyn)
Oxaprozin (e.g., Daypro)
Oxyphenbutazone (e.g., Tandearil)
Phenylbutazone (e.g., Butazolidin)
Piroxicam (e.g., Feldene)
Sulindac (e.g., Clinoril)
Suprofen (e.g., Suprol)
Tenoxicam (e.g., Mobiflex)
Tiaprofenic acid (e.g., Surgam)
Tolmetin (e.g., Tolectin)
Zomepirac (e.g., Zomax)

Also tell your health care professional if you are allergic to any other substances, such as foods, preservatives, or dyes.

## Pregnancy—

- *For aspirin:* Studies in humans have not shown that aspirin causes birth defects. However, aspirin has caused birth defects in animal studies.

  Some reports have suggested that too much use of aspirin late in pregnancy may cause a decrease in the newborn's weight and possible death of the fetus or newborn baby. However, the mothers in these reports had been taking much larger amounts of aspirin than are usually recommended. Studies of mothers taking aspirin in the doses that are usually recommended did not show these unwanted effects.

  Regular use of aspirin late in pregnancy may cause unwanted effects on the heart or blood flow in the fetus or in the newborn baby. Also, use of aspirin during the last 2 weeks of pregnancy may cause bleeding problems in the fetus before or during delivery or in the newborn baby. In addition, too much use of aspirin during the last 3 months of pregnancy may increase the length of pregnancy, prolong labor, cause other problems during delivery, or cause severe bleeding in the mother before, during, or after delivery. *Do not take aspirin during the last 3 months of pregnancy unless it has been ordered by your doctor.*

- *For orphenadrine:* Orphenadrine has not been reported to cause birth defects or other problems in humans.

**Breast-feeding**—This medicine has not been shown to cause problems in nursing babies. However, aspirin passes into the breast milk. Also, caffeine passes into the breast milk in small amounts. It is not known whether orphenadrine passes into the breast milk.

**Children**—*Do not give a medicine containing aspirin to a child or a teenager with a fever or other symptoms of a virus infection, especially flu or chickenpox, without first discussing its use with your child's doctor.* This is very important because aspirin may cause a serious illness called Reye's syndrome in children with fever caused by a virus infection, especially flu or chickenpox. Children who do not have a virus infection may also be more sensitive to the effects of aspirin, especially if they have a fever or have lost large amounts of body fluid because of vomiting, diarrhea, or sweating. This may increase the chance of side effects during treatment.

There is no specific information about the use of orphenadrine in children.

**Older adults**—Elderly people are especially sensitive to the effects of aspirin. This may increase the chance of side effects during treatment.

There is no specific information about the use of orphenadrine in the elderly.

**Other medicines**—Although certain medicines should not be used together at all, in other cases two different medicines may be used together even if an interaction might occur. In these cases, your doctor may want to change the dose, or other precautions may be necessary. When you are taking orphenadrine and aspirin combination, it is especially important that your health care professional know if you are taking any of the following:

- Anticoagulants (blood thinners) or
- Carbenicillin by injection (e.g., Geopen) or
- Cefamandole (e.g., Mandol) or
- Cefoperazone (e.g., Cefobid) or
- Cefotetan (e.g., Cefotan) or
- Dipyridamole (e.g., Persantine) or
- Divalproex (e.g., Depakote) or
- Heparin or
- Medicine for inflammation or pain, except narcotics, or
- Moxalactam (e.g., Moxam) or
- Pentoxifylline (e.g., Trental) or
- Plicamycin (e.g., Mithracin) or
- Ticarcillin (e.g., Ticar) or
- Valproic acid (e.g., Depakene)—Taking these medicines together with aspirin may increase the chance of bleeding
- Anticholinergics (medicine for abdominal or stomach spasms or cramps) or
- Central nervous system (CNS) depressants or
- Methotrexate (e.g., Mexate) or
- Tricyclic antidepressants (amitriptyline [e.g., Elavil], amoxapine [e.g., Asendin], clomipramine [e.g., Anafranil], desipramine [e.g., Pertofrane], doxepin [e.g., Sinequan], imipramine [e.g., Tofranil], nortriptyline [e.g., Aventyl], protriptyline [e.g., Vivactil], trimipramine [e.g., Surmontil]) or
- Vancomycin (e.g., Vancocin)—The chance of side effects may be increased
- Antidiabetics, oral (diabetes medicine you take by mouth)—Aspirin may increase the effects of the antidiabetic medicine; a change in dose may be needed if aspirin is taken regularly
- Probenecid (e.g., Benemid) or
- Sulfinpyrazone (e.g., Anturane)—Aspirin can keep these medicines from working properly for treating gout; also, taking aspirin together with sulfinpyrazone may increase the chance of bleeding
- Urinary alkalizers (medicine that makes the urine less acid, such as acetazolamide [e.g., Diamox], dichlorphenamide [e.g., Daranide], methazolamide [e.g., Neptazane], potassium or sodium citrate and/or citric acid)—These medicines may make aspirin less effective by causing it to be removed from the body more quickly
- Zidovudine (e.g., AZT; Retrovir)—Aspirin may increase the blood levels of zidovudine, which increases the chance of serious side effects

**Other medical problems**—The presence of other medical problems may affect the use of orphenadrine and aspirin combination. Make sure you tell your doctor if you have any other medical problems, especially:

- Anemia or
- Overactive thyroid or
- Stomach ulcer or other stomach problems—Aspirin may make your condition worse
- Asthma, allergies, and nasal polyps, history of or
- Glucose-6-phosphate dehydrogenase (G6PD) deficiency or
- Kidney disease or
- Liver disease—The chance of side effects may be increased
- Disease of the digestive tract, especially esophagus disease or intestinal blockage, or
- Enlarged prostate or

- Fast or irregular heartbeat or
- Glaucoma or
- Myasthenia gravis or
- Urinary tract blockage—Orphenadrine has side effects that may be harmful to people with these conditions
- Gout—Aspirin can make this condition worse and can also lessen the effects of some medicines used to treat gout
- Heart disease—The chance of some side effects may be increased. Also, the caffeine present in this combination medicine can make your condition worse
- Hemophilia or other bleeding problems or
- Vitamin K deficiency—Aspirin may increase the chance of bleeding

## Proper Use of This Medicine

*Take this medicine with food or a full glass (8 ounces) of water* to lessen stomach irritation.

*Do not take this medicine if it has a strong vinegar-like odor.* This odor means the aspirin in it is breaking down. If you have any questions about this, check with your health care professional.

*Do not take more of this medicine than your doctor ordered* to lessen the chance of side effects or overdose.

**Dosing**—The dose of orphenadrine and aspirin combination medicine will be different for different people. *Follow your doctor's orders or the directions on the label.* The following information includes only the average doses of the combination medicine. *If your dose is different, do not change it* unless your doctor tells you to do so.

- For *oral* dosage forms (tablets):
  —For muscle pain and stiffness:
    - Adults and teenagers—One or two tablets containing 25 milligrams (mg) of orphenadrine and 385 mg of aspirin, or one-half or one tablet containing 50 mg of orphenadrine and 770 mg of aspirin, three or four times a day.
    - Children—Dose must be determined by your doctor.

**Missed dose**—If you miss a dose of this medicine and remember within an hour or so of the missed dose, take it right away. But if you do not remember until later, skip the missed dose and go back to your regular dosing schedule. Do not double doses.

**Storage**—To store this medicine:
- Keep out of the reach of children. Overdose of aspirin is especially dangerous in young children.
- Store away from heat and direct light.
- Do not store this medicine in the bathroom, near the kitchen sink, or in other damp places. Heat or moisture may cause the medicine to break down.
- Do not keep outdated medicine or medicine no longer needed. Be sure that any discarded medicine is out of the reach of children.

## Precautions While Using This Medicine

If you will be taking this medicine for a long time (for example, more than a few weeks), your doctor should check your progress at regular visits.

*Check the labels of all nonprescription (over-the-counter [OTC]) and prescription medicines you now take.* If any contain orphenadrine or aspirin or other salicylates be especially careful, since taking them while taking this medicine may lead to overdose. If you have any questions about this, check with your health care professional.

Too much use of acetaminophen or certain other medicines together with the aspirin in this combination medicine may increase the chance of unwanted effects. The risk depends on how much of each medicine you take every day, and on how long you take the medicines together. If your doctor directs you to take these medicines together on a regular basis, follow his or her directions carefully. However, do not take acetaminophen or any of the following medicines together with this combination medicine for more than a few days, unless your doctor has directed you to do so and is following your progress:

Diclofenac (e.g., Voltaren)
Diflunisal (e.g., Dolobid)
Etodolac (e.g., Lodine)
Fenoprofen (e.g., Nalfon)
Floctafenine (e.g., Idarac)
Flurbiprofen, oral (e.g., Ansaid)
Ibuprofen (e.g., Motrin)
Indomethacin (e.g., Indocin)
Ketoprofen (e.g., Orudis)
Ketorolac (e.g., Toradol)
Meclofenamate (e.g., Meclomen)
Mefenamic acid (e.g., Ponstel)
Nabumetone (e.g., Relafen)
Naproxen (e.g., Naprosyn)
Oxaprozin (e.g., Daypro)
Phenylbutazone (e.g., Butazolidin)
Piroxicam (e.g., Feldene)
Sulindac (e.g., Clinoril)
Tenoxicam (e.g., Mobiflex)
Tiaprofenic acid (e.g., Surgam)
Tolmetin (e.g., Tolectin)

For *diabetic patients:*

- The aspirin in this combination medicine may cause false urine sugar test results if you are regularly taking 6 or more of the regular-strength tablets or 3 or more of the double-strength tablets of this medicine a day. Smaller doses or occasional use of aspirin usually will not affect urine sugar tests. If you have any questions about this, check with your health care professional especially if your diabetes is not well controlled.

Do not take this medicine for 5 days before any surgery, including dental surgery, unless otherwise directed by your medical doctor or dentist. Taking aspirin during this time may cause bleeding problems.

The orphenadrine in this combination medicine may add to the effects of alcohol and other CNS depressants (medicines that slow down the nervous system, possibly causing drowsiness). Some examples of CNS depressants are antihistamines or medicine for hay fever, other allergies, or colds; sedatives, tranquilizers, or sleeping medicine; prescription pain medicine or narcotics; barbiturates; medicine for seizures; other muscle relaxants; or anesthetics, including some dental anesthetics. Also, stomach problems may be more likely to occur if you drink alcoholic beverages while you are taking aspirin. *Do not drink alcoholic beverages, and check with your doctor before taking any of the medicines listed above, while you are using this medicine.*

This medicine may cause some people to have blurred vision or to become drowsy, dizzy, lightheaded, faint, or less alert than they are normally. *Make sure you know how you react to this medicine before you drive, use machines, or do anything else that could be dangerous if you are dizzy or are not alert.*

Dryness of the mouth may occur while you are taking this medicine. For temporary relief, use sugarless candy or gum, melt bits of ice in your mouth, or use a saliva substitute. However, if dry mouth continues for more than 2 weeks, check with your dentist. Continuing dryness of the mouth may increase the chance of dental disease, including tooth decay, gum disease, and fungus infections.

*If you think that you or someone else may have taken an overdose of this medicine, get emergency help at once.* Taking an overdose of this medicine may cause unconsciousness or death. Signs of overdose include convulsions (seizures), hearing loss, confusion, ringing or buzzing in the ears, severe drowsiness or tiredness, severe excitement or nervousness, and fast or deep breathing.

---

### Side Effects of This Medicine

Along with its needed effects, a medicine may cause some unwanted effects. Although not all of these side effects may occur, if they do occur they may need medical attention.

*Get emergency help immediately if any of the following symptoms of overdose occur:*

Any loss of hearing; bloody urine; confusion; convulsions (seizures); diarrhea; dizziness or lightheadedness (severe); drowsiness (severe); excitement or nervousness (severe);

fast or deep breathing; hallucinations (seeing, hearing, or feeling things that are not there); headache (severe or continuing); increased sweating; nausea or vomiting (severe or continuing); ringing or buzzing in the ears (continuing); uncontrollable flapping movements of the hands, especially in elderly patients; unexplained fever; unusual thirst; vision problems

*Symptoms of overdose in children*

Changes in behavior; drowsiness or tiredness (severe); fast or deep breathing

Also, check with your doctor as soon as possible if any of the following side effects occur:

*Less common or rare*

Abdominal or stomach pain, cramping, or burning (severe); bloody or black, tarry stools; decreased urination; eye pain; fainting; fast or pounding heartbeat; shortness of breath, troubled breathing, tightness in chest, or wheezing; skin rash, hives, itching, or redness; sores, ulcers, or white spots on lips or in mouth; swollen and/or painful glands; unusual bleeding or bruising; unusual tiredness or weakness; vomiting of blood or material that looks like coffee grounds

Other side effects may occur that usually do not need medical attention. These side effects may go away during treatment as your body adjusts to the medicine. However, check with your doctor if any of the following side effects continue or are bothersome:

*More common*

Abdominal or stomach cramps, pain, or discomfort (mild to moderate); dryness of mouth; heartburn or indigestion; nausea or vomiting (mild)

*Less common*

Blurred or double vision or other vision problems; confusion; constipation; difficult urination; dizziness or lightheadedness; drowsiness; excitement, nervousness, or restlessness; headache; muscle weakness; trembling; unusually large pupils of eyes

Other side effects not listed above may also occur in some patients. If you notice any other effects, check with your doctor.

---

Revised: July 1990
Interim revision: 08/11/94

---

# OVULATION PREDICTION TEST KITS FOR HOME USE

Some commonly used brand names are:

**In the U.S.—**

| | |
|---|---|
| Answer Ovulation | Fortel |
| Clearplan Easy | OvuGen |
| Color Ovulation Test | OvuKIT |
| Conceive Ovulation Predictor | OvuQUICK |
| First Response | Q-test |

**In Canada—**

| | |
|---|---|
| Clearplan Easy | Ovukit |
| First Response | OvuQuick |

### Description

Ovulation prediction kits are used to help a woman know when she is most likely to ovulate. This is helpful in timing sexual intercourse for becoming pregnant. It may be useful for couples who are having problems conceiving or are concerned about the timing of a pregnancy. A medical doctor may also recommend the use of this type of kit for timing artificial insemination or for fertility problems.

---

*These tests are not intended for contraceptive (birth control) use.*

Ovulation is the release of an egg from the ovary. It normally occurs once a month in about the middle of the menstrual cycle. The egg can be fertilized only for about 48 hours (24 hours is best), so this is the only time during the menstrual cycle that a woman can become pregnant. Ovulation is controlled by luteinizing hormone (LH). The amount of LH present in the blood and urine is very small during most of the menstrual cycle but rises suddenly for a short time near the middle of the menstrual cycle. This sharp rise, the LH surge, usually causes ovulation within about 30 hours. A woman is most likely to become pregnant if she has sexual intercourse within the first 24 hours after detecting the LH surge.

Ovulation prediction test kits test for this large amount of LH in the urine. A change in color of the test pad or liquid will occur if enough LH is in the urine. Correctly using an ovulation prediction test kit is more accurate for predicting ovulation than measuring daily basal body temperature.

## Before Using This Test Kit

It is important to get the best results possible from ovulation prediction test kits while you are using them. Therefore, the following should be considered by you and possibly by your doctor before you decide to use these test kits:

**Diet**—Drinking large amounts of fluids such as water or alcohol can dilute your urine. This may interfere with test results and lead to improper timing of intercourse.

**Medicines**—Certain medicines may affect the results of your testing. Check with your doctor if you are taking any medicines, especially:

- Anticonvulsants (seizure medicine) or
- Birth control pills or
- Estrogens (female hormones) or
- Medicine for mental problems or
- Menotropins or
- Progestins (another type of female hormone)—The use of these medicines may interfere with testing for the rise in LH that comes before ovulation and could result in improper timing of intercourse
- Clomiphene—Clomiphene changes the pattern of LH release; your doctor may recommend a different way to use the test kits

**Medical conditions**—The presence of other medical conditions may affect the results of your testing. Check with your doctor if you have any medical conditions, especially:

- Cysts of the ovaries or
- Decreased function of the ovaries
- Endometriosis or
- Menopause (change of life) or
- Pregnancy or
- Thyroid disease or
- Urinary tract infection—These conditions may interfere with testing for the rise in LH that comes before ovulation and could result in improper timing of intercourse

Also, if you have vision problems (such as color-blindness or poor vision), you will need someone to help you in reading your test results.

## Proper Use of This Test Kit

Ovulation prediction test kits test for a large amount of LH in the urine. A change in color of the test pad or liquid will occur if enough LH is in the urine.

These kits contain enough chemicals to perform 6 to 9 tests. The woman tests her urine daily, usually starting 2 to 3 days before ovulation is expected, according to her usual menstrual cycle length. If your menstrual cycles are unpredictable or irregular, ask your doctor about the best time to perform the tests.

To use:

- Your doctor may give you instructions on using the kit. If not, follow the test kit instructions carefully. The printed instructions on the proper use of ovulation prediction kits may be different for each brand.
- Collect a urine sample according to the written package instructions or your doctor's instructions. If you do not have time to test your urine right away, it may be stored according to the test kit instructions. Refrigeration of the urine may interfere with the test results.
- Choose a well-lighted area with normal room temperature and humidity. Perform the test on a clean, dry working surface with a cold water faucet nearby. You will also need a watch, timer, or clock that can measure in seconds.
- Be careful not to touch the testing areas. Skin oils or perspiration may affect the test results. It is also important that you use clean, dry test kit materials. Traces of old test chemicals or soaps may affect test reactions if materials are reused.
- At the end of the timing period compare the color of the test to the color chart on the package.
- Record your test results to discuss with your health care professional.

**Storage**—To store this product:

- Keep out of the reach of children. Test chemicals can be poisonous if swallowed.
- Store the kit in a cool, dry place, away from heat, moisture, and direct sunlight. Heat-exposed or chilled test kits will not work properly.
- Keep the product from freezing.
- Before purchasing, check the date printed on the package that tells you when the kit is too old to use (expiration date). Do not use an outdated test kit. Outdated test kits will not work properly.
- Discard used tests in the trash. Liquids may be poured down the drain or flushed in the toilet.

## About Your Test Results

Your best chance of becoming pregnant is by having intercourse or being artificially inseminated within 24 hours of detecting the LH surge. Each cycle may have a slightly different time of ovulation, or ovulation may not even occur in some cycles. Couples who have problems conceiving should always consult a doctor for advice and medical evaluation, especially if it takes longer than 6 to 12 months for the woman to become pregnant.

If you have any other questions about your results or the use of ovulation prediction test kits, ask your health care professional. Also, most kits provide a toll-free number for advice on using the kits.

Revised: 10/08/91
Interim revision: 07/05/94

# OXAMNIQUINE   Systemic†

A commonly used brand name in the U.S. is Vansil.

†Not commercially available in Canada.

## Description

Oxamniquine (ox-AM-ni-kwin) is used to treat a certain kind of worm infection (blood fluke), also known as snail fever, Manson's schistosomiasis (shis-toe-soe-MYE-a-siss), or bilharziasis (bil-har-ZYE-a-siss). It will not work for other kinds of worm infections (for example, pinworms or roundworms).

Oxamniquine is available only with your doctor's prescription, in the following dosage form:

*Oral*
- Capsules (U.S.)

## Before Using This Medicine

In deciding to use a medicine, the risks of taking the medicine must be weighed against the good it will do. This is a decision you and your doctor will make. For oxamniquine, the following should be considered:

**Allergies**—Tell your doctor if you have ever had any unusual or allergic reaction to oxamniquine. Also tell your health care professional if you are allergic to any other substances, such as foods, preservatives, or dyes.

**Pregnancy**—Studies have not been done in humans. Studies in animals have shown that oxamniquine may harm the unborn animal when it is given in high doses. However, there have been no reports of problems with the pregnancies or babies of pregnant women who took oxamniquine.

**Breast-feeding**—It is not known whether oxamniquine passes into the breast milk. However, this medicine has not been reported to cause problems in nursing babies.

**Children**—This medicine has been used in children, and, in effective doses, has not been shown to cause different side effects or problems in children than it does in adults.

**Older adults**—Many medicines have not been studied specifically in older people. Therefore, it may not be known whether they work exactly the same way they do in younger adults or if they cause different side effects or problems in older people. There is no specific information comparing use of oxamniquine in the elderly with use in other age groups.

**Other medicines**—Although certain medicines should not be used together at all, in other cases two different medicines may be used together even if an interaction might occur. In these cases, your doctor may want to change the dose, or other precautions may be necessary. Tell your health care professional if you are taking any other prescription or nonprescription (over-the-counter [OTC]) medicine.

**Other medical problems**—The presence of other medical problems may affect the use of oxamniquine. Make sure you tell your doctor if you have any other medical problems, especially:
- History of epilepsy or other medical problems that cause convulsions—Patients with a history of epilepsy may be more likely to have side effects

## Proper Use of This Medicine

No special preparations (for example, special diets, fasting, other medicines, laxatives, or enemas) are necessary before, during, or immediately after taking oxamniquine.

*Take this medicine after meals to lessen the chance of side effects* such as stomach upset, drowsiness, or dizziness, unless otherwise directed by your doctor.

To help clear up your infection completely, *take this medicine exactly as directed by your doctor for the full time of treatment. Do not miss any doses.*

**Dosing**—The dose of oxamniquine will be different for different patients. *Follow your doctor's orders or the directions on the label.* The following information includes only the average doses of oxamniquine. *If your dose is different, do not change it* unless your doctor tells you to do so.
- For *oral* dosage form (capsules):
  —For East, North, or South African snail fever:
    - Adults and children—Dose is based on body weight and must be determined by your doctor.

The usual dose is 15 milligrams (mg) per kilogram (kg) (6.8 mg per pound) of body weight two times a day for one, two, or three days.

—For West African and Western Hemisphere snail fever:

- Adults and children weighing 30 kg (66 pounds) and over—Dose is based on body weight and must be determined by your doctor. The usual dose is 15 mg per kg (6.8 mg per pound) of body weight as a single dose.

- Children weighing up to 30 kg (66 pounds)—Dose is based on body weight and must be determined by your doctor. The usual dose is 10 mg per kg (4.5 mg per pound) of body weight taken twice a day, two to eight hours apart.

**Missed dose**—If you miss a dose of this medicine, take it as soon as possible. However, if it is almost time for your next dose, skip the missed dose and go back to your regular dosing schedule. Do not double doses.

**Storage**—To store this medicine:

- Keep out of the reach of children.
- Store away from heat and direct light.
- Do not store in the bathroom, near the kitchen sink, or in other damp places. Heat or moisture may cause the medicine to break down.
- Do not keep outdated medicine or medicine no longer needed. Be sure that any discarded medicine is out of the reach of children.

---

## Precautions While Using This Medicine

It is important that your doctor check your progress at regular visits.

If your symptoms do not improve after you take this medicine for the full time of treatment, or if they become worse, check with your doctor.

This medicine may cause some people to become dizzy, drowsy, or less alert than they are normally. *Make sure you know how you react to this medicine before you drive, use machines, or do anything else that could be dangerous if you are dizzy or are not alert.* If these reactions are especially bothersome, check with your doctor.

---

## Side Effects of This Medicine

Along with its needed effects, a medicine may cause some unwanted effects. Although not all of these side effects may occur, if they do occur they may need medical attention.

*Check with your doctor immediately* if any of the following side effects occur:

*Rare*

Convulsions (seizures); fever; hallucinations (seeing, hearing, or feeling things that are not there); skin rash or hives

Other side effects may occur that usually do not need medical attention. These side effects may go away during treatment as your body adjusts to the medicine. However, check with your doctor if any of the following side effects continue or are bothersome:

*More common*

Dizziness; drowsiness; headache

*Less common*

Abdominal or stomach pain; diarrhea; loss of appetite; nausea or vomiting

This medicine may cause the urine to turn reddish orange. This side effect does not require medical attention.

Other side effects not listed above may also occur in some patients. If you notice any other effects, check with your doctor.

Revised: 01/19/93
Interim revision: 07/21/94

---

# OXICONAZOLE    Topical†

A commonly used brand name in the U.S. is Oxistat.

†Not commercially available in Canada.

---

## Description

Oxiconazole (ox-i-KON-a-zole) is used to treat infections caused by a fungus. It works by killing the fungus or preventing its growth.

Oxiconazole is applied to the skin to treat:

- ringworm of the body (tinea corporis);
- ringworm of the foot (tinea pedis; athlete's foot); and
- ringworm of the groin (tinea cruris; jock itch).

Oxiconazole is available only with your doctor's prescription, in the following dosage forms:

*Topical*

- Cream (U.S.)
- Lotion (U.S.)

---

## Before Using This Medicine

In deciding to use a medicine, the risks of using the medicine must be weighed against the good it will do.

This is a decision you and your doctor will make. For oxiconazole, the following should be considered:

**Allergies**—Tell your doctor if you have ever had any unusual or allergic reaction to oxiconazole. Also tell your health care professional if you are allergic to any other substances, such as foods, preservatives, or dyes.

**Pregnancy**—Oxiconazole has not been studied in pregnant women. However, this medication has not been shown to cause birth defects or other problems in animal studies.

**Breast-feeding**—Topical oxiconazole passes into breast milk. Mothers who are using this medicine and who wish to breast-feed should discuss this with their doctor.

**Children**—Although there is no specific information comparing use of topical oxiconazole in children with use in other age groups, this medicine is not expected to cause different side effects or problems in children than it does in adults.

**Older adults**—Many medicines have not been studied specifically in older people. Therefore, it may not be known whether they work exactly the same way they do in younger adults. Although there is no specific information comparing use of topical oxiconazole in the elderly with use in other age groups, this medicine is not expected to cause different side effects or problems in older people than it does in younger adults.

**Other medicines**—Although certain medicines should not be used together at all, in other cases two different medicines may be used together even if an interaction might occur. In these cases, your doctor may want to change the dose, or other precautions may be necessary. Tell your health care professional if you are using any other topical prescription or nonprescription (over-the-counter [OTC]) medicine that is to be applied to the same area of the skin.

## Proper Use of This Medicine

Apply enough oxiconazole to cover the affected and surrounding skin areas and rub in gently.

*Keep this medicine away from the eyes.* Also, do not use it in the vagina.

To help clear up your infection completely, *it is very important that you keep using oxiconazole for the full time of treatment,* even if your symptoms begin to clear up after a few days. Since fungus infections may be very slow to clear up, you may have to continue using this medicine every day for several weeks or more. If you stop using this medicine too soon, your symptoms may return. *Do not miss any doses.*

**Dosing**—The dose of topical oxiconazole will be different for different patients. *Follow your doctor's orders or the directions on the label.* The following information includes only the average doses of topical oxiconazole. *If your dose is different, do not change it* unless your doctor tells you to do so.

*The number of doses you use each day, the time allowed between doses, and the length of time you use the medicine depend on the medical problem for which you are using topical oxiconazole.*

- For *cream* or *lotion* dosage form:
  —For ringworm of the body or groin:
  - Adults and children—Use 1 or 2 times a day for at least 2 weeks.
  —For athlete's foot:
  - Adults and children—Use 1 or 2 times a day for at least 4 weeks.

**Missed dose**—If you miss a dose of this medicine, use it as soon as possible. However, if it is almost time for your next dose, skip the missed dose and go back to your regular dosing schedule.

**Storage**—To store this medicine:
- Keep out of the reach of children.
- Store away from heat and direct light.
- Keep the medicine from freezing. Do not refrigerate.
- Do not keep outdated medicine or medicine no longer needed. Be sure that any discarded medicine is out of the reach of children.

## Precautions While Using This Medicine

If your skin problem does not improve within 2 to 4 weeks, or if it becomes worse, check with your doctor.

*To help clear up your infection completely and to help make sure it does not return, good health habits are also required.* The following measures will help reduce chaffing and irritation and will also help keep the area cool and dry.

- *For patient using oxiconazole for ringworm of the groin:*
  —Avoid wearing underwear that is tight-fitting or made from synthetic materials (for example, rayon or nylon). Instead, wear loose-fitting, cotton underwear.
  —Use a bland, absorbent powder (for example, talcum powder) or an antifungal powder on the skin. It is best to use the powder between the times you use oxiconazole.
- *For patients using oxiconazole for ringworm of the foot:*
  —Carefully dry the feet, especially between the toes, after bathing.
  —Avoid wearing socks made from wool or synthetic materials (for example, rayon or nylon). Instead, wear clean, cotton socks and change them daily or more often if the feet sweat a lot.
  —Wear sandals or other well-ventilated shoes.
  —Use a bland, absorbent powder (for example, talcum powder) or an antifungal powder between the toes, on the feet, and in socks and shoes 1 or 2 times a day. It is best to use the powder between the times you use oxiconazole.

If you have any questions about these measures, check with your health care professional.

## Side Effects of This Medicine

Along with its needed effects, a medicine may cause some unwanted effects. Although not all of these side effects may occur, if they do occur they may need medical attention.

Check with your doctor as soon as possible if the following side effect occurs:

*Rare*
Rash

Other side effects may occur that usually do not need medical attention. These side effects may go away during treatment as your body adjusts to the medicine. However, check with your doctor if any of the following side effects continue or are bothersome:

*Less common*
Burning, stinging, itching, redness, or other sign of irritation not present before use of this medicine

Other side effects not listed above may also occur in some patients. If you notice any other effects, check with your doctor.

Revised: 07/06/93

# OXTRIPHYLLINE AND GUAIFENESIN   Systemic

Some commonly used brand names are:
**In the U.S.—**
Brondelate                                    Theocon
Generic name product may also be available.
**In Canada—**
Choledyl Expectorant

## Description

Oxtriphylline (ox-TRYE-fi-lin) and guaifenesin (gwye-FEN-e-sin) combination is used to treat the symptoms of bronchial asthma, chronic bronchitis, emphysema, and other lung diseases. This medicine relieves cough, wheezing, shortness of breath, and troubled breathing. It works by opening up the bronchial tubes (air passages) of the lungs and increasing the flow of air through them.

This medicine is available only with your doctor's prescription, in the following dosage forms:

*Oral*
• Elixir (U.S. and Canada)

## Before Using This Medicine

In deciding to use a medicine, the risks of taking the medicine must be weighed against the good it will do. This is a decision you and your doctor will make. For oxtriphylline and guaifenesin combination, the following should be considered:

**Allergies**—Tell your doctor if you have ever had any unusual or allergic reaction to aminophylline, caffeine, dyphylline, oxtriphylline, theobromine, or theophylline. Also tell your health care professional if you are allergic to any other substances, such as foods, preservatives, or dyes.

**Diet**—Make certain your health care professional knows if you are on any special diet, such as a low-sodium or low-sugar diet or a high-protein, low-carbohydrate or low-protein, high-carbohydrate diet. A high-protein, low-carbohydrate diet may decrease the effects of oxtriphylline; a low-protein, high-carbohydrate diet may increase the effects of oxtriphylline.

Avoid eating or drinking large amounts of caffeine-containing foods or beverages, such as chocolate, cocoa, tea, coffee, and cola drinks, because they may increase the central nervous system (CNS) stimulant effects of oxtriphylline.

Also, eating charcoal broiled foods every day while taking oxtriphylline may keep this medicine from working properly.

**Pregnancy**—Studies on birth defects have not been done in humans. However, some studies in animals have shown that oxtriphylline causes birth defects when given in doses many times the human dose. Also, use of oxtriphylline during pregnancy may cause unwanted effects such as fast heartbeat, jitteriness, irritability, gagging, vomiting, and breathing problems in the newborn infant. Guaifenesin has not been shown to cause birth defects or other problems in humans.

**Breast-feeding**—Theophylline passes into the breast milk and may cause irritability, fretfulness, or trouble in sleeping in babies of mothers taking oxtriphylline. Guaifenesin has not been reported to cause problems in nursing babies.

**Children**—The side effects of oxtriphylline are more likely to occur in newborn infants, who are usually more sensitive to the effects of this medicine.

Although there is no specific information about the use of guaifenesin in children, it is not expected to cause different side effects or problems in children than it does in adults.

**Older adults**—The side effects of oxtriphylline are more likely to occur in elderly patients, who are usually more sensitive than younger adults to the effects of this medicine.

Although there is no specific information about the use of guaifenesin in the elderly, it is not expected to cause different side effects or problems in older people than it does in younger adults.

**Other medicines**—Although certain medicines should not be used together at all, in other cases two different medicines may be used together even if an interaction might occur. In these cases, your doctor may want to change the dose, or other precautions may be necessary. When you are taking oxtriphylline and guaifenesin combination, it is especially important that your health care professional know if you are taking any of the following:

- Beta-blockers (acebutolol [e.g., Sectral], atenolol [e.g., Tenormin], betaxolol [e.g., Betoptic, Kerlone], bisoprolol [e.g., Zebeta], carteolol [e.g., Cartrol], labetalol [e.g., Normodyne], levobunolol [e.g., Betagan], metoprolol [e.g., Lopressor], nadolol [e.g., Corgard], oxprenolol [e.g., Trasicor], penbutolol [e.g., Levatol], pindolol [e.g., Visken], propranolol [e.g., Inderal], sotalol [e.g., Sotacor], timolol [e.g., Blocadren, Timoptic])—Use of these medicines with oxtriphylline may prevent either the beta-blocker or oxtriphylline from working properly
- Cimetidine (e.g., Tagamet) or
- Ciprofloxacin (e.g., Cipro) or
- Erythromycin (e.g., E-Mycin) or
- Nicotine chewing gum (e.g., Nicorette) or
- Norfloxacin (e.g., Noroxin) or
- Ranitidine (e.g., Zantac) or
- Troleandomycin (e.g., TAO)—These medicines may increase the effects of oxtriphylline
- Phenytoin (e.g., Dilantin)—The effects of phenytoin may be decreased by oxtriphylline
- Smoking tobacco or marijuana—If you smoke or have smoked (tobacco or marijuana) regularly within the last 2 years, the amount of medicine you need may vary, depending on how much and how recently you have smoked

**Other medical problems**—The presence of other medical problems may affect the use of oxtriphylline and guaifenesin combination. Make sure you tell your doctor if you have any other medical problems, especially:

- Alcohol abuse (or history of) or
- Fever or
- Liver disease or
- Respiratory infections, such as influenza (flu)—The effects of oxtriphylline may be increased
- Diarrhea—The absorption of oxtriphylline may be decreased; therefore, the effects of this medicine may be decreased
- Enlarged prostate or
- Heart disease or
- High blood pressure or
- Stomach ulcer (or history of) or other stomach problems—Oxtriphylline may make the condition worse
- Fibrocystic breast disease—Symptoms of this disease may be increased by oxtriphylline
- Overactive thyroid—The effects of oxtriphylline may be decreased

## Proper Use of This Medicine

*This medicine works best when taken with a glass of water on an empty stomach* (either 30 minutes to 1 hour before meals or 2 hours after meals) since that way it will get into the blood sooner. However, in some cases your doctor may want you to take this medicine with meals or right after meals to lessen stomach upset. If you have any questions about how you should be taking this medicine, check with your doctor.

*Take this medicine only as directed by your doctor.* Do not take more of it, do not take it more often, and do not take it for a longer time than your doctor ordered. To do so may increase the chance of serious side effects.

*In order for this medicine to help your medical problem, it must be taken every day in regularly spaced doses as ordered by your doctor.* This is necessary to keep a constant amount of the medicine in the blood. To help keep the amount constant, do not miss any doses.

**Dosing**—When you are taking oxtriphylline and guaifenesin combination, it is very important that you get the exact amount of medicine that you need. The dose of this medicine will be different for different patients. Your doctor will determine the proper dose of the oxtriphylline and guaifenesin combination for you. *Follow your doctor's orders or the directions on the label.*

After you begin taking oxtriphylline and guaifenesin combination, it is very important that your doctor check your blood level of theophylline at regular intervals to find out if your dose of oxtriphylline and guaifenesin combination needs to be changed. *Do not change your dose of this medicine* unless your doctor tells you to do so.

The number of teaspoonfuls of elixir that you take depends on the strength of the medicine.

**Missed dose**—If you miss a dose of this medicine, take it as soon as possible. However, if it is almost time for your next dose, skip the missed dose and go back to your regular dosing schedule. Do not double doses.

**Storage**—To store this medicine:
- Keep out of the reach of children.
- Store away from heat and direct light.
- Do not store the tablet form of this medicine in the bathroom, near the kitchen sink, or in other damp places. Heat or moisture may cause the medicine to break down.
- Keep the liquid form of this medicine from freezing.
- Do not keep outdated medicine or medicine no longer needed. Be sure that any discarded medicine is out of the reach of children.

## Precautions While Using This Medicine

Your doctor should check your progress at regular visits, especially for the first few weeks after you begin using this medicine. A blood test may be taken to help your doctor decide whether the dose of this medicine should be changed.

The oxtriphylline in this medicine may add to the central nervous system stimulant effects of caffeine-containing foods or beverages such as chocolate, cocoa, tea, coffee, and cola drinks. *Avoid eating or drinking large amounts of these foods or beverages while taking this medicine.* If you have any questions about this, check with your doctor.

Do not eat charcoal-broiled foods every day while taking this medicine since these foods may keep the medicine from working properly.

*Check with your doctor at once if you develop symptoms of influenza (flu) or a fever* since either of these may increase the chance of side effects with this medicine.

Also, *check with your doctor if diarrhea occurs* because the dose of this medicine may need to be changed.

## Side Effects of This Medicine

Along with its needed effects, a medicine may cause some unwanted effects. Although not all of these side effects may occur, if they do occur they may need medical attention.

Check with your doctor as soon as possible if any of the following side effects occur:

*Less common*
  Heartburn and/or vomiting

*Symptoms of overdose*
  Bloody or black, tarry stools; confusion or change in behavior; convulsions (seizures); diarrhea; dizziness or lightheadedness; fast breathing; fast, pounding, or irregular heartbeat; flushing or redness of face; headache; increased urination; irritability; loss of appetite; muscle twitching; nausea (continuing or severe) or vomiting; stomach cramps or pain; trembling; trouble in sleeping; unusual tiredness or weakness; vomiting blood or material that looks like coffee grounds

Other side effects may occur that usually do not need medical attention. These side effects may go away during treatment as your body adjusts to the medicine. However, check with your doctor if any of the following side effects continue or are bothersome:

*More common*
  Nausea; nervousness or restlessness

Other side effects not listed above may also occur in some patients. If you notice any other effects, check with your doctor.

Revised: September 1990
Interim revision: 09/02/94

---

# OXYBUTYNIN   Systemic

A commonly used brand name in the U.S. and Canada is Ditropan. Generic name product may also be available in the U.S.

## Description

Oxybutynin (ox-i-BYOO-ti-nin) belongs to the group of medicines called antispasmodics. It helps decrease muscle spasms of the bladder and the frequent urge to urinate caused by these spasms.

Oxybutynin is available only with your doctor's prescription, in the following dosage forms:

*Oral*
  • Syrup (U.S. and Canada)
  • Tablets (U.S. and Canada)

## Before Using This Medicine

In deciding to use a medicine, the risks of taking the medicine must be weighed against the good it will do. This is a decision you and your doctor will make. For oxybutynin, the following should be considered:

**Allergies**—Tell your doctor if you have ever had any unusual or allergic reaction to oxybutynin. Also tell your health care professional if you are allergic to any other substances, such as foods, preservatives, or dyes.

**Pregnancy**—Oxybutynin has not been studied in pregnant women. However, it has not been shown to cause birth defects or other problems in animal studies.

**Breast-feeding**—Oxybutynin has not been reported to cause problems in nursing babies. However, since this medicine tends to decrease the secretions of the body, it is possible that the flow of breast milk may be reduced in some patients.

**Children**—There is no specific information about the use of oxybutynin in children under 5 years of age. In older children, oxybutynin is not expected to cause different side effects or problems than it does in adults.

**Older adults**—Elderly people are especially sensitive to the effects of oxybutynin. This may increase the chance of side effects during treatment.

**Other medicines**—Although certain medicines should not be used together at all, in other cases two different medicines may be used together even if an interaction might occur. In these cases, your doctor may want to change the dose, or other precautions may be necessary. When you are taking oxybutynin, it is especially important that your health care professional know if you are taking any of the following:

  • Amantadine (e.g., Symmetrel) or
  • Anticholinergics (medicine for abdominal or stomach spasms or cramps) or
  • Antidepressants (medicine for depression) or
  • Antidyskinetics (medicine for Parkinson's disease or other conditions affecting control of muscles) or
  • Antihistamines or
  • Antipsychotics (medicine for mental illness) or

- Buclizine (e.g., Bucladin) or
- Carbamazepine (e.g., Tegretol) or
- Cyclizine (e.g., Marezine) or
- Cyclobenzaprine (e.g., Flexeril) or
- Disopyramide (e.g., Norpace) or
- Flavoxate (e.g., Urispas) or
- Ipratropium (e.g., Atrovent) or
- Meclizine (e.g., Antivert) or
- Methylphenidate (e.g., Ritalin) or
- Orphenadrine (e.g., Norflex) or
- Procainamide (e.g., Pronestyl) or
- Promethazine (e.g., Phenergan) or
- Quinidine (e.g., Quinidex) or
- Trimeprazine (e.g., Temaril)—Taking oxybutynin with these medicines may increase the effects of either medicine

**Other medical problems**—The presence of other medical problems may affect the use of oxybutynin. Make sure you tell your doctor if you have any other medical problems, especially:

- Bleeding (severe)—Oxybutynin may increase heart rate, which may make this condition worse
- Colitis (severe) or
- Dryness of mouth (severe and continuing) or
- Enlarged prostate or
- Glaucoma or
- Heart disease or
- Hiatal hernia or
- High blood pressure (hypertension) or
- Intestinal blockage or other intestinal or stomach problems or
- Myasthenia gravis or
- Toxemia of pregnancy or
- Urinary tract blockage or problems with urination—Oxybutynin may make these conditions worse
- Kidney disease or
- Liver disease—Higher blood levels of oxybutynin may occur, which increases the chance of side effects
- Overactive thyroid—Oxybutynin may further increase heart rate

## Proper Use of This Medicine

This medicine is usually taken with water on an empty stomach. However, your doctor may want you to take it with food or milk to lessen stomach upset.

*Take this medicine only as directed.* Do not take more of it, do not take it more often, and do not take it for a longer time than your doctor ordered. To do so may increase the chance of side effects.

**Dosing**—The dose of oxybutynin will be different for different patients. *Follow your doctor's orders or the directions on the label.* The following information includes only the average doses of oxybutynin. *If your dose is different, do not change it* unless your doctor tells you to do so.

- For *oral* dosage forms (syrup or tablets):
  —For treatment of bladder problems:
  - Adults and children 12 years of age and over— 5 milligrams (mg) two or three times a day.
  - Children up to 5 years of age—Use and dose have not been determined.

- Children 5 to 12 years of age—5 mg two or three times a day. The dose is usually not more than 15 mg a day.

**Missed dose**—If you miss a dose of this medicine, take it as soon as possible. However, if it is almost time for your next dose, skip the missed dose and go back to your regular dosing schedule. Do not double doses.

**Storage**—To store this medicine:
- Keep out of the reach of children.
- Store away from heat and direct light.
- Do not store the tablet form of this medicine in the bathroom, near the kitchen sink, or in other damp places. Heat or moisture may cause the medicine to break down.
- Keep the syrup form of this medicine from freezing.
- Do not keep outdated medicine or medicine no longer needed. Be sure that any discarded medicine is out of the reach of children.

## Precautions While Using This Medicine

This medicine will add to the effects of alcohol and other CNS depressants (medicines that slow down the nervous system, possibly causing drowsiness). Some examples of CNS depressants are antihistamines or medicine for hay fever, other allergies, or colds; sedatives, tranquilizers, or sleeping medicine; prescription pain medicine or narcotics; barbiturates; medicine for seizures; muscle relaxants; or anesthetics, including some dental anesthetics. *Check with your doctor before taking any of the above while you are using this medicine.*

This medicine may cause your eyes to become more sensitive to light than they are normally. Wearing sunglasses and avoiding too much exposure to bright light may help lessen the discomfort.

This medicine may cause some people to become drowsy or have blurred vision. *Make sure you know how you react to this medicine before you drive, use machines, or do anything else that could be dangerous if you are not alert or able to see well.*

Oxybutynin may make you sweat less, causing your body temperature to increase. *Use extra care not to become overheated during exercise or hot weather while you are taking this medicine,* since overheating may result in heat stroke. Also, hot baths or saunas may make you feel dizzy or faint while you are taking this medicine.

Your mouth, nose, and throat may feel very dry while you are taking this medicine. For temporary relief of mouth dryness, use sugarless candy or gum, melt bits of ice in your mouth, or use a saliva substitute. However, if your mouth continues to feel dry for more than 2 weeks, check with your medical doctor or dentist. Continuing dryness of the mouth may increase the chance of dental disease, including tooth decay, gum disease, and fungus infections.

## Side Effects of This Medicine

Along with its needed effects, a medicine may cause some unwanted effects. Although not all of these side effects may occur, if they do occur they may need medical attention.

Check with your doctor as soon as possible if any of the following side effects occur:

*Rare*

Eye pain; skin rash or hives

*Symptoms of overdose*

Clumsiness or unsteadiness; confusion; dizziness; drowsiness (severe); fast heartbeat; fever; flushing or redness of face; hallucinations (seeing, hearing, or feeling things that are not there); shortness of breath or troubled breathing; unusual excitement, nervousness, restlessness, or irritability

Other side effects may occur that usually do not need medical attention. These side effects may go away during treatment as your body adjusts to the medicine. However, check with your doctor if any of the following side effects continue or are bothersome:

*More common*

Constipation; decreased sweating; drowsiness; dryness of mouth, nose, and throat

*Less common or rare*

Blurred vision; decreased flow of breast milk; decreased sexual ability; difficult urination; difficulty in swallowing; headache; increased sensitivity of eyes to light; nausea or vomiting; trouble in sleeping; unusual tiredness or weakness

Other side effects not listed above may also occur in some patients. If you notice any other effects, check with your doctor.

---

Revised: 06/16/93

---

# OXYMETAZOLINE   Nasal

Some commonly used brand names are:

**In the U.S.—**

| | |
|---|---|
| Afrin Cherry Scented Nasal Spray | Neo-Synephrine 12 Hour Nasal Spray |
| Afrin Children's Strength Nose Drops | Neo-Synephrine 12 Hour Nasal Spray Pump |
| Afrin Extra Moisturizing Nasal Decongestant Spray | Nostrilla Long-Acting Nasal Decongestant |
| Afrin Menthol Nasal Spray | NTZ Long Acting Decongestant Nasal Spray |
| Afrin Nasal Spray | NTZ Long Acting Decongestant Nose Drops |
| Afrin Nose Drops | Vicks Sinex Long-Acting 12-Hour Formula Decongestant Nasal Spray |
| Afrin Spray Pump | |
| Cheracol Nasal Spray | |
| Cheracol Nasal Spray Pump Cherry Scented | |
| Dristan 12-Hr Nasal Spray | Vicks Sinex Long-Acting 12-Hour Formula Decongestant Ultra Fine Mist |
| Duramist Plus Up To 12 Hours Decongestant Nasal Spray | |
| Duration 12 Hour Nasal Spray | 4-Way Long Lasting Nasal Spray |
| Duration 12 Hour Nasal Spray Pump | |

**In Canada—**

| | |
|---|---|
| Nafrine Decongestant Nasal Drops | Nafrine Decongestant Pediatric Nasal Spray/ Drops |
| Nafrine Decongestant Nasal Spray | |

## Description

Oxymetazoline (ox-i-met-AZ-oh-leen) is used for the temporary relief of nasal (of the nose) congestion or stuffiness caused by hay fever or other allergies, colds, or sinus trouble.

This medicine may also be used for other conditions as determined by your doctor.

This medicine is available without a prescription; however, your doctor may have special instructions on the proper use or dose for your medical condition.

Oxymetazoline is available in the following dosage forms:

*Nasal*

- Nasal drops (U.S. and Canada)
- Nasal spray (U.S. and Canada)

## Before Using This Medicine

If you are using this medicine without a prescription, carefully read and follow any precautions on the label. For oxymetazoline, the following should be considered:

**Allergies—**Tell your doctor if you have ever had any unusual or allergic reaction to oxymetazoline or any other nasal decongestant. Also tell your health care professional if you are allergic to any other substances, such as foods, preservatives, or dyes.

**Pregnancy—**The medication may be absorbed into the body. However, oxymetazoline has not been shown to cause birth defects or other problems in humans.

**Breast-feeding—**Oxymetazoline may be absorbed into the body. However, oxymetazoline has not been reported to cause problems in nursing babies.

**Children—**Children may be especially sensitive to the effects of oxymetazoline. This may increase the chance of side effects during treatment.

**Older adults—**Many medicines have not been tested in older people. Therefore, it may not be known whether they work exactly the same way they do in younger adults or if they cause different side effects or problems in older people. There is no specific information about the use of oxymetazoline in the elderly.

**Other medicines**—Although certain medicines should not be used together at all, in other cases two different medicines may be used together even if an interaction might occur. In these cases, your doctor may want to change the dose, or other precautions may be necessary. When you are using oxymetazoline, it is especially important that your health care professional know if you are taking any other prescription or nonprescription (over-the-counter [OTC]) medicine.

**Other medical problems**—The presence of other medical problems may affect the use of oxymetazoline. Make sure you tell your doctor if you have any other medical problems, especially:

- Diabetes mellitus (sugar diabetes)
- Heart or blood vessel disease or
- High blood pressure—Oxymetazoline may make the condition worse
- Overactive thyroid

## Proper Use of This Medicine

To use the *nose drops:*

- Blow your nose gently. Tilt the head back while standing or sitting up, or lie down on a bed and hang the head over the side. Place the drops into each nostril and keep the head tilted back for a few minutes to allow the medicine to spread throughout the nose.
- Rinse the dropper with hot water and dry with a clean tissue. Replace the cap right after use.
- To avoid spreading the infection, do not use the container for more than one person.

To use the *nose spray:*

- Blow your nose gently. With the head upright, spray the medicine into each nostril. Sniff briskly while squeezing the bottle quickly and firmly. For best results, spray once into each nostril, wait 3 to 5 minutes to allow the medicine to work, then blow the nose gently and thoroughly. Repeat until the complete dose is used.
- Rinse the tip of the spray bottle with hot water, taking care not to suck water into the bottle, and dry with a clean tissue. Replace the cap right after use.
- To avoid spreading the infection, do not use the container for more than one person.

*Use this medicine only as directed.* Do not use more of it, do not use it more often, and do not use it for longer than 3 days without first checking with your doctor. To do so may make your runny or stuffy nose worse and may also increase the chance of side effects.

**Dosing**—The dose of oxymetazoline will be different for different patients. *Follow your doctor's orders or the directions on the label.* The following information includes only the average doses of oxymetazoline. *If your dose is different, do not change it* unless your doctor tells you to do so.

- For *nasal* dosage form (nose drops or spray):
  —For nasal congestion or stuffiness:
  - Adults and children 6 years of age and older—Use 2 or 3 drops or sprays of 0.05% solution in each nostril two times a day, morning and evening.
  - Children 2 to 6 years of age—Use 2 or 3 drops of 0.025% solution in each nostril two times a day, morning and evening.
  - Children up to 2 years of age—Use and dose must be determined by your doctor.

**Missed dose**—If you are using this medicine on a regular schedule and you miss a dose, use it right away if you remember within an hour or so of the missed dose. However, if you do not remember until later, skip the missed dose and go back to your regular dosing schedule. Do not double doses.

**Storage**—To store this medicine:

- Keep out of the reach of children.
- Store away from heat and direct light.
- Keep the medicine from freezing.
- Do not keep outdated medicine or medicine no longer needed. Be sure that any discarded medicine is out of the reach of children.

## Side Effects of This Medicine

Along with its needed effects, a medicine may cause some unwanted effects. Although not all of these side effects may occur, if they do occur they may need medical attention.

When this medicine is used for short periods of time at low doses, side effects usually are rare. However, check with your doctor as soon as possible if any of the following occur:

Increase in runny or stuffy nose

*Symptoms of too much medicine being absorbed into the body*

Fast, irregular, or pounding heartbeat; headache or lightheadedness; nervousness; trembling; trouble in sleeping

The above side effects are more likely to occur in children because there is a greater chance in children that too much of this medicine may be absorbed into the body.

Other side effects may occur that usually do not need medical attention. These side effects may go away during

treatment as your body adjusts to the medicine. However, check with your health care professional if any of the following side effects continue or are bothersome:

Burning, dryness, or stinging inside of nose; sneezing

Other side effects not listed above may also occur in some patients. If you notice any other effects, check with your health care professional.

Revised: 04/19/94

---

# OXYMETAZOLINE   Ophthalmic

Some commonly used brand names are:

**In the U.S.—**
OcuClear
Visine L.R.

**In Canada—**
OcuClear

## Description

Oxymetazoline (ox-i-met-AZ-oh-leen) is used to relieve redness due to minor eye irritations, such as those caused by colds, dust, wind, smog, pollen, swimming, or wearing contact lenses.

Oxymetazoline is available without a prescription; however, your doctor may have special instructions on the proper use of this medicine for your medical condition.

Oxymetazoline is available in the following dosage form:
*Ophthalmic*
• Ophthalmic solution (eye drops) (U.S. and Canada)

## Before Using This Medicine

If you are taking this medicine without a prescription, carefully read and follow any precautions on the label. For ophthalmic oxymetazoline, the following should be considered:

**Allergies**—Tell your doctor if you have ever had any unusual or allergic reaction to oxymetazoline or to any other decongestant used in the eye. Also tell your health care provider if you are allergic to any other substances, such as preservatives.

**Pregnancy**—Studies in humans have not shown that oxymetazoline causes birth defects or other problems in humans.

**Breast-feeding**—Oxymetazoline may be absorbed into the body. However, oxymetazoline has not been shown to cause problems in nursing babies.

**Children**—Check with your doctor before using oxymetazoline eye drops in children up to 6 years of age. Eye redness in children can occur with illnesses, such as allergies, fevers, colds, and measles, that may require medical attention.

**Older adults**—Many medicines have not been studied specifically in older people. Therefore, it may not be known whether they work exactly the same way they do in younger adults or if they cause different side effects or problems in older people. There is no specific information comparing use of oxymetazoline in the elderly with use in other age groups.

**Other medicines**—Although certain medicines should not be used together at all, in other cases two different medicines may be used together even if an interaction might occur. In these cases, your doctor may want to change the dose, or other precautions may be necessary. Tell your health care provider if you are using any other prescription or nonprescription (over-the-counter [OTC]) medicine.

**Other medical problems**—The presence of other medical problems may affect the use of ophthalmic oxymetazoline. Make sure you tell your doctor if you have any other medical problems, especially:

• Eye disease, infection, or injury—This medicine may mask the symptoms of these conditions
• Heart or blood vessel disease or
• High blood pressure or
• Overactive thyroid—If absorbed into the body, this medicine may cause side effects that may make the medical problem worse
• Use of soft contact lenses—Because of the preservative in this medicine, some eye conditions may get worse if this medicine is used on top of soft contact lenses

## Proper Use of This Medicine

Do not use oxymetazoline ophthalmic solution if it becomes cloudy or changes color.

To use:

• First, wash your hands. With the middle finger, apply pressure to the inside corner of the eye (and continue to apply pressure for 1 or 2 minutes after the medicine has been placed in the eye). Tilt the head back and with the index finger of the same hand, pull the lower eyelid away from the eye to form a pouch. Drop the medicine into the pouch and gently close the eyes. Do not blink. Keep the eyes closed for 1 or 2 minutes to allow the medicine to be absorbed.
• To keep the medicine as germ-free as possible, do not touch the applicator tip to any surface (including the eye). Also, keep the container tightly closed.

---

*Use this medicine only as directed.* Do not use more of it, do not use it more often, and do not use it for more than 72 hours, unless otherwise directed by your doctor. To do so may make your eye irritation worse and may also increase the chance of side effects.

**Dosing**—The dose of ophthalmic oxymetazoline will be different for different patients. *Follow your doctor's orders or the directions on the label.* The following information includes only the average doses of ophthalmic oxymetazoline. *If your dose is different, do not change it* unless your doctor tells you to do so.

- For *ophthalmic solution (eye drops)* dosage form:
  —For eye redness:
    - Adults and children 6 years of age and older— Use one drop in the eye every six hours.
    - Children up to 6 years of age—Use and dose must be determined by your doctor.

**Storage**—To store this medicine:
- Keep out of the reach of children.
- Store away from heat and direct light.
- Keep the medicine from freezing.
- Do not keep outdated medicine or medicine no longer needed. Be sure that any discarded medicine is out of the reach of children.

## Precautions While Using This Medicine

*If eye pain or change in vision occurs or if redness or irritation of the eye continues, gets worse, or lasts for more than 72 hours, stop using the medicine and check with your doctor.*

## Side Effects of This Medicine

Along with its needed effects, a medicine may cause some unwanted effects. Although not all of these side effects may occur, if they do occur they may need medical attention.

When this medicine is used for short periods of time at low doses, side effects usually are rare.

Check with your doctor as soon as possible if any of the following side effects occur:

*With overuse or long-term use*
  Increase in irritation or redness of eyes
*Symptoms of too much medicine being absorbed into the body*
  Fast, irregular, or pounding heartbeat; headache or light-headedness; nervousness; trembling; trouble in sleeping

Other side effects not listed above may also occur in some patients. If you notice any other effects, check with your doctor.

Revised: 04/29/92
Interim revision: 02/17/94

---

# OXYTOCIN Systemic

Some commonly used brand names are:
**In the U.S.—**
  Pitocin                    Syntocinon
  Generic name product may also be available.
**In Canada—**
  Syntocinon

## Description

Oxytocin (ox-i-TOE-sin) is a hormone used to help start or continue labor and to control bleeding after delivery. It is also sometimes used to help milk secretion in breast-feeding.

Oxytocin may also be used for other conditions as determined by your doctor.

*In general, oxytocin should not be used to start labor unless there are specific medical reasons.* Be sure you have discussed this with your doctor before receiving this medicine.

Oxytocin is available only with your doctor's prescription, in the following dosage forms:
  *Nasal*
    - Solution (U.S. and Canada)
  *Parenteral*
    - Injection (U.S. and Canada)

## Before Using This Medicine

In deciding to use a medicine, the risks of taking the medicine must be weighed against the good it will do. This is a decision you and your doctor will make. For oxytocin, the following should be considered:

**Allergies**—Tell your doctor if you have ever had any unusual or allergic reaction to oxytocin. Also tell your health care professional if you are allergic to any other substances, such as foods, preservatives, or dyes.

**Breast-feeding**—Although very small amounts of this medicine pass into breast milk, it has not been reported to cause problems in nursing babies.

**Other medicines**—Although certain medicines should not be used together at all, in other cases two different medicines may be used together even if an interaction might occur. In these cases, your doctor may want to change the dose, or other precautions may be necessary. Tell your health care professional if you are taking any other prescription or nonprescription (over-the-counter [OTC]) medicine.

**Other medical problems**—The presence of other medical problems may affect the use of oxytocin. Make sure you tell your doctor if you have any other medical problems, especially:

- Heart disease
- Hypertension
- Kidney disease

## Proper Use of This Medicine

For patients using the *nasal spray* form of this medicine:

- This medicine usually comes with directions for use. Read them carefully before using.

**Dosing**—The dose of oxytocin will be different for different patients. *Follow your doctor's orders*. The following information includes only the average doses of oxytocin.

- For *nasal* dosage form:
  —For increasing milk production in breast feeding:
  - Adults—One spray into one or both nostrils two or three minutes before nursing or pumping milk from breasts.
- For *injection* dosage form:
  —For helping to start or continue labor:
  - Adults—At first, 0.5 to 2 milliunits per minute slowly injected into a vein. Then, your doctor may increase the dose every fifteen to sixty minutes as needed.
  —For treating incomplete abortion, causing abortion, or controlling bleeding after an abortion:
  - Adults—10 units injected slowly into a vein.
  —For helping to control bleeding after delivery:
  - Adults—10 units injected into a muscle or slowly into a vein.

**Storage**—To store this medicine:

- Keep out of the reach of children.
- Store away from heat and direct light.
- Protect the medicine from freezing.
- Do not keep outdated medicine or medicine no longer needed. Be sure that any discarded medicine is out of the reach of children.

## Precautions While Using This Medicine

Oxytocin nasal spray may not help milk secretion in some breast-feeding women. Call your doctor if this medicine is not working.

## Side Effects of This Medicine

Oxytocin can be very useful for helping labor. However, there are certain risks with using it. Oxytocin causes contractions of the uterus. In women who are unusually sensitive to its effects, these contractions may become too strong. In rare cases, this may lead to tearing of the uterus. Also, if contractions are too strong, the supply of blood and oxygen to the fetus may be decreased.

Oxytocin has been reported to cause irregular heartbeat and increase bleeding after delivery in some women. It has also been reported to cause jaundice in some newborn infants.

Along with its needed effects, a medicine may cause some unwanted effects. Although not all of these side effects may occur, if they do occur they may need medical attention:

*Rare (with use of injection)*
Confusion; convulsions (seizures); difficulty in breathing; dizziness; fast or irregular heartbeat; headache (continuing or severe); hives; pelvic or abdominal pain (severe); skin rash or itching; vaginal bleeding (increased or continuing); weakness; weight gain (rapid)

*Rare (with use of nasal spray)*
Convulsions (seizures); mental disturbances; unexpected bleeding or contractions of the uterus

Other side effects may occur that usually do not need medical attention. However, check with your doctor if any of the following side effects continue or are bothersome:

*Rare (with use of injection)*
Nausea; vomiting

*Rare (with use of nasal spray)*
Nasal irritation; runny nose; tearing of the eyes

Other side effects not listed above may also occur in some patients. If you notice any other effects, check with your doctor.

## Additional information

Once a medicine has been approved for marketing for a certain use, experience may show that it is also useful for other medical problems. Although this use is not included in product labeling, oxytocin is used in certain patients for the following:

- Testing the ability of the placenta to support a pregnancy

Other than the above information, there is no additional information relating to proper use, precautions, or side effects for this use.

Revised: 07/14/93
Interim revision: 06/30/94

# PACLITAXEL    Systemic

A commonly used brand name in the U.S. and Canada is Taxol.

## Description

Paclitaxel (pak-li-TAX-el) belongs to the group of medicines called antineoplastics. It is used to treat cancer of the ovary.

Paclitaxel interferes with the growth of cancer cells, which are eventually destroyed. Since the growth of normal body cells may also be affected by paclitaxel, other effects will also occur. Some of these may be serious and must be reported to your doctor. Other effects may not be serious but may cause concern. Some effects may not occur for months or years after the medicine is used.

Paclitaxel may also be used to treat other conditions as determined by your doctor.

Before you begin treatment with paclitaxel, you and your doctor should talk about the good this medicine will do as well as the risks of using it.

Paclitaxel is to be administered only by or under the immediate supervision of your doctor. It is available in the following dosage form:

*Parenteral*
- Injection (U.S. and Canada)

## Before Using This Medicine

In deciding to use a medicine, the risks of taking the medicine must be weighed against the good it will do. This is a decision you and your doctor will make. For paclitaxel, the following should be considered:

**Allergies**—Tell your doctor if you have ever had any unusual or allergic reaction to paclitaxel.

**Pregnancy**—Tell your doctor if you are pregnant or if you intend to become pregnant. Studies in rats and rabbits have shown that paclitaxel causes miscarriages and deaths of the fetus, as well as problems in the mother.

Be sure that you have discussed this with your doctor before taking this medicine. It is best to use some kind of birth control while you are receiving paclitaxel. Tell your doctor right away if you think you have become pregnant while receiving paclitaxel.

**Breast-feeding**—It is not known whether paclitaxel passes into breast milk. However, because this medicine may cause serious side effects, breast-feeding is generally not recommended while you are receiving it.

**Children**—There is no specific information comparing use of paclitaxel in children with use in other age groups.

**Older adults**—This medicine has been tested in a limited number of patients and has not been shown to cause different side effects or problems in older people than it does in younger adults.

**Other medicines**—Although certain medicines should not be used together at all, in other cases two different medicines may be used together even if an interaction might occur. In these cases, your doctor may want to change the dose, or other precautions may be necessary. When you are receiving paclitaxel, it is especially important that your health care professional know if you are taking any of the following:
- Amphotericin B by injection (e.g., Fungizone) or
- Antithyroid agents (medicine for overactive thyroid) or
- Azathioprine (e.g., Imuran) or
- Chloramphenicol (e.g., Chloromycetin) or
- Colchicine or
- Flucytosine (e.g., Ancobon) or
- Ganciclovir (e.g., Cytovene) or
- Interferon (e.g., Intron A, Roferon-A) or
- Plicamycin (e.g., Mithracin) or
- Zidovudine (e.g., AZT, Retrovir) or
- If you have ever been treated with x-rays or cancer medicines—Paclitaxel may increase the effects of these medicines or radiation therapy on the blood

**Other medical problems**—The presence of other medical problems may affect the use of paclitaxel. Make sure you tell your doctor if you have any other medical problems, especially:
- Chickenpox (including recent exposure) or
- Herpes zoster (shingles)—Risk of severe disease affecting other parts of the body
- Heart rhythm problems—May be made worse by paclitaxel
- Infection—Paclitaxel may decrease your body's ability to fight infection

## Proper Use of This Medicine

This medicine often causes nausea and vomiting, which is usually mild. However, it is very important that you continue to receive the medicine even if you begin to feel ill. Ask your health care professional for ways to lessen these effects.

**Dosing**—The dose of paclitaxel will be different for different patients. The dose that is used may depend on a number of things, including what the medicine is being used for, the patient's size, and whether or not other medicines are also being taken. *If you are receiving paclitaxel at home, follow your doctor's orders or the directions on the label.* If you have any questions about the proper dose of paclitaxel, ask your doctor.

## Precautions While Using This Medicine

*It is very important that your doctor check your progress at regular visits* to make sure that this medicine is working properly and to check for unwanted effects.

While you are being treated with paclitaxel, and after you stop treatment with it, *do not have any immunizations (vaccinations) without your doctor's approval.* Paclitaxel may lower your body's resistance and there is a chance you might get the infection the immunization is meant to prevent. In addition, other persons living in your household should not take oral polio vaccine since there is a chance they could pass the polio virus on to you. Also, avoid persons who have taken oral polio vaccine. Do not get close to them and do not stay in the same room with them for very long. If you cannot take these precautions, you should consider wearing a protective face mask that covers the nose and mouth.

Paclitaxel can temporarily lower the number of white blood cells in your blood, increasing the chance of getting an infection. It can also lower the number of platelets, which are necessary for proper blood clotting. If this occurs, there are certain precautions you can take, especially when your blood count is low, to reduce the risk of infection or bleeding:

- If you can, avoid people with infections. *Check with your doctor immediately* if you think you are getting an infection or if you get a fever or chills, cough or hoarseness, lower back or side pain, or painful or difficult urination.
- *Check with your doctor immediately* if you notice any unusual bleeding or bruising; black, tarry stools; blood in urine or stools; or pinpoint red spots on your skin.
- Be careful when using a regular toothbrush, dental floss, or toothpick. Your medical doctor, dentist, or nurse may recommend other ways to clean your teeth and gums. Check with your medical doctor before having any dental work done.
- Do not touch your eyes or the inside of your nose unless you have just washed your hands and have not touched anything else in the meantime.
- Be careful not to cut yourself when you are using sharp objects such as a safety razor or fingernail or toenail cutters.
- Avoid contact sports or other situations where bruising or injury could occur.

## Side Effects of This Medicine

Along with its needed effects, a medicine may cause some unwanted effects. Some side effects will have signs or symptoms that you can see or feel. Your doctor may watch for others by doing certain tests.

Also, because of the way these medicines act on the body, there is a chance that they might cause other unwanted effects that may not occur until months or years after the medicine is used. These delayed effects may include certain types of cancer. Discuss these possible effects with your doctor.

*Check with your doctor immediately* if any of the following side effects occur:

*More common*

   Cough or hoarseness; fever or chills; lower back or side pain; painful or difficult urination

*Less common*

   Black, tarry stools; blood in urine or stools; pinpoint red spots on skin; unusual bleeding or bruising

*Rare*

   Shortness of breath (severe); skin reaction (severe)

Check with your doctor as soon as possible if any of the following side effects occur:

*More common*

   Flushing of face; shortness of breath; skin rash or itching

*Rare*

   Pain or redness at place of injection; sores in mouth and on lips (usually get better within 7 days after treatment)

This medicine may also cause the following side effects that your doctor will watch out for:

*More common*

   Anemia; low white blood cell count; low platelet count in blood

*Less common*

   Low blood pressure; slow heartbeat; effects on liver

Other side effects may occur that usually do not need medical attention. These side effects may go away during treatment as your body adjusts to the medicine. Also, your health care professional may be able to tell you about ways to prevent or reduce some of these side effects. Check with your health care professional if any of the following side effects continue or are bothersome or if you have any questions about them:

*More common*

   Diarrhea; nausea and vomiting; numbness, burning, or tingling in hands or feet; pain in joints or muscles, especially in arms or legs (begins 2 to 3 days after treatment and may last up to 5 days)

This medicine usually causes a temporary and total loss of hair (including eyebrows, eyelashes, and pubic hair) about 2 to 3 weeks after treatment begins. After treatment with paclitaxel has ended, normal hair growth should return.

Other side effects not listed above may also occur in some patients. If you notice any other effects, check with your doctor.

Revised: 09/15/93
Interim revision: 07/05/94

# PAMIDRONATE  Systemic

A commonly used brand name in the U.S. and Canada is Aredia. Another commonly used name is APD.

## Description

Pamidronate (pa-mi-DROE-nate) is used to treat hypercalcemia (too much calcium in the blood) that may occur with some types of cancer. This medicine may be used for other conditions as determined by your doctor.

This medicine is to be administered only by or under the supervision of your doctor. It is available in the following dosage form:

*Parenteral*
- Injection (U.S. and Canada)

## Before Receiving This Medicine

In deciding to use a medicine, the risks of receiving the medicine must be weighed against the good it will do. This is a decision you and your doctor will make. For pamidronate, the following should be considered:

**Allergies**—Tell your doctor if you have ever had any unusual or allergic reaction to pamidronate or etidronate. Also tell your health care professional if you are allergic to any other substances, such as foods, preservatives, or dyes.

**Pregnancy**—Studies have not been done in humans. However, studies in rats given higher doses of oral pamidronate have shown that the medicine may decrease fertility, increase the length of pregnancy, and cause death of the baby rat.

**Breast-feeding**—It is not known if pamidronate passes into breast milk.

**Children**—Studies on this medicine have been done only in adult patients, and there is no specific information comparing use of pamidronate in children with use in other age groups.

**Older adults**—When pamidronate is given along with a large amount of fluids, older people tend to retain (keep) the excess fluid.

**Other medicines**—Although certain medicines should not be used together at all, in other cases two different medicines may be used together even if an interaction might occur. In these cases, your doctor may want to change the dose, or other precautions may be necessary. When you are receiving pamidronate, it is especially important that your health care professional know if you are taking any of the following:
- Calcium-containing preparations or
- Vitamin D–containing preparations—Use with pamidronate may keep pamidronate from working properly

**Other medical problems**—The presence of other medical problems may affect the use of pamidronate. Make sure you tell your doctor if you have any other medical problems, especially:
- Heart problems—The increased amount of fluid may make this condition worse
- Kidney problems—Pamidronate may build up in the bloodstream, which may increase the chance of unwanted effects

## Proper Use of This Medicine

**Dosing**—The dose of pamidronate will be different for different patients. *Follow your doctor's orders.* The following information includes only the average doses of pamidronate.
- For *injectable* dosage form:
  —For treating hypercalcemia (too much calcium in the blood):
  - Adults: 30 to 90 mg in a solution to be given over 4 to 24 hours into a vein.
  - Children: Use is not recommended.

## Precautions While Receiving This Medicine

It is important that your doctor check your progress at regular visits after you have received pamidronate. If your condition has improved, your progress must still be checked. The results of laboratory tests or the occurrence of certain symptoms will tell your doctor if your condition is coming back and a second treatment is needed.

For patients using this medicine for *hypercalcemia (too much calcium in the blood):*
- Your doctor may want you to follow a low-calcium diet. If you have any questions about this, check with your doctor.

## Side Effects of This Medicine

Along with its needed effects, a medicine may cause some unwanted effects. Although not all of these side effects may occur, if they do occur they may need medical attention.

Check with your doctor as soon as possible if any of the following side effects occur:

*More common*
　Abdominal cramps; chills; confusion; fever; muscle spasms; sore throat
Note: Abdominal cramps, confusion, and muscle spasms are less common when pamidronate is given in doses of 60 mg or less.

Other side effects may occur that usually do not need medical attention. These side effects may go away during treatment as your body adjusts to the medicine. However, check with your doctor if any of the following side effects continue or are bothersome:

*More common—at higher doses*
　Nausea; pain and swelling at place of injection

*Less common*
  Muscle stiffness

Other side effects not listed above may also occur in some patients. If you notice any other effects, check with your doctor.

---

## Additional Information

Once a medicine has been approved for marketing for a certain use, experience may show that it is also useful for other medical problems. Although these uses are not included in product labeling, pamidronate is used in certain patients with the following medical conditions:

- Bone metastases
- Paget's disease of bone

Other than the above information, there is no additional information relating to proper use, precautions, or side effects for these uses.

---

Revised: 06/02/93

---

# PANCREATIN, PEPSIN, BILE SALTS, HYOSCYAMINE, ATROPINE, SCOPOLAMINE, AND PHENOBARBITAL   Systemic

A commonly used brand name in the U.S. and Canada is Donnazyme.

## Description

Pancreatin (PAN-kree-a-tin), pepsin (PEP-sin), bile salts, hyoscyamine (hye-oh-SYE-a-meen), atropine (A-troe-peen), scopolamine (skoe-POL-a-meen), and phenobarbital (fee-noe-BAR-bi-tal) combination is used to relieve indigestion in certain conditions in which the body does not produce enough of the enzymes needed for the complete digestion of food.

This medicine is available only with your doctor's prescription, in the following dosage form:

*Oral*
  - Tablets (U.S. and Canada)

## Before Using This Medicine

In deciding to use a medicine, the risks of taking the medicine must be weighed against the good it will do. This is a decision you and your doctor will make. For this combination medicine, the following should be considered:

**Allergies**—Tell your doctor if you have ever had any unusual or allergic reaction to any of the belladonna alkaloids such as atropine, hyoscyamine, or scopolamine; to pancrelipase, pancreatin, or beef or pork products; or to barbiturates. Also tell your health care professional if you are allergic to any other substances, such as foods, preservatives, or dyes.

**Pregnancy**—Studies have not been done in either humans or animals.

**Breast-feeding**—This medicine has not been reported to cause problems in nursing babies. However, the chance always exists since traces of the belladonna alkaloids and phenobarbital (contained in this combination medicine) pass into the breast milk. Also, because the belladonna alkaloids tend to decrease the secretions of the body, it is possible that the flow of breast milk may be reduced in some patients.

**Children**—Children are especially sensitive to the effects of belladonna alkaloids and barbiturates (contained in this combination medicine). This may increase the chance of side effects during treatment.

**Older adults**—Confusion or memory loss, drowsiness, unusual excitement or agitation may be more likely to occur in the elderly, who are usually more sensitive than younger adults to the effects of belladonna alkaloids and barbiturates (contained in this combination medicine).

**Other medicines**—Although certain medicines should not be used together at all, in other cases two different medicines may be used together even if an interaction might occur. In these cases, your doctor may want to change the dose, or other precautions may be necessary. When you are taking this combination medicine, it is especially important that your health care professional know if you are taking any of the following:

- Alcohol or
- Central nervous system (CNS) depressants—Taking this combination medicine with CNS depressants may increase the effects of either medicine
- Antacids or
- Diarrhea medicine containing kaolin or attapulgite—Use of these medicines with this combination medicine may prevent this combination medicine from working properly; these medicines and this combination medicine should be taken 2 hours apart
- Anticoagulants, coumarin- or indandione-type (blood thinners) or
- Digitalis glycosides (heart medicine) or
- Ketoconazole (e.g., Nizoral)—Use of digitalis glycosides, anticoagulants, or ketoconazole with this combination medicine may prevent the digitalis glycoside, anticoagulant, or ketoconazole from working properly
- Potassium chloride (e.g., Kay Ciel)—Use of potassium chloride with this combination medicine may make stomach and intestine problems caused by potassium worse

**Other medical problems**—The presence of other medical problems may affect the use of this combination medicine. Make sure you tell your doctor if you have any other medical problems, especially:

---

- Bleeding (severe)—The belladonna alkaloids in this combination medicine may increase heart rate, which may make this condition worse
- Colitis or
- Difficult urination or problems with urination or
- Dryness of mouth (severe and continuing) or
- Enlarged prostate or
- Fast heartbeat or
- Glaucoma or
- Heart disease or
- Hernia or
- High blood pressure (hypertension) or
- Intestinal blockage or other intestinal or stomach problems or
- Myasthenia gravis or
- Porphyria (or history of) or
- Urinary tract blockage—This combination medicine may make these conditions worse
- Drug abuse or history of—The phenobarbital in this combination may be habit-forming
- Kidney disease or
- Liver disease—Higher blood levels of this combination medicine may occur, which increases the chance of side effects
- Overactive thyroid—The belladonna alkaloids in this combination medicine may further increase heart rate

## Proper Use of This Medicine

Take this medicine with or after meals unless otherwise directed by your doctor.

*Take this medicine only as directed by your doctor.* Do not take more or less of it, do not take it more often, and do not take it for a longer period of time than your doctor ordered. If too much is used, it may increase the chance of side effects and it may also become habit-forming.

*Importance of diet*—When prescribing this medicine for your condition, your doctor may also prescribe a personal diet for you. Follow carefully the special diet your doctor gave you. This is most important and necessary for the medicine to work properly and to avoid indigestion.

*Swallow the tablets without chewing*, to avoid mouth irritation.

**Dosing**—The dose of this combination medicine will be different for different patients. *Follow your doctor's orders or the directions on the label.* The following information includes only the average dose of this combination medicine. *If your dose is different, do not change it* unless your doctor tells you to do so.

- To help digestion:
  —For *oral* dosage form (tablets):
    - Adults and teenagers—Two tablets after meals. Your doctor may change your dose if needed.
    - Children—Dose must be determined by your doctor.

**Missed dose**—If you miss a dose of this medicine, take it as soon as possible. However, if it is almost time for your next dose, skip the missed dose and go back to your regular dosing schedule. Do not double doses.

**Storage**—To store this medicine:
- Keep out of the reach of children. Overdose is especially dangerous in young children.
- Store away from heat and direct light.
- Do not store the tablet form of this medicine in the bathroom, near the kitchen sink, or in other damp places. The heat or moisture may cause the medicine to break down.
- Do not keep outdated medicine or medicine no longer needed. Be sure that any discarded medicine is out of the reach of children.

## Precautions While Using This Medicine

This medicine will add to the effects of alcohol and other CNS depressants (medicines that slow down the nervous system, possibly causing drowsiness). Some examples of CNS depressants are antihistamines or medicine for hay fever, other allergies, or colds; sedatives, tranquilizers, or sleeping medicine; prescription pain medicine or narcotics; barbiturates; medicine for seizures; muscle relaxants; or anesthetics, including some dental anesthetics. *Check with your doctor before taking any of the above while you are using this medicine.*

This medicine may cause your eyes to become more sensitive to light than they are normally. Wearing sunglasses and avoiding too much exposure to bright light may help lessen the discomfort from bright light.

This medicine may cause some people to have blurred vision or to become drowsy, dizzy, or less alert than they are normally. *Make sure you know how you react to this medicine before you drive, use machines, or do anything else that could be dangerous if you are dizzy or are not alert and able to see well.*

Belladonna alkaloids will often make you sweat less, causing your body temperature to increase. *Use extra care not to become overheated during exercise or hot weather while you are taking this medicine,* since overheating may result in heat stroke. Also, hot baths or saunas may make you feel dizzy or faint while you are taking this medicine.

The belladonna alkaloids in this medicine may cause dryness of the mouth, nose, and throat. For temporary relief of mouth dryness, use sugarless candy or gum, melt bits of ice in your mouth, or use a saliva substitute. However, if your mouth continues to feel dry for more than 2 weeks, check with your medical doctor or dentist. Continuing dryness of the mouth may increase the chance of dental disease, including tooth decay, gum disease, and fungus infections.

## Side Effects of This Medicine

Along with its needed effects, a medicine may cause some unwanted effects. Although not all of these side effects appear very often, when they do occur they may require medical attention.

Check with your doctor as soon as possible if any of the following side effects occur:

*Rare*

Blood in urine; diarrhea; eye pain; joint pain; nausea or vomiting; skin rash or hives; sore throat and fever; stomach cramps or pain; swelling of feet or lower legs; unusual bleeding or bruising; yellow eyes or skin

*Symptoms of overdose*

Clumsiness, unsteadiness, or staggering; confusion (especially in the elderly); dizziness; fever; flushing or redness of face; hallucinations (seeing, hearing, or feeling things that are not there); shortness of breath or troubled breathing; slow or fast heartbeat; unusual excitement, nervousness, restlessness, or irritability

Other side effects may occur that usually do not need medical attention. These side effects may go away during treatment as your body adjusts to the medicine. However,

check with your doctor if any of the following side effects continue or are bothersome:

*More common*

Constipation; decreased sweating; drowsiness; dryness of mouth, nose, and throat

*Less common or rare*

Blurred vision; decreased flow of breast milk; decreased sexual ability; difficult urination (especially in older men); difficulty in swallowing; headache; increased sensitivity of eyes to light; trouble in sleeping; unusual tiredness or weakness

Other side effects not listed above may also occur in some patients. If you notice any other effects, check with your doctor.

Revised: 04/15/92
Interim revision: 08/01/94

---

# PANCRELIPASE    Systemic

Some commonly used brand names are:

**In the U.S.—**

| | |
|---|---|
| Cotazym | Pancrease MT 10 |
| Cotazym-S | Pancrease MT 16 |
| Enzymase-16 | Protilase |
| Ilozyme | Ultrase MT 12 |
| Ku-Zyme HP | Ultrase MT 20 |
| Pancoate | Viokase |
| Pancrease | Zymase |
| Pancrease MT 4 | |

**In Canada—**

| | |
|---|---|
| Cotazym | Pancrease |
| Cotazym-65 B | Pancrease MT 4 |
| Cotazym E.C.S. 8 | Pancrease MT 10 |
| Cotazym E.C.S. 20 | Pancrease MT 16 |

Another commonly used name is lipancreatin.

## Description

Pancrelipase (pan-kre-LI-pase) is used to help digestion in certain conditions in which the pancreas is not working properly. It may also be used for other conditions as determined by your doctor.

Pancrelipase contains the enzymes needed for the digestion of proteins, starches, and fats.

Pancrelipase is available only with your doctor's prescription, in the following dosage forms:

*Oral*

• Capsules (U.S. and Canada)
• Delayed-release capsules (U.S. and Canada)
• Powder (U.S.)
• Tablets (U.S.)

## Before Using This Medicine

In deciding to use a medicine, the risks of taking the medicine must be weighed against the good it will do.

This is a decision you and your doctor will make. For pancrelipase, the following should be considered:

**Allergies**—Tell your doctor if you have ever had any unusual or allergic reaction to pancrelipase, pancreatin, or pork products. Also tell your health care professional if you are allergic to any other substances, such as foods, preservatives, or dyes.

**Pregnancy**—Studies have not been done in either humans or animals.

**Breast-feeding**—Pancrelipase has not been reported to cause problems in nursing babies.

**Children**—This medicine has been tested in children 6 months of age or older and has not been shown to cause different side effects or problems than it does in adults.

**Older adults**—Many medicines have not been studied specifically in older people. Therefore, it may not be known whether they work exactly the same way they do in younger adults. Although there is no specific information comparing use of pancrelipase in the elderly with use in other age groups, this medicine is not expected to cause different side effects or problems in older people than it does in younger adults.

**Other medicines**—Although certain medicines should not be used together at all, in other cases two different medicines may be used together even if an interaction might occur. In these cases, your doctor may want to change the dose, or other precautions may be necessary. Tell your health care professional if you are taking any other prescription or nonprescription (over-the-counter [OTC]) medicine.

**Other medical problems**—The presence of other medical problems may affect the use of pancrelipase. Make sure

you tell your doctor if you have any other medical problems, especially:

- Pancreatitis (sudden, severe inflammation of the pancreas)—Pancrelipase may make this condition worse

## Proper Use of This Medicine

Take this medicine before or with meals and snacks, unless otherwise directed by your doctor.

*When prescribing this medicine for your condition, your doctor may also prescribe a personal diet for you. Follow carefully the special diet your doctor gave you.* This is most important and necessary for the medicine to work properly and to avoid indigestion.

For patients taking the *tablet form* of this medicine:

- *Swallow the tablets quickly with some liquid, without chewing*, to avoid mouth irritation.

For patients taking the *capsules containing the enteric-coated spheres:*

- Swallow the capsule whole.
- Do not crush, break, or chew before swallowing.
- When given to children, the capsule may be opened and sprinkled on a small amount of liquid or soft food that can be swallowed without chewing, such as applesauce or gelatin. However, it should not be mixed with alkaline foods, such as milk and ice cream, which may reduce its effect.

**Dosing**—The dose of pancrelipase will be different for different patients. *Follow your doctor's orders or the directions on the label.* The following information includes only the average doses of pancrelipase. *If your dose is different, do not change it* unless your doctor tells you to do so.

- To help digestion:
  —For *oral* dosage form (capsules):
  - Older adults, adults, and teenagers—One to three capsules before or with meals and snacks. Your doctor may change your dose if needed.
  - Children—The contents of one to three capsules sprinkled on food at each meal. Your doctor may change your dose if needed.
  —For *oral* dosage form (delayed-release capsules):
  - Olders adults, adults, and teenagers—One to two capsules before or with meals and snacks. Your doctor may change your dose if needed.
  - Children—The contents of one to two capsules with meals. Your doctor may change your dose if needed. You should take the contents of the capsules with a liquid or a small amount of a soft food that you do not have to chew.
  —For *oral* dosage form (powder):
  - Older adults, adults, and teenagers—1/4 teaspoonful (0.7 gram) with meals and snacks. Your doctor may change your dose if needed.
  - Children—1/4 teaspoonful with meals. Your doctor may change your dose if needed.

—For *oral* dosage form (tablets):
- Older adults, adults, and teenagers—One to three tablets before or with meals and snacks. Your doctor may change your dose if needed.
- Children—One to two tablets with meals.

**Missed dose**—If you miss a dose of this medicine, take it as soon as possible. However, if it is almost time for your next dose, skip the missed dose and go back to your regular dosing schedule. Do not double doses.

**Storage**—To store this medicine:
- Keep out of the reach of children.
- Store away from heat and direct light.
- Do not store the capsule, powder, or tablet form of this medicine in the bathroom, near the kitchen sink, or in other damp places. Heat or moisture may cause the medicine to break down.
- Do not keep outdated medicine or medicine no longer needed. Be sure that any discarded medicine is out of the reach of children.

## Precautions While Using This Medicine

Your doctor may recommend that you take pancrelipase with another medicine, such as certain antacids or anti-ulcer medicines. However, antacids that contain calcium carbonate and/or magnesium hydroxide may not let the pancrelipase work properly and should be avoided.

Do not change brands or dosage forms of pancrelipase without first checking with your doctor. Different products may not work in the same way. If you refill your medicine and it looks different, check with your pharmacist.

For patients taking the *capsules containing the powder:*
- If the capsules are opened to mix with food, be careful not to breathe in the powder. To do so may cause harmful effects such as stuffy nose, shortness of breath, troubled breathing, wheezing, or tightness in chest.

For patients taking the *powder form* of this medicine:
- Avoid breathing in the powder. To do so may cause harmful effects such as stuffy nose, shortness of breath, troubled breathing, wheezing, or tightness in chest.

## Side Effects of This Medicine

Along with its needed effects, a medicine may cause some unwanted effects. Although not all of these side effects may occur, if they do occur they may need medical attention.

Check with your doctor as soon as possible if any of the following side effects occur:

*Rare*
   Skin rash or hives

*With high doses*
> Diarrhea; intestinal blockage; nausea; stomach cramps or pain

*With very high doses*
> Blood in urine; joint pain; swelling of feet or lower legs

*With powder dosage form or powder from opened capsules—if breathed in*
> Shortness of breath; stuffy nose; tightness in chest; troubled breathing; wheezing

*With tablets—if held in mouth*
> Irritation of the mouth

Other side effects not listed above may also occur in some patients. If you notice any other effects, check with your doctor.

---

Revised: 02/13/92
Interim revision: 08/01/94

---

# PANTOTHENIC ACID    (Vitamin B$_5$)    Systemic†

Other commonly used names are vitamin B$_5$ and calcium pantothenate. Generic name product may also be available in the U.S.

---

†Not commercially available in Canada.

---

## Description

Vitamins (VYE-ta-mins) are compounds that you *must* have for growth and health. They are needed in only small amounts and are usually available in the foods that you eat. Pantothenic acid (vitamin B$_5$) is necessary for normal metabolism.

No problems have been found that are due to a lack of pantothenic acid alone. However, a lack of one B vitamin usually goes along with a lack of others, so pantothenic acid is often included in B complex products.

Claims that pantothenic acid is effective for treatment of nerve damage, breathing problems, itching and other skin problems, and poisoning with some other drugs; for getting rid of or preventing gray hair; for preventing arthritis, allergies, and birth defects; or for improving mental ability have not been proven.

Pantothenic acid is available without a prescription. However, it may be a good idea to check with your doctor before taking any on your own. If you take more than you need, it will simply be lost from your body.

This vitamin is available in the following dosage forms:

*Oral*
> Calcium pantothenate
> • Tablets (U.S.)
> Pantothenic acid
> • Capsules (U.S.)
> • Oral solution (U.S.)
> • Tablets (U.S.)
> • Extended-release tablets (U.S.)

---

## Importance of Diet

Vitamin supplements should be taken only if you cannot get enough vitamins in your diet; however, some diets may not contain all of the vitamins you need. You may not be getting enough vitamins because of rapid weight loss, unusual diets (such as some reducing diets in which choice of foods is very limited), prolonged intravenous feeding, or malnutrition. A balanced diet should provide all the vitamins you normally need.

In order to get enough vitamins and minerals in your diet, it is important that you eat a balanced and varied diet. Follow carefully any diet program your doctor may recommend. For your specific vitamin and/or mineral needs, ask your doctor or dietitian for a list of appropriate foods.

Pantothenic acid is found in various foods including peas and beans (except green beans), lean meat, poultry, fish, and whole-grain cereals. Little pantothenic acid is lost from foods with ordinary cooking.

Vitamins alone will not take the place of a good diet and will not provide energy. Your body also needs other substances found in food—protein, minerals, carbohydrates, and fat.

In some cases, it may not be possible for you to get enough food to supply you with the proper vitamins. In other cases, the amount of vitamins you need may be increased above normal. Therefore, a vitamin supplement may be needed.

Experts have developed a list of recommended dietary allowances (RDA) for most of the vitamins. The RDA are not an exact number but a general idea of how much you need. They do not cover amounts needed for problems caused by a serious lack of vitamins. Because lack of pantothenic acid is so rare, there are no RDA for this vitamin. However, it is thought that 4 to 7 mg for adults and adolescents and 3 to 4 mg of pantothenic acid for children is enough.

---

## Before Using This Dietary Supplement

If you are taking this dietary supplement without a prescription, carefully read and follow any precautions on the label. For pantothenic acid, the following should be considered:

**Allergies**—Tell your health care professional if you are allergic to any substances, such as foods, preservatives, or dyes.

**Pregnancy**—It is especially important that you are receiving enough vitamins when you become pregnant and that you continue to receive the right amount of vitamins throughout your pregnancy. The healthy growth and development of the fetus depend on a steady supply of nutrients from the mother. However, taking large amounts of a nutritional supplement during pregnancy may be harmful to the mother and/or fetus and should be avoided.

**Breast-feeding**—It is especially important that you receive the right amounts of vitamins so that your baby will also get the vitamins needed to grow properly. However, taking large amounts of a nutritional supplement while breast-feeding may be harmful to the mother and/or baby and should be avoided.

**Children**—Normal daily requirements vary according to age. It is especially important that children receive enough vitamins in their diet for healthy growth and development. There is no specific information about the use of pantothenic acid in children in doses higher than the normal daily requirements.

**Older adults**—It is important that older people continue to receive enough vitamins in their diet for good health. There is no specific information about the use of pantothenic acid in older people in doses higher than the normal daily requirements.

**Other medicines or dietary supplements**—Although certain medicines or dietary supplements should not be used together at all, in other cases two different medicines or dietary supplements may be used together even if an interaction might occur. In these cases, your doctor may want to change the dose, or other precautions may be necessary. Tell your health care professional if you are taking any other prescription, nonprescription (over-the-counter [OTC]) medicine, or dietary supplements.

## Proper Use of This Dietary Supplement

Some people believe that taking very large doses of vitamins (called megadoses or megavitamin therapy) is useful for treating certain medical problems. Studies have not proven this. Large doses should be taken only under the direction of your doctor after need has been identified.

**Dosing**—The dose of pantothenic acid for prevention of pantothenic acid deficiency is based on daily recommended intake. See the *Importance of Diet* section for daily recommended intake for pantothenic acid.

**Missed dose**—If you miss taking a vitamin for one or more days there is no cause for concern, since it takes some time for your body to become seriously low in vitamins. However, if your doctor has recommended that you take this vitamin, try to remember to take it as directed every day.

**Storage**—To store this dietary supplement:

- Keep out of the reach of children.
- Store away from heat and direct light.
- Do not store in the bathroom, near the kitchen sink, or in other damp places. Heat or moisture may cause the dietary supplement to break down.
- Do not keep outdated dietary supplements or those no longer needed. Be sure that any discarded dietary supplement is out of the reach of children.

## Side Effects of This Dietary Supplement

Along with its needed effects, a dietary supplement may cause some unwanted effects. Although pantothenic acid does not usually cause any side effects, check with your doctor if you notice any unusual effects while you are taking it.

Revised: 07/16/92
Interim revision: 08/15/94

# PAPAVERINE    Intracavernosal

## Description

Papaverine (pa-PAV-er-een) belongs to the group of medicines called vasodilators. Vasodilators cause blood vessels to expand, thereby increasing blood flow. Papaverine is used to produce erections in some impotent men. When papaverine is injected into the penis (intracavernosal), it increases blood flow to the penis, which results in an erection.

Papaverine injection should not be used as a sexual aid by men who are not impotent. If the medicine is not used properly, permanent damage to the penis and loss of the ability to have erections could result.

Papaverine is available only with your doctor's prescription, in the following dosage form:

*Parenteral*
- Injection (U.S. and Canada)

## Before Using This Medicine

In deciding to use a medicine, the risks of taking the medicine must be weighed against the good it will do.

This is a decision you and your doctor will make. For papaverine, the following should be considered:

**Allergies**—Tell your doctor if you have ever had any unusual or allergic reaction to papaverine. Also tell your health care professional if you are allergic to any other substances, such as foods, preservatives, or dyes.

**Older adults**—Many medicines have not been studied specifically in older people. Therefore, it may not be known whether they work exactly the same way they do in younger adults or if they cause different side effects or problems in older people. Although there is no specific information comparing the use of papaverine for impotence in the elderly with use in other age groups, this medicine is not expected to cause different side effects or problems in older people than it does in younger adults.

**Other medicines**—Although certain medicines should not be used together at all, in other cases two different medicines may be used together even if an interaction might occur. In these cases, your doctor may want to change the dose, or other precautions may be necessary. Tell your health care professional if you are taking any other prescription or nonprescription (over-the-counter [OTC]) medicine.

**Other medical problems**—The presence of other medical problems may affect the use of papaverine. Make sure you tell your doctor if you have any other medical problems, especially:

- Bleeding problems—These conditions increase the risk of bleeding at the place of injection
- Liver disease—Papaverine can cause liver damage when it is given in ways that allow it to get into the bloodstream (by mouth or by injection into a muscle, a vein, or an artery); when papaverine is given by intracavernosal injection, liver damage is much less likely because the medicine enters the bloodstream very slowly
- Priapism (history of) or
- Sickle cell disease—Patients with these conditions have an increased risk of priapism (erection lasting longer than 4 hours) while using papaverine

---

## Proper Use of This Medicine

To give papaverine injection:

- Cleanse the injection site with alcohol. Using a sterile needle, *inject the medicine slowly and directly into the base of the penis as instructed by your doctor. Papaverine should not be injected just under the skin.* The injection is usually not painful, although you may feel some tingling in the tip of your penis. If the injection is very painful or you notice bruising or swelling at the place of injection, that means you have been injecting the medicine under the skin. Stop, withdraw the needle, and reposition it properly before continuing with the injection.
- After you have completed the injection, put pressure on the place of injection to prevent bruising. Then massage your penis as instructed by your doctor. This helps the medicine spread to all parts of the penis, so that it will work better.

This medicine usually begins to work in about 10 minutes. You should attempt intercourse within 2 hours after injecting the medicine.

**Dosing**—The dose of papaverine will be different for different patients. *Follow your doctor's orders or the directions on the label.* The following information includes only the average doses of papaverine. *If your dose is different, do not change it* unless your doctor tells you to do so.

- For *injection* dosage form:
  —For the treatment of impotence:
  - Adults—30 to 60 milligrams (mg) injected very slowly into the area of your penis as directed by your doctor. Allow one or two minutes to completely inject the dose. Do not inject more than one dose in a day. Also, do not use this medicine more than two days in a row or more than three times a week.

**Storage**—To store this medicine:
- Keep out of the reach of children.
- Store away from heat and direct light.
- Keep the medicine from freezing.

---

## Precautions While Using This Medicine

*Use papaverine injection exactly as directed by your doctor.* Do not use more of it and do not use it more often than ordered. If too much is used, the erection may become so strong that it lasts too long and does not reverse when it should. This condition is called priapism, and it can be very dangerous. If the effect is not reversed, the blood supply to the penis may be cut off and permanent damage may occur.

*Contact your doctor immediately if the erection lasts for longer than 4 hours or if it becomes painful.* This may be a sign of priapism and must be treated right away to prevent permanent damage.

If you notice bleeding at the site when you inject papaverine, put pressure on the spot until the bleeding stops. If it doesn't stop, check with your doctor.

It is important for you to examine your penis regularly. Check with your doctor if you find a lump where the medicine has been injected or if you notice that your penis is becoming curved. These may be signs that unwanted tissue is growing (called fibrosis), which should be seen by your doctor.

---

## Side Effects of This Medicine

Along with its needed effects, a medicine may cause some unwanted effects. Although not all of these side effects may occur, if they do occur they may need medical attention.

*Check with your doctor immediately* if the following side effect occurs:
  *Rare*
    Erection continuing for more than 4 hours, or painful erection

Check with your doctor as soon as possible if the following side effects occur:

*Rare*

Dizziness; lumps in the penis

Other side effects may occur that usually do not need medical attention. These side effects may go away during treatment as your body adjusts to the medicine. However, check with your doctor if any of the following side effects continue or are bothersome:

*Less common or rare*

Bruising or bleeding at place of injection; burning (mild) along penis; difficulty in ejaculating; swelling at place of injection

Papaverine injected into the penis may cause tingling at the tip of the penis. This is no cause for concern.

Other side effects not listed above may also occur in some patients. If you notice any other effects, check with your doctor.

Revised: 08/06/92
Interim revision: 06/07/94

---

# PAPAVERINE Systemic

Some commonly used brand names are:

**In the U.S.—**

| | |
|---|---|
| Cerespan | Pavagen |
| Genabid | Pavarine |
| Pavabid | Pavased |
| Pavabid HP | Pavatine |
| Pavacels | Pavatym |
| Pavacot | Paverolan |

Generic name product may also be available in the U.S. and Canada.

## Description

Papaverine (pa-PAV-er-een) belongs to the group of medicines called vasodilators. Vasodilators cause blood vessels to expand, thereby increasing blood flow. This medicine is used to treat problems resulting from poor blood circulation.

Papaverine is available only with your doctor's prescription, in the following dosage forms:

*Oral*
• Extended-release capsules (U.S.)
• Tablets (U.S. and Canada)

*Parenteral*
• Injection (U.S. and Canada)

## Before Using This Medicine

In deciding to use a medicine, the risks of taking the medicine must be weighed against the good it will do. This is a decision you and your doctor will make. For papaverine, the following should be considered:

**Allergies**—Tell your doctor if you have ever had any unusual or allergic reaction to papaverine. Also tell your health care professional if you are allergic to any other substances, such as foods, preservatives, or dyes.

**Pregnancy**—Studies on effects in pregnancy have not been done in either humans or animals.

**Breast-feeding**—It is not known whether papaverine passes into the breast milk. However, this medicine has not been reported to cause problems in nursing babies.

**Children**—Although there is no specific information comparing use of papaverine in children with use in other age groups, this medicine is not expected to cause different side effects or problems in children than it does in adults.

**Older adults**—Papaverine may reduce tolerance to cold temperatures in elderly patients.

**Other medicines**—Although certain medicines should not be used together at all, in other cases two different medicines may be used together even if an interaction might occur. In these cases, your doctor may want to change the dose, or other precautions may be necessary. Tell your health care professional if you are taking any other prescription or nonprescription (over-the-counter [OTC]) medicine, or if you smoke.

**Other medical problems**—The presence of other medical problems may affect the use of papaverine. Make sure you tell your doctor if you have any other medical problems, especially:
• Angina (chest pain) or
• Glaucoma or
• Heart disease or
• Myocardial infarction ("heart attack"), recent, or
• Stroke, recent—The chance of unwanted effects may be increased

## Proper Use of This Medicine

If this medicine upsets your stomach, it may be taken with meals, milk, or antacids.

For patients taking the *extended-release capsule* form of this medicine:
• Swallow the capsules whole. Do not crush, break, or chew before swallowing. However, if the capsule is too large to swallow, you may mix the contents with jam or jelly and swallow without chewing.

**Dosing**—The dose of papaverine will be different for different patients. *Follow your doctor's orders or the directions on the label.* The following information includes only the average doses of papaverine. *If your dose is*

*different, do not change it* unless your doctor tells you to do so:

- For *oral* dosage form (extended-release capsules):
  —Adults: 150 milligrams (mg) every twelve hours. The dose may be increased to 150 mg every eight hours or 300 mg every twelve hours.
- For *oral* dosage form (tablets):
  —Adults: 100 to 300 mg three to five times a day.
- For *injection* dosage form:
  —Adults: 30 to 120 mg every three hours injected slowly into the muscle or vein.
  —Children: 1.5 mg per kilogram (0.68 mg per pound) of body weight four times a day injected into the muscle or vein.

**Missed dose**—If you miss a dose of this medicine, take it as soon as you remember. However, if it is almost time for the next dose, skip the missed dose and go back to your regular dosing schedule. Do not double doses.

**Storage**—To store this medicine:

- Keep out of the reach of children.
- Store away from heat and direct light.
- Do not store in the bathroom, near the kitchen sink, or in other damp places. Heat or moisture may cause the medicine to break down.
- Do not keep outdated medicine or medicine no longer needed. Be sure that any discarded medicine is out of the reach of children.

## Precautions While Using This Medicine

It may take some time for this medicine to work. If you feel that the medicine is not working, do not stop taking it on your own. Instead, check with your doctor.

The helpful effects of this medicine may be decreased if you smoke. If you have any questions about this, check with your doctor.

*Dizziness may occur, especially when you get up from a lying or sitting position or climb stairs. Getting up slowly may help.* If this problem continues or gets worse, check with your doctor.

## Side Effects of This Medicine

Along with its needed effects, a medicine may cause some unwanted effects. Although not all of these side effects may occur, if they do occur they may need medical attention.

Check with your doctor as soon as possible if any of the following side effects occur:

*Symptoms of overdose*
   Blurred or double vision; drowsiness; weakness

*Rare*
   Yellow eyes or skin

Other side effects may occur after papaverine is given by injection. Check with your doctor if you notice any redness, swelling, or pain at the place of injection.

Other side effects that usually do not need medical attention may occur soon after an injection of this medicine. They usually go away after a little while. However, check with your doctor if any of the following side effects continue or are bothersome:

   Deep breathing; dizziness; fast heartbeat; flushing of face

Other side effects not listed above may also occur in some patients. If you notice any other effects, check with your doctor.

Revised: 04/13/93

---

# PARALDEHYDE   Systemic

A commonly used brand name in the U.S. is Paral.

Generic name product may also be available in the U.S. and Canada.

## Description

Paraldehyde (par-AL-de-hyde) is used to treat certain convulsive disorders. It also has been used in the treatment of alcoholism and in the treatment of nervous and mental conditions to calm or relax patients who are nervous or tense and to produce sleep. However, this medicine has generally been replaced by safer and more effective medicines for the treatment of alcoholism and in the treatment of nervous and mental conditions.

This medicine is available only with your doctor's prescription, in the following dosage forms:

*Oral*
- Oral liquid (U.S. and Canada)

*Parenteral*
- Injection (Canada)

*Rectal*
- Rectal liquid (U.S. and Canada)

## Before Using This Medicine

In deciding to use a medicine, the risks of taking the medicine must be weighed against the good it will do.

This is a decision you and your doctor will make. For paraldehyde, the following should be considered:

**Allergies**—Tell your doctor if you have ever had any unusual or allergic reaction to paraldehyde. Also tell your health care professional if you are allergic to any other substances, such as foods, preservatives, or dyes.

**Pregnancy**—Paraldehyde crosses the placenta. Studies on birth defects have not been done in either humans or animals. Use of paraldehyde during labor may cause breathing problems in the newborn infant.

**Breast-feeding**—Paraldehyde has not been reported to cause problems in nursing babies.

**Children**—Although there is no specific information comparing use of paraldehyde in children with use in other age groups, this medicine is not expected to cause different side effects or problems in children than it does in adults.

**Older adults**—Many medicines have not been studied specifically in older people. Therefore, it may not be known whether they work exactly the same way they do in younger adults or if they cause different side effects or problems in older people. There is no specific information comparing use of paraldehyde in the elderly with use in other age groups.

**Other medicines**—Although certain medicines should not be used together at all, in other cases 2 different medicines may be used together even if an interaction might occur. In these cases, your doctor may want to change the dose, or other precautions may be necessary. When you are taking paraldehyde, it is especially important that your health care professional know if you are taking any of the following:
- Central nervous system (CNS) depressants (medicine that causes drowsiness) or
- Tricyclic antidepressants (medicine for depression)—CNS depressant effects may be increased
- Disulfiram (e.g., Antabuse)—Higher blood levels of paraldehyde may occur, increasing the chance of side effects

**Other medical problems**—The presence of other medical problems may affect the use of paraldehyde. Make sure you tell your doctor if you have any other medical problems, especially:
- Alcohol abuse (or history of) or
- Drug abuse or dependence (or history of)—Dependence on paraldehyde may develop
- Colitis—Paraldehyde used rectally may make the condition worse.
- Emphysema, asthma, bronchitis, or other chronic lung disease, or
- Liver disease—Higher blood levels of paraldehyde may occur, increasing the chance of side effects
- Gastroenteritis (stomach flu) or
- Stomach ulcer—Paraldehyde taken by mouth may make the condition worse.

## Proper Use of This Medicine

*Use this medicine only as directed by your doctor.* Do not use more of it, do not use it more often, and do not use it for a longer time than your doctor ordered. If too much is used, the medicine may become habit-forming.

*Do not use if liquid turns brownish in color or if it has a strong vinegar-like odor,* since this means the paraldehyde is breaking down. If you have any questions about this, check with your health care professional.

For patients taking this medicine *by mouth:*
- *Do not use a plastic spoon, plastic glass, or any other plastic container to take this medicine,* since paraldehyde may react with the plastic. Use a metal spoon or glass container.
- *Take this medicine mixed in a glass of milk or iced fruit juice* to improve the taste and odor and to lessen stomach upset.

For patients using this medicine *rectally:*
- *Do not use paraldehyde in any plastic container* since it may react with the plastic.
- Before using paraldehyde rectally, make sure you understand exactly how to use it. Paraldehyde may need to be diluted. If you have any questions about this, check with your health care professional.

Keep this medicine away from the eyes and avoid getting it on the skin and clothing.

Keep this medicine away from heat, open flame, and sparks.

**Dosing**—The dose of paraldehyde will be different for different patients. *Follow your doctor's orders or the directions on the label.* The following information includes only the average doses of paraldehyde. *If your dose is different, do not change it* unless your doctor tells you to do so.

The amount of paraldehyde that you take depends on the strength of the medicine. Also, *the number of doses you take each day, the time allowed between doses, and the length of time you take the medicine depend on the medical problem for which you are taking paraldehyde.*
- For *oral and rectal* dosage forms (liquid):
  —Adults: Dose must be determined by your doctor.
  —Children: Dose is based on body weight, and must be determined by the doctor.
- For *injection* dosage form:
  —Adults: Dose must be determined by your doctor. It will be injected into a muscle or a vein.
  —Children: Dose is based on body weight, and must be determined by the doctor.

**Missed dose**—If you are taking this medicine regularly (for example, every day) and you miss a dose, take it right away if you remember within an hour or so of the missed dose. However, if you do not remember until later, skip the missed dose and go back to your regular dosing schedule. Do not double doses.

**Storage**—To store this medicine:
- Keep out of the reach of children.
- Store away from heat and direct light.
- Keep the medicine from freezing.
- Do not keep outdated medicine or medicine no longer needed. Be sure that any discarded medicine is out of the reach of children.

## Precautions While Using This Medicine

If you will be using this medicine regularly for a long time:
- Your doctor should check your progress at regular visits.
- Do not stop using it without first checking with your doctor. Your doctor may want you to reduce gradually the amount you are using before stopping completely.

This medicine will add to the effects of alcohol and other CNS depressants (medicines that slow down the nervous system, possibly causing drowsiness). Some examples of CNS depressants are antihistamines or medicine for hay fever, other allergies, or colds; sedatives, tranquilizers, or sleeping medicine; prescription pain medicine or narcotics; barbiturates; medicine for seizures; muscle relaxants; or anesthetics, including some dental anesthetics. *Check with your doctor before taking any of the above while you are using this medicine.*

Before you have any medical tests, tell the medical doctor in charge that you are taking this medicine. The results of some tests, such as the metyrapone test and the phentolamine test, may be affected by this medicine.

*If you think you or someone else may have taken an overdose of this medicine, get emergency help at once.* Taking an overdose of paraldehyde or taking alcohol or other CNS depressants with paraldehyde may lead to unconsciousness and possibly death. Some signs of an overdose are confusion, muscle tremors, nausea or vomiting (continuing or severe), severe stomach cramps, severe weakness, shortness of breath or slow or troubled breathing, and slow heartbeat.

This medicine may cause some people to become drowsy or less alert than they are normally. Even if taken at bedtime, it may cause some people to feel drowsy or less alert on arising. *Make sure you know how you react to this medicine before you drive, use machines, or do anything else that could be dangerous if you are not alert.*

## Side Effects of This Medicine

Along with its needed effects, a medicine may cause some unwanted effects. Although not all of these side effects may occur, if they do occur they may need medical attention.

Check with your doctor as soon as possible if any of the following side effects occur:
*More common*
Coughing (with injection only); skin rash
*Less common*
Redness, swelling, or pain at injection site
*With long-term use*
Yellow eyes or skin
*Symptoms of overdose*
Cloudy urine; confusion; decreased urination; fast and deep breathing; muscle tremors; nausea or vomiting (continuing or severe); nervousness, restlessness, or irritability; shortness of breath or slow or troubled breathing; slow heartbeat; stomach cramps (severe); weakness (severe)

Other side effects may occur that usually do not need medical attention. These side effects may go away during treatment as your body adjusts to the medicine. However, check with your doctor if any of the following side effects continue or are bothersome:
*More common*
Drowsiness; nausea or vomiting (when taken by mouth); stomach pain (when taken by mouth); unpleasant breath odor
*Less common*
Clumsiness or unsteadiness; dizziness; "hangover" effect

After you stop using this medicine, your body may need time to adjust. The length of time this takes depends on the amount of medicine you were using and how long you used it. During this period of time check with your doctor if you notice any of the following side effects:
Convulsions (seizures); hallucinations (seeing, hearing, or feeling things that are not there); increased sweating; muscle cramps; nausea and vomiting; stomach cramps; trembling

Paraldehyde will cause your breath to have a strong unpleasant odor. This effect will last until about one day after you have stopped using this medicine.

Other side effects not listed above may also occur in some patients. If you notice any other effects, check with your doctor.

Revised: 03/19/93

# PAROXETINE Systemic

A commonly used brand names in the U.S. and Canada is Paxil.

## Description

Paroxetine (pa-ROX-uh-teen) is used to treat mental depression.

This medicine is available only with your doctor's prescription, in the following dosage form:

*Oral*
- Tablets (U.S. and Canada)

## Before Using This Medicine

In deciding to use a medicine, the risks of taking the medicine must be weighed against the good it will do. This is a decision you and your doctor will make. For paroxetine, the following should be considered:

**Allergies**—Tell your doctor if you have ever had any unusual or allergic reaction to paroxetine. Also tell your health care professional if you are allergic to any other substances, such as foods, preservatives, or dyes.

**Pregnancy**—Studies have not been done in pregnant women. However, studies in animals have shown that paroxetine may cause miscarriages and decreased survival rates of offspring when given in doses many times the usual human dose. Before taking this medicine, make sure your doctor knows if you are pregnant or if you may become pregnant.

**Breast-feeding**—Paroxetine passes into the breast milk. However, this medicine has not been reported to cause problems in nursing babies.

**Children**—Studies on this medicine have been done only in adult patients, and there is no specific information comparing use of paroxetine in children with use in other age groups.

**Older adults**—In studies done to date that have included elderly people, paroxetine did not cause different side effects or problems in older people than it did in younger adults.

**Other medicines**—Although certain medicines should not be used together at all, in other cases two different medicines may be used together even if an interaction might occur. In these cases, your doctor may want to change the dose, or other precautions may be necessary. When you are taking paroxetine, it is especially important that your health care professional know if you are taking any of the following:
- Monoamine oxidase (MAO) inhibitors (furazolidone l[e.g., Furoxone], isocarboxazid [e.g., Marplan], phenelzine [e.g., Nardil], procarbazine [e.g., Matulane], selegiline [e.g., Eldepryl], tranylcypromine [e.g., Parnate]—Taking paroxetine while you are taking or within 2 weeks of taking MAO inhibitors may cause confusion, agitation, restlessness, stomach or intestinal symptoms, sudden high body temperature, extremely high blood pressure, and severe convulsions; at least 14 days should be allowed between stopping treatment with one medicine and starting treatment with the other
- Tryptophan—Taking this medicine while you are taking paroxetine may increase the risk of serious side effects
- Warfarin (e.g., Coumadin)—Taking this medicine together with paroxetine may cause bleeding problems; your doctor may need to adjust the dosage of either medicine

**Other medical problems**—The presence of other medical problems may affect the use of paroxetine. Make sure you tell your doctor if you have any other medical problems, especially:
- Drug abuse or dependence (or history of)—Because paroxetine is a new medicine, it is not known if it could become habit-forming, causing mental or physical dependence
- Kidney disease, severe, or
- Liver disease, severe—Higher blood levels of paroxetine may occur, increasing the chance of side effects
- Seizures, history of—The risk of seizures may be increased

## Proper Use of This Medicine

*Take this medicine only as directed by your doctor* to benefit your condition as much as possible. Do not take more of it, do not take it more often, and do not take it for a longer time than your doctor ordered.

*You may have to take paroxetine for up to 4 weeks or longer before you begin to feel better.* Your doctor should check your progress at regular visits during this time.

Paroxetine may be taken with or without food or on a full or empty stomach. However, if your doctor tells you to take the medicine a certain way, take it exactly as directed.

**Dosing**—The dose of paroxetine will be different for different patients. *Follow your doctor's orders or the directions on the label.* The following information includes only the average doses of paroxetine. *If your dose is different, do not change it* unless your doctor tells you to do so.
- For *oral* dosage form (tablets):
  —For treatment of depression:
    - Adults—At first, 20 milligrams (mg) once a day, usually taken in the morning. Your doctor may increase your dose if needed. However, the dose is usually not more than 50 mg a day.
    - Children—Use and dose must be determined by your doctor.
    - Older adults—At first, 10 mg once a day, usually taken in the morning. Your doctor may increase your dose if needed. However, the dose is usually not more than 40 mg a day.

**Missed dose**—If you miss a dose of this medicine, take it as soon as possible. However, if it is almost time for your next dose, skip the missed dose and go back to your regular dosing schedule. Do not double doses.

**Storage**—To store this medicine:
- Keep out of the reach of children.
- Store away from heat and direct light.
- Do not store in the bathroom, near the kitchen sink, or in other damp places. Heat or moisture may cause the medicine to break down.
- Do not keep outdated medicine or medicine no longer needed. Be sure that any discarded medicine is out of the reach of children.

---

## Precautions While Using This Medicine

It is important that your doctor check your progress at regular visits, to allow for changes in your dose and to help reduce any side effects.

Do not stop taking this medicine without first checking with your doctor. Your doctor may want you to gradually reduce the amount you are taking before stopping completely. This is to decrease the chance of side effects.

This medicine could possibly add to the effects of alcohol and other CNS depressants (medicines that cause drowsiness). Some examples of CNS depressants are antihistamines or medicine for hay fever, other allergies, or colds; sedatives, tranquilizers, or sleeping medicine; prescription pain medicine or narcotics; barbiturates; medicine for seizures; muscle relaxants; or anesthetics, including some dental anesthetics. *Check with your doctor before taking any of the above while you are using this medicine.*

Paroxetine may cause some people to become drowsy or have blurred vision. *Make sure you know how you react to this medicine before you drive, use machines, or do anything else that could be dangerous if you are not alert or able to see clearly.*

*Dizziness, lightheadedness, or fainting may occur,* especially when you get up from a lying or sitting position. Getting up slowly may help. If this problem continues or gets worse, check with your doctor.

*This medicine may cause dryness of the mouth. For temporary relief, use sugarless gum or candy, melt bits of ice in your mouth, or use a saliva substitute.* However, if your mouth continues to feel dry for more than 2 weeks, check with your medical doctor or dentist. Continuing dryness of the mouth may increase the chance of dental disease, including tooth decay, gum disease, and fungus infections.

---

## Side Effects of This Medicine

Along with its needed effects, a medicine may cause some unwanted effects. Although not all of these side effects

may occur, if they do occur they may need medical attention.

Check with your doctor as soon as possible if any of the following side effects occur:

*Less common*
Agitation; lightheadedness or fainting; muscle pain or weakness; rash

*Rare*
Absence of or decrease in body movements; diarrhea; difficulty in speaking; drowsiness; dryness of mouth; fever; inability to move eyes; incomplete, sudden, or unusual body or facial movements; increased sweating; increased thirst; lack of energy; mood or behavior changes; overactive reflexes; racing heartbeat; restlessness; shivering or shaking; talking, feeling, and acting with excitement and activity you cannot control

*Symptoms of overdose*
Drowsiness (severe); dryness of mouth (severe); irritability; large pupils; nausea (severe); racing heartbeat; tremor (severe); vomiting (severe)

Other side effects may occur that usually do not need medical attention. These side effects may go away during treatment as your body adjusts to the medicine. However, check with your doctor if any of the following side effects continue or are bothersome:

*More common*
Constipation; decreased sexual ability; dizziness; headache; nausea; problems in urinating; tremor; trouble in sleeping; unusual tiredness or weakness; vomiting

*Less common*
Anxiety or nervousness; blurred vision; change in your sense of taste; decreased or increased appetite; decreased sexual desire; fast or irregular heartbeat; tingling, burning, or prickly sensations; weight loss or gain

After you stop using this medicine, your body may need time to adjust. The length of time this takes depends on the amount of medicine you were using and how long you used it. During this period of time check with your doctor if you notice any of the following side effects:

Agitation, confusion, or restlessness; diarrhea; dizziness or lightheadedness; headache; increased sweating; muscle pain; nausea or vomiting; runny nose; tremor; trouble in sleeping; unusual tiredness or weakness; vision changes

Other side effects not listed above may also occur in some patients. If you notice any other effects, check with your doctor.

---

Developed: 08/22/94

---

# PEGADEMASE Systemic†

A commonly used brand name in the U.S. is Adagen.
Other commonly used names are PEG-ADA and PEG-adenosine deaminase.

---

†Not commercially available in Canada.

---

## Description

Pegademase contains an enzyme called adenosine deaminase (ADA). It is used to treat children who do not have a properly developed immune system because of a lack of ADA in the body.

Pegademase is to be given only by or under the supervision of your doctor. It is available in the following dosage form:

*Parenteral*
- Injection (U.S.)

## Before Using This Medicine

In deciding to use a medicine, the risks of taking the medicine must be weighed against the good it will do. This is a decision you and your doctor will make. For pegademase, the following should be considered:

**Allergies**—Tell your doctor if you have ever had any unusual or allergic reaction to pegademase. Also tell your health care professional if you are allergic to any other substances, such as foods, preservatives, or dyes.

**Other medicines**—Although certain medicines should not be used together at all, in other cases two different medicines may be used together even if an interaction might occur. In these cases, your doctor may want to change the dose, or other precautions may be necessary. When you are receiving pegademase, it is especially important that your health care professional know if you are taking any other medicine.

**Other medical problems**—The presence of other medical problems may affect the use of pegademase. Make sure you tell your doctor if you have any other medical problems, especially:
- Blood clotting problems—Injection may cause bleeding

## Proper Use of This Medicine

**Dosing**—The dose of pegademase will be different for different patients. *Follow your doctor's orders or the directions on the label.* The following information includes only the average doses of pegademase.
- For *injection* dosage form:
  - —For treatment of lack of ADA:
    - Children—Dose is based on body weight and must be determined by your doctor. The usual dose is 10 to 20 Units per kilogram (kg) (4.55 to 9.09 Units per pound) of body weight, injected into a muscle once a week. *If you are receiving pegademase at home, follow your doctor's orders or the directions on the label.* If you have any questions about the proper dose of pegademase, ask your doctor.

If you miss getting a dose of this medicine, get it as soon as possible.

## Precautions While Using This Medicine

It is very important that you continue to receive treatment with pegademase. Treatment must be continued for life. Do not stop treatment with pegademase without checking with your doctor. If regular treatment is not continued, the immune system will break down and serious infections may occur.

## Side Effects of This Medicine

Along with its needed effects, a medicine may cause some unwanted effects. Pegademase does not usually cause any side effects. However, check with your doctor if pain at the place of injection occurs and continues or is bothersome.

Other side effects not listed above may also occur in some patients. If you notice any other effects, check with your doctor.

---

Revised: 09/90
Interim revision: 07/11/94

---

# PEMOLINE Systemic

Some commonly used brand names are:
**In the U.S.—**
    Cylert
    Cylert Chewable
**In Canada—**
    Cylert

## Description

Pemoline (PEM-oh-leen) belongs to the group of medicines called central nervous system (CNS) stimulants. It is used to treat children with attention-deficit hyperactivity disorder (ADHD).

Pemoline increases attention and decreases restlessness in children who are overactive, cannot concentrate for very long or are easily distracted, and are emotionally unstable. This medicine is used as part of a total treatment program that also includes social, educational, and psychological treatment.

Pemoline is available only with your doctor's prescription, in the following dosage forms:

Oral
- Tablets (U.S. and Canada)
- Chewable tablets (U.S.)

## Before Using This Medicine

In deciding to use a medicine, the risks of taking the medicine must be weighed against the good it will do. This is a decision you and your doctor will make. For pemoline, the following should be considered:

**Allergies**—Tell your doctor if you have ever had any unusual or allergic reaction to pemoline. Also tell your health care professional if you are allergic to any other substances, such as foods, preservatives, or dyes.

**Pregnancy**—Pemoline has not been shown to cause birth defects or other problems in humans. However, studies in animals given large doses of pemoline have shown that pemoline causes an increase in stillbirths and decreased survival of the offspring after birth.

**Breast-feeding**—It is not known if pemoline is excreted in breast milk.

**Children**—Slowed growth rate in children who received pemoline for a long period of time have been reported. Some doctors recommend drug-free periods during treatment with pemoline.

**Other medicines**—Although certain medicines should not be used together at all, in other cases 2 different medicines may be used together even if an interaction might occur. In these cases, your doctor may want to change the dose, or other precautions may be necessary. Tell your health care professional if you are taking any other prescription or nonprescription (over-the-counter [OTC]) medicine.

**Other medical problems**—The presence of other medical problems may affect the use of pemoline. Make sure you tell your doctor if you have any other medical problems, especially:
- Gilles de la Tourette's disorder or other tics or
- Mental illness (severe) or
- Liver disease—Pemoline may make the condition worse
- Kidney disease—Higher blood levels of pemoline may occur, increasing the chance of side effects

## Proper Use of This Medicine

For patients taking the chewable tablet form of this medicine:
- These tablets must be chewed before swallowing. Do not swallow whole.

Sometimes this medicine must be taken for 3 to 4 weeks before improvement is noticed.

Take pemoline only as directed by your doctor. Do not take more of it, do not take it more often, and do not take it for a longer time than your doctor ordered. If too much is taken, it may become habit-forming.

**Dosing**—The dose of pemoline will be different for different patients. Follow your doctor's orders or the directions on the label. The following information includes only the average doses of pemoline. If your dose is different, do not change it unless your doctor tells you to do so.

The number of tablets that you take depends on the strength of the medicine. Also, the number of doses you take each day, the time allowed between doses, and the length of time you take the medicine depend on the medical problem for which you are taking pemoline.

- For oral or chewable dosage forms (tablets):
  —Children 6 years of age and over: To start, 37.5 milligrams (mg) every morning. Your doctor may increase your dose if needed. However, the dose is usually not more than 112.5 mg a day.
  —Children up to 6 years of age: Dose must be determined by the doctor.

**Missed dose**—If you miss a dose of this medicine, take it as soon as possible. Then go back to your regular dosing schedule. But if you do not remember the missed dose until the next day, skip it and go back to your regular dosing schedule. Do not double doses.

**Storage**—To store this medicine:
- Keep out of the reach of children.
- Store away from heat and direct light.
- Do not store in the bathroom, near the kitchen sink, or in other damp places. Heat or moisture may cause the medicine to break down.
- Do not keep outdated medicine or medicine no longer needed. Be sure that any discarded medicine is out of the reach of children.

## Precautions While Using This Medicine

Your doctor should check your progress at regular visits to make sure that this medicine does not cause unwanted effects.

If you will be taking this medicine in large doses for a long time, do not stop taking it without first checking with your doctor. Your doctor may want you to reduce gradually the amount you are taking before stopping completely.

This medicine may cause some people to become dizzy or less alert than they are normally. Make sure you know how you react to this medicine before you ride a bicycle or do anything else that could be dangerous if you are dizzy or are not alert.

If you have been using this medicine for a long time and you think you may have become mentally or physically

*dependent on it, check with your doctor.* Some signs of dependence on pemoline are:
- a strong desire or need to continue taking the medicine.
- a need to increase the dose to receive the effects of the medicine.
- withdrawal side effects (for example, mental depression, unusual behavior, or unusual tiredness or weakness) occurring after the medicine is stopped.

## Side Effects of This Medicine

Along with their needed effects, medicines like pemoline, when used for a long time, have been reported to slow the growth rate of children. Some doctors recommend drug-free periods during treatment with pemoline. Pemoline may also cause unwanted effects on behavior in children with severe emotional problems.

Although not all of these side effects may occur, if they do occur they may need medical attention.

Check with your doctor as soon as possible if any of the following side effects occur:

*Rare*
Yellow eyes or skin

*Symptoms of overdose*
Agitation; confusion; convulsions (seizures); false sense of well-being; fast heartbeat; hallucinations (seeing, hearing, or feeling things that are not there); headache (severe); high blood pressure; high fever with sweating; large pupils; muscle trembling or twitching; nervousness or restlessness; uncontrolled movements of the eyes or other parts of the body; vomiting

Other side effects may occur that usually do not need medical attention. These side effects may go away during treatment as your body adjusts to the medicine. However, check with your doctor if any of the following side effects continue or are bothersome:

*More common*
Loss of appetite; trouble in sleeping; weight loss

*Less common*
Dizziness; drowsiness; increased irritability; mental depression; nausea; skin rash; stomach ache

After you stop using this medicine, your body may need time to adjust. The length of time this takes depends on the amount of medicine you were using and how long you used it. During this period of time check with your doctor if you notice any of the following side effects:

Mental depression (severe); unusual behavior; unusual tiredness or weakness

Other side effects not listed above may also occur in some patients. If you notice any other effects, check with your doctor.

Revised: 04/16/93

---

# PENICILLAMINE  Systemic

Some commonly used brand names in the U.S. and Canada are Cuprimine and Depen.

## Description

Penicillamine (pen-i-SILL-a-meen) is used in the treatment of medical problems such as Wilson's disease (too much copper in the body) and rheumatoid arthritis. Also, it is used to prevent kidney stones. Penicillamine may also be used for other conditions as determined by your doctor.

In addition to the helpful effects of this medicine, it has side effects that can be very serious. Before you take penicillamine, be sure that you have discussed the use of it with your doctor.

This medicine is available only with your doctor's prescription, in the following dosage forms:

*Oral*
- Capsules (U.S. and Canada)
- Tablets (U.S. and Canada)

## Before Using This Medicine

In deciding to use a medicine, the risks of taking the medicine must be weighed against the good it will do. This is a decision you and your doctor will make. For penicillamine, the following should be considered:

**Allergies**—Tell your doctor if you have ever had any unusual or allergic reaction to penicillin or to penicillamine. Also tell your health care professional if you are allergic to any other substances, such as foods, preservatives, or dyes.

**Pregnancy**—Penicillamine may cause birth defects if taken during pregnancy.

**Breast-feeding**—It is not known whether penicillamine passes into breast milk.

**Children**—Although there is no specific information about the use of penicillamine in children, it is not expected to cause different side effects or problems in children than it does in adults.

**Older adults**—Sore throat and fever, with or without chills; sores, ulcers, or white spots on the lips or in the mouth; shortness of breath, troubled breathing, tightness in the chest, and/or wheezing; swollen and/or painful glands; black, tarry stools; blood in urine or stools; pinpoint red spots on skin; cough or hoarseness; lower back or side pain; painful or difficult urination; unusual bleeding or bruising; and unusual tiredness or weakness may be especially likely to occur in elderly patients, who are usually more sensitive than younger adults to some of the effects of penicillamine.

**Other medicines**—Although certain medicines should not be used together at all, in other cases two different medicines may be used together even if an interaction might occur. In these cases, your doctor may want to change the dose, or other precautions may be necessary. When you are taking penicillamine, it is important that your health care professional know if you are taking *any* other prescription or nonprescription (over-the-counter [OTC]) medicine, especially:

- Gold compounds (e.g., Ridaura) or
- Phenylbutazone (e.g., Cotylbutazone)—The chance of serious side effects may be increased

**Other medical problems**—The presence of other medical problems may affect the use of penicillamine. Make sure you tell your doctor if you have any other medical problems, especially:

- Blood disease caused by penicillamine treatment, history of, or
- Kidney disease or history of (only for patients with rheumatoid arthritis)—The chance of side effects may be increased

---

## Proper Use of This Medicine

Since penicillamine is taken in different ways for different medical problems, it is very important that you understand exactly why you are taking this medicine and how to take it. See below for information on specific medical problems. If you have any questions about this, check with your doctor.

For patients taking this medicine to *prevent kidney stones:*

- You should drink 2 full glasses (8 ounces each) of water at bedtime and another 2 full glasses (8 ounces each) during the night.
- It is very important that you follow any special instructions from your doctor, such as following a low-methionine diet. If you have any questions about this, check with your doctor.

For patients taking this medicine for *rheumatoid arthritis:*

- Take this medicine on an empty stomach (at least 1 hour before meals or 2 hours after meals) and at least 1 hour before or after any other food, milk, or medicine.
- After you begin taking this medicine, 2 to 3 months may pass before you feel its effects. It is very important that you keep taking the medicine, even if you do not feel better, in order to give it time to work.

For patients taking this medicine for *Wilson's disease:*

- Take this medicine on an empty stomach (at least ½ to 1 hour before meals or 2 hours after meals).

- It is very important that you follow any special instructions from your doctor, such as following a low-copper diet. If you have any questions about this, check with your doctor.
- After you begin taking this medicine, 1 to 3 months may pass before you notice any improvement in your condition.

For patients taking this medicine for *lead poisoning:*

- Take this medicine on an empty stomach (2 hours before meals or at least 3 hours after meals).

For *all patients:*

- *Take this medicine regularly as directed. Do not stop taking it without first checking with your doctor,* since stopping the medicine and then restarting it may increase the possibility of side effects.

**Dosing**—The dose of penicillamine will be different for different patients. *Follow your doctor's orders or the directions on the label.* The following information includes only the average doses of penicillamine. *If your dose is different, do not change it* unless your doctor tells you to do so.

- For *oral* dosage form (capsules or tablets):
  —For Wilson's disease (too much copper in the body):
    - Adults and teenagers—At first, 250 milligrams (mg) four times a day. After a while, your doctor may need to increase the dose, depending on the amount of copper in your urine. Most people do not need more than 2000 mg a day (two 250-mg capsules or tablets four times a day).
    - Children—At first, 250 mg a day. After a while, your doctor may need to increase the dose, depending on the amount of copper in your urine. Older children may need the same dose as adults.
  —For rheumatoid arthritis:
    - Adults—At first, 125 or 250 mg once a day. Your doctor may increase the dose after a few months, depending on how well the medicine is working and whether it causes any side effects. The largest dose is not more than 1500 mg a day (two 250-mg capsules or tablets three times a day).
    - Children—Use and dose must be determined by your doctor.
  —For preventing kidney stones:
    - Adults—At first, 500 mg (two 250-mg capsules or tablets) four times a day. After a while, your doctor may need to change the dose, depending on the results of your urine tests. Some people may need as much as 4000 mg a day (four 250-mg capsules or tablets four times a day).
    - Children—The dose is based on body weight and must be determined by your doctor. At first, 7.5 mg per kilogram (kg) (about 3.5 mg per pound) of body weight four times a day. After a while, your doctor may need to change the dose, depending on the results of your urine tests.

**Missed dose**—If you miss a dose of this medicine and your dosing schedule is:

- One dose a day—Take the missed dose as soon as possible. But if you do not remember the missed dose until the next day, skip the missed dose and go back to your regular dosing schedule. Do not double the next day's dose.
- Two doses a day—Take the missed dose as soon as possible. However, if it is almost time for your next dose, skip the missed dose and go back to your regular dosing schedule. Do not double doses.
- More than two doses a day—If you remember within an hour or so of the missed dose, take it right away. But if you do not remember until later, skip the missed dose and go back to your regular dosing schedule. Do not double doses.

If you have any questions about this, check with your doctor.

**Storage**—To store this medicine:

- Keep out of the reach of children.
- Store away from heat and direct light.
- Do not store this medicine in the bathroom, near the kitchen sink, or in other damp places. Heat or moisture may cause the medicine to break down.
- Do not keep outdated medicine or medicine no longer needed. Be sure that any discarded medicine is out of the reach of children.

## Precautions While Using This Medicine

Your doctor should check your progress at regular visits to make sure that this medicine does not cause unwanted effects.

Before having any kind of surgery (including dental surgery), tell the medical doctor or dentist in charge that you are taking this medicine.

If you are taking iron preparations, or vitamin preparations containing iron, do not take them within 2 hours of the time you take this medicine. Taking the 2 medicines too close together may keep the penicillamine from working properly.

## Side Effects of This Medicine

Along with its needed effects, a medicine may cause some unwanted effects. Although not all of these side effects may occur, if they do occur they may need medical attention.

Check with your doctor as soon as possible if any of the following side effects occur:

*More common*
   Fever; joint pain; skin rash, hives, or itching; swollen and/or painful glands; ulcers, sores, or white spots on lips or in mouth

*Less common*
   Bloody or cloudy urine; shortness of breath, troubled breathing, tightness in chest, or wheezing; sore throat and fever with or without chills; swelling of face, feet, or lower legs; unusual bleeding or bruising; unusual tiredness or weakness; weight gain

*Rare*
   Abdominal or stomach pain (severe); blisters on skin; bloody or black, tarry stools; chest pain; coughing or hoarseness; dark urine; difficulty in breathing, chewing, talking, or swallowing; eye pain, blurred or double vision, or any change in vision; general feeling of discomfort or illness or weakness; lower back or side pain; muscle weakness; painful or difficult urination; pale stools; pinpoint red spots on skin; redness, tenderness, itching, burning, or peeling of skin; red or irritated eyes; red, thick, or scaly skin; ringing or buzzing in the ears; spitting blood; yellow eyes or skin

Other side effects may occur that usually do not need medical attention. These side effects may go away during treatment as your body adjusts to the medicine. However, check with your doctor if any of the following side effects continue or are bothersome:

*More common*
   Diarrhea; lessening or loss of taste sense; loss of appetite; nausea or vomiting; stomach pain (mild)

Other side effects not listed above may also occur in some patients. If you notice any other effects, check with your doctor.

Revised: July 1990
Interim revision: 09/01/94

---

# PENICILLINS   Systemic

Some commonly used brand names are:

**In the U.S.—**

| | | |
|---|---|---|
| Amoxil[1] | Ledercillin VK[13] | Pfizerpen-AS[12] |
| Bactocill[11] | Mezlin[9] | Pipracil[14] |
| Beepen-VK[13] | Nafcil[10] | Polycillin[2] |
| Betapen-VK[13] | Nallpen[10] | Polycillin-N[2] |
| Bicillin L-A[12] | Omnipen[2] | Polymox[1] |
| Cloxapen[5] | Omnipen-N[2] | Principen[2] |
| Crysticillin 300 A.S.[12] | Pathocil[6] | Prostaphlin[11] |
| Dynapen[6] | Pentids[12] | Spectrobid[3] |
| Dycill[6] | Pen Vee K[13] | Staphcillin[8] |
| Geocillin[4] | Permapen[12] | |
| Geopen[4] | Pfizerpen[12] | |

| |
|---|
| Tegopen[5] |
| Ticar[17] |
| Totacillin[2] |
| Totacillin-N[2] |
| Trimox[1] |
| Unipen[10] |
| V-Cillin K[13] |
| Veetids[13] |
| Wycillin[12] |
| Wymox[1] |

**In Canada—**

| | |
|---|---|
| Amoxil[1] | Nu-Amoxi[1] |
| Ampicin[2] | Nu-Ampi[2] |
| Apo-Amoxi[1] | Nu-Cloxi[5] |
| Apo-Ampi[2] | Nu-Pen-VK[13] |
| Apo-Cloxi[5] | Orbenin[5] |
| Apo-Pen VK[13] | Penbritin[2] |
| Ayercillin[12] | Penglobe[3] |
| Bicillin L-A[12] | Pen-Vee[13] |
| Fluclox[7] | Pipracil[14] |
| Geopen Oral[4] | Pondocillin[15] |
| Ledercillin VK[13] | PVF[13] |
| Megacillin[12] | PVF K[13] |
| Nadopen-V[13] | Pyopen[4] |
| Nadopen-V 200[13] | Selexid[16] |
| Nadopen-V 400[13] | Tegopen[5] |
| Novamoxin[1] | Ticar[17] |
| Novo-Ampicillin[2] | Unipen[10] |
| Novo-Cloxin[5] | V-Cillin K[13] |
| Novo-Pen-VK[13] | Wycillin[12] |

Note: For quick reference, the following penicillins are numbered to match the corresponding brand names.

This information applies to the following medicines:

1. Amoxicillin (a-mox-i-SILL-in)‡
2. Ampicillin (am-pi-SILL-in)‡
3. Bacampicillin (ba-kam-pi-SILL-in)
4. Carbenicillin (kar-ben-i-SILL-in)
5. Cloxacillin (klox-a-SILL-in)‡
6. Dicloxacillin (dye-klox-a-SILL-in)†‡
7. Flucloxacillin (floo-klox-a-SILL-in)*
8. Methicillin (meth-i-SILL-in)†
9. Mezlocillin (mez-loe-SILL-in)†
10. Nafcillin (naf-SILL-in)‡
11. Oxacillin (ox-a-SILL-in)†‡
12. Penicillin G (pen-i-SILL-in)‡
13. Penicillin V‡
14. Piperacillin (pi-PER-a-sill-in)
15. Pivampicillin (piv-am-pi-SILL-in)*
16. Pivmecillinam (piv-me-SILL-in-am)*
17. Ticarcillin (tye-kar-SILL-in)

---

*Not commercially available in the U.S.
†Not commercially available in Canada.
‡Generic name product may also be available in the U.S.
§Generic name product may also be available in Canada.

---

# Description

Penicillins are used to treat infections caused by bacteria. They work by killing the bacteria or preventing their growth.

There are several different kinds of penicillins. Each is used to treat different kinds of infections. One kind of penicillin usually may not be used in place of another. In addition, penicillins are used to treat bacterial infections in many different parts of the body. They are sometimes given with other antibacterial medicines (antibiotics). Some of the penicillins may also be used for other problems as determined by your doctor. However, none of the penicillins will work for colds, flu, or other virus infections.

Penicillins are available only with your doctor's prescription, in the following dosage forms:

*Oral*

Amoxicillin
- Capsules (U.S. and Canada)
- Oral suspension (U.S. and Canada)
- Chewable tablets (U.S. and Canada)

Ampicillin
- Capsules (U.S. and Canada)
- Oral suspension (U.S. and Canada)

Bacampicillin
- Oral suspension (U.S.)
- Tablets (U.S. and Canada)

Carbenicillin
- Tablets (U.S. and Canada)

Cloxacillin
- Capsules (U.S. and Canada)
- Oral solution (U.S. and Canada)

Dicloxacillin
- Capsules (U.S.)
- Oral suspension (U.S.)

Flucloxacillin
- Capsules (Canada)
- Oral suspension (Canada)

Nafcillin
- Capsules (U.S.)
- Tablets (U.S.)

Oxacillin
- Capsules (U.S.)
- Oral solution (U.S.)

Penicillin G Benzathine
- Oral suspension (Canada)

Penicillin G Potassium
- Oral solution (U.S.)
- Tablets (U.S. and Canada)

Penicillin V Benzathine
- Oral suspension (Canada)

Penicillin V Potassium
- Oral solution (U.S. and Canada)
- Tablets (U.S. and Canada)

Pivampicillin
- Oral suspension (Canada)
- Tablets (Canada)

Pivmecillinam
- Tablets (Canada)

*Parenteral*

Ampicillin
- Injection (U.S. and Canada)

Carbenicillin
- Injection (U.S. and Canada)

Cloxacillin
- Injection (Canada)

Methicillin
- Injection (U.S.)

Mezlocillin
- Injection (U.S.)

Nafcillin
- Injection (U.S. and Canada)

Oxacillin
- Injection (U.S.)

Penicillin G Benzathine
- Injection (U.S. and Canada)

Penicillin G Potassium
- Injection (U.S. and Canada)

Penicillin G Procaine
- Injection (U.S. and Canada)

Penicillin G Sodium
- Injection (U.S. and Canada)

Piperacillin
- Injection (U.S. and Canada)

Ticarcillin
- Injection (U.S. and Canada)

## Before Using This Medicine

In deciding to use a medicine, the risks of taking the medicine must be weighed against the good it will do. This is a decision you and your doctor will make. For penicillins, the following should be considered:

**Allergies**—Tell your doctor if you have ever had any unusual or allergic reaction to any of the penicillins or cephalosporins. Also tell your health care professional if you are allergic to any other substances, such as foods, preservatives, or dyes, or procaine (e.g., Novocain) or other ester-type anesthetics (medicines that cause numbing) if you are receiving penicillin G procaine.

**Diet**—Make certain your health care professional knows if you are on a low-sodium (low-salt) diet. Some of these medicines contain enough sodium to cause problems in some people.

**Pregnancy**—Penicillins have not been studied in pregnant women. However, penicillins have been widely used in pregnant women and have not been shown to cause birth defects or other problems in animal studies.

**Breast-feeding**—Penicillins pass into the breast milk. Even though only small amounts may pass into breast milk, allergic reactions, diarrhea, fungus infections, and skin rash may occur in nursing babies.

**Children**—Many penicillins have been used in children and, in effective doses, are not expected to cause different side effects or problems in children than they do in adults.

**Older adults**—Penicillins have been used in the elderly and have not been shown to cause different side effects or problems in older people than they do in younger adults.

**Other medicines**—Although certain medicines should not be used together at all, in other cases two different medicines may be used together even if an interaction might occur. In these cases, your doctor may want to change the dose, or other precautions may be necessary. When you are taking a penicillin, it is especially important that your health care professional know if you are taking any of the following:

- Acetaminophen (e.g., Tylenol) (with long-term, high-dose use) or
- Amiodarone (e.g., Cordarone) or
- Anabolic steroids (nandrolone [e.g., Anabolin], oxandrolone [e.g., Anavar], oxymetholone [e.g., Anadrol], stanozolol [e.g., Winstrol]) or
- Androgens (male hormones) or
- Antithyroid agents (medicine for overactive thyroid) or
- Carmustine (e.g., BiCNU) or
- Chloroquine (e.g., Aralen) or
- Dantrolene (e.g., Dantrium) or
- Daunorubicin (e.g., Cerubidine) or
- Disulfiram (e.g., Antabuse) or
- Divalproex (e.g., Depakote) or
- Estrogens (female hormones) or
- Etretinate (e.g., Tegison) or
- Gold salts (medicine for arthritis) or
- Hydroxychloroquine (e.g., Plaquenil) or
- Mercaptopurine (e.g., Purinethol) or
- Methotrexate (e.g., Mexate) or

- Methyldopa (e.g., Aldomet) or
- Naltrexone (e.g., Trexan) (with long-term, high-dose use) or
- Oral contraceptives (birth control pills) containing estrogen or
- Other anti-infectives by mouth or by injection (medicine for infection) or
- Phenothiazines (acetophenazine [e.g., Tindal], chlorpromazine [e.g., Thorazine], fluphenazine [e.g., Prolixin], mesoridazine [e.g., Serentil], perphenazine [e.g., Trilafon], prochlorperazine [e.g., Compazine], promazine [e.g., Sparine], promethazine [e.g., Phenergan], thioridazine [e.g., Mellaril], trifluoperazine [e.g., Stelazine], triflupromazine [e.g., Vesprin], trimeprazine [e.g., Temaril]) or
- Plicamycin (e.g., Mithracin) or
- Valproic acid (e.g., Depakene)—These medicines may increase the chance of liver damage if taken with cloxacillin, dicloxacillin, flucloxacillin, mezlocillin, nafcillin, oxacillin, or piperacillin

- Amiloride (e.g., Midamor) or
- Benazepril (e.g., Lotensin) or
- Captopril (e.g., Capoten) or
- Enalapril (e.g., Vasotec) or
- Fosinopril (e.g., Monopril) or
- Lisinopril (e.g., Prinivil, Zestril) or
- Potassium-containing medicine or
- Quinapril (e.g., Accupril) or
- Ramipril (e.g., Altace) or
- Spironolactone (e.g., Aldactone) or
- Triamterene (e.g., Dyrenium)—Use of these medicines with penicillin G by injection may cause an increase in side effects

- Anticoagulants (blood thinners) or
- Dipyridamole (e.g., Persantine) or
- Divalproex (e.g., Depakote) or
- Heparin (e.g., Panheprin) or
- Inflammation or pain medicine (except narcotics) or
- Pentoxifylline (e.g., Trental) or
- Plicamycin (e.g., Mithracin) or
- Sulfinpyrazone (e.g., Anturane) or
- Valproic acid (e.g., Depakene)—Use of these medicines with high doses of carbenicillin, piperacillin, or ticarcillin may increase the chance of bleeding

- Cloramphenicol (e.g., Chloromycetin) or
- Erythromycins (e.g., E.E.S., E-Mycin, ERYC) or
- Sulfonamides (e.g., Gantanol, Gantrisin) or
- Tetracyclines (e.g., Achromycin, Minocin, Vibramycin)—Use of these medicines with penicillins may prevent the penicillin from working properly

- Cholestyramine (e.g., Questran) or
- Colestipol (e.g., Colestid)—Use of these medicines with oral penicillin G may prevent penicillin G from working properly

- Oral contraceptives (birth control pills) containing estrogen—Use of ampicillin, amoxicillin, or penicillin V with estrogen-containing oral contraceptives may prevent oral contraceptives from working properly, increasing the chance of pregnancy

- Methotrexate (e.g., Mexate)—Use of methotrexate with penicillins may increase the chance of side effects of methotrexate

- Probenecid (e.g., Benemid)—Probenecid causes penicillins to build up in the blood. This may increase the chance of side effects. However, your doctor may want to give you probenecid with a penicillin to treat some infections

**Other medical problems**—The presence of other medical problems may affect the use of penicillins. Make sure you tell your doctor if you have any other medical problems, especially:

- Allergy, general (such as asthma, eczema, hay fever, hives), history of—Patients with a history of general allergies may be more likely to have a severe reaction to penicillins
- Bleeding problems, history of—Patients with a history of bleeding problems may be more likely to have bleeding when receiving carbenicillin, piperacillin, or ticarcillin
- Congestive heart failure (CHF) or
- High blood pressure—Large doses of carbenicillin or ticarcillin may make these conditions worse, because these medicines contains a large amount of salt
- Cystic fibrosis—Patients with cystic fibrosis may have an increased chance of fever and skin rash when receiving piperacillin
- Kidney disease—Patients with kidney disease may have an increased chance of side effects
- Mononucleosis ("mono")—Patients with mononucleosis may have an increased chance of skin rash when receiving ampicillin, bacampicillin, or pivampicillin
- Stomach or intestinal disease, history of (especially colitis, including colitis caused by antibiotics)—Patients with a history of stomach or intestinal disease may be more likely to develop colitis while taking penicillins

## Proper Use of This Medicine

Penicillins (except bacampicillin tablets, amoxicillin, penicillin V, pivampicillin, and pivmecillinam) are best taken with a full glass (8 ounces) of water on an empty stomach (either 1 hour before or 2 hours after meals) unless otherwise directed by your doctor.

For patients taking *amoxicillin, penicillin V, pivampicillin, and pivmecillinam:*

- Amoxicillin, penicillin V, pivampicillin, and pivmecillinam may be taken on a full or empty stomach.
- The *liquid form of amoxicillin* may also be taken by itself or mixed with formulas, milk, fruit juice, water, ginger ale, or other cold drinks. If mixed with other liquids, take immediately after mixing. Be sure to drink all the liquid to get the full dose of medicine.

For patients taking *bacampicillin:*

- The liquid form of this medicine is best taken with a full glass (8 ounces) of water on an empty stomach (either 1 hour before or 2 hours after meals) unless otherwise directed by your doctor.
- The tablet form of this medicine may be taken on a full or empty stomach.

For patients taking *penicillin G by mouth:*

- Do not drink acidic fruit juices (for example, orange or grapefruit juice) or other acidic beverages within 1 hour of taking penicillin G since this may keep the medicine from working properly.

For patients taking the *oral liquid form of penicillins:*

- This medicine is to be taken by mouth even if it comes in a dropper bottle. If this medicine does not come in a dropper bottle, use a specially marked measuring spoon or other device to measure each dose accurately. The average household teaspoon may not hold the right amount of liquid.
- Do not use after the expiration date on the label. The medicine may not work properly after that date. If you have any questions about this, check with your pharmacist.

For patients taking the *chewable tablet form of amoxicillin:*

- Tablets should be chewed or crushed before they are swallowed.

To help clear up your infection completely, *keep taking this medicine for the full time of treatment*, even if you begin to feel better after a few days. *If you have a "strep" infection, you should keep taking this medicine for at least 10 days. This is especially important in "strep" infections. Serious heart problems could develop later* if your infection is not cleared up completely. Also, if you stop taking this medicine too soon, your symptoms may return.

This medicine works best when there is a constant amount in the blood or urine. *To help keep the amount constant, do not miss any doses. Also, it is best to take the doses at evenly spaced times, day and night.* For example, if you are to take 4 doses a day, the doses should be spaced about 6 hours apart. If this interferes with your sleep or other daily activities, or if you need help in planning the best times to take your medicine, check with your health care professional.

**Dosing**—The dose of these medicines will be different for different patients. *Follow your doctor's orders or the directions on the label.* The following information includes only the average doses of these medicines. *If your dose is different, do not change it* unless your doctor tells you to do so.

The number of tablets or teaspoonfuls of suspension that you take depends on the strength of the medicine. Also, *the number of doses you take each day, the time allowed between doses, and the length of time you take the medicine depend on the medical problem for which you are taking a penicillin.*

*For amoxicillin*

- For bacterial infections:
  —For *oral* dosage forms (capsules, chewable tablets, and oral suspension):
    - Adults, teenagers, and children weighing more than 20 kilograms (kg) (44 pounds)—250 to 500 milligrams (mg) every eight hours.
    - Infants and children weighing 8 to 20 kg (17 to 44 pounds): Dose is based on body weight and must be determined by your doctor. The usual dose is 6.7 to 13.3 mg per kg (3 to 6 mg per pound) of body weight every eight hours.
    - Infants weighing 6 to 8 kg (13 to 17 pounds): 50 to 100 mg every eight hours.
    - Infants weighing up to 6 kg (13 pounds): 25 to 50 mg every eight hours.

*For ampicillin*
- For bacterial infections:
  —For *oral* dosage forms (capsules and oral suspension):
  - Adults, teenagers, and children weighing more than 20 kilograms (kg) (44 pounds)—250 to 500 milligrams (mg) every six hours.
  - Infants and children weighing up to 20 kg (44 pounds)—Dose is based on body weight and must be determined by your doctor. The usual dose is 12.5 to 25 mg per kg (5.7 to 11.4 mg per pound) of body weight every six hours; or 16.7 to 33.3 mg per kg (7.6 to 15 mg per pound) of body weight every eight hours.
  —For *injection* dosage form:
  - Adults, teenagers, and children weighing more than 20 kg (44 pounds)—250 to 500 mg, injected into a vein or muscle every three to six hours.
  - Infants and children weighing up to 20 kg (44 pounds)—Dose is based on body weight and must be determined by your doctor. The usual dose is 12.5 mg per kg (5.7 mg per pound) of body weight, injected into a vein or muscle every six hours.

*For bacampicillin*
- For bacterial infections:
  —For *oral* dosage forms (oral suspension and tablets):
  - Adults, teenagers, and children weighing more than 25 kilograms (kg) (55 pounds)—400 to 800 milligrams (mg) every twelve hours.
  - Children weighing up to 25 kg (55 pounds)—Bacampicillin tablets are not recommended for use in children weighing up to 25 kg (55 pounds). The dose of the oral suspension is based on body weight and must be determined by your doctor. The usual dose is 12.5 to 25 mg per kg (5.7 to 11.4 mg per pound) of body weight every twelve hours.

*For carbenicillin*
- For bacterial infections:
  —For *oral* dosage form (tablets):
  - Adults and teenagers—500 milligrams (mg) to 1 gram every six hours.
  - Children—Dose must be determined by your doctor.
  —For *injection* dosage form:
  - Adults and teenagers—Dose is based on body weight and must be determined by your doctor. The usual dose is 50 to 83.3 mg per kilogram (kg) (22.8 to 37.9 mg per pound) of body weight, injected into a vein or muscle every four hours.
  - Older infants and children—Dose is based on body weight and must be determined by your doctor. The usual dose 16.7 to 75 mg per kg (7.6 to 34 mg per pound) of body weight, injected into a vein or muscle every four to six hours.

*For cloxacillin*
- For bacterial infections:
  —For *oral* dosage form (capsules and oral solution):
  - Adults, teenagers, and children weighing more than 20 kilograms (kg) (44 pounds)—250 to 500 milligrams (mg) every six hours.
  - Infants and children weighing up to 20 kg (44 pounds)—Dose is based on body weight and must be determined by your doctor. The usual dose is 6.25 to 12.5 mg per kg (2.8 to 5.7 mg per pound) of body weight every six hours.
  —For *injection* dosage form:
  - Adults, teenagers, and children weighing more than 20 kg—250 to 500 mg, injected into a vein every six hours.
  - Infants and children weighing up to 20 kg (44 pounds)—Dose is based on body weight and must be determined by your doctor. The usual dose is 6.25 to 12.5 mg per kg (2.8 to 5.7 mg per pound) of body weight, injected into a vein every six hours.

*For dicloxacillin*
- For bacterial infections:
  —For *oral* dosage form (capsules and oral suspension):
  - Adults, teenagers, and children weighing more than 40 kilograms (kg) (88 pounds)—125 to 250 milligrams (mg) every six hours.
  - Infants and children weighing up to 40 kg (88 pounds)—Dose is based on body weight and must be determined by your doctor. The usual dose is 3.1 to 6.2 mg per kg (1.4 to 2.8 mg per pound) of body weight every six hours.

*For flucloxacillin*
- For bacterial infections:
  —For *oral* dosage form (capsules and oral suspension):
  - Adults, teenagers, and children more than 12 years of age and weighing more than 40 kilograms (kg) (88 pounds)—250 to 500 milligrams (mg) every six hours.
  - Children less than 12 years of age and weighing up to 40 kg (88 pounds)—125 to 250 mg every six hours; or 6.25 to 12.5 mg per kg (2.8 to 5.7 mg per pound) of body weight every six hours.
  - Infants up to 6 months of age—Dose is based on body weight and must be determined by your doctor. The usual dose is 6.25 mg per kg (2.8 mg per pound) of body weight every six hours.

*For methicillin*
- For bacterial infections:
  —For *injection* dosage form:
  - Adults, teenagers, and children weighing more than 40 kilograms (kg) (88 pounds)—1 gram injected into a muscle every four to six hours; or 1 gram injected into a vein every six hours.

• Children weighing up to 40 kg (88 pounds)—Dose is based on body weight and must be determined by your doctor. The usual dose is 25 milligrams (mg) per kg (11.4 mg per pound) of body weight, injected into a vein or muscle every six hours.

*For mezlocillin*
• For bacterial infections:
  —For *injection* dosage form:
    • Adults and teenagers—Dose is based on body weight and must be determined by your doctor. The usual dose 33.3 to 87.5 milligrams (mg) per kilogram (kg) (15.1 to 39.8 mg per pound) of body weight, injected into a vein or muscle every four to six hours; or 3 to 4 grams every four to six hours.
    • Infants over 1 month of age and children up to 12 years of age—Dose is based on body weight and must be determined by your doctor. The usual dose is 50 mg per kg (22.7 mg per pound) of body weight, injected into a vein or muscle every four hours.

*For nafcillin*
• For bacterial infections:
  —For *oral* dosage form (capsules and tablets):
    • Adults and teenagers—250 milligrams (mg) to 1 gram every four to six hours.
    • Older infants and children—Dose is based on body weight and must be determined by your doctor. The usual dose is 6.25 to 12.5 mg per kilogram (kg) (2.8 to 5.7 mg per pound) of body weight every six hours.
    • Newborns—Dose is based on body weight and must be determined by your doctor. The usual dose is 10 mg per kg (4.5 mg per pound) of body weight every six to eight hours.
  —For *injection* dosage form:
    • Adults and teenagers—500 mg to 2 grams injected into a vein or muscle every four to six hours.
    • Infants and children—Dose is based on body weight and must be determined by your doctor. The usual dose is 10 to 25 mg per kg (4.5 to 11.4 mg per pound) of body weight, injected into a muscle every twelve hours; or 10 to 40 mg per kg (4.5 to 18.2 mg per pound) of body weight, injected into a vein every four to eight hours.

*For oxacillin*
• For bacterial infections:
  —For *oral* dosage form (capsules and oral solution):
    • Adults, teenagers, and children weighing more than 40 kilograms (kg) (88 pounds)—500 milligrams (mg) to 1 gram every four to six hours.
    • Children weighing up to 40 kg (88 pounds)—Dose is based on body weight and must be determined by your doctor. The usual dose is 12.5 to 25 mg per kg (5.7 to 11.4 mg per pound) of body weight every six hours.

—For *injection* dosage form:
  • Adults, teenagers, and children weighing more than 40 kg (88 pounds)—250 mg to 1 gram injected into a vein or muscle every four to six hours.
  • Children weighing up to 40 kg (88 pounds)—Dose is based on body weight and must be determined by your doctor. The usual dose is 12.5 to 25 mg per kg (5.7 to 11.4 mg per pound) of body weight, injected into a vein or muscle every four to six hours.
  • Premature infants and newborns—Dose is based on body weight and must be determined by your doctor. The usual dose is 6.25 mg per kg (2.8 mg per pound) of body weight, injected into a vein or muscle every six hours.

*For penicillin G*
• For bacterial infections:
  —For *oral* dosage form (oral solution, oral suspension, and tablets):
    • Adults and teenagers—200,000 to 500,000 Units (125 to 312 milligrams [mg]) every four to six hours.
    • Infants and children less than 12 years of age—Dose is based on body weight and must be determined by your doctor. The usual dose is 4167 to 30,000 Units per kilogram (kg) (189 to 13,636 Units per pound) of body weight every four to eight hours.
  —For *benzathine injection* dosage form:
    • Adults and teenagers—1,200,000 to 2,400,000 Units injected into a muscle as a single dose.
    • Infants and children—300,000 to 1,200,000 Units injected into a muscle as a single dose; or 50,000 Units per kg (22,727 Units per pound) of body weight injected into a muscle as a single dose.
  —For *injection* dosage forms (potassium and sodium salts):
    • Adults and teenagers—1,000,000 to 5,000,000 Units, injected into a vein or muscle every four to six hours.
    • Older infants and children—Dose is based on body weight and must be determined by your doctor. The usual dose is 8333 to 25,000 Units per kg (3788 to 11,363 Units per pound) of body weight, injected into a vein or muscle every four to six hours.
    • Premature infants and newborns—Dose is based on body weight and must be determined by your doctor. The usual dose is 30,000 Units per kg (13,636 Units per pound) of body weight, injected into a vein or muscle every twelve hours.
  —For *procaine injection* dosage form:
    • Adults and teenagers—600,000 to 1,200,000 Units injected into a muscle once a day.
    • Children—Dose is based on body weight and must be determined by your doctor. The usual

dose is 50,000 Units per kg (22,727 Units per pound) of body weight, injected into a muscle once a day.

*For penicillin V*

- For bacterial infections:

—For the *benzathine salt oral* dosage form (oral solution):

- Adults and teenagers—200,000 to 500,000 Units every six to eight hours.
- Children—100,000 to 250,000 Units every six to eight hours.

—For the *potassium salt oral* dosage forms (oral solution, oral suspension, and tablets):

- Adults and teenagers—125 to 500 milligrams (mg) every six to eight hours.
- Children—Dose is based on body weight and must be determined by your doctor. The usual dose is 2.5 to 16.7 mg per kilogram (kg) (1.1 to 7.6 mg per pound) of body weight every four to eight hours.

*For piperacillin*

- For bacterial infections:

—For *injection* dosage form:

- Adults and teenagers—3 to 4 grams, injected into a vein or muscle every four to six hours.
- Infants and children—Dose must be determined by your doctor.

*For pivampicillin*

- For bacterial infections:

—For *oral* dosage form (oral suspension):

- Adults, teenagers, and children 10 years of age and older—525 to 1050 milligrams (mg) two times a day.
- Children 7 to 10 years of age—350 mg two times a day.
- Children 4 to 6 years of age—262.5 mg two times a day.
- Children 1 to 3 years of age—175 mg two times a day.
- Infants 3 to 12 months of age—Dose is based on body weight and must be determined by your doctor. The usual dose is 20 to 30 mg per kilogram (kg) (9.1 to 13.6 mg per pound) of body weight two times a day.

—For *oral* dosage form (tablets):

- Adults, teenagers, and children 10 years of age and older—500 mg to 1 gram two times a day.
- Children up to 10 years of age—Dose must be determined by your doctor.

*For pivmecillinam*

- For bacterial infections:

—For *oral* dosage form (tablets):

- Adults, teenagers, and children weighing more than 40 kilograms (kg) (88 pounds)—200 milligrams (mg) two to four times a day for three days.

- Children up to 40 kg (88 pounds)—Dose must be determined by your doctor.

*For ticarcillin*

- For bacterial infections:

—For *injection* dosage form:

- Adults, teenagers, and children weighing more than 40 kilograms (kg) (88 pounds)—3 grams injected into a vein every four hours; or 4 grams injected into a vein every six hours.
- Children up to 40 kg (88 pounds)—Dose is based on body weight and must be determined by your doctor. The usual dose is 33.3 to 75 milligrams (mg) per kg (15 to 34 mg per pound) of body weight, injected into a vein every four to six hours.

**Missed dose**—If you miss a dose of this medicine, take it as soon as possible. This will help to keep a constant amount of medicine in the blood or urine. However, if it is almost time for your next dose, skip the missed dose and go back to your regular dosing schedule. Do not double doses.

**Storage**—To store this medicine:

- Keep out of the reach of children.
- Store away from heat and direct light.
- Do not store the capsule or tablet form of penicillins in the bathroom, near the kitchen sink, or in other damp places. Heat or moisture may cause the medicine to break down.
- Store the oral liquid form of penicillins in the refrigerator because heat will cause this medicine to break down. However, keep the medicine from freezing. Follow the directions on the label.
- Do not keep outdated medicine or medicine no longer needed. Be sure that any discarded medicine is out of the reach of children.

## Precautions While Using This Medicine

If your symptoms do not improve within a few days, or if they become worse, check with your doctor.

Penicillins may cause diarrhea in some patients.

- *Check with your doctor if severe diarrhea occurs.* Severe diarrhea may be a sign of a serious side effect. *Do not take any diarrhea medicine without first checking with your doctor.* Diarrhea medicines may make your diarrhea worse or make it last longer.
- For mild diarrhea, diarrhea medicine containing kaolin or attapulgite (e.g., Kaopectate tablets, Diasorb) may be taken. However, other kinds of diarrhea medicine should not be taken. They may make your diarrhea worse or make it last longer.
- If you have any questions about this or if mild diarrhea continues or gets worse, check with your health care professional.

*Oral contraceptives (birth control pills) containing estrogen may not work properly if you take them while you are taking ampicillin, amoxicillin, or penicillin V.*

*Unplanned pregnancies may occur. You should use a different or additional means of birth control while you are taking any of these penicillins.* If you have any questions about this, check with your health care professional.

For *diabetic patients:*

*   *Penicillins may cause false test results with some urine sugar tests.* Check with your doctor before changing your diet or the dosage of your diabetes medicine.

Before you have any medical tests, tell the doctor in charge that you are taking this medicine. The results of some tests may be affected by this medicine.

## Side Effects of This Medicine

Along with its needed effects, a medicine may cause some unwanted effects. Although not all of these side effects may occur, if they do occur they may need medical attention.

*Stop taking this medicine and get emergency help immediately* if any of the following side effects occur:

*Less common*

Fast or irregular breathing; fever; joint pain; lightheadedness or fainting (sudden); puffiness or swelling around the face; red, scaly skin; shortness of breath; skin rash, hives, itching

In addition to the side effects mentioned above, *check with your doctor immediately* if any of the following side effects occur:

*Rare*

Abdominal or stomach cramps and pain (severe); abdominal tenderness; convulsions (seizures); decreased amount of urine; diarrhea (watery and severe), which may also be bloody; mental depression; nausea and vomiting; pain at place of injection; sore throat and fever; unusual bleeding or bruising; yellow eyes or skin

Note: Some of the above side effects (severe abdominal or stomach cramps and pain, and watery and severe diarrhea, which may also be bloody) may also occur

up to several weeks after you stop taking any of these medicines.

*Rare—For penicillin G procaine only*

Agitation or combativeness; anxiety; confusion; fear of impending death; feeling, hearing, or seeing things that are not real

Other side effects may occur that usually do not need medical attention. These side effects may go away during treatment as your body adjusts to the medicine. However, check with your doctor if any of the following side effects continue or are bothersome:

*More common*

Diarrhea (mild); headache; sore mouth or tongue; vaginal itching and discharge; white patches in the mouth and/or on the tongue

Other side effects not listed above may also occur in some patients. If you notice any other effects, check with your doctor.

## Additional Information

Once a medicine has been approved for marketing for a certain use, experience may show that it is also useful for other medical problems. Although these uses are not included in product labeling, penicillins are used in certain patients with the following medical conditions:

*   Chlamydia infections in pregnant women—Amoxicillin and ampicillin
*   Gas gangrene—Penicillin G
*   *Helicobacter pylori*-associated gastritis or peptic ulcer disease—Amoxicillin
*   Leptospirosis—Ampicillin and penicillin G
*   Lyme disease—Amoxicillin and penicillin V
*   Typhoid fever—Amoxicillin and ampicillin

Other than the above information, there is no additional information relating to proper use, precautions, or side effects for these uses.

Revised: 08/25/94

# PENICILLINS AND BETA-LACTAMASE INHIBITORS    Systemic

Some commonly used brand names are:

**In the U.S.—**

| | |
|---|---|
| Augmentin[1] | Unasyn[2] |
| Timentin[4] | Zosyn[3] |

**In Canada—**

| | |
|---|---|
| Clavulin-250[1] | Clavulin-500F[1] |
| Clavulin-125F[1] | Tazocin[3] |
| Clavulin-250F[1] | Timentin[4] |

Note: For quick reference, the following penicillins and beta-lactamase inhibitors are numbered to match the corresponding brand names.

This information applies to the following medicines:

1.  Amoxicillin and Clavulanate (a-mox-i-SILL-in and klav-yoo-LAN-ate)
2.  Ampicillin and Sulbactam (am-pi-SILL-in and sul-BAK-tam)†
3.  Piperacillin and Tazobactam (pi-PER-a-sill-in and ta-zoe-BAK-tam)
4.  Ticarcillin and Clavulanate (tye-kar-SILL-in and klav-yoo-LAN-ate)

†Not commercially available in Canada.

## Description

Penicillins and beta-lactamase inhibitors are used to treat infections caused by bacteria. They work by killing the bacteria or preventing their growth. The beta-lactamase inhibitor is added to the penicillin to protect the penicillin from certain substances (enzymes) that will destroy the penicillin before it can kill the bacteria.

There are several different kinds of penicillins. Each is used to treat different kinds of infections. One kind of penicillin usually may not be used in place of another. In addition, penicillins are used to treat bacterial infections in many different parts of the body. They are sometimes given with other antibacterial medicines. Some of the penicillins may also be used for other problems as determined by your doctor. However, none of the penicillins will work for colds, flu, or other virus infections.

Penicillins are available only with your doctor's prescription, in the following dosage forms:

*Oral*

Amoxicillin and Clavulanate
- Oral suspension (U.S. and Canada)
- Tablets (U.S. and Canada)
- Chewable tablets (U.S.)

*Parenteral*

Ampicillin and Sulbactam
- Injection (U.S.)
Piperacillin and Tazobactam
- Injection (U.S.)
Ticarcillin and Clavulanate
- Injection (U.S. and Canada)

## Before Using This Medicine

In deciding to use a medicine, the risks of taking the medicine must be weighed against the good it will do. This is a decision you and your doctor will make. For penicillins, the following should be considered:

**Allergies**—Tell your doctor if you have ever had any unusual or allergic reaction to any of the penicillins, cephalosporins, or beta-lactamase inhibitors. Also tell your health care professional if you are allergic to any other substances, such as foods, preservatives, or dyes.

**Diet**—Tell your doctor if you are on a low-sodium (low-salt) diet. Some of these medicines contain enough sodium to cause problems in some people.

**Pregnancy**—Penicillins and beta-lactamase inhibitors have not been studied in pregnant women. However, penicillins have not been shown to cause birth defects or other problems in animal studies.

**Breast-feeding**—Penicillins and sulbactam, a beta-lactamase inhibitor, pass into the breast milk. Even though only small amounts may pass into breast milk, allergic reactions, diarrhea, fungus infections, and skin rash may occur in nursing babies.

**Children**—Penicillins and beta-lactamase inhibitors have been used in children and, in effective doses, are not expected to cause different side effects or problems in children than they do in adults.

**Older adults**—Penicillins and beta-lactamase inhibitors have been used in the elderly and have not been shown to cause different side effects or problems in older people than they do in younger adults.

**Other medicines**—Although certain medicines should not be used together at all, in other cases two different medicines may be used together even if an interaction might occur. In these cases, your doctor may want to change the dose, or other precautions may be necessary. When you are taking a penicillin and beta-lactamase inhibitor combination, it is especially important that your health care professional know if you are taking any of the following:

- Anticoagulants (blood thinners) or
- Dipyridamole (e.g., Persantine) or
- Divalproex (e.g., Depakote) or
- Heparin (e.g., Panheprin) or
- Inflammation or pain medicine (except narcotics) or
- Pentoxifylline (e.g., Trental) or
- Plicamycin (e.g., Mithracin) or
- Sulfinpyrazone (e.g., Anturane) or
- Valproic acid (e.g., Depakene)—Use of these medicines with piperacillin and tazobactam combination or with ticarcillin and clavulanate combination may increase the chance of bleeding
- Probenecid (e.g., Benemid)—Probenecid causes penicillins, sulbactam, and tazobactam to build up in the blood. This may increase the chance of side effects. However, your doctor may want to give you probenecid with a penicillin and beta-lactamase inhibitor combination to treat some infections

**Other medical problems**—The presence of other medical problems may affect the use of penicillin and beta-lactamase inhibitor combinations. Make sure you tell your doctor if you have any other medical problems, especially:

- Allergies or a history of allergies, such as asthma, eczema, hay fever, or hives—Patients with a history of allergies may be more likely to have a severe allergic reaction to a penicillin and beta-lactamase inhibitor combination
- Bleeding problems, history of—Patients with a history of bleeding problems may be more likely to have bleeding when receiving piperacillin and tazobactam combination or ticarcillin and clavulanate combination
- Congestive heart failure (CHF) or
- High blood pressure—Large doses of ticarcillin and clavulanate combination may make these conditions worse, because this medicine contains a large amount of salt
- Cystic fibrosis—Patients with cystic fibrosis may have an increased chance of fever and skin rash when receiving piperacillin and tazobactam combination
- Kidney disease—Patients with kidney disease may have an increased chance of side effects
- Mononucleosis ("mono")—Patients with mononucleosis may have an increased chance of skin rash when receiving ampicillin and sulbactam combination
- Stomach or intestinal disease, history of (especially colitis, including colitis caused by antibiotics)—Patients with a history of stomach or intestinal disease may be more likely to develop colitis while taking penicillins and beta-lactamase inhibitors

## Proper Use of This Medicine

Amoxicillin and clavulanate combination may be taken on a full or empty stomach. Taking amoxicillin and clavulanate combination with food may decrease the chance of diarrhea, nausea, and vomiting.

For patients taking the *oral liquid form of amoxicillin and clavulanate combination:*

- Use a specially marked measuring spoon or other device to measure each dose accurately. The average household teaspoon may not hold the right amount of liquid.
- Do not use after the expiration date on the label. The medicine may not work properly after that date. If you have any questions about this, check with your pharmacist.

For patients taking the *chewable tablet form of amoxicillin and clavulanate combination:*

- Tablets should be chewed or crushed before they are swallowed.

To help clear up your infection completely, *keep taking this medicine for the full time of treatment*, even if you begin to feel better after a few days.

This medicine works best when there is a constant amount in the blood or urine. *To help keep the amount constant, do not miss any doses. Also, it is best to take the doses at evenly spaced times, day and night.* For example, if you are to take 4 doses a day, the doses should be spaced about 6 hours apart. If this interferes with your sleep or other daily activities, or if you need help in planning the best times to take your medicine, check with your health care professional.

**Dosing**—The dose of these medicines will be different for different patients. *Follow your doctor's orders or the directions on the label.* The following information includes only the average doses of these medicines. *If your dose is different, do not change it* unless your doctor tells you to do so.

The number of tablets or teaspoonfuls of suspension that you take depends on the strength of the medicine. Also, *the number of doses you take each day, the time allowed between doses, and the length of time you take the medicine depend on the medical problem for which you are taking a penicillin and beta-lactamase inhibitor combination.*

*For amoxicillin and clavulanate combination*

- For bacterial infections:
  —For *oral* dosage forms (chewable tablets and suspension):
  - Adults, teenagers, and children weighing more than 40 kilograms (kg) (88 pounds)—250 to 500 milligrams (mg) of amoxicillin, in combination with 62.5 to 125 mg of clavulanate, every eight hours for seven to ten days.
  - Infants and children weighing up to 40 kg (88 pounds)—6.7 to 13.3 mg of amoxicillin per kg (3 to 6 mg per pound) of body weight, in combination with 1.7 to 3.3 mg of clavulanate per kg (0.8 to 1.5 mg per pound) of body weight, every eight hours for seven to ten days.

—For *oral* dosage form (tablets):
- Adults, teenagers, and children weighing more than 40 kg (88 pounds)—250 to 500 mg of amoxicillin, in combination with 125 mg of clavulanate, every eight hours for seven to ten days.
- Infants and children weighing up to 40 kg (88 pounds)—6.7 to 13.3 mg of amoxicillin per kg (3 to 6 mg per pound) of body weight, in combination with 1.7 to 3.3 mg of clavulanate per kg (0.8 to 1.5 mg per pound) of body weight, every eight hours for seven to ten days.

*For ampicillin and sulbactam combination*

- For bacterial infections:
  —For *injection* dosage form:
  - Adults and teenagers—1 to 2 grams of ampicillin, in combination with 500 milligrams (mg) to 1 gram of sulbactam, injected into a vein or a muscle every six hours.
  - Children up to 12 years of age—Use and dose must be determined by your doctor.

*For piperacillin and tazobactam combination*

- For bacterial infections:
  —For *injection* dosage form:
  - Adults and teenagers—3 to 4 grams of piperacillin, in combination with 0.375 to 0.5 grams of tazobactam, injected into a vein every six to eight hours for seven to ten days.
  - Children up to 12 years of age—Use and dose must be determined by your doctor.

*For ticarcillin and clavulanate combination*

- For bacterial infections:
  —For *injection* dosage form:
  - Adults and teenagers weighing 60 kilograms (kg) (132 pounds) or more—3 grams of ticarcillin, in combination with 100 milligrams (mg) of clavulanate, injected into a vein every four to six hours.
  - Adults and teenagers weighing less than 60 kg (132 pounds)—33.3 to 75 mg of ticarcillin per kg (15 to 34.1 mg per pound) of body weight, in combination with 1.1 to 2.5 mg of clavulanate per kg (0.5 to 1.1 mg per pound) of body weight, injected into a vein every four to six hours.
  - Infants and children 1 month to 12 years of age—50 mg of ticarcillin per kg (22.7 mg per pound) of body weight, in combination with 1.7 mg of clavulanate per kg (0.8 mg per pound) of body weight, injected into a vein every four to six hours.

**Missed dose**—If you miss a dose of this medicine, take it as soon as possible. This will help to keep a constant amount of medicine in the blood or urine. However, if it is almost time for your next dose, skip the missed dose and go back to your regular dosing schedule. Do not double doses.

**Storage**—To store this medicine:

- Keep out of the reach of children.
- Store away from heat and direct light.
- Do not store capsules or tablets in the bathroom, near the kitchen sink, or in other damp places. Heat or moisture may cause the medicine to break down.
- Store the oral liquid form of penicillins in the refrigerator because heat will cause this medicine to break down. However, keep the medicine from freezing. Follow the directions on the label.
- Do not keep outdated medicine or medicine no longer needed. Be sure that any discarded medicine is out of the reach of children.

## Precautions While Using This Medicine

If your symptoms do not improve within a few days, or if they become worse, check with your doctor.

Penicillins may cause diarrhea in some patients.

- *Check with your doctor if severe diarrhea occurs.* Severe diarrhea may be a sign of a serious side effect. *Do not take any diarrhea medicine.* Diarrhea medicines may make your diarrhea worse or make it last longer.
- For mild diarrhea, diarrhea medicine containing kaolin or attapulgite (e.g., Kaopectate tablets, Diasorb) may be taken. However, other kinds of diarrhea medicine should not be taken. They may make your diarrhea worse or make it last longer.
- If you have any questions about this or if mild diarrhea continues or gets worse, check with your health care professional.

For *diabetic patients:*

- *Penicillin and beta-lactamase inhibitor combinations may cause false test results with some urine sugar tests.* Check with your doctor before changing your diet or the dosage of your diabetes medicine.

Before you have any medical tests, tell the doctor in charge that you are taking this medicine. The results of some tests may be affected by this medicine.

## Side Effects of This Medicine

Along with its needed effects, a medicine may cause some unwanted effects. Although not all of these side effects may occur, if they do occur they may need medical attention.

*Stop taking this medicine and get emergency help immediately* if any of the following side effects occur:

*Less common*

Fast or irregular breathing; fever; joint pain; lightheadedness or fainting (sudden); puffiness or swelling around the face; shortness of breath; skin rash, hives, itching

In addition to the side effects mentioned above, *check with your doctor immediately* if any of the following side effects occur:

*Rare*

Abdominal or stomach cramps and pain (severe); convulsions (seizures); diarrhea (watery and severe), which may also be bloody; pain at place of injection; sore throat and fever; unusual bleeding or bruising

Note: Some of the above side effects (severe abdominal or stomach cramps and pain, and watery and severe diarrhea, which may also be bloody) may also occur up to several weeks after you stop taking any of these medicines.

Other side effects may occur that usually do not need medical attention. These side effects may go away during treatment as your body adjusts to the medicine. However, check with your doctor if any of the following side effects continue or are bothersome:

*More common*

Diarrhea (mild); headache; nausea or vomiting; sore mouth or tongue; stomach pain; vaginal itching and discharge; white patches in the mouth and/or on the tongue

Other side effects not listed above may also occur in some patients. If you notice any other effects, check with your doctor.

Developed: 07/29/94

---

# PENTAGASTRIN Diagnostic

A commonly used brand name in the U.S. and Canada is Peptavlon.

## Description

Pentagastrin (pen-ta-GAS-trin) is a testing agent used to help diagnose problems or disease of the stomach. This test determines how much acid your stomach produces.

How the test is done: The dose of pentagastrin is based on body weight and must be determined by your doctor. The pentagastrin is injected beneath the skin. Ten or 15 minutes later, the contents of the stomach are emptied and tested for the amount of the contents and the amount of acid in the contents. The procedure may be repeated several times.

Pentagastrin is used only under the supervision of a doctor. It is available in the following dosage form:

*Parenteral*

- Injection (U.S. and Canada)

## Before Having This Test

In deciding to use a diagnostic test, any risks of the test must be weighed against the good it will do. This is a decision you and your doctor will make. Also, test results may be affected by other things. For pentagastrin, the following should be considered:

**Allergies**—Tell your doctor if you have ever had any unusual or allergic reaction to pentagastrin. Also tell your health care professional if you are allergic to any other substances, such as foods, preservatives, or dyes.

**Pregnancy**—Studies on effects in pregnancy have not been done in either humans or animals.

**Breast-feeding**—It is not known whether pentagastrin passes into the breast milk. Although most medicines pass into breast milk in small amounts, many of them may be used safely while breast-feeding. Mothers who are receiving this diagnostic test and wish to breast-feed should discuss this with their doctor.

**Children**—Studies on this medicine have been done only in adult patients, and there is no specific information comparing use of pentagastrin in children with use in other age groups.

**Older adults**—Many medicines have not been studied specifically in older people. Therefore, it may not be known whether they work exactly the same way they do in younger adults or if they cause different side effects or problems in older people. There is no specific information comparing use of pentagastrin in the elderly with use in other age groups.

**Other medicines**—Although certain medicines should not be used together at all, in other cases two different medicines may be used together even if an interaction might occur. In these cases, your doctor may want to change the dose, or other precautions may be necessary. When you will be given pentagastrin, it is especially important that your health care professional know if you are taking any of the following:

- Antacids or
- Anticholinergics (medicine for abdominal or stomach spasms or cramps) or
- Cimetidine (e.g., Tagamet) or
- Famotidine (e.g., Pepcid) or
- Nizatidine (e.g., Axid) or
- Omeprazole (e.g., Prilosec) or
- Ranitidine (e.g., Zantac)—These medicines decrease the effect that pentagastrin has on the production of stomach acid, and the test may not work

**Other medical problems**—The presence of other medical problems may affect the use of pentagastrin. Make sure you tell your doctor if you have any other medical problems, especially:

- Gallbladder problems or
- Liver disease or
- Pancreatitis (inflammation of the pancreas) (severe) or
- Stomach ulcer (severe or bleeding)—Pentagastrin may make these conditions worse

## Preparation For This Test

Unless otherwise directed by your doctor:

- Do not eat anything beginning the night before and do not drink anything for at least four hours before the test. Having food or liquid in the stomach may affect the interpretation of the test results.
- Do not take antacids on the morning of the test. To do so may decrease the effect of pentagastrin and affect the test results.
- For 24 hours before the test, do not take any anticholinergics (medicine for abdominal or stomach spasms or cramps), cimetidine, famotidine, nizatidine, ranitidine, or any other medicine that decreases stomach acid. Do not take omeprazole for 96 hours (4 days) before the test.

## Side Effects of This Medicine

Along with its needed effects, pentagastrin may cause some unwanted effects. Although the side effects usually are rare, when they do occur they may require medical attention.

*Check with your health care professional immediately* if either of the following side effects occurs:

*Rare*

Skin rash or hives

Other side effects may occur that usually do not need medical attention. These side effects should go away as the effects of the medicine wear off. However, check with your doctor if any of the following side effects continue or are bothersome:

*More common (usually disappear within 15 minutes after injection)*

Gas; nausea or vomiting; stomach pain; urge to have bowel movement

*Less common or rare*

Blurred vision; chills; dizziness, faintness, or lightheadedness; drowsiness; fast heartbeat; feeling of heaviness of arms and legs; headache; increased sweating; numbness, tingling, pain, or weakness in hands or feet; shortness of breath; unusual tiredness; unusual warmth or flushing of skin

Other side effects not listed above may also occur in some patients. If you notice any other effects, check with your doctor.

Revised: 07/14/93
Interim revision: 07/01/94

# PENTAMIDINE    Inhalation

Some commonly used brand names are:

**In the U.S.—**
NebuPent

**In Canada—**
Pentacarinat
Pneumopent

## Description

Pentamidine (pen-TAM-i-deen) is used to try to prevent *Pneumocystis* (noo-moe-SISS-tis) *carinii* pneumonia (PCP), a very serious type of pneumonia. This type of pneumonia occurs commonly in patients whose immune systems are not working normally, such as patients with acquired immune deficiency syndrome (AIDS). Inhaled pentamidine does not prevent illness in parts of the body outside the lungs. This medicine may also be used for other conditions as determined by your doctor.

Pentamidine is available only with your doctor's prescription, in the following dosage form:

*Inhalation*
- Inhalation solution (U.S. and Canada)

## Before Using This Medicine

In deciding to use a medicine, the risks of taking the medicine must be weighed against the good it will do. This is a decision you and your doctor will make. For pentamidine inhalation, the following should be considered:

**Allergies**—Tell your doctor if you have ever had any unusual or allergic reaction to pentamidine inhalation. Also tell your health care professional if you are allergic to any other substances, such as foods, preservatives, or dyes.

**Pregnancy**—Studies on birth defects have not been done in humans. However, studies in rabbits, given doses by injection much larger than humans would absorb into their bloodstream through the lungs, have shown an increase in miscarriages and bone defects in the fetus.

**Breast-feeding**—It is not known whether pentamidine passes into breast milk. However, pentamidine has not been reported to cause problems in nursing babies.

**Children**—Studies on this medicine have been done only in adult patients, and there is no specific information comparing use of pentamidine inhalation in children with use in other age groups. However, pentamidine inhalation is recommended in children 5 years of age and older who cannot tolerate other medicines.

**Older adults**—Many medicines have not been studied specifically in older people. Therefore, it may not be known whether they work exactly the same way they do in younger adults or if they cause different side effects or problems in older people. There is no specific information comparing use of pentamidine inhalation in the elderly with use in other age groups.

**Other medicines**—Although certain medicines should not be used together at all, in other cases two different medicines may be used together even if an interaction might occur. In these cases, your doctor may want to change the dose, or other precautions may be necessary. Tell your health care professional if you are taking any other prescription or nonprescription (over-the-counter [OTC]) medicine.

**Other medical problems**—The presence of other medical problems may affect the use of pentamidine inhalation. Make sure you tell your doctor if you have any other medical problems, especially:

- Asthma—Patients with asthma may have an increase in coughing or difficulty in breathing while receiving pentamidine inhalation

## Proper Use of This Medicine

To help prevent the development or return of pneumocystis pneumonia, you must receive pentamidine inhalation on a regular basis, even if you are feeling well.

**Dosing**—The dose of pentamidine inhalation will be different for different patients. *Follow your doctor's orders or the directions on the label.* The following information includes only the average doses of pentamidine inhalation. *If your dose is different, do not change it* unless your doctor tells you to do so.

- For the *inhalation* dosage form:
  —For the prevention of *Pneumocystis carinii* pneumonia (PCP):
  - Adults and children 5 years of age and older— 300 milligrams (mg) by oral inhalation once every four weeks.
  - Children younger than 5 years of age—Use and dose must be determined by your doctor.

**Missed dose**—If you miss a dose of this medicine, receive your treatment as soon as possible.

## Precautions While Using This Medicine

If you are also using the inhalation form of a bronchodilator (medicine used to help relieve breathing problems), use the pentamidine inhalation at least 5 to 10 minutes after the bronchodilator, unless otherwise directed by your doctor. This will help to reduce the possibility of side effects. Do not use the bronchodilator or any medicine other than pentamidine in the nebulizer.

A bitter or metallic taste may occur during use of this medicine. Sucking on a hard candy after each treatment can help reduce this problem.

Cigarette smoking can increase the chance of coughing and difficulty in breathing during pentamidine inhalation therapy.

## Side Effects of This Medicine

On rare occasions, pneumocystis infections have occurred in parts of the body outside the lungs in patients receiving pentamidine inhalation therapy. You should discuss this possible problem with your doctor.

Along with its needed effects, a medicine may cause some unwanted effects. Although not all of these side effects may occur, if they do occur they may need medical attention.

*Check with your health care professional immediately* if any of the following side effects occur:

*More common*
> Burning pain, dryness, or sensation of lump in throat; chest pain or congestion; coughing; difficulty in breathing; difficulty in swallowing; skin rash; wheezing

*Rare*
> Nausea and vomiting; pain in upper abdomen, possibly radiating to the back; pain in side of chest (severe); shortness of breath (sudden and severe)

*Rare—with daily treatment doses only*
> Anxiety; chills; cold sweats; cool, pale skin; decreased urination; headache; increased hunger; loss of appetite; nausea and vomiting; nervousness; shakiness; stomach pain; unusual tiredness

Other side effects not listed above may also occur in some patients. If you notice any other effects, check with your doctor.

---

Revised: 03/03/92
Interim revision: 03/28/94

---

# PENTAMIDINE   Systemic

Some commonly used brand names are:

**In the U.S.—**
Pentam 300

**In Canada—**
Pentacarinat

Generic name product may also be available.

## Description

Pentamidine (pen-TAM-i-deen) is used to treat *Pneumocystis* (noo-moe-SISS-tis) *carinii* pneumonia (PCP), a very serious kind of pneumonia. This kind of pneumonia occurs commonly in patients whose immune system is not working normally, such as cancer patients, transplant patients, and patients with acquired immune deficiency syndrome (AIDS). In addition, your doctor may prescribe pentamidine for some other medical problems caused by protozoa. This medicine may also be used for other conditions as determined by your doctor.

Pentamidine may cause some serious side effects. Before you begin treatment with pentamidine, you and your doctor should talk about the good this medicine will do as well as the risks of using it.

Pentamidine is to be administered only by or under the immediate supervision of your doctor. It is available in the following dosage form:

*Parenteral*
• Injection (U.S. and Canada)

## Before Receiving This Medicine

In deciding to use a medicine, the risks of taking the medicine must be weighed against the good it will do. This is a decision you and your doctor will make. For pentamidine, the following should be considered:

**Allergies**—Tell your doctor if you have ever had any unusual or allergic reaction to pentamidine. Also tell your health care professional if you are allergic to any other substances, such as foods, preservatives, or dyes.

**Diet**—Make certain your health care professional knows if you are on a low-sodium, low-sugar, or any other special diet. Since most medicines contain more than their active ingredient, some products may have to be avoided.

**Pregnancy**—Pentamidine has not been studied in pregnant women. However, studies in rabbits have shown an increase in miscarriages and bone defects in the fetus.

**Breast-feeding**—It is not known whether pentamidine passes into breast milk. However, because of the risk of side effects in the newborn, breast-feeding is not recommended during treatment with this medicine.

**Children**—Although pentamidine has not been widely used in children, this medicine is not expected to cause different side effects or problems in children than it does in adults.

**Older adults**—Many medicines have not been studied specifically in older people. Therefore, it may not be known whether they work exactly the same way they do in younger adults or if they cause different side effects or problems in older people. There is no specific information comparing use of pentamidine in the elderly with use in other age groups.

**Other medicines**—Although certain medicines should not be used together at all, in other cases two different medicines may be used together even if an interaction might occur. In these cases, your doctor may want to change the dose, or other precautions may be necessary. When

you are receiving pentamidine, it is especially important that your health care professional know if you are taking any of the following:

- Amphotericin B by injection (e.g., Fungizone) or
- Antithyroid agents (medicine for overactive thyroid) or
- Azathioprine (e.g., Imuran) or
- Chloramphenicol (e.g., Chloromycetin) or
- Colchicine or
- Cyclophosphamide (e.g., Cytoxan) or
- Flucytosine (e.g., Ancobon) or
- Ganciclovir (e.g., Cytovene) or
- Interferon (e.g., Intron A, Roferon-A) or
- Mercaptopurine (e.g., Purinethol) or
- X-ray treatment or
- Zidovudine (e.g., AZT, Retrovir) or
- If you have ever been treated with x-rays or cancer medicine—When taken with pentamidine, these medicines may increase the chance of damage to your blood cells
- Carmustine (e.g., BiCNU) or
- Cisplatin (e.g., Platinol) or
- Combination pain medicine containing acetaminophen and aspirin (e.g., Excedrin) or other salicylates (with large amounts taken regularly) or
- Cyclosporine (e.g., Sandimmune) or
- Deferoxamine (e.g., Desferal) (with long-term use) or
- Foscarnet (e.g., Foscavir) or
- Gold salts (medicine for arthritis) or
- Inflammation or pain medicine (except narcotics) or
- Lithium (e.g., Lithane) or
- Other anti-infectives by mouth or by injection (medicine for infection) or
- Penicillamine (e.g., Cuprimine) or
- Streptozocin (e.g., Zanosar) or
- Tiopronin (e.g., Thiola)—When taken with pentamidine, these medicines may increase the chance of kidney damage
- Didanosine (e.g., ddI, Videx)—When taken with pentamidine, didanosine may increase the chance of pancreatitis (inflammation of the pancreas)
- Methotrexate (e.g., Mexate) or
- Plicamycin (e.g., Mithracin)—When taken with pentamidine, these medicines may increase the chance of damage to your blood cells and your kidneys

**Other medical problems**—The presence of other medical problems may affect the use of pentamidine. Make sure you tell your doctor if you have any other medical problems, especially:

- Anemia or
- Bleeding disorders (history of) or
- Heart disease or
- Hypotension (low blood pressure) or
- Kidney disease or
- Liver disease—Pentamidine may make these conditions worse
- Diabetes mellitus (sugar diabetes) or
- Hypoglycemia (low blood sugar)—Pentamidine may increase or decrease blood sugar levels and may disturb control of sugar diabetes

## Proper Use of This Medicine

To help clear up your infection completely, *pentamidine must be given for the full time of treatment,* even if you begin to feel better after a few days. Also, this medicine works best when there is a constant amount in the blood.

To help keep the amount constant, pentamidine must be given on a regular schedule.

**Dosing**—The dose of pentamidine will be different for different patients. *Follow your doctor's orders or the directions on the label.* The following information includes only the average doses of pentamidine. *If your dose is different, do not change it* unless your doctor tells you to do so.

- For *injection* dosage form:
  —For *Pneumocystis carinii* pneumonia (PCP):
    - Adults and children—Dose is based on body weight and must be determined by your doctor. The usual dose is 4 milligrams (mg) per kilogram (kg) (1.8 mg per pound) of body weight given once a day for fourteen to twenty-one days. This dose is injected slowly into a vein over a one- to two-hour period of time.

## Precautions While Using This Medicine

*Some patients may develop sudden, severe low blood pressure after a dose of pentamidine. Therefore, you should be lying down while you are receiving this medicine.* Also, your doctor may want to check your blood pressure while you are receiving a pentamidine injection and several times after the dose has been given until your blood pressure is stable.

Pentamidine can lower the number of white blood cells in your blood, increasing the chance of your getting certain infections. It can also lower the number of platelets, which are necessary for proper blood clotting. If these problems occur, there are certain precautions you can take to reduce the risk of infection or bleeding:

- *Check with your doctor immediately* if you think you are getting a cold or any other infection.
- *Check with your doctor immediately* if you notice any unusual bleeding or bruising.
- Be careful when using regular toothbrushes, dental floss, or toothpicks. Your medical doctor, dentist, or nurse may recommend other ways to clean your teeth and gums. Check with your health care professional before having any dental work done.
- Avoid using a safety razor. Use an electric shaver instead. Also, be careful when using fingernail or toenail cutters.

## Side Effects of This Medicine

Pentamidine may cause some serious side effects, including heart problems, low blood pressure, low or high blood sugar, and other blood problems. *You and your doctor should discuss the good this medicine will do as well as the risks of receiving it.*

Along with its needed effects, a medicine may cause some unwanted effects. Although not all of these side effects may occur, if they do occur they may need medical attention.

*Check with your health care professional immediately* if any of the following side effects occur:

*More common*

Decrease in urination; sore throat and fever; unusual bleeding or bruising

*Signs of diabetes mellitus or high blood sugar*

Drowsiness; flushed, dry skin; fruit-like breath odor; increased thirst; increased urination; loss of appetite

*Signs of low blood sugar*

Anxiety; chills; cold sweats; cool, pale skin; headache; increased hunger; nausea; nervousness; shakiness

*Signs of low blood pressure*

Blurred vision; confusion; dizziness; fainting or light-headedness; unusual tiredness or weakness

Note: *Signs of diabetes mellitus or high blood sugar, or signs of low blood sugar* may also occur up to several months after you stop receiving this medicine.

*Less common*

Fast or irregular pulse; fever; nausea and vomiting; pain in upper abdomen; pain, redness, and/or hardness at place of injection; skin rash, redness, or itching

Other side effects may occur that usually do not need medical attention. These side effects may go away during treatment as your body adjusts to the medicine. However, check with your doctor if any of the following side effects continue or are bothersome:

*More common*

Diarrhea; loss of appetite; nausea and vomiting

Stomach problems, such as nausea and vomiting, or loss of appetite, are common minor side effects seen in pentamidine treatment. However, if you have these problems, and at the same time have sharp pain in the upper abdomen, or an unusual decrease in the amount of urine, check with your doctor immediately.

Pentamidine may also cause an unpleasant metallic taste. This side effect is to be expected and does not require medical attention.

Other side effects not listed above may also occur in some patients. If you notice any other effects, check with your doctor.

---

## Additional Information

Once a medicine has been approved for marketing for a certain use, experience may show that it is also useful for other medical problems. Although these uses are not included in product labeling, pentamidine is used in certain patients with the following medical conditions:

- Leishmaniasis, cutaneous
- Leishmaniasis, visceral (kala-azar)
- Trypanosomiasis, African (African sleeping sickness)

If you are living in or will be traveling to an area where there is a chance of getting kala-azar or African sleeping sickness, the following measures will help to prevent reinfection with either disease:

- If possible, sleep under fine-mesh netting to avoid being bitten by sandflies (which carry kala-azar) or tsetse flies (which carry African sleeping sickness).
- Wear long-sleeved shirts or blouses and long trousers to protect your arms and legs, especially at dusk or during evening hours when sandflies are out. Since tsetse flies can bite through thin clothing, it is best to wear clothing made from fairly heavy material to protect arms and legs.
- Apply insect repellant to uncovered areas of the skin when sandflies or tsetse flies are out.

Other than the above information, there is no additional information relating to proper use, precautions, or side effects for these uses.

---

Revised: 05/27/94

---

# PENTOSTATIN    Systemic

A commonly used brand name in the U.S. and Canada is Nipent. Other commonly used names are 2'-deoxycoformycin and 2'DCF.

---

## Description

Pentostatin (PEN-toe-stat-in) belongs to the group of medicines called antimetabolites. It is used to treat hairy cell leukemia.

Pentostatin interferes with the growth of cancer cells, which are eventually destroyed. Since the growth of normal body cells may also be affected by pentostatin, other effects will also occur. Some of these may be serious and must be reported to your doctor. Other effects may not be serious but may cause concern. Some effects may not occur for months or years after the medicine is used.

Before you begin treatment with pentostatin, you and your doctor should talk about the good this medicine will do as well as the risks of using it.

Pentostatin is to be administered only by or under the immediate supervision of your doctor. It is available in the following dosage form:

*Parenteral*

- Injection (U.S. and Canada)

## Before Using This Medicine

In deciding to use a medicine, the risks of taking the medicine must be weighed against the good it will do. This is a decision you and your doctor will make. For pentostatin, the following should be considered:

**Allergies**—Tell your doctor if you have ever had any unusual or allergic reaction to pentostatin.

**Pregnancy**—There is a chance that this medicine may cause birth defects if either the male or female is taking it at the time of conception or if it is taken during pregnancy. Pentostatin has been shown to cause birth defects in rats and mice. In addition, many cancer medicines may cause sterility which could be permanent. Although sterility has not been reported with this medicine, it does occur in animals and the possibility should be kept in mind.

Be sure that you have discussed this with your doctor before taking this medicine. It is best to use some kind of birth control while you are receiving pentostatin. Tell your doctor right away if you think you have become pregnant while receiving pentostatin.

**Breast-feeding**—It is not known whether pentostatin passes into breast milk. However, because this medicine may cause serious side effects, breast-feeding is generally not recommended while you are receiving it.

**Children**—There is no specific information comparing use of pentostatin in children with use in other age groups.

**Older adults**—Many medicines have not been studied specifically in older people. Therefore, it may not be known whether they work exactly the same way they do in younger adults. Although there is no specific information comparing use of pentostatin in the elderly with use in other adults, this medicine is not expected to cause different side effects or problems in older people than it does in younger adults.

**Other medicines**—Although certain medicines should not be used together at all, in other cases two different medicines may be used together even if an interaction might occur. In these cases, your doctor may want to change the dose, or other precautions may be necessary. When you are receiving pentostatin, it is especially important that your health care professional know if you are taking any of the following:
- Amphotericin B by injection (e.g., Fungizone) or
- Antithyroid agents (medicine for overactive thyroid) or
- Azathioprine (e.g., Imuran) or
- Chloramphenicol (e.g., Chloromycetin) or
- Colchicine or
- Flucytosine (e.g., Ancobon) or
- Ganciclovir (e.g., Cytovene) or
- Interferon (e.g., Intron A, Roferon-A) or
- Plicamycin (e.g., Mithracin) or
- Zidovudine (e.g., AZT, Retrovir) or
- If you have ever been treated with x-rays or cancer medicines—Pentostatin may increase the effects of these medicines or radiation therapy on the blood

- Probenecid (e.g., Benemid) or
- Sulfinpyrazone (e.g., Anturane)—Pentostatin may raise the amount of uric acid in the blood. Since these medicines are used to lower uric acid levels, they may not be as effective in patients receiving pentostatin

**Other medical problems**—The presence of other medical problems may affect the use of pentostatin. Make sure you tell your doctor if you have any other medical problems, especially:
- Chickenpox (including recent exposure) or
- Herpes zoster (shingles)—Risk of severe disease affecting other parts of the body
- Gout (history of) or
- Kidney stones (history of)—Pentostatin may increase levels of uric acid in the body, which can cause gout or kidney stones
- Infection—Pentostatin may decrease your body's ability to fight infection
- Kidney disease—Effects of pentostatin may be increased because of slower removal from the body

## Proper Use of This Medicine

This medicine often causes nausea and vomiting. However, it is very important that you continue to receive the medicine even if you begin to feel ill. Ask your health care professional for ways to lessen these effects.

**Dosing**—The dose of pentostatin will be different for different patients. The dose that is used may depend on a number of things, including what the medicine is being used for, the patient's size, and whether or not other medicines are also being taken. *If you are receiving pentostatin at home, follow your doctor's orders or the directions on the label.* If you have any questions about the proper dose of pentostatin, ask your doctor.

## Precautions While Using This Medicine

*It is very important that your doctor check your progress at regular visits* to make sure that this medicine is working properly and to check for unwanted effects.

While you are being treated with pentostatin, and after you stop treatment with it, *do not have any immunizations (vaccinations) without your doctor's approval.* Pentostatin may lower your body's resistance and there is a chance you might get the infection the immunization is meant to prevent. In addition, other persons living in your household should not take oral polio vaccine since there is a chance they could pass the polio virus on to you. Also, avoid persons who have taken oral polio vaccine. Do not get close to them and do not stay in the same room with them for very long. If you cannot take these precautions, you should consider wearing a protective face mask that covers the nose and mouth.

Pentostatin can lower the number of white blood cells in your blood temporarily, increasing the chance of getting an infection. It can also lower the number of platelets, which are necessary for proper blood clotting. If this occurs, there are certain precautions you can take, especially when your blood count is low, to reduce the risk of infection or bleeding:

- If you can, avoid people with infections. *Check with your doctor immediately* if you think you are getting an infection or if you get a fever or chills, cough or hoarseness, lower back or side pain, or painful or difficult urination.
- *Check with your doctor immediately* if you notice any unusual bleeding or bruising; black, tarry stools; blood in urine or stools; or pinpoint red spots on your skin.
- Be careful when using a regular toothbrush, dental floss, or toothpick. Your medical doctor, dentist, or nurse may recommend other ways to clean your teeth and gums. Check with your medical doctor before having any dental work done.
- Do not touch your eyes or the inside of your nose unless you have just washed your hands and have not touched anything else in the meantime.
- Be careful not to cut yourself when you are using sharp objects such as a safety razor or fingernail or toenail cutters.
- Avoid contact sports or other situations where bruising or injury could occur.

## Side Effects of This Medicine

Along with its needed effects, a medicine may cause some unwanted effects. Some side effects will have signs or symptoms that you can see or feel. Your doctor may watch for others by doing certain tests.

Also, because of the way these medicines act on the body, there is a chance that they might cause other unwanted effects that may not occur until months or years after the medicine is used. These delayed effects may include certain types of cancer. Discuss these possible effects with your doctor.

*Check with your doctor or nurse immediately* if any of the following side effects occur:

*More common*

Cough or hoarseness; fever or chills; lower back or side pain; painful or difficult urination

*Less common*

Black, tarry stools; blood in urine or stools; chest pain; pinpoint red spots on skin; unusual bleeding or bruising

Check with your health care professional as soon as possible if any of the following side effects occur:

*More common*

Pain; skin rash or itching (sudden); unusual tiredness

*Less common*

Anxiety or nervousness; changes in vision; confusion; cramps in lower legs; mental depression; nosebleed; numbness or tingling of hands or feet; shortness of breath; sleepiness; sore, red eyes; sores in mouth or on lips; stomach pain; swelling of feet or lower legs; trouble in sleeping

This medicine may also cause the following side effects that your doctor will watch for:

*More common*

Anemia; liver problems; low platelet counts

*Less common*

Kidney problems

Other side effects may occur that usually do not need medical attention. These side effects may go away during treatment as your body adjusts to the medicine. Also, your health care professional may be able to tell you about ways to prevent or reduce some of these side effects. Check with your health care professional if any of the following side effects continue or are bothersome or if you have any questions about them:

*More common*

Diarrhea; headache; loss of appetite; muscle pain; nausea and vomiting; skin rash

*Less common*

Back pain; bloating or gas; constipation; dry skin; general feeling of discomfort or illness; itching; joint pain; weakness; weight loss

Other side effects not listed above may also occur in some patients. If you notice any other effects, check with your doctor.

Revised: 05/06/93
Interim revision: 06/30/94

# PENTOXIFYLLINE   Systemic

A commonly used brand name in the U.S. and Canada is Trental. Another commonly used name is oxypentifylline.

## Description

Pentoxifylline (pen-tox-IF-i-lin) improves the flow of blood through blood vessels. It is used to reduce leg pain caused by poor blood circulation. Pentoxifylline makes it possible to walk farther before having to rest because of leg cramps.

Pentoxifylline is available only with your doctor's prescription, in the following dosage form:

*Oral*

- Extended-release tablets (U.S. and Canada)

## Before Using This Medicine

In deciding to use a medicine, the risks of taking the medicine must be weighed against the good it will do.

This is a decision you and your doctor will make. For pentoxifylline, the following should be considered:

**Allergies**—Tell your doctor if you have ever had any unusual or allergic reaction to pentoxifylline or to other xanthines such as aminophylline, caffeine, dyphylline, ethylenediamine (contained in aminophylline), oxtriphylline, theobromine, or theophylline. Also tell your health care professional if you are allergic to any other substances, such as foods, preservatives, or dyes.

**Pregnancy**—Pentoxifylline has not been studied in pregnant women. Studies in animals have not shown that it causes birth defects. However, at very high doses it has caused other harmful effects. Before taking this medicine, make sure your doctor knows if you are pregnant or if you may become pregnant.

**Breast-feeding**—Pentoxifylline passes into breast milk. The medicine has not been reported to cause problems in nursing babies. However, pentoxifylline has caused noncancerous tumors in animals when given for a long time in doses much larger than those used in humans. Therefore, your doctor may not want you to breast-feed while taking it. Be sure that you discuss the risks and benefits of this medicine with your doctor.

**Children**—Studies on this medicine have been done only in adult patients, and there is no specific information comparing use of pentoxifylline in children with use in other age groups.

**Older adults**—Side effects may be more likely to occur in the elderly, who are usually more sensitive than younger adults to the effects of pentoxifylline.

**Other medicines**—Although certain medicines should not be used together at all, in other cases two different medicines may be used together even if an interaction might occur. In these cases, your doctor may want to change the dose, or other precautions may be necessary. When you are taking pentoxifylline, it is important that your health care professional know if you are taking any other prescription or nonprescription (over-the-counter [OTC]) medicine, or if you smoke tobacco.

**Other medical problems**—The presence of other medical problems may affect the use of pentoxifylline. Make sure you tell your doctor if you have any other medical problems, especially:

- Any condition in which there is a risk of bleeding (e.g., recent stroke)—Pentoxifylline may make the condition worse
- Kidney disease or
- Liver disease—The chance of side effects may be increased

## Proper Use of This Medicine

Swallow the tablet whole. Do not crush, break, or chew it before swallowing.

*Pentoxifylline should be taken with meals to lessen the chance of stomach upset.* Taking an antacid with the medicine may also help.

**Dosing**—The dose of pentoxifylline will be different for different patients. *Follow your doctor's orders or the directions on the label.* The following information includes only the average doses of pentoxifylline. *If your dose is different, do not change it* unless your doctor tells you to do so.

- For *oral* dosage form (extended-release tablets):
  —For peripheral vascular disease (circulation problems):
    - Adults—400 milligrams (mg) two to three times a day, taken with meals.
    - Children—Use must be determined by your doctor.

**Missed dose**—If you miss a dose of this medicine, take it as soon as possible. However, if it is almost time for your next dose, skip the missed dose and go back to your regular dosing schedule. Do not double doses.

**Storage**—To store this medicine:
- Keep out of the reach of children.
- Store away from heat and direct light.
- Do not store in the bathroom, near the kitchen sink, or in other damp places. Heat or moisture may cause the medicine to break down.
- Do not keep outdated medicine or medicine no longer needed. Be sure that any discarded medicine is out of the reach of children.

## Precautions While Using This Medicine

It may take several weeks for this medicine to work. If you feel that pentoxifylline is not working, do not stop taking it on your own. Instead, check with your doctor.

Smoking tobacco may worsen your condition since nicotine may further narrow your blood vessels. Therefore, it is best to avoid smoking.

## Side Effects of This Medicine

Along with its needed effects, a medicine may cause some unwanted effects. Although not all of these side effects may occur, if they do occur they may need medical attention.

Check with your doctor as soon as possible if any of the following side effects occur:

*Rare*
   Chest pain; irregular heartbeat

*Signs and symptoms of overdose (in the order in which they may occur)*
   Drowsiness; flushing; faintness; unusual excitement; convulsions (seizures)

Other side effects may occur that usually do not need medical attention. These side effects may go away during treatment as your body adjusts to the medicine. However,

check with your doctor if any of the following side effects continue or are bothersome:

*Less common*

Dizziness; headache; nausea or vomiting; stomach discomfort

Other side effects not listed above may also occur in some patients. If you notice any other effects, check with your doctor.

---

Revised: 07/13/93

---

# PERFLUBRON    Diagnostic†

A commonly used brand name in the U.S. is Imagent GI.
Another commonly used name is perfluorooctylbromide.

---

†Not commercially available in Canada.

---

## Description

Perflubron (per-FLOO-bron) is a contrast agent. Contrast agents are used to help provide a clear picture during magnetic resonance imaging (MRI). MRI is a special kind of diagnostic procedure. It uses magnets and computers to create images or "pictures" of certain areas inside the body. Unlike x-rays, it does not involve radiation.

Perflubron is taken by mouth before MRI to darken bowel (intestines) images, which may help the doctor diagnose problems or diseases of the bowel.

Perflubron is to be used only by or under the supervision of a doctor. It is available in the following dosage form:

*Oral*

• Solution (U.S.)

---

## Before Having This Test

In deciding to use a diagnostic test, any risks of the test must be weighed against the good it will do. This is a decision you and your doctor will make. Also, test results may be affected by other things. For perflubron, the following should be considered:

**Allergies**—Tell your doctor if you have ever had any unusual or allergic reaction to contrast agents such as perflubron. Also, tell your doctor if you are allergic to any other substances, such as foods, preservatives, or dyes.

**Pregnancy**—Studies have not been done in humans or animals. Also, it is not known if the magnetic field used in MRI has any effect on the development of the fetus. Be sure you have discussed this with your doctor.

**Breast-feeding**—It is not known if perflubron passes into the breast milk.

**Children**—Although there is no specific information comparing use of perflubron in children wth use in other age groups, this agent is not expected to cause different side effects or problems in children than it does in adults.

**Older adults**—This medicine has been tested and has not been shown to cause different side effects or problems in older people than it does in younger adults.

**Other medical problems**—The presence of other medical problems may affect the use of perflubron. Make sure you tell your doctor if you have any other medical problems, especially:

• Blockage or perforation of the bowel—Either of these conditions may allow perflubron to be absorbed into the body and possibly increase the risk of side effects

---

## Preparation for This Test

Your doctor may have special instructions for you in preparation for your test, depending on the type of test. If you have not received such instructions or if you do not understand them, check with your doctor in advance.

Your doctor may tell you not to eat for at least 4 hours before this test. This is to make it easier for you to drink all of the perflubron solution.

---

## Precautions After Having This Test

This agent may cause some leakage from the rectum. The use of absorbent pads may be necessary to prevent soiling of clothing and embarrassment.

---

## Side Effects of This Diagnostic Agent

Perflubron commonly causes some side effects shortly after it is given. Usually they last for only a short while. However, check with your doctor if any of the following side effects continue or are bothersome:

*More common*

Abdominal or stomach fullness; diarrhea; loss of control of bowels; nausea and vomiting; oily taste in mouth

---

© 1994   The United States Pharmacopeial Convention, Inc.

*Less common*
   Abdominal or stomach pain; rectal gas; rectal leakage of
      the solution of perflubron
*Rare*
   Chills; dizziness; flushing or redness of skin; headache;
      numb mouth; trembling

Other side effects not listed above may also occur in some
patients. If you notice any other effects, check with your
doctor.

Developed: 01/25/94

# PERGOLIDE Systemic

A commonly used brand name in the U.S. and Canada is Permax.

## Description

Pergolide (PER-go-lide) belongs to the group of medicines known as ergot alkaloids. It is used with levodopa
or with carbidopa and levodopa combination to treat people who have Parkinson's disease. It works by stimulating
certain parts of the central nervous system (CNS) that
are involved in this disease.

Pergolide is available only with your doctor's prescription,
in the following dosage form:
*Oral*
   • Tablets (U.S. and Canada)

## Before Using This Medicine

In deciding to use a medicine, the risks of taking the
medicine must be weighed against the good it will do.
This is a decision you and your doctor will make. For
pergolide, the following should be considered:

**Allergies**—Tell your doctor if you have ever had any unusual or allergic reaction to pergolide or other ergot medicines such as ergotamine. Also tell your health care
professional if you are allergic to any other substances,
such as foods, preservatives, or dyes.

**Pregnancy**—Studies have not been done in pregnant
women. However, pergolide has not been shown to cause
birth defects or other problems in animal studies.

**Breast-feeding**—This medicine may stop milk from being
produced.

**Children**—Studies on this medicine have been done only
in adult patients, and there is no specific information
about its use in children.

**Older adults**—This medicine has been tested and has not
been shown to cause different side effects or problems
in older people than it does in younger adults.

**Other medicines**—Although certain medicines should not
be used together at all, in other cases 2 different medicines may be used together even if an interaction might
occur. In these cases, your doctor may want to change
the dose, or other precautions may be necessary. When
you are taking pergolide, it is especially important that
your health care professional know if you are taking any
other prescription or nonprescription (over-the-counter
[OTC]) medicine.

**Other medical problems**—The presence of other medical
problems may affect the use of pergolide. Make sure you
tell your doctor if you have any other medical problems,
especially:
   • Heart disease or
   • Mental problems (history of)—Pergolide may make the
      condition worse

## Proper Use of This Medicine

If pergolide upsets your stomach, it may be taken with
meals. If stomach upset continues, check with your doctor.

**Dosing**—The dose of pergolide will be different for different patients. *Follow your doctor's orders or the directions on the label.* The following information includes
only the average doses of pergolide. *If your dose is different, do not change it* unless your doctor tells you to
do so.

The number of tablets that you take depends on the
strength of the medicine. Also, *the number of doses you
take each day, the time allowed between doses, and the
length of time you take the medicine depend on the medical problem for which you are taking pergolide.*

   • For *oral* dosage form (tablets):
      —Adults: 50 micrograms a day for the first two days.
      The dose may be increased every three days as
      needed. However, the usual dose is not more than
      5000 micrograms.

**Missed dose**—If you miss a dose of this medicine, take
it as soon as you remember it. However, if it is almost
time for your next dose, skip the missed dose and go back
to your regular dosing schedule. Do not double doses.

**Storage**—To store this medicine:
   • Keep out of the reach of children.
   • Store away from heat and direct light.
   • Do not store in the bathroom, near the kitchen sink,
      or in other damp places. Heat or moisture may cause
      the medicine to break down.
   • Do not keep outdated medicine or medicine no longer
      needed. Be sure that any discarded medicine is out
      of the reach of children.

## Precautions While Using This Medicine

It is important that your doctor check your progress at regular visits, to make sure that this medicine is working and to check for unwanted effects.

This medicine may cause some people to become drowsy, dizzy, or less alert than they are normally. *Make sure you know how you react to this medicine before you drive, use machines, or do anything else that could be dangerous if you are dizzy or are not alert.*

Dizziness, lightheadedness, or fainting may occur after the first doses of pergolide, especially when you get up from a lying or sitting position. Getting up slowly may help. Taking the first dose at bedtime or when you are able to lie down may also lessen problems. If the problem continues or gets worse, check with your doctor.

Pergolide may cause dryness of the mouth. For temporary relief, use sugarless candy or gum, melt bits of ice in your mouth, or use a saliva substitute. However, if your mouth continues to feel dry for more than 2 weeks, check with your medical doctor or dentist. Continuing dryness of the mouth may increase the chance of dental disease, including tooth decay, gum disease, and fungus infections.

It may take several weeks for pergolide to work. Do not stop taking this medicine or reduce the amount you are taking without first checking with your doctor.

## Side Effects of This Medicine

Along with its needed effects, a medicine may cause some unwanted effects. Although not all of these side effects may occur, if they do occur they may need medical attention.

*Check with your doctor immediately* if any of the following side effects occur:

*Rare*

 Chest pain (severe); convulsions (seizures); fainting; fast heartbeat; headache (severe or continuing); increased sweating; nausea and vomiting (continuing or severe); nervousness; unexplained shortness of breath; vision changes, such as blurred vision or temporary blindness; weakness (sudden)

Also, check with your doctor as soon as possible if any of the following side effects occur:

*More common*

 Confusion; hallucinations (seeing, hearing, or feeling things that are not there); pain or burning while urinating; uncontrolled movements of the body, such as the face, tongue, arms, hands, head, and upper body

*Less common*

 High blood pressure

Other side effects may occur that usually do not need medical attention. These side effects may go away during treatment as your body adjusts to the medicine. However, check with your doctor if any of the following side effects continue or are bothersome:

*More common*

 Abdominal or stomach pain; constipation; dizziness or lightheadedness, especially when getting up from a lying or sitting position; drowsiness; lower back pain; nausea; runny nose; weakness

*Less common*

 Chills; diarrhea; dryness of mouth; loss of appetite; swelling of the face; vomiting

Other side effects not listed above may also occur in some patients. If you notice any other effects, check with your doctor.

Revised: 03/19/93

---

# PERMETHRIN    Topical

A commonly used brand name in the U.S. and Canada is Nix Cream Rinse.

## Description

Permethrin (per-METH-rin) is used to treat head lice infections. It acts by destroying both the lice and their eggs.

This medicine is available in the following dosage form:

*Topical*
 • Lotion (U.S. and Canada)

## Before Using This Medicine

If you are using this medicine without a prescription, carefully read any precautions on the label. For topical permethrin, the following should be considered:

**Allergies**—Tell your doctor if you have ever had any unusual or allergic reaction to permethrin; to other synthetic pyrethroids, such as those found in household insecticides; to pyrethrins or chrysanthemums; or to veterinary insecticides containing permethrin. Also tell your health care professional if you are allergic to any other substances, such as preservatives or dyes.

**Pregnancy**—Permethrin has not been studied in pregnant women. However, this medication has not been shown to cause birth defects or other problems in animal studies.

**Breast-feeding**—It is not known whether permethrin passes into the breast milk. However, animal studies have shown that permethrin can cause tumors. Be sure you have discussed the risks and benefits of the medicine with your doctor.

**Children**—Studies on this medicine have been done only in adult patients, and there is no specific information comparing use of topical permethrin in children with use in other age groups.

**Older adults**—Many medicines have not been studied specifically in older people. Therefore, it may not be known whether they work exactly the same way they do in younger adults or if they cause different side effects or problems in older people. There is no specific information comparing use of topical permethrin in the elderly with use in other age groups.

**Other medicines**—Although certain medicines should not be used together at all, in other cases two different medicines may be used together even if an interaction might occur. In these cases, your doctor may want to change the dose, or other precautions may be necessary. Tell your health care professional if you are using any other prescription or nonprescription (over-the-counter [OTC]) medicine that is to be applied to the hair and scalp.

**Other medical problems**—The presence of other medical problems may affect the use of topical permethrin. Make sure you tell your doctor if you have other medical problems, especially:

- Severe inflammation of the scalp—Use of permethrin may make the condition worse

## Proper Use of This Medicine

*Keep this medicine away from the eyes.* If you accidentally get some in your eyes, flush them thoroughly with water at once.

Permethrin lotion comes in a container that holds only one treatment. Use as much of the medicine as you need and discard any remaining lotion properly.

To use:

- Shampoo the hair and scalp using regular shampoo.
- Thoroughly rinse and towel dry the hair and scalp.
- Allow hair to air dry for a few minutes.
- Shake the permethrin lotion well before applying.
- Thoroughly wet the hair and scalp with the permethrin lotion. Be sure to cover the areas behind the ears and on the back of the neck also. Allow the lotion to remain in place for 10 minutes.
- Then, rinse the hair and scalp thoroughly and dry with a clean towel.
- When the hair is dry, you may want to comb the hair with a fine-toothed comb to remove any remaining nits (eggs) or nit shells.

Head lice can be easily transferred from one person to another by direct contact with clothing, hats, scarves, bedding, towels, washcloths, hairbrushes and combs, or hairs from infected persons. Therefore, *all members of your household should be examined for head lice and should receive treatment if they are found to be infected.* If you have any questions about this, check with your doctor.

**Dosing**—*Follow your doctor's orders or the directions on the label.* The following information includes only the average dose of permethrin. *If your dose is different, do not change it* unless your doctor tells you to do so.

- For *topical* dosage form (lotion):
  —For head lice:
    - Adults and children 2 years of age and older— Apply to the hair and scalp one time.
    - Children up to 2 years of age—Use and dose must be determined by your doctor.

**Storage**—To store this medicine:

- Keep out of the reach of children.
- Store away from heat and direct light.
- Keep this medicine from freezing. Do not refrigerate.
- Do not keep outdated medicine or medicine no longer needed. Be sure that any discarded medicine is out of the reach of children.

## Precautions While Using This Medicine

To prevent reinfection or spreading of the infection to other people, good health habits are required. These include the following:

- Machine wash all clothing (including hats, scarves, and coats), bedding, towels, and washcloths in very hot water and dry them by using the hot cycle of a dryer for at least 20 minutes. Clothing or bedding that cannot be washed should be dry cleaned or sealed in an airtight plastic bag for 2 weeks.
- Shampoo all wigs and hairpieces.
- Wash all hairbrushes and combs in very hot soapy water (above 130 °F) for 5 to 10 minutes and do not share them with other people.
- Clean the house or room by thoroughly vacuuming upholstered furniture, rugs, and floors.
- Wash all toys in very hot soapy water (above 130 °F) for 5 to 10 minutes or seal in an airtight plastic bag for 2 weeks. This is especially important for stuffed toys used on the bed.

## Side Effects of This Medicine

Along with its needed effects, a medicine may cause some unwanted effects. Although not all of these side effects may occur, if they do occur they may need medical attention.

Check with your doctor if any of the following side effects continue or are bothersome:

*Less common or rare*

Burning, itching, numbness, rash, redness, stinging, swelling, or tingling of the scalp

Other side effects not listed above may also occur in some patients. If you notice any other effects, check with your doctor.

Revised: 07/25/94

---

# PERPHENAZINE AND AMITRIPTYLINE   Systemic

Some commonly used brand names are:

**In the U.S.—**

| | |
|---|---|
| Etrafon | Etrafon-Forte |
| Etrafon-A | Triavil |

Generic name product may also be available.

**In Canada—**

| | |
|---|---|
| Elavil Plus | |
| Etrafon | Etrafon-F |
| Etrafon-A | PMS Levazine |
| Etrafon-D | Triavil |

## Description

Perphenazine (per-FEN-a-zeen) and amitriptyline (a-mee-TRIP-ti-leen) combination is used to treat certain mental and emotional conditions.

This combination is available only with your doctor's prescription, in the following dosage form:

*Oral*
• Tablets (U.S. and Canada).

## Before Using This Medicine

In deciding to use a medicine, the risks of taking the medicine must be weighed against the good it will do. This is a decision you and your doctor will make. For perphenazine and amitriptyline combination, the following should be considered:

**Allergies**—Tell your doctor if you have ever had any unusual or allergic reaction to perphenazine (e.g., Trilafon) or other phenothiazines (such as acetophenazine [e.g., Tindal], chlorpromazine [e.g., Thorazine], fluphenazine [e.g., Prolixin], mesoridazine [e.g., Serentil], prochlorperazine [e.g., Compazine], promazine [e.g., Sparine], promethazine [e.g., Phenergan], thioridazine [e.g., Mellaril], trifluoperazine [e.g., Stelazine], triflupromazine [e.g., Vesprin], trimeprazine [e.g., Temaril]) or to amitriptyline (e.g., Elavil) or other tricyclic antidepressants (such as amoxapine [e.g., Asendin], clomipramine [e.g., Anafranil], desipramine [e.g., Pertofrane], doxepin [e.g., Sinequan], imipramine [e.g., Tofranil], nortriptyline [e.g., Aventyl], protriptyline [e.g., Vivactil], trimipramine [e.g., Surmontil]). Also tell your health care professional if you are allergic to any other substances, such as foods, preservatives, or dyes.

**Pregnancy**—Studies have not been done in pregnant women. However, perphenazine and amitriptyline combination has not been shown to cause birth defects in animal studies. Side effects such as jaundice and muscle tremors have occurred in some newborn babies when their mothers received other phenothiazines during pregnancy.

**Breast-feeding**—Perphenazine and amitriptyline combination passes into the breast milk and may cause drowsiness and other unwanted effects in nursing babies.

**Children**—Certain side effects, such as muscle spasms of the face, neck, and back, tic-like or twitching movements, inability to move the eyes, twisting of the body, or weakness of the arms and legs, are more likely to occur in children, who are usually more sensitive than adults to some of the side effects of perphenazine and amitriptyline combination.

**Older adults**—Confusion, vision problems, dizziness or fainting, drowsiness, dryness of mouth, constipation, problems in urinating, trembling of the hands and fingers, and symptoms of tardive dyskinesia (such as uncontrolled movements of the mouth, tongue, jaw, arms, and/or legs) are especially likely to occur in elderly patients. Older patients are usually more sensitive than younger adults to the effects of perphenazine and amitriptyline combination.

**Other medicines**—Although certain medicines should not be used together at all, in other cases 2 different medicines may be used together even if an interaction might occur. In these cases, your doctor may want to change the dose, or other precautions may be necessary. When you are taking perphenazine and amitriptyline combination, it is especially important that your health care professional know if you are taking any of the following:

• Amphetamines or
• Appetite suppressants (diet pills) or
• Medicine for asthma or other breathing problems or
• Medicine for colds, sinus problems, or hay fever or other allergies (including nose drops and sprays)—Using these medicines with perphenazine and amitriptyline combination may increase the risk of serious effects on the heart
• Antithyroid agents (medicine for overactive thyroid) or
• Cimetidine (e.g., Tagamet) or
• Methyldopa (e.g., Aldomet) or
• Metoclopramide (e.g., Reglan) or
• Metyrosine (e.g., Demser) or
• Pemoline (e.g., Cylert) or

- Pimozide (e.g., Orap) or
- Promethazine (e.g., Phenergan) or
- Rauwolfia alkaloids (alseroxylon [e.g., Rauwiloid], deserpidine [e.g., Harmonyl], rauwolfia serpentina [e.g., Raudixin], reserpine [e.g., Serpasil]) or
- Trimeprazine (e.g., Temaril)—Taking these medicines with perphenazine and amitriptyline combination may increase the risk of serious side effects
- Central nervous system (CNS) depressants (medicines that cause drowsiness)—Taking these medicines with perphenazine and amitriptyline combination may increase the CNS depressant effects
- Epinephrine (e.g., Adrenalin)—Severe low blood pressure (hypotension) and fast heartbeat may occur if epinephrine is used with perphenazine and amitriptyline combination
- Levodopa (e.g., Dopar)—Perphenazine may prevent levodopa from working properly in the treatment of Parkinson's disease
- Lithium (e.g., Lithane)—The amount of medicine you need to take may change
- Metrizamide—When this dye is used for myelograms during the use of perphenazine and amitriptyline combination, there is an increased risk of seizures
- Monoamine oxidase (MAO) inhibitors (furazolidone [e.g., Furoxone], isocarboxazid [e.g., Marplan], phenelzine [e.g., Nardil], procarbazine [e.g., Matulane], selegiline [e.g., Eldepryl], tranylcypromine [e.g., Parnate])—Taking amitriptyline while you are taking or within 2 weeks of taking monoamine oxidase (MAO) inhibitors may cause sudden high body temperature, extremely high blood pressure, and severe convulsions; however, sometimes certain of these medicines may be used together under close supervision by your doctor

**Other medical problems**—The presence of other medical problems may affect the use of perphenazine and amitriptyline combination. Make sure you tell your doctor if you have any other medical problems, especially:

- Alcohol abuse—Certain side effects such as heat stroke may be more likely to occur
- Asthma (history of) or other lung disease or
- Bipolar disorder (manic-depressive illness) or
- Blood disease or
- Breast cancer or
- Difficult urination or
- Enlarged prostate or
- Epilepsy or other seizure disorders or
- Glaucoma or
- Heart or blood vessel disease or
- Mental illness (severe) or
- Parkinson's disease or
- Stomach or intestinal problems—Perphenazine and amitriptyline combination may make the condition worse
- Kidney disease or
- Liver disease—Higher blood levels of perphenazine and amitriptyline may occur, increasing the chance of side effects
- Overactive thyroid—Perphenazine and amitriptyline combination may cause an increased chance of serious effects on the heart
- Reye's syndrome—There may be an increased chance of unwanted effects on the liver

## Proper Use of This Medicine

To lessen stomach upset, take this medicine immediately after meals or with food, unless your doctor has told you to take it on an empty stomach.

*Do not take more of this medicine and do not take it more often than your doctor ordered.* This is particularly important for elderly patients, since they are more sensitive to the effects of this medicine.

*Sometimes perphenazine and amitriptyline combination must be taken for several weeks before its full effect is reached.*

**Dosing**—The dose of perphenazine and amitriptyline combination will be different for different patients. *Follow your doctor's orders or the directions on the label.* The following information includes only the average doses of perphenazine and amitriptyline combination. *If your dose is different, do not change it* unless your doctor tells you to do so.

The number of tablets that you take depends on the strength of the medicine. Also, *the number of doses you take each day, the time allowed between doses, and the length of time you take the medicine depend on your special needs.*

- For *oral* dosage form (tablets):
  —For certain mental and emotional conditions:
    - Adults—At first, 1 tablet taken three or four times a day. Your doctor may increase your dose if needed.
    - Children—Use and dose must be determined by your doctor.

**Missed dose**—If you miss a dose of this medicine, take it as soon as possible. However, if it is within 2 hours of your next dose, skip the missed dose and go back to your regular dosing schedule. Do not double doses.

**Storage**—To store this medicine:

- Keep out of the reach of children. Overdose of perphenazine and amitriptyline combination is especially dangerous in young children.
- Store away from heat and direct light.
- Do not store in the bathroom, near the kitchen sink, or in other damp places. Heat or moisture may cause the medicine to break down.
- Do not keep outdated medicine or medicine no longer needed. Be sure that any discarded medicine is out of the reach of children.

## Precautions While Using This Medicine

Your doctor should check your progress at regular visits to allow dose adjustments and help reduce side effects.

*Do not stop taking this medicine without first checking with your doctor.* Your doctor may want you to reduce gradually the amount you are taking before stopping completely. This is to prevent side effects and to prevent your condition from becoming worse.

Do not take this medicine within two hours of taking antacids or medicine for diarrhea. Taking these products too close together may make this medicine less effective.

This medicine will add to the effects of alcohol and other CNS depressants (medicines that cause drowsiness). Some examples of CNS depressants are antihistamines or medicine for hay fever, other allergies, or colds; sedatives, tranquilizers, or sleeping medicine; prescription pain medicine or narcotics barbiturates; medicine for seizures; or anesthetics, including some dental anesthetics. *Check with your doctor before taking any of the above while you are using this medicine.*

*Before having any kind of surgery, dental treatment, or emergency treatment, tell the medical doctor or dentist in charge that you are taking this medicine.* Taking perphenazine and amitriptyline combination together with medicines that are used during surgery or dental or emergency treatments may increase the CNS depressant effects.

This medicine may cause some people to become drowsy or less alert than they are normally, especially during the first few weeks of treatment. Even if this medicine is taken only at bedtime, it may cause some people to feel drowsy or less alert on arising. *Make sure you know how you react to this medicine before you drive, use machines, or do anything else that could be dangerous if you are not alert.*

*Dizziness, lightheadedness, or fainting may occur,* especially when you get up from a lying or sitting position. Getting up slowly may help. If the problem continues or gets worse, check with your doctor.

This medicine may make you sweat less, causing your body temperature to increase. *Use extra care not to become overheated during exercise or hot weather while you are taking this medicine,* since overheating may result in heat stroke. Also, hot baths or saunas may make you feel dizzy or faint.

Perphenazine and amitriptyline combination may cause dryness of the mouth. For temporary relief, use sugarless gum or candy, melt bits of ice in your mouth, or use a saliva substitute. However, if your mouth continues to feel dry for more than 2 weeks, check with your medical doctor or dentist. Continuing dryness of the mouth may increase the chance of dental disease, including tooth decay, gum disease, and fungus infections.

Perphenazine may cause your skin to be more sensitive to sunlight than it is normally. Exposure to sunlight, even for brief periods of time, may cause a skin rash, itching, redness or other discoloration of the skin, or a severe sunburn. When you begin taking this medicine:

- Stay out of direct sunlight, especially between the hours of 10:00 a.m. and 3:00 p.m., if possible.
- Wear protective clothing, including a hat. Also, wear sunglasses.

- Apply a sun block product that has a skin protection factor (SPF) of at least 15. Some patients may require a product with a higher SPF number, especially if they have a fair complexion. If you have any questions about this, check with your health care professional.
- Apply a sun block lipstick that has an SPF of at least 15 to protect your lips.
- Do not use a sunlamp or tanning bed or booth.

*If you have a severe reaction from the sun, check with your doctor.*

## Side Effects of This Medicine

Along with its needed effects, perphenazine (included in this combination medicine) can sometimes cause serious side effects. Tardive dyskinesia (a movement disorder) may occur and may not go away after you stop using the medicine. Signs of tardive dyskinesia include fine, worm-like movements of the tongue, or other uncontrolled movements of the mouth, tongue, cheeks, jaw, or arms and legs. Other serious but rare side effects may also occur. These include severe muscle stiffness, fever, unusual tiredness or weakness, fast heartbeat, difficult breathing, increased sweating, loss of bladder control, and seizures (neuroleptic malignant syndrome). *You and your doctor should discuss the good this medicine will do as well as the risks of taking it.*

*Stop taking this medicine and get emergency help immediately* if any of the following side effects occur:

*Rare*
  Convulsions (seizures); difficulty in breathing; fast heartbeat; fever; high or low blood pressure; increased sweating; loss of bladder control; muscle stiffness (severe); unusual tiredness or weakness; unusually pale skin

Also, check with your doctor as soon as possible if any of the following side effects occur:

*More common*
  Blurred vision or any change in vision; difficulty in speaking or swallowing; fainting; inability to move eyes; lip smacking or puckering; loss of balance control; mask-like face; muscle spasms, especially of face, neck, and back; nervousness, restlessness, or need to keep moving; puffing of cheeks; rapid or fine, worm-like movements of tongue; shuffling walk; stiffness of arms and legs; trembling and shaking of fingers and hands; tic-like or twitching movements; twisting movements of body; uncontrolled chewing movements; uncontrolled movements of arms or legs; weakness of arms and legs

*Less common*
  Confusion; constipation; difficult urination; eye pain; hallucinations (seeing, hearing, or feeling things that are not there); increased skin sensitivity to sun; shakiness; slow pulse or irregular heartbeat

*Rare*
  Abdominal or stomach pain; aching muscles or joints; back or leg pain; fever and chills; hair loss; hot, dry skin or lack of sweating; irritability; loss of appetite; muscle weakness or twitching; nausea, vomiting, or

diarrhea; nosebleeds; prolonged, painful, inappropriate penile erection; ringing, buzzing, or other unexplained noises in ears; skin discoloration; skin rash and itching; sore throat and fever; swelling of face and tongue; swelling of testicles; unusual bleeding or bruising; yellow eyes or skin

*Symptoms of overdose*

Agitation; confusion; convulsions (seizures); drowsiness (severe); enlarged pupils; fast, slow, or irregular heartbeat; fever; hallucinations (seeing, hearing, or feeling things that are not there); shortness of breath or troubled breathing; unusual tiredness or weakness (severe); vomiting (severe)

Other side effects may occur that usually do not need medical attention. These side effects may go away during treatment as your body adjusts to the medicine. However, check with your doctor if any of the following side effects continue or are bothersome:

*More common*

Decreased sweating; dizziness; drowsiness; dryness of mouth; headache; increased appetite for sweets; nasal congestion; tiredness or weakness (mild); unpleasant taste; weight gain (unusual)

*Less common*

Changes in menstrual period; decreased sexual ability; heartburn; increased sweating; swelling or pain in breasts or unusual secretion of milk

After you stop using this medicine, your body may need time to adjust. The length of time this takes depends on the amount of medicine you are using and how long you used it. During this time, check with your doctor if you notice any of the following symptoms:

Dizziness; nausea or vomiting; stomach pain; trembling of fingers and hands; symptoms of tardive dyskinesia, including lip smacking or puckering, puffing of cheeks, rapid or fine, worm-like movements of tongue, uncontrolled chewing movements, or uncontrolled movements of arms or legs

Other side effects may occur if the medicine is stopped suddenly or stopped after long-term treatment. Check with your doctor if you notice any of the following symptoms:

Diarrhea; headache; irritability; restlessness; trouble in sleeping, with vivid dreams; unusual excitement

Other side effects not listed above may also occur in some patients. If you notice any other effects, check with your doctor.

---

Revised: 01/27/92
Interim revision: 08/09/94

---

# PHENACEMIDE Systemic†

Some commonly used brand names are:

**In the U.S.—**
  Phenurone
**Other—**
  Epiclase
  Phetylureum
Another commonly used name is phenacetylcarbamide.

---

†Not commercially available in Canada.

---

## Description

Phenacemide (fe-NASS-e-mide) is used to control certain seizures in the treatment of epilepsy. This medicine acts on the central nervous system (CNS) to reduce the number and severity of seizures.

Phenacemide is available only with your doctor's prescription in the following dosage form:

*Oral*
• Tablets (U.S.)

---

## Before Using This Medicine

In deciding to use a medicine, the risks of taking the medicine must be weighed against the good it will do.

This is a decision you and your doctor will make. For phenacemide, the following should be considered:

**Allergies**—Tell your doctor if you have ever had any unusual or allergic reaction to phenacemide or any other anticonvulsant medicines in the past. Also tell your health care professional if you are allergic to any other substances, such as foods, preservatives, or dyes.

**Pregnancy**—Phenacemide has been reported to cause birth defects when taken by the mother during pregnancy. However, this medicine may be necessary to control seizures in some pregnant patients. Be sure you have discussed this with your doctor. In addition, when taken during pregnancy, phenacemide may cause a bleeding problem in the mother during delivery and in the newborn. This may be prevented by giving vitamin K to the mother 1 month before and during delivery, and to the baby immediately after birth.

**Breast-feeding**—It is not known whether this medicine passes into breast milk.

**Children**—Although there is no specific information comparing use of phenacemide in children with use in other age groups, this medicine is not expected to cause different side effects or problems than it does in adults.

**Older adults**—Many medicines have not been studied specifically in older people. Therefore, it may not be known whether they work exactly the same way they do in younger adults. Although there is no specific information comparing use of phenacemide in the elderly with use in other age groups, this medicine is not expected to cause different side effects or problems in older people than it does in younger adults.

**Other medicines**—Although certain medicines should not be used together at all, in other cases 2 different medicines may be used together even if an interaction might occur. In these cases, your doctor may want to change the dose, or other precautions may be necessary. When you are taking phenacemide, it is especially important that your health care professional know if you are taking the following:

- Other anticonvulsants—Use of phenacemide may increase the chance of serious side effects

**Other medical problems**—The presence of other medical problems may affect the use of phenacemide. Make sure you tell your doctor if you have any other medical problems, especially:

- Blood disease or
- Kidney disease or
- Liver disease or
- Personality disorder (mental illness)—Phenacemide may make the condition worse

---

## Proper Use of This Medicine

To control your medical problem, *take this medicine every day* exactly as ordered by your doctor. Do not take more or less of it than your doctor ordered. To help you remember to take the medicine at the correct times, try to get into the habit of taking it at the same times each day.

**Dosing**—The dose of phenacemide will be different for different patients. *Follow your doctor's orders or the directions on the label.* The following information includes only the average doses of phenacemide. *If your dose is different, do not change it* unless your doctor tells you to do so:

- Adults—Oral, to start, 500 milligrams three times a day. After one week, your doctor may add an additional 500 milligram dose to be taken upon arising if needed. In the third week, your doctor may add another 500 milligram dose to be taken at bedtime if needed. Your doctor may increase your dose further. However, the dose is usually not more than 5000 milligrams a day.
- Children 5 years of age and older—Oral, to start, 250 milligrams three times a day. The doctor may increase the dose further. However, the dose is usually not more than 1500 milligrams a day.
- Children up to 5 years of age—Dose must be determined by the doctor.

**Missed dose**—If you miss a dose of this medicine, take it as soon as possible. However, if it is almost time for your next dose, skip the missed dose and go back to your regular dosing schedule. Do not double doses.

**Storage**—To store this medicine:

- Keep out of the reach of children.
- Store away from heat and direct light.
- Do not store in the bathroom, near the kitchen sink, or in other damp places. Heat or moisture may cause the medicine to break down.
- Do not keep outdated medicine or medicine no longer needed. Be sure that any discarded medicine is out of the reach of children.

---

## Precautions While Using This Medicine

*Your doctor should check your progress at regular visits*, especially during the first few months of treatment with this medicine. During this time, the amount of medicine you are taking may have to be changed often to meet your individual needs.

If you have been taking phenacemide regularly, do not stop taking it without first checking with your doctor. Your doctor may want you to decrease gradually the amount you are taking before stopping completely. This will help reduce the possibility of seizures.

*Be sure to tell your doctor as soon as possible if you have a sore throat, fever, or general feeling of tiredness, or if you notice any unusual bleeding or bruising,* such as reddish or purplish spots on skin, or recurring nosebleeds or bleeding gums.

*Also, be sure to tell your doctor as soon as possible if you or your family notice any changes in your behavior or mood,* such as aggressiveness, depression, or a decreased interest in your surroundings.

This medicine will add to the effects of alcohol and other CNS depressants (medicines that slow down the nervous system, possibly causing drowsiness). Some examples of CNS depressants are antihistamines or medicine for hay fever, other allergies, or colds; sedatives, tranquilizers, or sleeping medicine; prescription pain medicine or narcotics; barbiturates; other medicine for seizures; muscle relaxants; or anesthetics, including some dental anesthetics. *Check with your doctor before taking any of the above while you are using this medicine.*

This medicine may cause some people to become dizzy or drowsy. *Make sure your know how you react to this medicine before you drive, use machines, or do anything else that could be dangerous if you are dizzy or are not alert.*

---

## Side Effects of This Medicine

Phenacemide may cause some serious side effects, including behavior or mental changes, blood problems, liver problems, or kidney problems. You and your doctor should discuss the good this medicine will do as well as the risks of receiving it.

Check with your doctor as soon as possible if any of the following side effects occur:

*More common*
  Behavior or mood changes

---

© 1994   The United States Pharmacopeial Convention, Inc.

*Rare*

Blood in urine; dark-colored urine; difficulty in breathing, shortness of breath, wheezing, or tightness in chest; drowsiness; flu-like symptoms (fever with or without chills, headache, body ache); nausea or vomiting; skin rash; sore throat and fever; swelling of face, feet, or lower legs; swollen or painful glands; unusual bleeding or bruising; unusual tiredness or weakness; weight gain; white spots, sores, or ulcers on lips, or in mouth or throat; yellow eyes or skin

*Symptoms of overdose (in the order in which they may occur)*

Unusual excitement, nervousness, or irritability; clumsiness or unsteadiness; drowsiness (severe)

Other side effects may occur that usually do not need medical attention. These side effects may go away during treatment as your body adjusts to the medicine. However, check with your doctor if any of the following side effects continue or are bothersome:

*More common*

Drowsiness; headache; loss of appetite

*Less common or rare*

Dizziness; fever; muscle pain; pounding heartbeat; tingling, burning, or prickly sensations; trouble in sleeping; unusual tiredness or weakness; weight loss

Other side effects not listed above may also occur in some patients. If you notice any other effects, check with your doctor.

Revised: 03/09/93

---

# PHENAZOPYRIDINE  Systemic

Some commonly used brand names are:

**In the U.S.—**

| | |
|---|---|
| Azo-Standard | Pyridiate |
| Baridium | Pyridium |
| Eridium | Urodine |
| Geridium | Urogesic |
| Phenazodine | Viridium |

Generic name product may also be available.

**In Canada—**

| | |
|---|---|
| Phenazo | Pyridium |

## Description

Phenazopyridine (fen-az-oh-PEER-i-deen) is used to relieve the pain, burning, and discomfort caused by infection or irritation of the urinary tract. It is not an antibiotic and will not cure the infection itself.

In the U.S., phenazopyridine is available only with your doctor's prescription. In Canada, it is available without a prescription. It is available in the following dosage form:

*Oral*

- Tablets (U.S. and Canada)

## Before Using This Medicine

In deciding to use a medicine, the risks of taking the medicine must be weighed against the good it will do. This is a decision you and your doctor will make. For phenazopyridine, the following should be considered:

**Allergies**—Tell your doctor if you have ever had any unusual or allergic reaction to phenazopyridine. Also tell your health care professional if you are allergic to any other substances, such as foods, preservatives, or dyes.

**Pregnancy**—Phenazopyridine has not been studied in pregnant women. However, phenazopyridine has not been shown to cause birth defects in animal studies.

**Breast-feeding**—It is not known whether phenazopyridine passes into the breast milk. However, phenazopyridine has not been reported to cause problems in nursing babies.

**Children**—Although there is no specific information comparing use of phenazopyridine in children with use in other age groups, it is not expected to cause different side effects or problems in children than it does in adults.

**Older adults**—Many medicines have not been studied specifically in older people. Therefore, it may not be known whether they work exactly the same way they do in younger adults. Although there is no specific information comparing use of phenazopyridine in the elderly with use in other age groups, this medicine is not expected to cause different side effects or problems in older people than it does in younger adults.

**Other medicines**—Although certain medicines should not be used together at all, in other cases two different medicines may be used together even if an interaction might occur. In these cases, your doctor may want to change the dose, or other precautions may be necessary. Tell your health care professional if you are taking any other prescription or nonprescription (over-the-counter [OTC]) medicine.

**Other medical problems**—The presence of other medical problems may affect the use of phenazopyridine. Make sure you tell your doctor if you have any other medical problems, especially:

- Glucose-6-phosphate dehydrogenase (G6PD) deficiency or
- Hepatitis or
- Kidney disease—The chance of side effects may be increased.

## Proper Use of This Medicine

This medicine is best taken with food or after eating a meal or a snack to lessen stomach upset.

*Do not use any leftover medicine for future urinary tract problems without first checking with your doctor.* An infection may require additional medicine.

**Dosing**—The dose of phenazopyridine will be different for different patients. *Follow your doctor's orders or the directions on the label.* The following information includes only the average doses of phenazopyridine. *If your dose is different, do not change it* unless your doctor tells you to do so.

- For *oral* dosage form (tablets):
  —For relieving pain, burning, and discomfort in the urinary tract:
    - Adults and teenagers—200 milligrams (mg) three times a day.
    - Children—The dose is based on body weight and must be determined by your doctor. The usual dose is 4 mg per kilogram (kg) (about 1.8 mg per pound) of body weight three times a day.

**Missed dose**—If you miss a dose of this medicine, take it as soon as you remember. However, if it is almost time for your next dose, skip the missed dose and go back to your regular dosing schedule. Do not double doses.

**Storage**—To store this medicine:
- Keep out of the reach of children.
- Store away from heat and direct light.
- Do not store this medicine in the bathroom, near the kitchen sink, or in other damp places. Heat or moisture may cause the medicine to break down.
- Do not keep outdated medicine or medicine no longer needed. Be sure that any discarded medicine is out of the reach of children.

## Precautions While Using This Medicine

*Check with your doctor if symptoms such as bloody urine, difficult or painful urination, frequent urge to urinate, or sudden decrease in the amount of urine appear or become worse while you are taking this medicine.*

*Phenazopyridine causes the urine to turn reddish orange.* This is to be expected while you are using it. This effect is harmless and will go away after you stop taking the medicine. Also, the medicine may stain clothing.

For *patients who wear soft contact lenses:*
- It is best not to wear soft contact lenses while being treated with this medicine. Phenazopyridine may cause discoloration or staining of contact lenses. It may not be possible to remove the stain.

For *diabetic patients:*
- This medicine may cause false test results with urine sugar tests and urine ketone tests. If you have any questions about this, check with your health care professional, especially if your diabetes is not well controlled.

Before you have any medical tests, tell the person in charge that you are taking this medicine. The results of some tests may be affected by this medicine.

## Side Effects of This Medicine

Along with its needed effects, a medicine may cause some unwanted effects. Although not all of these side effects may occur, if they do occur they may need medical attention.

Check with your doctor as soon as possible if any of the following side effects occur:

*Rare*

Blue or blue-purple color of skin; fever and confusion; shortness of breath, tightness in chest, wheezing, or troubled breathing; skin rash; sudden decrease in the amount of urine; swelling of face, fingers, feet, and/or lower legs; unusual tiredness or weakness; weight gain; yellow eyes or skin

Other side effects may occur that usually do not need medical attention. These side effects may go away during treatment as your body adjusts to the medicine. However, check with your doctor if any of the following side effects continue or are bothersome:

*Less common or rare*

Dizziness; headache; indigestion; stomach cramps or pain

Other side effects not listed above may also occur in some patients. If you notice any other effects, check with your doctor.

Revised: 06/08/92
Interim revision: 08/24/94

# PHENOLSULFONPHTHALEIN    Diagnostic

Some commonly used names are phenol red and PSP.

## Description

Phenolsulfonphthalein (fee-nole-sul-fon-THAY-leen) is used as a test to help diagnose problems or disease of the kidneys. This test determines how well your kidneys are working.

Phenolsulfonphthalein passes out of the body almost entirely in the urine. Measuring the amount of phenolsulfonphthalein in the urine can help the doctor determine if the kidneys are working properly.

How test is done: After you have emptied your bladder, phenolsulfonphthalein will be given by injection. Then you will be asked to empty your bladder into a container one or more times after the medicine is given. The amount of this medicine in your urine will be measured. Then the results of the test will be studied. The way the phenolsulfonphthalein test is done may be different for different patients. Some patients may have the phenolsulfonphthalein injected into a vein, others, into a muscle.

It is very important that you *empty the bladder completely* and collect all the urine when you are asked to do so. If any urine is left behind or lost, it will change the results of the test.

Phenolsulfonphthalein is to be used only under the supervision of a doctor. It is available in the following dosage form:

*Parenteral*
- Injection (U.S.)

## Before Having This Test

In deciding to use a diagnostic test, any risks of the test must be weighed against the good it will do. This is a decision you and your doctor will make. Also, test results may be affected by other things. For phenolsulfonphthalein, the following should be considered:

**Allergies**—Tell your doctor if you have ever had any unusual or allergic reaction to phenolsulfonphthalein. Also tell your doctor if you are allergic to any other substances, such as foods, preservatives, or dyes.

**Pregnancy**—Studies have not been done in either humans or animals.

**Breast-feeding**—It is not known whether phenolsulfonphthalein passes into the breast milk. This medicine has not been reported to cause problems in nursing babies.

**Children**—Although there is no specific information comparing use of phenolsulfonphthalein in children with use in other age groups, phenolsulfonphthalein is not expected to cause different side effects or problems in children than it does in adults.

**Older adults**—Many medicines have not been studied specifically in older people. Therefore, it may not be known whether they work exactly the same way they do in younger adults. Although there is no specific information comparing use of phenolsulfonphthalein in the elderly with use in other age groups, this medicine is not expected to cause different side effects or problems in older people than it does in younger adults.

**Other medicines**—Although certain medicines should not be used together at all, in other cases two different medicines may be used together even if an interaction might occur. In these cases, your doctor may want to change the dose, or other precautions may be necessary. When you are taking phenolsulfonphthalein, it is especially important that your health care professional know if you are taking any of the following:

- Aspirin or other salicylates or
- Atropine or
- Diuretics (water pills) or
- Penicillins or
- Probenecid (e.g., Benemid) or
- Sulfinpyrazone (e.g., Anturane) or
- Sulfonamides (sulfa medicine)—Use of any of these medicines at the same time as phenolsulfonphthalein may affect the test results

**Other medical problems**—The presence of other medical problems may affect the use of phenolsulfonphthalein. Make sure you tell your doctor if you have any other medical problems, especially:

- Gout or
- Liver disease or
- Multiple myeloma (a kind of cancer)—These conditions may affect how fast the body gets rid of the phenolsulfonphthalein
- Heart or blood vessel disease or
- Kidney disease (severe)—Patients with these conditions are at greater risk of becoming ill because of the large amount of liquids that must be taken for this test

## Preparation for This Test

Your doctor will ask you to drink a certain amount of water a little while before this test is done. *Follow your doctor's instructions carefully.* Otherwise, this test may not work and may have to be done again.

## Side Effects of This Medicine

Along with its needed effects, a medicine may cause some unwanted effects. Although this medicine usually does not cause any side effects, *tell your health care professional immediately if you notice wheezing or skin rash or itching shortly after it is given.*

Other side effects not listed above may also occur in some patients. If you notice any other effects, check with your doctor.

Revised: 10/07/91
Interim revision: 05/24/94

# PHENOTHIAZINES   Systemic

Some commonly used brand names are:

**In the U.S.—**

| | |
|---|---|
| Compa-Z[9] | Prozine-50[10] |
| Compazine[9] | Serentil[4] |
| Compazine Spansule[9] | Serentil Concentrate[4] |
| Cotranzine[9] | Sparine[10] |
| Levoprome[5] | Stelazine[14] |
| Mellaril[13] | Stelazine Concentrate[14] |
| Mellaril Concentrate[13] | Thorazine[2] |
| Mellaril-S[13] | Thorazine Concentrate[2] |
| Ormazine[2] | Thorazine Spansule[2] |
| Permitil[3] | Thor-Prom[2] |
| Permitil Concentrate[3] | Tindal[1] |
| Primazine[10] | Trilafon[7] |
| Prolixin[3] | Trilafon Concentrate[7] |
| Prolixin Concentrate[3] | Ultrazine-10[9] |
| Prolixin Decanoate[3] | Vesprin[15] |
| Prolixin Enanthate[3] | |

**In Canada—**

| | |
|---|---|
| Apo-Fluphenazine[3] | Novo-Ridazine[13] |
| Apo-Perphenazine[7] | Nozinan[5] |
| Apo-Thioridazine[13] | Nozinan Liquid[5] |
| Apo-Trifluoperazine[14] | Nozinan Oral Drops[5] |
| Chlorpromanyl-5[2] | PMS Perphenazine[7] |
| Chlorpromanyl-20[2] | PMS Prochlorperazine[9] |
| Chlorpromanyl-40[2] | PMS Thioridazine[13] |
| Dartal[11] | PMS Trifluoperazine[14] |
| Largactil[2] | Prorazin[9] |
| Largactil Liquid[2] | Solazine[14] |
| Largactil Oral Drops[2] | Stelazine[14] |
| Majeptil[12] | Stelazine Concentrate[14] |
| Mellaril[13] | Stemetil[9] |
| Modecate[3] | Stemetil Liquid[9] |
| Modecate Concentrate[3] | Permitil[3] |
| Moditen Enanthate[3] | Piportil L₄[8] |
| Moditen HCl[3] | Serentil[4] |
| Moditen HCl-H.P.[3] | Terfluzine[14] |
| Neuleptil[6] | Terfluzine Concentrate[14] |
| Novo-Chlorpromazine[2] | Trilafon[7] |
| Novo-Flurazine[14] | Trilafon Concentrate[7] |

Note: For quick reference, the following phenothiazines are numbered to match the corresponding brand names.

This information applies to the following medicines:

1. Acetophenazine (a-set-oh-FEN-a-zeen)†
2. Chlorpromazine (klor-PROE-ma-zeen)‡§
3. Fluphenazine (floo-FEN-a-zeen)‡
4. Mesoridazine (mez-oh-RID-a-zeen)
5. Methotrimeprazine (meth-oh-trim-EP-ra-zeen)
6. Pericyazine (pair-ee-SYE-a-zeen)*
7. Perphenazine (per-FEN-a-zeen)‡§
8. Pipotiazine (pip-oh-TYE-a-zeen)*
9. Prochlorperazine (proe-klor-PAIR-a-zeen)‡§
10. Promazine (PROE-ma-zeen)‡§
11. Thiopropazate (thye-oh-PROE-pa-zayt)*
12. Thioproperazine (thye-oh-proe-PAIR-a-zeen)*
13. Thioridazine (thye-oh-RID-a-zeen)‡
14. Trifluoperazine (trye-floo-oh-PAIR-a-zeen)‡
15. Triflupromazine (trye-floo-PROE-ma-zeen)†

Note: This information does *not* apply to Ethopropazine, Promethazine, Propiomazine, and Trimeprazine.

---

*Not commercially available in the U.S.
†Not commercially available in Canada.
‡Generic name product may also be available in the U.S.
§Generic name product may also be available in Canada.

## Description

Phenothiazines (FEE-noe-THYE-a-zeens) are used to treat nervous, mental, and emotional disorders. Some are used also to control anxiety or agitation in certain patients, severe nausea and vomiting, severe hiccups, and moderate to severe pain in some hospitalized patients. Chlorpromazine is also used in the treatment of certain types of porphyria, and with other medicines in the treatment of tetanus. Phenothiazines may also be used for other conditions as determined by your doctor.

Phenothiazines are available only with your doctor's prescription in the following dosage forms:

*Oral*

Acetophenazine
- Tablets (U.S.)

Chlorpromazine
- Extended-release capsules (U.S.)
- Oral concentrate (U.S. and Canada)
- Syrup (U.S. and Canada)
- Tablets (U.S. and Canada)

Fluphenazine
- Elixir (U.S. and Canada)
- Oral solution (U.S.)
- Tablets (U.S. and Canada)

Mesoridazine
- Oral solution (U.S.)
- Tablets (U.S. and Canada)

Methotrimeprazine
- Oral solution (Canada)
- Syrup (Canada)
- Tablets (Canada)

Pericyazine
- Capsules (Canada)
- Oral solution (Canada)

Perphenazine
- Oral solution (U.S. and Canada)
- Syrup (Canada)
- Tablets (U.S. and Canada)

Prochlorperazine
- Extended-release capsules (U.S.)
- Syrup (U.S. and Canada)
- Tablets (U.S. and Canada)

Promazine
- Tablets (U.S.)

Thiopropazate
- Tablets (Canada)

Thioproperazine
- Tablets (Canada)

Thioridazine
- Oral solution (U.S. and Canada)
- Oral suspension (U.S. and Canada)
- Tablets (U.S. and Canada)

Trifluoperazine
- Oral solution (U.S. and Canada)
- Syrup (Canada)
- Tablets (U.S. and Canada)

*Parenteral*

Chlorpromazine
- Injection (U.S. and Canada)

Fluphenazine
- Injection (U.S. and Canada)

---

© 1994   The United States Pharmacopeial Convention, Inc.

Mesoridazine
- Injection (U.S.)

Methotrimeprazine
- Injection (U.S. and Canada)

Perphenazine
- Injection (U.S. and Canada)

Pipotiazine
- Injection (Canada)

Prochlorperazine
- Injection (U.S. and Canada)

Promazine
- Injection (U.S. and Canada)

Trifluoperazine
- Injection (U.S. and Canada)

Triflupromazine
- Injection (U.S.)

*Rectal*

Chlorpromazine
- Suppositories (U.S. and Canada)

Prochlorperazine
- Suppositories (U.S. and Canada)

## Before Using This Medicine

In deciding to use a medicine, the risks of taking the medicine must be weighed against the good it will do. This is a decision you and your doctor will make. For phenothiazines, the following should be considered:

**Allergies**—Tell your doctor if you have ever had any unusual or allergic reaction to phenothiazines. Also tell your health care professional if you are allergic to any other substances, such as foods, preservatives, or dyes.

**Pregnancy**—Although studies have not been done in pregnant women, some side effects, such as jaundice and muscle tremors and other movement disorders, have occurred in a few newborns whose mothers received phenothiazines close to the time of delivery. Studies in animals have shown that chlorpromazine and trifluoperazine, given in doses many times the usual human dose, may cause birth defects.

**Breast-feeding**—Phenothiazines pass into the breast milk and may cause drowsiness and a greater chance of unusual muscle movement in the nursing baby.

**Children**—Certain side effects, such as muscle spasms of the face, neck, and back, tic-like or twitching movements, inability to move the eyes, twisting of the body, or weakness of the arms and legs, are more likely to occur in children, especially those with severe illness or dehydration. Children are usually more sensitive than adults to some of the side effects of phenothiazines.

**Older adults**—Constipation, dizziness or fainting, drowsiness, dryness of mouth, trembling of the hands and fingers, and symptoms of tardive dyskinesia (such as rapid, worm-like movements of the tongue or any other uncontrolled movements of the mouth, tongue, or jaw, and/or arms and legs) are especially likely to occur in elderly patients, who are usually more sensitive than younger adults to the effects of phenothiazines.

**Other medicines**—Although certain medicines should not be used together at all, in other cases 2 different medicines may be used together even if an interaction might occur. In these cases, your doctor may want to change the dose, or other precautions may be necessary. When you are taking phenothiazines, it is especially important that your health care professional know if you are taking any of the following:
- Amantadine (e.g., Symmetrel) or
- Antihypertensives (high blood pressure medicine) or
- Bromocriptine (e.g., Parlodel) or
- Deferoxamine (e.g., Desferal) or
- Diuretics (water pills) or
- Levobunolol (e.g., Betagan) or
- Medicine for heart disease or
- Metipranolol (e.g., OptiPranolol) or
- Nabilone (e.g., Cesamet) (with high doses) or
- Narcotic pain medicine or
- Nimodipine (e.g., Nimotop) or
- Other antipsychotics (medicine for mental illness) or
- Pentamidine (e.g., Pentam) or
- Pimozide (e.g., Orap) or
- Promethazine (e.g., Phenergan) or
- Trimeprazine (e.g., Temaril)—Severe low blood pressure may occur
- Antidepressants (medicine for depression)—The risk of serious side effects may be increased
- Antithyroid agents (medicine for overactive thyroid) or
- Central nervous system (CNS) depressants (medicines that cause drowsiness)—There may be an increased chance of blood problems
- Epinephrine (e.g., Adrenalin)—Severe low blood pressure and fast heartbeat may occur
- Levodopa (e.g., Dopar)—Phenothiazines may prevent levodopa from working properly in the treatment of Parkinson's disease
- Lithium (e.g., Lithane, Lithizine)—The amount of medicine you need to take may change
- Methyldopa (e.g., Aldomet) or
- Metoclopramide (e.g., Reglan) or
- Metyrosine (e.g. Demser) or
- Pemoline (e.g., Cylert) or
- Rauwolfia alkaloids (alseroxylon [e.g., Rauwiloid], deserpidine [e.g., Harmonyl], rauwolfia serpentina [e.g., Raudixin], reserpine [e.g., Serpasil])—Taking these medicines with phenothiazines may increase the chance and severity of certain side effects
- Metrizamide—When this dye is used for myelograms, the risk of seizures may be increased

**Other medical problems**—The presence of other medical problems may affect the use of phenothiazines. Make sure you tell your doctor if you have any other medical problems, especially:
- Alcohol abuse—Certain side effects such as heat stroke may be more likely to occur
- Blood disease or
- Breast cancer or
- Difficult urination or
- Enlarged prostate or
- Glaucoma or
- Heart or blood vessel disease or
- Lung disease or
- Parkinson's disease or
- Seizure disorders or

- Stomach ulcers—Phenothiazines may make the condition worse
- Liver disease—Higher blood levels of phenothiazines may occur, increasing the chance of side effects
- Reye's syndrome—There may be an increased chance of unwanted effects on the liver

## Proper Use of This Medicine

For patients taking this medicine *by mouth:*

- This medicine may be taken with food or a full glass (8 ounces) of water or milk to reduce stomach irritation.
- *If your medicine comes in a dropper bottle,* measure each dose with the special dropper provided with your prescription and dilute it in ½ a glass (4 ounces) of orange or grapefruit juice or water.
- If you are taking the *extended-release capsule form* of this medicine, each dose should be swallowed whole. Do not break, crush, or chew before swallowing.

For patients using the *suppository form* of this medicine:

- If the suppository is too soft to insert, chill it in the refrigerator for 30 minutes or run cold water over it before removing the foil wrapper.
- To insert the suppository: First remove the foil wrapper and moisten the suppository with cold water. Lie down on your side and use your finger to push the suppository well up into the rectum.

*Do not take more of this medicine and do not take it more often than your doctor ordered.* This is particularly important for children or elderly patients, since they may react very strongly to this medicine.

*Sometimes this medicine must be taken for several weeks before its full effect is reached when it is used to treat mental and emotional conditions.*

**Dosing**—The dose of phenothiazines will be different for different patients. *Follow your doctor's orders or the directions on the label.* The following information includes only the average doses of phenothiazines. *If your dose is different, do not change it* unless your doctor tells you to do so.

The number of capsules, tablets, or teaspoonfuls of elixir, solution, suspension, or syrup that you take, or the number of injections you receive or suppositories that you use, depends on the strength of the medicine. Also, *the number of doses you use each day, the time allowed between doses, and the length of time you take the medicine depend on the medical problem for which you are taking phenothiazines.*

*For acetophenazine*

- For *oral* dosage form (tablets):
  - —For nervous, mental, or emotional disorders:
    - Adults and teenagers—20 milligrams (mg) three times a day. Your doctor may change your dose if needed.

- Children up to 12 years of age—Dose must be determined by your doctor.

*For chlorpromazine*

- For *oral extended-release capsule* dosage form:
  - —For nervous, mental, or emotional disorders:
    - Adults—30 to 300 milligrams (mg) one to three times a day. Your doctor may increase your dose if needed. However, the dose is usually not more than 1000 mg a day.
    - Children—This dosage form is not recommended for use in children.
- For *oral concentrate, syrup, or tablet* dosage forms:
  - —For nervous, mental, or emotional disorders:
    - Adults and teenagers—At first, 10 to 25 mg two to four times a day. Your doctor may increase your dose if needed. However, the dose is usually not more than 1000 mg a day.
    - Children up to 6 months of age—Dose must be determined by your doctor.
    - Children 6 months of age and older—Dose is based on body weight or size, and must be determined by your doctor. The usual dose is 0.55 mg per kilogram (kg) (0.25 mg per pound) of body weight, every four to six hours.
  - —For nausea and vomiting:
    - Adults and teenagers—10 to 25 mg every four hours as needed.
    - Children up to 6 months of age—Dose must be determined by your doctor.
    - Children 6 months of age and older—Dose is based on body weight or size, and must be determined by your doctor. The usual dose is 0.55 mg per kg (0.25 mg per pound) of body weight, every four to six hours.
  - —For sedation before surgery:
    - Adults and teenagers—25 to 50 mg two to three hours before surgery.
    - Children—Dose is based on body weight or size, and must be determined by your doctor. The usual dose is 0.55 mg per kg (0.25 mg per pound) of body weight, two or three hours before surgery.
  - —For treatment of hiccups:
    - Adults and teenagers—25 to 50 mg three or four times a day.
    - Children—Dose must be determined by your doctor.
  - —For porphyria:
    - Adults and teenagers—25 to 50 mg three or four times a day.
    - Children—Use and dose must be determined by your doctor.
- For *injection* dosage form:
  - —For severe nervous, mental, or emotional disorders:
    - Adults—At first, 25 to 50 mg, injected into a muscle. The dose may be repeated in one hour,

and every three to twelve hours thereafter. Your doctor may increase your dose if needed.
- Children up to 6 months of age—Dose must be determined by your doctor.
- Children 6 months of age and over—Dose is based on body weight or size and must be determined by your doctor. The usual dose is 0.55 mg per kg (0.25 mg per pound) of body weight, injected into a muscle every six to eight hours as needed.

—For nausea and vomiting:
- Adults—At first, 25 mg injected into a muscle. The dose may be increased to 25 to 50 mg every three to four hours if needed.
- Children up to 6 months of age—Dose must be determined by your doctor.
- Children 6 months of age and over—Dose is based on body weight or size and must be determined by your doctor. The usual dose is 0.55 mg per kg (0.25 mg per pound) of body weight, injected into a muscle every six to eight hours as needed.

—For nausea and vomiting during surgery:
- Adults—At first, 12.5 mg injected into a muscle. The dose may be repeated if needed. Or, up to 25 mg, diluted and injected slowly into a vein.
- Children—Dose is based on body weight or size and must be determined by your doctor. The usual dose is 0.275 mg per kg (0.125 mg per pound) of body weight, injected into a muscle, or diluted and injected slowly into a vein.

—For sedation before surgery:
- Adults—12.5 to 25 mg, injected into a muscle one or two hours before surgery.
- Children—Dose is based on body weight and must be determined by your doctor. The usual dose is 0.55 mg per kg (0.25 mg per pound) of body weight, injected into a muscle one to two hours before surgery.

—For treatment of hiccups:
- Adults—25 to 50 mg, injected into a muscle three or four times a day. Or, 25 to 50 mg diluted and injected slowly into a vein.
- Children—Dose must be determined by your doctor.

—For porphyria:
- Adults—25 mg injected into a muscle every six or eight hours.
- Children—Dose must be determined by your doctor.

—For tetanus:
- Adults—25 to 50 mg, injected into a muscle three or four times a day. Or, 25 to 50 mg, diluted and injected slowly into a vein. Your doctor may increase your dose if needed.
- Children—Dose is based on body weight and must be determined by your doctor. The usual

dose is 0.55 mg per kg (0.25 mg per pound) of body weight, injected into a muscle every six to eight hours. Or, 0.55 mg per kg (0.25 mg per pound) of body weight, diluted and injected slowly into a vein.

- For *rectal* dosage form (suppositories):
—For nausea and vomiting:
- Adults and teenagers—50 to 100 mg, inserted into the rectum every six to eight hours as needed.
- Children up to 6 months of age—Dose must be determined by your doctor.
- Children 6 months of age and over—Dose is based on body weight and must be determined by your doctor. The usual dose is 1 mg per kg (0.45 mg per pound) of body weight, inserted into the rectum every six to eight hours as needed.

*For fluphenazine*
- For *oral* dosage form (elixir, solution, or tablets):
—For nervous, mental, or emotional disorders:
- Adults—At first, 2.5 to 10 milligrams (mg) a day, taken in smaller doses every six to eight hours during the day. Your doctor may increase your dose if needed. However, the dose is usually not more than 20 mg a day.
- Children—0.25 to 0.75 mg one to four times a day.
- Older adults—1 to 2.5 mg a day. Your doctor may increase your dose if needed.
- For *long-acting decanoate injection* dosage form:
—For nervous, mental, or emotional disorders:
- Adults—At first, 12.5 to 25 mg, injected into a muscle or under the skin every one to three weeks. Your doctor may increase your dose if needed. However, the dose is usually not more than 100 mg.
- Children 5 to 12 years of age—3.125 to 12.5 mg, injected into a muscle or under the skin every one to three weeks.
- Children 12 years of age and over—At first, 6.25 to 18.75 mg a week, injected into a muscle or under the skin. Your doctor may increase your dose if needed. However, the dose is usually not more than 25 mg every one to three weeks.
- For *long-acting enanthate injection* dosage form:
—For nervous, mental, or emotional disorders:
- Adults and teenagers—25 mg, injected into a muscle or under the skin every one to three weeks. Your doctor may increase your dose if needed. However, the dose is usually not more than 100 mg.
- Children up to 12 years of age—Dose must be determined by your doctor.
- For *short-acting hydrochloride injection* dosage form:
—For nervous, mental, or emotional disorders:
- Adults and teenagers—1.25 to 2.5 mg, injected into a muscle every six to eight hours. Your doctor may increase your dose if needed. However, the dose is usually not more than 10 mg a day.

• Children up to 12 years of age—Dose must be determined by your doctor.

• Older adults—1 to 2.5 mg a day, injected into a muscle. Your doctor may increase your dose if needed.

*For mesoridazine*
• For *oral* dosage form (solution or tablets):
—For nervous, mental, or emotional disorders:
• Adults and teenagers—30 to 150 milligrams (mg), taken in smaller doses two or three times during the day.
• Children up to 12 years of age—Dose must be determined by your doctor.

• For *injection* dosage form:
—For nervous, mental, or emotional disorders:
• Adults and teenagers—25 mg injected into a muscle. The dose may be repeated in thirty to sixty minutes if needed.
• Children up to 12 years of age—Dose must be determined by your doctor.

*For methotrimeprazine*
• For *oral* dosage form (solution, syrup, or tablets):
—For nervous, mental, or emotional disorders:
• Adults and teenagers—At first, 6 to 75 milligrams (mg) a day, taken in smaller doses two or three times a day with meals. Your doctor may increase your dose if needed.
• Children—Dose is based on body weight and must be determined by your doctor. At first, the usual dose is 0.25 mg per kilogram (kg) (0.11 mg per pound) of body weight a day, taken in smaller doses two or three times a day with meals. Your doctor may increase your dose if needed.

—For pain:
• Adults and teenagers—At first, 6 to 25 mg a day, taken in smaller doses three times a day with meals. For more severe pain, 50 to 75 mg a day, taken in smaller doses two or three times a day with meals. Your doctor may increase your dose if needed.
• Children—Dose is based on body weight and must be determined by your doctor. At first, the usual dose is 0.25 mg per kg (0.11 mg per pound) of body weight a day, taken in smaller doses two or three times a day with meals. Your doctor may increase your dose if needed. However, the dose is usually not more than 40 mg a day.

—For sedation before surgery:
• Adults and teenagers—At first, 6 to 25 mg a day, taken in smaller doses three times a day with meals. Your doctor may increase your dose if needed.
• Children—Dose is based on body weight and must be determined by your doctor. At first, the usual dose is 0.25 mg per kg (0.11 mg per pound) of body weight a day, taken in smaller doses two or three times a day with meals. Your doctor

may increase your dose if needed. However, the dose is usually not more than 40 mg a day.

• For *injection* dosage form:
—For nervous, mental, or emotional disorders:
• Adults and teenagers—At first, 10 to 20 mg, injected into a muscle every four to six hours. Your doctor may increase your dose if needed.
• Children—Dose must be determined by your doctor.

—For pain:
• Adults and teenagers—At first, 2.5 to 20 mg, injected into a muscle. Your doctor may increase your dose if needed.
• Children—Dose is based on body weight and must be determined by your doctor. The usual dose is 0.062 to 0.125 mg per kg (0.028 to 0.057 mg per pound) of body weight, injected into a muscle.
• Older adults—At first, 5 to 10 mg injected into a muscle every four to six hours. Your doctor may increase your dose if needed.

—For sedation before surgery:
• Adults and teenagers—2 to 20 mg, injected into a muscle forty-five minutes to three hours before surgery.
• Children—Dose must be determined by your doctor.

*For pericyazine*
• For *oral* dosage form (capsules or solution):
—For nervous, mental, or emotional disorders:
• Adults—At first, 5 to 20 milligrams (mg) taken in the morning, and 10 to 40 mg taken in the evening. Your doctor may change your dose if needed.
• Children 5 years of age and over—2.5 to 10 mg taken in the morning, and 5 to 30 mg taken in the evening.
• Older adults—At first, 5 mg a day. Your doctor may increase your dose if needed. However, the dose is usually not more than 30 mg a day.

*For perphenazine*
• For *oral solution* dosage form:
—For nervous, mental, or emotional disorders in hospitalized patients:
• Adults and teenagers—8 to 16 milligrams (mg) two to four times a day.
• Children up to 12 years of age—Dose must be determined by your doctor.

• For *oral syrup* dosage form:
—For nervous, mental, or emotional disorders:
• Adults and teenagers—2 to 16 mg two to four times a day.
• Children up to 12 years of age—Dose must be determined by your doctor.

—For nausea and vomiting:
  • Adults and teenagers—2 to 4 mg two to four times a day.
  • Children up to 12 years of age—Dose must be determined by your doctor.
• For *oral tablet* dosage form:
  —For nervous, mental, or emotional disorders:
  • Adults and teenagers—4 to 16 mg two to four times a day.
  • Children up to 12 years of age—Dose must be determined by your doctor.
  —For nausea and vomiting:
  • Adults and teenagers—8 to 16 mg a day, taken in smaller doses during the day. Your doctor will lower your dose as soon as possible.
  • Children up to 12 years of age—Dose must be determined by your doctor.
• For *injection* dosage form:
  —For nervous, mental, or emotional disorders:
  • Adults and teenagers—5 to 10 mg injected into a muscle every six hours. Hospitalized patients may need higher doses.
  • Children up to 12 years of age—Dose must be determined by your doctor.
  —For nausea and vomiting:
  • Adults and teenagers—At first, 5 mg injected into a muscle, or diluted and injected slowly into a vein. Your doctor may increase your dose if needed.
  • Children up to 12 years of age—Dose must be determined by your doctor.

*For pipotiazine*
• For *injection* dosage form:
  —For nervous, mental, or emotional disorders:
  • Adults and teenagers—At first, 50 to 100 milligrams (mg) injected into a muscle. Your doctor may increase your dose if needed. However, the dose is usually not more than 150 mg every four weeks.
  • Children up to 12 years of age—Dose must be determined by your doctor.

*For prochlorperazine*
• For *oral syrup* dosage form:
  —For nervous, mental, or emotional disorders:
  • Adults and teenagers—At first, 5 to 10 milligrams (mg) three or four times a day. Your doctor may increase your dose if needed. However, the dose is usually not more than 150 mg a day.
  • Children up to 2 years of age—Dose must be determined by your doctor.
  • Children 2 to 12 years of age—2.5 mg two or three times a day.
  —For nausea and vomiting:
  • Adults and teenagers—5 to 10 mg three or four times a day.

  • Children—Dose is based on body weight and must be determined by your doctor. The usual dose is 2.5 mg taken one to three times a day. For children 2 to 5 years of age, the dose is usually not more than 20 mg a day. For children 6 to 12 years of age, the dose is usually not more than 25 mg a day.
  —For anxiety:
  • Adults and teenagers—5 mg three or four times a day. This dose is usually not taken for longer than twelve weeks.
  • Children—Dose must be determined by your doctor.
• For *oral extended-release capsule* dosage form:
  —For nervous, mental, or emotional disorders:
  • Adults and teenagers—At first, 5 to 10 mg every three or four hours. Your doctor may increase your dose if needed. However, the dose is usually not more than 150 mg a day.
  • Children—This dosage form is not recommended for use in children.
  —For nausea and vomiting:
  • Adults and teenagers—15 to 30 mg once a day in the morning, or 10 mg taken every twelve hours. Your doctor may increase your dose if needed. However, the dose is usually not more than 40 mg a day.
  • Children—This dosage form is not recommended for use in children.
  —For anxiety:
  • Adults and teenagers—15 mg once a day in the morning, or 10 mg taken every twelve hours. This dose is usually not taken for longer than twelve weeks.
  • Children—This dosage form is not recommended for use in children.
• For *oral tablet* dosage form:
  —For nervous, mental, or emotional disorders:
  • Adults and teenagers—5 to 10 mg three or four times a day. Your doctor may increase your dose if needed. However, the dose is usually not more than 150 mg a day.
  • Children—The tablet dosage form is often not suitable for use in children. The syrup dosage form is usually recommended.
  —For nausea and vomiting:
  • Adults and teenagers—5 to 10 mg three or four times a day.
  • Children—The tablet dosage form is often not suitable for use in children. The syrup dosage form is usually recommended.
  —For anxiety:
  • Adults and teenagers—5 mg three or four times a day. This dose is usually not taken for longer than twelve weeks.

• Children—The tablet dosage form is often not suitable for use in children. The syrup dosage form is usually recommended.
• For *injection* dosage form:
—For nervous, mental, or emotional disorders:
• Adults and teenagers—At first, 10 to 20 mg injected into a muscle. The dose may be repeated every two to four hours if needed for up to four doses. Later, the dose is usually 10 to 20 mg every four to six hours. However, the dose is usually not more than 200 mg a day.
• Children up to 2 years of age—Dose must be determined by your doctor.
• Children 2 to 12 years of age—Dose is based on body weight and must be determined by your doctor. The usual dose is 0.132 mg per kilogram (kg) (0.06 mg per pound) of body weight, injected into a muscle. However, the dose for children 2 to 5 years of age is usually not more than 20 mg a day. The dose for children 6 to 12 years of age is usually not more than 25 mg a day.
—For nausea and vomiting:
• Adults and teenagers—5 to 10 mg, injected into a muscle every three to four hours as needed. Or, 2.5 to 10 mg injected slowly into a vein. The dose is usually not more than 40 mg a day.
• Children up to 2 years of age—Dose must be determined by your doctor.
• Children 2 to 12 years of age—Dose is based on body weight and must be determined by your doctor. The usual dose is 0.132 mg per kg (0.06 mg per pound) of body weight, injected into a muscle. However, the dose for children 2 to 5 years of age is usually not more than 20 mg a day. The dose for children 6 to 12 years of age is usually not more than 25 mg a day.
—For nausea and vomiting in surgery:
• Adults and teenagers—5 to 10 mg, injected into a muscle. Or, up to 20 mg injected slowly into a vein. The dose is usually not more than 40 mg a day.
• Children—Dose must be determined by your doctor.
—For anxiety:
• Adults and teenagers—5 to 10 mg injected into a muscle every three to four hours. Or, 2.5 to 10 mg injected slowly into a vein. The dose is usually not more than 40 mg a day.
• Children up to 2 years of age—Dose must be determined by your doctor.
• Children 2 to 12 years of age—Dose is based on body weight and must be determined by your doctor. The usual dose is 0.132 mg per kg (0.06 mg per pound) of body weight, injected into a muscle. However, the dose for children 2 to 5 years of age is usually not more than 20 mg a day. The dose for children 6 to 12 years of age is usually not more than 25 mg a day.

• For *rectal* dosage form (suppositories):
—For nervous, mental, or emotional disorders:
• Adults and teenagers—10 mg inserted into the rectum three or four times a day. Your doctor may increase your dose if needed.
• Children—Dose must be determined by your doctor.
—For nausea and vomiting:
• Adults and teenagers—25 mg inserted into the rectum two times a day.
• Children up to 2 years of age—Dose must be determined by your doctor.
• Children 2 to 12 years of age—Dose is based on body weight and must be determined by your doctor. The usual dose is 2.5 mg inserted into the rectum one to three times a day. The dose in children 2 to 5 years of age is usually not more than 20 mg a day. The dose for children 6 to 12 years of age is usually not more than 25 mg a day.

*For promazine*
• For *oral* dosage form (tablets):
—For nervous, mental, or emotional disorders:
• Adults—10 to 200 milligrams (mg) every four to six hours.
• Children up to 12 years of age—Dose must be determined by your doctor.
• Children 12 years of age and over—10 to 25 mg every four to six hours.
• For *injection* dosage form:
—For nervous, mental, or emotional disorders:
• Adults—At first, 50 to 150 mg injected into a muscle, or diluted and injected into a vein. Later, 10 to 200 mg, injected into a muscle or vein, every four to six hours.
• Children up to 12 years of age—Dose must be determined by your doctor.
• Children 12 years of age and over—10 to 25 mg, injected into a muscle, every four to six hours.

*For thiopropazate*
• For *oral* dosage form (tablets):
—For nervous, mental, or emotional disorders:
• Adults and teenagers—At first, 10 milligrams (mg) three times a day. Your doctor may increase your dose if needed. However, the dose is usually not more than 100 mg a day.
• Children—Dose must be determined by your doctor.

*For thioproperazine*
• For *oral* dosage form (tablets):
—For nervous, mental, or emotional disorders:
• Adults and teenagers—At first, 5 milligrams (mg) a day. Your doctor may increase your dose if needed.

- Children—Dose must be determined by your doctor.

*For thioridazine*
- For *oral* dosage form (suspension, solution, or tablets):
  —For nervous, mental, or emotional disorders:
  - Adults and teenagers—At first, 25 to 100 milligrams (mg) three times a day. Your doctor may increase your dose if needed. However, the dose is usually not more than 800 mg a day.
  - Children up to 2 years of age—Dose must be determined by your doctor.
  - Children 2 to 12 years of age—Dose is based on body weight or size and must be determined by your doctor. The usual dose is 10 to 25 mg two or three times a day.

*For trifluoperazine*
- For *oral* dosage form (solution, syrup, or tablets):
  —For nervous, mental, or emotional disorders:
  - Adults and teenagers—At first, 2 to 5 milligrams (mg) two times a day. Your doctor may increase your dose if needed. However, the dose is usually not more than 40 mg a day.
  - Children up to 6 years of age—Dose must be determined by your doctor.
  - Children 6 years of age and over—1 mg one or two times a day.
  —For anxiety:
  - Adults and teenagers—1 to 2 mg a day. Your doctor may increase your dose if needed. However, the dose is usually not more than 6 mg a day, and is usually not taken for longer than twelve weeks.
  - Children—Dose must be determined by your doctor.
- For *injection* dosage form:
  —For nervous, mental, or emotional disorders:
  - Adults and teenagers—1 to 2 mg, injected into a muscle every four to six hours as needed. However, the dose is usually not more than 10 mg a day.
  - Children up to 6 years of age—Dose must be determined by your doctor.
  - Children 6 years of age and over—1 mg injected into a muscle one or two times a day.

*For triflupromazine*
- For *injection* dosage form:
  —For nervous, mental, or emotional disorders:
  - Adults and teenagers—60 milligrams (mg) injected into a muscle as needed. However, the dose is usually not more than 150 mg a day.
  - Children up to 2½ years of age—Dose must be determined by your doctor.
  - Children 2½ years of age and over—Dose is based on body weight and must be determined

by your doctor. The usual dose is 0.2 to 0.25 mg per kilogram (kg) (0.09 to 0.11 mg per pound) of body weight, injected into a muscle. However, the dose is usually not more than 10 mg a day.
  —For nausea and vomiting:
  - Adults and teenagers—5 to 15 mg injected into a muscle every four hours, or 1 mg injected into a vein as needed. Your doctor may increase your dose if needed. However, the dose is usually not more than 60 mg a day injected into a muscle, or 3 mg a day injected into a vein.
  - Children up to 2½ years of age—Dose must be determined by your doctor.
  - Children 2½ years of age and over—Dose is based on body weight and must be determined by your doctor. The usual dose is 0.2 to 0.25 mg per kg (0.09 to 0.11 mg per pound) of body weight, injected into a muscle. However, the dose is usually not more than 10 mg a day.

**Missed dose**—If you miss a dose of this medicine and your dosing schedule is:
- One dose a day: Take the missed dose as soon as possible. Then go back to your regular dosing schedule. However, if you do not remember the missed dose until the next day, skip it and go back to your regular dosing schedule. Do not double doses.
- More than one dose a day: If you remember within an hour or so of the missed dose, take it right away. However, if you do not remember until later, skip the missed dose and go back to your regular dosing schedule. Do not double doses.

If you have any questions about this, check with your doctor.

**Storage**—To store this medicine:
- Keep out of the reach of children.
- Store away from heat and direct light.
- Do not store the capsule or tablet form of this medicine in the bathroom, near the kitchen sink, or in other damp places. Heat or moisture may cause the medicine to break down.
- Keep the liquid form of this medicine from freezing.
- Do not keep outdated medicine or medicine no longer needed. Be sure that any discarded medicine is out of the reach of children.

---

## Precautions While Using This Medicine

Your doctor should check your progress at regular visits, especially during the first few months of treatment with this medicine. This will allow your dosage to be changed if necessary to meet your needs.

*Do not stop taking this medicine without first checking with your doctor.* Your doctor may want you to reduce gradually the amount you are taking before stopping completely. This is to prevent side effects and to keep your condition from becoming worse.

Do not take this medicine within two hours of taking antacids or medicine for diarrhea. Taking these products too close together may make this medicine less effective.

This medicine will add to the effects of alcohol and other CNS depressants (medicines that slow down the nervous system, possibly causing drowsiness). Some examples of CNS depressants are antihistamines or medicine for hay fever, other allergies, or colds; sedatives, tranquilizers, or sleeping medicine; prescription pain medicine or narcotics; barbiturates; medicine for seizures; muscle relaxants; or anesthetics, including some dental anesthetics. *Check with your doctor before taking any of the above while you are using this medicine.*

Before using any prescription or over-the-counter (OTC) medicine for colds or allergies, check with your doctor. These medicines may increase the chance of heat stroke or other unwanted effects, such as dizziness, dry mouth, blurred vision, and constipation, while you are taking a phenothiazine.

Before you have any medical tests, tell the medical doctor in charge that you are taking this medicine. The results of some tests (such as electrocardiogram [ECG] readings, certain pregnancy tests, the metyrapone test, and urine bilirubin tests) may be affected by this medicine.

*Before having any kind of surgery, dental treatment, or emergency treatment, tell the medical doctor or dentist in charge that you are using this medicine.*

This medicine may cause some people to become drowsy or less alert than they are normally. Even if this medicine is taken only at bedtime, it may cause some people to feel drowsy or less alert on arising. *Make sure you know how you react to this medicine before you drive, use machines, or do anything else that could be dangerous if you are not alert.*

Phenothiazines may cause blurred vision, difficulty in reading, or other changes in vision, especially during the first few weeks of treatment. Do not drive, use machines, or do anything else that could be dangerous if you are not able to see well. *If the problem continues or gets worse, check with your doctor.*

*Dizziness, lightheadedness, or fainting may occur,* especially when you get up from a lying or sitting position. Getting up slowly may help. If the problem continues or gets worse, check with your doctor.

This medicine may make you sweat less, causing your body temperature to increase. *Use extra care not to become overheated during exercise or hot weather while you are taking this medicine,* since overheating may result in heat stroke. Also, hot baths or saunas may make you feel dizzy or faint while you are taking this medicine.

This medicine may also make you more sensitive to cold temperatures. Dress warmly during cold weather. Be careful during prolonged exposure to cold, such as in winter sports or swimming in cold water.

*Phenothiazines may cause dryness of the mouth. For temporary relief, use sugarless candy or gum, melt bits*

*of ice in your mouth, or use a saliva substitute.* However, if your mouth continues to feel dry for more than 2 weeks, check with your medical doctor or dentist. Continuing dryness of the mouth may increase the chance of dental disease, including tooth decay, gum disease, and fungus infections.

Phenothiazines may cause your skin to be more sensitive to sunlight than it is normally. Exposure to sunlight, even for brief periods of time, may cause a skin rash, itching, redness or other discoloration of the skin, or a severe sunburn. When you begin taking this medicine:

- Stay out of direct sunlight, especially between the hours of 10:00 a.m. and 3:00 p.m., if possible.
- Wear protective clothing, including a hat. Also, wear sunglasses.
- Apply a sun block product that has a skin protection factor (SPF) of at least 15. Some patients may require a product with a higher SPF number, especially if they have a fair complexion. If you have any questions about this, check with your health care professional.
- Apply a sun block lipstick that has an SPF of at least 15 to protect your lips.
- Do not use a sunlamp or tanning bed or booth.

*If you have a severe reaction from the sun, check with your doctor.*

Phenothiazines may cause your eyes to be more sensitive to sunlight than they are normally. Exposure to sunlight over a period of time (several months to years) may cause blurred vision, change in color vision, or difficulty in seeing at night. When you go out during the daylight hours, even on cloudy days, wear sunglasses that block ultraviolet (UV) light. Ordinary sunglasses may not protect your eyes. If you have any questions about the kind of sunglasses to wear, check with your medical doctor or eye doctor.

*If you are taking a liquid form of this medicine,* avoid getting it on your skin or clothing because it may cause a skin rash or other irritation.

If you are receiving this medicine by injection:

- The effects of the long-acting injection form of this medicine may last for up to 12 weeks. *The precautions and side effects information for this medicine applies during this time.*

## Side Effects of This Medicine

Along with their needed effects, phenothiazines can sometimes cause serious side effects. Tardive dyskinesia (a movement disorder) may occur and may not go away after you stop using the medicine. Signs of tardive dyskinesia include fine, worm-like movements of the tongue, or other uncontrolled movements of the mouth, tongue, cheeks, jaw, or arms and legs. Other serious but rare side effects may also occur. These include severe muscle stiffness, fever, unusual tiredness or weakness, fast heartbeat, difficult breathing, increased sweating, loss of bladder control, and seizures (neuroleptic malignant syndrome).

*You and your doctor should discuss the good this medicine will do as well as the risks of taking it.*

*Stop taking this medicine and check with your doctor immediately* if any of the following side effects occur:

*Rare*

Convulsions (seizures); difficult or fast breathing; fast heartbeat or irregular pulse; fever; high or low blood pressure; increased sweating; loss of bladder control; muscle stiffness (severe); unusually pale skin; unusual tiredness or weakness

*Check with your doctor immediately* if any of the following side effects occur:

*More common*

Lip smacking or puckering; puffing of cheeks; rapid or fine, worm-like movements of tongue; uncontrolled chewing movements; uncontrolled movements of arms or legs

Also, check with your doctor as soon as possible if any of the following side effects occur:

*More common*

Blurred vision, change in color vision, or difficulty in seeing at night; difficulty in speaking or swallowing; fainting; inability to move eyes; loss of balance control; mask-like face; muscle spasms (especially of face, neck, and back); restlessness or need to keep moving; shuffling walk; stiffness of arms or legs; tic-like or twitching movements; trembling and shaking of hands and fingers; twisting movements of body; weakness of arms and legs

*Less common*

Difficulty in urinating; skin rash; sunburn (severe)

*Rare*

Abdominal or stomach pains; aching muscles and joints; confusion; fever and chills; hot, dry skin or lack of sweating; muscle weakness; nausea, vomiting, or diarrhea; painful, inappropriate penile erection (continuing); skin discoloration (tan or blue-gray); skin itching (severe); sore throat and fever; unusual bleeding or bruising; yellow eyes or skin

Other side effects may occur that usually do not need medical attention. These side effects may go away during treatment as your body adjusts to the medicine. However, check with your doctor if any of the following side effects continue or are bothersome:

*More common*

Constipation; decreased sweating; dizziness; drowsiness; dryness of mouth; nasal congestion

*Less common*

Changes in menstrual period; decreased sexual ability; increased sensitivity of skin to sunlight (skin rash, itching, redness or other discoloration of skin, or severe sunburn); swelling or pain in breasts; unusual secretion of milk; weight gain (unusual)

After you stop using this medicine, your body may need time to adjust. The length of time this takes depends on the amount of medicine you are using and how long you used it. During this time, check with your doctor if you notice dizziness, nausea and vomiting, stomach pain, trembling of the fingers and hands, or any of the following symptoms of tardive dyskinesia:

Lip smacking or puckering; puffing of cheeks; rapid or fine, worm-like movements of tongue; uncontrolled chewing movements; uncontrolled movements of arms or legs

Although not all of the side effects listed above have been reported for all of these medicines, they have been reported for at least one of them. However, since all of the phenothiazines are very similar, any of the above side effects may occur with any of these medicines.

Other side effects not listed above may also occur in some patients. If you notice any other effects, check with your doctor.

## Additional Information

Once a medicine has been approved for marketing for a certain use, experience may show that it is also useful for other medical problems. Although these uses are not included in product labeling, phenothiazines are used in certain patients with the following medical conditions:

- Chronic neurogenic pain (certain continuing pain conditions)
- Huntington's chorea (hereditary movement disorder)

Other than the above information, there is no additional information relating to proper use, precautions, or side effects for these uses.

Revised: 03/16/92
Interim revision: 08/23/94

# PHENOXYBENZAMINE  Systemic

A commonly used brand name in the U.S. is Dibenzyline.

## Description

Phenoxybenzamine (fen-ox-ee-BEN-za-meen) belongs to the general class of medicines called antihypertensives. It is used to treat high blood pressure (hypertension) due to a disease called pheochromocytoma.

Phenoxybenzamine blocks the effects of certain chemicals in the body. When these chemicals are present in large amounts, they cause high blood pressure.

Phenoxybenzamine may also be used for other conditions as determined by your doctor.

Phenoxybenzamine is available only with your doctor's prescription, in the following dosage form:

*Oral*
- Capsules (U.S.)

## Before Using This Medicine

In deciding to use a medicine, the risks of taking the medicine must be weighed against the good it will do. This is a decision you and your doctor will make. For phenoxybenzamine, the following should be considered:

**Allergies**—Tell your doctor if you have ever had any unusual or allergic reaction to phenoxybenzamine. Also, tell your health care professional if you are allergic to any other substances, such as foods, preservatives, or dyes.

**Pregnancy**—Phenoxybenzamine has not been studied in pregnant women or animals. Make sure your doctor knows if you are pregnant or if you may become pregnant before taking phenoxybenzamine.

**Breast-feeding**—It is not known whether phenoxybenzamine passes into breast milk. However, this medicine has not been reported to cause problems in nursing babies.

**Children**—Although there is no specific information about the use of phenoxybenzamine in children, it is not expected to cause different side effects or problems in children than it does in adults.

**Older adults**—Dizziness or lightheadedness may be more likely to occur in the elderly, who are more sensitive to the effects of phenoxybenzamine. In addition, phenoxybenzamine may reduce tolerance to cold temperatures in elderly patients.

**Other medicines**—Although certain medicines should not be used together at all, in other cases two different medicines may be used together even if an interaction might occur. In these cases, your doctor may want to change the dose, or other precautions may be necessary. Tell your health care professional if you are taking any other prescription or nonprescription (over-the-counter [OTC]) medicine.

**Other medical problems**—The presence of other medical problems may affect the use of phenoxybenzamine. Make sure you tell your doctor if you have any other medical problems, especially:
- Angina (chest pain) or
- Heart or blood vessel disease—Some kinds may be worsened by phenoxybenzamine
- Kidney disease—Effects may be increased
- Lung infection—Symptoms such as stuffy nose may be worsened
- Recent heart attack or stroke—Lowering blood pressure may make problems resulting from stroke or heart attack worse

## Proper Use of This Medicine

To help you remember to take your medicine, try to get into the habit of taking it at the same time each day.

**Dosing**—The dose of phenoxybenzamine will be different for different patients. *Follow your doctor's orders or the directions on the label.* The following information includes only the average doses of phenoxybenzamine. *If your dose is different, do not change it* unless your doctor tells you to do so.
- For *oral* dosage form (capsules):
  —For high blood pressure caused by pheochromocytoma:
    - Adults—At first, 10 milligrams (mg) two times a day. Then, your doctor may increase your dose to 20 to 40 mg two or three times a day.
    - Children—Dose is based on body weight and must be determined by your doctor. The usual starting dose is 0.2 mg per kilogram (kg) (0.09 mg per pound) of body weight taken once a day. Then, your doctor may increase your dose to 0.4 to 1.2 mg per kg (0.18 to 0.55 mg per pound) of body weight a day. This is divided into three or four doses.

**Missed dose**—If you miss a dose of this medicine, take it as soon as you remember. However, if it is almost time for your next dose, skip the missed dose and go back to your regular dosing schedule. Do not double doses.

**Storage**—To store this medicine:
- Keep out of the reach of children.
- Store away from heat and direct light.
- Do not store in the bathroom, near the kitchen sink, or in other damp places. Heat or moisture may cause the medicine to break down.
- Do not keep outdated medicine or medicine no longer needed. Be sure that any discarded medicine is out of the reach of children.

## Precautions While Using This Medicine

It is important that your doctor check your progress at regular visits to make sure that this medicine is working properly and to check for unwanted effects.

*Do not take other medicines unless they have been discussed with your doctor.* This especially includes over-the-counter (nonprescription) medicines for appetite control, asthma, colds, cough, hay fever, or sinus problems, since they may interfere with the effects of this medicine.

Phenoxybenzamine may cause some people to become dizzy, drowsy, or less alert than they are normally. This is more likely to happen when you begin to take it or when you increase the amount of medicine you are taking. *Make sure you know how you react to this medicine before you drive, use machines, or do anything else that could be dangerous if you are dizzy or not alert.*

*Dizziness, lightheadedness, or fainting may occur, especially when you get up from a lying or sitting position. Getting up slowly may help,* but if the problem continues or gets worse, check with your doctor.

The dizziness, lightheadedness, or fainting is also more likely to occur if you drink alcohol, stand for a long time, exercise, or if the weather is hot. *While you are taking this medicine, be careful in the amount of alcohol you drink. Also, use extra care during exercise or hot weather or if you must stand for a long time.*

Before having any kind of surgery (including dental surgery) or emergency treatment, *tell the medical doctor or dentist in charge that you are using this medicine.*

Phenoxybenzamine may cause dryness of the mouth, nose, and throat. For temporary relief of mouth dryness, use sugarless candy or gum, melt bits of ice in your mouth, or use a saliva substitute. However, if dry mouth continues for more than 2 weeks, check with your medical doctor or dentist. Continuing dryness of the mouth may increase the chance of dental disease, including tooth decay, gum disease, and fungus infections.

## Side Effects of This Medicine

In rats and mice, phenoxybenzamine has been found to increase the risk of development of malignant tumors. It is not known if phenoxybenzamine increases the chance of tumors in humans.

Along with its needed effects, a medicine may cause some unwanted effects. The following side effects may go away as your body adjusts to the medicine. However, check with your doctor if any of these effects continue or are bothersome:

*More common*
    Dizziness or lightheadedness, especially when getting up from a lying or sitting position; fast heartbeat; pinpoint pupils; stuffy nose

*Less common*
    Confusion; drowsiness; dryness of mouth; headache; lack of energy; sexual problems in males; unusual tiredness or weakness

Other side effects not listed above may also occur in some patients. If you notice any other effects, check with your doctor.

## Additional Information

Once a medicine has been approved for marketing for a certain use, experience may show that it is also useful for other medical problems. Although this use is not included in product labeling, phenoxybenzamine is used in certain patients with the following medical condition:

• Benign prostatic hypertrophy

Other than the above information, there is no additional information relating to proper use, precautions, or side effects for this use.

Revised: 09/20/92
Interim revision: 07/20/94

# PHENTOLAMINE AND PAPAVERINE    Intracavernosal

Some commonly used brand names for phentolamine are:
**In the U.S.—**
    Regitine
    Generic name product may also be available.
**In Canada—**
    Rogitine
    Generic name product may also be available.

## Description

Phentolamine (fen-TOLE-a-meen) given by injection causes blood vessels to expand, thereby increasing blood flow. When it is used in combination with papaverine (pa-PAV-er-een), another medicine that has this effect, and is injected into the penis (intracavernosal), it increases blood flow to the penis, which results in an erection. This combination is used to treat some men who are impotent.

This medicine should not be used as a sexual aid by men who are not impotent. If the medicine is not used properly, permanent damage to the penis and loss of the ability to have erections could result.

Phentolamine and papaverine are available only with your doctor's prescription, in the following dosage form:
*Parenteral*
    • Injection (U.S. and Canada)

## Before Using This Medicine

In deciding to use a medicine, the risks of taking the medicine must be weighed against the good it will do. This is a decision you and your doctor will make. For papaverine and phentolamine, the following should be considered:

**Allergies**—Tell your doctor if you have ever had any unusual or allergic reaction to papaverine or phentolamine. Also tell your health care professional if you are allergic to any other substances, such as foods, preservatives, or dyes.

**Older adults**—Many medicines have not been studied specifically in older people. Therefore, it may not be known whether they work exactly the same way they do in younger adults or if they cause different side effects or problems in older people. Although there is no specific information comparing the use of phentolamine and papaverine for impotence in the elderly, it is not expected to cause different side effects or problems in older people than it does in younger adults.

**Other medicines**—Although certain medicines should not be used together at all, in other cases two different medicines may be used together even if an interaction might occur. In these cases, your doctor may want to change the dose, or other precautions may be necessary. Tell your health care professional if you are taking any other prescription or nonprescription (over-the-counter [OTC]) medicine.

**Other medical problems**—The presence of other medical problems may affect the use of papaverine and phentolamine. Make sure you tell your doctor if you have any other medical problems, especially:
- Bleeding problems—These conditions increase the risk of bleeding at the place of injection
- Liver disease—Papaverine can cause liver damage when it is given in ways that allow it to get into the bloodstream (by mouth or by injection into a muscle, a vein, or an artery); when papaverine is given by intracavernosal injection, liver damage is much less likely because the medicine enters the bloodstream very slowly
- Priapism (history of) or
- Sickle cell disease—Patients with these conditions have an increased risk of priapism (erection lasting longer than 4 hours) while using papaverine and phentolamine

## Proper Use of This Medicine

To give the injection:
- Cleanse the injection site with alcohol. Using a sterile needle, *inject the medicine slowly and directly into the base of the penis as instructed by your doctor. It should not be injected just under the skin.* The injection is usually not painful, although you may feel some tingling in the tip of your penis. If the injection is very painful or you notice bruising or swelling at the place of injection, that means you are injecting the medicine under the skin. Stop, withdraw the needle, and reposition it properly before continuing with the injection.

- After you have completed the injection, put pressure on the place of injection to prevent bruising. Then massage your penis as instructed by your doctor. This helps the medicine spread to all parts of the penis, so that it will work better.

This medicine usually begins to work in about 10 minutes. You should attempt intercourse within 2 hours after injecting the medicine.

**Dosing**—The dose of phentolamine will be different for different patients. *Follow your doctor's orders or the directions on the label.* The following information includes only the average doses of phentolamine. *If your dose is different, do not change it* unless your doctor tells you to do so.
- For *injection* dosage form:
  —For the treatment of impotence:
    - Adults—First, add one milliliter (mL) of sterile water for injection to the phentolamine powder. Second, mix 0.5 to 1 milligram (mg) (0.1 to 0.2 mL) of phentolamine injection with 30 to 60 mg of papaverine injection in your syringe. Inject this medicine very slowly into the area of your penis as directed by your doctor. Allow one or two minutes to completely inject the dose. Do not inject more than one dose in a day. Also, do not use this medicine more than two days in a row or more than three times a week.

**Storage**—To store this medicine:
- Keep out of the reach of children.
- Store away from heat and direct light.
- Keep the medicine from freezing.

## Precautions While Using This Medicine

*Use the injection exactly as directed by your doctor.* Do not use more of it and do not use it more often than ordered. If too much is used, the erection may become so strong that it lasts too long and does not reverse when it should. This condition is called priapism, and it can be very dangerous. If the effect is not reversed, the blood supply to the penis may be cut off and permanent damage may occur.

*Contact your doctor immediately if the erection lasts for longer than 4 hours or if it becomes painful.* This may be a sign of priapism and must be treated right away to prevent permanent damage.

If you notice bleeding at the site when you inject the medicine, put pressure on the spot until the bleeding stops. If it doesn't stop, check with your doctor.

It is important for you to examine your penis regularly. Check with your doctor if you find a lump where the medicine has been injected or if you notice that your penis is becoming curved. These may be signs that unwanted tissue is growing (called fibrosis), which should be seen by your doctor.

## Side Effects of This Medicine

Along with its needed effects, a medicine may cause some unwanted effects. Although not all of these side effects may occur, if they do occur they may need medical attention.

*Check with your doctor immediately* if the following side effects occur:

*Rare*

Erection continuing for more than 4 hours, or painful erection

Check with your doctor as soon as possible if the following side effects occur:

*Rare*

Dizziness; lumps in the penis

Other side effects may occur that usually do not need medical attention. These side effects may go away during treatment as your body adjusts to the medicine. However, check with your doctor if any of the following side effects continue or are bothersome:

*Less common or rare*

Bruising or bleeding at place of injection; burning (mild) along penis; difficulty in ejaculating; swelling at place of injection

Phentolamine and papaverine injected into the penis may cause tingling at the tip of the penis. This is no cause for concern.

Other side effects not listed above may also occur in some patients. If you notice any other effects, check with your doctor.

---

Revised: 09/20/92
Interim revision: 06/07/94

---

# PHENYLEPHRINE   Nasal

Some commonly used brand names are:

**In the U.S.**

| | |
|---|---|
| Alconefrin Nasal Drops 12 | Neo-Synephrine Pediatric |
| Alconefrin Nasal Drops 25 | Nasal Drops |
| Alconefrin Nasal Drops 50 | Nostril Spray Pump |
| Alconefrin Nasal Spray 25 | Nostril Spray Pump Mild |
| Doktors | Rhinall |
| Duration | Rhinall-10 Children's Flavored |
| Neo-Synephrine Nasal Drops | Nose Drops |
| Neo-Synephrine Nasal Jelly | Vicks Sinex |
| Neo-Synephrine Nasal Spray | |

Generic name product may also be available.

**In Canada**

Neo-Synephrine Nasal Drops        Neo-Synephrine Nasal Spray

## Description

Phenylephrine (fen-ill-EF-rin) is used for the temporary relief of congestion or stuffiness in the nose caused by hay fever or other allergies, colds, or sinus trouble. It may also be used in ear infections to relieve congestion.

This medicine may also be used for other conditions as determined by your doctor.

This medicine is available without a prescription; however, your doctor may have special instructions on the proper use or dose for your medical condition.

Phenylephrine is available in the following dosage forms:

*Nasal*

- Nasal jelly (U.S.)
- Nasal drops (U.S. and Canada)
- Nasal spray (U.S. and Canada)

## Before Using This Medicine

If you are using this medicine without a prescription, carefully read and follow any precautions on the label.

For nasal phenylephrine, the following should be considered:

**Allergies**—Tell your doctor if you have ever had any unusual or allergic reaction to phenylephrine or to any other nasal decongestant. Also tell your health care professional if you are allergic to any other substances, such as foods, preservatives, or dyes.

**Pregnancy**—Nasal phenylephrine may be absorbed into the body. However, nasal phenylephrine has not been shown to cause birth defects or other problems in humans.

**Breast-feeding**—Nasal phenylephrine may be absorbed into the body. However, it is not known whether phenylephrine passes into the breast milk. This medicine has not been reported to cause problems in nursing babies.

**Children**—Children may be especially sensitive to the effects of nasal phenylephrine. This may increase the chance of side effects during treatment.

**Older adults**—Many medicines have not been studied specifically in older people. Therefore, it may not be known whether they work exactly the same way they do in younger adults or if they cause different side effects or problems in older people. There is no specific information comparing use of nasal phenylephrine in the elderly with use in other age groups.

**Other medicines**—Although certain medicines should not be used together at all, in other cases two different medicines may be used together even if an interaction might occur. In these cases, your doctor may want to change the dose, or other precautions may be necessary. Tell your health care professional if you are using any other prescription or nonprescription (over-the-counter [OTC]) medicine.

**Other medical problems**—The presence of other medical problems may affect the use of nasal phenylephrine. Make sure you tell your doctor if you have any other medical problems, especially:

- Diabetes mellitus (sugar diabetes) or
- Heart or blood vessel disease or
- High blood pressure or
- Overactive thyroid—Nasal phenylephrine may make the condition worse

## Proper Use of This Medicine

To use the *nose drops:*

- Blow your nose gently. Tilt the head back while standing or sitting up, or lie down on a bed and hang head over the side. Place the drops into each nostril and keep the head tilted back for a few minutes to allow the medicine to spread throughout the nose.
- Rinse the dropper with hot water and dry with a clean tissue. Replace the cap right after use.
- To avoid spreading the infection, do not use the container for more than one person.

To use the *nose spray:*

- Blow your nose gently. With the head upright, spray the medicine into each nostril. Sniff briskly while squeezing the bottle quickly and firmly. For best results, spray once or twice into each nostril and wait 3 to 5 minutes to allow the medicine to work. Then, blow your nose gently and thoroughly. Repeat until the complete dose is used.
- Rinse the tip of the spray bottle with hot water, taking care not to suck water into the bottle, and dry with a clean tissue. Replace the cap right after use.
- To avoid spreading the infection, do not use the container for more than one person.

To use the *nose jelly:*

- Blow your nose gently. Wash your hands before applying the medicine. With your finger, place a small amount of jelly (about the size of a pea) up each nostril. Sniff it well back into the nose.
- Wipe the tip of the tube with a clean, damp tissue and replace the cap right after use.

*Use this medicine only as directed.* Do not use more of it, do not use it more often, and do not use it for longer than 3 days without first checking with your doctor. To do so may make your runny or stuffy nose worse and may also increase the chance of side effects.

**Dosing**—The dose of nasal phenylephrine will be different for different patients. *Follow your doctor's orders or the directions on the label.* The following information includes only the average doses of nasal phenylephrine. *If your dose is different, do not change it* unless your doctor tells you to do so.

- For stuffy nose:

  —For *nose jelly* dosage form:

  - Adults—Use a small amount in the nose every three or four hours as needed.

- Children—Use is not recommended.

—For *nose drops* dosage form:

- Adults and children 12 years of age and older—Use two or three drops of a 0.25 to 0.5% solution in the nose every four hours as needed.
- Children 6 to 12 years of age—Use two or three drops of a 0.25% solution in the nose every four hours as needed.
- Children 2 to 6 years of age—Use two or three drops of a 0.125 or 0.16% solution in the nose every four hours as needed.
- Children up to 2 years of age—Use and dose must be determined by your doctor.

—For *nose spray* dosage form:

- Adults and children 12 years of age and older—Use two or three sprays of a 0.25 to 0.5% solution in the nose every four hours as needed.
- Children 6 to 12 years of age—Use two or three sprays of a 0.25% solution in the nose every four hours as needed.
- Children up to 6 years of age—Use and dose must be determined by your doctor.

**Missed dose**—If you are using this medicine on a regular schedule and you miss a dose, use it right away if you remember within an hour or so of the missed dose. However, if you do not remember until later, skip the missed dose and go back to your regular dosing schedule. Do not double doses.

**Storage**—To store this medicine:

- Keep out of the reach of children.
- Store away from heat and direct light.
- Keep the medicine from freezing.
- Do not keep outdated medicine or medicine no longer needed. Be sure that any discarded medicine is out of the reach of children.

## Side Effects of This Medicine

Along with its needed effects, a medicine may cause some unwanted effects. Although not all of these side effects may occur, if they do occur they may need medical attention.

When this medicine is used for short periods of time at low doses, side effects usually are rare. However, check with your doctor as soon as possible if any of the following occur:

Increase in runny or stuffy nose

*Symptoms of too much medicine being absorbed into the body*

Fast, irregular, or pounding heartbeat; headache or dizziness; increased sweating; nervousness; paleness; trembling; trouble in sleeping

Note: The above side effects are more likely to occur in children because there is a greater chance that too much of this medicine may be absorbed into the body.

Other side effects may occur that usually do not need medical attention. These side effects may go away during

treatment as your body adjusts to the medicine. However, check with your health care professional if any of the following side effects continue or are bothersome:

Burning, dryness, or stinging of inside of nose

Other side effects not listed above may also occur in some patients. If you notice any other effects, check with your health care professional.

Revised: 05/16/94

---

# PHENYLEPHRINE   Ophthalmic

Some commonly used brand names are:

**In the U.S.—**

| | |
|---|---|
| Ak-Dilate | Ocugestrin |
| Ak-Nefrin | Ocu-Phrin Sterile Eye Drops |
| Dilatair | Ocu-Phrin Sterile Ophthalmic |
| I-Phrine | Solution |
| Isopto Frin | Prefrin Liquifilm |
| Mydfrin | Relief Eye Drops for Red Eyes |
| Neo-Synephrine | |

Generic name product may also be available.

**In Canada—**

| | |
|---|---|
| Ak-Dilate | Prefrin Liquifilm |
| Minims Phenylephrine | Spersaphrine |
| Mydfrin | |

## Description

Ophthalmic phenylephrine (fen-ill-EF-rin) in strengths of 2.5 and 10% is used to dilate (enlarge) the pupil. It is used before eye examinations, before and after eye surgery, and to treat certain eye conditions. These preparations are available only with your doctor's prescription.

Ophthalmic phenylephrine in the strength of 0.12% is used to relieve redness due to minor irritations of the eye, such as those caused by allergy, dust, smoke, wind, and other irritants. This preparation is available without a prescription; however, your doctor may have special instructions on the proper use of phenylephrine for your eye problem.

Phenylephrine is available in the following dosage form:

*Ophthalmic*
- Ophthalmic solution (eye drops) (U.S. and Canada)

## Before Using This Medicine

In deciding to use a medicine, the risks of taking the medicine must be weighed against the good it will do. This is a decision you and your doctor will make. For phenylephrine, the following should be considered:

**Allergies**—Tell your doctor if you have ever had any unusual or allergic reaction to phenylephrine or to sulfites. Also tell your health care professional if you are allergic to any other substances, such as preservatives.

**Pregnancy**—Ophthalmic phenylephrine may be absorbed into the body. However, studies on effects in pregnancy have not been done in either humans or animals.

**Breast-feeding**—Ophthalmic phenylephrine may be absorbed into the mother's body. However, it is not known whether phenylephrine passes into the breast milk. This medicine has not been reported to cause problems in nursing babies.

**Children**—Children may be especially sensitive to the effects of phenylephrine. This may increase the chance of side effects during treatment. In addition, the 10% strength is not recommended for use in infants. Also, the 2.5 and 10% strengths are not recommended for use in low birth weight infants.

**Older adults**—Repeated use of 2.5 or 10% phenylephrine may increase the chance of problems during treatment with this medicine. In addition, heart and blood vessel problems have occurred more often in elderly patients than in younger adults.

**Other medicines**—Although certain medicines should not be used together at all, in other cases two different medicines may be used together even if an interaction might occur. In these cases, your doctor may want to change the dose, or other precautions may be necessary. Tell your health care professional if you are using any other prescription or nonprescription (over-the-counter [OTC]) medicine.

**Other medical problems**—The presence of other medical problems may affect the use of phenylephrine. Make sure you tell your doctor if you have any other medical problems, especially:

- Diabetes mellitus (sugar diabetes) or
- Heart or blood vessel disease or
- High blood pressure—The 2.5 and 10% strengths of phenylephrine may make the condition worse
- Idiopathic orthostatic hypotension (low blood pressure of a certain kind)—Use of this medicine may cause a large increase in blood pressure to occur

## Proper Use of This Medicine

Do not use if the solution turns brown or becomes cloudy.

To use:

- First, wash your hands. With the middle finger, apply pressure to the inside corner of the eye (and continue to apply pressure for 2 or 3 minutes after the medicine has been placed in the eye). Tilt the head back and with the index finger of the same hand, pull the lower eyelid away from eye to form a pouch. Drop the medicine into the pouch and gently close the eyes. Do not blink. Keep the eyes closed for 1 or 2 minutes to allow the medicine to be absorbed.

- Immediately after using the eye drops, wash your hands to remove any medicine that may be on them.
- To keep the medicine as germ-free as possible, do not touch the applicator tip to any surface (including the eye). Also, keep the container tightly closed.

For patients using the *2.5 or 10% eye drops:*

- *It is very important that you use this medicine only as directed.* Do not use more of it and do not use it more often than your doctor ordered. To do so may increase the chance of too much medicine being absorbed into the body and the chance of side effects. *This is especially important when this medicine is used in children or in patients with heart disease or high blood pressure,* since high doses of this medicine may cause an irregular heartbeat and an increase in blood pressure.

**Dosing**—The dose of ophthalmic phenylephrine will be different for different patients. *Follow your doctor's orders or the directions on the label.* The following information includes only the average doses of ophthalmic phenylephrine. *If your dose is different, do not change it* unless your doctor tells you to do so.

- For *ophthalmic solution (eye drops)* dosage form:
  —For eye redness:
    - Adults and children—Use one drop of 0.12% solution every three or four hours as needed.
  —For eye exams:
    - Adults and children—Use one drop of 2.5% solution. Depending on the eye test to be done, it will take from fifteen minutes to one or two hours for the medicine to work before you can have the eye test.
  —For use before eye surgery:
    - Adults and children—Use one drop of 2.5 or 10% solution thirty to sixty minutes before the start of eye surgery.
  —For certain eye conditions:
    - Adults and children—Depending on the eye condition being treated, your doctor may tell you to use one drop of 2.5 or 10% solution in the eye from once a day to three times a day.

**Missed dose**—If you are using the 2.5 or 10% eye drops and you miss a dose of this medicine, apply it as soon as possible. However, if it is almost time for your next dose, skip the missed dose and go back to your regular dosing schedule. Do not double doses.

**Storage**—To store this medicine:

- Keep out of the reach of children.
- Store away from heat and direct light.
- Keep the medicine from freezing.

- Do not keep outdated medicine or medicine no longer needed. Be sure that any discarded medicine is out of the reach of children.

---

## Precautions While Using This Medicine

*If eye pain or change in vision occurs or if redness or irritation of the eye continues, gets worse, or lasts for more than 72 hours, stop using the medicine and check with your doctor.*

For patients using the *2.5 or 10% eye drops:*

- After you apply this medicine to your eyes, your pupils will become unusually large. This will cause your eyes to become more sensitive to light than they are normally. *When you go out during the daylight hours, even on cloudy days, wear sunglasses that block ultraviolet (UV) light to protect your eyes from sunlight and other bright lights.* Ordinary sunglasses may not protect your eyes. If you have any questions about the kind of sunglasses to wear, check with your doctor. Also, if this effect continues for longer than 12 hours after you have stopped using this medicine, check with your doctor.

---

## Side Effects of This Medicine

Along with its needed effects, a medicine may cause some unwanted effects. Although not all of these side effects may occur, if they do occur they may need medical attention.

Check with your doctor as soon as possible if any of the following side effects occur:

*Symptoms of too much medicine being absorbed into the body—Less common with 10% solution; rare with 2.5% or weaker solution*

Dizziness; fast, irregular, or pounding heartbeat; increased sweating; increase in blood pressure; paleness; trembling

Other side effects may occur that usually do not need medical attention. These side effects may go away during treatment as your body adjusts to the medicine. However, check with your doctor if any of the following side effects continue or are bothersome:

*More common with 2.5 or 10% solution*

Burning or stinging of eyes; headache or browache; sensitivity of eyes to light; watering of eyes

*Less common*

Eye irritation not present before use of this medicine

Other side effects not listed above may also occur in some patients. If you notice any other effects, check with your doctor.

---

Revised: 05/14/92
Interim revision: 02/17/94

---

# PHENYLPROPANOLAMINE Systemic†

Some commonly used brand names are:

**In the U.S.—**

Acutrim 16 Hour
Acutrim Late Day
Acutrim II Maximum
  Strength
Control
Dexatrim Maximum Strength
  Caplets
Dexatrim Maximum Strength
  Capsules

Dexatrim Maximum Strength
  Tablets
Diet-Aid Maximum Strength
Efed II Yellow
Phenyldrine
Prolamine
Propagest

Generic name product may also be available.

Another commonly used name is PPA.

†Not commercially available in Canada.

## Description

Phenylpropanolamine (fen-ill-proe-pa-NOLE-a-meen), commonly known as PPA, is used as a nasal decongestant or as an appetite suppressant. It acts on many different parts of the body. PPA produces effects that may be helpful or harmful. This depends on a patient's individual condition and response and the amount of medicine taken.

Phenylpropanolamine clears nasal congestion (stuffy nose) by narrowing or constricting the blood vessels. However, this same action may cause an increase in blood pressure in patients who have hypertension (high blood pressure).

Phenylpropanolamine also decreases appetite. However, the way PPA and similar medicines do this is unclear. Stimulation of the central nervous system (CNS) may be a major reason. Phenylpropanolamine in combination with dieting, exercise, and changes in eating habits can help obese patients lose weight. However, this appetite-reducing effect is only temporary, and is useful only for the first few weeks of dieting until new eating habits are established.

Phenylpropanolamine has caused serious side effects (even death) when too much was taken.

There are a number of products on the market that contain only phenylpropanolamine. Other products contain PPA along with added ingredients. The information that follows is for PPA alone. There may be additional information for the combination products. Read the label of the product you are using. If you have questions or if you want more information about the other ingredients, check with your health care professional.

Some preparations containing PPA are available only with your doctor's prescription. Others are available without a prescription; however, your doctor may have special instructions on the proper use of this medicine.

Phenylpropanolamine is available in the following dosage forms:

*Oral*
- Capsules (U.S.)
- Extended-release capsules (U.S.)
- Tablets (U.S.)
- Extended-release tablets (U.S.)

## Before Using This Medicine

If you are taking this medicine without a prescription, carefully read and follow any precautions on the label. For phenylpropanolamine, the following should be considered:

**Allergies**—Tell your doctor if you have ever had any unusual or allergic reaction to phenylpropanolamine or to amphetamine, dextroamphetamine, ephedrine, epinephrine, isoproterenol, metaproterenol, methamphetamine, norepinephrine, phenylephrine, pseudoephedrine, or terbutaline. Also tell your health care professional if you are allergic to any other substances, such as foods, preservatives, or dyes.

**Pregnancy**—Phenylpropanolamine has not been shown to cause birth defects in humans. However, women who take phenylpropanolamine in the weeks following delivery may be more likely to suffer mental or mood changes.

**Breast-feeding**—Phenylpropanolamine has not been reported to cause problems in nursing babies.

**Children**—Mental changes may be more likely to occur in young children taking phenylpropanolamine than in adults. Phenylpropanolamine should not be used for weight control in children under the age of 12 years. Children 12 to 18 years old should not take phenylpropanolamine for weight control unless its use is ordered and supervised by a doctor.

**Older adults**—Many medicines have not been studied specifically in older people. Therefore, it may not be known whether they work exactly the same way they do in younger adults or if they cause different side effects or problems in older people. There is no specific information comparing use of phenylpropanolamine in the elderly with use in other age groups.

**Other medicines**—Although certain medicines should not be used together at all, in other cases 2 different medicines may be used together even if an interaction might occur. In these cases, your doctor may want to change the dose, or other precautions may be necessary. When you are taking phenylpropanolamine, it is especially important that your health care professional know if you are taking any of the following:

- Amantadine (e.g., Symmetrel) or
- Amphetamines or
- Caffeine (e.g., NoDoz) or
- Chlophedianol (e.g., Ulone) or
- Cocaine or
- Medicine for asthma or other breathing problems or
- Methylphenidate (e.g., Ritalin) or
- Nabilone (e.g., Cesamet) or
- Other appetite suppressants (diet pills) or
- Other medicine for colds, sinus problems, or hay fever or other allergies (including nose drops or sprays) or

- Pemoline (e.g., Cylert)—Using these medicines while taking phenylpropanolamine may cause severe nervousness, irritability, trouble in sleeping, or possibly irregular heartbeat or seizures
- Beta-blockers (acebutolol [e.g., Sectral], atenolol [e.g., Tenormin], betaxolol [e.g., Kerlone], carteolol [e.g., Cartrol], labetalol [e.g., Normodyne], metoprolol [e.g., Lopressor], nadolol [e.g., Corgard], oxprenolol [e.g., Trasicor], penbutolol [e.g., Levatol], pindolol [e.g., Visken], propranolol [e.g., Inderal], sotalol [e.g., Sotacor], timolol [e.g., Blocadren])—Taking these medicines with phenylpropanolamine may cause serious high blood pressure (hypertension) and other effects on the heart
- Digitalis glycosides (heart medicine)—Changes in the rhythm of your heart may occur
- Monoamine oxidase (MAO) inhibitors (furazolidone [e.g., Furoxone], isocarboxazid [e.g., Marplan], phenelzine [e.g., Nardil], procarbazine [e.g., Matulane], selegiline [e.g., Eldepryl], tranylcypromine [e.g., Parnate])—Taking phenylpropanolamine while you are taking or within 2 weeks of taking MAO inhibitors may cause sudden high body temperature, extremely high blood pressure, and severe convulsions; at least 14 days should be allowed between stopping treatment with one medicine and starting treatment with the other
- Rauwolfia alkaloids (alseroxylon [e.g., Rauwiloid], deserpidine [e.g., Harmonyl], rauwolfia serpentina [e.g., Raudixin], reserpine [e.g., Serpasil])—Phenylpropanolamine may not work properly when taken with rauwolfia alkaloids

**Other medical problems**—The presence of other medical problems may affect the use of phenylpropanolamine. Make sure you tell your doctor if you have any other medical problems, especially:

- Diabetes mellitus (sugar diabetes)—Use of phenylpropanolamine may cause an increase in blood glucose levels
- Enlarged prostate or
- Glaucoma or
- High blood pressure—Use of phenylpropanolamine may make the condition worse
- Heart or blood vessel disease (including a history of heart attack or stroke) or
- Overactive thyroid—Serious effects on the heart may occur
- Mental illness, history of—Use of phenylpropanolamine may cause the mental illness to return

## Proper Use of This Medicine

For patients taking an *extended-release form* of this medicine:

- Swallow the capsule or tablet whole. Do not crush, break, or chew before swallowing.
- Take with a full glass (at least 8 ounces) of water.
- If taking only one dose of this medicine a day, take it in the morning around 10 a.m.

*Take phenylpropanolamine (PPA) only as directed.* Do not take more of it, do not take it more often, and do not take it for a longer time than directed. To do so may increase the chance of side effects.

For patients taking this medicine *as an appetite suppressant:*

- *Do not take this medicine for longer than a few weeks without your doctor's permission.*

If PPA causes trouble in sleeping, take the last dose for each day a few hours before bedtime.

**Dosing**—The dose of phenylpropanolamine will be different for different patients. *Follow your doctor's orders or the directions on the label.* The following information includes only the average doses of phenylpropanolamine. *If your dose is different, do not change it* unless your doctor tells you to do so.

The number of capsules or tablets that you take depends on the strength of the medicine. Also, *the number of doses you take each day, the time allowed between doses, and the length of time you take the medicine depend on the medical problem for which you are taking phenylpropanolamine.*

- For appetite control:
  - —For *oral* dosage forms (capsules and tablets):
    - Adults—25 mg three times a day. Do not take more than 75 mg in twenty-four hours.
    - Children 12 to 18 years of age—Use and dose must be determined by your doctor.
    - Children up to 12 years of age—Use is not recommended.
  - —For *long-acting* dosage forms (extended-release capsules and tablets):
    - Adults—75 mg taken once a day in the morning around 10 a.m.
    - Children 12 to 18 years of age—Use and dose must be determined by your doctor.
    - Children up to 12 years of age—Use is not recommended.
- For stuffy nose:
  - —For *capsule and tablet* dosage forms:
    - Adults and children 12 to 18 years of age—25 mg every four hours as needed. Do not take more than 150 mg in twenty-four hours.
    - Children 6 to 12 years of age—12.5 mg every four hours as needed. Do not take more than 75 mg in twenty-four hours.
    - Children 2 to 6 years of age—6.25 mg every four hours as needed. Do not take more than 37.5 mg in twenty-four hours.
    - Children up to 2 years of age—Use and dose must be determined by your doctor.
  - —For *extended-release capsule* dosage form:
    - Adults—75 mg every twelve hours.
    - Children—Use and dose must be determined by your doctor.

**Missed dose**—For patients taking phenylpropanolamine *for nasal congestion:* If you miss a dose, take it as soon as possible. However, if it is within 2 hours (or 12 hours for extended-release forms) of your next dose, skip the missed dose and go back to your regular dosing schedule. Do not double doses.

**Storage**—To store this medicine:

- Keep out of the reach of children.
- Store away from heat and direct light.
- Do not store in the bathroom, near the kitchen sink, or in other damp places. Heat or moisture may cause the medicine to break down.
- Do not keep outdated medicine or medicine no longer needed. Be sure that any discarded medicine is out of the reach of children.

## Precautions While Using This Medicine

Do not drink large amounts of caffeine-containing coffee, tea, or colas while you are taking this medicine. To do so may cause unwanted effects.

This medicine may cause some people to become dizzy. *Make sure you know how you react to this medicine before you drive, use machines, or do anything else that could be dangerous if you are dizzy or not alert.*

For patients taking this medicine *for nasal congestion:*

- *If cold symptoms do not improve within 7 days or if you also have a high fever, check with your doctor.* These signs may mean that you have other medical problems.

## Side Effects of This Medicine

Along with its needed effects, a medicine may cause some unwanted effects. Although not all of these side effects may occur, if they do occur they may need medical attention.

Check with your doctor as soon as possible if any of the following side effects occur:

*Rare*
  Headache (severe); increased blood pressure; painful or difficult urination; tightness in chest

*Early symptoms of overdose*
  Abdominal or stomach pain; fast, pounding, or irregular heartbeat; headache (severe); increased sweating not caused by exercise; nausea and vomiting (severe); nervousness (severe); restlessness (severe)

*Late symptoms of overdose*
  Confusion; convulsions (seizures); fast breathing; fast and irregular pulse; hallucinations (seeing, hearing, or feeling things that are not there); hostile behavior; muscle trembling

Other side effects may occur that usually do not need medical attention. These side effects may go away during treatment as your body adjusts to the medicine. However, check with your doctor if any of the following side effects continue or are bothersome:

*Less common—more common with high doses*
  Dizziness; dryness of nose or mouth; false sense of well-being; headache (mild); nausea (mild); nervousness (mild); restlessness (mild); trouble in sleeping

Other side effects not listed above may also occur in some patients. If you notice any other effects, check with your doctor.

## Additional Information

Once a medicine has been approved for marketing for a certain use, experience may show that it is also useful for other medical problems. Although this use is not included in product labeling, phenylpropanolamine is used in certain patients with the following medical condition:

- Urinary stress incontinence (loss of bladder control when you cough, sneeze, or laugh)

Other than the above information, there is no additional information relating to proper use, precautions, or side effects for this use.

Revised: 06/21/94

# PHOSPHATES   Systemic

Some commonly used brand names are:

**In the U.S.—**
K-Phos M. F.[2]          Neutra-Phos[2]
K-Phos Neutral[2]        Neutra-Phos-K[1]
K-Phos No. 2[2]          Uro-KP-Neutral[2]
K-Phos Original[1]

**In Canada—**
Uro-KP-Neutral[2]

Note: For quick reference, the following phosphates are numbered to match the corresponding brand names.

This information applies to the following medicines:
1. Potassium Phosphates (poe-TASS-ee-um FOS-fates)[‡§]
2. Potassium and Sodium (SOE-dee-um) Phosphates
3. Sodium Phosphates[†‡]

†Not commercially available in Canada.
‡Generic name product may also be available in the U.S.
§Generic name product may also be available in Canada.

## Description

Phosphates are used as dietary supplements for patients who are unable to get enough phosphorus in their regular diet, usually because of certain illnesses or diseases. Phosphate is the drug form (salt) of phosphorus. Some phosphates are used to make the urine more acid, which helps treat certain urinary tract infections. Some phosphates are used to prevent the formation of calcium stones in the urinary tract.

Some of these preparations are available only with your doctor's prescription. Others are available without a prescription; however, your doctor may have special instructions on the proper dose of this medicine for your medical condition. You should take phosphates only under the supervision of your doctor.

Phosphates are available in the following dosage forms:

*Oral*
Potassium Phosphates
- Capsules for solution (U.S.)
- Powder for solution (U.S.)
- Tablets for solution (U.S.)
Potassium and Sodium Phosphates
- Capsules for solution (U.S.)
- Powder for solution (U.S.)
- Tablets for solution (U.S. and Canada)

*Parenteral*
Potassium Phosphates
- Injection (U.S. and Canada)
Sodium Phosphates
- Injection (U.S.)

## Importance of Diet

Many nutritionists recommend that, if possible, people should get all the phosphorus they need from foods. However, many people do not get enough phosphorus from food. For example, people on weight-loss diets may consume too little food to provide enough phosphorus. Others may lose phosphorus from the body because of illness or treatment with certain medicines. For such people, a phosphate supplement, given under your physician's care, is important.

In order to get enough vitamins and minerals in your diet, it is important that you eat a balanced and varied diet. Follow carefully any diet program your doctor may recommend. For your specific vitamin and/or mineral needs, ask your doctor for a list of appropriate foods.

The best dietary sources of phosphorus include dairy products, meat, poultry, fish, and cereal products.

Experts have developed a list of recommended dietary allowances (RDA) for most of the vitamins and some minerals. The RDA are not an exact number but a general idea of how much you need. They do not cover amounts needed for problems caused by a serious lack of vitamins or minerals.

The RDA for phosphorus are:
- Infants and children—
  Birth to 6 months of age: 400 mg per day.
  6 months to 1 year of age: 500 mg per day.
  1 to 10 years of age: 800 mg per day.
- Adolescent and adult males—
  11 to 24 years of age: 1200 mg per day.
  25 years of age and over: 800 mg per day.
- Adolescent and adult females—
  11 to 24 years of age: 1200 mg per day.
  25 years of age and over: 800 mg per day.
- Pregnant females—1200 mg per day.
- Breast-feeding females—1200 mg per day.

Remember:
- The total amount of phosphorus that you get every day includes what you get from food *and* what you may take as a supplement. Read the labels of processed foods, products such as certain soft drinks may contain phosphorus.
- Your total intake of phosphorus need not be greater than the recommended amounts, unless ordered by your doctor. In some cases, excessive amounts of phosphorus may be harmful.

## Before Using This Medicine

In deciding to use a medicine, the risks of taking the medicine must be weighed against the good it will do. This is a decision you and your doctor will make. For phosphates the following should be considered:

**Allergies**—Tell your doctor if you have ever had any unusual or allergic reaction to potassium, sodium, or phosphates. Also, tell your health care professional if you are allergic to any other substances, such as foods, preservatives, or dyes.

**Pregnancy**—It is especially important that you are receiving enough vitamins and minerals when you become pregnant and that you continue to receive the right amount of vitamins and minerals throughout your pregnancy. The healthy growth and development of the fetus depend on a steady supply of nutrients from the mother. However, taking large amounts of a nutritional supplement in pregnancy may be harmful to the mother and/or fetus and should be avoided.

**Breast-feeding**—It is especially important that you receive the right amount of vitamins and minerals so that your baby will also get the vitamins and minerals needed to grow properly. However, taking large amounts of a nutritional supplement while breast-feeding may be harmful to the mother and/or baby and should be avoided.

**Children**—Although there is no specific information comparing use of oral phosphates in children with use in other age groups, these medicines are not expected to cause different side effects in children than they do in adults. However, use of enemas that contain phosphates in children has resulted in high blood levels of phosphorus.

**Older adults**—Many medicines have not been studied specifically in older people. Therefore, it may not be known whether they work exactly the same way they do in younger adults or if they cause different side effects or problems in older people. There is no specific information

comparing use of phosphates in the elderly with use in other age groups.

**Other medicines**—Although certain medicines should not be used together at all, in other cases two different medicines may be used together even if an interaction might occur. In these cases, your doctor may want to change the dose, or other precautions may be necessary. When you are taking phosphates, it is especially important that your health care professional know if you are taking any of the following:

- Adrenocorticoids (cortisone-like medicine)—Use with sodium-containing phosphates may increase the risk of edema
- Amiloride (e.g., Midamor) or
- Captopril or
- Cyclosporine
- Digitalis glycosides (heart medicine) or
- Enalapril (e.g., Vasotec) or
- Heparin (e.g., Panheprin), with long-term use, or
- Lisinopril (e.g., Prinivil; Zestril) or
- Medicine for inflammation or pain (except narcotics) or
- Other potassium-containing medicine or
- Salt substitutes, low-salt foods, or milk or
- Spironolactone (e.g., Aldactone) or
- Triamterene (e.g., Dyrenium)—Use with potassium-containing phosphates may increase the risk of hyperkalemia (too much potassium in the blood), possibly leading to serious side effects
- Antacids—Use with phosphates may prevent the phosphate from working properly
- Calcium-containing medicine, including antacids and calcium supplements—Use with phosphates may prevent the phosphate from working properly; calcium deposits may form in tissues
- Phosphate-containing medications, other, including phosphate enemas—Use with sodium or potassium phophates may cause high blood levels of phosphorus which may increase the chance of side effects
- Sodium-containing medicines (other)—Use with sodium phosphates may cause your body to retain (keep) water

**Other medical problems**—The presence of other medical problems may affect the use of phosphates. Make sure you tell your doctor if you have any other medical problems, especially:

- Dehydration or
- Underactive adrenal glands—Potassium-containing phosphates may increase the risk of hyperkalemia (too much potassium in the blood)
- Edema (swelling in feet or lower legs or fluid in lungs) or
- High blood pressure or
- Liver disease or
- Toxemia of pregnancy—Sodium-containing phosphates may make these conditions worse
- Burns, severe or
- Heart disease or
- Pancreatitis (inflammation of the pancreas) or
- Rickets or
- Softening of bones or
- Underactive parathyroid glands—Sodium- or potassium-containing phosphates may make these conditions worse
- High blood levels of phosphate (hyperphosphatemia)—Use of phosphates may make this condition worse

- Infected kidney stones—Phosphates may make this condition worse
- Kidney disease—Sodium-containing phosphates may make this condition worse; potassium-containing phosphates may increase the risk of hyperkalemia (too much potassium in the blood)
- Myotonia congenita—Potassium-containing phosphates may increase the risk of hyperkalemia (too much potassium in the blood), and make this condition worse

## Proper Use of This Medicine

For patients taking the *tablet form* of this medicine:

- *Do not swallow the tablet.* Before taking, dissolve the tablet in ¾ to 1 glass (6 to 8 ounces) of water. Let the tablet soak in water for 2 to 5 minutes and then stir until completely dissolved.

For patients using the *capsule form* of this medicine:

- *Do not swallow the capsule.* Before taking, mix the contents of 1 capsule in one-third glass (about 2½ ounces) of water or juice or the contents of 2 capsules in two-thirds glass (about 5 ounces) of water and stir well until dissolved.

For patients using the *powder form* of this medicine:

- Add the entire contents of 1 bottle (2¼ ounces) to enough warm water to make 1 gallon of solution *or* the contents of one packet to enough warm water to make 1/3 of a glass (about 2.5 ounces) of solution. Shake the container for 2 or 3 minutes or until all the powder is dissolved.
- Do not dilute solution further.
- This solution may be chilled to improve the flavor; do not allow it to freeze.
- Discard unused solution after 60 days.

*Take this medicine immediately after meals or with food* to lessen possible stomach upset or laxative action.

To help prevent kidney stones, *drink at least a full glass (8 ounces) of water every hour during waking hours,* unless otherwise directed by your doctor.

*Take this medicine only as directed.* Do not take more of it and do not take it more often than recommended on the label, unless otherwise directed by your doctor.

**Dosing**—The dose of these single or combination medicines will be different for different patients. *Follow your doctor's orders or the directions on the label.* The following information includes only the average doses of these medicines. *If your dose is different, do not change it* unless your doctor tells you to do so.

The number of teaspoonfuls or ounces of prepared solution that you drink depends on the equivalent amount of phophorus contained in the product. Also, *the number of doses you take each day, the time allowed between doses, and the length of time you take the medicine depend on the medical problem for which you are taking the single or combination medicine.*

*For potassium phosphates*

- For *tablets for oral solution* dosage form:
  —To replace phosphorus lost by the body or to make the urine more acid or to prevent the formation of kidney stones in the urinary tract:
  - Adults and teenagers: The equivalent of 228 milligrams (mg) of phosphorus (2 tablets) dissolved in six to eight ounces of water four times a day, with meals and at bedtime.
  —To replace phosphorus lost by the body:
  - Children over 4 years of age: The equivalent of 228 mg of phosphorus (2 tablets) dissolved in six to eight ounces of water four times a day, with meals and at bedtime.
  - Children up to 4 years of age: The dose must be determined by your doctor.

- For *capsules for oral solution* dosage form:
  —To replace phosphorus lost by the body:
  - Adults, teenagers, and children over 4 years of age: The equivalent of 250 mg of phosphorus (contents of 1 capsule) dissolved in two and one-half ounces of water or juice four times a day, after meals and at bedtime.
  - Children up to 4 years of age: Dose must be determined by your doctor.

- For *powder for oral solution* dosage form:
  —To replace phosphorus lost by the body:
  - Adults, teenagers, and children over 4 years of age: The equivalent of 250 mg of phosphorus dissolved in two and one-half ounces of water four times a day, after meals and at bedtime.
  - Children up to 4 years of age: Dose must be determined by your doctor.

*For potassium and sodium phosphates*

- For *tablets for oral solution* dosage form:
  —To replace phosphorus lost by the body or to make the urine more acid or to prevent the fomation of kidney stones in the urinary tract:
  - Adults and teenagers: The equivalent of 250 milligrams (mg) of phosphorus dissolved in eight ounces of water four times a day, after meals and at bedtime.
  —To replace phosphorus lost by the body:
  - Children over 4 years of age: The equivalent of 250 mg of phosphorus dissolved in eight ounces of water four times a day, after meals and at bedtime.
  - Children up to 4 years of age: Dose must be determined by your doctor.

- For *capsules for oral solution* dosage form:
  —To replace phosphorus lost by the body:
  - Adults, teenagers, and children over 4 years of age: The equivalent of 250 mg of phosphorus (the contents of 1 capsule) dissolved in two and one-half ounces of water or juice four times a day, after meals and at bedtime.

- Children up to 4 years of age: Dose must be determined by your doctor.

- For *powder for oral solution* dosage form:
  —To replace phosphorus lost by the body:
  - Adults, teenagers, and children over 4 years of age: The equivalent of 250 mg of phosphorus dissolved in two and one-half ounces of water four times a day, after meals and at bedtime.
  - Children up to 4 years of age: Dose must be determined by your doctor.

- For *tablets for oral solution* dosage form:
  —To replace phosphorus lost by the body:
  - Adults, teenagers, and children over 4 years of age: The equivalent of 250 mg of phosphorus (1 tablet) dissolved in eight ounces of water four times a day.
  - Children up to 4 years of age: Dose must be determined by your doctor.

**Missed dose**—If you miss a dose of this medicine, take it as soon as possible. However, if it is within 1 or 2 hours of your next dose, skip the missed dose and go back to your regular dosing schedule. Do not double doses.

**Storage**—To store this medicine:

- Keep out of the reach of children.
- Store away from heat and direct light.
- Do not store the capsule, tablet, or powder form of this medicine in the bathroom, near the kitchen sink, or in other damp places. Heat or moisture may cause the medicine to break down.
- Keep the liquid form of this medicine from freezing.
- Do not keep outdated medicine or medicine no longer needed. Be sure that any discarded medicine is out of the reach of children.

## Precautions While Using This Medicine

Your doctor should check your progress at regular visits to make sure that this medicine does not cause unwanted effects.

*Do not take iron supplements within 1 to 2 hours of taking this medicine.* To do so may keep the iron from working properly.

*For patients taking potassium phosphate-containing medicines:*

- Check with your doctor before starting any strenuous physical exercise, especially if you are out of condition and are taking other medication. Exercise and certain medicines may increase the amount of potassium in the blood.

For patients on a *potassium-restricted diet:*

- This medicine may contain a large amount of potassium. If you have any questions about this, check with your health care professional.

- Do not use salt substitutes and low-salt milk unless told to do so by your doctor. They may contain potassium.

*For patients on a sodium-restricted diet:*

- This medicine may contain a large amount of sodium. If you have any questions about this, check with your health care professional.

## Side Effects of This Medicine

Along with its needed effects, a medicine may cause some unwanted effects. Although not all of these side effects may occur, if they do occur they may need medical attention.

Check with your doctor as soon as possible if any of the following side effects occur:

*Less common or rare*

Confusion; convulsions (seizures); decrease in amount of urine or in frequency of urination; fast, slow, or irregular heartbeat; headache or dizziness; increased thirst; muscle cramps; numbness, tingling, pain, or weakness in hands or feet; numbness or tingling around lips; shortness of breath or troubled breathing; swelling of feet or lower legs; tremor; unexplained anxiety; unusual tiredness or weakness; weakness or heaviness of legs; weight gain

Other side effects may occur that usually do not need medical attention. These side effects may go away during treatment as your body adjusts to the medicine. However, check with your doctor if any of the following side effects continue or are bothersome:

Diarrhea; nausea or vomiting; stomach pain

Other side effects not listed above may also occur in some patients. If you notice any other effects, check with your doctor.

---

Revised: 04/16/92
Interim revision: 08/30/94

---

# PHYSOSTIGMINE   Ophthalmic†

Some commonly used brand names in the U.S. are Eserine Salicylate, Eserine Sulfate, and Isopto Eserine.

Generic name product may also be available in the U.S.

---

†Not commercially available in Canada.

---

## Description

Physostigmine (fi-zoe-STIG-meen) is used to treat certain types of glaucoma.

This medicine is available only with your doctor's prescription, in the following dosage forms:

*Ophthalmic*
- Ophthalmic ointment (U.S.)
- Ophthalmic solution (eye drops) (U.S.)

## Before Using This Medicine

In deciding to use a medicine, the risks of taking the medicine must be weighed against the good it will do. This is a decision you and your doctor will make. For physostigmine, the following should be considered:

**Allergies**—Tell your doctor if you have ever had any unusual or allergic reaction to physostigmine. Also tell your health care professional if you are allergic to any other substances, such as preservatives.

**Pregnancy**—Ophthalmic physostigmine may be absorbed into the body. However, studies on effects in pregnancy have not been done in either humans or animals.

**Breast-feeding**—Ophthalmic physostigmine may be absorbed into the mother's body. However, physostigmine has not been reported to cause problems in nursing babies.

**Children**—Although there is no specific information comparing use of this medicine in children with use in other age groups, it is not expected to cause different side effects or problems in children than it does in adults.

**Older adults**—Many medicines have not been studied specifically in older people. Therefore, it may not be known whether they work exactly the same way they do in younger adults or if they cause different side effects or problems in older people. Although there is no specific information comparing use of physostigmine in the elderly with use in other age groups, it is not expected to cause different side effects or problems in older people than it does in younger adults.

**Other medicines**—Although certain medicines should not be used together at all, in other cases two different medicines may be used together even if an interaction might occur. In these cases, your doctor may want to change the dose, or other precautions may be necessary. Tell your health care professional if you are using any other prescription or nonprescription (over-the-counter [OTC]) medicine.

**Other medical problems**—The presence of other medical problems may affect the use of physostigmine. Make sure you tell your doctor if you have any other medical problems, especially:

- Eye disease or problems (other)—Physostigmine may make the condition worse

## Proper Use of This Medicine

To use the *ophthalmic solution (eye drops) form* of this medicine:

- Do not use if the solution becomes discolored.
- First, wash your hands. With the middle finger, apply pressure to the inside corner of the eye (and continue to apply pressure for 1 or 2 minutes after the medicine has been placed in the eye). Tilt the head back and with the index finger of the same hand, pull the lower eyelid away from the eye to form a pouch. Drop the medicine into the pouch and gently close the eyes. Do not blink. Keep the eyes closed for 1 or 2 minutes to allow the medicine to be absorbed.
- Immediately after using the eye drops, wash your hands to remove any medicine that may be on them.
- To keep the medicine as germ-free as possible, do not touch the applicator tip to any surface (including the eye). Also, keep the container tightly closed.

To use the *ointment form* of this medicine:

- First, wash your hands. Pull the lower eyelid away from the eye to form a pouch. Squeeze a thin strip of ointment into the pouch. A 1-cm (approximately 1/3-inch) strip of ointment is usually enough unless otherwise directed by your doctor. Gently close the eyes and keep them closed for 1 or 2 minutes to allow the medicine to be absorbed.
- Immediately after using the eye ointment, wash your hands to remove any medicine that may be on them.
- To keep the medicine as germ-free as possible, do not touch the applicator tip to any surface (including the eye). After using the eye ointment, wipe the tip of the ointment tube with a clean tissue and keep the tube tightly closed.

*Use this medicine only as directed.* Do not use more of it and do not use it more often than your doctor ordered. To do so may increase the chance of too much medicine being absorbed into the body and the chance of side effects.

**Dosing**—The dose of ophthalmic physostigmine will be different for different patients. *Follow your doctor's orders or the directions on the label.* The following information includes only the average doses of ophthalmic physostigmine. *If your dose is different, do not change it* unless your doctor tells you to do so.

*The number of doses you use each day, the time allowed between doses, and the length of time you use the medicine depend on the medical problem for which you are using ophthalmic physostigmine.*

- For glaucoma:
  - —For *ophthalmic ointment* dosage form:
    - Adults and children—Use in each eye one to three times a day.
  - —For *ophthalmic solution (eye drops)* dosage form:
    - Adults and children—One drop in each eye up to four times a day.

**Missed dose**—If you miss a dose of this medicine and your dosing schedule is:

- One dose a day—Apply the missed dose as soon as possible. However, if you do not remember the missed dose until the next day, skip the missed dose and go back to your regular dosing schedule. Do not double doses.
- More than one dose a day—Apply the missed dose as soon as possible. However, if it is almost time for your next dose, skip the missed dose and go back to your regular dosing schedule. Do not double doses.

**Storage**—To store this medicine:

- Keep out of the reach of children.
- Store away from heat and direct light.
- Keep the medicine from freezing.
- Do not keep outdated medicine or medicine no longer needed. Be sure that any discarded medicine is out of the reach of children.

## Precautions While Using This Medicine

Your doctor should check your eye pressure at regular visits.

For a short time after you apply this medicine, your vision may be blurred or there may be a change in your near or distant vision, especially at night. *Make sure your vision is clear before you drive, use machines, or do anything else that could be dangerous if you are not able to see well.*

## Side Effects of This Medicine

Along with its needed effects, a medicine may cause some unwanted effects. Although not all of these side effects may occur, if they do occur they may need medical attention.

Check with your doctor as soon as possible if any of the following side effects occur:

> *Symptoms of too much medicine being absorbed into the body*
>
> Increased sweating; loss of bladder control; muscle weakness; nausea, vomiting, diarrhea, or stomach cramps or pain; shortness of breath, tightness in chest, or wheezing; slow or irregular heartbeat; unusual tiredness or weakness; watering of mouth

Other side effects may occur that usually do not need medical attention. These side effects may go away during treatment as your body adjusts to the medicine. However, check with your doctor if any of the following side effects continue or are bothersome:

*More common*
> Blurred vision or change in near or distant vision; eye pain

*Less common*
> Burning, redness, stinging, or other eye irritation; headache or browache; twitching of eyelids; watering of eyes

Other side effects not listed above may also occur in some patients. If you notice any other effects, check with your doctor.

Revised: 07/01/93

# PILOCARPINE   Ophthalmic

Some commonly used brand names are:

**In the U.S.—**

| | |
|---|---|
| Adsorbocarpine | Pilocar |
| Akarpine | Pilokair |
| I-Pilocarpine | Pilopine HS |
| Isopto Carpine | Piloptic-1 |
| Ocu-Carpine | Piloptic-2 |
| Ocusert Pilo-20 | Piloptic-4 |
| Ocusert Pilo-40 | Pilostat |
| Pilagan | Spectro-Pilo |

Generic name product may also be available.

**In Canada—**

| | |
|---|---|
| Isopto Carpine | Pilopine HS |
| Minims Pilocarpine | Pilostat |
| Miocarpine | P.V. Carpine Liquifilm |
| Ocusert Pilo-20 | Spersacarpine |
| Ocusert Pilo-40 | |

## Description

Pilocarpine (pye-loe-KAR-peen) is used to treat glaucoma and other eye conditions.

This medicine is available only with your doctor's prescription, in the following dosage forms:

*Ophthalmic*
- Ocular system (eye insert) (U.S. and Canada)
- Ophthalmic gel (eye gel) (U.S. and Canada)
- Ophthalmic solution (eye drops) (U.S. and Canada)

## Before Using This Medicine

In deciding to use a medicine, the risks of taking the medicine must be weighed against the good it will do. This is a decision you and your doctor will make. For pilocarpine, the following should be considered:

**Allergies**—Tell your doctor if you have ever had any unusual or allergic reaction to pilocarpine. Also tell your health care professional if you are allergic to any other substances, such as preservatives

**Pregnancy**—Ophthalmic pilocarpine may be absorbed into the body. However, studies on effects in pregnancy have not been done in either humans or animals.

**Breast-feeding**—Ophthalmic pilocarpine may be absorbed into the body. However, it is not known whether pilocarpine passes into the breast milk. Although most medicines pass into breast milk in small amounts, many of them may be used safely while breast-feeding. Mothers who are using this medicine and who wish to breast-feed should discuss this with their doctor.

**Children**—Although there is no specific information comparing use of this medicine in children with use in other age groups, pilocarpine is not expected to cause different side effects or problems in children than it does in adults.

**Older adults**—Many medicines have not been studied specifically in older people. Therefore, it may not be known whether they work exactly the same way they do in younger adults or if they cause different side effects or problems in older people. Although there is no specific information comparing use of pilocarpine in the elderly with use in other age groups, this medicine is not expected to cause different side effects or problems in older people than it does in younger adults.

**Other medicines**—Although certain medicines should not be used together at all, in other cases two different medicines may be used together even if an interaction might occur. In these cases, your doctor may want to change the dose, or other precautions may be necessary. Tell your health care professional if you are using any other prescription or nonprescription (over-the-counter [OTC]) medicine.

**Other medical problems**—The presence of other medical problems may affect the use of pilocarpine. Make sure you tell your doctor if you have any other medical problems, especially:
- Asthma or
- Eye disease or problems (other)—Pilocarpine may make the condition worse

## Proper Use of This Medicine

To use the *eye drop form* of pilocarpine:
- First, wash your hands. With the middle finger, apply pressure to the inside corner of the eye (and continue to apply pressure for 1 or 2 minutes after the medicine has been placed in the eye). Tilt the head back and with the index finger of the same hand, pull the lower eyelid away from the eye to form a pouch. Drop the medicine into the pouch and gently close the eyes. Do not blink. Keep the eyes closed for 1 or 2 minutes to allow the medicine to be absorbed.

- Immediately after using the eye drops, wash your hands to remove any medicine that may be on them.
- To keep the medicine as germ-free as possible, do not touch the applicator tip to any surface (including the eye). Also, keep the container tightly closed.

To use the *eye gel form* of pilocarpine:

- First, wash your hands. Pull the lower eyelid away from the eye to form a pouch. Squeeze a thin strip of gel into the pouch. A 1½-cm (approximately ½-inch) strip of gel is usually enough unless otherwise directed by your doctor. Gently close the eyes and keep them closed for 1 or 2 minutes to allow the medicine to be absorbed.
- Immediately after using the eye gel, wash your hands to remove any medicine that may be on them.
- To keep the medicine as germ-free as possible, do not touch the applicator tip to any surface (including the eye). After using the eye gel, wipe the tip of the gel tube with a clean tissue and keep the tube tightly closed.

To use the *eye insert form* of pilocarpine:

- This medicine usually comes with patient directions. Read them carefully before using this medicine.
- If you think this medicine unit may be damaged, do not use it. If you have any questions about this, check with your health care professional.
- If the unit seems to be releasing too much medicine into your eye, remove it and replace with a new unit. If you have any questions about this, check with your doctor.

*Use this medicine only as directed.* Do not use more of it and do not use it more often than your doctor ordered. To do so may increase the chance of too much medicine being absorbed into the body and the chance of side effects.

**Dosing**—The dose of ophthalmic pilocarpine will be different for different patients. *Follow the doctor's orders or the directions on the label.* The following information includes only the average doses of ophthalmic pilocarpine. *If your dose is different, do not change it unless your doctor tells you to do so.*

*The number of doses you use each day, the time allowed between doses, and the length of time you use the medicine depend on the medical problem for which you are using ophthalmic pilocarpine.*

- For *eye insert* dosage form:
  —For glaucoma:
    • Adults and children—Insert one ocular system every seven days.
    • Infants—Use is generally not recommended.
- For *eye gel* dosage form:
  —For glaucoma:
    • Adults and adolescents—Use once a day at bedtime.
    • Children—Use is generally not recommended.

- For *eye drop* dosage form:
  —For chronic glaucoma:
    • Adults and children—One drop one to four times a day.
  —For acute angle-closure glaucoma:
    • Adults and children—One drop every five to ten minutes for three to six doses. Then one drop every one to three hours until eye pressure is reduced.

**Missed dose**—

- For patients using the *eye drop form* of pilocarpine: If you miss a dose of this medicine, apply it as soon as possible. However, if it is almost time for your next dose, skip the missed dose and go back to your regular dosing schedule. Do not double doses.
- For patients using the *eye gel form* of pilocarpine: If you miss a dose of this medicine, apply it as soon as possible. However, if you do not remember the missed dose until the next day, skip the missed dose and go back to your regular dosing schedule. Do not double doses.
- For patients using the *eye insert form* of pilocarpine: If you forget to replace the eye insert at the proper time, replace it as soon as possible. Then go back to your regular dosing schedule.

**Storage**—To store this medicine:

- Keep out of the reach of children.
- Store away from heat and direct light.
- Store the eye system form of this medicine in the refrigerator. However, keep the medicine from freezing.
- Store the 5-gram size of the gel form of this medicine in the refrigerator. Store the 3.5-gram size at room temperature.
- Keep the gel or solution form of this medicine from freezing.
- Do not keep outdated medicine or medicine no longer needed. Be sure that any discarded medicine is out of the reach of children.

## Precautions While Using This Medicine

Your doctor should check your eye pressure at regular visits.

For patients using the *eye drop or gel form* of this medicine:

- For a short time after you apply this medicine, your vision may be blurred or there may be a change in your near or far vision, especially at night. *Make sure your vision is clear before you drive, use machines, or do anything else that could be dangerous if you are not able to see well.*

For patients using the *eye insert form* of this medicine:

- For the first several hours after you insert this unit in the eye, your vision may be blurred or there may be a change in your near or far vision, especially at night. Therefore, insert this unit in the eye at bedtime, unless otherwise directed by your doctor. If this unit is inserted in the eye at any other time of the day, *make sure your vision is clear before you drive, use machines, or do anything else that could be dangerous if you are not able to see well.*

## Side Effects of This Medicine

Along with its needed effects, a medicine may cause some unwanted effects. Although not all of these side effects may occur, if they do occur they may need medical attention.

Check with your doctor as soon as possible if any of the following side effects occur:

*Symptoms of too much medicine being absorbed into the body*

   Increased sweating; muscle tremors; nausea, vomiting, or diarrhea; troubled breathing or wheezing; watering of mouth

*Less common or rare*
   Eye pain

Other side effects may occur that usually do not need medical attention. These side effects may go away during treatment as your body adjusts to the medicine. However, check with your doctor if any of the following side effects continue or are bothersome:

*More common*
   Blurred vision or change in near or far vision; decrease in night vision
*Less common*
   Eye irritation; headache or browache

Other side effects not listed above may also occur in some patients. If you notice any other effects, check with your doctor.

Revised: 07/01/93

# PIMOZIDE  Systemic

A commonly used brand name in the U.S. and Canada is Orap.

## Description

Pimozide (PIM-oh-zide) is used to treat the symptoms of Tourette's syndrome. It is meant only for patients with severe symptoms who cannot take or have not been helped by other medicine.

Pimozide works in the central nervous system to help control the vocal outbursts and uncontrolled, repeated movements of the body (tics) that interfere with normal life. It will not completely cure the tics, but will help to reduce their number and severity.

Pimozide may also be used for other conditions as determined by your doctor.

This medicine is available only with your doctor's prescription, in the following dosage form:
*Oral*
   • Tablets (U.S. and Canada)

## Before Using This Medicine

In deciding to use a medicine, the risks of taking the medicine must be weighed against the good it will do. This is a decision you and your doctor will make. For pimozide, the following should be considered:

**Allergies**—Tell your doctor if you have ever had any unusual or allergic reaction to pimozide, haloperidol, loxapine, molindone, phenothiazines, or thioxanthenes. Also tell your health care professional if you are allergic to any other substances, such as foods, preservatives, or dyes.

**Pregnancy**—Studies in rats and rabbits given more than the usual human dose of pimozide have shown fewer pregnancies, slowed development of the fetus, and toxic effects in the mother and fetus.

**Breast-feeding**—It is not known whether pimozide passes into breast milk.

**Children**—Children are especially sensitive to the effects of pimozide. This may increase the chance of side effects during treatment. Pimozide should not be used in children for any medical problem other than Tourette's syndrome.

**Older adults**—Constipation, dizziness or fainting, drowsiness, dryness of mouth, and trembling of the hands and fingers, and symptoms of tardive dyskinesia (such as rapid, worm-like movements of the tongue or any other uncontrolled movements of the mouth, tongue, or jaw, and/or arms and legs) may be especially likely to occur in the elderly, who are usually more sensitive than younger adults to the effects of pimozide.

**Other medicines**—Although certain medicines should not be used together at all, in other cases 2 different medicines may be used together even if an interaction might occur. In these cases, your doctor may want to change the dose, or other precautions may be necessary. When you are taking pimozide, it is especially important that your health care professional know if you are taking any of the following:
   • Amoxapine (e.g., Asendin) or
   • Methyldopa (e.g., Aldomet) or
   • Metoclopramide (e.g., Reglan) or
   • Metyrosine (e.g., Demser) or
   • Promethazine (e.g., Phenergan) or

- Rauwolfia alkaloids (alseroxylon [e.g., Rauwiloid], deserpidine [e.g., Harmonyl], rauwolfia serpentina [e.g., Raudixin], reserpine [e.g., Serpasil]) or
- Trimeprazine (e.g., Temaril)—Taking these medicines with pimozide may increase the chance of serious side effects
- Amphetamines or
- Methylphenidate (e.g., Ritalin) or
- Pemoline (e.g., Cylert)—Taking these medicines with pimozide may cover up the cause of tics
- Anticholinergics (medicine for abdominal or stomach spasms or cramps)—Taking these medicines with pimozide may cause an increased chance of certain side effects, such as dryness of mouth, constipation, and unusual excitement
- Antipsychotics (medicine for mental illness) or
- Disopyramide (e.g., Norpace) or
- Maprotiline (e.g., Ludiomil) or
- Procainamide (e.g., Pronestyl) or
- Quinidine (e.g., Quinidex) or
- Tricyclic antidepressants (medicine for depression)—Taking these medicines with pimozide may increase the chance of serious effects on the rhythm of your heart
- Central nervous system (CNS) depressants—Using these medicines with pimozide may increase the CNS depressant effects

**Other medical problems**—The presence of other medical problems may affect the use of pimozide. Make sure you tell your doctor if you have any other medical problems, especially:

- Breast cancer (history of) or
- Heart disease—Pimozide may make the condition worse
- Kidney disease or
- Liver disease—Higher blood levels of pimozide may occur, increasing the chance of side effects
- Tics other than those caused by Tourette's syndrome—Pimozide should not be used because of the risk of serious side effects

## Proper Use of This Medicine

*Use pimozide only as directed by your doctor.* Do not use more of it, do not use it more often, and do not use it for a longer time than your doctor ordered. To do so may increase the chance of side effects.

**Dosing**—The dose of pimozide will be different for different patients. *Follow your doctor's orders or the directions on the label.* The following information includes only the average doses of pimozide. *If your dose is different, do not change it* unless your doctor tells you to do so.

The number of tablets that you take depends on the strength of the medicine. Also, *the number of doses you take each day, the time allowed between doses, and the length of time you take the medicine depend on the medical problem for which you are using pimozide.*

- For *oral* dosage form (tablets):
  —Adults and adolescents: To start, 1 to 2 milligrams (mg) a day. Your doctor may increase your dose if needed. However, the dose is usually not more than 10 mg a day.

—Children up to 12 years of age: Dose must be determined by the doctor.

**Missed dose**—If you miss a dose of this medicine, take it as soon as possible. Then take any remaining doses for that day at regularly spaced times. Do not double doses.

**Storage**—To store this medicine:

- Keep out of the reach of children.
- Store away from heat and direct light.
- Do not store in the bathroom, near the kitchen sink, or in other damp places. Heat or moisture may cause the medicine to break down.
- Do not keep outdated medicine or medicine no longer needed. Be sure that any discarded medicine is out of the reach of children.

## Precautions While Using This Medicine

Your doctor should check your progress at regular visits, especially during the first few months of treatment with this medicine. The amount of pimozide you take may be changed often to meet the needs of your condition and to help avoid unwanted effects.

*Do not suddenly stop taking this medicine without first checking with your doctor.* Your doctor may want you to reduce gradually the amount you are taking before stopping completely. This will allow your body time to adjust and help to avoid worsening of your medical condition.

This medicine will add to the effects of alcohol and other CNS depressants (medicines that slow down the nervous system, possibly causing drowsiness). Some examples of CNS depressants are antihistamines or medicine for hay fever, other allergies, or colds; sedatives, tranquilizers, or sleeping medicine; prescription pain medicine or narcotics; barbiturates; medicine for seizures; muscle relaxants; or anesthetics, including some dental anesthetics. *Check with your doctor before taking any of the above while you are using this medicine.*

This medicine may cause some people to become drowsy or less alert or to have blurred vision or muscle stiffness, especially as the amount of medicine is increased. Even if you take pimozide at bedtime, you may feel drowsy or less alert on arising. *Make sure you know how you react to this medicine before you drive, use machines, or do anything else that could be dangerous if you are not alert or able to see well or if you do not have good muscle control.*

Although not a problem for many patients, dizziness, lightheadedness, or fainting may occur, especially when you get up from a sitting or lying position. Getting up slowly may help. If the problem continues or gets worse, check with your doctor.

*Before having any kind of surgery, dental treatment, or emergency treatment, tell the medical doctor or dentist in charge that you are using this medicine.* Taking pimozide together with medicines that are used during surgery or dental or emergency treatment may increase the CNS depressant effects.

Pimozide may cause dryness of the mouth. For temporary relief, use sugarless gum or candy, melt bits of ice in your mouth, or use a saliva substitute. However, if your mouth continues to feel dry for more than 2 weeks, check with your medical doctor or dentist. Continuing dryness of the mouth may increase the chance of dental disease, including tooth decay, gum disease, and fungus infections.

## Side Effects of This Medicine

Along with its needed effects, pimozide can sometimes cause serious side effects. Tardive dyskinesia (a movement disorder) may occur and may not go away after you stop using the medicine. Signs of tardive dyskinesia include fine, worm-like movements of the tongue, or other uncontrolled movements of the mouth, tongue, cheeks, jaw, or arms and legs. Other serious but rare side effects may also occur. These include severe muscle stiffness, fever, unusual tiredness or weakness, fast heartbeat, difficult breathing, increased sweating, loss of bladder control, and seizures (neuroleptic malignant syndrome). *You and your doctor should discuss the good this medicine will do as well as the risks of taking it.*

*Stop taking pimozide and get emergency help immediately* if any of the following side effects occur:

*Rare*
> Convulsions (seizures); difficult or fast breathing; fast heartbeat or irregular pulse; fever (high); high or low (irregular) blood pressure; increased sweating; loss of bladder control; muscle stiffness (severe); tiredness or weakness; unusually pale skin

*Symptoms of overdose*
> Drowsiness or dizziness (severe); muscle trembling, jerking, or stiffness (severe); troubled breathing (severe); uncontrolled movements (severe); unusual tiredness or weakness (severe)

Check with your doctor as soon as possible if any of the following side effects occur:

*More common*
> Difficulty in speaking or swallowing; loss of balance control; mask-like face; mood or behavior changes; rest-lessness or need to keep moving; shuffling walk; slowed movements; stiffness of arms and legs; trembling and shaking of fingers and hands

*Less common or rare*
> Inability to move eyes; increased blinking or spasms of eyelid; lip smacking or puckering; muscle spasms, especially of the face, neck, or back; puffing of cheeks; rapid or worm-like movements of tongue; sore throat and fever; uncontrolled chewing movements; uncontrolled twisting movements of neck, trunk, arms, or legs; unusual bleeding or bruising; unusual facial expressions or body positions; yellow eyes or skin

Other side effects may occur that usually do not need medical attention. These side effects may go away during treatment as your body adjusts to the medicine. However, check with your doctor if any of the following side effects continue or are bothersome:

*More common*
> Blurred vision or other vision problems; constipation; dizziness, lightheadedness, or fainting (especially when getting up from a lying or sitting position); drowsiness; dryness of mouth; skin rash, itching, or discoloration; swelling or soreness of breasts; unusual secretion of milk

*Less common*
> Decreased sexual ability; diarrhea; headache; loss of appetite and weight; mental depression; nausea or vomiting; swelling of the face

After you stop using pimozide, it may still produce some side effects that need attention. During this period of time, check with your doctor as soon as possible if you notice any of the following side effects:

> Lip smacking or puckering; puffing of cheeks; rapid or worm-like movements of the tongue; uncontrolled chewing movements; uncontrolled movements of the arms and legs

Other side effects not listed above may also occur in some patients. If you notice any other effects, check with your doctor.

---

Revised: 04/16/93

---

# PIPERAZINE  Systemic

A commonly used brand name in Canada is Entacyl.
Generic name product may also be available in the U.S.

## Description

Piperazine (PI-per-a-zeen) belongs to the family of medicines called anthelmintics (ant-hel-MIN-tiks). Anthelmintics are used in the treatment of worm infections.

Piperazine is used to treat:
- common roundworms (ascariasis) and
- pinworms (enterobiasis; oxyuriasis).

Piperazine works by paralyzing the worms. They are then passed in the stool.

Piperazine is available only with your doctor's prescription, in the following dosage forms:

*Oral*
- Granules for oral solution (Canada)
- Oral suspension (Canada)
- Tablets (U.S.)

## Before Using This Medicine

In deciding to use a medicine, the risks of taking the medicine must be weighed against the good it will do. This is a decision you and your doctor will make. For piperazine, the following should be considered:

**Allergies**—Tell your doctor if you have ever had any unusual or allergic reaction to piperazine or ethylenediamine. Also tell your health care professional if you are allergic to any other substances, such as foods, preservatives, or dyes.

**Pregnancy**—Piperazine has not been studied in pregnant women. Piperazine has not been shown to cause birth defects or other problems in animal studies. However, piperazine, taken by mouth, may be changed within the body into a substance that may cause cancer. Before taking piperazine, make sure your doctor knows if you are pregnant or if you may become pregnant.

**Breast-feeding**—Although it is not known whether piperazine passes into the breast milk, piperazine has not been reported to cause problems in nursing babies.

**Children**—Children may be especially sensitive to the effects of piperazine. This may increase the chance of side effects during treatment.

**Older adults**—Many medicines have not been studied specifically in older people. Therefore, it may not be known whether they work exactly the same way they do in younger adults or if they cause different side effects or problems in older people. There is no specific information comparing use of piperazine in the elderly with use in other age groups.

**Other medicines**—Although certain medicines should not be used together at all, in other cases two different medicines may be used together even if an interaction might occur. In these cases, your doctor may want to change the dose, or other precautions may be necessary. When you are taking piperazine, it is especially important that your health care professional know if you are taking any of the following:
- Phenothiazines (acetophenazine [e.g., Tindal], chlorpromazine [e.g., Thorazine], fluphenazine [e.g., Prolixin], mesoridazine [e.g., Serentil], perphenazine[e.g., Trilafon], prochlorperazine [e.g., Compazine], promazine [e.g., Sparine], promethazine [e.g., Phenergan], thioridazine [e.g., Mellaril], trifluoperazine [e.g., Stelazine], triflupromazine [e.g., Vesprin], trimeprazine [e.g., Temaril])—Taking piperazine and a phenothiazine together may increase the risk of convulsions
- Pyrantel (e.g., Antiminth)—Taking piperazine and pyrantel together may decrease the effects of piperazine

**Other medical problems**—The presence of other medical problems may affect the use of piperazine. Make sure you tell your doctor if you have any other medical problems, especially:
- Kidney disease or
- Liver disease—Patients with kidney or liver disease may have an increased chance of side effects
- Seizure disorder, especially a history of epilepsy—Piperazine may make the condition worse

## Proper Use of This Medicine

No special preparation (for example, special diet, fasting, other medicines, laxatives, or enemas) are necessary before, during, or immediately after you take piperazine.

Piperazine may be taken with or without food or on a full or empty stomach. However, if your doctor tells you to take the medicine a certain way, take it exactly as directed.

For patients taking the *granules for oral solution form* of piperazine:
- Dissolve the contents of 1 packet of granules in 57 mL (about 2 ounces) of water, milk, or fruit juice.
- Be sure to drink all of the liquid to get the full dose of medicine.

*Take this medicine only as directed.* Do not take more of it and do not take it more often than your doctor ordered. To do so may increase the chance of serious side effects.

To help clear up your infection completely, *take this medicine in regularly spaced doses as ordered by your doctor.* In some infections a second treatment with this medicine may be required to clear up the infection completely. *Do not miss any doses.*

For patients taking piperazine for *pinworms:*
- Pinworms may be easily passed from one person to another, especially among persons in the same household. Therefore, all household members may have to be treated at the same time to prevent their infection or reinfection.

**Dosing**—The dose of piperazine will be different for different patients. *Follow your doctor's orders or the directions on the label.* The following information includes only the average doses of piperazine. *If your dose is different, do not change it* unless your doctor tells you to do so.

The number of tablets or teaspoonfuls of solution or suspension of the medicine that you take depends on the strength of the medicine. Also, *the number of doses you take each day, the time allowed between doses, and the length of time you take the medicine depend on the medical problem for which you are taking piperazine.*
- For *oral suspension* or *granules for oral solution* dosage form:
  —For common roundworms or pinworms:
    - Adults and children over 14 years of age— 1.8 grams of oral suspension or 2 grams of granules for oral solution three times a day for one

day. Treatment may need to be repeated in two weeks.

- Children—Dose is based on age and/or body weight. Treatment may need to be repeated in two weeks.

    —Up to 2 years of age: 600 milligrams (mg) of oral suspension three times a day for one day.

    —2 to 8 years of age: 1.2 grams of oral suspension two times a day or 2 grams of granules for oral solution once a day, for one day.

    —8 to 14 years of age: 1.2 grams of oral suspension three times a day or 2 grams of granules for oral solution two times a day, for one day.

- For *tablet* dosage form:
  —For common roundworms:
    - Adults—3.5 grams (piperazine hexahydrate) per day for two days in a row. Treatment may need to be repeated in one week.
    - Children—Dose is based on body weight and must be determined by your doctor. However, the usual dose is 75 mg (piperazine hexahydrate) per kilogram (34 mg per pound) of body weight per day for two days in a row. Treatment may need to be repeated in one week.
  —For pinworms:
    - Adults and children—Dose is based on body weight and must be determined by your doctor. However, the usual dose is 65 mg (piperazine hexahydrate) per kilogram (29.5 mg per pound) of body weight per day for seven days in a row. Treatment may need to be repeated in one week.

**Missed dose**—If you miss a dose of this medicine, take it as soon as possible. However, if it is almost time for your next dose, skip the missed dose and go back to your regular dosing schedule. Do not double doses.

**Storage**—To store this medicine:
- Keep out of the reach of children. Overdose of piperazine is very dangerous in young children.
- Store away from heat and direct light.
- Do not store in the bathroom, near the kitchen sink, or in other damp places. Heat or moisture may cause the medicine to break down.
- Keep the liquid form of this medicine from freezing.
- Do not keep outdated medicine or medicine no longer needed. Be sure that any discarded medicine is out of the reach of children.

## Precautions While Using This Medicine

It is important that your doctor check your progress after treatment. This is to make sure that the infection is cleared up completely, and to allow your doctor to check for any unwanted effects.

If your symptoms do not improve after you have taken this medicine for the full course of treatment, or if they become worse, check with your doctor.

For patients taking piperazine for *pinworms*:
- In some patients, pinworms may return after treatment with piperazine. Washing (not shaking) all bedding and nightclothes (pajamas) after treatment may help to prevent this.

## Side Effects of This Medicine

Along with its needed effects, a medicine may cause some unwanted effects. Although not all of these side effects may occur, if they do occur they may need medical attention.

*Check with your doctor immediately* if any of the following side effects occur:
*Rare*
  Fever, joint pain, skin rash, or itching
*Symptoms of overdose*
  Convulsions (seizures); difficulty in breathing; muscle weakness

Other side effects may occur that usually do not need medical attention. These side effects may go away during treatment as your body adjusts to the medicine. However, check with your doctor if any of the following side effects continue or are bothersome:

*Less common*
  Abdominal or stomach cramps or pain; diarrhea; dizziness; drowsiness; headache; muscle weakness; nausea or vomiting; tremors

Other side effects not listed above may also occur in some patients. If you notice any other effects, check with your doctor.

Revised: 08/02/93

# PLICAMYCIN    Systemic†

A commonly used brand name in the U.S. is Mithracin.
Another commonly used name is mithramycin.

---

†Not commercially available in Canada.

---

## Description

Plicamycin (plye-ka-MYE-sin) belongs to the group of medicines known as antineoplastics. It may be used to treat certain types of cancer. It is also used to treat hypercalcemia or hypercalciuria (too much calcium in the blood or urine) that may occur with some types of cancer.

Plicamycin may also be used for other conditions as determined by your doctor.

Plicamycin is to be administered by or under the immediate care of your doctor. It is available only with a prescription, in the following dosage form:

*Parenteral*
- Injection (U.S.)

---

## Before Receiving This Medicine

Plicamycin is a very strong medicine. In addition to its helpful effects in treating your medical problem, it has side effects that could be very serious. Before you receive this medicine, be sure that you have discussed its use with your doctor.

In deciding to use a medicine, the risks of taking the medicine must be weighed against the good it will do. This is a decision you and your doctor will make. For plicamycin, the following should be considered:

**Allergies**—Tell your doctor if you have ever had any unusual or allergic reaction to plicamycin. Also tell your health care professional if you are allergic to any other substances, such as foods, preservatives, or dyes.

**Pregnancy**—Plicamycin is not recommended for use during pregnancy. There is a possibility that it may be harmful to the fetus.

**Breast-feeding**—It is not known whether plicamycin passes into the breast milk.

**Children**—Studies on this medicine have not been done in children; however, plicamycin can cause serious side effects in any patient. Therefore, it is especially important that you discuss with the child's doctor the good that this medicine may do as well as the risks of using it.

**Older adults**—Many medicines have not been studied specifically in older people. Therefore, it may not be known whether they work exactly the same way they do in younger adults or if they cause different side effects or problems in older people. There is no specific information

comparing use of plicamycin in the elderly with use in other age groups.

**Other medicines**—Although certain medicines should not be used together at all, in other cases two different medicines may be used together even if an interaction might occur. In these cases, your doctor may want to change the dose, or other precautions may be necessary. Tell your health care professional if you are taking *any* other medicines or are having x-ray treatments.

**Other medical problems**—The presence of other medical problems may affect the use of plicamycin. Make sure you tell your doctor if you have any other medical problems, especially:

- Bleeding problems—Use of plicamycin may increase the risk of bleeding
- Blood disease or
- Kidney disease or
- Liver disease—Use of plicamycin may make these conditions worse
- Chickenpox (including recent exposure) or
- Herpes zoster (shingles)—Use of plicamycin may make your reaction to either of these conditions worse

---

## Proper Use of This Medicine

Plicamycin sometimes causes nausea, vomiting, and loss of appetite. However, it is very important that you continue to receive the medicine, even if you begin to feel ill. If you have any questions about this, check with your doctor.

**Dosing**—The dose of plicamycin will be different for different patients. The dose is based on body weight and will be determined by your doctor. *Follow your doctor's orders.* The following information includes only the average doses of plicamycin.

- For *injection* dosage form:
  —To treat cancer:
   - Adults and children—The dose that is used may depend on a number of things, including what the medicine is being used for, the patient's weight, and whether or not other medicines are also being taken. *If you are receiving plicamycin at home, follow your doctor's orders or the directions on the label.* If you have any questions about the proper dose of plicamycin, ask your doctor.
  —To treat hypercalcemia or hypercalciuria (too much calcium in the blood or urine):
   - Adults—The dose is based on body weight and must be determined by your doctor. At first, the usual dose is 15 to 25 micrograms (mcg) per kg (6.8 to 11.4 mcg per pound) of body weight a day, injected slowly into a vein. The dose is given over a period of four to six hours once a day for

---

three to four days. Your doctor may repeat the treatment if needed.
- Children—Dose must be determined by your doctor.

## Precautions After Receiving This Medicine

It is very important that your doctor check your progress daily while you are receiving plicamycin to make sure that this medicine does not cause unwanted effects.

Your doctor may want you to follow a low-calcium, low–vitamin D diet. If you have any questions about this, check with your doctor.

*Do not take aspirin or large amounts of any other preparations containing aspirin, other salicylates, or acetaminophen without first checking with your doctor.* These medicines may increase the effects of plicamycin.

While you are being treated with plicamycin, and after you stop treatment with it, *do not have any immunizations (vaccinations) without your doctor's approval.* Plicamycin may lower your body's resistance and there is a chance you might get the infection the immunization is meant to prevent. In addition, other persons living in your household should not take or have recently taken oral polio vaccine since there is a chance they could pass the polio virus on to you. Also, avoid other persons who have taken oral polio vaccine. Do not get close to them, and do not stay in the same room with them for very long. If you cannot take these precautions, you should consider wearing a protective face mask that covers the nose and mouth.

Plicamycin can lower the number of white blood cells in your blood temporarily, increasing the chance of getting an infection. It can also lower the number of platelets, which are necessary for proper blood clotting. If this occurs, there are certain precautions your doctor may ask you to take, especially when your blood count is low, to reduce the risk of infection of bleeding:
- If you can, avoid people with infections. *Check with your doctor immediately* if you think you are getting an infection or if you get a fever or chills.
- *Check with your doctor immediately* if you notice any unusual bleeding or bruising.
- Be careful when using a regular toothbrush, dental floss, or toothpick. Your medical doctor, dentist, or nurse may recommend other ways to clean your teeth and gums. Check with your medical doctor before having any dental work done.
- Do not touch your eyes or the inside of your nose unless you have just washed your hands and have not touched anything else in the meantime.
- Be careful not to cut yourself when you are using sharp objects such as a safety razor or fingernail or toenail cutters.
- Avoid contact sports or other situations where bruising or injury could occur.

## Side Effects of This Medicine

Along with its needed effects, a medicine may cause some unwanted effects. Although not all of these side effects may occur, if they do occur they may need medical attention.

*Check with your doctor or nurse immediately* if any of the following side effects occur:

*Less common*
Muscle and abdominal cramps

*Symptoms of overdose*
Bloody or black, tarry stools; flushing or redness or swelling of face; nosebleed; skin rash or small red spots on skin; sore throat and fever; unusual bleeding or bruising; vomiting of blood; yellow eyes or skin

Other side effects may occur that usually do not need medical attention. These side effects may go away during treatment as your body adjusts to the medicine. However, check with your doctor if any of the following side effects continue or are bothersome:

*More common*
Diarrhea; irritation or soreness of mouth; loss of appetite; nausea or vomiting—may occur 1 to 2 hours after the injection is started and continue for 12 to 24 hours

*Less common*
Drowsiness; fever; headache; mental depression; pain, redness, soreness, or swelling at place of injection; unusual tiredness or weakness

After you stop using plicamycin, it may still produce some side effects that need attention. During this period of time check with your doctor if you notice any of the following side effects:

Bloody or black, tarry stools; nosebleed; sore throat and fever; unusual bleeding or bruising; vomiting of blood

Other side effects not listed above may also occur in some patients. If you notice any other effects, check with your doctor.

## Additional Information

Once a medicine has been approved for marketing for a certain use, experience may show that it is also useful for other medical problems. Although this use is not included in product labeling, plicamycin is used in certain patients with the following medical condition:
- Paget's disease of the bone

Other than the above information, there is no additional information relating to proper use, precautions, or side effects for these uses.

Revised: 09/14/92
Interim revision: 08/02/94

# PNEUMOCOCCAL VACCINE POLYVALENT   Systemic

Some commonly used brand names are:

**In the U.S.—**
Pneumovax 23
Pnu-Imune 23

**In Canada—**
Pneumovax 23

## Description

Pneumococcal (NEU-mo-KOK-al) vaccine polyvalent is an active immunizing agent used to prevent infection by pneumococcal bacteria. It works by causing your body to produce its own protection (antibodies) against the disease.

The following information applies only to the polyvalent 23 pneumococcal vaccine. Other polyvalent pneumococcal vaccines may be available in countries other than the U.S.

Pneumococcal infection can cause serious problems, such as pneumonia, which affects the lungs; meningitis, which affects the brain; bacteremia, which is a severe infection in the blood; and possibly death. These problems are more likely to occur in older adults and persons with certain diseases or conditions that make them more susceptible to a pneumococcal infection or more apt to develop serious problems from a pneumococcal infection.

Immunization against pneumococcal disease is recommended for:

- older adults, especially those 50 years of age and older.
- adults and children 2 years of age or older with chronic illnesses.
- persons with human immunodeficiency virus (HIV) infection, either with or without symptoms.
- persons with spleen problems or without spleens and persons who are to have their spleens removed.
- persons with sickle cell disease.
- persons who are waiting for organ transplants.
- persons who will be treated with x-rays or cancer medicines.
- persons in nursing homes and orphanages.
- persons who will be traveling outside the U.S. and who have certain diseases or conditions that make them more susceptible to pneumococcal infection or more likely to develop serious problems from pneumococcal infection.
- persons who are bedridden.

Immunization against pneumococcal infection is not recommended for infants and children younger than 2 years of age, because these persons cannot produce enough antibodies to the vaccine to protect them against a pneumococcal infection.

Pneumococcal vaccine is usually given only once to each person. Additional injections are not given, except in special cases, because of the possibility of more frequent and more severe side effects.

This vaccine is to be administered only by or under the supervision of your doctor or other health care professional. It is available in the following dosage form:

*Parenteral*
- Injection (U.S. and Canada)

## Before Receiving This Vaccine

In deciding to use a medicine, the risks of taking the medicine must be weighed against the good it will do. This is a decision you and your doctor will make. For pneumococcal vaccine, the following should be considered:

**Allergies**—Tell your doctor if you have ever had any unusual or allergic reaction to pneumococcal vaccine. Also tell your health care professional if you are allergic to any other substances, such as preservatives (especially thimerosal).

**Pregnancy**—Studies on effects in pregnancy have not been done in either humans or animals. However, if the vaccine is needed, it should be given after the first three months of pregnancy and only to women who have certain diseases or conditions that make them more susceptible to a pneumococcal infection or more likely to develop serious problems from a pneumococcal infection.

**Breast-feeding**—It is not known whether pneumococcal vaccine passes into the breast milk. Although most medicines pass into breast milk in small amounts, many of them may be used safely while breast-feeding. Mothers who are receiving this vaccine and who wish to breast-feed should discuss this with their doctor.

**Children**—Use of pneumococcal vaccine is not recommended in infants and children younger than 2 years of age. In children 2 years of age and older, this vaccine is not expected to cause different side effects or problems than it does in adults.

**Older adults**—Many medicines have not been studied specifically in older people. Therefore, it may not be known whether they work exactly the same way they do in younger adults. Although there is no specific information comparing use of pneumococcal vaccine in the elderly with use in other age groups, this vaccine is not expected to cause different side effects or problems in older people than it does in younger adults.

**Other medicines**—Although certain medicines should not be used together at all, in other cases two different medicines may be used together even if an interaction might occur. In these cases, your doctor may want to change the dose, or other precautions may be necessary. Before you receive pneumococcal vaccine, it is especially important that your health care professional know if you have received any of the following:

- Pneumococcal vaccine injection of any kind in the past— May increase the chance and severity of side effects

**Other medical problems**—The presence of other medical problems may affect the use of pneumococcal vaccine. Make sure you tell your doctor if you have any other medical problems, especially:

- Severe illness with fever—The symptoms of the illness may be confused with possible side effects of the vaccine
- Thrombocytopenic purpura (blood disorder)—Use of pneumococcal vaccine may make the condition worse

## Proper Use of This Vaccine

**Dosing**—The dose of pneumococcal vaccine will be different for different patients. The following information includes only the average doses of pneumococcal vaccine.

- For *injection* dosage form:
  - —For prevention of pneumococcal pneumonia:
    - Adults and children 2 years of age and older— One dose injected under the skin or into a muscle.
    - Children up to 2 years of age—Use is not recommended.

## Precautions After Receiving This Vaccine

*If you have more than one doctor, be sure they all know that you have received pneumococcal vaccine polyvalent 23 so that they can put the information in your medical records.* This vaccine is usually given only once to each person, except in special cases.

## Side Effects of This Vaccine

Along with its needed effects, a medicine may cause some unwanted effects. Although not all of these side effects may occur, if they do occur they may need medical attention.

*Get emergency help immediately* if any of the following side effects occur:

*Symptoms of allergic reaction*
Difficulty in breathing or swallowing; hives; itching, especially of feet or hands; reddening of skin, especially around ears; swelling of eyes, face, or inside of nose; unusual tiredness or weakness (sudden and severe)

Check with your doctor as soon as possible if the following side effect occurs:

*Rare*
Fever over 102 °F (39 °C)

Other side effects may occur that usually do not need medical attention. However, check with your doctor if any of the following side effects continue or are bothersome:

*More common*
Redness, soreness, hard lump, swelling, or pain at place of injection

*Less common or rare*
Aches or pain in joints or muscles; fever of 101 °F (38.3 °C) or less; skin rash; swollen glands; unusual tiredness or weakness; vague feeling of bodily discomfort

Side effects may be more common and more severe if this is not the first time you have received pneumococcal vaccine. Check with your doctor as soon as possible if you do have a severe reaction.

Other side effects not listed above may also occur in some patients. If you notice any other effects, check with your doctor.

Revised: 07/12/94

# PODOPHYLLUM  Topical

Some commonly used brand names in the U.S. are Podocon-25 and Podofin.

## Description

Podophyllum (pode-oh-FILL-um) is used to remove benign (not cancer) growths, such as certain kinds of warts. It works by destroying the tissue of the growth.

A few hours after podophyllum is applied to a wart, the wart becomes blanched (loses all color). In 24 to 48 hours, the medicine causes death of the tissue. After about 72 hours, the wart begins to slough or come off and gradually disappears.

Podophyllum is usually applied only in a doctor's office because it is a poison and can cause serious side effects if not used properly. However, your doctor may ask you to apply this medicine at home. If you do apply it at home, be sure you understand exactly how to use it.

Podophyllum is available only with your doctor's prescription, in the following dosage form:

*Topical*
- Topical solution (U.S.)

## Before Using This Medicine

In deciding to use a medicine, the risks of using the medicine must be weighed against the good it will do.

This is a decision you and your doctor will make. For podophyllum, the following should be considered:

**Allergies**—Tell your doctor if you have ever had any unusual or allergic reaction to podophyllum or benzoin. Also tell your health care professional if you are allergic to any other substances, such as preservatives or dyes.

**Pregnancy**—Topical podophyllum is absorbed through the skin. It should not be used during pregnancy, since it may cause birth defects or other harmful effects in the fetus.

**Breast-feeding**—Topical podophyllum is absorbed through the skin. However, it is not known whether topical podophyllum passes into breast milk. Although most medicines pass into breast milk in small amounts, many of them may be used safely while breast-feeding. Mothers who are using this medicine and who wish to breast-feed should discuss this with their doctor.

**Children**—Although there is no specific information comparing use of topical podophyllum in children with use in other age groups, this medicine is not expected to cause different side effects or problems in children than it does in adults.

**Older adults**—Many medicines have not been studied specifically in older people. Therefore, it may not be known whether they work exactly the same way they do in younger adults. Although there is no specific information comparing use of topical podophyllum in the elderly with use in other age groups, this medicine is not expected to cause different side effects or problems in older people than it does in younger adults.

**Other medicines**—Although certain medicines should not be used together at all, in other cases two different medicines may be used together even if an interaction might occur. In these cases, your doctor may want to change the dose, or other precautions may be necessary. Tell your health care professional if you are using any other prescription or nonprescription (over-the-counter [OTC]) medicine.

**Other medical problems**—The presence of other medical problems may affect the use of podophyllum. Make sure you tell your doctor if you have any other medical problems, especially:

- Crumbling or bleeding warts or warts that have recently had surgery on them—Using podophyllum on these warts may increase the chance of absorption of the medicine through the skin

## Proper Use of This Medicine

*Podophyllum is a poison. Keep it away from the mouth because it is harmful if swallowed.*

Also, *keep podophyllum away from the eyes and other mucous membranes,* such as the inside of the nose, mouth, or vagina. This medicine may cause severe irritation. If you get some in your eyes, immediately flush the eyes with water for 15 minutes. If you get some on your normal skin, thoroughly wash the skin with soap and water to remove the medicine. However, if this medicine contains tincture of benzoin, it may be removed more easily from the skin by swabbing with rubbing alcohol.

This medicine may contain alcohol and therefore may be flammable. *Do not use near heat, near open flame, or while smoking.*

*Use podophyllum only as directed.* Do not use more of it, do not use it more often, and do not use it for a longer time than your doctor ordered. To do so may increase the chance of too much medicine being absorbed into the body and the chance of side effects.

*Do not use podophyllum on moles or birthmarks.* To do so may cause severe irritation.

Also, *do not apply this medicine to crumbling or bleeding warts or to warts that have recently had surgery on them.* To do so may increase the chance of absorption through the skin.

*To use:*

- Podophyllum can cause severe irritation of normal skin. Therefore, apply petrolatum around the affected area before you apply podophyllum, and/or apply talcum powder to the treated area immediately after you apply podophyllum. This is to prevent the medicine from spreading to the normal skin.
- Use a toothpick or a cotton-tipped or glass applicator to apply this medicine. Apply 1 drop at a time, allowing time for drying between drops, until the affected area is covered.
- After podophyllum is applied, allow it to remain on the affected area for 1 to 6 hours as directed by your doctor. Then, remove the medicine by thoroughly washing the affected area with soap and water. If this medicine contains tincture of benzoin, it may be removed more easily by swabbing the affected area with rubbing alcohol. However, this may be more irritating than washing with soap and water.
- Immediately after applying this medicine, wash your hands to remove any medicine that may be on them.

**Dosing**—The dose of topical podophyllum will be different for different patients. *Follow your doctor's orders or the directions on the label.* The following information includes only the average doses of topical podophyllum. *If your dose is different, do not change it unless your doctor tells you to do so.*

- *For topical solution* dosage form:
  —For venereal warts:
  - Adults and children—Apply to the affected area(s) of the skin and leave on the skin for one to six hours. Treatment may be repeated every week for up to four weeks.
  —For other warts or benign growths:
  - Adults and children—Apply to the affected area(s) of the skin once a day.

**Missed dose**—If you miss a dose of this medicine, apply it as soon as possible. Then go back to your regular dosing schedule.

**Storage**—To store this medicine:

- Keep out of the reach of children.
- Store away from heat and direct light.
- Do not store in the bathroom, near the kitchen sink, or in other damp places. Heat or moisture may cause the medicine to break down.
- Do not keep outdated medicine or medicine no longer needed. Be sure that any discarded medicine is out of the reach of children.

## Side Effects of This Medicine

Along with its needed effects, a medicine may cause some unwanted effects. Although not all of these side effects may occur, if they do occur they may need medical attention.

*Check with your doctor immediately* if any of the following side effects occur:

*Early symptoms of too much medicine being absorbed into the body*

Abdominal or stomach pain; clumsiness or unsteadiness; confusion; decreased or loss of reflexes; diarrhea (may be severe and continuing); excitement, irritability, or nervousness; hallucinations (seeing, hearing, or feeling things that are not there); muscle weakness; nausea or vomiting; sore throat and fever; unusual bleeding or bruising

*Late symptoms of too much medicine being absorbed into the body*

Constipation; convulsions (seizures); difficult or painful urination; difficulty in breathing; dizziness or lightheadedness, especially when getting up from a lying or sitting position; drowsiness; fast heartbeat; numbness, tingling, pain, or weakness in hands or feet (may not occur for about 2 weeks after medicine is used); pain in upper abdomen or stomach (mild, dull, and continuing)

Also, check with your doctor as soon as possible if any of the following side effects occur:

Burning, redness, or other irritation of affected area; skin rash or itching

Other side effects not listed above may also occur in some patients. If you notice any other effects, check with your doctor.

Revised: 08/15/94

# POLIOVIRUS VACCINE    Systemic

Some commonly used brand names are:

**In the U.S.—**

| | |
|---|---|
| Ipol[2] | Orimune[3] |

Other commonly used names are:

| | |
|---|---|
| enhanced-potency IPV[2] | Sabin vaccine[3] |
| IPV[1] | Salk vaccine[1] |
| N-IPV[2] | TOPV[3] |
| OPV[3] | |

Note: For quick reference, the following poliovirus vaccines are numbered to match the corresponding brand names.

This information applies to the following medicines:

1. Poliovirus Vaccine Inactivated‡§
2. Poliovirus Vaccine Inactivated Enhanced Potency‡§
3. Poliovirus Vaccine Live Oral§

‡Generic name product may also be available in the U.S.
§Generic name product may also be available in Canada.

## Description

Poliovirus (POE-lee-oh VYE-russ) vaccine is an active immunizing agent used to prevent poliomyelitis (polio). It works by causing your body to produce its own protection (antibodies) against the virus that causes polio.

There are two types of polio vaccine that are given by injection, poliovirus vaccine inactivated (IPV) and poliovirus vaccine inactivated enhanced potency (enhanced-potency IPV). The type of vaccine that is given by mouth is called poliovirus vaccine live oral (OPV).

Polio is a very serious infection that causes paralysis of the muscles, including the muscles that enable you to walk and breathe. A polio infection may leave a person unable to breathe without the help of an iron lung, unable to walk without leg braces, or confined to a wheelchair. There is no cure for polio.

Immunization against polio is recommended for all infants from age 6 to 12 weeks, all children, all adolescents up to 18 years of age, and certain adults, including:

- Persons traveling outside the U.S. to countries where polio is uncontrolled, whether or not they have been vaccinated against polio in the past.
- All adults who may be exposed to polio, whether or not they have been vaccinated against polio in the past.
- Adults who have not been vaccinated or who have not had the complete series of vaccinations against polio and who live in households in which children are to be given the oral polio vaccine (OPV).
- Employees in day-care centers and group homes for children, such as orphanages.
- Employees in medical facilities, such as hospitals and doctors' offices.
- Laboratory workers handling samples that may contain polioviruses.

Immunization against polio is not recommended for infants younger than 6 weeks of age, because antibodies they received from their mothers before birth may interfere with the effectiveness of the vaccine. Infants who were immunized against polio before 6 weeks of age should receive the complete series of polio immunization.

This vaccine is to be administered only by or under the supervision of your doctor or other health care professional. It is available in the following dosage forms:

*Oral*
- Oral solution (U.S. and Canada)

*Parenteral*
- Injection (U.S. and Canada)

## Before Receiving This Vaccine

For a while after you are immunized, there is a very small risk (1 in 5 million) that any persons living in your household who have not yet been immunized against polio or who have or had an immune deficiency condition may develop poliomyelitis (polio) from being around you. Talk to your doctor if you have any questions about this.

In deciding to use a medicine, the risks of taking the medicine must be weighed against the good it will do. This is a decision you and your doctor will make. For polio vaccine, the following should be considered:

**Allergies**—Tell your doctor if you have ever had any unusual or allergic reaction to polio vaccine or to neomycin, penicillin, polymyxin B, or streptomycin. The polio vaccines available in the U.S. may contain neomycin, polymyxin B, and/or streptomycin. The polio vaccines available in Canada may contain neomycin, penicillin, polymyxin B, and/or streptomycin. Also tell your health care professional if you are allergic to any other substances, such as foods, preservatives, or dyes.

**Diet**—Make certain your health care professional knows if you are on any special diet, such as a low-sugar diet, because the oral solution form of polio vaccine may be given to you on a sugar cube.

**Pregnancy**—Studies on effects in pregnancy have not been done in either humans or animals. However, this vaccine has not been shown to cause birth defects or other problems in humans. Although it is not recommended for all pregnant women, polio vaccine is given to pregnant women at great risk of catching polio.

**Breast-feeding**—Polio vaccine has not been reported to cause problems in nursing babies.

**Children**—Use is not recommended for infants up to 6 weeks of age. For infants and children 6 weeks of age and older, polio vaccine is not expected to cause different side effects or problems than it does in adults.

**Older adults**—Many medicines have not been studied specifically in older people. Therefore, it may not be known whether they work exactly the same way they do in younger adults. Although there is no specific information comparing use of polio vaccine in the elderly with use in other age groups, this vaccine is not expected to cause different side effects or problems in older persons than it does in younger adults.

**Other medicines**—Although certain medicines should not be used together at all, in other cases two different medicines may be used together even if an interaction might occur. In these cases, your doctor may want to change the dose, or other precautions may be necessary. Before you receive polio vaccine, it is especially important that your health care professional know if you are receiving or have received any of the following:

- Cancer medicines or
- Corticosteroids (e.g., cortisone-like medicines) or
- Radiation therapy—May reduce the useful effect of the vaccine

**Other medical problems**—The presence of other medical problems may affect the use of polio vaccine. Make sure you tell your doctor if you have any other medical problems, especially:

- Diarrhea or
- Virus infection or
- Vomiting—The condition may reduce the useful effect of the vaccine
- Fever or
- Illness (moderate or severe) or
- Weakness (severe)—The symptoms of the condition may be confused with possible side effects of the vaccine
- Immune deficiency condition (or family history of)—The condition may increase the chance of side effects of the vaccine

## Proper Use of This Vaccine

**Dosing**—The dose of polio vaccine will be different for different patients. The following information includes only the average doses of polio vaccine.

- For prevention of polio:
  - For *enhanced-potency IPV injection* dosage form:
    - Adults and children 6 years of age and older—One dose is given at your first visit, then a second dose is given four to eight weeks later. A third dose is given six to twelve months after the second dose. The doses are injected under the skin.
    - Infants and children 6 weeks to 6 years of age—One dose is given at your first visit, then a second dose is given four to eight weeks later. A third dose is given six to twelve months after the second dose. A booster dose is given at four to six years of age only if the third dose was given before the child's fourth birthday. The doses are injected under the skin.
  - For *IPV injection* dosage form:
    - Adults and children 18 years of age and older—One dose is given every four to eight weeks for a total of three doses. A fourth dose is given six to twelve months after the third dose. The doses are injected under the skin.
    - Children 6 weeks to 18 years of age—One dose is given every four to eight weeks for a total of three doses. A fourth dose is given six to twelve months after the third dose. A booster dose is given at four to six years of age only if the fourth dose was given before the child's fourth birthday.

Booster doses are given every five years until the child is eighteen years of age. The doses are injected under the skin.

—For *OPV oral* dosage form:

• Adults and children 18 years of age and older—Use and dose must be determined by your doctor.

• Infants and children 6 weeks to 18 years of age—One dose is given at your first visit, then a second dose is given six to eight weeks later. A third dose is given eight to twelve months after the second dose. A booster dose is given at four to six years of age only if the third dose was given before the child's fourth birthday. The doses are taken by mouth.

## Precautions After Receiving This Vaccine

Tell your doctor that you have received this vaccine if you are to receive any other live virus vaccines within 1 month after receiving this vaccine.

## Side Effects of This Vaccine

In very rare instances (approximately 1 case in 3.2 million doses), healthy persons who have taken the oral vaccine (OPV) and healthy persons who are close contacts of adults or children who have taken OPV have been infected by the polio virus and have become paralyzed. No paralysis caused by polio infection has occurred with the injected vaccine (IPV) since 1955.

Along with its needed effects, a vaccine may cause some unwanted effects. Although not all of these side effects may occur, if they do occur they may need medical attention.

*Get emergency help immediately* if any of the following side effects occur:

*Symptoms of allergic reaction*

Difficulty in breathing or swallowing; hives; itching, especially of feet or hands; reddening of skin, especially around ears; swelling of eyes, face, or inside of nose; unusual tiredness or weakness (sudden and severe)

Other side effects may occur that usually do not need medical attention. However, check with your doctor if any of the following side effects continue or are bothersome:

*Less common*

Fever over 101.3 °F (38.5 °C) (with injection); itching or skin rash (with injection); redness, soreness, hard lump, tenderness, or pain at the place of injection (with injection)

Other side effects not listed above may also occur in some patients. If you notice any other effects, check with your doctor.

Revised: 07/12/94

# POLYETHYLENE GLYCOL AND ELECTROLYTES   Local

Some commonly used brand names are:

**In the U.S.—**

| | |
|---|---|
| Colovage | GoLYTELY |
| Colyte | Nulytely |
| Colyte-flavored | OCL |

**In Canada—**

| | |
|---|---|
| Colyte | Peglyte |
| GoLYTELY | |

## Description

The polyethylene glycol (pol-ee-ETH-i-leen GLYE-col) (PEG) and electrolytes solution is used to clean the colon (large bowel or lower intestine) before certain tests or surgery of the colon. The PEG-electrolyte solution is usually taken by mouth. However, sometimes it is given in the hospital through a nasogastric tube (a tube inserted through the nose).

The PEG-electrolyte solution acts like a laxative. It causes liquid stools or mild diarrhea. In this way, it flushes all solid material from the colon, so the doctor can have a clear view of the colon.

The PEG-electrolyte solution is available only with your doctor's prescription. It is available in the following dosage forms:

*Oral*

• Oral solution (U.S. and Canada)
• Powder for oral solution (U.S. and Canada)

## Before Using This Medicine

In deciding to use a medicine, the risks of taking the medicine must be weighed against the good it will do. This is a decision you and your doctor will make. For the PEG-electrolyte solution, the following should be considered:

**Allergies**—Tell your doctor if you have ever had any unusual or allergic reaction to PEG. Also tell your health care professional if you are allergic to any other substances, such as foods, preservatives, or dyes.

**Pregnancy**—Studies on effects in pregnancy have not been done in either humans or animals. Before taking the PEG-electrolyte solution or having a colon examination, make sure your doctor knows if you are pregnant.

**Breast-feeding**—The PEG-electrolyte solution has not been reported to cause problems in nursing babies.

**Children**—Although there is no specific information comparing use of PEG-electrolyte solution in children with use in other age groups, this medicine is not expected to cause different side effects or problems in children than it does in adults.

**Older adults**—This medicine has been tested and has not been shown to cause different side effects or problems in older people than it does in younger adults.

**Other medicines**—Although certain medicines should not be used together at all, in other cases two different medicines may be used together even if an interaction might occur. In these cases, your doctor may want to change the dose, or other precautions may be necessary. Tell your health care professional if you are taking any of the following:

- Any other oral medicines—Any medicines taken within 1 hour of the PEG-electrolyte solution may be flushed from the body and not have an effect

**Other medical problems**—The presence of other medical problems may affect the use of PEG-electrolyte solution. Make sure you tell your doctor if you have any other medical problems, especially:

- Blockage or obstruction of the intestine or
- Paralytic ileus or
- Perforated bowel or
- Toxic colitis or
- Toxic megacolon—PEG-electrolyte solution may make these conditions worse; in some cases the colon may rip open or tear

## Proper Use of This Medicine

Your doctor may have special instructions for you, depending on the type of test you are going to have. If you have not received such instructions or if you do not understand them, check with your doctor in advance.

*Take the PEG-electrolyte solution exactly as directed.* Otherwise, the test you are going to have may not work and may have to be done again.

*Do not eat anything for at least 3 hours before taking the PEG-electrolyte solution.* If you do so, the colon may not get completely clean. If you are drinking the PEG-electrolyte solution the evening before the test, you may drink clear liquids (e.g., water, ginger ale, decaffeinated cola, decaffeinated tea, broth, gelatin) up until the time of the test. However, check first with your doctor.

For patients *using the powder form of this medicine:*

- *The powder must be mixed with water before it is used.* Add lukewarm water to the fill mark on the bottle.
- *Shake well* until all the ingredients are dissolved.
- Do not add any other ingredients, such as flavoring, to the solution.

- After you mix the solution, you must use it within 48 hours.

**Dosing**—*Follow your doctor's orders or the directions on the label.* The following information includes only the usual amount taken of PEG-electrolyte solution. *If your dose is different, do not change it* unless your doctor tells you to do so:

- Drink one full glass (8 ounces) of the PEG-electrolyte solution *rapidly* every 10 minutes. If you sip small amounts of the solution, it will not work as well.
- It will take close to 3 hours to drink all of the PEG-electrolyte solution. The first bowel movement may start an hour or so after you start drinking the solution. *Continue drinking all the solution to get the best results,* unless otherwise directed by your doctor.

**Storage**—To store this medicine:

- Keep out of the reach of children.
- Store away from heat and direct light.
- Store the solution in the refrigerator to improve the taste. However, keep the medicine from freezing.
- Do not keep any leftover solution. Be sure that any discarded medicine is out of the reach of children.

## Side Effects of This Medicine

Along with its needed effects, a medicine may cause some unwanted effects. Although not all of these side effects may occur, if they do occur they may need medical attention.

Check with your doctor as soon as possible if the following side effect occurs:

*Rare*

Skin rash

Other side effects may occur that usually do not need medical attention. These side effects may go away as your body adjusts to the medicine. However, check with your health care professional if any of the following side effects continue or are bothersome:

*More common*

Bloating; nausea

*Less common*

Abdominal or stomach cramps; irritation of the anus; vomiting

Other side effects not listed above may also occur in some patients. If you notice any other effects, check with your health care professional.

Revised: 10/05/92

# POTASSIUM IODIDE  Systemic

Some commonly used brand names are:

**In the U.S.—**
  Pima
  Generic name product may also be available.
**In Canada—**
  Thyro-Block*
Other commonly used names are KI and SSKI.

---

*Not commercially available in the U.S.; however, potassium iodide tablets are available to government and public health organizations for use in radiation emergencies.

---

## Description

Potassium iodide (poe-TAS-ee-um EYE-oh-dide) is used to treat overactive thyroid and to protect the thyroid gland from the effects of radiation from inhaled or swallowed radioactive iodine. It may be used before and after administration of medicine containing radioactive iodine or after accidental exposure to radioactive iodine (for example, from nuclear power plant accidents that involved release of radioactivity to the environment). It may also be used for other problems as determined by your doctor.

Potassium iodide is taken by mouth. It may be taken as an oral solution, syrup, uncoated tablet, or enteric-coated tablet. However, the enteric-coated tablet form may cause serious side effects and its use is generally not recommended.

Some brands of the oral solution are available without a prescription. Use them only as directed by state or local public health authorities in case of a radiation emergency. Other forms and strengths of potassium iodide are available only with your doctor's prescription.

Potassium iodide is available in the following dosage forms:

*Oral*
  • Enteric-coated tablets (U.S.)
  • Oral solution (U.S.)
  • Syrup (U.S.)
  • Tablets (Canada)

## Before Using This Medicine

In deciding to use a medicine, the risks of taking the medicine must be weighed against the good it will do. This is a decision you and your doctor will make. For potassium iodide, the following should be considered:

**Allergies**—Tell your doctor if you have ever had any unusual or allergic reaction to potassium iodide, iodine, or iodine-containing foods. Also tell your health care professional if you are allergic to any substances, such as foods, preservatives, or dyes.

**Pregnancy**—Taking potassium during pregnancy may cause thyroid problems or goiter in the newborn infant.

**Breast-feeding**—Potassium iodide passes into the breast milk and may cause skin rash and thyroid problems in nursing babies.

**Children**—Potassium iodide may cause skin rash and thyroid problems in infants.

**Older adults**—Many medicines have not been studied specifically in older people. Therefore, it may not be known whether they work exactly the same way they do in younger adults. Although there is no specific information comparing use of potassium iodide in the elderly with use in other age groups, this medicine is not expected to cause different side effects or problems in older people than in younger adults.

**Other medicines**—Although certain medicines should not be used together at all, in other cases two different medicines may be used together even if an interaction might occur. In these cases, your doctor may want to change the dose, or other precautions may be necessary. When you are taking potassium iodide, it is especially important that your health care professional know if you are taking any of the following:

  • Amiloride (e.g., Midamor) or
  • Spironolactone (e.g., Aldactone) or
  • Triamterene (e.g., Dyrenium)—Use of these medicines with potassium iodide may increase the amount of potassium in the blood and increase the chance of side effects
  • Antithyroid agents (medicine for overactive thyroid) or
  • Lithium (e.g., Lithane)—Use of these medicines with potassium iodide may increase the chance of side effects

**Other medical problems**—The presence of other medical problems may affect the use of potassium iodide. Make sure you tell your doctor if you have any other medical problems, especially:

  • High blood levels of potassium (hyperkalemia) or
  • Myotonia congenita or
  • Tuberculosis—Potassium iodine may make these conditions worse
  • Kidney disease—May cause an increase of potassium in the blood
  • Overactive thyroid (unless you are taking this medicine for this medical problem)—Prolonged use of potassium iodine may be harmful to the thyroid gland

## Proper Use of This Medicine

For patients taking this medicine for *radiation exposure:*
  • Take this medicine only when directed to do so by state or local public health authorities.
  • Take this medicine once a day for 10 days, unless otherwise directed by public health authorities. *Do not take more of it and do not take it more often than directed.* Taking more of the medicine will not protect you better and may result in a greater chance of side effects.

If potassium iodide upsets your stomach, *take it after meals or with food or milk* unless otherwise directed by your doctor. If stomach upset (nausea, vomiting, stomach pain, or diarrhea) continues, check with your doctor.

For patients taking the *oral solution form* of this medicine:

- This medicine is to be taken by mouth even if it comes in a dropper bottle.
- Do not use if solution turns brownish yellow.
- Take potassium iodide in a full glass (8 ounces) of water or in fruit juice, milk, or broth to improve the taste and lessen stomach upset. Be sure to drink all of the liquid to get the full dose of medicine.
- If crystals form in potassium iodide solution, they may be dissolved by warming the closed container of solution in warm water and then gently shaking the container.

For patients taking the *uncoated tablet form* of this medicine:

- Before taking, dissolve each tablet in ½ glass (4 ounces) of water or milk. Be sure to drink all of the liquid to get the full dose of medicine.

**Dosing**—The dose of potassium iodide will be different for different patients. *Follow your doctor's orders or the directions on the label.* The following information includes only the average doses of potassium iodide. *If your dose is different, do not change it* unless your doctor tells you to do so.

The amount of solution or syrup or the number of tablets you take depends on the strength of the medicine. Also, *the number of doses you take each day, the time allowed between doses, and the length of time you take the medicine depend on the medical problem for which you are taking potassium iodide.*

- For *solution* dosage form:
  —To treat overactive thyroid (hyperthyroidism):
  - Adults and teenagers—250 milligrams (mg) (0.25 milliliters [mL]) three times a day.
  - Children—Use and dose must be determined by your doctor.
  —To protect the thyroid gland against radiation exposure:
  - Adults and teenagers—100 to 150 mg (0.1 to 0.15 mL) twenty-four hours before receiving or being exposed to radioactive iodine. Then, once a day for three to ten days after receiving or being exposed to radioactive iodine.
  - Children up to 1 year of age—65 mg (0.065 mL) once a day for ten days after receiving or being exposed to radioactive iodine.
  - Children 1 year of age or older—130 mg (0.13 mL) once a day for ten days after receiving or being exposed to radioactive iodine.
- For *syrup* dosage form:
  —To protect the thyroid gland against radiation exposure:
  - Adults and teenagers—100 to 150 mg (about 1.5 to 2.3 mL) twenty-four hours before receiving or being exposed to radioactive iodine. Then, once

a day for three to ten days after receiving or being exposed to radioactive iodine.
  - Children up to 1 year of age—65 mg (1 mL) once a day for ten days after receiving or being exposed to radioactive iodine.
  - Children 1 year of age or older—130 mg (2 mL) once a day for ten days after receiving or being exposed to radioactive iodine.
- For *tablet* dosage form:
  —To protect the thyroid gland against radiation exposure:
  - Adults and teenagers—100 to 150 mg twenty-four hours before receiving or being exposed to radioactive iodine. Then, once a day for three to ten days after receiving or being exposed to radioactive iodine.
  - Children up to 1 year of age—65 mg once a day for ten days after receiving or being exposed to radioactive iodine.
  - Children 1 year of age and older—130 mg a day for ten days after receiving or being exposed to radioactive iodine.

**Missed dose**—If you miss a dose of this medicine, take it as soon as possible. However, if it is almost time for your next dose, skip the missed dose and go back to your regular dosing schedule. Do not double doses.

**Storage**—To store this medicine:

- Keep out of the reach of children.
- Store away from heat and direct light.
- Do not store the tablet form of this medicine in the bathroom, near the kitchen sink, or in other damp places. Heat or moisture may cause the medicine to break down.
- Keep the oral liquid forms of this medicine from freezing. Do not refrigerate.
- Do not keep outdated medicine or medicine no longer needed. Be sure that any discarded medicine is out of the reach of children.

## Precautions While Using This Medicine

Your doctor should check your progress at regular visits to make sure that this medicine does not cause unwanted effects.

For patients on a low-potassium diet:

- *This medicine contains potassium.* Check with your health care professional before you take this medicine.

## Side Effects of This Medicine

Along with its needed effects, a medicine may cause some unwanted effects. Although not all of these side effects may occur, if they do occur they may need medical attention. When this medicine is used for a short time at low doses, side effects usually are rare.

Check with your doctor as soon as possible if any of the following side effects occur:

*Less common*

Hives; joint pain; swelling of arms, face, legs, lips, tongue, and/or throat; swelling of lymph glands

*With long-term use*

Burning of mouth or throat; confusion; headache (severe); increased watering of mouth; irregular heartbeat; metallic taste; numbness, tingling, pain or weakness in hands or feet; soreness of teeth and gums; sores on skin; symptoms of head cold; unusual tiredness; weakness or heaviness of legs

Other side effects may occur that usually do not need medical attention. These side effects may go away during treatment as your body adjusts to the medicine. However, check with your doctor if any of the following side effects continue or are bothersome:

*Less common*

Diarrhea; nausea or vomiting; stomach pain

Other side effects not listed above may also occur in some patients. If you notice any other effects, check with your doctor.

## Additional Information

Once a medicine has been approved for marketing for a certain use, experience may show that it is also useful for other medical problems. Although these uses are not included in product labeling, potassium iodide is used in certain patients with the following medical conditions:

- To prepare the thyroid gland before a thyroid operation
- Iodine deficiency
- Certain skin conditions caused by fungus

In addition to the above information, for patients taking this medicine for a fungus infection:

- *Keep taking it for the full course of treatment,* even if you begin to feel better after a few days. This will help clear up your infection completely. *Do not miss any doses.*

Other than the above information, there is no additional information relating to proper use, precautions, or side effects for these uses.

Revised: 04/14/92
Interim revision: 08/26/94

# POTASSIUM SUPPLEMENTS   Systemic

Some commonly used brand names are:

**In the U.S.—**

| | |
|---|---|
| Cena-K[5] | Klor-Con/25 Powder[5] |
| Effer-K[4] | Klorvess[3] |
| Gen-K[5] | Klorvess Effervescent |
| K + 10[5] |     Granules[3] |
| Kaochlor 10%[5] | Klorvess 10% Liquid[5] |
| Kaochlor-Eff[6] | Klotrix[5] |
| Kaochlor S-F 10%[5] | K-Lyte[2] |
| Kaon[7] | K-Lyte/Cl[3] |
| Kaon-Cl[5] | K-Lyte/Cl 50[3] |
| Kaon-Cl-10[5] | K-Lyte/Cl Powder[5] |
| Kaon-Cl 20% Liquid[5] | K-Lyte DS[4] |
| Kato[5] | K-Norm[5] |
| Kay Ciel[5] | Kolyum[8] |
| Kaylixir[7] | K-Tab[5] |
| K + Care[5] | Micro-K[5] |
| K + Care ET[2] | Micro-K 10[5] |
| K-Dur[5] | Micro-K LS[5] |
| K-G Elixir[7] | Potage[5] |
| K-Ide[2,5] | Potasalan[5] |
| K-Lease[5] | Rum-K[5] |
| K-Lor[5] | Slow-K[5] |
| Klor-Con 8[5] | Ten-K[5] |
| Klor-Con 10[5] | Tri-K[10] |
| Klor-Con/EF[2] | Twin-K[9] |
| Klor-Con Powder[5] | |

**In Canada—**

| | |
|---|---|
| Apo-K[5] | K-Lyte[2] |
| K-10[5] | K-Lyte/Cl[5] |
| Kalium Durules[5] | Micro-K[5] |
| Kaochlor-10[5] | Micro-K 10[5] |
| Kaochlor-20[5] | Neo-K[3] |
| Kaon[7] | Novolente-K[5] |
| KCL 5%[5] | Potassium-Rougier[7] |
| K-Dur[5] | Potassium-Sandoz[3] |
| K-Long[5] | Roychlor-10%[5] |
| K-Lor[5] | Slow-K[5] |
| Klor-Con/EF[2] | |

Note: For quick reference, the following potassium supplements are numbered to match the corresponding brand names.

This information applies to the following medicines:

1. Potassium Acetate (poe-TAS-ee-um AS-a-tate)‡§
2. Potassium Bicarbonate (bi-KAR-bo-nate)
3. Potassium Bicarbonate and Potassium Chloride (KLOR-ide)
4. Potassium Bicarbonate and Potassium Citrate (SIH-trayt)†
5. Potassium Chloride‡§
6. Potassium Chloride, Potassium Bicarbonate, and Potassium Citrate†
7. Potassium Gluconate (GLOO-ko-nate)‡
8. Potassium Gluconate and Potassium Chloride†
9. Potassium Gluconate and Potassium Citrate†
10. Trikates (TRI-kates)‡

†Not commercially available in Canada.
‡Generic name product may be available in the U.S.
§Generic name product may be available in Canada.

## Description

Potassium is needed to maintain good health. Although a balanced diet usually supplies all the potassium a person needs, potassium supplements may be needed by patients who do not have enough potassium in their regular diet or have lost too much potassium because of illness or treatment with certain medicines.

There is no evidence that potassium supplements are useful in the treatment of high blood pressure.

Lack of potassium may cause muscle weakness, irregular heartbeat, mood changes, or nausea and vomiting.

Some forms of potassium may be available in stores without a prescription. Since too much potassium may cause health problems, you should take potassium supplements only if directed by your doctor. Potassium supplements are available with your doctor's prescription in the following dosage forms:

*Oral*

Potassium Bicarbonate
- Tablets for solution (U.S. and Canada)

Potassium Bicarbonate and Potassium Chloride
- Powder for solution (U.S. and Canada)
- Tablets for solution (U.S. and Canada)

Potassium Bicarbonate and Potassium Citrate
- Tablets for solution (U.S.)

Potassium Chloride
- Extended-release capsules (U.S. and Canada)
- Solution (U.S. and Canada)
- Powder for solution (U.S. and Canada)
- Powder for suspension (U.S.)
- Extended-release tablets (U.S. and Canada)

Potassium Chloride, Potassium Bicarbonate, and Potassium Citrate
- Tablets for solution (U.S.)

Potassium Gluconate
- Elixir (U.S. and Canada)
- Tablets (U.S.)

Potassium Gluconate and Potassium Chloride
- Solution (U.S.)
- Powder for solution (U.S.)

Potassium Gluconate and Potassium Citrate
- Solution (U.S.)

Trikates
- Solution (U.S.)

*Parenteral*

Potassium Acetate
- Injection (U.S. and Canada)

Potassium Chloride
- Concentrate for injection (U.S. and Canada)

---

## Importance of Diet

Many nutritionists recommend that, if possible, people get the potassium they need from the foods they eat. However, many people do not get enough potassium from their diets. For example, people on weight-loss diets may consume too little food to get enough potassium. Others may lose potassium from the body because of illness or treatment with certain medicines. For such people, a potassium supplement, given under a doctor's supervision, is important.

In order to get enough vitamins and minerals in your diet, it is important that you eat a balanced and varied diet. Follow carefully any diet program your doctor may recommend. For your specific vitamin and/or mineral needs, ask your doctor for a list of appropriate foods.

The following table includes some potassium-rich foods.

| Food (amount) | Milligrams of potassium | Milli-equivalents of potassium |
|---|---|---|
| Acorn squash, cooked (1 cup) | 896 | 23 |
| Potato with skin, baked (1 long) | 844 | 22 |
| Spinach, cooked (1 cup) | 838 | 21 |
| Lentils, cooked (1 cup) | 731 | 19 |
| Kidney beans, cooked (1 cup) | 713 | 18 |
| Split peas, cooked (1 cup) | 710 | 18 |
| White navy beans, cooked (1 cup) | 669 | 17 |
| Butternut squash, cooked (1 cup) | 583 | 15 |
| Watermelon (1/16) | 560 | 14 |
| Raisins (½ cup) | 553 | 14 |
| Yogurt, low-fat, plain (1 cup) | 531 | 14 |
| Orange juice, frozen (1 cup) | 503 | 13 |
| Brussel sprouts, cooked (1 cup) | 494 | 13 |
| Zucchini, cooked, sliced (1 cup) | 456 | 12 |
| Banana (medium) | 451 | 12 |
| Collards, frozen, cooked (1 cup) | 427 | 11 |
| Cantaloupe (¼) | 412 | 11 |
| Milk, low-fat 1% (1 cup) | 348 | 9 |
| Broccoli, frozen, cooked (1 cup) | 332 | 9 |

Experts have developed a list of recommended dietary allowances (RDA) for most of the vitamins and some minerals. The RDA are not an exact number but a general idea of how much you need. They do not cover amounts needed for problems caused by a serious lack of vitamins or minerals. Because lack of potassium is rare, there are no RDA for this mineral. However, it is thought that 1600 to 2000 mg (40 to 50 mEq) per day for adults is adequate.

Remember:

- The total amount of potassium that you get every day includes what you get from food *and* what you may take as a supplement. Read the labels of processed foods. Many foods now have added potassium.

- Your total intake of potassium should not be greater than the recommended amounts, unless ordered by your doctor. In some cases, too much potassium may cause muscle weakness, confusion, irregular heartbeat, or difficult breathing.

---

## Before Using This Medicine

In deciding to use a medicine, the risks of taking the medicine must be weighed against the good it will do. This is a decision you and your doctor will make. For potassium supplements, the following should be considered:

**Allergies**—Tell your doctor if you have ever had any unusual or allergic reaction to potassium preparations. Also tell your health care professional if you are allergic to any other substances, such as foods, preservatives, or dyes.

**Pregnancy**—Potassium supplements have not been shown to cause problems in humans.

**Breast-feeding**—Potassium supplements pass into breast milk. However, this medicine has not been reported to cause problems in nursing babies.

**Children**—Although there is no specific information comparing use of potassium supplements in children with use in other age groups, they are not expected to cause different side effects or problems in children than they do in adults.

**Older adults**—Many medicines have not been studied specifically in older people. Therefore, it may not be known whether they work exactly the same way they do in younger adults. Although there is no specific information comparing use of potassium supplements in the elderly with use in other age groups, they are not expected to cause different side effects or problems in older people than they do in younger adults.

Older adults may be at a greater risk of developing high blood levels of potassium (hyperkalemia).

**Other medicines**—Although certain medicines should not be used together at all, in other cases two different medicines may be used together even if an interaction might occur. In these cases, your doctor may want to change the dose, or other precautions may be necessary. When you are taking potassium supplements, it is especially important that your health care professional know if you are taking any of the following:

- Amantadine (e.g., Symmetrel) or
- Anticholinergics (medicine for abdominal or stomach spasms or cramps) or
- Antidepressants (medicine for depression) or
- Antidyskinetics (medicine for Parkinson's disease or other conditions affecting control of muscles) or
- Antihistamines or
- Antipsychotic medicine (medicine for mental illness) or
- Buclizine (e.g., Bucladin) or
- Carbamazepine (e.g., Tegretol) or
- Cyclizine (e.g., Marezine) or
- Cyclobenzaprine (e.g., Flexeril) or
- Disopyramide (e.g., Norpace) or
- Flavoxate (e.g., Urispas) or
- Ipratropium (e.g., Atrovent) or
- Meclizine (e.g., Antivert) or
- Methylphenidate (e.g., Ritalin) or
- Orphenadrine (e.g., Norflex) or
- Oxybutynin (e.g., Ditropan) or
- Procainamide (e.g., Pronestyl) or
- Promethazine (e.g., Phenergan) or
- Quinidine (e.g., Quinidex) or
- Trimeprazine (e.g., Temaril)—Use with potassium supplements may cause or worsen certain stomach or intestine problems
- Angiotensin-converting enzyme (ACE) inhibitors (benazepril [e.g., Lotensin], captopril [e.g., Capoten], enalapril [e.g., Vasotec], fosinopril [e.g., Monotril], lisinopril [e.g., Prinivil, Zestril], quinapril [e.g., Accupril], ramipril [e.g., Altace]) or
- Amiloride (e.g., Midamor) or
- Beta-adrenergic blocking agents (acebutolol [e.g., Sectral], atenolol [e.g., Tenormin], betaxolol [e.g., Kerlone], carteolol [e.g., Cartrol], labetalol [e.g., Normodyne], metoprolol [e.g., Lopressor], nadolol [e.g., Corgard], oxprenolol [e.g., Trasicor], penbutolol [e.g., Levatol],

pindolol [e.g., Visken], propranolol [e.g., Inderal], sotalol [e.g., Sotacor], timolol [e.g., Blocadren]) or
- Heparin (e.g., Panheprin) or
- Inflammation or pain medicine (except narcotics) or
- Potassium-containing medicines (other) or
- Salt substitutes, low-salt foods, or milk or
- Spironolactone (e.g., Aldactone) or
- Triamterene (e.g., Dyrenium)—Use with potassium supplements may further increase potassium blood levels, which may cause or worsen heart problems
- Digitalis glycosides (heart medicine)—Use with potassium supplements may make heart problems worse
- Thiazide diuretics (water pills)—If you have been taking a potassium supplement and a thiazide diuretic together, stopping the thiazide diuretic may cause hyperkalemia (high blood levels of potassium)

**Other medical problems**—The presence of other medical problems may affect the use of potassium supplements. Make sure you tell your doctor if you have any other medical problems, especially:

- Addison's disease (underactive adrenal glands) or
- Dehydration (excessive loss of body water, continuing or severe)
- Diabetes mellitus or
- Kidney disease—Potassium supplements may increase the risk of hyperkalemia (high blood levels of potassium), which may worsen or cause heart problems in patients with these conditions
- Diarrhea (continuing or severe)—The loss of fluid in combination with potassium supplements may cause kidney problems, which may increase the risk of hyperkalemia (high blood levels of potassium)
- Heart disease—Potassium supplements may make this condition worse
- Intestinal or esophageal blockage—Potassium supplements may damage the intestines
- Stomach ulcer—Potassium supplements may make this condition worse

## Proper Use of This Medicine

For patients taking the *liquid form* of this medicine:
- This medicine *must be diluted* in at least one-half glass (4 ounces) of cold water or juice to reduce its possible stomach-irritating or laxative effect.
- If you are on a salt (sodium)-restricted diet, check with your doctor before using tomato juice to dilute your medicine. Tomato juice has a high salt content.

For patients taking the *soluble granule, soluble powder, or soluble tablet form* of this medicine:
- This medicine must be completely dissolved in at least one-half glass (4 ounces) of cold water or juice to reduce its possible stomach-irritating or laxative effect.
- Allow any "fizzing" to stop before taking the dissolved medicine.
- If you are on a salt (sodium)-restricted diet, check with your doctor before using tomato juice to dilute your medicine. Tomato juice has a high salt content.

For patients taking the *extended-release tablet form* of this medicine:

- Swallow the tablets whole with a full (8-ounce) glass of water. Do not chew or suck on the tablet.
- Some tablets may be broken or crushed and sprinkled on applesauce or other soft food. However, check with your health care professional first, since this should not be done for most tablets.
- If you have trouble swallowing tablets or if they seem to stick in your throat, check with your doctor. When this medicine is not properly released, it can cause irritation that may lead to ulcers.

For patients taking the *extended-release capsule form* of this medicine:

- Do not crush or chew the capsule. Swallow the capsule whole with a full (8-ounce) glass of water.
- Some capsules may be opened and the contents sprinkled on applesauce or other soft food. However, check with your health care professional first, since this should not be done for most capsules.

*Take this medicine immediately after meals or with food to lessen possible stomach upset or laxative action.*

*Take this medicine only as directed by your doctor.* Do not take more of it, do not take it more often, and do not take it for a longer time than your doctor ordered. *This is especially important if you are also taking both diuretics (water pills) and digitalis medicines for your heart.*

**Dosing**—The dose of these single or combination medicines will be different for different patients. *Follow your doctor's orders or the directions on the label.* The following information includes only the average dose of these medicines. *If your dose is different, do not change it unless your doctor tells you to do so.*

The number of ounces of solution that you drink, or the number of tablets or capsules you take, depends on the strength of the medicine. Also, *the number of doses you take each day, the time allowed between doses, and the length of time you take the medicine depend on the medical problem for which you are taking the single or combination medicine.*

*For potassium bicarbonate*

- For *oral* dosage form (tablets for solution):
  —To replace potassium lost by the body:
    - Adults and teenagers—25 to 50 milliequivalents (mEq) dissolved in one-half to one glass of cold water, taken one or two times a day. Your doctor may change the dose if needed. However, most people will not take more than 100 mEq a day.
    - Children—Dose must be determined by your doctor.

*For potassium bicarbonate and potassium chloride*

- For *oral* dosage form (granules for solution):
  —To replace potassium lost by the body:
    - Adults and teenagers—20 milliequivalents (mEq) dissolved in one-half to one glass of cold water, taken one or two times a day. Your doctor may change the dose if needed. However, most people will not take more than 100 mEq a day.
    - Children—Dose must be determined by your doctor.

- For *oral* dosage form (tablets for solution):
  —To replace potassium lost by the body:
    - Adults and teenagers—20, 25, or 50 mEq dissolved in one-half to one glass of cold water, taken one or two times a day. Your doctor may change the dose if needed. However, most people will not take more than 100 mEq a day.
    - Children—Dose must be determined by your doctor.

*For potassium bicarbonate and potassium citrate*

- For *oral* dosage form (tablets for solution):
  —To replace potassium lost by the body:
    - Adults and teenagers—25 or 50 milliequivalents (mEq) dissolved in one-half to one glass of cold water, taken one or two times a day. Your doctor may change the dose if needed. However, most people will not take more than 100 mEq a day.
    - Children—Dose must be determined by your doctor.

*For potassium chloride*

- For *oral* dosage form (extended-release capsules):
  —To replace potassium lost by the body:
    - Adults and teenagers—40 to 100 milliequivalents (mEq) a day, divided into two or three smaller doses during the day. Your doctor may change the dose if needed. However, most people will not take more than 100 mEq a day.
  —To prevent potassium loss:
    - Adults and teenagers—16 to 24 mEq a day, divided into two or three smaller doses during the day. Your doctor may change the dose if needed. However, most people will not take more than 100 mEq a day.
    - Children—Dose must be determined by your doctor.

- For *oral* dosage form (liquid for solution):
  —To replace potassium lost by the body:
    - Adults and teenagers—20 mEq mixed into one-half glass of cold water or juice, taken one to four times a day. Your doctor may change the dose if needed. However, most people will not take more than 100 mEq a day.
    - Children—Dose is based on body weight and must be determined by your doctor. The usual dose is 1 to 3 mEq of potassium per kilogram (kg) (0.45 to 1.36 mEq per pound) of body weight taken in smaller doses during the day. The solution should be well mixed in water or juice.

- For *oral* dosage form (powder for solution):
  —To replace potassium lost by the body:
  - Adults and teenagers—15 to 25 mEq dissolved in four to six ounces of cold water, taken two or four times a day. Your doctor may change the dose if needed. However, most people will not take more than 100 mEq a day.
  - Children—Dose is based on body weight and must be determined by your doctor. The usual dose is 1 to 3 mEq per kg (0.45 to 1.36 mEq per pound) of body weight taken in smaller doses during the day. The solution should be mixed into water or juice.
- For *oral* dosage form (powder for suspension):
  —To replace potassium lost by the body:
  - Adults and teenagers—20 mEq dissolved in two to six ounces of cold water, taken one to five times a day. Your doctor may change the dose if needed. However, most people will not take more than 100 mEq a day.
  - Children—Dose must be determined by your doctor.
- For *oral* dosage form (extended-release tablets):
  —To replace potassium lost by the body:
  - Adults and teenagers—6.7 to 20 mEq taken three times a day. However, most people will not take more than 100 mEq a day.
  - Children—Dose must be determined by your doctor.

*For potassium chloride, potassium bicarbonate and potassium citrate*
- For *oral* dosage form (tablets for solution):
  —To replace potassium lost by the body:
  - Adults and teenagers—20 milliequivalents (mEq) dissolved in one-half to one glass of cold water, taken one to four times a day. Your doctor may change the dose if needed. However, most people will not take more than 100 mEq a day.
  - Children—Dose must be determined by your doctor.

*For potassium gluconate*
- For *oral* dosage form (liquid for solution):
  —To replace potassium lost by the body:
  - Adults and teenagers—20 milliequivalents (mEq) mixed into one-half glass of cold water or juice, taken two to four times a day. Your doctor may change the dose if needed. However, most people will not take more than 100 mEq a day.
  - Children—Dose is based on body weight and must be determined by your doctor. The usual dose is 2 to 3 mEq per kilogram (kg) (0.9 to 1.36 mEq per pound) of body weight a day, taken in smaller doses during the day. The solution should be completely mixed into water or juice.

- For *oral* dosage form (tablets):
  —To replace potassium lost by the body:
  - Adults and teenagers—5 to 10 mEq taken two to four times a day. However, most people will not take more than 100 mEq a day.
  - Children—Dose must be determined by your doctor.

*For potassium gluconate and potassium chloride*
- For *oral* dosage form (liquid for solution):
  —To replace potassium lost by the body:
  - Adults and teenagers—20 milliequivalents (mEq) diluted in 2 tablespoonfuls or more of cold water or juice, taken two to four times a day. Your doctor may change the dose if needed. However, most people will not take more than 100 mEq a day.
  - Children—Dose is based on body weight and must be determined by your doctor. The usual dose is 2 to 3 mEq per kilogram (kg) (0.9 to 1.36 mEq per pound) of body weight taken in smaller doses during the day. The solution should be well mixed into water or juice.
- For *oral* dosage form (powder for solution):
  —To replace potassium lost by the body:
  - Adults and teenagers—20 mEq mixed in 2 tablespoonfuls or more of cold water or juice taken two to four times a day. Your doctor may change the dose if needed. However, most people will not take more than 100 mEq a day.
  - Children—Dose is base on body weight and must be determined by your doctor. The usual dose is 2 to 3 mEq per kg (0.9 to 1.36 mEq per pound) of body weight taken in smaller doses during the day. The solution should be well mixed into water or juice.

*For potassium gluconate and potassium citrate*
- For *oral* dosage form (liquid for solution):
  —To replace potassium lost by the body:
  - Adults and teenagers—20 milliequivalents (mEq) mixed into one-half glass of cold water or juice, taken two to four times a day. Your doctor may change the dose if needed. However, most people will not take more than 100 mEq a day.
  - Children—Dose is based on body weight and must be determined by your doctor. The usual dose is 2 to 3 mEq per kg (0.9 to 1.36 mEq per pound) of body weight taken in smaller doses during the day. The solution should be well mixed into water or juice.

*For trikates*
- For *oral* dosage form (liquid for solution):
  —To replace potassium lost by the body:
  - Adults and teenagers—15 milliequivalents (mEq) mixed into one-half glass of cold water or juice, taken three or four times a day. Your doctor may change the dose if needed. However,

most people will not take more than 100 mEq a day.

• Children—Dose is based on body weight and must be determined by your doctor. The usual dose is 2 to 3 mEq per kilogram (kg) (0.9 to 1.36 mEq per pound) of body weight taken in smaller doses during the day. The solution should be well mixed into water or juice.

**Missed dose**—If you miss a dose of this medicine and remember within 2 hours, take the missed dose right away with food or liquids. Then go back to your regular dosing schedule. However, if you do not remember until later, skip the missed dose and go back to your regular dosing schedule. Do not double doses.

**Storage**—To store this medicine:
• Keep out of the reach of children.
• Store away from heat and direct light.
• Do not store in the bathroom, near the kitchen sink, or in other damp places. Heat or moisture may cause the medicine to break down.
• Keep the liquid form of this medicine from freezing.
• Do not keep outdated medicine or medicine no longer needed. Be sure that any discarded medicine is out of the reach of children.

## Precautions While Using This Medicine

Your doctor should check your progress at regular visits to make sure the medicine is working properly and that possible side effects are avoided. Laboratory tests may be necessary.

*Do not use salt substitutes, eat low-sodium foods, especially some breads and canned foods, or drink low-sodium milk unless you are told to do so by your doctor, since these products may contain potassium. It is important to read the labels carefully on all low-sodium food products.*

Check with your doctor before starting any physical exercise program, especially if you are out of condition and are taking any other medicine. Exercise and certain medicines may increase the amount of potassium in the blood.

*Check with your doctor at once if you notice blackish stools or other signs of stomach or intestinal bleeding.*

This medicine may cause such a condition to become worse, especially when taken in tablet form.

## Side Effects of This Medicine

Along with its needed effects, a medicine may cause some unwanted effects. Although not all of these side effects may occur, if they do occur they may need medical attention.

*Stop taking this medicine and check with your doctor immediately if any of the following side effects occur:*
  *Less common*
    Confusion; irregular or slow heartbeat; numbness or tingling in hands, feet, or lips; shortness of breath or difficult breathing; unexplained anxiety; unusual tiredness or weakness; weakness or heaviness of legs

Also, check with your doctor if any of the following side effects occur:
  *Rare*
    Abdominal or stomach pain, cramping, or soreness (continuing); chest or throat pain, especially when swallowing; stools with signs of blood (red or black color)

Other side effects may occur that usually do not need medical attention. These side effects may go away during treatment as your body adjusts to the medicine. However, check with your doctor if any of the following side effects continue or are bothersome:
  *More common*
    Diarrhea; nausea; stomach pain, discomfort, or gas (mild); vomiting

Sometimes you may see what appears to be a whole tablet in the stool after taking certain extended-release potassium chloride tablets. This is to be expected. Your body has absorbed the potassium from the tablet and the shell is then expelled.

Other side effects not listed above may also occur in some patients. If you notice any other effects, check with your doctor.

Revised: 07/16/92
Interim revision: 08/29/94

# PRAZIQUANTEL   Systemic†

A commonly used brand name in the U.S. is Biltricide.
Another brand name is Cysticide.

†Not commercially available in Canada.

## Description

Praziquantel (pray-zi-KWON-tel) belongs to the family of medicines called anthelmintics (ant-hel-MIN-tiks).

Anthelmintics are used in the treatment of worm infections.

Praziquantel is used to treat blood fluke infections. These are also known as snail fever, schistosomiasis (shis-toe-soe-MYE-a-siss), or bilharziasis (bil-har-ZYE-a-siss). Praziquantel may also be used for other worm infections as determined by your doctor. However, it will not work for pinworms or other roundworms.

Praziquantel works by causing severe spasms and paralysis of the worms' muscles. Some kinds of worms are then passed in the stool. However, you may not notice them since they are sometimes completely destroyed in the intestine.

Praziquantel is available only with your doctor's prescription, in the following dosage form:

*Oral*
- Tablets (U.S.)

## Before Using This Medicine

In deciding to use a medicine, the risks of taking the medicine must be weighed against the good it will do. This is a decision you and your doctor will make. For praziquantel, the following should be considered:

**Allergies**—Tell your doctor if you have ever had any unusual or allergic reaction to praziquantel. Also tell your health care professional if you are allergic to any other substances, such as foods, preservatives, or dyes.

**Pregnancy**—Studies have not been done in humans. Studies in rats and rabbits given up to 40 times the usual human dose have not shown that praziquantel causes birth defects. However, praziquantel has been shown to cause a greater chance of miscarriage in rats given 3 times the human dose.

**Breast-feeding**—Praziquantel passes into the breast milk. You should stop breast-feeding on the day you begin taking praziquantel. Do not restart breast-feeding until 72 hours after treatment is completed. During this time the breast milk should be squeezed out or sucked out with a breast pump and thrown away.

**Children**—This medicine has been tested in a limited number of children 4 years of age or older and, in effective doses, has not been reported to cause different side effects or problems in children over 4 years of age than it does in adults.

**Older adults**—Many medicines have not been studied specifically in older people. Therefore, it may not be known whether they work exactly the same way they do in younger adults or if they cause different side effects or problems in older people. There is no specific information comparing use of praziquantel in the elderly with use in other age groups.

**Other medicines**—Although certain medicines should not be used together at all, in other cases two different medicines may be used together even if an interaction might occur. In these cases, your doctor may want to change the dose, or other precautions may be necessary. Tell your health care professional if you are taking any other prescription or nonprescription (over-the-counter [OTC]) medicine.

**Other medical problems**—The presence of other medical problems may affect the use of praziquantel. Make sure

you tell your doctor if you have any other medical problems, especially:
- Liver disease—Patients with moderate to severe liver disease may have an increased chance of side effects
- Worm cysts in the eye—The death of worm cysts in the eye caused by praziquantel may cause damage to the eyes

## Proper Use of This Medicine

No special preparations (for example, special diets, fasting, other medicines, laxatives, or enemas) are necessary before, during, or immediately after taking praziquantel.

Praziquantel has a bitter taste that may cause gagging or vomiting. The bitter taste may be more noticeable if the tablets are held in the mouth or chewed. Therefore, *do not chew praziquantel tablets.* Swallow them whole with a small amount of liquid during meals.

To help clear up your infection completely, *take this medicine exactly as directed by your doctor for the full time of treatment. Do not miss any doses.*

**Dosing**—The dose of praziquantel will be different for different patients. *Follow your doctor's orders or the directions on the label.* The following information includes only the average doses of praziquantel. *If your dose is different, do not change it* unless your doctor tells you to do so.

*The number of doses you take each day, the time allowed between doses, and the length of time you take the medicine depend on the medical problem for which you are taking praziquantel.*

- For the treatment of clonorchiasis (Chinese or Oriental liver fluke) and opisthorchiasis (liver flukes):
  —Adults and children 4 years of age and older: Dose is based on body weight and will be determined by your doctor. This dose is taken three times a day for one day.
  —Children up to 4 years of age: Dose must be determined by the doctor.

- For the treatment of schistosomiasis:
  —Adults and children 4 years of age and older: Dose is based on body weight and will be determined by your doctor. This dose is taken two or three times a day for one day.
  —Children up to 4 years of age: Dose must be determined by the doctor.

**Missed dose**—If you do miss a dose of this medicine, take it as soon as possible. However, if it is almost time for your next dose, skip the missed dose and go back to your regular dosing schedule. Do not double doses.

**Storage**—To store this medicine:
- Keep out of the reach of children.
- Store away from heat and direct light.
- Do not store in the bathroom, near the kitchen sink, or in other damp places. Heat or moisture may cause the medicine to break down.

- Do not keep outdated medicine or medicine no longer needed. Be sure that any discarded medicine is out of the reach of children.

## Precautions While Using This Medicine

It is important that your doctor check your progress after treatment. This is to make sure that the infection is cleared up completely.

If your symptoms do not improve after you have taken this medicine for the full time of treatment, or if they become worse, check with your doctor.

This medicine may cause some people to become dizzy, drowsy, or less alert than they are normally. If any of these side effects occur, *do not drive, use machines, or do anything else that could be dangerous if you are dizzy or are not alert* while you are taking praziquantel and for 24 hours after you stop taking it.

## Side Effects of This Medicine

Along with its needed effects, a medicine may cause some unwanted effects. The following side effects may go away during treatment as your body adjusts to the medicine. However, check with your doctor if any of the following side effects continue or are bothersome:

*More common*
  Abdominal or stomach cramps or pain; bloody diarrhea; dizziness; drowsiness; fever; headache; increased

sweating; loss of appetite; general feeling of discomfort or illness; nausea or vomiting

*Less common*
  Skin rash, hives, or itching

Other side effects not listed above may also occur in some patients. If you notice any other effects, check with your doctor.

## Additional Information

Once a medicine has been approved for marketing for a certain use, experience may show that it is also useful for other medical problems. Although these uses are not included in product labeling, praziquantel is used in certain patients with the following medical conditions:

- Some kinds of fluke infections
- Some kinds of tapeworm infections

Other than the above information, there is no additional information relating to proper use, precautions, or side effects for these uses.

Revised: 03/23/93

# PRAZOSIN  Systemic

A commonly used brand name in the U.S. and Canada is Minipress. Generic name product may also be available.

## Description

Prazosin (PRA-zoe-sin) belongs to the general class of medicines called antihypertensives. It is used to treat high blood pressure (hypertension).

High blood pressure adds to the work load of the heart and arteries. If it continues for a long time, the heart and arteries may not function properly. This can damage the blood vessels of the brain, heart, and kidneys, resulting in a stroke, heart failure, or kidney failure. High blood pressure may also increase the risk of heart attacks. These problems may be less likely to occur if blood pressure is controlled.

Prazosin works by relaxing blood vessels so that blood passes through them more easily. This helps to lower blood pressure.

Prazosin may also be used for other conditions as determined by your doctor.

Prazosin is available only with your doctor's prescription, in the following dosage forms:

*Oral*
- Capsules (U.S.)
- Tablets (Canada)

## Before Using This Medicine

In deciding to use a medicine, the risks of taking the medicine must be weighed against the good it will do. This is a decision you and your doctor will make. For prazosin, the following should be considered:

**Allergies**—Tell your doctor if you have ever had any unusual or allergic reaction to prazosin, doxazosin, or terazosin. Also tell your health care professional if you are allergic to any other substance, such as foods, preservatives, or dyes.

**Pregnancy**—Limited use of prazosin to control high blood pressure in pregnant women has not shown that prazosin causes birth defects or other problems. Studies in animals given many times the highest recommended human dose of prazosin also have not shown that prazosin causes birth defects. However, in rats given many times the highest recommended human dose, lower birth weights were seen.

**Breast-feeding**—Prazosin passes into breast milk in small amounts. However, it has not been reported to cause problems in nursing babies.

**Children**—Studies on this medicine have been done only in adult patients, and there is no specific information comparing use of prazosin in children with use in other age groups.

**Older adults**—Dizziness, lightheadedness, or fainting (especially when getting up from a lying or sitting position) may be more likely to occur in the elderly, who are more sensitive to the effects of prazosin. In addition, prazosin may reduce tolerance to cold temperatures in elderly patients.

**Other medicines**—Although certain medicines should not be used together at all, in other cases two different medicines may be used together even if an interaction might occur. In these cases, your doctor may want to change the dose, or other precautions may be necessary. Tell your health care professional if you are taking any other prescription or nonprescription (over-the-counter [OTC]) medicine.

**Other medical problems**—The presence of other medical problems may affect the use of prazosin. Make sure you tell your doctor if you have any other medical problems, especially:

- Angina (chest pain) or
- Heart disease (severe)—Prazosin may make these conditions worse
- Kidney disease—Possible increased sensitivity to the effects of prazosin

## Proper Use of This Medicine

For patients *taking this medicine for high blood pressure:*

- In addition to the use of the medicine your doctor has prescribed, treatment for your high blood pressure may include weight control and care in the types of foods you eat, especially foods high in sodium. Your doctor will tell you which of these are most important for you. You should check with your doctor before changing your diet.
- Many patients who have high blood pressure will not notice any signs of the problem. In fact, many may feel normal. It is very important that you *take your medicine exactly as directed* and that you keep your appointments with your doctor even if you feel well.
- Remember that prazosin will not cure your high blood pressure but it does help control it. Therefore, you must continue to take it as directed if you expect to lower your blood pressure and keep it down. *You may have to take high blood pressure medicine for the rest of your life.* If high blood pressure is not treated, it can cause serious problems such as heart failure, blood vessel disease, stroke, or kidney disease.

To help you remember to take your medicine, try to get into the habit of taking it at the same time each day.

**Dosing**—The dose of prazosin will be different for different patients. *Follow your doctor's orders or the directions on the label.* The following information includes only the average doses of prazosin. *If your dose is different, do not change it* unless your doctor tells you to do so.

The number of capsules or tablets that you take depends on the strength of the medicine.

- For *oral* dosage form (capsules or tablets):
  —For high blood pressure:
  - Adults—At first, 0.5 or 1 milligram (mg) two or three times a day. Then, your doctor will slowly increase your dose to 6 to 15 mg a day. This is divided into two or three doses.
  - Children—Dose is based on body weight and must be determined by your doctor. The usual dose is 50 to 400 micrograms (mcg) (0.05 to 0.4 mg) per kilogram of body weight (22.73 to 181.2 mcg per pound [0.023 to 0.18 mg per pound]) a day. This is divided into two or three doses.

**Missed dose**—If you miss a dose of this medicine, take it as soon as possible. However, if it is almost time for your next dose, skip the missed dose and go back to your regular dosing schedule. Do not double doses.

**Storage**—To store this medicine:

- Keep out of the reach of children.
- Store away from heat and direct light.
- Do not store in the bathroom, near the kitchen sink, or in other damp places. Heat or moisture may cause the medicine to break down.
- Do not keep outdated medicine or medicine no longer needed. Be sure that any discarded medicine is out of the reach of children.

## Precautions While Using This Medicine

It is important that your doctor check your progress at regular visits to make sure that this medicine is working properly.

For patients *taking this medicine for high blood pressure:*

- *Do not take other medicines unless they have been discussed with your doctor.* This especially includes over-the-counter (nonprescription) medicines for appetite control, asthma, colds, cough, hay fever, or sinus problems, since they may tend to make prazosin less effective.

Dizziness, lightheadedness, or sudden fainting may occur after you take this medicine, especially when you get up from a lying or sitting position. These effects are more likely to occur when you take the first dose of this medicine. Taking the first dose at bedtime may prevent problems. However, *be especially careful if you need to get up during the night.* These effects may also occur with any doses you take after the first dose. Getting up slowly may help lessen this problem. *If you feel dizzy, lie down so that you do not faint.* Then sit for a few moments before standing to prevent the dizziness from returning.

The dizziness, lightheadedness, or fainting is more likely to occur if you drink alcohol, stand for a long time, exercise, or if the weather is hot. *While you are taking this medicine, be careful to limit the amount of alcohol you drink. Also, use extra care during exercise or hot weather or if you must stand for a long time.*

Prazosin may cause some people to become drowsy or less alert than they are normally. *Make sure you know how you react to this medicine before you drive, use machines, or do anything else that could be dangerous if you are dizzy, drowsy, or are not alert.* After you have taken several doses of this medicine, these effects should lessen.

## Side Effects of This Medicine

Along with its needed effects, a medicine may cause some unwanted effects. Although not all of these side effects may occur, if they do occur they may need medical attention.

Check with your doctor as soon as possible if any of the following side effects occur:

*More common*
> Dizziness or lightheadedness, especially when getting up from a lying or sitting position; fainting (sudden)

*Less common*
> Loss of bladder control; pounding heartbeat; swelling of feet or lower legs

*Rare*
> Chest pain; painful inappropriate erection of penis (continuing); shortness of breath

Other side effects may occur that usually do not need medical attention. These side effects may go away during treatment as your body adjusts to the medicine. However,

check with your doctor if any of the following side effects continue or are bothersome:

*More common*
> Drowsiness; headache; lack of energy

*Less common*
> Dryness of mouth; nervousness; unusual tiredness or weakness

*Rare*
> Frequent urge to urinate; nausea

Other side effects not listed above may also occur in some patients. If you notice any other effects, check with your doctor.

## Additional Information

Once a medicine has been approved for marketing for a certain use, experience may show that it is also useful for other medical problems. Although these uses are not included in product labeling, prazosin is used in certain patients with the following medical conditions:

- Congestive heart failure
- Ergot alkaloid poisoning
- Pheochromocytoma
- Raynaud's disease
- Benign enlargement of the prostate

For patients taking this medicine for *benign enlargement of the prostate*:

- Prazosin will not shrink the size of your prostate, but it does help to relieve the symptoms.

Other than the above information, there is no additional information relating to proper use, precautions, or side effects for these uses.

Revised: 08/02/94

# PRAZOSIN AND POLYTHIAZIDE Systemic†

A commonly used brand name in the U.S. is Minizide.

†Not commercially available in Canada.

## Description

Prazosin (PRA-zoe-sin) and polythiazide (pol-i-THYE-a-zide) combination is used in the treatment of high blood pressure (hypertension).

High blood pressure adds to the workload of the heart and arteries. If it continues for a long time, the heart and arteries may not function properly. This can damage the blood vessels of the brain, heart, and kidneys resulting in a stroke, heart failure, or kidney failure. High blood pressure may also increase the risk of heart attacks. These

problems may be less likely to occur if blood pressure is controlled.

Prazosin works by relaxing blood vessels so that blood passes through them more easily. The polythiazide in this combination is a thiazide diuretic (water pill) that helps to reduce the amount of water in the body by increasing the flow of urine. Both of these actions help to lower blood pressure.

This medicine is available only with your doctor's prescription, in the following dosage form:

*Oral*
- Capsules (U.S.)

## Before Using This Medicine

In deciding to use a medicine, the risks of taking the medicine must be weighed against the good it will do. This is a decision you and your doctor will make. For prazosin and polythiazide, the following should be considered:

**Allergies**—Tell your doctor if you have ever had any unusual or allergic reaction to prazosin, sulfonamides (sulfa drugs), bumetanide, furosemide, acetazolamide, dichlorphenamide, methazolamide, or any of the thiazide diuretics. Also tell your health care professional if you are allergic to any other substance, such as foods, preservatives, or dyes.

**Pregnancy**—When polythiazide (contained in this combination medicine) is used during pregnancy, it may cause side effects including jaundice, blood problems, and low potassium in the newborn infant. The combination of prazosin and polythiazide has not been shown to cause birth defects.

**Breast-feeding**—Polythiazide passes into breast milk. Prazosin passes into breast milk in small amounts. However, prazosin and polythiazide combination has not been reported to cause problems in nursing babies.

**Children**—Although there is no specific information about the use of this medicine in children, it is not expected to cause different side effects or problems in children than it does in adults. However, extra caution may be necessary in infants with jaundice, because these medicines can make the condition worse.

**Older adults**—Dizziness, lightheadedness, or fainting or symptoms of too much potassium loss may be more likely to occur in the elderly, who are more sensitive to the effects of prazosin and polythiazide. In addition, this medicine may reduce tolerance to cold temperatures in elderly patients.

**Other medicines**—Although certain medicines should not be used together at all, in other cases two different medicines may be used together even if an interaction might occur. In these cases, your doctor may want to change the dose, or other precautions may be necessary. When you are taking prazosin and polythiazide, it is especially important that your health care professional know if you are taking any of the following:

- Cholestyramine or
- Colestipol—Use with thiazide diuretics may prevent the diuretic from working properly; take the diuretic at least 1 hour before or 4 hours after cholestyramine or colestipol
- Digitalis glycosides (heart medicine)—Polythiazide may cause low potassium in the blood, which can lead to symptoms of digitalis toxicity
- Lithium (e.g., Lithane)—Risk of lithium overdose, even at usual doses, may be increased

**Other medical problems**—The presence of other medical problems may affect the use of prazosin and polythiazide.

Make sure you tell your doctor if you have any other medical problems, especially:

- Angina (chest pain) or
- Heart disease (severe)—Prazosin may make these conditions worse
- Diabetes mellitus (sugar diabetes)—Polythiazide may increase the amount of sugar in the blood
- Gout (history of) or
- Lupus erythematosus (history of) or
- Pancreatitis (inflammation of the pancreas)—Thiazide diuretics may make these conditions worse
- Kidney disease—Effects of this combination medicine may be increased because of increased sensitivity to the effects of prazosin and slower removal of polythiazide from the body. If kidney disease is severe, polythiazide may not work
- Liver disease—If polythiazide causes loss of too much water from the body, liver disease can become much worse

## Proper Use of This Medicine

In addition to the use of the medicine your doctor has prescribed, treatment for your high blood pressure may include weight control and care in the types of foods you eat, especially foods high in sodium. Your doctor will tell you which of these are most important for you. You should check with your doctor before changing your diet.

Many patients who have high blood pressure will not notice any signs of the problem. In fact, many may feel normal. It is very important that you *take your medicine exactly as directed* and that you keep your appointments with your doctor even if you feel well.

Remember that this medicine will not cure your high blood pressure but it does help control it. Therefore, you must continue to take it as directed if you expect to lower your blood pressure and keep it down. *You may have to take high blood pressure medicine for the rest of your life.* If high blood pressure is not treated, it can cause serious problems such as heart failure, blood vessel disease, stroke, or kidney disease.

This medicine may cause you to have an unusual feeling of tiredness when you begin to take it. You may also notice an increase in the amount of urine or in your frequency of urination. After taking the medicine for a while, these effects should lessen.

It is best to plan your dose or doses according to a schedule that will least affect your personal activities and sleep. Ask your health care professional to help you plan the best time to take this medicine.

To help you remember to take your medicine, try to get into the habit of taking it at the same time each day.

**Dosing**—The dose of prazosin and polythiazide combination will be different for different patients. *Follow your doctor's orders or the directions on the label.* The following information includes only the average doses of prazosin and polythiazide combination. *If your dose is different, do not change it* unless your doctor tells you to do so.

The number of capsules that you take depends on the strength of the medicine.

- For *oral* dosage form (capsules):
  —For high blood pressure:
    - Adults—1 capsule two or three times a day.
    - Children—Dose must be determined by your doctor.

**Missed dose**—If you miss a dose of this medicine, take it as soon as possible. However, if it is almost time for your next dose, skip the missed dose and go back to your regular dosing schedule. Do not double doses.

**Storage**—To store this medicine:

- Keep out of the reach of children.
- Store away from heat and direct light.
- Do not store in the bathroom, near the kitchen sink, or in other damp places. Heat or moisture may cause the medicine to break down.
- Do not keep outdated medicine or medicine no longer needed. Be sure that any discarded medicine is out of the reach of children.

## Precautions While Using This Medicine

It is important that your doctor check your progress at regular visits to make sure this medicine is working properly.

*Do not take other medicines unless they have been discussed with your doctor.* This especially includes over-the-counter (nonprescription) medicine for appetite control, asthma, colds, cough, hay fever, or sinus problems, since they may tend to increase your blood pressure.

This medicine may cause a loss of potassium from your body.

- To help prevent this, your doctor may want you to:
  —eat or drink foods that have a high potassium content (for example, orange or other citrus fruit juices), or
  —take a potassium supplement, or
  —take another medicine to help prevent the loss of the potassium in the first place.
- It is very important to follow these directions. Also, it is important not to change your diet on your own. This is more important if you are already on a special diet (as for diabetes), or if you are taking a potassium supplement or a medicine to reduce potassium loss. Extra potassium may not be necessary and, in some cases, too much potassium could be harmful.

Check with your doctor if you become sick and have severe or continuing vomiting or diarrhea. These problems may cause you to lose additional water and potassium.

Dizziness, lightheadedness, or sudden fainting may occur after you take this medicine, especially when you get up from a lying or sitting position. These effects are more likely to occur when you take the first dose of this medicine. Taking the first dose at bedtime may prevent problems. However, *be especially careful if you need to get up during the night*. These effects may also occur with any doses you take after the first dose. Getting up slowly may help lessen this problem. *If you feel dizzy, lie down so that you do not faint*. Then sit for a few moments before standing to prevent the dizziness from returning.

*Make sure you know how you react to this medicine before you drive, use machines, or do anything else that could be dangerous if you are dizzy or are not alert.* After you have taken several doses of this medicine, these effects should lessen.

The dizziness, lightheadedness, or fainting is also more likely to occur if you drink alcohol, stand for a long time, exercise, or if the weather is hot. *While you are taking this medicine, be careful to limit the amount of alcohol you drink. Also, use extra care during exercise or hot weather or if you must stand for a long time.*

For *diabetic patients*:

- Polythiazide (contained in this combination medicine) may raise blood sugar levels. While you are using this medicine, be especially careful in testing for sugar in your blood or urine. If you have any questions about this, check with your doctor.

Some people who take this medicine may become more sensitive to sunlight than they are normally. Exposure to sunlight, even for brief periods of time, may cause a skin rash, itching, redness or other discoloration of the skin, or a severe sunburn. When you begin taking this medicine:

- Stay out of direct sunlight, especially between the hours of 10:00 a.m. and 3:00 p.m., if possible.
- Wear protective clothing, including a hat and sunglasses.
- Apply a sun block product that has a skin protection factor (SPF) of at least 15. Some patients may require a product with a higher SPF number, especially if they have a fair complexion. If you have any questions about this, check with your health care professional.
- Do not use a sunlamp or tanning bed or booth.
- Apply a sun block lipstick that has an SPF of at least 15 to protect your lips.

If you have a severe reaction from the sun, check with your doctor.

## Side Effects of This Medicine

Along with its needed effects, a medicine may cause some unwanted effects. Although not all of these side effects may occur, if they do occur they may need medical attention.

Check with your doctor as soon as possible if any of the following side effects occur, especially since some of them may mean that your body is losing too much potassium:

*Signs and symptoms of too much potassium loss*

Dryness of mouth (severe); increased thirst; irregular heartbeat (continuing); mood or mental changes; muscle cramps or pain; nausea or vomiting; unusual tiredness or weakness; weak pulse

*Signs and symptoms of too much sodium loss*

Confusion; convulsions; decreased mental activity; irritability; muscle cramps; unusual tiredness or weakness

*More common*

Dizziness or lightheadedness, especially when getting up from a lying or sitting position; sudden fainting

*Less common*

Inability to control urination; irregular heartbeat; pounding heartbeat; swelling of feet or lower legs; weight gain

*Rare*

Black, tarry stools; blood in urine or stools; chest pain; cough or hoarseness; fever or chills; joint pain; lower back or side pain; painful or difficult urination; painful, inappropriate erection of penis, continuing; pinpoint red spots on skin; shortness of breath; skin rash

or hives; stomach pain (severe) with nausea and vomiting; unusual bleeding or bruising; yellow eyes or skin

Other side effects may occur that usually do not need medical attention. These side effects may go away during treatment as your body adjusts to the medicine. However, check with your doctor if any of the following side effects continue or are bothersome:

*Less common*

Decreased sexual ability; diarrhea; drowsiness; headache; increased sensitivity of skin to sunlight; lack of energy; loss of appetite; nervousness; stomach upset or pain

*Rare*

Frequent urge to urinate; nausea

Other side effects not listed above may also occur in some patients. If you notice any other effects, check with your doctor.

---

Revised: 07/21/92
Interim revision: 07/20/94

---

# PREGNANCY TEST KITS FOR HOME USE

Some commonly used brand names are:

**In the U.S.—**

| | |
|---|---|
| Advance | e.p.t. Quick Stick |
| Answer | Fact Plus |
| Answer Plus | First Response |
| Answer Plus II | Fortel Midstream |
| Answer Quick & Simple | Fortel Plus |
| Clearblue Easy | Q-test |
| Daisy 2 | SureCell hCG-Urine Test |

**In Canada—**

Clearblue Easy

## Description

Pregnancy test kits may be purchased without a prescription for use in the home. The materials in the kit are designed to detect a hormone, human chorionic gonadotropin (HCG), in the urine.

HCG is produced by the fertilized egg (ovum) when it implants in the woman's uterus, and can be found in the urine 1 to 2 weeks after the fertilized ovum is implanted in the uterus. HCG helps make the hormones necessary for pregnancy and disappears from the woman's urine and blood when pregnancy is over. Therefore, it is seen as a way to tell when pregnancy has occurred.

Test kits can usually detect a pregnancy as early as 1 day after the first missed period should have started. Many kits contain enough materials for 2 tests, and advise that a second test be performed 7 days later if the first test is negative.

It is important to have the pregnancy confirmed by a health care professional as soon as a woman thinks she

is pregnant. The pregnancy due date should be determined. Early prenatal care benefits both the mother and baby by checking for possible problems in the pregnancy. Also, women should avoid drugs, tobacco, alcohol, x-rays, and other treatments that can be harmful to the fetus.

---

## Before Using This Test Kit

It is important to get the correct result from a home pregnancy test kit. Therefore, the following should be considered by you and possibly your doctor before you decide to use one of these test kits:

**Medicines**—Certain medicines may affect your pregnancy test and cause a false result. Check with your doctor if you are taking any medicines, especially:

- Anticonvulsants (seizure medicine)
- Medicine for mental problems

**Medical conditions**—The presence of certain medical conditions may affect your pregnancy test and cause a false test result. Check with your doctor if you have any medical conditions, especially:

- Abortion (incomplete or recent)
- Cancer
- Certain problems of the ovaries
- Delivery of a baby (recent)
- Endometriosis
- Menopause (change of life)
- Pregnancy (abnormal or tubal)
- Thyroid disease
- Urinary tract infection

---

© 1994 The United States Pharmacopeial Convention, Inc.

Also, if you have vision problems (such as color-blindness or poor vision), you will need someone to help you in reading your test results

---

## Proper Use of This Test Kit

Check the expiration date printed on the package before purchasing. Do not use an outdated test kit. Outdated test kits will not work properly.

To use:

- Read and follow the test kit instructions carefully. Be careful not to skip or rush any steps.
- Collect a urine sample in a clean, dry container according to the written package instructions. Pregnancy tests are best done on the first morning urine.
- Choose a well-lighted area with normal room temperature and humidity. Perform the test on a clean, dry working surface with a cold water faucet nearby. You will also need a watch, timer, or clock that can measure in seconds.
- Be careful not to touch the areas of the kit where you will put urine. Skin oils or perspiration may affect the test results. It is also important that you use clean, dry test materials. If no container comes with the test kit, use one that is clean and dry. Traces of old test chemicals or soaps may affect test reactions if materials are reused.
- At the end of the timing period, compare the color of the test with the color chart on the package. The test colors will begin to fade after this period has passed or as the test paper begins to dry.
- Record your test results and the date you did the test, to discuss your results with your doctor.

## Storage—To store this product:

- Keep out of the reach of children. Test kit chemicals can be poisonous if swallowed.
- Store these test kits in their original containers. Keep the container tightly closed.
- Keep in a cool, dry place, away from heat, humidity (such as the bathroom or shower area), and direct sunlight. Heat-exposed test kits will not work properly.
- Do not refrigerate this product. Keep the kit from freezing.
- Discard used tests in the trash. Liquids may be poured down the drain or flushed in the toilet. Be sure that any discarded test kit is out of the reach of children.

---

## About Your Test Results

Notify your doctor if the pregnancy test is positive, so that you can begin regular prenatal care.

If the test is negative, retest your urine after 7 days. If the test results are still negative after the second test and you still have not started your menstrual period, you should still see your doctor.

If you have any other questions about your results or about the use of pregnancy test kits, ask your health care professional. Also, most kits have a toll-free number for advice on using them.

---

Revised: 07/20/93
Interim revision: 06/30/94

---

# PRIMAQUINE    Systemic

Generic name product may be available in the U.S. and Canada.

## Description

Primaquine (PRIM-a-kween) belongs to the group of medicines called antiprotozoals. It is used in the treatment of malaria.

Primaquine is available only with your doctor's prescription, in the following dosage form:

*Oral*
- Tablets (U.S. and Canada)

## Before Using This Medicine

In deciding to use a medicine, the risks of taking the medicine must be weighed against the good it will do.

This is a decision you and your doctor will make. For primaquine, the following should be considered:

**Allergies**—Tell your doctor if you have ever had any unusual or allergic reaction to primaquine or iodoquinol (e.g., Yodoxin). Also tell your health care professional if you are allergic to any other substances, such as foods, preservatives, or dyes.

**Pregnancy**—Primaquine is not recommended for use during pregnancy.

**Breast-feeding**—It is not known if primaquine is excreted in breast milk. However, primaquine has not been reported to cause problems in nursing babies.

**Children**—Although there is no specific information comparing use of primaquine in children with use in other age groups, this medicine is not expected to cause different side effects or problems in children than it does in adults.

**Older adults**—Many medicines have not been studied specifically in older people. Therefore, it may not be known whether they work exactly the same way they do in younger adults or if they cause different side effects or problems in older people. There is no specific information comparing use of primaquine in the elderly with use in other age groups.

**Other medicines**—Although certain medicines should not be used together at all, in other cases two different medicines may be used together even if an interaction might occur. In these cases, your doctor may want to change the dose, or other precautions may be necessary. When you are taking primaquine it is especially important that your health care professional know if you are taking any of the following:

- Acetohydroxamic acid (e.g., Lithostat) or
- Antidiabetics, oral (diabetes medicine you take by mouth) or
- Dapsone or
- Furazolidone (e.g., Furoxone) or
- Methyldopa (e.g., Aldomet) or
- Nitrofurantoin (e.g., Furadantin) or
- Procainamide (e.g., Pronestyl) or
- Quinacrine (e.g., Atabrine) or
- Quinidine (e.g., Quinidex) or
- Quinine (e.g., Quinamm) or
- Sulfonamides (sulfa medicine) or
- Sulfoxone (e.g., Diasone) or
- Vitamin K (e.g., AquaMEPHYTON, Synkayvite)—Taking these medicines with primaquine may increase the chance of side effects affecting the blood

**Other medical problems**—The presence of other medical problems may affect the use of primaquine. Make sure you tell your doctor if you have any other medical problems, especially:

- Family or personal history of favism or hemolytic anemia or
- Glucose-6-phosphate dehydrogenase (G6PD) deficiency or
- Nicotinamide adenine dinucleotide (NADH) methemoglobin reductase deficiency—Patients with any of these medical problems who take primaquine may have an increased chance of side effects affecting the blood

## Proper Use of This Medicine

*If this medicine upsets your stomach, it may be taken with meals or antacids.* If stomach upset (nausea, vomiting, or stomach pain) continues, check with your doctor.

If you are taking primaquine for malaria, *keep taking it for the full time of treatment* to help prevent or completely clear up the infection. *Do not miss any doses.*

**Dosing**—The dose of primaquine will be different for different patients. *Follow your doctor's orders or the directions on the label.* The following information includes only the average doses of primaquine. *If your dose is different, do not change it* unless your doctor tells you to do so.

The number of tablets that you take depends on the strength of the medicine. Also, *the number of doses you take each day, the time allowed between doses, and the length of time you take the medicine depend on the medical problem for which you are taking primaquine.*

- For the *treatment of malaria*:
  —Adults and older children: 26.3 mg of primaquine phosphate (which equals 15 mg of primaquine base) once a day for fourteen days.
  —Younger children: Dose is based on body weight and must be determined by the doctor.

**Missed dose**—If you do miss a dose of this medicine, take it as soon as possible. However, if it is almost time for your next dose, skip the missed dose and go back to your regular dosing schedule. Do not double doses.

**Storage**—To store this medicine:
- Keep out of the reach of children.
- Store away from heat and direct light.
- Do not store in the bathroom, near the kitchen sink, or in other damp places. Heat or moisture may cause the medicine to break down.
- Do not keep outdated medicine or medicine no longer needed. Be sure that any discarded medicine is out of the reach of children.

## Precautions While Using This Medicine

Your doctor should check your progress at regular visits to make sure that primaquine is not causing blood problems.

## Side Effects of This Medicine

Along with its needed effects, a medicine may cause some unwanted effects. Although not all of these side effects may occur, if they do occur they may need medical attention.

*Check with your doctor immediately* if any of the following side effects occur:

*More common*
  Back, leg, or stomach pains; dark urine; fever; loss of appetite; pale skin; unusual tiredness or weakness

*Less common*
  Bluish fingernails, lips, or skin; dizziness or lightheadedness; difficulty breathing

*Rare*
  Sore throat and fever

Other side effects may occur that usually do not need medical attention. These side effects may go away during treatment as your body adjusts to the medicine. However, check with your doctor if any of the following side effects continue or are bothersome:

*More common*
  Nausea or vomiting; stomach pain or cramps

Other side effects not listed above may also occur in some patients. If you notice any other effects, check with your doctor.

## Additional Information

Once a medicine has been approved for marketing for a certain use, experience may show that it is also useful for other medical problems. Although this use is not included in product labeling, primaquine is used in certain patients with the following medical condition:

- *Pneumocystis carinii* pneumonia (PCP)

Other than the above information, there is no additional information relating to proper use, precautions, or side effects for this use.

Revised: 01/19/93

---

# PRIMIDONE Systemic

Some commonly used brand names are:

**In the U.S.—**
Myidone
Mysoline
Generic name product may also be available.

**In Canada—**
Apo-Primidone          PMS Primidone
Mysoline               Sertan
Generic name product may also be available.

## Description

Primidone (PRYE-mih-done) belongs to the group of medicines called anticonvulsants. It is used in the treatment of epilepsy to manage certain types of seizures. Primidone may be used alone or in combination with other anticonvulsants. It acts by controlling nerve impulses in the brain.

Primidone is available only with your doctor's prescription, in the following dosage forms:

*Oral*
- Suspension (U.S.)
- Tablets (U.S. and Canada)
- Chewable tablets (Canada)

## Before Using This Medicine

In deciding to use a medicine, the risks of taking the medicine must be weighed against the good it will do. This is a decision you and your doctor will make. For primidone, the following should be considered:

**Allergies**—Tell your doctor if you have ever had any unusual or allergic reaction to primidone or to any barbiturate medicine (for example, amobarbital, butabarbital, pentobarbital, phenobarbital, secobarbital). Also tell your health care professional if you are allergic to any other substances, such as foods, preservatives, or dyes.

**Pregnancy**—Although most mothers who take medicine for seizure control deliver normal babies, there are reports of increased birth defects when these medicines are used during pregnancy. Newborns whose mothers were taking primidone during pregnancy have been reported to have bleeding problems. It is not definitely known if any of these medicines are the cause of such problems.

**Breast-feeding**—Primidone passes into the breast milk and may cause unusual drowsiness in nursing babies. It may be necessary for you to take another medicine or to stop breast-feeding during treatment. Be sure you have discussed the risks and benefits of the medicine with your doctor.

**Children**—Unusual excitement or restlessness may occur in children, who are usually more sensitive than adults to these effects of primidone.

**Older adults**—Unusual excitement or restlessness may occur in elderly patients, who are usually more sensitive than younger adults to these effects of primidone.

**Other medicines**—Although certain medicines should not be used together at all, in other cases 2 different medicines may be used together even if an interaction might occur. In these cases, your doctor may want to change the dose, or other precautions may be necessary. When you are taking primidone it is especially important that your health care professional know if you are taking any of the following:

- Adrenocorticoids (cortisone-like medicines) or
- Anticoagulants (blood thinners)—Use with primidone may decrease the effects of these medications, and the amount of medicine you need to take may change
- Central nervous system (CNS) depressants (medicine that causes drowsiness)—Using these medicines with primidone may increase the CNS and other depressant effects
- Oral contraceptives (birth control pills) containing estrogen—Primidone may decrease the effectiveness of these oral contraceptives, and you may need to change to a different type of birth control
- Other anticonvulsants (seizure medicine)—A change in the pattern of seizures may occur; close monitoring of blood levels of both medications is recommended. Use of valproic acid with primidone may cause increased CNS depression and other serious side effects
- Monoamine oxidase (MAO) inhibitors (furazolidone [e.g., Furoxone], isocarboxazid [e.g., Marplan], phenelzine [e.g., Nardil], procarbazine [e.g., Matulane], selegiline [e.g., Eldepryl], tranylcypromine [e.g., Parnate])—Taking primidone while you are taking or within 2 weeks of taking monoamine oxidase (MAO) inhibitors may prolong the effects of primidone and may change the pattern of seizures

**Other medical problems**—The presence of other medical problems may affect the use of primidone. Make sure

you tell your doctor if you have any other medical problems, especially:

- Asthma, emphysema, or chronic lung disease—Primidone may cause serious problems in breathing
- Hyperactivity (in children) or
- Kidney disease or
- Liver disease—Primidone may make the condition worse
- Porphyria—Primidone should not be used when this medical problem exists because it may make the condition worse

## Proper Use of This Medicine

*Take primidone every day in regularly spaced doses as ordered by your doctor.* This will provide the proper amount of medicine needed to prevent seizures.

**Dosing**—The dose of primidone will be different for different patients. *Follow your doctor's orders or the directions on the label.* The following information includes only the average doses of primidone. *If your dose is different, do not change it* unless your doctor tells you to do so.

The number of tablets or teaspoonfuls of suspension that you take depends on the strength of the medicine. Also, *the number of doses you take each day, the time allowed between doses, and the length of time you take the medicine depend on your special needs.*

- For *oral* dosage forms (chewable tablets, tablets or suspension):
  - —For epilepsy:
    - Adults, teenagers, and children 8 years of age or older—At first, 100 or 125 milligrams (mg) once a day at bedtime. Your doctor may increase your dose if needed. However, the dose is usually not more than 2000 mg a day.
    - Children up to 8 years of age—At first, 50 mg once a day at bedtime. Your doctor may increase your dose if needed.

**Missed dose**—If you miss a dose of this medicine, take it as soon as possible. However, if it is within an hour of your next dose, skip the missed dose and go back to your regular dosing schedule. Do not double doses.

**Storage**—To store this medicine:

- Keep out of the reach of children.
- Store away from heat and direct light.
- Do not store the tablet form of this medicine in the bathroom, near the kitchen sink, or in other damp places. Heat or moisture may cause the medicine to break down.
- Keep the liquid form of this medicine from freezing.
- Do not keep outdated medicine or medicine no longer needed. Be sure that any discarded medicine is out of the reach of children.

## Precautions While Using This Medicine

It is very important that your doctor check your progress at regular visits, especially during the first few months of treatment with primidone. This will allow your doctor to adjust the amount of medicine you are taking to meet your needs.

If you have been taking primidone regularly for several weeks, you should not suddenly stop taking it. Your doctor may want you to reduce gradually the amount you are taking before stopping completely.

Before you have any medical tests, tell the medical doctor in charge that you are taking this medicine. The results of some tests (such as the metyrapone and phentolamine tests) may be affected by this medicine.

Before having any kind of surgery, dental treatment, or emergency treatment, tell the medical doctor or dentist in charge that you are using this medicine.

This medicine will add to the effects of alcohol and other CNS depressants (medicines that cause drowsiness). Some examples of CNS depressants are antihistamines or medicine for hay fever, other allergies, or colds; sedatives, tranquilizers, or sleeping medicine; prescription pain medicine or narcotics; barbiturates; medicine for seizures; muscle relaxants; or anesthetics, including some dental anesthetics. *Check with your doctor before taking any of the above while you are using this medicine.*

Primidone may cause some people to become dizzy, lightheaded, drowsy, or less alert than they are normally. Even if taken at bedtime, it may cause some people to feel drowsy or less alert on arising. *Make sure you know how you react to this medicine before you drive, use machines, or do anything else that could be dangerous if you are dizzy or are not alert.*

*Oral contraceptives (birth control pills) containing estrogen may not work properly if you take them while you are taking primidone. Unplanned pregnancies may occur. You should use a different or additional means of birth control while you are taking primidone.* If you have any questions about this, check with your health care professional.

## Side Effects of This Medicine

Along with its needed effects, a medicine may cause some unwanted effects. Although not all of these side effects may occur, if they do occur they may need medical attention.

Check with your doctor if any of the following side effects occur:

*Less common*
> Unusual excitement or restlessness (especially in children and in the elderly)

*Rare*
> Skin rash; unusual tiredness or weakness

*Symptoms of overdose*
> Confusion; continuous, uncontrolled back-and-forth and/or rolling eye movements; double vision; shortness of breath or troubled breathing

Other side effects may occur that usually do not need medical attention. These side effects may go away during treatment as your body adjusts to the medicine. However, check with your doctor if any of the following side effects continue or are bothersome:

*More common*
Clumsiness or unsteadiness; dizziness

*Less common*
Decreased sexual ability; drowsiness; loss of appetite; mood or mental changes; nausea or vomiting

Other side effects not listed above may also occur in some patients. If you notice any other effects, check with your doctor.

## Additional Information

Once a medicine has been approved for marketing for a certain use, experience may show that it is also useful for other medical problems. Although this use is not included in product labeling, primidone is used in certain patients with the following medical conditions:

- Essential tremor

Other than the above information, there is no additional information relating to proper use, precautions, or side effects for these uses.

Revised: 01/27/92
Interim revision: 08/16/94

# PROBENECID    Systemic

Some commonly used brand names are:

**In the U.S.—**
Benemid                    Probalan
Generic name product may also be available.

**In Canada—**
Benemid                    Benuryl

## Description

Probenecid (proe-BEN-e-sid) is used in the treatment of chronic gout or gouty arthritis. These conditions are caused by too much uric acid in the blood. The medicine works by removing the extra uric acid from the body. Probenecid does not cure gout, but after you have been taking it for a few months it will help prevent gout attacks. This medicine will help prevent gout attacks only as long as you continue to take it.

Probenecid is also used to prevent or treat other medical problems that may occur if too much uric acid is present in the body.

Probenecid is sometimes used with certain kinds of antibiotics to make them more effective in the treatment of infections.

Probenecid is available only with your doctor's prescription, in the following dosage form:

*Oral*
- Tablets (U.S. and Canada)

## Before Using This Medicine

In deciding to use a medicine, the risks of taking the medicine must be weighed against the good it will do. This is a decision you and your doctor will make. For probenecid, the following should be considered:

**Allergies**—Tell your doctor if you have ever had any unusual or allergic reaction to probenecid. Also tell your health care professional if you are allergic to any other substances, such as foods, preservatives, or dyes.

**Pregnancy**—Probenecid has not been shown to cause birth defects or other problems in humans.

**Breast-feeding**—Probenecid has not been reported to cause problems in nursing babies.

**Children**—Probenecid has been tested in children 2 to 14 years of age for use together with antibiotics. It has not been shown to cause different side effects or problems than it does in adults. Studies on the effects of probenecid in patients with gout have been done only in adults. Gout is very rare in children.

**Older adults**—Many medicines have not been studied specifically in older people. Therefore, it may not be known whether they work exactly the same way they do in younger adults. There is no specific information comparing use of probenecid in the elderly with use in other age groups.

**Other medicines**—Although certain medicines should not be used together at all, in other cases two different medicines may be used together even if an interaction might occur. In these cases, your doctor may want to change the dose, or other precautions may be necessary. When you are taking probenecid, it is especially important that your health care professional know if you are taking any of the following:

- Antineoplastics (cancer medicine)—The chance of serious side effects may be increased
- Aspirin or other salicylates—These medicines may keep probenecid from working properly for treating gout, depending on the amount of aspirin or other salicylate that you take and how often you take it
- Heparin—Probenecid may increase the effects of heparin, which increases the chance of side effects
- Indomethacin (e.g., Indocin) or
- Ketoprofen (e.g., Orudis) or

- Methotrexate (e.g., Mexate)—Probenecid may increase the blood levels of these medicines, which increases the chance of side effects
- Medicine for infection, including tuberculosis or virus infection—Probenecid may increase the blood levels of many of these medicines. In some cases, this is a desired effect and probenecid may be used to help the other medicine work better. However, the chance of side effects is sometimes also increased
- Nitrofurantoin (e.g., Furadantin)—Probenecid may keep nitrofurantoin from working properly
- Zidovudine (e.g., AZT, Retrovir)—Probenecid increases the blood level of zidovudine and may allow lower doses of zidovudine to be used. However, the chance of side effects is also increased

**Other medical problems**—The presence of other medical problems may affect the use of probenecid. Make sure you tell your doctor if you have any other medical problems, especially:

- Blood disease or
- Cancer being treated by antineoplastics (cancer medicine) or radiation (x-rays) or
- Kidney disease or stones (or history of) or
- Stomach ulcer (history of)—The chance of side effects may be increased

---

## Proper Use of This Medicine

If probenecid upsets your stomach, it may be taken with food. If this does not work, an antacid may be taken. If stomach upset (nausea, vomiting, or loss of appetite) continues, check with your doctor.

For patients taking probenecid *for gout:*

- After you begin to take probenecid, gout attacks may continue to occur for a while. However, if you take this medicine regularly as directed by your doctor, the attacks will gradually become less frequent and less painful than before. After you have been taking probenecid for several months, they may stop completely.
- This medicine will help prevent gout attacks but it will not relieve an attack that has already started. *Even if you take another medicine for gout attacks, continue to take this medicine also.* If you have any questions about this, check with your doctor.

For patients taking probenecid *for gout or to help remove uric acid from the body:*

- When you first begin taking probenecid, the amount of uric acid in the kidneys is greatly increased. This may cause kidney stones or other kidney problems in some people. To help prevent this, your doctor may want you to drink at least 10 to 12 full glasses (8 ounces each) of fluids each day, or to take another medicine to make your urine less acid. It is important that you follow your doctor's instructions very carefully.

**Dosing**—The dose of probenecid will be different for different patients. *Follow your doctor's orders or the directions on the label.* The following information includes only the average doses of probenecid. *If your dose is different, do not change it* unless your doctor tells you to do so.

- *For treating gout or removing uric acid from the body:*
  —Adults: 250 mg (one-half of a 500-mg tablet) two times a day for about one week, then 500 mg (one tablet) two times a day for a few weeks. After this, the dose will depend on the amount of uric acid in your blood or urine. Most people need 2, 3, or 4 tablets a day, but some people may need higher doses.
  —Children: It is not likely that probenecid will be needed to treat gout or to remove uric acid from the body in children. If a child needs this medicine, however, the dose would have to be determined by the doctor.
- *For helping antibiotics work better:*
  —Adults: The amount of probenecid will depend on the condition being treated. Sometimes, only one dose of 2 tablets is needed. Other times, the dose will be 1 tablet four times a day.
  —Children: The dose will have to be determined by the doctor. It depends on the child's weight, as well as on the condition being treated. Older children and teenagers may need the same amount as adults.

**Missed dose**—If you are taking probenecid regularly and you miss a dose, take the missed dose as soon as possible. However, if you do not remember until it is almost time for the next dose, skip the missed dose and go back to your regular dosing schedule. Do not double doses.

**Storage**—To store this medicine:

- Keep out of the reach of children.
- Store away from heat and direct light.
- Do not store this medicine in the bathroom, near the kitchen sink, or in other damp places. Heat or moisture may cause the medicine to break down.
- Do not keep outdated medicine or medicine no longer needed. Be sure that any discarded medicine is out of the reach of children.

---

## Precautions While Using This Medicine

If you will be taking probenecid for more than a few weeks, your doctor should check your progress at regular visits.

Before you have any medical tests, tell the person in charge that you are taking this medicine. The results of some tests may be affected by probenecid.

For *diabetic patients:*

- Probenecid may cause false test results with copper sulfate urine sugar tests (Clinitest®), but not with glucose enzymatic urine sugar tests (Clinistix®). If you have any questions about this, check with your health care professional.

---

For patients taking probenecid *for gout or to help remove uric acid from the body:*

- Taking aspirin or other salicylates may lessen the effects of probenecid. This will depend on the dose of aspirin or other salicylate that you take, and on how often you take it. Also, drinking too much alcohol may increase the amount of uric acid in the blood and lessen the effects of this medicine. Therefore, *do not take aspirin or other salicylates or drink alcoholic beverages while taking this medicine,* unless you have first checked with your doctor.

## Side Effects of This Medicine

Along with its needed effects, a medicine may cause some unwanted effects. Although not all of these side effects may occur, if they do occur they may need medical attention.

The following side effects may mean that you are having an allergic reaction to this medicine. *Check with your doctor immediately* if any of the following side effects occur:

*Rare*

Fast or irregular breathing; puffiness or swellings of the eyelids or around the eyes; shortness of breath, troubled breathing, tightness in chest, or wheezing; changes in the skin color of the face occurring together with any of the other side effects listed here; or skin rash, hives, or itching occurring together with any of the other side effects listed here

Also, check with your doctor as soon as possible if any of the following side effects occur:

*Less common*

Bloody urine; difficult or painful urination; lower back or side pain (especially if severe or sharp); skin rash, hives, or itching (occurring without other signs of an allergic reaction)

*Rare*

Cloudy urine; cough or hoarseness; fast or irregular breathing; fever; pain in back and/or ribs; sores, ulcers, or white spots on lips or in mouth; sore throat and fever with or without chills; sudden decrease in the amount of urine; swelling of face, fingers, feet, and/or lower legs; swollen and/or painful glands; unusual bleeding or bruising; unusual tiredness or weakness; yellow eyes or skin; weight gain

Other side effects may occur that usually do not need medical attention. These side effects may go away during treatment as your body adjusts to the medicine. However, check with your doctor if any of the following side effects continue or are bothersome:

*More common*

Headache; joint pain, redness, or swelling; loss of appetite; nausea or vomiting (mild)

*Less common*

Dizziness; flushing or redness of face (occurring without any signs of an allergic reaction); frequent urge to urinate; sore gums

Other side effects not listed above may also occur in some patients. If you notice any other effects, check with your doctor.

Revised: 09/01/92

# PROBENECID AND COLCHICINE  Systemic

Some commonly used brand names are:

**In the U.S.—**
ColBenemid          Proben-C
Col-Probenecid
Generic name product may also be available.

## Description

Probenecid (proe-BEN-e-sid) and colchicine (KOL-chi-seen) combination is used to treat gout or gouty arthritis.

The probenecid in this medicine helps to prevent gout attacks by removing extra uric acid from the body. The colchicine in this medicine also helps to prevent gout attacks. Although colchicine may also be used to relieve an attack of gout, this requires more colchicine than this combination medicine contains. Probenecid and colchicine combination does not cure gout. This medicine will help prevent gout attacks only as long as you continue to take it.

Probenecid and colchicine combination is available only with your doctor's prescription, in the following dosage form:

*Oral*
- Tablets (U.S.)

## Before Using This Medicine

In deciding to use a medicine, the risks of taking the medicine must be weighed against the good it will do. This is a decision you and your doctor will make. For probenecid and colchicine combination, the following should be considered:

**Allergies**—Tell your doctor if you have ever had any unusual or allergic reaction to probenecid or to colchicine. Also tell your health care professional if you are allergic to any other substances, such as foods, preservatives, or dyes.

**Pregnancy**—Probenecid has not been shown to cause birth defects or other problems in humans. Although studies with colchicine have not been done in pregnant women, some reports have suggested that use of colchicine during pregnancy can cause harm to the fetus. Also, studies in animals have shown that colchicine causes birth defects. Therefore, do not begin taking this medicine during pregnancy, and do not become pregnant while taking it, unless you have first discussed this problem with your doctor. Also, check with your doctor immediately if you suspect that you have become pregnant while taking this medicine.

**Breast-feeding**—This medicine has not been reported to cause problems in nursing babies.

**Children**—Studies on this combination medicine have been done only in adult patients, and there is no specific information about its use in children.

**Older adults**—Elderly people are especially sensitive to the effects of colchicine. This may increase the chance of side effects during treatment.

There is no specific information comparing use of probenecid in the elderly with use in other age groups.

**Other medicines**—Although certain medicines should not be used together at all, in other cases two different medicines may be used together even if an interaction might occur. In these cases, your doctor may want to change the dose, or other precautions may be necessary. When you are taking probenecid and colchicine combination, it is especially important that your health care professional know if you are taking any of the following:

- Amphotericin B by injection (e.g., Fungizone) or
- Antineoplastics (cancer medicine) or
- Antithyroid agents (medicine for overactive thyroid) or
- Azathioprine (e.g., Imuran) or
- Cyclophosphamide (e.g., Cytoxan) or
- Flucytosine (e.g., Ancobon) or
- Ganciclovir (e.g., Cytovene) or
- Interferon (e.g., Intron A, Roferon-A) or
- Mercaptopurine (e.g., Purinethol) or
- Methotrexate (e.g., Mexate) or
- Phenylbutazone (e.g., Butazolidin) or
- Plicamycin (e.g., Mithracin) or
- Zidovudine (e.g., AZT, Retrovir)—Taking any of these medicines together with colchicine may increase the chance of serious side effects. Also, the chance of serious side effects may be increased when antineoplastics (cancer medicine), methotrexate, phenylbutazone, or zidovudine are taken together with probenecid
- Aspirin or other salicylates, including bismuth subsalicylate (e.g., Pepto-Bismol)—These medicines may keep probenecid from working properly for treating gout, depending on the amount of aspirin or other salicylate that you take and how often you take it
- Heparin—Probenecid may increase the effects of heparin, which increases the chance of side effects
- Indomethacin (e.g., Indocin) or
- Ketoprofen (e.g., Orudis)—Probenecid may increase the blood levels of these medicines, which increases the chance of side effects

- Medicine for infection, including tuberculosis or virus infection—Probenecid may increase the blood levels of many of these medicines, which may increase the chance of side effects. Also, the chance of serious side effects may be increased when some of these medicines are taken together with colchicine
- Nitrofurantoin (e.g., Furadantin)—Probenecid may keep nitrofurantoin from working properly

**Other medical problems**—The presence of other medical problems may affect the use of probenecid and colchicine combination. Make sure you tell your doctor if you have any other medical problems, especially:

- Alcohol abuse or
- Blood disease or
- Cancer being treated by antineoplastics (cancer medicine) or radiation (x-rays) or
- Heart disease (severe) or
- Intestinal disease (severe) or
- Kidney disease or stones (or history of) or
- Liver disease or
- Stomach ulcer or other stomach problems (or history of)— The chance of serious side effects may be increased

## Proper Use of This Medicine

If this medicine upsets your stomach, it may be taken with food. If this does not work, an antacid may be taken. If stomach upset (nausea, vomiting, loss of appetite, or stomach pain) continues, check with your doctor.

Take this medicine only as directed by your doctor. Do not take more of it and do not take it more often than your doctor ordered. The colchicine in this combination medicine may cause serious side effects if too much is taken.

After you begin to take this medicine, gout attacks may continue to occur for a while. However, if you take this medicine regularly as directed by your doctor, the attacks will gradually become less frequent and less painful than before. After you have been taking this medicine for several months, they may stop completely.

This medicine will help prevent gout attacks but it will not relieve an attack that has already started. *Even if you take another medicine for gout attacks, continue to take this medicine also.*

When you first begin taking this medicine, the amount of uric acid in the kidneys is greatly increased. This may cause kidney stones or other kidney problems in some people. To help prevent this, your doctor may want you to drink at least 10 to 12 full glasses (8 ounces each) of fluids each day, or to take another medicine to make your urine less acid. It is important that you follow your doctor's instructions very carefully.

**Dosing**—The dose of probenecid and colchicine combination will be different for different patients. *Follow your doctor's orders or the directions on the label.* The following information includes only the average doses of this medicine. *If your dose is different, do not change it* unless your doctor tells you to do so.

- For *oral* dosage form (tablets):
  —For preventing gout attacks:
    - Adults—One tablet a day for one week, then one tablet twice a day. If you are still having a lot of gout attacks a month after you start taking two tablets a day, your doctor may direct you to increase the dose.
    - Children—Dose must be determined by your doctor.

**Missed dose**—If you miss a dose of this medicine, take it as soon as possible. However, if it is almost time for your next dose, skip the missed dose and go back to your regular dosing schedule. Do not double doses.

**Storage**—To store this medicine:

- Keep out of the reach of children.
- Store away from heat and direct light.
- Do not store this medicine in the bathroom, near the kitchen sink, or in other damp places. Heat or moisture may cause the medicine to break down.
- Do not keep outdated medicine or medicine no longer needed. Be sure that any discarded medicine is out of the reach of children.

---

## Precautions While Using This Medicine

Your doctor should check your progress at regular visits while you are taking this medicine.

Before you have any medical tests, tell the person in charge that you are taking this medicine. The results of some tests may be affected by probenecid or by colchicine.

For *diabetic patients:*

- The probenecid in this combination medicine may cause false test results with copper sulfate urine sugar tests (e.g., Clinitest®), but not with glucose enzymatic urine sugar tests (e.g., Clinistix®). If you have any questions about this, check with your health care professional.

Taking aspirin or other salicylates may lessen the effects of the probenecid in this combination medicine. This will depend on the dose of aspirin or other salicylate that you take, and on how often you take it. Also, drinking large amounts of alcoholic beverages may increase the chance of stomach problems and may increase the amount of uric acid in your blood. *Therefore, do not take aspirin or other salicylates or drink alcoholic beverages while you are taking this medicine,* unless you have first checked with your doctor.

For patients taking 4 tablets or more of this medicine a day:

- *Stop taking this medicine immediately and check with your doctor as soon as possible if severe diarrhea, nausea or vomiting, or stomach pain occurs while you are taking this medicine.*

## Side Effects of This Medicine

Along with its needed effects, a medicine may cause some unwanted effects. Although not all of these side effects may occur, if they do occur they may need medical attention.

The following side effects may mean that you are having an allergic reaction to this medicine. *Check with your doctor immediately* if any of the following side effects occur:

*Rare*

Fast or irregular breathing; puffiness or swelling of the eyelids or around the eyes; shortness of breath, troubled breathing, tightness in chest, or wheezing; changes in the skin color of the face occurring together with any of the other side effects listed here; or skin rash, hives, or itching occurring together with any of the other side effects listed here

*Also check with your doctor immediately* if any of the following side effects occur:

*Symptoms of overdose*

Bloody urine; burning feeling in stomach, throat, or skin; convulsions (seizures); diarrhea (severe or bloody); fever; mood or mental changes; muscle weakness (severe); nausea or vomiting (severe and continuing); sudden decrease in amount of urine; troubled or difficult breathing

Also, check with your doctor as soon as possible if any of the following side effects occur:

*Less common*

Difficult or painful urination; lower back or side pain (especially if severe or sharp); skin rash, hives, or itching (occurring without other signs of an allergic reaction)

*Rare*

Black or tarry stools; cloudy urine; cough or hoarseness; fast or irregular breathing; numbness, tingling, pain, or weakness in hands or feet; pinpoint red spots on skin; sores, ulcers, or white spots on lips or in mouth; sore throat, fever, and chills; sudden decrease in the amount of urine; swelling of face, fingers, feet, and/or lower legs; swollen and/or painful glands; unusual bleeding or bruising; unusual tiredness or weakness; yellow eyes or skin; weight gain

Other side effects may occur that usually do not need medical attention. These side effects may go away during treatment as your body adjusts to the medicine. However, check with your doctor if any of the following side effects continue or are bothersome:

*More common*

Diarrhea (mild); headache; loss of appetite; nausea or vomiting (mild); stomach pain

*Less common*

Dizziness; flushing or redness of face (occurring without any signs of an allergic reaction); frequent urge to urinate; sore gums; unusual loss of hair

Other side effects not listed above may also occur in some patients. If you notice any other effects, check with your doctor.

Revised: 09/09/92
Interim revision: 08/27/94

---

# PROBUCOL Systemic

Some commonly used brand names are:

**In the U.S.—**
Lorelco

**In Canada—**
Lorelco

**Other—**

| | |
|---|---|
| Bifenabid | Panesclerina |
| Lesterol | Superlipid |
| Lurselle | |

## Description

Probucol (PROE-byoo-kole) is used to lower levels of cholesterol (a fat-like substance) in the blood. This may help prevent medical problems caused by cholesterol clogging the blood vessels.

Probucol is available only with your doctor's prescription, in the following dosage form:

*Oral*
- Tablets (U.S. and Canada)

## Before Using This Medicine

In deciding to use a medicine, the risks of taking the medicine must be weighed against the good it will do. This is a decision you and your doctor will make. For probucol, the following should be considered:

**Allergies**—Tell your doctor if you have ever had any unusual or allergic reaction to probucol. Also tell your health care professional if you are allergic to any other substances, such as foods, preservatives, or dyes.

**Diet**—Before prescribing medicine for your condition, your doctor will probably try to control your condition by prescribing a personal diet for you. Such a diet may be low in fats, sugars, and/or cholesterol. Many people are able to control their condition by carefully following their doctor's orders for proper diet and exercise. Medicine is prescribed only when additional help is needed and is effective only when a schedule of diet and exercise is properly followed.

Also, this medicine is less effective if you are greatly overweight. It may be very important for you to go on a reducing diet. However, check with your doctor before going on any diet.

Make certain your health care professional know if you are on a low-sodium, low-sugar, or any other special diet.

**Pregnancy**—Probucol has not been studied in pregnant women. However, it has not been shown to cause birth defects or other problems in rats or rabbits.

**Breast-feeding**—It is not known whether probucol passes into the breast milk. However, this medicine is not recommended for use during breast-feeding because it may cause unwanted effects in nursing babies.

**Children**—There is no specific information about the use of probucol in children. However, use is not recommended in children under 2 years of age since cholesterol is needed for normal development.

**Older adults**—Many medicines have not been studied specifically in older people. Therefore, it may not be known whether they work exactly the same way they do in younger adults or if they cause different side effects or problems in older people. There is no specific information comparing use of probucol in the elderly with use in other age groups.

**Other medicines**—Although certain medicines should not be used together at all, in other cases two different medicines may be used together even if an interaction might occur. In these cases, your doctor may want to change the dose, or other precautions may be necessary. Tell your health care professional if you are taking any other prescription or nonprescription (over-the-counter [OTC]) medicine.

**Other medical problems**—The presence of other medical problems may affect the use of probucol. Make sure you tell your doctor if you have any other medical problems, especially:
- Gallbladder disease or gallstones or
- Heart disease—Probucol may make these conditions worse
- Liver disease—Higher blood levels of probucol may result, which may increase the chance of side effects

## Proper Use of This Medicine

Many patients who have high cholesterol levels will not notice any signs of the problem. In fact, many may feel normal. *Take this medicine exactly as directed by your doctor, even though you may feel well.* Try not to miss any doses and do not take more medicine than your doctor ordered.

Remember that this medicine will not cure your condition but it does help control it. Therefore, you must continue to take it as directed if you expect to keep your cholesterol levels down.

*Follow carefully the special diet your doctor gave you.* This is the most important part of controlling your condition, and is necessary if the medicine is to work properly.

This medicine works better when taken with meals.

**Dosing**—The dose of probucol will be different for different patients. *Follow your doctor's orders or the directions on the label.* The following information includes only the average doses of probucol. *If your dose is different, do not change it* unless your doctor tells you to do so:

- The number of tablets that you take depends on the strength of the medicine.
- For *oral* dosage form (tablets):
  —Adults: 500 milligrams two times a day taken with the morning and evening meals.
  —Children:
  • Up to 2 years of age—Use is not recommended.
  • 2 years of age and over—Dose must be determined by your doctor.

**Missed dose**—If you miss a dose of this medicine, take it as soon as possible. However, if it is almost time for your next dose, skip the missed dose and go back to your regular dosing schedule. Do not double doses.

**Storage**—To store this medicine:

- Keep out of the reach of children.
- Store away from heat and direct light.
- Do not store in the bathroom, near the kitchen sink, or in other damp places. Heat or moisture may cause the medicine to break down.
- Do not keep outdated medicine or medicine no longer needed. Be sure that any discarded medicine is out of the reach of children.

## Precautions While Using This Medicine

*It is very important that your doctor check your progress at regular visits.* This will allow your doctor to see if the medicine is working properly to lower your cholesterol levels and to decide if you should continue to take it.

*Do not stop taking this medicine without first checking with your doctor.* When you stop taking this medicine, your blood fat levels may increase again. Your doctor may want you to follow a special diet to help prevent this.

## Side Effects of This Medicine

Along with its needed effects, a medicine may cause some unwanted effects. Although not all of these side effects may occur, if they do occur they may need medical attention.

Check with your doctor as soon as possible if any of the following side effects occur:

*More common*
Dizziness or fainting; fast or irregular heartbeat
*Rare*
Swellings on face, hands, or feet, or in mouth; unusual bleeding or bruising; unusual tiredness or weakness

Other side effects may occur that usually do not need medical attention. These side effects may go away during treatment as your body adjusts to the medicine. However, check with your doctor if any of the following side effects continue or are bothersome:

*More common*
Bloating; diarrhea; nausea and vomiting; stomach pain
*Less common*
Headache; numbness or tingling of fingers, toes, or face

Other side effects not listed above may also occur in some patients. If you notice any other effects, check with your doctor.

Revised: 04/13/93

---

# PROCAINAMIDE    Systemic

Some commonly used brand names are:

**In the U.S.—**

| | |
|---|---|
| Procan SR | Pronestyl |
| Promine | Pronestyl-SR |

Generic name product may also be available.

**In Canada—**

| | |
|---|---|
| Procan SR | Pronestyl-SR |
| Pronestyl | |

Generic name product may also be available.

## Description

Procainamide (proe-KANE-a-mide) is used to correct irregular heartbeats to a normal rhythm and to slow an overactive heart. This allows the heart to work more efficiently. Procainamide produces its beneficial effects by slowing nerve impulses in the heart and reducing sensitivity of heart tissues.

Procainamide is available only with your doctor's prescription, in the following dosage forms:

*Oral*
- Capsules (U.S. and Canada)
- Tablets (U.S.)
- Extended-release tablets (U.S. and Canada)

*Parenteral*
- Injection (U.S. and Canada)

## Before Using This Medicine

In deciding to use a medicine, the risks of taking the medicine must be weighed against the good it will do. This is a decision you and your doctor will make. For procainamide, the following should be considered:

**Allergies**—Tell your doctor if you have ever had any unusual or allergic reaction to procainamide, procaine, or any other "caine-type" medicine. Also tell your health care professional if you are allergic to any other substance, such as foods, preservatives, or dyes.

**Pregnancy**—Procainamide has not been studied in pregnant women. However, it has been used in some pregnant women and has not been shown to cause problems. Before taking this medicine, make sure your doctor knows if you are pregnant or if you may become pregnant.

**Breast-feeding**—Procainamide passes into breast milk.

**Children**—Procainamide has been used in a limited number of children. In effective doses, the medicine has not been shown to cause different side effects or problems than it does in adults.

**Older adults**—Dizziness or lightheadedness is more likely to occur in the elderly, who are usually more sensitive to the effects of this medicine.

**Other medicines**—Although certain medicines should not be used together at all, in other cases two different medicines may be used together even if an interaction might occur. In these cases, your doctor may want to change the dose, or other precautions may be necessary. When you are taking procainamide, it is especially important that your health care professional know if you are taking any of the following:
- Antiarrhythmics (medicines for heart rhythm problems), other—Effects on the heart may be increased
- Antihypertensives (high blood pressure medicine)—Effects on blood pressure may be increased
- Antimyasthenics (ambenonium [e.g., Mytelase], neostigmine [e.g., Prostigmin], pyridostigmine [e.g., Mestinon])—Effects may be blocked by procainamide
- Pimozide (e.g., Orap)—May increase the risk of heart rhythm problems

**Other medical problems**—The presence of other medical problems may affect the use of procainamide. Make sure you tell your doctor if you have any other medical problems, especially:
- Asthma—Possible allergic reaction
- Kidney disease or
- Liver disease—Effects may be increased because of slower removal of procainamide from the body

- Lupus erythematosus (history of)—Procainamide may cause the condition to become active
- Myasthenia gravis—Procainamide may increase muscle weakness

## Proper Use of This Medicine

*Take procainamide exactly as directed by your doctor,* even though you may feel well. Do not take more medicine than ordered.

Procainamide should be taken with a glass of water on an empty stomach 1 hour before or 2 hours after meals so that it will be absorbed more quickly. However, to lessen stomach upset, your doctor may want you to take the medicine with food or milk.

For patients taking the *extended-release tablets:*
- Swallow the tablet whole without breaking, crushing, or chewing it.

This medicine works best when there is a constant amount in the blood. *To help keep the amount constant, do not miss any doses. Also, it is best to take the doses at evenly spaced times day and night.* For example, if you are to take 6 doses a day, the doses should be spaced about 4 hours apart. If this interferes with your sleep or other daily activities, or if you need help in planning the best times to take your medicine, check with your health care professional.

**Dosing**—The dose of procainamide will be different for different patients. *Follow your doctor's orders or the directions on the label.* The following information includes only the average doses of procainamide. *If your dose is different, do not change it* unless your doctor tells you to do so.

The number of capsules or tablets that you take depends on the strength of the medicine.
- For *regular (short-acting) oral* dosage forms (capsules or tablets):
  —For atrial arrhythmias (fast or irregular heartbeat):
    - Adults—500 milligrams (mg) to 1000 mg (1 gram) every four to six hours.
    - Children—12.5 mg per kilogram (5.68 mg per pound) of body weight four times a day.
  —For ventricular arrhythmias (fast or irregular heartbeat):
    - Adults—50 mg per kilogram (22.73 mg per pound) of body weight per day divided into eight doses taken every three hours.
    - Children—12.5 mg per kilogram (5.68 mg per pound) of body weight four times a day.
- For *long-acting oral* dosage form (extended-release tablets):
  —For atrial arrhythmias (fast or irregular heartbeat):
    - Adults—1000 mg (1 gram) every six hours.
    - Children—Use is not recommended.

—For ventricular arrhythmias (fast or irregular heartbeat):
- Adults—50 mg per kilogram (22.73 mg per pound) of body weight per day divided into four doses taken every six hours.

- For *injection* dosage form:
—For arrhythmias (fast or irregular heartbeat):
- Adults—
—*First few doses:* May be given intramuscularly (into the muscle) at 50 mg per kilogram (22.73 mg per pound) of body weight per day in divided doses every three hours; or may be given intravenously (into the vein) by slowly injecting 100 mg (mixed in fluid) every five minutes or infusing 500 to 600 mg (mixed in fluid) over a twenty-five to thirty minute period.
—*Doses after the first few doses:* 2 to 6 mg (mixed in fluid) per minute infused into the vein.
- Children—Dose must be determined by your doctor.

**Missed dose**—If you miss a dose of this medicine and remember within 2 hours (4 hours if you are taking the long-acting tablets), take it as soon as possible. However, if you do not remember until later, skip the missed dose and go back to your regular dosing schedule. Do not double doses.

**Storage**—To store this medicine:
- Keep out of the reach of children.
- Store away from heat and direct light.
- Do not store in the bathroom, refrigerator, near the kitchen sink, or in other damp places. Moisture usually present in these areas may cause the medicine to break down. Keep the container tightly closed and store in a dry place.
- Do not keep outdated medicine or medicine no longer needed. Be sure that any discarded medicine is out of the reach of children.

---

## Precautions While Using This Medicine

It is important that your doctor check your progress at regular visits to make sure the medicine is working properly. This will allow necessary changes in the amount of medicine you are taking, which also may help reduce side effects.

*Do not stop taking this medicine without first checking with your doctor.* Stopping it suddenly may cause a serious change in the activity of your heart. Your doctor may want you to reduce gradually the amount you are taking before stopping completely.

*Before having any kind of surgery (including dental surgery) or emergency treatment, tell the medical doctor or dentist in charge that you are taking this medicine.*

Your doctor may want you to carry a medical identification card or bracelet stating that you are taking this medicine.

Dizziness or lightheadedness may occur, especially in elderly patients and when large doses are used. *Elderly patients should use extra care to avoid falling. Make sure you know how you react to this medicine before you drive, use machines, or do anything else that could be dangerous if you are dizzy or are not alert.*

Tell the doctor in charge that you are taking this medicine before you have any medical tests. The results of some tests may be affected by this medicine.

---

## Side Effects of This Medicine

Along with its needed effects, a medicine may cause some unwanted effects. Although not all of these side effects may occur, if they do occur they may need medical attention.

Check with your doctor as soon as possible if any of the following side effects occur:
*Less common*
Fever and chills; joint pain or swelling; pains with breathing; skin rash or itching
*Rare*
Confusion; fever or sore mouth, gums, or throat; hallucinations (seeing, hearing, or feeling things that are not there); mental depression; unusual bleeding or bruising; unusual tiredness or weakness
*Signs and symptoms of overdose*
Confusion; decrease in urination; dizziness (severe) or fainting; drowsiness; fast or irregular heartbeat; nausea and vomiting

Other side effects may occur that usually do not need medical attention. These side effects may go away during treatment as your body adjusts to the medicine. However, check with your doctor if any of the following side effects continue or are bothersome:
*More common*
Diarrhea; loss of appetite
*Less common*
Dizziness or lightheadedness

The medicine in the extended-release tablets is contained in a special wax form (matrix). The medicine is slowly released, after which the wax matrix passes out of the body. Sometimes it may be seen in the stool. This is normal and is no cause for concern.

Other side effects not listed above may also occur in some patients. If you notice any other effects, check with your doctor.

---

Revised: 08/04/93

---

# PROCARBAZINE  Systemic

Some commonly used brand names are:
**In the U.S.**
   Matulane
**In Canada**
   Natulan

## Description

Procarbazine (pro-KAR-ba-zeen) belongs to the group of medicines known as alkylating agents. It is used to treat some kinds of cancer.

Procarbazine is thought to interfere with the growth of cancer cells which are eventually destroyed. It also blocks the action of a chemical substance in the central nervous system called monoamine oxidase (MAO), but this is probably not related to its effect against cancer. Since the growth of normal body cells may also be affected by procarbazine, other effects will also occur. Some of these may be serious and must be reported to your doctor. Other effects, like hair loss, may not be serious but may cause concern. Some effects may not occur for months or years after the medicine is used.

Before you begin treatment with procarbazine, you and your doctor should talk about the good this medicine will do as well as the risks of using it.

Procarbazine is available only with your doctor's prescription, in the following dosage form:
*Oral*
   • Capsules (U.S. and Canada)

## Before Using This Medicine

In deciding to use a medicine, the risks of taking the medicine must be weighed against the good it will do. This is a decision you and your doctor will make. For procarbazine, the following should be considered:

**Allergies**—Tell your doctor if you have ever had any unusual or allergic reaction to procarbazine.

**Pregnancy**—Tell your doctor if you are pregnant or if you intend to have children. This medicine may cause birth defects or premature birth if either the male or female is taking it at the time of conception or if it is taken during pregnancy. Procarbazine causes birth defects frequently in animals. In addition, many cancer medicines may cause sterility which could be permanent. Although sterility has not been reported with this medicine, procarbazine does affect production of sperm and the possibility should be kept in mind.

Be sure that you have discussed this with your doctor before taking this medicine. It is best to use some kind of birth control while you are taking procarbazine. Tell your doctor right away if you think you have become pregnant while taking procarbazine.

**Breast-feeding**—Tell your doctor if you are breast-feeding or if you intend to breast-feed during treatment with this medicine. Because procarbazine may cause serious side effects, breast-feeding is generally not recommended while you are taking it.

**Children**—Although there is no specific information about the use of procarbazine in children, it is not expected to cause different side effects or problems in children than it does in adults.

**Older adults**—Side effects may be more likely to occur in elderly patients, who are usually more sensitive to the effects of procarbazine.

**Other medicines**—Although certain medicines should not be used together at all, in other cases two different medicines may be used together even if an interaction might occur. In these cases, your doctor may want to change the dose, or other precautions may be necessary. When you are taking procarbazine, it is especially important that your health care professional know if you are taking any of the following:

• Amantadine (e.g., Symmetrel) or
• Anticholinergics (medicine to help reduce stomach acid and for abdominal or stomach spasms or cramps) or
• Antidiabetics, oral (diabetes medicine you take by mouth) or
• Antidyskinetics (medicine for Parkinson's disease or other conditions affecting control of muscles) or
• Antihistamines or
• Antipsychotics (medicine for mental illness) or
• Buclizine (e.g., Bucladin) or
• Central nervous system (CNS) depressants or
• Cyclizine (e.g., Marezine) or
• Disopyramide (e.g., Norpace) or
• Flavoxate (e.g., Urispas) or
• Insulin or
• Ipratropium (e.g., Atrovent) or
• Meclizine (e.g., Antivert) or
• Orphenadrine (e.g., Norflex) or
• Oxybutynin (e.g., Ditropen) or
• Procainamide (e.g., Pronestyl) or
• Promethazine (e.g., Phenergan) or
• Quinidine (e.g., Quinidex) or
• Trimeprazine (e.g., Temaril)—Effects of these medicines may be increased by procarbazine

• Amphetamines or
• Appetite suppressants (diet pills) or
• Dextromethorphan (e.g., Delsym) or
• Levodopa (e.g., Dopar) or
• Medicine for asthma or other breathing problems or
• Medicine for colds, sinus problems, or hay fever or other allergies (including nose drops or sprays) or
• Methyldopa (e.g., Aldomet) or
• Methylphenidate (e.g., Ritalin) or
• Narcotic pain medicine—Taking any of these medicines while you are taking or within 2 weeks of taking procarbazine may cause a severe high blood pressure reaction

• Amphotericin B by injection (e.g., Fungizone) or
• Antithyroid agents (medicine for overactive thyroid) or
• Azathioprine (e.g., Imuran) or
• Chloramphenicol (e.g., Chloromycetin) or
• Colchicine or
• Flucytosine (e.g., Ancobon) or

- Interferon (e.g., Intron A, Roferon-A) or
- Plicamycin (e.g., Mithracin) or
- Zidovudine (e.g., Retrovir) or
- If you have ever been treated with x-rays or cancer medicines—Procarbazine may increase the effects of these medicines or radiation therapy on the blood
- Buspirone (e.g., BuSpar)—Risk of increased blood pressure
- Carbamazepine (e.g., Tegretol) or
- Cyclobenzaprine (e.g., Flexeril) or
- Maprotiline (e.g., Ludiomil) or
- Monoamine oxidase (MAO) inhibitors (furazolidone [e.g., Furoxone], isocarboxazid [e.g., Marplan], pargyline [e.g., Eutonyl], phenelzine [e.g., Nardil], procarbazine [e.g., Matulane], tranylcypromine [e.g., Parnate]) or
- Tricyclic antidepressants (amitriptyline [e.g., Elavil], amoxapine [e.g., Asendin], clomipramine [e.g., Anafranil], desipramine [e.g., Pertofrane], doxepin [e.g., Sinequan], imipramine [e.g., Tofranil], nortriptyline [e.g., Aventyl], protriptyline [e.g., Vivactil], trimipramine [e.g., Surmontil])—Taking procarbazine while you are taking or within 2 weeks of taking any of these medicines may cause a severe high blood pressure reaction
- Cocaine—Use of cocaine while you are taking or within 2 weeks of taking procarbazine may cause a severe high blood pressure reaction
- Fluoxetine (e.g., Prozac)—Taking this medicine while you are taking or within 2 weeks of taking procarbazine may cause a severe high blood pressure reaction or may lead to confusion, agitation, restlessness, and stomach problems
- Guanadrel (e.g., Hylorel) or
- Guanethidine (e.g., Ismelin) or
- Rauwolfia alkaloids (alseroxylon [e.g., Rauwiloid], deserpidine [e.g., Harmonyl], rauwolfia serpentina [e.g., Raudixin], reserpine [e.g., Serpasil])—Taking these medicines while you are taking or within 1 week of taking procarbazine may cause a severe high blood pressure reaction

**Other medical problems**—The presence of other medical problems may affect the use of procarbazine. Make sure you tell your doctor if you have any other medical problems, especially:
- Alcoholism
- Angina (chest pain) or
- Heart or blood vessel disease or
- Heart attack or stroke (recent)—Lowered blood pressure caused by procarbazine may make problems associated with some of these conditions worse
- Chickenpox (including recent exposure) or
- Herpes zoster (shingles)—Risk of severe disease affecting other parts of the body
- Diabetes mellitus (sugar diabetes)—Procarbazine may change the amount of diabetes medicine needed
- Epilepsy—Procarbazine may change the seizures
- Headaches (severe or frequent)—You may not realize when a severe headache is caused by a dangerous reaction to procarbazine
- Infection—Procarbazine can reduce immunity to infection
- Kidney disease—Effects may be increased because of slower removal of procarbazine from the body
- Liver disease—Procarbazine can cause severe liver disease to become much worse

- Mental illness (or history of)—Some cases of mental illness may be worsened
- Overactive thyroid—Increased risk of dangerous reaction to procarbazine
- Parkinson's disease—May be worsened
- Pheochromocytoma—Blood pressure may be affected

## Proper Use of This Medicine

*Use this medicine only as directed by your doctor.* Do not use more or less of it and do not use it more often than your doctor ordered. The exact amount of medicine you need has been carefully worked out. Taking too much may increase the chance of side effects while taking too little may not improve your condition.

Procarbazine is sometimes given together with certain other medicines. If you are using a combination of medicines, make sure that you take each one at the right time and do not mix them. Ask your health care professional to help you plan a way to take your medicines at the right times.

Procarbazine commonly causes nausea and vomiting. Even if you begin to feel ill, *do not stop using this medicine without first checking with your doctor.* Ask your health care professional for ways to lessen these effects.

If you vomit shortly after taking a dose of procarbazine, check with your doctor. You will be told whether to take the dose again or to wait until the next scheduled dose.

**Dosing**—The dose of procarbazine will be different for different patients. The dose that is used may depend on a number of things, including what the medicine is being used for, the patient's weight, and whether or not other medicines are also being taken. *If you are taking procarbazine at home, follow your doctor's orders or the directions on the label.* If you have any questions about the proper dose of procarbazine, ask your doctor.

**Missed dose**—If you miss a dose of this medicine and you remember it within a few hours, take it as soon as you remember it. However, if several hours have passed or if it is almost time for the next dose, skip the missed dose and go back to your regular dosing schedule and check with your doctor. Do not double doses.

**Storage**—To store this medicine:
- Keep out of the reach of children.
- Store away from heat and direct light.
- Do not store in the bathroom, near the kitchen sink, or in other damp places. Heat or moisture may cause the medicine to break down.
- Do not keep outdated medicine or medicine no longer needed. Be sure that any discarded medicine is out of the reach of children.

## Precautions While Using This Medicine

*It is very important that your doctor check your progress at regular visits* to make sure that this medicine is working properly and to check for unwanted effects.

*Check with your doctor or hospital emergency room immediately if severe headache, stiff neck, chest pains, fast heartbeat, or nausea and vomiting occur* while you are taking this medicine. These may be symptoms of a serious high blood pressure reaction that should have a doctor's attention.

When taken with certain foods, drinks, or other medicines, procarbazine can cause very dangerous reactions such as sudden high blood pressure. To avoid such reactions, *obey the following rules of caution:*

- Do not eat foods that have a high tyramine content (most common in foods that are aged or fermented to increase their flavor), such as cheeses, yeast or meat extracts, fava or broad bean pods, smoked or pickled meat, poultry, or fish, fermented sausage (bologna, pepperoni, salami, and summer sausage) or other unfresh meat, or any overripe fruit. If a list of these foods and beverages is not given to you, ask your health care professional to provide one.
- Do not drink alcoholic beverages or alcohol-free or reduced-alcohol beer or wine.
- Do not eat or drink large amounts of caffeine-containing food or beverages, such as chocolate, coffee, tea, or cola.
- Do not take any other medicine unless approved or prescribed by your doctor. This especially includes over-the-counter (OTC) or nonprescription medicine such as that for colds (including nose drops or sprays), cough, asthma, hay fever, appetite control; "keep awake" products; or products that make you sleepy.

*After you stop using this medicine you must continue to obey the rules of caution* concerning food, drink, and other medication for at least 2 weeks since procarbazine may continue to react with certain foods or other medicines for up to 14 days after you stop taking it.

This medicine will add to the effects of alcohol and other CNS depressants (medicines that slow down the nervous system, possibly causing drowsiness). Some examples of CNS depressants are antihistamines or medicine for hay fever, other allergies, or colds; sedatives, tranquilizers, or sleeping medicine; prescription pain medicine or narcotics; barbiturates; medicine for seizures; muscle relaxants; or anesthetics, including some dental anesthetics. *Check with your doctor before taking any of the above while you are using this medicine.*

*This medicine may cause some people to become drowsy or less alert than they are normally. Make sure you know how you react to this medicine before you drive, use machines, or do anything else that could be dangerous if you are not alert.*

While you are being treated with procarbazine, and after you stop treatment with it, *do not have any immunizations (vaccinations) without your doctor's approval.* Procarbazine may lower your body's resistance and there is a chance you might get the infection the immunization is meant to prevent. In addition, other persons living in your household should not take or should not have recently taken oral polio vaccine since there is a chance

they could pass the polio virus on to you. Also, avoid persons who have taken oral polio vaccine. Do not get close to them and do not stay in the same room with them for very long. If you cannot take these precautions, you should consider wearing a protective face mask that covers the nose and mouth.

Procarbazine can lower the number of white blood cells in your blood temporarily, increasing the chance of getting an infection. It can also lower the number of platelets, which are necessary for proper blood clotting. If this occurs, there are certain precautions you can take, especially when your blood count is low, to reduce the risk of infection or bleeding:

- If you can, avoid people with infections. *Check with your doctor immediately* if you think you are getting an infection or if you get a fever or chills, cough or hoarseness, lower back or side pain, or painful or difficult urination.
- *Check with your doctor immediately* if you notice any unusual bleeding or bruising; black, tarry stools; blood in urine or stools; or pinpoint red spots on your skin.
- Be careful when using a regular toothbrush, dental floss, or toothpick. Your medical doctor, dentist, or nurse may recommend other ways to clean your teeth and gums. Check with your medical doctor before having any dental work done.
- Do not touch your eyes or the inside of your nose unless you have just washed your hands and have not touched anything else in the meantime.
- Be careful not to cut yourself when you are using sharp objects such as a safety razor or fingernail or toenail cutters.
- Avoid contact sports or other situations where bruising or injury could occur.

For *diabetic patients*:
- Procarbazine may affect blood sugar levels. While you are using this medicine, be especially careful in testing for sugar in your blood or urine.

*If you are going to have surgery (including dental surgery) or emergency treatment tell the medical doctor or dentist in charge that you are using this medicine or have used it within the past 2 weeks.*

Your doctor may want you to carry an identification card stating that you are using this medicine.

## Side Effects of This Medicine

Along with their needed effects, medicines like procarbazine can sometimes cause unwanted effects such as blood problems, loss of hair, high blood pressure reactions, and other side effects. These and others are described below. Also, because of the way these medicines act on the body, there is a chance that they might cause other unwanted effects that may not occur until months or years after the medicine is used. These delayed effects may include certain types of cancer, such as leukemia. Discuss these possible effects with your doctor.

Although not all of these side effects may occur, if they do occur they may need medical attention.

*Stop taking this medicine and check with your doctor immediately* if the following side effects occur. If your doctor is not available, go to the nearest hospital emergency room.

*Rare*

Chest pain (severe); enlarged pupils of eyes; fast or slow heartbeat; headache (severe); increased sensitivity of eyes to light; increased sweating (possibly with fever or cold, clammy skin); stiff or sore neck

*Check with your doctor immediately* if any of the following side effects occur:

*Less common*

Black, tarry stools; blood in urine or stools; bloody vomit; cough or hoarseness; fever or chills; lower back or side pain; painful or difficult urination; pinpoint red spots on skin; unusual bleeding or bruising

Check with your doctor as soon as possible if any of the following side effects occur:

*More common*

Confusion; convulsions (seizures); cough; hallucinations (seeing, hearing, or feeling things that are not there); missing menstrual periods; shortness of breath; thickening of bronchial secretions; tiredness or weakness (continuing)

*Less common*

Diarrhea; sores in mouth and on lips; tingling or numbness of fingers or toes; unsteadiness or awkwardness; yellow eyes or skin

*Rare*

Fainting; skin rash, hives, or itching; wheezing

Other side effects may occur that usually do not need medical attention. These side effects may go away during treatment as your body adjusts to the medicine. Also, your health care professional may be able to tell you about ways to prevent or reduce some of these side effects. Check with your health care professional if any of the following side effects continue or are bothersome or if you have any questions about them:

*More common*

Drowsiness; muscle or joint pain; muscle twitching; nausea and vomiting; nervousness; nightmares; trouble in sleeping; unusual tiredness or weakness

*Less common*

Constipation; darkening of skin; difficulty in swallowing; dizziness or lightheadedness when getting up from a lying or sitting position; dry mouth; feeling of warmth and redness in face; headache; loss of appetite; mental depression

This medicine may cause a temporary loss of hair in some people. After treatment with procarbazine has ended, normal hair growth should return.

Other side effects not listed above may also occur in some patients. If you notice any other effects, check with your doctor.

---

Revised: August 1990
Interim revision: 08/05/93; 06/30/94

---

# PROGESTINS  Systemic

Some commonly used brand names are:

**In the U.S.—**

| | |
|---|---|
| Amen[2] | Micronor[4] |
| Aygestin[4] | Norlutate[4] |
| Curretab[2] | Norlutin[4] |
| Cycrin[2] | Nor-QD[4] |
| Depo-Provera[2] | Ovrette[5] |
| Gesterol 50[6] | Pro-Depo[1] |
| Hy/Gestrone[1] | Prodrox[1] |
| Hylutin[1] | Pro-Span[1] |
| Megace[3] | Provera[2] |

**In Canada—**

| | |
|---|---|
| Depo-Provera[2] | |
| Megace[3] | Norlutate[4] |
| Micronor[4] | PMS-Progesterone[6] |
| | Provera[2] |

Another commonly used name is norethisterone.

Note: For quick reference, the following progestins are numbered to match the corresponding brand names.

This information applies to the following medicines:

1. Hydroxyprogesterone (hye-drox-ee-proe-JESS-te-rone)†‡
2. Medroxyprogesterone (me-DROX-ee-proe-JESS-te-rone)‡
3. Megestrol (me-JESS-trole)‡
4. Norethindrone (nor-eth-IN-drone)
5. Norgestrel (nor-JESS-trel)†
6. Progesterone (proe-JESS-ter-one)‡

---

†Not commercially available in Canada.
‡Generic name product may also be available in the U.S.

---

## Description

Progestins (proe-JESS-tins) are sometimes called female hormones. They are produced by the body and are necessary during the childbearing years for the development of the milk-producing glands, and for the proper regulation of the menstrual cycle.

Progestins are prescribed for several reasons:

- for the proper regulation of the menstrual cycle.
- to treat a certain type of disorder of the uterus known as endometriosis.
- to prevent pregnancy, when used in birth-control pills.
- to help treat selected cases of cancer of the breast, kidney, or uterus.
- for testing the body's production of certain hormones.

Progestins may also be used for other conditions as determined by your doctor.

Progestins should not be used in pregnancy tests or in most cases of threatened miscarriage, since there have been some reports that these medications may cause harmful effects on the fetus. However, progesterone is sometimes used in a few patients to treat a certain type of infertility. These patients are given progesterone because their bodies do not produce enough natural progesterone to support a pregnancy. Progesterone is used if this problem has not responded well to other types of treatment.

To make the use of a progestin as safe and reliable as possible, you should understand how and when to take it and what effects may be expected. A paper with information for the patient may be given to you with your filled prescription, and will provide many details concerning most uses of this medicine. Read this paper carefully and ask your health care professional if you need additional information or explanation.

Progestins are available only with your doctor's prescription, in the following dosage forms:

*Oral*
Medroxyprogesterone
- Tablets (U.S. and Canada)
Megestrol
- Tablets (U.S. and Canada)
Norethindrone
- Tablets (U.S. and Canada)
Norgestrel
- Tablets (U.S.)

*Parenteral*
Hydroxyprogesterone
- Injection (U.S.)
Medroxyprogesterone
- Injection (U.S. and Canada)
Progesterone
- Injection (U.S. and Canada)

*Rectal*
Progesterone
- Suppositories

*Vaginal*
Progesterone
- Suppositories

## Before Using This Medicine

In deciding to use a medicine, the risks of taking the medicine must be weighed against the good it will do. This is a decision you and your doctor will make. For progestins, the following should be considered:

**Allergies**—Tell your doctor if you have ever had any unusual or allergic reaction to progestins. Also tell your health care professional if you are allergic to any other substances, such as foods, preservatives, or dyes.

**Pregnancy**—Progestins are not recommended for use during pregnancy since there have been some reports that these medications may cause harmful effects on the fetus.

However, progesterone is sometimes used in a few patients to treat a certain type of infertility. These patients are given progesterone because their bodies do not produce enough natural progesterone to support a pregnancy. Progesterone is used if this problem has not responded well to other types of treatment.

**Breast-feeding**—Progestins pass into the breast milk and may cause unwanted effects in the nursing baby. It may be necessary for you to take another medicine or to stop breast-feeding during treatment.

**Children**—Studies on this medicine have been done only in adults, and there is no specific information about its use in children.

**Older adults**—This medicine has been tested and has not been shown to cause different side effects or problems in older people than it does in younger adults.

**Other medicines**—Although certain medicines should not be used together at all, in other cases two different medicines may be used together even if an interaction might occur. In these cases, your doctor may want to change the dose, or other precautions may be necessary. When you are taking a progestin, it is especially important that your health care professional know if you are taking any of the following:
- Bromocriptine (e.g., Parlodel)

**Other medical problems**—The presence of other medical problems may affect the use of progestins. Make sure you tell your doctor if you have any other medical problems, especially:
- Asthma
- Blood clots (or history of)
- Cancer (or history of)
- Changes in vaginal bleeding
- Diabetes mellitus (sugar diabetes)
- Epilepsy
- Heart or circulation disease
- High blood cholesterol
- Kidney disease
- Liver or gallbladder disease
- Mental depression (or history of)
- Migraine headaches
- Stroke (or history of)

## Proper Use of This Medicine

*Take this medicine only as directed by your doctor. Do not take more of it and do not take it for a longer time than your doctor ordered.* To do so may increase the chance of side effects. Try to take the medicine at the same time each day to reduce the possibility of side effects and to allow it to work better. When used for birth control, this medicine should be taken every day of the year, with doses taken 24 hours apart without interruption.

*For patients using the rectal suppository form of this medicine:*

- If the suppository is too soft to insert, chill it in the refrigerator for 30 minutes.
- To insert the suppository: Moisten the suppository with cold water. Lie down on your side and use your finger to push the suppository well up into the rectum.

*For patients using the vaginal suppository form of this medicine:*

- Use as directed by your doctor.

**Dosing**—The dose of these medicines will be different for different patients. *Follow your doctor's orders or the directions on the label.* The following information includes only the average doses of these medicines. *If your dose is different, do not change it* unless your doctor tells you to do so.

The number of tablets, injections, or suppositories that you take, receive, or use depends on the strength of the medicine. Also, *the number of doses you take or use each day, the time allowed between doses, and the length of time you take or use the medicine depend on the medical problem for which you are taking progestins.*

*For hydroxyprogesterone*

- For *injection* dosage form:

  —For starting the menstrual cycle (amenorrhea) or controlling unusual and heavy bleeding of the uterus (dysfunctional uterine bleeding):

  - Adults and teenagers—At first, 375 milligrams (mg) injected into a muscle as a single dose. Depending on your response, your doctor may want you to receive another dose in four or twenty-one days. Then, you will receive another dose every twenty-eight days for four more months.

  —For testing the amount of estrogen produced:

  - Adults and teenagers—250 mg injected into a muscle as a single dose once a month for two months.

  —For treating cancer of the uterus:

  - Adults and teenagers—1 gram injected into a muscle one to seven times a week for up to twelve weeks.

  —For treating unusual menstrual cycles:

  - Adults and teenagers—250 or 375 mg injected into a muscle as a single dose. Your doctor may also want you to use another hormone called estrogen. Depending on your response, your doctor may want you to receive an additional dose in four or twenty-one days. Then, you will receive another dose every twenty-eight days if needed.

*For medroxyprogesterone*

- For *oral* dosage form (tablets):

  —For starting the menstrual cycle (amenorrhea) or controlling unusual and heavy bleeding of the uterus (dysfunctional uterine bleeding):

  - Adults or teenagers—5 to 10 milligrams (mg) a day for five to ten days. Your treatment will probably begin on Day 16 or Day 21 (counting from the beginning of your last period).

  —For treating unusual menstrual cycles:

  - Adults or teenagers—10 mg daily for ten or thirteen days. Your treatment will probably begin on Day 13 through Day 16 (counting from the beginning of your last period). Your doctor may also want you to use another hormone called estrogen.

- For *injection* dosage form:

  —For treating cancer of the uterus or kidneys:

  - Adults and teenagers—At first, 400 to 1000 milligrams (mg) injected into a muscle as a single dose once a week. Then, your doctor may lower your dose to 400 mg once a month.

  —For preventing pregnancy:

  - Adults and teenagers—150 mg injected into a muscle every three months.

*For megestrol*

- For *oral* dosage form (tablets):

  —For treating cancer of the breast:

  - Adults and teenagers—40 milligrams (mg) four times a day for two or more months.

  —For treating cancer of the uterus:

  - Adults and teenagers—10 to 80 mg four times a day for two or more months.

*For norethindrone (base)*

- For *oral* dosage form (tablets):

  —For starting the menstrual cycle (amenorrhea) or controlling unusual and heavy bleeding of the uterus (dysfunctional uterine bleeding):

  - Adults or teenagers—5 to 20 milligrams (mg) a day from Day 5 through Day 25 (counting from the first day of the last menstrual cycle).

  —For treating endometriosis:

  - Adults or teenagers—At first, 10 mg a day for two weeks. Then, your doctor may increase your dose slowly to 30 mg a day for six to nine months. Let your doctor know if your menstrual period starts. Your doctor may want you to stop taking the medicine for a short period of time.

  —For preventing pregnancy:

  - Adults or teenagers—0.35 mg every day without interruption beginning on Day 1 of your menstrual cycle.

*For norethindrone acetate*

- For *oral* dosage form (tablets):

  —For starting the menstrual cycle (amenorrhea) or controlling unusual and heavy bleeding of the uterus (dysfunctional uterine bleeding):

  - Adults or teenagers—2.5 to 10 milligrams (mg) a day from Day 5 through Day 25 (counting from the first day of the last menstrual cycle).

  —For treating endometriosis:

  - Adults or teenagers—At first, 5 mg a day for two weeks. Then, your doctor may increase your dose slowly to 15 mg a day for six to nine months. Let your doctor know if your menstrual period starts. Your doctor may want you to stop taking the medicine for a short period of time.

*For norgestrel*

—For preventing pregnancy:

• Adults or teenagers—75 micrograms (mcg) every day without interruption beginning on Day 1 of your menstrual cycle.

*For progesterone*

• For *injection* dosage form:

—For starting the menstrual cycle (amenorrhea) or controlling unusual and heavy bleeding of the uterus (dysfunctional uterine bleeding):

• Adults or teenagers—50 to 100 milligrams (mg) injected into a muscle as a single dose. Or, your doctor may want you to receive 5 to 10 mg injected into a muscle a day for six to eight days. Your doctor may want you to take another hormone called estrogen first. If your menstrual period starts, your doctor will want you to stop taking the medicine.

—For maintaining a pregnancy (at ovulation and at the beginning of pregnancy)

• Adults or teenagers—12.5 mg injected into a muscle a day at the time of ovulation for up to two weeks. If needed, your doctor may want you to receive the medicine for up to eleven weeks.

• For *suppositories* dosage form (rectal or vaginal):

—For maintaining a pregnancy (at ovulation and at the beginning of pregnancy):

• Adults or teenagers—25 mg (one suppository) inserted into the rectum or the vagina two times a day at the time of ovulation for up to two weeks. If needed, your doctor may want you to receive the medicine for up to eleven weeks.

**Missed dose**—If you miss a dose of this medicine:

• If you are *not* taking this medicine for birth control, take the missed dose as soon as possible. However, if it is almost time for your next dose, skip the missed dose and go back to your regular dosing schedule. Do not double doses.

• *If you are taking this medicine for birth control,* the safest thing to do when you miss 1 day's dose is to stop taking the medicine immediately and use another method of birth control until your period begins or until your doctor determines that you are not pregnant. This procedure is different from the one used after missed doses of birth control tablets that contain more than one hormone.

**Storage**—To store this medicine:

• Keep out of the reach of children.

• Store away from heat and direct light.

• Do not store in the bathroom medicine cabinet because the heat or moisture may cause the medicine to break down.

• Keep the injectable form of this medicine from freezing.

• Do not keep outdated medicine or medicine no longer needed. Be sure that any discarded medicine is out of the reach of children.

---

## Precautions While Using This Medicine

*It is very important that your doctor check your progress at regular visits.* This will allow your dosage to be adjusted to your changing needs, and will allow any unwanted effects to be detected. These visits will usually be every 6 to 12 months, but some doctors require them more often.

Check with your doctor right away:

• if vaginal bleeding continues for an unusually long time.

• if your menstrual period has not started within 45 days of your last period.

• *if you suspect that you may have become pregnant. You should stop taking this medicine immediately,* since there have been some reports that these medications may cause harmful effects on the fetus when used during pregnancy. However, progesterone is sometimes used during early pregnancy to treat a certain type of infertility.

If you are scheduled for any laboratory tests, tell your doctor that you are taking a progestin.

In some patients, tenderness, swelling, or bleeding of the gums may occur. Brushing and flossing your teeth carefully and regularly and massaging your gums may help prevent this. See your dentist regularly to have your teeth cleaned. Check with your medical doctor or dentist if you have any questions about how to take care of your teeth and gums, or if you notice any tenderness, swelling, or bleeding of your gums.

If you are taking this medicine for birth control:

• *When you begin to use birth control tablets,* your body will require time to adjust before pregnancy will be prevented; therefore, you should *use a second method of birth control for at least the first 3 weeks to ensure full protection.*

• Since one of the most important factors in the proper use of birth control tablets is taking every dose exactly on schedule, you should make sure you never run out of tablets. Therefore, always keep 1 extra month's supply of tablets on hand. To keep the extra month's supply from becoming too old, use it next, after the pills now being used, and replace the extra supply each month on a regular schedule. The tablets will keep well when kept dry and at room temperature (light will fade some tablet colors but will not change the tablets' effect).

• Keep the tablets in the container in which you received them. Most containers aid you in keeping track of dosage schedule.

• Your doctor has prescribed this medicine only for you after studying your health record and the results of your physical examination. Use of the tablets by other persons may be dangerous because of differences in health and body make-up. Therefore, do not give your birth control tablets to anyone else, and do not take tablets prescribed for someone else. Also, check with your doctor before taking any leftover birth control tablets from an old prescription, especially after a pregnancy. This medicine may be dangerous if your health has changed since your last physical examination.

## Side Effects of This Medicine

Along with their needed effects, progestins sometimes cause some unwanted effects such as blood clots, heart attacks, and strokes, and problems of the liver and eyes. Although these effects are rare, they can be very serious and may cause death.

The following side effects may be caused by blood clots. Although not all of these side effects may occur, if they do occur they need immediate medical attention. *Get emergency help immediately* if any of the following side effects occur:

> Headache (severe or sudden); loss of coordination (sudden); loss of vision or change in vision (sudden); pains in chest, groin, or leg (especially in calf of leg); shortness of breath (sudden); slurred speech (sudden); weakness, numbness, or pain in arm or leg

Also, check with your doctor as soon as possible if any of the following side effects occur:

*More common*

> Changes in vaginal bleeding (spotting, breakthrough bleeding, prolonged or complete stoppage of bleeding)

*Less common or rare*

> Bulging eyes; discharge from breasts; double vision; loss of vision (gradual, partial, or complete); mental depression; pains in stomach, side, or abdomen; skin rash or itching; yellow eyes or skin

Other side effects may occur that usually do not need medical attention. These side effects may go away during treatment as your body adjusts to the medicine. However, check with your doctor if any of the following side effects continue or are bothersome:

*More common*

> Changes in appetite; changes in weight; pain or irritation at injection site (with progesterone); swelling of ankles and feet; unusual tiredness or weakness

*Less common or rare*

> Acne; brown, blotchy spots on exposed skin; fever; increased body and facial hair; increased breast tenderness; nausea; some loss of scalp hair; trouble in sleeping

Other side effects not listed above may also occur in some patients. If you notice any other effects, check with your doctor.

Revised: September 1990
Interim revision: 08/16/93; 07/06/94

# PROGUANIL    Systemic*

A commonly used brand name in Canada is Paludrine.

*Not commercially available in the U.S.

## Description

Proguanil (pro-GWAN-il) is used to prevent malaria. It works by killing the malaria parasites or preventing their growth.

This medicine may be given together with another medicine to prevent malaria infection.

Proguanil is available only with your doctor's prescription, in the following dosage form:

*Oral*
- Tablets (Canada and United Kingdom)

## Before Using This Medicine

In deciding to use a medicine, the risks of taking the medicine must be weighed against the good it will do.

This is a decision you and your doctor will make. For proguanil, the following should be considered:

**Allergies**—Tell your doctor if you have ever had any unusual or allergic reaction to proguanil. Also tell your health care professional if you are allergic to any other substances, such as foods, preservatives, or dyes.

**Pregnancy**—Proguanil has not been shown to cause birth defects or other problems in humans.

**Breast-feeding**—Proguanil passes into the breast milk. This medicine has not been reported to cause problems in nursing babies. However, the amount of proguanil that passes into breast milk is not sufficient to protect the infant from malaria.

**Children**—Although there is no specific information comparing use of proguanil in children with use in other age groups, this medicine is not expected to cause different side effects or problems in children than it does in adults.

**Older adults**—Many medicines have not been studied specifically in older people. Therefore, it may not be known

whether they work exactly the same way they do in younger adults or if they cause different side effects or problems in older people. There is no specific information comparing use of proguanil in the elderly with use in other age groups.

**Other medicines**—Although certain medicines should not be used together at all, in other cases two different medicines may be used together even if an interaction might occur. In these cases, your doctor may want to change the dose, or other precautions may be necessary. Tell your health care professional if you are taking any other prescription or nonprescription (over-the-counter [OTC]) medicine.

**Other medical problems**—The presence of other medical problems may affect the use of proguanil. Make sure you tell your doctor if you have any other medical problems, especially:

- Kidney problems, severe—Patients with kidney problems may have an increased chance of side effects.

## Proper Use of This Medicine

Take proguanil with a glass of water after meals to lessen possible stomach upset, unless otherwise directed by your doctor.

For young children, proguanil may be given by crushing the tablet and mixing it with milk, honey, or jam.

You may start taking proguanil at least 24 hours before you arrive in an area where there is a chance of getting malaria. This will allow your body to absorb enough medicine to fight the malaria parasites. Also, keep taking this medicine every day while you are in an area where malaria occurs and take it every day for 4 weeks after you leave the area.

No medicine will protect you completely from malaria. However, to protect yourself as completely as possible, *keep taking this medicine for the full time your doctor ordered.*

**Dosing**—The dose of proguanil will be different for different patients. *Follow your doctor's orders or the directions on the label.* The following information includes only the average doses of proguanil. *If your dose is different, do not change it* unless your doctor tells you to do so.

- For *oral* dosage form (tablets):
  —For prevention of malaria:
    - Adults and children over 12 years of age—200 milligrams (mg) (2 tablets), taken after meals, beginning at least twenty-four hours before arrival in an area where malaria occurs. Take the same dose every day while staying in the area, and every day for four weeks after leaving the area.
    - Children up to 1 year of age—25 mg (1/4 tablet), taken after meals, beginning at least twenty-four hours before arrival in an area where malaria occurs. Take the same dose every

day while staying in the area, and every day for four weeks after leaving the area.
- Children 1 to 4 years of age—50 mg (1/2 tablet), taken after meals, beginning at least twenty-four hours before arrival in an area where malaria occurs. Take the same dose every day while staying in the area, and every day for four weeks after leaving the area.
- Children 5 to 8 years of age—75 to 100 mg (3/4 to 1 tablet), taken after meals, beginning at least twenty-four hours before arrival in an area where malaria occurs. Take the same dose every day while staying in the area, and every day for four weeks after leaving the area.
- Children 9 to 12 years of age—100 to 150 mg (1 to 1½ tablets), taken after meals, beginning at least twenty-four hours before arrival in an area where malaria occurs. Take the same dose every day while staying in the area, and every day for four weeks after leaving the area.

**Missed dose**—If you miss a dose of this medicine, take it as soon as possible. However, if it is almost time for your next dose, skip the missed dose and go back to your regular dosing schedule. Do not double doses.

**Storage**—To store this medicine:
- Keep out of the reach of children.
- Store away from heat and direct light.
- Do not store in the bathroom, near the kitchen sink, or in other damp places. Heat or moisture may cause the medicine to break down.
- Do not keep outdated medicine or medicine no longer needed. Be sure that any discarded medicine is out of the reach of children.

## Precautions While Using This Medicine

Malaria is spread by the bites of certain kinds of infected female mosquitoes. If you are living in, or will be traveling to, an area where there is a chance of getting malaria, the following mosquito-control measures will help to prevent infection:

- If possible, avoid going out between dusk and dawn because it is at these times when mosquitoes most commonly bite.
- Wear long-sleeved shirts and long trousers to protect your arms and legs, especially from dusk through dawn when mosquitoes are out.
- Apply insect repellant, preferably one containing diethyltoluamide (DEET), to uncovered areas of the skin, especially from dusk through dawn when mosquitoes are out.
- If possible, sleep in a screened or air-conditioned room or under mosquito netting sprayed with insecticide to avoid being bitten by malaria-carrying mosquitoes.
- Use mosquito coils or sprays to kill mosquitoes in living and sleeping quarters during evening and night-time hours.

If fever or "flu-like" symptoms develop during your travels or within a year (especially within the first 2 months) after you leave an area where malaria occurs, *check with your doctor immediately.*

## Side Effects of This Medicine

Along with its needed effects, a medicine may cause some unwanted effects. Although not all of these side effects may occur, if they do occur they may need medical attention.

Check with your doctor as soon as possible if any of the following side effects occur:

*Rare*
Skin rash or itching
*Symptoms of overdose*
Abdominal or stomach pain; bloody urine

Other side effects may occur that usually do not need medical attention. These side effects may go away during treatment as your body adjusts to the medicine. However, check with your doctor if any of the following side effects continue or are bothersome:

*More common*
Diarrhea; headache; loss of appetite; mouth sores or ulcers; nausea; vomiting
*Less common or rare*
Temporary hair loss

Other side effects not listed above may also occur in some patients. If you notice any other effects, check with your doctor.

Developed: 04/18/94

---

# PROPAFENONE   Systemic

A commonly used brand name in the U.S. and Canada is Rythmol.

## Description

Propafenone (proe-pa-FEEN-none) belongs to the group of medicines known as antiarrhythmics. It is used to correct irregular heartbeats to a normal rhythm.

Propafenone produces its helpful effects by slowing nerve impulses in the heart and making the heart tissue less sensitive.

There is a chance that propafenone may cause new or make worse existing heart rhythm problems when it is used. Since similar medicines have been shown to cause severe problems in some patients, propafenone is only used to treat serious heart rhythm problems. Discuss this possible effect with your doctor.

This medicine is available only with your doctor's prescription, in the following dosage form:

*Oral*
• Tablets (U.S. and Canada)

## Before Using This Medicine

In deciding to use a medicine, the risks of taking the medicine must be weighed against the good it will do. This is a decision you and your doctor will make. For propafenone, the following should be considered:

**Allergies**—Tell your doctor if you have ever had any unusual or allergic reaction to propafenone. Also tell your health care professional if you are allergic to any other substances, such as foods, preservatives, or dyes.

**Pregnancy**—Propafenone has not been studied in pregnant women. Although this medicine has not been shown to cause birth defects in animal studies, it has been shown to reduce fertility in monkeys, dogs, and rabbits. In addition, in rats it caused decreased growth in the infant and deaths of mothers and infants. Before taking propafenone, make sure your doctor knows if you are pregnant or if you may become pregnant.

**Breast-feeding**—Propafenone passes into breast milk. However, this medicine has not been reported to cause problems in nursing babies.

**Children**—Propafenone can cause serious side effects in any patient. Therefore, it is especially important that you discuss with the child's doctor the good that this medicine may do as well as the risks of using it.

**Older adults**—Many medicines have not been studied specifically in older people. Therefore, it may not be known whether they work exactly the same way they do in younger adults or if they cause different side effects or problems in older people. There is no specific information comparing use of propafenone in the elderly with use in other age groups.

**Other medicines**—Although certain medicines should not be used together at all, in other cases two different medicines may be used together even if an interaction might occur. In these cases, your doctor may want to change the dose, or other precautions may be necessary. When you are taking propafenone it is especially important that your health care professional know if you are taking either of the following:

• Digoxin (e.g., Lanoxin) or
• Warfarin (e.g., Coumadin)—Effects of these medicines may be increased when used with propafenone

**Other medical problems**—The presence of other medical problems may affect the use of propafenone. Make sure

you tell your doctor if you have any other medical problems, especially:

- Asthma or
- Bronchitis or
- Emphysema—Propafenone can increase trouble in breathing
- Bradycardia (unusually slow heartbeat)—There is a risk of further decreased heart function
- Congestive heart failure—Propafenone may make this condition worse
- Kidney disease or
- Liver disease—Effects of propafenone may be increased because of slower removal from the body
- Recent heart attack—Risk of irregular heartbeat may be increased
- If you have a pacemaker—Propafenone may interfere with the pacemaker and require more careful follow-up by the doctor

## Proper Use of This Medicine

*Take propafenone exactly as directed by your doctor,* even though you may feel well. Do not take more or less of it than your doctor ordered.

This medicine works best when there is a constant amount in the blood. *To help keep the amount constant, do not miss any doses. Also, it is best to take each dose at evenly spaced times day and night.* For example, if you are to take 3 doses a day, doses should be spaced about 8 hours apart. If you need help in planning the best times to take your medicine, check with your health care professional.

**Dosing**—The dose of propafenone will be different for different patients. *Follow your doctor's orders or the directions on the label.* The following information includes only the average doses of propafenone. *If your dose is different, do not change it* unless your doctor tells you to do so:

- The number of tablets that you take depends on the strength of the medicine.
- For *oral* dosage forms (tablets):

  —Adults: 150 milligrams every eight hours; may be increased to 225 milligrams every eight hours or 300 mg every twelve hours; up to 300 mg every eight hours.

**Missed dose**—If you do miss a dose of propafenone and remember within 4 hours, take it as soon as possible. However, if you do not remember until later, skip the missed dose and go back to your regular dosing schedule. Do not double doses.

**Storage**—To store this medicine:

- Keep out of the reach of children.
- Store away from heat and direct light.

- Do not store in the bathroom, near the kitchen sink, or in other damp places. Heat or moisture may cause the medicine to break down.
- Do not keep outdated medicine or medicine no longer needed. Be sure that any discarded medicine is out of the reach of children.

## Precautions While Using This Medicine

It is important that your doctor check your progress at regular visits to make sure the medicine is working properly. This will allow changes to be made in the amount of medicine you are taking, if necessary.

Your doctor may want you to carry a medical identification card or bracelet stating that you are using this medicine.

*Before having any kind of surgery (including dental surgery) or emergency treatment, tell the medical doctor or dentist in charge that you are taking this medicine.*

Propafenone may cause some people to become dizzy or lightheaded. Make sure you know how you react to this medicine before you drive, use machines, or do anything else that could be dangerous if you are dizzy.

## Side Effects of This Medicine

Along with its needed effects, a medicine may cause some unwanted effects. Although not all of these side effects may occur, if they do occur they may need medical attention.

Check with your doctor as soon as possible if any of the following side effects occur:

*More common*
    Fast or irregular heartbeat

*Less common*
    Chest pain; shortness of breath; swelling of feet or lower legs

*Rare*
    Fever or chills; joint pain; low blood pressure; slow heartbeat; trembling or shaking

Other side effects may occur that usually do not need medical attention. These side effects may go away during treatment as your body adjusts to the medicine. However, check with your doctor if any of the following side effects continue or are bothersome:

*More common*
    Change in taste or bitter or metallic taste; dizziness

*Less common*

    Blurred vision; constipation or diarrhea; dryness of mouth; headache; nausea and/or vomiting; skin rash; unusual tiredness or weakness

Other side effects not listed above may also occur in some patients. If you notice any other effects, check with your doctor.

Revised: 10/07/92

---

# PROPIOMAZINE   Systemic†

A commonly used brand name in the U.S. is Largon.

    †Not commercially available in Canada.

## Description

Propiomazine (proe-pee-OH-ma-zeen) is used to produce sleepiness or drowsiness and to relieve anxiety before or during surgery or certain procedures. It is also used with analgesics (pain medicine) during labor to produce drowsiness and relieve anxiety.

*Propiomazine is given only by or under the immediate supervision of a medical doctor or dentist trained to use this medicine.* If you will be receiving propiomazine during surgery, your doctor or anesthesiologist will give you the medicine and closely follow your progress.

Propiomazine is available in the following dosage form:

*Parenteral*

* Injection (U.S.)

## Before Receiving This Medicine

In deciding to use a medicine, the risks of taking the medicine must be weighed against the good it will do. This is a decision you and your doctor will make. For propiomazine, the following should be considered:

**Allergies**—Tell your doctor if you have ever had any unusual or allergic reaction to propiomazine or to other phenothiazines (such as acetophenazine, chlorpromazine, fluphenazine, mesoridazine, perphenazine, prochlorperazine, promazine, promethazine, thioridazine, trifluoperazine, triflupromazine, trimeprazine). Also tell your health care professional if you are allergic to any other substances, such as foods, preservatives, or dyes.

**Pregnancy**—Propiomazine has not been shown to cause problems in pregnant women.

**Breast-feeding**—Propiomazine has not been reported to cause problems in nursing babies.

**Children**—Although there is no specific information comparing use of propiomazine in children with use in other age groups, this medicine is not expected to cause different side effects or problems in children than it does in adults.

**Older adults**—Many medicines have not been studied specifically in older people. Therefore, it may not be known whether they work exactly the same way they do in younger adults or if they cause different side effects or problems in older people. There is no specific information comparing use of propiomazine in the elderly with use in other age groups.

**Other medicines**—Although certain medicines should not be used together at all, in other cases 2 different medicines may be used together even if an interaction might occur. In these cases, your doctor may want to change the dose, or other precautions may be necessary. When you are taking propiomazine, it is especially important that your health care professional know if you are taking any of the following:

* Central nervous system (CNS) depressants (medicine that causes drowsiness) or
* Tricyclic antidepressants (medicine for depression)—Taking these medicines with propiomazine will cause an increase in CNS depressant effects

## Proper Use of This Medicine

**Dosing**—The dose of propiomazine will be different for different patients. Your doctor will decide on the right amount for you. The dose will depend on:

* Your age;
* Your general physical condition;
* The kind of surgery you are having; and
* Other medicines you are taking or will receive before and during surgery or labor.

## Precautions After Receiving This Medicine

For patients going home within 24 hours after receiving propiomazine:

* Propiomazine may cause some people to feel drowsy, tired, or weak for up to one or two days after it has been given. It may also cause problems with coordination and one's ability to think. Therefore, *do not drive, use machines, or do other things that could be dangerous if you are not alert* until the effects of the medicine have disappeared or until the day after receiving propiomazine, whichever period of time is longer.
* *Do not drink alcoholic beverages or take other CNS depressants (medicines that slow down the nervous system, possibly causing drowsiness) for about*

---

*24 hours after you have received propiomazine, unless otherwise directed by your doctor.* To do so may add to the effects of the medicine. Some examples of CNS depressants are antihistamines or medicine for hay fever, other allergies, or colds; other sedatives, tranquilizers, or sleeping medicine; prescription pain medicine or narcotics; medicine for seizures; and muscle relaxants.

## Side Effects of This Medicine

Along with its needed effects, a medicine may cause some unwanted effects. Although not all of these side effects may occur, if they do occur they may need medical attention.

*Check with your doctor immediately* if any of the following side effects occur:

*Rare*

Convulsions (seizures); difficult or unusually fast breathing; fast or irregular heartbeat or pulse; fever (high); high or low blood pressure; loss of bladder control; muscle stiffness (severe); unusual increase in sweating; unusually pale skin; unusual tiredness or weakness

Also, check with your doctor as soon as possible if the following side effect occurs:

Redness, swelling, or pain at place of injection

Other side effects may occur that usually do not need medical attention. The following side effects may go away as the effects of propiomazine wear off. However, check with your doctor if any of the following side effects continue or are bothersome:

*More common*

Dizziness; drowsiness (prolonged); dryness of mouth

*Less common*

Confusion; diarrhea; nausea or vomiting; restlessness; skin rash; stomach pain

Other side effects not listed above may also occur in some patients. If you notice any other effects, check with your doctor.

Revised: 04/16/93
Interim revision: 07/26/94

---

# PROTIRELIN    Diagnostic

A commonly used brand name in the U.S. and Canada is Relefact TRH.

## Description

Protirelin (proe-TYE-re-lin) is used to test the response of the anterior pituitary gland in people who may have certain medical conditions involving the thyroid gland. Testing with this medicine may help to identify the problem or may ensure that the dose of medicine being used is correct.

Protirelin stimulates release of a hormone called thyroid-stimulating hormone or TSH from the anterior pituitary gland. TSH then stimulates the thyroid gland. By measuring the amount of TSH in the blood after protirelin is given, the doctor can determine how well the anterior pituitary is working.

How test is done: First, a sample of your blood is taken. Then protirelin is given by injection by your doctor. The dose of protirelin may be different for different patients. Adults are usually given 500 micrograms (mcg) injected into a vein. The dose for children is based on body weight and must be determined by your doctor. A little while after the dose is given, one or more blood samples are taken. Then the results of the test are studied. You will be asked to lie down before, during, and for 15 minutes after the test. This is to prevent dizziness and possible fainting.

Protirelin is to be used only under the supervision of a doctor. It is available in the following dosage form:

*Parenteral*
• Injection (U.S. and Canada)

---

## Before Having This Test

In deciding to use a diagnostic test, any risks of the test must be weighed against the good it will do. This is a decision you and your doctor will make. Also, test results may be affected by other things. For protirelin, the following should be considered:

**Allergies**—Tell your doctor if you have ever had any unusual or allergic reaction to protirelin. Also tell your health care professional if you are allergic to any other substances, such as foods, preservatives, or dyes.

**Pregnancy**—Studies have not been done in humans. However, studies in rabbits have shown that protirelin increases the chance of death of the fetus when given in doses 1½ and 6 times the human dose.

**Breast-feeding**—Protirelin has not been reported to cause problems in nursing babies. However, it may cause extra swelling of the breasts and leaking of milk for up to 2 or 3 days after it is given.

**Children**—This medicine has been tested in children and, in effective doses, has not been shown to cause different side effects or problems in children than it does in adults.

**Older adults**—This medicine has been tested and has not been shown to cause different side effects or problems in older people than it does in younger adults.

**Other medicines**—Although certain medicines should not be used together at all, in other cases two different medicines may be used together even if an interaction might occur. In these cases, your doctor may want to change the dose, or other precautions may be necessary. Tell your health care professional if you are taking any other prescription or nonprescription (over-the-counter [OTC]) medicine.

**Other medical problems**—The presence of other medical problems may affect the use of protirelin. Make sure you tell your doctor if you have any other medical problems, especially:
- Heart or blood vessel disease or
- High blood pressure or
- Stroke (history of)—Sudden changes in blood pressure caused by protirelin may put patients with these conditions at greater risk
- Kidney disease—Test results may be affected if patient has kidney disease

## Preparation for This Test

Your doctor may ask you not to eat for several hours before the test or to eat a low-fat meal before the test. This will not be necessary for all patients. If it is necessary for you, *follow your doctor's instructions carefully*. Otherwise, this test may not work and may have to be done again.

## Side Effects of This Medicine

Along with its needed effects, a medicine may cause some unwanted effects. Check with your health care professional as soon as possible if either of the following side effects occurs:

*Rare*
Fainting
*For patients with pituitary tumors—Rare*
Loss of vision (temporary)

Protirelin commonly causes some side effects just after it is given. Usually they last for only a few minutes. However, check with your doctor if any of the following side effects continue or are bothersome:

*More common*
Flushing or redness of skin; frequent urge to urinate; headache (sometimes severe); lightheadedness; nausea; stomach pain; unpleasant taste in mouth or dryness of mouth
*Less common*
Anxiety; drowsiness; pressure in the chest or tightness in throat; sweating; tingling

Other side effects not listed above may also occur in some patients. If you notice any other effects, check with your doctor.

Revised: 09/19/91
Interim revision: 07/05/94

# PSEUDOEPHEDRINE    Systemic

Some commonly used brand names are:

**In the U.S.—**

| | |
|---|---|
| Cenafed | Myfedrine |
| Chlor-Trimeton Non-Drowsy Decongestant 4 Hour | Novafed |
| | PediaCare Infants' Oral Decongestant Drops |
| Decofed | |
| Dorcol Children's Decongestant Liquid | Pseudo |
| | Pseudogest |
| Drixoral Non-Drowsy Formula | Sudafed |
| Efidac/24 | Sudafed Liquid, Children's |
| Genaphed | Sudafed 12 Hour |
| Halofed | Sufedrin |
| Halofed Adult Strength | |

Generic name product may also be available.

**In Canada—**

| | |
|---|---|
| Balminil Decongestant Syrup | Robidrine |
| Benylin Decongestant | Sudafed |
| Eltor 120 | Sudafed 12 Hour |
| Maxenal | |

Generic name product may also be available.

## Description

Pseudoephedrine (soo-doe-e-FED-rin) is used to relieve nasal or sinus congestion caused by the common cold, sinusitis, and hay fever and other respiratory allergies. It is also used to relieve ear congestion caused by ear inflammation or infection.

Some of these preparations are available only with your doctor's prescription. Others are available without a prescription; however, your doctor may have special instructions on the proper dose of pseudoephedrine for your medical condition.

Pseudoephedrine is available in the following dosage forms:

*Oral*
- Capsules (Canada)
- Extended-release capsules (U.S. and Canada)
- Oral solution (U.S.)
- Syrup (U.S. and Canada)
- Tablets (U.S. and Canada)
- Extended-release tablets (U.S. and Canada)

## Before Using This Medicine

If you are taking this medicine without a prescription, carefully read and follow any precautions on the label. For pseudoephedrine, the following should be considered:

**Allergies**—Tell your doctor if you have ever had any unusual or allergic reaction to pseudoephedrine or similar medicines, such as albuterol, amphetamines, ephedrine, epinephrine, isoproterenol, metaproterenol, norepinephrine, phenylephrine, phenylpropanolamine, or terbutaline. Also tell your health care professional if you are allergic to any other substances, such as foods, preservatives, or dyes.

**Pregnancy**—Studies on birth defects have not been done in humans. Pseudoephedrine has not been shown to cause birth defects in animal studies. However, studies in animals have shown that pseudoephedrine causes a reduction in average weight, length, and rate of bone formation in the animal fetus.

**Breast-feeding**—Pseudoephedrine passes into breast milk and may cause unwanted effects in nursing babies (especially newborn and premature babies).

**Children**—Pseudoephedrine may be more likely to cause side effects in infants, especially newborn and premature infants, than in older children and adults.

**Older adults**—Many medicines have not been studied specifically in older people. Therefore, it may not be known whether they work exactly the same way they do in younger adults or if they cause different side effects or problems in older people. There is no specific information comparing use of pseudoephedrine in the elderly with use in other age groups.

**Other medicines**—Although certain medicines should not be used together at all, in other cases two different medicines may be used together even if an interaction might occur. In these cases, your doctor may want to change the dose, or other precautions may be necessary. When you are taking pseudoephedrine, it is especially important that your health care professional knows if you are taking any of the following:

- Beta-blockers (acebutolol [e.g., Sectral], atenolol [e.g., Tenormin], betaxolol [e.g., Kerlone], bisoprolol [e.g., Zebeta], carteolol [e.g., Cartrol], labetalol [e.g., Normodyne], metoprolol [e.g., Lopressor], nadolol [e.g., Corgard], oxprenolol [e.g., Trasicor], penbutolol [e.g., Levatol], pindolol [e.g., Visken], propranolol [e.g., Inderal], sotalol [e.g., Sotacor], timolol [e.g., Blocadren])—Pseudoephedrine may decrease the effect of these medicines; also, taking pseudoephedrine with beta-blockers may increase the chance of side effects
- Cocaine—Using cocaine with pseudoephedrine may increase the effects of either one of these medicines on the heart and increase the chance of side effects
- Monoamine oxidase (MAO) inhibitors (furazolidone [e.g., Furoxone], isocarboxazid [e.g., Marplan], phenelzine [e.g., Nardil], procarbazine [e.g., Matulane], selegiline [e.g., Eldepryl], tranylcypromine [e.g., Parnate])—Taking pseudoephedrine while you are taking or within 2 weeks of taking monoamine oxidase (MAO) inhibitors may increase the chance of serious side effects

**Other medical problems**—The presence of other medical problems may affect the use of pseudoephedrine. Make sure you tell your doctor if you have any other medical problems, especially:

- Diabetes mellitus (sugar diabetes)
- Enlarged prostate or
- Heart or blood vessel disease or
- High blood pressure—Pseudoephedrine may make the condition worse
- Overactive thyroid

## Proper Use of This Medicine

For patients taking *pseudoephedrine extended-release capsules:*
- Swallow the capsule whole. However, if the capsule is too large to swallow, you may mix the contents of the capsule with jam or jelly and swallow without chewing.
- Do not crush or chew before swallowing.

For patients taking *pseudoephedrine extended-release tablets:*
- Swallow the tablet whole.
- Do not break, crush, or chew before swallowing.

To help prevent trouble in sleeping, *take the last dose of pseudoephedrine for each day a few hours before bedtime.* If you have any questions about this, check with your doctor.

*Take this medicine only as directed.* Do not take more of it, do not take it more often, and do not take it for a longer period of time than recommended on the label (usually 7 days), unless otherwise directed by your doctor. To do so may increase the chance of side effects.

**Dosing**—The dose of pseudoephedrine will be different for different patients. *Follow your doctor's orders or the directions on the label.* The following information includes only the average doses of pseudoephedrine. *If your dose is different, do not change it* unless your doctor tells you to do so.

The number of capsules, tablets, or teaspoonfuls of solution or syrup that you take each day depends on the strength of the medicine. Also, the time between doses depends on whether you are taking a short-acting or long-acting form of pseudoephedrine.

- For nasal or sinus congestion:
  —For *regular (short-acting) oral* dosage form (capsules, oral solution, syrup, or tablets):
  - Adults and children 12 years of age and older—60 milligrams (mg) every four to six hours. Do not take more than 240 mg in twenty-four hours.
  - Children 6 to 12 years of age—30 mg every four to six hours. Do not take more than 120 mg in twenty-four hours.
  - Children 2 to 6 years of age—15 mg every four to six hours. Do not take more than 60 mg in twenty-four hours.
  - Children up to 2 years of age—Use and dose must be determined by your doctor.

—For *long-acting oral* dosage form (extended-release capsules or extended-release tablets):

- Adults and children 12 years of age and older—120 mg every 12 hours, or 240 mg every 24 hours. Do not take more than 240 mg in twenty-four hours.
- Children up to 12 years of age—Use is not recommended.

**Missed dose**—If you miss a dose of this medicine and you remember within an hour or so of the missed dose, take it right away. However, if you do not remember until later, skip the missed dose and go back to your regular dosing schedule. Do not double doses.

**Storage**—To store this medicine:

- Keep out of the reach of children.
- Store away from heat and direct light.
- Do not store the capsule or tablet form of this medicine in the bathroom, near the kitchen sink, or in other damp places. Heat or moisture may cause the medicine to break down.
- Keep the liquid form of this medicine from freezing.
- Do not keep outdated medicine or medicine no longer needed. Be sure that any discarded medicine is out of the reach of children.

## Precautions While Using This Medicine

*If symptoms do not improve within 7 days or if you also have a high fever, check with your doctor* since these signs may mean that you have other medical problems.

## Side Effects of This Medicine

Along with its needed effects, a medicine may cause some unwanted effects. Although not all of these side effects may occur, if they do occur they may need medical attention.

Check with your doctor as soon as possible if any of the following side effects occur:

*Rare—more common with high doses*

Convulsions (seizures); hallucinations (seeing, hearing, or feeling things that are not there); irregular or slow heartbeat; shortness of breath or troubled breathing

*Symptoms of overdose*

Convulsions (seizures); fast breathing; hallucinations (seeing, hearing, or feeling things that are not there); increase in blood pressure; irregular heartbeat (continuing); shortness of breath or troubled breathing (severe or continuing); slow or fast heartbeat (severe or continuing); unusual nervousness, restlessness, or excitement

Other side effects may occur that usually do not need medical attention. These side effects may go away during treatment as your body adjusts to the medicine. However, check with your health care professional if any of the following side effects continue or are bothersome:

*More common*

Nervousness; restlessness; trouble in sleeping

*Less common*

Difficult or painful urination; dizziness or lightheadedness; fast or pounding heartbeat; headache; increased sweating; nausea or vomiting; trembling; troubled breathing; unusual paleness; weakness

Other side effects not listed above may also occur in some patients. If you notice any other effects, check with your health care professional.

Revised: 04/19/94

---

# PYRANTEL   Oral

Some commonly used brand names are:

**In the U.S.—**

Antiminth                     Reese's Pinworm Medicine

Generic name product may also be available.

**In Canada—**

Combantrin

**Other—**

Aut                          Lombriareu
Cobantril                    Trilombrin
Helmex

## Description

Pyrantel (pi-RAN-tel) belongs to the family of medicines called anthelmintics (ant-hel-MIN-tiks). Anthelmintics are used in the treatment of worm infections.

Pyrantel is used to treat:

- common roundworms (ascariasis);
- pinworms (enterobiasis; oxyuriasis); and
- more than one worm infection at a time.

This medicine may also be used for other worm infections as determined by your doctor.

Pyrantel works by paralyzing the worms. They are then passed in the stool.

Pyrantel is available in the following dosage forms:

*Oral*

- Oral suspension (U.S. and Canada)
- Tablets (Canada)

## Before Using This Medicine

In deciding to use a medicine, the risks of taking the medicine must be weighed against the good it will do.

This is a decision you and your doctor will make. For pyrantel, the following should be considered:

**Allergies**—Tell your doctor if you have ever had any unusual or allergic reaction to pyrantel. Also tell your health care professional if you are allergic to any other substances, such as foods, preservatives, or dyes.

**Pregnancy**—Studies have not been done in pregnant women. However, pyrantel has not been reported to cause birth defects or other problems in animal studies.

**Breast-feeding**—Only small amounts of pyrantel are absorbed into the body. Pyrantel has not been reported to cause problems in nursing babies.

**Children**—This medicine has been tested in a limited number of children 2 years of age or older and, in effective doses, has not been reported to cause different side effects or problems in children than it does in adults.

**Older adults**—Many medicines have not been studied specifically in older people. Therefore, it may not be known whether they work exactly the same way they do in younger adults or if they cause different side effects or problems in older people. There is no specific information comparing use of pyrantel in the elderly with use in other age groups.

**Other medicines**—Although certain medicines should not be used together at all, in other cases two different medicines may be used together even if an interaction might occur. In these cases, your doctor may want to change the dose, or other precautions may be necessary. When you are taking pyrantel, it is especially important that your health care professional know if you are taking any of the following:
- Piperazine (e.g., Entacyl)—Using pyrantel and piperazine together may decrease the effectiveness of pyrantel

## Proper Use of This Medicine

No special preparations (for example, special diets, fasting, other medicines, laxatives, or enemas) are necessary before, during, or immediately after you take pyrantel.

For patients taking pyrantel *oral suspension:*
- Use a specially marked measuring spoon or other device to measure each dose accurately. The average household teaspoon may not hold the right amount of liquid.

To help clear up your infection completely, *take this medicine exactly as directed by your doctor.* In some infections a second dose of this medicine may be required to clear up the infection completely.

For patients taking pyrantel for *pinworms:*
- Pinworms may be easily passed from one person to another, especially among persons in the same household. Therefore, all household members may have to be treated at the same time to prevent their infection or reinfection. Also, all household members may have to be treated again in 2 to 3 weeks to clear up the infection completely.

**Dosing**—The dose of pyrantel will be different for different patients. *Follow your doctor's orders or the directions on the label.* The following information includes only the average doses of pyrantel. *If your dose is different, do not change it* unless your doctor tells you to do so.

The number of tablets or teaspoonfuls of suspension that you take depends on the strength of the medicine. Also, *the number of doses you take each day, the time allowed between doses, and the length of time you take the medicine depend on the medical problem for which you are taking pyrantel.*
- For *oral* dosage forms (oral suspension or tablets):
  —Adults and children 2 years of age and older: Dose is based on body weight and will be determined by your doctor. It is taken as a single dose and may need to be repeated in two to three weeks.

**Storage**—To store this medicine:
- Keep out of the reach of children.
- Store away from heat and direct light.
- Keep the liquid form of this medicine from freezing.
- Do not keep outdated medicine or medicine no longer needed. Be sure that any discarded medicine is out of the reach of children.

## Precautions While Using This Medicine

If your symptoms do not improve within a few days, or if they become worse, check with your doctor.

This medicine may cause some people to become dizzy, drowsy, or less alert than they are normally. *Make sure you know how you react to this medicine before you drive, use machines, or do anything else that could be dangerous if you are dizzy or are not alert.* If these reactions are especially bothersome, check with your doctor.

For patients taking pyrantel for *pinworms:*
- In some patients, pinworms may return after treatment with pyrantel. Washing (not shaking) all bedding and nightclothes (pajamas) after treatment may help to prevent this.
- Some doctors may also recommend other measures to help keep your infection from returning. If you have any questions about this, check with your doctor.

## Side Effects of This Medicine

Along with its needed effects, a medicine may cause some unwanted effects. Although not all of these side effects may occur, if they do occur they may need medical attention.

*Check with your doctor as soon as possible* if any of the following side effects occur:
*Rare*
  Skin rash

Other side effects may occur that usually do not need medical attention. These side effects may go away during

treatment as your body adjusts to the medicine. However, check with your doctor if any of the following side effects continue or are bothersome:

*Less common*
   Abdominal or stomach cramps or pain; diarrhea; dizziness; drowsiness; headache; loss of appetite; nausea or vomiting; trouble in sleeping

Other side effects not listed above may also occur in some patients. If you notice any other effects, check with your doctor.

## Additional Information

Once a medicine has been approved for marketing for a certain use, experience may show that it is also useful for other medical problems. Although this use is not included in product labeling, pyrantel is used in certain patients with the following medical condition:

• Hookworm infection

For patients taking this medicine for *hookworm infection:*

• Anemia (iron-poor blood) may occur in patients with hookworm infections. Therefore, your doctor may want you to take iron supplements to help clear up the anemia. If so, it is important to take iron every day while you are being treated for hookworms. Do not miss any doses. Your doctor may also want you to keep taking iron supplements for up to 6 months after you stop taking pyrantel. If you have any questions about this, check with your doctor.

Other than the above information, there is no additional information relating to proper use, precautions, or side effects for this use.

Revised: 01/19/93

# PYRAZINAMIDE    Systemic

Some commonly used brand names in Canada are pms-Pyrazinamide and Tebrazid.
Available in the U.S. as generic name product.

## Description

Pyrazinamide (peer-a-ZIN-a-mide) belongs to the family of medicines called anti-infectives. It is used, along with other medicines, to treat tuberculosis (TB).

*To help clear up your tuberculosis (TB) completely, you must keep taking this medicine for the full time of treatment, even if you begin to feel better. This is very important. It is also important that you do not miss any doses.*

Pyrazinamide is available only with your doctor's prescription, in the following dosage form:

*Oral*
   • Tablets (U.S. and Canada)

## Before Using This Medicine

In deciding to use a medicine, the risks of taking the medicine must be weighed against the good it will do. This is a decision you and your doctor will make. For pyrazinamide, the following should be considered:

**Allergies**—Tell your doctor if you have ever had any unusual or allergic reaction to pyrazinamide or to ethionamide (e.g., Trecator-SC), isoniazid (e.g., INH, Nydrazid), or niacin (e.g., Nicobid, nicotinic acid). Also tell your health care professional if you are allergic to any other substances, such as foods, preservatives, or dyes.

**Pregnancy**—Studies on effects in pregnancy have not been done in either humans or animals.

**Breast-feeding**—Pyrazinamide passes into the breast milk in small amounts.

**Children**—Pyrazinamide has been used in children and, in effective doses, has not been reported to cause different side effects or problems in children than it does in adults.

**Older adults**—Many medicines have not been studied specifically in older people. Therefore, it may not be known whether they work exactly the same way they do in younger adults. Although there is no specific information comparing pyrazinamide in the elderly with use in other age groups, this medicine is not expected to cause different side effects or problems in older people than it does in younger adults.

**Other medicines**—Although certain medicines should not be used together at all, in other cases two different medicines may be used together even if an interaction might occur. In these cases, your doctor may want to change the dose, or other precautions may be necessary. Tell your health care professional if you are taking any other prescription or nonprescription (over-the-counter [OTC]) medicine.

**Other medical problems**—The presence of other medical problems may affect the use of pyrazinamide. Make sure you tell your doctor if you have any other medical problems, especially:

• Gout (history of)—Pyrazinamide may worsen or cause a gout attack in patients with a history of gout
• Liver disease (severe)—Patients with severe liver disease who take pyrazinamide may have an increase in side effects

## Proper Use of This Medicine

To help clear up your TB completely, *it is important that you keep taking this medicine for the full time of treatment,* even if you begin to feel better after a few weeks. *It is important that you do not miss any doses.*

**Dosing**—The dose of pyrazinamide will be different for different patients. *Follow your doctor's orders or the directions on the label.* The following information includes only the average doses of pyrazinamide. *If your dose is different, do not change it* unless your doctor tells you to do so.

- For *oral* dosage form (tablets):
  —For tuberculosis (TB):
    - Adults and children—Dose is based on body weight. The usual dose is 15 to 30 milligrams (mg) of pyrazinamide per kilogram (kg) (6.8 to 13.6 mg per pound) of body weight once a day; or 50 to 70 mg per kg (22.7 to 31.8 mg per pound) two times a week or three times a week, depending on the schedule your doctor chooses for you. This medicine must be taken along with other medicines used to treat TB.

**Missed dose**—If you do miss a dose of this medicine, take it as soon as possible. However, if it is almost time for your next dose, skip the missed dose and go back to your regular dosing schedule. Do not double doses.

**Storage**—To store this medicine:
- Keep out of the reach of children.
- Store away from heat and direct light.
- Do not store in the bathroom, near the kitchen sink, or in other damp places. Heat or moisture may cause the medicine to break down.
- Do not keep outdated medicine or medicine no longer needed. Be sure that any discarded medicine is out of the reach of children.

## Precautions While Using This Medicine

It is very important that your doctor check your progress at regular visits.

If your symptoms do not improve within 2 to 3 weeks, or if they become worse, check with your doctor.

For diabetic patients:
- *This medicine may cause false test results with urine ketone tests.* Check with your doctor before changing your diet or the dosage of your diabetes medicine.

## Side Effects of This Medicine

Along with its needed effects, a medicine may cause some unwanted effects. Although not all of these side effects may occur, if they do occur they may need medical attention.

*Check with your doctor immediately* if any of the following side effects occur:

*More common*
  Pain in large and small joints
*Rare*
  Loss of appetite; pain and swelling of joints, especially big toe, ankle, and knee; tense, hot skin over affected joints; unusual tiredness or weakness; yellow eyes or skin

Other side effects may occur that usually do not need medical attention. These side effects may go away during treatment as your body adjusts to the medicine. However, check with your doctor if any of the following side effects continue or are bothersome:

*Rare*
  Itching; skin rash

Other side effects not listed above may also occur in some patients. If you notice any other effects, check with your doctor.

Revised: 05/02/94

# PYRETHRINS AND PIPERONYL BUTOXIDE    Topical

Some commonly used brand names are:

**In the U.S.—**

| | |
|---|---|
| A-200 Gel Concentrate | Pyrinyl |
| A-200 Shampoo Concentrate | R & C |
| Barc | Rid |
| Blue | Tisit |
| Licetrol | Tisit Blue |
| Pronto Lice Killing Shampoo | Tisit Shampoo |
| Kit | Triple X |

**In Canada—**
  R & C

## Description

Medicine containing pyrethrins (pye-REE-thrins) is used to treat head, body, and pubic lice infections. This medicine is absorbed by the lice and destroys them by acting on their nervous systems. It does not affect humans in this way. The piperonyl butoxide (pye-PEER-i-nil byoo-TOX-ide) is included to make the pyrethrins more effective in killing the lice. This combination medicine is known as a pediculicide (pe-DIK-yoo-li-side).

This medicine is available without a prescription; however, your doctor may have special instructions on the proper use of this medicine for your medical condition.

Pyrethrins and piperonyl butoxide combination medicine is available in the following dosage forms:

*Topical*
- Gel (U.S.)
- Solution shampoo (U.S. and Canada)
- Topical solution (U.S.)

## Before Using This Medicine

If you are using this medicine without a prescription, carefully read and follow any precautions on the label. For pyrethrins and piperonyl butoxide combination, the following should be considered:

**Allergies**—Tell your doctor if you have ever had any unusual or allergic reaction to pyrethrins, piperonyl butoxide, ragweed, chrysanthemum plants, or kerosene or other petroleum products. Also tell your health care professional if you are allergic to any other substances, such as preservatives or dyes.

**Pregnancy**—Pyrethrins and piperonyl butoxide may be absorbed through the skin. However, this medicine has not been shown to cause birth defects or other problems in humans when used on the skin.

**Breast-feeding**—Pyrethrins and piperonyl butoxide combination may be absorbed through the mother's skin. It is not known whether pyrethrins and piperonyl butoxide combination passes into the breast milk. Although most medicines pass into breast milk in small amounts, many of them may be used safely while breast-feeding. Mothers who are using this medicine and who wish to breast-feed should discuss this with their doctor.

**Children**—Although there is no specific information comparing use of pyrethrins and piperonyl butoxide combination in children with use in other age groups, this medicine is not expected to cause different side effects or problems in children than it does in adults.

**Older adults**—Many medicines have not been studied specifically in older people. Therefore, it may not be known whether they work exactly the same way they do in younger adults. Although there is no specific information comparing use of pyrethrins and piperonyl butoxide combination medicine in the elderly with use in other age groups, this medicine is not expected to cause different side effects or problems in older people than it does in younger adults.

**Other medical problems**—The presence of other medical problems may affect the use of pyrethrins and piperonyl butoxide combination. Make sure you tell your doctor if you have any other medical problems, especially:
- Inflammation of the skin (severe)—Use of pyrethrins and piperonyl butoxide combination may make the condition worse

## Proper Use of This Medicine

Pyrethrins and piperonyl butoxide combination medicine usually comes with patient directions. Read them carefully before using this medicine.

*Use this medicine only as directed. Do not use more of it and do not use it more often than recommended on the label.* To do so may increase the chance of absorption through the skin and the chance of side effects.

*Keep pyrethrins and piperonyl butoxide combination medicine away from the mouth and do not inhale it. This medicine is harmful if swallowed or inhaled.*

*To lessen the chance of inhaling this medicine, apply it in a well-ventilated room* (for example, one with free flowing air or with a fan turned on).

*Keep this medicine away from the eyes and other mucous membranes, such as the inside of the nose, mouth, or vagina, because it may cause irritation.* If you accidentally get some in your eyes, flush them thoroughly with water at once.

*Do not apply this medicine to the eyelashes or eyebrows.* If they become infected with lice, check with your doctor.

To use the *gel or solution form* of this medicine:
- Apply enough medicine to thoroughly wet the dry hair and scalp or skin. Allow the medicine to remain on the affected areas for exactly 10 minutes.
- Then, thoroughly wash the affected areas with warm water and soap or regular shampoo. Rinse thoroughly and dry with a clean towel.

To use the *shampoo form* of this medicine:
- Apply enough medicine to thoroughly wet the dry hair and scalp or skin. Allow the medicine to remain on the affected areas for exactly 10 minutes.
- Then use a small amount of water and work shampoo into the hair and scalp or skin until a lather forms. Rinse thoroughly and dry with a clean towel.

After rinsing and drying, use a nit removal comb (special fine-toothed comb, usually included with this medicine) to remove the dead lice and eggs (nits) from hair.

Immediately after using this medicine, wash your hands to remove any medicine that may be on them.

This medicine should be used again in 7 to 10 days after the first treatment in order to kill any newly hatched lice.

Lice can easily move from one person to another by close body contact. This can happen also by direct contact with such things as clothing, hats, scarves, bedding, towels, washcloths, hairbrushes and combs, or the hair of infected persons. Therefore, *all members of your household should be examined for lice and receive treatment if they are found to be infected.*

To use this medicine for *pubic (crab) lice:*
- Your sexual partner may also need to be treated, since the infection may spread to persons in close contact. If your partner is not being treated or if you

have any questions about this, check with your doctor.

**Dosing**—The dose of pyrethrins and piperonyl butoxide combination will be different for different patients. *Follow your doctor's orders or the directions on the label.* The following information includes only the average doses of pyrethrins and piperonyl butoxide combination. *If your dose is different, do not change it* unless your doctor tells you to do so.

- For *topical* dosage forms (gel, solution shampoo, and topical solution):
  —For head, body, or pubic lice:
    - Adults and children—Use one time, then repeat one time in seven to ten days.

**Storage**—To store this medicine:

- Keep out of the reach of children.
- Store away from heat and direct light.
- Keep the medicine from freezing.
- Do not keep outdated medicine or medicine no longer needed. Be sure that any discarded medicine is out of the reach of children.

## Precautions While Using This Medicine

To prevent reinfection or spreading of the infection to other people, good health habits are also required. These include the following:

- For *head lice*
  —Machine wash all clothing (including hats, scarves, and coats), bedding, towels, and washcloths in very hot water and dry them by using the hot cycle of a dryer for at least 20 minutes. Clothing or bedding that cannot be washed should be dry-cleaned or sealed in a plastic bag for 2 weeks.
  —Shampoo all wigs and hairpieces.
  —Wash all hairbrushes and combs in very hot soapy water (above 130 °F) for 5 to 10 minutes and do not share them with other people.

- —Clean the house or room by thoroughly vacuuming upholstered furniture, rugs, and floors.
- For *body lice*
  —Machine wash all clothing, bedding, towels, and washcloths in very hot water and dry them by using the hot cycle of a dryer for at least 20 minutes. Clothing or bedding that cannot be washed should be dry-cleaned or sealed in a plastic bag for 2 weeks.
  —Clean the house or room by thoroughly vacuuming upholstered furniture, rugs, and floors.
- For *pubic lice*
  —Machine wash all clothing (especially underwear), bedding, towels, and washcloths in very hot water and dry them by using the hot cycle of a dryer for at least 20 minutes. Clothing or bedding that cannot be washed should be dry-cleaned or sealed in a plastic bag for 2 weeks.
  —Scrub toilet seats frequently.

## Side Effects of This Medicine

Along with its needed effects, a medicine may cause some unwanted effects. Although not all of these side effects may occur, if they do occur they may need medical attention.

Check with your doctor as soon as possible if any of the following side effects occur:

*Less common or rare*
  Skin irritation not present before use of this medicine; skin rash or infection; sneezing (sudden attacks of); stuffy or runny nose; wheezing or difficulty in breathing

Other side effects not listed above may also occur in some patients. If you notice any other effects, check with your health care professional.

Revised: 07/26/93
Interim revision: 02/18/94

# PYRIDOXINE (Vitamin B₆)  Systemic

Some commonly used brand names are:

**In the U.S.—**

| | |
|---|---|
| Beesix | Pyri |
| Doxine | Rodex |
| Nestrex | Vitabee 6 |

Generic name product may also be available.

**In Canada—**
Generic name product is available.

## Description

Vitamins (VYE-ta-mins) are compounds that you *must* have for growth and health. They are needed in small amounts only and are usually available in the foods that you eat. Pyridoxine (peer-i-DOX-een) (vitamin B₆) is necessary for normal metabolism.

Patients with the following conditions may be more likely to have a deficiency of pyridoxine:

- Alcoholism
- Burns
- Diarrhea
- Dialysis
- Heart disease
- Intestinal problems
- Liver disease

- Overactive thyroid
- Stress, long-term illness, or serious injury
- Surgical removal of stomach

In addition, infants receiving unfortified formulas such as evaporated milk may need additional pyridoxine.

If any of the above apply to you, you should take pyridoxine only on the advice of your doctor after need has been established.

Lack of pyridoxine may lead to anemia (weak blood), nerve damage, seizures, skin problems, and sores in the mouth. Your doctor may treat these problems by prescribing pyridoxine for you.

Claims that pyridoxine is effective for treatment of acne and other skin problems, alcohol intoxication, asthma, hemorrhoids, kidney stones, mental problems, migraine headaches, morning sickness, and menstrual problems, or to stimulate appetite or milk production have not been proven.

Oral forms of pyridoxine are available without a prescription. However, it may be a good idea to check with your doctor before taking any on your own.

Pyridoxine is available in the following dosage forms:

*Oral*
- Extended-release capsules (U.S.)
- Tablets (U.S. and Canada)
- Extended-release tablets (U.S.)

*Parenteral*
- Injection (U.S. and Canada)

---

## Importance of Diet

Vitamin supplements should be taken only if you cannot get enough vitamins in your diet; however, some diets may not contain all of the vitamins you need. You may not be getting enough vitamins because of rapid weight loss, unusual diets (such as some reducing diets in which choice of foods is very limited), prolonged intravenous feeding, or malnutrition. A balanced diet should provide all the vitamins you normally need.

In order to get enough vitamins and minerals in your diet, it is important that you eat a balanced and varied diet. Follow carefully any diet program your doctor may recommend. For your specific vitamin and/or mineral needs, ask your doctor or dietitian for a list of appropriate foods.

Pyridoxine is found in various foods, including meats, bananas, lima beans, egg yolks, peanuts, and whole-grain cereals. Pyridoxine is not lost from food during ordinary cooking, although some other forms of vitamin B$_6$ are.

Vitamins alone will not take the place of a good diet and will not provide energy. Your body also needs other substances found in food such as protein, minerals, carbohydrates, and fat. Vitamins themselves often cannot work without the presence of other foods.

In some cases, it may not be possible for you to get enough food to supply you with the proper vitamins. In other cases, the amount of vitamins you need may be increased above normal. Therefore, a vitamin supplement may be needed.

Experts have developed a list of recommended dietary allowances (RDA) for most of the vitamins. The RDA are not an exact number but a general idea of how much you need. They do not cover amounts needed for problems caused by a serious lack of vitamins.

The RDA for pyridoxine are:
- Infants and children—
    Birth to 6 months of age: 0.3 milligrams (mg) per day.
    6 months to 1 year of age: 0.6 mg per day.
    1 to 3 years of age: 1 mg per day.
    4 to 6 years of age: 1.1 mg per day.
    7 to 10 years of age: 1.4 mg per day.
- Adolescent and adult males—
    11 to 14 years of age: 1.7 mg per day.
    15 years of age and over: 2 mg per day.
- Adolescent and adult females—
    11 to 14 years of age: 1.4 mg per day.
    15 to 18 years of age: 1.5 mg per day.
    19 years of age and over: 1.6 mg per day.
- Pregnant females—2.2 mg per day.
- Breast-feeding females—2.1 mg per day.

Remember:
- The total amount of each vitamin that you get every day includes what you get from the foods that you eat *and* what you may take as a supplement.
- This total amount should not be greater than the RDA, unless ordered by your doctor.

---

## Before Using This Dietary Supplement

If you are taking this dietary supplement without a prescription, carefully read and follow any precautions on the label. For pyridoxine, the following should be considered:

**Allergies**—Tell your doctor if you have ever had any unusual or allergic reaction to pyridoxine. Also tell your health care professional if you are allergic to any other substances, such as foods, preservatives, or dyes.

**Pregnancy**—It is especially important that you are receiving enough vitamins when you become pregnant and that you continue to receive the right amount of vitamins throughout your pregnancy. The healthy growth and development of the fetus depend on a steady supply of nutrients from the mother. However, excessive doses of pyridoxine taken during pregnancy may cause the infant to become dependent on pyridoxine.

**Breast-feeding**—It is especially important that you receive the right amounts of vitamins so that your baby will also get the vitamins needed to grow properly. You should also check with your doctor if you are giving your baby an unfortified formula. In that case, the baby must get the vitamins needed some other way. However, taking large amounts of a dietary supplement while breast-feeding may be harmful to the mother and/or baby and should be avoided.

**Children**—Normal daily requirements vary according to age. It is especially important that children receive enough vitamins in their diet for healthy growth and development. Although there is no specific information about the use of pyridoxine in children in doses higher than the normal daily requirements, it is not expected to cause different side effects or problems in children than in adults.

**Older adults**—It is important that older people continue to receive enough vitamins in their diet for good health. Although there is no specific information about the use of pyridoxine in older people in doses higher than the normal daily requirements, it is not expected to cause different side effects or problems in older people than in younger adults.

**Medicines or other dietary supplements**—Although certain medicines or dietary supplements should not be used together at all, in other cases they may be used together even if an interaction might occur. In these cases, your doctor may want to change the dose, or other precautions may be necessary. When you are taking pyridoxine, it is especially important that your health care professional know if you are taking the following:

- Levodopa (e.g., Larodopa)—Use with pyridoxine may prevent the levodopa from working properly

## Proper Use of This Dietary Supplement

Do not take more than the recommended daily amount. Taking too much pyridoxine may cause harmful effects, such as nerve damage, which may appear as clumsiness, or numbness of hands or feet. Some people believe that taking very large doses of vitamins (called megadoses or megavitamin therapy) is useful for treating certain medical problems. Studies have not proven this. Large doses should be taken only under the direction of your doctor after need has been identified.

To use the *extended-release capsule form* of this dietary supplement:

- Swallow the capsule whole.

- Do not crush, break, or chew before swallowing.
- If the capsule is too large to swallow, you may mix the contents of the capsule with jam or jelly and swallow without chewing.

To use the *extended-release tablet form* of this dietary supplement:

- Swallow the tablet whole.
- Do not crush, break, or chew before swallowing.

**Dosing**— The dose of pyridoxine for prevention of pyridoxine deficiency is based on the Recommended Dietary Allowances (RDA). See the *Importance of Diet* section for the RDA for pyridoxine.

**Missed dose**—If you miss taking a vitamin for 1 or more days there is no cause for concern, since it takes some time for your body to become seriously low in vitamins. However, if your doctor has recommended that you take this vitamin, try to remember to take it as directed every day.

**Storage**—To store this dietary supplement:

- Keep out of the reach of children.
- Store away from heat and direct light.
- Do not store the capsule or tablet form of this medicine in the bathroom, near the kitchen sink, or in other damp places. Heat or moisture may cause the dietary supplement to break down.
- Do not keep outdated dietary supplements or those no longer needed. Be sure that any discarded medicine is out of the reach of children.

## Side Effects of This Dietary Supplement

Along with its needed effects, a dietary supplement may cause some unwanted effects. Although pyridoxine does not usually cause any side effects at usual doses, check with your doctor as soon as possible if you notice either of the following side effects:

*With large doses*
    Clumsiness; numbness of hands or feet

Also check with your doctor if you notice any other unusual effects while you are taking pyridoxine.

Revised: 09/21/92
Interim revision: 08/22/94

# PYRIMETHAMINE  Systemic

A commonly used brand name in the U.S. and Canada is Daraprim.

## Description

Pyrimethamine (peer-i-METH-a-meen) is an antiprotozoal (an-tee-proe-toe-ZOE-al) medicine. Antiprotozoals

work by killing protozoa (tiny, one-celled animals) or preventing their growth. Some protozoa are parasites that can cause many different kinds of infections in the body.

This medicine is used with one or more other medicines to treat malaria and toxoplasmosis (tok-soe-plaz-MOE-siss). This medicine may also be used for other problems as determined by your doctor.

Pyrimethamine is available only with your doctor's prescription, in the following dosage form:

*Oral*
- Tablets (U.S. and Canada)

## Before Using This Medicine

In deciding to use a medicine, the risks of taking the medicine must be weighed against the good it will do. This is a decision you and your doctor will make. For pyrimethamine, the following should be considered:

**Allergies**—Tell your doctor if you have ever had any unusual or allergic reaction to pyrimethamine. Also tell your health care professional if you are allergic to any other substances, such as foods, preservatives, or dyes.

**Pregnancy**—Studies in humans have not shown that pyrimethamine causes birth defects. Also, use in pregnant women has not shown pyrimethamine to cause birth defects. However, use is not generally recommended during the first 3 to 4 months of pregnancy. Studies in animals have shown that pyrimethamine may cause birth defects, anemia, or other problems, especially when given in large doses.

**Breast-feeding**—Pyrimethamine passes into the breast milk. However, problems in nursing babies have not been reported.

**Children**—Pyrimethamine has been used in children and, in effective doses, has not been shown to cause different side effects or problems in children than it does in adults.

**Older adults**—Many medicines have not been studied specifically in older people. Therefore, it may not be known whether they work exactly the same way they do in younger adults or if they cause different side effects or problems in older people. There is no specific information comparing use of pyrimethamine in the elderly with use in other age groups.

**Other medicines**—Although certain medicines should not be used together at all, in other cases two different medicines may be used together even if an interaction might occur. In these cases, your doctor may want to change the dose, or other precautions may be necessary. When you are taking pyrimethamine, it is especially important that your health care professional know if you are taking any of the following:

- Amphotericin B by injection (e.g., Fungizone) or
- Antineoplastics (cancer medicine) or
- Antithyroid agents (medicine for overactive thyroid) or
- Azathioprine (e.g., Imuran) or
- Chloramphenicol (e.g., Chloromycetin) or
- Colchicine or
- Cyclophosphamide (e.g., Cytoxan) or
- Flucytosine (e.g., Ancobon) or
- Ganciclovir (e.g., Cytovene) or
- Interferon (e.g., Intron A, Roferon-A) or

- Mercaptopurine (e.g., Purinethol) or
- Methotrexate (e.g., Mexate) or
- Plicamycin (e.g., Mithracin) or
- Zidovudine (e.g., AZT, Retrovir)—Use of these medicines together with pyrimethamine may increase the chance of side effects affecting the blood

**Other medical problems**—The presence of other medical problems may affect the use of pyrimethamine. Make sure you tell your doctor if you have any other medical problems, especially:

- Anemia or other blood problems—High doses of pyrimethamine may make these conditions worse
- Liver disease—Patients with liver disease may have an increased chance of side effects
- Seizure disorders, such as epilepsy—High doses of pyrimethamine may increase the chance of convulsions (seizures)

## Proper Use of This Medicine

*Keep this medicine out of the reach of children.* Overdose is especially dangerous.

If this medicine upsets your stomach or causes vomiting, it may be taken with meals or a snack.

If you are taking this medicine to *treat malaria*, take the number of tablets your doctor told you to take (up to 3) once, as a single dose, along with other medicine your doctor gave you. If you develop a fever and are not near a medical facility, and are taking this medicine to treat what you think may possibly be malaria, take the number of tablets your doctor told you to take (up to 3) once, as a single dose.

This medicine works best when you take it on a regular schedule. If you are to take 2 doses a day, one dose may be taken with breakfast and the other one with the evening meal. *Make sure that you do not miss any doses.* If you have any questions about this, check with your health care professional.

**Dosing**—The dose of pyrimethamine will be different for different patients. *Follow your doctor's orders or the directions on the label.* The following information includes only the average doses of pyrimethamine. *If your dose is different, do not change it* unless your doctor tells you to do so.

*The number of doses you take each day, the time allowed between doses, and the length of time you take the medicine depend on the medical problem for which you are taking pyrimethamine.*

- For the treatment of *malaria*:

  —Adults and adolescents: 75 milligrams of pyrimethamine together with 1.5 grams of sulfadoxine as a single dose. These 2 medicines may also be taken with other medicine. This will be determined by your doctor.

  —Children: Dose is based on body weight and will be determined by the doctor. Pyrimethamine taken together with other medicines.

- For the treatment of *toxoplasmosis*:
  —Adults and adolescents: 25 to 200 milligrams of pyrimethamine taken together with other medicines for several weeks. The proper dose for you must be determined by the doctor.
  —Children: Dose is based on body weight and must be determined by the doctor.

**Missed dose**—If you do miss a dose of this medicine, take it as soon as possible. This will help to keep you taking your medicine on a regular schedule. However, if it is almost time for your next dose, skip the missed dose and go back to your regular dosing schedule. Do not double doses.

**Storage**—To store this medicine:

- Keep out of the reach of children. Overdose is very dangerous.
- Store away from heat and direct light.
- Do not store in the bathroom, near the kitchen sink, or in other damp places. Heat or moisture may cause the medicine to break down.
- Do not keep outdated medicine or medicine no longer needed. Be sure that any discarded medicine is out of the reach of children.

## Precautions While Using This Medicine

*It is very important that your doctor check you at regular visits* for any blood problems that may be caused by this medicine, especially if you will be taking this medicine in high doses for toxoplasmosis.

If your symptoms do not improve within a few days or if they become worse, check with your doctor.

If this medicine causes anemia, your doctor may want you to take leucovorin (e.g., folinic acid, Wellcovorin) to help clear up the anemia. If so, it is important to take the leucovorin every day while you are taking this medicine. Do not miss any doses.

Pyrimethamine, especially in high doses, may cause blood problems. These problems may result in a greater chance of certain infections, slow healing, and bleeding of the gums. Therefore, you should be careful when using regular toothbrushes, dental floss, and toothpicks. Dental work should be delayed until your blood counts have returned to normal. Check with your medical doctor or dentist if you have any questions about proper oral hygiene (mouth care) during treatment.

## Side Effects of This Medicine

Along with its needed effects, a medicine may cause some unwanted effects. Although not all of these side effects may occur, if they do occur they may need medical attention.

*Check with your doctor immediately* if any of the following side effects occur:

*More common with high doses*

Change in or loss of taste; fever and sore throat; soreness, swelling, or burning of tongue; unusual bleeding or bruising; unusual tiredness or weakness

*Rare*

Skin rash

*Symptoms of overdose*

Abdominal or stomach pain; convulsions (seizures); increased excitability; vomiting (severe and continuing)

Other side effects may occur that usually do not need medical attention. These side effects may go away during treatment as your body adjusts to the medicine. However, check with your doctor if either of the following side effects continues or is bothersome:

*More common with high doses*

Diarrhea; loss of appetite; nausea; vomiting

Other side effects not listed above may also occur in some patients. If you notice any other effects, check with your doctor.

## Additional Information

Once a medicine has been approved for marketing for a certain use, experience may show that it is also useful for other medical problems. Although these uses are not included in product labeling, pyrimethamine is used in certain patients with the following medical conditions:

- Isosporiasis (treatment and prevention)
- *Pneumocystis carinii* pneumonia (treatment)

For patients taking this medicine for *Pneumocystis carinii* pneumonia:

- Pyrimethamine is used in combination with other medicines for mild to moderate pneumonia in patients who cannot take standard treatment.

Other than the above information, there is no additional information relating to proper use, precautions, or side effects for these uses.

Revised: 01/19/93

# PYRITHIONE   Topical

Some commonly used brand names are:

**In the U.S.—**

| | |
|---|---|
| Danex | Head & Shoulders |
| DHS Zinc Dandruff Shampoo | Antidandruff Lotion |
| Head & Shoulders | Shampoo 2 in 1 (Complete |
| Antidandruff Cream | Dandruff Shampoo plus |
| Shampoo Normal to Dry | Conditioner in One) |
| Formula | Formula |
| Head & Shoulders | Head & Shoulders Dry Scalp |
| Antidandruff Cream | Conditioning Formula |
| Shampoo Normal to Oily | Lotion Shampoo |
| Formula | Head & Shoulders Dry Scalp |
| Head & Shoulders | Regular Formula Lotion |
| Antidandruff Lotion | Shampoo |
| Shampoo Normal to Dry | Head & Shoulders Dry Scalp |
| Formula | 2 in 1 (Dry Scalp Shampoo |
| Head & Shoulders | Plus Conditioner in One) |
| Antidandruff Lotion | Formula Lotion Shampoo |
| Shampoo Normal to Oily | Sebex |
| Formula | Sebulon |
| | Zincon Dandruff Lotion |
| | Shampoo |
| | ZNP Bar Shampoo |
| | ZNP Shampoo |

**In Canada—**

| | |
|---|---|
| Dan-Gard | Sebulon |

## Description

Pyrithione (peer-i-THYE-one) is used to help control the symptoms of dandruff and seborrheic dermatitis of the scalp.

This medicine is available without a prescription; however, your doctor may have special instructions on the proper use of this medicine for your medical condition.

Pyrithione is available in the following dosage forms:

*Topical*
- Bar shampoo (U.S.)
- Cream shampoo (U.S.)
- Lotion shampoo (U.S. and Canada)

## Before Using This Medicine

If you are using this medicine without a prescription, carefully read and follow any precautions on the label. For pyrithione, the following should be considered:

**Allergies**—Tell your doctor if you have ever had any unusual or allergic reaction to pyrithione. Also tell your health care professional if you are allergic to any other substances, such as preservatives or dyes.

**Pregnancy**—Pyrithione has not been shown to cause birth defects or other problems in humans.

**Breast-feeding**—Pyrithione has not been reported to cause problems in nursing babies.

**Children**—Although there is no specific information comparing use of pyrithione in children with use in other age groups, this medicine is not expected to cause different side effects or problems in children than it does in adults.

**Older adults**—Many medicines have not been studied specifically in older people. Therefore, it may not be known whether they work exactly the same way they do in younger adults. Although there is no specific information comparing use of pyrithione in the elderly with use in other age groups, this medicine is not expected to cause different side effects or problems in older people than it does in younger adults.

**Other medicines**—Although certain medicines should not be used together at all, in other cases two different medicines may be used together even if an interaction might occur. In these cases, your doctor may want to change the dose, or other precautions may be necessary. Tell your health care professional if you are using any other topical prescription or nonprescription (over-the-counter [OTC]) medicine that is to be applied to the same area of the skin.

## Proper Use of This Medicine

For best results, use this medicine at least 2 times a week or as directed by your doctor.

To use:
- Before applying this shampoo, wet the hair and scalp with lukewarm water.
- Apply enough shampoo to the scalp to work up a lather and rub in well, then rinse.
- Apply the shampoo again and rinse thoroughly.

*Keep this medicine away from the eyes.* If you should accidentally get some in your eyes, flush them thoroughly with water.

**Dosing**—The dose of pyrithione will be different for different patients. *Follow your doctor's orders or the directions on the label.* The following information includes only the average dose of pyrithione. *If your dose is different, do not change it* unless your doctor tells you to do so:

- For *topical* dosage forms (bar shampoo, cream shampoo, and lotion shampoo):

    —For dandruff and seborrheic dermatitis of the scalp:

    - Adults and children—Use as a shampoo on the scalp 2 times a week.

**Missed dose**—If you miss a dose of this medicine, use it as soon as possible. However, if it is almost time for your next dose, skip the missed dose and go back to your regular dosing schedule.

**Storage**—To store this medicine:
- Keep out of the reach of children.
- Store away from heat and direct light.
- Keep the medicine from freezing.

- Do not keep outdated medicine or medicine no longer needed. Be sure that any discarded medicine is out of the reach of children.

## Precautions While Using This Medicine

If your condition does not get better after regular use of this medicine, or if it gets worse, check with your doctor.

## Side Effects of This Medicine

Along with its needed effects, a medicine may cause some unwanted effects. Although not all of these side effects may occur, if they do occur they may need medical attention.

Check with your doctor as soon as possible if the following side effect occurs:

*Less common or rare*
  Irritation of skin

Other side effects not listed above may also occur in some patients. If you notice any other effects, check with your health care professional.

Revised: 07/26/93

# PYRVINIUM   Oral*

A commonly used brand name in Canada is Vanquin.
Another commonly used name is viprynium.

*Not commercially available in the U.S.

## Description

Pyrvinium (peer-VIN-ee-um) is used to treat pinworms (enterobiasis). It will not work for other types of worm infections (for example, roundworms or tapeworms).

Pyrvinium is available only with your doctor's prescription, in the following dosage forms:

*Oral*
  - Oral suspension (Canada)

## Before Using This Medicine

In deciding to use a medicine, the risks of taking the medicine must be weighed against the good it will do. This is a decision you and your doctor will make. For pyrvinium, the following should be considered:

**Allergies**—Tell your doctor if you have ever had any unusual or allergic reaction to pyrvinium. Also tell your health care professional if you are allergic to any other substances, such as foods, preservatives, or dyes.

**Pregnancy**—Pyrvinium has not been studied in pregnant women or animals. However, pyrvinium has not been reported to cause birth defects or other problems in humans.

**Breast-feeding**—Pyrvinium has not been reported to cause problems in nursing babies.

**Children**—Pyrvinium has been studied in children and, in effective doses, has not been reported to cause different side effects or problems in children than it does in adults. However, because of limited experience, caution is recommended in children weighing less than 10 kilograms (22 pounds). Older children are more likely to have stomach upset after receiving large doses.

**Older adults**—Many medicines have not been studied specifically in older people. Therefore, it may not be known whether they work exactly the same way they do in younger adults. Although there is no specific information comparing use of pyrvinium in the elderly with use in other age groups, this medicine is not expected to cause different side effects or problems in older people than it does in younger adults.

**Other medicines**—Although certain medicines should not be used together at all, in other cases two different medicines may be used together even if an interaction might occur. In these cases, your doctor may want to change the dose, or other precautions may be necessary. Tell your health care professional if you are taking any other prescription or nonprescription (over-the-counter [OTC]) medicine.

**Other medical problems**—The presence of other medical problems may affect the use of pyrvinium. Make sure you tell your doctor if you have any other medical problems, especially:

  - Inflammatory bowel disease—Patients with inflammatory bowel disease may have an increased chance of side effects

## Proper Use of This Medicine

No special preparations (for example, special diets, fasting, other medicines, laxatives, or enemas) are necessary before, during, or immediately after you take pyrvinium.

Use a specially marked measuring spoon or other device to measure each dose accurately. The average household teaspoon may not hold the right amount of liquid.

Pinworms may be easily passed from one person to another, especially among persons in the same household. Therefore, all household members may have to be treated at the same time to prevent their infection or reinfection. Also, all household members may have to be treated again in 2 to 3 weeks to clear up the infection completely. Make sure each family member takes the correct amount, since the dose may be different for each person.

To help clear up your infection completely, *take this medicine exactly as directed by your doctor*. Read the instructions on the label and follow them carefully. The amount of medicine you need is based on your weight. You must take the exact amount if the medicine is going to work. A second course of pyrvinium is usually required to clear up the infection completely.

**Dosing**—The dose of pyrvinium will be different for different patients. *Follow your doctor's orders or the directions on the label.* The following information includes only the average doses of pyrvinium. *If your dose is different, do not change it* unless your doctor tells you to do so.

- For the *oral suspension* dosage form:
  —Adults and children: Dose is based on body weight and will be determined by your doctor. It is taken as a single dose and is repeated in 2 to 3 weeks.

**Storage**—To store this medicine:
- Keep out of the reach of children.
- Store away from heat and direct light.
- Do not store in the bathroom, near the kitchen sink, or in other damp places. Heat or moisture may cause the medicine to break down.
- Do not freeze oral suspension.
- Do not keep outdated medicine or medicine no longer needed. Be sure that any discarded medicine is out of the reach of children.

## Precautions While Using This Medicine

If your symptoms do not improve within a few days, or if they become worse, check with your doctor.

Pyrvinium may cause your skin to be more sensitive to sunlight than it is normally. Exposure to sunlight, even for brief periods of time, may cause a skin rash, itching, redness or other discoloration of the skin, or a severe sunburn. For a day or two after taking this medicine:

- Stay out of direct sunlight, especially between the hours of 10:00 a.m. and 3:00 p.m., if possible.
- Wear protective clothing, including a hat. Also, wear sunglasses.
- Apply a sun block product that has a skin protection factor (SPF) of at least 15. Some patients may require a product with a higher SPF number, especially if they have a fair complexion. If you have

any questions about this, check with your health care professional.

- Apply a sunblock lipstick that has an SPF of at least 15 to protect your lips.
- Do not use a sunlamp or tanning bed or booth.

*If you have a severe reaction from the sun, check with your doctor.*

In some patients, pinworms may return after treatment with pyrvinium. Washing (not shaking) all bedding and nightclothes (pajamas) after treatment may help to prevent this. Some doctors may also recommend other measures to help keep your infection from returning. If you have any questions about this, check with your doctor.

## Side Effects of This Medicine

Along with its needed effects, a medicine may cause some unwanted effects. Although not all of these side effects may occur, if they do occur they may need medical attention.

Check with your doctor as soon as possible if the following side effect occurs:

*Rare*
Skin rash

Other side effects may occur that usually do not need medical attention. These side effects may go away during treatment as your body adjusts to the medicine. However, check with your doctor if any of the following side effects continue or are bothersome:

*Rare*
Diarrhea; increased sensitivity of skin to sunlight; nausea and vomiting; stomach cramps

This medicine is a dye and will *color your stools red*. This color is not harmful and will disappear in a few days. Pyrvinium may also stain clothing red. If vomiting occurs, the vomit will be red in color.

Other side effects not listed above may also occur in some patients. If you notice any other effects, check with your doctor.

---

Revised: 01/19/93

# QUINACRINE   Systemic

A commonly used brand name in the U.S. and Canada is Atabrine. Another commonly used name is mepacrine.

## Description

Quinacrine (KWIN-a-kreen) is used to treat giardiasis (jee-ar-DYE-a-siss), a protozoal infection of the intestinal tract. This medicine may also be used for other conditions as determined by your doctor.

Quinacrine is available only with your doctor's prescription, in the following dosage form:

*Oral*
- Tablets (U.S. and Canada)

## Before Using This Medicine

In deciding to use a medicine, the risks of taking the medicine must be weighed against the good it will do. This is a decision you and your doctor will make. For quinacrine, the following should be considered:

**Allergies**—Tell your doctor if you have ever had any unusual or allergic reaction to quinacrine. Also tell your health care professional if you are allergic to any other substances, such as foods, preservatives, or dyes.

**Pregnancy**—Use of quinacrine to treat giardiasis in a pregnant woman should be delayed until after delivery as long as the woman is not experiencing symptoms of the disease.

**Breast-feeding**—Quinacrine is excreted in breast milk. However, quinacrine has not been reported to cause problems in nursing babies.

**Children**—Quinacrine can cause serious side effects in any patient. Therefore, it is especially important that you discuss with the child's doctor the good that this medicine may do as well as the risks of using it.

**Older adults**—Many medicines have not been studied specifically in older people. Therefore, it may not be known whether they work exactly the same way they do in younger adults. Although there is no specific information comparing use of quinacrine in the elderly with use in other age groups, this medicine is not expected to cause different side effects or problems in older people than it does in younger adults.

**Other medicines**—Although certain medicines should not be used together at all, in other cases two different medicines may be used together even if an interaction might occur. In these cases, your doctor may want to change the dose, or other precautions may be necessary. When you are taking quinacrine, it is especially important that your health care professional know if you are taking any of the following:
- Primaquine—Use with quinacrine may increase the chance of side effects from primaquine

**Other medical problems**—The presence of other medical problems may affect the use of quinacrine. Make sure you tell your doctor if you have any other medical problems, especially:
- Mental illness (severe) (history of)—Quinacrine may cause mood or other mental changes in some patients
- Porphyria—Quinacrine may make porphyria worse
- Psoriasis—Quinacrine may cause an attack of psoriasis or make psoriasis worse

## Proper Use of This Medicine

Quinacrine is best taken after meals with a full glass (8 ounces) of water, tea, or fruit juice, unless otherwise directed by your doctor.

For patients *unable to swallow tablets or unable to tolerate bitter taste:*
- The tablets may be crushed and mixed with jam, honey, or chocolate syrup or placed in empty gelatin capsules to cover up the bitter taste. Be sure to take all the food so that you get the full dose of medicine.

To help clear up your infection completely, *keep taking quinacrine for the full time of treatment,* even if you begin to feel better after a few days. If you stop taking this medicine too soon, your symptoms may return. *Do not miss any doses.*

**Dosing**—The dose of quinacrine will be different for different patients. *Follow your doctor's orders or the directions on the label.* The following information includes only the average doses of quinacrine. *If your dose is different, do not change it* unless your doctor tells you to do so.
- For the *tablet* dosage form:
  —Adults and older children: 100 milligrams three times a day for five to seven days.
  —Younger children: Dose is based on body weight and will be determined by the doctor. The dose is taken three times a day for five to seven days.

**Missed dose**—If you do miss a dose of this medicine, take it as soon as possible. However, if it is almost time for your next dose, skip the missed dose and go back to your regular dosing schedule. Do not double doses.

**Storage**—To store this medicine:
- Keep out of the reach of children.
- Store away from heat and direct light.
- Do not store in the bathroom, near the kitchen sink, or in other damp places. Heat or moisture may cause the medicine to break down.
- Do not keep outdated medicine or medicine no longer needed. Be sure that any discarded medicine is out of the reach of children.

## Precautions While Using This Medicine

It is important that your doctor check your progress at different times. This is to check whether or not the infection is cleared up completely.

If your symptoms do not improve within a few days, or if they become worse, check with your doctor.

Quinacrine may cause some people to become dizzy. *Make sure you know how you react to this medicine before you drive, use machines, or do anything else that could be dangerous if you are dizzy or are not alert.* If this reaction is especially bothersome, check with your doctor.

## Side Effects of This Medicine

Along with its needed effects, a medicine may cause some unwanted effects. Although not all of these side effects may occur, if they do occur they may need medical attention. When this medicine is used for a short time, side effects are not generally serious. However, if this medicine is used for a long time and/or in high doses, other more serious side effects may occur.

*Check with your doctor immediately* if any of the following side effects occur:

*Less common*

Hallucinations (seeing, hearing, or feeling things that are not there); irritability; mood or other mental changes; nervousness; nightmares; skin rash, redness, itching, or peeling

*Symptoms of overdose*

Convulsions (seizures); fainting; irregular heartbeat

Other side effects may occur that usually do not need medical attention. These side effects may go away during treatment as your body adjusts to the medicine. However, check with your doctor if any of the following side effects continue or are bothersome:

*More common*

Abdominal or stomach cramps; diarrhea; dizziness; headache; loss of appetite; nausea or vomiting

Quinacrine is a dye-like medicine and commonly causes *yellow discoloration of the skin or urine.* This side effect is only *temporary* and will go away when you stop taking this medicine.

Other side effects not listed above may also occur in some patients. If you notice any other effects, check with your doctor.

## Additional Information

Once a medicine has been approved for marketing for a certain use, experience may show that it is also useful for other medical problems. Although this use is not included in product labeling, quinacrine is used in certain patients with the following medical condition:

• Discoid lupus erythematosus

Other than the above information, there is no additional information relating to proper use, precautions, or side effects for this use.

Revised: 02/01/93

# QUINIDINE   Systemic

Some commonly used brand names are:

**In the U.S.—**

| | |
|---|---|
| Cardioquin | Quinalan |
| Cin-Quin | Quinidex Extentabs |
| Duraquin | Quinora |
| Quinaglute Dura-tabs | |

Generic name product may also be available.

**In Canada—**

| | |
|---|---|
| Apo-Quinidine | Quinaglute Dura-tabs |
| Cardioquin | Quinate |
| Novoquinidin | Quinidex Extentabs |

Generic name product may also be available.

## Description

Quinidine (KWIN-i-deen) is used to correct certain irregular heartbeats to a normal rhythm and to slow an overactive heart. The injection dosage form is also used to treat malaria.

Quinidine acts directly on the heart tissues to make them less responsive. It also slows impulses along special nerve networks to the heart. This allows the heart to work more efficiently.

Do not confuse this medicine with *quinine*, which, although related, has different medical uses.

Quinidine is available only with your doctor's prescription, in the following dosage forms:

*Oral*

• Capsules (U.S.)
• Tablets (U.S. and Canada)
• Extended-release tablets (U.S. and Canada)

*Parenteral*

• Injection (U.S. and Canada)

## Before Using This Medicine

In deciding to use a medicine, the risks of taking the medicine must be weighed against the good it will do. This is a decision you and your doctor will make. For quinidine, the following should be considered:

**Allergies**—Tell your doctor if you have ever had any unusual or allergic reaction to quinidine or quinine. Also tell your health care professional if you are allergic to any other substance, such as foods, preservatives, or dyes.

**Pregnancy**—Studies on effects in pregnancy have not been done in either humans or animals. However, a closely related medicine, quinine, has been shown to cause birth defects of the nervous system, fingers, and toes, and decreased hearing in the infant. Quinine also may cause contractions of the uterus.

**Breast-feeding**—Quinidine passes into breast milk. However, it has not been reported to cause problems in nursing babies.

**Children**—Studies on this medicine have been done only in adult patients, and there is no specific information comparing use of quinidine in children with use in other age groups. Use of the extended-release tablets in children is not recommended.

**Older adults**—Many medicines have not been studied specifically in older people. Therefore, it may not be known whether they work exactly the same way they do in younger adults. Although there is no specific information comparing use of quinidine in the elderly with use in other age groups, this medicine is not expected to cause different side effects or problems in older people than it does in younger adults.

**Other medicines**—Although certain medicines should not be used together at all, in other cases two different medicines may be used together even if an interaction might occur. In these cases, your doctor may want to change the dose, or other precautions may be necessary. When you are taking quinidine, it is especially important that your health care professional knows if you are taking any of the following:

- Anticoagulants (blood thinners)—Risk of bleeding may be increased
- Other heart medicine (especially digoxin)—Effects on the heart may be increased
- Pimozide (e.g., Orap)—Risk of heart rhythm problems may be increased
- Urinary alkalizers (medicine that makes the urine less acid, such as acetazolamide [e.g., Diamox], calcium- and/or magnesium-containing antacids, dichlorphenamide [e.g., Daranide], methazolamide [e.g., Neptazane], potassium or sodium citrate and/or citric acid, sodium bicarbonate [baking soda])—Effects may be increased because levels of quinidine in the body may be increased

**Other medical problems**—The presence of other medical problems may affect the use of quinidine. Make sure you tell your doctor if you have any other medical problems, especially:

- Asthma or emphysema—Possible allergic reaction
- Blood disease
- Infection
- Kidney disease or
- Liver disease—Effects may be increased because of slower removal of quinidine from the body
- Myasthenia gravis—Muscle weakness may be increased
- Overactive thyroid
- Psoriasis

## Proper Use of This Medicine

Take quinidine with a full glass (8 ounces) of water on an empty stomach 1 hour before or 2 hours after meals so that it will be absorbed more quickly. However, to lessen stomach upset, your doctor may want you to take the medicine with food or milk.

For patients taking the *extended-release tablet* form of this medicine:

- Swallow the tablets whole.
- Do not break, crush, or chew before swallowing.

*Take quinidine exactly as directed by your doctor even though you may feel well.* Do not take more medicine than ordered and do not miss any doses.

**Dosing**—The dose of quinidine will be different for different patients. *Follow your doctor's orders or the directions on the label.* The following information includes only the average doses of quinidine. *If your dose is different, do not change it* unless your doctor tells you to do so.

The number of capsules or tablets that you take depends on the strength of the medicine. Also, *the number of doses you take each day, the time allowed between doses, and the length of time you take the medicine depend on the medical problem for which you are taking quinidine.* When you first begin to take quinidine for irregular heartbeat, you may need to take a higher number of doses each day. This depends on what type of irregular heartbeat you have and will be determined by your doctor.

- For *regular (short-acting) oral* dosage forms (capsules and tablets):
  —For irregular heartbeat:
    - Adults—200 to 650 milligrams (mg) two to four times a day.
    - Children—6 to 8.25 mg per kilogram (kg) (2.73 to 3.75 mg per pound) of body weight five times a day.
- For *long-acting oral* dosage forms (tablets):
  —For irregular heartbeat:
    - Adults—300 to 660 mg every six to twelve hours.
    - Children—Use is not recommended.
- For *injection* dosage form:
  —For irregular heartbeat:
    - Adults—400 to 600 mg injected into the muscle every two hours. Or, 600 to 800 mg in a solution and injected into a vein.
    - Children—Dose must be determined by your doctor.
  —For malaria:
    - Adults—10 mg per kg (4.54 mg per pound) of body weight in a solution and injected slowly into a vein over one to two hours. Then, 0.02 mg per kg (0.009 mg per pound) of body weight per minute is given. Or, 12 to 24 mg per kg (5.45 to 10.91 mg per pound) of body weight in a solution

and injected slowly into a vein over a four hour period every eight hours.
- Children—Dose must be determined by your doctor.

**Missed dose**—If you miss a dose of this medicine and remember within 2 hours of the missed dose, take it as soon as possible. However, if you do not remember until later, skip the missed dose and go back to your regular dosing schedule. Do not double doses.

**Storage**—To store this medicine:
- Keep out of the reach of children.
- Store away from heat and direct light.
- Do not store in the bathroom, near the kitchen sink, or in other damp places. Heat or moisture may cause the medicine to break down.
- Do not keep outdated medicine or medicine no longer needed. Be sure that any discarded medicine is out of the reach of children.

## Precautions While Using This Medicine

It is very important that your doctor check your progress at regular visits to make sure that the quinidine is working properly and does not cause unwanted effects.

*Do not stop taking this medicine without first checking with your doctor,* to avoid possible worsening of your condition.

*Before having any kind of surgery (including dental surgery) or emergency treatment, tell the medical doctor or dentist in charge that you are taking this medicine.*

Your doctor may want you to carry a medical identification card or bracelet stating that you are using this medicine.

*Some people who are unusually sensitive to this medicine may have side effects after the first dose or first few doses.* Check with your doctor right away if the following side effects occur: breathing difficulty, changes in vision, dizziness, fever, headache, ringing in ears, or skin rash.

## Side Effects of This Medicine

Along with its needed effects, a medicine may cause some unwanted effects. Although not all of these side effects may occur, if they do occur they may need medical attention.

*Check with your doctor immediately* if any of the following side effects occur:

*Less common*

Blurred vision or any change in vision; dizziness, light-headedness, or fainting; fever; headache (severe); ringing or buzzing in the ears or any loss of hearing; skin rash, hives, or itching; wheezing, shortness of breath, or troubled breathing

*Rare*

Fast heartbeat; unusual bleeding or bruising; unusual tiredness or weakness

Other side effects may occur that usually do not need medical attention. These side effects may go away during treatment as your body adjusts to the medicine. However, check with your doctor if any of the following side effects continue or are bothersome:

*More common*

Bitter taste; diarrhea; flushing of skin with itching; loss of appetite; nausea or vomiting; stomach pain or cramping

*Less common*

Confusion

Other side effects not listed above may also occur in some patients. If you notice any other effects, check with your doctor.

Revised: 03/24/94

---

# QUININE   Systemic

Some commonly used brand names are:

**In the U.S.—**

| | |
|---|---|
| Legatrin | Quindan |
| Quin-260 | Quiphile |
| Quin-amino | Q-vel |
| Quinamm | |

Generic name product may also be available.

**In Canada—**

Novoquinine

Generic name product may also be available.

## Description

Quinine (KWYE-nine) is used to treat malaria. This medicine is usually given with one or more other medicines for malaria.

Quinine is also used to prevent and treat nighttime leg cramps. It may also be used for other problems as determined by your doctor. Do not confuse quinine with *quinidine*, a different medicine that is used for heart problems.

Some quinine products for use in nighttime leg cramps are available only with your doctor's prescription; others are available without a prescription.

Quinine is available in the following dosage forms:
*Oral*
- Capsules (U.S. and Canada)
- Tablets (U.S.)

---

## Before Using This Medicine

In deciding to use a medicine, the risks of taking the medicine must be weighed against the good it will do. This is a decision you and your doctor will make. For quinine, the following should be considered:

**Allergies**—Tell your doctor if you have ever had any unusual or allergic reaction to quinine, quinidine (e.g., Quinidex), or to dietary items that contain quinine, such as tonic water or bitter lemon. Also tell your health care professional if you are allergic to any other substances, such as foods, preservatives, or dyes.

**Pregnancy**—Quinine has been used for the treatment of malaria in pregnant women. Treatment is important because if a pregnant woman gets malaria, there is an increased chance of premature births, stillbirths, and abortion. However, quinine has been shown to cause birth defects in rabbits and guinea pigs and has also been shown to cause rare birth defects, stillbirths, and other problems in humans. In addition, quinine has been shown to cause miscarriage when taken in large amounts.

**Breast-feeding**—Quinine passes into the breast milk in small amounts. However, this medicine has not been reported to cause problems in nursing babies.

**Children**—This medicine has been used to treat malaria in children and, in effective doses, has not been shown to cause different side effects or problems in children than it does in adults.

**Older adults**—Many medicines have not been studied specifically in older people. Therefore, it may not be known whether they work exactly the same way they do in younger adults or if they cause different side effects or problems in older people. There is no specific information comparing use of quinine in the elderly with use in other age groups.

**Other medicines**—Although certain medicines should not be used together at all, in other cases two different medicines may be used together even if an interaction might occur. In these cases, your doctor may want to change the dose, or other precautions may be necessary. When you are taking quinine, it is especially important that your health care professional know if you are taking the following:

- Mefloquine (e.g., Larium)—Use of mefloquine with quinine may increase the chance of side effects

**Other medical problems**—The presence of other medical problems may affect the use of quinine. Make sure you tell your doctor if you have any other medical problems, especially:

- Blackwater fever, history of, or
- Glucose-6-phosphate dehydrogenase (G6PD) deficiency or

- Purpura, or history of (purplish or brownish red discoloration of skin)—Patients with a history of blackwater fever, G6PD deficiency, or purpura may have an increased risk of side effects affecting the blood
- Heart disease—Quinine can cause side effects of the heart, usually at higher doses
- Hypoglycemia—Quinine may cause low blood sugar
- Myasthenia gravis—Quinine may increase muscle weakness in patients with myasthenia gravis

---

## Proper Use of This Medicine

*Take this medicine only as directed. Do not take more of it, do not take it more often, and do not take it for a longer time than recommended on the label,* unless otherwise directed by your doctor. To do so may increase the chance of side effects.

*Take this medicine with or after meals* to lessen possible stomach upset, unless otherwise directed by your doctor. If you are to take this medicine at bedtime, take it with a snack or with a glass of water, milk, or other beverage.

For patients *taking quinine for malaria:*

- To help clear up your infection completely, *keep taking this medicine for the full time of treatment,* even if you begin to feel better after a few days. If you stop taking this medicine too soon, your symptoms may return. *Do not miss any doses.*

**Dosing**—The dose of quinine will be different for different patients. *Follow your doctor's orders or the directions on the label.* The following information includes only the average doses of quinine. *If your dose is different, do not change it* unless your doctor tells you to do so.

The number of capsules or tablets that you take depends on the strength of the medicine. Also, *the number of doses you take each day, the time allowed between doses, and the length of time you take the medicine depend on the medical problem for which you are taking quinine.*

- For treatment of *malaria:*
  —Adults and older children: 600 to 650 mg every eight hours for at least three days. This medicine must be taken with other medicine to treat malaria.
  —Younger children: Dose must be determined by the doctor.
- For prevention and treatment of *leg cramps:*
  —Adults: 200 to 300 mg taken at bedtime.
  —Children: Dose has not been determined.

**Missed dose**—If you do miss a dose of this medicine, take it as soon as possible. However, if it is almost time for your next dose, skip the missed dose and go back to your regular dosing schedule. Do not double doses.

**Storage**—To store this medicine:
- Keep out of the reach of children.
- Store away from heat and direct light.
- Do not store in the bathroom, near the kitchen sink, or in other damp places. Heat or moisture may cause the medicine to break down.

- Do not keep outdated medicine or medicine no longer needed. Be sure that any discarded medicine is out of the reach of children.

## Precautions While Using This Medicine

Quinine may cause blurred vision or a change in color vision. *Make sure you know how you react to this medicine before you drive, use machines, or do anything else that could be dangerous if you are not able to see well.* If these reactions are especially bothersome, check with your doctor.

## Side Effects of This Medicine

Along with its needed effects, a medicine may cause some unwanted effects. Although not all of these side effects may occur, if they do occur they may need medical attention.

*Check with your doctor immediately* if any of the following side effects occur:

*Rare*

Anxiety; back, leg, or stomach pains; cold sweats; cool, pale skin; fever and chills; headache; increased hunger; loss of appetite; muscle aches; nausea and vomiting; nervousness; pale skin; pale stools; shakiness; skin rash,

redness, hives, or itching; sore throat and fever; stomach pain; sweating; unusual bleeding or bruising; unusual tiredness or weakness; wheezing, shortness of breath, or difficult breathing; yellow skin and eyes

*Signs and symptoms of overdose*

Blindness; confusion; convulsions (seizures); decreased vision; irregular heartbeat; lightheadedness

Other side effects may occur that usually do not need medical attention. These side effects may go away during treatment as your body adjusts to the medicine. However, check with your doctor if any of the following side effects continue or are bothersome:

*More common*

Abdominal or stomach cramps or pain; blurred vision or change in color vision; diarrhea; headache (severe); nausea and vomiting; ringing or buzzing in ears or loss of hearing (usually temporary)

Other side effects not listed above may also occur in some patients. If you notice any other effects, check with your doctor.

Revised: 02/23/93

# RABIES IMMUNE GLOBULIN  Systemic

Some commonly used brand names in the U.S. and Canada are Hyperab and Imogam.
Generic name product may also be available.
Other commonly used names are HRIG and RIG.

## Description

Rabies immune globulin (RAY-beez im-MUNE GLOB-yoo-lin) is used along with rabies vaccine to prevent infection caused by the rabies virus. Rabies immune globulin works by giving your body the antibodies it needs to protect it against the rabies virus. This is called passive protection. This passive protection lasts long enough to protect your body until your body can produce its own antibodies against the rabies virus.

Rabies immune globulin is given to persons who have been exposed (for example, by a bite, scratch, or lick) to an animal that is known, or thought, to have rabies. This is called post-exposure prophylaxis. Rabies immune globulin is used only in persons who have never before received the rabies vaccine.

Rabies infection is a serious, and often fatal, infection. In the U.S., rabies in wild animals, especially raccoons, skunks, and bats, accounts for most cases of rabies passed on to humans, pets, and other domestic animals. In Canada, the animals most often infected with rabies are foxes, skunks, bats, dogs, and cats. Horses, swine, and cattle also have been known to become infected with rabies. In much of the rest of the world, including Latin America, Africa, and Asia, dogs account for most cases of rabies passed on to humans.

If you are being (or will be) treated for a possible rabies infection while traveling outside of the U.S. or Canada, contact your doctor as soon as you return to the U.S. or Canada, since it may be necessary for you to have additional treatment.

Rabies immune globulin is to be administered only by or under the supervision of your doctor or other health care professional. It is available in the following dosage form:

*Parenteral*
- Injection (U.S. and Canada)

## Before Receiving This Medicine

In deciding to use a medicine, the risks of using the medicine must be weighed against the good it will do. This is a decision you and your doctor will make. For rabies immune globulin, the following should be considered:

**Allergies**—Tell your doctor if you have ever had any unusual or allergic reaction to rabies immune globulin or any other kind of human immune globulin. Also tell your health care professional if you are allergic to any other substances, such as foods, thimerosal or other preservatives, or dyes.

**Pregnancy**—Studies on effects in pregnancy have not been done in either humans or animals. However, the use of rabies immune globulin in pregnant women has not been reported to cause problems.

**Breast-feeding**—Rabies immune globulin has not been reported to cause problems in nursing babies.

**Children**—Although there is no specific information comparing use of rabies immune globulin in children with use in other age groups, this medicine is not expected to cause different side effects or problems in children than it does in adults.

**Older adults**—Many medicines have not been studied specifically in older people. Therefore, it may not be known whether they work exactly the same way they do in younger adults or if they cause different side effects or problems in older people. There is no specific information comparing use of rabies immune globulin in the elderly with use in other age groups.

**Other medical problems**—The presence of other medical problems may affect the use of rabies immune globulin. Make sure you tell your doctor if you have any other medical problems, especially:
- Immunoglobulin A (IgA) deficiencies—Rabies immune globulin may cause an allergic reaction to occur

## Proper Use of This Medicine

**Dosing**—The dose of rabies immune globulin will be different for different patients. The following information includes only the average dose of rabies immune globulin.
- *For injection* dosage form:
  —For preventing rabies infection:
    - Adults and children—The dose is based on body weight and must be determined by your doctor. The usual dose is 20 International Units (IU) per kilogram (kg) (9.1 IU per pound) of body weight. This medicine is injected into the buttocks (gluteal) muscle and may also be injected around the areas of any wounds caused by the animal with rabies. This medicine is usually used on the first day of your rabies treatment along with the first dose of rabies vaccine. If this medicine is not used on the first day, it may be used any day up through the seventh day of your rabies treatment.

## Side Effects of This Medicine

Along with its needed effects, a medicine may cause some unwanted effects. The following side effects may occur, but usually do not need medical attention. However, check with your doctor if any of the following side effects continue or are bothersome:

*Less common*

Fever; pain, soreness, tenderness, or stiffness of the muscles at the place(s) of injection—may last for several hours after the injection(s)

Other side effects not listed above may also occur in some patients. If you notice any other effects, check with your doctor.

---

Developed: 08/31/94

---

# RABIES VACCINE   Systemic

Some commonly used brand names are:

**In the U.S.—**

Imovax[2]                                    Imovax I.D.[2]

Other commonly used names are:

HDCV[2]                                       RVA[1]

Note: For quick reference, the following rabies vaccines are numbered to match the corresponding brand names.

This information applies to the following vaccines:

1. Rabies Vaccine Adsorbed[†‡]
2. Rabies Vaccine, Human Diploid Cell[§]

---

[†]Not commercially available in Canada.
[‡]Generic name product may also be available in the U.S.
[§]Generic name product may also be available in Canada.

---

## Description

Rabies (RAY-beez) Vaccine is an active immunizing agent used to prevent infection caused by the rabies virus. The vaccine works by causing your body to produce its own protection (antibodies) against the rabies virus.

Rabies vaccine is used in two ways. Rabies vaccine is given to persons who have been exposed (for example, by a bite, scratch, or lick) to a animal that is known, or thought, to have rabies. This is called post-exposure prophylaxis. Rabies vaccine may also be given ahead of time to persons who have a high risk of getting infected with rabies virus. These persons include veterinarians, animal handlers, travelers who will spend more than 1 month in countries having a high rate of rabies infection, and persons who live, work, or take vacations in wild areas of the country where they are likely to come into contact with wild animals. This is called pre-exposure prophylaxis.

Rabies infection is a serious, and often fatal, infection. In the U.S., rabies in wild animals, especially raccoons, skunks, and bats, accounts for most cases of rabies passed on to humans, pets, and other domestic animals. In Canada, the animals most often infected with rabies are foxes, skunks, bats, dogs, and cats. Horses, swine, and cattle also have been known to become infected with rabies. In much of the rest of the world, including Latin America, Africa, and Asia, dogs account for most cases of rabies passed on to humans.

If you are being (or will be) treated for a possible rabies infection while traveling outside of the U.S. or Canada, contact your doctor as soon as you return to the U.S. or Canada, since it may be necessary for you to have additional treatment.

This vaccine is to be administered only by or under the supervision of your doctor or other health care professional. It is available in the following dosage form:

*Parenteral*

• Injection (U.S. and Canada)

---

## Before Receiving This Vaccine

In deciding to use a vaccine, the risks of using the vaccine must be weighed against the good it will do. This is a decision you and your doctor will make. For rabies vaccine, the following should be considered:

**Allergies**—Tell your doctor if you have ever had any unusual or allergic reaction to rabies vaccine, or to cow (bovine) serum, human albumin, kanamycin, monkey proteins, neomycin, polymyxin B, or thimerosal, since some of these may also be present in the vaccine. Also tell your health care professional if you are allergic to any other substances, such as foods, preservatives, or dyes.

**Pregnancy**—Studies on effects in pregnancy have not been done in either humans or animals. However, the use of rabies vaccine in pregnant women has not been reported to cause problems.

**Breast-feeding**—Rabies vaccine has not been reported to cause problems in nursing babies.

**Children**—This vaccine is not expected to cause different side effects or problems in children than it does in adults.

**Older adults**—Many vaccines have not been studied specifically in older people. Therefore, it may not be known whether they work exactly the same way they do in younger adults or if they cause different side effects or problems in older people. There is no specific information comparing use of rabies vaccine in the elderly with use in other age groups.

**Other medicines**—Although certain medicines should not be used together at all, in other cases two different medicines may be used together even if an interaction might occur. In these cases, your doctor may want to change the dose, or other precautions may be necessary. While you are receiving rabies vaccine, it is especially important that your health care professional know if you are taking any of the following:

• Cancer medicines or
• Corticosteroids (i.e., cortisone-like medicines) or

- Medicine to prevent malaria, such as chloroquine (Aralen), hydroxychloroquine (Plaquenil), or mefloquine (Lariam), or
- Radiation therapy—These treatments may reduce the useful effect of the vaccine

**Other medical problems**—The presence of other medical problems may affect the use of rabies vaccine. Make sure you tell your doctor if you have any other medical problems, especially:

- Illness, severe, with fever—The symptoms of the condition may be confused with the possible side effects of the vaccine
- Immune deficiency condition (or family history of)—May decrease the useful effects of the vaccine

## Proper Use of This Vaccine

In order for rabies vaccine to work properly, *it is very important that you do not miss any doses.* Keep your appointments with your doctor.

**Dosing**—The dose of rabies vaccine will be different for different patients. The number of injections and the time between injections depend on the reason for which you are receiving rabies vaccine.

*For rabies vaccine adsorbed*

- For *injection* dosage form:
  —For post-exposure prophylaxis if you have never received rabies vaccine before:
  - Adults and children—One dose on the first day, then one dose three, seven, fourteen, and twenty-eight days later for a total of five doses. The vaccine is injected into the muscle (deltoid) in the upper arm. Very young or small children may have the vaccine injected into the upper leg (thigh) muscle. On the first day, you will also receive an injection of another medicine (rabies immune globulin).
  —For post-exposure prophylaxis if you have received rabies vaccine before:
  - Adults and children—One dose on the first day, then one dose three days later for a total of two doses. The vaccine is injected into the muscle (deltoid) in the upper arm. Very young or small children may have the vaccine injected into the upper leg (thigh) muscle.
  —For pre-exposure prophylaxis if you have never received rabies vaccine before:
  - Adults and children—One dose on the first day, then one dose seven and twenty-one or twenty-eight days later for a total of three doses. The vaccine is injected into the muscle (deltoid) in the upper arm. Very young or small children may have the vaccine injected into the upper leg (thigh) muscle.
  —For pre-exposure prophylaxis if you have received rabies vaccine before (also known as a booster dose):
  - Adults and children—One dose injected into the muscle (deltoid) in the upper arm. Very young

or small children may have the vaccine injected into the upper leg (thigh) muscle.

*For rabies vaccine, human diploid cell*

- For *injection* dosage form:
  —For post-exposure prophylaxis if you have never received rabies vaccine before:
  - Adults and children—One dose on the first day, then one dose three, seven, fourteen, and twenty-eight days later for a total of five doses. The vaccine is injected into the muscle (deltoid) in the upper arm. Very young or small children may have the vaccine injected into the upper leg (thigh) muscle. On the first day, you will also receive an injection of another medicine (rabies immune globulin).
  —For post-exposure prophylaxis if you have received rabies vaccine before:
  - Adults and children—One dose on the first day, then one dose three days later for a total of two doses. The vaccine is injected into the muscle (deltoid) in the upper arm. Very young or small children may have the vaccine injected into the upper leg (thigh) muscle.
  —For pre-exposure prophylaxis if you have never received rabies vaccine before:
  - Adults and children—One dose on the first day, then one dose seven and twenty-one or twenty-eight days later for a total of three doses. The vaccine is injected into, or under the skin of, the muscle (deltoid) in the upper arm. Very young or small children may have the vaccine injected into the upper leg (thigh) muscle.
  —For pre-exposure prophylaxis if you have received rabies vaccine before (also known as a booster dose):
  - Adults and children—One dose injected into, or under the skin of, the muscle (deltoid) in the upper arm. Very young or small children may have the vaccine injected into the upper leg (thigh) muscle.

**Missed dose**—If you miss a dose of this vaccine, *contact your doctor as soon as possible.*

## Precautions While Receiving This Vaccine

This vaccine may cause some people to become dizzy. Make sure you know how you react to this vaccine before you drive, use machines, or do anything else that could be dangerous if you are dizzy.

## Side Effects of This Vaccine

Along with its needed effects, a vaccine may cause some unwanted effects. Although not all of these side effects may occur, if they do occur they may need medical attention.

Check with your doctor as soon as possible if either of the following side effects occur:

*Rare*

Hives or skin rash

Other side effects may occur that usually do not need medical attention. These side effects may go away during treatment as your body adjusts to the vaccine. However, check with your doctor if any of the following side effects continue or are bothersome:

*More common*

Chills; dizziness; fever; general feeling of discomfort or illness; headache; itching, pain, redness, or swelling at the place of injection; muscle or joint aches; nausea; stomach or abdomen pain; tiredness or weakness

Other side effects not listed above may also occur in some patients. If you notice any other effects, check with your doctor.

Developed: 08/31/94

---

# RADIOPAQUE AGENTS    Diagnostic

This information applies to the following medicines:
1. Diatrizoates (dye-a-tri-ZOE-ates)
2. Iodipamide (eye-oh-DI-pa-mide)
3. Iohexol (eye-oh-HEX-ole)
4. Iopamidol (eye-oh-PA-mi-dole)
5. Iothalamate (eye-oh-thal-A-mate)
6. Ioversol (eye-oh-VER-sole)
7. Ioxaglate (eye-OX-a-glate)
8. Metrizamide (me-TRI-za-mide)

## Description

Radiopaque agents are drugs used to help diagnose certain medical problems. They contain iodine, which absorbs x-rays. Depending on how they are given, radiopaque agents build up in a particular area of the body. The resulting high level of iodine allows the x-rays to make a "picture" of the area.

The radiopaque agents are used in the diagnosis of:

- Biliary tract problems—Diatrizoates, Iodipamide, Iohexol, Iothalamate
- Blood vessel diseases—Diatrizoates, Iohexol, Iopamidol, Iothalamate, Ioversol, Ioxaglate, Metrizamide
- Blood vessel diseases of the brain—Diatrizoates, Iohexol, Iopamidol, Iothalamate, Ioversol, Ioxaglate
- Blood vessel diseases of the heart—Diatrizoates, Iohexol, Iopamidol, Iothalamate, Ioversol, Ioxaglate, Metrizamide
- Brain diseases and tumors—Diatrizoates, Iohexol, Iopamidol, Iothalamate, Ioversol, Ioxaglate, Metrizamide
- Breast lesions—Diatrizoates
- Heart disease—Diatrizoates, Iohexol, Iopamidol, Iothalamate, Ioversol, Ioxaglate, Metrizamide
- Impaired flow of cerebrospinal fluid in brain—Iohexol, Iopamidol, Metrizamide
- Kidney diseases—Diatrizoates, Iothalamate, Ioversol, Ioxaglate
- Joint diseases—Diatrizoates, Iohexol, Iothalamate, Ioxaglate, Metrizamide
- Liver diseases—Diatrizoates, Iohexol, Iothalamate, Ioversol, Ioxaglate
- Pancreas disease—Diatrizoates, Iohexol, Iothalamate, Ioversol, Ioxaglate
- Spinal disk diseases—Diatrizoates
- Spleen diseases—Diatrizoates, Iothalamate
- Stomach and intestinal problems—Diatrizoates, Iohexol
- Urinary tract problems—Diatrizoates, Iohexol, Iopamidol, Iothalamate, Ioversol, Ioxaglate, Metrizamide

Radiopaque agents are taken by mouth or given by enema or injection. X-rays are then used to check if there are any problems with the stomach, intestines, kidneys, or other parts of the body.

Some radiopaque agents, such as iohexol, iopamidol, and metrizamide are given by injection into the spinal canal. X-rays are then used to help diagnose problems or diseases in the head, spinal canal, and nervous system.

The doses of radiopaque agents will be different for different patients and depend on the type of test. The strength of the solution is determined by how much iodine it contains. Different tests will require a different strength and amount of solution depending on the age of the patient, the contrast needed, and the x-ray equipment used.

Radiopaque agents are to be used only by or under the direct supervision of a doctor.

## Before Having This Test

In deciding to use a diagnostic test, any risks of the test must be weighed against the good it will do. This is a decision you and your doctor will make. Also, test results may be affected by other things. For radiopaque agents, the following should be considered:

**Allergies**—Tell your doctor if you have ever had any unusual or allergic reaction to iodine, to products containing iodine (for example, iodine-containing foods such as seafood, cabbage, kale, rape [turnip-like vegetable], turnips, or iodized salt), or to any radiopaque agent. Also tell your doctor if you are allergic to any other substance, such as sulfites or other preservatives.

**Pregnancy**—Studies have not been done in humans with most of the radiopaque agents. However, iohexol, iopamidol, iothalamate, ioversol, ioxaglate, and metrizamide have not been shown to cause birth defects or other problems in animal studies. Some of the radiopaque agents, such as diatrizoates have, on rare occasions, caused hypothyroidism (underactive thyroid) in the baby when they were taken late in the pregnancy. Also, x-rays of the abdomen are usually not recommended during pregnancy. This is to avoid exposing the fetus to radiation. Be sure you have discussed this with your doctor.

**Breast-feeding**—Although some of these radiopaque agents pass into the breast milk, they have not been shown to cause problems in nursing babies. However, it may be necessary for you to stop breast-feeding temporarily after receiving a radiopaque agent. Be sure you have discussed this with your doctor.

**Children**—Children, especially those with other medical problems, may be especially sensitive to the effects of radiopaque agents. This may increase the chance of side effects.

**Older adults**—Elderly people are especially sensitive to the effects of radiopaque agents. This may increase the chance of side effects.

**Other medical problems**—The presence of other medical problems may affect the use of radiopaque agents. Make sure you tell your doctor if you have any other medical problems, especially:

- Asthma, hay fever, or other allergies (history of)—If you have a history of these conditions, the risk of having a reaction, such as an allergic reaction to the radiopaque agent, is greater
- Diabetes mellitus (sugar diabetes)—There is a greater risk of having kidney problems
- High blood pressure (severe) or
- Pheochromocytoma (PCC)—Injection of the radiopaque agent may cause a dangerous rise in blood pressure
- Kidney disease (severe)—More serious kidney problems may develop; also, the radiopaque agent may build up in the body and cause side effects
- Liver disease—The radiopaque agent may build up in the body and cause side effects
- Multiple myeloma (bone cancer)—Serious kidney problems may develop in patients with this condition
- Overactive thyroid—A sudden increase in symptoms, such as fast heartbeat or palpitations, unusual tiredness or weakness, nervousness, excessive sweating, or muscle weakness may occur
- Sickle cell disease—The radiopaque agent may promote the formation of abnormal blood cells

## Preparation For This Test

Your doctor may have special instructions for you in preparation for your test. He or she might prescribe a special diet or use of a laxative, depending on the type of test.

If you have not received such instructions or if you do not understand them, check with your doctor in advance.

For some tests your doctor may tell you not to eat for several hours before having the test. This is to prevent any food from coming back up and entering your lungs during the test. You may be allowed to drink small amounts of clear liquids; however, check first with your doctor.

## Precautions After Having This Test

Make sure your doctor knows if you are planning to have any thyroid tests in the near future. Even after several weeks or months the results of the thyroid test may be affected by the iodine in this agent.

## Side Effects of This Medicine

Along with their needed effects, radiopaque agents can sometimes cause serious effects such as severe allergic reactions or heart problems. These effects may occur almost immediately or a few minutes after the radiopaque agent is given. Although these serious side effects appear only rarely, your health care professional will be prepared to give you immediate medical attention if needed. If you have any questions about this, check with your doctor.

Check with your doctor as soon as possible if the following side effects occur:

*With injection into the spinal canal*
*Rare*
    Hallucinations (seeing hearing, or feeling things that are not there); paralysis of one side of body or of legs and arms

Other side effects may occur that usually do not need medical attention. These side effects may go away as your body adjusts to this agent. However, check with your doctor if any of the following side effects continue or are bothersome:

*With oral or rectal use*
*Less common*
    Diarrhea or laxative effect
*With injection into a vein or an artery*
*More common*
    Unusual warmth and flushing of skin
*Less common*
    Chills; dizziness or lightheadedness; headache; nausea or vomiting; pain or burning at the place of injection; sweating; unusual or metallic taste; unusual thirst
*With injection into the spinal canal*
*More common*
    Backache; dizziness; headache (mild to moderate); nausea and vomiting (mild to moderate); stiffness of neck
*Less common or rare*
    Difficult urination; drowsiness; headache (severe); increased sensitivity of eyes to light; increased sweating; loss of appetite; ringing or buzzing in ears; unusual tiredness or weakenss

Not all of the side effects listed above have been reported for each of these agents, but they have been reported for at least one of them. There are some similarities among these agents, so many of the above side effects may occur with any of them.

Other side effects not listed above may also occur in some patients. If you notice any other effects, check with your doctor.

Revised: August 1990
Interim revision: 05/23/94

# RADIOPAQUE AGENTS    Diagnostic, Mucosal

This information applies to the following medicines:
1. Diatrizoate and Iodipamide (dye-a-tri-ZOE-ate and eye-oh-DI-pa-mide)
2. Diatrizoates
3. Iohexol (eye-oh-HEX-ole)
4. Iothalamate (eye-oh-thal-A-mate)
5. Ioxaglate (eye-OX-a-glate)

## Description

Radiopaque agents are drugs used to help diagnose certain medical problems. They contain iodine, which absorbs x-rays. Depending on how the radiopaque agent is given, it builds up in certain areas of the body. The resulting high level of iodine allows the x-rays to make a "picture" of the area.

The mucosal radiopaque agents are used in the diagnosis of:

• Urinary tract diseases—Diatrizoates, Iohexol, Iothalamate
• Uterus and fallopian tube diseases—Diatrizoate and Iodipamide, Diatrizoates, Iohexol, Ioxaglate

A catheter or syringe is used to put the solution of the radiopaque agent into the bladder or ureters to help diagnose problems or diseases of the kidneys or other areas of the urinary tract. It may also be placed into the uterus and fallopian tubes to help diagnose problems or disease of those organs. After the test is done, the patient expels most of the solution by urinating (after bladder or ureter studies) or from the vagina (after uterine or fallopian tube studies).

The doses of radiopaque agents will be different for different patients and depend on the type of test. The strength of the solution is determined by how much iodine it contains. Different tests will require a different strength and amount of solution depending on the age of the patient, the contrast needed, and the x-ray equipment used. Also, for tests of the kidneys and other areas of the urinary tract, the amount of solution to be used depends on the size of the bladder.

Radiopaque agents are to be used only by or under the supervision of a doctor.

## Before Having This Test

In deciding to use a diagnostic test, any risks of the test must be weighed against the good it will do. This is a decision you and your doctor will make. Also, test results may be affected by other things. For radiopaque agents the following should be considered:

Allergies—Tell your doctor if you have ever had any unusual or allergic reaction to iodine, to products containing iodine (for example, iodine-containing foods, such as seafoods, cabbage, kale, rape [turnip-like vegetable], turnips, or iodized salt), or to other radiopaque agents. Also tell your doctor if you are allergic to any other substance, such as sulfites or other preservatives.

Pregnancy—Studies on effects in pregnancy when radiopaque agents are instilled into the bladder or ureters have not been done in women. Studies in animals have been done only with iothalamate, which has not been shown to cause birth defects or other problems.

Diagnostic tests of the uterus and fallopian tubes using radiopaque agents are not recommended during pregnancy or for at least 6 months after a pregnancy has ended. The test may cause other problems, such as infection in the uterus.

Also, radiopaque agents containing iodine have, on rare occasions, caused hypothyroidism (underactive thyroid) in the baby when they were injected late in the pregnancy. In addition, x-rays of the abdomen during pregnancy may have harmful effects on the fetus. Make sure your doctor knows if you are pregnant or if you suspect that you may be pregnant when you are to receive this radiopaque agent.

Breast-feeding—Although small amounts of radiopaque agents are absorbed into the body and may pass into the breast milk, these agents have not been shown to cause problems in nursing babies.

Children—Although there is no specific information about the use of radiopaque agents in children they are not expected to cause different side effects or problems in children than they do in adults when used in the bladder or ureters. There is no specific information about the use of radiopaque agents in children for studies of the uterus or fallopian tubes.

Older adults—Many medicines have not been tested in older people. Therefore, it may not be known whether they work exactly the same way they do in younger adults. Although there is no specific information about the use of radiopaque agents for instillation into the bladder or ureters or into the uterus and fallopian tubes in the elderly, they are not expected to cause different side effects or problems in older people than they do in younger adults.

**Other medical problems**—The presence of other medical problems may affect the use of radiopaque agents. Make sure you tell your doctor if you have any other medical problems, especially:

- Asthma, hay fever, or other allergies (history of)—If you have a history of these conditions, there is a greater chance of having a reaction, such as an allergic reaction, to the radiopaque agent
- Enlarged prostate or
- Kidney disease (severe)—There may be blockage that makes it difficult or impossible to put the solution of the radiopaque agent into the bladder or ureters
- Genital tract infection or
- Urinary tract infection—The risk of complications is greater in patients with these conditions
- Pelvic inflammatory disease (severe)—The condition may be aggravated by this test

## Preparation for This Test

Your doctor may have special instructions for you in preparation for your test, such as the need for a special diet or for a laxative, enema, or vaginal douche depending on the kind of test you are having done. If you have not received such instructions or if you do not understand them, check with your doctor in advance.

For your comfort and for best test results, you may be instructed to urinate just before the procedure.

## Precautions After Having This Test

Make sure your doctor knows if you are planning to have any thyroid tests in the near future. Even after several weeks the results of the thyroid test may be affected by the iodine in this agent.

## Side Effects of This Medicine

Along with its needed effects, radiopaque agents can cause serious side effects such as allergic reactions. These effects may occur almost immediately or a few minutes after the radiopaque agent is given. Although these serious side effects appear only rarely, your health care professional will be prepared to give you immediate medical attention if needed. If you have any questions about this, check with your doctor.

*Check with your health care professional immediately* if any of the following side effects occur:

*Less common*
   Abdominal or stomach pain and discomfort (severe); backache

Other side effects may occur that usually do not need medical attention. These side effects should go away as the effects of the radiopaque agent wear off. However, check with your doctor if any of the following side effects continue or are bothersome:

*More common*
   Abdominal or stomach pain and discomfort
*Less common*
   Chills; fever; nausea and vomiting

Other side effects not listed above may also occur in some patients. If you notice any other effects, check with your doctor.

Revised: August 1990
Interim revision: 05/23/94

---

# RADIOPHARMACEUTICALS   Diagnostic

This information applies to the following medicines when used for diagnosis:

1. Ammonia N 13 (a-MOE-nya)
2. Cyanocobalamin Co 57 (sye-an-oh-koe-BAL-a-min)
3. Ferrous Citrate Fe 59 (FER-us SI-trate)
4. Fludeoxyglucose F 18 (flu-dee-ox-ee-GLOO-kose)
5. Gallium Citrate Ga 67 (GAL-ee-um)
6. Indium In 111 Oxyquinoline (IN-dee-um ox-i-KWIN-oh-leen)
7. Indium In 111 Pentetate (PEN-te-tate)
8. Indium In 111 Satumomab Pendetide
9. Iobenguane, Radioiodinated
10. Iodohippurate Sodium I 123 (eye-oh-doe-HIP-yoor-ate SOE-dee-um)
11. Iodohippurate Sodium I 131
12. Iofetamine I 123 (eye-oh-FET-a-meen)
13. Iothalamate Sodium I 125 (eye-oh-thal-A-mate)
14. Krypton Kr 81m (KRIP-tonn)
15. Radioiodinated Albumin (ray-dee-oh-EYE-oh-din-nay-ted al-BYOO-min)
16. Rubidium Rb 82 (roo-BID-ee-um)
17. Sodium Chromate Cr 51 (KROE-mate)
18. Sodium Iodide I 123 (EYE-oh-dyed)
19. Sodium Iodide I 131
20. Sodium Pertechnetate Tc 99m (per-TEK-ne-tate)
21. Technetium Tc 99m Albumin (tek-NEE-see-um al-BYOO-min)
22. Technetium Tc 99m Albumin Aggregated
23. Technetium Tc 99m Albumin Colloid
24. Technetium Tc 99m Disofenin (DYE-so-fen-in)
25. Technetium Tc 99m Exametazime (ex-a-MET-a-zeem)
26. Technetium Tc 99m Gluceptate (gloo-SEP-tate)
27. Technetium Tc 99m Lidofenin (lye-doe-FEN-in)
28. Technetium Tc 99m Mebrofenin (ME-bro-fen-in)
29. Technetium Tc 99m Medronate (ME-droe-nate)
30. Technetium Tc 99m Mertiatide (meer-TYE-a-tide)
31. Technetium Tc 99m Oxidronate (OX-i-dron-ate)
32. Technetium Tc 99m Pentetate (PEN-te-tate)
33. Technetium Tc 99m Pyrophosphate (peer-oh-FOS-fate)
34. Technetium Tc 99m (Pyro- and trimeta-) Phosphates
35. Technetium Tc 99m Sestamibi (SES-ta-mi-bi)
36. Technetium Tc 99m Succimer (SUX-sim-mer)
37. Technetium Tc 99m Sulfur Colloid
38. Technetium Tc 99m Teboroxime (te-boe-ROX-eem)
39. Thallous Chloride Tl 201 (THA-luss KLOR-ide)
40. Xenon Xe 127 (ZEE-non)
41. Xenon Xe 133

# Description

Radiopharmaceuticals (ray-dee-oh-far-ma-SOO-ti-kals) are agents used to diagnose certain medical problems or treat certain diseases. They may be given to the patient in several different ways. For example, they may be given by mouth, given by injection, or placed into the eye or into the bladder.

These radiopharmaceuticals are used in the diagnosis of:

- Abscess and infection—Gallium Citrate Ga 67, Indium In 111 Oxyquinoline
- Biliary tract blockage—Technetium Tc 99m Disofenin, Technetium Tc 99m Lidofenin, Technetium Tc 99m Mebrofenin
- Blood volume studies—Radioiodinated Albumin, Sodium Chromate Cr 51
- Blood vessel diseases—Sodium Pertechnetate Tc 99m
- Blood vessel diseases of the brain—Ammonia N 13, Iofetamine I 123, Technetium Tc 99m Exametazime, Xenon Xe 133
- Bone diseases—Technetium Tc 99m Medronate, Technetium Tc 99m Oxidronate, Technetium Tc 99m Pyrophosphate, Technetium Tc 99m (Pyro- and trimeta-) Phosphates
- Bone marrow diseases—Sodium Chromate Cr 51, Technetium Tc 99m Albumin Colloid, Technetium Tc 99m Sulfur Colloid
- Brain diseases and tumors—Fludeoxyglucose F 18, Iofetamine I 123, Sodium Pertechnetate Tc 99m, Technetium Tc 99m Exametazime, Technetium Tc 99m Gluceptate, Technetium Tc 99m Pentetate
- Cancer; tumors—Fludeoxyglucose F 18, Gallium Citrate Ga 67, Indium In 111 Satumomab Pendetide, Radioiodinated Iobenguane
- Disorders of iron metabolism and absorption—Ferrous Citrate Fe 59
- Heart disease—Ammonia N 13, Fludeoxyglucose F 18, Rubidium Rb 82, Sodium Pertechnetate Tc 99m, Technetium Tc 99m Albumin, Technetium Tc 99m Sestamibi, Technetium Tc 99m Teboroxime, Thallous Chloride Tl 201
- Heart muscle damage (infarct)—Ammonia N 13, Fludeoxyglucose F 18, Rubidium Rb 82, Technetium Tc 99m Pyrophosphate, Technetium Tc 99m (Pyro- and trimeta-) Phosphates, Technetium Tc 99m Sestamibi, Technetium Tc 99m Teboroxime, Thallous Chloride Tl 201
- Impaired flow of cerebrospinal fluid in brain—Indium In 111 Pentetate
- Kidney diseases—Iodohippurate Sodium I 123, Iodohippurate Sodium I 131, Iothalamate Sodium I 125, Technetium Tc 99m Gluceptate, Technetium Tc 99m Mertiatide, Technetium Tc 99m Pentetate, Technetium Tc 99m Succimer
- Liver diseases—Ammonia N 13, Fludeoxyglucose F 18, Technetium Tc 99m Albumin Colloid, Technetium Tc 99m Disofenin, Technetium Tc 99m Lidofenin, Technetium Tc 99m Mebrofenin, Technetium Tc 99m Sulfur Colloid

- Lung diseases—Krypton Kr 81m, Technetium Tc 99m Albumin Aggregated, Technetium Tc 99m Pentetate, Xenon Xe 127, Xenon Xe 133
- Parathyroid diseases; parathyroid cancer—Technetium Tc 99m Sestamibi, Thallous Chloride Tl 201
- Pernicious anemia; improper absorption of vitamin $B_{12}$ from intestines—Cyanocobalamin Co 57
- Red blood cell diseases—Sodium Chromate Cr 51
- Salivary gland diseases—Sodium Pertechnetate Tc 99m
- Spleen diseases—Sodium Chromate Cr 51, Technetium Tc 99m Albumin Colloid, Technetium Tc 99m Sulfur Colloid
- Stomach and intestinal bleeding—Sodium Chromate Cr 51, Sodium Pertechnetate Tc 99m, Technetium Tc 99m (Pyro- and trimeta-) Phosphates, Technetium Tc 99m Sulfur Colloid
- Stomach problems—Technetium Tc 99m Sulfur Colloid
- Tear duct blockage—Sodium Pertechnetate Tc 99m
- Thyroid diseases; thyroid cancer—Fludeoxyglucose F 18, Radioiodinated Iobenguane, Sodium Iodide I 123, Sodium Iodide I 131, Sodium Pertechnetate Tc 99m, Technetium Tc 99m Sestamibi
- Urinary bladder diseases—Sodium Pertechnetate Tc 99m

Radiopharmaceuticals are radioactive agents. However, when small amounts are used, the radiation your body receives is very low and is considered safe. When larger amounts of these agents are given to treat disease, there may be different effects on the body.

When radiopharmaceuticals are used to help diagnose medical problems, only small amounts are given to the patient. The radiopharmaceutical then passes through, or is taken up by, an organ of the body (which organ depends on what radiopharmaceutical is used and how it has been given). Then the radioactivity is detected, and pictures are produced, by special imaging equipment. These pictures allow the nuclear medicine doctor to study how the organ is working and to detect cancer or tumors that may be present in the organ.

Some radiopharmaceuticals are used in larger amounts to treat certain kinds of cancer and other diseases. In those cases, the radioactive agent is taken up in the cancerous area and destroys the affected tissue. *The information that follows applies only to radiopharmaceuticals when used in small amounts to diagnose medical problems.*

The dosages of radiopharmaceuticals that are used to diagnose medical problems will be different for different patients and depend on the type of test. The amount of radioactivity of a radiopharmaceutical is expressed in units called becquerels or curies. Radiopharmaceutical dosages given may be as small as 0.185 megabecquerels (5 microcuries) or as high as 1295 megabecquerels

(35 millicuries). The radiation received from these dosages may be about the same as, or even less than, the radiation received from an x-ray study of the same organ.

Radiopharmaceuticals are to be given only by or under the direct supervision of a doctor with specialized training in nuclear medicine.

## Before Having This Test

In deciding to use a diagnostic test, any risks of the test must be weighed against the good it will do. This is a decision you and your doctor will make. Also, test results may be affected by other things. For radiopharmaceuticals, the following should be considered:

**Allergies**—If you will be receiving albumin in the form of radioiodinated albumin, technetium Tc 99m albumin aggregated, technetium Tc 99m albumin colloid, or technetium Tc 99m albumin for your test, tell your doctor if you have ever had any unusual or allergic reaction to products containing human serum albumin.

Also tell your doctor if you are allergic to any other substance, such as foods, preservatives, or dyes.

**Pregnancy**—Radiopharmaceuticals usually are not recommended for use during pregnancy. This is to avoid exposing the fetus to radiation. Some radiopharmaceuticals may be used for diagnostic tests in pregnant women, but it is necessary to inform your doctor if you are pregnant so the doctor may reduce the radiation dose to the baby. This is especially important with radiopharmaceuticals that contain radioactive iodine, which can go to the baby's thyroid gland and, in high enough amounts, may cause thyroid damage. Be sure you have discussed this with your doctor.

**Breast-feeding**—Some radiopharmaceuticals pass into the breast milk and may expose the baby to radiation. If you must receive a radiopharmaceutical, it may be necessary for you to stop breast-feeding for some time after receiving it. Be sure you have discussed this with your doctor.

**Children**—For most radiopharmaceuticals, the amount of radiation used for a diagnostic test is very low and considered safe. However, be sure you have discussed with your doctor the benefit versus the risk of exposing your child to radiation.

**Older adults**—Many medicines have not been studied specifically in older people. Therefore, it may not be known whether they work exactly the same way they do in younger adults or if they cause different side effects or problems in older people. Although there is no specific information comparing use of most radiopharmaceuticals in the elderly with use in other age groups, problems would not be expected to occur. However, it is a good idea to check with your doctor if you notice any unusual effects after receiving a radiopharmaceutical.

**Other medicines**—Although certain medicines should not be used together at all, in other cases two different medicines may be used together even if an interaction might

occur. In these cases, your doctor may want to change the dose, or other precautions may be necessary. When you are going to receive a radiopharmaceutical, it is especially important that your doctor know if you are taking any other prescription or nonprescription (over-the-counter [OTC]) medicine.

In addition, if you will be receiving radioactive iodine (sodium iodide I 123, sodium iodide I 131) or sodium pertechnetate Tc 99m for a thyroid test, it is especially important that your doctor know if you have been taking iodine through other medicine or foods. For example, the results of your test may be affected if:

- You are taking iodine-containing medicines, including certain multivitamins and cough syrups.
- You eat large amounts of iodine-containing foods, such as iodized salt, seafood, cabbage, kale, rape (turnip-like vegetable), or turnips.
- You have had an x-ray test recently for which you were given a special dye that contained iodine.

**Other medical problems**—The presence of other medical problems may affect the use of radiopharmaceuticals. Make sure you tell your doctor if you have any other medical problems.

## Preparation for This Test

The nuclear medicine doctor may have special instructions for you in preparation for your test. For example, before some tests you must fast for several hours, or the results of the test may be affected. For other tests you should drink plenty of liquids. If you do not understand the instructions you receive or if you have not received any instructions, check with the nuclear medicine doctor in advance.

## Precautions After Having This Test

There are usually no special precautions to observe for radiopharmaceuticals when they are used in small amounts for diagnosis.

Some radiopharmaceuticals may accumulate in your bladder. Therefore, to increase the flow of urine and lessen the amount of radiation to your bladder, your doctor may instruct you to drink plenty of liquids and urinate often after certain tests.

For patients receiving *radioactive iodine (iodohippurate sodium I 123, iodohippurate sodium I 131, iofetamine I 123, iothalamate I 125, radioiodinated albumin, or radioiodinated iobenguane)*:

- Make sure your doctor knows if you are planning to have any future thyroid tests. Even after several weeks, the results of the thyroid test may be affected by the iodine solution that may be given before the radiopharmaceutical.

## Side Effects of This Medicine

Along with its needed effects, a medicine may cause some unwanted effects. When radiopharmaceuticals are used in very small doses to study an organ of the body, side effects are rare and usually involve an allergic reaction. These effects may occur almost immediately or a few minutes after the radiopharmaceutical is given. It may be helpful to note the time when you first notice any side effect. Your doctor, nuclear medicine physician and/or technologist, or nurse will be prepared to give you immediate medical attention if needed.

*Check with your doctor or nurse immediately* if any of the following side effects occur:

*Rare*

Chills; difficulty breathing; drowsiness (severe); fainting; fast heartbeat; fever; flushing or redness of skin; head-ache (severe); nausea or vomiting; skin rash, hives, or itching; stomach pain; swelling of throat, hands, or feet

Other side effects not listed above may also occur in some patients. If you notice any other effects, note the time when they start and check with your doctor.

---

Revised: 08/30/94

---

# RAUWOLFIA ALKALOIDS    Systemic

Some commonly used brand names are:

**In the U.S.—**

| | |
|---|---|
| Harmonyl[1] | Rauverid[2] |
| Raudixin[2] | Serpalan[3] |
| Rauval[2] | Wolfina[2] |

**In Canada—**

| | |
|---|---|
| Novoreserpine[3] | Serpasil[3] |
| Reserfia[3] | |

Note: For quick reference, the following rauwolfia alkaloids are numbered to match the corresponding brand names.

This information applies to the following medicines:

1. Deserpidine (de-SER-pi-deen)[†]
2. Rauwolfia Serpentina (rah-WOOL-fee-a ser-pen-TEE-na)[†‡]
3. Reserpine (re-SER-peen)[‡]

[†]Not commercially available in Canada.

[‡]Generic product may also be available in the U.S.

## Description

Rauwolfia alkaloids belong to the general class of medicines called antihypertensives. They are used to treat high blood pressure (hypertension).

High blood pressure adds to the workload of the heart and arteries. If it continues for a long time, the heart and arteries may not function properly. This can damage the blood vessels of the brain, heart, and kidneys, resulting in a stroke, heart failure, or kidney failure. High blood pressure may also increase the risk of heart attacks. These problems may be less likely to occur if blood pressure is controlled.

Rauwolfia alkaloids work by controlling nerve impulses along certain nerve pathways. As a result, they act on the heart and blood vessels to lower blood pressure.

Rauwolfia alkaloids may also be used to treat other conditions as determined by your doctor.

These medicines are available only with your doctor's prescription, in the following dosage forms:

*Oral*

Deserpidine
• Tablets (U.S.)
Rauwolfia Serpentina
• Tablets (U.S.)
Reserpine
• Tablets (U.S. and Canada)

## Before Using This Medicine

In deciding to use a medicine, the risks of taking the medicine must be weighed against the good it will do. This is a decision you and your doctor will make. For rauwolfia alkaloids, the following should be considered:

**Allergies**—Tell your doctor if you have ever had any unusual or allergic reaction to rauwolfia alkaloids. Also tell your health care professional if you are allergic to any other substance, such as foods, preservatives, or dyes.

**Pregnancy**—Rauwolfia alkaloids have not been studied in pregnant women. However, too much use of rauwolfia alkaloids during pregnancy may cause unwanted effects (difficult breathing, low temperature, loss of appetite) in the baby. In rats, use of rauwolfia alkaloids during pregnancy causes birth defects and in guinea pigs decreases newborn survival rates. Before taking this medicine, make sure your doctor knows if you are pregnant or if you may become pregnant.

**Breast-feeding**—Rauwolfia alkaloids pass into breast milk and may cause unwanted effects (difficult breathing, low temperature, loss of appetite) in infants of mothers taking large doses of this medicine. Be sure you have discussed this with your doctor before taking this medicine.

**Children**—Although there is no specific information comparing use of rauwolfia alkaloids in children with use in other age groups, rauwolfia alkaloids are not expected to cause different side effects or problems in children than they do in adults.

**Older adults**—Many medicines have not been studied specifically in older people. Therefore, it may not be known whether they work exactly the same way they do in younger adults. Although there is no specific information comparing use of rauwolfia alkaloids in the elderly with use in other age groups, dizziness or drowsiness may be more likely to occur in the elderly, who are more sensitive to the effects of rauwolfia alkaloids.

**Other medicines**—Although certain medicines should not be used together at all, in other cases two different medicines may be used together even if an interaction might occur. In these cases, your doctor may want to change the dose, or other precautions may be necessary. When you are taking rauwolfia alkaloids, it is especially important that your health care professional know if you are taking any of the following:

- Monoamine oxidase (MAO) inhibitors (furazolidone [e.g., Furoxone], isocarboxazid [e.g., Marplan], phenelzine [e.g., Nardil], procarbazine [e.g., Matulane], selegiline [e.g., Eldepryl], tranylcypromine [e.g., Parnate])—Taking a rauwolfia alkaloid while you are taking or within 2 weeks of taking MAO inhibitors may increase the risk of central nervous system depression or may cause a severe high blood pressure reaction

**Other medical problems**—The presence of other medical problems may affect the use of rauwolfia alkaloids. Make sure you tell your doctor if you have any other medical problems, especially:

- Allergies or other breathing problems such as asthma—Rauwolfia alkaloids can cause breathing problems
- Epilepsy
- Gallstones or
- Stomach ulcer or
- Ulcerative colitis—Rauwolfia alkaloids increase activity of the stomach, which may make the condition worse
- Heart disease—Rauwolfia alkaloids can cause heart rhythm problems or slow heartbeat
- Kidney disease—Some patients may not do well when blood pressure is lowered by rauwolfia alkaloids
- Mental depression (or history of)—Rauwolfia alkaloids cause mental depression
- Parkinson's disease—Rauwolfia alkaloids can cause parkinsonism-like effects
- Pheochromocytoma

## Proper Use of This Medicine

For patients taking this medicine *for high blood pressure*:

- In addition to the use of the medicine your doctor has prescribed, treatment for your high blood pressure may include weight control and care in the types of foods you eat, especially foods high in sodium. Your doctor will tell you which of these are most important for you. You should check with your doctor before changing your diet.
- Many patients who have high blood pressure will not notice any signs of the problem. In fact, many may feel normal. It is very important that you *take your medicine exactly as directed* and that you keep your appointments with your doctor even if you feel well.
- Remember that this medicine will not cure your high blood pressure but it does help control it. Therefore, you must continue to take it as directed if you expect to lower your blood pressure and keep it down. *You may have to take high blood pressure medicine for the rest of your life.* If high blood pressure is not treated, it can cause serious problems such as heart failure, blood vessel disease, stroke, or kidney disease.

To help you remember to take your medicine, try to get into the habit of taking it at the same time each day.

This medicine is sometimes given together with certain other medicines. If you are using a combination of drugs, make sure that you take each medicine at the proper time and do not mix them. Ask your health care professional to help you plan a way to remember to take your medicines at the right times.

If this medicine upsets your stomach, it may be taken with meals or milk. If stomach upset (nausea, vomiting, stomach cramps or pain) continues or gets worse, check with your doctor.

**Dosing**—The dose of these medicines will be different for different patients. *Follow your doctor's orders or the directions on the label.* The following information includes only the average doses of these medicines. *If your dose is different, do not change it* unless your doctor tells you to do so.

The number of tablets that you take depends on the strength of the medicine.

*For deserpidine*

- For *oral* dosage form (tablets):
  —For high blood pressure:
    - Adults—250 to 500 micrograms (mcg) a day. This may be taken as a single dose or divided into two doses.
    - Children—Dose must be determined by your doctor.

*For rauwolfia serpentina*

- For *oral* dosage form (tablets):
  —For high blood pressure:
    - Adults—50 to 200 milligrams (mg) a day. This may be taken as a single dose or divided into two doses.
    - Children—Dose must be determined by your doctor.

*For reserpine*

- For *oral* dosage form (tablets):
  —For high blood pressure:
    - Adults—100 to 250 micrograms (mcg) a day.
    - Children—Dose is based on body weight and must be determined by your doctor. The usual dose is 5 to 20 mcg per kilogram (kg) (2.27 to 9.1 mcg per pound) of body weight a day. This may be taken as a single dose or divided into two doses.

**Missed dose**—If you miss a dose of this medicine, do not take the missed dose at all and do not double the next one. Instead, go back to your regular dosing schedule.

**Storage**—To store this medicine:

- Keep out of the reach of children.
- Store away from heat and direct light.

- Do not store in the bathroom, near the kitchen sink, or in other damp places. Heat or moisture may cause the medicine to break down.
- Do not keep outdated medicine or medicine no longer needed. Be sure that any discarded medicine is out of the reach of children.

## Precautions While Using This Medicine

It is important that your doctor check your progress at regular visits to make sure that this medicine is working properly.

For patients taking this medicine *for high blood pressure*:

- *Do not take other medicines unless they have been discussed with your doctor.* This especially includes over-the-counter (nonprescription) medicines for appetite control, asthma, colds, cough, hay fever, or sinus problems, since they may tend to increase your blood pressure.

Before having any kind of surgery (including dental surgery) or emergency treatment, *tell the medical doctor or dentist in charge that you are taking this medicine.*

In some patients, this medicine may cause mental depression. *Tell your doctor right away:*

- if you or anyone else notices unusual changes in your mood.
- if you start having early-morning sleeplessness or unusually vivid dreams or nightmares.

This medicine will add to the effects of alcohol and other CNS depressants (medicines that slow down the nervous system, possibly causing drowsiness). Some examples of CNS depressants are antihistamines or medicine for hay fever, other allergies, or colds; sedatives, tranquilizers, or sleeping medicine; prescription pain medicine or narcotics; barbiturates; medicine for seizures; muscle relaxants; or anesthetics, including some dental anesthetics. *Check with your doctor before taking any of the above while you are using this medicine.*

This medicine may cause some people to become drowsy or less alert than they are normally. This is more likely to happen when you begin to take it or when you increase the amount of medicine you are taking. *Make sure you know how you react to this medicine before you drive, use machines, or do anything else that could be dangerous if you are not alert.*

This medicine may cause dryness of the mouth. For temporary relief, use sugarless candy or gum, melt bits of ice in your mouth, or use a saliva substitute. However, if dry mouth continues for more than 2 weeks, check with your medical doctor or dentist. Continuing dryness of the mouth may increase the chance of dental disease, including tooth decay, gum disease, and fungus infections.

This medicine often causes stuffiness in the nose. However, do not use nasal decongestant medicines without first checking with your health care professional.

## Side Effects of This Medicine

Suggestions that rauwolfia alkaloids may increase the risk of breast cancer occurring later have not been proven. However, rats and mice given 100 to 300 times the human dose had an increased number of tumors.

Along with its needed effects, a medicine may cause some unwanted effects. Although not all of these side effects may occur, if they do occur they may need medical attention.

*Check with your doctor immediately* if any of the following side effects occur:

*Less common*

Drowsiness or faintness; impotence or decreased sexual interest; lack of energy or weakness; mental depression or inability to concentrate; nervousness or anxiety; vivid dreams or nightmares or early-morning sleeplessness

Check with your doctor as soon as possible if any of the following side effects occur:

*More common*

Dizziness

*Less common*

Black, tarry stools; bloody vomit; chest pain; headache; irregular heartbeat; shortness of breath; slow heartbeat; stomach cramps or pain

*Rare*

Painful or difficult urination; skin rash or itching; stiffness; trembling and shaking of hands and fingers; unusual bleeding or bruising

*Signs and symptoms of overdose*

Dizziness or drowsiness (severe); flushing of skin; pinpoint pupils of eyes; slow pulse

Other side effects may occur that usually do not need medical attention. These side effects may go away during treatment as your body adjusts to the medicine. However, check with your doctor if any of the following side effects continue or are bothersome:

*More common*

Diarrhea; dryness of mouth; loss of appetite; nausea and vomiting; stuffy nose

*Less common*

Swelling of feet and lower legs

After you stop using this medicine, it may still produce some side effects that need attention. During this period of time *check with your doctor immediately* if you notice any of the following side effects:

Drowsiness or faintness; impotence or decreased sexual interest; irregular or slow heartbeat; lack of energy or weakness; mental depression or inability to concentrate; nervousness or anxiety; vivid dreams or nightmares or early-morning sleeplessness

Other side effects not listed above may also occur in some patients. If you notice any other effects, check with your doctor.

## Additional Information

Once a medicine has been approved for marketing for a certain use, experience may show that it is also useful for other medical problems. Although this use is not included in product labeling, reserpine is used in certain patients with the following medical condition:

- Raynaud's disease

Other than the above information, there is no additional information relating to proper use, precautions, or side effects for these uses.

---

Revised: 07/28/92
Interim revision: 07/20/94

---

# RAUWOLFIA ALKALOIDS AND THIAZIDE DIURETICS    Systemic

Some commonly used brand names are:

**In the U.S.—**

| | |
|---|---|
| Demi-Regroton[5] | Mallopres[6] |
| Diupres[4] | Metatensin[10] |
| Diurese-R[10] | Naquival[10] |
| Diurigen with Reserpine[4] | Oreticyl[1] |
| Diutensen-R[8] | Oreticyl Forte[1] |
| Enduronyl[2] | Rauzide[3] |
| Enduronyl Forte[2] | Regroton[5] |
| Hydropine[7] | Renese-R[9] |
| Hydropine H.P.[7] | Salazide[7] |
| Hydropres[6] | Salutensin[7] |
| Hydrosine[6] | Salutensin-Demi[7] |
| Hydrotensin[6] | |

**In Canada—**

| | |
|---|---|
| Dureticyl[2] | Salutensin[7] |
| Hydropres[6] | |

Note: For quick reference, the following rauwolfia alkaloids and thiazide diuretics are numbered to match the corresponding brand names.

This information applies to the following medicines:

1. Deserpidine (de-SER-pi-deen) and Hydrochlorothiazide (hye-droe-klor-oh-THYE-a-zide)†
2. Deserpidine and Methyclothiazide (meth-i-kloe-THYE-a-zide)‡
3. Rauwolfia Serpentina (rah-WOOL-fee-a ser-pen-TEE-na) and Bendroflumethiazide (ben-droe-floo-meth-EYE-a-zide)†
4. Reserpine (re-SER-peen) and Chlorothiazide (klor-oh-THYE-a-zide)†‡
5. Reserpine and Chlorthalidone (klor-THAL-i-done)†
6. Reserpine and Hydrochlorothiazide‡
7. Reserpine and Hydroflumethiazide (hye-droe-floo-meth-EYE-a-zide)‡
8. Reserpine and Methyclothiazide†
9. Reserpine and Polythiazide (pol-i-THYE-a-zide)†
10. Reserpine and Trichlormethiazide (trye-klor-meth-EYE-a-zide)†‡

---

†Not commercially available in Canada.
‡Generic name product may also be available in the U.S.

---

## Description

Rauwolfia alkaloid and thiazide diuretic combinations are used in the treatment of high blood pressure (hypertension).

High blood pressure adds to the workload of the heart and arteries. If it continues for a long time, the heart and arteries may not function properly. This can damage the blood vessels of the brain, heart, and kidneys, resulting in a stroke, heart failure, or kidney failure. High blood pressure may also increase the risk of heart attacks. These problems may be less likely to occur if blood pressure is controlled.

Rauwolfia alkaloids work by controlling nerve impulses along certain nerve pathways. As a result, they act on the heart and blood vessels to lower blood pressure. Thiazide diuretics help to reduce the amount of water in the body by increasing the flow of urine. This also helps to lower blood pressure.

These medicines are available only with your doctor's prescription, in the following dosage forms:

*Oral*

Deserpidine and Hydrochlorothiazide
- Tablets (U.S.)

Deserpidine and Methyclothiazide
- Tablets (U.S. and Canada)

Rauwolfia Serpentina and Bendroflumethiazide
- Tablets (U.S.)

Reserpine and Chlorothiazide
- Tablets (U.S.)

Reserpine and Chlorthalidone
- Tablets (U.S.)

Reserpine and Hydrochlorothiazide
- Tablets (U.S. and Canada)

Reserpine and Hydroflumethiazide
- Tablets (U.S. and Canada)

Reserpine and Methyclothiazide
- Tablets (U.S.)

Reserpine and Polythiazide
- Tablets (U.S.)

Reserpine and Trichlormethiazide
- Tablets (U.S.)

---

## Before Using This Medicine

In deciding to use a medicine, the risks of taking the medicine must be weighed against the good it will do. This is a decision you and your doctor will make. For rauwolfia alkaloids and thiazide diuretics, the following should be considered:

**Allergies**—Tell your doctor if you have ever had any unusual or allergic reaction to sulfonamides (sulfa drugs), thiazide diuretics (water pills), or rauwolfia alkaloids. Also tell your health care professional if you are allergic to any other substance, such as foods, preservatives, or dyes.

**Pregnancy**—Too much use of thiazide diuretics (contained in this combination medicine) during pregnancy may cause unwanted effects including jaundice, blood problems, and low potassium in the baby. Too much use of rauwolfia alkaloids may cause difficult breathing, low temperature, and loss of appetite in the baby. This medicine has not been shown to cause birth defects in humans. In rats, use of rauwolfia alkaloids during pregnancy decreases newborn survival rates. Be sure that you have discussed this with your doctor before taking this medicine.

**Breast-feeding**—Rauwolfia alkaloids pass into breast milk and may cause unwanted effects (difficult breathing, low temperature, loss of appetite) in infants of mothers taking it in large doses. Thiazide diuretics also pass into breast milk. Be sure you have discussed this with your doctor before taking this medicine.

**Children**—Although there is no specific information comparing use of these medicines in children with use in other age groups, these medicines are not expected to cause different side effects or problems in children than they do in adults.

**Older adults**—Many medicines have not been studied specifically in older people. Therefore, it may not be known whether they work exactly the same way they do in younger adults. Although there is no specific information comparing use of rauwolfia alkaloid and thiazide diuretic combinations in the elderly with use in other age groups, this medicine is not expected to cause different side effects or problems in older people than it does in younger adults. However, drowsiness, dizziness, or faintness or symptoms of too much potassium loss may be more likely to occur in the elderly, who are more sensitive to the effects of rauwolfia alkaloids and thiazide diuretics.

**Other medicines**—Although certain medicines should not be used together at all, in other cases two different medicines may be used together even if an interaction might occur. In these cases, your doctor may want to change the dose, or other precautions may be necessary. When you are taking rauwolfia alkaloids and thiazide diuretics, it is especially important that your health care professional know if you are taking any of the following:

- Cholestyramine or
- Colestipol—Use with thiazide diuretics may prevent the diuretic from working properly; take the diuretic at least 1 hour before or 4 hours after cholestyramine or colestipol
- Digitalis glycosides (heart medicine)—Thiazide diuretics may cause low potassium in the blood, which can lead to symptoms of digitalis toxicity
- Lithium (e.g., Lithane)—Risk of lithium overdose, even at usual doses, may be increased
- Monoamine oxidase (MAO) inhibitors (furazolidone [e.g., Furoxone], isocarboxazid [e.g., Marplan], phenelzine [e.g., Nardil], procarbazine [e.g., Matulane], selegiline [e.g., Eldepryl], tranylcypromine [e.g., Parnate])—Taking a rauwolfia alkaloid while you are taking or within 2 weeks of taking MAO inhibitors may increase the risk of central nervous system depression or may cause a severe high blood pressure reaction

**Other medical problems**—The presence of other medical problems may affect the use of rauwolfia alkaloids and thiazide diuretics. Make sure you tell your doctor if you have any other medical problems, especially:

- Allergies or other breathing problems such as asthma—Rauwolfia alkaloids can cause breathing problems
- Diabetes mellitus (sugar diabetes)—Thiazide diuretics may change the amount of diabetes medicine needed
- Epilepsy
- Gallstones or
- Stomach ulcer or
- Ulcerative colitis—Rauwolfia alkaloids increase activity of the stomach, which may make the condition worse
- Gout (history of)—Thiazide diuretics may increase the amount of uric acid in the blood, which can lead to gout
- Heart disease—Rauwolfia alkaloids can cause heart rhythm problems or slow heartbeat
- Kidney disease—Some patients may not do well when blood pressure is lowered by this medicine. If kidney disease is severe, thiazide diuretics may not work
- Liver disease—If thiazide diuretics cause loss of too much water from the body, liver disease can become much worse
- Lupus erythematosus (history of)—Thiazide diuretics may worsen the condition
- Mental depression (or history of)—Rauwolfia alkaloids cause mental depression
- Pancreatitis (inflammation of pancreas)
- Parkinson's disease—Rauwolfia alkaloids can cause parkinsonism-like effects
- Pheochromocytoma

## Proper Use of This Medicine

In addition to the use of the medicine your doctor has prescribed, treatment for your high blood pressure may include weight control and care in the types of foods you eat, especially foods high in sodium. Your doctor will tell you which of these are most important for you. You should check with your doctor before changing your diet.

Many patients who have high blood pressure will not notice any signs of the problem. In fact, many may feel normal. It is very important that you *take your medicine exactly as directed* and that you keep your appointments with your doctor even if you feel well.

Remember that this medicine will not cure your high blood pressure but it does help control it. Therefore, you must continue to take it as directed if you expect to lower your blood pressure and keep it down. *You may have to take high blood pressure medicine for the rest of your life.* If high blood pressure is not treated, it can cause serious problems such as heart failure, blood vessel disease, stroke, or kidney disease.

This medicine may cause you to have an unusual feeling of tiredness when you begin to take it. You may also notice an increase in the amount of urine or in your frequency of urination. After you have taken the medicine for a while, these effects should lessen. In general, to keep the increase in urine from affecting your sleep:

- If you are to take a single dose a day, take it in the morning after breakfast.

- If you are to take more than one dose a day, take the last dose no later than 6 p.m., unless otherwise directed by your doctor.

However, it is best to plan your dose or doses according to a schedule that will least affect your personal activities and sleep. Ask your health care professional to help you plan the best time to take this medicine.

To help you remember to take your medicine, try to get into the habit of taking it at the same time each day.

If this medicine upsets your stomach, it may be taken with meals or milk. If stomach upset (nausea, vomiting, stomach pain or cramps) continues, check with your doctor.

**Dosing**—The dose of these medicines will be different for different patients. *Follow your doctor's orders or the directions on the label.* The following information includes only the average doses of these medicines. *If your dose is different, do not change it* unless your doctor tells you to do so.

*For deserpidine and hydrochlorothiazide combination*
- For *oral* dosage form (tablets):
  —For high blood pressure:
    - Adults—1 tablet two times a day.
    - Children—Dose must be determined by your doctor.

*For deserpidine and methyclothiazide combination*
- For *oral* dosage form (tablets):
  —For high blood pressure:
    - Adults—One-half to 1 tablet a day.
    - Children—Dose must be determined by your doctor.

*For rauwolfia serpentina and bendroflumethiazide combination*
- For *oral* dosage form (tablets):
  —For high blood pressure:
    - Adults—1 to 4 tablets a day.
    - Children—Dose must be determined by your doctor.

*For reserpine and chlorothiazide combination*
- For *oral* dosage form (tablets):
  —For high blood pressure:
    - Adults—1 or 2 tablets one or two times a day.
    - Children—Dose must be determined by your doctor.

*For reserpine and chlorthalidone combination*
- For *oral* dosage form (tablets):
  —For high blood pressure:
    - Adults—1 or 2 tablets once a day.
    - Children—Dose must be determined by your doctor.

*For reserpine and hydrochlorothiazide combination*
- For *oral* dosage form (tablets):
  —For high blood pressure:
    - Adults—1 tablet one to four times a day.
    - Children—Dose must be determined by your doctor.

*For reserpine and hydroflumethiazide combination*
- For *oral* dosage form (tablets):
  —For high blood pressure:
    - Adults—1 tablet one or two times a day.
    - Children—Dose must be determined by your doctor.

*For reserpine and methyclothiazide combination*
- For *oral* dosage form (tablets):
  —For high blood pressure:
    - Adults—1 to 4 tablets a day.
    - Children—Dose must be determined by your doctor.

*For reserpine and polythiazide combination*
- For *oral* dosage form (tablets):
  —For high blood pressure:
    - Adults—One-half to 2 tablets a day.
    - Children—Dose must be determined by your doctor.

*For reserpine and trichlormethiazide combination*
- For *oral* dosage form (tablets):
  —For high blood pressure:
    - Adults—1 or 2 tablets a day. This may be taken as a single dose or divided into smaller doses.
    - Children—Dose must be determined by your doctor.

**Missed dose**—If you miss a dose of this medicine, take it as soon as possible. However, if it is almost time for your next dose, skip the missed dose and go back to your regular dosing schedule. Do not double doses.

**Storage**—To store this medicine:
- Keep out of the reach of children.
- Store away from heat and direct light.
- Do not store in the bathroom, near the kitchen sink, or in other damp places. Heat or moisture may cause the medicine to break down.
- Do not keep outdated medicine or medicine no longer needed. Be sure that any discarded medicine is out of the reach of children.

## Precautions While Using This Medicine

It is important that your doctor check your progress at regular visits to make sure that this medicine is working properly.

*Do not take other medicines unless they have been discussed with your doctor.* This especially includes over-the-counter (nonprescription) medicines for appetite control, asthma, colds, cough, hay fever, or sinus problems, since they may tend to increase your blood pressure.

Before having any kind of surgery (including dental surgery), or emergency treatment, *tell the medical doctor or dentist in charge that you are taking this medicine.*

This medicine may cause a loss of potassium from your body.

- To help prevent this, your doctor may want you to:
  —eat or drink foods that have a high potassium content (for example, orange or other citrus fruit juices), or
  —take a potassium supplement, or
  —take another medicine to help prevent the loss of the potassium in the first place.
- It is very important to follow these directions. Also, it is important not to change your diet on your own. This is more important if you are already on a special diet (as for diabetes), or if you are taking a potassium supplement or a medicine to reduce potassium loss. Extra potassium may not be necessary and, in some cases, too much potassium could be harmful.

Check with your doctor if you become sick and have severe or continuing vomiting or diarrhea. These problems may cause you to lose additional water and potassium.

This medicine may cause some people to become drowsy or less alert than they are normally. This is more likely to happen when you begin to take it or when you increase the amount of medicine you are taking. *Make sure you know how you react to this medicine before you drive, use machines, or do anything else that could be dangerous if you are not alert.*

*Dizziness, lightheadedness, or fainting may occur, especially when you get up from a lying or sitting position.* This is more likely to occur in the morning. Getting up slowly may help. When you get up from lying down, sit on the edge of the bed with your feet dangling for 1 or 2 minutes. Then stand up slowly. If the problem continues or gets worse, check with your doctor.

The dizziness, lightheadedness, or fainting is also more likely to occur if you drink alcohol, stand for a long time, exercise, or if the weather is hot. *While you are taking this medicine, be careful to limit the amount of alcohol you drink. Also, use extra care during exercise or hot weather or if you must stand for a long time.*

In some patients, this medicine may cause mental depression. *Tell your doctor right away:*
- if you or anyone else notices unusual changes in your moods.
- if you start having early-morning sleeplessness or unusually vivid dreams or nightmares.

This medicine will add to the effects of alcohol and other CNS depressants (medicines that slow down the nervous system, possibly causing drowsiness). Some examples of CNS depressants are antihistamines or medicine for hay fever, other allergies, or colds; sedatives, tranquilizers, or sleeping medicine; prescription pain medicine or narcotics; barbiturates; medicine for seizures; muscle relaxants; or anesthetics, including dental anesthetics. *Check with your doctor before taking any of the above while you are taking this medicine.*

For *diabetic patients*:
- This medicine may raise blood sugar levels. While you are using this medicine, be especially careful in testing for sugar in your urine. If you have any questions about this, check with your doctor.

Some people who take this medicine may become more sensitive to sunlight than they are normally. Exposure to sunlight, even for brief periods of time, may cause severe sunburn; skin rash, redness, itching, or discoloration; or vision changes. When you begin taking this medicine:
- Stay out of direct sunlight, especially between the hours of 10:00 a.m. and 3:00 p.m., if possible.
- Wear protective clothing, including a hat and sunglasses.
- Apply a sun block product that has a skin protection factor (SPF) of at least 15. Some patients may require a product with a higher SPF number, especially if they have a fair complexion. If you have any questions about this, check with your health care professional.
- Do not use a sunlamp or tanning bed or booth.

If you have a severe reaction from the sun, check with your doctor.

This medicine often causes stuffiness in the nose. However, do not use nasal decongestant medicines without first checking with your health care professional.

This medicine may cause dryness of the mouth. For temporary relief, use sugarless candy or gum, melt bits of ice in your mouth, or use a saliva substitute. However, if dry mouth continues for more than 2 weeks, check with your medical doctor or dentist. Continuing dryness of the mouth may increase the chance of dental disease, including tooth decay, gum disease, and fungus infections.

---

## Side Effects of This Medicine

Suggestions that rauwolfia alkaloids may increase the risk of breast cancer occurring later have not been proven. However, rats and mice given 100 to 300 times the human dose had an increased risk of tumors.

Along with its needed effects, a medicine may cause some unwanted effects. Although not all of these side effects may occur, if they do occur they may need medical attention.

*Check with your doctor immediately if any of the following side effects occur:*

*Less common*

Drowsiness or faintness; impotence or decreased sexual interest; lack of energy or weakness; mental depression or inability to concentrate; nervousness or anxiety; vivid dreams or nightmares or early-morning sleeplessness

Check with your doctor as soon as possible if any of the following side effects occur:

*Less common*

Black, tarry stools; bloody vomit; chest pain; headache; irregular or slow heartbeat; joint pain; shortness of breath

*Rare*

Painful or difficult urination; skin rash or itching; sore throat and fever; stiffness; stomach pain (severe) with nausea and vomiting; trembling and shaking of hands and fingers; unusual bleeding or bruising; yellow eyes or skin

*Symptoms of too much potassium loss or overdose*

Dry mouth; increased thirst; muscle cramps or pain; nausea or vomiting

*Other signs and symptoms of overdose*

Dizziness or drowsiness, severe; flushing of skin; pinpoint pupils of eyes; slow pulse

Other side effects may occur that usually do not need medical attention. These side effects may go away during treatment as your body adjusts to the medicine. However, check with your doctor if any of the following side effects continue or are bothersome:

*More common*

Diarrhea; dizziness, especially when getting up from a lying or sitting position; loss of appetite; stuffy nose

After you stop using this medicine, it may still produce some side effects that need attention. During this period of time *check with your doctor immediately* if you notice any of the following side effects:

Drowsiness or faintness; impotence or decreased sexual interest; irregular or slow heartbeat; lack of energy or weakness; mental depression or inability to concentrate; nervousness or anxiety; vivid dreams or nightmares or early-morning sleeplessness

Other side effects not listed above may also occur in some patients. If you notice any other effects, check with your doctor.

---

Revised: 09/22/92
Interim revision: 07/20/94

---

# RESERPINE, HYDRALAZINE, AND HYDROCHLOROTHIAZIDE   Systemic

Some commonly used brand names are:

**In the U.S.—**

| | |
|---|---|
| Cam-Ap-Es | Ser-Ap-Es |
| Cherapas | Serpazide |
| Ser-A-Gen | Tri-Hydroserpine |
| Seralazide | Unipres |

Generic name product may also be available.

**In Canada—**

Ser-Ap-Es

## Description

Reserpine (re-SER-peen), hydralazine (hye-DRAL-a-zeen), and hydrochlorothiazide (hye-droe-KLOR-oh-THYE-a-zide) combinations are used to treat high blood pressure (hypertension).

High blood pressure adds to the workload of the heart and arteries. If it continues for a long time, the heart and arteries may not function properly. This can damage the blood vessels of the brain, heart, and kidneys, resulting in a stroke, heart failure, or kidney failure. High blood pressure may also increase the risk of heart attacks. These problems may be less likely to occur if blood pressure is controlled.

Reserpine works by controlling nerve impulses along certain nerve pathways. As a result, it acts on the heart and blood vessels to lower blood pressure. Hydralazine works by relaxing blood vessels and increasing the supply of blood to the heart while reducing its work load. Hydrochlorothiazide is a thiazide diuretic (water pill) that helps to reduce the amount of water in the body by increasing the flow of urine. This also helps to lower blood pressure.

This medicine is available only with your doctor's prescription, in the following dosage form:

*Oral*
- Tablets (U.S. and Canada)

---

## Before Using This Medicine

In deciding to use a medicine, the risks of taking the medicine must be weighed against the good it will do. This is a decision you and your doctor will make. For reserpine, hydralazine, and hydrochlorothiazide, the following should be considered:

**Allergies**—Tell your doctor if you have ever had any unusual or allergic reaction to hydralazine, sulfonamides (sulfa drugs), thiazide diuretics (water pills), or rauwolfia alkaloids. Also tell your health care professional if you are allergic to any other substances, such as foods, preservatives, or dyes.

**Pregnancy**—Too much use of reserpine and hydrochlorothiazide during pregnancy may cause unwanted effects (jaundice, blood problems, low potassium, difficult breathing, low temperatures, and loss of appetite) in the baby. In rats, rauwolfia alkaloids (like reserpine) decrease newborn survival rates.

Studies with hydralazine have not been done in humans. However, studies in mice have shown that hydralazine causes birth defects (cleft palate, defects in head and face bones); these birth defects may also occur in rabbits, but do not occur in rats. Be sure that you have discussed this with your doctor before taking this medicine.

**Breast-feeding**—Reserpine passes into breast milk and may cause unwanted effects (difficult breathing, low temperature, loss of appetite) in infants of mothers taking large doses of it. Hydrochlorothiazide also passes into breast milk. Be sure you have discussed this with your doctor before taking this medicine.

**Children**—Although there is no specific information comparing use of this medicine in children with use in other age groups, this medicine is not expected to cause different side effects or problems in children than it does in adults.

**Older adults**—Many medicines have not been studied specifically in older people. Therefore, it may not be known whether they work exactly the same way they do in younger adults. Although there is no specific information comparing use of reserpine, hydralazine, and hydrochlorothiazide combination in the elderly with use in other age groups, this medicine is not expected to cause different side effects or problems in older people than it does in younger adults. However, drowsiness, dizziness, or faintness, or symptoms of too much potassium loss may be more likely to occur in the elderly, who are usually more sensitive to the effects of this medicine. Also, this medicine may reduce tolerance to cold temperatures in elderly patients.

**Other medicines**—Although certain medicines should not be used together at all, in other cases two different medicines may be used together even if an interaction might occur. In these cases, your doctor may want to change the dose, or other precautions may be necessary. When you are taking this medicine, it is especially important that your health care professional know if you are taking any of the following:

- Cholestyramine or
- Colestipol—Use with thiazide diuretics may prevent the diuretic from working properly; take the diuretic at least 1 hour before or 4 hours after cholestyramine or colestipol
- Diazoxide (e.g., Proglycem)—Effect on blood pressure may be increased
- Digitalis glycosides (heart medicine)—Hydrochlorothiazide may cause low potassium in the blood, which can lead to symptoms of digitalis toxicity
- Lithium (e.g., Lithane)—Risk of lithium overdose, even at usual doses, may be increased
- Monoamine oxidase (MAO) inhibitors (furazolidone [e.g., Furoxone], isocarboxazid [e.g., Marplan], phenelzine [e.g., Nardil], procarbazine [e.g., Matulane], selegiline [e.g., Eldepryl], tranylcypromine [e.g., Parnate])—Taking a rauwolfia alkaloid while you are taking or within 2 weeks of taking MAO inhibitors may increase the risk of central nervous system depression or may cause a severe high blood pressure reaction

**Other medical problems**—The presence of other medical problems may affect the use of this medicine. Make sure you tell your doctor if you have any other medical problems, especially:

- Allergies or other breathing problems such as asthma—Reserpine can cause breathing problems
- Diabetes mellitus (sugar diabetes)—Hydrochlorothiazide may change the amount of diabetes medicine needed
- Epilepsy
- Gallstones or
- Stomach ulcer or
- Ulcerative colitis—Reserpine increases activity of the stomach, which may make the condition worse
- Gout (history of)—Hydrochlorothiazide may increase the amount of uric acid in the blood, which can lead to gout
- Heart disease—Reserpine can cause heart rhythm problems or slow heartbeat. Lowering blood pressure may worsen some conditions
- Kidney disease—Some patients may not do well when blood pressure is lowered by this medicine. Effects of hydralazine may be increased because of slower removal from the body. If kidney disease is severe, hydrochlorothiazide may not work
- Liver disease—If hydrochlorothiazide causes loss of too much water from the body, liver disease can become much worse
- Lupus erythematosus (history of)—Hydrochlorothiazide may worsen the condition
- Mental depression (or history of)—Reserpine causes mental depression
- Pancreatitis (inflammation of pancreas)
- Parkinson's disease—Reserpine can cause parkinsonism-like effects
- Pheochromocytoma
- Stroke (recent)—Lowering blood pressure may make problems resulting from this condition worse

## Proper Use of This Medicine

In addition to the use of the medicine your doctor has prescribed, treatment for your high blood pressure may include weight control and care in the types of foods you eat, especially foods high in sodium. Your doctor will tell you which of these are most important for you. You should check with your doctor before changing your diet.

Many patients who have high blood pressure will not notice any signs of the problem. In fact, many may feel normal. It is very important that you *take your medicine exactly as directed* and that you keep your appointments with your doctor even if you feel well.

Remember that this medicine will not cure your high blood pressure but it does help control it. Therefore, you must continue to take it as directed if you expect to lower your blood pressure and keep it down. *You may have to take high blood pressure medicine for the rest of your life.* If high blood pressure is not treated, it can cause serious problems such as heart failure, blood vessel disease, stroke, or kidney disease.

This medicine may cause you to have an unusual feeling of tiredness when you begin to take it. You may also notice an increase in the amount of urine or in your frequency of urination. After you have taken the medicine for a while, these effects should lessen. In general, to keep the increase in urine from affecting your sleep:

- If you are to take a single dose a day, take it in the morning after breakfast.

- If you are to take more than one dose a day, take the last dose no later than 6 p.m., unless otherwise directed by your doctor.

However, it is best to plan your dose or doses according to a schedule that will least affect your personal activities and sleep. Ask your health care professional to help you plan the best time to take this medicine.

To help you remember to take your medicine, try to get into the habit of taking it at the same time each day.

If this medicine upsets your stomach, it may be taken with meals or milk. If stomach upset (nausea, vomiting, stomach pain or cramps) continues, check with your doctor.

**Dosing**—The dose of reserpine, hydralazine, and hydrochlorothiazide combination will be different for different patients. *Follow your doctor's orders or the directions on the label.* The following information includes only the average doses of reserpine, hydralazine, and hydrochlorothiazide combination. *If your dose is different, do not change it* unless your doctor tells you to do so.

- For *oral* dosage form (tablets):
  —For high blood pressure:
    - Adults—1 or 2 tablets three times a day.
    - Children—Use and dose must be determined by your doctor.

**Missed dose**—If you miss a dose of this medicine, take it as soon as possible. However, if it is almost time for your next dose, skip the missed dose and go back to your regular dosing schedule. Do not double doses.

**Storage**—To store this medicine:
- Keep out of the reach of children.
- Store away from heat and direct light.
- Do not store in the bathroom, near the kitchen sink, or in other damp places. Heat or moisture may cause the medicine to break down.
- Do not keep outdated medicine or medicine no longer needed. Be sure that any discarded medicine is out of the reach of children.

## Precautions While Using This Medicine

It is important that your doctor check your progress at regular visits to make sure that this medicine is working properly.

*Do not take other medicines unless they have been discussed with your doctor.* This especially includes over-the-counter (nonprescription) medicines for appetite control, asthma, colds, cough, hay fever, or sinus problems, since they may tend to increase your blood pressure.

Before having any kind of surgery (including dental surgery), or emergency treatment, *make sure the medical doctor or dentist in charge knows that you are taking this medicine.*

This medicine may cause some people to have headaches or to feel dizzy or drowsy. *Make sure you know how you react to this medicine before you drive, use machines, or do anything else that could be dangerous if you are dizzy or are not alert.*

*Dizziness, lightheadedness, or fainting may occur, especially when you get up from a lying or sitting position.* This is more likely to occur in the morning. *Getting up slowly may help.* When you get up from lying down, sit on the edge of the bed with your feet dangling for 1 or 2 minutes. Then stand up slowly. If the problem continues or gets worse, check with your doctor.

The dizziness, lightheadedness, or fainting is also more likely to occur if you drink alcohol, stand for a long time, exercise, or if the weather is hot. *While you are taking this medicine, be careful to limit the amount of alcohol you drink. Also, use extra care during exercise or hot weather or if you must stand for a long time.*

In some patients, this medicine may cause mental depression. *Tell your doctor right away:*
- if you or anyone else notices unusual changes in your mood.
- if you start having early-morning sleeplessness or unusually vivid dreams or nightmares.

This medicine will add to the effects of alcohol and other CNS depressants (medicines that slow down the nervous system, possibly causing drowsiness). Some examples of CNS depressants are antihistamines or medicine for hay fever, other allergies, or colds; sedatives, tranquilizers, or sleeping medicine; prescription pain medicine or narcotics; barbiturates; medicine for seizures; muscle relaxants; or anesthetics, including dental anesthetics. *Check with your doctor before taking any of the above while you are taking this medicine.*

This medicine may cause a loss of potassium from your body.
- To help prevent this, your doctor may want you to:
  —eat or drink foods that have a high potassium content (for example, orange or other citrus fruit juices), or
  —take a potassium supplement, or
  —take another medicine to help prevent the loss of the potassium in the first place.
- It is very important to follow these directions. Also, it is important not to change your diet on your own. This is more important if you are already on a special diet (as for diabetes), or if you are taking a potassium supplement or a medicine to reduce potassium loss. Extra potassium may not be necessary and, in some cases, too much potassium could be harmful.

Check with your doctor if you become sick and have severe or continuing nausea, vomiting, or diarrhea. These problems may cause you to lose additional water and potassium.

For *diabetic patients:*
- This medicine may raise blood sugar levels. While you are using this medicine, be especially careful in

testing for sugar in your urine. If you have any questions about this, check with your doctor.

Some people who take this medicine may become more sensitive to sunlight than they are normally. Exposure to sunlight, even for brief periods of time, may cause severe sunburn; skin rash, redness, itching, or discoloration; or vision changes. When you begin taking this medicine:

- Stay out of direct sunlight, especially between the hours of 10:00 a.m. and 3:00 p.m., if possible.
- Wear protective clothing, including a hat and sunglasses.
- Apply a sun block product that has a skin protection factor (SPF) of at least 15. Some patients may require a product with a higher SPF number, especially if they have a fair complexion. If you have any questions about this, check with your health care professional.
- Do not use a sunlamp or tanning bed or booth.

If you have a severe reaction from the sun, check with your doctor.

This medicine often causes stuffiness in the nose. However, do not use nasal decongestant medicines without first checking with your health care professional.

This medicine may cause dryness of the mouth. For temporary relief, use sugarless candy or gum, melt bits of ice in your mouth, or use a saliva substitute. However, if dry mouth continues for more than 2 weeks, check with your medical doctor or dentist. Continuing dryness of the mouth may increase the chance of dental disease, including tooth decay, gum disease, and fungus infections.

## Side Effects of This Medicine

Suggestions that rauwolfia alkaloids may increase the risk of breast cancer occurring later have not been proven. However, rats and mice given 100 to 300 times the human dose had an increased number of tumors.

Along with its needed effects, a medicine may cause some unwanted effects. Although not all of these side effects may occur, if they do occur they may need medical attention.

*Check with your doctor immediately* if any of the following side effects occur:

*More common*

General feeling of discomfort or illness or weakness

*Less common*

Drowsiness or faintness; impotence or decreased sexual interest; lack of energy or weakness; mental depression or inability to concentrate; nervousness or anxiety; vivid dreams or nightmares or early-morning sleeplessness

Check with your doctor as soon as possible if any of the following side effects occur:

*Signs and symptoms of too much potassium loss*

Dryness of mouth; increased thirst; irregular heartbeat; mood or mental changes; muscle cramps or pain; weak pulse

*Signs and symptoms of too much sodium loss*

Confusion; convulsions; decreased mental activity; irritability; muscle cramps; unusual tiredness or weakness

*Less common*

Black, tarry stools; blisters on skin; bloody vomit; chest pain; fever and sore throat; headache; irregular heartbeat; joint pain; numbness, tingling, pain, or weakness in hands or feet; shortness of breath; skin rash or itching; slow heartbeat; stomach cramps or pain; swelling of lymph glands

*Rare*

Lower back or side pain; painful or difficult urination; stiffness; stomach pain (severe) with nausea and vomiting; trembling and shaking of hands and fingers; unusual bleeding or bruising; yellow eyes or skin

*Signs and symptoms of overdose*

Dizziness or drowsiness (severe); dryness of mouth; flushing of skin; increased thirst; muscle cramps or pain; nausea or vomiting (severe); pinpoint pupils of eyes; slow pulse

Other side effects may occur that usually do not need medical attention. These side effects may go away during treatment as your body adjusts to the medicine. However, check with your doctor if any of the following side effects continue or are bothersome:

*More common*

Diarrhea; dizziness, especially when getting up from a lying or sitting position; loss of appetite; nausea or vomiting; stuffy nose

*Less common*

Constipation; flushing or redness of skin; increased sensitivity of skin to sunlight; swelling of feet and lower legs; watering or irritated eyes

After you stop using this medicine, it may still produce some side effects that need attention. During this period of time *check with your doctor immediately* if you notice any of the following side effects:

Drowsiness or faintness; general feeling of discomfort or illness or weakness; impotence or decreased sexual interest; irregular heartbeat; mental depression or inability to concentrate; nervousness or anxiety; vivid dreams or nightmares or early-morning sleeplessness

Other side effects not listed above may also occur in some patients. If you notice any other effects, check with your doctor.

Revised: 09/22/92
Interim revision: 07/20/94

# RESORCINOL   Topical

A commonly used brand name in the U.S. is RA.

## Description

Resorcinol (re-SOR-si-nole) is used to treat acne, seborrheic dermatitis, eczema, psoriasis, and other skin disorders. It is also used to treat corns, calluses, and warts.

Resorcinol works by helping to remove hard, scaly, or roughened skin.

Some of these preparations are available only with your doctor's prescription. Others are available without a prescription; however, your doctor may have special instructions on the proper use of resorcinol for your medical condition.

Resorcinol is available in the following dosage forms:

*Topical*
- Lotion (U.S.)
- Ointment (U.S. and Canada)

## Before Using This Medicine

If you are using this medicine without a prescription, carefully read and follow any precautions on the label. For resorcinol, the following should be considered:

**Allergies**—Tell your doctor if you have ever had any unusual or allergic reaction to resorcinol. Also tell your health care professional if you are allergic to any other substances, such as preservatives or dyes.

**Pregnancy**—Resorcinol may be absorbed through the mother's skin. However, topical resorcinol has not been shown to cause birth defects or other problems in humans.

**Breast-feeding**—This medicine may be absorbed through the mother's skin. However, topical resorcinol has not been reported to cause problems in nursing babies.

**Children**—Resorcinol may be absorbed through the skin and should not be used on large areas of the bodies of infants and children. In addition, resorcinol should not be used on wounds, since doing so may cause a blood disease called methemoglobinemia.

**Older adults**—Many medicines have not been studied specifically in older people. Therefore, it may not be known whether they work exactly the same way they do in younger adults. Although there is no specific information comparing use of resorcinol in the elderly with use in other age groups, this medicine is not expected to cause different side effects or problems in older people than it does in younger adults.

**Other medicines**—Although certain medicines should not be used together at all, in other cases two different medicines may be used together even if an interaction might occur. In these cases, your doctor may want to change the dose, or other precautions may be necessary. Tell your health care professional if you are using any other prescription or nonprescription (over-the-counter [OTC]) medicine.

## Proper Use of This Medicine

*It is very important that you use this medicine only as directed.* Do not use more of it, do not use it more often, and do not use it for a longer time than your doctor ordered. To do so may increase the chance of absorption through the skin and the chance of resorcinol poisoning.

Apply enough resorcinol to cover the affected areas, and rub in gently.

Immediately after using this medicine, wash your hands to remove any medicine that may be on them.

*Keep this medicine away from the eyes.* If you should accidentally get some in your eyes, flush them thoroughly with water.

**Dosing**—The dose of resorcinol will be different for different patients. *Follow your doctor's orders or the directions on the label.* The following information includes only the average doses of resorcinol. *If your dose is different, do not change it* unless your doctor tells you to do so.

- For *lotion* dosage form:
  —For acne, seborrheic dermatitis, eczema, or psoriasis:
    - Adults and children—Use as needed.
- For *ointment* dosage form:
  —For acne, seborrheic dermatitis, eczema, psoriasis, corns, calluses, or warts:
    - Adults and children—Use and dose must be determined by the doctor.

**Missed dose**—If you miss a dose of this medicine, apply it as soon as possible. However, if it is almost time for your next dose, skip the missed dose and go back to your regular dosing schedule. Do not double doses.

**Storage**—To store this medicine:
- Keep out of the reach of children.
- Store away from heat and direct light.
- Keep the medicine from freezing.
- Do not keep outdated medicine or medicine no longer needed. Be sure that any discarded medicine is out of the reach of children.

## Precautions While Using This Medicine

*When using resorcinol, do not use any of the following preparations on the same affected area as this medicine,* unless otherwise directed by your doctor:

Abrasive soaps or cleansers
Alcohol-containing preparations

Any other topical acne preparation or preparation containing a peeling agent (for example, benzoyl peroxide, salicylic acid, sulfur, or tretinoin [vitamin A acid])
Cosmetics or soaps that dry the skin
Medicated cosmetics
Other topical medicine for the skin

To use any of the above preparations on the same affected area as resorcinol may cause severe irritation of the skin.

*This medicine may darken light-colored hair.*

---

## Side Effects of This Medicine

Along with its needed effects, a medicine may cause some unwanted effects. Although not all of these side effects may occur, if they do occur they may need medical attention.

Check with your doctor as soon as possible if any of the following side effects occur:

*Less common or rare*
Skin irritation not present before use of this medicine

*Symptoms of resorcinol poisoning*
Diarrhea, nausea, stomach pain, or vomiting; dizziness; drowsiness; headache (severe or continuing); nervousness or restlessness; slow heartbeat, shortness of breath, or troubled breathing; sweating; unusual tiredness or weakness

Other side effects may occur that usually do not need medical attention. These side effects may go away during treatment as your body adjusts to the medicine. However, check with your doctor if the following side effect continues or is bothersome:

*More common*
Redness and peeling of skin (may occur after a few days)

Other side effects not listed above may also occur in some patients. If you notice any other effects, check with your doctor.

---

Revised: 07/26/93

---

# RESORCINOL AND SULFUR   Topical

Some commonly used brand names are:
**In the U.S.—**
Acnomel Acne Cream
Bensulfoid Cream
Clearasil Adult Care
  Medicated Blemish Cream
Clearasil Adult Care
  Medicated Blemish Stick
Night Cast Special Formula
  Mask-lotion
Rezamid Acne Treatment
Sulforcin

**In Canada—**
Acne-Aid Gel
Acnomel Cake
Acnomel Cream
Acnomel Vanishing Cream
Rezamid Lotion

---

## Description

Resorcinol and sulfur (re-SOR-si-nole and SUL-fur) combination is used to treat acne and similar skin conditions.

This medicine is available without a prescription; however, your doctor may have special instructions on the proper use of this medicine for your medical condition.

Resorcinol and sulfur combination is available in the following dosage forms:

*Topical*
- Cake (Canada)
- Cream (U.S. and Canada)
- Gel (Canada)
- Lotion (U.S. and Canada)
- Stick (U.S.)

---

## Before Using This Medicine

If you are using this medicine without a prescription, carefully read and follow any precautions on the label.

For resorcinol and sulfur combination, the following should be considered:

**Allergies**—Tell your doctor if you have ever had any unusual or allergic reaction to resorcinol or sulfur. Also tell your health care professional if you are allergic to any other substances, such as preservatives or dyes.

**Pregnancy**—Resorcinol may be absorbed through the mother's skin. However, topical resorcinol and sulfur combination has not been shown to cause birth defects or other problems in humans.

**Breast-feeding**—Resorcinol may be absorbed through the mother's skin. However, topical resorcinol and sulfur combination has not been reported to cause problems in nursing babies.

**Children**—Resorcinol may be absorbed through the skin and should not be used on large areas of the bodies of infants and children. In addition, resorcinol should not be used on wounds, since doing so may cause a blood disease called methemoglobinemia.

**Older adults**—Many medicines have not been studied specifically in older people. Therefore, it may not be known whether they work exactly the same way they do in younger adults or if they cause different side effects or problems in older people. There is no specific information comparing use of resorcinol and sulfur in the elderly with use in other age groups.

**Other medicines**—Although certain medicines should not be used together at all, in other cases two different medicines may be used together even if an interaction might occur. In these cases, your doctor may want to change

---

the dose, or other precautions may be necessary. Tell your health care professional if you are using any other prescription or nonprescription (over-the-counter [OTC]) medicine.

## Proper Use of This Medicine

*Use this medicine only as directed.* Do not use more of it and do not use it more often than recommended on the label, unless otherwise directed by your doctor. To do so may increase the chance of absorption through the skin and the chance of resorcinol poisoning.

Before using this medicine, wash the affected areas thoroughly and gently pat dry. Then apply a small amount to the affected areas and spread on gently, but do not rub in.

Immediately after using this medicine, wash your hands to remove any medicine that may be on them.

*Keep this medicine away from the eyes.* If you should accidentally get some in your eyes, flush them thoroughly with water.

**Dosing**—The dose of resorcinol and sulfur combination will be different for different patients. *Follow your doctor's orders or the directions on the label.* The following information includes only the average doses of resorcinol and sulfur combination. *If your dose is different, do not change it* unless your doctor tells you to do so.

- For acne and similar skin conditions:
  —For *cake* dosage form:
  - Adults and children—Use two or three times a day.
  —For *cream* dosage form:
  - Adults and children—Use one to three times a day.
  —For *gel and stick* dosage forms:
  - Adults and children—Use as needed.
  —For *lotion* dosage form:
  - Adults and children—Use two times a day.

**Missed dose**—If you miss a dose of this medicine, apply it as soon as possible. However, if it is almost time for your next dose, skip the missed dose and go back to your regular dosing schedule. Do not double doses.

**Storage**—To store this medicine:
- Keep out of the reach of children.
- Store away from heat and direct light.
- Keep the medicine from freezing.
- Do not keep outdated medicine or medicine no longer needed. Be sure that any discarded medicine is out of the reach of children.

## Precautions While Using This Medicine

*When using resorcinol and sulfur combination, do not use any of the following preparations on the same af-* fected area as this medicine, unless otherwise directed by your doctor:
  Abrasive soaps or cleansers
  Alcohol-containing preparations
  Any other topical acne preparation or preparation containing a peeling agent (for example, benzoyl peroxide, salicylic acid, or tretinoin [vitamin A acid])
  Cosmetics or soaps that dry the skin
  Medicated cosmetics
  Other topical medicine for the skin

To use any of the above preparations on the same affected area as this medicine may cause severe irritation of the skin.

*Do not use any topical mercury-containing preparation, such as ammoniated mercury ointment, on the same affected area as this medicine.* To do so may cause a foul odor, may be irritating to the skin, and may stain the skin black. If you have any questions about this, check with your health care professional.

This medicine (depending on the product you are using) may darken light-colored hair. If you have any questions about this, check with your health care professional.

## Side Effects of This Medicine

Along with its needed effects, a medicine may cause some unwanted effects. Although not all of these side effects may occur, if they do occur they may need medical attention.

Check with your doctor as soon as possible if the following side effect occurs:

*Less common or rare*
  Skin irritation not present before use of this medicine

*Symptoms of resorcinol poisoning*
  Diarrhea, nausea, stomach pain, or vomiting; dizziness; drowsiness; headache (severe or continuing); nervousness or restlessness; slow heartbeat, shortness of breath, or troubled breathing; sweating; unusual tiredness or weakness

Other side effects may occur that usually do not need medical attention. However, check with your health care professional if the following side effects continue or are bothersome:

*More common*
  Redness and peeling of skin (may occur after a few days)
*Less common*
  Unusual dryness of skin

Other side effects not listed above may also occur in some patients. If you notice any other effects, check with your health care professional.

Revised: 07/26/93

# RH₀(D) IMMUNE GLOBULIN    Systemic

Some commonly used brand names are:

**In the U.S.—**

Gamulin Rh               MICRhoGAM
HypRho-D Full Dose       Mini-Gamulin Rh
HypRho-D Mini-Dose       RhoGAM

**In Canada—**

HypRho-D Full Dose       WinRho SD

Other commonly used names are anti-D gammaglobulin; anti-D (Rh₀) immunoglobulin; anti-Rh immunoglobulin; anti-Rh₀(D); D(Rh₀) immune globulin; RhD immune globulin; Rh immune globulin; Rh-IG; and Rh₀(D) immune human globulin.

## Description

Rh₀(D) immune globulin is used to prevent your body from interacting with any of your baby's blood that may get into your blood system while you are pregnant or during the delivery of your baby. If your blood type is Rh₀(D) negative and your baby's blood type is Rh₀(D) positive, your body may produce a defense (antibodies) against Rh₀(D) positive blood. These antibodies usually will not cause a problem if this is your first pregnancy, unless you have had a blood transfusion in the past and have already developed these antibodies. However, if you have other Rh₀(D) positive babies in the future, these antibodies may try to destroy the blood of the future babies. If this occurs, it is a very serious condition. Babies born with this condition may need to have their blood replaced.

Rh₀(D) immune globulin may also be used if you have recently received a transfusion that contained Rh₀(D) positive blood and your blood type is Rh₀(D) negative.

Rh₀(D) immune globulin is to be administered only by or under the supervision of your doctor or other health care professional. It is available in the following dosage form:

*Parenteral*

- Injection (U.S. and Canada)

## Before Using This Medicine

In deciding to use a medicine, the risks of using the medicine must be weighed against the good it will do. This is a decision you and your doctor will make. For Rh₀(D) immune globulin, the following should be considered:

**Allergies**—Tell your doctor if you have ever had any unusual or allergic reaction to Rh₀(D) immune globulin, any other kind of human immune globulin, or to thimerosal. Also tell your health care professional if you are allergic to any other substances, such as foods, preservatives, or dyes.

**Pregnancy**— Studies on effects in pregnancy have not been done in either humans or animals. However, this medicine has been used in pregnant women and has not been shown to cause birth defects or other problems.

**Breast-feeding**—Rh₀(D) immune globulin has not been reported to cause problems in nursing babies.

**Children**—Studies on this medicine have been done only in adult patients and there is no specific information comparing use of Rh₀(D) immune globulin in children with use in other age groups.

**Other medical problems**—The presence of other medical problems may affect the use of Rh₀(D) immune globulin. Make sure you tell your doctor if you have any other medical problems, especially:

- Immunoglobulin A (IgA) deficiencies—Rh₀(D) immune globulin may cause an allergic reaction to occur

## Proper Use of This Medicine

**Dosing**—The dose of Rh₀(D) immune globulin will be different for different patients. The following information includes only the average dose of Rh₀(D) immune globulin.

- *For injection* dosage form:

  —To prevent your body from producing antibodies against Rh₀(D) positive blood:

  - Adults and children—One or more injections, depending on how much Rh₀(D) positive blood has gotten into your blood system. The medicine may be used during your pregnancy, within 72 hours after your baby is born, at the end of an incomplete pregnancy (abortion, miscarriage), or after a transfusion. The medicine is usually injected into a muscle, although it may be injected into a vein.

## Side Effects of This Medicine

Along with its needed effects, a medicine may cause some unwanted effects. The following side effects may occur and usually do not need medical attention. However, check with your doctor if either of the following side effects continue or are bothersome:

*Less common*

Fever; soreness at the place of injection

Other side effects not listed above may also occur in some patients. If you notice any other effects, check with your doctor.

Developed: 08/31/94

# RIBAVIRIN   Systemic

Some commonly used brand names are:

**In the U.S.—**
Virazole

**In Canada—**
Virazole

**Other—**
Virazid

Another commonly used name is tribavirin.

## Description

Ribavirin (rye-ba-VYE-rin) is used to treat severe virus pneumonia in infants and young children. It is given by oral inhalation (breathing in the medicine as a fine mist through the mouth), using a special nebulizer (sprayer) attached to an oxygen hood or tent or face mask.

This medicine may also be used for other virus infections as determined by your doctor. However, it will not work for certain viruses, such as the common cold.

Ribavirin is to be administered only by or under the immediate supervision of your doctor, in the following dosage form:

*Inhalation*
- For inhalation solution (U.S. and Canada)

## Before Receiving This Medicine

In deciding to use a medicine, the risks of taking the medicine must be weighed against the good it will do. This is a decision you and your doctor will make. For ribavirin, the following should be considered:

**Allergies**—Tell your doctor if you or your child has ever had any unusual or allergic reaction to ribavirin for inhalation. Also tell your health care professional if you or your child is allergic to any other substances, such as foods, preservatives, or dyes.

**Pregnancy**—Ribavirin for inhalation is not usually prescribed for teenagers or adults. However, women who are pregnant or may become pregnant may be exposed to ribavirin that is given off in the air if they spend time at the patient's bedside while ribavirin is being given. Although studies have not been done in humans, ribavirin has been shown to cause birth defects and other problems in certain animal studies. Be sure you have discussed this with your doctor.

**Breast-feeding**—Ribavirin for inhalation is not usually prescribed for teenagers or adults. However, ribavirin passes into the breast milk of animals and has been shown to cause problems in nursing animals and their young.

**Children**—This medicine has been tested in children, and, when used as it should be and in effective doses, has not been shown to cause serious side effects or problems.

**Older adults**—Ribavirin for inhalation is not usually prescribed for use in elderly patients.

## Proper Use of This Medicine

To help clear up your infection completely, *ribavirin must be given for the full time of treatment,* even if you or your child begins to feel better after a few days. Also, this medicine works best when there is a constant amount in the lungs. To help keep the amount constant, ribavirin must be given on a regular or continuous schedule.

**Dosing**—The dose of ribavirin will be different for different patients. *Follow your doctor's orders or the directions.* The following information includes only the average doses of ribavirin. *If your dose is different, do not change it* unless your doctor tells you to do so.

- For the *inhalation* dosage form:
  - —For treatment of respiratory syncytial virus (RSV) infection:
    - Adults and teenagers—Dose has not been determined since this medicine is not usually prescribed for teenagers or adults.
    - Infants and children—Dose must be determined by the doctor.

## Side Effects of This Medicine

Along with its needed effects, a medicine may cause some unwanted effects. The following side effects may go away during treatment as your body adjusts to the medicine. However, check with your doctor if any of the following side effects continue or are bothersome:

*Rare*
Headache; itching, redness, or swelling of eye; skin rash or irritation

Other side effects not listed above may also occur in some patients. If you notice any other effects, check with your doctor.

## Additional Information

Once a medicine has been approved for marketing for a certain use, experience may show that it is also useful for other medical problems. Although these uses are not included in product labeling, ribavirin is used in certain patients with the following medical conditions:

- Influenza A and B (given by aerosol inhalation)
- Lassa fever (either given orally or by injection)

For patients taking this medicine by mouth or injection for *Lassa fever:*

- *Check with your doctor immediately* if any of the following side effects occur:
  *More common*
  Unusual tiredness and weakness
- Other side effects may occur that usually do not need medical attention. The following side effects may go away during treatment as your body adjusts to the medicine. However, check with your doctor if any

of the following side effects continue or are bothersome:

*Less common*
Headache; loss of appetite; nausea; trouble in sleeping; unusual tiredness or weakness

Other than the above information, there is no additional information relating to proper use, precautions, or side effects for these uses.

Revised: 02/23/93
Interim revision: 06/08/94

# RIBOFLAVIN    (Vitamin B₂)    Systemic

Generic name product is available in the U.S. and Canada.

## Description

Vitamins (VYE-ta-mins) are compounds that you *must* have for growth and health. They are needed in small amounts only and are usually available in the foods that you eat. Riboflavin (RYE-boe-flay-vin) (vitamin B₂) is necessary for normal metabolism.

Lack of riboflavin may lead to itching and burning eyes, sensitivity of eyes to light, sore tongue, itching and peeling skin on the nose and scrotum, and sores in the mouth. Your doctor may treat this condition by prescribing riboflavin for you.

Patients with the following conditions may be more likely to have a deficiency of riboflavin:

- Alcoholism
- Burns
- Cancer
- Diarrhea (continuing)
- Fever (continuing)
- Illness (continuing)
- Infection
- Intestinal diseases
- Liver disease
- Overactive thyroid
- Serious injury
- Stress (continuing)
- Surgical removal of stomach

In addition, riboflavin may be given to infants with high blood levels of bilirubin (hyperbilirubinemia).

If any of the above apply to you, you should take riboflavin supplements only on the advice of your doctor after need has been established.

Claims that riboflavin is effective for treatment of acne, some kinds of anemia (weak blood), migraine headaches, and muscle cramps have not been proven.

Oral forms of riboflavin are available without a prescription. However, it may be a good idea to check with your doctor before taking riboflavin on your own. If you take more than you need, it will simply be lost from your body.

Riboflavin is available in the following dosage form:
*Oral*
- Tablets (U.S. and Canada)

## Importance of Diet

Vitamin supplements should be taken only if you cannot get enough vitamins in your diet; however, some diets may not contain all of the vitamins you need. You may not be getting enough vitamins because of rapid weight loss, unusual diets (such as some reducing diets in which choice of foods is very limited), prolonged intravenous feeding, or malnutrition. A balanced diet should provide all the vitamins you normally need.

In order to get enough vitamins and minerals in your diet, it is important that you eat a balanced and varied diet. Follow carefully any diet program your doctor may recommend. For your specific vitamin and/or mineral needs, ask your doctor for a list of appropriate foods.

Riboflavin is found in various foods, including milk and dairy products, fish, meats, green leafy vegetables, and whole grain and enriched cereals and bread. It is best to eat fresh fruits and vegetables whenever possible since they contain the most vitamins. Food processing may destroy some of the vitamins, although little riboflavin is lost from foods during ordinary cooking.

Vitamins alone will not take the place of a good diet and will not provide energy. Your body also needs other substances found in food such as protein, minerals, carbohydrates, and fat. Vitamins themselves often cannot work without the presence of other foods.

In some cases it may not be possible for you to get enough food to supply you with the proper vitamins. In other cases, the amount of vitamins you need may be increased above normal. Therefore, a vitamin supplement may be needed.

Experts have developed a list of recommended dietary allowances (RDA) for most of the vitamins. The RDA are not an exact number but a general idea of how much you need. They do not cover amounts needed for problems caused by a serious lack of vitamins.

The RDA for riboflavin are:

- Infants and children—
  Birth to 6 months of age: 0.4 milligrams (mg) per day.
  6 months to 1 year of age: 0.5 mg per day.
  1 to 3 years of age: 0.8 mg per day.
  4 to 6 years of age: 1.1 mg per day.
  7 to 10 years of age: 1.2 mg per day.
- Adolescent and adult males—
  11 to 14 years of age: 1.5 mg per day.
  15 to 18 years of age: 1.8 mg per day.
  19 to 50 years of age: 1.7 mg per day.
  51 years of age and over: 1.4 mg per day.
- Adolescent and adult females—
  11 to 50 years of age: 1.3 mg per day.
  51 years of age and over: 1.2 mg per day.
- Pregnant females: 1.6 mg per day.
- Breast-feeding females:
  First 6 months: 1.6 mg per day.
  Second 6 months: 1.7 mg per day.

Remember:

- The total amount of each vitamin that you get every day includes what you get from the foods that you eat *and* what you may take as a supplement.
- Your total amount should not be greater than the RDA, unless ordered by your doctor.

## Before Using This Dietary Supplement

If you are taking this dietary supplement without a prescription, carefully read and follow any precautions on the label. For riboflavin, the following should be considered:

**Allergies**—Tell your health care professional if you are allergic to any substances, such as foods, preservatives, or dyes.

**Pregnancy**—It is especially important that you are receiving enough vitamins when you become pregnant and that you continue to receive the right amounts of vitamins throughout your pregnancy. The healthy growth and development of the fetus depend on a steady supply of nutrients from the mother. However, taking large amounts of a dietary supplement in pregnancy may be harmful to the mother and/or fetus and should be avoided.

**Breast-feeding**—It is especially important that you receive the right amounts of vitamins so that your baby will also get the vitamins needed to grow properly. However, taking large amounts of a dietary supplement while breast-feeding may be harmful to the mother and/or baby and should be avoided.

**Children**—Normal daily requirements vary according to age. It is especially important that children receive enough vitamins in their diet for healthy growth and development. Although there is no specific information about the use of riboflavin in children in doses higher than the normal daily requirements, it is not expected to cause different side effects or problems in children than in adults.

**Older adults**—It is important that older people continue to receive enough vitamins in their diet for good health. Although there is no specific information about the use of riboflavin in older people in doses higher than the normal daily requirements, it is not expected to cause different side effects or problems in older people than in younger adults.

**Other medicines or dietary supplements**—Although certain medicines or dietary supplements should not be used together at all, in other cases two different medicines or dietary supplements may be used together even if an interaction might occur. In these cases, your doctor may want to change the dose, or other precautions may be necessary. Tell your health care professional if you are taking any other dietary supplements or prescription or nonprescription (over-the-counter [OTC]) medicine.

## Proper Use of This Dietary Supplement

Some people believe that taking very large doses of vitamins (called megadoses or megavitamin therapy) is useful for treating certain medical problems. Studies have not proven this. Large doses should be taken only under the direction of your doctor after need has been identified.

**Dosing**—The dose of riboflavin for prevention of riboflavin deficiency is based on the Recommended Dietary Allowances (RDA). See the *Importance of Diet* section for the RDA for riboflavin.

**Missed dose**—If you miss taking a vitamin for 1 or more days there is no cause for concern, since it takes some time for your body to become seriously low in vitamins. However, if your doctor has recommended that you take this vitamin, try to remember to take it as directed every day.

**Storage**—To store this dietary supplement:

- Keep out of the reach of children.
- Store away from heat and direct light.
- Do not store in the bathroom, near the kitchen sink, or in other damp places. Heat or moisture may cause the dietary supplement to break down.
- Do not keep outdated dietary supplements or those no longer needed. Be sure that any discarded dietary supplement is out of the reach of children.

## Side Effects of This Dietary Supplement

Along with its needed effects, a dietary supplement may cause some unwanted effects. Riboflavin may cause urine to have a more yellow color than normal, especially if large doses are taken. This is to be expected and is no cause for alarm. Usually, however, riboflavin does not cause any side effects. Check with your doctor if you notice any other unusual effects while you are using it.

---

Revised: 08/22/92
Interim revision: 07/29/94

---

# RIFABUTIN    Systemic

A commonly used brand name in the U.S. and Canada is Mycobutin.

## Description

Rifabutin (rif-a-BUE-tin) is used to help prevent *Mycobacterium avium* complex (MAC) disease from causing disease throughout the body in patients with advanced human immunodeficiency virus (HIV) infection. MAC is an infection caused by two similar bacteria, *Mycobacterium avium* and *Mycobacterium intracellulare*. *Mycobacterium avium* is more common in patients with HIV infection. MAC may also occur in other patients whose immune system is not working properly. Symptoms of MAC in people with acquired immunodeficiency syndrome (AIDS) include fever, night sweats, chills, weight loss, and weakness. Rifabutin will not work for colds, flu, or most other infections.

Rifabutin is available only with your doctor's prescription, in the following dosage form:

   *Oral*
     • Capsules (U.S. and Canada)

## Before Using This Medicine

In deciding to use a medicine, the risks of taking the medicine must be weighed against the good it will do. This is a decision you and your doctor will make. For rifabutin, the following should be considered:

**Allergies**—Tell your doctor if you have ever had any unusual or allergic reaction to rifabutin or rifampin. Also tell your health care professional if you are allergic to any other substances, such as foods, preservatives, or dyes.

**Pregnancy**—Rifabutin has not been studied in pregnant women. However, studies in animals have shown that rifabutin causes birth defects. Before you take this medicine, make sure your doctor knows if you are pregnant or if you may become pregnant.

**Breast-feeding**—It is not known whether rifabutin passes into the breast milk. However, if your baby does not have the AIDS virus, there is a chance that you could pass the virus to your baby by breast-feeding. Talk to your doctor first if you are thinking about breast-feeding your baby.

**Children**—Studies on this medicine have only been done in adult patients, and there is no specific information comparing use of rifabutin in children with use in other age groups. However, studies are being done to determine the best dose for children.

**Older adults**—Many medicines have not been studied specifically in older people. Therefore, it may not be known whether they work exactly the same way they do in younger adults. Although there is no specific information comparing use of rifabutin in the elderly with use in other age groups, this medicine is not expected to cause different side effects or problems in older people than it does in younger adults.

**Other medicines**—Although certain medicines should not be used together at all, in other cases two different medicines may be used together even if an interaction might occur. In these cases, your doctor may want to change the dose, or other precautions may be necessary. When you are taking rifabutin, it is especially important that your health care professional know if you are taking any of the following:

   • Zidovudine (e.g., AZT, Retrovir)—Use of rifabutin with zidovudine may lower the amount of zidovudine in the blood

**Other medical problems**—The presence of other medical problems may affect the use of rifabutin. Make sure you tell your doctor if you have any other medical problems, especially:

   • Active tuberculosis—Patients with active tuberculosis (TB) who need to take rifabutin *must* also take other medicines to cure their TB. Rifabutin used alone may cause TB germs to develop a resistance to other medicines. This may make future treatment of TB very difficult

## Proper Use of This Medicine

Rifabutin may be taken on an empty stomach (either 1 hour before or 2 hours after a meal). However, if this medicine upsets your stomach, you may want to take it with food.

For *patients unable to swallow capsules:*

   • The contents of the capsules may be mixed with applesauce. Be sure to take all the food to get the full dose of medicine.

To help prevent MAC disease, *it is very important that you keep taking this medicine for the full time of treatment.* You may have to take it every day for many months. *It is important that you do not miss any doses.*

**Dosing**—The dose of rifabutin may be different for different patients. *Follow your doctor's orders or the directions on the label.* The following information includes only the average doses of rifabutin. *If your dose is different, do not change it* unless your doctor tells you to do so.

- For *oral* dosage forms (capsules):
  —For the prevention of *Mycobacterium avium* complex (MAC):
  - Adults and teenagers—300 milligrams (mg) once a day, or 150 mg two times a day.
  - Children—Use and dose must be determined by your doctor.

**Missed dose**—If you miss a dose of this medicine, take it as soon as possible. However, if it is almost time for your next dose, skip the missed dose and go back to your regular dosing schedule. Do not double doses. *If this medicine is taken on an irregular schedule, side effects may occur more often and may be more serious than usual.* If you have any questions about this, check with your health care professional.

**Storage**—To store this medicine:
- Keep out of the reach of children.
- Store away from heat and direct light.
- Do not store in the bathroom, near the kitchen sink, or in other damp places. Heat or moisture may cause the medicine to break down.
- Do not keep outdated medicine or medicine no longer needed. Be sure that any discarded medicine is out of the reach of children.

## Precautions While Using This Medicine

*It is very important that your doctor check your progress at regular visits.*

Rifabutin will cause your urine, stool, saliva, skin, sputum, sweat, and tears to turn reddish orange to reddish brown. This is to be expected while you are taking this medicine. This effect may cause soft contact lenses to become permanently discolored. Standard cleaning solutions may not take out all the discoloration. Therefore, *it is best not to wear soft contact lenses while taking this medicine.* Hard contact lenses are not discolored by rifabutin. If you have any questions about this, check with your doctor.

## Side Effects of This Medicine

Along with its needed effects, a medicine may cause some unwanted effects. Although not all of these side effects may occur, if they do occur they may need medical attention.

*Check with your doctor immediately* if any of the following side effects occur:

*More common*
  Skin rash

*Rare*
  Change in taste; eye pain; fever and sore throat; joint pain; loss of vision; muscle pain; yellow skin

Other side effects may occur that usually do not need medical attention. These side effects may go away during treatment as your body adjusts to the medicine. However, check with your doctor if any of the following side effects continue or are bothersome:

*More common*
  Nausea; vomiting

This medicine commonly causes reddish orange to reddish brown discoloration of urine, stools, saliva, skin, sputum, sweat, and tears. This side effect does not usually need medical attention. However, tears that have been discolored by this medicine may also discolor soft contact lenses (see *Precautions While Using This Medicine*).

Other side effects not listed above may also occur in some patients. If you notice any other effects, check with your doctor.

Revised: 06/22/94

# RIFAMPIN  Systemic

Some commonly used brand names are:

**In the U.S.—**
Rifadin                    Rimactane
Rifadin IV
**In Canada—**
Rifadin                    Rofact
Rimactane

Another commonly used name is rifampicin.

## Description

Rifampin (rif-AM-pin) is used to treat certain bacterial infections.

Rifampin is used with other medicines to treat tuberculosis (TB). Rifampin is also taken alone by patients who may carry meningitis bacteria in their nose and throat (without feeling sick) and may spread these bacteria to others. This medicine may also be used for other problems as determined by your doctor. However, rifampin will not work for colds, flu, or other virus infections.

*To help clear up your tuberculosis (TB) completely, you must keep taking this medicine for the full time of treatment, even if you begin to feel better. This is very important. It is also important that you do not miss any doses.*

Rifampin is available only with your doctor's prescription, in the following dosage forms:

*Oral*
- Capsules (U.S. and Canada)

*Parenteral*
- Injection (U.S.)

## Before Using This Medicine

In deciding to use a medicine, the risks of taking the medicine must be weighed against the good it will do. This is a decision you and your doctor will make. For rifampin, the following should be considered:

**Allergies**—Tell your doctor if you have ever had any unusual or allergic reaction to rifampin. Also tell your health care professional if you are allergic to any other substances, such as foods, preservatives, or dyes.

**Pregnancy**—Pregnant women with tuberculosis (TB) should be treated with TB medicines, including rifampin. Rarely, rifampin has caused bleeding in newborn babies and mothers when it was taken during the last weeks of pregnancy. Studies in rodents have shown that rifampin given in high doses causes birth defects, usually backbone problems (spina bifida) and cleft palate.

**Breast-feeding**—Rifampin passes into the breast milk. However, rifampin has not been reported to cause problems in nursing babies.

**Children**—This medicine has been tested in children and, in effective doses, has not been shown to cause different side effects or problems in children than it does in adults.

**Older adults**—Many medicines have not been studied specifically in older people. Therefore, it may not be known whether they work exactly the same way they do in younger adults. Although there is no specific information comparing use of rifampin in the elderly with use in other age groups, this medicine is not expected to cause different side effects or problems in older people than it does in younger adults.

**Other medicines**—Although certain medicines should not be used together at all, in other cases two different medicines may be used together even if an interaction might occur. In these cases, your doctor may want to change the dose, or other precautions may be necessary. When you are taking rifampin, it is especially important that your health care professional know if you are taking any of the following:
- Acetaminophen (e.g., Tylenol) (with long-term, high-dose use) or
- Amiodarone (e.g., Cordarone) or
- Anabolic steroids (nandrolone [e.g., Anabolin], oxandrolone [e.g., Anavar], oxymetholone [e.g., Anadrol], stanozolol [e.g., Winstrol]) or
- Androgens (male hormones) or
- Antithyroid agents (medicine for overactive thyroid) or
- Carbamazepine (e.g., Tegretol) or
- Carmustine (e.g., BiCNU) or
- Chloroquine (e.g., Aralen) or
- Dantrolene (e.g., Dantrium) or
- Daunorubicin (e.g., Cerubidine) or
- Disulfiram (e.g., Antabuse) or
- Divalproex (e.g., Depakote) or
- Etretinate (e.g., Tegison) or
- Gold salts (medicine for arthritis) or
- Hydroxychloroquine (e.g., Plaquenil) or
- Isoniazid (e.g., INH, Nydrazid) or
- Mercaptopurine (e.g., Purinethol) or
- Methotrexate (e.g., Mexate) or
- Methyldopa (e.g., Aldomet) or
- Naltrexone (e.g., Trexan) (with long-term, high-dose use) or
- Other anti-infectives by mouth or by injection (medicine for infection) or
- Phenothiazines (acetophenazine [e.g., Tindal], chlorpromazine [e.g., Thorazine], fluphenazine [e.g., Prolixin], mesoridazine [e.g., Serentil], perphenazine [e.g., Trilafon], prochlorperazine [e.g., Compazine], promazine [e.g., Sparine], promethazine [e.g., Phenergan], thioridazine [e.g., Mellaril], trifluoperazine [e.g., Stelazine], triflupromazine [e.g., Vesprin], trimeprazine [e.g., Temaril]) or
- Plicamycin (e.g., Mithracin) or
- Valproic acid (e.g., Depakene)—These medicines may increase the chance of liver damage if taken with rifampin
- Anticoagulants (blood thinners) or
- Aminophylline (e.g., Somophyllin) or
- Antidiabetics, oral (diabetes medicine you take by mouth), or
- Chloramphenicol or
- Corticosteroids (cortisone-like medicine) or
- Digitalis glycosides (heart medicine) or
- Disopyramide (e.g., Norpace) or
- Fluconazole (e.g., Diflucan) or
- Itraconazole (e.g., Sporanox) or
- Ketoconazole (e.g., Nizoral) or
- Methadone (e.g., Dolophine) or
- Mexiletine (e.g., Mexitil) or
- Oxtriphylline (e.g., Choledyl) or
- Quinidine (e.g., Quinidex) or
- Theophylline (e.g., Theo-dur, Somophyllin-T) or
- Tocainide (e.g., Tonocard) or
- Verapamil (e.g., Calan)—Rifampin may decrease the effects of these medicines
- Estramustine (e.g., EMCYT) or
- Estrogens (female hormones) or
- Oral contraceptives (birth control pills) containing estrogen or
- Phenytoin (e.g., Dilantin)—Rifampin may decrease the effects of these medicines. If you are taking oral contraceptives, this may increase the chance of pregnancy. These medicines may also increase the chance of liver damage if taken with rifampin

**Other medical problems**—The presence of other medical problems may affect the use of rifampin. Make sure you tell your doctor if you have any other medical problems, especially:

- Alcohol abuse (or history of) or
- Liver disease—There may be an increased chance of side effects affecting the liver in patients with a history of alcohol abuse or liver disease

## Proper Use of This Medicine

Rifampin is best taken with a full glass (8 ounces) of water on an empty stomach (either 1 hour before or 2 hours after a meal). However, if this medicine upsets your stomach, your doctor may want you to take it with food.

For *patients unable to swallow capsules:*

- Contents of the capsules may be mixed with applesauce or jelly. Be sure to take all the food to get the full dose of medicine.
- Your pharmacist can prepare an oral liquid form of this medicine if needed. The liquid form may be kept at room temperature or in the refrigerator. Follow the directions on the label. Shake the bottle well before using. Do not use after the expiration date on the label. The medicine may not work properly after that date. In addition, use a specially marked measuring spoon or other device to measure each dose accurately. The average household teaspoon may not hold the right amount of liquid.

*To help clear up your tuberculosis (TB) completely, it is very important that you keep taking this medicine for the full time of treatment,* even if you begin to feel better after a few weeks. You may have to take it every day for as long as 1 to 2 years or more. *It is important that you do not miss any doses.*

**Dosing**—The dose of rifampin will be different for different patients. *Follow your doctor's orders or the directions on the label.* The following information includes only the average doses of rifampin. *If your dose is different, do not change it* unless your doctor tells you to do so.

The number of capsules that you take depends on the strength of the medicine. Also, *the number of doses you take each day, the time allowed between doses, and the length of time you take the medicine depend on the medical problem for which you are taking rifampin.*

- For *oral* dosage form (capsules) and *injection* dosage form:

—For the treatment of tuberculosis (TB):

- Adults and older children—600 milligrams (mg) once a day. Your doctor may instruct you to take 600 mg two times a week or three times a week. Rifampin must be taken with other medicines to treat tuberculosis.
- Infants and children—Dose is based on body weight and will be determined by your doctor. Rifampin is usually taken once a day. Your doctor may instruct you to take rifampin two times a week or three times a week. Rifampin must be taken with other medicines to treat tuberculosis.

—For the treatment of patients in contact with the meningitis bacteria:

- Adults and older children—600 mg two times a day for two days.
- Infants and children—Dose is based on body weight and will be determined by your doctor. The medicine is taken twice a day for two days.

**Missed dose**—If you do miss a dose of this medicine, take it as soon as possible. However, if it is almost time for your next dose, skip the missed dose and go back to your regular dosing schedule. Do not double doses. *If this medicine is taken on an irregular schedule, side effects may occur more often and may be more serious than usual.* If you have any questions about this, check with your health care professional.

**Storage**—To store the capsule form of this medicine:

- Keep out of the reach of children.
- Store away from heat and direct light.
- Do not store in the bathroom, near the kitchen sink, or in other damp places. Heat or moisture may cause the medicine to break down.
- Do not keep outdated medicine or medicine no longer needed. Be sure that any discarded medicine is out of the reach of children.

## Precautions While Using This Medicine

*It is very important that your doctor check your progress at regular visits.*

If your symptoms do not improve within 2 to 3 weeks, or if they become worse, check with your doctor.

*Oral contraceptives (birth control pills) containing estrogen may not work properly if you take them while you are taking rifampin. Unplanned pregnancies may occur. You should use a different means of birth control while you are taking rifampin.* If you have any questions about this, check with your health care professional.

Liver problems may be more likely to occur if you drink alcoholic beverages regularly while you are taking this medicine. Also, the regular use of alcohol may keep this medicine from working properly. Therefore, *you should not drink alcoholic beverages while you are taking this medicine.*

*If this medicine causes you to feel very tired or very weak or causes a loss of appetite, nausea, or vomiting, stop taking it and check with your doctor immediately.* These may be early warning signs of more serious problems that could develop later.

Rifampin will cause the urine, stool, saliva, sputum, sweat, and tears to turn reddish orange to reddish brown. This is to be expected while you are taking this medicine. This effect may cause soft contact lenses to become permanently discolored. Standard cleaning solutions may not take out all the discoloration. Therefore, *it is best not to wear soft contact lenses while taking this medicine.* Hard contact lenses are not discolored by rifampin. If you have any questions about this, check with your doctor.

© 1994   The United States Pharmacopeial Convention, Inc.

Rifampin can lower the number of white blood cells in your blood temporarily, increasing the chance of getting an infection. It can also lower the number of platelets, which are necessary for proper blood clotting. These problems may result in a greater chance of getting certain infections, slow healing, and bleeding of the gums. Be careful when using a regular toothbrush, dental floss, or a toothpick. Dental work should be delayed until your blood counts have returned to normal. Check with your medical doctor or dentist if you have any questions about proper oral hygiene (mouth care) during treatment.

Before you have any medical tests, tell the doctor in charge that you are taking this medicine. The results of some tests may be affected by this medicine.

## Side Effects of This Medicine

Along with its needed effects, a medicine may cause some unwanted effects. Although not all of these side effects may occur, if they do occur they may need medical attention.

*Check with your doctor immediately* if any of the following side effects occur:

*Less common*

Chills; difficult breathing; dizziness; fever; headache; itching; muscle and bone pain; shivering; skin rash and redness

*Rare*

Bloody or cloudy urine; greatly decreased frequency of urination or amount of urine; loss of appetite; nausea or vomiting; sore throat; unusual bleeding or bruising; unusual tiredness or weakness; yellow eyes or skin

*Signs and symptoms of overdose*

Itching over the whole body; mental changes; reddish orange color of skin, mouth, and eyeballs; swelling around the eyes or the whole face

Other side effects may occur that usually do not need medical attention. These side effects may go away during treatment as your body adjusts to the medicine. However, check with your doctor if any of the following side effects continue or are bothersome:

*More common*

Diarrhea; stomach cramps

*Less common*

Sore mouth or tongue

This medicine commonly causes reddish orange to reddish brown discoloration of urine, stool, saliva, sputum, sweat, and tears. This side effect does not usually need medical attention.

Other side effects not listed above may also occur in some patients. If you notice any other effects, check with your doctor.

## Additional Information

Once a medicine has been approved for marketing for a certain use, experience may show that it is also useful for other medical problems. Although these uses are not included in product labeling, rifampin is used in certain patients with the following medical conditions:

• Atypical mycobacterial infections, such as *Mycobacterium avium* complex (MAC)
• Leprosy (Hansen's disease)
• Prevention of *Haemophilus influenzae* infection
• Treatment of serious staphylococcal infections

Other than the above information, there is no additional information relating to proper use, precautions, or side effects for these uses.

Revised: 06/22/94

# RIFAMPIN AND ISONIAZID Systemic†

A commonly used brand name in the U.S. is Rifamate.
Another commonly used name is rifampicin and isoniazid.

†Not commercially available in Canada.

## Description

Rifampin (rif-AM-pin) and isoniazid (eye-soe-NYE-a-zid) is a combination antibiotic and anti-infective medicine. It is used to treat tuberculosis (TB). It may be taken alone or with one or more other medicines for TB.

*To help clear up your tuberculosis (TB) completely, you must keep taking this medicine for the full time of treatment, even if you begin to feel better. This is very important. It is also important that you do not miss any doses.*

Rifampin and isoniazid combination is available only with your doctor's prescription, in the following dosage form:

*Oral*

• Capsules (U.S.)

## Before Using This Medicine

In deciding to use a medicine, the risks of taking the medicine must be weighed against the good it will do. This is a decision you and your doctor will make. For rifampin and isoniazid combination, the following should be considered:

**Allergies**—Tell your doctor if you have ever had any unusual or allergic reaction to ethionamide (e.g., Trecator-SC), pyrazinamide, niacin (e.g., Nicobid, nicotinic acid), rifampin (e.g., Rifadin), or isoniazid (e.g., INH, Nydrazid). Also tell your health care professional if you are allergic to any other substances, such as foods, preservatives, or dyes.

**Pregnancy**—Pregnant women with tuberculosis (TB) should be treated with TB medicines, including isoniazid and rifampin. Rifampin and isoniazid combination has not been shown to cause birth defects or other problems in humans. However, rifampin has rarely caused bleeding in newborn babies and mothers when it was taken during the last weeks of pregnancy. Also, studies in rodents have shown that rifampin given in high doses causes birth defects, usually backbone problems (spina bifida) and cleft palate.

**Breast-feeding**—Rifampin and isoniazid both pass into the breast milk. However, rifampin and isoniazid have not been reported to cause problems in nursing babies.

**Children**—Rifampin and isoniazid combination is not recommended for use in children.

**Older adults**—Dark urine and yellowing of the eyes or skin are more likely to occur in patients over 50 years of age who are taking isoniazid-containing medicines.

**Other medicines**—Although certain medicines should not be used together at all, in other cases two different medicines may be used together even if an interaction might occur. In these cases, your doctor may want to change the dose, or other precautions may be necessary. When you are taking rifampin and isoniazid combination, it is especially important that your health care professional knows if you are taking any of the following:

- Acetaminophen (e.g., Tylenol) (with long-term, high-dose use) or
- Amiodarone (e.g., Cordarone) or
- Anabolic steroids (nandrolone [e.g., Anabolin], oxandrolone [e.g., Anavar], oxymetholone [e.g., Anadrol], stanozolol [e.g., Winstrol]) or
- Androgens (male hormones) or
- Antithyroid agents (medicine for overactive thyroid) or
- Carbamazepine (e.g., Tegretol) or
- Carmustine (e.g., BiCNU) or
- Chloroquine (e.g., Aralen) or
- Dantrolene (e.g., Dantrium) or
- Daunorubicin (e.g., Cerubidine) or
- Disulfiram (e.g., Antabuse) or
- Divalproex (e.g., Depakote) or
- Etretinate (e.g., Tegison) or
- Gold salts (medicine for arthritis) or
- Hydroxychloroquine (e.g., Plaquenil) or
- Mercaptopurine (e.g., Purinethol) or
- Methyldopa (e.g., Aldomet) or
- Naltrexone (e.g., Trexan) (with long-term, high-dose use) or
- Other anti-infectives by mouth or by injection (medicine for infection) or
- Phenothiazines (acetophenazine [e.g., Tindal], chlorpromazine [e.g., Thorazine], fluphenazine [e.g., Prolixin], mesoridazine [e.g., Serentil], perphenazine [e.g., Trilafon], prochlorperazine [e.g., Compazine], promazine [e.g., Sparine], promethazine [e.g., Phenergan], thioridazine

[e.g., Mellaril], trifluoperazine [e.g., Stelazine], triflupromazine [e.g., Vesprin], trimeprazine [e.g., Temaril]) or
- Plicamycin (e.g., Mithracin) or
- Valproic acid (e.g., Depakene)—These medicines may increase the chance of liver damage if taken with rifampin and isoniazid combination
- Aminophylline (e.g., Somophyllin) or
- Anticoagulants (blood thinners) or
- Antidiabetics, oral (diabetes medicine you take by mouth) or
- Chloramphenicol or
- Corticosteroids (cortisone-like medicine) or
- Digitalis glycosides (heart medicine) or
- Disopyramide (e.g., Norpace) or
- Estramustine (e.g., EMCYT) or
- Fluconazole (e.g., Diflucan) or
- Itraconazole (e.g., Sporanox) or
- Ketoconazole (e.g., Nizoral) or
- Methadone (e.g., Dolophine) or
- Methotrexate (e.g., Mexate) or
- Mexiletine (e.g., Mexitil) or
- Oxtriphylline (e.g., Choledyl) or
- Quinidine (e.g., Quinidex) or
- Theophylline (e.g., Theo-dur, Somophyllin-T) or
- Tocainide (e.g., Tonocard) or
- Verapamil (e.g., Calan)—Rifampin and isoniazid combination may decrease the effects of these medicines
- Disulfiram (e.g., Antabuse)—This medicine may increase the chance of liver damage and side effects, such as dizziness, lack of coordination, irritability, and inability to sleep
- Estrogens (female hormones) or
- Oral contraceptives (birth control pills) containing estrogen or
- Phenytoin (e.g., Dilantin)—Rifampin and isoniazid combination may decrease the effects of these medicines. If you are taking oral contraceptives, this may increase the chance of pregnancy. These medicines may also increase the chance of liver damage if taken with rifampin and isoniazid combination

**Other medical problems**—The presence of other medical problems may affect the use of rifampin and isoniazid combination. Make sure you tell your doctor if you have any other medical problems, especially:

- Alcohol abuse (or history of) or
- Liver disease—There may be an increased chance of getting hepatitis if you take this medicine and drink alcohol daily
- Convulsive disorders such as seizures or epilepsy—Rifampin and isoniazid combination may increase the frequency of seizures (convulsions) in some patients
- Kidney disease (severe)—There may be an increased chance of side effects in patients with severe kidney disease

## Proper Use of This Medicine

If this medicine upsets your stomach, take it with food. Antacids may also help. However, do not take aluminum-containing antacids within 1 hour of the time you take rifampin and isoniazid combination. They may keep this medicine from working properly.

*To help clear up your tuberculosis (TB) completely, it is very important that you keep taking this medicine for the full time of treatment*, even if you begin to feel better after a few weeks. You may have to take it every day for as long as 1 to 2 years or more. *It is important that you do not miss any doses.*

Your doctor may also want you to take pyridoxine (e.g., Hexa-Betalin, vitamin $B_6$) every day to help prevent or lessen some of the side effects of isoniazid. If it is needed, *it is very important to take pyridoxine every day along with this medicine. Do not miss any doses.*

**Dosing**—The dose of rifampin and isoniazid combination will be different for different patients. *Follow your doctor's orders or the directions on the label.* The following information includes only the average doses of rifampin and isoniazid combination. *If your dose is different, do not change it* unless your doctor tells you to do so.

- For the *oral* dosage form (tablets):
  —For the treatment of tuberculosis:
  - Adults and older children—600 milligrams (mg) of rifampin and 300 mg of isoniazid once a day.
  - Children—This medicine is not recommended for use in children.

**Missed dose**—If you do miss a dose of this medicine, take it as soon as possible. However, if it is almost time for your next dose, skip the missed dose and go back to your regular dosing schedule. Do not double doses. *If rifampin and isoniazid combination is taken on an irregular schedule, side effects may occur more often and may be more serious than usual.* If you have any questions about this, check with your health care professional.

**Storage**—To store this medicine:
- Keep out of the reach of children.
- Store away from heat and direct light.
- Do not store in the bathroom, near the kitchen sink, or in other damp places. Heat or moisture may cause the medicine to break down.
- Do not keep outdated medicine or medicine no longer needed. Be sure that any discarded medicine is out of the reach of children.

## Precautions While Using This Medicine

*It is very important that your doctor check your progress at regular visits.* In addition, you should *check with your doctor immediately if blurred vision or loss of vision, with or without eye pain, occurs during treatment.* He or she may want you to have your eyes checked by an ophthalmologist (eye doctor).

If your symptoms do not improve within 2 to 3 weeks, or if they become worse, check with your doctor.

*Oral contraceptives (birth control pills) containing estrogen may not work properly if you take them while you are taking rifampin and isoniazid combination. Unplanned pregnancies may occur. You should use a different means of birth control while you are taking this medicine.* If you have any questions about this, check with your health care professional.

Liver problems may be more likely to occur if you drink alcoholic beverages regularly while you are taking this medicine. Also, the regular use of alcohol may keep this medicine from working properly. Therefore, *you should strictly limit the amount of alcoholic beverages you drink while you are taking this medicine.*

Certain foods such as cheese (Swiss or Cheshire) or fish (tuna, skipjack, or Sardinella) may rarely cause reactions in some patients taking isoniazid-containing medicines. Check with your doctor if redness or itching of the skin, hot feeling, fast or pounding heartbeat, sweating, chills or clammy feeling, headache, or lightheadedness occurs while you are taking this medicine.

This medicine will cause the urine, stool, saliva, sputum, sweat, and tears to turn reddish orange to reddish brown. This is to be expected while you are taking this medicine. This effect may cause soft contact lenses to become permanently discolored. Standard cleaning solutions may not take out all the discoloration. Therefore, *it is best not to wear soft contact lenses while taking this medicine.* Hard contact lenses are not discolored by this medicine. If you have any questions about this, check with your doctor.

*If this medicine causes you to feel very tired or very weak; or causes clumsiness; unsteadiness; a loss of appetite; nausea; numbness, tingling, burning, or pain in the hands and feet; or vomiting, stop taking it and check with your doctor immediately.* These may be early warning symptoms of more serious liver or nerve problems that could develop later.

Rifampin and isoniazid combination may cause blood problems. These problems may result in a greater chance of certain infections, slow healing, and bleeding of the gums. Therefore, you should be careful when using regular toothbrushes, dental floss, and toothpicks. Dental work should be delayed until your blood counts have returned to normal. Check with your medical doctor or dentist if you have any questions about proper oral hygiene (mouth care) during treatment.

## Side Effects of This Medicine

Along with its needed effects, a medicine may cause some unwanted effects. Although not all of these side effects may occur, if they do occur they may need medical attention.

*Check with your doctor immediately* if any of the following side effects occur:

*More common*

Clumsiness or unsteadiness; dark urine; loss of appetite; nausea or vomiting; numbness, tingling, burning, or pain in hands and feet; unusual tiredness or weakness; yellow eyes or skin

*Less common*

Chills; difficult breathing; dizziness; fever; headache; itching; muscle and bone pain; shivering; skin rash and redness

*Rare*

Bloody or cloudy urine; blurred vision or loss of vision, with or without eye pain; convulsions (seizures); depression; greatly decreased frequency of urination or amount of urine; joint pain; mood or mental changes; sore throat; unusual bruising or bleeding

Other side effects may occur that usually do not need medical attention. These side effects may go away during treatment as your body adjusts to the medicine. However, check with your doctor if any of the following side effects continue or are bothersome:

*More common*

Diarrhea; stomach cramps or upset

*Less common*

Sore mouth or tongue

This medicine commonly causes reddish orange to reddish brown discoloration of urine, stool, saliva, sputum, sweat, and tears. This side effect does not usually require medical attention.

Dark urine and yellowing of the eyes or skin (signs of liver problems) are more likely to occur in patients over 50 years of age.

Other side effects not listed above may also occur in some patients. If you notice any other effects, check with your doctor.

Revised: 05/02/94

---

# RIMANTADINE  Systemic†

A commonly used brand name in the U.S. in Flumadine.

†Not commercially available in Canada.

## Description

Rimantadine (ri-MAN-ta-deen) is an antiviral. It is used to prevent or treat certain influenza (flu) infections (type A). It may be given alone or along with flu shots. Rimantadine will not work for colds, other types of flu, or other virus infections.

Rimantadine is available only with your doctor's prescription, in the following dosage forms:

*Oral*
- Syrup (U.S.)
- Tablets (U.S.)

## Before Using This Medicine

In deciding to use a medicine, the risks of taking the medicine must be weighed against the good it will do. This is a decision you and your doctor will make. For rimantadine, the following should be considered:

**Allergies**—Tell your doctor if you have ever had any unusual or allergic reaction to rimantadine or amantadine. Also tell your health care professional if you are allergic to any other substances, such as foods, preservatives, or dyes.

**Pregnancy**—Studies have not been done in humans. However, studies in some animals have shown that rimantadine is harmful to the fetus and causes birth defects.

**Breast-feeding**—It is not known if rimantadine passes into breast milk. Although most medicines pass into breast milk in small amounts, many of them may be used safely while breast-feeding. Mothers who are taking this medicine and who wish to breast-feed should discuss this with their doctor.

**Children**—This medicine has been tested in children over one year of age and has not been shown to cause different side effects or problems in these children than it does in adults. There is no specific information comparing the use of rimantadine in children under one year of age with use in other age groups.

**Older adults**—Elderly people are especially sensitive to the effects of rimantadine. Difficulty in sleeping, difficulty in concentrating, dizziness, headache, nervousness, and weakness may be especially likely to occur. Stomach pain, nausea, vomiting, and loss of appetite may also occur.

**Other medicines**—Although certain medicines should not be used together at all, in other cases two different medicines may be used together even if an interaction might occur. In these cases, your doctor may want to change the dose, or other precautions may be necessary. Tell your health care professional if you are taking any other prescription or nonprescription (over-the-counter [OTC]) medicine.

**Other medical problems**—The presence of other medical problems may affect the use of rimantadine. Make sure you tell your doctor if you have any other medical problems, especially:

- Epilepsy or other seizures (history of)—Rimantadine may increase the frequency of convulsions (seizures) in patients with a seizure disorder
- Kidney disease—Rimantadine is removed from the body by the kidneys; patients with severe kidney disease will need to receive a lower dose of rimantadine
- Liver disease—Patients with severe liver disease may need to receive a lower dose of rimantadine

## Proper Use of This Medicine

Talk to your doctor about the *possibility of getting a flu shot* if you have not had one yet.

This medicine is *best taken before exposure, or as soon as possible after exposure,* to people who have the flu.

To help keep yourself from getting the flu, *keep taking this medicine for the full time of treatment.*

If you already have the flu, *continue taking this medicine for the full time of treatment even if you begin to feel better after a few days.* This will help to clear up your infection completely. If you stop taking this medicine too soon, your symptoms may return. This medicine should be taken for at least 5 to 7 days.

This medicine works best when there is a constant amount in the blood. *To help keep the amount constant, do not miss any doses. Also, it is best to take the doses at evenly spaced times day and night.*

If you are using the oral liquid form of rimantadine, use a specially marked measuring spoon or other device to measure each dose accurately. The average household teaspoon may not hold the right amount of liquid.

**Dosing**—The dose of rimantadine will be different for different patients. *Follow your doctor's orders or the directions on the label.* The following information includes only the average doses of rimantadine. Your dose may be different if you have kidney disease or liver disease. *If your dose is different, do not change it* unless your doctor tells you to do so.

- For *oral* dosage forms (syrup, tablets):
  —For the prevention or treatment of flu:
    - Elderly adults—100 milligrams (mg) once a day.
    - Adults and children 10 years of age and older—100 mg two times a day.
    - Children up to 10 years of age—5 mg per kilogram (2.3 mg per pound) of body weight once a day. Children in this age group should not receive more than 150 mg a day.

**Missed dose**—If you do miss a dose of this medicine, take it as soon as possible. This will help to keep a constant amount of medicine in the blood. However, if it is almost time for your next dose, skip the missed dose and go back to your regular dosing schedule. Do not double doses.

**Storage**—To store this medicine:
- Keep out of the reach of children.
- Store away from heat and direct light.
- Keep the syrup form of this medicine from freezing.
- Do not keep outdated medicine or medicine no longer needed. Be sure that any discarded medicine is out of the reach of children.

## Precautions While Using This Medicine

This medicine may cause some people to become dizzy or confused, or to have trouble concentrating. *Make sure you know how you react to this medicine before you drive, use machines, or do anything else that could be dangerous if you are dizzy or confused.* If these reactions are especially bothersome, check with your doctor.

If your symptoms do not improve within a few days, or if they become worse, check with your doctor.

## Side Effects of This Medicine

Along with its needed effects, a medicine may cause some unwanted effects. Although not all of these side effects may occur, if they do occur they may need medical attention.

Side effects may occur that usually do not need medical attention. These side effects may go away during treatment as your body adjusts to the medicine. However, check with your doctor if any of the following side effects continue or are bothersome:

*Less common*
  Difficulty in concentrating; dizziness; dryness of mouth; headache; loss of appetite; nausea; nervousness; stomach pain; trouble in sleeping; unusual tiredness; vomiting

Other side effects not listed above may also occur in some patients. If you notice any other effects, check with your doctor.

Developed: 03/29/94

# RITODRINE   Systemic

A commonly used brand name in the U.S. and Canada is Yutopar. Generic name product may be available in the U.S.

## Description

Ritodrine (RI-toe-dreen) is used to stop premature labor. It is available only with your doctor's prescription and is to be administered only by or under the supervision of your doctor.

Ritodrine is available in the following dosage forms:
*Oral*
- Tablets (U.S. and Canada)
*Parenteral*
- Injection (U.S. and Canada)

## Before Using This Medicine

In deciding to use a medicine, the risks of taking the medicine must be weighed against the good it will do.

This is a decision you and your doctor will make. For ritodrine, the following should be considered:

**Allergies**—Tell your doctor if you have ever had any unusual or allergic reaction to ritodrine. Also tell your health care professional if you are allergic to any other substances, such as foods, preservatives, or dyes.

**Other medicines**—Although certain medicines should not be used together at all, in other cases two different medicines may be used together even if an interaction might occur. In these cases, your doctor may want to change the dose, or other precautions may be necessary. When you are taking ritodrine, it is especially important that your health care professional know if you are taking any of the following:

- Corticosteroids (cortisone-like medicines)—There is an increased chance of fluid in the lungs when these medicines and ritodrine are used together
- Beta-adrenergic blocking agents (acebutolol [e.g., Sectral], atenolol [e.g., Tenormin], betaxolol [e.g., Kerlone], carteolol [e.g., Cartrol], labetalol [e.g., Normodyne], metoprolol [e.g., Lopressor], nadolol [e.g., Corgard], oxprenolol [e.g., Trasicor], penbutolol [e.g., Levatol], pindolol [e.g., Visken], propranolol [e.g., Inderal], sotalol [e.g., Sotacor], timolol [e.g., Blocadren])—Ritodrine may be less effective if it is used with any of these medicines

**Other medical problems**—The presence of other medical problems may affect the use of ritodrine. Make sure you tell your doctor if you have any other medical problems, especially:

- Asthma
- Diabetes mellitus (sugar diabetes)—Ritodrine may make this condition worse
- Heart disease or
- Overactive thyroid—Use of ritodrine may cause serious effects on the heart, including irregular heartbeat
- High blood pressure (hypertension)
- Migraine headaches (or history of)—Rarely, use of ritodrine may cause problems with blood circulation in the brain

## Proper Use of This Medicine

**Dosing**—The dose of ritodrine will be different for different women. *Follow your doctor's orders or the directions on the label.* The following information includes only the average doses of ritodrine. *If your dose is different, do not change it* unless your doctor tells you to do so.

- For *injection* dosage forms:
  —Adults: 50 to 350 micrograms per minute, injected into a vein.
- For *oral* dosage forms (tablets):
  —Adults: In the first twenty-four hours after the doctor stops your intravenous ritodrine, your dose may be as high as 10 milligrams (mg) every two hours. After that, the dose is usually 10 to 20 mg every four to six hours. Your doctor may want you to take oral ritodrine up until it is time for you to deliver your baby.

**Missed dose**—If you miss a dose of this medicine and remember within an hour or so of the missed dose, take it right away. However, if you do not remember until later, skip the missed dose and go back to your regular dosing schedule. Do not double doses.

**Storage**—To store this medicine:
- Keep out of the reach of children.
- Store away from heat and direct light.
- Do not store in the bathroom, near the kitchen sink, or in other damp places. Heat or moisture may cause the medicine to break down.
- Do not keep outdated medicine or medicine no longer needed. Be sure that any discarded medicine is out of the reach of children.

## Precautions While Using This Medicine

*Check with your doctor right away if your contractions begin again or your water breaks.*

*Do not take other medicines unless they have been discussed with your doctor.* This especially includes over-the-counter (nonprescription) medicines for appetite control, asthma, colds, cough, hay fever, or sinus problems since they may increase the unwanted effects of this medicine.

## Side Effects of This Medicine

Along with its needed effects, a medicine may cause some unwanted effects. Although not all of these side effects may occur, if they do occur they may need medical attention.

*Tell your health care professional immediately* if either of the following side effects occurs while you are receiving this medicine by injection:

*Rare*
Chest pain or tightness; shortness of breath

Check with your health care professional as soon as possible if the following side effects occur:

*More common*
Fast or irregular heartbeat
*Rare*
Yellow eyes or skin
*Symptoms of overdose*
Fast or irregular heartbeat (severe); nausea or vomiting (severe); nervousness or trembling (severe); shortness of breath (severe)

Other side effects may occur that usually do not need medical attention. These side effects may go away during treatment as your body adjusts to the medicine. However, check with your doctor if any of the following side effects continue or are bothersome:

*More common*
Trembling

*Less common*

    Anxiety; emotional upset; headache—more common with injection; jitteriness, nervousness, or restlessness; nausea and vomiting; reddened skin—injection only; skin rash

Other side effects not listed above may also occur in some patients. If you notice any other effects, check with your doctor.

Revised: 07/28/93

---

# RUBELLA VIRUS VACCINE LIVE    Systemic

A commonly used brand name in the U.S. and Canada is Meruvax II. Generic name product may also be available.

## Description

Rubella (rue-BELL-a) Virus Vaccine Live is an active immunizing agent used to prevent infection by the rubella virus. It works by causing your body to produce its own protection (antibodies) against the virus.

The following information applies only to the Wistar RA 27/3 strain of rubella vaccine. Different types of rubella vaccines may be available in countries other than the U.S. and Canada.

Rubella (also known as German measles) is a serious infection that causes miscarriages, stillbirths, or birth defects in unborn babies when pregnant women get the disease. While immunization against rubella is recommended for everyone, it is especially important for women of child-bearing age.

Immunization against rubella is also important for employees in medical facilities, persons in colleges and in the military, persons traveling outside the U.S., children of pregnant women who have not yet received their own rubella immunization, and all children 12 months of age and older, including school-age children.

Immunization against rubella is not recommended for infants younger than 12 months of age, because antibodies they received from their mothers before birth may interfere with the effectiveness of the vaccine. Children who were immunized against rubella before 12 months of age should be immunized again.

If the rubella vaccine is going to be given in a combination immunization that includes measles vaccine, the child to be immunized should be at least 15 months old to make sure the measles vaccine is effective.

You can be considered to be immune to rubella only if you received rubella vaccine on or after your first birthday and have the medical record to prove it or if you have had a blood test showing immunity to rubella. A past history of having a rubella infection is not used to prove immunity, because the signs of rubella infection are not reliable enough to be certain that you have had the disease.

Since vaccination with rubella vaccine may not provide protection for everyone, you may want to ask your doctor to check your immunity to the rubella virus 6 to 8 weeks following your vaccination. This may be especially important if you are a woman of child-bearing age who intends to become pregnant in the future.

This vaccine is to be administered only by or under the supervision of your doctor or other health care professional. It is available in the following dosage form:

*Parenteral*
- Injection (U.S. and Canada)

## Before Receiving This Vaccine

In deciding to use a medicine, the risks of taking the medicine must be weighed against the good it will do. This is a decision you and your doctor will make. For rubella vaccine, the following should be considered:

**Allergies**—Tell your doctor if you have ever had any unusual or allergic reaction to rubella vaccine or to the antibiotic neomycin or polymyxin B. Also tell your health care professional if you are allergic to any other substances, such as preservatives.

**Pregnancy**—Tell your doctor if you are pregnant or if you may become pregnant within 3 months after receiving this vaccine. Although studies have not been done in either humans or animals, use during pregnancy is not recommended, because rubella vaccine crosses the placenta. However, the Centers for Disease Control observed over 200 women who received the vaccine within 3 months before or after becoming pregnant and those women gave birth to normal babies.

**Breast-feeding**—Rubella vaccine may pass into the breast milk and may cause mild rubella infection in nursing babies. However, studies have not shown that this infection causes any problems.

**Children**—Use is not recommended for infants younger than 12 months of age. This medicine has been tested in older infants and children and, in effective doses, has not been shown to cause different side effects or problems than it does in adults.

**Other medicines**—Although certain medicines should not be used together at all, in other cases two different medicines may be used together even if an interaction might occur. In these cases, your doctor may want to change the dose, or other precautions may be necessary. Before you receive rubella vaccine, it is especially important that your health care professional know if you have received any of the following:

- Cancer medicines or
- Corticosteroids (e.g., cortisone-like medicines) or
- Radiation therapy—May reduce the useful effect of the vaccine

**Other medical problems**—The presence of other medical problems may affect the use of rubella vaccine. Make sure you tell your doctor if you have any other medical problems, especially:

- Immune deficiency condition (or family history of)—Condition may increase the chance and severity of side effects of the vaccine and/or may decrease the useful effects of the vaccine
- Severe illness with fever—The symptoms of the condition may be confused with the possible side effects of the vaccine
- Tuberculosis—Use of rubella vaccine may interfere with the tuberculin skin test

## Proper Use of This Vaccine

**Dosing**—The dose of rubella vaccine will be different for different patients. The following information includes only the average dose of rubella vaccine.

- For *injection* dosage form:
  —For prevention of rubella:
  - Adults and children 12 months of age and older—One dose injected under the skin.
  - Children up to 12 months of age—Use is not recommended.

## Precautions After Receiving This Vaccine

*Do not become pregnant for 3 months after receiving rubella vaccine without first checking with your doctor.* There is a chance that this vaccine may cause birth defects.

Tell your doctor that you have received this vaccine:

- if you are to receive a tuberculin skin test within 8 weeks after receiving this vaccine. The results of the test may be affected by this vaccine.
- if you are to receive any other live virus vaccines within 1 month after receiving this vaccine.
- if you are to receive blood transfusions or other blood products within 2 weeks after receiving this vaccine.
- if you are to receive gamma globulin or other globulins within 2 weeks after receiving this vaccine.

## Side Effects of This Vaccine

Along with its needed effects, a vaccine may cause some unwanted effects. Although not all of these side effects may occur, if they do occur they may need medical attention.

*Get emergency help immediately* if any of the following side effects occur:

*Symptoms of allergic reaction*
> Difficulty in breathing or swallowing; hives; itching, especially of feet or hands; reddening of skin, especially around ears; swelling of eyes, face, or inside of nose; unusual tiredness or weakness (sudden and severe)

Check with your doctor as soon as possible if any of the following side effects occur:

*Less common*
> Pain or tenderness of eyes

*Rare*
> Bruising or purple spots on skin; confusion; convulsions (seizures); headache (severe or continuing); pain, numbness, or tingling of hands, arms, legs, or feet; stiff neck; unusual irritability; vomiting

Other side effects may occur that usually do not need medical attention. However, check with your doctor if any of the following side effects continue or are bothersome:

*More common*
> Burning or stinging at place of injection; skin rash; swelling of glands in neck

*Less common*
> Aches or pain in joints; headache (mild), sore throat, runny nose, or fever; itching, swelling, redness, tenderness, or hard lump at place of injection; nausea; vague feeling of bodily discomfort

The above side effects (especially aches or pain in joints) are more likely to occur in adults, particularly women.

Some of the above side effects may not occur until 1 to 4 weeks after immunization and usually last less than 1 week.

Check with your doctor as soon as possible if any of the following side effects occur:

> Pain, numbness, or tingling of hands, arms, legs, or feet; pain or tenderness of eyes

In addition, check with your doctor if any of the following side effects continue or are bothersome:

> Headache (mild), sore throat, runny nose, or fever; swelling of glands in neck; vague feeling of bodily discomfort

Also, aches or pain in joints may not occur until 1 to 10 weeks after immunization and usually last less than 1 week. Check with your doctor if either of these side effects continues or is bothersome.

Other side effects not listed above may also occur in some patients. If you notice any other effects, check with your doctor.

Revised: 07/12/94

# SALICYLATES   Systemic

Some commonly used brand names are:

**In the U.S.—**

| | |
|---|---|
| Amigesic[8] | Magan[7] |
| Anacin[2] | Magnaprin[3] |
| APAC Improved[2] | Magnaprin Arthritis Strength[3] |
| Arthritis Pain Formula[3] | Maprin[3] |
| Arthropan[5] | Maprin I-B[3] |
| Ascriptin[3] | Measurin[1] |
| Ascriptin A/D[3] | Mobidin[7] |
| Aspergum[1] | Mono-Gesic[8] |
| Bayer Aspirin[1] | Norwich Aspirin[1] |
| Buffaprin[3] | P-A-C Revised Formula[2] |
| Bufferin[3] | Salcylic Acid[8] |
| Buffinol[3] | Salflex[8] |
| Cama Arthritis Pain Reliever[3] | Salgesic[8] |
| Diagen[8] | Salsitab[8] |
| Disalcid[8] | St. Joseph Adult Chewable |
| Doan's[7] | Aspirin[1] |
| Easprin[1] | Therapy Bayer[1] |
| Ecotrin[1] | Tricosal[6] |
| Empirin[1] | Trilisate[6] |
| Halfprin[1] | Uracel[9] |
| 8-Hour Bayer Timed-Release[1] | ZORprin[1] |

**In Canada—**

| | |
|---|---|
| Anacin[2] | Doan's[7] |
| APF Arthritic Pain Formula[3] | Dodd's Pills[9] |
| Apo-Asa[1] | Ecotrin[1] |
| Apo-Asen[1] | Entrophen[1] |
| Arthrinol[1] | Headstart[1] |
| Arthrisin[1] | Instantine[2] |
| Artria S.R.[1] | Nervine[2] |
| Aspergum[1] | Novasen[1] |
| Aspirin[1] | Riphen[1] |
| Astrin[1] | Sal-Adult[1] |
| Back-Ese[7] | Sal-Infant[1] |
| Bayer Timed-Release Arthritic | 217 Strong[2] |
| Pain Formula[1] | Supasa[1] |
| Bufferin[3] | 217[2] |
| C2[2] | Triaphen[1] |
| C2 Buffered[4] | Trilisate[6] |
| Coryphen[1] | |

Other commonly used names are:

| | |
|---|---|
| acetylsalicylic acid[1] | choline magnesium |
| ASA[1]# | trisalicylate[6] |
| | salicylsalicylic acid[8] |

Note: For quick reference, the following salicylates are numbered to match the corresponding brand names.

This information applies to the following medicines:

1. Aspirin (AS-pir-in)‡§#
2. Aspirin and Caffeine (kaf-EEN)‡
3. Buffered Aspirin‡#**
4. Buffered Aspirin and Caffeine*#
5. Choline Salicylate (KOE-leen sa-LI-si-late)
6. Choline and Magnesium (mag-NEE-zhum) Salicylates
7. Magnesium Salicylate
8. Salsalate (SAL-sa-late)‡
9. Sodium Salicylate‡

---

*Not commercially available in the U.S.
‡Generic name product may also be available in the U.S.
§Generic name product may also be available in Canada.
*#Aspirin* is a brand name in Canada; acetylsalicylic acid is the generic name. ASA, a commonly used designation for aspirin (or acetylsalicylic acid) in both the U.S. and Canada, is the term used in Canadian product labeling.
**Some of the buffered aspirin products may be identified on the label as Aspirin (ASA), Alumina, and Magnesia.

## Description

Salicylates are used to relieve pain and reduce fever. Most salicylates are also used to relieve some symptoms caused by arthritis (rheumatism), such as swelling, stiffness, and joint pain. However, they do not cure arthritis and will help you only as long as you continue to take them.

Aspirin may also be used to lessen the chance of heart attack, stroke, or other problems that may occur when a blood vessel is blocked by blood clots. Aspirin helps prevent dangerous blood clots from forming. However, this effect of aspirin may increase the chance of serious bleeding in some people. Therefore, aspirin should be used for this purpose only when your doctor decides, after studying your medical condition and history, that the danger of blood clots is greater than the risk of bleeding. *Do not take aspirin to prevent blood clots or a heart attack unless it has been ordered by your doctor.*

Salicylates may also be used for other conditions as determined by your doctor.

The caffeine present in some of these products may provide additional relief of headache pain or faster pain relief.

Some salicylates are available only with your medical doctor's or dentist's prescription. Others are available without a prescription; however, your medical doctor or dentist may have special instructions on the proper dose of these medicines for your medical condition.

These medicines are available in the following dosage forms:

*Oral*

Aspirin
- Capsules (U.S.)
- Delayed-release (enteric-coated) capsules (Canada)
- Tablets (U.S. and Canada)
- Chewable tablets (U.S. and Canada)
- Chewing gum tablets (U.S. and Canada)
- Delayed-release (enteric-coated) tablets (U.S. and Canada)
- Dispersible tablets (Canada)
- Extended-release tablets (U.S. and Canada)

Aspirin and Caffeine
- Capsules (Canada)
- Tablets (U.S. and Canada)

Buffered Aspirin
- Tablets (U.S. and Canada)

Buffered Aspirin and Caffeine
- Tablets (Canada)

Choline Salicylate
- Oral solution (U.S.)

Choline and Magnesium Salicylates
- Oral solution (U.S.)
- Tablets (U.S. and Canada)

Magnesium Salicylate
- Tablets (U.S. and Canada)

Salsalate
- Capsules (U.S.)
- Tablets (U.S.)

Sodium Salicylate
- Tablets (U.S. and Canada)
- Delayed-release (enteric-coated) tablets (U.S.)

*Rectal*

Aspirin
- Suppositories (U.S. and Canada)

---

## Before Using This Medicine

If you are taking this medicine without a prescription, carefully read and follow any precautions on the label. For salicylates, the following should be considered:

**Allergies**—Tell your doctor if you have ever had any unusual or allergic reaction to aspirin or other salicylates, including methyl salicylate (oil of wintergreen), or to any of the following medicines:

Diclofenac (e.g., Voltaren)
Diflunisal (e.g., Dolobid)
Fenoprofen (e.g., Nalfon)
Floctafenine (e.g., Idarac)
Flurbiprofen, oral (e.g., Ansaid)
Ibuprofen (e.g., Motrin)
Indomethacin (e.g., Indocin)
Ketoprofen (e.g., Orudis)
Ketorolac (e.g., Toradol)
Meclofenamate (e.g., Meclomen)
Mefenamic acid (e.g., Ponstel)
Naproxen (e.g., Naprosyn)
Oxyphenbutazone (e.g., Tandearil)
Phenylbutazone (e.g., Butazolidin)
Piroxicam (e.g., Feldene)
Sulindac (e.g., Clinoril)
Suprofen (e.g., Suprol)
Tiaprofenic acid (e.g., Surgam)
Tolmetin (e.g., Tolectin)
Zomepirac (e.g., Zomax)

Also tell your health care professional if you are allergic to any other substances, such as foods, preservatives, or dyes.

**Diet**—Make certain your health care professional knows if you are on a low-sodium diet. Regular use of large amounts of sodium salicylate (as for arthritis) can add a large amount of sodium to your diet. Sodium salicylate contains 46 mg of sodium in each 325-mg tablet and 92 mg of sodium in each 650-mg tablet.

**Pregnancy**—Salicylates have not been shown to cause birth defects in humans. Studies on birth defects in humans have been done with aspirin but not with other salicylates. However, salicylates caused birth defects in animal studies.

Some reports have suggested that too much use of aspirin late in pregnancy may cause a decrease in the newborn's weight and possible death of the fetus or newborn infant. However, the mothers in these reports had been taking much larger amounts of aspirin than are usually recommended. Studies of mothers taking aspirin in the doses that are usually recommended did not show these unwanted effects. However, there is a chance that regular use of salicylates late in pregnancy may cause unwanted effects on the heart or blood flow in the fetus or in the newborn infant.

Use of salicylates, especially aspirin, during the last 2 weeks of pregnancy may cause bleeding problems in the fetus before or during delivery or in the newborn infant. Also, too much use of salicylates during the last 3 months of pregnancy may increase the length of pregnancy, prolong labor, cause other problems during delivery, or cause severe bleeding in the mother before, during, or after delivery. *Do not take aspirin during the last 3 months of pregnancy unless it has been ordered by your doctor.*

Studies in humans have not shown that caffeine (present in some aspirin products) causes birth defects. However, studies in animals have shown that caffeine causes birth defects when given in very large doses (amounts equal to those present in 12 to 24 cups of coffee a day).

**Breast-feeding**—Salicylates pass into the breast milk. Although salicylates have not been reported to cause problems in nursing babies, it is possible that problems may occur if large amounts are taken regularly, as for arthritis (rheumatism).

Caffeine passes into the breast milk in small amounts.

**Children**—*Do not give aspirin or other salicylates to a child or a teenager with a fever or other symptoms of a virus infection, especially flu or chickenpox, without first discussing its use with your child's doctor.* This is very important because salicylates may cause a serious illness called Reye's syndrome in children and teenagers with fever caused by a virus infection, especially flu or chickenpox.

Some children may need to take aspirin or another salicylate regularly (as for arthritis). However, your child's doctor may want to stop the medicine for a while if a fever or other symptoms of a virus infection occur. Discuss this with your child's doctor, so that you will know ahead of time what to do if your child gets sick.

Children who do not have a virus infection may also be more sensitive to the effects of salicylates, especially if they have a fever or have lost large amounts of body fluid because of vomiting, diarrhea, or sweating. This may increase the chance of side effects during treatment.

**Older adults**—Elderly people are especially sensitive to the effects of salicylates. This may increase the chance of side effects during treatment.

**Other medicines**—Although certain medicines should not be used together at all, in other cases two different medicines may be used together even if an interaction might occur. In these cases, your doctor may want to change the dose, or other precautions may be necessary. When you are taking a salicylate, it is especially important that your health care professional know if you are taking any of the following:

- Anticoagulants (blood thinners) or
- Carbenicillin by injection (e.g., Geopen) or

- Cefamandole (e.g., Mandol) or
- Cefoperazone (e.g., Cefobid) or
- Cefotetan (e.g., Cefotan) or
- Dipyridamole (e.g., Persantine) or
- Divalproex (e.g., Depakote) or
- Heparin or
- Medicine for inflammation or pain, except narcotics, or
- Moxalactam (e.g., Moxam) or
- Pentoxifylline (e.g., Trental) or
- Plicamycin (e.g., Mithracin) or
- Ticarcillin (e.g., Ticar) or
- Valproic acid (e.g., Depakene)—Taking these medicines together with a salicylate, especially aspirin, may increase the chance of bleeding
- Antidiabetics, oral (diabetes medicine you take by mouth)— Salicylates may increase the effects of the antidiabetic medicine; a change in dose may be needed if a salicylate is taken regularly
- Ketoconazole (e.g., Nizoral) or
- Tetracyclines (medicine for infection), taken by mouth— The antacids present in buffered aspirin products can keep the ketoconazole or tetracycline from working properly if taken too close to them. Also, the magnesium present in choline and magnesium salicylates (e.g., Trilisate) or magnesium salicylate (e.g., Doan's) can keep the tetracycline from working properly if taken too close to it
- Methotrexate (e.g., Mexate) or
- Vancomycin (e.g., Vancocin)—The chance of serious side effects may be increased
- Probenecid (e.g., Benemid)—Salicylates can keep probenecid from working properly for treating gout
- Sulfinpyrazone (e.g., Anturane)—Salicylates can keep sulfinpyrazone from working properly for treating gout; also, taking a salicylate, especially aspirin, with sulfinpyrazone may increase the chance of bleeding
- Urinary alkalizers (medicine that makes the urine less acid, such as acetazolamide [e.g., Diamox], calcium- and/or magnesium-containing antacids, dichlorphenamide [e.g., Daranide], methazolamide [e.g., Neptazane], potassium or sodium citrate and/or citric acid, sodium bicarbonate [baking soda])—These medicines may make the salicylate less effective by causing it to be removed from the body more quickly
- Zidovudine (e.g., AZT, Retrovir)—Aspirin may increase the blood levels of zidovudine, which increases the chance of serious side effects

**Other medical problems**—The presence of other medical problems may affect the use of salicylates. Make sure you tell your doctor if you have any other medical problems, especially:

- Anemia or
- Overactive thyroid or
- Stomach ulcer or other stomach problems—Salicylates may make your condition worse
- Asthma, allergies, and nasal polyps (history of) or
- Glucose-6-phosphate dehydrogenase (G6PD) deficiency or
- High blood pressure (hypertension) or
- Kidney disease or
- Liver disease—The chance of side effects may be increased.
- Gout—Salicylates can make this condition worse and can also lessen the effects of some medicines used to treat gout

- Heart disease—The chance of some side effects may be increased. Also, the caffeine present in some aspirin products can make some kinds of heart disease worse
- Hemophilia or other bleeding problems—The chance of bleeding may be increased, especially with aspirin

## Proper Use of This Medicine

*Take this medicine after meals or with food* (except for enteric-coated capsules or tablets and aspirin suppositories) to lessen stomach irritation.

*Take tablet or capsule forms of this medicine with a full glass (8 ounces) of water.* Also, do not lie down for about 15 to 30 minutes after swallowing the medicine. This helps to prevent irritation that may lead to trouble in swallowing.

For patients taking *aspirin (including buffered aspirin and/or products containing caffeine):*

- *Do not use any product that contains aspirin if it has a strong, vinegar-like odor.* This odor means the medicine is breaking down. If you have any questions about this, check with your health care professional.
- If you are to take any medicine that contains aspirin within 7 days after having your tonsils removed, a tooth pulled, or other dental or mouth surgery, be sure to swallow the aspirin whole. Do not chew aspirin during this time.
- Do not place any medicine that contains aspirin directly on a tooth or gum surface. This may cause a burn.
- There are several different forms of aspirin or buffered aspirin tablets. If you are using:
  —*chewable aspirin tablets,* they may be chewed, dissolved in liquid, crushed, or swallowed whole.
  —*dispersible aspirin tablets,* they are to be dissolved in the mouth before swallowing. If your mouth is too dry, sip a little water to help dissolve the medicine.
  —*delayed-release (enteric-coated) aspirin tablets,* they must be swallowed whole. Do not crush them or break them up before taking.
  —*extended-release (long-acting) aspirin tablets,* check with your pharmacist as to how they should be taken. Some may be broken up (but must not be crushed) before swallowing if you cannot swallow them whole. Others should not be broken up and must be swallowed whole.

To use *aspirin suppositories:*

- If the suppository is too soft to insert, chill it in the refrigerator for 30 minutes or run cold water over it before removing the foil wrapper.
- To insert the suppository: First remove the foil wrapper and moisten the suppository with cold water. Lie down on your side and use your finger to push the suppository well up into the rectum.

To take *choline and magnesium salicylates (e.g., Tril-isate) oral solution:*

- The liquid may be mixed with fruit juice just before taking.
- Drink a full glass (8 ounces) of water after taking the medicine.

To take *enteric-coated sodium salicylate tablets:*

- The tablets must be swallowed whole. Do not crush them or break them up before taking.

Unless otherwise directed by your medical doctor or dentist:

- Do not take more of this medicine than recommended on the label, to lessen the chance of side effects.
- Children up to 12 years of age should not take this medicine more than 5 times a day.

*When used for arthritis (rheumatism), this medicine must be taken regularly as ordered by your doctor in order for it to help you.* Up to 2 to 3 weeks or longer may pass before you feel the full effects of this medicine.

**Missed dose**—If your medical doctor or dentist has ordered you to take this medicine according to a regular schedule and you miss a dose, take it as soon as you remember. However, if it is almost time for your next dose, skip the missed dose and go back to your regular dosing schedule. Do not double doses.

**Storage**—To store this medicine:

- Keep out of the reach of children. Overdose is very dangerous in young children.
- Store away from heat and direct light.
- Do not store tablets or capsules in the bathroom, near the kitchen sink, or in other damp places. Heat or moisture may cause the medicine to break down.
- Keep liquid forms of this medicine from freezing.
- Store aspirin suppositories in a cool place. It is usually best to keep them in the refrigerator, but keep them from freezing.
- Do not keep outdated medicine or medicine no longer needed. Be sure that any discarded medicine is out of the reach of children.

## Precautions While Using This Medicine

*Check the labels of all nonprescription (over-the-counter [OTC]) and prescription medicines you now take.* If any contain aspirin or other salicylates, including bismuth subsalicylate (e.g., Pepto-Bismol), be especially careful. Also, be especially careful if you regularly use a shampoo or other medicine for your skin that contains salicylic acid or any other salicylate. Using other salicylate-containing products while taking this medicine may lead to overdose. If you have any questions about this, check with your health care professional.

If you will be taking salicylates for a long time (more than 5 days in a row for children or 10 days in a row for

adults) or in large amounts, *your doctor should check your progress at regular visits.*

Check with your medical doctor or dentist:

- If you are taking this medicine to relieve pain and the pain lasts for more than 10 days (5 days for children) or if the pain gets worse, if new symptoms occur, or if redness or swelling is present. These could be signs of a serious condition that needs medical or dental treatment.
- If you are taking this medicine to bring down a fever, and the fever lasts for more than 3 days or returns, if the fever gets worse, if new symptoms occur, or if redness or swelling is present. These could be signs of a serious condition that needs treatment.
- If you are taking this medicine for a sore throat, and the sore throat is very painful, lasts for more than 2 days, or occurs together with or is followed by fever, headache, skin rash, nausea, or vomiting.
- If you are taking this medicine regularly, as for arthritis (rheumatism), and you notice a ringing or buzzing in your ears or severe or continuing headaches. These are often the first signs that too much salicylate is being taken. Your doctor may want to change the amount of medicine you are taking every day.

For patients taking *aspirin to lessen the chance of heart attack, stroke, or other problems caused by blood clots:*

- *Take only the amount of aspirin ordered by your doctor.* If you need a medicine to relieve pain, a fever, or arthritis, your doctor may not want you to take extra aspirin. It is a good idea to discuss this with your doctor, so that you will know ahead of time what medicine to take.
- *Do not stop taking this medicine for any reason without first checking with the doctor who directed you to take it.*

Taking certain other medicines together with a salicylate may increase the chance of unwanted effects. The risk will depend on how much of each medicine you take every day, and on how long you take the medicines together. If your doctor directs you to take these medicines together on a regular basis, follow his or her directions carefully. However, *do not take any of the following medicines together with a salicylate for more than a few days, unless your doctor has directed you to do so and is following your progress:*

Acetaminophen (e.g., Tylenol)
Diclofenac (e.g., Voltaren)
Diflunisal (e.g., Dolobid)
Fenoprofen (e.g., Nalfon)
Floctafenine (e.g., Idarac)
Flurbiprofen, oral (e.g., Ansaid)
Ibuprofen (e.g., Motrin)
Indomethacin (e.g., Indocin)
Ketoprofen (e.g., Orudis)
Ketorolac (e.g., Toradol)
Meclofenamate (e.g., Meclomen)
Mefenamic acid (e.g., Ponstel)
Naproxen (e.g., Naprosyn)
Phenylbutazone (e.g., Butazolidin)

Piroxicam (e.g., Feldene)
Sulindac (e.g., Clinoril)
Tiaprofenic acid (e.g., Surgam)
Tolmetin (e.g., Tolectin)

For *diabetic patients:*

- False urine sugar test results may occur if you are regularly taking large amounts of salicylates, such as:

    —*Aspirin:* 8 or more 325-mg (5-grain), or 4 or more 500-mg or 650-mg (10-grain), or 3 or more 800-mg (or higher strength), doses a day.

    —*Buffered aspirin or*
    —*Sodium salicylate:* 8 or more 325-mg (5-grain), or 4 or more 500-mg or 650-mg (10-grain), doses a day.

    —*Choline salicylate:* 4 or more teaspoonfuls (each teaspoonful containing 870 mg) a day.

    —*Choline and magnesium salicylates:* 5 or more 500-mg tablets or teaspoonfuls, 4 or more 750-mg tablets, or 2 or more 1000-mg tablets, a day.

    —*Magnesium salicylate:* 7 or more 325-mg, or 4 or more 500-mg (or higher strength), tablets a day.

    —*Salsalate:* 4 or more 500-mg doses, or 3 or more 750-mg doses, a day.

- Smaller doses or occasional use of salicylates usually will not affect urine sugar tests. However, check with your health care professional (especially if your diabetes is not well-controlled) if:

    —you are not sure how much salicylate you are taking every day.

    —you notice any change in your urine sugar test results.

    —you have any other questions about this possible problem.

Do not take aspirin for 5 days before any surgery, including dental surgery, unless otherwise directed by your medical doctor or dentist. Taking aspirin during this time may cause bleeding problems.

For patients taking *buffered aspirin, choline and magnesium salicylates (e.g., Trilisate), or magnesium salicylate (e.g., Doan's):*

- If you are also taking a tetracycline antibiotic, do not take the 2 medicines within 3 to 4 hours of each other. Taking them too close together may prevent the tetracycline from being absorbed by your body.

- If you are also taking ketoconazole, do not take buffered aspirin within 3 hours of the ketoconazole. Taking them too close together may prevent the ketoconazole from being absorbed by your body.

- If you have any questions about this, check with your health care professional.

If you are taking a laxative containing cellulose, take the salicylate at least 2 hours before or after you take the laxative. Taking these medicines too close together may lessen the effects of the salicylate.

For patients taking this medicine by mouth:

- Stomach problems may be more likely to occur if you drink alcoholic beverages while being treated with this medicine, especially if you are taking it in high doses or for a long time. Check with your doctor if you have any questions about this.

For patients using *aspirin suppositories:*

- Aspirin suppositories may cause irritation of the rectum. Check with your doctor if this occurs.

Salicylates may interfere with the results of some medical tests. Before you have any medical tests, tell the doctor in charge if you have taken any of these medicines within the past week. If possible, it is best to check with the doctor first, to find out whether the medicine may be taken during the week before the test.

For patients taking one of the products that contains *caffeine:*

- Caffeine may interfere with the result of a test that uses dipyridamole (e.g., Persantine) to help find out how well your blood is flowing through certain blood vessels. Therefore, you should not have any caffeine for at least 4 hours before the test.

*If you think that you or anyone else may have taken an overdose, get emergency help at once.* Taking an overdose of these medicines may cause unconsciousness or death. Signs of overdose include convulsions (seizures), hearing loss, confusion, ringing or buzzing in the ears, severe drowsiness or tiredness, severe excitement or nervousness, and fast or deep breathing.

## Side Effects of This Medicine

Along with its needed effects, a medicine may cause some unwanted effects. When this medicine is used for short periods of time at low doses, side effects usually are rare. Although not all of the following side effects may occur, if they do occur they may need medical attention.

*Get emergency help immediately* if any of the following side effects occur:

Any loss of hearing; bloody urine; confusion; convulsions (seizures); diarrhea (severe or continuing); difficulty in swallowing; dizziness, lightheadedness, or feeling faint (severe); drowsiness (severe); excitement or nervousness (severe); fast or deep breathing; flushing, redness, or other change in skin color; hallucinations (seeing, hearing, or feeling things that are not there); increased sweating; increased thirst; nausea or vomiting (severe or continuing); shortness of breath, troubled breathing, tightness in chest, or wheezing; stomach pain (severe or continuing); swelling of eyelids, face, or lips; unexplained fever; uncontrollable flapping movements of the hands (especially in elderly patients); vision problems

*Symptoms of overdose in children*

Changes in behavior; drowsiness or tiredness (severe); fast or deep breathing

Also, check with your doctor as soon as possible if any of the following side effects occur:

*Less common or rare*

Abdominal or stomach pain, cramping, or burning (severe); bloody or black, tarry stools; headache (severe or continuing); ringing or buzzing in ears (continuing); skin rash, hives, or itching; unusual tiredness or weakness; vomiting of blood or material that looks like coffee grounds

Other side effects may occur that usually do not need medical attention. These side effects may go away during treatment as your body adjusts to the medicine. However, check with your health care professional if any of the following side effects continue or are bothersome:

*More common*
Abdominal or stomach cramps, pain, or discomfort (mild to moderate); heartburn or indigestion; nausea or vomiting

*Less common*
Trouble in sleeping, nervousness, or jitters (only for products containing caffeine)

Other side effects not listed above may also occur in some patients. If you notice any other effects, check with your doctor.

Revised: August 1990

---

# SALICYLIC ACID    Topical

Some commonly used brand names are:

**In the U.S.—**

Antinea
Buf-Puf Acne Cleansing Bar with Vitamin E
Calicylic Creme
Clearasil Clearstick Maximum Strength Topical Solution
Clearasil Clearstick Regular Strength Topical Solution
Clearasil Double Textured Pads Maximum Strength
Clearasil Double Textured Pads Regular Strength
Clearasil Medicated Deep Cleanser Topical Solution
Clear Away
Clear by Design Medicated Cleansing Pads
Compound W Gel
Compound W Liquid
Duofilm
Duoplant Topical Solution
Freezone
Gordofilm
Hydrisalic
Ionax Astringent Skin Cleanser Topical Solution
Ionil Plus Shampoo
Ionil Shampoo
Keralyt
Keratex Gel
Lactisol
Listerex Golden Scrub Lotion
Listerex Herbal Scrub Lotion
Mediplast
Noxzema Anti-Acne Gel
Noxzema Anti-Acne Pads Maximum Strength
Noxzema Anti-Acne Pads Regular Strength
Occlusal-HP Topical Solution
Occlusal Topical Solution
Off-Ezy Topical Solution Corn & Callus Remover Kit
Off-Ezy Topical Solution Wart Removal Kit
Oxy Clean Medicated Cleanser
Oxy Clean Medicated Pads Maximum Strength
Oxy Clean Medicated Pads Regular Strength

Oxy Clean Medicated Pads Sensitive Skin
Oxy Night Watch Maximum Strength Lotion
Oxy Night Watch Sensitive Skin Lotion
Paplex
Paplex Ultra
Propa pH Medicated Acne Cream Maximum Strength
Propa pH Medicated Cleansing Pads Maximum Strength
Propa pH Medicated Cleansing Pads Sensitive Skin
Propa pH Perfectly Clear Skin Cleanser Topical Solution Normal/Combination Skin
Propa pH Perfectly Clear Skin Cleanser Topical Solution Oily Skin
Propa pH Perfectly Clear Skin Cleanser Topical Solution Sensitive Skin Formula
P&S
Salac
Salacid
Sal-Acid Plaster
Salactic Film Topical Solution
Sal-Clens Plus Shampoo
Sal-Clens Shampoo
Saligel
Salonil
Sal-Plant Gel Topical Solution
Sebucare
Stri-Dex Dual Textured Pads Maximum Strength
Stri-Dex Dual Textured Pads Regular Strength
Stri-Dex Dual Textured Pads Sensitive Skin
Stri-Dex Maximum Strength Pads
Stri-Dex Regular Strength Pads
Stri-Dex Super Scrub Pads
Trans-Plantar
Trans-Ver-Sal
Verukan-HP Topical Solution
Verukan Topical Solution

Viranol
Viranol Ultra

Wart-Off Topical Solution
X-Seb

Generic name product may also be available.

**In Canada—**

Compound W Gel
Compound W Liquid
Cuplex Gel
Occlusal-HP Topical Solution
Occlusal Topical Solution
Oxy Clean Extra Strength Medicated Pads
Oxy Clean Extra Strength Cleanser Topical Solution
Oxy Clean Medicated Soap
Oxy Clean Regular Strength Medicated Cleanser Topical Solution
Oxy Clean Regular Strength Medicated Pads

Oxy Clean Sensitive Skin Cleanser Topical Solution
Oxy Clean Sensitive Skin Pads
Oxy Night Watch Night Time Acne Medication Extra Strength Lotion
Oxy Night Watch Night Time Acne Medication Regular Strength Lotion
Oxy Sensitive Skin Vanishing Formula Lotion
Salac
Tersac Cleansing Gel
Trans-Ver-Sal

## Description

Salicylic acid (sal-i-SILL-ik AS-id) is used to treat many skin disorders, such as acne, dandruff, psoriasis, seborrheic dermatitis of the skin and scalp, calluses, corns, common warts, and plantar warts, depending on the dosage form and strength of the preparation.

Some of these preparations are available only with your doctor's prescription. Others are available without a prescription; however, your doctor may have special instructions on the proper use of salicylic acid for your medical condition.

Salicylic acid is available in the following dosage forms:

*Topical*
- Cream (U.S.)
- Gel (U.S. and Canada)
- Lotion (U.S. and Canada)
- Ointment (U.S.)
- Pads (U.S. and Canada)
- Plaster (U.S. and Canada)
- Shampoo (U.S.)
- Soap (U.S. and Canada)
- Topical solution (U.S. and Canada)

## Before Using This Medicine

If you are using this medicine without a prescription, carefully read and follow any precautions on the label. For salicylic acid, the following should be considered:

**Allergies**—Tell your doctor if you have ever had any unusual or allergic reaction to salicylic acid. Also tell your health care professional if you are allergic to any other substances, such as preservatives or dyes.

**Pregnancy**—This medicine may be absorbed through the mother's skin. Salicylic acid has not been studied in pregnant women. However, studies in animals have shown that salicylic acid causes birth defects when given orally in doses about 6 times the highest dose recommended for topical use in humans. Before using this medicine, make sure your doctor knows if you are pregnant or if you may become pregnant, especially if you will be using salicylic acid on large areas of your body.

**Breast-feeding**—Salicylic acid may be absorbed through the mother's skin. However, topical salicylic acid has not been reported to cause problems in nursing babies.

**Children**—Young children may be at increased risk of unwanted effects because of increased absorption of salicylic acid through the skin. Also, young children may be more likely to get skin irritation from salicylic acid. Salicylic acid should not be applied to large areas of the body, used for long periods of time, or used under occlusive dressing (air-tight covering, such as kitchen plastic wrap) in infants and children.

**Older adults**—Elderly people are more likely to have age-related blood vessel disease. This may increase the chance of problems during treatment with this medicine.

**Other medicines**—Although certain medicines should not be used together at all, in other cases two different medicines may be used together even if an interaction might occur. In these cases, your doctor may want to change the dose, or other precautions may be necessary. Tell your health care professional if you are using any other prescription or nonprescription (over-the-counter [OTC]) medicine.

**Other medical problems**—The presence of other medical problems may affect the use of salicylic acid, especially if you are using a 5% or stronger salicylic acid preparation. Make sure you tell your doctor if you have any other medical problems, especially:

- Blood vessel disease
- Diabetes mellitus (sugar diabetes)—Use of this medicine may cause severe redness or ulceration, especially on the hands or feet
- Inflammation, irritation, or infection of the skin—Use of this medicine may cause severe irritation if applied to inflamed, irritated, or infected area of the skin

## Proper Use of This Medicine

*It is very important that you use this medicine only as directed.* Do not use more of it, do not use it more often, and do not use it for a longer time than recommended on the label, unless otherwise directed by your doctor. To do so may increase the chance of absorption through the skin and the chance of salicylic acid poisoning.

If your doctor has ordered an occlusive dressing (airtight covering, such as kitchen plastic wrap) to be applied over this medicine, make sure you know how to apply it. Since an occlusive dressing will increase the amount of medicine absorbed through your skin and the possibility of salicylic acid poisoning, use it only as directed. If you have any questions about this, check with your doctor.

*Keep this medicine away from the eyes and other mucous membranes,* such as the mouth and inside of the nose. If you should accidentally get some in your eyes or on other mucous membranes, immediately flush them with water for 15 minutes.

To use the *cream, lotion, or ointment form* of salicylic acid:

- Apply enough medicine to cover the affected area, and rub in gently.

To use the *gel form* of salicylic acid:

- Before using salicylic acid gel, apply wet packs to the affected areas for at least 5 minutes. If you have any questions about this, check with your health care professional.
- Apply enough gel to cover the affected areas, and rub in gently.

To use the *pad form* of salicylic acid:

- Wipe the pad over the affected areas.
- Do not rinse off medicine after treatment.

To use the *plaster form* of salicylic acid for warts, corns, or calluses:

- This medicine comes with patient instructions. Read them carefully before using.
- *Do not use this medicine on irritated skin or on any area that is infected or reddened. Also, do not use this medicine if you are a diabetic or if you have poor blood circulation.*
- *Do not use this medicine on warts with hair growing from them or on warts on the face, in or on the genital (sex) organs, or inside the nose or mouth. Also do not use on moles or birthmarks.* To do so may cause severe irritation.
- Wash the area to be treated and dry thoroughly. Warts may be soaked in warm water for 5 minutes before drying.
- Cut the plaster to fit the wart, corn, or callus and apply.
- For corns and calluses:
  —Repeat every 48 hours as needed for up to 14 days, or as directed by your doctor, until the corn or callus is removed.
  —Corns or calluses may be soaked in warm water for 5 minutes to help in their removal.

- For warts:
  - —Depending on the product, either:
    - Apply plaster and repeat every 48 hours as needed, or
    - Apply plaster at bedtime, leave in place for at least 8 hours, remove plaster in the morning, and repeat every 24 hours as needed.
  - —Repeat for up to 12 weeks as needed, or as directed by your doctor, until wart is removed.
- If discomfort gets worse during treatment or continues after treatment, or if the wart spreads, check with your doctor.

To use the *shampoo form* of salicylic acid:

- Before applying this medicine, wet the hair and scalp with lukewarm water. Apply enough medicine to work up a lather and rub well into the scalp for 2 or 3 minutes, then rinse. Apply the medicine again and rinse thoroughly.

To use the *soap form* of salicylic acid:

- Work up a lather with the soap, using hot water, and scrub the entire affected area with a washcloth or facial sponge or mitt.
- If you are to use this soap in a foot bath, work up rich suds in hot water and soak the feet for 10 to 15 minutes. Then pat dry without rinsing.

To use the *topical solution form* of salicylic acid for acne:

- Wet a cotton ball or pad with the topical solution and wipe the affected areas.
- Do not rinse off medicine after treatment.

To use the *topical solution form* of salicylic acid for warts, corns, or calluses:

- This medicine comes with patient instructions. Read them carefully before using.
- *This medicine is flammable. Do not use it near heat or open flame or while smoking.*
- *Do not use this medicine on irritated skin or on any area that is infected or reddened. Also, do not use this medicine if you are a diabetic or if you have poor blood circulation.*
- *Do not use this medicine on warts with hair growing from them or on warts on the face, in or on the genital (sex) organs, or inside the nose or mouth. Also do not use on moles or birthmarks.* To do so may cause severe irritation.
- Avoid breathing in the vapors from the medicine.
- Wash the area to be treated and dry thoroughly. Warts may be soaked in warm water for 5 minutes before drying.
- Apply the medicine one drop at a time to completely cover each wart, corn, or callus. Let dry.
- For warts—Repeat one or two times a day as needed for up to 12 weeks, or as directed by your doctor, until wart is removed.
- For corns and calluses—Repeat one or two times a day as needed for up to 14 days, or as directed by your doctor, until the corn or callus is removed.

- Corns and calluses may be soaked in warm water for 5 minutes to help in their removal.
- If discomfort gets worse during treatment or continues after treatment, or if the wart spreads, check with your doctor.

Unless your hands are being treated, wash them immediately after applying this medicine to remove any medicine that may be on them.

**Dosing**—The dose of salicylic acid will be different for different patients. *Follow your doctor's orders or the directions on the label.* The following information includes only the average doses of salicylic acid. *If your dose is different, do not change it* unless your doctor tells you to do so.

- For *cream* dosage form:
  - —For corns and calluses:
    - Adults and children—Use the 2 to 10% cream as needed. Use the 25 to 60% cream one time every three to five days.
- For *gel* dosage form:
  - —For acne:
    - Adults and children—Use the 0.5 to 5% gel one time a day.
  - —For psoriasis:
    - Adults and children—Use the 5% gel one time a day.
  - —For common warts:
    - Adults and children—Use the 5 to 26% gel one time a day.
- For *lotion* dosage form:
  - —For acne:
    - Adults and children—Use the 1 to 2% lotion one to three times a day.
  - —For dandruff and antiseborrhic dermatitis of the scalp:
    - Adults and children—Use the 1.8 to 2% lotion on the scalp one or two times a day.
- For *ointment* dosage form:
  - —For acne:
    - Adults and children—Use the 3 to 6% ointment as needed.
  - —For psoriasis and seborrheic dermatitis:
    - Adults and children—Use the 3 to 10% ointment as needed.
  - —For common warts:
    - Adults and children—Use the 3 to 10% ointment as needed. Use the 25 to 60% ointment one time every three to five days.
- For *pads* dosage form:
  - —For acne:
    - Adults and children—Use one to three times a day.

- For *plaster* dosage form:
  —For corns, calluses, common warts, or plantar warts:
  - Adults and children—Use one time a day or one time every other day.
- For *shampoo* dosage form:
  —For dandruff or seborrheic dermatitis of the scalp:
  - Adults and children—Use on the scalp one or two times a week.
- For *soap* dosage form:
  —For acne:
  - Adults and children—Use as needed.
- For *topical solution* dosage form:
  —For acne:
  - Adults and children—Use the 0.5 to 2% topical solution one to three times a day.
  —For common warts and plantar warts:
  - Adults and children—Use the 5 to 27% topical solution one or two times a day.
  —For corns and calluses:
  - Adults and children—Use the 12 to 27% topical solution one or two times a day.

**Missed dose**—If you miss a dose of this medicine, apply it as soon as possible. However, if it is almost time for your next dose, skip the missed dose and go back to your regular dosing schedule.

**Storage**—To store this medicine:
- Keep out of the reach of children.
- Store away from heat and direct light.
- Keep the medicine from freezing.
- Do not keep outdated medicine or medicine no longer needed. Be sure that any discarded medicine is out of the reach of children.

---

## Precautions While Using This Medicine

*When using salicylic acid, do not use any of the following preparations on the same affected area as this medicine, unless otherwise directed by your doctor:*

Abrasive soaps or cleansers
Alcohol-containing preparations
Any other topical acne preparation or preparation containing a peeling agent (for example, benzoyl peroxide, resorcinol, sulfur, or tretinoin [vitamin A acid])
Cosmetics or soaps that dry the skin
Medicated cosmetics
Other topical medicine for the skin

To use any of the above preparations on the same affected area as salicylic acid may cause severe irritation of the skin.

---

## Side Effects of This Medicine

Along with its needed effects, a medicine may cause some unwanted effects. Although not all of these side effects may occur, if they do occur they may need medical attention.

Check with your doctor as soon as possible if any of the following side effects occur:

*Less common or rare*
  Skin irritation not present before use of this medicine (moderate or severe)

*Symptoms of salicylic acid poisoning*
  Confusion; dizziness; headache (severe or continuing); rapid breathing; ringing or buzzing in ears (continuing)

Other side effects may occur that usually do not need medical attention. However, check with your doctor if any of the following side effects continue or are bothersome:

*More common*
  Skin irritation not present before use of this medicine (mild); stinging

Other side effects not listed above may also occur in some patients. If you notice any other effects, check with your health care professional.

Revised: 07/26/93

---

# SALICYLIC ACID AND SULFUR  Topical

Some commonly used brand names are:

**In the U.S.—**

Acno
Acnotex
Aveeno Cleansing Bar
Creamy SS Shampoo
Fostex Regular Strength Medicated Cleansing Bar
Fostex Regular Strength Medicated Cleansing Cream (for face and scalp)
Meted Maximum Strength Anti-Dandruff Shampoo with Conditioners
Night Cast Regular Formula Mask-lotion
Pernox Lemon Medicated Scrub Cleanser

Pernox Lotion Lathering Abradant Scrub Cleanser
Pernox Lotion Lathering Scrub Cleanser
Pernox Regular Medicated Scrub Cleanser
Sastid (AL) Scrub
Sastid Plain Shampoo and Acne Wash
Sastid Soap
Sebasorb Liquid
Sebex
Sebulex Antiseborrheic Treatment and Conditioning Shampoo
Sebulex Antiseborrheic Treatment Shampoo

Sebulex Cream Medicated Shampoo
Sebulex Medicated Dandruff Shampoo with Conditioners
Sebulex Regular Medicated Dandruff Shampoo

Generic name product may also be available.

**In Canada—**

Aveeno Acne Bar
Fostex Medicated Cleansing Bar
Fostex Medicated Cleansing Cream (for face and scalp)
Fostex Medicated Cleansing Liquid
Meted Maximum Strength Anti-Dandruff Shampoo with Conditioners
Night Cast R

Therac Lotion
Vanseb Cream Dandruff Shampoo
Vanseb Lotion Dandruff Shampoo

Pernox Lemon Medicated Scrub Cleanser
Pernox Regular Medicated Scrub Cleanser
Sastid Soap
Sebulex Conditioning Suspension Shampoo
Sebulex Lotion Shampoo
Sebulex Medicated Shampoo
Sulsal Soap

## Description

Salicylic acid (sal-i-SILL-ik AS-id) and sulfur (SUL-fur) combination is used to treat acne and other skin disorders and dandruff and other scalp disorders, such as seborrheic dermatitis.

This medicine is available without a prescription; however, your doctor may have special instructions on the proper use of this medicine for your medical condition.

Salicylic acid and sulfur combination is available in the following dosage forms:

*Topical*
- Cleansing cream (U.S. and Canada)
- Lotion (U.S. and Canada)
- Cleansing lotion (U.S. and Canada)
- Cream shampoo (U.S. and Canada)
- Lotion shampoo (U.S. and Canada)
- Suspension shampoo (U.S. and Canada)
- Bar soap (U.S. and Canada)
- Cleansing suspension (U.S. and Canada)
- Topical suspension (U.S.)

## Before Using This Medicine

If you are using this medicine without a prescription, carefully read and follow any precautions on the label. For salicylic acid and sulfur combination, the following should be considered:

**Allergies**—Tell your doctor if you have ever had any unusual or allergic reaction to salicylic acid or sulfur. Also tell your health care professional if you are allergic to any other substances, such as preservatives or dyes.

**Pregnancy**—Salicylic acid and sulfur combination has not been studied in pregnant women. However, for the individual medicines:

- *Salicylic acid*—Salicylic acid may be absorbed through the mother's skin. Studies with topical salicylic acid have not been done in humans. However, studies in animals have shown that salicylic acid causes birth defects when given orally in doses about 6 times the highest dose recommended for topical use in humans.
- *Sulfur*—Topical sulfur has not been shown to cause birth defects or other problems in humans.

Before using this medicine, make sure your doctor knows if you are pregnant or if you may become pregnant.

**Breast-feeding**—Salicylic acid may be absorbed through the mother's skin. However, topical salicylic acid and sulfur combination has not been reported to cause problems in nursing babies.

**Children**—Young children may be at increased risk of unwanted effects because of increased absorption of salicylic acid through the skin. Products containing salicylic acid should not be applied to large areas of the body or used for long periods of time in infants and children.

**Older adults**—Many medicines have not been studied specifically in older people. Therefore, it may not be known whether they work exactly the same way they do in younger adults or if they cause different side effects or problems in older people. There is no specific information comparing use of salicylic acid and sulfur combination in the elderly with use in other age groups.

**Other medicines**—Although certain medicines should not be used together at all, in other cases two different medicines may be used together even if an interaction might occur. In these cases, your doctor may want to change the dose, or other precautions may be necessary. Tell your health care professional if you are using any other topical prescription or nonprescription (over-the-counter [OTC]) medicine that is to be applied to the same area of the skin.

## Proper Use of This Medicine

*Use this medicine only as directed.* Do not use more of it and do not use it more often than recommended on the label, unless otherwise directed by your doctor.

Immediately after using this medicine, wash your hands to remove any medicine that may be on them.

*Keep this medicine away from the eyes.* If you should accidentally get some in your eyes, flush them thoroughly with water.

To use the *skin cleanser form* of this medicine:
- After wetting the skin, apply this medicine with your fingertips or a wet sponge and rub in gently to work up a lather. Then rinse thoroughly and pat dry.

To use the *lotion or topical suspension form* of this medicine:
- Apply a small amount of this medicine to the affected areas, and rub in gently.

To use the *shampoo form* of this medicine:
- Wet the hair and scalp with lukewarm water. Then apply enough medicine to work up a lather and rub into the scalp. Continue rubbing the lather into the scalp for several minutes or allow it to remain on the scalp for about 5 minutes, depending on the product being used, then rinse. Apply the medicine again and rinse thoroughly.

To use the *bar soap form* of this medicine:
- After wetting the skin, use this medicine to wash the face and other affected areas. Then rinse thoroughly and pat dry.

**Dosing**—The dose of salicylic acid and sulfur combination will be different for different patients. *Follow your doctor's orders or the directions on the label.* The following information includes only the average doses of salicylic acid and sulfur combination. *If your dose is different, do not change it* unless your doctor tells you to do so.

- For acne or oily skin:
  —For *bar soap and cleansing cream* dosage forms:
    - Adults and children—Use on the skin two or three times a day.

—For *cleansing suspension, lotion, and topical suspension* dosage forms:
  - Adults and children—Use on the skin one or two times a day.
—For *cleansing lotion* dosage form:
  - Adults and children—Use on the skin one to three times a day.
- For dandruff and seborrheic dermatitis of the scalp:
  —For *cream shampoo, lotion shampoo, and suspension shampoo* dosage forms:
    - Adults and children—Use on the scalp one or two times a week.

**Missed dose**—If you miss a dose of this medicine, apply or use it as soon as possible. However, if it is almost time for your next dose, skip the missed dose and go back to your regular dosing schedule.

**Storage**—To store this medicine:
- Keep out of the reach of children.
- Store away from heat and direct light.
- Keep the medicine from freezing.
- Do not keep outdated medicine or medicine no longer needed. Be sure that any discarded medicine is out of the reach of children.

## Precautions While Using This Medicine

*When using salicylic acid and sulfur combination medicine, do not use any of the following preparations on the same affected area as this medicine,* unless otherwise directed by your doctor:
  Abrasive soaps or cleansers
  Alcohol-containing preparations
  Any other topical acne preparation or preparation containing a peeling agent (for example, benzoyl peroxide, resorcinol, or tretinoin [vitamin A acid])
  Cosmetics or soaps that dry the skin
  Medicated cosmetics
  Other topical medicine for the skin

To use any of the above preparations on the same affected area as salicylic acid and sulfur combination medicine may cause severe irritation of the skin.

*Do not use any topical mercury-containing preparation, such as ammoniated mercury ointment, on the same affected area as this medicine.* To do so may cause a foul odor, may be irritating to the skin, and may stain the skin black. If you have any questions about this, check with your health care professional.

Taking large doses of aspirin or other salicylates (including diflunisal) while using topical salicylic acid (contained in this medicine) may lead to overdose. If you have any questions about this, check with your health care professional.

## Side Effects of This Medicine

Along with its needed effects, a medicine may cause some unwanted effects. Although not all of these side effects may occur, if they do occur they may need medical attention.

Check with your doctor as soon as possible if the following side effect occurs:
  Skin irritation not present before use of this medicine

Other side effects may occur that usually do not need medical attention. However, check with your health care professional if the following side effects continue or are bothersome:
  Redness and peeling of skin (may occur after a few days); unusual dryness of skin

Other side effects not listed above may also occur in some patients. If you notice any other effects, check with your health care professional.

Revised: 07/26/93

---

# SALICYLIC ACID, SULFUR, AND COAL TAR   Topical

Some commonly used brand names are:

**In the U.S.—**
  Sebex-T Tar Shampoo          Vanseb-T
  Sebutone

**In Canada—**
  Sebutone

## Description

Salicylic acid (sal-i-SILL-ik AS-id), sulfur (SUL-fur), and coal tar combination is used to treat dandruff, seborrheic dermatitis, and psoriasis of the scalp.

This medicine is available without a prescription; however, your doctor may have special instructions on the proper use of this medicine for your medical condition.

Salicylic acid, sulfur, and coal tar combination is available in the following dosage forms:

*Topical*
  - Cream shampoo (U.S.)
  - Lotion shampoo (U.S. and Canada)

## Before Using This Medicine

If you are using this medicine without a prescription, carefully read and follow any precautions on the label. For salicylic acid, sulfur, and coal tar combination, the following should be considered:

**Allergies**—Tell your doctor if you have ever had any unusual or allergic reaction to salicylic acid, sulfur, or coal tar. Also tell your health care professional if you are allergic to any other substances, such as preservatives or dyes.

**Pregnancy**—Salicylic acid, sulfur, and coal tar combination has not been studied in pregnant women. However, for the individual medicines:

- *Salicylic acid*—Salicylic acid may be absorbed through the mother's skin. Studies with topical salicylic acid have not been done in humans. However, studies in animals have shown that salicylic acid causes birth defects when given orally in doses about 6 times the highest dose recommended for topical use in humans.
- *Sulfur*—Sulfur has not been shown to cause birth defects or other problems in humans.
- *Coal tar*—Studies with coal tar on effects in pregnancy have not been done in either humans or animals.

**Breast-feeding**—Salicylic acid may be absorbed through the mother's skin. However, topical salicylic acid, sulfur, and coal tar combination has not been reported to cause problems in nursing babies.

**Children**—Young children may be at increased risk of unwanted effects because of increased absorption of salicylic acid through the skin. Medicines containing salicylic acid should not be applied to large areas of the body or used for long periods of time in infants and children.

**Older adults**—Many medicines have not been studied specifically in older people. Therefore, it may not be known whether they work exactly the same way they do in younger adults or if they cause different side effects or problems in older people. There is no specific information comparing use of salicylic acid, sulfur, and coal tar combination medicine in the elderly with use in other age groups.

**Other medicines**—Although certain medicines should not be used together at all, in other cases two different medicines may be used together even if an interaction might occur. In these cases, your doctor may want to change the dose, or other precautions may be necessary. Tell your health care professional if you are using any other topical prescription or nonprescription (over-the-counter [OTC]) medicine that is to be applied to the same area of the skin.

## Proper Use of This Medicine

*Use this medicine only as directed.* Do not use it more often than recommended on the label, unless otherwise directed by your doctor.

*Keep this medicine away from the eyes.* If you should accidentally get some in your eyes, flush them thoroughly with water.

Before using this medicine, wet the hair and scalp with lukewarm water. Then apply a generous amount to the scalp and work up a rich lather. Rub the lather into the scalp for 5 minutes, then rinse. Apply the medicine again and rinse thoroughly.

Immediately after using this medicine, wash your hands to remove any medicine that may be on them.

**Dosing**—The dose of salicylic acid, sulfur, and coal tar combination will be different for different patients. *Follow your doctor's orders or the directions on the label.* The following information includes only the average doses of salicylic acid, sulfur, and coal tar combination. *If your dose is different, do not change it* unless your doctor tells you to do so.

- For dandruff, seborrheic dermatitis, and psoriasis of the scalp:
    —For *cream shampoo and lotion shampoo* dosage forms:
    - Adults and children—Use on the scalp one or two times a week.

**Missed dose**—If you miss a dose of this medicine, apply it as soon as possible. However, if it is almost time for your next dose, skip the missed dose and go back to your regular dosing schedule.

**Storage**—To store this medicine:

- Keep out of the reach of children.
- Store away from heat and direct light.
- Keep the medicine from freezing.
- Do not keep outdated medicine or medicine no longer needed. Be sure that any discarded medicine is out of the reach of children.

## Precautions While Using This Medicine

*Do not use any topical mercury-containing preparation, such as ammoniated mercury ointment, on the same affected area as this medicine.* To do so may cause a foul odor, may be irritating to the skin, and may stain the skin black. If you have any questions about this, check with your health care professional.

This medicine may temporarily discolor blond, bleached, or tinted hair.

## Side Effects of This Medicine

In animal studies, coal tar (contained in this combination medicine) has been shown to increase the chance of skin cancer.

Along with its needed effects, a medicine may cause some unwanted effects. Although not all of these side effects may occur, if they do occur they may need medical attention.

Check with your doctor as soon as possible if the following side effect occurs:

Skin irritation not present before use of this medicine

Other side effects not listed above may also occur in some patients. If you notice any other effects, check with your health care professional.

Revised: 07/26/93

---

# SELEGILINE  Systemic

Some commonly used brand names are:

**In the U.S.—**
  Eldepryl

**In Canada—**
  Eldepryl                                SD Deprenyl

**Other—**
  Jumex                                   Movergan
  Jumexal                                 Procythol
  Juprenil

Other commonly used names are deprenil and deprenyl.

## Description

Selegiline (seh-LEDGE-ah-leen) is used in combination with levodopa or levodopa and carbidopa combination to treat Parkinson's disease, sometimes called shaking palsy or paralysis agitans. This medicine works to increase and extend the effects of levodopa, and may help to slow the progress of Parkinson's disease.

Selegiline is available only with your doctor's prescription, in the following dosage form:

*Oral*
• Tablets (U.S. and Canada)

## Before Using This Medicine

In deciding to use a medicine, the risks of taking the medicine must be weighed against the good it will do. This is a decision you and your doctor will make. For selegiline, the following should be considered:

**Allergies**—Tell your doctor if you have ever had any unusual or allergic reaction to selegiline. Also tell your health care professional if you are allergic to any other substances, such as foods, preservatives, or dyes.

**Pregnancy**—Selegiline has not been studied in pregnant women. However, this medicine has not been shown to cause birth defects or other problems in animal studies.

**Breast-feeding**—It is not known whether selegiline passes into the breast milk.

**Children**—Studies on this medicine have been done only in adult patients and there is no specific information about its use in children. Therefore, be sure to discuss with your doctor the use of this medicine in children.

**Older adults**—In studies done to date that included elderly people, selegiline did not cause different side effects or problems in older people than it did in younger adults.

**Other medicines**—Although certain medicines should not be used together at all, in other cases 2 different medicines may be used together even if an interaction might occur. In these cases, your doctor may want to change the dose, or other precautions may be necessary. When you are taking selegiline, it is especially important that your health care professional know if you are taking any of the following:

• Fluoxetine (e.g., Prozac) or
• Meperidine (e.g., Demerol)—Using these medicines together may increase the chance of serious side effects

**Other medical problems**—The presence of other medical problems may affect the use of selegiline. Make sure you tell your doctor if you have any other medical problems, especially:

• Stomach ulcer (history of)—Selegiline may make the condition worse

## Proper Use of This Medicine

*Take this medicine only as directed by your doctor.* Do not take more of it, do not take it more often, and do not take it for a longer time than your doctor ordered.

**Dosing**—The dose of selegiline will be different for different patients. Your doctor will determine the proper dose of selegiline for you. *Follow your doctor's orders or the directions on the label.*

For the treatment of Parkinson's disease, the usual dose of selegiline is 5 mg two times a day, taken with breakfast and lunch. Some patients may need less than this.

**Missed dose**—If you miss a dose of this medicine, take it as soon as possible. However, if you do not remember the missed dose until late afternoon or evening, skip the missed dose and go back to your regular dosing schedule. Do not double doses.

**Storage**—To store this medicine:
• Keep out of the reach of children.
• Store away from heat and direct light.
• Do not store in the bathroom, near the kitchen sink, or in other damp places. Heat or moisture may cause the medicine to break down.

---

- Do not keep outdated medicine or medicine no longer needed. Be sure that any discarded medicine is out of the reach of children.

## Precautions While Using This Medicine

When selegiline is taken at doses of 10 mg or less per day for the treatment of Parkinson's disease, there are no restrictions on food or beverages you eat or drink. However, the chance exists that dangerous reactions, such as sudden high blood pressure, may occur if doses higher than those used for Parkinson's disease are taken with certain foods, beverages, or other medicines. These foods, beverages, and medicines include:

- Foods that have a high tyramine content (most common in foods that are aged or fermented to increase their flavor), such as cheeses; fava or broad bean pods; yeast or meat extracts; smoked or pickled meat, poultry, or fish; fermented sausage (bologna, pepperoni, salami, summer sausage) or other fermented meat; sauerkraut; or any overripe fruit. If a list of these foods and beverages is not given to you, ask your health care professional to provide one.
- Alcoholic beverages or alcohol-free or reduced-alcohol beer and wine.
- Large amounts of caffeine-containing food or beverages such as coffee, tea, cola, or chocolate.
- Any other medicine unless approved or prescribed by your doctor. This especially includes nonprescription (over-the-counter [OTC]) medicine, such as that for colds (including nose drops or sprays), cough, asthma, hay fever, and appetite control; "keep awake" products; or products that make you sleepy.

Also, for at least 2 weeks after you stop taking this medicine, these foods, beverages, and other medicines may continue to react with selegiline if it was taken in doses higher than those usually used for Parkinson's disease.

Check with your doctor or hospital emergency room immediately if severe headache, stiff neck, chest pains, fast heartbeat, or nausea and vomiting occur while you are taking this medicine. These may be symptoms of a serious side effect that should have a doctor's attention.

Dizziness, lightheadedness, or fainting may occur, especially when you get up from a lying or sitting position. Getting up slowly may help. If the problem continues or gets worse, check with your doctor.

Selegiline may cause dryness of the mouth. For temporary relief, use sugarless candy or gum, melt bits of ice in your mouth, or use a saliva substitute. However, if your mouth continues to feel dry for more than 2 weeks, check with your medical doctor or dentist. Continuing dryness of the mouth may increase the chance of dental disease, including tooth decay, gum disease, and fungus infections.

## Side Effects of This Medicine

When you start taking selegiline in addition to levodopa or carbidopa and levodopa combination, you may experience an increase in side effects. If this occurs, your doctor may gradually reduce the amount of levodopa or carbidopa and levodopa combination you take.

Along with its needed effects, a medicine may cause some unwanted effects. Although not all of these side effects may occur, if they do occur they may need medical attention.

*Stop taking this medicine and get emergency help immediately* if any of the following side effects occur:

*Symptoms of unusually high blood pressure (caused by reaction of higher than usual doses of selegiline with restricted foods or medicines)*

Chest pain (severe); enlarged pupils; fast or slow heartbeat; headache (severe); increased sensitivity of eyes to light; increased sweating (possibly with fever or cold, clammy skin); nausea and vomiting (severe); stiff or sore neck

Check with your doctor as soon as possible if any of the following side effects occur:

*More common*

Increase in unusual movements of body; mood or other mental changes

*Less common or rare*

Bloody or black, tarry stools; severe stomach pain; or vomiting of blood or material that looks like coffee grounds; difficulty in speaking; loss of balance control; uncontrolled movements, especially of face, neck, and back; restlessness or desire to keep moving; or twisting movements of body; difficult or frequent urination; dizziness or lightheadedness, especially when getting up from a lying or sitting position; hallucinations (seeing, hearing, or feeling things that are not there); irregular heartbeat; lip smacking or puckering, puffing of cheeks, rapid or worm-like movements of tongue, uncontrolled chewing movements, uncontrolled movements of arms and legs; swelling of feet or lower legs; wheezing, difficulty in breathing, or tightness in chest

*Symptoms of overdose*

Agitation or irritability; chest pain; convulsions (seizures); difficulty opening mouth or lockjaw; dizziness (severe) or fainting; fast or irregular pulse (continuing); high fever; high or low blood pressure; increased sweating (possibly with fever or cold, clammy skin); severe spasm where the head and heels are bent backward and the body arched forward; troubled breathing

Other side effects may occur that usually do not need medical attention. These side effects may go away during treatment as your body adjusts to the medicine. However, check with your doctor if any of the following side effects continue or are bothersome:

*More common*

Abdominal or stomach pain; dizziness or feeling faint; dryness of mouth; nausea or vomiting; trouble in sleeping

*Less common or rare*

Anxiety, nervousness, or restlessness; blurred or double vision; body ache or back or leg pain; burning of lips, mouth, or throat; chills; constipation or diarrhea; drowsiness; headache; heartburn; high or low blood pressure; inability to move; slow or difficult urination; frequent urge to urinate; increased sensitivity of skin to light; increased sweating; irritability (temporary); loss of appetite or weight loss; memory problems; muscle cramps or numbness of fingers or toes; pounding or fast heartbeat; red, raised, or itchy skin; ringing or buzzing in ears; slowed movements; uncontrolled closing of eyelids; taste changes; unusual feeling of well-being; unusual tiredness or weakness

*With doses higher than 10 mg a day*

Clenching, gnashing, or grinding teeth; sudden jerky movements of body

Other side effects not listed above may also occur in some patients. If you notice any other effects, check with your doctor.

Revised: 09/30/92

# SELENIUM SULFIDE   Topical

Some commonly used brand names are:

**In the U.S.—**
Exsel Lotion Shampoo
Glo-Sel
Head & Shoulders Intensive Treatment Conditioning Formula Dandruff Lotion Shampoo
Head & Shoulders Intensive Treatment Regular Formula Dandruff Lotion Shampoo
Head & Shoulders Intensive Treatment 2 in 1 (Persistent Dandruff Shampoo plus Conditioner in One)
Formula Dandruff Lotion Shampoo
Selsun
Selsun Blue Dry Formula
Selsun Blue Extra Conditioning Formula
Selsun Blue Extra Medicated Formula
Selsun Blue Oily Formula
Selsun Blue Regular Formula

Generic name product may also be available.

**In Canada—**
Selsun
Selsun Blue
Selsun Blue Extra Conditioning Formula
Versel Lotion

## Description

Selenium sulfide (se-LEE-nee-um SUL-fide) 1% and 2.5% strengths are used on the scalp to help control the symptoms of dandruff and seborrheic dermatitis.

Selenium sulfide 2.5% strength is used also on the body to treat tinea versicolor (a type of fungus infection of the skin).

In the United States, the 2.5% strength is available only with your doctor's prescription. The 1% strength is available without a prescription; however, your doctor may have special instructions on the proper use of this medicine for your medical problem.

Selenium sulfide is available in the following dosage form:

*Topical*
• Lotion (U.S. and Canada)

## Before Using This Medicine

If you are using this medicine without a prescription, carefully read and follow any precautions on the label. For selenium sulfide, the following should be considered:

**Allergies—**Tell your doctor if you have ever had any unusual or allergic reaction to selenium sulfide. Also tell your health care professional if you are allergic to any other substances, such as preservatives or dyes.

**Pregnancy—**
• *For use on the scalp:* Selenium sulfide has not been shown to cause birth defects or other problems in humans.
• *For use on the body:* Selenium sulfide should not be used if you are pregnant or if you may become pregnant. The medicine may be absorbed into your body and may affect your baby.

**Breast-feeding—**Selenium sulfide has not been reported to cause problems in nursing babies.

**Children—**There is no specific information comparing use of selenium sulfide in infants and children with use in other age groups; however, this medicine is not expected to cause different side effects or problems in children than it does in adults.

**Older adults—**Many medicines have not been studied specifically in older people. Therefore, it may not be known whether they work exactly the same way they do in younger adults. Although there is no specific information comparing use of selenium sulfide in the elderly with use in other age groups, this medicine is not expected to cause different side effects or problems in older people than it does in younger adults.

**Other medicines—**Although certain medicines should not be used together at all, in other cases two different medicines may be used together even if an interaction might occur. In these cases, your doctor may want to change the dose, or other precautions may be necessary. Tell your health care professional if you are using any other topical prescription or nonprescription (over-the-counter [OTC]) medicine that is to be applied to the same area of the skin.

**Other medical problems—**The presence of other medical problems may affect the use of selenium sulfide. Make sure you tell your doctor if you have any other medical problems, especially:
• Blistered, raw, or oozing areas on your scalp or body—Use of this medicine on these areas may increase the chance of absorption through the skin

## Proper Use of This Medicine

*If you are using the 2.5% strength of selenium sulfide: Use this medicine only as directed.* Do not use it more often than recommended on the label, unless otherwise directed by your doctor.

*If you are using the 1% strength of selenium sulfide:* For best results, use this medicine at least 2 times a week or as directed by your doctor.

To use selenium sulfide for *dandruff or seborrheic dermatitis of the scalp:*

- Before using this medicine, wet the hair and scalp with lukewarm water.
- Apply enough medicine (1 or 2 teaspoonfuls) to the scalp to work up a lather. Allow the lather to remain on the scalp for 2 to 3 minutes, then rinse.
- Apply the medicine again and rinse well.
- If this medicine is used on light or blond, gray, or chemically treated (bleached, tinted, permanent-waved) hair, rinse your hair well for at least 5 minutes after using the medicine to lessen the chance of hair discoloration.
- After treatment, wash your hands well.

To use selenium sulfide for *tinea versicolor of the body:*

- Apply the medicine to the affected areas of your body, except for your face and genitals (sex organs).
- Work up a lather using a small amount of water.
- Allow the medicine to remain on your skin for 10 minutes.
- Rinse your body well to remove all the medicine.

*Do not use this medicine if blistered, raw, or oozing areas are present on your scalp or the area of your body that is to be treated,* unless otherwise directed by your doctor.

*Keep this medicine away from the eyes.* If you should accidentally get some in your eyes, flush them thoroughly with water.

**Dosing**—The dose of selenium sulfide will be different for different patients. *Follow your doctor's orders or the directions on the label.* The following information includes only the average doses of selenium sulfide. *If your dose is different, do not change it* unless your doctor tells you to do so.

- For *lotion* dosage form:
  - —For dandruff or seborrheic dermatitis:
    - Adults and children—If you are using the 1% lotion, use on the scalp two times a week. If you are using the 2.5% lotion, use on the scalp two times a week for two weeks, then use one time a week or less often.

  - Infants—Use and dose must be determined by your doctor.
  - —For tinea versicolor:
    - Adults and children—Use the 2.5% lotion on the body one time a day for seven days.
    - Infants—Use and dose must be determined by your doctor.

**Missed dose**—If you miss a dose of this medicine, use it as soon as possible. However, if it is almost time for your next dose, skip the missed dose and go back to your regular dosing schedule.

**Storage**—To store this medicine:

- Keep out of the reach of children.
- Store away from heat and direct light.
- Keep the medicine from freezing.
- Do not keep outdated medicine or medicine no longer needed. Be sure that any discarded medicine is out of the reach of children.

## Precautions While Using This Medicine

If your condition does not get better after regular use of this medicine, or if it gets worse, check with your doctor.

## Side Effects of This Medicine

Along with its needed effects, a medicine may cause some unwanted effects. Although not all of these side effects may occur, if they do occur they may need medical attention.

Check with your doctor as soon as possible if the following side effect occurs:

*Less common or rare*
    Skin irritation

Other side effects may occur that usually do not need medical attention. Check with your health care professional if any of the following side effects continue or are bothersome:

*More common*
    Unusual dryness or oiliness of hair or scalp
*Less common*
    Increase in normal hair loss

Other side effects not listed above may also occur in some patients. If you notice any other effects, check with your health care professional.

Revised: 07/26/93

# SELENIUM SUPPLEMENTS    Systemic

Some commonly used brand names are:
**In the U.S.—**
    Sele-Pak[1]
    Selepen[1]
Note: For quick reference, the following (family name) are numbered to match the corresponding brand names.
This information applies to the following medicines:
1. Selenious Acid (se-LEE-nee-us as-id)†‡
2. Selenium (se-LEE-nee-um)‡§

---

†Not commercially available in Canada.
‡Generic name product may also be available in the U.S.
§Generic name product may also be available in Canada.

---

## Description

Selenium supplements are used to prevent or treat selenium deficiency.

The body needs selenium for normal growth and health. For patients who are unable to get enough selenium in their regular diet or who have need for more selenium, selenium supplements may be necessary.

Lack of selenium may lead to changes in fingernails, muscle weakness, and heart problems.

Selenium deficiency in the United States is rare. Patients receiving total parenteral nutrition (TPN) for long periods of time may need selenium. Selenium deficiency is a problem in areas of the world where the soil contains little selenium.

Although selenium is being used to prevent certain types of cancer, there is not enough information to show that this is effective.

Some selenium preparations are available only with your doctor's prescription. Others are available without a prescription; however, your doctor may have special instructions on the proper use and dose for your condition.

Selenium supplements are available as part of a multivitamin/mineral complex or alone in the following dosage forms:

*Oral*
    Selenium
      • Tablets (U.S. and Canada)

*Parenteral*
    Selenious Acid
      • Injection (U.S.)

## Importance of Diet

Many nutritionists recommend that, if possible, people should get all the selenium they need from foods. However, some people do not get enough selenium from their diets. For such people, a selenium supplement is important.

In order to get enough vitamins and minerals in your regular diet, it is important that you eat a balanced and varied diet. Follow carefully any diet program your doctor may recommend. For your specific vitamin and/or mineral needs, ask your doctor or dietitian for a list of appropriate foods.

Selenium is found in seafood, liver, lean red meat, and grains grown in soil that is rich in selenium.

Experts have developed a list of recommended dietary allowances (RDA) of selenium. The RDA are not an exact number but a general idea of how much you need every day. They do not cover amounts needed for problems caused by a serious lack of selenium.

The RDA for selenium are as follows:
• Infants and children—
    Birth to 6 months of age: 10 micrograms (mcg) a day.
    6 months to 1 year of age: 15 mcg a day.
    1 to 6 years of age: 20 mcg a day.
    7 to 10 years of age: 30 mcg a day.
• Adolescent and adult males—
    11 to 14 years of age: 40 mcg a day.
    15 to 18 years of age: 50 mcg a day.
    19 years of age and over: 70 mcg a day.
• Adolescent and adult females—
    11 to 14 years of age: 45 mcg a day.
    15 to 18 years of age: 50 mcg a day.
    19 years of age and over: 55 mcg a day.
• Pregnant females—65 mcg a day.
• Breast-feeding females—75 mcg a day.

Remember:
• The total amount of selenium that you get every day includes what you get from the food that you eat *and* what you may take as a supplement.
• This total amount should not be greater than the RDA, unless ordered by your doctor.

## Before Using This Dietary Supplement

If you are taking this dietary supplement without a prescription, carefully read and follow any precautions on the label. For selenium supplements, the following should be considered:

**Allergies**—Tell your doctor if you have ever had any unusual or allergic reaction to selenious acid or selenium. Also tell your health care professional if you are allergic to any other substances, such as foods, preservatives, or dyes.

**Pregnancy**—It is especially important that you are receiving enough vitamins and minerals when you become pregnant and that you continue to receive the right amount of vitamins and minerals throughout your pregnancy. The healthy growth and development of the fetus depend on a steady supply of nutrients from the mother. However, taking large amounts of a dietary supplement in pregnancy may be harmful to the mother and/or fetus and should be avoided.

**Breast-feeding**—It is important that you receive the right amounts of vitamins and minerals so that your baby will also get the vitamins and minerals needed to grow properly. However, taking large amounts of a dietary supplement while breast-feeding may be harmful to the mother and/or baby and should be avoided.

**Children**—It is especially important that children receive enough selenium in their diet for healthy growth and development. Although there is no specific information comparing use of selenium in children with use in other age groups, this medicine is not expected to cause different side effects or problems in children than it does in adults.

**Older adults**—It is important that older people continue to receive enough selenium in their daily diets.

**Medicines or dietary supplements**—Although certain medicines should not be used together at all, in other cases or dietary supplements may be used together even if an interaction might occur. In these cases, your doctor may want to change the dose, or other precautions may be necessary. Tell your health care professional if you are taking any other dietary supplement or any nonprescription (over-the-counter [OTC]) or prescription medicine.

## Proper Use of This Dietary Supplement

Some people believe that taking very large doses of a vitamin or mineral (called megadoses) is useful for treating certain medical problems. Studies have not proven this. Large doses should be taken only under the direction of your doctor after need has been identified.

**Dosing**—The dose of selenium for prevention of selenium deficiency is based on the Recommended Dietary Allowances (RDA). See the *Importance of Diet* section for the RDA for selenium.

**Missed dose**—If you miss taking selenium supplements for one or more days there is no cause for concern, since it takes some time for your body to become seriously low in selenium. However, if your doctor has recommended that you take selenium, try to remember to take it as directed every day.

**Storage**—To store this dietary supplement:

• Keep out of the reach of children.

• Store away from heat and direct light.

• Do not store in the bathroom, near the kitchen sink, or in other damp places. Heat or moisture may cause the dietary supplement to break down.

• Keep the dietary supplement from freezing. Do not refrigerate.

• Do not keep outdated dietary supplement or those no longer needed. Be sure that any discarded dietary supplement is out of the reach of children.

## Side Effects of This Dietary Supplement

Along with its needed effects, a dietary supplement may cause some unwanted effects. Although selenium supplements have not been reported to cause any side effects, check with your doctor immediately if any of the following side effects occur as a result of an overdose:

*Symptoms of overdose*
> Diarrhea; fingernail weakening; garlic odor of breath and sweat; hair loss; irritability; itching of skin; metallic taste; nausea and vomiting; unusual tiredness and weakness

Other side effects not listed above may also occur in some patients. If you notice any other effects, check with your doctor.

Revised: 04/16/92
Interim revisions: 06/06/92; 08/15/94

# SERTRALINE    Systemic

A commonly used brand name in the U.S. and Canada is Zoloft.

## Description

Sertraline (SER-tral-leen) is used to treat mental depression.

This medicine is available only with your doctor's prescription, in the following dosage form:
*Oral*
• Capsules (Canada)
• Tablets (U.S.)

## Before Using This Medicine

In deciding to use a medicine, the risks of taking the medicine must be weighed against the good it will do. This is a decision you and your doctor will make. For sertraline, the following should be considered:

**Allergies**—Tell your doctor if you have ever had any unusual or allergic reaction to sertraline. Also tell your health care professional if you are allergic to any other substances, such as foods, preservatives, or dyes.

**Pregnancy**—Studies have not been done in pregnant women. However, studies in animals have shown that sertraline may cause delayed development and decreased survival rates of offspring when given in doses many times the usual human dose. Before taking this medicine, make sure your doctor knows if you are pregnant or if you may become pregnant.

**Breast-feeding**—It is not known whether sertraline is excreted in breast milk.

**Children**—Studies on this medicine have been done only in adult patients, and there is no specific information comparing use of sertraline in children with use in other age groups.

**Older adults**—In studies done to date that have included elderly people, sertraline did not cause different side effects or problems in older people than it did in younger adults.

**Other medicines**—Although certain medicines should not be used together at all, in other cases two different medicines may be used together even if an interaction might occur. In these cases, your doctor may want to change the dose, or other precautions may be necessary. When you are taking sertraline, it is especially important that your health care professional know if you are taking any of the following:

- Digitoxin (e.g., Crystodigin) or
- Warfarin (e.g., Coumadin)—Higher or lower blood levels of these medicines or sertraline may occur, which may increase the chance of unwanted effects; your doctor may need to change the dose of either these medicines or sertraline
- Monoamine oxidase (MAO) inhibitors (furazolidone [e.g., Furoxone], isocarboxazid [e.g., Marplan], phenelzine [e.g., Nardil], procarbazine [e.g., Matulane], selegiline [e.g., Eldepryl], tranylcypromine [e.g., Parnate])—Taking sertraline while you are taking or within 2 weeks of taking MAO inhibitors may cause confusion, agitation, restlessness, stomach or intestinal symptoms, sudden high body temperature, extremely high blood pressure, and severe convulsions; at least 14 days should be allowed between stopping treatment with one medicine and starting treatment with the other

**Other medical problems**—The presence of other medical problems may affect the use of sertraline. Make sure you tell your doctor if you have any other medical problems, especially:

- Drug abuse or dependence (or history of)—Because sertraline is a new drug, it is not known if it could become habit-forming, causing mental or physical dependence
- Kidney disease, severe, or
- Liver disease—Higher blood levels of sertraline may occur, increasing the chance of side effects

## Proper Use of This Medicine

*Take this medicine only as directed by your doctor,* to benefit your condition as much as possible. Do not take more of it, do not take it more often, and do not take it for a longer time than your doctor ordered.

*You may have to take sertraline for up to 4 weeks or longer before you begin to feel better.* Your doctor should check your progress at regular visits during this time.

This medicine should always be taken at the same time in relation to meals and snacks to make sure that it is absorbed in the same way.

**Dosing**—The dose of sertraline will be different for different patients. *Follow your doctor's orders or the directions on the label.* The following information includes only the average doses of sertraline. *If your dose is different, do not change it* unless your doctor tells you to do so.

- The number of capsules or tablets that you take depends on the strength of the medicine and the medical problem for which you are taking sertraline.
- For *oral* dosage forms (capsules or tablets):
  —Adults: To start, usually 50 milligrams once a day, taken either in the morning or evening. Your doctor may gradually increase your dose if needed.
  —Children: Dose must be determined by the doctor.
  —Older adults: To start, usually 12.5 to 25 milligrams once a day, taken either in the morning or evening. Your doctor may gradually increase your dose if needed.

**Missed dose**—Because sertraline may be given to different patients at different times of the day, you and your doctor should discuss what to do about any missed doses.

**Storage**—To store this medicine:

- Keep out of the reach of children.
- Store away from heat and direct light.
- Do not store in the bathroom, near the kitchen sink, or in other damp places. Heat or moisture may cause the medicine to break down.
- Do not keep outdated medicine or medicine no longer needed. Be sure that any discarded medicine is out of the reach of children.

## Precautions While Using This Medicine

It is important that your doctor check your progress at regular visits, to allow for changes in your dose and to help reduce any side effects.

This medicine could possibly add to the effects of alcohol and other CNS depressants (medicines that slow down the nervous system, possibly causing drowsiness). Some examples of CNS depressants are antihistamines or medicine for hay fever, other allergies, or colds; sedatives, tranquilizers, or sleeping medicine; prescription pain medicine or narcotics; barbiturates; medicine for seizures; muscle relaxants; or anesthetics, including some dental anesthetics. *Check with your doctor before taking any of the above while you are using this medicine.*

This medicine may cause some people to become drowsy. *Make sure you know how you react to sertraline before you drive, use machines, or do anything else that could be dangerous if you are not alert.*

*This medicine may cause dryness of the mouth. For temporary relief, use sugarless gum or candy, melt bits of ice in your mouth, or use a saliva substitute.* However, if your mouth continues to feel dry for more than 2 weeks, check with your medical doctor or dentist. Continuing dryness of the mouth may increase the chance of dental disease, including tooth decay, gum disease, and fungus infections.

## Side Effects of This Medicine

Along with its needed effects, a medicine may cause some unwanted effects. Although not all of these side effects may occur, if they do occur they may need medical attention.

Check with your doctor as soon as possible if any of the following side effects occur:

*Less common or rare*

Fast talking and excited feelings or actions that are out of control; fever; skin rash, hives, or itching

Other side effects may occur that usually do not need medical attention. These side effects may go away during treatment as your body adjusts to the medicine. However, check with your doctor if any of the following side effects continue or are bothersome:

*More common*

Decreased appetite or weight loss; decreased sexual drive or ability; diarrhea; drowsiness; dryness of mouth; headache; nausea; stomach or abdominal cramps, gas, or pain; tiredness or weakness; tremor; trouble in sleeping

*Less common*

Anxiety, agitation, nervousness or restlessness; changes in vision, including blurred vision; constipation; fast or irregular heartbeat; flushing or redness of skin, with feeling of warmth or heat; increased appetite; vomiting

Other side effects not listed above may also occur in some patients. If you notice any other effects, check with your doctor.

Revised: 03/19/93

# SILVER SULFADIAZINE    Topical

Some commonly used brand names are:

**In the U.S.—**

| | |
|---|---|
| Flint SSD | SSD |
| Sildimac | SSD AF |
| Silvadene | Thermazene |

**In Canada—**
Flamazine

## Description

Silver sulfadiazine (SILL-ver sul-fa-DYE-a-zeen), a sulfa medicine, is used to prevent and treat bacterial or fungus infections. It works by killing the fungus or bacteria.

Silver sulfadiazine cream is applied to the skin and/or burned area(s) to prevent and treat bacterial or fungus infections that may occur in burns. This medicine may also be used for other problems as determined by your doctor.

Other medicines are used along with this medicine for burns. Patients with severe burns or burns over a large area of the body must be treated in a hospital.

Silver sulfadiazine is available only with your doctor's prescription, in the following dosage form:

*Topical*
• Cream (U.S. and Canada)

## Before Using This Medicine

In deciding to use a medicine, the risks of using the medicine must be weighed against the good it will do.

This is a decision you and your doctor will make. For silver sulfadiazine, the following should be considered:

**Allergies**—Tell your doctor if you have ever had any unusual or allergic reaction to silver sulfadiazine or to any of the following medicines:

• Acetazolamide (e.g., Diamox)
• Antidiabetics, oral (diabetes medicine you take by mouth)
• Dichlorphenamide (e.g., Daranide)
• Furosemide (e.g., Lasix)
• Methazolamide (e.g., Neptazane)
• Sulfonamides, other (sulfa medicine)
• Thiazide diuretics (water pills)

Also tell your health care professional if you are allergic to any other substances, such as preservatives or dyes.

**Pregnancy**—Studies have not been done in humans. However, sulfa medicines may increase the chance of liver problems in newborn infants. Silver sulfadiazine has not been shown to cause birth defects or other problems in studies in rabbits treated with 3 to 10 times the usual amount of silver sulfadiazine.

**Breast-feeding**—It is not known whether silver sulfadiazine applied to the skin and/or burns passes into the breast milk. However, silver sulfadiazine may be absorbed into the body when used on skin and/or burns. Sulfa medicines given by mouth do pass into the breast milk. They may cause liver problems, anemia (iron-poor blood), and other unwanted effects in nursing babies, especially those with glucose-6-phosphate dehydrogenase deficiency (lack of G6PD enzyme). Therefore, caution is recommended when using this medicine in nursing women.

**Children**—Use is not recommended in premature or newborn infants up to 1 month of age. Sulfa medicines may cause liver problems in these infants. Although there is no specific information comparing use of silver sulfadiazine in older infants and children with use in other age groups, this medicine is not expected to cause different side effects or problems in older infants and children than it does in adults.

**Older adults**—Many medicines have not been studied specifically in older people. Therefore, it may not be known whether they work exactly the same way they do in younger adults or if they cause different side effects or problems in older people. There is no specific information comparing use of silver sulfadiazine in the elderly with use in other age groups.

**Other medicines**—Although certain medicines should not be used together at all, in other cases two different medicines may be used together even if an interaction might occur. In these cases, your doctor may want to change the dose, or other precautions may be necessary. When you are taking silver sulfadiazine, it is especially important that your health care professional know if you are taking any of the following:

- Collagenase (e.g., Santyl) or
- Papain (e.g., Panafil) or
- Sutilains (e.g., Travase)—Silver sulfadiazine may prevent these enzymes from working properly

**Other medical problems**—The presence of other medical problems may affect the use of silver sulfadiazine. Make sure you tell your doctor if you have any other medical problems, especially:

- Blood problems or
- Glucose-6-phosphate dehydrogenase deficiency (lack of G6PD enzyme)—Use of this medicine may cause blood problems or make them worse
- Kidney disease or
- Liver disease—In persons with these conditions, use may result in higher blood levels of this medicine; a smaller dose may be needed
- Porphyria—Use of this medicine may result in a severe attack of porphyria

## Proper Use of This Medicine

*This medicine should not be used on premature or newborn infants up to 1 month of age,* unless otherwise directed by your doctor. It may cause liver problems in these infants.

To use:

- Before applying this medicine, cleanse the affected area(s). Remove dead or burned skin and other debris.
- Wear a sterile glove to apply this medicine. Apply a thin layer (about 1/16 inch) of silver sulfadiazine to the affected area(s). Keep the affected area(s) covered with the medicine at all times.

- If this medicine is rubbed off the affected area(s) by moving around or if it is washed off during bathing, showering, or the use of a whirlpool bath, reapply the medicine.
- After this medicine has been applied, the treated area(s) may be covered with a dressing or left uncovered as desired.

To help clear up your skin and/or burn infection completely, *keep using silver sulfadiazine for the full time of treatment.* You should keep using this medicine until the burned area has healed or is ready for skin grafting. *Do not miss any doses.*

**Dosing**—The dose of silver sulfadiazine will be different for different patients. *Follow your doctor's orders or the directions on the label.* The following information includes only the average doses of silver sulfadiazine. *If your dose is different, do not change it* unless your doctor tells you to do so.

- For *topical* dosage form (cream):
  —For burn wound infections:
    - Adults and children 1 month of age and older— Use one or two times a day.
    - Premature and newborn infants up to 1 month of age—Use and dose must be determined by the doctor.

**Missed dose**—If you miss a dose of this medicine, apply it as soon as possible. However, if it is almost time for your next dose, skip the missed dose and go back to your regular dosing schedule.

**Storage**—To store this medicine:

- Keep out of the reach of children.
- Store away from heat and direct light.
- Keep the medicine from freezing.
- Do not keep outdated medicine or medicine no longer needed. Be sure that any discarded medicine is out of the reach of children.

## Precautions While Using This Medicine

It is important that your doctor check your progress at regular visits.

If your skin infection or burn does not improve within a few days or weeks (for more serious burns or burns over larger areas), or if it becomes worse, check with your doctor.

This medicine may rarely stain skin brownish gray.

## Side Effects of This Medicine

Along with its needed effects, a medicine may cause some unwanted effects. Although not all of these side effects may occur, if they do occur they may need medical attention.

Check with your doctor as soon as possible if the following side effect occurs:

*Rare*

Increased sensitivity of skin to sunlight, especially in patients with burns on large areas

Other side effects may occur that usually do not need medical attention. These side effects may go away during treatment as your body adjusts to the medicine. However, check with your doctor if any of the following side effects continue or are bothersome:

*More common*

Burning feeling on treated area(s)

*Less common or rare*

Brownish-gray skin discoloration; itching or skin rash

Other side effects not listed above may also occur in some patients. If you notice any other effects, check with your doctor.

Revised: 07/26/93

# SIMETHICONE   Oral

Some commonly used brand names are:

**In the U.S.—**

| | |
|---|---|
| Extra Strength Gas-X | Mylanta Gas Maximum |
| Gas Relief | Strength |
| Gas-X | Mylanta Gas Regular Strength |
| Maximum Strength Gas Relief | Mylicon Drops |
| Maximum Strength Phazyme | Phazyme |
| Mylanta Gas | |

Generic name product may also be available.

**In Canada**

| | |
|---|---|
| Ovol | Phazyme 55 |
| Ovol-40 | Phazyme 95 |
| Ovol-80 | |

## Description

Simethicone (si-METH-i-kone) is used to relieve the painful symptoms of too much gas in the stomach and intestines.

Simethicone may also be used for other conditions as determined by your doctor.

Simethicone is available without a prescription; however, your doctor may have special instructions on the proper use and dose for your medical problem. It is available in the following dosage forms:

*Oral*

- Capsules (U.S.)
- Oral suspension (U.S. and Canada)
- Tablets (U.S. and Canada)
- Chewable tablets (U.S. and Canada)

## Before Using This Medicine

In deciding to use a medicine, the risks of taking the medicine must be weighed against the good it will do. This is a decision you and your doctor will make. For simethicone, the following should be considered:

**Allergies**—Tell your doctor if you have ever had any unusual or allergic reaction to simethicone. Also tell your health care professional if you are allergic to any other substances, such as foods, preservatives, or dyes.

**Diet**—Avoid foods that seem to increase gas. Chew food thoroughly and slowly. Reduce air swallowing by avoiding

fizzy, carbonated drinks. Do not smoke before meals. Develop regular bowel habits and exercise regularly. Make certain your health care professional knows if you are on a low-sodium, low-sugar, or any other special diet. Most medicines contain more than their active ingredient.

**Pregnancy**—Simethicone is not absorbed into the body and is not likely to cause problems.

**Breast-feeding**—Simethicone has not been reported to cause problems in nursing babies.

**Children**—This medicine has been tested in children and, in effective doses, has not been shown to cause different side effects or problems than it does in adults.

**Older adults**—Many medicines have not been studied specifically in older people. Therefore, it may not be known whether they work exactly the same way they do in younger adults. There is no specific information comparing use of simethicone in the elderly with use in other age groups.

## Proper Use of This Medicine

For effective use of simethicone:

- Follow your doctor's instructions if this medicine was prescribed.
- Follow the manufacturer's package directions if you are treating yourself.

*Take this medicine after meals and at bedtime for best results.*

For patients taking the *chewable tablet* form of this medicine:

- It is important that you chew the tablets thoroughly before you swallow them. This is to allow the medicine to work faster and more completely.

For patients taking the *oral liquid* form of this medicine:

- This medicine is to be taken by mouth even if it comes in a dropper bottle. The amount you should take is to be measured with the specially marked dropper.

© 1994   The United States Pharmacopeial Convention, Inc.

**Dosing**—The dose of simethicone will be different for different patients. *Follow your doctor's orders or the directions on the label.* The following information includes only the average doses of simethicone. *If your dose is different, do not change it* unless your doctor tells you to do so.

- For symptoms of too much gas:
  - —For *oral* dosage forms (capsules or tablets):
    - Adults and children 12 years of age and older— 40 to 125 milligrams (mg) four times a day, after meals and at bedtime. The dose should not be more than 500 mg in 24 hours.
    - Children up to 12 years of age—Dose must be determined by the doctor.
  - —For *oral* dosage form (suspension):
    - Adults and children 12 years of age and older— 40 mg four times a day, before meals and at bedtime. The dose should not be more than 500 mg in 24 hours.
    - Children up to 12 years of age—Dose must be determined by the doctor.

**Missed dose**—If you must take this medicine regularly and you miss a dose, take it as soon as possible. However, if it is almost time for your next dose, skip the missed dose and go back to your regular dosing schedule. Do not double doses.

**Storage**—To store this medicine:
- Keep out of the reach of children.
- Store away from heat and direct light.
- Do not store the tablet form of this medicine in the bathroom, near the kitchen sink, or in other damp places. Heat or moisture may cause the medicine to break down.
- Keep the liquid form of this medicine from freezing.
- Do not keep outdated medicine or medicine no longer needed. Be sure that any discarded medicine is out of the reach of children.

## Side Effects of This Medicine

There have not been any common or important side effects reported with this medicine. However, if you notice any side effects, check with your doctor.

## Additional Information

Once a medicine has been approved for marketing for a certain use, experience may show that it is also useful for other medical problems. Although these uses are not included in product labeling, simethicone is used in certain patients before the following tests:
- Before a gastroscopy
- Before a radiography of the bowel

Other than the above information, there is no additional information relating to proper use, precautions, or side effects for these uses.

Revised: 06/16/93

# SKELETAL MUSCLE RELAXANTS  Systemic

Some commonly used brand names are:

**In the U.S.—**

| | |
|---|---|
| Carbacot[5] | Robaxin[5] |
| Delaxin[5] | Robomol[5] |
| Maolate[2] | Skelaxin[4] |
| Marbaxin[5] | Skelex[5] |
| Paraflex[3] | Sodol[1] |
| Parafon Forte DSC[3] | Soma[1] |
| Rela[1] | Soprodol[1] |
| Robamol[5] | Soridol[1] |

**In Canada—**
Robaxin[5]
Soma[1]

Note: For quick reference, the following skeletal muscle relaxants are numbered to match the corresponding brand names.

This information applies to the following medicines:

1. Carisoprodol (kar-eye-soe-PROE-dole)‡
2. Chlorphenesin (klor-FEN-e-sin)
3. Chlorzoxazone (klor-ZOX-a-zone)‡
4. Metaxalone (me-TAX-a-lone)
5. Methocarbamol (meth-oh-KAR-ba-mole)‡

This information does *not* apply to Baclofen, Cyclobenzaprine, Dantrolene, Diazepam, or Orphenadrine.

‡Generic name product may also be available in the U.S.

## Description

Skeletal muscle relaxants are used to relax certain muscles in your body and relieve the pain and discomfort caused by strains, sprains, or other injury to your muscles. However, these medicines do not take the place of rest, exercise or physical therapy, or other treatment that your doctor may recommend for your medical problem. Methocarbamol also has been used to relieve some of the muscle problems caused by tetanus.

Skeletal muscle relaxants act in the central nervous system (CNS) to produce their muscle relaxant effects. Their actions in the CNS may also produce some of their side effects.

In the U.S., these medicines are available only with your doctor's prescription. In Canada, some of these medicines are available without a prescription.

These medicines are available in the following dosage forms:

*Oral*
  Carisoprodol
  - Tablets (U.S. and Canada)

Chlorphenesin
  • Tablets (U.S.)
Chlorzoxazone
  • Tablets (U.S.)
Metaxalone
  • Tablets (U.S.)
Methocarbamol
  • Tablets (U.S. and Canada)

*Parenteral*

Methocarbamol
  • Injection (U.S. and Canada)

## Before Using This Medicine

In deciding to use a medicine, the risks of taking the medicine must be weighed against the good it will do. This is a decision you and your doctor will make. For the skeletal muscle relaxants, the following should be considered:

**Allergies**—Tell your doctor if you have ever had any unusual or allergic reaction to any of the skeletal muscle relaxants or to carbromal, mebutamate, meprobamate (e.g., Equanil), or tybamate. Also tell your health care professional if you are allergic to any other substances, such as foods, preservatives, or dyes.

**Pregnancy**—Although skeletal muscle relaxants have not been shown to cause birth defects or other problems, studies on birth defects have not been done in pregnant women. Studies in animals with metaxalone have not shown that it causes birth defects.

**Breast-feeding**—Carisoprodol passes into the breast milk and may cause drowsiness or stomach upset in nursing babies. Chlorphenesin, chlorzoxazone, metaxalone, and methocarbamol have not been shown to cause problems in nursing babies. However, methocarbamol passes into the breast milk in small amounts. It is not known whether chlorphenesin, chlorzoxazone, or metaxalone passes into the breast milk.

**Children**—Chlorzoxazone has been tested in children and has not been shown to cause different side effects or problems than it does in adults.

Although there is no specific information about the use of carisoprodol in children, it is not expected to cause different side effects or problems in children than it does in adults.

There is no specific information about the use of other skeletal muscle relaxants in children.

**Older adults**—Many medicines have not been tested in older people. Therefore, it may not be known whether they work exactly the same way they do in younger adults or if they cause different side effects or problems in older people. There is no specific information about the use of skeletal muscle relaxants in the elderly.

**Other medicines**—Although certain medicines should not be used together at all, in other cases two different medicines may be used together even if an interaction might occur. In these cases, your doctor may want to change

the dose, or other precautions may be necessary. When you are taking a skeletal muscle relaxant, it is especially important that your health care professional know if you are taking any of the following:

  • Central nervous system (CNS) depressants or
  • Tricyclic antidepressants (amitriptyline [e.g., Elavil], amoxapine [e.g., Asendin], clomipramine [e.g., Anafranil], desipramine [e.g., Pertofrane], doxepin [e.g., Sinequan], imipramine [e.g., Tofranil], nortriptyline [e.g., Aventyl], protriptyline [e.g., Vivactil], trimipramine [e.g., Surmontil])—The chance of side effects may be increased

**Other medical problems**—The presence of other medical problems may affect the use of a skeletal muscle relaxant. Make sure you tell your doctor if you have any other medical problems, especially:

  • Allergies, history of, or
  • Blood disease caused by an allergy or reaction to any other medicine, history of, or
  • Drug abuse or dependence, or history of, or
  • Kidney disease or
  • Liver disease or
  • Porphyria—Depending on which of the skeletal muscle relaxants you take, the chance of side effects may be increased; your doctor can choose a muscle relaxant that is less likely to cause problems
  • Epilepsy—Convulsions may be more likely to occur if methocarbamol is given by injection

## Proper Use of This Medicine

Chlorzoxazone, metaxalone, or methocarbamol tablets may be crushed and mixed with a little food or liquid if needed to make the tablets easier to swallow.

**Missed dose**—If you miss a dose of this medicine and remember within an hour or so of the missed dose, take it right away. But if you do not remember until later, skip the missed dose and go back to your regular dosing schedule. Do not double doses.

**Storage**—To store this medicine:

  • Keep out of the reach of children.
  • Store away from heat and direct light.
  • Do not store this medicine in the bathroom, near the kitchen sink, or in other damp places. Heat or moisture may cause the medicine to break down.
  • Do not keep outdated medicine or medicine no longer needed. Be sure that any discarded medicine is out of the reach of children.

## Precautions While Using This Medicine

If you will be taking this medicine for a long time (for example, more than a few weeks), your doctor should check your progress at regular visits.

This medicine will add to the effects of alcohol and other CNS depressants (medicines that slow down the nervous system, possibly causing drowsiness). Some examples of CNS depressants are antihistamines or medicine for hay fever, other allergies, or colds; sedatives, tranquilizers, or sleeping medicine; prescription pain medicine or narcotics; barbiturates; medicine for seizures; other muscle relaxants; or anesthetics, including some dental anesthetics. *Do not drink alcoholic beverages, and check with your doctor before taking any of the medicines listed above, while you are using this medicine.*

Skeletal muscle relaxants may cause blurred vision or clumsiness or unsteadiness in some people. They may also cause some people to feel drowsy, dizzy, lightheaded, faint, or less alert than they are normally. *Make sure you know how you react to this medicine before you drive, use machines, or do anything else that could be dangerous if you are dizzy or are not alert, well-coordinated, and able to see well.*

For *diabetic patients:*

- Metaxalone (e.g., Skelaxin) may cause false test results with one type of test for sugar in your urine. If your urine sugar test shows an unusually large amount of sugar, or if you have any questions about this, check with your health care professional. This is especially important if your diabetes is not well controlled.

## Side Effects of This Medicine

Along with its needed effects, a medicine may cause some unwanted effects. Although not all of these side effects may occur, if they do occur they may need medical attention.

Check with your doctor as soon as possible if any of the following side effects occur:

*Less common*

Fainting; fast heartbeat; fever; hive-like swellings (large) on face, eyelids, mouth, lips, and/or tongue; mental depression; shortness of breath, troubled breathing, tightness in chest, and/or wheezing; skin rash, hives, itching, or redness; slow heartbeat (methocarbamol injection only); stinging or burning of eyes; stuffy nose and red or bloodshot eyes

*Rare*

Blood in urine; bloody or black, tarry stools; convulsions (seizures) (methocarbamol injection only); cough or hoarseness; fast or irregular breathing; lower back or side pain; muscle cramps or pain (not present before treatment or more painful than before treatment); painful or difficult urination; pain, tenderness, heat,

redness, or swelling over a blood vessel (vein) in arm or leg (methocarbamol injection only); pinpoint red spots on skin; puffiness or swelling of the eyelids or around the eyes; sores, ulcers, or white spots on lips or in mouth; sore throat and fever with or without chills; swollen and/or painful glands; unusual bruising or bleeding; unusual tiredness or weakness; vomiting of blood or material that looks like coffee grounds; yellow eyes or skin

Other side effects may occur that usually do not need medical attention. These side effects may go away during treatment as your body adjusts to the medicine. However, check with your doctor if any of the following side effects continue or are bothersome:

*More common*

Blurred or double vision or any change in vision; dizziness or lightheadedness; drowsiness

*Less common or rare*

Abdominal or stomach cramps or pain; clumsiness or unsteadiness; confusion; constipation; diarrhea; excitement, nervousness, restlessness, or irritability; flushing or redness of face; headache; heartburn; hiccups; muscle weakness; nausea or vomiting; pain or peeling of skin at place of injection (methocarbamol only); trembling; trouble in sleeping; uncontrolled movements of eyes (methocarbamol injection only)

Although not all of the side effects listed above have been reported for all of these medicines, they have been reported for at least one of them. However, since all of these skeletal muscle relaxants have similar effects, it is possible that any of the above side effects may occur with any of these medicines.

In addition to the other side effects listed above, chlorzoxazone may cause your urine to turn orange or reddish purple. Methocarbamol may cause your urine to turn black, brown, or green. This effect is harmless and will go away when you stop taking the medicine. However, if you have any questions about this, check with your doctor.

Other side effects not listed above may also occur in some patients. If you notice any other effects, check with your doctor.

Revised: August 1990
Interim revision: 08/17/93

# SODIUM BENZOATE AND SODIUM PHENYLACETATE    Systemic†

A commonly used brand name in the U.S. is Ucephan.

†Not commercially available in Canada.

## Description

Sodium benzoate (SOE-dee-um BEN-zo-ate) and sodium phenylacetate (fen-ill-AH-seh-tate) combination is used to treat a condition caused by too much ammonia in the blood (hyperammonemia). This medicine works by causing less ammonia to be produced by the body.

Ammonia is formed from the breakdown of protein in the body. If the ammonia cannot be removed by the body, then a buildup may cause serious unwanted effects.

Sodium benzoate and sodium phenylacetate combination is available only with your doctor's prescription in the following dosage form:

*Oral*
- Oral solution (U.S.)

## Before Using This Medicine

In deciding to use a medicine, the risks of taking the medicine must be weighed against the good it will do. This is a decision you and your doctor will make. For sodium benzoate and sodium phenylacetate combination, the following should be considered:

**Allergies**—Tell your doctor if you have ever had any unusual or allergic reaction to sodium benzoate or sodium phenylacetate. Also tell your health care professional if you are allergic to any other substances, such as foods, preservatives, or dyes.

**Pregnancy**—Sodium benzoate and sodium phenylacetate combination has not been studied in pregnant women or animals.

**Breast-feeding**—It is not known whether sodium benzoate and sodium phenylacetate combination passes into the breast milk. Although most medicines pass into breast milk in small amounts, many of them may be used safely while breast-feeding. Mothers who are taking this medicine and who wish to breast-feed should discuss this with their doctor.

**Children**—Sodium benzoate and sodium phenylacetate may cause serious unwanted effects if given to infants of low birthweight.

**Older adults**—Many medicines have not been studied specifically in older people. Therefore, it may not be known whether they work exactly the same way they do in younger adults or if they cause different side effects or problems in older people. There is no specific information comparing the use of sodium benzoate and sodium phenylacetate in the elderly with use in other age groups.

**Other medicines**—Although certain medicines should not be used together at all, in other cases two different medicines may be used together even if an interaction might occur. In these cases, your doctor may want to change the dose, or other precautions may be necessary. When you are taking sodium benzoate and sodium phenylacetate combination, it is especially important that your health care professional know if you are taking the following:
- Penicillins—Use with penicillins may keep the sodium benzoate and sodium phenylacetate combination from working properly

**Other medical problems**—The presence of other medical problems may affect the use of sodium benzoate and sodium phenylacetate combination. Make sure you tell your doctor if you have any other medical problems, especially:
- Edema (swelling) or
- Heart disease or
- Kidney disease or
- Toxemia of pregnancy—Increased retention of water may make these conditions worse

## Proper Use of This Medicine

This medicine should be added to infant formula or milk and given immediately after mixing. Sodium benzoate and sodium phenylacetate should not be mixed with other beverages (especially acidic beverages such as tea or coffee), since they may cause the medicine to separate out.

Take this medicine with meals.

It is important that you follow any special instructions from your doctor, such as following a low protein diet. If you have any questions about this, check with your doctor.

**Dosing**—The dose of this combination medicine will be different for different patients. *Follow your doctor's orders or the directions on the label.* The following information includes only the average dose of this combination medicine. *If your dose is different, do not change it* unless your doctor tells you to do so.
- For *oral* dosage form (solution):
  —Treatment of too much ammonia in the blood:
    - Adults and children—The dose is based on body weight and must be determined by the doctor. It is usually 2.5 milliliters (mL) per kilogram (1.1 mL per pound) a day, given in three to six divided doses. The dose is usually no more than 100 mL a day.

**Missed dose**—If you miss a dose of this medicine, take it as soon as possible. However, if it is almost time for your next dose, skip the missed dose and go back to your regular dosing schedule. Do not double doses.

**Storage**—To store this medicine:
- Keep out of the reach of children.
- Store away from heat and direct light.
- Do not store in the bathroom, near the kitchen sink, or in other damp places. Heat or moisture may cause the medicine to break down.
- Keep the medicine from freezing. Do not refrigerate.
- Do not keep outdated medicine or medicine no longer needed. Be sure that any discarded medicine is out of the reach of children.

## Precautions While Using This Medicine

Your doctor should check your progress at regular visits to make sure that this medicine is working properly.

## Side Effects of This Medicine

Along with its needed effects, a medicine may cause some unwanted effects. Although not all of these side effects may occur, if they do occur they may need medical attention.

*Stop taking this medicine and get emergency help immediately* if any of the following side effects occur:

*Symptoms of overdose*
> Continual vomiting; feeling of faintness; rapid fall in blood pressure; shortness of breath or troubled breathing; unusual drowsiness; unusual irritability

Other side effects may occur that usually do not need medical attention. These side effects may go away during treatment as your body adjusts to the medicine. However, check with your doctor if either of the following side effects continue or are bothersome:

*More common*
> Nausea or vomiting

Other side effects not listed above may also occur in some patients. If you notice any other effects, check with your doctor.

Revised: 07/15/93

---

# SODIUM BICARBONATE  Systemic

Some commonly used brand names are:

**In the U.S.—**
| | |
|---|---|
| Arm and Hammer | Citrocarbonate |
| Pure Baking Soda | Soda Mint |
| Bell/ans | |

Generic name product may also be available.

**In Canada—**
Citrocarbonate

Generic name product may also be available.

## Description

Sodium bicarbonate (SOE-dee-um bye-KAR-boe-nate), also known as baking soda, is used to relieve heartburn, sour stomach, or acid indigestion by neutralizing excess stomach acid. When used for this purpose, it is said to belong to the group of medicines called antacids. It may be used to treat the symptoms of stomach or duodenal ulcers. Sodium bicarbonate is also used to make the blood and urine more alkaline in certain conditions.

*Antacids should not be given to young children (up to 6 years of age) unless prescribed by their doctor.* Since children cannot usually describe their symptoms very well, a doctor should check the child before giving this medicine. The child may have a condition that needs other treatment. If so, antacids will not help and may even cause unwanted effects or make the condition worse.

Sodium bicarbonate for oral use is available without a prescription; however, your doctor may have special instructions on the proper use and dose for your medical problem. Sodium bicarbonate is available in the following dosage forms:

*Oral*
- Effervescent powder (U.S. and Canada)
- Oral powder (U.S. and Canada)
- Tablets (U.S. and Canada)

*Parenteral*
- Injection (U.S. and Canada)

## Before Using This Medicine

If you are taking this medicine without a prescription, carefully read and follow any precautions on the label. For sodium bicarbonate, the following should be considered:

**Allergies**—Tell your doctor if you have ever had any unusual or allergic reaction to sodium bicarbonate. Also tell your health care professional if you are allergic to any other substances, such as foods, preservatives, or dyes.

**Pregnancy**—Sodium bicarbonate is absorbed by the body and although it has not been shown to cause problems, the chance always exists. In addition, medicines containing sodium should usually be avoided if you tend to retain (keep) body water.

**Breast-feeding**—It is not known whether sodium bicarbonate passes into the breast milk. However, this medicine has not been reported to cause problems in nursing babies.

**Children**—Antacids should not be given to young children (up to 6 years of age) unless prescribed by a physician.

This medicine may not help and may even worsen some conditions, so make sure that your child's problem should be treated with this medicine before you use it.

**Older adults**—Many medicines have not been studied specifically in older people. Therefore, it may not be known whether they work exactly the same way they do in younger adults or if they cause different side effects or problems in older people. There is no specific information comparing use of sodium bicarbonate in the elderly with use in other age groups.

**Other medicines**—Although certain medicines should not be used together at all, in other cases two different medicines may be used together even if an interaction might occur. In these cases, your doctor may want to change the dose, or other precautions may be necessary. When you are taking sodium bicarbonate, it is especially important that your health care professional know if you are taking any of the following:

- Ketoconazole (e.g., Nizoral) or
- Tetracyclines (medicine for infection) taken by mouth— Use with sodium bicarbonate may result in lower blood levels of these medicines, possibly decreasing their effectiveness
- Mecamylamine (e.g., Inversine)—Use with sodium bicarbonate may increase the effects of mecamylamine
- Methenamine (e.g., Mandelamine)—Use with sodium bicarbonate may reduce the effects of methenamine

**Other medical problems**—The presence of other medical problems may affect the use of sodium bicarbonate. Make sure you tell your doctor if you have any other medical problems, especially:

- Appendicitis or
- Intestinal or rectal bleeding—Oral forms of sodium bicarbonate may make these conditions worse
- Edema (swelling of feet or lower legs) or
- Heart disease or
- High blood pressure (hypertension)
- Kidney disease or
- Liver disease or
- Problems with urination or
- Toxemia of pregnancy—Sodium bicarbonate may cause the body to retain (keep) water, which may make these conditions worse

## Proper Use of This Medicine

For safe and effective use of sodium bicarbonate:

- Follow your doctor's instructions if this medicine was prescribed.
- Follow the manufacturer's package directions if you are treating yourself.

For patients *taking this medicine for a stomach ulcer:*

- *Take it exactly as directed and for the full time of treatment as ordered by your doctor,* to obtain maximum relief of your symptoms.
- Take it 1 and 3 hours after meals and at bedtime for best results, unless otherwise directed by your doctor.

**Dosing**—The dose of sodium bicarbonate will be different for different patients. *Follow your doctor's orders or the directions on the label.* The following information includes only the average doses of this medicine. *If your dose is different, do not change it* unless your doctor tells you to do so.

The number of teaspoonfuls of powder or of tablets you take depends on the strength of the medicine. *Also, the number of doses you take each day, the time allowed between doses, and the length of time you take the medicine depends on the medical problem for which you are taking sodium bicarbonate.*

- For *sodium bicarbonate* effervescent powder:
  —To relieve heartburn or sour stomach:
  - Adults and teenagers—3.9 to 10 grams (1 to 2½ teaspoonfuls) in a glass of cold water after meals. However, the dose is usually not more than 19.5 grams (5 teaspoonfuls) a day.
  - Children up to 6 years of age—Dose must be determined by your doctor.
  - Children 6 to 12 years of age—1 to 1.9 grams (¼ to ½ teaspoonful) in a glass of cold water after meals.

- For *sodium bicarbonate* powder:
  —To relieve heartburn or sour stomach:
  - Adults and teenagers—One-half teaspoonful in a glass of water every two hours. Your doctor may change the dose if needed.
  - Children—Dose must be determined by your doctor.
  —To make the urine more alkaline (less acidic):
  - Adults and teenagers—One teaspoonful in a glass of water every four hours. Your doctor may change the dose if needed. However, the dose is usually not more than 4 teaspoonfuls a day.
  - Children—Dose must be determined by your doctor.

- For *sodium bicarbonate* tablets:
  —To relieve heartburn or sour stomach:
  - Adults and teenagers—325 milligrams (mg) to 2 grams one to four times a day.
  - Children up to 6 years of age—Dose must be determined by your doctor.
  - Children 6 to 12 years of age—The dose is 520 mg. The dose may be repeated in thirty minutes.
  —To make the urine more alkaline (less acidic):
  - Adults and teenagers—At first, four grams, then 1 to 2 grams every four hours. However, the dose is usually not more than 16 grams a day.
  - Children—The dose is based on body weight and must be determined by your doctor. The usual dose is 23 to 230 mg per kilogram (kg) (10.5 to 105 mg per pound) of body weight a day. Your doctor may change the dose if needed.

**Missed dose**—If you must take this medicine regularly and you miss a dose, take it as soon as possible. However, if it is almost time for your next dose, skip the missed dose and go back to your regular dosing schedule. Do not double doses.

**Storage**—To store this medicine:

- Keep out of the reach of children.
- Store away from heat and direct light.
- Do not store the powder or tablet form of this medicine in the bathroom, near the kitchen sink, or in other damp places. Heat or moisture may cause the medicine to break down.
- Do not keep outdated medicine or medicine no longer needed. Be sure that any discarded medicine is out of the reach of children.

---

## Precautions While Using This Medicine

If this medicine has been ordered by your doctor and if you will be taking it regularly for a long time, your doctor should check your progress at regular visits. This is to make sure the medicine does not cause unwanted effects.

*Do not take sodium bicarbonate:*

- *Within 1 to 2 hours of taking other medicine by mouth.* To do so may keep the other medicine from working properly.
- *For a long period of time.* To do so may increase the chance of side effects.

For patients on a *sodium-restricted diet*:

- This medicine contains a large amount of sodium. If you have any questions about this, check with your health care professional.

For patients *taking this medicine as an antacid*:

- *Do not take this medicine if you have any signs of appendicitis* (such as stomach or lower abdominal pain, cramping, bloating, soreness, nausea, or vomiting). Instead, check with your doctor as soon as possible.

- *Do not take this medicine with large amounts of milk or milk products.* To do so may increase the chance of side effects.
- *Do not take sodium bicarbonate for more than 2 weeks* or if the problem comes back often. Instead, check with your doctor. Antacids should be used only for occasional relief, unless otherwise directed by your doctor.

### Side Effects of This Medicine

Along with its needed effects, a medicine may cause some unwanted effects. Although the following side effects occur very rarely when this medicine is taken as recommended, they may be more likely to occur if it is taken:

- In large doses.
- For a long time.
- By patients with kidney disease.

Check with your doctor as soon as possible if any of the following side effects occur:

Frequent urge to urinate; headache (continuing); loss of appetite (continuing); mood or mental changes; muscle pain or twitching; nausea or vomiting; nervousness or restlessness; slow breathing; swelling of feet or lower legs; unpleasant taste; unusual tiredness or weakness

Other side effects may occur that usually do not need medical attention. These side effects may go away during treatment as your body adjusts to the medicine. However, check with your doctor if any of the following side effects continue or are bothersome:

*Less common*
Increased thirst; stomach cramps

Other side effects not listed above may also occur in some patients. If you notice any other effects, check with your doctor.

---

Revised: 02/03/92
Interim revision: 08/10/94

---

# SODIUM CHLORIDE    Intra-amniotic

## Description

Sodium chloride (SOE-dee-um KLOR-ide) as a 20% solution is given by injection into the uterus to cause abortion. It is to be administered only by or under the immediate care of your doctor. It is available in the following dosage form:

*Parenteral*
- Injection (U.S. and Canada)

## Before Receiving This Medicine

In deciding to use a medicine, the risks of taking the medicine must be weighed against the good it will do.

This is a decision you and your doctor will make. For sodium chloride, the following should be considered:

**Allergies**—Tell your doctor if you have ever had any unusual or allergic reaction to sodium chloride. Also, tell your health care professional if you are allergic to any other substances, such as foods, preservatives, or dyes.

**Teenagers**—Although there is no specific information comparing use of sodium chloride in adolescent females with use in other age groups, this medicine is not expected to cause different side effects or problems in adolescent females than it does in adults.

**Other medicines**—Although certain medicines should not be used together at all, in other cases two different medicines may be used together even if an interaction might occur. In these cases, your doctor may want to change the dose, or other precautions may be necessary. Tell your health care professional if you are taking any other prescription or nonprescription (over-the-counter [OTC]) medicine.

**Other medical problems**—The presence of other medical problems may affect the use of sodium chloride. Make sure you tell your doctor if you have any other medical problems, especially:

- Bleeding problems
- Epilepsy
- Fibroid tumors of the uterus
- Heart or blood vessel disease
- High blood pressure (hypertension)
- Kidney disease

## Proper Use of This Medicine

Unless otherwise directed by your doctor, drink at least 2 liters (about 2 quarts) of fluids the day that this procedure is to be done.

**Dosing**—The dose of sodium chloride will be different for different patients. *Follow your doctor's orders.* The medicine will be given by your doctor in a health care setting, such as a hospital or clinic. The following information includes only the average doses of sodium chloride.

- For *injection* dosage form:
  —For causing abortion:
    • Adults and teenagers—200 to 250 milliliters (mL) injected through the abdomen into the uterus after the same amount of fluid has been taken out of the bag around the fetus (amniotic sac). The injection may be repeated 48 hours after the first dose if needed.

## Side Effects of This Medicine

Along with its needed effects, a medicine may cause some unwanted effects. Although not all of these effects may occur, if they do occur they may need medical attention.

*Check with your health care professional immediately* if any of the following side effects occur during the time that the injection is being given:

*Less common*
    Burning pain in lower abdomen; confusion; feeling of heat; feeling of warmth in lips and tongue; headache (severe); nervousness; numbness of the fingertips; pain in lower back, pelvis, or stomach; ringing in the ears; thirst (sudden) or salty taste

Other side effects may occur that usually do not need medical attention. These side effects usually go away after the medicine is stopped. However, let the health care professional know if either of the following side effects continues or is bothersome:

*More common*
    Fever; flushing or redness of face

After the procedure is completed, this procedure may still produce some side effects that need medical attention. Check with your doctor if you notice any of the following side effects:

    Chills or shivering; fever; foul-smelling vaginal discharge; increase in bleeding from the uterus; pain in lower abdomen

Other side effects not listed above may also occur in some patients. If you notice any other effects, check with your health care professional.

Revised: 07/28/93
Interim revision: 06/21/94

# SODIUM FLUORIDE    Systemic

## Description

Some commonly used brand names are:

**In the U.S.—**

| | |
|---|---|
| Fluoritab | Karidium |
| Fluorodex | Luride |
| Flura | Luride-SF |
| Flura-Drops | Pediaflor |

Generic name product may also be available.

**In Canada—**

| | |
|---|---|
| Fluor-A-Day | Pedi-Dent |
| Fluotic | Solu-Flur |
| Karidium | |

## Description

Fluoride has been found to be helpful in reducing the number of cavities in the teeth. It is usually present naturally in drinking water. However, some areas of the country do not have a high enough level in the water to prevent cavities. To make up for this, extra fluorides may be added to the diet. Some children may require both dietary fluorides and topical fluoride treatments by the dentist. Use of a fluoride toothpaste or rinse may be helpful as well.

Taking fluorides does not replace good dental habits. These include eating a good diet, brushing and flossing teeth often, and having regular dental checkups.

Fluoride may also be used for other conditions as determined by your medical doctor or dentist.

This medicine is available only with your medical doctor's or dentist's prescription, in the following dosage forms:

*Oral*
- Oral solution (U.S. and Canada)
- Tablets (U.S. and Canada)
- Chewable tablets (U.S. and Canada)

## Importance of Diet

Nutritionists recommend that, if possible, people should get all the fluoride they need from foods and/or drinking water that has fluoride added to it. However, some people do not get enough fluoride from their diets. For these people, a fluoride supplement may be necessary.

In order to get enough vitamins and minerals in your regular diet, it is important that you eat a balanced and varied diet. Follow carefully any diet program your doctor may recommend. For your specific vitamin and/or minerals needs, ask your doctor for a list of appropriate foods.

Experts have developed a list of recommended dietary allowances (RDA) for most vitamins and some minerals. The RDA are not an exact number but a general idea of how much you need. They do not cover amounts needed for problems caused by a serious lack of vitamins and minerals. There are no RDA for fluoride. The following intakes are thought to be plenty for most individuals:

- Infants and children—
  Birth to 6 months of age: 0.1 to 0.5 mg a day.
  1 to 3 years of age: 0.5 to 1.5 mg a day.
  4 to 6 years of age: 1 to 2.5 mg a day.
  7 to 10 years of age: 1.5 to 2.5 mg a day.
- Adolescent and adult men and women: 1.5 to 4 mg a day.

People get needed fluoride from fish that are eaten with their bones, tea, and drinking water that has fluoride added to it. Food that is cooked in water containing fluoride or in Teflon-coated pans also provides fluoride. However, foods cooking in aluminum pans provide less fluoride.

Remember:
- The total amount of fluoride you get every day includes what you get from the foods and beverages that you eat and what you may take as a supplement.
- This total amount *should not* be greater than the above recommendations, unless ordered by your doctor. Taking too much fluoride can cause serious problems to the teeth and bones.

## Before Using This Medicine

In deciding to use a medicine, the risks of taking the medicine must be weighed against the good it will do. This is a decision you and your medical doctor or dentist will make. For sodium fluoride, the following should be considered:

**Allergies**—Tell your medical doctor, dentist, and pharmacist if you are allergic to any other substances, such as foods, preservatives, or dyes.

**Pregnancy**—Sodium fluoride occurs naturally in water and has not been shown to cause problems in infants of mothers who drank fluoridated water or took appropriate doses of supplements.

**Breast-feeding**—Small amounts of sodium fluoride pass into breast milk.

**Children**—Doses of sodium fluoride that are too large or are taken for a long time may cause bone problems and teeth discoloration in children.

**Older adults**—Older people are more likely to have joint pain, kidney problems, or stomach ulcers which may be made worse by taking large doses of sodium fluoride. You should check with your doctor.

**Other medicines**—Although certain medicines should not be used together at all, in other cases two different medicines may be used together even if an interaction might occur. In these cases, your medical doctor or dentist may want to change the dose, or other precautions may be necessary. Tell your medical doctor, dentist, and pharmacist if you are taking/using any other prescription or nonprescription (over-the-counter [OTC]) medicine.

**Other medical problems**—The presence of other medical problems may affect the use of sodium fluoride. Make sure you tell your medical doctor or dentist if you have any other medical problems, especially:
- Brown, white, or black discoloration of teeth or
- Joint pain or
- Kidney problems (severe) or
- Stomach ulcer—Sodium fluoride may make these conditions worse

## Proper Use of This Medicine

*Take this medicine only as directed by your medical doctor or dentist*. Do not take more of it and do not take it more often than ordered. Taking too much fluoride over a period of time may cause unwanted effects.

For patients taking the *chewable tablet form* of this medicine:
- Tablets should be chewed or crushed before they are swallowed.
- This medicine works best if it is taken at bedtime, after the teeth have been thoroughly brushed. Do not eat or drink for at least 15 minutes after taking sodium fluoride.

For patients taking the *oral liquid form* of this medicine:
- This medicine is to be taken by mouth even though it comes in a dropper bottle. The amount to be taken is to be measured with the specially marked dropper.

© 1994   The United States Pharmacopeial Convention, Inc.

- *Always store this medicine in the original plastic container*. Fluoride will affect glass and should not be stored in glass containers.
- This medicine may be dropped directly into the mouth or mixed with cereal, fruit juice, or other food. However, if this medicine is mixed with foods or beverages that contain calcium, the amount of sodium fluoride that is absorbed may be reduced.

**Dosing**—The dose of sodium fluoride will be different for different patients. *Follow your doctor's orders or the directions on the label*. The following information includes only the average doses of sodium fluoride. *If your dose is different, do not change it* unless your doctor tells you to do so.

The amount of solution or the number of tablets you take depends on the strength of the medicine. Also, *the number of doses you take each day, the time allowed between doses, and the length of time you take the medicine depend on the medical problem for which you are taking sodium fluoride*.

- For *oral* dosage form (solution, tablets, or chewable tablets):
    —To prevent cavities in the teeth (where there is not enough fluoride in the water):
    - Children—Dose is based on the amount of fluoride in drinking water in your area. Dose is also based on the child's age and must be determined by your doctor.

**Storage**—To store this medicine:

- Keep out of the reach of children, since overdose is especially dangerous in children.
- Store away from heat and direct light.
- Do not store in the bathroom, near the kitchen sink, or in other damp places. Heat or moisture may cause the medicine to break down.
- Protect the oral liquid from freezing.
- Do not keep outdated medicine or medicine no longer needed. Be sure that any discarded medicine is out of the reach of children.

---

## Precautions While Using This Medicine

The level of fluoride present in the water is different in different parts of the U.S. If you move to another area, check with a medical doctor or dentist in the new area as soon as possible to see if this medicine is still needed or if the dose needs to be changed. Also, check with your medical doctor or dentist if you change infant feeding habits (e.g., breast-feeding to infant formula), drinking water (e.g., city water to nonfluoridated bottled water), or filtration (e.g., tap water to filtered tap water).

Do not take calcium supplements or aluminum hydroxide–containing products and sodium fluoride at the same time. It is best to space doses of these two products 2 hours apart, to get the full benefit from each medicine.

*Inform your medical doctor or dentist as soon as possible if you notice white, brown, or black spots on the teeth*. These are signs of too much fluoride in children when it is given during periods of tooth development.

---

## Side Effects of This Medicine

Along with its needed effects, a medicine may cause some unwanted effects. Although not all of these side effects may occur, if they do occur they may need medical attention.

Check with your doctor as soon as possible if any of the following side effects occur(s):

Sores in mouth and on lips (rare)

Sodium fluoride in drinking water or taken as a supplement does not usually cause any side effects. However, *taking an overdose of fluoride may cause serious problems*.

*Stop taking this medicine and check with your medical doctor or dentist immediately* if any of the following side effects occur, as they may be symptoms of severe overdose:

Black, tarry stools; bloody vomit; diarrhea; drowsiness; faintness; increased watering of mouth; nausea or vomiting; shallow breathing; stomach cramps or pain; tremors; unusual excitement; watery eyes; weakness

Check with your medical doctor or dentist as soon as possible if the following side effects occur, as some may be early symptoms of possible chronic overdose:

Pain and aching of bones; stiffness; white, brown, or black discoloration of teeth—occur only during periods of tooth development in children

Other side effects not listed above may also occur in some patients. If you notice any other effects, check with your medical doctor or dentist.

---

Revised: 07/17/92
Interim revision: 08/24/94

# SODIUM IODIDE  Systemic†

A commonly used brand name in the U.S. is Iodopen.
Generic name product may also be available.

†Not commercially available in Canada.

## Description

Sodium iodide is used to prevent or treat iodine deficiency.

The body needs iodine for normal growth and health. For patients who are unable to get enough iodine in their regular diet or who have a need for more iodine, sodium iodide may be necessary.

Iodine deficiency in the United States is rare because iodine is added to table salt. Most people get enough salt from the foods they eat, without adding salt to their meals. Iodine deficiency is a problem in other areas of the world.

Lack of iodine may lead to thyroid problems, mental problems, hearing loss, and goiter.

Sodium iodide is available by itself only as an injection, which is given by your doctor or under your doctor's supervision. Some multivitamin/mineral preparations that contain sodium iodide are available without your doctor's prescription.

Sodium iodide is available in the following dosage form:

*Parenteral*
Sodium Iodide
• Injection (U.S.)

## Importance of Diet

Nutritionists recommend that, if possible, people should get all the iodine they need from foods. However, some people may not get enough iodine from their diets. Others may need more iodine than normal. For such people, an iodine supplement is important.

In order to get enough vitamins and minerals in your diet, it is important that you eat a balanced and varied diet. Follow carefully any diet program your doctor may recommend. For your specific vitamin and/or mineral needs, ask your doctor for a list of appropriate foods.

Iodine is found in various foods, including seafood, small amounts of iodized salt, and vegetables grown in iodine-rich soils. Iodine-containing mist from the ocean is another important source of iodine, since iodine is absorbed by the skin. Iodized salt provides 76 mcg of iodine per gram of salt.

Experts have developed a list of recommended dietary allowances (RDA) for most vitamins and some minerals. The RDA are not an exact number but a general idea of how much you need. They do not cover amounts needed for problems caused by a serious lack of vitmains and minerals.

The RDA for iodine are:
Infants and children—
Birth to 6 months of age: 40 micrograms (mcg) a day.
6 months to 1 year of age: 50 mcg a day.
1 to 3 years of age: 70 mcg a day.
4 to 6 years of age: 90 mcg a day.
7 to 10 years of age: 120 mcg a day.
Adolescent and adult males—150 mcg a day.
Adolescent and adult females—150 mcg a day.
Pregnant females—175 mcg a day.
Breast-feeding females—200 mcg a day.

Remember:
• The total amount of iodine that you get every day includes what you get from the foods that you eat *and* what you may take as a supplement.
• This total amount should not be greater than the RDA, unless ordered by your doctor.

## Before Using This Medicine

In deciding to use a medicine, the risks of taking the medicine must be weighed against the good it will do. This is a decision you and your doctor will make. For sodium iodide, the following should be considered:

**Allergies**—Tell your doctor if you have ever had any unusual or allergic reaction to iodine, iodine-containing foods, or sodium iodide. Also tell your health care professional if you are allergic to any other substances, such as foods, preservatives, or dyes.

**Pregnancy**—It is especially important that you are receiving enough vitamins and minerals when you become pregnant and that you continue to receive the right amount of vitamins and minerals throughout your pregnancy. The healthy growth and development of the fetus depend on a steady supply of nutrients from the mother. A deficiency of iodine in the mother may cause nerve or growth problems for the fetus. Taking high doses of sodium iodide may cause thyroid problems or goiter in the newborn infant.

**Breast-feeding**—It is important that you receive the right amounts of vitamins and minerals so that your baby will also get the vitamins and minerals needed to grow properly. Taking high doses of sodium iodide may cause skin rash and thyroid problems in nursing babies.

**Children**—It is especially important that children receive enough iodine in their diet for healthy growth and development. However, high doses of sodium iodide may cause skin rash and thyroid problems in infants.

**Older adults**—It is important that older people continue to receive enough iodine in their daily diets.

**Other medicines**—Although certain medicines should not be used together at all, in other cases two different medicines may be used together even if an interaction might occur. In these cases, your doctor may want to change the dose, or other precautions may be necessary. When you are taking sodium iodide, it is especially important that your health care professional know if you are taking any of the following:

- Antithyroid agents (medicine for overactive thyroid)—These medicines may prevent sodium iodide from working properly
- Iodine-containing medicines, other—Use of these medicines with sodium iodide may increase blood levels of iodine, which may increase the chance of side effects
- Lithium (e.g., Lithane)—Use of this medicine with sodium iodide may increase the chance of side effects

**Other medical problems**—The presence of other medical problems may affect the use of sodium iodide. Make sure you tell your doctor if you have any other medical problems, especially:

- Kidney disease—Use of sodium iodide may increase the amount of iodine in the blood and increase the chance of side effects
- Thyroid disease—This condition may increase the chance of side effects of sodium iodide
- Tuberculosis—Use of sodium iodide may make this condition worse

## Proper Use of This Medicine

Some people believe that taking very large doses of a vitamin or mineral (called megadoses) is useful for treating certain medical problems. Studies have not proven this. Large doses should be taken only under the direction of your doctor after need has been identified.

**Dosing**—The dose of sodium iodide for prevention of iodine deficiency is based on the Recommended Dietary Allowances (RDA). See the *Importance of Diet* section for the RDA for iodine.

**Missed dose**—If you miss taking sodium iodide for one or more days there is no cause for concern, since it takes some time for your body to become seriously low in iodine. However, if your doctor has recommended that you take iodine try to remember to use it as directed every day.

**Storage**—To store this medicine:

- Keep out of the reach of children.
- Store away from heat and direct light.
- Do not store in the bathroom, near the kitchen sink, or in other damp places. Heat or moisture may cause the medicine to break down.
- Keep the medicine from freezing. Do not refrigerate.
- Do not keep outdated medicine or medicine no longer needed. Be sure that any discarded medicine is out of the reach of children.

## Precautions While Using This Medicine

Many other products contain iodine. For example, iodine is absorbed through the skin from some skin cleansers (e.g., povidone-iodine). It may be especially important that infants and small children not receive large amounts of iodine. Check with your doctor before using any other products that contain iodine while you are using this medicine.

## Side Effects of This Medicine

Along with its needed effects, a medicine may cause some unwanted effects. Although not all of these side effects may occur, if they do occur they may need medical attention. When this medicine is used at low doses, side effects are rare.

Check with your doctor as soon as possible if any of the following side effects occur:

*Less common*
Hives; joint pain; swelling of arms, face, legs, lips, tongue, and/or throat; swelling of lymph glands

*With long-term use*
Burning of mouth or throat; headache (severe); increased watering of mouth; metallic taste; skin sores; soreness of teeth and gums; stomach irritation

Other side effects not listed above may also occur in some patients. If you notice any other effects, check with your doctor.

## Additional Information

Once a medicine has been approved for marketing for a certain use, experience may show that it is also useful for other medical problems. Although this use is not included in product labeling, injections of sodium iodide are used in certain patients with the following medical condition:

- Thyrotoxicosis crisis (severe overactive thyroid)

Other than the above information, there is no additional information relating to proper use, precautions, or side effects for this use.

Revised: 02/26/92
Interim revision: 08/19/94

# SODIUM IODIDE I 131    Therapeutic

## Description

Sodium iodide (EYE-oh-dyed) I 131, also called radio-active iodine or radioiodide, is a radiopharmaceutical (ray-dee-oh-far-ma-SOO-ti-kal). Radiopharmaceuticals are radioactive agents, which may be used to diagnose some diseases by studying the function of the body's organs or to treat certain diseases.

Sodium iodide I 131 is used to treat an overactive thyroid gland and certain kinds of thyroid cancer. It is taken up mainly by the thyroid gland. In the treatment of hyperactive thyroid gland, radiation from the radioactive iodine damages the thyroid gland to bring its activity back down to normal. Larger doses of radioiodide are usually used after thyroid cancer surgery to destroy any remaining diseased thyroid tissue.

When very small doses are given, a measure of the radioactivity taken up by the gland helps your doctor decide whether your thyroid gland is working properly. Also, an image of the organ on paper or a computer printout can be provided.

*The information that follows applies only to the use of sodium iodide I 131 in treating an overactive or cancerous thyroid gland.*

Sodium iodide I 131 is to be given only by or under the direct supervision of a doctor with specialized training in nuclear medicine or radiation oncology. It is available in the following dosage forms:

*Oral*
- Capsules (U.S. and Canada)
- Solution (U.S. and Canada)

## Before Using This Medicine

In deciding to use a medicine, the risks of taking the medicine must be weighed against the good it will do. This is a decision you and your doctor will make. For sodium iodide I 131, the following should be considered:

**Diet**—If you eat large amounts of iodine-containing foods, such as iodized salt and seafoods, or cabbage, kale, rape (turnip-like vegetable), or turnips, the iodine contained in these foods will reduce the amount of this radiopharmaceutical that your thyroid gland will accept. Avoid these foods for at least 2 to 4 weeks weeks before the treatment with radioiodide.

**Pregnancy**—Sodium iodide I 131 should not be used during pregnancy. This is to avoid exposing the fetus to radiation. Also, it may cause the newborn baby to have an underactive thyroid gland. A pregnancy test may be done prior to treatment with radioactive iodine. Be sure you have discussed this with your doctor.

**Breast-feeding**—Sodium iodide I 131 passes into the breast milk and may cause unwanted effects, such as underactive thyroid, in the nursing baby. If you must receive this radiopharmaceutical, it will be necessary for you to stop breast-feeding several weeks before treatment. Be sure you have discussed this with your doctor.

**Children**—Children and teenagers are especially sensitive to the effects of radiation. This may increase the chance of side effects during and after treatment.

**Older adults**—Sodium iodide I 131 has been used in older people and has not been shown to cause different side effects or problems in older people than it does in younger adults.

**Other medicines/tests**—Tell your doctor if you have had an x-ray test recently for which you were given a radiopaque agent that contained iodine. The iodine contained in the radiopaque agent will reduce the amount of sodium iodide I 131 that your thyroid gland will accept. Also, tell your doctor if you are taking any other prescription or nonprescription (over-the-counter [OTC]) medicine.

**Other medical problems**—The presence of other medical problems may affect the use of sodium iodide I 131. Make sure you tell your doctor if you have any other medical problems, especially:

- Diarrhea or
- Vomiting—The radioactive iodine will be present in the diarrhea and vomit and put you and others at a higher risk of radiation contamination; also, some of the dose will be lost, making the treatment less effective
- Iodine deficiency—This condition may cause the thyroid gland to take up more of the sodium iodide I 131 than it would normally
- Kidney disease—Kidney disease may cause the radioiodide to stay in the body longer than usual, which may increase the risk of side effects
- If you have heart disease and are receiving sodium iodide I 131 to treat an overactive thyroid—The radiation may worsen the thyroid condition if antithyroid medicine and/or beta-blockers, such as propranolol, are not given before and after treatment

## Proper Use of This Medicine

Your doctor may have special instructions for you to get ready for your treatment. If you have not received such instructions or you do not understand them, check with your doctor ahead of time.

**Dosing**—The doses of radiopharmaceuticals will be different for different patients and for the different types of treatments. The amount of radioactivity of a radiopharmaceutical is expressed in units called becquerels or curies. The usual adult dose of radioiodide to treat an overactive thyroid gland is 148 to 370 megabecquerels (4 to 10 millicuries). The usual amount of radioiodide to treat cancer of the thyroid is much larger, 1.85 to 7.4 gigabecquerels (50 to 200 millicuries). The dose you receive depends on your size and age. The amount of radiation received by specific areas of the body to treat a disease is many times higher than that received from any diagnostic test, such as x-rays and nuclear medicine scans. Doses may need to be repeated, depending on the kind of disease you have and how your body is responding to treatment.

## Precautions After Using This Medicine

There are no special precautions when this medicine is used in very small doses to help study the function of the thyroid. However, if you are receiving sodium iodide I 131 for an overactive thyroid or cancer of the thyroid, your doctor may tell you to *follow some or all of these guidelines for 48 to 96 hours* after receiving the medicine, to help reduce the chance of contaminating other persons:

- *Do not kiss anyone, or handle or use another person's eating or drinking utensils, toothbrush, or bathroom glass.*
- *Do not have sex.*
- *Do not sit close to others and do not hold children in your lap for long periods of time.*
- Sleep alone.
- *Wash the tub and sink after each use (including after brushing teeth).*
- *Wash your hands after using or cleaning the toilet.*
- Use a separate towel and washcloth.
- Wash your clothes, bed linens, and eating utensils separately.
- Sodium iodide I 131 is passed in the urine. To prevent contamination of your home, *flush the toilet twice after you urinate.*

To increase the flow of urine and lessen the amount of radioactive iodine in your body, drink plenty of liquids and urinate often.

## Side Effects of This Medicine

Studies have not shown that sodium iodide I 131 increases the chance of cancer or other long-term problems. When used to treat an overactive thyroid gland or cancer of the thyroid, sodium iodide I 131 may cause the patient to have an underactive thyroid gland after treatment. Before receiving this medicine, be sure you have discussed its use with your doctor.

Along with its needed effects, a medicine may cause some unwanted effects. Although not all of these side effects may occur, if they do occur they may need medical attention.

When this medicine is used in very small doses to help study the function of the gland, side effects are rare. However, check with your doctor as soon as possible if any of the following side effects occur after treatment for overactive thyroid or cancer of the thyroid:

*After treatment of overactive thyroid or cancer of the thyroid*
  *Symptoms of an underactive thyroid*
  Changes in menstrual periods; clumsiness; coldness; drowsiness; dry, puffy skin; headache; listlessness; muscle aches; thinning of hair (temporary)—may occur 2 to 3 months after treatment; unusual tiredness or weakness; weight gain

*Rare*
  *After treatment of overactive thyroid*
  Excessive sweating; fast heartbeat; fever; palpitations; unusual irritability; unusual tiredness
  *After treatment of cancer of the thyroid*
  Black, tarry stools; blood in urine or stools; cough or hoarseness; fever or chills; lower back or side pain; painful or difficult urination; pinpoint red spots on skin; unusual bleeding or bruising

Other side effects may occur that usually do not need medical attention. These side effects may go away during treatment as your body adjusts to the medicine. However, check with your doctor if any of the following side effects continue or are bothersome:

*Less common*
  *After treatment of overactive thyroid or cancer of the thyroid*
  Neck tenderness or swelling; sore throat
  *After treatment of cancer of the thyroid*
  Loss of taste (temporary); nausea and vomiting (temporary); tenderness of salivary glands

Other side effects not listed above may also occur in some patients. If you notice any other effects, check with your doctor.

---

Revised: 09/02/94

---

# SODIUM PHOSPHATE P 32  Therapeutic

## Description

Sodium phosphate (SOE-dee-um FOS-fate) P 32 is a radiopharmaceutical (ray-dee-oh-far-ma-SOO-ti-kal). Radiopharmaceuticals are radioactive agents that may be used to treat certain diseases or to study the activity of the body's organs.

Sodium phosphate P 32 is used to treat certain kinds of cancer. In this case, the radioactive agent builds up in the cancerous area and destroys the affected tissue. This radiopharmaceutical may also be used for other conditions as determined by your doctor.

Sodium phosphate P 32 is to be given only by or under the direct supervision of a doctor with specialized training

---

© 1994   The United States Pharmacopeial Convention, Inc.

in nuclear medicine. It is available in the following dosage form:

*Parenteral*
- Solution (U.S. and Canada)

## Before Using This Medicine

In deciding to use a medicine, the risks of taking the medicine must be weighed against the good it will do. This is a decision you and your doctor will make. For sodium phosphate P 32, the following should be considered:

**Allergies**—Tell your doctor if you have ever had any unusual or allergic reaction to sodium phosphate P 32. Also tell your doctor if you are allergic to any other substances, such as foods, preservatives, or dyes.

**Pregnancy**—Studies have not been done in either humans or animals. However, to avoid exposing the fetus to radiation, sodium phosphate P 32 is not recommended for use during pregnancy. Be sure you have discussed this with your doctor.

**Breast-feeding**—Sodium phosphate may pass into the breast milk. If you must receive this radiopharmaceutical, it will be necessary for you to stop breast-feeding during treatment. Be sure you have discussed this with your doctor.

**Children**—Studies on this medicine have been done only in adult patients, and there is no specific information about its use in children. However, children are especially sensitive to the effects of radiation. This may increase the chance of side effects during and after treatment.

**Older adults**—Older adults are especially sensitive to the effects of radiation. This may increase the chance of side effects during and after treatment.

**Other medicines**—Although certain medicines should not be used together at all, in other cases two different medicines may be used together even if an interaction might occur. In these cases, your doctor may want to change the dose, or other precautions may be necessary. When you are receiving sodium phosphate P 32, it is especially important that your doctor know if you are taking any other prescription or nonprescription (over-the-counter [OTC]) medicine.

**Other medical problems**—The presence of other medical problems may affect the use of sodium phosphate P 32. Make sure you tell your doctor if you have any other medical problems.

## Proper Use of This Medicine

Your doctor may have special instructions for you in preparation for your treatment. If you do not understand them or if you have not received such instructions, check with your doctor in advance.

**Dosing**—The doses of radiopharmaceuticals will be different for different patients and for the different types of treatments. The amount of radioactivity of a radiopharmaceutical is expressed in units called becquerels or curies. Usual adult doses of sodium phosphate P 32 range from 37 megabecquerels (1 millicurie) to 185 megabecquerels (5 millicuries). The dose you receive depends on your size, age, and blood test measurements (blood counts). The amount of radiation received by the body to treat a disease is many times higher than from any diagnostic test, such as x-rays and nuclear medicine scans. Repeated doses may be necessary, depending on the kind of disease you have and how your body is responding to treatment.

## Side Effects of This Medicine

Along with its needed effects, a medicine may cause some unwanted effects. When sodium phosphate P 32 is used at recommended doses, side effects usually are rare. However, blood problems, such as anemia or a decrease in the number of white blood cells, may occur in some patients.

Also, the following side effects may occur in patients with bone cancer receiving sodium phosphate P 32 for the relief of bone pain:

*More common*
Diarrhea, fever, nausea, vomiting

Other side effects not listed above may also occur in some patients. If you notice any other effects, check with your doctor.

Revised: 07/16/93

# SODIUM THIOSULFATE  Systemic

A commonly used brand name in the U.S. and Canada for the antidote kit containing sodium thiosulfate is Cyanide Antidote Package. Generic name product may also be available.

## Description

Sodium thiosulfate (thye-oh-SUL-fate) may be used to lessen some of the side effects of cisplatin (a cancer medicine). It is also used with another medicine in the emergency treatment of cyanide poisoning.

Sodium thiosulfate is to be administered only by or under the immediate supervision of your doctor. It is available in the following dosage form:

*Parenteral*
- Injection (U.S. and Canada)

## Before Receiving This Medicine

In deciding to use a medicine, the risks of taking the medicine must be weighed against the good it will do. This is a decision you and your doctor will make. When sodium thiosulfate is to be used to lessen the side effects of cancer medicine, the following should be considered:

**Allergies**—Tell your doctor if you have ever had any unusual or allergic reaction to sodium thiosulfate. Also tell your health care professional if you are allergic to any other substances, such as foods, preservatives, or dyes.

**Pregnancy**—Studies on effects in pregnancy have not been done in humans or animals.

**Breast-feeding**—It is not known whether sodium thiosulfate passes into breast milk. Although most medicines pass into breast milk in small amounts, many of them may be used safely while breast-feeding. Mothers who receive this medicine and who wish to breast-feed should discuss this with their doctor.

**Children**—Although there is no specific information comparing use of sodium thiosulfate in children with use in other age groups, this medicine is not expected to cause different side effects or problems in children than it does in adults.

**Older adults**—Many medicines have not been studied specifically in older people. Therefore, it may not be known whether they work exactly the same way they do in younger adults. Although there is no specific information comparing the use of sodium thiosulfate in the elderly with use in other age groups, this medicine is not expected to cause different side effects or problems in older people than it does in younger adults.

**Other medicines**—Although certain medicines should not be used together at all, in other cases two different medicines may be used together even if an interaction might occur. In these cases, your doctor may want to change the dose, or other precautions may be necessary. Tell your health care professional if you are taking any other prescription or nonprescription (over-the-counter [OTC]) medicine.

**Other medical problems**—The presence of other medical problems may affect the use of sodium thiosulfate. Make sure you tell your doctor if you have any other medical problems, especially:

- Edema (swelling of feet or lower legs) or
- Heart disease or
- High blood pressure (hypertension) or
- Kidney disease or
- Liver disease or

- Toxemia of pregnancy—Sodium thiosulfate may cause the body to retain (keep) water, which may make these conditions worse

## Proper Use of This Medicine

**Dosing**—The dose of sodium thiosulfate will be different for different patients. The following information includes only the average doses of sodium thiosulfate.

- For *injection* dosage form:
  - —For use with cisplatin (a cancer medicine):
    - Adults and teenagers—The first dose, given just before the cancer medicine, is usually 4 grams per square meter of body surface area, injected into a vein. The second dose is started at the same time as the cancer medicine. It is usually 12 grams per square meter of body surface area, injected into a vein over a period of six hours.
  - —For cyanide poisoning:
    - Adults and teenagers—The usual dose is 12.5 grams injected into a vein at a rate of 0.625 to 1.25 grams (2.5 to 5 milliliters [mL]) per minute.
    - Children—The usual dose is 412.5 milligrams (mg) per kilogram (kg) (187 mg per pound) of body weight or 7 grams per square meter of body surface area injected into a vein at a rate of 0.625 to 1.25 grams (2.5 to 5 mL) per minute.

## Side Effects of This Medicine

Along with its needed effects, a medicine may cause some unwanted effects. Although not all of these side effects may occur, if they do occur they may need medical attention.

*Check with your doctor immediately* if any of the following side effects occur:

*Symptoms of overdose*

Agitation; blurred vision; hallucinations (seeing, hearing, or feeling things that are not there); mental changes; muscle cramps; nausea and vomiting; pain in the joints; ringing in the ears

Other side effects not listed above may also occur in some patients. If you notice any other effects, check with your doctor.

Developed: 03/30/94

# SPECTINOMYCIN Systemic

A commonly used brand name in the U.S. and Canada is Trobicin.

## Description

Spectinomycin (spek-ti-noe-MYE-sin) is used to treat most types of gonorrhea. It is given by injection into a muscle. It is sometimes given with other medicines for gonorrhea and related infections.

Spectinomycin may be used in patients who are allergic to penicillins, cephalosporins, or probenecid (e.g., Benemid). This medicine is also used to treat recent sexual partners of patients who have gonorrhea. However, spectinomycin will not work for gonorrhea of the throat, syphilis, colds, flu, or other virus infections.

Spectinomycin is available only with your doctor's prescription, in the following dosage form:

*Parenteral*
- Injection (U.S. and Canada)

## Before Receiving This Medicine

In deciding to use a medicine, the risks of taking the medicine must be weighed against the good it will do. This is a decision you and your doctor will make. For spectinomycin, the following should be considered:

**Allergies**—Tell your doctor if you have ever had any unusual or allergic reaction to spectinomycin. Also tell your health care professional if you are allergic to any other substances, such as foods, preservatives, or dyes.

**Pregnancy**—Studies have not been done in humans. However, spectinomycin has been recommended for the treatment of gonorrhea and related infections in pregnant patients who are allergic to penicillins, cephalosporins, or probenecid (e.g., Benemid). In addition, studies in animals have not shown that spectinomycin causes birth defects or other problems.

**Breast-feeding**—It is not known if spectinomycin passes into breast milk. However, spectinomycin has not been reported to cause problems in nursing babies.

**Children**—This medicine has been used in a limited number of children. In effective doses, the medicine has not been shown to cause different side effects or problems than it does in adults. However, use in infants is not recommended.

**Older adults**—Many medicines have not been studied specifically in older people. Therefore, it may not be known whether they work exactly the same way they do in younger adults. Although there is no specific information comparing use of spectinomycin in the elderly with use in other age groups, this medicine is not expected to cause different side effects or problems in older people than it does in younger adults.

**Other medicines**—Although certain medicines should not be used together at all, in other cases two different medicines may be used together even if an interaction might occur. In these cases, your doctor may want to change the dose, or other precautions may be necessary. Tell your health care professional if you are taking any other prescription or nonprescription (over-the-counter [OTC]) medicine.

## Proper Use of This Medicine

Spectinomycin is given by injection into a muscle. To help clear up your gonorrhea completely, usually only one dose is needed. However, in some infections a second dose of this medicine may be required.

Gonorrhea and related infections are spread by having sex with an infected partner. Therefore, it may be desirable that the male sexual partner wear a condom (prophylactic) during intercourse to prevent infection. Also, it may be necessary for your partner to be treated at the same time you are being treated. This will help to avoid passing the infection back and forth.

**Dosing**—The dose of spectinomycin will be different for different patients. The following information includes only the average doses of spectinomycin.
- For *cervical, rectal, or urethral gonorrhea*:
  —Adults and children 45 kilograms of body weight (99 pounds) and over: 2 grams injected into a muscle as a single dose.
  —Children up to 45 kilograms of body weight (99 pounds): 40 milligrams per kilogram of body weight injected into a muscle as a single dose.
  —Infants: Use is not recommended.

## Precautions After Receiving This Medicine

If your symptoms do not improve within a few days, or if they become worse, check with your doctor.

This medicine may cause some people to become dizzy. *Make sure you know how you react to this medicine before you drive, use machines, or do anything else that could be dangerous if you are dizzy.* If this reaction is especially bothersome, check with your doctor.

## Side Effects of This Medicine

Along with its needed effects, a medicine may cause some unwanted effects. Although not all of these side effects may occur, if they do occur they may need medical attention.

Check with your doctor as soon as possible if any of the following side effects occur:
*Rare*
   Chills or fever; itching or redness of the skin

Other side effects may occur that usually do not need medical attention. These side effects may go away during treatment as your body adjusts to the medicine. However, check with your doctor if any of these effects continue or are bothersome:

*Less common*
  Dizziness; nausea and vomiting; pain at the place of injection; stomach cramps

Other side effects not listed above may also occur in some patients. If you notice any other effects, check with your doctor.

---

Revised: 02/23/93

---

# SPERMICIDES     Vaginal

Some commonly used brand names are:

**In the U.S.—**

| | |
|---|---|
| Because[2] | Koromex Crystal Clear Gel[2] |
| Conceptrol Contraceptive | Koromex Foam[2] |
|    Inserts[2] | Koromex Jelly[2] |
| Conceptrol Gel[2] | Ortho-Creme[2] |
| Delfen[2] | Ortho-Gynol[3] |
| Emko[2] | Pre-Fil[2] |
| Encare[2] | Ramses Crystal Clear Gel[2] |
| Gynol II Extra Strength | Semicid[2] |
|    Contraceptive Jelly[2] | Shur-Seal[2] |
| Gynol II Original Formula | Today[2] |
|    Contraceptive Jelly[2] | VCF[2] |
| Koromex Cream[3] | |

**In Canada—**

| | |
|---|---|
| Delfen[2] | Ramses Contraceptive Foam[2] |
| Emko[2] | Ramses Contraceptive Vaginal |
| Ortho-Gynol[3] |    Jelly[2] |
| Pharmatex[1] | Today[2] |

Note: For quick reference, the following spermicides are numbered to match the corresponding brand names.

This information applies to the following medicines:
  1. Benzalkonium (benz-al-KOE-nee-um) Chloride*
  2. Nonoxynol (no-NOX-i-nole) 9
  3. Octoxynol (awk-TOX-i-nole) 9

---

*Not commercially available in the U.S.

---

## Description

Vaginal spermicides are a type of contraceptive (birth control). These products are inserted into the vagina *before* any genital contact occurs or sexual intercourse begins. They work by damaging and killing sperm in the vagina. Therefore, sperm are not able to travel from the vagina into the uterus and fallopian tubes, where fertilization usually takes place.

Vaginal spermicides when used alone are much less effective in preventing pregnancy than birth control pills or the IUD or spermicides used with another form of birth control such as the condom, cervical cap, diaphragm, or sponge. *Studies have shown that when spermicides are used alone, pregnancy usually occurs in 21 of each 100 women during the first year of spermicide use.* The number of pregnancies is reduced when spermicides are used with another method, especially the condom. Discuss with a doctor what your options are for birth control and the risks and benefits of each method.

*Laboratory studies* have shown that nonoxynol 9 kills or stops the growth of the AIDS virus (HIV) and herpes simplex I and II viruses. It was also shown to be effective against other types of organisms that cause gonorrhea, chlamydia, syphilis, trichomoniasis, and other sexually transmitted diseases (venereal disease, VD, STDs). Benzalkonium chloride also killed the AIDS virus in laboratory studies. Although this has *not* been proven in *human* studies, some scientists *believe* that if spermicides are put into the vagina or on the inside and outside of a latex (rubber) condom, they *may* kill these germs before they are able to come in contact with the vagina or rectum (lower bowel).

The most effective way to protect yourself against STDs (such as AIDS) is by abstinence (not having sexual intercourse) or by having one partner you can be sure is not already infected or is not going to get an STD. However, if either of these methods is not likely or possible, using latex (rubber) condoms with a spermicide is the best way of protecting yourself.

The use of a spermicide is recommended even when you are using nonbarrier methods of birth control such as birth control pills (the Pill) or intrauterine devices (IUDs), since these do not offer any protection from STDs.

The safety of using spermicides in the rectum (lower bowel), anus, or rectal area is not known. However, no side effects or problems have been reported that are different from those reported for use in the vagina.

Vaginal spermicides are available without a prescription, in the following dosage forms:

*Vaginal*
  Benzalkonium chloride
    • Suppositories (Canada)
  Nonoxynol 9
    • Cream (U.S. and Canada)
    • Film (U.S.)
    • Foam (U.S. and Canada)
    • Gel (U.S.)
    • Jelly (U.S. and Canada)
    • Sponge (U.S. and Canada)
    • Suppositories (U.S.)
  Octoxynol 9
    • Cream (U.S.)
    • Jelly (U.S. and Canada)

---

## Before Using This Medicine

In deciding to use vaginal spermicides, the risks of using them must be weighed against the good they will do. This is a decision you and possibly your doctor will make. The following information may help you in making your decision:

**Allergies**—If you have ever had any unusual or allergic reaction to benzalkonium chloride, nonoxynol 9, or octoxynol 9, it is best to check with your doctor before using vaginal spermicides.

**Pregnancy**—Many studies have shown that the use of vaginal spermicides does not increase the risk of birth defects or miscarriage.

**Breast-feeding**—It is not known if vaginal spermicides pass into breast milk in humans. However, their use has not been reported to cause problems in nursing babies.

**Adolescents**—These products have been used by teenagers and have not been shown to cause different side effects or problems than they do in adults. However, some younger users may need extra counseling and information on the importance of using spermicides exactly as they are supposed to be used so they will work properly.

**Other medicines**—Although certain medicines should not be used together at all, in other cases 2 different medicines may be used together even if an interaction might occur. In these cases, your doctor may want you to use the spermicide differently or other precautions may be necessary. When using vaginal spermicides, it is especially important that your health care professional know if you are using any of the following:

- Salicylates used on the skin (e.g., some types of ointments for muscle aches) or
- Sulfonamides (sulfa medicine) for use in the vagina or
- Chemicals or substances such as aluminum, citrate, cotton, hydrogen peroxide, lanolin, iodides, nitrates, permanganates, some forms of silver, soaps, detergents, or tartrates—Benzalkonium chloride may not work if it comes in direct contact with these as well as many other chemicals
- Vaginal medicines, douches, or rinsing—For spermicides to work properly to prevent pregnancy, they must stay in contact with the sperm in the vagina for at least 6 or 8 hours (depending upon which brand of spermicide you use) after sexual intercourse. *Vaginal douching is not necessary after use of these medicines.* Douching too soon (even with just water) may stop the spermicide from working. Washing or rinsing the vaginal or rectal area may also make the spermicide ineffective in helping to prevent sexually transmitted diseases

**Medical problems**—The presence of certain medical problems may affect the use of vaginal spermicides. Since in some cases spermicides should not be used, check with your doctor if you have any of the following:

- Allergies, irritations, or infections of the genitals—Using vaginal spermicides may cause moderate to severe irritation in these conditions. Also, benzalkonium suppositories may be less effective in women with vaginal infections

- Conditions or medical problems where it is important that pregnancy does not occur—Vaginal spermicides when used alone are much less effective than birth control pills or the IUD or spermicides used with another form of birth control such as the condom, cervical cap, diaphragm, or sponge. Discuss with your doctor what your options are for birth control and the risks and benefits of each method.
- During the menstrual period or
- Recent childbirth or abortion or
- Toxic-shock syndrome (history of)—The cervical cap, contraceptive sponge, or diaphragm should not be used in these cases because there is an increased risk of toxic-shock syndrome; your doctor may recommend that you use condoms with a spermicide instead during your menstrual period
- Sores on the genitals (sex organs) or
- Irritation of the vagina—It is not known whether spermicides can cause breaks in the skin that could increase the chances of getting a sexually transmitted disease, especially AIDS. Discuss this with a doctor if you have any questions

*If you develop any medical problem or begin using any new medicine* (prescription or nonprescription) while you are using this medicine, you may want to check with your doctor.

## Proper Use of This Medicine

It is very important that the spermicide be placed properly in the vagina. It should be put deep into the vagina, directly on the cervix (opening to the uterus). The written instructions about how the product container and the applicator work, how much spermicide to use each time, and how long each application remains effective may be different for each product. Make sure you carefully read and follow the instructions that come with each product.

*Make sure the spermicide you choose is labeled as being safe for use with latex diaphragms, cervical caps, or condoms.* Otherwise, it may cause the diaphragm, cervical cap, or condom to weaken and leak or even break during intercourse. If there is a leak or break during intercourse, it may be a good idea for a female partner to immediately place more spermicide in the vagina.

Spermicides, especially gels and jellies, provide some lubrication during sexual intercourse. *If you need an extra lubricant, make sure it is a water-based product safe for use with condoms, cervical caps, or diaphragms.* Oil-based products such as hand, face, or body cream; petroleum jelly; cooking oils or shortenings; or baby oil should *not* be used because they weaken the latex rubber. (Even some products that easily rinse away with water are oil-based and should not be used.) Use of oil-based products increases the chances of the condom breaking during sexual intercourse. These products can also cause the rubber in cervical caps or diaphragms to break down faster and wear out sooner.

*For patients using spermicides with a cervical cap:*
- *To be most effective at preventing pregnancy, the cervical cap must always be used with a spermicide.* Both must be used every time you have sexual intercourse.

- Before inserting the cervical cap, inspect it for holes, tears, or cracks. If there are holes or defects, the cervical cap will not work effectively, even with a spermicide. It must be replaced.
- Before you put the cap over the cervix (opening to the uterus), a spermicide cream, foam, gel, or jelly should be put into the cup of the cap. Follow the manufacturer's directions on how long before sexual intercourse you may apply the spermicide. Fill the cap one-third full with spermicide.
- To insert the cervical cap, squeeze the rim between your thumb and forefinger so that it is narrow enough to fit into the vagina. While in a comfortable position, push the cervical cap as deeply into the vagina as it will go. Release the rim and press it into place around the cervix with your finger. The rim should be round again and be directly on the cervix. The cap is held onto the cervix by suction.
- Some doctors may recommend that you put more spermicide into the vagina each time you repeat sexual intercourse using a cervical cap. You should also check to make sure the cap is in the proper position on the cervix before and after each time you have intercourse. You may wear the cervical cap for up to 48 hours (2 days).
- *Do not remove the cap if it has been less than 8 hours since the last time you had sexual intercourse.* For the cervical cap to be most effective at preventing pregnancy, it must remain in the vagina for at least 8 hours after sexual intercourse.
- To remove the cervical cap, use 1 or 2 fingers to push the rim away from the cervix. This will break the suction seal with the cervix. Then gently pull the cap out of the vagina.

*For patients using spermicides with condoms:*
- Condoms do not have to be used with spermicides, but the spermicide may provide a back-up in case the condom breaks or leaks.
- Spread some spermicide on the outside of the condom, after it is unrolled over the penis. It is even more important that a female partner also use a spermicide inside the vagina.
- Each time you repeat intercourse, a new condom must be used. *Condoms should never be reused.* Spermicide should also be applied outside of the new condom. A female partner must also put more spermicide in the vagina for each time she has intercourse.

*For patients using spermicides with a diaphragm:*
- *To be most effective at preventing pregnancy, diaphragms must always be used with a spermicide.* Some women may choose to insert a diaphragm every night, to avoid the chance of unprotected sexual intercourse and unplanned pregnancy happening.
- Inspect the diaphragm for holes by holding it up to a light. If there are holes or defects, the diaphragm will not work effectively, even with a spermicide. It must be replaced.

- Before you put the diaphragm over the cervix (opening to the uterus), a spermicide cream, foam, gel, or jelly should be put into the cup of the diaphragm. Follow the manufacturer's directions on how much spermicide to use and how long before sexual intercourse you may apply the spermicide. Also, spread some spermicide all around the rim of the diaphragm that will be touching the cervix. Some doctors also advise spreading more spermicide on the outside of the cup of the diaphragm.
- To insert the diaphragm, squeeze the rim between your thumb and forefinger so that it is narrow enough to fit into the vagina. While in a comfortable position, push the diaphragm as deeply into the vagina as it will go. (Some women use a special applicator that makes it easier to insert the diaphragm.) Release the rim. The diaphragm rim should be round again and be directly on the cervix.
- Each time you repeat sexual intercourse, you should put more spermicide into the vagina. *Do not remove the diaphragm if it has been less than 6 or 8 hours (depending upon which brand of spermicide you use) since the last sexual intercourse.* For the diaphragm to be most effective at preventing pregnancy, it must remain in the vagina for at least 6 or 8 hours (depending upon which brand of spermicide you use) after sexual intercourse. Be careful not to move the diaphragm out of place while you are applying more spermicide.
- Do not wear the diaphragm for more than 24 hours, since doing so increases the risk of getting toxic-shock syndrome or a urinary tract (bladder) infection.
- To remove the diaphragm, hook one finger over the rim nearest the front. Pull the diaphragm downward and out of the vagina.

*For patients using the contraceptive sponge:*
- Before the sponge is inserted, activate the spermicide by wetting the sponge with clean water and squeezing it. When you insert the sponge, it should be very wet and foamy when it is squeezed.
- Fold the sponge in half so that the dimple side is facing up and the removal loop is facing down. Carefully insert the sponge into the vagina. Push it deeply into the vagina so that the dimple side fits directly onto the cervix (the opening to the uterus) and the removal loop is on the side of the sponge that faces out of the vagina.
- It is not necessary to use more spermicide during the 24 hours the sponge is in the correct position in the vagina, regardless of how many times you have sexual intercourse. You may also bathe or swim while the sponge is in the vagina.
- *For the sponge to be most effective at preventing pregnancy, it must remain in the vagina for at least 6 hours after the last intercourse. Do not wear the sponge for longer than 30 hours, since doing so increases the risk of getting toxic-shock syndrome.*

- Sometimes the sponge can move from its proper place during urination or a bowel movement. If the sponge moves away from its proper place on the cervix but does not come out of the vagina, use one finger to move it back into place. If the sponge comes completely out of the vagina, discard it. Then immediately wet a new sponge and insert it. Using a new sponge is necessary only if it has been less than 6 hours since the last sexual intercourse.
- To remove the contraceptive sponge, hook one finger through the removal loop and gently pull the sponge out of the vagina. *Contact a doctor immediately if you have problems removing the sponge.* Examples are tearing of the sponge or loop, breaking off pieces of the sponge in the vagina, or scratching or injuring the vagina. The chances of your getting toxic-shock syndrome may be increased if any of these things happen.

**Dosing**—*Follow your doctor's orders or the directions on the label.* The following information includes the usual way that spermicides are used.

*For benzalkonium chloride*
- For preventing pregnancy:
—For *vaginal suppositories* dosage form:
- Adults and teenagers:
—For use alone: One suppository inserted into the vagina at least ten minutes but not longer than four hours before each time you have sexual intercourse.
—For use with a diaphragm: After the diaphragm with spermicide has been placed into the vagina, insert one suppository at least ten minutes but not longer than four hours before each time you have sexual intercourse. Also, insert another suppository before sexual intercourse if six hours have passed since you inserted the diaphragm.

*For nonoxynol 9*
- For preventing pregnancy:
—For *vaginal cream* dosage form:
- Adults and teenagers:
—For use alone: One applicatorful of a 5% cream inserted into the vagina just before each time you have sexual intercourse.
—For use with a diaphragm: One applicatorful of a 2 or 5% cream inserted into the cup of the diaphragm. Spread more spermicide along the rim of the diaphragm. Insert the diaphragm into the vagina just before but not longer than six hours before sexual intercourse. Also, insert one applicatorful just before each time you have intercourse or if six hours have passed since you inserted the diaphragm.
—For *vaginal film* dosage form:
- Adults and teenagers—One film inserted into the vagina from five to fifteen minutes (but not longer than one and one-half hours) before each time you have sexual intercourse.
—For *vaginal foam* dosage form:
- Adults and teenagers:
—For use alone: One applicatorful inserted into the vagina just before but not longer than one hour before each time you have sexual intercourse.
—For use with a diaphragm: One applicatorful inserted into either the vagina or into the cup of the diaphragm, depending on the product. Spread more spermicide along the rim of the diaphragm. Insert the diaphragm into the vagina just before but not longer than one hour before sexual intercourse. Also, insert another applicatorful into the vagina just before but not longer than one hour before each time you have sexual intercourse.
—For *vaginal gel* dosage form:
- Adults and teenagers:
—For use alone: One applicatorful of a 4 or 5% gel inserted into the vagina just before each time you have sexual intercourse. The contraceptive effect of the 4% gel will last for one hour.
—For use with a diaphragm: One or two teaspoonfuls (depending on the product) or one packet of gel is placed into the cup of the diaphragm. Spread more spermicide along the rim of the diaphragm. Insert the diaphragm into the vagina just before or up to six hours before sexual intercourse. Also, insert another applicatorful or packet into the vagina before each time you have sexual intercourse or if six hours have passed since you inserted the diaphragm.
—For *vaginal jelly* dosage form:
- Adults and teenagers:
—For use alone: One applicatorful of 3 or 5% jelly inserted into the vagina just before each time you have sexual intercourse. The contraceptive effect of the 3% jelly will last one hour.
—For use with a diaphragm: One applicatorful or two teaspoonfuls of jelly (depending on the product) placed into the cup of the diaphragm. Spread more spermicide along the rim of the diaphragm. Insert the diaphragm into the vagina just before but not longer than six hours before sexual intercourse. Also, insert another applicatorful before each time you have sexual intercourse or if six hours have passed since you inserted the diaphragm.
—For *vaginal sponge* dosage form:
- Adults and teenagers:
—For use alone: One sponge inserted into the vagina no more than twenty-four hours before sexual intercourse.

—For *vaginal suppositories* dosage form:
- Adults and teenagers:
  —For use alone: One suppository inserted into the vagina from ten to fifteen minutes (depending on the product) but not longer than one hour before each time you have sexual intercourse.
- Adults and teenagers:
  —For use with a diaphragm: After the diaphragm with spermicide has been placed into the vagina, insert one suppository into the vagina from ten to fifteen minutes (depending on the product) but not longer than one hour before sexual intercourse. Also, insert another suppository before each time you have sexual intercourse or if six hours have passed since you have inserted the diaphragm.

*For octoxynol 9*
- For preventing pregnancy:
  —For *vaginal cream* dosage form:
  - Adults and teenagers:
    —For use with a diaphragm: Two teaspoonfuls placed into the cup of the diaphragm. Spread more spermicide along the rim of the diaphragm. Insert the diaphragm into the vagina just before but not longer than six hours before sexual intercourse. Also, insert one applicatorful of the vaginal cream just before each time you have sexual intercourse or if six hours have passed since you inserted the diaphragm.
  —For *vaginal jelly* dosage form:
  - Adults and teenagers:
    —For use with a diaphragm: One applicatorful placed into the cup of the diaphragm. Spread more spermicide along the rim of the diaphragm. Insert the diaphragm into the vagina just before but not longer than six hours before sexual intercourse. Also, insert another applicatorful just before each time you have sexual intercourse or if six hours have passed since you inserted the diaphragm.

**Storage**—To store this medicine:
- Keep out of the reach of children.
- Store away from heat and direct light.
- Do not store in the bathroom, near the kitchen sink, or in other damp places. Heat or moisture may cause the medicine to break down.
- Do not refrigerate.
- Do not keep outdated products or products no longer needed. Be sure that any discarded products are out of the reach of children.

## Precautions While Using This Medicine

During use of spermicides, either partner may notice burning, stinging, warmth, itching, or other irritation of the skin, sex organs, anus, or rectum. Using a weaker strength of vaginal spermicide or one with different ingredients may be necessary. If you are using benzalkonium chloride suppositories, it may help to wet them before they are inserted into the vagina. If any of these effects continue after you have changed products, you may have an allergy to these products or an infection and should contact a doctor as soon as possible.

## Side Effects of This Medicine

Along with its needed effects, a medicine may cause some unwanted effects. Although not all of these side effects may occur, if they do occur they may need medical attention.

Check with a doctor *immediately* if any of the following side effects occur:
> *Rare*
> *For the cervical cap, contraceptive sponge, or diaphragm only*
> Signs of **toxic-shock syndrome** such as:
>> Chills; confusion; dizziness; fever; lightheadedness; muscle aches; sunburn-like rash that is followed by peeling of the skin; unusual redness of the inside of the nose, mouth, throat, vagina, or insides of the eyelids

Also, check with a doctor as soon as possible if any of the following side effects occur:
> *Rare*
> *For females and males*
> Skin rash, redness, irritation, or itching that does not subside or go away within a short period of time
> *For females only*
> Signs of *urinary tract infection or vaginal allergy or infection such as:*
>> Cloudy or bloody urine; increased frequency of urination; pain in the bladder or lower abdomen; pain on urination; thick, white, or curd-like vaginal discharge—with use of the cervical cap, contraceptive sponge, or diaphragm only; vaginal irritation, redness, rash, dryness, or whitish discharge

Other side effects may occur that usually do not need medical attention. However, check with a doctor if any of the following side effects continue or are bothersome:
> *Less common*
> Vaginal discharge (temporary)—for creams, foams, and suppositories; vaginal dryness or odor

Also, either partner may notice burning, stinging, warmth, itching, or other irritation of the skin, sex organs, anus, or rectum. Using a weaker strength of vaginal spermicide or one with different ingredients may be necessary. If you are using benzalkonium chloride suppositories, it may help to wet them before they are inserted into the vagina. If any of these effects continue after you have changed products, it is possible that you may have an infection and you should contact a doctor as soon as possible.

Other side effects not listed above may also occur in some people. If you notice any other effects, check with your doctor.

Revised: 07/28/93
Interim revision: 06/30/94

# STREPTOZOCIN  Systemic

A commonly used brand name in the U.S. and Canada is Zanosar.

## Description

Streptozocin (strep-toe-ZOE-sin) belongs to the group of medicines known as alkylating agents. It is used to treat cancer of the pancreas.

Streptozocin seems to interfere with the growth of cancer cells, which are eventually destroyed. It also directly affects the way the pancreas works. Since the growth of normal body cells may also be affected by streptozocin, other effects will also occur. Some of these may be serious and must be reported to your doctor. Other effects may not be serious but may cause concern. Some effects may not occur for months or years after the medicine is used.

Before you begin treatment with streptozocin, you and your doctor should talk about the good this medicine will do as well as the risks of using it.

Streptozocin is to be given only by or under the immediate supervision of your doctor. It is available in the following dosage form:

*Parenteral*
- Injection (U.S. and Canada)

## Before Using This Medicine

In deciding to use a medicine, the risks of taking the medicine must be weighed against the good it will do. This is a decision you and your doctor will make. For streptozocin, the following should be considered:

**Allergies**—Tell your doctor if you have ever had any unusual or allergic reaction to streptozocin.

**Pregnancy**—Tell your doctor if you are pregnant or if you intend to have children. There is a chance that this medicine may cause birth defects if either the male or the female is receiving it at the time of conception or if it is taken during pregnancy. Studies in rats and rabbits have shown that streptozocin causes birth defects or miscarriage. In addition, many cancer medicines may cause sterility which could be permanent. Although this has not been reported with this medicine, the possibility should be kept in mind.

Be sure that you have discussed this with your doctor before receiving this medicine. It is best to use some kind of birth control while you are receiving streptozocin. Tell your doctor right away if you think you have become pregnant while receiving streptozocin.

**Breast-feeding**—Tell your doctor if you are breast-feeding or if you intend to breast-feed during treatment with this medicine. Because streptozocin may cause serious side effects, breast-feeding is generally not recommended while you are receiving it.

**Children**—There is no specific information comparing use of streptozocin in children with use in other age groups.

**Older adults**—Many medicines have not been studied specifically in older people. Therefore, it may not be known whether they work exactly the same way they do in younger adults or if they cause different side effects or problems in older people. There is no specific information comparing use of streptozocin in the elderly with use in other age groups.

**Other medicines**—Although certain medicines should not be used together at all, in other cases two different medicines may be used together even if an interaction might occur. In these cases, your doctor may want to change the dose, or other precautions may be necessary. When you are receiving streptozocin, it is especially important that your health care professional know if you are taking any of the following:

- Anti-infectives by mouth or by injection (medicine for infection) or
- Carmustine (e.g., BiCNU) or
- Cisplatin (e.g., Platinol) or
- Combination pain medicine containing acetaminophen and aspirin (e.g., Excedrin) or other salicylates (with large amounts taken regularly) or
- Cyclosporine (e.g., Sandimmune) or
- Deferoxamine (e.g., Desferal) (with long-term use) or
- Gold salts (medicine for arthritis) or
- Inflammation or pain medicine except narcotics or
- Lithium (e.g., Lithane) or
- Methotrexate (e.g., Mexate) or
- Penicillamine (e.g., Cuprimine) or
- Plicamycin (e.g., Mithracin) or
- Tiopronin (e.g., Thiola)—Increased risk of harmful effects on the kidney
- Phenytoin (e.g., Dilantin)—May interfere with the effects of streptozocin

**Other medical problems**—The presence of other medical problems may affect the use of streptozocin. Make sure

you tell your doctor if you have any other medical problems, especially:

- Chickenpox (including recent exposure) or
- Herpes zoster (shingles)—Risk of severe disease affecting other parts of the body
- Diabetes mellitus (sugar diabetes)—May be worsened
- Infection—Streptozocin can decrease your body's ability to fight infection
- Kidney disease or
- Liver disease—Effects of streptozocin may be increased because of slower removal from the body

## Proper Use of This Medicine

While you are receiving streptozocin, your doctor may want you to drink extra fluids so that you will pass more urine. This will help prevent kidney problems and keep your kidneys working well.

This medicine usually causes nausea and vomiting, which may be severe. However, it is very important that you continue to receive the medicine, even if you begin to feel ill. Ask your health care professional for ways to lessen these effects.

**Dosing**—The dose of streptozocin will be different for different patients. The dose that is used may depend on a number of things, including what the medicine is being used for, the patient's size, and whether or not other medicines are also being taken. *If you are receiving streptozocin at home, follow your doctor's orders or the directions on the label.* If you have any questions about the proper dose of streptozocin, ask your doctor.

## Precautions While Using This Medicine

*It is very important that your doctor check your progress at regular visits* to make sure that this medicine is working properly and to check for any unwanted effects.

While you are being treated with streptozocin, and after you stop treatment with it, *do not have any immunizations (vaccinations) without your doctor's approval.* Streptozocin may lower your body's resistance and there is a chance you might get the infection the immunization is meant to prevent. In addition, other people living in your household should not take oral polio vaccine since there is a chance they could pass the polio virus on to you. Also, avoid persons who have recently taken oral polio vaccine. Do not get close to them and do not stay in the same room with them for very long. If you cannot take these precautions, you should consider wearing a protective face mask that covers the nose and mouth.

If streptozocin accidentally seeps out of the vein into which it is injected, it may damage some tissues and cause scarring. *Tell the health care professional right away if you notice redness, pain, or swelling at the place of injection.*

## Side Effects of This Medicine

Along with their needed effects, medicines like streptozocin can sometimes cause unwanted effects such as kidney problems and other side effects. These and others are described below. Also, because of the way these medicines act on the body, there is a chance that they might cause other unwanted effects that may not occur until months or years after the medicine is used. These delayed effects may include certain types of cancer, such as leukemia. Streptozocin has been shown to cause tumors (some cancerous) in animals. Discuss these possible effects with your doctor.

Although not all of these side effects may occur, if they do occur they may need medical attention.

*Check with your health care professional immediately* if any of the following side effects occur shortly after the medicine is given:

*Less common*

Anxiety, nervousness, or shakiness; chills, cold sweats, or cool, pale skin; drowsiness or unusual tiredness or weakness; fast pulse; headache; pain or redness at place of injection; unusual hunger

*Check with your doctor immediately* if the following side effects occur any time while you are being treated with this medicine:

*Rare*

Black, tarry stools; blood in urine or stools; cough or hoarseness; fever or chills; lower back or side pain; painful or difficult urination; pinpoint red spots on skin; unusual bleeding or bruising

Check with your health care professional as soon as possible if any of the following side effects occur:

*More common*

Swelling of feet or lower legs; unusual decrease in urination

Other side effects may occur that usually do not need medical attention. These side effects may go away during treatment as your body adjusts to the medicine. Also, your health care professional may be able to tell you about ways to prevent or reduce some of these side effects. Check with your health care professional if any of the following side effects continue or are bothersome or if you have any questions about them:

*More common*

Nausea and vomiting (usually occurs within 2 to 4 hours after receiving dose and may be severe)

*Less common*

Diarrhea

After you stop receiving streptozocin, your body may need time to adjust. The length of time this takes depends on the amount of medicine you were using and how long you used it. During this period of time, check with your doctor if you notice either of the following side effects:

*More common*

Decrease in urination; swelling of feet or lower legs

Other side effects not listed above may also occur in some patients. If you notice any other effects, check with your doctor.

Revised: 08/26/92
Interim revision: 06/30/94

---

# STRONTIUM 89 CHLORIDE   Therapeutic

A commonly used brand name in the U.S. and Canada is Metastron.

## Description

Strontium 89 chloride (STRON-shee-um KLOR-ide) is a radiopharmaceutical (ray-dee-oh-far-ma-SOO-ti-kal). Radiopharmaceuticals are radioactive agents that may be used to diagnose some diseases by studying the function of the body's organs or to treat certain diseases.

Strontium 89 chloride is used to help relieve the bone pain that may occur with certain kinds of cancer. The radioactive strontium is taken up in the bone cancer area and gives off radiation that helps provide relief of pain.

Strontium 89 chloride is to be given only by or under the direct supervision of a doctor with specialized training in nuclear medicine or radiation oncology. It is available in the following dosage form:

*Parenteral*

• Injection (U.S. and Canada)

## Before Using This Medicine

In deciding to use a medicine, the risks of receiving the medicine must be weighed against the good it will do. This is a decision you and your doctor will make. For strontium 89 chloride, the following should be considered:

**Allergies**—Tell your doctor if you have ever had any unusual or allergic reaction to bone tumor–seeking medicines, like strontium 89 chloride. Also tell your doctor if you are allergic to any other substances, such as foods, preservatives, or dyes.

**Pregnancy**—Studies have not been done in either humans or animals. However, to avoid exposing the fetus to radiation, strontium 89 chloride is not recommended for use during pregnancy. Be sure you have discussed this with your doctor.

**Breast-feeding**—Strontium 89 chloride may pass into the breast milk. If you must receive this radiopharmaceutical, it will be necessary for you to stop breast-feeding. Be sure you have discussed this with your doctor.

**Children**—Studies on this medicine have been done only in adult patients, and there is no specific information about its use in children.

**Older adults**—Strontium 89 chloride has been used in older people and has not been shown to cause different side effects or problems in older people than it does in younger adults.

**Other medicines**—Although certain medicines should not be used together at all, in other cases two different medicines may be used together even if an interaction might occur. In these cases, your doctor may want to change the dose, or other precautions may be necessary. When you are receiving strontium 89 chloride, it is especially important that your doctor know if you are taking any of the following:

• Calcium-containing medicines—These medicines may keep the strontium 89 chloride from being taken up by the bone
• If you have ever been treated with x-rays or cancer medicines—Cancer medicines or radiation therapy may increase the harmful effects of strontium 89 chloride on the bone marrow

**Other medical problems**—The presence of other medical problems may affect the use of strontium 89 chloride. Make sure you tell your doctor if you have any other medical problems.

## Proper Use of This Medicine

Your doctor may have special instructions for you to follow to get ready for your treatment. If you do not understand them or if you have not received such instructions, check with your doctor in advance.

If you have a problem controlling your bladder, tell your doctor before receiving strontium 89 chloride. Special precautions will need to be taken to prevent contamination of clothing, bed linen, and the environment.

**Dosing**—The doses of radiopharmaceuticals will be different for different patients and for the different types of treatments. The amount of radioactivity of a radiopharmaceutical is expressed in units called becquerels or curies. The usual adult dose of strontium 89 chloride is 148 megabecquerels (4 millicuries). The dose you receive depends on your size, age, and blood test measurements (blood counts). The amount of radiation received by specific areas of the body to treat a disease is many times higher than from any diagnostic test, such as x-rays and nuclear medicine scans. Repeated doses may be necessary, depending on the kind of disease you have and how your body is responding to treatment.

---

## Precautions After Using This Medicine

*It is very important that your doctor check your progress at regular visits* to make sure that this medicine is working properly and to check for unwanted effects. You may need to have blood tests done regularly.

*Follow these guidelines for 1 week* after receiving strontium 89 chloride, to help reduce the chance of contaminating other persons or the environment:

- *Use a normal toilet, if available, instead of a urinal.*
- *Strontium 89 chloride is passed in the urine and feces. To prevent contamination of your home environment, flush the toilet twice after using.*
- *Wipe any spilled urine with a tissue and flush it away.*
- *Wash your hands after using or cleaning the toilet.*
- Wash your clothes and bed linens immediately if they become soiled with your urine or blood. Wash them separately from other clothes.
- *If you cut yourself, wash away any spilled blood.*

Strontium 89 chloride can temporarily lower the number of white blood cells in your blood, increasing the chance of getting an infection. It can also lower the number of platelets, which are necessary for proper blood clotting. If *your blood count becomes abnormally low*, there are certain precautions you can take, to reduce the risk of infection or bleeding, such as:

- With abnormally low white blood cell counts—
  - —If you can, avoid people with infections. *Check with your doctor immediately* if you think you are getting an infection or if you get a fever or chills, cough or hoarseness, lower back or side pain, or painful or difficult urination.
  - —Be careful when using a regular toothbrush, dental floss, or toothpick. Your medical doctor, dentist, or nurse may recommend other ways to clean your teeth and gums. Check with your medical doctor before having any dental work done.

—Do not touch your eyes or the inside of your nose unless you have just washed your hands and have not touched anything else in the meantime.

- With abnormally low platelet blood counts—
  - —Be careful not to cut yourself when you are using sharp objects such as a safety razor or fingernail or toenail cutters.
  - —Avoid contact sports or other situations where bruising or injury could occur.

---

## Side Effects of This Medicine

Along with its needed effects, a medicine may cause some unwanted effects. When strontium 89 chloride is used at recommended doses, side effects usually are rare. However, blood problems, such as a decrease in the number of white blood cells or platelets, may occur in some patients.

*Check with your doctor immediately* if any of the following side effects occur:

*Rare*

Black, tarry stools; blood in urine or stools; cough or hoarseness; fever or chills; lower back or side pain; painful or difficult urination; pinpoint red spots on skin; unusual bleeding or bruising

Other side effects may occur that usually do not need medical attention. These side effects may go away after treatment as your body adjusts to the medicine. Check with your doctor if any of the following side effects continue or are bothersome or if you have any questions about them:

*More common*

Flushing; increase in bone pain

Other side effects not listed above may also occur in some patients. If you notice any other effects, check with your doctor.

---

Developed: 06/23/94

---

# SUCCIMER Systemic†

A commonly used brand name in the U.S. is Chemet.
Other commonly used names are dimercaptosuccinic acid and DMSA.

†Not commercially available in Canada.

---

## Description

Succimer (SUX-i-mer) is used to remove excess lead from the body. It is used to treat acute lead poisoning, especially in small children.

Succimer combines with lead in the bloodstream. The combination of lead and succimer is then removed from the body by the kidneys. By removing the excess lead, the medicine lessens damage to various organs and tissues of the body.

*Oral*

Capsules (U.S.)

## Before Using This Medicine

In deciding to use a medicine, the risks of taking the medicine must be weighed against the good it will do. This is a decision you and your doctor will make. For succimer, the following should be considered:

**Allergies**—Tell your doctor if you have ever had any unusual or allergic reaction to succimer. Also, tell your health care professional if you are allergic to any other substances, such as foods, preservatives, or dyes.

**Pregnancy**—Studies have not been done in humans. However, some studies in animals have shown that succimer causes birth defects.

**Breast-feeding**—It is not known whether succimer is excreted in breast milk.

**Children**—This medicine has been tested in children over the age of 1 year and, in effective doses, has not been shown to cause different side effects or problems than it does in adults.

**Older adults**—Many medicines have not been studied specifically in older people. Therefore, it may not be known whether they work exactly the same way they do in younger adults or if they cause different side effects or problems in older people. There is no specific information comparing use of succimer in the elderly with use in other age groups.

**Other medical problems**—The presence of other medical problems may affect the use of succimer. Make sure you tell your doctor if you have any other medical problems, especially:

• Dehydration or
• Kidney disease—Higher blood levels of succimer may result and your doctor may need to change your dose

## Proper Use of This Medicine

Children who have too much lead in their bodies should be removed from the lead-containing environment (for example, home, school, or other areas where the child has been exposed to lead) until the lead has been removed from the environment.

Your doctor may want to put your child in the hospital while he or she is receiving succimer. This will allow the doctor to check your child's condition while the lead can be removed from the child's environment.

When opening your bottle of succimer, you may notice an unpleasant odor. However, this is a normal odor for these capsules and does not affect the medicine's working properly.

If the capsules cannot be swallowed, the contents of the capsule may be sprinkled on food and eaten immediately. The contents may also be given on a spoon and followed by a fruit drink.

**Dosing**—The dose of succimer will be different for different patients. *Follow your doctor's orders or the directions on the label.*

• For the *oral* dosage form (capsules):
  —For treatment of lead poisoning:
  • For adults and children 12 years of age and older—Dose is based on body weight. The usual dose is 10 milligrams (mg) of succimer per kilogram (4.5 mg per pound) of body weight every eight hours for five days.
  • For children up to 12 years of age—Dose is based on body weight. The usual dose is 10 mg of succimer per kilogram (4.5 mg per pound) of body weight every eight hours for five days. The same dose is then given every twelve hours for the next fourteen days, for a total of nineteen days of therapy.

**Missed dose**—If you miss a dose of this medicine, take it as soon as possible. However, if it is almost time for your next dose, skip the missed dose and go back to your regular dosing schedule. Do not double doses.

**Storage**—To store this medicine:
• Keep out of the reach of children.
• Store away from heat and direct light.
• Do not store in the bathroom, near the kitchen sink, or in other damp places. Heat or moisture may cause the medicine to break down.
• Keep the medicine from freezing. Do not refrigerate.
• Do not keep outdated medicine or medicine no longer needed. Be sure that any discarded medicine is out of the reach of children.

## Precautions While Using This Medicine

*It is important that your doctor check your progress at regular visits* to make sure that this medicine is working properly and to prevent unwanted effects. Certain blood and urine tests must be done regularly to make sure you are taking the correct dose of succimer.

## Side Effects of This Medicine

Along with its needed effects, a medicine may cause some unwanted effects. Although not all of these side effects may occur, if they do occur they may need medical attention.

Check with your doctor as soon as possible if the following side effect occurs:

*Less common*
  Fever and chills

Other side effects may occur that usually do not need medical attention. These side effects may go away during treatment as your body adjusts to the medicine. However, check with your doctor if any of the following side effects continue or are bothersome:

*More common*
Diarrhea; loose stools; loss of appetite; nausea and vomiting; skin rash

Succimer may cause your urine, sweat, and feces to have an unpleasant odor.

Other side effects not listed above may also occur in some patients. If you notice any other effects, check with your doctor.

Revised: 06/22/93

# SUCRALFATE   Oral

Some commonly used brand names are:

**In the U.S.—**
Carafate

**In Canada—**
Sulcrate

## Description

Sucralfate (soo-KRAL-fate) is used to treat and prevent duodenal ulcers. This medicine may also be used for other conditions as determined by your doctor.

Sucralfate works by forming a "barrier" or "coating" over the ulcer. This protects the ulcer from the acid of the stomach, allowing it to heal. Sucralfate contains an aluminum salt.

This medicine is available only with your doctor's prescription, in the following dosage form:

*Oral*
- Oral suspension (U.S. and Canada)
- Tablets (U.S. and Canada)

## Before Using This Medicine

In deciding to use a medicine, the risks of taking the medicine must be weighed against the good it will do. This is a decision you and your doctor will make. For sucralfate, the following should be considered:

**Allergies**—Tell your doctor if you have ever had any unusual or allergic reaction to sucralfate. Also, tell your health care professional if you are allergic to any other substances, such as foods, preservatives, or dyes.

**Pregnancy**—Studies have not been done in humans. However, sucralfate has not been shown to cause birth defects or other problems in animal studies.

**Breast-feeding**—Sucralfate has not been shown to cause problems in nursing babies.

**Children**—This medicine has been tested in a limited number of children. In effective doses, the medicine has not been shown to cause different side effects or problems than it does in adults.

**Older adults**—Many medicines have not been studied specifically in older people. Therefore, it may not be known whether they work exactly the same way they do in younger adults. Although there is no specific information comparing the use of sucralfate in the elderly with use in other age groups, this medicine is not expected to cause different side effects or problems in older people than it does in younger adults.

**Other medicines**—Although certain medicines should not be used together at all, in other cases two different medicines may be used together even if an interaction might occur. In these cases, your doctor may want to change the dose, or other precautions may be necessary. When you are taking sucralfate, it is especially important that your health care professional know if you are taking the following:

- Ciprofloxacin or
- Digoxin or
- Norfloxacin or
- Ofloxacin or
- Phenytoin or
- Theophylline—Sucralfate may prevent these medicines from working properly

**Other medical problems**—The presence of other medical problems may affect the use of sucralfate. Make sure you tell your doctor if you have any other medical problems, especially:

- Gastrointestinal tract obstruction disease—Sucralfate may bind with other foods and drugs and cause obstruction of the gastrointestinal tract
- Kidney failure—Use may lead to a toxic increase of aluminum blood levels

## Proper Use of This Medicine

Sucralfate is best taken with water on an empty stomach 1 hour before meals and at bedtime, unless otherwise directed by your doctor.

Take this medicine for the full time of treatment, even if you begin to feel better. Also, it is important that you keep your doctor's appointments for check-ups so that your doctor will be better able to tell you when to stop taking this medicine.

**Dosing**—The dose of sucralfate will be different for different patients. *Follow your doctor's orders or the directions on the label.* The following information includes only the average doses of sucralfate. *If your dose is different, do not change it* unless your doctor tells you to do so.

The number of tablets or teaspoonfuls of suspension that you take depends on the strength of the medicine. Also, *the number of doses you take each day, the time allowed between doses, and the length of time you take the medicine depend on the medical problem for which you are taking sucralfate.*

- For *oral* dosage form (suspension):
  - —To treat duodenal ulcers:
    - Adults and teenagers—One gram four times a day, one hour before each meal and at bedtime. Some people may take two grams two times a day, when they wake up and at bedtime on an empty stomach.
    - Children—Dose must be determined by your doctor.
- For *oral* dosage form (tablets):
  - —To treat duodenal ulcers:
    - Adults and teenagers—One gram four times a day, one hour before each meal and at bedtime.
    - Children—Dose must be determined by your doctor.
  - —To prevent duodenal ulcers:
    - Adults and teenagers—One gram two times a day on an empty stomach.
    - Children—Dose must be determined by your doctor.

**Missed dose**—If you miss a dose of this medicine, take it as soon as possible. However, if it is almost time for your next dose, skip the missed dose and go back to your regular dosing schedule. Do not double doses.

**Storage**—To store this medicine:
- Keep out of the reach of children.
- Store away from heat and direct light.
- Do not store in the bathroom, near the kitchen sink, or in other damp places. Heat or moisture may cause the medicine to break down.
- Keep the liquid form of this medicine from freezing. Do not refrigerate.
- Do not keep outdated medicine or medicine no longer needed. Be sure that any discarded medicine is out of the reach of children.

## Precautions While Using This Medicine

Antacids may be taken with sucralfate to help relieve any stomach pain, unless your doctor has told you not to use them. *However, antacids should not be taken within 30 minutes before or after sucralfate.* Taking these medicines too close together may keep sucralfate from working properly.

## Side Effects of This Medicine

Along with its needed effects, a medicine may cause some unwanted effects. Some side effects may occur that usually do not need medical attention. These side effects may go away during treatment as your body adjusts to the medicine. *Check with your doctor immediately* if any of the following side effects occur:

*Signs of aluminum toxicity*
   Drowsiness; convulsions (seizures)

Check with your doctor as soon as possible if any of the following side effects continue or are bothersome:

*More common*
   Constipation
*Less common or rare*
   Backache; diarrhea; dizziness or lightheadedness; dryness of mouth; indigestion; nausea; skin rash, hives, or itching; stomach cramps or pain

Other side effects not listed above may also occur in some patients. If you notice any other effects, check with your doctor.

## Additional Information

Once a medicine has been approved for marketing for a certain use, experience may show that it is also useful for other medical problems. Although these uses are not included in product labeling, sucralfate is used in certain patients with the following medical conditions:

- Gastric ulcers
- Gastroesophageal reflux disease (a condition in which stomach acid washes back into the esophagus)
- Stomach or intestinal ulcers resulting from stress or trauma damage or from damage caused by medication used to treat rheumatoid arthritis

Other than the above information, there is no additional information relating to proper use, precautions, or side effects for these uses.

Revised: 03/24/92
Interim revision: 08/17/94

# SULCONAZOLE    Topical†

A commonly used brand name in the U.S. is Exelderm.

†Not commercially available in Canada.

## Description

Sulconazole (sul-KON-a-zole) is used to treat infections caused by a fungus. It works by killing the fungus or preventing its growth.

Sulconazole is applied to the skin to treat the following:
- ringworm of the body (tinea corporis);
- ringworm of the foot (tinea pedis; athlete's foot);
- ringworm of the groin (tinea cruris; jock itch);
- "sun fungus" (tinea versicolor; pityriasis versicolor).

Sulconazole may also be used for other conditions as determined by your doctor.

Topical sulconazole is available only with your doctor's prescription in the following dosage forms:

*Topical*
- Cream (U.S.)
- Solution (U.S.)

## Before Using This Medicine

In deciding to use a medicine, the risks of taking the medicine must be weighed against the good it will do. This is a decision you and your doctor will make. For sulconazole, the following should be considered:

**Allergies**—Tell your doctor if you have ever had any unusual or allergic reaction to sulconazole or other antifungals such as miconazole (e.g., Micatin) or econazole (e.g., Spectazole). Also tell your health care professional if you are allergic to any other substances such as foods, preservatives, or dyes.

**Pregnancy**—Topical sulconazole has not been studied in pregnant women. However, studies in animals have shown that sulconazole when taken by mouth causes unwanted effects such as death of the fetus or difficult labor. Before you use this medicine, make sure your doctor knows if you are pregnant or if you may become pregnant.

**Breast-feeding**—It is not known whether topical sulconazole passes into the breast milk. Although most medicines pass into breast milk in small amounts, many of them may be used safely while breast-feeding. Mothers who are using this medicine and who wish to breast-feed should discuss this with their doctor.

**Children**—Studies on this medicine have been done only in adult patients, and there is no specific information comparing use of sulconazole in children with use in other age groups.

**Older adults**—Many medicines have not been studied specifically in older people. Therefore, it may not be known whether they work exactly the same way they do in younger adults. Although there is no specific information comparing use of topical sulconazole in the elderly with use in other age groups, this medicine is not expected to cause different side effects or problems in older people than it does in younger adults.

**Other medicines**—Although certain medicines should not be used together at all, in other cases two different medicines may be used together even if an interaction might occur. In these cases, your doctor may want to change the dose, or other precautions may be necessary. Tell your health care professional if you are using any other topical prescription or nonprescription (over-the-counter [OTC]) medicine that is to be applied to the same area of the skin.

## Proper Use of This Medicine

Apply enough sulconazole to cover the affected and surrounding skin areas, and rub in gently.

*Keep this medicine away from the eyes.*

When sulconazole is used to treat certain types of fungus infections of the skin, occlusive dressing (airtight covering, such as kitchen plastic wrap) should *not* be applied over the medicine. To do so may irritate the skin. *Do not apply an airtight covering over this medicine unless you have been directed to do so by your doctor.*

To help clear up your infection completely, *it is very important that you keep using sulconazole for the full time of treatment,* even if your symptoms begin to clear up after a few days. Since fungus infections may be very slow to clear up, you may have to continue using this medicine every day for several weeks or more. If you stop using this medicine too soon, your symptoms may return.

Do not miss any doses.

**Dosing**—The dose of sulconazole will be different for different patients. *Follow your doctor's orders or the directions on the label.* The following information includes only the average doses of topical sulconazole. *If your dose is different, do not change it* unless your doctor tells you to do so.

*The number of doses you use each day, the time allowed between doses, and the length of time you use the medicine depend on the medical problem for which you are using topical sulconazole.*
- For *topical cream* dosage form:
  —For ringworm of the body or ringworm of the groin or "sun fungus":
    - Adults—Use one or two times a day for at least three weeks.
    - Children—Use and dose must be determined by your doctor.
  —For athlete's foot:
    - Adults—Use two times a day for at least four weeks.
    - Children—Use and dose must be determined by your doctor.
- For *topical solution* dosage form:
  —For ringworm of the body or ringworm of the groin or "sun fungus":
    - Adults—Use one or two times a day for at least three weeks.
    - Children—Use and dose must be determined by your doctor.

**Missed dose**—If you miss a dose of this medicine, apply it as soon as possible. However, if it is almost time for your next dose, skip the missed dose and go back to your regular dosing schedule.

**Storage**—To store this medicine:

- Keep out of the reach of children.
- Store away from heat and direct light.
- Keep the medicine from freezing. Do not refrigerate.
- Do not keep outdated medicine or medicine no longer needed. Be sure that any discarded medicine is out of the reach of children.

## Precautions While Using This Medicine

If your skin problem does not improve within 4 to 6 weeks or if it becomes worse, check with your doctor.

*To help clear up your infection completely and to help make sure it does not return, good health habits are also required.* The following measures will help reduce chaffing and irritation and will also help keep the area cool and dry:

- For patients using sulconazole for *ringworm of the groin (tinea cruris; jock itch):*
  —Avoid wearing underwear that is tight-fitting or made from synthetic materials (for example, rayon or nylon). Instead, wear loose-fitting, cotton underwear.
- For patients using sulconazole for *ringworm of the foot (tinea pedis; athlete's foot):*
  —Carefully dry the feet, especially between the toes, after bathing.
  —Avoid wearing socks made from wool or synthetic materials (for example, rayon or nylon). Instead wear clean, cotton socks and change them daily or more often if the feet sweat a lot.
  —Wear sandals or other well-ventilated shoes.
- For patients using sulconazole for *ringworm of the body (tinea corporis):*
  —Carefully dry yourself after bathing.

—Avoid too much heat and humidity if possible.
—Wear well-ventilated, loose-fitting clothing.

If you have any questions about these measures, check with your health care professional.

## Side Effects of This Medicine

Along with its needed effects, a medicine may cause some unwanted effects. Although not all of these side effects may occur, if they do occur they may need medical attention.

Check with your doctor as soon as possible if any of the following side effects occur:

*Less common*

Burning or stinging, itching, redness of the skin, or other signs of irritation not present before use of this medicine

Other side effects not listed above may also rarely occur. If you notice any other effects, check with your doctor.

## Additional Information

Once a medicine has been approved for marketing for a certain use, experience may show that it is also useful for other medical problems. Although this use is not included in product labeling, sulconazole is used in certain patients with the following medical condition:

- Cutaneous candidiasis

Other than the above information, there is no additional information relating to proper use, precautions, or side effects for this use.

Developed: 03/29/94

# SULFADOXINE AND PYRIMETHAMINE  Systemic

A commonly used brand name in the U.S. and Canada is Fansidar.

## Description

Sulfadoxine (sul-fa-DOX-een), a sulfa medicine, and pyrimethamine (peer-i-METH-a-meen) combination is used to treat malaria. This medicine may also be used to prevent malaria in people who are living in, or will be traveling to, an area where there is a chance of getting malaria. Sulfadoxine and pyrimethamine combination may also be taken with other medicines for malaria, or may be used for other problems as determined by your doctor.

Since sulfadoxine and pyrimethamine combination may cause some serious side effects, it is usually used only to prevent or treat serious malaria infections in areas where it is known that other medicines may not work.

This medicine is available only with your doctor's prescription, in the following dosage form:

*Oral*
- Tablets (U.S. and Canada)

## Before Using This Medicine

In deciding to use a medicine, the risks of taking the medicine must be weighed against the good it will do. This is a decision you and your doctor will make. For sulfadoxine and pyrimethamine combination, the following should be considered:

**Allergies**—Tell your doctor if you have ever had any unusual or allergic reaction to sulfa medicines, furosemide (e.g., Lasix) or thiazide diuretics (water pills), oral antidiabetics (diabetes medicine you take by mouth), glaucoma medicine you take by mouth (acetazolamide [e.g., Diamox], dichlorphenamide [e.g., Daranide], methazolamide [e.g., Neptazane]), or pyrimethamine (e.g., Daraprim). Also tell your health care professional if you are allergic to any other substances, such as foods, preservatives, or dyes.

**Pregnancy**—Studies have not been done in pregnant women. However, use is not recommended during pregnancy. Studies in rats have shown that sulfadoxine and pyrimethamine combination may cause birth defects and anemia. Also, women who travel to an area where there is a chance of getting malaria, and who may be taking sulfadoxine and pyrimethamine combination, should not become pregnant.

**Breast-feeding**—Sulfadoxine and pyrimethamine pass into the breast milk. This medicine is not recommended for use during breast-feeding. It may cause liver problems, anemia, and other unwanted effects in nursing babies.

**Children**—Sulfadoxine and pyrimethamine combination should not be used in infants up to 2 months of age.

**Older adults**—Many medicines have not been studied specifically in older people. Therefore, it may not be known whether they work exactly the same way they do in younger adults or if they cause different side effects or problems in older people. There is no specific information comparing use of sulfadoxine and pyrimethamine combination in the elderly with use in other age groups.

**Other medicines**—Although certain medicines should not be used together at all, in other cases two different medicines may be used together even if an interaction might occur. In these cases, your doctor may want to change the dose, or other precautions may be necessary. When you are taking sulfadoxine and pyrimethamine combination, it is especially important that your health care professional know if you are taking any of the following:

- Acetaminophen (e.g., Tylenol) (with long-term, high-dose use) or
- Amiodarone (e.g., Cordarone) or
- Anabolic steroids (dromostanolone [e.g., Drolban], ethylestrenol [e.g., Maxibolin], nandrolone [e.g., Anabolin], oxandrolone [e.g., Anavar], oxymetholone [e.g., Anadrol], stanozolol [e.g., Winstrol]) or
- Androgens (male hormones) or
- Carbamazepine (e.g., Tegretol) or
- Carmustine (e.g., BiCNU) or
- Chloroquine (e.g., Aralen) or
- Dantrolene (e.g., Dantrium) or
- Daunorubicin (e.g., Cerubidine) or
- Disulfiram (e.g., Antabuse) or
- Divalproex (e.g., Depakote) or
- Estrogens (female hormones) or
- Etretinate (e.g., Tegison) or
- Gold salts (medicine for arthritis) or
- Hydroxychloroquine (e.g., Plaquenil) or
- Naltrexone (e.g., Trexan) (with long-term, high-dose use) or
- Oral contraceptives (birth control pills) containing estrogen or

- Other anti-infectives by mouth or by injection (medicine for infection) or
- Phenothiazines (acetophenazine [e.g., Tindal], chlorpromazine [e.g., Thorazine], fluphenazine [e.g., Prolixin], mesoridazine [e.g., Serentil], perphenazine [e.g., Trilafon], prochlorperazine [e.g., Compazine], promazine [e.g., Sparine], promethazine [e.g., Phenergan], thioridazine [e.g., Mellaril], trifluoperazine [e.g., Stelazine], triflupromazine [e.g., Vesprin], trimeprazine [e.g., Temaril]) or
- Phenytoin (e.g., Dilantin) or
- Valproic acid (e.g., Depakene)—Use of sulfadoxine and pyrimethamine combination with these medicines may increase the chance of side effects affecting the liver
- Acetohydroxamic acid (e.g., Lithostat) or
- Amphotericin B by injection (e.g., Fungizone) or
- Antidiabetics, oral (diabetes medicine you take by mouth) or
- Antineoplastics (cancer medicine) or
- Azathioprine (e.g., Imuran) or
- Chloramphenicol (e.g., Chloromycetin) or
- Colchicine or
- Cyclophosphamide (e.g., Cytoxan) or
- Dapsone or
- Flucytosine (e.g., Ancobon) or
- Furazolidone (e.g., Furoxone) or
- Ganciclovir (e.g., Cytovene) or
- Interferon (e.g., Intron A, Roferon-A) or
- Nitrofurantoin (e.g., Furadantin) or
- Primaquine or
- Procainamide (e.g., Pronestyl) or
- Quinidine (e.g., Quinidex) or
- Quinine (e.g., Quinamm) or
- Sulfoxone (e.g., Diasone) or
- Vitamin K (e.g., AquaMEPHYTON, Synkayvite) or
- Zidovudine (e.g., AZT, Retrovir)—Use of sulfadoxine and pyrimethamine combination with these medicines may increase the chance of side effects affecting the blood
- Antithyroid agents (medicine for overactive thyroid) or
- Mercaptopurine (e.g., Purinethol) or
- Methotrexate (e.g., Mexate) or
- Methyldopa (e.g., Aldomet) or
- Plicamycin (e.g., Mithracin)—Use of sulfadoxine and pyrimethamine combination with these medicines may increase the chance of side effects affecting the liver and the blood

**Other medical problems**—The presence of other medical problems may affect the use of sulfadoxine and pyrimethamine combination. Make sure you tell your doctor if you have any other medical problems, especially:

- Anemia or other blood problems—Patients with these problems may have an increase in side effects involving the blood
- Kidney disease or
- Liver disease—Patients with kidney and/or liver disease may have an increased chance of side effects
- Porphyria—This medicine may cause an attack of porphyria
- Seizure disorders, such as epilepsy—High doses of this medicine may increase the chance of convulsions (seizures)

## Proper Use of This Medicine

*Do not give this medicine to infants under 2 months of age* unless otherwise directed by your doctor. Also, *keep this medicine out of the reach of children.* Overdose is especially dangerous in children.

*Sulfa-containing medicines are best taken with a full glass (8 ounces) of water. Several additional glasses of water should be taken every day,* unless otherwise directed by your doctor. Drinking extra water will help to prevent some unwanted effects (e.g., kidney stones) of this medicine. If this medicine upsets your stomach or causes vomiting, it may be taken with meals or a snack.

For patients taking this medicine *to prevent malaria:*

- Your doctor may want you to start taking this medicine 1 to 2 weeks before you travel to an area where there is a chance of getting malaria. This will help you to see how you react to the medicine. Also, it will allow time for your doctor to change your medicine if you have a reaction to this medicine.
- Also, you should keep taking this medicine while you are in the area and for 4 weeks after you leave the area. No medicine will protect you completely from malaria. However, to protect you as completely as possible, *it is important that you keep taking this medicine for the full time your doctor ordered.* Also, if fever develops during your travels or within 2 months after you leave the area, *check with your doctor immediately.*
- This medicine works best when you take it on a regular schedule. For example, if you are to take it once a week, it is best to take it on the same day each week. *Do not miss any doses.* If you have any questions about this, check with your health care professional.

For patients taking this medicine *to treat malaria:*

- To help clear up your infection completely, *take this medicine exactly as directed by your doctor.*

For patients taking this medicine *to self-treat presumptive malaria:*

- After you take this medicine to self-treat presumptive malaria, you should continue to take your other medicine for malaria once a week.

**Dosing**—The dose of sulfadoxine and pyrimethamine combination will be different for different patients. *Follow your doctor's orders or the directions on the label.* The following information includes only the average doses of sulfadoxine and pyrimethamine combination. *If your dose is different, do not change it* unless your doctor tells you to do so.

- For *treatment* of malaria:
  —Adults and teenagers: 3 tablets as a single dose on the third day of quinine therapy.
  —Children: Dose is based on body weight and must be determined by your doctor.
- For *self-treatment of presumed malaria*:
  —Adults and teenagers: 3 tablets as a single dose when you get a fever and medical care is not available.

—Children: Dose is based on body weight and must be determined by your doctor. The dose may range from ¼ tablet to 3 tablets taken as a single dose.

- For *prevention* of malaria:
  —Adults and teenagers: 1 tablet once every seven days, or 2 tablets once every fourteen days.
  —Children: Dose is based on body weight and must be determined by your doctor. The dose may range from ½ tablet to ¾ tablet taken once every seven days, or ¼ tablet to 1½ tablets taken once every fourteen days.

**Missed dose**—For patients taking this medicine *to prevent malaria:* If you do miss a dose of this medicine, take it as soon as possible. This will help to keep you taking your medicine on a regular schedule. However, if it is almost time for your next dose, skip the missed dose and go back to your regular dosing schedule. Do not double doses.

**Storage**—To store this medicine:

- Keep out of the reach of children. Overdose of sulfadoxine and pyrimethamine combination is very dangerous in children.
- Store away from heat and direct light.
- Do not store in the bathroom, near the kitchen sink, or in other damp places. Heat or moisture may cause the medicine to break down.
- Do not keep outdated medicine or medicine no longer needed. Be sure that any discarded medicine is out of the reach of children.

## Precautions While Using This Medicine

*If this medicine causes skin rash, itching, redness, sores in the mouth or on the genitals (sex organs), or sore throat, check with your doctor immediately.* These may be early warning signs of more serious skin or related problems that could develop later.

Malaria is spread by mosquitoes. If you are living in, or will be traveling to, an area where there is a chance of getting malaria, the following mosquito-control measures will help to prevent infection:

- If possible, sleep under mosquito netting to avoid being bitten by malaria-carrying mosquitoes.
- Wear long-sleeved shirts or blouses and long trousers to protect your arms and legs, especially from dusk through dawn when mosquitoes are out.
- Apply mosquito repellant to uncovered areas of the skin from dusk through dawn when mosquitoes are out.

For patients taking this medicine *to prevent malaria:*

- *It is very important that your doctor check your progress at regular visits.* This medicine may cause blood problems, especially if it is taken for a long time.
- If this medicine causes anemia, your doctor may want you to take leucovorin (e.g., folinic acid, Wellcovorin) to help clear up the anemia. If so, it is

important to take the leucovorin every day while you are taking this medicine. Do not miss any doses.

- Sulfadoxine and pyrimethamine combination may cause blood problems. These problems may result in a greater chance of certain infections, slow healing, and bleeding of the gums. Therefore, you should be careful when using regular toothbrushes, dental floss, and toothpicks. Dental work should be delayed until your blood counts have returned to normal. Check with your medical doctor or dentist if you have any questions about proper oral hygiene (mouth care) during treatment.

- Sulfadoxine and pyrimethamine combination may cause your skin to be more sensitive to sunlight than it is normally. Exposure to sunlight, even for brief periods of time, may cause a skin rash, itching, redness or other discoloration of the skin, or a severe sunburn. When you begin taking this medicine:

—Stay out of direct sunlight, especially between the hours of 10:00 a.m. and 3:00 p.m., if possible.

—Wear protective clothing, including a hat. Also, wear sunglasses.

—Apply a sun block product that has a skin protection factor (SPF) of at least 15. Some patients may require a product with a higher SPF number, especially if they have a fair complexion. If you have any questions about this, check with your health care professional.

—Apply a sun block lipstick that has an SPF of at least 15 to protect your lips.

—Do not use a sunlamp or tanning bed or booth.

*If you have a severe reaction from the sun, check with your doctor.*

For patients taking this medicine *to self-treat presumed malaria:*

- Seek medical help as soon as possible, especially if your symptoms do not improve within 48 hours.

## Side Effects of This Medicine

Along with its needed effects, a medicine may cause some unwanted effects. Although not all of these side effects may occur, if they do occur they may need medical attention.

*Check with your doctor immediately* if any of the following side effects occur:

*More common*

Change in or loss of taste; fever and sore throat; skin rash; soreness, redness, swelling, burning, or stinging of

tongue; unusual bleeding or bruising; unusual tiredness or weakness

*Less common*

Aching of joints and muscles; redness, blistering, peeling, or loosening of skin; yellow eyes or skin

*Rare*

Blood in urine; lower back pain; pain or burning while urinating; swelling of front part of neck

*Symptoms of overdose*

Bleeding or bruising (severe); clumsiness or unsteadiness; convulsions (seizures); loss of appetite (severe); sore throat and fever (severe); tiredness or weakness (severe); trembling; vomiting (severe)

Also, check with your doctor as soon as possible if the following side effect occurs:

*More common*

Increased sensitivity of skin to sunlight

Other side effects may occur that usually do not need medical attention. These side effects may go away during treatment as your body adjusts to the medicine. However, check with your doctor if any of the following side effects continue or are bothersome:

*More common*

Diarrhea; headache; nausea or vomiting; nervousness; stomach pain

Other side effects not listed above may also occur in some patients. If you notice any other effects, check with your doctor.

## Additional Information

Once a medicine has been approved for marketing for a certain use, experience may show that it is also useful for other medical problems. Although this use is not included in product labeling, sulfadoxine and pyrimethamine combination is used in certain patients with the following medical condition:

- Isosporiasis (prevention)

Other than the above information, there is no additional information relating to proper use, precautions, or side effects for this use.

Revised: 02/23/93

# SULFAMETHOXAZOLE AND TRIMETHOPRIM   Systemic

Some commonly used brand names are:

**In the U.S.—**

| | |
|---|---|
| Bactrim | Sulfatrim |
| Bactrim DS | Sulfatrim DS |
| Cotrim | Sulfoxaprim |
| Cotrim DS | Sulfoxaprim DS |
| Septra | Triazole |
| Septra DS | Triazole DS |
| Sulfamethoprim | Trimeth-Sulfa |
| Sulfamethoprim DS | Trisulfam |
| Sulfaprim | Uroplus DS |
| Sulfaprim DS | Uroplus SS |

Generic name product may also be available.

**In Canada—**

| | |
|---|---|
| Apo-Sulfatrim | Nu-Cotrimox |
| Apo-Sulfatrim DS | Nu-Cotrimox DS |
| Bactrim | Roubac |
| Bactrim DS | Septra |
| Novotrimel | Septra DS |
| Novotrimel DS | |

Some other commonly used names are cotrimoxazole and SMZ-TMP.

## Description

Sulfamethoxazole and trimethoprim (sul-fa-meth-OX-a-zole and trye-METH-oh-prim) combination is used to treat infections, such as bronchitis, middle ear infection, urinary tract infection, and traveler's diarrhea. It is also used for the prevention and treatment of *Pneumocystis carinii* pneumonia (PCP). It will not work for colds, flu, or other virus infections. It may also be used for other conditions as determined by your doctor.

Sulfamethoxazole and trimethoprim combination is available only with your doctor's prescription, in the following dosage forms:

*Oral*
- Oral suspension (U.S. and Canada)
- Tablets (U.S. and Canada)

*Parenteral*
- Injection (U.S. and Canada)

## Before Using This Medicine

In deciding to use a medicine, the risks of taking the medicine must be weighed against the good it will do. This is a decision you and your doctor will make. For sulfamethoxazole and trimethoprim combination, the following should be considered:

**Allergies—**Tell your doctor if you have ever had any unusual or allergic reaction to sulfa medicines, furosemide (e.g., Lasix) or thiazide diuretics (water pills), oral antidiabetics (diabetes medicine you take by mouth), glaucoma medicine you take by mouth (for example, acetazolamide [e.g., Diamox], dichlorphenamide [e.g., Daranide], methazolamide [e.g., Neptazane]), or trimethoprim (e.g., Trimpex). Also tell your health care professional if you are allergic to any other substances, such as foods, preservatives, or dyes.

**Pregnancy—**Sulfamethoxazole and trimethoprim combination has not been reported to cause birth defects or other problems in humans. However, studies in mice, rats, and rabbits have shown that some sulfonamides cause birth defects, including cleft palate and bone problems. Studies in rabbits have also shown that trimethoprim causes birth defects, as well as a decrease in the number of successful pregnancies.

**Breast-feeding—**Sulfamethoxazole and trimethoprim pass into the breast milk. This medicine is not recommended for use during breast-feeding. It may cause liver problems, anemia, and other unwanted effects in nursing babies, especially those with glucose-6-phosphate dehydrogenase (G6PD) deficiency.

**Children—**This medicine should not be given to infants under 2 months of age unless directed by the child's doctor, because it may cause brain problems.

**Older adults—**Elderly people are especially sensitive to the effects of sulfamethoxazole and trimethoprim combination. Severe skin problems and blood problems may be more likely to occur in the elderly. These problems may also be more likely to occur in patients who are taking diuretics (water pills) along with this medicine.

**Other medicines—**Although certain medicines should not be used together at all, in other cases two different medicines may be used together even if an interaction might occur. In these cases, your doctor may want to change the dose, or other precautions may be necessary. When you are taking sulfamethoxazole and trimethoprim combination, it is especially important that your health care professional knows if you are taking any of the following:

- Acetaminophen (e.g., Tylenol) (with long-term, high-dose use) or
- Amiodarone (e.g., Cordarone) or
- Anabolic steroids (nandrolone [e.g., Anabolin], oxandrolone [e.g., Anavar], oxymetholone [e.g., Anadrol], stanozolol [e.g., Winstrol]) or
- Androgens (male hormones) or
- Antithyroid agents (medicine for overactive thyroid) or
- Carbamazepine (e.g., Tegretol) or
- Carmustine (e.g., BiCNU) or
- Chloroquine (e.g., Aralen) or
- Dantrolene (e.g., Dantrium) or
- Daunorubicin (e.g., Cerubidine) or
- Disulfiram (e.g., Antabuse) or
- Divalproex (e.g., Depakote) or
- Estrogens (female hormones) or
- Etretinate (e.g., Tegison) or
- Gold salts (medicine for arthritis) or
- Hydroxychloroquine (e.g., Plaquenil) or
- Mercaptopurine (e.g., Purinethol) or
- Naltrexone (e.g., Trexan) (with long-term, high-dose use) or
- Oral contraceptives (birth control pills) containing estrogens or
- Other anti-infectives by mouth or by injection (medicine for infection) or
- Phenothiazines (acetophenazine [e.g., Tindal], chlorpromazine [e.g., Thorazine], fluphenazine [e.g., Prolixin], mesoridazine [e.g., Serentil], perphenazine [e.g., Trilafon], prochlorperazine [e.g., Compazine], promazine [e.g.,

Sparine], promethazine [e.g., Phenergan], thioridazine [e.g., Mellaril], trifluoperazine [e.g., Stelazine], triflupromazine [e.g., Vesprin], trimeprazine [e.g., Temaril]) or
- Plicamycin (e.g., Mithracin) or
- Valproic acid (e.g., Depakene)—Use of sulfamethoxazole and trimethoprim combination with these medicines may increase the chance of side effects affecting the liver
- Acetohydroxamic acid (e.g., Lithostat) or
- Dapsone or
- Furazolidone (e.g., Furoxone) or
- Nitrofurantoin (e.g., Furadantin) or
- Primaquine or
- Procainamide (e.g., Pronestyl) or
- Quinidine (e.g., Quinidex) or
- Quinine (e.g., Quinamm)—Use of sulfamethoxazole and trimethoprim combination with these medicines may increase the chance of side effects affecting the blood
- Anticoagulants (blood thinners) or
- Ethotoin (e.g., Peganone) or
- Mephenytoin (e.g., Mesantoin)—Use of sulfamethoxazole and trimethoprim combination with these medicines may increase the chance of side effects of these medicines
- Antidiabetics, oral (diabetes medicine you take by mouth)—Use of oral antidiabetics with sulfamethoxazole and trimethoprim combination may increase the chance of side effects affecting the blood and/or the side effects of the oral antidiabetics
- Methenamine (e.g., Mandelamine)—Use of methenamine with sulfamethoxazole and trimethoprim combination may increase the chance of side effects of the sulfamethoxazole
- Methotrexate (e.g., Mexate) or
- Phenytoin (e.g., Dilantin)—Use of these medicines with sulfamethoxazole and trimethoprim combination may increase the chance of side effects affecting the liver and/or the side effects of these medicines
- Methyldopa (e.g., Aldomet)—Use of methyldopa with sulfamethoxazole and trimethoprim combination may increase the chance of side effects affecting the liver and/or the blood

**Other medical problems**—The presence of other medical problems may affect the use of sulfamethoxazole and trimethoprim combination. Make sure you tell your doctor if you have any other medical problems, especially:
- Anemia or other blood problems or
- Glucose-6-phosphate dehydrogenase (G6PD) deficiency—Patients with these problems may have an increase in side effects affecting the blood
- Kidney disease or
- Liver disease—Patients with kidney and/or liver disease may have an increased chance of side effects
- Porphyria—This medicine may bring on an attack of porphyria

## Proper Use of This Medicine

*Sulfamethoxazole and trimethoprim combination is best taken with a full glass (8 ounces) of water. Several additional glasses of water should be taken every day,* unless otherwise directed by your doctor. Drinking extra water will help to prevent some unwanted effects of sulfonamides.

For patients taking the *oral liquid form* of this medicine:
- Use a specially marked measuring spoon or other device to measure each dose accurately. The average household teaspoon may not hold the right amount of liquid.

To help clear up your infection completely, *keep taking this medicine for the full time of treatment,* even if you begin to feel better after a few days. If you stop taking this medicine too soon, your symptoms may return.

This medicine works best when there is a constant amount in the blood or urine. *To help keep the amount constant, do not miss any doses. Also, it is best to take the doses at evenly spaced times day and night.* For example, if you are to take 4 doses a day, the doses should be spaced about 6 hours apart. If this interferes with your sleep or other daily activities, or if you need help in planning the best times to take your medicine, check with your health care professional.

**Dosing**—The dose of sulfamethoxazole and trimethoprim combination will be different for different patients. *Follow your doctor's orders or the directions on the label.* The following information includes only the average doses of sulfamethoxazole and trimethoprim combination. *If your dose is different, do not change it* unless your doctor tells you to do so.

The number of tablets or teaspoonfuls of suspension that you take depends on the strength of the medicine. Also, *the number of doses you take each day, the time allowed between doses, and the length of time you take the medicine depend on the medical problem for which you are taking sulfamethoxazole and trimethoprim combination.*

- For *oral* dosage forms (suspension, tablets):
  —For bacterial infections:
    - Adults and children over 40 kilograms (kg) of body weight (88 pounds)—160 milligrams (mg) of trimethoprim and 800 mg of sulfamethoxazole every twelve hours.
    - Infants younger than 2 months of age—Use and dose must be determined by your doctor.
    - Infants 2 months of age and older and children up to 40 kg of weight (88 pounds)—Dose is based on body weight. The usual dose is 4 to 6 mg of trimethoprim and 20 to 30 mg of sulfamethoxazole per kg (1.8 to 2.7 mg of trimethoprim and 9.1 to 13.6 mg of sulfamethoxazole per pound) of body weight every twelve hours.
  —For the treatment of *Pneumocystis carinii* pneumonia (PCP):
    - Adults and children older than 2 months—Dose is based on body weight. The usual dose is 3.75 to 5 mg of trimethoprim and 18.75 to 25 mg of sulfamethoxazole per kg (1.7 to 2.3 mg of trimethoprim and 8.5 to 11.4 mg of sulfamethoxazole per pound) of body weight every six hours.

—For the prevention of *Pneumocystis carinii* pneumonia (PCP):

- Adults and teenagers—160 mg of trimethoprim and 800 mg of sulfamethoxazole one or two times a day.
- Infants and children 1 month of age and older—Dose is based on body size and must be determined by your doctor. There are several dosing regimens available that your doctor may choose from. One dosing regimen is 75 mg of trimethoprim and 375 mg of sulfamethoxazole per square meter of body surface ($m^2$) three times a week on consecutive days (e.g., Monday, Tuesday, Wednesday).

- For *injection* dosage form:
  —For bacterial infections:
  - Adults and children older than 2 months—The usual total daily dose is 8 to 10 mg of trimethoprim and 40 to 50 mg of sulfamethoxazole per kg (3.6 to 4.5 mg of trimethoprim and 18.2 to 22.7 mg of sulfamethoxazole per pound) of body weight. This total daily dose may be divided up and injected into a vein every six, eight, or twelve hours.
  - Infants younger than 2 months of age—Use and dose must be determined by your doctor.
  —For the treatment of *Pneumocystis carinii* pneumonia (PCP):
  - Adults and children older than 2 months—The usual dose is 3.75 to 5 mg of trimethoprim and 18.75 to 25 mg of sulfamethoxazole per kg (1.7 to 2.3 mg of trimethoprim and 8.5 to 11.4 mg of sulfamethoxazole per pound) of body weight. This is injected into a vein every six hours.
  - Infants younger than 2 months of age—Use and dose must be determined by your doctor.

**Missed dose**—If you miss a dose of this medicine, take it as soon as possible. This will help to keep a constant amount of medicine in the blood or urine. However, if it is almost time for your next dose, skip the missed dose and go back to your regular dosing schedule. Do not double doses.

**Storage**—To store this medicine:

- Keep out of the reach of children.
- Store away from heat and direct light.
- Do not store the tablet form of this medicine in the bathroom, near the kitchen sink, or in other damp places. Heat or moisture may cause the medicine to break down.
- Keep the oral liquid form of this medicine from freezing.
- Do not keep outdated medicine or medicine no longer needed. Be sure that any discarded medicine is out of the reach of children.

## Precautions While Using This Medicine

*It is very important that your doctor check your progress at regular visits.* This medicine may cause blood problems, especially if it is taken for a long time.

If your symptoms do not improve within a few days, or if they become worse, check with your doctor.

Sulfamethoxazole and trimethoprim combination may cause blood problems. These problems may result in a greater chance of certain infections, slow healing, and bleeding of the gums. Therefore, you should be careful when using regular toothbrushes, dental floss, and toothpicks. Dental work should be delayed until your blood counts have returned to normal. Check with your medical doctor or dentist if you have any questions about proper oral hygiene (mouth care) during treatment.

Sulfamethoxazole and trimethoprim combination may cause your skin to be more sensitive to sunlight than it is normally. Exposure to sunlight, even for brief periods of time, may cause a skin rash, itching, redness or other discoloration of the skin, or a severe sunburn. When you begin taking this medicine:

- Stay out of direct sunlight, especially between the hours of 10:00 a.m. and 3:00 p.m., if possible.
- Wear protective clothing, including a hat. Also, wear sunglasses.
- Apply a sun block product that has a skin protection factor (SPF) of at least 15. Some patients may require a product with a higher SPF number, especially if they have a fair complexion. If you have any questions about this, check with your health care professional.
- Apply a sun block lipstick that has an SPF of at least 15 to protect your lips.
- Do not use a sunlamp or tanning bed or booth.

*If you have a severe reaction from the sun, check with your doctor.*

This medicine may also cause some people to become dizzy. *Make sure you know how you react to this medicine before you drive, use machines, or do anything else that could be dangerous if you are dizzy or are not alert.* If this reaction is especially bothersome, check with your doctor.

## Side Effects of This Medicine

Along with its needed effects, a medicine may cause some unwanted effects. Although not all of these side effects may occur, if they do occur they may need medical attention.

*Check with your doctor immediately* if any of the following side effects occur:

*More common*
   Itching; skin rash

*Less common*
   Aching of joints and muscles; difficulty in swallowing; pale skin; redness, blistering, peeling, or loosening of

---

skin; sore throat and fever; unusual bleeding or bruising; unusual tiredness or weakness; yellow eyes or skin

*Rare*

Blood in urine; bluish fingernails, lips, or skin; difficult breathing; greatly increased or decreased frequency of urination or amount of urine; increased thirst; lower back pain; pain or burning while urinating; swelling of front part of neck

Also, check with your doctor as soon as possible if the following side effect occurs:

*More common*

Increased sensitivity of skin to sunlight

Other side effects may occur that usually do not need medical attention. These side effects may go away during treatment as your body adjusts to the medicine. However, check with your doctor if any of the following side effects continue or are bothersome:

*More common*

Diarrhea; dizziness; headache; loss of appetite; nausea or vomiting

Other side effects not listed above may also occur in some patients. If you notice any other effects, check with your doctor.

## Additional Information

Once a medicine has been approved for marketing for a certain use, experience may show that it is also useful for other medical problems. Although these uses are not included in product labeling, sulfamethoxazole and trimethoprim combination is used in certain patients with the following medical conditions:

- Bile infections
- Bone and joint infections
- Sexually transmitted diseases, such as gonorrhea
- Sinus infections
- Urinary tract infections (for prevention)

Other than the above information, there is no additional information relating to proper use, precautions, or side effects for these uses.

Revised: 09/30/92
Interim revision(s): 03/17/94; 05/20/94

# SULFAPYRIDINE    Systemic

A commonly used brand name in Canada is Dagenan.
Generic name product may also be available in the U.S. and Canada.

## Description

Sulfapyridine (sul-fa-PEER-i-deen) is a sulfa medicine. It is used to help control dermatitis herpetiformis (Duhring's disease), a skin problem. It may also be used for other problems as determined by your doctor. However, this medicine will not work for any kind of infection as other sulfa medicines do.

This medicine may cause some serious side effects. *Before using this medicine, be sure to talk to your doctor about these problems, as well as the good this medicine will do.*

Sulfapyridine is available only with your doctor's prescription, in the following dosage form:

*Oral*

- Tablets (U.S. and Canada)

## Before Using This Medicine

In deciding to use a medicine, the risks of taking the medicine must be weighed against the good it will do. This is a decision you and your doctor will make. For sulfapyridine, the following should be considered:

**Allergies**—Tell your doctor if you have ever had any unusual or allergic reaction to sulfa medicines, furosemide

(e.g., Lasix) or thiazide diuretics (water pills), oral antidiabetics (diabetes medicine you take by mouth), glaucoma medicine you take by mouth (acetazolamide [e.g., Diamox], dichlorphenamide [e.g., Daranide], methazolamide [e.g., Neptazane]), or pyrimethamine (e.g., Daraprim). Also tell your health care professional if you are allergic to any other substances, such as foods, preservatives, or dyes.

**Pregnancy**—Studies have not been done in humans. Studies in rats and mice have shown that some sulfa medicines, given by mouth in high doses, cause birth defects, including cleft palate and bone problems. In addition, sulfa medicines may cause liver problems in newborn infants. Therefore, use is not recommended during pregnancy.

**Breast-feeding**—Sulfapyridine passes into the breast milk. This medicine may cause liver problems in nursing babies. In addition, it may cause blood problems in nursing babies with glucose-6-phosphate dehydrogenase (G6PD) deficiency (lack of G6PD enzyme). Therefore, use is not recommended in nursing women.

**Children**—Use of this medicine is not recommended since dermatitis herpetiformis usually does not occur in children.

**Older adults**—Many medicines have not been studied specifically in older people. Therefore, it may not be known whether they work exactly the same way they do in younger adults or if they cause different side effects or problems in older people. There is no specific information comparing the use of sulfapyridine in the elderly with use in other age groups.

**Other medicines**—Although certain medicines should not be used together at all, in other cases two different medicines may be used together even if an interaction might occur. In these cases, your doctor may want to change the dose, or other precautions may be necessary. When you are taking sulfapyridine, it is especially important that your health care professional know if you are taking any of the following:

- Acetaminophen (e.g., Tylenol) (with long-term, high-dose use) or
- Amiodarone (e.g., Cordarone) or
- Anabolic steroids (nandrolone [e.g., Anabolin], oxandrolone [e.g., Anavar], oxymetholone [e.g., Anadrol], stanozolol [e.g., Winstrol]) or
- Androgens (male hormones) or
- Antithyroid agents (medicine for overactive thyroid) or
- Carbamazepine (e.g., Tegretol) or
- Carmustine (e.g., BiCNU) or
- Chloroquine (e.g., Aralen) or
- Dantrolene (e.g., Dantrium) or
- Daunorubicin (e.g., Cerubidine) or
- Disulfiram (e.g., Antabuse) or
- Divalproex (e.g., Depakote) or
- Estrogens (female hormones) or
- Etretinate (e.g., Tegison) or
- Gold salts (medicine for arthritis) or
- Hydroxychloroquine (e.g., Plaquenil) or
- Mercaptopurine (e.g., Purinethol) or
- Naltrexone (e.g., Trexan) (with long-term, high-dose use) or
- Oral contraceptives (birth control pills) containing estrogen or
- Other anti-infectives by mouth or by injection (medicine for infection) or
- Phenothiazines (acetophenazine [e.g., Tindal], chlorpromazine [e.g., Thorazine], fluphenazine [e.g., Prolixin], mesoridazine [e.g., Serentil], perphenazine [e.g., Trilafon], prochlorperazine [e.g., Compazine], promazine [e.g., Sparine], promethazine [e.g., Phenergan], thioridazine [e.g., Mellaril], trifluoperazine [e.g., Stelazine], triflupromazine [e.g., Vesprin], trimeprazine [e.g., Temaril]) or
- Plicamycin (e.g., Mithracin) or
- Valproic acid (e.g., Depakene)—Use of sulfapyridine with these medicines may increase the chance of side effects affecting the liver
- Acetohydroxamic acid (e.g., Lithostat) or
- Dapsone or
- Furazolidone (e.g., Furoxone) or
- Nitrofurantoin (e.g., Furadantin) or
- Primaquine or
- Procainamide (e.g., Pronestyl) or
- Quinidine (e.g., Quinidex) or
- Quinine (e.g., Quinamm) or
- Sulfoxone (e.g., Diasone) or
- Vitamin K (e.g., AquaMEPHYTON, Synkayvite)—Use of sulfapyridine with these medicines may increase the chance of side effects affecting the blood
- Anticoagulants (blood thinners) or
- Ethotoin (e.g., Peganone) or

- Mephenytoin (e.g., Mesantoin)—Use of sulfapyridine with these medicines may increase the chance of side effects of these medicines
- Antidiabetics, oral (diabetes medicine you take by mouth)—Use of oral antidiabetics with sulfapyridine may increase the chance of side effects affecting the blood and/or the side effects or oral antidiabetics
- Methotrexate (e.g., Mexate)—Use of methotrexate with sulfapyridine may increase the chance of side effects affecting the liver and/or the side effects of methotrexate
- Methyldopa (e.g., Aldomet)—Use of methyldopa with sulfapyridine may increase the chance of side effects affecting the liver and/or the blood
- Phenytoin (e.g., Dilantin)—Use of phenytoin with sulfapyridine may increase the chance of side effects affecting the liver and/or the side effects of phenytoin

**Other medical problems**—The presence of other medical problems may affect the use of sulfapyridine. Make sure you tell your doctor if you have any other medical problems, especially:

- Blood problems or
- Glucose-6-phosphate dehydrogenase deficiency (lack of G6PD enzyme)—Patients with these problems may have an increase in side effects affecting the blood
- Kidney disease or
- Liver disease—Patients with kidney disease or liver disease may have an increased chance of side effects
- Porphyria—Use of sulfapyridine may cause an attack of porphyria

## Proper Use of This Medicine

*Each dose of sulfapyridine should be taken with a full glass (8 ounces) of water. Several additional glasses of water should be taken every day,* unless otherwise directed by your doctor. Drinking extra water will help to prevent some unwanted effects (e.g., kidney stones) of the sulfa medicine.

For patients taking sulfapyridine *for dermatitis herpetiformis:*

- Your doctor may want you to follow a strict, gluten-free diet.
- You may have to use this medicine regularly for 6 months to a year before you can reduce the dose of sulfapyridine or stop it altogether. If you have any questions about this, check with your doctor.

**Dosing**—The dose of sulfapyridine will be different for different patients. *Follow your doctor's orders or the directions on the label.* The following information includes only the average doses of sulfapyridine. Your dose may be different if you have kidney disease. *If your dose is different, do not change it* unless your doctor tells you to do so.

- For *dermatitis herpetiformis:*
  —Adults and adolescents: 250 milligrams to 1 gram four times a day until improvement occurs. After improvement has occurred, the dose should then be reduced by 250 to 500 milligrams every three days until there are no symptoms; that dose should be taken once daily.

—Children: Use is not recommended, because children usually do not get this condition.

**Missed dose**—For patients taking sulfapyridine *for dermatitis herpetiformis:* You may skip a missed dose if this does not make your symptoms return or get worse. If your symptoms do return or get worse, take the missed dose as soon as possible. Then go back to your regular dosing schedule.

**Storage**—To store this medicine:
- Keep out of the reach of children.
- Store away from heat and direct light.
- Do not store in the bathroom, near the kitchen sink, or in other damp places. Heat or moisture may cause the medicine to break down.
- Do not keep outdated medicine or medicine no longer needed. Be sure that any discarded medicine is out of the reach of children.

## Precautions While Using This Medicine

*It is very important that your doctor check your progress at regular visits.* This medicine may cause blood problems, especially if it is taken for a long time.

If your symptoms do not improve within a few days, or if they become worse, check with your doctor.

Sulfapyridine may cause blood problems. These problems may result in a greater chance of certain infections, slow healing, and bleeding of the gums. Therefore, you should be careful when using regular toothbrushes, dental floss, and toothpicks. Dental work should be delayed until your blood counts have returned to normal. Check with your medical doctor or dentist if you have any questions about proper oral hygiene (mouth care) during treatment.

Sulfapyridine may cause your skin to be more sensitive to sunlight than it is normally. Exposure to sunlight, even for brief periods of time, may cause a skin rash, itching, redness or other discoloration of the skin, or a severe sunburn. When you begin taking this medicine:
- Stay out of direct sunlight, especially between the hours of 10:00 A.M. and 3:00 P.M., if possible.
- Wear protective clothing, including a hat. Also, wear sunglasses.
- Apply a sun block product that has a skin protection factor (SPF) of at least 15. Some patients may require a product with a higher SPF number, especially if they have a fair complexion. If you have any questions about this, check with your health care professional.
- Apply a sun block lipstick that has an SPF of at least 15 to protect your lips.
- Do not use a sunlamp or tanning bed or booth.

You may still be more sensitive to sunlight or sunlamps for many months after stopping this medicine. *If you have a severe reaction from the sun, check with your doctor.*

Tell the doctor in charge that you are taking this medicine before you have any medical tests. The results of the bentiromide (e.g., Chymex) test for pancreas function are affected by this medicine.

## Side Effects of This Medicine

Along with its needed effects, a medicine may cause some unwanted effects. Although not all of these side effects may occur, if they do occur they may need medical attention.

*Check with your doctor immediately* if any of the following side effects occur:
*More common*
    Fever; headache (continuing); itching; skin rash
*Less common*
    Aching of joints and muscles; difficulty in swallowing; pale skin; redness, blistering, peeling, or loosening of skin; sore throat; unusual bleeding or bruising; unusual tiredness or weakness; yellow eyes or skin
*Rare*
    Blood in urine; lower back pain; pain or burning while urinating; swelling of front part of neck

Also, check with your doctor as soon as possible if the following side effect occurs:
*More common*
    Increased sensitivity of skin to sunlight

Other side effects may occur that usually do not need medical attention. These side effects may go away during treatment as your body adjusts to the medicine. However, check with your doctor if any of the following side effects continue or are bothersome:
*More common*
    Diarrhea; loss of appetite; nausea or vomiting

Other side effects not listed above may also occur in some patients. If you notice any other effects, check with your doctor.

## Additional Information

Once a medicine has been approved for marketing for a certain use, experience may show that it is also useful for other medical problems. Although these uses are not included in product labeling, sulfapyridine is used in certain patients with the following medical conditions:
- Pemphigoid
- Pyoderma gangrenosum
- Subcorneal pustular dermatitis

Other than the above information, there is no additional information relating to proper use, precautions, or side effects for these uses.

Revised: 02/01/93

# SULFASALAZINE  Systemic

Some commonly used brand names are:

**In the U.S.—**
Azulfidine                Azulfidine EN-Tabs
Generic name product may also be available.

**In Canada—**
PMS Sulfasalazine        Salazopyrin EN-Tabs
PMS Sulfasalazine E.C.   S.A.S.-500
Salazopyrin              S.A.S. Enteric-500
Generic name product may also be available.

Other commonly used names are salazosulfapyridine and salicylazo-sulfapyridine.

## Description

Sulfasalazine (sul-fa-SAL-a-zeen), a sulfa medicine, is used to prevent and treat inflammatory bowel disease, such as ulcerative colitis. It works inside the bowel by helping to reduce the inflammation and other symptoms of the disease. Sulfasalazine is sometimes given with other medicines to treat inflammatory bowel disease. However, this medicine will not work for all kinds of infection the way other sulfa medicines do.

Sulfasalazine is available only with your doctor's prescription, in the following dosage forms:

*Oral*
- Enteric-coated tablets (U.S. and Canada)
- Oral suspension (U.S.)
- Tablets (U.S. and Canada)

## Before Using This Medicine

In deciding to use a medicine, the risks of taking the medicine must be weighed against the good it will do. This is a decision you and your doctor will make. For sulfasalazine, the following should be considered:

**Allergies**—Tell your doctor if you have ever had any unusual or allergic reaction to any of the sulfa medicines, furosemide (e.g., Lasix) or thiazide diuretics (water pills), oral antidiabetics (diabetes medicine you take by mouth), glaucoma medicine you take by mouth (for example, acetazolamide [e.g., Diamox], dichlorphenamide [e.g., Daranide], methazolamide [e.g., Neptazane]), or salicylates (for example, aspirin). Also tell your health care professional if you are allergic to any other substances, such as foods, preservatives, or dyes.

**Pregnancy**—Studies have not been done in humans. However, reports on women who took sulfasalazine during pregnancy have not shown that it causes birth defects or other problems. In addition, sulfasalazine has not been shown to cause birth defects in studies in rats and rabbits given doses of up to 6 times the human dose.

**Breast-feeding**—Sulfa medicines pass into the breast milk in small amounts. They may cause unwanted effects in nursing babies with glucose-6-phosphate dehydrogenase (G6PD) deficiency.

**Children**—Sulfasalazine should not be used in children up to 2 years of age because it may cause brain problems.

However, sulfasalazine has not been shown to cause different side effects or problems in children over the age of 2 than it does in adults.

**Older adults**—Many medicines have not been studied specifically in older people. Therefore, it may not be known whether they work exactly the same way they do in younger adults or if they cause different side effects or problems in older people. There is no specific information comparing use of sulfasalazine in the elderly with use in other age groups.

**Other medicines**—Although certain medicines should not be used together at all, in other cases two different medicines may be used together even if an interaction might occur. In these cases, your doctor may want to change the dose, or other precautions may be necessary. When you are taking sulfasalazine, it is especially important that your health care professional know if you are taking any of the following:

- Acetaminophen (e.g., Tylenol) (with long-term, high-dose use) or
- Amiodarone (e.g., Cordarone) or
- Anabolic steroids (nandrolone [e.g., Anabolin], oxandrolone [e.g., Anavar], oxymetholone [e.g., Anadrol], stanozolol [e.g., Winstrol]) or
- Androgens (male hormones) or
- Antithyroid agents (medicine for overactive thyroid) or
- Carbamazepine (e.g., Tegretol) or
- Carmustine (e.g., BiCNU) or
- Chloroquine (e.g., Aralen) or
- Dantrolene (e.g., Dantrium) or
- Daunorubicin (e.g., Cerubidine) or
- Disulfiram (e.g., Antabuse) or
- Divalproex (e.g., Depakote) or
- Estrogens (female hormones) or
- Etretinate (e.g., Tegison) or
- Gold salts (medicine for arthritis) or
- Hydroxychloroquine (e.g., Plaquenil) or
- Mercaptopurine (e.g., Purinethol) or
- Naltrexone (e.g., Trexan) (with long-term, high-dose use) or
- Oral contraceptives (birth control pills) containing estrogen or
- Other anti-infectives by mouth or by injection (medicine for infection) or
- Phenothiazines (acetophenazine [e.g., Tindal], chlorpromazine [e.g., Thorazine], fluphenazine [e.g., Prolixin], mesoridazine [e.g., Serentil], perphenazine [e.g., Trilafon], prochlorperazine [e.g., Compazine], promazine [e.g., Sparine], promethazine [e.g., Phenergan], thioridazine [e.g., Mellaril], trifluoperazine [e.g., Stelazine], triflupromazine [e.g., Vesprin], trimeprazine [e.g., Temaril]) or
- Plicamycin (e.g., Mithracin) or
- Valproic acid (e.g., Depakene)—Use of sulfasalazine with these medicines may increase the chance of side effects affecting the liver
- Acetohydroxamic acid (e.g., Lithostat) or
- Dapsone or
- Furazolidone (e.g., Furoxone) or
- Nitrofurantoin (e.g., Furadantin) or
- Primaquine or

- Procainamide (e.g., Pronestyl) or
- Quinidine (e.g., Quinidex) or
- Quinine (e.g., Quinamm) or
- Sulfoxone (e.g., Diasone) or
- Vitamin K (e.g., AquaMEPHYTON, Synkayvite)—Use of sulfasalazine with these medicines may increase the chance of side effects affecting the blood
- Anticoagulants (blood thinners) or
- Ethotoin (e.g., Peganone) or
- Mephenytoin (e.g., Mesantoin)—Use of sulfasalazine with these medicines may increase the chance of side effects of these medicines
- Antidiabetics, oral (diabetes medicine you take by mouth)—Use of oral antidiabetics with sulfasalazine may increase the chance of side effects affecting the blood and/or the side effects or oral antidiabetics
- Methotrexate (e.g., Mexate)—Use of methotrexate with sulfasalazine may increase the chance of side effects affecting the liver and/or the side effects of methotrexate
- Methyldopa (e.g., Aldomet)—Use of methyldopa with sulfasalazine may increase the chance of side effects affecting the liver and/or the blood
- Phenytoin (e.g., Dilantin)—Use of phenytoin with sulfasalazine may increase the chance of side effects affecting the liver and/or the side effects of phenytoin

**Other medical problems**—The presence of other medical problems may affect the use of sulfasalazine. Make sure you tell your doctor if you have any other medical problems, especially:

- Blood problems or
- Glucose-6-phosphate dehydrogenase deficiency (lack of G6PD enzyme)—Patients with these problems may have an increase in side effects affecting the blood
- Kidney disease or
- Liver disease—Patients with kidney disease or liver disease may have an increased chance of side effects
- Porphyria—Use of sulfasalazine may cause an attack of porphyria

## Proper Use of This Medicine

*Do not give sulfasalazine to infants up to 2 years of age,* unless otherwise directed by your doctor. It may cause brain problems.

Sulfasalazine is best taken after meals or with food to lessen stomach upset. If stomach upset continues or is bothersome, check with your doctor.

*Each dose of sulfasalazine should also be taken with a full glass (8 ounces) of water. Several additional glasses of water should be taken every day,* unless otherwise directed by your doctor. Drinking extra water will help to prevent some unwanted effects (e.g., kidney stones) of the sulfa medicine.

For patients taking the *enteric-coated tablet form* of this medicine:
- Swallow tablets whole. Do not break or crush.

*Keep taking this medicine for the full time of treatment,* even if you begin to feel better after a few days. *Do not miss any doses.*

**Dosing**—The dose of sulfasalazine will be different for different patients. *Follow your doctor's orders or the directions on the label.* The following information includes only the average doses of sulfasalazine. *If your dose is different, do not change it* unless your doctor tells you to do so.

The number of tablets or teaspoonfuls of oral suspension that you take depends on the strength of the medicine. Also, *the number of doses you take each day, the time allowed between doses, and the length of time you take the medicine depend on the medical problem for which you are taking sulfasalazine.*

- For *oral* dosage forms (oral suspension, tablets, enteric-coated tablets):
  —For prevention or treatment of inflammatory bowel disease:
  - Adults—To start, 500 milligrams (mg) to 1000 mg (1 gram) every six to eight hours. Your doctor may then decrease the dose to 500 mg every six hours. After a time, your doctor may change your dose as needed.
  - Children 2 years of age and over—Dose is based on body weight and must be determined by your doctor.
    —To start, the dose is usually:
    - 6.7 to 10 mg per kilogram (kg) (3.05 to 4.55 mg per pound) of body weight every four hours or
    - 10 to 15 mg per kg (4.55 to 6.82 mg per pound) of body weight every six hours or
    - 13.3 to 20 mg per kg (6.05 to 9.09 mg per pound) of body weight every eight hours.
    —Then, the dose is usually 7.5 mg per kg (3.41 mg per pound) of body weight every six hours.
  - Infants and children less than 2 years of age—Use is not recommended.

**Missed dose**—If you do miss a dose of this medicine, take it as soon as possible. However, if it is almost time for your next dose, skip the missed dose and go back to your regular dosing schedule. Do not double doses.

**Storage**—To store this medicine:
- Keep out of the reach of children.
- Store away from heat and direct light.
- Do not store the tablet form of this medicine in the bathroom, near the kitchen sink, or in other damp places. Heat or moisture may cause the medicine to break down.
- Keep the oral liquid form of this medicine from freezing.
- Do not keep outdated medicine or medicine no longer needed. Be sure that any discarded medicine is out of the reach of children.

# Precautions While Using This Medicine

*It is very important that your doctor check your progress at regular visits.* This medicine may cause blood problems, especially if it is taken for a long time.

If your symptoms (including diarrhea) do not improve within a month or 2, or if they become worse, check with your doctor.

Sulfasalazine may cause blood problems. These problems may result in a greater chance of certain infections, slow healing, and bleeding of the gums. Therefore, you should be careful when using regular toothbrushes, dental floss, and toothpicks. Dental work should be delayed until your blood counts have returned to normal. Check with your medical doctor or dentist if you have any questions about proper oral hygiene (mouth care) during treatment.

Sulfasalazine may cause your skin to be more sensitive to sunlight than it is normally. Exposure to sunlight, even for brief periods of time, may cause a skin rash, itching, redness or other discoloration of the skin, or a severe sunburn. When you begin taking this medicine:

- Stay out of direct sunlight, especially between the hours of 10:00 a.m. and 3:00 p.m., if possible.
- Wear protective clothing, including a hat. Also, wear sunglasses.
- Apply a sun block product that has a skin protection factor (SPF) of at least 15. Some patients may require a product with a higher SPF number, especially if they have a fair complexion. If you have any questions about this, check with your health care professional.
- Apply a sun block lipstick that has an SPF of at least 15 to protect your lips.
- Do not use a sunlamp or tanning bed or booth.

*If you have a severe reaction from the sun, check with your doctor.*

This medicine may also cause some people to become dizzy. *Make sure you know how you react to this medicine before you drive, use machines, or do anything else that could be dangerous if you are dizzy.* If this reaction is especially bothersome, check with your doctor.

Before you have any medical tests, tell the doctor in charge that you are taking this medicine. The results of the bentiromide (e.g., Chymex) test for pancreas function are affected by this medicine.

# Side Effects of This Medicine

Along with its needed effects, a medicine may cause some unwanted effects. Although not all of these side effects may occur, if they do occur they may need medical attention.

*Check with your doctor immediately* if any of the following side effects occur:

*More common*
Aching of joints and muscles; headache (continuing); itching; skin rash

*Less common*
Back, leg, or stomach pains; difficulty in swallowing; fever and sore throat; pale skin; redness, blistering, peeling, or loosening of skin; unusual bleeding or bruising; unusual tiredness or weakness; yellow eyes or skin

*Rare*
Bloody diarrhea, fever, and rash; cough; difficult breathing

Also, check with your doctor as soon as possible if the following side effect occurs:

*More common*
Increased sensitivity of skin to sunlight

Other side effects may occur that usually do not need medical attention. These side effects may go away during treatment as your body adjusts to the medicine. However, check with your doctor if any of the following side effects continue or are bothersome:

*More common*
Abdominal or stomach pain or upset; diarrhea; dizziness; loss of appetite; nausea or vomiting

In some patients this medicine may also cause the urine or skin to become orange-yellow. This side effect does not need medical attention.

Other side effects not listed above may also occur in some patients. If you notice any other effects, check with your doctor.

# Additional Information

Once a medicine has been approved for marketing for a certain use, experience may show that it is also useful for other medical problems. Although these uses are not included in product labeling, sulfasalazine is used in certain patients with the following medical conditions:

- Ankylosing spondylitis
- Rheumatoid arthritis

Other than the above information, there is no additional information relating to proper use, precautions, or side effects for these uses.

Annual revision: 08/22/91
Interim revision: 07/20/94

# SULFINPYRAZONE   Systemic

Some commonly used brand names are:
**In the U.S.—**
    Anturane
    Generic name product may also be available.
**In Canada—**
    Anturan                              Novopyrazone
    Apo-Sulfinpyrazone

## Description

Sulfinpyrazone (sul-fin-PEER-a-zone) is used in the treatment of chronic gout (gouty arthritis), which is caused by too much uric acid in the blood. The medicine works by removing the extra uric acid from the body. Sulfinpyrazone does not cure gout, but after you have been taking it for a few months it may help prevent gout attacks. This medicine will help prevent gout attacks only as long as you continue to take it.

Sulfinpyrazone is sometimes used to prevent or treat other medical problems that may occur if too much uric acid is present in the body.

Sulfinpyrazone may also be used for other conditions as determined by your doctor.

Sulfinpyrazone is available only with your doctor's prescription, in the following dosage forms:

*Oral*
- Capsules (U.S.)
- Tablets (U.S. and Canada)

## Before Using This Medicine

In deciding to use a medicine, the risks of taking the medicine must be weighed against the good it will do. This is a decision you and your doctor will make. For sulfinpyrazone, the following should be considered:

**Allergies**—Tell your doctor if you have ever had any unusual or allergic reaction to sulfinpyrazone or to aspirin, oxyphenbutazone (e.g., Tandearil), or phenylbutazone (e.g., Butazolidin), or other anti-inflammatory analgesics (medicines used for pain and/or inflammation). Also tell your health care professional if you are allergic to any other substances, such as foods, preservatives, or dyes.

**Pregnancy**—Sulfinpyrazone has not been reported to cause problems in humans.

**Breast-feeding**—It is not known whether sulfinpyrazone passes into the breast milk.

**Children**—Studies on this medicine have been done only in adult patients, and there is no specific information comparing use of sulfinpyrazone in children with use in other age groups.

**Older adults**—Many medicines have not been studied specifically in older people. Therefore, it may not be known whether they work exactly the same way they do in younger adults or if they cause different side effects or problems in older people. There is no specific information comparing use of sulfinpyrazone in the elderly with use in other age groups.

**Other medicines**—Although certain medicines should not be used together at all, in other cases two different medicines may be used together even if an interaction might occur. In these cases, your doctor may want to change the dose, or other precautions may be necessary. When you are taking sulfinpyrazone, it is especially important that your health care professional know if you are taking any of the following:
- Anticoagulants (blood thinners) or
- Carbenicillin by injection (e.g., Geopen) or
- Cefamandole (e.g., Mandol) or
- Cefoperazone (e.g., Cefobid) or
- Cefotetan (e.g., Cefotan) or
- Dipyridamole (e.g., Persantine) or
- Divalproex (e.g., Depakote) or
- Heparin (e.g., Panheprin) or
- Inflammation or pain medicine, except narcotics, or
- Moxalactam (e.g., Moxam) or
- Pentoxifylline (e.g., Trental) or
- Plicamycin (e.g., Mithracin) or
- Ticarcillin (e.g., Ticar) or
- Valproic acid (e.g., Depakene)—Use of these medicines together with sulfinpyrazone may increase the chance of bleeding
- Antineoplastics (cancer medicine)—The chance of serious side effects may be increased
- Aspirin or other salicylates, including bismuth subsalicylate (e.g., Pepto Bismol)—These medicines may keep sulfinpyrazone from working properly in treating gout, depending on the amount of aspirin or other salicylate that you take and how often you take it. Taking sulfinpyrazone and aspirin together may also increase the chance of bleeding
- Nitrofurantoin (e.g., Furadantin)—Sulfinpyrazone may keep nitrofurantoin from working properly

**Other medical problems**—The presence of other medical problems may affect the use of sulfinpyrazone. Make sure you tell your doctor if you have any other medical problems, especially:
- Blood disease (or history of) or
- Cancer being treated by antineoplastics (cancer medicine) or radiation (x-rays) or
- Kidney stones (or history of) or other kidney disease or
- Stomach ulcer or other stomach or intestinal problems (or history of)—The chance of serious side effects may be increased; also, sulfinpyrazone may not work properly for treating gout if some kinds of kidney disease are present

## Proper Use of This Medicine

*If sulfinpyrazone upsets your stomach, it may be taken with food.* If this does not work, an antacid may be taken. If stomach upset (nausea, vomiting, or stomach pain) continues, check with your doctor.

*In order for sulfinpyrazone to help you, it must be taken regularly as ordered by your doctor.*

When you first begin taking sulfinpyrazone, the amount of uric acid in the kidneys is greatly increased. This may cause kidney stones in some people. To help prevent this, your doctor may want you to drink at least 10 to 12 full glasses (8 ounces each) of fluids each day, or to take another medicine to make your urine less acid. *It is important that you follow your doctor's instructions very carefully.*

For patients taking sulfinpyrazone for *gout:*

- After you begin to take sulfinpyrazone, gout attacks may continue to occur for a while. However, if you take this medicine regularly as directed by your doctor, the attacks will gradually become less frequent and less painful. After you have been taking sulfinpyrazone for several months, they may stop completely.
- Sulfinpyrazone helps to prevent gout attacks. It will not relieve an attack that has already started. *Even if you take another medicine for gout attacks, continue to take this medicine also.*

**Dosing**—The dose of sulfinpyrazone will be different for different patients. *Follow your doctor's orders or the directions on the label.* The following information includes only the average doses of sulfinpyrazone. *If your dose is different, do not change it* unless your doctor tells you to do so.

- *For treating gout or removing uric acid from the body:*
  —Adults: The starting dose of sulfinpyrazone is usually 100 mg or 200 mg a day (one-half of a 100-mg tablet two times a day, one 100-mg tablet one or two times a day, or one 200-mg capsule or tablet once a day). Then, the dose is usually increased by 100 mg or 200 mg every few days, up to 800 mg a day. Starting with a low dose and increasing the dose gradually helps prevent kidney stones and other side effects. After a while, the dose may be changed again, depending on the amount of uric acid in your blood or urine.
  —Children: It is not likely that sulfinpyrazone will be needed to treat gout or remove uric acid from the body in children. However, if a child needs this medicine, the dose would have to be determined by the doctor.

**Missed dose**—If you miss a dose of this medicine, take it as soon as possible. However, if is almost time for your next dose, skip the missed dose and go back to your regular dosing schedule. Do not double doses.

**Storage**—To store this medicine:

- Keep out of the reach of children.
- Store away from heat and direct light.
- Do not store this medicine in the bathroom, near the kitchen sink, or in other damp places. Heat or moisture may cause the medicine to break down.
- Do not keep outdated medicine or medicine no longer needed. Be sure that any discarded medicine is out of the reach of children.

## Precautions While Using This Medicine

Your doctor should check your progress at regular visits to make sure that this medicine does not cause unwanted effects.

Before you have any medical tests, tell the person in charge that you are taking this medicine. The results of some tests may be affected by sulfinpyrazone.

For patients taking sulfinpyrazone for *gout or to help remove uric acid from the body:*

- Taking aspirin or other salicylates may lessen the effects of sulfinpyrazone. This will depend on the dose of aspirin or other salicylate that you take, and on how often you take it. Also, drinking too much alcohol may increase the amount of uric acid in the blood and lessen the effects of sulfinpyrazone. Therefore, *do not take aspirin or other salicylates or drink alcoholic beverages while taking this medicine,* unless you have first checked with your doctor.

## Side Effects of This Medicine

Along with its needed effects, a medicine may cause some unwanted effects. Although not all of these side effects may occur, if they do occur they may need medical attention.

*Check with your doctor immediately* if any of the following side effects occur:

*Rare*

Shortness of breath, troubled breathing, tightness in chest, and/or wheezing; sores, ulcers, or white spots on lips or in mouth; sore throat and fever with or without chills; swollen and/or painful glands; unusual bleeding or bruising

*Symptoms of overdose*

Clumsiness or unsteadiness; convulsions (seizures); diarrhea; nausea or vomiting (severe or continuing); stomach pain (severe or continuing); difficulty in breathing

Also, check with your doctor as soon as possible if any of the following side effects occur:

*More common*

Lower back and/or side pain; painful urination (possibly with blood)

*Less common*

Skin rash

*Rare*

Bloody or black, tarry stools; fever; increased blood pressure; pinpoint red spots on skin; sudden decrease in amount of urine; swelling of face, fingers, feet, and/or lower legs; unusual tiredness or weakness; vomiting of blood or material that looks like coffee grounds; weight gain

Other side effects may occur that usually do not need medical attention. These side effects may go away during treatment as your body adjusts to the medicine. However,

check with your doctor if any of the following side effects continue or are bothersome:

*More common*

Joint pain, redness, and/or swelling; nausea or vomiting; stomach pain

Other side effects not listed above may also occur in some patients. If you notice any other effects, check with your doctor.

Revised: 01/19/93

---

# SULFONAMIDES    Ophthalmic

Some commonly used brand names are:

**In the U.S.—**

| | |
|---|---|
| Ak-Sulf[1] | Sodium Sulamyd[1] |
| Bleph-10[1] | Spectro-Sulf[1] |
| Cetamide[1] | Steri-Units Sulfacetamide[1] |
| Gantrisin[2] | Sulf-10[1] |
| Isopto-Cetamide[1] | Sulfair[1] |
| I-Sulfacet[1] | Sulfair 10[1] |
| Ocu-Sul-10[1] | Sulfair 15[1] |
| Ocu-Sul-15[1] | Sulfair Forte[1] |
| Ocu-Sul-30[1] | Sulfamide[1] |
| Ocusulf-10[1] | Sulten-10[1] |
| Ophthacet[1] | |

**In Canada—**

| | |
|---|---|
| Ak-Sulf[1] | Isopto-Cetamide[1] |
| Bleph-10[1] | Sodium Sulamyd[1] |
| Cetamide[1] | Sulfex[1] |

Another commonly used name for sulfisoxazole is sulfafurazole.

Note: For quick reference, the following sulfonamides are numbered to match the corresponding brand names.

This information applies to the following medicines:

1. Sulfacetamide (sul-fa-SEE-ta-mide)‡
2. Sulfisoxazole (sul-fi-SOX-a-zole)

‡Generic name product may may also be available in the U.S.

---

## Description

Sulfonamides (sul-FON-a-mides) or sulfa medicines belong to the family of medicines called anti-infectives. Sulfonamide ophthalmic preparations are used to treat infections of the eye.

Sulfonamides are available only with your doctor's prescription, in the following dosage forms:

*Ophthalmic*

Sulfacetamide
- Ophthalmic ointment (U.S. and Canada)
- Ophthalmic solution (eye drops) (U.S. and Canada)

Sulfisoxazole
- Ophthalmic ointment (U.S.)
- Ophthalmic solution (eye drops) (U.S.)

---

## Before Using This Medicine

In deciding to use a medicine, the risks of using the medicine must be weighed against the good it will do. This is a decision you and your doctor will make. For sulfonamide ophthalmic preparations, the following should be considered:

**Allergies**—Tell your doctor if you have ever had any unusual or allergic reaction to any of the sulfa medicines;

furosemide (e.g., Lasix) or thiazide diuretics (water pills); oral antidiabetics (diabetes medicine you take by mouth); or glaucoma medicine you take by mouth (for example, acetazolamide [e.g., Diamox], dichlorphenamide [e.g., Daranide], or methazolamide [e.g., Neptazane]). Also tell your health care professional if you are allergic to any other substances, such as preservatives.

**Pregnancy**—Sulfonamide ophthalmic preparations have not been shown to cause birth defects or other problems in humans.

**Breast-feeding**—Sulfonamide ophthalmic preparations have not been reported to cause problems in nursing babies.

**Children**—Studies on sulfonamide ophthalmic preparations have been done only in adult patients, and there is no specific information comparing use in children with use in other age groups.

**Older adults**—Many medicines have not been studied specifically in older people. Therefore, it may not be known whether they work exactly the same way they do in younger adults or if they cause different side effects or problems in older people. There is no specific information comparing use of sulfonamides in the elderly with use in other age groups.

**Other medicines**—Although certain medicines should not be used together at all, in other cases two different medicines may be used together even if an interaction might occur. In these cases, your doctor may want to change the dose, or other precautions may be necessary. When you are taking sulfonamide ophthalmic preparations, it is especially important that your health care professional know if you are using any of the following:

- Silver preparations, such as silver nitrate or mild silver protein for the eye—Sulfonamide ophthalmic preparations should not be used with silver ophthalmic preparations, since a chemical reaction may occur.

---

## Proper Use of This Medicine

For patients using the *eye drop form* of sulfonamides:

- The bottle is only partially full to provide proper drop control.
- To use:

  —First, wash your hands. Then tilt the head back and pull the lower eyelid away from the eye to form a pouch. Drop the medicine into the pouch and gently close the eyes. Do not blink. Keep the eyes closed for 1 or 2 minutes to allow the medicine to come into contact with the infection.

—If you think you did not get the drop of medicine into your eye properly, use another drop.

—To keep the medicine as germ-free as possible, do not touch the applicator tip to any surface (including the eye). Also, keep the container tightly closed.

For patients using the *eye ointment form* of sulfonamides:
- To use:
  —First, wash your hands. Then pull the lower eyelid away from the eye to form a pouch. Squeeze a thin strip of ointment into the pouch. A 1.25- to 2.5-cm (approximately ½- to 1-inch) strip of ointment is usually enough unless otherwise directed by your doctor. Gently close the eyes and keep them closed for 1 or 2 minutes to allow the medicine to come into contact with the infection.

  —To keep the medicine as germ-free as possible, do not touch the applicator tip to any surface (including the eye). After using sulfonamides eye ointment, wipe the tip of the ointment tube with a clean tissue and keep the tube tightly closed.

To help clear up your infection completely, *keep using this medicine for the full time of treatment,* even if your symptoms have disappeared. *Do not miss any doses.*

**Dosing**—The dose of ophthalmic sulfonamides will be different for different patients. *Follow your doctor's orders or the directions on the label.* The following information includes only the average doses of ophthalmic sulfonamides. *If your dose is different, do not change it* unless your doctor tells you to do so.

*The number of doses you use each day, the time allowed between doses, and the length of time you use the medicine depend on the medical problem for which you are using ophthalmic sulfonamides.*

*For sulfacetamide*
- For eye infections:
  —For *ophthalmic* dosage forms (ointment):
    - Adults and adolescents—Use four times a day and at bedtime.
    - Children—Use and dose must be determined by your doctor.
  —For *ophthalmic* dosage forms (solution):
    - Adults and adolescents—One drop every one to three hours during the day and less often during the night.
    - Children—Use and dose must be determined by your doctor.

*For sulfisoxazole*
- For eye infections:
  —For *ophthalmic* dosage forms (ointment):
    - Adults and children—Use one to three times a day and at bedtime.
  —For *ophthalmic* dosage forms (solution):
    - Adults and adolescents—One drop three or more times a day.
    - Children—
      —Infants up to 2 months of age: Use and dose must be determined by your doctor.
      —Infants and children 2 months of age and older: One drop three or more times a day.

**Missed dose**—If you miss a dose of this medicine, apply it as soon as possible. However, if it is almost time for your next dose, skip the missed dose and go back to your regular dosing schedule.

**Storage**—To store this medicine:
- Keep out of the reach of children.
- Store away from heat and direct light.
- Keep sulfacetamide eye drops in a cool place. Keep all dosage forms of these medicines from freezing.
- Do not keep outdated medicine or medicine no longer needed. Be sure that any discarded medicine is out of the reach of children.

## Precautions While Using This Medicine

After application, eye ointments usually cause your vision to blur for a few minutes.

After application of this medicine to the eye, occasional stinging or burning may be expected.

If your symptoms do not improve within a few days, or if they become worse, check with your doctor.

## Side Effects of This Medicine

Along with its needed effects, a medicine may cause some unwanted effects. Although not all of these side effects may occur, if they do occur they may need medical attention.

Check with your doctor as soon as possible if any of the following side effects occur:

*More common*
　Itching, redness, swelling, or other sign of irritation not present before use of this medicine

Other side effects not listed above may also occur in some patients. If you notice any other effects, check with your doctor.

Revised: 07/01/93

# SULFONAMIDES    Systemic

Some commonly used brand names are:

**In the U.S.—**

| | |
|---|---|
| Gantanol[4] | Renoquid[1] |
| Gantrisin[5] | Thiosulfil Forte[3] |

**In Canada—**

| | |
|---|---|
| Apo-Sulfamethoxazole[4] | Novosoxazole[5] |
| Gantanol[4] | |

Another commonly used name for sulfisoxazole is sulfafurazole.

Note: For quick reference, the following sulfonamides are numbered to match the corresponding brand names.

This information applies to the following medicines:

1. Sulfacytine (sul-fa-SYE-teen)[†]
2. Sulfadiazine (sul-fa-DYE-a-zeen)[†‡]
3. Sulfamethizole (sul-fa-METH-a-zole)[†]
4. Sulfamethoxazole (sul-fa-meth-OX-a-zole)[‡]
5. Sulfisoxazole (sul-fi-SOX-a-zole)[‡§]

---

[†]Not commercially available in Canada.
[‡]Generic name product may also be available in the U.S.
[§]Generic name product may also be available in Canada.

---

## Description

Sulfonamides (sul-FON-a-mides) or sulfa medicines are used to treat infections. They will not work for colds, flu, or other virus infections.

Sulfonamides are available only with your doctor's prescription, in the following dosage forms:

*Oral*

Sulfacytine
- Tablets (U.S.)

Sulfadiazine
- Tablets (U.S.)

Sulfamethizole
- Tablets (U.S.)

Sulfamethoxazole
- Oral suspension (U.S.)
- Tablets (U.S. and Canada)

Sulfisoxazole
- Oral suspension (U.S.)
- Syrup (U.S.)
- Tablets (U.S. and Canada)

---

## Before Using This Medicine

In deciding to use a medicine, the risks of taking the medicine must be weighed against the good it will do. This is a decision you and your doctor will make. For sulfonamides, the following should be considered:

**Allergies**—Tell your doctor if you have ever had any unusual or allergic reaction to sulfa medicines, furosemide (e.g., Lasix) or thiazide diuretics (water pills), oral antidiabetics (diabetes medicine you take by mouth), glaucoma medicine you take by mouth (for example, acetazolamide [e.g., Diamox], dichlorphenamide [e.g., Daranide], or methazolamide [e.g., Neptazane]). Also tell your health care professional if you are allergic to any other substances, such as foods, preservatives, or dyes.

**Pregnancy**—Studies have not been done in pregnant women. However, studies in mice, rats, and rabbits have shown that some sulfonamides cause birth defects, including cleft palate and bone problems.

**Breast-feeding**—Sulfonamides pass into the breast milk. This medicine is not recommended for use during breast-feeding. It may cause liver problems, anemia, and other unwanted effects in nursing babies, especially those with glucose-6-phosphate dehydrogenase (G6PD) deficiency.

**Children**—Sulfonamides should not be given to infants under 2 months of age unless directed by the child's doctor, because they may cause brain problems. Sulfacytine should not be given to children up to the age of 14.

**Older adults**—Elderly people are especially sensitive to the effects of sulfonamides. Severe skin problems and blood problems may be more likely to occur in the elderly. These problems may also be more likely to occur in patients who are taking diuretics (water pills) along with this medicine.

**Other medicines**—Although certain medicines should not be used together at all, in other cases two different medicines may be used together even if an interaction might occur. In these cases, your doctor may want to change the dose, or other precautions may be necessary. When you are taking sulfonamides, it is especially important that your health care professional knows if you are taking any of the following:

- Acetaminophen (e.g., Tylenol) (with long-term, high-dose use) or
- Amiodarone (e.g., Cordarone) or
- Anabolic steroids (nandrolone [e.g., Anabolin], oxandrolone [e.g., Anavar], oxymetholone [e.g., Anadrol], stanozolol [e.g., Winstrol]) or
- Androgens (male hormones) or
- Antithyroid agents (medicine for overactive thyroid) or
- Carbamazepine (e.g., Tegretol) or
- Carmustine (e.g., BiCNU) or
- Chloroquine (e.g., Aralen) or
- Dantrolene (e.g., Dantrium) or
- Daunorubicin (e.g., Cerubidine) or
- Disulfiram (e.g., Antabuse) or
- Divalproex (e.g., Depakote) or
- Estrogens (female hormones) or
- Etretinate (e.g., Tegison) or
- Gold salts (medicine for arthritis) or
- Hydroxychloroquine (e.g., Plaquenil) or
- Mercaptopurine (e.g., Purinethol) or
- Naltrexone (e.g., Trexan) (with long-term, high-dose use) or
- Oral contraceptives (birth control pills) containing estrogens or
- Other anti-infectives by mouth or by injection (medicine for infection) or
- Phenothiazines (acetophenazine [e.g., Tindal], chlorpromazine [e.g., Thorazine], fluphenazine [e.g., Prolixin], mesoridazine [e.g., Serentil], perphenazine [e.g., Trilafon], prochlorperazine [e.g., Compazine], promazine [e.g., Sparine], promethazine [e.g., Phenergan], thioridazine

[e.g., Mellaril], trifluoperazine [e.g., Stelazine], triflu-promazine [e.g., Vesprin], trimeprazine [e.g., Temaril]) or

- Plicamycin (e.g., Mithracin) or
- Valproic acid (e.g., Depakene)—Use of sulfonamides with these medicines may increase the chance of side effects affecting the liver
- Acetohydroxamic acid (e.g., Lithostat) or
- Dapsone or
- Furazolidone (e.g., Furoxone) or
- Nitrofurantoin (e.g., Furadantin) or
- Primaquine or
- Procainamide (e.g., Pronestyl) or
- Quinidine (e.g., Quinidex) or
- Quinine (e.g., Quinamm) or
- Sulfoxone (e.g., Diasone)—Use of sulfonamides with these medicines may increase the chance of side effects affecting the blood
- Anticoagulants (blood thinners) or
- Ethotoin (e.g., Peganone) or
- Mephenytoin (e.g., Mesantoin)—Use of sulfonamides with these medicines may increase the chance of side effects of these medicines
- Antidiabetics, oral (diabetes medicine you take by mouth)—Use of oral antidiabetics with sulfonamides may increase the chance of side effects affecting the blood and/or the side effects of oral antidiabetics
- Methenamine (e.g., Mandelamine)—Use of this medicine with sulfonamides may increase the chance of side effects of sulfonamides
- Methotrexate (e.g., Mexate) or
- Phenytoin (e.g., Dilantin)—Use of these medicines with sulfonamides may increase the chance of side effects affecting the liver and/or the side effects of these medicines
- Methyldopa (e.g., Aldomet)—Use of methyldopa with sulfonamides may increase the chance of side effects affecting the liver and/or the blood

**Other medical problems**—The presence of other medical problems may affect the use of sulfonamides. Make sure you tell your doctor if you have any other medical problems, especially:

- Anemia or other blood problems or
- Glucose-6-phosphate dehydrogenase (G6PD) deficiency—Patients with these problems may have an increase in side effects affecting the blood
- Kidney disease or
- Liver disease—Patients with kidney and/or liver disease may have an increased chance of side effects
- Porphyria—This medicine may bring on an attack of porphyria

## Proper Use of This Medicine

*Sulfonamides are best taken with a full glass (8 ounces) of water. Several additional glasses of water should be taken every day,* unless otherwise directed by your doctor. Drinking extra water will help to prevent some unwanted effects (e.g., kidney stones) of sulfonamides.

For patients taking the *oral liquid form* of this medicine:

- Use a specially marked measuring spoon or other device to measure each dose accurately. The average household teaspoon may not hold the right amount of liquid.

To help clear up your infection completely, *keep taking this medicine for the full time of treatment,* even if you begin to feel better after a few days. If you stop taking this medicine too soon, your symptoms may return.

This medicine works best when there is a constant amount in the blood or urine. *To help keep the amount constant, do not miss any doses. Also, it is best to take the doses at evenly spaced times day and night.* For example, if you are to take 4 doses a day, the doses should be spaced about 6 hours apart. If this interferes with your sleep or other daily activities, or if you need help in planning the best times to take your medicine, check with your health care professional.

**Dosing**—The dose of these medicines will be different for different patients. *Follow your doctor's orders or the directions on the label.* The following information includes only the average doses of these medicines. *If your dose is different, do not change it* unless your doctor tells you to do so.

*For sulfacytine*

- For *tablet* dosage form:
  —For bacterial infections:
    - Adults and children 14 years of age and older—500 milligrams (mg) for the first dose, then 250 mg every six hours.
    - Children up to age 14—Use and dose must be determined by your doctor.

*For sulfadiazine*

- For *tablet* dosage form:
  —For bacterial infections:
    - Adults and teenagers—2 to 4 grams for the first dose, then 1 gram every four to six hours.
    - Children up to 2 months of age—Use and dose must be determined by your doctor.
    - Children 2 months of age and older—Dose is based on body weight. The usual dose is 75 milligrams (mg) per kilogram (kg) (34 mg per pound) of body weight for the first dose, then 37.5 mg per kg (17 mg per pound) of body weight every six hours, or 25 mg per kg (11.4 mg per pound) of body weight every four hours.

*For sulfamethizole*

- For *tablet* dosage form:
  —For bacterial infections:
    - Adults and teenagers—500 milligrams (mg) to 1 gram every six to eight hours.
    - Children up to 2 months of age—Use and dose must be determined by your doctor.
    - Children 2 months of age and older—Dose is based on body weight. The usual dose is 7.5 to 11.25 mg per kilogram (kg) (3.4 to 5.1 mg per pound) of body weight every six hours.

*For sulfamethoxazole*

- For *suspension or tablet* dosage forms:
  —For bacterial or protozoal infections:
    - Adults and teenagers—2 grams for the first dose, then 1 gram every eight to twelve hours.

- Children up to 2 months of age—Use and dose must be determined by your doctor.
- Children 2 months of age and older—Dose is based on body weight. The usual dose is 50 to 60 milligrams (mg) per kilogram (kg) (22.7 to 27.3 mg per pound) of body weight for the first dose, then 25 to 30 mg per kg (11.4 to 13.6 mg per pound) of body weight every twelve hours.

*For sulfisoxazole*
- For *suspension, syrup, or tablet* dosage forms:
  —For bacterial or protozoal infections:
  - Adults and teenagers—2 to 4 grams for the first dose, then 750 milligrams (mg) to 1.5 grams every four hours; or 1 to 2 grams every six hours.
  - Children up to 2 months of age—Use and dose must be determined by your doctor.
  - Children 2 months of age and older—Dose is based on body weight. The usual dose is 75 mg per kilogram (kg) (34 mg per pound) of body weight for the first dose, then 25 mg every per kg (11.4 mg per pound) of body weight every four hours, or 37.5 mg per kg (17 mg per pound) of body weight every six hours.

**Missed dose**—If you miss a dose of this medicine, take it as soon as possible. This will help to keep a constant amount of medicine in the blood or urine. However, if it is almost time for your next dose, skip the missed dose and go back to your regular dosing schedule. Do not double doses.

**Storage**—To store this medicine:
- Keep out of the reach of children.
- Store away from heat and direct light.
- Do not store the tablet form of this medicine in the bathroom, near the kitchen sink, or in other damp places. Heat or moisture may cause the medicine to break down.
- Keep the oral liquid forms of this medicine from freezing.
- Do not keep outdated medicine or medicine no longer needed. Be sure that any discarded medicine is out of the reach of children.

---

## Precautions While Using This Medicine

*It is very important that your doctor check your progress at regular visits.* This medicine may cause blood problems, especially if it is taken for a long time.

If your symptoms do not improve within a few days, or if they become worse, check with your doctor.

Sulfonamides may cause blood problems. These problems may result in a greater chance of certain infections, slow healing, and bleeding of the gums. Therefore, you should be careful when using regular toothbrushes, dental floss, and toothpicks. Dental work should be delayed until your blood counts have returned to normal. Check with your medical doctor or dentist if you have any questions about proper oral hygiene (mouth care) during treatment.

Sulfonamides may cause your skin to be more sensitive to sunlight than it is normally. Exposure to sunlight, even for brief periods of time, may cause a skin rash, itching, redness or other discoloration of the skin, or a severe sunburn. When you begin taking this medicine:
- Stay out of direct sunlight, especially between the hours of 10:00 a.m. and 3:00 p.m., if possible.
- Wear protective clothing, including a hat. Also, wear sunglasses.
- Apply a sun block product that has a skin protection factor (SPF) of at least 15. Some patients may require a product with a higher SPF number, especially if they have a fair complexion. If you have any questions about this, check with your health care professional.
- Apply a sun block lipstick that has an SPF of at least 15 to protect your lips.
- Do not use a sunlamp or tanning bed or booth.

*If you have a severe reaction from the sun, check with your doctor.*

This medicine may also cause some people to become dizzy. *Make sure you know how you react to this medicine before you drive, use machines, or do anything else that could be dangerous if you are dizzy or are not alert.* If this reaction is especially bothersome, check with your doctor.

---

## Side Effects of This Medicine

Along with its needed effects, a medicine may cause some unwanted effects. Although not all of these side effects may occur, if they do occur they may need medical attention.

*Check with your doctor immediately* if any of the following side effects occur:

*More common*
  Itching; skin rash

*Less common*
  Aching of joints and muscles; difficulty in swallowing; pale skin; redness, blistering, peeling, or loosening of skin; sore throat and fever; unusual bleeding or bruising; unusual tiredness or weakness; yellow eyes or skin

*Rare*
  Blood in urine; greatly increased or decreased frequency of urination or amount of urine; increased thirst; lower back pain; pain or burning while urinating; swelling of front part of neck

Also, check with your doctor as soon as possible if the following side effect occurs:

*More common*
  Increased sensitivity of skin to sunlight

Other side effects may occur that usually do not need medical attention. These side effects may go away during treatment as your body adjusts to the medicine. However,

---

check with your doctor if any of the following side effects continue or are bothersome:

*More common*

Diarrhea; dizziness; headache; loss of appetite; nausea or vomiting; tiredness

Other side effects not listed above may also occur in some patients. If you notice any other effects, check with your doctor.

Revised: 10/10/92
Interim revision: 03/28/94

# SULFONAMIDES  Vaginal

Some commonly used brand names are:

**In the U.S.—**
AVC[1]
Sulfa-Gyn[3]
Sulnac[3]
Sultrin[3]
Trysul[3]
V.V.S.[3]
Vagitrol[1]

**In Canada—**
AVC[2]
Sultrin[3]

Another commonly used name for triple sulfa is sulfathiazole, sulfacetamide, and sulfabenzamide.

Note: For quick reference, the following vaginal sulfonamides are numbered to match the corresponding brand names.

This information applies to the following medicines:

1. Sulfanilamide (sul-fa-NILL-a-mide)
2. Sulfanilamide, Aminacrine (am-in-AK-rin), and Allantoin (al-AN-toyn)*
3. Triple Sulfa (TRI-pel SUL-fa)‡

*Not commercially available in the U.S.
‡Generic name product may also be available in the U.S.

## Description

Sulfonamides (sul-FON-a-mides), or sulfa medicines, are used to treat bacterial infections. They work by killing bacteria or preventing their growth.

Vaginal sulfonamides are used to treat bacterial infections. These medicines may also be used for other problems as determined by your doctor.

Vaginal sulfonamides are available only with your doctor's prescription, in the following dosage forms:

*Vaginal*

Sulfanilamide
• Cream (U.S.)
• Suppositories (U.S.)
Sulfanilamide, Aminacrine, and Allantoin
• Cream (Canada)
• Suppositories (Canada)
Triple Sulfa
• Cream (U.S. and Canada)
• Tablets (U.S.)

## Before Using This Medicine

In deciding to use a medicine, the risks of using the medicine must be weighed against the good it will do.

This is a decision you and your doctor will make. For vaginal sulfonamides, the following should be considered:

**Allergies**—Tell your doctor if you have ever had any unusual or allergic reaction to any of the sulfa medicines, furosemide (e.g., Lasix) or thiazide diuretics (water pills), oral antidiabetics (diabetes medicine you take by mouth), or glaucoma medicine you take by mouth (for example, acetazolamide [e.g., Diamox], dichlorphenamide [e.g., Daranide], or methazolamide [e.g., Neptazane]). Also tell your health care professional if you are allergic to any other substances, such as foods, preservatives, or dyes.

**Pregnancy**—Studies have not been done in humans. However, vaginal sulfonamides are absorbed through the vagina into the bloodstream and appear in the bloodstream of the fetus. Studies in rats and mice given high doses by mouth have shown that certain sulfonamides cause birth defects.

**Breast-feeding**—Vaginal sulfonamides are absorbed through the vagina into the bloodstream and pass into the breast milk. Use is not recommended in nursing mothers. Vaginal sulfonamides may cause liver problems in nursing babies. These medicines may also cause anemia in nursing babies with glucose-6-phosphate dehydrogenase (G6PD) deficiency.

**Children**—Studies on this medicine have been done only in adult patients and there is no specific information comparing the use of vaginal sulfonamides in children with use in other age groups.

**Older adults**—Many medicines have not been studied specifically in older people. Therefore, it may not be known whether they work exactly the same way they do in younger adults or if they cause different side effects or problems in older people. There is no specific information comparing the use of vaginal sulfonamides in the elderly with use in other age groups.

**Other medicines**—Although certain medicines should not be used together at all, in other cases two different medicines may be used together even if an interaction might occur. In these cases, your doctor may want to change the dose, or other precautions may be necessary. Tell your health care professional if you are taking or using any other prescription or nonprescription (over-the-counter [OTC]) medicine.

**Other medical problems**—The presence of other medical problems may affect the use of vaginal sulfonamides. Make sure you tell your doctor if you have any other medical problems, especially:

- Glucose-6-phosphate dehydrogenase (G6PD) deficiency—Anemia (a blood problem) can occur if sulfonamides are used
- Kidney disease
- Porphyria—Sulfonamides can cause porphyria attacks

## Proper Use of This Medicine

Vaginal sulfonamides usually come with patient directions. Read them carefully before using this medicine.

This medicine is usually inserted into the vagina with an applicator. However, if you are pregnant, check with your doctor before using the applicator.

To help clear up your infection completely, *it is very important that you keep using this medicine for the full time of treatment*, even if your symptoms begin to clear up after a few days. If you stop using this medicine too soon, your symptoms may return. *Do not miss any doses.* Also, *do not stop using this medicine if your menstrual period starts during the time of treatment.*

**Dosing**—The dose of these medicines will be different for different patients. *Follow your doctor's orders or the directions on the label.* The following information includes only the average doses of these medicines. *If your dose is different, do not change it* unless your doctor tells you to do so.

*For sulfanilamide*

- For *vaginal cream* dosage form:
  —For bacterial infections:
    - Adults and teenagers—One applicatorful (approximately 6 grams) inserted into the vagina one or two times a day for thirty days. Use when you wake up and/or just before you go to bed.
    - Children—Dose must be determined by your doctor.
- For *vaginal suppositories* dosage form:
  —For bacterial infections:
    - Adults and teenagers—One suppository inserted into the vagina one or two times a day for thirty days. Use when you wake up and/or just before you go to bed.
    - Children—Dose must be determined by your doctor.

*For sulfanilamide, aminacrine, and allantoin*

- For *vaginal cream* dosage form:
  —For bacterial infections:
    - Adults and teenagers—One applicatorful (approximately 6 grams) inserted into the vagina one or two times a day. Use when you wake up and/or just before you go to bed.
    - Children—Dose must be determined by your doctor.

- For *vaginal suppositories* dosage form:
  —For bacterial infections:
    - Adults and teenagers—One suppository inserted into the vagina one or two times a day for thirty days. Use when you wake up and/or just before you go to bed.
    - Children—Dose must be determined by your doctor.

*For triple sulfa*

- For *vaginal cream* dosage form:
  —For bacterial infections:
    - Adults and teenagers—At first, one applicatorful (approximately 4 to 5 grams) inserted into the vagina two times a day for four to six days. Then, your doctor may lower your dose to one-half to one-quarter applicatorful two times a day. Use when you wake up and just before you go to bed.
    - Children—Dose must be determined by your doctor.
- For *vaginal tablets* dosage form:
  —For bacterial infections:
    - Adults and teenagers—One tablet inserted into the vagina two times a day for ten days. Use when you wake up and just before you go to bed.
    - Children—Dose must be determined by your doctor.

**Missed dose**—If you miss a dose of this medicine, insert it as soon as possible. However, if it is almost time for your next dose, skip the missed dose and go back to your regular dosing schedule.

**Storage**—To store this medicine:

- Keep out of the reach of children.
- Store away from heat and direct light.
- Do not store the vaginal tablet or vaginal suppository form of this medicine in the bathroom, near the kitchen sink, or in other damp places. Heat or moisture may cause the medicine to break down.
- Keep the vaginal cream and vaginal suppository forms of this medicine from freezing.
- Do not keep outdated medicine or medicine no longer needed. Be sure that any discarded medicine is out of the reach of children.

## Precautions While Using This Medicine

If your symptoms do not improve within a few days, or if they become worse, check with your doctor.

Vaginal medicines usually will slowly work their way out of the vagina during treatment. Also, aminacrine-containing vaginal sulfonamides may stain underclothing. To keep the medicine from soiling or staining your clothing, a sanitary napkin may be worn. Minipads, clean paper tissues, or paper diapers may also be used. However, the use of tampons is not recommended since they may soak up too much of the medicine. In addition, tampons may be more likely to slip out of the vagina if you use them during treatment with this medicine.

*To help clear up your infection completely and to help make sure it does not return, good health habits are also required.*

- Wear cotton panties (or panties or pantyhose with cotton crotches) instead of synthetic (for example, nylon or rayon) underclothes.
- Wear only freshly washed underclothes.

If you have any questions about this, check with your health care professional.

Many vaginal infections are spread by sexual intercourse. The male sexual partner may carry the fungus or other organism in his reproductive tract. Therefore, it may be desirable that your partner wear a condom (prophylactic) during intercourse to keep the infection from returning. Also, it may be necessary for your partner to be treated at the same time you are being treated to avoid passing the infection back and forth. In addition, *do not stop using this medicine if you have intercourse during treatment.*

Some patients who use vaginal medicines may prefer to use a douche for cleansing purposes before inserting the next dose of medicine. Some doctors recommend a vinegar and water or other douche. However, others do not recommend douching at all. If you do use a douche, *do not overfill the vagina with douche solution.* To do so may force the solution up into the uterus (womb) and may cause inflammation or infection. Also, *do not douche if you are pregnant since this may harm the fetus.* If you have any questions about this or which douche products are best for you, check with your health care professional.

## Side Effects of This Medicine

Studies in rats have shown that long-term use of sulfonamides may cause cancer of the thyroid gland. In addition, studies in rats have shown that sulfonamides may increase the chance of goiters (noncancerous tumors of the thyroid gland).

Along with its needed effects, a medicine may cause some unwanted effects. Although not all of these side effects may occur, if they do occur they may need medical attention.

*Check with your doctor immediately* if any of the following side effects occur:

*Less common*
Itching, burning, skin rash, redness, swelling, or other sign of irritation not present before use of this medicine

Other side effects may occur that usually do not need medical attention. These side effects may go away during treatment as your body adjusts to the medicine. However, check with your doctor if either of the following side effects continues or is bothersome:

*Less common or rare*
Rash or irritation of penis of sexual partner

Other side effects not listed above may also occur in some patients. If you notice any other effects, check with your doctor.

Revised: 07/22/92
Interim revision: 06/15/94

# SULFONAMIDES AND PHENAZOPYRIDINE Systemic

Some commonly used brand names are:

**In the U.S.—**
Azo Gantanol[1]
Azo Gantrisin[2]
Azo-Sulfamethoxazole[1]

Azo-Sulfisoxazole[2]
Azo-Truxazole[2]
Sul-Azo[2]

**In Canada—**
Azo Gantrisin[2]

Note: For quick reference, the following sulfonamides and phenazopyridine combinations are numbered to match the corresponding brand names.

This information applies to the following medicines:

1. Sulfamethoxazole (sul-fa-meth-OX-a-zole) and Phenazopyridine (fen-az-oh-PEER-i-deen)[†‡]
2. Sulfisoxazole (sul-fi-SOX-a-zole) and Phenazopyridine[‡]

[†]Not commercially available in Canada.
[‡]Generic name product may also be available in the U.S.

## Description

Sulfonamides and phenazopyridine, combination products containing a sulfa medicine and a urinary pain reliever, are used to treat infections of the urinary tract and to help relieve the pain, burning, and irritation of these infections.

Sulfonamides and phenazopyridine combinations are available only with your doctor's prescription, in the following dosage forms:

*Oral*
Sulfamethoxazole and Phenazopyridine
- Tablets (U.S.)
Sulfisoxazole and Phenazopyridine
- Tablets (U.S. and Canada)

## Before Using This Medicine

In deciding to use a medicine, the risks of taking the medicine must be weighed against the good it will do. This is a decision you and your doctor will make. For sulfonamides and phenazopyridine, the following should be considered:

**Allergies—**Tell your doctor if you have ever had any unusual or allergic reaction to any of the sulfa medicines, furosemide (e.g., Lasix) or thiazide diuretics (water pills), oral antidiabetics (diabetes medicine you take by mouth), glaucoma medicine you take by mouth (for example, acetazolamide [e.g., Diamox], dichlorphenamide [e.g., Daranide], or methazolamide [e.g., Neptazane]), or phenazopyridine (e.g., Pyridium). Also tell your health care professional if you are allergic to any other substances, such as foods, preservatives, or dyes.

**Pregnancy**—Studies have not been done in humans. Studies in mice, rats, and rabbits have shown that some sulfonamides cause birth defects, including cleft palate and bone problems. In addition, sulfa medicines may cause liver problems in newborn infants. Therefore, use is not recommended during pregnancy. Phenazopyridine has not been shown to cause birth defects in animal studies.

**Breast-feeding**—Sulfonamides pass into the breast milk. This medicine is not recommended for use during breast-feeding. It may cause liver problems, anemia, and other unwanted effects in nursing babies, especially those with glucose-6-phosphate dehydrogenase (G6PD) deficiency.

**Children**—This medicine has been tested in a limited number of children 12 years of age or older. In effective doses, the medicine has not been shown to cause different side effects or problems in children than it does in adults.

**Older adults**—Elderly people are especially sensitive to the effects of sulfonamides. Severe skin problems and blood problems may be more likely to occur in the elderly. These problems may also be more likely to occur in patients who are taking diuretics (water pills) along with this medicine.

**Other medicines**—Although certain medicines should not be used together at all, in other cases two different medicines may be used together even if an interaction might occur. In these cases, your doctor may want to change the dose, or other precautions may be necessary. When you are taking sulfonamides and phenazopyridine, it is especially important that your health care professional know if you are taking any of the following:

- Acetaminophen (e.g., Tylenol) (with long-term, high-dose use) or
- Amiodarone (e.g., Cordarone) or
- Anabolic steroids (nandrolone [e.g., Anabolin], oxandrolone [e.g., Anavar], oxymetholone [e.g., Anadrol], stanozolol [e.g., Winstrol]) or
- Androgens (male hormones) or
- Antithyroid agents (medicine for overactive thyroid) or
- Carbamazepine (e.g., Tegretol) or
- Carmustine (e.g., BiCNU) or
- Chloroquine (e.g., Aralen) or
- Dantrolene (e.g., Dantrium) or
- Daunorubicin (e.g., Cerubidine) or
- Disulfiram (e.g., Antabuse) or
- Divalproex (e.g., Depakote) or
- Estrogens (female hormones) or
- Etretinate (e.g., Tegison) or
- Gold salts (medicine for arthritis) or
- Hydroxychloroquine (e.g., Plaquenil) or
- Mercaptopurine (e.g., Purinethol) or
- Naltrexone (e.g., Trexan) (with long-term, high-dose use) or

- Oral contraceptives (birth control pills) containing estrogen or
- Other anti-infectives by mouth or by injection (medicine for infection) or
- Phenothiazines (acetophenazine [e.g., Tindal], chlorpromazine [e.g., Thorazine], fluphenazine [e.g., Prolixin], mesoridazine [e.g., Serentil], perphenazine [e.g., Trilafon], prochlorperazine [e.g., Compazine], promazine [e.g., Sparine], promethazine [e.g., Phenergan], thioridazine [e.g., Mellaril], trifluoperazine [e.g., Stelazine], triflupromazine [e.g., Vesprin], trimeprazine [e.g., Temaril]) or
- Plicamycin (e.g., Mithracin) or
- Valproic acid (e.g., Depakene)—Use of sulfonamides and phenazopyridine combination with these medicines may increase the chance of side effects affecting the liver
- Acetohydroxamic acid (e.g., Lithostat) or
- Dapsone or
- Furazolidone (e.g., Furoxone) or
- Nitrofurantoin (e.g., Furadantin) or
- Primaquine or
- Procainamide (e.g., Pronestyl) or
- Quinidine (e.g., Quinidex) or
- Quinine (e.g., Quinamm) or
- Sulfoxone (e.g., Diasone) or
- Vitamin K (e.g., AquaMEPHYTON, Synkayvite)—Use of sulfonamides and phenazopyridine combination with these medicines may increase the chance of side effects affecting the blood
- Anticoagulants (blood thinners) or
- Ethotoin (e.g., Peganone) or
- Heparin or
- Mephenytoin (e.g., Mesantoin)—Use of sulfonamides and phenazopyridine combination with these medicines may increase the chance of side effects of these medicines
- Antidiabetics, oral (diabetes medicine you take by mouth)—Use of oral antidiabetics with sulfonamides and phenazopyridine combination may increase the chance of side effects affecting the blood and/or the side effects of oral antidiabetics
- Methenamine (e.g., Mandelamine) or
- Methenamine-containing medicines (e.g., Urised)—Use of these medicines with sulfonamides and phenazopyridine combination may increase the chance of side effects of the sulfonamides
- Methotrexate (e.g., Mexate)—Use of methotrexate with sulfonamides and phenazopyridine combination may increase the chance of side effects affecting the liver and/or the side effects of methotrexate
- Methyldopa (e.g., Aldomet)—Use of methyldopa with sulfonamides and phenazopyridine combination may increase the chance of side effects affecting the liver and/or the blood
- Phenytoin (e.g., Dilantin)—Use of phenytoin with sulfonamides and phenazopyridine combination may increase the chance of side effects affecting the liver and/or the side effects of phenytoin

**Other medical problems**—The presence of other medical problems may affect the use of sulfonamides and phenazopyridine. Make sure you tell your doctor if you have any other medical problems, especially:

- Anemia or other blood problems or
- Glucose-6-phosphate dehydrogenase deficiency (lack of G6PD enzyme)—Patients with these problems may have an increase in side effects affecting the blood

- Hepatitis or other liver disease or
- Kidney disease—Patients with kidney disease or liver disease may have an increased chance of side effects
- Porphyria—Use of sulfonamides may bring on an attack of porphyria

## Proper Use of This Medicine

*Sulfonamides and phenazopyridine combinations are best taken with a full glass (8 ounces) of water. Several additional glasses of water should be taken every day,* unless otherwise directed by your doctor. Drinking extra water will help to prevent some unwanted effects (e.g., kidney stones) of the sulfonamide. This medicine may be taken with meals or following meals if it upsets your stomach.

To help clear up your infection completely, *keep taking this medicine for the full time of treatment,* even if you begin to feel better after a few days. If you stop taking this medicine too soon, your symptoms may return.

This medicine works best when there is a constant amount in the urine. *To help keep the amount constant, do not miss any doses. Also, it is best to take the doses at evenly spaced times, day and night.* For example, if you are to take 4 doses a day, the doses should be spaced about 6 hours apart. If this interferes with your sleep or other daily activities, or if you need help in planning the best times to take your medicine, check with your health care professional.

**Dosing**—The dose of sulfonamides and phenazopyridine combination may be different for different patients. *Follow your doctor's orders or the directions on the label.* The following information includes only the average doses of sulfonamides and phenazopyridine combination. Your dose may be different if you have kidney disease. *If your dose is different, do not change it* unless your doctor tells you to do so.

- For *sulfamethoxazole and phenazopyridine combination*:
  —Adults and children 12 years of age and older: 2 grams of sulfamethoxazole and 400 mg of phenazopyridine for the first dose, then 1 gram of sulfamethoxazole and 200 mg of phenazopyridine every twelve hours for up to two days.
  —Children up to 12 years of age: This medication is not recommended.
- For *sulfisoxazole and phenazopyridine combination*:
  —Adults and children 12 years of age and older: 2 to 3 grams of sulfisoxazole and 200 to 300 mg of phenazopyridine for the first dose, then 1 gram of sulfisoxazole and 100 mg of phenazopyridine every twelve hours for up to two days.
  —Children up to 12 years of age: This medication is not recommended.

**Missed dose**—If you miss a dose of this medicine, take it as soon as possible. This will help to keep a constant amount of medicine in the urine. However, if it is almost time for your next dose, skip the missed dose and go back to your regular dosing schedule. Do not double doses.

**Storage**—To store this medicine:
- Keep out of the reach of children.
- Store away from heat and direct light.
- Do not store in the bathroom, near the kitchen sink, or in other damp places. Heat or moisture may cause the medicine to break down.
- Do not keep outdated medicine or medicine no longer needed. Be sure that any discarded medicine is out of the reach of children.

## Precautions While Using This Medicine

If your symptoms do not improve within a few days, or if they become worse, check with your doctor.

Sulfonamides may cause blood problems. These problems may result in a greater chance of certain infections, slow healing, and bleeding of the gums. Therefore, you should be careful when using regular toothbrushes, dental floss, and toothpicks. Dental work should be delayed until your blood counts have returned to normal. Check with your medical doctor or dentist if you have any questions about proper oral hygiene (mouth care) during treatment.

Sulfonamides may cause your skin to be more sensitive to sunlight than it is normally. Exposure to sunlight, even for brief periods of time, may cause a skin rash, itching, redness or other discoloration of the skin, or a severe sunburn. When you begin taking this medicine:

- Stay out of direct sunlight, especially between the hours of 10:00 a.m. and 3:00 p.m., if possible.
- Wear protective clothing, including a hat. Also, wear sunglasses.
- Apply a sun block product that has a skin protection factor (SPF) of at least 15. Some patients may require a product with a higher SPF number, especially if they have a fair complexion. If you have any questions about this, check with your health care professional.
- Apply a sun block lipstick that has an SPF of at least 15 to protect your lips.
- Do not use a sunlamp or tanning bed or booth.

*If you have a severe reaction, check with your doctor.*

This medicine may also cause some people to become dizzy. *Make sure you know how you react to this medicine before you drive, use machines, or do anything else that could be dangerous if you are dizzy or are not alert.* If this reaction is especially bothersome, check with your doctor.

*This medicine causes the urine to turn reddish orange.* This is to be expected while you are using this medicine and is not harmful. Also, the medicine may stain clothing. If you have any questions about removing the stain, check with your health care professional.

For diabetic patients:

- *This medicine may cause false test results with some urine sugar tests and urine ketone tests.* Check with your doctor before changing your diet or the dosage of your diabetes medicine.

## Side Effects of This Medicine

Along with its needed effects, a medicine may cause some unwanted effects. Although not all of these side effects may occur, if they do occur they may need medical attention.

*Check with your doctor immediately* if any of the following side effects occur:

*More common*
> Itching; skin rash

*Less common*
> Aching of joints and muscles; blue or blue-purple discoloration of skin; difficulty in swallowing; pale skin; redness, blistering, peeling, or loosening of skin; shortness of breath; sore throat and fever; unusual bleeding or bruising; unusual tiredness or weakness; yellow eyes or skin

*Rare*
> Blood in urine; greatly increased or decreased frequency of urination or amount of urine; increased thirst; lower back pain; pain or burning while urinating; swelling of front part of neck

In addition to the side effects listed above, check with your doctor as soon as possible if the following side effect occurs:

*More common*
> Increased sensitivity of skin to sunlight

Other side effects may occur that usually do not need medical attention. These side effects may go away during treatment as your body adjusts to the medicine. However, check with your doctor if any of the following side effects continue or are bothersome:

*More common*
> Diarrhea; dizziness; headache; loss of appetite; nausea or vomiting; tiredness

*Less common*
> Indigestion; stomach cramps or pain

This medicine causes the urine to become reddish orange. This side effect does not require medical attention.

Other side effects not listed above may also occur in some patients. If you notice any other effects, check with your doctor.

Revised: 02/01/93

---

# SULFUR    Topical

Some commonly used brand names are:

**In the U.S.—**

| | |
|---|---|
| Cuticura Ointment | Fostril Lotion |
| Finac | Lotio Alsulfa |
| Fostex Regular Strength Medicated Cover-Up | Sulpho-Lac |

Generic name product may also be available.

**In Canada—**

| | |
|---|---|
| Fostex CM | Fostril Cream |

Generic name product may also be available.

## Description

Sulfur (SUL-fur) is used to treat many kinds of skin disorders. Sulfur cream, lotion, ointment, and bar soap are used to treat acne. Sulfur ointment is used to treat seborrheic dermatitis and scabies. Sulfur may also be used for other conditions as determined by your doctor.

Some of these preparations are available only with your doctor's prescription. Others are available without a prescription; however, your doctor may have special instructions on the proper use of sulfur for your medical condition.

Sulfur is available in the following dosage forms:

*Topical*
- Cream (U.S. and Canada)
- Lotion (U.S.)
- Ointment (U.S.)
- Bar soap (U.S. and Canada)

## Before Using This Medicine

If you are using this medicine without a prescription, carefully read and follow any precautions on the label. For topical sulfur preparations, the following should be considered:

**Allergies**—Tell your doctor if you have ever had any unusual or allergic reaction to sulfur. Also tell your health care professional if you are allergic to any other substances, such as preservatives or dyes.

**Pregnancy**—Topical sulfur has not been shown to cause birth defects or other problems in humans.

**Breast-feeding**—Topical sulfur has not been reported to cause problems in nursing babies.

**Children**—Although there is no specific information comparing use of this medicine in children with use in other age groups, this medicine is not expected to cause different side effects or problems in children than it does in adults.

**Older adults**—Many medicines have not been studied specifically in older people. Therefore, it may not be known whether they work exactly the same way they do in younger adults or if they cause different side effects or problems in older people. Although there is no specific information comparing use of sulfur in the elderly with use in other age groups, this medicine is not expected to cause different side effects or problems in older people than it does in younger adults.

**Other medicines**—Although certain medicines should not be used together at all, in other cases two different medicines may be used together even if an interaction might occur. In these cases, your doctor may want to change the dose, or other precautions may be necessary. Tell your health care professional if you are using any other topical prescription or nonprescription (over-the-counter [OTC]) medicine that is to be applied to the same area of the skin.

## Proper Use of This Medicine

*Use this medicine only as directed.* Do not use it more often and do not use it for a longer period of time than recommended on the label, unless otherwise directed by your doctor.

*Keep this medicine away from the eyes.* If you should accidentally get some in your eyes, flush them thoroughly with water.

To use the *cream or lotion form* of this medicine:

- Before applying the medicine, wash the affected areas with soap and water and dry thoroughly. Then apply enough medicine to cover the affected areas and rub in gently.

To use the *ointment form* of this medicine for *seborrheic dermatitis:*

- Before applying the medicine, wash the affected areas with soap and water and dry thoroughly. Then apply enough medicine to cover the affected areas and rub in gently.

To use the *ointment form* of this medicine for *scabies:*

- Before applying the medicine, wash your entire body with soap and water and dry thoroughly.
- At bedtime, apply enough medicine to cover your entire body from the neck down and rub in gently. Leave the medicine on your body for 24 hours.
- Before applying the medicine again, you may wash your entire body.
- 24 hours after the last treatment with this medicine, it is important that you thoroughly wash your entire body again.

To use the *soap form* of this medicine:

- Work up a rich lather with the soap, using warm water. Wash the affected areas and rinse thoroughly.

Apply again, and rub in gently for a few minutes. Remove excess lather with a towel or tissue without rinsing.

**Dosing**—The dose of topical sulfur will be different for different patients. *Follow your doctor's orders or the directions on the label.* The following information includes only the average doses of topical sulfur. *If your dose is different, do not change it* unless your doctor tells you to do so.

- For acne:
  —For *cream and bar soap* dosage forms:
    - Adults and children—Use on the skin as needed.
  —For *lotion* dosage form:
    - Adults and children—Use two or three times a day.
  —For *ointment* dosage form:
    - Adults and children—Use the 0.5% ointment on the skin as needed.
- For seborrheic dermatitis:
  —For *ointment* dosage form:
    - Adults and children—Use the 5 to 10% ointment one or two times a day.
- For scabies:
  —For *ointment* dosage form:
    - Adults and children—Use the 6% ointment each night for three nights.

**Missed dose**—If you miss a dose of this medicine, use it as soon as possible. However, if it is almost time for your next dose, skip the missed dose and go back to your regular dosing schedule.

**Storage**—To store this medicine:

- Keep out of the reach of children.
- Store away from heat and direct light.
- Keep the cream, lotion, and ointment forms of this medicine from freezing.
- Do not keep outdated medicine or medicine no longer needed. Be sure that any discarded medicine is out of the reach of children.

## Precautions While Using This Medicine

*When using sulfur, do not use any of the following preparations on the same affected area as this medicine,* unless otherwise directed by your doctor:

Abrasive soaps or cleansers
Alcohol-containing preparations
Any other topical acne preparation or preparation containing a peeling agent (for example, benzoyl peroxide, resorcinol, salicylic acid, or tretinoin [vitamin A acid])
Cosmetics or soaps that dry the skin
Medicated cosmetics
Other topical medicine for the skin

To use any of the above preparations on the same affected area as sulfur may cause severe irritation of the skin.

*Do not use any topical mercury-containing preparation, such as ammoniated mercury ointment, on the same area as this medicine*. To do so may cause a foul odor, may be irritating to the skin, and may stain the skin black. If you have any questions about this, check with your health care professional.

## Side Effects of This Medicine

Along with its needed effects, a medicine may cause some unwanted effects. Although not all of these side effects may occur, if they do occur they may need medical attention.

Check with your doctor as soon as possible if the following side effect occurs:

Skin irritation not present before use of this medicine

Other side effects may occur that usually do not need medical attention. However, check with your health care professional if the following side effect continues or is bothersome:

Redness and peeling of skin (may occur after a few days)

Other side effects not listed above may also occur in some patients. If you notice any other effects, check with your health care professional.

Revised: 10/28/93

---

# SULFURATED LIME    Topical

Some commonly used brand names are:
**In the U.S.—**
Vlemasque
Generic name product may also be available.
**In Canada—**
Vlemasque
Another commonly used name is Vleminckx's solution.

## Description

Sulfurated (SUL-fur-ay-ted) lime is used to treat acne, scabies, and other skin disorders, such as seborrheic dermatitis and pustular infections.

This medicine is available without a prescription; however, your doctor may have special instructions on the proper use of this medicine for your medical problem.

Sulfurated lime is available in the following dosage forms:

*Topical*
- Mask (U.S. and Canada)
- Topical solution (U.S.)

## Before Using This Medicine

If you are using this medicine without a prescription, carefully read and follow any precautions on the label. For sulfurated lime, the following should be considered:

**Allergies**—Tell your doctor if you have ever had any unusual or allergic reaction to sulfurated lime. Also tell your health care professional if you are allergic to any other substances, such as preservatives or dyes.

**Pregnancy**—Sulfurated lime has not been shown to cause birth defects or other problems in humans.

**Breast-feeding**—Sulfurated lime has not been reported to cause problems in nursing babies.

**Children**—Although there is no specific information comparing use of sulfurated lime in children with use in other

age groups, this medicine is not expected to cause different side effects or problems in children than it does in adults.

**Older adults**—Many medicines have not been studied specifically in older people. Therefore, it may not be known whether they work exactly the same way they do in younger adults or if they cause different side effects or problems in older people. There is no specific information comparing use of sulfurated lime in the elderly with use in other age groups.

**Other medicines**—Although certain medicines should not be used together at all, in other cases two different medicines may be used together even if an interaction might occur. In these cases, your doctor may want to change the dose, or other precautions may be necessary. Tell your health care professional if you are using any other topical prescription or nonprescription (over-the-counter [OTC]) medicine that is to be applied to the same area of the skin.

## Proper Use of This Medicine

*Use this medicine only as directed.* Do not use more of it, do not use it more often, and do not use it for a longer period of time than recommended on the label, unless otherwise directed by your doctor.

*Keep this medicine away from the eyes.* If you should accidentally get some in your eyes, flush them thoroughly with water.

To use the *topical solution form* of sulfurated lime for wet dressings, as a soak, or in a bath:

- Sulfurated lime solution must be diluted before you use it on your skin for wet dressings, as a soak, or in a bath. The directions may say to dilute to 1:9 or 1:32. To dilute to 1:9 means that for every 1 part of sulfurated lime you add 9 parts of water. (If you are using cupfuls, for example, you would add 9 cupfuls of water to 1 cupful of sulfurated lime.) In the same way, if the directions say 1:32, for every 1 part of sulfurated lime you add 32 parts of water. Make sure you understand exactly how you should use this solution. If you have any questions about this, check with your health care professional.

- Before diluting and/or applying this solution, remove all jewelry and metallic ornaments, since the solution may discolor metals. Also, avoid getting this solution on metal spoons or bath fixtures.

To use the *mask form* of sulfurated lime:

- Apply a generous amount of this medicine over the entire face and neck, unless otherwise directed by your doctor.
- Allow the medicine to remain on the affected areas for 20 to 25 minutes.
- Remove the medicine with lukewarm water, using a gentle circular motion. Then, pat the skin dry.

**Dosing**—The dose of sulfurated lime will be different for different patients. *Follow your doctor's orders or the directions on the label.* The following information includes only the average doses of sulfurated lime. *If your dose is different, do not change it* unless your doctor tells you to do so.

- For *mask* dosage form:
  —For acne:
    - Adults and children—Use once a day.
- For *topical solution* dosage form:
  —For acne, seborrheic dermatitis, and pustular infections:
    - Adults and children—Use as a diluted solution (1:32 to 1:9) one or two times a day.
  —For scabies:
    - Adults and children—Use as a diluted solution (1:9) one or two times a day for three days.

**Missed dose**—If you miss a dose of this medicine, apply it as soon as possible. However, if it is almost time for your next dose, skip the missed dose and go back to your regular dosing schedule.

**Storage**—To store this medicine:

- Keep out of the reach of children.
- Store away from heat and direct light.
- Keep the medicine from freezing.
- Do not keep outdated medicine or medicine no longer needed. Be sure that any discarded medicine is out of the reach of children.

## Precautions While Using This Medicine

*When using sulfurated lime, do not use any of the following preparations on the same affected area as this medicine,* unless otherwise directed by your doctor:

    Abrasive soaps or cleansers
    Alcohol-containing preparations
    Any other topical acne preparation or preparation containing a peeling agent (for example, benzoyl peroxide, resorcinol, salicylic acid, sulfur, or tretinoin [vitamin A acid])
    Cosmetics or soaps that dry the skin
    Medicated cosmetics
    Other topical medicine for the skin

To use any of the above preparations on the same affected area as sulfurated lime may cause severe irritation of the skin.

*Do not use any topical mercury-containing preparation, such as ammoniated mercury ointment on the same affected area as this medicine.* To do so may cause a foul odor, may be irritating to the skin, and may stain the skin black. If you have any questions about this, check with your doctor.

## Side Effects of This Medicine

Along with its needed effects, a medicine may cause some unwanted effects. Although not all of these side effects may occur, if they do occur they may need medical attention.

Check with your doctor as soon as possible if the following side effect occurs:

    Skin irritation not present before use of this medicine

Other side effects may occur that usually do not need medical attention. However, check with your health care professional if the following side effects continue or are bothersome:

    Redness and peeling of skin (may occur after a few days); unusual dryness of skin

Other side effects not listed above may also occur in some patients. If you notice any other effects, check with your health care professional.

Revised: 09/28/93

# SUMATRIPTAN  Systemic

A commonly used brand name in the U.S. and Canada is Imitrex.

## Description

Sumatriptan (soo-ma-TRIP-tan) is used to treat severe migraine headaches. Many people find that their headaches go away completely after they take sumatriptan. Other people find that their headaches are much less painful, and that they are able to go back to their normal activities even though their headaches are not completely gone. Sumatriptan often relieves other symptoms that occur together with a migraine headache, such as nausea, vomiting, sensitivity to light, and sensitivity to sound.

Sumatriptan is not an ordinary pain reliever. It will not relieve any kind of pain other than migraine headaches. This medicine is usually used for people whose headaches are not relieved by acetaminophen, aspirin, or other pain relievers.

Sumatriptan is available only with your doctor's prescription, in the following dosage forms:

*Oral*
- Tablets (Canada)

*Parenteral*
- Injection (U.S. and Canada)

## Before Using This Medicine

In deciding to use a medicine, the risks of using the medicine must be weighed against the good it will do. This is a decision you and your doctor will make. For sumatriptan, the following should be considered:

**Allergies**—Tell your doctor if you have ever had any unusual or allergic reaction to sumatriptan. Also tell your health care professional if you are allergic to any other substances, such as foods, preservatives, or dyes.

**Pregnancy**—Sumatriptan has not been studied in pregnant women. However, in some animal studies, sumatriptan caused harmful effects on the fetus. These unwanted effects usually occurred when sumatriptan was given in amounts that were large enough to cause harmful effects in the mother.

**Breast-feeding**—It is not known whether sumatriptan passes into human breast milk. However, it has been found in the breast milk of animals. Breast-feeding mothers should discuss the risks and benefits of this medicine with their doctors.

**Children**—Studies on this medicine have been done only in adult patients, and there is no specific information comparing use of sumatriptan in children with use in other age groups.

**Teenagers**—Studies on this medicine have been done only in patients 18 years of age or older, and there is no specific information comparing use of sumatriptan in younger teenagers with use in other age groups.

**Older adults**—This medicine has been tested in a limited number of patients between 60 and 65 years of age. It did not cause different side effects or problems in these patients than it did in younger adults. However, there is no specific information comparing use of sumatriptan in patients older than 65 years of age with use in younger adults.

**Other medicines**—Although certain medicines should not be used together at all, in other cases two different medicines may be used together even if an interaction might occur. In these cases, your doctor may want to change the dose, or other precautions may be necessary. Tell your health care professional if you are taking any other prescription or nonprescription (over-the-counter [OTC]) medicine, especially other prescription medicine for migraine headaches, or if you smoke tobacco.

**Other medical problems**—The presence of other medical problems may affect the use of sumatriptan. Make sure you tell your doctor if you have any other medical problems, especially:

- Angina (chest pain) or
- Fast or irregular heartbeat or
- Heart or blood vessel disease or
- High blood pressure or
- Kidney disease or
- Liver disease or
- Stroke (history of)—The chance of side effects may be increased

## Proper Use of This Medicine

To relieve your migraine as soon as possible, use sumatriptan at the first sign that the headache is coming. If you get warning signals of a coming migraine (an aura), you may use the medicine before the headache pain actually starts. However, even if you do not use sumatriptan until your migraine has been present for several hours, the medicine will still work.

Lying down in a quiet, dark room for a while after you use this medicine may help relieve your migraine.

If you are not much better in 1 or 2 hours after an injection of sumatriptan, or in 2 to 4 hours after a tablet is taken, *do not use any more of this medicine for the same migraine*. A migraine that is not relieved by the first dose of sumatriptan probably will not be relieved by a second dose, either. Ask your doctor ahead of time about other medicine to be taken if sumatriptan does not work. However, even if sumatriptan does not relieve one migraine, it may still relieve the next one.

If you feel much better after a dose of sumatriptan, but your headache comes back or gets worse after a while, you may use more sumatriptan. However, *use this medicine only as directed by your doctor. Do not use more of it, and do not use it more often, than directed*. Using too much sumatriptan may increase the chance of side effects.

Your doctor may direct you to take another medicine to help prevent headaches. *It is important that you follow your doctor's directions, even if your headaches continue to occur.* Headache-preventing medicines may take several weeks to start working. Even after they do start working, your headaches may not go away completely. However, your headaches should occur less often, and they should be less severe and easier to relieve. This can reduce the amount of sumatriptan or pain relievers that you need. If you do not notice any improvement after several weeks of headache-preventing treatment, check with your doctor.

For patients taking *sumatriptan tablets*:
- Sumatriptan tablets are to be swallowed whole. *Do not break, crush, or chew the tablets before swallowing them.*

For patients using *sumatriptan injection*:
- This medicine comes with patient directions. *Read them carefully before using the medicine,* and check with your health care professional if you have any questions.
- Your health care professional will teach you how to inject yourself with the medicine. *Be sure to follow the directions carefully. Check with your health care professional if you have any problems using the medicine.*
- After you have finished injecting the medicine, be sure to follow the precautions in the patient directions about safely discarding the empty cartridge and the needle. Always return the empty cartridge and needle to their container before discarding them. Do not throw away the autoinjector unit, because refills are available.

**Dosing**—The dose of sumatriptan will be different for different patients. *Follow your doctor's orders or the directions on the label.* The following information includes only the average doses of sumatriptan. *If your dose is different, do not change it* unless your doctor tells you to do so.
- For *oral* dosage form (tablets):
  —For migraine headaches:
   - Adults—One 100-milligram (mg) tablet. Another 100-mg tablet may be taken one or two times more, if necessary, if the migraine comes back after being relieved. *Do not take more than three 100-mg tablets in any twenty-four-hour period.*
   - Children—Use and dose must be determined by your doctor.
- For *parenteral* dosage form (injection):
  —For migraine headaches:
   - Adults—6 mg. One more 6-mg dose may be injected, if necessary, if the migraine comes back after being relieved. However, the second injection should not be given any sooner than one hour after the first one. *Do not use more than two 6-mg injections in forty-eight hours (two days).*
   - Children—Use and dose must be determined by your doctor.

**Storage**—To store this medicine:
- Keep out of the reach of children since overdose is especially dangerous in children.
- Store away from heat and direct light.
- Do not store tablets in the bathroom, near the kitchen sink, or in other damp places. Heat or moisture may cause the medicine to break down.
- Keep the injection form of sumatriptan from freezing.
- Do not keep outdated medicine or medicine no longer needed. Be sure that any discarded medicine is out of the reach of children.

## Precautions While Using This Medicine

Check with your doctor if you have used sumatriptan for 3 headaches, and have not had good relief. Also, check with your doctor if your migraine headaches are worse, or if they are occurring more often, than before you started using sumatriptan.

Drinking alcoholic beverages can make headaches worse or cause new headaches to occur. People who suffer from severe headaches should probably avoid alcoholic beverages, especially during a headache.

Some people feel drowsy or dizzy during or after a migraine, or after taking sumatriptan to relieve a migraine. As long as you are feeling drowsy or dizzy, *do not drive, use machines, or do anything else that could be dangerous if you are dizzy or are not alert.*

## Side Effects of This Medicine

Along with its needed effects, a medicine may cause some unwanted effects. Most side effects of sumatriptan are milder and occur less often with the tablets than with the injection. Although not all of these side effects may occur, if they do occur they may need medical attention.

*Stop using this medicine and check with your doctor immediately if any of the following side effects occur:*
   *Rare*
      Chest pain (severe); swelling of eyelids, face, or lips; wheezing

*Check with your doctor right away if any of the following side effects continue for more than 1 hour.* Even if they go away in less than 1 hour, *check with your doctor before using any more sumatriptan if any of the following side effects occur:*
   *Less common*
      Chest pain (mild); heaviness, tightness, or pressure in chest and/or neck

Also check with your doctor as soon as possible if any of the following side effects occur:
   *Less common*
      Difficulty in swallowing; pounding heartbeat; skin rash or bumps on skin

Other side effects may occur that usually do not need medical attention. Some of the following effects, such as nausea, vomiting, drowsiness, dizziness, and general feeling of illness or tiredness often occur during or after a migraine, even when sumatriptan has not been used. Most of the side effects caused by sumatriptan go away within a short time (less than 1 hour after an injection or 2 hours after a tablet). However, check with your doctor if any of the following side effects continue or are bothersome:

*More common*

Burning, pain, or redness at place of injection; feeling of burning, warmth, heat, numbness, tightness, or tingling; discomfort in jaw, mouth, tongue, throat, nose,

or sinuses; dizziness; drowsiness; feeling cold, "strange," or weak; flushing; lightheadedness; muscle aches, cramps, or stiffness; nausea or vomiting

*Less common or rare*

Anxiety; general feeling of illness or tiredness; vision changes

Other side effects not listed above may also occur in some patients. If you notice any other effects, check with your doctor.

Revised: 07/01/93

# TACRINE Systemic†

A commonly used brand name in the U.S. is Cognex.
Other commonly used names are THA and tetrahydroaminoacridine.

†Not commercially available in Canada.

## Description

Tacrine (TA-crin) is used to treat the symptoms of mild to moderate Alzheimer's disease. Tacrine will not cure Alzheimer's disease, and it will not stop the disease from getting worse. However, tacrine can improve thinking ability in some patients with Alzheimer's disease.

In Alzheimer's disease, many chemical changes take place in the brain. One of the earliest and biggest changes is that there is less of a chemical messenger called acetylcholine (ACh). ACh helps the brain to work properly. Tacrine slows the breakdown of ACh, so it can build up and have a greater effect. However, as Alzheimer's disease gets worse, there will be less and less ACh, so tacrine may not work as well.

Tacrine may cause liver problems. You must have blood tests regularly while taking this medicine to see if the medicine is affecting your liver.

This medicine is available only with your doctor's prescription, in the following dosage form:

*Oral*
- Capsules (U.S.)

## Before Using This Medicine

In deciding to use a medicine, the risks of taking the medicine must be weighed against the good it will do. This is a decision you and your doctor will make. For tacrine the following should be considered:

**Allergies**—Tell your doctor if you have ever had any unusual or allergic reaction to tacrine or to wound antiseptics (e.g., Akrinol, Panflavin, Monacrin). Also tell your health care professional if you are allergic to any other substances, such as foods, preservatives, or dyes.

**Pregnancy**—Studies on effects in pregnancy have not been done in either humans or animals.

**Breast-feeding**—It is not known whether tacrine passes into breast milk. However, use of tacrine is not recommended in nursing mothers.

**Older adults**—Studies on tacrine have been done only in middle-aged and older patients. Information on the effects of tacrine is based on these patients.

**Other medicines**—Although certain medicines should not be used together at all, in other cases two different medicines may be used together even if an interaction might occur. In these cases, your doctor may want to change the dose, or other precautions may be necessary. When you are taking tacrine, it is especially important that your health care professional know if you are taking any of the following:

- Cimetidine (e.g., Tagamet)—Cimetidine may cause higher blood levels of tacrine, which may increase the chance of side effects
- Inflammation or pain medicine, except narcotics—Stomach irritation may be increased
- Neuromuscular blocking agents (medicines used in surgery to relax muscles)—Tacrine may increase the effects of these medicines; your doctor may change the dose of tacrine before you have surgery.
- Smoking tobacco—Smoking may cause lower blood levels of tacrine, which may decrease the effects of tacrine; if you smoke, your doctor may need to change the dose of tacrine
- Theophylline (e.g., Theo-Dur, Uniphyl)—Tacrine may cause higher blood levels of theophylline, which may increase the chance of side effects; your doctor may need to change the dose of theophylline

**Other medical problems**—The presence of other medical problems may affect the use of tacrine. Make sure you tell your doctor if you have any other medical problems, especially:

- Asthma (or history of) or
- Heart problems, including slow heartbeat or hypotension (low blood pressure), or
- Intestinal blockage or
- Liver disease (or history of) or
- Parkinson's disease or
- Stomach ulcer (or history of) or
- Urinary tract blockage or difficult urination—Tacrine may make these conditions worse
- Brain disease, other, or
- Epilepsy or history of seizures or
- Head injury with loss of consciousness—Tacrine may cause seizures

## Proper Use of This Medicine

*Take this medicine only as directed by your doctor.* Do not take more or less of it, and do not take it more or less often than your doctor ordered. Taking too much may increase the chance of side effects, while taking too little may not improve your condition.

Tacrine is best taken on an empty stomach (1 hour before or 2 hours after meals). However, if this medicine upsets your stomach, your doctor may want you to take it with food.

Tacrine seems to work best when it is taken at regularly spaced times, usually four times a day.

**Dosing**—The dose of tacrine will be different for different patients. *Follow your doctor's orders or the directions on the label.* The following information includes only the average doses of tacrine. *If your dose is different, do not change it* unless your doctor tells you to do so.

* For *oral* dosage form (capsules):
  —For treatment of Alzheimer's disease:
  * Adults—To start, 10 milligrams (mg) four times a day. Your doctor may increase your dose gradually if you are doing well on this medicine and your liver tests are normal. However, the dose is usually not more than 40 mg four times a day.

**Missed dose**—If you miss a dose of this medicine, take it as soon as possible. However, if it is within 2 hours of your next dose, skip the missed dose and go back to your regular dosing schedule. Do not double doses.

**Storage**—To store this medicine:
* Keep out of the reach of children.
* Store away from heat and direct light.
* Do not store in the bathroom, near the kitchen sink, or in other damp places. Heat or moisture may cause the medicine to break down.
* Do not keep outdated medicine or medicine no longer needed. Be sure that any discarded medicine is out of the reach of children.

---

## Precautions While Using This Medicine

It is important that your doctor check your progress at regular visits. Also, you must have your blood tested every week for at least 18 weeks when you first start using tacrine, and every week for at least 6 weeks every time your dose is increased to see if this medicine is affecting your liver. If all of these blood tests are normal, you will still need regular testing, but then your doctor may decide to do the tests less often.

Tell your doctor if your symptoms get worse, or if you notice any new symptoms.

Before you have any kind of surgery, dental treatment, or emergency treatment, tell the medical doctor or dentist in charge that you are taking this medicine. Taking tacrine together with medicines that are sometimes used during surgery or dental or emergency treatments may increase the effects of these medicines.

Tacrine may cause some people to become dizzy, clumsy, or unsteady. Make sure you know how you react to this medicine before you do anything that could be dangerous if you are dizzy, clumsy, or unsteady.

*Do not stop taking this medicine or decrease your dose without first checking with your doctor.* Stopping this medicine suddenly or decreasing the dose by a large amount may cause mental or behavior changes.

If you think you or someone else may have taken an overdose of tacrine, get emergency help at once. Taking an overdose of tacrine may lead to seizures or shock. Some signs of shock are large pupils, irregular breathing, and fast weak pulse. Other signs of an overdose are severe nausea and vomiting, increasing muscle weakness, greatly increased sweating, and greatly increased watering of the mouth.

## Side Effects of This Medicine

Along with its needed effects, a medicine may cause some unwanted effects. Some side effects will have signs or symptoms that you can see or feel. Your doctor may watch for others by doing certain tests

Tacrine may cause some serious side effects, including liver problems. You and your doctor should discuss the good this medicine will do as well as the risks of receiving it.

*Check with your doctor as soon as possible if any of the following side effects occur:*

*More common*
Clumsiness or unsteadiness; diarrhea; loss of appetite; nausea; vomiting

*Less common*
Fainting; fast or pounding heartbeat; fever; high or low blood pressure; skin rash; slow heartbeat

*Rare*
Aggression, irritability, or nervousness; change in stool color; convulsions (seizures); cough, tightness in chest, troubled breathing, or wheezing; stiffness of arms or legs, slow movement, or trembling and shaking of hands and fingers; trouble in urinating; yellow eyes or skin

*Symptoms of overdose*
Convulsions (seizures); greatly increased sweating; greatly increased watering of mouth; increasing muscle weakness; low blood pressure; nausea (severe); shock (fast weak pulse, irregular breathing, large pupils); slow heartbeat; vomiting (severe)

This medicine may also cause the following side effect that your doctor will watch for:

*More common*
Liver problems

Other side effects may occur that usually do not need medical attention. These side effects may go away during treatment as your body adjusts to the medicine. However, check with your doctor if any of the following side effects continue or are bothersome:

*More common*
Abdominal or stomach pain or cramping; dizziness; headache; indigestion; muscle aches or pain

*Less common*
Belching; fast breathing; flushing of skin; general feeling of discomfort or illness; increased sweating; increased urination; increased watering of eyes; increased watering of mouth; runny nose; swelling of feet or lower legs; trouble in sleeping

Other side effects not listed above may also occur in some patients. If you notice any other effects, check with your doctor.

---

Developed: 08/05/94

---

© 1994   The United States Pharmacopeial Convention, Inc.

# TAMOXIFEN   Systemic

Some commonly used brand names are:

**In the U.S.—**
    Nolvadex

**In Canada—**

| | |
|---|---|
| Alpha-Tamoxifen | Novo-Tamoxifen |
| Med Tamoxifen | Tamofen |
| Nolvadex | Tamone |
| Nolvadex-D | Tamoplex |

## Description

Tamoxifen (ta-MOX-i-fen) is a medicine that blocks the effects of the hormone estrogen in the body. It is used to treat breast cancer in women or men.

The exact way that tamoxifen works against cancer is not known but it may be related to the way it blocks the effects of estrogen on the body.

Before you begin treatment with tamoxifen, you and your doctor should talk about the good this medicine will do as well as the risks of using it.

Tamoxifen is available only with your doctor's prescription, in the following dosage forms:

*Oral*
- Tablets (U.S. and Canada)
- Enteric-coated tablets (Canada)

## Before Using This Medicine

In deciding to use a medicine, the risks of taking the medicine must be weighed against the good it will do. This is a decision you and your doctor will make. For tamoxifen, the following should be considered:

**Allergies**—Tell your doctor if you have ever had any unusual or allergic reaction to tamoxifen.

**Pregnancy**—Tell your doctor if you are pregnant or if you intend to become pregnant. Tamoxifen use in women has been shown to cause miscarriages, birth defects, death of the fetus, and vaginal bleeding. Studies in rats and rabbits have also shown that tamoxifen causes miscarriages, death of the fetus, and slowed learning. Studies in animals have also shown that tamoxifen may cause some of the same problems as an estrogen called diethylstilbestrol (DES). DES causes genital tract problems and, rarely, an increased risk of cancer of the cervix or vagina in daughters of women who took it during their pregnancy; it is not known whether tamoxifen causes these same problems.

Be sure that you have discussed this with your doctor before taking this medicine. It is best to use some kind of birth control while you are taking tamoxifen and for about two months after you stop taking it. However, do not use oral contraceptives ("the Pill") since they may interfere with this medicine. Tell your doctor right away if you think you have become pregnant while taking tamoxifen.

**Breast-feeding**—Because this medicine may cause serious side effects, breast-feeding is generally not recommended while you are taking it.

**Older adults**—Many medicines have not been studied specifically in older people. Therefore, it may not be known whether they work exactly the same way they do in younger adults. Although there is no specific information comparing use of tamoxifen in the elderly with use in other age groups, this medicine is not expected to cause different side effects or problems in older people than it does in younger adults.

**Other medicines**—Although certain medicines should not be used together at all, in other cases two different medicines may be used together even if an interaction might occur. In these cases, your doctor may want to change the dose, or other precautions may be necessary. Tell your health care professional if you are taking any other prescription or nonprescription (over-the-counter [OTC]) medicine.

**Other medical problems**—The presence of other medical problems may affect the use of tamoxifen. Make sure you tell your doctor if you have any other medical problems, especially:
- Cataracts or other eye problems—Tamoxifen may also cause these problems
- High cholesterol levels in the blood—Tamoxifen can increase cholesterol levels

## Proper Use of This Medicine

*Use this medicine only as directed by your doctor.* Do not use more or less of it, and do not use it more often than your doctor ordered. The exact amount of medicine you need has been carefully worked out. Taking too much may increase the chance of side effects, while taking too little may not improve your condition.

For patients taking *enteric-coated tamoxifen tablets:*
- The tablets must be swallowed whole. Do not crush them or break them up before taking.

Tamoxifen sometimes causes mild nausea and vomiting. However, it may have to be taken for several weeks or months to be effective. Even if you begin to feel ill, *do not stop using this medicine without first checking with your doctor.* Ask your health care professional for ways to lessen these effects.

If you vomit shortly after taking a dose of tamoxifen, check with your doctor. You will be told whether to take the dose again or to wait until the next scheduled dose.

**Dosing**—The dose of tamoxifen will be different for different patients. *Follow your doctor's orders or the directions on the label.* The following information includes only the average doses of tamoxifen. *If your dose is different, do not change it* unless your doctor tells you to do so.

- For *oral* dosage forms (tablets or enteric-coated tablets):
  —For breast cancer in women or men:
    - Adults—10 to 20 milligrams (mg) two times a day, in the morning and evening.

**Missed dose**—If you miss a dose of this medicine, do not take the missed dose at all and do not double the next one. Instead, go back to your regular dosing schedule and check with your doctor.

**Storage**—To store this medicine:
- Keep out of the reach of children.
- Store away from heat and direct light.
- Do not store in the bathroom, near the kitchen sink, or in other damp places. Heat or moisture may cause the medicine to break down.
- Do not keep outdated medicine or medicine no longer needed. Be sure that any discarded medicine is out of the reach of children.

## Precautions While Using This Medicine

*It is very important that your doctor check your progress at regular visits* to make sure that this medicine is working properly and to check for unwanted effects.

For women: Tamoxifen may make you more fertile. It is best to use some type of birth control while you are taking it. However, do not use oral contraceptives (the "Pill") since they may change the effects of tamoxifen. Tell your doctor right away if you think you have become pregnant while taking this medicine.

For patients taking *enteric-coated tamoxifen tablets:*
- If you are also taking an antacid, take this medicine at least 1 or 2 hours before or after taking the antacid. Taking the two medicines too close together may cause the enteric coating to dissolve too early. This may increase the risk of unwanted effects from tamoxifen.

## Side Effects of This Medicine

Along with its needed effects, a medicine may cause some unwanted effects. Some side effects will have signs or symptoms that you can see or feel. Your doctor will watch for others by doing certain tests.

Also, because of the way this medicine acts on the body, there is a chance that it might cause other unwanted effects that may not occur until months or years after the medicine is used. Tamoxifen has been reported to increase the chance of cancer of the uterus (womb) in some women taking it. It also causes liver cancer in rats.

In addition, tamoxifen has been reported to cause cataracts and other eye problems. Discuss these possible effects with your doctor.

Check with your doctor as soon as possible if any of the following side effects occur:

*For both females and males*

*Less common or rare*

Blurred vision; confusion; pain or swelling in legs; shortness of breath; weakness or sleepiness; yellow eyes or skin

*For females only*

*Less common or rare*

Change in vaginal discharge; pain or feeling of pressure in pelvis; vaginal bleeding

This medicine may also cause the following side effect that your doctor will watch for:

*For both females and males*

*Less common or rare*

Cataracts in the eyes or other eye problems; liver problems

Other side effects may occur that usually do not need medical attention. These side effects may go away during treatment as your body adjusts to the medicine. Also, your health care professional may be able to tell you about ways to prevent or reduce some of these side effects. Check with your health care professional if any of the following side effects continue or are bothersome or if you have any questions about them:

*For both females and males*

*Less common*

Bone pain; headache; nausea and/or vomiting (mild); skin rash or dryness

*For females only*

*More common*

Hot flashes; weight gain

*Less common*

Changes in menstrual period; itching in genital area; vaginal discharge

*For males only*

*Less common*

Impotence or decreased sexual interest

Other side effects not listed above may also occur in some patients. If you notice any other effects, check with your doctor.

Revised: 08/12/94

# TERAZOSIN  Systemic

A commonly used brand name in the U.S. and Canada is Hytrin.

## Description

Terazosin (ter-AY-zoe-sin) is used to treat high blood pressure (hypertension).

High blood pressure adds to the work load of the heart and arteries. If it continues for a long time, the heart and arteries may not function properly. This can damage the blood vessels of the brain, heart, and kidneys, resulting in a stroke, heart failure, or kidney failure. High blood pressure may also increase the risk of heart attacks. These problems may be less likely to occur if blood pressure is controlled.

Terazosin helps to lower blood pressure by relaxing blood vessels so that blood passes through them more easily.

Terazosin is also used to treat benign enlargement of the prostate (benign prostatic hyperplasia [BPH]). Benign enlargement of the prostate is a problem that can occur in men as they get older. The prostate gland is located below the bladder. As the prostate gland enlarges, certain muscles in the gland may become tight and get in the way of the tube that drains urine from the bladder. This can cause problems in urinating, such as a need to urinate often, a weak stream when urinating, or a feeling of not being able to empty the bladder completely.

Terazosin helps relax the muscles in the prostate and the opening of the bladder. This may help increase the flow of urine and/or decrease the symptoms. However, terazosin will not help shrink the prostate. The prostate may continue to grow. This may cause the symptoms to become worse over time. Therefore, even though terazosin may lessen the problems caused by enlarged prostate now, surgery still may be needed in the future.

Terazosin is available only with your doctor's prescription, in the following dosage form:

*Oral*
- Tablets (U.S. and Canada)

## Before Using This Medicine

In deciding to use a medicine, the risks of taking the medicine must be weighed against the good it will do. This is a decision you and your doctor will make. For terazosin, the following should be considered:

**Allergies**—Tell your doctor if you have ever had any unusual or allergic reaction to terazosin, prazosin, or doxazosin. Also tell your health care professional if you are allergic to any other substances, such as foods, preservatives, or dyes.

**Pregnancy**—Studies have not been done in humans. Studies in animals given many times the highest recommended human dose have not shown that terazosin causes birth defects. However, these studies have shown a decrease in successful pregnancies.

**Breast-feeding**—It is not known whether terazosin passes into breast milk. Although most medicines pass into breast milk in small amounts, many of them may be used safely while breast-feeding. Mothers who are taking this medicine and who wish to breast-feed should discuss this with their doctor.

**Children**—Studies on this medicine have been done only in adult patients, and there is no specific information comparing use of terazosin in children with use in other age groups.

**Older adults**—Dizziness, lightheadedness, or fainting (especially when getting up from a lying or sitting position) may be more likely to occur in the elderly, who are more sensitive to the effects of terazosin.

**Other medicines**—Although certain medicines should not be used together at all, in other cases two different medicines may be used together even if an interaction might occur. In these cases, your doctor may want to change the dose, or other precautions may be necessary. Tell your health care professional if you are taking any other prescription or nonprescription (over-the-counter [OTC]) medicine.

**Other medical problems**—The presence of other medical problems may affect the use of terazosin. Make sure you tell your doctor if you have any other medical problems, especially:
- Angina (chest pain)—Terazosin may make this condition worse
- Heart disease (severe)—Terazosin may make this condition worse
- Kidney disease—Possible increased sensitivity to the effects of terazosin

## Proper Use of This Medicine

For patients *taking this medicine for high blood pressure:*
- In addition to the use of the medicine your doctor has prescribed, treatment for your high blood pressure may include weight control and care in the types of foods you eat, especially foods high in sodium. Your doctor will tell you which of these are most important for you. You should check with your doctor before changing your diet.
- Many patients who have high blood pressure will not notice any signs of the problem. In fact, many may feel normal. It is very important that you *take your medicine exactly as directed* and that you keep your appointments with your doctor even if you feel well.
- Remember that terazosin will not cure your high blood pressure but it does help control it. Therefore, you must continue to take it as directed if you expect to lower your blood pressure and keep it down. *You may have to take high blood pressure medicine for the rest of your life.* If high blood pressure is not

© 1994  The United States Pharmacopeial Convention, Inc.

treated, it can cause serious problems such as heart failure, blood vessel disease, stroke, or kidney disease.

For patients *taking this medicine for benign enlargement of the prostate:*

- Remember that terazosin will not shrink the size of your prostate but it does help to relieve the symptoms.
- It may take up to 6 weeks before your symptoms get better.

To help you remember to take your medicine, try to get into the habit of taking it at the same time each day.

**Dosing**—The dose of terazosin will be different for different patients. *Follow your doctor's orders or the directions on the label.* The following information includes only the average doses of terazosin. *If your dose is different, do not change it* unless your doctor tells you to do so.

The number of tablets that you take depends on the strength of the medicine.

- For *oral* dosage form (tablets):
  —For benign enlargement of the prostate:
  - Adults—At first, 1 milligram (mg) taken at bedtime. Then, 5 to 10 mg once a day.
  —For high blood pressure:
  - Adults—At first, 1 mg taken at bedtime. Then, 1 to 5 mg once a day.
  - Children—Use and dose must be determined by your doctor.

**Missed dose**—If you miss a dose of this medicine, take it as soon as possible the same day. However, if you do not remember the missed dose until the next day, skip the missed dose and go back to your regular dosing schedule. Do not double doses.

**Storage**—To store this medicine:

- Keep out of the reach of children.
- Store away from heat and direct light.
- Do not store in the bathroom, near the kitchen sink, or in other damp places. Heat or moisture may cause the medicine to break down.
- Do not keep outdated medicine or medicine no longer needed. Be sure that any discarded medicine is out of the reach of children.

## Precautions While Using This Medicine

It is important that your doctor check your progress at regular visits to make sure that this medicine is working properly.

For patients *taking this medicine for high blood pressure:*

- *Do not take other medicines unless they have been discussed with your doctor.* This especially includes over-the-counter (nonprescription) medicines for appetite control, asthma, colds, cough, hay fever, or sinus problems, since they may tend to increase your blood pressure.

Dizziness, lightheadedness, or sudden fainting may occur after you take this medicine, especially when you get up from a lying or sitting position. These effects are more likely to occur when you take the first dose of this medicine. Taking the first dose at bedtime may prevent problems. However, *be especially careful if you need to get up during the night*. These effects may also occur with any doses you take after the first dose. Getting up slowly may help lessen this problem. *If you feel dizzy, lie down so that you do not faint.* Then sit for a few moments before standing to prevent the dizziness from returning.

The dizziness, lightheadedness, or fainting is more likely to occur if you drink alcohol, stand for long periods of time, exercise, or if the weather is hot. *While you are taking this medicine, be careful to limit the amount of alcohol you drink. Also, use extra care during exercise or hot weather or if you must stand for long periods of time.*

Terazosin may cause some people to become drowsy or less alert than they are normally. *Make sure you know how you react to this medicine before you drive, use machines, or do anything else that could be dangerous if you are dizzy, drowsy, or are not alert.* After you have taken several doses of this medicine, these effects should lessen.

## Side Effects of This Medicine

Along with its needed effects, a medicine may cause some unwanted effects. Although not all of these side effects may occur, if they do occur they may need medical attention.

Check with your doctor as soon as possible if any of the following side effects occur:

*More common*
    Dizziness

*Less common*
    Chest pain; dizziness or lightheadedness when getting up from a lying or sitting position; fainting (sudden); fast or irregular heartbeat; pounding heartbeat; shortness of breath; swelling of feet or lower legs

*Rare*
    Weight gain

Other side effects may occur that usually do not need medical attention. These side effects may go away during treatment as your body adjusts to the medicine. However, check with your doctor if any of the following side effects continue or are bothersome:

*More common*
  Headache; unusual tiredness or weakness
*Less common*
  Back or joint pain; blurred vision; drowsiness; nausea and vomiting; stuffy nose

Other side effects not listed above may also occur in some patients. If you notice any other effects, check with your doctor.

Revised: 06/26/92
Interim revision: 07/08/94

# TERBINAFINE    Topical†

A commonly used brand name in the U.S. is Lamisil.

†Not commercially available in Canada.

## Description

Terbinafine (TER-bin-a-feen) is used to treat infections caused by a fungus. It works by killing the fungus or preventing its growth.

Terbinafine is applied to the skin to treat:
  • ringworm of the body (tinea corporis);
  • ringworm of the foot (tinea pedis; athlete's foot); and
  • ringworm of the groin (tinea cruris; jock itch).

Terbinafine is available only with your doctor's prescription, in the following dosage form:

*Topical*
  • Cream (U.S.)

## Before Using This Medicine

In deciding to use a medicine, the risks of using the medicine must be weighed against the good it will do. This is a decision you and your doctor will make. For terbinafine, the following should be considered:

**Allergies**—Tell your doctor if you have ever had any unusual or allergic reaction to terbinafine. Also tell your health care professional if you are allergic to any other substances, such as foods, preservatives, or dyes.

**Pregnancy**—Terbinafine has not been studied in pregnant women. However, terbinafine has not been shown to cause birth defects or other problems in animal studies.

**Breast-feeding**—Oral terbinafine passes into the breast milk. It is not known whether topical terbinafine passes into breast milk. Although most medicines pass into breast milk in small amounts, many of them may be used safely while breast-feeding. Mothers who are using this medicine and who wish to breast-feed should discuss this with their doctor.

**Children**—Studies on this medicine have been done only in adult patients, and there is no specific information comparing use of terbinafine in children under the age of 12 with use in other age groups.

**Older adults**—Many medicines have not been studied specifically in older people. Therefore, it may not be known whether they work exactly the same way they do in younger adults. Although there is no specific information comparing use of terbinafine in the elderly with use in other age groups, this medicine is not expected to cause different side effects or problems in older people than it does in younger adults.

**Other medicines**—Although certain medicines should not be used together at all, in other cases two different medicines may be used together even if an interaction might occur. In these cases, your doctor may want to change the dose, or other precautions may be necessary. Tell your health care professional if you are using any other topical prescription or nonprescription (over-the-counter [OTC]) medicine that is to be applied to the same area of the skin.

## Proper Use of This Medicine

Apply enough terbinafine to cover the affected and surrounding skin areas and rub in gently.

*Keep this medicine away from the eyes.*

*Do not apply an occlusive dressing (airtight covering, such as a tight bandage or plastic kitchen wrap) over this medicine* unless you have been directed to do so by your doctor.

**Dosing**—The dose of terbinafine will be different for different patients. *Follow your doctor's orders or the directions on the label.* The following information includes only the average doses of terbinafine. *If your dose is different, do not change it* unless your doctor tells you to do so:

*The number of doses you use each day, the time allowed between doses, and the length of time you use the medicine depend on the medical problem for which you are using terbinafine.*
  • For *topical* dosage form (cream):
    —For tinea corporis or tinea cruris:
      • Adults and children 12 years of age and over— Use one or two times a day.
      • Infants and children up to 12 years of age— Use and dose must be determined by your doctor.

—For tinea pedis:
- Adults and children 12 years of age and over—Use two times a day.
- Infants and children up to 12 years of age—Use and dose must be determined by your doctor.

To help clear up your infection completely, it *is very important that you keep using terbinafine for the full time of treatment,* even if your symptoms begin to clear up after a few days. Since fungus infections may be very slow to clear up, you may have to continue using this medicine every day for several weeks or more. If you stop using this medicine too soon, your symptoms may return. *Do not miss any doses.*

**Missed dose**—If you do miss a dose of this medicine, apply it as soon as possible. However, if it is almost time for your next dose, skip the missed dose and go back to your regular dosing schedule.

**Storage**—To store this medicine:
- Keep out of the reach of children.
- Store away from heat and direct light.
- Keep the medicine from freezing.
- Do not keep outdated medicine or medicine no longer needed. Be sure that any discarded medicine is out of the reach of children.

---

## Precautions While Using This Medicine

If your skin problem does not improve within 4 weeks, or if it becomes worse, check with your doctor.

*To help clear up your infection completely and to help make sure it does not return, good health habits are also needed.* The following measures will help reduce chafing and irritation and will also help keep the area cool and dry.

- *For patients using terbinafine for ringworm of the body:*
  —Carefully dry yourself after bathing.
  —Avoid too much heat and humidity if possible. Try to keep moisture from building up on affected areas of the body.
  —Wear well-ventilated, loose-fitting clothing.
  —Use a bland, absorbent powder (for example, talcum powder) once or twice a day. Be sure to use the powder after terbinafine cream has been applied and has disappeared into the skin.

- *For patients using terbinafine for ringworm of the groin:*
  —Avoid wearing underwear that is tight-fitting or made from synthetic (man-made) materials (for example, rayon or nylon). Instead, wear loose-fitting, cotton underwear.
  —Use a bland, absorbent powder (for example, talcum powder) on the skin. It is best to use the powder between the times you use terbinafine.

- *For patients using terbinafine for ringworm of the foot:*
  —Carefully dry the feet, especially between the toes, after bathing.
  —Avoid wearing socks made from wool or synthetic materials (for example, rayon or nylon). Instead, wear clean, cotton socks and change them daily or more often if the feet sweat a lot.
  —Wear sandals or well-ventilated shoes (for example, shoes with holes).
  —Use a bland, absorbent powder (for example, talcum powder) between the toes, on the feet, and in socks and shoes once or twice a day. It is best to use the powder between the times you use terbinafine.

If you have any questions about these measures, check with your health care professional.

## Side Effects of This Medicine

Along with its needed effects, a medicine may cause some unwanted effects. Although not all of these side effects may occur, if they do occur they may need medical attention.

Check with your health care professional as soon as possible if any of the following side effects occur:

*Rare*

Redness, itching, burning, blistering, swelling, oozing, or other signs of skin irritation not present before use of this medicine

Other side effects not listed above may also occur in some patients. If you notice any other effects, check with your doctor.

---

Revised: 07/29/93

---

# TERIPARATIDE   Systemic†

A commonly used brand name in the U.S. is Parathar.

†Not commercially available in Canada.

## Description

Teriparatide (terr-ih-PAR-a-tyd) is synthetic human parathyroid hormone used by injection as a test to help diagnose problems of the parathyroid gland. This test determines whether you have hypoparathyroidism or a type of pseudohypoparathyroidism.

How this test is done: Before the medicine is given, at least three blood and urine samples will be collected and tested. The dose of teriparatide, which is based on body weight, is injected into an arm vein over a 10-minute period. Then more blood and urine samples are collected and tested. Teriparatide causes changes in the amounts of certain chemicals in the urine. These changes will help determine which hypoparathyroid problem you have.

Teriparatide is to be used only by or under the supervision of a doctor, in the following dosage form:

*Parenteral*
- Injection (U.S.)

## Before Having This Test

In deciding to use a diagnostic test, any risks of the test must be weighed against the good it will do. This is a decision you and your doctor will make. For teriparatide, the following should be considered:

**Allergies**—Tell your doctor if you have ever had any unusual or allergic reaction to peptides, gelatin, or teriparatide. Also tell your health care professional if you are allergic to any other substances, such as foods, preservatives, or dyes.

**Pregnancy**—Teriparatide has not been shown to cause birth defects or other problems in humans.

**Breast-feeding**—It is not known whether teriparatide passes into the breast milk. However, teriparatide is not recommended during breast-feeding, because it may cause unwanted effects in nursing babies.

**Children**—This medicine has not been shown to cause different side effects or problems in children over 3 years of age than it does in adults.

**Older adults**—Many medicines have not been studied specifically in older people. Therefore, it may not be known whether they work exactly the same way they do in younger adults. Although there is no specific information comparing use of teriparatide in the elderly with use in other age groups, this medicine is not expected to cause different side effects or problems in older people than it does in younger adults.

**Other medicines**—Although certain medicines should not be used together at all, in other cases two different medicines may be used together even if an interaction might occur. In these cases, your doctor may want to change the dose, or other precautions may be necessary. Tell your health care professional if you are taking any other prescription or nonprescription (over-the-counter [OTC]) medicine.

## Preparation for This Test

*Follow your doctor's instructions carefully.* Otherwise, this test may not work well and may have to be done again.

Unless otherwise directed by your doctor:
- Do not eat or drink anything but water after 8:00 p.m. the night before the test. Food may affect the test results.
- Starting about 2½ hours before the test, drink about 6 or 7 ounces of water every 30 minutes until the test is finished. This is to be sure there is enough urine for testing.

## Side Effects of This Medicine

Along with its needed effects, a medicine may cause some unwanted effects. Check with your doctor as soon as possible if any of the following side effects occur:

*Symptoms of overdose*
    Constipation; headache; loss of appetite; muscle weakness

Other side effects may occur that usually do not need medical attention. These side effects may go away after the test as your body adjusts to the medicine. However, check with your doctor if any of the following side effects continue or are bothersome:

*Rare*
    Abdominal or stomach cramps; diarrhea; metallic taste; nausea; pain at the place of injection during or following injection; tingling feeling in hands and feet; urge for bowel movement

Other side effects not listed above may also occur in some patients. If you notice any other effects, check with your doctor.

Revised: 06/22/92
Interim revision: 06/15/94

# TESTOLACTONE    Systemic†

A commonly used brand name in the U.S. is Teslac.

†Not commercially available in Canada.

## Description

Testolactone (tess-toe-LAK-tone) belongs to the general group of medicines called antineoplastics. It is used to treat some cases of breast cancer in females.

Testolactone is available only with your doctor's prescription, in the following dosage form:

*Oral*

- Tablets (U.S.)

## Before Using This Medicine

In deciding to use a medicine, the risks of taking the medicine must be weighed against the good it will do. This is a decision you and your doctor will make. For testolactone, the following should be considered:

**Allergies**—Tell your doctor if you have ever had any unusual or allergic reaction to testolactone.

**Pregnancy**—Studies have not been done in humans. However, studies in rats at doses 2.5 to 7.5 times the human dose have shown that testolactone causes an increase in the number of fetus and infant deaths and abnormal growth.

**Breast-feeding**—It is not known whether testolactone passes into breast milk. However, this medicine has not been reported to cause problems in nursing babies.

**Older adults**—Many medicines have not been studied specifically in older people. Therefore, it may not be known whether they work exactly the same way they do in younger adults or if they cause different side effects or problems in older people. There is no specific information comparing use of testolactone in the elderly with use in other age groups.

**Other medicines**—Although certain medicines should not be used together at all, in other cases two different medicines may be used together even if an interaction might occur. In these cases, your doctor may want to change the dose, or other precautions may be necessary. Tell your health care professional if you are taking any other prescription or nonprescription (over-the-counter [OTC]) medicine.

**Other medical problems**—The presence of other medical problems may affect the use of testolactone. Make sure you tell your doctor if you have any other medical problems, especially:

- Heart or kidney disease

## Proper Use of This Medicine

*Use this medicine only as directed by your doctor.* Do not use more or less of it, and do not use it more often than your doctor ordered. The exact amount of medicine you need has been carefully worked out. Taking too much may increase the chance of side effects, while taking too little may not improve your condition.

Testolactone sometimes causes nausea and vomiting. However, it may have to be taken for several weeks or months to be effective. Even if you begin to feel ill, *do not stop using this medicine without first checking with your doctor*. Ask your health care professional for ways to lessen these effects.

If you vomit shortly after taking a dose of testolactone, check with your doctor. You will be told whether to take the dose again or to wait until the next scheduled dose.

**Dosing**—The dose of testolactone will be different for different patients. The dose that is used may depend on a number of things, including what the medicine is being used for and whether or not other medicines are also being taken. *If you are taking testolactone at home, follow your doctor's orders or the directions on the label*. If you have any questions about the proper dose of testolactone, ask your doctor.

**Missed dose**—If you miss a dose of this medicine, take it as soon as you remember. However, if it is almost time for the next dose, skip the missed dose and go back to your regular dosing schedule. Do not double doses. If you miss two or more doses in a row, check with your doctor.

**Storage**—To store this medicine:

- Keep out of the reach of children.
- Store away from heat and direct light.
- Do not store in the bathroom, near the kitchen sink, or in other damp places. Heat or moisture may cause the medicine to break down.
- Do not keep outdated medicine or medicine no longer needed. Be sure that any discarded medicine is out of the reach of children.

## Precautions While Using This Medicine

*It is very important that your doctor check your progress at regular visits* to make sure that this medicine is working properly and to check for unwanted effects.

## Side Effects of This Medicine

Along with its needed effects, a medicine may cause some unwanted effects. Although not all of these side effects may occur, if they do occur they may need medical attention.

Check with your doctor as soon as possible if the following side effect occurs:

*Less common*
    Numbness or tingling of fingers, toes, or face

Other side effects may occur that usually do not need medical attention. These side effects may go away during treatment as your body adjusts to the medicine. Also, your health care professional may be able to tell you about ways to prevent or reduce some of these side effects. Check with your health care professional if any of the following side effects continue or are bothersome or if you have any questions about them:

*Less common*
  Diarrhea; loss of appetite; nausea or vomiting; pain or swelling in feet or lower legs; swelling or redness of tongue

Other side effects not listed above may also occur in some patients. If you notice any other effects, check with your doctor.

Revised: 08/04/92
Interim revision: 06/30/94

# TETANUS TOXOID  Systemic

## Description

Tetanus (TET-n-us) Toxoid is used to prevent tetanus (also known as lockjaw). Tetanus is a serious illness that causes convulsions (seizures) and severe muscle spasms that can be strong enough to cause bone fractures of the spine. Tetanus causes death in 30 to 40 percent of cases.

Immunization against tetanus is recommended for all infants 6 to 8 weeks of age and older, all children, and all adults. Immunization against tetanus consists first of a series of either 3 or 4 injections, depending on which type of tetanus toxoid you receive. In addition, it is very important that you get a booster injection every 10 years for the rest of your life. Also, if you get a wound that is unclean or hard to clean, you may need an emergency booster injection if it has been more than 5 years since your last booster. In recent years, two-thirds of all tetanus cases have been in persons 50 years of age and older. A tetanus infection in the past does not make you immune to tetanus in the future.

This vaccine is to be administered only by or under the supervision of your doctor or other health care professional. It is available in the following dosage form:

*Parenteral*
  • Injection (U.S. and Canada)

## Before Receiving This Vaccine

In deciding to receive this vaccine, the risks of receiving the vaccine must be weighed against the good it will do. This is a decision you and your doctor will make. For tetanus toxoid, the following should be considered:

**Allergies**—Tell your doctor if you have ever had any unusual or allergic reaction to tetanus toxoid. Also tell your health care professional if you are allergic to any other substances, such as preservatives (especially thimerosal).

**Pregnancy**—This vaccine has not been shown to cause birth defects or other problems in humans. Vaccination of a pregnant woman can prevent her newborn baby from getting tetanus at birth.

**Breast-feeding**—Tetanus toxoid has not been reported to cause problems in nursing babies.

**Children**—Use is not recommended for infants up to 6 weeks of age. For infants and children 6 weeks of age and older, tetanus toxoid is not expected to cause different side effects or problems than it does in adults.

**Older adults**—This vaccine is not expected to cause different side effects or problems in older people than it does in younger adults. However, the vaccine may be slightly less effective in older persons than in younger adults.

**Other medicines**—Although certain medicines should not be used together at all, in other cases two different medicines may be used together even if an interaction might occur. In these cases, your doctor may want to change the dose, or other precautions may be necessary. Before you receive tetanus toxoid, it is especially important that your health care professional know if you are using any prescription or nonprescription (over-the-counter [OTC]) medicine.

**Other medical problems**—The presence of other medical problems may affect the use of tetanus toxoid. Make sure you tell your doctor if you have any other medical problems, especially:
  • A severe reaction or a fever greater than 103 °F (39.4 °C) following a previous dose of tetanus toxoid—May increase the chance of side effects with future doses of tetanus toxoid; be sure your doctor knows about this before you receive the next dose of tetanus toxoid
  • Bronchitis, pneumonia, or other illness involving lungs or bronchial tubes, or
  • Severe illness with fever—Possible side effects from tetanus toxoid may be confused with the symptoms of the condition

## Proper Use of This Vaccine

**Dosing**—The dose of tetanus toxoid will be different for different patients. The following information includes only the average doses of tetanus toxoid.
  • For *injection* dosage forms:
    —For prevention of tetanus (lockjaw):
      • Adults, children, and infants 6 weeks of age and older—One dose is given at your first visit, then a second dose is given four to eight weeks later. Depending on the product given, you may receive a third dose four to eight weeks after the second dose, and a fourth dose six to twelve months after that; or you may receive a third dose six to twelve months after the second dose.

Everyone should receive a booster dose every ten years. The doses are injected under the skin or into a muscle. In addition, if you get a wound that is unclean or hard to clean, you may need an emergency booster injection if it has been more than 5 years since your last booster dose.

## Side Effects of This Vaccine

Along with its needed effects, a vaccine may cause some unwanted effects. Although not all of these side effects may occur, if they do occur they may need medical attention.

*Get emergency help immediately* if any of the following side effects occur:

*Symptoms of allergic reaction*
Difficulty in breathing or swallowing; hives; itching, especially of feet or hands; reddening of skin, especially around ears; swelling of eyes, face, or inside of nose; unusual tiredness or weakness (sudden and severe)

Check with your doctor as soon as possible if any of the following side effects occur:

*Rare*
Confusion; convulsions (seizures); fever over 103 °F (39.4 °C); headache (severe or continuing); sleepiness

(excessive); swelling, blistering, or pain at place of injection (severe or continuing); swelling of glands in armpit; unusual irritability; vomiting (severe or continuing)

Other side effects may occur that usually do not need medical attention. However, check with your doctor if any of the following side effects continue or are bothersome:

*More common*
Redness or hard lump at place of injection

*Less common*
Chills, fever, irritability, or unusual tiredness; pain, tenderness, itching, or swelling at place of injection; skin rash

Other side effects not listed above may also occur in some patients. If you notice any other effects, check with your doctor.

Revised: 07/12/94

---

# TETRACYCLINES  Ophthalmic

Some commonly used brand names are:

**In the U.S.—**
Achromycin[2]
Aureomycin[1]

**In Canada—**
Achromycin[2]
Aureomycin[1]

Note: For quick reference, the following tetracyclines are numbered to match the corresponding brand names.

This information applies to the following medicines:
1. Chlortetracycline (klor-te-tra-SYE-kleen)
2. Tetracycline (te-tra-SYE-kleen)

## Description

Tetracyclines belong to the family of medicines called antibiotics. Tetracycline ophthalmic preparations are used to treat infections of the eye. They may also be used along with other medicines that are taken by mouth for infections of the eye.

Tetracyclines are available only with your doctor's prescription, in the following dosage forms:

*Ophthalmic*
Chlortetracycline
• Ophthalmic ointment (U.S. and Canada)
Tetracycline
• Ophthalmic ointment (U.S. and Canada)
• Ophthalmic suspension (eye drops) (U.S.)

## Before Using This Medicine

In deciding to use a medicine, the risks of using the medicine must be weighed against the good it will do. This is a decision you and your doctor will make. For tetracycline ophthalmic preparations, the following should be considered:

**Allergies**—Tell your doctor if you have ever had any unusual or allergic reaction to tetracycline or chlortetracycline or to any related antibiotics, such as demeclocycline (e.g., Declomycin), doxycycline (e.g., Vibramycin), methacycline (e.g., Rondomycin), minocycline (e.g., Minocin), or oxytetracycline (e.g., Terramycin). Also tell your health care professional if you are allergic to any other substances, such as preservatives.

**Pregnancy**—Tetracycline ophthalmic preparations have not been shown to cause birth defects or other problems in humans.

**Breast-feeding**—Tetracycline ophthalmic preparations have not been reported to cause problems in nursing babies.

**Children**—Although there is no specific information comparing use of ophthalmic tetracyclines in children with use in other age groups, they are not expected to cause different side effects or problems in children than they do in adults.

**Older adults**—Many medicines have not been studied specifically in older people. Therefore, it may not be known whether they work exactly the same way they do in younger adults or if they cause different side effects or problems in older people. There is no specific information comparing use of tetracyclines in the elderly with use in other age groups.

**Other medicines**—Although certain medicines should not be used together at all, in other cases two different medicines may be used together even if an interaction might occur. In these cases, your doctor may want to change the dose, or other precautions may be necessary. Tell your health care professional if you are using any other prescription or nonprescription (over-the-counter [OTC]) medicine that is to be used in the eye.

## Proper Use of This Medicine

For patients using the *eye drop form* of tetracyclines:

* The bottle is only partially full to provide proper drop control.
* To use:
  —First, wash your hands. Then tilt the head back and pull the lower eyelid away from the eye to form a pouch. Drop the medicine into the pouch and gently close the eyes. Do not blink. Keep the eyes closed for 1 or 2 minutes to allow the medicine to come into contact with the infection.
  —If you think you did not get the drop of medicine into your eye properly, use another drop.
  —To keep the medicine as germ-free as possible, do not touch the applicator tip to any surface (including the eye). Also, keep the container tightly closed.

For patients using the *eye ointment form* of tetracyclines:

* To use:
  —First, wash your hands. Then pull the lower eyelid away from the eye to form a pouch. Squeeze a thin strip of ointment into the pouch. A 1-cm (approximately ⅓-inch) strip of ointment is usually enough unless otherwise directed by your doctor. Gently close the eyes and keep them closed for 1 or 2 minutes to allow the medicine to come into contact with the infection.
  —To keep the medicine as germ-free as possible, do not touch the applicator tip to any surface (including the eye). After using tetracyclines eye ointment, wipe the tip of the ointment tube with a clean tissue and keep the tube tightly closed.

To help clear up your infection completely, *keep using this medicine for the full time of treatment,* even if your symptoms have disappeared. *Do not miss any doses.*

**Dosing**—The dose of ophthalmic tetracyclines will be different for different patients. *Follow your doctor's orders or the directions on the label.* The following information includes only the average doses of ophthalmic tetracyclines. *If your dose is different, do not change it unless your doctor tells you to do so.*

*The number of doses you use each day, the time allowed between doses, and the length of time you use the medicine depend on the medical problem for which you are using ophthalmic tetracyclines.*

* For eye infections:
  —For *ophthalmic ointment* dosage forms:
    * Adults and children—Use every two to four hours.
  —For *ophthalmic suspension* dosage form:
    * Adults and children—One drop every six to twelve hours.

**Missed dose**—If you miss a dose of this medicine, apply it as soon as possible. However, if it is almost time for your next application, skip the missed dose and go back to your regular dosing schedule.

**Storage**—To store this medicine:

* Keep out of the reach of children.
* Store away from heat and direct light.
* Keep the medicine from freezing.
* Do not keep outdated medicine or medicine no longer needed. Be sure that any discarded medicine is out of the reach of children.

## Precautions While Using This Medicine

After application, this medicine usually causes your vision to blur for a few minutes.

If your symptoms do not improve within a few days, or if they become worse, check with your doctor.

## Side Effects of This Medicine

There have not been any common or important side effects reported with this medicine. However, if you notice any unusual effects, check with your doctor.

Revised: 07/01/93

# TETRACYCLINES    Systemic

Some commonly used brand names are:

**In the U.S.—**

| | |
|---|---|
| Achromycin[5] | Panmycin[5] |
| Achromycin V[5] | Robitet[5] |
| Declomycin[1] | Sumycin[5] |
| Doryx[2] | Terramycin[4] |
| Doxy[2] | Tetracyn[5] |
| Doxy-Caps[2] | Tija[4] |
| Minocin[3] | Vibramycin[2] |
| Monodox[2] | Vibra-Tabs[2] |

**In Canada—**

| | |
|---|---|
| Achromycin[5] | Minocin[3] |
| Achromycin V[5] | Novodoxylin[2] |
| Apo-Doxy[2] | Novotetra[2] |
| Apo-Tetra[5] | Nu-Tetra[5] |
| Declomycin[1] | Tetracyn[5] |
| Doryx[2] | Vibramycin[2] |
| Doxycin[2] | Vibra-Tabs[2] |

Note: For quick reference, the following tetracyclines are numbered to match the corresponding brand names.

This information applies to the following medicines:

1. Demeclocycline (dem-e-kloe-SYE-kleen)
2. Doxycycline (dox-i-SYE-kleen)‡
3. Minocycline (mi-noe-SYE-kleen)‡
4. Oxytetracycline (ox-i-te-tra-SYE-kleen)‡
5. Tetracycline (te-tra-SYE-kleen)‡

‡Generic name product may also be available in the U.S.

## Description

Tetracyclines are used to treat infections and to help control acne. Demeclocycline and doxycycline may also be used for other problems as determined by your doctor. Tetracyclines will not work for colds, flu, or other virus infections.

Tetracyclines are available only with your doctor's prescription, in the following dosage forms:

*Oral*

Demeclocycline
  • Capsules (U.S.)
  • Tablets (U.S. and Canada)
Doxycycline
  • Capsules (U.S. and Canada)
  • Delayed-release capsules (U.S. and Canada)
  • Oral suspension (U.S.)
  • Tablets (U.S. and Canada)
Minocycline
  • Capsules (U.S. and Canada)
  • Oral suspension (U.S.)
  • Tablets (U.S.)
Oxytetracycline
  • Capsules (U.S.)
Tetracycline
  • Capsules (U.S. and Canada)
  • Oral suspension (U.S. and Canada)
  • Tablets (U.S. and Canada)

*Parenteral*

Doxycycline
  • Injection (U.S. and Canada)
Minocycline
  • Injection (U.S.)
Oxytetracycline
  • Injection (U.S.)
Tetracycline
  • Injection (U.S. and Canada)

## Before Using This Medicine

In deciding to use a medicine, the risks of taking the medicine must be weighed against the good it will do. This is a decision you and your doctor will make. For tetracyclines, the following should be considered:

**Allergies**—Tell your doctor if you have ever had any unusual or allergic reaction to any of the tetracyclines or combination medicines containing a tetracycline. Also tell your health care professional if you are allergic to any other substances, such as foods, preservatives, or dyes. In addition, if you are going to be given oxytetracycline or tetracycline by injection, tell your doctor if you have ever had an unusual or allergic reaction to "caine-type" anesthetics.

**Pregnancy**—Use is not recommended during the last half of pregnancy. Tetracyclines may cause the unborn infant's teeth to become discolored and may slow down the growth of the infant's teeth and bones if they are taken during that time. In addition, liver problems may occur in pregnant women, especially those receiving high doses by injection into a vein.

**Breast-feeding**—Use is not recommended since tetracyclines pass into the breast milk. They may cause the nursing baby's teeth to become discolored and may slow down the growth of the baby's teeth and bones. They may also cause increased sensitivity of nursing babies' skin to sunlight and fungus infections of the mouth and vagina. In addition, minocycline may cause dizziness, lightheadedness, or unsteadiness in nursing babies.

**Children**—Tetracyclines may cause permanent discoloration of teeth and slow down the growth of bones. These medicines should not be given to children up to 8 years of age unless directed by the child's doctor.

**Older adults**—Many medicines have not been studied specifically in older people. Therefore, it may not be known whether they work exactly the same way they do in younger adults or if they cause different side effects or problems in older people. There is no specific information comparing use of tetracyclines in the elderly with use in other age groups.

**Other medicines**—Although certain medicines should not be used together at all, in other cases two different medicines may be used together even if an interaction might occur. In these cases, your doctor may want to change the dose, or other precautions may be necessary. When you are taking tetracyclines, it is especially important that your health care professional know if you are taking any of the following:
  • Antacids or
  • Calcium supplements such as calcium carbonate or
  • Cholestyramine (e.g., Questran) or

- Choline and magnesium salicylates (e.g., Trilisate) or
- Colestipol (e.g., Colestid) or
- Iron-containing medicine or
- Laxatives (magnesium-containing) or
- Magnesium salicylate (e.g., Magan)—Use of these medicines with tetracyclines may decrease the effect of tetracyclines
- Oral contraceptives (birth control pills) containing estrogen—Use of birth control pills with tetracyclines may decrease the effect of the birth control pills and increase the chance of unwanted pregnancy

**Other medical problems**—The presence of other medical problems may affect the use of tetracyclines. Make sure you tell your doctor if you have any other medical problems, especially:

- Diabetes insipidus (water diabetes)—Demeclocycline may make the condition worse
- Kidney disease (does not apply to doxycycline or minocycline)—Patients with kidney disease may have an increased chance of side effects
- Liver disease—Patients with liver disease may have an increased chance of side effects if they use doxycycline or minocycline

## Proper Use of This Medicine

*Do not give tetracyclines to infants or children up to 8 years of age* unless directed by your doctor. Tetracyclines may cause permanently discolored teeth and other problems in this age group.

Do not take milk, milk formulas, or other dairy products within 1 to 2 hours of the time you take tetracyclines (except doxycycline and minocycline) by mouth. They may keep this medicine from working properly.

*If this medicine has changed color or tastes or looks different, has become outdated (old), has been stored incorrectly (too warm or too damp area or place), do not use it.* To do so may cause *serious side effects*. Discard the medicine. If you have any questions about this, check with your health care professional.

Tetracyclines should be taken with a full glass (8 ounces) of water to prevent irritation of the esophagus (tube between the throat and stomach) or stomach. In addition, most tetracyclines (except doxycycline and minocycline) are best taken on an empty stomach (either 1 hour before or 2 hours after meals). However, if this medicine upsets your stomach, your doctor may want you to take it with food.

For patients taking the *oral liquid form* of this medicine:

- Use a specially marked measuring spoon or other device to measure each dose accurately. The average household teaspoon may not hold the right amount of liquid.
- Do not use after the expiration date on the label since the medicine may not work properly after that date. Check with your pharmacist if you have any questions about this.

For patients taking *doxycycline or minocycline:*

- These medicines may be taken with food or milk if they upset your stomach.
- Swallow the capsule (with enteric-coated pellets) form of doxycycline whole. Do not break or crush.

To help clear up your infection completely, *keep taking this medicine for the full time of treatment*, even if you begin to feel better after a few days. If you stop taking this medicine too soon, your symptoms may return.

This medicine works best when there is a constant amount in the blood or urine. *To help keep the amount constant, do not miss any doses. Also, it is best to take the doses at evenly spaced times day and night.* For example, if you are to take 4 doses a day, the doses should be spaced about 6 hours apart. If this interferes with your sleep or other daily activities, or if you need help in planning the best times to take your medicine, check with your health care professional.

**Dosing**—The dose of these medicines will be different for different patients. *Follow your doctor's orders or the directions on the label.* The following information includes only the average doses of these medicines. *If your dose is different, do not change it* unless your doctor tells you to do so.

The number of capsules, tablets or teaspoonfuls of suspension that you take depends on the strength of the medicine. Also, *the number of doses you take each day, the time allowed between doses, and the length of time you take the medicine depend on the medical problem for which you are taking a tetracycline.*

*For demeclocycline*

- For *oral* dosage forms (capsules, tablets):
  —For bacterial or protozoal infections:
  - Adults and teenagers—150 milligrams (mg) every six hours; or 300 mg every twelve hours.
  - Infants and children up to 8 years of age—Tetracyclines are usually not used in young children because tetracyclines can permanently stain teeth.
  - Children 8 years of age and older—Dose is based on body weight. The usual dose is 1.65 to 3.3 mg per kilogram (kg) (0.8 to 1.5 mg per pound) of body weight every six hours; or 3.3 to 6.6 mg per kg (1.5 to 3 mg per pound) of body weight every twelve hours.

*For doxycycline*

- For *oral* dosage forms (capsules, suspension, and tablets):
  —For bacterial or protozoal infections:
  - Adults and children over 45 kilograms (kg) of body weight (99 pounds)—100 milligrams (mg) every twelve hours the first day, then 100 to 200 mg once a day or 50 to 100 mg every twelve hours.

- Infants and children up to 8 years of age—Tetracyclines are usually not used in young children because tetracyclines can permanently stain teeth.

- Children 45 kg of body weight (99 pounds) and less—Dose is based on body weight. The usual dose is 2.2 mg per kg (1 mg per pound) of body weight the first day, then 2.2 to 4.4 mg per kg (1 to 2 mg per pound) of body weight once a day; or 1.1 to 2.2 mg per kg (0.5 to 1 mg per pound) of body weight every twelve hours.

—For the prevention of malaria:

- Adults and teenagers—100 mg once a day. You should take the first dose one or two days before travel to an area where malaria may occur, continue taking the medicine every day throughout travel, and for four weeks after you leave the malarious area.

- Children over 8 years of age—Dose is based on body weight. The usual dose is 2 mg per kg (0.9 mg per pound) of body weight once a day. You should take the first dose one or two days before travel to an area where malaria may occur, continue taking the medicine every day throughout travel, and for four weeks after you leave the malarious area.

- Infants and children up to 8 years of age—Tetracyclines are usually not used in young children because tetracyclines can permanently stain teeth.

- For *injection* dosage form:

—For bacterial or protozoal infections:

- Adults and children over 45 kg of body weight (99 pounds)—200 mg injected into a vein once a day; or 100 mg injected into a vein every twelve hours the first day, then 100 to 200 mg injected into a vein once a day. Another dose is 50 to 100 mg every twelve hours.

- Infants and children up to 8 years of age—Tetracyclines are usually not used in young children because tetracyclines can permanently stain teeth.

- Children 45 kg of body weight (99 pounds) and less—Dose is based on body weight. The usual dose is 4.4 mg per kg (2 mg per pound) of body weight injected into a vein once a day; or 2.2 mg per kg (1 mg per pound) of body weight injected into a vein every twelve hours the first day, then 2.2 to 4.4 mg per kg (1 to 2 mg per pound) of body weight once a day, or 1.1 to 2.2 per kg (0.5 to 1 mg per pound) of body weight every twelve hours.

### For minocycline

- For *oral* dosage forms (capsules, suspension, and tablets):

—For bacterial or protozoal infections:

- Adults and teenagers—200 milligrams (mg) at first, then 100 mg every twelve hours; or 100 to 200 mg at first, then 50 mg every six hours.

- Infants and children up to 8 years of age—Tetracyclines are usually not used in young children because tetracyclines can permanently stain teeth.

- Children 8 years of age and over—Dose is based on body weight. The usual dose is 4 mg per kilogram (kg) (1.8 mg per pound) of body weight at first, then 2 mg per kg (0.9 mg per pound) of body weight every twelve hours.

- For *injection* dosage form:

—For bacterial or protozoal infections:

- Adults and teenagers—200 mg at first, then 100 mg every twelve hours, injected into a vein.

- Infants and children up to 8 years of age—Tetracyclines are usually not used in young children because tetracyclines can permanently stain teeth.

- Children 8 years of age and over—Dose is based on body weight. The usual dose is 4 mg per kg (1.8 mg per pound) of body weight at first, then 2 mg per kg (0.9 mg per pound) of body weight every twelve hours, injected into a vein.

### For oxytetracycline

- For *oral* dosage form (capsules):

—For bacterial or protozoal infections:

- Adults and teenagers—250 to 500 milligrams (mg) every six hours.

- Infants and children up to 8 years of age—Tetracyclines are usually not used in young children because tetracyclines can permanently stain teeth.

- Children 8 years of age and over—Dose is based on body weight. The usual dose is 6.25 to 12.5 mg per kilogram (kg) (2.8 to 5.7 mg per pound) of body weight every six hours.

- For *injection* dosage form (muscle injection):

—For bacterial or protozoal infections:

- Adults and teenagers—100 mg every eight hours; or 150 mg every twelve hours; or 250 mg once a day, injected into a muscle.

- Infants and children up to 8 years of age—Tetracyclines are usually not used in young children because tetracyclines can permanently stain teeth.

- Children 8 years of age and over—Dose is based on body weight. The usual dose is 5 to 8.3 mg per kg (2.3 to 3.8 mg per pound) of body weight every eight hours; or 7.5 to 12.5 mg per kg (3.4 to 5.7 mg per pound) of body weight every twelve hours, injected into a muscle.

- For *injection* dosage form (vein injection):

—For bacterial or protozoal infections:

- Adults and teenagers—250 to 500 mg injected into a vein every twelve hours.

- Infants and children up to 8 years of age—Tetracyclines are usually not used in young children because tetracyclines can permanently stain teeth.
- Children 8 years of age and over—Dose is based on body weight. The usual dose is 5 to 10 mg per kg (2.3 to 4.5 mg per pound) of body weight, injected into a vein, every twelve hours.

*For tetracycline*
- For *oral* dosage forms (capsules, suspension, and tablets):
  —For bacterial or protozoal infections:
  - Adults and teenagers—250 to 500 milligrams (mg) every six hours; or 500 mg to 1 gram every twelve hours.
  - Infants and children up to 8 years of age—Tetracyclines are usually not used in young children because tetracyclines can permanently stain teeth.
  - Children 8 years of age and over—Dose is based on body weight. The usual dose is 6.25 to 12.5 mg per kilogram (kg) (2.8 to 5.7 mg per pound) of body weight every six hours; or 12.5 to 25 mg per kg (5.7 to 11.4 mg per pound) of body weight every twelve hours.
- For *injection* dosage form:
  —For bacterial or protozoal infections:
  - Adults and teenagers—100 mg every eight hours; or 150 mg every twelve hours; or 250 mg once a day, injected into a muscle.
  - Infants and children up to 8 years of age—Tetracyclines are usually not used in young children because tetracyclines can permanently stain teeth.
  - Children 8 years of age and over—Dose is based on body weight. The usual dose is 5 to 8.3 mg per kg (2.3 to 3.8 mg per pound) of body weight every eight hours; or 7.5 to 12.5 mg per kg (3.4 to 5.7 mg per pound) of body weight every twelve hours, injected into a muscle.

**Missed dose**—If you miss a dose of this medicine, take it as soon as possible. This will help to keep a constant amount of medicine in the blood or urine. However, if it is almost time for your next dose, skip the missed dose and go back to your regular dosing schedule. Do not double doses.

**Storage**—To store this medicine:
- Keep out of the reach of children.
- Store away from heat and direct light.
- Do not store the capsule or tablet form of this medicine in the bathroom, near the kitchen sink, or in other damp places. Heat or moisture may cause the medicine to break down.
- Keep the oral liquid forms of this medicine from freezing.

- Do not keep outdated medicine or medicine no longer needed. Be sure that any discarded medicine is out of the reach of children.

## Precautions While Using This Medicine

If your symptoms do not improve within a few days (or a few weeks or months for acne patients), or if they become worse, check with your doctor.

*Do not take antacids; calcium supplements* such as calcium carbonate; *choline and magnesium salicylates combination (e.g., Trilisate); magnesium salicylate (e.g., Magan); magnesium-containing laxatives* such as Epsom salt; *or sodium bicarbonate* (baking soda) within 1 to 2 hours of the time you take any of the tetracyclines by mouth. In addition, *do not take iron preparations* (including vitamin preparations that contain iron) within 2 to 3 hours of the time you take tetracyclines by mouth. To do so may keep this medicine from working properly.

*Oral contraceptives (birth control pills) containing estrogen may not work properly if you take them while you are taking tetracyclines. Unplanned pregnancies may occur. You should use a different or additional means of birth control while you are taking tetracyclines.* If you have any questions about this, check with your health care professional.

Before having surgery (including dental surgery) with a general anesthetic, tell the medical doctor or dentist in charge that you are taking a tetracycline. This does not apply to doxycycline, however.

Tetracyclines may cause your skin to be more sensitive to sunlight than it is normally. Exposure to sunlight, even for brief periods of time, may cause a skin rash, itching, redness or other discoloration of the skin, or a severe sunburn. When you begin taking this medicine:
- Stay out of direct sunlight, especially between the hours of 10:00 a.m. and 3:00 p.m., if possible.
- Wear protective clothing, including a hat. Also, wear sunglasses.
- Apply a sun block product that has a skin protection factor (SPF) of at least 15. Some patients may require a product with a higher SPF number, especially if they have a fair complexion. If you have any questions about this, check with your health care professional.
- Apply a sun block lipstick that has an SPF of at least 15 to protect your lips.
- Do not use a sunlamp or tanning bed or booth.

You may still be more sensitive to sunlight or sunlamps for 2 weeks to several months or more after stopping this medicine. *If you have a severe reaction, check with your doctor.*

For patients taking *minocycline:*
- Minocycline may also cause some people to become dizzy, lightheaded, or unsteady. *Make sure you know how you react to this medicine before you drive, use*

*machines, or do anything else that could be dangerous if you are dizzy or are not alert.* If these reactions are especially bothersome, check with your doctor.

## Side Effects of This Medicine

Along with its needed effects, a medicine may cause some unwanted effects. In some infants and children, tetracyclines may cause the teeth to become discolored. Even though this may not happen right away, check with your doctor as soon as possible if you notice this effect or if you have any questions about it.

*For all tetracyclines*
   *More common*
      Increased sensitivity of skin to sunlight (rare with minocycline)
   *Rare*
      Abdominal pain; bulging fontanel (soft spot on head) of infants; headache; loss of appetite; nausea and vomiting; yellowing skin; visual changes
*For demeclocycline only*
   *Less common*
      Greatly increased frequency of urination or amount of urine; increased thirst; unusual tiredness or weakness
*For minocycline only*
   *Less common*
      Pigmentation (darker color or discoloration) of skin and mucous membranes

Other side effects may occur that usually do not need medical attention. These side effects may go away during treatment as your body adjusts to the medicine. However, check with your doctor if any of the following side effects continue or are bothersome:

*For all tetracyclines*
   *More common*
      Cramps or burning of the stomach; diarrhea; nausea or vomiting
   *Less common*
      Itching of the rectal or genital (sex organ) areas; sore mouth or tongue

*For minocycline only*
   *More common*
      Dizziness, lightheadedness, or unsteadiness

In some patients tetracyclines may cause the tongue to become darkened or discolored. This effect is only temporary and will go away when you stop taking this medicine.

Other side effects not listed above may also occur in some patients. If you notice any other effects, check with your doctor.

## Additional Information

Once a medicine has been approved for marketing for a certain use, experience may show that it is also useful for other medical problems. Although these uses are not included in product labeling, tetracyclines are used in certain patients with the following medical conditions:

• Syndrome of inappropriate antidiuretic hormone (SIADH) (for demeclocycline)
• Traveler's diarrhea (for doxycyline)

For patients taking this medicine for *SIADH:*

• Some doctors may prescribe demeclocycline for certain patients who retain (keep) more body water than usual. Although demeclocycline works like a diuretic (water pill) in these patients, it will not work that way in other patients who may need a diuretic.

For patients taking this medicine for *Traveler's diarrhea:*

• Some doctors may prescribe doxycycline by mouth to help prevent or treat traveler's diarrhea. It is usually given daily for three weeks to prevent traveler's diarrhea. If you have any questions about this, check with your doctor.

Other than the above information, there is no additional information relating to proper use, precautions, or side effects for these uses.

Revised: 08/30/92
Interim revision(s): 03/18/94; 05/26/94

# TETRACYCLINES   Topical

Some commonly used brand names are:
**In the U.S.—**
   Aureomycin[1]           Meclan[2]
   Achromycin[3]           Topicycline[3]
**In Canada—**
   Achromycin[3]
   Aureomycin[1]
Note: For quick reference, the following tetracyclines are numbered to match the corresponding brand names.
This information applies to the following medicines:
1. Chlortetracycline (klor-te-tra-SYE-kleen)
2. Meclocycline (me-kloe-SYE-kleen)
3. Tetracycline (te-tra-SYE-kleen)

## Description

Tetracyclines belong to the family of medicines called antibiotics. The topical ointment forms are used to treat infections of the skin. Meclocycline cream and the topical liquid form of tetracycline are used to help control acne. They may be used alone or with one or more other medicines that are applied to the skin or taken by mouth for acne.

Topical ointment forms of the tetracyclines are available without a prescription; however, your doctor may have special instructions on the proper use of these medicines for your medical problem. Meclocycline cream and the topical liquid form of tetracycline are available only with your doctor's prescription.

Topical tetracycline is available in the following dosage forms:

*Topical*

Chlortetracycline
- Ointment (U.S. and Canada)

Meclocycline
- Cream (U.S.)

Tetracycline
- Ointment (U.S. and Canada)
- Topical solution (U.S.)

---

## Before Using This Medicine

In deciding to use a medicine, the risks of using the medicine must be weighed against the good it will do. This is a decision you and your doctor will make. For topical tetracyclines, the following should be considered:

**Allergies**—Tell your doctor if you have ever had any unusual or allergic reaction to topical tetracyclines or to any related antibiotics, such as chlortetracycline for the eye (e.g., Aureomycin); demeclocycline (e.g., Declomycin); doxycycline (e.g., Vibramycin); methacycline (e.g., Rondomycin); minocycline (e.g., Minocin); oxytetracycline (e.g., Terramycin); or tetracycline by mouth or by injection (e.g., Achromycin). In addition, if you are to use the cream form of meclocycline, tell your doctor if you have ever had any unusual or allergic reaction to formaldehyde. Also tell your health care professional if you are allergic to any other substances, such as preservatives or dyes.

**Pregnancy**—Studies have not been done in humans. In studies in rats and rabbits, chlortetracycline and tetracycline topical preparations have not been shown to cause birth defects or other problems. However, studies in rabbits have shown meclocycline to cause a slight delay in bone formation.

**Breast-feeding**—It is not known whether tetracycline topical preparations pass into breast milk. Although most medicines pass into breast milk in small amounts, many of them may be used safely while breast-feeding. Mothers who are using any of these medicines and who wish to breast-feed should discuss this with their doctor.

**Children**—Tetracycline topical solution has been tested on a limited number of children 11 years of age or older and has not been shown to cause different side effects or problems in children than it does in adults. Although there is no specific information about the use of topical chlortetracycline or topical meclocycline in children, they are not expected to cause different side effects or problems in children than they do in adults.

**Older adults**—Many medicines have not been tested in older people. Therefore, it may not be known whether they work exactly the same way they do in younger adults or if they cause different side effects or problems in older

people. There is no specific information about the use of topical tetracyclines in the elderly.

**Other medicines**—Although certain medicines should not be used together at all, in other cases two different medicines may be used together even if an interaction might occur. In these cases, your doctor may want to change the dose, or other precautions may be necessary. When you are using topical tetracyclines, it is important that your health care professional knows if you are using any other topical prescription or nonprescription (over-the-counter [OTC]) medicine that is to be applied to the same area of the skin.

---

## Proper Use of This Medicine

For patients using the *cream form or topical liquid form* of this medicine for acne:

- The cream or topical liquid form of this medicine will not cure your acne. However, to help keep your acne under control, *keep using this medicine for the full time of treatment,* even if your symptoms begin to clear up after a few days. You may have to continue using this medicine every day for months or even longer in some cases. If you stop using this medicine too soon, your symptoms may return. *It is important that you do not miss any doses.*

For patients using the *cream form* of this medicine for acne:

- Do not get this medicine on your clothing since it may stain.
- Before applying this medicine, thoroughly wash the affected area with warm water and soap, rinse well, and pat dry.
- To use:
  —Apply a thin film of medicine, using enough to cover the affected area lightly. *You should apply the medicine to the whole area usually affected by acne, not just to the pimples themselves.* This will help keep new pimples from breaking out.
  —Do not get this medicine in the eyes, nose, mouth, or on other mucous membranes. Spread the medicine away from these areas when applying.

For patients using the *topical liquid form* of this medicine for acne:

- Do not get this medicine on your clothing since it may stain.
- This medicine usually comes with patient instructions. Read these instructions carefully before using this medicine.
- The liquid form contains alcohol and is flammable. *Do not use near heat, near open flame, or while smoking.*
- Do not use after the expiration date on the label. The medicine may not work properly. Check with your pharmacist if you have any questions about this.
- The presence of the floating plastic plug in the liquid means that the medicine has been mixed properly. *Do not remove the plastic plug.*

- It is important that you do not use this medicine more often than your doctor ordered. It may cause your skin to become too dry or irritated.
- Before applying this medicine, thoroughly wash the affected area with warm water and soap, rinse well, and pat dry. After washing or shaving, it is best to wait 30 minutes before applying this medicine. The alcohol in it may irritate freshly washed or shaved skin.
- You should avoid washing the acne-affected areas too often. This may dry your skin and make your acne worse. Washing with a mild, bland soap 2 or 3 times a day should be enough, unless you have oily skin. If you have any questions about this, check with your doctor.
- To use:

  —This medicine comes in a bottle with an applicator tip that may be used to apply the medicine directly to the skin. Use the applicator with a dabbing motion instead of a rolling motion (not like a roll-on deodorant, for example). Tilt the bottle and press the tip firmly against your skin. If needed, you can make the medicine flow faster from the applicator tip by slightly increasing the pressure against the skin. If the medicine flows too fast, use less pressure.

  —Apply a generous amount of medicine, using enough so that the skin feels wet all over. After applying the medicine with the applicator, use your fingertips to spread the medicine around evenly and rub it into your skin. A second coat may be needed to completely cover the affected areas. Be sure to wash the medicine off your hands afterward.

  —*You should apply the medicine to the whole area usually affected by acne, not just to the pimples themselves.* This will help keep new pimples from breaking out.

  —Since this medicine contains alcohol, it will sting or burn. Therefore, *do not get this medicine in the eyes, nose, mouth, or on other mucous membranes.* Spread the medicine away from these areas when applying. If this medicine does get in the eyes, wash them out immediately, but carefully, with large amounts of cool tap water. If your eyes still burn or are painful, check with your doctor.

- The bottle contains about an 8-week supply of medicine if used only on the face and neck or about a 4-week supply if used on the face and neck plus other affected areas.

For patients using the *topical ointment form* of this medicine:

- To help clear up your infection completely, *keep using this medicine for the full time of treatment,* even if your symptoms begin to clear up after a few days. If you stop using this medicine too soon, your symptoms may return. *Do not miss any doses.*
- Do not get this medicine on your clothing since it may stain.

- If you are using this medicine without a prescription, do not use it to treat deep wounds, puncture wounds, or serious burns without first checking with your health care professional.
- Do not get this medicine in the eyes.
- Before applying this medicine, thoroughly wash the affected area with warm water and soap, rinse well, and dry completely.
- After applying this medicine, you may cover the treated area with a gauze dressing if you wish.

**Dosing**—The dose of these medicines will be different for different patients. *Follow your doctor's orders or the directions on the label.* The following information includes only the average doses of these medicines. *If your dose is different, do not change it* unless your doctor tells you to do so.

*For chlortetracycline*
- For *ointment* dosage form:
  —For skin infections:
    - Adults and children—Use one or two times a day.

*For meclocycline*
- For *cream* dosage form:
  —For acne:
    - Adults and children—Use two times a day, morning and evening.

*For tetracycline*
- For *ointment* dosage form:
  —For skin infections:
    - Adults and children—Use one or two times a day.
- For *topical solution* dosage form:
  —For acne:
    - Adults and children over 11 years of age—Use two times a day, morning and evening.
    - Infants and children up to 11 years of age—Use and dose must be determined by the doctor.

**Missed dose**—If you miss a dose of this medicine, apply it as soon as possible. However, if it is almost time for your next dose, skip the missed dose and go back to your regular dosing schedule.

**Storage**—To store this medicine:
- Keep out of the reach of children.
- Store away from heat and direct light.
- Keep the medicine from freezing.
- Do not keep outdated medicine or medicine no longer needed. Be sure that any discarded medicine is out of the reach of children.

---

## Precautions While Using This Medicine

For patients using either the *cream form or the topical liquid form* of this medicine for acne:

- Some people may notice improvement in their acne within 4 to 6 weeks. However, if there is no improvement in your acne after you have used this medicine for 6 to 8 weeks or if it becomes worse, check with your health care professional. The treatment of acne may take up to 8 to 12 weeks before full improvement is seen.

- If your doctor has ordered another medicine to be applied to the skin along with this medicine, it is best to wait at least 1 hour before you apply the second medicine. This may help keep your skin from becoming too irritated. Also, if the medicines are used too close together, they may not work properly.
- The liquid form of this medicine may also cause the skin to become unusually dry, even with normal use. If this occurs, check with your doctor.
- This medicine may cause faint yellowing of the skin, especially around hair roots. This may be more easily seen in people with light complexions. The color may be removed by washing. However, the medicine should be left on the skin as long as possible. Do not wash immediately after applying the medicine. To do so will keep the medicine from working properly. If the yellow color is bothersome during the daytime, the medicine may be applied after school or work and again at bedtime, unless otherwise directed by your doctor.
- Treated areas of the skin may glow bright yellow under "black" (ultraviolet or UV) light such as that used in some discos. To help reduce or avoid this, apply the medicine later in the evening or wash it off before exposure to "black" light.
- You may continue to use cosmetics (make-up) while you are using this medicine for acne. However, it is best to use only "water-base" cosmetics. Also, it is best not to use cosmetics too heavily or too often. They may make your acne worse. If you have any questions about this, check with your doctor.

For patients using the *topical ointment form* of this medicine:

- If your skin infection does not improve within 2 weeks, or if it becomes worse, check with your health care professional.

## Side Effects of This Medicine

Along with its needed effects, a medicine may cause some unwanted effects. Although not all of these side effects may occur, if they do occur they may need medical attention.

Check with your doctor as soon as possible if any of the following side effects occur:

*Less common*
　　Pain, redness, swelling, or other sign of irritation not present before use of this medicine

Other side effects may occur that usually do not need medical attention. These side effects may go away during treatment as your body adjusts to the medicine. However, check with your doctor if any of the following side effects continue or are bothersome:

*More common—For topical liquid form only*
　　Dry or scaly skin; stinging or burning feeling
*More common—For cream and topical liquid forms only*
　　Faint yellowing of the skin, especially around hair roots

Other side effects not listed above may also occur in some patients. If you notice any other effects, check with your doctor.

Revised: 10/27/93

# THEOPHYLLINE, EPHEDRINE, GUAIFENESIN, AND PHENOBARBITAL　Systemic†

Some commonly used brand names are:

**In the U.S.—**
　　Bronkolixir　　　　　　Guiaphed
　　Bronkotabs　　　　　　Mudrane GG

†Not commercially available in Canada.

## Description

Theophylline, ephedrine, guaifenesin, and phenobarbital (fee-noe-BAR-bi-tal) combination is used to treat the symptoms of bronchial asthma, chronic bronchitis, emphysema, and other lung diseases. This medicine relieves cough, wheezing, shortness of breath, and troubled breathing. It works by opening up the bronchial tubes (air passages) of the lungs and increasing the flow of air through them.

Some of these preparations are available only with your doctor's prescription. Others are available without a prescription; however, your doctor may have special instructions on the proper use of this medicine for your medical condition.

Theophylline, ephedrine, guaifenesin, and phenobarbital combination is available in the following dosage forms:

*Oral*
- Elixir (U.S.)
- Tablets (U.S.)

## Before Using This Medicine

If you are taking this medicine without a prescription, carefully read and follow any precautions on the label.

For theophylline, ephedrine, guaifenesin, and phenobarbital combination medicine, the following should be considered:

**Allergies**—Tell your doctor if you have ever had any unusual or allergic reaction to aminophylline, caffeine, dyphylline, oxtriphylline, theobromine, or theophylline; ephedrine or medicines like ephedrine such as albuterol, amphetamines, epinephrine, isoproterenol, metaproterenol, norepinephrine, phenylephrine, phenylpropanolamine, pseudoephedrine, or terbutaline; or phenobarbital or other barbiturates. Also tell your health care professional if you are allergic to any other substances, such as foods, preservatives, or dyes.

**Diet**—Make certain your health care professional knows if you are on any special diet, such as a low-sodium or low-sugar diet or a high-protein, low-carbohydrate or low-protein, high-carbohydrate diet. A high-protein, low-carbohydrate diet may decrease the effects of theophylline; a low-protein, high-carbohydrate diet may increase the effects of theophylline.

Avoid eating or drinking large amounts of caffeine-containing foods or beverages, such as chocolate, cocoa, tea, coffee, and cola drinks, because they may increase the central nervous system (CNS) stimulant effects of theophylline.

Also, eating charcoal broiled foods every day while taking theophylline may keep this medicine from working properly.

**Pregnancy**—Studies with theophylline on birth defects has not been done in humans. However, some studies in animals have shown that theophylline causes birth defects when given in doses many times the human dose. Also, use of theophylline during pregnancy may cause unwanted effects such as fast heartbeat, jitteriness, irritability, gagging, vomiting, and breathing problems in the newborn infant.

Studies with ephedrine on birth defects have not been done in either humans or animals.

Phenobarbital taken during pregnancy has been shown to increase the chance of birth defects in humans. Also, taking phenobarbital regularly during the last 3 months of pregnancy may cause the baby to become dependent on the medicine. This may lead to withdrawal side effects in the baby after birth. In addition, one study in humans has suggested that phenobarbital taken during pregnancy may increase the chance of brain tumors in the baby.

Guaifenesin has not been shown to cause birth defects or other problems in humans.

**Breast-feeding**—Theophylline, ephedrine, and phenobarbital pass into the breast milk and may cause unwanted effects such as drowsiness, irritability, fretfulness, or trouble in sleeping in babies of mothers taking this medicine. Guaifenesin has not been reported to cause problems in nursing babies.

**Children**—Newborn infants may be especially sensitive to the effects of theophylline, ephedrine, guaifenesin, and phenobarbital combination medicine. This may increase the chance of side effects during treatment.

**Older adults**—Elderly people 55 years of age or older may be especially sensitive to the effects of theophylline, ephedrine, guaifenesin, and phenobarbital combination medicine. This may increase the chance of side effects during treatment.

**Other medicines**—Although certain medicines should not be used together at all, in other cases two different medicines may be used together even if an interaction might occur. In these cases, your doctor may want to change the dose, or other precautions may be necessary. When you are taking theophylline, ephedrine, guaifenesin, and phenobarbital combination medicine, it is especially important that your health care professional know if you are taking any of the following:

- Anticoagulants (blood thinners) or
- Corticosteroids (cortisone-like medicines) or
- Corticotropin—The effects of these medicines may be decreased by the phenobarbital in this combination medicine
- Beta-blockers (acebutolol [e.g., Sectral], atenolol [e.g., Tenormin], betaxolol [e.g., Betoptic, Kerlone], bisoprolol [e.g., Zebeta], carteolol [e.g., Cartrol], labetalol [e.g., Normodyne], levobunolol [e.g., Betagan], metoprolol [e.g., Lopressor], nadolol [e.g., Corgard], oxprenolol [e.g., Trasicor], penbutolol [e.g., Levatol], pindolol [e.g., Visken], propranolol [e.g., Inderal], sotalol [e.g., Sotacor], timolol [e.g., Blocadren, Timoptic])—Use of these medicines with this combination medicine may prevent either the beta-blocker or this combination medicine from working properly
- Central nervous system (CNS) depressants—The effects of these medicines or the phenobarbital in this combination medicine may be increased
- Cimetidine (e.g., Tagamet) or
- Ciprofloxacin (e.g., Cipro) or
- Erythromycin (e.g., E-Mycin) or
- Nicotine chewing gum (e.g., Nicorette) or
- Norfloxacin (e.g., Noroxin) or
- Ranitidine (e.g., Zantac) or
- Troleandomycin (e.g., TAO)—These medicines may increase the effects of theophylline
- Cocaine or
- Ergoloid mesylates (e.g., Hydergine) or
- Ergotamine (e.g., Gynergen)—The effects of these medicines on the heart and blood vessels may be increased by ephedrine
- Digitalis glycosides (heart medicine)—Use of digitalis glycosides with this combination medicine may increase the chance of irregular heartbeat
- Monoamine oxidase (MAO) inhibitors (furazolidone [e.g., Furoxone], isocarboxazid [e.g., Marplan], phenelzine [e.g., Nardil], procarbazine [e.g., Matulane], tranylcypromine [e.g., Parnate])—Taking ephedrine while you are taking or within 2 weeks of taking monoamine oxidase (MAO) inhibitors may increase the chance of serious side effects
- Oral contraceptives (birth control pills) containing estrogen—Phenobarbital may decrease the birth control effects of these medicines; use of another method of birth control may be necessary while you are taking this combination medicine

- Phenytoin—The effects of phenytoin may be decreased by theophylline
- Smoking tobacco or marijuana—If you smoke or have smoked (tobacco or marijuana) regularly within the last 2 years, the amount of medicine you need may vary, depending on how much and how recently you have smoked

**Other medical problems**—The presence of other medical problems may affect the use of theophylline, ephedrine, guaifenesin, and phenobarbital combination medicine. Make sure you tell your doctor if you have any other medical problems, especially:

- Alcohol abuse or
- Fever or
- Liver disease or
- Respiratory infections, such as influenza (flu)—The effects of theophylline may be increased
- Diabetes mellitus (sugar diabetes)—Ephedrine may make the condition worse; your doctor may need to change the dose of your diabetes medicine
- Diarrhea—The absorption of theophylline may be decreased; therefore, the effects of this medicine may be decreased
- Enlarged prostate or
- Heart or blood vessel disease or
- High blood pressure or
- Hyperactivity (in children) or
- Stomach ulcer (or history of) or other stomach problems or
- Underactive adrenal gland—This combination medicine may make the condition worse
- Fibrocystic breast disease—Symptoms of this disease may be increased by theophylline
- Kidney disease—The effects of phenobarbital may be increased
- Overactive thyroid—The effects of theophylline may be decreased
- Pain—Phenobarbital may cause unusual excitement in the presence of pain
- Porphyria (or history of)—Phenobarbital may make the symptoms of this disease worse

## Proper Use of This Medicine

*This medicine works best when taken with a glass of water on an empty stomach* (either 30 minutes to 1 hour before meals or 2 hours after meals) since that way it will get into the blood sooner. However, in some cases your doctor may want you to take this medicine with meals or right after meals to lessen stomach upset. If you have any questions about how you should be taking this medicine, check with your doctor.

*Take this medicine only as directed.* Do not take more of it and do not take it more often than recommended on the label, unless otherwise directed by your doctor. To do so may increase the chance of serious side effects. Also, if too much is taken, the phenobarbital in this medicine may become habit-forming.

*In order for this medicine to help your medical problem, it must be taken every day in regularly spaced doses as recommended.* This is necessary to keep a constant amount of this medicine in the blood. To help keep the amount constant, do not miss any doses.

**Dosing**—The dose of theophylline, ephedrine, guaifenesin, and phenobarbital combination will be different for different patients. *Follow your doctor's orders or the directions on the label.* The following information includes only the average doses of theophylline, ephedrine, guaifenesin, and phenobarbital combination. *If your dose is different, do not change it* unless your doctor tells you to do so.

The number of tablets or teaspoonfuls of elixir that you take depends on the strength of the medicine. Also, *the number of doses you take each day, the time allowed between doses, and the length of time you take the medicine depend on the medical problem for which you are taking theophylline, ephedrine, guaifenesin, and phenobarbital combination.*

- For symptoms of bronchial asthma, chronic bronchitis, emphysema, or other lung disease:
  —For *elixir* dosage form:
  - Adults—10 milliliters (mL) (2 teaspoonfuls) four times a day or 15 mL (3 teaspoonfuls) three or four times a day, depending on which product you are taking.
  - Children—Dose must be determined by your doctor.
  —For *tablet* dosage form:
  - Adults—One tablet four or five times a day or one or two tablets three or four times a day, depending on which product you are taking.
  - Children—Dose must be determined by your doctor.

**Missed dose**—If you miss a dose of this medicine, take it as soon as possible. However, if it is almost time for your next dose, skip the missed dose and go back to your regular dosing schedule. Do not double doses.

**Storage**—To store this medicine:
- Keep out of the reach of children.
- Store away from heat and direct light.
- Do not store the tablet form of this medicine in the bathroom, near the kitchen sink, or in other damp places. Heat or moisture may cause the medicine to break down.
- Keep the liquid form of this medicine from freezing.
- Do not keep outdated medicine or medicine no longer needed. Be sure that any discarded medicine is out of the reach of children.

## Precautions While Using This Medicine

The theophylline in this medicine may add to the central nervous system (CNS) stimulant effects of caffeine-containing foods or beverages such as chocolate, cocoa, tea, coffee, and cola drinks. *Avoid eating or drinking large amounts of these foods or beverages while taking this medicine.* If you have any questions about this, check with your doctor.

The phenobarbital in this medicine will add to the effects of alcohol and other CNS depressants (medicines that slow down the nervous system, possibly causing drowsiness). Some examples of CNS depressants are antihistamines or medicine for hay fever, other allergies, or colds; sedatives, tranquilizers, or sleeping medicine; prescription pain medicine or narcotics; other barbiturates; medicine for seizures; muscle relaxants; or anesthetics, including some dental anesthetics. *Check with your doctor before taking any of the above while you are using this medicine.*

Do not eat charcoal-broiled foods every day while taking this medicine since these foods may keep the medicine from working properly.

*Check with your doctor at once if you develop symptoms of influenza (flu) or a fever*, since either of these may increase the chance of side effects with this medicine.

Also, *check with your doctor if diarrhea occurs* because the dose of this medicine may need to be changed.

This medicine may cause some people to become dizzy, lightheaded, drowsy, or less alert than they are normally. *Make sure you know how you react to this medicine before you drive, use machines, or do anything else that could be dangerous if you are dizzy or are not alert.*

## Side Effects of This Medicine

Along with its needed effects, a medicine may cause some unwanted effects. Although not all of these side effects may occur, if they do occur they may need medical attention.

Check with your doctor as soon as possible if any of the following side effects occur:

*Less common*
Heartburn and/or vomiting

*Symptoms of overdose*
Bloody or black, tarry stools; chest pain; convulsions (seizures); diarrhea; dizziness or lightheadedness; fast, pounding, or irregular heartbeat; hallucinations (seeing, hearing, or feeling things that are not there); increase or decrease in blood pressure; irritability; loss of appetite; mood or mental changes; muscle twitching; nausea (continuing or severe) or vomiting; stomach cramps or pain; trembling; trouble in sleeping; unusual tiredness or weakness; vomiting blood or material that looks like coffee grounds

Other side effects may occur that usually do not need medical attention. These side effects may go away during treatment as your body adjusts to the medicine. However, check with your health care professional if any of the following side effects continue or are bothersome:

*More common*
Drowsiness; headache; nausea; nervousness or restlessness

*Less common*
Difficult or painful urination; feeling of warmth; flushing or redness of face

Other side effects not listed above may also occur in some patients. If you notice any other effects, check with your doctor.

Revised: October 1990
Interim revision: 09/02/94

# THEOPHYLLINE, EPHEDRINE, AND HYDROXYZINE    Systemic†

Some commonly used brand names are:

**In the U.S.—**
Ami Rax                 Marax-DF
Hydrophed               Theomax DF
Marax
Generic name product may also be available.

†Not commercially available in Canada.

## Description

Theophylline (thee-OFF-i-lin), ephedrine (e-FED-rin), and hydroxyzine (hye-DROX-i-zeen) combination medicine is used to treat the symptoms of bronchial asthma, chronic bronchitis, emphysema, and other lung diseases. This medicine relieves cough, wheezing, shortness of breath, and troubled breathing. It works by opening up the bronchial tubes (air passages) of the lungs and increasing the flow of air through them.

This medicine is available only with your doctor's prescription, in the following dosage forms:

*Oral*
• Syrup (U.S.)
• Tablets (U.S.)

## Before Using This Medicine

In deciding to use a medicine, the risks of taking the medicine must be weighed against the good it will do. This is a decision you and your doctor will make. For theophylline, ephedrine, and hydroxyzine combination medicine, the following should be considered:

**Allergies**—Tell your doctor if you have ever had any unusual or allergic reaction to aminophylline, caffeine, dyphylline, oxtriphylline, theobromine, or theophylline; ephedrine or medicines like ephedrine such as albuterol, amphetamines, epinephrine, isoproterenol, metaproterenol, norepinephrine, phenylephrine, phenylpropanolamine, pseudoephedrine, or terbutaline; or hydroxyzine.

Also tell your health care professional if you are allergic to any other substances, such as foods, preservatives, or dyes.

**Diet**—Make certain your health care professional knows if you are on any special diet, such as a low-sodium or low-sugar diet or a high-protein, low-carbohydrate or low-protein, high-carbohydrate diet. A high-protein, low-carbohydrate diet may decrease the effects of theophylline; a low-protein, high-carbohydrate diet may increase the effects of theophylline.

Avoid eating or drinking large amounts of caffeine-containing foods or beverages, such as chocolate, cocoa, tea, coffee, and cola drinks, because they may increase the central nervous system (CNS) stimulant effects of theophylline.

Also, eating charcoal broiled foods every day while taking theophylline may keep this medicine from working properly.

**Pregnancy**—Studies with theophylline on birth defects have not been done in humans. However, some studies in animals have shown that theophylline causes birth defects when given in doses many times the human dose. Also, use of theophylline during pregnancy may cause unwanted effects such as fast heartbeat, jitteriness, irritability, gagging, vomiting, and breathing problems in the newborn infant.

Studies with ephedrine on birth defects have not been done in either humans or animals.

Hydroxyzine is not recommended during the first months of pregnancy because it has been shown to cause birth defects in rats when given in doses up to many times the usual human dose.

**Breast-feeding**—Theophylline and ephedrine pass into the breast milk and may cause unwanted effects such as irritability, fretfulness, or trouble in sleeping in babies of mothers taking this medicine. Hydroxyzine has not been reported to cause problems in nursing babies.

**Children**—Theophylline, ephedrine, and hydroxyzine combination medicine is not recommended for use in children up to 2 years of age. Although there is no specific information about the use of theophylline, ephedrine, and hydroxyzine combination medicine in children 2 years of age and older, it is not expected to cause different side effects or problems in these children than it does in adults.

**Older adults**—Elderly people 55 years of age or older may be especially sensitive to the effects of theophylline, ephedrine, and hydroxyzine combination medicine. This may increase the chance of side effects during treatment.

**Other medicines**—Although certain medicines should not be used together at all, in other cases two different medicines may be used together even if an interaction might occur. In these cases, your doctor may want to change the dose, or other precautions may be necessary. When you are taking theophylline, ephedrine, and hydroxyzine combination medicine, it is especially important that your

health care professional know if you are taking any of the following:

- Beta-blockers (acebutolol [e.g., Sectral], atenolol [e.g., Tenormin], betaxolol [e.g., Betoptic, Kerlone], bisoprolol [e.g., Zebeta], carteolol [e.g., Cartrol], labetalol [e.g., Normodyne], levobunolol [e.g., Betagan], metoprolol [e.g., Lopressor], nadolol [e.g., Corgard], oxprenolol [e.g., Trasicor], penbutolol [e.g., Levatol], pindolol [e.g., Visken], propranolol [e.g., Inderal], sotalol [e.g., Sotacor], timolol [e.g., Blocadren, Timoptic])—Use of these medicines with this combination medicine may prevent either the beta-blocker or this medicine from working properly
- Central nervous system (CNS) depressants—The effects of these medicines or hydroxyzine may be increased
- Cimetidine (e.g., Tagamet) or
- Ciprofloxacin (e.g., Cipro) or
- Erythromycin (e.g., E-Mycin) or
- Nicotine chewing gum (e.g., Nicorette) or
- Norfloxacin (e.g., Noroxin) or
- Ranitidine (e.g., Zantac) or
- Troleandomycin (e.g., TAO)—These medicines may increase the effects of theophylline
- Cocaine or
- Ergoloid mesylates (e.g., Hydergine) or
- Ergotamine (e.g., Gynergen)—The effects of these medicines on the heart and blood vessels may be increased by ephedrine
- Digitalis glycosides (heart medicine)—Use of these medicines with ephedrine may increase the chance of irregular heartbeat
- Monoamine oxidase (MAO) inhibitors (furazolidone [e.g., Furoxone], isocarboxazid [e.g., Marplan], phenelzine [e.g., Nardil], procarbazine [e.g., Matulane], tranylcypromine [e.g., Parnate])—Taking ephedrine while you are taking or within 2 weeks of taking monoamine oxidase (MAO) inhibitors may increase the chance of serious side effects
- Phenytoin—The effects of phenytoin may be decreased by theophylline
- Smoking tobacco or marijuana—If you smoke or have smoked (tobacco or marijuana) regularly within the last 2 years, the amount of medicine you need may vary, depending on how much and how recently you have smoked

**Other medical problems**—The presence of other medical problems may affect the use of theophylline, ephedrine, and hydroxyzine combination medicine. Make sure you tell your doctor if you have any other medical problems, especially:

- Alcohol abuse or
- Fever or
- Liver disease or
- Respiratory infections, such as influenza (flu)—The effects of theophylline may be increased
- Diabetes mellitus (sugar diabetes)—Ephedrine may make the condition worse; your doctor may need to change the dose of your diabetes medicine
- Diarrhea—The absorption of theophylline may be decreased; therefore, the effects of this medicine may be decreased
- Enlarged prostate or
- Heart or blood vessel disease or
- High blood pressure or
- Stomach ulcer (or history of) or other stomach problems—This combination medicine may make the condition worse

- Fibrocystic breast disease—Symptoms of this disease may be increased by theophylline
- Overactive thyroid—The effects of theophylline may be decreased

## Proper Use of This Medicine

*This medicine works best when taken with a glass of water on an empty stomach* (either 30 minutes to 1 hour before meals or 2 hours after meals) since that way it will get into the blood sooner. However, in some cases your doctor may want you to take this medicine with meals or right after meals to lessen stomach upset. If you have any questions about how you should be taking this medicine, check with your doctor.

*Take this medicine only as directed.* Do not take more of it and do not take it more often than your doctor ordered. To do so may increase the chance of serious side effects.

*In order for this medicine to help your medical problem, it must be taken every day in regularly spaced doses as ordered by your doctor.* This is necessary to keep a constant amount of this medicine in the blood. To help keep the amount constant, do not miss any doses.

**Dosing**—The dose of theophylline, ephedrine, and hydroxyzine combination will be different for different patients. *Follow your doctor's orders or the directions on the label.* The following information includes only the average doses of theophylline, ephedrine, and hydroxyzine combination. *If your dose is different, do not change it* unless your doctor tells you to do so.

- For symptoms of bronchial asthma, chronic bronchitis, emphysema, or other lung disease:
  —For *syrup* dosage form:
    - Adults—20 milliliters (mL) (4 teaspoonfuls) two to four times a day.
    - Children 5 years of age and over—5 mL (1 teaspoonful) three or four times a day.
    - Children 2 to 5 years of age—2.5 to 5 mL (½ to 1 teaspoonful) three or four times a day.
    - Children up to 2 years of age—Use is not recommended.
  —For *tablet* dosage form:
    - Adults—One tablet two to four times a day.
    - Children 5 years of age and over: One-half tablet two to four times a day.
    - Children up to 5 years of age: Use is not recommended.

**Missed dose**—If you miss a dose of this medicine, take it as soon as possible. However, if it is almost time for your next dose, skip the missed dose and go back to your regular dosing schedule. Do not double doses.

**Storage**—To store this medicine:
- Keep out of the reach of children.
- Store away from heat and direct light.
- Do not store the tablet form of this medicine in the bathroom, near the kitchen sink, or in other damp places. Heat or moisture may cause the medicine to break down.
- Keep the syrup form of this medicine from freezing.
- Do not keep outdated medicine or medicine no longer needed. Be sure that any discarded medicine is out of the reach of children.

## Precautions While Using This Medicine

The theophylline in this medicine may add to the central nervous system stimulant effects of caffeine-containing foods or beverages such as chocolate, cocoa, tea, coffee, and cola drinks. *Avoid eating or drinking large amounts of these foods or beverages while taking this medicine.* If you have any questions about this, check with your doctor.

The hydroxyzine in this medicine will add to the effects of alcohol and CNS depressants (medicines that slow down the nervous system, possibly causing drowsiness). Some examples of CNS depressants are antihistamines or medicine for hay fever, other allergies, or colds; sedatives, tranquilizers, or sleeping medicine; prescription pain medicine or narcotics; barbiturates; medicine for seizures; muscle relaxants; or anesthetics, including dental anesthetics. *Check with your doctor before taking any of the above while you are taking this medicine.*

Do not eat charcoal-broiled foods every day while taking this medicine since these foods may keep the medicine from working properly.

*Check with your doctor at once if you develop symptoms of influenza (flu) or a fever*, since either of these may increase the chance of side effects with this medicine.

Also, *check with your doctor if diarrhea occurs* because the dose of this medicine may need to be changed.

This medicine may cause some people to become dizzy, lightheaded, drowsy, or less alert than they are normally. *Make sure you know how you react to this medicine before you drive, use machines, or do anything else that could be dangerous if you are dizzy or are not alert.*

## Side Effects of This Medicine

Along with its needed effects, a medicine may cause some unwanted effects. Although not all of these side effects may occur, if they do occur they may need medical attention.

Check with your doctor as soon as possible if any of the following side effects occur:

*Less common*
   Heartburn and/or vomiting
*Symptoms of overdose*
   Bloody or black, tarry stools; chest pain; convulsions (seizures); diarrhea; dizziness or lightheadedness; fast, pounding, or irregular heartbeat; hallucinations (seeing, hearing, or feeling things that are not there); increase or decrease in blood pressure; irritability; loss of appetite; mood or mental changes; muscle twitching; nausea (continuing or severe) or vomiting; stomach

cramps or pain; trembling; trouble in sleeping; unusual tiredness or weakness; vomiting blood or material that looks like coffee grounds

Other side effects may occur that usually do not need medical attention. These side effects may go away during treatment as your body adjusts to the medicine. However, check with your doctor if any of the following side effects continue or are bothersome:

*More common*
   Drowsiness; headache; nausea; nervousness or restlessness

*Less common*
   Difficult or painful urination; feeling of warmth; flushing or redness of face

Other side effects not listed above may also occur in some patients. If you notice any other effects, check with your doctor.

Revised: October 1990
Interim revision: 09/02/94

---

# THEOPHYLLINE, EPHEDRINE, AND PHENOBARBITAL   Systemic†

Some commonly used brand names are:

**In the U.S.—**
   Tedrigen
   Theodrine
   Theofedral
   Theophedrital
   Theotal

   Generic name product may also be available.

†Not commercially available in Canada.

## Description

Theophylline (thee-OFF-i-lin), ephedrine (e-FED-rin), and phenobarbital (fee-noe-BAR-bi-tal) combination is used to treat the symptoms of bronchial asthma, asthmatic bronchitis, and other lung diseases. This medicine relieves cough, wheezing, shortness of breath, and troubled breathing. It works by opening up the bronchial tubes (air passages) of the lungs and increasing the flow of air through them.

Some preparations of this medicine are available only with your doctor's prescription. Others are available without a prescription; however, your doctor may have special instructions on the proper dose of this medicine for your medical condition.

Theophylline, ephedrine, and phenobarbital combination is available in the following dosage forms:

*Oral*
   • Tablets (U.S.)

## Before Using This Medicine

If you are taking this medicine without a prescription, carefully read and follow any precautions on the label. For theophylline, ephedrine, and phenobarbital combination medicine, the following should be considered:

**Allergies**—Tell your doctor if you have ever had any unusual or allergic reaction to aminophylline, caffeine, dyphylline, oxtriphylline, theobromine, or theophylline; to ephedrine or medicines like ephedrine such as albuterol, amphetamines, epinephrine, isoproterenol, metaproterenol, norepinephrine, phenylephrine, phenylpropanolamine, pseudoephedrine, or terbutaline; or to phenobarbital or other barbiturates. Also tell your health care professional if you are allergic to any other substances, such as foods, preservatives, or dyes.

**Diet**—Make certain your health care professional knows if you are on any special diet, such as a low-sodium or low-sugar diet or a high-protein, low-carbohydrate or low-protein, high-carbohydrate diet. A high-protein, low-carbohydrate diet may decrease the effects of theophylline; a low-protein, high-carbohydrate diet may increase the effects of theophylline.

Avoid eating or drinking large amounts of caffeine-containing foods or beverages, such as chocolate, cocoa, tea, coffee, and cola drinks, because they may increase the central nervous system (CNS) stimulant effects of theophylline.

Also, eating charcoal broiled foods every day while taking theophylline may keep this medicine from working properly.

**Pregnancy**—Studies with theophylline on birth defects have not been done in humans. However, some studies in animals have shown that theophylline causes birth defects when given in doses many times the human dose. Also, use of theophylline during pregnancy may cause unwanted effects such as fast heartbeat, jitteriness, irritability, gagging, vomiting, and breathing problems in the newborn infant.

Studies with ephedrine on birth defects have not been done in either humans or animals.

Phenobarbital taken during pregnancy has been shown to increase the chance of birth defects in humans. Also, taking phenobarbital regularly during the last 3 months of pregnancy may cause the baby to become dependent on the medicine. This may lead to withdrawal side effects in the baby after birth. In addition, one study in humans has suggested that phenobarbital taken during pregnancy may increase the chance of brain tumors in the baby.

**Breast-feeding**—Theophylline, ephedrine, and phenobarbital pass into the breast milk and may cause unwanted effects such as drowsiness, irritability, fretfulness, or trouble in sleeping in nursing babies of mothers taking this medicine.

**Children**—Newborn infants may be especially sensitive to the effects of theophylline, ephedrine, and phenobarbital combination medicine. This may increase the chance of side effects during treatment.

**Older adults**—Elderly people 55 years of age or older may be especially sensitive to the effects of theophylline, ephedrine, and phenobarbital combination medicine. This may increase the chance of side effects during treatment.

**Other medicines**—Although certain medicines should not be used together at all, in other cases two different medicines may be used together even if an interaction might occur. In these cases, your doctor may want to change the dose, or other precautions may be necessary. When you are taking theophylline, ephedrine, and phenobarbital combination medicine, it is especially important that your health care professional know if you are taking any of the following:

- Anticoagulants (blood thinners) or
- Corticosteroids (cortisone-like medicines) or
- Corticotropin—The effects of these medicines may be decreased by phenobarbital
- Beta-blockers (acebutolol [e.g., Sectral], atenolol [e.g., Tenormin], betaxolol [e.g., Betoptic, Kerlone], bisoprolol [e.g., Zebeta], carteolol [e.g., Cartrol], labetalol [e.g., Normodyne], levobunolol [e.g., Betagan], metoprolol [e.g., Lopressor], nadolol [e.g., Corgard], oxprenolol [e.g., Trasicor], penbutolol [e.g., Levatol], pindolol [e.g., Visken], propranolol [e.g., Inderal], sotalol [e.g., Sotacor], timolol [e.g., Blocadren, Timoptic])—Use of these medicines with this combination medicine may prevent either the beta-blocker or this combination medicine from working properly
- Central nervous system (CNS) depressants—The effects of these medicines or phenobarbital may be increased
- Cimetidine (e.g., Tagamet) or
- Ciprofloxacin (e.g., Cipro) or
- Erythromycin (e.g., E-Mycin) or
- Nicotine chewing gum (e.g., Nicorette) or
- Norfloxacin (e.g., Noroxin) or
- Ranitidine (e.g., Zantac) or
- Troleandomycin (e.g., TAO)—These medicines may increase the effects of theophylline
- Cocaine or
- Ergoloid mesylates (e.g., Hydergine) or
- Ergotamine (e.g., Gynergen)—The effects of these medicines on the heart and blood vessels may be increased by ephedrine
- Digitalis glycosides (heart medicine)—Use of digitalis glycosides with this combination medicine may increase the chance of irregular heartbeat
- Monoamine oxidase (MAO) inhibitors (furazolidone [e.g., Furoxone], isocarboxazid [e.g., Marplan], phenelzine [e.g., Nardil], procarbazine [e.g., Matulane], tranylcypromine [e.g., Parnate])—Taking ephedrine while you are taking or within 2 weeks of taking monoamine oxidase (MAO) inhibitors may increase the chance of serious side effects
- Oral contraceptives (birth control pills) containing estrogen—Phenobarbital may decrease the birth control effects of these medicines; use of another method of birth control may be necessary while you are taking this combination medicine
- Phenytoin—The effects of phenytoin may be decreased by theophylline

- Smoking tobacco or marijuana—If you smoke or have smoked (tobacco or marijuana) regularly within the last 2 years, the amount of medicine you need may vary, depending on how much and how recently you have smoked

**Other medical problems**—The presence of other medical problems may affect the use of theophylline, ephedrine, and phenobarbital combination medicine. Make sure you tell your doctor if you have any other medical problems, especially:

- Alcohol abuse or
- Fever or
- Liver disease or
- Respiratory infections, such as influenza (flu)—The effects of theophylline may be increased
- Diabetes mellitus (sugar diabetes)—Ephedrine may make the condition worse; your doctor may need to change the dose of your diabetes medicine
- Diarrhea—The absorption of theophylline may be decreased; therefore, the effects of this medicine may be decreased
- Enlarged prostate or
- Heart or blood vessel disease or
- High blood pressure or
- Hyperactivity (in children) or
- Stomach ulcer (or history of) or other stomach problems or
- Underactive adrenal gland—This combination medicine may make the condition worse
- Fibrocystic breast disease—Symptoms of this disease may be increased by theophylline
- Kidney disease—The effects of phenobarbital may be increased
- Overactive thyroid—The effects of theophylline may be decreased
- Pain—Phenobarbital may cause unusual excitement in the presence of pain
- Porphyria (or history of)—Phenobarbital may make the symptoms of this disease worse

---

## Proper Use of This Medicine

*This medicine works best when taken with a glass of water on an empty stomach* (either 30 minutes to 1 hour before meals or 2 hours after meals) since that way it will get into the blood sooner. However, in some cases your doctor may want you to take this medicine with meals or right after meals to lessen stomach upset. If you have any questions about how you should be taking this medicine, check with your doctor.

*Take this medicine only as directed.* Do not take more of it and do not take it more often than recommended on the label, unless otherwise directed by your doctor. To do so may increase the chance of serious side effects. Also, if too much is taken, the phenobarbital in this medicine may become habit-forming.

*In order for this medicine to help your medical problem, it must be taken every day in regularly spaced doses as recommended.* This is necessary to keep a constant amount of this medicine in the blood. To help keep the amount constant, do not miss any doses.

**Dosing**—The dose of theophylline, ephedrine, and phenobarbital combination will be different for different patients. *Follow your doctor's orders or the directions on the label.* The following information includes only the average doses of theophylline, ephedrine, and phenobarbital combination. *If your dose is different, do not change it* unless your doctor tells you to do so.

The number of tablets that you take depends on the strength of the medicine. Also, *the number of doses you take each day, the time allowed between doses, and the length of time you take the medicine depend on the medical problem for which you are taking theophylline, ephedrine, and phenobarbital combination.*

- For *oral* dosage form (tablets):
  —For symptoms of bronchial asthma, chronic bronchitis, emphysema, or other lung disease:
    - Adults—One or two tablets every four hours.
    - Children 6 to 12 years of age—One-half to one tablet every four hours.
    - Children up to 6 years of age—Dose must be determined by your doctor.

**Missed dose**—If you miss a dose of this medicine, take it as soon as possible. However, if it is almost time for your next dose, skip the missed dose and go back to your regular dosing schedule. Do not double doses.

**Storage**—To store this medicine:
- Keep out of the reach of children.
- Store away from heat and direct light.
- Do not store the tablet form of this medicine in the bathroom, near the kitchen sink, or in other damp places. Heat or moisture may cause the medicine to break down.
- Do not keep outdated medicine or medicine no longer needed. Be sure that any discarded medicine is out of the reach of children.

## Precautions While Using This Medicine

The theophylline in this medicine may add to the central nervous system stimulant effects of caffeine-containing foods or beverages such as chocolate, cocoa, tea, coffee, and cola drinks. *Avoid eating or drinking large amounts of these foods or beverages while taking this medicine.* If you have any questions about this, check with your doctor.

The phenobarbital in this combination medicine will add to the effects of alcohol and other CNS depressants (medicines that slow down the nervous system, possibly caus-

ing drowsiness). Some examples of CNS depressants are antihistamines or medicine for hay fever, other allergies, or colds; sedatives, tranquilizers, or sleeping medicine; prescription pain medicine or narcotics; other barbiturates; medicine for seizures; muscle relaxants; or anesthetics, including some dental anesthetics. *Check with your doctor before taking any of the above while you are using this medicine.*

Do not eat charcoal-broiled foods every day while taking this medicine since these foods may keep the medicine from working properly.

*Check with your doctor at once if you develop symptoms of influenza (flu) or a fever* since either of these may increase the chance of side effects with this medicine.

Also, *check with your doctor if diarrhea occurs* because the dose of this medicine may need to be changed.

This medicine may cause some people to become dizzy, lightheaded, drowsy, or less alert than they are normally. *Make sure you know how you react to this medicine before you drive, use machines, or do anything else that could be dangerous if you are dizzy or are not alert.*

## Side Effects of This Medicine

Along with its needed effects, a medicine may cause some unwanted effects. Although not all of these side effects may occur, if they do occur they may need medical attention.

Check with your doctor as soon as possible if any of the following side effects occur:

*Less common*
  Heartburn and/or vomiting

*Symptoms of overdose*
  Bloody or black, tarry stools; chest pain; convulsions (seizures); diarrhea; dizziness or lightheadedness; fast, pounding, or irregular heartbeat; hallucinations (seeing, hearing, or feeling things that are not there); increase or decrease in blood pressure; irritability; loss of appetite; mood or mental changes; muscle twitching; nausea (continuing or severe) or vomiting; stomach cramps or pain; trembling; trouble in sleeping; unusual tiredness or weakness; vomiting blood or material that looks like coffee grounds

Other side effects may occur that usually do not need medical attention. These side effects may go away during treatment as your body adjusts to the medicine. However, check with your health care professional if any of the following side effects continue or are bothersome:

*More common*

Drowsiness; headache; nausea; nervousness or restlessness

*Less common*

Difficult or painful urination; feeling of warmth; flushing or redness of face

Other side effects not listed above may also occur in some patients. If you notice any other effects, check with your doctor.

---

Revised: October 1990
Interim revision: 09/02/94

---

# THEOPHYLLINE AND GUAIFENESIN    Systemic†

Some commonly used brand names are:

**In the U.S.—**

| | |
|---|---|
| Asbron G | Mudrane GG-2 |
| Asbron G Inlay-Tabs | Quibron |
| Bronchial | Quibron-300 |
| Broncomar GG | Slo-Phyllin GG |
| Ed-Bron G | Synophylate-GG |
| Elixophyllin-GG | Theolate |
| Equibron G | Uni-Bronchial |
| Glyceryl-T | |

Generic name product may also be available.

Another commonly used name is theophylline and glyceryl guaiacolate.

†Not commercially available in Canada.

---

## Description

Theophylline (thee-OFF-i-lin) and guaifenesin (gwye-FEN-e-sin) combination is used to treat the symptoms of bronchial asthma, chronic bronchitis, emphysema, and other lung diseases. This medicine relieves cough, wheezing, shortness of breath, and troubled breathing. It works by opening up the bronchial tubes (air passages) of the lungs and increasing the flow of air through them.

This medicine is available only with your doctor's prescription, in the following dosage forms:

*Oral*

- Capsules (U.S.)
- Elixir (U.S.)
- Oral solution (U.S.)
- Syrup (U.S.)
- Tablets (U.S.)

## Before Using This Medicine

In deciding to use a medicine, the risks of taking the medicine must be weighed against the good it will do. This is a decision you and your doctor will make. For theophylline and guaifenesin combination medicine, the following should be considered:

**Allergies**—Tell your doctor if you have ever had any unusual or allergic reaction to aminophylline, caffeine, dyphylline, oxtriphylline, theobromine, or theophylline. Also tell your health care professional if you are allergic to any other substances, such as foods, preservatives, or dyes.

**Diet**—Make certain your health care professional knows if you are on any special diet, such as a low-sodium or low-sugar diet or a high-protein, low-carbohydrate or low-protein, high-carbohydrate diet. A high-protein, low-carbohydrate diet may decrease the effects of theophylline; a low-protein, high-carbohydrate diet may increase the effects of theophylline.

Avoid eating or drinking large amounts of caffeine-containing foods or beverages, such as chocolate, cocoa, tea, coffee, and cola drinks, because they may increase the central nervous system (CNS) stimulant effects of theophylline.

Also, eating charcoal broiled foods every day while taking theophylline may keep this medicine from working properly.

**Pregnancy**—Studies on birth defects have not been done in humans. However, some studies in animals have shown that theophylline causes birth defects when given in doses many times the human dose. Also, use of theophylline during pregnancy may cause unwanted effects such as fast heartbeat, jitteriness, irritability, gagging, vomiting, and breathing problems in the newborn infant. Guaifenesin has not been shown to cause birth defects or other problems in humans.

**Breast-feeding**—Theophylline passes into the breast milk and may cause irritability, fretfulness, or trouble in sleeping in babies of mothers taking this medicine. Guaifenesin has not been reported to cause problems in nursing babies.

**Children**—The side effects of theophylline are more likely to occur in newborn infants, who are usually more sensitive to the effects of this medicine.

Although there is no specific information about the use of guaifenesin in children, it is not expected to cause different side effects or problems in children than it does in adults.

**Older adults**—The side effects of theophylline are more likely to occur in elderly patients 55 years of age and older, who are usually more sensitive than younger adults to the effects of this medicine.

Although there is no specific information about the use of guaifenesin in the elderly, it is not expected to cause different side effects or problems in older people than it does in younger adults.

**Other medicines**—Although certain medicines should not be used together at all, in other cases two different medicines may be used together even if an interaction might occur. In these cases, your doctor may want to change the dose, or other precautions may be necessary. When you are taking theophylline and guaifenesin combination medicine, it is especially important that your health care professional know if you are taking any of the following:

- Beta-blockers (acebutolol [e.g., Sectral], atenolol [e.g., Tenormin], betaxolol [e.g., Betoptic, Kerlone], bisoprolol [e.g., Zebeta], carteolol [e.g., Cartrol], labetalol [e.g., Normodyne], levobunolol [e.g., Betagan], metoprolol [e.g., Lopressor], nadolol [e.g., Corgard], oxprenolol [e.g., Trasicor], penbutolol [e.g., Levatol], pindolol [e.g., Visken], propranolol [e.g., Inderal], sotalol [e.g., Sotacor], timolol [e.g., Blocadren, Timoptic])—Use of these medicines with theophylline may prevent either the beta-blocker or theophylline from working properly
- Cimetidine (e.g., Tagamet) or
- Ciprofloxacin (e.g., Cipro) or
- Erythromycin (e.g., E-Mycin) or
- Nicotine chewing gum (e.g., Nicorette) or
- Norfloxacin (e.g., Noroxin) or
- Ranitidine (e.g., Zantac) or
- Troleandomycin (e.g., TAO)—These medicines may increase the effects of theophylline
- Phenytoin (e.g., Dilantin)—The effects of phenytoin may be decreased by theophylline
- Smoking tobacco or marijuana—If you smoke or have smoked (tobacco or marijuana) regularly within the last 2 years, the amount of medicine you need may vary, depending on how much and how recently you have smoked

**Other medical problems**—The presence of other medical problems may affect the use of theophylline and guaifenesin combination medicine. Make sure you tell your doctor if you have any other medical problems, especially:

- Alcohol abuse or
- Fever or
- Liver disease or
- Respiratory infections, such as influenza (flu)—The effects of theophylline may be increased
- Diarrhea—The absorption of theophylline may be decreased; therefore, the effects of this medicine may be decreased
- Enlarged prostate or
- Heart disease or
- High blood pressure or
- Stomach ulcer (or history of) or other stomach problems—Theophylline may make the condition worse
- Fibrocystic breast disease—Symptoms of this disease may be increased by theophylline
- Overactive thyroid—The effects of theophylline may be decreased

## Proper Use of This Medicine

*This medicine works best when taken with a glass of water on an empty stomach* (either 30 minutes to 1 hour before meals or 2 hours after meals) since that way it will get into the blood sooner. However, in some cases your doctor may want you to take this medicine with meals or right after meals to lessen stomach upset. If you

have any questions about how you should be taking this medicine, check with your doctor.

*Take this medicine only as directed.* Do not take more of it, do not take it more often, and do not take it for a longer time than your doctor ordered. To do so may increase the chance of serious side effects.

*In order for this medicine to help your medical problem, it must be taken every day in regularly spaced doses as ordered by your doctor.* This is necessary to keep a constant amount of this medicine in the blood. To help keep the amount constant, do not miss any doses.

**Dosing**—When you are taking theophylline and guaifenesin combination, it is very important that you get the exact amount of medicine that you need. The dose of this medicine will be different for different patients. Your doctor will determine the proper dose of the theophylline and guaifenesin combination for you. *Follow your doctor's orders or the directions on the label.*

After you begin taking theophylline and guaifenesin combination, it is very important that your doctor check your blood level of theophylline at regular intervals to find out if your dose of theophylline and guaifenesin combination needs to be changed. *Do not change your dose of theophylline and guaifenesin combination* unless your doctor tells you to do so.

The number of capsules or tablets or teaspoonfuls of elixir, solution, or syrup that you take depends on the strength of the medicine.

**Missed dose**—If you miss a dose of this medicine, take it as soon as possible. However, if it is almost time for your next dose, skip the missed dose and go back to your regular dosing schedule. Do not double doses.

**Storage**—To store this medicine:

- Keep out of the reach of children.
- Store away from heat and direct light.
- Do not store the capsule or tablet form of this medicine in the bathroom, near the kitchen sink, or in other damp places. Heat or moisture may cause the medicine to break down.
- Keep the liquid form of this medicine from freezing.
- Do not keep outdated medicine or medicine no longer needed. Be sure that any discarded medicine is out of the reach of children.

## Precautions While Using This Medicine

Your doctor should check your progress at regular visits, especially for the first few weeks after you begin taking this medicine. A blood test may be taken to help your doctor decide whether the dose of this medicine should be changed.

The theophylline in this medicine may add to the central nervous system stimulant effects of caffeine-containing foods or beverages such as chocolate, cocoa, tea, coffee, and cola drinks. *Avoid eating or drinking large amounts of these foods or beverages while taking this medicine.*

If you have any questions about this, check with your doctor.

Do not eat charcoal-broiled foods every day while taking this medicine since these foods may keep the medicine from working properly.

*Check with your doctor at once if you develop symptoms of influenza (flu) or a fever* since either of these may increase the chance of side effects with this medicine.

Also, *check with your doctor if diarrhea occurs* because the dose of this medicine may need to be changed.

---

## Side Effects of This Medicine

Along with its needed effects, a medicine may cause some unwanted effects. Although not all of these side effects may occur, if they do occur they may need medical attention.

Check with your doctor as soon as possible if any of the following side effects occur:

*Less common*
   Heartburn and/or vomiting

*Symptoms of overdose of theophylline*
   Bloody or black, tarry stools; confusion or change in behavior; convulsions (seizures); diarrhea; dizziness or lightheadedness; fast breathing; fast, pounding, or irregular heartbeat; flushing or redness of face; headache; increased urination; irritability; loss of appetite; muscle twitching; nausea (continuing or severe) or vomiting; stomach cramps or pain; trembling; trouble in sleeping; unusual tiredness or weakness; vomiting blood or material that looks like coffee grounds

Other side effects may occur that usually do not need medical attention. These side effects may go away during treatment as your body adjusts to the medicine. However, check with your doctor if any of the following side effects continue or are bothersome:

*More common*
   Nausea; nervousness or restlessness

Other side effects not listed above may also occur in some patients. If you notice any other effects, check with your doctor.

---

Revised: October 1990
Interim revision: 09/02/94

---

# THIABENDAZOLE   Systemic†

Some commonly used brand names are:
**In the U.S.**
   Mintezol
**Other**
   Foldan                    Triasox
   Minzolum

---

†Not commercially available in Canada.

---

## Description

Thiabendazole (thye-a-BEN-da-zole) belongs to the family of medicines called anthelmintics (ant-hel-MIN-tiks). Anthelmintics are medicines used in the treatment of worm infections.

Thiabendazole is used to treat:
   • creeping eruption (cutaneous larva migrans);
   • pork worms (trichinosis);
   • threadworms (strongyloidiasis); and
   • visceral larva migrans (toxocariasis).

This medicine may also be used for other worm infections as determined by your doctor.

Thiabendazole is available only with your doctor's prescription, in the following dosage forms:
*Oral*
   • Chewable tablets (U.S.)
   • Oral suspension (U.S.)

## Before Using This Medicine

In deciding to use a medicine, the risks of taking the medicine must be weighed against the good it will do. This is a decision you and your doctor will make. For thiabendazole, the following should be considered:

**Allergies**—Tell your doctor if you have ever had any unusual or allergic reaction to thiabendazole. Also tell your health care professional if you are allergic to any other substances, such as foods, preservatives, or dyes.

**Pregnancy**—Studies have not been done in humans. In addition, thiabendazole has not been shown to cause birth defects or other problems in studies in rabbits, rats, and mice given 2½ to 15 times the usual human dose. However, another study in mice given 10 times the usual human dose has shown that thiabendazole causes cleft palate (a split in the roof of the mouth) and bone defects.

**Breast-feeding**—It is not known whether thiabendazole passes into human breast milk. However, this medicine has not been reported to cause problems in nursing babies.

**Children**—This medicine has been tested in children over 13.6 kg of body weight (30 pounds). In effective doses, it has not been reported to cause different side effects or problems in children than it does in adults.

**Older adults**—Many medicines have not been studied specifically in older people. Therefore, it may not be known

whether they work exactly the same way they do in younger adults or if they cause different side effects or problems in older people. There is no specific information comparing use of thiabendazole in the elderly with use in other age groups.

**Other medicines**—Although certain medicines should not be used together at all, in other cases two different medicines may be used together even if an interaction might occur. In these cases, your doctor may want to change the dose, or other precautions may be necessary. When you are taking thiabendazole, it is especially important that your health care professional know if you are taking any of the following:

- Theophylline—Patients taking thiabendazole and theophylline together may have an increased chance of theophylline side effects

**Other medical problems**—The presence of other medical problems may affect the use of thiabendazole. Make sure you tell your doctor if you have any other medical problems, especially:

- Kidney disease or
- Liver disease—Patients with kidney and/or liver disease may have an increased chance of side effects

## Proper Use of This Medicine

No special preparations (for example, special diets, fasting, other medicines, laxatives, or enemas) are necessary before, during, or immediately after treatment with thiabendazole.

Thiabendazole is best taken after meals (breakfast and evening meal). This helps to prevent some common side effects such as nausea, vomiting, dizziness, or loss of appetite.

Doctors may also prescribe a corticosteroid (a cortisone-like medicine) for certain patients with *pork worms (trichinosis)*, especially for those with severe symptoms. This is to help reduce the inflammation caused by the pork worm larvae. If your doctor prescribes these 2 medicines together, it is important to take the corticosteroid along with thiabendazole. Take them exactly as directed by your doctor. Do not miss any doses.

For patients taking the *oral liquid form* of thiabendazole:

- Use a specially marked measuring spoon or other device to measure each dose accurately. The average household teaspoon may not hold the right amount of liquid.

For patients taking the *chewable tablet form* of thiabendazole:

- Tablets should be chewed or crushed before they are swallowed.

To help clear up your infection completely, *take this medicine exactly as directed by your doctor for the full time of treatment*. In some patients a second course of this medicine may be required to clear up the infection completely. *Do not miss any doses.*

**Dosing**—The dose of thiabendazole will be different for different patients. *Follow your doctor's orders or the directions on the label*. The following information includes only the average doses of thiabendazole. *If your dose is different, do not change it* unless your doctor tells you to do so.

The number of tablets or teaspoonfuls of suspension that you take depends on the strength of the medicine. Also, *the number of doses you take each day, the time allowed between doses, and the length of time you take the medicine depend on the medical problem for which you are taking thiabendazole.*

- For *oral* dosage forms (oral suspension or tablets):
  —Adults and children over 13.6 kilograms (30 pounds) of body weight:
- For *cutaneous larva migrans* and *strongyloidiasis*: Dose is based on body weight and will be determined by your doctor. The dose is taken two times a day for two days.
- For *trichinosis*: Dose is based on body weight and will be determined by your doctor. The dose is taken two times a day for two to four days.
- For *visceral larva migrans*: Dose is based on body weight and will be determined by your doctor. The dose is taken two times a day for five to seven days.
  —Children up to 13.6 kilograms (30 pounds) of body weight: Dose must be determined by the doctor.

**Missed dose**—If you do miss a dose of this medicine, take it as soon as possible. However, if it is almost time for your next dose, skip the missed dose and go back to your regular dosing schedule. Do not double doses.

**Storage**—To store this medicine:

- Keep out of the reach of children.
- Store away from heat and direct light.
- Do not store the chewable tablet form of this medicine in the bathroom, near the kitchen sink, or in other damp places. Heat or moisture may cause the medicine to break down.
- Keep the oral liquid form of this medicine from freezing.
- Do not keep outdated medicine or medicine no longer needed. Be sure that any discarded medicine is out of the reach of children.

## Precautions While Using This Medicine

It is important that your doctor check your progress at regular visits. This is to make sure that the infection is cleared up completely.

Thiabendazole may cause blurred vision or yellow vision. It may also cause some people to become dizzy, drowsy, or less alert than they are normally. *Make sure you know how you react to this medicine before you drive, use machines, or do anything else that could be dangerous if you are dizzy or are not alert or able to see well.* If these reactions are especially bothersome, check with your doctor.

Good health habits are required to help prevent reinfection. These include the following:

- For creeping eruption (cutaneous larva migrans) or visceral larva migrans (toxocariasis):
    - —Keep dogs and cats off beaches and bathing areas.
    - —Treat household pets for worms (deworm) regularly.
    - —Cover children's sandboxes when not being used.

    These measures help to prevent contamination of the sand or soil by worm larvae from the animals' wastes. This helps to keep children from picking up the larvae when they put their hands in their mouths after touching contaminated sand or soil.

- For pork worms (trichinosis):
    - —Cook all pork, pork-containing products, and game at not less than 140 °F (60 °C) until well done (not pink in the center) before eating. This will kill any trichinosis larvae that may be in the meat.

---

## Side Effects of This Medicine

Along with its needed effects, a medicine may cause some unwanted effects. Although not all of these side effects may occur, if they do occur they may need medical attention.

*Check with your doctor immediately* if any of the following side effects occur:

*More common*
Confusion; diarrhea (severe); hallucinations (seeing, hearing, and feeling things that are not there); irritability; loss of appetite; nausea and vomiting (severe); numbness or tingling in the hands or feet

*Less common*
Skin rash or itching

In addition to the side effects mentioned above, check with your doctor as soon as possible if any of the following side effects occur:

*Rare*
Aching of joints and muscles; blurred or yellow vision; chills; convulsions (seizures); dark urine; fever; lower back pain; pain or burning while urinating; pale stools; redness, blistering, peeling, or loosening of skin; unusual feeling in the eyes; unusual tiredness or weakness; yellow eyes and skin

Other side effects may occur that usually do not need medical attention. These side effects may go away during treatment as your body adjusts to the medicine. However, check with your doctor if any of the following side effects continue or are bothersome:

*More common*
Dizziness; drowsiness; dryness of eyes and mouth; headache; ringing or buzzing in the ears

This medicine may cause the urine to have an asparagus-like or other unusual odor while you are taking it and for about 24 hours after you stop taking it. This side effect does not need medical attention.

Other side effects not listed above may also occur in some patients. If you notice any other effects, check with your doctor.

---

## Additional Information

Once a medicine has been approved for marketing for a certain use, experience may show that it is also useful for other medical problems. Although these uses are not included in product labeling, thiabendazole is used in certain patients with the following medical conditions:

- Capillariasis
- Dracunculiasis
- Trichostrongyliasis

Other than the above information, there is no additional information relating to proper use, precautions, or side effects for these uses.

---

Revised: 02/01/93

---

# THIABENDAZOLE    Topical*†

*Not commercially available in the U.S.
†Not commercially available in Canada.

---

## Description

Thiabendazole (thye-a-BEN-da-zole) belongs to the family of medicines called anthelmintics (ant-hel-MIN-tiks). Anthelmintics are medicines used in the treatment of worm infections.

Thiabendazole topical preparations are used to treat a skin disease called cutaneous larva migrans (creeping eruption). Cutaneous larva migrans is caused by dog and cat hookworm larvae. These larvae cause slowly moving burrows or tunnels in the skin. This may result in itching, redness, or inflammation around the end of the burrows or tunnels.

Thiabendazole is available only with your doctor's prescription, in the following dosage form:

*Topical*
- Topical suspension

## Before Using This Medicine

In deciding to use a medicine, the risks of using the medicine must be weighed against the good it will do.

---

© 1994   The United States Pharmacopeial Convention, Inc.

This is a decision you and your doctor will make. For topical thiabendazole, the following should be considered:

**Allergies**—Tell your doctor if you have ever had any unusual or allergic reaction to thiabendazole. Also tell your health care professional if you are allergic to any other substances, such as preservatives or dyes.

**Pregnancy**—Thiabendazole may be absorbed through the skin. However, thiabendazole topical preparations have not been shown to cause birth defects or other problems in humans.

**Breast-feeding**—Thiabendazole may be absorbed through the mother's skin. However, thiabendazole topical preparations have not been shown to cause problems in nursing babies.

**Children**—Although there is no specific information comparing the use of thiabendazole in children with use in other age groups, this medicine is not expected to cause different side effects or problems in children than it does in adults.

**Older adults**—Many medicines have not been studied specifically in older people, Therefore, it may not be known whether they work exactly the same way they do in younger adults. Although there is no specific information comparing the use of thiabendazole in the elderly with use in other age groups, this medicine is not expected to cause different side effects or problems in older people than it does in younger adults.

**Other medicines**—Although certain medicines should not be used together at all, in other cases two different medicines may be used together even if an interaction might occur. In these cases, your doctor may want to change the dose, or other precautions may be necessary. Tell your health care professional if you are using any other topical prescription or nonprescription (over-the-counter [OTC]) medicine that is to be applied to the same area of the skin.

## Proper Use of This Medicine

Apply thiabendazole directly to, and about 5 to 7.5 cm (2 to 3 inches) around, the slowly moving end of each burrow or tunnel being made by the larva of the worm in the skin.

To help clear up your infection completely, *use this medicine exactly as directed by your doctor for the full time of treatment. Do not miss any doses.*

**Dosing**—The dose of topical thiabendazole will be different for different patients. *Follow your doctor's orders or the directions on the label.* The following information includes only the average doses of topical thiabendazole. *If your dose is different, do not change it* unless your doctor tells you to do so.
- For *topical* dosage form (suspension):
  —For cutaneous larva migrans:
    - Adults and children—Use two to four times a day for two to seven days.

**Missed dose**—If you miss a dose of this medicine, apply it as soon as possible. However, if it is almost time for your next dose, skip the missed dose and go back to your regular dosing schedule.

**Storage**—To store this medicine:
- Keep out of the reach of children.
- Store away from heat and direct light.
- Keep the medicine from freezing.
- Do not keep outdated medicine or medicine no longer needed. Be sure that any discarded medicine is out of the reach of children.

## Precautions While Using This Medicine

If your skin problem does not improve within a few days, or if the burrow or tunnel continues to get longer, check with your doctor.

## Side Effects of This Medicine

There have not been any common or important side effects reported with this medicine when used on the skin. However, if you notice any side effects, check with your doctor.

Revised: 09/28/93
Interim revision: 05/31/94

# THIAMINE (Vitamin B₁) Systemic

Some commonly used brand names are:
**In the U.S.—**
Biamine
Generic name product may also be available.

**In Canada—**
Betaxin                     Bewon
Generic name product may also be available.

## Description

Vitamins (VYE-ta-mins) are compounds that you *must* have for growth and health. They are needed in small amounts only and are usually available in the foods that you eat. Thiamine (THYE-a-min) (vitamin B₁) is necessary for normal metabolism.

Patients with the following conditions may be more likely to have a deficiency of thiamine:

- Alcoholism
- Burns
- Diarrhea (continuing)
- Fever (continuing)
- Illness (continuing)
- Intestinal disease
- Liver disease
- Overactive thyroid
- Stress (continuing)
- Surgical removal of stomach

Also, the following groups of people may have a deficiency of thiamine:

- Patients using an artificial kidney (on hemodialysis)
- Individuals who do heavy manual labor on a daily basis

If any of the above apply to you, you should take thiamine supplements only on the advice of your doctor after need has been established.

Lack of thiamine may lead to a condition called beriberi. Signs of beriberi include loss of appetite, constipation, muscle weakness, pain or tingling in arms or legs, and possible swelling of feet or lower legs. In addition, if severe, lack of thiamine may cause mental depression, memory problems, weakness, shortness of breath, and fast heartbeat. Your doctor may treat this by prescribing thiamine for you.

Thiamine may also be used for other conditions as determined by your doctor.

Claims that thiamine is effective for treatment of skin problems, chronic diarrhea, tiredness, mental problems, multiple sclerosis, nerve problems, and ulcerative colitis (a disease of the intestines), or as an insect repellant or to stimulate appetite have not been proven.

Oral forms of thiamine are available without a prescription. However, it may be a good idea to check with your doctor before taking thiamine on your own.

Thiamine is available in the following dosage forms:

*Oral*
- Elixir (Canada)
- Tablets (U.S. and Canada)

*Parenteral*
- Injection (U.S. and Canada)

## Importance of Diet

Vitamin supplements should be taken only if you cannot get enough vitamins in your diet; however, some diets may not contain all of the vitamins you need. You may not be getting enough vitamins because of rapid weight loss, unusual diets (such as some reducing diets in which choice of foods is limited), prolonged intravenous feeding, or malnutrition. A balanced diet should provide all the vitamins you normally need.

In order to get enough vitamins and minerals in your diet, it is important that you eat a balanced and varied diet. Follow carefully any diet program your doctor may recommend. For your specific vitamin and/or mineral needs, ask your doctor or dietitian for a list of appropriate foods.

Thiamine is found in various foods, including cereals (whole-grain and enriched), peas, beans, nuts, and meats (especially pork and beef). Some thiamine in foods is lost with cooking.

Vitamins alone will not take the place of a good diet and will not provide energy. Your body also needs other substances found in food such as protein, minerals, carbohydrates, and fat. Vitamins themselves often cannot work without the presence of other foods.

In some cases, it may not be possible for you to get enough food to supply you with the proper vitamins. In other cases, the amount of vitamins you need may be increased above normal. Therefore, a vitamin supplement may be needed.

Experts have developed a list of recommended dietary allowances (RDA) for most of the vitamins. The RDA are not an exact number but a general idea of how much you need. They do not cover amounts needed for problems caused by a serious lack of vitamins.

The RDA for thiamine are:

- Infants and children—
  Birth to 6 months of age: 0.3 milligrams (mg) per day.
  6 months to 1 year of age: 0.4 mg per day.
  1 to 3 years of age: 0.7 mg per day.
  4 to 6 years of age: 0.9 mg per day.
  7 to 10 years of age: 1 mg per day.
- Adolescent and adult males—
  11 to 14 years of age: 1.1 mg per day.
  15 to 50 years of age: 1.5 mg per day.
  51 years of age and over: 1.2 mg per day.
- Adolescent and adult females—
  11 to 50 years of age: 1.1 mg per day.
  51 years of age and over: 1 mg per day.
- Pregnant females—1.5 mg per day.
- Breast-feeding females—1.6 mg per day.

Remember:

- The total amount of each vitamin that you get every day includes what you get from the foods that you eat *and* what you may take as a supplement.
- Your total amount should not be greater than the RDA, unless ordered by your doctor.

## Before Using This Dietary Supplement

If you are taking this dietary supplement without a prescription, carefully read and follow any precautions on the label. For thiamine, the following should be considered:

**Allergies**—Tell your doctor if you have ever had any unusual or allergic reaction to thiamine. Also tell your health care professional if you are allergic to any other substances, such as foods, preservatives, or dyes.

**Pregnancy**—It is especially important that you are receiving enough vitamins when you become pregnant and that you continue to receive the right amount of vitamins throughout your pregnancy. The healthy growth and development of the fetus depend on a steady supply of nutrients from the mother. However, taking large amounts of a dietary supplement in pregnancy may be harmful to the mother and/or fetus and should be avoided.

**Breast-feeding**—It is especially important that you receive the right amounts of vitamins so that your baby will also get the vitamins needed to grow properly. However, taking large amounts of a dietary supplement while breast-feeding may be harmful to the mother and/or baby and should be avoided.

**Children**—Normal daily requirements vary according to age. It is especially important that children receive enough vitamins in their diet for healthy growth and development. Although there is no specific information about the use of thiamine in children in doses higher than the normal daily requirements, it is not expected to cause different side effects or problems in children than in adults.

**Older adults**—It is important that older people continue to receive enough vitamins in their diet for good health. Studies have shown that older adults may have lower blood levels of thiamine than younger adults. Your doctor may recommend that you take a vitamin supplement that contains thiamine.

**Medicines or other dietary supplements**—Although certain medicines or dietary supplements should not be used together at all, in other cases they may be used together even if an interaction might occur. In these cases, your doctor may want to change the dose, or other precautions may be necessary. Tell your health care professional if you are taking any other dietary supplement or prescription or nonprescription (over-the-counter [OTC]) medicine.

## Proper Use of This Dietary Supplement

Some people believe that taking very large doses of vitamins (called megadoses or megavitamin therapy) is useful for treating certain medical problems. Studies have not proven this. Large doses should be taken only under the direction of your doctor after need has been identified.

**Dosing**—The dose of thiamine for prevention of thiamine deficiency is based on the Recommended Dietary Allowances (RDA). See the *Importance of Diet* section for the RDA for thiamine.

**Missed dose**—If you miss taking a vitamin for 1 or more days there is no cause for concern, since it takes some time for your body to become seriously low in vitamins. However, if your doctor has recommended that you take this vitamin, try to remember to take it as directed every day.

**Storage**—To store this dietary supplement:
- Keep out of the reach of children.
- Store away from heat and direct light.
- Do not store in the bathroom, near the kitchen sink, or in other damp places. Heat or moisture may cause the dietary supplement to break down.
- Keep the oral liquid form of this dietary supplement from freezing.
- Do not keep outdated dietary supplements or those no longer needed. Be sure that any discarded dietary supplement is out of the reach of children.

## Side Effects of This Dietary Supplement

Along with its needed effects, a dietary supplement may cause some unwanted effects. Although not all of these side effects may occur, if they do occur they may need medical attention.

*Check with your doctor immediately* if any of the following side effects occur:
> *Rare—Soon after receiving injection only*
>> Coughing; difficulty in swallowing; hives; itching of skin; swelling of face, lips, or eyelids; wheezing or difficulty in breathing

Other side effects not listed above may also occur in some patients. If you notice any other effects, check with your doctor.

## Additional Information

Once a medicine or dietary supplement has been approved for marketing for a certain use, experience may show that it is also useful for other medical problems. Although this use is not included in product labeling, thiamine is used in certain patients with the following medical conditions:
- Enzyme deficiency diseases such as encephalomyelopathy, maple syrup urine disease, pyruvate carboxylase, and hyperalaninemia

Other than the above information, there is no additional information relating to proper use, precautions, or side effects for these uses.

Revised: 06/24/92
Interim revision: 07/29/94

# THIETHYLPERAZINE   Systemic

Some commonly used brand names are:

**In the U.S.—**
  Norzine                          Torecan

**In Canada—**
  Torecan

## Description

Thiethylperazine (thye-eth-il-PER-a-zeen) is a pheno-thiazine medicine. It is used to treat nausea and vomiting.

This medicine is available only with your doctor's prescription in the following dosage forms:

*Oral*
  • Tablets (U.S. and Canada)

*Parenteral*
  • Injection (U.S. and Canada)

*Rectal*
  • Suppositories (U.S.)

## Before Using This Medicine

In deciding to use a medicine, the risks of taking the medicine must be weighed against the good it will do. This is a decision you and your doctor will make. For thiethylperazine, the following should be considered:

**Allergies**—Tell your doctor if you have ever had any unusual or allergic reaction to thiethylperazine or other phenothiazine medicines. Also tell your health care professional if you are allergic to any other substances, such as foods, preservatives, or dyes.

**Pregnancy**—Thiethylperazine is not recommended during pregnancy. Other phenothiazine medicines have been reported to cause unwanted effects, such as jaundice and muscle tremors and other movement disorders, in newborn babies whose mothers took these medicines during pregnancy.

**Breast-feeding**—It is not known if thiethylperazine passes into the breast milk. However, thiethylperazine is not recommended for use during breast-feeding because there is the chance that it may cause unwanted effects in nursing babies.

**Children**—Children are usually more sensitive than adults to the effects of phenothiazine medicines such as thiethylperazine. Certain side effects, such as muscle spasms of the face, neck, and back, tic-like or twitching movements, inability to move the eyes, twisting of the body, or weakness of the arms and legs, are more likely to occur in children, especially those with severe illness or dehydration.

**Older adults**—Elderly patients are usually more sensitive to the effects of phenothiazine medicines such as thiethylperazine. Confusion; difficult or painful urination; dizziness; drowsiness; feeling faint; or dryness of mouth, nose, or throat may be more likely to occur in elderly patients. Also, nightmares or unusual excitement, nervousness, restlessness, or irritability may be more likely to occur in elderly patients. In addition, uncontrolled movements may be more likely to occur in elderly patients taking thiethylperazine.

**Other medicines**—Although certain medicines should not be used together at all, in other cases two different medicines may be used together even if an interaction might occur. In these cases, your doctor may want to change the dose, or other precautions may be necessary. When you are taking thiethylperazine, it is especially important that your health care professional know if you are taking any of the following:

  • Amoxapine (e.g., Asendin) or
  • Antipsychotics (medicine for mental illness) or
  • Methyldopa (e.g., Aldomet) or
  • Metoclopramide (e.g., Reglan) or
  • Metyrosine (e.g., Demser) or
  • Pemoline (e.g., Cylert) or
  • Pimozide (e.g., Orap) or
  • Promethazine (e.g., Phenergan) or
  • Rauwolfia alkaloids (alseroxylon [e.g., Rauwiloid], deserpidine [e.g., Harmonyl], rauwolfia serpentina [e.g., Raudixin], reserpine [e.g., Serpasil]) or
  • Trimeprazine (e.g., Temaril)—Side effects of these medicines, such as uncontrolled body movements, may become more severe and frequent if they are used together with thiethylperazine
  • Central nervous system (CNS) depressants (medicine that causes drowsiness) or
  • Tricyclic antidepressants (medicine for depression)—CNS depressant effects of these medicines or thiethylperazine, such as drowsiness, may be increased in severity; also, taking maprotiline or tricyclic antidepressants may cause some side effects of these medicines, such as dryness of mouth, to become more severe
  • Contrast agents, injected into spinal canal—If you are having an x-ray test of the head, spinal canal, or nervous system for which you are going to receive an injection into the spinal canal, thiethylperazine may increase your chance of having seizures
  • Epinephrine—Side effects, such as low blood pressure and fast or racing heartbeat, may occur more often or may be more severe
  • Levodopa—When used together with thiethylperazine, the levodopa may not work as it should
  • Quinidine—Unwanted effects on the heart may occur or become more severe

**Other medical problems**—The presence of other medical problems may affect the use of thiethylperazine. Make sure you tell your doctor if you have any other medical problems, especially:

  • Alcohol abuse—This medicine, if taken together with alcohol, may lower the blood pressure and cause CNS depressant effects, such as severe drowsiness
  • Asthma attack or
  • Other lung diseases—Thiethylperazine may cause secretions to become thick so that it might be difficult to cough them up, for example, during an asthma attack

- Blood disease or
- Heart or blood vessel disease—These medicines may cause more serious conditions to develop
- Difficult urination or
- Enlarged prostate—This medicine may cause urinary problems to get worse
- Glaucoma—This medicine may cause an increase in inner eye pressure
- Liver disease—Thiethylperazine may accumulate in the body, increasing the chance of side effects, such as muscle spasms
- Parkinson's disease or
- Seizure disorders—The chance of thiethylperazine causing seizures or uncontrolled movements is greater when these conditions are present

## Proper Use of This Medicine

Thiethylperazine is used only to relieve or prevent nausea and vomiting. *Use it only as directed. Do not use more of it and do not use it more often than your doctor ordered.* To do so may increase the chance of side effects.

For patients *taking this medicine by mouth:*

- This medicine may be taken with food or a full glass (8 ounces) of water or milk to reduce stomach irritation.

For patients using the *suppository form of this medicine:*

- To insert suppository: First, remove foil wrapper and moisten the suppository with cold water. Lie down on your side and use your finger to push the suppository well up into the rectum. If the suppository is too soft to insert, chill it in the refrigerator for 30 minutes or run cold water over it before removing the foil wrapper.

**Dosing**—The dose of thiethylperazine will be different for different patients. *Follow your doctor's orders or the directions on the label.* The following information includes only the average doses of thiethylperazine. *If your dose is different, do not change it* unless your doctor tells you to do so.

*The number of doses you take each day, the time allowed between doses, and the length of time you take the medicine depend on the medical problem for which you are taking thiethylperazine.*

- For nausea and vomiting:
  —For *oral* dosage form (tablets):
  - Adults—10 milligrams (mg) one to three times a day.
  - Children—Use and dose must be determined by your doctor.
  —For *injection* dosage form:
  - Adults—10 mg one to three times a day, injected into a muscle.
  - Children—Use and dose must be determined by your doctor.
  —For *rectal* dosage form (suppositories):
  - Adults—10 mg one to three times a day.

- Children—Use and dose must be determined by your doctor.

**Missed dose**—If you are taking this medicine regularly and you miss a dose, take it as soon as possible. However, if it is almost time for your next dose, skip the missed dose and go back to your regular dosing schedule. Do not double doses.

**Storage**—To store this medicine:

- Keep out of the reach of children, since overdose may be very dangerous in children.
- Store away from heat and direct light.
- Do not store the tablet form of this medicine in the bathroom medicine cabinet, near the kitchen sink, or in other damp places. Heat or moisture may cause the medicine to break down.
- Do not keep outdated medicine or medicine no longer needed. Be sure that any discarded medicine is out of the reach of children.

## Precautions While Using This Medicine

If you are going to be taking this medicine for a long time, your doctor should check your progress at regular visits, especially during the first few months of treatment with this medicine. This will allow your dosage to be changed if necessary to meet your needs.

Thiethylperazine will add to the effects of alcohol and other CNS depressants (medicines that slow down the nervous system, possibly causing drowsiness). Some examples of CNS depressants are antihistamines or medicine for hay fever, other allergies, or colds; sedatives, tranquilizers, or sleeping medicine; prescription pain medicine or narcotics; barbiturates; medicine for seizures; muscle relaxants; or anesthetics, including some dental anesthetics. *Check with your doctor before taking any of the above while you are using this medicine.*

This medicine may cause some people to have blurred vision or to become dizzy, lightheaded, drowsy, or less alert than they are normally. *Make sure you know how you react to this medicine before you drive, use machines, or do anything else that could be dangerous if you are dizzy or are not alert or able to see well.*

*Dizziness, lightheadedness, or fainting may occur,* especially when you get up from a lying or sitting position. Getting up slowly may help. If the problem continues or gets worse, check with your doctor.

When using thiethylperazine on a regular basis, make sure your doctor knows if you are taking large amounts of aspirin or other salicylates at the same time (as for arthritis or rheumatism). Effects of too much aspirin, such as ringing in the ears, may be covered up by this medicine.

Thiethylperazine may cause dryness of the mouth, nose, and throat. For temporary relief of mouth dryness, use sugarless candy or gum, melt bits of ice in your mouth, or use a saliva substitute. However, if your mouth continues to feel dry for more than 2 weeks, check with your medical doctor or dentist. Continuing dryness of the mouth may increase the chance of dental disease, including tooth decay, gum disease, and fungus infections.

## Side Effects of This Medicine

Along with its needed effects, a medicine may cause some unwanted effects. Although not all of these side effects may occur, if they do occur they may need medical attention.

*Check with your doctor immediately* if any of the following side effects occur:

*Less common or rare*

Lip smacking or puckering; puffing of cheeks; rapid or fine, worm-like movements of tongue; uncontrolled chewing movements; uncontrolled movements of arms or legs

Also, check with your doctor as soon as possible if any of the following side effects occur:

*Less common or rare*

Abdominal or stomach pains; aching muscles and joints; blurred vision, change in color vision, or difficulty in seeing at night; confusion (especially in the elderly); convulsions (seizures); difficulty in speaking or swallowing; fast heartbeat; fever and chills; inability to move eyes; loss of balance control; mask-like face; muscle spasms (especially of face, neck, and back);

nausea, vomiting, or diarrhea; shuffling walk; skin itching (severe); sore throat and fever; stiffness of arms or legs; swelling of arms, hands, and face; tic-like or twitching movements; trembling and shaking of hands and fingers; twisting movements of body; unusual bleeding or bruising; unusual tiredness or weakness; weakness of arms and legs; yellow eyes or skin

Other side effects may occur that usually do not need medical attention. These side effects may go away during treatment as your body adjusts to the medicine. However, check with your doctor if any of the following side effects continue or are bothersome:

*More common*

Drowsiness or dizziness

*Less common or rare*

Constipation; decreased sweating; dryness of mouth, nose and throat; feeling faint; fever; headache; lightheadedness; nightmares (continuing); ringing or buzzing in ears; skin rash; unusual excitement, nervousness, restlessness, or irritability

Other side effects not listed above may also occur in some patients. If you notice any other effects, check with your doctor.

Revised: 06/17/93

# THIOGUANINE    Systemic

A commonly used brand name in Canada is Lanvis.
Generic name product available in the U.S.

## Description

Thioguanine (thye-oh-GWON-een) belongs to the group of medicines known as antimetabolites. It is used to treat some kinds of cancer.

Thioguanine interferes with the growth of cancer cells, which are eventually destroyed. Since the growth of normal body cells may also be affected by thioguanine, other effects will also occur. Some of these may be serious and must be reported to your doctor. Other effects may not be serious but may cause concern. Some effects may not occur for months or years after the medicine is used.

Before you begin treatment with thioguanine, you and your doctor should talk about the good this medicine will do as well as the risks of using it.

Thioguanine is available only with your doctor's prescription, in the following dosage form:

*Oral*

• Tablets (U.S. and Canada)

## Before Using This Medicine

In deciding to use a medicine, the risks of taking the medicine must be weighed against the good it will do. This is a decision you and your doctor will make. For thioguanine, the following should be considered:

**Allergies**—Tell your doctor if you have ever had any unusual or allergic reaction to thioguanine.

**Pregnancy**—Tell your doctor if you are pregnant or if you intend to have children. There is a chance that this medicine may cause birth defects if either the male or female is taking it at the time of conception or if it is taken during pregnancy. In addition, many cancer medicines may cause sterility which could be permanent. Although this has not been reported with this medicine, the possibility should be kept in mind.

Be sure that you have discussed this with your doctor before taking this medicine. It is best to use some kind of birth control while you are taking thioguanine. Tell your doctor right away if you think you have become pregnant while taking thioguanine.

**Breast-feeding**—Tell your doctor if you are breast-feeding or if you intend to breast-feed during treatment with this medicine. Because thioguanine may cause serious side effects, breast-feeding is generally not recommended while you are receiving it.

**Children**—Although there is no specific information about the use of thioguanine in children, it is not expected to cause different side effects or problems in children than it does in adults.

**Older adults**—Many medicines have not been tested in older people. Therefore, it may not be known whether they work exactly the same way they do in younger adults or if they cause different side effects or problems in older people. There is no specific information about the use of thioguanine in the elderly.

**Other medicines**—Although certain medicines should not be used together at all, in other cases two different medicines may be used together even if an interaction might occur. In these cases, your doctor may want to change the dose, or other precautions may be necessary. When you are taking thioguanine, it is especially important that your health care professional know if you are taking any of the following:

- Antithyroid agents (medicine for overactive thyroid) or
- Azathioprine (e.g., Imuran) or
- Chloramphenicol (e.g., Chloromycetin) or
- Colchicine or
- Flucytosine (e.g., Ancobon) or
- Interferon (e.g., Intron A, Roferon-A) or
- Plicamycin (e.g., Mithracin) or
- Zidovudine (e.g., Retrovir) or
- If you have ever been treated with x-rays or cancer medicines—Thioguanine may increase the effects of these medicines or radiation therapy on the blood
- Probenecid (e.g., Benemid) or
- Sulfinpyrazone (e.g., Anturane)—Thioguanine may increase the concentration of uric acid in the blood, which these medicines are used to lower

**Other medical problems**—The presence of other medical problems may affect the use of thioguanine. Make sure you tell your doctor if you have any other medical problems, especially:

- Chickenpox (including recent exposure) or
- Herpes zoster (shingles)—Risk of severe disease affecting other parts of the body
- Gout (history of) or
- Kidney stones (history of)—Thioguanine may increase levels of uric acid in the body, which can cause gout or kidney stones
- Infection—Thioguanine can reduce immunity to infection
- Kidney disease or
- Liver disease—Effects may be increased because of slower removal of thioguanine from the body

## Proper Use of This Medicine

*Take this medicine only as directed by your doctor.* Do not take more or less of it, and do not take it more often than your doctor ordered. The exact amount of medicine you need has been carefully worked out. Taking too much may increase the chance of side effects, while taking too little may not improve your condition.

Thioguanine is sometimes given together with certain other medicines. If you are using a combination of medicines, make sure that you take each one at the right time and do not mix them. Ask your health care professional to help you plan a way to take your medicine at the right times.

While you are using thioguanine, your doctor may want you to drink extra fluids so that you will pass more urine. This will help prevent kidney problems and keep your kidneys working well.

Thioguanine sometimes causes nausea and vomiting. However, it is very important that you continue to take this medicine, even if you begin to feel ill. *Do not stop taking this medicine without first checking with your doctor.* Ask your health care professional for ways to lessen these effects.

If you vomit shortly after taking a dose of thioguanine, check with your doctor. You will be told whether to take the dose again or to wait until the next scheduled dose.

**Dosing**—The dose of thioguanine will be different for different patients. The dose that is used may depend on a number of things, including what the medicine is being used for, the patient's weight, and whether or not other medicines are also being taken. *If you are taking thioguanine at home, follow your doctor's orders or the directions on the label.* If you have any questions about the proper dose of thioguanine, ask your doctor.

**Missed dose**—If you miss a dose of this medicine, do not take the missed dose at all and do not double the next one. Instead, go back to your regular dosing schedule and check with your doctor.

**Storage**—To store this medicine:

- Keep out of the reach of children.
- Store away from heat and direct light.
- Do not store in the bathroom, near the kitchen sink, or in other damp places. Heat or moisture may cause the medicine to break down.
- Do not keep outdated medicine or medicine no longer needed. Be sure that any discarded medicine is out of the reach of children.

## Precautions While Using This Medicine

*It is very important that your doctor check your progress at regular visits* to make sure that this medicine is working properly and to check for unwanted effects.

While you are being treated with thioguanine, and after you stop treatment with it, *do not have any immunizations (vaccinations) without your doctor's approval.* Thioguanine may lower your body's resistance and there is a chance you might get the infection the immunization is meant to prevent. Other people living in your household should not take or should not have recently taken oral polio vaccine since there is a chance they could pass the polio virus on to you. Also, avoid other persons who have taken oral polio vaccine. Do not get close to them and do not stay in the same room with them for very long. If you cannot take these precautions, you should consider wearing a protective face mask that covers the nose and mouth.

Thioguanine can lower the number of white blood cells in your blood temporarily, increasing the chance of getting an infection. It can also lower the number of platelets, which are necessary for proper blood clotting. If this occurs, there are certain precautions you can take, especially when your blood count is low, to reduce the risk of infection or bleeding:

- If you can, avoid people with infections. *Check with your doctor immediately* if you think you are getting an infection or if you get a fever or chills, cough or hoarseness, lower back or side pain, or painful or difficult urination.
- *Check with your doctor immediately* if you notice any unusual bleeding or bruising; black, tarry stools; blood in urine or stools; or pinpoint red spots on your skin.
- Be careful when using a regular toothbrush, dental floss, or toothpick. Your medical doctor, dentist, or nurse may recommend other ways to clean your teeth and gums. Check with your medical doctor before having any dental work done.
- Do not touch your eyes or the inside of your nose unless you have just washed your hands and have not touched anything else in the meantime.
- Be careful not to cut yourself when you are using sharp objects such as a safety razor or fingernail or toenail cutters.
- Avoid contact sports or other situations where bruising or injury could occur.

## Side Effects of This Medicine

Along with their needed effects, medicines like thioguanine can sometimes cause unwanted effects such as blood problems and other side effects. These and others are described below. Also, because of the way these medicines act on the body, there is a chance that they might cause other unwanted effects that may not occur until months or years after the medicine is used. These delayed effects may include certain types of cancer, such as leukemia. Discuss these possible effects with your doctor.

Although not all of these side effects may occur, if they do occur they may need medical attention.

*Check with your doctor immediately* if any of the following side effects occur:

*Less common*
Black, tarry stools; blood in urine or stools; cough or hoarseness; fever or chills; lower back or side pain; painful or difficult urination; pinpoint red spots on skin; unusual bleeding or bruising

Check with your doctor as soon as possible if any of the following side effects occur:

*Less common*
Joint pain; swelling of feet or lower legs; unsteadiness when walking

*Rare*
Sores in mouth and on lips; yellow eyes or skin

Other side effects may occur that usually do not need medical attention. These side effects may go away during treatment as your body adjusts to the medicine. Also, your health care professional may be able to tell you about ways to prevent or reduce some of these side effects. Check with your health care professional if any of the following side effects continue or are bothersome or if you have any questions about them:

*Less common*
Diarrhea; loss of appetite; nausea and vomiting; skin rash or itching

After you stop taking thioguanine, it may still produce some side effects that need attention. During this period of time, check with your doctor if you notice any of the following side effects:

Black, tarry stools; blood in urine or stools; cough or hoarseness; fever or chills; lower back or side pain; painful or difficult urination; pinpoint red spots on skin; unusual bleeding or bruising

Other side effects not listed above may also occur in some patients. If you notice any other effects, check with your doctor.

Revised: 09/90
Interim revision(s): 08/11/93; 07/05/94

# THIOTEPA   Systemic

Generic name product available in the U.S. and Canada.

## Description

Thiotepa (thye-oh-TEP-a) belongs to the group of medicines called alkylating agents. It is used to treat some kinds of cancer.

Thiotepa interferes with the growth of cancer cells, which are eventually destroyed. Since the growth of normal body cells may also be affected by thiotepa, other effects will also occur. Some of these may be serious and must be reported to your doctor. Other effects, like hair loss, may not be serious but may cause concern. Some effects do not occur for months or years after the medicine is used.

Before you begin treatment with thiotepa, you and your doctor should talk about the good this medicine will do as well as the risks of using it.

Thiotepa is to be administered only by or under the immediate supervision of your doctor. It is available in the following dosage form:

*Parenteral*
- Injection (U.S. and Canada)

## Before Using This Medicine

In deciding to use a medicine, the risks of taking the medicine must be weighed against the good it will do. This is a decision you and your doctor will make. For thiotepa, the following should be considered:

**Allergies**—Tell your doctor if you have ever had any unusual or allergic reaction to thiotepa.

**Pregnancy**—Tell your doctor if you are pregnant or if you intend to have children. There is a chance that this medicine may cause birth defects if either the male or female is using it at the time of conception or if it is used during pregnancy. Studies have shown that thiotepa causes birth defects in humans. In addition, many cancer medicines may cause sterility which could be permanent. Although this is uncommon with this medicine, the possibility should be kept in mind.

Be sure that you have discussed this with your doctor before using this medicine. It is best to use some kind of birth control while you are receiving thiotepa. Tell your doctor right away if you think you have become pregnant while receiving thiotepa.

**Breast-feeding**—Tell your doctor if you intend to breast-feed. Because this medicine may cause serious side effects, breast-feeding is generally not recommended while you are receiving it. It is not known whether thiotepa passes into the breast milk.

**Children**—There is no specific information about the use of thiotepa in children.

**Older adults**—Many medicines have not been tested in older people. Therefore, it may not be known whether they work exactly the same way they do in younger adults or if they cause different side effects or problems in older people. There is no specific information about the use of thiotepa in the elderly.

**Other medicines**—Although certain medicines should not be used together at all, in other cases two different medicines may be used together even if an interaction might occur. In these cases, your doctor may want to change the dose, or other precautions may be necessary. When you are receiving thiotepa, it is especially important that your health care professional know if you are taking any of the following:

- Antithyroid agents (medicine for overactive thyroid) or
- Azathioprine (e.g., Imuran) or
- Chloramphenicol (e.g., Chloromycetin) or
- Colchicine or
- Flucytosine (e.g., Ancobon) or

- Interferon (e.g., Intron A, Roferon-A) or
- Plicamycin (e.g., Mithracin) or
- Zidovudine (e.g., Retrovir) or
- If you have ever been treated with x-rays or cancer medicines—Thiotepa may increase the effects of these medicines or radiation therapy on the blood
- Probenecid (e.g., Benemid) or
- Sulfinpyrazone (e.g., Anturane)—Thiotepa may increase the concentration of uric acid in the blood, which these medicines are used to lower

**Other medical problems**—The presence of other medical problems may affect the use of thiotepa. Make sure you tell your doctor if you have any other medical problems, especially:

- Chickenpox (including recent exposure) or
- Herpes zoster (shingles)—Risk of severe disease affecting other parts of the body
- Gout (history of) or
- Kidney stones (history of)—Thiotepa may increase levels of uric acid in the body, which can cause gout or kidney stones
- Infection—Thiotepa can reduce immunity to infection
- Kidney disease or
- Liver disease—Effects may be increased because of slower removal of thiotepa from the body

## Proper Use of This Medicine

While you are using thiotepa, your doctor may want you to drink extra fluids so that you will pass more urine. This will help prevent kidney problems and keep your kidneys working well.

Thiotepa sometimes causes nausea, vomiting, and loss of appetite. However, it is very important that you continue to receive the medicine, even if you begin to feel ill. Ask your health care professional for ways to lessen these effects.

**Dosing**—The dose of thiotepa will be different for different patients. The dose that is used may depend on a number of things, including what the medicine is being used for, the patient's weight, and whether or not other medicines are also being taken. *If you are receiving thiotepa at home, follow your doctor's orders or the directions on the label.* If you have any questions about the proper dose of thiotepa, ask your doctor.

## Precautions While Using This Medicine

*It is very important that your doctor check your progress at regular visits* to make sure that this medicine is working properly and to check for unwanted effects.

Before having any kind of surgery, including dental surgery, make sure the medical doctor or dentist in charge knows that you are taking this medicine.

While you are being treated with thiotepa, and after you stop treatment with it, *do not have any immunizations (vaccinations) without your doctor's approval.* Thiotepa may lower your body's resistance and there is a chance you might get the infection the immunization is meant to prevent. Other people living in your household should not take or should not have recently taken oral polio vaccine since there is a chance they could pass the polio virus on to you. Also, avoid other persons who have taken oral polio vaccine. Do not get close to them and do not stay in the same room with them for very long. If you cannot take these precautions, you should consider wearing a protective face mask that covers the nose and mouth.

Thiotepa can lower the number of white blood cells in your blood temporarily, increasing the chance of getting an infection. It can also lower the number of platelets, which are necessary for proper blood clotting. If this occurs, there are certain precautions you can take, especially when your blood count is low, to reduce the risk of infection or bleeding:

- If you can, avoid people with infections. *Check with your doctor immediately* if you think you are getting an infection or if you get a fever or chills, cough or hoarseness, lower back or side pain, or painful or difficult urination.
- *Check with your doctor immediately* if you notice any unusual bleeding or bruising; black, tarry stools; blood in urine or stools; or pinpoint red spots on your skin.
- Be careful when using a regular toothbrush, dental floss, or toothpick. Your medical doctor, dentist, or nurse may recommend other ways to clean your teeth and gums. Check with your medical doctor before having any dental work done.
- Do not touch your eyes or the inside of your nose unless you have just washed your hands and have not touched anything else in the meantime.
- Be careful not to cut yourself when you are using sharp objects such as a safety razor or fingernail or toenail cutters.
- Avoid contact sports or other situations where bruising or injury could occur.

---

## Side Effects of This Medicine

Along with their needed effects, medicines like thiotepa can sometimes cause unwanted effects such as blood problems, loss of hair, and other side effects. These and others are described below. Also, because of the way these medicines act on the body, there is a chance that they might cause other unwanted effects that may not occur until months or years after the medicine is used. These delayed effects may include certain types of cancer, such as leukemia. Discuss these possible effects with your doctor.

Although not all of these side effects may occur, if they do occur they may need medical attention.

*Check with your doctor or nurse immediately* if any of the following side effects occur:

*Less common*
  Black, tarry stools; blood in urine or stools; cough or hoarseness; fever or chills; lower back or side pain; painful or difficult urination; pinpoint red spots on skin; unusual bleeding or bruising

*Rare*
  Skin rash; tightness of throat; wheezing

Check with your health care professional as soon as possible if any of the following side effects occur:

*Less common*
  Joint pain; pain at place of injection or instillation; swelling of feet or lower legs

*Rare*
  Sores in mouth and on lips

Other side effects may occur that usually do not need medical attention. These side effects may go away during treatment as your body adjusts to the medicine. Also, your health care professional may be able to tell you about ways to prevent or reduce some of these side effects. Check with your health care professional if any of the following side effects continue or are bothersome or if you have any questions about them:

*Less common*
  Dizziness; hives; loss of appetite; missing menstrual periods; nausea and vomiting

This medicine may cause a temporary loss of hair in some people. After treatment with thiotepa has ended, normal hair growth should return.

After you stop receiving thiotepa, it may still produce some side effects that need attention. During this period of time, check with your doctor if you notice any of the following:

  Black, tarry stools; blood in urine or stools; cough or hoarseness; fever or chills; lower back or side pain; painful or difficult urination; pinpoint red spots on skin; unusual bleeding or bruising

Other side effects not listed above may also occur in some patients. If you notice any other effects, check with your doctor.

---

Revised: 09/90
Interim revision(s): 08/11/93; 07/05/94

# THIOXANTHENES   Systemic

Some commonly used brand names are:

**In the U.S.—**
Navane[3]
Taractan[1]

Thiothixene HCl Intensol[3]

**In Canada—**
Fluanxol[2]
Fluanxol Depot[2]

Navane[3]

Note: For quick reference, the following thioxanthenes are numbered to match the corresponding brand names.

This information applies to the following medicines:

1. Chlorprothixene (klor-proe-THIX-een)†
2. Flupenthixol (floo-pen-THIX-ole)*
3. Thiothixene (thye-oh-THIX-een)‡

---

*Not commercially available in the U.S.
†Not commercially available in Canada.
‡Generic name product may also be available in the U.S.

---

## Description

This medicine belongs to the family of medicines known as thioxanthenes (thye-oh-ZAN-theens). It is used in the treatment of nervous, mental, and emotional conditions. Improvement in such conditions is thought to result from the effect of the medicine on nerve pathways in specific areas of the brain.

Thioxanthene medicines are available only with your doctor's prescription, in the following dosage forms:

*Oral*

Chlorprothixene
• Suspension (U.S.)
• Tablets (U.S.)
Flupenthixol
• Tablets (Canada)
Thiothixene
• Capsules (U.S. and Canada)
• Solution (U.S.)

*Parenteral*

Chlorprothixene
• Injection (U.S.)
Flupenthixol
• Injection (Canada)
Thiothixene
• Injection (U.S.)

## Before Using This Medicine

In deciding to use a medicine, the risks of taking the medicine must be weighed against the good it will do. This is a decision you and your doctor will make. For thioxanthenes, the following should be considered:

**Allergies**—Tell your doctor if you have ever had any unusual or allergic reaction to thioxanthene or to phenothiazine medicines. Also tell your health care professional if you are allergic to any other substances, such as foods, preservatives, or dyes.

**Pregnancy**—Studies have not been done in pregnant women. Although animal studies have not shown that thioxanthenes cause birth defects, the studies have shown that these medicines cause a decrease in fertility and fewer successful pregnancies.

**Breast-feeding**—It is not known if thioxanthenes pass into the breast milk. However, similar medicines for nervous, mental, or emotional conditions do pass into breast milk and may cause drowsiness and increase the risk of other problems in the nursing baby. Be sure you have discussed the risks and benefits of this medicine with your doctor.

**Children**—Certain side effects, such as muscle spasms of the face, neck, and back, tic-like or twitching movements, inability to move the eyes, twisting of the body, or weakness of the arms and legs, are more likely to occur in children, who are usually more sensitive than adults to the side effects of thioxanthenes.

**Older adults**—Constipation, dizziness or fainting, drowsiness, dryness of mouth, trembling of the hands and fingers, and symptoms of tardive dyskinesia (such as rapid, worm-like movements of the tongue or any other uncontrolled movements of the mouth, tongue, or jaw, and/or arms and legs) are especially likely to occur in elderly patients, who are usually more sensitive than younger adults to the effects of thioxanthenes.

**Other medicines**—Although certain medicines should not be used together at all, in other cases 2 different medicines may be used together even if an interaction might occur. In these cases, your doctor may want to change the dose, or other precautions may be necessary. When you are taking thioxanthenes, it is especially important that your health care professional know if you are taking any of the following:

• Amoxapine (e.g., Asendin) or
• Methyldopa (e.g., Aldomet) or
• Metoclopramide (e.g., Reglan) or
• Metyrosine (e.g., Demser) or
• Other antipsychotics (medicine for mental illness) or
• Pemoline (e.g., Cylert) or
• Pimozide (e.g., Orap) or
• Promethazine (e.g., Phenergan) or
• Rauwolfia alkaloids (alseroxylon [e.g., Rauwiloid], deserpidine [e.g., Harmonyl], rauwolfia serpentina [e.g., Raudixin], reserpine [e.g., Serpasil]) or
• Trimeprazine (e.g., Temaril)—Taking these medicines with thioxanthenes may increase the chance and severity of certain side effects
• Central nervous system (CNS) depressants (medicine that causes drowsiness) or
• Tricyclic antidepressants (medicine for depression)—Taking these medicines with thioxanthenes may add to the CNS depressant effects
• Epinephrine (e.g., Adrenalin)—Severe low blood pressure (hypotension) and fast heartbeat may occur if epinephrine is used with thioxanthenes
• Levodopa (e.g., Sinemet)—Thioxanthenes may keep levodopa from working properly in the treatment of Parkinson's disease
• Quinidine (e.g., Quinidex)—Unwanted effects on your heart may occur

**Other medical problems**—The presence of other medical problems may affect the use of thioxanthenes. Make sure you tell your doctor if you have any other medical problems, especially:

- Alcohol abuse—Drinking alcohol will add to the central nervous system (CNS) depressant effects of thioxanthenes
- Blood disease or
- Enlarged prostate or
- Glaucoma or
- Heart or blood vessel disease or
- Lung disease or
- Parkinson's disease or
- Stomach ulcers or
- Urination problems—Thioxanthenes may make the condition worse
- Liver disease—Higher blood levels of thioxanthenes may occur, increasing the chance of side effects
- Reye's syndrome—The risk of liver problems may be increased
- Seizure disorders—The risk of seizures may be increased

## Proper Use of This Medicine

This medicine may be taken with food or a full glass (8 ounces) of water or milk to reduce stomach irritation.

For patients taking *thiothixene oral solution:*

- This medicine must be diluted before you take it. Just before taking, measure the dose with the specially marked dropper. Mix the medicine with a full glass of water, milk, tomato or fruit juice, soup, or carbonated beverage.

*Do not take more of this medicine or take it more often than your doctor ordered.* This is particularly important when this medicine is given to children, since they may react very strongly to its effects.

*Sometimes this medicine must be taken for several weeks before its full effect is reached.*

**Dosing**—The dose of these medicines will be different for different patients. *Follow your doctor's orders or the directions on the label.* The following information includes only the average doses of these medicines. *If your dose is different, do not change it* unless your doctor tells you to do so.

The number of capsules or tablets or the amount of liquid that you take depends on the strength of the medicine. Also, the number of doses you take each day, the time allowed between doses, and the length of time you take the medicine depend on the medical problem for which you are taking thioxanthenes.

*For chlorprothixene*

- For treatment of psychosis:
  - —*Oral* dosage forms (suspension or tablets):
    - Adults and teenagers—25 to 50 milligrams (mg) three or four times a day.
    - Children 6 to 12 years of age—10 to 25 mg three or four times a day.
    - Children up to 6 years of age—Use and dose must be determined by your doctor.

- —*Injection* dosage form:
  - Adults and teenagers—25 to 50 mg, injected into a muscle, three or four times a day.
  - Children up to 12 years of age—Use and dose must be determined by your doctor.

*For flupenthixol*

- For treatment of psychosis:
  - —*Oral* dosage form (tablets):
    - Adults—To start, 1 milligram (mg) three times a day. Your doctor may increase your dose if needed, depending on your condition.
    - Children— Use and dose must be determined by your doctor.
  - —*Long-acting injection* dosage form:
    - Adults—To start, 20 to 40 milligrams (mg) injected into a muscle. Your doctor will determine whether your dose needs to be changed, depending on your condition.
    - Children—Use and dose must be determined by your doctor.

*For thiothixene*

- For treatment of psychosis:
  - —*Oral* dosage forms (capsules and solution):
    - Adults and teenagers—To start, 2 milligrams (mg) three times a day, or 5 mg two times a day. Your doctor may increase your dose if needed. However, the dose is usually not more than 60 mg a day.
    - Children up to 12 years of age—Use and dose must be determined by your doctor.
  - —*Injection* dosage form:
    - Adults and teenagers—4 milligrams (mg), injected into a muscle, two to four times a day. Your doctor may increase your dose if needed. However, the dose is usually not more than 30 mg a day.
    - Children up to 12 years of age—Use and dose must be determined by your doctor.

**Missed dose**—If you miss a dose of this medicine, take it as soon as possible. However, if it is within 2 hours of your next dose, skip the missed dose and go back to your regular dosing schedule. Do not double doses.

**Storage**—To store this medicine:

- Keep out of the reach of children.
- Store away from heat and direct light.
- Do not store the capsule or tablet form of this medicine in the bathroom, near the kitchen sink, or in other damp places. Heat or moisture may cause the medicine to break down.
- Keep the liquid form of this medicine from freezing.
- Do not keep outdated medicine or medicine no longer needed. Be sure that any discarded medicine is out of the reach of children.

## Precautions While Using This Medicine

Your doctor should check your progress at regular visits. This will allow the dosage of the medicine to be adjusted when necessary and also will reduce the possibility of side effects.

Do not stop taking this medicine without first checking with your doctor. Your doctor may want you to gradually reduce the amount you are taking before stopping completely. This is to prevent side effects and to prevent your condition from becoming worse.

This medicine will add to the effects of alcohol and other CNS depressants (medicines that slow down the nervous system, possibly causing drowsiness). Some examples of CNS depressants are antihistamines or medicine for hay fever, other allergies, or colds; sedatives, tranquilizers, or sleeping medicine; prescription pain medicine or narcotics; barbiturates; medicine for seizures; muscle relaxants; or anesthetics, including some dental anesthetics. *Check with your doctor before taking any such depressants while you are using this medicine.*

Do not take this medicine within an hour of taking antacids or medicine for diarrhea. Taking them too close together may make this medicine less effective.

*Before having any kind of surgery, dental treatment, or emergency treatment, tell the medical doctor or dentist in charge that you are using this medicine.* Taking thioxanthenes together with medicines that are used during surgery or dental or emergency treatments may increase the CNS depressant effects.

This medicine may cause some people to become drowsy or less alert than they are normally, especially during the first few weeks the medicine is being taken. Even if you take this medicine only at bedtime, you may feel drowsy or less alert on arising. *Make sure you know how you react to this medicine before you drive, use machines, or do anything else that could be dangerous if you are not alert.*

*Dizziness, lightheadedness, or fainting may occur while you are taking this medicine,* especially when you get up from a lying or sitting position. Getting up slowly may help. If the problem continues or gets worse, check with your doctor.

This medicine may make you sweat less, causing your body temperature to increase. *Use extra care not to become overheated during exercise or hot weather while you are taking this medicine,* since overheating may result in heat stroke. Also, hot baths or saunas may make you feel dizzy or faint while you are taking this medicine.

Thioxanthenes may cause your skin to be more sensitive to sunlight than it is normally. Exposure to sunlight, even for brief periods of time, may cause a skin rash, itching, redness or other discoloration of the skin, or a severe sunburn. When you begin taking this medicine:

- Stay out of direct sunlight, especially between the hours of 10:00 a.m. and 3:00 p.m., if possible.
- Wear protective clothing, including a hat. Also, wear sunglasses.
- Apply a sun block product that has a skin protection factor (SPF) of at least 15. Some patients may require a product with a higher SPF number, especially if they have a fair complexion. If you have any questions about this, check with your health care professional.
- Apply a sun block lipstick that has an SPF of at least 15 to protect your lips.
- Do not use a sunlamp or tanning bed or booth.

*If you have a severe reaction from the sun, check with your doctor.*

This medicine may cause dryness of the mouth. For temporary relief, use sugarless gum or candy, melt bits of ice in your mouth, or use a saliva substitute. However, if your mouth continues to feel dry for more than 2 weeks, check with your medical doctor or dentist. Continuing dryness of the mouth may increase the chance of dental disease, including tooth decay, gum disease, and fungus infections.

If you are taking a liquid form of this medicine, *try to avoid spilling it on your skin or clothing.* Skin rash and irritation have been caused by similar medicines.

If you are receiving this medicine by injection:

- The effects of the long-acting injection form of this medicine may last for up to 3 weeks. *The precautions and side effects information for this medicine applies during this period of time.*

## Side Effects of This Medicine

Along with their needed effects, thioxanthenes can sometimes cause serious side effects. Tardive dyskinesia (a movement disorder) may occur and may not go away after you stop using the medicine. Signs of tardive dyskinesia include fine, worm-like movements of the tongue, or other uncontrolled movements of the mouth, tongue, cheeks, jaw, or arms and legs. Other serious but rare side effects may also occur. Some of these side effects, including severe muscle stiffness, fever, unusual tiredness or weakness, fast heartbeat, difficult breathing, increased sweating, loss of bladder control, and seizures, may be the sign of a condition called neuroleptic malignant syndrome. *You and your doctor should discuss the good this medicine will do as well as the risks of taking it.*

Although not all of these side effects may occur, if they do occur they may need medical attention.

*Stop taking this medicine and get emergency help immediately* if any of the following side effects occur:

*Rare*

Convulsions (seizures); difficulty in breathing; fast heartbeat; high fever; high or low (irregular) blood pressure; increased sweating; loss of bladder control; muscle stiffness (severe); unusually pale skin; unusual tiredness

Also, check with your doctor as soon as possible if any of the following side effects occur:

*More common*

Difficulty in talking or swallowing; inability to move eyes; lip smacking or puckering; loss of balance control; mask-like face; muscle spasms, especially of the neck and back;

puffing of cheeks; rapid or worm-like movements of tongue; restlessness or need to keep moving (severe); shuffling walk; stiffness of arms and legs; trembling and shaking of fingers and hands; twisting movements of body; uncontrolled chewing movements; uncontrolled movements of the arms and legs

*Less common*

Blurred vision or other eye problems; difficult urination; fainting; skin discoloration; skin rash

*Rare*

Hot, dry skin or lack of sweating; increased blinking or spasms of eyelid; muscle weakness; sore throat and fever; uncontrolled twisting movements of neck, trunk, arms, or legs; unusual bleeding or bruising; unusual facial expressions or body positions; yellow eyes or skin

*Symptoms of overdose*

Difficulty in breathing (severe); dizziness (severe); drowsiness (severe); muscle trembling, jerking, stiffness, or uncontrolled movements (severe); small pupils; unusual excitement; unusual tiredness or weakness (severe)

Other side effects may occur that usually do not need medical attention. These side effects may go away during treatment as your body adjusts to the medicine. However, check with your doctor if any of the following side effects continue or are bothersome:

*More common*

Constipation; decreased sweating; dizziness, lightheadedness, or fainting; drowsiness (mild); dryness of mouth; increased appetite and weight; increased sensitivity of skin to sunlight (skin rash, itching, redness or other discoloration of skin, or severe sunburn); stuffy nose

*Less common*

Changes in menstrual period; decreased sexual ability; swelling of breasts (in males and females); unusual secretion of milk

After you stop taking this medicine your body may need time to adjust, especially if you took this medicine in high doses or for a long time. If you stop taking it too quickly, the following withdrawal effects may occur and should be reported to your doctor:

Dizziness; nausea and vomiting; stomach pain; trembling of fingers and hands; uncontrolled, continuing movements of mouth, tongue, or jaw

Although not all of the side effects listed above have been reported for all thioxanthenes, they have been reported for at least one of them. However, since these medicines are very similar, any of the above side effects may occur with any of them.

Other side effects not listed above may also occur in some patients. If you notice any other effects, check with your doctor.

Revised: 06/17/93

# THROMBOLYTIC AGENTS   Systemic

Some commonly used brand names are:

**In the U.S.—**
Abbokinase[4]
Abbokinase Open-Cath[4]
Activase[1]

Eminase[2]
Kabikinase[3]
Streptase[3]

**In Canada—**
Abbokinase[4]
Abbokinase Open-Cath[4]
Activase rt-PA[1]

Lysatec rt-PA[1]
Streptase[3]

Other commonly used names are:

Anisoylated plasminogen-streptokinase activator complex[2]
APSAC[2]

Tissue-type plasminogen activator (recombinant)[1]
t-PA[1]
rt-PA[1]

Note: For quick reference, the following thrombolytic agents are numbered to match the corresponding brand names.

This information applies to the following medicines:

1. Alteplase, Recombinant (AL-ti-plase)
2. Anistreplase (an-EYE-strep-lase)†
3. Streptokinase (strep-toe-KYE-nase)
4. Urokinase (yoor-oh-KYE-nase)

†Not commercially available in Canada.

## Description

Thrombolytic agents are used to dissolve blood clots that have formed in certain blood vessels. These medicines are usually used when a blood clot seriously lessens the flow of blood to certain parts of the body.

Thrombolytic agents are also used to dissolve blood clots that form in tubes that are placed into the body. The tubes allow treatments (such as dialysis or injections into a vein) to be given over a long period of time.

These medicines are to be given only by or under the direct supervision of a doctor.

These medicines are available in the following dosage forms:

*Parenteral*

Alteplase, Recombinant
• Injection (U.S. and Canada)
Anistreplase
• Injection (U.S.)
Streptokinase
• Injection (U.S. and Canada)
Urokinase
• Injection (U.S. and Canada)

## Before Receiving This Medicine

In deciding to use a medicine, the risks of using the medicine must be weighed against the good it will do. This is a decision you and your doctor will make. For thrombolytic agents, the following should be considered:

**Allergies**—Tell your doctor if you have ever had any unusual or allergic reaction to alteplase, anistreplase, streptokinase, or urokinase. Also tell your health care professional if you are allergic to any other substances, such as foods, preservatives, or dyes.

**Pregnancy**—Tell your doctor if you are pregnant or if you have recently delivered a baby.

There is a slight chance that use of a thrombolytic agent during the first five months of pregnancy may cause a miscarriage. However, both streptokinase and urokinase have been used in pregnant women and have not been reported to cause this problem. Also, studies in pregnant women (for streptokinase) and studies in animals (for urokinase) have not shown that these medicines cause either miscarriage or harm to the fetus (including birth defects). Studies on birth defects with alteplase and anistreplase have not been done in either pregnant women or animals.

**Breast-feeding**—It is not known whether thrombolytic agents pass into the breast milk. Although most medicines pass into breast milk in small amounts, many of them may be used safely while breast-feeding. Mothers who are taking any of these medicines and who wish to breast-feed should discuss this with their doctor.

**Children**—These medicines have been tested in children and, in effective doses, have not been shown to cause different side effects or problems than they do in adults.

**Older adults**—The need for treatment with a thrombolytic agent (instead of other kinds of treatment) may be increased in elderly patients with blood clots. However, the chance of bleeding may also be increased. It is especially important that you discuss the use of this medicine with your doctor.

**Other medicines**—Although certain medicines should not be used together at all, in other cases two different medicines may be used together even if an interaction might occur. In these cases, your doctor may want to change the dose, or other precautions may be necessary. Before you receive a thrombolytic agent, it is especially important that your doctor know if you are taking any of the following:

- Anticoagulants (blood thinners) or
- Aspirin or
- Cefamandole (e.g., Mandol) or
- Cefoperazone (e.g., Cefobid) or
- Cefotetan (e.g., Cefotan) or
- Divalproex (e.g., Depakote) or
- Enoxaparin (e.g., Lovenox) or
- Heparin or
- Indomethacin (e.g., Indocin) or
- Inflammation or pain medicine (except narcotics) or
- Phenylbutazone (e.g., Butazolidin) or
- Plicamycin (e.g., Mithracin) or
- Sulfinpyrazone (e.g., Anturane) or
- Ticlopidine (e.g., Ticlid) or
- Valproic acid (e.g., Depakene)—The chance of bleeding may be increased

Also, tell your doctor if you have had an injection of anistreplase or streptokinase within the past year. If you have, these medicines may not work properly if they are given to you again. Your doctor may decide to use alteplase or urokinase instead.

**Other medical problems or recent childbirth**—The presence of other medical problems or recent delivery of a child may affect the use of thrombolytic agents. Make sure you tell your doctor if you have any other medical problems, especially:

- Blood disease, bleeding problems, or a history of bleeding in any part of the body or
- Brain disease or tumor or
- Colitis or stomach ulcer (or history of) or
- Heart or blood vessel disease or
- High blood pressure or
- Liver disease (severe) or
- Stroke (or history of) or
- Tuberculosis (TB) (active)—The chance of serious bleeding may be increased
- Streptococcal ("strep") infection (recent)—Anistreplase or streptokinase may not work properly after a streptococcal infection; your doctor may decide to use a different thrombolytic agent

Also, tell your doctor if you have recently had any of the following conditions:

- Falls or blows to the body or head or any other injury or
- Injections into a blood vessel or
- Placement of any tube into the body or
- Surgery, including dental surgery—The chance of serious bleeding may be increased

If you have recently delivered a baby, use of these medicines may cause serious bleeding.

---

## Proper Use of This Medicine

**Dosing**—The dose of these medicines will be different for different patients. The dose you receive will depend on the medicine you receive and will be based on the condition for which you are receiving the medicine. In some cases, the dose will also depend on your body weight.

---

## Precautions While Receiving This Medicine

Thrombolytic agents can cause bleeding that usually is not serious. However, serious bleeding may occur in some people. *To help prevent serious bleeding, carefully follow any instructions given by your health care professional. Also, move around as little as possible, and do not get out of bed on your own, unless your health care professional tells you it is all right to do so.*

---

## Side Effects of This Medicine

Along with its needed effects, a medicine may cause some unwanted effects. Although not all of these side effects may occur, if they do occur they may need medical attention.

*Tell your health care professional immediately if any of the following side effects occur:*

*More common*

    Bleeding or oozing from cuts, gums, or around the place of injection; fever

---

*Less common or rare*

Bruising; changes in facial skin color; confusion; double vision; fast or irregular breathing; flushing or redness of skin; headache (mild); muscle pain (mild); nausea; shortness of breath, troubled breathing, tightness in chest, and/or wheezing; skin rash, hives, or itching; swelling of eyes, face, lips, or tongue; trouble in speaking; weakness in arms or legs

*Symptoms of bleeding inside the body*

Abdominal or stomach pain or swelling; back pain or backaches; blood in urine; bloody or black, tarry stools; constipation; coughing up blood; dizziness; headaches (sudden, severe, or continuing); joint pain, stiffness, or swelling; muscle pain or stiffness (severe or continuing); nosebleeds; unexpected or unusually heavy bleeding from vagina; vomiting of blood or material that looks like coffee grounds

Other side effects not listed above may also occur in some patients. If you notice any other effects, check with your doctor.

Revised: 09/01/94

---

# THYROID HORMONES     Systemic

Some commonly used brand names are:

**In the U.S.—**

| | |
|---|---|
| Armour Thyroid[5] | Synthroid[1] |
| Cytomel[2] | Thyrar[5] |
| Levo-T[1] | Thyroid Strong[5] |
| Levothroid[1] | Thyrolar[3] |
| Levoxine[1] | Westhroid[5] |

**In Canada—**

| | |
|---|---|
| Cytomel[2] | PMS-Levothyroxine Sodium[1] |
| Eltroxin[1] | Synthroid[1] |

Note: For quick reference, the following thyroid hormones are numbered to match the corresponding brand names.

This information applies to the following medicines:

1. Levothyroxine (lee-voe-thye-ROX-een)‡
2. Liothyronine (lye-oh-THYE-roe-neen)‡
3. Liotrix (LYE-oh-trix)†
4. Thyroglobulin (thye-roe-GLOB-yoo-lin)*†
5. Thyroid (THYE-roid)‡§

Note: This information does *not* apply to Thyrotropin.

*Not commercially available in the U.S.
†Not commercially available in Canada.
‡Generic name product may also be available in the U.S.
§Generic name product may also be available in Canada.

---

## Description

Thyroid medicines belong to the general group of medicines called hormones. They are used when the thyroid gland does not produce enough hormone. They are also used to help decrease the size of enlarged thyroid glands (known as goiter) and to treat thyroid cancer.

These medicines are available only with your doctor's prescription, in the following dosage forms:

*Oral*

Levothyroxine
- Tablets (U.S. and Canada)

Liothyronine
- Tablets (U.S. and Canada)

Liotrix
- Tablets (U.S.)

Thyroglobulin
- Tablets

Thyroid
- Tablets (U.S. and Canada)
- Enteric-coated tablets (U.S.)

*Parenteral*

Levothyroxine
- Injection (U.S. and Canada)

---

## Before Using This Medicine

In deciding to use a medicine, the risks of taking the medicine must be weighed against the good it will do. This is a decision you and your doctor will make. For thyroid hormones, the following should be considered:

**Allergies**—Tell your doctor if you have ever had any unusual or allergic reaction to thyroid hormones. Also tell your health care professional if you are allergic to any other substances, such as foods, preservatives, or dyes.

**Pregnancy**—It is essential that your baby receive the right amount of thyroid for normal development. You may need to take different amounts while you are pregnant. In addition, you may respond differently than usual to some tests. Your doctor should check your progress at regular visits while you are pregnant.

**Breast-feeding**—Use of proper amounts of thyroid hormones by mothers has not been shown to cause problems in nursing babies.

**Children**—Thyroid hormones have been tested in children and have not been shown to cause different side effects or problems in children than they do in adults.

**Older adults**—This medicine has been tested and has not been shown to cause different side effects or problems in older people than it does in younger adults. However, a different dose may be needed in the elderly. Therefore, it is important to take the medicine only as directed by the doctor.

**Other medicines**—Although certain medicines should not be used together at all, in other cases two different medicines may be used together even if an interaction might occur. In these cases, your doctor may want to change the dose, or other precautions may be necessary. When you are taking thyroid hormones, it is especially important that

---

your health care professional know if you are taking any of the following:

- Amphetamines
- Anticoagulants (blood thinners)
- Appetite suppressants (diet pills)
- Cholestyramine (e.g., Questran)
- Colestipol (e.g., Colestid)
- Medicine for asthma or other breathing problems
- Medicine for colds, sinus problems, or hay fever or other allergies (including nose drops or sprays)

**Other medical problems**—The presence of other medical problems may affect the use of thyroid hormones. Make sure you tell your doctor if you have any other medical problems especially:

- Diabetes mellitus (sugar diabetes)
- Hardening of the arteries
- Heart disease
- High blood pressure
- Overactive thyroid (history of)
- Underactive adrenal gland
- Underactive pituitary gland

## Proper Use of This Medicine

*Use this medicine only as directed by your doctor.* Do not use more or less of it, and do not use it more often than your doctor ordered. Your doctor has prescribed the exact amount your body needs and if you take different amounts, you may experience symptoms of an overactive or under-active thyroid. Take it at the same time each day to make sure it always has the same effect.

If your condition is due to a lack of thyroid hormone, you may have to take this medicine for the rest of your life. It is very important that you *do not stop taking this medicine without first checking with your doctor.*

**Dosing**—The dose of these medicines will be different for different patients. *Follow your doctor's orders or the directions on the label.* The following information includes only the average doses of these medicines. *If your dose is different, do not change it* unless your doctor tells you to do so.

The number of tablets that you take depends on the strength of the medicine. The amount of thyroid hormone that you need to take every day depends on the results of your thyroid tests. However, treatment is usually started with lower doses that are increased a little at a time until you are taking the full amount. This helps prevent side effects.

*For levothyroxine*

- For *oral* dosage form (tablets):
  —For replacing the thyroid hormone:
    - Adults and teenagers—At first, 0.0125 to 0.05 milligrams (mg) once a day. Then, your doctor may increase your dose a little at a time to 0.075 to 0.125 mg a day. The dose is usually no higher than 0.15 mg once a day.
    - Children less than 6 months of age—The dose is based on body weight and must be determined

by your doctor. The usual dose is 0.025 to 0.05 mg once a day.
    - Children 6 months to 12 months of age—The dose is based on body weight and must be determined by your doctor. The usual dose is 0.05 to 0.075 mg once a day.
    - Children 1 to 5 years of age—The dose is based on body weight and must be determined by your doctor. The usual dose is 0.075 to 0.1 mg once a day.
    - Children 6 to 10 years of age—The dose is based on body weight and must be determined by your doctor. The usual dose is 0.1 to 0.15 mg once a day.
    - Children over 10 years of age—The dose is based on body weight and must be determined by your doctor. The usual dose is 0.15 to 0.2 mg once a day.
- For *injection* dosage form:
  —For replacing the thyroid hormone:
    - Adults and teenagers—50 to 100 micrograms (mcg) injected into a muscle or into a vein once a day. People with very serious conditions caused by too little thyroid hormone may need higher doses.
    - Children less than 6 months of age—The dose is based on body weight and must be determined by your doctor. The usual dose is 0.019 to 0.038 mg once a day.
    - Children 6 months to 12 months of age—The dose is based on body weight and must be determined by your doctor. The usual dose is 0.038 to 0.056 mg once a day.
    - Children 1 to 5 years of age—The dose is based on body weight and must be determined by your doctor. The usual dose is 0.056 to 0.075 mg once a day.
    - Children 6 to 10 years of age—The dose is based on body weight and must be determined by your doctor. The usual dose is 0.075 to 0.113 mg once a day.
    - Children over 10 years of age—The dose is based on body weight and must be determined by your doctor. The usual dose is 0.113 to 0.15 mg once a day.

*For liothyronine sodium*

- For *oral* dosage form (tablets):
  —For replacing the thyroid hormone:
    - Adults and teenagers—At first, 25 micrograms (mcg) a day. Some patients with very serious conditions caused by too little thyroid hormone may need to take only 2.5 to 5 mcg a day at first. Also, some patients with heart disease or the elderly may need lower doses at first. Then, your doctor may increase your dose a little at a time to up to 50 mcg a day if needed. Your doctor may want you to divide your dose into smaller amounts that are taken two or more times a day.

—For treating a large thyroid gland (goiter):
- Adults—At first, 5 mcg a day. Some patients with heart disease or the elderly may need lower doses at first. Then, your doctor may increase your dose a little at a time to 50 to 100 mcg a day.

*For liotrix (levothyroxine and liothyronine combination)*
- For *oral* dosage form (tablets):
  —For replacing the thyroid hormone:
  - Adults, teenagers, and children—At first, 50 micrograms (mcg) of levothyroxine and 12.5 mcg of liothyronine once a day. Some people with very serious conditions caused by too little thyroid hormone may need only 12.5 mcg of levothyroxine and 3.1 mcg of liothyronine once a day. Also, some elderly patients may need lower doses at first. Then, your doctor may want to increase your dose a little at a time to up to 100 mcg of levothyroxine and 25 mcg of liothyronine.

*For thyroglobulin*
- For *oral* dosage form (tablets):
  —For replacing the thyroid hormone:
  - Adults, teenagers, and children—At first, 32 milligrams (mg) a day. Some people with very serious conditions caused by too little thyroid hormone may need to take only 16 to 32 mg a day at first. Then, the doctor may want you to increase your dose a little at a time to 65 to 160 mg a day.

*For thyroid*
- For *oral* dosage form (tablets):
  —For replacing thyroid hormone:
  - Adults, teenagers, and children—60 milligrams (mg) a day. Some people with very serious conditions caused by too little thyroid hormone may need to take only 15 mg a day at first. Also, some elderly patients may need lower doses at first. Then, your doctor may want to increase your dose a little at a time to 60 to 120 mg a day.

**Missed dose**—If you miss a dose of this medicine, take it as soon as possible. However, if it is almost time for your next dose, skip the missed dose and go back to your regular dosing schedule. Do not double doses. If you miss 2 or more doses in a row or if you have any questions about this, check with your doctor.

**Storage**—To store this medicine:
- Keep out of the reach of children.
- Store away from heat and direct light.
- Do not store in the bathroom, near the kitchen sink, or in other damp places. Heat or moisture may cause the medicine to break down.
- Do not keep outdated medicine or medicine no longer needed. Be sure that any discarded medicine is out of the reach of children.

## Precautions While Using This Medicine

*It is very important that your doctor check your progress at regular visits*, to make sure that this medicine is working properly.

If you have certain kinds of heart disease, this medicine may cause chest pain or shortness of breath when you exert yourself. If these occur, do not overdo exercise or physical work. If you have any questions about this, check with your doctor.

Before having any kind of surgery (including dental surgery) or emergency treatment, *tell the medical doctor or dentist in charge that you are taking this medicine*.

Do not take any other medicine unless prescribed by your doctor. Some medicines may increase or decrease the effects of thyroid on your body and cause problems in controlling your condition. Also, thyroid hormones may change the effects of other medicines.

## Side Effects of This Medicine

Along with its needed effects, a medicine may cause some unwanted effects. Although not all of these side effects may occur, if they do occur they may need medical attention.

Check with your doctor as soon as possible if any of the following side effects occur since they may indicate an overdose or an allergic reaction:

*Rare*

Headache (severe) in children; skin rash or hives

*Signs and symptoms of overdose*

Chest pain; fast or irregular heartbeat; shortness of breath

For patients taking this medicine for underactive thyroid:
- This medicine usually takes several weeks to have a noticeable effect on your condition. Until it begins to work, you may experience no change in your symptoms. Check with your doctor if the following symptoms continue:

Clumsiness; coldness; constipation; dry, puffy skin; listlessness; muscle aches; sleepiness; tiredness; weakness; weight gain

Other effects may occur if the dose of the medicine is not exactly right. These side effects will go away when the dose is corrected. Check with your doctor if any of the following symptoms occur:

Changes in appetite; changes in menstrual periods; diarrhea; fever; hand tremors; headache; increased sensitivity to heat; irritability; leg cramps; nervousness; sweating; trouble in sleeping; vomiting; weight loss

Other side effects not listed above may also occur in some patients. If you notice any other effects, check with your doctor.

Revised: 05/22/92
Interim revision: 07/25/94

# THYROTROPIN Systemic

A commonly used brand name in the U.S. and Canada is Thytropar.

## Description

Thyrotropin (thye-roe-TROE-pin) is used in a test to determine how well your thyroid is working. It may also be used for other conditions as determined by your doctor.

Thyrotropin is to be administered only by or under the immediate supervision of your doctor. It is available in the following dosage form:

*Parenteral*
- Injection (U.S. and Canada)

## Before Using This Medicine

In deciding to use a medicine, the risks of taking the medicine must be weighed against the good it will do. This is a decision you and your doctor will make. For thyrotropin, the following should be considered:

**Allergies**—Tell your doctor if you have ever received thyrotropin or ever had any unusual or allergic reaction to thyrotropin. Also tell your health care professional if you are allergic to any other substances, such as foods, preservatives, or dyes.

**Pregnancy**—Studies on effects in pregnancy have not been done in either humans or animals.

**Breast-feeding**—It is not known whether thyrotropin passes into breast milk. However, this medicine has not been reported to cause problems in nursing babies.

**Children**—This medicine has been tested in children and has not been shown to cause different side effects or problems than it does in adults.

**Older adults**—Many medicines have not been studied specifically in the elderly. Therefore, it may not be known whether they work exactly the same way they do in younger adults. Although, there is no specific information comparing the use of thyrotropin in the elderly with use in other age groups, this medicine is not expected to cause different side effects or problems in older people than it does in younger adults.

**Other medicines**—Although certain medicines should not be used together at all, in other cases two different medicines may be used together even if an interaction might occur. In these cases, your doctor may want to change the dose, or other precautions may be necessary. When you are receiving thyrotropin, it is especially important that your health care professional know if you are taking any of the following:
- Thyroid hormones—You may not respond as strongly to thyrotropin if you have been taking thyroid hormones regularly

**Other medical problems**—The presence of other medical problems may affect the use of thyrotropin. Make sure you tell your doctor if you have any other medical problems, especially:
- Hardening of the arteries or
- Heart disease or
- High blood pressure—Thyrotropin increases body metabolism and causes the heart to work harder, which may make these conditions worse
- Untreated underactive adrenal gland or
- Untreated underactive pituitary gland—Use of thyrotropin may severely worsen these conditions

## Proper Use of This Medicine

For your doctor to properly treat your medical condition, *you must receive every dose of this medicine*. After the last dose, the doctor may want to perform certain tests that are very important.

**Dosing**—The dose of thyrotropin will be different for different patients. *Follow your doctor's orders*. The following information includes only the average doses of thyrotropin.
- For *injection* dosage form:
  —For testing the thyroid gland:
    - Adults and children—10 International Units (IU) injected under the skin or into a muscle once a day for one to three days. If thyroid testing is being done after surgery, this medicine will usually be given for three to seven days.

## Side Effects of This Medicine

Along with its needed effects, a medicine may cause some unwanted effects. Although not all of these side effects may occur, if they do occur they may need medical attention.

*Check with your doctor immediately* if any of the following side effects occur:
> *Rare—more common in patients who have received thyrotropin previously*
>> Faintness; itching; redness or swelling at place of injection; skin rash; tightness of throat; wheezing

Other effects may occur if the dose of the medicine is not exactly right. Check with your doctor as soon as possible if any of the following symptoms occur:
> Chest pain; fast or irregular heartbeat; irritability; nervousness; shortness of breath; sweating

Other side effects may occur that usually do not need medical attention. These side effects may go away during treatment as your body adjusts to the medicine. However,

check with your doctor if any of the following side effects continue or are bothersome:

*More common*

Flushing of face; frequent urge to urinate; headache; nausea and vomiting; stomach discomfort

Other side effects not listed above may also occur in some patients. If you notice any other effects, check with your doctor.

Revised: 01/31/92
Interim revision: 06/21/94

---

# TICLOPIDINE   Systemic

A commonly used brand name in the U.S. and Canada is Ticlid.

## Description

Ticlopidine (tye-KLOE-pi-deen) is used to lower the chance of having a stroke. It is given to people who have already had a stroke and to people with certain medical problems that may lead to a stroke. Because ticlopidine can cause serious side effects, especially during the first 3 months of treatment, it is used mostly for people who cannot take aspirin to prevent strokes.

A stroke may occur when a blood vessel in the brain is blocked by a blood clot. Ticlopidine lessens the chance that a harmful blood clot will form, by preventing certain cells in the blood from clumping together. This effect of ticlopidine may also increase the chance of serious bleeding in some people.

This medicine is available in the following dosage forms:

*Oral*

• Tablets (U.S. and Canada)

## Before Using This Medicine

In deciding to use a medicine, the risks of taking the medicine must be weighed against the good it will do. This is a decision you and your doctor will make. For ticlopidine, the following should be considered:

**Allergies**—Tell your doctor if you have ever had any unusual or allergic reaction to ticlopidine. Also tell your health care professional if you are allergic to any other substances, such as foods, preservatives, or dyes.

**Pregnancy**—Studies with ticlopidine have not been done in pregnant women. This medicine did not cause birth defects in animal studies. However, it caused other unwanted effects in animal studies when it was given in amounts that were large enough to cause harmful effects in the mother.

**Breast-feeding**—It is not known whether ticlopidine passes into the breast milk.

**Children**—There is no specific information comparing use of ticlopidine in children with use in other age groups.

**Older adults**—This medicine has been tested and has not been shown to cause different side effects or problems in older people than it does in younger adults.

**Other medicines**—Although certain medicines should not be used together at all, in other cases two different medicines may be used together even if an interaction might occur. In these cases, your doctor may want to change the dose, or other precautions may be necessary. When you are taking ticlopidine, it is especially important that your health care professional know if you are taking any of the following:

• Anticoagulants (blood thinners) or
• Aspirin or
• Heparin (e.g., Hepalean, Liquaemin)—The chance of serious bleeding may be increased

**Other medical problems**—The presence of other medical problems may affect the use of ticlopidine. Make sure you tell your doctor if you have any other medical problems, especially:

• Blood disease—The chance of serious side effects may be increased
• Blood clotting problems, such as hemophilia, or
• Liver disease (severe) or
• Stomach ulcers—The chance of serious bleeding may be increased
• Kidney disease (severe)—Ticlopidine is removed from the body more slowly when the kidneys are not working properly. This may increase the chance of side effects.

## Proper Use of This Medicine

Ticlopidine should be taken with food. This increases the amount of medicine that is absorbed into the body. It may also lessen the chance of stomach upset.

Take this medicine only as directed by your doctor. Ticlopidine will not work properly if you take less of it than directed. Taking more ticlopidine than directed may increase the chance of serious side effects without increasing the helpful effects.

**Dosing**—*Follow your doctor's orders or the directions on the label.* The following dose was used, and found effective, in studies. However, some people may need a different dose. *If your dose is different, do not change it* unless your doctor tells you to do so:

• For adults—1 tablet (250 mg) two times a day, with food.
• For children—It is not likely that ticlopidine would be used to help prevent strokes in children. If a child needs this medicine, however, the dose would have to be determined by the doctor.

**Missed dose**—If you miss a dose of this medicine, take it as soon as possible. However, if it is almost time for your next dose, skip the missed dose and go back to your regular dosing schedule. Do not double doses.

**Storage**—To store this medicine:

- Keep out of the reach of children.
- Store away from heat and direct light.
- Do not store in the bathroom, near the kitchen sink, or in other damp places. Heat or moisture may cause the medicine to break down.
- Do not keep outdated medicine or medicine no longer needed. Be sure that any discarded medicine is out of the reach of children.

## Precautions While Using This Medicine

*It is very important that blood tests be done every 2 weeks for the first 3 months of treatment with ticlopidine.* The tests are needed to find out whether certain side effects are occurring. Finding these side effects early helps to prevent them from becoming serious. Your doctor will arrange for the blood tests to be done. *Be sure that you do not miss any appointments for these tests.* You will probably not need to have your blood tested so often after the first 3 months of treatment, because the side effects are less likely to occur after that time.

*Tell all medical doctors, dentists, nurses, and pharmacists you go to that you are taking this medicine.* Ticlopidine may increase the risk of serious bleeding during an operation or some kinds of dental work. Therefore, treatment may have to be stopped about 10 days to 2 weeks before the operation or dental work is done.

Ticlopidine may cause serious bleeding, especially after an injury. Sometimes, bleeding inside the body can occur without your knowing about it. Ask your doctor whether there are certain activities you should avoid while taking this medicine (for example, sports that can cause injuries). *Also, check with your doctor immediately if you are injured while being treated with this medicine.*

*Check with your doctor immediately if you notice any of the following side effects:*

- Bruising or bleeding, especially bleeding that is hard to stop.
- Any sign of infection, such as fever, chills, or sore throat.
- Sores, ulcers, or white spots in the mouth.

After you stop taking ticlopidine, the chance of bleeding may continue for 1 or 2 weeks. During this period of time, continue to follow the same precautions that you followed while you were taking the medicine.

## Side Effects of This Medicine

Along with its needed effects, a medicine may cause some unwanted effects. Although not all of these side effects may occur, if they do occur they may need medical attention.

*Check with your doctor immediately* if any of the following side effects occur:

*Less common or rare*

Abdominal or stomach pain (severe) or swelling; back pain; blood in eyes; blood in urine; bloody or black, tarry stools; bruising or purple areas on skin; coughing up blood; decreased alertness; dizziness; fever, chills, or sore throat; headache (severe or continuing); joint pain or swelling; nosebleeds; pinpoint red spots on skin; sores, ulcers, or white spots in mouth; paralysis or problems with coordination; stammering or other difficulty in speaking; unusually heavy bleeding or oozing from cuts or wounds; unusually heavy or unexpected menstrual bleeding; vomiting of blood or material that looks like coffee grounds

Also, check with your doctor as soon as possible if any of the following side effects occur:

*More common*

Skin rash

*Less common or rare*

Hives or itching of skin; ringing or buzzing in ears; yellow eyes or skin

Other side effects may occur that usually do not need medical attention. These side effects may go away during treatment as your body adjusts to the medicine. However, check with your doctor if any of the following side effects continue or are bothersome:

*More common*

Abdominal or stomach pain (mild); bloating or gas; diarrhea; nausea

*Less common*

Indigestion; vomiting

Other side effects not listed above may also occur in some patients. If you notice any other effects, check with your doctor.

Revised: 07/22/92

# TIOPRONIN  Systemic†

In the U.S.—
　Thiola

Other—
| | |
|---|---|
| Capen | Sutilan |
| Captimer | Thiosol |
| Epatiol | Tioglis |
| Mucolysin | Vincol |

†Not commercially available in Canada.

## Description

Tiopronin (tye-oh-PRO-nin) is used to prevent kidney stones, which may develop due to too much cystine in the urine (cystinuria). This medicine works by removing the extra cystine from the body.

In addition to the helpful effects of this medicine, it has side effects that can be very serious. Before you take tiopronin, be sure that you have discussed its use with your doctor.

Tiopronin is available only with your doctor's prescription, in the following dosage form:

*Oral*
- Tablets (U.S.)

## Before Using This Medicine

In deciding to use a medicine, the risks of taking the medicine must be weighed against the good it will do. This is a decision you and your doctor will make. For tiopronin, the following should be considered:

**Allergies**—Tell your doctor if you have ever had any unusual or allergic reaction to penicillamine or tiopronin. Also tell your health care professional if you are allergic to any other substances, such as foods, preservatives, or dyes.

**Diet**—It is important that you follow any special instructions from your doctor, such as following a low-methionine diet. Methionine is found in animal proteins such as milk, eggs, cheese, and fish. Also, make certain your health care professional knows if you are on any special diet, such as a low-sodium or low-sugar diet.

**Pregnancy**—Studies have not been done in humans. However, studies in animals have shown that tiopronin may cause problems during pregnancy and harmful effects on the fetus.

**Breast-feeding**—Tiopronin may pass into the breast milk. This medicine is not recommended during breast-feeding because it may cause unwanted effects in nursing babies.

**Children**—Although there is no specific information comparing use of tiopronin in children with use in other age groups, this medicine is not expected to cause different side effects or problems in children than it does in adults.

**Older adults**—Many medicines have not been studied specifically in older people. Therefore, it may not be known whether they work exactly the same way they do in younger adults or if they cause different side effects or problems in older people. Although there is no specific information comparing the use of tiopronin in the elderly with use in other age groups, this medicine is not expected to cause different side effects or problems in older people than it does in younger adults.

**Other medicines**—Although certain medicines should not be used together at all, in other cases two different medicines may be used together even if an interaction might occur. In these cases, your doctor may want to change the dose, or other precautions may be necessary. Tell your health care professional if you are taking any other prescription or nonprescription (over-the-counter [OTC]) medicine.

**Other medical problems**—The presence of other medical problems may affect the use of tiopronin. Make sure you tell your doctor if you have any other medical problems, especially:
- Blood problems (or a history of) or
- Kidney disease (or a history of) or
- Liver disease—Tiopronin may make these conditions worse

## Proper Use of This Medicine

Take this medicine on an empty stomach (at least 30 minutes before meals or 2 hours after meals).

You should drink 2 full glasses (8 ounces each) of water with each meal and at bedtime. You should also drink another 2 full glasses during the night.

It is important that you follow any special instructions from your doctor, such as following a low-methionine diet. Methionine is found in animal proteins such as milk, eggs, cheese, and fish. If you have any questions about this, check with your doctor.

*Take this medicine regularly as directed. Do not stop taking it without first checking with your doctor,* since stopping the medicine and then restarting it may increase the chance of side effects.

**Dosing**—The dose of tiopronin will be different for different patients. *Follow your doctor's orders or the directions on the label.* The following information includes only the average doses of tiopronin. *If your dose is different, do not change it* unless your doctor tells you to do so.
- For *oral* dosage form (tablets):
　—To prevent kidney stones:
　　- Adults—To start, 800 milligrams (mg) a day, divided into three doses. Your doctor may change your dose if needed.
　　- Children up to 9 years of age—Dose must be determined by your doctor.

- Children 9 years and older—Dose is based on body weight and must be determined by your doctor. The usual dose to start is 15 mg per kilogram (kg) (6.8 mg per pound) of body weight a day, divided into three doses. Your doctor may change your dose if needed.

**Missed dose**—If you miss a dose of this medicine, take it as soon as possible. However, if it is almost time for your next dose, skip the missed dose and go back to your regular dosing schedule. Do not double doses.

**Storage**—To store this medicine:
- Keep out of the reach of children.
- Store away from heat and direct light.
- Do not store in the bathroom, near the kitchen sink, or in other damp places. Heat or moisture may cause the medicine to break down.
- Do not keep outdated medicine or medicine no longer needed. Be sure that any discarded medicine is out of the reach of children.

## Precautions While Using This Medicine

Your doctor should check your progress at regular visits to make sure that this medicine is working properly and does not cause unwanted effects.

## Side Effects of This Medicine

Along with its needed effects, a medicine may cause some unwanted effects. Although not all of these side effects may occur, if they do occur they may need medical attention.

*Check with your doctor immediately* if any of the following side effects occur:

*More common*
Yellow skin or eyes

*Less common*
Muscle pain; sore throat and fever; unusual bleeding or bruising

Check with your doctor as soon as possible if any of the following side effects occur:

*More common*
Pain, swelling, or tenderness of the skin; skin rash, hives or itching; ulcers or sores in mouth

*Less common*
Bloody or cloudy urine; chills; difficulty in breathing; high blood pressure; hoarseness; joint pain; swelling of feet or lower legs; tenderness of glands; unusual bleeding

*Rare*
Chest pain; cough; difficulty in chewing, talking, or swallowing; double vision; general feeling of discomfort, illness, or weakness; muscle weakness; spitting up blood; swelling of lymph glands

Other side effects may occur that usually do not need medical attention. These side effects may go away during treatment as your body adjusts to the medicine. However, check with your doctor if any of the following side effects continue or are bothersome:

*More common*
Abdominal or stomach pain; bloating or gas; diarrhea or soft stools; loss of appetite; nausea and vomiting; warts; wrinkling or peeling or unusually dry skin

*Less common*
Changes in taste or smell

Other side effects not listed above may also occur in some patients. If you notice any other effects, check with your doctor.

Revised: 05/19/92
Interim revision: 08/09/94

# TOBRAMYCIN   Ophthalmic

A commonly used brand name in the U.S. and Canada is Tobrex. Generic name product may also be available in the U.S.

## Description

Ophthalmic tobramycin (toe-bra-MYE-sin) is used in the eye to treat bacterial infections of the eye. Tobramycin works by killing bacteria.

Ophthalmic tobramycin may be used alone or with other medicines for eye infections. Either the drops or ointment form of this medicine may be used alone during the day. In addition, both forms may be used together, with the drops being used during the day and the ointment at night.

Tobramycin ophthalmic preparations are available only with your doctor's prescription, in the following dosage forms:

*Ophthalmic*
- Ophthalmic ointment (U.S. and Canada)
- Ophthalmic solution (eye drops) (U.S. and Canada)

## Before Using This Medicine

In deciding to use a medicine, the risks of using the medicine must be weighed against the good it will do. This is a decision you and your doctor will make. For ophthalmic tobramycin, the following should be considered:

**Allergies**—Tell your doctor if you have ever had any unusual or allergic reaction to ophthalmic tobramycin or to any related medicines, such as amikacin (e.g., Amikin), gentamicin (e.g., Garamycin), kanamycin (e.g., Kantrex), neomycin (e.g., Mycifradin), netilmicin (e.g., Netromycin), streptomycin, or tobramycin by injection (e.g., Nebcin). Also tell your health care professional if you are allergic to any other substances, such as preservatives.

**Pregnancy**—Studies have not been done in humans. However, tobramycin ophthalmic preparations have not been shown to cause birth defects or other problems in animals given high doses.

**Breast-feeding**—Tobramycin ophthalmic preparations may be absorbed into the eye. However, tobramycin is unlikely to pass into the breast milk in large amounts and little would be absorbed by the infant. Therefore, this medicine is unlikely to cause serious problems in nursing babies.

**Children**—This medicine has been tested in children and, in effective doses, has not been shown to cause different side effects or problems than it does in adults.

**Older adults**—Many medicines have not been studied specifically in older people. Therefore, it may not be known whether they work exactly the same way they do in younger adults or if they cause different side effects or problems in older people. There is no specific information comparing use of ophthalmic tobramycin in the elderly with use in other age groups.

**Other medicines**—Although certain medicines should not be used together at all, in other cases two different medicines may be used together even if an interaction might occur. In these cases, your doctor may want to change the dose, or other precautions may be necessary. Tell your health care professional if you are using any other prescription or nonprescription (over-the-counter [OTC]) medicine that is to be used in the eye.

---

## Proper Use of This Medicine

For patients using tobramycin *ophthalmic solution (eye drops)*:

- The bottle is only partially full to provide proper drop control.
- To use:
   — First, wash your hands. Tilt the head back and with the index finger of one hand, press gently on the skin just beneath the lower eyelid and pull the lower eyelid away from the eye to make a space. Drop the medicine into this space. Let go of the eyelid and gently close the eyes. Do not blink. Keep the eyes closed for 1 or 2 minutes, to allow the medicine to come into contact with the infection.
   —If you think you did not get the drop of medicine into your eye properly, use another drop.
   —To keep the medicine as germ-free as possible, do not touch the applicator tip to any surface (including the eye). Also, keep the container tightly closed.

- If your doctor ordered two different ophthalmic solutions to be used together, wait at least 5 minutes between the times you apply the medicines. This will help to keep the second medicine from "washing out" the first one.

For patients using tobramycin *ophthalmic ointment (eye ointment)*:

- To use:
   —First, wash your hands. Tilt the head back and with the index finger of one hand, press gently on the skin just beneath the lower eyelid and pull the lower eyelid away from the eye to make a space. Squeeze a thin strip of ointment into this space. A 1.25-cm (approximately ½-inch) strip of ointment is usually enough unless otherwise directed by your doctor. Let go of the eyelid and gently close the eyes and keep them closed for 1 or 2 minutes, to allow the medicine to come into contact with the infection.
   —To keep the medicine as germ-free as possible, do not touch the applicator tip to any surface (including the eye). After using tobramycin eye ointment, wipe the tip of the ointment tube with a clean tissue and keep the tube tightly closed.

To help clear up your eye infection completely, *keep using tobramycin for the full time of treatment*, even if your symptoms have disappeared. *Do not miss any doses*.

**Dosing**—The dose of ophthalmic tobramycin will be different for different patients. *Follow your doctor's orders or the directions on the label*. The following information includes only the average dose of ophthalmic tobramycin. *If your dose is different, do not change it* unless your doctor tells you to do so.

*The number of doses you use each day, the time allowed between doses, and the length of time you use the medicine depend on the medical problem for which you are using ophthalmic tobramycin.*

- For *ophthalmic ointment* dosage forms:
   —For mild to moderate infections:
     - Adults and children—Use every eight to twelve hours.
   —For severe infections:
     - Adults and children—Use every three to four hours until improvement occurs.
- For *ophthalmic solution (eye drops)* dosage forms:
   —For mild to moderate infections:
     - Adults and children—One drop every four hours.
   —For severe infections:
     - Adults and children—One drop every hour until improvement occurs.

**Missed dose**—If you miss a dose of this medicine, use it as soon as possible. However, if it is almost time for your next dose, skip the missed dose and go back to your regular dosing schedule.

**Storage**—To store this medicine:
- Keep out of the reach of children.
- Store away from heat and direct light.
- Keep the medicine from freezing.
- Do not keep outdated medicine or medicine no longer needed. Be sure that any discarded medicine is out of the reach of children.

## Precautions While Using This Medicine

If your eye infection does not improve within a few days, or if it becomes worse, check with your doctor.

## Side Effects of This Medicine

Along with its needed effects, a medicine may cause some unwanted effects. Although not all of these side effects may occur, if they do occur they may need medical attention.

*Check with your doctor immediately* if any of the following side effects occur:

*Less common*
Itching, redness, swelling, or other sign of eye or eyelid irritation not present before use of this medicine

*Symptoms of overdose*
Increased watering of the eyes; itching, redness, or swelling of the eyes or eyelids

Other side effects may occur that usually do not need medical attention. These side effects may go away during treatment as your body adjusts to the medicine. However, check with your doctor if either of the following side effects continues or is bothersome:

*Less common*
Burning or stinging of the eyes

Eye ointments usually cause your vision to blur for a few minutes after application.

Other side effects not listed above may also occur in some patients. If you notice any other effects, check with your doctor.

Revised: 07/01/93
Interim revision: 09/30/93

---

# TOCAINIDE  Systemic

A commonly used brand name in the U.S. and Canada is Tonocard.

## Description

Tocainide (toe-KAY-nide) belongs to the group of medicines known as antiarrhythmics. It is used to correct irregular heartbeats to a normal rhythm.

Tocainide produces its helpful effects by slowing nerve impulses in the heart and making the heart tissue less sensitive.

Tocainide is available only with your doctor's prescription, in the following dosage form:

*Oral*
- Tablets (U.S. and Canada)

## Before Using This Medicine

In deciding to use a medicine, the risks of taking the medicine must be weighed against the good it will do. This is a decision you and your doctor will make. For tocainide, the following should be considered:

**Allergies**—Tell your doctor if you have ever had any unusual or allergic reaction to tocainide or anesthetics. Also tell your health care professional if you are allergic to any other substances, such as foods, preservatives, or dyes.

**Pregnancy**—Tocainide has not been shown to cause birth defects or other problems in humans. Studies in animals have shown that high doses of tocainide may increase the possibility of death in the animal fetus, although it has not been shown to cause birth defects.

**Breast-feeding**—It is not known whether tocainide passes into breast milk. However, this medicine has not been reported to cause problems in nursing babies.

**Children**—Studies on this medicine have been done only in adult patients and there is no specific information comparing use of tocainide in children with use in other age groups.

**Older adults**—Dizziness or lightheadedness may be more likely to occur in the elderly, who are usually more sensitive to the effects of tocainide.

**Other medicines**—Although certain medicines should not be used together at all, in other cases two different medicines may be used together even if an interaction might occur. In these cases, your doctor may want to change the dose, or other precautions may be necessary. Tell your health care professional if you are taking any other prescription or nonprescription (over-the-counter [OTC]) medicine.

**Other medical problems**—The presence of other medical problems may affect the use of tocainide. Make sure you tell your doctor if you have any other medical problems, especially:
- Congestive heart failure—Tocainide may make this condition worse

- Kidney disease or
- Liver disease—Effects may be increased because of slower removal of tocainide from the body

## Proper Use of This Medicine

*Take tocainide exactly as directed by your doctor*, even though you may feel well. Do not take more medicine than ordered.

If tocainide upsets your stomach, your doctor may advise you to take it with food or milk.

This medicine works best when there is a constant amount in the blood. *To help keep the amount constant, do not miss any doses. Also, it is best to take the doses at evenly spaced times day and night.* For example, if you are to take 3 doses a day, the doses should be spaced about 8 hours apart. If this interferes with your sleep or other daily activities, or if you need help in planning the best times to take your medicine, check with your health care professional.

**Dosing**—The dose of tocainide will be different for different patients. *Follow your doctor's orders or the directions on the label.* The following information includes only the average doses of tocainide. *If your dose is different, do not change it* unless your doctor tells you to do so.

The number of tablets that you take depends on the strength of the medicine.

- For *oral* dosage form (tablets):
  —For irregular heartbeat:
    - Adults—At first, 400 milligrams (mg) every eight hours. Then, your doctor may increase your dose up to 600 mg three times a day.
    - Children—Use and dose must be determined by your doctor.

**Missed dose**—If you miss a dose of tocainide and remember within 4 hours, take it as soon as possible. Then go back to your regular dosing schedule. However, if you do not remember until later, skip the missed dose and go back to your regular dosing schedule. Do not double doses.

**Storage**—To store this medicine:
- Keep out of the reach of children.
- Store away from heat and direct light.
- Do not store in the bathroom, near the kitchen sink, or in other damp places. Heat or moisture may cause the medicine to break down.
- Do not keep outdated medicine or medicine no longer needed. Be sure that any discarded medicine is out of the reach of children.

## Precautions While Using This Medicine

It is important that your doctor check your progress at regular visits to make sure the medicine is working properly. This will allow changes to be made in the amount of medicine you are taking, if necessary.

Your doctor may want you to carry a medical identification card or bracelet stating that you are using this medicine.

Tocainide may cause some people to become dizzy, lightheaded, or less alert than they are normally. *Make sure you know how you react to this medicine before you drive, use machines, or do anything else that could be dangerous if you are dizzy or are not alert.*

*Before having any kind of surgery (including dental surgery) or emergency treatment, tell the medical doctor or dentist in charge that you are taking this medicine.*

## Side Effects of This Medicine

Along with its needed effects, a medicine may cause some unwanted effects. Although not all of these side effects may occur, if they do occur they may need medical attention.

Check with your doctor as soon as possible if any of the following side effects occur:

*Less common*
  Trembling or shaking
*Rare*
  Blisters on skin; cough or shortness of breath; fever or chills; irregular heartbeats; peeling or scaling of skin; skin rash (severe); sores in mouth; unusual bleeding or bruising

Other side effects may occur that usually do not need medical attention. These side effects may go away during treatment as your body adjusts to the medicine. However, check with your doctor if any of the following side effects continue or are bothersome:

*More common*
  Dizziness or lightheadedness; loss of appetite; nausea
*Less common*
  Blurred vision; confusion; headache; nervousness; numbness or tingling of fingers and toes; skin rash; sweating; vomiting

Other side effects not listed above may also occur in some patients. If you notice any other effects, check with your doctor.

Revised: 08/06/92
Interim revision: 07/20/94

# TOLNAFTATE    Topical

Some commonly used brand names are:

**In the U.S.—**

| | |
|---|---|
| Aftate for Athlete's Foot Aerosol Spray Liquid | Tinactin Aerosol Liquid |
| Aftate for Athlete's Foot Aerosol Spray Powder | Tinactin Aerosol Powder |
| Aftate for Athlete's Foot Gel | Tinactin Antifungal Deodorant Powder Aerosol |
| Aftate for Athlete's Foot Sprinkle Powder | Tinactin Cream |
| Aftate for Jock Itch Aerosol Spray Powder | Tinactin Jock Itch Cream |
| Aftate for Jock Itch Gel | Tinactin Jock Itch Spray Powder |
| Aftate for Jock Itch Sprinkle Powder | Tinactin Powder |
| Genaspore Cream | Tinactin Solution |
| NP-27 Cream | Ting Antifungal Cream |
| NP-27 Cream | Ting Antifungal Powder |
| NP-27 Solution | Ting Antifungal Spray Liquid |
| NP-27 Spray Powder | Ting Antifungal Spray Powder |
| | Zeasorb-AF Powder |

Generic name product may also be available.

**In Canada—**

| | |
|---|---|
| Pitrex Cream | Tinactin Jock Itch Cream |
| Tinactin Aerosol Liquid | Tinactin Plus Aerosol Powder |
| Tinactin Aerosol Powder | Tinactin Plus Powder |
| Tinactin Cream | Tinactin Powder |
| Tinactin Jock Itch Aerosol Powder | Tinactin Solution |

## Description

Tolnaftate (tole-NAF-tate) belongs to the group of medicines called antifungals. It is used to treat some types of fungus infections. It may also be used together with medicines taken by mouth for fungus infections.

Tolnaftate is available without a prescription; however, your doctor may have special instructions on the proper use of tolnaftate for your medical problem.

Tolnaftate is available in the following dosage forms:

*Topical*
- Aerosol powder (U.S. and Canada)
- Aerosol solution (U.S. and Canada)
- Cream (U.S. and Canada)
- Gel (U.S.)
- Powder (U.S. and Canada)
- Topical solution (U.S. and Canada)

## Before Using This Medicine

If you are taking this medicine without a prescription, carefully read and follow any precautions on the label. For tolnaftate, the following should be considered:

**Allergies**—Tell your doctor if you have ever had any unusual or allergic reaction to tolnaftate. Also tell your health care professional if you are allergic to any other substances, such as preservatives or dyes.

**Pregnancy**—Tolnaftate topical preparations have not been shown to cause birth defects or other problems in humans.

**Breast-feeding**—Tolnaftate topical preparations have not been reported to cause problems in nursing babies.

**Children**—Tolnaftate should not be used on children up to 2 years of age, unless otherwise directed by your doctor. Although there is no specific information comparing use of tolnaftate in children 2 years of age and older with use in other age groups, this medicine is not expected to cause different side effects or problems in children 2 years of age and older than it does in adults.

**Older adults**—Many medicines have not been studied specifically in older people. Therefore, it may not be known whether they work exactly the same way they do in younger adults or if they cause different side effects or problems in older people. There is no specific information comparing use of tolnaftate in the elderly with use in other age groups.

**Other medicines**—Although certain medicines should not be used together at all, in other cases two different medicines may be used together even if an interaction might occur. In these cases, your doctor may want to change the dose, or other precautions may be necessary. Tell your health care professional if you are using any other topical prescription or nonprescription (over-the-counter [OTC]) medicine that is to be applied to the same area of the skin.

## Proper Use of This Medicine

Before applying tolnaftate, wash the affected area and dry thoroughly. Then apply enough medicine to cover the affected area.

*Keep this medicine away from the eyes.*

For patients using the *powder form* of this medicine:
- If the powder is used on the feet, sprinkle it between toes, on feet, and in socks and shoes.

For patients using the *aerosol powder form* of this medicine:
- Shake well before using.
- From a distance of 6 to 10 inches, spray the powder on the affected areas. If it is used on the feet, spray it between toes, on feet, and in socks and shoes.
- Do not inhale the powder.
- Do not use near heat, near open flame, or while smoking.

For patients using the *solution form* of this medicine:
- If tolnaftate solution becomes a solid, it may be dissolved by warming the closed container of medicine in warm water.

For patients using the *aerosol solution form* of this medicine:
- Shake well before using.
- From a distance of 6 inches, spray the solution on the affected areas. If it is used on the feet, spray between toes and on feet.
- Do not inhale the vapors from the spray.

- Do not use near heat, near open flame, or while smoking.

To help clear up your infection completely, *keep using this medicine for 2 weeks after burning, itching, or other symptoms have disappeared,* unless otherwise directed by your doctor. *Do not miss any doses.*

**Dosing**—The dose of tolnaftate will be different for different patients. *Follow your doctor's orders or the directions on the label.* The following information includes only the average dose of tolnaftate. *If your dose is different, do not change it* unless your doctor tells you to do so.

- For *topical* dosage forms (aerosol powder, aerosol solution, cream, gel, powder, or topical solution):
  —For fungus infections:
    - Adults and children 2 years of age and over—Apply to the affected area(s) of the skin two times a day.
    - Children up to 2 years of age—Use is not recommended except under the advice and supervision of your doctor.

**Missed dose**—If you miss a dose of this medicine, apply it as soon as possible. Then go back to your regular dosing schedule.

**Storage**—To store this medicine:

- Keep out of the reach of children.
- Store away from heat and direct light.
- Do not store the powder form of this medicine in the bathroom, near the kitchen sink, or in other damp places. Heat or moisture may cause the medicine to break down.
- Keep the medicine from freezing.

- Do not puncture, break, or burn the aerosol powder or aerosol solution container.
- Do not keep outdated medicine or medicine no longer needed. Be sure that any discarded medicine is out of the reach of children.

## Precautions While Using This Medicine

If your skin problem does not improve within 4 weeks, or if it becomes worse, check with your health care professional.

To help prevent reinfection after the period of treatment with this medicine, the powder or spray powder form of this medicine may be used each day after bathing and carefully drying the affected area.

## Side Effects of This Medicine

Along with its needed effects, a medicine may cause some unwanted effects. Although not all of these side effects may occur, if they do occur they may need medical attention.

Check with your health care professional as soon as possible if the following side effect occurs:

Skin irritation not present before use of this medicine

When you apply the aerosol solution form of this medicine, a mild temporary stinging may be expected.

Other side effects not listed above may also occur in some patients. If you notice any other effects, check with your health care professional.

Revised: 11/05/91
Interim revision: 08/10/94

# TRAZODONE    Systemic

Some commonly used brand names are:

**In the U.S.—**
Desyrel                    Trialodine
Trazon
Generic name product may also be available.

**In Canada—**
Desyrel

## Description

Trazodone (TRAZ-oh-done) belongs to the group of medicines known as antidepressants or "mood elevators." It is used to relieve mental depression and depression that sometimes occurs with anxiety.

Trazodone is available only with your doctor's prescription, in the following dosage form:

*Oral*
- Tablets (U.S. and Canada)

## Before Using This Medicine

In deciding to use a medicine, the risks of taking the medicine must be weighed against the good it will do. This is a decision you and your doctor will make. For trazodone, the following should be considered:

**Allergies**—Tell your doctor if you have ever had any unusual or allergic reaction to trazodone. Also tell your health care professional if you are allergic to any other substances, such as foods, preservatives, or dyes.

**Pregnancy**—Studies have not been done in pregnant women. However, studies in animals have shown that trazodone causes birth defects and a decrease in the number of successful pregnancies when given in doses many times larger than human doses.

**Breast-feeding**—Trazodone passes into breast milk.

**Children**—Studies on this medicine have been done only in adult patients, and there is no specific information comparing use of trazodone in children with use in other age groups.

**Older adults**—Drowsiness, dizziness, confusion, vision problems, dryness of mouth, and constipation may be more likely to occur in the elderly, who are usually more sensitive to the effects of trazodone.

**Other medicines**—Although certain medicines should not be used together at all, in other cases two different medicines may be used together even if an interaction might occur. In these cases, your doctor may want to change the dose, or other precautions may be necessary. When you are taking trazodone, it is especially important that your health care professional know if you are taking any of the following:

- Antihypertensives (high blood pressure medicine)—Taking these medicines with trazodone may result in low blood pressure (hypotension); the amount of medicine you need to take may change
- Central nervous system (CNS) depressants (medicine that causes drowsiness) or
- Tricyclic antidepressants (medicine for depression)—Taking these medicines with trazodone may add to the CNS depressant effects

**Other medical problems**—The presence of other medical problems may affect the use of trazodone. Make sure you tell your doctor if you have any other medical problems, especially:

- Alcohol abuse (or history of)—Drinking alcohol with trazodone will increase the central nervous system (CNS) depressant effects
- Heart disease—Trazodone may make the condition worse
- Kidney disease or
- Liver disease—Higher blood levels of trazodone may occur, increasing the chance of side effects

## Proper Use of This Medicine

To lessen stomach upset and to reduce dizziness and lightheadedness, take this medicine with or shortly after a meal or light snack, even for a daily bedtime dose, unless your doctor has told you to take it on an empty stomach.

*Take trazodone only as directed by your doctor,* to benefit your condition as much as possible.

*Sometimes trazodone must be taken for up to 4 weeks before you begin to feel better,* although most people notice improvement within 2 weeks.

**Dosing**—The dose of trazodone will be different for different patients. *Follow your doctor's orders or the directions on the label.* The following information includes only the average doses of trazodone. *If your dose is different, do not change it* unless your doctor tells you to do so:

- Adults—Oral, to start, 50 milligrams per dose taken three times a day, or 75 milligrams per dose taken two times a day. Your doctor may increase your dose if needed.

- Children 6 to 18 years of age—Oral. Your doctor will tell you what dose to take based on your body weight.
- Children up to 6 years of age—Dose must be determined by the doctor.
- Elderly patients—Oral, to start, 25 milligrams per dose taken three times a day. Your doctor may increase your dose if needed.

**Missed dose**—If you miss a dose of this medicine, take it as soon as possible. However, if it is within 4 hours of your next dose, skip the missed dose and go back to your regular dosing schedule. Do not double doses.

**Storage**—To store this medicine:

- Keep out of the reach of children.
- Store away from heat and direct light.
- Do not store in the bathroom, near the kitchen sink, or in other damp places. Heat or moisture may cause the medicine to break down.
- Do not keep outdated medicine or medicine no longer needed. Be sure that any discarded medicine is out of the reach of children.

## Precautions While Using This Medicine

It is very important that your doctor check your progress at regular visits. This will allow your doctor to check the medicine's effects and to change the dose if needed.

*Do not stop taking this medicine without first checking with your doctor.* To prevent a possible return of your medical problem, your doctor may want you to reduce gradually the amount of medicine you are using before you stop completely.

*Before having any kind of surgery, dental treatment, or emergency treatment, tell the medical doctor or dentist in charge that you are using this medicine.* Taking trazodone together with medicines that are used during surgery or dental or emergency treatments may increase the CNS depressant effects.

This medicine will add to the effects of alcohol and other CNS depressants (medicines that slow down the nervous system, possibly causing drowsiness). Some examples of CNS depressants are antihistamines or medicine for hay fever, other allergies, or colds; sedatives, tranquilizers, or sleeping medicine; prescription pain medicine or narcotics; barbiturates; medicine for seizures; muscle relaxants; or anesthetics, including some dental anesthetics. *Check with your doctor before taking any of the above while you are using this medicine.*

This medicine may cause some people to become drowsy or less alert than they are normally. *Make sure you know how you react to this medicine before you drive, use machines, or do anything else that could be dangerous if you are not alert.*

*Dizziness, lightheadedness, or fainting may occur,* especially when you get up from a lying or sitting position. Getting up slowly may help. If this problem continues or gets worse, check with your doctor.

Trazodone may cause dryness of the mouth. For temporary relief, use sugarless gum or candy, melt bits of ice in your mouth, or use a saliva substitute. However, if your mouth continues to feel dry for more than 2 weeks, check with your medical doctor or dentist. Continuing dryness of the mouth may increase the chance of dental disease, including tooth decay, gum disease, and fungus infections.

## Side Effects of This Medicine

Along with its needed effects, a medicine may cause some unwanted effects. Although not all of these side effects may occur, if they do occur they may need medical attention.

*Stop taking this medicine and check with your doctor immediately* if the following side effect occurs:

*Rare*

Painful, inappropriate erection of the penis, continuing

Also, check with your doctor as soon as possible if any of the following side effects occur:

*Less common*

Confusion; muscle tremors

*Rare*

Fainting; fast or slow heartbeat; skin rash; unusual excitement

*Symptoms of overdose*

Drowsiness; loss of muscle coordination; nausea and vomiting

Other side effects may occur that usually do not need medical attention. These side effects may go away during treatment as your body adjusts to the medicine. However, check with your doctor if any of the following side effects continue or are bothersome:

*More common*

Dizziness or lightheadedness; drowsiness; dryness of mouth (usually mild); headache; nausea and vomiting; unpleasant taste

*Less common*

Blurred vision; constipation; diarrhea; muscle aches or pains; unusual tiredness or weakness

Other side effects not listed above may also occur in some patients. If you notice any other effects, check with your doctor.

Revised: 01/13/93

# TRETINOIN    Topical

Some commonly used brand names are:

**In the U.S.—**
Retin-A
Retin-A Regimen Kit

**In Canada—**
Retin-A               Stieva-A Forte
Stieva-A              Vitamin A Acid

Another commonly used name is retinoic acid.

## Description

Tretinoin (TRET-i-noyn) is used to treat certain types of acne. It may also be used to treat other skin diseases as determined by your doctor.

Although tretinoin is being used to treat skin that has been damaged by long time exposure to sunlight, there is not enough information to show that this treatment is safe and effective.

Tretinoin is available only with your doctor's prescription, in the following dosage forms:

*Topical*
- Cream (U.S. and Canada)
- Gel (U.S. and Canada)
- Topical solution (U.S. and Canada)

## Before Using This Medicine

In deciding to use a medicine, the risks of taking the medicine must be weighed against the good it will do. This is a decision you and your doctor will make. For tretinoin, the following should be considered:

**Allergies**—Tell your doctor if you have ever had any unusual or allergic reaction to etretinate, isotretinoin, tretinoin, or vitamin A preparations. Also tell your health care professional if you are allergic to any other substances, such as preservatives or dyes.

**Pregnancy**—Tretinoin has not been studied in pregnant women. Topical tretinoin has been shown to cause some delayed bone development in some animal fetuses. Before using this medicine, make sure your doctor knows if you are pregnant or if you may become pregnant.

**Breast-feeding**—It is not known whether tretinoin passes into the breast milk. However, this medicine has not been reported to cause problems in nursing babies.

**Children**—Studies on this medicine have been done only in adult patients, and there is no specific information comparing use of this medicine in children with use in other age groups.

**Older adults**—Many medicines have not been studied specifically in older people. Therefore, it may not be known whether they work exactly the same way they do in younger adults or if they cause different side effects or problems in older people. There is no specific information

comparing use of tretinoin in the elderly with use in other age groups.

**Other medicines**—Although certain medicines should not be used together at all, in other cases two different medicines may be used together even if an interaction might occur. In these cases, your doctor may want to change the dose, or other precautions may be necessary. Tell your health care professional if you are using any other topical prescription or nonprescription (over-the-counter [OTC]) medicine that is to be applied to the same area of the skin.

**Other medical problems**—The presence of other medical problems may affect the use of tretinoin. Make sure you tell your doctor if you have any other medical problems, especially:

- Eczema or
- Sunburn—Use of this medicine may cause or increase the irritation associated with these problems

## Proper Use of This Medicine

*It is very important that you use this medicine only as directed.* Do not use more of it, do not use it more often, and do not use it for a longer time than your doctor ordered. To do so may cause irritation of the skin.

*Do not apply this medicine to windburned or sunburned skin or on open wounds.*

*Do not use this medicine in or around the eyes or mouth, or inside of the nose.* Spread the medicine away from these areas when applying.

This medicine usually comes with patient directions. Read them carefully before using the medicine.

Before applying tretinoin, wash the skin with a mild or nonallergic type of soap and warm water; then gently pat dry. Wait 20 to 30 minutes before applying this medicine to make sure the skin is completely dry.

To use the *cream or gel form* of this medicine:

- Apply enough medicine to cover the affected areas, and rub in gently.

To use the *solution form* of this medicine:

- Using your fingertips, a gauze pad, or a cotton swab, apply enough tretinoin solution to cover the affected areas. If you use a gauze pad or a cotton swab for applying the medicine, avoid getting it too wet, to prevent the medicine from running into areas not intended for treatment.

**Dosing**—The dose of topical tretinoin will be different for different patients. *Follow your doctor's orders or the directions on the label.* The following information includes only the average dose of topical tretinoin. *If your dose is different, do not change it* unless your doctor tells you to do so.

- For *topical* dosage forms (cream, gel, or solution):
  —For acne:
  - Adults, teenagers, and children—Apply to the affected area(s) of the skin once a day, at bedtime.

**Missed dose**—If you miss a dose of this medicine, skip the missed dose and go back to your regular dosing schedule. Do not double doses.

**Storage**—To store this medicine:

- Keep out of the reach of children.
- Store away from heat and direct light.
- Keep the medicine from freezing.
- Do not keep outdated medicine or medicine no longer needed. Be sure that any discarded medicine is out of the reach of children.

## Precautions While Using This Medicine

During the first 2 or 3 weeks you are using tretinoin, your acne may seem to get worse before it gets better. However, you should not stop using tretinoin unless irritation or other symptoms become severe. If you have any questions about this, check with your doctor.

You should avoid washing your face too often. Washing it with a mild bland soap 2 or 3 times a day should be enough, unless you are otherwise directed by your doctor.

*When using tretinoin, do not use any of the following preparations on the same affected area as this medicine,* unless otherwise directed by your doctor:

Abrasive soaps or cleansers
Alcohol-containing preparations
Any other topical acne preparation or preparation containing a peeling agent (for example, benzoyl peroxide, resorcinol, salicylic acid, or sulfur)
Cosmetics or soaps that dry the skin
Medicated cosmetics
Other topical medicine for the skin

To use any of the above preparations on the same affected area as tretinoin may cause severe irritation of the skin.

You may use cosmetics (nonmedicated) while being treated with tretinoin, unless otherwise directed by your doctor. However, the areas to be treated must be washed thoroughly before the medicine is applied.

During treatment with this medicine, *avoid exposing the treated areas to too much sunlight or overuse of a sunlamp,* since the skin may be more prone to sunburn.

If exposure to too much sunlight cannot be avoided while you are using this medicine, use sunscreen preparations or wear protective clothing over the treated areas.

Some people who use this medicine may become more sensitive to wind and cold temperatures than they are normally. *When you first begin using this medicine, use protection against wind or cold until you see how you react.* If you notice severe skin irritation, check with your doctor.

## Side Effects of This Medicine

In some animal studies, tretinoin has been shown to cause skin tumors to develop faster when the treated area is exposed to ultraviolet light (sunlight or artificial sunlight of a sunlamp). It is not known if tretinoin causes skin tumors to develop faster in humans.

Along with its needed effects, a medicine may cause some unwanted effects. Although not all of these side effects may occur, if they do occur they may need medical attention.

Check with your doctor as soon as possible if any of the following side effects occur:

Blistering, crusting, severe burning or redness, or swelling of skin; darkening or lightening of the treated skin

Other side effects may occur that usually do not need medical attention. These side effects may go away during treatment as your body adjusts to the medicine. However, check with your doctor if any of the following side effects continue or are bothersome:

Feeling of warmth on skin; peeling of skin (may occur after a few days); stinging (mild) or redness of skin

The side effects of tretinoin will go away after you stop using the medicine. However, the side effect of darkening or lightening of the skin may take several months before it goes away.

Other side effects not listed above may also occur in some patients. If you notice any other effects, check with your doctor.

Revised: 01/15/92
Interim revision: 07/06/94

---

# TRIENTINE   Systemic†

A commonly used brand name in the U.S. is Syprine.

Another commonly used name is trien.

†Not commercially available in Canada.

## Description

Trientine (TRYE-en-teen) is used to treat Wilson's disease, a disease in which there is too much copper in the body.

This medicine combines with excess copper in the body and may prevent your body from absorbing the copper in the foods you eat. Removing copper from the body prevents damage to the liver, brain, and other organs. The combination of copper and trientine is then easily removed by the kidneys and it passes from the body in urine.

Trientine is available only with your doctor's prescription, in the following dosage form:

*Oral*
• Capsules (U.S.)

## Before Using This Medicine

In deciding to use a medicine, the risks of taking the medicine must be weighed against the good it will do. This is a decision you and your doctor will make. For trientine, the following should be considered:

**Pregnancy**—Trientine has not been shown to cause birth defects or other problems in humans. However, it has been shown to cause birth defects in rats.

**Breast-feeding**—It is not known whether trientine passes into the breast milk. This medicine has not been reported to cause problems in nursing babies.

**Children**—Anemia is especially likely to occur in children during treatment with trientine.

**Older adults**—Many medicines have not been studied specifically in older people. Therefore, it may not be known whether they work exactly the same way they do in younger adults or if they cause different side effects or problems in older people. There is no specific information comparing use of trientine in the elderly with use in other age groups.

**Other medicines**—Although certain medicines should not be used together at all, in other cases two different medicines may be used together even if an interaction might occur. In these cases, your doctor may want to change the dose, or other precautions may be necessary. When you are taking trientine, it is especially important that your health care professional know if you are taking:

• Copper supplements or
• Iron supplements or other medicine containing minerals (contained in some vitamin combination products)—Use of these medicines with trientine may decrease the effects of trientine; iron supplements or other medicines containing minerals should be given 2 hours before or after trientine

**Other medical problems**—The presence of other medical problems may affect the use of trientine. Make sure you tell your doctor if you have any other medical problems, especially:

• Iron-deficiency—Trientine may make this condition worse

## Proper Use of This Medicine

Take trientine with water. The capsule should be swallowed whole. It must not be opened, crushed, or chewed.

*Take this medicine on an empty stomach (at least 1 hour before or 2 hours after meals) and at least 1 hour before or after any other medicine, food, or milk.* This will allow trientine to be better absorbed by your body.

Trientine will not cure Wilson's disease, but it will help remove the excess copper from your body. Therefore, *you must continue to take this medicine regularly, as directed. You may have to take trientine for the rest of your life.* If Wilson's disease is not treated continually, it can cause severe liver damage and can cause death. *Do not stop taking this medicine without first checking with your doctor.*

*It is very important for you to follow any special instructions from your doctor, such as following a low-copper diet.* You may need to avoid foods known to be high in copper, such as chocolate, mushrooms, liver, molasses, broccoli, cereals enriched with copper, shellfish, organ meats, and nuts. If you have any questions about this, check with your doctor.

*Take this medicine only as directed by your doctor.* Do not take more or less of it and do not take it more often than your doctor ordered. If too much is used, it may increase the chance of side effects.

**Dosing**—The dose of trientine will be different for different patients. *Follow your doctor's orders or the directions on the label.*
- For *oral* dosage form (capsules):
  —For Wilson's disease:
  - Adults and teenagers—The usual dose is 750 milligrams (mg) to 1.25 grams a day. The dose may be divided into two to four smaller doses.
  - Children—The usual dose is 500 to 750 mg a day. The dose may be divided into two to four smaller doses.

**Missed dose**—If you miss a dose of this medicine, double the next dose. Do not make up more than one missed dose at a time.

**Storage**—To store this medicine:
- Keep out of the reach of children.
- Store sealed, unopened bottles of trientine in the refrigerator, but not in the freezer. Before opening a sealed bottle, let it stand at room temperature for about 6 hours. Keep it at room temperature after opening it.
- Do not store in the bathroom, near the kitchen sink, or in other damp places. Heat or moisture may cause the medicine to break down.
- Do not keep outdated medicine or medicine no longer needed. Be sure that any discarded medicine is out of the reach of children.

## Precautions While Using This Medicine

*Your doctor should check your progress at regular visits* to make sure trientine is working properly and to check for unwanted effects. Laboratory tests may be needed. This will allow your doctor to change your dose, if necessary.

During the first month of treatment, you may need to take your temperature each night. *Tell your doctor if you develop a fever or skin rash.*

*Do not take copper or iron preparations or any other mineral supplements within 2 hours of taking trientine.* This includes any vitamin preparation that contains minerals.

If a capsule breaks open and the contents touch your skin, wash the area right away with water. Trientine may cause a rash.

## Side Effects of This Medicine

Along with its needed effects, a medicine may cause some unwanted effects. Although not all of these side effects may occur, if they do occur they may need medical attention.

Check with your doctor as soon as possible if any of the following side effects occur:

*More common—Symptoms of anemia*
  Unusually pale skin; unusual tiredness
  Note: The above signs of anemia are more likely to occur in children, menstruating women, and pregnant women, who usually need more iron than other patients. If these signs appear during trientine treatment, your doctor will need to do some tests.

*Rare*
  Fever; general feeling of discomfort, illness, or weakness; joint pain; skin rash, blisters, hives, or itching; swollen glands

Other side effects not listed above may also occur in some patients. If you notice any other effects, check with your doctor.

Revised: 09/17/92
Interim revision(s): 04/29/94

# TRIFLURIDINE    Ophthalmic

A commonly used brand name in the U.S. and Canada is Viroptic. Another commonly used name is trifluorothymidine.

## Description

Trifluridine (trye-FLURE-i-deen) ophthalmic preparations are used to treat virus infections of the eye.

Trifluridine is available only with your doctor's prescription, in the following dosage form:

*Ophthalmic*
- Ophthalmic solution (eye drops) (U.S. and Canada)

## Before Using This Medicine

In deciding to use a medicine, the risks of using the medicine must be weighed against the good it will do. This is a decision you and your doctor will make. For trifluridine, the following should be considered:

**Allergies**—Tell your doctor if you have ever had any unusual or allergic reaction to trifluridine. Also tell your health care professional if you are allergic to any other substances, such as preservatives.

**Pregnancy**—Studies have not been done in humans. When injected into developing chick embryos, trifluridine has been shown to cause birth defects. However, studies in rats and rabbits have not shown that trifluridine causes birth defects, although it did cause delayed bone formation in rats and rabbits and death in unborn rabbits.

**Breast-feeding**—It is unlikely that trifluridine, used in the eyes, is absorbed into the mother's body and passes into the breast milk. In addition, trifluridine has not been reported to cause problems in nursing babies.

**Children**—Although there is no specific information comparing the use of trifluridine in children with use in other age groups, it is not expected to cause different side effects or problems in children than it does in adults.

**Older adults**—Many medicines have not been studied specifically in older people. Therefore, it may not be known whether they work exactly the same way they do in younger adults or if they cause different side effects or problems in older people. There is no specific information comparing the use of trifluridine in the elderly with use in other age groups.

**Other medicines**—Although certain medicines should not be used together at all, in other cases two different medicines may be used together even if an interaction might occur. In these cases, your doctor may want to change the dose, or other precautions may be necessary. Tell your health care professional if you are using any other prescription or nonprescription (over-the-counter [OTC]) medicine that is to be used in the eye.

## Proper Use of This Medicine

The bottle is only partially full to provide proper drop control.

To use:
- First, wash your hands. Then tilt the head back and pull the lower eyelid away from the eye to form a pouch. Drop the medicine into the pouch and gently close the eyes. Do not blink. Keep the eyes closed for 1 or 2 minutes to allow the medicine to come into contact with the infection.

- If you think you did not get the drop of medicine into your eye properly, use another drop.
- To keep the medicine as germ-free as possible, do not touch the applicator tip to any surface (including the eye). Also, keep the container tightly closed.

*Do not use this medicine more often or for a longer time than your doctor ordered*. To do so may cause problems in the eyes. If you have any questions about this, check with your doctor.

To help clear up your infection completely, *keep using this medicine for the full time of treatment*, even if your symptoms have disappeared. *Do not miss any doses*.

**Dosing**—The dose of ophthalmic trifluridine will be different for different patients. *Follow your doctor's orders or the directions on the label.* The following information includes only the average doses of ophthalmic trifluridine. *If your dose is different, do not change it unless your doctor tells you to do so.*

*The number of doses you use each day, the time allowed between doses, and the length of time you use the medicine depend on the medical problem for which you are using ophthalmic trifluridine.*

- For *ophthalmic solution* dosage forms:
  - For virus eye infection:
    - Adults and children—One drop every two hours while you are awake. After healing has occurred, the dose may be reduced for seven more days to one drop every four hours (at least 5 doses a day) while you are awake.

**Missed dose**—If you miss a dose of this medicine, apply it as soon as possible. However, if it is almost time for your next dose, skip the missed dose and go back to your regular dosing schedule.

**Storage**—To store this medicine:
- Keep out of the reach of children.
- Store in the refrigerator because heat will cause this medicine to break down. However, keep the medicine from freezing. Follow the directions on the label.
- Do not keep outdated medicine or medicine no longer needed. Be sure that any discarded medicine is out of the reach of children.

## Precautions While Using This Medicine

It is very important that you keep your appointment with your doctor. If your symptoms become worse, check with your doctor sooner.

## Side Effects of This Medicine

Along with its needed effects, a medicine may cause some unwanted effects. Although not all of these side effects may occur, if they do occur they may need medical attention.

Check with your doctor as soon as possible if any of the following side effects occur:

*Rare*

Blurred vision or other change in vision; dryness of eye; irritation of eye; itching, redness, swelling, or other sign of irritation not present before use of this medicine

Other side effects may occur that usually do not need medical attention. These side effects may go away during treatment as your body adjusts to the medicine. However,

check with your doctor if either of the following side effects continues or is bothersome:

*More common*

Burning or stinging

Other side effects not listed above may also occur in some patients. If you notice any other effects, check with your doctor.

Revised: 07/01/93

---

# TRILOSTANE Systemic†

A commonly used brand name in the U.S. is Modrastane.

†Not commercially available in Canada.

## Description

Trilostane (TRYE-loe-stane) is used in the treatment of Cushing's syndrome. It is normally used in short-term treatment until permanent therapy is possible.

In Cushing's syndrome, the adrenal gland overproduces steroids. Although steroids are important for various functions of the body, too much can cause problems. Trilostane reduces the amount of steroids produced by the adrenal gland.

Trilostane is available only with your doctor's prescription, in the following dosage form:

*Oral*

• Capsules (U.S.)

## Before Using This Medicine

In deciding to use a medicine, the risks of taking the medicine must be weighed against the good it will do. This is a decision you and your doctor will make. For trilostane, the following should be considered:

**Allergies**—Tell your doctor if you have ever had any unusual or allergic reaction to trilostane. Also tell your health care professional if you are allergic to any other substance, such as foods, preservatives, or dyes.

**Pregnancy**—Use of trilostane is not recommended during pregnancy. It has been shown to cause serious problems, including miscarriage, in humans. Trilostane has also been shown to cause birth defects in animals.

**Breast-feeding**—It is not known whether trilostane passes into breast milk. However, this medicine has not been reported to cause problems in nursing babies.

**Children**—There is no specific information about the use of trilostane in children.

**Older adults**—Many medicines have not been tested in older people. Therefore, it may not be known whether they work exactly the same way they do in younger adults or if they cause different side effects or problems in older people. There is no specific information about the use of trilostane in the elderly.

**Other medicines**—Although certain medicines should not be used together at all, in other cases two different medicines may be used together even if an interaction might occur. In these cases, your doctor may want to change the dose, or other precautions may be necessary. When you are taking trilostane, it is especially important that your health care professional know if you are taking any other prescription or nonprescription (over-the-counter [OTC]) medicine.

**Other medical problems**—The presence of other medical problems may affect the use of trilostane. Make sure you tell your doctor if you have any other medical problems, especially:

• Infection or
• Injury (recent serious)—Trilostane may weaken the body's normal defenses
• Kidney disease
• Liver disease

## Proper Use of This Medicine

*Take trilostane only as directed by your doctor.* Do not take more or less of it, and do not take it more often than your doctor ordered.

**Dosing**—The dose of trilostane will be different for different patients. *Follow your doctor's orders or the directions on the label.* The following information includes only the average doses of trilostane. *If your dose is different, do not change it* unless your doctor tells you to do so.

• For *oral* dosage form (capsules):
  —For Cushing's syndrome:
    • Adults—To start, 30 milligrams (mg) four times a day. Your doctor may increase the dose

every three to four days as needed. However, the dose is usually not more than 90 mg four times a day.

- Children—Dose must be determined by your doctor.

**Missed dose**—If you miss a dose of this medicine, take it as soon as possible. However, if it is almost time for your next dose, skip the missed dose and go back to your regular dosing schedule. Do not double doses.

**Storage**—To store this medicine:

- Keep out of the reach of children.
- Store away from heat and direct light.
- Do not store in the bathroom, near the kitchen sink, or in other damp places. Heat or moisture may cause the medicine to break down.
- Do not keep outdated medicine or medicine no longer needed. Be sure that any discarded medicine is out of the reach of children.

## Precautions While Using This Medicine

*It is very important that your doctor check your progress at regular visits* to make sure that trilostane is working properly and does not cause unwanted effects.

*Check with your doctor right away if you get an injury, infection, or illness of any kind.* This medicine may weaken your body's normal defenses.

*Before having any kind of surgery (including dental surgery) or emergency treatment, tell the medical doctor or dentist in charge that you are taking trilostane.*

Your doctor may want you to carry a medical identification card or wear a bracelet stating that you are taking this medicine.

## Side Effects of This Medicine

Along with its needed effects, a medicine may cause some unwanted effects. Although not all of these side effects may occur, if they do occur they may need medical attention.

Check with your doctor as soon as possible if any of the following side effects occur:
*Rare*
    Darkening of skin; drowsiness or tiredness; loss of appetite; mental depression; skin rash; vomiting

Other side effects may occur that usually do not need medical attention. These side effects may go away during treatment as your body adjusts to the medicine. However, check with your health care professional if any of the following side effects continue or are bothersome:
*More common*
    Diarrhea; stomach pain or cramps
*Less common*
    Aching muscles; belching or bloating; burning mouth or nose; dizziness or lightheadedness; fever; flushing; headache; increase in salivation; nausea; watery eyes

Other side effects not listed above may also occur in some patients. If you notice any other effects, check with your doctor.

Revised: 09/90
Interim revision: 07/05/94

---

# TRIMETHOBENZAMIDE    Systemic†

Some commonly used brand names are:
**In the U.S.—**

| | |
|---|---|
| Arrestin | T-Gen |
| Benzacot | Ticon |
| Bio-Gan | Tigan |
| Stemetic | Tiject-20 |
| Tebamide | Triban |
| Tegamide | Tribenzagan |

Generic name product may also be available.

†Not commercially available in Canada.

## Description

Trimethobenzamide (trye-meth-oh-BEN-za-mide) is used to treat nausea and vomiting.

This medicine is available only with your doctor's prescription in the following dosage forms:
*Oral*
- Capsules (U.S.)

*Parenteral*
- Injection (U.S.)

*Rectal*
- Suppositories (U.S.)

## Before Using This Medicine

In deciding to use a medicine, the risks of taking the medicine must be weighed against the good it will do. This is a decision you and your doctor will make. For trimethobenzamide, the following should be considered:

**Allergies**—Tell your doctor if you have ever had any unusual or allergic reaction to trimethobenzamide, or if you are allergic or sensitive to benzocaine or other local anesthetics (the suppository form of this medicine contains benzocaine). Also tell your health care professional if you are allergic to any other substances, such as foods, preservatives, or dyes.

© 1994    The United States Pharmacopeial Convention, Inc.

**Pregnancy**—Studies have not been done in pregnant women. However, although studies in animals have not shown that trimethobenzamide causes birth defects, it has been shown to increase the chance of a miscarriage.

**Breast-feeding**—It is not known whether trimethobenzamide passes into breast milk. Although most medicines pass into breast milk in small amounts, many of them may be used safely while breast-feeding. Mothers who are taking this medicine and who wish to breast-feed should discuss this with their doctor.

**Children**—This medicine should not be used to treat nausea and vomiting in children unless otherwise directed by your doctor. Some side effects may be more serious in children.

**Older adults**—Many medicines have not been studied specifically in older people. Therefore, it may not be known whether they work exactly the same way they do in younger adults or if they cause different side effects or problems in older people. There is no specific information comparing use of trimethobenzamide in the elderly with use in other age groups.

**Other medicines**—Although certain medicines should not be used together at all, in other cases 2 different medicines may be used together even if an interaction might occur. In these cases, your doctor may want to change the dose, or other precautions may be necessary. When you are using trimethobenzamide, it is especially important that your health care professional know if you are taking any of the following:

- Central nervous system (CNS) depressants (medicine that causes drowsiness) or
- Tricyclic antidepressants (medicine for depression)—Taking these medicines with trimethobenzamide may cause increased CNS depressant or other serious effects

**Other medical problems**—The presence of other medical problems may affect the use of trimethobenzamide. Make sure you tell your doctor if you have any other medical problems, especially:

- High fever or
- Intestinal infection—Using trimethobenzamide may result in serious side effects

## Proper Use of This Medicine

Do not use this medicine to treat nausea and vomiting in children unless otherwise directed by your doctor. If you are giving this medicine to a child, be especially careful not to give more than is prescribed since side effects may be more serious in children.

Trimethobenzamide is used only to relieve or prevent nausea and vomiting. Use it only as directed. Do not use more of it and do not use it more often than your doctor ordered. To do so may increase the chance of side effects.

To insert the *rectal suppository form* of this medicine:

- First, remove foil wrapper and moisten the suppository with cold water. Lie down on your side and use your finger to push the suppository well up into the rectum. If the suppository is too soft to insert, chill

it in the refrigerator for 30 minutes or run cold water over it before removing the foil wrapper.
- Wash your hands with soap and water.

**Dosing**—The dose of trimethobenzamide will be different for different patients. *Follow your doctor's orders or the directions on the label.* The following information includes only the average doses of trimethobenzamide. *If your dose is different, do not change it* unless your doctor tells you to do so.

The number of capsules that you take, or suppositories that you use, depends on the strength of the medicine. Also, *the number of doses you take each day, the time allowed between doses, and the length of time you take the medicine depend on the medical problem for which you are taking trimethobenzamide.*

- For *oral* dosage form (capsules):
  —For nausea and vomiting:
    - Adults and children 12 years of age and older—250 milligrams (mg) three or four times a day as needed.
    - Children—Dose is based on body weight and must be determined by your doctor. The usual dose is 15 mg per kilogram (6.8 mg per pound). The dose is usually not more than 200 mg three or four times a day as needed.
- For *rectal* dosage form (suppositories):
  —For nausea and vomiting:
    - Adults and children 12 years of age and older—200 mg three or four times a day as needed.
    - Children—Dose is based on body weight and must be determined by your doctor. The usual dose is 15 mg per kilogram (6.8 mg per pound). The dose is usually not more than 200 mg three or four times a day as needed.
- For *injection* dosage form:
  —For nausea and vomiting:
    - Adults and children 12 years of age and older—200 mg three or four times a day as needed, injected into a muscle.
    - Children—Dose must be determined by your doctor.

**Missed dose**—If you must use this medicine regularly and you miss a dose, use it as soon as possible. However, if it is almost time for your next dose, skip the missed dose and go back to your regular dosing schedule. Do not double doses.

**Storage**—To store this medicine:

- Keep out of the reach of children.
- Store away from heat and direct light.
- Do not store the capsule form of this medicine in the bathroom, near the kitchen sink, or in other damp places. Heat or moisture may cause the medicine to break down.
- Do not keep outdated medicine or medicine no longer needed. Be sure that any discarded medicine is out of the reach of children.

## Precautions While Using This Medicine

Trimethobenzamide will add to the effects of alcohol and other CNS depressants (medicines that slow down the nervous system, possibly causing drowsiness). Some examples of CNS depressants are antihistamines or medicine for hay fever, other allergies, or colds; sedatives, tranquilizers, or sleeping medicine; prescription pain medicine or narcotics; barbiturates; medicine for seizures; muscle relaxants; or anesthetics, including some dental anesthetics. *Check with your doctor before taking any of the above while you are using this medicine.*

This medicine may cause some people to become dizzy, lightheaded, drowsy, or less alert than they are normally. *Make sure you know how you react to this medicine before you drive, use machines, or do anything else that could be dangerous if you are dizzy or are not alert.*

When using trimethobenzamide on a regular basis, make sure your doctor knows if you are taking large amounts of aspirin or other salicylates at the same time (as for arthritis or rheumatism). Effects of too much aspirin, such as ringing in the ears, may be covered up by this medicine.

## Side Effects of This Medicine

Along with its needed effects, a medicine may cause some unwanted effects. Although not all of these side effects may occur, if they do occur they may need medical attention.

Check with your doctor as soon as possible if any of the following side effects occur:

*Rare*

Body spasm, with head and heels bent backward and body bowed forward; convulsions (seizures); mental depression; shakiness or tremors; skin rash; sore throat and fever; unusual tiredness; vomiting (severe or continuing); yellow eyes or skin

Other side effects may occur that usually do not need medical attention. These side effects may go away during treatment as your body adjusts to the medicine. However, check with your doctor if any of the following side effects continue or are bothersome:

*More common*

Drowsiness

*Less common*

Blurred vision; diarrhea; dizziness; headache; muscle cramps

Other side effects not listed above may also occur in some patients. If you notice any other effects, check with your doctor.

Revised: 05/12/93

# TRIMETHOPRIM  Systemic

Some commonly used brand names are:

**In the U.S.—**

Proloprim                    Trimpex

Generic name product may also be available.

**In Canada**

Proloprim

## Description

Trimethoprim (trye-METH-oh-prim) is used to treat infections of the urinary tract. It may also be used for other problems as determined by your doctor. It will not work for colds, flu, or other virus infections.

Trimethoprim is available only with your doctor's prescription, in the following dosage form:

*Oral*

• Tablets (U.S. and Canada)

## Before Using This Medicine

In deciding to use a medicine, the risks of taking the medicine must be weighed against the good it will do. This is a decision you and your doctor will make. For trimethoprim, the following should be considered:

**Allergies**—Tell your doctor if you have ever had any unusual or allergic reaction to trimethoprim. Also tell your health care professional if you are allergic to any other substances, such as foods, preservatives, or dyes.

**Pregnancy**—Studies have not been done in humans. Studies in rats have shown that trimethoprim causes birth defects. Studies in rabbits have shown that trimethoprim causes a decrease in the number of successful pregnancies. However, in the few reports where trimethoprim was taken by pregnant women, trimethoprim has not been reported to cause birth defects or other problems in humans.

**Breast-feeding**—Trimethoprim passes into the breast milk. However, this medicine has not been reported to cause serious problems in nursing babies.

**Children**—This medicine has been used in a limited number of children 2 months of age or older, and tested in children 12 years of age or older. In effective doses, the medicine has not been shown to cause different side effects or problems in children than it does in adults.

**Older adults**—Elderly people may be more sensitive to the effects of trimethoprim. Blood problems may be more likely to occur in elderly patients who are taking diuretics (water pills) along with this medicine.

**Other medicines**—Although certain medicines should not be used together at all, in other cases two different medicines may be used together even if an interaction might occur. In these cases, your doctor may want to change the dose, or other precautions may be necessary. When you are taking trimethoprim, it is especially important that your health care professional know if you are taking any of the following:

- Anticonvulsants (seizure medicine) or
- Methotrexate (e.g., Mexate) or
- Pyrimethamine (e.g., Daraprim) or
- Triamterene (e.g., Dyrenium)—Use of these medicines with trimethoprim may increase the chance of side effects effecting the blood

**Other medical problems**—The presence of other medical problems may affect the use of trimethoprim. Make sure you tell your doctor if you have any other medical problems, especially:

- Anemia—Patients with anemia may have an increased chance of side effects affecting the blood
- Kidney disease—Patients with kidney disease may have an increased chance of side effects

## Proper Use of This Medicine

*Do not give this medicine to infants or children under 12 years of age* unless otherwise directed by your doctor.

Trimethoprim may be taken on an empty stomach or, if it upsets your stomach, it may be taken with food.

To help clear up your infection completely, *keep taking this medicine for the full time of treatment* even if you begin to feel better after a few days. If you stop taking this medicine too soon, your symptoms may return.

This medicine works best when there is a constant amount in the body. *To help keep the amount constant, do not miss any doses. Also, it is best to take the doses at evenly spaced times day and night.* For example, if you are to take 2 doses a day, the doses should be spaced about 12 hours apart. If this interferes with your sleep or other daily activities, or if you need help in planning the best times to take your medicine, check with your health care professional.

**Dosing**—The dose of trimethoprim will be different for different patients. *Follow your doctor's orders or the directions on the label.* The following information includes only the average doses of trimethoprim. Your dose may be different if you have kidney disease. *If your dose is different, do not change it* unless your doctor tells you to do so.

The number of tablets that you take depends on the strength of the medicine. Also, *the number of doses you take each day, the time allowed between doses, and the length of time you take the medicine depend on the medical problem for which you are taking trimethoprim.*

- For the *treatment of urinary tract infections:*
  —Adults and children 12 years of age and older: 100 milligrams every twelve hours for ten days, or 200 milligrams once a day for ten days.
  —Children up to 12 years of age: Dose must be determined by the doctor.

**Missed dose**—If you do miss a dose of this medicine, take it as soon as possible. This will help to keep a constant amount of medicine in the body. However, if it is almost time for your next dose, skip the missed dose and go back to your regular dosing schedule. Do not double doses.

**Storage**—To store this medicine:

- Keep out of the reach of children.
- Store away from heat and direct light.
- Do not store in the bathroom, near the kitchen sink, or in other damp places. Heat or moisture may cause the medicine to break down.
- Do not keep outdated medicine or medicine no longer needed. Be sure that any discarded medicine is out of the reach of children.

## Precautions While Using This Medicine

It is important that your doctor check your progress at regular visits if you will be taking this medicine for a long time. This will allow your doctor to check for any unwanted effects that may be caused by this medicine.

If your symptoms do not improve within a few days, or if they become worse, check with your doctor.

If this medicine causes anemia, your doctor may want you to take folic acid (a vitamin) every day to help clear up the anemia. If so, it is important to take folic acid every day along with this medicine; do not miss any doses.

Trimethoprim may cause blood problems. These problems may result in a greater chance of certain infections, slow healing, and bleeding of the gums. Therefore, you should be careful when using regular toothbrushes, dental floss, and toothpicks. Dental work should be delayed until your blood counts have returned to normal. Check with your medical doctor or dentist if you have any questions about proper oral hygiene (mouth care) during treatment.

## Side Effects of This Medicine

Along with its needed effects, a medicine may cause some unwanted effects. Although not all of these side effects may occur, if they do occur they may need medical attention.

*Check with your doctor immediately* if any of the following side effects occur:

*Rare*

Bluish fingernails, lips, or skin; difficult breathing; headache; general feeling of discomfort or illness; nausea; neck stiffness; pale skin; skin rash or itching; sore throat and fever; unusual bleeding or bruising; unusual tiredness or weakness; signs of Stevens-Johnson syndrome, such as aching joints and muscles; redness, blistering, peeling, or loosening of skin; unusual tiredness or weakness

Other side effects may occur that usually do not need medical attention. These side effects may go away during treatment as your body adjusts to the medicine. However, check with your doctor if any of the following side effects continue or are bothersome:

*Less common*
 Diarrhea; headache; loss of appetite; nausea or vomiting; stomach cramps or pain

Other side effects not listed above may also occur in some patients. If you notice any other effects, check with your doctor.

---

## Additional Information

Once a medicine has been approved for marketing for a certain use, experience may show that it is also useful for other medical problems. Although these uses are not included in product labeling, trimethoprim is used in certain patients for the following medical conditions:

- Prevention of urinary tract infections
- Treatment of *Pneumocystis carinii* pneumonia (PCP)

For patients taking this medicine for *prevention of urinary tract infections*:

- Your doctor may have prescribed this medicine to *prevent* infections of the urinary tract. It is usually given once a day and may be given for a long time for this purpose. If you have any questions about this, check with your doctor.

Other than the above information, there is no additional information relating to proper use, precautions, or side effects for these uses.

---

Revised: 02/23/93

---

# TRIMETREXATE   Systemic

A commonly used brand name in the U.S. and Canada is NeuTrexin.

## Description

Trimetrexate (tre-me-TREX-ate) is used, together with leucovorin (loo-koe-VOR-in), to treat *Pneumocystis* (noo-moe-SISS-tis) *carinii* pneumonia (PCP), a very serious kind of pneumonia. This kind of pneumonia occurs commonly in patients whose immune system is not working normally, such as cancer patients, transplant patients, and patients with acquired immune deficiency syndrome (AIDS).

Trimetrexate may cause some serious side effects. To prevent these effects, *you must take another medicine, leucovorin, together with trimetrexate*, and for three days after you stop taking trimetrexate. Before you begin treatment with trimetrexate, you and your doctor should talk about the good this medicine will do as well as the risks of using it.

Trimetrexate is to be administered only by or under the immediate supervision of your doctor. It is available in the following dosage form:

*Parenteral*
- Injection (U.S. and Canada)

## Before Using This Medicine

In deciding to use a medicine, the risks of using the medicine must be weighed against the good it will do. This is a decision you and your doctor will make. For trimetrexate, the following should be considered:

**Allergies**—Tell your doctor if you have ever had any unusual or allergic reaction to trimetrexate. Also tell your health care professional if you are allergic to any other substances, such as foods, preservatives, or dyes.

**Pregnancy**—Use of trimetrexate during pregnancy should be avoided whenever possible since trimetrexate has caused birth defects and death of the fetus in animal studies. The use of birth control is recommended during trimetrexate therapy. Be sure to tell your doctor if you are pregnant or if you need advice about birth control.

**Breast-feeding**—It is not known if trimetrexate passes into breast milk. However, breast-feeding should be stopped during treatment with this medicine because trimetrexate may cause serious unwanted effects in nursing babies.

**Children**—This medicine has been tested in a limited number of children younger than 18 years of age. Trimetrexate can cause serious side effects in any patient. However, in effective doses, the medicine has not been shown to cause different side effects or problems in children than it does in adults.

**Older adults**—Many medicines have not been studied specifically in older people. Therefore, it may not be known whether they work exactly the same way they do in younger adults or if they cause different side effects or problems in older people. There is no specific information comparing use of trimetrexate in the elderly with use in other age groups.

**Other medicines**—Although certain medicines should not be used together at all, in other cases 2 different medicines may be used together even if an interaction might occur. In these cases, your doctor may want to change the dose, or other precautions may be necessary. When you are taking trimetrexate, it is especially important that your health care professional knows if you are taking any of the following:

- Alcohol or
- Cimetidine (e.g., Tagamet) or
- Diltiazem (e.g., Cardizem) or
- Disulfiram (e.g., Antabuse) or
- Divalproex (e.g., Depakote) or
- Erythromycins (medicine for infection) or
- Isoniazid (e.g., INH, Nydrazid) or
- Oral contraceptives (birth control pills) containing estrogen or
- Quinine (e.g., Quinamm) or
- Ranitidine (e.g., Zantac) or
- Valproic acid (e.g., Depakene) or
- Verapamil (e.g., Calan)—Use of these medicines with trimetrexate may increase the chance of trimetrexate side effects
- Amphotericin B by injection (e.g., Fungizone) or
- Antineoplastics (cancer medicine) or
- Antithyroid agents (medicine for overactive thyroid) or
- Azathioprine (e.g., Imuran) or
- Colchicine or
- Cyclophosphamide (e.g., Cytoxan) or
- Flucytosine (e.g., Ancobon) or
- Ganciclovir (e.g., Cytovene) or
- Interferon (e.g., Intron A, Roferon-A) or
- Mercaptopurine (e.g., Purinethol) or
- Methotrexate (e.g., Mexate) or
- Plicamycin (e.g., Mithracin) or
- Zidovudine (e.g., AZT, Retrovir)—Receiving trimetrexate while you are using these medicines may make side effects affecting the blood worse
- Chloramphenicol (e.g., Chloromycetin)—Use of chloramphenicol with trimetrexate may increase the chance of side effects from trimetrexate

**Other medical problems**—The presence of other medical problems may affect the use of trimetrexate. Make sure you tell your doctor if you have any other medical problems, especially:

- Anemia or
- Low platelet count or
- Low white blood cell count—Trimetrexate may make any blood diseases that you have worse

## Proper Use of This Medicine

When you take leucovorin:

- *Leucovorin must be taken with trimetrexate* to help prevent very serious unwanted effects. Leucovorin should be taken during trimetrexate treatment and for 3 days after trimetrexate is stopped.
- *Take oral leucovorin exactly as directed by your doctor.* Do not take more of it, do not take it more often, and do not take it for a longer time than your doctor ordered. Also, do not stop taking this medicine without checking with your doctor first.
- Oral leucovorin works best when there is a constant amount in the blood. *To help keep the amount constant, do not miss any doses.* If you need help in planning the best times to take your medicine, check with your health care professional.

**Dosing**—The doses of trimetrexate and of leucovorin will be different for different patients. *Follow your doctor's orders or the directions on the label.* The following information includes only the average doses of trimetrexate and leucovorin. *If your doses are different, do not change them* unless your doctor tells you to do so:

*For trimetrexate*
- For the treatment of *Pneumocystis carinii* pneumonia:
  —For *injection* dosage form:
    • Adults—45 milligrams (mg) per square meter of body surface area (mg/m$^2$) injected into a vein once a day for twenty-one days. Your doctor will check your blood counts and may change your dose based on these counts.
    • Children and teenagers—Use and dose must be determined by your doctor.

*For leucovorin*
- For the treatment of *Pneumocystis carinii* pneumonia:
  —For the *oral or injection* dosage forms:
    • Adults—20 mg per square meter of body surface area (mg/m$^2$) taken by mouth or injected into a vein every six hours for twenty-four days. Your doctor will check your blood counts and may change your dose based on these counts.
    • Children and teenagers—Use and dose must be determined by your doctor.

**Missed dose**—If you miss a dose of leucovorin, take it as soon as possible. This will help to keep a constant amount of medicine in the blood. However, if it is almost time for your next dose, skip the missed dose and go back to your regular dosing schedule. Do not double doses.

**Storage**—To store leucovorin:
- Keep out of the reach of children.
- Store away from heat and direct light.
- Do not store in the bathroom, near the kitchen sink, or in other damp places. Heat or moisture may cause the medicine to break down.
- Do not keep outdated medicine or medicine no longer needed. Be sure that any discarded medicine is out of the reach of children.

## Precautions While Using This Medicine

If your symptoms do not improve within a few days, or if they become worse, check with your doctor.

*It is very important that your doctor check your progress at regular visits* to make sure that this medicine is working properly and to check for unwanted effects.

Trimetrexate can lower the number of white blood cells in your blood temporarily, increasing your chance of getting an infection. It can also lower the number of platelets, which are necessary for proper blood clotting. If this occurs, there are certain precautions you can take, especially when your blood count is low, to reduce the risk of infection or bleeding:

- If you can, avoid people with infections. *Check with your doctor immediately* if you think you are getting an infection or if you get a fever or chills, cough or hoarseness, lower back or side pain, or painful or difficult urination.
- *Check with your doctor immediately* if you notice any unusual bleeding or bruising; black, tarry stools; blood in urine or stools; or pinpoint red spots on your skin.
- Be careful when using a regular toothbrush, dental floss, or toothpick. Your medical doctor, dentist, or nurse may recommend other ways to clean your teeth and gums. Check with your medical doctor before having any dental work done.
- Be careful not to cut yourself when you are using sharp objects such as a safety razor or fingernail or toenail cutters.

## Side Effects of This Medicine

Along with its needed effects, a medicine may cause some unwanted effects. Although not all of these side effects may occur, if they do occur they may need medical attention.

*Check with your doctor immediately* if any of the following side effects occur:

*More common*
Fever and sore throat

*Less common*
Unusual bleeding or bruising

*Rare*
Fever; mouth sores or ulcers; skin rash and itching; unusual tiredness or weakness

Other side effects may occur that usually do not need medical attention. These side effects may go away during treatment as your body adjusts to the medicine. However, check with your doctor if any of the following side effects continue or are bothersome:

*Less common*
Confusion; nausea and vomiting; stomach pain

Other side effects not listed above may also occur in some patients. If you notice any other effects, check with your doctor.

Developed: 04/15/94

---

# TRIOXSALEN    Systemic

A commonly used brand name in the U.S. and Canada is Trisoralen. Another commonly used name is trioxysalen.

## Description

Trioxsalen (trye-OX-sa-len) belongs to the group of medicines called psoralens. It is used along with ultraviolet light (found in sunlight and some special lamps) in a treatment called psoralen plus ultraviolet light A (PUVA) to treat vitiligo, a disease in which skin color is lost. Trioxsalen may also be used for other conditions as determined by your doctor.

Trioxsalen is available only with your doctor's prescription, in the following dosage form:

*Oral*
- Tablets (U.S. and Canada)

## Before Using This Medicine

Trioxsalen is a very strong medicine that increases the skin's sensitivity to sunlight. In addition to causing serious sunburns if not properly used, it has been reported to increase the chance of skin cancer and cataracts. Also, like too much sunlight, PUVA can cause premature aging of the skin. Therefore, trioxsalen should be used only as directed and it should *not* be used simply for suntanning.

Before using this medicine, be sure that you have discussed its use with your doctor.

In deciding to use a medicine, the risks of taking the medicine must be weighed against the good it will do. This is a decision you and your doctor will make. For trioxsalen, the following should be considered:

**Allergies**—Tell your doctor if you have ever had any unusual or allergic reaction to trioxsalen. Also tell your health care professional if you are allergic to any other substances, such as preservatives or dyes.

**Pregnancy**—Studies have not been done in either humans or animals.

**Breast-feeding**—Trioxsalen has not been reported to cause problems in nursing babies.

**Children**—Although there is no specific information comparing use of trioxsalen in children with use in other age groups, this medicine is not expected to cause different side effects or problems in children than it does in adults.

**Older adults**—Many medicines have not been studied specifically in older people. Therefore, it may not be known whether they work exactly the same way they do in younger adults or if they cause different side effects or problems in older people. There is no specific information

comparing use of trioxsalen in the elderly with use in other age groups.

**Other medicines**—Although certain medicines should not be used together at all, in other cases two different medicines may be used together even if an interaction might occur. In these cases, your doctor may want to change the dose, or other precautions may be necessary. Tell your health care professional if you are using any other prescription or nonprescription (over-the-counter [OTC]) medicine.

**Other medical problems**—The presence of other medical problems may affect the use of trioxsalen. Make sure you tell your doctor if you have any other medical problems, especially:

- Allergy to sunlight (family history of) or
- Lupus erythematosus or
- Porphyria or
- Other conditions that make you more sensitive to light— This medicine will make the condition worse
- Eye problems, such as cataracts or loss of the lens of the eyes—Use of this medicine may make your cataracts or other eye problems worse; having no lens in your eye may increase the side effects of this medicine
- Heart or blood vessel disease (severe)—The heat from the light treatment may make the condition worse
- Infection or
- Stomach problems—Use of this medicine may make the condition worse
- Melanoma or other skin cancer (history of) or
- Recent treatment with x-rays or cancer medicines or plans to have x-rays in the near future—May increase your chance of skin cancer

## Proper Use of This Medicine

This medicine may take several weeks or months to help your condition. *Do not increase the amount of trioxsalen you are taking or spend extra time in the sunlight or under an ultraviolet lamp.* This will not make the medicine act any more quickly and may result in a serious burn.

If this medicine upsets your stomach, it may be taken with meals or milk.

**Dosing**—The dose of trioxsalen will be different for different patients. *Follow your doctor's orders or the directions on the label.* The following information includes only the average doses of trioxsalen. *If your dose is different, do not change it* unless your doctor tells you to do so.

*The number of doses you take each day, the time allowed between doses, and the length of time you take the medicine depend on the medical problem for which you are taking trioxsalen.*

- For *oral* dosage form (tablets):
  —For vitiligo:
    - Adults and children 12 years of age and over— 20 to 40 milligrams (mg) taken two to four hours before ultraviolet light A (UVA) exposure. This treatment (trioxsalen and UVA) is given two or

three times a week with the treatments spaced at least forty-eight hours apart.
    - Children up to 12 years of age—Dose must be determined by your doctor.
  —For increasing tolerance to sunlight or increasing color of the skin:
    - Adults and children 12 years of age and over— 20 to 40 mg taken two hours before ultraviolet light A (UVA) exposure. This treatment (trioxsalen and UVA) is given two or three times a week with the treatments spaced at least forty-eight hours apart.
    - Children up to 12 years of age—Dose must be determined by your doctor.

**Missed dose**—If you are late in taking, or miss taking, a dose of this medicine, notify your doctor so your light treatment can be rescheduled. Remember that exposure to sunlight or ultraviolet light must take place 2 to 4 hours *after* you take the medicine or it will not work. If you have any questions about this, check with your doctor.

**Storage**—To store this medicine:

- Keep out of the reach of children.
- Store away from heat and direct light.
- Do not store in the bathroom, near the kitchen sink, or in other damp places. Heat or moisture may cause the medicine to break down.
- Do not keep outdated medicine or medicine no longer needed. Be sure that any discarded medicine is out of the reach of children.

## Precautions While Using This Medicine

Your doctor should check your progress at regular visits to make sure this medicine is working and that it does not cause unwanted effects. Eye examinations should be included.

This medicine increases the sensitivity of your skin and lips to sunlight. Therefore, *exposure to the sun, even through window glass or on a cloudy day, could cause a serious burn.* If you must go out during the daylight hours:

- *Before each treatment, cover your skin for at least 24 hours* by wearing protective clothing, such as long-sleeved shirts, full-length slacks, wide-brimmed hat, and gloves. In addition, *protect your lips with a special sun block lipstick that has a skin protection factor of at least 15.* Check with your doctor before using sun block products on other parts of your body before a treatment, since sun block products should not be used on the areas of your skin that are to be treated.
- *After each treatment, cover your skin for at least 8 hours* by wearing protective clothing. In addition, use a sun block product that has a skin protection factor of at least 15 on your lips and on those areas of your body that cannot be covered.

If you have any questions about this, check with your health care professional.

Your skin may continue to be sensitive to sunlight for some time after treatment with this medicine. Use extra caution for at least 48 hours following each treatment if you plan to spend any time in the sun. Do not sunbathe during this time.

*For 24 hours after you take each dose of trioxsalen, your eyes should be protected during daylight hours with special wraparound sunglasses that totally block or absorb ultraviolet light* (ordinary sunglasses are not adequate). This is to prevent cataracts. Your doctor will tell you what kind of sunglasses to use. These glasses should be worn even in indirect light, such as light coming through window glass or on a cloudy day.

Eating certain foods while you are taking trixosalen may increase your skin's sensitivity to sunlight. To help prevent this, avoid eating limes, figs, parsley, parsnips, mustard, carrots, and celery while you are being treated with this medicine.

This medicine may cause your skin to become dry or itchy. *However, check with your doctor before applying anything to your skin to treat this problem.*

## Side Effects of This Medicine

Along with its needed effects, a medicine may cause some unwanted effects. Although not all of these side effects may occur, if they do occur they may need medical attention.

*Check with your doctor immediately* if you think you have taken an overdose or if any of the following side effects occur, since they may indicate a serious burn:

> Blistering and peeling of skin; reddened, sore skin; swelling, especially of feet or lower legs

Other side effects may occur that usually do not need medical attention. These side effects may go away during treatment as your body adjusts to the medicine. However, check with your doctor if any of the following side effects continue for more than 48 hours or are bothersome:

> *More common*
>> Itching of skin; nausea

> *Less common*
>> Dizziness; headache; mental depression; nervousness; trouble in sleeping

There is an increased risk of developing skin cancer after use of trioxsalen. You should check your body regularly and show your doctor any skin sores that do not heal, new skin growths, and skin growths that have changed in the way they look or feel.

Premature aging of the skin may occur as a result of prolonged trioxsalen therapy. This effect is permanent and is similar to what happens when a person sunbathes for long periods of time.

Other side effects not listed above may also occur in some patients. If you notice any other effects, check with your doctor.

## Additional Information

Once a medicine has been approved for marketing for a certain use, experience may show that it is also useful for other medical problems. Although this use is not included in product labeling, trioxsalen is used in certain patients with the following medical condition:

- Psoriasis

Other than the above information, there is no additional information relating to proper use, precautions, or side effects for this use.

Revised: 07/25/94

# TROPICAMIDE    Ophthalmic

Some commonly used brand names are:
**In the U.S.—**
> I-Picamide                Ocu-Tropic
> Mydriacyl                 Spectro-Cyl
> Mydriafair                Tropicacyl
> Generic name product may also be available.

**In Canada—**
> Minims Tropicamide        Tropicacyl
> Mydriacyl

## Description

Tropicamide (troe-PIK-a-mide) is used to dilate (enlarge) the pupil so that the doctor can see into the back of your eye. It is used before eye examinations, such as cyclo-plegic refraction and examination of the fundus of the eye. Tropicamide may also be used before and after eye surgery.

This medicine is available only with your doctor's prescription, in the following dosage form:
> *Ophthalmic*
>> • Ophthalmic solution (eye drops) (U.S. and Canada)

## Before Using This Medicine

In deciding to use a medicine, the risks of taking the medicine must be weighed against the good it will do.

This is a decision you and your doctor will make. For tropicamide, the following should be considered:

**Allergies**—Tell your doctor if you have ever had any unusual or allergic reaction to tropicamide. Also tell your health care professional if you are allergic to any other substances, such as preservatives.

**Pregnancy**—Studies on effects in pregnancy have not been done in either humans or animals.

**Breast-feeding**—Tropicamide has not been reported to cause problems in nursing babies.

**Children**—Infants and young children and children with blond hair or blue eyes may be especially sensitive to the effects of tropicamide. This may increase the chance or severity of some of the side effects during treatment.

**Older adults**—Elderly people are especially sensitive to the effects of tropicamide. This may increase the chance of side effects during treatment.

**Other medicines**—Although certain medicines should not be used together at all, in other cases two different medicines may be used together even if an interaction might occur. In these cases, your doctor may want to change the dose, or other precautions may be necessary. Tell your health care professional if you are using any other prescription or nonprescription (over-the-counter [OTC]) medicine.

**Other medical problems**—The presence of other medical problems may affect the use of tropicamide. Make sure you tell your doctor if you have any other medical problems, especially:
- Brain damage (in children) or
- Down's syndrome (mongolism) (in children and adults) or
- Glaucoma or
- Spastic paralysis (in children)—Tropicamide may make the condition worse.

## Proper Use of This Medicine

To use:
- First, wash your hands. Tilt the head back and with the index finger of one hand, press gently on the skin just beneath the lower eyelid and pull the lower eyelid away from the eye to make a space. Drop the medicine into this space. Let go of the eyelid and gently close the eyes. Do not blink. Keep the eyes closed and apply pressure to the inner corner of the eye with your finger for 2 or 3 minutes, to allow the medicine to be absorbed by the eye. *This is especially important in infants.*
- Immediately after using the eye drops, wash your hands to remove any medicine that may be on them. If you are using the eye drops for an infant or child, be sure to wash the infant's or child's hands also, and do not let any of the medicine get in the infant's or child's mouth.
- To keep the medicine as germ-free as possible, do not touch the applicator tip to any surface (including the eye). Also, keep the container tightly closed.

*Use this medicine only as directed.* Do not use more of it and do not use it more often than your doctor ordered. To do so may increase the chance of too much medicine being absorbed into the body and the chance of side effects.

**Dosing**—The dose of tropicamide will be different for different patients. *Follow your doctor's orders or the directions on the label.* The following information includes only the average doses of tropicamide. If your dose is different, do not change it unless your doctor tells you to do so.
- For *ophthalmic solution (eye drops)* dosage form:
  —For cycloplegic refraction (eye examination):
    - Adults—One drop of 1% solution, repeated once in five minutes.
    - Children—One drop of 0.5 to 1% solution, repeated once in five minutes.
  —For examination of fundus of eye:
    - Adults and children—One drop of 0.5% solution fifteen to twenty minutes before examination.

## Precautions While Using This Medicine

After this medicine is applied to your eyes:
- Your pupils will become unusually large and you will have blurring of vision, especially for close objects. *Make sure your vision is clear before you drive, use machines, or do anything else that could be dangerous if you are not able to see well.*
- Your eyes will become more sensitive to light than they are normally. When you go out during the daylight hours, even on cloudy days, *wear sunglasses that block ultraviolet (UV) light to protect your eyes from sunlight and other bright lights.* Ordinary sunglasses may not protect your eyes. If you have any questions about the kind of sunglasses to wear, check with your doctor.
- If these effects continue for longer than 24 hours after the medicine is used, check with your doctor.

## Side Effects of This Medicine

Along with its needed effects, a medicine may cause some unwanted effects. Although not all of these side effects may occur, if they do occur they may need medical attention.

Check with your doctor as soon as possible if any of the following side effects occur:
*Symptoms of too much medicine being absorbed into the body*
  Clumsiness or unsteadiness; confusion; fast heartbeat; flushing or redness of face; hallucinations (seeing, hearing, or feeling things that are not there); increased thirst or dryness of mouth; skin rash; slurred speech; swollen stomach in infants; unusual behavior, especially in children; unusual drowsiness, tiredness, or weakness

Other side effects may occur that usually do not need medical attention. These side effects may go away during treatment as your body adjusts to the medicine. However, check with your doctor if any of the following side effects continue or are bothersome:

*More common*

Blurred vision; headache; sensitivity of eyes to light; stinging of the eye when the medicine is applied

Other side effects not listed above may also occur in some patients. If you notice any other effects, check with your doctor.

Revised: 11/22/93

---

# TYPHOID VACCINE LIVE ORAL   Systemic†

A commonly used brand name in the U.S. is Vivotif Berna.

†Not commercially available in Canada.

## Description

Typhoid (TYE-foid) fever is a serious disease that can cause death. It is caused by a germ called *Salmonella typhi*, and is spread most often through infected food or water. Typhoid may also be spread by close person-to-person contact with infected persons (such as occurs with persons living in the same household). Some infected persons do not appear to be sick, but they can still spread the germ to others.

Typhoid fever is very rare in the U.S. and other areas of the world that have good water and sewage (waste) systems. However, it is a problem in parts of the world that do not have such systems. If you are traveling to certain countries or remote (out-of-the-way) areas, typhoid vaccine will help protect you from typhoid fever. The U.S. Centers for Disease Control (CDC) currently recommend caution in the following areas of the world:

• Africa
• Asia
• Latin America

Typhoid vaccine taken by mouth helps prevent typhoid fever, but does not provide 100% protection. Therefore, it is very important to avoid infected persons and food and water that may be infected, even if you have taken the vaccine.

To get the best possible protection against typhoid, you should complete the vaccine dosing schedule (all 4 doses of the vaccine) at least 1 week before travel to areas where you may be exposed to typhoid.

If you will be traveling regularly to parts of the world where typhoid is a problem, you should get a booster (repeat) dose of the vaccine every 5 years.

Typhoid vaccine is available only from a health care professional, in the following dosage form:

*Oral*
• Enteric-coated capsules (U.S.)

## Before Using This Vaccine

In deciding to use a medicine, the risks of taking the medicine must be weighed against the good it will do. This is a decision you and your doctor will make. For typhoid vaccine, the following should be considered:

**Allergies**—Tell your doctor if you have ever had any unusual or allergic reaction to typhoid vaccine. Also tell your health care professional if you are allergic to any other substances, such as foods, preservatives, or dyes. This vaccine contains sucrose and lactose, and the vaccine bacteria are grown in a mixture containing beef.

**Pregnancy**—Studies on effects in pregnancy have not been done in either humans or animals. Before taking this medicine, make sure your doctor knows if you are pregnant or if you may become pregnant.

**Breast-feeding**—It is not known whether typhoid vaccine passes into the breast milk. However, this vaccine has not been reported to cause problems in nursing babies.

**Children**—Typhoid vaccine is not recommended for infants and children up to 6 years of age. Although there is no specific information comparing use of typhoid vaccine in children 6 years of age and over with use in other age groups, this vaccine is not expected to cause different side effects or problems in these children than it does in adults.

**Older adults**—Many medicines have not been studied specifically in older people. Therefore, it may not be known whether they work exactly the same way they do in younger adults. Although there is no specific information comparing use of typhoid vaccine in the elderly with use in other age groups, this vaccine is not expected to cause different side effects or problems in older people than it does in younger adults.

**Other medicines**—Although certain medicines should not be used together at all, in other cases two different medicines may be used together even if an interaction might occur. In these cases, your doctor may want to change the dose, or other precautions may be necessary. When you are taking typhoid vaccine, it is especially important

---

© 1994   The United States Pharmacopeial Convention, Inc.

that your health care professional know if you are taking any of the following:

- Anti-infectives by mouth or by injection (medicine for infection) or
- Antimalarials (medicine for malaria)—These medicines may reduce the useful effect of the typhoid vaccine
- Treatment with x-rays, cancer medicines, or high doses of steroids—Treatment may increase the action of the vaccine, causing an increase in vaccine side effects, or treatment may block the useful effect of the vaccine

**Other medical problems**—The presence of other medical problems may affect the use of typhoid vaccine. Make sure you tell your doctor if you have any other medical problems, especially:

- Diarrhea or
- Fever or
- Other illness (severe) or
- Stomach or intestinal illness (severe) or
- Vomiting—The condition may reduce the useful effect of the vaccine
- Immune deficiency condition, including HIV or AIDS— The condition may increase the chance of side effects of the vaccine

## Proper Use of This Vaccine

*It is important that all 4 doses of the vaccine be taken exactly as directed.* If all the doses are not taken or if doses are not taken at the correct times, the vaccine may not work properly.

The vaccine capsules are meant to dissolve in the intestines. Therefore, they should be inspected to make sure that they are not broken or cracked when you take them. If any are broken or cracked, you will need to replace them.

Typhoid vaccine must be stored in the refrigerator at a temperature between 2 and 8 °C (35.6 and 46.4 °F) at all times. If the vaccine is left at room temperature, it will lose its effectiveness. Therefore, remember to replace unused vaccine in the refrigerator between doses.

Each dose of the vaccine should be taken approximately 1 hour before a meal. Take with a cold or lukewarm drink that has a temperature that does not exceed body temperature, e.g., 37 °C (98.6 °F).

Swallow the capsule whole. Do not chew it before swallowing. Also swallow the capsule as soon as possible after you place it in your mouth.

**Dosing**—*Follow your doctor's orders or the directions on the label.* The following information includes only the average dose of typhoid vaccine. *If your dose is different, do not change it* unless your doctor tells you to do so:

- Take 1 capsule by mouth every other day for a total of 4 doses.

**Missed dose**—If you miss a dose of this medicine and you remember it on the day it should be taken, take it as directed. However, if you do not remember the missed dose until the next day, take the missed dose at that time and reschedule your every-other-day doses from then. *It is important that this vaccine be taken exactly as directed so it can give you the most protection against typhoid fever.*

**Storage**—To store this medicine:

- Keep out of the reach of children.
- *Store in the refrigerator at all times.* However, keep the medicine from freezing.
- Do not keep outdated medicine or medicine no longer needed. Be sure that any discarded medicine is out of the reach of children.

## Precautions While Using This Medicine

Tell your doctor that you have taken this vaccine:

- If you are to receive any other live vaccines within 1 month after taking this vaccine.

## Side Effects of This Vaccine

Along with its needed effects, a medicine may cause some unwanted effects. Although not all of these side effects may occur, if they do occur they may need medical attention.

*Get emergency help immediately* if any of the following side effects occur:

*Symptoms of allergic reaction*
  Difficulty in breathing or swallowing; hives; itching, especially of feet or hands; reddening of skin, especially around ears; swelling of eyes, face, or inside of nose; unusual tiredness or weakness (sudden and severe)

Other side effects may occur that usually do not need medical attention. These side effects may go away during treatment as your body adjusts to the medicine. However, check with your doctor if any of the following side effects continue or are bothersome:

*Less common or rare*
  Diarrhea; fever; hives; nausea; skin rash; stomach cramps or pain; vomiting

Other side effects not listed above may also occur in some patients. If you notice any other effects, check with your doctor.

Revised: 07/22/92

# UNDECYLENIC ACID, COMPOUND   Topical

Some commonly used brand names are:

**In the U.S.—**

| | |
|---|---|
| Caldesene Medicated Powder | Desenex Antifungal Ointment |
| Cruex Antifungal Cream | Desenex Antifungal |
| Cruex Antifungal Powder | Penetrating Foam |
| Cruex Antifungal Spray | Desenex Antifungal Powder |
| Powder | Desenex Antifungal Spray |
| Decylenes Powder | Powder |
| Desenex Antifungal Cream | Gordochom Solution |
| Desenex Antifungal Liquid | |

**In Canada—**

| | |
|---|---|
| Cruex Aerosol Powder | Desenex Foam |
| Cruex Cream | Desenex Ointment |
| Cruex Powder | Desenex Powder |
| Desenex Aerosol Powder | Desenex Solution |

## Description

Compound undecylenic acid (un-de-sill-ENN-ik AS-id) belongs to the group of medicines called antifungals. It is used to treat some types of fungus infections. However, compound undecylenic acid generally has been replaced by newer and more effective medicines for the treatment of fungus infections.

Compound undecylenic acid is available without a prescription; however, your doctor may have special instructions on the proper use of this medicine for your medical condition.

Compound undecylenic acid is available in the following dosage forms:

*Topical*
- Aerosol foam (U.S. and Canada)
- Aerosol powder (U.S. and Canada)
- Cream (U.S. and Canada)
- Ointment (U.S. and Canada)
- Powder (U.S. and Canada)
- Solution (U.S. and Canada)

## Before Using This Medicine

If you are taking this medicine without a prescription, carefully read and follow any precautions on the label. For compound undecylenic acid, the following should be considered:

**Allergies**—Tell your doctor if you have ever had any unusual or allergic reaction to compound undecylenic acid. Also tell your health care professional if you are allergic to any other substances, such as preservatives or dyes.

**Pregnancy**—Compound undecylenic acid topical preparations have not been shown to cause birth defects or other problems in humans.

**Breast-feeding**—Compound undecylenic acid topical preparations have not been reported to cause problems in nursing babies.

**Children**—Compound undecylenic acid should not be used on children up to 2 years of age, unless otherwise directed by your doctor. Although there is no specific information comparing use of compound undecylenic acid topical preparations in children 2 years of age and older with use in other age groups, this medicine is not expected to cause different side effects or problems in children 2 years of age and older than it does in adults.

**Older adults**—Many medicines have not been studied specifically in older people. Therefore, it may not be known whether they work exactly the same way they do in younger adults or if they cause different side effects or problems in older people. There is no specific information comparing use of compound undecylenic acid in the elderly with use in other age groups.

**Other medicines**—Although certain medicines should not be used together at all, in other cases two different medicines may be used together even if an interaction might occur. In these cases, your doctor may want to change the dose, or other precautions may be necessary. Tell your health care professional if you are using any other topical prescription or nonprescription (over-the-counter [OTC]) medicine that is to be applied to the same area of the skin.

## Proper Use of This Medicine

Before applying compound undecylenic acid, wash the affected and surrounding areas, and dry thoroughly. Then apply enough medicine to cover these areas.

*Keep this medicine away from the eyes.*

For patients using the *cream form* of this medicine:
- Apply cream generously to affected and surrounding areas. Rub in well.
- Do not use on pus-containing sores or on badly broken skin.

For patients using the *powder form* of this medicine:
- If the powder is used on the feet, sprinkle it between toes, on feet, and in socks and shoes.

For patients using the *aerosol powder or aerosol foam form* of this medicine:
- From a distance of 4 to 6 inches, spray the affected and surrounding areas. If the medicine is used on the feet, spray it between the toes also. The powder may also be sprayed in socks and shoes.
- Do not use this medicine around the eyes, nose, or mouth.
- Do not inhale the aerosol.
- Do not use near heat, near open flame, or while smoking.

To help clear up your infection completely, *keep using this medicine for 2 weeks after burning, itching, or other symptoms have disappeared,* unless otherwise directed by your doctor. *Do not miss any doses.*

**Dosing**—The dose of topical compound undecylenic acid will be different for different patients. *Follow your doctor's orders or the directions on the label.* The following information includes only the average doses of topical compound undecylenic acid. *If your dose is different, do not change it unless your doctor tells you to do so.*

- For fungus infections:
  —For *aerosol foam, aerosol powder, ointment, powder,* or *solution* dosage forms:
  - Adults and children 2 years of age and over—Apply to the affected area(s) of the skin two times a day.
  - Children up to 2 years of age—Use is not recommended.
  —For *cream* dosage form:
  - Adults and children—Apply to the affected area(s) of the skin as often as necessary.

**Missed dose**—If you miss a dose of this medicine, apply it as soon as possible. Then go back to your regular dosing schedule.

**Storage**—To store this medicine:
- Keep out of the reach of children.
- Store away from heat and direct light.
- Do not store the powder form of this medicine in the bathroom, near the kitchen sink, or in other damp places. Heat or moisture may cause the medicine to break down.
- Keep the aerosol foam, aerosol powder, cream, ointment, and solution forms of this medicine from freezing.
- Do not puncture, break, or burn the aerosol foam or powder container.

- Do not keep outdated medicine or medicine no longer needed. Be sure that any discarded medicine is out of the reach of children.

## Precautions While Using This Medicine

If your skin problem does not improve within 4 weeks, or if it becomes worse, check with your health care professional.

To help prevent reinfection after the period of treatment with this medicine, the powder or spray powder form of this medicine may be used each day after bathing and careful drying.

## Side Effects of This Medicine

Along with its needed effects, a medicine may cause some unwanted effects. Although not all of these side effects may occur, if they do occur they may need medical attention.

Check with your health care professional as soon as possible if the following side effect occurs:

Skin irritation not present before use of this medicine

Other side effects not listed above may also occur in some patients. If you notice any other effects, check with your health care professional.

Revised: 07/25/94

---

# URACIL MUSTARD      Systemic†

Generic name product available in the U.S.

†Not commercially available in Canada.

## Description

Uracil (YOOR-a-sill) mustard belongs to the group of medicines known as alkylating agents. It is used to treat some kinds of cancer as well as some noncancerous conditions.

Uracil mustard interferes with the growth of cancer cells, which are eventually destroyed. Since the growth of normal body cells may also be affected by uracil mustard, other effects will also occur. Some of these may be serious and must be reported to your doctor. Other effects, such as hair loss, may not be serious but may cause concern. Some effects may not occur for months or years after the medicine is used.

Before you begin treatment with uracil mustard, you and your doctor should talk about the good this medicine will do as well as the risks of using it.

Uracil mustard is available only with your doctor's prescription, in the following dosage form:

*Oral*
- Capsules (U.S.)

## Before Using This Medicine

In deciding to use a medicine, the risks of taking the medicine must be weighed against the good it will do. This is a decision you and your doctor will make. For uracil mustard, the following should be considered:

**Allergies**—Tell your doctor if you have ever had any unusual or allergic reaction to uracil mustard.

**Pregnancy**—Tell your doctor if you are pregnant or if you intend to have children. This medicine may cause birth defects if either the male or female is taking it at the time of conception or if it is taken during pregnancy. In addition, many cancer medicines may cause sterility which could be permanent. Although sterility has not been reported with this medicine, the possibility should be kept in mind.

Be sure that you have discussed this with your doctor before taking this medicine. It is best to use some kind of birth control while you are taking uracil mustard. Tell your doctor right away if you think you have become pregnant while taking uracil mustard.

**Breast-feeding**—Tell your doctor if you are breast-feeding or if you intend to breast-feed during treatment with this medicine. Because uracil mustard may cause serious side effects, breast-feeding is generally not recommended while you are receiving it.

**Children**—Although there is no specific information about the use of uracil mustard in children, it is not expected to cause different side effects or problems in children than it does in adults.

**Older adults**—Many medicines have not been tested in older people. Therefore, it may not be known whether they work exactly the same way they do in younger adults or if they cause different side effects or problems in older people. There is no specific information about the use of uracil mustard in the elderly.

**Other medicines**—Although certain medicines should not be used together at all, in other cases two different medicines may be used together even if an interaction might occur. In these cases, your doctor may want to change the dose, or other precautions may be necessary. When you are taking uracil mustard, it is especially important that your health care professional know if you are taking any of the following:

- Amphotericin B by injection (e.g., Fungizone) or
- Antithyroid agents (medicine for overactive thyroid) or
- Azathioprine (e.g., Imuran) or
- Chloramphenicol (e.g., Chloromycetin) or
- Colchicine or
- Flucytosine (e.g., Ancobon) or
- Interferon (e.g., Intron A, Roferon-A) or
- Plicamycin (e.g., Mithracin) or
- Zidovudine (e.g., Retrovir) or
- If you have ever been treated with x-rays or cancer medicines—Uracil mustard may increase the effects of these medicines or radiation therapy on the blood
- Probenecid (e.g., Benemid) or
- Sulfinpyrazone (e.g., Anturane)—Uracil mustard may increase the concentration of uric acid in the blood, which these medicines are used to lower

**Other medical problems**—The presence of other medical problems may affect the use of uracil mustard. Make sure you tell your doctor if you have any other medical problems, especially:

- Chickenpox (including recent exposure) or
- Herpes zoster (shingles)—Risk of severe disease affecting other parts of the body
- Gout (history of) or
- Kidney stones (history of)—Uracil mustard may increase levels of uric acid in the body, which can cause gout or kidney stones
- Infection—Uracil mustard can reduce immunity to infection
- Kidney disease
- Liver disease

## Proper Use of This Medicine

*Use this medicine only as directed by your doctor.* Do not use more or less of it, and do not use it more often than your doctor ordered. The exact amount of medicine you need has been carefully worked out. Taking too much may increase the chance of side effects, while taking too little may not improve your condition.

While you are using this medicine, your doctor may want you to drink extra fluids so that you will pass more urine. This will help prevent kidney problems and keep your kidneys working well.

Uracil mustard often causes nausea and vomiting. Even if you begin to feel ill, *do not stop using this medicine without first checking with your doctor.* Ask your health care professional for ways to lessen these effects.

If you vomit shortly after taking a dose of uracil mustard, check with your doctor. You will be told whether to take the dose again or to wait until the next scheduled dose.

**Dosing**—The dose of uracil mustard will be different for different patients. The dose that is used may depend on a number of things, including what the medicine is being used for, the patient's weight, and whether or not other medicines are also being taken. *If you are taking uracil mustard at home, follow your doctor's orders or the directions on the label.* If you have any questions about the proper dose of uracil mustard, ask your doctor.

**Missed dose**—If you miss a dose of this medicine, skip the missed dose and go back to your regular dosing schedule. Do not double doses.

**Storage**—To store this medicine:

- Keep out of the reach of children.
- Store away from heat and direct light.
- Do not store in the bathroom, near the kitchen sink, or in other damp places. Heat or moisture may cause the medicine to break down.
- Do not keep outdated medicine or medicine no longer needed. Be sure that any discarded medicine is out of the reach of children.

## Precautions While Using This Medicine

*It is very important that your doctor check your progress at regular visits* to make sure that this medicine is working properly and to check for unwanted effects.

While you are being treated with uracil mustard, and after you stop treatment with it, *do not have any immunizations (vaccinations) without your doctor's approval.* Uracil mustard may lower your body's resistance and there is a chance you might get the infection the immunization is meant to prevent. Other people living in your household should not take or should not have recently taken oral polio vaccine since there is a chance they could pass the polio virus on to you. Also, avoid other persons who have taken oral polio vaccine. Do not get close to them and do not stay in the same room with them for very long. If you cannot take these precautions, you should consider wearing a protective face mask that covers the nose and mouth.

Uracil mustard can lower the number of white blood cells in your blood temporarily, increasing the chance of getting an infection. It can also lower the number of platelets, which are necessary for proper blood clotting. If this occurs, there are certain precautions you can take, especially when your blood count is low, to reduce the risk of infection or bleeding:

- If you can, avoid people with infections. *Check with your doctor immediately* if you think you are getting an infection or if you get a fever or chills, cough or hoarseness, lower back or side pain, or painful or difficult urination.

- *Check with your doctor immediately* if you notice any unusual bleeding or bruising; black, tarry stools; blood in urine or stools; or pinpoint red spots on your skin.

- Be careful when using a regular toothbrush, dental floss, or toothpick. Your medical doctor, dentist, or nurse may recommend other ways to clean your teeth and gums. Check with your medical doctor before having any dental work done.

- Do not touch your eyes or the inside of your nose unless you have just washed your hands and have not touched anything else in the meantime.

- Be careful not to cut yourself when you are using sharp objects such as a safety razor or fingernail or toenail cutters.

- Avoid contact sports or other situations where bruising or injury could occur.

## Side Effects of This Medicine

Along with their needed effects medicines like uracil mustard can sometimes cause unwanted effects such as blood problems, loss of hair, and other side effects. These and others are described below. Also, because of the way these medicines act on the body, there is a chance that they might cause other unwanted effects that may not occur until months or years after the medicine is used. These delayed effects may include certain types of cancer, such as leukemia. Discuss these possible effects with your doctor.

Although not all of the side effects may occur, if they do occur they may need medical attention.

*Check with your doctor immediately* if any of the following side effects occur:

*Less common*

Black, tarry stools; blood in urine or stools; cough or hoarseness; fever or chills; lower back or side pain; painful or difficult urination; pinpoint red spots on skin; unusual bleeding or bruising

Check with your doctor as soon as possible if any of the following side effects occur:

*Less common*

Joint pain; swelling of feet or lower legs

*Rare*

Sores in mouth and on lips; yellow eyes or skin

Other side effects may occur that usually do not need medical attention. These side effects may go away during treatment as your body adjusts to the medicine. Also, your health care professional may be able to tell you about ways to prevent or reduce some of these side effects. Check with your health care professional if any of the following side effects continue or are bothersome or if you have any questions about them:

*More common*

Diarrhea; nausea or vomiting

*Less common*

Darkening of the skin; irritability; mental depression; nervousness; skin rash and itching

This medicine may cause a temporary loss of hair in some people. After treatment with uracil mustard has ended, normal hair growth should return.

After you stop taking uracil mustard, it may still produce some side effects that need attention. During this period of time, check with your doctor if you notice any of the following:

Black, tarry stools; blood in urine or stools; cough or hoarseness; fever or chills; lower back or side pain; painful or difficult urination; pinpoint red spots on skin; unusual bleeding or bruising

Other side effects not listed above may also occur in some patients. If you notice any other effects, check with your doctor.

Revised: 09/90
Interim revision(s): 08/11/93; 06/30/94

# UREA    Intra-amniotic

A commonly used brand name in the U.S. is Ureaphil.
Another commonly used name is carbamide.

## Description

Intra-amniotic urea (yoor-EE-a) is given by injection into the uterus to cause abortion. It is to be administered only by or under the immediate care of your doctor. It is available in the following dosage form:

*Parenteral*
- Injection (U.S.)

## Before Receiving This Medicine

In deciding to use a medicine, the risks of taking the medicine must be weighed against the good it will do. This is a decision you and your doctor will make. For urea, the following should be considered:

**Allergies**—Tell your doctor if you have ever had any unusual or allergic reaction to urea. Also tell your health care professional if you are allergic to any other substances, such as foods, preservatives, or dyes.

**Teenagers**—Although there is no specific information comparing use of urea in teenagers with use in other age groups, this medicine is not expected to cause different side effects or problems in teenagers than it does in adults.

**Other medicines**—Although certain medicines should not be used together at all, in other cases two different medicines may be used together even if an interaction might occur. In these cases, your doctor may want to change the dose, or other precautions may be necessary. Tell your health care professional if you are taking any other prescription or nonprescription (over-the-counter [OTC]) medicine.

**Other medical problems**—The presence of other medical problems may affect the use of urea. Make sure you tell your doctor if you have any other medical problems, especially:
- Diabetes mellitus (sugar diabetes)
- Fibroid tumors of the uterus
- Kidney disease
- Liver disease
- Sickle cell disease

## Proper Use of This Medicine

During the abortion procedure, you should drink fluids to help prevent your body from losing too much water.

**Dosing**—The dose of urea will be different for different patients. *Follow your doctor's orders.* The dose will be given by your doctor in a health care setting, such as a hospital or clinic. The following information includes only the average doses of urea.

- For *injection* dosage form:
  —For causing abortion:
    - Adults and teenagers—Up to 250 milliliters (mL) injected through the abdomen into the uterus after the same amount of fluid is taken out of the bag around the fetus (amniotic sac). The injection may be repeated 48 hours after the first dose if needed.

## Side Effects of This Medicine

Along with its needed effects, a medicine may cause some unwanted effects. Although not all of these side effects may occur, if they do occur they may need medical attention.

*Check with your health care professional immediately if either of the following side effects occurs during the time that the injection is being given:*
> Pain in lower abdomen; weakness

Check with your health care professional as soon as possible if any of the following side effects occur:
> *Rare*
> Confusion; irregular heartbeat; muscle cramps or pain; numbness, tingling, pain, or weakness in hands or feet; unusual tiredness or weakness; weakness and heaviness of legs

Other side effects may occur that usually do not need medical attention. However, check with your health care professional if any of the following side effects continue or are bothersome:
> *More common*
> Nausea or vomiting
> *Less common or rare*
> Headache

After the procedure is completed, this procedure may still produce some side effects that need medical attention. Check with your doctor if you notice any of the following side effects:
> Chills or shivering; fever; foul-smelling vaginal discharge; increase in bleeding of the uterus; pain in lower abdomen

Other side effects not listed above may also occur in some patients. If you notice any other effects, check with your health care professional.

Revised: 08/18/93
Interim revision: 06/21/94

# URINE GLUCOSE AND KETONE TEST KITS FOR HOME USE

Some commonly used brand names are:

**In the U.S.—**
Acetest[3]
Biotel/diabetes[2]
Chemstrip K[3]
Chemstrip uG[2]
Chemstrip uGK[4]
Clinistix[2]
Clinitest[1]
Diastix[2]
Glucose & Ketone Urine Test[4]
Keto-diastix[4]
KetoStix[3]
Tes-tape[2]

**In Canada—**
Acetest[3]
Chemstrip uGK[4]
Clinistix[2]
Clinitest[1]
Diastix[2]
Keto-diastix[4]
KetoStix[3]
Tes-tape[2]

Note: For quick reference, the following urine glucose and ketone test kits for home use are numbered to match the corresponding brand names.

This information applies to the following medicines:
1. Copper Reduction Urine Glucose Test
2. Glucose Oxidase Urine Glucose Test
3. Nitroprusside Urine Ketone Test
4. Urine Glucose and Ketone (Combined) Test

## Description

Diabetes mellitus (sugar diabetes) is a condition that causes problems in controlling the amount of sugar (glucose) in the blood. This is because the pancreas gland does not work properly to make enough insulin to allow the body to handle glucose the right way. Normally, insulin helps glucose enter body cells so it can be used for energy. It also helps the body store extra nutrients and release them for energy when needed. If there is not enough insulin, the unused glucose builds up in the blood. Some of this extra glucose will be passed into the urine. Having extra glucose in the blood for many years causes damage to blood vessels and nerves. Eventually, the body organs (especially the eyes, heart, kidneys, and lower limbs) are damaged. People with diabetes who carefully control their condition may be less likely to develop these problems.

When body cells are not able to use glucose because of the shortage of insulin, they use stored fats instead. Abnormally fast use of fats causes a buildup of their breakdown product, ketones, in the blood. The ketones make the blood more acid, resulting in a condition called ketoacidosis. The combined ketone and acid condition is poisonous to the brain, causing the patient to become confused and drowsy. Coma and death may follow if the problem is not corrected.

Patients with diabetes are taught to test their urine or blood for glucose and ketones as part of a program to manage their diabetes. Blood tests for glucose are considered by most doctors to be the best way to monitor diabetes. Urine tests are mostly used by patients who do not need insulin to control their diabetes and patients whose disease is stable, or those who are not able to take blood samples. These tests may also be used in addition to blood tests when monitoring must be done often, such as on sick days.

Testing for ketones is important when blood or urine tests are high for glucose, or when a patient is sick or cannot eat. Ketone testing is especially important during pregnancy, because insulin needs change rapidly and ketones are damaging to the fetus. Some products test for glucose and ketones on the same strip.

## Before Using This Test Kit

It is important to get the best results possible from these urine tests. Therefore, the following should be considered by you and your diabetes care provider before choosing which urine test is the best for you or what adjustments may be needed when you are testing your urine:

**Diet**—Foods that color the urine may make the test colors harder to read. Check the urine sample for unusual color when test results are not what you expect.

**Medicines**—Certain medicines may affect the results of your testing. When a new medicine is prescribed for you, ask your diabetes care provider about possible problems with the test you usually use. Also, make sure you tell your diabetes care provider about any medicines you may use.

Medicines that color the urine may make the test colors harder to read. Check the urine sample for unusual color when your urine test results are not what you expect.

Many medicines (including nonprescription products such as vitamins, aspirin, and iron) may cause false test results, especially with certain tablet products.

**Other medical problems**—The presence of certain medical problems may affect the results of your testing. Check with your diabetes care provider if you have any other medical conditions, including:

- Vision problems—If you are color-blind or have poor vision, you will need someone to help you in reading your test results

## Proper Use of This Test

Usually your diabetes care provider (doctor, nurse, or diabetes educator) will help you choose and learn to use a test product. Some tests are more sensitive, easier to use, or more likely to be affected by other medicines and conditions. The test product should be matched to your needs.

Once the choice of a urine test is made by the diabetes care provider or teacher, you should use it at the planned times, as often as instructed. This may be 4 or more times a day for some patients. Doing the test often allows for better control of your diabetes.

Buy only the product recommended by your doctor or diabetes specialist or center. Do not switch products without the advice of one of these professionals. The printed instructions on the proper use of these urine test kits are different for each product. You could get confusing results with a different product until you learn its proper use.

To use:

- Wash and dry your hands.
- Collect a urine sample in a clean, dry container according to the written package instructions or your diabetes specialist's instructions. Do not refrigerate the urine or let it stand for more than one-half hour (30 minutes) before testing it.
- Choose a well-lighted area with normal room temperature and humidity, with a clean, dry working surface to perform the test. You will also need a watch, timer, or clock that can measure in seconds and a cold water faucet nearby.
- Wash and dry your hands before handling the test materials. Be careful not to touch the testing areas. Skin oils or perspiration may affect the test chemicals and cause a false result. It is also important that you use clean, dry test kit materials. Traces of old test chemicals or soaps can cause false test results. Reused containers or droppers should be rinsed with distilled water and allowed to dry between uses.
- Read and follow the test kit instructions carefully. Soon after you take out a test strip, tablet, or piece of tape, close the container.
- For test strips, dip the strip in the urine for one second and tap it on the edge of the container to remove the extra urine. You may also hold the strip directly in your urine stream to wet the test areas.
- Compare the color of the test strip to the color chart on the package at the end of the timing period. You may hold the strip right next to the color chart. The color should be the same on all of the wet area.
- When you are using tests that require drops of urine to be put into a test tube, hold the dropper straight up and down. Carefully count the water and urine drops as you drop them in the test tube. Place the test tube in its holder and wait for any boiling to stop. (After the boiling stops, the test tube will still be hot, so be careful not to burn your fingers.)
- 15 seconds after boiling has stopped, read the test results by matching the color of the urine in the test tube with the proper color chart. You may want to hold the color chart right next to the test tube. If

your test kit has more than one method, make sure to use the correct color chart, based on the number of drops you use.
- For *Acetest*, allow each drop to soak into the tablet and read the test at 15 seconds.
- Do the test control, if one is recommended in the package instructions.
- Record your test results.

**Storage**—To store these products:

- Keep out of the reach of children. Test kit chemicals can be poisonous if swallowed.
- Store these test kits in their original containers. Keep the container tightly closed. Recap the test product container immediately after use.
- Keep in a cool, dry place, away from heat, humidity (such as the bathroom or shower area), and direct sunlight. Heat-exposed test kits will not work properly.
- Do not put test kits in the refrigerator. Keep the product from freezing.
- Check the expiration date printed on the package before purchasing. Do not use an outdated test kit. Outdated test kits will not work correctly.
- Do not use tablets or strips that have changed color or are falling apart. This is a sign that they are no longer good and will not give correct results.
- Unused liquids may be poured down the drain. Any urine or tests with urine in them should be flushed in the toilet. Be sure that any discarded test kit is out of the reach of children.

## About Your Test Results

After you have your urine test results, you should write them in a log book or diary, along with any other problems you may be having. Your diabetes care providers can then give you any advice you will need to help you best control your diabetes.

Use the guidelines (rules) that your doctor has given you on what to do when your results show that your diabetes is not under the proper control. Usually these rules involve adjustments in your diet, medicines, or exercise. Depending upon your diabetes control program, you may be able to make some of these adjustments or handle some problems by yourself or at home with telephone advice from your doctor's office. However, some problems are serious enough that you will need to see your doctor to get your diabetes under control again.

Notify your doctor, nurse, or diabetes educator if you are not sure of your test results for any reason. Your control of your diabetes depends on your understanding of diabetes and its treatment as well as the decisions you make every day.

Having high levels of glucose in your urine (or blood) and finding ketones in your urine may indicate a hidden illness or infection. Prompt notification of your doctor is important to get additional treatment to regain control of your condition, and to avoid complications.

If you have any other questions about your results or the use of diabetic urine test kits, ask your diabetes care provider or pharmacist. Also, most kits have a toll-free number advice to call for advice.

Revised: 10/26/92
Interim revision: 07/12/94

# UROFOLLITROPIN    Systemic

A commonly used brand name in the U.S. and Canada is Metrodin. Other commonly used names are follicle-stimulating hormone and FSH.

## Description

Urofollitropin (YOO-roe-fall-ee-troe-pin) is a fertility drug that is identical to the hormone called follicle-stimulating hormone (FSH) that is produced naturally by the pituitary gland.

FSH is primarily responsible for stimulating growth of the ovarian follicle, which includes the developing egg, the cells surrounding the egg that produce the hormones needed to support a pregnancy, and the fluid around the egg. As the ovarian follicle grows, an increasing amount of the hormone estrogen (ESS-troe-jen) is produced by the cells in the follicle and released into the bloodstream. Estrogen causes the endometrium (lining of the uterus) to thicken before ovulation occurs. The higher blood levels of estrogen will also provide a cue to the hypothalamus and pituitary gland to slow the production and release of FSH.

Another pituitary hormone, luteinizing hormone (LH), also helps to increase the amount of estrogen produced by the follicle cells. However, the main function of LH is to cause ovulation. The sharp rise in the blood level of LH that triggers ovulation is sometimes called the LH surge. After ovulation, the group of hormone-producing follicle cells become what is called the corpus luteum and will produce estrogen and large amounts of another hormone, progesterone (proe-JESS-ter-one). Progesterone causes the endometrium to mature so that it can support the egg after it is fertilized. If implantation of a fertilized egg does not occur, the levels of estrogen and progesterone decrease and the endometrium sloughs off (e.g., menstruation occurs).

Urofollitropin is usually given in combination with human chorionic gonadotropin (hCG). The actions of hCG are almost identical to those of LH. It is given to simulate the natural LH surge. This results in predictable ovulation.

Urofollitropin is often used in women who have low levels of FSH and too-high levels of LH. Women with polycystic ovary syndrome usually have hormone levels such as this and are treated with urofollitropin to make up for the low amounts of FSH. Many women being treated with urofollitropin have already tried clomiphene (e.g., Serophene) and have not been able to conceive yet. Urofollitropin may also be used to cause the ovary to produce several follicles, which can then be harvested for use in gamete intrafallopian transfer (GIFT) or in vitro fertilization (IVF).

Urofollitropin is to be given only by or under the supervision of your doctor. It is available in the following dosage form:

*Parenteral*
  • Injection (U.S. and Canada)

## Before Receiving This Medicine

In deciding to use a medicine, the risks of taking the medicine must be weighed against the good it will do. This is a decision you and your doctor will make. For urofollitropin, the following should be considered:

**Allergies**—Tell your doctor if you have ever had any unusual or allergic reaction to urofollitropin. Also tell your health care professional if you are allergic to any other substances, such as foods, preservatives, or dyes.

**Pregnancy**—If you become pregnant as a result of using this medicine, there is an increased chance of a multiple pregnancy.

**Other medicines**—Although certain medicines should not be used together at all, in other cases two different medicines may be used together even if an interaction might occur. In these cases, your doctor may want to change the dose, or other precautions may be necessary. Tell your health care professional if you are taking any other prescription or nonprescription (over-the-counter [OTC]) medicine.

**Other medical problems**—The presence of other medical problems may affect the use of urofollitropin. Make sure you tell your doctor if you have any other medical problems, especially:
  • Cyst on ovary—Urofollitropin can cause further growth of cysts on the ovary
  • Unusual vaginal bleeding—Some irregular vaginal bleeding is a sign that the endometrium is growing too rapidly, possibly of endometrial cancer, or some hormone imbalances; the increases in estrogen production caused by urofollitropin can make these problems worse. If a hormonal imbalance is present, it should be treated before the beginning of menotropins therapy

## Proper Use of This Medicine

**Dosing**—The dose of urofollitropin will be different for different patients. *Follow your doctor's orders or the directions on the label.* The following information includes only the average doses of urofollitropin. *If your dose is different, do not change it* unless your doctor tells you to do so.

- For *injection* dosage form:
  —For becoming pregnant while having a condition called polycystic ovary syndrome:
  - Adults—75 Units injected into a muscle once a day for seven or more days. Usually, another medicine called chorionic gonadotropin (hCG) will be given the day after the last dose. If needed, your doctor may then increase your dose of urofollitropin to 150 Units a day for another seven or more days.
  —For becoming pregnant while using other pregnancy methods (assisted reproductive technology [ART]):
  - Adults—150 Units injected into a muscle once a day. Your treatment will probably begin on Day 2 or Day 3 after your menstrual period begins. Usually, another medicine called chorionic gonadotropin (hCG) will be given the day after the last dose.

## Precautions While Receiving This Medicine

*It is very important that your doctor check your progress at regular visits* to make sure that the medicine is working properly and to check for unwanted effects. Your doctor will likely want to monitor the development of the ovarian follicle(s) by measuring the amount of estrogen in your bloodstream and by checking the size of the follicle(s) with ultrasound examinations.

If your doctor has asked you to record your basal body temperature (BBT) daily, make sure that you do this every day. It is important that intercourse take place around the time of ovulation to give you the best chance of becoming pregnant.

## Side Effects of This Medicine

Along with its needed effects, a medicine may cause some unwanted effects. Although not all of these side effects may occur, if they do occur they may need medical attention.

Check with your doctor as soon as possible if any of the following side effects occur:

*More common*
　Abdominal or pelvic pain; bloating (mild); redness, pain, or swelling at the injection site

*Less common or rare*
　Abdominal or stomach pain (severe); bloating (moderate to severe); decreased amount of urine; feeling of indigestion; fever and chills; nausea, vomiting, or diarrhea (continuing or severe); pelvic pain (severe); shortness of breath; skin rash or hives; swelling of lower legs; weight gain (rapid)

Other side effects may occur that usually do not need medical attention. These side effects may go away during treatment as your body adjusts to the medicine. However, check with your doctor if any of the following side effects continue or are bothersome:

*Less common or rare*
　Breast tenderness; diarrhea (mild); nausea; vomiting

After you stop using this medicine, your body may need time to adjust. The length of time this takes depends on the amount of medicine you were using and how long you used it. During this period of time check with your doctor if you notice any of the following side effects:

　Abdominal or stomach pain (severe); bloating (moderate to severe); decreased amount of urine; feeling of indigestion; nausea, vomiting, or diarrhea (continuing or severe); pelvic pain (severe); shortness of breath; swelling of lower legs; weight gain (rapid)

Other side effects not listed above may also occur in some patients. If you notice any other effects, check with your doctor.

Revised: 07/08/92
Interim revision: 06/30/94

# URSODIOL  Systemic

Some commonly used brand names are:
**In the U.S.—**
　Actigall
**In Canada—**
　Ursofalk
Another commonly used name is ursodeoxycholic acid.

## Description

Ursodiol (ur-so-DYE-ole) is used in the treatment of gallstone disease. It is taken by mouth to dissolve the gallstones.

Ursodiol is used in patients who do not need to have their gallbladder removed or in those in whom surgery should be avoided because of other medical problems. However, ursodiol works only in those patients whose gallstones are made of cholesterol and works best when these stones are small and of the "floating" type.

Ursodiol is available only with your doctor's prescription, in the following dosage form:
*Oral*
- Capsules (U.S. and Canada)

## Before Using This Medicine

In deciding to use a medicine, the risks of taking the medicine must be weighed against the good it will do. This is a decision you and your doctor will make. For ursodiol, the following should be considered:

**Allergies**—Tell your doctor if you have ever had any unusual or allergic reaction to ursodiol or other products containing bile acids.

**Diet**—It is thought that body weight and the kind of diet the patient follows may affect how fast the stones dissolve and whether new stones will form. However, check with your doctor before going on any diet.

**Pregnancy**—Ursodiol has not been studied in pregnant women. However, ursodiol has not been shown to cause birth defects or other problems in animal studies.

**Breast-feeding**—It is not known whether ursodiol passes into the breast milk. Although most medicines pass into breast milk in small amounts, many of them may be used safely while breast-feeding. Mothers who are taking this medicine and who wish to breast-feed should discuss this with their doctor.

**Children**—Although there is no specific information comparing use of ursodiol in children with use in other age groups, this medicine is not expected to cause different side effects or problems in children than it does in adults.

**Older adults**—Many medicines have not been studied specifically in older people. Therefore, it may not be known whether they work exactly the same way they do in younger adults. Although there is no specific information comparing use of ursodiol in the elderly with use in other age groups, this medicine is not expected to cause different side effects or problems in older people than it does in younger adults.

**Other medicines**—Although certain medicines should not be used together at all, in other cases 2 different medicines may be used together even if an interaction might occur. In these cases, your doctor may want to change the dose, or other precautions may be necessary. Tell your health care professional if you are taking any other prescription or nonprescription (over-the-counter [OTC]) medicine.

**Other medical problems**—The presence of other medical problems may affect the use of ursodiol. Make sure you tell your doctor if you have any other medical problems, especially:
- Biliary tract problems or
- Pancreatitis (inflammation of pancreas)—These conditions may make it necessary to have surgery since treatment with ursodiol would take too long

## Proper Use of This Medicine

Take ursodiol with meals for best results, unless otherwise directed by your doctor.

*Take ursodiol for the full time of treatment, even if you begin to feel better.* If you stop taking this medicine too soon, the gallstones may not dissolve as fast or may not dissolve at all.

**Dosing**—The dose of ursodiol will be different for different patients. *Follow your doctor's orders or the directions on the label.* The following information includes only the average doses of ursodiol. *If your dose is different, do not change it unless your doctor tells you to do so.*

The number of capsules that you take depends on the strength of the medicine. Also, *the number of doses you take each day, the time allowed between doses, and the length of time you take the medicine depend on the medical problem for which you are taking ursodiol.*
- For *oral* dosage form (capsules):
  —For gallstone disease:
    - Adults and children 12 years of age and older— The dose is based on body weight and must be determined by your doctor. The usual dose is 8 to 10 milligrams (mg) per kilogram (kg) (3.6 to 4.5 mg per pound) of body weight a day, divided into two or three doses. Each dose is usually taken with a meal.
    - Children up to 12 years of age—Use and dose must be determined by your doctor.

**Missed dose**—If you miss a dose of this medicine, take it as soon as possible or double your next dose.

**Storage**—To store this medicine:
- Keep out of the reach of children.
- Store away from heat and direct light.
- Do not store in the bathroom, near the kitchen sink, or in other damp places. Heat or moisture may cause the medicine to break down.
- Do not keep outdated medicine or medicine no longer needed. Be sure that any discarded medicine is out of the reach of children.

## Precautions While Using This Medicine

*It is important that your doctor check your progress at regular visits. Laboratory tests will have to be done every few months* while you are taking this medicine to make sure that the gallstones are dissolving and your liver is working properly.

Do not take aluminum-containing antacids (e.g., ALternaGEL, Maalox) while taking ursodiol. To do so may keep ursodiol from working properly. Before using an antacid, check with your health care professional.

*Check with your doctor immediately if severe abdominal or stomach pain, especially toward the upper right side, and severe nausea and vomiting occur.* These symptoms may mean that you have other medical problems or that your gallstone condition needs your doctor's attention.

## Side Effects of This Medicine

Along with its needed effects, a medicine may cause some unwanted effects. The following side effect may go away during treatment as your body adjusts to the medicine. However, check with your doctor if it continues or is bothersome:

*Less common or rare*
Diarrhea

Other side effects not listed above may also occur in some patients. If you notice any other effects, check with your doctor.

## Additional Information

Once a medicine has been approved for marketing for a certain use, experience may show that it is also useful for other medical problems. Although these uses are not included in product labeling, ursodiol is used in certain patients with the following medical conditions:

- Chronic liver disease
- Risk of gallstones (in patients who are in a weight-reduction program)
- Liver transplant (to help reduce the risk of rejection)

There is no additional information relating to proper use, precautions, or side effects for these uses.

Revised: 07/26/94

# VALPROIC ACID    Systemic

Some commonly used brand names are:

**In the U.S.—**

Depakene[2]                    Depakote Sprinkle[1]
Depakote[1]                    Myproic Acid[2]

**In Canada—**

Depakene[2]
Epival[1]

Note: For quick reference, the following medicines are numbered to match the corresponding brand names.

This information applies to the following medicines:

1. Divalproex (dye-VAL-pro-ex)
2. Valproic Acid (val-PRO-ic acid)‡

‡Generic name product may also be available in the U.S.

## Description

Valproic acid and divalproex belong to the group of medicines called anticonvulsants. They are used to control certain types of seizures in the treatment of epilepsy. Valproic acid and divalproex may be used alone or with other seizure medicine.

Divalproex forms valproic acid in the body. Therefore, the following information applies to both medicines.

This medicine is available only with your doctor's prescription, in the following dosage forms:

*Oral*

Divalproex
  • Delayed-release capsules (U.S.)
  • Delayed-release tablets (U.S. and Canada)
Valproic Acid
  • Capsules (U.S. and Canada)
  • Syrup (U.S. and Canada)

## Before Using This Medicine

In deciding to use a medicine, the risks of taking the medicine must be weighed against the good it will do. This is a decision you and your doctor will make. For valproic acid and divalproex, the following should be considered:

**Allergies**—Tell your doctor if you have ever had any unusual or allergic reaction to divalproex or valproic acid. Also tell your health care professional if you are allergic to any other substances, such as foods or dyes.

**Pregnancy**—Valproic acid and divalproex have been reported to cause birth defects when taken by the mother during the first 3 months of pregnancy. Also, animal studies have shown that valproic acid causes birth defects when taken in doses several times greater than doses used in humans. However, these medicines may be necessary to control seizures in some pregnant patients. Be sure you have discussed this with your doctor.

**Breast-feeding**—Valproic acid and divalproex pass into the breast milk, but their effect on the nursing baby is not known. It may be necessary for you to take another medicine or to stop breast-feeding during treatment with

valproic acid or divalproex. Be sure you have discussed the risks and benefits of this medicine with your doctor.

**Children**—Abdominal or stomach cramps, nausea or vomiting, tiredness or weakness, and yellow eyes or skin may be especially likely to occur in children, who are usually more sensitive to the effects of valproic acid and divalproex. Children up to 2 years of age and those taking more than 1 medicine for seizure control may be more likely to develop serious side effects.

**Older adults**—Elderly people are especially sensitive to the effects of valproic acid or divalproex. This may increase the chance of side effects during treatment.

**Other medicines**—Although certain medicines should not be used together at all, in other cases 2 different medicines may be used together even if an interaction might occur. In these cases, your doctor may want to change the dose, or other precautions may be necessary. When you are taking valproic acid or divalproex, it is especially important that your health care professional knows if you are taking any of the following:

  • Acetaminophen (e.g., Tylenol) (with long-term, high-dose use) or
  • Amiodarone (e.g., Cordarone) or
  • Anabolic steroids (nandrolone [e.g., Anabolin], oxandrolone [e.g., Anavar], oxymetholone [e.g., Anadrol], stanozolol [e.g., Winstrol]) or
  • Androgens (male hormones) or
  • Anti-infectives by mouth or injection (medicine for infection) or
  • Antithyroid agents (medicine for overactive thyroid) or
  • Barbiturates or
  • Carbamazepine (e.g., Tegretol) or
  • Carmustine (e.g., BiCNU) or
  • Chloroquine (e.g., Aralen) or
  • Dantrolene (e.g., Dantrium) or
  • Daunorubicin (e.g., Cerubidine) or
  • Disulfiram (e.g., Antabuse) or
  • Estrogens (female hormones) or
  • Etretinate (e.g., Tegison) or
  • Gold salts (medicine for arthritis) or
  • Hydroxychloroquine (e.g., Plaquenil) or
  • Mercaptopurine (e.g., Purinethol) or
  • Methotrexate (e.g., Mexate) or
  • Methyldopa (e.g., Aldomet) or
  • Naltrexone (e.g., Trexan) (with long-term, high-dose use) or
  • Oral contraceptives (birth control pills) containing estrogen or
  • Phenothiazines (acetophenazine [e.g., Tindal], chlorpromazine [e.g., Thorazine], fluphenazine [e.g., Prolixin], mesoridazine [e.g., Serentil], perphenazine [e.g., Trilafon], prochlorperazine [e.g., Compazine], promazine [e.g., Sparine], promethazine [e.g., Phenergan], thioridazine [e.g., Mellaril], trifluoperazine [e.g., Stelazine], triflupromazine [e.g., Vesprin], trimeprazine [e.g., Temaril]) or
  • Plicamycin (e.g., Mithracin)—There is an increased risk of serious side effects to the liver

- Central nervous system (CNS) depressants (medicine that causes drowsiness) or
- Tricyclic antidepressants (medicine for depression)—Valproic acid and divalproex may increase CNS depressant effects
- Carbenicillin by injection (e.g., Geopen)
- Dipyridamole (e.g., Persantine) or
- Inflammation or pain medicine, except narcotics, or
- Pentoxifylline (e.g., Trental) or
- Sulfinpyrazone (e.g., Anturane) or
- Ticarcillin (e.g., Ticar)—Valproic acid or divalproex may increase the chance of bleeding because of decreased blood clotting ability; the potential of aspirin, medicine for inflammation or pain, or sulfinpyrazone to cause stomach ulcer and bleeding may also increase the chance of bleeding in patients taking valproic acid or divalproex
- Heparin—There is an increased risk of side effects that may cause bleeding
- Mefloquine—The amount of valproic acid or divalproex that you need to take may change
- Other anticonvulsants (medicine for seizures)—There is an increased risk of seizures

**Other medical problems**—The presence of other medical problems may affect the use of valproic acid or divalproex. Make sure you tell your doctor if you have any other medical problems, especially:

- Blood disease or
- Brain disease or
- Kidney disease—There is an increased risk of serious side effects
- Liver disease—Valproic acid or divalproex may make the condition worse

## Proper Use of This Medicine

For patients taking *the capsule form* of valproic acid:

- Swallow the capsule whole without chewing or breaking. This is to prevent irritation of the mouth or throat.

For patients taking *the delayed-release capsule form* of divalproex:

- Swallow the capsule whole, or sprinkle the contents on a small amount of soft food such as applesauce or pudding and swallow without chewing.

For patients taking *the delayed-release tablet form* of this medicine:

- Swallow the tablet whole without chewing, breaking, or crushing. This is to prevent damage to the special coating that helps lessen irritation of the stomach.

For patients taking *the syrup form* of this medicine:

- The syrup may be mixed with any liquid or added to food for a better taste.

This medicine may be taken with meals or snacks to reduce stomach upset.

*This medicine must be taken exactly as directed* by your doctor to prevent seizures and lessen the possibility of side effects.

**Dosing**—The dose of valproic acid or divalproex will be different for different patients. *Follow your doctor's orders or the directions on the label.* The following information includes only the average doses of valproic acid or divalproex. *If your dose is different, do not change it* unless your doctor tells you to do so.

- The number of capsules or tablets or teaspoonfuls of syrup that you take depends on the strength of the medicine. Also, *the number of doses you take each day, the time allowed between doses, and the length of time you take the medicine depend on the medical problem for which you are using valproic acid or divalproex.*
- If valproic acid or divalproex is the only medicine you are taking for seizures:

  —Adults and adolescents: Dose is based on body weight. The usual dose is 5 to 15 milligrams per kilogram (2.3 to 6.9 milligrams per pound) of body weight to start. Your doctor may increase your dose gradually every week by 5 to 10 milligrams per kilogram of body weight if needed. However, the dose is usually not more than 60 milligrams per kilogram of body weight a day. If the total dose a day is greater than 250 milligrams, it is usually divided into smaller doses and taken two or more times during the day.

  —Children 1 to 12 years of age: Dose is based on body weight. The usual dose is 15 to 45 milligrams per kilogram (6.9 to 20.7 milligrams per pound) of body weight to start. The doctor may increase the dose gradually every week by 5 to 10 milligrams per kilogram of body weight if needed.

- If you are taking more than one medicine for seizures:

  —Adults and adolescents: Dose is based on body weight. The usual dose is 10 to 30 milligrams per kilogram (4.6 to 13.8 milligrams per pound) of body weight to start. Your doctor may increase your dose gradually every week by 5 to 10 milligrams per kilogram of body weight if needed. If the total dose a day is greater than 250 milligrams, it is usually divided into smaller doses and taken two or more times during the day.

  —Children 1 to 12 years of age: Dose is based on body weight. The usual dose is 30 to 100 milligrams per kilogram (13.8 to 45.5 milligrams per pound) of body weight.

**Missed dose**—If you miss a dose of this medicine, and your dosing schedule is:

- One dose a day—Take the missed dose as soon as possible. However, if you do not remember until the next day, skip the missed dose and go back to your regular dosing schedule. Do not double doses.
- Two or more doses a day—If you remember within 6 hours of the missed dose, take it right away. Then take the rest of the doses for that day at equally spaced times. Do not double doses.

If you have any questions about this, check with your doctor.

**Storage**—To store this medicine:
- Keep out of the reach of children.
- Store away from heat and direct light.
- Do not store the capsule or tablet form of this medicine in the bathroom, near the kitchen sink, or in other damp places. Heat or moisture may cause the medicine to break down.
- Keep the syrup form of this medicine from freezing.
- Do not keep outdated medicine or medicine no longer needed. Be sure that any discarded medicine is out of the reach of children.

## Precautions While Using This Medicine

*Your doctor should check your progress at regular visits,* especially for the first few months you take this medicine. This is necessary to allow dose adjustments and to reduce any unwanted effects.

*Do not stop taking valproic acid or divalproex without first checking with your doctor.* Your doctor may want you to gradually reduce the amount you are taking before stopping completely. Stopping the medicine suddenly may cause you to have seizures again.

Before you have any medical tests, tell the doctor in charge that you are taking this medicine. The results of the metyrapone and thyroid function tests may be affected by this medicine.

*Before having any kind of surgery, dental treatment, or emergency treatment, tell the medical doctor or dentist in charge that you are taking this medicine.* Valproic acid or divalproex may change the time it takes your blood to clot, which may increase the chance of bleeding. Also, taking valproic acid or divalproex together with medicines that are used during surgery or dental or emergency treatments may increase the CNS depressant effects.

Valproic acid and divalproex will add to the effects of alcohol and other CNS depressants (medicines that slow down the nervous system, possibly causing drowsiness). Some examples of CNS depressants are antihistamines or medicine for hay fever, other allergies, or colds; sedatives, tranquilizers, or sleeping medicine; prescription pain medicine or narcotics; barbiturates; medicine for seizures; muscle relaxants; or anesthetics, including some dental anesthetics. *Check with your doctor before taking any of the above while you are using this medicine.*

For diabetic patients:
- This medicine may interfere with urine tests for ketones and give false-positive results.

Your doctor may want you to carry a medical identification card or bracelet stating that you are taking this medicine.

This medicine may cause some people to become drowsy or less alert than they are normally. *Make sure you know how you react to this medicine before you drive, use machines, or do anything else that could be dangerous if you are not alert.*

## Side Effects of This Medicine

Along with its needed effects, a medicine may cause some unwanted effects. Although not all of these side effects may occur, if they do occur they may need medical attention.

Check with your doctor as soon as possible if any of the following side effects occur:

*Less common*
Abdominal or stomach cramps (severe); behavioral, mood, or mental changes; continuous, uncontrolled back-and-forth and/or rolling eye movements; double vision; increase in seizures; loss of appetite; nausea or vomiting (continuing); spots before eyes; swelling of face; tiredness and weakness; unusual bleeding or bruising; yellow eyes or skin

Other side effects may occur that usually do not need medical attention. These side effects may go away during treatment as your body adjusts to the medicine. However, check with your doctor if any of the following side effects continue or are bothersome:

*More common*
Abdominal or stomach cramps (mild); change in menstrual periods; diarrhea; hair loss; indigestion; loss of appetite; nausea and vomiting; trembling of hands and arms; unusual weight loss or gain

*Less common or rare*
Clumsiness or unsteadiness; constipation; dizziness; drowsiness; headache; skin rash; unusual excitement, restlessness, or irritability

Other side effects not listed above may also occur in some patients. If you notice any other effects, check with your doctor.

## Additional Information

Once a medicine has been approved for marketing for a certain use, experience may show that it is also useful for other medical problems. Although these uses are not included in product labeling, valproic acid and divalproex are used in certain patients with the following medical condition:
- Bipolar disorder (manic-depressive illness)

Other than the above information, there is no additional information relating to proper use, precautions, or side effects for this use.

Revised: 03/09/93
Interim revision: 11/04/93

© 1994   The United States Pharmacopeial Convention, Inc.

# VANCOMYCIN  Oral

A commonly used brand name in the U.S. and Canada is Vancocin.

## Description

Vancomycin (van-koe-MYE-sin) belongs to the family of medicines called antibiotics. Antibiotics are medicines used in the treatment of infections caused by bacteria.

Vancomycin is taken by mouth to treat a certain type of diarrhea or colitis (an inflammation of the large intestine) caused by a certain type of bacteria. Vancomycin will not work for colds, flu, or other virus infections. Vancomycin may also be used for other conditions as determined by your doctor.

Vancomycin is available only with your doctor's prescription, in the following dosage forms:

*Oral*
- Capsules (U.S. and Canada)
- Oral solution (U.S.)

## Before Using This Medicine

In deciding to use a medicine, the risks of taking the medicine must be weighed against the good it will do. This is a decision you and your doctor will make. For oral vancomycin, the following should be considered:

**Allergies**—Tell your doctor if you have ever had any unusual or allergic reaction to oral vancomycin. Also tell your health care professional if you are allergic to any other substances, such as foods, preservatives, or dyes.

**Pregnancy**—Studies with oral vancomycin have not been done in either humans or animals.

**Breast-feeding**—Vancomycin passes into the breast milk. However, when taken by mouth, only small amounts of vancomycin are absorbed into the mother's body. In addition, vancomycin is not absorbed very much from the digestive tract (stomach and intestines) of the nursing infant.

**Children**—Although there is no specific information comparing use of oral vancomycin in children with use in other age groups, this medicine is not expected to cause different side effects or problems in children than it does in adults.

**Older adults**—Many medicines have not been studied specifically in older people. Therefore, it may not be known whether they work exactly the same way they do in younger adults. Although there is no specific information comparing use of oral vancomycin in the elderly with use in other age groups, this medicine is not expected to cause different side effects or problems in older people than it does in younger adults.

**Other medicines**—Although certain medicines should not be used together at all, in other cases two different medicines may be used together even if an interaction might occur. In these cases, your doctor may want to change

the dose, or other precautions may be necessary. When you are taking oral vancomycin, it is especially important that your health care professional know if you are taking any of the following:

- Cholestyramine (e.g., Questran) or
- Colestipol (e.g., Colestid)—Use of these medicines with oral vancomycin may decrease the effects of oral vancomycin; oral vancomycin and these medicines should be taken several hours apart

**Other medical problems**—The presence of other medical problems may affect the use of oral vancomycin. Make sure you tell your doctor if you have any other medical problems, especially:

- Kidney disease, severe, or
- Other inflammatory bowel disorders—Patients with these medical problems may have an increased chance of side effects

## Proper Use of This Medicine

For patients taking the *oral liquid form* of vancomycin:

- Use a specially marked measuring spoon or other device to measure each dose accurately. The average household teaspoon may not hold the right amount of liquid.
- Do not use after the expiration date on the label. The medicine may not work properly after that date. Check with your pharmacist if you have any questions about this.

To help clear up your colitis completely, *keep taking this medicine for the full time of treatment,* even if you begin to feel better after a few days. If you stop taking this medicine too soon, your symptoms may return. *Do not miss any doses.*

**Dosing**—The dose of oral vancomycin will be different for different patients. *Follow your doctor's orders or the directions on the label.* The following information includes only the average doses of oral vancomycin. *If your dose is different, do not change it* unless your doctor tells you to do so.

The number of capsules or teaspoonfuls of solution that you take depends on the strength of the medicine. Also, *the number of doses you take each day, the time allowed between doses, and the length of time you take the medicine depend on the medical problem for which you are taking oral vancomycin.*

- For *oral* dosage forms (capsules, oral solution):
  —For treatment of colitis or severe diarrhea:
  - Adults and teenagers—125 to 500 milligrams (mg) every six hours for five to ten days.
  - Children—Dose is based on body weight and must be determined by the doctor. The usual dose is 10 mg per kilogram (kg) of body weight (4.5 mg per pound), up to 125 mg. This dose is taken every six hours for five to ten days.

**Missed dose**—If you miss a dose of this medicine, take it as soon as possible. However, if it is almost time for your next dose, skip the missed dose and go back to your regular dosing schedule. Do not double doses.

**Storage**—To store this medicine:
- Keep out of the reach of children.
- Store away from heat and direct light.
- Do not store the capsule form of this medicine in the bathroom, near the kitchen sink, or in other damp places. Heat or moisture may cause the medicine to break down.
- Store the oral liquid form of vancomycin in the refrigerator because heat will cause this medicine to break down. However, keep the medicine from freezing. Follow the directions on the label.
- Do not keep outdated medicine or medicine no longer needed. Be sure that any discarded medicine is out of the reach of children.

## Precautions While Using This Medicine

It is important that your doctor check your progress during and after treatment. This is to make sure that the colitis is cleared up completely.

If the symptoms of your colitis do not improve within a few days, or if they become worse, check with your doctor.

*If your doctor orders cholestyramine or colestipol for your colitis, do not take vancomycin by mouth within 3 to 4 hours of taking either of these medicines.* To do so may keep vancomycin from working properly.

*If you are taking this medicine for diarrhea caused by other antibiotics, do not take any other diarrhea medicine* without first checking with your health care professional. Medicines for diarrhea may make your diarrhea worse or make it last longer.

## Side Effects of This Medicine

Along with its needed effects, a medicine may cause some unwanted effects. Although not all of these side effects may occur, if they do occur they may need medical attention.

*Check with your doctor immediately* if the following side effect occurs:

*Rare*
   Skin rash

Other side effects may occur that usually do not need medical attention. These side effects may go away during treatment as your body adjusts to the medicine. However, check with your doctor if any of the following side effects continue or are bothersome:

*More common*
   Bitter or unpleasant taste; mouth irritation; nausea or vomiting

Other side effects not listed above may also occur in some patients. If you notice any other effects, check with your doctor.

Revised: 08/10/94

---

# VANCOMYCIN   Systemic

Some commonly used brand names are:

**In the U.S.—**
   Lyphocin                    Vancoled
   Vancocin
   Generic name product may also be available.

**In Canada—**
   Vancocin

## Description

Vancomycin (van-koe-MYE-sin) belongs to the family of medicines called antibiotics. Antibiotics are medicines used in the treatment of infections caused by bacteria. They work by killing bacteria or preventing their growth. Vancomycin will not work for colds, flu, or other virus infections.

Vancomycin is used to treat infections in many different parts of the body. It is sometimes given with other antibiotics. Vancomycin is also used in patients with heart valve disease (e.g., rheumatic fever) or prosthetic (artificial) heart valves who are allergic to penicillin. This medicine is used to prevent endocarditis (inflammation of the lining of the heart) in these patients who are having dental work or surgery done on the upper respiratory tract (for example, nose or throat). Vancomycin may also be used for other conditions as determined by your doctor.

Vancomycin given by injection is usually used for serious infections in which other medicines may not work. However, this medicine may also cause some serious side effects, including damage to your hearing and kidneys. These side effects may be more likely to occur in elderly patients. You and your doctor should talk about the good this medicine will do as well as the risks of receiving it.

Vancomycin is available only with your doctor's prescription, in the following dosage form:

*Parenteral*
- Injection (U.S. and Canada)

## Before Receiving This Medicine

In deciding to use a medicine, the risks of taking the medicine must be weighed against the good it will do.

This is a decision you and your doctor will make. For vancomycin, the following should be considered:

**Allergies**—Tell your doctor if you have ever had any unusual or allergic reaction to vancomycin. Also tell your health care professional if you are allergic to any other substances, such as foods, preservatives, or dyes.

**Pregnancy**—Vancomycin has not been reported to cause hearing loss or kidney damage in the infants of women given vancomycin during their second or third trimesters of pregnancy. It has also not been reported to cause birth defects in animal studies.

**Breast-feeding**—Vancomycin passes into breast milk. However, this medicine has not been reported to cause problems in nursing babies.

**Children**—Vancomycin can cause serious side effects in any patient. Therefore, it is especially important that you discuss with the child's doctor the good that this medicine will do as well as the risks of using it.

**Older adults**—Elderly people may be especially sensitive to the effects of vancomycin. This may increase the chance of hearing or kidney damage.

**Other medicines**—Although certain medicines should not be used together at all, in other cases two different medicines may be used together even if an interaction might occur. In these cases, your doctor may want to change the dose, or other precautions may be necessary. When you are receiving vancomycin, it is especially important that your health care professional knows if you are taking any of the following:

- Aminoglycosides by injection (amikacin [e.g., Amikin], gentamicin [e.g., Garamycin], kanamycin [e.g., Kantrex], neomycin [e.g., Mycifradin], netilmicin [e.g., Netromycin], streptomycin, tobramycin [e.g., Nebcin]) or
- Amphotericin B by injection (e.g., Fungizone) or
- Bacitracin by injection or
- Bumetanide by injection (e.g., Bumex) or
- Capreomycin (e.g., Capastat) or
- Cisplatin (e.g., Platinol) or
- Cyclosporine (e.g., Sandimmune) or
- Ethacrynic acid by injection (e.g., Edecrin) or
- Furosemide by injection (e.g., Lasix) or
- Paromomycin (e.g., Humatin) or
- Polymyxins, especially colistimethate (e.g., Coly-Mycin M) and polymyxin B (e.g., Aerosporin) or
- Streptozocin (e.g., Zanosar)—Use of these medicines with vancomycin may increase the chance of side effects

**Other medical problems**—The presence of other medical problems may affect the use of vancomycin. Make sure you tell your doctor if you have any other medical problems, especially:

- Kidney disease or
- Loss of hearing, or deafness, history of—Patients with kidney disease or a history of hearing loss or deafness may have an increased chance of side effects

## Proper Use of This Medicine

Some medicines given by injection may sometimes be given at home to patients who do not need to be in the hospital for the full time of treatment. If you are receiving this medicine at home, *make sure you clearly understand and carefully follow your doctor's instructions*.

To help clear up your infection completely, *vancomycin must be given for the full time of treatment*, even if you begin to feel better after a few days. Also, this medicine works best when there is a constant amount in the blood or stool. To help keep the amount constant, vancomycin must be given on a regular schedule.

**Dosing**—The dose of vancomycin will be different for different patients. *Follow your doctor's orders or the directions on the label*. The following information includes only the average doses of vancomycin. *If your dose is different, do not change it* unless your doctor tells you to do so.

- For *injection* dosage form:
    —For the prevention of heart infection in patients who have heart valve problems and are allergic to penicillin:
    - Adults and teenagers—1 gram injected into a vein one hour before dental work or surgery, and 1 gram injected into a vein 8 hours after the first dose.
    - Children—20 milligrams (mg) per kilogram (kg) (9.1 mg per pound) of body weight injected into a vein one hour before a dental procedure or surgery, and 20 mg per kg (9.1 mg per pound) of body weight injected into a vein 8 hours after the first dose.
    —For treatment of bacterial infections:
    - Adults and teenagers—7.5 mg per kg (3.4 mg per pound) of body weight, or 500 mg, injected into a vein every six hours; or 15 mg per kg (6.8 mg per pound) of body weight, or 1 gram, injected into a vein every twelve hours.
    - Children—10 mg per kg (4.5 mg per pound) of body weight injected into a vein every six hours; or 20 mg per kg (9.1 mg per pound) of body weight injected into a vein every twelve hours.
    - Newborns and infants 1 week to 1 month of age—15 mg per kg (6.8 mg per pound) of body weight injected into a vein at first, then 10 mg per kg (4.5 mg per pound) of body weight injected into a vein every eight hours.
    - Newborns up to 1 week of age—15 mg per kg (6.8 mg per pound) of body weight injected into a vein at first, then 10 mg per kg (4.5 mg per pound) of body weight injected into a vein every twelve hours.

## Side Effects of This Medicine

Along with its needed effects, a medicine may cause some unwanted effects. Although not all of these side effects may occur, if they do occur they may need medical attention.

*Check with your health care professional immediately* if any of the following side effects occur:

*Less common*

Change in the frequency of urination or amount of urine; difficulty in breathing; drowsiness; increased thirst; loss of appetite; nausea or vomiting; weakness

*Rare*

Loss of hearing; ringing or buzzing or a feeling of fullness in the ears

Note: The above side effects may also occur up to several weeks after you stop receiving this medicine.

*Symptoms of "red-neck syndrome"—Rare*

Chills or fever; fainting; fast heartbeat; itching; nausea or vomiting; rash or redness of the face, base of neck, upper body, back, and arms; tingling; unpleasant taste

Note: Symptoms of the "red-neck syndrome" are more common when vancomycin is given by direct or rapid injection.

The above side effects, except the "red-neck syndrome," are more likely to occur in the elderly, who are usually more sensitive to the effects of vancomycin.

Other side effects not listed above may also occur in some patients. If you notice any other effects, check with your doctor.

Revised: 09/20/92
Interim revision: 03/28/94

---

# VASOPRESSIN   Systemic

Some commonly used brand names are:

**In the U.S.—**
Pitressin
Generic name product may also be available.

**In Canada—**
Pitressin                                    Pressyn

## Description

Vasopressin (vay-soe-PRESS-in) is a hormone naturally produced by your body. It is necessary to maintain good health. Lack of vasopressin causes your body to lose too much water.

Vasopressin is used to control the frequent urination, increased thirst, and loss of water associated with diabetes insipidus (water diabetes).

Vasopressin also may be used for other conditions as determined by your doctor.

This medicine is available only with your doctor's prescription, in the following dosage form:

*Parenteral*
• Injection (U.S. and Canada)

## Before Receiving This Medicine

In deciding to use a medicine, the risks of taking the medicine must be weighed against the good it will do. This is a decision you and your doctor will make. For vasopressin, the following should be considered:

**Allergies**—Tell your doctor if you have ever had any unusual or allergic reaction to vasopressin. Also tell your health care professional if you are allergic to any other substances, such as foods, preservatives, or dyes.

**Pregnancy**—Vasopressin has not been shown to cause birth defects or other problems in humans.

**Breast-feeding**—Vasopressin has not been reported to cause problems in nursing babies.

**Children**—Children may be especially sensitive to the effects of vasopressin. This may increase the chance of side effects during treatment.

**Older adults**—Many medicines have not been studied specifically in older people. Therefore, it may not be known whether they work exactly the same way they do in younger adults or if they cause different side effects or problems in older people. Although there is no specific information comparing the use of vasopressin in the elderly with use in other age groups, the elderly may be more sensitive to its effects.

**Other medicines**—Although certain medicines should not be used together at all, in other cases two different medicines may be used together even if an interaction might occur. In these cases, your doctor may want to change the dose, or other precautions may be necessary. Tell your health care professional if you are taking any other prescription or nonprescription (over-the-counter [OTC]) medicine.

**Other medical problems**—The presence of other medical problems may affect the use of vasopressin. Make sure you tell your doctor if you have any other medical problems, especially:

• Asthma or
• Epilepsy or
• Heart disease or
• Kidney disease or
• Migraine headaches—If fluid retention (keeping more body water) caused by vasopressin occurs too fast, these conditions may be worsened
• Heart or blood vessel disease—Vasopressin can cause chest pain or a heart attack; it can also increase blood pressure

## Proper Use of This Medicine

*Use this medicine only as directed.* Do not use more of it and do not use it more often than your doctor ordered. To do so may increase the chance of side effects.

**Dosing**—The dose of vasopressin will be different for different patients. *Follow your doctor's orders or the directions on the label.* The following information includes only the average doses of vasopressin. *If your dose is different, do not change it* unless your doctor tells you to do so.

- For *injection* dosage form:
  - —For controlling water loss when urinating too often (diabetes insipidus):
    - Adults and teenagers—5 to 10 Units injected into a muscle or under the skin two or three times a day as needed.
    - Children—2.5 to 10 Units injected into a muscle or under the skin three or four times a day.

**Missed dose**—If you miss a dose of this medicine, use it as soon as possible. However, if it is almost time for your next dose, skip the missed dose and go back to your regular dosing schedule. Do not double doses.

**Storage**—To store this medicine:

- Keep out of the reach of children.
- Store away from heat and direct light.
- Keep from freezing.
- Do not keep outdated medicine or medicine no longer needed. Be sure that any discarded medicine is out of the reach of children.

## Side Effects of This Medicine

Along with its needed effects, a medicine may cause some unwanted effects. Although not all of these effects may occur, if they do occur they may need medical attention.

*Check with your doctor immediately* if any of the following side effects occur since they may be signs or symptoms of an allergic reaction or overdose:

*Rare*

Chest pain; coma; confusion; convulsions (seizures); drowsiness; fever; headache (continuing); problems with urination; redness of skin; skin rash, hives, or itching; swelling of face, feet, hands, or mouth; weight gain; wheezing or troubled breathing

Other side effects may occur that usually do not need medical attention. These side effects may go away during treatment as your body adjusts to the medicine. However, check with your doctor if any of the following side effects continue or are bothersome:

*Less common*

Abdominal or stomach cramps; belching; diarrhea; dizziness or lightheadedness; increased sweating; increased urge for bowel movement; nausea or vomiting; pale skin; passage of gas; "pounding" in head; trembling; white-colored area around mouth

Other side effects not listed above may also occur in some patients. If you notice any other effects, check with your doctor.

Revised: 08/26/93
Interim revision: 06/30/94

---

# VIDARABINE    Ophthalmic

A commonly used brand name in the U.S. and Canada is Vira-A. Other commonly used names are arabinoside and ara-A.

## Description

Vidarabine (vye-DARE-a-been) ophthalmic preparations are used to treat virus infections of the eye.

Vidarabine is available only with your doctor's prescription, in the following dosage form:

*Ophthalmic*
- Ophthalmic ointment (U.S. and Canada)

## Before Using This Medicine

In deciding to use a medicine, the risks of using the medicine must be weighed against the good it will do. This is a decision you and your doctor will make. For vidarabine, the following should be considered:

**Allergies**—Tell your doctor if you have ever had any unusual or allergic reaction to vidarabine. Also tell your health care professional if you are allergic to any other substances, such as preservatives.

**Pregnancy**—Studies have not been done in humans. Studies in rats and rabbits have shown that vidarabine, given by injection, causes birth defects. In addition, studies in rabbits have shown that vidarabine, applied as a 10% ointment to the skin, may cause birth defects or other problems. However, these doses are much higher than those used in the eyes of humans. Therefore, the chance that vidarabine ophthalmic ointment would cause birth defects or other problems in humans is very small.

**Breast-feeding**—It is not known whether vidarabine, applied to the eyes, is absorbed into the body and passes into the breast milk. Although most medicines pass into breast milk in small amounts, many of them may be used safely while breast-feeding. Mothers who are taking this medicine and who wish to breast-feed should discuss this with their doctor.

---

© 1994   The United States Pharmacopeial Convention, Inc.

**Children**—Although there is no specific information comparing use of vidarabine in children with use in other age groups, it is not expected to cause different side effects or problems in children than it does in adults.

**Older adults**—Many medicines have not been studied specifically in older people. Therefore, it may not be known whether they work exactly the same way they do in younger adults or if they cause different side effects or problems in older people. There is no specific information comparing use of vidarabine in the elderly with use in other age groups.

**Other medicines**—Although certain medicines should not be used together at all, in other cases two different medicines may be used together even if an interaction might occur. In these cases, your doctor may want to change the dose, or other precautions may be necessary. Tell your health care professional if you are using any other prescription or nonprescription (over-the-counter [OTC]) medicine in your eyes.

## Proper Use of This Medicine

To use:

- First, wash your hands. Then pull the lower eyelid away from the eye to form a pouch. Squeeze a thin strip of ointment into the pouch. A 1.25-cm (approximately ½-inch) strip of ointment is usually enough unless otherwise directed by your doctor. Gently close the eyes and keep them closed for 1 or 2 minutes to allow the medicine to come into contact with the infection.
- To keep the medicine as germ-free as possible, do not touch the applicator tip to any surface (including the eye). After using vidarabine eye ointment, wipe the tip of the ointment tube with a clean tissue and keep the tube tightly closed.

*Do not use this medicine more often or for a longer time than your doctor ordered.* To do so may cause problems in the eyes. If you have any questions about this, check with your doctor.

To help clear up your infection completely, *keep using this medicine for the full time of treatment,* even if your symptoms have disappeared. *Do not miss any doses.*

**Dosing**—The dose of ophthalmic vidarabine will be different for different patients. *Follow your doctor's orders or the directions on the label.* The following information includes only the average doses of ophthalmic vidarabine. *If your dose is different, do not change it* unless your doctor tells you to do so.

*The number of doses you use each day, the time allowed between doses, and the length of time you use the medicine depend on the medical problem for which you are using ophthalmic vidarabine.*

- For *ophthalmic ointment* dosage forms:
  —For virus eye infection:
    - Adults and children—Use in each eye every three hours (five times a day). After healing has occurred, the dose may be reduced to two times a day for seven days more.

**Missed dose**—If you miss a dose of this medicine, apply it as soon as possible. However, if it is almost time for your next dose, skip the missed dose and go back to your regular dosing schedule.

**Storage**—To store this medicine:

- Keep out of the reach of children.
- Store away from heat and direct light.
- Keep the medicine from freezing.
- Do not keep outdated medicine or medicine no longer needed. Be sure that any discarded medicine is out of the reach of children.

## Precautions While Using This Medicine

After application, eye ointments usually cause your vision to blur for a few minutes.

It is very important that you keep your appointments with your doctor. If your symptoms become worse, check with your doctor sooner.

This medicine may cause your eyes to become more sensitive to light than they are normally. Wearing sunglasses and avoiding too much exposure to bright light may help lessen the discomfort.

## Side Effects of This Medicine

Along with its needed effects, a medicine may cause some unwanted effects. Although not all of these side effects may occur, if they do occur they may need medical attention.

Check with your doctor as soon as possible if any of the following side effects occur:

Increased sensitivity of eyes to light; itching, redness, swelling, pain, burning, or other sign of irritation not present before use of this medicine

Other side effects may occur that usually do not need medical attention. These side effects may go away during treatment as your body adjusts to the medicine. However, check with your doctor if either of the following side effects continues or is bothersome:

Excess flow of tears; feeling of something in the eye

Other side effects not listed above may also occur in some patients. If you notice any other effects, check with your doctor.

Revised: 07/01/93

---

# VINBLASTINE    Systemic

**In the U.S.—**
  Velban
  Velsar
  Generic name product may also be available.
**In Canada—**
  Velbe

## Description

Vinblastine (vin-BLAS-teen) belongs to the group of medicines known as antineoplastic agents. It is used to treat some kinds of cancer as well as some noncancerous conditions.

Vinblastine interferes with the growth of cancer cells, which are eventually destroyed. Since the growth of normal body cells may also be affected by vinblastine, other effects will also occur. Some of these may be serious and must be reported to your doctor. Other effects, such as hair loss, may not be serious but may cause concern. Some effects do not occur for months or years after the medicine is used.

Before you begin treatment with vinblastine, you and your doctor should talk about the good this medicine will do as well as the risks of using it.

Vinblastine is to be administered only by or under the immediate supervision of your doctor. It is available in the following dosage form:

*Parenteral*
  • Injection (U.S. and Canada)

## Before Using This Medicine

In deciding to use a medicine, the risks of taking the medicine must be weighed against the good it will do. This is a decision you and your doctor will make. For vinblastine, the following should be considered:

**Allergies**—Tell your doctor if you have ever had any unusual or allergic reaction to vinblastine.

**Pregnancy**—Tell your doctor if you are pregnant or if you intend to have children. This medicine may cause birth defects if either the male or female is taking it at the time of conception or if it is taken during pregnancy. In addition, many cancer medicines may cause sterility which could be permanent. Although sterility has not been reported with this medicine, vinblastine may interfere with production of sperm and the possibility should be kept in mind.

Be sure that you have discussed this with your doctor before receiving this medicine. It is best to use some kind of birth control while you are receiving vinblastine. Tell your doctor right away if you think you have become pregnant while receiving vinblastine.

**Breast-feeding**—Tell your doctor if you are breast-feeding or if you intend to breast-feed during treatment with this medicine. Because vinblastine may cause serious side effects, breast-feeding is generally not recommended while you are receiving it.

**Children**—This medicine has been tested in children and has not been shown to cause different side effects or problems than it does in adults.

**Older adults**—Many medicines have not been tested in older people. Therefore, it may not be known whether they work exactly the same way they do in younger adults or if they cause different side effects or problems in older people. There is no specific information about the use of vinblastine in the elderly.

**Other medicines**—Although certain medicines should not be used together at all, in other cases two different medicines may be used together even if an interaction might occur. In these cases, your doctor may want to change the dose, or other precautions may be necessary. When you are receiving vinblastine, it is especially important that your health care professional know if you are taking any of the following:

  • Amphotericin B by injection (e.g., Fungizone) or
  • Antithyroid agents (medicine for overactive thyroid) or
  • Azathioprine (e.g., Imuran) or
  • Chloramphenicol (e.g., Chloromycetin) or
  • Colchicine or
  • Flucytosine (e.g., Ancobon) or
  • Interferon (e.g., Intron A, Roferon-A) or
  • Plicamycin (e.g., Mithracin) or
  • Zidovudine (e.g., Retrovir) or
  • If you have ever been treated with x-rays or cancer medicines—Vinblastine may increase the effects of these medicines or radiation therapy on the blood
  • Probenecid (e.g., Benemid) or
  • Sulfinpyrazone (e.g., Anturane)—Vinblastine may increase the concentration of uric acid in the blood, which these medicines are used to lower

**Other medical problems**—The presence of other medical problems may affect the use of vinblastine. Make sure you tell your doctor if you have any other medical problems, especially:

  • Chickenpox (including recent exposure) or
  • Herpes zoster (shingles)—Risk of severe disease affecting other parts of the body
  • Gout (history of) or
  • Kidney stones (history of)—Vinblastine may increase levels of uric acid in the body, which can cause gout or kidney stones
  • Infection—Vinblastine can reduce immunity to infection
  • Liver disease—Effects may be increased because of slower removal of vinblastine from the body

## Proper Use of This Medicine

Vinblastine is sometimes given together with certain other medicines. If you are using a combination of medicines, it is important that you receive each one at the proper time. If you are taking some of these medicines by mouth, ask your health care professional to help you plan a way to take them at the right times.

While you are using this medicine, your doctor may want you to drink extra fluids so that you will pass more urine. This will help prevent kidney problems and keep your kidneys working well.

Vinblastine sometimes causes nausea and vomiting. However, it is very important that you continue to receive the medicine, even if you begin to feel ill. Ask your health care professional for ways to lessen these effects.

**Dosing**—The dose of vinblastine will be different for different patients. The dose that is used may depend on a number of things, including what the medicine is being used for, the patient's weight or size, and whether or not other medicines are also being taken. *If you are receiving vinblastine at home, follow your doctor's orders or the directions on the label.* If you have any questions about the proper dose of vinblastine, ask your doctor.

## Precautions While Using This Medicine

*It is very important that your doctor check your progress at regular visits* to make sure that this medicine is working properly and to check for unwanted effects.

While you are being treated with vinblastine, and after you stop treatment with it, *do not have any immunizations (vaccinations) without your doctor's approval.* Vinblastine may lower your body's resistance and there is a chance you might get the infection the immunization is meant to prevent. Other people living in your household should not take oral polio vaccine since there is a chance they could pass the polio virus on to you. Also, avoid persons who have taken oral polio vaccine. Do not get close to them, and do not stay in the same room with them for very long. If you cannot take these precautions, you should consider wearing a protective face mask that covers the nose and mouth.

Vinblastine can temporarily lower the number of white blood cells in your blood, increasing the chance of getting an infection. It can also lower the number of platelets, which are necessary for proper blood clotting. If this occurs, there are certain precautions you can take, especially when your blood count is low, to reduce the risk of infection or bleeding:

- If you can, avoid people with infections. *Check with your doctor immediately* if you think you are getting an infection or if you get a fever or chills, cough or hoarseness, lower back or side pain, or painful or difficult urination.
- *Check with your doctor immediately* if you notice any unusual bleeding or bruising; black, tarry stools; blood in urine or stools; or pinpoint red spots on your skin.
- Be careful when using a regular toothbrush, dental floss, or toothpick. Your medical doctor, dentist, or nurse may recommend other ways to clean your teeth and gums. Check with your medical doctor before having any dental work done.

- Do not touch your eyes or the inside of your nose unless you have just washed your hands and have not touched anything else in the meantime.
- Be careful not to cut yourself when you are using sharp objects such as a safety razor or fingernail or toenail cutters.
- Avoid contact sports or other situations where bruising or injury could occur.

If vinblastine accidentally seeps out of the vein into which it is injected, it may damage the skin and cause some scarring. *Tell the doctor or nurse right away if you notice redness, pain, or swelling at the place of injection.*

## Side Effects of This Medicine

Along with their needed effects medicines like vinblastine can sometimes cause unwanted effects such as blood problems, loss of hair, and other side effects. These and others are described below. Also, because of the way these medicines act on the body, there is a chance that they might cause other unwanted effects that may not occur until months or years after the medicine is used. These delayed effects may include certain types of cancer, such as leukemia. Discuss these possible effects with your doctor.

Although not all of these side effects may occur, if they do occur they may need medical attention.

*Check with your doctor or nurse immediately* if any of the following side effects occur:

*Less common*

Cough or hoarseness; fever or chills; lower back or side pain; painful or difficult urination; pain or redness at place of injection

*Rare*

Black, tarry stools; blood in urine or stools; pinpoint red spots on skin; unusual bleeding or bruising

Check with your health care professional as soon as possible if any of the following side effects occur:

*Less common*

Joint pain; sores in mouth and on lips; swelling of feet or lower legs

*Rare*

Difficulty in walking; dizziness; double vision; drooping eyelids; headache; jaw pain; mental depression; numbness or tingling in fingers and toes; pain in fingers and toes; pain in testicles; weakness

Other side effects may occur that usually do not need medical attention. These side effects may go away during treatment as your body adjusts to the medicine. Also, your health care professional may be able to tell you about ways to prevent or reduce some of these side effects. Check with your health care professional if any of the following side effects continue or are bothersome or if you have any questions about them:

*Less common*
Muscle pain; nausea and vomiting

This medicine often causes a temporary loss of hair. After treatment with vinblastine has ended, or sometimes even during treatment, normal hair growth should return.

Other side effects not listed above may also occur in some patients. If you notice any other effects, check with your doctor.

Revised: 09/90
Interim revision(s): 08/02/93; 07/05/94

# VINCRISTINE  Systemic

Some commonly used brand names are:

**In the U.S.—**
Oncovin
Vincasar PFS
Vincrex
Generic name product may also be available.

**In Canada—**
Oncovin

## Description

Vincristine (vin-KRIS-teen) belongs to the group of medicines known as antineoplastic agents. It is used to treat some kinds of cancer as well as some noncancerous conditions.

Vincristine interferes with the growth of cancer cells, which are eventually destroyed. Since the growth of normal body cells may also be affected by vincristine, other effects will also occur. Some of these may be serious and must be reported to your doctor. Other effects, such as hair loss, may not be serious but may cause concern. Some effects may not occur for months or years after the medicine is used.

Before you begin treatment with vincristine, you and your doctor should talk about the good this medicine will do as well as the risks of using it.

Vincristine is to be administered only by or under the immediate supervision of your doctor. It is available in the following dosage form:

*Parenteral*
• Injection (U.S. and Canada)

## Before Using This Medicine

In deciding to use a medicine, the risks of taking the medicine must be weighed against the good it will do. This is a decision you and your doctor will make. For vincristine, the following should be considered:

**Allergies**—Tell your doctor if you have ever had any unusual or allergic reaction to vincristine.

**Pregnancy**—Tell your doctor if you are pregnant or if you intend to have children. There is a chance that this medicine may cause birth defects if either the male or female is taking it at the time of conception or if it is taken during pregnancy. Vincristine causes birth defects and death of the fetus in animals. In addition, many cancer medicines may cause sterility, which could be permanent. Although sterility has not been reported with this medicine, the possibility should be kept in mind.

Be sure that you have discussed this with your doctor before receiving this medicine. It is best to use some kind of birth control while you are receiving vincristine. Tell your doctor right away if you think you have become pregnant while receiving vincristine.

**Breast-feeding**—Tell your doctor if you are breast-feeding or if you intend to breast-feed during treatment with this medicine. Because vincristine may cause serious side effects, breast-feeding is generally not recommended while you are receiving it.

**Children**—This medicine has been tested in children and has not been shown to cause different side effects or problems than it does in adults.

**Older adults**—Nervous system effects may be more likely to occur in the elderly, who are usually more sensitive to the effects of vincristine.

**Other medicines**—Although certain medicines should not be used together at all, in other cases two different medicines may be used together even if an interaction might occur. In these cases, your doctor may want to change the dose, or other precautions may be necessary. When you are receiving vincristine, it is especially important that your health care professional know if you are taking any of the following:

• Probenecid (e.g., Benemid) or
• Sulfinpyrazone (e.g., Anturane)—Vincristine may increase the concentration of uric acid in the blood, which these medicines are used to lower
• If you have ever been treated with x-rays or cancer medicines—Vincristine may increase the effects of these medicines or radiation therapy on the blood

**Other medical problems**—The presence of other medical problems may affect the use of vincristine. Make sure you tell your doctor if you have any other medical problems, especially:

• Chickenpox (including recent exposure) or
• Herpes zoster (shingles)—Risk of severe disease affecting other parts of the body

- Gout (history of) or
- Kidney stones (history of)—Vincristine may increase levels of uric acid in the body, which can cause gout or kidney stones
- Infection—Vincristine can reduce immunity to infection
- Liver disease—Effects may be increased because of slower removal of vincristine from the body
- Nerve or muscle disease—May be worsened

## Proper Use of This Medicine

Vincristine is often given together with certain other medicines. If you are using a combination of medicines, it is important that you receive each one at the proper time. If you are taking some of these medicines by mouth, ask your health care professional to help you plan a way to take them at the right times.

While you are using this medicine, it may be necessary to drink extra fluids so that you will pass more urine. This will help prevent kidney problems and keep your kidneys working well. Ask your doctor if this is necessary for you.

This medicine sometimes causes nausea and vomiting. However, it is very important that you continue to receive the medicine, even if you begin to feel ill. Ask your health care professional for ways to lessen these effects.

Vincristine frequently causes constipation and stomach cramps. Your doctor may want you to take a laxative. However, do not decide to take these medicines on your own without first checking with your doctor.

**Dosing**—The dose of vincristine will be different for different patients. The dose that is used may depend on a number of things, including what the medicine is being used for, the patient's weight or size, and whether or not other medicines are also being taken. *If you are receiving vincristine at home, follow your doctor's orders or the directions on the label.* If you have any questions about the proper dose of vincristine, ask your doctor.

## Precautions While Using This Medicine

*It is very important that your doctor check your progress at regular visits* to make sure that vincristine is working properly and to check for unwanted effects.

While you are being treated with vincristine, and after you stop treatment with it, *do not have any immunizations (vaccinations) without your doctor's approval.* Vincristine may lower your body's resistance and there is a chance you might get the infection the immunization is meant to prevent. Other people living in your household should not take or should not have recently taken oral polio vaccine since there is a chance they could pass the polio virus on to you. Also, avoid other persons who have taken oral polio vaccine. Do not get close to them, and do not stay in the same room with them for very long. If you cannot take these precautions, you should consider wearing a protective face mask that covers the nose and mouth.

If vincristine accidentally seeps out of the vein into which it is injected, it may damage some tissues and cause scarring. *Tell the doctor or nurse right away if you notice redness, pain, or swelling at the place of injection.*

## Side Effects of This Medicine

Along with their needed effects, medicines like vincristine can sometimes cause unwanted effects such as blood problems, nervous system problems, loss of hair, and other side effects. These and others are described below. Also, because of the way these medicines act on the body, there is a chance that they might cause other unwanted effects that may not occur until months or years after the medicine is used. These delayed effects may include certain types of cancer, such as leukemia. Discuss these possible effects with your doctor.

Although not all of these side effects may occur, if they do occur they may need medical attention.

*Check with your doctor or nurse immediately* if the following side effects occur:

*Less common*
> Pain or redness at place of injection

*Rare*
> Black, tarry stools; blood in urine or stools; cough or hoarseness; fever or chills; pinpoint red spots on skin; unusual bleeding or bruising

Check with your health care professional as soon as possible if any of the following side effects occur:

*More common*
> Blurred or double vision; constipation; difficulty in walking; drooping eyelids; headache; jaw pain; joint pain; lower back or side pain; numbness or tingling in fingers and toes; pain in fingers and toes; pain in testicles; stomach cramps; swelling of feet or lower legs; weakness

*Less common*
> Agitation; bed-wetting; confusion; convulsions (seizures); decrease or increase in urination; dizziness or lightheadedness when getting up from a lying or sitting position; hallucinations (seeing, hearing, or feeling things that are not there); lack of sweating; loss of appetite; mental depression; painful or difficult urination; trouble in sleeping; unconsciousness

*Rare*
> Sores in mouth and on lips

Other side effects may occur that usually do not need medical attention. These side effects may go away during treatment as your body adjusts to the medicine. Also, your health care professional may be able to tell you about ways to prevent or reduce some of these side effects. Check with your health care professional if any of the following side effects continue or are bothersome or if you have any questions about them:

*Less common*

    Bloating; diarrhea; loss of weight; nausea and vomiting; skin rash

This medicine often causes a temporary loss of hair. After treatment with vincristine has ended, or sometimes even during treatment, normal hair growth should return.

Other side effects not listed above may also occur in some patients. If you notice any other effects, check with your doctor.

---

Revised: 09/90
Interim revision(s): 08/11/93; 07/05/94

---

# VITAMIN A    Systemic

A commonly used brand name in the U.S. and Canada is Aquasol A. Another commonly used name is retinol.

Generic name product may also be available in the U.S. and Canada.

## Description

Vitamins (VYE-ta-mins) are compounds that you *must* have for growth and health. They are needed in small amounts only and are usually available in the foods that you eat. Vitamin A is needed for night vision and for growth of skin, bones, and male and female reproductive organs. In pregnant women vitamin A is necessary for the growth of a healthy fetus.

Lack of vitamin A may lead to a rare condition called night blindness (problems seeing in the dark), as well as dry eyes, eye infections, skin problems, and slowed growth. Your doctor may treat these problems by prescribing vitamin A for you.

Increased need for vitamin A may occur in patients with the following conditions:

- Diarrhea
- Eye diseases
- Intestine diseases
- Infections (continuing or chronic)
- Measles
- Pancreas disease
- Stomach removal
- Stress (continuing)

In addition, infants receiving unfortified formula may need vitamin A supplements.

Vitamin A absorption will be decreased in any condition in which fat is poorly absorbed.

Increased need for vitamin A should be determined by your health care professional.

Claims that vitamin A is effective for treatment of conditions such as acne or lung diseases, or for treatment of eye problems, wounds, or dry or wrinkled skin not caused by lack of vitamin A have not been proven. Although vitamin A is being used to prevent certain types of cancer, some experts feel there is not enough information to show that this is effective, particularly in well-nourished individuals.

Some strengths of vitamin A are available only with a prescription. Others are available without a prescription.

Vitamin A is available in the following dosage forms:

*Oral*

- Capsules (U.S. and Canada)
- Oral solution (U.S.)
- Tablets (U.S.)

*Parenteral*

- Injection (U.S.)

## Importance of Diet

For good health, it is important that you eat a balanced and varied diet. Follow carefully any diet program your health care professional may recommend. For your specific dietary vitamin and/or mineral needs, ask your health care professional for a list of appropriate foods. If you think that you are not getting enough vitamins and/or minerals in your diet, you may choose to take a dietary supplement.

Vitamin A is found in various foods including yellow-orange fruits and vegetables; dark green, leafy vegetables; vitamin A-fortified milk; liver; and margarine. Vitamin A comes in two different forms, retinols and beta-carotene. Retinols are found in foods that come from animals (meat, milk, eggs). The form of vitamin A found in plants is called beta-carotene (which is converted to vitamin A in the body). Food processing may destroy some of the vitamins. For example, freezing may reduce the amount of vitamin A in foods.

Vitamins alone will not take the place of a good diet and will not provide energy. Your body needs other substances found in food, such as protein, minerals, carbohydrates, and fat. Vitamins themselves often cannot work without the presence of other foods. For example, small amounts

---

    

of fat are needed so that vitamin A can be absorbed into the body.

The daily amount of vitamin A needed is defined in several different ways.

*For U.S.—*

- RDA (Recommended Dietary Allowances) are used to determine the amount of vitamins and minerals needed to provide for adequate nutrition in most healthy persons.
- DVs (Daily Values) are used on food labels and show the percent of the daily amount of each nutrient that a serving of food provides.
- DRVs (Daily Reference Values) are used to determine DVs but do not appear on the labels themselves. DRVs are used for fat, carbohydrate, protein, and fiber and are based on the number of calories consumed per day.
- RDIs (Reference Daily Intakes) are also used to determine DVs but do not appear on food labels either. RDIs are used for vitamins and minerals and are based on the RDA. RDI replaces the previous designation of USRDA (United States Recommended Daily Allowances).

*For Canada—*

- RNI (Recommended Nutrient Intakes) are used to determine the amounts of vitamins, minerals, and protein needed to provide adequate nutrition and lessen the risk of chronic disease.

In the past, the RDA for vitamin A have been expressed in Units. This term Units has been replaced by retinol equivalents (RE) or micrograms (mcg) of retinol, with 1 RE equal to 1 mcg of retinol. This was done to better describe the two forms of vitamin A, retinol and beta-carotene. One RE of vitamin A is equal to 3.33 Units of retinol and 10 Units of beta-carotene. Some products available have not changed their labels and continue to be labeled in Units.

Normal daily recommended intakes for vitamin A are generally defined according to age or condition and to the form of vitamin A as follows:

| Age or Condition | Form of Vitamin A | | |
|---|---|---|---|
| | RE or mcg of Retinol | Amount in Units as Retinol | Amount in Units as a Combination of Retinol and Beta-carotene* |
| Infants and children | | | |
| Birth to 3 years | 375–400 | 1250–1330 | 1875–2000 |
| 4 to 6 years | 500 | 1665 | 2500 |
| 7 to 10 years | 700 | 2330 | 3500 |

| Age or Condition | Form of Vitamin A | | |
|---|---|---|---|
| | RE or mcg of Retinol | Amount in Units as Retinol | Amount in Units as a Combination of Retinol and Beta-carotene* |
| Adolescent and adult males | 800–1000 | 2665–3330 | 4000–5000 |
| Adolescent and adult females | 800 | 2665 | 4000 |
| Pregnant females | 800–900 | 2665–3000 | 4000–4500 |
| Breast-feeding females | 1200–1300 | 4000–4330 | 6000–6500 |

*Based on 1980 recommended dietary allowances (RDA) for vitamin A in the diet that is a combination of retinol and beta-carotene.

## Before Using This Dietary Supplement

If you are taking this dietary supplement without a prescription, carefully read and follow any precautions on the label. For vitamin A, the following should be considered:

**Allergies**—Tell your health care professional if you have ever had any unusual or allergic reaction to vitamin A. Also tell your health care professional if you are allergic to any other substances, such as foods, preservatives, or dyes.

**Pregnancy**—It is especially important that you are receiving enough vitamins when you become pregnant and that you continue to receive the right amount of vitamins throughout your pregnancy. It is recommended that you receive 800 retinol equivalents (RE) (2665 Units) to 900 RE (3000 Units) a day during pregnancy. The healthy growth and development of the fetus depend on a steady supply of nutrients from the mother.

However, taking too much vitamin A (more than 1800 RE [6000 Units] during pregnancy can also cause harmful effects such as birth defects or slow or reduced growth in the child.

**Breast-feeding**—It is especially important that you receive the right amounts of vitamins so that your baby will also get the vitamins needed to grow properly. It is recommended that you receive 1200 RE (4000 Units) to 1300 RE (4330 Units) a day while breast-feeding. However, taking large amounts of a dietary supplement while breast-feeding may be harmful to the mother and/or baby and should be avoided.

**Children**—Problems in humans have not been reported with intake of normal daily recommended intakes. However, side effects from high doses and/or prolonged use of vitamin A are more likely to occur in young children than adults.

**Older adults**—Problems in humans have not been reported with intake of normal daily recommended intakes. However, some studies have shown that the elderly may be at risk of high blood levels of vitamin A with long-term use.

**Dental**—High doses and/or prolonged use of vitamin A may cause bleeding from the gums; dry or sore mouth; or drying, cracking, or peeling of the lips.

**Medicines or other dietary supplements**—Although certain medicines or dietary supplements should not be used together at all, in other cases they may be used together even if an interaction might occur. In these cases, your health care professional may want to change the dose, or other precautions may be necessary. When you are taking vitamin A, it is especially important that your health care professional know if you are taking any of the following:

- Etretinate or
- Isotretinoin (e.g., Accutane)—Use with vitamin A may cause high blood levels of vitamin A, which may increase the chance of side effects

**Other medical problems**—The presence of other medical problems may affect the use of vitamin A. Make sure you tell your health care professional if you have any other medical problems, especially:

- Alcohol abuse (or history of) or
- Liver disease—Vitamin A use may make liver problems worse
- Kidney disease—May cause high blood levels of vitamin A, which may increase the chance of side effects

## Proper Use of This Dietary Supplement

**Dosing**—The amount of vitamin A to meet normal daily recommended intakes will be different for different patients. The following information includes only the average amounts of vitamin A.

- For *oral* dosage form (capsules, tablets, oral solution):
  —To prevent deficiency, the amount taken by mouth is based on normal daily recommended intakes:
  - Adults—
    —Adolescent and adult males: 800 RE (2665 Units) to 1000 RE (3330 Units).
    —Adolescent and adult females: 800 RE (2665 Units).
    —Pregnant females: 800 RE (2665 Units) to 900 RE (3000 Units).
    —Breast-feeding females: 1200 RE (4000 Units) to 1300 RE (4330 Units).

- Children—
  —Birth to 3 years: 375 RE (1250 Units) to 400 RE (1330 Units).
  —4 to 6 years: 500 RE (1665 Units).
  —7 to 10 years: 700 RE (2330 Units).

—To treat deficiency:

- Adults—Treatment dose is determined by prescriber for each individual based on severity of deficiency. The following dose has been determined for xerophthalmia (eye disease)—Oral, 7500 to 15,000 RE (25,000 to 50,000 Units) a day.
- Children—Treatment dose is determined by prescriber for each individual based of severity of deficiency. The following dosages have been determined:
  —Measles
  - For children 6 months to 1 year of age: Oral, 30,000 RE (100,000 Units) as a single dose.
  - For children 1 year of age and older: Oral, 60,000 RE (200,000 Units) as a single dose.
  —Xerophthalmia (eye disease)
  - For children 6 months to 1 year of age: Oral, 30,000 RE (100,000 Units) as a single dose, the same dose being repeated the next day and again at 4 weeks.
  - For children 1 year of age and older: Oral, 60,000 RE (200,000 Units) as a single dose, the same dose being repeated the next day and again at 4 weeks.

Note: Vitamin A is used in measles and xerophthalmia only when vitamin A deficiency is a problem as determined by your health care professional. Vitamin A deficiency occurs in malnutrition or in certain disease states.

**Missed dose**—If you miss taking a vitamin for one or more days there is no cause for concern, since it takes some time for your body to become seriously low in vitamins. However, if your health care professional has recommended that you take this vitamin, try to remember to take it as directed every day.

For patients taking the *oral liquid form* of vitamin A:

- This preparation is to be taken by mouth even though it comes in a dropper bottle.
- This dietary supplement may be dropped directly into the mouth or mixed with cereal, fruit juice, or other food.

**Storage**—To store this dietary supplement:

- Keep out of the reach of children.
- Store away from heat and direct light.
- Do not store in the bathroom, near the kitchen sink or in other damp places. Heat or moisture may cause the dietary supplement to break down.
- Keep the oral liquid form of this dietary supplement from freezing.

- Do not keep outdated dietary supplements or those no longer needed. Be sure that any discarded dietary supplement is out of the reach of children.

## Precautions While Using This Dietary Supplement

Vitamin A is stored in the body; therefore, when you take more than the body needs, it will build up in the body. This may lead to poisoning and even death. Problems are more likely to occur in:

- Adults taking 7500 RE (25,000 Units) a day for 8 months in a row, or 450,000 RE (1,500,000 Units) all at once; or
- Children taking 5400 RE (18,000 Units) to 15,000 RE (50,000 Units) a day for several months in a row, or 22,5000 RE (75,000 Units) to 105,100 RE (350,000 Units) all at once.
- Pregnant women taking more than 1800 RE (6000 Units) a day.

Remember that the total amount of vitamin A you get every day includes what you get from foods that you eat and what you take as a supplement.

## Side Effects of This Dietary Supplement

Along with its needed effects, a dietary supplement may cause some unwanted effects. Vitamin A does not usually cause any side effects at normal recommended doses.

*However, taking large amounts of vitamin A over a period of time may cause some unwanted effects that can be serious. Check with your health care professional immediately if any of the following side effects occur, since they may be signs of sudden overdose:*

Bleeding from gums or sore mouth; bulging soft spot on head (in babies); confusion or unusual excitement; diarrhea; dizziness or drowsiness; double vision; headache (severe); irritability (severe); peeling of skin, especially on lips and palms; vomiting (severe)

Check with your health care professional as soon as possible if any of the following side effects occur, since they may also be signs of gradual overdose:

Bone or joint pain; convulsions (seizures); drying or cracking of skin or lips; dry mouth; fever; general feeling of discomfort or illness or weakness; headache; increased sensitivity of skin to sunlight; increase in frequency of urination, especially at night, or in amount of urine; irritability; loss of appetite; loss of hair; stomach pain; unusual tiredness; vomiting; yellow-orange patches on soles of feet, palms of hands, or skin around nose and lips

Other side effects not listed above may also occur in some patients. If you notice any other effects, check with your health care professional.

Revised: 07/29/94

---

# VITAMIN B₁₂   Systemic

Some commonly used brand names are:

**In the U.S.—**

| | |
|---|---|
| Alphamine[2] | Hydrobexan[2] |
| Cobex[1] | Hydro-Cobex[2] |
| Crystamine[1] | Hydro-Crysti-12[2] |
| Crysti-12[1] | LA-12[2] |
| Cyanoject[1] | Rubesol-1000[1] |
| Cyomin[1] | Rubramin PC[1] |

**In Canada—**

| | |
|---|---|
| Anacobin[1] | Rubion[1] |
| Bedoz[1] | Rubramin[1] |

Note: For quick reference, the following vitamin b₁₂ are numbered to match the corresponding brand names.

This information applies to the following medicines:

1. Cyanocobalamin (sye-an-oh-koe-BAL-a-min)†
2. Hydroxocobalamin (hye-drox-oh-koe-BAL-a-min)†‡

---

†Not commercially available in Canada.
‡Generic name product may also be available in the U.S.

## Description

Vitamins (VYE-ta-mins) are compounds that you *must* have for growth and health. They are needed in small amounts only and are usually available in the foods that you eat. Vitamin B₁₂ is necessary for healthy blood. Cyanocobalamin and hydroxocobalamin are man-made forms of vitamin B₁₂.

Some people have a medical problem called pernicious anemia in which vitamin B₁₂ is not absorbed from the intestine. Others may have a badly diseased intestine or have had a large part of their stomach or intestine removed, so that vitamin B₁₂ cannot be absorbed. These people need to receive vitamin B₁₂ by injection.

Patients with the following conditions also may be more likely to have a deficiency of vitamin B₁₂:

- Alcoholism
- Anemia, hemolytic
- Fever (continuing)
- Genetic disorders such as homocystinuria and/or methylmalonic aciduria
- Intestine diseases
- Infections (continuing or chronic)
- Kidney disease
- Liver disease
- Pancreas disease
- Stomach disease
- Stress (continuing)
- Worm infections

If any of these conditions apply to you, you should take vitamin B₁₂ supplements only on the advice of your doctor after need has been established.

Lack of vitamin B$_{12}$ may lead to anemia (weak blood), stomach problems, and nerve damage. Your doctor may treat this by prescribing vitamin B$_{12}$ for you.

Claims that vitamin B$_{12}$ is effective for treatment of various conditions such as aging, allergies, eye problems, slow growth, poor appetite or malnutrition, skin problems, tiredness, mental problems, sterility, thyroid disease, and nerve diseases have not been proven. Many of these treatments involve large and expensive amounts of vitamins.

Some strengths of the B vitamins are available only with your doctor's prescription. Others are available without a prescription. However, it may be a good idea to check with your doctor before taking vitamin B$_{12}$ on your own.

Vitamin B$_{12}$ is available in the following dosage forms:

*Oral*
Cyanocobalamin
- Tablets (U.S. and Canada)

*Parenteral*
Cyanocobalamin
- Injection (U.S. and Canada)
Hydroxocobalamin
- Injection (U.S.)

---

## Importance of Diet

Vitamin supplements should be taken only if you cannot get enough vitamins in your diet; however, some diets may not contain all of the vitamins you need. This may occur with rapid weight loss, unusual diets such as some reducing diets in which choice of foods is very limited, or strict vegetarian (vegan-vegetarian) or macrobiotic diets, prolonged intravenous feeding, or malnutrition. A balanced diet should provide all the vitamins you normally need.

In order to get enough vitamins and minerals in your diet, it is important that you eat a balanced and varied diet. Follow carefully any diet program your doctor may recommend. For your specific vitamin and/or mineral needs, ask your doctor or dietitian for a list of appropriate foods.

Vitamin B$_{12}$ is found in various foods, including fish, egg yolk, milk, and fermented cheeses. It is *not* found in any vegetables. Ordinary cooking probably does not destroy the vitamin B$_{12}$ in food.

Vitamins alone will not take the place of a good diet and will not provide energy. Your body also needs other substances found in food, such as protein, minerals, carbohydrates, and fat. Vitamins themselves often cannot work without the presence of other foods.

In some cases, it may not be possible for you to get enough food to supply you with the proper vitamins. In other cases, the amount of vitamins you need may be increased above normal. Therefore, a vitamin supplement may be needed.

Experts have developed a list of recommended dietary allowances (RDA) for most of the vitamins. The RDA are not an exact number but a general idea of how much you need. They do not cover amounts needed for problems caused by a serious lack of vitamins.

The RDA for vitamin B$_{12}$ are:
- Infants and children—
    Birth to 6 months of age: 0.3 micrograms (mcg) per day.
    6 months to 1 year of age: 0.5 mcg per day.
    1 to 3 years of age: 0.7 mcg per day.
    4 to 6 years of age: 1 mcg per day.
    7 to 10 years of age: 1.4 mcg per day.
- Adolescent and adult males—11 years of age and over: 2 mcg per day.
- Adolescent and adult females—11 years of age and over: 2 mcg per day.
- Pregnant females—2.2 mcg per day.
- Breast-feeding females—2.6 mcg per day.

Remember:
- The total amount of each vitamin that you get every day includes what you get from the foods that you eat *and* what you may take as a supplement.
- Your total amount should not be greater than the RDA, unless ordered by your doctor.

---

## Before Using This Dietary Supplement

If you are taking this medicine without a prescription, carefully read and follow any precautions on the label. For vitamin B$_{12}$, the following should be considered:

**Allergies**—Tell your doctor if you have ever had any unusual or allergic reaction to vitamin B$_{12}$. Also, tell your health care professional if you are allergic to any other substances, such as foods, preservatives, or dyes.

**Pregnancy**—It is especially important that you are receiving enough vitamins when you become pregnant and that you continue to receive the right amount of vitamins throughout your pregnancy. Healthy fetal growth and development depend on a steady supply of nutrients from mother to fetus. However, taking large amounts of a dietary supplement in pregnancy may be harmful to the mother and/or fetus and should be avoided.

You may need vitamin B$_{12}$ supplements if you are a strict vegetarian (vegan-vegetarian). Too little vitamin B$_{12}$ can cause harmful effects such as anemia or nervous system injury.

**Breast-feeding**—It is especially important that you receive the right amounts of vitamins so that your baby will also get the vitamins needed to grow properly. If you are a strict vegetarian, your baby may not be getting the vitamin B$_{12}$ needed. However, taking large amounts of a dietary supplement while breast-feeding may be harmful to the mother and/or baby and should be avoided.

**Children**—Normal daily requirements vary according to age. It is especially important that children receive enough vitamins in their diet for healthy growth and development.

**Older adults**—It is important that older people continue to receive enough vitamins in their diet for good health.

**Medicines or other dietary supplements**—Although certain medicines or dietary supplement should not be used together at all, in other cases they may be used together even if an interaction might occur. In these cases, your doctor may want to change the dose, or other precautions may be necessary. Tell your health care professional if you are taking any other dietary supplement or any prescription or nonprescription (over-the-counter [OTC]) medicine.

**Other medical problems**—The presence of other medical problems may affect the use of vitamin B$_{12}$. Make sure you tell your doctor if you have any other medical problems, especially:

- Leber's disease (an eye disease)—Vitamin B$_{12}$ may make this condition worse

## Proper Use of This Dietary Supplement

Some people believe that taking very large doses of vitamins (called megadoses or megavitamin therapy) is useful for treating certain medical problems. Studies have not proven this. Large doses should be taken only under the direction of your doctor after need has been identified.

*For patients receiving vitamin B$_{12}$ by injection for pernicious anemia or if part of the stomach or intestine has been removed:*

- You will have to receive treatment for the rest of your life. You must continue to receive this medicine even if you feel well, in order to prevent future problems.

**Dosing**—The dose of vitamin B$_{12}$ for prevention of vitamin B$_{12}$ deficiency is based on the Recommended Dietary Allowances (RDA). See the *Importance of Diet* section for the RDA for vitamin B$_{12}$.

**Missed dose**—If you miss taking a vitamin for one or more days there is no cause for concern, since it takes some time for your body to become seriously low in vitamins. However, if your doctor has recommended that you take this vitamin, try to remember to take it as directed.

**Storage**—To store this dietary supplement:

- Keep out of the reach of children.
- Store away from heat and direct light.
- Do not store in the bathroom, near the kitchen sink, or in other damp places. Heat or moisture may cause the dietary supplement to break down.
- Do not keep outdated dietary supplement or those no longer needed. Be sure that any discarded dietary supplement is out of the reach of children.

## Side Effects of This Dietary Supplement

Along with its needed effects, a dietary supplement may cause some unwanted effects. Cyanocobalamin or hydroxocobalamin do not usually cause any side effects. *However, check with your doctor immediately* if any of the following side effects occur:

*Rare—soon after receiving injection only*
Skin rash or itching; wheezing

Check with your doctor as soon as possible if either of the following side effects continues or is bothersome:

*Less common*
Diarrhea; itching of skin

Other side effects not listed above may also occur in some patients. If you notice any other effects, check with your health care professional.

Revised: 01/29/92
Interim revision(s): 06/02/92; 08/16/94

# VITAMIN D and Related Compounds  Systemic

Some commonly used brand names are:

**In the U.S.—**

| | |
|---|---|
| Calciferol[5] | DHT Intensol[4] |
| Calcijex[3] | Drisdol[5] |
| Calderol[2] | Hytakerol[4] |
| Deltalin[5] | Rocaltrol[3] |
| DHT[4] | |

**In Canada—**

| | |
|---|---|
| Calciferol[5] | Ostoforte[5] |
| Drisdol[5] | Radiostol Forte[5] |
| Hytakerol[4] | Rocaltrol[3] |
| One-Alpha[1] | |

Note: For quick reference, the following vitamin D and related compounds are numbered to match the corresponding brand names.

This information applies to the following medicines:

1. Alfacalcidol (al-fa-KAL-si-dol)*
2. Calcifediol (kal-si-fe-DYE-ole)†
3. Calcitriol (kal-si-TRYE-ole)
4. Dihydrotachysterol (dye-hye-droh-tak-ISS-ter-ole)
5. Ergocalciferol (er-goe-kal-SIF-e-role)‡

*Not commercially available in the U.S.
†Not commercially available in Canada.
‡Generic name product may also be available in the U.S.

# Description

Vitamins (VYE-ta-mins) are compounds that you *must* have for growth and health. They are needed in small amounts only and are available in the foods that you eat. Vitamin D is necessary for strong bones and teeth.

Lack of vitamin D may lead to a condition called rickets, especially in children, in which bones and teeth are weak. In adults it may cause a condition called osteomalacia, in which calcium is lost from bones so that they become weak. Your doctor may treat these problems by prescribing vitamin D for you. Vitamin D is also sometimes used to treat other diseases in which calcium is not used properly by the body.

Ergocalciferol is the form of vitamin D used in vitamin supplements.

Patients with the following conditions may be more likely to have a deficiency of vitamin D:
Alcoholism
Intestine diseases
Kidney disease
Liver disease
Pancreas disease
Surgical removal of stomach

In addition, individuals and breast-fed infants who lack exposure to sunlight, as well as dark-skinned individuals, may be more likely to have a vitamin D deficiency.

If any of the above apply to you, you should take vitamin D supplements only on the advice of your doctor after need has been established.

Alfacalcidol, calcifediol, calcitriol, and dihydrotachysterol are forms of vitamin D used to treat hypocalcemia (not enough calcium in the blood). Alfacalcidol, calcifediol, and calcitriol are also used to treat certain types of bone disease that may occur with kidney disease in patients who are undergoing kidney dialysis.

Claims that vitamin D is effective for treatment of arthritis and prevention of nearsightedness or nerve problems have not been proven. Some psoriasis patients may benefit from vitamin D supplements; however, controlled studies have not been performed.

Some strengths of ergocalciferol and all strengths of alfacalcidol, calcifediol, calcitriol, and dihydrotachysterol are available only with your doctor's prescription. Other strengths of ergocalciferol are available without a prescription. However, it may be a good idea to check with your doctor before taking vitamin D on your own. *Taking large amounts over long periods may cause serious unwanted effects.*

Vitamin D and related compounds are available in the following dosage forms:

*Oral*
Alfacalcidol
- Capsules (Canada)
- Oral solution (Canada)

Calcifediol
- Capsules (U.S.)
Calcitriol
- Capsules (U.S. and Canada)
Dihydrotachysterol
- Capsules (U.S. and Canada)
- Oral solution (U.S.)
- Tablets (U.S.)
Ergocalciferol
- Capsules (U.S. and Canada)
- Oral solution (U.S. and Canada)
- Tablets (U.S. and Canada)

*Parenteral*
Calcitriol
- Injection (U.S. and Canada)
Ergocalciferol
- Injection (U.S. and Canada)

# Importance of Diet

*For dietary supplement use only:*
- Dietary supplements should be taken only if you cannot get enough vitamins in your diet; however, some diets may not contain all of the vitamins you need. This may occur with rapid weight loss, unusual diets (such as strict vegetarian or macrobiotic diets that do not include milk or reducing diets in which choice of foods is very limited), prolonged intravenous feeding, or malnutrition. A balanced diet should provide all the vitamins you normally need.

In order to get enough vitamins and minerals in your diet, it is important that you eat a balanced and varied diet. Follow carefully any diet program your doctor may recommend. For your specific vitamin and/or mineral needs, ask your doctor or dietitian for a list of appropriate foods.

Vitamin D is found naturally only in fish and fish-liver oils. However, it is also found in milk (vitamin D–fortified). Cooking does not affect the vitamin D in foods. Vitamin D is sometimes called the "sunshine vitamin" since it is made in your skin when you are exposed to sunlight. If you eat a balanced diet and get outside in the sunshine at least 1.5 to 2 hours a week, you should be getting all the vitamin D you need.

Vitamins alone will not take the place of a good diet and will not provide energy. Your body also needs other substances found in food such as protein, minerals, carbohydrates, and fat. Vitamins themselves often cannot work without the presence of other foods. For example, fat is needed so that vitamin D can be absorbed into the body.

In some cases, it may not be possible for you to get enough food to supply you with the proper vitamins. In other cases, the amount of vitamins you need may be increased above normal. Therefore, a vitamin supplement may be needed.

Experts have developed a list of recommended dietary allowances (RDA) for most of the vitamins. The RDA

---

are not an exact number but a general idea of how much you need. They do not cover amounts needed for problems caused by a serious lack of vitamins.

In the past, the RDA for vitamin D have been expressed in Units (U). This term has been replaced by micrograms (mcg) of vitamin D.

The RDA for vitamin D are:

- Infants and children—
    Birth to 6 months of age: 7.5 micrograms (mcg) (300 Units) per day.
    6 months to 10 years of age: 10 mcg (400 Units) per day.
- Adolescent and adult males—
    11 to 25 years of age: 10 mcg (400 Units) per day.
    25 years of age and over: 5 mcg (200 Units) per day.
- Adolescent and adult females—
    11 to 25 years of age: 10 mcg (400 Units) per day.
    25 years of age and over: 5 mcg (200 Units) per day.
- Pregnant females—10 mcg (400 Units) per day.
- Breast-feeding females—10 mcg (400 Units) per day.

Remember:

- The total amount of each vitamin that you get every day includes what you get from the foods that you eat *and* what you may take as a supplement.
- Your total amount should not be greater than the RDA, unless ordered by your doctor. *Taking too much vitamin D over a period of time may cause harmful effects.*

## Before Using This Dietary Supplement

If you are taking this dietary supplement without a prescription, carefully read and follow any precautions on the label. For vitamin D and related compounds, the following should be considered:

**Allergies**—Tell your doctor if you have ever had any unusual or allergic reaction to alfacalcidol, calcifediol, calcitriol, dihydrotachysterol, or ergocalciferol. Also, tell your health care professional if you are allergic to any other substances, such as foods, preservatives, or dyes.

**Pregnancy**—It is especially important that you are receiving enough vitamin D when you become pregnant and that you continue to receive the right amounts of vitamins throughout your pregnancy. The healthy growth and development of the fetus depend on a steady supply of nutrients from the mother.

You may need vitamin D supplements if you are a strict vegetarian (vegan-vegetarian) and/or have little exposure to sunlight and do not drink vitamin D-fortified milk.

Taking too much alfacalcidol, calcifediol, calcitriol, dihydrotachysterol, or ergocalciferol can also be harmful to the fetus. Taking more than your doctor has recommended can cause your baby to be more sensitive than

usual to its effects, can cause problems with a gland called the parathyroid, and can cause a defect in the baby's heart.

**Breast-feeding**—It is especially important that you receive the right amounts of vitamins so that your baby will also get the vitamins needed to grow properly. Infants who are totally breast-fed and have little exposure to the sun may require vitamin D supplementation. However, taking large amounts of a dietary supplement while breast-feeding may be harmful to the mother and/or baby and should be avoided.

Only small amounts of alfacalcidol, calcifediol, calcitriol, or dihydrotachysterol pass into breast milk and these amounts have not been reported to cause problems in nursing babies.

**Children**—Normal daily requirements vary according to age. It is especially important that children receive enough vitamins in their diet for healthy growth and development. Some studies have shown that infants who are totally breast-fed, especially with dark-skinned mothers, and have little exposure to sunlight may be at risk of vitamin D deficiency. Your doctor may prescribe a vitamin/mineral supplement that contains vitamin D. Some infants may be sensitive to even small amounts of alfacalcidol, calcifediol, calcitriol, dihydrotachysterol, or ergocalciferol. Also, children may show slowed growth when receiving large doses of alfacalcidol, calcifediol, calcitriol, dihydrotachysterol, or ergocalciferol for a long time.

**Older adults**—It is important that older people continue to receive enough vitamins in their diet for good health. Studies have shown that older adults may have lower blood levels of vitamin D than younger adults, especially those who have little exposure to sunlight. Your doctor may recommend that you take a vitamin supplement that contains vitamin D.

**Medicines or other dietary supplements**—Although certain medicines or dietary supplements should not be used together at all, in other cases they may be used together even if an interaction might occur. In these cases, your doctor may want to change the dose, or other precautions may be necessary. When you are taking vitamin D and related compounds it is especially important that your health care professional know if you are taking any of the following:

- Antacids containing magnesium—Use of these products with any vitamin D–related compound may result in high blood levels of magnesium, especially in patients with kidney disease
- Calcium-containing preparations or
- Thiazide diuretics (water pills)—Use of these medicines with vitamin D may cause high blood levels of calcium and increase the chance of side effects
- Vitamin D and related compounds, other—Use of vitamin D with a related compound may cause high blood levels of vitamin D and increase the chance of side effects.

**Other medical problems**—The presence of other medical problems may affect the use of vitamin D and related compounds. Make sure you tell your doctor if you have any other medical problems, especially:

- Heart or blood vessel disease—Alfacalcidol, calcifediol, calcitriol, or dihydrotachysterol may cause hypercalcemia (high blood levels of calcium), which may make these conditions worse
- Kidney disease—High blood levels of alfacalcidol, calcifediol, calcitriol, dihydrotachysterol, or ergocalciferol may result, which may increase the chance of side effects
- Sarcoidosis—May increase sensitivity to alfacalcidol, calcifediol, calcitriol, dihydrotachysterol, or ergocalciferol and increase the chance of side effects

## Proper Use of This Dietary Supplement

*For use as a dietary supplement:*

- *Do not take more than the recommended daily amount.* Vitamin D is stored in the body, and taking too much over a period of time can cause poisoning and even death. Some people believe that taking very large doses of vitamins (called megadoses or megavitamin therapy) is useful for treating certain medical problems. Studies have not proven this. Large doses should be taken only under the direction of your doctor after need has been identified.

If you have any questions about this, check with your health care professional.

For patients taking the *oral liquid form* of this dietary supplement:

- This preparation should be taken by mouth even though it comes in a dropper bottle.
- This dietary supplement may be dropped directly into the mouth or mixed with cereal, fruit juice, or other food.

*While you are taking alfacalcidol, calcifediol, calcitriol, or dihydrotachysterol,* your doctor may want you to follow a special diet or take a calcium supplement. Be sure to follow instructions carefully. If you are already taking a calcium supplement or any medicine containing calcium, make sure your doctor knows.

**Dosing**—The dose of these vitamin D and related compounds will be different for different patients. *Follow your doctor's orders or the directions on the label.* The following information includes only the average doses of these medicines. *If your dose is different, do not change it* unless your doctor tells you to do so.

The number of milliliters (mL) of solution that you take, or the number of capsules or tablets you take, depends on the strength of the medicine. Also, *the number of doses you take each day, the time allowed between doses, and the length of time you take the medicine depend on the medical problem for which you are taking the combination medicine.*

*For alfacalcidol*

- To treat diseases in which calcium is not used properly by the body or to treat bone disease in kidney patients undergoing kidney dialysis:
  —For *oral* dosage form (capsules):
  - Adults and teenagers—At first, 1 microgram (mcg) a day. Your doctor may change your dose

if needed. However, most people will take not more than 3 mcg a day.
  —For *oral* dosage form (solution):
  - Adults and teenagers—At first, 1 mcg a day. Your doctor may change your dose if needed. However, most people will take not more than 3 mcg a day.
  - Children—0.25 mcg a day.

*For calcifediol*

- To treat diseases in which calcium is not used properly by the body or to treat bone disease in kidney patients undergoing kidney dialysis:
  —For *oral* dosage form (capsules):
  - Adults, teenagers, and children over 10 years of age—At first, 300 to 350 micrograms (mcg) a week, taken in divided doses either once a day or every other day. Your doctor may change your dose if needed.
  - Children up to 2 years of age—20 to 50 mcg a day.
  - Children 2 to 10 years of age—50 mcg a day.

*For calcitriol*

- To treat diseases in which calcium is not used properly by the body or to treat bone disease in kidney patients undergoing kidney dialysis:
  —For *oral* dosage form (capsules):
  - Adults, teenagers, and children—At first, 0.25 micrograms (mcg) a day. Your doctor may change your dose if needed.
  —For *injection* dosage form:
  - Adults and teenagers—At first, 0.5 mcg injected into a vein three times a week. Your doctor may change your dose if needed.
  - Children—Use and dose must be determined by your doctor.

*For dihydrotachysterol*

- To treat diseases in which calcium is not used properly by the body:
  —For *oral* dosage forms (capsules, solution, or tablets):
  - Adults and teenagers—At first, 100 micrograms (mcg) to 2.5 milligrams (mg) a day. Your doctor may change your dose if needed.
  - Children—At first, 1 to 5 mg a day. Your doctor may change your dose if needed.

*For ergocalciferol*

- To treat vitamin D deficiency and diseases in which calcium and phosphate are not used properly by the body:
  —For *oral* dosage forms (capsules, solution, or tablets):
  - Adults and teenagers—At first, 1000 to 500,000 Units a day. The doctor may change your dose if needed.
  - Children—At first, 1000 to 200,000 Units a day. The doctor may change your dose if needed.

—For *injection* dosage form:
  - Adults, teenagers, and children—Dose must be determined by your doctor. Some patients may receive 10,000 Units injected into a muscle once a day.

**Missed dose—**
  - *For use as a dietary supplement:* If you miss taking a dietary supplement for one or more days there is no cause for concern, since it takes some time for your body to become seriously low in vitamins. However, if your doctor has recommended that you take this dietary supplement, try to remember to take it as directed every day.
  - If you are taking this medicine for a reason other than as a dietary supplement and you miss a dose and your dosing schedule is:
    —One dose every other day: Take the missed dose as soon as possible if you remember it on the day it should be taken. However, if you do not remember the missed dose until the next day, take it at that time. Then skip a day and start your dosing schedule again. Do not double doses.
    —One dose a day: Take the missed dose as soon as possible. Then go back to your regular dosing schedule. However, if you do not remember the missed dose until the next day, skip the missed dose and go back to your regular dosing schedule. Do not double doses.
    —More than one dose a day: Take the missed dose as soon as possible. Then go back to your regular dosing schedule. However, if it is almost time for your next dose, skip the missed dose and go back to your regular dosing schedule. Do not double doses.

If you have any questions about this, check with your doctor.

**Storage**—To store this dietary supplement:
  - Keep out of the reach of children.
  - Store away from heat and direct light.
  - Do not store in the bathroom, near the kitchen sink, or in other damp places. Heat or moisture may cause the dietary supplement to break down.
  - Keep the oral liquid form of the dietary supplement from freezing.
  - Do not keep outdated dietary supplements or those no longer needed. Be sure that any discarded dietary supplement is out of the reach of children.

## Precautions While Using This Dietary Supplement

If you are taking this medicine for a reason other than as a dietary supplement, *your doctor should check your progress at regular visits* to make sure that it does not cause unwanted effects.

Do not take any nonprescription (over-the-counter [OTC]) medicine or dietary supplement that contains calcium, phosphorus, or vitamin D while you are taking any of these dietary supplements unless you have been told to do so by your doctor. The extra calcium, phosphorus, or vitamin D may increase the chance of side effects.

*Do not take antacids or other medicines containing magnesium while you are taking any of these medicines. Taking these medicines together may cause unwanted effects.*

## Side Effects of This Dietary Supplement

Along with its needed effects, a dietary supplement may cause some unwanted effects. Alfacalcidol, calcifediol, calcitriol, dihydrotachysterol, and ergocalciferol do not usually cause any side effects when taken as directed. However, *taking large amounts over a period of time may cause some unwanted effects that can be serious.*

*Check with your doctor immediately* if any of the following effects occur:
  *Late symptoms of severe overdose*
    High blood pressure; irregular heartbeat; stomach pain (severe)

Check with your doctor as soon as possible if any of the following effects occur:
  *Early symptoms of overdose*
    Constipation (especially in children or adolescents); diarrhea; dryness of mouth; headache (continuing); increased thirst; increase in frequency of urination, especially at night, or in amount of urine; loss of appetite; metallic taste; nausea or vomiting (especially in children or adolescents); unusual tiredness or weakness
  *Late symptoms of overdose*
    Bone pain; cloudy urine; drowsiness; increased sensitivity of eyes to light or irritation of eyes; itching of skin; mood or mental changes; muscle pain; nausea or vomiting; weight loss

Other side effects not listed above may also occur in some patients. If you notice any other effects, check with your doctor.

Revised: 08/03/92
Interim revision(s): 08/18/92; 09/03/94

# VITAMIN E   Systemic

Some commonly used brand names are:

**In the U.S.—**

| | |
|---|---|
| Amino-Opti-E | E-400 I.U. in a Water Soluble |
| Aquasol E | Base |
| E-Complex-600 | E-Vitamin Succinate |
| E-200 I.U. Softgels | Liqui-E |
| E-1000 I.U. Softgels | Pheryl-E |
| | Vita Plus E |

Generic name product may also be available.

**In Canada—**

| | |
|---|---|
| Aquasol E | Webber Vitamin E |

Generic name product may also be available.

Another commonly used name is alpha tocopherol.

## Description

Vitamins (VYE-ta-mins) are compounds that you *must* have for growth and health. They are needed in only small amounts and are available in the foods that you eat. Vitamin E prevents a chemical reaction called oxidation, which can sometimes result in harmful effects in your body. It is also important for the proper function of nerves and muscles.

Patients with the following conditions may be more likely to have a deficiency of vitamin E:

Intestine disease
Liver disease
Pancreas disease
Surgical removal of stomach

If any of the above apply to you, you should take vitamin E supplements only on the advice of your doctor after need has been established.

Infants who are receiving a formula that is not fortified with vitamin E may be likely to have a vitamin E deficiency. Also, diets high in polyunsaturated fatty acids may increase your need for vitamin E.

Claims that vitamin E is effective for treatment of cancer and for prevention or treatment of acne, aging, loss of hair, bee stings, liver spots on the hands, bursitis, diaper rash, frostbite, stomach ulcer, heart attacks, labor pains, certain blood diseases, miscarriage, muscular dystrophy, poor posture, sexual impotence, sterility, infertility, menopause, sunburn, and lung damage from air pollution have not been proven. Although vitamin E is being used to prevent certain types of cancer, there is not enough information to show that this is effective.

Vitamin E is available without a prescription. However, it may be a good idea to check with your doctor before taking vitamin E on your own. Lack of vitamin E is extremely rare, except in people who have a disease in which it is not absorbed into the body.

If you are using vitamin E for reasons other than as a vitamin supplement, most of the following information will not apply to you.

Vitamin E is available in the following dosage forms:

*Oral*

- Capsules (U.S. and Canada)
- Oral solution (U.S. and Canada)
- Tablets (U.S.)
- Chewable tablets (U.S.)

## Importance of Diet

Vitamin supplements should be taken only if you cannot get enough vitamins in your diet; however, intravenous feeding solutions may not contain enough vitamin E and may cause your body to become low in vitamin E if they are used for a long time.

In order to get enough vitamins and minerals in your diet, it is important that you eat a balanced and varied diet. Follow carefully any diet program your doctor may recommend. For your specific vitamin and/or mineral needs, ask your doctor or dietitian for a list of appropriate foods.

Vitamin E is found in various foods including vegetable oils (corn, cottonseed, soybean, safflower), wheat germ, whole-grain cereals, and green leafy vegetables. Cooking and storage may destroy some of the vitamin E in foods.

Vitamin supplements alone will not take the place of a good diet and will not provide energy. Your body also needs other substances found in food such as protein, minerals, carbohydrates, and fat. Vitamins themselves often cannot work without the presence of other foods. For example, small amounts of fat are needed so that vitamin E can be absorbed into the body.

In some cases, it may not be possible for you to get enough food to supply you with the proper vitamins. In other cases, the amount of vitamins you need may be increased above normal. Therefore, a vitamin supplement may be needed. However, lack of vitamin E is very rare.

Experts have developed Recommended Dietary Allowances (RDA) for vitamins and other nutrients based on the amount you need for good health. RDA cover the needs of most healthy people. They do not cover the needs of those who require extra vitamins or nutrients because of disease or serious lack of good nutrition. RDA should not be thought of as the amount of vitamins or other nutrients you need every day. Instead, they are the amounts you should eat on an average over time.

Vitamin E is available in various forms, including *d*- or *dl*-alpha tocopheryl acetate, *d*- or *dl*-alpha tocopherol, and *d*- or *dl*-alpha tocopheryl acid succinate. In the past, the RDA for vitamin E have been expressed in Units. This term has been replaced by alpha tocopherol equivalents (alpha-TE) or milligrams (mg) of *d*-alpha tocopherol. One Unit is equivalent to 1 mg of *dl*-alpha tocopherol acetate or 0.6 mg *d*-alpha tocopherol. Most products available in stores continue to be labeled in Units.

The RDAs for vitamin E are:
- Infants and children—
    Birth to 6 months of age: 3 mg alpha-TE (5 Units) per day.
    6 months to 1 year of age: 4 mg alpha-TE (6.7 Units) per day.
    1 to 3 years of age: 6 mg alpha-TE (10 Units) per day.
    4 to 10 years of age: 7 mg alpha-TE (11.7 Units) per day.
- Adolescent and adult males—11 years of age and over: 10 mg alpha-TE (16.7 Units) per day.
- Adolescent and adult females—11 years of age and over: 8 mg alpha-TE (13 Units) per day.
- Pregnant females—10 mg alpha-TE (16.7 Units) per day.
- Breast-feeding females—
    First 6 months: 12 mg alpha-TE (20 Units) per day.
    Second 6 months: 11 mg alpha-TE (18 Units) per day.

Remember:
- The total amount of each vitamin that you get every day includes what you get from the foods that you eat *and* what you may take as a supplement.
- The total amount you get, averaged over several days, should not be greater than twice the RDA, unless ordered by your doctor. Taking more than 400 Units of vitamin E a day over a period of time may cause nausea, stomach cramps, or muscle weakness.

## Before Using This Dietary Supplement

If you are taking this dietary supplement without a prescription, carefully read and follow any precautions on the label. For vitamin E, the following should be considered:

**Allergies**—Tell your doctor if you have ever had any unusual or allergic reaction to vitamin E. Also, tell your health care professional if you are allergic to any other substances, such as foods, preservatives, or dyes.

**Pregnancy**—It is especially important that you are receiving enough vitamins when you become pregnant and that you continue to receive the right amount of vitamins throughout your pregnancy. The healthy growth and development of the fetus depend on a steady supply of nutrients from the mother. However, taking large amounts of a dietary supplement during pregnancy may be harmful and should be avoided.

**Breast-feeding**—It is especially important that you receive the right amounts of vitamins so that your baby will also get the vitamins needed to grow properly. You should also check with your doctor if you are giving your baby an unfortified formula. In that case, the baby must get the vitamins needed some other way. However, taking large amounts of a dietary supplement while breast-feeding may be harmful to the mother and/or baby and should be avoided.

**Children**—Normal daily requirements vary according to age. It is especially important that children receive enough vitamins in their diet for healthy growth and development. You should check with your doctor if you are giving your baby an unfortified formula. In that case, the baby must get the vitamins needed some other way. Some studies have shown that premature infants may have low levels of vitamin E. Your doctor may recommend a vitamin E supplement.

**Older adults**—It is important that older people continue to receive enough vitamins in their diet for good health. Although there is no specific information about the use of vitamin E in older people in doses higher than the normal daily requirements, it is not expected to cause different side effects or problems in older people than in younger adults.

**Medicines or other dietary supplements**—Although certain medicines or dietary supplements should not be used together at all, in other cases they may be used together even if an interaction might occur. In these cases, your doctor may want to change the dose, or other precautions may be necessary. Tell your health care professional if you are taking any other prescription or nonprescription (over-the-counter [OTC]) medicine.

**Other medical problems**—The presence of other medical problems may affect the use of vitamin E. Make sure you tell your doctor if you have any other medical problems, especially:
- Bleeding problems—Vitamin E may make this condition worse

## Proper Use of This Dietary Supplement

Do not take more than the recommended daily amount. Vitamin E is stored in the body, and taking more than 400 Units a day over a period of time may cause harmful effects. Some of these effects are described below. Some people believe that taking very large doses of vitamins (called megadoses or megavitamin therapy) is useful for treating certain medical problems. Studies have not proven this. Large doses should be taken only under the direction of your doctor after need has been identified.

For patients taking the *oral liquid form of this dietary supplement:*

- This preparation should be taken by mouth even though it comes in a dropper bottle.
- This dietary supplement may be dropped directly into the mouth or mixed with cereal, fruit juice, or other food.

**Dosing**—The dose of vitamin E for prevention of vitamin E deficiency is based on the Recommended Dietary Allowances (RDA). See the *Importance of Diet* section for the RDA for Vitamin E.

**Missed dose**—If you miss taking a vitamin for one or more days there is no cause for concern, since it takes some time for your body to become seriously low in vitamins. However, if your doctor has recommended that you take this vitamin, try to remember to take it as directed every day.

**Storage**—To store this dietary supplement:

- Keep out of the reach of children.
- Store away from heat and direct light.
- Do not store in the bathroom, near the kitchen sink, or in other damp places. Heat or moisture may cause the dietary supplement to break down.

- Keep the oral liquid form of this dietary supplement from freezing.
- Do not keep outdated dietary supplements or those no longer needed. Be sure that any discarded dietary supplement is out of the reach of children.

## Side Effects of This Dietary Supplement

Along with its needed effects, a dietary supplement may cause some unwanted effects. When used for short periods of time at recommended doses, vitamin E usually does not cause any side effects. However, check with your doctor as soon as possible if any of the following side effects occur:

*With doses greater than 400 Units a day and long-term use*

Blurred vision; diarrhea; dizziness; headache; nausea or stomach cramps; unusual tiredness or weakness

Other side effects not listed above may also occur in some patients. If you notice any other effects, check with your doctor.

Revised: 06/22/93
Interim revision: 07/20/94

# VITAMIN K   Systemic

Some commonly used brand names are:
**In the U.S.—**
AquaMEPHYTON[2]
Konakion[2]
Mephyton[2]
Synkayvite[1]
Note: For quick reference, the following corticosteroids are numbered to match the corresponding brand names.
Another commonly used name is phytomenadione.
This information applies to the following medicines:
1. Menadiol (men-a-DYE-ole)†
2. Phytonadione (fye-toe-na-DYE-one)§

†Not commercially available in Canada.
§Generic name product may also be available in Canada.

## Description

Vitamins (VYE-ta-mins) are compounds that you *must* have for growth and health. They are needed in only small amounts and are usually available in the foods that you eat. Vitamin K is necessary for normal clotting of the blood.

Vitamin K is found in various foods including green leafy vegetables, meat, and dairy products. If you eat a balanced diet containing these foods, you should be getting all the vitamin K you need. Little vitamin K is lost from foods with ordinary cooking.

Lack of vitamin K is rare but may lead to problems with blood clotting and increased bleeding. Your doctor may treat this by prescribing vitamin K for you.

Vitamin K is routinely given to newborn infants to prevent bleeding problems.

This medicine is available only with your doctor's prescription, in the following dosage forms:
*Oral*
Menadiol
- Tablets (U.S.)
Phytonadione
- Tablets (U.S.)
*Parenteral*
Menadiol
- Injection (U.S.)
Phytonadione
- Injection (U.S. and Canada)

## Before Using This Medicine

In deciding to use a medicine, the risks of taking the medicine must be weighed against the good it will do. This is a decision you and your doctor will make. For vitamin K, the following should be considered:

**Allergies**—Tell your doctor if you have ever had any unusual or allergic reaction to vitamin K. Also tell your

health care professional if you are allergic to any other substances, such as foods, preservatives, or dyes.

**Pregnancy**—Vitamin K has not been reported to cause birth defects or other problems in humans.

**Breast-feeding**—Vitamin K taken by the mother has not been reported to cause problems in nursing babies. You should also check with your doctor if you are giving your baby an unfortified formula. In that case, the baby must get the vitamins needed some other way.

**Children**—Children may be especially sensitive to the effects of vitamin K, especially menadiol. This may increase the chance of side effects during treatment.

**Older adults**—Many medicines have not been tested in older people. Therefore, it may not be known whether they work exactly the same way they do in younger adults or if they cause different side effects or problems in older people. There is no specific information about the use of vitamin K in the elderly.

**Other medicines**—Although certain medicines should not be used together at all, in other cases two different medicines may be used together even if an interaction might occur. In these cases, your doctor may want to change the dose, or other precautions may be necessary. When you are taking vitamin K, it is especially important that your health care professional know if you are taking any of the following:

- Acetohydroxamic acid (e.g., Lithostat) or
- Antidiabetics, oral (diabetes medicine you take by mouth) or
- Dapsone or
- Furazolidone (e.g., Furoxone) or
- Methyldopa (e.g., Aldomet) or
- Nitrofurantoin (e.g., Furadantin) or
- Primaquine or
- Procainamide (e.g., Pronestyl) or
- Quinidine (e.g., Quinidex) or
- Quinine (e.g., Quinamm) or
- Sulfonamides (sulfa medicine) or
- Sulfoxone (e.g., Diasone)—The chance of a serious side effect may be increased, especially with menadiol
- Anticoagulants (blood thinners)—Vitamin K decreases the effects of these medicines and is sometimes used to treat bleeding caused by anticoagulants; however, anyone receiving an anticoagulant should not take any supplement that contains vitamin K (alone or in combination with other vitamins or nutrients) unless it has been ordered by their doctor

**Other medical problems**—The presence of other medical problems may affect the use of vitamin K. Make sure you tell your doctor if you have any other medical problems, especially:

- Cystic fibrosis or
- Diarrhea (prolonged) or
- Intestinal problems—These conditions may interfere with absorption of vitamin K into the body when it is taken by mouth; higher doses may be needed, or the medicine may have to be injected
- Glucose-6-phosphate dehydrogenase (G6PD) deficiency or
- Liver disease—The chance of unwanted effects may be increased

## Proper Use of This Medicine

*Take this medicine only as directed by your doctor.* Do not take more or less of it, do not take it more often, and do not take it for a longer time than your doctor ordered. To do so may cause serious unwanted effects such as blood clotting problems.

*Your doctor should check your progress at regular visits.* A blood test must be taken regularly to see how fast your blood is clotting. This will help your doctor decide how much medicine you need.

**Dosing**—The dose of these medicines will be different for different patients. *Follow your doctor's orders or the directions on the label.* The following information includes only the average doses of these medicines. *If your dose is different, do not change it* unless your doctor tells you to do so.

The number of tablets or injections that you take depends on the strength of the medicine. Also, *the number of doses you take each day, the time allowed between doses, and the length of time you take the medicine depend on the medical problem for which you are taking the medicine.*

*For menadiol*

- For *oral* dosage form (tablets):
  —For problems with blood clotting or increased bleeding, or for dietary supplementation:
  - Adults and children—The usual dose is 5 to 10 milligrams (mg) a day.
- For *injection* dosage form:
  —For problems with blood clotting or increased bleeding, or for dietary supplementation:
  - Adults and children—The usual dose is 5 to 15 mg, injected into a muscle or under the skin, one or two times a day.

*For phytonadione*

- For *oral* dosage form (tablets):
  —For problems with blood clotting or increased bleeding, or for dietary supplementation:
  - Adults and teenagers—The usual dose is 2.5 to 25 milligrams (mg). The dose may be repeated after twelve to forty-eight hours, if needed.
  - Children—The usual dose is 5 to 10 mg.
- For *injection* dosage form:
  —For problems with blood clotting or increased bleeding, or for dietary supplementation:
  - Adults and teenagers receiving solid food—The usual dose is 2 to 25 mg, injected into a muscle or under the skin. The dose may be repeated, if needed.
  - Adults and teenagers receiving total parenteral nutrition (TPN)—The usual dose is 5 to 10 mg, injected into a muscle, once a week.
  - Children receiving solid food—The usual dose is 5 to 10 mg injected into a muscle or under the skin.

• Children receiving TPN—The usual dose is 2 to 5 mg, injected into a muscle, once a week.

• Infants receiving solid food—The usual dose is 1 to 2 mg injected into a muscle or under the skin.

• Infants receiving milk substitutes or breast milk—The dose is based on the amount of vitamin K in the infant's diet and must be determined by your doctor.

—For prevention of bleeding in newborns: The usual dose is 0.5 to 1 mg, injected into a muscle or under the skin, right after delivery. The dose may be repeated after six to eight hours, if needed.

**Missed dose**—If you miss a dose of this medicine, take it as soon as possible. However, if it is almost time for your next dose, skip the missed dose and go back to your regular dosing schedule. Do not double doses. *Tell your doctor about any doses you miss.*

**Storage**—To store this medicine:

• Keep out of the reach of children.

• Store away from heat and direct light.

• Do not store in the bathroom, near the kitchen sink, or in other damp places. Heat or moisture may cause the medicine to break down.

• Do not keep outdated medicine or medicine no longer needed. Be sure that any discarded medicine is out of the reach of children.

## Precautions While Using This Medicine

*Tell all medical doctors and dentists you go to that you are taking this medicine.*

*Always check with your health care professional before you start or stop taking any other medicine.* This includes any nonprescription (over-the-counter [OTC]) medicine, even aspirin. Other medicines may change the way this medicine affects your body.

## Side Effects of This Medicine

Along with its needed effects, a medicine may cause some unwanted effects. Although vitamin K does not usually cause side effects that need medical attention, check with your doctor if any of the following side effects continue or are bothersome:

*Less common*

Flushing of face; redness, pain, or swelling at place of injection; unusual taste

Other side effects not listed above may also occur in some patients. If you notice any other effects, check with your doctor.

Annual revision: August 1990
Interim revision: 07/20/94

---

# VITAMINS AND FLUORIDE    Systemic

Some commonly used brand names are:

**In the U.S.—**

| | |
|---|---|
| Adeflor[1] | Poly-Vi-Flor[1] |
| Cari-Tab[2] | Tri-Vi-Flor[2] |
| Mulvidren-F[1] | Vi-Daylin/F[1] |

**In Canada—**

| | |
|---|---|
| Adeflor[1] | Tri-Vi-Flor[2] |
| Poly-Vi-Flor[1] | |

Note: For quick reference, the following vitamins and fluoride combinations are numbered to match the corresponding brand names.

This information applies to the following medicines:

1. Multiple Vitamins and Fluoride
2. Vitamins A, D, and C and Fluoride

## Description

This medicine is a combination of vitamins and fluoride. Vitamins are used when the daily diet does not include enough of the vitamins needed for good health.

Fluoride has been found to be helpful in reducing the number of cavities in the teeth. It is usually present naturally in drinking water. However, some areas of the country do not have a high enough level of fluoride in the water. To make up for this, extra fluorides may be added to the diet. Some children may require both dietary fluorides and fluoride treatments by the dentist. Use of a fluoride toothpaste or rinse may be helpful, as well.

Taking fluorides does not replace good dental habits. These include eating a good diet, brushing and flossing teeth frequently, and having regular dental checkups.

This medicine is available only with your medical doctor's or dentist's prescription, in the following dosage forms:

*Oral*

• Oral solution (U.S. and Canada)
• Chewable Tablets (U.S. and Canada)

## Before Using This Dietary Supplement

In deciding to use a dietary supplement, the risks of taking the dietary supplement must be weighed against the good it will do. This is a decision you and your medical doctor or dentist will make. For multiple vitamins and fluoride, the following should be considered:

**Allergies**—Tell your medical doctor or dentist if you have ever had any unusual or allergic reactions to fluoride. Also, tell your medical doctor, dentist, and pharmacist if you are allergic to any other substances, such as foods, preservatives, or dyes.

**Pregnancy**—Fluoride occurs naturally in water and has not been shown to cause problems in infants of mothers who drank fluoridated water or took recommended doses of supplements.

**Breast-feeding**—Small amounts of fluoride pass into breast milk; however, problems have not been documented with normal intake.

**Children**—Doses of fluoride that are too large or are taken for a long time may cause bone problems and teeth discoloration in children.

**Older adults**—This dietary supplement has not been shown to cause different side effects or problems in older people than it does in younger adults.

**Medicines or other dietary supplements**—Although certain medicines or dietary supplements should not be used together at all, in other cases they may be used together even if an interaction might occur. In these cases, your medical doctor or dentist may want to change the dose, or other precautions may be necessary. When you are taking multiple vitamins and fluoride it is especially important that your medical doctor or dentist, and pharmacist know if you are taking any of the following:

- Anticoagulants, coumarin- or indandione-derivative (blood thinners)—Use with vitamin K (in the multiple vitamins and fluoride preparations) may prevent the anticoagulant from working properly
- Iron supplements—Use with vitamin E (in the multiple vitamins and fluoride preparation) may prevent the iron supplement from working properly
- Vitamin D and related compounds—Use with vitamin D (in the multiple vitamins and fluoride preparations) may cause high blood levels of vitamin D, which may increase the chance of side effects

**Other medical problems**—The presence of other medical problems may affect the use of multiple vitamins and fluoride. Make sure you tell your medical doctor or dentist if you have any other medical problems, especially:

- Dental fluorosis (teeth discoloration)—Fluorides may make this condition worse

## Proper Use of This Dietary Supplement

*Take this dietary supplement only as directed by your medical doctor or dentist.* Do not take more of it and do not take it more often than ordered. Taking too much fluoride and some vitamins (especially vitamins A and D) over a period of time may cause unwanted effects.

Do not take multiple vitamins and fluoride products at the same time as taking foods that contain calcium. It is best to space them 1 to 2 hours apart, to get the full benefit from the medicine.

For patients taking the *chewable tablet form* of this dietary supplement:

- Tablets should be chewed or crushed before they are swallowed.
- This dietary supplement works best if it is taken at bedtime, after the teeth have been thoroughly brushed.

For patients taking the *oral liquid form of* this dietary supplement:

- This dietary supplement is to be taken by mouth even though it comes in a dropper bottle. The amount to be taken is to be measured with the specially marked dropper.
- *Always store this dietary supplement in the original plastic container.* It has been designed to give you the correct dose. Also, fluoride will interact with glass and should not be stored in glass containers.
- This dietary supplement may be dropped directly into the mouth or mixed with cereal, fruit juice, or other food.

**Missed dose**—If you miss a dose of this dietary supplement, take it as soon as you remember. However, if it is almost time for the next dose, skip the missed dose and go back to your regular dosing schedule. Do not double doses.

**Storage**—To store this dietary supplement:

- Keep this dietary supplement out of the reach of children, since overdose is especially dangerous in children.
- Store away from heat and direct light.
- Do not store in the bathroom, near the kitchen sink, or in other damp places. Heat or moisture may cause the dietary supplement to break down.
- Protect the oral solution from freezing.
- Do not keep outdated dietary supplements or those no longer needed. Be sure that any discarded dietary supplement is out of the reach of children.

## Precautions While Using This Dietary Supplement

The level of fluoride present in the water is different in different parts of the country. If you move to another area, check with a medical doctor or dentist in the new area as soon as possible to see if this medicine is still needed or if the dose needs to be changed. Also, check with your medical doctor or dentist if you change infant feeding habits (e.g., breast-feeding to infant formula), drinking water (e.g., city water to nonfluoridated bottled water), or filtering systems (e.g., tap water to filtered tap water).

*Inform your medical doctor or dentist as soon as possible if you notice white, brown, or black spots on the teeth.* These are signs of too much fluoride.

## Side Effects of This Dietary Supplement

Along with its needed effects, a dietary supplement may cause some unwanted effects. Although not all of these side effects may occur, if they do occur they may need medical attention.

When the correct amount of this dietary supplement is used, side effects usually are rare. However, *taking an overdose of fluoride may cause serious problems.*

*Stop taking this dietary supplement and check with your medical doctor immediately* if any of the following side effects occur, as they may be signs of severe fluoride overdose:

> Black, tarry stools; bloody vomit; diarrhea; drowsiness; faintness; increased watering of mouth; nausea or vomiting; shallow breathing; stomach cramps or pain; tremors; unusual excitement; watery eyes; weakness

Check with your medical doctor or dentist as soon as possible if the following side effects occur, as some may be early signs of possible chronic fluoride overdose:

> Pain and aching of bones; skin rash; sores in the mouth and on the lips; stiffness; white, brown, or black discoloration of teeth

Other side effects not listed above may also occur in some patients. If you notice any other effects, check with your medical doctor or dentist.

---

Revised: September 1990
Interim revision: 08/21/92

---

# XYLOMETAZOLINE    Nasal

Some commonly used brand names are:

**In the U.S.—**
Chlorohist-LA
Neo-Synephrine II Long
    Acting Nasal Spray Adult
    Strength
Neo-Synephrine II Long
    Acting Nose Drops Adult
    Strength

Otrivin Nasal Drops
Otrivin Nasal Spray
Otrivin Pediatric Nasal Drops

Generic name product may also be available.

**In Canada—**
Otrivin Nasal Drops
Otrivin Nasal Spray
Otrivin Pediatric Nasal Drops

Otrivin Pediatric Nasal Spray
Otrivin With Metered-Dose
    Pump

## Description

Xylometazoline (zye-loe-met-AZ-oh-leen) is used for the temporary relief of congestion or stuffiness in the nose caused by hay fever or other allergies, colds, or sinus trouble.

This medicine may also be used for other conditions as determined by your doctor.

This medicine is available without a prescription; however, your doctor may have special instructions on the proper use or dose for your medical condition.

Xylometazoline is available in the following dosage forms:
*Nasal*
  • Nasal drops (U.S. and Canada)
  • Nasal spray (U.S. and Canada)

## Before Using This Medicine

If you are using this medicine without a prescription, carefully read and follow any precautions on the label. For xylometazoline, the following should be considered:

**Allergies**—Tell your doctor if you have ever had any unusual or allergic reaction to xylometazoline or to any of the other nasal decongestants. Also tell your health care professional if you are allergic to any other substances, such as foods, preservatives, or dyes.

**Pregnancy**—Xylometazoline may be absorbed into the body. However, xylometazoline has not been shown to cause birth defects or other problems in humans.

**Breast-feeding**—Xylometazoline may be absorbed into the body. However, xylometazoline has not been reported to cause problems in nursing babies.

**Children**—Children may be especially sensitive to the effects of xylometazoline. This may increase the chance of side effects during treatment.

**Older adults**—Many medicines have not been studied specifically in older people. Therefore, it may not be known whether they work exactly the same way they do in younger adults or if they cause different side effects or problems in older people. There is no specific information

comparing use of xylometazoline in the elderly with use in other age groups.

**Other medicines**—Although certain medicines should not be used together at all, in other cases two different medicines may be used together even if an interaction might occur. In these cases, your doctor may want to change the dose, or other precautions may be necessary. Tell your health care professional if you are taking any other prescription or nonprescription (over-the-counter [OTC]) medicine.

**Other medical problems**—The presence of other medical problems may affect the use of xylometazoline. Make sure you tell your doctor if you have any other medical problems, especially:
  • Diabetes mellitus (sugar diabetes)
  • Heart or blood vessel disease or
  • High blood pressure—Xylometazoline may make the condition worse
  • Overactive thyroid

## Proper Use of This Medicine

To use the *nose drops*:
  • Blow your nose gently. Tilt the head back while standing or sitting up. Place the drops into each nostril and immediately bend head forward toward the knees for a few seconds to allow the medicine to spread throughout the nose.
  • Rinse the dropper with hot water and dry with a clean tissue. Replace the cap right after use.

To use the *nose spray*:
  • Blow your nose gently. With the head upright, spray the medicine into each nostril. Sniff briskly while squeezing the bottle quickly and firmly. For best results, spray once into each nostril, wait 3 to 5 minutes to allow the medicine to work, then blow your nose gently and thoroughly. Repeat until the complete dose is used.
  • Rinse the tip of the spray bottle with hot water taking care not to suck water into the bottle, and dry with a clean tissue. Replace the cap right after use.

To avoid spreading the infection, do not use the container for more than one person.

*Use this medicine only as directed.* Do not use more of it, do not use it more often, and do not use it for longer than 3 days, unless otherwise directed by your doctor. To do so may make your runny or stuffy nose worse and may also increase the chance of side effects.

**Dosing**—The dose of nasal xylometazoline will be different for different patients. *Follow your doctor's orders or the directions on the label.* The following information includes only the average doses of nasal xylometazoline. *If your dose is different, do not change it* unless your doctor tells you to do so.

- For stuffy nose:
  - —For *nose drops* dosage form:
    - Adults and children 12 years of age and older—Use two or three drops of a 0.05 to 0.1% solution in each nostril every eight to ten hours as needed.
    - Children 2 to 12 years of age—Use two or three drops of a 0.05% solution in each nostril every eight to ten hours as needed.
    - Children up to 2 years of age—Use and dose must be determined by your doctor.
  - —For *nose spray* dosage form:
    - Adults and children 12 years of age and older—Use two or three sprays of a 0.05 to 0.1% solution in each nostril every eight to ten hours as needed.
    - Children up to 12 years of age—Use and dose must be determined by your doctor.

**Missed dose**—If you miss a dose of this medicine and you remember within an hour or so of the missed dose, use it right away. However, if you do not remember until later, skip the missed dose and go back to your regular dosing schedule. Do not double doses.

**Storage**—To store this medicine:

- Keep out of the reach of children.
- Store away from heat and direct light.
- Keep the medicine from freezing.
- Do not keep outdated medicine or medicine no longer needed. Be sure that any discarded medicine is out of the reach of children.

## Side Effects of This Medicine

Along with its needed effects, a medicine may cause some unwanted effects. Although not all of these side effects may occur, if they do occur they may need medical attention.

When this medicine is used for short periods of time at low doses, side effects usually are rare. However, check with your doctor as soon as possible if any of the following occur:

Increase in runny or stuffy nose

*Symptoms of too much medicine being absorbed into the body*

Blurred vision; headache or lightheadedness; nervousness; pounding, irregular, or fast heartbeat; trouble in sleeping

Other side effects may occur that usually do not need medical attention. These side effects may go away during treatment as your body adjusts to the medicine. However, check with your health care professional if any of the following side effects continue or are bothersome:

Burning, dryness, or stinging of inside of nose; sneezing

Other side effects not listed above may also occur in some patients. If you notice any other effects, check with your health care professional.

Revised: 05/16/94

# YELLOW FEVER VACCINE   Systemic

A commonly used brand name in the U.S. is YF-Vax.
Generic name product may be available in Canada.

## Description

Yellow Fever Vaccine is used to prevent infection by the yellow fever virus. It works by causing your body to produce its own protection (antibodies) against the virus.

Vaccination against yellow fever is recommended for all persons 9 months of age and older who are traveling to or living in areas of Africa, South America, or other countries where there is yellow fever infection and for people who are traveling to countries that require yellow fever immunization (certificate of vaccination). It is also needed by other people who might come into contact with the yellow fever virus.

Infants 6 to 9 months of age and pregnant women should be vaccinated only if they must travel to areas where there is an epidemic of yellow fever and they cannot be protected from mosquito bites.

Infants 4 to 6 months of age may be vaccinated only if there is a high risk of getting yellow fever infection.

Vaccination against yellow fever is not recommended for infants younger than 4 months of age because they have an increased chance of getting serious side effects from the vaccine.

The certificate of vaccination for yellow fever is valid for 10 years beginning 10 days after the first vaccination, or on the date of the second vaccination if within 10 years of the first injection.

Yellow fever vaccine is given only at authorized Yellow Fever Vaccination Centers. The location of these centers can be obtained from your state, province, and local health departments.

The vaccine is available in the following dosage form:

*Parenteral*
- Injection (U.S. and Canada)

## Before Using This Medicine

In deciding to use a medicine, the risks of taking the medicine must be weighed against the good it will do. This is a decision you and your doctor will make. For yellow fever vaccine, the following should be considered:

**Allergies**—Tell your doctor if you have ever had any unusual or allergic reaction to yellow fever vaccine. Also tell your doctor if you are allergic to any other substances, such as foods (especially eggs and chicken), preservatives, or dyes. The yellow fever vaccine available in the U.S. and Canada is grown in chick embryo cell culture so it may contain egg or chicken protein.

If you are allergic to eggs or chicken, your doctor may have to do a skin test before giving you the vaccine. However, if you need the vaccine because of international travel requirements, not because you are traveling to a country where there is a high risk of getting yellow fever, you may ask your doctor for a waiver letter stating the reason why you cannot be vaccinated.

**Pregnancy**—Yellow fever vaccine may cause birth defects. Therefore, it is not recommended for use in pregnant women, especially in the first 3 months of pregnancy, unless they are at high risk of getting yellow fever. Pregnant women who have not already been immunized are generally advised to postpone their travel and vaccination until after giving birth.

If travel to high-risk areas cannot be postponed, pregnant women should be vaccinated. The chance of getting serious problems from infection with yellow fever in those areas is much greater than the chance of getting a serious side effect from the vaccine for both the mother and the fetus.

However, a pregnant woman who needs the vaccine because of international travel requirements, not because she is traveling to a country where there is a high risk of getting yellow fever, may ask the doctor for a waiver letter (official-looking on letterhead stationery) stating why she cannot be vaccinated.

**Breast-feeding**—Yellow fever vaccine has not been shown to cause problems in nursing babies.

**Children**—Yellow fever vaccine is recommended for children 9 months of age or older if they are traveling to, or living in, areas where there is yellow fever infection, or if they are traveling to areas that require yellow fever immunization (certificate of vaccination). In special cases, such as high-risk exposure, yellow fever vaccine may be given to children 4 to 9 months of age. However, the vaccine is not recommended for infants younger than 4 months of age, because of an increased chance of serious side effects.

**Other medicines**—Although certain medicines should not be used together at all, in other cases two different medicines may be used together even if an interaction might occur. In these cases, your doctor may want to change the dose, or other precautions may be necessary. Before you receive yellow fever vaccine, it is especially important that your doctor know if you have received any of the following:

- Treatment with x-rays or medicines that may lower the body's protection against infection such as those used for organ transplants (e.g., cyclosporine), cancer medicines, or corticosteroids—May decrease the useful effect of yellow fever vaccine

**Other medical problems**—The presence of other medical problems may affect the use of yellow fever vaccine. Make sure you tell your doctor if you have any other medical problems, especially:

- Immune deficiency condition (or family history of)—The condition may decrease the useful effect of the vaccine or may increase the risk and severity of side effects

• Serious illness with fever—The symptoms of the illness may be confused with the possible side effects of the vaccine

## Side Effects of This Medicine

Along with its needed effects, a vaccine may cause some unwanted effects. Although not all of these side effects may occur, if they do occur they may need medical attention.

*Get emergency help immediately* if any of the following side effects occur:

*Rare*

Confusion; convulsions (seizures); coughing; difficulty in breathing or swallowing; fast heartbeat; feeling of burning, crawling, or tingling of skin; nervousness or irritability; reddening of skin; severe headache; skin rash or itching; sneezing; stiff neck; throbbing in the ears; unusual tiredness or weakness; vomiting

Other side effects may occur that usually do not need medical attention. These side effects may go away during treatment as your body adjusts to the medicine. However, check with your doctor if any of the following side effects continue or are bothersome:

*Less common*

Low fever; mild headache; muscle pain; pain at place of injection

Other side effects not listed above may also occur in some patients. If you notice any other effects, check with your doctor.

Developed: 11/22/93

# YOHIMBINE   Systemic

Some commonly used brand names are:

**In the U.S.—**

| | |
|---|---|
| Actibine | Yocon |
| Aphrodyne | Yohimar |
| Baron-X | Yohimex |
| Dayto Himbin | Yoman |
| Prohim | Yovital |
| Thybine | |

Generic name product may also be available.

**In Canada—**

| | |
|---|---|
| PMS-Yohimbine | Yocon |

Generic name product may also be available.

## Description

Yohimbine (yo-HIM-been) is used to treat men who are impotent (not able to have sex). It is taken by mouth to help produce erections.

The way yohimbine works is not known for sure. It is thought, however, to work by increasing the body's production of certain chemicals that help produce erections. It does not work in all men who are impotent.

Yohimbine is available only with your doctor's prescription, in the following dosage form:

*Oral*

• Tablets (U.S. and Canada)

## Before Using This Medicine

In deciding to use a medicine, the risks of taking the medicine must be weighed against the good it will do. This is a decision you and your doctor will make. For yohimbine, the following should be considered:

**Allergies**—Tell your doctor if you have ever had any unusual or allergic reaction to yohimbine or any of the rauwolfia alkaloids, such as deserpidine (e.g, Harmonyl), rauwolfia serpentina (e.g., Raudixin), or reserpine (e.g., Serpalan). Also tell your health care professional if you are allergic to any other substances, such as foods, preservatives, or dyes.

**Older adults**—Many medicines have not been studied specifically in older people. Therefore, it may not be known whether they work exactly the same way they do in younger adults. Although there is no specific information comparing use of yohimbine in the elderly with use in other age groups, this medicine has been used in some elderly patients and has not been shown to cause different side effects or problems in older people than it does in younger adults.

**Other medicines**—Although certain medicines should not be used together at all, in other cases two different medicines may be used together even if an interaction might occur. In these cases, your doctor may want to change the dose, or other precautions may be necessary. Tell your health care professional if you are taking any other prescription or nonprescription (over-the-counter [OTC]) medicine.

**Other medical problems**—The presence of other medical problems may affect the use of yohimbine. Make sure you tell your doctor if you have any other medical problems, especially:

• Angina pectoris or
• Depression or
• Other psychiatric illness or
• Heart disease or
• High blood pressure or
• Kidney disease—Yohimbine may make these conditions worse

• Liver disease—Effects of yohimbine may be increased because of slower removal from the body

## Proper Use of This Medicine

This medicine usually begins to work about 2 to 3 weeks after you begin to take it.

**Dosing**—The dose of yohimbine will be different for different patients. *Follow your doctor's orders or the directions on the label.* The following information includes only the average doses of yohimbine. *If your dose is different, do not change it* unless your doctor tells you to do so.

The number of tablets that you take depends on the strength of the medicine.

- For *oral* dosage form (tablets):
  —For treating impotence:
  - Adults—5.4 to 6 milligrams (mg) three times a day.

**Missed dose**—If you miss a dose of this medicine, take it as soon as possible. However, if it is almost time for your next dose, skip the missed dose and go back to your regular dosing schedule. Do not double doses.

**Storage**—To store this medicine:
- Keep out of the reach of children.
- Store away from heat and direct light.
- Do not store in the bathroom, near the kitchen sink, or in other damp places. Heat or moisture may cause the medicine to break down.
- Keep the medicine from freezing. Do not refrigerate.
- Do not keep outdated medicine or medicine no longer needed. Be sure that any discarded medicine is out of the reach of children.

## Precautions While Using This Medicine

It is important that your doctor check your progress at regular visits to make sure that this medicine is working properly.

Use yohimbine exactly as directed by your doctor. Do not use more of it and do not use it more often than ordered. If too much is used, the risk of side effects such as fast heartbeat and high blood pressure is increased.

## Side Effects of This Medicine

Along with its needed effects, a medicine may cause some unwanted effects. Although not all of these side effects may occur, if they do occur they may need medical attention.

*Check with your doctor as soon as possible if any of the following side effects occur:*
    *Less common*
        Fast heartbeat; increased blood pressure

Other side effects may occur that usually do not need medical attention. These side effects may go away during treatment as your body adjusts to the medicine. However, check with your doctor if any of the following side effects continue or are bothersome:
    *Less common*
        Dizziness; headache; irritability; nervousness or restlessness
    *Rare*
        Nausea and vomiting; skin flushing; sweating; tremor

Other side effects not listed above may also occur in some patients. If you notice any other effects, check with your doctor.

Revised: 10/24/92
Interim revision: 07/05/94

# ZALCITABINE  Systemic

A commonly used brand name in the U.S. and Canada is HIVID. Another commonly used name is ddC.

## Description

Zalcitabine (zal-SITE-a-been) (also known as ddC) is used in the treatment of the infection caused by the human immunodeficiency virus (HIV). HIV is the virus that causes acquired immune deficiency syndrome (AIDS).

Zalcitabine (ddC) will not cure or prevent HIV infection or AIDS; however, it helps keep HIV from reproducing and appears to slow down the destruction of the immune system. This may help delay the development of problems usually related to AIDS or HIV disease. Zalcitabine will not keep you from spreading HIV to other people. People who receive this medicine may continue to have other problems usually related to AIDS or HIV disease.

Zalcitabine may cause some serious side effects, including peripheral neuropathy (a problem involving the nerves). Symptoms of peripheral neuropathy include tingling, burning, numbness, or pain in the hands or feet. Zalcitabine may also cause pancreatitis (inflammation of the pancreas). Symptoms of pancreatitis include stomach pain, and nausea and vomiting. *Check with your doctor if any new health problems or symptoms occur while you are taking zalcitabine.*

Zalcitabine is available only with your doctor's prescription, in the following dosage form:

*Oral*
- Tablets (U.S. and Canada)

## Before Using This Medicine

In deciding to use a medicine, the risks of taking the medicine must be weighed against the good it will do. This is a decision you and your doctor will make. For zalcitabine, the following should be considered:

**Allergies**—Tell your doctor if you have ever had any unusual or allergic reaction to zalcitabine. Also tell your health care professional if you are allergic to any other substances, such as foods, preservatives, or dyes.

**Pregnancy**—Zalcitabine has not been studied in pregnant women. However, studies in animals have shown that zalcitabine causes birth defects when given in very high doses. Before taking this medicine, make sure your doctor knows if you are pregnant or if you may become pregnant.

**Breast-feeding**—It is not known whether zalcitabine passes into the breast milk. However, if your baby does not already have the AIDS virus, there is a chance that you could pass it to your baby by breast-feeding. Talk to your doctor first if you are thinking about breast-feeding your baby.

**Children**—Zalcitabine can cause serious side effects in any patient. Therefore, it is especially important that you

discuss with your child's doctor the good that this medicine may do as well as the risks of using it. Your child must be seen frequently and your child's progress carefully followed by the doctor while the child is taking zalcitabine.

**Older adults**—Zalcitabine has not been studied specifically in older people. Therefore, it is not known whether it causes different side effects or problems in the elderly than it does in younger adults.

**Other medicines**—Although certain medicines should not be used together at all, in other cases two different medicines may be used together even if an interaction might occur. In these cases, your doctor may want to change the dose, or other precautions may be necessary. When you are taking zalcitabine, it is especially important that your health care professional know if you are taking any of the following:

- Alcohol or
- Asparaginase (e.g., Elspar) or
- Azathioprine (e.g., Imuran) or
- Estrogens (female hormones) or
- Furosemide (e.g., Lasix) or
- Methyldopa (e.g., Aldomet) or
- Pentamidine by injection (e.g., Pentam, Pentacarinat) or
- Sulfonamides (e.g., Bactrim, Septra) or
- Sulindac (e.g., Clinoril) or
- Tetracyclines or
- Thiazide diuretics (water pills) (e.g., Diuril, Hydrodiuril) or
- Valproic acid (e.g., Depakote)—Use of these medicines with zalcitabine may increase the chance of pancreatitis (inflammation of the pancreas)
- Aminoglycosides by injection (amikacin [e.g., Amikin], gentamicin [e.g., Garamycin], kanamycin [e.g., Kantrex], neomycin [e.g., Mycifradin], netilmicin [e.g., Netromycin], streptomycin, tobramycin [e.g., Nebcin]) or
- Amphotericin B (e.g., Fungizone) or
- Foscarnet (e.g., Foscavir)—Use of these medicines with zalcitabine may increase the chance of side effects
- Chloramphenicol (e.g., Chloromycetin) or
- Cisplatin (e.g., Platinol) or
- Dapsone (e.g., Avlosulfon) or
- Didanosine (e.g. Videx) or
- Ethambutol (e.g., Myambutol) or
- Ethionamide (e.g., Trecator-SC) or
- Hydralazine (e.g., Apresoline) or
- Isoniazid (e.g., Nydrazid) or
- Lithium (e.g., Eskalith, Lithobid) or
- Metronidazole (e.g., Flagyl) or
- Nitrous oxide or
- Phenytoin (e.g., Dilantin) or
- Stavudine (e.g., d4T) or
- Vincristine (e.g., Oncovin)—Use of these medicines with zalcitabine may increase the chance of peripheral neuropathy (tingling, burning, numbness, or pain in your hands or feet)
- Nitrofurantoin (e.g., Furadantin, Macrodantin)—Use of nitrofurantoin with zalcitabine may increase the chance of side effects, including peripheral neuropathy (tingling, burning, numbness, or pain in your hands or feet) and pancreatitis (inflammation of the pancreas)

**Other medical problems**—The presence of other medical problems may affect the use of zalcitabine. Make sure you tell your doctor if you have any other medical problems, especially:

- Alcohol abuse or
- Increased blood triglycerides (or a history of) or
- Pancreatitis (or a history of)—Patients with these medical problems may be at increased risk of pancreatitis (inflammation of the pancreas)
- Alcohol abuse, history of, or
- Liver disease—Zalcitabine may make liver disease worse in patients with liver disease or a history of alcohol abuse
- Kidney disease—Patients with kidney disease may have an increased chance of side effects
- Peripheral neuropathy—Zalcitabine may make this condition worse

## Proper Use of This Medicine

*Take this medicine exactly as directed by your doctor.* Do not take more of it, do not take it more often, and do not take it for a longer time than your doctor ordered. Also, do not stop taking this medicine without checking with your doctor first.

*Keep taking zalcitabine for the full time of treatment,* even if you begin to feel better.

This medicine works best when there is a constant amount in the blood. *To help keep the amount constant, do not miss any doses.* If you need help in planning the best times to take your medicine, check with your health care professional.

Only take medicine that your doctor has prescribed specifically for you. Do not share your medicine with others.

**Dosing**—The dose of zalcitabine will be different for different patients. *Follow your doctor's orders or the directions on the label.* The following information includes only the average doses of zalcitabine. Your dose may be different if you have kidney disease. *If your dose is different, do not change it* unless your doctor tells you to do so:

- For *oral* dosage form (tablets):
  - —For treatment of HIV infection:
    - Adults and children 13 years of age and older— 0.75 milligrams (mg), together with 200 mg of zidovudine, every eight hours.
    - Children up to 12 years of age—Use and dose are based on body weight and must be determined by your doctor.

**Missed dose**—If you miss a dose of this medicine, take it as soon as possible. However, if it is almost time for your next dose, skip the missed dose and go back to your regular dosing schedule. Do not double doses.

**Storage**—To store this medicine:

- Keep out of the reach of children.
- Store away from heat and direct light.

- Do not store in the bathroom, near the kitchen sink, or in other damp places. Heat or moisture may cause the medicine to break down.
- Do not keep outdated medicine or medicine no longer needed. Be sure that any discarded medicine is out of the reach of children.

## Precautions While Using This Medicine

*It is very important that your doctor check your progress at regular visits.*

*Do not take any other medicines without checking with your doctor first.* To do so may increase the chance of side effects from zalcitabine.

HIV may be acquired from or spread to other people through infected body fluids, including blood, vaginal fluid, or semen. *If you are infected, it is best to avoid any sexual activity involving an exchange of body fluids with other people. If you do have sex, always wear (or have your partner wear) a condom ("rubber"). Only use condoms made of latex, and use them every time you have vaginal, anal, or oral sex.* The use of a spermicide (such as nonoxynol-9) may also help prevent transmission of HIV if it is not irritating to the vagina, rectum, or mouth. Spermicides have been shown to kill HIV in lab tests. Do not use oil-based jelly, cold cream, baby oil, or shortening as a lubricant—these products can cause the condom to break. Lubricants without oil, such as *K-Y Jelly*, are recommended. Women may wish to carry their own condoms. Birth control pills and diaphragms will help protect against pregnancy, but they will not prevent someone from giving or getting the AIDS virus. *If you inject drugs,* get help to stop. *Do not share needles or equipment with anyone.* In some cities, more than half of the drug users are infected, and sharing even 1 needle or syringe can spread the virus. If you have any questions about this, check with your health care professional.

## Side Effects of This Medicine

Along with its needed effects, a medicine may cause some unwanted effects. Although not all of these side effects may occur, if they do occur they may need medical attention.

*Check with your doctor immediately* if any of the following side effects occur:

*More common*

Tingling, burning, numbness, or pain in the hands, arms, feet, or legs

*Less common*

Fever; joint pain; muscle pain; skin rash; ulcers in the mouth and throat

*Rare*

Fever and sore throat; nausea and vomiting; stomach pain (severe)

Other side effects may occur that usually do not need medical attention. These side effects may go away during treatment as your body adjusts to the medicine. However, check with your doctor if any of the following side effects continue or are bothersome:

*Less common*
    Diarrhea; headache

Other side effects not listed above may also occur in some patients. If you notice any other effects, check with your doctor.

Revised: 06/22/94

---

# ZIDOVUDINE  Systemic

Some commonly used brand names are:
**In the U.S.—**
    Retrovir
**In Canada—**
    Apo-Zidovudine          Retrovir
    Novo-AZT
Another commonly used name is AZT.

## Description

Zidovudine (zye-DOE-vue-deen) (also known as AZT) is used in the treatment of the infection caused by the human immunodeficiency virus (HIV). HIV is the virus responsible for acquired immune deficiency syndrome (AIDS). Zidovudine is also used to slow the progression of disease in patients infected with HIV who have early symptoms or no symptoms at all.

Zidovudine will not cure or prevent HIV infection or AIDS; however, it helps keep HIV from reproducing and appears to slow down the destruction of the immune system. This may help delay the development of problems usually related to AIDS or HIV disease. Zidovudine will not keep you from spreading HIV to other people. People who receive this medicine may continue to have the problems usually related to AIDS or HIV disease.

Zidovudine may cause some serious side effects, including bone marrow problems. Symptoms of bone marrow problems include fever, chills, or sore throat; pale skin; and unusual tiredness or weakness. These problems may require blood transfusions or temporarily stopping treatment with zidovudine. *Check with your doctor if any new health problems or symptoms occur while you are taking zidovudine.*

Zidovudine is available only with your doctor's prescription, in the following dosage forms:
*Oral*
  • Capsules (U.S. and Canada)
  • Syrup (U.S. and Canada)
*Parenteral*
  • Injection (U.S. and Canada)

## Before Using This Medicine

In deciding to use a medicine, the risks of taking the medicine must be weighed against the good it will do.

This is a decision you and your doctor will make. For zidovudine, the following should be considered:

**Allergies—**Tell your doctor if you have ever had any unusual or allergic reaction to zidovudine. Also tell your health care professional if you are allergic to any other substances, such as foods, preservatives, or dyes.

**Pregnancy—**Zidovudine crosses the placenta. Studies in pregnant women have not been completed. However, zidovudine has been shown to decrease the chance of passing HIV to your baby during pregnancy and at birth. Zidovudine has not been shown to cause birth defects in studies in rats and rabbits given this medicine by mouth in doses many times larger than the human dose.

**Breast-feeding—**It is not known whether zidovudine passes into the breast milk. However, if your baby does not have the AIDS virus, there is a chance that you could pass it to your baby by breast-feeding. Talk to your doctor first if you are thinking about breast-feeding your baby.

**Children—**Zidovudine can cause serious side effects in any patient. Therefore, it is especially important that you discuss with your child's doctor the good that this medicine may do as well as the risks of using it. Your child must be carefully followed, and frequently seen, by the doctor while he or she is taking zidovudine.

**Older adults—**Zidovudine has not been studied specifically in older people. Therefore, it is not known whether it causes different side effects or problems in the elderly than it does in younger adults.

**Other medicines—**Although certain medicines should not be used together at all, in other cases 2 different medicines may be used together even if an interaction might occur. In these cases, your doctor may want to change the dose, or other precautions may be necessary. When you are taking zidovudine, it is especially important that your health care professional know if you are taking any of the following:
  • Amphotericin B by injection (e.g., Fungizone) or
  • Antineoplastics (cancer medicine) or
  • Antithyroid agents (medicine for overactive thyroid) or
  • Azathioprine (e.g., Imuran) or
  • Chloramphenicol (e.g., Chloromycetin) or
  • Colchicine or
  • Cyclophosphamide (e.g., Cytoxan) or
  • Flucytosine (e.g., Ancobon) or

- Ganciclovir (e.g., Cytovene) or
- Interferon (e.g., Intron A, Roferon-A) or
- Mercaptopurine (e.g., Purinethol) or
- Methotrexate (e.g., Mexate) or
- Plicamycin (e.g., Mithracin)—Caution should be used if these medicines and zidovudine are used together; taking zidovudine while you are using or receiving these medicines may make anemia and other blood problems worse
- Clarithromycin (e.g., Biaxin)—Clarithromycin may decrease the amount of zidovudine in the blood
- Probenecid (e.g., Benemid)—Probenecid may increase the amount of zidovudine in the blood, increasing the chance of side effects

**Other medical problems**—The presence of other medical problems may affect the use of zidovudine. Make sure you tell your doctor if you have any other medical problems, especially:

- Anemia or other blood problems—Zidovudine may make these conditions worse
- Liver disease—Patients with liver disease may have an increase in side effects from zidovudine
- Low amounts of folic acid or vitamin $B_{12}$ in the blood—Zidovudine may worsen anemia caused by a decrease of folic acid or vitamin $B_{12}$

## Proper Use of This Medicine

Patient information sheets about zidovudine are available. Read this information carefully.

*Take this medicine exactly as directed by your doctor.* Do not take more of it, do not take it more often, and do not take it for a longer time than your doctor ordered. Also, do not stop taking this medicine without checking with your doctor first.

*Keep taking zidovudine for the full time of treatment,* even if you begin to feel better.

For patients using *zidovudine syrup:*

- Use a specially marked measuring spoon or other device to measure each dose accurately. The average household teaspoon may not hold the right amount of liquid.

This medicine works best when there is a constant amount in the blood. *To help keep the amount constant, do not miss any doses.* If you need help in planning the best times to take your medicine, check with your health care professional.

**Dosing**—The dose of zidovudine will be different for different patients. *Follow your doctor's orders or the directions on the label.* The following information includes only the average doses of zidovudine. *If your dose is different, do not change it* unless your doctor tells you to do so.

- For the treatment of HIV infection:
  —For *oral* dosage forms (capsules and syrup):
  - Adults and teenagers—100 milligrams (mg) every four hours for a total of 500 or 600 mg a day.

  - Children 3 months to 12 years of age—Dose is based on body size and must be determined by your doctor.
  —For *injection* dosage form:
  - Adults and teenagers—Dose is based on body weight and must be determined by your doctor. The usual dose is 1 to 2 mg per kilogram (0.45 to 0.9 mg per pound) of body weight, injected slowly into a vein every four hours around the clock. The injection dosage form is given until you can take zidovudine by mouth.
  - Children 3 months to 12 years of age—Dose is based on body size and must be determined by your doctor.

**Missed dose**—If you do miss a dose of this medicine, take it as soon as possible. However, if it is almost time for your next dose, skip the missed dose and go back to your regular dosing schedule. Do not double doses.

**Storage**—To store this medicine:

- Keep out of the reach of children.
- Store away from heat and direct light.
- Do not store in the bathroom, near the kitchen sink, or in other damp places. Heat or moisture may cause the medicine to break down.
- Do not keep outdated medicine or medicine no longer needed. Be sure that any discarded medicine is out of the reach of children.

## Precautions While Using This Medicine

*It is very important that your doctor check your progress at regular visits.* This medicine may cause blood problems.

*Do not take any other medicines without checking with your doctor first.* To do so may increase the chance of side effects from zidovudine.

Zidovudine may cause blood problems. These problems may result in a greater chance of certain infections and slow healing. Therefore, you should be careful when using regular toothbrushes, dental floss, and toothpicks not to damage your gums. Check with your medical doctor or dentist if you have any questions about proper oral hygiene (mouth care) during treatment.

HIV may be acquired from or spread to other people through infected body fluids, including blood, vaginal fluid, or semen. *If you are infected, it is best to avoid any sexual activity involving an exchange of body fluids with other people. If you do have sex, always wear (or have your partner wear) a condom ("rubber"). Only use condoms made of latex, and use them every time you have vaginal, anal, or oral sex.* The use of a spermicide (such as nonoxynol-9) may also help prevent the spread of HIV if it is not irritating to the vagina, rectum, or mouth. Spermicides have been shown to kill HIV in lab tests. Do not use oil-based jelly, cold cream, baby oil, or shortening as a lubricant—these products can cause the condom to break. Lubricants without oil, such as *K-Y*

*Jelly*, are recommended. Women may wish to carry their own condoms. Birth control pills and diaphragms will help protect against pregnancy, but they will not prevent someone from giving or getting the AIDS virus. *If you inject drugs*, get help to stop. *Do not share needles with anyone.* In some cities, more than half of the drug users are infected, and sharing even 1 needle can spread the virus. If you have any questions about this, check with your health care professional.

## Side Effects of This Medicine

Along with its needed effects, a medicine may cause some unwanted effects. Although not all of these side effects may occur, if they do occur they may need medical attention.

*Check with your doctor immediately* if any of the following side effects occur:

*More common*
Fever, chills, or sore throat; pale skin; unusual tiredness or weakness
Note: The above side effects may also occur up to weeks or months after you stop taking this medicine.

*Rare*
Abdominal discomfort; confusion; convulsions (seizures); general feeling of discomfort; loss of appetite; mood or mental changes; muscle tenderness and weakness; nausea

Other side effects may occur that usually do not need medical attention. These side effects may go away during treatment as your body adjusts to the medicine. However, check with your doctor if any of the following side effects continue or are bothersome:

*More common*
Headache (severe); muscle soreness; nausea; trouble in sleeping

*Less common*
Bluish-brown colored bands on nails

Other side effects not listed above may also occur in some patients. If you notice any other effects, check with your doctor.

## Additional Information

Once a medicine has been approved for marketing for a certain use, experience may show that it is also useful for other medical problems. Although this use is not included in product labeling, zidovudine is used in certain patients with the following medical condition:

- Human immunodeficiency virus (HIV) infection due to occupational exposure (possible prevention of)

Other than the above information, there is no additional information relating to proper use, precautions, or side effects for this use.

Revised: 06/22/94

# ZINC SUPPLEMENTS     Systemic

Some commonly used brand names are:
**In the U.S.—**
Orazinc[3]              Zincate[3]
Verazinc[3]            Zinkaps-220[3]
Zinc-220[3]

**In Canada—**
PMS Egozinc[3]
Note: For quick reference, the following zinc supplements are numbered to match the corresponding brand names.
This information applies to the following medicines:
1. Zinc Chloride (zink KLOR-ide)[†‡]
2. Zinc Gluconate (GLOO-coh-nate)[‡§]
3. Zinc Sulfate (SUL-fate)[‡§]

[†]Not commercially available in Canada.
[‡]Generic name product may also be available in the U.S.
[§]Generic name product may also be available in Canada.

## Description

Zinc supplements are used to prevent or treat zinc deficiency.

The body needs zinc for normal growth and health. For patients who are unable to get enough zinc in their regular diet or who have a need for more zinc, zinc supplements may be necessary. They are generally taken by mouth but some patients may have to receive them by injection.

Zinc supplements may be used for other conditions as determined by your doctor.

Lack of zinc may lead to poor night vision and wound-healing, a decrease in sense of taste and smell, a reduced ability to fight infections, and poor development of reproductive organs.

Patients with the following conditions may be more likely to have a deficiency of zinc:

- Acrodermatitis enteropathica (a lack of absorption of zinc from the intestine)
- Alcoholism
- Burns
- Diabetes mellitus (sugar diabetes)
- Down's syndrome
- Eating disorders
- Intestine diseases
- Infections (continuing or chronic)
- Kidney disease

- Liver disease
- Pancreas disease
- Sickle cell disease
- Skin disorders
- Stomach removal
- Stress (continuing)
- Thalassemia
- Trauma (prolonged)

In addition, premature infants may need additional zinc.

If any of the above apply to you, you should take zinc supplements only on the advice of your doctor after need has been established.

Claims that zinc is effective in preventing vision loss in the elderly have not been proven. Zinc has not been proven effective in the treatment of porphyria.

Some zinc preparations are available only with your doctor's prescription. Others are available without a prescription; however, your doctor may have special instructions on the proper use and dose for your condition.

Zinc supplements are available in the following dosage forms:

*Oral*
    Zinc Gluconate
        • Tablets (U.S. and Canada)
    Zinc Sulfate
        • Capsules (U.S. and Canada)
        • Tablets (U.S.)
*Parenteral*
    Zinc Chloride
        • Injection (U.S.)
    Zinc Sulfate
        • Injection (U.S. and Canada)

## Importance of Diet

Many nutritionists recommend that, if possible, people should get all the zinc they need from foods. However, some people do not get enough zinc from their diet. For example, people on weight-loss diets may consume too little food to provide enough zinc. Others may need more zinc than normal. For such people, a zinc supplement is important.

In order to get enough vitamins and minerals in your regular diet, it is important that you eat a balanced and varied diet. Follow carefully any diet program your doctor or dietitian may recommend. For your specific vitamin and/or mineral needs, ask your doctor for a list of appropriate foods.

Zinc is found in various foods, including lean red meats, seafoods (especially herring and oysters), peas, and beans. Zinc is also found in whole grains; however, large amounts of whole-grains have been found to decrease the amount of zinc that is absorbed. Additional zinc may be added to the diet through treated (galvanized) cookware. Foods stored in uncoated tin cans may cause less zinc to be available for absorption from food.

Experts have developed a list of Recommended Dietary Allowances (RDA) of zinc. The RDA are not an exact number but a general idea of how much you need every day. They do not cover amounts needed for problems caused by a serious lack of zinc.

The RDA for zinc are:
- Infants and children—
  Birth to 1 year of age: 5 mg per day.
  1 to 10 years of age: 10 mg per day.
- Adolescent and adult males—11 years of age and over: 15 mg per day.
- Adolescent and adult females—11 years of age and over: 12 mg per day.
- Pregnant females—15 mg per day.
- Breast-feeding females—
  First 6 months: 19 mg per day.
  Second 6 months: 16 mg per day.

Remember:
- The total amount of zinc that you get every day includes what you get from the foods that you eat *and* what you may take as a supplement.
- This total amount should not be greater than the RDA, unless ordered by your doctor.

## Before Using This Dietary Supplement

If you are taking this dietary supplement without a prescription, carefully read and follow any precautions on the label. For zinc supplements, the following should be considered:

**Allergies**—Tell your health care professional if you are allergic to any substances, such as foods, preservatives, or dyes.

**Pregnancy**—It is especially important that you are receiving enough vitamins and minerals when you become pregnant and that you continue to receive the right amount of vitamins and minerals throughout your pregnancy. The healthy growth and development of the fetus depend on a steady supply of nutrients from the mother. There is evidence that low blood levels of zinc may lead to problems in pregnancy or defects in the baby. However, taking large amounts of a dietary supplement in pregnancy may be harmful to the mother and/or fetus and should be avoided.

**Breast-feeding**—It is important that you receive the right amounts of vitamins and minerals so that your baby will also get the vitamins and minerals needed to grow properly. However, taking large amounts of a dietary supplement while breast-feeding may be harmful to the mother and/or baby and should be avoided.

**Children**—It is especially important that children receive enough zinc in their diet for healthy growth and development. Although there is no specific information comparing use of zinc in children with use in other age groups, this medicine is not expected to cause different side effects or problems in children than it does in adults.

**Older adults**—It is important that older people continue to receive enough zinc in their daily diets. There is some evidence that the elderly may be at risk of becoming deficient in zinc due to poor food selection, decreased absorption of zinc by the body, or medicines that decrease absorption of zinc or increase loss of zinc from the body.

**Medicines or other dietary supplements**—Although certain medicines or dietary supplements should not be used together at all, in other cases they may be used together even if an interaction might occur. In these cases, your doctor may want to change the dose, or other precautions may be necessary. When you are taking zinc supplements, it is especially important that your health care professional know if you are taking any of the following:

- Copper supplements or
- Penicillamine and other medicines that bind with metals or
- Tetracycline (medicine for infection)—Use with zinc supplements may cause these medicines to be less effective; zinc supplements should be given at least 2 hours after copper supplements, penicillamine, or tetracycline
- Iron supplements—Use with zinc supplements may cause the zinc to be less effective; zinc supplements should be given at least 2 hours after iron supplements

**Other medical problems**—The presence of other medical problems may affect the use of zinc supplements. Make sure you tell your doctor if you have any other medical problems, especially:

- Copper deficiency—Zinc supplements may make this condition worse

## Proper Use of This Dietary Supplement

Zinc supplements are most effective if they are taken at least 1 hour before or 2 hours after meals. However, if zinc supplements cause stomach upset, they may be taken with a meal. You should tell your doctor if you are taking your zinc supplement with meals.

Some people believe that taking very large doses of a vitamin or mineral (called megadoses) is useful for treating certain medical problems. Studies have not proven this. Large doses should be taken only under the direction of your doctor after need has been identified.

**Dosing**—The dose of zinc for prevention of zinc deficiency is based on the Recommended Dietary Allowances (RDA). See the *Importance of Diet* section for the RDA for zinc.

**Missed dose**—If you miss taking zinc supplements for one or more days there is no cause for concern, since it takes some time for your body to become seriously low in zinc. However, if your doctor has recommended that you take zinc, try to remember to take it as directed every day.

**Storage**—To store this dietary supplement:

- Keep out of the reach of children.
- Store away from heat and direct light.
- Do not store in the bathroom, near the kitchen sink, or in other damp places. Heat or moisture may cause the dietary supplement to break down.
- Keep the dietary supplement from freezing. Do not refrigerate.
- Do not keep outdated dietary supplements or those no longer needed. Be sure that any discarded dietary supplement is out of the reach of children.

## Precautions While Using This Dietary Supplement

When zinc combines with certain foods it may not be absorbed into your body and it will do you no good. If you are taking zinc, the following foods should be avoided or taken 2 hours after you take zinc:

- Bran
- Fiber-containing foods
- Phosphorus-containing foods such as milk or poultry
- Whole-grain breads and cereals

Do not take zinc supplements and copper, iron, or phosphorus supplements at the same time. It is best to space doses of these products 2 hours apart, to get the full benefit from each dietary supplement.

## Side Effects of This Dietary Supplement

Along with its needed effects, a dietary supplement may cause some unwanted effects. Although not all of these side effects may occur, if they do occur they may need medical attention.

Check with your doctor as soon as possible if any of the following side effects occur:

*Rare—With large doses*

Chills; continuing ulcers or sores in mouth or throat; fever; heartburn; indigestion; nausea; sore throat; unusual tiredness or weakness

*Symptoms of overdose*

Chest pain; dizziness; fainting; shortness of breath; vomiting; yellow eyes or skin

Other side effects not listed above may also occur in some patients. If you notice any other effects, check with your doctor.

## Additional Information

Once a medicine or dietary supplement has been approved for marketing for a certain use, experience may show that it is also useful for other medical problems.

Although this use is not included in product labeling, zinc supplements are used in certain patients with the following medical condition:

- Wilson's disease (a disease of too much copper in the body)

Other than the above information, there is no additional information relating to proper use, precautions, or side effects for this use.

Revised: 02/03/92
Interim revision(s): 08/21/92; 08/18/94

# ZOLPIDEM   Systemic†

A commonly used brand name in the U.S. is Ambien.

†Not commercially available in Canada.

## Description

Zolpidem (ZOLE-pi-dem) belongs to the group of medicines called central nervous system (CNS) depressants (medicines that slow down the nervous system). Zolpidem is used to treat insomnia (trouble in sleeping). In general, when sleep medicines are used every night for a long time, they may lose their effectiveness. In most cases, sleep medicines should be used only for short periods of time, such as 1 or 2 days, and generally for no longer than 1 or 2 weeks.

This medicine is available only with your doctor's prescription, in the following dosage form:

*Oral*
- Tablets (U.S.)

## Before Using This Medicine

Sleep medicines may cause a special type of memory loss or "amnesia". When this occurs, a person does not remember what has happened during the several hours between use of the medicine and the time when its effects wear off. This is usually not a problem since most people fall asleep after taking the medicine. In most instances, memory problems can be avoided by taking zolpidem only when you are able to get a full night's sleep (7 to 8 hours) before you need to be active again. Be sure to talk to your doctor if you think you are having memory problems.

In deciding to use a medicine, the risks of taking the medicine must be weighed against the good it will do. This is a decision you and your doctor will make. For zolpidem, the following should be considered:

**Allergies**—Tell your doctor if you have ever had any unusual or allergic reaction to zolpidem. Also tell your health care professional if you are allergic to any other substances, such as foods, preservatives, or dyes.

**Pregnancy**—Zolpidem has not been studied in pregnant women. However, studies in pregnant animals have shown that zolpidem slows down the development of the offspring when given to the mother in doses many times the human dose. Before taking this medicine, make sure your doctor knows if you are pregnant or if you may become pregnant.

**Breast-feeding**—Although zolpidem passes into breast milk, it has not been reported to cause problems in nursing babies.

**Children**—Studies on this medicine have been done only in adult patients, and there is no specific information comparing use of zolpidem in children with use in other age groups.

**Older adults**—Confusion and falling are more likely to occur in the elderly, who are usually more sensitive than younger adults to the effects of zolpidem.

**Other medicines**—Although certain medicines should not be used together at all, in other cases two different medicines may be used together even if an interaction might occur. In these cases, your doctor may want to change the dose, or other precautions may be necessary. When you are taking zolpidem, it is especially important that your health care professional know if you are taking any of the following:

- Other central nervous system (CNS) depressants (medicines that cause drowsiness) or
- Tricyclic antidepressants (amitriptyline [e.g., Elavil], amoxapine [e.g., Asendin], clomipramine [e.g., Anafranil], desipramine [e.g., Pertofrane], doxepin [e.g., Sinequan], imipramine [e.g., Tofranil], nortriptyline [e.g., Aventyl], protriptyline [e.g., Vivactil], trimipramine [e.g., Surmontil])—The CNS depressant effects of either these medicines or zolpidem may be increased, possibly leading to unwanted effects

**Other medical problems**—The presence of other medical problems may affect the use of zolpidem. Make sure you tell your doctor if you have any other medical problems, especially:

- Alcohol abuse (or history of) or
- Drug abuse or dependence (or history of)—Dependence on zolpidem may develop
- Emphysema, asthma, bronchitis, or other chronic lung disease or
- Mental depression or
- Sleep apnea (temporary stopping of breathing during sleep)—Zolpidem may make these conditions worse
- Kidney disease or
- Liver disease—Higher blood levels of zolpidem may result, increasing the chance of side effects

## Proper Use of This Medicine

*Take this medicine only as directed by your doctor.* Do not take more of it, do not take it more often, and do not take it for a longer time than your doctor ordered. If too much is taken, it may become habit-forming (causing mental or physical dependence).

Take zolpidem just before going to bed, when you are ready to go to sleep. This medicine works very quickly to put you to sleep.

*Do not take this medicine when your schedule does not permit you to get a full night's sleep (7 to 8 hours).* If you must wake up before this, you may continue to feel drowsy and may experience memory problems, because the effects of the medicine have not had time to wear off.

Zolpidem may be taken with or without food or on a full or empty stomach. It may work faster if you take it on an empty stomach. However, if your doctor tells you to take the medicine a certain way, take it exactly as directed.

**Dosing**—The dose of zolpidem will be different for different patients. *Follow your doctor's orders or the directions on the label.* The following information includes only the average doses of zolpidem. *If your dose is different, do not change it* unless your doctor tells you to do so.

The number of tablets that you take depends on the strength of the medicine.

- For *oral* dosage form (tablets):
  —For the treatment of insomnia (trouble in sleeping):
    - Adults—10 milligrams (mg) at bedtime.
    - Older adults—5 mg at bedtime.
    - Children up to 18 years of age—Use and dose must be determined by the doctor.

**Missed dose**—If you miss a dose of this medicine, skip the missed dose and go back to your regular dosing schedule. Do not double doses.

**Storage**—To store this medicine:
- Keep out of the reach of children.
- Store away from heat and direct light.
- Do not store in the bathroom, near the kitchen sink, or in other damp places. Heat or moisture may cause the medicine to break down.
- Do not keep outdated medicine or medicine no longer needed. Be sure that any discarded medicine is out of the reach of children.

## Precautions While Using This Medicine

If you think you need to take zolpidem for more than 7 to 10 days, be sure to discuss it with your doctor. Insomnia that lasts longer than this may be a sign of another medical problem.

This medicine will add to the effects of alcohol and other CNS depressants (medicines that slow down the nervous system, possibly causing drowsiness). Some examples of CNS depressants are antihistamines or medicine for hay fever, other allergies, or colds; sedatives, tranquilizers, or sleeping medicine; prescription pain medicine or narcotics; barbiturates; medicine for seizures; muscle relaxants; or anesthetics, including some dental anesthetics. *Check with your doctor before taking any of the above while you are using this medicine.*

This medicine may cause some people, especially older persons, to become drowsy, dizzy, lightheaded, clumsy or unsteady, or less alert than they are normally. Even though zolpidem is taken at bedtime, it may cause some people to feel drowsy or less alert on arising. Also, this medicine may cause double vision or other vision problems. *Make sure you know how you react to zolpidem before you drive, use machines, or do anything else that could be dangerous if you are dizzy, or are not alert or able to see well.*

If you develop any unusual and strange thoughts or behavior while you are taking zolpidem, be sure to discuss it with your doctor. Some changes that have occurred in people taking this medicine are like those seen in people who drink alcohol and then act in a manner that is not normal. Other changes may be more unusual and extreme, such as confusion, hallucinations (seeing, hearing, or feeling things that are not there), and unusual excitement, nervousness, or irritability.

If you will be taking zolpidem for a long time, do not stop taking it without first checking with your doctor. Your doctor may want you to reduce gradually the amount you are taking before stopping completely. Stopping this medicine suddenly may cause withdrawal side effects.

After taking zolpidem for insomnia, you may have difficulty sleeping (rebound insomnia) for the first few nights after you stop taking it.

*If you think you or someone else may have taken an overdose of this medicine, get emergency help at once.* Taking an overdose of zolpidem or taking alcohol or other CNS depressants with zolpidem may lead to breathing problems and unconsciousness. Some signs of an overdose are severe drowsiness, severe nausea or vomiting, staggering, and troubled breathing.

## Side Effects of This Medicine

Along with its needed effects, a medicine may cause some unwanted effects. Although not all of these side effects may occur, if they do occur they may need medical attention.

*Check with your doctor as soon as possible if any of the following side effects occur:*

*Less common*
    Clumsiness or unsteadiness; confusion—more common in older adults; mental depression

*Rare*

Dizziness, lightheadedness, or fainting; falling—more common in older adults; fast heartbeat; hallucinations (seeing, hearing, or feeling things that are not there); skin rash; swelling of face; trouble in sleeping; unusual excitement, nervousness, or irritability; wheezing or difficulty in breathing

*Symptoms of overdose*

Clumsiness or unsteadiness (severe); dizziness (severe); double vision or other vision problems; drowsiness (severe); nausea (severe); troubled breathing; slow heartbeat; vomiting (severe)

Other side effects may occur that usually do not need medical attention. These side effects may go away during treatment as your body adjusts to the medicine. However, check with your doctor if any of the following side effects continue or are bothersome:

*Less common*

Abdominal or stomach pain; daytime drowsiness; diarrhea; double vision or other vision problems; drugged feelings; dryness of mouth; general feeling of discomfort or illness; headache; memory problems; nausea; nightmares or unusual dreams; vomiting

After you stop using this medicine, your body may need time to adjust. The length of time this takes depends on the amount of medicine you were using and how long you used it. During this time check with your doctor if you notice any of the following side effects:

Abdominal or stomach cramps or discomfort; agitation, nervousness, or feelings of panic; convulsions (seizures); flushing; lightheadedness; muscle cramps; nausea; sweating; tremors; uncontrolled crying; unusual tiredness or weakness; vomiting; worsening of mental or emotional problems

Other side effects not listed above may also occur in some patients. If you notice any other effects, check with your doctor.

Developed: 06/29/94

# Glossary

**Abdomen**—The body area between the chest and pelvis.

**Abortifacient**—Medicine that causes abortion.

**Abrade**—Scrape or rub away the outer cover or layer of a part.

**Absorption**—Passing into the body; incorporation of substances into or across tissues of the body, for example, digested food into the blood from the small intestine, or poisons through the skin.

**Achlorhydria**—Absence of acid that normally would be found in the stomach.

**Acidifier, urinary**—Medicine that makes the urine more acidic.

**Acidosis**—Too much acidity or loss of alkalinity in the body fluids and tissues.

**Acromegaly**—Enlargement of the face, hands, and feet because of too much growth hormone.

**Acute**—Sharp or intense; describes a condition that begins suddenly, has severe symptoms, and usually lasts a short time.

**Addison's disease**—Disease caused by not enough secretion of corticosteroid hormones by the adrenal glands; causes weakness, salt loss, and low blood pressure.

**Adhesion**—The union by connective tissue of two parts that are normally separate (such as parts of a joint).

**Adjunct**—An additional or secondary treatment that is helpful but is not necessary to treatment of a particular condition; not effective for that condition if used alone.

**Adjuvant**—1. A substance added to or used with another substance to assist its action. 2. Something that assists or enhances the effectiveness of medical treatment.

**Adrenal cortex**—Outer layer of tissue of the adrenal gland, which produces corticosteroid hormones.

**Adrenal glands**—Two organs located next to the kidneys. They produce the hormones epinephrine and norepinephrine and corticosteroid hormones, such as cortisol.

**Adrenaline**—See epinephrine.

**Adrenal medulla**—Inner part of the adrenal gland, which produces epinephrine and norepinephrine.

**Adrenocorticoids**—See corticosteroids.

**Aerosol**—Suspension of very small liquid or solid particles in compressed gas; drugs in aerosol form are dispensed in the form of a mist by releasing the gas.

**African sleeping sickness**—See Trypanosomiasis, African.

**Agent**—A force or substance capable of causing a change.

**Agoraphobia**—Fear of public places or open spaces.

**Agranulocytosis**—Disorder in which there is a severe decrease in the number of granulocytes normally present in the blood.

**AIDS (acquired immunodeficiency syndrome)**—Disease caused by human immunodeficiency virus (HIV). The disease results in a breakdown of the body's immune system, which makes a person more likely to get some other infections and some forms of cancer.

**Alcohol-abuse deterrent**—Medicine used to help alcoholics avoid the use of alcohol.

**Alkaline**—Having a pH of more than 7. Opposite of acidic.

**Alkalizer, urinary**—Medicine that makes the urine more alkaline.

**Alkalosis**—Too much alkalinity or loss of acidity in the body fluids and tissues.

**Alopecia**—Loss or absence of hair from areas where it normally is present; baldness.

**Altitude sickness agent**—Medicine used to prevent or lessen some of the effects of high altitude on the body.

**Alzheimer's disease**—Progressive disorder of thinking and other mental processes, usually beginning in late middle age.

**Aminoglycosides**—A class of chemically related antibiotics used to treat some serious types of bacterial infections.

**Anabolic steroids**—Synthetic forms of male hormones.

**Analgesic**—Medicine that relieves pain without causing unconsciousness.

**Anaphylaxis**—Sudden, severe allergic reaction.

**Androgen**—Substance, such as testosterone, that stimulates development of male characteristics.

**Anemia**—Reduction, to below normal, of hemoglobin in the blood.

**Anesthesiologist**—A physician who is qualified to give an anesthetic and other medicines to a patient before and during surgery.

**Anesthetic**—Medicine that causes a loss of feeling or sensation, especially of pain, sometimes through loss of consciousness.

**Aneurysm**—Abnormal dilatation or saclike swelling of an artery, vein, or the heart.

**Angina**—Pain, tightness, or feeling of heaviness in the chest, due mostly to lack of oxygen for the heart muscle. The pain may be felt in the left shoulder, jaw, or arm instead of or in addition to the chest. Symptoms often occur during exercise.

**Angioedema**—Allergic condition marked by continuing swelling and severe itching of areas of the skin.

**Anorexia**—Loss of appetite for food.

**Anoxia**—Absence of oxygen. The term is sometimes incorrectly used for hypoxia, which means an abnormally low amount of oxygen in the body.

**Antacid**—Medicine used to neutralize excess acid in the stomach.

**Antagonist**—Drug or other substance that blocks or works against the action of another.

**Anthelmintic**—Medicine used to destroy or expel intestinal worms.

**Antiacne agent**—Medicine used to treat acne.

**Antianemic**—Agent that prevents or corrects anemia.

**Antianginal**—Medicine used to prevent or treat angina attacks.

**Antianxiety agent**—Medicine used to treat excessive nervousness, tension, or anxiety.

**Antiarrhythmic**—Medicine used to treat irregular heartbeats.

**Antiasthmatic**—Medicine used to treat asthma.

**Antibacterial**—Medicine that kills or stops the growth of bacteria.

**Antibiotic**—Chemical substance used to treat infections.

**Antibody**—Special kind of blood protein that helps the body fight infection.

**Antibulimic**—Medicine used to treat bulimia.

**Anticholelithic**—Medicine used to dissolve gallstones.

**Anticoagulant**—Medicine used to prevent formation of blood clots in the blood vessels.

**Anticonvulsant**—Medicine used to prevent or treat convulsions (seizures).

**Antidepressant**—Medicine used to treat mental depression.

**Antidiabetic agent**—Medicine used to control blood sugar levels in patients with diabetes mellitus (sugar diabetes).

**Antidiarrheal**—Medicine used to treat diarrhea.

**Antidiuretic**—Medicine used to decrease formation of urine (for example, in patients with diabetes insipidus).

**Antidote**—Medicine used to prevent or treat harmful effects of another medicine or a poison.

**Antidyskinetic**—Medicine used to help treat the loss of muscle control caused by certain diseases or by some other medicines.

**Antidysmenorrheal**—Medicine used to treat menstrual cramps.

**Antiemetic**—Medicine used to prevent or treat nausea and vomiting.

**Antiendometriotic**—Medicine used to treat endometriosis.

**Antienuretic**—Medicine used to help prevent bedwetting.

**Antifibrotic**—Medicine used to treat fibrosis.

**Antiflatulent**—Medicine used to help relieve excess gas in the stomach or intestines.

**Antifungal**—Medicine used to treat infections caused by a fungus.

**Antiglaucoma agent**—Medicine used to treat glaucoma.

**Antigout agent**—Medicine used to prevent or relieve gout attacks.

**Antihemorrhagic**—Medicine used to prevent or help stop serious bleeding.

**Antihistamine**—Medicine used to prevent or relieve the symptoms of allergies (such as hay fever).

**Antihypercalcemic**—Medicine used to help lower the amount of calcium in the blood.

**Antihyperlipidemic**—Medicine used to help lower high levels of lipids in the blood.

**Antihyperphosphatemic**—Medicine used to help lower the amount of phosphate in the blood.

**Antihypertensive**—Medicine used to treat high blood pressure.

**Antihyperuricemic**—Medicine used to prevent or treat gout or other medical problems caused by too much uric acid in the blood.

**Antihypocalcemic**—Medicine used to increase calcium blood levels in patients with too little calcium.

**Antihypoglycemic**—Medicine used to increase blood sugar levels in patients with low blood sugar.

**Antihypokalemic**—Medicine used to increase potassium blood levels in patients with too little potassium.

**Anti-infective**—Medicine used to treat infection.

**Anti-inflammatory**—Medicine used to relieve pain, swelling, and other symptoms of inflammation.

**Anti-inflammatory, nonsteroidal**—An anti-inflammatory medicine that is not a cortisone-like medicine.

**Anti-inflammatory, steroidal**—A cortisone-like anti-inflammatory medicine.

**Antimetabolite**—Medicine that interferes with the normal processes within cells, preventing their growth.

**Antimuscarinic**—Medicine used to block the effects of a certain chemical in the body; often used to reduce smooth muscle spasms, especially abdominal or stomach cramps or spasms.

**Antimyasthenic**—Medicine used to treat myasthenia gravis.

**Antimyotonic**—Medicine used to prevent or relieve nighttime leg cramps or muscle spasms.

**Antineoplastic**—Medicine used to treat cancer.

**Antineuralgic**—Medicine used to treat neuralgia.

**Antiprotozoal**—Medicine used to treat infections caused by protozoa.

**Antipsoriatic**—Medicine used to treat psoriasis.

**Antipsychotic**—Medicine used to treat certain nervous, mental, and emotional conditions.

**Antipyretic**—Medicine used to reduce fever.

**Antirheumatic**—Medicine used to treat arthritis (rheumatism).

**Antirosacea**—Medicine used to treat rosacea.

**Antiseborrheic**—Medicine used to treat dandruff and seborrhea.

**Antiseptic**—Medicine that stops the growth of germs. Used on the surface of the skin to prevent infections in cuts, scrapes, and wounds.

**Antispasmodic**—Medicine used to reduce smooth muscle spasms (for example, stomach, intestinal, or urinary tract spasms).

**Antispastic**—Medicine used to treat muscle spasms.

**Antithyroid agent**—Medicine used to treat an overactive thyroid gland.

**Antitremor agent**—Medicine used to treat tremors (trembling or shaking).

**Antitubercular**—Medicine used to treat tuberculosis (TB).

**Antitussive**—Medicine used to relieve cough.

**Antiulcer agent**—Medicine used to treat stomach and duodenal ulcers.

**Antivertigo agent**—Medicine used to prevent dizziness.

**Antiviral**—Medicine used to treat infections caused by a virus.

**Anus**—The opening at the end of the digestive tract through which bowel contents are passed.

**Anxiety**—An emotional state with apprehension, worry, or tension in reaction to real or imagined danger or dread of a situation; accompanied by sweating, increased pulse, trembling, weakness, and fatigue.

**Apnea**—Temporary absence of breathing.

**Apoplexy**—See Stroke.

**Appendicitis**—Inflammation of the appendix.

**Appetite stimulant**—Medicine used to help increase the desire for food.

**Appetite suppressant**—Medicine used in weight control programs to help decrease the desire for food.

**Arrhythmia**—Abnormal heart rhythm.

**Arteritis, temporal**—Inflammatory disease of arteries, usually of the head; occurs in older people.

**Arthralgia**—Pain in a joint.

**Arthritis, rheumatoid**—Chronic disease, especially of the joints, marked by pain and swelling.

**Ascites**—Accumulation of fluid in the abdominal cavity.

**Asthma**—Disease marked by inflammation of the bronchial tubes (air passages). During an attack, air passages become constricted, causing wheezing and difficult breathing. Attacks may be brought on by allergens, virus infection, cold air, or exercise.

**Atherosclerosis**—Common disease of the arteries in which artery walls thicken and harden.

**Avoid**—To keep away from deliberately.

**Bacteremia**—Presence of bacteria in the blood.

**Bacterium**—Tiny, one-celled organism. Different types of bacteria are responsible for a number of diseases and infections.

**Bancroft's filariasis**—Disease transmitted by mosquitos in which an infection with the filarial worm occurs. Affects the lymph system, producing inflammation.

**Beriberi**—Disorder caused by too little vitamin $B_1$ (thiamine), marked by an accumulation of fluid in the body, extreme weight loss, inflammation of nerves, or paralysis.

**Bile**—Thick fluid produced by the liver and stored in the gallbladder. Bile helps in the digestion of fats.

**Bile duct**—Tubular passage which carries bile from the liver to the gallbladder, or from the gallbladder to the intestine.

**Bilharziasis**—See Schistosomiasis.

**Biliary**—Relating to bile, the bile duct, or the gallbladder.

**Bilirubin**—The bile pigment that is orange-colored or yellow; an excess in the blood may cause jaundice.

**Bipolar disorder**—Severe mental illness marked by repeated episodes of depression and mania. Also called *manic-depressive illness.*

**Bisexual**—One who is sexually attracted to both sexes.

**Black fever**—See Leishmaniasis, visceral.

**Blackwater fever**—Condition, marked by dark urine, rarely seen as a complication of malaria.

**Bone marrow**—Soft material filling the cavities of bones.

**Bone marrow depression**—Condition in which the production of red blood cells, leukocytes, or platelets by the red bone marrow is decreased.

**Bone resorption inhibitor**—Medicine used to prevent or treat certain types of bone disorders, such as Paget's disease of the bone; helps prevent bone loss.

**Bowel disease, inflammatory, suppressant**—Medicine used to treat certain intestinal disorders, such as colitis.

**Bradycardia**—Slow heart rate, usually less than 60 beats per minute.

**Bronchitis**—Inflammation of the bronchial tubes (air passages) of the lungs.

**Bronchodilator**—Medicine used to open up the bronchial tubes (air passages) of the lungs to increase the flow of air through them.

**Buccal**—Relating to the cheek. A buccal medicine is taken by placing it in the pocket between the cheek and the gum and letting it slowly dissolve.

**Bulimia**—Disturbance in eating behavior marked by bouts of excessive eating followed by self-induced vomiting and diarrhea, hard exercise, or fasting.

**Bursa**—Small fluid-filled sac present where body parts move over one another (such as in a joint) to help reduce friction.

**Bursitis**—Inflammation of a bursa.

**Candidiasis of the mouth**—Overgrowth of the yeast *Candida* in the mouth marked by white patches on the tongue or inside the mouth. Also called *thrush* or *white mouth*.

**Candidiasis of the vagina**—Yeast infection of the vagina caused by the yeast *Candida;* associated with itching, burning, and a cheesy or curd-like white discharge.

**Cardiac**—Relating to the heart.

**Cardiac arrhythmia**—Irregularity or loss of the normal rhythm of the heartbeat.

**Cardiac load–reducing agent**—Medicine used to ease the workload of the heart by allowing the blood to flow through the blood vessels more easily.

**Cardiotonic**—Medicine used to improve the strength and efficiency of the heart.

**Caries, dental**—Tooth decay, sometimes causing pain, leading to the crumbling of the tooth. Also called *cavities*.

**Cataract**—An opacity (cloudiness) in the eye lens that impairs vision or causes blindness.

**Catheter**—Tube inserted into a small opening in the body so that fluids can be put in or taken out.

**Caustic**—Burning or corrosive agent; irritating and destructive to living tissue.

**Cavity**—1. Hollow space within the body. 2. Hole in a tooth, caused by dental caries.

**Central nervous system**—Part of the nervous system that is composed of the brain and spinal cord.

**Cerebral palsy**—Permanent disorder of motor weakness and loss of coordination due to damage to the brain.

**Cervix**—Lower end or necklike opening of the uterus to the vagina.

**Chemotherapy**—Treatment of illness or disease by chemical agents. The term most commonly refers to the use of drugs to treat cancer.

**Chickenpox**—See Varicella.

**Chlamydia**—A family of microorganisms that cause a variety of diseases in humans. One form is transmitted by sexual contact.

**Cholesterol**—Fatlike substance made by the liver but also absorbed from the diet; found only in animal tissues. Too much blood cholesterol is associated with several potential health risks, especially atherosclerosis (hardening of the arteries).

**Chromosome**—The structure in the cell nucleus that contains the DNA; in humans, there are normally 46.

**Chronic**—Describes a condition of long duration, which is often of gradual onset and may involve very slow changes. Note that the term "chronic" has nothing to do with how serious the condition is.

**Cirrhosis**—Chronic liver disease marked by destruction of its cells and abnormal tissue growth.

**Clitoris**—Small, erectile body, being a part of the female external sex organs.

**CNS**—See Central nervous system.

**Cold sores**—See Herpes simplex.

**Colic**—Waves of sudden severe abdominal pain, which are usually separated by relatively pain-free intervals.

**Colitis**—Inflammation of the colon (bowel).

**Colony stimulating factor**—Protein that stimulates the production of one or more kinds of cells made in the bone marrow.

**Colostomy**—Operation in which part of the colon (bowel) is brought through the abdominal wall to create an artificial opening. The contents of the intestine are discharged through the opening, bypassing the rest of the intestines.

**Coma**—State of unconsciousness from which the patient cannot be aroused.

**Coma, hepatic**—Disturbances in mental function and the nervous system caused by severe liver disease.

**Condom**—Thin sheath or cover worn over the penis during sexual intercourse to prevent pregnancy or infection; made of latex (rubber) or animal intestine.

**Congestive heart failure**—Condition resulting from inability of the heart to pump strongly enough to maintain adequate blood flow; characterized by breathlessness and edema.

**Conjunctiva**—Delicate mucous membrane covering the front of the eye and the inside of the eyelid.

**Conjunctivitis**—Inflammation of the conjunctiva.

**Constriction**—Squeezing together and becoming narrower or smaller, such as constriction of blood vessels or eye pupils.

**Contagious disease**—Disease that can be transmitted from one person to another.

**Contamination**—The introduction of germs or unclean material into or on normally sterile substances or objects.

**Contraceptive**—Medicine or device used to prevent pregnancy.

**Contraction**—A shortening or tightening, as in the normal function of muscles.

**Convulsion**—Sudden involuntary contraction or series of jerkings of muscles.

**Corticosteroids**—Group of cortisone-like hormones that are secreted by the adrenal cortex and are critical to the body. The two major groups of corticosteroids are glucocorticoids, which affect fat and body metabolism, and mineralocorticoids, which regulate salt/water balance. Also called *adrenocorticoids*.

**Cortisol**—Natural hormone produced by the adrenal cortex, important for carbohydrate, protein, and fat metabolism and for the normal response to stress; synthetic cortisol (hydrocortisone) is used to treat inflammations, allergies, collagen diseases, rheumatic disorders, and adrenal failure.

**Cot death**—See Sudden infant death syndrome (SIDS).

**Cowpox**—See Vaccinia.

**Creutzfeldt-Jakob disease**—Rare disease, probably caused by a slow-acting virus that affects the brain and nervous system.

**Crib death**—See Sudden infant death syndrome (SIDS).

**Crohn's disease**—Chronic, inflammatory disease of the digestive tract, usually the lower small intestine.

**Croup**—Inflammation and blockage of the larynx (voice box) in young children.

**Crystalluria**—Crystals in the urine.

**Cushing's syndrome**—Condition in which the adrenal gland produces too much cortisone-like hormone, leading to weight gain, round face, and high blood pressure.

**Cycloplegia**—Paralysis of certain eye muscles; can be induced by medication for certain eye examinations.

**Cycloplegic**—Medicine used to induce cycloplegia.

**Cyst**—Abnormal sac or closed cavity filled with liquid or semisolid matter.

**Cystic**—Marked by cysts.

**Cystic fibrosis**—Hereditary disease of children and young adults which predominately affects the lungs. Exocrine glands do not function normally, and excess mucus is produced.

**Cystine**—An amino acid found in most proteins; it is produced by the digestion of the protein.

**Cystitis, interstitial**—Inflammation of the bladder, predominantly in women, with frequent urge to urinate and painful urination.

**Cytomegalovirus**—One of a group of viruses. One form may be sexually transmitted and can be fatal in patients with weakened immune systems.

**Cytoplasm**—The contents of a cell outside the nucleus.

**Cytotoxic agent**—Chemical that kills cells or stops cell division; used to treat cancer.

**Decongestant, nasal**—Medicine used to help relieve nasal congestion (stuffy nose).

**Decongestant, ophthalmic**—Medicine used in the eye to relieve redness, burning, itching, or other irritation.

**Decubitus**—The position taken in lying down.

**Decubitus ulcer**—Bedsore; damage to the skin and underlying tissues caused by constant pressure.

**Dental**—Related to the teeth and gums.

**Depression, mental**—Condition marked by deep sadness; associated with lack of any pleasurable interest in life. Other symptoms include disturbances in sleep, appetite, and concentration, and difficulty in performing day-to-day tasks.

**Dermatitis herpetiformis**—Skin disease marked by sores and itching.

**Dermatitis, seborrheic**—Type of eczema found on the scalp and face.

**Dermatomyositis**—Inflammatory disorder of the skin and underlying tissues, including breakdown of muscle fibers.

**Diabetes insipidus**—Disorder in which the patient produces large amounts of dilute urine and is constantly thirsty. Also called *water diabetes*.

**Diabetes mellitus**—Disorder in which the body cannot process sugars to release energy; either the body does not produce enough insulin or the body tissues are unable to use the insulin present. This leads to too much sugar in the blood (hyperglycemia). Also called *sugar diabetes*.

**Diagnose**—Find out the cause or nature of a disorder by examination and laboratory tests.

**Diagnostic procedure**—A process carried out to determine the cause or nature of a condition, disease, or disorder.

**Dialysis, renal**—Artificial technique for removing waste materials or poisons from the blood when the kidneys are not working properly.

**Digestant**—Agent that will help in digestion.

**Diplopia**—Awareness of two images of a single object at one time; double vision.

**Diuretic**—Medicine used to increase the amount of urine produced by helping the kidneys get rid of water and salt. Also called *water pill*.

**Diverticulitis**—Inflammation of a diverticulum in the intestinal tract.

**Diverticulum**—Sac or pouch opening from a canal or cavity.

**DNA**—Deoxyribonucleic acid; the genetic material that controls heredity. DNA is located in the cell nucleus.

**Down syndrome**—Mental retardation associated with the presence of an extra chromosome 21. Patients with Down syndrome are marked physically by a round head, flat nose, slightly slanted eyes, and short stature. Also called *mongolism*.

**Duct**—Tube or channel, especially one that serves to carry secretions from a gland.

**Dumdum fever**—See Leishmaniasis, visceral.

**Duodenal ulcer**—Open sore in that part of the small intestine closest to the stomach.

**Duodenum**—First of the three parts of the small intestine.

**Dyskinesia**—Refers to abnormal, involuntary movement or a defect in voluntary movement.

**Dyspnea**—Shortness of breath; difficult breathing.

**Eczema**—Inflammation of the skin, marked by itching and rash.

**Edema**—Swelling of body tissue due to accumulation of fluids, usually first noticed in the feet or lower legs.

**Eighth-cranial-nerve disease**—Disease of the eighth cranial nerve, serving the inner ear; results in dizziness, loss of balance, loss of hearing, nausea, or vomiting.

**Electrolyte**—In medical use, chemicals (ions) in body fluids that are needed for normal functioning of the body. Body electrolytes include bicarbonate, chloride, sodium, potassium, etc.

**Embolism**—Sudden blocking of a blood vessel by a blood clot or foreign substances carried to the place of obstruction by the blood.

**Embryo**—In humans, a developing fertilized egg within the uterus (womb) from about two to eight weeks after fertilization.

**Emergency**—Extremely serious unexpected or sudden happening or situation that calls for immediate action.

**Emollient**—Substance that soothes and softens an irritated surface, such as the skin.

**Emphysema**—Lung condition in which destructive changes occur in the air spaces; air is not exchanged normally during the process of breathing in and out.

**Encephalitis**—Inflammation of the brain.

**Encephalopathy**—Any degenerative disease of the brain; caused by many different medical conditions.

**Endocarditis**—Inflammation of the lining of the heart, leading to fever, heart murmurs, and heart failure.

**Endocrine gland**—A gland that has no duct; releases its secretion directly into the blood.

**Endometriosis**—Condition in which material similar to the lining of the uterus (womb) appears at other sites within the pelvic cavity, causing pain and bleeding.

**Enteric coating**—Coating on tablets which allows them to pass through the stomach unchanged before being broken up in the intestine and being absorbed. Used to protect the stomach from the medicine and/or the medicine from the stomach's acid.

**Enteritis**—Inflammation of the small intestine, usually causing diarrhea.

**Enuresis**—Urinating while asleep (bedwetting).

**Enzyme**—Type of protein produced by cells that may bring about or speed up a normal chemical reaction in the body.

**Eosinophil**—One type of white blood cells readily stained by the dye eosin; important in allergic reactions and parasitic infections.

**Eosinophilia**—Condition in which the number of eosinophils in the blood is abnormally high.

**Epidural space**—Area in the spinal column into which medicines (usually for pain) can be administered.

**Epilepsy**—Any of a group of brain disorders featuring sudden attacks of seizures and other symptoms.

**Epinephrine**—Hormone secreted by the adrenal medulla. It stimulates the heart, constricts blood vessels, and relaxes some smooth muscles. Also called *adrenaline*.

**EPO**—See erythropoietin.

**Ergot alkaloids**—A class of medicines that cause narrowing of blood vessels; used to treat migraine headaches, and to reduce bleeding in childbirth.

**Erythropoietin**—Hormone secreted by the kidney. It controls the production of red blood cells by the bone marrow; also available as a synthetic drug (EPO).

**Esophagus**—The part of the digestive tract connecting the pharynx to the stomach.

**Estrogen**—Principal female sex hormone necessary for the normal sexual development of the female; during the menstrual cycle, its actions help prepare for possible pregnancy. Estrogen is often used to treat discomforts of menopause.

**Exocrine gland**—Any gland that discharges its secretion through a duct that opens on a surface (not into the blood).

**Exophthalmos**—Thrusting forward of the eyeballs in their sockets giving the appearance of the eyes sticking out too far; commonly associated with hyperthyroidism.

**Expectorant**—Medicine used to help remove mucus or phlegm in the lungs by coughing or spitting it up.

**Extrapyramidal symptoms**—Movement disorders occurring with certain diseases or with use of certain drugs, including trembling and shaking of hands and fingers, twisting movements of the body, shuffling walk, and stiffness of arms or legs.

**Familial Mediterranean fever**—Inherited condition involving inflammation of the lining of the chest, abdomen, and joints. Also called *recurrent polyserositis*.

**Fasciculation**—Small, spontaneous contraction of a few muscle fibers, which is visible through the skin; muscular twitching.

**Favism**—Inherited condition resulting from sensitivity to broad (fava) beans; marked by fever, vomiting, diarrhea, and acute destruction of red blood cells.

**Fertility**—Capacity to bring about the start of pregnancy.

**Fertilization**—Union of an ovum with a sperm.

**Fetus**—In humans, a developing baby within the uterus (womb) from about the beginning of the third month of pregnancy.

**Fibrocystic**—Having benign (noncancerous) tumors of connective tissue.

**Fibroid tumor**—A noncancerous tumor of the uterus formed of fibrous or fully developed connective tissue.

**Fibrosis**—Condition in which the skin and underlying tissues tighten and become less flexible.

**Fistula**—Abnormal tubelike passage connecting two internal organs or one that leads from an abscess or internal organ to the body surface.

**Flatulence**—Excessive amount of air or gas in the stomach or intestine.

**Flu**—See Influenza.

**Flushing**—Temporary redness of the face and/or neck.

**Fungus**—Any of a group of simple organisms, including molds and yeasts.

**Fungus infection**—Infection caused by a fungus. Some common fungus infections are tinea pedis (athlete's foot), tinea capitis (ringworm of the scalp), tinea cruris (ringworm of the groin or jock itch), and mouth or vaginal candidiasis (yeast infections).

**Gait**—Manner of walk.

**Gamma globulin**—The portion of the blood that contains most of the antibodies associated with the body's immunity to infection.

**Gastric**—Relating to the stomach.

**Gastric acid secretion inhibitor**—Medicine used to decrease the amount of acid produced by the stomach.

**Gastroenteritis**—Inflammation of the stomach and intestine.

**Gastroesophageal reflux**—Backward flow into the esophagus of the contents of the stomach and duodenum. The condition is often characterized by "heartburn."

**Generic**—General in nature; relating to an entire group or class. In relation to medicines, the general name of a drug substance; not owned by one specific group as would be true for a trademark or brand name.

**Genital**—1. Relating to the organs concerned with reproduction; the sexual organs. 2. Relating to reproduction.

**Genital warts**—Small growths found on the genitals or around the anus; caused by a virus. The disease may be transmitted by sexual contact.

**Gilles de la Tourette syndrome**—See Tourette's disorder.

**Gingiva**—Gums.

**Gingival hyperplasia**—Overgrowth of the gums.

**Gingivitis**—Inflammation of the gums.

**Glandular fever**—See Mononucleosis.

**Glaucoma**—Condition of abnormally high pressure in the eye; may lead to loss of vision if not treated.

**Glomeruli**—Clusters of capillaries in the nephrons of the kidney that act as filters of the blood.

**Glomerulonephritis**—Inflammation of the glomeruli of the kidney not directly caused by infection.

**Glucose-6-phosphate dehydrogenase (G6PD) deficiency**—Lack of or reduced amounts of an enzyme (glucose-6-phosphate dehydrogenase) that helps the breakdown of certain sugar compounds in the body.

**Gluten**—Type of protein found primarily in wheat and rye.

**Goiter**—Enlargement of the thyroid gland that causes the neck to swell. Condition usually results from a lack of iodine or overactivity of the thyroid gland.

**Gonadotropin**—Any hormone that stimulates the activities of the ovaries or testes.

**Gonorrhea**—An infectious disease, usually transmitted by sexual contact. It causes infection in the genital organs in both men and women, and may also result in systemic disease.

**Gout**—Disease in which too much uric acid builds up in the blood and joints, leading to inflammation of the joints.

**Granulation**—Small, fleshy outgrowths on the healing surface of a wound or ulcer; a normal stage in healing.

**Granulocyte**—A class of white blood cell.

**Granulocytopenia**—Abnormal reduction of the number of granulocytes in the blood; agranulocytosis.

**Granuloma**—A growth or mass of granulation tissue produced in response to chronic infection, inflammation, a foreign body, or to unknown causes.

**Graves' disease**—Disorder that causes thyrotoxicosis, goiter, and exophthalmos. Also called *exophthalmic goiter*.

**Groin**—The area between the abdomen and thigh.

**Guillain-Barré syndrome**—Nerve disease marked by sudden numbness and weakness in the limbs that may progress to complete paralysis.

**Gynecomastia**—Excessive development of the breasts in the male.

**Hair follicle**—Sheath of tissue surrounding a hair root.

**Hansen's disease**—See Leprosy.

**Hartnup disease**—Hereditary disease in which the body has trouble processing certain chemicals, leading to mental retardation, rough skin, and problems with muscle coordination.

**Heart attack**—See Myocardial infarction.

**Hematuria**—Presence of blood or red blood cells in the urine.

**Hemoglobin**—Iron-containing substance found in red blood cells that transports oxygen from the lungs to the tissues of the body.

**Hemolytic anemia**—Type of anemia resulting from breakdown of red blood cells.

**Hemophilia**—Hereditary disease in males in which blood clotting is delayed, leading to excessive and uncontrolled bleeding even after minor injuries.

**Hemorrhoids**—Enlarged veins in the walls of the anus. Also called *piles*.

**Hepatic**—Relating to the liver.

**Hepatitis**—Inflammation of the liver.

**Hernia, hiatal**—Condition in which the stomach passes partly into the chest through the opening for the esophagus in the diaphragm.

**Herpes simplex**—The virus that causes "cold sores." These are an inflammation of the skin resulting in small, painful blisters. Infection may occur either in or around the mouth or, in the case of genital herpes, on the genitals (sex organs).

**Herpes zoster**—An infectious disease usually marked by pain and blisters along one nerve, often on the face, chest, stomach, or back. The infection is caused by the virus that also causes chickenpox. Also called *shingles*.

**Heterosexual**—One who is sexually attracted to persons of the opposite sex.

**High blood pressure**—See Hypertension.

**Hirsutism**—Adult male pattern of hair growth in women.

**HIV (human immunodeficiency virus)**—Virus that causes AIDS.

**Hodgkin's disease**—Malignant condition marked by swelling of the lymph nodes, with weight loss and fever.

**Homosexual**—One who is sexually attracted to persons of the same sex.

**Hormone**—Substance produced in one part of the body (such as a gland), which then passes into the bloodstream and travels to other organs or tissues, where it carries out its effect.

**Hot flashes**—Sensations of heat of the face, neck, and upper body, often accompanied by sweating and flushing; commonly associated with menopause.

**Hydrocortisone**—See cortisol.

**Hyperactivity**—Abnormally increased activity.

**Hypercalcemia**—Too much calcium in the blood.

**Hypercalciuria**—Too much calcium in the urine.

**Hypercholesterolemia**—Excessive amount of cholesterol in the blood.

**Hyperglycemia**—Abnormally high blood sugar.

**Hyperkalemia**—Abnormally high amount of potassium in the blood.

**Hyperkeratosis**—Overgrowth or thickening of the outer horny layer of the skin.

**Hyperlipidemia**—General term for an abnormally high level of any or all of the lipids in the blood.

**Hyperphosphatemia**—Too much phosphate in the blood.

**Hypersensitivity**—Condition in which the body has an abnormally increased reaction to a foreign substance.

**Hypertension**—Blood pressure in the arteries (blood vessels) that is higher than normal for the patient's age group. Hypertension may lead to a number of serious health problems. Also called *high blood pressure*.

**Hyperthermia**—Abnormally high body temperature.

**Hyperthyroidism**—Excessive secretion of thyroid hormones by the thyroid gland, causing thyrotoxicosis.

**Hypocalcemia**—Too little calcium in the blood.

**Hypoglycemia**—Abnormally low blood sugar.

**Hypokalemia**—Abnormally low amount of potassium in the blood.

**Hypotension, orthostatic**—Excessive fall in blood pressure that occurs when standing or upon standing up.

**Hypothalamus**—Area of the brain that controls many body functions, including body temperature, certain metabolic and endocrine processes, and some activities of the nervous system.

**Hypothermia**—Abnormally low body temperature.

**Hypothyroidism**—Condition caused by thyroid hormone deficiency, which results in a decrease in metabolism.

**Hypoxia**—Broad term meaning intake of oxygen or its use by the body is inadequate.

**Ileostomy**—Operation in which the ileum is brought through the abdominal wall to create an artificial opening. The contents of the intestine are discharged through the opening, bypassing the colon (bowel).

**Ileum**—Last of the three portions of the small intestine.

**Immune deficiency condition**—Lack of immune response to protect against infectious disease.

**Immune system**—Complex network of the body that defends against foreign substances or organisms that may harm the body.

**Immunizing agent, active**—Agent that causes the body to produce its own antibodies for protection against certain infections.

**Immunocompromised**—Decreased natural immunity caused by irradiation, certain medicine or diseases, or other conditions.

**Immunosuppressant**—Medicine that reduces the body's natural immunity.

**Impair**—To cause to decrease, weaken, or damage, usually because of injury or disease.

**Impetigo**—Contagious bacterial skin infection common in babies and children in which skin redness develops into blisters that break and form a thick crust.

**Implant**—1. Special form of medicine, often a small pellet or rod, that is inserted into the body or beneath the skin so that the medicine will be released continuously over a period of time. 2. To insert or graft material or an object into a body site. 3. Material or an object inserted into a body site, such as a lens implant or a breast implant. 4. Action of a fertilized ovum becoming attached or embedded in the uterus.

**Impotence**—Difficulty or inability of a male to have or maintain an erection of the penis.

**Incontinence**—Inability to control natural passage of urine or of bowel movements.

**Induce**—To cause or bring about.

**Infertility**—Medical condition which results in the difficulty or inability of a woman to become pregnant or of a man to cause pregnancy.

**Inflammation**—Pain, redness, swelling, and heat in a part of the body, usually in response to injury or illness.

**Influenza**—Highly contagious respiratory virus infection, marked by coughing, headache, chills, fever, muscle pain, and general weakness. Also called *flu*.

**Ingredient**—One of the parts or substances that make up a mixture or compound.

**Inhalation**—1. Act of drawing in the breath or drawing air into the lungs. 2. Medicine that is used when breathed (inhaled) into the lungs. Some inhalations work locally in the lungs, while others produce their effects elsewhere in the body.

**Inhibitor**—Substance that prevents a process or reaction.

**Inner ear**—Inner portion of the ear; a liquid filled system of cavities and ducts that make up the organs of hearing and balance.

**Insomnia**—Inability to sleep or remain asleep.

**Insulin**—Hormone that increases the efficiency with which the body uses sugar. Injections of insulin are used in the treatment and control of diabetes mellitus (sugar diabetes).

**Intra-amniotic**—Within the sac that contains the fetus and amniotic fluid.

**Intra-arterial**—Within an artery.

**Intracavernosal**—Into the corpus cavernosa (cavities in the penis that, when filled with blood, produce an erection).

**Intracavitary**—Into a body cavity (for example, the chest cavity or bladder).

**Intramuscular**—Into a muscle.

**Intrauterine device (IUD)**—Small plastic or metal device placed in the uterus (womb) to prevent pregnancy.

**Intravenous**—Into a vein.

**Ion**—Atom or group of atoms carrying an electric charge.

**Irrigation**—Washing of a body cavity or wound with a stream of sterile water or a solution of a medicine.

**Ischemia**—Condition caused by inadequate blood flow to a part of the body; usually caused by constriction or blocking of blood vessels that supply the part of the body affected.

**Jaundice**—Yellowing of the eyes and skin due to excess bilirubin in the blood.

**Jock itch**—Ringworm of the groin.

**Kala-azar**—See Leishmaniasis, visceral.

**Kaposi's sarcoma**—Malignant tumor of blood vessels; often appears in the skin. One form occurs in immunocompromised patients, for example, transplant recipients and AIDS patients.

**Keratolytic**—Medicine used to soften hardened areas of the skin, such as warts.

**Ketoacidosis**—Type of acidosis associated with diabetes.

**Lactation**—Secretion of breast milk.

**Larva**—The immature form of life of some insects and other animal groups that hatch from eggs.

**Larynx**—Organ that serves as a passage for air from the pharynx to the lungs; it contains the vocal cords.

**Laxative**—Medicine used to encourage bowel movements.

**Laxative, bulk-forming**—Laxative that acts by absorbing liquid and swelling to form a soft, bulky stool. The bowel is then stimulated normally by the presence of the bulky mass.

**Laxative, hyperosmotic**—Laxative that acts by drawing water into the bowel from surrounding body tissues. This provides a soft stool mass and increased bowel action.

**Laxative, lubricant**—Laxative that acts by coating the bowel and the stool mass with a waterproof film. This keeps moisture in the stool. The stool remains soft and its passage is made easier.

**Laxative, stimulant**—Laxative that acts directly on the intestinal wall. The direct stimulation increases the muscle contractions that move the stool mass along. Also called *contact laxative*.

**Laxative, stool softener**—Laxative that acts by helping liquids mix into the stool and prevent dry, hard stool masses. The stool remains soft and its passage is made easier. Also called *emollient laxative*.

**Legionnaires' disease**—Lung infection caused by a certain bacterium.

**Leishmaniasis, visceral**—Tropical disease, transmitted by sandfly bites, which causes liver and spleen enlargement, anemia, weight loss, and fever. Also called *black fever, Dumdum fever,* or *kala-azar*.

**Lennox-Gastaut syndrome**—Type of childhood epilepsy.

**Leprosy**—Chronic infectious disease characterized by lesions, especially in the skin and nerves, leading to loss of feeling, paralysis in the hands and feet and deformity. Also called *Hansen's disease*.

**Leukemia**—Disease of the blood and bone marrow in which too many white blood cells are produced, resulting in anemia, bleeding, and low resistance to infections.

**Leukocyte**—White blood cell.

**Leukoderma**—See Vitiligo.

**Leukopenia**—Abnormal reduction in the total number of leukocytes in the blood.

**Lipid**—Term applied generally to dietary fat or fatlike substances not soluble in water.

**Local effect**—Affecting only the area to which something is being applied.

**Lugol's solution**—Transparent, deep brown liquid containing iodine and potassium iodide.

**Lupus**—See Lupus erythematosus, systemic.

**Lupus erythematosus, systemic**—Chronic inflammatory disease most often affecting the skin, joints, and various internal organs. Also called *lupus* or *SLE* (systemic lupus erythematosus).

**Lymph**—Fluid that bathes the tissues. It is formed in tissue spaces in all parts of the body and circulated by the lymphatic system.

**Lymphatic system**—Network of vessels that conveys lymph from the spaces between the cells of the body back to the bloodstream.

**Lymph node**—A small rounded body found at intervals along the lymphatic system. The nodes act as filters for the lymph by keeping bacteria and other foreign particles from entering the bloodstream. They also produce lymphocytes.

**Lymphocyte**—Any of a number of white blood cells found in the blood, lymph, and lymphatic tissues. They are involved in immunity.

**Lymphoma**—Malignant tumor of lymph nodes or tissue.

**Lyse**—To cause breakdown. In cells, damage or rupture of the membrane results in destruction of the cell.

**Macrobiotic**—Vegetarian diet consisting mostly of whole grains.

**Malaria**—Tropical blood infection caused by a protozoa; symptoms include chills, fever, sweats, headaches, and anemia. Malaria is spread to humans by the bite of an infected mosquito.

**Malignant**—Describing a condition that becomes continually worse if untreated; also used to mean cancerous.

**Malnutrition**—Condition caused by unbalanced or insufficient diet.

**Mammogram**—X-ray picture of the breast.

**Mania**—Mental state in which fast talking and excited feelings or actions are out of control.

**Mast cells**—Cells in the connective tissue that store histamine; they release substances that bring about inflammation and produce signs of allergic reactions.

**Mastocytosis**—Accumulation of too many mast cells in tissues.

**Mediate**—To bring about or accomplish indirectly.

**Megavitamin therapy**—Taking very large doses of vitamins to prevent or treat certain medical problems.

**Melanoma**—Highly malignant cancer tumor, usually occurring on the skin.

**Meniere's disease**—Disease affecting the inner ear that is characterized by ringing in the ears, hearing loss, and dizziness.

**Meningitis**—Inflammation of the tissues that surround the brain and spinal cord.

**Menopause**—The time in a woman's life when the ovaries no longer produce an egg cell at regular times and menstruation stops.

**Methemoglobin**—Substance formed when hemoglobin has been oxidized; in this form, hemoglobin cannot act as an oxygen carrier.

**Methemoglobinemia**—Presence of methemoglobin in the blood.

**Middle ear**—Chamber of the ear lying behind the eardrum and containing the structures that conduct sound.

**Migraine**—Throbbing headache, usually affecting one side of the head; often accompanied by nausea, vomiting, and sensitivity to light.

**Miotic**—Medicine used in the eye that causes the pupil to constrict (become smaller).

**Mongolism**—See Down syndrome.

**Mono**—See Mononucleosis.

**Monoclonal**—Derived from a single cell; related to production of drugs by genetic engineering, such as monoclonal antibodies.

**Mononucleosis**—Infectious viral disease occurring mostly in adolescents and young adults, marked by fever, sore throat, swelling of the lymph nodes in the neck and armpits, and by severe fatigue. Also called *mono* or *glandular fever*.

**Motility**—Ability to move without outside aid, force, or cause.

**Motor**—Relating to structures that bring about movement, such as nerves and muscles.

**Mucolytic**—Medicine that breaks down or dissolves mucus.

**Mucosal**—Relating to the mucous membrane.

**Mucous membrane**—Moist layer of tissue surrounding or lining many body structures and cavities, including the mouth, lips, inside of nose, anus, and vagina.

**Mucus**—Thick fluid produced by the mucous membranes and glands.

**Multiple sclerosis (MS)**—Chronic, inflammatory nerve disease marked by weakness, unsteadiness, shakiness, and speech and vision problems.

**Myasthenia gravis**—Chronic disease marked by abnormal weakness, and sometimes paralysis, of certain muscles.

**Mydriatic**—Medicine used in the eye that causes the pupil to dilate (become larger).

**Myelogram**—X-ray picture of the spinal cord.

**Myeloma, multiple**—Cancerous bone marrow disease.

**Myocardial infarction**—Interruption of blood supply to the heart, leading to sudden, severe chest pain, and damage to the heart muscle. Also called *heart attack*.

**Myocardial reinfarction prophylactic**—Medicine used to help prevent additional heart attacks in patients who have already had one attack.

**Myotonia congenita**—Hereditary muscle disorder marked by difficulty in relaxing a muscle or releasing a grip after any strong effort.

**Narcolepsy**—Extreme tendency to fall asleep suddenly.

**Nasal**—Relating to the nose.

**Nasogastric (NG) tube**—Tube that is inserted through the nose, down the throat, and into the stomach. It may be used to remove fluid or gas from the stomach or to administer medicine, food, fluid, or nutrients to the patient.

**Nebulizer**—Instrument that administers liquid in the form of a fine spray.

**Necrosis**—Death of tissue, cells, or a part of a structure or organ, surrounded by healthy parts.

**Neoplasm**—New and abnormal growth of tissue in or on a part of the body, in which the multiplication of cells is uncontrolled and progressive. Also called *tumor*.

**Nephron**—Unit of the kidney that acts as a filter of the blood in forming urine.

**Neuralgia**—Severe stabbing or throbbing pain along the course of one or more nerves.

**Neuralgia, trigeminal**—Severe burning or stabbing pain along certain nerves in the face. Also called *tic douloureux*.

**Neuritis, optic**—Disease of the nerves in the eye.

**Neuritis, peripheral**—Inflammation of terminal nerves or the nerve endings, usually associated with pain, muscle wasting, and loss of reflexes.

**Neutropenia**—Abnormally small number of neutrophils in the blood.

**Neutrophil**—The most common type of granulocyte; important in the body's protection against infection.

**Nodule**—Small, rounded mass, lump, or swelling.

**Nonsuppurative**—Not discharging pus.

**NSAID (nonsteroidal anti-inflammatory drug)**—See Anti-inflammatory, nonsteroidal.

**Nucleus**—The part of the cell that contains the chromosomes.

**Nystagmus**—Rapid, rhythmic, involuntary movements of the eyeball; may be from side to side, up and down, or around.

**Obesity**—Excess accumulation of fat in the body along with an increase in body weight that exceeds the healthy range for the body's frame.

**Obstetrics**—Field of medicine concerned with the care of women during pregnancy and childbirth.

**Obstruction**—Something that blocks or closes up a passage or structure.

**Occlusive dressing**—Dressing (such as plastic kitchen wrap) that completely cuts off air to the skin.

**Occult**—Concealed, hidden, or of unknown cause; cannot be seen by the human eye; detectable only by microscope or chemical testing, as for occult blood in the stools or feces.

**Ophthalmic**—Relating to the eye.

**Opioid**—1. Any synthetic narcotic with opium-like actions; not derived from opium. 2. Natural chemicals that produce opium-like effects by acting at the same cell sites where opium exerts action.

**Oral**—Relating to the mouth.

**Orchitis**—Inflammation of the testis.

**Osteitis deformans**—See Paget's disease.

**Osteomalacia**—Softening of the bones due to lack of vitamin D.

**Osteoporosis**—Loss of calcium from bone tissue, resulting in bones that are brittle and easily fractured.

**OTC (over the counter)**—Refers to medicine or devices available without a prescription.

**Otic**—Relating to the ear.

**Otitis media**—Inflammation of the middle ear.

**Ototoxicity**—Having a harmful effect on the organs or nerves of the ear concerned with hearing and balance.

**Ovary**—Female sex organ that produces egg cells and sex hormones. The two ovaries are in the lower abdomen, one on each side.

**Overactive thyroid**—See hyperthyroidism.

**Ovulation**—Process by which an ovum is released from the ovary. In human menstruating females, this usually occurs once a month.

**Ovum**—Mature female sex or reproductive cell, or egg cell. It is capable of developing into a new organism if fertilized.

**Paget's disease**—Chronic bone disease, marked by thickening of the bones and severe pain. Also called *osteitis deformans*.

**Pancreatitis**—Inflammation of the pancreas.

**Pancytopenia**—Reduction in the number of red cells, all types of white cells, and platelets in the blood.

**Paralysis agitans**—See Parkinson's disease.

**Parathyroid glands**—Four small bodies situated beside the thyroid gland; secrete parathyroid hormone that regulates calcium and phosphorus metabolism.

**Parenteral**—Any method of administering medicine when the medicine cannot be given by mouth; most often refers to injecting a medicine into the body using a needle and syringe.

**Parkinsonism**—See Parkinson's disease.

**Parkinson's disease**—Brain disease marked by tremor (shaking), stiffness, and difficulty in moving. Also called *Parkinsonism, paralysis agitans,* or *shaking palsy*.

**Patent ductus arteriosus (PDA)**—Condition in babies in which an important blood vessel adjacent to the heart fails to close as it should, resulting in faulty circulation and serious health problems.

**Pediculicide**—Medicine that kills lice.

**Pediculosis**—Infestation of the body, pubis, or scalp with lice.

**Pellagra**—Disease caused by too little niacin, which results in scaly skin, diarrhea, and mental depression.

**Pemphigus**—Skin disease marked by successive outbreaks of blisters.

**Peptic ulcer**—Open sore in esophagus, stomach, or duodenum.

**Peritoneum**—Membrane sac lining the abdominal wall and covering the liver, stomach, spleen, gallbladder, and intestines.

**Peritonitis**—Inflammation of the peritoneum.

**Peyronie's disease**—Dense, fiber-like growth in the penis, which can be felt as an irregular hard lump, and which usually causes bending and pain when the penis is erect.

**Pharynx**—Space just behind the mouth that serves as a passageway for food from the mouth to the esophagus and for air from the nose and mouth to the larynx.

**Phenol**—Substance used as a preservative for some injectable medicines.

**Pheochromocytoma**—Tumor of the adrenal medulla.

**Phlebitis**—Inflammation of a vein.

**Phlegm**—Thick mucus produced in the respiratory passages.

**Piles**—See Hemorrhoids.

**Pituitary gland**—Pea-sized body located at the base of the skull. It produces a number of hormones that are essential to normal body growth and functioning.

**Placebo**—Medicine that, unknown to the patient, has no active medicinal substance; its use may relieve or improve a condition because the patient believes it will. Also called *sugar pill*.

**Plaque, dental**—Mixture of saliva, bacteria, and carbohydrates that forms on the teeth, leading to caries (cavities) and gum disease.

**Platelet**—Small, disk-shaped body found in the blood that plays an important role in blood clotting.

**Platelet aggregation inhibitor**—Medicine used to help prevent the platelets in the blood from clumping together. This effect reduces the chance of heart attack or stroke in certain patients.

**Pleura**—Membrane covering the lungs and lining the chest cavity.

**Pneumococcal**—Relating to certain bacteria that cause pneumonia.

**Pneumocystis carinii**—Organism that causes pneumocystis carinii pneumonia.

**Pneumocystis carinii pneumonia**—A pulmonary disease of infants and weakened persons, including those with AIDS or those receiving drugs that weaken the immune system.

**Polymorphous light eruption**—A skin problem in certain people, which results from exposure to sunlight.

**Polymyalgia rheumatica**—A rheumatic disease, most common in elderly patients, which causes aching and stiffness in the shoulders and hips.

**Polyp**—Tumor or mass of tissue attached with a stalk or broad base; found in cavities such as the nose, uterus, or rectum.

**Porphyria**—A group of uncommon, usually inherited diseases of defective porphyrin metabolism.

**Porphyrin**—One of a number of pigments occurring in living organisms throughout nature; porphyrins are constituents of bile pigment, hemoglobin, and certain enzymes.

**Prevent**—To stop or to keep from happening.

**Priapism**—Prolonged abnormal, painful erection of the penis.

**Proctitis**—Inflammation of the rectum.

**Progesterone**—Natural steroid hormone responsible for preparing the uterus for pregnancy. If fertilization occurs, progesterone's actions carry on or maintain the pregnancy.

**Progestin**—A natural or synthetic hormone that has progesterone-like actions.

**Prolactin**—Hormone secreted by the pituitary gland that stimulates and maintains milk flow in women following childbirth.

**Prolactinoma**—A pituitary tumor; results in secretion of excess prolactin.

**Prophylactic**—1. Agent or medicine used to prevent the occurrence of a specific condition. 2. Condom.

**Prostate**—Gland surrounding the neck of the male urethra just below the base of the bladder. It secretes a fluid that constitutes a major portion of the semen.

**Prosthesis**—Any artificial substitute for a missing body part.

**Protozoa**—Tiny, one-celled animals; some cause diseases in humans.

**Psoralen**—Chemical found in plants and used in certain perfumes and medicines. Exposure to a psoralen and then to sunlight may increase the risk of severe burning.

**Psoriasis**—Chronic skin disease marked by itchy, scaly, red patches.

**Psychosis**—Severe mental illness marked by loss of contact with reality, often involving delusions, hallucinations, and disordered thinking.

**Purpura**—Condition marked by bleeding into the skin; skin rash or spots are first red, darken to purple, then fade to brownish-yellow.

**PUVA**—Treatment for psoriasis by use of a psoralen, such as methoxsalen or trioxsalen, and long-wave ultraviolet light.

**Rachischisis**—See Spina bifida.

**Radiopaque agent**—Substance that makes it easier to see an area of the body with x-rays. Radiopaque agents are used to help diagnose a variety of medical problems.

**Radiopharmaceutical**—Radioactive agent used to diagnose certain medical problems or treat certain diseases.

**Raynaud's syndrome**—Condition marked by paleness, numbness, and discomfort in the fingers when they are exposed to cold.

**Rectal**—Relating to the rectum.

**Renal**—Relating to the kidneys.

**Reye's syndrome**—Serious disease affecting the liver and brain that sometimes occurs after a virus infection, such as influenza or chickenpox. It occurs most often in young children and teenagers. The first sign of Reye's syndrome is usually severe, prolonged vomiting.

**Rheumatic heart disease**—Heart disease marked by scarring and chronic inflammation of the heart and its valves, occurring after rheumatic fever.

**Rhinitis**—Inflammation of the mucous membrane inside the nose.

**Rickets**—Bone disease usually caused by too little vitamin D, resulting in soft and malformed bones.

**Ringworm**—See Tinea.

**Risk**—The possibility of injury or of suffering harm.

**River blindness**—Tropical disease produced by infection with worms of the Onchocerca type. The condition usually causes severe itching and may cause blindness. Also called *Roble's disease, blinding filarial disease,* and *craw-craw.*

**Rosacea**—Skin disease of the face, usually in middle-aged and older persons. Also called *adult acne*.

**Sarcoidosis**—Chronic disorder in which the lymph nodes in many parts of the body are enlarged, and small fleshy swellings develop in the lungs, liver, and spleen.

**Scabicide**—Medicine used to treat scabies (itch mite) infection.

**Scabies**—Contagious dermatitis caused by a mite burrowing into the skin; characterized by tiny skin eruptions and severe itching.

**Schistosomiasis**—Tropical infection in which worms enter the skin from infested water and settle in the bladder or intestines, causing inflammation and scarring. Also called *bilharziasis*.

**Schizophrenia**—Severe mental disorder in which thinking, mood, and behavior are disturbed.

**Scintigram**—Image obtained by detecting radiation emitted from a radiopharmaceutical introduced into the body.

**Scleroderma**—Chronic disease first characterized by hardening, thickening, and shrinking of the skin; later, certain organs also are affected.

**Scotoma**—Area of decreased vision or total loss of vision in a part of the visual field; blind spot.

**Scrotum**—Sac that holds the testes (male sex glands).

**Scurvy**—Disease caused by a deficiency of vitamin C (ascorbic acid), marked by bleeding gums, bleeding beneath the skin, and body weakness.

**Sebaceous gland**—Skin gland that secretes sebum.

**Seborrhea**—Skin condition caused by the excess release of sebum from the sebaceous glands, accompanied by dandruff and oily skin.

**Sebum**—Fatty secretion produced by sebaceous (oil) glands of the skin.

**Secretion**—1. Process in which a gland in the body or on the surface of the body releases a substance for use. 2. The substance released by the gland.

**Sedative-hypnotic**—Medicine used to treat excessive nervousness, restlessness, or insomnia.

**Sedation**—A profoundly relaxed or calmed state.

**Seizure**—A sudden attack or convulsion, as in epilepsy or other disorders.

**Semen**—Fluid released from the penis at sexual climax. It is made up of sperm suspended in secretions from the reproductive tract.

**Severe**—Of a great degree, such as very serious pain or distress.

**Shaking palsy**—See Parkinson's disease.

**Shingles**—See Herpes zoster.

**Shock**—Severe disruption of cellular metabolism associated with reduced blood volume and blood pressure too low to supply adequate blood to the tissues.

**Shunt**—Surgical tube used to transfer blood or other fluid from one part of the body to another.

**SIADH (secretion of inappropriate antidiuretic hormone) syndrome**—Disease in which the body retains (keeps) more fluid than normal.

**Sickle cell anemia**—Hereditary disorder that predominantly affects blacks; caused by abnormal hemoglobin. The name comes from the sickle-shaped red blood cells found in the blood of patients.

**Sinusitis**—Inflammation of a sinus.

**Sjögren's syndrome**—Condition usually occurring in older women, marked by dry eyes, dry mouth, and rheumatoid arthritis.

**Skeletal muscle relaxant**—Medicine used to relax certain muscles and help relieve the pain and discomfort caused by strains, sprains, or other injury to the muscles.

**SLE**—See Lupus erythematosus, systemic.

**Soluble**—Able to be dissolved in a fluid.

**Spasticity**—Increase in normal muscular tone, causing stiff, awkward movements.

**Spastic paralysis**—Paralysis marked by muscle rigidity or spasticity in the part of the body that is paralyzed.

**Sperm**—Mature male reproductive or sex cell.

**Spermicide**—Substance that kills sperm.

**Spina bifida**—Birth defect in which the infant's spinal cord is partially exposed through a hole in the backbone. Also called *rachischisis*.

**Stenosis**—Abnormal narrowing of a passage or duct of the body.

**Sterility**—1. Inability to produce offspring. 2. The state of being free of living microorganisms.

**Stimulant, respiratory**—Medicine used to stimulate breathing.

**Stomatitis**—Inflammation of the mucous membrane of the mouth.

**Streptokinase**—Enzyme that dissolves blood clots.

**Stroke**—Very serious event which occurs when an artery to the brain becomes clogged by a blood clot or bursts and causes hemorrhage. Stroke can effect speech, memory behavior, and other life patterns, and may result in paralysis. Also called *apoplexy*.

**Stye**—Infection of one or more sebaceous glands of the eyelid, marked by swelling.

**Subcutaneous**—Under the skin.

**Sublingual**—Under the tongue. A sublingual medicine is taken by placing it under the tongue and letting it slowly dissolve.

**Sudden infant death syndrome (SIDS)**—Death of an infant, usually while asleep, from an unknown cause. Also called *crib death* or *cot death*.

**Sugar diabetes**—See Diabetes mellitus.

**Sugar pill**—See Placebo.

**Sulfite**—Type of preservative; causes allergic reactions, such as asthma, in sensitive patients.

**Sunscreen**—Substance, usually a cream or lotion, that blocks ultraviolet light and helps prevent sunburn when applied to the skin.

**Suppository**—Mass of medicated material shaped for insertion into the rectum, vagina, or urethra. Suppository is solid at room temperature but melts at body temperature.

**Suppressant**—Medicine that stops an action or condition.

**Suspension**—A form of medicine in which the drug is mixed with a liquid but is not dissolved in it. When left standing, particles settle at the bottom of the liquid and the top portion turns clear. When shaken it is ready for use.

**Syncope**—Sudden loss of consciousness due to inadequate blood flow to the brain; fainting.

**Syphilis**—An infectious disease, usually transmitted by sexual contact. The three stages of the disease may be separated by months or years.

**Syringe**—Device used to inject liquids into the body, remove material from a part of the body, or wash out a body cavity.

**Systemic**—For general effects throughout the body; applies to most medicines when taken by mouth or given by injection.

**Tachycardia**—Abnormal rapid beating of the heart, usually at a rate over 100 beats per minute in adults.

**Temporomandibular joint (TMJ)**—Hinge that connects the lower jaw to the skull.

**Tendinitis**—Inflammation of a tendon.

**Teratogenic**—Causing abnormal development in an embryo or fetus resulting in birth defects.

**Testosterone**—Principal male sex hormone.

**Tetany**—Condition marked by spasm and twitching of the muscles, particularly those of the hands, feet, and face; caused by a decrease in the calcium ion concentration in the blood.

**Therapeutic**—Relating to the treatment of a specific condition.

**Thimerosal**—Chemical used as a preservative in some medicines, and as an antiseptic and disinfectant.

**Thrombolytic agent**—Substance that dissolves blood clots.

**Thrombophlebitis**—Inflammation of a vein accompanied by the formation of a blood clot.

**Thrombus**—Blood clot that obstructs a blood vessel or a cavity of the heart.

**Thrush**—See Candidiasis of the mouth.

**Thyroid gland**—Gland in the lower front of the neck. It releases thyroid hormones, which control body metabolism.

**Thyrotoxicosis**—Condition resulting from excessive amounts of thyroid hormones in the blood, causing increased metabolism, fast heartbeat, tremors, nervousness, and increased sweating.

**Tic**—Repeated involuntary movement or spasm of a muscle.

**Tic douloureux**—See Neuralgia, trigeminal.

**Tinea**—Fungus infection of the surface of the skin, particularly the scalp, feet, and nails. Also called *ringworm*.

**Tone**—The slight, continuous tension present in resting muscles.

**Topical**—For local effects when applied directly to the skin.

**Tourette's disorder**—Condition usually marked with motor tics (jerking movements) and vocal tics (grunts, sniffs). Also called *Gilles de la Tourette syndrome*.

**Toxemia**—Blood poisoning caused by bacterial production of toxins.

**Toxemia of pregnancy**—Condition occurring in pregnant women marked by hypertension, edema, excess protein in the urine, convulsions, and possibly coma.

**Toxic**—Poisonous; related to or caused by a toxin or poison.

**Toxin**—A substance produced by an animal or plant that is poisonous to another organism.

**Toxoplasmosis**—Disease caused by a blood protozoan, usually transmitted to humans from cats or by eating raw meat; generally the symptoms are mild and self-limited.

**Tracheostomy**—A surgical opening through the throat into the trachea (windpipe) to bypass an obstruction to breathing.

**Tranquilizer**—Medicine that produces a calming effect. It is used to relieve mental anxiety and tension.

**Transdermal**—A means of administering medicine into the body by use of skin patches or disks, or ointment; medicine contained in the patch or disk or the ointment is absorbed through the skin.

**Trichomoniasis**—Infection of the vagina resulting in inflammation of genital tissues and discharge. It can be passed on to males.

**Triglyceride**—A molecular form in which fats are present in food and the body; triglycerides are stored in the body as fat.

**Trypanosome fever**—See Trypanosomiasis, African.

**Trypanosomiasis, African**—Tropical disease, transmitted by tsetse fly bites, which causes fever, headache, and chills, followed by enlarged lymph nodes and anemia. Months or even years later, the disease affects the central nervous system, causing drowsiness and lethargy, coma, and death. Also called *African sleeping sickness*.

**Tuberculosis (TB)**—Infectious disease which may affect any organ but most commonly the lungs; symptoms include fever, night sweats, weight loss, and spitting up blood.

**Tumor**—Abnormal growth or enlargement in or on a part of the body.

**Tyramine**—Chemical present in many foods and beverages. Its structure and action in the body are similar to epinephrine.

**Ulcer**—Open sore or break in the skin or mucous membrane; often fails to heal and is accompanied by inflammation.

**Ulcerative colitis**—Chronic, recurrent inflammation and ulceration of the colon.

**Ulceration**—1. Formation or development of an ulcer. 2. Condition of an area marked with ulcers loosely associated with one another.

**Underactive thyroid**—See hypothyroidism.

**Ureter**—Tube through which urine passes from the kidney to the bladder.

**Urethra**—Tube through which urine passes from the bladder to the outside of the body.

**Urticaria**—Hives; an eruption of itching wheals on the skin.

**Vaccine**—Medicine given by mouth or by injection to produce immunity to a certain infection.

**Vaccinia**—The skin and sometimes body reactions associated with smallpox vaccine. Also called *cowpox*.

**Vaginal**—Relating to the vagina.

**Varicella**—Very infectious virus disease marked by fever and itchy rash that develops into blisters and then scabs. Also called *chickenpox*.

**Vascular**—Relating to the blood vessels.

**Vasodilator**—Medicine that dilates the blood vessels, permitting increased blood flow.

**Ventricular fibrillation**—Life-threatening condition of fine, quivering, irregular movements of many individual muscle fibers of the ventricular muscle; replaces the normal heart beat and interrupts pumping function.

**Ventricle**—A small cavity, such as one of the two lower chambers of the heart or one of the several cavities of the brain.

**Vertigo**—Sensation of whirling motion or dizziness, either of oneself or of one's surroundings.

**Veterinary**—Relating to animals and their diseases and treatment.

**Virus**—Any of a group of simple microbes too small to be seen by a light microscope. They can grow and reproduce only in living cells. Many cause diseases in humans, including the common cold.

**Vitiligo**—Condition in which some areas of skin lose pigment and turn white. Also called *leukoderma*.

**von Willebrand's disease**—Hereditary blood disease in which blood clotting is delayed, leading to excessive and uncontrolled bleeding even after minor injuries.

**Water diabetes**—See Diabetes insipidus.

**Water pill**—See Diuretic.

**Wheal**—Temporary, small, raised area of the skin, usually accompanied by itching or burning; welt.

**Wheezing**—A whistling sound made when there is difficulty in breathing.

**White mouth**—See Candidiasis of the mouth.

**Wilson's disease**—Inborn defect in the body's ability to process copper. Too much copper may lead to jaundice, cirrhosis, mental retardation, or symptoms like those of Parkinson's disease.

**Zollinger-Ellison syndrome**—Disorder in which the stomach produces too much acid, leading to ulcers.

# Appendix I

## GENERAL INFORMATION ABOUT USE OF MEDICINES

Information about the proper use of medicines is of two types. One type is drug specific and applies to a certain medicine or group of medicines only. The other type is general in nature and applies to the use of any medicine.

The information that follows is general in nature. For your own safety, health, and well-being, however, it is important that you learn about the proper use of your specific medicines as well. You can get this information from your health care professional, or find it in the individual listings of this book.

### Before Using Your Medicine

Before you use any medicine, your health care professional should be told:

—if you have ever had an allergic or unusual reaction to any medicine, food, or other substance, such as yellow dye or sulfites.

—if you are on a low-salt, low-sugar, or any other special diet. Most medicines contain more than their active ingredient, and many liquid medicines contain alcohol.

—*if you are pregnant or if you plan to become pregnant.* Certain medicines may cause birth defects or other problems in the unborn child. For other medicines, safe use during pregnancy has not been established. *The use of any medicine during pregnancy must be carefully considered* and should be discussed with a health care professional.

—*if you are breast-feeding.* Some medicines may pass into the breast milk and cause unwanted effects in the baby.

—*if you are now taking or have taken any medicines or dietary supplements in the recent past.* Do not forget over-the-counter (nonprescription) medicines such as pain relievers, laxatives, and antacids or dietary supplements.

—*if you have any medical problems* other than the one(s) for which your medicine was prescribed.

—*if you have difficulty remembering things or reading labels.*

### Storage of Your Medicine

*It is important to store your medicines properly. Guidelines for proper storage include:*

• *Keep out of the reach of children.*
• Keep medicines in their original containers.

• Store away from heat and direct light.
• Do not store capsules or tablets in the bathroom, near the kitchen sink, or in other damp places. Heat or moisture may cause the medicine to break down. Also, do not leave the cotton plug in a medicine container that has been opened, since it may draw moisture into the container.
• Keep liquid medicines from freezing.
• Do not store medicines in the refrigerator unless directed to do so.
• Do not leave your medicines in an automobile for long periods of time.
• Do not keep outdated medicine or medicine that is no longer needed. Be sure that any discarded medicine is out of the reach of children.

### Proper Use of Your Medicine

Take medicine only as directed, at the right time, and for the full length of your prescribed treatment. If you are using an over-the-counter (nonprescription) medicine, follow the directions on the label unless otherwise directed by your health care professional. If you feel that your medicine is not working for you, check with your health care professional.

Unless your pharmacist has packaged different medicines together in a "bubble-pack," different medicines should never be mixed in one container. It is best to keep your medicines tightly capped in their original containers when not in use. Do not remove the label since directions for use and other important information may appear on it.

To avoid mistakes, do not take medicine in the dark. Always read the label before taking, especially noting the expiration date and any directions for use.

**For oral (by mouth) medicines:**

• In general, it is best to take oral medicines with a full glass of water. However, follow your health care professional's directions. Some medicines should be taken with food, while others should be taken on an empty stomach.
• When taking most long-acting forms of a medicine, each dose should be swallowed whole. Do not break, crush, or chew before swallowing unless you have been specifically told that it is all right to do so.
• If you are taking liquid medicines, you should consider using a specially marked measuring spoon or other device to measure each dose accurately. Ask

your pharmacist about these devices. The average household teaspoon may not hold the right amount of liquid.

- Oral medicine may come in a number of different dosage forms, such as tablets, capsules, and liquids. If you have trouble swallowing the dosage form prescribed for you, check with your health care professional. Another dosage form that you can swallow more easily may be available.
- Child-resistant caps on medicine containers have decreased greatly the number of accidental poisonings that occur each year. Use of these caps is required by law. However, if you find it hard to open such caps, you may ask your pharmacist for a regular, easier-to-open cap. He or she can provide you with a regular cap if you request it. However, you must make this request each time you get a prescription filled.

**For skin patches:**
- Apply the patch to a clean, dry skin area with little or no hair and free of scars, cuts, or irritation. Remove the previous patch before applying a new one.
- Apply a new patch if the first one becomes loose or falls off.
- Apply each patch to a different area of skin to prevent skin irritation or other problems.
- Do not try to trim or cut the adhesive patch to adjust the dosage. Check with your health care professional if you think the medicine is not working as it should.

**For inhalers:**
- Medicines that come in inhalers usually come with patient directions. *Read the directions carefully before using the medicine.* If you do not understand the directions, or if you are not sure how to use the inhaler, check with your health care professional.
- Since different types of inhalers may be used in different ways, it is very important to follow carefully the directions given to you.

**For ophthalmic (eye) drops:**
- To prevent contamination, do not let the tip of the eye drop applicator touch any surface (including the eye) and keep the container tightly closed.
- The bottle may not be full; this is to provide proper drop control.
- How to apply: First, wash your hands. Tilt your head back and, with the index finger, pull the lower eyelid away from the eye to form a pouch. Drop the medicine into the pouch and gently close your eyes. Do not blink. Keep your eyes closed for 1 to 2 minutes.
- If your medicine is for glaucoma or inflammation of the eye: Follow the directions for application that are listed above. However, immediately after placing the drops in your eye, apply pressure to the inside corner of the eye with your middle finger. Continue

to apply pressure for 1 to 2 minutes after the medicine has been placed in the eye. This will help prevent the medicine from being absorbed into the body and causing side effects.
- After applying the eye drops, wash your hands to remove any medicine.

**For ophthalmic (eye) ointments:**
- To prevent contamination of the eye ointment, do not let the tip of the applicator touch any surface (including the eye). After using, wipe the tip of the ointment tube with a clean tissue and keep the tube tightly closed.
- How to apply: First, wash your hands. Pull the lower eyelid away from the eye to form a pouch. Squeeze a thin strip of ointment into the pouch. A 1-cm (approximately ⅓-inch) strip of ointment is usually enough unless otherwise directed. Gently close your eyes and keep them closed for 1 to 2 minutes.
- After applying the eye ointment, wash your hands to remove any medicine.

**For nasal (nose) drops:**
- How to use: Blow your nose gently, without squeezing. Tilt your head back while standing or sitting up, or lie down on your back on a bed and hang your head over the side. Place the drops into each nostril and keep your head tilted back for a few minutes to allow the medicine to spread throughout the nose.
- Rinse the dropper with hot water and dry with a clean tissue. Replace the cap right after use. To avoid the spread of infection, do not use the container for more than one person.

**For nasal (nose) spray:**
- How to use: Blow your nose gently, without squeezing. With your head upright, spray the medicine into each nostril. Sniff briskly while squeezing the bottle quickly and firmly.
- Rinse the tip of the spray bottle with hot water, taking care not to suck water into the bottle, and dry with a clean tissue. Replace the cap right after cleaning. To avoid the spread of infection, do not use the container for more than one person.

**For otic (ear) drops:**
- To prevent contamination of the ear drops, do not touch the applicator tip to any surface (including the ear).
- The bottle may not be full; this is to provide proper drop control.
- How to apply: First, wash your hands. Lie down or tilt your head so the ear that the medicine will go into is facing up. For adults, gently pull the ear lobe up and back to straighten the ear canal. (For children, gently pull the ear lobe down and back to straighten the ear canal). Drop the medicine into the ear canal. Keep the ear facing up for several minutes to allow the medicine to run to the bottom of the

ear canal. A sterile cotton plug may be gently inserted into the ear opening to prevent the medicine from leaking out.

- Do not rinse the dropper after use. Wipe the tip of the dropper with a clean tissue and keep the container tightly closed.

**For rectal suppositories:**

- How to insert suppository: First, wash your hands. Remove the foil wrapper and moisten the suppository with water. Lie down on your side. Push the suppository well up into the rectum with your finger. If the suppository is too soft to insert, chill it in the refrigerator for 30 minutes or run cold water over it before removing the foil wrapper.
- Wash your hands after you have inserted the suppository.

**For rectal cream or ointment:**

- Bathe and dry the rectal area. Apply a small amount of cream or ointment and rub it in gently.
- If your health care professional wants you to insert the medicine into the rectum: First, attach the plastic applicator tip onto the opened tube. Insert the applicator tip into the rectum and gently squeeze the tube to deliver the cream. Remove the applicator tip from the tube and wash with hot, soapy water. Replace the cap of the tube after use.
- Wash your hands after you have inserted the medicine.

**For vaginal medicines:**

- How to insert the medicine: First, wash your hands. Use the special applicator. Follow any special directions that are provided by the manufacturer. However, if you are pregnant, check with your health care professional before using the applicator to insert the medicine.
- Lie on your back, with your knees drawn up. Using the applicator, insert the medicine into the vagina as far as you can without using force or causing discomfort. Release the medicine by pushing on the plunger. Wait several minutes before getting up.
- Wash the applicator and your hands with soap and warm water.

## Precautions While Using Your Medicine

*Never give your medicine to anyone else.* It has been prescribed for your personal medical problem and may not be the correct treatment for or may even be harmful to another person.

Many medicines should not be taken with other medicines or with alcoholic beverages. Follow your health care professional's directions to help avoid problems.

Before having any kind of surgery (including dental surgery) or emergency treatment, tell the physician or dentist about any medicine you are taking.

*If you think you have taken an overdose of any medicine or if a child has taken a medicine by accident:* Call your poison control center or your health care professional at once. Keep those telephone numbers handy. Also, keep a bottle of Ipecac Syrup safely stored in your home in case you are told to cause vomiting. Read the directions on the label of Ipecac Syrup before using.

## Side Effects of Your Medicine

Along with its intended effects, a medicine may cause some unwanted effects. Some of these side effects may need medical attention, while others may not. It is important for you to know what side effects may occur and what you should do if you notice signs of them. Check with your health care professional about the possible side effects of the medicines you are taking, or if you notice any unusual reactions or side effects.

## Additional Information

It is a good idea for you to learn both the generic and brand names of your medicine and even to write them down and keep them for future use.

Many prescriptions may not be refilled until your pharmacist checks with your health care professional. *To save time, do not wait until you have run out of medicine before requesting a refill.* This is especially important if you must take your medicine every day.

*When traveling:*

- Carry your medicine with you rather than putting it in your checked luggage. Checked luggage may get lost or misplaced or may be stored in very cold or very hot areas.
- Make sure a source of medicine is available where you are traveling, or take a large enough supply to last during your visit. It is also a good idea to take a copy of your written prescription with you.

If you want more information about your medicines, ask your health care professional. *Do not be embarrassed to ask questions* about any medicine you are taking. To help you remember, it may be helpful to write down any questions and bring them with you on your next visit to your health care professional.

# AVOIDING MEDICINE MISHAPS

## Tips Against Tampering

Over-the-counter (OTC) or nonprescription medicines are now packaged so that it will be easier to notice signs of tampering. A tamper-evident package is required either to be unique so that it cannot be copied easily, or to have a barrier or indicator (that has an identifying characteristic, such as a pattern, picture, or logo) that will be easily noticed if it is broken. For two-piece, unsealed, hard gelatin capsules, two tamper-evident features are required. Improved packaging also includes the use of special wrappers, seals, or caps on the outer and/or inner containers, or sealing each dose in its own pouch.

Even with such packaging, however, no system is completely safe. It is important that you do your part by checking for signs of tampering whenever you buy or use a medicine.

The following information may help you detect possible signs of tampering.

### Protecting yourself

General common sense suggestions include the following:

• When buying a drug product, *consider* the dosage form (for example, capsules, tablets, syrup), the type of packaging, and the tamper-evident features. Ask yourself: Would it be easy for someone to tamper with this product? Will I be able to determine whether or not this product has been tampered with?

• *Look very carefully* at the outer packaging of the drug product before you buy it. After you buy it, also check the inner packaging as soon as possible.

• If the medicine has a protective packaging feature, it should be described in the labeling. This description is required to be placed so that it will not be affected if the feature is broken or missing. If the feature is broken or missing, *do not buy or use* the product. If you have already purchased the product, return it to the store. Always be sure to tell someone in charge about any problems.

• *Do not take* medicines that show even the slightest signs of tampering or don't seem quite right.

• Never take medicines in the dark or in poor lighting. *Read* the label and check each dose of medicine before you take it.

### What to look for

#### Packaging

• Are there breaks, cracks, or holes in the outer or inner wrapping or protective cover or seal?

• Does the outer or inner covering appear to have been disturbed, unwrapped, or replaced?

• Does a plastic or other shrink band (tight-fitting wrap) around the top of the bottle appear distorted or stretched, as though it had been rolled down and then

put back into place? Is the band missing? Has the band been slit and retaped?

• Is the bottom of the container intact?

• Does the container appear to be too full or not full enough?

• Is the cap on tight?

• Are there bits of paper or glue stuck on the rim of the container that make it seem the container once had a bottle seal?

• Is the cotton plug or filler in the bottle torn, sticky, or stained, or does it appear to have been taken out and put back?

• Do eye drops have a protective seal? All eye drops must be sealed when they are made, in order to keep them germ-free. Do not use if there is any sign of a broken or removed seal.

• Check the bottom as well as the top of a tube. Is the tube properly sealed? Metal tubes crimped up from the bottom like a tube of toothpaste should be firmly sealed.

• Are the expiration date, lot number, and other information the same on both the container and its outer wrapping or box?

#### Liquids

• Is the medicine the usual color? Thickness?

• Is a normally clear liquid cloudy or colored?

• Are there particles (small pieces) in the bottom of the bottle or floating in the solution? For some liquids, called suspensions, floating particles are normal.

• Does the medicine have a strange or different taste or odor (for example, bleach, acid, gasoline-like, or other pungent or sharp odor)? Do not taste the medicine if it has a strange odor.

#### Tablets

• Do the tablets look different than they usually do? Do they have unusual spots or markings? If they normally are shiny and smooth, are some dull or rough? Is there anything unusual about the color?

• Are the tablets all the same size and thickness?

• If there is printing on the tablets, do they all have the same imprint? Is the imprint missing from any?

• Do the tablets have a strange or different odor or taste?

• Are any of the tablets broken?

#### Capsules

• Do the capsules look different than they usually do? Are any cracked or dented? Are they all the same size and color?

• Do they have their normal shiny appearance or are some dull or have fingerprints on them as though they have been handled?

• Are the capsules all the same length?

• If there is printing on the capsules, do they all have the same imprint? Is the imprint missing from any? Do the imprints all line up the same way?

• Do the capsules have an unexpected or unusual odor or taste?

**Tubes and jars** (ointments, creams, pastes, etc.)

• Does the product or container look different than usual?

• Are ointments and creams smooth and non-gritty? Have they separated?

Be a wise consumer. Look for signs of tampering before you buy a medicine and again each time you take a dose. Also, pay attention to the daily news in order to learn about any reported tampering.

It is important to understand that a change in the appearance or condition of a product may not mean that the package has been tampered with. The manufacturer may have changed the color of a medicine or its packaging. Also, the product may be breaking down with age or it may have had rough or unusual handling in shipping. In addition, some minor product variations may be normal.

Whenever you suspect that something is unusual about a medicine or its packaging, take it to your pharmacist. He or she is familiar with most products and their packaging. If there are serious concerns or problems, your pharmacist should report it to the USP Drug Product Problem Reporting Program (USP DPPR) at 1-800-638-6725, or other appropriate authorities.

## Unintentional Poisoning

According to information provided by the American Association of Poison Control Centers, nearly one million children 6 years of age and under were unintentionally poisoned in 1993; 27 children 6 years of age and younger died as a result of poisoning.

Adults also may be unintentionally poisoned. This happens most often through carelessness or lack of information. For example, the sleepy adult who takes a medicine in the dark and winds up getting the wrong one, or the adult who decides to take the medicine prescribed for a friend to treat "the same symptoms."

Drug poisoning from an unintentional overdose is 1 type of accidental poisoning that contributes to these figures. Other causes include household chemical poisoning from unintentional ingestion or contact, and inhaled poisoning—for example, carbon monoxide, usually from a car.

### Children are ready victims

The natural curiosity of children makes them ready victims of poisoning. Children explore everywhere and investigate their environment. What they find frequently goes into their mouths. They do not understand danger and possibly cannot read warning labels.

Accidental poisoning from medicine is especially dangerous in small children because the strength of most medicines that may be ingested is often based on their use in adults. Even a small quantity of an adult dose can sometimes poison a child.

### Preventing poisoning from medicines

• Store medicines out of the sight and reach of children, preferably in a locked cabinet—not in the bathroom medicine cabinet or in a food cabinet.

• If you have children living with you or only as occasional guests, you should have child-resistant caps on your medicine containers. These will help to ensure that an accidental poisoning does not occur in your home. Always store your medicines in a secure place.

• Adults who have difficulty opening child-resistant closures may request traditional, easy-to-open packaging for their medicines.

• Always replace lids and return medicines to their storage place after use, even if you will be using them again soon.

• If you are called to the telephone or to answer the door while you are taking medicine, take the container with you or put the medicine out of the reach of small children. Children act quickly—usually when no one is watching.

• Date medicines when purchased and clean out your medicines periodically. Discard prescription medicines that are past their expiration or "beyond use" date. As medicines grow old, the chemicals in them may change. In general, medicines that do not have an expiration date should not be kept for more than 1 year. Carefully discard any medicines so that children cannot get them. Rinse containers well before discarding in the trash.

• Take only those medicines prescribed for you and give medicines only to those for whom prescribed. A medicine that worked well for one person may harm another.

• It is best to keep all medicines in their original containers with their labels intact. The label contains valuable information for taking the medicine properly. Also, in case of accidental poisoning, it is important to know the ingredients in a drug product and any emergency instructions from the manufacturer. While prescription medicines usually do not list ingredients, information on the label makes it possible for your pharmacist to identify the contents.

• Ask your pharmacist to include on the label the number of tablets or capsules that he or she put in the container. In case of poisoning, it may be important to know roughly how many tablets or capsules were taken.

• Do not trust your memory—read the label before using the medicine, and take it as directed.

• If a medicine container has no label or the label has been defaced so that you are not absolutely sure what it says, do not use it.

• Turn on a light when taking or giving medicines at night or in a dark room.

• Label medicine containers with poison symbols, especially if you have children, individuals with poor vision, or other persons in your home who cannot read well.

• Teach children that medicine is not candy by calling each medicine by its proper name.

• Do not take medicines in front of children. They may wish to imitate you.

• Communicate these safety rules to any babysitters you have and remember them if you babysit or are visiting a house with children. Children are naturally curious and can get into a pocketbook, briefcase, or overnight bag that contains medicines.

### What to do if a poisoning happens

*Remember:*

• There may be no immediate, significant symptoms or warning signs, particularly in a child.

• Nothing you can give will work equally well in all cases of poisoning. In fact, one "antidote" may counteract the effects of another.

• Many poisons act quickly, leaving little time for treatment.

*Therefore:*

• If you think someone has swallowed medicine or a household product, and the person is unconscious, having seizures (convulsions), or is not breathing, immediately call for an ambulance. Otherwise, do not wait

to see what effect the poison will have or if symptoms of overdose develop, immediately call a Poison Control Center (listed in the white pages of your telephone book under "Poison Control" or inside the front cover with other emergency numbers). These numbers should be posted beside every telephone in the house, as should those of your pharmacist, the police, the fire department, and ambulance services. (Some poison control centers have TTY capability for the deaf. Check with your local center if you or someone in your family requires this service.)

• Have the container with you when you call so you can read the label on the product for ingredients.

• Describe what, when, and how much was taken and the age and condition of the person poisoned—for example, if the person is vomiting, choking, drowsy, shows a change in color or temperature of skin, is conscious or unconscious, or is convulsing.

• *Do not induce vomiting* unless instructed by medical personnel. *Do not induce vomiting or force liquids* into a person who is convulsing, unconscious, or very drowsy.

• Stay calm and in control of the situation.

Keep a bottle of Ipecac Syrup stored in a secure place in your home for emergency use. It is available at pharmacies in 1 ounce bottles without prescription. Ipecac Syrup is often recommended to induce vomiting in cases of poisoning.

Activated Charcoal also is sometimes recommended in certain types of poisoning and you may wish to add a supply to your emergency medicines. It is available without a prescription. Before using this medicine for poisoning, however, call a poison control center for advice.

# GETTING THE MOST OUT OF YOUR MEDICINES

To get the most out of your medicines, there are certain things that you must do. Although your health care professionals will be working with you, you also have a responsibility for your own health.

## Communicating With Your Health Care Provider

Communication between you and your health care professional is central to good medical care. Your health care professional needs to know about you, your medical history, and your current problems. In turn, you need to understand the recommendations he or she is making and what you will need to do to follow the treatment. You will have to ask questions—and answer some too. Communication is a two-way street.

### Giving information

To provide effective care, your health care professional needs to know some details about your past and present

medical history. In discussing these details, you should always be completely open and honest. Your health professional's diagnosis and treatment will be based in part on the information that you provide. A complete list of the details that should be included in in a full medical history is provided below.

### "Medical history" checklist

A "medical history" checklist covers the following information:

• All the serious illnesses you have ever had and the approximate dates.

• Your current symptoms, if any.

• **All** the medicines and dietary supplements you are taking or have taken in the recent past. This includes prescription and nonprescription medicines (such as pain relievers, antacids, laxatives, and cold medicines, etc.) and home remedies. This is especially important if you are seeing more than one health care professional; if you are having surgery, including dental or emergency treatment; or if you get your medicines from more than one source.

• **Any** allergies or sensitivities to medicines, foods, or other substances.

• Your smoking, drinking, and exercise habits.

• Any recent changes in your lifestyle or personal habits. New job? Retired? Change of residence? Death in family? Married? Divorced? Other?

• Any special diet you are on—low-sugar, low-sodium, low-fat, or a diet to lose or gain weight.

• If you are pregnant, plan to become pregnant, or if you are breast-feeding.

• All the vaccinations and vaccination boosters you have had, with dates if possible.

• Any operations you have had, including dental and those performed on an outpatient basis, and any accidents that have required hospitalization.

• Illnesses or conditions that run in your family.

• Cause of death of closest relatives.

Remember, be sure to tell your health care professional at each visit if there have been any changes since your last visit.

Many health care professionals have a standard "medical history" form they will ask you to fill out when they see you for the first time. Some may ask the questions and write down the answers for you. If you will be visiting a health care professional for the first time, prepare yourself before you go by thinking about the questions that might be asked and jotting down the answers—including dates—so that you will not forget an important detail. Once your "medical history" is in the files, subsequent visits will take less time.

You will have to supply each health care provider you see—every time you see one—with complete information about what happened since your last visit. It is important that your records are updated so he or she can make sound recommendations for your continued treatment, or treatment of any new problems.

It will simplify things if you develop a "medical history" file at home for yourself and each family member for whom you are responsible. Setting up the file will take time. However, once it is established, you need only to keep it up-to-date and remember to take it with you when you see a health care professional. This will be easier than having to repeat the information each time and running the risk of confusing or forgetting details.

It is also a good idea to carry in your wallet a card that summarizes your chronic medical conditions, the medicines you are taking, and your allergies and drug sensitivities. You should keep this card as up-to-date as possible. Many pharmacists provide these cards as a service.

*Getting information*

For your health care professional to be able to serve you well, you must communicate all that you know about your present health condition at every visit. In order to benefit from the advice for which you have paid, your health care professional must communicate full instructions for your care. More importantly, you must understand completely everything that he or she tells you. Do not be embarrassed to ask questions, or to ask him or her to explain again any instruction or detail that you do not understand. Then it is up to you to carry out those instructions precisely. If there is a failure in any part of this system, you will pay an even higher price—physically and financially—for your health care.

Your health care professional may provide instructions to you in written form. If he or she does not, you may want to write them down or ask the health care professional to write them down for you. If you do not have time to jot down everything while you are still with your health care professional, sit down in the waiting room before you leave and write down the information while it is still fresh in your mind and you can still ask questions. If you have been given a prescription, ask for written information about the drug and how to take it. Your pharmacist can also answer questions when you have your prescription filled.

*What you need to know about your medicines*

There are a number of things that you should know about each medicine you are taking. These include:

• The medicine's generic and brand name.

• How it will help you and the expected results. How it makes you feel. How long it takes to begin working.

• How much to take at one time.

• How often to take the medicine.

• How long it will be necessary to take the medicine.

• When to take it. Before, during, after meals? At bedtime? At any other special times?

• How to take it. With water? With fruit juice? How much?

• What to do if you forget to take it (miss a dose).

• Foods, drinks, or other medicines that you should not take while taking the medicine.

• Restrictions on activities while taking the medicine. May I drive a car or operate other motor vehicles?

• Possible side effects. What to do if they appear. How to minimize the side effects. How soon they will go away.

• When to seek help if there are problems.

• How long to wait before reporting no change in symptoms.

• How to store the medicine.

• The expiration date.

• The cost of the medicine.

• How to have your prescription refilled, if necessary.

## Other information

Following are some other issues and information that you may want to consider:

- Ask your health care professional about the ingredients in the medicines (both prescription and over-the-counter [OTC]) you are taking and whether there may be a conflict with other medicines. Your health care professional can help you avoid dangerous combinations or drug products that contain ingredients to which you are allergic or sensitive.

- Ask your health care professional for help in developing a system for taking your medicines properly, particularly if you are taking a number of them on a daily basis. (When you are a patient in a hospital, ask for instructions before you are discharged.) Do not hesitate or be embarrassed to ask questions or ask for help.

- If you are over 60 years of age, ask your health care professional if the dose of the medicine prescribed is right for you. Some medicines should be given in lower doses to certain older individuals.

- If you are taking several different medicines, ask your health care professional if all of them are necessary for you. You should take only those medicines that you need.

- Medicines should be kept in the container they came in. If this is not possible when you are at work or away from home, ask your pharmacist to provide or recommend a container to transport your medicines safely. The use of "pill boxes" can also cause some problems, such as broken or chipped tablets, mistaking one medicine for another, and even interactions between the medicine and the metal of these boxes.

- Some people have trouble taking tablets or capsules. Your health care professional will know if another dosage form is available, and if tablets or capsule contents can be taken in a liquid. If this is an ongoing problem, ask your prescriber to write the prescription for the dosage form you can take most comfortably.

- Child-resistant caps are required by law on most prescription medicines for oral use to protect children from accidental poisoning. These containers are designed so that children will have difficulty opening them. Since many adults also find these containers hard to open, the law allows consumers to request traditional, easy-to-open packaging for their drugs. If you do not use child-resistant packaging, make sure that your medicines are stored where small children cannot see or reach them. If you use child-resistant containers, ask your pharmacist to show you how to open them.

Consumer education is one of the most important responsibilities of your health care professional. To supplement what you learn during your visit, ask if there is any written information about your medicines that you can take home with you. Your health care professional may also have available various reference books or computerized drug information that you can consult for details about precautions, side effects, and proper use of your medicines.

# Your Health Care Team

Your health care team will be made up of several different health care professionals. Each of these individuals will play an important part in the overall provision of your health care. It is important that you understand the roles of each of these providers and what you should be able to expect from each of them.

## Your dentist

In addition to providing care and maintenance of your mouth, teeth, and gums, your dentist is also an essential member of your overall health care team since your oral health and general health often affect one another.

In providing dental treatment, your dentist should base his or her decisions upon an extensive knowledge of your current condition and past medical and dental history. Because the dentist is a prescriber of medications, it is very important that he or she is aware of your **full** medical and dental history. A complete medical and dental history should include the information that is listed in the "Medical history checklist" section above. Even if you do not consider this information important, you should inform your dentist as fully as possible.

In the treatment of any dental/oral problem your dentist should make every effort to inform you as fully as possible about the nature of the problem. He or she should explain why this problem has occurred, the advantages and disadvantages of available treatments (including no treatment), and what types of preventive measures can be employed to avoid future problems. These measures may include periodic visits to the dentist, and a general awareness of the manner in which dental and overall health may affect one another. In any type of treatment, your dentist should always allow you to ask questions, and should be willing to answer them to your satisfaction.

In selecting a dentist, it is important to keep in mind the role of the dentist as a member of the health care team, and the extent of the information that he or she should be asking for and providing. There are also several practical issues that you should consider, such as:

- Is the dentist a specialist or general practitioner?
- What are the office hours?
- Is the dentist or his/her associates available after office hours by phone? In emergencies, will you be able to contact a dentist?
- What is the office policy on cancellations?
- What types of payment are accepted at the office?
- What is the office policy on x-ray procedures?
- Is the dentist willing to work with other medical and/or dental specialists that you may be seeing?

Your dentist should be an integral part of your health care team. In treating problems and providing general maintenance of your oral health, your dentist should base decisions upon a full dental and medical history. He or she should also be willing to answer any questions that you have regarding your oral health, any medications prescribed, and preventive measures to avoid future problems.

### Your nurse

Depending upon the setting, type of therapy being administered, and state regulations, the role of the nurse in your health care team may vary. Registered nurses practice in diverse health care settings, such as hospitals, outpatient clinics or physicians' offices, schools, workplaces, homes, and long-term care facilities like nursing homes and retirement centers. Some nurses, including certified nurse practitioners and midwives, hold a master's degree in nursing and may assume the role of primary health care professional, either in practice by themselves or in joint practices with physicians. In most states, nurse practitioners may prescribe selected medications. Clinical nurse specialists also have a master's degree in nursing and specialize in a particular area of health care. In some hospitals, long-term care facilities, and out-patient care settings, licensed practical nurses (LPNs) have certain responsibilities in administering medication to patients. LPNs usually work under the supervision of a RN or physician. Nursing aides assist RNs and LPNs with different kinds of patient care activities. In most places where people receive health care, RNs may be the primary source of information for drug therapies and other medical treatments. It is important that you be aware of the roles and responsibilities of the nurses participating in your health care.

Professional nurses participate with other health professionals, such as physicians and pharmacists, to ensure that your medication therapy is safe and effective and to monitor any effects (both desired and negative) from the medication. You may be admitted to the hospital so that nurses can administer medications and monitor your response to therapy. In hospitals or long-term care facilities, nurses are responsible for administering your medications in their proper dosage form and dose, and at correct time intervals, as well as monitoring your response to these medications. At home or in outpatient settings, nurses should ensure that you have the proper information and support of others, if needed, to get the medication and take it as prescribed. When nurses administer medication, they should explain why you are receiving this medication, how it works, any possible side effects, special precautions or actions that you must take while using the medication, and any potential interactions with other medications.

If you experience any side effects or symptoms from a medication, you should always tell your health care provider. It is important that these reactions be detected before they become serious or permanent. You can seek advice about possible ways to minimize these side effects from your nurse. Your health care professional should also be made aware of any additional medical problems or conditions (such as pregnancy) that you may have, since these can also affect the safety and effectiveness of a medication.

The professional nurse is someone who can help to clarify drug information. In most health care settings, nurses are accessible and can answer your questions or direct you to others who can assist you. Professional nurses are skilled in the process of patient teaching. To make sure that patients learn important information about their health problem and its treatment, RNs often use a combination of teaching methods, such as verbal instruction, written materials, demonstration, and audio-visual instructions. Above all, professional nurses should teach at a pace and level that are appropriate for you. RNs can also help you design a medication schedule that fits your lifestyle and may be less likely to cause unwanted side effects.

### Your pharmacist

Your pharmacist is an important member of your health care team. In addition to performing traditional services, such as dispensing medications, your pharmacist can help you understand your medications and how to take them safely and effectively. By keeping accurate and up-to-date records and monitoring your use of medications, your pharmacist can help to protect you from improper medication therapy, unwanted side effects, and dangerous drug interactions. Because your pharmacist can play a vital role in protecting and improving your health, you should seek a pharmacist who will provide these services.

To provide you with the best possible care, your pharmacist should be informed about your current condition and medication history. Your personal medication history should include the information that is listed in the "Medical history checklist" section above. Your pharmacist should also be aware of any special packaging needs that you may have (such as child-resistant or easy-to-open containers). Your pharmacist should keep accurate and up-to-date records that contain this information. If you visit a new pharmacy that does not have access to your medication records, it is important that you inform that pharmacist as fully as possible about your medical history or provide him or her with a copy of your medication records from your previous pharmacy. In general, in order to get the most out of your pharmacy services, it is best to get all of your medications (including OTCs) from the same pharmacy.

Your pharmacist should be a knowledgeable and approachable source of information about your medications. Some of the information that your pharmacist should explain to you about your medications is listed in the "What you need to know about your medicines" section above. Ideally, this information should also be provided in written form, so that you may refer to it later if you have any questions or problems. The pharmacist should always be willing to answer any questions that you have regarding your medications, and should also be willing to contact your physician or other health care professionals (dentist, nurses, etc.) on your behalf if necessary.

Your pharmacist can also help you with information on the costs of your medicines. Many medicines are available from more than one company. They may have equal effects, but may have different costs. Your insurance company, HMO, or other third-party payment group may reimburse you for only some of these medications or only for part of their costs. Your pharmacist will be able to tell you which of these medications are covered by your payment plan or which cost less.

In selecting a pharmacist, it is important that you understand the role of the pharmacist as a member of your health care team and the extent of information that he or she should be asking for and providing. Because pharmacies can offer different types of services and have different policies regarding patient information, some of the issues that you should consider in selecting a pharmacist also relate to the pharmacy where that person practices. There are several issues regarding the pharmacist and pharmacy that you should consider, such as:

- Does the pharmacy offer written information that you can take home? Home delivery?
- Are you able to talk to your pharmacist without other people hearing you?
- Can the pharmacist be reached easily by phone? In an emergency, is a pharmacist available twenty-four hours (including weekends and holidays) by phone?
- What types of payment are accepted in the pharmacy?
- Does the pharmacy accept your HMO or third-party payment plan?
- Does the pharmacy offer any specialized services, such as diabetes education?

You should select your pharmacist and pharmacy as carefully as you select your physician, and stay with the same pharmacy so that all of your medication records are in the same place. This will help to ensure that your records are accurate and up-to-date and will allow you to develop a beneficial relationship with your pharmacist.

### Your physician

One of the most important health care decisions that you will make is your choice of a personal physician. The physician is central to your health care team, and is responsible for helping you maintain your overall health. In addition to detecting and treating ailments or adverse conditions, your physician and his or her coworkers should also serve as primary sources of health care information. Because the physician plays such an important role in your overall health care, it is important that you understand the full range of the physician's role as health care and information provider.

In providing any type of treatment or counseling, your physician should base his or her decisions upon an extensive knowledge of your current condition and past medical history. A complete medical history should include the information that is listed in the "Medical history checklist" section above. Your physician should keep accurate and comprehensive medical records containing this information. Because your treatment (and your health) is dependent upon a full disclosure of your medical history, as well as any factors that may currently be affecting your health (i.e., stress, smoking, drug use, etc.), it is important that you inform your physician as fully as possible, even if you might not consider this information important.

It is important that you inform your personal physician of any other physicians (such as specialists or subspecialists), dentists, or other health care professionals that you are seeing. You should also inform your physician of the pharmacy that you use or intend to use, so that he or she can contact the pharmacist if necessary.

In treating any health problem, your physician should make every effort to help you understand completely the nature of the problem and its treatment. He or she should take the time to explain the problem, why it may have occurred, and what preventive measures (if any) can be taken to avoid it in the future. Your physician should explain fully the reasons for any prescribed treatment. He or she should also be willing to discuss alternative therapies, especially if you are uncomfortable with the one that has been prescribed. Your physician should always be willing to answer all of your questions to your satisfaction.

In selecting a physician, you should look for one who will provide a full range of services. Asking for a full medical history and providing complete information about your treatment and medications are some of these services. There are several other issues that you may want to consider. Does your physician:

- Consult peers with specialty training for difficult problems?
- Inquire about your general health as well as specific problems?
- Have a good working relationship with your pharmacist? With the nurses and staff at his/her office?
- Periodically have you bring in bottles or labels from all of the medications (prescription and nonprescription) that you are taking or have at home?
- Periodically check the status of your vaccinations?

You may also want to consider your physician's medical credentials. Your local medical society should be able to provide specific facts about your physician's training, experience, and membership in professional societies.

One of the most important issues in contemporary health care is that of cost and payment. Your physician should be sensitive to the costs of your treatment and the manner in which you intend to pay for this and related medications. If you belong to an HMO or third-party payment plan, be sure that your physician is aware of your involvement in the plan. You should also be aware of the different types of payment that are accepted at the physician's office.

In prescribing medications, your physician should take into account the manner in which you intend to pay for your drugs, and should be aware of any specific concerns regarding the costs of your treatment and medication. He or she should also explain why brand or generic medication may be preferable in certain situations.

In selecting a physician, there are also several practical issues and matters of convenience that you should consider, such as:

- Is the office convenient to your home or work?
- What are the office hours?
- Is your physician or his/her associates or partners available (twenty-four hours) by phone? In emergencies, will you be able to contact a physician?
- Are you able to arrange appointments to fit your schedule? What is the office policy on cancellations?
- Is the physician well regarded in the community? Does he or she have a reputation for listening to patients and answering questions?
- Does the physician have admitting privileges at a hospital of your preference?
- Does he/she participate in your health plan?

In addition to the considerations already mentioned, your physician should be sensitive to the special concerns of treating the elderly. Older patients can present disease processes differently from younger adults, can react differently to certain drugs and dosages, and may have preexisting conditions that require special treatments to be prescribed.

There are also several special issues to consider in your selection of a pediatrician or family physician. If your child is not old enough to understand all instructions and information, it is important that your child's physician explain to you any information pertaining to the nature of a problem and all instructions for medications. When your child is of school age, the physician should speak directly to the child as well, asking and answering questions, and providing information about cause and prevention of medical problems and the use of medications. He or she should choose a dosage form and dose that is appropriate for your child's age and explain what to do if your child has certain symptoms, such as fever, vomiting, etc. (including the amount and type of medicine to give, if any, and when to call him or her for advice).

Your physician should be a primary source of information about your health and any medications that you are taking. In providing treatment for medical problems or conditions, the physician should base decisions upon a full medical history and be willing to answer any questions that you have regarding your health, treatment, and medications.

## Managing Your Medicines

To get the full benefit and reduce risks in taking your prescribed medicines, it is important to take the right medicine and dose at correct time intervals for the length of time prescribed. Bad effects can result from taking too much or too little of a medicine, or taking it too often or not often enough.

### Establishing a system

Whether you are taking one or several medicines, you should develop a system for taking them. It can be just as difficult to remember whether you took your once-a-day medicine as it can be to keep track of a number of medicines that need to be taken several times a day. Many medicines also have special instructions that can further complicate proper use.

Establish a way of knowing whether you took your medicines properly, then make that a part of your daily routine. If you take 1 or 2 medicines a day, you may only need to take them at the same time that you perform some other regular task, such as brushing your teeth or getting dressed.

For most people, a check-off record can also be a handy way of managing multiple medicines. Keep your medicine record in a handy, visible place next to where you take your medicines. Check off each dose as you take it. If you miss a dose, make a note about what happened and what you did on the back of the record or the bottom of the sheet.

Be sure to note any unwanted effects or anything unusual that you think may be connected with your medicines. Also note if a medicine does not do what you expect. Remember that some medicines take a while before they start having a noticeable effect.

If you keep a check-off record faithfully, you will know for sure whether or not you took your medicine. You will also have a complete record for your health care professionals to review when you visit them again. This information can help them determine if the medicine is working properly or causing unwanted side effects, or whether adjustments should be made in your medicines and/or doses.

If your medicines or the instructions for taking them are changed, correct your record or make a new one. Keep the old record until you are sure you or your health care professionals no longer need that information.

You might want to color code your medicine containers to help tell them apart. If you are having trouble reading labels or if you are color-blind, codes that can be recognized by touch (rubber bands, a cotton ball, or a piece of emery board, for instance) can be attached to the container. If you code your medicines, be sure these identifications are included on any medicine record you use. If necessary, ask your pharmacist to type medicine labels in large letters for easier reading.

A check-off list is not the only method to record medicine use. If this system does not work for you, ask your health care professional to help you develop an alternative. Be sure he or she knows all the medicines prescribed for you and any nonprescription medicines you take regularly, the hours you usually eat your meals, and any special diet you are following.

### Informed management

Your medicines have been prescribed for you and your condition. Ask your health care professional what benefits to expect, what side effects may occur, and when to report any side effects. If your symptoms go away, do not decide you are well and stop taking your medicine. If you stop too soon, the symptoms may come back. Finish all of the medicine if you have been told to do so. However, if you develop diarrhea or other unpleasant side effects, do not continue with the medicine just because you were told to finish it. Call your health care professional and report these effects. A change in dose or in the kind of medicine you are taking may be necessary.

When you are given a prescription for a medicine, ask the person who wrote it to explain it to you. For example, does "four times a day" mean one in the morning, one at noon, one in the evening, and one at bedtime; or does it mean every six hours around the clock? When a prescription says "take as needed," ask how close together the doses can be taken and what the maximum number of doses you can take in one day should be. Does "take with liquids" mean with water, milk, or something else? Are there some liquids that should avoided? What does "take with food" mean? At every meal time (some people must eat six meals a day), or with a snack? Do not trust your memory—have the instructions written down. To follow the instructions for taking your medicines, you must understand exactly what the prescriber wants you to do in order to "take as directed."

When the pharmacist dispenses your medicine, you have another opportunity to clarify information or to ask other questions. Before you leave, check the label on your medicine to be sure it matches the prescription and your understanding of what you are to do. If it does not, ask more questions.

The key to getting the most from your prescribed treatments is following instructions accurately and intelligently. If you have questions or doubts about the prescribed treatment, do not decide not to take the medicine or fail to follow the prescribed regimen. Discuss your questions and doubts with your health care professional.

The time and effort put into setting up a system to manage your medicines and establish a routine for taking them will pay off by relieving anxiety and helping you get the most from your prescribed treatment.

## Taking Your Medicine

To take medicines safely and get the greatest benefit from them, it is important to establish regular habits so that you are less likely to make mistakes.

Before taking any medicine, read the label and any accompanying information. You can also consult books to learn more about the medicine. If you have unanswered questions, check with your health care professional.

The label on the container of a prescription medicine should bear your first and last name; the name of the prescriber; the pharmacy address and telephone number; the prescription number; the date of dispensing; and directions for use. Some states or provinces may have additional requirements. If the name of the drug product is not on the label, ask the pharmacist to include the brand (if any) and generic names. An expiration date may also appear. All of this information is important in identifying your medicines and using them properly. The labels on containers should never be removed and all medicines should be kept in their original containers.

Some tips for taking medicines safely and accurately include the following:

- Read the label of each medicine container three times:
  —before you remove it from its storage place,
  —before you take the lid off the container to remove the dose, and
  —before you replace the container in its storage place.
- Never take medicines in the dark, even if you think you know exactly where to find them.
- Use standard measuring devices to take your medicines (the household teaspoon, cup, or glass vary widely in the amount they hold). Ask your pharmacist for help with measuring.
- Set bottles and boxes of medicines on a clear area, well back from the edge of the surface to prevent containers and/or caps from being knocked to the floor.
- When pouring liquid medicines, pick up the container with the label against the palm of your hand to protect it from being stained by dripping medicine.
- Wipe off the top and neck of bottles of liquid medicines to keep labels from being obscured, and to make it less likely that the lid will stick.
- Shake all liquid suspensions of drug products before pouring so that ingredients are mixed thoroughly.
- If you are to take medicine with water, take a full, 8 ounce glassful, not just enough to get it down. Too little liquid with some medicines can prevent the medicine from working properly, and can cause throat irritation if the medicine does not get completely to the stomach.
- To avoid accidental confusion of lids, labels, and medicines, replace the lid on one container before opening another.
- When you are interrupted while taking your medicine, take the container with you or put the medicine up out of the reach of small children. It only takes a second for them to take an overdose. When you return, check the label of the medicine to be sure you have the right one before taking it.
- Only crush tablets or open capsules to take with food or beverages if your health care professional has told you that this will not affect the way the medicine works. If you have difficulty swallowing a tablet or capsule, check with your health care professional about the availability of a different dosage form.
- Follow any diet instructions or other treatment measures prescribed by your health care professional.
- If at any point you realize you have taken the wrong medicine or the wrong amount, call your health care

professional immediately. In an emergency, call your local emergency number.

When you have finished taking your medicines, mark it down immediately on your medication calendar to avoid "double dosing." Also, make notes of any unusual changes in your body: change in weight, color or amount of urine, perspiration, or sputum; your pulse, temperature, or any other items you may have been instructed to observe for your condition or your medicine.

Try to take your medicines on time, but a half hour early or late will usually not upset your schedule. If you are more than several hours late and are getting close to your next scheduled dose, check any instructions that were given to you by your health care professional. If you did not receive instructions for what to do about a missed dose, check with your health care professional. You may also find missed dose information in the entries included in this book.

When your medicines are being managed by someone else (for example, when you are a patient in a hospital or nursing home), question what is happening to you and communicate what you know about your previous drug therapy or any other treatments. If you know you always take 1, not 2, of a certain tablet, say so and ask that your record be checked before you take the medicine. If you think you are receiving the wrong treatment or medication, do not hesitate to say so. You should always remain involved in your own therapy.

Many hospitals and nursing homes now offer counseling in medicine management as part of their discharge planning for patients. If you or a family member are getting ready to come home, ask your health care professional if you can be part of such instruction.

## The "Expiration Date" on Medicine Labels

To assure that a drug product meets applicable standards of identity, strength, quality, and purity at the time of use, an "expiration date" is added by the manufacturer to the label of most prescription and nonprescription drug products.

The expiration date on a drug product is valid only as long as the product is stored in the original, unopened container under the storage conditions specified by the manufacturer. Among other things, drugs can be affected by humidity, temperature, light, and even air. A medicine taken after the expiration date may have changed in potency or may have formed harmful material as it deteriorates. In other instances, contamination with germs may have occurred. The safest rule is not to use any medicine beyond the expiration date.

### Preventing deterioration

A drug begins to deteriorate the minute it is made. This rate of deterioration is factored in by the manufacturer in calculating the expiration date. Keeping the drug product in the container supplied by the pharmacist helps slow down deterioration. Storing the drug in the prescribed manner—for example, in a light-resistant container or in a cool, dry place (not the bathroom medicine cabinet)—also helps. The need for medicines to be kept in their containers and stored properly cannot be overstressed.

Patients sometimes ask their health care professionals to prescribe a large quantity of a particular medicine in order to "economize." Although this may be all right in some cases, this practice may backfire. If you have a large supply of your medicine and it deteriorates before you can use it all, or if your doctor changes your medicine, you may lose out.

Sometimes deterioration can be recognized by physical changes in the drug, such as a change in odor or appearance. For example, aspirin tablets develop a vinegar odor when they break down. These changes are not true of all drugs, however, and the absence of physical changes should not be assumed to mean that no deterioration has occurred.

Some liquid medicines mixed at the pharmacy will have a "beyond use" date on the label. This is an expiration date that is calculated from the date of preparation in the pharmacy. This is a definite date, after which you should discard any of the medicine that remains.

If your prescription medicines do not bear an "expiration" or "beyond use" date, your dispensing pharmacist is the best person to advise you about how long they can be safely utilized.

# ABOUT THE MEDICINES YOU ARE TAKING

## New Drugs—From Idea to Marketplace

To be sold legitimately in the United States, new drugs must pass through a rigorous system of approval specified in the Food, Drug, and Cosmetic Act and supervised by the Food and Drug Administration (FDA). Except for certain drugs subject to other regulatory provisions, no new drug for human use may be marketed in this country unless FDA has approved a "New Drug Application" (NDA) for it.

### The idea

The creation of a new drug usually starts with an idea. Most likely that idea results from the study of a disease or group of symptoms. Ideas can also come from observations of clinical research. This may involve many years of study, or the idea may occur from an accidental discovery in a research laboratory. Some may be coincidental discoveries, as in the case of penicillin.

Idea development takes place most often in the laboratory of a pharmaceutical company, but may also happen in laboratories at research institutions like the National Institutes of Health, at medical centers and universities, or in the laboratory of a chemical company.

### Animal testing

The idea for a new drug is first tested on animals to help determine how toxic the substance may be. Most drugs interfere in some way with normal body functions. These animal studies are designed to discover the degree of that interference and the extent of the toxic effects.

After successful animal testing, perhaps over several years, the sponsors of the new drug apply to the FDA for an Investigational New Drug (IND) application. This status allows the drug to be tested in humans. As part of their request, the sponsoring manufacturer must submit the results of the animal studies, plus a detailed outline of the proposed human testing and information about the researchers that will be involved.

### Human testing

Drug testing in humans usually consists of three consecutive phases. "Informed consent" must be secured from all volunteers participating in this testing.

Phase I testing is most often done on young, healthy adults. This testing is done on a relatively small number of subjects, generally between 20 and 80. Its purpose is to learn more about the biochemistry of the drug: how it acts on the body, and how the body reacts to it. The procedure differs for some drugs, however. For example, Phase I testing of drugs used to treat cancer involves actual patients with the disease from the beginning of testing.

During Phase II, small controlled clinical studies are designed to test the effectiveness and relative safety of the drug. These are done on closely monitored patients who have the disease for which the drug is being tested. Their numbers seldom go beyond 100 to 200 patients. Some volunteers for Phase II testing who have severely complicating conditions may be excluded.

A "control" group of people of comparable physical and disease types is used to do double-blind, controlled experiments for most drugs. These are conducted by medical investigators thoroughly familiar with the disease and this type of research. In a double-blind experiment, the patient, the health care provider, and other personnel do not know whether the patient is receiving the drug being tested, another active drug, or no medicine at all (a placebo or "sugar pill"). This helps eliminate bias and assures the accuracy of results. The findings of these tests are statistically analyzed to determine whether they are "significant" or due to chance alone.

Phase III consists of larger studies. This testing is performed after effectiveness of the drug has been established and is intended to gather additional evidence of effectiveness for specific uses of the drug. These studies also help discover adverse drug reactions that may occur with the drug. Phase III studies involve a few hundred to several thousand patients who have the disease the drug is intended to treat.

Patients with additional diseases or those receiving other therapy may be included in later Phase II and Phase III studies. They would be expected to be representative of certain segments of the population who would receive the drug following approval for marketing.

### Final approval

When a sponsor believes the investigational studies on a drug have shown it to be safe and effective in treating specific conditions, a New Drug Application (NDA) is submitted to FDA. This application is accompanied by all the documentation from the company's research, including complete records of all the animal and human testing. This documentation can run to many thousands of pages.

The NDA application and its documentation must then be reviewed by FDA physicians, pharmacologists, chemists, statisticians, and other professionals experienced in evaluating new drugs. Proposed labeling information for the physician and pharmacist is also screened for accuracy, completeness, and conformity to FDA-approved wording.

Regulations call for the FDA to review an NDA within 180 days. This period may be extended and actually takes an average of 2 to 3 years. When all research phases are considered, the actual time it takes from idea to marketplace may be 8 to 10 years or even longer. However, for drugs representing major therapeutic advances, FDA may "fast-track" the approval process to try to get those drugs to patients who need them as soon as possible.

### After approval

After a drug is marketed, the manufacturer must inform the FDA of any unexpected side effects or toxicity that comes to its attention. Consumers and health care professionals have an important role in helping to identify any previously unreported effects. If new evidence indicates that the drug may present an "imminent hazard," the FDA can withdraw approval for marketing or add new information to the drug's labeling at any time.

## Generic drugs

After a new drug is approved for marketing, a patent will generally protect the financial interests of the drug's developer for a number of years. The traditional protection period is for 17 years. In reality, however, the period is much less due to the extended period of time needed to gain approval before marketing can begin. Recognizing that a considerable part of a drug's patent life may be tied up in the approval process, in 1984 Congress passed a law providing patent extension for drugs whose commercial sale may have been unduly delayed by the approval process.

Any manufacturer can apply for permission to produce and market a drug after the patent for the drug has expired. Following a procedure called an Abbreviated New Drug Application (ANDA), the applicant must show that its product is bioequivalent to the originator's product. Although the extensive clinical testing the originator had to complete during the drug's development does not have to be repeated, comparative testing between the products must be done to ensure that they will be therapeutically equivalent.

## Drug Names

Every drug must have a nonproprietary name; a name that is available for each manufacturer to use. These names are commonly called generic names.

The FDA requires that the generic name of a drug product be placed on its labeling. However, manufacturers often coin brand (trade) names to use in promoting their products. In general, brand names are shorter, catchier, and easier to use than the corresponding generic name. The brand name manufacturer will then emphasize its brand name (which cannot be used by anyone else) in its advertising and other promotions. In many instances, the consumer may not recognize that a drug being sold under one particular brand name is indeed available under other brand names or by generic name. Ask your pharmacist if you have any questions about the names of your medicines.

## Drug Quality

After an NDA or an ANDA has been approved for a product, the manufacturer must then meet all requirements relating to production. These include current Good Manufacturing Practice regulations of the Food and Drug Administration (FDA) and any applicable standards relating to strength, quality, purity, packaging, and labeling that are established by the *United States Pharmacopeia* (USP).

Simply placing a brand name on a label does not assure the quality of the product inside the container. Rather, the quality of a product depends on the manufacturer's ability to create a value product consistently from batch to batch.

Routine product testing by the manufacturer is required by the Good Manufacturing Practice regulations of the FDA (the FDA itself does not routinely test all products, except in cases where there is a suspicion that something might be wrong). In addition to governmental requirements, drug products must meet public standards of strength, quality, and purity that are published in the USP. In order to market their products, all manufacturers in the United States must meet USP-established standards unless they specifically choose not to meet the standards for a particular product. In this case, that product's label must state that it is "not USP" and how it differs from USP standards (this occurs very rarely).

## Differences in Drug Products

Although standards to ensure strength, quality, purity, and bioequivalence exist for drug products, the standards allow for variations in certain factors that may produce other differences from product to product. These product variations may be important to some patients, since not all patients are "equivalent." For example, the size, shape, and coating may vary and, therefore, be harder or easier for some patients to swallow; an oral liquid will taste good to some patients and awful to others; one manufacturer may use lactose as an inactive ingredient in its product while a therapeutically equivalent product may use some other inactive ingredient; one product may contain sugar or alcohol while another product may not.

In deciding to use one therapeutically equivalent product over another, consumers should keep the following in mind:

- Consider convenience factors of drug products (for example, ease of taking a particular dosage form).
- Don't overlook the convenience of the package. The package must protect the drug in accordance with USP requirements, but packages can be quite different in their ease of carrying, storing, opening, and measuring.
- If you have a known allergy or any type of dietary restriction, you need to be aware of the pharmaceutic or "inactive" ingredients that may be present in medicines you have to take. These inactive ingredients may vary from product to product.
- Price is always a consideration. The price difference between products (e.g., different brands, or brands versus generics) may be a major factor in the overall price of a prescription. Talk to your pharmacist about price considerations. Some states require that the pharmacist dispense exactly what is prescribed. However, other states allow the pharmacist to dispense less expensive medicines when appropriate.

Aside from differences in the drug product, there are many other factors that may influence the effectiveness of a medicine. For example, your diet, body chemistry, medical conditions, or other drugs you are taking may affect how much of a dose of a particular medicine gets into the body.

For the majority of drugs, slight differences in the amount of drug made available to the body will not make any therapeutic difference. For other drugs, the precise amount that gets into the body is more critical. For example, some heart or epilepsy medicines may create problems for the patient if the dose delivered to the body varies for some reason.

For those drugs that fall in the critical category, it is a good idea to stay on the specific product you started on. Changes should only be made after consultation with the health care professional who prescribed the medicine for you. If you feel that a certain batch of your medicine is more potent or does not work as well as other batches, or if you have other questions, check with your health care professional.

# Appendix II

## USP PEOPLE 1990–1995

### OFFICERS

**Mark Novitch, M.D.,** *President*, Washington, DC
**Donald R. Bennett, M.D., Ph.D.,** *Vice-President*, Chicago, IL
**John T. Fay, Jr., Ph.D.,** *Treasurer*, San Clemente, CA
**Arthur Hull Hayes, Jr., M.D.,** *Past President*, New Rochelle, NY
**Jerome A. Halperin,** *Secretary*, Rockville, MD

### BOARD OF TRUSTEES

**James T. Doluisio, Ph.D.**[1], *Chair*, Austin, TX
**Donald R. Bennett, M.D., Ph.D.,** *ex officio*, Chicago, IL
**John V. Bergen, Ph.D.**[2], *Vice Chair*, Villanova, PA
**Edwin D. Bransome, Jr., M.D.**[3], Augusta, GA
**Jordan L. Cohen, Ph.D.**[1], Lexington, KY
**J. Richard Crout, M.D.**[3], Rockville, MD
**John T. Fay, Jr., Ph.D.,** *ex officio*, San Clemente, CA
**Arthur Hull Hayes, Jr., M.D.,** *ex officio*, New Rochelle, NY
**Joseph A. Mollica, Ph.D.**[2], Wilmington, DE
**Grace Powers Monaco, J.D.**[4], Washington, DC
**Mark Novitch, M.D.,** *ex officio*, Washington, DC

### GENERAL COMMITTEE OF REVISION

**Jerome A. Halperin**[5], *Executive Director, USPC, Chairman*
**Lee T. Grady, Ph.D.**[5], *Director, Drug Standards Division*
**Keith W. Johnson**[5], *Director, Drug Information Division*
**Loyd V. Allen, Jr., Ph.D.,** Oklahoma City, OK
**Jerry R. Allison, Ph.D.,** New Brunswick, NJ
**Thomas J. Ambrosio, Ph.D.,** Somerville, NJ
**Gregory E. Amidon, Ph.D.,** Kalamazoo, MI
**Norman W. Atwater, Ph.D.,** Hopewell, NJ
**Henry L. Avallone, B.Sc.,** North Brunswick, NJ
**Leonard C. Bailey, Ph.D.,** Piscataway, NJ
**John A. Belis, M.D.,** Hershey, PA
**Leslie Z. Benet, Ph.D.,** San Francisco, CA
**Judy P. Boehlert, Ph.D.,** Nutley, NJ
**James C. Boylan, Ph.D.,** Abbott Park, IL
**Lynn R. Brady, Ph.D.**[6], (1990–1992), Seattle, WA
**R. Edward Branson, Ph.D.,** Beltsville, MD
**William H. Briner, Capt., B.S.,** Durham, NC
**Stephen R. Byrn, Ph.D.,** West Lafayette, IN
**Peter R. Byron, Ph.D.,** Richmond, VA
**Herbert S. Carlin, D.Sc.,** Florham Park, NJ
**Dennis L. Casey, Ph.D.,** Raritan, NJ
**Lester Chafetz, Ph.D.,** Kansas City, MO
**Virginia C. Chamberlain, Ph.D.,** Rockville, MD
**Wei-Wei, Chang, Ph.D.,** (1992–), Morris Plains, NJ
**Mary Beth Chenault, B.S.,** Harrisonburg, VA

[1]Representing pharmacy.
[2]At large.
[3]Representing medicine.
[4]Public member.
[5]12601 Twinbrook Parkway, Rockville, MD 20852.
[6]Deceased.

**Zak T. Chowhan, Ph.D.,** Palo Alto, CA
**Sebastian G. Ciancio, D.D.S.,** Buffalo, NY
**Murray S. Cooper, Ph.D.,** Islamorada, FL
**Lloyd E. Davis, Ph.D., D.V.M.,** Urbana, IL
**Leon Ellenbogen, Ph.D.,** Clifton, NJ
**R. Michael Enzinger, Ph.D.,** (1990–1992), Kalamazoo, MI
**Clyde R. Erskine, B.S., M.B.A.,** Newtown Square, PA
**Edward A. Fitzgerald, Ph.D.,** Bethesda, MD
**Everett Flanigan, Ph.D.,** Kankakee, IL
**Klaus G. Florey, Ph.D.,** Princeton, NJ
**Thomas S. Foster, Pharm.D.,** Lexington, KY
**Joseph F. Gallelli, Ph.D.,** Bethesda, MD
**Robert L. Garnick, Ph.D.,** So. San Francisco, CA
**Douglas D. Glover, M.D., R.Ph.,** Morgantown, WV
**Alan M. Goldberg, Ph.D.,** Baltimore, MD
**Burton J. Goldstein, M.D.,** Williams Island, FL
**Dennis K. J. Gorecki, Ph.D.,** Saskatoon, Saskatchewan, Canada
**Michael J. Groves, Ph.D.,** Lake Forest, IL
**Robert M. Guthrie, M.D.,** Columbus, OH
**Samir A. Hanna, Ph.D.,** Lawrenceville, NJ
**Stanley L. Hem, Ph.D.,** West Lafayette, IN
**Joy Hochstadt, Ph.D.,** New York, NY
**David W. Hughes, Ph.D.,** (1990–1993), Nepean, Ontario, Canada
**Norman C. Jamieson, Ph.D.,** St. Louis, MO
**Richard D. Johnson, Pharm.D., Ph.D.,** Kansas City, MO
**Judith K. Jones, M.D., Ph.D.,** Arlington, VA
**Stanley A. Kaplan, Ph.D.,** Baltimore, MD
**Herbert E. Kaufman, M.D.,** New Orleans, LA
**Donald Kaye, M.D.,** Philadelphia, PA
**Paul E. Kennedy, Ph.D.,** West Conshohocken, PA
**Jay S. Keystone, M.D.,** Toronto, Ontario, Canada
**Rosalyn C. King, Pharm.D., M.P.H.,** Silver Spring, MD
**Gordon L. Klein, M.D.** Galveston, TX
**Joseph E. Knapp, Ph.D.,** Pittsburgh, PA
**John B. Landis, Ph.D.,** (1990–1992), Kalamazoo, MI
**Thomas P. Layloff, Ph.D.,** St. Louis, MO
**Lewis J. Leeson, Ph.D.,** Summit, NJ
**John W. Levchuk, Ph.D.,** Rockville, MD
**Robert D. Lindeman, M.D.,** Albuquerque, NM
**Charles H. Lochmüller, Ph.D.,** Durham, NC
**Edward G. Lovering, Ph.D.,** Nepean, Ontario, Canada
**Catherine M. MacLeod, M.D.,** Chicago, IL
**Carol S. Marcus, Ph.D., M.D.,** Torrance, CA
**Tibor I. Matula, Ph.D.,** (1993–), Ottawa, Ontario, Canada
**Thomas Medwick, Ph.D.,** Piscataway, NJ
**Robert F. Morrissey, Ph.D.,** New Brunswick, NJ
**Terry E. Munson, B.S.,** Fairfax, VA
**Harold S. Nelson, M.D.,** Denver, CO
**Wendel L. Nelson, Ph.D.,** Seattle, WA
**Maria I. New, M.D.,** New York, NY
**Sharon C. Northup, Ph.D.,** Round Lake, IL
**Jeffery L. Otto, Ph.D.,** (1992–), Broomfield, CO
**Garnet E. Peck, Ph.D.,** West Lafayette, IN
**Robert V. Petersen, Ph.D.,** Salt Lake City, UT

Rosemary C. Polomano, R.N., M.S.N., Philadelphia, PA
Thomas P. Reinders, Pharm.D., Richmond, VA
Christopher T. Rhodes, Ph.D., West Kingston, RI
Joseph R. Robinson, Ph.D., Madison, WI
Lary A. Robinson, M.D., Tampa, FL
David B. Roll, Ph.D., Salt Lake City, UT
Theodore J. Roseman, Ph.D., Round Lake, IL
Sanford H. Roth, M.D., Phoenix, AZ
Leonard P. Rybak, M.D., Springfield, IL
Ronald J. Sawchuk, Ph.D., Minneapolis, MN
Gordon D. Schiff, M.D., Chicago, IL
Andrew J. Schmitz, Jr., M.S.[6], (1990–1992), Huntington, NY
Ralph F. Shangraw, Ph.D., Baltimore, MD
Albert L. Sheffer, M.D., Boston, MA
Eli Shefter, Ph.D., San Diego, CA
Eric B. Sheinin, Ph.D., Rockville, MD
Robert L. Siegle, M.D., San Antonio, TX
Edward B. Silberstein, M.D., Cincinnati, OH
Joseph E. Sinsheimer, Ph.D., Ann Arbor, MI
Marilyn Dix Smith, Ph.D., Dayton, NJ
Burton E. Sobel, M.D., St. Louis, MO
E. John Staba, Ph.D., Minneapolis, MN
Robert S. Stern, M.D., Boston, MA
James T. Stewart, Ph.D., Athens, GA
Henry S. I. Tan, Ph.D., Cincinnati, OH
Theodore G. Tong, Pharm.D., Tucson, AZ
Salvatore J. Turco, Pharm.D., Philadelphia, PA
Clarence T. Ueda, Pharm.D., Ph.D., Omaha, NE
Elizabeth B. Vadas, Ph.D., Pointe Claire-Dorval, Quebec, Canada
Huib J. M. van de Donk, Ph.D., Bilthoven, The Netherlands
Stanley van den Noort, M.D., Irvine, CA
Vincent S. Venturella, Ph.D., Murray Hill, NJ
Robert E. Vestal, M.D., Boise, ID
James A. Visconti, Ph.D., Columbus, OH
Edward W. Voss, Jr., Ph.D., Urbana, IL
Philip D. Walson, M.D., Columbus, OH
Paul F. White, Ph.D., M.D., Dallas, TX
Robert G. Wolfangel, Ph.D., St. Louis, MO
Manfred E. Wolff, Ph.D., San Diego, CA
Wesley E. Workman, Ph.D., (1992–), St. Louis, MO
Linda R. Wuhl, Ph.D., (1993–), Thousand Oaks, CA
John W. Yarbro, M.D., Springfield, IL
George Zografi, Ph.D., Madison, WI

## EXECUTIVE COMMITTEE OF REVISION (1993–1994)

Jerome A. Halperin, *Chair*

Norman W. Atwater, Ph.D.
Clyde R. Erskine, B.S., M.B.A.
Burton J. Goldstein, M.D.
Robert V. Petersen, Ph.D.
Robert S. Stern, M.D.
Paul F. White, Ph.D., M.D.

## DRUG INFORMATION DIVISION EXECUTIVE COMMITTEE (1993–1994)

Herbert S. Carlin, D.Sc., *Chair*

James C. Boylan, Ph.D.
Sebastian G. Ciancio, D.D.S.
Lloyd E. Davis, D.V.M., Ph.D.
Jay S. Keystone, M.D.
Robert D. Lindeman, M.D.
Maria I. New, M.D.
Rosemary C. Polomano, R.N., M.S.N.
Thomas P. Reinders, Pharm.D.
Gordon D. Schiff, M.D.
Albert L. Sheffer, M.D.
Theodore G. Tong, Pharm.D.
Robert E. Vestal, M.D.
John W. Yarbro, M.D., Ph.D.

## DRUG STANDARDS DIVISION EXECUTIVE COMMITTEE (1993–1994)

James T. Stewart, Ph.D. *Chair*

Jerry R. Allison, Ph.D.
Judy P. Boehlert, Ph.D.
Capt. William H. Briner, B.S.
Herbert S. Carlin, D.Sc.
Lester Chafetz, Ph.D.
Zak T. Chowhan, Ph.D.
Murray S. Cooper, Ph.D.
Klaus G. Florey, Ph.D.
Joseph F. Gallelli, Ph.D.
Robert L. Garnick, Ph.D.
Thomas P. Layloff, Ph.D.
Lewis J. Leeson, Ph.D.
Thomas Medwick, Ph.D.
Robert F. Morrissey, Ph.D.
Sharon C. Northup, Ph.D.
Ralph F. Shangraw, Ph.D.

## DRUG NOMENCLATURE COMMITTEE (1993–1994)

Herbert S. Carlin, D.Sc., *Chair*

William M. Heller, Ph.D., *Consultant/Advisor*
Lester Chafetz, Ph.D.
Lloyd E. Davis, D.V.M., Ph.D.
Everett Flanigan, Ph.D.
Douglas D. Glover, M.D.
Richard D. Johnson, Pharm.D., Ph.D.
Edward G. Lovering, Ph.D.
Rosemary C. Polomano, R.N., M.S.N.
Thomas P. Reinders, Pharm.D.
Eric B. Sheinin, Ph.D.
Philip D. Walson, M.D.

# DRUG INFORMATION DIVISION ADVISORY PANELS

Members who serve as Chairs are listed first.

The information presented in this text represents an ongoing review of the drugs contained herein and represents a consensus of various viewpoints expressed. The individuals listed below have served on the USP Advisory Panels for the 1993–1994 revision period and have contributed to the development of the 1995 USP DI database. Such listing does not imply that these individuals have reviewed all of the material in this text or that they individually agree with all statements contained herein.

## Anesthesiology

Paul F. White, Ph.D., M.D., *Chair*, Dallas, TX; David R. Bevan, M.B., FFARCS, MRCP, Vancouver, British Columbia; Eugene Y. Cheng, M.D., Milwaukee, WI; Charles J. Coté, M.D., Chicago, IL; Robert Feinstein, M.D., St. Louis, MO; Peter S.A. Glass, M.D., Durham, NC; Michael B. Howie, M.D., Columbus, OH; Beverly A. Krause, C.R.N.A., M.S., St. Louis, MO; Carl Lynch, III, M.D., Ph.D., Charlottesville, VA; Carl Rosow, M.D., Ph.D., Boston, MA; Peter S. Sebel, M.B., Ph.D., Atlanta, GA; Walter L. Way, M.D., Greenbrae, CA; Matthew B. Weinger, M.D., San Diego, CA; Richard Weiskopf, M.D., San Francisco, CA; David H. Wong, Pharm.D., M.D., Long Beach, CA

## Cardiovascular and Renal Drugs

Burton E. Sobel, M.D., *Chair*, St. Louis, MO; William P. Baker, M.D., Ph.D., Bethesda, MD; Nils U. Bang, M.D., Indianapolis, IN; Emmanuel L. Bravo, M.D., Cleveland, OH; Mary Jo Burgess, M.D., Salt Lake City, UT; James H. Chesebro, M.D., Boston, MA; Peter Corr, Ph.D., St. Louis, MO; Dwain L. Eckberg, M.D., Richmond, VA; Ruth Eshleman, Ph.D., W. Kingston, RI; William H. Frishman, M.D., Bronx, NY; Edward D. Frohlich, M.D., New Orleans, LA; Martha Hill, Ph.D., R.N., Baltimore, MD; Norman M. Kaplan, M.D., Dallas, TX; Michael Lesch, M.D., Detroit, MI; Manuel Martinez-Maldonado, M.D., Decatur, GA; Patrick A. McKee, M.D., Oklahoma City, OK; Dan M. Roden, M.D., Nashville, TN; Michael R. Rosen, M.D., New York, NY; Jane Schultz, R.N., B.S.N., Rochester, MN; Robert L. Talbert, Pharm.D., San Antonio, TX; Raymond L. Woosley, M.D., Ph.D., Washington, DC

## Clinical Immunology/Allergy/Rheumatology

Albert L. Sheffer, M.D., *Chair*, Boston, MA; John A. Anderson, M.D., Detroit, MI; Emil Bardana, Jr., M.D., Portland, OR; John Baum, M.D., Rochester, NY; Debra Danoff, M.D., Montreal, Quebec; Daniel G. de Jesus, M.D., Ph.D., Vanier, Ontario; Elliott F. Ellis, M.D., Jacksonville, FL; Patricia A. Fraser, M.D., Boston, MA; Frederick E. Hargreave, M.D., Hamilton, Ontario; Evelyn V. Hess, M.D., Cincinnati, OH; Jean M. Jackson, M.D., Boston, MA; Stephen R. Kaplan, M.D., Buffalo, NY; Sandra M. Koehler, Milwaukee, WI; Richard A. Moscicki, M.D., Newton, MA; Shirley Murphy, M.D., Albuquerque, NM; Gary S. Rachelefsky, M.D., Los Angeles, CA; Robert E. Reisman, M.D., Buffalo, NY; Robert L. Rubin, Ph.D., La Jolla, CA; Daniel J. Stechschulte, M.D., Kansas City, KS; Virginia S. Taggert, Bethesda, MD; Joseph A. Tami, Pharm.D., San Antonio, TX; John H. Toogood, M.D., London, Ontario; Martin D. Valentine, M.D., Baltimore, MD; Michael Weinblatt, M.D., Boston, MA; Dennis Michael Williams, Pharm.D., Chapel Hill, NC; Stewart Wong, Ph.D., Annandale, VA

## Clinical Toxicology/Substance Abuse

Theodore G. Tong, Pharm.D., *Chair*, Tucson, AZ; John Ambre, M.D., Ph.D., Chicago, IL; Usoa E. Busto, Pharm.D., Toronto, Ontario; Darryl Inaba, Pharm.D., San Francisco, CA; Edward P. Krenzelok, Pharm.D., Pittsburgh, PA; Michael Montagne, Ph.D., Boston, MA; Sven A. Normann, Pharm.D., Tampa, FL; Gary M. Oderda, Pharm.D., Salt Lake City, UT; Paul Pentel, M.D., Minneapolis, MN; Rose Ann Soloway, R.N., Washington, DC; Daniel A. Spyker, M.D., Ph.D., Rockville, MD; Anthony R. Temple, M.D., Ft. Washington, PA; Anthony Tommasello, Pharm.D., Baltimore, MD; Joseph C. Veltri, Pharm.D., Salt Lake City, UT; William A. Watson, Pharm.D., Kansas City, MO

## Consumer Interest/Health Education

Gordon D. Schiff, M.D., *Chair*, Chicago, IL; Michael J. Ackerman, Ph.D., Bethesda, MD; Barbara Aranda-Naranjo, R.N., San Antonio, TX; Frank J. Ascione, Pharm.D., Ph.D., Ann Arbor, MI; Judith I. Brown, Silver Spring, MD; Jose Camacho, Austin, TX; Margaret A. Charters, Ph.D., Syracuse, NY; Jennifer Cross, San Francisco, CA; William G. Harless, Ph.D., Bethesda, MD; Louis H. Kompare, Lake Buena Vista, FL; Margo Kroshus, R.N., B.S.N., Rochester, MN; Marilyn Lister, Wakefield, Quebec; Margaret Lueders, Seattle, WA; Frederick S. Mayer, R.Ph., M.P.H., Sausalito, CA; Nancy Milio, Ph.D., Chapel Hill, NC; Irving Rubin, Port Washington, NY; T. Donald Rucker, Ph.D., River Forest, IL; Stephen B. Soumerai, Sc.D., Boston, MA; Carol A. Vetter, Rockville, MD

## Critical Care Medicine

Catherine M. MacLeod, M.D., *Chair*, Chicago, IL; William Banner, Jr., M.D., Salt Lake City, UT; Philip S. Barie, M.D., New York, NY; Thomas P. Bleck, M.D., Charlottesville, VA; Roger C. Bone, M.D., Toledo, OH; Susan S. Fish, Pharm.D., Boston, MA; Edgar R. Gonzalez, Pharm.D., Richmond, VA; Robert Gottesman, Rockville, MD; John W. Hoyt, M.D., Pittsburgh, PA; Sheldon A. Magder, M.D., Montreal, Quebec; Joseph E. Parrillo, M.D., Chicago, IL; Sharon Peters, M.D., St. John's, Newfoundland; Domenic A. Sica, M.D., Richmond, VA; Martin G. Tweeddale, M.B., Ph.D., Vancouver, British Columbia

## Dentistry

Sebastian G. Ciancio, D.D.S., *Chair*, Buffalo, NY; Donald F. Adams, D.D.S., Portland, OR; Karen A. Baker, M.S. Pharm., Iowa City, IA; Stephen A. Cooper, D.M.D., Ph.D., Philadelphia, PA; Frederick A. Curro, D.M.D., Ph.D., Jersey City, NJ; Paul J. Desjardins, D.M.D., Ph.D., Newark, NJ; Tommy W. Gage, D.D.S., Ph.D., Dallas, TX; Stephen F. Goodman, D.D.S., New York, NY; Daniel A. Haas, D.D.S., Ph.D., Toronto, Ontario; Richard E. Hall, D.D.S., Ph.D., Buffalo,

NY; Lireka P. Joseph, Dr.P.H., Rockville, MD; Janice Lieberman, Fort Lee, NJ; Laurie Lisowski, Lewiston, NY; Clarence L. Trummel, D.D.S., Ph.D., Farmington, CT; Joel M. Weaver, II, D.D.S., Ph.D., Columbus, OH; Clifford W. Whall, Jr., Ph.D., Chicago, IL; Raymond P. White, Jr., D.D.S., Ph.D., Chapel Hill, NC; Ray C. Williams, D.M.D., Boston, MA

**Dermatology**
Robert S. Stern, M.D., *Chair*, Boston, MA; Beatrice B. Abrams, Ph.D., Somerville, NJ; Richard D. Baughman, M.D., Hanover, NH; Michael Bigby, M.D., Boston, MA; Janice T. Chussil, R.N., M.S.N., Portland, OR; Stuart Maddin, M.D., Vancouver, British Columbia; Milton Orkin, M.D., Robbinsdale, MN; Neil H. Shear, M.D., Toronto, Ontario; Edgar Benton Smith, M.D., Galveston, TX; Dennis P. West, M.S. Pharm., Lincolnshire, IL; Gail M. Zimmerman, Portland, OR

**Diagnostic Agents—Nonradioactive**
Robert L. Siegle, M.D., *Chair*, San Antonio, TX; Kaizer Aziz, Ph.D., Rockville, MD; Robert C. Brasch, M.D., San Francisco, CA; Nicholas Harry Malakis, M.D., Bethesda, MD; Robert F. Mattrey, M.D., San Diego, CA; James A. Nelson, M.D., Seattle, WA; Jovitas Skucas, M.D., Rochester, NY; Gerald L. Wolf, Ph.D., M.D., Charlestown, MA

**Drug Information Science**
James A. Visconti, Ph.D., *Chair*, Columbus, OH; Marie A. Abate, Pharm.D., Morgantown, WV; Ann B. Amerson, Pharm.D., Lexington, KY; Philip O. Anderson, Pharm.D., San Diego, CA; Danial E. Baker, Pharm.D., Spokane, WA; C. David Butler, Pharm.D., M.B.A., Naperville, IL; Linda L. Hart, Pharm.D., Saddle River, NJ; Edward J. Huth, M.D., Philadelphia, PA; John M. Kessler, Pharm.D., Chapel Hill, NC; R. David Lauper, Pharm.D., Emeryville, CA; Domingo R. Martinez, Pharm.D., Birmingham, AL; William F. McGhan, Pharm.D., Ph.D., Philadelphia, PA; John K. Murdoch, B.Sc.Phm., Toronto, Ontario; Kurt A. Proctor, Ph.D., Alexandria, VA; Arnauld F. Scafidi, M.D., M.P.H., Rockville, MD; John A. Scarlett, M.D., Austin, TX; Gary H. Smith, Pharm.D., Tucson, AZ; Dennis F. Thompson, Pharm.D., Oklahoma City, OK; William G. Troutman, Pharm.D., Albuquerque, NM; Lee A. Wanke, M.S., Houston, TX

**Drug Utilization Review**
Judith K. Jones, M.D., Ph.D., *Chair*, Arlington, VA; John F. Beary, III., M.D., Washington, DC; James L. Blackburn, Pharm.D., Saskatoon, Saskatchewan; Richard S. Blum, M.D., East Hills, NY; Amy Cooper-Outlaw, Pharm.D., Stone Mountain, GA; Joseph W. Cranston, Jr., Ph.D., Chicago, IL; W. Gary Erwin, Pharm.D., Philadelphia, PA; Jere E. Goyan, Ph.D., Saddle River, NJ; Duane M. Kirking, Ph.D., Ann Arbor, MI; Karen E. Koch, Pharm.D., Tupelo, MS; Aida A. LeRoy, Pharm.D., Arlington, VA; Jerome Levine, M.D., Baltimore, MD; Richard W. Lindsay, M.D., Charlottesville, VA; M. Laurie Mashford, M.D., Melbourne, Victoria, Australia; Deborah M. Nadzam, R.N., Ph.D., Oakbrook Terrace, IL; William Z. Potter, M.D., Ph.D., Bethesda, MD; Louise R. Rodriquez, M.S., Washington, DC; Stephen P. Spielberg, M.D., Ph.D., West Point, PA; Suzan M. Streichenwein, M.D., Houston, TX; Brian L. Strom, M.D., Philadelphia, PA; Michael Weintraub, M.D., Rockville, MD; Antonio Carlos Zanini, M.D., Ph.D., Sao Paulo, Brazil

**Endocrinology**
Maria I. New, M.D., *Chair*, New York, NY; Ronald D. Brown, M.D., Oklahoma City, OK; R. Keith Campbell, Pharm.D., Pullman, WA; David S. Cooper, M.D., Baltimore, MD; Betty J. Dong, Pharm.D., San Francisco, CA; Andrea Dunaif, M.D., New York, NY; Anke A. Ehrhardt, Ph.D., New York, NY; Nadir R. Farid, M.D., Durham, N.C.; John G. Haddad, Jr., M.D., Philadelphia, PA; Michael M. Kaplan, M.D., Southfield, MI; Harold E. Lebovitz, M.D., Brooklyn, NY; Marvin E. Levin, M.D., Chesterfield, MO; Marvin M. Lipman, M.D., Scarsdale, NY; Barbara J. Maschak-Carey, R.N., M.S.N., Philadelphia, PA; James C. Melby, M.D., Boston, MA; Walter J. Meyer, III., M.D., Galveston, TX; Rita Nemchik, R.N., M.S., C.D.E., Florence, NJ; Daniel A. Notterman, M.D., New York, NY; Ron Gershon Rosenfeld, M.D., Stanford, CA; Paul Saenger, M.D., Bronx, NY; Leonard Wartofsky, M.D., Washington, DC

**Family Practice**
Robert M. Guthrie, M.D., *Chair*, Columbus, OH; Jack A. Brose, D.O., Athens, OH; Jannet M. Carmichael, Pharm.D., Reno, NV; Jacqueline A. Chadwick, M.D., Scottsdale, AZ; Mark E. Clasen, M.D., Ph.D., Dayton, OH; Lloyd P. Haskell, M.D., West Borough, MA; Luis A. Izquierdo-Mora, M.D., Rio Piedras, PR; Edward L. Langston, M.D., Houston, TX; Stephen T. O'Brien, M.D., Enfield, CT; Charles D. Ponte, Pharm.D., Morgantown, WV; Jack M. Rosenberg, Pharm.D., Ph.D., Brooklyn, NY; John F. Sangster, M.D., London, Ontario; Theodore L. Yarboro, Sr., M.D., M.P.H., Sharon, PA

**Gastroenterology**
Gordon L. Klein, M.D., *Chair*, Galveston, TX; Karl E. Anderson, M.D., Galveston, TX; William Balistreri, M.D., Cincinnati, OH; Paul Bass, Ph.D., Madison, WI; Rosemary R. Berardi, Pharm.D., Ann Arbor, MI; Raymond F. Burk, M.D., Nashville, TN; Thomas Q. Garvey, III, M.D., Potomac, MD; Donald J. Glotzer, M.D., Boston, MA; Flavio Habal, M.D., Toronto, Ontario; Paul E. Hyman, M.D., Torrance, CA; Bernard Mehl, D.P.S., New York, NY; William J. Snape, Jr., M.D., Torrance, CA; Ronald D. Soltis, M.D., Minneapolis, MN; C. Noel Williams, M.D., Halifax, Nova Scotia; Hyman J. Zimmerman, M.D., Bethesda, MD

**Geriatrics**
Robert E. Vestal, M.D., *Chair*, Boise, ID; Darrell R. Abernethy, M.D., Washington, DC; William B. Abrams, M.D., West Point, PA; Jerry Avorn, M.D., Boston, MA; Robert A. Blouin, Pharm.D., Lexington, KY; S. George Carruthers, M.D., Halifax, Nova Scotia; Lynn E. Chaitovitz, Rockville, MD; Terry Fulmer, R.N., Ph.D., New York, NY; Philip P. Gerbino, Pharm.D., Philadelphia, PA; Pearl S. German, Sc.D., Baltimore, MD; David J. Greenblatt, M.D., Boston, MA; Martin D. Higbee, Pharm.D., Tucson, AZ; Brian B. Hoffman, M.D., Palo Alto, CA; J. Edward Jackson, M.D., San Diego, CA; Joseph V. Levy, Ph.D., San Francisco, CA; Paul A. Mitenko, M.D., FRCPC, Nanaimo, British Columbia; John E. Morley, M.B., B.Ch., St. Louis, MO; Jay Roberts, Ph.D., Philadelphia, PA; Louis J. Rubenstein, R.Ph., Alexandria, VA; Janice B. Schwartz, M.D., San Francisco, CA; Alexander M.M. Shepherd, M.D., San Antonio, TX; William Simonson, Pharm.D., Portland, OR; Daniel S. Sitar, Ph.D., Winnipeg, Manitoba; Mary K. Walker, R.N., Ph.D., Lexington, KY; Alastair J. J. Wood, M.D., Nashville, TN

## Hematologic and Neoplastic Disease
John W. Yarbro, M.D., Ph.D., *Chair*, Springfield, IL; Joseph S. Bailes, M.D., McAllen, TX; Laurence H. Baker, D.O., Ann Arbor, MI; Barbara D. Blumberg-Carnes, Albuquerque, NM; Helene G. Brown, B.S., Los Angeles, CA; Nora L. Burnham, Pharm.D., Princeton, NJ; William J. Dana, Pharm.D., Houston, TX; Connie Henke-Yarbro, R.N., B.S.N., Springfield, IL; William H. Hryniuk, M.D., San Diego, CA; B. J. Kennedy, M.D., Minneapolis, MN; Barnett Kramer, M.D., Rockville, MD; Michael J. Mastrangelo, M.D., Philadelphia, PA; David S. Rosenthal, M.D., Cambridge, MA; Richard L. Schilsky, M.D., Chicago, IL; Rowena N. Schwartz, Pharm.D., Pittsburgh, PA; Roy L. Silverstein, M.D., New York, NY; Samuel G. Taylor, IV, M.D., Chicago, IL; Raymond B. Weiss, M.D., Washington, DC

## Infectious Disease Therapy
Donald Kaye, M.D., *Chair*, Philadelphia, PA; Robert Austrian, M.D., Philadelphia, PA; C. Glenn Cobbs, M.D., Birmingham, AL; Joseph W. Cranston, Jr., Ph.D., Chicago, IL; John J. Dennehy, M.D., Danville, PA; Courtney V. Fletcher, Pharm. D., Minneapolis, MN; Earl H. Freimer, M.D., Toledo, OH; Marc LeBel, Pharm.D., Quebec, Quebec; John D. Nelson, M.D., Dallas, TX; Lindsay E. Nicolle, M.D., Winnipeg, Manitoba; Alvin Novick, M.D., New Haven, CT; Charles G. Prober, M.D., Stanford, CA; Douglas D. Richman, M.D., San Diego, CA; Spotswood L. Spruance, M.D., Salt Lake City, UT; Roy T. Steigbigel, M.D., Stony Brook, NY; Paul F. Wehrle, M.D., San Clemente, CA

## International Health
Rosalyn C. King, Pharm.D., M.P.H., *Chair*, Silver Spring, MD; Walter M. Batts, Rockville, MD; Eugenie Brown, Pharm.D., Kingston, Jamaica; Alan Cheung, Pharm.D., M.P.H., Washington, DC; Mary Couper, M.D., Geneva, Switzerland; Gabriel Daniel, Washington, DC; S. Albert Edwards, Pharm.D., Lincolnshire, IL; Enrique Fefer, Ph.D., Washington, DC; Peter H. M. Fontilus, Curacao, Netherlands Antilles; Gan Ee Kiang, Penang, Malaysia; Marcellus Grace, Ph.D., New Orleans, LA; George B. Griffenhagen, Washington, DC; Margareta Helling-Borda, Geneva, Switzerland; Thomas Langston, Silver Spring, MD; Thomas Lapnet-Moustapha, Yaounde, Cameroon; David Lee, B.A., M.D., Arlington, VA; Aissatov Lo, Ka-Olack, Senegal; Stuart M. MacLeod, M.D., Hamilton, Ontario; Russell E. Morgan, Jr., Dr.P.H., Chevy Chase, MD; David Ofori-Adjei, M.D., Accra, Ghana; S. Ofosu-Amaah, M.D., New York, NY; James Rankin, Arlington, VA; Olikoye Ransome-Kuti, M.D., Lagos, Nigeria; Budiono Santoso, M.D., Ph.D., Yogyakarta, Indonesia; Carmen Selva, Ph.D., Madrid, Spain; Valentin Vinogradov, Moscow, Russia; Fela Viso-Gurovich, Mexico City, Mexico; William B. Walsh, M.D., Chevy Chase, MD; Lawrence C. Weaver, Ph.D., Minneapolis, MN; Albert I. Wertheimer, Ph.D., Glen Allen, VA

## Neurology
Stanley van den Noort, M.D., *Chair*, Irvine, CA; William T. Beaver, M.D., Washington, DC; Elizabeth U. Blalock, M.D., Anaheim, CA; James C. Cloyd, Pharm.D., Minneapolis, MN; David M. Dawson, M.D., West Roxbury, MA; Kevin Farrell, M.D., Vancouver, British Columbia; Kathleen M. Foley, M.D., New York, NY; Anthony E. Lang, M.D., Toronto, Ontario; Ira T. Lott, M.D., Orange, CA; James R. Nelson, M.D., La Jolla, CA; J. Kiffin Penry, M.D., Winston-Salem, NC; Neil H. Raskin, M.D., San Francisco, CA; Alfred J. Spiro, M.D., Bronx, NY; M. DiAnn Turek, R.N., Holt, MI

## Nursing Practice
Rosemary C. Polomano, R.N., M.S.N., *Chair*, Philadelpia, PA; Mecca S. Cranley, R.N., Ph.D., Buffalo, NY; Jan M. Ellerhorst-Ryan, R.N., M.S.N., Cincinnati, OH; Linda Felver, Ph.D., R.N., Portland, OR; Hector Hugo Gonzalez, R.N., Ph.D., San Antonio, TX; Mary Harper, R.N., Ph.D., Rockville, MD; Ada K. Jacox, R.N., Ph.D., Baltimore, MD; Patricia Kummeth, R.N., M.S., Rochester, MN; Ida M. Martinson, R.N., Ph.D., San Francisco, CA; Carol P. Patton, R.N., Ph.D., J.D., Detroit, MI; Ginette A. Pepper, R.N., Ph.D., Englewood, CO; Geraldine A. Peterson, R.N., M.A., Potomac, MD; Linda C. Pugh, R.N., Ph.D., York, PA; Sharon S. Rising, R.N., C.N.M., Cheshire, CT; Marjorie Ann Spiro, R.N., B.S., C.S.N., Scarsdale, NY

## Nutrition and Electrolytes
Robert D. Lindeman, M.D., *Chair*, Albuquerque, NM; Hans Fisher, Ph.D., New Brunswick, NJ; Walter H. Glinsmann, M.D., Washington, DC; Helen Andrews Guthrie, M.S., Ph.D., State College, PA; Steven B. Heymsfield, M.D., New York, NY; K. N. Jeejeebhoy, M.D., Toronto, Ontario; Leslie M. Klevay, M.D., Grand Forks, ND; Linda S. Knox, M.S.N., Philadelphia, PA; Bonnie Liebman, M.S., Washington, DC; Sudesh K. Mahajan, M.D., Grosse Point Woods, MI; Craig J. McClain, M.D., Lexington, KY; Jay M. Mirtallo, M.S., Columbus, OH; Sohrab Mobarhan, M.D., Maywood, IL; Robert M. Russell, M.D., Boston, MA; Harold H. Sandstead, M.D., Galveston, TX; William J. Stone, M.D., Nashville, TN; Carlos A. Vaamonde, M.D., Miami, FL; Stanley Wallach, M.D., New York, NY

## Obstetrics and Gynecology
Douglas D. Glover, M.D., *Chair*, Morgantown, WV; Rudi Ansbacher, M.D., Ann Arbor, MI; Florence Comite, M.D., New Haven, CT; James W. Daly, M.D., Columbia, MO; Marilynn C. Frederiksen, M.D., Chicago, IL; Charles B. Hammond, M.D., Durham, NC; Barbara A. Hayes, M.A., New Rochelle, NY; Art Jacknowitz, Pharm.D., Morgantown, WV; William J. Ledger, M.D., New York, NY; Andre-Marie Leroux, M.D., Ottawa, Ontario; William A. Nahhas, M.D., Dayton, OH; Warren N. Otterson, M.D., Shreveport, LA; Samuel A. Pasquale, M.D., New Brunswick, NJ; Johanna Perlmutter, M.D., Boston, MA; Robert W. Rebar, M.D., Cincinnati, OH; Richard H. Reindollar, M.D., Boston, MA; G. Millard Simmons, M.D., Morgantown, WV; J. Benjamin Younger, M.D., Birmingham, AL

## Ophthalmology
Herbert E. Kaufman, M.D., *Chair*, New Orleans, LA; Steven R. Abel, Pharm.D., Indianapolis, IN; Jules Baum, M.D., Boston, MA; Lee R. Duffner, M.D., Miami, FL; David L. Epstein, M.D., Durham, NC; Allan J. Flach, Pharm.D., M.D., Corte Madera, CA; Vincent H. L. Lee, Ph.D., Los Angeles, CA; Steven M. Podos, M.D., New York, NY; Kirk R. Wilhelmus, M.D., Houston, TX; Thom J. Zimmerman, M.D., Ph.D., Louisville, KY

## Otorhinolaryngology
Leonard P. Rybak, M.D., Ph.D., *Chair*, Springfield, IL; Robert E. Brummett, Ph.D., Portland, OR; Robert A. Dobie, M.D., San Antonio, TX; Linda J. Gardiner, M.D., Fort Myers, FL; David Hilding, M.D., Price, UT; David B. Hom, M.D., Minneapolis, MN; Helen F. Krause, M.D., Pittsburgh, PA; Richard L. Mabry, M.D., Dallas, TX; Lawrence J. Marentette, M.D., Ann Arbor, MI; Robert A. Mickel, M.D., Ph.D., San Francisco, CA; Randal A. Otto, M.D., San Antonio, TX;

Richard W. Waguespack, M.D., Birmingham, AL; William R. Wilson, M.D., Washington, DC

## Parasitic Disease

Jay S. Keystone, M.D., *Chair*, Toronto, Ontario; Michele Barry, M.D., New Haven, CT; Frank J. Bia, M.D., M.P.H., Guilford, CT; David Botero, M.D., Medellin, Colombia; David O. Freedman, M.D., Birmingham, AL; Elaine C. Jong, M.D., Seattle, WA; Dennis D. Juranek, M.D., Atlanta, GA; Donald J. Krogstad, M.D., New Orleans, LA; Douglas W. MacPherson, M.D., Hamilton, Ontario; Edward K. Markell, M.D., Berkeley, CA; Theodore Nash, M.D., Bethesda, MD; Murray Wittner, M.D., Bronx, NY

## Patient Counseling (Ad Hoc)

Frank J. Ascione, Pharm.D., Ph.D., *Chair*, Ann Arbor, MI; John E. Arradondo, M.D., Houston, TX; Candace Barnett, Atlanta, GA; Karin Bolte, Washington, DC; Allan H. Bruckheim, M.D., Harrison, NY; Mark Clasen, M.D., Ph.D., Dayton, OH; Amy Cooper-Outlaw, Pharm.D., Stone Mountain, GA; Frederick A. Curro, D.M.D., Ph.D., Jersey City, NJ; Robin DiMatteo, Ph.D., Riverside, CA; Diane B. Ginsburg, Austin, TX; Denise Grimes, R.N., Jackson, MI; Richard Herrier, Tucson, AZ; Barry Kass, R.Ph., Boston, MA; Thomas Kellenberger, Pharm.D., Montvale, NJ; Alice Kimball, Darnestown, MD; Pat Kramer, Bismarck, ND; Patti Kummeth, R.N., Rochester, MN; Ken Leibowitz, Philadelphia, PA; Colleen Lum Lung, R.N., Denver, CO; Louise Matte, Quebec, Canada; Scotti Milley, Richmond, VA; Constance Pavlides, R.N., D.N.Sc., Rockville, MD; Lisa Tedesco, Ph.D., Ann Arbor, MI

## Pediatric Anesthesiology (Ad Hoc)

Charles J. Coté, M.D., *Chair*, Chicago, IL, J. Michael Badgwell, M.D., Lubbock, TX; Barbara Brandon, M.D., Pittsburgh, PA; Ryan Cook, M.D., Pittsburgh, PA; John J. Downes, M.D., Philadelphia, PA; Dennis Fisher, M.D., San Francisco, CA; John E. Forestner, M.D., Fort Worth, TX; Helen W. Karl, M.D., Seattle, WA; Harry G. G. Kingston, M.B., Portland, OR; Anne Marie Lynn, M.D., Seattle, WA; Mark Shriner, M.D. Philadelphia, PA; Victoria Simpson, M.D., Ph.D., Denver, CO; Meb Watcha, M.D., St. Louis, MO

## Pediatrics

Philip D. Walson, M.D., *Chair*, Columbus, OH; Susan Alpert, Ph.D., M.D., Rockville, MD; Jacob V. Aranda, M.D., Ph.D., Montreal, Quebec; Cheston M. Berlin, Jr., M.D., Hershey, PA; Nancy Jo Braden, M.D., Phoenix, AZ; Patricia J. Bush, Ph.D., Washington, DC; Marion J. Finkel, M.D., Morris Township, NJ; George S. Goldstein, M.D., Briarcliff Manor, NY; Ralph E. Kauffman, M.D., Detroit, MI; Gideon Koren, M.D., Toronto, Ontario; Joan M. Korth-Bradley, Pharm.D., Ph.D., Philadelphia, PA; Richard Leff, Pharm.D., Kansas City, KS; Carolyn Lund, R.N., M.S., San Francisco, CA; Wayne Snodgrass, M.D., Galveston, TX; Celia A. Viets, M.D., Ottawa, Canada; John T. Wilson, M.D., Shreveport, LA; Sumner J. Yaffe, M.D., Bethesda, MD; Karin E. Zenk, Pharm.D., Irvine, CA

## Pharmacy Practice

Thomas P. Reinders, Pharm.D., *Chair*, Richmond, VA; Olya Duzey, M.S., Big Rapids, MI; Yves Gariepy, B.Sc.Pharm., Quebec, Quebec; Ned Heltzer, M.S., New Castle, DE; Lester S. Hosto, B.S., Little Rock, AR; Martin J. Jinks, Pharm.D., Pullman, WA; Frederick Klein, B.S., Montvale, NJ; Calvin H. Knowlton, Ph.D., Lumberton, NJ; Patricia

A. Kramer, B.S., Bismarck, ND; Dennis McCallum, Pharm.D., Minneapolis, MN; Shirley P. McKee, B.S., Houston, TX; William A. McLean, Pharm.D., Ottawa, Ontario; Gladys Montañez, B.S., Santurce, PR; Donald L. Moore, B.S., Kokomo, IN; John E. Ogden, M.S., Washington, DC; Henry A. Palmer, Ph.D., Storrs, CT; Lorie G. Rice, B.A., M.P.H., San Francisco, CA; Mike R. Sather, M.S., Albuquerque, NM; Albert Sebok, B.S., Hudson, OH; William E. Smith, Pharm.D., Ph.D., Boston, MA; Susan East Torrico, B.S., Orlando, FL; J. Richard Wuest, Pharm.D., Cincinnati, OH; Glenn Y. Yokoyama, Pharm.D., Pasadena, CA

## Psychiatric Disease

Burton J. Goldstein, M.D., *Chair*, Williams Island, FL; Magda Campbell, M.D., New York, NY; Alex A. Cardoni, M.S. Pharm., Hartford, CT; James L. Claghorn, M.D., Houston, TX; N. Michael Davis, M.S., Miami, FL; Larry Ereshefsky, Pharm.D., San Antonio, TX; W. Edwin Fann, M.D., Houston, TX; Alan J. Gelenberg, M.D., Tucson, AZ; Tracy R. Gordy, M.D., Austin, TX; Paul Grof, M.D., Ottawa, Ontario; Russell T. Joffe, M.D., Toronto, Ontario; Harriet P. Lefley, Ph.D., Miami, FL; Nathan Rawls, Pharm.D., Memphis, TN; Ruth Robinson, Saskatoon, Saskatchewan; Matthew V. Rudorfer, M.D., Rockville, MD; Karen A. Theesen, Pharm.D., Omaha, NE

## Pulmonary Disease

Harold S. Nelson, M.D., *Chair*, Denver, CO; Richard C. Ahrens, M.D., Iowa City, IA; Eugene R. Bleecker, M.D., Baltimore, MD; William W. Busse, M.D., Madison, WI; Christopher Fanta, M.D., Boston, MA; Mary K. Garcia, R.N., Sugarland, TX; Nicholas Gross, M.D., Hines, IL; Leslie Hendeles, Pharm.D., Gainesville, FL; Elliot Israel, M.D., Boston, MA; Susan Janson-Bjerklie, R.N., Ph.D., San Francisco, CA; John W. Jenne, M.D., Hines, IL; H. William Kelly, Pharm.D., Albuquerque, NM; James P. Kemp, M.D., San Diego, CA; Henry Levison, M.D., Toronto, Ontario; Gail Shapiro, M.D., Seattle, WA; Stanley J. Szefler, M.D., Denver, CO

## Radiopharmaceuticals

Carol S. Marcus, Ph.D., M.D., *Chair*, Torrance, CA; Capt. William H. Briner, B.S., Durham, NC; Ronald J. Callahan, Ph.D., Boston, MA; Janet F. Eary, M.D., Seattle, WA; Joanna S. Fowler, Ph.D., Upton, NY; David L. Gilday, M.D., Toronto, Ontario; David A. Goodwin, M.D., Palo Alto, CA; David L. Laven, N.Ph., C.R.Ph., FASCP, Bay Pines, FL; Andrea H. McGuire, M.D., Des Moines, IA; Peter Paras, Ph.D., Rockville, MD; Barry A. Siegel, M.D., St. Louis, MO; Edward B. Silberstein, M.D., Cincinnati, OH; Dennis P. Swanson, M.S., Pittsburgh, PA; Mathew L. Thakur, Ph.D., Philadelphia, PA; Henry N. Wellman, M.D., Indianapolis, IN

## Surgical Drugs and Devices

Lary A. Robinson, M.D., *Chair*, Tampa, FL; Gregory Alexander, M.D., Rockville, MD; Norman D. Anderson, M.D., Baltimore, MD; Alan R. Dimick, M.D., Birmingham, AL; Jack Hirsh, M.D., Hamilton, Ontario; Manucher J. Javid, M.D., Madison, WI; Henry J. Mann, Pharm.D., Bloomington, MN; Kurt M. W. Niemann, M.D., Birmingham, AL; Robert P. Rapp, Pharm.D., Lexington, KY; Ronald Rubin, M.D., West Newton, MA

## Urology

John A. Belis, M.D., *Chair*, Hershey, PA; Culley C. Carson, M.D., Chapel Hill, NC; Richard A. Cohen, M.D., Red Bank,

NJ; B. J. Reid Czarapata, R.N., North Potomac, MD; Jean B. de Kernion, M.D., Los Angeles, CA; Warren Heston, Ph.D., New York, NY; Mark V. Jarowenko, M.D., Hershey, PA; Mary Lee, Pharm.D., Chicago, IL; Marguerite C. Lippert, M.D., Charlottesville, VA; Penelope A. Longhurst, Ph.D., Philadelphia, PA; Tom F. Lue, M.D., San Francisco, CA; Michael G. Mawhinney, Ph.D., Morgantown, WV; Martin G. McLoughlin, M.D., Vancouver, British Columbia; Randall G. Rowland, M.D., Ph.D., Indianapolis, IN; J. Patrick Spirnak, M.D., Cleveland, OH; William F. Tarry, M.D., Morgantown, WV; Keith N. Van Arsdalen, M.D., Philadelphia, PA

**Veterinary Medicine**

Lloyd E. Davis, D.V.M., Ph.D., *Chair*, Urbana, IL; Arthur L. Aronson, D.V.M., Ph.D., Raleigh, NC; Gordon W. Brumbaugh, D.V.M., Ph.D., College Station, TX; Peter Conlon, D.V.M., Ph.D., Guelph, Ontario; Gordon L. Coppoc, D.V.M., Ph.D., West Lafayette, IN; Sidney A. Ewing, D.V.M., Ph.D., Stillwater, OK; Stuart D. Forney, M.S., Fort Collins, CO; William G. Huber, D.V.M., Ph.D., Sun City West, AZ; Vernon Corey Langston, D.V.M., Ph.D., Mississippi State, MS; Mark G. Papich, D.V.M., Raleigh, NC; John W. Paul, D.V.M., Somerville, NJ; Thomas E. Powers, D.V.M., Ph.D., Columbus, OH; Charles R. Short, D.V.M., Ph.D., Baton Rouge, LA; Richard H. Teske, D.V.M., Ph.D., Rockville, MD; Jeffrey R. Wilcke, D.V.M., M.S., Blacksburg, VA

# DRUG INFORMATION DIVISION ADDITIONAL CONTRIBUTORS

The information presented in this text represents an ongoing review of the drugs contained herein and represents a consensus of various viewpoints expressed. In addition to the individuals listed below, many schools, associations, pharmaceutical companies, and governmental agencies have provided comment or otherwise contributed to the development of the 1995 USP DI data base. Such listing does not imply that these individuals have reviewed all of the material in this text or that they individually agree with all statements contained herein.

Donald I. Abrams, M.D., San Francisco, CA
Jonathan Abrams, M.D., Albuquerque, NM
Bruce H. Ackerman, Pharm.D., Philadelphia, PA
N. Franklin Adkinson, M.D., Baltimore, MD
Allen C. Alfrey, M.D., Denver, CO
Joanne Allard, M.D., Toronto, Ontario, Canada
Carmen Allegra, M.D., Bethesda, MD
Mike Apley, D.V.M., Greeley, CO
Martin Bacon, M.D., Bethesda, MD
José M. Ballester, M.D., La Habana, Cuba
Rick Barbarash, Pharm.D., St. Louis, MO
Patsy Barnett, Pharm.D., Birmingham, AL
LuAnne Barron, Birmingham, AL
Robert W. Beightol, Pharm.D., Roanoke, VA
William Bell, M.D., Baltimore, MD
Gladys Bendahan Barchilón, Barcelona, Spain
Patricia Bennett, B.S.Pharm., Cincinnati, OH
David L. Benowitz, M.D., San Francisco, CA
Byron S. Berlin, M.D., Lansing, MI
Frederick A. Berry, M.D., Charlottesville, VA
Ernest Beutler, M.D., La Jolla, CA
Christine A. Bezouska, M.D., Morgantown, WV
S. Bruce Binder, M.D., Ph.D., Dayton, OH
Martin Black, M.D., Philadelphia, PA
Laura Boehnke, Pharm.D., Houston, TX
Halcy Bohen, Ph.D., Washington, DC
Wayne E. Bradley, Duluth, GA
Michael Brady, M.D., Columbus, OH
Edward L. Braud, M.D., Springfield, IL
Robert E. Braun, D.D.S., Buffalo, NY
Kenneth Bridges, M.D., Boston, MA
Paul J. Brown, M.D., Bedford, NH
Louis Buttino, Jr., M.D., Dayton, OH
Wesley G. Byerly, Pharm.D., Winston-Salem, NC

Karim A. Calis, Pharm.D., Bethesda, MD
Mary E. Carman, Ottawa, Ontario
Charles C.J. Carpenter, M.D., Providence, RI
Peggy Carver, M.D., Ann Arbor, MI
Marcel Casavant, M.D., Columbus, OH
Bruce A. Chabner, M.D., Bethesda, MD
Erin S. Champagne, D.V.M., Blacksburg, VA
Chih Wen Chang, Pharm.D., Maywood, IL
Te-Wen Chang, M.D., Boston, MA
Kenneth R. Chapman, M.D., Toronto, Ontario
Bruce D. Cheson, M.D., Bethesda, MD
Henry Chilton, Pharm.D., Winston-Salem, NC
Frank Chytil, Ph.D., Nashville, TN
Scott B. Citino, D.V.M., Yulee, FL
Cyril R. Clarke, Ph.D., Stillwater, OK
Jackson Como, M.D., Birmingham, AL
Betsy Jane Cooper, M.D., Washington, DC
James W. Cooper, Ph.D., Athens, GA
Deborah Cotton, M.D., Boston, MA
Fred F. Cowan, Ph.D., Portland, OR
Donald W. Cox, M.D., Morgantown, WV
Mark V. Crisman, D.V.M., Blacksburg, VA
Craig Darby, R.Ph., Twinsburg, OH
Michael Davidson, D.V.M., Raleigh, NC
Ann J. Davis, M.D., Boston, MA
Janet Davis, M.D., Miami, FL
Ken Davis, M.D., New York, NY
Thomas D. DeCillis, North Port, FL
Carel P. de Haseth, Ph.D., Netherland Antilles
Daniel Deykin, M.D., Boston, MA
Nick Diamant, M.D., Toronto, Ontario Canada
Annette Dickinson, Ph.D., Washington, DC
Barry D. Dickinson, Ph.D., Chicago, IL
Christine Z. Dickinson, M.D., Royal Oak, MI

John B. DiMarco, M.D., Ph.D., Charlottesville, VA
James E. Doherty, M.D., Little Rock, AR
Donald C. Doll, M.D., Columbia, MO
Jerry Dolovich, M.D., Hamilton, Ontario
R. Gordon Douglas, M.D., Rahway, NJ
Ed Drea, Pharm.D., Phoenix, AZ
Bonnie Driggers, R.N., Portland, OR
Marion Dugdale, M.D., Memphis, TN
Carol Duncan, R.N., Portland, OR
Suzanne Eastman, M.S., R.Ph., Columbus, OH
John E. Edwards, Jr., M.D., Torrance, CA
Robert Edwards, Pharm.D., Columbus, OH
Lawrence H. Einhorn, M.D., Indianapolis, IN
Augustin Escalante, M.D., Downey, CA
Gary Euler, Dr.P.H., Atlanta, GA
William Fant, Pharm.D., Cincinnati, OH
Martin N. Farlow, M.D., Indianapolis, IN
R. Edward Faught, M.D., Birmingham, AL
David S. Fedson, M.D., Charlottesville, VA
John P. Feighner, La Mesa, CA
James M. Ferguson, M.D., Salt Lake City, UT
Paul Ferrell, M.D., Bethesda, MD
Anne Gilbert Feuer, R.Ph., Cincinnati, OH
Suzanne Fields, Pharm.D., San Antonio, TX
J.R. Fontilus, M.D., Netherland Antilles
Tammy Fox, R.Ph., Fairfield, OH
Charles W. Francis, M.D., Rochester, NY
Ruth Francis-Floyd, D.V.M., Gainesville, FL
Rudolph M. Franklin, M.D., New Orleans, LA
H. H. Frey, Berlin, Germany
Dorothy Friedberg, M.D., New York, NY
Alan Friedman, M.D., New York, NY
José P.B. Gallardo, R.Ph., Iowa City, IA
Gloria Garber, R.Ph., Cincinnati, OH
Arthur Garson, M.D., Durham, NC
S. Gauthier, M.D., Montreal, PQ, Canada
Edward Genton, M.D., New Orleans, LA
Anne A. Gershon, M.D., New York, NY
Larry N. Gever, Pharm.D., Cranbury, NJ
Michael J. Glade, Ph.D., Chicago, IL
Charles J. Glueck, M.D., Cincinnati, OH
Maryanne Godlewski-Vagnini, R.Ph., Brooklyn, NY
Lewis Goldfrank, M.D., New York, NY
J. Max Goodson, D.D.S., Ph.D., Boston, MA
Fred Gordin, M.D., Washington, DC
John D. Grabenstein, M.S., Fort Sam Houston, TX
Roni Grad, M.D., Albuquerque, NM
Nina M. Graves, Pharm.D., Minneapolis, MN
Terri Graves Davidson, Pharm.D., Atlanta, GA
David Green, M.D., Chicago, IL
Harry Green, M.D., Evansville, IN
Martin D. Green, M.D., Rockville, MD
Philip C. Greig, M.D., Durham, NC
Vincent Habiyambere, M.D., Geneva, Switzerland
Angela M. Hadbavny, Pharm.D., Pittsburgh, PA
Benjamin F. Hammond, D.D.S., Ph.D., Philadelphia, PA
Kenneth R. Hande, M.D., Nashville, TN
Edward A. Hartshorn, Ph.D., League City, TX
Robert C. Hastings, M.D., Carville, LA
William E. Hathaway, Denver, CO
Frederick G. Hayden, M.D., Charlottesville, VA
Cleopatra L. Hazel, Pharm.D., Netherland Antilles
Murk-Hein Heinemann, M.D., New York, NY
Peter Hellyer, D.V.M., Raleigh, NC

Bryan N. Henderson, II, D.D.S., Dallas, TX
William Herbert, M.D., Durham, NC
Barbara Herwaldt, M.D., Atlanta, GA
Monto Ho, M.D., Pittsburgh, PA
Vincent C. Ho, M.D., British Columbia, Canada
M.E. Hoar, Springfield, MA
Robert Hodgeman, M.S., R.Ph., Cincinnati, OH
Gary N. Holland, M.D., Los Angeles, CA
Richard A. Holmes, M.D., Columbia, MO
William Hopkins, Pharm.D., Atlanta, GA
Richard B. Hornick, M.D., Orlando, FL
Raymond W. Houde, M.D., New York, NY
Colin W. Howden, M.D., Columbia, SC
Walter T. Hughes, M.D., Memphis, TN
B. Thomas Hutchinson, M.D., Boston, MA
John Iazzetta, Pharm.D., Toronto, Ontario, Canada
Rodney D. Ice, Ph.D., Atlanta, GA
Frederick Jacobsen, M.D., Washington, DC
Mark Jacobson, M.D., San Francisco, CA
Robert Jacobson, M.D., Carville, LA
Ann L. Janer, M.S., Auburn, AL
Janet P. Jaramilla, Pharm.D., Chicago, IL
James W. Jefferson, M.D., Madison, WI
Alan Jenkins, M.D., Charlottesville, VA
Leslye Johnson, Ph.D., Bethesda, MD
Joseph L. Jorizzo, M.D., Winston-Salem, NC
Gunnar Juliusson, M.D., Ph.D., Huddinge, Sweden
Hugh F. Kabat, Ph.D., Albuquerque, NM
James Kahn, M.D., San Francisco, CA
Alan Kanada, Pharm.D., Denver, CO
John J. Kavanagh, M.D., Houston, TX
Michael J. Keating, M.D., Houston, TX
Michael Kelley, M.D., Columbus, OH
David C. Kem, M.D., Oklahoma City, OK
N. David Kennedy, R.Ph., Washington, DC
Joseph M. Khoury, M.D., Bethesda, MD
Agnes V. Klein, M.D., Vanier, Ontario
Anne Klibanski, M.D., Boston, MA
Sandra Knowles, B.Pharm., Toronto, Ontario, Canada
John Koepke, Pharm.D., Columbus, OH
Joseph A. Kovacs, M.D., Bethesda, MD
Paul A. Krusinski, M.D., Burlington, VT
Paul B. Kuehn, Ph.D., Woodinville, WA
R.W. Kuncl, M.D., Baltimore, MD
Thomas L. Kurt, M.D., Dallas, TX
Lyle Laird, Pharm.D., San Antonio, TX
John S. Lambert, M.D., Rochester, NY
John R. LaMontagne, Bethesda, MD
Michael Lange, M.D., New York, NY
Victor J. Lanzotti, M.D., Springfield, IL
P. Reed Larsen, M.D., Boston, MA
Eugene Laska, M.D., Orangeburg, NY
Oscar L. Laskin, M.D., East Hanover, NJ
John Laszlo, M.D., Atlanta, GA
Belle Lee, Pharm.D., San Francisco, CA
Ilo E. Leppik, M.D., Minneapolis, MN
Raymond Levy, London, England
Richard A. Lewis, M.D., Houston, TX
William Lieber, M.D., Waterbury, CT
Charles Liebow, II, D.D.S., Ph.D., Buffalo, NY
Christopher D. Lind, M.D., Nashville, TN
Charles H. Livengood, III, M.D., Durham, NC
Don M. Long, M.D., Ph.D., Baltimore, MD
Julio R. Lopez, M.D., Martinez, CA

Colleen Lum Lung, R.N., Denver, CO
Howard I. Maibach, M.D., San Francisco, CA
Marilyn Manco-Johnson, Denver, CO
Victor J. Marder, M.D., Rochester, NY
Joseph E. Margarone, II, D.D.S., Buffalo, NY
Maurie Markman, M.D., Cleveland, OH
Jon Markovitz, M.D., Phoenix, AZ
William C. Matthews, M.D., San Diego, CA
Harry R. Maxon, III, M.D., Cincinnati, OH
Alice Lorraine McAfee, Pharm.D., San Pedro, CA
Lisa Y. McDonald, Pharm.D., Emeryville, CA
Norman L. McElroy, San Jose, CA
Charles McGrath, D.V.M., Blacksburg, VA
Ross E. McKinney, M.D., Durham, NC
Anne McNulty, M.D., Waterbury, CT
Wallace B. Mendelson, M.D. Cleveland, OH
Dean D. Metcalfe, M.D., Bethesda, MD
Donald Miller, Pharm.D., Fargo, ND
John Mills, M.D., Fairfield, Victoria, Australia
Joel S. Mindel, M.D., Ph.D., New York, NY
Bernard L. Mirkin, M.D., Chicago, IL
Janet L. Mitchell, M.D., New York, NY
John R. Modlin, M.D., Hanover, NH
C. Craig Moldenhauer, M.D., San Diego, CA
Garreth A. Moore, Blacksburg, VA
Mary E. Mortensen, M.D., Columbus, OH
Robyn Mueller, R.Ph., Cincinnati, OH
R.I. Ogilvie, M.D., Toronto, Ontario
Linda K. Ohri, Pharm.D., Omaha, NE
James M. Oleske, M.D., Newark, NJ
Robert O'Mara, M.D., Rochester, NY
Michael J. O'Neill, R.Ph., Twinsburg, OH
Walter A. Orenstein, M.D., Atlanta, GA
James R. Oster, M.D., Miami, FL
Judith M. Ozbun, R.Ph., M.S., Fargo, ND
David C. Pang, Ph.D., Chicago, IL
Michael F. Para, M.D., Columbus, OH
Satyapal R. Pareddy, B.Pharm., Brooklyn, NY
Robert C. Park, M.D., Washington, DC
William W. Parmly, M.D., San Francisco, CA
Albert Patterson, Hines, IL
James A. Pederson, M.D., Oklahoma City, OK
Ronald Peterson, M.D., Ph.D., Rochester, MN
Melenie Petropoulos, R.Ph., Twinsburg, OH
Lawrence D. Piro, M.D., La Jolla, CA
Philip A. Pizzo, M.D., Bethesda, MD
Christopher V. Plowe, M.D., Bethesda, MD
Therese Poirier, Pharm.D., Pittsburgh, PA
Michael A. Polis, M.D., Bethesda, MD
James A. Ponto, R.Ph., Iowa City, IA
Carol M. Proudfit, Ph.D., Chicago, IL
Nixa Ramos, Arecibo, Puerto Rico
Norbert P. Rapoza, Ph.D., Chicago, IL
Gary Raskob, M.Sc., Oklahoma City, OK
Terry D. Rees, D.D.S., Dallas, TX
Alfred J. Remillard, Pharm.D., Saskatoon, Saskatchewan, Canada
David Robertson, M.D., Nashville, TN
Robert Roberts, M.D., Houston, TX
Daniel C. Robinson, Pharm.D., Los Angeles, CA
John E. Roney, R.Ph., Cincinnati, OH
Jeff Rosner, R.Ph., Twinsburg, OH
Douglas S. Ross, M.D., Boston, MA
Phillip J. Rubin, M.D., Phoenix, AZ

Michael S. Saag, M.D., Birmingham, AL
Henry S. Sacks, Ph.D., M.D., New York, NY
Sharon Safrin, M.D., San Francisco, CA
Evelyn Salerno, Pharm.D., Hialeah, FL
Hugh A. Sampson, Jr., M.D., Baltimore, MD
Subbiah Sangiah, D.V.M., Ph.D., Stillwater, OK
Victor M. Santana, Memphis, TN
Belinda Sartor, M.D., Shreveport, LA
Donald C. Sawyer, East Lansing, MI
Elliot Schecter, M.D., Oklahoma City, OK
Udo P. Schmiedl, M.D., Ph.D., Seattle, WA
Gabriel Schmunis, M.D., Washington, DC
Steven M. Schnittman, M.D., Rockville, MD
George Schuster, M.D., Augusta, GA
Stephen Schuster, M.D., Philadelphia, PA
Dorothy Schwartz-Porsche, Berlin, Germany
Douglas A. Sears, Tenafly, NJ
Jerome Seidenfeld, Ph.D., Chicago, IL
Charles F. Seifert, Pharm.D., Oklahoma City, OK
Allen Shaughnessy, Pharm.D., Harrisburg, PA
Donald J. Sherrard, M.D., Seattle, WA
Yvonne M. Shevchuk, Pharm.D., Saskatoon, Saskatchewan, Canada
Harold M. Silverman, Pharm.D., Silver Spring, MD
Irv Siven, M.D., New York, NY
Barry H. Smith, M.D., Ph.D., New York, NY
Dance Smith, Pharm.D., Ft. Steilacoom, WA
Geralynn B. Smith, M.S., Detroit, MI
John R. Smith, M.S., Ph.D., Portland, OR
Steven J. Smith, Ph.D., Chicago, IL
Elliott M. Sogol, Ph.D., Research Triangle Park, NC
Nicholas Soter, M.D., New York, NY
William Speliacy, M.D., Tampa, FL
Joan Stachnik, Chicago, IL
William Steers, M.D., Charlottesville, VA
John J. Stern, M.D., Philadelphia, PA
Irwin Strathman, M.D., Lutz, FL
Kris Strohbehn, M.D., Boston, MA
David Stuhr, Denver, CO
Alan Sugar, M.D., Boston, MA
Linda Gore Sutherland, Pharm.D., Laramie, WY
Sandra Tailor, Pharm.D., Toronto, Ontario, Canada
David A. Taylor, M.D., Morgantown, WV
Mary E. Teresi, Iowa City, IA
Cheryl Nunn Thompson, Chicago, IL
John C. Thurman, D.V.M., Urbana, IL
Roger C. Toffle, M.D., Morgantown, WV
Douglas M. Tollefsen, M.D., St. Louis, MO
Eric J. Topol, M.D., Ann Arbor, MI
Jayme Trott, Pharm.D., San Antonio, TX
Donald G. Vidt, M.D., Cleveland, OH
Richard Vogel, D.D.S., Newark, NJ
Georgia Vogelsang, M.D., Baltimore, MD
Paul A. Volberding, M.D., San Francisco, CA
Andrea Wall, R.Ph., Cincinnati, OH
William Warner, Ph.D., New York, NY
Michael Weber, M.D., Irvine, CA
Krisantha Weerasuriya, M.D., Geneva, Switzerland
G. John Weir, M.D., Marshfield, WI
Timothy E. Welty, Pharm.D., Cincinnati, OH
Stanford Wessler, M.D., Rye, NY
Carolyn Westhoff, New York, NY
John White, Pharm.D., Spokane, WA
Richard J. Whitley, M.D., Birmingham, AL

Catherine Wilfert, M.D., Durham, NC
Robert G. Wolfangel, Ph.D., St. Louis, MO
M. Michael Wolfe, M.D., Boston, MA
William Wonderlin, Ph.D., Morgantown, WV
Richard J. Wood, M.D., Boston, MA
Curtis Wright, M.D., Rockville, MD

Catharine Wuest, R.Ph., Cincinnati, OH
Robert Yarchoan, M.D., Bethesda, MD
Stephanie Zarus, Pharm.D., Philadelphia, PA
John M. Zajecka, M.D., Chicago, IL
Frederic J. Zucchero, M.A., R.Ph., Chesterfield, MO
Jane R. Zucker, Atlanta, GA

# HEADQUARTERS STAFF

## DRUG INFORMATION DIVISION

**Director:** Keith W. Johnson

**Assistant Director:** Georgie M. Cathey

**Administrative Staff:** Jaime A. Ramirez *(Administrative Assistant)*, Albert Crucillo, Mayra L. Rios

**Senior Drug Information Specialists:** Sandra Lee Boyer, Nancy Lee Dashiell, Debra A. Edwards, Esther H. Klein *(Supervisor)*, Angela Méndez Mayo *(Spanish Publications Coordinator)*

**Drug Information Specialists:** Katherine M. Bennett, Joyce Carpenter, Ann Corken, Jymeann King, Doris Lee *(Supervisor)*, Robin Schermerhorn, Denise Seldon, Daniel W. Seyoum

**Veterinary Drug Information Specialist:** Amy Neal

**Coordinator, Patient Counseling and Education Programs:** Stacy M. Hartranft

**Computer Applications:** Richard Allen *(Programmer)*, Bernard G. Silverstein *(Computer Applications Specialist)*

**Publications Development Staff:** Diana M. Blais *(Manager)*, Anne M. Lawrence *(Associate)*, Dorothy Raymond *(Assistant)*, Darcy Schwartz *(Assistant)*

**Library Services:** Florence A. Hogan *(Manager)*, Terri Rikhy *(Assistant)*, Madeleine Welsch

**Research Associate, International Programs:** David D. Housley

**Research Assistant:** Annamarie J. Sibik

**Consultants:** Janet Elgert, Lourdes de Gonzalez, David W. Hughes, S. Ramakrishnan Iyer, Wanda Janicki, Kate Phelan, Marcelo Vernengo

**Scholar in Residence:** Patricia J. Bush, Georgetown University

**Student Interns/Externs:** Robyn Dubinsky, University of Missouri at Kansas City; Rachel Ellis, Nottingham University, England; Kevin Garey, Dalhousie University, Nova Scotia; Bereket Melaku, Howard University; Kavita Nair, University of Toledo; Ken Rogers, University of Arizona; Yván Sánchez-Huamaní, National University of Trujillo, Peru

**Visiting Scholars:** Giulia Cingolani, Rome, Italy; Elena Oshkalova, Moscow, Russian Federation; Svetlana Udotova, Moscow, Russian Federation

## USP ADMINISTRATIVE STAFF

**Executive Director:** Jerome A. Halperin
**Associate Executive Director:** Joseph G. Valentino

**Assistant Executive Director for Professional and Public Affairs:** Jacqueline L. Eng
**Director, Finance:** Abe Brauner
**Director, Operations:** J. Robert Strang
**Director, Personnel:** Arlene Bloom
**Director, Fulfillment/Facilities:** Drew J. Lutz
**Legal:** Kim Keller (Staff Attorney), John Lindow (Associate Legal Counsel for Business Affairs), Colleen Ottoson (Staff Attorney)

## DRUG STANDARDS DIVISION

**Director:** Lee T. Grady

**Assistant Directors:** Charles H. Barnstein *(Revision)*, Barbara B. Hubert, *(Scientific Administration)*, Robert H. King *(Technical Services)*

**Senior Scientists:** Roger Dabbah, V. Srinivasan, William W. Wright

**Scientists:** Frank P. Barletta, Vivian A. Gray, W. Larry Paul

**Senior Scientific Associate:** Todd L. Cecil

**Technical Editors:** Ann K. Ferguson, Melissa M. Smith

**Supervisor of Administration:** Anju K. Malhotra

**Support Staff:** Patricia Barnhill, Glenna Etherton, Theresa H. Lee, Cecilia Luna, Maureen Rawson, Ernestene Williams

**Drug Research and Testing Laboratory:** Richard F. Lindauer *(Director)*

**Hazard Communications:** Linda Shear

**Consultants:** J. Joseph Belson, Zorach R. Glaser, Martin Golden, Aubrey S. Outschoorn

## MARKETING

**Director:** Joan Blitman

**Senior Product Manager:** Mark A. Sohasky *(Electronic Information)*

**Product Manager:** Kathleen Bagas *(Publications)*

**Marketing Associates:** Jennifer C. Glenn, Dana L. McCullah, Steven Saars

**Marketing Representative:** Susan M. Williams *(Electronic Applications)*

**Marketing Communications Manager:** Derek Rice

**Marketing Research Analyst:** Deborah King

## PUBLICATION SERVICES

**Acting Director:** Gail M. Oring

**Managing Editors:** A. V. Precup *(USP DI)*, Sandra Boynton *(USP-NF)*

# MEMBERS OF THE USPC AND THE INSTITUTIONS AND ORGANIZATIONS REPRESENTED
## as of March 15, 1994

*University of Arizona, College of Pharmacy:* Michael Mayersohn, Ph.D.
*Arizona Pharmacy Association:* Edward Armstrong

## Arkansas
*University of Arkansas for Medical Sciences, College of Pharmacy:* Kenneth G. Nelson, Ph.D.
*Arkansas Pharmacists Association:* Norman Canterbury, P.D.

## California
*Loma Linda University Medical Center:* Ralph Cutler, M.D.
*Stanford University School of Medicine:* Brian B. Hoffman, M.D.
*University of California, Davis, School of Medicine:* Larry Stark, Ph.D.
*University of California, San Diego, School of Medicine:* Harold J. Simon, M.D., Ph.D.
*University of California, San Francisco, School of Medicine:* Walter L. Way, M.D.
*University of Southern California, School of Medicine:* Wayne R. Bidlack, Ph.D.
*University of California, San Francisco, School of Pharmacy:* Richard H. Guy, Ph.D.
*University of Southern California, School of Pharmacy:* Robert T. Koda, Pharm.D., Ph.D.
*University of the Pacific, School of Pharmacy:* Alice Jean Matuszak, Ph.D.
*California Pharmacists Association:* Robert P. Marshall, Pharm.D.

## Colorado
*University of Colorado School of Pharmacy:* Merrick Lee Shively, Ph.D.
*Colorado Pharmacists Association:* Thomas G. Arthur, R.Ph.

## Connecticut
*University of Connecticut, School of Medicine:* Paul F. Davern
*University of Connecticut, School of Pharmacy:* Karl A. Nieforth, Ph.D.
*Connecticut Pharmaceutical Association:* Henry A. Palmer, Ph.D.

## Delaware
*Delaware Pharmaceutical Society:* Charles J. O'Connor
*Medical Society of Delaware:* John M. Levinson, M.D.

## District of Columbia
*George Washington University:* Janet Elgert-Madison, Pharm.D.
*Georgetown University, School of Medicine:* Arthur Raines, Ph.D.
*Howard University, College of Medicine:* Sonya K. Sobrian, Ph.D.
*Howard University, College of Pharmacy & Pharmacal Sciences:* Wendell T. Hill, Jr., Pharm.D.

## Florida
*Southeastern College of Pharmacy:* William D. Hardigan, Ph.D.
*University of Florida, College of Medicine:* Thomas F. Muther, Ph.D.
*University of Florida, College of Pharmacy:* Michael A. Schwartz, Ph.D.
*University of South Florida, College of Medicine:* Joseph J. Krzanowski, Jr., Ph.D.
*Florida Pharmacy Association:* "Red" Camp

## Georgia
*Medical College of Georgia, School of Medicine:* David W. Hawkins, Pharm.D.
*Mercer University School of Medicine:* W. Douglas Skelton, M.D.
*Mercer University, Southern School of Pharmacy:* Hewitt W. Matthews, Ph.D.
*Morehouse School of Medicine:* Ralph W. Trottier, Jr., Ph.D., J.D.
*University of Georgia, College of Pharmacy:* Stuart Feldman, Ph.D.
*Medical Association of Georgia:* E. D. Bransome, Jr., M.D.
*Georgia Pharmaceutical Association, Inc.:* Larry R. Braden

## Idaho
*Idaho State University, College of Pharmacy:* Eugene I. Isaacson, Ph.D.
*Idaho State Pharmaceutical Association:* Doris Denney

## Illinois
*Chicago Medical School/University of Health Sciences:* Velayudhan Nair, Ph.D., D.Sc.
*Loyola University of Chicago, Stritch School of Medicine:* Erwin Coyne, Ph.D.
*Northwestern University Medical School:* Marilynn C. Frederiksen, M.D.

*Rush Medical College of Rush University:* Paul G. Pierpaoli, M.S.
*Southern Illinois University, School of Medicine:* Leonard Rybak, M.D., Ph.D.
*University of Chicago, Pritzker School of Medicine:* Patrick T. Horn, M.D., Ph.D.
*University of Illinois, College of Medicine:* Marten M. Kernis, Ph.D.
*University of Illinois, College of Pharmacy:* Henri R. Manasse, Jr., Ph.D.
*Chicago College of Pharmacy:* David J. Slatkin, Ph.D.
*Illinois Pharmacists Association:* Ronald W. Gottrich
*Illinois State Medical Society:* Vincent A. Costanzo, Jr., M.D.

## Indiana
*Butler University, College of Pharmacy:* Wagar H. Bhatti, Ph.D.
*Purdue University, School of Pharmacy and Pharmacal Sciences:* Garnet E. Peck, Ph.D.
*Indiana State Medical Association:* Edward Langston, R.Ph., M.D.

## Iowa
*Drake University, College of Pharmacy:* Sidney L. Finn, Ph.D.
*University of Iowa, College of Medicine:* John E. Kasik, M.D., Ph.D.
*University of Iowa, College of Pharmacy:* Robert A. Wiley, Ph.D.
*Iowa Pharmacists Association:* Steve C. Firman, R.Ph.

## Kansas
*University of Kansas, School of Pharmacy:* Prof. Christopher Riley
*Kansas Pharmacists Association:* Robert R. Williams

## Kentucky
*University of Kentucky, College of Medicine:* John M. Carney, Ph.D.
*University of Kentucky, College of Pharmacy:* Patrick P. DeLuca, Ph.D.
*University of Louisville, School of Medicine:* Peter P. Rowell, Ph.D.
*Kentucky Medical Association:* Ellsworth C. Seeley, M.D.
*Kentucky Pharmacists Association:* Chester L. Parker, Pharm.D.

## Louisiana
*Louisiana State University School of Medicine in New Orleans:* Paul L. Kirkendol, Ph.D.
*Northeast Louisiana University, School of Pharmacy:* William M. Bourn, Ph.D.
*Tulane University, School of Medicine:* Floyd R. Domer, Ph.D.
*Xavier University of Louisiana:* Barry A. Bleidt, Ph.D., R.Ph.
*Louisiana State Medical Society:* Henry W. Jolly, Jr., M.D.
*Louisiana Pharmacists Association:* Mona J. Davis

## Maryland
*Johns Hopkins University, School of Medicine:* E. Robert Feroli, Jr., Pharm.D.
*University of Maryland, School of Medicine:* Edson X. Albuquerque, M.D., Ph.D.
*Uniformed Services University of the Health Sciences, F. Edward Hebert School of Medicine:* Louis R. Cantilena, Jr., M.D., Ph.D.
*University of Maryland, Baltimore, School of Pharmacy:* Larry L. Augsburger, Ph.D.
*Medical and Chirurgical Faculty of the State of Maryland:* Frederick Wilhelm, M.D.
*Maryland Pharmacists Association:* Nicholas C. Lykos, P.D.

## Massachusetts
*Boston Univeristy, School or Medicine:* J. Worth Estes, M.D.
*Harvard Medical School:* Peter Goldman, M.D.
*Massachusetts College of Pharmacy and Allied Health Sciences:* David A. Williams, Ph.D.
*Northeastern University, College of Pharmacy and Allied Health Professions:* John L. Neumeyer, Ph.D.
*Tufts University, School of Medicine:* John Mazzullo, M.D.
*University of Massachusetts Medical School:* Brian Johnson, M.D.
*Massachusetts Medical Society:* Errol Green, M.D.

## Michigan
*Ferris State University, School of Pharmacy:* Gerald W.A. Slywka, Ph.D.
*Michigan State University, College of Human Medicine:* John Penner, M.D.
*University of Michigan, College of Pharmacy:* Ara G. Paul, Ph.D.
*University of Michigan Medical Center:* Jeoffrey K. Stross, M.D.
*Wayne State University, School of Medicine:* Ralph E. Kauffman, M.D.

*Wayne State University, College of Pharmacy and Allied Health Professions:* Janardan B. Nagwekar, Ph.D.
*Michigan Pharmacists Association:* Patrick L. McKercher, Ph.D.

**Minnesota**
*Mayo Medical School:* James J. Lipsky, M.D.
*University of Minnesota, College of Pharmacy:* E. John Staba, Ph.D.
*University of Minnesota Medical School, Minneapolis:* Jack W. Miller, Ph.D.
*Minnesota Medical Association:* Harold Seim, M.D.
*Minnesota Pharmacists Association:* Arnold D. Delger

**Mississippi**
*University of Mississippi, School of Medicine:* James L. Achord, M.D.
*University of Mississippi, School of Pharmacy:* Robert W. Cleary, Ph.D.
*Mississippi State Medical Association:* Charles L. Mathews
*Mississippi Pharmacists Association:* Mike Kelly

**Missouri**
*St. Louis College of Pharmacy:* John W. Zuzack, Ph.D.
*St. Louis University, School of Medicine:* Alvin H. Gold, Ph.D.
*University of Missouri, Columbia, School of Medicine:* John W. Yarbro, M.D.
*University of Missouri-Kansas City, School of Medicine:* Paul Cuddy, Pharm.D.
*University of Missouri, Kansas City, School of Pharmacy:* Lester Chafetz, Ph.D.
*Washington University, School of Medicine:* H. Mitchell Perry, Jr., M.D.
*Missouri Pharmaceutical Association:* George L. Oestreich

**Montana**
*The University of Montana, School of Pharmacy & Allied Health Sciences:* David S. Forbes, Ph.D.

**Nebraska**
*Creighton University, School of Medicine:* Michael C. Makoid, Ph.D.
*Creighton University School of Pharmacy and Allied Health Professions:* Kenneth R. Keefner, Ph.D.
*University of Nebraska, College of Medicine:* Manuchair Ebadi, Ph.D.
*University of Nebraska, College of Pharmacy:* Clarence T. Ueda, Pharm.D., Ph.D.
*Nebraska Pharmacists Association:* Rex C. Higley, R.P.

**Nevada**
*Nevada Pharmacists Association:* Steven P. Bradford

**New Hampshire**
*Dartmouth Medical School:* James J. Kresel, Ph.D.
*New Hampshire Pharmaceutical Association:* William J. Lancaster, P.D.

**New Jersey**
*University of Medicine and Dentistry of New Jersey, New Jersey Medical School:* Sheldon B. Gertner, Ph.D.
*Rutgers, The State University of New Jersey, College of Pharmacy:* John L. Colaizzi, Ph.D.
*Medical Society of New Jersey:* Joseph N. Micale, M.D.
*New Jersey Pharmaceutical Association:* Stephen J. Csubak, Ph.D.

**New Mexico**
*University of New Mexico, College of Pharmacy:* William M. Hadley, Ph.D.
*New Mexico Pharmaceutical Association:* Hugh Kabat, Ph.D.

**New York**
*Albert Einstein College of Medicine of Yeshiva University:* Walter G. Levine, Ph.D.
*City University of New York, Mt. Sinai School of Medicine:* Joel S. Mindel, M.D., Ph.D.
*Columbia University College of Physicians and Surgeons:* Michael R. Rosen, M.D.
*Cornell University Medical College:* Lorraine J. Gudas, Ph.D.
*Long Island University, Arnold and Marie Schwartz College of Pharmacy and Health Sciences:* Jack M. Rosenberg, Ph.D.
*New York Medical College:* Mario A. Inchiosa, Jr., Ph.D.
*New York University School of Medicine:* Norman Altzuler, Ph.D.

*State University of New York, Buffalo, School of Medicine:* Robert J. McIsaac, Ph.D.
*State University of New York, Buffalo, School of Pharmacy:* Robert M. Cooper
*State University of New York, Health Science Center, Syracuse:* Oliver M. Brown, Ph.D.
*St. John's University, College of Pharmacy and Allied Health Professions:* Albert A. Belmonte, Ph.D.
*Union University, Albany College of Pharmacy:* David W. Newton, Ph.D.
*University of Rochester, School of Medicine and Dentistry:* Michael Weintraub, M.D., Ph.D.
*Medical Society of the State of New York:* Richard S. Blum, M.D.
*Pharmaceutical Society of the State of New York:* Bruce Moden

**North Carolina**
*Bowman Gray School of Medicine, Wake Forest University:* Jack W. Strandhoy, Ph.D.
*Campbell University, School of Pharmacy:* Antoine Al-Achi, Ph.D.
*Duke University Medical Center:* William J. Murray, M.D., Ph.D.
*East Carolina University, School of Medicine:* A-R.A. Abdel-Rahman, Ph.D.
*University of North Carolina, Chapel Hill, School of Medicine:* George Hatfield, Ph.D.
*University of North Carolina, Chapel Hill, School of Pharmacy:* Richard J. Kowalsky, Pharm.D.
*North Carolina Pharmaceutical Association:* George H. Cocolas, Ph.D.
*North Carolina Medical Society:* T. Reginald Harris, M.D.

**North Dakota**
*University of North Dakota, School of Medicine:* David W. Hein, Ph.D.
*North Dakota State University, College of Pharmacy:* William M. Henderson, Ph.D.
*North Dakota Medical Association:* Vernon E. Wagner
*North Dakota Pharmaceutical Association:* William H. Shelver, Ph.D.

**Ohio**
*Case Western Reserve University, School of Medicine:* Kenneth A. Scott, Ph.D.
*Medical College of Ohio at Toledo:* R. Douglas Wilkerson, Ph.D.
*Northeastern Ohio University, College of Medicine:* Ralph E. Berggren, M.D.
*Ohio Northern University, College of Pharmacy:* Joseph Theodore, Ph.D.
*Ohio State University, College of Medicine:* Robert Guthrie, M.D.
*Ohio State University, College of Pharmacy:* Michael C. Gerald, Ph.D.
*University of Cincinnati, College of Medicine:* Leonard T. Sigell, Ph.D.
*University of Cincinnati, College of Pharmacy:* Henry S.I. Tan, Ph.D.
*University of Toledo, College of Pharmacy:* Norman F. Billups, Ph.D.
*Wright State University, School of Medicine:* John O. Lindower, M.D., Ph.D.
*Ohio State Medical Association:* Janet K. Bixel, M.D.
*Ohio State Pharmaceutical Association:* J. Richard Wuest, Pharm.D.

**Oklahoma**
*University of Oklahoma College of Medicine:* Ronald D. Brown, M.D.
*Southwestern Oklahoma State University, School of Pharmacy:* W. Steven Pray, Ph.D.
*University of Oklahoma, College of Pharmacy:* Loyd V. Allen, Jr., Ph.D.
*Oklahoma State Medical Association:* Clinton Nicholas Corder, M.D., Ph.D.
*Oklahoma Pharmaceutical Association:* Carl D. Lyons

**Oregon**
*Oregon Health Sciences University, School of Medicine:* Hall Downes, M.D., Ph.D.
*Oregon State University, College of Pharmacy:* Randall L. Vanderveen, Ph.D.

**Pennsylvania**
*Duquesne University, School of Pharmacy:* Lawrence H. Block, Ph.D.
*Hahnemann University, School of Medicine:* Vincent J. Zarro, M.D., Ph.D.
*Medical College of Pennsylvania:* Athole G. McNeil Jacobi, M.D.
*Pennsylvania State University, College of Medicine:* John D. Connor, Ph.D.

*Philadelphia College of Pharmacy and Science:* Alfonso R. Gennaro, Ph.D.
*Temple University, School of Medicine:* Ronald J. Tallarida, Ph.D.
*Temple University, School of Pharmacy:* Murray Tuckerman, Ph.D.
*University of Pennsylvania, School of Medicine:* Marilyn E. Hess, Ph.D.
*University of Pittsburgh, School of Pharmacy:* Terrence L. Schwinghammer, Pharm.D.
*Pennsylvania Medical Society:* Benjamin Calesnick, M.D.
*Pennsylvania Pharmaceutical Association:* Joseph A. Mosso, R.Ph.

**Puerto Rico**
*Universidad Central del Caribe, School of Medicine:* Jesús Santos-Martínez, Ph.D.
*University of Puerto Rico, College of Pharmacy:* Benjamin P. de Gracia, Ph.D.
*University of Puerto Rico, School of Medicine:* Walmor C. De Mello, M.D., Ph.D.

**Rhode Island**
*Brown University Program in Medicine:* Darrell R. Abernethy, M.D., Ph.D.
*University of Rhode Island, College of Pharmacy:* Thomas E. Needham, Ph.D.

**South Carolina**
*Medical University of South Carolina, College of Medicine:* Herman B. Daniell, Ph.D.
*Medical University of South Carolina, College of Pharmacy:* Paul J. Niebergall, Ph.D.
*University of South Carolina, College of Pharmacy:* Robert L. Beamer, Ph.D.

**South Dakota**
*South Dakota State University, College of Pharmacy:* Gary S. Chappell, Ph.D.
*South Dakota State Medical Association:* Robert D. Johnson
*South Dakota Pharmaceutical Association:* James Powers

**Tennessee**
*East Tennessee State University, Quillen College of Medicine:* Ernest A. Daigneault, Ph.D.
*Meharry Medical College, School of Medicine:* Dolores C. Shockley, Ph.D.
*University of Tennessee, College of Medicine:* Murray Heimberg, M.D., Ph.D.
*University of Tennessee, College of Pharmacy:* Dick R. Gourley, Pharm.D.
*Vanderbilt University, School of Medicine:* David H. Robertson, M.D.
*Tennessee Pharmacists Association:* Roger L. Davis, Pharm.D.

**Texas**
*Texas A & M University, College of Medicine:* Marsha A. Raebel, Pharm.D.
*Texas Southern University, College of Pharmacy and Health Sciences:* Eugene Hickman, Ph.D.
*University of Houston, College of Pharmacy:* Mustafa Lokhandwala, Ph.D.
*University of Texas, Austin, College of Pharmacy:* James T. Doluisio, Ph.D.
*University of Texas, Medical Branch at Galveston:* George T. Bryan, M.D.
*University of Texas Medical School, Houston:* Jacques E. Chelly, M.D., Ph.D.
*University of Texas Medical School, San Antonio:* Alexander M.M. Shepherd, M.D., Ph.D.
*Texas Medical Association:* Robert H. Barr, M.D.
*Texas Pharmaceutical Association:* Shirley McKee, R.Ph.

**Utah**
*University of Utah, College of Pharmacy:* David B. Roll, Ph.D.
*Utah Pharmaceutical Association:* Robert V. Peterson, Ph.D.
*Utah Medical Association:* David A. Hilding, M.D.

**Vermont**
*University of Vermont, College of Medicine:* John J. McCormack, Ph.D.
*Vermont Pharmacists Association:* Frederick Dobson

**Virginia**
*Medical College of Hampton Roads:* William J. Cooke, Ph.D.
*Medical College of Virginia/Virginia Commonwealth University, School of Pharmacy:* William H. Barr, Pharm.D., Ph.D.
*Medical Society of Virginia:* Richard W. Lindsay, M.D.
*University of Virginia, School of Medicine:* Peyton E. Weary, M.D.
*Virginia Pharmaceutical Association:* Daniel A. Herbert

**Washington**
*Unversity of Washington, School of Pharmacy:* Wendel L. Nelson, Ph.D.
*Washington State University, College of Pharmacy:* Martin J. Jinks, Pharm.D.
*Washington State Pharmacists Association:* Danial E. Baker

**West Virginia**
*Marshall University, School of Medicine:* John L. Szarek, Ph.D.
*West Virginia University, School of Medicine:* Douglas D. Glover, M.D.
*West Virginia University Medical Center, School of Pharmacy:* Arthur I. Jacknowitz, Pharm.D.

**Wisconsin**
*Medical College of Wisconsin:* Garrett J. Gross, Ph.D.
*University of Wisconsin, Madison, School of Pharmacy:* Chester A. Bond, Pharm.D.
*University of Wisconsin Medical School, Madison:* Joseph M. Benforado, M.D.
*State Medical Society of Wisconsin:* Thomas L. Adams, CAE
*Wisconsin Pharmacists Association:* Dennis Dziczkowski, R.Ph.

**Wyoming**
*University of Wyoming, School of Pharmacy:* Kenneth F. Nelson, Ph.D.
*Wyoming Medical Society:* R. W. Johnson, Jr.
*Wyoming Pharmaceutical Association:* Linda G. Sutherland

## Members-at-Large

Norman W. Atwater, Ph.D., Hopewell, NJ
Cheston M. Berlin, Jr., M.D., The Milton S. Hershey Medical Center
Fred S. Brinkley, Jr., Texas State Board of Pharmacy
Herbert S. Carlin, D.Sc., Califon, NJ
Jordan Cohen, Ph.D., College of Pharmacy, University of Kentucky
John L. Cova, Ph.D., Health Insurance Association of America
Enrique Fefer, Ph.D., Pan American Health Organization
Leroy Fevang, Canadian Pharmaceutical Association
Klaus G. Florey, Ph.D., Princeton, NJ
Lester Hosto, Ph.D., Arkansas State Board of Pharmacy
Jay S. Keystone, M.D., Toronto General Hospital
Calvin M. Kunin, M.D., Ohio State University
Marvin Lipman, M.D., Scarsdale, NY
Joseph A. Mollica, Ph.D., Montcharin, DE
Stuart L. Nightingale, M.D., Food and Drug Administration
Daniel A. Nona, Ph.D., The American Council on Pharmaceutical Education
Mark Novitch, M.D., Kalamazoo, MI
Charles A. Pergola, SmithKline Beecham Consumer Brands
Donald O. Schiffman, Ph.D., Genealogy Unlimited
Carl E. Trinca, Ph.D., American Association of Colleges of Pharmacy

## Members-at-Large (representing other countries that provide legal status to *USP* or *NF*)

Prof. T. D. Arias, Estafeta Universitaria, Panama, Republica De Panama
Keith Bailey, Ph.D., Canadian Bureau of Drug Research
Quintin L. Kintanar, M.D., Ph.D., Department of Health, Metro Manila, Philippines
Marcelo Jorge Vernego, Ph.D., Buenos Aires, Argentina

## Members-at-Large (Public)

Clement Bezold, Ph.D., Alternative Futures Association
Alexander Grant, Food and Drug Administration
Grace Powers Monaco, J.D., Washington, DC
Paul G. Rogers, National Council on Patient Information and Education
Frances M. West, J.D., Wilmington, DE

**Ex-Officio Members**

Joseph M. Benforado, M.D., Madison, WI
Joseph P. Buckley, Ph.D., Houston, TX
Estelle G. Cohen, M.A., Baltimore, MD
Leo E. Hollister, M.D., Houston, TX
Paul F. Parker, D.Sc., Lexington, KY

**Committee Chairmen**

*Credentials Committee:* Peyton E. Weary, M.D.
*Nominating Committee for the General Committee of Revision:* Walter L. Way, M.D.
*Nominating Committee for Officers and Trustees:* Joseph M. Benforado, M.D.

*Resolutions Committee:* J. Richard Crout, M.D.
*General Committee of Revision:* Jerome A. Halperin
*Constitution and Bylaws Committee:* John V. Bergen, Ph.D.

**Honorary Members**

George F. Archambault, Pharm.D., J.D., Bethesda, MD
William J. Kinnard, Jr., Ph.D., Baltimore, MD
Lloyd C. Miller, Ph.D., Escondido, CA
John H. Moyer, M.D., D.Sc., Palmyra, PA
John A. Owen, Jr., M.D., Charlottesville, VA
Harry C. Shirkey, M.D., Cincinnati, OH
Linwood F. Tice, D.Sc., Philadelphia, PA

# Appendix III

## ADDITIONAL PRODUCTS AND USES

The following information is new information not included in the text of this book. It has not gone through the USP DI review process. Refer to the Glossary for definitions of medical and technical terms.

| GENERIC NAME (*Brand name*) | DOSAGE FORM(S) | USE | COMMENTS |
|---|---|---|---|
| Acenocoumarol (*Sintrom* [Canada]) | Tablets | Anticoagulant | For general information that may apply to all coumarin-derivative anticoagulants, see *Anticoagulants (Systemic)* |
| Acetazolamide (Generic [U.S.]) | Tablets | Antiglaucoma agent; Anticonvulsant, in epilepsy | Available generically |
| Acitretin (*Soriatane* [Canada]) | Capsules | Antipsoriatic, for psoriasis | Canadian drug product |
| Amsacrine (*Amsa P-D* [Canada]) | Injection | Antineoplastic, for leukemia | Canadian drug product |
| Anileridine (*Leritine* [Canada]) | Tablets Injection | Analgesic, for moderate to severe pain | An opioid analgesic<br>For general information that may apply to all opioid analgesics, see *Narcotic Analgesics—For Pain Relief (Systemic)* |
| Benzydamine Hydrochloride (*Tantum* [Canada]) | Oral Topical Solution | Analgesic (oral-local), for mouth and throat pain | Canadian drug product |
| Betamethasone Dipropionate (*Occlucort* [Canada]) | Lotion | Corticosteroid (topical); Anti-inflammatory, steroidal (topical), for skin disorders | Canadian brand name product |
| Betamethasone Disodium Phosphate (*Betnesol* [Canada]) | Dental Pellets | Corticosteroid (topical); Anti-inflammatory (steroidal), for mouth ulcers | Dosage form available in Canada; for use in the mouth<br>For general information that may apply to this medication see *Corticosteroids—Medium to Very High Potency (Topical)* |
| Betaxolol Hydrochloride (*Betoptic S* [Canada]) | Ophthalmic Suspension | Antiglaucoma agent | Now available in Canada |
| Budesonide (*Entocort* [Canada]) | Tablets for Suspension | Inflammatory suppressant, for bowel disease | Additional dosage form |
| Bufexamac (*Norfemac* [Canada]; *Parfenac* [Canada]) | Cream Ointment | Anti-inflammatory (nonsteroidal), for skin or rectal inflammation | Canadian drug products |
| Butorphanol Tartrate (*Stadol NS* [U.S.]) | Nasal Solution | Analgesic | Additional dosage form |
| Calcipotriene (*Dovonex* [U.S.]) | Topical Ointment | Antipsoriatic, for psoriasis | U.S. drug product |
| Calcium Acetate (Generic [U.S.]) | Tablets | Antihyperphosphatemic, for lowering blood phosphate levels | Available generically |

© 1994   The United States Pharmacopeial Convention, Inc.

**Additional Products and Uses** *(continued)*

| GENERIC NAME (*Brand name*) | DOSAGE FORM(S) | USE | COMMENTS |
|---|---|---|---|
| Calcium Polycarbophil (*FiberNorm* [U.S.]) | Tablets | Laxative; Antidiarrheal | Additional brand name product; OTC |
| Carboxymethylcellulose (*Cellufresh* [U.S.]; *Celluvisc* [U.S.]) | Ophthalmic Solution | Protectant (ophthalmic); Artificial tears | Additional brand name products; OTC |
| Cervical Cap, Cavity-rim (*Prentif* [U.S.]) | | Contraceptive | Cervical cap should be left in place a minimum of 8 hours after last act of intercourse. May be left in place for 48 hours after initial insertion<br><br>Additional contraceptive cream or jelly is not necessary prior to repeat acts of intercourse. However, proper cervical cap placement should be confirmed before and after each act of intercourse |
| Chlorhexidine Gluconate (*PerioGard* [U.S.]) | Oral Rinse | Antibacterial (dental) | Additional brand name product |
| Chlorpheniramine Maleate, Phenylephrine Hydrochloride, and Acetaminophen (*Dristan Cold* [U.S.]) | Tablets | Antihistamine-decongestant-analgesic, for cough and cold symptoms and other upper respiratory problems | Additional brand name product; OTC |
| Chlorpheniramine Maleate, Phenylephrine Hydrochloride, Codeine Phosphate, and Ammonium Chloride (*Statuss Expectorant* [U.S.]) | Oral Solution | Antihistamine-decongestant-antitussive-expectorant, for cough and cold symptoms and other upper respiratory problems | Additional combination product; contains 5% alcohol; Schedule V<br>For general information that may apply to this medication, see *Cough/Cold Combinations (Systemic)* |
| Chlorpheniramine Maleate, Phenylephrine Hydrochloride, and Hydrocodone Bitartrate (*Endal-HD Plus* [U.S.]) | Oral Solution | Antihistamine-decongestant-antitussive, for cough and cold symptoms and other upper respiratory problems | Additional brand name product; alcohol free; Schedule III |
| Chlorpheniramine Maleate, Phenylpropanolamine Hydrochloride, Dextromethorphan Hydrobromide, and Acetaminophen (*Contac-C Cold Care Formula Caplets* [Canada]) | Tablets | Antihistamine-decongestant-antitussive-analgesic, for cough and cold symptoms and other upper respiratory problems | Canadian brand name product; OTC |
| Chlorpheniramine Maleate, Phenylpropanolamine Hydrochloride, and Aspirin (*BC Cold Powder* [U.S.]) | for Oral Solution | Antihistamine-decongestant-analgesic, for cough and cold symptoms and other upper respiratory problems | Additional brand name product; OTC |
| Chlorpheniramine Maleate, Phenyltoloxamine Citrate, Phenylephrine Hydrochloride, and Phenylpropanolamine Hydrochloride (*Par Decon* [U.S.]) | Extended-release Tablets | Antihistamine-decongestant, for cough and cold symptoms and other upper respiratory problems | Additional brand name product |

**Additional Products and Uses** (continued)

| GENERIC NAME (Brand name) | DOSAGE FORM(S) | USE | COMMENTS |
|---|---|---|---|
| Chlorpheniramine Maleate and Pseudoephedrine Hydrochloride (*Children's NyQuil* [U.S.]) | Oral Solution | Antihistamine-decongestant, for cough and cold symptoms and other upper respiratory problems | Additional brand name product; OTC |
| Chlorpheniramine Maleate, Pseudoephedrine Hydrochloride, and Acetaminophen (*Tylenol Allergy Sinus Gelcaps* [U.S.]) | Tablets | Antihistamine-decongestant-analgesic, for cough and cold symptoms and other respiratory problems | Additional brand name product; OTC |
| Chlorpheniramine Maleate, Pseudoephedrine Hydrochloride, and Dextromethorphan Hydrobromide (*Triaminic DM Night time for Children* [Canada]) | Syrup | Antihistamine-decongestant-antitussive, for cough and cold symptoms and other upper respiratory problems | Canadian brand name product; OTC |
| Chlorpheniramine Maleate, Pseudoephedrine Hydrochloride, Dextromethorphan Hydrobromide, and Acetaminophen (*Comtrex Multi-Symptom Hot Flu Relief* [U.S.]; *Dristan Cold and Flu* [U.S.]; *TheraFlu Nighttime Maximum Strength* [U.S.]) | for Oral Solution | Antihistamine-decongestant-antitussive-analgesic, for cough and cold symptoms and other upper respiratory problems | Additional brand name products; OTC |
| Choline Salicylate and Cetyl-dimethyl-benzyl-ammonium Chloride (*Teejel* [Canada]) | Gel | Analgesic (oral-local), for teething or mouth pain | Contains 39% alcohol<br>Should not be used by patients who cannot take other salicylates |
| Clioquinol and Flumethasone Pivalate (*Locacorten Vioform* [Canada]) | Cream<br>Ointment | Antibacterial-antifungal-corticosteroid (topical), for skin inflammation, infection, and itching | Canadian combination products<br>For general information that may apply to this combination, see *Clioquinol and Hydrocortisone (Topical)* |
| Clioquinol and Flumethasone Pivalate (*Locacorten Vioform* [Canada]) | Otic Solution | Antibacterial-antifungal-corticosteroid (otic), for ear infections | Canadian combination product<br>For general information that may apply to all otic corticosteroids, see *Corticosteroids (Otic)* |
| Clobazam (*Frisium* [Canada]) | Tablets | Anticonvulsant | Canadian drug product |
| Clomiphene Citrate (Generic [U.S.]) | Tablets | Antiestrogenic agent | Available generically |
| Cyproterone Acetate (*Androcur* [Canada]) | Tablets<br>Injection | Antineoplastic, for prostate cancer | Canadian drug product |
| Debrisoquine Sulfate (*Declinax* [Canada]) | Tablets | Antihypertensive | Canadian drug product |
| Dextromethorphan Hydrobromide (*Calmylin #1* [Canada]) | Syrup | Antitussive | Canadian brand name product |
| Dextromethorphan Hydrobromide and Guaifenesin (*Benylin DM-E* [Canada]) | Syrup | Antitussive-expectorant | Canadian brand name product; alcohol 5%; OTC |

## Additional Products and Uses *(continued)*

| GENERIC NAME<br>*(Brand name)* | DOSAGE<br>FORM(S) | USE | COMMENTS |
|---|---|---|---|
| Diethylamine Salicylate (*Algesal* [Canada]) | Cream | Analgesic (topical), for muscle and joint pain | Caution required in patients who cannot take other salicylates |
| Diphenhydramine Hydrochloride, Dextromethorphan Hydrobromide, and Ammonium Chloride (*Calmylin #4* [Canada]) | Oral Solution | Antihistamine-antitussive-expectorant, for cough and cold symptoms and other upper respiratory problems | Canadian brand name product |
| Diphenhydramine Hydrochloride, Pseudoephedrine Hydrochloride, and Acetaminophen (*Benadryl Allergy/Sinus Headache Caplets* [U.S.]) | Tablets | Antihistamine-decongestant-analgesic, for cough and cold symptoms and other upper respiratory problems | Additional brand name product; OTC |
| Dipyridamole and Aspirin (*Asasantine* [Canada]) | Capsules | Platelet aggregation inhibitor | For general information that may apply to this combination, see *Dipyridamole (Therapeutic)* and *Salicylates (Systemic)* |
| Domperidone (*Motilium* [Canada]) | Tablets | Stomach and intestine stimulant; Antiemetic, drug-related | Canadian drug product |
| Enalapril Maleate and Hydrochlorothiazide (*Vaseretic* [Canada]) | Tablets | Antihypertensive | Canadian brand name product |
| Enteral Nutrition Formula, Disease-specific (*Respalor* [U.S.]) | Oral Solution | Nutritional supplement, for nutritional deficiency | U.S. product |
| Enteral Nutrition Formula, Polymeric (*Sustacal Plus* [U.S.]) | Oral Solution | Nutritional supplement, for nutritional deficiency | U.S. product |
| Epirubicin Hydrochloride<br><br>(*Pharmorubicin PFS* [Canada])<br>(*Pharmorubicin RDF* [Canada]) | <br><br>Injection<br>for injection | Antineoplastic, for several kinds of cancer | Canadian drug product |
| Erythromycin<br>(*E/Gel* [U.S.]; *Emgel* [U.S.])<br>(*Theramycin Z* [U.S.])<br>(Generic [U.S.]) | Topical:<br>Gel<br>Solution<br>Gel | Antiacne agent (topical) | <br>Additional brand name products<br><br>Available generically |
| Estrogens, Conjugated (*Mannest* [U.S.]) | Tablets | Estrogen replacement therapy; Antineoplastic, for breast or prostate cancer; Osteoporosis prophylactic | Additional brand name product |
| Flumazenil (*Romazicon* [U.S.]; *Anexate* [Canada]) | Injection | Reversal agent for sedation or toxicity caused by benzodiazepines | U.S. and Canadian drug product |
| Fluocinonide (Generic [U.S.]) | Ointment | Corticosteroid (topical); Anti-inflammatory, steroidal (topical), for skin disorders | Available generically |
| Fluocinonide, Procinonide, and Ciprocinonide (*Trisyn* [Canada]) | Cream | Corticosteroid (topical); Anti-inflammatory (steroidal), for skin disorders | For general information that may apply to all topical corticosteroids, see *Corticosteroids—Medium to Very High Potency (Topical)* |

**Additional Products and Uses** (continued)

| GENERIC NAME (Brand name) | DOSAGE FORM(S) | USE | COMMENTS |
|---|---|---|---|
| Fluoxetine (*Prozac* [Canada]) | Capsules | Antibulimic | Additional use in Canada |
| Fluspirilene (*Imap* [Canada]; *Imap Forte* [Canada]) | Injection | Antipsychotic | Canadian drug product |
| Framycetin Sulfate (*Soframycin* [Canada]) | Ophthalmic Ointment Ophthalmic Solution | Antibacterial (ophthalmic), for eye infections | Canadian drug product Belongs to the group of *Streptomyces*-derived antibiotics (including neomycin, paromomycin, kanamycin) |
| Framycetin Sulfate (*Sofra-Tulle* [Canada]) | Impregnated Gauze | Antibacterial (topical), for skin or burn infections | Canadian drug product Belongs to the group of *Streptomyces*-derived antibiotics (including neomycin, paromomycin, kanamycin) |
| Framycetin Sulfate and Gramicidin (*Soframycin* [Canada]) | Ointment | Antibacterial (topical), for skin or burn infections | Canadian combination product |
| Framycetin Sulfate, Gramicidin, and Dexamethasone (*Sofracort Eye-Ear Drops* and *Sofracort Eye-Ear Ointment* [Canada]) | Ophthalmic Ointment Ophthalmic Solution | Antibacterial-adrenocorticoid (ophthalmic), for eye infections | Canadian combination product |
| Framycetin Sulfate, Gramicidin, and Dexamethasone (*Sofracort Eye-Ear Drops* and *Sofracort Eye-Ear Ointment* [Canada]) | Otic Ointment Otic Solution | Antibacterial-corticosteroid (otic), for ear infections | Canadian combination product |
| Fusidic Acid (*Fucidin* [Canada]) | for Injection Oral Suspension Tablets | Antibacterial (systemic), for infections in many different parts of the body | Canadian drug product |
| Fusidic Acid (*Fucidin* [Canada]) | Cream Impregnated Gauze Ointment | Antibacterial (topical), for skin or burn infections | Canadian drug product |
| Gabapentin (*Neurontin* [U.S.]) | Capsules | Anticonvulsant, in epilepsy | U.S. drug product |
| Glipizide (*Glucotrol XL* [U.S.]) | Extended-release Tablets | Antidiabetic | Additional dosage form; tablets should not be chewed, divided, or crushed |
| Gonadorelin Acetate (*Lutrepulse* [U.S.]) | for Injection | Hormone, for treatment of infertility | Additional FDA-approved use Intended for use only with *Lutrepulse* pump |
| Goserelin Acetate (*Zoladex* [U.S. and Canada]) | Implant | Hormone, for treatment of endometriosis | Additional FDA-approved use; also approved in Canada |
| Granisetron (*Kytril* [U.S.]) | Injection | Antiemetic, following cancer chemotherapy | U.S. drug product |
| Guaifensin (*Calmylin Expectorant* [Canada]) | Syrup | Expectorant | Canadian brand name product |
| Histrelin (*Supprelin* [U.S.]) | Injection | Hormone-like agent for treatment of premature puberty | U.S. drug product |

## Additional Products and Uses *(continued)*

| GENERIC NAME<br>*(Brand name)* | DOSAGE FORM(S) | USE | COMMENTS |
|---|---|---|---|
| Hydrocortisone (*Anusol-HC 2.5%* [U.S.]; *Prevex HC* [Canada]) | Cream | Corticosteroid (topical); Anti-inflammatory, steroidal (topical), for skin disorders | U.S. and Canadian brand name products |
| Hydrocortisone Acetate (*Gynecort 10* [U.S.]; *Lanacort 10* [U.S.]) | Cream | Corticosteroid (topical); Anti-inflammatory, steroidal (topical), for skin disorders | Additional brand name products; OTC |
| Hydrocortisone and Urea (*Sential* [Canada]) | Cream | Corticosteroid (topical); Anti-inflammatory, steroidal (topical), for skin disorders | Canadian brand name product<br>For general information that may apply to this medication, see *Corticosteroids—Low Potency (Topical)* |
| Interferon, Alfa-2b, recombinant (*Intron A* [Canada]) | | Antineoplastic, for leukemia or skin cancer<br>Hepatitis treatment | Additional HPB-approved uses |
| | Injection<br>for Injection | | Additional dosage form in Canada |
| Interferon, Beta-1b (*Betaseron* [U.S.]) | for Injection | Immunomodulator, for multiple sclerosis | U.S. drug product |
| Isosorbide Dinitrate (*Coradur* [Canada]) | Extended-release Tablets | Antianginal | Canadian brand name product |
| Isotretinoin (*Isotrex* [Canada]) | Gel | Antiacne agent (topical) | Canadian brand name product |
| Ketotifen Fumarate (*Zaditen* [Canada]) | Syrup<br>Tablets | Antiallergic (systemic); Asthma prophylactic in children | Canadian drug product |
| Leuprolide Acetate | | Hormone-like agent for treatment of premature puberty | Additional FDA-approved use; additional brand name products |
| (*Lupron Depot-Ped* [U.S.])<br>(*Lupron for Pediatric Use* [U.S.]) | for Injection<br>Injection | | |
| Levobunolol Hydrochloride (Generic [U.S.]) | Ophthalmic Solution | Antiglaucoma agent | Now available generically |
| Levocabastine (*Livostin* [Canada]) | Nasal Suspension | Antihistamine (nasal); Antiallergic (nasal) | Canadian drug product |
| Levodopa and Benserazide (*Prolopa* [Canada]) | Capsules | Antidyskinetic, for symptoms of Parkinson's disease | Canadian drug product |
| Liothyronine Sodium (*Triostat* [U.S.]) | Injection | Thyroid hormone | Additional dosage form |
| Loperamide Hydrochloride | | Antidiarrheal | Additional brand name products; OTC |
| (*Kaopectate II Caplets* [U.S.])<br>(*Pepto Diarrhea Control* [U.S.])<br>(Generic [U.S.]) | Tablets<br>Oral Solution<br>Capsules | | Contains 5.25% alcohol<br>Available generically |

**Additional Products and Uses** *(continued)*

| GENERIC NAME (*Brand name*) | DOSAGE FORM(S) | USE | COMMENTS |
|---|---|---|---|
| Megestrol Acetate (*Megace Oral Suspension* [U.S.]) | Suspension | Antianoretic, for anorexia, weight loss, and wasting in AIDS | Additional FDA-approved uses; additional dosage form<br>Contraindicated in pregnancy<br>Plastic cup with 10 mL and 20 mL markings is provided |
| Melphalan Hydrochloride (*Alkeran* [U.S.]) | for Injection | Antineoplastic, for multiple myeloma | Additional dosage form |
| Mesalamine | | Inflammatory suppressant, for bowel disease | Another name is aminosalicylic acid |
| (*Asacol* [U.S. and Canada]) | Delayed-release Tablets | | Additional dosage form in the U.S.; enteric-coated tablets |
| (*Pentasa* [U.S.]) | Extended-release Capsules | | Additional dosage form |
| Metformin Hydrochloride (*Glucophage* [Canada]) | Tablets | Antidiabetic | Canadian drug product<br>Metformin should be taken with food or meals to help prevent upset stomach |
| Methotrexate (*Rheumatrex* [Canada]) | Tablets | Antirheumatic, for rheumatoid arthritis | Approved in Canada for rheumatoid arthritis |
| Methyldopa (*Nu-Medopa* [Canada]) | Tablets | Antihypertensive | Canadian brand name product |
| Metoprolol Tartrate (*Nu-Metop* [Canada]) | Tablets | Antianginal; Antihypertensive; Myocardial reinfarction prophylactic | Canadian brand name product |
| Metronidazole and Nystatin (*Flagystatin* [Canada]) | Vaginal Cream<br>Vaginal Suppositories<br>Vaginal Tablets | Antiprotozoal-antifungal (vaginal), for yeast infections or trichomoniasis | Canadian combination products |
| Nafarelin Acetate (*Synarel* [U.S.]) | Nasal Solution | Hormone-like agent for treatment of premature puberty | Additional FDA-approved use |
| Nicotinamide (*Papulex* [Canada]) | Gel | Antiacne agent (topical) | Canadian drug product |
| Nilutamide (*Anandron* [Canada]) | Tablets | Antineoplastic, for prostate cancer | Canadian drug product |
| Nitrofurantoin (*Macrobid* [U.S.]) | Extended-release Capsules | Antibacterial (systemic), for urinary tract infections | Additional dosage form |
| Ondansetron | | | |
| (*Zofran* [U.S.]) | Tablets | Antiemetic, following cancer chemotherapy | Additional dosage form |
| (*Zofran* [Canada]) | Injection<br>Tablets | Antiemetic, following cancer chemotherapy or radiation therapy | Now available in Canada |
| Paclitaxel (*Taxol* [U.S. and Canada]) | Injection | Antineoplastic, for breast cancer | Additional FDA- and HPB-approved use |
| Pegaspargase (*Oncaspar* [U.S.]) | Injection | Antineoplastic, for leukemia | U.S. drug product<br>Also known as PEG-L-asparaginase |

## Additional Products and Uses *(continued)*

| GENERIC NAME<br>*(Brand name)* | DOSAGE FORM(S) | USE | COMMENTS |
|---|---|---|---|
| Permethrin<br>(*Elimite* [U.S.]; *Nix Dermal Cream* [Canada]) | Cream | Scabicide, for scabies | Additional brand name products |
| (*Nix Creme Rinse* [U.S. and Canada]) | Lotion | Pediculicide, for head lice | OTC in U.S.; formerly Rx<br>Now available in Canada<br>Note—Permethrin 0.5% is used also as a repellant in the form of a contact spray for clothing (not skin) to prevent the bites of ixodid ticks. The bites of ixodid ticks infected with *Borrelia burgdorferi* cause Lyme disease |
| Pheniramine Maleate, Phenylephrine Hydrochloride, and Dextromethorphan Hydrobromide (*NeoCitran DM Coughs & Colds* [Canada]) | for Oral Solution | Antihistamine-decongestant-antitussive, for cough and cold symptoms and other upper respiratory problems | Canadian brand name product; OTC |
| Pheniramine Maleate, Pyrilamine Maleate, Phenylephrine Hydrochloride, Phenylpropanolamine Hydrochloride, and Hydrocodone Bitartrate (*Statuss Green* [U.S.]) | Oral Solution | Antihistamine-decongestant-antitussive, for cough and cold symptoms and other upper respiratory problems | Additional brand name product; contains 5% alcohol; Schedule III |
| Phenylephrine Hydrochloride, Phenylpropanolamine Hydrochloride, and Guaifenesin (*Despec* [U.S.]) | Oral Solution | Decongestant-expectorant, for cough and cold symptoms and other upper respiratory problems | Additional brand name product |
| Phenylpropanolamine Hydrochloride, Dextromethorphan Hydrobromide, and Guaifenesin (*Triaminic DM Daytime* [Canada]) | Oral Solution | Decongestant-antitussive-expectorant, for cough and cold symptoms and other upper respiratory problems | Canadian brand name product; for pediatric use |
| Phenylpropanolamine Hydrochloride and Guaifenesin | | Decongestant-expectorant, for cough and cold symptoms and other upper respiratory problems | Additional brand name products |
| (*Despec* [U.S.]) | Extended-release Capsules | | |
| (*Stamoist LA* [U.S.]; *ULR-LA* [U.S.]) | Extended-release Tablets | | |
| Pilocarpine Hydrochloride (*Salagen* [U.S.]) | Tablets | Cholinergic, for dry mouth caused by radiation treatment for cancer of the head and neck | Additional dosage form |
| Pizotyline Hydrogen Maleate (*Sandomigran* [Canada]; *Sandomigran DS* [Canada]) | Tablets | Migraine headache preventive | Dosage should be decreased gradually over 2-weeks before stopping the medicine completely, to prevent rebound headache |
| Podofilox (*Condylox* [U.S.]) | Topical solution | Cytotoxic (topical), for venereal warts | U.S. drug product |

**Additional Products and Uses** (*continued*)

| GENERIC NAME (*Brand name*) | DOSAGE FORM(S) | USE | COMMENTS |
|---|---|---|---|
| Polymyxin B Sulfate (*Aerosporin* [U.S.]) | for Ophthalmic Solution | Antibacterial, for certain eye infections | U.S. drug product; additional dosage form |
| Progesterone (*Progestasert* [U.S.]) | Intrauterine System | Contraceptive (intrauterine-local) | Patient informed consent forms must be completed before insertion of the system |
| Pseudoephedrine Hydrochloride and Acetaminophen (*Bayer Select Maximum Strength Sinus Pain Relief Caplets* [U.S.]; *Tylenol Sinus Maximum Strength Gel-caps* [U.S.]) | Tablets | Decongestant-analgesic, for congestion and headache caused by sinusitis, colds, or allergies | Additional brand name products; OTC |
| Pseudoephedrine Hydrochloride, Codeine Phosphate, and Guaifenesin (*Calmylin Codeine* [Canada]) | Oral Solution | Decongestant-antitussive-expectorant, for cough and cold symptoms and other upper respiratory problems | Canadian brand name product |
| Pseudoephedrine Hydrochloride and Dextromethorphan Hydrobromide | | Decongestant-antitussive, for cough and cold symptoms and other upper respiratory problems | U.S. and Canadian brand name products |
| (*Benylin DM-D* [Canada]; *Children's Benylin DM-D* [Canada]) | Syrup | | Alcohol free; OTC |
| (*Calmylin #2* [Canada]) | Oral Solution | | |
| (*Calmylin Pediatric* [Canada]) | Syrup | | |
| (*Robitussin Maximum Strength Cough and Cold* [U.S.]) | Oral Solution | | Additional dosage form; OTC |
| Pseudoephedrine Hydrochloride, Dextromethorphan Hydrobromide, and Acetaminophen | | Decongestant-antitussive-analgesic, for cough and cold symptoms and other upper respiratory problems | OTC |
| (*Dristan Juice Mix-in Cold, Flu, and Cough* [U.S.]) | for Oral Solution | | Additional dosage form |
| (*Tylenol Cold No Drowsiness Formula Gelcaps* [U.S.]) | Tablets | | Additional brand name product |
| Pseudoephedrine Hydrochloride, Dextromethorphan Hydrobromide, Guaifenesin, and Acetaminophen | Oral solution | Decongestant-antitussive-expectorant-analgesic, for cough and cold symptoms and other upper respiratory problems | U.S. and Canadian brand name products |
| (*Calmylin Cough & Cold* [Canada]) | | | |
| (*DayQuil Non-Drowsy Cold/Flu* [U.S.]) | | | OTC |
| Pseudoephedrine Hydrochloride and Guaifenesin (*Stamoist E* [U.S.]; *GuaiMAX-D* [U.S.]) | Extended-release Tablets | Decongestant-expectorant, for cough and cold symptoms and other upper respiratory problems | Additional brand name products |
| Pseudoephedrine Hydrochloride and Ibuprofen (*Dimetapp Sinus Caplets* [U.S.]) | Tablets | Decongestant-analgesic, for congestion and headache caused by sinusitis, colds, or allergies | Additional brand name product; OTC |

## Additional Products and Uses (continued)

| GENERIC NAME (Brand name) | DOSAGE FORM(S) | USE | COMMENTS |
|---|---|---|---|
| Pyrethrins and Piperonyl Butoxide (*Lice-Enz Foam and Comb Lice Killing Shampoo Kit* [U.S.]) | Solution Shampoo | Pediculicide, for head lice | Additional brand name product; OTC |
| Pyrithione (*Theraplex Z* [U.S.]) | Lotion Shampoo | Antiseborrheic (topical), for dandruff and other scalp disorders | Additional brand name product |
| Risperidone (*Risperdal* [U.S. and Canada]) | Tablets | Antipsychotic | U.S. and Canadian drug product |
| Salicylic Acid and Sulfur (*Diasporal Cream* [U.S.]) | Cream | Antiacne agent (topical) | Additional brand name product; additional dosage form; OTC |
| Salmeterol Xinafoate (*Serevent* [U.S.]) | Inhalation Aerosol | Bronchodilator | U.S. drug product |
| Sulfadiazine and Trimethoprim (*Coptin* [Canada]) | Tablets Oral Suspension | Antibacterial (systemic), for urinary tract infections | Canadian combination products For general information that may apply to this combination, see *Sulfamethoxazole and Trimethoprim (Systemic)* |
| Tacrolimus (*Prograf* [U.S.]) | Capsules Injection | Immunosuppressant after transplant surgery | U.S. drug product |
| Teniposide (*Vumon* [U.S. and Canada]) | Injection | Antineoplastic, for several kinds of cancer | U.S. and Canadian drug product |
| Testosterone (*Testopel* [U.S.]) | Pellets | Androgen, for treatment of androgen deficiency and delayed puberty in boys | Additional dosage form |
| Timolol Maleate (*Timoptic-XE* [U.S.]) | Ophthalmic Gel-forming Solution | Antiglaucoma agent | Additional dosage form; additional brand name product |
| Tioconazole (*Trosyd Dermal Cream* [Canada]) | Cream | Antifungal (topical), for treatment of ringworm of the body, jock itch, athlete's foot, sun fungus, or other skin fungus infections | Canadian drug product |
| Torsemide (*Demadex* [U.S.]) | Tablets Injection | Diuretic; Antihypertensive | U.S. drug product |
| Triethanolamine Salicylate (*Myoflex* [Canada]; *Royflex* [Canada]) | Cream | Analgesic (topical), for muscle and joint pain | Should not be used by patients who cannot take other salicylates |
| Triprolidine Hydrochloride and Pseudoephedrine Hydrochloride (*Atrofed* [U.S.]) | Tablets | Antihistamine-decongestant, for upper respiratory problems caused by colds or allergies | Additional brand name product; OTC |
| Triprolidine Hydrochloride, Pseudoephedrine Hydrochloride, and Codeine Phosphate (*Cotridin* [Canada]) | Syrup | Antihistamine-decongestant-antitussive, for cough and cold symptoms and other upper respiratory problems | Canadian brand name product |

**Additional Products and Uses** (*continued*)

| GENERIC NAME (*Brand name*) | DOSAGE FORM(S) | USE | COMMENTS |
|---|---|---|---|
| Triprolidine Hydrochloride, Pseudo-ephedrine Hydrochloride, Codeine Phosphate, and Guaifenesin (*Cotridin Expectorant* [Canada]) | Oral Solution | Antihistamine-decongestant-antitussive-expectorant, for cough and cold symptoms and other upper respiratory problems | Canadian brand name product |
| Venlafaxine (*Effexor* [U.S.]) | Tablets | Antidepressant | U.S. drug product |
| Vindesine Sulfate (*Eldisine* [Canada]) | for Injection | Antineoplastic, for leukemia | Canadian drug product |
| Warfarin (*Coumadin* [U.S.]) | Tablets USP | Anticoagulant, to prevent blood clots after heart valve replacement | Additional FDA-approved use |

# Appendix IV

## ATHLETES PRECAUTIONS

### Banned Substances and the Athlete

Since the beginning of organized competition, athletes have tried to gain every possible advantage over their competitors. Sometimes this competitive edge is gained fairly by training harder or developing new and improved methods. Recently, however, many athletes have tried to gain an advantage through the use of substances that affect the body in ways that can improve athletic performance. Called ergogenic aids, these substances can be drugs, herbal products, or materials that are produced by the body. Ergogenic aids can be defined as any natural or man-made substance that can increase strength, endurance, or flexibility. In the United States, the increasing use of ergogenic aids and the drug-related deaths of several well-known athletes have led the National Collegiate Athletic Association (NCAA) and United States Olympic Committee (USOC) to monitor more closely the use of drugs and other ergogenic aids by athletes. The NCAA and USOC have established lists of banned substances, as well as education and testing programs. The use of substances that are on these lists is illegal by NCAA and USOC rules, and can result in an athlete being disqualified from an event and other penalties. In most cases, banned substances are also used in doses that are much higher than those recommended by health professionals, and can cause dangerous and even permanent or life-threatening side effects.

The brief descriptions of banned substances that are listed below have been compiled using information in the USP DI database, NCAA and USOC publications, and other sources. The lists that follow these descriptions are unofficial and, due to the sometimes rapid changes in the NCAA and USOC lists, may be incomplete or inaccurate. These lists are meant to be an example of the kinds of substances that may be banned, and should not be used in the place of the USOC or NCAA lists. Before using or advising an athlete to use a substance, always check with the appropriate governing body. The NCAA Drug-Testing/Education Program phone number is 913-339-1906; the USOC Drug Education Program toll-free hotline number is 1-800-233-0393. Both of these lists are constantly updated to address any changes in the drug use patterns of athletes.

### What Athletes Should Know About Banned Substances and Use of Medications

Athletes should always check with the appropriate governing body for their sport before taking **any** medicines or substances. Even medicines that a physician may prescribe for common conditions such as allergies may contain a substance that is banned by the NCAA or USOC. Nonprescription, or over-the-counter (OTC), medicines may also be banned. It is important that athletes check with the appropriate governing body for their sport to be sure that a substance is not banned. A medicine that may work equally well and is not banned can often be substituted for a banned one.

The NCAA and USOC maintain different lists of banned substances, and have different rules regarding procedures, drug testing, and violations. Also, there are different lists of banned substances for some USOC sports or events; and the NCAA riflery list contains some substances that are not included in the rest of the NCAA list. Athletes should always know the different drugs that are banned for their sport or event, and should consult the governing body for their sport before taking any substances that could be banned.

Once it is determined that a drug is not banned, it should be taken exactly as recommended by the health care professional. Patients should always feel free to ask any questions about their medicines or treatment. Athletes may also want to ask about any possible effect that taking a medicine can have on their status with the NCAA or USOC, and if any changes should be made in their training or competition schedule. Athletes should always know what medicines they are taking and why they were prescribed, as well as any special warnings or instructions, potential drug interactions, and/or possible side effects that they can cause.

### Classes of NCAA and/or USOC Banned Substances

#### Stimulants:

Central nervous system (CNS) stimulants include a wide range of drugs in many dosage forms. Some stimulants, such as amphetamines, are used to treat children with attention-deficit hyperactivity disorder (ADHD) and people who have narcolepsy. Because stimulants can increase the heart rate and flow of blood and oxygen, they are often used by athletes to quicken reaction times, heighten alertness, and reduce fatigue. However, the abuse of these substances can cause dangerous reactions in the athlete's body. During normal exercise or competition, some of the athlete's bodily functions (such as heart rate and blood pressure) can be increased to very stressful levels. With stimulant use, these functions can be pushed to dangerously high levels that can result in stroke, heartbeat irregularities, and heart attack. When taken in unusually high doses, some common stimulants (caffeine, for example) are considered toxic and can even cause death. When stimulants are taken to relieve fatigue, the body's natural warning signals can be covered up. This can place the athlete at greater risk of injury and dangerous reactions, including heat exhaustion and collapse. Athletes also take stimulants for the mental effects that they believe these drugs can have, such as increased competitiveness, aggressiveness, and self-confidence. These effects can also place the athlete at a greater risk of injury. Stimulants can also cause depression and thought disorders.

Some banned stimulants can be found in common products, such as cough/cold medications. Some herbal products (teas, some dietary supplements) may also contain banned substances, such as ephedrine. Athletes should always check to be sure that even common products do not contain stimulants that are banned by the NCAA and/or USOC.

**Caffeine** is one of the most widely used and often abused stimulants in the world. It is found in many common products, including coffee, tea, chocolate, some sodas, and many common medications. Caffeine can be dangerous when taken at very high doses, and the NCAA and USOC ban certain levels of caffeine use. The NCAA prohibits urinary concentrations of caffeine that exceed 15 micrograms/mL; the USOC limit is 12 micrograms/mL.

The following stimulants may be banned by the NCAA and/or USOC (listed by generic name with examples of commonly used brand names in parentheses):

- Amphetamine
- Amphetamine and Dextroamphetamine Resin Complex (e.g., Biphetamine)
- Benzphetamine (e.g., Didrex)
- Caffeine (e.g., NoDoz)
- Caffeine, Citrated
- Cocaine
- Dextroamphetamine (e.g., Dexedrine)
- Diethylpropion (e.g., Tenuate)
- Ephedrine
- Isoproterenol (e.g., Isuprel)
- Metaproterenol (e.g., Alupent, Metaprel)
- Methamphetamine (e.g., Desoxyn)
- Methylphenidate (e.g., Ritalin)
- Pemoline (e.g., Cylert)
- Phendimetrazine (e.g., Anorex)
- Phentermine (e.g., Fastin)
- Phenylpropanolamine (e.g., Dexatrim)
- Pseudoephedrine (e.g., Sudafed)

## Beta-blockers:

Beta-adrenergic blocking agents, commonly called beta-blockers, are used to treat high blood pressure and chest pain, to prevent additional heart attacks in heart attack patients, and for a number of other conditions, such as irregular heartbeat and migraine headaches. Ophthalmic beta-blockers are used in the eye to treat glaucoma.

Some forms of beta-blockers are used by athletes in certain sports (mainly the shooting events) because they lower the heart rate, which steadies the nerves (and trigger finger). It has even been suggested that shooters' heart rates can be so slowed by beta-blockers that they are able to shoot between heartbeats. Use of these drugs can give the athlete an unfair advantage, and is banned for all riflery competition by the NCAA. The USOC permits the use of ophthalmic beta-blockers, and tests for beta-blocker abuse in the following events (this list is subject to change): archery, biathlon, bobsled, diving, equestrian, fencing, figure skating, gymnastics, luge, modern pentathlon (shooting), sailing, shooting, and ski jumping.

The following beta-blockers may be banned by the NCAA and/or USOC (listed by generic name):

- Acebutolol (e.g., Sectral)
- Alprenolol (e.g., Aptin)
- Atenolol (e.g., Tenormin)
- Betaxolol* (e.g., Kerlone)

- Atenolol and Chlorthalidone (e.g., Tenoretic)
- Labetolol and Hydrochlorothiazide (e.g., Normozide)
- Metoprolol (e.g., Lopressor)
- Metoprolol and Hydrochlorothiazide (e.g., Lopressor HCT)
- Nadolol (e.g., Corgard)
- Nadolol and Bendroflumethiazide (e.g., Corzide)
- Oxprenolol (e.g., Trasicor)
- Pindolol (e.g., Visken)
- Pindolol and Hydrochlorothiazide (e.g., Viskazide)
- Propranolol (e.g., Inderal)
- Propranolol and Hydrochlorothiazide (e.g., Inderide)
- Sotalol (e.g., Sotacor)
- Timolol* (e.g., Blocadren)
- Timolol and Hydrochlorothiazide (.e,g, Timolide)

*Ophthalmic use of these drugs is allowed by the USOC; any use is banned by the NCAA.

## Diuretics:

Diuretics act on the kidneys to increase the flow of urine. They are commonly used to reduce the amount of water in the body. Diuretics are often used to treat high blood pressure, and may be used for other conditions as well. Athletes use diuretics to lose weight rapidly. The rapid flushing of water from the body, however, can result in harmful effects such as dehydration, muscle cramps, and exhaustion. Athletes also take diuretics to reduce the concentrations of other banned substances in their urine. Use of diuretics is banned by both the NCAA and USOC.

The following diuretics may be banned by the NCAA and/or USOC (listed by generic name):

- Acetazolamide (e.g., Diamox)
- Amiloride (e.g., Midamor)
- Bendroflumethiazide (e.g., Naturetin)
- Benzthiazide (e.g., Exna)
- Bumetanide (e.g., Bumex)
- Chlorothiazide (e.g., Diuril)
- Chlorthalidone (e.g., Hygroton)
- Cyclothiazide (e.g., Anhydron)
- Ethacrynic Acid (e.g., Edecrin)
- Furosemide (e.g., Lasix)
- Hydrochlorothiazide (e.g., HydroDIURIL)
- Hydroflumethiazide (e.g., Saluron)
- Indapamide (e.g., Lozol)
- Methyclothiazide (e.g., Aquatensin)
- Metolazone (e.g., Zaroxolyn)
- Polythiazide (e.g., Renese)
- Quinethazone (e.g., Hydromox)
- Spironolactone (e.g., Aldactone)
- Triamterene (e.g., Dyrenium)
- Trichlormethiazide (e.g., Metahydrin)

## Blood Doping:

Blood doping is the practice of administering blood or blood-related products to an athlete to enhance his or her performance. Blood doping is usually practiced by endurance athletes, who expect the additional red blood cells (which carry oxygen) to increase their endurance. An unnecessary transfusion can place the athlete at risk of side effects such as allergic reaction, bacterial contamination, and hepatitis. The manipulation of the blood, especially the process of adding red blood cells (or "red blood cell packing"), creates serious risks due to the high red blood cell concentration that may result. The endurance athlete's concentration of red blood cells can rise due to fluid loss during competition. Adding even more red blood cells through doping can cause the blood to thicken. As the blood thickens the athlete is at increasing risk of blood clotting, stroke, and heart failure. Using additional (unneeded) blood is similar to using any other performance-enhancing aid, and the process of blood doping is banned by both the NCAA and USOC.

## Peptide Hormones and Analogs:

Peptide hormones carry messages between organs in the body. Man-made versions of these substances are called analogs. The peptide hormones and analogs most abused by athletes are those that cause the release of growth-related chemicals in the body. When they are produced naturally, these substances act in a positive manner upon the body (stimulating growth and muscle mass, for instance). When these effects are unnecessarily produced by a man-made substance, however, they upset the body's chemical balance, and can cause dangerous and long-term side effects.

**Human growth hormone** (GH) is produced by the pituitary gland and is needed for growth in children. If a child fails to grow normally because his or her body is not producing enough GH, this substance may be used to stimulate growth. The analogs of GH are called somatrem and somatropin. Athletes use GH and its analogs in the same manner as anabolic steroids. They believe that these substances will increase strength and muscle mass, stimulate growth, and strengthen the tendons and ligaments. Because it acts on the pituitary gland, however, GH stimulates the growth of other tissues and organs as well. This can result in very dangerous side effects. These effects can include the development of diabetes; abnormal growth of the bones and internal organs such as the heart, kidneys, and liver; hardening of the arteries; and high blood pressure. Leukemia has also been reported in several short-stature children who were treated with GH.

GH, and other analogs with similar effects, such as chorionic gonadotropin and corticotropin (ACTH), and growth hormone releasing factor, are banned by the NCAA and USOC.

**Erythropoietin (EPO)** is produced by the body (mainly in the kidneys) and causes the bone marrow to produce red blood cells. **Epoetin** is a man-made version of erythropoietin, and is used to treat or prevent anemia (a disease caused by a lack of red blood cells). Athletes take epoetin to increase levels of red blood cells in hopes of increasing their endurance. With use of these substances, however, the athlete's red blood cell concentration may rise above acceptable and safe levels. The thickening of the blood that can result may cause blood clotting, stroke, and heart failure. There is evidence that links the use of epoetin to the heart attack-related deaths of several endurance athletes. Use of epoetin in this manner is equivalent to blood doping, and is banned by both the NCAA and USOC.

## Anabolic Steroids:

Anabolic steroids are analogs of **testosterone**, a naturally produced male sex hormone (an androgen) that stimulates the growth of reproductive and body tissue, protein synthesis, and the development of male traits. Accepted medical uses for these drugs include helping patients gain weight following a severe illness, injury, or continuing infection, if they have failed to gain or maintain normal weight, or for patients with AIDS wasting syndrome; as well as treatment of certain types of anemia, certain kinds of breast cancer (in women), and hereditary angioedema.

Athletes take anabolic steroids because they believe that these drugs will increase the growth and development of muscle mass and strength. Whether steroids produce these effects is a subject of debate in the medical and athletic communities, and has yet to be definitely proven or disproven. When used for this purpose, however, steroids are usually taken in dangerously high doses that can exceed recommended doses by ten to one-hundred times.

When taken in very high doses, steroids often have serious and sometimes permanent side effects that include tumors of the liver, liver cancer, and liver disease; as well as premature heart disease. Steroid use in young males may result in stunted growth; enlarged penis; increased frequency of erections; severe acne; unnatural hair growth; and unexplained darkening of the skin. In adult males, side effects can include enlargement of breasts or breast soreness; enlargement of the prostate gland; frequent or continuing erections; frequent urge to urinate; increased and inappropriate aggressiveness and sexual appetite ("roid rage"); kidney dysfunction; premature baldness; and reduction of the testicles. Adult females may be subject to side effects that include abnormal menstrual cycles; enlargement of the clitoris; and the development of masculine traits such as deepening of the voice, unnatural hair growth on the face and body, and/or hair loss.

The following androgens and anabolic steroids are banned by the NCAA and/or USOC (listed by generic name):
- Fluoxymesterone (e.g., Halotestin)
- Methyltestosterone (e.g., Oreton)
- Nandrolone (e.g., Durabolin)
- Oxandrolone (e.g., Anavar)
- Oxymetholone (e.g., Anadrol)
- Stanozolol (e.g., Winstrol)

## Other Banned Classes and Substances:

Some recreational drugs, such as **marijuana** and **heroin,** are banned by the NCAA. Because these substances are not believed to improve performance, they are not banned by the USOC (although marijuana is banned by the national governing bodies of some sports). **Cocaine,** which some may consider a recreational drug, is banned as a stimulant and local anesthetic by the NCAA and USOC. Several other drugs, such as **LSD, PCP, mescaline,** and **angel dust,** are not believed to improve performance and are not banned. Both the NCAA and USOC, however, strongly discourage the use of these substances. **Alcohol** is banned for all riflery events by the NCAA, but is not banned by the USOC (it may be banned by national governing bodies of particular sports, such as the rifle events). Use of any **tobacco** product (smoked and smokeless) by players, coaches, or officials is now banned during all NCAA games and practices.

**Corticosteroids** are anti-inflammatory drugs that may be produced by the body or man-made. Corticosteroids are not banned by the NCAA. However, corticosteroids that you take by mouth or inject into the muscle or vein are banned by the USOC. Use of topical and inhaled corticosteroids is not banned by the USOC. Local or intra-articular injections of these substances for medical purposes is also not banned. However, permission to compete while using them in this manner must be requested before the event by a letter from the team doctor, and granted by the USOC or International Olympic Committee (IOC) Medical Commission (whichever is responsible for testing at the particular event).

The following corticosteroids (when taken by mouth or injected) may be banned or require official permission for use by USOC athletes (listed by generic name):
- Betamethasone (e.g., Celestone)
- Corticotropin (e.g., Acthar)

- Cortisone (e.g., Cortone)
- Dexamethasone (e.g., Decadron)
- Hydrocortisone (e.g., Cortef, Solu-Cortef)
- Methylprednisolone (e.g., Depo-Medrol, Medrol)
- Paramethasone (e.g., Haldrone)
- Prednisolone (e.g., Delta-cortef, Hydeltrasol)
- Prednisone (e.g., Meticorten)
- Triamcinolone (e.g., Aristocort)

Certain types of **local anesthetics** may contain other drugs that are banned by the NCAA and USOC. The use of topical local anesthetics is permitted by both bodies, but there are certain restrictions placed upon their use by injection.

The following local anesthetics may be banned by the NCAA and/or USOC (listed by generic name):

- Bupivacaine (e.g., Marcaine)
- Chloroprocaine (e.g., Nesacaine)
- Cocaine
- Etidocaine (e.g., Duranest-MPF)
- Lidocaine (e.g., Xylocaine)
- Mepivacaine (e.g., Carbocaine)
- Prilocaine (e.g., Citanest Plain)
- Procaine (e.g., Novocain)
- Propoxycaine and Procaine (e.g., Ravocaine and Novocain with Neo-Cobefrin)

**Note: The lists of drugs that are included above are unofficial and are not meant to be used as a substitute for NCAA and/or USOC banned substance information. The only way to be sure if a substance is banned for a particular sport or event is to consult the appropriate governing body.**